Inflammation

Basic Principles and
Clinical Correlates

Third Edition

Inflammation
Basic Principles and Clinical Correlates
=== *Third Edition* ===

Editors

John I. Gallin, M.D.
Director, Warren G. Magnuson Clinical Center
National Institutes of Health
Bethesda, Maryland

Ralph Snyderman, M.D.
Chancellor for Health Affairs
James B. Duke Professor of Medicine
Duke University Medical Center
President and CEO, Duke University Health System
Durham, North Carolina

Associate Editors

Douglas T. Fearon, M.D.
Wellcome Trust Research Professor of Medicine
University of Cambridge School of Clinical Medicine
Cambridge, United Kingdom

Barton F. Haynes, M.D.
Fredric M. Hanes Professor and Chair
Department of Medicine
Duke University School of Medicine
Durham, North Carolina

Carl Nathan, M.D.
R. A. Rees Pritchett Professor of Microbiology
Professor, Microbiology, Immunology and Medicine
Chairman, Department of Microbiology and Immunology
Joan and Sanford I. Weill Medical College of Cornell University
New York, New York

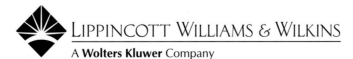
LIPPINCOTT WILLIAMS & WILKINS
A **Wolters Kluwer** Company
Philadelphia • Baltimore • New York • London
Buenos Aires • Hong Kong • Sydney • Tokyo

Acquisitions Editor: Jonathan Pine
Developmental Editor: Anne Snyder
Manufacturing Manager: Tim Reynolds
Production Manager: Liane Carita
Production Editor: Mary Ann McLaughlin
Cover Designer: Cambria Kahoud
Indexer: Susan Thomas
Compositor: Lippincott Williams & Wilkins Electronic Production
Printer: Maple Vail

Library of Congress Cataloging-in-Publication Data
Inflammation : basic principles and clinical correlates / editors,
   John I. Gallin, Ralph Snyderman : associate editors, Douglas T. Fearon, Barton F. Haynes, Carl
Nathan. —3rd ed.
     p. cm.
   Includes bibliographical references and index.
   ISBN 0397517599
   1. Inflammation. I. Gallin, John I. II. Snyderman, Ralph.
   [DNLM: 1. Inflammation—immunology. 2. Inflammation—physiopathology.
QZ 150 I435 1999]
RB131.I519 1999
616′.0473—dc21
DNLM/DLC
for Library of Congress   98-40681
                                                       CIP

In Memory of Ira M. Goldstein, M.D.

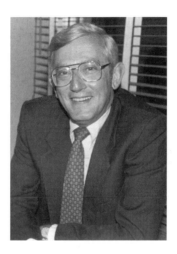

On December 2, 1992, Ira M. Goldstein, M.D., a co-founding editor of *Inflammation: Basic Principles and Clinical Correlates*, died of metastatic lung cancer. Ira Goldstein's shockingly premature death stunned the community of scientists and clinicians interested in inflammation and related diseases. He had a remarkable talent for doing everything in a seemingly effortless fashion. He was gifted with brilliant skills as a clinician, teacher, scientist, administrator, and editor. Ira Goldstein's optimism, joy for life, attention to detail, tireless energy, engaging personality, and caring relationships with his colleagues created a delightful atmosphere for the authors and co-editors of the first two editions of *Inflammation*. He was an accomplished investigator in many aspects of inflammation, with his research moving effortlessly between such diverse areas as the cell biology of neutrophils, to the description of new aspects of the complement pathway, to the study of leukotrienes. He made pioneering contributions in each of these areas. The outstanding quality and praise for the first two editions of *Inflammation* reflect his commitment to excellence. In addition to Ira Goldstein's immediate family, we, the founding editors of *Inflammation*, were robbed too early of a brilliant friend and colleague. We dedicate the third edition of *Inflammation* to Ira M. Goldstein's memory.

John I. Gallin
Ralph Snyderman

Contents

Part III: Cellular Mechanisms

Contributors

Donald C. Anderson, M.D.
Professor
Department of Pediatrics
Baylor College of Medicine
Houston, Texas
Vice President and Chief Scientific Officer
Pharmacia and Upjohn, Inc.
301 Henrietta Street
Kalamazoo, Michigan 49007

Mark Anderson, Ph.D.
The Magainin Research Institute
and Magainin Pharmaceuticals Inc.
5110 Campus Drive
Plymouth Meeting, Pennsylvania 19462

Grant J. Anhalt, M.D.
Professor and Acting Chairman
Department of Dermatology
Johns Hopkins University,
    School of Medicine
720 Rutland Avenue, Ross Room 771
Baltimore, Maryland 21205
Johns Hopkins Hospital
600 N. Wolfe Street
Baltimore, Maryland 21205

Douglas A. Arenberg, M.D.
Assistant Professor
Department of Internal Medicine—
    Pulmonary
University of Michigan Medical School
6301 MSRB III
Ann Arbor, Michigan 48109

Myriam A. Armant, Ph.D.
Post Doctoral Fellow
Laboratory of Parasitic Diseases
National Institutes of Health
9000 Rockville Pike
Bethesda, Maryland 20892

K. Frank Austen, M.D.
Theodore B. Bayles Professor of Medicine
Harvard Medical School
Director, Inflammation and Allergic Diseases
    Research Section
Department of Medicine and Division of
    Rheumatology, Immunology, and Allergy
Brigham and Women's Hospital
75 Francis Street
Boston, Massachusetts 02115

Erika A. Bach, Ph.D.
Postdoctoral Fellow
Department of Pathology
Center for Immunology
Washington University School of Medicine
660 South Euclid Avenue, Box 8118
St. Louis, Missouri 63110
Department of Genetics
Harvard Medical School
200 Longwood Avenue
Boston, Massachusetts 02115

Marco Baggiolini, M.D.
Professor
Director, Theodor-Kocher Institute
University of Bern
Freiestrasse 1
CH-3012 Bern, Switzerland

Dorothy F. Bainton, M.D.
Vice Chancellor
Department of Academic Affairs
University of California, San Francisco
513 Parnassus Avenue, Rm. S-115
San Francisico, California 94143-0400

Eric T. Baldwin, Ph.D.
Research Scientist
Pharmacia and Upjohn, Inc.
301 Henrietta Street
Kalamazoo, Michigan 49007

Carol Beadling, Ph.D.
Division of Immunology, LC907
Cornell University Medical College
1300 York Avenue
New York, New York 10021

Giorgio Berton, M.D.
Full Professor
Department of Pathology, Section of
*   General Pathology*
University of Verona
8 Strada Le Grazie
Verona, Italy 37134

Nina Bhardwaj, M.D., Ph.D.
Assistant Professor, Associate Physician
Laboratory of Cellular Physiology and
*   Immunology*
The Rockefeller University
1230 York Avenue
New York, New York 10021
Associate Professor
Department of Medicine
Hospital for Special Surgery
525 East 68th Street
New York, New York 10021

Martin J. Blaser, M.D.
Addison B. Scoville Professor of Medicine
Department of Medicine
Director, Division of Infectious Diseases
Vanderbilt University School of Medicine
A3310 Medical Center North
Nashville, Tennessee 37232

Salah Chettibi, Ph.D.
Senior Research Fellow
School of Biological Sciences
Manchester University
3.239 Stopford Building
Oxford Road
Manchester M13 9PT United Kingdom

Kelvin Cooper, Ph.D.
Senior Executive Director, Candidate Synthesis,
*   Enhancement and Evaluation*
Pfizer Central Research
Pfizer Inc.
558 Eastern Point Road
Groton, Connecticut 06340

Neil R. Cooper, M.D.
Professor
Department of Immunology
The Scripps Research Institute
10550 N. Torrey Pines Road
La Jolla, California 92037

John J. Costa, M.D.
Department of Medicine and Pathology
Beth Israel Hospital Deaconess Medical Center
Harvard Medical School
330 Brookline Avenue
Boston, Massachusetts 02215

Ramzi S. Cotran, M.D.
F.B. Mallory Professor of Pathology
Department of Pathology
Harvard Medical School
25 Shattuck Street
Boston, Massachusetts 02115
Chairman, Department of Pathology
Brigham and Women's Hospital and
*   Children's Hospital*
75 Francis Street
Boston, Massachusetts 02115

Bruce N. Cronstein, M.D.
Professor of Medicine and Pathology
New York University Medical Center
550 First Avenue
New York, New York 10016

Ronald G. Crystal, M.D.
Department of Pulmonary and
*   Critical Care Medicine*
The New York Hospital–
*   Cornell University Medical Center*
520 East 70th Street
Starr 505
New York, New York 10021

Khavar J. Dar, M.D.
Division of Pulmonary and
*   Critical Care Medicine*
The New York Hospital–
*   Cornell Medical Center*
520 East 70th Street, Suite 505
New York, New York 10021

Thomas E. DeCoursey, Ph.D.
Professor
Department of Molecular Biophysics and
*   Physiology*
Rush Presbyterian St. Luke's Medical Center
1653 West Congress Parkway
Chicago, Illinois 60612

René de Waal Malefyt, Ph.D.
Department of Immunobiology
DNAX Research Institute
901 California Avenue
Palo Alto, California 94304

Beatrice Dewald, Ph.D.
Theodor-Kocher Institute
University of Bern
Freiestrasse 1
CH-3012 Bern, Switzerland

Betty Diamond, M.D.
Professor
Microbiology and Immunology and Medicine
Albert Einstein College of Medicine
1300 Morris Park Avenue, Forch Building,
*   Room 405*
Bronx, New York 10461

Charles A. Dinarello, M.D.
Professor of Medicine
Department of Medicine
University of Colorado School of Medicine
4200 East Ninth Avenue
Denver, Colorado 80262

Peter Q. Eichacker, M.D.
Critical Care Medicine Department
National Institutes of Health
Building 10, Room 7D43
9000 Rockville Pike
Bethesda, Maryland 20892

Peter Elsbach, M.D.
Professor
Departments of Medicine and Microbiology
New York University School of Medicine
550 First Avenue
New York, New York 10016

R. Alan B. Ezekowitz, M.B.Ch.B., D.Phil.
Charles Wilder Professor of Pediatrics
Harvard Medical School
Chief, Pediatric Service
Laboratory of Developmental Immunology
Massachusetts General Hospital
15 Parkman Street- WAC 731
Boston, Massachusetts 02114

Douglas T. Fearon, M.D.
Wellcome Trust Research Professor of Medicine
University of Cambridge School of Clinical
*   Medicine*
Department of Medicine
Wellcome Trust Immunology Unit
Hills Road
Cambridge CB2 2SP, United Kingdom

Marc Feldmann, Ph.D., F.R.C.P., F.R.C.Path
Professor
Cytokine and Cellular Immunology Division
Kennedy Institute of Rheumatology
1 Aspenlea Road
Hammersmith
London W6 8LH United Kingdom

Mark W. J. Ferguson, B.Sc., B.D.S., Ph.D.,
**   F.F.D., F.D.S.**
Professor
School of Biological Sciences
University of Manchester
3.239 Stopford Building
Manchester M13 9PT, United Kingdom

Iain P. Fraser, M.B.Ch.B., D.Phil.
Laboratory of Developmental Immunology
Massachusetts General Hospital
Jackson 14/GRJ 1402
55 Fruit Street
Boston, Massachusetts 02114

Bradley D. Freeman, M.D.
Assistant Professor
Department of Surgery
Washington University Medical Center
660 South Euclid Avenue
St. Louis, Missouri 63110

John I. Gallin, M.D.
Director, Warren G. Magnuson Clinical Center
National Institutes of Health
Building 10, Room 2C146, MSC 1504
10 Center Drive
Bethesda, Maryland 20892-1504

Berhane Ghebrehiwet, D.V.M., D.Sc.
Professor
Department of Medicine
State University of New York at Stony Brook
Health Sciences Center, T16-040
Stony Brook, New York 11794

Siamon Gordon, M.B., Ch.B., Ph.D.
Professor
Department of Cellular Pathology
Sir William Dunn School of Pathology
University of Oxford
South Parks Road
Oxford OX1 3RE, United Kingdom

Richard D. Granstein, M.D.
Professor and Chairman
Department of Dermatology
Weill College of Medicine of Cornell University
Dermatologist-in-Chief
New York Hospital
525 East 68th Street, Room F340
New York, New York 10021

Steven Greenberg, M.D.
Assistant Professor
Departments of Medicine and Pharmacology
Columbia University
630 West 168 Street
New York, New York 10032

Richard J. Griffiths, Ph.D.
Department of Respiratory, Allergy,
*   Immunology, Inflammation, Infectious Diseases*
Pfizer Central Research Division
Pfizer Inc.
558 Eastern Point Road
Groton, Connecticut 06340

Sergio Grinstein, Ph.D.
Professor
Department of Biochemistry
University of Toronto
College Street and University Avenue
Toronto, Ontario M5S 1A8, Canada
Head, Department of Cell Biology
Hospital for Sick Children
555 University Avenue
Toronto, Ontario M5G 1X8, Canada

Laura P. Hale, M.D., Ph.D.
Assistant Professor
Department of Pathology
Duke University Medical Center, 2608
181B Medical Sciences Research Building
Durham, North Carolina 27710

Yusuf A. Hannun, M.D.
Ralph Hirschmann Professor and Chair
Departments of Medicine and Biochemistry
Medical University of South Carolina
171 Ashley Street
Charleston, South Carolina 29425

David M. Harlan, M.D.
Associate Professor
Department of Medicine
Uniformed Services University of the
*   Health Sciences*
4301 Jones Bridge Road
Bethesda, Maryland 20814-4799
Staff Endocrinologist
Department of Internal Medicine
National Naval Medical Center
8901 Wisconsin Avenue
Bethesda, Maryland 20889

Barton F. Haynes, M.D.
Frederic M. Hanes Professor and Chair
Department of Medicine
Duke University School of Medicine
1102 Duke Hospital, Box 3703
Durham, North Carolina 27710

Steven M. Holland, M.D.
NIAID Investigator
Laboratory of Host Defenses
National Institute of Allergy and Infectious Diseases
National Institutes of Health
10 Center Drive, MSC 1886
Bethesda, Maryland 20892

Elizabeth Leef Jacobson, M.D.
Assistant Professor
Department of Medicine
Cornell University Medical School
Associate Attending Physician
The New York Hospital
525 East 68th Street
New York, New York 10021

Charles A. Janeway, Jr., M.D.
Professor
Section of Immunobiology
Yale University School of Medicine
Howard Hughes Medical Institute
Post Office Box 208011
New Haven, Connecticut 06510

Kusumam Joseph, Ph.D.
Instructor
Department of Medicine
Medical University of South Carolina
171 Ashley Avenue
Charleston, South Carolina 29425

Carl H. June, M.D.
Professor
Department of Medicine and
*   Molecular and Cell Biology*
Uniformed Services University of
*   the Health Sciences*
Director, Immune Reconstitution Program
Henry M. Jackson Foundation for the
*   Advancement of Military Medicine*
US Military HIV Research Program
Immune Cell Biology Program, Code 61
Naval Medical Research Institute
8901 Wisconsin Avenue
Bethesda, Maryland 20889-5607

Andrew H. Kang, M.D.
Professor
Department of Medicine
University of Tennessee, Memphis
956 Court Avenue, G326
Memphis, Tennessee 38163

Allen P. Kaplan, M.D.
Professor
Department of Medicine
Medical University of South Carolina
171 Ashley Avenue
Charleston, South Carolina 29425

Daniel H. Kaplan, M.D.
Center for Immunology and
*   Department of Pathology*
Washington University School of Medicine
660 South Euclid Avenue
St. Louis, Missouri 63110

Arthur F. Kavanaugh, M.D.
Associate Professor
Department of Internal Medicine
The University of Texas Southwestern
  Medical Center
5323 Harry Hines Boulevard
Dallas, Texas 75235-8577
Chief of Rheumatology
Veterans Administration North Texas
  Health Care System
4500 South Lancaster
Dallas, Texas 75216

Kenneth S. Kilgore, Ph.D.
Assistant Research Scientist
Department of Pharmacology
University of Michigan Medical School
1301 Medical Science Research Building III
Ann Arbor, Michigan 48109-0632

Takashi Kei Kishimoto, Ph.D.
Associate Director, Biology
Boehringer Ingelheim Pharmaceuticals, Inc.
900 Ridgebury Road
Ridgefield, Connecticut 06877-0368

Seymour J. Klebanoff, M.D., Ph.D.
Professor
Department of Medicine
University of Washington School of Medicine
I-104E Health Sciences Building, Box 357185
Seattle, Washington 98195

Amy D. Klion, M.D.
Staff Physician
Laboratory of Parasitic Diseases
National Institutes of Health
9000 Rockville Pike
Bethesda, Maryland 20892

Gary A. Koretzky, M.D., Ph.D.
Department of Internal Medicine
College of Medicine
University of Iowa
540 EMRB
Iowa City, Iowa 52242
Rheumatologist
University of Iowa, Hospitals and Clinics
Iowa City, Iowa 52242

Irving Kushner, M.D.
Professor
Departments of Medicine and Pathology
Case Western Reserve University
10900 Euclid Avenue
Cleveland, Ohio 44106
Department of Medicine
MetroHealth Medical Center
2500 MetroHealth Drive
Cleveland, Ohio 44109

Bing K. Lam, Ph.D.
Department of Medicine
Harvard Medical School
Division of Rheumatology,
  Immunology, and Allergy
Brigham and Women's Hospital
1 Jimmy Fund Way
Boston, Massachusetts 02115

Kong-Peng Lam, Ph.D.
Assistant Professor
Institute of Molecular and Cell Biology
The National University of Singapore
30 Medical Drive
S 117609 Singapore

Gerald Sylvan Lazarus, M.D.
Professor
Department of Dermatology
University of California, Davis
  School of Medicine
4860 Y Street, Suite 3400
Sacramento, California 95817

Kelvin P. Lee, M.D.
Head, Immune Regulation Branch
Immune Cell Biology Program, Code 06
Naval Medical Research Institute
Associate Professor, Department of Medicine
Uniformed Services University of
  the Health Sciences
8901 Wisconsin Avenue, Building 17, Room 214
Bethesda, Maryland 20889

Thomas L. Leto, Ph.D.
Senior Investigator
Laboratory of Host Defenses
National Institute of Allergy and Infectious
  Diseases
National Institutes of Health
Building 10, Room 11N106
10 Medical Center Drive
Bethesda, Maryland 20892

Norman L. Letvin, M.D.
Professor of Medicine
Harvard Medical School
Chief, Division of Viral Pathogenesis
Department of Medicine
Beth Israel Deaconess Medical Center
330 Brookline Avenue, RE-113
Boston, Massachusetts 02215

Ofer Levy, M.D., Ph.D.
Resident in Medicine
Department of Medicine
The Children's Hospital
300 Longwood Avenue
Boston, Massachusetts 02115

Peter E. Lipsky, M.D.
Professor
Department of Internal Medicine
University of Texas Southwestern
    Medical Center at Dallas
5323 Harry Hines Boulevard
Dallas, Texas 75235
Chief, Rheumatic Diseases Division
Parkland Memorial Hospital
5201 Harry Hines Boulevard
Dallas, Texas 75235

Benedict R. Lucchesi, M.D., Ph.D.
Professor
Department of Pharmacology
University of Michigan Medical School
1301C Medical Science Research Building III
Ann Arbor, Michigan 48109-0632

Ian A. MacNeil, M.D.
Staff Scientist
ARIAD Pharmaceuticals, Inc.
26 Landsdowne Street
Cambridge, Massachusetts 02139

Anthony M. Manning, Ph.D.
Senior Director, Immunology and Preclinical
    Development
Signal Pharmaceuticals, Inc.
5555 Oberlin Drive
San Diego, California 92121

Aaron J. Marcus, M.D.
Professor of Medicine and Pathology
Cornell University Medical College
1300 York Avenue
New York, New York 10021
Chief, Hematology/Oncology
Department of Veterans Affairs
    Medical Center
423 East 23rd Street
New York, New York 10010

Shaun R. McColl, Ph.D.
Senior Lecturer
Department of Microbiology
    and Immunology
University of Adelaide
Frome Road
Adelaide, South Australia, 5005 Australia

Thomas M. McIntyre, Ph.D.
Department of Medicine
CVRTI
University of Utah
95 S. 2000 E.
Salt Lake City, Utah 84112

Dean D. Metcalfe, M.D.
Chief, Laboratory of Allergic Diseases
National Institute of Allergy and
    Infectious Diseases
National Institutes of Health
Building 10, Room 11C205
10 Center Drive, MSC 1881
Bethesda, Maryland 20892-1881

Donald Metcalf, M.D.
Professor Emeritus
Division of Cancer and Haematology
The Walter and Eliza Hall Institute of
    Medical Research
P.O. Royal Melbourne Hospital
3050, Victoria, Australia

Maria Cristina Mingari, Ph.D.
Associate Professor
Dipartimento Oncologia
    Clinica e Sperimentale
Università degli Studi di Genova
Deputy Director
Laboratorio di Immunopatologia
Centro di Biotecnologie Avanzate
L.go R. Benzi, 10
16132 Genova, Italy

Eeva Moilanen, M.D., Ph.D.
Assistant Professor
Department of Pharmacology
University of Tampere
PO Box 607
33101 Tampere, Finland
Department of Clinical Chemistry
Tampere University Hospital
P.O. Box 2000
33521 Tampere, Finland

Salvador Moncada, M.D., Ph.D., F.R.C.P.,
    F.R.S.
Director, The Wolfson Institute for
    Biomedical Research
University College of London
140 Tottenham Court Road
London W1P 9LN, United Kingdom

Lorenzo Moretta, M.D.
Full Professor of
    General Pathology
Dipartimento di Medicina Sperimentale
Università degli Studi di Genova
Director, Immunopathology Laboratories
Laboratorio di Immunopatologia
Centro Biotecnologie Avanzate
L.go R. Benzi, 10
16132 Genova, Italy

Bernhard Moser, Ph.D.
Theodor-Kocher Institute
University of Bern
Freiestrasse 1
CH-3012 Bern, Switzerland

William A. Muller, M.D., Ph.D.
Associate Professor
Attending Staff
Department of Pathology
Weill Medical College of Cornell University
1300 York Avenue
New York, New York 10021

Henry W. Murray, M.D.
Professor and Associate Chairman
Department of Medicine
Cornell University Medical College
Attending Physician
The New York Hospital
1300 York Avenue
New York, New York 10021

Paul Henri Naccache, Ph.D.
Professor
Department of Medicine
Le Centre de Recherche en Rhumatologie et
*   Immunologie*
Université Laval
Centre Hospitalier de l'Université Laval
2705 Boulevard Laurier
Ste-Foy, Québec G1V 4G2, Canada

Yoshitaka Nakazawa, M.D.
Department of Medicine—
*   Division of Pulmonary and Critical Care*
*   Medicine, Allergy & Clinical Immunology*
Medical University of South Carolina
96 Jonathan Lucas Street, P.O. Box 250623
Charleston, South Carolina 29425

Charles Natanson, M.D.
Senior Investigator
Critical Care Medicine Department
National Institutes of Health
Building 10, Room 7D43
9000 Rockville Pike
Bethesda, Maryland 20892

Carl Nathan, M.D.
R. A. Rees Pritchett Professor of Microbiology
Professor, Microbiology, Immunology and
*   Medicine*
Chairman
Department of Microbiology and Immunology
Joan and Sanford I. Weill Medical College
*   of Cornell University*
1300 York Avenue
New York, New York 10021

Gunnar Nilsson, Ph.D.
Associate Professor
Department of Genetics and Pathology
Uppsala University
Uppsala, Sweden 75185

Hossein Carlos Nousari, M.D.
Chief Resident
Department of Dermatology
Johns Hopkins University, School of Medicine
720 Rutland Avenue, Room 771
Baltimore, Maryland 21205

Thomas B. Nutman, M.D.
Head, Helminth Immunology Section
Laboratory of Parasitic Diseases
National Institute of Allergy and
*   Infectious Diseases*
National Institutes of Health
Building 4, Room 126
Bethesda, Maryland 20892

Lina M. Obeid, M.D.
Boyle Professor
Departments of Medicine and Biochemistry
Medical University of South Carolina
P.O. Box 250779
770 MUSC Complex, Suite 143
Charleston, South Carolina 29425

Halina Offner, Ph.D.
Professor
Department of Neurology
Oregon Health Sciences University
Neuroimmunologist
Neuroimmunology Research R&D-31
VA Medical Center
3710 South West US Veterans Hospital Road
Portland, Oregon 97201

Drew M. Pardoll, M.D., Ph.D.
Professor
Department of Oncology
Johns Hopkins University School of Medicine
720 Rutland Avenue, Ross 364
Baltimore, Maryland 21205-2196

Dhavalkumar D. Patel, M.D., Ph.D.
Assistant Professor
Departments of Medicine
*   and Immunology*
Duke University School of Medicine
Box 3258, DUMC
Durham, North Carolina 27710
Senior Staff
Department of Medicine
Duke University Medical Center
Erwin Road
Durham, North Carolina 27710

John F. Penrose, M.D.
Assistant Professor
Department of Medicine
Harvard Medical School
Associate Physician
Department of Medicine
Division of Rheumatology, Immunology,
  and Allergy
Brigham and Women's Hospital
Smith Building, Room 626
1 Jimmy Fund Way
Boston, Massachusetts 02115

Jeffrey L. Platt, M.D.
Professor
Departments of Surgery,
  Immunology, and Pediatrics
Mayo Clinic
Room 2-66 Medical Sciences Building
Rochester, Minnesota 55905

Arnold E. Postlethwaite, M.D.
Professor and Director
Division of Connective Tissue Diseases
Department of Medicine
The University of Tennessee, Memphis
956 Court Avenue, Room G326
Memphis, Tennessee 38163
Staff Physician
Department of Medical Services
Veterans Affairs Medical Center
1030 Jefferson Avenue
Memphis, Tennessee 38104

Stephen M. Prescott, M.D.
Professor of Internal Medicine
Senior Director for Research
Huntsman Cancer Institute
University of Utah
18N. 2030 E, Room 4220
Salt Lake City, Utah 84112

Klaus Rajewsky, M.D.
Professor of Molecular Genetics
Institute for Genetics
University of Cologne
Weyertal 121
D-50931 Cologne, Germany

Anjana Rao, Ph.D.
Professor
Department of Pathology
Harvard Medical School
Senior Investigator,
  The Center for Blood Research
200 Longwood Avenue
Boston, Massachusetts 02115

Sesha Reddigari, M.D.
Enzyme Research Laboratories
South Bend, Indiana 46601

Lisa A. Robinson, M.D., F.R.C.P.C.
Fellow, Pediatric Nephrology
Department of Pediatrics
Duke University Medical Center
Box 3959
Durham, North Carolina 27710

Sergio Romagnani, M.D.
Professor and Head
Institute of Internal Medicine and
  Immunoallergology
University of Florence
Viale Morgagni 85
Firenze-50134, Italy

Helene F. Rosenberg, M.D.
Laboratory of Host Defenses
National Institute of Allergy and
  Infectious Diseases
National Institutes of Health
Building 10, Room 11N104
9000 Rockville Pike
Bethesda, Maryland 20892

Russell Ross, Ph.D.
Professor of Pathology
Director, Center for Vascular Biology
Department of Pathology
University of Washington
  School of Medicine
Box 357470
Seattle, Washington 98195-7470

Donald A. Rowley, M.D.
Professor
Department of Pathology
The University of Chicago, MC 1089
5841 South Maryland Avenue
Chicago, Illinois 60637

Erkki Ruoslahti, M.D., Ph.D.
President and Chief Executive Officer
La Jolla Cancer Research Center
The Burnham Institute
10901 North Torrey Pines Road
La Jolla, California 92037

Debra L. Rzewnicki, B.S.
Case Western University at
MetroHealth Medical Center
2500 MetroHealth Drive
Cleveland, Ohio 44109

Richard I. Schiff, M.D., Ph.D.
Director, Clinical Immunology
Miami Children's Hospital
3100 SW 62nd Avenue
Miami, Florida 33155

Jörn E. Schmitz, M.D.
Instructor
Department of Medicine
Harvard Medical School
Division of Viral Pathogenesis
Beth Israel Deaconess Medical Center
P.O. Box 15732
Boston, Massachusetts 02215

Hans Schreiber, M.D., Ph.D.
Department of Pathology
Division of Biological Sciences
The University of Chicago, MC 109
5841 South Maryland Avenue
Chicago, Illinois 60637

Robert D. Schreiber, Ph.D.
Alumni Endowed Professor
Department of Pathology
Washington University School of
*   Medicine*
660 South Euclid Avenue, Box 8118
St. Louis, Missouri 63110

Charles N. Serhan, Ph.D.
Professor of Anaesthesia, (Biochemistry and
*   Molecular Pharmacology)*
Department of Anaesthesia
Harvard Medical School
Director, Center for Experimental Therapeutics
*   and Reperfusion Injury*
Brigham and Women's Hospital
75 Francis Street
Boston, Massachusetts 02115

Robert S. Sherwin, M.D.
C.N.H. Long Professor of Internal
*   Medicine*
Section of Endocrinology
Department of Internal Medicine
Yale University School of Medicine
333 Cedar Street
New Haven, Connecticut 06510

Yoji Shibayama
Research Scientist
Nippon Zoki Pharmaceuticals Co.
442-1 Kinashi, Yashiro
Kato, Hyogo 673-1461 Japan

Henry J. Showell
Senior Research Fellow
Genomics, Targets and Cancer Research
Central Research Division
Pfizer Inc.
558 Eastern Point Road
Groton, Connecticut 06340

Michael Silverberg, M.D.
The Division of Pulmonary and
*   Critical Care Medicine,*
*   Allergy and Clinical Immunology*
Medical University of South Carolina
171 Ashley Avenue
Charleston, South Carolina 29425

Roy L. Silverstein, M.D.
Chief, Division of Hematology and
*   Medical Oncology*
Department of Medicine
New York Presbyterian Hospital
Mark W. Pismantier Professor of Medicine
Department of Medicine
Weill Medical College of Cornell University
1300 York Avenue
New York, New York 10021

Phillip D. Smith, M.D.
Professor
Departments of Medicine and
*   Microbiology*
Division of Gastroenterology and Hepatology
University of Alabama School of Medicine and
Medical Service, VA Medical Center
703 South 19th Street
Birmingham, Alabama 35294

Kendall A. Smith, M.D.
Professor
Department of Medicine
Cornell University Medical College
1300 York Avenue
New York, New York 10021
Chief, Division of Immunology
New York Presbyterian Hospital
East 68th Street
New York, New York 10021

Ralph Snyderman, M.D.
Chancellor for Health Affairs
James B. Duke Professor of Medicine
Duke University Medical Center
President and Chief Executive Officer,
*   Duke University Health System*
DUMC 3701
Durham, North Carolina 27710

Jonathan Sprent, M.D., Ph.D.
Department of Immunology, IMM4
The Scripps Research Institute
10550 N. Torrey Pines Road
La Jolla, California 92037

Robyn L. Stanfield, Ph.D.
Assistant Professor
Department of Molecular Biology
The Scripps Research Institute
10550 North Torrey Pines Road
La Jolla, California 92037

Douglas A. Steeber, Ph.D.
Assistant Research Professor
Department of Immunology
Duke University Medical Center
Box 3010
Durham, North Carolina 27710

Ralph M. Steinman, M.D.
Professor and Senior Physician
Laboratory of Cellular Physiology and
*   Immunology*
The Rockefeller University
1230 York Avenue
New York, New York 10021

Thomas P. Stossel, M.D.
American Cancer Society Professor
Department of Medicine
Harvard Medical School
Co-Director, Hematology Division
Brigham and Women's Hospital
221 Longwood Avenue
Boston, Massachusetts 02115

Robert M. Strieter, M.D.
Professor
Internal Medicine–Pulmonary
University of Michigan Medical School
Professor
University of Michigan Health System
3916 Taubman Center
Ann Arbor, Michigan 48109

John S. Sundy, M.D., Ph.D.
Associate in Medicine
Department of Medicine
Duke University Medical Center
Box 3258
Durham, North Carolina 27710
Physician, Department of Medicine
Duke Hospital
Durham, North Carolina 27710

Charles D. Surh, Ph.D.
Assistant Professor
Department of Immunology, IMM26
The Scripps Research Institute
10550 North Torrey Pines Road
La Jolla, California 92037

Thomas F. Tedder, Ph.D.
Professor and Chair
Department of Immunology
Duke University Medical Center,
Box 3010
Durham, North Carolina 27710

Robert F. Todd III, M.D., Ph.D.
Professor of Internal Medicine
Chief, Division of Hematology/Oncology
Department of Internal Medicine
University of Michigan Medical School
1500 East Medical Center Drive
Ann Arbor, Michigan 48109-0948

Kevin J. Tracey, M.D., F.A.C.S.
Professor
The Picower Institute for Medical Research
North Shore University Hospital (Surgery)
350 Community Drive
Manhasset, New York 11030-3816

Giorgio Trinchieri, M.D.
Professor and Chairman
Immunology Program
The Wistar Institute
3601 Spruce Street
Philadelphia, Pennsylvania 19104

Ronald J. Uhing, Ph.D.
COVANCE Biotechnology Services Inc.
Senior Scientist
6051 George Watts Hill Drive
Research Triangle Park, North Carolina 27709

Arthur A. Vandenbark, M.D.
Professor
Departments of Neurology and Molecular
*   Microbiology and Immunology*
Oregon Health Sciences University
Neuroimmunology Research R&D-31
Veterans Administration Medical Center
Portland Veterans Administration Medical Center
3181 South West US Veterans Hospital Road
Portland, Oregon 97201

Sharon M. Wahl, Ph.D.
Chief, Oral Infection and Immunity Branch
National Institute of Dental Research
National Institutes of Health
30 Convent Drive, MSC 4352
Bethesda, Maryland 20892-4352

Haichao Wang, Ph.D.
Surgical Resident
Department of Emergency Medicine
North Shore University Hospital
New York University
* School of Medicine*
Manhasset, New York 11030

Howard L. Weiner, M.D.
Robert L. Krok Professor of Neurology
Harvard Medical School
Center for Neurologic Diseases
Brigham and Women's Hospital
Harvard Medical School
77 Avenue Louis Pasteur, HIM 730
Boston, Massachusetts 02115

Jerrold Weiss, Ph.D.
Professor
Departments of Medicine
* and Microbiology*
University of Iowa College of Medicine
200 Hawkins Drive
Iowa City, Iowa 52246

Brendan Whittle, Ph.D., D.Sc.
William Harvey Research Institute
St. Bartholomew's and The Royal London School
* of Medicine*
Charterhouse Square
London EC1M 6BQ, United Kingdom

Ian A. Wilson, D.Phil.
Professor
Department of Molecular Biology
Skaggs Institute for Chemical
* Biology*
The Scripps Research Institute
10550 North Torrey Pines Road
La Jolla, California 92037

Samuel D. Wright, Ph.D.
Executive Director
Department of Lipid Biochemistry
Merck Research Laboratories
PO Box 2000, R80W-250
Rahway, New Jersey 07065

Gisele Zandman-Goddard, M.D.
Research Fellow
Division of Rheumatology
Department of Medicine
Albert Einstein College of Medicine
1300 Morris Park Avenue
Bronx, New York 10461
Instructor in Medicine, Senior Staff Physician
Department of Medicine
Sheba Medical Center
Tel Hashomer
Israel

Michael Zasloff, M.D., Ph.D.
President
The Magainin Research Institute
Magainin Pharmaceuticals Inc.
5110 Campus Drive
Plymouth Meeting, Pennsylvania 19462

Guy A. Zimmerman, M.D.
Professor
Department of Medicine
Nora Eccles Harrison Cardiovascular Research
* and Training Institute*
University of Utah
95 S. 2000 E.
Salt Lake City, Utah 84112

Mark J. Zoller, Ph.D.
Vice President Research—Molecular Biology
ARIAD Pharmaceuticals, Inc
26 Landsdowne Street
Cambridge, Massachusetts 02139

Preface

The inflammatory process is vital to the survival of all complex organisms, and its functions play a profound role in health and disease. Despite its importance to diverse areas of research and clinical medicine, when we initially conceived the first edition of *Inflammation,* there were no comprehensive textbooks that encompassed the entire subject in a contemporary manner. Published in 1988, the first edition of *Inflammation* was assembled to fill this void. It served as an advanced text that was designed to be of use to students, fellows, and physicians of differing backgrounds, as well as a reference for scientists. As such, it appealed to medical and graduate students and research fellows, as well as to primary investigators and clinical subspecialists interested in infectious diseases, clinical immunology, rheumatology, dermatology, pathology, and hematology-oncology.

The second edition, substantially revised and published in 1992, broadened the scope of the text with considerable new information about cytokines, signal transduction, and emerging therapeutic modulation of inflammation. Over the past seven years, there has been an explosion in our understanding of the immune system and its relationship to the inflammatory process. In addition, signal transduction, mechanisms of cellular adhesion, angiogenesis, and wound healing have been far more broadly defined. The field of cytokines and their receptors has been enhanced dramatically through the use of molecular genetics and cellular technologies. Not only has our understanding of cytokine biology grown, but its relevance to human diseases, particularly AIDS, has been entraordinary. The power of advances in biomedical research has impacted inflammation research so profoundly that the text has been almost entirely rewritten, with many chapters and authors added. Given the great increase in the scope of *Inflammation,* three associate editors were enlisted to add expertise in vital new areas.

This volume will be important to many research and clinical subspecialties. Each chapter is written by an individual actively engaged in research underlying the information detailed in the chapter. Some areas are controversial, and varying opinions may be represented therein. These chapters reflect the rapidly evolving nature of the field, and we urge the reader to view these topics with a critical eye. The field of inflammation is amongst the most active areas of research progress. Our hope is that the third edition of *Inflammation* reflects this exciting new understanding of the inflammatory process. It is our intention that the book will not only teach the basic principles of inflammation, but will also prepare readers for the rapid changes that will continue to occur in the future.

John I. Gallin
Ralph Snyderman

Acknowledgments

John Gallin thanks Maggi Stakem for hours of help overseeing the manuscripts for this project.

Ralph Snyderman thanks Vicki Saito and Ethel Byron for their most valuable help.

Barton Haynes thanks Kim R. McClammey for assistance in managing manuscript correspondence.

Carl Nathan thanks Lester Grant, MD, DPhil, editor of "The Inflammatory Process," for introducing him to science in general and inflammation in particular from 1960 to 1966, and Christine Sinclair-Prince, administrator, for her help and counsel through this and many other projects.

Inflammation: Basic Principles and Clinical Correlates,
3rd ed., edited by John I. Gallin and Ralph Snyderman.
Lippincott Williams & Wilkins, Philadelphia © 1999.

Overview

John I. Gallin and Ralph Snyderman

Inflammation normally is a localized, protective response to trauma or microbial invasion that destroys, dilutes, or walls-off the injurious agent and the injured tissue. It is characterized in the acute form by the classic signs of pain *(dolor)*, heat *(calor)*, redness *(rubor)*, swelling *(tumor)*, and loss of function *(functio laesa)*. Microscopically, it involves a complex series of events, including dilation of arterioles, capillaries, and venules, with increased permeability and blood flow; exudation of fluids, including plasma proteins; and leukocytic migration into the inflammatory focus.

Diseases characterized by inflammation are an important cause of morbidity and mortality in humans. Commonly, inflammation occurs as a defensive response to invasion of the host by foreign, particularly microbial, material. Responses to mechanical trauma, toxins, and neoplasia also may result in inflammatory reactions. The accumulation and subsequent activation of leukocytes are central events in the pathogenesis of most forms of inflammation. Deficiencies of inflammation compromise the host. Excessive inflammation caused by abnormal recognition of host tissue as foreign or prolongation of the inflammatory process may lead to inflammatory diseases as diverse as diabetes, atherosclerosis, Alzheimer's disease, cataracts, reperfusion injury, and cancer; to postinfectious syndromes such as in infectious meningitis and rheumatic fever; and to rheumatic diseases such as systemic lupus erythematosus and rheumatoid arthritis. The centrality of the inflammatory response in these varied disease processes makes its regulation a major element in the prevention, control, or cure of human disease. Ongoing research into the normal and pathologic mechanisms that generate and regulate the inflammatory response is needed, because many of these processes remain poorly understood.

Major strides since the second edition of *Inflammation* provide a strong foundation for a detailed model of leukocyte accumulation at sites of inflammation. Soluble chemotactic and leukocyte-activating molecules have been identified and characterized, and receptors for new and previously characterized soluble mediators have been cloned. Significant advances have occurred in understanding the molecular events that lead to leukocyte activation by bacterial peptides, lipopolysaccharides, and complement fragments. The advances made in understanding signaling cascades in inflammatory cells provide numerous targets for future pharmacologic modifications of the inflammatory response. The molecular processes of cell adhesion, locomotion, and generation of substances toxic to microorganisms or host tissues are understood in greater detail, providing a much clearer picture of how an inflammatory response occurs. The rolling interaction between leukocytes and the endothelium allows the leukocyte to sensitively identify inflammatory mediators, especially interleukin-8 and other chemokines, which activate additional adhesive processes mediated by cooperative interactions among selectins, integrins, and their ligands. The mechanisms by which leukocytes move to endothelial junctions, where they emigrate through the endothelium without damaging the integrity of the endothelial barrier, has been greatly clarified.

The restoration of homeostasis after an inflammatory insult leads to cessation of leukocyte influx into the site and to rapid removal of the leukocytes present. This late phase of inflammation is still poorly understood at a molecular level, although some advances have occurred. Other progress in understanding the resolution of inflammation includes development of sensitive assays for detecting phagocytosis of apoptotic cells. Information about how inflammatory cells accumulate in tissues and the mechanisms whereby such cells are stimulated to damage tissues should provide insights into the pathogenesis of human diseases and provide clues for developing more rational forms of therapy.

Most forms of acute and chronic inflammation are amplified and propagated as a result of the recruitment of humoral and cellular components of the immune system. Immunologically mediated elimination of foreign material proceeds through a series of integrated steps. The material to be eliminated (i.e., antigen) is recognized as foreign by specific or nonspecific means. Specific recognition is mediated by immunoglobulins (i.e., antibodies) or by receptors on T lymphocytes that bind to specific determinants (i.e., epitopes). Nonspecific forms of recognition (i.e., recognition of denatured proteins or endotoxins) are mediated directly by the alternative complement pathway or by phagocytes. Binding of a recognition component of the immune system to an antigen usually activates an amplification system, initiating production of proinflammatory substances. These mediators alter blood flow, increase vascular permeability, augment adherence of circulating leukocytes to vascular endothelium, promote migration of leukocytes into tissues, and stimulate leukocytes to destroy the inciting agent.

Destruction of antigens by immune mechanisms is mediated by phagocytic cells. Such cells may migrate freely or may exist at fixed tissue sites as components of the mononuclear phagocyte system. Macrophages and related cells (e.g., Kupffer cells, type A synovial lining cells) are central components of this system. Destruction of antigens outside of the mononuclear phagocyte system usually takes place in tissue spaces and is mediated by polymorphonuclear leukocytes (i.e., neutrophils) or monocytes, which are recruited from circulating blood. Immune processes are probably ongoing and, in most instances, lead to the elimination of antigens without producing clinically detectable inflammation. Development of clinically apparent inflammation indicates that the immune system has encountered an unusually large amount of antigen, antigen in an unusual location, or antigen that was difficult to digest. In some diseases (e.g., rheumatoid arthritis), the inciting agent is unknown or may be related to normal host tissue components. In other disorders (e.g., systemic lupus erythematosus), inherent or acquired immunoregulatory abnormalities may contribute to the sustained nature of the inflammatory process.

Inflammation and tissue injury on an immune basis characterize a wide variety of human diseases. Although little is known about the causes of these disorders, considerable progress has been made in understanding their pathogenesis. A convenient way of classifying immunologically induced inflammation is shown in Table 1.

ALLERGIC OR REAGINIC INFLAMMATION

Certain types of antigens have a propensity for stimulating production of immunoglobulin E antibodies in genetically susceptible persons. IgE antibodies bind nonspecifically through their Fc regions to receptors on basophils and mast cells. Subsequent attachment of antigens to the Fab portions of such cell-bound IgE antibodies causes mast cells and basophils to secrete contents of their cytoplasmic granules (e.g., histamine) and to synthesize and secrete biologically active products of arachidonic acid (e.g., leukotrienes). These mediators alter blood flow, increase vascular permeability, and constrict bronchial smooth muscle. Reaginic reactions are responsible for allergic phenomena such as urticaria, seasonal rhinitis, asthma, and when large amounts of allergens gain access to the circulation, systemic anaphylaxis.

INFLAMMATION MEDIATED BY CYTOTOXIC ANTIBODIES

Severe tissue injury can result from the binding of complement-fixing antibodies to cells. Recognition by antibodies of antigens on circulating erythrocytes, platelets, or leukocytes can lead to complement activation and deposition of complement fragments (e.g., C3b) on the surfaces of these cells. Macrophages of the mononuclear phagocyte system express plasma membrane receptors for the Fc portion of immunoglobulin G and for C3b; these macrophages also eliminate from the circulation particles coated with these proteins. Phagocytes also have membrane-bound mannose receptors, scavenger receptors, and lipopolysaccharide receptors, and they can directly ingest some invading pathogens by binding bacteria-specific carbohydrate and lipid molecules.

Extravascularly, binding of complement-fixing antibodies to cells or to extracellular structures (e.g., basement membrane) activates the complement cascade and

TABLE 1. *Immunopathologic processes*

Type of inflammation	Immune recognition component	Soluble mediator	Inflammatory response	Disease/ example
Reagenic/allergic	IgE	Basophil and mast cell products (i.e., histamine, arachidonate metabolites)	Immediate flare and wheal; smooth muscle constriction	Atopy; anaphylaxis
Cytotoxic antibody	IgG, IgM	Complement	Lysis or phagocytosis of circulating antigens; acute inflammation in tissues	Autoimmune hemolytic anemia; thrombocytopenia associated with lupus erythematosus
Immune complex	IgG, IgM	Complement	Accumulation of PMNs and macrophages	Rheumatoid arthritis; lupus erythematosus
Delayed hypersensitivity	T lymphocytes	Cytokines	Mononuclear cell infiltrate	Tuberculosis; sarcoidosis; polymyositis; granulomatosis; vasculitis

Adapted from ref. 1.

leads to binding of complement fragments to the antigen and to generation of mediators of inflammation. Cleavage products derived from C4, C3, and C5 (i.e., C4a, C3a, and C5a) increase vascular permeability and induce vascular stasis. C5a is a potent chemotactic factor that attracts granulocytes and macrophages. Accumulation of inflammatory cells and direct complement-mediated lysis destroy tissues coated with antibody. Goodpasture's syndrome is a dramatic example of a human disease that results from the deposition of antibodies onto glomerular and pulmonary basement membranes. Many common rheumatologic disorders are characterized by the development of antibodies to cells. Systemic lupus erythematosus, for example, frequently is accompanied by autoimmune hemolytic anemia and immune-mediated thrombocytopenia.

INFLAMMATION MEDIATED BY IMMUNE COMPLEXES

Inflammation due to deposition of immune complexes in tissues is a common feature of numerous rheumatic disorders. The combination of IgM or IgG antibodies with antigen is followed by activation of complement and the generation of several complement-derived peptides with proinflammatory activity. C3a and C5a, for example, enhance vascular permeability, contract smooth muscle, and degranulate mast cells. C5a also is a potent chemotactic factor and prompts accumulation of inflammatory cells at sites of immune complex formation or deposition. Other chemokines and cytokines, such as interleukins, amplify and modulate the inflammatory process. Key advances since the second edition of *Inflammation* include identification of the CC and CXC chemokine families, demonstration of extensive sharing of receptors by different chemokines, identification of functional interactions among multiple mediators, appreciation for extensive use of GTPase-associated receptors in leukocyte signaling, and early development of specific inhibitors of inflammation.

Polymorphonuclear leukocytes and mononuclear phagocytes recognize immune complexes by means of their surface receptors for C3b and IgG. Suitable ligand-receptor interactions ultimately lead to phagocytosis. When the amount of immune complexes deposited locally is not great, phagocytic cells ingest and degrade the complexes without causing tissue destruction. However, if the amount of immune complexes is great or if they are enmeshed in the basement membrane of blood vessels, leukocytes are incapable of completely ingesting and digesting the inflammatory stimulus. They instead adhere to immune complexes and degranulate, releasing a portion of their lysosomal contents. Binding of immune complexes to phagocytes also activates a respiratory burst and causes the cells to release toxic oxygen metabolites and proinflammatory cytokines. These events frequently

disrupt the integrity of blood vessels and lead to hemorrhagic necrosis and local tissue destruction.

When a large amount of antigen gains access to the circulation (e.g., after administration of heterologous serum), it can initiate a serum sickness reaction. As antibody is produced, antigen-antibody complexes form in the great antigen excess. Such complexes do not activate complement efficiently and may circulate harmlessly. As antibody production increases, however, immune complexes develop a lower ratio of antigen to antibody, thereby increasing their ability to activate complement. These complexes may deposit in the walls of small blood vessels, where they initiate inflammatory reactions by the mechanisms described earlier. Deposition of antigen in glomerular basement membrane can lead to the formation of immune complexes at that site. Alternatively, certain complexes may be phagocytosed by mesangial cells in the glomerulus. In either case, complement is deposited, and inflammation ensues. Associated with immune complex–mediated inflammation are leukocytic vasculitis (i.e., palpable purpuric skin lesions), arthritis, glomerulitis, and fever. Rheumatoid arthritis has many characteristics of a local immune complex reaction, whereas systemic erythematosus has many clinical features of serum sickness.

DELAYED-TYPE HYPERSENSITIVITY REACTIONS

When antigen is recognized by receptors on T lymphocytes, a delayed-type hypersensitivity reaction (i.e., inflammation mediated by mononuclear leukocytes) may be stimulated. The term *delayed-type hypersensitivity* reflects the kinetics of inflammation after deposition of antigen in the skin. Whereas allergic reactions occur within seconds to minutes and immune complex–mediated reactions occur within several to 24 hours, delayed-type hypersensitivity reactions peak at 48 to 72 hours after deposition of antigen. In delayed hypersensitivity reactions, antigen is encountered and processed by macrophages. The processed form of antigen is "presented" to T lymphocytes that contain receptors for the antigen and for Ia antigens (i.e., class II major histocompatibility complex antigen) on the macrophage. Binding of the processed antigen to T lymphocytes leads to the production of lymphokines (e.g., interleukin-2, interferon-γ, lymphocyte-derived chemotactic factor) and monokines (e.g., interleukin-1). Lymphokines and monokines, collectively called cytokines, are important mediators of inflammatory responses by virtue of their ability to attract and activate neutrophils, macrophages, and other lymphocytes. Macrophages ingest and degrade antigen in most cases.

Delayed-type hypersensitivity reactions appear to be particularly important for the destruction of many intracellular parasites, tumor cells, and viruses. Lesions typical of delayed-type hypersensitivity reactions are seen in human diseases such as tuberculosis, sarcoidosis, and polymyositis.

The importance of the inflammatory response for host defense has been recognized for more than a century. During the past decade, however, dramatic advances have been made in understanding the precise biochemical and cellular mechanisms that regulate this process. Inflammatory processes play a central role in mediating immune host defense and wound healing, but they also participate in the pathogenesis of many diseases. Better control of this complex inflammatory system offers a great challenge and opportunity for medical research. The following chapters summarize our understanding of inflammation and its clinical consequences.

REFERENCE

1. Snyderman R. Mechanisms of inflammation and tissue destruction in the rheumatic diseases. In: Wyngaarden JB, Smith LH Jr, eds. *Cecil's textbook of medicine,* 17th ed. Philadelphia: WB Saunders, 1985;1898–1906.

Inflammation: Basic Principles and Clinical Correlates,
3rd ed., edited by John I. Gallin and Ralph Snyderman.
Lippincott Williams & Wilkins, Philadelphia © 1999.

CHAPTER 1

Inflammation: Historical Perspectives

Ramzi S. Cotran

These are heady times for inflammation research. Besides advances made possible by the molecular revolution, it is now clear that inflammatory injury underlies some of the most prevalent and devastating diseases, such as atherosclerosis and perhaps Alzheimer's disease. In addition, the mechanisms regulating inflammatory events—from the acute cellular responses to fibroplasia and regeneration—overlap with those underlying normal and abnormal development and cancer. The increased understanding of molecular pathways has galvanized a mushrooming biotechnology effort focused on the holy grail of therapy: the discovery of agents that preserve the "salutary" effects of inflammation—first stated by John Hunter in 1793—and prevent its harmful effects.

Inflammation has had a long and colorful history, intimately linked to the history of wounds, wars, and infections. Majno captures these ancient times in his marvelous book, *The Healing Hand: Man and Wound in the Ancient World* (1), with descriptions of inflammation long before the cardinal signs of rubor, tumor, calor, and dolor were stamped by Celsius in the 1st century. Similarly, much has been written about the advances of the 19th and early 20th centuries: the classic descriptions of Cohnheim of the vascular and cellular events in thin, transparent membranes *in vivo* (2); the discovery of phagocytosis by Metchnikoff (3); proof of the role of antibodies by Ehrlich (4); and development of the concept of endogenous mediation of inflammation by Lewis in 1927 (5).

However, after that period, inflammation was largely forgotten, and it was not until the early 1960s that the new era of investigation began. Much of the progress has come from developments in fields such as immunology, cell biology, biochemistry, and molecular biology. Advances

specific to inflammation arose from a familiar pattern in biomedical research—a sequence of bold hypotheses, based on relatively crude experiments, which lead to technologic breakthroughs largely stimulated by such hypotheses, which further pushed the envelope. With this perspective, I recount some of the stories of inflammation research for which I was an eyewitness, participant, or passerby, with apologies to those who think that other examples are more worthy.

MEDIATORS: FROM MENKIN, BOYDEN, AND BEYOND

The concept of the chemical mediation of inflammation is ascribed to Sir Thomas Lewis' ingenious and characteristically simple experiments on the "triple response" elicited in the skin of the forearm by firm stroking (5). He postulated that the release of a humoral histamine-like substance (H substance) by injured tissue was the cause of the dull red line, which he ascribed to vasodilatation, and of the wheal, which he attributed to increased vascular permeability.

Lewis' work opened the door, and a small number of investigators entered. Their aim was to identify in normal, inflamed, and injured tissue the putative mediators of the local response in inflammation—increased vascular permeability and leukocyte influx—and the systemic effects, mainly pyrexia and leukocytosis. Their efforts were heroic, but the tools were primitive; the biochemical methods were crude; and there were few reliable pharmacologic antagonists, no available antibodies, and few reproducible methods with which to study the events. The only remotely quantitative technique was the estimation of leakage of an intravenously injected diazo dye (i.e., trypan or Evans blue), which binds to serum albumin after intradermal injections of substances in rabbits, guinea pigs, and rats. All else required detailed histologic studies.

R. S. Cotran: Pathology Departments of Harvard Medical School, Brigham and Women's Hospital and Children's Hospital, Boston, Massachusetts 02115.

The dominant figure of that time was Valy Menkin (6). Menkin published scores of papers and several monographs describing inflammatory activities in extracts that he derived from pleural exudates of rabbits and dogs injected with turpentine or croton oil. The most famous of the extracts was *leukotaxine*, which increased capillary permeability and caused migration of polymorphonuclear leukocytes, but he also reported *necrosin*, which was toxic to cells, *pyrexin*, which caused fever, and *growth-promoting factors*, which he thought were significant in the reparative reaction. Menkin's work was much maligned, largely because of the crudity of the substances injected and lack of specificity (7). Nevertheless, by today's measure, his concepts were very close to the mark. His diagrams (see Fig. 22 in reference 7) showing an irritant acting on a cell to induce "injury" and the elaboration of a variety of mediators with overlapping functions is strikingly similar to numerous drawings of similar events throughout this book. Menkin also predicted the importance of proteolysis and suggested adding it to the four cardinal signs as a *biochemical feature* of inflammation. More than anyone else in those days, he kept the flame of inflammation investigation alive.

The 1960s brought improved chemical methods, more sophisticated biochemists, and dissection of the complement, kinin, and coagulation systems. In the search for components of these systems that caused inflammation, the gold standard remained trypan blue leakage, although its use had been made more quantitative or supplemented by measurement of the escape of injected radiolabeled albumin into test sites. However, there was always the problem of whether a mediator, no matter how pure, produced its effects directly when injected into the skin or through activation of another mediator system, such as mast cell degranulation and histamine release. Some mediators, such as the anaphylatoxins, turned out to function indirectly. This uncertainty continued to plague investigators through later years and delayed acceptance of molecules that eventually turned out to be of enormous importance. When Dvorak's group first reported a vasopermeability factor (VPF) derived from cultured cancer cells (8), the "experts" thought that such conditioned media acted by releasing histamine or activating complement or by some other secondary mechanism. Ultimately, VPF was identified as a direct permeability-enhancing factor and as a vascular endothelial growth factor (VEGF), the hottest contender for *the* angiogenesis factor.

Many early workers searched for chemotaxins as mediators of leukocyte emigration, usually in histologic sections after injection of substances in skin. In 1962, it was Boyden who turned the early fishing expeditions for chemotactic agents into an international sport (9). In Boyden's original micropore filter chambers, leukocytes were placed in one compartment of a chamber, separated by a porous filter membrane from a second compartment into which a putative chemotactic substance is placed. If a chemotactic influence existed, the leukocytes crawled across the pores of the filter, and quantitation was done by counting the cells on the stained filter membrane or in the second chamber. The Boyden technique was initially criticized because it could not discriminate between chemotaxis and accelerated random locomotion of cells (i.e., chemokinesis), and alternate direct microscopic observation methods were devised. Nevertheless, the Boyden chamber was critical in that it allowed identification of substances that acted directly on leukocytes, and it was instrumental in the discovery of chemotactic peptides from bacteria and chemotactic products of the complement (10) and other mediator system. Later, similar chambers were used to study chemotaxis and migration in a variety of other cell types.

Other techniques, sometimes by serendipity, fueled the mediator search. Because many inflammatory mediators cause smooth muscle contraction and relaxation, techniques designed to study smooth muscle had a major impact on the discovery of mediators critical to inflammation. Slow-reacting substance of anaphylaxis (SRS) was described as a small acidic lipid that causes the slow and prolonged contraction of guinea pig ileum (10a), and much later, an endothelium-derived relaxation factor (EDRF) was delineated as an endothelial product that was required for vasodilation produced by acetylcholine in vessel segments *in vitro* (11). The former was a forerunner of the leukotrienes and the latter of nitric oxide, and the rest is history.

What cells make mediators? Because of histamine, mast cells were long suspected, and the plasma-derived systems came to attention in the 1960s. However, other cellular sources remained unclear. Menkin admitted that he did not know which cells produced the mediators in his extracts. One-half century later, all sets of leukocytes, platelets, endothelium, all types of connective tissues cells, and even epithelial cells are known to elaborate mediators. The pendulum swings as to which is most important. It was once only the leukocytes, but modern literature extols the importance of the mediators released by parenchymal cells—liver, renal tubule, keratinocytes—in acute and chronic inflammation; these concepts were barely imagined 10 years ago. For example, tubular epithelial cells, once thought to be interesting only to micropuncture jocks, are at the center of renal inflammation, and some believe they are as relevant as leukocytes to the genesis of renal fibrosis (12).

ENTER THE ENDOTHELIUM

One of the major advances of inflammation research has been the "discovery" of the endothelium. In historical terms, the story of discovery is recent, barely 25 years old, and it is worth retelling, because it highlights the paradigm of how hypotheses beget techniques that beget new concepts and create a new field of research (12a). In the late 1950s, there was virtually no endothelial research. A slender book by Altschule, published in 1954, summarized the field and has fewer references on endothelium than appear today in a month (13). Altschule, an anatomist, had spent a career studying endothelium, but he confessed in the book's preface, "I have not tempted to camouflage the dryness of my topic; it would be a mistake however if endothelium were hidden under the bushel of academic exclusiveness." He argued that blood vessels are primarily endothelial tubes, and "therefore, it may be postulated that the endothelium has a great importance in our life and if there is failure will cause death of any of us." The view that endothelium was an inert tissue was perpetrated by physiologists, presumably on the basis of experiments that showed that vascular permeability was similar in live and dead animals.

The first hint in the early 1960s was found by electron microscopy (EM). Palade described the fine structure of endothelium, discovered the pinocytotic vesicles, and suggested that vesicles ferried fluid and solutes across the endothelial barrier (14). For the next 35 years, the issue of what pinocytotic vesicles ferry and whether they represent the small or large pore of physiologists, or both, has been controversial. Fortunately, studies by Schnitzer, a pupil of Palade, have given much credence to the importance of endothelial vesicals and their role in endothelial physiology (15).

It was natural to extend ultrastructural studies to inflammation, and a small group of experimental pathologists from other fields became new students of endothelial research. Majno, learning EM with Palade at the Rockefeller Institute, used carbon black and EM to show that histamine and other mediators caused increased vascular permeability by forming intercellular gaps in venules (16). [This observation stood the test of time for more than 35 years. However, even this idea is being challenged by reports that increased *transcytosis*, rather than intercellular junctions, accounts for leakage (17). This story is still unfolding, and both probably occur, but my heart is still with junctions!] Marchesi, working as a student in Florey's laboratory at Oxford, showed beautiful pictures of neutrophils squeezing between endothelial cells and across intercellular junctions (18). Even this truism is being threatened by descriptions of neutrophils crossing the endothelium through the cytoplasm (19). Karnovsky discovered that horseradish peroxidase could be made a visible marker by EM (20), and several others used markers to examine the ultrastructural basis of inflammatory events. But for these descriptive EM studies, however, the endothelium remained dormant.

The next phase was the most critical in launching the field. It was sparked by conceptual advances in the form of hypotheses that ascribed a central role for endothelial cells in the two most common serious diseases of humans. The first was the "reaction to injury" hypothesis of atherosclerosis, put forth by Ross and his associates,

which focused on endothelial "injury" as the initiating event in atherosclerosis (21). The theory had great merit and was supported by studies of smooth muscle cultures and the demonstration of platelet-derived growth factors. However, what really put it to the test were rather crude experiments in which endothelial cells of the entire aorta of rabbits (and later of rats) were injured by an inflated balloon (22), resulting in thickenings resembling atherosclerosis. This balloon model became the staple for atherosclerosis research, and, it is said, ballooned many a cardiovascular career.

The second hypothesis was Folkman's targeting of tumor angiogenesis and therefore endothelial proliferation as a critical event in tumor growth (23). This was based first on simple Menkin-like *in vivo* experiments, in which tumor-conditioned medium was injected locally and observations of increased vascularization made. Some "experts" were again skeptical, claiming the changes represented vasodilatation and were nonspecific.

These two hypotheses stimulated the then relatively small group of enthusiasts to commit to endothelial research. An informal "Blood Vessel Club" was formed, fashioned along the Kinin and Complement clubs, and met annually on the Sunday before the start of the FASEB meetings. It became clear that the field needed methods for growing endothelium in culture. The issue was "nonnegotiable," and the challenge was on.

Previous attempts to culture endothelial cells from a variety of sources had very limited success. However, most of these attempts were done *in vacuo* "to study" the endothelium, and that few were driven by hypotheses or end points. Most concluded that endothelium in culture "turns into fibroblasts," and the researchers apparently quit. Maruyama had some success with cultures derived from trypsin-infused umbilical cord veins, but the endothelial nature of the cells remained in doubt (24). Jaffe et al. (25) and Gimbrone et al. (26) subsequently pursued experiments with umbilical cord veins, but they used special culture conditions and collagenase rather than trypsin to harvest more viable endothelial cells, and applied modern criteria (e.g., Weibel-Palade bodies by EM, von Willebrand factor staining by immunofluorescence) to establish cellular identity. They showed their results at the inaugural meeting of the Blood Vessel Club, which to many of us also inaugurated the new era of vascular biology.

The explosion of endothelial research in the 1970s and 1980s established the now well-known multifunctional nature of endothelial cells and their roles in pathophysiology. The research also led to the paradigm of "endothelial activation" as an important event in inflammation (12a). Endothelial activation is a term used by light and electron microscopists to describe the morphologic changes in endothelium that accompanied delayed hypersensitivity reactions—hypertrophy of endothelial cells, which acquire a plump, cuboidal appearance and protrude into the lumen, a marked increase in biosynthetic organelles seen by EM, and increased vascular permeability. About 40 years ago, Gell suggested that such activation may be related to the presence of sensitized cells or their products, although the nature of the activation process and the specific signals that induce it were unknown (28).

Three sets of studies in the early 1980s supported the concept of endothelial activation: induction of the surface expression of major histocompatibility (MHC) complex class II antigens by interferon-γ in cultured human endothelial cells (28) and demonstrations that endotoxin (29), interleukin-1, and tumor necrosis factor (TNF) (30) increase tissue factor-like procoagulant activity in cultured endothelium and that these cytokines cause enhanced adhesion of leukocytes on endothelium (32). The leukocyte adhesion studies led to the identification and cloning of the first endothelial-specific adhesion molecule, ELAM-1 (now called E-selectin) and to understanding of leukocyte-endothelial adhesion. Powerful immunologic and molecular techniques contributed to the phenomenal progress in endothelial research, but the initial driving force came from two hypotheses based on simple experiments and one enormously enabling technology.

THE YIN AND YANG OF LEUKOCYTES

The yin and yang of leukocytes, as soldiers meant to protect against invaders but also able to provoke great damage, is elegantly told on a backdrop of *Casablanca* in Weissman's historical perspective in the second edition of this book (33). Leukocyte-induced injury has become established as a mechanism of disease in a variety of disorders, from acute asthma and reperfusion injury to chronic transplant rejection and atherosclerosis. Much has been learned in the past decade about the mediators, adhesion molecules, specific chemokines, receptors, signal transduction mechanisms, and toxic leukocyte products that lead to defensive and injurious effects of leukocytes. However, beyond the dialogue on whether "pus" is good or bad for you, clear-cut evidence for the yin and yang properties is relatively recent. We know, for example, how potentially lethal is the factory of macrophages, but the first International Conference on Mononuclear Phagocytes organized by Ralph van Furth and Zanvil Cohn in the beautiful Dutch town of Leiden in 1970—a landmark for the macrophage crowd—added little to this and mostly examined the good side of macrophages. It was that first Leiden Conference that led to the new nomenclature of the mononuclear phagocyte system (34). Not until the fourth Leiden Conference in 1984, did the subject of macrophage secretory products peak.

On the yin side, work in animals contributed to the field, but some of the seminal discoveries came from the bedside to the bench through studies on patients with rel-atively rare disorders of leukocyte function. A dramatic example (see Chapter 41) is provided by chronic granulomatous disease, first recognized as a distinct clinical entity in 1957 (35). It was relatively quickly identified by a series of studies, converging from various sources, as a leukocyte microbicidal defect caused by the inability of leukocytes to respond with a burst of oxidative activity accompanying phagocytosis and failure of the H_2O_2-myeloperoxidase-halide-killing mechanism (36).

Another important story is the discovery of the defects in leukocyte adhesion, such as the leukocyte adhesion disease (LAD-1) (37). The outlines of the historical sequence of events leading to its discovery reviewed previously (37), are fascinating. In the 1970s, several patients were described who suffered from recurrent bacterial infections of the skin, periodontal tissues, and upper respiratory tract, sometimes with a fatal outcome. An article in 1980 reported that a neutrophil surface protein of 110 kd was absent in one such infant and that such neutrophils did not adhere to glass (38). In 1982, neutrophils from another such patient showed absence of a normal granulocyte surface glycoprotein of 150 kd (GP150), which was present in reduced amounts in cells from both parents (39), and in 1984, a patient with similar abnormalities was shown to have a deficiency of a neutrophil surface protein of 138 kd (GP138) (40). These patients sparked a flurry of activity to identify the defective proteins, largely by using monoclonal antibodies available from somewhat unrelated work on leukocyte differentiation antigens and lymphocyte interactions. When the dust settled, the defect underlying this disease became clear: deficient synthesis of the common β subunit of the $\alpha_1\beta_2$ integrins (e.g., LFA-1/MAC-1, P150) and impairments in adhesion, phagocytosis, and other functions that ensue (41). By binding to intercellular adhesion molecule-1 (ICAM-1) on endothelium, lymphocyte function antigen-1 (LFA-1) and membrane attack complex-1 (MAC-1) play a critical role in firm adhesion to endothelium as a prelude to emigration, and abrogation of these molecules by antibodies or in genetic-engineered mice results in disturbance of leukocyte functions, including adhesion. In contrast to LAD-1, LAD-2 was uncovered by examining patients with recurrent infections (not exhibiting a β_2 defect), after the identification of selectins as adhesion molecules, and was traced to a defect in fucosylation that interferes with the expression of sialylated oligosaccharides, the ligands for selectins (43).

BACK TO *IN VIVO*

It is an axiom that the relevance of the multitude of genes and molecules being discovered—in terms of their role in physiology and disease—will depend on where, when, and how they act in the complex events that occur in the whole organism. Inflammation research, which is in large part driven by the need for understanding for perfect therapy, therefore requires *in vivo* experimental models.

In vivo models dominated inflammation research in the premolecular days. Cohnheim's experiments in frog's tongues defined the vascular and cellular events in inflammation; Metchnikoff discovered the defensive function of leukocytes in starfish larvae; and Lewis used human skin to show chemical mediation. However, models have also been important more recently. In the 1960s, no models were more in style than those of experimental glomerulonephritis, perfected by Frank Dixon and his many pupils (44). They were fairly decisive in documenting the role of immune complexes, antibodies to fixed antigens, complement components, neutrophils, and later, monocytes in the immunologic inflammatory injury. Despite the structural and physiologic complexity of the glomerulus, glomerular injury is readily quantifiable functionally by the presence of proteinuria, and the model was one of the gold standards for studying the effects of mediators and their antagonists. Over the years, new models were developed for acute inflammation, such as ischemia reperfusion and chronic fibrosing inflammation in a variety of organs; these have been enormously helpful in assessing the roles of molecules uncovered from *in vitro* work and a variety of therapeutically promising antagonists.

It is ironic that variations of some of the oldest methods have been resurrected. An industry has grown to examine the inflamed microcirculation in thin, transparent membranes—á la Cohnheim—armed with lasers, computers, fluorescent labels, and exquisite photographic techniques. The roles of specific adhesion molecules and chemokines in every minute step of leukocyte extravasation of every leukocyte type, from rolling, to tethering, to semifirm and firm adhesion, to emigration, is being dissected by such methods (see Chapters 37–40).

The transgenic techniques—knock-outs, knock-ins, over-expressors—have been as much a boon to inflammation as they have to other fields. The power and pitfalls of the transgenic technology have been discussed elsewhere, but from the view of inflammation, two points can be made. First, although the mouse has the most exhaustively studied immune system, it has not been a target of inflammation research, and few of the standard models using rats, guinea pigs, and rabbits have been developed for mice. Methods to induce reproducible and quantifiable renal, pulmonary, cutaneous, and cerebral inflammation are few, as are models for more chronic inflammatory responses, and much work must be done to develop and characterize new models to ensure maximal benefits for this technology. Second, there has never been a greater need for traditional experimentalists—morphologists, pathologists, physiologists, and cell and molecular biologists—who can interpret the *in vivo* findings and design experiments to pursue pathogenetic mechanisms suggested by these powerful tools. To quote Nobel Laureate Michael Brown in not too dissimilar a context, "Ironically, what's happening now is the PhDs, especially because of all these gene manipulation experiments, can knock out genes in mice, and suddenly the mouse gets sick. The PhDs have no idea why the mouse is sick, so they need to come to their MD friends to try to tell them why this mouse is sick. It's ironic that the same kind of clinical acumen is now needed to diagnose a mouse as it is a person" (45). This is the time for experimentalists, such as those who toiled with inflammation in premolecular days, to join "the back to *in vivo*" crusade, using modern tools, as all the genes come home.

REFERENCES

1. Majno G. *The healing hand:* man and wound in the ancient world. Cambridge, MA: Harvard University Press, 1975.
2. Cohnheim J. *Lectures in general pathology* [translated by McKee AD from the German], 2nd ed, vol 1. London: New Sydenham Society, 1889.
3. Heifets L. Centennial of Metchnikoff's discovery. *J Reticuloendothel Soc* 1982;31:381.
4. Silverstein AM. History of Immunology. In: Paul W, ed. *Fundamental immunology.* New York: Raven Press, 1992:23–40.
5. Lewis T. The blood vessels of the human skin and their responses. London: Shaw & Sons, 1927.
6. Menkin V. Modern views on inflammation. *Int Arch Allergy* 1953;4:131–168.
7. Moon VH, Menkin V. Letters. *Science* 1952;115:382–384.
8. Senger DR, Galli SJ, Dvorak AM, Perruzzi CA, Harvey VS, Dvorak HF. Tumor cells secrete a vascular permeability factor that promotes accumulation of ascites fluid. *Science* 1983;219:983–985.
9. Boyden S. The chemotactic effects of mixtures of antigen and antibody on polymorphonuclear leukocytes. *J Exp Med* 1962;115:453.
10. Snyderman R, Phillips J, Mergenhagen SE. Polymorphonuclear leukocyte chemotactic activity in rabbit serum and guinea pig serum treated with immune complexes: evidence for C5a as the major chemotactic factor. *Infect Immun* 1970;1:521.
10a. Feldberg W, Kellaway CH. Liberation of histamine and formation of lysolecithin-like substance by cobra venom. *J Phys* 1938;94:187.
11. Furchgott RF, Zawadski JV. The obligatory role of endothelial cells in the relaxation of arterial smooth muscle by acetylcholine. *Nature* 1980;288:373.
12. Palmer BF. The renal tubule in the progression of chronic renal failure. *J Invest Med* 1997;45:346.
12a. Cotran RS. New roles for the endothelium in inflammation and immunity. *Am J Pathol* 1987;129:407–413.
13. Altschul R. *Endothelium:* its development, *morphology, function, and pathology.* New York: Macmillan, 1954.
14. Palade GE. Transport in quanta across the endothelium of blood capillaries. *Anat Rec* 1960;136:254–264.
15. Schnitzer J, Allard J, Oh P. NEM inhibits transcytosis, endocytosis, and capillary permeability: implication of caveolae fusion in endothelia. *Am J Physiol* 1995;268:H48–H55.
16. Majno G, Palade GE. Studies on inflammation. II. The site of action of histamine and serotonin on vascular permeability: An electron microscopic study. *J Biophys Biochem Cytol (J Cell Biol)* 1961;11:571–605.
17. Feng D, Nagy J, Hipp J, Dvorak H, Dvorak A. Vesiculo-vacuolar organelles and the regulation of venule permeability to macromolecules by VPF, histamine, and serotonin. *J Exp Med* 1996;183:1981.
18. Marchesi VT. The site of leukocyte emigration during inflammation. *Q J Exp Physiol* 1961;46:115.
19. Feng D, Nagy JA, Pyne K, Dvorak HF, Dvorak AM. Neutrophils emigrate from venules by a transendothelial pathway in response to FMLP. *J Exp Med* 1998;187:903.
20. Karnovsky MJ. The ultrastructural basis of capillary permeability studied with horseradish peroxidase. *J Cell Biol* 1967;35:213–236.

21. Ross R, Glomset JA. I. The pathogenesis of atherosclerosis. *N Engl J Med* 1976;295:420–425.
22. Baumgartner HR, Stemerman MB, Spaet TH. Adhesion of blood platelets to subendothelial surface: Distinct from adhesion to collagen. *Experientia* 1971;27:283–285.
23. Folkman J, Merler E, Abernathy C, Williams G. Isolation of a tumor factor responsible for angiogenesis. *J Exp Med* 1971;133:275–288.
24. Maruyama Y. The human endothelial cell in culture. *Z Zellforshung Mikro Anat* 1963;60:69.
25. Jaffe EA, Nachman RL, Becker CG. Culture of human endothelial cells derived from umbilical veins: identification by morphological and immunologic criteria. *J Clin Invest* 1973;52:2745–2758.
26. Gimbrone MA Jr, Cotran RS, Folkman J. Human vascular endothelial cells in culture: Growth and DNA synthesis. *J Cell Biol* 1974;60: 673–682.
27. Reference moved in text.
28. Gell PGH. Cytologic events in hypersensitivity reactions, cellular, and humoral aspects of hypersensitivity states. In: Lawrence HS, ed. *xxx*. New York: Harper & Row, 1959:43–66.
29. Pober JS, Gimbrone MA Jr, Cotran RS, et al. Ia expression by vascular endothelium is inducible by activated T cells and by human τ interferon. *J Exp Med* 1983;157:1339–1353.
30. Colucci M, Balconi G, Lorenzet R, et al. Cultured human endothelial cells generate tissue factor in response to endotoxin. *J Clin Invest* 1983;71:1893–1896.
31. Reference deleted in text.
32. Bevilacqua MP, Pober JS, Wheeler ME, Cotran RS, Gimbrone MA Jr. Interleukin-1 acts on cultured human vascular endothelial cells to increase the adhesion of polymorphonuclear leukocytes, monocytes, and related cell lines. *J Clin Invest* 1985;76:2003–2011.
33. Weissman G. Inflammation historical perspectives. In: Gallin JI, Goldstein JM. Snyderman R, eds. Inflammation: Basic Principles and Clinical Correlates, 2nd ed. New York: Raven Press, 1992:5–13.
34. Van Furth R, Cohn ZA, Hirsch JG, Humphrey JH, Spector WG. *Bull World Health Organ* 1972;46:845–852.
35. Berendes H, Bridges RA, Good RA. Fatal granulomatosis of childhood: the clinical study of a new syndrome. *Minn Med* 1951;40:309–312.
36. Johnson RB Jr, Keele BB Jr, Misra HP, et al. The role of superoxide anion generation in phagocytic bactericidal activity. Studies with normal and chronic granulomatous disease leukocytes. *J Clin Invest* 1975;55:1357–1372.
37. Schmalstieg FC. Discovery of the leukocyte adherence defect—a historical perspective. *Semin Hematol* 1993;30:66–71.
38. Crowley CA, Curnutte JT, Rosin RE, Andre-Schwartz J, Gallin JI, et al. An inherited abnormality of neutrophil adhesion: its genetic transmission and its association with a missing protein. *N Engl J Med* 1980;302:1163–1168.
39. Arnaout MA, Pitt J, Cohen HJ, Melamed J, Rosen FS, Colten HR. Deficiency of a granulocyte-membrane glycoprotein (GP150) in a boy with recurrent bacterial infections. *N Engl J Med* 1982;306:693–699.
40. Anderson DC, Schmalstieg FC, Arnaout MA, Kohls S, Tosi MF, et al. Abnormalities of polymorphonuclear leukocyte function associated with a heritable deficiency of a high molecular weight surface glycoproteins (GP138): common relationship to diminished cell adherence. *J Clin Invest* 1984;74:536–551.
41. Anderson DC, Springer TA. Leukocyte adhesion deficiency: an inherited defect in the Mac-1, LFA-1, and p150,95 glycoproteins. *Annu Rev Med* 1987;38:175–194.
42. Reference deleted in text.
43. Etzioni A, Frydman M, Pollak S, Avidor I, Phillips ML, et al. Brief report: recurrent severe infections caused by a novel leukocyte adhesion deficiency. *N Engl J Med* 1992;327:1789.
44. Dixon FJ, Feldman JD, Vasquez J. Experimental glomerulonephritis: the pathogenesis of a laboratory model resembling the spectrum of human glomerulonephritis. *Am J Med* 1961;44:493.
45. Brown MS. In The J.I.M. [interview]. *J Invest Med* 1996;44:14–23.

PART I

Cellular Components of Inflammation

Inflammation: Basic Principles and Clinical Correlates,
3rd ed., edited by John I. Gallin and Ralph Snyderman.
Lippincott Williams & Wilkins, Philadelphia © 1999.

CHAPTER 2

Developmental Biology of Neutrophils and Eosinophils

Dorothy Ford Bainton

The ability of each type of leukocyte to perform its special function depends on the synthesis of particular chemical substances during its maturation. Certain leukocytes (e.g., neutrophils, eosinophils) synthesize proteins at regular intervals early in their maturation in bone marrow and store them for days as large cytoplasmic granules (1–3). When appropriately stimulated, these cells can move from blood to tissues, and within seconds, the granules may release their contents into an endocytic vacuole or, by fusion with the plasma membrane, to the exterior of the cell. Their major function in inflammatory processes is usually accomplished by endocytosis ("eating") or exocytosis ("secreting") (4).

These cells are produced in the bone marrow; this hemopoietic factory weighs about 2600 g, which is about 4.5% of body weight of a normal adult. Although widely distributed within the various bones, the marrow is an organ larger than the liver, which weighs about 1500 g. About 55% to 60% of bone marrow is dedicated to the production of one cell type, the neutrophil. The normal ratio of neutrophils to erythroid cells is 2:1 to 3:1. Developing eosinophils constitute about 3% of the bone marrow. The cellularity of bone marrow varies greatly with age; cells constitute 75% of the marrow in the young, 50% in young adults, and 25% in the elderly, although there is great variability among individuals of a given age (5,6). Bone marrow is a highly proliferative tissue, and mitoses are normally observed in 10 to 25 per 1,000 nucleated cells (7).

Approximately 100 billion neutrophils enter and leave the circulation daily in normal adults (8,9). The normal sites of destruction of neutrophils have yet to be defined. Many observations suggest that there may be a random

loss of granulocytes into the tissues. In a study by Jamuar and Cronkite (10), neutrophils of mice were not found in transit through vascular endothelium nor in extravascular spaces. Granulocytes did concentrate in the spleen and presumably were destroyed there. The role of Kupffer cells in eliminating aging and apoptotic neutrophils was investigated in rats (11) after an injection of bacteria. Apoptotic neutrophils were found in Kupffer cells of the liver but were rare in spleen, lung, or blood. The results establish that, in rats under conditions of bacteremia, Kupffer cells are responsible for the rapid clearance of neutrophils.

Three major compartments of differentiation in the bone marrow have been established: the most primitive compartment of pluripotent stem cells, committed cells, and maturing cells. The third and most familiar stage of hemopoiesis consists of cells identifiable by morphologic features (e.g., a characteristic nuclear configuration, presence of obvious cytoplasmic granules). These cells are fully mature leukocytes or those undergoing the last few divisions leading to maturity. This chapter examines this third stage of development of neutrophils and eosinophils.

NEUTROPHILS

In the normal adult human, the life of polymorphonuclear neutrophils (PMNs) is spent in three environments: bone marrow, blood, and tissues. Bone marrow is the site of the important processes of proliferation and terminal maturation of neutrophilic granulocytes (myeloblast → PMNs). Proliferation, consisting of approximately five divisions, takes place only during the first three stages of neutrophil maturation (i.e., blast, promyelocyte, and myelocyte). After the myelocyte stage, the cells become end cells (i.e., no longer capable of mitosis) and enter a large

D. F. Bainton: Pathology Department, University of California at San Francisco, San Francisco, California 94143.

storage pool. About 5 days later, they are released into the blood, where they circulate for about 10 hours. Their fate after they have migrated to tissues is unknown, but they probably live for only 1 or 2 days (4).

Light Microscopy and Peroxidase Histochemistry of Neutrophils in Bone Marrow and Blood Smears

Figure 2-1 shows the stages of neutrophil maturation (2,4). The myeloblast is a relatively undifferentiated cell with a large, oval nucleus, sizable nucleoli, and few or no granules. It originates from a precursor pool of stem cells and is followed by the promyelocyte and myelocyte stages, during which two distinct types of granules are formed. The first type, the azurophil or primary granule, is formed during the promyelocyte stage and contains peroxidase. The second type, the specific or secondary granule, is formed later during the myelocyte stage and is peroxidase negative. In Figure 2-1, the azurophil is shown as a solid, black granule, and the specific granule is shown as a light granule. The metamyelocyte and band forms are nonsecretory, nonproliferating stages leading to the mature PMN, which contains both types of gran-

ules in the proportions of 33% azurophils and 67% specifics. The times spent in the various stages were determined by isotope-labeling techniques (12). No mitoses occur after the myelocyte stage.

A few comments are necessary to clarify the relation between azurophil granules and specific granules. Around the turn of the 20th century, it was proposed that the granules produced during the promyelocyte stage (which stain azurophilic [reddish purple]) change, "ripen," or differentiate into specific granules. Such a change would explain why the large, metachromatic, reddish-purple azurophils, so prominent in the early neutrophil precursors in Wright-stained smears of normal bone marrow, are no longer observed after the myelocyte stage. A loss of metachromasia during maturation accounts for the change in appearance of the azurophils. Increasing concentration of their contents at the myelocyte stage may lead to decreased absorption of dye molecules and lessening metachromasia, particularly if stainable acid mucosubstances form complexes with basic proteins (13). The indisputable electron microscopic demonstration (2) that large ($\approx$500 nm), peroxidase-positive azurophil granules persist in mature PMNs leaves lit-

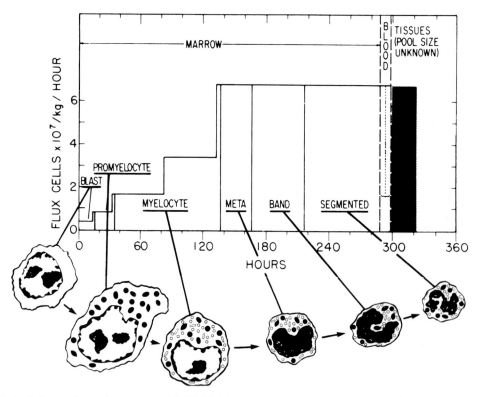

FIG. 2-1. Polymorphonuclear neutrophil (PMN) lifespan and stages of maturation. Of every 100 nucleated cells in bone marrow, 2% are myeloblasts, 5% are promyelocytes, 12% are myelocytes, 22% are metamyelocytes and bands, and 20% are mature PMNs, yielding a total of about 60% developing PMNs. The times indicated for the various compartments were obtained by isotope-labeling techniques (12). The ordinate shows the flux through each compartment, and the abscissa shows the time in each compartment. The stepwise increase in cell numbers through the dividing compartments represents serial divisions. No mitoses occur after the myelocyte stage. (From ref. 2, with permission.)

tle doubt that the fairly prominent violet granules visible by light microscopy in mature cells on Wright-stained smears are azurophils whose staining characteristics have altered during maturation. It follows that the most reliable method for visualizing azurophil granules on smears (using the light microscope) is to stain the cells for peroxidase. Because most of the specific granules are in a size range ($\approx$200 nm) at the limit of resolution of the light microscope, they probably cannot be distinguished individually, but they are responsible for the pink background color of neutrophils during and after the myelocyte stage.

The nucleus of the mature neutrophil is segmented into three to five interconnected lobes. The physiologic purpose of nuclear segmentation is unknown. Campbell et al. (14) tested the role of cytoskeletal elements in the process and determined that neither microtubule inhibitor nocodazole nor the microfilament inhibitor cytochalasin D prevented the nuclear segmentation. Using fluorescence *in situ* hybridization of whole chromosome probes, they determined that chromosomes are randomly distributed among the nuclear lobes. Some mature neutrophils of females have drumsticks or club-shaped nuclear appendages. These appendages are thought to contain an inactivated X chromosome. One study, in which an X-chromosome–specific nucleic acid probe was used to detect the position of the X chromosomes in leukocyte nuclei by *in situ* hybridization, provided the first direct evidence of X chromosomal material in the drumstick structures (15).

Stages of Neutrophil Differentiation Determined by Electron Microscopy and Peroxidase Cytochemistry

All of the following observations were derived from specimens of normal human bone marrow and from blood tested for peroxidase. The dense enzyme reaction product served as a marker and stabilizer of azurophil granules (2,16–18).

Myeloblast

The earliest cell is a relatively undifferentiated cell with a high nuclear to cytoplasmic ratio and prominent nucleoli. It contains reaction product for peroxidase within the rough-surfaced endoplasmic reticulum (RER) and Golgi cisternae, and sometimes it contains immature peroxidase-positive azurophil granules.

Polymorphonuclear Neutrophil Promyelocyte

The PMN promyelocyte stage of maturation (Fig. 2-2) is characterized by the production and accumulation of a large population of peroxidase-positive granules that vary in contour and size; most are spherical ($\approx$500 nm), but there are also ellipsoid, crystalline forms and small granules connected by filaments (Fig. 2-3). Peroxidase is present throughout the secretory apparatus of the promyelo-

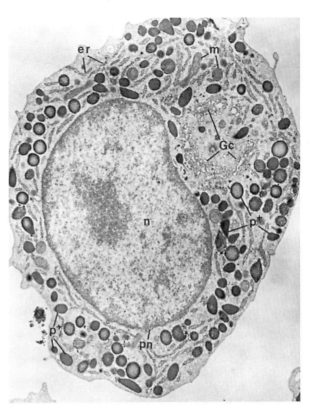

FIG. 2-2. Electron micrograph of a neutrophilic promyelocyte reacted for peroxidase from normal human bone marrow. This cell is the largest of the neutrophilic series. It has a sizable, slightly indented nucleus (n), a prominent Golgi region, and cytoplasm packed with dense, peroxidase-positive azurophil granules (p$^+$) of various shapes and sizes. Peroxidase reaction product is visible in less concentrated form within all compartments of the secretory apparatus. No reaction product is apparent in the cytoplasmic matrix, mitochondria (m), or nucleus (n). er, endoplasmic reticulum; pn, perinuclear cisterna; Gc, Golgi cisternae. ×13,000. (From ref. 2.)

cyte—in cisternae of the RER, in all Golgi cisternae and some vesicles, and in all forming granules. Its presence in these compartments at this stage indicates that it is synthesized and packaged into storage granules by the pathway defined for other secretory proteins (RER → Golgi complex via vesicles → granules).

Hiatal Cell

Peroxidase abruptly disappears from RER and Golgi cisternae at the end of the promyelocyte stage; at this point, the production of azurophil granules ceases, and the myelocyte stage and production of the peroxidase-negative specific granules begin. However, cells with the nuclear configuration of the myelocyte and lacking peroxidase in the RER or Golgi cisternae often contain mature azurophil granules but no specific granules, and they have large Golgi complexes containing no forming granules of either type. Such cells are presumed to exist in a hiatus between the two waves of granule formation (20).

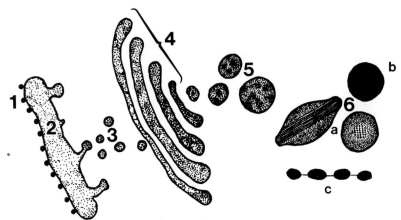

FIG. 2-3. Hypothetical steps involved in the formation of azurophil granules in normal neutrophilic promyelocytes. Peroxidase reaction product has been observed in increasing concentrations within the rough-surfaced endoplasmic reticulum (RER), Golgi cisternae, and azurophil granules, indicating that in general the pathway of secretion and condensation of this enzyme conforms to that of secretory proteins in the pancreas and in other cell types. These steps include synthesis on bound ribosomes (1), segregation within RER cisternae (2), pinching off of vesicles from transitional elements of the RER and their transfer to the Golgi complex through junctional vesicles (3), packing and concentration of the enzyme within the Golgi cisternae and the formation of Golgi-derived vesicles (4), aggregation of smaller vesicles into large, immature azurophil granules (5), and condensation to produce the azurophil granules (6). Azurophil granules occur in two main forms. Most are spherical (b), with dense homogeneous matrices; others are ellipsoid, with crystalline substructures (a). Round granule profiles with a central periodicity are presumed to represent ellipsoids cut perpendicular to the crystal axis (right). A third form (c) is distinguished by their small size and the fact that they are interconnected by microtrabeculae (19).

Polymorphonuclear Neutrophil Myelocyte

The myelocyte stage (Fig. 2-4) is characterized by the production and accumulation of the peroxidase-negative specific (secondary) granules. The only peroxidase-positive elements at this stage are the azurophil granules. The specific granules are formed by the Golgi complex (Fig. 2-5). They vary in size and shape (see Figs. 2-4 and 2-5), but they are typically spherical (≈200 nm) or rod shaped (130 × 1,000 nm). Kinetic studies of human

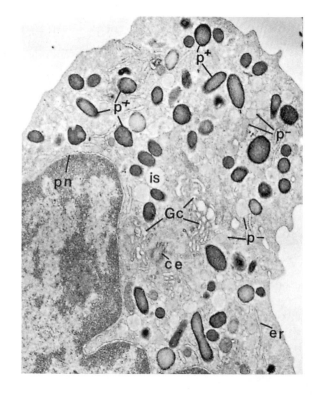

FIG. 2-4. Neutrophilic myelocyte reacted for peroxidase. At this stage, the cell is smaller than the promyelocyte (see Fig. 2-2), the nucleus is more indented, and the cytoplasm contains two different types of granule: large, peroxidase-positive azurophils (p+) and the generally smaller specific granules (p−), which do not stain for peroxidase. A number of immature specific granules (is)—larger, less compact, and more irregular in contour than mature granules—appear in the Golgi region. Peroxidase reaction product is present only in azurophil granules (p+) and not in the rough-surfaced endoplasmic reticulum (er), perinuclear cisterna (pn), or Golgi cisternae (Gc). This finding is in keeping with the fact that azurophil granule production has ceased and only peroxidase-negative specific granules are produced during the myelocyte stage. ce, centriole. ×16,000.

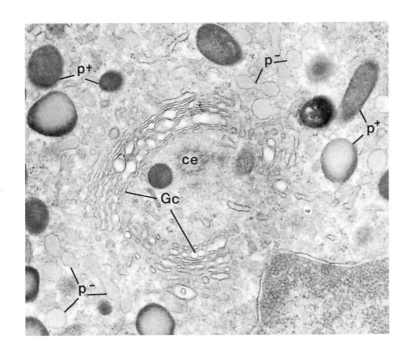

FIG. 2-5. Golgi region of a neutrophilic myelocyte reacted for peroxidase. As in Figure 2-4, peroxidase reaction product is found in azurophils (p⁺) but not in specific granules (p⁻). The stacked, smooth-surfaced Golgi cisternae (Gc) are oriented around the centriole (ce). ×23,000.

myelocytes (12) indicate that about three divisions occur at this stage of maturation. Mitoses can be observed (Fig. 2-6), and the two types of granules appear to be distributed to the daughter cells in fairly equal numbers.

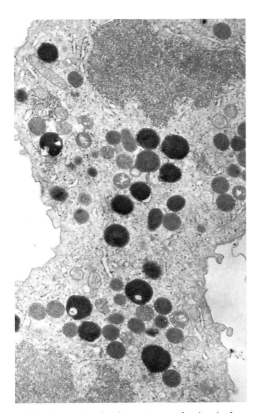

FIG. 2-6. Myelocyte in the late stage of mitosis from rabbit bone marrow. This myelocyte is in telophase. The granules are being relatively equally distributed to the daughter cells. ×17,000.

Later Stages of Differentiation in Bone Marrow

The metamyelocyte, band, and mature PMN are nondividing, nonsecretory stages identifiable by their nuclear morphology, mixed granule population, small Golgi regions, and accumulation of glycogen particles. In the mature PMN, the smaller, peroxidase-negative specific granules are twice as abundant as the peroxidase-positive azurophils (Fig. 2-7). On average, a thin-section cell profile has 200 to 300 granules.

The data on human PMNs indicate that the peroxidase-positive azurophils and peroxidase-negative specific granules are separate populations of granules that are chemically distinct from the time of their formation and that both are present in the mature PMN. Specific granules become more numerous than azurophils during the myelocyte stage because azurophil formation ceases after the promyelocyte stage, the number of azurophils per cell is reduced by mitoses, and specific granules continue to be produced by daughter myelocyte generations. Bainton and Farquhar (1) have provided a more detailed explanation.

Microperoxisomes are present from the promyelocyte stage through mature PMNs (21). Microperoxisomes are small, membrane-bound vesicles that contain catalase. Although this enzyme is known to destroy peroxide (H_2O_2), its exact function in leukocytes has yet to be determined. Additional changes that occur during the course of differentiation in regard to surface markers, cytoskeleton elements, and other organelles have been reviewed elsewhere (22). Changes in cell-surface carbohydrates, glycoproteins, glycolipids, and human leukocyte antigens (HLA) occur during maturation. For example, the densities of membrane HLA-A, -B, and -C antigens decrease with granulocyte maturation. Some

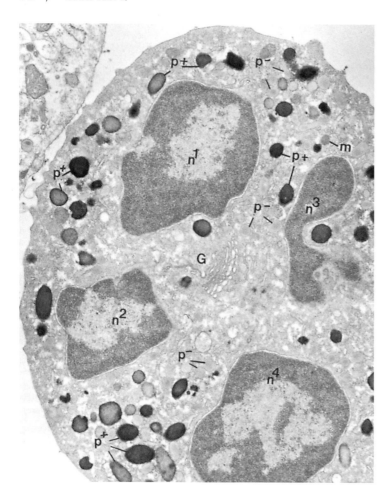

FIG. 2-7. Mature polymorphonuclear neutrophils from normal human bone marrow reacted for peroxidase. The cytoplasm is filled with granules of the two basic types: the small, pale, peroxidase-negative granules (p⁻) and the large, dense, peroxidase-positive granules (p⁺). The nucleus is condensed and lobulated (n¹ through n⁴), the Golgi region (G) is small and without any forming granules, the rough-surfaced endoplasmic reticulum is scant, and mitochondria (m) are few. ×21,000.

surface antigens appear during PMN maturation. The development of chemotactic and recognition capabilities parallels the acquisition of certain membrane receptors.

Fc receptors are not present or are poorly expressed on progenitors younger than myelocytes, whereas more than 90% of mature PMNs have Fc receptors. Mature PMNs possess at least two classes of receptors for fragments of the complement component C3, called CRI and CR3. Formyl peptide receptors are not detectable in myeloblasts but gradually emerge through later stages of neutrophil maturation (23). Other maturation changes occur in cytoskeletal elements and biophysical features such as deformability and surface charge (22).

Heterogeneity of Neutrophil Granules

The initial classification into two major types of granules was based on their content of myeloperoxidase. However, the granules can be further subdivided on the basis of other proteins, as summarized by Borregaard and Cowland (24). Four distinct populations (Table 2-1) have been identified by cytochemical, immunocytochemical, and cell fractionation procedures: azurophil, specific, gelatinase, and secretory granules.

Azurophil granules are known to contain myeloperoxidase, an antibacterial enzyme (25), and other numerous antimicrobial agents, lysozyme, and lysosomal enzymes (2,26,27). Elastase (28–30) and proteinase-3 (31,32) colocalize with some peroxidase-positive granules. Egesten et al. (30) found proteinase-3 (PR-3) was associated with the crystalline structure within azurophil granules. Lysozyme has been demonstrated in both types of granules (33–36). Many of the bactericidal factors such as defensins (37–39), azurophil-derived bacterial factors (ADBF) (40), and bactericidal permeability–increasing protein (BPI) (41), which were previously called phagocytin or cationic proteins, have been found in some azurophil granules. It is now known (42) that, of the 10 antimicrobial proteins of known sequence in the azurophil granule of human PMNs, two are thought to be unique in primary structure (lysozyme and BPI), whereas the remaining eight fall into two families of four members each: the family of defensins (which comprise 30% to 50% of granule protein) and cathepsin G, elastase, PR-3, and azurocidin. Collectively, these latter four proteins could be called "serprocidins" to denote that they represent, or are closely related to, serine proteases with microbicidal activity (42,43). Little is known about the membranes of azurophil granules (44–46). We had

TABLE 2-1. *Content of human neutrophil granules and secretory vesicles*

Azurophil granules	Specific granules	Gelatinase granules	Secretory vesicles
Membrane	**Membrane**	**Membrane**	**Membrane**
CD63	CD11b	CD11b	Alkaline phosphatase
CD68	Cd15 antigens	Cytochrome b_{558}	CR1
V-type H$^+$-ATPase	CD66	Diacylglycerol-deacylating	Cytochrome b_{558}
	CD67	enzyme	CD11b
	Cytochrome b_{558}	FMLP-R	CD14
	FMLP-R	SCAMP	CD16[a]
	Fibronectin-R	Urokinase-type plasminogen	FMLP-R
	G-protein subunit	activator-R	SCAMP
	Laminin-R	VAMP-2	Urokinase-type
	NB-1 antigen	V-type H$^+$-ATPase	plasminogen activator-R
	19-kd protein		V-type H$^+$-ATPase
	155-kd protein		VAMP-2
	Rap1, Rap2		CD10, CD13, CD45[a]
	SCAMP		C1q-receptor[a]
	Thrombospondin-R		DAF[a]
	TNF-R		
	Urokinase-type plasminogen activator-R		
	VAMP-2		
	Vitronectin-R		
Matrix	**Matrix**	**Matrix**	**Matrix**
Acid β-glycerophosphatase	β_2-Microglobulin	Acetyltransferase	Plasma proteins (including albumin and tetranectin)
Acid mucopolysaccharide	Collagenase	β_2-Microglobulin	
α_1-Antitrypsin	Gelatinase	Gelatinase	
α-Mannosidase	hCAP-18	Lysozyme	
Azurocidin/CAP37/ heparin-binding protein	Histaminase		
Bactericidal permeability increasing protein	Heparanase		
β-Glycerophosphatase	Lactoferrin		
β-Glucuronidase	Lysozyme		
Cathepsins	NGAL		
Defensins	Urokinase-type plasminogen activator		
Elastase	Sialidase		
Lysozyme	SGP28		
Myeloperoxidase	Vitamin B$_{12}$-binding protein		
N-acetyl-β-glucosaminidase			
Proteinase-3			
Sialidase			
Ubiquitin-protein			

[a]This localization is based on kinetics of upregulation in response to stimulation with inflammatory mediators but has not yet been demonstrated by subcellular localization by immunocytochemistry.

anticipated that the lysosome-associated membrane proteins (LAMPs) would be found there, but such was not the case (47). LAMPs were absent in all identified granule populations, but were consistently found in the membranes of vesicles, multivesicular bodies (MVB), and multilaminar compartment (MLC), which are identified by their content of concentric arrays of internal membranes. The latter compartment has not been previously described in this cell type and is illustrated in Figure 2-8.

Specific granules, which by definition do not contain peroxidase, contain lysozyme (33–36), lactoferrin (26, 48–50), B$_{12}$-binding proteins (51), and others (52) (see Table 2-1). The limiting membrane of the specific granules and/or other intracellular vesicles serves as a reser-

voir of receptors and other proteins involved in adherence (49,53,54), signal transduction (55), and functional activation of microbicidal pathways (56). For example, Singer et al. (54) gathered data that indicate that four types of extracellular matrix receptors (laminin, C3bi/fibrinogen, fibronectin, and vitronectin) are located in specific granules and suggested the term *adhesomes*.

Gelatinase granules are a subgroup of small, peroxidase-negative specific granules. They are defined by their high content of gelatinase (24,27,57,58).

Secretory granules were originally discovered as highly mobilizable intracellular vesicles that contain alkaline phosphatase on their luminal surface (59,60). Although many studies have assumed that alkaline phos-

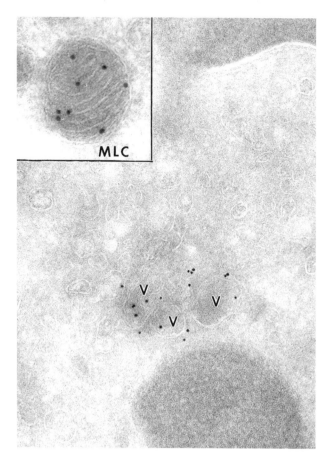

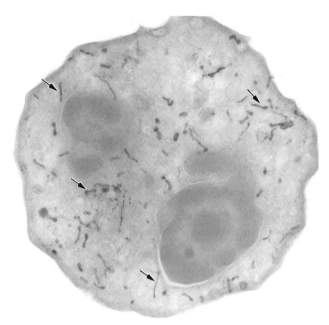

FIG. 2-9. Electron micrograph of a thick section of unstimulated neutrophils from cells incubated for the cytochemical detection of AlkPase activity. AlkPase activity was found primarily in slender rod-shaped organelles *(arrows)*. (From ref. 61, with permission.)

FIG. 2-8. In mature neutrophils, lysosome-associated membrane protein-2 is absent from granules and mainly found in vesicles (V), typical multivesicular bodies, and a distinct organelle, the multilaminar compartment (MLC) *(see inset)*. ×52,000; inset ×100,000.

phatase was a plasma membrane marker, it seems instead to be in a cytoplasmic organelle, distinguishable from azurophil-, specific-, and gelatinase-containing granules, which is easily mobilized to the surface (59,61,62). These alkaline phosphatase–containing compartments are short, rod-shaped organelles (Fig. 2-9) that rapidly undergo a dramatic reorganization on stimulation. In unstimulated neutrophils, most activity is intracellular, but after stimulation, essentially all of the activity becomes associated with the cell surface (61). The presence of plasma proteins, such as albumin, in secretory vesicles that are secreted as these vesicles fuse with the plasma membrane is of unknown significance (62).

Pertaining to the plasma membrane, L-selectin (63) and P-selectin glycoprotein ligand-1 (64,65) are found on the tips of neutrophil microvilli in resting neutrophils. Figure 2-10 demonstrates the localization of L-selectin by immunogold procedure.

Borregaard and Cowland (24) hypothesized that there is no specific sorting of proteins to individual subsets and that all granule proteins that are synthesized at the same time localize to the same granules. Formal proof that no

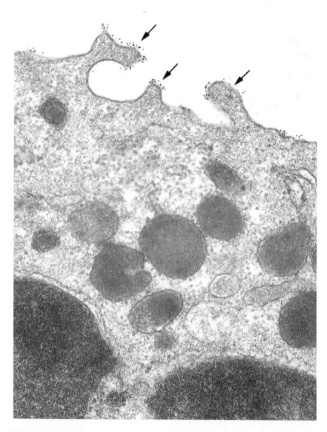

FIG. 2-10. L-selectin on tips of microvilli *(arrows)* of neutrophil plasma membrane. ×45,000.

targeting is required was achieved by the analysis of the granule protein neutrophil gelatinase–associated lipocalin (NGAL). NGAL is synthesized at the same stage as lactoferrin and colocalizes with lactoferrin in specific granules. When NGAL was transfected into HL-60 cells, NGAL was synthesized at the same time as myeloperoxidase and colocalized in azurophil granules (66). They believe this implies that differences in protein content that define the different subsets of granules result from differences in the biosynthetic window of the various granule proteins in relation to maturation (Fig. 2-11). Mature neutrophils are capable of synthesizing and secreting interleukin-1 and tumor necrosis factor X (67). Wheeler et al. (68) showed that bacterial infection can induce nitric oxide synthase in human neutrophils.

Degranulation

Neutrophils can secrete their specific and azurophil granules independently (69–73). Although both types of granules empty into the intracellular phagocytic vacuoles, the specific granules are particularly accessible for extracellular release, and there are marked differences in mobilization among the granule subsets (27). As a rule, the azurophil granule population is the least mobilizable when it comes to extracellular release of its contents (24). The hierarchy of mobilization seems to be

secretory vesicles, gelatinase granules, and specific granules (60). This phenomenon has also been observed *in vivo* during diapedesis and migration into skin windows (74). In resting neutrophils, the cytochrome b_{558} subunits are located in the membranes of specific granules, gelatinase granules, and secretory vesicles (see Table 2-1). Cell activation leads to fusion of these organelles with the plasma membrane and the association with certain cytosol complexes (75). The generation of reactive oxygen metabolites essential for microbicidal activity also depends on the contribution of the azurophil granule myeloperoxidase in the phagocytic vacuole (25,75). Patients after burn injury express a deficiency of the important cytosolic phagocyte oxidase components P47-phox and P67-phox (76).

Granule Abnormalities

Some well-documented examples of pathologic PMN granulations have been reported, and each can be classified as a selective abnormality of one granule type or the other. In an attempt to unify the results of pathologic studies of PMN granules in hereditary or acquired (usually leukemic) disease states, we have proposed the classification shown in Table 2-2 (77). Additional abnormalities of neutrophils are described elsewhere (25,78).

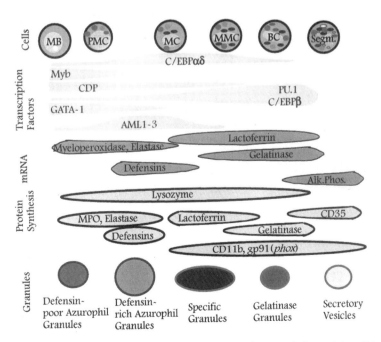

FIG. 2-11. Granules defined by timing of biosynthesis of their characteristic proteins. It is hypothesized that the granules formed at any given stage of maturation of neutrophil precursors are composed of the granule proteins synthesized at that time. The different subsets of granules identified are the result of differences in the biosynthetic windows of the various granule proteins during maturation and not the result of specific sorting between individual granule subsets. (From ref. 24, with permission.)

TABLE 2-2. *Proposed classification of neutrophil granule abnormalities*[a]

I. Abnormalities of azurophil granules
  A. Quantitative
    1. None
    2. Fewer than normal
    3. More than normal
  B. Qualitative
    1. Contents of granule incomplete
      Examples: hereditary peroxidase deficiency (see Fig. 2-12)
    2. Abnormal variants
      Examples: Auer bodies (see Fig. 2-13), Chediak-Higashi syndrome (see Fig. 2-14), drug-induced changes (see Fig. 2-16)
II. Abnormalities of specific granules
  A. Quantitative
    1. None
    2. Fewer than normal
    3. More than normal
  B. Qualitative
    1. Contents of granule are incomplete
    2. Abnormal variants

[a]Modified from ref. 77.

Abnormalities of Azurophil Granules

Quantitative Abnormalities

The circulating PMN sometimes contains smaller or larger than normal numbers of azurophils, or this whole granule population may be missing. Some mature PMNs lack azurophil granules in certain leukemic states, in acute myelogenous leukemia (AML) (79,80), and in the blastic crisis of chronic myelogenous leukemia (CML) (81). A study (82) of the neutrophilic cells of six children with severe congenital neutropenia and repeated, life-threatening infections described several abnormalities, including the defective synthesis or degeneration of azurophil (primary) granules, an absence or marked deficiency of specific (secondary) granules, and autophagia. This disease has been called *congenital dysgranulopoietic neutropenia*.

Qualitative Abnormalities

Contents of some granules are incomplete. In some instances, azurophil granules may be formed, but they may lack one or more enzymes or other substances. In hereditary myeloperoxidase deficiency, the azurophil granules of neutrophils and monocytes (83,84), but not of eosinophils or basophils, lack peroxidase (Fig. 2-12).

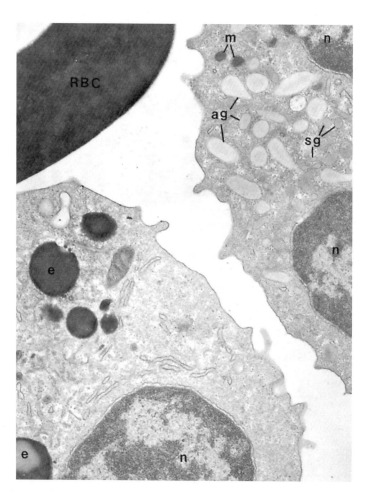

FIG. 2-12. Neutrophilic polymorphonuclear neutrophils reacted for peroxidase from the blood of a patient with hereditary peroxidase deficiency. Both types of granules are present: the large azurophils (ag), pale because of the absence of peroxidase, and the small specific granules (sg). Neutrophils and monocytes are devoid of the enzyme, whereas eosinophil and basophil granules are positive. Observe the peroxidase in an eosinophil granule (e) and the density of the adjacent red blood cell. m, mitochondria; n, nucleus. ×14,000.

This deficiency occurs in 1 of 2,000 to 5,000 persons (85,86) and is not usually associated with clinical abnormalities. It has been shown (87) that, although not detectable enzymatically, peroxidase can be demonstrated by immunologic methods in the neutrophils of individuals with the deficiency. Molecular analysis of the cells from peroxidase-deficient families have documented some heterogenous disorders of translation (88,89). Peroxidase deficiency has also been observed in refractory anemia (90), in preleukemia (91,92), and in the blastic crisis of CML (81). In each of these examples of peroxidase deficiency, both types of granule are present and apparently normal, and only the enzyme peroxidase is absent; however, in the hereditary deficiency, all of the neutrophils are peroxidase negative, whereas in the refractory anemias and leukemias (92,93), the percentage of peroxidase-negative PMN varies. PMNs lacking peroxidase were observed in AML (79,92–94) and in cases of "blast cell transformation" of CML (81). This abnormality, when present, affected 8% to 70% of the circulating PMNs. It has been hypothesized that the deficient PMN may originate from the leukemic precursors (94). Gulley et al. (95) reported high neutrophil peroxidase activity in patients with megaloblastic anemia.

Abnormal variants occur. Auer bodies, found in the immature cells of some patients with AML, are abnormally large, elongated, azurophil granules containing peroxidase, lysosomal enzymes, and large crystalline inclusions (80,96–98). Although the presence of Auer bodies is usually associated with acute myeloid leukemias, a small percentage have been observed in M5 monocytic leukemia (99). Although similar to normal azurophil granules in content and staining properties, Auer bodies are abnormal because of their gigantic size (Fig. 2-13). Auer body formation in leukemic blasts and promyelocytes differs markedly from the normal secretory process of azurophil granule formation in that Golgi cisternae contain very little peroxidase (80,97).

More Auer bodies can be detected on smears of bone marrow and blood from patients with AML when special stains (i.e., peroxidase, chloroacetate esterase, acid phosphatase, or Sudan black) are applied than when Romanovsky stain alone is used. Not all Auer bodies exhibit all these staining characteristics at the same time (77). Hanker et al. (100) modified the Graham and Karnovsky stain for peroxidase (3,3′-diaminobenzidine and H_2O_2 at pH 7.3 to 7.6) by staining afterward with $Cu(NO_3)_2$. Not surprisingly, this stain reveals additional reactive organelles (i.e., phi bodies) on smears from patients with AML. The term *phi body* was originally introduced to describe the shape of catalase-positive rods in the excretory ducts of mouse salivary glands. Because Auer originally described variably shaped abnormal organelles in leukemia, many hematologists feel that the peroxidase-positive organelles seen in AML leukocytes should be referred to as variants of Auer bodies and not

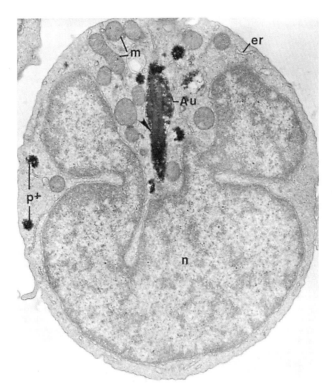

FIG. 2-13. Peroxidase localization in an abnormal immature cell from a patient with acute myelogenous leukemia. Notice the Auer body (Au) with its crystalline inclusion *(arrowhead)* and a matrix containing peroxidase. A few small reactive granules (p^+) are also present. n, nucleus; m, mitochondria; er, rough-surfaced endoplasmic reticulum. ×10,000.

as phi bodies (77). It has been suggested that Auer rod formation is an occasional but normal phenomenon in fetal hematopoiesis (101). This observation should be confirmed in other laboratories. Auer rodlike inclusions also may be seen at the light microscopic level in certain B-cell malignancies, but they are peroxidase negative (102).

The Chediak-Higashi anomaly or syndrome, a rare autosomal recessive disease, is characterized by oculocutaneous albinism, increased susceptibility to infection, and the presence of abnormally large, lysosome-like organelles in most granule-containing cells. The large inclusions in the PMNs of individuals with Chediak-Higashi syndrome have proved to be enormous abnormal azurophil granules (103–105). Normal azurophil granules form early in PMN maturation, but they then fuse to form megagranules; later, during the myelocyte stage, normal specific granules form. The mature, circulating PMN contains the abnormal azurophil and normal specific granules (Fig. 2-14). The contents of specific granules may also be present in the megagranules (105,106). Giant, peroxidase-positive granules have been observed in the PMNs of a patient with neutrophil dysfunction (107). These granules were structurally similar to those seen in Chediak-Higashi syndrome, but the PMNs were biochemically different in that there was

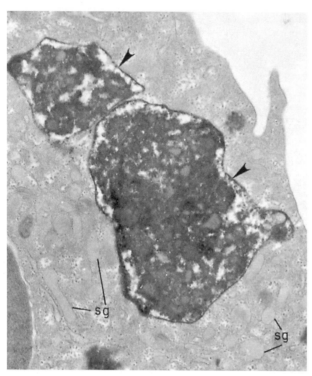

FIG. 2-14. Peroxidase localization in a polymorphonuclear neutrophil from a patient with Chediak-Higashi syndrome. The megagranules are peroxidase positive *(arrowheads)*, and the specific granules (sg) appear normal. ×17,500.

defective activation of the respiratory burst. Ganz et al. (108) demonstrated the absence of elastase and cathepsin G, along with normal defensin content, in patients with the Chediak-Higashi syndrome. Barbosa et al. (109) identified the Chediak-Higashi syndrome defective gene as *LYST,* which encodes a protein with multiple phosphorylation sites.

In 1974, giant round granules in leukemic cells were observed on Wright-stained smears from two patients with AML (110). Because this acquired morphologic abnormality closely mimicked the giant round granules seen in the Chediak-Higashi anomaly, it was called the pseudo-Chediak-Higashi anomaly of acute leukemia (111,112). In bone marrow from three patients with AML, we observed enormous, round, pink inclusions resembling ingested erythrocytes in blasts and promyelocytes. Analysis by electron microscopy and peroxidase cytochemistry showed that these inclusions were large, membrane-bound, peroxidase-positive granules with homogeneous content. We believe that they correspond to the abnormal granules of pseudo-Chediak-Higashi anomaly. Like the Auer rods also seen in AML, these granules appear to be an abnormal variant of peroxidase-positive azurophil granules. Their lack of azurophilia results from the absence of sulfated glycosaminoglycans (113).

In certain inflammatory disorders, morphologic changes may occur in peripheral blood neutrophils. The best-known alteration is the "shift to the left," which denotes the presence of bands, metamyelocytes, and sometimes myelocytes in the circulating blood. The mature PMN may also show certain cytoplasmic modifications, including "toxic" granules, which stain more prominently than those of normal neutrophils; light blue, amorphous inclusion bodies called Dohle bodies; and vacuoles. Toxic granules are azurophils that stain abnormally by light microscopy (114) but that are indistinguishable from normal azurophils by electron microscopy. Dohle bodies are not granules; they have been defined as several rows of RER. They stain as blue bodies in the cytoplasm because of the ribosomes bound to the membrane of the RER (Fig. 2-15). Functional studies of toxic neutrophils have revealed decreases in chemotaxis and in phagocytic and intracellular bactericidal activities (115,116). Increased numbers of lipid bodies have been observed in inflammatory reactions (117), and other inclusion bodies can be seen in certain hereditary conditions (118–120).

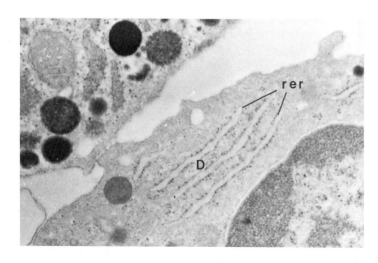

FIG. 2-15. A portion of a polymorphonuclear neutrophil depicts a Dohle body (D), consisting of three stacks of rough-surfaced endoplasmic reticulum (rer). It stains blue as seen by light microscopy because of the concentration of ribosomes. ×20,000.

An acquired azurophil granule abnormality has been observed in neutrophils of patients with amiodarone pulmonary toxicity (121). As can be seen in Figure 2-16, some of the peroxidase-positive azurophil granules contain lamellar inclusions as have been found in other cell types. The target antigen of anticytoplasmic antibodies circulating in Wegener's granulomatosis has been shown to be proteinase-3, located in azurophil granules (31,32,122,123,124).

Abnormalities of Specific Granules

Quantitative Abnormalities

The three quantitative abnormalities of azurophil granules apply to specific granules as well: circulating PMNs may have smaller or larger than normal quantities of these granules, or they may lack them entirely. The absence of specific granules was first observed in 1974 (125), in a 14-year-old boy with no leukocyte alkaline phosphatase and with recurrent infection. More cases have since been reported (126–134). These patients have an abnormality that affects production of specific granules and their protein contents, and they have at least two

additional proteins (i.e., gelatinase and defensins) (108,132,133). Parmley et al. (132) also noticed abnormalities in the peroxidase-positive granules of these patients. In congenital dysgranulocytic neutropenia, specific granules may be absent or markedly decreased in number.

The absence or paucity of specific granules in the more mature segmented neutrophils of certain leukemic patients warrants comment. It appears that cytoplasmic development in these cells has ceased after the promyelocytic stage, whereas nuclear maturation has progressed in a fairly normal fashion. The absence of certain normal organelles from mature neutrophils of patients with acute leukemia has been documented by electron microscopy and cytochemistry. For example, we demonstrated the absence of specific granules in neutrophils from patients with AML (79). We also observed these abnormal neutrophils quite frequently in acute myeloid leukemia with maturation (i.e., the M2 variety) and in certain cases of hematopoietic dysplasia. After treatment of acute promyelocyte leukemia with all-*trans*-retinoic acid, Miyauchi et al. (135) observed aberrant peroxidase-positive granules, including Auer rods, becoming normal, although they lacked the specific (secondary) peroxidase-negative population. Repine et al. (136) reported a case of leukemia in which PMNs were deficient in all granules.

Qualitative Abnormalities

The contents of some granules are incomplete. The specific granules are present in fairly normal numbers in all PMNs of patients with CML (81,137). Two hematologic conditions are associated with a consistent decrease in alkaline phosphatase: CML and paroxysmal nocturnal hemoglobinuria (PNH) (138). In CML, alkaline phosphatase mRNA is undetectable, but in PNH, normal or high levels of its mRNA are present. The latter finding supports the concept of a deficit in the anchorage to the membrane through the glycolipid pathway (138). Studies (139) have shown that the neutrophils of patients with AML lack, or are markedly deficient in, lactoferrin, a substance found exclusively in the specific granule. Parmley et al. (140) described a patient with a defect in complex carbohydrate staining that involved primary and secondary granules.

It is unknown why diabetes is associated with a high susceptibility to infection. Li et al. (141) showed that two major antibacterial proteins, lysozyme and lactoferrin, can specifically bind glucose-modified proteins bearing advanced glycosylation end products (AGEs). Exposure to AGE-modified proteins inhibits the enzymatic and bacterial activity of lysozyme and blocks the bacterial agglutination and bacterial killing activities of lactoferrin.

No reports of abnormal variants of specific granules have been published.

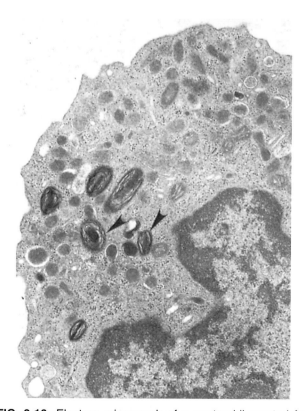

FIG. 2-16. Electron micrograph of a neutrophil reacted for peroxidase from a patient with amiodarone pulmonary toxicity. Lamellar membranes have peroxidase-positive granules *(arrowheads)*. ×30,000.

In Vitro Experiments on Neutrophil Maturation

Cell Lines

Several human acute myeloid leukemia cell lines have become available, as reviewed by Lubbert and Koeffler (142). A cell line, HL-60, was established from the peripheral blood of a patient with acute promyelocytic leukemia (143). It has maintained continuous growth for years in suspension culture without added conditioned medium or colony-stimulating factor, and it is tumorigenic in athymic nude mice. Most unstimulated HL-60 cells have promyelocytic morphologic and histochemical characteristics, and 4% to 15% of them show morphologic characteristics of the more mature myeloid cells: myelocytes, metamyelocytes, band forms, and PMNs. Many investigators are using the HL-60 cell line to analyze the detailed events of early myeloid differentiation, particularly in studies with inducers of differentiation (142). No specific granules have been seen (144), and no mRNA for lactoferrin has been detected (145). When myeloperoxidase was localized on HL-60 cells and compared with normal cells, it was found that HL 60 cells had little or no peroxidase in their Golgi cisternae and that the granules that were formed varied greatly from those synthesized *in vivo* (146).

Enucleated Degranulated Polymorphonuclear Neutrophils

Roos et al. (147) described the preparation of cytoplasts—vesicles of neutrophil cytoplasm surrounded by plasma membrane and devoid of granules and nucleus. These cytoplasts ingested and killed *Staphylococcus aureus,* proving that neither nucleus nor granules are essential for killing these bacteria. Additional work by Petrequin et al. (148), demonstrating some fusion of granule membranes with the plasma membrane of cytoplasts, suggests that degranulation occurs during cytoplast preparation and that specific granule membranes can be found on the surface. Malawista et al. (149) studied inhibitors of nitric oxide synthase in cytokineplasts.

EOSINOPHILS

Light Microscopy of Eosinophils in Bone Marrow and Blood Smears

The earliest identifiable form of eosinophilic leukocyte is a late myeloblast or early promyelocyte. This cell is about 15 μm in diameter and has a large nucleus containing nucleoli and a few granules in intensely basophilic cytoplasm. The later eosinophilic promyelocyte is similar but has less prominent nucleoli and more granules. Although a few of these granules may stain blue or azure, most are acidophilic.

The myelocyte, 18 to 20 μm in diameter, is the largest cell of the development series. It has many more specific (eosinophilic) granules than does the promyelocyte, and its nucleoli are difficult to discern. The metamyelocyte is somewhat smaller than the myelocyte and has an indented nucleus. The cytoplasm is tightly packed with eosinophilic granules, but they are somewhat less numerous than in the myelocyte. The band form resembles the metamyelocyte, except that the nucleus has further matured and is shaped like a slightly bent rod.

The fully mature eosinophilic leukocyte has a lobed nucleus, and its cytoplasm is filled with larger eosinophilic granules whose rims stain for peroxidase and Sudan black. The nucleus is almost always bilobed, although trilobed forms are sometimes seen. Multilobed nuclei, comparable to those of adult neutrophils, are rare (150). Eosinophils are susceptible to mechanical damage during the preparation of blood smears. It has been suggested that eosinophilic precursors may degranulate during maturation (151). Lipid bodies may be found in eosinophils (152) and in neutrophils.

Determination by Electron Microscopy and Cytochemistry

Early Stages: Promyelocyte and Myelocyte

When eosinophils of the promyelocyte (Fig. 2-17) and myelocyte (Fig. 2-18) stages are stained for peroxidase, reaction product is seen within all cisternae of the RER, including transitional elements, and the perinuclear cisterna, clusters of smooth vesicles at the periphery of the Golgi complex, all cisternae of the Golgi complex, and all immature and mature specific granules (3). The mature granules are completely filled with reaction product except in areas occupied by crystals.

Later Stages: Metamyelocyte, Band, and Mature Cell

In the later stages of development, after granule formation has ceased, the eosinophil contains few of the organelles associated with the synthesis and packaging of secretory proteins. RER is sparse or virtually nonexistent, and the Golgi complex is small and inconspicuous. The cytoplasm of the mature eosinophil (Fig. 2-19) contains primarily granules and glycogen. Most of the granules are specific granules with crystals, which are usually centrally located.

After the myelocyte stage, peroxidase is not detectable in the endoplasmic reticulum or Golgi elements of the eosinophil by any of the enzyme procedures. It is demonstrable only in the matrix of granules, as are the lysosomal enzymes (3).

Mature human eosinophils contain two populations of granules (153). About 5% of the large granules are primary granules identified by the presence of the Charcot-Leyden crystal protein (154–156), the presence of eosinophil peroxidase (157), but not crystalline core.

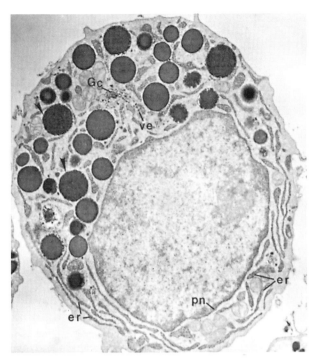

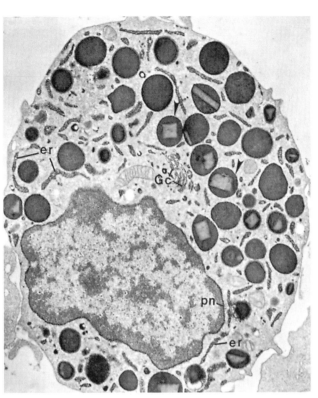

FIG. 2-17. Human eosinophilic promyelocyte from a preparation incubated for peroxidase. Reaction product appears as a dark flocculent precipitate that fills the entire rough-surfaced endoplasmic reticulum (er), including the perinuclear cisterna (pn), clusters of smooth vesicles (ve) at the periphery of the Golgi complex, all of the cisternae of the Golgi complex (Gc), and all the immature granules in the Golgi region and in the peripheral cytoplasm. The immature granules *(arrowheads)* are large and lack the distinctive crystalline bar of mature eosinophil granules. ×10,000.

FIG. 2-18. Human eosinophilic myelocyte incubated for peroxidase. Because peroxidase is still being synthesized, reaction product is present in the rough-surfaced endoplasmic reticulum (er), the perinuclear cisterna (pn), Golgi elements (Gc), and granules. Many of the granules contain a crystalline bar *(arrowheads)*. In mature granules, reaction product is not present in the area occupied by the crystalline bar, which stands out sharply against the dark background provided by the remainder of the reactive granule. ×10,000.

Dvorak et al., (154) refer to these granules as unicompartmental. The second granule populations (95%) are bicompartmental (matrix with a crystalline core) and store a number of eosinophil proteins. These include eosinophil peroxidase, major basic protein (MBP) (154,158), eosinophil-derived neurotoxin (EDN) (158), eosinophil peroxidase, tumor necrosis factor α (159), transforming growth factor α (TGF-α) (160) and granulocyte-macrophage colony-stimulating factor (GM-CSF) (161). MPB is confined to the central crystalline core (Fig. 2-20), as is GM-CSF. The remainder of the proteins are present in the matrix compartment. Lysosomal enzymes are also present in the matrix of the crystalloid granules (3).

Granule Contents

Eosinophil peroxidase is genetically and biochemically distinct from neutrophil peroxidase, and it appears to play no role in the bactericidal activity of eosinophils (162). Eosinophils have much less bactericidal activity than do neutrophils (163). Immunocytochemical evidence indicates that the specific granules of eosinophils are true per-

oxisomes in that they also contain catalase (164), two enzymes of peroxisomal lipid β-oxidation (enoyl-CoA hydratase and ketoacyl-CoA thiolase [165]), and a flavoprotein (acyl-CoA oxidase [166]). All of these substances have been found in the matrix of the granule and not in the crystalloid of the granule. Lectins have also been identified in eosinophil granules, heaviest in the crystalloids (167).

The eosinophil granule also contains several basic proteins: MBP, an eosinophil cationic protein, and EDN (158). More than one half of the granule protein is the MBP, which constitutes the crystalline core of the granule (see Fig. 2-20). It is cytotoxic to parasites and to normal mammalian cells and induces histamine release from basophils and mast cells. The other two cationic proteins are found in the matrix of the granule (158). Studies have shown that eosinophil cationic protein can cause the formation of transmembrane pores and may thereby cause membrane damage (168). The amino acid sequences of eosinophil cationic protein are remarkably homologous with those of EDN, and both sequences show striking homology with those of ribonuclease (169,170). Eosinophils also synthesize proteoglycans (171).

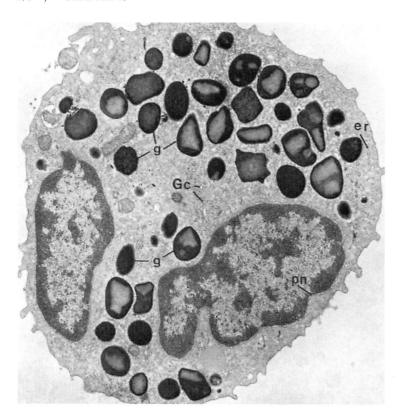

FIG. 2-19. Human mature eosinophil incubated for peroxidase. Reaction product is present only in granules (g). The rough-surfaced endoplasmic reticulum (er), including the perinuclear cisterna (pn) and the Golgi cisternae (Gc), does not contain reaction product. Most of the granules contain the distinctive crystalline bar. ×8000.

Charcot-Leyden crystals, bipyramidal crystals observed in fluids in association with eosinophilic inflammatory reactions, possess lysophospholipase activity and comprise 7% to 10% of total eosinophil protein (155). Human basophils also contain the Charcot-Leyden crystal protein (172).

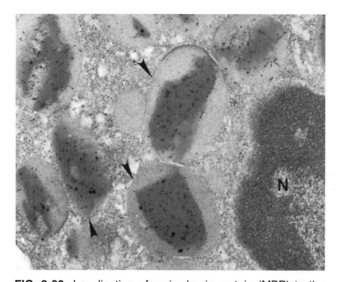

FIG. 2-20. Localization of major basic protein (MBP) to the core of the eosinophil granule. Sections stained with affinity-purified rabbit anti-human MBP and GCP-goat anti-rabbit immunoglobulin G show localization of gold particles over the cores of many eosinophil granules (arrowheads). (From ref. 158, with permission.)

Granule Abnormalities

Inherited Abnormalities of Eosinophils

Although rare, there are four known inherited abnormalities of eosinophils:

1. The absence of peroxidase and phospholipids in eosinophils is an autosomal recessive defect that produces no signs of disease (173–175).
2. In Chediak-Higashi syndrome (103,104), almost all granulated cells, including eosinophils, contain large abnormal granules.
3. A family was found to have gray inclusions in eosinophils and basophils; the abnormality showed autosomal dominance and had no clinical effects. Electron microscopy revealed cytoplasmic crystals and curved lamellar bodies in the cells (176).
4. Neutrophil specific granule deficiency, previously discussed, also involves eosinophils (177).

Acquired Abnormalities of Eosinophils

Several gross morphologic or cytochemical abnormalities of eosinophils have been observed in leukemias and dysplasias and in association with benign eosinophilias.

Cytochemistry of Abnormal Eosinophils in Leukemias

In a cytochemical study of eosinophils in acute leukemia (178), the cells were considered normal when they did not show toluidine blue metachromasia or positivity for alkaline phosphatase, chloroacetate esterase, Astra blue, or periodic acid–Schiff (PAS) but did show positivity for peroxidase and Sudan black and moderate reactivity for naphthol-AS or α-naphthyl esterase. The observation of chloroacetate esterase activity in some abnormal eosinophils is of particular interest in view of the subsequent finding that abnormal marrow eosinophils in acute myelomonocytic leukemia (AMML) are associated with the inversion of chromosome 16 (179). Most of the patients studied had a higher than normal percentage of immature eosinophils containing a mixture of eosinophilic and basophilic granules. The eosinophilic granules showed abnormal reactivity for chloroacetate esterase and PAS. Electron microscopy revealed that none of the granules had well-formed central crystalloids. Studies have proven that the inversion of chromosome 16 is also present in these abnormal eosinophils (180).

A fairly common abnormality seen in patients with CML is the presence of basophilic and eosinophilic granules in eosinophilic myelocytes and, occasionally, in mature eosinophils (181). Because, under normal circumstances, eosinophilic and basophilic granules can be viewed as mutually exclusive markers of the respective granulocytic lineages, the presence of both markers in CML cells has been considered a sign of lineage infidelity. This concept deserves further study.

Degranulated and Light Density Eosinophils Associated with Eosinophilia

There is an expanding clinical spectrum of multisystem diseases associated with eosinophilia (182). The idiopathic hypereosinophilic syndrome (HES) (183) is characterized by persistent eosinophilia of 1500 eosinophils/mm³ for at least 6 months or death before 6 months with signs and symptoms of HES; lack of evidence for parasitic, allergic, or other recognized causes of eosinophilia despite careful evaluation; and signs and symptoms of organ system involvement or dysfunction directly related to eosinophilia or unexplained in the given clinical setting. Eosinophils with fewer granules than are normal or usual can be detected in the blood of patients with a wide variety of eosinophilic disorders (184–186). Other features observed are metabolic abnormalities of eosinophils (187), heterogeneity of granule shape and content (78,152,153), and lipid inclusions (78,152,153).

Dramatic eosinophilia was a striking component of the newly recognized tryptophan-induced eosinophilia-myalgia syndrome (188–190). A chromosome translocation from B-cell acute lymphocytic leukemia with eosinophilia has been linked to the activation of the interleukin-3 gene (191).

Intranuclear Crystalloids Associated with Abnormal Granules in Eosinophilic Leukocytes

Eosinophils with abnormal granules and intranuclear crystalloids were observed in a 2-year-old girl with chronic benign neutropenia (192). The father had the same morphologic abnormality but was asymptomatic and had normal leukocyte counts.

Acquired Eosinophil Nuclear Anomaly

Acquired eosinophil nuclear anomaly is also called pseudo-Pelger-Huet anomaly. Incomplete segmentation of the nucleus of mature eosinophils is seen in AML (193) and myelodysplasia (194).

In Vitro Experiments on Eosinophilic Differentiation

The HL-60 leukemic cell line can be induced by specific chemical agents to produce mature cells of the neutrophilic or macrophage lineage. These cells can also differentiate to eosinophils and eosinophilic precursors when cultured under mildly alkaline conditions (pH 7.6 to 7.8) for 7 days without refeeding (195). When stained with Wright-Giemsa, new cytoplasmic granules appear blue in the least mature of these cells and red in the most mature cells. Most of the cells contain the eosinophil MBP, the Charcot-Leyden crystal protein (lysophospholipase), and eosinophil peroxidase. Examination of finely banded chromosomes from these cells has revealed translocation break points at q22 on chromosome 16 and q23 on the other homologue; abnormalities in this region of the long arm of 16 are a characteristic finding in AMML with abnormal bone marrow eosinophils. Like the bone marrow eosinophils in patients with this disease, the HL-60 eosinophil granules contain material reactive for chloroacetate esterase and PAS and rarely have crystalloid inclusions.

The HL-60 cell line appears to be suitable for investigating eosinophilopoiesis in vitro and may be especially useful for the study of the abnormal eosinophils seen in certain malignant conditions (195). In eosinophils that differentiated from umbilical cord blood progenitors cultured in the presence of interleukin-5, unicompartmental, MBP-rich secondary granules that were devoid of matrix compartments and eosinophil peroxidase developed. Dvorak et al. (154) commented on the morphologic similarity to the eosinophil-deficient granules of patients with that deficiency.

Distribution of Mature Eosinophils in Blood and Tissues

The turnover time of circulating eosinophils in the rat, as determined by use of tritiated thymidine, is 4.5 days (196). The tissue lifespan of eosinophils was estimated to be 2 to 4 days in this study and 8 to 12 days in another (197). When blood eosinophils are cultured in the presence of T-cell–conditioned medium, they can survive for 3 weeks or more (184). Eosinophils can also be maintained in vitro by coculture with endothelial cells (198).

In a kinetic study of radiolabeled eosinophils in patients with eosinophilia, the mean blood half-life of the cells was 44 hours (199).

Eosinophils are found throughout body tissues and cavities but are most prominent in the gastrointestinal tract. The content of eosinophils in the bowel wall varies; it is usually greatest in the colon. Almost all eosinophils of the alimentary canal are found in the lamina propria and submucosa (150).

Blood and tissue eosinophilia are characteristic of certain types of allergic and parasitic conditions. Interleukin-5 may be an important mediator of eosinophilic response to parasites (200,201). It is less well recognized that peripheral blood eosinophilia accompanies a wide variety of carcinomas arising from mucin-secreting epithelium (i.e., bronchus, gut, pancreas, and uterus) and Hodgkin's disease. In this regard, it is of interest that a tumor-derived eosinophilopoietic factor has been extracted from a metastatic pulmonary carcinoma of a patient with an eosinophilic leukemoid reaction (202). TGF-α production by tissue-infiltrating eosinophils and eosinophils in the hypereosinophilic syndrome has been demonstrated (203). Walsh reviewed eosinophil accumulation, activation, fate, and apoptosis (204,205).

Eosinopenia occurs with acute stress or inflammation. Certain chemotactic substances (e.g., *N*-formylmethionyl-leucyl-phenylalanine) have been shown to produce an eosinopenic response in experiments (206,207), but the relevance of this eosinopenic response to acute inflammation is unknown. Considerable progress is being made in the areas of synthesis and storage of cytokines in human eosinophils (208) and in the area of chemokines specific for certain types of leukocytes (209).

REFERENCES

1. Bainton DF, Farquhar MG. Origin of granules in polymorphonuclear leukocytes: two types derived from opposite faces of the Golgi complex in developing granulocytes. *J Cell Biol* 1966;28:277–301.
2. Bainton DF, Ullyot JL, Farquhar MG. The development of neutrophilic polymorphonuclear leukocytes in human bone marrow: origin and content of azurophil and specific granules. *J Exp Med* 1971; 134:907–934.
3. Bainton DF, Farquhar MG. Segregation and packaging of granule enzymes in eosinophilic leukocytes. *J Cell Biol* 1970;45:54–73.
4. Bainton DF. The cells of inflammation: a general view. In: Weissman G, ed. *The cell biology of inflammation,* vol 2. New York: Elsevier/North-Holland, 1980:1–25.
5. Hartsock RJ, Smith EB, Petty CS. Normal variations with aging of the amount of hematopoietic tissue in bone marrow from the anterior iliac crest: a study made from 177 cases of sudden death examined by necropsy. *Am J Clin Pathol* 1965;43:326–334.
6. Bartl R, Frisch B, Burkhardt R, eds. *Bone marrow biopsies revisited: a new dimension for haematologic malignancies,* 2nd revised ed. New York: Karger, 1985.
7. Wulffraat NM, deWaal FC, Stamhuis IH, Broekema GJ, Loonen AH. Bone marrow mitotic index: a methodological study. *Acta Haematol (Basel)* 1985;73:89–92.
8. Dancey JT, Deubelbeiss KA, Harker LA, Finch CA. Neutrophil kinetics in man. *J Clin Invest* 1976;58:705–715.
9. Walker RI, Willemze R. Neutrophil kinetics and the regulation of granulopoiesis. *Rev Infect Dis* 1980;2:282–292.
10. Jamuar MP, Cronkite EP. The fate of granulocytes. *Exp Hematol* 1980; 8:884–894.
11. Shi J, Fujieda H, Kokubo Y, Wake K. Apoptosis of neutrophils and their elimination by Kupffer cells in rat liver. *Hepatology* 1996;5:1256–1263.
12. Cronkite EP, Vincent PC. Granulocytopoiesis. *Ser Haematol* 1969;2: 3–43.
13. Hardin JH, Spicer SS. Ultrastructural localization of dialyzed iron-reactive mucosubstance in rabbit heterophils, basophils, and eosinophils. *J Cell Biol* 1971;48:368–386.
14. Campbell MS, Lovell MA, Gorbsky GJ. Stability of nuclear segments in human neutrophils and evidence role for microfilaments or microtubules in their genesis during differentiation of HL60 myelocytes. *J Leukoc Biol* 1995;58:659–666.
15. Hochstenbach PFR, Scheres JMJC, Hustinx TWJ, Wieringa B. Demonstration of X chromatin in drumstick-like nuclear appendages of leukocytes by in situ hybridization on blood smears. *Histochemistry* 1986;84:383–386.
16. Ackerman GA, Clark MA. Ultrastructural localization of peroxidase activity in normal human bone marrow cells. *Z Zellforsch* 1971;117: 463–475.
17. Brederoo P, van der Meulen J, Daems WT. Ultrastructural localization of peroxidase activity in developing neutrophil granulocytes from human bone marrow. *Histochemistry* 1986;84:445–453.
18. Breton-Gorius J, Guichard J. Etude au microscope electronique de la localisation des peroxydases dane les cellules de la moelle osseuse humaines. *Nouv Rev Fr Hematol* 1969;9:678–687.
19. Pryzwansky KB, Breton-Gorius J. Identification of a subpopulation of primary granules in human neutrophils based upon maturation and distribution: study by transmission electron microscopy cytochemistry and high voltage electron microscopy of whole cell preparations. *Lab Invest* 1985;53:664–671.
20. Bainton DF. Differentiation of human neutrophilic granulocytes: normal and abnormal. In: Greenwalt TJ, Jamieson GA, eds. *The granulocyte:* function and clinical utilization. New York: Alan R Liss, 1977: 1–27.
21. Breton-Gorius J, Coquin Y, Guichard J. Cytochemical distinction between azurophils and catalase-containing granules in leukocytes. *Lab Invest* 1978;38:21–34.
22. Wallace PJ, Packman CH, Lichtman MA. Maturation-associated changes in the peripheral cytoplasm of human neutrophils: a review. *Exp Hematol* 1987;15:34–45.
23. Sullivan R, Griffin JD, Malech HL. Acquisition of formyl peptide receptors during normal human myeloid differentiation. *Blood* 1987;70:1222–1224.
24. Borregaard N, Cowland BJ. Granules of the human neutrophilic polymorphonuclear leukocyte. *Blood* 1997;89:3503–3521.
25. Klebanoff SJ, Clark RA, eds. *The neutrophil:* function and clinical disorders. New York: North-Holland, 1978:556–557.
26. Bretz U, Baggiolini M. Biochemical and morphological characterization of azurophil and specific granules of human neutrophilic polymorphonuclear leukocytes. *J Cell Biol* 1974;63:251–269.
27. Borregaard N, Lollike K, Kjeldsen L, et al. Human neutrophil granules and secretory vesicles. *Eur J Haematol* 1993;51:187–198.
28. Damiano VV, Kucich U, Murer E, Laudenslager N, Weinbaum G. Ultrastructural quantitation of peroxidase- and elastase-containing granules in human neutrophils. *Am J Pathol* 1988;131:235–245.
29. Cramer EM, Beesley JE, Pulford KA, Breton-Gorius J, Mason DY. Colocalization of elastase and myeloperoxidase in human blood and bone marrow neutrophils using a monoclonal antibody and immunogold. *Am J Pathol* 1989;134:1275–1284.
30. Egesten A, Breton-Gorius J, Guichard J, Gullberg U, Olsson I. The heterogeneity of azurophil granules in neutrophil promyelocytes: immunogold localization of myeloperoxidase, cathepsin G, elastase, proteinase 3, and bactericidal/permeability increasing protein. *Blood* 1994;83:2985–2994.
31. Calafat J, Goldschmeding R, Ringeling PL, Janssen H, vanderSchoot CE. In situ localization by double-labeling immunoelectron microscopy of anti-neutrophil cytoplasmic autoantibodies in neutrophils and monocytes. *Blood* 1990;75:242–250.
32. Csernok E, Ludemann J, Gross WL, Bainton DF. Ultrastructural localization of proteinase 3, the target antigen of anticytoplasmic antibodies circulating in Wegener's granulomatosis. *Am J Pathol* 1990;137: 1113–1120.
33. Cramer EM, Breton-Gorius J. Ultrastructural localization of lysozyme

in human neutrophils by immunogold. *J Leukoc Biol* 1987;41: 242–247.

34. Livesey SA, Buescher ES, Krannig GL, Harrison DS, Linner JG, Choivetti R. Human neutrophil granule heterogeneity: immunolocalization studies using cryofixed, dried and embedded specimens. *Scanning Microsc* 1989;3:231–240.

35. Mutasa HC. Combination of diaminobenzidine staining and immunogold labeling: a novel technical approach to identify lysozyme in human neutrophil cells. *Eur J Cell Biol* 1989;49:319–325.

36. Peretz R, Shaft D, Yaari A, Nir E. Distinct intracellular lysozyme content in normal granulocytes and monocytes: a quantitative immunoperoxidase and ultrastructural immunogold study. *J Histochem Cytochem* 1994;42:1471–1477.

37. Rice WG, Ganz T, Kinkade JM Jr, Selsted ME, Lehrer RI, Parmley RT. Defensin-rich dense granules of human neutrophils. *Blood* 1987; 70:757–765.

38. Ganz T, Selsted ME, Szklarek D, et al. Defensins: natural peptide antibiotics of human neutrophils. *J Clin Invest* 1985;76:1427–1435.

39. Lehrer RI, Ganz T, Selsted ME. Defensins: endogenous antibiotic peptides of animal cells. *Cell* 1991;64:229–230.

40. Gabay JE, Heiple JM, Cohn ZA, Nathan CF. Subcellular location and properties of bactericidal factors from human neutrophils. *J Exp Med* 1986;164:1407–1421.

41. Weiss J, Olsson I. Cellular and subcellular localization of the bactericidal/permeability-increasing protein of neutrophils. *Blood* 1987;69: 652–659.

42. Gabay JE, Scott RW, Campanelli D, et al. Antibiotic proteins of human polymorphonuclear leukocytes. *Proc Natl Acad Sci USA* 1989;86: 5610–5614.

43. Spitznagel JK. Antibiotic proteins of human neutrophils. *J Clin Invest* 1990;86:1381–1386.

44. Kuijpers TW, Tool ATJ, van der Schoot CE, et al. Membrane surface antigen expression on neutrophils: a reappraisal of the use of surface markers for neutrophil activation. *Blood* 1991;78:4:1105–1111.

45. Saito N, Pulford KAF, Breton-Gorius J, Massé J-M, Mason DY, Cramer EM. Ultrastructural localization of the CD68 macrophage-associated antigen in human blood neutrophils and monocytes. *Am J Pathol* 1991;139:5:1053–1059.

46. Cham BP, Gerrard JM, Bainton DF. Granulophysin is located in the membranes of azurophilic granules in human neutrophil and mobilizes to the plasma membrane following cell stimulation. *Am J Pathol* 1994;144:1369–1380.

47. Cieutat A-M, Lobel P, August JT, et al. Azurophilic granules of human neutrophilic leukocytes are deficient in lysosome-associated membrane proteins but retain the mannose 6-phosphate recognition. *Blood* 1998;91:1044–1058.

48. Cramer E, Pryzwansky KB, Villeval J-L, Testa U, Breton-Gorius J. Ultrastructural localization of lactoferrin and myeloperoxidase in human neutrophils by immunogold. *Blood* 1985;65:423–432.

49. Bainton DF, Miller LJ, Kishimoto TK, Springer TA. Leukocyte adhesion receptors are stored in peroxidase-negative granules of human neutrophils. *J Exp Med* 1987;166:1641–1653.

50. Esaguy N, Aguas AP, Silva MT. High-resolution localization of lactoferrin in human neutrophils: labeling of secondary granules and cell heterogeneity. *J Leukoc Biol* 1989;46:51–62.

51. Kane SP, Peters TJ. Analytical subcellular fractionation of human granulocytes with reference to the localization of vitamin B_{12}-binding proteins. *Clin Sci Mol Med* 1975;49:171–182.

52. Bjerrum OW, Bjerrum OJ, Borregaard N. Beta$_2$-microglobulin in neutrophils: an intragranular protein. *J Immunol* 1987;138:3913–3917.

53. Yoon PS, Boxer LA, Mayo LA, Yang AY, Wicha MS. Human neutrophil laminin receptors: activation-dependent receptor expression. *J Immunol* 1987;138:259–265.

54. Singer II, Scott S, Kawka DW, Kazazis DM. Adhesomes: specific granules containing receptors for laminin, C3bi/fibrinogen, fibronectin, and vitronectin in human polymorphonuclear leukocytes and monocytes. *J Cell Biol* 1989;109:3169–3182.

55. Rotrosen D, Gallin JI, Spiegel AM, Malech HL. Subcellular localization of $G_i\alpha$ in human neutrophils. *J Biol Chem* 1988;263: 10958–10964.

56. Roos D, de Boer M, Kuribayashi F, et al. Mutations in the X-linked and autosomal recessive forms of chronic granulomatous disease. *Blood* 1996;87:5:1663–1681.

57. Dewald B, Bretz U, Baggiolini M. Release of gelatinase from a novel secretory compartment of human neutrophils. *J Clin Invest* 1982;70: 518–525.

58. Kjelsen L, Bainton DF, Sengelov H, Borregaard N. Structural and functional heterogeneity among peroxidase-negative granules in human neutrophils: identification of a distinct gelatinase-containing granule subset by combined immunocytochemistry and subcellular fractionation. *Blood* 1993;82:10:3183–3191.

59. Borregaard N, Christensen L, Bejerrum OW, Birgens HS, Clemmensen I. Identification of a highly mobilizable subset of human neutrophil intracellular vesicles that contains tetranectin and latent alkaline phosphatase. *J Clin Invest* 1990;85:408–416.

60. Borregaard N. Current concepts about neutrophil granule physiology. *Curr Opin Hematol* 1996;3:11–20.

61. Robinson JM, Kobayashi T. A novel intracellular compartment with unusual secretory properties in human neutrophils. *J Cell Biol* 1991;113:743–756.

62. Borregaard N, Sengelov H, Kjeldsen L, Johnsen AH, Nielsen MH. Stimulus-dependent exocytosis of plasma proteins from human neutrophils. *J Cell Biol* 1991;115:257a.

63. Borregaard N, Kjeldsen L, Sengelov H, et al. Changes in subcellular localization and surface expression of L-selectin, alkaline phosphatase, and Mac-1 in human neutrophils during stimulation with inflammatory mediators. *J Leukoc Biol* 1994;56:80–87.

64. Moore KL, Patel KD, Bruehl RE, et al. P-selectin glycoprotein ligand-1 mediates rolling of human neutrophils on P-selectin. *J Cell Biol* 1995;128:4:661–671.

65. Bruehl RE, Moore KL, Lorant DE, et al. Leukocyte activation induces surface redistribution of P-selectin glycoprotein ligand-1. *J Leukoc Biol* 1997;61:489–499.

66. Le Cabec V, Cowland JB, Calafat J, Borregaard N. Targeting of proteins to granule subsets is determined by timing and not by sorting: the specific granule protein NGAL is localized to azurophil granules when expressed in HL-60 cells. *Proc Natl Acad of Sci USA* 1996;93:6454–6457.

67. Dubravec DB, Spriggs DR, Mannick JA, Rodrick ML. Circulating human peripheral blood granulocytes synthesize and secrete tumor necrosis factor. *Proc Natl Acad Sci USA* 1990;87:6758–6761.

68. Wheeler MA, Smith SD, Garcia-Cardena G, Nathan CF, Weiss RM, Sessa WC. Bacterial infection induces nitric oxide synthase in human neutrophils. *J Clin Invest* 1997;99:1:110–116.

69. Wright DG, Bralove DA, Gallin JI. The differential mobilization of human neutrophil granules: effects of phorbol myristate acetate and ionophore A23187. *Am J Pathol* 1977;87:273–284.

70. Pryzwansky KB, MacRae EK, Spitznagel JK, Cooney MH. Early degranulation of human neutrophils: immunocytochemical studies of surface and intracellular phagocytic events. *Cell* 1979;18:1025–1033.

71. Wright DG, Gallin JI. Secretory responses of human neutrophils:exocytosis of specific (secondary) granules by human neutrophils during adherence in vitro and during exudation in vivo. *J Immunol* 1979; 123:285–294.

72. Baggiolini M, Dewald B. Exocytosis by neutrophils. In: Snyderman R, ed. *Regulation of leukocyte function.* New York: Plenum Press, 1984:221–246.

73. Wilson E, Rice WG, Kinkade JM Jr, Merrill AH Jr, Arnold RR, Lambeth JD. Protein kinase C inhibition by sphingoid long chain bases: effects on secretion in human neutrophils. *Arch Biochem Biophys* 1987;259:204–214.

74. Sengelov H, Follin P, Kjeldsen L, Lollike K, Dahlgren C, Borregaard N. Mobilization of granules and secretory vesicles during in vivo exudation of human neutrophils. *J Immunol* 1995;154:8:4157–4165.

75. Roos D, de Boer M, Kuribayashi K, et al. Mutations in the X-linked and autosomal recessive forms of chronic granulomatous disease. *J Am Soc Hematol* 1996;87:1663–1681.

76. Rosenthal J, Thurman GW, Cusack N, Peterson VM, Malech HL, Ambruso DR. Neutrophils from patients after burn injury express a deficiency of the oxidase components p47-phox and p67-phox. *Blood* 1996;88:4321–4329.

77. Bainton DF. Selective abnormalities of azurophil and specific granules of human neutrophilic leukocytes. *Fed Proc* 1981; 40:1443–1450.

78. Zucker-Franklin D, Greaves MF, Grossi CE, Marmont AM. *Atlas of blood cells:* function and pathology. Philadelphia: Lea & Febiger, 1981:276–284.

79. Bainton DF. Abnormal neutrophils in acute myelogenous leukemia:

identification of subpopulations based on analysis of azurophil and specific granules. *Blood Cells* 1975;1:191–199.

80. Bainton DF, Friedlander LM, Shohet SB. Abnormalities in granule formation in acute myelogenous leukemia. *Blood* 1977;49:693–704.

81. Ullyot JL, Bainton DF. Azurophil and specific granules of blood neutrophils in chronic myelogenous leukemia: an ultrastructural and cytochemical analysis. *Blood* 1974;44:469–482.

82. Parmley RT, Crist WM, Ragab AH, et al. Congenital dysgranulopoietic neutropenia. *Blood* 1980;56:465–475.

83. Lehrer RI, Cline MJ. Leukocyte myeloperoxidase deficiency and disseminated candidiasis: the role of myeloperoxidase in resistance to Candida infection. *J Clin Invest* 1969;48:1478–1488.

84. Breton Gorius J, Coquin MY, Guichard J. Activities peroxydasiques de certaines granulations des neutrophils dans deux cas de deficit congenital en myeloperoxidase. *C R Acad Sci [D]* 1975;280:1753–1756.

85. Kitahara M, Eyre HJ, Simonian Y, Atkin C, Hasstedt SJ. Hereditary myeloperoxidase deficiency. *Blood* 1981;57:888–893.

86. Parry MF, Root RK, Metcalf JA, Delaney KK, Kaplow LS, Richard WJ. Myeloperoxidase deficiency. *Ann Intern Med* 1981;95:293–301.

87. Ross DW, Kaplow LS. Myeloperoxidase deficiency: increased sensitivity for immunocytochemical compared to cytochemical detection of enzyme. *Arch Pathol Lab Med* 1985;109:1005–1006.

88. Nauseef WM. Posttranslational processing of a human myeloid lysosomal protein, myeloperoxidase. *Blood* 1987;70:1143–1150.

89. Tobler A, Selsted ME, Miller CW, et al. Evidence for a pretranslational defect in hereditary and acquired myeloperoxidase deficiency. *Blood* 1989;73:1980–1986.

90. Lehrer RI, Goldberg LS, Apple MA, Rosenthal NP. Refractory megaloblastic anemia with myeloperoxidase and deficient neutrophils. *Ann Intern Med* 1972;76:447–453.

91. Breton-Gorius J, Houssay D, Dryfux B. Partial myeloperoxidase deficiency in a case of preleukemia. *Br J Haematol* 1975;30:273–278.

92. Davey FR, Erber WN, Gatter KC, Mason DY. Abnormal neutrophils in acute myeloid leukemia and myelodysplastic syndrome. *Hum Pathol* 1988;19:454–459.

93. Catovsky D, Galton DAG, Robinson J. Myeloperoxidase-deficient neutrophils in acute myeloid leukaemia. *Scand J Haematol* 1972;9:142–148.

94. Bendix-Hansen K, Nielsen HK. Myeloperoxidase-deficient polymorphonuclear leucocytes (IV): relation to FAB-classification in acute myeloid leukaemia. *Scand J Haematol* 1985;35:174–177.

95. Gulley ML, Bentley SA, Ross DW. Neutrophil myeloperoxidase measurement uncovers masked megaloblastic anemia. *Blood* 1990;76:1004–1007.

96. Beckstead JH, Halverson PS, Ries CA, Bainton DF. Enzyme histochemistry and immunohistochemistry on biopsy specimens of pathologic human bone marrow. *Blood* 1981;57:1088–1098.

97. Breton-Gorius J, Houssay D. Auer bodies in acute promyelocytic leukemia: demonstration of their fine structure and peroxidase localization. *Lab Invest* 1973;28:135–141.

98. Tulliez M, Breton-Gorius J. Three types of Auer bodies in acute leukemia. *Lab Invest* 1979;41:419–426.

99. Hassan HT, Rees JKH. Auer bodies in acute myeloid leukemia patients. *Pathol Res Pract* 1990;186:293–295.

100. Hanker JS, Laszlo J, Moore JO. The light microscopic demonstration of hydroperoxidase-positive Phi bodies and rods in leukocytes in acute myeloid leukemia. *Histochemistry* 1978;58:241–252.

101. Newburger PE, Novak TJ, McCaffrey RP. Eosinophilic cytoplasmic inclusions in fetal leukocytes: are Auer bodies a recapitulation of fetal morphology? *Blood* 1983;61:593–595.

102. Juneja HS, Rajaraman S, Alperin JB, Bainton DF. Auer rodlike inclusions in prolymphocytic leukemia. *Acta Haematol* 1987;77:115–119.

103. Davis WC, Douglas SD. Defective granule formation and function in the Chediak-Higashi syndrome in man and animals. *Semin Hematol* 1972;9:431–450.

104. Oliver C, Essner E. Formation of anomalous lysosomes in monocytes, neutrophils, and eosinophils from bone marrow of mice with Chediak-Higashi syndrome. *J Lab Invest* 1975;32:17–27.

105. Rausch PG, Pryzwansky KB, Spitznagel JK. Immunocytochemical identification of azurophilic and specific granule markers in the giant granules of Chediak-Higashi neutrophils. *N Engl J Med* 1978;298:694–698.

106. Gale PF, Parkin JL, Quie PG, Pettit RE, Nelson RP, Brunning RD. Leukocyte granulation abnormality associated with normal neutrophil function and neurologic impairment. *Am J Clin Pathol* 1986;86:33–49.

107. Newburger PE, Robinson JM, Pryzwansky KB, Rosoff PM, Greenberger JS, Tauber AI. Human neutrophil dysfunction with giant granules and defective activation of the respiratory burst. *Blood* 1983;61:1247–1257.

108. Ganz T, Metcalf JA, Gallin JI, Boxer LA, Lehrer RI. Microbicidal/cytotoxic proteins of neutrophils are deficient in two disorders: Chediak-Higashi syndrome and "specific" granule deficiency. *J Clin Invest* 1988;82:552–556.

109. Barbosa MD, Nguyen QA, Tchernev VT, et al. Identification of the homologous beige and Chediak-Higashi syndrome genes. *Nature* 1996;382:262–265.

110. VanSlyck EJ, Rebuck JW. Pseudo-Chediak-Higashi anomaly in acute leukemia: a significant morphologic corollary? *Am J Clin Pathol* 1974;62:673–678.

111. Gorman AM, O'Connell LG. Pseudo-Chediak-Higashi anomaly in acute leukemia. *Am J Clin Pathol* 1976;65:1030–1031.

112. Efrati P, Nir E, Kaplan H, Dvilanski A. Pseudo-Chediak-Higashi anomaly in acute myeloid leukaemia: an electron microscopical study. *Acta Haematol (Basel)* 1979;61:264–271.

113. Dittman WA, Kramer RJ, Bainton DF. Electron microscopic and peroxidase cytochemical analysis of pink pseudo-Chediak-Higashi granules in acute myelogenous leukemia. *Cancer Res* 1980;40:4473–4481.

114. McCall CE, Katayama I, Cotran RS, Finland M. Lysosomal ultrastructural changes in human "toxic" neutrophils during bacterial infection. *J Exp Med* 1969;129:267–293.

115. McCall CE, Caves J, Cooper R, DeChatelet L. Functional characteristics of human toxic neutrophils. *J Infect Dis* 1971;124:68–75.

116. McCall CE, DeChatelet LR, Cooper MR, Shannon C. Human toxic neutrophils. III. Metabolic characteristics. *J Infect Dis* 1973;127:26–33.

117. Weller PF, Ackerman SJ, Nicholson-Weller A, Dvorak AM. Cytoplasmic lipid bodies of human neutrophilic leukocytes. *Am J Pathol* 1989;135:947–959.

118. Peterson LC, Rao KV, Crosson JT, White JG. Fechtner syndrome—a variant of Alport's syndrome with leukocyte inclusions and macrothrombocytopenia. *Blood* 1985;65:397–406.

119. Heynen MJ, Blockmans D, Verwilghen RL, Vermylen J. Congenital macrothrombocytopenia, leucocyte inclusions deafness and proteinuria: functional and electron microscopic observations on platelets and megakaryocytes. *Br J Haematol* 1988;70:441–448.

120. Greinacher A, Mueller-Eckhardt C. Hereditary types of thrombocytopenia with giant platelets and inclusion bodies in the leukocytes. *Blut* 1990;60:53–60.

121. Dake MD, Madison JM, Montgomery CK, et al. Electron microscopic demonstration of lysosomal inclusion bodies in lung, liver, lymph nodes, and blood leukocytes of patients with amiodarone pulmonary toxicity. *Am J Med* 1985;78:506–512.

122. Burkholder L, Bainton DF. Auto-antigens in Wegener's granulomatosis. *Blood* 1990;75:1588–1589.

123. Stummann WA, Kjeldsen L, Borregaard N, Ullman S, Jacobsen S, Halberg P. The diversity of perinuclear antineutrophil cytoplasmic antibodies (pANCA) antigens. *Clin Exp Immunol* 1995;101(Suppl 1):15–17.

124. Gilligan HM, Bredy B, Brady HR, et al. Antineutrophil cytoplasmic autoantibodies interact with primary granule constituents on the surface of apoptotic neutrophils in the absence of neutrophil priming. *J Exp Med* 1996;184:2231–2241.

125. Strauss RG, Bove KE, Jones JF, Mauer AM, Filginiti VA. An anomaly of neutrophil morphology with impaired function. *N Engl J Med* 1974;290:478–484.

126. Boxer LA, Blackwood RA. Leukocyte disorders: quantitative and qualitative disorders of the neutrophils, part 1. *Pediatr Rev* 1996;17:19–28.

127. Boxer LA, Blackwood RA. Leukocyte disorders: quantitative and qualitative disorders of the neutrophils, part 2. *Pediatr Rev* 1996;17:47–50.

128. Komiyama A, Morosawa H, Nakahata T, Miyagawa Y, Akabene T. Abnormal neutrophil maturation in a neutrophil defect with morphologic abnormality and impaired function. *J Pediatr* 1979;94:19–25.

129. Breton-Gorius J, Mason DY, Buriot D, Vilde JL, Griscelli C. Lactoferrin deficiency as a consequence of a lack of specific granules in neutrophils from a patient with recurrent infections: detection by immunoperoxidase staining for lactoferrin and cytochemical electron microscopy. *Am J Pathol* 1980;99:413–428.

130. Gallin JI. Neutrophil specific granule deficiency. *Annu Rev Med* 1985;36:263–274.

131. Malech HL, Gallin JI. Neutrophils in human diseases. *N Engl J Med* 1987;317:687–694.

132. Parmley RT, Gilbert CS, Boxer LA. Abnormal peroxidase-positive granules in "specific granule" deficiency. *Blood* 1989;73:838–844.

133. Lomax KJ, Gallin JI, Rotrosen D, et al. Selective defect in myeloid cell lactoferrin gene expression in neutrophil specific granule deficiency. *J Clin Invest* 1989;83:514–519.

134. Johnston JJ, Boxer LA, Berliner N. Correlation of messenger RNA levels with protein defects in specific granule deficiency. *Blood* 1992; 80:2088.

135. Miyauchi J, Ohyashiki K, Inatomi Y, Toyama K. Neutrophil secondary-granule deficiency as a hallmark of all-trans retinoic acid-induced differentiation of acute promyelocytic leukemia cells. *Blood* 1997;90:2:803 813.

136. Repine JE, Clawson CC, Brunning RD. Abnormal pattern of bactericidal activity of neutrophils deficient in granules, myeloperoxidase, and alkaline phosphatase. *J Lab Clin Med* 1976;88:788–795.

137. Thiele J, Timmer J, Jansen B, Zankovich R, Fischer R. Ultrastructure of neutrophilic granulopoiesis in the bone marrow of patients with chronic myeloid leukemia (CML): a morphometric study with special emphasis on azurophil (primary) and specific (secondary) granules. *Virchows Arch (Cell Pathol)* 1990;59:125–131.

138. Rambaldi A, Terao M, Bettoni S, et al. Differences in the expression of alkaline phosphatase mRNA in chronic myelogenous leukemia and paroxysmal nocturnal hemoglobinuria polymorphonuclear leukocytes. *Blood* 1989;73:1113–1115.

139. Odeberg H, Olofsson T, Olsson I. Primary and secondary granule contents and bactericidal capability of neutrophils in acute leukaemia. *Blood Cells* 1976;2:543–551.

140. Parmley RT, Tzeng DY, Baehner RL, Boxer LA. Abnormal distribution of complex carbohydrates in neutrophils of a patient with lactoferrin deficiency. *Blood* 1983;62:538–548.

141. Li YM, Tan AX, Vlassara H. Antibacterial activity of lysozyme and lactoferrin is inhibited by binding of advanced glycation-modified proteins to a conserved motif. *Nat Med* 1995;1:1057–1061.

142. Lübbert M, Koeffler HP. Myeloid cell lines: tools for studying differentiation of normal and abnormal hematopoietic cells. *Blood Rev* 1988;2:121–133.

143. Gallagher R, Collins S, Trujillo J, et al. Characterization of the continuous differentiating myeloid cell line (HL-60) from a patient with acute promyelocytic leukemia. *Blood* 1979;54:713–733.

144. Lübbert M, Herrmann F, Koeffler HP. Expression and regulation of myeloid-specific genes in normal and leukemic myeloid cells. *Blood* 1991;77:909–924.

145. Rado TA, Wei X, Benz EJ Jr. Isolation of lactoferrin cDNA from a human myeloid library and expression of mRNA during normal and leukemic myelopoiesis. *Blood* 1987;70:989–993.

146. Bainton DF. HL-60 cells have abnormal myeloperoxidase transport and packaging. *Exp Hematol* 1988;16:150–158.

147. Roos D, Voetman AA, Meerhof LJ. Functional activity of enucleated human polymorphonuclear leukocytes. *J Cell Biol* 1983;97:368–377.

148. Petrequin PR, Todd RF III, Smolen JE, Boxer LA. Expression of specific granule markers on the cell surface of neutrophil cytoplasts. *Blood* 1986;67:1119–1125.

149. Malawista SE, Montgomery RR, Van Blaricom G. Microbial killing by human neutrophil cytokineplasts: similar suppressive effects of reversible and irreversible inhibitors of nitric oxide synthase. *J Leukoc Biol* 1996;60:6:753–757.

150. Archer RK. *The eosinophil leucocytes.* Oxford: Blackwell Scientific Publications, 1963.

151. Butterfield JH, Ackerman SJ, Scott RE, Pierre RV, Gleich GJ. Evidence for secretion of human eosinophil granule major basic protein and Charcot-Leyden crystal protein during eosinophil maturation. *Exp Hematol* 1984;12:163–170.

152. Weller PF, Monahan-Earley RA, Dvorak HF, Dvorak AM. Cytoplasmic lipid bodies of human eosinophils. *Am J Pathol* 1991;138: 141–148.

153. Dvorak AM, Ackerman SJ, Weller PF. Subcellular morphological and biochemistry of eosinophils. In: Harris JR, ed. *Blood cell biochemistry*, vol 2. *Megakaryocytes, platelets, macrophages, and eosinophils.* New York: Plenum Press, 1990;237–344.

154. Dvorak AM, Furitsu T, Estrella P, Letourneau L, Ishizaka T, Ackerman J. Ultrastructural localization of major basic protein in the human eosinophil lineage in vitro. *J Histochem Cytochem* 1994;42:1443–1451.

155. Weller PF, Bach DS, Austen KF. Biochemical characterization of human eosinophil Charcot-Leyden crystal protein (lysophospholipase). *J Biol Chem* 1984;259:15100–15105.

156. Dvorak AM, Letourneau L, Login GR, Weller PF, Ackerman SJ. Ultrastructural localization of the Charcot-Leyden crystal protein (lysophospholipase) to a distinct crystalloid-free granule population in mature human eosinophils. *Blood* 1988;72:150–158.

157. Calafat J, Janssen H, Knol EF, Weller PF, Egesten A. Ultrastructural localization of Charcot-Leyden crystal protein in human eosinophils and basophils. *Eur J Haematol* 1997;58:56–66.

158. Peters MS, Rodriguez M, Gleich GJ. Localization of human eosinophil granule major basic protein, eosinophil cationic protein, and eosinophil-derived neurotoxin by immunoelectron microscopy. *Lab Invest* 1986;54:656–662.

159. Waltraud JB, Weller PF, Tzizik DM, Galli SJ, Dvorak AM. Ultrastructural immunogold localization of tumor necrosis factor-α to the matrix compartment of eosinophil secondary granules in patients with idiopathic hypereosinophilic syndrome. *J Histochem Cytochem* 1993; 41:1611–1615.

160. Egesten A, Calafat J, Knol EF, Janssen H, Walz TM. Subcellular localization of transforming growth factor-α in human eosinophil granulocytes. *Blood* 1996;87:3910–3918.

161. Levi-Schaffer F, Lacy P, Severs NJ, et al. Association of granulocyte-macrophage colony-stimulating factor with the crystalloid granules of human eosinophils. *Blood* 1995;85:2579–2586.

162. Bujak JS, Root RK. The role of peroxidase in the bactericidal activity of human blood eosinophils. *Blood* 1974;43:727–736.

163. Yazdanbakhsh M, Eckmann CM, Bot AA, Roos D. Bactericidal action of eosinophils from normal human blood. *Infect Immun* 1986;53:192–198.

164. Iozzo RV, MacDonald, GH, Wight TN. Immunoelectron microscopic localization of catalase in human eosinophilic leukocytes. *J Histochem Cytochem* 1982;30:697–701.

165. Yokota S, Deimann W, Hashimoto T, Fahimi HD. Immunocytochemical localization of two peroxisomal enzymes of lipid-oxidation in specific granules of rat eosinophils. *Histochemistry* 1983;78:425–433.

166. Yokota S, Deimann W, Hashimoto T, Fahimi HD. Specific granules of rat eosinophils contain peroxisomal acyl-CoA oxidase: possible involvement in production of H_2O_2. *Histochem J* 1984;16:573–577.

167. Eguchi M, Ozawa T, Suda J, Sugita K, Furukawa T. Lectins for electron microscopic distinction of eosinophils from other blood cells. *J Histochem Cytochem* 1989;37:743–749.

168. Young JD-E, Peterson CGB, Venge P, Cohn ZA. Mechanism of membrane damage mediated by human eosinophil cationic protein. *Nature* 1986;321:613–616.

169. Gleich GJ, Loegering DA, Bell MP, Checkel JL, Ackerman SJ, McKean DJ. Biochemical and functional similarities between human eosinophil-derived neurotoxin and eosinophil cationic protein: homology with ribonuclease. *Proc Natl Acad Sci USA* 1986;83:3146–3150.

170. Rosenberg HF, Ackerman SJ, Tenen DG. Human eosinophil cationic protein: molecular cloning of a cytotoxin and helminthotoxin with ribonuclease activity. *J Exp Med* 1989;170:163–176.

171. Rothenberg ME, Pomerantz JL, Owen WF Jr, et al. Characterization of a human eosinophil proteoglycan, and augmentation of its biosynthesis and size by interleukin 3, interleukin 5, and granulocyte/macrophage colony stimulating factor. *J Biol Chem* 1988;263:13901–13908.

172. Dvorak AM, MacGlashan DW, Warner JA, et al. Localization of Charcot-Leyden crystal protein in individual morphological phenotypes of human basophils stimulated by f-met peptide. *Clin Exp Allergy* 1997; 27:452–474.

173. Presentey B. Ultrastructure of human eosinophils genetically lacking peroxidase. *Acta Haematol (Basel)* 1984;71:334–340.

174. Zabucchi G, Soranzo MR, Menegazzi R, et al. Eosinophil peroxidase deficiency: morphological and immunocytochemical studies of the eosinophil-specific granules. *Blood* 1992;80:2903.

175. Romano M, Patriarca P, Melo C, Baralle FE, Dri P. Hereditary eosinophil peroxidase deficiency: immunochemical and spectroscopic studies and evidence for a compound heterozygosity of the defect. *Proc Natl Acad Sci USA* 1994;91:12496–12500.

176. Tracey R, Smith H. An inherited anomaly of human eosinophils and basophils. *Blood Cells* 1978;4:291–298.

177. Rosenberg HF, Gallin JI. Neutrophil-specific granule deficiency includes eosinophils. *Blood* 1993;82:1:268–273.

178. Liso V, Troccoli G, Specchia G, Magno M. Cytochemical "normal" and "abnormal" eosinophils in acute leukemias. *Am J Hematol* 1977; 2:123–131.

179. LeBeau MM, Larson RA, Bitter MA, Vardiman JW, Golomb HM, Rowley JD. Association of an inversion of chromosome 16 with abnormal marrow eosinophils in acute myelomonocytic leukemia. *N Engl J Med* 1983;309:630–636.

180. Haferlach T, Winkemann M, Loffler H, et al. The abnormal eosinophils are part of the leukemic cell population in acute myelomonocytic leukemia with abnormal eosinophils (AML M4Eo) and carry the pericentric inversion 16: a combination of May-Grunwald-Giemsa staining and fluorescence in situ hybridization. *Blood* 1996;87:2459–2463.

181. Mlynek M-L, Leder L-D. Lineage infidelity in chronic myeloid leukemia: demonstration and significance of hybridoid leukocytes. *Virchows Arch* 1986;51:107–114.

182. Kaufman LD, Gleich GJ. The expanding clinical spectrum of multisystem disease associated with eosinophilia [Editorial and comment]. *Arch Dermatol* 1997;133:225–227.

183. Harley JB. Clinical manifestations of patients with hypereosinophilic syndrome. *Ann Intern Med* 1982;97:78–92.

184. Spry CJF. Synthesis and secretion of eosinophil granule substances. *Immunol Today* 1985;6:332–335.

185. Caulfield JP, Hein A, Rothenberg ME, et al. A morphometric study of normodense and hypodense human eosinophils that are derived in vivo and in vitro. *Am J Pathol* 1990:137:27–41.

186. Owen WF, Petersen J, Sheff DM, et al. Hypodense eosinophils and interleukin 5 activity in the blood of patients with the eosinophilia-myalgia syndrome. *Am J Med* 1990;88:542–546.

187. Pincus SH, Schooley WR, DiNapoli AM, Broder S. Metabolic heterogeneity of eosinophils from normal and hypereosinophilic patients. *Blood* 1981;58:1175–1181.

188. Jaffe I, Kopelman R, Baird R, Grossman M, Hays A. Eosinophilic fasciitis associated with the eosinophilia-myalgia syndrome. *Am J Med* 1990;88:542–546.

189. Jimenez SA, Varga J. The eosinophilia-myalgia syndrome. *West J Med* 1990;153:322–323.

190. Mayeno AN, Lin F, Foote CS, Loegering DA, Ames MM, Hedberg CW, Gleich GJ. Characterization of "Peak E," a novel amino acid associated with eosinophilia-myalgia syndrome. *Science* 1990;250:1707–1708.

191. Meeker TC, Hardy D, Willman C, Hogan T, Abrams J. Activation of the interleukin-3 gene by chromosome translocation in acute lymphocytic leukemia with eosinophilia. *Blood* 1990;76:285–289.

192. Parmley RT, Crist WM, Roper M, Takagi M, Austin RL. Intranuclear crystalloids associated with abnormal granules in eosinophilic leukocytes. *Blood* 1981;58:1134–1140.

193. Chilosi M, Fossaluzza V, Tosato F. Eosinophilic acquired Pelger-Hut anomaly in acute myeloblastic leukemia. *Acta Haematol (Basel)* 1979;61:198–202.

194. Fossaluzza V, Tosato F. Acquired Pelger-Huet anomaly limited to eosinophils. *Acta Haematol (Basel)* 1980;63:295.

195. Fischkoff SA, Pollak A, Gleich GJ, Testa JR, Misawa S, Reber TJ. Eosinophilic differentiation of the human promyelocytic leukemia cell line, HL-60. *J Exp Med* 1984;160:179–196.

196. Cohen NS, LoBue J, Gordon AS. Mechanisms of leukocyte production and release. VIII. Eosinophil and neutrophil kinetics in rats. *Scand J Haematol* 1967;4:339–350.

197. Osgood EE. Culture of human marrow; length of life of the neutrophils, eosinophils and basophils of normal blood as determined by comparative cultures and sternal marrow from healthy persons. *JAMA* 1937;109:933–936.

198. Rothenberg ME, Owen WF Jr, Silberstein DS, Soberman RJ, Austen KF, Stevens RL. Eosinophils cocultured with endothelial cells have increased survival and functional properties. *Science* 1987;237:645–647.

199. Dale DC, Hubert RT, Fauci A. Eosinophil kinetics in the hypereosinophilic syndrome. *J Lab Clin Med* 1976;3:487–495.

200. Coffman RL, Seymour BWP, Hudak S, Jackson J, Rennick D. Antibody to interleukin-5 inhibits helminth-induced eosinophilia in mice. *Science* 1989;245:308–310.

201. Rennick DM, Thompson-Snipes L, Coffman RL, Seymour BWP, Jackson JD, Hudak S. In vivo administration of antibody to interleukin-5 inhibits increased generation of eosinophils and their progenitors in bone marrow of parasitized mice. *Blood* 1990; 76:312–316.

202. Slungaard A, Ascensao J, Zanjani E, Jacob HS. Pulmonary carcinoma with eosinophilia: demonstration of a tumor-derived eosinophilopoietic factor. *N Engl J Med* 1983;309:778–781.

203. Wong DTW, Weller PF, Galli SJ, et al. Human eosinophils express transforming growth factor. *J Exp Med* 1990;172:673–681.

204. Walsh GM. Mechanisms of human eosinophil survival and apoptosis. *Clin Exp Allergy* 1997;27:482–487.

205. Walsh GM. Human eosinophils: their accumulation, activation and fate. *Br J Haematol* 1997;97:701–709.

206. Bass DA. Behavior of eosinophil leukocytes in acute inflammation. II. Eosinophil dynamics during acute inflammation. *J Clin Invest* 1975;56:870–879.

207. Bass DA, Gonwa TA, Szejda P, Cousart MS, De Chatelet LR, McCall CE. Eosinopenia of acute infection: production of eosinopenia by chemotactic factors of acute inflammation. *J Clin Invest* 1980;65: 1265–1271.

208. Moqbel R. Synthesis and storage of regulatory cytokines in human eosinophils. *Adv Exp Med Biol* 1996;409:287–294.

209. Rollins BJ. Chemokines. *Blood* 1997;90:909–928.

Inflammation: Basic Principles and Clinical Correlates,
3rd ed., edited by John I. Gallin and Ralph Snyderman.
Lippincott Williams & Wilkins, Philadelphia © 1999.

CHAPTER 3

Development and Distribution of Mononuclear Phagocytes:

Relevance to Inflammation

Siamon Gordon

Resident macrophages are a family of long-lived, specialized phagocytic and secretory cells that are widely distributed throughout host tissues in the absence of inflammation. Their presence in skin, lung, liver, gut, and the nervous system, as well as in hemopoietic and lymphoid organs, constitutes an early warning system to protect the host against exogenous agents, including infectious organisms. These cells are able to react selectively to abnormalities that arise within the host, such as during ischemia or a metabolic disturbance, and to initiate an inflammatory and repair process. If local responses are insufficient to remove or counteract the initiating stimulus, macrophages and other cells can mobilize other leukocytes, especially polymorphonuclear cells (PMNs) from blood by activating local endothelium and by production of a range of chemokines, cytokines, and lipid mediators of acute inflammation. Monocytes and lymphoid cells are also recruited and, if the stimulus persists, give rise to a chronic inflammatory process in which, depending on helper T-lymphocyte activation, the local and recruited macrophages can acquire enhanced microbicidal activity. Macrophages elicited by a nonimmune irritant or activated by an immunologically specific stimulus display common features that set them apart from resident cells and express distinctive properties.

An important concept in considering the role of the macrophages in inducing, amplifying, and limiting inflammation is the importance of phenotypic heterogeneity in relation to macrophages' life history and their tissue microenvironment. Heterogeneity is reflected in the varied profiles of plasma membrane receptors by which the cells interact with their environment and the complex regulation of their biosynthetic and secretory responses to different stimuli.

Macrophages are not unique in many of their functions, which overlap with those of PMNs and other myeloid and lymphoid cells. Dendritic cells share a common origin with macrophages and are specialized to process and present antigens to naive T lymphocytes. Macrophages interact with all other leukocytes, including mast cells and natural killer (NK) cells, and with lymphoid cells to regulate their own activities and those of other cells. Nonhemopoietic cells in their local environment, whether endothelial, epithelial, mesenchymal, or neuroendocrine, are profoundly affected by macrophage products and subtly affect properties of the ever-adaptable macrophages. By virtue of their tissue distribution and ability to produce or respond to local and circulating mediators, macrophages orchestrate many of the systemic responses associated with inflammation.

Overall, the cells of the macrophage system provide a unique, nonredundant role in tissue homeostasis, contributing to classic and modified forms of inflammation in diseases such as atherosclerosis and neurodegeneration. As key cells involved in the pathogenesis of immune, infectious, and other disease processes, they provide important targets for drug treatment. Appreciation of their varied roles in inflammation permits a more selective approach to inhibition or stimulation of cells locally or systemically within the host.

S. Gordon: Sir William Dunn School of Pathology, Oxford, United Kingdom.

Metchnikoff, a comparative zoologist, drew attention to the role of phagocytic cells in host defense and inflammation in simpler, multicellular organisms. Subsequently, their role in many species was studied *in situ* by morphologic means, by cell isolation, and in cell culture. Development of monoclonal antibodies provided a powerful impetus to delineate their differentiation, distribution, and responses *in vivo*. *In situ* hybridization makes it possible to localize mRNA for protein products at sites of expression, and sensitive polymerase chain reaction (PCR) technology detects macrophages activities in small amounts of material. Gene knock-out methodology applied to experimental animals has provided a powerful approach for validating postulated functions and discovering unexpected aspects of their role in inflammation.

Many other chapters in this volume deal with topics relevant to our understanding of the contribution of macrophages to inflammation. This chapter considers their development and differentiation in tissues, their key properties relevant to migration and responses, and implications of their regional and functional heterogeneity for understanding inflammation.

DEVELOPMENT AND DISTRIBUTION WITHIN THE HOST

Ontogeny

The earliest CD34+ progenitors of hemopoietic cells, and possibly of endothelial cells, can be found in the paraaortic region of the developing embryo. Primitive erythropoiesis in the yolk sac is accompanied by the first generation of intravascular monocytes and by macrophages in the vessel wall. Physical association between mature, stromal-type macrophages and clusters of erythroblasts, giving rise to anucleate erythrocytes and switching their globin chain production, is a striking feature of subsequent hemopoiesis in the fetal liver. The sites of hemopoiesis, expanding to include production of PMNs, shift to the spleen and bone marrow before birth. The bone marrow becomes the major site of postnatal production of all hemopoietic cells, including different myeloid and lymphoid cells.

From mid-gestation, macrophages are widely distributed throughout the mesenchyme of developing organs; monocytes invade the developing nervous system and ingest apoptotic neurons before differentiating into immature and then highly ramified mature microglia. Their phagocytic activity is widespread throughout the organism and includes disposal of erythroid nuclei and apoptotic cells of all types. The role for macrophages in tissue remodeling is prominent in the developing limb bud and in cartilaginous bone. Other, poorly understood cell-cell interactions involve nonphagocytic adhesion receptors such as EbR, a divalent cation-dependent receptor for erythroblasts and hemopoietic cells, and sialoadhesin, a sialic acid-binding lectin, and may mediate trophic, growth-regulatory functions.

Resident Macrophages in the Normal Adult

Most macrophages in the tissues of the adult derive from circulating monocytes, constitutively recruited by unknown mechanisms (Fig. 3-1). The bone marrow contains small numbers of proliferating precursors and immature and morphologically recognizable monocytes. More differentiated, mature macrophages form part of the stromal microenvironment and are implicated in the production and differentiation of other hemopoietic cells, especially erythroid and myeloid cells. In selected tissues such as lung, mature macrophages retain some ability to divide, although in most tissues, the cells become terminally differentiated. Despite losing the ability to proliferate, these resident macrophages retain active RNA and protein synthesis and turn over slowly. Inflammatory stimuli enhance recruitment from blood and bone marrow to local sites; these cells can proliferate *in situ* and have a shortened life span, the result of induced apoptosis, necrosis, or both. Resident and other mature macrophages in tissues clear dying macrophages and other cells in their environment.

Our understanding of macrophage distribution in tissues and of their lineage relationships has benefited greatly from the development of membrane antigen markers of differentiation such as F4/80 and macrosialin (CD68). The murine F4/80 antigen is a plasma membrane glycoprotein of unknown function, with a novel chimeric structure, a large extracellular portion consisting of multiple epidermal growth factor–like domains, and a seven-transmembrane domain that is homologous to the secretin peptide–receptor family. It is expressed during differentiation as the promonocytic cells become adherent, is weakly present on monocytes, and is then highly expressed in many tissue macrophages (Fig. 3-2). F4/80 is an excellent marker for macrophages in development, in brain, and in nonlymphoid organs such as liver and gut; it is sparsely present on alveolar macrophages and absent on macrophages in T-lymphocyte–dependent areas, in splenic white pulp and elsewhere. A human homologue, EMR1, has been defined, but because there is no monoclonal antibody available, its expression in human tissues remains unknown.

Macrosialin (antigen FA-11) was defined in mouse as a predominantly intracellular (late-endosomal) glycoprotein; cloning studies showed it to be homologous to human CD68, defined by a panel of monoclonal antibodies, and a macrophage-restricted member of the LAMP (lysosome-associated membrane protein) family, by virtue of an extracellular mucin-like domain. Macrosialin is a panmacrophage marker present in all tissue macrophages, dendritic cells, and osteoclasts, members of the extended macrophage family that include cells in which F4/80 antigen is downregulated or absent. Macrosialin has one known ligand, oxidized low-density lipoprotein, although others are likely, and it is present in tissues as different glycoforms, apparently dependent on phagocytic and inflammatory stimuli.

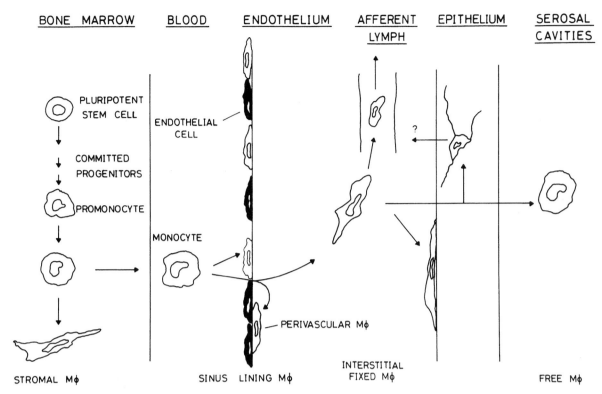

BONE MARROW   BLOOD   ENDOTHELIUM   AFFERENT LYMPH   EPITHELIUM   SEROSAL CAVITIES

PLURIPOTENT STEM CELL

ENDOTHELIAL CELL

COMMITTED PROGENITORS

PROMONOCYTE

MONOCYTE

PERIVASCULAR Mφ

STROMAL Mφ   SINUS LINING Mφ   INTERSTITIAL FIXED Mφ   FREE Mφ

FIG. 3-1. Differentiation of macrophages and distribution pathway in tissues. Schematic representation of origin in bone marrow, with local differentiation into stromal macrophages or delivery to blood. After circulating, the monocyte adopts a sinus-lining position, as in liver, or migrates across endothelium. Resident macrophages associate with endothelium or epithelium (Langerhans cells illustrated); traffic into serosal cavities (free macrophages) or become interstitial fixed cells. Resident macrophages respond to circulating or tissue stimuli to initiate inflammatory changes in endothelium and leukocyte recruitment. Stimulated macrophages and newly recruited monocytes that differentiate into macrophages drain into afferent lymph; antigen or adjuvant-stimulated Langerhans cells also deliver antigens to secondary lymphoid organs. Based on immunocytochemical studies with the murine differentiation marker, F4/80.

The origin, differentiation, migration, and functions of dendritic cells (DCs) are discussed elsewhere in this volume; their relationship to monocyte-derived cells is addressed here. *In vivo*, human monocytes can be induced by appropriate culture additions to differentiate into macrophage-like cells (i.e., macrophage colony-stimulating factor, granulocyte-macrophage colony-stimulating factor [GM-CSF] or interleukin-4 [IL-4] alone) or into immature DC (i.e., IL-4 plus GM-CSF) or mature DCs (plus lipopolysaccharide [LPS], tumor necrosis factor α [TNF-α] or monocyte-derived conditioned medium). Early changes are reversible; later differences between macrophages and dendritic-like cells apparently not. In the mouse, blood mononuclear cell-derived Langerhans cells express F4/80, which they lose after an antigenic stimulus as cells migrate in afferent lymph to draining lymph nodes to become DC; TNF-α contributes to their migration. Although macrophages express abundant FA-11–positive intracellular organelles, DCs downregulate their expression of FA-11 to a single dotlike structure, in keeping with downregulation of other endocytic organelles as their antigen-presenting function matures.

The expression pattern of F4/80 makes it possible to construct a putative migration pathway for resident macrophages (see Fig. 3-1). An intimate relationship exists between macrophages and endothelial cells; in organs such as liver, Kupffer cells (F4/80+ macrophages) are distinct but closely apposed to other sinusoidal endothelial cells (F4/80−). Elsewhere, F4/80+ plasma membrane processes envelop small blood vessels (e.g., some pericytes, perivascular macrophages in the central nervous system [CNS]). Macrophages are widely distributed in mesenchymal tissues but also associate with epithelia, lying beneath basement membrane (e.g., tubules in renal medulla) or entering simple (e.g., submaxillary gland duct) or complex epithelia (e.g., bladder, Langerhans cells in skin). This distribution pattern suggests a precisely controlled migration pathway after monocyte diapedesis.

Stromal macrophages in fetal liver and bone marrow are strongly F4/80−. In secondary lymphoid organs, there is considerable microheterogeneity of macrophage phenotype. For example, normal spleen contains distinct macrophages subpopulations in the red pulp (F4/80−),

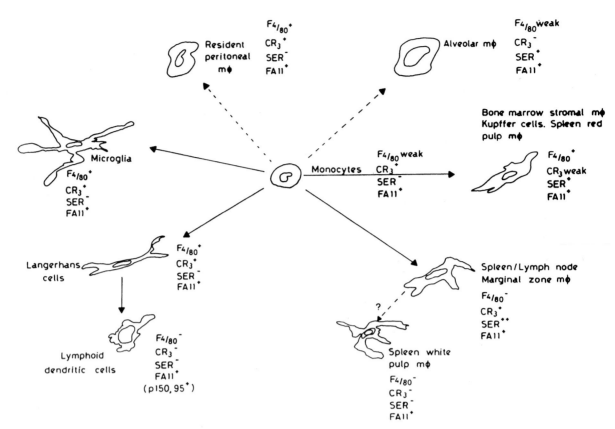

FIG. 3-2. Phenotypic heterogeneity of resident macrophages in different tissues. Monocytes give rise to distinctive macrophage populations in lymphohemopoietic organs, liver (Kupffer cells), lung, skin (Langerhans cells), nervous system (microglia), serosal cavities and other sites, not shown. Alveolar and peritoneal macrophages are relatively autonomous, once established. Based on studies of the following murine marker antigens; F4/80, CR3 (type 3 complement receptor), SER (sheep erythrocyte receptor, also known as sialoadhesin) and FA-11 (macrosialin, homologue of CD68). Notice the micro-heterogeneity within spleen and lymph node, and relationship to myeloid-type dendritic cells. Inflammatory and immunologic stimuli induce migration of macrophages and DC; newly recruited monocytes adopt similar properties as they enter local sites, such as the central nervous system and become difficult to distinguish from locally activated macrophages.

marginal zone (F4/80⁻, FA–11⁺), and white pulp (F4/80⁻, FA–11⁻). Other antigenic markers, including sialoadhesin, are selectively present on marginal zone macrophages. Studies have implicated sialoadhesin in the binding of the mannose receptor (MR) cysteine-rich domain and in the capture and transport of mannosylated immunogens.

All serosal cavities contain F4/80⁻ macrophages as resident cells; peritoneal macrophages in mouse, for example, provide a useful source for study in the normal and stimulated animal after monocytes are recruited from blood by intraperitoneal injection of an inflammatory agent such as thioglycolate broth. Resident peritoneal macrophages turn over slowly within the peritoneal cavity, probably involving local sources on the mesentery ("milk spots"), and emigrate rapidly to draining lymph nodes after intraperitoneal inflammation.

The nervous system is a good example of local differentiation and altered responsiveness to inflammatory stimuli. After recruitment during development, microglia remain in the neuropil throughout adult life. Cell recruitment and turnover are low, although there is variation at particular sites such as the posterior pituitary, where microglia are responsive to salt loading and take up local hormones by intimate interactions with neurosecretory cells. Microglia differ from macrophages in the choroid plexus, cerebrospinal fluid, and meninges in their altered responses to local inflammatory stimuli.

Analysis of gene knock-out models in the mouse has contributed to our understanding of macrophage heterogeneity in different microanatomic sites. A naturally occurring colony-stimulating factor-1 (CSF-1) deficiency, the osteopetrotic (op/op) mutation, established that osteoclasts share critical dependence on this growth factor with selected macrophages. In particular, op/op animals contain reduced levels of circulating monocytes, resident peritoneal macrophages, alveolar macrophages, and Kupffer

MONONUCLEAR PHAGOCYTES AND INFLAMMATION / 39

cells, whereas Langerhans cells and DCs are unaffected; the marginal zone macrophage population is absent. Members of the TNF-α/lymphotoxin family have also been implicated in macrophage subpopulations and in complex abnormalitieσ οφ λψμπηοιδ αρχηιτεχτυρε. ΔNA–βινδ–ινγ προτεινσ (ε.γ., Πυ.–1, FOS, members of the NF-κB family) also influence macrophage, osteoclast, and DC differentiation, as revealed by knock-out experiments.

Recruitment and Immune Activation of Macrophages *In Vivo*

The mechanisms of induced recruitment of monocytes and of other circulating white blood cells are better understood than those of constitutive entry into tissues. The roles of selectins, β$_2$-integrins, CD31, and other adhesion molecules and of locally acting chemokines and cytokines have been established mainly by studies of PMNs and lymphoid cells in humans (e.g., leukocyte adhesion deficiency) and in experimental models using blocking antibodies or knock-out animals. Adhesion molecules relevant to monocyte recruitment after inflammatory and metabolic stimuli include CD44, vascular cell adhesion molecule (VCAM), β$_1$ and other integrins, and CD14; novel, monocyte-specific molecules are still being described, and ligands for these molecules are also less well defined. Examples of homotypic (e.g., CD31) and heterotypic (e.g., lymphocyte function antigen-1 plus intercellular adhesion molecule) interactions have been reported. Subsequent migration within tissues after diapedesis may involve different surface molecules, production of proteolytic enzymes, and chemokines more or less selective for macrophages. The role of macrophage chemotactic protein-1 and its receptor can be studied in knock-out animals; other G-protein–coupled chemokine receptors are being defined in macrophages and related cells and in relation to novel monokines (Table 3-1). Migration arrest and localization of macrophages may depend on cell- or matrix-bound chemokines.

The properties of recruited, elicited, and activated macrophages compared with those of resident macrophages depend on the particular microenvironment and immune activation pathway. *In vivo*, the response of macrophages to foreign bodies or infectious microbes such as mycobacteria illustrates the heterogeneity of macrophages observable in granulomas. These discrete collections of recruited macrophages vary in their turnover and interactions with other myeloid, lymphoid, and connective tissue elements. Lesions can be highly dynamic, with recruitment and proliferation balanced by apoptosis, necrosis, and emigration. Macrophages in granulomas often fuse to form polykaryons and may display the distinctive morphology of epithelioid cells, with less evident phagocytic organelles, and the features of secretory cells.

Although recently recruited macrophages can initially be readily identified, the cells adapt to their local environment and acquire properties of previously resident macrophages. For example, in the CNS, the microglia undergo changes resembling those of less differentiated, more recently recruited macrophages as they undergo reactivation by local inflammatory stimuli. It becomes difficult to distinguish between recruited and resident cells by morphology and marker analysis. This is especially true in other tissues, where local differentiation of macrophages can be less marked than in the nervous system. Although further migration of DCs and recirculation of lymphocytes are well-described, the emigratory capacity of macrophages is more limited to draining lymph nodes or into body cavities.

PROPERTIES OF MACROPHAGES

Much has been learned in the past two decades about the molecules that underlie macrophage cellular functions, mainly by studies with isolated primary cells and with cell lines. The nature and diversity of these molecules are summarized to highlight principles, and their roles in specialized functions of macrophages are addressed, with particular reference to inflammation.

Plasma Membrane Receptors and Phagocytosis

Table 3-1 lists selected receptors that mediate the recognition of phagocytic targets, including pathogens, by opsonic and nonopsonic mechanisms. Macrophages express collectin receptors able to interact with C1q and mannose-binding protein (MBP) and receptors for surfactant proteins such as SP-D. Other receptors include the well-known Fc and complement receptors (CR), especially CR3; lectins, such as the mannose receptor (MR); and another pattern-recognition receptor, the type-A scavenger receptor (SR-A).

The zipper mechanism of phagocytosis was postulated on the basis of early studies with FcR and CR. Various receptors can mediate cellular cytotoxicity and contribute to immunoregulation and phagocytosis. The MR, a glycoprotein with multiple C-type lectin domains, plays a role in immune induction by antigen transport, mediated through its cysteine-rich domain. As a lectin, it shares some properties with MBP, a soluble, hepatocyte-derived, acute-phase reactant, which also interacts with the complement cascade. The SR-A interacts with a range of polyanionic ligands (e.g., acetylated low-density lipo-protein, LPS, lipoteichoic acid), mediating their endocytosis and degradation; it contributes to phagocytosis of apoptotic thymocytes, although the ligands are undefined. *In vivo*, it protects the host against LPS-induced, CD14-mediated septic shock, as shown in experiments with SR-A knock-out mice. Other scavenger receptors such as MARCO (macrophage

TABLE 3-1. *Selected macrophage plasma membrane receptors and ligands*

Receptor	Ligands	Functions	Comments
FcR (several)	IgG, IgE	Opsonic phagocytosis ADCC Release inflammatory mediators	Ig superfamily FcR can downregulate hypersensitivity
CR3	iC3B, ICAM-1, promiscuous	Opsonic phagocytosis Nonopsonic phagocytosis Migration (?), adhesion Macrophage activation	β_2-integrin may not signal secretion of mediators; promotes neutrophil apoptosis; essential for granuloma formation
Macrophage mannose receptor (MR)	Lectin: mannosyl glycoconjugates, cysteine-rich domains, ligands in secondary lymphoid organs	Endocytosis, phagocytosis and secretion; antigen capture and transport	Multiple C-type carbohydrate recognition domains; downregulated by IFN-γ; upregulated by IL-4, IL-13.
C1qR	C1q, collectins (mannose binding protein, surfactant protein-D)	Opsonic (?)	Ligands lectins with collagenous sequences
Scavenger receptor (SR-A)	Selected polyanions, LPS, lipoteichoic acid	Endocytosis, phagocytosis, adhesion	Collagenous trimeric molecules (2 isoforms), resembling, but distinct from MARCO, a more restricted SR-A; protects host against LPS; upregulated by CSF-1
CD36 (SR-B)	Thrombospondin	Adhesion, phagocytosis	Apoptotic cell clearance with VnR
AGE R	Advanced glycosylation products	Endocytosis, cytokine release	Interacts with nonenzymatically glucosylated proteins (e.g., diabetes)
CD14	LPS-binding protein	Transduces LPS signaling (?), TNF-α release	GPI-linked, septic shock, soluble form
VLA 1,2,4,5,6 VnR (CD51)	Matrix/coagulation components, laminin, fibrogen Vitronectin	Adhesion/migration	Several β_1 and possibly β_3 integrins $\alpha_v\beta_e$
CD31	Endothelial cells, platelets	Diapedesis	Homophilic IgSF
CD44	Hyaluronic acid	Adhesion, migration	Hematopoietic variant
L-selectin	Lectin: sialyl-Lewis x antigen	Rolling on inflamed endothelium	Monocytes also express ligand for E- and P-selectins
Sialoadhesin	Lectin: Neu Acα2$\rightarrow$3 Gal β1$\rightarrow$3Gal NAc on sialoproteins and gangliosides	Interactions with hematopoietic cells incl. T lymphocytes and PMN	IgSF expressed by stromal and granuloma macrophages; down-regulated by IFN-γ, IL-4, IL-13.
Chemokine receptors CCR1	MIP-1α, RANTES, MCP-3	Recruitment and migration monocytes	Seven-transmembrane spanners, G-protein–linked
CCR2a/b	MCP-1,2,3,4	Same as above	Same as above
CCR3	Eotaxin, MCP-3,4, RANTES	Same: regulation of haemopoiesis	
CCR5	RANTES, MIP-1α, β	Same as above: and HIV-1 coreceptor	Same as above
CXCR4	SDF-1α	Same as above	Same as above
CX3CR1	Fractalkine	Same: adhesion	Attached to cell surface by stalk
Cytokine receptors M-CSF		Growth, differentiation of macrophages and osteoclasts, endocytosis	IgSF, macrophage-restricted FMS
GM-CSF		Growth, differentiation of macrophages and dendritic cells	Hematopoietin receptor superfamily (low- and high-affinity polypeptides)
IFN-γ		Activation macrophages MHC class II ag ↑, induction iNOS respiratory burst	Regulation by T_H1 cells; two polypeptides
IL-4		Alternate differentiation and activation, fusion	Regulation by T_H2 cells, related to IL-13 receptor, which has similar effects
TNF-α		Granuloma formation, antimicrobial activity, tissue injury	Two polypeptides (P75, P55)
IL-10		Deactivation, antiinflammatory	Regulation by T_H2 cells and stimulated macrophages
α_2-Macroglobulin	Clearance proteinases	Not macrophage specific	
Urokinase		Localization proteolysis, endocytosis	
Transferrin	Transferrin	Endocytosis (Fc^{2+})	
Peptides	Substance P, VIP, bradykinin, C5a, C3a	Modulation of inflammatory functions	Often not well defined on macrophages; several are seven transmembrane molecules

ADCC, antibody-dependent cellular cytotoxicity; IFN, interferon; IL, interleukin; LPS, lipopolysaccharide; CSF, colony-stimulating factor; PMN, polymorphonuclear cells; TNF, tumor necrosis factor; MCP, macrophage chemotatic protein; MIP, macrophage inflammatory protein.

receptor collagenous domain) and CD36 may have related functions.

Growth Factors and Cytokines

Macrophages express restricted (e.g., CSF-1, GM-CSF) and general receptors (e.g., interferon-γ [IFN-γ], TNF-α) for cytokines that regulate their growth, differentiation, recruitment, migration, and activation. Signaling pathways in macrophages have on the whole received less attention than they deserve; although it is likely that cell-specific responses are determined at the level of the plasma membrane receptors and by combinations of DNA-binding transcription factors, rather than by unique signalling pathways. Kinases and phosphatases, lipids, and transcription inhibitors (e.g., IkB) that determine cytoplasmic versus nuclear localization have all been shown to be important in macrophage signaling, as in other cells. The regulation of immune activation is complex.

Adhesion Molecules

In addition to the adhesion molecules implicated in cell recruitment, various molecules mediate other types of regulated cellular interactions. Sialoadhesin, for example, is selectively induced or downregulated on macrophages by cytokines and other factors; it binds sialylated ligands on inflammatory PMNs and other cells. SR-A can also mediate EDTA-resistant adhesion *in vitro* to undefined serum ligands, compared with CR3, which interacts with C3-derived proteins by divalent cation-dependent mechanisms.

Proteinases and Antiproteinases

Neutral proteinases (e.g., urokinase) produced by macrophages themselves or other cells can bind directly to macrophages receptors and therefore limit proteolysis to pericellular sites. Other receptors (e.g., for α_2-macroglobulin) clear a range of proteolytic enzymes by endocytosis and targeting to lysosomes.

Peptides

Bioactive peptides such as substance P, vasoactive intestinal peptide (VIP) and those generated by complement (e.g., C3a, C5a) and kinin cascade activation (e.g., bradykinin) have binding sites on macrophages and may influence their migration and function. Receptors for a range of chemokines are listed in Table 3-1. Macrophages express a wide range of seven-transmembrane–spanning G-protein–linked molecules for chemokine and peptides; F4/80 may mediate analogous functions for unknown extracellular ligands.

Endocytosis and Targeting of Lysosomes

Several receptors contain internalization motifs for targeting to endosomes and lysosomes. CD68 is enriched in late endosomal and phagosomal membranes; complex remodeling of glycoforms is mediated by phagocytic uptake through selective receptors. Exogenous macromolecules are taken up and processed for major histocompatibility complex (MHC) class II–dependent antigen presentation and interact with newly synthesized MHC molecules, possibly in distinct compartments. The fate of infectious microorganisms is partly determined by the uptake receptors and involves complex interactions between the host cell vacuolar system and the intracellular pathogen. Persistence of foreign particulates, including microbial wall derivatives within lysosomes, is a potent stimulus for continued responses by macrophages and perpetuation of inflammation.

Biosynthesis and Secretion

Table 3-2 illustrates the variety of macromolecules and other products that macrophages are able to release in response to stimulation. These include relatively abundant enzymes such as lysozyme, an antimicrobial product, and molecules involved in host defense, inflammation, and repair; cytokines such as TNF-α, IL-1, IL-6, IL-10, and IL-12; neutral proteinases implicated in coagulation, fibrinolysis, and tissue catabolism; arachidonates; and reactive oxygen and nitrogen metabolites.

Specificity and regulation of production vary greatly *in vivo* and can differ from that observed *in vitro*. For example, lysozyme is strikingly downregulated on most resident macrophages *in situ* but can be induced by infectious and phagocytic stimuli; only subpopulations of activated macrophages express mRNA for TNF-α, IL-1, and IL-6. Reverse transcriptase PCR and *in situ* hybridization should be combined with improved immunochemical methods to localize and determine the relevance of present widely used detection methods. The role of selective stimuli, signaling pathways, transcriptional control of gene expression, and posttranslational modifications that determine the production and release of molecules needs much more attention. Examples of selective processing, such as TNF-α by plasma membrane metalloproteinases, offer potential targets for novel inhibitors.

Several products act synergistically on particular targets, such as small blood vessels, to regulate angiogenesis; others, such as TNF-α, act on a range of target cells and induce pleiotropic responses. A group of products can be produced coordinately, such as the different proteinases, urokinase, collagenase, and elastase; others are independently regulated, such as α_1-antitrypsin, or are

TABLE 3-2. *Selected macrophage-derived secretory products*

Product	Functions	Comments
Enzymes		
Lysozyme	Antimicrobial	Constitutive *in vitro*, inducible *in vivo*; myelomonocytic and Paneth cells
Urokinase	Plasminogen activation and fibrinolysis, neutral proteinase activation	Inducible by macrophage activation and phagocytosis, cytokines
Collagenase	Connective tissue catabolism	Inducible
Elastase		
Angiotensin-converting enzyme	Pressor	Steroid inducible
Acid hydrolases (many)	Lysosomal digestion	Mainly intracellular
Cytokines		
IL-1(β) ⎤	Multiple local and systemic host defense functions (e.g., endothelium, leukocytes, connective tissue)	Endogenous pyrogen, tissue injury, weight loss, superinducible
TNF-α ⎦		
IFN-α/β	Antiviral, immune modulation	
IL-6	Acute phase response	
IL-10	Inhibitor proinflammatory cytokines and APC functions	Also product of T_H2 cells
IL-12, IL-18	Stimulate IFN-γ production by NK and helper T cells	
FGF	Fibroblast growth	
TGF-β	Inhibitor activation of macrophages and other targets	
GM-CSF	Granulocyte, macrophage, and dendritic cell growth and differentiation	
IL-8	Granulocyte chemoattractant	Chemokine family (also other C-X-C)
MIP-1α/β	Chemoattractant, hematopoietic regulator	Chemokine family
MCP-1	Monocyte recruitment	Chemokine family (also other C-C)
RANTES	Recruitment of monocytes and helper T cells	
MDC	Chemotactic for DC and NK cells	
Complement proteins		
Most components: classic and alternative pathway	Local opsonization and complement activation	Other sources (e.g., liver)
Coagulation factors, including tissue factor	Local initiation and regulation clotting	Other major sources
Adhesion, matrix molecules: fibronectin, thrombospondin, proteoglycan	Localization, migration; modulation of cellular interactions and phagocytosis	Other major sources
Transport proteins: transferrin, B_{12}-binding protein, apolipoprotein E	Transport iron, vitamin, lipid	Other sources
α₂-Macroglobulin	Proteinase inhibitor	
Bioactive lipids		
Cyclooxygenase, lipoxygenase, products of arachidonate	Mediators of inflammation (e.g., effects on leukocytes, small vessels)	Macrophage has high-level arachidonate in membranes, therefore potent source
Platelet-activating factor	Platelet activation	
Reactive oxygen intermediates		
Superoxide anion, hydrogen peroxide, singlet oxygen, hydroxyl radicals	Killing and stasis of microorganisms and cells by activated macrophages	Tissue injury, modulated by radical scavengers
Reactive nitrogen intermediates		
Nitric oxide, nitrites, nitrates	Killing of microbial, parasitic, and cellular targets by IFN-γ–activated macrophages	iNOS inducible, compared with low levels of NOS; constitutive in other tissues. NO not readily detectable in human monocyte or macrophage culture systems
Defensins		
Polypeptides	Antibacterial	Produced only by some macrophages and by polymorphonuclear leukocytes and Paneth cells

APC, antigen-presenting cells; CSF, colony-stimulating factor; DC, dendritic cells; FGF, fibroblast growth factor; GM, granulocyte-macrophage; IFN, interferon; IL, interleukin; MCP, membrane cofactor protein; MIP, macrophage inflammatory protein; NK, natural killer; NOS, nitric oxide synthase; RANTES, chemokine (regulated on activation, normally T-cell expressed and secreted).

temporally distinct, such as IL-12 and IL-10. Studies have emphasized products that can be released into the cellular environment or act close to the cell surface. Less is known about intracellular enzymes, such as Interleukin 1 converting enzyme (ICE)–related proteases and caspases involved in apoptosis of macrophages and proteases involved in MHC class I–linked antigen processing.

PHENOTYPIC HETEROGENEITY OF MACROPHAGES AND IMMUNE REGULATION

Properties of Resident, Elicited, and *In Vivo* Activated Peritoneal Macrophages

The peritoneal cavity of the mouse yields macrophages with strikingly different characteristics when resident cells (i.e., no stimulus) are compared with elicited macrophages (i.e., thioglycolate broth or biogel polyacrylamide beads) and immune-activated macrophages (e.g., after bacille Calmette-Guérin [BCG] infection) (Fig. 3-3). Thioglycolate broth ("Brewer's complete") provides a vigorous immunologically nonspecific stimulus for recruitment of PMNs (peak, 18 hours) and monocytes (peak, 3 to 5 days); the recruited macrophages exceed the resident, reactivated cells and express a higher proliferative response to growth factors. Dying (apoptotic?) PMN are phagocytosed by macrophages, which also become loaded with poorly degradable constituents of the broth (agar?), which accumulate in lysosomes. Recruited and reactivated resident macrophages are stimulated to emigrate rapidly to draining lymph nodes.

Thioglycolate broth therefore provides a combination of inflammatory recruitment and local phagocytic stimulation; the concept of a two-stage activation mechanism was in part derived from early studies of plasminogen activator production by thioglycolate compared with LPS-elicited macrophages, with or without an additional

phagocytic stimulus *in vitro*. Subsequently, my colleagues and I used a different stimulus to elicit peritoneal macrophages; biogel polyacrylamide beads are too large to ingest and, depending on size, evoke good yields of myelomonocytic cells that lack the inclusions previously described. These macrophages adhere well, although more transiently than thioglycolate-produced macrophages, and they provide good models for further stimulation *in vitro* and for confocal microscopic study of cellular responses, particularly endocytosis and phagocytosis.

The biogel-elicited peritoneal macrophages have been useful for demonstrating altered expression of macrosialin glycoforms after an inflammatory stimulus and after phagocytosis of zymosan by specific receptors. BCG infection, with or without specific intraperitoneal antigen challenge, yields immunologically activated peritoneal macrophages. These macrophages express higher levels of MHC II antigens, spontaneously release nitric oxide (NO) in culture, and can be triggered to produce H_2O_2 by LPS, unlike elicited or resident cells. Figure 3-3 illustrates some of the properties that differentiate these

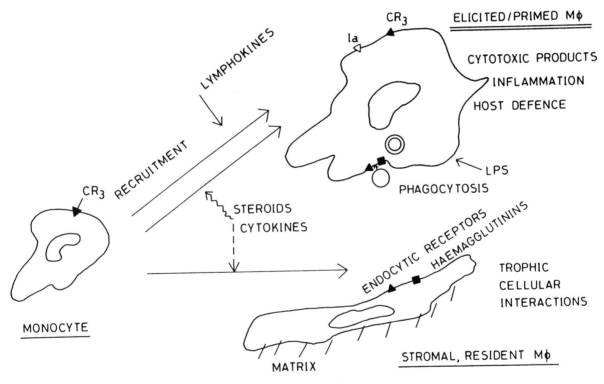

FIG. 3-3. Heterogeneity of resident and newly recruited macrophages. Monocytes give rise to resident macrophages constitutively, in the absence of an inflammatory stimulus. In bone marrow, for example, stromal-type mature macrophages associate with developing blood cells, through cell adhesion molecules (hemagglutinins such as sialoadhesin and the erythroblast receptor, possibly VCAM), mediating poorly characterized trophic interactions. They associate with matrix elements in stroma and are actively endocytic and phagocytic. In response to inflammatory or immune stimuli, monocytes are recruited to tissues in increased numbers, and display common and distinct (elicited or primed) properties, depending on exposure of the latter to lymphokines such as IFN-γ, which induce Ia (MHC II antigens). These cells mediate inflammatory and host defense functions by release of cytotoxic products and phagocytosis. CR3 expression, important in cell recruitment and phagocytosis, is retained on newly recruited monocytes and is often downregulated on stromal-type resident macrophages.

recruited macrophages from resident macrophages in tissue populations. Induction of MHC II and the ability to generate reactive oxygen and nitrogen metabolites can be replicated by treating macrophages (resident or elicited) with IFN-γ *in vitro* before further challenge with LPS. Bone marrow culture–derived macrophages or macrophage-like cell lines can be used for similar studies; however, prior growth and differentiation in CSF-1 or GM-CSF, for example, may alter the cells' responses, and cell lines often lack elements of whichever pathway is under study in addition to manifesting differences attributable to growth.

The effects of cytokines such as IFN-γ, IL-4 or IL-13, and IL-10 on the phenotype of elicited murine peritoneal macrophages have been studied to gain insight into modulation of macrophages activation by these key regulators. It is possible to define a spectrum of effects in which IFN-γ (activation) and IL-10 (deactivation) are at opposite poles, and IL-4 or IL-13 induce a distinctive, alternate pathway of activation (Fig. 3-4 and Table 3-3). One of the reasons for this classification, rather than the more common grouping together of IL-10 and IL-4 as deactivators, is that IL-4 and IL-13, which have many overlapping activities, induce MHC class II antigens and are less potent inhibitors of NO and proinflammatory cytokine production, such as TNF-α, than IL-10. IL-4 and IL-13 enhance macrophage endocytic activity, in parallel with induction of humoral responses.

Properties of Human Blood Monocyte Culture-Derived Macrophages

The monocyte culture system can replicate many of the concepts previously described, but there are interesting differences. Freshly isolated human monocytes (Ficoll-Hypaque and adherence) express high respiratory burst activity on challenge and spread rapidly on artificial substrata. They resemble biogel-elicited peritoneal mouse macrophages in their immaturity and respond to adhesion and cytokine stimuli by further differentiation *in vitro*, acquiring several endocytic receptors such as MR. Human monocytes gradually lose the ability to release

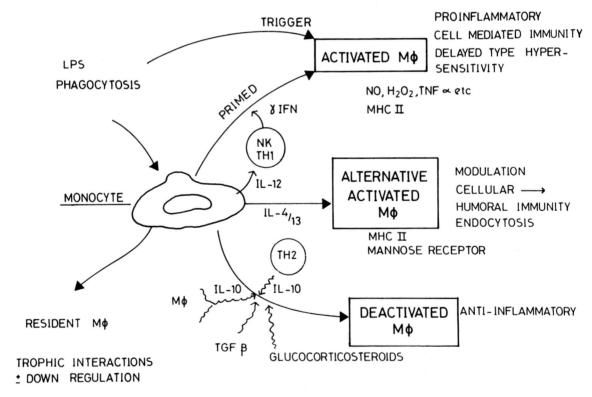

FIG. 3-4. Modulation of macrophage activation. Monocyte-macrophages interact with microbial and other stimuli by releasing cytokines such as IL-12 and IL-10, which regulate their activation phenotype directly or indirectly, through NK and T-helper lymphocyte subsets. The activation spectrum can vary from activation, IFN-γ–dependent priming that underlies proinflammatory effects, cell-mediated immunity, and delayed-type hypersensitivity, to deactivation, mediated by IL-10. IL-4 and IL-13 (T$_H$2-type cytokines) induce an alternative activation phenotype with upregulation of MHCII and mannose receptor, consistent with a switch from cellular to humoral immunity, and enhanced endocytosis.

TABLE 3-3. *Regulation of macrophage phenotypes by T$_H$1- and T$_H$2-type cytokines*

	T$_H$1 type	T$_H$2 types		Significance
	IFN-γ	IL-4/13	IL-10	
MHC II (Ia)	++^{a}	+	—	Immune cell interactions
Respiratory burst	++	(−)	—	⎡Cell-mediated immunity
nitric oxide	++	(−)	—	⎣Tissue injury
TNF-α, IL-1, IL-6	++	(−)	—	Proinflammatory
Mannosyl receptor	—	++	0	Phagocytosis/endocytosis (e.g., antigens)
Growth	—	+	0	Local growth of macrophages in immune lesions
Fusion	0	++	0	Giant cell formation, granulomas (e.g., tuberculosis)
Growth factor secretion	—	++	+	Healing of lesions

IFN, interferon; IL, interleukin; MHC, major histocompatibility complex; TNF, tumor necrosis factor.
^{a}++, strongly upregulated; +, upregulated; —, inhibition; (−), partial inhibition

H$_2$O$_2$, and it has been difficult to demonstrate significant NO production, perhaps an artifact of *in vitro* culture, because activated human tissue macrophages can express inducible nitric oxide synthase (iNOS), as in lung tissue. Monocytes start out with higher levels of MHC II antigen, which can be maintained or upregulated by IFN-γ and IL-4 or IL-13. Another striking feature is their enhanced ability to form polykaryons *in vitro*, in response to IL-4 or IL-13, especially in the presence of human serum. The presence of human serum, which contains factors required for *in vitro* differentiation, unlike fetal bovine serum, introduces an artifactual component, which may mimic *in vivo* changes in plasma constituents resulting from inflammation and coagulation.

The trend in cell culture experimentation is toward increasing use of defined media or the use of minimal amounts of undefined human serum components. In certain respects, freshly isolated monocytes resemble recruited and activated macrophages *in vivo* more than *in vitro* culture-differentiated cells do. Apart from the culture environment (e.g., substratum, serum), macrophages themselves produce IL-10 and transforming growth factors (e.g., transforming growth factor β [TGF-β]), which modulate their responses to other cytokines. The use of combinations of IL-4, GM-CSF, and TNF-α can give rise to dendritic-like cells in culture, unlike use of single cytokines. Other molecules, such as IL-3, KIT, FMS, FLT3, and their cognate ligands, are able to modulate mononuclear cell growth and differentiation *in vitro*. The role of myeloid-specific transcription factors in differential gene expression during monocyte differentiation *in vitro* is poorly understood.

Further Complexity of Cellular Interactions and Activation of Macrophages

The analysis of gene knock-out and mutant animals has confirmed the *in vivo* importance of several of the molecules previously implicated in macrophages activation and inflammatory functions. These include IFN-γ and its receptor in mice and humans, IL-12, IL-10, TNF-α and related molecules, iNOS, phagocyte oxidase (phox) GP91, TGF-β, macrophage elastase, and natural resistance-associated macrophage protein (NRAMP). Cytokines are involved in the macrophage activation pathway through IFN-γ via (IL-12, IL-18), and the regulation of macrophages effector activities by autocrine and paracrine interactions is highly complex. Low-molecular-weight downregulators of macrophages include glucocorticoids and prostaglandins; cytokine downregulators include IL-10, TGF-β, and IFN-α/β. Targeted disruption of genes in macrophages and their subpopulations can further pinpoint their specific contributions to various immune and inflammatory disorders.

RELEVANCE OF MICROANATOMIC HETEROGENEITY OF MACROPHAGES TO INFLAMMATION

While emphasizing the common features of recruited or activated macrophages in local and systemic inflammatory responses, we should also explore the possible relevance of regional anatomic differences in determining the nature of tissue injury, host reactions, and repair. These concepts can be illustrated by a few examples.

Contribution of Local Macrophages to Systemic Responses

Disseminated acute or chronic diseases can induce increased numbers of locally activated and recruited macrophages to modulate key elements of the host systemic response through their secretory products and local interactions. Targets and responses include the hypothalamic-pituitary-adrenal axis, hepatocytes (i.e., acute and sustained metabolic responses), cardiovascular system (i.e., alterations in local blood flow, cardiac output and vascular permeability), enhanced muscle and adipocyte catabolism, and hemopoietic-lymphoid reactions to injury.

Most macrophage products are limited to short-range actions before they are inhibited or destroyed. Circulating cytokines such as IL-6 can reach more distant targets, perhaps even across the blood-brain barrier; within the CNS, there may be local sources from macrophages and other cells of candidate mediators such as IL-1, TNF-α, and lipid metabolites. Resident macrophages are present at key interfaces with blood (i.e., liver and spleen marginal zone), tissue fluids (i.e., choroid plexus with the cerebrospinal fluid); and lymph (i.e., intestine and lymph nodes). They associate intimately with neurons, endocrine-producing cells (e.g., posterior pituitary, adrenal gland), hepatocytes, gut and bronchial epithelium, and developing hemopoietic cells. Interactions of T cells and macrophages can generate migration-inhibition factor, which participates in neuroendocrine regulatory networks. In kidney, resident macrophages form part of the juxtaglomerular complex, are closely apposed to tubular epithelial cells, and may contribute to fluid balance, pressor activity, and the host response to hypoxia. Macrophages adjacent to vessel walls can influence vascular permeability through effects on endothelial cells and their junctions, and modulate capillary growth through local angiogenic regulators. Pericellular proteolysis and generation of bioactive peptides from activation of coagulation, complement, and kinase cascades are regulated by potent antiproteinases, including those derived from macrophages themselves (e.g., α$_1$-antitrypsin, α$_2$-macroglobulin, endopeptidases or exopeptidases such as angiotensin-converting enzyme). Although other sources of plasma proteins such as hepatocytes may predominate systemically, local concentrations of macrophage-derived products can be significant in confined microenvironments.

Central Nervous System

The parenchymal cell of the CNS, the neuropil, exerts a powerful antiinflammatory effect that downregulates the recruitment of PMNs after local injury by excitotoxin or LPS injection. If the stimulus persists, local reactivation of microglia and vascular changes follow, and monocytes can be recruited after a long period. PMNs can be recruited even later and contribute to breakdown in the blood-brain barrier. The nature of the inhibition by the neuropil, which is developmentally regulated, is unknown and apparently not caused by endothelial cell hyporesponsiveness to cytokine stimuli or failure to produce chemokines; direct injection of chemokines known to be active systemically fails to initiate cell recruitment within the CNS.

Monocytes retain their ability to enter the CNS; T lymphocytes only follow once activated. Reversal of antiinflammatory effects can be accompanied by upregulation of MHC expression on microglia. Astrocytes, which can be induced to express molecules similar to those of macrophages or microglia, may complement microglial function. Macrophage-derived products such as NO can exert potent effects on neurons, and macrophage plasma membrane receptors such as SR-A, which are upregulated in brain by local inflammatory stimuli such as LPS, can interact with β-amyloid fibrils in chronic degenerative and inflammatory processes. The macrophages in the meninges and choroid plexus resemble systemic macrophages in their responses to infection.

Liver

Kupffer and sinusoidal endothelial cells rapidly clear pathogens and macromolecules, including mannose-terminated lysosomal hydrolases and SR ligands from the circulation. As resident macrophages, Kupffer cells express only limited antimicrobial resistance; H$_2$O$_2$ production may be downregulated, perhaps because of repeated exposure to gut-derived LPS. Initial host resistance to fast-growing organisms such as *Listeria monocytogenes* depends on rapid recruitment of other myelomonocytic cells, which express microbial and cytocidal activities, and NK cells, which produce IFN-γ. Later resistance depends on the acquired immune response and the activities of newly recruited and activated macrophages. Pathogens such as *Listeria* rapidly invade hepatocytes and macrophages. It is presumed that Kupffer cell-derived cytokines such as IL-6, TNF-α, and other inflammatory mediators act directly on hepatocytes in the acute-phase reaction (i.e., C-reactive protein production) or in more prolonged metabolic responses to infection (i.e., fibrinogen and complement protein production). Macrophage-derived products may be produced by newly recruited monocytes and locally activated Kupffer cells.

Gut

Epithelial and mucus barriers provide a first line of defense; resident macrophages are abundant in the adjacent lamina propria all the way down the small and large intestine. Their properties are poorly defined but include uptake of pathogens and absorbed toxins, including LPS, because they express SR-A. Recruited PMNs and monocytes are important in acute and chronic inflammatory bowel disease; the latter are markedly exacerbated by the lack of IL-10 to downregulate macrophage and T$_H$1-lymphocyte responses. Macrophages (FA-11$^+$) may play a role in antigen uptake through Peyer's patches, subsequent to M-cell transport. Paneth cells are intriguing, specialized epithelial cells found at the base of small intestine crypts, are rich in granules containing lysozyme and defensins, and express TNF-α, although clearly lacking myeloid surface antigens. Macrophages themselves are well placed to interact with blood vessels, lymphatics, and nerves in the lamina propria, and together with Paneth cells, they may influence turnover, regeneration, and secretory functions of gut epithelium.

Lung

Alveolar macrophages are directly and chronically exposed to airborne particulates, pollutants, and antigens. As resident cells, they differ from other macrophages in their rounded morphology and surface phenotype (e.g., low CR3, high SR-A and MR). They express lysozyme constitutively, perhaps the result of repeated phagocytic stimulation. After an airway stimulus, the initial response of intraepithelial DCs is extremely rapid. These cells migrate to draining lymphoid tissues, where they are able to present antigen to naive T lymphocytes. Alveolar macrophages are potent suppressors of T-cell activation, in part through NO production. Recruited monocytes (CR3$^+$) infiltrate the pulmonary interstitium, which also contains distinct resident macrophages, and may enter the alveolar space. Local production of macrophage products can influence smooth muscle and bronchial epithelium in the airway. Resident and recruited macrophages express receptors for surfactant proteins and play a role in their clearance, together with associated lipids, and in the local defense against infections. Granulomatous inflammation is a feature of pulmonary tuberculosis, and antigen challenge through the airway can result in delayed-type hypersensitivity, massive cell death, and local tissue destruction.

Large Arteries

As an example of a modified, chronic inflammatory disease process, atherosclerosis results from the recruitment of monocytes and their local uptake of excess oxidized and modified lipoproteins in the vessel wall. This process is selective for monocytes compared with PMNs, and recruitment of macrophages overshadows that of T lymphocytes. Macrophages differentiate into foam cells, accumulate low-density lipoproteins by various scavenger receptors, and secrete cytokines such as TNF-α and proteinases that influence the composition and fate of the plaque. CSF-1 is important in promoting lesion development by enhancing monocyte recruitment and retention, in part by enhanced expression of SR-A as shown in knock-out models. Local macrophages interact with other cells and extracellular components by poorly characterized, mainly T-cell–independent mechanisms. Their functions include the clearance of apoptotic cells, including macrophages themselves. Apolipoprotein E, produced by local macrophages, also plays an important protective role in murine models of atherosclerosis.

ACKNOWLEDGMENTS

Work in the author's laboratory supported by grants from the Medical Research Council, Arthritis and Rheumatism Research Council, and The Wellcome Trust. I thank Christine Holt for help in preparing the manuscript.

SUGGESTED READING

Books

Gordon S, section ed. The myeloid system, sect 26. In: Herzenberg LA, Weir DM, Herzenberg LA, and Blackwell C, eds. *Weir's handbook of experimental immunology,* 5th ed, vol IV. *The integrated immune system.* London: Blackwell Scientific Publications, 1997;153–175.

Horton MA, ed. *Blood cell biochemistry,* vol 5. *Macrophages and related cells.* New York: Plenum Press, 1993.

Lewis C, McGee JO'D, eds. *The macrophage.* Oxford, UK: IRL Press, 1992.

Phagocytosis. *Trends in cell biology.* 1995;15:85–142.

Van Furth R, ed. *Mononuclear phagocytes. Biology of monocytes and macrophages.* Dordrect, The Netherlands: Kluwer, 1992. (Also see earlier volumes of Leiden Conferences).

Zembala M, Asherson GL, eds. *Human monocytes.* London: Academic Press, 1989.

Selected Reviews

Bach EA, Aguet M, Schreiber RD. The IFNγ receptor: a paradigm for cytokine receptor signalling. *Annu Rev Imunol* 1997;15:563–91.

Bacon KB, Schall TJ. Chemokines as mediators of allergic inflammation. *Int Arch Allergy Immunol* 1996;109:97–109.

Daeron M. Fc receptor biology. *Annu Rev Immunol* 1997;15:203–234.

Gordon S. Overview: the myeloid system. In: Herzenberg LA, Weir DM, Herzenberg LA, and Blackwell C, eds. *Weir's handbook of experimental immunology,* 5th ed, vol IV. *The integrated immune system.* Cambridge, MA: Blackwell Science, 1997;1–9.

Gordon S, Hughes DA. Macrophages and their origins: heterogeneity in relation to tissue microenvironment. In: Lipscomb M, Russell S, eds. *Lung macrophages and dendritic cells.* New York: Marcel Dekker, 1997:3–31.

Gordon S. Mononuclear phagocyte system and tissue homeostasis. In: *Oxford textbook of medicine,* 1995;84–95.

Gordon S, Lawson L, Rabinowitz S, Crocker PR, Morris L, Perry VH. Antigen markers of macrophage differentiation in murine tissues. In: Russell S, Gordon S, eds. *Macrophage biology and activation,* vol 181. Berlin: Springer-Verlag, 1992:1–37.

Greaves DR, Bacon KB, Dairaghi DJ, Schall TJ. In: Thomson A, ed. *Cytokines handbook,* 3rd ed. London: Academic Press, 1997.

Greenberg S, Silverstein SC. Phagocytosis. In: Paul W, ed. *Fundamental immunology,* 3rd ed. New York: Raven Press, 1993:941–964.

MacMicking J, Xie, Q-W, Nathan C. Nitric oxide and macrophage function. *Annu Rev Immunol* 1997;15:323–350.

McKnight AJ, Gordon S. EGF-TM7: a novel subfamily of seven-transmembrane-region leukocyte cell-surface molecules. *Immunol Today* 1996;17:283–287.

McKnight AJ, Gordon S. Membrane molecules as markers of murine macrophage differentiation. *Adv Immunol* 1998;68:271–314.

Medzhitov R, Janeway CA Jr. Innate Immunity: impact on the adaptive immune response. *Curr Opin Immunol* 1997;9:4–9.

Pearson AM. Scavenger receptors in innate immunity. *Curr Opin Immunol* 1996;8:20–28.

Perry VH, Andersson P-B, Gordon S. Macrophages and inflammation in the central nervous system. *Trends Neurosci* 1993;16:268–273.

Pontow SE, Kery V, Stahl PD. Mannose receptor. *Int Rev Cytol* 1992; 137B:221–244.

Premack BA, Schall TJ. Chemokine receptors: gateways to inflammation and infection. *Nat Med* 1996;2:1174–1178.

Ravetch JV. Fc receptors. *Curr Opin Immunol* 1997;9:121–125.

Rollins B. Chemokines. *Blood* 1997;90:909–928.

Trinchieri G. Cytokines acting on or secreted by mononuclear phagocytes during intracellular infection (IL-10, IL-12, IFN-γ). *Curr Opin Immunol* 1997;9:17–23.

Wiktor-Jedrzejczak W, Gordon S. Cytokine regulation of the M system using the colony stimulating factor-1 deficient op/op mouse. *Physiol Rev* 1996;76:927–947.

Selected Papers

Allen LA, Aderem A. Molecular definition of distinct cytoskeletal structures involved in complement- and Fc receptor-mediated phagocytosis in macrophages. *J Exp Med* 1996;184:627–637.

Bell MD, Lopez-Gonzalez R, Lawson LJ, et al. Upregulation of the macrophage scavenger receptor in response to different forms of injury in the CNS. *J Neurocytol* 1994;23:605–613.

Crocker PR, Mucklow S, Bouckson V, et al. Sialoadhesin, a macrophage-specific adhesion molecule for haemopoietic cells with 17 immunoglobulin-like domains. *EMBO J* 1994;13:4490–4503.

Crowley MT, Costello PS, Fitzer-Attas, CJ et al. A critical role for Syk in signal transduction and phagocytosis mediated by Fcγ receptors on macrophages. *J Exp Med* 1997;186:1027–1039.

Dalton DK, Pitts-Meek S, Keshav S, Figari IS, Bardley A, Stewart TA. Multiple defects of immune cell function in mice with disrupted interferon-γ genes. *Science* 1993;259:1739–1742.

de Villiers W, Fraser IP, Hughes DA, Doyle AG, Gordon S. M-CSF selectively enhances macrophage scavenger receptor expression and function. *J Exp Med* 1994;180:705–709.

Fraser IP, Hughes DA, Gordon S. Divalent cation-independent macrophage adhesion inhibited by monoclonal antibody to murine scavenger receptor. *Nature* 1993;364:343–346.

Gruenheid S, Pinner E, Desjardins M, Gros P. Natural resistance to infection with intracellular pathogens: the Nramp1 protein is recruited to the membrane of the phagosome. *J Exp Med* 1997;185:717–730.

Havell EA. Production of tumor necrosis factor during murine listeriosis. *J Immunol* 1987;139:4225–4231.

Haworth R, Platt N, Keshav S, et al. The Macrophage Scavenger Receptor Type A (SR-A) is expressed by activated macrophages and protects the host against lethal endotoxic shock. *J Exp Med* 1997;186:1431–1439.

Haziot A, Ferrero E, Kontgen F, et al. Resistance to endotoxin shock and reduced dissemination of gram-negative bacteria in CD14-deficient mice. *Immunity* 1996;4:407–414.

Holness CL, da Silva RP, Fawcett J, Gordon S, Simmons DL. Macrosialin, a mouse macrophage restricted glycoprotein, is a member of the lamp/lgp family. *J Biol Chem* 1993;268:9661–9666.

Keshav S, Chung L-P, Milon G, Gordon S. Lysozyme is an inducible marker of macrophage activation in murine tissues as demonstrated by in situ hybridization. *J Exp Med* 1991;174:1049–1058.

Kindler V, Sappino A-P, Grau GE, Piguet P-F, Vassalli P. The inducing role of tumor necrosis factor in the development of bactericidal granulomas during BCG infection. *Cell* 1989;56:731–740.

Martinez-Pomares L, Kosco-Vilbois M, Darley E, et al. Fc chimeric protein containing the cysteine-rich domain of the murine mannose receptor binds to macrophages from splenic marginal zone and lymph node subcapsular sinus, and to germinal centres. *J Exp Med* 1996;184: 1927–1937.

Platt N, Suzuki H, Kurihara Y, Kodama T, Gordon S. Role for the Class A macrophage scavenger receptor in the phagocytosis of apoptotic thymocytes. *Proc Natl Acad Sci USA* 1996;93:12456–12460.

Rabinowitz S, Gordon S. Macrosialin, a macrophage-restricted membrane sialoprotein differentially glycosylated in response to inflammatory stimuli. *J Exp Med* 1991;174:827–836.

Ren Y, Silverstein RL, Allen J, Savill J. CD36 gene transfer confers capacity for phagocytosis of cells undergoing apoptosis. *J Exp Med* 1995;181: 1857–1862.

Rosen H, Gordon S. Monoclonal antibody to the murine type 3 complement receptor inhibits adhesion of myelomonocytic cells *in vitro* and inflammatory cell recruitment in vivo. *J Exp Med* 1987;166:1685–1701.

Stein M, Keshav S, Harris N, Gordon S. IL-4 potently enhances murine macrophage mannose receptor activity: a marker of alternative immune macrophage activation. *J Exp Med* 1992;176:287–293.

Inflammation: Basic Principles and Clinical Correlates, 3rd ed., edited by John I. Gallin and Ralph Snyderman. Lippincott Williams & Wilkins, Philadelphia © 1999.

CHAPTER 4

Dendritic Cells

Ralph M. Steinman and Nina Bhardwaj

IMMUNOSTIMULATORY PROPERTIES OF DENDRITIC CELLS

Dendritic cells (DCs) are distinctive antigen-presenting cells (APCs), as illustrated by three main functional features. DCs are potent APCs. The T-cell responses *in vitro* and *in vivo* are strong, and to achieve this, relatively small numbers of DCs and small amounts of antigen or superantigen are required (1–3). DCs induce primary immune T-cell responses to antigens that have not been previously encountered (4–6). The T cells initially exhibit markers of naive lymphocytes and are induced to develop into helper and cytolytic (killer) cells (3,7,8). After activation by DCs, T cells interact efficiently with other APCs. DCs are physiologic or nature's adjuvants, able to prime CD4-positive (9–13) and CD8-positive (14–19) T cells *in vivo*. DCs are distributed *in vivo* in a way that maximizes antigen capture and T-cell encounter.

FEATURES OF MATURE DENDRITIC CELLS

Maturation

The ability of dendritic cells to process antigens and prime naive T cells develops sequentially, a process commonly referred to as *maturation.* DCs that reside in tissues are "immature" in that they do not have potent stimulatory activity for T cells. After isolation from tissues or organs (e.g., skin, spleen), they rapidly undergo maturation in culture. Maturation is typically marked by a coordinate series of changes. These include the upregulation of major histocompatibility complex (MHC) and co-stimulator molecules (20,21). Human DCs acquire restricted sets of cell surface markers such as CD83 (22) and p55 (23). The mature DCs that have been isolated from many different tissues and species display a consistent group of features (Fig. 4-1), which readily discriminate DCs from other leukocytes.

Morphology

As in the case of other myeloid cells, morphology is useful for identifying DCs. DCs extend large sheetlike processes, also called veils or lamellipodia, in several directions from the cell body. The processes continually form and retract in the living state. These nonpolarized movements are unlike that seen in any other leukocyte. When spun onto slides, cells exhibit spiny or dendritic processes (Fig. 4-2) and an irregularly shaped nucleus.

Although these cytologic features are not as diagnostic as the stained granules of eosinophils or basophils, the morphology of DCs has been sufficiently distinctive to allow their identification and purification in many settings. The main tissues that have been used for the study of DCs are human blood; afferent lymph from several species; skin from mice, monkeys, and humans; lymphoid organs from mice, rats, and humans; and airways and lung, especially in the rat. The unusual morphology of DCs has been used to establish methods to generate large numbers of DCs from proliferating and nonproliferating progenitors in mice and humans.

Phenotype

The surface phenotype of DCs, usually assessed by fluorescence-activated cell sorter (FACS) procedures, is distinctive. MHC products, especially MHC class II (e.g., human leukocyte antigen [HLA]-DP, -DQ, -DR), are abundant. Quantitative binding studies indicate more than 10^6 binding sites per cell for monoclonal anti–class II antibodies (24) or for superantigens (3). DCs express many of the known accessory molecules for T cells such as CD40, CD54, CD58, CD80, and CD86 (25–30). These

R. M. Steinman and N. Bhardwaj: Laboratory of Cellular Physiology and Immunology, The Rockefeller University, New York, New York 10021.

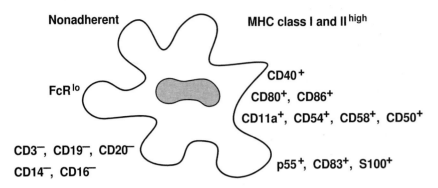

Nonadherent

MHC class I and II high

CD40 +

CD80 +, **CD86** +

FcR lo

CD11a +, **CD54** +, **CD58** +, **CD50** +

CD3 −, **CD19** −, **CD20** −

CD14 −, **CD16** −

p55 +, **CD83** +, **S100** +

FIG. 4-1. Features of mature dendritic cells.

molecules contribute to the efficiency with which DCs bind and co-stimulate T cells (28,31). The interaction is bidirectional in the sense that T-cell binding leads to changes in the DC and the T cell. This is especially true for CD40 on DCs. After interaction with CD40-L on activated T cells, the DCs maintain viability and produce large amounts of IL-12 (27,32,33). Certain key markers for other leukocytes are missing from DCs, such as CD14 for macrophages, CD16 for natural killer cells, and CD19 and CD20 for B cells. Mature DCs also have little or no Fc or C3 receptors, whether this is assessed by binding of monoclonal antibodies (mAbs) or immune complexes

(27,28,30). However, FcεR may be expressed by mature DCs and to a similar extent as by basophils (34).

Cell-specific markers for DCs have been difficult to identify. Lineage-restricted markers are also rare for the other pathways of myeloid differentiation (e.g., macrophages, neutrophils, eosinophils). Nonetheless, a group of three antigens is useful for identifying human DCs. These are two cytoplasmic proteins called S100b (35,36) and p55 (23) and an immunoglobulin superfamily member, CD83 (22), that is expressed on the cell surface. These are not perfectly cell specific; S100b and p55 are abundant in neural tissue, where DCs are rare. How-

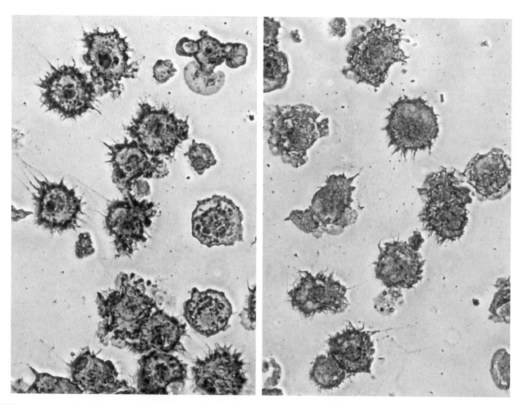

FIG. 4-2. Appearance of dendritic cells in cytospins after immunoperoxidase labeling. **Left:** Major histocompatibility complex class II. **Right:** p55, a presumptive actin-bundling protein.

ever, among leukocytes, mature DCs are the main cells that express S100b, p55, and CD83. The functions of these molecules are not yet known.

FEATURES OF IMMATURE DENDRITIC CELLS

Definitions

The DCs that normally reside in most tissues (e.g., skin, spleen, lymph nodes) are immature in the sense that the cells do not have potent stimulatory activity for T cells. This immaturity is associated with lower or absent levels of several surface molecules. Surface MHC class II molecules can be 10 times lower on immature than on mature DCs, and there may be little or no CD40, CD54, or CD86. The latter three accessory molecules are the ones that typically are expressed at much higher levels on mature DCs relative to other leukocytes.

The prototype immature DC is the epidermal Langerhans cell (24,26,37–39). Although weak at T-cell stimulation, immature DCs seem precommitted to become DCs and cannot be diverted to become macrophages, even if exposed to macrophage colony-stimulating factor (M-CSF) (29,38).

Maturation of DCs occurs rapidly in cultures of bulk leukocytes from skin, lung, blood, and spleen (24,40,41). Cytokines from other cells presumably contribute to this maturation, as becomes evident if the immature DCs are purified before culture. Purified molecules like granulocyte-macrophage colony-stimulating factor (GM-CSF) sometimes suffice for maturation, as in the case of mouse Langerhans cells (38,39), but a monocyte conditioned medium often is more efficient (41). This conditioned medium is obtained by plating T-depleted mononuclear cells on plates that are coated with human immunoglobulin. The medium is rich in cytokines and chemokines, including interleukin-1 (IL-1), IL-6, interferon (IFN), tumor necrosis factor (TNF), RANTES (i.e., regulated on activation, normally T-cell expressed and secreted), macrophage inflammatory proteins (MIP-1α) (42).

To illustrate, mature DCs are not readily identified in fresh human blood. If blood mononuclear cells are cultured for 2 days, it is possible to isolate a small fraction (0.5% of total cells) of mature dendritic cells (41,43). If immature DCs are purified from fresh blood as MHC class II–positive cells that lack lineage specific markers, the cells mature into typical DCs after culture in monocyte-conditioned medium (41,43).

Stimuli for Maturation

The driving forces for DC development have been studied in a number of systems. TNF-α (44) and CD40-L (27) are important stimuli. DCs have very high levels of all members of the NF-κB/REL family of transcriptional control proteins (45). NF-κB factors drive the expression of many genes that are involved in inflammation and immunity, and NF-κB is activated by signalling through the TNF receptor family.

Another pathway that can be activated by the TNF-receptor family is the release of ceramide from sphingomyelin. Ceramide can mediate many of the typical changes that occur during DC maturation, including a decrease in endocytosis and upregulation of T-cell stimulatory function (46).

Major Histocompatibility Class II–Rich Compartments or MIICS

An important feature of the immature DC is the presence of large amounts of MHC class II gene products within intracellular endocytic vacuoles called MHC II–rich compartments (MIICs) (47–49). Compared with other leukocytes, immature DCs are unusually rich in MIICs. These vacuoles also express lysosome-associated membrane glycoproteins (LAMPs), cathepsins, and the HLA-DM products that are involved in editing the peptides that bind to MHC class II molecules.

It is presumed that MIICs are important sites in which intact antigens are cleaved to peptides that bind to MHC class II products. During maturation, the MIICs seem to discharge high levels of MHC class II–peptide complexes onto the cell surface, giving rise to the mature DC phenotype with abundant surface MHC class II molecules and only few intracellular lysosomes (50). When immature DCs are isolated from bone marrow or skin, the cells are at first loaded with MIICs that colabel for LAMP or H-2DM. Within 6 to 8 hours, the cells have many peripheral vacuoles that label for MHC class II products but lack LAMPs. These MHC class II–rich, nonlysosomal vacuoles are called CIIVs. By 12 hours, most of the MHC class II product is on the cell surface, where the molecules exhibit very slow turnover (50).

The presence of MIICs helps to explain the fact that immature DCs are the stage of DC development that is the most active at capturing proteins for presentation to T cells (51,52). In effect, DCs segregate in time the two major components of successful antigen presentation: the capture of antigens for processing and binding to MHC products to be recognized by T cells and the expression and use of surface adhesion and costimulatory molecules that increase T-cell responses.

GENERATION OF LARGE NUMBERS OF DENDRITIC CELLS FROM PROLIFERATING PROGENITORS

Much of the original work on immature and mature DCs required their separation from other leukocytes, especially macrophages. This separation has been demanding because DCs are a trace cell type. In human blood (e.g., fresh blood or after 2 days of culture), immature DCs are outnumbered by monocytes by 20 to 50 : 1.

Newer methods are available to derive DCs in much larger numbers from progenitors. This is making the study of DCs more feasible and has even led to the development of protocols to use DCs in active immunotherapy for tumor and viral antigens.

The first successes in generating DCs from proliferating progenitors involved the use of mouse blood (53) and marrow (29) and human CD34+ cells in cord blood (44) and marrow (54). On addition of GM-CSF or of GM-CSF plus tumor necrosis factor alpha (TNF-α), distinctive proliferating cell aggregates appeared in the culture. In these cultures, it is important to rinse away aggregates of proliferating granulocytes to observe the growing DCs. The latter aggregates attach to the adherent stroma and become covered with the veil-like projections of DCs. When the aggregates are dislodged into subcultures, mature nonproliferating DCs are released. Cells within the proliferating DC aggregates are immature. The cells have some phagocytic activity, are full of intracellular MIICs, and have lower levels of surface MHC class II products and CD86 (26,55).

More than one pathway of DC development is likely to be taking place in suspension cultures of human CD34+ cells (56). One involves the rapid formation of CD14−, CD1a+ cells that have several markers found in epidermal Langerhans cells. These markers include Birbeck granules (i.e., tennis-racquet–shaped granules that acquire endocytic tracers), the lymphocyte-activated gene-1 (LAG-1) antigen that is associated with Birbeck granules (57), and the E-cadherin molecule that may help position Langerhans cells in contact with keratinocytes (58). During the development of Langerhans cells from CD34+ progenitors, there is little or no expression of nonspecific esterase, and endocytic activity is expressed only for a limited period (56,59). The CD34+ progenitors for Langerhans cells (LCs) also express the cutaneous lymphocyte antigen (CLA) (60) and very likely give rise to homogeneous DC-type colonies in standard colony culture systems (61).

A second pathway develops from CD34+, CLA− progenitors and proceeds through a CD14+, CD1a− intermediate. The progeny are more like DCs in other compartments such as the dermis. The cells express CD13, CD33, and CD36 but lack LAG-1 and E-cadherin. Cells in this CD14 pathway express nonspecific esterase and pino-cytic activity for prolonged periods until the mature CD14−, nonspecific esterase-negative DC is produced. Within this pathway are bipotential progenitors that can become macrophages or DCs, depending on the applied cytokines, M-CSF and GM-CSF, respectively (56,62). A novel function with respect to B cells has been identified for the DCs derived from this pathway. They have the capacity to bind immune complexes and induce resting B cells to synthesize immunoglobulin M in the presence of CD40-L (59,63). These cells possibly correspond to the DCs described in germinal centers (64).

More recently, a third pathway of DC development has been proposed by Shortman and colleagues. This pathway gives rise to "lymphoid DCs," so called because they are thought to develop from progenitors that also give rise to T cells, B cells, and natural killer cells but not myeloid cells. The pathway uses IL-3 rather than GM-CSF (65), and the DCs express low levels of phagocyte markers such as CD11b and CD33.

GENERATION OF LARGE NUMBERS OF DENDRITIC CELLS FROM NONPROLIFERATING PROGENITORS

Monocytes in human blood give rise to firmly adherent and actively phagocytic macrophages on prolonged culture, especially in M-CSF. The macrophages have high levels of CD14 and Fc receptors and low levels of MHC products and accessory molecules.

An alternative differentiation pathway has been identified whereby monocytes give rise to typical mature DCs (Fig. 4-3). It was once thought that monocytes were unipotential. However, studies demonstrate that these cells have the ability to develop into macrophages or DCs. Differentiation into DCs requires a prolonged and complex set of culture conditions. In an initial step, the monocytes are "primed" by culture in GM-CSF and in IL-4 or IL-13 for 6 to 7 days (2,66). The cells begin to express some of the features of DCs, especially low levels of CD14 and CD115, and higher levels of MHC class II products, CD86, and T-cell stimulatory activity. If the cytokines are removed, however, the cells revert back to firmly adherent, less stimulatory cells. If the primed cells are exposed to a monocyte-conditioned medium, full and stable differentia-

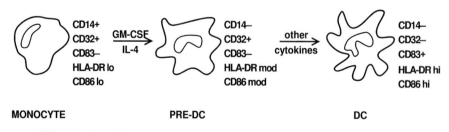

FIG. 4-3. Cytokine-driven differentiation of monocytes into dendritic cells.

tion to DCs takes place (20,21). MHC class II, CD86, and T-cell stimulation rises further, CD14 and CD115 become undetectable, the DC restricted markers CD83 and p55 are expressed, CD1a is lost, and CD25 becomes abundant. The physiologic counterpart for this monocyte pathway is unknown, but one possibility is that this pathway provides DCs in the spleen and afferent lymph, which are known to turn over at substantial rates *in vivo* (67).

Monocyte-derived DCs are the most potent immuno-stimulatory cells that have been described. Reproducibly, very strong stimulation of the mixed leukocyte reaction takes place at DC and T-cell ratios of 1 : 1000 (20,21). The DCs efficiently present viral antigens to autologous CD8+ T cells as well.

Cytokine-activated DCs can be generated entirely in the presence of human products, and their phenotype is stable for days *in vitro*. These features make the cells strong candidates for manipulating the human immune response in what might be called active immunotherapy. If the DCs are charged with clinically relevant antigens, such as those in tumors and in chronic viral infections (e.g., cytomegalovirus [CMV], Epstein-Barr virus [EBV], human immunodeficiency virus type 1 [HIV-1], and human papilloma virus infections), it should be possible to initiate strong T-cell–mediated immunity *in vivo* in the form of helper- and killer-type responses.

THE DENDRITIC CELL SYSTEM

Distribution

DCs are widely distributed *in vivo*. Cells that were initially given different names (Fig. 4-4) are now known to express all the essential features of DCs. The cells include Langerhans cells of the epidermis and other stratified squamous epithelia (e.g., vagina, ectocervix, pharynx, esophagus, anus); veiled cells within afferent lymphatics; interstitial dendritic cells of most organs such as heart, kidney, and dermis but not brain; and interdigitating cells in the T-cell areas of peripheral lymphoid organs like spleen, lymph nodes, and mucosa-associated lymphoid tissue. All these cells can express the cytologic features of DCs: weak Fc receptors, nonadherence to plastic, and very high levels of MHC class II and T-cell stimulatory function. All express restricted antigens such as S100b, CD83, and p55. DCs in different compartments may develop from different progenitors, such as the Langerhans cells from CLA+, CD34+ cells.

Migration

DCs in different compartments can be connected by migration (see Fig. 4-4). Cells from the skin and heart can move into the afferent lymph or blood, respectively, and then migrate to the T-cell areas of the draining peripheral lymphoid organs. DCs that are isolated from lymph, lymphoid tissue, or marrow progenitors, on reinfusion, home to the T-cell areas (53,68–70). During migration, the DCs also mature in phenotype, expressing higher levels of MHC class II molecules and CD86 (71).

There may be more than one origin for DCs in the T-cell areas of lymphoid organs. Langerhans cells may only leave the skin to move to the T-cell area on application of a stimulus such as a contact allergen or transplantation. Many Langerhans cells are seen in lymph nodes in aller-

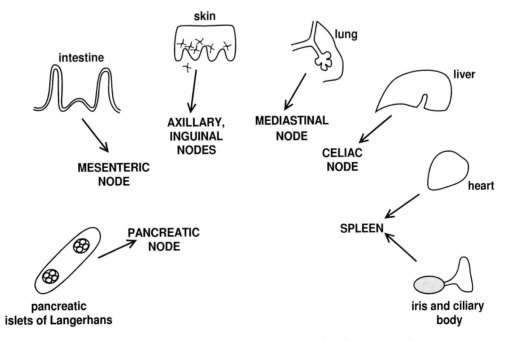

FIG. 4-4. Some members of a dendritic cell system of antigen-presenting cells.

gic lymphadenitis (72). Cells from interstitial spaces such as those in the dermis may continually traffic through the blood and afferent lymph to the T-cell areas, and they stop only if T cells are identified that are specific for presented antigens and superantigens. Shortman proposed a separate pathway for DC development that gave rise to "lymphoid DCs" (73,74). This pathway lacks myeloid markers such as CD11b, CD14, and CD33. Lymphoid DCs can express FAS-L and can regulate CD4$^+$ T-cell responses by FAS-mediated killing (75). Lymphoid DCs in the T-cell areas also express high levels of MHC class II–self peptide complexes (76). Some T-cell area DCs therefore may not originate as antigen-bearing, immunizing cells from the periphery but may instead comprise resident self-antigen–presenting cells for the induction of FAS-mediated tolerance.

Antigen Capture

If antigens are administered into the skin, muscles, or blood and different populations of APCs isolated, the DCs are the major cell type that has captured the antigen in a form that is stimulatory for antigen-specific T cells (1,10,77–81). Foreign and self antigens are efficiently presented by DCs *in vivo*.

This has led to the idea that DCs represent a widely distributed system that is designed to capture antigens and then migrate with the antigen to T-cell areas (82,83). The corresponding T cells then can be selected from the recirculating repertoire of immunocompetent lymphocytes and activated.

SPECIALIZATIONS OF DENDRITIC CELLS

The mechanism underlying the immunogenicity of DCs cannot be ascribed to a single feature. Initially, immunologists believed that IL-1 was all that was required to activate lymphocytes during antigen presentation. However, mature DCs do not produce IL-1, and their function is not blocked by neutralizing anti-IL-1 antibodies (84). Instead there are many specializations related to three broad functions: antigen capture, processing, and presentation; membrane-bound and soluble accessory molecules for T-cell stimulation; and several properties *in vivo* (Fig. 4-5).

Antigen Handling

It has been assumed that antigen-nonspecific cells such as DCs would have to capture antigens solely through bulk mechanisms. DCs, especially immature DCS, use macropinocytosis to incorporate large volumes of extracellular fluid (52). However, several receptors have been identified on DCs that may enhance antigen uptake more specifically. Two examples are multilectin-

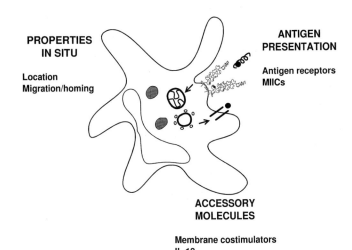

FIG. 4-5. Three groups of specializations of dendritic cells.

type molecules, called the macrophage mannose receptor (MMR) and DEC-205 (52,85). These have 8 and 10 contiguous, C-type lectin domains, and both can mediate adsorptive endocytosis in coated pits (85,86).

For the MMR, it is evident that mannosylated proteins serve as ligands, and for DEC-205, specific antibodies have been used as surrogate ligands, because native ligands have yet to be identified. When these ligands are presented as antigens by DCs to T cells, mannosylated BSA is a much more potent antigen than bovine serum albumin (BSA), and anti-DEC immunoglobulins are much more potent than nonbinding immunoglobulins (52,85). Receptors such as MMR and DEC-205 may provide means for selective targeting of antigens to DCs *in vivo*.

Certain populations of immature DCs can express Fc receptors and use these to efficiently present immune complexes. Fcγ (2) and Fcε (34,87) receptors have been identified on DCs.

Immature DCs contain high numbers of MIICs. These are regarded as compartments that facilitate peptide formation and loading onto newly synthesized MHC class II products. MIICs are multilamellar or multivesicular compartments that contain cathepsins and HLA-DM products. Cathepsins presumably generate peptides from incoming antigens, and HLA-DM facilitates peptide exchange, particularly with the CLIP peptide from the invariant chain.

The intracellular machinery for assembling MHC class I peptide complexes has yet to be studied in detail in DCs. However, DCs are potent APCs for presentation on MHC class I products, including allo-MHC, tumor, and viral peptides. It is worth commenting on the differences wherein CD4$^+$ and CD8$^+$ recall responses can be elicited from human T cells *in vitro*. It is quite straightforward to elicit recall responses in human CD4$^+$ T cells. Individuals exposed to or vaccinated against bacille Calmette-Guérin or tetanus toxoid have peripheral blood mononuclear cells that demonstrate strong CD4+ T-cell proliferation in response to antigen challenge *in vitro*. However, even though most humans are exposed to influenza virus, EBV, CMV and other antigens that are presented on MHC class I products, it is difficult to elicit a strong recall response from CD8+ peripheral blood mononuclear cells. It is often necessary to repetitively stimulate the cells and add exogenous cytokines. One of the obstacles may be the need for the antigen to access MHC class I products on DCs. Access to MHC class II products takes place more readily through endocytosis.

Cytotoxic T lymphocytes generally recognize antigens that are localized in the cytoplasm of the target cell, processed and presented as peptide-MHC class I complexes. This is commonly referred to as the endogenous or classic pathway for class I restricted antigen presentation. When suitably charged with viral peptides, DCs elicit strong CD8+ T-cell responses in purified CD8+ T cells. The responses include extensive proliferation, cytokine production, and the development of killer function (88). In the case of influenza, nonreplicating virus and replicating virus are presented (89). The virus is inactivated by heating at 56°C for 30 minutes or with ultraviolet light. These treatments block viral replication but not the hemagglutinating (binding) and hemolytic (fusogenic) activities of influenza. Therefore, it is likely that virions are delivered to the cytoplasm of the DC, but that extensive new protein synthesis is not required to generate the number of peptides needed for CD8+ T-cell activation. Live replicating and inactivated influenza viruses probably are processed through the endogenous pathway. There is evidence for an exogenous pathway in DCs whereby antigens that are not expected to gain access to the cytoplasm are presented on MHC class I molecules. Influenza-infected macrophages that are undergoing apoptosis can be phagocytosed by uninfected DCs, which subsequently induce virus-specific cytotoxic T lymphocytes (90). This is a potentially important pathway, because DCs may be able to acquire antigens from cells that are dying by apoptosis within tumors, transplants, self tissue, and cells during infection.

Accessory or Costimulatory Molecules and Interleukin-12

DCs express cell adhesion molecules (ICAM-1/CD54, ICAM-3/CD50), lymphocyte function antigens (LFA-1/CD11a, LFA-2/CD2, LFA-3/CD58) and B7 molecules (B7-1/CD80, B7-2/CD86). These molecules mediate T-cell binding and stimulation, and antibodies to their corresponding ligands block DC-mediated responses *in vitro* (28,31). A distinctive feature of DCs is the rapidity and extent to which accessory molecules are expressed when DCs mature in culture (26) and *in vivo* (71,91).

DCs are a major source of IL-12, a cytokine that is critical for the development of type 1 helper T cells (T_H1).

Unlike macrophages, where lipopolysaccharide and organisms constitute triggers for IL-12 production, the main signal for DCs seems to be T cells (92,93). The mechanism involves CD40 on the DC and CD40-L on the T cell (32,33). CD40 is expressed during DC maturation, and CD40-L increases on activation of the T cell. As the immune response proceeds, IL-12 can be made in large amounts and skew the response toward the T_H1 phenotype (92,93).

In Vivo Properties

DCs are found at several body surfaces. In addition to skin and stratified squamous epithelia, DCs are distributed throughout the surfaces of the respiratory (94,95), intestinal (96,97), and even iris-ciliary body (98) epithelia. The cells are best visualized in tangential sections through these epithelia (94,95,97). DCs are also found beneath the surfaces of mucosa-associated lymphoid tissues, such as the adenoid (99), tonsil (100), and Peyer's patch (101). Antigen-transporting M cells are found in the epithelium that overlies these lymphoid organs (102), so that the M cells deliver antigens directly to underlying DCs.

DCs can migrate into the afferent lymph to the lymph node but are not found in efferent lymph. Presumably, DCs that traffic to the T-cell areas are short lived except when a cognate T cell is identified. The T cell could then maintain DC viability in the lymphoid organ through CD40 triggering (27). The stimuli for DC migration into lymph are unknown, but there are several reports that lipopolysaccharide and possibly TNF-α trigger migration of DCs in rodents (103,104).

Factors that target the movement of DCs from tissues to the T-cell areas need to be defined. Two sets of small polypeptides are attracting attention: chemokines and certain polypeptides such as calcitonin gene-related peptide (CGRP) that are usually studied in the context of metabolism. DCs can respond to chemokines and can even produce unique chemokines (105). CGRP and other polypeptides can be found at nerve terminals that abut DCs *in vivo* (106).

DENDRITIC CELLS IN SOME INFLAMMATORY CONDITIONS

Rheumatoid Arthritis and Autoimmunity

DCs are found in relatively high numbers in the synovial exudates of rheumatoid arthritis but not other arthritides (107,108). The function of these cells in the exudate is unclear, but it has been proposed that, within the synovial lining, DCs are critical in presenting autoantigens to T cells (109). Rheumatoid synovial fluids are rich in GM-CSF, IL-4, IL-6, and TNF-α, among other cytokines (110), and these may contribute to DC maturation *in situ*.

DCs have also been detected in significant numbers in the dermis of psoriatic skin (111). Unlike their counterparts in normal skin, epidermal and dermal DCs express high levels of MHC class II and co-stimulator molecules such as CD86 and CD83 *in situ*. These findings suggest that DCs are activated and undergo maturation within the skin. DCs isolated from skin reportedly induce autologous T-cell proliferation and a T_H1 profile of cytokine production (i.e., IL-2 and IFNγ) (112). As for RA, it has been speculated that the DCs stimulate autoreactive T cells through antigen-presentation in rheumatoid arthritis.

DCs may present autoantigens *in situ* and perhaps maintain peripheral tolerance. Kurtz et al. reported that peptides from renal cells are expressed primarily on MHC class I products of marrow-derived APCs in the draining lymph node (113). Inaba et al. directly documented the expression of high levels of MHC class II–self peptide complexes on DCs from the T-cell areas of lymphoid organs (76). DCs in lymphoid organs may be responsible for generating immunity to foreign antigens, but DCs (perhaps different subsets) may also be involved in maintaining peripheral tolerance to autoantigens.

Induction of Allograft Rejection

Because DCs are potent stimulators of the mixed leukocyte reaction, attention initially was given to the elimination of DCs from allografts as a mechanism for avoiding graft rejection. This can be achieved with small endocrine grafts in rodents (114,115), but it is not likely to be successful in larger grafts, which probably would have peptides that, because of genetic polymorphism, are different from the recipient's peptides. These could be presented on host APCs, setting up a condition of chronic delayed-type hypersensitivity. DCs are prevalent in delayed-type hypersensitivity infiltrates (116), and host DCs would probably populate most organ grafts.

Immune Responses in the Lung

The lung, like the gut, is chronically exposed to foreign proteins in the environment. DCs can be isolated from both organs (94,117), but chronic cell-mediated immunity does not occur in either. There is evidence that lung and intestinal macrophages are suppressing the function of DCs (118) and that suppression can be bypassed by the addition of GM-CSF, at least *in vitro* (40).

Nonetheless, several antigens, when administered through the airway, elicit a rapid and substantial immigration of DCs into the epithelium (119). The cells do not emerge into the alveolar spaces but are found in the epithelium, presumably to pick up antigens and move through the lymph to the mediastinal lymph nodes. The acute influx of DCs into the lung can be as rapid or even more rapid than the influx of neutrophils (119).

Contact Allergy

Contact allergens are among the most potent stimuli of cell-mediated immunity. Skin may lack suppressive macrophages, in contrast to lung and gut. On the other hand, the application of contact allergens may induce the migration of DCs into the afferent lymph (120,121) and the maturation of DCs (i.e., an increase in cell size and MHC class II expression) (122). If the contact allergen is a fluorescent compound such as fluorescein isothiocyanate (FITC), DCs with FITC are found in the draining lymph node 8 to 24 hours after application (123,124). It is of interest that chemicals that do not induce contact allergy do not induce DC migration and maturation (125), so the latter events seem critical in inducing allergy.

Leishmaniasis

Leishmania major organisms have been visualized in dermal DCs in the mouse and in the T-cell areas of draining lymph nodes (126). The implication is that DCs can internalize and present *Leishmania* antigens. It is unknown whether DCs have an antimicrobial apparatus to control parasite replication, but the number of organisms per cell is not large.

Human Immunodeficiency Virus Type 1 Infection

Much evidence indicates that HIV-1 infection is a battleground. The virus replicates continually, even during the chronic, clinically asymptomatic phases of the disease. However, the level of plasma viremia can remain constant for long periods, and evidence for robust $CD8^+$ T-cell responses exists. *In vitro*, HIV-1 replicates actively in certain mixtures of DCs and $CD4^+$ T cells (127–129), and DCs can elicit strong responses in HIV-1 specific $CD8^+$ T cells. The DCs may control both sides of the HIV-1 battleground: replication in concert with $CD4^+$ T cells and resistance in concert with $CD8^+$ T cells. Presentation by DCs to $CD8^+$ T cells may not require replicating infectious virus, and it is known that most of the virus that is made during HIV-1 infection is nonreplicating (130).

Critical sites for HIV-1 replication may be at mucosal surfaces. In the adenoid (99) and tonsil (100), infected syncytia derived from DCs have been visualized, especially during the chronic asymptomatic phase of infection.

REFERENCES

1. Crowley M, Inaba K, Steinman RM. Dendritic cells are the principal cells in mouse spleen bearing immunogenic fragments of foreign proteins. *J Exp Med* 1990;172:383–386.
2. Sallusto F, Lanzavecchia A. Efficient presentation of soluble antigen by cultured human dendritic cells is maintained by granulocyte/macrophage colony-stimulating factor plus interleukin 4 and downregulated by tumor necrosis factor α. *J Exp Med* 1994;179:1109–1118.

3. Bhardwaj N, Young JW, Nisanian AJ, Baggers J, Steinman RM. Small amounts of superantigen, when presented on dendritic cells, are sufficient to initiate T cell responses. *J Exp Med* 1993;178:633–642.

4. Steinman RM, Witmer MD. Lymphoid dendritic cells are potent stimulators of the primary mixed leukocyte reaction in mice. *Proc Natl Acad Sci USA* 1978;75:5132–5136.

5. Inaba K, Steinman RM. Protein-specific helper T lymphocyte formation initiated by dendritic cells. *Science* 1985;229:475–479.

6. Inaba K, Steinman RM. Resting and sensitized T lymphocytes exhibit distinct stimulatory [antigen-presenting cell] requirements for growth and lymphokine release. *J Exp Med* 1984;160:1717–1735.

7. Seder RA, Paul WE, Davis MM, Fazekas de St Groth B. The presence of interleukin 4 during in vitro priming determines the lymphokine-producing potential of CD4+ T cells from T cell receptor transgenic mice. *J Exp Med* 1992;176:1091–1098.

8. Croft M, Duncan DD, Swain SL. Response of naive antigen-specific CD4+ T cells in vitro: characteristics and antigen-presenting cell requirements. *J Exp Med* 1992;176:1431–1437.

9. Inaba K, Metlay JP, Crowley MT, Steinman RM. Dendritic cells pulsed with protein antigens in vitro can prime antigen-specific, MHC-restricted T cells in situ. *J Exp Med* 1990;172:631–640.

10. Liu LM, MacPherson GG. Antigen acquisition by dendritic cells: intestinal dendritic cells acquire antigen administered orally and can prime naive T cells in vivo. *J Exp Med* 1993;177:1299–1307.

11. Sornasse T, Flamand V, DeBecker G, et al. Antigen-pulsed dendritic cells can efficiently induce an antibody response in vivo. *J Exp Med* 1992;175:15–21.

12. Havenith CEG, Breedijk AJ, Betjes MGH, Calame W, Beelen RHJ, Hoefsmit ECM. T cell priming in situ by intratracheally instilled antigen-pulsed dendritic cells. *Am J Respir Cell Mol Biol* 1993;8:319–324.

13. Flamand V, Sornasse T, Thielemans K, et al. Murine dendritic cells pulsed in vitro with tumor antigen induce tumor resistance in vivo. *Eur J Immunol* 1994;24:605–610.

14. Porgador A, Gilboa E. Bone marrow-generated dendritic cells pulsed with a class I–restricted peptide are potent inducers of cytotoxic T lymphocytes. *J Exp Med* 1995;182:255–260.

15. Zitvogel L, Mayordomo JI, Tjandrawan T, et al. Therapy of murine tumors with tumor peptide pulsed dendritic cells: dependence on T-cells, B7 costimulation, and Th1-associated cytokines. *J Exp Med* 1996;183:87–97.

16. Celluzzi CM, Mayordomo JI, Storkus WJ, Lotze MT, Falo Jr. LD. Peptide-pulsed dendritic cells induce antigen-specific, CTL-mediated protective tumor immunity. *J Exp Med* 1996;183:283–287.

17. Paglia P, Chiodoni C, Rodolfo M, Colombo MP. Murine dendritic cells loaded *in vitro* with soluble protein prime CTL against tumor antigen *in vivo*. *J Exp Med* 1996;183:317–322.

18. Mayordomo JI, Zorina T, Storkus WJ, et al. Bone marrow-derived dendritic cells pulsed with synthetic tumour peptides elicit protective and therapeutic antitumour immunity. *Nat Med* 1995;1:1297–1302.

19. Boczkowski D, Nair SK, Snyder D, Gilboa E. Dendritic cells pulsed with RNA are potent antigen-presenting cells in vitro and in vivo. *J Exp Med* 1996;184:465–472.

20. Bender A, Sapp M, Schuler G, Steinman RM, Bhardwaj N. Improved methods for the generation of dendritic cells from nonproliferating progenitors in human blood. *J Immunol Methods* 1996;196:121–135.

21. Romani N, Reider D, Heuer M, et al. Generation of mature dendritic cells from human blood: An improved method with special regard to clinical applicability. *J Immunol Methods* 1996;196:137–151.

22. Zhou L-J, Tedder TF. Human blood dendritic cells selectively express CD83, a member of the immunoglobulin superfamily. *J Immunol* 1995;154:3821–3835.

23. Mosialos G, Birkenbach M, Ayehunie S, et al. Circulating human dendritic cells differentially express high levels of a 55-kd actin-bundling protein. *Am J Pathol* 1996;148:593–600.

24. Schuler G, Steinman RM. Murine epidermal Langerhans cells mature into potent immunostimulatory dendritic cells in vitro. *J Exp Med* 1985;161:526–546.

25. Larsen CP, Ritchie SC, Pearson TC, Linsley PS, Lowry RP. Functional expression of the costimulatory molecule, B7/BB1, on murine dendritic cell populations. *J Exp Med* 1992;176:1215–1220.

26. Inaba K, Witmer-Pack M, Inaba M, et al. The tissue distribution of the B7-2 costimulator in mice: abundant expression on dendritic cells in situ and during maturation in vitro. *J Exp Med* 1994;180:1849–1860.

27. Caux C, Massacrier C, Vanbervliet B, et al. Activation of human dendritic cells through CD40 cross-linking. *J Exp Med* 1994;180:1263–1272.

28. Caux C, Vanbervliet B, Massacrier C, Azuma M, Okumura K, Lanier LL, Banchereau J. B70/B7-2 is identical to CD86 and is the major functional ligand for CD28 expressed on human dendritic cells. *J Exp Med* 1994;180:1841–1847.

29. Inaba K, Inaba M, Romani N, et al. Generation of large numbers of dendritic cells from mouse bone marrow cultures supplemented with granulocyte/macrophage colony-stimulating factor. *J Exp Med* 1992;176:1693–1702.

30. Freudenthal PS, Steinman RM. The distinct surface of human blood dendritic cells, as observed after an improved isolation method. *Proc Natl Acad Sci USA* 1990;87:7698–7702.

31. Young JW, Koulova L, Soergel SA, Clark EA, Steinman RM, Dupont B. The B7/BB1 antigen provides one of several costimulatory signals for the activation of CD4+ T lymphocytes by human blood dendritic cells in vitro. *J Clin Invest* 1992;90:229–237.

32. Koch F, Stanzl U, Jennewien P, et al. High level IL-12 production by murine dendritic cells: upregulation via MHC class II and CD40 molecules and downregulation by IL-4 and IL-10. *J Exp Med* 1996;184:741–747.

33. Cella M, Scheidegger D, Palmer-Lehmann K, Lane P, Lanzavecchia A, Alber G. Ligation of CD40 on dendritic cells triggers production of high levels of interleukin-12 and enhances T cell stimulatory capacity: T-T help via APC activation. *J Exp Med* 1996;184:747–752.

34. Maurer D, Fiebiger E, Ebner C, et al. Peripheral blood dendritic cells express FcεR1 as a complex composed of FcεR1α- and FcεR1 gamma-chains and can use this receptor for IgE-mediated allergen presentation. *J Immunol* 1996;157:607–616.

35. Takahashi K, Isobe T, Ohtsuki Y, Sonobe H, Takeda I, Akagi T. Immunohistochemical localization and distribution of S-100 proteins in the human lymphoreticular system. *Am J Pathol* 1984;116:497–503.

36. Takahashi K, Yamaguchi H, Ishizeki J, Nakajima T, Nakazata Y. Immunohistochemical and immunoelectron microscopic localization of S-100 protein in the interdigitating reticulum cells of the human lymph node. *Virchows Arch B Cell Pathol* 1981;37:125–135.

37. Inaba K, Schuler G, Witmer MD, Valinsky J, Atassi B, Steinman RM. The immunologic properties of purified Langerhans cells: distinct requirements for the stimulation of unprimed and sensitized T lymphocytes. *J Exp Med* 1986;164:605–613.

38. Witmer-Pack MD, Olivier W, Valinsky J, Schuler G, Steinman RM. Granulocyte/macrophage colony-stimulating factor is essential for the viability and function of cultured murine epidermal Langerhans cells. *J Exp Med* 1987;166:1484–1498.

39. Heufler C, Koch F, Schuler G. Granulocyte/macrophage colony-stimulating factor and interleukin 1 mediate the maturation of murine epidermal Langerhans cells into potent immunostimulatory dendritic cells. *J Exp Med* 1988;167:700–705.

40. Bilyk N, Holt PG. Inhibition of the immunosuppressive activity of resident pulmonary alveolar macrophages by granulocyte/macrophage colony-stimulating factor. *J Exp Med* 1993;177:1773–1777.

41. O'Doherty U, Steinman RM, Peng M, et al. Dendritic cells freshly isolated from human blood express CD4 and mature into typical immunostimulatory dendritic cells after culture in monocyte-conditioned medium. *J Exp Med* 1993;178:1067–1078.

42. Reddy A, Sapp M, Feldman M, Subklewe M, Bhardwaj N. A monocyte conditioned medium is more effective than defined cytokines in mediating the terminal maturation of human dendritic cells. *Blood* 1997;90:3640–3646.

43. O'Doherty U, Peng M, Gezelter S, et al. Human blood contains two subsets of dendritic cells, one immunologically mature, and the other immature. *Immunology* 1994;82:487–493.

44. Caux C, Dezutter-Dambuyant C, Schmitt D, Banchereau J. GM-CSF and TNF-α cooperate in the generation of dendritic Langerhans cells. *Nature* 1992;360:258–261.

45. Granelli-Piperno A, Pope M, Inaba K, Steinman RM. Coexpression of REL and SP1 transcription factors in HIV-1 induced, dendritic cell–T cell syncytia. *Proc Natl Acad Sci USA* 1995;92:10944–10948.

46. Sallusto F, Nicolo C, De Maria R, Corinti S, Testi R. Ceramide inhibits antigen uptake and presentation by dendritic cells. *J Exp Med* 1996;184:2411–2416.

47. Kleijmeer MJ, Oorschot VMJ, Geuze HJ. Human resident Langerhans

cells display a lysosomal compartment enriched in MHC class II. *J Invest Dermatol* 1994;103:516–523.

48. Kleijmeer MJ, Ossevoort MA, Van Veen CJH, et al. MHC class II compartments and the kinetics of antigen presentation in activated mouse spleen dendritic cells. *J Immunol* 1995;154:5715–5724.

49. Nijman HW, Kleijmeer MJ, Ossevoort MA, et al. Antigen capture and MHC class II compartments of freshly isolated and cultured human blood dendritic cells. *J Exp Med* 1995;182:163–174.

50. Pierre P, Turley SJ, Gatti E, et al. Developmental regulation of MHC class II transport in mouse dendritic cells. *Nature* 1997;388:787–792.

51. Romani N, Koide S, Crowley M, et al. Presentation of exogenous protein antigens by dendritic cells to T cell clones: intact protein is presented best by immature, epidermal Langerhans cells. *J Exp Med* 1989;169:1169–1178.

52. Sallusto F, Lanzavecchia A. Dendritic cells use macropinocytosis and the mannose receptor to concentrate antigen in the MHC class II compartment: downregulation by cytokines and bacterial products. *J Exp Med* 1995;182:389–400.

53. Inaba K, Steinman RM, Witmer-Pack M, et al. Identification of proliferating dendritic cell precursors in mouse blood. *J Exp Med* 1992; 175:1157–1167.

54. Szabolcs P, Moore MAS, Young JW. Expansion of immunostimulatory dendritic cells among the myeloid progeny of human CD34+ bone marrow precursors cultured with c-*kit* ligand, granulocyte-macrophage colony-stimulating factor, and TNF-α. *J Immunol* 1995;154: 5851–5861.

55. Inaba K, Inaba M, Naito M, Steinman RM. Dendritic cell progenitors phagocytose particulates, including bacillus Calmette-Guérin organisms, and sensitize mice to mycobacterial antigens in vivo. *J Exp Med* 1993;178:479–488.

56. Caux C, Vanbervliet B, Massacrier C, et al. CD34+ hematopoietic progenitors from human cord blood differentiate along two independent dendritic cell pathways in response to GM-CSF + TNF-α. *J Exp Med* 1996;184:695–706.

57. Kashihara M, Ueda M, Horiguchi Y, Furukawa F, Hanaoka M, Imamura S. A monoclonal antibody specifically reactive to human Langerhans cells. *J Invest Dermatol* 1986;87:602–607.

58. Tang A, Amagai M, Granger LG, Stanley JR, Udey MC. Adhesion of epidermal Langerhans cells to keratinocytes mediated by E-cadherin. *Nature* 1993;361:82–85.

59. Caux C, Massacrier C, Vanbervliet B, et al. CD34+ hematopoietic progenitors from human cord blood differentiate along two independent dendritic cell pathways in response to GM-CSF+TNF-α: II. Functional analysis. *JEM* 1996;184:695–706.

60. Strunk D, Egger C, Leitner G, Hanau D, Stingl G. A skin homing molecule defines the Langerhans cells progenitor in human peripheral blood. *J Exp Med* 1997;185:1131–1136.

61. Young JW, Szabolcs P, Moore MAS. Identification of dendritic cell colony-forming units among normal CD34+ bone marrow progenitors that are expanded by c-*kit* ligand and yield pure dendritic cell colonies in the presence of granulocyte/macrophage colony-stimulating factor and tumor necrosis factor α. *J Exp Med* 1995;182:1111–1120.

62. Szabolcs P, Avigan D, Gezelter S, et al. Dendritic cells and macrophages can mature independently from a human bone marrow-derived, post-CFU intermediate. *Blood* 1996;87:4520–4530.

63. Dubois B, Vanbervliet B, Fayette J, et al. Dendritic cells enhance growth and differentiation of CD40-activated B lymphocytes. *J Exp Med* 1997;185:941–951.

64. Grouard G, Durand I, Filgueira L, Banchereau J, Liu Y-J. Dendritic cells capable of stimulating T cells in germinal centres. *Nature* 1996; 384:364–367.

65. Saunders D, Lucas K, Ismaili J, et al. Dendritic cell development in culture from thymic precursor cells in the absence of granulocyte/ macrophage colony-stimulating factor. *J Exp Med* 1996;184:2185–2196.

66. Romani N, Gruner S, Brang D, et al. Proliferating dendritic cell progenitors in human blood. *J Exp Med* 1994;180:83–93.

67. Steinman RM, Lustig DS, Cohn ZA. Identification of a novel cell type in peripheral lymphoid organs of mice. III. Functional properties in vivo. *J Exp Med* 1974;139:1431–1445.

68. Austyn JM, Kupiec-Weglinski JW, Hankins DF, Morris PJ. Migration patterns of dendritic cells in the mouse: homing to T cell-dependent areas of spleen and binding within marginal zone. *J Exp Med* 1988; 167:646–651.

69. Fossum S. Lymph-borne dendritic leucocytes do not recirculate, but enter the lymph node paracortex to become interdigitating cells. *Scand J Immunol* 1989;27:97–105.

70. Kudo S, Matsuno K, Ezaki T, Ogawa M. A novel migration pathway for rat dendritic cells from the blood: hepatic sinusoids-lymph translocation. *J Exp Med* 1997;185:777–784.

71. Larsen CP, Steinman RM, Witmer-Pack M, Hankins DF, Morris PJ, Austyn JM. Migration and maturation of Langerhans cells in skin transplants and explants. *J Exp Med* 1990;172:1483–1493.

72. van den Oord JJ, De Wolf-Peeters C, de Vos R, Desmet VJ. The paracortical area in dermatopathic lymphadenitis and other reactive conditions of the lymph node. *Virchows Arch B Cell Pathol* 1984;45: 289–299.

73. Ardavin C, Wu L, Li C, Shortman K. Thymic dendritic cells and T cells develop simultaneously in the thymus from a common precursor population. *Nature* 1993;362:761–763.

74. Vremec D, Zorbas M, Scollay R, et al. The surface phenotype of dendritic cells purified from mouse thymus and spleen: investigation of the CD8 expression by a subpopulation of dendritic cells. *J Exp Med* 1992;176:47–58.

75. Suss G, Shortman K. A subclass of dendritic cells kills CD4 T cells via Fas/Fas-ligand induced apoptosis. *J Exp Med* 1996;183:1789–1796.

76. Inaba K, Pack M, Inaba M, Sakuta H, Isdell F, Steinman RM. High levels of an MHC II self-peptide complex on dendritic cells from lymph node. *JEM* 1997;186:665–672.

77. Kyewski BA, Fathman CG, Rouse RV. Intrathymic presentation of circulating non-MHC antigens by medullary dendritic cells. An antigen-dependent microenviroment for T cell differentiation. *J Exp Med* 1986;163:231–246.

78. Bujdoso R, Hopkins J, Dutia BM, Young P, McConnell I. Characterization of sheep afferent lymph dendritic cells and their role in antigen carriage. *J Exp Med* 1989;170:1285–1302.

79. Guery J-C, Adorini L. Dendritic cells are the most efficient in presenting endogenous naturally processed self-epitopes to class II–restricted T cells. *J Immunol* 1995;154:536–544.

80. Xia W, Pinto CE, Kradin RL. The antigen-presenting activities of Ia-dendritic cells shift dynamically from lung to lymph node after an airway challenge with soluble antigen. *J Exp Med* 1995;181:1275–1283.

81. Guery J-C, Ria F, Adorini L. Dendritic cells but not B cells present antigenic complexes to class II–restricted T cells after administration of protein in adjuvant. *J Exp Med* 1996;183:751–757.

82. Steinman RM, Nussenzweig MC. Dendritic cells: features and functions. *Immunol Rev* 1980;53:127–147.

83. Steinman RM. The dendritic cell system and its role in immunogenicity. *Annu Rev Immunol* 1991;9:271–296.

84. Bhardwaj N, Lau LL, Friedman SM, Crow MK, Steinman RM. Interleukin 1 production during accessory cell-dependent mitogenesis of T lymphocytes. *J Exp Med* 1989;169:1121–1136.

85. Jiang W, Swiggard WJ, Heufler C, et al. The receptor DEC-205 expressed by dendritic cells and thymic epithelial cells is involved in antigen processing. *Nature* 1995;375:151–155.

86. Stahl P, Schlesinger PH, Sigardson E, Rodman JS, Lee YC. Receptor-mediated pinocytosis of mannose glycoconjugates by macrophages: Characterization and evidence for receptor recycling. *Cell* 1980;19: 207–215.

87. Wang B, Rieger A, Kilgus O, et al. Epidermal Langerhans cells from normal human skin bind monomeric IgE via FcεRI. *J Exp Med* 1992; 175:1353–1365.

88. Bhardwaj N, Bender A, Gonzalez N, Bui LK, Garrett MC, Steinman RM. Influenza virus-infected dendritic cells stimulate strong proliferative and cytolytic responses from human CD8+ T cells. *J Clin Invest* 1994;94:797–807.

89. Bender A, Bui LK, Feldman MAV, Larsson M, Bhardwaj N. Inactivated influenza virus, when presented on dendritic cells, elicits human CD8+ cytolytic T cell responses. *J Exp Med* 1995;182:1663–1671.

90. Albert ML, Sauter B, Bhardwaj N. Dendritic cells acquire antigens from apoptotic cells and induce class I–restricted CTL responses. *Nature* 1998;392:86–89.

91. Larsen CP, Ritchie SC, Hendrix R, et al. Regulation of immunostimulatory function and costimulatory molecule [B7-1 and B7-2] expression on murine dendritic cells. *J Immunol* 1994;152:5208–5219.

92. Macatonia SE, Hosken NA, Litton M, et al. Dendritic cells produce IL-12 and direct the development of Th1 cells from naive CD4+ T cells. *J Immunol* 1995;154:5071–5079.

93. Heufler C, Koch F, Stanzl U, et al. Interleukin-12 is produced by den-

dritic cells and mediates T helper 1 development as well as interferon-gamma production by T helper 1 cells. *Eur J Immunol* 1996;26:659–668.

94. Holt PG, Schon-Hegrad MA, Oliver J. MHC class II antigen-bearing dendritic cells in pulmonary tissues of the rat: regulation of antigen presentation activity by endogenous macrophage populations. *J Exp Med* 1987;167:262–274.

95. Holt PG, Schon-Hegrad MA, Oliver J, Holt BJ, McMenamin PG. A contiguous network of dendritic antigen presenting cells within the respiratory epithelium. *Int Arch Allergy Appl Immunol* 1990;91: 155–159.

96. Mayrhofer G, Pugh CW, Barclay AN. The distribution, ontogeny and origin in the rat of Ia-positive cells with dendritic morphology and of Ia antigen in epithelia, with special reference to the intestine. *Eur J Immunol* 1983;13:112–122.

97. Maric I, Holt PG, Perdue MH, Bienenstock J. Class II MHC antigen [Ia]-bearing dendritic cells in the epithelium of the rat intestine. *J Immunol* 1996;156:1408–1414.

98. McMenamin PG, Holthouse I, Holt PG. Class II major histocompatibility complex (Ia) antigen-bearing dendritic cells within the iris and ciliary body of the rat eye: distribution, phenotype and relation to retinal microglia. *Immunology* 1992;77:385–393.

99. Frankel SS, Wenig BM, Burke AP, et al. Replication of HIV-1 in dendritic cell-derived syncytia at the mucosal surface of the adenoid. *Science* 1996;272:115–117.

100. Frankel SS, Tenner-Racz K, Racz P, et al. Active replication of HIV-1 in the lymphoepithelial regions of the nasopharyngeal and palatine tonsils. *Am J Pathol* 1997;151:89–96.

101. Kelsall BL, Strober W. Distinct populations of dendritic cells are present in the subepithelial dome and T cell regions of the murine Peyer's Patch. *J Exp Med* 1996;183:237–247.

102. Neutra MR, Pringault E, Kraehenbuhl J-P. Antigen sampling across epithelial barriers and induction of mucosal immune responses. *Annu Rev Immunol* 1996;14:275–300.

103. Roake JA, Rao AS, Morris PJ, Larsen CP, Hankins DF, Austyn JM. Dendritic cell loss from non-lymphoid tissues following systemic administration of lipopolysaccharide, tumour necrosis factor, and interleukin-1. *J Exp Med* 1995;181:2237–2248.

104. MacPherson GG, Jenkins CD, Stein MJ, Edwards C. Endotoxin-mediated dendritic cell release from the intestine: characterization of released dendritic cells and TNF dependence. *J Immunol* 1995;154: 1317–1322.

105. Adema GJ, Hartgers F, Verstraten R, et al. DC-CK1, a dendritic cell specific C-C chemokine highly expressed in tonsils preferentially attracts naive T cells. *Nature* 1997;387:713–717.

106. Hosoi J, Murphy GF, Egan CL, et al. Regulation of Langerhans cell function by nerves containing calcitonin gene-related peptide. *Nature* 1993;363:159–162.

107. Zvaifler NJ, Steinman RM, Kaplan G, Lau LL, Rivelis M. Identification of immunostimulatory dendritic cells in the synovial effusions of patients with rheumatoid arthritis. *J Clin Invest* 1985;76:789–800.

108. Thomas R, Davis LS, Lipsky PE. Rheumatoid synovium is enriched in mature antigen-presenting dendritic cells. *J Immunol* 1994;152: 2613–2623.

109. Thomas R, Quinn C. Functional differentiation of dendritic cells in rheumatoid arthritis. *J Immunol* 1996;156:3074–3086.

110. Klareskog L, Ronnelid J, Holm G. Immunopathogenesis and immunotherapy in rheumatoid arthritis: an area in transition. *J Intern Med* 1995;238:191–206.

111. Nestle FO, Zheng X-G, Thompson CB, Turka LA, Nickoloff BJ. Characterization of dermal dendritic cells obtained from normal human skin reveals phenotypic and functionally distinctive subsets. *J Immunol* 1993;151:6535–6545.

112. Nestle FO, Turka LA, Nickoloff BJ. Characterization of dermal dendritic cells in psoriasis: autostimulation of T lymphocytes and induction of Th1 type cytokines. *J Clin Invest* 1994;94:202–209.

113. Kurts C, Heath WR, Carbone FR, Allison J, Miller JFAP, Kosaka H. Constitutive class I–restricted exogenous presentation of self antigens in vivo. *J Exp Med* 1996;184:923–930.

114. Faustman DL, Steinman RM, Gebel HM, Hauptfeld V, Davie JM, Lacy PE. Prevention of rejection of murine islet allografts by pretreatment with anti-dendritic cell antibody. *Proc Natl Acad Sci USA* 1984;81:3864–3868.

115. Iwai H, Kuma S-I, Inaba MM, Good RA, Yamashita T, Kumazawa T, Ikehara S. Acceptance of murine thyroid allografts by pretreatment of anti-Ia antibody or anti-dendritic cell antibody in vitro. *Transplantation* 1989;47:45–49.

116. Kaplan G, Nusrat A, Witmer MD, Nath I, Cohn ZA. Distribution and turnover of Langerhans cells during delayed immune responses in human skin. *J Exp Med* 1987;165:763–776.

117. Pavli P, Hume DA, Van de Pol E, Doe WF. Dendritic cells, the main antigen-presenting cells of the human colonic lamina propria. *Immunology* 1993;78:132–141.

118. Holt PG, Oliver J, Bilyk N, McMenamin C, McMenamin PG, Kraal G, Thepen T. Downregulation of the antigen presenting cell function[s] of pulmonary dendritic cells in vivo by resident alveolar macrophages. *J Exp Med* 1993;177:397–407.

119. McWilliam AS, Nelson D, Thomas JA, Holt PG. Rapid dendritic cell recruitment is a hallmark of the acute inflammatory response at mucosal surfaces. *J Exp Med* 1994;179:1331–1336.

120. Silberberg-Sinakin I, Thorbecke GJ, Baer RL, Rosenthal SA, Berezowsky V. Antigen-bearing Langerhans cells in skin, dermal lymphatics and in lymph nodes. *Cell Immunol* 1976;25:137–151.

121. Lens JW, Drexhage HA, Benson W, Balfour BM. A study of cells present in lymph draining from a contact allergic reaction in pigs sensitized to DNFB. *Immunology* 1983;49:415–422.

122. Enk AH, Angeloni VL, Udey SI. An essential role for Langerhans cell-derived IL-1 beta in the initiation of primary immune responses in skin. *J Immunol* 1993;150:3698–3704.

123. Macatonia SE, Knight SC, Edwards AJ, Griffiths S, Fryer P. Localization of antigen on lymph node dendritic cells after exposure to the contact sensitizer fluorescein isothiocyanate. *J Exp Med* 1987;166: 1654–1667.

124. Kripke ML, Munn CG, Jeevan A, Tang J-M, Bucana C. Evidence that cutaneous antigen-presenting cells migrate to regional lymph nodes during contact sensitization. *J Immunol* 1990;145:2833–2838.

125. Weinlich G, Sepp N, Koch F, Schuler G, Romani N. Evidence that Langerhans cells rapidly disappear from the epidermis in response to contact sensitizers but not to tolerogens/nonsensitizers. *Arch Dermatol Res* 1989;281:556.

126. Moll H, Fuchs H, Blank C, Rollinghoff M. Langerhans cells transport *Leishmania major* from the infected skin to the draining lymph node for presentation to antigen-specific T cells. *Eur J Immunol* 1993;23: 1595–1601.

127. Pope M, Betjes MGH, Romani N, et al. Conjugates of dendritic cells and memory T lymphocytes from skin facilitate productive infection with HIV-1. *Cell* 1994;78:389–398.

128. Pope M, Gezelter S, Gallo N, Hoffman L, Steinman RM. Low levels of HIV-1 in cutaneous dendritic cells initiate a productive infection upon binding to memory CD4+ T cells. *J Exp Med* 1995;182:2045–2056.

129. Cameron P, Pope M, Granelli-Piperno A, Steinman RM. Dendritic cells and the replication of HIV-1. *J Leukoc Biol* 1996;59:158–171.

130. Piatak M, Saag MS, Yang LC, et al. High levels of HIV-1 in plasma during all stages of infection determined by competitive PCR. *Science* 1993;259:1749–1754.

Inflammation: Basic Principles and Clinical Correlates,
3rd ed., edited by John I. Gallin and Ralph Snyderman.
Published by Lippincott Williams & Wilkins, Philadelphia 1999.

CHAPTER 5

Eosinophils

Helene F. Rosenberg

The eosinophilic leukocyte is a cell of the granulocyte lineage with a unique and distinctive morphology. Paul Ehrlich (1854–1915) described eosinophils as cells so richly endowed with granules that their entire protoplasm stained violet (1) and later speculated that the granules were secretory in nature (2). Little else about the eosinophil can be said with such assurance, because research has uncovered many intriguing and unexpected features of this enigmatic cell. Findings have challenged the nearly universally accepted view of eosinophils as providing host defense against helminthic parasites (3–6). Many excellent publications have provided extensive reviews of eosinophil structure, function, and physiology (7–24). The basic, undisputed findings about eosinophils are covered briefly in this chapter. This information serves as an introduction to the more substantial coverage of the novel and controversial issues in this area of inflammation research.

STRUCTURE, FUNCTION AND PHYSIOLOGY: THE BASICS

Life of an Eosinophilic Leukocyte

Eosinophils are derived from pluripotent precursor cells that mature and differentiate in approximately 5 days within the bone marrow, progressing through a continuum of defined morphologic stages under the direction of three eosinophilopoietic cytokines, interleukin-3 (IL-3), granulocyte-macrophage colony-stimulating factor (GM-CSF), and IL-5 (see Chapters 2 and 27). Mature, nondividing eosinophils are released into the circulation, where they persist for 3 to 26 hours before migration into the tissues. At any time, most eosinophils are found in the tissues, primarily within the lung and the gastrointestinal and genitourinary tracts, where they survive for several days.

When eosinophils are activated *in vivo* or by *in vitro* manipulations, they respond with directed migration toward attracting stimuli (i.e., chemotaxis), by releasing the contents of storage granules (i.e., degranulation), and by the production of reactive oxygen metabolites (i.e., oxidative burst). Although capable of phagocytosis, eosinophils are not as efficient at this process as neutrophils; eosinophils generally release the contents of their secretory granules onto targets in the extracellular space. The eosinophil responses to activation are similar to those described more thoroughly for neutrophils and are considered as individual subjects in Chapters 45, 46, 47, 48, and 50; aspects unique to eosinophil physiology and function are considered in subsequent sections.

Eosinophilia results from increased production and release of mature eosinophils from the bone marrow, accompanied by a decreased rate of cell death, or apoptosis, in the periphery. Blood and tissue eosinophilia have been associated with allergic inflammation, with asthma and bronchial hyperreactivity, and with end-organ damage characteristic of chronic parasitic infection and idiopathic syndromes. Although the detrimental sequelae of eosinophilia and eosinophil activation have been extensively characterized, the potential beneficial features of these cells and their degranulation products have yet to be fully realized.

Morphology

Eosinophils are characteristically slightly larger and denser than neutrophils and have bilobed nuclei and large cytoplasmic granules that stain with eosin and other acidic dyes (Fig. 5-1). Several distinct cytoplasmic structures have been identified (25,26). Most prominent are the specific granules (Fig. 5-2), which are the storage

H. F. Rosenberg: Laboratory of Host Defenses, National Institute of Allergy and Infectious Diseases, National Institutes of Health, Bethesda, Maryland 20892.

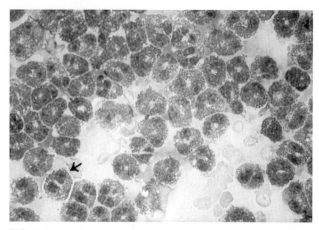

FIG. 5-1. Light microscopic view of human peripheral blood eosinophils prepared with Giemsa stain. The characteristic bilobed nucleus and individually stained granules can be seen in the cell *(arrowhead).* (Courtesy of Joseph B. Domachowske, M.D. Dept. of Pediatrics, SUNY Health Science Center at Syracuse, Syracuse, NY)

sites for the four major secretory effector proteins and various enzymes and cytokines (Table 5-1). Primary granules contain the Charcot-Leyden crystal protein. The lipid bodies, which are non–membrane-bound organelles containing arachidonic acid, cyclooxygenase, and 5-lipoxygenase, may be the principal sites of prostaglandin and leukotriene synthesis in the eosinophil (27). Also described are vesiculotubular structures that contain the cytochrome b_{558} component of the NADPH oxidase, the

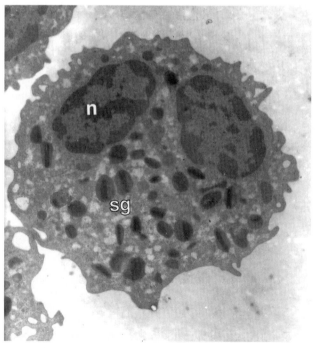

FIG. 5-2. Electron microscopic view of a human peripheral blood eosinophil. The nucleus (n) and specific granules (sg) are identified. (Courtesy of Arne Egesten, M.D., Dept. of Medicine, Lund University, Lund, Sweden)

TABLE 5-1. *Secreted mediators from eosinophilic leukocytes*

Major granule proteins
Eosinophil peroxidase
Major basic protein
Eosinophil cationic protein
Eosinophil-derived neurotoxin
Charcot-Leyden crystal protein
Lipid mediators
Platelet-activating factor
Leukotriene C_4
Prostaglandins
Thromboxane
Cytokines
Interleukin-1α
Interleukin-3
Interleukin-5
Granulocyte-macrophage colony-stimulating factor
Interleukin-6
Interleukin-8
T-cell growth factor α
T-cell growth factor β1
Tumor necrosis factor α
Macrophage inflammatory peptide-1α
Enzymes and Peptides
Arylsulfatase
Histaminase
Acid phosphatase

source of microbicidal superoxide produced on eosinophil activation. A group of smaller granules containing acid phosphatase and arylsulfatase have been described in tissue eosinophils.

Major Granule Proteins

Because the specific granules are the visual hallmark of the eosinophil, it is perhaps not surprising that the cationic granule components have historically received the lion's share of attention (28,29). These proteins are released into the extracellular space on eosinophil activation and degranulation, and they represent the bullets by which these cells exert many of the detrimental (and possibly beneficial) effects. Major basic protein (MBP) is a small, cationic protein found in the core of the specific granule that has been characterized as a broad-spectrum cytotoxin, primarily as a potent antiparasitic agent in *in vitro* cytotoxicity assays (30). Several groups have provided evidence suggesting that MBP contributes directly to airway hyperreactivity and damage to respiratory epithelial cells seen in cases of bronchial asthma (28,30). Other activities attributed to MBP include induction of histamine release from basophils and mast cells and superoxide production from isolated human neutrophils (31). MBP has no characterized enzymatic activity, and its mechanism of action remains unknown, although receptor-mediated neutrophil activation has been suggested (32).

Eosinophil peroxidase (EPO) catalyzes the conversion of hydrogen peroxide to hydrogen halides and has a spectrum of *in vitro* cytotoxicity that is very similar to that of MBP. Klebanoff and Coombs (33) showed that EPO has antiviral activity against clinical isolates of human immunodeficiency virus type 1 (HIV-1).

Eosinophil cationic protein (ECP) is similarly cationic and cytotoxic to parasites and mammalian cells *in vitro*, whereas eosinophil-derived neurotoxin (EDN) is structurally related to ECP but shares few of its cytotoxic properties, except the nonphysiologic neurotoxicity for which is was named (34). EDN and ECP are members of the ribonuclease A superfamily, and both proteins have ribonuclease activity (EDN > ECP), although the cytotoxicity of ECP was shown to operate independently of its ribonuclease activity (35,36). The evolutionary analysis of these proteins demonstrated that the genes encoding EDN and ECP are incorporating nonsilent mutations at rates exceeding those of all other functional coding sequences studied in primates, while retaining the structural and catalytic elements necessary for ribonuclease activity (37). Mosimann et al. reported the x-ray crystallographic structure of EDN (38); our understanding of the relationship between the ribonuclease activity and function of these two granule proteins is just beginning to evolve (39,40).

Charcot-Leyden Crystal Protein

A major constituent of the eosinophil (7% to 10% of the total protein), this primary granule protein was identified by Weller et al. (41) as the eosinophil lysophospholipase, suggesting a role for Charcot-Leyden crystal protein (CLC) in lipid and membrane metabolism. Although there has been some discussion about the precise localization of this protein in the eosinophil, it appears to be associated with the primary granules in resting cells (42) and can be detected at the nuclear and cytoplasmic membranes on eosinophil activation. The x-ray crystallographic structure of CLC has been reported, demonstrating the similarities between CLC and the β-galactoside–binding proteins known as galectins (43). CLC can bind specifically to β-galactoside sugars (43,44), and its genomic structure is similar to those of the galectin genes (45). The existence and identity of a natural ligand for CLC have not yet been reported.

Lipid Mediators and Cytokines

The esterified arachidonic acid stored in the cytoplasmic lipid bodies can serve as precursor molecules for the two major lipid mediators synthesized and released by eosinophils. Synthesis of the lipid mediators by the $5'$-lipoxygenase pathway is regulated by intracellular calcium. The major product of this pathway in the eosinophil is leukotriene C_4 (LTC_4), which mediates bronchoconstriction, vasoconstriction, and smooth muscle contrac-

tion (46). Platelet-activating factor (PAF) is another major secretory product of activated eosinophils, which mediates activation of platelets, neutrophils, eosinophils, and likewise induces bronchoconstriction (47,48). Production of various prostaglandins and thromboxane B_2 by eosinophils has also been reported. These factors are discussed in Chapters 22 and 23. Mature eosinophils also synthesize and secrete proinflammatory and antiinflammatory cytokines, as listed among the secreted mediators in Table 5-1. T_H1- and T_H2-type cytokines have been identified as eosinophil secretion products (49,50), and among those that have been studied, the cytokines produced by eosinophils are stored within the cytoplasmic specific granules. Several examples are discussed here and in Chapters 28 and 29.

Membrane Proteins

As befits a cell with multiple functions, eosinophils express several classes of membrane proteins and receptors (Table 5-2). Eosinophils maintain immunoglobulin Fc receptors for immunoglobulins A, E, and G. Eosinophils mediate several IgE-dependent functions, expressing low-affinity IgE receptors (FcϵRII, or CD23 (51)) and in atopic individuals, high-affinity IgE recep-

TABLE 5-2. *Major eosinophil receptors*

Growth factors and cytokines
Interleukin-3
Granulocyte-macrophage colony-stimulating factor
Interleukin-5
Interleukin-2
Interferon-γ
Tumor necrosis factor α
Chemokines
RANTES
MIP-1α
Interleukin-8
Eotaxin
Macrophage chemotactic protein-2, -3, -4
Adhesion
CD11a/CD18 (LFA-1)
CD11b/CD18 (MAC-1, CR3)
CD11c/CD18 (P150, 95)
Very late antigen-4
L-selectin
Lipid mediators
Platelet-activating factor
Leukotriene B_4
Complement components
C5a
C3b/C4b
C1q
CR1
Immunoglobulin Fc receptors
FcαR (IgA)
Fcγ (IgG)
FcϵRI (IgE)
FcϵRII (IgE)

tors (FcεRI) are also present (52–57). Studies have documented that the high-affinity receptor binds IgE and mediates the release of EPO from activated eosinophils (58). Human eosinophils also express two distinct IgG receptors; the high-affinity FcγRI (CD64) and low affinity FcγRII (CDw32) have been characterized, although CDw32 predominates under physiologic conditions. De Andres et al. (59) demonstrated that murine eosinophils have no IgE receptors and do not bind IgE; the oxidative burst in these cells is mediated by binding of IgG. Further information on these receptors can be found in Chapter 18.

Seven-transmembrane G-protein–coupled chemokine receptors have been identified in eosinophils, including receptors for RANTES ("regulated on activation, normally T-cell expressed and secreted"), macrophage inflammatory proteins 1α (MIP-1α), macrophage chemotactic protein-2 (MCP-2), MCP-3, IL-8, N-formyl-methionyl-leucyl-phenylalanine, and eotaxin; these receptors are promiscuous, responding to one or more chemokines within a given class (60–65) (see Chapter 41). Eosinophils also express receptors for the complement component C5a, lipid mediators PAF and LTB_4, and β_2-adrenergic agonists. The cytokines most closely associated with eosinophil differentiation, IL-3, GM-CSF, and IL-5, have high-affinity heterodimeric receptors on the eosinophil cell surface, which are discussed subsequently and in Chapter 29.

Six β integrins have been identified as eosinophil cell surface antigens, including β_2-integrins CD11a/CD18 (LFA-1), CD11b/CD18 (MAC-1, CR3), CD11c/CD18 (P150,95); the β_1-integrins VLA-4 and VLA-6; and one β_7-integrin (66–72); eosinophils also express L-selectin (see Chapters 38 and 39). Eosinophils express FAS receptor and CD69, both implicated in apoptosis (73–78), and human leukocyte antigen DR (HLA-DR), suggesting a role for eosinophils in antigen presentation (79,80).

Eosinophils and Disease

The diseases associated with peripheral blood or tissue eosinophilia are listed in Table 5-3. Many of these diseases are allergic (e.g., atopic dermatitis, urticaria, bronchospasm) or potentially allergic (e.g., eosinophilia-myalgia syndrome) in nature and feature the detrimental aspects of the eosinophil. The hypereosinophilic syndrome, reviewed by Weller and Bubley (81) and by Bain (82), is a nonmalignant disorder of eosinophil production whose cause is incompletely understood but whose sequelae likewise feature the more unpleasant aspects of eosinophil function. The role of the eosinophil in parasitic infection, once heralded as host defense, is now a subject of great controversy (3–6). Several of these disorders are considered in the following sections and in Chapters 56, 57, 58, and 67.

TABLE 5-3. *Diseases associated with peripheral blood or tissue eosinophilia*

Parasitic diseases
Helminth infections
Visceral larval migrans
Tropical eosinophilia
Dermatologic diseases
Atopic dermatitis
Urticaria
Immunodeficiencies
Hyper-IgE (Job's) syndrome
Wiskott-Aldrich syndrome
Rheumatologic diseases
Hypersensitivity vasculitis
Eosinophilic fasciitis
Myeloproliferative and neoplastic diseases
Idiopathic hypereosinophilic syndrome (IHES)
Kimura disease
Eosinophil leukemia
Hodgkin's disease
Gastrointestinal diseases
Inflammatory bowel disease
Eosinophilic gastroenteritis
Respiratory diseases
Asthma
Allergic rhinitis
Eosinophilic pneumonia
Loeffler's syndrome
Aspergillosis
Viral disease
Human immunodeficiency virus-1
Respiratory syncytial virus
Graft-versus-host disease
Drug or toxin reactions
Cytokine therapies (e.g., interleukin-2, granulocyte-macrophage colony-stimulating factor)
Toxic oil syndrome
Eosinophilia-myalgia syndrome

CURRENT CONCEPTS AND CONTROVERSIES

Interleukin-5, Eosinophils, and the Pathogenesis of Bronchial Hyperreactivity

IL-5, a chemokine derived primarily from type 2 helper T lymphocytes (T_H2), has well-established growth-enhancing and chemoattractant properties, whose effects in humans are relatively specific to the eosinophil lineage (83–86). Elevated concentrations of IL-5 have been detected in sera of individuals with a number of eosinophil-associated diseases, including parasitic infection (4,87), Hodgkin's disease (88), hypereosinophilic syndrome (81), and eosinophilia-myalgia syndrome (89), and IL-5 has been shown to support terminal growth and differentiation of eosinophils in culture (90).

The role of IL-5 in the pathogenesis of bronchial asthma has been a topic of significant interest. Although eosinophils were present in increased numbers in peripheral blood and bronchial washings from asthmatics, their ability to initiate the pathophysiologic responses characteristic of this disorder was somewhat controversial. The role of IL-5 and, by extension, of eosinophils in the pathogenesis of bronchial asthma has been addressed *in vivo* through several different experimental approaches.

The availability of an anti-IL-5 neutralizing monoclonal antibody (87) enabled several groups to evaluate bronchial hyperreactivity in the context of ablated IL-5. Using a model of allergic inflammation in which sensitized animals are challenged with aerosolized ovalbumin, Egan et al. (91), Gulbenkian et al. (92), and Hamelmann et al. (93) demonstrated that the eosinophilic lung inflammation ordinarily observed in this response was directly dependent on the presence of IL-5 in murine and guinea pig models. Mauser et al. (94) extended these studies to primates (cynomolgus monkeys) that had been sensitized to *Ascaris suum* antigens, demonstrating that pulmonary eosinophilia and airway hyperreactivity were eliminated in the absence of IL-5. Iwamoto et al. (95) showed that IL-12 prevents the IL-5-mediated eosinophil recruitment in a sensitized mouse model of pulmonary inflammation.

Approaching this question from another direction, three independent groups have reported the development of four distinct IL-5–producing transgenic mice. The first of these models, developed by Tominaga et al. (96) and Dent et al. (97) employed relatively nonspecific gene promoters. Both groups reported marked eosinophilia in blood and bone marrow and eosinophil infiltration in nearly all somatic tissues. A subsequent report using the first of these two mice described increased bronchial hyperreactivity in the transgenics compared with normal controls (98); a similar study by Lefort et al. (99) yielded contradictory results. Subsequently, Lee et al. (100) developed a transgenic mouse in which production of IL-5 is regulated by elements from the CD3δ gene; this model was designed to create a more physiologic type of IL-5 production limited to T cells. This model was also characterized by peripheral blood eosinophilia, in this case derived from extramedullary hematopoiesis, with eosinophilic infiltrates in virtually all somatic tissues. To address the question of bronchial hyperreactivity, Lee et al. (101) have since developed another transgenic mouse model, with gene expression directed by the promoter of the rat lung Clara cell secretory protein CC10, providing tissue-specific expression of IL-5.

Perhaps most convincing are the studies done with IL-5 deficient (knock-out) mice. Kopf et al. (6) observed that, although these mice did not develop peripheral blood eosinophilia in response to helminth infection, their peripheral blood eosinophil counts at baseline were normal, and the cells were of normal morphology. Foster et al. (102) compared the responses of these mice to sensitization and ovalbumin challenge. Not only was the eosinophilia, hyperreactivity, and lung damage that normally accompanies this procedure abolished in these deficient mice, restoration of deficient IL-5 production (within airway epithelial cells) restored this pathologic response. Although some may quibble with the production of IL-5 in an exogenous, non–T-lymphocyte source, this study provides a dramatic demonstration of the pivotal role of IL-5 in a defined model of reactive airway disease. As a result of these and related studies, IL-5 has been identified as a potential target for antiinflammatory therapy (103,104).

Interleukin-4, Eosinophils, and Antitumor Activity

Over the years, a number of clinical researchers have remarked on the correlation between improved prognosis and the presence of eosinophilic infiltrates in solid tumor tissues (105–107). The possibility that eosinophils might exert their cytotoxicity in a directed fashion emerged from the work of Tepper et al. (108,109) and Golumbek et al. (110) in their studies of the antitumor properties of the chemokine, IL-4. Tepper et al. (108) observed that IL-4 transfected clones of the mammary adenocarcinoma K485 were unable to proliferate in a murine host *in vivo*, with an overwhelming eosinophilic cellular infiltrate observed at the site of the aborted tumor. Studies in immunodeficient strains demonstrated that the IL-4–mediated effect was in fact eosinophil-dependent and did not require T, natural killer, or mast cell participation (109,111). Golumbek et al. (110) likewise demonstrated T-cell–independent rejection of IL-4 secreting experimental tumors and went on to report the development of CD8+ T-cell–dependent systemic immunity that was also effective at tumor rejection.

Although the specific mechanisms by which IL-4 induces eosinophil accumulation have not been clarified, IL-4 has been shown to promote the adherence of eosinophils to endothelial cells (112), potentially through endothelial cell expression of vascular cell adhesion molecule-1 (VCAM-1) (111). Production of the novel eosinophil-specific chemokine, eotaxin, has been identified as a component of the response to IL-4 secreting murine tumors (113). The participation of additional chemokines, perhaps produced locally by endothelial and fibroblast cells in response to IL-4, is a reasonable hypothesis.

Given the specificity and efficiency with which eosinophils mediate the destruction of IL-4 secreting tumors, it is not surprising that studies focused on targeting tumors with IL-4 encoding retroviral expression vectors are already in progress (111).

Eotaxin: A Novel Eosinophil Chemoattractant

Despite the discovery of eotaxin just a few years ago, there has been significant progress in characterizing the biochemical and physiologic properties of this novel chemokine. Initially isolated from bronchiolar fluid from sensitized guinea pigs, eotaxin was identified as an 8- to 9-kd protein with an amino acid sequence most closely related to the CC chemokines, human MCP-1, -2, and -3

(114). Guinea pig, mouse, and human orthologs of eotaxin have been cloned and sequenced (113,115–118). Human eotaxin functions as a strong and specific eosinophil chemoattractant *in vitro* and *in vivo* (114,117), and specific seven-transmembrane receptors expressed by murine (119) and human (115,120,121) eosinophils have been identified. The human eotaxin receptor expressed on eosinophils, CCR3, is shared with the chemokines RANTES and MCP-2, -3, and -4 (122,123). Alkhatib et al. (124) demonstrated that CCR3 can serve as a coreceptor for entry of macrophage-tropic strains of HIV-1, an activity inhibited by eotaxin; CCR3 may behave as a coreceptor in the observed HIV-1 infection of CD4+ eosinophils (125).

Several studies have addressed the physiologic role assumed by eotaxin in human and rodent experimental systems. In their earliest study, Griffiths-Johnson et al. (126) demonstrated that intradermal injection of eotaxin elicited eosinophilic infiltration and that aerosol exposure resulted in eosinophil accumulation in the guinea pig lung. Rothenberg et al. (118) demonstrated constitutive expression of eotaxin mRNA in guinea pig lung, and Lilly et al. (127) reported that eotaxin mRNA expression in cells of human pulmonary epithelial cell lines stimulated with tumor necrosis factor α (TNF-α) and IL-1β, a response that was suppressed by glucocorticoid administration. Human eotaxin has been shown to activate eosinophils, inducing calcium mobilization, production of reactive oxygen species, and upregulation of CD11b through pertussis-sensitive signaling pathways (128–130), and eotaxin mRNA has been detected in lesions characteristic of inflammatory bowel disease (117).

Results obtained with eotaxin-deficient (knock-out) mice were intriguing (131). Although targeted disruption of the murine eotaxin gene did reduce the tissue eosinophilia in response to antigen challenge, perhaps more striking was the observation that eotaxin-null mice had reduced numbers of peripheral blood eosinophils at baseline, even though this was surprisingly not the case with the IL-5 knock-out mouse discussed previously. It is possible that eotaxin plays a more central role in regulating hematopoiesis than previously suspected.

Work has extended the field beyond eosinophils. Yamada et al. (132) reported that eotaxin is also a chemoattractant for human basophils. Forsmann et al. (133) identified yet another CC chemokine, which they have named eotaxin-2 on the basis of its functional (rather than structural) similarity to the preexisting protein. Similar to eotaxin, eotaxin-2 is a chemoattractant for eosinophils and basophils, mediating its effects through the chemokine receptor CCR3.

Cytokines Produced by Eosinophils

Despite their designation as nonsynthetic or end cells, peripheral blood eosinophils synthesize, store, and secrete a vast array of primarily T_H2-cytokines, which are listed in Table 5-2 (49,50,134–139). Several groups have undertaken experiments designed to evaluate the biologic role of eosinophil-derived cytokines. Del Pozo et al. (140) and Weller et al. (79) demonstrated production of IL-1α in murine and human eosinophils, respectively. One of the major activities defined for IL-1 is as a co-stimulator for T_H2 lymphocytes in conjunction with antigen-presenting cells, providing support for eosinophils as active participants in this process. Wong et al. (141) and Todd et al. (142) have demonstrated that eosinophils also express transforming growth factor α (TGF-α), a potential stimulus for collagen synthesis in the rabbit skin wound model. Several groups have detected one or more of the three eosinophilopoietic cytokines—IL-3, IL-5, and GM-CSF—from eosinophils treated with a variety of stimuli (143–146), suggesting the potential for autocrine-induced differentiation and sustained viability.

These findings, among others, suggest functions for eosinophil-derived cytokines. The significance (or redundancy) of this response awaits further analysis in *in vivo* experimental systems.

Hematopoiesis, Signal Transduction, and the Transcription of Eosinophil-Specific Genes

Eosinophils develop from committed precursors in the bone marrow, proceeding through a continuum of morphologically defined stages before their release into the circulation (see Chapter 2). Although the roles of IL-3, GM-CSF, and IL-5 in mediating eosinophil maturation and differentiation have been well documented, the transcriptional events promoted by these cytokines that ultimately create the unique morphology and characteristics of the eosinophil lineage remain elusive.

Signal Transduction through the Interleukin-5 Receptor

Eosinophils express high affinity, heterodimeric receptors for IL-5, composed of a specific α subunit combined with a β subunit shared with IL-3 and GM-CSF. Although binding of IL-5 to its receptor in heterologous systems has been found to initiate a cascade of events including phosphorylation of tyrosine residues of proteins of the RAS and Janus kinase (JAK/STAT) pathway, it is not clear exactly how much of this information reflects the situation within the eosinophil (147–150). In human eosinophils, three specific tyrosine kinases of the JAK/STAT pathway—LYN, SYK, and JAK2 (151–153) have been identified as participants in signal transduction from the IL-5 receptor. Similarly, IL-5 has been shown to induce activation of RAF, RAS, MAPK, and MAPKK in human eosinophils (147,151), similar (but perhaps not identical) to what has been observed in other cell types.

Although progress has been made toward identifying signal transduction events taking place within the eosinophil, none of the elements identified so far are unique to this cell type. However, Caldenhoven et al. (154) reported the molecular cloning of STAT3-β, a naturally occurring isoform of the STAT3 response element, from an eosinophil cDNA library. Like STAT3, STAT3-β was phosphorylated in response to IL-5, and served to inhibit the protranscriptional activity of STAT3. The role of STAT3-β and its potential specificity to the eosinophil lineage, is a promising development.

Model Systems for the Study of Eosinophilopoiesis

Although bone marrow progenitors represent the most physiologic source of eosinophil precursors, the difficulties inherent in obtaining these cells in adequate number and with sufficient purity has spurred researchers in the direction of hematopoietic model systems. Perhaps the most successful of these is the cord blood system, originating with the observation that mononuclear cells isolated from blood from human umbilical cords can differentiate into phenotypically mature eosinophils when stimulated with conditioned medium or cytokines. Dvorak et al. (155) provided an extensive analysis of the growth conditions promoting eosinophil maturation. Butterfield et al. (156) demonstrated that cord blood cells stimulated with murine thymocyte-conditioned medium synthesize the four major granule proteins, and Walsh et al. (157) identified and characterized their functional receptors.

We (158,159) and others (160) have shown that CD34+ progenitor cells isolated from peripheral blood can also be induced to develop along the eosinophil lineage. After several days growth in the presence of IL-3, stem cell factor, IL-5, and GM-CSF, the differentiating cells transcribed mRNA encoding all four major granule proteins and CLC (158). As CD34+ progenitor cells are present in constant numbers and are readily isolated from virtually all normal donors, this system for studying eosinophil development certainly warrants further investigation.

Over the years, several cell lines that mimic one or more aspects of normal eosinophil development have been established. Cells of the clone 15 cell line, developed by Fischkoff et al. (161,162) as a subline from the human promyelocytic cell line, HL-60 (163), can be induced to synthesize eosinophil-specific proteins (162), to respond to specific chemotactic stimuli (164,165), and to express cell surface receptors for IL-5 (166,167). The subline HL-60-3-5-c, developed by Tomonaga et al. (168), has similar properties. An independent cell line, EoL, was established from cells from an individual with eosinophilic leukemia (169). Unlike the HL-60–derived cell lines, reports document that the EoL cells have a limited program of differentiation and respond to multiple stimuli by differentiating only into eosinophilic cells;

these results suggest that cells of the EoL lines represent more committed, more matured eosinophil progenitors. Paul et al. (170,171) described a novel cell line, AML14, and its derivative, AML14.3D10, the latter of which can differentiate into eosinophilic myelocytes in the absence of cytokine stimulation. AML14.3D10 expresses all the major granule proteins and the receptor for IL-5, but when induced with all-trans-retinoic acid, the cells appear to differentiate into cells with markers and receptors characteristic of mature neutrophils. This finding is intriguing in and of itself and may ultimately shed some light on elements of coordinate regulation of eosinophil and neutrophil differentiation (172).

Characterization of Eosinophil Gene Promoters

Traditionally, the isolation of putative lineage-specific transcription factors begins with the characterization of lineage-specific gene promoters. Functional promoters of several eosinophil-specific and near-specific genes have been identified, including those for eosinophil peroxidase (173,174), Charcot-Leyden crystal protein (175), and MBP (176). Each of these promoters includes consensus binding sites for numerous characterized transcription factors, although the functional significance of these sites remains to be elucidated. Further progress has been made on the functional promoter for the IL-5 receptor α chain gene (177), in which a cis-acting enhancer element, EOS-1, has been defined (178). Regulated expression of the genes encoding EDN and ECP depends on an enhancer element (or elements) present within the first and only intron of each gene (179,180); although much of the enhancer activity was mediated by a consensus-binding site for the pleiotropic transcription factor NFAT-1, no supershift was observed with anti-NFAT-1 antisera, suggesting that this activity is mediated by a distinct, perhaps related transcription factor binding at this site (180). Further studies on these gene promoters may provide insight into the unique transcriptional events that may or may not be occurring during eosinophil differentiation; the possibility of posttranscriptional regulation of gene expression should also be considered.

Eosinophil-Specific Recruitment: Very Late Antigen-4 and Vascular Cell Adhesion Molecule-1

How are eosinophils (and not neutrophils) specifically recruited from the bloodstream to sites of allergic inflammation? Although discriminating chemoattractants may provide part of the explanation, several groups have focused on elucidating the specific interactions between eosinophils and endothelial cells. Eosinophils, like neutrophils, adhere to vascular endothelial cells through a multistep process, beginning with selectin-mediated rolling and followed by the activation-dependent association between eosinophil CD11b-CD18 cell surface antigen and intercellular adhesion molecule-1 (ICAM-1) of the endothelial cells (66–72). However, in individuals with leukocyte antigen CD18 deficiency, a disorder characterized by impaired neutrophil adhesion and migration, eosinophils can still be found within inflammatory lesions (181); these results suggest that an alternative mechanism of recruitment is at work.

This mechanism has been characterized and involves the eosinophil surface β_1-integrin very late antigen-4 (VLA-4). VLA-4 has been detected in eosinophils from normal and eosinophilic donors, but it cannot be found on neutrophils (182–186). VLA-4 mediates eosinophil binding to VCAM-1 and to fibronectin (187), and blockade of VLA-4 and CD18 binding resulted in total inhibition of eosinophil adherence to vascular endothelial cells (66). IL-4 increases the expression of VCAM-1 on vascular endothelial cells and promotes VLA-4 plus VCAM-1–mediated eosinophil adherence (186,188), which may in part explain the overwhelmingly eosinophilic nature of the infiltrates observed at the sites of IL-4 secreting experimental tumors (117).

Eosinophils as Antigen-Presenting Cells

The topic of eosinophils as antigen-presenting cells has emerged as an intriguing field of study. Lucey et al. (80) were the first to report that mature peripheral blood eosinophils from normal and eosinophilic donors, which at baseline do not express major histocompatibility complex (MHC) class II proteins, could be induced to synthesize and display the MHC class II molecule, HLA-DR, when cultured with GM-CSF. Other studies followed, including the demonstration that HLA-DR$^+$ eosinophils functioned as antigen-presenting cells, stimulating antigen-specific T-cell proliferation in *in vitro* experimental systems (79,189) and the extension of these observations to murine eosinophils (190). Hansel et al. (191) demonstrated that eosinophils isolated from sputum from asthmatic patients expressed HLA-DR without exogenous cytokine stimulation; Beninati et al. (192) reported similar findings from eosinophils from individuals with chronic eosinophilic pneumonia, as did Sedgewick et al. (193) from airway eosinophils isolated from allergic patients subjected to antigen challenge. Mawhorter et al. (194) demonstrated that peripheral blood eosinophils induced to express HLA-DR in culture with GM-CSF functioned as accessory cells for the presentation of staphylococcal superantigens, although with lesser efficiency than that displayed by macrophages.

Although several groups have documented that cytokine-stimulated HLA-DR$^+$ eosinophils can function as antigen-presenting cells *in vitro*, whether this actually happens *in vivo* remains unclear, particularly in light of the eosinophil's relative inefficiency at phagocytosis, the first step in antigen processing. Does the eosinophil have some as yet undiscovered specific uptake system,

permitting it to process and present a unique subset of peptide antigens? Does the HLA-DR complex have functions aside from those of antigen presentation? Answers to these questions may ultimately clarify some of these issues.

Eosinophils, Apoptosis, and Control of the Inflammatory Response

Apoptosis has been characterized as a form of programmed cell death with distinct morphologic and biochemical changes, including cell shrinkage, formation of pyknotic nuclei accompanied by discrete nicks within chromosomal DNA, and loss of nucleoli. In contrast to necrosis, a process characterized by uncontrolled degradation, apoptosis provides a mechanism by which dying cells can be phagocytosed without dispersing their contents, thereby limiting the local inflammatory response.

Eosinophils, as terminally differentiated cells, rapidly undergo apoptosis in culture in the absence of stimulating cytokines (73–78). When cultured with IL-5, IL-3, or GM-CSF (or some combination), eosinophil apoptosis is inhibited (73), an effect mediated by their specific receptors. The shared β subunit of the IL-5/IL-3/GM-CSF receptor interacts with Lyn and Syk, two tyrosine kinases participating in the transmission of cytokine-stimulated anti-apoptotic signals in eosinophils (195). Apoptotic eosinophils, similar to neutrophils, are ingested by macrophages through a distinct mechanism involving macrophage surface proteins CD36 and $\alpha_v\beta_3$ (196).

In addition to the cytokine-minus default pathway, eosinophil apoptosis can be initiated directly through activation of the cell surface protein known as the FAS receptor (CD95) (197,198). Stimulation with FAS receptor-specific monoclonal antibody accelerates eosinophil death in culture, overcoming the effects of IL-5, IL-3, or GM-CSF (199), and absence of FAS receptors has been suggested as a cause for eosinophilia (197). Similarly, Walsh et al. (200) have demonstrated that monoclonal antibody directed against CD69, a type II membrane antigen expressed on cytokine-stimulated eosinophils, also induced eosinophil apoptosis, overcoming the anti-apoptotic effects of GM-CSF. Other agents identified as inducing eosinophil apoptosis include interferons-α and -γ (201), glucocorticoids (202–204), and TGF-β1 (205); there is one report suggesting that nitric oxide serves to prevent apoptosis in eosinophils cultured in the absence of cytokines (206). The role of the protooncogene *BCL2*, characterized as an anti-apoptotic regulator in neutrophils, is just beginning to be elucidated in the eosinophil (207).

Is eosinophil apoptosis a laboratory finding, or does it have specific significance to inflammatory disease? Several studies provide evidence in support of the latter hypothesis. In a study by Simon et al. (208), tissue from eosinophil-infiltrated nasal polyps was studied, and IL-5 was detected within the infiltrating lymphocytes, mast cells, and eosinophils. Administration of neutralizing anti-IL-5 monoclonal antibody resulted in induction of eosinophil apoptosis *in situ*. In the study by Tsyuki et al. (209), administration of anti-FAS receptor monoclonal antibody resulted in a decrease in the number of eosinophils recovered in bronchoalveolar lavage fluid and resolution of the inflammatory response. In a second study by Simon et al. (210), two individuals with hypereosinophilia—one with idiopathic HES and the other with HIV-1 infection—were identified with peripheral blood T cells that were without functional FAS receptors. These dysfunctional T cells promoted deregulation of eosinophil apoptosis through the unchallenged production of anti-apoptotic cytokines. This observed sequential dysregulation mechanism (75) is also supported by the work of Coyle et al. (211), who observed prolonged T_H2 cytokine production from T cells of IFN-γ receptor–deficient (knock-out) mice associated with a profound inability to resolve eosinophilic inflammation in the lungs.

Eosinophilia-Myalgia Syndrome

In the summer of 1989, eosinophils were in the news. A new clinical syndrome consisting of muscular pain accompanied by peripheral blood eosinophilia was described in three women in New Mexico, all of whom had recently ingested the over-the-counter dietary supplement, L-tryptophan (212–215). The association of this eosinophilia-myalgia syndrome (EMS) with consumption of L-tryptophan was supported by the results of two subsequent case-control studies (213,216), although these studies have been subject to significant criticism (217). Further epidemiologic studies suggested that L-tryptophan manufactured by a single supplier, Showa Denko KK of Japan, was the most likely etiologic agent (218–220). Chromatographic analysis of this product demonstrated that EMS was associated with ingestion of L-tryptophan that contained a contaminant peak E, later identified as 1,1′-ethylidenebis[tryptophan] (EBT) (221).

The Centers for Disease Control diagnostic criteria for EMS include peripheral blood eosinophil count greater than 1,000 cells/mm³, generalized debilitating myalgia, and no evidence of infection or neoplasm that would otherwise explain the clinical findings. Pathologic findings include perivascular infiltrates in the fascia, skeletal muscle, and dermis, consisting of primarily lymphocytes with some eosinophils. Fibroblast growth and collagen deposition have been observed in association with increasing concentrations of TGF-β1 (222). Glucocorticoid therapy has not been found to alter the natural course of the disease, and two long-term follow-up studies yielded completely contradicting results (223,224).

There have been a number of hypotheses concerning the pathophysiologic mechanism of EMS. Several groups have considered the possibility that L-tryptophan and or contaminants induce production of eosinophil chemoattractants by peripheral blood mononuclear cells, and there have been some reports invoking IL-5 (89,225,226). Others have suggested that the activities of these chemicals are directed at the fibroblasts and that the eosinophilia is an indirect result of the fibroblast-lymphocyte interactions. Still others have focused their attentions on 3-phenylamino alanine, another L-tryptophan contaminant that was implicated in an unrelated eosinophilia-related epidemic known as toxic oil syndrome (227–229).

These findings have not been without controversy. Perhaps the most profound element in question is this: Is EMS really related to tryptophan ingestion? Shapiro (217) offered an in-depth critique of the defects in the methodology and data analysis found in the original case-control studies. Can EMS truly be differentiated clinically and pathologically from eosinophilic fasciitis (230–232)? Many researchers think not. Was there really an epidemic, or was this a media-created blitz? Several articles present pro and con viewpoints (217,233–237).

The results with animal models have fueled the controversy (238). In rodent studies, administration of high doses of L-tryptophan resulted in some histopathologic changes, regardless of the source of the L-tryptophan and regardless of the presence or absence of EBT. Most intriguing is the observation that, in rodents, L-tryptophan administration did not induce a peripheral blood eosinophilia. Studies performed with rhesus monkeys, who tolerated 10 to 20 times the dose of L-tryptophan ingested by humans developing EMS, were found to develop no weakness, no myalgias, and no eosinophilia (238,239).

Eosinophils and Host Defense Against Helminthic Parasites

This remains among the most controversial topics in eosinophil research today. Although peripheral blood eosinophilia is elicited in response to parasitic infection (a response mediated by IL-5 (3,87,240), the role played by eosinophils in this response—major defenders, ancillary troops, or uninvolved bystanders—has been the subject of significant dispute. In 1973, Mahmoud et al. (241) reported the development of a rabbit anti-mouse eosinophil antiserum (AES) that did not cross-react with peripheral blood neutrophils. In a subsequent report, this group successfully used this antiserum to eliminate the peripheral blood eosinophilia accompanying infection of preimmunized mice with cercariae of *Schistosoma mansoni;* approximately twice as many schistosomula were recovered from lung and liver from mice treated with AES compared with normal rabbit serum control (242).

Similarly, Grove et al. (243) demonstrated a small (less than twofold) but statistically significant increase in muscle larvae in mice treated with AES before and after primary infection with *Trichinella spiralis;* AES had no effect on the rate of expulsion of larvae from the intestines. In an independent set of studies using antiserum prepared against guinea pig eosinophils (244), Gleich et al. (245) demonstrated a moderate (30%) increase in worms of *Trichostrongylus colubriformis* isolated from the intestines of AES-treated animals, which was interesting in hindsight in light of the dramatic reduction in number of eosinophils found in the inflammatory infiltrates (approximately 100-fold). A number of studies followed in which the capacity of human (but not murine) eosinophils to mediate the destruction of isolated parasites *in vitro* was examined (246,247), along with the relative potencies of the individual eosinophil granule proteins (248–250).

In 1989, Coffman et al. (87) reported the development of murine monoclonal antibodies directed against the eosinophil differentiating agent, IL-5. Shortly thereafter, Sher et al. (3) reported that, on ablation of eosinophils with this neutralizing monoclonal antibody, TRFK-5, the number of schistosomula recovered from ablated, preimmunized mice was no different from the nonablated controls. Herndon and Kayes (4) reported that eosinophil depletion with TRFK-5 also did not affect recovery of *Trichinella spiralis* larvae from muscle tissue. Similar results were obtained by Korenaga et al. (251) with respect to *Strongyloides* infection in mice, using another monoclonal antibody against IL-5. Freeman et al. (5) demonstrated that the peripheral blood eosinophilia characteristic of their IL-5 transgenic mice afforded no resistance to infection with *Schistosoma mansoni,* also in preimmunized mice, and Kopf et al. (6) demonstrated no difference in the handling of *Mesocestoides corti* by control or IL-5–deficient (knock-out) mice.

Why the discrepancy? The initial results, although statistically significant, did not show dramatic differences between AES-treated and control mice. The AESs themselves, although defined with respect to cross-reactivity with neutrophils, may have had uncharacterized and unexpected cross-reactivities *in vivo*, which may have provided the degree of immune dysfunction observed. Destruction of eosinophils *in situ* may have resulted in release of toxic mediators that altered the overall immune response; there is some evidence suggesting that eosinophil cationic proteins can alter lymphocyte function (4,252). However, it is also important to recognize that depletion of IL-5 may have other as yet uncharacterized effects *in vivo* that may ultimately lead to a reconsideration of the conclusions of the latter set of experiments.

A final point to consider is the possibility that this finding is species specific. Eosinophils from mice differ significantly from those isolated from humans. De

Andres et al. (59) demonstrated that mouse eosinophils do not have Fcε receptors for IgE. We demonstrated that the eosinophil ribonucleases EDN and ECP are the most rapidly evolving coding sequences known among primates (37); the amino acid sequences of the EDN/ECP-type ribonucleases identified as components of mouse (253) and rat (254,255) eosinophils differ dramatically from their human counterparts and may be of a completely distinct evolutionary lineage (256) with distinctly different functions. Folkard et al. (257) reported that eosinophils were of primary importance in resistance to reinfection with microfilariae of *Onchocerca lienalis* in experiments performed in mice in which eosinophils were ablated with the TRFK-5 anti-IL-5 monoclonal antibody. The controversy continues.

Eosinophils and RNA Viruses

Although eosinophils have not been traditionally associated with viral disease, this perception may be changing (258,259). There are two specific viral pathogens—HIV-1 and respiratory syncytial virus (RSV)—whose associations with eosinophils merit comment.

Eosinophils and Human Immunodeficiency Virus Type 1 Infection

Although the focus on HIV-1 disease has been on chemokines and coreceptors, several groups have commented on the enigmatic association of peripheral blood eosinophilia and HIV-1 infection. Harris (260) hypothesized that many of the common sequelae of HIV-1 disease (e.g., urticaria, peripheral neuropathy, cerebral atrophy) may be related to eosinophils and their degranulation products and highlighted the fact that infected individuals showing improvement with IL-2 therapy also demonstrated increased eosinophil counts and activation (261,262). Other studies, such as those by Scadden et al. (263), designed to determine the effectiveness of IL-3 therapy, demonstrated no change in viral activity despite an associated 2-fold to 59-fold increase in absolute eosinophil counts in the treated individuals. The two major studies of eosinophilia and HIV concluded that the cause and clinical significance of the eosinophilia remain unclear (264,265).

It is tempting to speculate on the role of eosinophils in host defense against this virus; Klebanoff and Coombs (33) demonstrated that activated peripheral blood eosinophils and eosinophil peroxidase alone were active against a clinical isolate of HIV-1, and our group demonstrated that eosinophils inhibited cellular transduction by a murine retrovirus through a mechanism that depends on the activity of the eosinophil ribonucleases (266). Eosinophils themselves can also be infected by HIV-1, as demonstrated by Lucey et al. (125).

Eosinophils and Respiratory Syncytial Virus

RSV, an enveloped, single-stranded RNA virus of the family Paramyxoviridae, is the most important respiratory pathogen in the newborn to 2-year-old age group (267). There are a number of intriguing associations between eosinophils, eosinophil granule proteins, asthma and allergic bronchospasm, and the pathogenesis of RSV disease. Several groups have shown that, during RSV infection, eosinophils are recruited to and degranulate into the lung parenchyma, and wheezing during RSV infection is associated with increased concentrations of ECP in respiratory secretions (268–273). Most dramatically, children vaccinated with a formalin-inactivated RSV vaccine who subsequently developed natural RSV infection had increased blood eosinophil counts (274), with massive eosinophil infiltrates observed in two post-mortem specimens (275).

Eosinophils have been uniformly perceived as the villains in RSV disease. We have considered the possibility that eosinophils, through their membrane lytic and ribonucleolytic secretory effectors, may provide a degree of host defense against these RNA viral pathogens and have shown that eosinophils can mediate the destruction of RSV virions *in vitro*, an effect that directly depends on the actions of the secreted eosinophil ribonucleases (276). The degree of host defense provided by eosinophils present in the respiratory tract awaits future study.

PATHS OF FUTURE EOSINOPHIL RESEARCH

The issues and questions facing those involved in eosinophil research have been discussed in this chapter, and the progress of recent years has been highlighted. However, the essential question still remains: What are eosinophils? Are eosinophils the perpetual helpers, the jacks-of-all-trades but masters of none? Are eosinophils the jacks-of-no-trade, vestigial remnants from the defunct immune system of an earlier vertebrate species? Would we be better off without them? Do eosinophils have unique and specific beneficial functions? Is peripheral blood eosinophilia a meaningful guide toward elucidating these functions, or is it a mere distraction? Future research may hold the answers to one or more of these questions.

REFERENCES

1. Ehrlich P. On the specific granulations of blood (translation). *Arch Anat Physiol* 1897;1:166.
2. Ehrlich P. Methodological contribution on the physiology and pathology of various forms of leukocytes (translation). *Z Klin Med* 1880;1:533.
3. Sher A, Coffman RL, Hieny S, Cheever AW. Ablation of eosinophil and IgE responses with anti-IL-5 or anti-IL-4 antibodies fails to affect immunity against *Schistosoma mansoni* in the mouse. *J Immunol* 1990;145:3911–3916.
4. Herndon FJ, Kayes SG. Depletion of eosinophils by anti-IL-5 mono-clonal antibody treatment of mice infected with *Trichinella spiralis* does not alter parasite burden or immunologic resistance to reinfection. *J Immunol* 1992;149:3642–3647.
5. Freeman GL, Tominaga A, Takatsu, K, Secor WE, Colley DG. Elevated innate peripheral blood eosinophilia fails to augment irradiated cercarial vaccine-induced resistance to Schistosoma mansoni in IL-5 transgenic mice. *J Parasitol* 1995;81:1010–1011.
6. Kopf M, Brombacher F, Hodgkin PD, et al. IL-5-deficient mice have a developmental defect in CD5⁺ B-1 cells and lack eosinophilia but have normal antibody and cytotoxic T cell responses. *Immunity* 1996;4:15–24.
7. Weller PF. The immunobiology of eosinophils. *N Engl J Med* 1991;324:1110–1118.
8. Makino S, Fukuda T. *Eosinophils: biological and clinical aspects.* Boca Raton, FL: CRC Press, 1993.
9. Capron M, Desreumaux P. Immunobiology of eosinophils in allergy and inflammation. *Res Immunol* 1997;148:29–33.
10. Wardlaw AJ. Eosinophils in the 1990s: new perspectives on their role in health and disease. *Postgrad Med J* 1994;70:536–552.
11. Weller PF. Cytokine regulation of eosinophil function. *Clin Immunol Immunopathol* 1992;62:S55–S59.
12. Weller PF. Eosinophils: structure and functions. *Curr Opin Immunol* 1994;6:85–90.
13. Spry CJF, Kay AB, Gleich GJ. Eosinophils 1992. *Immunol Today* 1992;13:384–387.
14. Silberstein DS. Eosinophil function in health and disease. *Crit Rev Oncol Hematol* 1995;19:47–77.
15. Wardlaw AJ, Moqbel R, Kay AB. Eosinophils: biology and role in disease. *Adv Immunol* 1995;60:151–266.
16. Gleich GJ. The eosinophil and bronchial asthma: current understanding. *J Allergy Clin Immunol* 1990;85:422–436.
17. Gleich GJ, Adolphson CR, Leiferman KM. The biology of the eosinophilic leukocyte. *Annu Rev Med* 1993;44:85–101.
18. Weller PF, Lim K, Wan HC, et al. Role of the eosinophil in allergic reactions. *Eur Respir J* 1996;9(Suppl 22):109s–115s.
19. Bignold LP. The eosinophil leukocyte: controversies of recruitment and function. *Experientia* 1995;51:317–327.
20. Walsh GM. Human eosinophils: their accumulation, activation and fate. *Br J Haematol* 1997;97:701–709.
21. Persson CG, Erjefalt JS, Andersson M, et al. Epithelium, microcirculation and eosinophils—new aspects of the allergic airway in vivo. *Allergy* 1997;52:241–255.
22. Desreumaux P, Capron M. Eosinophils in allergic reactions. *Curr Opin Immunol* 1996;8:790–795.
23. Martin LB, Kita H, Leiferman KM, Gleich GJ. Eosinophils in allergy: role in disease, degranulation and cytokines. *Int Arch Allergy Immunol* 1996;109:207–215.
24. Weller PF. Intercellular interactions in the recruitment and functions of human eosinophils. *Ann N Y Acad Sci* 1996;796:116–125.
25. Dvorak AM. Similarities in the ultrastructural morphology and developmental and secretory mechanisms of human basophils and eosinophils. *J Allergy Clin Immunol* 1994;94:1103–1134.
26. Dvorak AM, Ishizaka T. Human eosinophils in vitro: an ultrastructural morphology primer. *Histol Histopathol* 1994;9:339–374.
27. Weller PF, Dvorak AM. Lipid bodies: intracellular sites for eicosanoid formation. *J Allergy Clin Immunol* 1994;94:1151–1156.
28. Ackerman SJ. Characterization and functions of eosinophil granule proteins. In: Makino S, Fukuda T, eds. *Eosinophils:* biological and clinical aspects. Boca Raton, FL: CRC Press, 1993:33–74.
29. Hamann KJ, Barker RL, Ten RM, Gleich GJ. The molecular biology of eosinophil granule proteins. *Int Arch Allergy Appl Immunol* 1991;94:202–209.
30. Popken-Harris P, Thomas L, Oxvig C, Sottrup-Jensen L, Kubo H, Klein JS, Gleich GJ. Biochemical properties, activities and presence in biologic fluids of eosinophil granule major basic protein. *J Allergy Clin Immunol* 1994;94:1282–1289.
31. Moy JN, Gleich GJ, Thomas LL. Non-cytotoxic activation of neutrophils by eosinophil granule major basic protein: effect on superoxide anion generation and lysosomal enzyme release. *J Immunol* 1990;145:2626–2632.
32. Haskell MD, Moy JN, Gleich GJ, Thomas LL. Analysis of signaling events associated with activation of neutrophil superoxide anion production by eosinophil granule major basic protein. *Blood* 1995;86:4627–4637.

33. Klebanoff SJ, Coombs RW. Virucidal effect of stimulated eosinophils on human immunodeficiency virus type I. *AIDS Res Hum Retroviruses* 1996;12:25–29.

34. Durack DT, Ackerman SJ, Loegering DA, Gleich GJ. Purification of human eosinophil-derived neurotoxin *Proc Natl Acad Sci USA* 1981;78:5165–5169.

35. Molina HA, Kierszenbaum F, Hamann KJ, Gleich GJ. Toxic effects produced or mediated by human eosinophil granule components on *Trypanosoma cruzi*. *Am J Trop Med Hyg* 1988;38:327–334.

36. Rosenberg HF. Recombinant eosinophil cationic protein (ECP): ribonuclease activity is not essential for cytotoxicity. *J Biol Chem* 1995;270:7876–7881.

37. Rosenberg HF, Dyer KD, Tiffany HL, Gonzalez M. Rapid evolution of a unique family of primate ribonuclease genes. *Nat Genet* 1995;10: 219–223.

38. Mosimann SC, Newton DL, Youle RJ, James MN. X-ray crystallographic structure of recombinant eosinophil-derived neurotoxin at 1.83 A resolution. *J Mol Biol* 1996;260:540–552.

39. Rosenberg HF, Dyer KD. Eosinophil cationic protein and eosinophil-derived neurotoxin: evolution of novel function in a primate ribonuclease gene family. *J Biol Chem* 1995;270:21539–21544.

40. Rosenberg HF, Dyer KD. Diversity among the primate eosinophil-derived neurotoxin genes: a specific carboxy-terminal sequence is necessary for enhanced ribonuclease activity. *Nucl Acids Res (in press)*.

41. Weller PF, Bach DK, Austen KF. Biochemical characterization of human eosinophil Charcot-Leyden crystal protein (lysophospholipase). *J Biol Chem* 1984;259:15100–15105.

42. Dvorak AM, Letourneau L, Login GR, Weller PF, Ackerman SJ. Ultra-structural localization of the Charcot-Leyden crystal protein (lysophospholipase) to a distinct crystalloid-free granule population in mature human eosinophils. *Blood* 1988;72:150–158.

43. Leonidas DD, Elbert BL, Zhou Z, Leffler H, Ackerman SJ, Acharya KR. Crystal structure of human Charcot-Leyden crystal protein, and eosinophil lysophospholipase, identifies it as a new member of the carbohydrate-binding family of galectins. *Structure* 1995;3: 1379–1393.

44. Dyer KD, Rosenberg HF. Eosinophil Charcot-Leyden crystal protein binds to beta-galactoside sugars. *Life Sci* 1996;58:2073–2082.

45. Dyer KD, Handen JS, Rosenberg HF. The genomic structure of the human Charcot-Leyden crystal protein gene is analogous to those of the galectin genes. *Genomics* 1997;40:217–221.

46. Lewis RA, Austen KF. The biologically active leukotrienes: biosynthesis, metabolism, receptors and pharmacology. *J Clin Invest* 1984; 73:889–897.

47. Lee T, Denchan DJ, Malone B, Roddy LL, Wasserman SI. Increased biosynthesis of platelet activating factor in activated human eosinophils. *J Biol Chem* 1984;259:5226–5530.

48. Sugiura T, Mabuchi K, Ojima-Uchiyama A, et al. Synthesis and action of PAF in human eosinophils. *J Lipid Mediat* 1992;5:151–153.

49. Lucey DR, Clerici M, Shearer GM. Type 1 and type 2 cytokine dysregulation in human infectious, neoplastic and inflammatory diseases. *Clin Microbiol Rev* 1996;9:532–562.

50. Lamkhioued B, Gounni AS, Aldebert D, et al. Synthesis of type 1 (IFN gamma) and type 2 (IL-4, IL-5 and IL-10) cytokines by human eosinophils. *Ann N Y Acad Sci* 1996;796:203–208.

51. Capron M, Truong MJ, Aldebert D, et al. Heterogeneous expression of CD23 epitopes by eosinophils from patients. Relationships with IgE-mediated functions. *Eur J Immunol* 1991;21:2423–2429.

52. Gounni AS, Lamkhioued B, Ochiai K, et al. High-affinity IgE receptor on eosinophils is involved in defense against parasites. *Nature* 1994;367:183–186.

53. Gounni AS, Lamkhioued B, Delaport E, et al. The high-affinity IgE receptor on eosinophils: from allergy to parasites of from parasites to allergy? *J Allergy Clin Immunol* 1994;94:1214–1216.

54. Humbert M, Grant JA, Taborda-Barata L, et al. High-affinity IgE receptor (FcεRI)-bearing cells in bronchial biopsies from atopic and nonatopic asthma. *Am J Respir Crit Care Med* 1996;153:1931–1937.

55. Sihra BS, Kon OM, Grant JA, Kay AB. Expression of high-affinity IgE receptors on peripheral blood basophils, monocytes, and eosinophils in atopic and nonatopic subjects: relationship to total serum IgE concentrations. *J Allergy Clin Immunol* 1997;99:699–706.

56. Klubal R, Osterhoff B, Wang B, Kinet JP, Maurer D, Stingl G. The high-affinity receptor for IgE is the predominant IgE-binding structure in lesional skin of atopic dermatitis patients. *J Invest Dermatol* 1997;108:336–342.

57. Capron M, Gounni AS, Morita M, et al. Eosinophils: from low to high affinity immunoglobulin E receptors. *Allergy* 1995;50(Suppl 25): 20–23.

58. Khalife J, Capron M, Cesbron JY, et al. Role of specific IgE antibodies in peroxidase (EPO) release from human eosinophils. *J Immunol* 1986;137:1659–1664.

59. De Andres B, Rakasz E, Hagen M, et al. Lack of Fc epsilon receptors on murine eosinophils—implications for the functional significance of elevated IgE and eosinophils in parasitic infections. *Blood* 1997;89: 3826–3836.

60. Murphy PM. Chemokine receptors. *Annu Rev Immunol* 1994;12: 593–633.

61. Schroder JM, Noso N, Sticherling M, Christophers E. Role of eosinophil chemotactic CC chemokines in cutaneous inflammation. *J Leukoc Biol* 1996;59:1–5.

62. Kaplan AP, Kuna P, Reddigari SR. Chemokines and the allergic response. *Exp Dermatol* 1995;4:260–265.

63. Schroder JM, Kameyoshi Y, Christopher E. RANTES, a novel eoisnophil-chemotactic cytokine. *Ann N Y Acad Sci* 1994;725:91–103.

64. Alam R, Grant JA. The chemokines and the histamine-releasing factors: modulation of function of basophils, mast cells and eosinophils. *Chem Immunol* 1995;61:148–160.

65. Kita H, Gleich GJ. Chemokines active on eosinophils: potential roles in allergic inflammation. *J Exp Med* 1996;183:2421–2426.

66. Knol EF, Roos D. Mechanisms regulating eosinophil extravasation in asthma. *Eur Respir J* 1996;9(Suppl 22):136s–140s.

67. Henricks PAJ, Bloemen PGM, Nijkamp FP. Adhesion molecules and the recruitment of eosinophils to the airways. *Res Immunol* 1997;148: 18–28.

68. Resnick MB, Weller PF. Mechanisms of eosinophil recruitment. *Am J Respir Cell Mol Biol* 1993;8:349–355.

69. Foster CA. VCAM-1/alpha 4-integrin adhesion pathway: therapeutic target for allergic inflammatory disorders. *J Allergy Clin Immunol* 1996;98:S270–S277.

70. Lobb RR, Pepinsky B, Leone DR, Abraham WM. The role of alpha 4 integrins in lung pathophysiology. *Eur Respir J Suppl* 1996;22: 104S–108S.

71. Wardlaw AJ, Walsh GM, Symon FA. Adhesion interactions involved in eosinophil migration through vascular endothelium. *Ann N Y Acad Sci* 1996;796:124–137.

72. Bochner BS, Schleimer RP. The role of adhesion molecules in human eosinophil and basophil recruitment. *J Allergy Clin Immunol* 1994;94: 427–438.

73. Simon HU, Blaser K. Inhibition of programmed eosinophil death: a key pathogenic event for eosinophilia? *Immunol Today* 1995;16:53–55.

74. Walsh GM. Mechanisms of human eosinophil survival and apoptosis. *Clin Exp Allergy* 1997;27:482–487.

75. Simon HU. Molecular mechanisms of defective eosinophil apoptosis in diseases associated with eosinophilia. *Int Arch Allergy Immunol* 1997;113:206–208.

76. Yousefi S, Blaser K, Simon HU. Activation of signaling pathways and prevention of apoptosis by cytokines in eosinophils. *Int Arch Allergy Immunol* 1997;112:9–12.

77. Simon HU, Yousefi S, Blaser K. Tyrosine phosphorylation regulates activation and inhibition of apoptosis in human eosinophils and neutrophils. *Int Arch Allergy Immunol* 1995;107:338–339.

78. Haslett C, Savill JS, Whyte MK, Stern M, Dransfield I, Meagher LC. Granulocyte apoptosis and the control of inflammation. *Philos Trans R Soc London B Biol Sci* 1994;345:327–333.

79. Weller PF, Rand TH, Barrett T, Elovic A, Wong DTW, Finberg RW. Accessory cell function of human eosinophils: HLA-DR dependent MHC restricted antigen presentation and interleukin-1-alpha formation. *J Immunol* 1993;150:2554–2562.

80. Lucey DR, Nicholson-Weller A, Weller PF. Mature human eosinophils have the capacity to express HLA-DR. *Proc Natl Acad Sci USA* 1989; 86:1348–1351.

81. Weller PF, Bubley GJ. The idiopathic hypereosinophilic syndrome. *Blood* 1994;83:2759–2779.

82. Bain BJ. Eosinophilic leukaemias and the idiopathic hypereosinophilic syndrome. *Br J Haematol* 1996;95:2–9.

83. Mahanty S, Nutman TB. The biology of interleukin-5 and its receptor. *Cancer Invest* 1993;11:624–634.

84. Koike M, Takatsu K. IL-5 and its receptor: which role do they play in the immune response. *Int Arch Allergy Immunol* 1994;104:1–9.

85. Egan RW, Umland SP, Cuss RM, Chapman RW. Biology of interleukin-5 and it relevance to allergic disease. *Allergy* 1996;51:71–81.

86. Sanderson CJ. Interleukin-5, eosinophils and disease. *Blood* 1992;79:3101–3109.

87. Coffman RL, Seymour BWP, Hudak S, Jackson J, Rennick D. Antibody to interleukin-5 inhibits helminth-induced eosinophilia in mice. *Science* 1989;245:308–310.

88. Di Biagio E, Sanchez-Borges M, Desenne JJ, Suarez-Chacon R, Somoza R, Acquatella G. Eosinophilia in Hodgkin's disease: a role for interleukin-5. *Int Arch Allergy Immunol* 1996;110:244–251.

89. Owen WF, Petersen J, Sheff DM, et al. Hypodense eosinophils and interleukin 5 activity in the blood of patients with the eosinophilia-myalgia syndrome. *Proc Natl Acad Sci USA* 1990;87:8647–8651.

90. Yamaguchi Y, Hayashi Y, Sugama Y, et al. Highly purified murine interleukin-5 (IL-5) stimulates eosinophil function and prolongs in vitro survival. *J Exp Med* 1988;167:1737–1742.

91. Egan RW, Kreutner W, Watnick AS, Jones H, Chapman RW. Involvement of IL-5 in a murine model of allergic pulmonary inflammation: prophylactic and therapeutic effect of an anti-IL-5 antibody. *Am J Respir Cell Mol Biol* 1995;13:360–365.

92. Gulbenkian AR, Egan RW, Fernandez X, et al. Interleukin-5 modulates eosinophil accumulation in allergic guinea pig lung. *Am Rev Respir Dis* 1992;146:263–266.

93. Hamelmann E, Oshiba A, Loader J, et al. Antiinterleukin-5 antibody prevents airway hyperresponsiveness in a murine model of airway sensitization. *Am J Respir Crit Care Med* 1997;155:819–825.

94. Mauser PJ, Pitman AM, Fernandez X, et al. Effects of an antibody to interleukin-5 in a monkey model of asthma. *Am J Respir Crit Care Med* 1995;152:467–472.

95. Iwamoto I, Kumano K, Kasai M, Kurasawa K, Nakao A. Interleukin-12 prevents antigen-induced eosinophil recruitment into mouse airways. *Am J Respir Crit Care Med* 1996;154:1257–1260.

96. Tominaga A, Takaki S, Koyama N, et al. Transgenic mice expressing a B cell growth and differentiation factor gene (interleukin 5) develop eosinophilia and autoantibody production. *J Exp Med* 1991;173:429–437.

97. Dent LA, Strath M, Mellor AL, Sanderson CJ. Eosinophilia in transgenic mice expressing interleukin 5. *J Exp Med* 1990;172:1425–1431.

98. Iwamoto T, Takatsu K. Evaluation of airway hyperreactivity in interleukin-5 transgenic mice. *Int Arch Allergy Immunol* 1995;108(Suppl 1):28–30.

99. Lefort J, Bachelet CM, Leduc D, Vargaftig BB. Effect of antigen provocation of IL-5 transgenic mice on eosinophil mobilization and bronchial hyperresponsiveness. *J Allergy Clin Immunol* 1996;97:788–799.

100. Lee NA, McGarry MP, Larson KA, Horton MA, Kristensen AB, Lee JJ. Expression of IL-5 in thymocytes/T cells leads to the development of massive eosinophilia, extramedullary eosinophilopoiesis, and unique histopathologies. *J Immunol* 1997;158:1332–1344.

101. Lee JJ, McGarry MP, Farmer SC, et al. Interleukin-5 expression in the lung epithelium of transgenic mice leads to pulmonary changes pathognomonic of asthma. *J Exp Med* 1997;185:2143–2156.

102. Foster PS, Hogan SP, Ramsay AJ, Matthaei KI, Young IG. Interleukin 5 deficiency abolishes eosinophilia, airways hyperreactivity and lung damage in a mouse asthma model. *J Exp Med* 1996;183:195–201.

103. Takatsu K. Interleukin-5—immunological functions and therapeutic potential of a putative antagonist. *Biodrugs* 1997;8:33–45.

104. Devos R, Plaetinck G, Cornelis S, Guisez Y, van der Heyden J, Tavernier J. Interleukin-5 and its receptor: a drug target for eosinophilia associated with chronic allergic disease. *J Leukoc Biol* 1995;57:813–819.

105. Pretlow TP, Keith EF, Cryar AK, et al. Eosinophil infiltration of human colonic carcinomas as a prognostic indicator. *Cancer Res* 1983;43:2997–3000.

106. Yoon IL. The eosinophil and gastrointestinal carcinoma. *Am J Surg* 1959;97:195–201.

107. Kolb E, Muller E. Local responses in primary and secondary human lung cancers. II. Clinical correlations. *Br J Cancer* 1979;40:410–416.

108. Tepper RI, Pattengale PK, Leder P. Murine interleukin-4 displays potent antitumor activity in vivo. *Cell* 1989;57:503–512.

109. Tepper RI, Coffman RL, Leder P. An eosinophil-dependent mechanism for the antitumor effect of IL-4. *Science* 1992;257:548–551.

110. Golumbek PT, Lazenby AJ, Levitsky HI, et al. Treatment of established renal cancer by tumor cells engineered to secrete interleukin-4. *Science* 1991;254:713–716.

111. Tepper RI. The eosinophil-mediated antitumor activity of interleukin-4. *J Allergy Clin Immunol* 1994;94:1225–1231.

112. Schleimer RP, Sterbinsky SA, Kaiser J, et al. IL-4 induces adherence of human eosinophils and basophils but not neutrophils to endothelium. *J Immunol* 1992;148:1086–1092.

113. Rothenberg ME, Luster AD, Leder P. Murine eotaxin: an eosinophil chemoattractant inducible in endothelial cells and in interleukin 4-induced tumor suppression. *Proc Natl Acad Sci USA* 1995;92:8960–8964.

114. Jose PJ, Griffiths-Johnson DA, Collins PD, et al. Eotaxin: a potent eosinophil chemoattractant cytokine detected in a guinea pig model of allergic airways inflammation. *J Exp Med* 1994;179:881–887.

115. Kitaura M, Nakajima T, Imai T, et al. Molecular cloning of human eotaxin, an eosinophil-selective CC chemokine, and identification of a specific eosinophil eotaxin receptor, CC chemokine receptor 3. *J Biol Chem* 1996;271:7725–7730.

116. Ponath PD, Qin S, Ringler DJ, et al. Cloning of the human eosinophil chemoattractant, eotaxin. *J Clin Invest* 1996;97:604–612.

117. Garcia-Zepeda EA, Rothenberg ME, Ownbey RT, Celestin J, Leder P, Luster AD. Human eotaxin is a specific chemoattractant for eosinophil cells and provides a new mechanism to explain tissue eosinophilia. *Nat Med* 1996;2:449–456.

118. Rothenberg ME, Luster AD, Lilly CM, Drazen JM, Leder P. Constitutive and allergen-induced expression of eotaxin mRNA in the guinea pig lung. *J Exp Med* 1995;181:1211–1216.

119. Gao JL, Sen AI, Kitaura M, Yoshie O, Rothenberg ME, Murphy PM, Luster AD. Identification of a mouse eosinophil receptor for the CC chemokine eotaxin. *Biochem Biophys Res Commun* 1996;223:679–684.

120. Ponath PD, Qin S, Post TW, et al. Molecular cloning and characterization of a human eotaxin receptor expressed selectively on eosinophils. *J Exp Med* 1996;183:2437–2448.

121. Daugherty BL, Siciliano SJ, DeMartino JA, Malkowitz L, Sirotina A, Springer MS. Cloning, expression, and characterization of the human eosinophil eotaxin receptor. *J Exp Med* 1996;183:2349–2354.

122. Heath H, Qin S, Rao P, et al. The chemokine receptor usage by human eosinophils. *J Clin Invest* 1997;99:178–184.

123. Marleau S, Griffiths-Johnson DA, Collins PD, Bakhle YS, Williams TJ, Jose PJ. Human RANTES acts as a receptor antagonist for guinea pig eotaxin in vitro and in vivo. *J Immunol* 1996;157:4141–4146.

124. Alkhatib G, Berger EA, Murphy PM, Pease JE. Determinants of HIV-1 coreceptor function of CC chemokine receptor 3. *J Biol Chem* 1997;272:20420–20426.

125. Weller PF, Marshall WL, Lucey DR, Rand TH, Dvorak AM, Finberg RW. Infection, apoptosis, and killing of mature human eosinophils by human immunodeficiency virus-1. *Am J Respir Cell Mol Biol* 1995;13:610–620.

126. Griffiths-Johnson DA, Collins PD, Rossi AG, Jose PJ, Williams TJ. The chemokine, eotaxin, activates guinea-pig eosinophils in vitro and causes their accumulation in the lung in vivo. *Biochem Biophys Res Commun* 1993;197:1167–1172.

127. Lilly CM, Nakamura H, Kesselman H, et al. Expression of eotaxin by human lung epithelial cells. Induction by cytokines and inhibition by glucocorticoids. *J Clin Invest* 1997;99:1767–1773.

128. Tenscher K, Metzner B, Schopf E, Norgauer J, Czech W. Recombinant human eotaxin induces oxygen radical production, calcium mobilization, actin reorganization, and CD11b upregulation in human eosinophils via a pertussis toxin-sensitive heterotrimeric guanine nucleotide-binding protein. *Blood* 1996;88:3195–3199.

129. Elsner J, Hochstetter R, Kimmig D, Kapp A. Human eotaxin represents a potent activator of the respiratory burst of human eosinophils. *Eur J Immunol* 1996;26:1919–1925.

130. Rothenberg ME, Ownbey R, Mehlhop PD, et al. Eotaxin triggers eosinophil-selective chemotaxis and calcium flux via a distinct receptor and induces pulmonary eosinophilia in the presence of interleukin 5 in mice. *Mol Med* 1996;2:334–348.

131. Rothenberg ME, MacLean JA, Pearlman E, Luster AD, Leder P. Targeted disruption of the chemokine eotaxin partially reduces antigen-induced tissue eosinophilia. *J Exp Med* 1997;185:785–790.

132. Yamada H, Hirai K, Miyamasu M, et al. Eotaxin is a potent chemotaxin for human basophils. *Biochem Biophys Res Commun* 1997;231:365–368.

133. Forssmann U, Uguccioni M, Loetscher P, et al. Eotaxin-2, a novel CC chemokine that is selective for the chemokine receptor CCR3 and acts like eotaxin on human eosinophil and basophil leukocytes. *J Exp Med* 1997;185:2171–2176.

134. Moqbel R. Eosinophil-derived cytokines in allergic inflammation and asthma. *Ann N Y Acad Sci* 1996;796:209–217.

135. Moqbel R, Levi-Schaffer F, Kay AB. Cytokine generation by eosinophils. *J Allergy Clin Immunol* 1994;94:1183–1188.

136. Moqbel R. Synthesis and storage of regulatory cytokines in human eosinophils. *Adv Exp Med Biol* 1996;409:287–294.

137. Lamkhioued B, Aldebert D, Gounni AS, et al. Synthesis of cytokines by eosinophils and their regulation. *Int Arch Allergy Immunol* 1995; 107:122–123.

138. Kay AB, Barata L, Meng Q, Durham SR, Ying S. Eosinophils and eosinophil associated cytokines in allergic inflammation. *Int Arch Allergy Immunol* 1997;113:196–199.

139. Kita H. The eosinophil: a cytokine-producing cell? *J Allergy Clin Immunol* 1996;97:889–892.

140. Del Pozo V, De Andres B, Martin E, et al. Murine eosinophils and IL-1:alpha IL-1 mRNA detected by in situ hybridization: production and release of IL-1 from peritoneal eosinophils. *J Immunol* 1990;144: 3117–3122.

141. Wong DTW, Weller PF, Galli SJ, et al. Human eosinophils express transforming growth factor alpha. *J Exp Med* 1990;172:673–681.

142. Todd R, Donoff BR, Chiang T, et al. The eosinophil as a cellular source of transforming growth factor alpha in healing cutaneous wounds. *Am J Pathol* 1991;138:1307–1313.

143. Desreumaux P, Janan A, Dubucquoi S, et al. Synthesis of interleukin 5 by activated eosinophils in patients with eosinophilic heart diseases. *Blood* 1993;82:1553–1560.

144. Moqbel R, Hamid Q, Ying S, et al. Expression of mRNA and immunoreactivity for the granulocyte-macrophage colony-stimulating factor (GM-CSF) in activated human eosinophils. *J Exp Med* 1991;174:749–752.

145. Kita H, Ohnishi T, Okubo Y, Weiler D, Abrams JS, Gleich GJ. GM-CSF and interleukin 3 release from human peripheral blood eosinophils and neutrophils. *J Exp Med* 1991;174:743–748.

146. Broide H, Paine M, Firestein G. Eosinophils express interleukin 5 and granulocyte macrophage colony stimulating factor mRNA at sites of allergic inflammation. *J Clin Invest* 1992;90:1414–1424.

147. van der Bruggen T, Koenderman L. Signal transduction in eosinophils. *Clin Exp Allergy* 1996;26:880–891.

148. Koenderman L, van der Bruggen T, Schweizer RC, et al. Eosinophil priming by cytokines: from cellular signal to in vivo modulation. *Eur Respir J* 1996;9(Suppl 22):119s–125s.

149. Yousefi S, Blaser K, Simon HU. Activation of signaling pathways and prevention of apoptosis by cytokines in eosinophils. *Int Arch Allergy Immunol* 1997;112:9–12.

150. Quinn MT. Low molecular weight GTP-binding proteins and leukocyte signal transduction. *J Leukoc Biol* 1995;58:263–276.

151. Pazdrak K, Schreiber D, Forsythe P, Justement L, Alam R. The intracellular signal transduction mechanisms of interleukin 5 in eosinophils. *J Exp Med* 1995;181:1827–1834.

152. van der Bruggen T, Caldenhoven E, Kanders D, et al. IL-5 signaling in human eosinophils involves JAK2 tyrosine kinase and Stat1 alpha. *Blood* 1995;85:1442–1448.

153. Pazdrak K, Stafford S, Alam R. The activation of the JAK-Stat 1 signaling pathway by IL-5 in eosinophils. *J Immunol* 1995;155:397–402.

154. Caldenhoven E, van Dijk TB, Solari R, et al. STAT3 beta, a splice variant of transcription factor ATAT3, is a dominant negative regulator of transcription. *J Biol Chem* 1996;271:13221–13227.

155. Dvorak AM, Ishizaka T, Weller PF, Ackerman SJ. Ultrastructural contributions to the understanding of the cell biology of human eosinophils: mechanisms of growth factor-induced development, secretion, and resolution of released constituents from the microenvironment. In: Makino S, Fukuda T, eds. *Eosinophils:* biological and clinical aspects. Boca Raton, FL: CRC Press, 1993:13–32.

156. Butterfield JH, Kita H, Weller DA, et al. Eosinophil differentiation of human umbilical cord mononuclear cells and prolonged survival of mature eosinophils by murine EL-4 thymoma cell conditioned medium. *Cytokine* 1991;3:350–359.

157. Walsh GM, Hartnell A, Moqbel R, et al. Receptor expression and functional status of cultured human eosinophils derived from umbilical cord blood mononuclear cells. *Blood* 1990;76:105–111.

158. Rosenberg HF, Dyer KD, Li F. Characterization of eosinophils generated in vitro from CD34[+] peripheral blood progenitor cells. *Exp Hematol* 1996;24:888–893.

159. Tiffany HL, Li F, Rosenberg HF. Hyperglycosylation of eosinophil ribonucleases in a promyelocytic cell line and in differentiated peripheral blood progenitor cells. *J Leukoc Biol* 1995;58:49–54.

160. Shalit M, Sekhsaria S, Malech HL. Modulation of growth and differentiation of eosinophils from human peripheral blood CD34+ cells by IL-5 and other growth factors. *Cell Immunol* 1995;160:50–57.

161. Fischkoff SA, Pollak A, Gleich GJ, Testa JR, Misawa S, Reber T. Eosinophilic differentiation of the human promyelocytic leukemia cell line, HL-60. *J Exp Med* 1984;60:179–196.

162. Fischkoff SA. Graded increase in probability of eosinophilic differentiation of HL-60 promyelocytic leukemia cells induced by culture under alkaline conditions. *Leuk Res* 1988;12:679–686.

163. Gallagher R, Collins S, Trujillo J, et al. Characterization of the continuous differentiating myeloid cell line (HL-60) from a patient with acute promyelocytic leukemia. *Blood* 1979;54:713–733.

164. Howe RS, Fischkoff SA, Rossi RM, Lyttle CR. Chemotactic capabilities of HL-60 human myeloid leukemia cells differentiated to eosinophils. *Exp Hematol* 1990;18:299–303.

165. Xu Q, Leiva MC, Fischkoff SA, Handschumacher RE, Lyttle CR. Leukocyte chemotactic activity of cyclophilin. *J Biol Chem* 1992;267: 11968–11971.

166. Plaetinck G, van der Heyden J, Tavernier J, et al. Characterization of interleukin 5 receptors on eosinophilic sublines from human promyelocytic leukemia (HL-60) cells. *J Exp Med* 1990;172:683–691.

167. Tavernier J, Devos R, Cornelis S, et al. A human high affinity interleukin-5 receptor (IL5R) is composed of an IL5-specific alpha chain and a beta chain shared with the receptor for GM-CSF. *Cell* 1991;66: 1175–1184.

168. Tomonaga M, Gasson JC, Quan SG, Golde DW. Establishment of eosinophilic sublines from human promyelocytic leukemia (HL-60) cells: demonstration of multipotentiality and single lineage commitment of HL-60 stem cells. *Blood* 1986;67:1433–1441.

169. Morita M. Review: recent studies on a human eosinophilic leukemia cell line EoL as an experimental model of eosinophils. *Nippon Rinsho* 1993;51:712–717.

170. Paul CC, Ackerman SJ, Mahrer S, Tolbert M, Dvorak AM, Baumann MA. Cytokine induction of granule protein synthesis in an eosinophil-inducible human myeloid cell line, AML14. *J Leukoc Biol* 1994;56: 74–79.

171. Paul CC, Mahrer S, Tolbert M, et al. Changing the differentiation program of hematopoietic cells: retinoic acid-induced shift of eosinophil-committed cells to neutrophils. *Blood* 1995;86:3737–3744.

172. Rosenberg HF, Gallin JI. Neutrophil specific granule deficiency includes eosinophils: coordinate regulation of neutrophil and eosinophil granule protein biosynthesis. *Blood* 1993;82:268–273.

173. Yamaguchi Y, Zhang DE, Sun Z, et al. Functional characterization of the promoter for the gene encoding human eosinophil peroxidase. *J Biol Chem* 1994;269:19410–19419.

174. Yamaguchi Y, Tenen DG, Ackerman SJ. Transcriptional regulation of the human eosinophil peroxidase genes: characterization of a peroxidase promoter. *Int Arch Allergy Immunol* 1994;104(Suppl):30–31.

175. Gomolin HI, Yamaguchi Y, Paulpillai AV, Dvorak LA, Ackerman SJ, Tenen DG. Human eosinophil Charcot-Leyden crystal protein: cloning and characterization of a lysophospholipase gene promoter. *Blood* 1993;82:1868–1874.

176. Li MS, Sun L, Satoh T, Fisher LM, Spry CJ. Human eosinophil major basic protein, a mediator of allergic inflammation, is expressed by alternative splicing from two promoters. *Biochem J* 1995;305: 921–927.

177. Sun Z, Yergeau DA, Tuypens T, et al. Identification and characterization of a functional promoter region in the human eosinophil IL-5 receptor alpha subunit gene. *J Biol Chem* 1995;270:1462–1471.

178. Sun Z, Yergeau DA, Wong IC, et al. Interleukin-5 receptor alpha subunit gene regulation in human eosinophil development: identification of a unique *cis*-element that acts like an enhancer in regulating activity of the IL-5R alpha promoter. *Curr Top Microbiol Immunol* 1996; 211:173–187.

179. Tiffany HL, Handen JS, Rosenberg HF. Enhanced expression of the eosinophil-derived neurotoxin ribonuclease (RNS2) gene requires interaction between the promoter and intron. *J Biol Chem* 1996;271: 12387–12393.

180. Handen JS, Rosenberg HF. Intronic enhancer activity of the eosinophil-derived neurotoxin (RNS2) and eosinophil cationic protein (RNS3) genes is mediated by an NFAT-1 consensus binding sequence. *J Biol Chem* 1997;272:1665–1669.

181. Anderson DC, Schmalstieg FC, Finegold MJ, et al. The severe and moderate phenotypes of heritable Mac-1, LFA-1 deficiency: their quantitative definition and relation to leukocyte dysfunction and clinical features. *J Infect Dis* 1985;152:668–689.

182. Weller PF, Rand TH, Goelz SE, Chi-Rosso G, Lobb RJ. Human eosinophil adherence to vascular endothelium mediated by binding to VCAM-1 and ELAM-1. *Proc Natl Acad Sci USA* 1991;88:7430–7433.

183. Dobrina A, Menegazzi R, Carlos TM, et al. Mechanisms of eosinophil adherence to cultured vascular endothelial cells. *J Clin Invest* 1991; 88:20–26.

184. Walsh GM, Mermod JJ, Hartnell A, Kay AB, Wardlaw AJ. Human eosinophil, but not neutrophils adherence to IL-1-stimulated human umbilical vascular endothelial cells is alpha 4 beta 1 (very late antigen-4) dependent. *J Immunol* 1991;146:3419–3423.

185. Bochner BS, Luscinskas FW, Gimbrone MAJ, et al. Adhesion of human basophils, eosinophils, and neutrophils to interleukin-1-activated human vascular endothelial cells: contributions of endothelial cell adhesion molecules. *J Exp Med* 1991;173:1553–1557.

186. Schleimer RP, Sterbinsky SA, Kaiser J, et al. Interleukin-4 induces adherence of human eosinophils and basophils but not neutrophils to endothelium: association with expression of VCAM-1. *J Immunol* 1992;148:1086–1092.

187. Elices MJ, Osborn L, Takada Y, Crouse C, Luhowskyj S, Hemler ME, Lobb RR. VCAM-1 on activated endothelium interacts with the leukocyte integrin VLA-4 at a site distinct from the VLA-4/fibronectin binding site. *Cell* 1990;60:577–584.

188. Moser R, Fehr J, Bruijnzeel PL. IL-4 controls the selective endothelium-driven transmigration of eosinophils from allergic individuals. *J Immunol* 1992;149:4021–4028.

189. Hansel TT, deVries IJ, Carballido JM, et al. Induction and function of eosinophil intercellular adhesion molecule 1 and HLA-DR. *J Immunol* 1992;149:2130–2136.

190. Del Pozo V, De Andres B, Martin E, et al. Eosinophil as antigen-presenting cell: activation of T cell clones and T cell hybridoma by eosinophils after antigen processing. *Eur J Immunol* 1992;22:1919–1925.

191. Hansel TT, Braunstein JB, Walker C, et al. Sputum eosinophils from asthmatics express ICAm-1 and HLA-DR. *Clin Exp Immunol* 1991; 86:271–277.

192. Beninati W, Derdak S, Dixon PF, et al. Pulmonary eosinophils express HLA-DR in chronic eosinophilic pneumonia. *J Allergy Clin Immunol* 1993;92:442–449.

193. Sedgwick JB, Calhoun WJ, Vrtis RF, Bates ME, McAllister PK, Busse WW. Comparison of airway and blood eosinophil function after in vivo antigen challenge. *J Immunol* 1992;149:3710–3718.

194. Mawhorter SD, Kazura JW, Boom WH. Human eosinophils as antigen-presenting cells: relative efficiency for superantigen and antigen induced CD4+ T-cell proliferation. *Immunology* 1994;81:584–591.

195. Yousefi S, Hoessli DC, Blaser K, Mills GB, Simon HU. Requirement of Lyn and Syk tyrosine kinases for the prevention of apoptosis by cytokines in human eosinophils. *J Exp Med* 1996;183:1407–1414.

196. Stern M, Savill J, Haslett C. Human monocyte-derived macrophage phagocytosis of senescent eosinophils undergoing apoptosis. *Am J Pathol* 1996;149:911–921.

197. Hebestreit H, Yousefi S, Balatti I, et al. Expression and function of the Fas receptor on human blood and tissue eosinophils. *Eur J Immunol* 1996;26:1775–1778.

198. Druilhe A, Cai Z, Haile S, Chouaib S, Pretolani M. Fas-mediated apoptosis in cultured human eosinophils. *Blood* 1996;87:2822–2830.

199. Matsumoto K, Schleimer RP, Saito H, Iikura Y, Bochner BS. Induction of apoptosis in human eosinophils by anti-Fas antibody treatment in vitro. *Blood* 1995;86:1437–1443.

200. Walsh GM, Williamson ML, Symon FA, Willars GB, Wardlaw AJ. Ligation of CD69 induced apoptosis and cell death in human eosinophils cultured with granulocyte-macrophage colony-stimulating factor. *Blood* 1996;87:2815–2821.

201. Morita M, Lamkhioued B, Soussi Gounni A, et al. Induction by interferons of human eosinophil apoptosis and regulation by interleukin-3, granulocyte/macrophage colony stimulating factor and interleukin-5. *Eur Cytokine Netw* 1996;7:725–732.

202. Adachi T, Motojima S, Hirata A, et al. Eosinophil apoptosis caused by theophylline, glucocorticoids, and macrolides after stimulation with IL-5. *J Allergy Clin Immunol* 1996;98:S207–S215.

203. Woolley KL, Gibson PG, Carty K, Wilson AJ, Twaddell SH, Woolley MJ. Eosinophil apoptosis and resolution of airway inflammation in asthma. *Am J Respir Crit Care Med* 1996;154:237–243.

204. Meagher LC, Cousin JM, Seckl JR, Haslett C. Opposing effects of glucocorticoids on the rate of apoptosis in neutrophilic and eosinophilic granulocytes. *J Immunol* 1996;156:4422–4428.

205. Atsuka J, Fujisawa T, Iguchi K, Terada A, Kamiya H, Sakurai M. Inhibitory effect of transforming growth factor beta 1 on cytokine-enhanced eosinophil survival and degranulation. *Int Arch Allergy Immunol* 1995;108(Suppl 1):31–35.

206. Beauvais F, Michel L, Dubertret L. The nitric oxide donors, azide and hydroxylamine, inhibit the programmed cell death of cytokine-deprived human eosinophils. *FEBS Lett* 1995;361:229–232.

207. Ochiai K, Kagami M, Matsumura R, Tomioka H. IL-5 but not interferon-gamma (IFN-gamma) inhibits eosinophil apoptosis by up-regulation of bcl-2 expression. *Clin Exp Immunol* 1997;107:198–204.

208. Simon HU, Yousefi S, Schranz C, Schapowal A, Bachert C, Blaser K. Direct demonstration of delayed eosinophil apoptosis as a mechanism causing tissue eosinophilia. *J Immunol* 1997;158:3902–3908.

209. Tsuyuki S, Bertrand C, Erard F, et al. Activation of the Fas receptor on lung eosinophils leads to apoptosis and the resolution of eosinophilic inflammation of the airways. *J Clin Invest* 1995;96:2924–2931.

210. Simon HU, Yousefi S, Dommann-Scherrer CC, et al. Expansion of cytokine-producing CD4−CD8− T cells associated with abnormal Fas expression and hypereosinophilia. *J Exp Med* 1996;183:1071–82.

211. Coyle AJ, Tsuyuki S, Bertrand C, et al. Mice lacking the IFN-gamma receptor have impaired ability to resolve a lung eosinophilic inflammatory response associated with a prolonged capacity of T cells to exhibit a Th2 cytokine profile. *J Immunol* 1996;156:2680–2685.

212. Hertzman PA, Blevins WL, Mayer J, Greenfield B, Ting M, Gleich GJ. Association of the eosinophilia-myalgia syndrome with the ingestion of tryptophan. *N Engl J Med* 1990;322:869–873.

213. Eidson M, Philen RM, Sewell CM, Vorhees R, Kilbourne EM. L-tryptophan and eosinophilia-myalgia syndrome in New Mexico. *Lancet* 1990;355:645–648.

214. Swygert LA, Maes EF, Sewell LE, Miller L, Falk H, Kilbourne EM. Eosinophilia-myalgia syndrome: results of national surveillance. *JAMA* 1990;264:1698–1703.

215. Hibbs JR, Mittleman B, Hill P, Medsger TA. L-tryptophan-associated eosinophilic fasciitis prior to the 1989 eosinophilia-myalgia syndrome outbreak. *Arthritis Rheum* 1992;35:299–303.

216. Centers for Disease Control and Prevention. Eosinophilia-myalgia syndrome and L-tryptophan-containing products—New Mexico, Minnesota, Oregon and New York. *MMWR Morb Mortal Wkly Rep* 1989;38:785–788.

217. Shapiro S. Epidemiologic studies of the association of L-tryptophan with the eosinophilia-myalgia syndrome: a critique. *J Rheumatol* 1996;23(Suppl 46):44–59.

218. Slutsker L, Hoesly FC, Miller L, Williams LP, Watson JC, Fleming DW. Eosinophilia-myalgia syndrome associated with exposure to tryptophan from a single manufacturer. *JAMA* 1990;264:213–217.

219. Belongia EA, Hedberg CW, Gleich GJ, et al. An investigation of the cause of the eosinophilia myalgia syndrome associated with L-tryptophan use. *N Engl J Med* 1990;323:357–365.

220. Back EE, Henning KJ, Kallenbach LR, Brix KA, Gunn RA, Melius JM. Risk factors for developing eosinophilia-myalgia syndrome among L-tryptophan users in New York. *J Rheumatol* 1993;20:666–672.

221. Mayeno AN, Lin F, Foote CS, et al. Characterization of peak E, a novel amino acid associated with eosinophilia-myalgia syndrome. *Science* 1990;250:1707–1708.

222. Peltonen J, Varga J, Solberg S, Uitto J, Jiminez SA. Elevated expression of the genes for transforming growth factor beta 1 and type VI collagen in diffuse fasciitis associated with the eosinophilia-myalgia syndrome. *J Invest Dermatol* 1991;96:20–25.

223. Campbell DS, Morris PD, Silver RM. Eosinophilia-myalgia syndrome: a long-term follow-up study. *South Med J* 1995;88:953–958.

224. Hertzman PA, Clauw DJ, Kaufman LD, et al. The eosinophilia-myalgia syndrome: status of 205 patients and results of treatment two years after onset. *Ann Intern Med* 1995;122:851–855.

225. Yamaoka KA, Miyasaka N, Inuo G, et al. 1,1'-Ethylidenebis (tryptophan) (peak E) induces functional activation of human eosinophils

and interleukin-5 production from T lymphocytes: association of eosinophilia-myalgia syndrome with an L-tryptophan contaminant. *J Clin Immunol* 1994;14:50–60.

226. Jones MM, Vivado AK, Thomas PA, Waldschmidt TJ. Anti-IL-5 antibody ablates the eosinophilia induced by L-tryptophan administration in mice. *Arthritis Rheum Suppl* 1994;37:274.

227. Mayeno AN, Belongia EA, Lin F, Lundy SK, Gleich GJ. 3-(phenylamino) alanine, a novel aniline-derived amino acid associated with the eosinophilia-myalgia syndrome: a link to the toxic oil syndrome? *Mayo Clin Proc* 1992;67:1134–1139.

228. Kilbourne EM, Rigau-Perez JG, Heath CJ, et al. Clinical epidemiology of toxic-oil syndrome: manifestations of a new illness. *N Engl J Med* 1983;309:1408–1414.

229. Kilbourne EM, Bernert JT, Posada de la Paz M, et al. Chemical correlates of pathogenicity of oils related to the toxic oil syndrome epidemic in Spain. *Am J Epidemiol* 1988;127:1210–1227.

230. Doyle JA, Ginsburg WW. Eosinophilic fasciitis. *Med Clin North Am* 1989;73:1157–1166.

231. Martin RW, Duffy J, Lie JT. Eosinophilic fasciitis associated with use of L-tryptophan: a case control study and comparison of clinical and histopathologic features. *Mayo Clin Proc* 1991;66:892–898.

232. Jimenez SA, Varga J. The eosinophilia-myalgia syndrome and eosinophilic fasciitis. *Curr Opin Rheumatol* 1991;3:986–994.

233. Belongia EA, Mayeno AN, Osterholm MT. The eosinophilia-myalgia syndrome and tryptophan. *Annu Rev Nutr* 1992;12:235–256.

234. Spitzer WO, Haggerty JL, Berkson L, et al. Analysis of Centers for Disease control and prevention criteria for the eoisnophilia-myalgia syndrome in a geographically defined population. *J Rheumatol* 1996; 23(Suppl 46):73–80.

235. Kilbourne EM, Philen RM, Kamb ML, Falk H. Tryptophan produced by Showa Denko and epidemic eosinophilia-myalgia syndrome. *J Rheumatol* 1996;23(Suppl 46):81–88 [comment by Shapiro S. *J Rheumatol* 1996;23(suppl 46):89–91].

236. Sullivan EA, Staehling N, Philen RM. Eosinophilia-myalgia syndrome among the non-L-tryptophan users and pre-epidemic cases. *J Rheumatol* 1996;23:1784–1787.

237. Sternberg EM. Pathogenesis of L-tryptophan eosinophilia myalgia syndrome. *Adv Exp Med Biol* 1996;398:325–330.

238. Clauw DJ. Animal models of the eosinophilia-myalgia syndrome. *J Rheumatol* 1996;23(Suppl 46):93–98.

239. Anderson ST, Klein EC. Eosinophilic fasciitis in a rhesus macaque. *Arthritis Rheum* 1992;35:714–716.

240. Mawhorter SD. Eosinophilia caused by parasites. *Pediatr Ann* 1994; 23:409–413.

241. Mahmoud AAF, Kellermeyer RW, Warren KS. Production of monospecific rabbit antihuman eosinophil serums and demonstration of a blocking phenomenon. *N Engl J Med* 1974;290:417–420.

242. Mahmoud AAF, Warren KS, Peters PA. A role for the eosinophil in acquired resistance to Schistosoma mansoni infection as determined by antieosinophil serum. *J Exp Med* 1975;142:805–813.

243. Grove DI, Mahmoud AAF, Warren KS. Eosinophils and resistance to *Trichinella spiralis. J Exp Med* 1977;145:755–759.

244. Gleich GJ, Loegering DA, Olson GM. Reactivity of rabbit antiserum to guinea pig eosinophils. *J Immunol* 1975;115:950–954.

245. Gleich GJ, Olson GM, Herlich H. The effect of antiserum to eosinophils on susceptibility and acquired immunity of the guinea-pig to *Trichostrongylus colubriformis. Immunology* 1979;37:873–880.

246. Butterworth AE, Sturrock RF, Houba V, Mahmoud AA, Sher A, Rees PH. Eosinophils as mediators of antibody-dependent damage to schistosomula. *Nature* 1975;256:727–729.

247. Butterworth AE. Cell-mediated damage to helminths. *Adv Parasitol* 1984;23:143–158.

248. Hamann KJ, Barker RL, Loegering DA, Gleich GJ. Comparative toxicity of purified human eosinophil granule proteins for newborn larvae of *Trichinella spiralis. J Parasitol* 1987;73:523–529.

249. Ackerman SJ, Gleich GJ, Loegering DA, Richardson BA, Butterworth AE. Comparative toxicity of purified human eosinophil granule cationic proteins for schistosomula of *Schistosoma mansoni. Am J Trop Med Hyg* 1985;34:735–745.

250. Molina HA, Kierszenbaum F, Hamann KJ, Gleich GJ. Toxic effects produced or mediated by human eosinophil granule components on *Trypanosoma cruzi. Am J Trop Med Hyg* 1988;38:327–334.

251. Korenaga M, Hitoshi Y, Yamaguchi N, Sato Y, Takatsu K, Tada I. The role of interleukin-5 in protective immunity to Strongyloides venezuelensis infection in mice. *Immunology* 1991;72:502–507.

252. Peterson CGB, Skoog V, Venge P. Human eosinophil cationic proteins (ECP and EPX) and their suppressive effects on lymphocyte proliferation. *Immunobiology* 1986;171:1–13.

253. Larson KA, Olson EA, Madden BJ, Gleich GJ, Lee NA, Lee JJ. Two highly homologous ribonuclease genes expressed in mouse eosinophils identify a larger subgroup of the mammalian ribonuclease superfamily. *Proc Natl Acad Sci USA* 1996;93:12370–12375.

254. Watanabe M, Nittoh T, Suzuki T, Kitoh A, Mue S, Ohuchi K. Isolation and partial characterization of eosinophil granule proteins in rats: eosinophil cationic protein and major basic protein. *Int Arch Allergy Immunol* 1995;108:11–18.

255. Nittoh T, Hirakata M, Mue S, Ohuchi K. Identification of cDNA encoding rat eosinophil cationic protein/eosinophil-associated ribonuclease. *Biochem Biophys Acta* 1997;1351:42–46.

256. Batten D, Dyer KD, Domachowske JB, Rosenberg HF. Molecular cloning of four novel murine ribonuclease genes: unusual expansion within the ribonuclease A gene family. *Nucleic Acids Res* 1997;25: 4235–4239.

257. Folkard SG, Hogarth PJ, Taylor MJ, Bianco AE. Eosinophils are the major effector cells of immunity to microfilariae in a mouse model of onchocerciasis. *Parasitology* 1996;112:323–329.

258. Handzel ZT. Eosinophils, respiratory viruses and allergic asthma. *Isr J Med Sci* 1997;33:66–70.

259. Coyle AJ, Erard F, Bertrand C, Walti S, Pircher H, Le Gros G. Virus-specific CD8+ cells can switch to interleukin 5 production and induce airway eosinophilia. *J Exp Med* 1995;181:1229–1233.

260. Harris PJ. Eosinophils and AIDS. *Med Hypoth* 1994;43:75–76.

261. Silberstein DS, Schoof DD, Rodrick ML, et al. Activation of eosinophils in cancer patients treated with IL-2 and IL-2-generated lymphokine-activated killer cells. *J Immunol* 1989;142:2162–2167.

262. Kern P, Dietrich M. Eosinophil differentiating activity in sera of patients with AIDS under recombinant IL-2 substitution. *Blut* 1986;52:249–254.

263. Scadden DT, Levine JD, Bresnahan J, et al. In vivo effects of interleukin 3 in HIV type 1–infected patients with cytopenia. *AIDS Res Hum Retroviruses* 1995;11:731–740.

264. Cohen AJ, Steigbigel RT. Eosinophilia in patients infected with human immunodeficiency virus. *J Infect Dis* 1996;174:615–618.

265. Skiest DJ, Keiser P. Clinical significance of eosinophilia in HIV-infected individuals. *Am J Med* 1997;102:449–453.

266. Domachowske JB, Rosenberg HF. Eosinophils inhibit retroviral transduction of human target cells by a ribonuclease-dependent mechanism. *J Leukoc Biol* 1997;62:363–368.

267. Prober CG, Wang EEL. Reducing the morbidity of lower respiratory tract infections caused by respiratory syncytial virus: still no answer. *Pediatrics* 1997;99:472–475.

268. Garofalo R, Kimpen JLL, Welliver RC, Ogra PL. Eosinophil degranulation in the respiratory tract during naturally acquired respiratory syncytial virus infection. *J Pediatr* 1992;120:28–32.

269. Colocho Zelaya EA, Orvell C, Strannegard O. Eosinophil cationic protein in nasopharyngeal secretions and serum of infants infected with respiratory syncytial virus. *Pediatr Allergy Immunol* 1994;5: 100–106.

270. Sigurs N, Bjarnason R, Sigubergsson F. Eosinophil cationic protein in nasal secretion and in serum and myeloperoxidase in serum in respiratory syncytial virus. *Acta Paediatr* 1994;83:1151–1155.

271. Kimpen JL, Garofalo R, Welliver RC, Fujihara K, Ogra PL. An ultrastructural study of the interaction of human eosinophils with respiratory syncytial virus. *Pediatr Allergy Immunol* 1996;7:48–53.

272. Stark JM, Godding V, Sedgewick JB, Busse WW. Respiratory syncytial virus infection enhances neutrophil and eosinophil adhesion to cultured respiratory epithelial cells: roles of CD18 and intercellular adhesion molecule-1. *J Immunol* 1996;156:4774–4782.

273. Saito T, Deskin RW, Casola A, et al. Respiratory syncytial virus induces selective production of the chemokine RANTES by upper airway epithelial cells. *J Infect Dis* 1997;175:497–504.

274. Chin J, Maggoffin RL, Shearer LA, Schieble JH, Lennette EH. Field evaluation of a respiratory syncytial virus vaccine in a pediatric population. *Am J Epidemiol* 1969;89:449–463.

275. Kim HW, Canchola JG, Brandt CD, et al. Respiratory syncytial virus disease in infants despite prior administration of antigenic inactivated vaccine. *Am J Epidemiol* 1969;89:422–433.

276. Domachowske JB, Dyer KD, Bonville CA, Rosenberg HF. Recombinant human eosinophil-derived neurotoxin/RNase 2 functions as an effective antiviral agent against respiratory syncytial virus. *J Infec Dis* 1998;177:1458–1464.

Inflammation: Basic Principles and Clinical Correlates,
3rd ed., edited by John I. Gallin and Ralph Snyderman.
Published by Lippincott Williams & Wilkins, Philadelphia 1999.

CHAPTER 6

Platelets: Their Role in Hemostasis, Thrombosis, and Inflammation

Aaron J. Marcus

PLATELET MORPHOLOGY AND PLATELET PRODUCTION

Platelets are the keystone of the hemostatic arch. In contrast to the thrombocytes of birds (1) and reptiles (2), mammalian platelets are cytoplasmic fragments, devoid of nuclei, and are derived from megakaryocytes in the marrow. Megakaryocytes themselves originate from pluripotent stem cells of hematopoiesis (3). *In vitro* culture studies have shown that at least two stages of megakaryocyte progenitors can be demonstrated: the burst-forming unit-megakaryocyte and the colony-forming unit-megakaryocyte. Developmental stages of these progenitors are controlled by various cytokines. As the colony-forming unit-megakaryocyte matures, these cells become recognizable as such. An endomitotic process then leads to multilobulation of megakaryocyte nuclei. Under normal circumstances, megakaryocyte ploidy can range from 8N to 32N. However, platelet production and consumption are the main determinants of ploidy number.

The megakaryocyte cytoplasm fragments along demarcation membranes which are formed by enfolding of cytoplasmic membrane material. The size of the demarcation zones is the ultimate determinant of platelet size. When there is a demand for increased platelet production, the demarcation zones become larger. This is reflected in measurements of mean platelet volume (MPV), which is larger in thrombocytopenic states due to increased platelet consumption. The total mass of platelets in the circulation is the main determinant of platelet count. This is observed in platelet diseases such as the Bernard-Soulier syndrome and the May-Hegglin anomaly, wherein thrombocytopenia is accompanied by an increase in MPV (4). One third of circulating platelets are in the spleen (5).

It is possible to increase platelet production therapeutically through administration of recombinant human thrombopoietin or megakaryocyte growth and development factor. This material elevates the platelet count in a dose-dependent manner within 4 to 6 days after initiation of treatment (6).

Although platelets look somewhat uncomplicated on microscopic examination, this appearance is deceptive. The platelet is a functional entity, as evidenced by the critical roles it plays in hemostasis, coagulation, thrombosis, and as a participant in the inflammatory response. Platelets in the circulation appear to be passive, smooth discs, but on their surface they possess mechanisms for recognizing a site of injury that can trigger subsequent adhesion, spreading, activation, and release (5,7,8).

The discoid, circulating, "resting" platelet contains a circumferential band of microtubules that serves to maintain its discoid shape. The platelet membrane, which is the only cell plasma membrane derived from cytoplasmic components, contains invaginations. These form the surface-connected open canalicular system. The area beneath the plasma membrane, known as the sol-gel zone, contains abundant quantities of actin and myosin. In all likelihood, these proteins are critical for platelet shape change and spicule formation, which is part of the response to agonists inducing platelet activation (5). The platelet counterpart of endoplasmic reticulum is the dense tubular system, which is a reservoir for calcium storage. Other major platelet cytoplasmic components include mitochondria, peroxisomes, platelet α granules,

A.J. Marcus: Division of Hematology and Medical Oncology, Department of Medicine, Veterans Affairs Medical Center, New York, New York 10010.

This chapter is dedicated to the memory of Dr. Ira M. Goldstein.

and dense granules. Platelets also have abundant storage pools of glycogen.

A broad spectrum of proteins has been identified in platelet granules. It is controversial whether intracellular platelet proteins were adsorbed from plasma or were actively synthesized in the megakaryocyte. Probably both mechanisms play a role. For example, platelet albumin, fibrinogen, and immunoglobulin G (IgG) quantities seem to be proportionate to their plasma concentrations. Platelet factor-4 (the antiheparin protein), β-thromboglobulin, and von Willebrand's factor (vWF) do originate in the megakaryocyte. The platelet dense granule compartment contains adenosine diphosphate (ADP), adenosine triphosphate (ATP), serotonin, and calcium. ADP is the most important platelet agonist and recruiting agent in human plasma.

Platelets circulate for approximately 7 to 10 days. Normal platelet counts range from 150,000 to 440,000 per microliter. Normal platelets have a diameter of 3.6±0.7 μm. The platelet thickness is 0.9±0.3 μm, and the volume of the average platelet is 7.06±4.85 fL. When thrombopoiesis is increased, the MPV increases accordingly. This is a reflection of an increase in size of the megakaryocytes. It is generally accepted that MPV decreases as platelets age. Platelet α granules are the major determinants of platelet density, which varies about 5% among different subjects. Figure 6-1 depicts the major aspects of platelet morphology.

Despite major advances in comprehension of platelet biochemistry and function, one of the most important properties of platelets—maintenance of vascular integrity—is not understood. Yet, it forms the main basis for therapy with platelet transfusions. Acute thrombocytopenia usually is associated with spontaneous cutaneous and mucous membrane hemorrhage. It has been assumed that the hemorrhage is caused by loss of structural and functional integrity at the level of the vascular endothelium. This breakdown leads to increases in capillary fragility and permeability. The platelet components responsible for maintenance of vascular integrity have not been identified, and there is no explanation for their hypothetical mechanism of action. Only viable, intact platelets can halt thrombocytopenic bleeding, which suggests that the platelet "vascular integrity factor" is a metabolic entity.

Platelets also mediate clot retraction—a function that can be observed *in vitro*. Clot retraction requires ATP, glucose, and a highly consolidated coagulum as promoted by thrombin. The process of clot retraction may be mediated by an interaction between gpIIb/IIIa and the actin cytoskeleton. Cytoskeletal proteins such as talin and vinculin also appear to be involved in clot retraction. As anticipated, clot retraction is weak to absent in thrombasthenia, owing to a deficiency or absence of gpIIb/IIIa. Clot retraction is defective in thrombocytopenic states and during excessive fibrinolysis. In the latter condition, the retracted clot becomes liquefied *in vitro*.

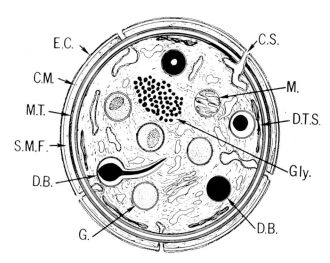

FIG. 6-1. Diagram of platelet ultrastructure in an equatorial plane. The peripheral zone, exterior to the plasma membrane, contains glycoprotein-rich material and is considered as glycocalyx (EC). The glycocalyx is the locale of platelet receptors for agonists and inhibitors. The glycocalyx is also the site of signal transduction. The platelet plasma membrane (CM) is a classic lipid bilayer with a unique phospholipoprotein component that can rearrange itself in response to agonist stimulation. This rearrangement confers coagulation-promoting properties on the activated platelet. The cell membrane and submembrane filament area (SMF) are the site of invaginations at specific sites. These invaginations comprise lining channels of the surface-connected open canalicular system (CA). The submembrane filaments are composed of actin from the membrane cytoskeleton.

In response to activation, a platelet surface membrane rearrangement occurs, forming the catalytic phospholipoprotein surface for assembly of activated coagulation proteins. This assembly does not take place on the surface of resting platelets. Also in response to activation, the platelet submembrane filaments form parallel structures that are the basis of filopodia or spicule formation—the "marker" for stimulated platelets.

The circumferential system of microtubules (MT) constitutes the entire cytoskeleton and it is proposed, although controversial, that the microtubule system is responsible for maintenance of the disk shape of unstimulated platelets. The platelet cytoplasm itself is also known as the sol-gel zone. It contains microfilaments, submembrane filaments, the circumferential band of microtubules, and glycogen. Other formed elements in the sol-gel zone include mitochrondia (M), dense bodies (DB), and lysosomes.

Platelet granules (G) are of two types. One is lysosomal, and those of the other type contain adhesive-type proteins and agonists that are released into the external milieu upon platelet activation. These include fibrinogen, von Willebrand's factor, thrombospondin, fibronectin, and P-selectin; P-selectin translocates to the platelet surface on activation. Also present are platelet factor-4, β-thromboglobulin, and platelet-derived growth factor (PDGF). In addition, transforming growth factor-β, coagulation factor V, plasma activator inhibitor-1 (PAI-1), protein S, and high-molecular-weight kininogen. The major agonists are adenosine diphosphate (ADP) and serotonin. The dense tubular system (DTS) and surface-connected canalicular system are actually membrane systems within the platelet that are counterparts of the sarcoplasmic reticulum in other cells. (From White JG. Platelet granule disorders. *Crit Rev Oncol Hematol* 1996;4:337, copyright CRC Press, Inc., Boca Raton, Florida, with permission.)

MECHANISMS OF HEMOSTASIS

The hemostatic process represents a series of physiologic and biochemical reactions that culminate in the arrest of hemorrhage from blood vessels that have been severed or mechanically traumatized. Hemostasis is accomplished by the interaction of three systems: components of the vasculature itself, including endothelial cells; blood platelets; and plasma proteins of the intrinsic and extrinsic coagulation systems (9,10). Qualitative or quantitative deficiencies in one of these systems can result in defective hemostasis or coagulation, or both, leading to a mild, moderate, or severe hemorrhagic diathesis (5,7).

The efficiency of the hemostatic process leads to a paradox: at sites of pathologic damage, such as a necrotic or fissured atherosclerotic plaque, these structures serve as agonists for unwanted activation of hemostasis and promotion of blood coagulation. This culminates in arterial or venous thrombosis at critical sites such as the coronary or cerebral circulation. Thrombosis therefore can be classified as a misdirected form of hemostasis. It is the major complication of atherosclerotic disease (8) and accounts for 50% of mortality in the United States, Europe, and Japan (11-13). Last year in the United States alone, there were 2,500,000 thrombotic episodes, leading to 600,000 deaths.

Primary Hemostasis

Interruption of blood vessel continuity evokes a series of responses which are defined as primary hemostasis. Initial events are modulated by exposed blood vessel components such as subendothelial matrix. Concomitantly, platelet adhesion and activation occur, but at this point proteins of the coagulation system are not directly involved. However, tissue factor may play an earlier role than previously anticipated (14). This sequence of events probably accounts for the clinical observation that the bleeding time in hemophilia is essentially normal, since it is not a platelet disorder per se.

As visualized in *ex vivo* studies, the vessel wall quickly retracts and platelets immediately adhere to subendothelium—especially the collagen component. vWF, both in the subendothelial matrix and from plasma, rapidly adsorbs to the site of damage and further mediates platelet adhesion through an interaction with the platelet glycoprotein Ib-IX-V receptor complex (5,15,16).

These events are accompanied by activation of gpIIb/IIIa on the platelet membrane (integrin $\alpha_{IIb}\beta_3$) (17,18). Activated platelets continue to spread and further adhere to the damaged vessel surface. They rapidly generate a releasate composed of a large variety of stored proteins, some of which serve as recruiting agents for platelets arriving at the injury site from the circulation. Platelet recruitment is the critical step in generation of a thrombus. The recruitment process ultimately promotes total occlusion of a vessel by the platelet thrombus. As mentioned, this early process is mediated in a major way by circulating vWF and by the vWF that is locally released from activated

platelets and endothelial cells. During high-shear-stress conditions, which occur in small vessels and in larger ones that have been partially occluded, vWF plays a critical role in generation of the platelet plug (15). In the setting described, continued local accumulation of activated platelets expands the physical dimensions of the thrombus through recruitment of additional platelets that arrive in the microenvironment (19,20).

The subendothelial collagen to which platelets initially adhere and on which they spread is a very strong agonist. (It meets this criterion because it induces about 65% platelet serotonin release *in vitro*.) The physiologic events initiated by platelet-collagen contact can be subdivided into four steps, as a working classification:

1. Biologically and biochemically active compounds that are mainly stored in intracellular platelet granules are secreted into the extracellular milieu. This is the classic platelet release reaction (5,16).
2. P-selectin, a platelet granule membrane glycoprotein, translocates to the platelet surface, where it mediates adhesion of activated platelets to neutrophils, monocytes, and certain lymphocyte subsets (21-24).
3. Activation of the platelet eicosanoid metabolic pathway commences with the appearance of free arachidonic acid (20 carbons, 4 double bonds), which is released from the platelet phospholipid compartment by the action of phospholipases (25-27). Free arachidonic acid is immediately oxygenated to form the labile, biologically active endoperoxide prostaglandin H_2 (PGH_2), a reaction catalyzed by prostaglandin-H endoperoxide synthase-1 (PGHS-1) (28). Isomerization of the endoperoxide to thromboxane A_2 is catalyzed by thromboxane synthase (29). Simultaneously, two compounds of unknown function are generated and released: 12-hydroxyheptadecatrienoic acid (HHTrE) and malondialdehyde (MDA). Importantly, initial cyclooxygenation of arachidonate as catalyzed by PGHS-1, the prerequisite for formation of all of these compounds, is completely inhibited by aspirin. This medication irreversibly acetylates the "active site" serine residue of cyclooxygenase at position 530 (30).

Unprocessed free arachidonate escapes from platelets and is metabolized by cells in the surrounding milieu, such as endothelium, neutrophils, and monocytes (lymphocytes do not process arachidonate). This phenomenon results in biosynthesis of new, biologically active compounds and illustrates the phenomenon of transcellular metabolism (see later discussion) (13,26,31). Platelets also contain an aspirin-insensitive cytoplasmic enzyme, 12-lipoxygenase, which processes remaining free platelet arachidonate to 12-hydroxyeicosatetraenoic acid (12-HETE). This hydroxy acid is produced in great abundance after aspirin ingestion because the acetylated cyclooxygenase cannot process the accumulating free arachidonate. The 12-HETE thus formed also leaves the platelet and metabolically interacts with other cells (e.g., neutrophils), leading to synthesis of new compounds (32).

4. The activated platelet undergoes a drastic transition in shape, from the smooth disk configuration of the resting state to a spiny sphere. This rearrangement results in more efficient platelet-platelet contact and adhesion. The shape change also produces a rearrangement of the platelet membrane phospholipoprotein compartment,

converting the platelet membrane into a highly efficient procoagulant surface (10). The shape change also permits optimal binding between the platelet membrane phospholipoprotein (not phospholipid) and activated coagulation factor X in the presence of activated factor V. Furthermore, the rearranged phospholipoprotein surface of the stimulated platelet activates factor VII via the extrinsic coagulation pathway. These events are summarized and depicted in Figure 6-2.

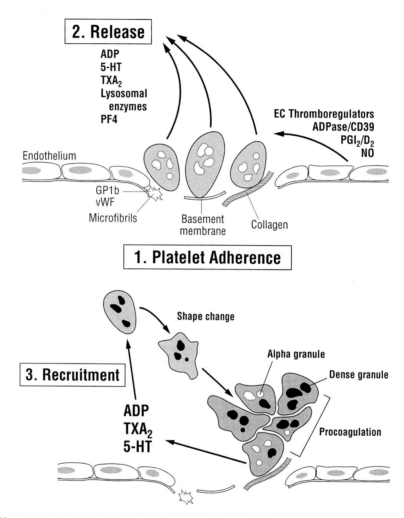

FIG. 6-2. Diagrammatic representation of the normal hemostatic process.

1, Platelet adherence begins. Exposure of subendothelium as a result of vascular injury causes immediate platelet adherence to collagen, basement membrane, and microfibrils in the presence of von Willebrand's factor and platelet glycoprotein Ib (GPIb).

2, Platelet release occurs. Collagen, a strong platelet agonist, induces release of adenosine diphosphate (ADP) and serotonin (5-HT) from dense granules. Several α granule proteins are also secreted. The eicosanoid thromboxane A_2 is formed enzymatically in platelets from released free arachidonate. Unmetabolized released arachidonate penetrates and is metabolized by other cell types in the microenvironment (33). Concomitant with adhesion and activation, endothelial cell defense mechanisms (thromboregulators) become functional and serve to limit the size of the thrombus.

3, Formation of the releasate initiates the recruitment phase of thrombin formation. ADP and thromboxane are the most important recruiting agents in the platelet releasate. Both 5-HT and thromboxane serve to induce vasoconstriction, thereby helping to consolidate the evolving thrombus and limiting the velocity of blood flow proximal to the thrombus. Components of the releasate serve to activate additional platelets arriving in the fluid phase. As the arriving platelets become activated, they undergo shape change and aggregate on the initial layer of adherent platelets. Phospholipoproteins on the platelet surface are now available for catalytic activation of proteins of the coagulation system.

The interactions described culminate in thrombin formation, an event that amplifies the initial activating steps described for collagen (see Fig. 6-2). Thrombin maximally activates platelets, which results in strong recruitment. The agonistic properties of thrombin are verified by the fact that this enzyme induces 90% serotonin release from platelets *in vitro*. The activating effect of thrombin induces maximal release, abundant eicosanoid formation, and the appearance of fibrin in both the interstices and outer portions of the platelet thrombus (see Fig. 6-2). The end result is total occlusion of the blood vessel, which now contains a hemostatic plug in completely impermeable form. This secondary "consolidation phase" completes the hemostatic process. The platelet plug represents a consolidated mass of microscopic particles which, in conjunction with fibrin strands, must pos-

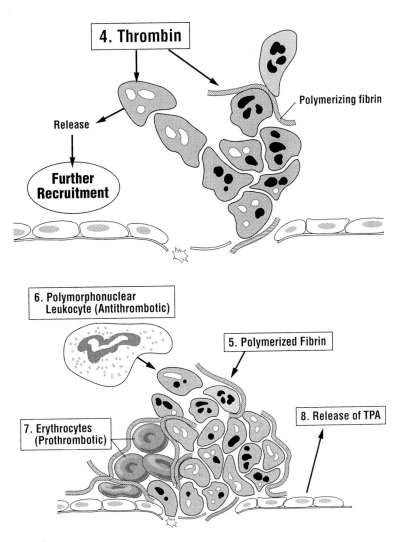

FIG. 6-2. *Continued*

4, Thrombin formation, the last stage of primary hemostasis, has important consequences that comprise the final steps of platelet thrombus development. Thrombin strongly induces further platelet activation, release and recruitment, as well as fibrin formation.

5, Fibrin strands begin to intercalate among activated platelets, and the entire thrombus becomes consolidated. The consolidated platelet thrombus is now virtually impermeable, and its multicellular nature is evident.

6, Polymorphonuclear leukocytes, which can be seen in close contact with platelets, serve an antithrombotic function in that they inhibit further platelet activation and recruitment (35).

7, Intact, metabolically viable erythrocytes are prothrombotic because they react to the presence of an activated platelet releasate with production of an unidentified material that increases platelet reactivity (34). Platelet-neutrophil contact is amplified by the adhesive glycoprotein, P-selectin, which interacts with its receptor on the neutrophil surface (22,23).

8, Formation of the platelet thrombus also signals initiation of the fibrinolytic process—that is, release of tissue plasminogen activator from endothelial cells (19).

sess enormous tensile strength to withstand the pressure of the circulation after it has occluded the blood vessel, either beneficially as a hemostatic plug or pathologically as a thrombus.

The Platelet Releasate: Components, Significance, and Methods of Study

Major components of the platelet releasate responsible for recruitment have already been discussed. From the standpoint of hemostasis and thrombosis, recruitment is the most important stage of platelet participation in vascular occlusion. Releasate constituents consolidate the thrombus and can also propagate it if intrinsic defense systems (thromboregulators) are overcome by the strength of the agonist (8,20).

In addition, as already described, components of the releasate such as free arachidonate and 12-HETE interact with other cells in the microenvironment by means of cell-cell interactions and transcellular metabolism. Released thromboxane serves as an agonist for vasoconstriction and platelet aggregation. It does not interact with cells other than platelets. ADP in the platelet releasate is metabolized by endothelial cell ecto-ADPase/CD39 (an example of thromboregulation). Calcium, originating from dense bodies, is prominent in the platelet releasate. This divalent cation may be important for calcium-requiring enzymes in the coagulation cascade or enzymes involved in crosslinking of deposited fibrin. Platelet-activating factor may promote platelet deposition in response to allergic injury (16).

Lysosomal enzymes are also secreted by platelets, although not in quantities comparable to leukocytes. Platelets are not inflammatory cells in the true sense. For example, in contrast to proinflammatory leukocytes, the platelet cannot generate an oxygen burst for production of superoxide. The platelet oxygen burst involves consumption of that element for oxygenation of arachidonic acid. Furthermore, platelets are not capable of engaging in true phagocytosis (i.e., they cannot produce a phagocytic vacuole). The contribution of platelets in inflammation is mainly in the form of substances they secrete. For example, platelets participate in the inflammatory process through transcellular metabolism of eicosanoid precursors and intermediates (13,25,33).

Platelet-released heparatinase cleaves surface glycosaminoglycans on endothelial cells to produce a fragment with antiproliferative properties. The transglutaminase, factor XIII, catalyzes peptide bonds between the γ-glutamyl residues and ε-amino groups of lysines to form stable crosslinks between fibrin in the interstices between platelets and fibrin surrounding the clot. Factor XIII can also cross-link fibronectin and α₂-antiplasmin to fibrin. Factor XIII is the only released cytoplasmic platelet protein; all others originate from granules. Platelet-derived growth factor (PDGF), which is secreted

from α granules, modulates growth and patterns of gene expression in cells of the vessel wall (11,12). PDGF also promotes the smooth muscle proliferation that occurs as a consequence of platelet–vessel wall interactions. Receptors for PDGF are transmembrane tyrosine kinase–type molecules. The connective tissue-activating peptide III is thought to be a precursor of β-thromboglobulin and is probably involved in fibroblast proliferation. It is structurally similar to platelet factor-4, and both belong to a protein class involved in growth control and the inflammatory response.

Transforming growth factor-β (TGF-β) is of platelet origin and is an important agonist for synthesis of extracellular matrix molecules and their receptors. TGF-β has a broad spectrum of effects on cell proliferation, being inhibitory in some instances and mitogenic in others. Platelets are the major source of thrombospondin, which plays a role in platelet aggregation, activation of TGF-β, and angiogenesis. Endothelial and smooth muscle cells also produce thrombospondin (16). Proteins involved in the coagulation cascade and in cell adhesion are also components of the platelet releasate, having originated in platelet α granules. As mentioned, plasma proteins are taken up by developing megakaryocytes and stored in α granules during maturation in the marrow. Examples are albumin and IgG, which can be detected in platelet α granules. However, their concentration is much lower than in plasma, so they probably were not biosynthesized in the developing megakaryocyte. These findings have confounded measurements of platelet-associated IgG in patients with thrombocytopenia (16).

In contrast, the quantity of factor V in platelet α granules is higher than can be explained by uptake from plasma. Platelet factor V is critical for assembly of coagulation proteins on the stimulated platelet surface. The finding of protein S in platelets is interesting because it is a cofactor for activity of activated protein C. Plasminogen activator inhibitor 1 (PAI-1), which is released from activated platelets, may be important for control of fibrinolytic activity in the microenvironment of a thrombus (16).

An unexpected component of the platelet releasate is the β-amyloid precursor protein (APP). This α-granule protein is a precursor of about 40 peptide residues identified in amyloid deposits in brain tissue of patients with Alzheimer's disease. APP belongs to the protease inhibitor family and can be released by proteolytic cleavage. As with other contents of the platelet releasate, one can ask whether APP plays a direct or indirect role in platelet function (16).

P-selectin is not a component of the platelet releasate. It is an α-granule membrane protein which, as mentioned, translocates to the platelet surface after activation (21-23). P-selectin binds specific carbohydrates and belongs to the same family as E- and L-selectin, which play a role in adhesive processes between leukocytes. P-selectin itself controls interactions of monocytes and neutrophils with platelets. Selectins are prototype systems for cell-cell interactions resulting in leukocyte recruitment in both hemostasis and thrombosis, as well as in the inflammatory response.

Adhesive proteins are also found in releasates from platelet α granules. Platelet vWF is synthesized in megakaryocytes and concentrated in platelets. The platelet form of vWF contains larger multimers, which are hemostatically more effective than smaller multimers. Fibronectin in platelets is present in alternatively spliced forms that are not found in plasma. This indicates that platelet fibronectin may play a role in matrix assembly. Vitronectin is found in low concentrations in platelets. PAI-1 binds to vitronectin, and both proteins are released in complex during platelet activation (16).

Platelet Activation and Recruitment as Studied in the Laboratory

The importance of the platelet releasate as a recruiting agent for other platelets and as a transport system for secreted platelet components that interact with other cells in the circulation has repeatedly been emphasized. If platelet activation and recruitment could be studied separately, the information would be more specific than that obtained from coincubation systems, as was demonstrated by Santos and Valles (34-36). Their novel system is demonstrated in Figure 6-3. Platelets alone, or platelets and other cells in combined suspension, are incubated in the presence of stirring to promote cell-cell contact. An agonist is added to this suspension, which is then inverted three times for 10 seconds. During the next 50 seconds, the tube is centrifuged and the cell-free releasate is removed for further testing. Components of the releasate are analyzed biochemically, and the releasate itself is used as an agonist for platelet-rich plasma (also stirred). By this method it is possible to separate and analyze the fluid phase of activated platelets for specific proteins and other released, biologically active compounds such as ADP, thromboxane, serotonin, and PDGF.

This system of study has revealed both basic and clinically applicable information. For example, on exposure to the fluid phase of activated platelets, erythrocytes release an aspirin-insensitive substance that promotes platelet reactivity. Interesting concepts have emerged from these results. Low-dose aspirin administration to patients with vascular diseases loses its protective effect with time. The low-dose aspirin must be supplemented with a therapeutic dose (325 mg) every 2 weeks (36). Neutrophils inhibit platelet reactivity when exposed to the releasate from activated platelets. Therefore, neutrophils accumulating at the site of a thrombus may exert a protective effect against its propagation (see Fig. 6-2) (34,35).

Role of G Proteins in Platelet Activation

The G protein group consists of an homologous array of guanine nucleotide—binding regulatory proteins. These proteins modulate interactions between receptors on the cell surface and effector molecules in the cell. The effectors are enzymes that generate second messages and also control movement through ion channels. In platelets, G proteins regulate adenylyl cyclase, phospholipase C, and phospholipase A_2. The G proteins are heterotrimeric and consist of α-, β-, and γ-subunits. The α-subunits are the most diverse and account for most of the activities of the G protein group. In resting cells, the α-subunit is bound to guanosine diphosphate (GDP). This complex associates with βγ-subunits. When the G protein instead binds guanosine triphosphate (GTP), activation results (Fig. 6-4). Receptor interaction with agonists such as thrombin is most efficient when G protein is in the heterotrimeric form. Platelet receptors that couple to G proteins include thrombin and the protease-activated receptor-2 (PAR-2). Others include those for epinephrine, thromboxane A_2, vasopressin, and platelet-activating fac-

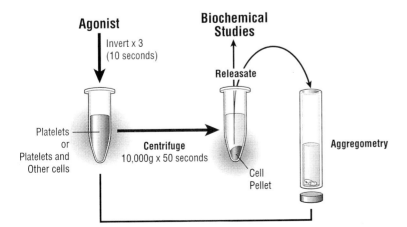

FIG. 6-3. System for separate evaluation of platelet activation (generating system, *left*) and recruitment (assay system, *right*). An agonist is added to the generating system in order to activate platelets alone or platelets plus other cells. A cell-free releasate is obtained after centrifugation of the generating system. This releasate is transferred to the assay system (platelet-rich plasma) for assessment of proaggregatory activity (recruiting properties) of the releasate and for biochemical studies to measure activation. These include studies of serotonin (5-HT) release, arachidonic acid release and metabolism, and agonistic or inhibitory properties of combined cell suspensions that were exposed to an agonist (34-36).

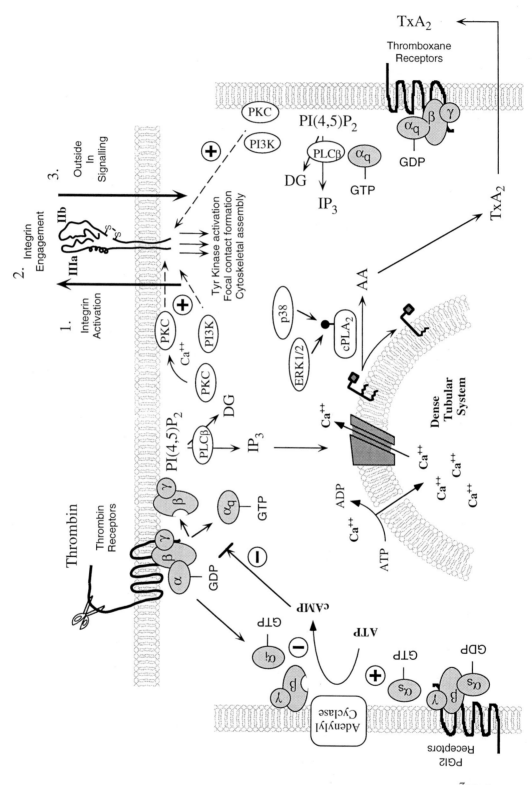

tor. When thrombin binds to and cleaves its receptor's N-terminus between residues Arg^{41} and Ser^{42}, a "tethered ligand" domain is exposed (i.e., the amino acid string, SFLLRN). It was research on thrombin receptors and PAR-2 that first led to the concept that a cleaveable cell surface receptor could initiate intracellular signaling. In the future, other proteases that can activate cells in a similar manner, through receptors on the cell surface, should be identified (37,38).

In platelets, adenylyl cyclase catalyzes formation of cyclic adenosine monophosphate (cAMP) from ATP. This promotes inhibition of platelet reactivity by blockade of calcium mobilization. Different types of G proteins can regulate adenylyl cyclase. Prostacyclin (PGI_2) from endothelial cells is another stimulus for adenylyl cyclase through the G protein G_s. Thrombin inhibits cAMP formation through the action of one of the forms of G_i that exist in platelets (37). Signal transduction during platelet activation is summarized and depicted in Figure 6-4.

Phosphorylation and Dephosphorylation Systems in Platelets

Levy-Toledano et al. (39) outlined several phosphorylation pathways occurring in the course of platelet activation:

1. Thrombin activates phospholipase C_β in a reaction stimulated by the heterotrimeric G_i subunit protein that is coupled to the seven-transmembrane domain receptor of thrombin. Phospholipase C acts on phosphatidylinositol 4,5-bisphosphate (PIP_2) in the membrane, leading to synthesis of the second messenger inositol-1,4,5-trisphosphate (IP_3), which mobilizes intracellular calcium, and diacylglyceride, which activates protein kinase C. The latter catalyzes phosphorylation of substrates at serine/threonine residues, such as myosin light chain (20 kd) and pleckstrin (47 kd). Hydrolysis of PIP_2 results from stimulation of phospholipase C_γ, which requires tyrosine kinase activity but is independent of G protein.

2. Thrombin increases levels of phosphotyrosines on several proteins. This function depends on integrin $\alpha_{IIb}\beta_3$ involvement and platelet aggregation. (Blockade of fibrinogen binding inhibits tyrosine phosphorylation). When platelets are tyrosine phosphorylated, there is activation and translocation of several nonreceptor protein-tyrosine kinases, such as the SRC family kinases (60 kd), SYK (72 kd), and FAK (125 kd). SYK also contains two SRC homology-2 (SH2) domains and one SH3 domain, which are involved in regulation of protein-protein interactions in platelets.

3. Platelet stimulation and activation of surface receptors results in activation of phosphoinositide 3-kinase. This important enzyme catalyzes phosphorylation of inositol phospholipids at the 3-position of the inositol ring (40,41). The phosphoinositide 3-kinase in platelets catalyzes formation of phosphatidylinositol 3,4-P_2 and phosphatidylinositol 3,4,5-P_3. These are important second messengers for platelet function (42).

4. Mitogen-activated protein kinase (MAP kinase) is an important signaling molecule that transfers receptor

FIG. 6-4. Pathways of signal transduction in response to platelet activation. When agonists bind to their receptors on the platelet membrane, several intracellular second messengers are activated. Phosphatidylinositol 4,5-bisphosphate (PIP_2) is hydrolyzed by phospholipase C_β (PLC_β) to generate inositol 1,4,5-trisphosphate (IP_3) and diacylglycerol (DG). PLC_β is activated by G protein, probably $G_{\beta\gamma}$ derived from G_i, in a manner that is sensitive to pertussis toxin. PLC_β is also activated in a pertussis toxin–resistant manner by a separate G protein, $G_{q\alpha}$ or $G11_\alpha$ or both. IP_3 releases calcium from the dense tubular system, resulting in an increase in free calcium concentration in the platelet cytosol. DG activates protein kinase C, which induces the platelet release reaction (inside-out signaling) and exposure of the fibrinogen receptor by reorientation of the gpIIb/IIIa complex. Fibrinogen binding to the gpIIb/IIIa complex (integrin engagement), is followed by outside-in signaling such as tyrosine kinase activation (43). The rise in cytosolic free calcium promotes arachidonic acid release as catalyzed by the cytosolic form of phospholipase A_2 ($cPLA_2$), culminating in thromboxane A_2 formation and release. Phospholipase A_2 may also be activated at the cell membrane by $G_{\beta\gamma}$ originating from one or more G proteins. The thromboxane A_2 formed from released arachidonate interacts with receptors on the platelet membrane, inducing further platelet activation. During the activation process, tyrosine kinases such as members of the SRC family are activated and phosphorylate a large variety of platelet proteins, many of which have not been precisely identified. In addition, focal contact formation occurs, as does cytoskeletal rearrangement (43). Tyrosine activation in platelets occurs at a later time than fibrinogen receptor exposure and platelet aggregation. The thrombin receptor is coupled to G proteins, as are the thromboxane and prostacyclin (PGI_2) receptors.

Platelet activation is always accompanied by a fall in cyclic adenosine monophosphate (cAMP). Elevations in cAMP block calcium mobilization, thereby inhibiting platelet reactivity (37). (Courtesy of Dr. Lawrence F. Brass.)

signals to multiple pathways. These pathways are used for signaling throughout the platelet cytoplasm. The MAP kinase pathway is stimulated by platelet agonist exposure. In this pathway, low-molecular-weight GTP-binding proteins such as RAS play a role.

Platelet protein kinases and phosphatases have an integrative activity and amplify signals induced by multiple receptors at the cell surface. Interactions among these kinases and phosphatases remain to be determined in detail, and their delineation will increase our comprehension of platelet phosphorylation and dephosphorylation systems. New information should emerge from gene knockout experiments, use of antibodies to the kinases and phosphatases, and development of highly specific inhibitors of individual kinases or phosphatases (39).

To summarize, on platelet activation an intracellular metabolic event (possibly protein kinase C activation) involves $\alpha_{IIb}\beta_3$, inducing its ability to engage fibrinogen on the extracellular domain of this receptor. This initiates an "outside-in" integrin signaling event through $\alpha_{IIb}\beta_3$, which is critical for platelet reactivity. Signaling proteins such as SYK and FAK become increasingly tyrosine phosphorylated, calcium is mobilized, calpain is activated, and the cytoskeleton undergoes reorganization (39) (see Fig. 6-4).

Integrin Signaling in Platelet Function

The integrin class of receptors is required for development of vascular and hematopoietic cells, angiogenesis, cell migration in response to injury, and assembly of extracellular matrix. The platelet integrin $\alpha_{IIb}\beta_3$ is mandatory for hemostasis (43). The outstanding work of Coller has led to development of a therapeutic agent that inhibits $\alpha_{IIb}\beta_3$ (17,18).

Integrins are composed of noncovalent $\alpha\beta$ heterodimers. Subunits consist of a large NH_2-terminal extracellular domain, a single domain that spans the membrane, and a COOH-terminal cytoplasmic tail. Numerous α- and β-subunits have been cloned, and there are at least 20 different $\alpha\beta$ pairings in various tissues. Although integrins were originally thought to function solely as adhesive proteins, it is now recognized that they play an equally important role as receptors in signaling. Shattil and Ginsberg (43) defined integrin signaling as the ability of these receptors to transmit biochemical messages in both directions across the cell surface.

Integrins can also regulate gene expression, cell growth and differentiation, and survival through the mechanism of outside-in signalling. Ligand-occupied and clustered integrins control both cell shape and organization of the cytoskeleton. In addition, ligand-engaged integrins can generate a broad spectrum of biochemical signals. Integrin-triggered reactions include activation of protein-tyrosine kinases such as pp60[SRC], pp125[FAK], and pp72[SYK]. They can also activate phosphatidylinositol 3-kinase and MAP kinases. These activation steps are initiated by means of other agonist receptors, such as those that interact with growth factors and cytokines. The initial focus of integrin signaling is topographic, on locations of the cell surface where cell-cell and cell-extracellular matrix contact takes place. These reactions involve alterations in cell shape, polarization, and motility—all of which are classified as "anchorage-dependent" changes (43).

Integrins have the capacity to promote extracellular effector responses as they undergo ligand engagement during activation. Binding of ligands is regulated by signaling mechanisms in the cell, a process called *integrin activation* or "inside-out signaling." By this means, intracellular signals are translated into extracellular activation.

The initial binding of soluble fibrinogen or vWF to $\alpha_{IIb}\beta_3$ is controlled by affinity modulation. When affinity is modified, it is implied that a structural change has occurred in the integrin heterodimer, resulting in stronger ligand binding. Various affinity states have been studied in integrins of several β classes, using soluble ligands that specifically induce cell activation. The different affinity states probably reflect conformational changes in and between receptor subunits. These ultimately influence the shape or accessibility of the ligand-binding interface.

Antithrombotic medications currently in use probably function by regulating the capacity of platelet-signaling mechanisms to initiate conformational changes in $\alpha_{IIb}\beta_3$. A high-affinity state may not always be beneficial. When there is high integrin affinity, migration can be blocked if substrate and integrin densities are also elevated. In addition, the ability of cells to assemble a fibronectin matrix is regulated by the activation state of integrins (43).

Integrins cluster or multimerize on the plasma membrane (44). Clusters of ligand-occupied integrins in adherent cells such as platelets, endothelial cells, and vascular smooth muscle can be observed by light microscopy. These clusters form small, focal complexes that assemble during activated platelet filopodial extension. Larger focal adhesions connect with actin stress fibers and assemble during late stages of platelet spreading. Filopodia and focal adhesions are regulated by the *rho* group of GTPases; they form a link between *rho* signaling and integrin function. Focal complexes and focal adhesions contain a broad spectrum of signaling molecules and cytoskeletal proteins. Assembly and disassembly of these complexes is essential for platelet reactivity and vascular cell migration.

The cytoplasmic domains of integrins are critical for integrin signaling because they interface with signaling components of the cell. Most integrin tails range from about 20 to 70 amino acid residues in size. If membrane-distal sequences of β cytoplasmic tails are mutated or truncated, integrin-initiated signaling and cytoskeletal organization are disrupted.

A large number of proteins can bind directly to integrin cytoplasmic tails (some to α tails, others to β tails) (43). Although many binding proteins have been identified, the role of this binding in cell function is unknown. Some binding proteins are part of the cytoskeletal compartment (α-actinin, filamin, talin), and others have kinase activity (pp125^{FAK}, integrin-linked kinase [ILK]). Some have guanine nucleotide exchange activity (cytohesin-1), and others function as adaptors (paxillin). Calrecticulin binds to the membrane-proximal portion of α cytoplasmic tails. This protein is found in several subcellular compartments and may be involved with other adhesion receptors and cytoskeletal proteins. Calrecticulin-null embryonic stem cells do not participate in integrin-mediated cell adhesion and calcium influx.

Integrin signaling also involves association of integrins with other transmembrane proteins. β$_3$ integrins interact with the integrin-associated protein, CD47. This could function in regulation of neutrophil phagocytosis in response to ligand agonists. CD9, CD63, and CD81 belong to the tetraspanin class of transmembrane proteins. When detergent extracts are prepared from some cells, the tetraspanins coprecipitate with integrins. These associations can be promoted by antibody crosslinking of integrins. Therefore, tetraspanins may be involved in regulation of integrin signaling and cell migration. Tetraspanins and integrins are also physically associated with phosphatidylinositol 4-kinase. This suggests a relation between integrins and phosphatidylinositol metabolism (43,44).

In some instances, β$_1$ integrins promote cell growth, and in others, they promote differentiation. Correlations have been made between growth promotion and the ability of β$_2$ integrins to activate the MAP kinase pathway through the adaptor, SHC. Formation of physical complexes with SHC correlates with associations between extracellular or transmembrane domains of the integrin α-subunit and caveolin. The latter protein may provide a supporting framework for signaling molecules (44).

In summary, the adhesive and signaling functions of integrins are very important for control of the reactivity of platelets and inflammatory cells. Specific roles have been identified for integrin signaling events in angiogenesis, cell migration during development, hemostasis, inflammation, and wound repair. Unwanted or uncontrolled integrin signaling is probably involved in the pathogenesis of occlusive vascular diseases and atherosclerosis, as well as angiogenesis in diseases such as diabetic retinopathy (43,44).

THROMBOREGULATION

Thromboregulation is defined as a group of processes by which circulating blood cells and cells of the vessel wall interact to regulate development of a thrombus. Most thromboregulatory activities occur in the setting of cell-cell interactions. The reactions are biochemical in nature and can result in formation of biologically active metabolites that could only have arisen through interactions between heterogeneous cell types in the vasculature (5,13,19,33,45,46).

Thromboregulators are mainly responsible for maintenance of blood fluidity *in vivo*. They prevent or reverse platelet accumulation, activation of coagulation factors, and the fibrin formation that these processes produce. These defense systems can be overwhelmed by vascular injury in the form of a fissured or fractured atherosclerotic plaque, disturbances in blood flow, or inactivation or destruction of cell-associated or fluid-phase thromboregulators. The fibrinolytic system also participates in thromboregulation by preventing excessive fibrin formation and enhancing its removal (5,8).

Currently known thromboregulators can be classified according to their chronologic modalities of action in relation to thrombin formation (Table 6-1). For example, the protein C–protein S natural anticoagulant system is operative *after* thrombin has formed at an injury site. Thrombin then enters the fluid phase of the microenvironment and binds thrombomodulin on the proximal endothelial cell surface. In arterial thrombosis, thromboregulatory mechanisms are nullified by the agonistic effect of injured tissue and tissue factor (14). Alternatively, these thromboregulatory mechanisms fail and the natural proclivity toward fibrin formation at the site of injury escapes regulation. The ADPase/CD39 system is operative very early in the hemostatic/thrombotic cascade.

Cell-Cell Interactions and Transcellular Metabolism

When the morphology of evolving thrombi was initially studied by light and electron microscopy, erythrocytes, neutrophils, and platelet components could be seen in close proximity (Fig. 6-5). These associations were initially interpreted as passive in nature. Cells other than platelets were not thought to be biochemical participants in the formation of a thrombus. However, both *in vitro* evidence and clinical correlations now support the con-

---

TABLE 6-1. *Classification of vascular thromboregulators*

Early thromboregulators
  (inhibit events preceding thrombin formation)
Nitric oxide (NO)
Eicosanoids (prostacyclin, PGD$_2$)
Endothelial cell ecto-ADPase/CD39
Late thromboregulators
  (exert effects after thrombin formation)
Antithrombin III
Endothelial cell/heparan proteoglycans
Tissue factor pathway inhibitor (TFPI)
Thrombomodulin–protein C–protein S pathway
Proteins of the fibrinolytic system

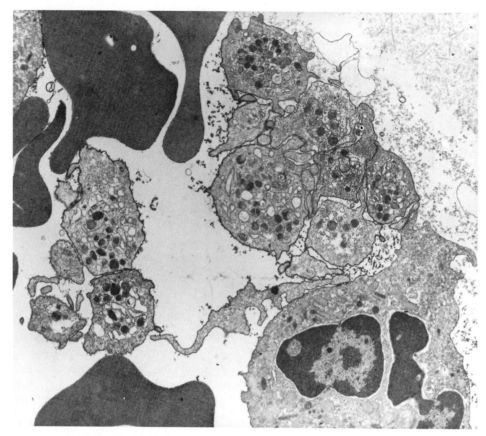

FIG. 6-5. Electron micrograph of an evolving thrombus after addition of adenosine diphosphate to whole blood. Platelets have partially degranulated and are in the process of forming an aggregate. Erythrocytes can be seen in close proximity and in some areas actually making contact with the platelet surface. Such erythrocytes, when exposed to activated platelets, release material that promotes platelet reactivity. A neutrophil can be seen in the lower right portion of the figure, also making contact with activated platelets. Neutrophils under these circumstances release material that inhibits platelet reactivity. These interactions are described in detail in the text and are comparable to sections 6 and 7 of Figure 6-2. (Courtesy of Dr. Dorothea Zucker-Franklin, Department of Medicine, New York University School of Medicine, New York, New York.)

cepts already mentioned: erythrocytes enhance platelet activation and recruitment (34,36), whereas neutrophils inhibit platelet reactivity and may play a role in limiting the size and extent of a thrombus (5,8,13,19,27,31,35).

These cell-cell interactions occur in addition to those described for platelets and endothelial cells (45-47). Besides direct metabolic interchange between cellular components of a thrombus, there is another form of cell communication via the eicosanoid pathway, known as *transcellular metabolism* (26,32,33,45,48). Studies of this pathway have been elegantly developed by Serhan et al., especially with regard to the lipoxin group of autacoids (25,26,48).

Initial studies of eicosanoids focused on arachidonic acid mobilization and metabolism in single cell types; this is summarized in Figure 6-6. It is now known that eicosanoid metabolism also takes place between different cell types in close proximity. Reactive eicosanoid precursors and reactive intermediates can traverse the fluid phase between neighboring cells, thereby giving rise to

biologically active metabolites with properties different from those normally synthesized by either cell alone. Cell-cell interactions and transcellular metabolism are important modalities for the amplification and generation of eicosanoid-derived inflammatory mediators, especially those catalyzed by lipoxygenase enzymes in various cells. All of these lipoxygenase-driven reactions are insensitive to aspirin and, in fact, are frequently enhanced after aspirin ingestion. These systems are of potential significance for hemostasis, thrombosis, and the inflammatory response (25,27,32,33,45). My colleagues and I have proposed a working classification of cell-cell interactions and transcellular biosynthesis in the eicosanoid pathway (49); this is shown in Table 6-2.

An example of type IA interactions is the utilization of platelet-derived endoperoxides by endothelial cells that have been pretreated with aspirin. This results in the formation of PGI_2 from released platelet endoperoxides (47). In type IB interactions, a cell cannot produce a precursor endogenously but can further process a precursor

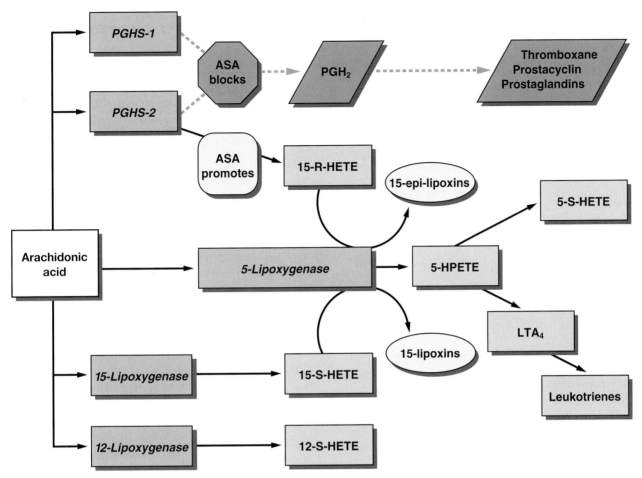

FIG. 6-6. In response to inflammatory or prothrombotic stimuli, arachidonic acid, an essential fatty acid, is released from cell membrane phospholipids. It is metabolized by two classes of oxygenases: prostaglandin-H endoperoxide synthases (PGHS-1 and -2, also known as cyclooxygenases) and lipoxygenases. PGHS-1 and -2 catalyze the insertion of two molecules of oxygen into arachidonic acid to form prostaglandin endoperoxide (PGH_2), which is then converted to thromboxane A_2 in platelets, prostacyclin (PGI_2) in endothelial cells, and other prostaglandins. Aspirin (ASA) completely blocks formation of PGH_2 and its metabolites by irreversibly acetylating serine in the active site of PGHS-1 and -2. However, in contrast to PGHS-1, PGHS-2, an independent gene product, retains its capacity to add one molecule of oxygen to the C15 position of arachidonic acid, even when acetylated. Aspirin-treated cells induced by inflammatory stimuli to express PGHS-2 therefore can produce the monohydroxy fatty acid (15R)-hydroxyeicosatetraenoic acid, or (15R)-HETE. The second class of oxygenases (5-, 12-, and 15-lipoxygenases) are insensitive to ASA. They catalyze the production of an abundance of the monohydroxy fatty acids (5S)-HETE, (12S)-HETE, and (15S)-HETE. When the enzyme activity of PGHS-1 and -2 is inhibited by ASA, more arachidonic acid is available for lipoxygenase metabolism (aspirin shunt). Various types of cells interact to metabolize (15S)-HETE and other lipoxygenase metabolites (by transcellular metabolism) to products including the lipoxins (25). (Modified from ref. 66, with permission.)

obtained from another stimulated cell. For example, the erythrocyte can transform leukotriene A_4, obtained from a stimulated neutrophil, to leukotriene B_4 (50). In addition, platelets can generate leukotriene C_4 from leukotriene A_4 (51). This reaction is of clinical significance because leukotriene C_4 production is not blocked by aspirin and this autacoid is a vasoconstrictor (13,19).

The type IIA reaction occurs when neutrophils and platelets are exposed to a common agonist, such as calcium ionophore A23187. Released platelet 12-HETE is used by activated neutrophils for production of (5S,12S)-diHETE (45). Of critical importance for understanding of type IIA reactions was the elucidation by Serhan of 5-lipoxygenase-initiated lipoxin synthesis (25,48): the 5-lipoxygenase from activated neutrophils and the 12-lipoxygenase from activated platelets promote the formation of lipoxins A_4 and B_4 (52). Just as neutrophils can convert platelet-derived 12-HETE into (5S,12S)-diHETE, so 5-HETE from activated neutrophils can be converted to (5S,12S)-diHETE by activated platelets. This interaction diverts neutrophil production of the proinflammatory molecule leukotriene B_4. These dihydroxy acid

TABLE 6-2. *Generation of new mediators via cell-cell interactions and transcellular metabolism in the eicosanoid pathway*

Type I:	**Common eicosanoid precursors can be shared by different cells.**
Type IA:	In addition to generating its own precursor, a cell can obtain the same compounds from another; more end product is thereby synthesized.
Type IB:	A cell cannot synthesize a precursor endogenously but can obtain it from a stimulated neighboring cell and use it for novel eicosanoid synthesis.
Type II:	**A cell can transform an eicosanoid from a neighboring cell into a new metabolite that neither cell alone can synthesize.**
Type IIA:	Both cells are activated by a common agonist.
Type IIB:	An activated cell produces an eicosanoid that an unstimulated cell in proximity can use for generating a new metabolite.
Type III:	**An intermediate or eicosanoid generated by one cell can serve as an agonist or inhibitor for biosynthesis of a different type of eicosanoid from a neighboring cell.**
	A leukotriene can serve as agonist for thromboxane production.

eicosanoids can serve as antiinflammatory compounds by an indirect mechanism (26).

In type IIB reactions, only one of the two cell types under study is activated. For example, if thrombin or collagen is added to a combined suspension of neutrophils and platelets, released platelet 12-HETE will be metabolized by the unstimulated neutrophils to 12,20-diHETE. (Thrombin and collagen do not activate neutrophils.)

In type III cell-cell interactions, eicosanoids themselves serve as agonists for production of other eicosanoids in a different cell type. For example, leukotrienes can serve as agonists for thromboxane release in perfused lung preparations (53).

Such developments in eicosanoid research have provided answers *in vitro* and *in vivo* for phenomena that could not be explained previously (27) (see Table 6-2). Furthermore, these reactions demonstrate a direct relation between thrombosis and the inflammatory response (25). As a result, comprehension of the involvement of eicosanoids in host response systems has been greatly amplified. Novel eicosanoids have been discovered, several receptors have been identified and cloned, and it is now understood that these lipid mediators are critical for signal transduction and cell-cell communication (25). Relations among precursors, intermediates, and end products in the eicosanoid pathways are depicted in Figure 6-6.

Blockade of Platelet Activation and Recruitment by Endothelial Cell Ecto-ADPase/CD39

As emphasized previously, appreciation of the importance of vascular cell-cell interactions and transcellular metabolism in thrombosis and inflammation has markedly increased in recent years (13,19,26,31). This is particularly pertinent with regard to platelets and endothelial cells. My colleagues and I currently hypothesize that endothelial cells control platelet reactivity by at least three mechanisms (see Table 6-1): a cell-associated

ecto-ADPase system and two fluid-phase reactants— eicosanoids such as PGI$_2$ and the relaxing factor nitric oxide (NO), which is generated by endothelium (54,55).

In previous work, we demonstrated inhibition of platelet aggregation by PGI$_2$ synthesized by aspirin-treated endothelial cells from platelet endoperoxides (47). We subsequently performed experiments in which NO production was neutralized by hemoglobin and both platelets and endothelial cells were treated with aspirin, resulting in total blockade of PGI$_2$ production. Biochemical and functional data indicated that these aspirin-treated, NO-deficient endothelial cells were actually inhibiting platelet function via a mechanism involving metabolism of ADP with consequent loss of this nucleotide's ability to induce platelet activation and platelet recruitment (56). We found that when aspirin-treated, washed platelets were stimulated by agonists in the presence of aspirin-treated endothelial cells, platelet aggregation and recruitment were inhibited (Fig. 6-7).

To establish whether ADPase activity was present on cultured human umbilical vein endothelial cells (HUVEC) and could account for their platelet-inhibitory properties, biochemical and functional assays were developed (56). Carbon 14–labeled ADP was incubated with aspirin-treated HUVEC for increasing periods. After removal of the cells, supernatants were examined for content of residual [^{14}C]ADP and its metabolites. In addition, the platelet-aggregating potential of supernatant fluid containing unmetabolized [^{14}C]ADP was examined. HUVEC induced a progressive decrease in [^{14}C]ADP concentration, which was paralleled by a loss of proaggregatory activity of the supernatant fluid. Thin-layer chromatography was performed with radiographic scans of the metabolites of [^{14}C]ADP after 5, 10, and 30 minutes of incubation with aspirin-treated HUVEC suspensions. At 5 minutes, ADP had fallen to account for 51% of total nucleotides, nucleosides, and bases. In addition, AMP (28%) and inosine (13%) were identified, together with trace quantities of adenosine, hypoxanthine, and

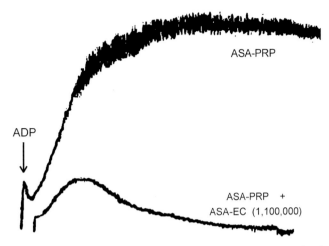

FIG. 6-7. Platelet-rich plasma from a donor who had ingested aspirin (ASA-PRP) was fully aggregated by adenosine diphosphate (ADP). In contrast, when this plasma was stimulated in the presence of 10^6 aspirin-treated endothelial cells (ASA-EC), the inhibited aggregation curve demonstrated a brief ascending limb, followed by reversal to baseline. This pattern of reversibility was reminiscent of previous experiments in which ADP released from platelets by agonists was intentionally removed by addition of purified apyrase. Subsequently, the endothelial cell membrane component responsible for the inhibition was shown to be an apyrase identical to CD39 (46,56).

adenine. After 30 minutes, inosine (85%) was the major [^{14}C]ADP metabolite and ADP itself was virtually absent. This absence of ADP correlated with total loss of aggregatory activity of the aspirin-treated endothelial cell supernatant. These studies indicated that ADP hydrolysis by endothelial cells is a major mechanism underlying their inhibitory effect on stimulated platelets (19,56).

The results suggested that the HUVEC ADPase is a membrane-associated ectonucleotidase of the E type (57). This was verified by calcium/magnesium dependence, the ineffectiveness of specific inhibitors of P-, F-, and V-type ATPases, and the capacity to metabolize both ATP and ADP but not AMP. These findings identified the human endothelial cell enzyme as an apyrase (ATP diphosphohydrolase, ATPDase, EC3.6.1.5).

Research on ectonucleotidases had always been encumbered by difficulties in isolation related to their low abundance, relatively high activity, and sensitivity to denaturing agents (46,57-62). In 1996, Handa and Guidotti purified and cloned a soluble ATPDase (apyrase) from potato tubers (63). Sequence analysis revealed 25% amino acid identity and 48% amino acid homology with human CD39. The latter, a lymphoid cell activation antigen, had been cloned and structurally characterized by Maliszewski et al. (64). CD39 is a cell-surface glycoprotein that is expressed in activated natural killer cells, B cells, and subsets of T cells. It has also been identified in some human endothelial cell lines (65). Based on these reports, we hypothesized that the human endothelial cell ecto-ADPase was identical to CD39.

Experimental data were developed which established identity between CD39 and the human endothelial cell ecto-ADPase (46,61,62). We tested whether antibodies against human CD39 would recognize ADPase on cultured HUVEC. Lysates from intact HUVEC were incubated with CD39 antibodies, and the resulting immunoprecipitates demonstrated ADPase activity in this assay system (46). When serial immunoprecipitation with a monoclonal antibody was used, more than 95% of the ADPase activity was removed from a purified HUVEC ADPase preparation. CD39 was responsible for more than 95% of the HUVEC ecto-ADPase activity.

Our hypothesis that the human endothelial cell ecto-ADPase was CD39 was further verified by transient transfection of COS cells with plasmids containing the human or murine CD39 sequence. Transfected COS cells acquired ADPase activity that was comparable to or greater than that of HUVEC. Microsomal membrane preparations from transfected COS cells also displayed ADPase activity.

We also compared human endothelial cell mRNA with recombinant human CD39 cDNA. Endothelial cell mRNA was analyzed by reverse transcriptase–polymerase chain reaction (RT-PCR) using four separate primer pairs derived from the original sequence of human CD39 (64). Emphasis was placed on the NH_2-terminal portion, which represents the enzymatic domain. Then, pHuCD39 cDNA was used for direct comparison of PCR product sizes. The PCR products of HUVEC and pHuCD39 were of similar size for each of four fragments spanning 1,144 of the 1,529 bp of the human CD39 coding sequence. Sequence analysis of gel-purified PCR products confirmed 100% identity between HUVEC CD39 and the published CD39 sequence (46).

Northern blot analyses using a probe derived from pHuCD39 cDNA revealed that mRNA for CD39 in human endothelial cells was expressed in the same band pattern as MP-1 cells. MP-1 is the Epstein-Barr virus–transformed B-cell line from which CD39 was originally cloned (64). The message from pHuCD39-transfected COS cells corresponded to the 1.9-kb cloned species.

We reasoned that if HUVEC ecto-ADPase and CD39 were identical, the CD39-bearing cells should induce blockade or reversal of platelet responsiveness to the agonist, ADP. This hypothesis was verified with the use of CD39-expressing cells, both endogenous (endothelial and MP-1) cells and COS cells transfected with pHuCD39 or its murine equivalent, pMuCD39. When any of these three types of cells was combined with platelet-rich plasma, platelet reactivity to 10 μmol/L ADP was reversed within

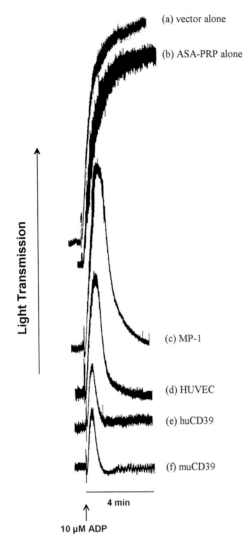

(a) vector alone

(b) ASA-PRP alone

Light Transmission

(c) MP-1

(d) HUVEC

(e) huCD39

(f) muCD39

4 min

↑
10 µM ADP

FIG. 6-8. Demonstration of blockade and reversal of platelet aggregation in response to adenosine diphosphate (ADP) by intact human umbilical vein endothelial cells (HUVEC), MP-1 cells from which CD39 was originally cloned, and COS cells transfected with full-length CD39. Aspirin-treated platelet-rich plasma (ASA-PRP) was stimulated with 10 µmol/L ADP, and the aggregation response was measured over a 4-minute period. Addition of COS cells transfected with vector alone resulted in a full aggregation response (**A**), indistinguishable from the response with ASA-PRP alone (**B**). **C**: MP-1 cells reversed the aggregation response. **D**: Intact HUVEC also reversed the aggregation response to ADP, to a slightly greater degree than did MP-1 cells. COS cells transfected with either pHuCD39 (**E**) or pMuCD39 (**F**) demonstrated an even greater inhibitory effect on platelet responsiveness than HUVEC. This correlated with their higher degree of biochemical ecto-ADPase activity (46).

60 seconds. MP-1 cells, which express both CD39 antigen and ecto-ADPase activity, also inhibited ADP-induced platelet aggregation (Fig. 6-8).

Results of these studies are particularly pertinent for the concept highlighted in this chapter—thromboregulation. The three known thromboregulators—eicosanoids, NO, and the ecto-ADPase—have important biologic properties that merit consideration for therapeutic intervention. Aspirin treatment does eliminate the prothrombotic action of thromboxane, but it also prevents formation of PGI$_2$, which limits its therapeutic effectiveness. NO is an aspirin-insensitive inhibitor of platelet function, but it is inhibited itself *in vitro* and *in vivo* by hemoglobin as it rapidly diffuses into erythrocytes.

In contrast, ecto-ADPase/CD39 is aspirin insensitive and completely inhibits platelet reactivity, even when eicosanoid formation and NO production are blocked. An emerging concept in vascular biology is that ADPase/CD39 is an effective physiologic and constitutively expressed endothelial cell inhibitor of platelet reactivity. ADPase/CD39 may form the nidus for a new class of antithromboerapeutic agents. Figure 6-9 illustrates the possible mode of action of ecto-ADPase/CD39.

Summary and Future Perspectives

This chapter has emphasized that thrombosis and atherosclerosis are essentially multicellular processes, the course of which may be modulated by varying degrees of cell contact, activation, and secretion. During the development of occlusive vascular diseases, thrombotic and proinflammatory events are biochemically linked as parts of host defense mechanisms. Functional, biochemical, and molecular biologic determinations of the interactions among cell components of thrombi and fluid-phase reactants have yielded new information relevant to the pathogenesis of thrombosis and the inflammatory response.

This information presents new therapeutic opportunities. Upregulation of endogenous ecto-ADPase/CD39 would be advantageous, as would its development as an antithrombotic agent to be administered *in vivo*. Therapeutic agents to complement aspirin administration as currently employed should prove fruitful. A "global" multicellular approach toward prevention and treatment of vascular occlusion may be conceptually more complicated than traditional unicellular modalities, but it may offer more antithrombotic potential and greater safety.

ACKNOWLEDGMENT

The author wishes to thank Dr. M. Johan Broekman for critical review of the manuscript. Research in our laboratory was supported in part by a Merit Review grant from the Department of Veterans Affairs, and by National Institutes of Health grants HL 47073, HL 46403, and the Isadore Rosenfeld Heart Foundation.

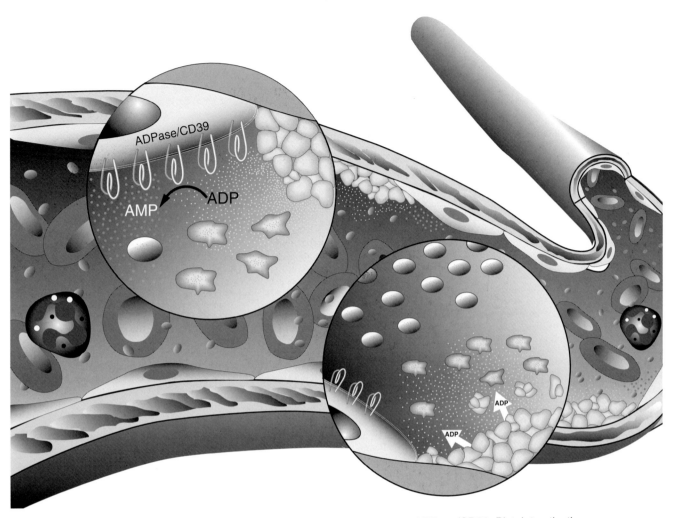

FIG. 6-9. Depiction of thromboregulation by endothelial cell ecto-ADPase/CD39. Platelet activation on or proximal to a site of vascular injury induces secretion of adenosine diphosphate (ADP) from platelet dense granules (*inset, lower right*). Released ADP activates and thereby recruits additional platelets arriving in the local microenvironment into the evolving thrombus (20). Activation and recruitment of platelets in proximity to endothelial cells is inhibited by metabolism of released ADP to adenosine monophosphate (AMP) by endothelial cell ecto-ADPase/CD39. These platelets return to an unstimulated state, thereby limiting thrombus formation (*inset, upper left*). Ecto-ADPase/CD39 has been identified and functionally characterized as a physiologic, constitutively expressed thromboregulator (46,56).

REFERENCES

1. Dieterlen-Lievre F. Birds. In: Rowley AF, Ratcliffe NA, eds. *Vertebrate blood cells.* Cambridge: Cambridge University Press, 1988:257–336.
2. Sypek J, Borysenko M. Reptiles. In: Rowley AF, Ratcliffe NA, eds. *Vertebrate blood cells.* Cambridge: Cambridge University Press, 1988: 211–256.
3. Isenberg WM, Bainton DF. Megakaryocyte and platelet structure. In: Hoffman R, Benz EJ Jr, Shattil SJ, Furie B, Cohen HJ, Silberstein LE, eds. *Hematology: Basic principles and practice,* 2nd ed. New York: Churchill Livingstone, 1995:1516–1524.
4. Brandt JT. Overview of hemostasis. In: McClatchey KD, ed. *Clinical laboratory medicine.* Baltimore: Williams & Wilkins, 1994:1045–1062.
5. Marcus AJ. Platelets and their disorders. In: Ratnoff OD, Forbes CD, eds. *Disorders of Hemostasis,* 3rd ed. Philadelphia: WB Saunders, 1996:79–137.
6. Kaushansky K. Thrombopoietin: Platelets on demand? *Ann Intern Med* 1997;126:731–733.
7. Ware JA, Coller BS. Platelet morphology, biochemistry, and function. In: Beutler E, Lichtman MA, Coller BS, Kipps TJ, eds. *Williams hematology,* 5th ed. New York: McGraw-Hill, 1995:1161–1201.
8. Marcus AJ. Platelet activation. In: Fuster V, Ross R, Topol EJ, eds. *Atherosclerosis and coronary artery disease,* vol 1. Philadelphia: Lippincott-Raven, 1996:607–637.
9. Marcus AJ, Zucker-Franklin D, Safier LB, et al. Studies on human platelet granules and membranes. *J Clin Invest* 1966;45:14–28.
10. Nesheim ME, Eid S, Mann KG. Assembly of the prothrombinase complex in the absence of prothrombin. *J Biol Chem* 1981;256:9874–9882.
11. Ross R. The pathogenesis of atherosclerosis: A perspective for the 1990s. *Nature* 1993;362:801–809.
12. Ross R. Cell biology of atherosclerosis. *Annu Rev Physiol* 1995;57: 791–804.
13. Marcus AJ, Hajjar DP. Vascular transcellular signalling. *J Lipid Res* 1993;34:2017–2032.
14. Taubman MB, Fallon JT, Schecter AD, et al. Tissue factor in the pathogenesis of atherosclerosis. *Thromb Haemost* 1997;78:200–204.

15. Ruggeri ZM. von Willebrand factor. *J Clin Invest* 1997;99:559–564.

16. Plow EF, Ginsberg MH. Molecular basis of platelet function. In: Hoffman R, Benz EJ Jr, Shattil SJ, Furie B, Cohen HJ, Silberstein LE, eds. *Hematology: Basic principles and practice,* 2nd ed. New York: Churchill Livingstone, 1995:1524–1535.

17. Jordan RE, Wagner CL, Mascelli MA, et al. Preclinical development of c7E3 Fab; a mouse/human chimeric monoclonal antibody fragment that inhibits platelet function by blockade of GPIIb/IIIa receptors with observations on the immunogenicity of c7E3 Fab in humans. In: Horton MA, ed. *Adhesion receptors as therapeutic targets.* Boca Raton, FL: CRC Press, 1996:281–305.

18. Coller BS. Platelet GPIIb/IIIa antagonists: The first anti-integrin receptor therapeutics. *J Clin Invest* 1997;99:1467–1471.

19. Marcus AJ, Safier LB. Thromboregulation: Multicellular modulation of platelet reactivity in hemostasis and thrombosis. *FASEB J* 1993;7:516–522.

20. Hagberg IA, Roald HE, Lyberg T. Platelet activation in flowing blood passing growing arterial thrombi. *Arterioscler Thromb Vasc Biol* 1997;17:1331–1336.

21. Berman CL, Yeo EL, Wencel-Drake JD, et al. A platelet alpha granule membrane protein that is associated with the plasma membrane after activation: Characterization and subcellular localization of platelet activation-dependent granule-external membrane protein. *J Clin Invest* 1986;78:130–137.

22. McEver RP. Leukocyte interactions mediated by selectins. *Thromb Haemost* 1991;66:80–87.

23. Frenette PS, Wagner DD. Insights into selectin function from knockout mice. *Thromb Haemost* 1997;78:60–64.

24. Bevilacqua MP, Nelson RM. Selectins. *J Clin Invest* 1993;91:379–387.

25. Serhan CN, Haeggstrom JZ, Leslie CC. Lipid mediator networks in cell signaling: Update and impact of cytokines. *FASEB J* 1996;10:1147–1158.

26. Serhan CN. Lipoxins and novel aspirin-triggered 15-epi-lipoxins (ATL): A jungle of cell-cell interactions or a therapeutic opportunity? *Prostaglandins* 1997;53:107–137.

27. Marcus AJ. Cellular interactions of platelets in thrombosis. In: Loscalzo J, Schafer AI, eds. *Thrombosis and hemorrhage.* Boston: Blackwell Scientific Publications, 1994:279–289.

28. Meade EA, Smith WL, DeWitt DL: Differential inhibition of prostaglandin endoperoxide synthase (cyclooxygenase) isozymes by aspirin and other non-steroidal anti-inflammatory drugs. *J Biol Chem* 1993;268:6610–6614.

29. Ohashi K, Ruan K-H, Kulmacz RJ, et al. Primary structure of human thromboxane synthase determined from the cDNA sequence. *J Biol Chem* 1992;267:789–793.

30. Smith WL. Prostanoid biosynthesis and mechanisms of action. *Am J Physiol* 1992;263:F181–F191.

31. Karim S, Habib A, Levy-Toledano S, et al. Cyclooxygenases-1 and -2 of endothelial cells utilize exogenous or endogenous arachidonic acid for transcellular production of thromboxane. *J Biol Chem* 1996;271:12042–12048.

32. Marcus AJ, Safier LB, Ullman HL, et al. Platelet-neutrophil interactions: (12S)-Hydroxyeicosatetraen-1,20-dioic acid, a new eicosanoid synthesized by unstimulated neutrophils from (12S)-20-dihydroxyeicosatetraenoic acid. *J Biol Chem* 1988;263:2223–2229.

33. Marcus AJ, Broekman MJ, Safier LB, et al. Formation of leukotrienes and other hydroxy acids during platelet-neutrophil interactions in vitro. *Biochem Biophys Res Commun* 1982;109:130–137.

34. Santos MT, Valles J, Marcus AJ, et al. Enhancement of platelet reactivity and modulation of eicosanoid production by intact erythrocytes. *J Clin Invest* 1991;87:571–580.

35. Valles J, Santos MT, Marcus AJ, et al. Down-regulation of human platelet reactivity by neutrophils: participation of lipoxygenase derivatives and adhesive proteins. *J Clin Invest* 1993;92:1357–1365.

36. Santos MT, Valles J, Aznar J, et al. Prothrombotic effects of erythrocytes on platelet reactivity: Reduction by aspirin. *Circulation* 1997;95:63–68.

37. Brass LF. Molecular basis for platelet activation. In: Hoffman R, Benz EJ Jr, Shattil SJ, Furie B, Cohen HJ, Silberstein LE, eds. *Hematology: Basic principles and practice,* 2nd ed. New York: Churchill Livingstone, 1995:1536–1552.

38. Brass LF, Molino M. Protease-activated G protein-coupled receptors on human platelets and endothelial cells. *Thromb Haemost* 1997;78:234–241.

39. Levy-Toledano S, Gallet C, Nadal F, et al. Phosphorylation and dephosphorylation mechanisms in platelet function: A tightly regulated balance. *Thromb Haemost* 1997;78:226–233.

40. Rittenhouse SE. Phosphoinositide 3-kinase activation and platelet function. *Blood* 1996;88:4401–4414.

41. Vanhaesebroeck B, Leevers SJ, Panayotou G, et al. Phosphoinositide 3-kinases: A conserved family of signal transducers. *Trends Biochem Sci* 1997;22:267–272.

42. Kucera GL, Rittenhouse SE. Human platelets form 3-phosphorylated phosphoinositides in response to alpha-thrombin, U46619, or GTP gamma S. *J Biol Chem* 1990;265:5345–5348.

43. Shattil SJ, Ginsberg MH. Perspectives series: Cell adhesion in vascular biology. Integrin signaling in vascular biology. *J Clin Invest* 1997;100:1–5.

44. Shattil SJ, Gao JB, Kashiwagi H. Not just another pretty face: Regulation of platelet function at the cytoplasmic face of integrin $\alpha_{IIb}\beta_3$. *Thromb Haemost* 1997;78:220–225.

45. Marcus AJ, Safier LB, Ullman HL, et al. 12S,20-Dihydroxyicosatetraenoic acid: A new icosanoid synthesized by neutrophils from 12S-hydroxyicosatetraenoic acid produced by thrombin- or collagen-stimulated platelets. *Proc Natl Acad Sci U S A* 1984;81:903–907.

46. Marcus AJ, Broekman MJ, Drosopoulos JHF, et al. The endothelial cell ecto-ADPase responsible for inhibition of platelet function is CD39. *J Clin Invest* 1997;99:1351–1360.

47. Marcus AJ, Weksler BB, Jaffe EA, et al. Synthesis of prostacyclin from platelet-derived endoperoxides by cultured human endothelial cells. *J Clin Invest* 1980;66:979–986.

48. Takano T, Fiore S, Maddox JF, et al. Aspirin-triggered 15-epi-lipoxin A4 (LXA4) and LXA4 stable analogues are potent inhibitors of acute inflammation: Evidence for anti-inflammatory receptors. *J Exp Med* 1997;185:1693–1704.

49. Marcus AJ. Eicosanoid interactions between platelets, endothelial cells, and neutrophils. *Methods Enzymol* 1990;187:585–598.

50. Fitzpatrick FA, Liggett W, McGee J, et al. Metabolism of leukotriene A4 by human erythrocytes: A novel cellular source of leukotriene B4. *J Biol Chem* 1984;259:11403–11407.

51. Maclouf J, Murphy RC. Transcellular metabolism of neutrophil-derived leukotriene A$_4$ by human platelets: A potential cellular source of leukotriene C$_4$. *J Biol Chem* 1988;263:174–181.

52. George JN, Nurden AT. Inherited disorders of the platelet membrane: Glanzman thrombasthenia, Bernard-Soulier syndrome, and other disorders. In: Colman RW, Hirsh J, Marder VJ, Salzman EW, eds. *Hemostasis and thrombosis: Basic principles and clinical practice,* 3rd ed. Philadelphia: JB Lippincott, 1994:652–672.

53. Piper PJ. Pharmacology of leukotrienes. *Br Med Bull* 1983;39:255–259.

54. Ignarro LJ, Buga GM, Chaudhuri G. EDRF generation and release from perfused bovine pulmonary artery and vein. *Eur J Pharmacol* 1988;149:79–88.

55. Broekman MJ, Eiroa AM, Marcus AJ. Inhibition of human platelet reactivity by endothelium-derived relaxing factor from human umbilical vein endothelial cells in suspension: Blockade of aggregation and secretion by an aspirin-insensitive mechanism. *Blood* 1991;78:1033–1040.

56. Marcus AJ, Safier LB, Hajjar KA, et al. Inhibition of platelet function by an aspirin-insensitive endothelial cell ADPase: Thromboregulation by endothelial cells. *J Clin Invest* 1991;88:1690–1696.

57. Plesner L. Ecto-ATPases: Identities and functions. *Int Rev Cytol* 1995;158:141–214.

58. Côté YP, Filep JG, Battistini B, et al. Characterization of ATP-diphosphohydrolase activities in the intima and media of the bovine aorta. *Biochim Biophys Acta* 1992;1139:133–142.

59. Strobel RS, Nagy AK, Knowles AF, et al. Chicken oviductal ecto-ATP-diphosphohydrolase: Purification and characterization. *J Biol Chem* 1996;271:16323–16331.

60. Vasconcelos EG, Ferreira ST, de Carvalho TMU, et al. Partial purification and immunohistochemical localization of ATP diphosphohydrolase from *Schistosoma mansoni:* Immunological cross-reactivities with potato apyrase and *Toxoplasma gondii* nucleoside triphosphate hydrolase. *J Biol Chem* 1996;271:22139–22145.

61. Kaczmarek E, Koziak K, Sévigny J, et al. Identification and characterization of CD39 vascular ATP diphosphohydrolase. *J Biol Chem* 1996;271:33116–33122.

62. Wang TF, Guidotti G. CD39 is an ecto-(Ca^{2+},Mg^{2+})-apyrase. *J Biol Chem* 1996;271:9898–9901.

63. Handa M, Guidotti G. Purification and cloning of a soluble ATP-diphosphohydrolase (apyrase) from potato tubers (*Solanum tuberosum*). *Biochem Biophys Res Commun* 1996;218:916–923.

64. Maliszewski CR, Delespesse GJ, Schoenborn MA, et al. The CD39 lymphoid cell activation antigen: Molecular cloning and structural characterization. *J Immunol* 1994;153:3574–3583.

65. Kansas GS, Wood GS, Tedder TF. Expression, distribution, and biochemistry of human CD39: Role in activation-associated homotypic adhesion of lymphocytes. *J Immunol* 1991;146:2235–2244.

66. Marcus AJ. Aspirin as prophylaxis against colorectal cancer. *N Engl J Med* 1995;333:656–658.

Inflammation: Basic Principles and Clinical Correlates,
3rd ed., edited by John I. Gallin and Ralph Snyderman.
Published by Lippincott Williams & Wilkins, Philadelphia 1999.

CHAPTER 7

Mast Cells and Basophils

Gunnar Nilsson, John J. Costa, and Dean D. Metcalfe

Mast cells and basophils are considered together because of their similarities in structure, content, and activation. Both types of cells contain multiple prominent granules (Fig. 7-1) that stain purple to red with blue aniline dyes, thus exhibiting metachromasia. This metachromasia is now attributed to highly sulfated proteoglycans within mast cell and basophil granules. Both cells synthesize and store histamine, cytokines, and proteases complexed to these proteoglycans within granules and produce lipid mediators and cytokines on stimulation. When these cells are activated, mediators are released and function in both the early initiation phase (vascular reaction and exudation) and the late phase (leukocyte accumulation and wound healing) of allergic inflammation. Physiologic activation resulting in mast cell and basophil degranulation frequently is initiated by antigens recognized by antigen-specific immunoglobulin E (IgE) bound to the high-affinity IgE receptor, designated FcεRI. Activation may also occur through other mechanisms, such as those involving complement or cytokines.

It is an attractive but probably oversimplistic idea that mast cells and basophils represent solely a host defense system that evolved as part of protective mechanisms directed against parasitic infections (1). This hypothesis that this is the only justification for this effector system appears no longer tenable. The body of information on the origin, differentiation, and biologic potential of basophils and mast cells now suggests that both cell types are more central to innate and acquired immune responses than previously believed (2,3). Today mast cells and basophils are considered to be well-engineered, multifunctional cells involved in multiple biologic processes.

They phagocytose particles, process antigen, produce cytokines, and release vasoactive substances, to name a few of their biologic capabilities. Mast cells and basophils exhibit an array of adhesion and immune-response receptors that empower both cell types with an advanced capability to react to multiple nonspecific and specific stimuli. These biologic characteristics and the locations of mast cells, particularly at sites where the internal and external environments meet, no doubt account for the tendency of investigators to implicate mast cells in host defense mechanisms against parasites (4) and bacteria (5-8) and in the genesis of disease states such as vasculitis (9) and fibrosis (10).

The characterization and cloning of stem cell factor (SCF), the ligand to a receptor encoded by the protooncogene *KIT*, has been of central importance for contemporary research in mast cell biology (11). SCF—also referred to as KIT ligand, Steel factor, or mast cell growth factor—is a central factor in mast cell growth, differentiation, survival, migration, adhesion, and degranulation. The availability of recombinant SCF has made it possible to culture human mast cells. This in turn has allowed the study of processes that control mast cell numbers and has provided a system to supply mast cells for studies on various aspects of mast cell biology. This review concentrates on presenting recent advances in the understanding of the origin, migration, development, and biologic functions of basophils and mast cells, adding to the considerable body of knowledge that exists on how such cells respond to activation.

DEVELOPMENT AND MATURATION

Basophil Development and Maturation

Basophils originate in humans from pluripotential CD34-positive cells (12,13). Basophils account for approximately 0.33% of nucleated cells in the marrow (14). They circulate in mature form and account for 0.5%

G. Nilsson: Department of Genetics and Pathology, Uppsala University, Uppsala, Sweden 75185. J.J. Costa: Department of Pathology, Beth Israel Hospital Deaconess Medical Center, Harvard Medical School, Boston, Massachusetts 02115. D.D. Metcalfe: Laboratory of Allergic Diseases, National Institute of Allergy and Infectious Diseases NIH, Bethesda, Maryland 20892-1881.

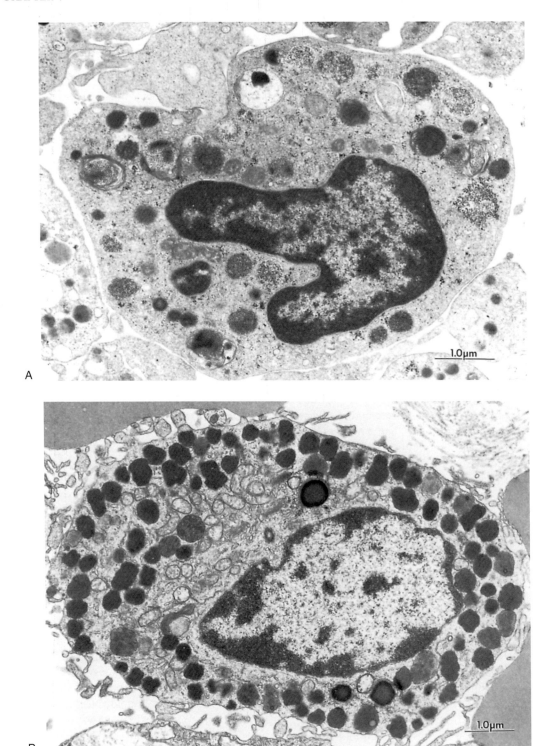

FIG. 7-1. Human peripheral blood basophil (**A**) (original magnification, ×21,585) and human lung mast cell (**B**) (original magnification, ×17,820), showing characteristic morphology.

to 1% of circulating leukocytes. Culture of human bone marrow in suspension in the presence of interleukin-3 (IL-3) gives rise to cultures in which 25% or more of the cells develop into basophils and the remainder consist of neutrophils, eosinophils, monocytes, and mast cells (15-17). The prominent role for IL-3 in basophil biology is supported by the demonstration of high-affinity binding sites for IL-3 on the mature human basophil (18) but not the mast cell surface (19).

Although IL-3 appears to be a major growth factor in the production of human basophils, other cytokines also contribute to their differentiation (20). Granulocyte-macrophage colony-stimulating factor (GM-CSF), but not G-CSF or M-CSF, encourages the growth of basophils from peripheral blood (21). IL-5 also stimulates the growth of metachromatic cells including basophils (15,22). Other factors may enhance the activity of basophil-promoting factors without having a direct effect on basophil differentiation. Nerve growth factor (NGF) is synergistic with GM-CSF (23,24), and transforming growth factor-β (TGF-β) is synergistic with IL-3, in the stimulation of metachromatic basophil-like cells (25). Differentiation of the human basophil-like cell line KU812 (26) is promoted by IL-3 (27) and also by IL-6 and tumor necrosis factor-α (TNF-α) (28).

Mast Cell Development and Maturation

The elucidation of the responsiveness and function of basophils has been facilitated by the ready availability of basophils in bone marrow and peripheral blood. Mast cells, on the other hand, are resident in tissues, a fact that has long complicated studies of their origin and function. Studies of mutant mice that were genetically deficient in mast cells (W/W^v and Sl/Sl^d mice) and their congenic normal littermates initially suggested that murine mast cells were derived from pluripotent hematopoietic cells in the bone marrow (29,30). W/W^v mice were known to have a defect within the mast cell precursor population, and Sl/Sl^d mice were known to have an abnormality in the tissue microenvironment that prevented mast cell survival and differentiation. It was later shown that the White spotting locus (W) encodes for KIT, a receptor with tyrosine kinase activity (31,32), and the Steel locus (Sl) encodes the ligand of this receptor (33-37), now commonly referred to as SCF. SCF is both released as a soluble growth factor and expressed on the surface of stromal cells (33,35). The membrane-bound form of SCF is determined by tissue-specific alternative splicing (38). Membrane-bound ligand may also play a role as a homing and adhesion molecule for hematopoietic progenitor cells and mast cells (38).

In vitro studies have confirmed the bone marrow origin of mouse mast cells and have led to the identification of factors that encourage murine mast cell proliferation, such as IL-3 (39). In addition to IL-3 and SCF, a number of other cytokines and growth factors have been described that promote or augment murine mast cell proliferation or differentiation (or both), including IL-4, IL-9, IL-10, and NGF (39-44). GM-CSF, on the other hand, inhibits the growth of IL-3–dependent mast cells (45), as does TGF-β and interferon α (IFN-α) (46).

The origin of human mast cells from CD34$^+$ progenitor cells was first shown *in vitro* using CD34$^+$-sorted cells (13) and later *in vivo* in bone marrow transplantation studies (47). The mast cell progenitor circulating in the blood not only is positive for CD34 but also expresses the receptor for SCF, KIT (CD117), and the low-affinity IgG receptor, FcγRII (CD32). It lacks expression of FcεRI (48), CD14, and CD17 (49). The earliest committed mast cell precursor from fetal murine liver cells is THY-1^{lo}, CKIT^{hi} (50). These data are consistent with the conclusion that mast cells do not originate from circulating basophils, monocytes, or lymphocytes but rather from a specific lineage within the hematopoietic system.

Studies in the early 1980s revealed that mouse mast cells differentiate when cultured with fibroblasts, as evidenced by heparin synthesis (51). Studies of cells using human bone marrow, umbilical cord blood, or fetal liver–derived cells cultured on murine 3T3 fibroblasts showed that the human mast cell also developed in similar cocultures (52,53). The growth factor from the 3T3 fibroblast thought to be responsible for this effect is now known to be SCF. In the presence of recombinant SCF, mast cells develop from human bone marrow (54,55), fetal liver (56), cord blood (57), and peripheral blood (55). These cultured human mast cells have granules containing tryptase that exhibit a variety of granule morphologies, including the scroll, mixed, reticular, dense-core, and homogeneous patterns found in mature human mast cells within tissues (13,58). The cultured SCF-dependent human mast cells express both α- and β-tryptase and contain both heparin and chondroitin sulfate (59). Furthermore, treatment of patients with SCF promotes human mast cell hyperplasia *in vivo* (60).

The discovery of SCF as a major mast cell growth factor has allowed further study of the growth and differentiation process of human mast cells and classification of the cytokines involved. Specific cytokines have been shown to differ in their effects on human and rodent mast cells. For instance, IL-3 is a growth factor for rodent mast cells and human basophils (15-17,39) but has a minimal direct effect on human mast cell proliferation (16,56,61). Similarly, IL-4 enhances mast cell growth in the presence of IL-3 in the rodent (44) but inhibits the SCF-dependent differentiation of human mast cells derived from fetal liver (62). Likewise, prolonged exposure to IL-3 has been reported to inhibit the SCF-dependent differentiation of human mast cells (63). IL-13, an interleukin with properties similar to those of IL-4, has effects similar to IL-4 on human mast cells (64). GM-CSF inhibits the development of mast cells from both mouse and human marrow (45,65).

FcεRI is one of the classic markers for mast cells. However, cultured mast cells may sometimes be negative for this receptor. Long-term cultures of mouse bone marrow yield a small subpopulation of mast cells that lack the high-affinity IgE receptor (66,67), and similar populations have been described in mast cells cultured from human bone marrow, fetal liver, and cord blood (59,68,69). The human mast cell line HMC-1, established from a patient with mast cell leukemia, also lacks the surface expression of FcεRI (70,71).

FcεRI expression on most mast cells occurs early in ontogeny, at stages in which mast cells are not yet fully granulated (72). IgE levels contribute to the expression of FcεRI. FcεRI expression on human basophils correlates with serum concentrations of IgE (73). IgE also enhances the expression of FcεRI on cells in culture (74), which in turn enhances their ability to release mediators after activation (75-77). Treatment of atopic patients with an antibody against IgE causes a downregulation of FcεRI expressed on basophils (78). IL-4 also has a direct effect on the expression of FcεRI on mast cells in culture (79).

Further studies on the regulation of FcεRI expression may be of importance to the development of future treatment strategies for allergic diseases. FcεRI α-chain–deficient mice, which have normal numbers of mast cells, cannot manifest allergen-induced IgE-dependent anaphylactic reactions (80). Downregulation of FcεRI may mitigate IgE-dependent allergic reactions while keeping other effector functions of mast cells and basophils intact.

Mast Cell Heterogeneity

Although mast cells in different tissues share many characteristics, they are not a homogenous population. The histochemical heterogeneity of murine mast cells was first documented by Enerbäck through variation in staining properties of mast cell granules in mast cell populations at different anatomic sites (81). Variation in fixation properties also provided the first experimental evidence of the existence of different populations of human mast cells (82). Human mast cells also exhibit variations in other characteristics, such as cell size, cytoplasmic granule ultrastructure, quantities of stored mediators, sensitivity to stimulation by various secretagogues, and susceptibility to various drugs (83,84) (Table 7-1).

One widely applied approach to characterize human mast cell subpopulations relies on characterization of the cytoplasmic granule protease content ("phenotype"). Evidence for the presence of two principal types of human mast cells is based on distinct protease expression patterns found in mast cells from different tissues (85,86). Some human mast cells contain tryptase, chymase, a cathepsin G–like protease, and carboxypeptidase (87,88). These cells are designated MC_{TC} because of their tryptase and chymase content; those designated MC_T contain only tryptase (89). Although MC_T predominate in the alveolar septa of the lung and in the small intestinal mucosa, MC_{TC} predominate in the skin and in the small intestinal submucosa (83) (Table 7-2). Therefore, in terms of tissue localization, the human MC_T corresponds most closely to the rodent mucosal mast cell, whereas the MC_{TC} corresponds most closely to the rodent connective tissue mast cell.

The influence of T-lymphocyte–derived cytokines on the differentiation of human mast cells has not been studied in detail. However, diseases that alter the functions or numbers of T cells in tissues are associated with alterations in mast cell subpopulations. The number of intestinal mucosal and submucosal M_{CT}, but not MC_{TC}, is reduced in patients with either congenital combined immunodeficiency or advanced human immunodeficiency virus infection, consistent with a T-cell–dependent requirement for generation and maintenance of normal populations of MC_T (90). Inflammatory diseases also

TABLE 7-1. *Characteristics of human mast cell subsets and basophils*

Features	MC_T	MC_{TC}	Basophil
Nucleus	Rounded without deeply divided lobes	Rounded without deeply divided lobes	Polymorphonuclear, lobulated
Granule structure	Discrete scrolls	Grating and lattices	Amorphous
FcεRI	Yes	Yes	Yes
Histamine	Yes	Yes	Yes
Neutral proteases	Tryptase	Tryptase, chymase, carboxypeptidase, cathepsin G	none identified
Proteoglycans	Heparin, chondroitin sulfate A and E	Heparin, chondroitin sulfate A and E	Chondroitin sulfate A
Lipid mediators	Prostaglandin D_2, leukotrienes B_4 and C_4	Prostaglandin D_2, leukotrienes B_4 and C_4	Leukotriene C_4
T-lymphocyte dependence	Yes	No	Yes
Growth and differentiation dependence	SCF	SCF	IL-3
Cytokine production profile	IL-4, IL-5, IL-6	IL-4	IL-4

MC_T, mast cells containing tryptase; MC_{TC}, mast cells containing tryptase and chymase; SCF, stem cell factor; IL, interleukin.

TABLE 7-2. *Mast cell numbers and tissue distribution of MC$_T$ and MC$_{TC}$*

Tissue	Mast cells (/mm^3)	MC$_T$ (%)	MC$_{TC}$ (%)
Skin (dermis)	3,100	12	88
Alveolar wall	26,600	93	7
Nasal mucosa			
Epithelium	700	100	0
Subepthelium	9,200	60	40
Small intestine			
Mucosa	21,000	98	2
Submucosa	8,600	12	88

yield insight into the regulation of mast cell populations. In synovium obtained from subjects with rheumatoid arthritis in whom mast cell hyperplasia has been documented, a mixture of MC$_{TC}$ and MC$_T$ is observed in areas of lymphocytic infiltration. MC$_{TC}$ are by far the predominant mast cell type in normal synovium (91,92).

Mast Cell Hyperplasia

The identification of factors that regulate mast cell growth has led to insights into diseases of mast cell hyperplasia, classified under systemic mastocytosis. There is some evidence that benign forms of this disease are in some cases associated with a local overproduction of SCF (93). Forms of the disease, especially those associated with hematologic disorders including dysmyelopoiesis, are associated with a mutation in the catalytic domain of *KIT* (94). Similar mutations have been demonstrated in both rodent and human established mast cell lines. These mutations promote ligand-independent autophosphorylation of the mutant receptor (95,96). This mutation in the catalytic domain alters the substrate specificity for the *KIT* receptor and induces degradation of src homology domain-containing protein tyrosine phosphatase (SHP)-1, a protein tyrosine phosphatase that acts as a negative regulator of signaling by KIT (97).

SURVIVAL AND APOPTOSIS

Programmed cell death, or *apoptosis,* is a process whereby cells die in a controlled manner in response to specific stimuli. Mast cells survive in tissues for several months, and their numbers under normal conditions are relatively constant (98). Human lung mast cells cocultured with fibroblasts remain viable, but cells in media alone do not survive; the fibroblast-derived survival factor is SCF (99). Cultured murine and human mast cells are therefore factor dependent. Mast cells undergo apoptosis on withdrawal of growth factors (100,101). This apoptosis is accompanied by condensation of chromatin, shrinkage of total cell volume, production of apoptotic bodies, and fragmentation of DNA.

Murine IL-3–dependent mast cells are "rescued" on withdrawal of IL-3 by the addition of SCF (100). This effect is prevented by the addition of TGF-β (102). The finding of SCF-mediated "rescue" from apoptosis of IL-3–deprived mast cells has been confirmed *in vivo* (103). Other factors also promote mast cell viability, including NGF (104,105). Insulin-like growth factor has been shown to prevent apoptosis in murine mast cells (106).

The ability of growth factors to promote cell survival by suppressing apoptosis is fundamental to their ability to promote cell proliferation and differentiation. Because mast cells reside mainly in extravascular tissues, it is reasonable to assume that regulation of their number is related to local control of mast cell proliferation or apoptosis, or both. The number of tissue mast cells is now believed to be regulated principally by SCF, which is produced by resident cells such as stromal cells, endothelial cells, fibroblasts, and keratinocytes (93,107,108). One approach to regulating mast cell numbers in tissues, then, is to regulate the local synthesis of SCF. Glucocorticoids delivered at sites of potential or ongoing tissue inflammation significantly reduce mast cell numbers (109-111). This has been shown to result from a direct effect of glucocorticoids on local SCF production, leading to mast cell apoptosis and a decrease in tissue mast cell numbers (112).

Another possible pathway for induction of mast cell apoptosis is through the interaction between FAS (CD95) and FAS ligand (113). Mast cells do express FAS. Certain mast cell lines, and a subset of normal cultured murine mast cells, are induced to undergo apoptosis after crosslinking of FAS with antibodies against FAS (114).

In contrast to mast cells, basophils have a relatively short life span. When put into culture, basophils die through mechanisms that are not yet understood. The life span of basophils is only partially prolonged by IL-3 or GM-CSF, and not at all by IL-4, G-CSF, or M-CSF (115). SCF does not have an effect on basophil survival (116). Basophils differentiated *in vitro* in the presence of IL-3 appear within 1 week in culture, peak at about 3 weeks, and then decline in cell number (16,56), suggesting apoptosis.

MEDIATORS

Mast cells and basophils both release and generate a heterogeneous group of mediators that differ in their potency and biologic activities. These mediators are both pleiotropic and redundant. That is, each mediator has more than one function, and mediators may overlap in their biologic effects. For instance, histamine alters vasopermeability and induces mucus secretion, properties it shares with leukotriene C$_4$ (LTC$_4$). These mediators may be categorized into three groups: preformed secretory granule–associated mediators, lipid-derived mediators, and cytokines.

Preformed Secretory Granule Mediators

Histamine

Histamine (2-(4-Imidazolyl)ethylamine) is the sole significant biogenic amine in human mast cells and basophils. Histamine is formed in mast cells and basophils from histidine through the action of histidine carboxylase (117). Histamine is stored in secretory granules at acidic pH at a level of 100 mmol/L (118,119), associated by ionic linkage with the carboxyl groups of proteins and proteoglycans. Approximately 3 to 8 pg histamine is found per mast cell isolated from human lung, skin, lymphoid tissue, or small intestine; and in circulating basophils, there is a concentration of about 1 pg per cell (120,121).

During degranulation, histamine is released and dissociated from the proteoglycan-protein complex by cation exchange with extracellular sodium at neutral pH. Extracellular histamine is metabolized within minutes of release to either methylhistamine or imidazole acetic acid. Some 4% to 10% of the methylhistamine is excreted. The remainder undergoes further degradation by monoamine oxidase to N-methylimidazole acetic acid. A small amount (about 2% to 3%) of histamine is secreted directly into the urine. The rapid metabolism of histamine suggests that under normal conditions it is destined to act near the site of its release.

Histamine has direct potent vasoactive and smooth muscle spasmogenic effects. The biologic effects of histamine are mediated through its interactions with cell-specific H_1, H_2, and H_3 receptors (122,123). Characterization of the biologic and physiologic activities mediated by these histamine receptors has resulted from the development of receptor-specific agonists and antagonists (124,125) (Table 7-3). The effects of histamine mediated by H_1 receptors include increased vasopermeability, vasodilatation, and contraction of bronchial and gastrointestinal smooth muscle. Gastric acid secretion by parietal cells and mucus secretion at various sites follow activation through H_2 receptors. A number of immunomodulatory effects mediated through H_2 receptors have also been described. These include inhibition of secretion from cytotoxic lymphocytes, neutrophils, and basophils and augmentation of suppression by T lymphocytes. Histamine activates endothelial cells via H_2 receptors to release prostacyclin (prostaglandin I_2, or PGI_2), a potent inhibitor of platelet aggregation. Neurotransmitter release in the central and peripheral nervous systems, as well as histamine formation in these regions, has been shown to be mediated through H_3 receptors.

Neutral Proteases

Mast cells in different species and at different stages of development express varied combinations of granule proteases. Proteases of the serine class are termed chymases when they have specificity for aromatic residues in the S1 site and tryptases when they have specificity for basic residues in the S1 site. The most prominent serine proteinase in human mast cells is tryptase; it is believed to be present in all human mast cells. Five highly homologous tryptases (one α- and four β-tryptases) have been cloned and sequenced (126-128). Tryptase is comprised of a tetramer of 134 kd with two subunits of 31 to 34 kd. Each chain possesses a single active site. Tryptase is stored in a complex with proteoglycan and is released in this complex. β-Tryptase homotetramers, but not α-tryptase homotetramers, are enzymatically active (59) owing to a mutation in the leader peptide of α-tryptase that precludes autoprocessing (129). The α form of human tryptase is the predominant type present in blood at baseline in normal individuals. This form is elevated in mastocytosis (130). Tryptase is not inhibited by the serine esterase inhibitors in plasma and tissues. The protease-proteoglycan complex (131), which stabilizes the active tetrameric form, may be destabilized by other proteins

TABLE 7-3. *Receptors, biologic effects and antagonists of histamine*

Receptor	Effects	Antagonists
H_1	Induces vascular permeability Dilates arterioles Stimulates intestinal and bronchial smooth muscle contraction	Ethanolamines Alkylamines Ethylenediamines Piperazines Phenothiazines Piperazines
H_2	Stimulates gastric output Stimulates mucus secretion Modulates immune response Stimulates endothelial cells	Burimamide Cimetidine Ranitidine Famotidine Nizatidine
H_3	Modulates neuroconduction	Thioperamide Impentamine Iodoproxyfan

such as antithrombin III. Tryptase cleaves fibrinogen, activates latent collagenase (132), hydrolyzes some neuropeptides, may cause mucus secretion, and may be mitogenic (133).

Human mast cell chymase is present in almost all of the mast cells of the skin and intestinal submucosa, but mast cells of the intestinal mucosa and lung fail to stain with monoclonal antibodies directed against this protease (85). Human chymase is a monomer of 30 kd, is not affected by heparin, and is inhibited by biologic inhibitors of serine proteases, such as α_1-antichymotrypsin and α_2-macroglobulin (134). Chymase appears to have a number of possible biologic functions. It converts angiotensin I to angiotensin II (135), degrades the basement membrane at the dermal-epidermal junction, stimulates mucus secretion, degrades neuropeptides, and converts a precursor of IL-1β to an active form (136).

Carboxypeptidase A is also stored in the mast cell granule complexed with proteoglycans. Carboxypeptidase A is a protein of 35 kd. It acts as a hydrolytic enzyme at neutral pH to cleave the peptide and ester bonds of the amino end of C-terminal aromatic amino acids in a manner similar to that of chymase. Chymase and carboxypeptidase A may complement each other's actions (137). Like chymase, carboxypeptidase A remains complexed with heparin in association with tryptase, where it presumably acts in the same capacity as its rodent counterpart. Human mast cell carboxypeptidase is associated with the MC$_{TC}$ (87). A cathepsin G neutral protease is also found in MC$_{TC}$ (88).

Proteoglycans

Proteoglycans are composed of a protein core with extended unbranched carbohydrate side chains (glycosaminoglycans) of repeating disaccharide subunits (138). Each disaccharide has between zero and, in the case of heparin, three sulfate groups which by virtue of their high charge bestow to the proteoglycan many of its characteristic physicochemical properties. These properties allow proteoglycans to act as extracellular mediators and as storage matrices for other preformed mediators that might otherwise have deleterious effects on the mast cell itself. For example, histamine is bound to the carboxyl groups of glucuronide and iduronic acid. Neutral proteases, chymases, and carboxypeptidases A and B, which are themselves highly cationic, bind to the anionic carboxyl and sulfate groups. The preformed mediators are released slowly from the proteoglycan during exocytosis by an ion-exchange mechanism. Proteoglycans therefore influence the rates of release of mediators from the secretory granule and, in some instances, their subsequent biologic function. Chymase, tryptase, and carboxypeptidase remain associated with heparin in the extracellular environment. More neutral molecules, such as histamine, are released rapidly from the storage matrix under physiologic conditions.

The central core of heparin has numerous serine-glycine repeating residues, making heparin a serglycin. Its structure contributes to protease resistance of the proteoglycan. The cores of mast cell proteoglycans are encoded by the same gene; their diversity is a posttranslational step involving the addition of various side chains to each molecule. A glycosaminoglycan is attached to each second or third serine residue by means of a GlcA-Gal-Gal-Xyl linkage. The disaccharide subunits are then α_{1-4}-linked and are composed of either glucuronic or iduronic acid and, in β_{1-4} linkage, glucosamine. Rat serosal mast cell proteoglycan heparin is approximately 750 kd, whereas human proteoglycan heparin is approximately 60 kd (138,139).

Lipid-derived Mediators

Activation of mast cells not only causes the release of preformed granule-associated mediators but initiates the *de novo* synthesis of lipid-derived substances. Of particular importance are the cyclooxygenase and lipoxygenase metabolites of arachidonic acid, because these products possess potent inflammatory activities. Phospholipase A$_2$ activation and the generation of arachidonic acid from phosphatidylcholine appears to be a common step in the activation pathway of the mast cell. Cyclooxygenase products include prostaglandins and thromboxanes; lipoxygenases generate leukotrienes (LTs), hydroperoxyeicosatetraenoic acids (HPETEs), and the reduced products of the HPETEs, hydroxyeicosatetraenoic acids (HETEs) (see Chapter 23).

The lipoxygenase pathway first forms 5-HPETE, which is subsequently converted into LTB$_4$ and the sulfidopeptide leukotrienes, LTC$_4$, LTD$_4$, and LTE$_4$. LTC$_4$ is derived from LTA$_4$ by the enzymic addition of glutathione. After it is released into the extracellular fluid, it is converted to LTD$_4$ and LTE$_4$ by the release of glutamic acid and glycine, respectively. Purified human mast cells produce more LTC$_4$ than LTB$_4$ (140,141). Leukotrienes induce a prolonged cutaneous wheal and flare response, stimulate prolonged bronchoconstriction (10 to 1,000 times as potent as histamine), enhance venular permeability, promote bronchial mucus secretion, and induce constriction of arterial, arteriolar, and intestinal smooth muscle (142). In placebo-controlled trials in patients with bronchial asthma, a cysteinyl leukotriene receptor blocker and a 5-lipoxygenase inhibitor both reduced measures of airways obstruction (142).

LTB$_4$ is derived from LTA$_4$ by the enzymatic addition of water. LTB$_4$ has potent chemotactic activity for neutrophils and eosinophils, enhances lysosomal enzyme release and augments superoxide anion production. It has also been suggested that LTB$_4$ modifies lymphocyte function by inducing specific suppressor lymphocytes and augmenting human natural cytotoxic cell activity.

PGD$_2$ is generated after the immunologic activation of human mast cells. It has been detected in dispersed and purified human pulmonary mast cells after IgE-mediated activation (143). PGD$_2$ is a potent inhibitor of platelet aggregation; it is chemokinetic for human neutrophils and, in conjunction with LTD$_4$, mediates accumulation of neutrophils in human skin. High levels of PGD$_2$ metabolites have been detected in urine of patients with mastocytosis, and PGD$_2$ is believed to contribute to hypotension in such patients. Inhibition of PGD$_2$ from rat connective-tissue mast cells with indomethacin had no effect on immunologic histamine release from rat or human mast cells. The addition of PGD$_2$ has the effect of enhancing histamine release by several different agents, including antigen.

Cytokines

Cytokines are glycoproteins that are synthesized and secreted by cells. In general, induction of cytokine genes occurs in response to cellular injury or activation, although there are also examples of constitutive cytokine production. Cytokines exert their biologic effects by interacting with specific cytokine receptors located on the surface of target cells. Cytokines as a group possess a broad spectrum of bioactivities, including regulatory functions in cell growth, tissue repair, inflammation, and the immune response. Cytokines are both pleiotropic (each having multiple functions) and redundant (more than one cytokine possessing a given bioactivity). *In vivo* these molecules do not exist in isolation but rather as a network through which the expression of one cytokine may be influenced by other cytokines and by noncytokine mediators.

The first demonstration of mast cell cytokine production was in mouse mast cells transformed with the Abelson murine leukemia virus. Several of these lines were found to contain mRNA for GM-CSF and to release bioactive GM-CSF (144). The presence of IL-4 message and bioactivity was then demonstrated in mouse mast cell lines derived from fetal liver that had been similarly transformed (145). In addition, IL-4 mRNA was detected in the original mast cell populations from which the transformed cell lines were derived, thus providing the first evidence that nontransformed mast cells were capable of cytokine synthesis.

At about the same time, other laboratories were examining the ability of mast cells to produce TNF-α, based on the observation that purified murine peritoneal mast cells were cytotoxic for specific target cells (146). It was soon appreciated that mast cell–mediated cytotoxicity and that of TNF-α displayed similar target cell specificity and kinetics of killing (147). Anti-TNF-α antibodies were then found to partially block cytotoxicity of mast cells derived from bone marrow. New protein synthesis was

not required for expression of this cytotoxicity. It was therefore suggested that mast cell natural cytotoxicity was mediated through a TNF-α–like molecule that was preformed and stored in the cytoplasmic granules. Several groups have now demonstrated the presence of TNF-α mRNA in long-term mouse mast cell lines, mast cells cultured from mouse marrow, mast cells cultured from normal human bone marrow, and purified mouse peritoneal mast cells (148-150). The low level of TNF-α message constitutively transcribed in unstimulated mast cells has been found to increase within 30 to 60 minutes after FcϵRI crosslinking. The FcϵRI-mediated induction of TNF-α mRNA is associated with an increase in the amount of cytotoxic activity present in both culture supernatants and cell lysates.

Since these initial observations, mouse mast cells have been shown to produce many additional cytokines, including IL-1, IL-2, IL-3, IL-4, IL-5, IL-6, GM-SCF, and IFN-γ. Murine mast cells also produce mRNA for macrophage inflammatory protein-1α (MIP-1α), MIP-1β, T cell activation gene (TCA)3, MARC, lymphotactin, and JE/monocyte chemotactic protein-1 (MCP-1), as well as IL-1, IL-4, and IL-6 bioactivity or protein, or both (151-153).

Studies of human mast cell cytokine production have been slower to emerge, in part because of the difficulty of obtaining highly purified preparations of human mast cells. Advances in technology that now permit isolation of significant numbers of mast cells from human tissues, along with techniques to clearly colocalize mast cell–specific markers and various cytokines in human biopsy specimens, have greatly extended knowledge of human mast cell cytokine production. Such studies have shown that human mast cells represent a potential source of many cytokines, including TNF-α, basic fibroblast growth factor (bFGF), IL-4, IL-5, IL-6, IL-8, IL-13, and IL-16 (2,154,155).

In accordance with the mouse data, several groups have demonstrated either *de novo* or enhanced cytokine production by human mast cells in response to IgE-dependent activation, an observation relevant to the pathogenesis of allergic inflammation. Stimulation of purified human skin mast cells with anti-IgE induced these cells to release TNF-α bioactivity (156). Challenge of human lung fragments with anti-IgE antibodies *in vitro* caused three resident cell populations (mast cells, tissue and alveolar macrophages, and bronchial epithelial cells) to express TNF-α by immunohistochemistry 4 hours later. No cells exhibited TNF-α immunoreactivity in specimens incubated with medium alone (157). Finally, the evidence from reverse transcriptase–polymerase chain reaction (RT-PCR) and enzyme-linked immunosorbent assay studies of preparations of at least 94% to 99% purity indicates that both SCF and anti-IgE induce human lung mast cells to produce TNF-α, with up to 150 pg TNF-α per 10^6 mast cells being generated into the supernatant within 4 hours (158).

In vitro studies have confirmed human mast cells as a potentially significant source of IL-5. RT-PCR and *in situ* hybridization of human lung mast cells revealed IgE-dependent expression of IL-5 mRNA, which persisted from 24 to 72 hours after activation (159). The strength of the IL-5 mRNA signal was positively correlated with the anti-IgE concentration used to activate the cells. Immunoreactive IL-5 could be detected by 8 hours after challenge in the culture supernatants (160).

Other investigators have documented enhanced mast cell cytokine expression in nasal or lung tissue from symptomatic atopic persons compared with nonallergic control subjects. Immunohistochemistry has been used to assess the distribution and identity of cells that express IL-4, IL-5, IL-6, and TNF-α in the airways of normal subjects and of those with mildly symptomatic atopic asthma (161). In biopsies of both normal and asthmatic airways, many cells stained for each of these four cytokines. Most of these cells were identified as mast cells by their tryptase content. The mean number of cells staining for TNF-α in biopsies of asthmatic airways was sevenfold higher than in normal airways, a finding that was found statistically to be highly significant. Furthermore, approximately twice as many mast cells were positive for TNF-α by immunohistochemistry in biopsies from asthmatic subjects. In both groups, the majority of the TNF-α–positive cells in the biopsies were mast cells. Immunohistochemical analysis also has revealed that some mast cells in nasal turbinate specimens from patients with allergic rhinitis or from nonatopic subjects display immunoreactivity for IL-4, IL-5, and IL-6 (162).

In situ hybridization and immunohistochemistry have been used to examine bronchial biopsies and cytospins of bronchoalveolar lavage fluid from mildly atopic asthmatic patients and nonatopic controls (163). In both the fluid and the biopsied tissues, approximately 15% of the IL-4– and IL-5–positive cells were identified as tryptase-positive mast cells (100). Biopsies from atopic asthmatics showed significantly increased percentages of tryptase-positive mast cells coexpressing IL-4 and IL-5 mRNA, but not IL-2 or IFN-γ, compared with biopsies from nonatopic controls (163).

The ability of basophils to serve as a source of multifunctional cytokines has also been studied. Mature human basophils isolated from peripheral blood release IL-4 in response to FcεRI-dependent activation. Such release is enhanced in basophils exposed to IL-3 but not in those exposed to IL-5, GM-CSF, or NGF (164-167). Stimulation of human basophils via FcεRI crosslinking also results in the release of IL-13. Basophil IL-13 synthesis is increased by preincubation with IL-3 (168).

IL-4 derived from mast cells and basophils at sites of allergic inflammation may play a role in T-cell differentiation toward a T_H2 phenotype. Since both human basophils and mast cells can express the CD40 ligand, it is possible these cells are able to contribute to IgE pro-

duction by promoting immunoglobulin class switching (169). Studies of human basophils have also demonstrated synthesis and secretion of MIP-1α. This observation raises the possibility of autocrine augmentation of effector cell function (170).

It is now clear that mast cells and basophils influence many important aspects of the pathogenesis of allergic inflammation via the elaboration of multifunctional cytokines. It is likely that the production of cytokines represents a critical link among the IgE-dependent mast cell activation that occurs immediately after allergen challenge in atopic subjects, the inflammation that develops during subsequent late-phase reactions to such provocation, and the persistent inflammation and associated tissue changes that are characteristic of chronic allergic disorders (2,3,154). Moreover, many of the clinically significant consequences of IgE-dependent reactions, both in the respiratory tract and in the skin, are now thought to reflect actions of leukocytes recruited to these sites during the late-phase reaction rather than direct effects of the mediators released by mast cells soon after antigen challenge (2,171).

Several lines of evidence derived from both clinical and animal studies suggest that the leukocyte infiltration associated with the late-phase reaction is a result of mast cell degranulation (2). Studies in mast cell–reconstituted mice have demonstrated that the influx of leukocytes at sites of IgE-dependent cutaneous reactions, which reaches maximal levels 6 to 12 hours after antigen challenge, is entirely mast cell–dependent (172). Furthermore, the injection of anti-TNF-α antiserum at sites of IgE-dependent cutaneous mast cell activation diminishes the observed leukocyte infiltration by about 50% (172).

Activation of mast cells through FcεRI initiates the allergic inflammatory response, in part through the release of TNF-α and IL-14, which influence the recruitment and function of additional effector cells. These recruited cells then contribute to further progression of the inflammatory response by providing additional sources of certain cytokines and other mediators that may not be produced by mast cells. Finally, mast cell activation may directly or indirectly promote the release of cytokines from certain resident cells in the respiratory tract, such as alveolar macrophages and bronchial epithelial cells.

ACTIVATION AND MEDIATOR RELEASE

Basophil and mast cell activation may be initiated when a multivalent antigen (allergen) interacts with its specific IgE antibody attached to the cell membrane via the high affinity receptor, FcεRI. Crosslinkage of IgE by the interaction of allergen with specific determinants on the Fab portion of the molecule brings the receptors into juxtaposition and initiates cell activation and mediator generation and release. Basophils and mast cells may also be activated by nonimmunologic stimuli induced by substances such as neuropeptides, basic compounds, complement components, and certain drugs such as opiates. Morphologically, degranulation produced by immunologic versus nonimmunologic stimulation appears similar, although the biochemical processes that lead to mediator release may differ (173). After degranulation, the cells regranulate after release of cytoplasmic granules and shedding of large amounts of membrane (174). This recovery process takes place 3 to 48 hours after activation (175,176).

Immunoglobulin E–mediated Activation

The FcεRI high-affinity receptor for IgE is a tetrameric protein complex consisting of the IgE-binding α chain, a single β chain, and two disulfide-linked γ chains (177). IgE binds to membranes or solubilized FcεRI with high affinity ($K_d = 10^{-10}$ mol/L). The binding is highly specific and cannot be inhibited by an excess of any other immunoglobulin. The binding of IgE occurs via the Fc region of the immunoglobulin in a 1 : 1 ratio. The Cε3 domain of the IgE-Fc region contains the principal site of interaction with the receptor (178). The minimal degree of crosslinking required for triggering of exocytosis involves dimers of the receptor (179). Maximal histamine release is obtained when 10% of the receptors are aggregated. A detectable response is achieved when approximately 100 receptors (out of 3×10^5 receptors per cell) are aggregated (180). Crosslinking of FcεRI on tyrosine residues of several proteins has been shown to induce phosphorylation within 5 to 15 seconds (181). The newly phosphorylated tyrosines promote the recruitment of more kinase molecules, probably by their SRC homology-2 (SH2) domains (182).

Basophils are also activated by an IgE-dependent histamine-releasing factor (183). This factor interacts with the IgE molecule, but only a subpopulation of atopic patients are responsive to this factor. The IgE molecules that interact with the factor are designated IgE+, and the remaining IgE molecules that do not interact with the factor are said to be IgE−. This HRF has now been cloned (184).

Activation Not Mediated by Immunoglobulin E

A family of polybasic molecules is known to stimulate exocytosis from mast cells. Members of this family include compound 48/80, mastoparan, polymyxin B, and polymers of basic amino acids (185). The polybasic secretagogues appear to release histamine by a common mechanism, and they share similar structural features essential for histamine-releasing activity. Other agents that induce histamine release from basophils or mast cells, or both, include opiates, contrast media, mellitin, bee venom peptide, dextran, lectins, and calcium iono-

phores (186). Mast cell degranulation is also induced by bacteria in mice (187). Degranulation is potentiated by adenosine (188). There are functional differences between mast cells and basophils in their response to specific stimuli (Table 7-4).

Several neuropeptides have been reported to cause histamine release from mast cells. These include substance P, calcitonin gene-related peptide, somatostatin, VIP, and neurotensin (189). Substance P has been shown to activate human skin mast cells (190,191). Substance P also differentially activates mediator pathways, stimulating cytokine (mRNA) production at concentrations less than that required to release histamine. The widespread distribution of these peptides in tissues, together with the localization of some mast cells in close proximity to nerve terminals, suggests a neurocrine–mast cell interaction (192).

The complement fragments C3a, C4a, and C5a are reported to cause basophil and mast cell degranulation and possibly have a role in anaphylactoid reactions. They are therefore known as anaphylatoxins (193). C3a and C5a selectively activate human skin mast cells, with no effect on human lung mast cells (194,195). The physiologic relevance of anaphylatoxins has not yet been established, although they have been suggested as the mechanism by which mast cells may be activated in immune complex–mediated diseases, reactions to iodinated contrast media, and certain adverse responses related to dialysis tubing.

A number of cytokines have been described that either augment histamine release or are direct agonists, especially for basophils. These factors are referred to as inflammatory cell–derived HRFs (196). Of the chemokines, monocyte chemotactic protein-1 (MCP-1) is the most effective. Chemokines induce histamine release with different efficacies: MCP-1 = MCP-3 > RANTES (regulated on activation, normal T-cell expressed) > MCP-2 > MIP-1α (197-202). Another member of the chemokines, IL-8, inhibits the release of histamine from basophils in response to certain stimuli (203). IL-1, IL-3, and GM-CSF directly acti-

TABLE 7-4. *Human basophil and mast cell secretagogues*

Secretagogue	Basophil	Lung mast cell	Skin mast cell
IgE-antigen	+	+	+
Substance P	+	−	+
Opiates	+	−	+
Platelet-activating factor	+	−	−
C3a	+	−	+
C5a	+	−	+
fMLP	+	−	−
Contrast media	+	+	−
Ionophores	+	+	+

fMLP, formyl-methionyl-leucyl-phenylalanine.

vate basophils, but they also prime these cells and thereby enhance their response to a second agonist (204,205). IL-5 has similar effects (206), as does NGF (207), which mediates its effect through the tyrosine kinase receptor A (TrkA) receptor expressed on basophils (208).

SCF induces histamine release from mast cells. SCF also augments IgE-dependent mediator release from human mast cells (209,210), and at high concentrations it directly promotes mediator release from human basophils *in vitro* (210). SCF also induces anaphylactic-type degranulation from human cutaneous mast cells *in vivo* (60). In contrast to their effects on basophils, chemokines do not appear to cause histamine release from human mast cells *in vitro* (211-213), although MIP-1α has been shown to cause mast cell degranulation *in vivo* (214).

Mast cells express the low-affinity IgG receptors, FcγRII and FcγRIII. Aggregation of FcγRIII in the murine system is followed by mast cell adhesion, degranulation, and an increase in TNF-α synthesis (215-217). Current evidence suggests that low-affinity receptors on murine mast cells may regulate high-affinity IgE receptor–mediated activation (218,219).

ADHESION AND ADHESION RECEPTORS

Cellular adhesion receptors provide a mechanism for transmission of signals within the microenvironment. Such signals are mediated by interactions between cells and extracellular matrix molecules or through cell-cell contact. They provide the means by which immature or mature cells are recruited to specific tissues, govern the movement of cells during inflammatory reactions, provide a means for communication among cells of distinct lineages, and allow cells to respond to a specific tissue environment. The cellular receptors governing the participation of mast cells and basophils in these respects are only partially characterized (2,220) (Table 7-5).

Basophils are attracted into extravascular inflammatory sites. An initial step in the recruitment of a circulating leukocyte is its adhesion to vascular endothelium. Cellular recruitment depends on the expression and function of cell adhesion molecules. These are grouped into families (integrins, immunoglobulin-like structures, selectins, and sialylated carbohydrate counterligands for selectins) based on shared structural characteristics and function. The adhesion of basophils to endothelial cells involves a number of counterreceptors that bind to adhesion molecules expressed on endothelial cells, such as intracellular adhesion molecule-1 (ICAM-1), vascular cell adhesion molecule-1 (VCAM-1), and E-selectin. Basophils have been shown to express β_1, β_2, and β_7 integrins along with sialylated surface ligands which are necessary for the attachment of basophils to the endothelium (221). IL-1 and TNF-α treatment of endothelial cell monolayers enhances their adhesiveness for basophils (222).

Basophil FcεRI aggregation results in increased basophil adherence to human endothelial cells (223). IL-3 treatment of basophils leads to a rapid and sustained increase in the cell surface expression of CD11b membrane attack complex-1 (MAC-1) (224). Since neither of these responses is observed with neutrophils, it is possible that exposure of basophils to low concentrations of antigen *in vivo* and local production of IL-3 during allergic reactions act in concert to promote basophil activation, adhesion to endothelium, and recruitment to extravascular sites of inflammation. An associated mechanism for basophil recruitment is the induction of the expression of VCAM-1 by IL-4 and IL-13 (225,226). In contrast to neutrophils, basophils (and eosinophils) express receptors for VCAM-1 ($\alpha_4\beta_1$ and $\alpha_4\beta_7$), thereby providing a selective recruitment of these cells.

In contrast to basophils, a surface receptor governing mast cell progenitor interactions with endothelial cells has not been defined. Mature mast cells exist exclusively within tissues under normal conditions. If it is assumed that mast cell distribution and heterogeneity relate to the biologic function of the cell, then to clearly understand the

TABLE 7-5. *Cell surface receptors on human mast cells and basophils*

Integrin	Cluster designation (CD)	Ligand	Basophil	Lung mast cell	Skin mast cell	Uterine mast cell
$\alpha_L\beta_2$	11a/18	ICAM-1,2	+	–	–	–
$\alpha_M\beta_2$	11b/18	C3bi, Fb	+	–	–	–
$\alpha_x\beta_2$	11c/18	Fb	+	–	–	–
$\alpha_2\beta_1$	49b/29	Lm, Co	nk	–	–	–
$\alpha_3\beta_1$	49c/29	Fn, Lm, Co	nk	nk	+	nk
$\alpha_4\beta_1$	49d/29	Fn, VCAM-1	+	+	+	+
$\alpha_5\beta_1$	49e/29	Fn	+	+	+	+
$\alpha_6\beta_1$	49f/29	Lm	–	–	–[a]	–
$\alpha_v\beta_3$	51/61	Vn, Fb	nk	+	+	+
$\alpha_4\beta_7$[b]	49d/-	Fn, VCAM-1	+	nk	nk	nk
$\alpha_E\beta_7$[b]	–/–		nk	nk	nk	nk

Co, collagen; Fb, fibrinogen; Fn, fibronectin; ICAM, intracellular adhesion molecule; Lm, laminin; nk, not known; VCAM, vascular cell adhesion molecule; Vn, vitronectin; +, molecules are present on most cells; -, molecules absent or found on few cells.
[a]Expression has been detected by immunohistochemistry of skin biopsies but not on purified skin mast cells.
[b]Expression has been shown on mouse bone marrow cultured mast cells.

basis of mast cell biology it is necessary to understand the interactions among mast cells, other cells, and the extracellular connective tissue matrix. Interactions between mast cells and extracellular matrix components such as collagen, fibronectin, laminin, and vitronectin are important for the migration of mast cells into tissues and their specific localization therein. Adhesion to extracellular matrix also affects the reactivity of mast cells. The composition of the extracellular matrix in a specific tissue determines the localization of mast cells. Cells bind to extracellular matrix proteins, for the most part through interactions with receptors belonging to the integrin family (227,228).

The mechanisms for recruitment of mast cell progenitors from the blood into tissues are not known. However, mast cells and T cells share at least some receptors involved in the homing and migration of T cells to the mucosa (229). For example, maturing mast cells initially express the Peyer's patch homing receptors lymphocyte Peyer's patch adhesion molecule (LPAM-1) ($\alpha_4\beta_7$) and LPAM-2 ($\alpha_4\beta_1$). Both could be involved in the localization of mast cells to the lamina propria (230-232). Once within the lamina propria, the $\alpha_E\beta_7$ integrin chain is expressed, which may allow the mast cells to be retained in this compartment.

Tissue mast cells are often found distributed adjacent to basement membranes. This observation led researchers to focus on the possibility that mast cells might bind to laminin, a component of basement membranes (233). Furthermore, human skin mast cells have been identified as being associated with laminin *in vivo* (234). Mast cells were found variably to adhere spontaneously to laminin or to attach after activation with phorbol migristate acetate (PMA) (233). These observations led to a search for a physiologic stimulus that would promote adhesion. Aggregation of the FcεRI receptor was found to be a potent physiologic stimulus to promote attachment, at a threefold log concentration of antigen less than that required to induce mast cell degranulation (235).

After the demonstration that mast cells interact with laminin, it was hypothesized that mast cells would also adhere to other matrix components; this was demonstrated for both fibronectin (236) and vitronectin (237). As with laminin, adherence to fibronectin required cell activation with PMA or occurred after aggregation of FcεRI. Mast cells also adhered to fibronectin after treatment with SCF (238) or stimulation through Fcγ receptors (239). Cultured human mast cells have been found to express the $\alpha_v\beta_3$ integrin and to attach to vitronectin (240).

The adhesion of mast cells to extracellular matrix proteins affects not only the localization but also the activation of these cells. Murine bone marrow–derived mast cells adhere spontaneously to vitronectin, an adhesion protein, leading to an increased proliferation (237). Spontaneous adhesion of mast cells to vitronectin is followed by the rapid phosphorylation of multiple intracellular proteins, including focal adhesion kinase (241). In addi-

tion to these effects, mast cell adhesion has been reported to enhance FcεRI-dependent mast cell histamine release (242) and to synergistically regulate FcεRI-induced tyrosine phosphorylation of focal adhesion kinase (243,244).

Most of the functional studies of adhesion mentioned used rodent mast cells. Studies of human mast cells have been more limited and have focused on the characterization of adhesion receptors expressed on mast cells (227,245,246) (see Table 7-5). Human lung, skin, heart, and uterine mast cells express surface antigens for ICAM-1 and are deficient in CD11a (leukocyte function-associated antigen-1, or LFA-1) and CD11b (MAC-1) (227). Uterine mast cells are also reported to express both CD11c (p150,95) and the β_2 subunit (CD18) (247), as well as the α and β subunits of the vitronectin receptor, CD51/CD61 ($\alpha_v\beta_3$), and VLA-4 ($\alpha_4\beta_1$, or CD49d/CD29).

Mast cells adhere not only to matrix but to other cells. The biologic consequences of these interactions may include presentation of specific growth factors and cell activation. Mast cells are known to adhere to fibroblasts *in vitro*. This adhesion is mediated through interactions between KIT expressed on mast cells and membrane-bound SCF expressed on the fibroblasts (248,249). This interaction is believed to promote mast cell differentiation and survival. Interdigitation of lymphocyte and mast cell membranes has been observed in inflamed tissues (250). Activated mast cells also form heterotypic aggregates with T lymphocytes *in vitro*. These observations suggest a functional relation between mast cells and lymphocytes that involves direct contact between these cells and an interaction that may regulate cell responsiveness in one or both populations. FcεRI aggregation–induced degranulation is augmented when bone marrow cultured BMCMC mast cells are cocultured with activated T cells. Anti-LFA-1/ICAM-1 antibody inhibits the aggregation-induced degranulation (251). Activated lymphocytes induce promoter activity of the TCA3 gene in mast cells after cell-cell contact (252).

MIGRATION AND ACCUMULATION

Basophil recruitment from the circulation into inflamed tissues requires interactions between the circulating basophil and the vascular endothelium. After transmigration, inflammatory cells must migrate toward a gradient of chemotaxins, either derived from resident cells or generated in the fluid phase, such as complement split products. Infiltration of basophils has been described in diseases such as allergic rhinitis and asthma (253,254). In the lung, basophil numbers may increase after introduction of an antigen (255). Factors that are basophil chemoattractants include IL-3 and GM-CSF (256,257); chemokines, with RANTES = MCP-3 > MCP-1 > MCP-1 > MIP-1α (198,199,258); the anaphylatoxins C3a and C5a (259); LTB$_4$; and platelet-activating factor (PAF) (256) (Table 7-6).

TABLE 7-6. *Mast cell and basophil chemoattractants*

Chemoattractant	Basophils	Rodent mast cells	HMC-1	HCMC	Pulmonary mast cells
SCF	−	+	+	+	+
TGF-β	nk	+	+	+	+
PDGF-AB	nk	+	nk	nk	nk
bFGF	nk	+	nk	nk	nk
VEGF	nk	+	nk	nk	nk
IL-3	+	+	-	−	−
IL-4	−	+[a]	nk	nk	nk
GM-CSF	+	nk	nk	nk	nk
IL-8	+	−	−	−	nk
MCP-1/MCAF	+	+	−	−	nk
MCP-2	+	nk	nk	nk	nk
MCP-3	+	nk	nk	nk	nk
MIP-1α	+	+[a]	−	−	nk
RANTES	+	+[a]	−	+	+
PF-4	nk	+[a]	nk	nk	nk
C3a	+	nk	+	+	nk
C5a	+	nk	+	+	nk
C1q	nk	+	nk	nk	nk
PAF	+	+	+	+	nk
LTB₄	+	nk	nk	nk	nk
Tumor-derived peptides	nk	+	nk	nk	nk
Laminin	nk	+	nk	nk	−
Fibronectin	nk	nk	nk	nk	+

bFGF, basic fibroblast growth factor; GM-CSF, granulocyte-macrophage colony-stimulating factor; HCMC, human cultured mast cells; HMC-1, human mast cell line 1; IL, interleukin; LTB₄, leukotriene B₄; MCAF, monocyte chemotactic and activating factor; MCP, monocyte chemotactic protein; MIP, macrophage inflammatory protein; nk, not known; PAF, platelet-activating factor; PDGF, platelet-derived growth factor; PF-4, platelet factor 4; RANTES, regulated on activation, normal T-cell expressed and secreted; SCF, stem cell factor; TGF-β, transforming growth factor β; VEGF, vascular endothelial cell growth factor.

[a]Cell migration observed only after activation

Mast cells also accumulate during inflammation, at least in part by redistribution and recruitment of neighboring mast cells. Such an accumulation of mast cells has been described to occur in asthma (260), hay fever (261,262), scleroderma (263), rheumatoid arthritis (264), and interstitial cystis (265); in transplant rejection (266); and in association with various tumors (267,268). No mast cells are found in the epithelial layer of the normal nasal mucosa. On provocation with specific antigen, an increase in the number of mast cells in the epithelium of allergic patients is observed (269). There is also an increase of mast cells in brush samples (262,270).

Cytokines responsible for this local increase in mast cell number presumably are secreted during the acute phase of inflammation by resident cells. One cytokine shown to be a chemoattractant for mast cells is SCF (271,272), which is produced by airway epithelial cells (273). SCF is one of the mast cell chemoattractants released after allergen provocation (274). TGF-β at low concentrations attracts mast cells (275). The chemokine RANTES is also a chemoattractant for human mast cells (272,276), although MCP-1, MIP-1α, and platelet factor-4 are active on murine mast cells (213). A number of angiogenic factors act as chemoattractants for murine mast cells (277) (see Table 7-6), as do the anaphylatoxins C3a and C5a (278), and C1q (279). PAF is a lipid-derived

mast cell attractant factor (280). Tumor cells also secrete peptides that act as mast cell chemotactic factors and are thus responsible for a local mast cell hyperplasia (281).

Extracellular matrix proteins similarly induce mast cell chemotaxis (see Table 7-6). Laminin is chemotactic for murine mast cells (282), as is fibronectin for human pulmonary mast cells (276). The mean velocity of BMCMC on laminin, fibronectin, and Matrigel was found to be similar to that of macrophages and averaged approximately 180 μm/hr (283).

MAST CELLS AND BASOPHILS IN INFLAMMATION

Acute inflammatory reactions are characterized by an influx of leukocytes (predominantly neutrophils), edema, and changes in the caliber and permeability of the microvasculature. Because many of these changes reflect, at least in part, the release of chemical mediators derived from injured tissues, mast cells have long been regarded as potentially important in the initiation and amplification of acute inflammatory responses (2). Similarly, basophils release histamine, potent mediator in the inflammatory response.

The involvement of basophils in allergic inflammation is supported by data showing basophilia in association with atopic diseases such as allergic rhinitis and asthma. This increase in basophil numbers is noted in nasal secretions, skin window studies, and intradermal skin test sites several hours after allergen challenge in allergic subjects (285). Basophils are recruited from the circulation to the nasal secretions, with the magnitude of this response correlating with the severity of the experimental antigen-induced nasal late-phase symptoms or the symptoms resulting from natural exposure to allergens (253). The presence of LTC_4 and the absence of PGD_2 synthesis help to implicate the basophil as the cell responsible for the late-phase reaction, because mast cells would also be expected to produce PGD_2, which is seen in the acute response. Similarly, studies using skin blister antigen challenge models have revealed an influx of basophils into the dermis (286).

Activation of basophils leads to increased expression of glycoprotein cell surface adhesion molecules and an increased adhesion to vascular endothelial cell surfaces. This adhesion is mediated by receptors of the CD18 integrins. The expression of CD18 receptors is increased after activation with IgE-specific antigen or anti-IgE (223). *In vitro* experiments demonstrate a dose-dependent increase in basophil adherence to vascular endothelial cells. This is observed at suboptimal concentrations that do not induce histamine release. In contrast, neutrophils and eosinophils are unaffected by a similar treatment, suggesting basophil-specific stimulation of adhesion. The activation of basophils by anti-IgE or antigen is accompanied by a transient *de novo* expression of the corresponding ligand, endothelial leukocyte adhesion molecule-1 (ELAM-1), on the surface of endothelial cells by TNF and IL-1 (222,287). In an inflammatory reaction, low concentrations of antigen, C5a, formyl-methionyl-leucyl-phenylalanine (fMLP), or PAF may result in a recruitment of basophils from the peripheral blood via their adhesion to vascular endothelium and subsequent chemotaxis to sites of tissue injury.

Mast cells are regarded as critical effector cells in the inflammatory reaction underlying immediate hypersensitivity. Numerous observations have also suggested the possibility that these cells contribute to other inflammatory and physiologic processes (2,288,289). The remarkable variety of mediators derived from mast cells and the recognition that mast cells release these mediators in response to stimulation by many different signals in addition to FcεRI aggregation have led to this conclusion. Furthermore, changes in mast cell number or state of degranulation at various anatomic sites have been observed in a number of innate, adaptive, and pathologic immune responses and in a large number of diseases or disease-related processes, including delayed hypersensitivity reactions (290,291), fibrosis (292), autoimmune pathology (293), inflammation in the rheumatoid synovium (91,294) inflammatory bowel diseases (295,296), and neoplasia (297).

Several lines of evidence suggest that mast cells may also participate in fibrotic processes. Some chronic allergic states in which repeated stimulation of mast cells has been demonstrated are associated with the development of some fibrosis–for example in allergic asthma (298), in the skin of patients with atopic dermatitis (299), and in the liver, spleen, and bone marrow of some patients with systemic mastocytosis (2). Many substances produced by mast cells have the ability to affect the connective tissue microenvironment, including heparin and tryptase (300-303). Tryptase from human mast cells induces fibroblast proliferation, activation, and migration *in vitro* (304,305). Cytokines produced by mast cells are also known for their fibrogenic activity. These include IL-4 (306), TNF-α, and TGF-β1 (307). Mast cells also produce bFGF, a growth factor for fibroblasts (308,309). Platelet-derived growth factor may influence fibroblast proliferation and has been found to be expressed by human basophil and mast cell lines (310,311). Finally, mast cells may synthesize basement membrane components (312).

The induction of new blood vessels (angiogenesis) is a fundamental part of several integrated biologic processes (e.g., wound healing, tumor growth) and has in part been related to mast cells (2,268). Several mast cell mediators exert modulatory effects on endothelial growth and function. Histamine stimulates corneal angiogenesis (313). Heparin, when introduced *in vivo,* also promotes new vessel formation. The antagonist of heparin, protamine sulfate, suppresses angiogenesis (314,315). The mast cell–derived cytokines and bFGF also influence angiogenesis.

The discovery that basophils and mast cells produce cytokines has expanded the role of these cells beyond that of simple effector cells to include possible functions as regulatory and modulatory elements of both inflammatory and immune responses. One example of this role in immunoregulation is the ability to influence IgE-synthesis by B lymphocytes. This is achieved by the expression of the CD40 ligand by basophils and mast cells (169), providing one of the signals required for IgE synthesis, and by the secretion of IL-4 (145,165,166,316) and IL-13 (168,317,318), which are involved in the switch to IgE synthesis.

SUMMARY

Both basophils and mast cells are hematopoietically-derived cells. Basophils circulate in the blood and are drawn into tissues when appropriately stimulated. Mast cells reach maturity within tissues. Both basophils and mast cells express a variety of surface receptors that allow them to migrate to specific tissue locations, interact with cells and tissues, and respond to activation molecules. Through the aggregation of FcεRI, mast cells and basophils are directed to release and generate a variety of proinflammatory molecules involved in the genesis and perpetuation of the allergic response. These cells, however, should not be considered only in this context. Their tissue distribution and ability to interact with other cells and with their environment through a wide variety of mechanisms support the concept that basophils and mast cells participate in both innate and acquired immunologic processes.

REFERENCES

1. Moqbel R, Pritchard DI. Parasites and allergy: Evidence for a cause and effect relationship. *Clin Exp Allergy* 1990;20:611–618.
2. Metcalfe DD, Baram D, Mekori YA. Mast cells. *Physiol Rev* 1997;77:1033–1079.
3. Nilsson G, Metcalfe DD. Contemporary issues in mast cell biology. *Allergy Asthma Proc* 1996;70:1759–1763.
4. Nutman TB. Mast cells and their role in parasitic helminth infection. In: Kaliner MA, Metcalfe DD, eds. *The mast cell in health and disease.* New York: Marcel Dekker, 1993:669–686.
5. Malaviya R, Ross EA, MacGregor JI, et al. Mast cell phagocytosis of FimH-expressing enterobacteria. *J Immunol* 1994;152:1907–1914.
6. Echtenacher B, Männel DN, Hültner L. Critical protective role of mast cells in a model of acute septic peritonitis. *Nature* 1996;381:75–77.
7. Malaviya R, Ikeda T, Ross E, Abraham SN. Mast cell modulation of neutrophil influx and bacterial clearance at sites of infection through TNF-α. *Nature* 1996;381:77–80.
8. Sylvestre DL, Ravetch JV. A dominant role for mast cell Fc receptors in the Arthus reaction. *Immunity* 1996;5:387–390.
9. Ramos BF, Qureshi R, Olsen KM, Jakschik BA. The importance of mast cells for the neutrophil influx in immune complex-induced peritonitis in mice. *J Immunol* 1990;145:1868–1873.
10. Gato T, Befus D, Low R, Bienestock J. Mast cell heterogeneity and hyperplasia in bleomycin-induced pulmonary fibrosis in rats. *Am Rev Respir Dis* 1984;130:797–802.
11. Galli SJ, Zsebo KM, Geissler EN. The kit ligand, stem cell factor. *Adv Immunol* 1994;55:1–96.
12. Metcalf D. The molecular control of cell division, differentiation, commitment, and maturation in hematopoietic cells. *Nature* 1989; 339:27–30.
13. Kirshenbaum AS, Kessler SW, Goff JP, Metcalfe DD. Demonstration of the origin of human mast cells from CD34+ bone marrow progenitor cells. *J Immunol* 1991;146:1410–1415.
14. Juhlin L. Basophil leukocyte differential in blood and bone marrow. *Acta Haematol* 1963;29:89–95.
15. Saito H, Hatake K, Dvorak AM, et al. Selective differentiation and proliferation of hematopoietic cells induced by recombinant human interleukins. *Proc Natl Acad Sci U S A* 1988;85:2288–2292.
16. Kirshenbaum AS, Goff JP, Dreskin SC, Irani AM, Schwartz LB, Metcalfe DD. IL-3-dependent growth of basophil-like cells and mast-like cells from human bone marrow. *J Immunol* 1989;142:2424–2429.
17. Valent P, Schmidt G, Besemer J, et al. Interleukin-3 is a differentiation factor for human basophils. *Blood* 1989;73:1763–1769.
18. Valent P, Besemer J, Muhm M, Majdic O, Lechner K, Bettelheim P. Interleukin-3 activates human blood basophils via high affinity binding sites. *Proc Natl Acad Sci U S A* 1989;86:5542–5546.
19. Valent P, Besemer J, Sillaber CH, et al. Failure to detect IL-3-binding sites on human mast cells. *J Immunol* 1990;145:3432–3437.
20. Denburg JA. Basophil and mast cell lineages in vitro and in vivo. *Blood* 1992;79:846–860.
21. Hutt-Taylor SR, Harnish D, Richardson M, Ishizaka T, Denburg JA. Sodium butyrate and a T lymphocyte cell line–derived differentiation factor induce basophilic differentiation of the human promyelocytic leukemia cell line HL-60. *Blood* 1988;71:209–215.
22. Denburg JA, Silver JE, Abrams JS. Interleukin-5 is a human basophilopoietin: Induction of histamine content and basophilic differentiation of HL-60 cells and of peripheral blood basophil-eosinophil progenitors. *Blood* 1991;77:1462–1468.
23. Matsuda H, Coughlin MD, Bienenstock J, Denburg JA. Nerve growth factor promotes human hemopoietic colony growth and differentiation. *Proc Natl Acad Sci U S A* 1988;85:6508–6512.
24. Tsuda T, Wong D, Dolovich J, Bienenstock J, Marshall J, Denburg JA.
25. Sillaber C, Geissler K, Scherrer R, et al. Type beta transforming growth factors promote interleukin-3 (IL-3)-dependent differentiation of human basophils but inhibit IL-3-dependent differentiation of human eosinophils. *Blood* 1992;80:1–8.
26. Kishi K. A new leukemia cell line with Philadelphia chromosome characterized as basophil precursors. *Leuk Res* 1985;9:381–390.
27. Valent P, Besemer J, Kishi K, et al. IL-3 promotes basophilic differentiation of KU812 cells through high affinity binding sites. *J Immunol* 1990;145:1885–1889.
28. Nilsson G, Carlsson M, Jones I, Ahlstedt S, Matsson P, Nilsson K. TNF-alpha and IL-6 induce differentiation in the human basophilic leukemia cell line KU812. *Immunology* 1994;81:73–78.
29. Kitamura Y, Go S, Hatanaka S. Decrease of mast cells in W/Wv mice and their increase by bone marrow transplantation. *Blood* 1978;52: 447–452.
30. Kitamura Y, Go S. Decreased production of mast cells in Sl/Sld anemic mice. *Blood* 1979;53:492–497.
31. Chabot B, Stephenson DA, Chapman VM, Besmer P, Bernstein A. The protooncogene *c-kit* encoding a transmembrane tyrosine kinase receptor maps to the mouse W locus. *Nature* 1988;335:88–89.
32. Geissler EN, Ryan MA, Housman DE. The dominant-white spotting (*W*) locus of the mouse encodes the *c-kit* protooncogene. *Cell* 1988; 55:185–192.
33. Anderson DM, Lyman SD, Baird A, et al. Molecular cloning of mast cell growth factor, a hematopoietin that is active in both membrane bound and soluble forms. *Cell* 1990;63:235–243.
34. Zsebo KM, Williams DA, Geissler EN, et al. Stem cell factor is encoded at the Sl locus of the mouse and is the ligand for the c-kit tyrosine kinase receptor. *Cell* 1990;63:213–224.
35. Flanagan JG, Leder P. The kit ligand: A cell surface molecule altered in Steel mutant fibroblasts. *Cell* 1990;63:185–194.
36. Williams DE, Eisenman J, Baird A, et al. Identification of a ligand for the c-kit proto-oncogene. *Cell* 1990;63:167–174.
37. Huang EJ, Nocka KH, Beier DR, et al. The hematopoietic growth factor KL is encoded by the Sl locus and is the ligand of the c-kit receptor, the gene product of the W locus. *Cell* 1990;63:225–233.
38. Flanagan JG, Chan D, Leder P. Transmembrane form of the kit ligand growth factor is determined by alternative splicing and is missing in the Sld mutant. *Cell* 1991;64:1025–1035.
39. Ihle JN, Keller JR, Oroszlan S, et al. Biologic properties of homogeneous interleukin-3: I. Demonstration of WEHI-3 growth factor activity, mast cell growth factor activity, p cell-stimulating factor activity, colony-stimulating factor activity, and histamine-producing cell-stimulating factor activity. *J Immunol* 1983;131:282–287.
40. Hultner L, Druez C, Moeller J, et al. Mast cell growth-enhancing activity (MEA) is structurally related and functionally identical to the novel mouse T cell growth factor P40/TCGFIII (interleukin 9). *Eur J Immunol* 1990;20:1413–1416.
41. Matsuda H, Kannan Y, Ushio H, et al. Nerve growth factor induces development of connective tissue-type mast cells in vitro from murine bone marrow cells. *J Exp Med* 1991;174:7–14.
42. Rottem M, Hull G, Metcalfe DD. Demonstration of differential effects of cytokines on mast cells derived from murine bone marrow and peripheral blood mononuclear cells. *Exp Hematol* 1994;22:1147–1155.
43. Thompson-Snipes L, Dhar V, Bond MW, Mosmann TR, Moore KW, Rennick DM. Interleukin 10: A novel stimulatory factor for mast cells and their progenitors. *J Exp Med* 1991;173:507–510.
44. Tsuji K, Nakahata T, Takagi M, et al. Effects of interleukin-3 and interleukin-4 on the development of "connective tissue-type" mast cells: Interleukin-3 supports their survival and interleukin-4 triggers and supports their proliferation synergistically with interleukin-3. *Blood* 1990;75:421–427.
45. Bressler RB, Thompson HL, Keffer JM, Metcalfe DD. Inhibition of the growth of IL-3-dependent mast cells from murine bone marrow by recombinant granulocyte macrophage-colony-stimulating factor. *J Immunol* 1989;143:135–140.
46. Broide DH, Wasserman SI, Alvaro GJ, Zvaifler NJ, Firestein GS. Transforming growth factor-beta 1 selectively inhibits IL-3-dependent mast cell proliferation without affecting mast cell function or differentiation. *J Immunol* 1989;143:1591–1597.
47. Födinger M, Fritsch G, Emminger W, et al. Origin of human mast

Synergistic effects of nerve growth factor and granulocyte-macrophage colony-stimulating factor on human basophilic cell differentiation. *Blood* 1991;77:971–979.

cells: Development from transplantated hematopoietic stem cells after allogeneic bone marrow transplantation. *Blood* 1994;84:2954–2959.

48. Rottem M, Okada T, Goff JP, Metcalfe DD. Mast cells cultured from the peripheral blood of normal donors and patients with mastocytosis originate from a CD34+ Fc(epsilon)RI(−) cell population. *Blood* 1994;84:2489–2496.

49. Agis H, Willheim M, Sperr WR, et al. Monocytes do not make mast cells when cultured in the presence of SCF: Characterization of the circulating mast cell progenitor as a c-kit+, CD34+, Ly−, CD14−, CD17−, colony-forming cell. *J Immunol* 1993;151:4221–4227.

50. Rodewald H-R, Dessing M, Dvorak AM, Galli SJ. Identification of a committed precursor for the mast cell lineage. *Science* 1996;271: 818–822.

51. Bland CE, Ginsburg H, Silbert JE, Metcalfe DD. Mouse heparin proteglycan: Synthesis by mast cell-fibroblast monolayers during lymphocyte-dependent mast cell proliferation. *J Biol Chem* 1982;257: 8661–8666.

52. Furitsu T, Saito H, Dvorak AM, et al. Development of human mast cells in vitro. *Proc Natl Acad Sci U S A* 1989;86:10039–10043.

53. Irani AA, Craig SS, Nilsson G, Ishizaka T, Schwartz LB. Characterization of human mast cells developed in vitro from fetal liver cells cocultured with murine 3T3 fibroblasts. *Immunology* 1992;77: 136–143.

54. Kirshenbaum AS, Goff JP, Kessler SW, Mican JM, Zsebo KM, Metcalfe DD. Effect of IL-3 and stem cell factor on the appearance of human basophils and mast cells from CD34+ pluripotent progenitor cells. *J Immunol* 1992;148:772–777.

55. Valent P, Spanblöchl E, Sperr WR, et al. Induction of differentiation of human mast cells from bone marrow and peripheral blood mononuclear cells by recombinant human stem cell factor/kit-ligand in long-term culture. *Blood* 1992;80:2237–2245.

56. Irani AA, Nilsson G, Miettinen U, et al. Recombinant human stem cell factor stimulates differentiation of mast cells from dispersed human fetal liver cells. *Blood* 1992;80:3009–3021.

57. Mitsui H, Furitsu T, Dvorak AM, et al. Development of human mast cells from umbilical cord blood cells by recombinant human and murine c-kit ligand. *Proc Natl Acad Sci U S A* 1993;90:735–739.

58. Dvorak AM, Mitsui H, Ishizaka T. Ultrastructural morphology of immature mast cells in sequential suspension cultures of human cord blood cells supplemented with c-kit ligand: Distinction from mature basophilic leukocytes undergoing secretion in the same cultures. *J Leukocyte Biol* 1993;54:465–485.

59. Nilsson G, Blom T, Harvima I, Kusche-Gullberg M, Nilsson K, Hellman L. Stem cell factor-dependent human cord blood derived mast cells express α- and β-tryptase, heparin and chondroitin sulphate. *Immunology* 1996;88:308–314.

60. Costa JJ, Demetri GD, Harrist TJ, et al. Recombinant human stem cell factor (kit ligand) promotes human mast cell and melanocyte hyperplasia and functional activation in vivo. *J Exp Med* 1996;183: 2681–2686.

61. Nilsson G, Irani AA, Ishizaka T, Schwartz LB. Human recombinant stem cell factor (SCF), the ligand for c-kit, induces development of human mast cells whereas IL-3 induces basophil-like cells from fetal liver cells (FLC). *FASEB J* 1992;6:A1722.

62. Nilsson G, Miettinen U, Ishizaka T, Irani AM, Schwartz LB. IL-4 inhibits the expression of Kit and tryptase during the stem cell factor-dependent development of human mast cells from fetal liver cells. *Blood* 1994;84:1519–1527.

63. Sillaber C, Sperr WR, Agis H, Spanblöchl E, Lechner K, Valent P. Inhibition of stem cell factor dependent formation of human mast cells by interleukin-3 and interleukin-4. *Int Arch Allergy Immunol* 1994;105:264–268.

64. Nilsson G, Nilsson K. Effects of IL-13 on immediate-early response gene expression, phenotype and differentiation of human mast cells: Comparision with IL-4. *Eur J Immunol* 1995;25:870–873.

65. Saito H, Ebisawa M, Tachimoto H, et al. Selective growth of human mast cells induced by steel factor, IL-6, and prostaglandin E$_2$ from cord blood mononuclear cells. *J Immunol* 1996;157:343–350.

66. Kinzer CA, Keegan AD, Paul WE. Identification of FcεRIneg mast cells in mouse bone marrow cultures: Use of a monoclonal anti-p61 antibody. *J Exp Med* 1995;182:575–579.

67. Ryan JJ, Kinzer CA, Paul WE. Mast cells lacking the high affinity immunoglobulin E receptor are deficient in Fc epsilon RI gamma messenger RNA. *J Exp Med* 1995;182:567–574.

68. Li L, Macpherson JJ, Adelstein S, et al. Conditioned media from a cell strain derived from a patient with mastocytosis induces preferential development of cells that possess high affinity IgE receptors and the granule proteases phenotype of mature cutaneous mast cells. *J Biol Chem* 1995;270:2258–2263.

69. Nilsson G, Forsberg K, Bodger MP, et al. Phenotypic characterization of stem cell factor dependent human fetal liver derived mast cells. *Immunology* 1993;79:325–330.

70. Nilsson G, Blom T, Kusche GM, et al. Phenotypic characterization of the human mast cell line HMC-1. *Scand J Immunol* 1994;39:489–498.

71. Butterfield JH, Weiler D, Dewald G, Gleich GJ. Establishment of an immature mast cell line from a patient with mast cell leukemia. *Leuk Res* 1988;12:345–355.

72. Thompson HL, Metcalfe DD, Kinet JP. Early expression of high-affinity receptor for immunoglobulin E (FcεRI) during differentiation of mouse mast cells and human basophils. *J Clin Invest* 1990;85: 1227–1233.

73. Conroy MC, Adkinson NF Jr, Lichtenstein LM. Measurements of IgE on human basophils: Relation to serum IgE and anti-IgE-induced histamine release. *J Immunol* 1977;118:1317–1321.

74. Furuichi K, Rivera J, Isersky C. The receptor for immunoglobulin E on rat basophilic leukemia cells: Effect of ligand binding on receptor expression. *Proc Natl Acad Sci U S A* 1985;82:1522–1527.

75. Hsu C, MacGlashan DW Jr. IgE antibody up-regulates high affinity IgE binding on murine bone marrow derived mast cells. *Immunol Lett* 1996;52:129–134.

76. Yamaguchi M, Lantz CS, Oettgen HC, et al. IgE enhances mouse mast cell FcεRI expression in vitro and in vivo: Evidence for a novel amplification mechanism in IgE-dependent reactions. *J Exp Med* 1997;185: 663–672.

77. Shaikh N, Rivera J, Hewlett BR, Stead RH, Zhu F-G, Marshall JS. Mast cell Fc-epsilon-RI expression in the rat intestinal mucosa and tongue is enhanced during *Nippostrongylus brasiliensis* infection and can be up-regulated by in vivo administration of IgE. *J Immunol* 1997; 158:3805–3812.

78. MacGlashan DW Jr, Bochner BS, Adelman DC, et al. Down-regulation of FcεRI expression on human basophils during in vivo treatment of atopic patients with anti-IgE antibody. *J Immunol* 1997;158: 1438–1445.

79. Toru H, Ra C, Nonoyama S, Suzuki K, Yata J-I, Nakahata T. Induction of the high-affinity IgE receptor (FcεRI) on human mast cells by IL-4. *Int Immunol* 1996;8:1367–1373.

80. Dombrowicz D, Flamand V, Brigman KK, Koller BH, Kinet JP. Abolition of anaphylaxis by targeted disruption of the high affinity immunoglobulin-E receptor alpha-chain gene. *Cell* 1993;75:969–976.

81. Enerbäck L. Mast cells in rat gastrointestinal mucosa: I. Effects of fixation. *Acta Pathol Microbiol Scand* 1966;66:289–302.

82. Strobel S, Miller HR, Ferguson A. Human intestinal mucosal mast cells: Evaluation of fixation and staining techniques. *J Clin Pathol* 1981;34:851–858.

83. Nilsson G, Schwartz LB. Mast cell heterogeneity: Structure and mediators. In: Busse WW, Holgate ST, eds. *Asthma and rhinitis.* Boston: Blackwell Science, 1995:195–208.

84. Church MK, Okayama Y, Bradding P. Functional mast-cell heterogeneity. In: Busse WW, Holgate ST, eds. *Asthma and rhinitis.* Boston: Blackwell Science, 1995:209–220.

85. Irani AA, Schechter NM, Craig SS, DeBlois G, Schwartz LB. Two types of human mast cells that have distinct neutral protease compositions. *Proc Natl Acad Sci U S A* 1986;83:4464–4468.

86. Schwartz LB, Irani AM, Roller K, Castells MC, Schechter NM. Quantitation of histamine, tryptase and chymase in dispersed human T and TC mast cells. *J Immunol* 1987;138:2611–2615.

87. Irani AA, Goldstein SM, Wintroub BU, Bradford T, Schwartz LB. Human mast cell carboxypeptidase: Selective localization to MC$_{TC}$ cells. *J Immunol* 1991;147:247–253.

88. Schechter NM, Irani AM, Sprows JL, Abernethy J, Wintroub B, Schwartz LB. Identification of a cathepsin G-like proteinase in the MC$_{TC}$ type of human mast cell. *J Immunol* 1990;145:2652–2661.

89. Irani AA, Bradford TR, Kepley CL, Schechter NM, Schwartz LB. Detection of MC$_T$ and MC$_{TC}$ types of human mast cells by immunohistochemistry using new monoclonal anti-tryptase and anti-chymase antibodies. *J Histochem Cytochem* 1989;37:1509–1515.

90. Irani AA, Craig SS, DeBlois G, Elson CO, Schechter NM, Schwartz LB. Deficiency of the tryptase-positive, chymase-negative mast cell

type in gastrointestinal mucosa of patients with defective T lymphocyte function. *J Immunol* 1987;138:4381–4386.

91. Malone DH, Irani AM, Schwartz LB, Barrett KE, Metcalfe DD. Mast cell numbers and histamine levels in synovial fluids from patients with diverse arthritis. *Arthritis Rheum* 1986;29:956–963.

92. Tetlow LC, Woolley DE. Distribution, activation and tryptase/chymase phenotype of mast cells in the rheumatoid lesion. *Ann Rheum Dis* 1995;54:549–555.

93. Longley BJ, Morganroth GS, Tyrrell L, et al. Altered metabolism of mast-cell growth factor (c-kit ligand) in cutaneous mastocytosis. *N Engl J Med* 1993;328:1302–1307.

94. Nagata H, Worobec AS, Oh CK, et al. Identification of a point mutation in the catalytic domain of the protooncogene c-kit in peripheral blood mononuclear cells of patients who have mastocytosis with an associated hematologic disorder. *Proc Natl Acad Sci U S A* 1995;92:10560–10564.

95. Tsujimura T, Furitsu T, Morimoto M, et al. Ligand-independent activation of C-Kit receptor tyrosine kinase in a murine mastocytoma cell line P-815 generated by a point mutation. *Blood* 1994;83:2619–2626.

96. Furitsu T, Tsujimura T, Tono T, et al. Identification of mutations in the coding sequence of the proto-oncogene c-kit in a human mast cell leukemia cell line causing ligand-independent activation of c-kit product. *J Clin Invest* 1993;92:1736–1744.

97. Piao X, Paulson R, van der Geer P, Pawson T, Bernstein A. Oncogenic mutation in the Kit receptor tyrosine kinase alters substrate specificity and induces degradation of the protein tyrosine phosphatase SHP-1. *Proc Natl Acad Sci U S A* 1996;93:14665–14669.

98. Garriga MM, Friedman M, Metcalfe DD. A survey of the number and distribution of mast cells in the skin of patients with mast cell disorders. *J Allergy Clin Immunol* 1988;82:425–430.

99. Levi-Schaffer F, Austen KF, Caulfield JP, Hein A, Gravellese PM, Stevens RL. Co-culture of human lung-derived mast cells with mouse 3T3 fibroblasts: Morphology and IgE-mediated release of histamine, prostaglandin D$_2$ and leukotrienes. *J Immunol* 1987;130:494–500.

100. Mekori YA, Oh CK, Metcalfe DD. IL-3-dependent murine mast cells undergo apoptosis on removal of IL-3: Prevention of apoptosis by c-kit ligand. *J Immunol* 1993;151:3775–3784.

101. Yanagida M, Fukamachi H, Ohgami K, et al. Effects of T-helper 2-type cytokines, interleukin-3 (IL-3), IL-4, IL-5, and IL-6 on the survival of cultured human mast cells. *Blood* 1995;86:3705–3714.

102. Mekori YA, Metcalfe DD. Transforming growth factor-beta prevents stem cell factor–mediated rescue of mast cells from apoptosis after IL-3 deprivation. *J Immunol* 1994;153:2194–2203.

103. Inemura A, Tsai M, Ando A, Wershil BK, Galli SJ. The c-kit ligand, stem cell factor, promotes mast cell survival by suppressing apoptosis. *Am J Pathol* 1994;144:321–328.

104. Horigome K, Bullock ED, Johnson EM. Effects of nerve growth factor on rat peritoneal mast cells: Survival promotion and immediate-early gene induction. *J Biol Chem* 1994;269:2695–2702.

105. Kawamoto K, Okada T, Kannan Y, Ushio H, Matsumoto M, Matsuda H. Nerve growth factor prevents apoptosis of rat peritoneal mast cells through the trk proto-oncogene receptor. *Blood* 1995;86:4638–4644.

106. Rodriguez-Tarduchy G, Collins MKL, Garcia I, Lopez-Rivas A. Insulin-like growth factor-I inhibits apoptosis in IL-3-dependent hematopoietic cells. *J Immunol* 1992;149:535–540.

107. Nocka K, Buck J, Levi E, Besmer P. Candidate ligand for the c-kit transmembrane kinase receptor: KL, a fibroblast derived growth factor stimulates mast cells and erythroid progenitors. *EMBO J* 1990;9:3287–3294.

108. Aye MT, Hashemi S, Leclair B, et al. Expression of stem cell factor and c-kit mRNA in cultured endothelial cells, monocytes and cloned human bone marrow stromal cells (CFU-RF). *Exp Hematol* 1992;20:523–527.

109. Lavker RM, Schechter NM. Cutaneous mast cell depletion results from topical corticosteroids usage. *J Immunol* 1985;135:2368–2373.

110. Pipkorn U, Hammarlund A, Enerbäck L. Prolonged treatment with topical glucocorticoids results in an inhibition of the allergen-induced weal-and-flare response and a reduction in skin mast cell numbers and histamine content. *Clin Exp Allergy* 1989;19:19–25.

111. Goldsmith P, McGarity B, Walls AF, Church MK, Milward-Sadler GH, Robertson DA. Corticosteroid treatment reduces mast cell numbers in inflammatory bowel disease. *Dig Dis Sci* 1990;35:1409–1413.

112. Finotto S, Mekori YA, Metcalfe DD. Glucocorticoids decrease tissue mast cell number by reducing the production of the c-kit ligand, stem

113. cell factor, by resident cells: In vitro and in vivo evidence in murine systems. *J Clin Invest* 1997;99:1721–1728.

113. Nagata S, Golstein P. The Fas death factor. *Science* 1995;267:1449–1456.

114. Hartmann K, Mekori YA, Metcalfe DD. FAS-/APO-1-mediated apoptosis in murine mast cells. *FASEB J* 1996;10:A1022.

115. Yamaguchi M, Hirai K, Morita Y, et al. Hemopoietic growth factors regulate the survival of human basophils in vitro. *Int Arch Allergy Immunol* 1992;97:322–329.

116. Dvorak AM, Seder RA, Paul WE, Morgan ES, Galli SJ. Effects of interleukin-3 with or without the c-kit ligand, stem cell factor, on the survival and cytoplasmic granule formation of mouse basophils and mast cells in vitro. *Am J Pathol* 1994;144:160–170.

117. Bauza MT, Lagunoff D. Histidine transport by isolated rat peritoneal mast cells. *Biochem Pharmacol* 1981;30:1271–1276.

118. Johnson RG, Carty SE, Fingerhoff BJ, Scarpa A. The internal pH of mast cell granules. *FEBS Lett* 1980;120:75–79.

119. Lagunoff D, Rickard A. Evidence for control of mast cell granule protease in situ by low pH. *Exp Cell Res* 1983;144:353–360.

120. Fox CC, Dvorak AM, Peters SP, Kagey-Sobotka A, Lichtenstein LM. Isolation and characterization of human intestinal mucosal mast cells. *J Immunol* 1985;135:483–491.

121. Schulman ESK-S A, MacGlashan DW Jr, Adkinson NF Jr, Peters SP, Schleimer RP, Lichtenstein LM. Heterogeneity of human mast cells. *J Immunol* 1983;131:1936–1941.

122. Black JW, Duncan WAM, Durant CJ, Ganellin CR, Parsons EM. Definition and antagonism of histamine H2-receptors. *Nature* 1972;236:385–390.

123. Arrang JM, Garbarg M, Schwartz JC. Highly potent and selective ligands for histamine H3-receptors. *Nature* 1983;302:832–837.

124. Cavanah DK, Casale TB. Histamine. In: Kaliner MA, Metcalfe DD, eds. *The mast cell in health and disease.* New York: Marcel Dekker, 1993:321–342.

125. Wood-Baker R. Histamine and its receptors. In: Busse WW, Holgate ST, eds. *Asthma and rhinitis.* Boston: Blackwell Science, 1994:791–800.

126. Miller JS, Westin EH, Schwartz LB. Cloning and characterization of complementary DNA for human tryptase. *J Clin Invest* 1989;84:1188–1195.

127. Miller JS, Moxley G, Schwartz LB. Cloning and characterization of a second complementary DNA for human tryptase. *J Clin Invest* 1990;86:864–870.

128. Vanderslice P, Ballinger SM, Tam EK, Goldstein SM, Craik CS, Caughey GH. Human mast cell tryptase: Multiple cDNAs and genes reveal a multigene serine protease family. *Proc Natl Acad Sci U S A* 1990;87:3811–3815.

129. Sakai K, Ren SL, Schwartz LB. A novel heparin-dependent processing pathway for human tryptase: Autocatalysis followed by activation with dipeptidyl peptidase I. *J Clin Invest* 1996;97:988–995.

130. Schwartz LB, Sakai K, Bradford TR, et al. The alpha form of human tryptase is the predominant type present in blood at baseline in normal subjects and is elevated in those with systemic mastocytosis. *J Clin Invest* 1995;96:2702–2710.

131. Alter SC, Metcalfe DD, Bradford TR, Schwartz LB. Regulation of human mast cell tryptase: Effects of enzyme concentration, ionic strength and the structure and negative charge density of polysaccharides. *Biochem J* 1987;248:821–827.

132. Gruber BL, Schwartz LB, Ramamurthy NS, Irani AM, Marchese MJ. Activation of latent rheumatoid synovial collagenase by human mast cell tryptase. *J Immunol* 1988;140:3936–3942.

133. Caughey GH. The structure and airway biology of mast cell proteinases. *Am J Respir Cell Mol Biol* 1991;4:387–394.

134. Schechter NM, Sprows JL, Schoenberger OL, Lazarus GS, Cooperman BS, Rubin H. Reaction of human skin chymotrypsin-like proteinase chymase with plasma proteinase inhibitors. *J Biol Chem* 1989;264:21308–21315.

135. Wintroub BU, Schechter NB, Lazarus GS, Kaempfer CE, Schwartz LB. Angiotensin 1 conversion by human and rat chymotryptic proteinasis. *J Invest Dermatol* 1984;83:336–339.

136. Mizutani H, Schechter N, Lazarus C, Black RA, Kupper TS. Rapid and specific conversion of precursor interleukin 1B (IL-1B) to an active IL-1 species by human mast cell chymase. *J Exp Med* 1991;174:821–825.

137. Schwartz LB, Riedel C, Schratz JJ, Austen KF. Localization of car-

boxypeptidase A to the macromolecular heparin proteoglycan-protein complex in secretory granules of rat serosal mast cells. *J Immunol* 1982;128:1128–1133.

138. Metcalfe DD, Lewis RA, Silbert JE, Rosenberg RD, Wasserman SI, Austen KF. Isolation and characterization of heparin from human lung. *J Clin Invest* 1979;64:1537–1543.

139. Woodbury RG, Everitt M, Sanada Y, Katunuma N, Lagunoff D, Neurath H. A major serine esterase in skeletal muscle: Evidence for its mast cell origin. *Proc Natl Acad Sci U S A* 1978;75:5311–5313.

140. Lewis RA, Austen KF, Soberman RJ. Leukotrienes and other products of the 5-lipoxygenase pathway: Biochemistry and relation to pathobiology in human disease. *N Engl J Med* 1990;323:645–655.

141. Peters SP, MacGlashan DW Jr, Schulman ES, et al. Arachidonic acid metabolism in purified human lung mast cells. *J Immunol* 1984;132:1972–1979.

142. Drazen JM, Austen KF. Leukotrienes and airway responses. *Am Rev Respir Dis* 1987;136:985–998.

143. Lewis RA, Austen KF. The biologically active leukotrienes: Biosynthesis, metabolism, receptors, functions and pharmacology. *J Clin Invest* 1984;73:889–897.

144. Chung SW, Wong PMC, Shen-Ong G, Ruscetti S, Ishizaka T, Eaves CJ. Production of granulocyte-macrophage colony-stimulating factor by Abelson virus-induced tumorigenic mast cell lines. *Blood* 1986;68:1074–1081.

145. Brown MA, Pierce JH, Watson CJ, Falco J, Ihle JN, Paul WE. B cell stimulatory factor-1/interleukin-4 mRNA is expressed by normal and transformed mast cells. *Cell* 1987;50:809–818.

146. Farram E, Nelson DS. Mouse mast cells as anti-tumor effector cells. *Cell Immunol* 1980;55:294–301.

147. Jadus MR, Schmunk G, Djeu JY, Parkman R. Morphology and lytic mechansims of interleukin 3-dependent natural cytotoxic cells: Tumor necrosis factor as a possible mediator. *J Immunol* 1986;137:2774–2783.

148. Gordon JR, Galli SJ. Mast cells as a source of both preformed and immunologically inducible TNF-alpha/cachectin. *Nature* 1990;346:274–276.

149. Steffen M, Abboud M, Potter GK, Yung YP, Moore MAS. Presence of tumour necrosis factor or a related factor in human basophil/mast cells. *Immunology* 1989;66:445–450.

150. Ohno I, Tanno Y, Yamauchi K, Takishima T. Gene expression and production of tumour necrosis factor by a rat basophilic leukaemia cell line (RBL-2H3) with IgE receptor triggering. *Immunology* 1990;70:88–93.

151. Plaut M, Pierce JH, Watson CJ, Hanley HJ, Nordan RP, Paul WE. Mast cell lines produce lymphokines in response to cross-linkage of FcεRI or to calcium ionophores. *Nature* 1989;339:64–67.

152. Burd PR, Rogers HW, Gordon JR, et al. Interleukin 3-dependent and -independent mast cells stimulated with IgE and antigen express multiple cytokines. *J Exp Med* 1989;170:245–257.

153. Rumsaeng V, Vliagoftis H, Oh CK, Metcalfe DD. Lymphotactin gene expression in mast cells following FcεRI aggregation: Modulation by TGF-β, dexamethasone, and cyclosporin A. *J Immunol* 1997;158:1353–1360.

154. Galli SJ, Costa JJ. Mast cell-leukocyte cytokine cascade in allergic inflammation. *Allergy* 1995;50:851–862.

155. Rumsaeng V, Cruikshank WW, Foster B, et al. Human mast cells produce the CD4+ T-lymphocyte chemoattractant factor, interleukin-16. *J Immunol* 1997;159:2904–2910.

156. Benyon RC, Bissonnette EY, Befus AD. Tumor necrosis factor-alpha dependent cytotoxicity of human skin mast cells is enhanced by anti-IgE antibodies. *J Immunol* 1991;147:2253–2258.

157. Ohkawara Y, Yamauchi K, Tanno Y, et al. Human lung mast cells and pulmonary macrophages produce tumor necrosis factor-alpha in sensitized lung tissue after IgE-receptor triggering. *Am J Respir Cell Mol Biol* 1992;7:385–392.

158. Okayama Y, Lau LCK, Church MK. TNF-α production by human lung mast cells in response to stimulation by stem cell factor and FcεRI cross-linkage. *Submitted for publication* 1997.

159. Okayama Y, Petitfrere C, Kassel O, et al. IgE-dependent expression of mRNA for IL-4 and IL-5 in human lung mast cells. *J Immunol* 1995;155:1796–1808.

160. Jaffe JS, Glaum MC, Raible DG, et al. Human lung mast cell IL-5 gene and protein expression: Temporal analysis of upregulation following IgE-mediated activation. *Am J Respir Cell Mol Biol* 1995;13:665–675.

161. Bradding P, Roberts JA, Britten KM, et al. Interleukin-4, -5, and -6 and tumor necrosis factor-alpha in normal and asthmatic airways: Evidence for the human mast cell as a source of these cytokines. *Am J Respir Cell Mol Biol* 1994;10:471–480.

162. Bradding P, Feather IH, Wilson S, et al. Immunolocalization of cytokines in the nasal mucosa of normal and perennial rhinitic subjects: The mast cell as a source of IL-4, IL-5, and IL-6 in human allergic mucosal inflammation. *J Immunol* 1993;151:3853–3865.

163. Ying S, Durham SR, Corrigan CJ, Hamid Q, Kay AB. Phenotype of cells expressing mRNA for TH2-type (interleukin 4 and interleukin 5) and TH1-type (interleukin 2 and interferon gamma) cytokines in bronchoalveolar lavage and bronchial biopsies from atopic asthmatic and normal control subjects. *Am J Respir Cell Mol Biol* 1995;12:477–487.

164. Arock M, Merle-Beral H, Dugas B, et al. IL-4 release by human leukemic and activated normal basophils. *J Immunol* 1993;151:1441–1447.

165. Brunner T, Heusser CH, Dahinden CA. Human peripheral blood basophils primed by interleukin 3 (IL-3) produce IL-4 in response to immunoglobulin E receptor stimulation. *J Exp Med* 1993;177:605–611.

166. MacGlashan D, White JM, Huang SK, Ono SJ, Schroeder JT, Lichtenstein LM. Secretion of IL-4 from human basophils: The relationship between IL-4 mRNA and protein in resting and stimulated basophils. *J Immunol* 1994;152:3006–3016.

167. MacGlashan D Jr, White JM, Huang SK, Ono SJ, Schroeder JT, Lichtenstein LM. Secretion of IL-4 from human basophils: The relationship between cytokine production and histamine release in mixed leukocyte cultures. *J Immunol* 1994;153:1808–1817.

168. Li H, Sim TC, Alam R. IL-13 released by and localized in human basophils. *J Immunol* 1996;156:4833–4838.

169. Gauchat JF, Henchoz S, Mazzei G, et al. Induction of human IgE synthesis in B-cells by mast cells and basophils. *Nature* 1993;365:340–343.

170. Li H, Sim TC, Grant JA, Alam R. The production of macrophage inflammatory protein-1 alpha by human basophils. *J Immunol* 1996;157:1207–1212.

171. Lemanske RFJ, Kaliner MA. Late phase allergic reactions. In: Middleton EJ, Reed CE, Ellis EF, Adkinson NF, Yuninger JW, Busse WW, eds. *Allergy: Principles and practice.* St. Louis: Mosby, 1993:320–361.

172. Wershil BK, Wang ZS, Gordon JR, Galli SJ. Recruitment of neutrophils during IgE-dependent cutaneous late phase reactions in the mouse is mast cell-dependent: Partial inhibition of the reaction with antiserum against tumor necrosis factor-alpha. *J Clin Invest* 1991;87:446–453.

173. Norman JC, Price LS, Ridley AJ, Koffer A. The small GTP-binding proteins, Rac and Rho, regulate cytoskeletal organization and exocytosis in mast cells by parallel pathways. *Mol Biol Cell* 1996;7:1429–1442.

174. Kobayasi T, Asboe-Hansen G. Degranulation and regranulation of human mast cells. *Acta Derm Venerol* 1969;49:369–381.

175. Dvorak AM, Schleimer RP, Lichtenstein LM. Morphologic mast cell cycles. *Cell Immunol* 1987;105:199–204.

176. Dvorak AM, Schleimer RP, Lichtenstein LM. Human mast cells synthesize new granules during recovery from degranulation: In vitro studies with mast cells purified from human lungs. *Blood* 1988;71:76–85.

177. Metzger H. The receptor with high affinity for IgE. *Immunol Rev* 1992;125:37–48.

178. Weetall M, Shopes B, Holowka D, Baird B. Mapping the site of interaction between murine IgE and its high affinity receptor with chimeric Ig. *J Immunol* 1990;145:3849–3854.

179. Segal DM, Taurog JD, Metzger H. Dimeric immunoglobulin E serves as a unit signal for mast cell degranulation. *Proc Natl Acad Sci U S A* 1977;74:2993–2997.

180. Menon AK, Holowka D, Baird B. Small oligomers of immunoglobulin E cause large-scale clustering of IgE receptors on the surface of rat basophilic leukemia cells. *J Cell Biol* 1984;98:577–583.

181. Razin E, Rivera J. Signal transduction in the activation of mast cells and basophils. *Immunol Today* 1995;16:370–373.

182. Hamawy MM, Mergenhagen SE, Siraganian RP. Protein tyrosine phosphorylation as a mechanism of signalling in mast cells and basophils. *Cell Signal* 1995;7:535–544.

183. MacDonald SM. Histamine releasing factors and IgE heterogeneity. In: Middleton E, Reed CE, Ellis EF, Adkinson NF, Yunginger JW, Busse WW, eds. *Allergy: Principles and practice.* St. Louis: Mosby, 1993:1–11.

184. MacDonald SM, Tafnar T, Langdon J, Lichtenstein LM. Molecular identification of an IgE-dependent histamine-releasing factor. *Science* 1995;269:688–690.

185. Lagunoff D, Martin TW, Read G. Agents that release histamine from mast cells. *Annu Rev Pharmacol Toxicol* 1983;23:331–351.

186. Peters SP. Mechanism of mast-cell activation. In: Busse WW, Holgate ST, eds. *Asthma and rhinitis.* Boston: Blackwell Science, 1995:221–230.

187. Malaviya R, Ross E, Jakschik BA, Abraham SN. Mast cell degraulation induced by type 1 fimbriated *Escherichia coli* in mice. *J Clin Invest* 1994;93:1645–1653.

188. Marquardt DL, Parker CW, Sullivan TJ. Potentiation of mast cell mediator release by adenosine. *J Immunol* 1978;120:871–878.

189. White MV. Mast cell secretagogues. In: Kaliner MA, Metcalfe DD, eds. *The mast cell in health and disease.* New York: Marcel Dekker, 1993:109–128.

190. Ali K, Leung KPB, Pearce FL, Hayes NA, Foreman JC. Comparision of the histamine-releasing action of substance P on mast cells and basophils from different species and tissues. *Int Arch Allergy Immunol* 1986;79:413–418.

191. Benyon RC, Lowman MA, Church MK. Human skin mast cells: their dispersion, purification and secretory characteristcs. *J Immunol* 1987;138:861–867.

192. Williams RM, Bienenstock J, Stead RH. Mast cells: The neuroimmune connection. In: Marone G, ed. *Human basophils and mast cells: Biological aspects.* Basel: Karger, 1995:208–235.

193. Hugli TE. The structural basis for anaphylatoxin and chemotactic functions of C3a, C4a, and C5a. *Crit Rev Immunol* 1981;2:321–366.

194. Schulman ES, Post TJ, Henson PM, Gicias PC. Differential effects of complement peptides, C5a and C5a des arg on human basophils and lung mast cell histamine release. *J Clin Invest* 1985;81:918–923.

195. El-Lati SG, Dahinden CA, Church MK. Complement peptides C3a- and C5a-induced mediator release from dissociated human skin mast cells. *J Invest Dermatol* 1994;102:803–806.

196. Kaplan AP, Reddigari S, Baeza M, Kuna P. Histamine releasing factors and cytokine-dependent activation of basophils and mast cells. *Adv Immunol* 1991;50:237–260.

197. Alam R, Lett BM, Forsythe PA, et al. Monocyte chemotactic and activating factor is a potent histamine-releasing factor for basophils. *J Clin Invest* 1992;89:723–728.

198. Alam R, Forsythe P, Stafford S, et al. Monocyte chemotactic protein-2, monocyte chemotactic protein-3, and fibroblast-induced cytokine: Three new chemokines induce chemotaxis and activation of basophils. *J Immunol* 1994;153:3155–3159.

199. Dahinden CA, Geiser T, Brunner T, et al. Monocyte chemotactic protein 3 is a most effective basophil- and eosinophil-activating chemokine. *J Exp Med* 1994;179:751–756.

200. Kuna P, Reddigari SR, Schall TJ, Rucinski D, Sadick M, Kaplan AP. Characterization of the human basophil response to cytokines, growth factors, and histamine releasing factors of the intercrine/chemokine family. *J Immunol* 1993;150:1932–1943.

201. Kuna P, Reddigari SR, Rucinski D, Oppenheim JJ, Kaplan AP. Monocyte chemotactic and activating factor is a potent histamine-releasing factor for human basophils. *J Exp Med* 1992;175:489–494.

202. Weber M, Uguccioni M, Ochensberger B, Baggiolonin M, Lewis I, Dahinden CA. Monocyte chemotactic protein MCP-2 activates human basophil and eosinophil leukocytes similar to MCP-3. *J Immunol* 1995;154:4166–4172.

203. Kuna P, Reddigari SR, Kornfeld D, Kaplan AP. IL-8 inhibits histamine release from human basophils induced by histamine-releasing factors, connective tissue activating peptide III, and IL-3. *J Immunol* 1991;147:1920–1924

204. Massey WA, Randall TC, Kagey-Sobotka A, et al. Recombinant human IL-1 alpha and -1 beta potentiates IgE-mediated histamine release from human basophils. *J Immunol* 1989;143:1875–1880.

205. Bischoff SC, de Weck AL, Dahinden C. Interleukin 3 and granulocyte/macrophage-colony-stimulating factor render human basophils responsive to low concentrations of complement component C3a. *Proc Natl Acad Sci U S A* 1991;87:6813–6817.

206. Bischoff SC, Brunner T, de Weck AL, Dahinden CA. Interleukin 5

207. Bischoff SC, Dahinden CA. Effect of nerve growth factor on the release of inflammatory mediators by mature human basophils. *Blood* 1992;79:2662–2669.

208. Bürgi B, Otten UH, Ochensberger B, et al. Basophil priming by neurotrophic factors: Activation through the trk receptor. *J Immunol* 1996;157:5582–5588.

209. Bischoff SC, Dahinden CA. c-Kit ligand: A unique potentiator of mediator release by human lung mast cells. *J Exp Med* 1992;175:237–244.

210. Columbo M, Horowitz EM, Botana LM, et al. The human recombinant c-kit receptor ligand, rhSCF, induces mediator release from human cutaneous mast cells and enhances IgE-dependent mediator release from both skin mast cells and peripheral blood basophils. *J Immunol* 1992;149:599–608.

211. Hartmann K, Beiglbock F, Czarnetzki BM, Zuberbier T. Effect of CC chemokines on mediator release from human skin mast cells and basophils. *Int Arch Allergy Immunol* 1995;108:224–230.

212. Freder W, Agis H, Semper H, et al. Differential response of human basophils and mast cells to recombinant chemokines. *Ann Hematol* 1995;70:251–258.

213. Taub D, Dastych J, Inamura N, et al. Bone marrow-derived murine mast cells migrate, but do not degranulate, in response to chemokines. *J Immunol* 1995;154:2393–2402.

214. Alam R, Kumar D, Andersonwalters D, Forsythe PA. Macrophage inflammatory protein-1 alpha and monocyte chemoattractant peptide-1 elicit immediate and late cutaneous reactions and activate murine mast cells in vivo. *J Immunol* 1994;152:1298–1303.

215. Katz RH, Raizman MB, Gartner CS, Scott HC, Benson AC, Austen KF. Secretory granule mediator release and generation of oxidative metabolites of arachidonic acid via Fc-IgG receptor bridging in mouse mast cells. *J Immunol* 1992;148:868–873.

216. Latour S, Bonnerot C, Fridman WH, Daron M. Induction of tumor necrosis factor-alpha production by mast cells via FcγR: Role of the FcγRIII γ-subunit. *J Immunol* 1992;149:2155–2162.

217. Dastych J, Hardison MC, Metcalfe DD. Aggregation of low affinity IgG receptors induces mast cell adherence to fibronectin: Requirement for the common FcR γ-chain. *J Immunol* 1997;158:1803–1809.

218. Daeron M, Latour S, Malbec O, Espinosa E, Pasmans S, Fridman WH. The same tyrosine-based inhibition motif, in the intracytoplasmic domain of Fc γ RIIB, regulates BCR-, TCR-, and FcR-dependent cell activation. *Immunity* 1995;3:635–646.

219. Daeron M, Malbec O, Latour S, Arock M, Fridman WH. Regulation of high-affinity IgE receptor-mediated mast cell activation by murine low-affinity IgG receptors. *J Clin Invest* 1995;95:577–585.

220. Hamawy MM, Mergenhagen SE, Siraganian RP. Adhesion molecules as regulators of mast-cell and basophil function. *Immunol Today* 1994; 15:62–66.

221. Bochner BS, Sterbinsky SA, Briskin M, Saini SS, Macglashan DW. Counter-receptors on human basophils for endothelial cell adhesion molecules. *J Immunol* 1996;157:844–850.

222. Bochner BS, Peachell PT, Brown KE, Schleimer RP. Adherence of human basophils to cultured umbilical vein vascular endothelial cells. *J Clin Invest* 1988;81:1355–1363.

223. Bochner BS, MacGlashan DW Jr, Maarcotte GV, Schleimer RP. IgE-dependent regulation of human basophil adherence to vascular endothelium. *J Immunol* 1989;142:3180–3186.

224. Bochner BS, McKelvey AA, Sterbinsky SA, et al. Interleukin-3 augments adhesiveness for endothelium and CD11b expression in human basophils but not neutrophils. *J Immunol* 1990;145:1832–1837.

225. Bochner BS, Klunk DA, Sterbinsky SA, Coffman RL, Schleimer RP. Interleukin-13 selectively induces vascular cell adhesion molecule-1 (VCAM-1) expression in human endothelial cells. *J Immunol* 1995; 154:799–803.

226. Schleimer RP, Sterbinsky SA, Kaiser J, et al. Interleukin-4 induces adherence of human eosinophils and basophils but not neutrophils to endothelium: association with expression of VCAM-1. *J Immunol* 1992;148:1086–1092.

227. Sperr WR, Agis H, Czerwenka K, et al. Differential expression of cell surface integrins on human mast cells and human basophils. *Ann Hematol* 1992;65:10–16.

228. Vliagoftis H, Metcalfe DD. Cell adhesion molecules in mast cell

modifies histamine release and leukotriene generation by human basophils in response to diverse agonists. *J Exp Med* 1990;172: 1577–1582.

adhesion and migration. In: Bochner B, ed. *Adhesion molecules in allergic diseases.* New York: Marcel Dekker, 1997:151–172.

229. Smith TJ, Weis JH. Mucosal T cells and mast cells share common adhesion receptors. *Immunol Today* 1996;17:60–63.

230. Gurish MF, Bell AF, Smith TJ, Ducharme LA, Wang RK, Weis JH. Expression of murine beta 7, alpha 4, and beta 1 integrin genes by rodent mast cells. *J Immunol* 1992;149:1964–1972.

231. Ducharme LA, Weis JH. Modulation of integrin expression during mast cell differentiation. *Eur J Immunol* 1992;22:2603–2607.

232. Smith TJ, Ducharme LA, Shaw SK, et al. Murine M290 integrin expression modulated by mast cell activation. *Immunity* 1994;1:393–403.

233. Thompson HL, Burbelo PD, Segui-Real B, Yamada Y, Metcalfe DD. Laminin promotes mast cell attachment. *J Immunol* 1989;143:2323–2327.

234. Walsh LJ, Kaminer MS, Lazarus GS, Lavker RM, Murphy GF. Role of laminin in localization of human dermal mast cells. *Lab Invest* 1991;65:433–440.

235. Thompson HL, Burbelo PD, Metcalfe DD. Regulation of adhesion of mouse bone marrow-derived mast cells to laminin. *J Immunol* 1990;145:3425–3431.

236. Dastych J, Costa JJ, Thompson HL, Metcalfe DD. Mast cell adhesion to fibronectin. *Immunology* 1991;73:478–484.

237. Bianchine PJ, Burd PR, Metcalfe DD. IL-3-dependent mast cells attach to plate-bound vitronectin: Demonstration of augmented proliferation in response to signals transduced via cell surface vitronectin receptors. *J Immunol* 1992;149:3665–3671.

238. Dastych J, Metcalfe DD. Stem cell factor induces mast cell adhesion to fibronectin. *J Immunol* 1994;152:213–219.

239. Dastych J, Hardison ML, Metcalfe DD. Aggregation of low affinity IgG receptors induces mast cell adherence to fibronectin: requirement for the common FcRγ-chain. *J Immunol* 1997;158:1803–1809.

240. Shimizu Y, Irani A, Brown EJ, Ashman LK, Schwartz LB. Human mast cells derived from fetal liver cells cultured with stem cell factor express a functional CD51/CD61 (alpha v beta 3) integrin. *Blood* 1995;86:930–939.

241. Bianchine PJ, Paolini R, Kinet J-P, Metcalfe DD. Mast cell adhesion to vitronectin is sufficient to phosphorylate focal adhesion kinase. *J Allergy Clin Immunol* 1994;93:226(380A).

242. Hamawy MM, Oliver C, Mergenhagen SE, Siraganian RP. Adherence of rat basophilic leukemia (RBL-2H3) cells to fibronectin-coated surfaces enhances secretion. *J Immunol* 1992;149:615–621.

243. Hamawy MM, Mergenhagen SE, Siraganian RP. Tyrosine phosphorylation of pp125FAK by the aggregation of high affinity immunoglobulin E receptors requires cell adherence. *J Biol Chem* 1993;268:6851–6854.

244. Hamawy MM, Mergenhagen SE, Siraganian RP. Cell adherence to fibronectin and the aggregation of the high affinity immunoglobulin E receptor synergistically regulate tyrosine phosphorylation of 105-115-kDa proteins. *J Biol Chem* 1993;268:5227–5233.

245. Guo CB, Kagey SA, Lichtenstein LM, Bochner BS. Immunophenotyping and functional analysis of purified human uterine mast cells. *Blood* 1992;79:708–712.

246. Sperr WR, Czerwenka K, Mundigler G, et al. Specific activation of human mast cells by the ligand for c-kit: Comparision between lung, uterus and heart mast cells. *Int Arch Allergy Immunol* 1993;102:170–175.

247. Columbo M, Bochner BS, Marone G. Human skin mast cells express functional beta(1), integrins that mediate adhesion to extracellular matrix proteins. *J Immunol* 1995;154:6058–6064.

248. Adachi S, Tsujimura T, Jippo T, et al. Inhibition of attachment between cultured mast cells and fibroblasts by phorbol 12-myristate 13-acetate and stem cell factor. *Exp Hematol* 1995;23:58–65.

249. Adachi S, Ebi Y, Nishikawa SI, et al. Necessity of extracellular domain of W (c-kit) receptors for attachment of murine cultured mast cells to fibroblasts. *Blood* 1992;79:650–656.

250. Friedman MM, Kaliner MM. In situ degranulation of human nasal mucosal mast cells: Ultrastructural features and cell-cell association. *J Allergy Clin Immunol* 1985;76:70–82.

251. Inamura N, Mekori YA, Bhattacharyya SP, Bianchine PJ, Metcalf DD. Induction and enhancement of FcεRI-dependent mast cell degranulation following coculture with activated T cells: dependency on ICAM-I- and leukocyte function-associated antigen (LFA)-I-mediated heterotypic aggregation. *J Immunol* 1998;160:4026–4033.

252. Oh CK, Metcalfe DD. Activated lymphocytes induce promoter activity of the TCA3 gene in mast cells following cell to cell contact. *Biochem Biophys Res Commun* 1996;221:510–514.

253. Bascom R, Wachs M, Naclerio RM, Pipkorn U, Galli SJ, Lichtenstein LM. Basophil influx occurs after nasal antigen challenge: Effects of topical corticosteroid pretreatment. *J Allergy Clin Immunol* 1988;81:580–590.

254. Koshino T, Arai Y, Miyamoto Y, et al. Mast cell and basophil number in the airway correlate with bronchial responsiveness of asthmatics. *Int Arch Allergy Immunol* 1995;107:378–379.

255. Guo CB, Liu MC, Galli SJ, Bochner BS, Kagey-Sobotka A, Lichtenstein LM. Identification of IgE-bearing cells in the late-phase response to antigen in the lung as basophils. *Am J Respir Cell Mol Biol* 1994;10:384–390.

256. Tanimoto Y, Takahashi K, Kimura I. Effects of cytokines on human basophil chemotaxis. *Clin Exp Allergy* 1992;22:1020–1025.

257. Yamaguchi M, Hirai K, Shoji S, et al. Haemopoietic growth factors induce human basophil migration in vitro. *Clin Exp Allergy* 1992;22:379–384.

258. Rot A, Krieger M, Brunner T, Bischoff SC, Schall TJ, Dahinden CA. RANTES and macrophage inflammatory protein 1 alpha induce the migration and activation of normal human eosinophil granulocytes. *J Exp Med* 1992;176:1489–1495.

259. Lett-Brown MA, Boetcher DA, Leonard EJ. Chemotactic responses of normal human basophils to C5a and to a lymphocyte-derived chemotactic factor. *J Immunol* 1976;117:246–252.

260. Laitinen LA, Laitinen A, Haahtela T. Airway mucosal inflammation even in patients with newly diagnosed asthma. *Am Rev Respir Dis* 1993;147:697–704.

261. Enerbck L, Pipkorn U, Granerus G. Intraepithelial migration of nasal mucosal mast cells in hay fever. *Int Arch Allergy Immunol* 1986;80:44–50.

262. Juliusson S, Pipkorn U, Karlsson G, Enerbäck L. Mast cells and eosinophils in the allergic mucosal response to allergen challenge: Changes in distribution and signs of activation in relation to symptoms. *J Allergy Clin Immunol* 1992;90:898–909.

263. Chanez P, Lacoste JY, Guillot B, et al. Mast cells' contribution to the fibrosing alveolitis of the scleroderma lung. *Am Rev Respir Dis* 1993;147:1497–1502.

264. Godfrey HP, Ilardi C, Engber W, Graziano FM. Quantification of human synovial mast cells in rheumatoid arthritis and other rheumatic diseases. *Arthritis Rheum* 1984;27:852–856.

265. Aldenborg F, Fall M, Enerbäck L. Proliferation and transepithelial migration of mucosal mast cells in interstitial cystitis. *Immunology* 1986;58:411–416.

266. Li Q, Raza AA, MacAulay MA, et al. The relationship of mast cells and their secreted products to the volume of fibrosis in posttransplant hearts. *Transplantation* 1992;53:1047–1051.

267. Baroni C. On the relationship of mast cells to various soft tissue tumours. *Br J Cancer* 1964;18:686–691.

268. Meininger CJ, Zetter BR. Mast cells and angiogenesis. *Semin Cancer Biol* 1992;3:73–79.

269. Fokkens WJ, Godthelp T, Holm AF, et al. Dynamics of mast cells in the nasal mucosa of patients with allergic rhinitis and non-allergic controls: A biopsy study. Clin Exp Allergy 1992;22:701–710.

270. Gibson PG, Allen CJ, Yang JP, et al. Intraepithelial mast cells in allergic and nonallergic asthma: Assessment using bronchial brushings. *Am Rev Respir Dis* 1993;148:80–86.

271. Meininger CJ, Yano H, Rottapel R, Bernstein A, Zsebo KM, Zetter BR. The c-kit receptor ligand functions as a mast cell chemoattractant. *Blood* 1992;79:958–963.

272. Nilsson G, Butterfield JH, Nilsson K, Siegbahn A. Stem cell factor is a chemotactic factor for human mast cells. *J Immunol* 1994;153:3717–3723.

273. Wen LP, Fahrni JA, Matsui S, Rosen GD. Airway epithelial cells produce stem cell factor. *Biochem Biophys Acta* 1996;1314:183–186.

274. Nilsson G, Hjertson M, Andersson M, Nilsson K, Siegbahn A. Mast cell chemotactic activity in nasal lavage from allergic patients. *J Allergy Clin Immunol* 1996;97:392A.

275. Gruber BL, Marchese MJ, Kew RR. Transforming growth factor-beta 1 mediates mast cell chemotaxis. *J Immunol* 1994;152:5860–5867.

276. Mattoli S, Ackerman V, Vittori E, Marini M. Mast cell chemotactic activity of RANTES. *Biochem Biophys Res Commun* 1995;209:316–321.

277. Gruber BL, Marchese MJ, Kew R. Angiogenic factors stimulate mast-cell migration. *Blood* 1995;86:2488–2493.

278. Nilsson G, Johnell M, Hammer CH, et al. C3a and C5a are chemo-

taxins for mast cells and act through distinct receptors via a pertussis toxin-sensitive signal transduction pathway. *J Immunol* 1996;157:1693–1698.

279. Ghebrehiwet B, Kew RR, Gruber BL, Marchese MJ, Peerschke E, Reid K. Murine mast cells express two types of C1q receptors that are involved in the induction of chemotaxis and chemokinesis. *J Immunol* 1995;155:2614–2619.

280. Nilsson G, Metcalfe DD, Taub DD. Platelet-activating factor is a mast cell chemotaxin. *Submitted for publication.*

281. Poole TJ, Zetter BR. Stimulation of rat peritoneal mast cell migration by tumor-derived peptides. *Cancer Res* 1983;43:5857–5861.

282. Thompson HL, Burbelo PD, Yamada Y, Kleinman HK, Metcalfe DD. Mast cells chemotax to laminin with enhancement after IgE-mediated activation. *J Immunol* 1989;143:4188–4192.

283. Thompson HL, Thomas L, Metcalfe DD. Murine mast cells attach to and migrate on laminin-coated, fibronectin-coated, and matrigel-coated surfaces in response to Fc-epsilon-RI-mediated signals. *Clin Exp Allergy* 1993;23:270–275.

284. Mitchell EB, Askenase PW. Basophils in human disease. *Clin Rev Allergy* 1983;1:427–438.

285. Naclerio RM, Proud D, Togias AG, et al. Inflammatory mediators in late antigen-induced rhinitis. *N Engl J Med* 1985;11:65–70.

286. Shalit M, Schwartz LB, Golzar N, et al. Release of histamine and tryptase in vivo after prolonged cutaneous challenge with allergen in humans. *J Immunol* 1988;141:821–826.

287. Bevilaqua MP, Pober JS, Mendrick DL, Cotran RS, Gimbrone MA Jr. Identification of an inducible endothelial leukocyte adhesion molecule. *Proc Natl Acad Sci U S A* 1987;84:9238–9242.

288. Purcell WM, Atterwill CK. Mast cells in neuroimmune function: Neurotoxicological and neuropharmacological perspectives. *Neurochem Res* 1995;20:521–532.

289. Brody D, Metcalfe DD. Mast cells: A unique and functional diversity. *Clin Exp Allergy* 1998 (*in press*).

290. Dvorak AM, Mihm MC Jr, Dvorak HF. Morphology of delayed-type hypersensitivity reactions in man: II. Ultrastructural alteration affecting the microvasculature and the tissue mast cells. *Lab Invest* 1976;34:179–191.

291. Takizawa H, Ohta K, Hirai K, et al. Mast cells are important in the development of hypersensitivity pneumonitis. *J Immunol* 1989;143:1982–1988.

292. Claman HN. Mast cells and fibrosis: Hints from graft-versus-host disease and scleroderma. In: Kaliner MA, Metcalfe DD, eds. *The mast cell in health and disease.* New York: Marcel Dekker, 1993:653–667.

293. Dietsch GM, Hinrichs DJ. The role of mast cells in the elicitation of experimental allergic encephalomyelitis. *J Immunol* 1989;142:1476–1481.

294. Gruber B, Poznansky M, Boss E, Partin J, Gorevic P, Kaplan AP. Characterization and functional studies of rheumatoid synovial mast cells: Activation by secretagogues, anti-IgE, and a histamine-releasing lymphokine. *Arthritis Rheum* 1986;29:944–955.

295. Marsh MN, Hinde J. Inflammatory component of celiac sprue mucosa: I. Mast cells, basophils and eosinophils. *Gastroenterology* 1985;89:92–101.

296. Sarin SK, Mahlotra V, Gupta SS, Karol A, Gaur SK, Anand BS. Significance of eosinophil and mast cell counts in rectal mucosal in ulcerative colitis. *Dig Dis Sci* 1987;32:363–367.

297. Hartveit FS, Thoresen S, Tangen M, Maartmann H. Mast cell changes and tumor dissemination in human breast carcinoma. *Invasion Metastasis* 1984;4:146–155.

298. Brewster CEP, Howarth PH, Djukanovic R, Wilson J, Holgate ST, Roche WR. Myofibroblasts and subepithelia fibrosis in bronchial asthma. *Am J Res Cell Mol Biol* 1990;3:507–511.

299. Leiferman KM, Ackerman SJ, Sampson HA, Haugen HS, Venencie PY, Gleich GJ. Dermal deposition of eosinophil-granule major basic protein in atopic dermatitis. *N Engl J Med* 1985;313:282–285.

300. Norrby K. Effect of heparin, histamine and serotonin on the density-dependent inhibition of replication in two fibroblastic cell lines. *Virchows Arch B Cell Pathol* 1973;15:75–93.

301. Sandberg H. Accelerated collagen formation and histamine. *Nature* 1962;194:183.

302. Yamashita Y, Nakagomi K, Takeda T, Hasegawa S, Misui Y. Effect of heparin on pulmonary fibroblasts and vascular cells. *Thorax* 1992;47:634–639.

303. Ferrao AV, Mason RM. The effect of heparin on cell proliferation and type-1 collagen synthesis by adult human dermal fibroblasts. *Biochem Biophys Acta* 1993;1180:225–230.

304. Ruoss SJ, Hartmann T, Caughey GH. Mast cell tryptase is a mitogen for cultured fibroblasts. *J Clin Invest* 1991;88:493–499.

305. Gruber BL, Kew RR, Jelaska A, et al. Human mast cells activate fibroblasts. *J Immunol* 1997;158:2310–2317.

306. Monroe JG, Haldar S, Prystowsky MB, Lammie P. Lymphokine regulation of inflammatory processes: Interleukin-4 stimulates fibroblast proliferation. *Clin Immunol Immunopathol* 1988;49:292–298.

307. Kovacs EH. Fibrogenic cytokines: The role of immune mediators in the development of scar tissue. *Immunol Today* 1991;12:17–23.

308. Reed JA, Albino AP, McNutt NS. Human cutaneous mast cells express basic fibroblast growth factor. *Lab Invest* 1995;72:215–222.

309. Qu ZH, Liebler JM, Powers MR, et al. Mast cells are a major source of basic fibroblast growth factor in chronic inflammation and cutaneous hemangioma. *Am J Pathol* 1995;147:564–573.

310. Forsberg K, Nilsson G, Ren ZP, Hellman L, Westermark B, Nistér M. Constitutive and inducible expression of PDGF in the human basophilic cell line KU 812. *Growth Factors* 1993;9:231–241.

311. Nilsson G, Svensson V, Nilsson K. Constitutive and inducible cytokine mRNA expression in the human mast cell line HMC-1. *Scand J Immunol* 1995;42:76–81.

312. Thompson HL, Burbelo PD, Gabriel G, Yamada Y, Metcalfe DD. Murine mast cells synthesize basement membrane components: A potential role in early fibrosis. *J Clin Invest* 1991;87:619–623.

313. Zauberman H, Michaelsson IC, Bergman F, Maurice DM. Stimulation of neovascularization of the cornea by biogenic amines. *Exp Eye Res* 1969;8:77–83.

314. Jakobsson A, Sorbo J, Norrby K. Protamine and mast-cell-mediated angiogenesis in the rat. *Int J Exp Pathol* 1990;71:209–217.

315. Norrby K, Sorbo J. Heparin enhances angiogenesis by a systemic mode of action. *Int J Exp Pathol* 1992;73:147–155.

316. Bradding P, Feather IH, Howarth PH, et al. Interleukin 4 is localized to and released by human mast cells. *J Exp Med* 1992;176:1381–1385.

317. Burd PR, Thompson WC, Max EE, Mills FC. Activated mast cells produce interleukin 13. *J Exp Med* 1995;181:1373–1380.

318. Ochensberger B, Daepp GC, Rihs S, Dahinden CA. Human blood basophils produce interleukin-13 in response to IgE-receptor-dependent and -independent activation. *Blood* 1996;88:3028–3037.

Inflammation: Basic Principles and Clinical Correlates,
3rd ed., edited by John I. Gallin and Ralph Snyderman.
Lippincott Williams & Wilkins, Philadelphia © 1999.

CHAPTER 8

Overview of Development and Function of Lymphocytes

Laura P. Hale and Barton F. Haynes

The inflammatory response against pathogens is mediated both by *innate* immune responses, which are not antigen-specific and do not involve immunologic memory, and by *antigen-specific* immune responses, which generate immunologic memory against the inciting agent. Innate immune responses directly induce effector functions to combat the pathogen and also enhance the activation of antigen-specific immune responses (1). Effector cells of the innate immune system include natural killer (NK) cells, neutrophils, eosinophils, basophils, mast cells, and professional antigen-presenting cells (APCs). Antigen-specific immune responses are mediated by T and B lymphocytes. The specificity of antigen-specific responses results from the repertoire of unique antigen receptors expressed on T and B lymphocytes. B lymphocytes are the precursors of antibody-secreting plasma cells, which mediate humoral immune responses. T lymphocytes mediate cellular immune responses and also regulate the function of B lymphocytes and macrophages through cellular interactions and the production of cytokines. The importance of T and B lymphocytes to the overall function of the immune system is reflected in the array of infectious diseases that occur when these cells are decreased or absent. If not treated, acquired immunodeficiency syndrome caused by human immunodeficiency virus infection and congenital immunodeficiency syndromes of T or B cells, or both, generally result in death from severe infections.

Each individual T or B lymphocyte expresses an antigen receptor that is uniquely capable of recognizing specific structural determinants (*epitopes*) on antigens. The diversity of antigen receptors is generated by combinatorial rearrangement of a variety of germ-line immunoglobulin (Ig) or T-cell receptor (TCR) gene segments; by random addition of nucleotides; and, in the case of Ig genes, by somatic mutation. This extraordinary antigen-receptor diversity ensures a broad immune repertoire and allows lymphocyte populations to respond to virtually any potentially pathogenic agent. Selective amplification of lymphocyte clones stimulated by exposure to an antigen allows the immune system to adapt the repertoire to respond to current pathogens and to develop immunologic "memory," which facilitates a rapid response on subsequent reexposure to the antigen.

This chapter presents an overview of the developmental ontogeny of lymphocytes in humans and the molecular and functional bases for the specificity and diversity of the immune response generated by T, B, and NK lymphocytes. This overview provides a framework for understanding the central role of lymphocytes in the initiation and propagation of inflammatory responses. Individual aspects of lymphocyte function are discussed in Chapters 9 (T-cell development), and 10 (B-cell development), 11 (NK lymphocytes), 12 (CD4 lymphocytes), and 13 (CD8 lymphocytes).

T LYMPHOCYTES

Antigen Recognition and Presentation

The antigen recognition system of T cells does not directly recognize structural determinants or epitopes on antigens in their native form. Instead, T cells recognize proteolytically processed peptide fragments of the antigens that are bound to polymorphic major histocompatibility complex (MHC) molecules on the surface of APCs. The process of thymic development and education of T lymphocytes selects for those cells with antigen receptors that react only with antigen bound to self MHC mole-

L. P. Hale and B. F. Haynes: Duke University Medical Center, Durham, North Carolina 27710.

cules. The antigen recognition capability of T cells is therefore defined to be *MHC-restricted*.

The process through which antigen-derived peptides are degraded and bound to self MHC molecules is known as *antigen processing*. Specialized pathways of antigen processing exist to deal with extracellular (exogenous) and intracellular (endogenous) antigens (2) (Fig. 8-1).

Extracellular antigens may be derived from foreign substances, bacteria, or viruses that have not yet gained access to the cell. Extracellular antigens are taken up via endocytosis or phagocytosis by specialized MHC class II–positive APCs such as macrophages, B cells, or dendritic cells. During processing, antigens are partially degraded and resulting peptide fragments are bound to MHC class II molecules trafficking through the same cellular compartments. Peptide–MHC class II complexes are brought to the cell surface of the APC for recognition by the TCRs of CD4-positive T lymphocytes. CD4+ helper T cells that are activated by the peptide–class II MHC complexes secrete cytokines, which ultimately activate and recruit either B cells or other T cells to participate in antigen-specific immune responses.

Alternatively, antigens may be synthesized within the cell as the result of infection by virus or other obligate intracellular pathogens or from alterations in normal cellular proteins generated by tumor cells (tumor antigens). In this case, peptides derived from proteolytic degradation of these intracellular proteins are loaded onto MHC class I molecules and then expressed on the surface of the APC for recognition by CD8+ cytotoxic T cells. Peptides derived from any protein generated within the cell, including those that do not normally appear on the cell surface, can bind to class I MHC molecules and thereby serve as stimuli for MHC class I–mediated cytotoxic T-cell responses.

A third mechanism of T-cell recognition occurs for antigens such as the lipid and glycolipid cell wall antigens from intracellular bacteria (e.g., *Mycobacterium tuberculosis*, *Mycobacterium leprosum*, *Listeria monocytogenes*). Bacterial lipid-containing antigens such as mycolic acid and lipoarabinomannan bind to the MHC-related CD1 cell surface molecules and are presented to certain antigen-specific T cells—either TCRαβ+ T cells lacking CD4 and CD8, or TCRγδ+ T cells (3,4).

The differential recognition of endogenous and exogenous antigens by different classes of T cells has important functional consequences. Antibody produced in response to B-cell stimulation by pathogen-activated CD4+ helper T cells binds to intact native extracellular antigen, thereby targeting the pathogen for destruction by phagocytic effector cells. Induction of CD8+ cytotoxic T cells specific for intracellular antigens allows the specific immune-mediated destruction of virus-infected cells and tumor cells, against which antibody alone may be inef-

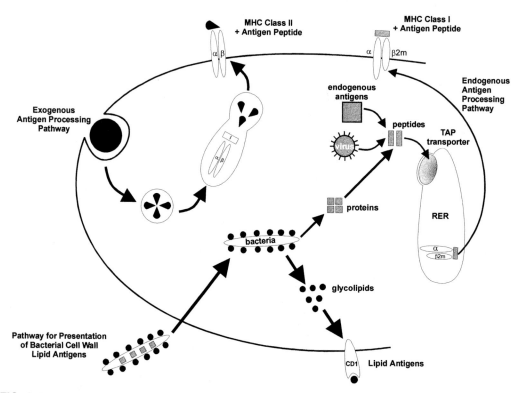

FIG. 8-1. Antigen processing and presentation pathways. Endogenous major histocompatibility complex (MHC) class I, exogenous MHC class II, and CD1 antigen presentation pathways are shown. (These pathways are reviewed in ref. 1).

fective. However, crosspriming (i.e., class I presentation of exogenous antigens or class II presentation of endogenous antigens) does occur and has been exploited for immunotherapy of experimental tumors (5-7).

T cells recognize conventional antigens as processed linear peptides bound to the antigen-binding groove of MHC molecules. However, certain unprocessed bacterial and retroviral products can bind MHC molecules at a location outside the antigen-binding groove. These *superantigens* also have specificity for TCR β-chain variable residues and bind the TCR at a site distinct from the conventional antigen-binding site. The binding of superantigens in this fashion can polyclonally stimulate entire families of T cells that share certain TCR β-chain variable sequences. The ability of superantigens to potentially stimulate up to 10% to 20% of T cells contributes to clinical syndromes such as toxic shock syndrome and may also be involved in the activation of certain autoimmune diseases (8).

T-Cell Receptors

The TCR for antigen is a multipeptide complex composed of the polymorphic heterodimeric αβ or γδ antigen receptor and the CD3 complex (Fig. 8-2). The polymorphic αβ antigen receptor is composed of both variable and constant regions; it contains two identical binding sites for antigen peptides bound by class I or class II MHC molecules. TCR variable regions encode the antigen binding sites, which are specified by combinations of V (variable), D (diversity), and J (joining) gene segments. Additional variability, generated by random addition of nucleotides at the junctions and by pairing of different α and β chains, easily accounts for the very large diversity of T-cell specificities within the immune system. The majority of T cells within the body bear αβ antigen receptors. The structure and patterns of gene rearrangement for γδ antigen receptors are similar to those for αβ receptors.

The CD3 complex contains γ, δ, and ε polypeptides, plus either a ζ$_2$ homodimer or a ζη heterodimer (see Fig. 8-2). The CD3 polypeptides are responsible for transducing signals generated by engagement of the polymorphic TCR, through interaction with cytoplasmic tyrosine kinases and other members of the cellular signal transduction machinery.

Functions of Mature T Cells

Helper T Cells

CD4$^+$ helper T cells (T$_H$ cells) recognize antigen in the context of MHC class II molecules. The specificity of

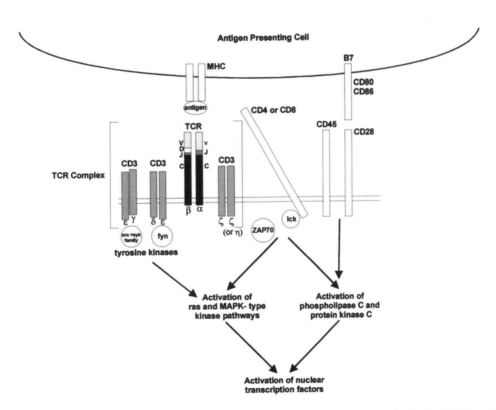

FIG. 8-2. T-cell antigen receptor (TCR) complex and signaling. Molecules included in the TCR are indicated. When antigen binds to the TCR, additional signaling molecules are recruited to the TCR complex (examples shown), generating an intricate signaling cascade that results in activation of nuclear transcription. (These processes are reviewed in refs. 51 and 53.)

CD4+ T cells for recognition of antigen peptides presented in this context derives from the ability of CD4 to serve as a nonpolymorphic ligand for MHC class II molecules (9) and to stabilize the TCR–MHC class II interaction. T_H cells were so named for their regulatory interactions with B lymphocytes and other immune cells. Through cytokine secretion and cell surface receptor–mediated interactions, T_H cells stimulate B cells to differentiate into antibody-producing plasma cells or into memory B cells. Similar T_H interactions with macrophages result in increased macrophage production of reactive oxygen intermediates, nitric oxide, and other factors that enhance the cytotoxic potential of these macrophages against viable intracellular organisms or phagocytosed antigens.

At least two general classes of T_H cells can be defined, based on their cytokine secretion profiles. T_H1 cells are characterized by production of interferon-γ (IFN-γ), interleukin-2 (IL-2), and tumor necrosis factor (TNF-β), cytokines that enhance macrophage reactivity and cellular immune responses. T_H2 cells produce IL-4, IL-5, IL-6, IL-10, and IL-13, cytokines that are important for activation of B cells or modulation of the activation states of macrophages. Although this separation of T_H functions is an oversimplification, it facilitates understanding of immune response patterns in a variety of induced and naturally occurring immune processes (see Chapter 12).

Cytotoxic T Cells

CD8+ cytotoxic T cells (CTLs) recognize antigen-derived peptides in the context of MHC class I molecules after antigen processing via the endogenous antigen-processing pathway. Their specificity relies on the ability of the CD8 molecule to bind directly to MHC class I molecules and to stabilize TCR interactions with APC MHC class I molecules, thereby maximizing antigen presentation events (10). After activation and terminal differentiation into CD8+ effector cells, CD8+ MHC class I–restricted CTLs are capable of inducing lysis of target cells bearing the appropriate antigen–MHC class I complex. CD8+ CTLs thus provide a major defense against a variety of intracellular pathogens such as viruses and intracellular bacteria (e.g., *Mycobacteria*, *Listeria*) and against tumor cells. CTLs can kill either by perforin-mediated lytic mechanisms or by induction of apoptosis of the target cell (11,12) (see Chapter 13).

T-Cell Development

Ontogeny of the Human Thymic Microenvironment

The thymic primordia arise from the endodermal lining of the third branchial pouches bilaterally at the fourth week of gestation. Cells obtained primarily from the third branchial clefts attach to the thymic primordia, investing them with an ectodermal lining. The thymic lobes then migrate caudally and medially, fuse along the midline, and descend to their definitive position in the anterior mediastinum by the end of the eighth week (Fig. 8-3) (13,14). A large increase in thymus size occurs when lymphoid precursors begin to populate the thymic rudiment in the eighth week (Figs. 8-4 and 8-5). The endodermally-derived thymic epithelial cells develop into a meshwork in intimate contact with the developing thymocytes. Adhesive interactions between thymocytes and thymic epithelial cells stimulate cytokine secretion and drive the activation and differentiation of both types of cells (15-18). Mesenchymal elements surrounding the developing thymus form a capsule and focally invaginate into the parenchyma, forming trabeculae that divide the thymus into lobules (see Fig. 8-3). Histologic distinction between cortical and medullary zones is first evident at 14 weeks. Hassall's bodies form in the thymic medulla between the 15th and 16th weeks of gestation (13). The definitive postnatal structure of the human thymus is clearly developed by 16 weeks of gestation. The size of the thymus grows progressively until about 12 months of age (19) but undergoes involution thereafter, a process characterized by fatty infiltration and replacement of thymic parenchyma by adipose tissue (14,20) (Fig. 8-6).

The thymic microenvironment provided by thymic stromal cells (epithelial cells, fibroblasts, dendritic cells, macrophages) and the extracellular matrix is critical for the maturation and differentiation of T cells. In human thymus, terminally differentiated medullary thymic epithelial cells form characteristic structures known as Hassall's bodies (Fig. 8-7). Interactions between developing thymocytes and the microenvironment occur through cell surface interactions and cytokines. The cell surface and cytokine expression profiles differ among stromal cells derived from different anatomic regions of the thymus (subcapsular cortex, cortex proper, and medulla), suggesting potentially different inductive effects of the microenvironment as immature thymocytes traffic from the subcapsular cortex, through the cortex, to the medulla, from which they exit into the periphery as mature T cells.

T-Lymphocyte Development

The thymus is composed of a cortex filled with proliferating immature thymocytes and a medulla containing more mature thymocytes, both within the epithelial/stromal cell network (see Fig. 8-7). Thymocyte precursors migrate from the bone marrow to the thymus, where they differentiate, undergo positive and negative selection, and mature into functional T lymphocytes. Passage through the thymus is required for initial development of a functional T-cell repertoire, as evidenced by the profound immune dysfunction seen in nude mice and in children with complete DiGeorge syndrome, conditions that are characterized by congenital absence of a normal thymus.

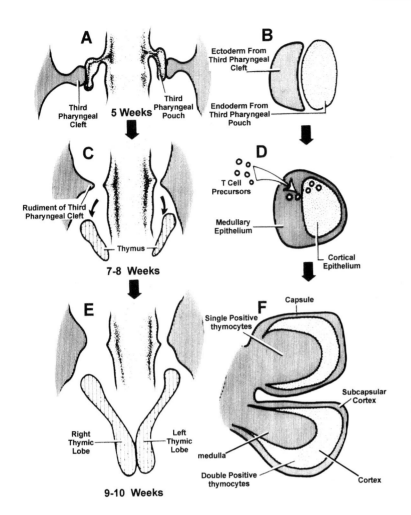

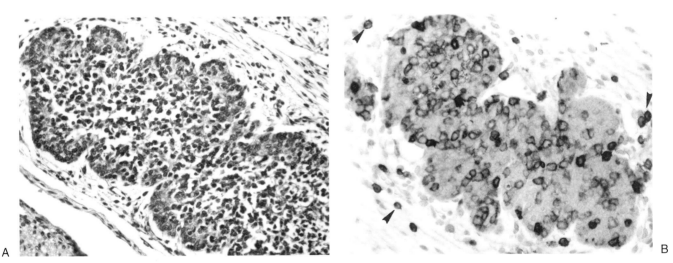

FIG. 8-3. Embryologic development of the human thymus. The anatomic derivation of the nonlymphoid components of the human thymus during fetal development is depicted in panels **A** through **C**. The corresponding contributions of each of the three germ layers to the thymic compartments at each developmental stage are shown in panels **D** through **F**.

FIG. 8-4. (**A**) Developing thymus in an 8-week human embryo (hematoxylin and eosin stain). (**B**) Colonization of the thymus by thymocyte precursors is highlighted by CD45 immunoperoxidase stain. Note the presence of CD45⁺ thymocyte precursors migrating through perithymic mesenchyme en route to the thymus (*arrowheads*). (**A** and **B**, original magnification, ×250).

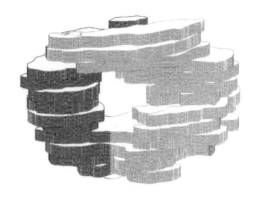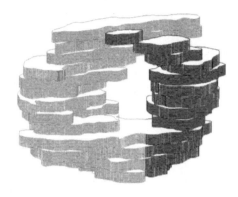

Anterior view   Posterior view

FIG. 8-5. Three-dimensional reconstruction of a normal 8.75-week fetal human thymus. Computer-assisted reconstruction of the thymus was performed by overlay of hematoxylin and eosin–stained serial sections obtained at a time just after seeding of the thymic microenvironment with bone marrow–derived stem cells. Thymic lobulation by invading blood vessels occurs at this stage. Differential dark and light shading is used to indicate the right and left lobes of the thymus, respectively, in both anterior (*left*) and posterior (*right*) views. Actual thymus size is 1 × 1 × 0.25 mm.

Thymopoiesis, defined as the balance between proliferation and apoptosis of thymocyte precursors, results in net production of functional mature T lymphocytes. Thymopoiesis decreases in adulthood due to thymic atrophy (20) (see Fig. 8-6). The function of the thymus was thought to be unimportant in the adult, because of the persistence of long-lived postthymic T-lymphocyte precursors in the periphery as well as the lack of obvious immune defects in adults and children thymectomized for treatment of myasthenia gravis. However, more recent studies have suggested that thymic function may be important in situations in which the peripheral T-cell pool is destroyed, as in HIV infection or after high-dose chemotherapy for treatment of malignancy (21). Although development of T cells in locations outside the thymus has been hypothesized, primarily on the basis of expression of enzymes important to TCR rearrangement (22,23), the contribution of extrathymic maturation to the functional T-cell pool has yet to be established. Focal thymopoiesis can be observed in some aged adults (see Fig. 8-6), but the contribution of this limited thymopoiesis to total immune function also is unclear. The cellular and molecular events that transpire during thymic atrophy and aging remain obscure, although defects in T-cell maturation and TCR rearrangement have been implicated in the process (24).

Surface Phenotypes of Maturing Thymocytes

The differentiation of bone marrow–derived precursors into mature T cells within the thymus occurs in a stepwise fashion. Cells at each maturation step can be identified by a specific complement of cell surface antigens and/or by patterns of gene rearrangement or expression. Developing thymocytes can be divided into three main subsets, based on their expression of cell surface and cytoplasmic differentiation antigens. In order of their appearance during differentiation, they are the triple-negative (CD4$^-$CD8$^-$CD3$^-$), double-positive (CD4$^+$CD8$^+$CD3/TCR^{lo}), and single-positive (CD4$^+$CD3^{hi}TCR^{hi} or CD8$^+$CD3^{hi}TCR^{hi}) subsets (25,26) (Fig. 8-8). Very low numbers of other transitional stages, characterized by expression of unique combinations of additional differentiation anti-

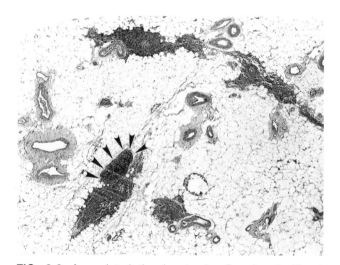

FIG. 8-6. Age-related thymic atrophy. Despite significant atrophy and fatty replacement, foci of normal thymopoiesis (*arrowheads*) are still present in this thymus tissue obtained from a 78-year-old woman. (Original magnification, ×25).

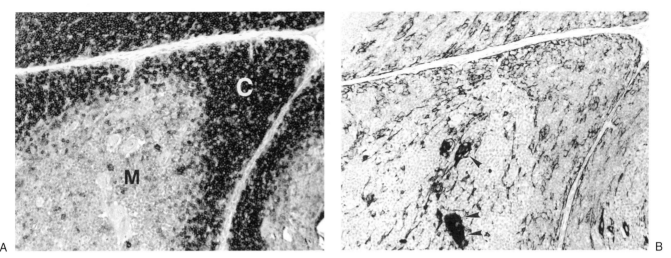

FIG. 8-7. Cellular organization within normal thymus. (**A**), CD1a stain. Immature T cells are located primarily within the cortex (C), whereas mature virgin T cells are located primarily within the medulla (M). (**B**) Cytokeratin stain. Thymic epithelial cells form a lacy network surrounding the thymocytes. Note the Hassall's bodies present in the medulla (*arrowheads*). (**A** and **B**, immunoperoxidase method; original magnification, ×170).

gens, have also been identified in murine and human thymocyte populations. For example, murine thymocytes undergoing differentiation from triple-negative to double-positive subsets pass through transitional stages progressively characterized by CD44+CD25−, CD44+CD25+, CD44−/loCD25+, and CD44−/loCD25− surface phenotypes and by expression of low levels of CD4 or CD8, or both (24,26-28). Although thymocytes with similar phenotypes have been identified in humans, the temporal order of progression within transitional stages of immature thymocytes has not been well established for human thymocytes.

T-Cell Receptor Rearrangements

TCR β-chain rearrangement begins to occur at the triple-negative thymocyte stage (26). Recombination of specific V, D, and J gene segments into a functional TCR β gene is targeted to specific recombination signal sequences, composed of conserved heptamer and nonamer motifs separated by random sequences of 12 or 23 bp that flank the individual gene segments. Introduction of double-stranded breaks at the recombination signal sequences requires activity of recombination-activating gene-1 and -2, *RAG1* and *RAG2* (29). Under normal con-

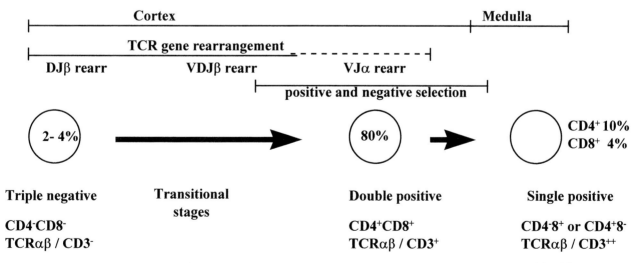

FIG. 8-8. T-lymphocyte differentiation within the thymus. Thymocyte subsets can be distinguished by their complement of cell surface antigens. The percentage of the total thymocyte population represented by each subset is indicated. TCR, T-cell receptor.

ditions, a recombinase complex containing RAG1 and RAG2 catalyzes site-specific cleavage coordinately at the junction of two coding segments (V and D or D and J) and their flanking recombination signal sequences, one of which has a 12-bp spacer and the other a 23-bp spacer. TCR gene cleavage by the recombinase generates blunt, $5'$ phosphorylated ends at the recombination signal sequence (signal ends). Hairpin ends are formed by the coding segments (coding ends) through nucleophilic attack of the $3'$-hydroxyl group onto the phosphate group of the opposite DNA strand. Signal ends are joined precisely, but TCR coding ends may be modified by addition or deletion of nucleotides, further adding to potential sequence diversity of the final rearranged TCR gene product. The recombination process is completed by ligation of the coding gene segments to assemble the TCR VDJ coding sequence. The combinatorial diversity generated by D to J and V to DJ joining and random association of rearranged α and β chains is at least 3×10^6, compared with 8×10^2 for $\gamma\delta$ antigen receptors. Additional potential diversity is generated in both $\alpha\beta$ and $\gamma\delta$ receptors through alternative joining of D gene segments (particularly for δ chains), junctional flexibility, and *N*-nucleotide addition by terminal deoxynucleotidyl transferase, for total potential diversities of 10^{15} and 10^{18}, respectively (30).

Productive rearrangement of the TCR β chain is required for progression to the double-positive thymocyte stage, a process known as *β selection*. The newly rearranged TCR β gene product is expressed on the cell surface in combination with a surrogate α chain (the pre-α chain) to form a pre-TCR (31). Cells expressing the pre-TCR show changes in expression of cell cycle control proteins, including hyperphosphorylation of retinoblastoma gene product (Rb), increased expression of cyclins A and B, downregulation of p27, increased activity of CDK2, induction of cdc2 activity, and progression through DNA synthesis (28). These changes favor the transition from the DNA synthesis (S) phase to the mitosis (M) phase of the cell cycle, resulting in proliferation and expansion of the β-selected thymocytes. Destabilization of the RAG2 recombinase protein resulting from phosphorylation by CDC2 kinase has been hypothesized to contribute to the ability of a productively rearranged TCR β gene to inhibit further rearrangement at the β locus (a process called *allelic exclusion*) (28,32). However, allelic exclusion still occurs in cells with mutant RAG2, which cannot be phosphorylated by CDC2 and therefore is constitutively expressed throughout the cell cycle (33); this suggests that additional controls regulate the process of allelic exclusion.

TCR α chain gene rearrangement occurs after β chain gene rearrangement; therefore, cells rearranging TCR α overlap primarily with the double-positive thymocyte subset. Cells that are unable to generate productive TCR rearrangements undergo apoptosis within the thymus in a process regulated by a p53-dependent checkpoint (34-36).

Thymic Selection

Once TCR gene rearrangements have been successfully accomplished, thymocytes undergo negative selection to remove autoreactive cells and positive selection to expand those cells that can respond to antigen in combination with autologous MHC molecules. Negative selection induces those T lymphocytes that express TCRs that are highly reactive with self peptide-MHC complexes to undergo apoptosis (37). Because the susceptibility of thymocytes to apoptosis has been shown to correlate with cellular levels of the B-cell lymphoma-2 (BCL-2) protein (38), regulation of this protein is critical for control of the negative selection process. Analysis of genes expressed in thymus after crosslinking of TCRs on double-positive thymocytes demonstrates upregulation of thymocyte production of IFN-γ, IL-1β, granulocyte-macrophage colony-stimulating factor (GM-CSF), IL-4, and TNF-α. These cytokines activate thymic stromal cells, and the resulting crosstalk has been hypothesized to provide the additional signals required for induction of thymocyte apoptosis (39). The majority of immature thymocytes undergo apoptosis in the thymus, as the result of thymocyte selection processes.

Positive selection leads to survival and clonal amplification of T cells that have appropriate interactions with MHC class I or class II molecules; it results in T-cell commitment to either the CD4$^+$ or the CD8$^+$ T-cell subsets (26). The cell surface density of each MHC-peptide complex present in the thymus influences the selection of CD4$^+$ thymocytes, with positive selection for ligands present in low density and negative selection for ligands present in high density (40). Thymic self peptides are also recognized during selection of CD8$^+$ T cells, generating a T-cell repertoire that is weakly self-reactive and deleting T cells that are strongly self-reactive (41). The ability of these weakly self-reactive cells to cross-react with other antigens provides the basis for the resulting diverse repertoire of specificities for both CD4$^+$ and CD8$^+$ T cells (41,42). For both CD4$^+$ and CD8$^+$ T cells, the affinity of the interaction between the TCR and its ligand and the ligand density determine the balance between positive and negative selection (43).

Cytokine Control of Thymocyte Maturation Events

IL-7 has been demonstrated to induce proliferation and differentiation of immature thymocytes and to promote thymic reconstitution after lethal irradiation and bone marrow transplantation (44). Anti-IL-7 antibodies inhibit both T- and B-cell development (45), and children with X-linked severe combined immunodeficiency syndrome, characterized by defects in the γ chain associated with multiple cytokine receptors including the IL-7 receptor, also show failure of both T- and B-cell development (46,47). *In vivo* experiments using TCR transgenic mice that were genetically deficient in the α chain of the IL-7 receptor confirmed that the IL-7R α chain controls expression of RAG1 and RAG2 and initiation of TCR gene rearrangement in triple-negative thymocytes (48). Additional *in vitro* experiments demonstrated that IL-7, which is expressed in the subcapsular region of the thymic cortex, is capable of promoting D-Jβ but not V-DJβ rearrangements of the TCR β gene in thymocyte precursors derived from murine fetal liver (45). These later data imply that intrathymic molecules regulating V-DJβ recombination are distinct from IL-7. The development of T cells from pluripotent hematopoietic stem cell precursors is also regulated by the induction and sequential activity of a variety of nuclear transcription factors, such as NF-κB, FOS, JUN, and MYC (49). These transcription factors influence transcription of developmentally specific genes directly (50).

T-Cell Activation

Through their TCRs, T lymphocytes recognize and bind to antigen-derived peptides complexed to MHC molecules. Antigen-dependent stimulation of the TCR results in a complex cascade of biochemical signaling events, with three possible outcomes: proliferation and clonal expansion, apoptosis, or anergy (unresponsiveness) (49). Evidence suggests that the net outcome of ligation of antigen receptors depends on the timing or other features of the physical recruitment of signaling pathways subsequent to TCR binding (51). The stimulus from the binding of the antigen-MHC complex to the TCR initiates the activation process but is not sufficient to induce proliferation. The avidity of TCR binding is enhanced by binding of the CD8 or CD4 accessory molecules to nonpolymorphic regions of the MHC class I or class II molecules, respectively (9,10). Physical juxtaposition of at least two TCRs (oligomerization) is necessary to initiate an activating TCR response. Additional costimulatory interactions, such as between B7.1/CD80 or B7.2/CD86 on the APC and CD28 on the T cell, are also required for T-cell proliferation to occur.

The binding of antigen-MHC molecules to the TCR and to CD4 or CD8 recruits lck and other protein-tyrosine kinases that phosphorylate TCR/CD3 components within immune receptor tyrosine-based activation motif (ITAM) regions. Surface expression of the CD45 tyrosine phosphatase is also required for proper coupling of TCR activation and the protein-tyrosine kinase signaling pathways (51,52). Phosphorylated ITAMs provide binding sites for other proteins containing SRC homology-2 (SH2) domains, such as ZAP-70, which are recruited to the TCR complex. The binding of these adaptor proteins

may serve as the primary mechanism for regulation of downstream signaling processes (51) (see Fig. 8-2). For example, differences in the relative abundance or affinity of adaptor molecules during T-cell development and maturation may influence the response generated by TCR ligation.

When fully activated, the TCR receptor complex transmits further signals via a cascade of signaling pathways (49,53) involving phospholipase C-γ, calcium mobilization, protein kinase C, calcium-dependent kinases and phosphatases, RAS, and mitogen-activated protein (MAP) kinase–type serine/threonine kinases (see Fig. 8-2). These signals ultimately result in the activation of the NFAT family and other transcription factors. Although signaling responses occur within seconds of TCR triggering, the biochemical changes associated with TCR activation occur over a period of hours and therefore may be subject to modification by other cellular regulatory pathways. The approximate time course of TCR activation pathways is as follows: secretion of cytokines, 2 hours; initiation of DNA replication, 24 hours; cell division, 48 hours; and differentiation into effector cells, days (51).

Engagement of the TCR without concomitant CD28 engagement results in anergy, a state of unresponsiveness to subsequent stimulation of the TCR. These cells exhibit defects in effector pathways downstream of the TCR (51), but the mechanisms of induction and regulation of the anergic state remain unclear.

Engagement of the TCR at critical times during T-cell development leads to apoptosis as a result of negative selection against self-reactive TCRs. Apoptosis also plays an important role in the regulation of peripheral T cells. As the original antigenic stimulus is successfully eliminated, it is important to prevent accumulation of excess numbers of responding lymphocytes. Therefore, TCR engagement is accompanied by upregulation of the CD95/FAS/APO-1 molecule. Ligation of CD95 results in activation of programmed cell death (apoptosis). The availability of CD95 ligand and cytokines within the microenvironment of the responding T cell plays a role in the regulation of apoptosis induced by TCR activation (53,54), but other mechanisms regulating this process are not well understood.

In the periphery during antigen-specific T-cell responses, most of the T cells participating in the immune response are eliminated, but a subset of these cells survive and differentiate into long-lived memory cells. Because memory T cells require less time to differentiate into effector T cells than do naive T cells, they provide an accelerated pathway for rejection of graft, allogeneic, or virally infected cells on reexposure to antigen (55-58). Memory T cells can generally be distinguished from naive T cells (but not from activated T cells) by their expression of the CD45RO isoform and higher levels of CD44.

B LYMPHOCYTES

B-Cell Receptors

The ultimate function of B lymphocytes is to produce antibodies, the mediators of the humoral immune response. Antibodies, which can be composed of any of five general isotypes of Ig, are soluble proteins that bind specifically to antigens or invading pathogens, inactivating them or targeting them for disposal by phagocytic cells of the reticuloendothelial system (or both). Membrane-bound Ig molecules also serve as the antigen-specific portion of the B-cell receptor for antigen (BCR). Ig BCRs, unlike TCRs, can recognize antigens in their native soluble or cell-bound forms. Prior antigen processing is not required for recognition of antigen by B lymphocytes.

Ig molecules of all Ig isotypes are made up of two heavy chains and two (κ or λ) light chains joined by multiple disulfide bonds (Fig. 8-9). Two antigen-binding sites are present on each Ig molecule, one at the N-terminal portion of each heavy chain–light chain complex. Cell-surface Ig also contains a spacer, a transmembrane region, and a cytoplasmic tail generated by alternative splicing. Five classes of Ig are defined by the type of heavy-chain constant regions expressed: μ, γ, α, δ, and ε constant regions give rise to IgM, IgG, IgA, IgD, and IgE molecules, respectively (59). The BCR also contains the Igα (CD79a) and Igβ (CD79b) molecules, which bear structural and functional similarities to the CD3 components of the TCR (60,61). Like CD3 for T cells, the Igα and Igβ molecules are necessary for surface expression of the BCR and for progression through the various stages of B-cell development (62). They function in transduction of signals generated by antigen binding to surface Ig through interaction with the BCR-associated family of SRC-related cytoplasmic tyrosine kinases (61) (see Fig. 8-9).

The specificity of BCRs, like that of TCRs, results from combinatorial diversity generated by a repertoire of V, D, and J gene segments and from somatic mutation. The estimated potential diversity of the human antibody repertoire, resulting from the numbers of germ-line Ig gene segments, combinatorial diversity, and junction-related diversity of the light and heavy Ig chains, is 10^{10} to 10^{11} different antibody molecules (63,64). The random and highly varied sequences of Ig variable regions increase the probability that B cells with receptors that bind to any given foreign antigen will be present in the total B-cell repertoire.

Two forms of Ig heavy chain are normally expressed on naive B cells: IgM and IgD. They contain, respectively, the μ and δ heavy-chain constant regions, designated C_μ and C_δ. IgD is generated by alternate splicing of the VDJ-$C_\mu C_\delta$ mRNA transcript. Therefore, the specificity of cell-surface IgD molecules is identical to that of the surface IgM molecules. IgD expression is switched off during the primary immune response to antigen, so that activated B cells are IgD-. Some of these activated B cells retain expression of IgM, but others switch to expression of IgG, IgA, or IgE through additional DNA rearrangement.

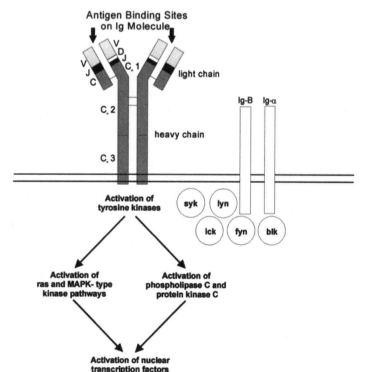

FIG. 8-9. B-cell antigen receptor (BCR) complex and signaling. The individual gene segments that constitute each immunoglobulin (Ig) molecule are indicated. When antigen binds to the Ig portion of the BCR, signal transduction occurs through the Igα/Igβ heterodimer, activating a complex signaling cascade with selected signaling molecules schematically represented. (This process is reviewed in refs. 60 and 65.)

The precise mechanisms regulating the isotype-switching process are not fully understood, but the cytokine milieu surrounding the switching B cell plays an important role in this process.

In addition to the BCR (composed of Ig, Igα, and Igβ), a coreceptor complex composed of CD19, CD21, and CD81 is also required for efficient signaling through the BCR (65). Ligation of the BCR results in CD19-mediated signal transduction through the LYN tyrosine kinase (66). The CD19-CD21-CD81 complex is particularly important for signaling under conditions of low antigen occupancy of BCRs (65).

B-Cell Development

Generation of Naive Mature B Cells

The site of B-cell maturation varies in different species. B cells mature in the bursa of Fabricus in chickens and in the kidney in fish (67). In humans, B lymphocytes are generated initially in the fetal liver, but development also occurs in bone marrow beginning at 8 to 10 weeks of gestation (63). The bone marrow becomes the primary site of B-cell generation late in the third trimester and continues so throughout postnatal life. B-cell development within the bone marrow requires both adhesion- and cytokine-mediated signals from bone marrow stromal cells. Although the stromal compartments of bone marrow are not well-defined anatomically compared with those of the thymus, microdomains with locally different inductive effects probably exist. Stromal cells that interact with developing B lymphocytes include bone-lining (endosteal) cells, reticular cells, adipocytes, macrophages, mast cells, and cells of the vascular walls (68). The bone marrow phase of B-cell development is also called the antigen-independent phase, because bone marrow selection processes are independent of the presence of antigen (Fig. 8-10).

Naive mature B cells migrate out of the bone marrow and traffic into secondary lymphoid organs such as lymph node, spleen, Peyer's patches/mucosa-associated lymphoid tissues (MALT), and tonsils. In the absence of encounter with antigen, these B cells may recirculate between the blood, lymph, and secondary lymphoid organs. However, those B lymphocytes whose antigen receptors encounter antigen are retained in the secondary lymphoid organs, where they are activated in association with antigen-specific T cells to differentiate into antibody-secreting plasma cells or memory B cells (Figs. 8-11 and 8-12).

Immunoglobulin Gene Rearrangements

The gene rearrangement processes used by B cells to generate a large repertoire of antigen-specific Ig receptors are analogous to those used by T cells to generate the antigen-specific TCRs. Ig heavy chains are encoded by V, D,

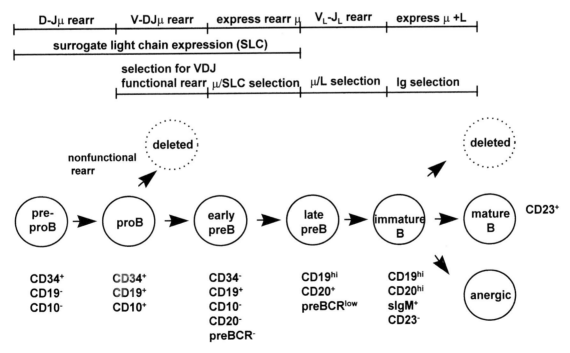

FIG. 8-10. Antigen-independent B-cell development. Stages of B-cell differentiation can be distinguished by the rearrangement status and expression of immunoglobulin (Ig) genes and by expression of cell-surface molecules. Immature B cells that receive strong signals from self ligands are deleted or become anergic. L, Ig light chain; μ, Ig heavy chain; BCR, B-cell receptor; rearr, rearrangement.

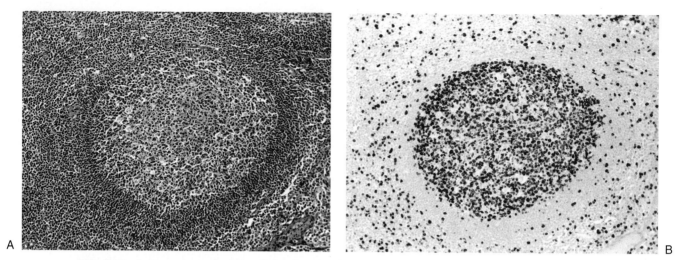

FIG. 8-11. Antigen-dependent B-cell development in germinal centers. (**A**) Differentiation to antibody-secreting plasma cells or to memory B cells occurs in germinal centers (hematoxylin and eosin stain). (**B**) Ki-67 immunoperoxidase stain highlights cells that are not in the G_0 phase of the cell cycle. (Original magnification, ×130).

J, and C (constant) segments. Light-chain genes contain V, J, and C segments. Ig gene rearrangements are regulated by RAG-1 and RAG-2. Ig gene rearrangement is coupled to expression of B-cell surface molecules and forms an ordered series of B-cell differentiation steps (see Fig. 8-

10) (63,69,70). Rearrangement at the heavy-chain locus occurs first. The order of heavy chain gene rearrangement is D-J, followed by V-DJ. Analogous to the β selection step in thymocytes, expression of a pre-BCR, composed of the product of a successfully rearranged Ig heavy-chain (μ)

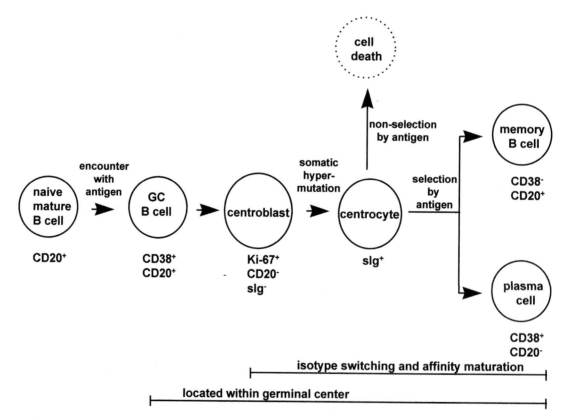

FIG. 8-12. Antigen-dependent B-cell development. The cell-surface molecules characteristic of each developmental stage are indicated. The Ki-67 antigen is expressed by mitotically active cells. GC, germinal center.

gene and a surrogate light-chain (λ15/VpreB) is required for development beyond the pre-B-cell stage (71). At each locus, the functional rearrangement of Ig genes on one chromosome inhibits rearrangement at the other locus (allelic exclusion). The κ light-chain genes rearrange after heavy-chain rearrangement has been successfully accomplished. The λ genes rearrange only if κ rearrangements on both chromosomes fail to lead to functional gene products. The random addition of nucleotides and imprecise joining of V, D, J, and C coding segments generate additional (junctional) diversity throughout the gene rearrangement process, at the cost of an increased number of nonfunctional rearrangements.

Control of B-Cell Maturation Events

Each step of the B-cell differentiation/maturation process is regulated by both cell-surface receptor–mediated and cytokine-mediated interactions. Adhesive interactions between lymphocyte function antigen-1 (LFA-1, or CD11a/CD18) on the earliest B-cell progenitors and vascular cell adhesion molecule-1 (VCAM-1, or CD106) on bone marrow stromal cells serve to facilitate the binding of KIT on the B-cell progenitor to its ligand, stem cell factor (SCF), on the stromal cells (72,73). This interaction results in tyrosine kinase activity that drives proliferation of the early pro-B cells. Late-stage pro-B cells express receptors for IL-7, which is produced by bone marrow stroma. IL-7 induces proliferation and survival of pro-B cells into the pre-B stage, where cells cease to express KIT and detach from the bone marrow stroma (70). IL-4, IL-5, and IL-6, among other cytokines, also have critical roles in maturation and activation of B cells (see Chapter 10) (50,68,72).

Germinal Center Reactions

Antigen- and T-cell–dependent B-cell reactions in secondary lymphoid tissues (lymph node, spleen, Peyer's patches) take place in structures known as germinal centers (see Fig. 8-11). Germinal centers contain two distinct populations of B lymphocytes: (a) the mitotically active Ig⁻ centroblasts, which give rise to (b) the nondividing Ig⁺ centrocytes. Germinal centers first appear 4 to 5 days after encounter with antigen. Within germinal centers, B lymphocytes interact with antigen on the surface of follicular dendritic cells and with T cells and are stimulated to undergo mutation of V, D, and J, coding segments (VDJ hypermutation) and selection, required for affinity maturation of antibody responses (74). Germinal center reactions are also necessary for development of B-cell immunologic memory (75,76). Although the majority of VDJ hypermutation events are point mutations (75), studies have shown that abundant RAG-1 and RAG-2 mRNA and protein are expressed in splenic and Peyer's patch germinal centers in mice (77), in association with abundant intermediate prod-

ucts of VDJ recombination (78). Abundant RAG-2 mRNA has also been found in normal lymph nodes in humans (79). The pattern of RAG expression correlates with the onset of μ-to-γ1 Ig class switching and with the accumulation of mutations in the Ig heavy chains of germinal center B cells. This raises the possibility that the VDJ rearrangements that occur within germinal centers may also play a role in modification of the antibody repertoire, followed by positive selection of cells expressing higher-affinity antibodies against foreign antigens (see Fig. 8-12).

Somatically-mutated BCRs generated within germinal centers may be high-affinity, low-affinity, or autoreactive. High-affinity mutants (centrocytes) pick up antigen, process it, and present it to germinal-center T cells. The germinal-center T cells are further stimulated to produce cytokines, including IL-4 and IL-10, and to upregulate their expression of the ligand for CD40 (CD40L, also named CO154), both of which favor proliferation and isotype switching of the high-affinity B cells. Cells bearing low-affinity and autoreactive BCRs are eliminated (80). The process of generating B cells that express Ig molecules with higher affinity for antigen through the processes of somatic mutation and selection within germinal centers is called *affinity maturation*.

B-Cell Activation

Antigen recognition and subsequent B-cell activation is mediated by the Ig portion of the BCR. Studies using anti-Ig antibodies have demonstrated that engagement of BCR provides an initial activation signal but by itself is insufficient to induce the massive proliferation and differentiation of B cells seen on physiologic encounter with antigen (81). Therefore, attention has been focused on other B-cell surface molecules that may also be involved in the B-cell activation process.

When the BCR binds antigen, BCR-antigen complexes undergo endocytosis and proteolytic processing, and antigen-derived peptides are reexpressed on the cell surface bound to MHC class II molecules (60). B cells then present the antigen to MHC class II–restricted T_H cells, activating the T_H cells to secrete cytokines and to express cell molecules associated with T-cell activation. Numerous studies have established that the cytokines secreted by activated T cells play a critical role in B-cell activation (see Chapter 12). However, the full effect of T cells cannot be reproduced with T-cell supernatants alone; it also requires intact T cells or T-cell membranes (82). These findings indicate that direct cell-cell contact with T-cell surface ligands is necessary to trigger further B-cell activation and differentiation to antibody-secreting plasma cells.

When antigen binds to the BCR, signaling occurs via the Igα and Igβ components of the BCR. These molecules interact cytoplasmically with BCR-associated tyrosine kinases and are themselves tyrosine phosphorylated as part of the biochemical signaling pathways activated by antigen binding (60). The activation of BCR-associated tyrosine kinases initiates a cascade of signaling events that amplifies the signal and propagates it to the nucleus. The activity of the BCR-associated tyrosine kinases can be further modulated by coreceptors such as CD19, CD21, and CD81, giving the cell the ability to fine-tune the level of signal generated by BCR ligation. For example, antigen complexed with complement can bind simultaneously to complement receptor CD21 and to the BCR, a process that recruits CD19 to the complex. Ligation of CD19 in addition to the BCR dramatically increases tyrosine phosphorylation and calcium flux, particularly in response to low levels of antigen (65).

Other modifiers of the BCR signaling response include the tyrosine phosphatase CD45 and transmembrane Ig superfamily member CD22. CD45 expression is necessary for the transition from immature to mature B cells and for optimal signaling through the BCR (60). CD22 is tyrosine phosphorylated during the activation cascade and may serve to recruit tyrosine kinases and phosphatases to the antigen receptor complex during BCR activation. The CD32 low-affinity Ig receptor (FcγRIIb1) expressed on B cells is a coreceptor that downregulates BCR signaling.

The involvement of coreceptors in the B-cell activation process has led to the concept that, as in TCR signaling, optimal BCR signaling involves the accumulation of a number of signaling molecules into a large complex. In this model, B-cell activation occurs when this complex reaches a critical threshold size or concentration of enzymes and signaling molecules. This model explains why coreceptors are not required when BCRs are extensively cross-linked, for example by using anti-Ig antibodies or multivalent antigens.

Initial activation of BCR-associated SRC-family tyrosine kinases results in waves of activation of additional tyrosine kinases, including FYN, LYN, BLK, LCK, and SYK. These molecules provide links to other second-messenger pathways, including the phospholipase C pathway, which results in protein kinase C activation and calcium mobilization; the phosphatidylinositol 3-kinase pathway; and the RAS pathway, which results in phosphorylation and activation of transcription factors (60,83) (see Fig. 8-9).

The CD40 molecule on B cells has been identified as a critical costimulatory molecule for B-cell differentiation. The CD40 ligand (CD40L, also named CD154) is a member of the TNFα family and is expressed on activated T cells. B cells stimulated via CD40/CD40L interactions demonstrate strong and long-lasting proliferation. Further crosslinking of the BCR leads to differentiation into antibody-secreting plasma cells. Isotype switching is induced by the balance of cytokines present in the surrounding milieu: IL-4 favors secretion of IgE, as does IL-13; IL-10 favors secretion of IgG$_1$ or IgG$_3$; and TGFβ favors secretion of IgA (82,84). The isotype switch is mediated by a DNA recombination process that moves the V(D)J gene segment adjacent to the heavy-chain gene segment for the switch isotype, eliminating the intervening DNA (85). Switches in Ig isotypes can produce an immune response tailored for the location of antigenic challenge (e.g., IgA specific for an antigen encountered in the MALT). The importance of CD40/CD40L interactions in class switching and in the overall immune response can be seen in patients with the hyper-IgM syndrome, which is characterized by mutations in CD40L. Although these patients make increased amounts of IgM, they lack appreciable amounts of IgG, IgA, and IgE and suffer from recurrent infections (86). Because CD40L also plays a role in both T-cell and monocyte activation, these patients also demonstrate defects in cell-mediated immunity.

In vitro culture of germinal-center (CD38$^+$CD20$^+$) B cells with IL-2, IL-10, and a source of CD40L results in differentiation into CD38$^-$CD20$^+$ memory B cells. During secondary immune responses, memory B cells can be activated in extrafollicular areas, giving rise to plasma cells and to new germinal centers. Cells similarly cultured in IL-2 and IL-10 but without CD40L become terminally differentiated plasma cells (82). Therefore, triggering by CD40 plays a critical role in control of the differentiation of germinal-center B cells toward memory cells or toward plasma cells.

B-cell activation has been best studied in the context of antigen-dependent activation of mature B cells. However, antigen-induced BCR crosslinking also occurs in pre-B cells and immature B cells. In these cases, BCR ligation results not in cellular activation but in negative selection and apoptosis or the induction of specific nonresponsiveness (tolerance) (69,87,88).

NATURAL KILLER CELLS

In addition to T and B lymphocytes, up to 10% of the circulating lymphocyte population is composed of large granular lymphocytes known as NK cells (30). NK cells were named for their ability to kill tumors in a non-MHC-restricted fashion without the need for prior activation by tumor antigens. NK cells arise in the bone marrow and share a common precursor with T lymphocytes (89). Although NK cells can develop within and traffic through the thymus, they do not rearrange or productively express a TCR, and they do not require the thymic microenvironment for maturation (90). NK cells are present in human fetal liver before formation of the thymic primordium (91).

NK cells express membrane CD2, CD16 (FcγRIII), and CD56 but do not express the TCR-CD3 complex. NK cells kill their target cells by both perforin- and apoptosis-related mechanisms and are believed to play a role in the elimination of virally infected cells (or tumor cells) early in infection, before activation and differentiation of CD8[+] cells into functional CTLs. The importance of NK cells in this regard is highlighted by case reports of severe and life-threatening viral infections in persons lacking NK cells (30,92,93). In addition to their cytolytic function, NK cells produce cytokines that regulate the immune response, inflammation, and hematopoiesis (94).

NK cells have been shown to express specialized cell-surface receptors that recognize MHC class I molecules expressed on normal cells. NK receptors come in two molecular forms, one that inhibits and one that activates NK responses. During NK development, cells adapt to recognize epitopes on self MHC class I (human leukocyte antigen [HLA]-A, -B, or -C) molecules. When NK receptors are engaged in the periphery, tyrosine-based inhibitory motifs in the cytoplasmic domains of the NK inhibitory receptors recruit SH2-containing protein-tyrosine phosphatases, resulting in inhibition of NK cytotoxicity (95). Cells that lack or express only low levels of MHC class I molecules fail to engage the inhibitory receptors sufficiently and therefore are targets for NK-mediated lysis. Allogeneic MHC molecules and self MHC molecules that have bound unusual peptides do not engage inhibitory receptors, allowing foreign or virally infected cells to be killed by NK cells (94,96). Since virally infected cells and tumor cells may also downregulate their expression of class I molecules, potentially allowing them to evade recognition by CTLs, NK-cell function plays a significant role in protection against these pathogens. Additional forms of NK receptors have been described that are identical to the inhibitory receptors in their extracellular domains but have shorter cytoplasmic tails; they are activated on binding to MHC class I molecules (94,97) (see Chapter 11).

SUMMARY

The human immune system is a complex yet versatile system that has evolved to protect the host against invasion from foreign pathogens by means of complex innate (NK) and antigen-specific (T and B) cell lineages. Inappropriate activation of either the innate or the antigen-specific arm of the immune system can result in harm to the host. Great strides in understanding of the mechanisms for normal development and activation of lymphocytes have been made in the 1990s. Because lymphocytes play a key role in the initiation and maintenance of inflammation, increased understanding of lymphopoiesis now provides a rational basis for the design and development of novel therapeutic strategies for the wide spectrum of inflammatory and immune-mediated disorders.

ACKNOWLEDGMENTS

This work was supported by grants from the U.S. Army Medical Research and Materiel Command (DAMD-94-J-4168 to LPH) and from the National Institutes of Health (CA28936 to BFH and AG16826 to LPH).

REFERENCES

1. Medzhitov R, Janeway CA Jr. Innate immunity: The virtues of a nonclonal system of recognition. *Cell* 1997;91:295–298.
2. Braciale TJ, Morrison LA, Sweetser MT, Sambrook J, Gething M-J, Braciale VL. Antigen presentation pathways to class I and class II MHC-restricted T lymphocytes. *Immunol Rev* 1987;98:95–114.
3. Beckman EM, Brenner MB. MHC class I-like, class II-like and CD1 molecules: Distinct roles in immunity. *Immunol Today* 1995;16:349–352.
4. Sieling PA, Chatterjee D, Porcelli SA, et al. CD1-restricted T cell recognition of microbial lipoglycan antigen. *Science* 1995;269:227–230.
5. Ashley DM, Sampson JH, Archer GE, Batra SK, Bigner DD, Hale LP. A genetically modified allogeneic cellular vaccine generates MHC class I-restricted cytotoxic responses against tumor-associated antigens and protects against CNS tumors in vivo. *J Neuroimmunol* 1997;78:34–46.
6. Yewdell JN, Bennink JR, Hosaka Y. Cells process exogenous antigen for recognition by cytotoxic T lymphocytes. *Science* 1988;239:637–640.
7. Jaraquemada D, Marti M, Long EO. An endogenous processing pathway in vaccinia virus-infected cells for presentation of antigen to class II-restricted T cells. *J Exp Med* 1990;172:947–954.
8. Huston DP. The biology of the immune system. *J Am Med Assoc* 1997;278:1804–1814.
9. Doyle C, Strominger JL. Interaction between CD4 and class II MHC molecules mediates cell adhesion. *Nature* 1988;330:256–259.
10. Norment AM, Salter RD, Parham P, Engelhard VH, Littman DR. Cell-cell adhesion mediated by CD8 and MHC class I molecules. *Nature* 1988;336:79–81.
11. Nagata S. Apoptosis by death factor. *Cell* 1997;88:355–365.
12. Sprent J, Tough DF, Sun S. Factors controlling the turnover of T memory cells. *Immunol Rev* 1997;156:79–85.
13. Lobach DF, Haynes BF. Ontogeny of the human thymus during fetal development. *J Clin Immunol* 1987;7:81–97.
14. Suster S, Rosai J. Histology of the normal thymus. *Am J Surg Pathol* 1990;14:284–303.
15. Haynes BF. Human thymic epithelium and T cell development: Current issues and future directions. *Thymus* 1990;16:143–157.
16. Denning SM, Kurtzberg J, Le PT, Tuck DT, Singer KH, Haynes BF. Human thymic epithelial cells directly induce activation of autologous immature thymocytes. *Proc Natl Acad Sci U S A* 1988;85:3125–3129.
17. Kurtzberg J, Denning SM, Nycum LM, Singer KH, Haynes BF. Immature human thymocytes can be driven to differentiate into nonlymphoid lineages by cytokines from thymic epithelial cells. *Proc Natl Acad Sci U S A* 1989;86:7575–7579.
18. Ritter MA, Boyd RL. Development in the thymus: It takes two to tango. *Immunol Today* 1993;14:462–468.
19. Steinmann GG, Klaus B, Muller-Hermelink H-K. The involution of the ageing thymic epithelium is independent of puberty: A morphometric study. *Scand J Immunol* 1985;22:563–575.
20. George AJ, Ritter MA. Thymic involution with ageing: Obsolescence or good housekeeping? *Immunol Today* 1996;17:267–272.
21. Mackall CL, Hakim FT, Gress RE. T-cell regeneration: All repertoires are not created equal. *Immunol Today* 1997;18:245–251.
22. Collins C, Norris S, McEntee, et al. RAG1, RAG2 and pre-T cell receptor α chain expression by adult human hepatic T cells: Evidence for extrathymic T cell maturation. *Eur J Immunol* 1996;26:3114–3118.
23. Lynch S, Kelleher D, McManus R, O'Farrelly C. RAG1 and RAG2 expression in human intestinal epithelium: Evidence of extrathymic T cell differentiation. *Eur J Immunol* 1995;25:1143–1147.
24. Aspinall R. Age-associated thymic atrophy in the mouse is due to a deficiency affecting rearrangement of the TCR during intrathymic T cell development. *J Immunol* 1997;158:3037–3045.
25. Haynes BF, Denning SM, Le PT, Singer KH. Human intrathymic T cell differentiation. *Semin Immunol* 1990;2:67–77.
26. Rothenberg EV. The development of functionally responsive T cells. *Adv Immunol* 1992;51:85–214.
27. Ismaili J, Antica M, Wi L. CD4 and CD8 expression and T cell antigen receptor gene rearrangement in early intrathymic precursor cells. *Eur J Immunol* 1996;26:731–737.

28. Hoffman ES, Passoni L, Crompton T, et al. Productive T-cell receptor β-chain gene rearrangement: Coincident regulation of cell cycle and clonality during development in vivo. *Genes Dev* 1996;10:948–962.

29. van Gent DC, McBlane JF, Ramsden DA, Sadofsky MJ, Hesse JE, Gellert M. Initiation of V(D)J recombination in a cell-free system. *Cell* 1995;81:925–934.

30. Kuby J. *Immunology,* 2nd ed. New York: WH Freeman, 1994.

31. Saint-Ruf C, Ungeweiss K, Groettrup M, Bruno L, Fehling HJ, von Boehmer H. Analysis and expression of a cloned pre-T cell receptor gene. *Science* 1994;266:1208–1212.

32. Lin W-C, Desiderio S. V(D)J recombination and the cell cycle. *Immunol Today* 1995;16:279–289.

33. Li Z, Dordai DI, Lee J, Desiderio S. A conserved degradation signal regulates RAG-2 accumulation during cell division and links V(D)J recombination to the cell cycle. *Immunity* 1996;5:575–589.

34. Nacht M, Strasser A, Chan YR, et al. Mutations in the p53 and SCID genes cooperate in tumorigenesis. *Genes Dev* 1996;10:2055–2066.

35. Guidos CJ, Williams CJ, Grandal I, Knowles G, Huang MTF, Danska JS. V(D)J recombination activates a p53-dependent DNA damage checkpoint in SCID lymphocyte precursors. *Genes Dev* 1996;10:2038–2054.

36. Jiang D, Lenardo MJ, Zuniga-Pflucker JC. P53 prevents maturation to the CD4+ CD8+ stage of thymocyte differentiation in the absence of T cell receptor rearrangement. *J Exp Med* 1996;183:1923–1928.

37. Suhr CD, Sprent J. T-cell apoptosis detected in situ during positive and negative selection in the thymus. *Nature* 1994;372:100–103.

38. Beneviste P, Cohen A. P53 protein is required for thymocyte apoptosis induced by adenosine deaminase deficiency. *Proc Natl Acad Sci U S A* 1995;92:8373–8377.

39. Lerner A, Clayton LK, Mizoguchi E, et al. Cross-linking of T cell receptors on double-positive thymocytes induces a cytokine-mediated stromal activation process linked to cell death. *EMBO J* 1996;15:5876–5887.

40. Fukui Y, Ishimoto T, Utsuyama M, et al. Positive and negative CD4+ thymocyte selection by a single MHC class II/peptide ligand affected by its expression level in the thymus. *Immunity* 1997;6:401–410.

41. Hu Q, Bazemore Walker CR, Girao C, et al. Specific recognition of thymic self-peptides induces the positive selection of cytotoxic T lymphocytes. *Immunity* 1997;7:221–231.

42. Tourne S, Miyazaki T, Oxenius A, et al. Selection of a broad repertoire of CD4+ T cells in H-2Ma0/0 mice. *Immunity* 1997;7:187–195.

43. Bevan MJ. In thymic selection, peptide diversity gives and takes away. *Immunity* 1997;7:175–178.

44. Bolotin E, Smogorzewska M, Smith S, Widmer M, Weinberg K. Enhancement of thymopoiesis after bone marrow transplant by in vivo interleukin-7. *Blood* 1996;88:1887–1894.

45. Tsuda S, Rieke S, Hashimoto Y, Nakauchi H, Takahama Y. IL-7 supports D-J but not V-DJ rearrangement of TCR-β gene in fetal liver progenitor cells. *J Immunol* 1996;156:3233–3242.

46. Noguchi M, Yi H, Rosenblatt HM, et al. Interleukin-2 receptor γ chain mutation results in X-linked severe combined immunodeficiency. *Cell* 1993;73:147–157.

47. Plum J, De Smedt M, Leclercq G, Verhasselt B, Vandekerckhove B. Interleukin-7 is a critical growth factor in early human T-cell development. *Blood* 1996;88:4239–4245.

48. Crompton T, Outram SV, Buckland J, Owen MJ. A transgenic T cell receptor restores thymocyte differentiation in interleukin-7 receptor α chain-deficient mice. *Eur J Immunol* 1997;27:100–104.

49. Berridge MJ. Lymphocyte activation in health and disease. *Crit Rev Immunol* 1997;17:155–178.

50. Fitzsimmons D, Hagman J. Regulation of gene expression at early stages of B-cell and T-cell differentiation. *Curr Opin Immunol* 1996;8:166–174.

51. Alberola-Ila J, Takaki S, Kerner JD, Perlmutter RM. Differential signaling by lymphocyte antigen receptors. *Ann Rev Immunol* 1997;15:125–154.

52. Koretzky GA, Kohmetscher MA, Kadleck T, Weiss A. Restoration of T cell receptor-mediated signal transduction by transfection of CD45 cDNA into CD45-deficient variant of the Jurkat cell line. *J Immunol* 1992;149:1138–1142.

53. Musci MA, Latinis KM, Koretzky GA. Signaling events in T lymphocytes leading to cellular activation or programmed cell death. *Clin Immunol Immunopathol* 1997;83:205–222.

54. Akbar AN, Salmon M. Cellular microenvironments and apoptosis: Tissue microenvironments control activated T-cell death. *Immunol Today* 1997;18:72–76.

55. Sprent J, Tough DF, Sun S. Factors controlling the turnover of T memory cells. *Immunol Rev* 1997;156:79–85.

56. Sprent J. Immunological memory. *Curr Opin Immunol* 1997;9:371–379.

57. Ahmed R, Gray D. Immunological memory and protective immunity: Understanding their relation. *Science* 1997;272:54–60.

58. Mullbacher A, Flynn K. Aspects of cytotoxic T cell memory. *Immunol Rev* 1997;150:113–127.

59. Haynes BF, Fauci AS. Introduction to the immune system. In: Fauci AS, Braunwald E, Isselbacher KJ, et al., eds. *Harrison's principles of internal medicine,* 14th ed. New York: McGraw-Hill, 1998:1753–1776.

60. Birkeland ML, Monroe JG. Biochemistry of antigen receptor signaling in mature and developing B lymphocytes. *Crit Rev Immunol* 1997;17:353–385.

61. Sanchez M, Misulovin Z, Burkhardt AL, et al. Signal transduction by immunoglobulin is mediated through Iga and Igb. *J Exp Med* 1993;178:1049–1055.

62. Hombach J, Tsubata T, Leclerq L, Stappert H, Reth M. Molecular components of the B-cell antigen receptor complex of the IgM class. *Nature* 1990;343:760–762.

63. Duchosal MA. B-cell development and differentiation. *Semin Hematol* 1997;34:2–12.

64. Milstein C, Neuberger MS. Maturation of the immune response. *Adv Protein Chem* 1996;49:451–485.

65. Fearon DT. The CD19/CR2/TAPA-1 complex, CD45, and signaling by the antigen receptor of B lymphocytes. *Curr Opin Immunol* 1993;5:341–348.

66. Fearon DT, Carter RH. The CD19/CR2/TAPA-1 complex of B lymphocytes: Linking natural to acquired immunity. *Ann Rev Immunol* 1995;13:127–149.

67. Willett CE, Zapata AG, Hopkins N, Steiner LA. Expression of zebrafish rag genes during early development identifies the thymus. *Develop Biol* 1997;182:331–341.

68. Opstelten D. B lymphocyte development and transcription regulation in vivo. *Adv Immunol* 1996;63:197–268.

69. Hayakawa K, Li Y-S, Wasserman R, Sauder S, Shinton S, Hardy RR. B lymphocyte developmental lineages. *Ann N Y Acad Sci* 1997;815:15–29.

70. Billips LG, Lassoued K, Nunez C, et al. Human B cell development. *Ann N Y Acad Sci* 1995;764:1–8.

71. Kitamura D, Kudo A, Schaal S, Muller W, Melchers F, Rajewsky K. A critical role of λ5 protein in B cell development. *Cell* 1992;69:823–831.

72. Takatsu K. Cytokines involved in B-cell differentiation and their sites of action. *Proc Soc Exp Biol Med* 1997;215:121–133.

73. Owen MJ, Venkitaraman AR. Signalling in lymphocyte development. *Curr Opin Immunol* 1996;8:191–198.

74. Kelsoe G. The germinal center: A crucible for lymphocyte selection. *Semin Immunol* 1996;8:179–184.

75. Kelsoe G. Life and death in germinal centers (redux). *Immunity* 1996;4:107–111.

76. Zheng B, Kelsoe G, Han S. Somatic diversification of antibody responses. *J Clin Immunol* 1996;16:1–11.

77. Han S, Zheng B, Schatz DG, Spanopoulo E, Kelsoe G. Neoteny in lymphocytes: Rag1 and Rag2 expression in germinal center B cells. *Science* 1996;274:2094–2097.

78. Han S, Dillon SR, Zheng B, Shimoda M, Schlissel MS, Kelsoe G. V(D)J recombinase activity in a subset of germinal center B lymphocytes. *Science* 1997;278:301–305.

79. Davis CM, McLaughlin TM, Watson TJ, et al. Normalization of the peripheral blood T cell receptor V-β repertoire after cultured postnatal human thymic transplantation in DiGeorge syndrome. *J Clin Immunol* 1997;17:167–175.

80. Shokat KM, Goodnow CC. Antigen-induced B cell death and elimination during germinal-centre immune responses. *Nature* 1995;375:334–338.

81. Bancherau J, Rousset F. Human B lymphocytes: Phenotype, proliferation, and differentiation. *Adv Immunol* 1992;52:125–262.

82. Bancherau J, Galibert L, Arpin C, Burdin N, Liu Y-J, Garrone P. Positive and negative selection of human B lymphocytes in vitro. *Ann N Y Acad Sci* 1997;815:237–245.

83. Cambier JC, Pleiman CM, Clark MR. Signal transduction by the B cell

antigen receptor and its coreceptor. *Ann Rev Immunol* 1994;12: 457–486.

84. Malisan F, Briere F, Bridon JM, et al. Interleukin-10 induces immunoglobulin G isotype switch recombination in human CD40-activated naive B lymphocytes. *J Exp Med* 1996;183:937–947.

85. Harriman W, Volk H, Defranoux N, Wabl M. Immunoglobulin class switch recombination. *Ann Rev Immunol* 1993;11:361–384.

86. Callard RE, Smith SH, Matthews DJ. Regulation of human B cell growth and differentiation: Lessons from the primary immunodeficiencies. *Chem Immunol* 1997;67:114–132.

87. Norvell A, Birkeland ML, Carman J, Sillman AL, Wechsler-Reya R, Monroe JG. Use of isolated immature-stage B cells to understand negative selection and tolerance induction at the molecular level. *Immunol Res* 1996;15:191–207.

88. Healy JI, Dolmetsch RE, Timmerman LA, et al. Different nuclear signals are activated by the B cell receptor during positive versus negative signaling. *Immunity* 1997;6:419–428.

89. Spits H, Lanier LL, Phillips JH. Development of human T and natural killer cells. *Blood* 1995;85:2654–2670.

90. Rodewald HR, Moingeon P, Lucich JL, Dosiou C, Lopez P, Reinherz EL. A population of early fetal thymocytes expressing FcγRII/III contains precursors of T lymphocytes and natural killer cells. *Cell* 1992;69: 139–150.

91. Phillips JH, Hori T, Nagler A, Bhat N, Spits H, Lanier LL. Ontogeny of human natural killer cells: Fetal NK cells mediate cytolytic function and express CD3ε,δ proteins. *J Exp Med* 1992;175:1055–1066.

92. Biron CA, Byron KS, Sullivan JL. Severe herpesvirus infections in an adolescent without natural killer cells. *N Engl J Med* 1989;320: 1731–1735.

93. Jawahar S, Moody C, Chan M, Finberg R, Geha R, Chatila T. Natural killer (NK) cell deficiency associated with an epitope-deficient Fc receptor type IIIA (CD16-II). *Clin Exp Immunol* 1996;103:408–413.

94. Moretta A, Bottino C, Vitale M, et al. Receptors for HLA class-I molecules in human natural killer cells. *Annu Rev Immunol* 1996;14: 619–648.

95. Lanier LL. Natural killer cell receptors and MHC class I interactions. *Curr Opin Immunol* 1997;9:126–131.

96. Lanier LL, Corliss B, Phillips JH. Arousal and inhibition of human NK cells. *Immunol Rev* 1997;155:145–154.

97. Moretta L, Mingari MC, Pende D, Bottino C, Biassoni R, Moretta A. The molecular basis of natural killer (NK) cell recognition and function. *J Clin Immunol* 1996;16:243–253.

Inflammation: Basic Principles and Clinical Correlates,
3rd ed., edited by John I. Gallin and Ralph Snyderman.
Lippincott Williams & Wilkins, Philadelphia © 1999.

CHAPTER 9

The Thymus and T-Cell Development

Charles D. Surh and Jonathan Sprent

The thymus is a bilobed structure situated above the heart in the anterior mediastinum. It is conspicuously large in infancy and up until the time of puberty (1-3). Thereafter, the thymus undergoes progressive atrophy until it is barely functional in old age. The main and perhaps sole function of the thymus is to produce T lymphocytes. In discussing how the thymus generates T cells, it is important to consider the antigen specificity of mature T cells.

In the peripheral lymphoid organs, most typical T cells express a diverse array of $\alpha\beta$ T-cell receptor (TCR) molecules and display specificity for foreign peptides bound to major histocompatibility complex (MHC) molecules. For these T cells the primary function of the thymus is to screen a large pool of precursor T cells and selectively export only those cells that are equipped to function optimally in the postthymic environment. At a population level, the T cells released from the thymus must display maximal reactivity for an almost infinite variety of foreign antigens but remain unresponsive to a multiplicity of self antigens. To meet these criteria, intrathymic precursors of mature T cells are subjected to a complex process of positive and negative selection based on their reactivity to MHC molecules and the self peptides bound to these molecules. Very few T cells survive thymic selection, and, as a result, more than 95% of thymocytes die *in situ.*

This chapter provides a brief overview of the various mechanisms and selection processes involved in the transformation of immature thymocytes into mature functional $\alpha\beta$ T cells. Because of space constraints, differentiation of the minor subset of thymocytes expressing $\gamma\delta$ TCR molecules is not discussed; these cells comprise less than 2% of thymocytes, and their function is still largely obscure. Although many of the studies of thymocyte dif-

ferentiation and selection have been done on mice, it is highly likely that the data are applicable to other species, including humans. An overview of human cell ontogeny and function can be found in Chapter 12.

SUBSETS OF THYMOCYTES

The expression of cell-surface CD4 and CD8 molecules divides thymocytes into four broad subsets (2-4). Cells lacking both CD4 and CD8 molecules form about 2% of total thymocytes. Although numerically few, these *double-negative* (DN) CD4$^-$CD8$^-$ thymocytes are highly important because they act as stem cell precursors for other thymocyte subsets. Most thymocytes (80% to 90%) show dual expression of CD4 and CD8 molecules, and most of these *double-positive* (DP) CD4$^+$CD8$^+$ cells express a low level of $\alpha\beta$ TCR molecules. DP cells are the main target cells for thymic selection; they give rise to typical mature T cells expressing either CD4 or CD8 molecules. These *single-positive* (SP) CD4$^+$CD8$^-$ and CD4$^-$CD8$^+$ cells express high levels of $\alpha\beta$ TCR molecules and are exported to the periphery to form the pool of mature T cells.

Although cell suspensions from thymus consist almost entirely of lymphocytes, histologic sections of thymus reveal a dense network of epithelial cells (5,6). The histology of the thymus is discussed in the next section.

ARCHITECTURE OF THE THYMUS

With conventional staining, the thymus in sections is divisible into two distinctive regions: the dark outer cortex and the pale inner medulla (Fig. 9-1*A*). In young animals, the cortex is large and makes up the bulk of the thymus. The cortex is densely packed with small, immature DP thymocytes (Fig. 9-1*B*), which reside within a network of epithelial cells expressing both class I and class II MHC molecules (Fig. 9-1*C,E,F*). As mentioned, DP

C.D. Surh and J. Sprent: Department of Immunology, The Scripps Research Institute, La Jolla, California 92037.

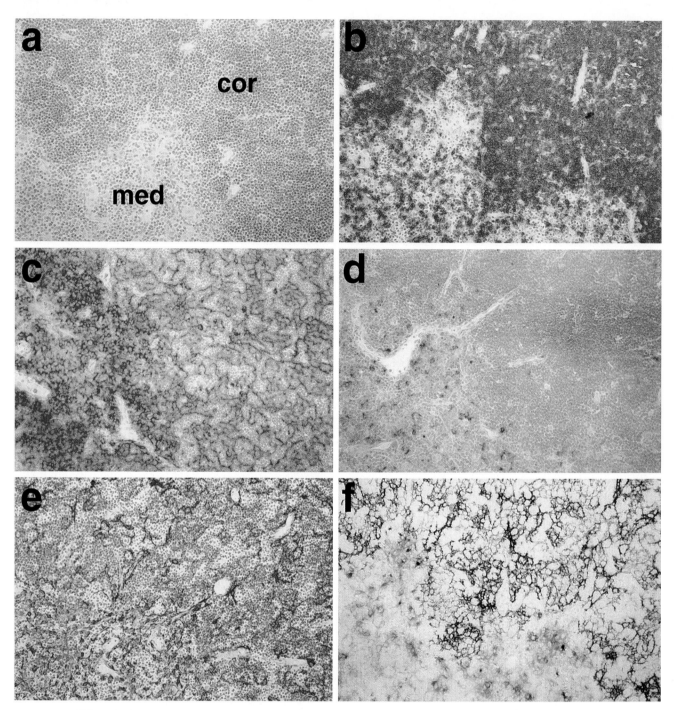

FIG. 9-1. Histologic views of adjacent frozen sections from a normal mouse thymus stained with various reagents. (**a**) Hematoxylin for nuclear staining, demonstrating that cell density is higher in the cortex (cor) than in the medulla (med). (**b**) An antibody to CD8: expression of CD8 on all double-positive (DP) cells in the cortex but on only a proportion of single-positive (SP) cells in the medulla leads to very dense staining of the cortex and scattered staining of the medulla. (**c**) An antibody to MHC class II molecules: the reticular pattern of staining in the cortex is restricted to epithelial cells; confluent staining in the medulla reflects staining of both epithelial cells and bone marrow–derived macrophages, B cells, and dendritic cells. (**d**) An antibody to dendritic cells, revealing scattered cells restricted to the medulla. (**e**) An antibody to cytokeratin, showing a network of epithelial cells in the cortex and a heterogeneous mixture of epithelial cells in the medulla. (**f**) Double staining with an antibody to cortical epithelial cells (blue) and a plant lectin, UEA-1, which binds to a subpopulation of medullary epithelial cells (red), revealing distinct phenotypic differences between cortical and medullary epithelial cells. (**a** through **f**, original magnification, ×200.)

cells arise from the small subset of DN cells; the latter are larger than DP cells and form a thin rim of cells beneath the outer capsule (Fig. 9-2).

The medulla contains few if any DP cells. It consists largely of SP cells enmeshed in a heterogeneous network of epithelial cells and bone marrow–derived antigen-presenting cells (APCs) such as dendritic cells and macrophages (see Fig. 9-1C–F). The majority of these nonlymphoid cells express a high density of MHC mole-cules; as discussed later, these cells play an important role in the induction of self-tolerance. The epithelial cells in the cortex and in the medulla are phenotypically distinct (see Fig. 9-1F), reflecting their different embryonic origins (see later discussion).

In addition to epithelial cells and APCs, a variety of other nonlymphoid cells in the thymus perform important functions. For example, mesenchyme-derived cells such as fibroblasts, which line the outer capsule of the thymus

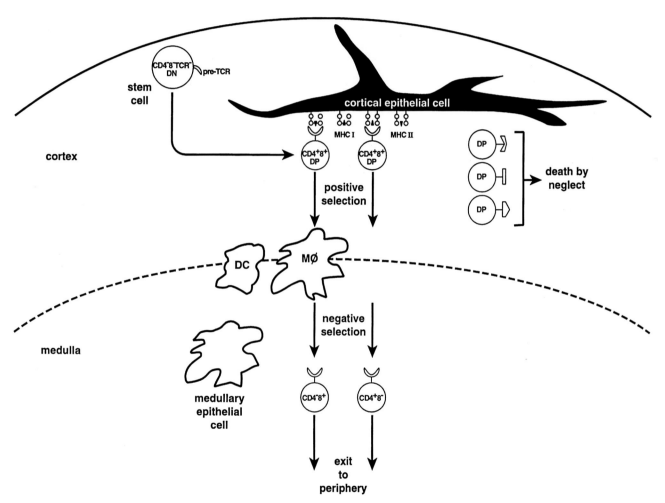

FIG. 9-2. Selection events in the thymus. Under the outer capsule, marrow-derived immature double-negative (DN) cells expressing the pre–T-cell receptor (pre-TCR) proliferate and differentiate into corti-cal double-positive (DP) cells expressing a low density of the αβ TCR. Through binding via TCR and CD4 or CD8 molecules, DP cells are screened for their ability to recognize peptide-bound major histo-compatibility complex (MHC) class I and II molecules displayed on cortical epithelial cells. Small num-bers of DP cells able to bind to MHC molecules with low affinity are rescued from "death by neglect" and undergo positive selection. The positively-selected DP cells migrate into the medulla and become either CD4+CD8− or CD4−CD8+ single-positive (SP) cells, depending on whether they are positively selected on class II or class I MHC molecules, respectively. On reaching the medulla, positively-selected cells encounter antigen-presenting cells (APC), such as dendritic cells (DC) and macrophages (MØ); these cells express MHC molecules loaded with peptides derived either from endogenous cellular pro-teins or from circulating self proteins entering the thymus from the bloodstream. T cells that bind to these self peptides with high affinity undergo negative selection (death) by apoptosis *in situ*. The combination of positive and negative selection allows maturation and export of only a small proportion of total thy-mocytes (1% to 2%); the remainder of the cells die *in situ*.

and form sheaths around blood vessels, appear to be necessary for the transformation of DN cells into DP cells (7). Macrophages are found scattered throughout the cortex and play a crucial role in phagocytosing nonselected thymocytes—that is, cells undergoing apoptosis from lack of positive selection (8) (Fig. 9-3).

ONTOGENY OF THE THYMUS

Thymic epithelial cells are derived from three embryonic sources—the ectoderm of the third branchial cleft, the endoderm of the third pharyngeal pouch, and the neural crest mesectoderm—which give rise to cortical

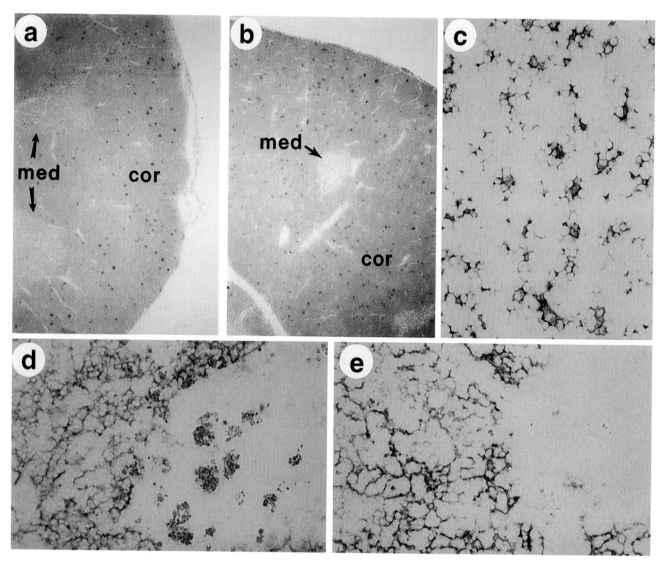

FIG. 9-3. *In situ* detection of apoptotic cells in thymus frozen sections detected by the terminal deoxynucleotidyl transferase-mediated dUTP-biotin nick end-labelling (TUNEL) staining method. **(a)** Normal thymus: stained cells are scattered throughout the cortex (cor) but are sparse in the medulla (med). **(b)** Major histocompatibility complex (MHC) class I–deficient, class II–deficient thymus: stained cells are present in the cortex at about the same frequency as in the normal mouse; the medulla is small, reflecting the paucity of mature T cells in MHC-deficient mice. **(c)** Cortex of normal thymus double stained for apoptotic cells (red) and for a macrophage marker (blue): almost all apoptotic cells are situated inside macrophages. **(d)** MHC class II H2-E+ TCR variable β-chain 5 (Vβ5) transgenic thymus double stained for apoptotic cells (red) and a marker on cortical epithelial cells (blue): large aggregates of apoptotic cells are apparent in the medulla. Here, Vβ5+ cells are undergoing negative selection to H2-E molecules plus endogenous mammary tumor virus (Mtv) antigens expressed in the medulla and corticomedullary junction. **(e)** H2-E- TCR Vβ5 transgenic thymus double stained as in **d**, reflecting the lack of negative selection in these mice; apoptotic cells are not visible in the medulla.

epithelial cells, medullary epithelial cells, and mesenchymal cells, respectively (9–11). In the mouse, the embryonic cells from these three sources assemble together at about gestation day 9 to form rudimentary thymic lobes; by day 14, the two lobes have migrated into the anterior mediastinum and fused to form the fetal thymus. During this migration and starting on day 11 or 12, the thymus is colonized by stem cells from the fetal liver. These cells differentiate rapidly into DN cells, which give rise to DP cells at about day 16; mature SP cells begin to appear on about day 18. Low levels of MHC expression are apparent in the cortex and medulla at about day 16 and increase progressively to reach adult levels by the time of birth.

EARLY STAGES OF THYMOCYTE DEVELOPMENT

In adult animals, constant production of T cells depends on continuous seeding of the thymus by small numbers of precursor cells from the bone marrow. Although the exact identity of thymic stem cells is

unclear, these cells are slightly more mature than pluripotent hematopoietic stem cells (12). The differentiation of thymic stem cells into DN cells and then into DP cells is highly complex and involves a series of steps associated with distinct changes in surface phenotype. The most immature cells in adult mouse thymus express CD4^{lo}, THY-1^{lo}, SCA-2$^+$, c-KIT$^+$, CD44$^+$, CD25$^-$ (Fig. 9-4), which is similar but not identical to the phenotype of hematopoietic stem cells in the bone marrow (12,13). These early thymic precursor cells are pluripotent in that they can give rise to both αβ and γδ T cells and also to B cells, natural killer (NK) cells, and dendritic cells. However, unlike hematopoietic stem cells, they cannot form macrophages or granulocytes. These precursor cells differentiate into cells with the phenotype CD4$^-$, THY-1^{hi}, SCA-2$^+$, c-KIT$^+$, CD44$^+$, CD25$^+$; they can no longer form B cells but continue to generate dendritic cells and low numbers of NK cells (14). Further differentiation into cells with a CD4$^-$, THY-1^{hi}, SCA-2$^-$, c-KIT$^-$, CD44$^-$, CD25$^+$ phenotype commits the cells to the T cell lineage, thus curtailing production of dendritic and NK cells. At

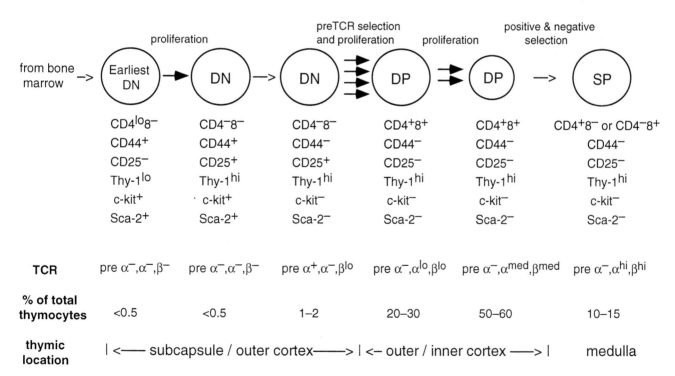

FIG. 9-4. Developmental stages of immature T cells in the mouse thymus. As indicated by the expression of various cell-surface markers, thymocytes exhibit specific phenotypes at different stages of differentiation. Two main steps are involved. First, expression of pre–T-cell receptor (pTCR) molecules during the late double-negative (DN) stage induces extensive proliferation and differentiation into αβ TCR^{lo} double-positive (DP) cells; this transition does not involve major histocompatibility complex (MHC) molecules. Second, at the DP stage, TCR-mediated contact with MHC molecules plus self peptides on cortical epithelial cells induces a small proportion of DP cells to undergo positive selection and maturation into SP cells; these cells are then subjected to negative selection through contact with bone marrow (BM)–derived antigen-presenting cells (APCs) and epithelial cells in the medulla. The figure shows the relative cell size, proportion, thymic location, and proliferative status of cells at different stages of differentiation.

this stage, the cells begin to rearrange the TCR γ, δ, and β genes; α gene rearrangement is delayed until the DP stage (see later discussion) (15).

The molecular mechanisms involved in attracting bone marrow precursor cells into the thymus and inducing their subsequent differentiation are yet to be fully defined. However, maturation and proliferation of the earliest precursor subsets of DN cells are known to depend on signaling through c-KIT and the common cytokine receptor γ chain (γ_c) (16,17). The protein-tyrosine kinase c-KIT is the receptor for stem cell factor (SCF), which is expressed by thymic stromal cells, and the γ_c chain is an integral part of various cytokine receptors. For thymocytes, these receptors bind cytokines such as interleukin-7 (IL-7) and, via kinases, induce activation of the Janus kinases-signal transducers and activators of transcription (JAK-STAT) transcription pathway (18). This pathway is highly important in the transformation of DN cells to DP cells, because mice deficient in either the γ_c chain or IL-7 have a marked (30-fold) reduction in thymic cellularity (17,19,20). A similar, although less profound (fivefold) reduction in thymic cellularity is seen in mice deficient in c-KIT (16). Significantly, however, mice deficient for both c-KIT and γ_c have a complete block in thymocyte development at the early DN stage (21). This developmental arrest is T-cell specific, because B-cell development is only mildly reduced. The thymuses of these double-knockout mice are extremely small and consist largely of residual THY-1⁻ stromal cells. Whether thymic aplasia in these mice is caused by the absence of thymus-seeding bone marrow precursor cells or by lack of expansion of these cells after thymus colonization (or both) remains to be determined.

After bone marrow precursor cells colonize the thymus and undergo initial proliferation and differentiation, the first critical developmental step involving a distinct selection process occurs at the point of transition from CD44⁻CD25⁺ DN to DP cells. In order for this transition to occur, DN cells must rearrange the variable β-chain (V_β) TCR genes in-frame and express a functional β chain on the cell surface (22). Successful V_β gene rearrangement suppresses further V_β rearrangement and also inhibits rearrangement at the TCR γ locus. During the DN-to-DP transition, the TCR β chain is expressed on the cell surface coupled with the pre-TCR (pTCR) α chain, a novel nonrearranging gene belonging to the immunoglobulin superfamily (23). The pTCR α chains form a heterodimer with TCR β chains and associate with CD3 chains to form the pre-TCR complex. Efficient transition of DN cells into the TCR⁺ DP stage depends initially on expression of the pTCR complex, because mutant mice deficient in any of the components of the pTCR complex have a complete or near-complete block of this step. Virtually no DP cells are found in mice deficient in the CD3 ε chain or in mice that are unable to rearrange TCR genes—for example, mice with the severe combined immunodeficiency (SCID) mutation or mice lacking the recombination-activating gene proteins (RAG-1 and RAG-2) that cause TCR gene rearrangement. Similarly, mice selectively deficient in either TCR β or the pTCR α chain show a 95% to 97% reduction in total DP cell counts (24-29).

Although the ligand for pTCR has yet to be defined, signaling through the pTCR and CD3 components is transmitted via the protein-tyrosine kinase p56^LCK (LCK). Whereas the CD3-associated ζ chains are crucial for signal transduction in mature T cells, signaling in immature thymocytes is controlled largely by CD3 ε chains. Therefore, mice deficient in ζ chains possess moderate numbers of DP thymocytes, but those deficient in CD3 ε have no DP cells (24,30). Significantly, the DN-to-DP transition can be induced artificially in the absence of the pTCR by signaling directly through CD3—for example, by injecting SCID mice or RAG⁻/⁻ mice with antibodies to CD3 ε (31,32). This finding confirms that CD3 components are expressed on the cell surface of DN cells and are capable of signal transduction in the absence of TCR β.

Signaling through the pTCR/CD3 complex is known to be mediated by LCK, because DP cell production is severely reduced in LCK-deficient mice (33). Likewise, anti–CD3 ε monoclonal antibody fails to induce DP cell development in RAG-deficient mice if these mice are also deficient in LCK (34). In the absence of LCK, another related SRC-family protein-tyrosine kinase, p59^FYN (FYN) can compensate for LCK, but only inefficiently. This molecule allows small numbers of DP cells to arise in LCK-deficient mice. However, complete abrogation of DP cell generation is observed in mice that are deficient in both LCK and FYN (35,36).

In addition to SRC-family protein-tyrosine kinases, members of the SYK family, notably SYK and ζ-associated protein-70 (ZAP-70), are required for the DN-to-DP transition. Very few DP cells are found in mice lacking both SYK and ZAP-70 (37). The downstream signaling events involved in the DN-to-DP transition are not yet clearly defined but appear to be mediated through the RAS proteins and mitogen-activated protein (MAP) kinases (38).

As immature DP cells make the transition to the DP stage, the cells cease production of pTCR α chains and begin to synthesize TCR α chains and to express TCR αβ complexes on the cell surface (see Fig. 9-4). As with immunoglobulin chains on B cells, TCR αβ chains are generated through random rearrangement of the variable (V), diversity (D), and joining (J) gene segments, by which a highly diverse TCR repertoire is generated. At this stage, DP cells bearing these receptors are subjected to positive selection.

POSITIVE SELECTION

To understand the requirement for positive selection (39–42), it must be recognized that the specificity of mature T cells is skewed toward recognition of foreign peptides presented by self MHC molecules. Because MHC molecules are highly polymorphic, the self MHC–restricted population of mature T cells in each person must be tailor-made for that individual. The task of the thymus is to screen a very large repertoire of DP cells for covert reactivity to the particular MHC molecules expressed in the thymus. DP cells displaying this specificity are allowed to survive and differentiate into mature T cells; most DP cells have no reactivity for the limited array of MHC molecules in the thymus, and these cells are allowed to die *in situ* ("death by neglect") (8). After removal of overtly autoaggressive cells (negative selection), the progeny of the cells undergoing positive selection retain "physiologic" reactivity for self MHC molecules in the postthymic environment. During T-cell recognition of antigens, these self molecules are ignored when they are associated with self peptides but are highly immunogenic when they are bound to foreign peptides.

A corollary of positive selection is that the fine specificity of DP cells for MHC molecules plus peptides is enormous and sufficient to encompass reactivity to all of the different MHC alleles expressed in the species as a whole. Examination of a panel of T-cell hybridomas prepared directly from DP cells has shown that the MHC specificity of immature T cells is indeed vast (43).

Positive selection of DP cells occurs in the cortex and reflects recognition of MHC-peptide complexes expressed on cortical epithelial cells. TCR-mediated binding to MHC-peptide complexes is thought to deliver a low-level signal that allows the cells to differentiate into mature T cells. Such signaling is augmented by CD4 or CD8 molecules, which act as coreceptors and bind to nonpolymorphic residues on the membrane-proximal domains of class II and class I MHC molecules, respectively. This interaction is also important for determining the CD4/CD8 phenotype of mature SP cells. CD4 stabilizes TCR interaction with class II molecules, thereby causing downregulation of CD8 molecules and promoting differentiation into CD4$^+$CD8$^-$ SP cells; conversely, CD8 strengthens TCR reactivity to class I molecules and induces development of CD4$^-$CD8$^+$ SP cells.

Demonstrating Positive Selection

Evidence that the specificity of mature T cells reflects positive selection came initially from studies with MHC-mismatched bone marrow chimeras and thymus-grafted mice (44-47). These experiments showed that the capacity of mature T cells to respond to foreign peptides was much more effective when these peptides were presented in the context of self rather than foreign MHC molecules. The key observation was that T cells differentiating in a chimeric thymus in which the radioresistant stromal cells (epithelial cells) were MHC^a and the bone marrow–derived cells were MHC^b showed self-MHC

restriction to MHC^a rather than MHC^b. Thus "self" appeared to be determined by the MHC molecules expressed on epithelial cells rather than by bone marrow-derived APCs. It was concluded that generation of a repertoire of self MHC^a–restricted T cells required a process of positive selection to MHC^a molecules in the thymus, presumably on epithelial cells. Further support for this notion came from studies with TCR transgenic mice (48). The significant finding here was that mice constructed from an MHC^a-restricted T-cell clone generated mature T cells only when the transgenic mice expressed MHC^a; with an MHC^b background, the thymus contained DP cells but these cells failed to differentiate into SP cells.

With normal (nontransgenic) mice, it was subsequently determined that mice expressing MHC class I molecules but lacking class II molecules (I$^+$II$^-$ mice) generate only mature CD8$^+$ and not CD4$^+$ cells (49,50). Conversely, only CD4$^+$ cells are found in I$^-$II$^+$ mice (51,52). Virtually no mature T cells occur in I$^-$II$^-$ mice (53).

Cell Types That Induce Positive Selection

There is now general agreement that positive selection is controlled largely (though perhaps not exclusively) by cortical epithelial cells. The most convincing evidence on this point was provided by the finding that MHC transgenic mice expressing MHC molecules solely on cortical epithelial cells showed normal positive selection (54,55). Similarly, positive selection was induced in a thymus reaggregation system in which purified DP thymocytes were aggregated in a three-dimensional network *in vitro* with dispersed populations of thymic epithelial cells (56). Positive selection in this model occurred with purified cortical epithelial cells but was very limited or undetectable with medullary epithelial cells or bone marrow–derived cells. Likewise, several other cell types, including primary epithelial cells from skin, gut, and salivary glands, failed to induce more than minimal positive selection in thymus reaggregation cultures (57,58).

Despite these findings, studies with other models suggest that the ability to promote positive selection is not an exclusive property of cortical epithelial cells. In one study, irradiation bone marrow chimeras constructed to express MHC class I molecules only on bone marrow–derived cells contained small numbers of CD8$^+$ SP cells, suggesting that bone marrow–derived cells do have a limited capacity to induce positive selection, at least for CD8$^+$ cells (59). In other studies, *in vitro*–established thymic epithelial cell lines were shown to induce positive selection when injected directly into the thymus (60,61). More surprisingly, MHC$^+$ fibroblasts were also found to induce positive selection on intrathymic injection, especially in a TCR transgenic line (62). Although these findings can be interpreted as evidence that cortical epithelial cells are not unique in their capacity to promote positive selection, it is striking that the other cell types induce positive selection only in the presence of cortical epithelial cells. One interpretation of these data is that positive selection is controlled by a separate set of accessory molecules expressed selectively on cortical epithelium and that "bystander" T-cell contact with these molecules allows weak but significant positive selection to MHC molecules expressed on other cells. Thus far, however, attempts to find unique accessory molecules on cortical epithelium have been unsuccessful.

Role of Peptide Diversity in Positive Selection

In the 1990s, the nature of the MHC-bound peptides required for positive selection came under close scrutiny (63,64). Currently, there are three views on the role of peptides in positive selection (63–65). In the first model, peptide recognition by immature T cells is highly specific, with the result that each TCR is selectable by only one or a few structurally-related peptides; here, T-cell diversity is ultimately a reflection of self peptide diversity. In the second hypothesis, positive selection is the result of low-affinity TCR interaction with a limited set of self peptides, each peptide being capable of selecting multiple specificities unrelated to the selecting peptide. According to the third theory, the main function of peptides is to stabilize MHC molecules (which are unstable without peptides) and allow TCR recognition of MHC epitopes rather than peptides (65). In this latter model, T-cell diversity is obtained by positive selection of cells capable of recognizing MHC molecules per se, followed by negative selection of T cells specific for self-peptide epitopes expressed on thymic epithelial cells or on APCs.

One of the earliest pieces of evidence that peptides play a role in positive selection came from the finding that MHC residues that interact solely with the bound peptide and not with the TCR were able to affect the fine specificity of positive selection (66,67). However, the relation between the peptide and the selected T cells could not be addressed until the advent of an ingenious *in vitro* system that uses fetal thymus from TCR transgenic mice bred onto a class I–deficient background. By adding peptides that rescue (stabilize) the expression of class I molecules in fetal thymic organ cultures, it was shown that positive selection of TCR transgenic T cells depends on both the type and the concentration of the peptides used. In one of the earliest studies with this system, Hogquist et al. (68,69) found that positive selection of CD8$^+$ TCR transgenic T cells specific for an ovalbumin (ova) peptide presented by MHC class I (K^b) molecules was most efficient with antagonist peptides—that is, with weak peptides that provided a suboptimal level of interaction with the TCR (70). Addition of agonist (antigenic) peptides in fetal thymic organ cultures induced either negative selection only or selection of anergic T cells that did not respond to the antigenic peptide. Moreover, no

selection was observed with unrelated null peptides, which bind to MHC but cannot activate or antagonize the transgenic T cells. In two other related studies, it was found that positive selection of CD8$^+$ T cells from another TCR transgenic line specific for lymphocytic choriomeningitis virus (LCMV) glycoprotein occurred on addition of low doses of agonist peptides, whereas high doses induced negative selection (71,72). As with anti-ova T cells, low-affinity variants of agonist peptides promoted positive selection but a null polyserine peptide was ineffective (71,72). However, in contrast to the anti-ova T cells, a moderate-agonist variant of the LCMV peptide induced positive selection of anti-LCMV TCR transgenic T cells over a wide range of concentrations without causing negative selection at high doses (69,73). Collectively, these data suggest that the role of peptides in positive selection is highly specific.

Despite these findings, other approaches do not support the view that the role of peptides is specific. First, positive selection of CD8$^+$ cells from a third TCR transgenic line (designated 2C) in fetal thymic organ cultures was found to be mediated by a variety of unrelated peptides, including polyserine null peptides (74). Second, with the use of a novel system involving intrathymic injection of adenoviruses containing minigene expression vectors, it was found that thymic MHC class II expression of agonist-variant peptides (i.e., peptides with no agonist or antagonist activity) could positively select CD4$^+$ T cells against both the agonist peptide and unrelated antigenic peptides (75). In this model, positive selection was also induced by an agonist peptide, although this finding may have reflected inefficient negative selection caused by lack of expression of the peptide on bone marrow–derived cells.

An alternative way of studying the role of peptides in thymic selection is to generate lines of mice that express only a single species of MHC-bound peptide. This has been accomplished in two ways. First, a transgenic line was generated that expressed a single peptide covalently bound to MHC class II molecules (76). Second, positive selection was examined in mice lacking MHC class II-like H2-M molecules; in these mice, the lack of H2-M molecules prevents dissociation of the invariant-chain class II-associated invariant chain peptides (CLIP) peptide from MHC class II molecules and thereby precludes class II molecules from binding other peptides (77-79). Although the bound peptides in these two types of mice were structurally different, positive selection of CD4$^+$ cells was clearly apparent. For both types of mice, expression of a single peptide on class II molecules led to the production of substantial numbers of CD4$^+$ cells (25% to 50% of normal); these CD4$^+$ cells were polyclonal in terms of TCR chain usage and responses to alloantigens (75–78). Subsequent analysis of the fine specificity of these CD4$^+$ cells showed that a single peptide was capable of positively selecting polyclonal T cells with multiple specificities for a wide variety of foreign peptides examined (79,80). More importantly, these CD4+ cells were reactive to peptides structurally unrelated to the selecting peptides. These findings do not support the view that peptides have a specific role in positive selection. Instead, the data suggest that there is no clear relation between the peptides inducing positive selection and those subsequently recognized by mature T cells.

Significantly, the CD4+ T-cell populations generated in mice expressing only single peptides were highly autoreactive to the diverse peptides expressed by syngeneic wild-type APCs (76–79). Precursor frequency measurements revealed that 65% to 75% of these CD4+ cells were autoreactive (76, 81–82). The implication is that, in the normal thymus, many of the T cells undergoing positive selection to individual self peptides subsequently undergo negative selection to other peptides. Therefore, if T cells undergoing positive selection to a single peptide were exposed during development to a normal array of self peptides on wild-type bone marrow–derived APCs, such contact would be expected in many of them and therefore greatly reduce the production of mature CD4+ cells. Studies with H2-M−/− mice reconstituted with stem cells derived from normal mice have shown that this is indeed the case. However, the fine specificity of the few CD4 cells generated in these chimeric mice is somewhat more restricted than for normal CD4+ cells (81–82). Therefore, generation of normal numbers of T cells with a diverse repertoire probably requires positive selection directed to multiple peptides.

In view of the conflicting data described here, the precise role of peptides in positive selection is still unclear. One important point is that the role of individual peptides in positive selection may be influenced by peptide concentration (83). Rare agonist peptides existing at a very low density may positively select T cells that can subsequently recognize foreign peptides resembling the selecting peptide. On the other hand, high concentrations of agonist peptides probably lead to negative rather than positive selection. By contrast, moderate to high concentrations of antagonist (weak) peptides may be optimal for induction of positive selection and may be capable of selecting multiple specificities unrelated to the selecting peptide. This situation presumably operates for positive selection directed to the CLIP peptide in H2-M−/− mice (see previous discussion). Here, promiscuous selection occurs presumably because the affinity threshold required for positive selection is low and favors selection of T cells on MHC residues with minimal recognition of the peptide. However, detailed information on the range of peptides controlling positive selection is still unavailable.

NEGATIVE SELECTION

As discussed, positive selection of DP thymocytes is considered to reflect low-level TCR signaling induced through contact with MHC-peptide complexes on cortical epithelial cells. During positive selection, the avidity of interaction between T cells and MHC-peptide complexes is presumed to be weak, with the result that subsequent contact with the selecting peptides in the peripheral lymphoid tissues is nonimmunogenic. However, some DP thymocytes inevitably display strong reactivity to MHC-peptide complexes. If these cells were allowed to leave the thymus, contact with the selecting MHC-peptide complexes in the periphery might induce overt activation of the cells and lead to autoimmune disease. Therefore, any DP cells displaying strong reactivity for MHC-peptide complexes in the thymus must be destroyed. As mentioned previously, this process of central tolerance or negative selection causes the cells to undergo apoptosis in situ. By definition, negative selection applies only to self antigens that enter the thymus from the periphery or are synthesized in situ. With the assumption that most self proteins are highly conserved and expressed in all cell types, one can envisage that the vast majority of self antigens are expressed in the thymus. Hence, most T cells with potential self-reactivity are probably tolerized (deleted) in the thymus rather than in the periphery. However, it is well accepted that a small proportion of self components fall into the category of tissue-specific proteins (e.g., myelin basic protein). Tolerization of T cells to these sequestered antigens is presumed to reflect various peripheral mechanisms (84–86).

Site of Negative Selection

The issue of whether negative selection occurs predominantly in the cortex or in the medulla is highly controversial (84,87). Evidence for negative selection in the cortex is provided by the finding that crossing of the male-antigen-specific HY TCR transgenic line to a male background induces disappearance of DP thymocytes and atrophy of the cortex (48). Likewise, it is well established that injection of normal mice with anti-TCR monoclonal antibody (88) or TCR transgenic mice with specific peptide (89) causes rapid onset of apoptosis in the cortex. Despite these findings, TCR expression in TCR transgenic mice often occurs abnormally early in ontogeny (48), so that deletion in the HY line could occur before differentiation into cortical DP cells. There is also the problem that destruction of DP cells after injection of antigen or anti-TCR monoclonal antibody could be largely stress related because of stimulation of mature postthymic T cells (90). Finally, a transgenic line in which MHC class II molecules were expressed selectively in cortical epithelium failed to show negative selection after antigen injection (55). In view of these concerns, the role of the cortex in physiologic negative selection remains unclear.

In contrast to the cortex, the medulla is relatively open to the circulation and is packed with bone-marrow–derived APCs, cells known to be important for tolerance induction

(84,87). It has long been argued that the medulla is an important site for negative selection (91). Direct evidence for negative selection in the medulla has come from the observation that apoptotic transferase-mediated dVTP-biotin nick end-labelling (TUNEL⁺) cells in variable B-chain 5 ($V_\beta5^+$) transgenic mice expressing endogenous mammary tumor virus (Mtv) 8,9 antigens are restricted to the medulla and corticomedullary junction (8) (see Fig. 9-3). This observation is consistent with the finding that negative selection of T cells specific for endogenous Mtv antigens occurs relatively late in thymocyte differentiation (92). An obvious problem with the medulla as a site for negative selection is that the great majority of T cells in the medulla are SP cells, cells thought to be beyond the stage of (central) tolerance induction. However, it is possible that early SP cells remain susceptible to tolerance for a brief period after reaching the medulla from the cortex. In support of this idea, it has been demonstrated that negative selection can affect a population of semimature heat stable antigen (HSA^hi) SP cells found in the medulla (93); by contrast, fully mature HSA^lo SP cells are resistant to negative selection.

Role of Costimulatory Molecules

Although it is generally agreed that negative selection requires costimulation (94–96), it is unclear which particular costimulatory molecules are involved. Many investigators have approached this issue by examining negative selection in mice lacking certain cell-surface molecules, including FAS (97,98), CD28 (99), CD30 (101), CD5 (102), the CD40 ligand (CD40L) (103), and the tumor necrosis factor receptor (TNFR) (105). For the most part, this approach has failed to demonstrate that any of these molecules are crucial for negative selection. Deletion of CD30 impairs anti-TCR monoclonal antibody–induced destruction of DP cells but does not prevent V_β deletion in response to endogenous Mtv antigens (101). V_β deletion is inhibited in CD40L⁻ mice, but this effect is not considered to indicate that CD40 provides direct costimulation for negative selection but rather that CD40L-CD40 interaction is important for maintaining expression of other costimulatory molecules (104). Particular attention has been focused on the role of FAS in negative selection (98,107). However, with the exception of one study on cortical deletion (107), most groups have concluded that FAS is not involved in central tolerance. Nevertheless, under defined conditions, FAS may indeed play a role in negative selection of HSA^hi medullary SP cells, especially for antigens expressed at a high level (93).

THYMIC SELECTION AND INTRACELLULAR SIGNALING

In considering the relation between positive and negative selection, the simplest idea is that positive selection is a consequence of weak TCR-mediated signaling, whereas negative selection reflects strong signaling. This difference in intensity of signaling may be a direct reflection of the relative affinities of TCR-MHC-peptide interactions. In discussing this issue, it is important to consider the consequences of stimulation of mature versus immature T cells.

For immature thymocytes, the upstream signaling events induced by TCR ligation appear to be much the same as for mature T cells (108–111). There may also be considerable overlap for downstream signaling because, as for stimulation of mature T cells, negative selection of immature T cells requires a combination of TCR ligation and costimulation (94–96,111). It seems likely that the diametrically opposite consequences of signaling in immature and mature T cells—death and stimulation, respectively—occur because immature T cells are unduly sensitive to certain end products of TCR-controlled signaling pathways, these mediators being toxic for immature T cells but not for mature T cells. An obvious problem with this line of reasoning is that TCR ligation of thymocytes can also have the opposite effect; that is, it can lead to augmented survival (positive selection) rather than death. A key issue, therefore, is whether the signaling events involved in positive and negative selection are quantitatively or qualitatively different (110). Although direct evidence on this issue is still sparse, it is clear that inactivation of the function of a number of different molecules involved in TCR-controlled signal transduction, including LCK (112), ZAP-70 (113), and the transcription factor interferon regulatory transcription factor (IRF-1) (114), can inhibit both positive and negative selection, presumably by reducing the overall intensity of signaling. However, inactivation of certain other molecules, such as intermediates in the MAP kinase pathway (115,116), inhibits positive selection but not negative selection. Similar effects can be induced by blocking the function of calcineurin with cyclosporine (CsA), although the effects of CsA on negative selection seem to be rather variable (117–119). In the case of CsA, it is of interest that negative selection of thymocytes becomes susceptible to inhibition by CsA when the dose of antigen (specific peptide) is reduced to a low level (111), suggesting that negative selection depends on calcineurin only when TCR signaling is moderate rather than strong. Finally, inactivation of certain transcription factors, such as NUR-77 (120,121) or particular caspases (122), blocks only negative and not positive selection, implying that these molecules are crucial for apoptosis but are not required for the cell maturation events involved in positive selection.

Ultimately, the choice for death or survival in thymic selection may reflect the relative intensity of signaling through one pathway versus another. For neurons, whether a cell survives or undergoes apoptosis seems to be determined by the dynamic balance between activation of extracellular regulating kinase (ERK) and Jun N-terminal kinase (JNK) (123). This balance could be crucial for influencing the relative proportion of a multiplicity of different molecules known to augment or impede apoptosis. These molecules include members of the BCL-2 family (124,125) and various FAS/TNFR-associated molecules (126–128).

EXPORT OF T CELLS FROM THE THYMUS

In terms of their phenotype, the T cells released from the thymus closely resemble the typical mature CD4+ and CD8+ cells found in the secondary lymphoid organs; in particular, recent thymic emigrants are essentially devoid of immature DP cells. Because of the massive attrition of immature T cells induced by thymic selection, the total number of mature T cells exported from the thymus is quite small. For instance, the thymus of a young mouse contains about 2×10^8 cells, but the rate of T-cell export from the thymus is only about 2×10^6 cells per day (4,129), and by 6 months of age thymic export is reduced by 10- to 20-fold. Therefore, only about 1% of the pool size is exported per day—and much less in late adult life. However, because naive T cells have a prolonged life span (129,130), in unmanipulated animals a slow, progressive production of new T cells by the thymus up until the time of puberty is sufficient to generate a large pool of mature T cells. After puberty, further production of new T cells is largely unnecessary: the thymus becomes redundant and atrophy ensues. Problems develop in adulthood only if the mature T-cell pool is depleted. However, there is no clear evidence that the thymus is subject to homeostatic mechanisms; depletion of mature T cells from the periphery does not augment the production of new T cells from the thymus. Replenishment after exposure to irradiation, cytotoxic drugs, or other insults that deplete the peripheral pool of naive T cells occurs only very slowly and depends critically on the presence of a functional thymus (131).

ACKNOWLEDGMENTS

We thank Ms. Barbara Marchand for typing the manuscript. This work was supported by grants CA38355, CA25803, AI21487, AI32068, AG01743, AI38385, and AI41079 from the United States Public Health Service. Publication no. 11300-IMM from the Scripps Research Institute.

REFERENCES

1. Miller JFAP, Osoba D. Current concepts of the immunological function of the thymus. *Physiol Rev* 1967;47:437–520.
2. Sprent J. T lymphocytes and the thymus. In: Paul WE, ed. *Fundamental Immunology,* vol 3. New York: Raven Press, 1993;75–110.
3. Fink PJ, Bevan MJ. Positive selection of thymocytes. *Adv Immunol* 1995;59:99–133.
4. Shortman K, Egerton M, Sprangrude GJ, Scollay R. The generation and fate of thymocytes. *Semin Immunol* 1990;2:3–12.
5. van Ewijk W. T-cell differentiation is influenced by thymic microenvironments. *Annu Rev Immunol* 1991;9:591–615.
6. Surh CD, Gao EK, Kosaka H, et al. Two subsets of epithelial cells in the thymic medulla. *J Exp Med* 1992;176:495–505.
7. Anderson G, Jenkinson EJ, Moore NC, Owen JJT. MHC class II-positive epithelium and mesenchyme cells are both required for T-cell development in the thymus. *Nature* 1993;362:70–73.
8. Surh CD, Sprent J. T-cell apoptosis detected *in situ* during positive and negative selection in the thymus. *Nature* 1994;372:100–103.
9. Auerbach R. Morphogenetic interactions in the development of the mouse thymus gland. *Dev Biol* 1960;2:271–284.
10. Cordier AC, Haumont SM. Development of thymus, parathyroids, and ultimo-branchial bodies in NMRI and nude mice. *Am J Anat* 1980;157:227–263.
11. Le Douarin N, Jotereau FV. Tracing of cells of the avian thymus through embryonic life in interspecific chimeras. *J Exp Med* 1975;142:17–40.
12. Shortman K, Wu L. Early T lymphocyte progenitors. *Annu Rev Immunol* 1996;14:29–47.
13. Wu L, Scollay R, Egerton M, Pearse M, Spangrude GJ, Shortman K. CD4 expressed on earliest T-lineage precursor cells in the adult murine thymus. *Nature* 1991;349:71–74.
14. Wu L, Li C-L, Shortman K. Thymic dendritic cell precursors: Relationship to the T lymphocyte lineage and phenotype of the dendritic cell progeny. *J Exp Med* 1996;184:903–911.
15. Petri HT, Livak F, Burtrum D, Mazel S. T cell receptor gene recombination patterns and mechanisms: Cell death, rescue, and T cell production. *J Exp Med* 1995;182:121–127.
16. Rodewald H-R, Kretzschmar K, Swat W, Takeda S. Intrathymically expressed c-kit ligand (stem cell factor) is a major factor driving expansion of very immature thymocytes *in vivo*. *Immunity* 1995;3:313–319.
17. Cao X, Shore EW, Hu-Li J, et al. Defective lymphoid development in mice lacking expression of the common cytokine receptor γ chain. *Immunity* 1995;2:223–238.
18. Ihle JN. Cytokine receptor signalling. *Nature* 1995;377:591–594.
19. Peschon JJ, Morrissey PJ, Grabstein KH, et al. Early lymphocyte expansion is severely impaired in interleukin 7 receptor-deficient mice. *J Exp Med* 1994;180:1955–1960.
20. von Freeden-Jeffry U, Vieira P, Lucian LA, McNeil T, Burdach SEG, Murray R. Lymphopenia in interleukin (IL)-7 gene-deleted mice identifies IL-7 as a nonredundant cytokine. *J Exp Med* 1995;181:1519–1526.
21. Rodewald H-R, Ogawa M, Haller C, Waskow C, DiSanto JP. Pro-thymocyte expansion by c-kit and the common cytokine receptor γ chain is essential for repertoire formation. *Immunity* 1997;6:265–272.
22. Fehling HJ, von Boehmer H. Early αβ T cell development in the thymus of normal and genetically altered mice. *Curr Opin Immunol* 1997;9:263–275.
23. von Boehmer H, Fehling HJ. Structure and function of the pre-T cell receptor. *Annu Rev Immunol* 1997;15:433–452.
24. Malissen M, Gillet A, Ardouin L, et al. Altered T cell development in mice with a targeted mutation of the CD3ε gene. *EMBO J* 1995;14:4641–4653.
25. Bosma GC, Custer RP, Bosma MJ. A severe combined immunodeficiency mutation in mice. *Nature* 1983;301:527–530.
26. Mombaerts P, Clarke AR, Rudnicki MA, et al. Mutations in T-cell antigen receptor genes α and β block thymocyte development at different stages. *Nature* 1992;360:225–231.
27. Shinkai Y, Rathbun G, Lam K-P, et al. RAG-2-deficient mice lack mature lymphocytes owing to inability to initiate V(D)J rearrangement. *Cell* 1992;68:855–867.
28. Mombaerts R, Iacomini J, Johnson RS, Herrup K, Tonegawa S, Papaioannou VE. RAG-1 deficient mice have no mature B and T lymphocytes. *Cell* 1992;68:869–877.
29. Fehling HJ, Krotkova A, Saint-Ruf C, von Boehmer H. Crucial role of the pre-T-cell receptor alpha gene in development of alpha beta but not gamma delta T cells. *Nature* 1995;375:795–8.
30. Love PE, Shore EW, Johnson MD, et al. T cell development in mice that lack the ζ chain of the T cell antigen receptor complex. *Science* 1993;261:918–921.
31. Levelt CN, Mombaers P, Iglesias A, Tonegawa S, Eichmann K. Restoration of early thymocyte differentiation in T cell receptor-β chain-deficient mutant mice by transmembrane signaling through CD3ε. *Proc Natl Acad Sci U S A* 1993;90:11401–11405.
32. Shinkai Y, Alt FW. CD3ε-mediated signals rescue the development of

CD4[+]8[+] thymocytes in RAG-2[-/-] mice in the absence of TCR β chain expression. *Int Immunol* 1994;6:995–1001.

33. Molina TJ, Kishihara K, Siderovski DP, et al. Profound block in thymocyte development in mice lacking p56[lck]. *Nature* 1992;357: 161–164.

34. Levelt CN, Mombaerts P, Wang B, et al. Regulation of thymocyte development through CD3: Functional dissociation between p56[lck] and CD3ζ in early thymic selection. *Immunity* 1995;3:215–222.

35. Groves T, Smiley P, Cooke MP, Forbush K, Perlmutter RM, Guidos CJ. Fyn can partially substitute for lck in T lymphocyte development. *Immunity* 1996;5:417–428.

36. van Oers NSC, Lowin-Kropf B, Finlay D, Connolly K, Weiss A. αβ T cell development is abolished in mice lacking both lck and fyn protein tyrosine kinases. *Immunity* 1996;5:429–436.

37. Cheng AM, Negishi I, Anderson SJ, et al. The Syk and ZAP-70 SH2-containing tyrosine kinases are implicated in pre-T cell receptor signalling. *Proc Natl Acad Sci U S A* 1997;94:9797–9801.

38. Crompton T, Gilmour KC, Owen MJ. The MAP kinase pathway controls differentiation from double-negative to double-positive thymocyte. *Cell* 1996;86:241–251.

39. Sprent J, Webb SR. Function and specificity of T-cell subsets in the mouse. *Adv Immunol* 1987;1987:39–133.

40. von Boehmer H. Positive selection of lymphocytes. *Cell* 1994;76: 219–228.

41. Robey E, Fowlkes BJ. Selective events in T cell development. *Annu Rev Immunol* 1994;12:675–705.

42. Jameson SC, Hogquist KA, Bevan MJ. Positive selection of thymocytes. *Annu Rev Immunol* 1995;13:93–126.

43. Zerrahn J, Held W, Raulet DH. The MHC reactivity of the T cell repertoire prior to positive and negative selection. *Cell* 1997;86:627–636.

44. Bevan MJ. In a radiation chimera host H-2 antigens determine the immune responsiveness of donor cytotoxic cells. *Nature* 1977;269: 417–418.

45. Sprent J. Restricted helper function of F1 hybrid T cells positively selected to heterologous erythrocytes in irradiation parental strain mice: II. Evidence for restriction affecting helper cell induction and T-B collaboration, both mapping to the K-end of the H-2 complex. *J Exp Med* 1978;147:1159–1174.

46. Fink PJ, Bevan MJ. H-2 antigens of the thymus determine lymphocyte specificity. *J Exp Med* 1978;148:766–775.

47. Zinkernagel RM, Callahan GN, Klein J, Dennert G. Cytotoxic T cells learn specificity for self H-2 during differentiation in the thymus. *Nature* 1979;271:251–253.

48. von Boehmer H. Developmental biology of T cells in T cell receptor transgenic mice. *Annu Rev Immunol* 1990;8:531–556.

49. Cosgrove D, Gray D, Dierich A, et al. Mice lacking MHC class II molecules. *Cell* 1991;66:1051–1066.

50. Grusby MJ, Johnson RS, Papaioannou VE, Glimcher LH. Depletion of CD4[+] T cells in major histocompatibility complex class II-deficient mice. *Science* 1991;20:1417–1420.

51. Zijlstra M, Bix M, Simister NE, MLJ, Raulet DH, Jaenisch R. β2-Microglobulin deficient mice lack CD4[-]8[+] cytotoxic T cells. *Nature* 1990;344:742–746.

52. Koller BH, Marrack P, Kappler JW, Smithies O. Normal development of mice deficient in β2M, MHC class I proteins and CD8[+] T cells. *Science* 1990;248:1227–1230.

53. Chan SH, Cosgrove D, Waltzinger C, Benoist C, Matis D. Another view of the selective model of thymocytes selection. *Cell* 1993;73:225–236.

54. Cosgrove D, Chan SH, Waltzinger C, Benoist C, Matis D. The thymic compartment responsible for positive selection of CD4[+] T cells. *Int Immunol* 1992;4:707–710.

55. Laufer TM, DeKoning J, Markowitz JS, Lo D, Glimcher LH. Unopposed positive selection and autoreactivity in mice expressing class II MHC only on thymic cortex. *Nature* 1996;383:81–85.

56. Jenkinson EJ, Anderson G, Owen JJT. Studies on T cell maturation on defined thymic stromal cell populations in vitro. *J Exp Med* 1992;176:845–853.

57. Anderson G, Owen JJT, Moore NC, Jenkinson EJ. Thymic epithelial cells provide unique signals for positive selection of CD4[+]CD8[+] thymocytes in vitro. *J Exp Med* 1994;179:2027–2031.

58. Ernst B, Surh CD, Sprent J. Bone marrow-derived cells fail to induce positive selection in thymus reaggregation cultures. *J Exp Med* 1996;183:1235–1240.

59. Bix M, Raulet D. Inefficient positive selection of T cells directed by haematopoietic cells. *Nature* 1992;359:330–333.

60. Vukmanovic S, Grandea III AG, Faas SJ, Knowles BB, Bevan MJ. Positive selection of T-lymphocytes induced by intrathymic injection of a thymic epithelial cell line. *Nature* 1992;359:729–732.

61. Hugo P, Kappler JW, Godfry DI, Marrack PC. A cell line that can induce thymocyte positive selection. *Nature* 1992;360:679–682.

62. Pawlowski T, Elliott JD, Loh DY, Staerz UD. Positive selection of T lymphocytes on fibroblasts. *Nature* 1993;364:642–645.

63. Bevan MJ, Hogquist KA, Jameson SC. Selecting the T cell receptor repertoire. *Science* 1994;264:796–797.

64. Hogquist KA, Jameson SC, Bevan MJ. The ligand for positive selection of T lymphocytes in the thymus. *Curr Opin Immunol* 1994;6:273–278.

65. Schumacher TN, Ploegh HL. Are MHC-bound peptides a nuisance for positive selection? *Immunity* 1994;1:721–723.

66. Nikolic-Zugic J, Bevan MJ. Role of self-peptides in positively selecting the T-cell repertoire. *Nature* 1990;344:65–67.

67. Sha W, Nelson CA, Newberry RD, et al. Positive selection of transgenic receptor-bearing thymocytes by K[b] antigen is altered by K[b] mutations that involve peptide binding. *Proc Natl Acad Sci U S A* 1990;87:6180–6190.

68. Hogquist KA, Jameson SC, Heath WR, et al. T cell receptor antagonist peptides induce positive selection. *Cell* 1994;76:17–27.

69. Hogquist KA, Jameson SC, Bevan MJ. Strong agonist ligands for the T cell receptor do not mediate positive selection of functional CD8[+] T cells. *Immunity* 1995;3:79–86.

70. Alam SM, Travers PJ, Wung JL, et al. T-cell-receptor affinity and thymocyte positive selection [see comments]. *Nature* 1996;381:616–620.

71. Ashton-Rickardt PG, Bandeira A, Delaney JR, et al. Evidence for an avidity model of T cell activation in the thymus. *Cell* 1994;73: 1041–1049.

72. Sebzda E, Wallace VA, Mayer J, Yeung RSM, Mak TW, Ohashi PS. Positive and negative thymocytes selection induced by different concentrations of a single peptide. *Science* 1994;263:1615–1618.

73. Sebzda E, Kundig TM, Thomson CT, et al. Mature T cell reactivity altered by peptide agonist that induces positive selection. *J Exp Med* 1996;183:1093–1104.

74. Pawlowski TJ, Singleton MD, Loh DY, Berg R, Staerz UD. Permissive recognition during positive selection. *Eur J Immunol* 1996;26: 851–857.

75. Nakano N, Rooke R, Benoist C, Mathis D. Positive selection of T cells induced by viral delivery of neopeptides to the thymus. *Science* 1997;275:678–683.

76. Ignatowicz L, Kappler J, Marrack P. The repertoire of T cells shaped by a single MHC/peptide ligand. *Cell* 1996;84:521–529.

77. Fung-Leung W-P, Surh CD, Liljedahl M, et al. Antigen presentation and T cell development in H2-M-deficient mice. *Science* 1996;271: 1278–1281.

78. Martin WD, Hicks GG, Mendiratta SK, Leva HI, Ruley HE, Van Kaer L. H2-M mutant mice are defective in the peptide loading of class II molecules, antigen presentation, and T cell repertoire selection. *Cell* 1996;84:543–550.

79. Miyazaki T, Wolf P, Tourne S, et al. Mice lacking H2-M complexes, enigmatic elements of the MHC class II peptide-loading pathway. *Cell* 1996;84:531–541.

80. Ignatowicz L, Rees W, Pacholczyk R, et al. T cells can be activated by peptides that are unrelated in sequence to their selecting peptide. *Immunity* 1997;7:179–186.

81. Tourne S, Miyazaki T, Oxenius A, et al. Selection of a broad repertoire of CD4[+] T cells in H2-Ma[0/0] mice. *Immunity* 1997;7:187–195.

82. Surh CD, Lee D-S, Fung-Leung W-P, Karlsson L, Sprent J. Thymic selection by a single MHC/peptide ligand produces a semidiverse repertoire of CD4[+] T cells. *Immunity* 1997;7:209–219.

83. Bevan MJ. In thymic selection, peptide diversity gives and takes away. *Immunity* 1997;7:175–178.

84. Sprent J, Webb SR. Intrathymic and extrathymic clonal deletion of T cells. *Cur Opin Immunol* 1995;7:196–205.

85. Miller JFAP. Autoantigen-induced deletion of peripheral self-reactive T cells. *Int Rev Immunol* 1995;13:107–114.

86. van Parijs L, Abbas AK. Role of Fas-mediated cell death in the regulation of immune responses. *Cur Opin Immunol* 1996;8:355–361.

87. Nossal GJV. Negative selection of lymphocytes. *Cell* 1994;76: 229–239.

88. Shi Y, Bissonnette RP, Parfrey N, Szalay M, Kubo RT, Green DR. In vivo administration of antibodies to the CD3-T cell receptor complex induces cell death (apoptosis) in immature thymocytes. *J Immunol* 1991;146:3340–3346.

89. Murphy KM, Heimberger AB, Loh DH. Induction by antigen of intrathymic apoptosis of CD4$^+$ CD8$^+$ TCR^{lo} thymocytes in vivo. *Science* 1990;250:1720–1723.

90. Jondal M, Okret S, McConkey D. Killing of immature CD4$^+$ CD8$^+$ thymocytes in vivo by anti-CD3 or 5'(N-ethyl)-carboxamide-adenosine is blocked by glucocorticoid receptor antagonist RU-486. *Eur J Immunol* 1993;23:1246–1250.

91. Lo D, Sprent J. Identity of cells that imprint H-2-restricted T-cell specificity in the thymus. *Nature* 1986;319:672–675.

92. White J, Herman A, Pullen AM, Kubo RT, Kappler JW, Marrack P. The Vβ-specific superantigen staphylococcal enterotoxin B: Stimulation of mature T cells and clonal deletion in neonatal mice. *Cell* 1989;56:27–35.

93. Kishimoto H, Sprent J. Negative selection in the thymus includes semimature T cells. *J Exp Med* 1997;185:263–271.

94. Page DM, Kane LP, Allison JP, Hedrick SM. Two signals are required for negative selection of CD4$^+$CD8$^+$ thymocytes. *J Immunol* 1993;151:1868–1880.

95. Aiba Y, Mazda O, Davis MM, Muramatsu S, Katsura Y. Requirement of a second signal from antigen presenting cells in the clonal deletion of immature T cells. *Int Immunol* 1994;6:1475–1483.

96. Punt JA, Osborne BA, Takahama Y, Sharrow SO, Singer A. Negative selection of CD4$^+$CD8$^+$ thymocytes by T cell receptor-induced apoptosis requires a costimulatory signal that can be provided by CD28. *J Exp Med* 1994;179:709–713.

97. Crispe IN. Fatal interactions: Fas-induced apoptosis of mature T cells. *Immunity* 1994;1:347–349.

98. Nagata S, Golstein P. The Fas death factor. *Science* 1995;267:1449–1456.

99. June CH, Bluestone JA, Nadler LM, Thompson CB. The B7 and CD28 receptor families. *Immunol Today* 1994;15:321–331.

100. Lenschow DJ, Walunas TL, Bluestone JA. CD28/B7 system of T cell co-stimulation. *Annu Rev Immunol* 1996;14:233–258.

101. Amakawa R, Hakem A, Kundig TM, et al. Impaired negative selection of T cells in Hodgkin's disease antigen CD30-deficient mice. *Cell* 1996;84:551–562.

102. Tarakhovsky A, Kanner SB, Hombach J, et al. A role for CD5 in TCR-mediated signal transduction and thymocyte selection. 1996;269:535.

103. Foy TM, Durie FH, Noelle RJ. The expansive role of CD40 and its ligand, gp39, in immunity. *Semin Immunol* 1994;6:259–266.

104. Foy TM, Page DM, Waldschmidt TJ, et al. An essential role for gp39, the ligand for CD40, in thymic selection. *J Exp Med* 1995;182:1377–1388.

105. Pfeffer K, Matsuyama T, Kundig TM, et al. Mice deficient for the 55 kd tumor necrosis factor receptor are resistant to endotoxic shock, yet succumb to *L. monocytogenes* infection. *Cell* 1993;73:457–467.

106. Erickson SL, de Sauvage FJ, Kikly K, et al. Decreased sensitivity to tumour-necrosis factor but normal T-cell development in TNF receptor-2-deficient mice. *Nature* 1994;372:560–563.

107. Castro JE, Listman JA, Jacobson BA, et al. Fas modulation of apoptosis during negative selection of thymocytes. *Immunity* 1996;5:617–627.

108. Chan AC, Desai DM, Weiss A. The role of protein tyrosine kinases and protein tyrosine phosphatases in T cell antigen receptor signal transduction. *Annu Rev Immunol* 1994;12:555–592.

109. Rothenberg E. Developmental biology of lymphocytes. *The Immunologist* 1995;3:172–175.

110. Alberola-Ila J, Takakt S, Kerner JD, Perlmutter R. Differential signaling by lymphocyte antigen receptors. *Annu Rev Immunol* 1997;15:125–154.

111. Kane LP, Hedrick S. A role for calcium influx in setting the threshold for CD4$^+$ CD8$^+$ thymocyte negative selection. *J Immunol* 1996;156:4594–4601.

112. Hashimoto K, Sohn SJ, Levin S, Tada T, Perlmutter RM, Nakayama T. Requirement for p56^{lck} tyrosine kinase activation in TCR-mediated thymic selection. *J Exp Med* 1996;184:931–943.

113. Negishi I, Motoyama N, Nakayama K, et al. Essential role for ZAP-70 in both positive and negative selection of thymocytes. *Nature* 1995;376:435–438.

114. Penninger JM, Sirard C, Mittrucker HW, et al. The interferon regulatory transcription factor IRF-1 controls positive and negative selection of CD3$^+$ thymocytes. *Immunity* 1997;7:243–254.

115. Swan KA, Alberola-Ila J, Gross JA, et al. Involvement of p21^{ras} distinguishes positive and negative selection in thymocytes. *EMBO J* 1995;14:276–285.

116. Alberola-Ila J, Hogquist KA, Swan KA, Bevan MJ, Perlmutter RM. Positive and negative selection invoke distinct signaling pathways. *J Exp Med* 1996;184:9–18.

117. Vasquez NJ, Kaye J, Hedrick SM. In vivo and in vitro clonal deletion of double positive thymocytes. *J Exp Med* 1992;175:1307–1316.

118. Curnow SJ, Schmidt-Verhulst A-M. The balance between deletion and activation of CD4$^+$ 8$^+$ thymocytes is controlled by T cell receptor-antigen interactions and is affected by cyclosporin A. *Eur J Immunol* 1994;24:2401–2409.

119. Urdahl DB, Pardoll DM, Jenkins MK. Cyclosporin A inhibits positive selection and delays negative selection in αβ TCR transgenic mice. *J Immunol* 1994;152:2853–2859.

120. Calnan BJ, Szychowski S, Chan FK, Cado D, Winoto A. A role for the orphan steroid receptor Nur77 in apoptosis accompanying antigen-induced negative selection. *Immunity* 1995;3:273–282.

121. Zhou T, Cheng J, Yang P, et al. Inhibition of Nur77/Nurr1 leads to inefficient clonal deletion of self-reactive T cells. *J Exp Med* 1996;183:1879–1892.

122. Clayton LK, Ghendler Y, Mizoguchi E, et al. T-cell receptor ligation by peptide/MHC induces activation of a caspase in immature thymocytes: The molecular basis of negative selection. *EMBO J* 1997;16:2282–2293.

123. Xia Z, Dickens M, Raingeaud J, Davis RJ, Greenberg ME. Opposing effects of ERK and JNK-p38 MAP kinases on apoptosis. *Science* 1995;270:1326–1331.

124. Cory S. Regulation of lymphocyte survival by the *bcl-2* gene family. *Annu Rev Immunol* 1995;13:513–544.

125. Yang E, Korsmeyer SJ. Molecular thanatopsis: A discourse on the Bcl2 family and cell death. *Blood* 1996;88:386–401.

126. Wallach D. Placing death under control. *Nature* 1997;388:123–126.

127. Barinaga M. Forging a path to cell death. *Science* 1997;273:735–737.

128. Nagata S. Apoptosis by death factor. *Cell* 1997;88:355–365.

129. Tough DF, Sprent J. Turnover of naive- and memory-phenotype T cells. *J Exp Med* 1994;179:1127–1135.

130. Sprent J. Immunological memory. *Curr Opin Immunol* 1997;9:371–379.

131. Mackall CL, Fleisher TA, Brown MR, et al. Age, thymopoiesis, and CD4+ T-lymphocyte regeneration after intensive chemotherapy. *N Engl J Med* 1995;332:143–149.

Inflammation: Basic Principles and Clinical Correlates,
3rd ed., edited by John I. Gallin and Ralph Snyderman.
Lippincott Williams & Wilkins, Philadelphia © 1999.

CHAPTER 10

B-Cell Development

Kong-Peng Lam and Klaus Rajewsky

One of the major players in immune responses against foreign antigens is the B lymphocyte–named after the sites in which it develops, namely the bone marrow in humans and mice and the bursa of Fabricius in chicken. B cells are responsible for the secretion of serum antibodies, or immunoglobulins (Ig), that can recognize and neutralize a vast array of foreign antigens.

The idea that the organism contains specific antibodies before encountering antigen was first conceived by Paul Ehrlich at the beginning of the century. Ehrlich's concept was subsequently abandoned but reappeared in the 1950s when Niels Jerne proposed that the organism possesses a specialized system of cells, the immune system, whose function is the production of a diverse repertoire of specific antibodies. This theory was subsequently developed by Burnet (1) and Talmage (2) into the *clonal selection theory*, which postulates that each lymphocyte is genetically committed to express an antibody of a distinct specificity as an antigen receptor on its surface. Cells encountering an antigen fitting to their receptors could clonally expand and subsequently differentiate into antibody-secreting cells. Early in ontogeny, receptor engagement by antigen (mostly self antigens in that case) would result in cell death, establishing immunologic tolerance.

Despite an enormous increase of knowledge about the immune system over the last decades, the clonal selection theory remains a central paradigm in immunology. However, as will become apparent from the discussion to follow, it is now understood that the antibody response is controlled by the interaction of the antibody-producing cells with regulatory cells of the immune system and, most importantly, that the B cells, *in response to antigenic stimulation,* are able to modify their receptor specificity to increase the efficiency of antigen binding or to escape autoreactivity–a concept not contained in, and indeed quite opposite to, the original concept of clonal selection.

OVERVIEW OF B-CELL DEVELOPMENT

All lymphocytes are derived from pluripotent hematopoietic stem cells by way of committed lymphoid progenitors. Once committed to the B lineage, B-cell progenitors differentiate into mature B lymphocytes in a series of distinct steps. Cells at various stages of differentiation can be distinguished by their cell-surface phenotype, their differential expression of intracellular genes, and the status of their Ig heavy-chain (IgH) and light-chain (IgL) gene rearrangements.

Overall, B-cell development can be broadly divided into two phases, as shown in Figure 10-1. The initial (which is thought to be antigen-independent) phase takes place mainly in the primary lymphoid organs (fetal liver and adult bone marrow). B-cell progenitors attempt to express a functional antibody in the form of surface immunoglobulin (sIg) on the cell. In doing so, they become immature B cells. Selected immature B cells then seed the periphery as naive mature B cells.

In the second phase of B-cell development, which takes place in the secondary lymphoid organs (e.g., spleen, lymph nodes), naive B cells encounter specific antigens and undergo clonal expansion. They differentiate into either memory B cells or antibody-secreting plasma cells. During this antigen-dependent phase of B-cell development, B lymphocytes can generate antibodies with higher affinities for antigens or with different effector functions through the processes of somatic hypermutation of Ig genes and IgH-chain isotype class switching, respectively.

The overall scheme of B-cell development is fairly well understood. Many details concerning the molecular and cellular mechanisms of B-cell generation, mainte-

K-P. Lam: Institute of Molecular and Cell Biology, The National University of Singapore, S 117609 Singapore.

K. Rajewsky: Institute for Genetics, University of Cologne, D-50931 Cologne, Germany.

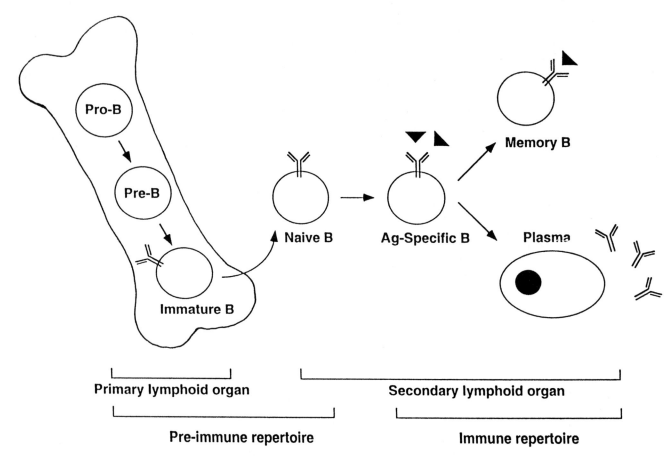

FIG. 10-1. Overview of B-cell development. In the adult, early B-cell development occurs in the bone marrow. B-cell progenitors (Pro-B) differentiate through a series of stages into surface immunoglobulin M (sIgM)–expressing immature B cells. Thereafter, B lymphocytes seed the peripheral lymphoid organs as sIgM+sIgD+ mature B cells. After encountering specific antigens, they differentiate into memory B cells or antibody-secreting plasma cells.

nance, and selection are now being discovered and are discussed in the following sections.

CELLULAR DEVELOPMENT OF B-LINEAGE CELLS FROM HEMATOPOIETIC STEM CELLS

Production of B lymphocytes is a dynamic process that involves continuous generation of these cells from progenitors. B cells are derived from pluripotent stem cells that also give rise to T cells and cells of the erythroid and myeloid lineages. B and T lymphocytes are thought to originate from a common lymphoid-committed stem cell that differentiates from the pluripotent stem cell in a process in which the transcription factors, IKAROS, PU.1, and transforming gene, myeloblastosis (MYB) may be critical (3,4). Mutant mice that lack early lymphoid-specific transcription factor (IKAROS) (5), PU.1 (6,7), or MYB (8) fail to generate any definitive B- or T-lymphocyte precursors, suggesting that genes regulated by these transcription factors may be involved in determining the fate of these stem cells. Because many other genes must

be temporally and specifically expressed for B lymphopoiesis to proceed, it is reasonable to assume that other transcription factors also play important regulatory roles in this differentiation process. Further development of cells along the B lineage seems to require the transcription factors enhancer binding transcription factor (E2A), early B factor (EBF), PAX-5 (B-cell lineage-specific activator protein, or BSAP), and sex-determining region Y box 4 (SOX-4) (9). Inactivation of E2A in mice (10,11) leads to a total lack of B cells, whereas inactivation of BSAP (12), EBF (13), or SOX-4 (14) arrests B-cell development at a very early stage in the bone marrow and fetal liver. The terminal stages of B-cell development in the peripheral lymphoid organs require additional transcription factors, such as B-cell specific transcription coactivator, or OCA-B, OBF-1 (BOB-1) (15,16), B-lymphocyte-induced maturation protein-1 (BLIMP-1) (17), and octamer binding transcription factor 2 (OCT-2) (18).

Committed B-cell progenitors migrate into a specialized cellular microenvironment, where they clonally expand. The elements of this microenvironment, known as the stroma, include adventitial cells, reticular cells, endothelial cells, fibroblasts, macrophages, and adipocytes, as well as the extracellular matrix. The homing of B-cell progenitors to the bone marrow stroma seems to depend on the chemokine stromal cell—derived factor-1 (SDF-1) (19). Cell-cell contact between B-cell progenitors and stromal cells, as well as cytokines secreted by stromal cells, is mandatory for the further development of B-lineage cells (20). Cytokines such as interleukin-3 (IL-3) and IL-7 stimulate the proliferation of B-cell progenitors (21), whereas others such as cyclic neutropenia factor, insulin-like growth factor-1 (22) stem cell factor, SCF (KIT) ligand (23), and fms-like tyrosine kinase (FLT-3) ligand (24) potentiate the differentiation of B-cell progenitors. Other factors in the microenvironment inhibit or limit B-cell development; these factors include interferon (25), transforming growth factor-β (26), and estrogen (27). Thus, B-cell generation is controlled by a multitude of factors produced by cells in the microenvironment in which B-cell development occurs. As shown by gene targeting experiments in mice, none of these factors by itself seems to be essential for this developmental process. Rather, it is their concerted action that optimizes B-cell development.

In the chicken, the main site of B-cell generation is the bursa of Fabricius. In the sheep, B-cell production takes place mainly in the ileal Peyer's patches. In these two species, B-cell generation is restricted primarily to a few weeks or months of postnatal life. In mouse and human, B-cell generation begins in embryonic life, first in the paraaortic tissue (28) and later in fetal liver and spleen (29). After birth, B-cell production shifts to the bone marrow, where it continues at a diminishing rate throughout life.

B-Cell and Pre-B-Cell Receptors

The first descendant of the lymphoid stem cell that is committed to the B lineage is termed a pro-B cell. From this stage onward, the cells begin to express B-lineage-specific genes and undergo a series of ordered somatic gene rearrangements, usually at the IgH-chain locus first and then at the loci-encoding IgL chains. This leads ultimately to the deposition of a membrane-bound antibody of class M (sIgM) on the surface of the cell, making it an immature B cell (see Fig. 10-1). Later, naive mature B cells express both sIgM and sIgD (reviewed by Rajewsky, 1996).

The existence of (monospecific) antibodies as antigen receptors on the surface of B cells was a central prediction of the clonal selection hypothesis of Burnet, explaining the selection of these cells by antigen. However, the IgM and IgD antibodies that are first expressed on B cells have short cytoplasmic tails, and it was not immediately clear how signals generated on antigen stimulation could be transmitted into the cells to effect the process of clonal selection. It is now known that sIg is part of the B-cell antigen receptor (BCR) complex, which also comprises the heterodimeric signal-transducing subunits, Igα and Igβ

(30) (Fig. 10-2). Cross-linking of BCR by antigens leads to the generation of signals via the immunoreceptor tyrosine-based activation motif (ITAM) in the cytoplasmic regions of the Igα/Igβ complex (31). These signals are further propagated into the cells by other cytoplasmic signaling molecules, such as the tyrosine kinase spleen tyrosine kinase (SYK) and the SRC family of tyrosine kinases [B lymphoid kinase (BLK), Bruton's tyrosine kinase (BTK), SRC-homology phosphatase 1 (SHP-1), FYN, LYN] and by various membrane-bound phosphatases such as CD45 and cytoplasmic phosphatases such as SHP-1 (32).

In addition to the signal from the BCR, B cells may also receive signals from other cell-surface molecules. These include CD19, which forms a complex with CD21, CD81, and LEU3 (33); CD22; CD23; CD38; and the type II Fcγ receptor (IgG receptor FcγRII). The CD19/CD21 complex augments BCR signaling, presumably by lowering the threshold required to activate antigen-specific B cells (34,35). In contrast, CD22 (36) and FcγRII may deliver an inhibition signal when cross-linked with the BCR. Other costimulatory molecules on the surface of B cells, such as B7.1 and B7.2 (37) and CD40 (38), interact with specific molecules on T cells to deliver additional signals to antigen-activated B lymphocytes. The final response of a B cell to an antigen depends on the interplay and integration of these various signaling pathways and on the stage of B-cell development.

At earlier stages of B-cell development, B-lymphocyte progenitors that already express an IgH chain but not yet an IgL chain carry a receptor structure on their surface which is called the pre-B-cell receptor (pBCR) (39). As shown in Figure 10-2, pBCR, like the BCR, contains IgH chains; however, instead of the classic IgL chains, these IgH chains are associated with "surrogate" IgL chains consisting of the λ5 and VpreB polypeptides (40). Like the BCR, pBCR contains the signal-transducing Igα/Igβ complex. As discussed later, the pBCR plays an important role in regulating the early stages of B-cell development.

Immunoglobulin Gene Rearrangements

Each B lymphocyte makes an antibody of a distinct specificity. In all higher vertebrates, this is achieved through a process of site-specific recombination in which the antibody variable regions are assembled during B-cell development from certain gene segments. These are the variable (V), diversity (D), and joining (J) segments for the IgH-chain locus and the V and J segments for the IgL-chain locus (41). In the chicken (42) and rabbit (43), the same V, D, and J genes are initially assembled in all B-cell progenitors. Diversification of the antibodies occurs later through gene conversion, whereby upstream V-region genes are used to replace the initially rearranged V gene. In mice and humans, numerous functional V, D, and J gene segments are present in both the IgH-chain locus and the two IgL-chain loci (κ and λ), and each develop-

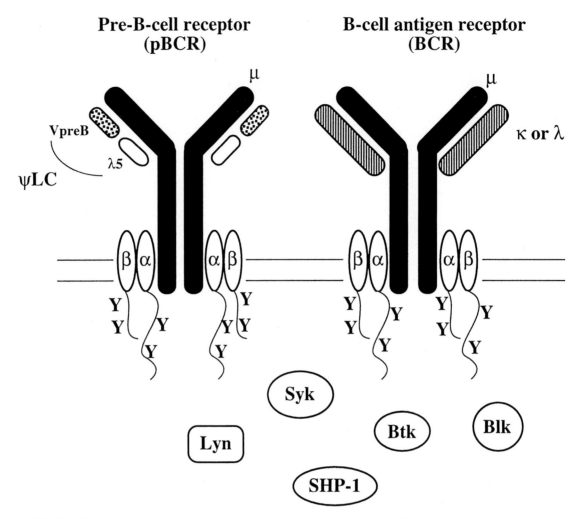

FIG. 10-2. The pre-B-cell receptor and B-cell antigen receptor associate with the signal-transducing heterodimer Igα/Igβ. Y-Y denotes the immunoreceptor tyrosine-based activation motif (ITAM). Signals from the antigen receptors are further propagated downstream by other signaling molecules such as the SYK and the SRC family of tyrosine kinases (FYN, LYN, BLK, and BTK), as well as by the phosphatase, SHP-1.

ing B cell combines a different set of these segments. This gives rise to a situation in which each cell expresses a distinct antibody from the beginning. This genetic basis of antibody generation explains how the immune system can contain antibodies of infinite specificities without having to encode each specificity in the germ line. It also directly fits the clonal selection theory, in that the interaction of an antigen with a cell-bound antibody of a particular specificity selects for B-cell clones committed to the production of antibodies of that specificity.

The V(D)J recombination reaction somatically assembles the various gene segments that together encode the variable regions of the IgH and IgL chains. It involves the introduction of DNA double-strand breaks at specific recognition signal sequences (RSS) adjacent to the V, D, and J elements (44), the resolution of intermediate recombination structures, and subsequent DNA double-strand break repair. The machinery responsible for V(D)J

recombination has not yet been fully elucidated, but it is clear that multiple components are required.

V(D)J recombination is initiated by the lymphoid-specific recombination-activating gene proteins-1 and -2 (RAG-1 and RAG-2) (45,46), which introduce DNA double-strand breaks at the base of the RSS (47,48). Recombination between the free ends involves the cellular mechanisms of DNA double-strand break repair, of which several components have been identified—namely the Ku heterodimer of 70-kd and 80-kd subunits (49), the DNA-dependent protein kinase (50), and the product of the X-ray-complementing Chinese hamster gene 4 (*XRCC4*) (51,52). Mutant mice and cell lines deficient in either of the latter two proteins exhibit impaired V(D)J recombination as well as impaired DNA double-strand break repair (53,54). Together with DNA ligase IV, these proteins mediate the joining step of the recombination process. In addition, the enzyme terminal deoxynucleotidyl transferase (TdT), when present, participates in V(D)J recombination, adding nontemplated nucleotides to the coding joints (55,56).

Even though B and T lymphocytes express the same V(D)J recombinase, variable-region genes in Ig loci are arranged only in B cells and those in T-cell receptor (TCR) loci only in T cells. Moreover, at different stages of development within the B lineage, V(D)J recombination occurs predominantly at either the IgH- or IgL-chain locus. Therefore, the control of V(D)J recombination at different gene loci (Ig or TCR) is tightly regulated with regard to cell type and stage specificity. This control is probably effected at the level of the accessibility of gene segments to the V(D)J recombinase (57). Although there is evidence that accessibility correlates with transcription and the pattern of DNA methylation of the gene segments involved (58,59), the precise mechanism by which this accessibility of variable-region gene segments to V(D)J recombination is controlled remains to be worked out.

Allelic Exclusion and the Ordered Model of Gene Rearrangement

In theory, both alleles of the Ig genes can be functionally assembled and expressed. However, in most cases, B cells carry functionally assembled IgH- and IgL-chain variable-region genes from only one allele and therefore express antibodies of a single unique specificity. This phenomenon is known as *allelic exclusion*. In order to explain allelic exclusion, Alt et al. postulated an "ordered" model of Ig rearrangement in which a regulated mechanism controls the recombination process (60). According to this model, based mainly on studies of Abelson virus–transformed pre-B cell lines, Ig gene recombination is first initiated at the IgH locus, beginning with a joining of D_H to J_H segments, after which there is a V_H-to-$D_H J_H$ rearrangement. If the $V_H D_H J_H$ joint is productive (i.e., in-frame), a μ heavy chain is expressed at the cell surface. This results in feedback inhibition of gene rearrangement at the second IgH allele, which is normally arrested at the $D_H J_H$ rearrangement stage, and initiation of gene rearrangement at the IgL-chain locus. However, if rearrangement at the first IgH allele results in a nonproductive (i.e., out-of-frame) joint, then V_H-to-$D_H J_H$ rearrangements at the second allele can proceed.

The central proposition of the ordered model of Ig gene rearrangement is that expression of a membrane-bound μ chain signals the shutdown of recombination at the second IgH allele. Studies of transgenic and knockout mice strongly support this notion. It has been shown that loss of IgH-chain allelic exclusion occurs in mice that are heterozygous for deletion of the membrane exon of the μ chain (61). Furthermore, expression of the membrane-bound form of an IgH chain but not of the secreted form in transgenic mice resulted in inhibition of rearrangement of the endogenous IgH genes (62).

IgH-chain allelic exclusion is maintained during the phase of IgL-chain gene rearrangement, when the RAG genes are reexpressed. This suggests that the feedback inhibition signal from the expressed IgH chain must be followed by a shutdown of accessibility of the second IgH locus for the VDJ recombinase. How such a mechanism operates remains a puzzle.

Checkpoints in B-Cell Development

B-cell development is a highly regulated process, and checkpoints exist (as shown in Fig. 10-3) during the early differentiation steps to ensure that only functional lymphocytes that are capable of responding to antigens seed the peripheral lymphoid organs. Studies with mutant mice indicate that much of the control of B-cell differentiation is centered on the expression of a pBCR and, later, a functional and nonautoreactive BCR (161).

Productive $V_H D_H J_H$ rearrangement of the IgH allele leads to the expression of membrane-bound μ chains in association with the components of the surrogate IgL chain, VpreB and $\lambda 5$ (40), and with the signal-transducing Igα/Igβ heterodimer (30). This complex, the pBCR (see Fig. 10-2), is necessary for further differentiation of B cells and marks a critical checkpoint in the progression of B-cell development. This fact has been demonstrated in the mouse by the targeted deletion in embryonic stem cells of the membrane exon of the μ IgH-chain gene (63), the gene encoding $\lambda 5$ (64), or the Igβ gene (65). These mutations, when transmitted into the germ line, abolish membrane expression of pBCR and lead to the arrest of B-cell differentiation at the pro-B cell stage. A similar effect is seen in various mouse mutants in which the Ig rearrangement process is impaired either by inactivation of the *RAG1* (66) or *RAG2* (67) genes or subunits of the DNA-dependent protein kinase, or by deletion of the J_H elements and IgH-chain Eμ enhancer, all of which indirectly affect pBCR formation. The block in B-cell development in RAG-deficient mice can be overcome by introduction of IgH-chain transgenes, which leads to differentiation of pro-B cells into pre-B cells, or of IgH and IgL-chain transgenes, which results in generation of B cells (68,69). Similarly, expression of an IgH-chain transgene in the J_H mutant background or an IgH and IgL-chain transgene in the $\lambda 5$ mutant (70) background can rescue B-cell development.

The pBCR is required for differentiation of pro-B cells into pre-B cells. Progenitor cells expressing this structure are drawn into proliferation, by an unknown signal, presumably over four to six generations. They downregulate RAG expression, so that the second IgH allele does not undergo further variable-region gene rearrangements. The cells then enter a resting state, that of the classic, small pre-B cells. Here, RAG is reexpressed, but recombination now is targeted to the IgL (κ and λ) loci, guaranteeing allelic exclusion at IgH (71). Overall, this part of the process of B-

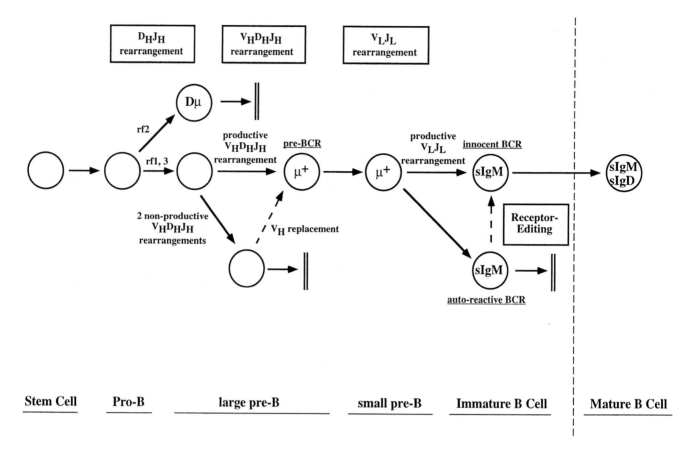

FIG. 10-3. General scheme of B-cell development in the adult bone marrow. The status of immunoglobulin (Ig) gene rearrangements at each step of the differentiation pathway and the checkpoints in B-cell development, marked by the expression of Dμ protein, pre-B-cell receptor (pBCR), and B-cell antigen receptor (BCR), are indicated. Pro-B cells begin a program of gene rearrangements at the Ig heavy (H) chain locus, starting with joining of D_H to J_H. This can occur in three different reading frames (rf). In the mouse, use of rf2 results in the expression of a truncated Dμ protein, and cells expressing this protein are counterselected. V_H-to-D_HJ_H rearrangements follow, and cells with a productive $V_HD_HJ_H$ joint express a μ IgH chain protein that, together with components of the surrogate light chain, VpreB and λ5, results in expression of a pBCR. The cell then progresses to the pre-B cell stage of differentiation. Cells with two nonproductive $V_HD_HJ_H$ joints are arrested in development but can be rescued by functional V_H gene recombinations into the nonfunctional $V_HD_HJ_H$ joint (V_H replacement). Subsequent productive rearrangement at the Ig light chain locus leads to expression of a BCR in the form of a surface immunoglobulin M (sIgM) on immature B cells. Autoreactive B cells are eliminated or undergo a process of receptor editing to revise the specificities of their BCR. Cells with a functional and nonautoreactive BCR exit into the peripheral pool as mature B cells expressing sIgM and sIgD.

cell generation allows the assembly of different IgL chains with the same IgH chain, within clones of pre-B cells arising from individual pBCR-expressing progenitors. Even within a given pre-B cell, the IgH chain expressed by the cell can be successively assembled with different IgL chains if the cell eliminates a V_LJ_L rearrangement it has acquired and substitutes another one for it. It is now clear that such secondary IgL-chain gene rearrangements occur frequently in pre-B cells (and also, as discussed later, in peripheral B cells in certain circumstances). These processes allow the cells to edit their BCR by replacing one IgL chain with another (72,73). In molecular terms, such *receptor editing* can be achieved in various ways. The V_LJ_L gene segment can be replaced, on the same chromosome,

by another segment through rearrangement and joining of an upstream V_L to a downstream J_L element (74). Alternatively, the Igκ locus can be inactivated by RAG-mediated, so-called recombining sequence (RS), eliminating the $C_κ$ gene in the locus. This allows the cell to undergo $V_κJ_κ$ rearrangements on the second Igκ allele or, if that is nonproductive, to rearrange V and J gene segments in the Igλ loci. Receptor editing, which can also involve the IgH locus through a process called V-gene replacement (75-77), is an important mechanism not only of antibody diversification but also, as discussed later, of immunologic tolerance in the B-cell compartment.

The expression of a functional BCR on successful V_LJ_L joining marks another critical checkpoint in B-cell development (see Fig. 10-3). B cells that are devoid of sIg are not found in the peripheral lymphoid organs. The most obvious explanation for this phenomenon is that a signal from the BCR is required to select the cells into the long-lived peripheral B-cell pool. The existence of such a hypothetical signal was suggested by an experiment in which the signaling capacity of the BCR was compromised by truncation of the cytoplasmic region of Igα (78). In this mutant mouse strain, B-cell development was most severely affected at the transition from immature to mature B cells, with a 100-fold decrease in the number of B cells in the periphery, compared with wild-type animals. It has now been shown that expression of a BCR is required not only for selection of B lymphocytes into the mature B-cell pool but also for their maintenance in the periphery (79). Ablation of sIg on mature B cells by inducible gene targeting leads to rapid cell death, indicating that B cells are continuously being selected for their ability to express a functional BCR. The overall picture suggests that signals from the BCR (or its precursor, the pBCR) are required not only for the progression of early B-cell development but also for the persistence of B lymphocytes in the periphery.

GENERATION AND SELECTION OF THE PRIMARY ANTIBODY REPERTOIRE AND COUNTERSELECTION OF AUTOREACTIVITY

The IgH variable-region genes are assembled from V, D, and J gene segments. In the human, there are approximately 50 functional V_H, 25 D_H, and 6 J_H gene segments; in mice, there are 100 or more V_H, 13 D_H, and 4 J_H gene segments. In principle, every D_H segment can be joined to every J_H element, and the resulting $D_H J_H$ segment can recombine with every V_H gene. This combinatorial joining process creates an enormous number of IgH-chain variable-region genes from a limited number of gene segments. Further diversification is achieved by variations in the recombination breakpoints during the joining process, which is achieved by the deletion of nucleotides and the addition of nontemplated nucleotides (N-region) at these breakpoints.

The IgL variable-region genes are assembled from V and J gene segments that are encoded at the Ig κ and λ loci. In humans, there are 32 functional $V_κ$ and 5 $J_κ$ gene segments, with an approximate equal number of $V_λ$ and $J_λ$ gene segments. In the mouse, there are approximately 140 $V_κ$, 4 $J_κ$, 3$V_λ$, and 3 $J_λ$ functional gene segments. As with the IgH variable-region genes, combinatorial joining between these V and J gene segments can create a diverse array of IgL-chain variable-region genes from a limited number of gene segments.

Assuming every IgH-chain variable region can potentially combine with every IgL-chain variable region to generate an antigen-binding site, the full potential repertoire of sites is obtained by multiplying the number of dif-

ferent V_H regions by the number of V_L regions. Such estimates yield values on the order of 10^{11} different antigen-binding sites—equal or beyond the number of B lymphocytes in the body (80). By far, most of this diversity resides in the third complementarity-determining region (CDR3) of the IgH chain, because it is generated by the joining process itself, which in this case uniquely involves three genetic elements (V_H, D_H, and J_H), and the addition of nontemplated nucleotides (N-region) at the recombination breakpoints. Therefore, the main determinants of binding-site diversity in the primary antibody repertoire are the CDR3s of the IgH chain and, to a lesser extent, the IgL chain of the antibody (80). As discussed later, this picture changes when antibodies are further diversified in T-cell-dependent immune responses through somatic hypermutation.

The primary antibody repertoire generated during Ig gene rearrangement is shaped and selected during B-cell differentiation, so that the available repertoire is much smaller than the theoretical value. The mechanisms of antibody diversification can themselves restrict the primary antibody repertoire. This is evident in the newborn mouse, where the absence of TdT expression in B cells during early ontogeny leads to variable-region gene rearrangements that lack N-region nucleotide insertions (81,82). Moreover, there is preferential recombination of V, D, and J elements at short sequence homologies (81,83), further restricting the primary antibody repertoire at this early developmental stage. Later on, diversity increases as a result of N-region addition at the D_H and, in humans, also at the $V_κ$-$J_κ$ border. Diversity of the antibody repertoire can also be restricted by the inability of certain IgH and IgL chains to associate with each other (72,84) and by the preferential use of certain germ-line V, D, and J elements, such as V_H genes located close to D segments (85).

The random Ig rearrangement process inevitably generates some antibodies that recognize self antigens; therefore, negative selection of autoreactive antibody specificities represents a second class of mechanisms that shape (and restrict) the primary antibody repertoire. Transgenic mice expressing transgene-encoded autoreactive antibodies in their B cells have proved particularly useful in the study of these mechanisms, including more recent "second-generation" transgenic mice, which carry the rearranged variable-region genes targeted into their physiologic position in the IgH and IgL loci (86). Two basic mechanisms of negative selection of autoreactivity have become apparent from the study of such animals: the revision of autoreactive receptors by secondary Ig gene rearrangements predominantly at the IgL loci (receptor editing) (72,73,87), and negative selection of the autoreactive cells themselves through the induction of apoptosis on BCR engagement by self antigen (88,89). Evidence suggests that in B-cell development in the bone marrow these two processes occur in succession. Cells initially attempt to get rid of autoreactive receptors through receptor diversification, and subsequently, if that process fails, they differentiate to a state that leads to death on encounter with autoantigen, as predicted by the clonal selection theory (90,91). A variant of the latter process is the induction of anergy, an antigen-unresponsive state, in newly generated autoreactive B cells on encounter with soluble (monovalent) autoantigen (92). Anergic B cells can leave the bone marrow and enter the peripheral B-cell pool, but they fail to compete with normal, nonanergic cells in populating the peripheral lymphoid organs and thus are also counterselected (93).

B-Cell Subsets

In both mouse and human, most of the peripheral B cells found in the spleen and lymph nodes (approximately 5×10^8 and 10^{11} cells, respectively) are IgM^+IgD^+ mature B cells. These conventional B cells are derived from precursors in the bone marrow. The majority of the conventional B cells also express CD23 and moderate levels of complement receptors 1 and 2 (CR1/CR2) in addition to the pan–B cell marker, CD19. In the mouse, these cells also express high levels of B220. Conventional B cells are able to recirculate among lymph, blood, and secondary lymphoid organs (e.g., lymph nodes, spleen, Peyer's patches). In the secondary lymphoid organs, they are found mostly in the primary follicles and in the mantle zone of the secondary follicles. A smaller fraction (5% to 10%) of the conventional B cells are found in the marginal zone and express lower levels of CD23 and IgD. Conventional B cells are involved mainly in primary immune responses to antigens and differentiate later into memory B cells or antibody-secreting plasma cells.

Work on the characterization of B cells found in human tonsils, a site of permanent antigen stimulation, has further identified various subsets of conventional B cells at different stages of activation and development (94). These include the naive $IgM^+IgD^+CD38^-$ follicular mantle B cells, the $IgM^+IgD^+CD38^+$ germinal-center founder cells, the IgD^-CD38^+ germinal-center cells, and the IgD^-CD38^- memory B cells. In addition, $Ig^-CD20^+CD38^{++}$ plasma cells can also be found in the tonsils. Memory B cells and plasma cells make up a minor fraction of the total B cells found in the mouse (see later discussion). In the human, the memory B-cell compartment may become as large as 40% of all B cells (151).

In addition, a minor subset of B cells distinguishable by a unique phenotype is also found in the periphery. These are the B-1 cells, which express cell surface markers such as CD5 and MAC-1 (CD11b) in addition to high levels of IgM, low levels of IgD and B220, and little or no CD23. In contrast to the conventional B cells, B-1 cells are generated early in ontogeny and appear to be self-replenishing throughout life (95).

B-1 cells are for the most part confined to the peritoneal and pleural cavities, where they are thought to participate in gut- and airway-associated immune responses (96). In the mouse, these cells secrete most of the natural IgM antibodies in the serum. Certain antibody specificities, often directed to bacterial antigens, are highly enriched in the B-1 cell population. It is believed that the secretion of low-affinity IgM antibodies by B-1 cells helps, in T-cell-dependent antibody response, to promote the formation of immune complexes that seem to play a role in the generation of germinal centers from conventional B cells. Therefore, B-1 cells are thought to form a first line of defense against invading pathogens, allowing time for a more specialized and high-affinity response to be developed by the conventional B cells (97).

Life Span and Trafficking of B Lymphocytes

Despite the fact that B cells are continuously generated in the bone marrow, most B cells in the peripheral immune system, whether conventional naive or memory B cells or cells of the B-1 subset, are resting, long-lived cells, with a life span on the order of weeks, months, or sometimes even years (98). A large fraction of the newly arising B cells in the bone marrow presumably never makes it into the stable peripheral B-cell pool and instead rapidly disappears. The basis on which some cells, but not others, are selected into the peripheral pool is presently unknown.

Mature conventional B lymphocytes are able to recirculate between the blood and the various lymphoid tissues, an important feature of the physiology of these cells in their constant search for target antigens in the body. Recirculation involves interactions of adhesion molecules on B cells with ligands on endothelial cells. This lymphocyte-homing process directs B-cell subsets to specialized microenvironments, where naive and memory B cells can effect their functions. The homing molecules found on B cells include CD44, L-selectin, and members of the integrin family such as $\alpha_4\beta_7$, $\alpha_4\beta_1$, and $\alpha_L\beta_2$ (lymphocyte function associated antigen-1, or LFA-1) (99).

B lymphocytes receive physiologic cues, in the form of chemokines secreted by other cell types, that direct their migration to specific lymphoid organs and compartments. Several proteins that bear resemblance to the well-characterized G-protein-coupled chemokine receptors have been shown to be expressed in B cells. These include Burkitt's lymphoma receptor 1 (BLR-1) (100), Epstein Barr virus induced molecule 1 (EBI-1) (BLR-2) (101). The significance of chemokines and chemokine-receptor interactions in directing the trafficking of B lymphocytes is evident in mutant mice that lack BLR-1 (102). These mice have impaired germinal-center formation, lack inguinal lymph nodes, and have few or no Peyer's patches. In addition, mutant B cells fail to migrate into B-cell follicles in the spleen. The ligand for BLR-1, B lymphocyte chemokine (BLC) (103), has been cloned on the basis of homology to other chemokines. Overall, the mechanisms by which chemokines participate in the control of B-cell development and differentiation are just beginning to be elucidated.

THE PRIMARY IMMUNE RESPONSE

In general, there are two types of B-cell immune responses to antigens: T-cell-independent responses and T-cell-dependent responses. The latter of which requires the induction of antigen-specific T-cell help. Induction of T-cell-independent antibody responses in both B-1 and conventional B cells requires cross-linking of their BCRs and coengagement of their coreceptors, which together stimulate cell proliferation and differentiation into antibody-secreting plasma cells (104,105). Multimeric antigens such as those found on bacterial cell surfaces can lead to such direct stimulation.

In contrast, the immune response to most protein antigens requires T-cell help. In this process, the B cells present antigens to T cells in order to solicit their help. B cells can pinocytose antigens or take antigens up by direct BCR-mediated endocytosis (106,107). The latter process is much more efficient, since antigen-specific B cells require an antigen concentration 10^3 to 10^4 times lower than that required by nonantigen-specific B cells for efficient antigen processing and presentation. *In vivo,* it is likely that B cells encounter antigens that are already complexed by natural antibody and components of the complement system. Such immune complexes, normally trapped on antigen-presenting cells such as the follicular dendritic cells (FDC), are then available for uptake by B lymphocytes via their BCR. Immune complexes are potent stimulators of B cells and greatly enhance their activation by co-ligating the BCR with a second B-cell surface complex involving the complement receptor (CR2) and CD19 (108).

In B cells, the antigen is processed and fragmented into peptides and presented by the cell's major histocompatibility complex (MHC) class II molecules to antigen-specific helper T cells (109). The T cells recognize the peptide-MHC complex via their TCR together with their CD4 coreceptor. Functional interaction between T and B cells requires cell-cell contact and involves multiple receptors and ligands on both cells. Activated B cells upregulate the costimulatory molecules B7.1 and B7.2, which deliver a second signal to functionally activate T cells via their CD28 molecule (37,110). This upregulates the expression of CD40 ligand (CD40L) on T cells, which further activates B cells via CD40-CD40L interaction (38). This latter signal is critical for the further development of immune responses such as immunoglobulin isotype class switching and the generation of B-cell memory.

AFFINITY MATURATION AND SOMATIC HYPERMUTATION

It has long been recognized that the antibodies produced in the course of an immune response show increasing affinity for antigens. This phenomenon is known as *affinity maturation* of the antibody response. The clonal selection theory of Burnet precisely describes the basis of affinity maturation of antibodies: antigens directly select for B-cell clones that compete most efficiently for binding to them. At the molecular level, affinity maturation of antibodies is associated with the process of *somatic hypermutation*, in which mutations are introduced at a high rate into the Ig variable-region genes (111). This was first recognized in the murine λ IgL chains by amino acid sequencing of antibodies selected on the basis of their improved binding to antigen (112). Subsequently, DNA sequence analyses of antibodies obtained early and late in the immune response revealed the accumulation of mutations in the Ig variable region as the response progressed. Furthermore, in response to a specific antigen, certain "key" mutations were repeatedly found that substantially increased the antibody's affinity for that antigen. The emerging picture indicates that the stepwise affinity maturation of antibodies corresponds to the stepwise introduction of mutations in their variable-region genes (113).

Somatic hypermutation acts to diversify the antibody repertoire at the mature B-cell stage and appears to target rearranged variable-region genes (114). During this process, point mutations and deletions or insertions of nucleotides occur (151), resulting in both silent and replacement mutational events. Both productive and nonproductive variable-region genes can be somatically mutated. The mutation rate has been estimated to be as high as 1 point mutation per 10^3 to 10^4 nucleotides per cell per generation (111).

The process responsible for the somatic hypermutation process has yet to be discovered, although there is good reason to believe that some form of error-prone DNA repair mechanism is involved (115). It appears that Ig genes must be actively transcribed to be targets for somatic hypermutation (116). Certain *cis*-acting DNA elements in the Ig locus (e.g., enhancers) and a promoter are necessary for the process to occur (117). In addition, studies suggest that genes other than rearranged Ig variable-region gene segments can be targets for the somatic hypermutation when they are associated as transgenes with the known *cis*-regulatory elements of the Ig locus (118). This suggests that there is no particular motif within the Ig variable-region genes that acts as a target for the mutation mechanism.

IMMUNOGLOBULIN HEAVY-CHAIN ISOTYPE CLASS SWITCHING

The carboxy-terminal domains of the IgH chain, which represent its constant (C) region, define the isotype or class of an antibody. Humans have nine different Ig isotypes: IgM; IgD; IgE; two IgA subtypes (IgA1 and IgA2); and four IgG subtypes (IgG1, IgG2, IgG3, and IgG4) (119). In mice, there are eight different Ig classes:

IgM, IgD, IgE, IgA, and four IgG subtypes (IgG1, IgG2a, IgG2b, and IgG3) (120). The different C regions are encoded by independent C-region genes located 3' of the rearranged $V_HD_HJ_H$ gene segment.

During the course of the humoral (antibody-based) immune response, B cells switch from production of antibodies of class M to those of class A, G, and E. This phenomenon is termed *Ig class switching*. At the molecular level, class switching is a nonhomologous, site-specific recombination event in which the initial $V_HD_HJ_H$ gene segment is juxtaposed to a new downstream C-region gene, resulting in the production of antibodies of the same specificity but with an IgH chain C region distinct from the μ and δ C regions initially expressed (121,122). Although the molecular mechanism of this type of recombination remains to be elucidated, it has been shown that the process involves repetitive sequences ("switch regions") located 5' of each C-region gene (123).

Class switching is a clonal, antigen-induced process that occurs after B-cell activation in the primary antibody response and during memory B-cell differentiation in germinal centers (see next section). Different Ig isotypes equip the antibodies with different effector functions, such as the ability to fix complement, cross the placenta, or bind Fc receptors that, when cross-linked, can trigger certain cellular reactions. In addition, the cytoplasmic portion of the C regions of IgA, IgE, and IgG are longer than those of IgM and IgD and are well conserved, suggesting that they may serve some important signaling function. Studies suggest that these regions may be important for efficient endocytosis and processing of antigens by B lymphocytes (124) and for generation and maintenance of memory B cells (125,126).

Ig class switching is regulated primarily by cytokines and through cell-cell contact between CD40 on B cells and CD40L on T cells. Mutations in CD40 or CD40L in humans (127-131) or in mice (132,133) results in a severe deficiency in all serum Igs except for IgM, a condition known in humans as X-linked hyper-IgM syndrome.

THE GERMINAL CENTER REACTION

The secondary lymphoid organs (lymph nodes, spleen, mucosa-associated lymphoid tissues) are organized into B-cell-rich follicles and T-cell-rich extrafollicular areas. In addition to the IgM⁺IgD⁺ naive recirculating B cells, the follicles also contain FDCs, which can trap antigens in the form of antibody-antigen immune complexes and retain them for long periods. The extrafollicular area contains helper T cells and the potent antigen-presenting interdigitating dendritic cells, which can activate the naive T cells (94).

In the absence of antigenic encounter, naive B cells recirculate through the blood and secondary lymphoid organs. Once they encounter specific antigens that are trapped by the FDCs, these passing B lymphocytes are retained within the secondary lymphoid tissues (134). During a T-cell-dependent humoral immune response, antigen-specific B cells are first activated in the extrafollicular areas that are rich in T cells and interdigitating dendritic cells. Activated B cells are recruited into the follicles, where they undergo intense proliferation and give rise to germinal centers (135,136).

The germinal center is divided into dark and light zones according to histologic staining. The dark zone consists mainly of proliferating B-cell blasts (centroblasts) and is the site where somatic hypermutation of Ig variable-region genes takes place (Fig. 10-4). Subsequently, B cells expressing mutated variable-region genes that encode high-affinity binding sites are selected by antigen-antibody complexes trapped on FDCs in the light zone of the germinal centers (137).

Sequencing of Ig variable-region genes from populations of purified germinal-center B cells and from cell populations or single cells picked from individual germinal centers on histologic sections has shown that somatic hypermutation takes place in the germinal centers (138-140). These and other experiments also indicate that the B cells that populate the germinal centers arise from only a few founder cells. Individual germinal centers often may be specific for a given antigen. In contrast, the follicular B cells surrounding the germinal centers are polyclonal in nature and express unmutated Ig variable-region genes.

In addition to somatic hypermutation of Ig variable-region genes, B cells also undergo IgH-chain isotype switching in the germinal center (141). Furthermore, in some germinal-center B cells, presumably cells in the light zone, RAG-1 and RAG-2 are upregulated (142,143) and secondary Ig gene rearrangements are initiated (144,145). It therefore seems that affinity maturation may involve not only somatic hypermutation and class switching but also receptor editing. Because the latter involves Ig gene rearrangements predominantly in the IgL loci, whereas the main determinant of antibody specificity seems to be the CDR3 of the IgH chain, it is conceivable that receptor editing can contribute to affinity maturation in a meaningful way.

A few weeks after the initial antigenic challenge, the germinal center shrinks and largely disappears.

Positive and Negative Selection of B Cells in the Germinal Center

Somatic hypermutation of Ig V-region genes can change the affinity and specificity of the BCR. Therefore, both positive and negative selection are required during the germinal center reaction to ensure that only high-affinity antigen-specific B cells are selected and that low-affinity mutants and cells acquiring altered specificities that include autoreactivities are counterselected. The mechanisms underlying this selection process are now beginning to be elucidated.

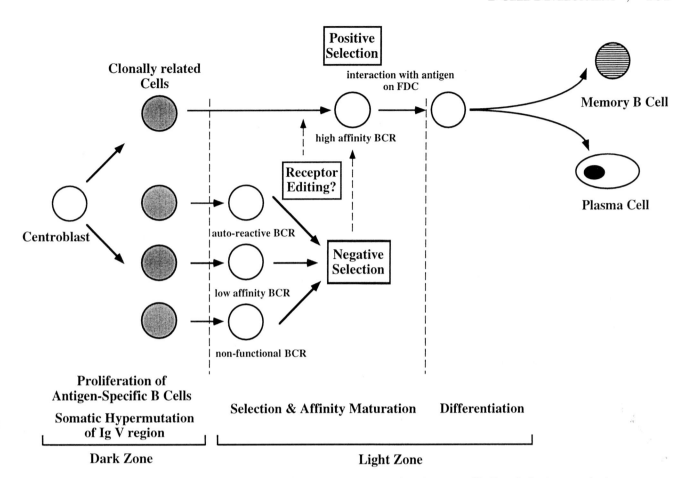

FIG. 10-4. General scheme of differentiation and selection of antigen-specific B cells in the germinal center (GC) of secondary lymphoid organs. After activation, antigen-specific B cells undergo cellular proliferation and somatic hypermutation of their immunoglobulin (Ig) variable (V)-region genes in the dark zone of the GC. This gives rise to clonally related B cells. Selection of B cells occurs in the light zone of the GC. The somatic hypermutation process can change the specificities of the B-cell receptor for antigen (BCR). Cells that recognize antigens trapped on follicular dendritic cells (FDC) with high affinity are positively selected. These cells interact with antigen-specific T cells and differentiate further into memory B cells or antibody-secreting plasma cells. Cells whose BCRs bind antigen with low affinity or whose BCRs became autoreactive or nonfunctional as a result of somatic hypermutation are negatively selected and are likely to undergo apoptosis. It is not known whether receptor editing may occur in the GC to allow these B cells another chance to express a high-affinity antigen-binding BCR.

Germinal-center B cells, unlike naive B cells, express low levels of B cell lymphoma gene 2 (BCL-2) (promoting cell survival) but high levels of apoptosis-inducing gene products such as CD95, transforming gene, myelocytomatosis (MYC), cellular tumor antigen (p53), and Bcl-2-associated X protein (BAX) (146). This reflects the fact that they are programmed to die unless they receive a survival signal. This provides a mechanism for the positive selection of high-affinity B cells. Cells expressing antibodies with improved affinities can compete more efficiently for antigens on FDCs, which they bind, process, and present to antigen-specific helper T cells. Delivery of T-cell-derived signals via CD40L-CD40 interaction subsequently selects the high-affinity mutants for survival, whereas B cells with low-affinity antibodies and those whose antibodies no longer bind antigen, or are otherwise crippled by mutations of their Ig variable

region, die of neglect (147,148). Competition among mutating B cells for antigen and T-cell help thus provides an efficient cellular mechanism for the selection of B cells expressing high-affinity antibodies.

A potential danger of the somatic hypermutation process in the germinal center is the generation of high-affinity autoreactive B cells. Experimental evidence suggests that such cells are actively eliminated by negative selection, based presumably on prolonged engagement of the antigen receptor in the absence of T-cell help (149).

After somatic hypermutation and selection, high-affinity germinal-center B cells can differentiate into either memory B cells or plasma cells. The former are the carriers of immunologic memory in the B-cell compartment; they enable the organism to mount an efficient, high-affinity response to an antigen previously encountered. Experiments suggest that the generation of memory B cells results from continual signaling via CD40 on positively selected germinal-center B cells (150). In the absence of such a signal, germinal-center B cells undergo terminal differentiation into antibody-secreting plasma cells.

Memory B Cells

In mice, memory B cells comprise only a minor subset of all the B cells present. However, in humans, these cells may comprise up to 40% of the B cells present. Memory B cells are typically recognized by their somatically mutated Ig variable region, and most, but not all, have undergone IgH-chain isotype class switching from IgM to IgA, IgE, or IgG. In the human, the CD27 antigen may represent a faithful surface marker of memory B cells (151).

Memory B cells are mostly resting, long-lived cells (152). It is believed that the life span of these cells depends on their occasional contact with the eliciting antigen. Studies indicate that memory B cells home preferentially to mucosal surfaces where they can rapidly respond to incoming pathogens (153). These cells can efficiently present antigens to T cells to initiate a robust secondary immune response. In this response, the majority of the memory B cells undergo proliferative expansion outside the germinal center, without further somatic hypermutation, and terminally differentiate into plasma cells (154). This ensures rapid generation of effector cells to efficiently eliminate pathogens. Some memory B cells, however, may reenter the germinal center pathway and go through further rounds of mutation and selection, further propagating and optimizing B-cell memory.

Antibody-Secreting Cells

This chapter does not cover plasma cell generation and physiology in any detail. The data indicate that plasma cells, like many other cells in the immune system (including most cells in the B-cell compartment), often have long life spans, explaining at least in part sustained antibody production after an antigenic stimulus over periods of weeks, months, and sometimes years (155).

MEDICAL ASPECTS

Because B lymphocytes are key participants in the initiation and effector phases of immune responses, dysregulation of their development and differentiation (described in this chapter for the physiologic condition) can result in immunodeficiency or autoimmunity. Several such human conditions have been identified, including X-linked hyper-IgM syndrome, caused by mutations in CD40 and CD40L (described earlier); human severe combined immunodeficiency syndrome, caused by RAG mutation (156); human X-linked agammaglobulinemia,

caused by mutations in the tyrosine kinase BTK (157); human autoimmune lymphoproliferative syndrome (158); and many others resulting from mutations in genes that regulate the generation or function of lymphocytes. These conditions are comprehensively reviewed by Fischer et al. (159) and Elkon and Marshak-Rothstein (160). Researchers are just beginning to understand the many ways in which B lymphocytes can be involved in states of disease in mouse and human.

REFERENCES

1. Burnet FM. *The clonal selection theory of acquired immunity.* Cambridge, UK: The University Press, 1959.
2. Talmage DW. Clonal selection theory. *Science* 1959;129:1643–1648.
3. Georgopoulous K. Transcriptional factors required for lymphoid lineage commitment. *Curr Opin Immunol* 1997;9:222–227.
4. Clevers HC, Grosschedl R. Transcriptional control of lymphoid development: Lessons from gene targeting. *Immunol Today* 1996;13:336–343.
5. Georgopoulos K, Bigby M, Wang J-H, et al. The ikaros gene is required for the development of all lymphoid lineages. *Cell* 1994;79:143–156.
6. McKercher SR, Torbett BE, Anderson KL, et al. Targeted disruption of the PU.1 gene results in multiple hematopoietic abnormalities. *EMBO J* 1996;15:5647–5658.
7. Scott E, Simon M, Anastasi J, Singh H. Requirement of the transcription factor PU.1 in the development of multiple hematopoietic lineages. *Science* 1994;265:1573–1577.
8. Mucenski M, Mclain K, Kier A, et al. A functional c-myb gene is required for normal murine fetal hematopoiesis. *Cell* 1991;65:677–689.
9. Dorshkind K. Transcriptional control points during lymphopoiesis. *Cell* 79:751–753.
10. Zhuang Y, Soriano P, Weintraub H. The helix-loop-helix gene E2A is required for B cell formation. *Cell* 1994;79:875–884.
11. Bain G, Maandag EC, Izon DS, et al. E2A proteins are required for proper B cell development and initiation of immunoglobulin gene rearrangements. *Cell* 1994;79:885–892.
12. Urbanek P, Wang ZQ, Fetka I, Wagner E, Busslinger M. Complete block of early B cell differentiation and altered patterning of the posterior midbrain in mice lacking Pax5/BSAP. *Cell* 1994;79:901–912.
13. Lin H, Grosschedl R. Failure of B-cell differentiation in mice lacking the transcription factor EBF. *Nature* 1995;376:263–267.
14. Schilham MW, Oosterwegel MA, Moerer P, et al. Defects in cardiac outflow tract formation and pro-B-lymphocyte expansion in mice lacking Sox-4. *Nature* 1996;380:711–714.
15. Nielsen PJ, Georgiev O, Lorenz B, Schaffner W. B lymphocytes are impaired in mice lacking the transcriptional coactivator Bob1/OCA-B/OBF1. *Eur J Immunol* 1996;26:3214–3218.
16. Kim U, Qin XF, Gong S, et al. The B-cell-specific transcription coactivator OCA-B/OBF-1/Bob-1 is essential for normal production of immunoglobulin isotypes. *Nature* 1996;383:542–547.
17. Turner C Jr, Mack DH, Davis MM. Blimp-1, a novel zinc finger-containing protein that can drive the maturation of B lymphocytes into immunoglobulin-secreting cells. *Cell* 1994;77:297–306.
18. Corcoran LM, Karvelas M, Nossal GJV, et al. Oct-2, although not required for early B cell development, is critical for later B cell maturation and for postnatal survival. *Genes Dev* 1993;7:570–582.
19. Nagasawa T, Hirota S, Tachibana K, et al. Defects of B cell lymphopoiesis and bone marrow myelopoiesis in mice lacking the CXC chemokine PBSF/SDF-1. *Nature* 1996;382:635–638.
20. Kincade PW, Lee G, Pietrangeli CE, Hayashi SI, Gimble JM. Cells and molecules that regulate B lymphopoiesis in bone marrow. *Annu Rev Immunol* 1989;7:111–143.
21. Dorshkind K. Regulation of hemopoiesis by bone marrow stromal cells and their products. *Annu Rev Immunol* 1990;8:111–137.
22. Landreth KS, Narayanan R, Dorshkind K. Insulin-like Growth Factor-1 regulates pro-B cell differentiation. *Blood* 1992;80:1207–1212.
23. Billips LG, Petitte D, Dorshkind K, Narayanan R, Chiu C-P, Landreth

KS. Differential roles of stromal cells, interleukin-7, and kit-ligand in the regulation of B lymphopoiesis. *Blood* 1992;79:1185–1192.

24. Hirayama F, Lyman SD, Clark SC, Ogawa M. The flt3 ligand supports proliferation of lymphohematopoietic progenitors and early B-lymphoid progenitors. *Blood* 1995;85:1762–1768.

25. Gimble JM, Medina K, Hudson J, Robinson M, Kincade PW. Modulation of lymphohematopoiesis in long-term cultures by gamma interferon: direct and indirect action on lymphoid and stromal cells. *Exp Hematol* 1993;21:224–230.

26. Lee G, Ellingsworth LR, Gillis S, Wall R, Kincade PW. Beta-transforming growth factors are potential regulators of B lymphopoiesis. *J Exp Med* 1987;166:1290–1299.

27. Medina KL, Smithson G, Kincade PW. Suppression of B lymphopoiesis during normal pregnancy. *J Exp Med* 1993;178:1507–1515.

28. Cumano A, Dieterlen-Lievre F, Godin I. Lymphoid potential, probed before circulation in mouse, is restricted to caudal intraembryonic splanchnopleura. *Cell* 1996;86:907–916.

29. Delassus S, Cumano A. Circulation of hematopoietic progenitors in the mouse embryo. *Immunity* 1996;4:97–106.

30. Reth M. Antigen receptors on B lymphocytes. *Annu Rev Immunol* 1992;10:97–121.

31. Reth M, Wienands J. Initiation and processing of signals from the B cell antigen receptor. *Annu Rev Immunol* 1997;15:453–479.

32. Satterthwaite A, Witte O. Genetic analysis of tyrosine kinase function in B cell development. *Annu Rev Immunol* 1996;14:131–154.

33. Fearon DT, Carter RH. The CD19/CR2/TAPA-1 complex of B lymphocytes: Linking natural to acquired immunity. *Annu Rev Immunol* 1995;13:127–149.

34. Tedder TF, Inaoki M, Sato S. The CD19-CD21 complex regulates signal transduction thresholds governing humoral immunity and autoimmunity. *Immunity* 1997;6:107–118.

35. Carter RH, Fearon DT. CD19: Lowering the threshold for antigen receptor stimulation of B lymphocytes. *Science* 1992;256:105–107.

36. Tedder TF, Tuscano J, Sato S, Kehrl JH. CD22, a B lymphocyte-specific adhesion molecule that regulates antigen receptor signaling. *Annu Rev Immunol* 1997;15:481–504.

37. Lenschow DJ, Walunas TL, Bluestone JA. CD28/B7 system of T cell costimulation. *Annu Rev Immunol* 1996;14:233–258.

38. Foy TM, Aruffo A, Bajorath J, Buhlmann JE, Noelle RJ. Immune regulation by CD40 and its ligand gp39. *Annu Rev Immunol* 1996;14:591–617.

39. Karasuyama H, Rolink A, Shinkai Y, Young F, Alt FW, Melchers F. The expression of Vpre-B/lambda 5 surrogate light chain in early bone marrow precursor B cells of normal and B cell-deficient mutant mice. *Cell* 1994;77:133–143.

40. Karasuyama H, Rolink A, Melchers F. Surrogate light chain in B cell development. *Adv Immunol* 1996;63:1–41.

41. Tonegawa S. Somatic generation of antibody diversity. *Nature* 1983;302:575–581.

42. Reynaud C, Anquez V, Dahan A, Weill J. A single rearrangement event generates most of the chicken Ig light chain diversity. *Cell* 1985;40:283–291.

43. Becker R, Knight K. Somatic diversification of Ig heavy chain VDJ genes: Evidence for somatic gene conversion in rabbits. *Cell* 1990;63:987–989.

44. Alt FW, Oltz EM, Young F, Gorman J, Taccioli G, Chen J. VDJ recombination. *Immunol Today* 1992;13:306–314.

45. Schatz DG, Oettinger MA, Baltimore D. The V(D)J recombination activating gene, RAG-1. *Cell* 1989;59:1035–1048.

46. Oettinger MA, Schatz DG, Gorka C, Baltimore D. RAG-1 and RAG-2, adjacent genes that synergistically activate V(D)J recombination. *Science* 1990;248:1517–1523.

47. Hiom K, Gellert M. A stable RAG1-RAG2-DNA complex that is active in V(D)J cleavage. *Cell* 1997;88:65–72.

48. Gellert M. Recent advances in understanding V(D)J recombination. *Adv Immunol* 1997;64:39–64.

49. Taccioli GE, Gottlieb TM, Blunt T, et al. Ku80: Product of the XRCC5 gene and its role in DNA repair and V(D)J recombination. *Science* 1994;265:1442–1445.

50. Blunt T, Finnie NJ, Taccioli GE, et al. Defective DNA-dependent protein kinase activity is linked to V(D)J recombination and DNA repair defects associated with the murine scid mutation. *Cell* 1995;80:813–823.

51. Li Z, Otevrel T, Gao Y, et al. The XRCC4 gene encodes a novel protein involved in DNA double-strand break repair and V(D)J recombination. *Cell* 1995;83:1079–1089.

52. Li Z, Alt FW. Identification of the XRCC4 gene: Complementation of the DSBR and V(D)J recombination defects of XR-1 cells. *Curr Top Microbiol Immunol* 1996;217:143–150.

53. Gu Y, Seidl KJ, Rathbun GA, et al. Growth retardation and leaky SCID phenotype of Ku70-deficient mice. *Immunity* 1997;7:653–665.

54. Nussenzweig A, Chen C, da Costa Soares V, et al. Requirement for Ku80 in growth and immunoglobulin V(D)J recombination. *Nature* 1996;382:551–555.

55. Komori T, Pricop L, Hatakeyama A, Bona CA, Alt FW. Repertoires of antigen receptors in Tdt congenitally deficient mice. *Int Rev Immunol* 1996;13:317–325.

56. Gilfillan S, Benoist C, Mathis D. Mice lacking terminal deoxynucleotidyl transferase: Adult mice with a fetal antigen receptor repertoire. *Immunol Rev* 1995;148:201–219.

57. Stanhope-Baker P, Hudson K, Schaffer A, Constantinescu A, Schissel M. Cell type specific chromatin structure determines the targeting of VDJ recombinase activity in vitro. *Cell* 1996;85:887–897.

58. Lichtenstein M, Keini G, Cedar H, Bergman Y. B cell-specific demethylation: A novel role for the intronic kappa chain enhancer sequence. *Cell* 1994;76:913–923.

59. Sleckman BP, Gorman JR, Alt FW. Accessibility control of antigen receptor variable-region gene assembly: Role of cis-acting elements. *Annu Rev Immunol* 1996;14:459–481.

60. Alt FW, Yancopoulos GD, Blackwell TK, et al. Ordered rearrangement of immunoglobulin heavy chain variable region segments. *EMBO J* 1984;3:1209–1219.

61. Kitamura D, Rajewsky K. Targeted disruption of mu chain membrane exon causes loss of heavy-chain allelic exclusion [see comments]. *Nature* 1992;356:154–156.

62. Nussenzweig MC, Shaw AC, Sinn E, et al. Allelic exclusion in transgenic mice that express the membrane form of immunoglobulin mu. *Science* 1987;236:816–819.

63. Kitamura D, Roes J, Kühn R, Rajewsky K. A B cell-deficient mouse by targeted disruption of the membrane exon of the immunoglobulin mu chain gene. *Nature* 1991;350:423–426.

64. Kitamura D, Kudo A, Schaal S, Müller W, Melchers F, Rajewsky K. A critical role of lambda 5 protein in B cell development. *Cell* 1992;69:823–831.

65. Gong S, Nussenzweig MC. Regulation of an early developmental checkpoint in the B cell pathway by Ig beta. *Science* 1996;272:411–414.

66. Mombaerts P, Iacomini J, Johnson RS, Herrup K, Tonegawa S. RAG-1 deficient mice have no mature B and T lymphocytes. *Cell* 1992;68:869–877.

67. Shinkai Y, Rathbun G, Lam KP, et al. RAG-2-deficient mice lack mature lymphocytes owing to inability to initiate V(D)J rearrangement. *Cell* 1992;68:855–867.

68. Spanopoulou E, Roman CA, Corcoran LM, et al. Functional immunoglobulin transgenes guide ordered B-cell differentiation in Rag-1-deficient mice. *Genes Dev* 1994;8:1030–1042.

69. Young F, Ardman B, Shinkai Y, et al. Influence of immunoglobulin heavy- and light-chain expression on B-cell differentiation. *Genes Dev* 1994;8:1043–1057.

70. Pelanda R, Schaal S, Torres RM, Rajewsky K. A prematurely expressed Ig(kappa) transgene, but not V(kappa)J(kappa) gene segment targeted into the Ig(kappa) locus, can rescue B cell development in lambda5-deficient mice. *Immunity* 1996;5:229–239.

71. Grawunder U, Leu TM, Schatz DG, et al. Down-regulation of RAG1 and RAG2 gene expression in preB cells after functional immunoglobulin heavy chain rearrangement. *Immunity* 1995;3:601–608.

72. Gay D, Saunders T, Camper S, Weigert M. Receptor editing: An approach by autoreactive B cells to escape tolerance. *J Exp Med* 1993;177:999–1008.

73. Tiegs SL, Russell DM, Nemazee D. Receptor editing in self-reactive bone marrow B cells. *J Exp Med* 1993;177:1009–1020.

74. Prak EL, Weigert M. Light chain replacement: A new model for antibody gene rearrangement. *J Exp Med* 1995;182:541–548.

75. Kleinfield R, Hardy RR, Tarlinton D, Dangl J, Herzenberg LA, Weigert M. Recombination between an expressed immunoglobulin heavy-chain gene and a germline variable gene segment in a Ly 1+ B-cell lymphoma. *Nature* 1986;322:843–846.

76. Reth M, Gehrmann P, Petrac E, Wiese P. A novel VH to VHDJH join-

ing mechanism in heavy-chain-negative (null) pre-B cells results in heavy-chain production. *Nature* 1986;322:840–842.

77. Chen C, Nagy Z, Prak EL, Weigert M. Immunoglobulin heavy chain gene replacement: A mechanism of receptor editing. *Immunity* 1995;3:747–755.

78. Torres RM, Flaswinkel H, Reth M, Rajewsky K. Aberrant B cell development and immune response in mice with a compromised BCR complex [see comments]. *Science* 1996;272:1804–1808.

79. Lam KP, Kühn R, Rajewsky K. In vivo ablation of surface immunoglobulin on mature B cells by inducible gene targeting results in rapid cell death [see comments]. *Cell* 1997;90:1073–1083.

80. Davis MM, Boniface JJ, Reich Z, et al. Ligand recognition by alpha-beta T cell receptors. *Annu Rev Immunol* 1998;16:523–544.

81. Gu H, Förster I, Rajewsky K. Sequence homologies, N sequence insertion and JH gene utilization in VHDJH joining: Implications for the joining mechanism and the ontogenetic timing of Ly1 B cell and B-CLL progenitor generation. *EMBO J* 1990;9:2133–2140.

82. Feeney AJ. Lack of N regions in fetal and neonatal mouse immuno-globulin V-D-J junctional sequences. *J Exp Med* 1990;172:1377–1390.

83. Gerstein RM, Lieber MR. Extent to which homology can constrain coding exon junctional diversity in V(D)J recombination. *Nature* 1993;363:625–627.

84. Grey HM, Mannik M. Specificity of recombination of H and L chains from human gamma-G-myeloma proteins. *J Exp Med* 1965;122:619–632.

85. Alt FW, Blackwell TK, Yancoupoulos GD. Development of the primary antibody repertoire. *Science* 1987;238:1079–1087.

86. Taki S, Meiering M, Rajewsky K. Targeted insertion of a variable region gene into the immunoglobulin heavy chain locus [see comments]. *Science* 1993;262:1268–1271.

87. Radic MZ, Erikson J, Litwin S, Weigert M. B lymphocytes may escape tolerance by revising their antigen receptors. *J Exp Med* 1993;177:1165–1173.

88. Hartley SB, Cooke MP, Fulcher DA, et al. Elimination of self-reactive B lymphocytes proceeds in two stages: Arrested development and cell death. *Cell* 1993;72:325–335.

89. Hartley SB, Crosbie J, Brink R, Kantor AB, Basten A, Goodnow CC. Elimination from peripheral lymphoid tissues of self-reactive B lymphocytes recognizing membrane-bound antigens. *Nature* 1991;353:765–769.

90. Pelanda R, Schwers S, Sonoda E, Torres RM, Nemazee D, Rajewsky K. Receptor editing in a transgenic mouse model: Site, efficiency, and role in B cell tolerance and antibody diversification. *Immunity* 1997;7:765–775.

91. Melamed D, Benschop RJ, Cambier JC, Nemazee D. Developmental regulation of B lymphocyte immune tolerance compartmentalizes clonal selection from receptor selection. *Cell* 1998;92:173–182.

92. Goodnow CC, Crosbie J, Adelstein S, et al. Altered immunoglobulin expression and functional silencing of self-reactive B lymphocytes in transgenic mice. *Nature* 1988;334:676–682.

93. Cyster JG, Hartley SB, Goodnow CC. Competition for follicular niches excludes self-reactive cells from the recirculating B-cell repertoire [see comments]. *Nature* 1994;371:389–395.

94. Liu Y-J, Bancheareau J. The paths and molecular controls of peripheral B-cell development. *Immunol Today* 1996;4:55–66.

95. Kantor AB, Herzenberg LA. Origins of B cell lineages. *Annu Rev Immunol* 1993;11:501–538.

96. Kroese FGM, Butcher EC, Stall AM, Lalor PA, Adam S, Herzenberg LA. Many of the IgA producing plasma cells in murine gut are derived from self-replenishing precursors in the peritoneal cavity. *Int Immunol* 1989;1:75–84.

97. Stall AM, Wells SM, Lam KP. B-1 cells: Unique origins and functions. *Semin Immunol* 1996;8:45–59.

98. Fulcher DA, Basten A. B cell life span: A review. *Immunol Cell Biol* 1997;75:446–455.

99. Butcher EC, Picker LJ. Lymphocyte homing and homeostasis. *Science* 1996;272:60–68.

100. Dobner T, Wolf I, Ernich T, Lipp M. Differentiation-specific expression of a novel G protein-coupled receptor from Burkitt's lymphoma. *Eur J Immunol* 1992;22:2795.

101. Birkenbach M, Josefsen K, Yalamanchili R, Lenoir G, Kieff E. Epstein-Barr virus-induced genes: First lymphocyte-specific G protein-coupled peptide receptors. *J Virol* 1993;67:2209–2220.

102. Förster R, Mattis AE, Kremmer E, Wolf E, Brem G, Lipp M. A puta-

tive chemokine receptor, BLR1, directs B cell migration to defined lymphoid organs and specific anatomic compartments of the spleen. *Cell* 1996;87:1037–1047.

103. Gunn MD, Ngo VN, Ansel KM, Ekland EH, Cyster JG, Williams LT. A B-cell-homing chemokine made in lymphoid follicles activates Burkitt's lymphoma receptor-1. *Nature* 1998;391:799–803.

104. Doody GM, Dempsey PW, Fearon DT. Activation of B lymphocytes: Integrating signals from CD19, CD22 and FcγRIIb1. *Curr Opin Immunol* 1996;8:378–382.

105. O'Rourke L, Tooze R, Fearon DT. Co-receptors of B lymphocytes. *Curr Opin Immunol* 1997;9:324–329.

106. Mitchell RN, Barnes KA, Grupp SA, et al. Intracellular targeting of antigens internalized by membrane immunoglobulin in B lympho-cytes. *J Exp Med* 1995;181:1705–1714.

107. Patel KJ, Neuberger MS. Antigen presentation by the B cell antigen receptor is driven by the alpha/beta sheath and occurs independently of its cytoplasmic tyrosines. *Cell* 1993;74:939–946.

108. Dempsey PW, Allison MED, Akkaraju S, Goodnow CC, T Fearon DT. C3d of complement as a molecular adjuvant: Bridging innate and acquired immunity. *Science* 1996;271:348–350.

109. Watts C. Capture and processing of exogenous antigens for presenta-tion on MHC molecules. *Annu Rev Immunol* 1997;15:821–850.

110. Lenschow DJ, Sperling AI, Cooke MP, et al. Differential up-regulation of the B7-1 and B7-2 costimulatory molecules after Ig receptor engagement by antigen. *J Immunol* 1994;153:1990–1997.

111. Wagner SD, Neuberger MS. Somatic hypermutation of immunoglob-ulin genes. *Annu Rev Immunol* 1996;14:441–457.

112. Weigert M, Cesari IM, Yankovich SJ, Cohn M. Variability in the lambda light chain sequences of mouse antibody. *Nature* 1970;228:1045–1047.

113. Kocks C, Rajewsky K. Stable expression and somatic hypermutation of antibody V regions in B-cell developmental pathways. *Annu Rev Immunol* 1989;7:537–59.

114. Gorski J, Rollini P, Mach B. Somatic mutations of immunoglobulin variable genes are restricted to the rearranged V gene. *Science* 1983;220:1179–1181.

115. Storb U. The molecular basis of somatic hypermutation of immunoglobulin genes. *Curr Opin Immunol* 1996;8:206–214.

116. Peters A, Storb U. Somatic hypermutation of immunoglobulin genes is linked to transcription initiation. *Immunity* 1996;4:57–65.

117. Betz A, Milstein C, Gonzalez-Fernandes R, Pannell R, Larson T, Neu-berger M. Elements regulating somatic hypermutation of an immunoglobulin κ gene: Critical role for the intron enhancer/matrix attachment region. *Cell* 1994;77:239–248.

118. Yelamos J, Klix N, Goyenechea B, et al. Targeting of non-Ig sequences in place of the V segment by somatic hypermutation. *Nature* 1995;376:225–229.

119. Hofker MH, Walter M-A, Cox DW. Complete physical map of the human immunoglobulin heavy chain constant region gene complex. *Proc Natl Acad Sci U S A* 1989;86:5567–5571.

120. Shimizu A, Takahashi N, Yaoita Y, Honjo T. Organization of the con-stant region gene family of the mouse immunoglobulin heavy chain. *Cell* 1982;28:499–506.

121. Stavnezer J. Antibody class switching. *Adv Immunol* 1996;61:79–145.

122. Coffman RL, Lebman DA, Rothman P. The mechanism and regulation of immunoglobulin isotype switching. *Adv Immunol* 1993;54:229–270.

123. Kataoka T, Miyata T, Honjo T. Repetitive sequences in class-switch recombination regions of immunoglobulin heavy chain genes. *Cell* 1981;23:357–368.

124. Knight AM, Lucocq JM, Prescott AR, Ponnambalam S, Watts C. Anti-gen endocytosis and presentation mediated by human IgG1 in the absence of the Igalpha/beta dimer. *EMBO J* 1997;16:3842–3888.

125. Kaisho T, Schwenk F, Rajewsky K. The roles of gamma1 heavy chain membrane expression and cytoplasmic tail in IgG1 responses. *Science* 1997;276:412–415.

126. Achatz G, Nitschke L, Lamers MC. Effect of transmembrane and cytoplasmic domains of IgE on the IgE response. *Science* 1997;276:409–411.

127. Allen RC, Armitage RJ, Conley ME, et al. CD40 ligand gene defects responsible for X-linked hyper-IgM syndrome. *Science* 1993;259:990–993.

128. DiSanto JP, Bonnefoy JY, Gauchat JF, Fischer A, de Saint Basile G. CD40 ligand mutations in X-linked immunodeficiency with hyper-IgM [see comments]. *Nature* 1993;361:541–543.

129. Farrington M, Grosmaire LS, Nonoyama S, et al. CD40 ligand expres-

sion is defective in a subset of patients with common variable immunodeficiency. *Proc Natl Acad Sci U S A* 1994;91:1099–1103.

130. Fuleihan R, Ramesh N, Loh R, et al. Defective expression of the CD40 ligand in X chromosome-linked immunoglobulin deficiency with normal or elevated IgM. *Proc Natl Acad Sci U S A* 1993;90:2170–2173.

131. Korthauer U, Graf D, Mages HW, et al. Defective expression of T-cell CD40 ligand causes X-linked immunodeficiency with hyper-IgM. *Nature* 1993;361:539–541.

132. Kawabe T, Naka T, Yoshida K, et al. The immune responses in CD40-deficient mice: Impaired immunoglobulin class switching and germinal center formation. *Immunity* 1994;1:167–178.

133. Xu J, Foy TM, Laman JD, et al. Mice deficient for the CD40 ligand. *Immunity* 1994;1:423–432.

134. Tew JG, Wu J, Qin D, Helm S, Burton GF, Szakal AK. Follicular dendritic cells and presentation of antigen and costimulatory signals to B cells. *Immunol Rev* 1997;156:39–52.

135. MacLennan IC. 1994. Germinal centers. *Annu Rev Immunol* 1994;12:117–139.

136. Liu YJ, Arpin C. Germinal center development. *Immunol Rev* 1997;156:111–126.

137. Kelsoe G. The germinal center: a crucible for lymphocyte selection. *Semin Immunol* 1996;8:179–184.

138. Küppers R, Zhao M, Hansmann ML, Rajewsky K. Tracing B cell development in human germinal centres by molecular analysis of single cells picked from histological sections. *EMBO J* 1993;12:4955–4967.

139. Jacob J, Kelsoe G, Rajewsky K, Weiss U. Intraclonal generation of antibody mutants in germinal centres. *Nature* 1991;354:389–392.

140. Berek C, Berger A, Apel M. Maturation of the immune response in germinal centers. *Cell* 1991;67:1121–1129.

141. Liu YJ, Malisan F, de Bouteiller O, et al. Within germinal centers, isotype switching of immunoglobulin genes occurs after the onset of somatic mutation. *Immunity* 1996;4:241–250.

142. Hikida M, Mori M, Takai T, Tomochika K, Hamatani K, Ohmori H. Reexpression of rag-1 and rag-2 genes in activated mature mouse B cells. *Science* 1996;274:2092–2094.

143. Han S, Zheng B, Schatz DG, Spanopoulou E, Kelsoe G. Neoteny in lymphocytes: RAG1 and RAG2 expression in germinal center B cells. *Science* 1996;274:2094–2097.

144. Papavasiliou F, Casellas R, Suh H, et al. V(D)J recombination in mature B cells: A mechanism for altering antibody responses [see comments]. *Science* 1997;278:298–301.

145. Han S, Dillon SR, Zheng B, Shimoda M, Schlissel MS, Kelsoe G. V(D)J recombinase activity in a subset of germinal center B lymphocytes [see comments]. *Science* 1997;278:301–305.

146. Martinez-Valdez H, Guret C, de Bouteiller O, Fugier I, Banchereau J, Liu YJ. Human germinal center B cells express the apoptosis-inducing genes Fas, c-myc, P53, and Bax but not the survival gene bcl-2. *J Exp Med* 1996;183:971–977.

147. Lagresle C, Mondiere P, Bella C, Krammer PH, Defrance T. Concurrent engagement of CD40 and the antigen receptor protects naive and memory human B cells from APO-1/Fas-mediated apoptosis. *J Exp Med* 1996;183:1377–1388.

148. Rathmell JC, Townsend SE, Xu JC, Flavell RA, Goodnow CC. Expansion or elimination of B cells in vivo: Dual roles for CD40- and Fas (CD95)-ligands modulated by the B cell antigen receptor. *Cell* 1996;87:319–329.

149. Galibert L, Burdin N, Barthelemy C, et al. Negative selection of human germinal center B cells by prolonged BCR cross-linking. *J Exp Med* 1996;183:2075–2085.

150. Arpin C, Dechanet J, Van Kooten C, et al. Generation of memory B cells and plasma cells in vitro. *Science* 1995;268:720–722.

151. Klein U, Goossens T, Fischer M, et al. Somatic hypermutation in normal and transformed human B cells. *Immunol Rev* 162:261–280.

152. Schittek B, Rajewsky K. Maintenance of B-cell memory by long-lived cells generated from proliferating precursors. *Nature* 1990;346:749–751.

153. Liu YJ, Barthelemy C, de Bouteiller O, Arpin C, Durand I, Banchereau J. Memory B cells from human tonsils colonize mucosal epithelium and directly present antigen to T cells by rapid up-regulation of B7-1 and B7-2. *Immunity* 1995;2:239–248.

154. Arpin C, Banchereau J, Liu YJ. Memory B cells are biased towards terminal differentiation: A strategy that may prevent repertoire freezing. *J Exp Med* 1997;186:931–940.

155. Mans RA, Thiel A, Radbruch A. Lifetime of plasma cells in the bone marrow. *Nature* 1997;388:133–134.

156. Schwarz K, Gauss GH, Ludwig L, et al. RAG mutations in human B cell-negative SCID. *Science* 1996;274:97–99.

157. Conley ME. Primary immunodeficiencies. *Immunol Today* 1995;16:313–315.

158. Rieux-Laucat F, LeDeist F, Hivroz C, et al. Mutations in Fas associated with human lymphoproliferative syndrome and autoimmunity. *Science* 1995;268:1347–1349.

159. Fischer A, Cavazzana-Calvo M, De Saint Basile G, et al. Naturally occurring primary deficiencies of the immune system. *Annu Rev Immunol* 1997;15:93–124.

160. Elkon KB, Marshak-Rothstein A. B cells in systemic autoimmune disease: Recent insights from Fas-deficient mice and men. *Curr Opin Immunol* 1996;8:852–859.

161. Rajewsky K. Selection and learning in the antibody system. *Nature* 1996;381:751–758.

Inflammation: Basic Principles and Clinical Correlates,
edited by John I. Gallin and Ralph Snyderman.
Lippincott Williams & Wilkins, Philadelphia © 1999.

CHAPTER 11

Natural Killer Cells

Lorenzo Moretta and Maria Cristina Mingari

Natural killer (NK) cells represent a discrete lymphoid population, substantially different from T or B lymphocytes in that they do not express or rearrange known receptors for antigen (i.e., T-cell receptors or surface immunoglobulins). NK cells account for up to 20% of peripheral blood lymphocytes and are phenotypically characterized by the surface expression of CD16 (the low-affinity receptor for the Fc portion of immunoglobulin G [IgG]) and of CD56, which is homologous to the neural cell adhesion molecule (NCAM). In contrast to resting T or B lymphocytes, NK cells are relatively large and are characterized by typical cytoplasmic azurophilic granules. Because of these morphologic features they have been called "large granular lymphocytes" (1).

NK cells were originally identified on a functional basis, as a background cytolytic activity in studies aimed at identifying antitumor responses. Lymphocytes from nonimmunized animals were found to lyse certain tumors. The effector cells responsible for this function were thought to represent a cell type distinct from T lymphocytes because their activity could be detected also in athymic mice and in mice with the severe combined immunodeficiency (SCID) mutation. Tumor-specific cytolytic T lymphocytes (CTLs) did not represent an exception to the rule of major histocompatibility complex (MHC) restriction in T-cell–mediated recognition (2,3), but studies of antitumor cytotoxicity exerted by peripheral lymphocytes indicated that both syngenic and allogenic tumor cells were killed (i.e., in a non-MHC-restricted fashion). Moreover, tumor cell lysis was mediated also by lymphocytes isolated from healthy, non–tumor-bearing animals. Further studies in humans indicated that peripheral blood lymphocytes isolated from any normal donor in the absence of deliberate immuniza-

tion were spontaneously cytolytic *in vitro* against various tumor cell lines and even against some fresh or cultured normal cells and hematopoietic cell precursors (4-9). The term *natural cytotoxicity* was therefore used to define this non-MHC-restricted, nonadaptive cellular cytotoxicity.

It is generally accepted that NK cells provide a first line of defense against tumors and certain viral infections (1). Triggering of NK cells results not only in the induction of their cytolytic activity but also in the production of cytokines that can exert a regulatory role in the immune response, inflammation, and hematopoiesis (10,11). The ability of NK cells to detect and lyse tumor cells but not normal cells has been interpreted to reflect the existence of multiple receptors for an altered pattern of ligand molecules on tumor cells. These poorly defined NK-cell functions and receptors were considered to be homogeneously expressed by virtually all NK cells rather than being distributed in a clonal fashion. More recently, however, a number of major advances have been made in the understanding of the functional properties of NK cells, and in particular the mechanisms by which NK cells lyse (or fail to lyse) given target cells (12-14). A number of putative receptors potentially involved in NK-cell triggering have been identified. More importantly, an inverse correlation has been established between the expression of surface MHC class I molecules on target cells and their susceptibility to NK-cell–mediated lysis (15,16). This suggested that MHC molecules can exert a protective role, sparing normal cells from NK-cell–mediated lysis. Lack of expression or masking of self MHC molecules, as may occur in virus-infected cells or tumor cells, would result in susceptibility to NK-cell–mediated lysis. These concepts were proposed by Kärre et al. in their "missing self" hypothesis (17,18). This hypothesis has now been confirmed and extended by experimental data in both mouse and human (12,13). In addition, success in cloning of NK cells in humans has been basic for the demonstration that NK cells display a clonal hetero-

---

L. Moretta and M. C. Mingari: University of Genova and Istituto Nazionale per la Ricerca sul Cancro, Centro Biotecnologie Avanzate, Genova, Italy.

geneity in their ability to recognize specific MHC molecules. This finding has led to the new concept that at least some NK cells can recognize allelic forms of MHC molecules by means of clonally distributed receptors.

This chapter discusses some of the general properties of NK cells, with special emphasis on recent results that have substantially changed the perception of these cells.

DEVELOPMENT OF NK CELLS

Commitment to the B- or T-cell lineage is characterized by irreversible rearrangement of the immunoglobulin (Ig) or T-cell receptor (TCR) genes, respectively. In contrast, NK cells do not rearrange Ig or TCR genes and can undergo phenotypic and functional maturation in athymic and SCID mice. Despite this "thymus independence" and the lack of TCR rearrangement, NK cells share a number of properties with T cells, and particularly with CD8-positive CTLs, including the expression of surface markers, the molecular mechanisms of target cell lysis, and the pattern of lymphokine production (1). This supports the notion that T and NK cells belong to related lineages, a relation that has been clarified by further data in mice and in humans. These data were obtained by analysis of lymphocyte differentiation during fetal ontogeny and by the development of in vitro systems that mimic in vivo environments necessary for NK- or T-cell maturation from precursors present in human postnatal thymus or fetal liver.

Although physiologic maturation of NK cells occurs in the bone marrow, a murine population has been identified in early fetal thymocytes that has the potential to differentiate toward either T- or NK-cell lineages, depending on the in vivo microenvironment (19). A predominant thymic population was detected at 14.5 days of gestation; these cells lacked both CD4 and CD8 antigens, but expressed FcγRII/III several days before the expression of TCR. When this population was maintained in a thymic microenvironment it underwent differentiation toward mature T cells, but when removed from the thymus it selectively generated functional NK cells in vivo as well as in vitro (19). These data clearly indicate that a typical marker of mature NK cells is expressed early during T-cell ontogeny. More importantly, they indicate that an immature thymocyte population gives rise to either T or NK cells depending on the microenvironment.

In agreement with these data, human postnatal thymocytes, characterized by the CD7+CD34+CD3−CD4−CD8−surface phenotype, were shown to undergo in vitro maturation toward T- or NK-cell lineages (20). Again, the pattern of maturation depended strictly on the type of microenvironment and stimuli provided. In early studies, growth of CD3−CD16+ NK cells with strong non-MHC-restricted cytolytic activity was obtained at both the population and the clonal level in the presence of exogenous interleukin-2 (IL-2) together with particu-

lar feeder cells represented by the H9 leukemia cell line. More recently, IL-15 was shown to induce optimal differentiation toward mature NK cells even in the absence of H9 feeder cells (21) (Fig. 11-1). The resulting NK cells expressed the human leukocyte antigen (HLA) class I–specific CD94/NKG2A inhibitory receptors (21) (see later discussion). These data clearly indicate that precursors of NK cells are present within the human thymus. A similar approach has been applied to the study of lymphoid precursors present in human liver isolated from embryos of 6 to 10 weeks' gestation (12).

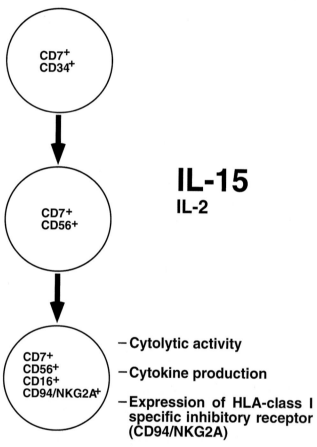

FIG. 11-1. Interleukin-15 (IL-15) induces maturation of CD7+CD34+ cell precursors into phenotypically and functionally mature natural killer (NK) cells. Early precursors isolated from bone marrow, peripheral blood, or thymus have been shown to give rise to NK cells in the presence of appropriate feeder cells and culture supplements. This figure illustrates the more recent finding that IL-15 is sufficient to induce maturation of CD7+CD34+ cells (isolated, in this case, from human thymus) toward phenotypically and functionally mature NK cells. IL-15 induces the expression of the inhibitory NK receptor (NKR) CD94/NKG2A, which has a broad human leukocyte antigen (HLA) class I specificity, but not of NKRs belonging to the immunoglobulin (Ig) superfamily. Expression of CD94/NKG2A is sufficient to prevent lysis of autologous target cells.

The precursors of CD3⁻CD16⁺ mature NK cells were found in a small subset of liver cells expressing the common leukocyte antigen CD45 (12).

Taken together, these data indicate that precursors capable of *in vitro* differentiation toward NK cells can be identified at as early as 6 weeks of gestation. In addition, although NK-cell maturation occurs primarily in the bone marrow after birth, these data show that precursors capable of differentiating toward NK cells are present in thymus. This is consistent with the concept that a common precursor undergoes maturation toward T or NK cells depending on the type of microenvironment at the maturation site. IL-15 appears to be sufficient to drive CD7⁺CD34⁺ precursors toward NK-cell maturation (21). However, it is predictable that other cytokines display a similar function. This assumption is based not only on the frequent redundancy of cytokine function but also on the finding that IL-15 induces maturation of NK cells expressing CD94/NKG2A but not those HLA class I–specific receptors belonging to the Ig superfamily (21) (see later discussion). This implies that other factors acting alone or in synergy with IL-15 are responsible for maturation of NK cells displaying a complete NK receptor (NKR) repertoire.

TISSUE DISTRIBUTION AND MIGRATION OF NK CELLS

Unlike T cells, in normal conditions NK cells are confined mostly to blood and spleen. Some NK cells can be detected in uterus, gut mucosa, and lung (1). In some pathologic conditions, such as viral or bacterial infection, they rapidly migrate to extravascular sites (22,23). In addition, NK cells have been detected in the mononuclear infiltrate of allografts in the early phase of rejection (24,25). The molecular mechanisms leading to NK-cell extravasation and recruitment into tissues have been defined only in part. NK cells express several adhesion molecules (e.g., β1 and β2 integrins) that allow attachment to endothelial cells and transmigration across endothelial monolayers (24). In addition, NK cells migrate in response to various chemotactic factors and cytokines, including tumor necrosis factor (TNF), IL-2, and IL-12 (27). The effects of different chemokines on NK-cell migration have also been documented. In addition to macrophage chemotactic protein-1 and -2 (MCP-1 and MCP-2); IL-8; macrophage inflammatory proteins-1α (MIP-1α); and the cytokine regulated on activation, normally T-cell expressed and secreted (RANTES), a new chemokine, lymphotactin (LpTn), has

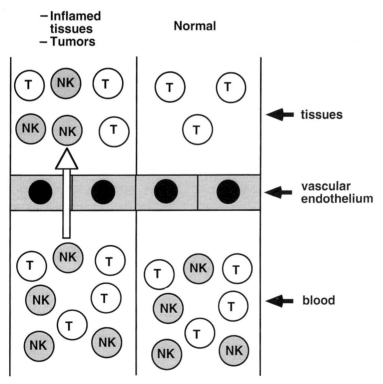

FIG. 11-2. Tissue distribution of natural killer (NK) cells in normal and inflamed tissues. In normal conditions, NK cells are mostly confined to peripheral blood (and spleen), whereas T cells recirculate in the lymph and traffic to various tissues. In the case of inflammation or tumor, NK cells can be detected in tissues and lymph nodes as a consequence of the production of various chemoattractants, cytokines, or chemokines that induce their extravasation.

been shown to exert a potent chemoattractant effect on NK cells (28). Whereas other chemokines attract diverse leukocyte types including monocytes, neutrophils, dendritic cells, and lymphocytes, LpTn is specific for the lymphoid lineage, primarily for T and NK cells.

In conclusion, a major difference in the tissue distribution of NK cells, compared with T cells, is that the latter physiologically traffic to normal tissues and recirculate in lymph and lymph nodes. In contrast, extravasation of NK cells requires signaling by chemotactic factors or chemokines (Fig. 11-2). This explains why NK cells are not found in normal lymph, lymph nodes, or most normal tissues. Detection of NK cells in these sites most likely reflects the occurrence of an inflammatory response (e.g., to infection) or the production (e.g., by tumor cells or activated macrophages) of cytokines that exert a chemoattractant effect on NK cells and determine their rapid recruitment.

RECOGNITION OF MHC CLASS I MOLECULES

Major progress has been made in understanding the mechanisms by which NK cells lyse or fail to lyse certain target cells. As indicated previously, an inverse correlation has been found between the expression of surface MHC class I molecules on target cells and their susceptibility to NK-cell–mediated lysis. This has led to the "missing self" hypothesis, which states that surface expression of MHC class I molecules can protect cells from NK lysis, whereas lack of such expression renders them susceptible to NK-mediated attack (17,18).

In accordance with this hypothesis, the NK-mediated lysis of MHC class I–negative target cells occurs *because* of the lack of self MHC molecules (17,18). This model implies that NK cells are generally activated by the interaction between triggering molecules expressed at the NK-cell surface and their ligands expressed on most nucleated cells. The MHC class I–specific NKR would exert an inhibitory effect on the activating signal that normally would lead to target cell lysis (Fig. 11-3).

In this manner, NK cells play a role complementary to that of CTLs, which are triggered on recognition of self MHC class I molecules loaded with foreign peptides. Some virus-infected cells and tumor cells downregulate the expression of single or multiple HLA alleles (29-32) (see later discussion), and in this context NK cells may play an important role by eliminating these MHC-negative cells. The "missing self" model does not exclude the possibility that normal cells expressing normal levels of MHC class I molecules may be susceptible to NK-mediated lysis. However, this can occur only with allogeneic cells carrying a mismatched MHC haplotype or with autologous cells in which MHC molecules are loaded with unusual (foreign) peptides. On the other hand, killing of normal autologous cells expressing normal levels of self MHC class I molecules has never been

observed, and loss of MHC class I molecules is sufficient to render cells susceptible to NK-cell–mediated lysis.

THE NK-CELL REPERTOIRE IN HUMANS

A precise understanding of NK-cell heterogeneity in humans became possible with the use of cloned NK cells. NK-cell clones, derived not only from different individuals but also from single donors, were found to display different patterns of cytotoxicity against allogeneic cells (35). These experiments indicated the existence of distinct groups of NK-cell clones characterized by different specificities. These groups of clones were analyzed for their ability to lyse phitohemag glutinin (PHA) blasts isolated from different members of representative families. These analyses provided clear evidence that the character "resistance to lysis" cosegregated with certain HLA haplotypes (12). At that time, evidence already existed as to the possible protective role of MHC class I molecules, but there were no data on the specific protective roles of various allelic forms of these molecules. These data provided the first evidence for the existence of a clonal heterogeneity in the ability of NK cells to recognize allelic forms of MHC molecules. Further suggestive evidence was obtained by the analysis of cell variants selectively lacking the expression of a given protective allele (12). The use of HLA class I–negative target cells transfected with HLA class I alleles provided a direct demonstration that these molecules represent the specific elements that protect cells from lysis by defined groups of NK clones (13).

Analysis of the protective effect of various HLA class I alleles indicated that all of the expressed HLA-C alleles functioned as protective elements mediated by two groups of NK clones, designated group 1 and group 2 (13). In the case of group 1 clones, the protective alleles included Cw2, Cw4, Cw5, and Cw6; in the case of group 2 clones, the protective alleles were represented by Cw1, Cw3, Cw7, and Cw8 (13,14). Comparison of the amino acid sequences of the HLA-C alleles indicated the existence of a dimorphism in residues 77 and 80 in pocket F of the $\alpha 1$ domain of HLA-C molecules. The HLA-C alleles recognized by group 1 clones have aspartic acid and lysine at these positions (Asn^{77} and Lys^{80}, respectively), whereas the HLA-C alleles recognized by group 2 NK clones are characterized by serine (Ser^{77}) and aspartic acid (Asn^{80}). Experiments in site-directed mutagenesis have confirmed the critical role of these residues in the protective effect (35).

HLA-C alleles have been shown to function as protective elements only for a fraction of NK-cell clones. On the other hand, the use of specific monoclonal antibodies (MAbs) to mask class I molecules on target cells has suggested that all clonogenic NK cells are actually specific for HLA class I molecules (14). These anti–class I MAbs induced lysis of resistant target cells by all clonogenic NK cells analyzed. They also induced lysis of normal autologous cells, suggesting that self class I molecules

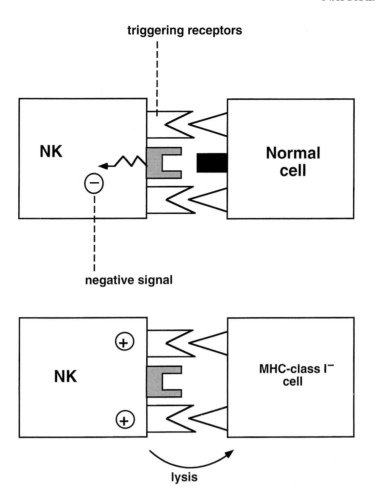

FIG. 11-3. The general mechanism of natural killer (NK)-cell activation and inactivation in target cell lysis. NK cells express a number of activating receptors that, on interaction with their ligands expressed on most nucleated cells, trigger NK cells to lyse target cells. These triggering molecules have been only partially identified, but it is generally accepted that multiple activating pathways may be involved. Such NK-cell triggering processes do not cause lysis of normal self cells, however, because of a fail-safe mechanism involving major histocompatibility complex (MHC) class I molecules expressed on normal cells (■) and specific inhibitory receptors expressed by NK cells (⊔). Cells that express normal levels of MHC class I molecules are protected from NK-mediated attack because those molecules interact with the NK receptor to generate a negative signal via activation of SHP phosphatase while inhibiting the triggering pathways. The lack of expression of MHC class I molecules that frequently occurs in tumor transformation or viral infections renders cells susceptible to NK-mediated lysis.

exert an important role by protecting normal cells from NK-cell–mediated autoreactivity. These data indicated that HLA class I molecules exert a general role in the protection from NK cells and that all NK cells are capable of recognizing one or more self MHC alleles.

MHC CLASS I–SPECIFIC INHIBITORY NK RECEPTORS

The finding that NK cells display a clonally distributed ability to recognize different HLA class I alleles implies the existence of NKRs responsible for this specific recognition. These NKRs were expected to be distributed in a clonal fashion and to mediate inhibition of NK-cell function.

NK Receptors Belonging to the Immunoglobulin Superfamily

The first identified NK-cell surface molecules displaying these properties were two glycoproteins of 58 kd, named p58.1 and p58.2 (CD158a and CD158b), respectively. MAb-mediated masking of p58 molecules led to lysis of protected, HLA class I–positive target cells. The p58.1 and p58.2 molecules were found to recognize two different groups of HLA-C alleles: Cw2, Cw4, Cw5, and Cw6 are recognized by p58.1, and Cw1, Cw3, Cw7, and Cw8 are recognized by p58.2 (36). The HLA-C alleles recognized by p58.1 share the aminoacidic positions Ser[77] and Asn[80], whereas those recognized by p58.2 have Asn[77] and Lys[80] (37). These amino acid positions are crucial for p58-mediated recognition, as shown by experiments of site-directed mutagenesis. Even a single amino acid substitution at position 77 or 80 is sufficient to render HLA-C molecules undetectable by p58+ NK-cell clones (37). Although only a fraction of NK cells (variable in different individuals) express p58 molecules, the ability to recognize HLA class I molecules is a common feature of all NK cells.

The use of p58- NK-cell clones allowed definition of other HLA class I allele specificities and, subsequently, identification of the receptors involved. These studies led to the discovery of additional receptors. For example, a 70-kd molecule was found to mediate recognition of HLA alleles belonging to the Bw4 supertypic specificity, and a 140-kd homodimer was found to mediate specific recognition of certain HLA-A alleles, including A3 and A11 (38). A role of the HLA class I–bound peptides in NK-mediated recognition has been shown in HLA-Bw4–specific NK clones. The simple binding of a peptide to HLA-B2705 was not sufficient to inhibit target-cell lysis, and only one of several peptides tested was able to confer protection. However, the limited polymorphism of NKR and the relatively low proportions of MHC molecules binding a given peptide under normal conditions would suggest a limited role for peptides in NK-mediated recognition. Perhaps only in particular situations in which a few peptides dominate the set of MHC-bound peptides (e.g., in some viral infections) does an effect on NKR-MHC interaction actually occur.

Molecular cloning of p58 molecules revealed new members of the Ig superfamily. They display some degree of sequence homology with the receptor for the human Fc portion of IgA and the mouse gp49 protein (31% and 33% homology in the extracellular portion, respectively) (39,40). P58 receptors are characterized by an extracellular region of 224 amino acids with two Ig-like domains, a transmembrane portion of 20 nonpolar amino acids, and a cytoplasmic region of variable length (76 to 84 amino acids) (Fig. 11-4). The extracellular portion contains two to four N-linked glycosylation sites. The HLA-C–specific p58 molecules are encoded by a multigene family located on chromosome 19 (39,40). Southern blot analysis revealed that the genes encoding for p58 molecules do not undergo somatic gene rearrangement. The cytoplasmic tail contains a typical motif characterized by two (V/I) XYXXL sequences, called the immunoreceptor tyrosine-based inhibitory motif (ITIM) (see Fig. 11-4). Cross-linking of p58 molecules induced by the ligand or by specific MAbs results in tyrosine phosphorylation and recruitment of the SRC homology (SH2) domain–containing tyrosine phosphatases (SHP). The effect of SHP is crucial for delivery of the negative signal that inhibits NK-cell–mediated cytotoxicity (41).

Cloning of the Bw4-specific p70 revealed a molecule displaying a high degree of sequence homology with p58 but characterized by three Ig-like domains (see Fig. 11-

4). Again, the p70-encoding gene was mapped onto chromosome 19. The HLA-A3, HLA-A11–specific p140 molecule is a homodimer formed by two receptors with three Ig-like domains linked by a disulphide bridge. It differs from p70 in about 50 amino acids in the extracellular portion. In addition, p140 receptors have a longer (95 amino acids) cytoplasmic tail (see Fig. 11-4).

NK Receptors Belonging to the C-type Lectin Superfamily

In mice, the inhibitory receptors for MHC class I molecules that have been characterized so far are represented by the Ly49 molecules, which do not belong to the Ig superfamily but are type II transmembrane proteins containing a C-type lectin domain. The type II protein CD94 has now been shown to be involved in MHC class I recognition also in humans. In early studies, CD94 molecules were described as inhibiting NKRs able to recognize operationally HLA-Bw6 alleles but not HLA-Bw4 alleles. More recently, the CD94 molecule has been shown to function as an HLA class I–specific inhibitory receptor characterized by a broad specificity, recognizing various HLA-A, -B, or -C alleles (38,42).

CD94 molecules are expressed on virtually all NK cells. Moreover, they are heterogeneous in function, since both inhibiting and activating forms of CD94 receptors have been described on different NK-cell clones. The inhibitory form of the CD94 receptor has now been shown to be formed by a heterodimeric complex with another type II protein characterized by intracytoplasmic ITIM motifs (42). Although the NKG2A-encoding cDNA was known, the corresponding molecule and its function were not identified for several years, until after NKG2A-specific MAbs were obtained in our laboratory (43).

The presence of a C-type lectin domain in CD94/NKG2A molecules suggests that a carbohydrate moiety, common to various class I alleles, may play at least a partial role in the binding of this receptor to HLA class I molecules. The broad specificity for HLA class I molecules displayed by CD94/NKG2A inhibitory receptors, together with the fact that they are expressed primarily by NK cells, which do not express receptors with a more defined specificity, suggests that these molecules may represent a receptor that evolved before the allotype-specific receptors such as p58, p70, and p140. The redundancy of receptors displaying similar specificities and functions may be important for sensing epitopes of MHC class I molecules and their possible modifications induced by virus infection or tumor transformation (Fig. 11-5). No inhibiting receptors belonging to the Ig superfamily that are specific for HLA-Bw6 or for the majority of HLA-A alleles have yet been identified. Therefore, redundancy of NKRs appears to be confined to certain HLA class I allotypes, and CD94/NKG2A may represent the only NKR available for recognition of all the remain-

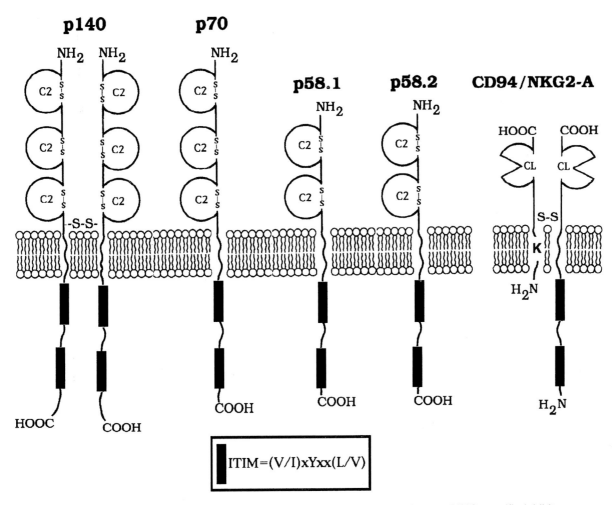

FIG. 11-4. MHC class I–specific inhibitory receptors in humans. The human MHC-specific inhibitory receptors belong to two distinct groups. The first group encompasses members of the immunoglobulin (Ig) superfamily; they are characterized by two or three Ig-like domains in the extracellular portion. The transmembrane region is composed of 20 nonpolar amino acids (aa), whereas the intracytoplasmic tail (76 to 95 aa long) is characterized by two immunoreceptor tyrosine-based inhibitory motifs (ITIM). The ITIMs recruit the SHP phosphatase, which is responsible for the inhibitory effect. This group of receptors recognize allelic forms of HLA class I molecules. For example, p58.1 and p58.2 specifically bind two distinct groups of HLA-C alleles, p70 recognizes HLA molecules sharing the Bw4 supertypic specificity, and p140 (a homodimer) displays specificity for some HLA-A alleles. The second group of receptors includes type II membrane proteins (i.e., those in which the COOH terminal is extracellular) associated in a heterodimeric form comprising CD94 and a member of the NKG2 family (NKG2A or NKG2B). This inhibitory receptor has a broader specificity for HLA class I alleles (although it preferentially recognizes certain alleles and binds poorly to others).

ing HLA-B and HLA-A alleles. CD94/NKG2A may represent a fundamental device to control NK-mediated autoreactivity.

Molecular Mechanisms of NK-Cell Activation

Although detailed information is available concerning the MHC class I–specific NKR, the nature of the triggering surface molecules involved in target cell recognition and lysis has long remained elusive. Most of the known triggering molecules are shared by T lymphocytes (1,13). A number of adhesion molecules not only mediate NK-cell adhesion to other cells but also transmit triggering signals that may lead to cell activation and triggering of the cytolytic machinery. In this context, it is possible that NK-cell triggering results from a number of interactions between adhesion molecules and their ligands (14). Release of inflammatory cytokines results in the *de novo* expression or upregulation of different adhesion molecules by different cell types. It is conceivable that the expression of an appropriate pattern of adhesion molecules by NK cells or of a

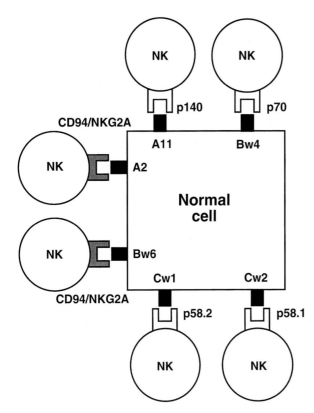

FIG. 11-5. Human natural killer (NK) cells display clonally distributed receptors for self human leukocyte antigen (HLA) class I alleles. In this representative donor with HLA haplotype HLA-A2, HLA-A11; HLA-B7 (Bw6), HLA-B27 (Bw4); HLA-Cw1, HLA-Cw2, each NK cell expresses at least one inhibitory receptor (NKR) interacting with a self HLA allele. The NKRs depicted in white are those belonging to the immunoglobulin (Ig) superfamily, which recognize allelic forms of HLA class I molecules. The CD94/NKG2A receptors (depicted in gray) display a broad specificity for class I molecules, although they preferentially recognize certain alleles (e.g., alleles of the Bw6 supertypic specificities). The receptors belonging to the Ig superfamily do not cover the whole set of HLA class I alleles and are not expressed by 100% of NK cells. Therefore, CD94/NKG2A may play an important role in recognition of various class I alleles and in inhibition of cytolysis by NK cells that lack NKRs belonging to the Ig superfamily.

high density of the corresponding ligands, or both, is responsible for NK-cell activation (14,44). Resting NK cells express CD2, CD11a/CD18 (lymphocyte function antigen-1, or LFA-1), CD49d/CD29 (very late activation antigen-4, or VLA-4). Cell activation results in upregulation of these molecules and in *de novo* expression of CD69, which mediates a potent NK-cell triggering. Several additional triggering surface molecules have now been identified, including the recently characterized NK$_r$46, which is strictly NK-cell specific and induces a strong NK-cell triggering (45). Although the natural ligand of this molecule has not been identified, mAbs against the molecule significantly inhibit lysis of

certain tumor target cells, suggesting a role for NK$_r$46 in NK-cell triggering during tumor cell lysis (46,47).

Activating forms of the inhibitory receptors belonging to the Ig superfamily also have been identified (14). Although these molecules are highly homologous to their corresponding inhibitory forms, they are different in their transmembrane and intracytoplasmic portions. The intracytoplasmic portion does not contain the ITIM motifs that are crucial for generation of inhibitory activity. A possible function of these receptors is to provide yet another pathway for optimal NK-cell triggering in the case of HLA class I–positive target cells (14,48). Another possibility (which does not exclude the previous interpretation) is that the activating form of the NKR may be triggered preferentially by HLA class I molecules that bind unusual peptides (e.g., viral or heat shock proteins). In this context, the amino acid sequences of the extracellular portions are highly homologous in inhibitory and activating forms, only a few differences having been detected.

A well-known triggering receptor expressed by NK cells is CD16, the low-affinity Fc receptor for IgG (1). IgG antibody–coated target cells trigger antibody-dependent cellular cytotoxicity (ADCC) and cytokine production. The latter can also be induced by IgG immune complexes. CD16 is associated with FcεRIγ and with CD3 ζ chains, which are involved in signal transduction. It is unclear whether CD16 can serve functions other than ADCC and, consequently, whether ligands different from IgG immune complexes can bind CD16.

Efficient NK-cell triggering also occurs in response to several cytokines, including IL-15, TNF-α, and IL-12, that are produced by activated macrophages at sites of inflammation. This triggering results in rapid production of interferon-γ (IFN-γ) after infection and before triggering of specific immune responses. The effect of IFN-γ may largely explain the important role of NK cells in the innate response to pathogens (1). In addition, at a later stage, IL-2 produced by T lymphocytes may substantially contribute to NK-cell triggering and to amplification of the immune response (1).

NK-CELL INVOLVEMENT IN ANTIVIRAL RESPONSES

It is well known that T lymphocytes, primarily MHC class I–restricted CD8$^+$ CTLs, play a major role in the control of viral infections. Some DNA viruses, however, have evolved strategies to interfere with the process of MHC presentation of viral peptides to CTLs. Advances in understanding of the mechanisms involved in antigen presentation have allowed the unraveling of several of the molecular mechanisms by which viruses accomplish this interference. However, although downregulation of cell-surface expression of MHC class I molecules prevents the CTL-mediated lysis of infected cells, it should also render them susceptible to NK-mediated lysis.

The first known example of viral protein interference with the MHC class I pathway was the E19 protein of adenovirus (49). Because the E19 molecule interacts with MHC class I molecules at the level of the endoplasmic reticulum (ER), class I molecules do not reach the cell surface but are retrieved from the Golgi apparatus together with E19 molecules. Not all of the HLA class I alleles bind equally well to E19, so that the protein preferentially inhibits the expression of certain alleles (thereby rendering cells susceptible to lysis by NK-cell subsets expressing appropriate NKRs).

Other viruses that inhibit MHC class I expression include members of the herpesvirus family. For example, the herpes simplex–encoded ICP47 molecule binds to transporters associated with antigen processing-1 and -2 (TAP-1 and TAP-2) in the cytosol and prevents the TAP-mediated binding and transport of peptides. The human cytomegalovirus (hCMV) employs several different strategies to inhibit HLA class I expression (49). The US6 glycoprotein resides in the ER and interferes with peptide translocation but not with binding of peptides to TAP molecules. US11 prevents the HLA class I heavy chains from leaving the ER compartment and shuttles them back into the cytosol, where they are degraded by proteasomes. US3 protein is expressed very early during hCMV infection, as early as virus-encoded transcription factors; it binds to class I molecules and prevents their export to the surface. Consequently, in the course of hCMV infection, HLA class I molecules are first retained and then degraded, suggesting that US3 represents the first line of viral interference, followed by US11 and possibly by other US proteins.

NK cells play an important role in controlling both HSV and hCMV infections. However, a potential mechanism to escape NK-cell recognition can be found in the expression of a β_2-binding protein with a structural homology to the MHC class I heavy chain. This protein, termed UL18, also binds peptides (50,51). Rather than interfering substantially with antigen presentation, unique long (UL) 18 has been shown to function by protecting hCMV-infected cells against NK-cell lysis (52). Experiments have shown that UL18 transfection into HLA class I–negative target cells confers on these cells resistance to NK-mediated lysis. The broad-specificity CD94/NKG2A receptor appears to be responsible for binding UL18 (52). Therefore, hCMV has evolved two complementary strategies to avoid identification of infected cells by both CTLs and NK cells. A corollary of the fact that hCMV has developed a mechanism for evading NK-mediated detection is that NK cells must represent an important component of the cell-mediated immune response to viral infection.

EXPRESSION OF NK RECEPTORS ON A T-CELL SUBSET

A subset of memory T cells, primarily CD8+ CTLs, have been found to express HLA class I–specific inhibitory

NKRs belonging to the Ig or C-type lectin superfamilies (53,54). These NKRs have been detected in both $\alpha\beta$ and $\gamma\delta$ T lymphocytes (53). Interaction of these receptors with their specific ligands leads to inhibition of CTL functions, including those mediated by the TCR pathway of activation (53).

The expression of HLA class I–specific inhibitory receptors poses an important question as to the actual significance of such inhibition. A possible explanation is that the expression of inhibitory NKRs represents a fail-safe mechanism that prevents autoimmunity, particularly for those CTLs that have acquired NK-like activity and could lyse normal cells. It is possible that the expression of NKRs parallels the acquisition of NK-like activity by the CTLs. The acquisition of NK-like activity probably reflects (at least in part) the de novo expression of triggering surface receptor molecules that mediate binding of CTLs to target cells and their subsequent activation. The expression of the inhibitory NKR would prevent CTL triggering. If this is indeed the case, it is conceivable that expression of both the set of activating molecules and the inhibitory NKR is induced by the same signal or signals. In this context it has recently been shown that both IL-15 and transforming growth factor-β (TGF-β) induce the de novo expression of CD94/NKG2A in superantigen or alloantigen triggered T cells (55,56). On the other hand, it is evident that expression of NKRs that work against the main function of CTLs—to eliminate cells that present foreign antigens—could be dangerous to the host in certain chronic viral infections or in antitumor responses. NKR-mediated inhibition may lead to a less efficient control of tumor growth or viral infection by virus-specific CTLs.

The fact that antigen-specific CTLs may simultaneously express TCRs and NKRs, both recognizing MHC class I molecules but mediating signals of opposite sign, offers new perspectives for a better understanding of the regulation of T-cell responses (57).

ACKNOWLEDGMENTS

This work was supported by grants awarded by the Associazione Italiana per la Ricerca sul Cancro (AIRC), Istituto Superiore di Sanità (ISS), Consiglio Nazionale delle Ricerche (CNR), Progetto Finalizzato ACRO, and Ministero dell Università e della Ricerca Scientifica e Tecnologica (MURST) to L. Moretta and grants by MURST and ISS to M. C. Mingari.

REFERENCES

1. Trinchieri G. Biology of natural killer cells. *Adv Immunol* 1989;47:187–376.
2. Zinkernagel RM, Doherty P. Immunological surveillance against altered self components by sensitized T lymphocytes in lymphochoriomeningitis. *Nature* 1974;251:457.
3. Trinchieri G, Aden D, Knowles BB. Cell-mediated cytotoxicity to SV40-specific tumor-associated antigens. *Nature* 1976;261:312.
4. Jondal M, Pross H. Surface markers on human B and T lymphocytes: VI. Cytotoxicity against cell lines as a functional marker for lymphocyte subpopulations. *Int J Cancer* 1975;15:596.

5. Matthews N, MacLaurin BP, Clarke GN. Characterization of the normal lymphocyte population cytolytic to Burkitt's lymphoma cells of the EB2 cell line. *J Exp Biol Med Sci* 1975;53:389.

6. Ortaldo JR, Oldham RK, Cannon GC, Herberman RB. Specificity of natural cytotoxic reactivity of normal human lymphocytes against a myeloid leukemia cell line. *J Natl Cancer Inst* 1977;59:77.

7. Peter HH, Pavie-Fischer J, Fridman WH, et al. Cell-mediated cytotoxicity in vitro of human lymphocytes against a tissue culture melanoma cell line (IGR3). *J Immunol* 1975;115:539.

8. Takasuki M, Mickey MR, Terasaki PI. Reactivity of lymphocytes from normal persons on cultured tumor cells. *Cancer Res* 1973;33:2898.

9. West WH, Cannon GB, Kay HD, Bonnard GD, Herberman RB. Natural cytotoxic reactivity of human lymphocytes against a myeloid cell line: Characterization of the effector cells. *J Immunol* 1977;118:355.

10. Trinchieri G. Natural killer cells wear different hats: Effector cells of innate resistance and regulatory cells of adoptive immunity and hematopoiesis. *Semin Immunol* 1995;7:83–88.

11. Bellone G, Valiante NM, Viale O, Ciccone E, Moretta L, Trinchieri G. Regulation of hematopoiesis in vitro by alloreactive natural killer cell clones. *J Exp Med* 1993;77:1117–1122.

12. Moretta L, Ciccone E, Moretta A, Höglund P, Öhlen C, Kärre K. Allorecognition by NK cells: Nonself or no self? *Immunol Today* 1992;13:300–306.

13. Moretta L, Ciccone E, Mingari MC, Biassoni R, Moretta A. Human NK cells: Origin, clonality, specificity and receptors. *Adv Immunol* 1994;55:341–380.

14. Moretta A, Bottino C, Vitale M, et al. Receptors for HLA class I molecules in human natural killer cells. *Annu Rev Immunol* 1996;14:619–648.

15. Ljunggren HG, Kärre K. Host resistance directed selectively against H-2–deficient lymphoma variants: Analysis of the mechanism. *J Exp Med* 1985;162:1745–1759.

16. Storkus WJ, Howell DN, Salter RD, Dawson JR, Cresswell P. NK susceptibility varies inversely with target cell class I HLA antigen expression. *J Immunol* 1987;138:1657–1659.

17. Ljunggren H-G, Kärre K. In search of the "missing self": MHC molecules and NK cell recognition. *Immunol Today* 1990;11:237–44.

18. Kärre K. An unexpected petition for pardon. *Curr Biol* 1992;2:613–616.

19. Rodewald HR, Moingeon P, Lucich JL, Dosiou C, Lopez P, Reinherz EL. A population of early fetal thymocytes expressing FcγRII/III contains precursors of T lymphocytes and natural killer cells. *Cell* 1992;69:139.

20. Mingari MC, Poggi A, Biassoni R, et al. In vitro proliferation and cloning of CD3-CD16+ cells from human thymocyte precursors. *J Exp Med* 1991;174:21–26.

21. Mingari MC, Vitale C, Cantoni C, et al. Interleukin-15-induced maturation of human natural killer cells from early thymic precursors: Selective expression of CD94/NKG2A as the only HLA-class I specific inhibitory receptor. *Eur J Immunol* (in press).

22. Sanchez MJ, Muench MO, Roncarolo MG, Lanier LL, Phillips JH. Identification of a common T/natural killer cell progenitor in human fetal liver. *J Exp Med* 1994;180:569–576.

23. McIntyre KW, Welsh RM. *J Exp Med* 1986;164:1667.

24. Su HC, Ishikawa R, Biron CA. *J Immunol* 1993;151:4874.

25. Nemlander A, Saksela E, Hayrj P. *Eur J Immunol* 1983;13:348.

26. Inverardi L, Samaja M, Motterlini R, Mangili F, Bender JR, Pardi R. *J Immunol* 1992;149:1416.

27. Allavena P, Paganin C, Martin Padura I, et al. *J Exp Med* 1991;173:439.

28. Bianchi G, Sironi M, Ghibaudi E, et al. *J Immunol* 1993;151:5135.

29. Allavena P, Paganin C, Zhou D, Bianchi G, Sozzani S, Mantovani A. *Blood* 1994;84:2261.

30. Bianchi G, Sozzani S, Zlotnik A, Mantovani A, Allavena P. Migratory response of human natural killer cells to lymphotactin. *Eur J Immunol* 1996;26:3238–3241.

31. Garrido F. MHC molecules in normal and neoplastic cells. *Int J Cancer* 1996;6:1–10.

32. Burgert HG, Maryanski HL, Kvist S. E3/19K protein of adenovirus type 2 inhibits lysis of cytolytic T lymphocytes by blocking cell-surface expression of histocompatibility class I antigens. *Proc Natl Acad Sci U S A* 1987;84:1356–1360.

33. Del Val M, Hengel H, Häcker H, et al. Cytomegalovirus prevents antigen presentation by blocking the transport of peptide-loaded major histocompatibility complex class I molecules into the medial-Golgi compartment. *J Exp Med* 1992;176:729–738.

34. Garrido F, Cabrera T, Lopez Nevot MA, Ruiz-Cabello F. HLA-class I antigens in human tumours. *Adv in Cancer Res* 1995;67:155–195.

35. Ciccone E, Pende D, Viale O, et al. Evidence of a natural killer (NK) cell repertoire for (allo)antigen recognition: Definition of five distinct NK-determined allospecificities in humans. *J Exp Med* 1992;175:709–718.

36. Moretta A, Vitale M, Bottino C, et al. P58 molecules as putative receptors for MHC class I molecules in human natural killer (NK) cells: Anti-p58 antibodies reconstitute lysis of MHC class I–protected cells in NK clones displaying different specificities. *J Exp Med* 1993;178:597–604.

37. Biassoni R, Falco M, Cambiaggi A, et al. Amino acid substitutions can influence the NK-mediated recognition of HLA-C molecules: Role of Serine-77 and lysine-80 in the target cell protection from lysis mediated by group 2 or group 1 NK clones. *J Exp Med* 1995;182:605–609.

38. Moretta A, Biassoni R, Bottino C, et al. Major histocompatibility complex class I–specific receptors on human natural killer and T lymphocytes. *Immunol Rev* 1997;155:105–117.

39. Wagtmann N, Biassoni R, Cantoni C, et al. Molecular clones of the p58 NK cell receptor reveal immunoglobulin related molecules with diversity in both the extra- and intracellular domains. *Immunity* 1995;2:439–449.

40. Colonna M, Samaridis J. Cloning of immunoglobulin-superfamily members associated with HLA-C and HLA-B recognition by human natural killer cells. *Science* 1995;268:405–408.

41. Olcese L, Lang P, Vély F, et al. Human and mouse natural killer cell inhibitory receptors recruit the PTP1C and PTP1D protein tyrosine phosphatase. *J Immunol* 1996;156:4531–4534.

42. Carretero M, Cantoni C, Bellón T, et al. The CD94 and NKG2-A C-type lectins covalently assemble to form a NK cell inhibitory receptor for HLA class I molecules. *Eur J Immunol* 1997;27:563–567.

43. Sivori S, Vitale M, Bottino C, et al. CD94 functions as a natural killer cell inhibitory receptor for different HLA-class-I alleles: Identification of the inhibitory form of CD94 by the use of novel monoclonal antibodies. *Eur J Immunol* 1996;26:2487–2492.

44. Lanier LL, Corliss B, Phillips JH. Arousal and inhibition of human NK cells. *Immunol Rev* 1997;155:145–154.

45. Sivori S, Vitale M, Morelli L, et al. p46, a novel natural killer cell-specific surface molecule which mediates cell activation. *J Exp Med* 1997;186(7):1129–1136.

46. Pessino A, Sivori S, Bottino C, et al. Molecular cloning of NKp46: a novel member of the immunoglobulin superfamily involved in triggering of Natural cytotoxicity. *J Exp Med* 1998;188:953:960.

47. Vitale M, Bottino C, Sivori S, et al. NKp44, a novel triggering surface molecule specifically expressed by activated Natural Killer cells is involved in non-MHC restricted tumor cell lysis. *J Exp Med* 1998;187:2065–2072.

48. Biassoni R, Cantoni C, Falco M, et al. The human Leukocyte Antigen (HLA)-C-specific "activatory" or "inhibitory" Natural Killer cell receptors display highly homologous extracellular domains but differ in their transmembrane and intracytoplasmic portions. *J Exp Med* 1996;183:645–650.

49. Fruh K, Ahn K, Peterson PA. Inhibition of MHC class I antigen presentation by viral proteins. *J Mol Med* 1997;75:18–27.

50. Beck S, Barrell BG. Human cytomegalovirus encodes a glycoprotein homologous to MHC class I antigens. *Nature* 1988;331:269–272.

51. Fahnestock MJ, Johnson JL, Feldman RM, Neveu JM, Lane WS, Bjorkman PJ. The MHC class I homolog encoded by human cytomegalovirus binds endogenous peptides. *Immunity* 1995;3:583–590.

52. Reyburn H, Mandelboim O, Valés-Goméz M, et al. Human NK cells: Their ligands, receptors and functions. *Immunol Rev* 1997;155:119–125.

53. Mingari MC, Vitale C, Cambiaggi A, et al. Cytolytic T lymphocytes displaying Natural Killer (NK)-like activity: Expression of NK-related functional receptors for HLA class I molecules (p58 and CD94) and inhibitory effect on the TCR-mediated target cell lysis or lymphokine production. *Int Immunol* 1995;7:697–703.

54. Mingari MC, Schiavetti F, Ponte M, et al. Human CD8+ T lymphocyte subsets that express HLA-class I specific inhibitory receptors represent oligoclonally or monoclonally expanded cell populations. *Proc Natl Acad Sci U S A* 1996;93:12433–12438.

55. Mingari MC, Ponte M, Bertone S, et al. HLA-class I-specific inhibitory receptors in human T lymphocytes. IL-15 induced expression of CD94/NKG2A in superantigen- or alloantigen-activated human T cells. *Proc Natl Acad Sci U S A* 1998;95:1172–1177.

56. Bertone S, Schiavetti F, Bellomo R, et al. Transforming growth factor-β–induced expression of CD94/NKG2A inhibitory receptors in human T lymphocytes. *Eur J Immunol* 1998;28:1–7.

57. Mingari MC, Moretta A, Moretta L. Regulation of KIR expression in human T lymphocytes. A safety mechanism which may impair protective T cell responses. *Immunol Today* 1998;19:153–157.

Inflammation: Basic Principles and Clinical Correlates,
3rd ed., edited by John I. Gallin and Ralph Snyderman.
Lippincott Williams & Wilkins, Philadelphia © 1999.

CHAPTER 12

CD4 Effector Cells

Sergio Romagnani

Infectious microorganisms, although able to elicit an immunologic response, have evolved numerous mechanisms for evading the consequences of immune aggression. Teleologically, attempts of microorganisms to colonize the host were continually held at bay by the process of natural selection, which in humans and other higher organisms continuously shaped and refined the mechanisms used by the immune system to defend against infection. In vertebrates, specialized types of specific immune responses have evolved in response to different microorganisms that allow their recognition and elimination or control. For example, viruses, which grow within the cytoplasm and the nucleus of the infected cell, can be eliminated only by killing their host cells. To this end, viral antigens synthesized within the infected cell are presented on the cell surface in association with class I major histocompatibility complex (MHC) molecules and recognized by CD8-positive (CD8$^+$) class I MHC-restricted cytotoxic T lymphocytes. Most other microbial antigens are endocytosed by antigen-presenting cells (APCs), such as macrophages, dendritic cells, and B lymphocytes; processed into the endosomes; and presented preferentially in association with class II MHC molecules to CD4$^+$ class II MHC-restricted helper T (T$_H$) cells. CD4$^+$ T cells collaborate with B lymphocytes for the production of antibodies that, with or without the collaboration of serum complement proteins, are able to challenge microbes living outside cells or neutralize their soluble toxic products (i.e., exotoxins). This branch of the specific T$_H$ cell-mediated immune response is known as *humoral immunity.*

Microbes such as mycobacteria can survive and multiply within macrophages despite the unfavorable life conditions provided by the background activity of proteolytic enzymes and other toxic substances produced by these cells. CD4$^+$ T$_H$ cells, responding to mycobacterial soluble antigens, can activate macrophages to produce reactive oxygen intermediates, nitric oxide, and tumor necrosis factor-α (TNF-α, which participate in destruction of the microbe. This branch of the specific T$_H$ cell-mediated immune response is known as *cellular immunity* or *cell-mediated immunity* (CMI). Because the occurrence of CMI can be revealed by demonstration of an indurative skin reaction, resulting from the accumulation of mononuclear cells and appearing 24 to 96 hours after the intradermal injection of antigen, it is also commonly defined as *delayed-type hypersensitivity* (DTH) reaction.

Most immune responses involve both branches of the immune system, humoral immunity and DTH, acting in concert. However, the two types of effector reactions may also be mutually exclusive in some conditions. In certain experimental models, suppression of DTH may be associated with increased levels of antibody production.

CHARACTERISTICS OF CD4$^+$ HELPER T-CELL SUBSETS

The mechanisms by which CD4$^+$ T$_H$ cells may be responsible for humoral immunity or CMI in response to different infectious agents or in the course of the same infection remained unclear until Mosmann et al. (1) provided evidence that repeated stimulation of murine CD4$^+$ T$_H$ lymphocytes *in vitro* with given antigens produced a restricted and stereotyped pattern of lymphokine production: type 1 (T$_H$1) and type 2 (T$_H$2). T$_H$1 cells produce interferon-γ (IFN-γ), interleukin-2 (IL-2), and TNF-β, which mediate macrophage activation and DTH reactions. The T$_H$2 cells produce IL-4, IL-5, IL-6, IL-10, and IL-13, which act as growth or differentiation factors for B cells, providing an explanation for the observed dichotomy of immune responses. Subsequently, a similar

S. Romagnani: Institute of Internal Medicine and Immunoallergology, University of Florence, Florence, Italy 50134.

heterogeneity in the cytokine profile was observed even among CD8$^+$ cytotoxic T cells (T$_C$1 and T$_C$2) (2) and among T cells expressing the $\gamma\delta$ antigen receptor (3).

T$_H$1 and T$_H$2 are not the only cytokine patterns possible. T cells expressing cytokines of both patterns have been designated T$_H$0, and additional patterns have been described among long-term clones (4). T$_H$0 cells probably represent a heterogenous population of partially differentiated effector cells consisting of multiple, discrete subsets that can secrete T$_H$1 and T$_H$2 cytokines (4). The cytokine response at effector level can remain mixed or can be induced to further differentiate into the T$_H$1 or T$_H$2 pathway under the influence of polarizing signals received from the microenvironment. Some studies, however, have demonstrated heterogeneity of cytokine synthesis at the single-cell level even in polarized T$_H$1 and T$_H$2 responses. Moreover, each of the cytokine genes seems to be under unique control, with distinct tendencies for concordant (e.g., IL-4 and IL-5) or discordant (e.g., IL-4 and IFN-γ) expression. On the basis of such results, the existence of T-cell subsets whose functional differences are determined by their cytokine profile has been questioned (5).

Two main series of findings, however, confirm the validity of the T$_H$1 and T$_H$2 paradigm. First, in many experimental models, induced and naturally occurring immune responses are characterized by a clear pattern of T$_H$1 or T$_H$2 predominance (6). Second, T-cell subsets comparable to murine T$_H$1 and T$_H$2 cells can be detected in a variety of chronic infectious or immunopathologic human disorders (7).

Classification of T$_H$1 and T$_H$2 cells as responsible for CMI and humoral immunity is an oversimplification. In addition to their ability to activate macrophages, T$_H$1 cells are able to promote the production of immunoglobulin G2a opsonizing and complement-fixing antibodies (2,4) (Table 12-1). It is more appropriate to consider T$_H$1 cells as effectors of phagocyte-dependent responses (4,8). However, some cytokines produced by T$_H$2 cells (e.g., IL-4, IL-10, IL-13) provide B-cell help for antibody production and inhibit several macrophage functions (2,4) (see Table 12-1). T$_H$2 cells may be considered as effectors of phagocyte-independent responses (4,8). In general, human T cells exhibit a less restricted cytokine profile than murine T cells. For example, IL-2, IL-6, IL-10, and IL-13 tend to segregate less clearly among human CD4$^+$ subsets than in the mouse (9). Nevertheless, human T$_H$1 and T$_H$2 clones

TABLE 12-1. *Main functional properties of murine T$_H$1 and T$_H$2 cells*

Property	T$_H$1	T$_H$2
Cytokine production		
IL-2	++	–
IFN-γ	++	–
TNF-β	++	–
TNF-α	++	+
GM-CSF	++	+
IL-3	++	++
IL-4	–	++
IL-5	–	++
IL-6	–	+
IL-9	–	++
IL-10	–	++
IL-13	–	++
B-cell help		
IgM	++	++
IgG1	+	++
IgG2a	++	+
IgE	–	++
Macrophage activation	++	–
Delayed-type hypersensitivity	++	–
Cytotoxicity	++	–
Antibody-dependent cell-mediated cytotoxicity	++	–
Inhibition of macrophage function	–	++
Eosinophil differentiation and activation	–	++
Mast cell growth	–	++

IFN, interferon; IL, interleukin; GM-SCF, granulocyte-macrophage colony-stimulating factor; Ig, immunoglobulin; +, positive; ++, strong; –, absent.
From ref. 7, with permission.

TABLE 12-2. *Main properties of human T$_H$1 and T$_H$2 cells*

Property	T$_H$1	T$_H$2
Cytokine secretion		
IFN-γ	+++	–
TNF-β	+++	–
IL-2	+++	+
TNF-α	+++	+
GM-CSF	++	++
IL-3	++	+++
IL-10	+	++
IL-13	++	+++
IL-4	–	+++
IL-5	–	+++
Cytolytic potential	+++	–
B-cell help for Ig synthesis		
IgE	–	+++
IgM, IgG, IgA		
At low T/B ratios	+++	++
At high T/B ratios	–	+++
Macrophage activation		
Induction of PCA	+++	–
TF production	+++	–
Surface expression		
LAG-3	+++	+/–
mIFN-γ	+	–
CCR5	+++	+/–
CXCR3	+++	++
CD30	+/–	+++
CCR3	–	+/–
CCR4	–	+
CCR8	–	+
CXCR4	+	+++

IFN, interferon; IL, interleukin; GM-SCF, granulocyte-macrophage colony-stimulating factor; LAG-3, lymphocyte activation gene-3 product; TF, tissue factor; TNF, tumor necrosis factor; PCA, procoagulant activity; –, absent; +/–, poor or transient; +, positive; ++, strong; +++, very strong.
From ref. 7, with permission.

also exhibit distinct functional properties and preferential expression of some activation markers. Th1 cells express the lymphocyte activation gene-3 (LAG-3), CD26, membrane IFN-γ (mIFN-γ) and the chemokine receptors CCR5 and CXCR3. Th2 cells preferentially express CD30 and the chemokine receptors CCR3, CCR4, and CCR8 (56). Moreover, the chemokine receptor CSCR4 is up-regulated by IL-4 and down-regulated by IFN-γ (Table 12-2) (57).

These findings and the results of studies performed on gene-targeted mice have shown that T_H1-dominated responses are highly protective against most microbes and usually eliminate them. However, if the microbe persists in

the body, the ongoing T_H1 response results in inflammatory tissue injury (Fig. 12-1). T_H2-dominated responses are usually observed during infections sustained by gastrointestinal nematodes (10). This type of response avoids the extensive inflammatory tissue injury that may result from challenging such complex parasites by T_H1 cells and macrophages. A switch to a T_H2-dominated response also can occur in the course of some immune responses against microbes when the T_H1 response cannot rapidly eradicate the infection. Some cytokines (e.g., IL-4, IL-10, IL-13) produced by T_H2 cells inhibit the development of T_H1 cells and inhibit the activity of T_H1 cells and macrophages,

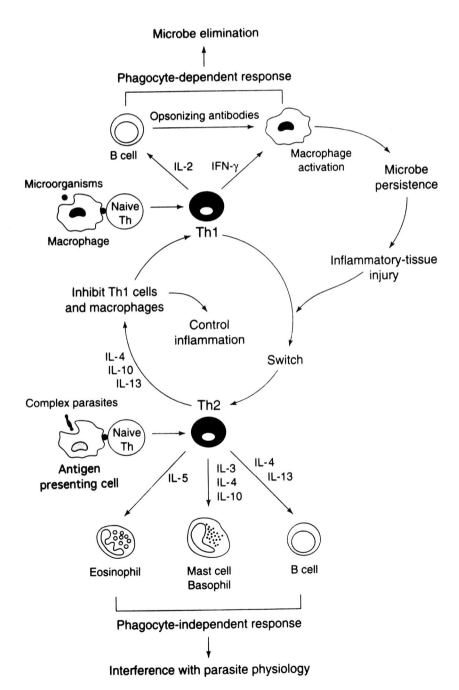

FIG. 12-1. The T_H1-T_H2 paradigm. Microbes, especially intracellular parasites, are challenged by T_H1 cells, which are able to promote the activation of macrophages through release of interferon (IFN)-γ and the production of opsonizing antibodies through release of interleukin (IL)-2 and IFN-γ. This phagocyte-dependent response usually promotes the microbe's elimination. If the microbe persists despite such a response, the inflammatory reaction triggered by T_H1 cells and macrophages can result in tissue injury. Large and complex parasites such as gastrointestinal nematodes, which cannot be rapidly eliminated by T_H1 cells because of their size, are challenged by T_H2 cells, which do not kill them but interfere with their physiology. The T_H2 cells inhibit the development and function of T_H1 cells through IL-4 and IL-10 and several macrophage functions through IL-4, IL-10, and IL-13. This phagocyte-independent response also may occur as a result of a "switch" during infections sustained by microbes that are not rapidly cleared by T_H1 cells, resulting in the control of dangerous inflammation. (From ref. 8, with permission.)

avoiding or reducing the inflammatory tissue injury that may be harmful to the host. These findings suggest that the most important physiologic function of T_H2 cells may be as regulators of immune responses (4,8,9) (see Fig. 12-1).

POLARIZED IMMUNE RESPONSES OF HELPER T-CELL SUBSETS

In the last few years, the factors responsible for the polarization of the specific immune response into a predominant T_H1 or T_H2 profile have been extensively investigated. Strong evidence suggests that T_H1 and T_H2 cells do not derive from distinct lineages; they instead develop from the same T_H-cell precursor under the influence of mechanisms acting at the level of antigen presentation (11). Environmental and genetic factors influence T_H1 or T_H2 differentiation by determining the predominance of a given cytokine in the microenvironment of the responding T_H cell (Fig. 12-2). The early presence of IL-4 is the most potent stimulus for T_H2 differentiation, whereas IL-12 and IFNs favor T_H1 development (12–15). Among the environmental factors, a role has been demonstrated for the site of antigen presentation, the physical form of immunogen, the type of adjuvant, and the dose of antigen (16). For example, potent adjuvants and many microbial products, particularly from intracellular bacteria (e.g., *Mycobacterium, Listeria*) and protozoa (e.g., *Toxoplasma*), induce T_H1-dominated responses because they stimulate IL-12 production. IFN-γ and IFN-α also favor T_H1 development by enhancing IL-12 secretion by macrophages or by maintaining the expression of functional IL-12 receptors on T_H cells (17).

The source of IL-4 and the mechanisms responsible for the early IL-4 production involved in the differentiation of naive T_H cells into T_H2 effectors are still unclear. Under certain circumstances, one such source may be a small subset of CD4-NK1.1$^+$ cells capable of recognizing antigens presented in association with the nonpolymorphic β2-microglobulin–associated molecule, CD1 (18). However, it is likely that T cells themselves produce small amounts of IL-4 from their initial activation and that the concentration of IL-4 that accumulates at the level of the T_H cell response increases with increasing lymphocyte activation. The inducing effect of IL-4 dominates other cytokines; if IL-4 levels reach a necessary threshold, differentiation of the T_H cell into the T_H2 phenotype occurs (16).

The genetic mechanisms that concur with the environmental factors in controlling the type of T_H cell differentiation remain elusive. Such mechanisms may act at the level of co-stimulatory molecules on APCs, the T-cell receptor repertoire, or the release of hormones in the microenvironment (see Fig. 12-2). A locus on murine chromosome 11, designated T-cell phenotype switch-1 *(Tps-1)*, may control the maintenance of IL-12 responsiveness and therefore the subsequent T_H1 or T_H2 response (19).

The molecular mechanisms by which IL-4 and IL-12 or IFN promote the development of naive T_H cells into T_H2

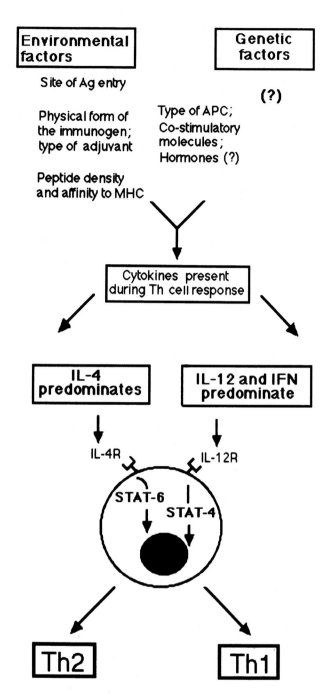

FIG. 12-2. Polarizing factors for T_H1 and T_H2 development. Environmental and genetic factors influence the development of T_H cells into T_H1 or T_H2 effectors by determining the early predominance of interleukin (IL)-4 or IL-12 plus interferon (IFN) during the T_H cell response. If IL-4 predominates, the STAT-4 intracellular signaling pathway is activated in the T_H cell, which promotes the production of IL-4 and T_H2 polarization; if IL-12 and IFN predominate, the STAT-6 pathway is activated, which promotes T_H1 development. Although some environmental factors influencing T_H1 or T_H2 development are well known, the genetic mechanisms involved remain unclear. A locus, called T-cell phenotype switch-1 (TPS-1), that maintains the IL-12 responsiveness of the T_H cell may be involved in the control of T_H1 and T_H2 development. (From ref. 8, with permission.)

or T$_H$1 effectors are being clarified. The binding of cytokines to their receptors typically results in receptor homodimerization or heterodimerization and triggers intracellular signals. One important component of cytokine signaling is specific transcriptional activation of target genes, which is rapid and does not require the synthesis of new proteins. Analysis of rapid transduction of signals to the nucleus has led to the identification and characterization of the JAK signal transducer and activator of transcription (STAT) signaling pathway (20). STAT factors are rapidly tyrosine phosphorylated after stimulation with cytokines and subsequently dimerize and translocate to the nucleus, where they can activate transcription. Six members of the STAT family, STAT-1 through STAT-6, have been identified and characterized. Among CD4$^+$ T cells, functional receptors for IL-12 appear restricted to recently activated, uncommitted cells and to T$_H$1 cells, and are lost on differentiated T$_H$2 cells. IL-12 activates STAT-1, STAT-3, and STAT-4. Of these, STAT-4 appears to be selectively activated by IL-12 (see Fig. 12-2), and targeting of the *STAT4* gene results in inhibition of T$_H$1 responses (21,22). However, signaling by IL-4 occurs through activation of STAT-6 (see Fig. 12-2), and knock-out of *STAT6* gene results in deficient T$_H$2 responses (23,24), the opposite of the IL-12 and *STAT4* knockouts. These data demonstrate that some cytokines, their associated receptors, and the STATs fulfill specific functions to generate protective immune responses against different infectious organisms and suggest that STATs may be useful targets for manipulating such responses.

More recently, other transcription factors, selectively expressed during the development of Th1 and Th2 cells, have been discovered. They include Hlx and ERM for Th1 cells and GATA-3 and the oncogene *c-maf* for Th2 cells (58).

EFFECTS OF HELPER T-CELL SUBSETS ON PHYSIOLOGIC CONDITIONS

T$_H$1- and T$_H$2-dominated responses provide different modalities of protection against exogenous offending agents. They also may play a critical role in the development or maintenance of other pathophysiologic conditions.

Infectious Diseases

Studies of the numerous animal models and the few studies of humans have revealed that the ability of a host to effectively eradicate an invading organism depends on the class of effector-specific immune response that is mounted. In general, T$_H$1 cells are more suitable for protection against intracellular parasites. The most impressive model is the infection of different mouse strains with *Leishmania major,* which provided evidence that resistance and susceptibility to this parasite are caused by a specific T$_H$1 or T$_H$2 response, respectively (25). Extracel-

lular parasites are best counteracted by a combination of T$_H$2- and T$_H$1-type cytokines (e.g., by T$_H$0 cells) (6). The optimal reaction against metazoan parasites is provided by T$_H$2 cells, which aggravate the activities of metazoan parasites once they have entered the body without making attempts to destroy them through T$_H$1-mediated responses that may be harmful to the host (10).

Fetal Transplantation Tolerance

It appears that T$_H$1-dependent effector mechanisms, such as DTH and cytotoxic T lymphocyte activity, play a central role in acute allograft rejection (26). However, the production of T$_H$2-type cytokines may be central to the induction and maintenance of allograft tolerance (27). Embryos are not rejected by the maternal immune system until the time of delivery despite the presence of paternal MHC antigens. This apparent paradox may be explained by a T$_H$2 switch at the level of maternofetal interface, which allows fetal survival by inhibiting T$_H$1 responses (28). The CD4$^+$ and CD8$^+$ T-cell clones generated from the decidua of women suffering from unexplained recurrent abortions showed significantly reduced IL-4 and IL-10 production compared with levels generated from the decidua of women with voluntary abortion (i.e., normal gestation) (59). Concentrations of progesterone comparable to those present at the maternofetal interface favor development of human T cells producing T$_H$2-type cytokines (29) and the production of leukemia inhibitory factor (LIF), which is enhanced by the T$_H$2-type cytokines IL-4, IL-10, and IL-13 (59). It is likely that progesterone-mediated production of T$_H$2 cytokines (which hamper fetus rejection by inhibiting T$_H$1 responses) and LIF (a cytokine essential for embryo implantation) contribute to the development and maintenance of successful pregnancy.

Immunodeficiency Diseases

Omenn's syndrome (OS) is a rare and severe combined immunodeficiency, characterized by hypereosinophilia and increased serum IgE levels. High numbers of CD4$^+$CD30$^+$ T cells were found in lymph nodes and skin of patients with OS, and most T-cell clones generated from circulating CD4$^+$CD30$^+$ T cells from OS patients showed a clear-cut T$_H$2 profile (30).

During human immunodeficiency virus (HIV) infection, a bias toward T$_H$2-like responses and therefore T$_H$1 inhibition may contribute to the loss of control of the immune system over the infection, resulting in progression to acquired immunodeficiency syndrome (AIDS) (31). Although evidence is lacking for a general massive alteration to a T$_H$2 pattern in HIV-infected individuals, large numbers of CD8$^+$CD30$^+$ T$_C$2-like clones, showing reduced cytolytic activity against HIV, were generated from subjects in advanced phases of HIV infection (32). Moreover, HIV replication was higher in established T$_H$2 clones (33) or IL-4–conditioned T-cell lines than in established T_H1 clones or IL-12–conditioned T-cell lines and associated with the release of enhanced concentrations of soluble CD30 (57). CD30 triggering on HIV-infected CD4$^+$ T cells promotes HIV replication, which is strongly inhibited by blockers of CD30/CD30L interactions (34).

Atopic Allergy

Several findings support the concept that atopic diseases result from T_H2-dominated responses to single or multiple environmental allergens:

Allergens preferentially expand T_H cells, showing a T_H2-like profile in atopic donors, whereas allergen-specific T cells in nonatopic donors are predominantly T_H1-like.

T_H2-like cells accumulate in the target organs of allergic patients.

Allergen challenge results in local activation and recruitment of allergen-specific T_H2-like cells.

Successful specific immunotherapy is associated with changes from a predominantly T_H2 to predominantly T_H1 profile of allergen-reactive T_H cells.

Allergen-reactive CD30$^+$ T_H2 cells are present in the circulation of allergic patients during seasonal allergen exposure.

CD4$^+$ T-cell clones generated from umbilical cord blood lymphocytes of newborns with atopic parents produce higher IL-4 concentrations than neonatal lymphocytes of newborns with nonatopic parents (35).

Genetic alterations of molecular mechanisms directly involved in IL-4 gene expression, deficient regulation by T_H2-inhibitory cytokines (IFN-α/γ and IL-12), or both may account for the preferential T_H2-type response to environmental allergens in atopic persons. An epidemiologic study found a highly significant inverse association between DTH to *Mycobacterium tuberculosis* and atopy among Japanese schoolchildren (36). This finding supports the view that the decline of tubercular infection and perhaps of other infections in childhood (with reduced production of T_H2-inhibitory cytokines) may contribute to the rising severity and prevalence of atopic disorders during past decades in developed countries (35).

Autoimmune and Other Immunopathologic Disorders

Accumulating evidence from animal models suggests that T_H1-type lymphokines are involved in the genesis of organ-specific autoimmune diseases, such as experimental autoimmune uveoretinitis, experimental allergic encephalomyelitis, or insulin-dependent diabetes mellitus (37–39). The data on human diseases favor a prevalent T_H1 lymphokine profile in the target organs of patients with organ-specific autoimmunity, such as autoimmune

TABLE 12-3. *Pathophysiologic conditions associated with prevalent T_H1 or T_H2 responses*

T_H1 cells
Protection against intracellular bacteria (6)
Type 1 diabetes mellitus (39)
Autoimmune thyroid diseases (40)
Multiple sclerosis (41)
Crohn's disease (42)
Helicobacter pylori–induced peptic ulcer (43)
Acute allograft rejection (26)
Unexplained recurrent abortions (59)

T_H2 cells
Protection against gastrointestinal nematodes (10)
Transplantation tolerance (27)
Successful pregnancy (28)
Omenn's syndrome (30)
Some idiopathic hypereosinophilic syndromes (45)
Vernal conjunctivitis (46)
Atopic disorders (35)
Progressive systemic scleroderma (44)
Sézary syndrome (47)
Chronic graft-versus-host disease
Cryptogenic fibrosing alveolitis (49)
Progression to acquired immunodeficiency syndrome from human immunodeficiency virus infection (31,33)

thyroid diseases and multiple sclerosis (40,41). T_H1 cell predominance and spontaneous IL-12 expression were also found in the guts of patients with Crohn's disease (42). Likewise, T_H1-like cells predominated in the gastric antrum of *Helicobacter pylori* (Hp)–infected patients with peptic ulcer, which appeared to be specific for Hp antigens (43). In contrast, T_H2-cell predominance and high CD30 expression were found in the skin of patients with chronic graft-versus-host disease and in those with progressive systemic sclerosis (44) (Table 12-3).

THERAPEUTIC IMPLICATIONS OF THE HELPER T-CELL SUBSET PARADIGM

The T_H1-T_H2 paradigm provides the basis for therapeutic strategies in the control of infectious diseases and the manipulation of immunopathologic reactions. Vaccines against infectious agents may be developed based on the use of selected peptides, antigens associated to selected adjuvants (including cytokines), or naked DNA, which seem to be able to induce preferential T_H1 responses (50–52). Deviation of established T_H1 or T_H2 responses may be attempted in conditions in which harmful T_H1 or T_H2 responses develop against environmental antigens or autoantigens, such as allergic or autoimmune disorders. Strategies for the treatment of allergic diseases may include tolerization, redirection of harmful allergen-specific T_H2 responses, or targeting T_H2 cells or T_H2-dependent effector molecules (35). Strategies for the therapy of autoimmune disorders may be based on the induction of tolerance by injection of modified autoantigen peptides (53), oral administration of autoantigens

(54), or induction of immune deviation by appropriate cytokines (55).

Since the concept of T_H1 and T_H2 cells was introduced, enormous progress in the knowledge of the physiology of $CD4^+$ T-cell effector cells has been achieved. T_H1 and T_H2 cells represent polarized forms of the $CD4^+$ T-cell effector response that occur under combined genetic and environmental conditions and that result in the selective production of different sets of cytokines. The T_H1-T_H2 paradigm provides a useful model for understanding the mechanisms of protection against infectious agents and the pathogenesis of several pathophysiologic conditions, and it represents the basis for the development of novel immunotherapeutic strategies.

ACKNOWLEDGMENTS

The experiments reported in this chapter have been performed by funds provided by Associated Italiana Ricerca Canero, Italian Ministry of Health (AIDS Project), Consiglio Nazionale Ricerche, and European Community.

REFERENCES

1. Mosmann TR, Cherwinski H, Bond MW, Giedlin MA, Coffman RL. Two types of murine T cell clone. I. Definition according to profiles of lymphokine activities and secreted proteins. *J Immunol* 1986;136: 2348–2357.
2. Mosmann TR, Sad S. The expanding universe of T-cell subsets: Th1, Th2 and more. *Immunol Today* 1996;17:138–146.
3. Ferrick DA, Schrenzel MD, Mulvania T, Hsieh B, Ferlin WG, Lepper H. Differential production of interferon-γ and interleukin-4 in response to Th1- and Th2-stimulating pathogens by T cells. *Nature* 1995; 373:255–257.
4. Abbas AK, Murphy KM, Sher A. Functional diversity of helper T lymphocytes. *Nature* 1996;383:787–793.
5. Kelso A. Th1 and Th2 subsets: paradigm lost? *Immunol Today* 1995; 16:374–379.
6. Daugelat S, Kaufmann SHE. Role of Th1 and Th2 cells in bacterial infections. *Chem Immunol* 1996;63:66–97.
7. Romagnani S. Lymphokine production by human T cells in disease states. *Annu Rev Immunol* 1994;12:227–257.
8. Romagnani S. Understanding the role of Th1 and Th2 cells in infection. *Trends Microbiol* 1996;4:463–466.
9. Romagnani S. *The Th1/Th2 paradigm in disease.* Austin: Landes Company, 1997.
10. Urban JF, Maliszewski CR, Madden KB, Katona IM, Finkelman FD. IL-4 treatment can cure established gastrointestinal nematode infections in immunocompetent and immunodeficient mice. *J Immunol* 1995;154:4675–4684.
11. Kamogawa Y, Minasi LE, Carding SR, Bottomly K, Flavell RA. The relationship of IL-4– and IFN-γ–producing T cells studied by lineage ablation of IL-4–producing cells. *Cell* 1993;75:985–995.
12. Swain SL, Weinberg AD, English M, Huston G. IL-4 directs the development of Th2-like helper effectors. *J Immunol* 1990;145:3796–3806.
13. Maggi E, Parronchi P, Manetti R. Reciprocal regulatory role of IFN-γ and IL-4 on the *in vitro* development of human Th1 and Th2 cells. *J Immunol* 1992;148:2142–2147.
14. Hsieh CS, Macatonia SE, Tripp CS, Wolf SF, O'Garra A, Murphy KM. Development of TH1 $CD4^+$ T cells through IL-12 produced by *Listeria*-induced macrophages. *Science* 1993;260:547–549.
15. Manetti R, Parronchi P, Giudizi MG, et al. Natural killer cell stimulatory factor (interleukin-12) induces T helper type 1 (Th1)-specific immune responses and inhibits the development of IL-4–producing Th cells. *J Exp Med*, 177:1199–1204.
16. Constant SL, Bottomly K. Induction of T_H1 and T_H2 $CD4^+$ T cell responses: the alternative approaches. *Annu Rev Immunol* 1997;15: 297–322.
17. Szabo S, Jacobson NG, Dighe AS, Gubler U, Murphy KM. Developmental commitment to the Th2 lineage by extinction of IL-12 signaling. *Immunity* 1995;2:665–675.
18. Yashimoto T, Bendelac A, Watson C, Hu-Li J, Paul WE. CD-1-specific, NK1.1^{pos} T cells play a key *in vivo* role in a Th2 response and in IgE production. *Science* 1995;270:1845–1847.
19. Gorham JD, Guler ML, Steen RG, et al. Genetic mapping of a locus controlling development of Th1/Th2 type responses. *Proc Natl Acad Sci USA* 1996;93:12467–12472.
20. Ivashkiv LB. Cytokines and STATs: how can signals achieve specificity? *Immunity* 1995;3:1–4.
21. Thierfelder WE, van Deursen JM, Yamamoto K, et al. Requirement for Stat4 in interleukin-12–mediated responses of natural killer and T cells. *Nature* 1996;382:171–174
22. Kaplan MH, Sun Y-L, Hoey T, Grusby MJ. Impaired IL-12 responses and enhanced development of Th2 cells in Stat4-deficient mice. *Nature* 1996;382:174–177.
23. Takeda K, Tanaka T, Shi W, et al. Essential role of Stat6 in IL-4 signalling. *Nature* 1996;380:627–630.
24. Shimoda K, van Deursen J, Sangster MY, et al. Lack of IL-4–induced Th2 response and IgE class switching in mice with disrupted Stat6 gene. *Nature* 1996;380:630–633.
25. Reiner SL, Locksley RM. The regulation of immunity to Leishmania Major. *Annu Rev Immunol* 1995;13:151–177.
26. D'Elios M, Josien R, Manghetti M, et al. Predominant Th1 cell infiltration in acute rejection episodes of human kidney grafts: evidence for correlation between *in vitro* IFN-γ production and degree of interstitial infiltration. *Kidney Int* 1997;51:1876–1884.
27. Dallman MJ. Cytokines and transplantation: Th1/Th2 regulation of the immune response to solid organ transplants in the adult. *Curr Opin Immunol* 1995;7:632–638.
28. Wegmann TG, Lin H, Guilbert L, Mossmann TR. Bidirectional cytokine interactions in the maternal-fetal relationship: is successful pregnancy a Th2 phenomenon? *Immunology Today* 1993;14:353–356.
29. Piccinni M-P, Giudizi M-G, Biagiotti R, et al. Progesterone favors the development of human T helper (Th) cells producing Th2-type cytokines and promotes both IL-4 production and membrane CD30 expression in established Th1 clones. *J Immunol* 1995;155:128–133.
30. Chilosi M, Facchetti F, Notarangelo LD, et al. CD30 cell expression and abnormal soluble CD30 serum accumulation in Omenn's syndrome: evidence for a Th2-mediated condition. *Eur J Immunol* 1996;26: 329–334.
31. Clerici M, Shearer GM. A Th1/Th2 switch is a critical step in the etiology of HIV infection. *Immunol Today* 1993;14:107–111.
32. Maggi E, Manetti R, Annunziato F, et al. Functional characterization and modulation of cytokine profile of CD8- T cell clones from HIV-infected individuals. *Blood* 1997;89:3672–3681.
33. Maggi E, Mazzetti M, Ravina A, et al. Ability of HIV to promote a Th1 to Th0 shift and to replicate preferentially in Th2 and Th0 cells. *Science* 1994;265:248–252.
34. Maggi E, Annunziato F, Manetti R, et al. Activation of HIV expression by CD30 triggering in $CD4^+$ T cells from HIV-infected individuals. *Immunity* 1995;3:251–255.
35. Romagnani S. Regulation of the development of type 2 T-helper cells in allergy. *Curr Opin Immunol* 1994;6:838–846.
36. Shirikawa T, Enomoto T, Shimazu S, Hopkin JM. The inverse association between tuberculin responses and atopic disorders. *Science* 1997; 275:77–79.
37. Druet P, Sheela R, Pelletier L. Th1 and Th2 cells in autoimmunity. *Chem Immunol* 1996;63:158–170.
38. Windhagen A, Nicholson LB, Weiner HL, Kuchroo VK, Hafler DA. Role of Th1 and Th2 cells in neurologic disorders. *Chem Immunol* 1996;63:181–186.
39. Liblau RS, Singer SM, McDevitt HO. Th1 and Th2 $CD4-$ T cells in the pathogenesis of organ-specific autoimmune diseases. *Immunol Today* 1995;16:34–38.
40. De Carli M, D'Elios MM, Mariotti S, et al. Cytolytic T cells with Th1-like cytokine profile predominate in retroorbital lymphocytic infiltrates of Graves' ophthalmopathy. *J Clin Endocrinol Metab* 1993;77: 1120–1124.

41. Brod S, Benjamin D, Hafler DA. Restricted T cell expression of IL2/IFN-γ mRNA in human inflammatory disease. *J Immunol* 1991; 147:810–815.

42. Parronchi P, Romagnani P, Annunziato F, et al. Type 1 T helper (Th1)-predominance and IL-12 expression in the gut of patients with Crohn's disease. *Am J Pathol* 1997;150:823–832.

43. D'Elios MM, Manghetti M, De Carli M, et al. Th1 effector cells specific for *Helicobacter pylori* in the gastric antrum of patients with peptic ulcer. *J Immunol* 1997;158:962–967.

44. Mavilia C, Scaletti C, Romagnani P, et al. Type 2 helper T (Th2) cell predominance and high CD30 expression in progressive systemic sclerosis. *Amer J Pathol* 1997;151:1751–1758.

45. Cogan E, Schandené L, Crusiaux A, Cochaux P, Velu T, Goldman M. Brief report: clonal proliferation of type 2 helper T cells in a man with the hypereosinophilic syndrome. *N Engl J Med* 1994;330:535–538.

46. Maggi E, Biswas P, Del Prete GF, et al. Accumulation of Th2-like helper T cells in the conjunctiva of patients with vernal conjunctivitis. *J Immunol* 1991;146:1169–1174.

47. Vowels BR, Lessin SR, Cassin M, Jaworsky C, Benoit B, Wolfe JT, Rook AH. Th2 cytokine mRNA expression in skin in cutaneous T-cell lymphoma. *J Invest Dermatol* 1994;103:669–673.

48. Ferrara JLM. Cytokine dysregulation as a mechanism of graft versus host disease. *Curr Opin Immunol* 1993;5:794–799.

49. Wallace WAH, Ramage EA, Lamb D, Howie SEM. A type 2 (Th2-like) pattern of immune response predominates in the pulmonary interstitium of patients with cryptogenic fibrosing alveolitis (CFA). *Clin Exp Immunol* 1995;101:436–441.

50. Tsitoura DC, Verhoef A, Gelder CM, O'Heir R, Lamb JR. Altered T cell ligands derived from a major house dust mite allergen enhance IFN-gamma but not IL-4 production by human CD4- T cells. *J Immunol* 1996;157:2160–2165.

51. Nash AD, Lofthouse SA, Barcham GJ, et al. Recombinant cytokines as immunological adjuvants. *Immunol Cell Biol* 1993;71:367–379.

52. Raz E, Tighe E, Sato Y, et al. Preferential induction of a Th1 immune response and inhibition of specific IgE antibody formation by plasmid DNA immunization. *Proc Natl Acad Sci USA* 1996;93:5141–5145.

53. Kuchroo VK, Greer JM, Kaul D, et al. A single TCR antagonist peptide inhibits experimental allergic encephalomyelitis mediated by a diverse T cell repertoire. *J Immunol* 1994;153:3326–3336.

54. Mitchison A, Sieper J. Immunological basis of oral tolerance. *Z Rheumatol* 1995;54:141–144.

55. Rocken M, Racke M, Shevach E. Interleukin 4–induced immune deviation as antigen-specific therapy for inflammatory autoimmune disease. *Immunol Today* 1996;17:225–231.

56. Bonecchi R, Bianchi G, Bordignon PP, et al. Differential expression of chemokine receptors and chemotactic responsiveness of type 1 T helper cells (Th1s) and Th2s. *J Exp Med* 1998;187:129–134.

57. Galli G, Annunziato F, Mavilia C, et al. Enhanced HIV expression during T helper 2-oriented responses due to the opposite regulatory effect of IL-4 and IFN-γ on Fusin/CXCR4. *Eur J Immunol* 1998;28:1–11.

58. Szabo SJ, Glimcher LH, Ho I-C. Genes that regulate interleukin-4 expression in T cells. *Curr Opin Immunol* 1997;9:776–781.

59. Piccinni M-P, Beloni L, Livi C, Maggi E, Scarselli G, Romagnani S. Role of type 2 T helper (Th2) cytokines and leukemia inhibitory factor (LIF) produced by decidual T cells in the development and maintenance of successful pregnancy. *Nature Med* 1998;4:1020–1024.

Inflammation: Basic Principles and Clinical Correlates,
3rd ed., edited by John I. Gallin and Ralph Snyderman.
Lippincott Williams & Wilkins, Philadelphia © 1999.

CHAPTER 13

CD8 Effector Cells

Norman L. Letvin and Jörn E. Schmitz

Compelling evidence suggests that CD8+ cytotoxic T lymphocytes (CTLs) play a central role in containing the spread of certain infectious pathogens (1–3), in controlling tumor growth (4,5) and in allograft rejection (6). Perhaps the strongest data indicating an important function for CTLs *in vivo* are derived from studies of virus replication during the period of primary infection in mice and humans (1,6–9). The transfer into naive mice of CD8+ lymphocyte populations from virus-immune syngeneic mice or cloned CD8+ virus-specific CTLs can block the initiation of certain viral infections in these mice. This antiviral effect can complement the protection afforded by antibody, as seen in influenza infection of mice (10,11), or can be the sole mechanism of protective immunity, as seen in lymphocytic choriomeningitis virus (LCMV) infection (12,13) of mice. In humans, the rapidity with which an influenza infection is cleared from the upper airways correlates with the potency of a CTL response (14) and the adoptive transfer of cytomegalovirus-specific CD8+ CTL clones can prevent infection with cytomegalovirus in a clinical posttransplantation setting (15).

Growing data support a role for CD8+ CTLs in containing certain bacterial and parasitic infections. The replication of intracellular bacteria such as *Listeria* and *Mycobacterium* species is limited by macrophages that are stimulated by cytokines produced by antigen-specific helper T cells. CD8+ CTLs also may play a part in controlling the replication of these bacteria (16,17). CD8+ CTLs play a central role in containing parasitic infections, including *Trypanosoma cruzi* in mice, *Theileria parva* in livestock, and malaria in a variety of animal models (18,19).

The concept of immune surveillance presupposes the existence of tumor-specific host lymphocytes that are capable of eliminating tumor cells as they arise in an individual. CTLs have been implicated in this process (20). Although few tumor-specific antigens have been defined, it is presumed that they exist (21). Lymphokine-activated tumor-associated T lymphocytes have been infused in clinical trials as novel anticancer therapies (22,23).

The first description of cytotoxic T lymphocytes in 1960 by Govaertz (24) involved the immune response elicited in the setting of allograft rejection. He showed that thoracic duct lymphocytes obtained from dogs after renal allograft exhibited cytopathicity specific for donor renal cells. The lymphocytes with cytopathic potential that are elicited by allogeneic tissue include CTLs. Numerous studies have shown that host lymphocytes infiltrating an allograft at the time of rejection include alloantigen-specific CTLs (25).

In this chapter, CD8+ CTLs refer to T-cell receptor (TCR) $\alpha\beta$ CTLs. Chapters 9 and 11 discuss CD8+ TCR $\gamma\delta$ cells and CD8+ natural killer cells.

INDUCTION OF CYTOTOXIC T LYMPHOCYTES

The earliest events leading to the initiation of a CTL response involve the transformation of self or foreign proteins into a form that can be recognized by these effector cells (26) (Fig. 13-1). Proteins that are actively synthesized in the cytosol of a cell are broken down to peptide fragments through the actions of proteases (27,28). The major protease involved in the generation of these peptides is the proteasome complex, a high-molecular-weight, multicatalytic molecule consisting of 28 20- to 30-kd subunits (29). The resulting peptide fragments are transported from the cytosol to the endoplasmic reticulum by the TAP transporter complex (30). These peptides then bind to major histocompatibility complex (MHC) class I heavy chains, and the peptide-MHC class I com-

N.L. Letvin and J.E. Schmitz: Harvard Medical School, Division of Viral Pathogenesis, Department of Medicine, Beth Israel Deaconess Medical Center, Boston, Massachusetts 02215.

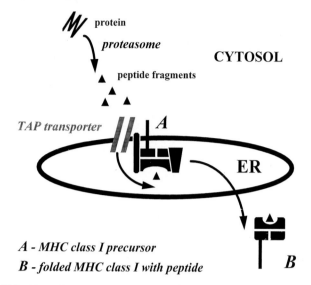

A - MHC class I precursor
B - folded MHC class I with peptide

FIG. 13-1. Degradation and processing pathway of antigens that bind to major histocompatibility complex (MHC) class I molecules. Proteins within the cytosol are degraded to peptide fragments by multienzyme protease complexes known as proteasomes. The peptides are transported by the TAP transporters into the lumen of the endoplasmic reticulum (ER). TAP-bound, partially folded MHC class I precursor molecules **(A)** bind specific peptides and fold to form functional MHC class I molecules **(B)**. A MHC class I molecule is released from its precursor molecule complex and delivered to the cell membrane.

ulum, and cell fragmentation. Two different cellular pathways can lead to these apoptotic events: a perforin- and granzyme-mediated secretory pathway and a ligand-induced and receptor-mediated nonsecretory pathway (Fig. 13-2).

On engagement of the TCRs of CTLs by the peptide–MHC class I molecules expressed on the surface of target cells, a signaling event is initiated that is associated with the synthesis of lytic granules. These granules contain perforin (37) and several serine proteases that are referred to as *granzymes* (38). Perforin, a molecule with significant homology to lytic components of complement, undergoes calcium-dependent polymerization after cell triggering, and in that form, it induces pore formation in target cells. Isolated perforin alone induces lysis but no DNA fragmentation in target cells (39). However, perforin-induced pores facilitate the entrance into cells of granzymes that then initiate apoptotic events.

Multiple members of the granzyme family of molecules have been defined in individual species. Granzyme B, a rapidly acting enzyme, has been implicated in the early events associated with killing; granzyme A activity is more slowly activated (40). These molecules synergistically induce DNA fragmentation in target cells (41). Although granzymes may initiate the apoptotic pathway directly, evidence suggests that certain granzymes can trigger this pathway through interactions with members

plexes are stabilized by β_2-microglobulin. The resulting trimolecular complexes move through the Golgi compartment to the cell surface, where they are expressed. It is in this form that antigen is recognized by CD8+ CTLs.

Resting CD8+ pre-CTLs are triggered by a highly specific TCR-mediated interaction with peptide–MHC class I complex expressed by cells (31). This interaction initiates interleukin-2 receptor (IL-2R) expression by the pre-CTLs, enabling the cells to expand after exposure to IL-2. IL-2 is produced endogenously by the CD8+ cells and by local CD4+ helper T lymphocytes. Other cytokines, including IL-7, and a second, co-stimulatory signal mediated by a CD28-B7 interaction can influence the maturation of CTLs (32,33).

MECHANISMS OF CELL KILLING

Although lymphocytes were first shown to be capable of killing other cells several decades ago (24), the cellular mechanisms employed in this killing process remained poorly understood until recently. On interaction with a CTL, susceptible target cells undergo apoptosis (34–36). Their chromatin condenses, their membranes bleb, and their DNA fragments. These events result in cell shrinkage, dilation of the endoplasmic retic-

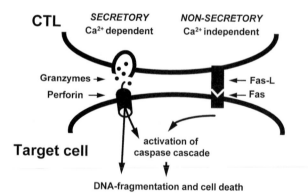

FIG. 13-2. Cytotoxic T lymphocyte (CTL)–mediated death pathways. CTLs employ two major pathways to induce cell death in target cells that present specific peptide fragments by major histocompatibility complex (MHC) class I molecules. The secretory pathway involves a Ca^{2+}-dependent secretion of perforin, a pore-forming molecule that inserts into the cell membrane of the target cell, and neutral serine proteases known as granzymes. Granzymes can directly induce DNA fragmentation, leading to cell death, or can activate the caspase cascade, which eventually leads to DNA fragmentation and cell death. The nonsecretory pathway does not involve Ca^{2+}. This pathway is mediated by ligand (FASL) expression on the cell surface of CTLs and cell surface receptor (FAS) expression on the target cell. Triggering of the FAS molecule induces activation of the caspase cascade, leading to DNA fragmentation and cell death.

of the interleukin-1β-converting (ICE) enzyme family of molecules known as *caspases* (42). Ten members of the caspase family of molecules have been defined in humans. Caspases 8 and 10 appear to initiate the activation cascade of caspases; caspases 3 and 7 are the executor caspase molecules in the nucleus of cells (43,44).

A second major pathway CTLs employ for killing target cells is initiated by the FAS ligand (FASL, CD95)–FAS interactions (34). FASL is a type II membrane protein whose expression is induced on CD8+ CTLs after TCR-initiated activation (45). Through binding to FAS, a transmembrane protein that is structurally homologous to the nerve growth factor receptors, a Ca^{2+}-independent initiation of apoptosis occurs (46). Like the granzyme molecules, FAS-FASL–induced cell death is executed through activation of ICE-family proteases (47,48).

Although these two major pathways mediate CTLs lysis of target cells, they do not represent the only mechanisms that CTLs employ to mediate their effector functions. In clearing viral infections, CTLs can secrete a variety of soluble factors that exert antiviral activity (32). Interferon-γ produced by CD8+ T cells suppresses the replication of a number of viruses. CD8+ lymphocyte-derived β-chemokines may contain human immunodeficiency virus type 1 (HIV-1) replication (49,50).

VIRUS ESCAPE FROM CYTOTOXIC T-CELL RECOGNITION

Perhaps the most compelling evidence for the *in vivo* importance of CTLs in containing virus spread comes from studies demonstrating that viruses with high mutation rates selectively mutate to avoid recognition by these effector cells. This phenomenon was first observed in studies of LCMV, a murine RNA virus with a high mutation rate and an exclusive dependence on CTLs for control of early infection (51). These studies were performed in transgenic mice in which LCMV recognition by CTLs is limited to a single glycoprotein epitope. The investigators demonstrated the rapid emergence of LCMV variants that were not susceptible to CTL lysis. The variants had selective amino acid alterations in epitopes recognized by CTLs.

In studies assessing HIV escape from CTLs *in vivo*, Phillips et al. (52) demonstrated fluctuations over time in the predominant gag protein epitope recognized in a limited number of HIV-infected patients. In HIV strains isolated several months later, they observed a clustering of gag amino acid sequence substitutions in this CTL epitope that affected gag-epitope recognition.

Other mechanisms can contribute to the ability of viruses to avoid clearance by CTL in the infected host. These mechanisms include virus sequestration in immunologically privileged sites, down-modulation of antigen-presenting cell MHC molecules, and induction of immunosuppression (53).

DETECTION OF CYTOTOXIC T CELLS

Evaluation of CTLs has depended on the use of cumbersome and technically challenging assays. The traditional approach for assaying CTLs involves measurement of released radioactive chromium (^{51}Cr) from radiolabeled, antigen-expressing target cells after a 4- to 6-hour incubation with the putative effector cells (54). Effector cells in such assays are expanded through *in vitro* restimulation. Because antigen can be recognized only by CTLs as peptide fragments bound to MHC class I molecules, antigen expression by target cells is accomplished by pulsing the target cells with specific peptide antigen or infecting those cells with a recombinant live vector such as vaccinia virus that expresses antigen in a form that allows it to be processed in the MHC class I pathway. Using this type of assay, effector cells can be fractionated to determine the phenotype of the cytotoxic cell subpopulation. The precise genetic restriction on the effector cell–target cell interactions can also be determined by assessing the ability of an effector cell to lyse a variety of genetically distinct, antigen-expressing target cells. The drawbacks of this assay include the usual requirement for *in vitro* restimulation of effector cells, the reliance on radioactive isotopes, and its nonquantitative nature.

Several detection systems have been developed that overcome many of the drawbacks inherent in the standard ^{51}Cr-release assay. To bypass the requirement for using radioactivity in detecting CTLs, the assays measure interferon-γ production by lymphocytes after exposure to antigen (55). CTL precursor frequency assays also are employed to allow precise quantitation of CTL responses (56). However, the standard ^{51}Cr-release assays, interferon-γ production assays, and CTL precursor frequency assays all suffer from the same limitation—they cannot be readily applied to large numbers of experimental subjects by routine clinical laboratories.

The most successful quantitative approaches to studying lymphocytes that have gained acceptance in clinical settings have relied on the use of immunophenotyping and flow cytometry. Because CTLs recognize peptide fragments of antigen bound to MHC class I molecules, it had been suggested that a fluorescent-labeled peptide–MHC class I complex might be capable of binding to epitope-specific CTL populations and providing a means of detecting these cells using flow cytometric technology. Although studies have suggested that the on-off rate of such complexes is too rapid to allow their use for this purpose, it has been demonstrated that fluorescent-labeled tetrameric complexes of peptide-MHC class I molecules can be used to label CTL subpopulations, facilitating their analysis by flow cytometry (57). This

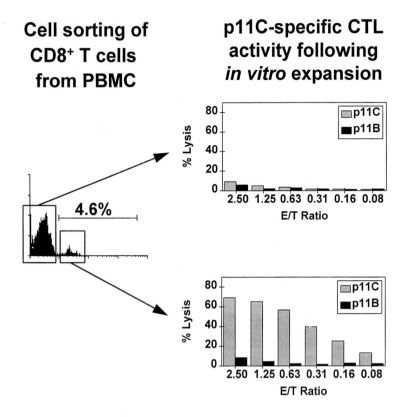

Cell sorting of CD8⁺ T cells from PBMC

p11C-specific CTL activity following *in vitro* expansion

FIG. 13-3. Functional characterization of the rhesus monkey class I/p11C peptide tetrameric complex–binding cytotoxic T lymphocytes from simian immunodeficiency virus (SIV)–infected rhesus monkeys. CD8⁺ T cells were stained with the fluorescein isothiocyanate–coupled tetrameric complex and sorted into fractions of negatively and positively binding cells. These cells were expanded by antigen nonspecific stimulation in *in vitro* cultures and evaluated for their p11C (SIV gag peptide)–specific killing of autologous lymphoblastoid B cells. The irrelevant p11B peptide was used as a control. The tetrameric complex–binding lymphocytes show significant p11C-specific lysis, even at very low effector to target ratios (E/T ratio).

technology provides a powerful new approach for studying antigen-specific CTLs (Fig. 13-3).

PHENOTYPIC CHARACTERISTICS OF CYTOTOXIC T CELLS

Much has been learned about the biology of CTLs through their immunophenotypic characterization. CD8+CD4– T cells evolve after thymic maturation from a common precursor cell, the CD8+CD4+ T cell. Before encountering specific antigens, CD8+ T cells are quiescent or naive and exhibit little or no expression of cell surface molecules associated with activation (e.g., HLA-DR, CD25, CD71) or adhesion (e.g., CD11a, CD49d, CD54, CD58) (58). At this time in their ontogeny, CD8+ T cells are characterized by relatively high cell surface expression of the RA isoform of the CD45 molecule and high-density expression of the L-selectin, CD62L (59). After activation, CD8+ T cells upregulate the expression of activation- and adhesion-associated molecules (60) and downregulate expression of the CD62L molecule (59). The CD45RA isoform on the cell surface is gradually decreased and replaced by expression of the CD45RO isoform. However, the CD45RA isoform is eventually reexpressed on CD8 T cells that are deprived from further antigen stimulation. Therefore, the CD45RA/CD45RO naive-memory paradigm must be taken with caution, because investigations have suggested that subsets of CD45RA+CD8+ T cells might not be

naive T cells (61). On the other hand, high levels of cell surface expression of activation or adhesion molecules on CD8+ T cells do not necessarily indicate that these cells will have an increased functional activity (62,63).

CYTOTOXIC T-CELL–INDUCED PATHOLOGY

Although CTLs are important components of the host immune response, they occasionally mediate tissue damage. The classic example of this phenomenon is the laboratory model of viral immunopathogenesis in the LCMV-infected mouse, in which the CTLs responsible for viral clearance cause a severe leptomeningitis in infected animals (64). Chronic active hepatitis in hepatitis B virus–infected humans is mediated in part by CTL-induced damage of liner parenchymal cells (65). Even in HIV-induced disease, HIV-specific CTLs can be detected in lungs of individuals with lymphocytic alveolitis, an HIV-related disorder frequently observed before the onset of opportunistic infections (66).

REFERENCES

1. Riddell SR, Gilbert MJ, Greenberg PD. CD8⁺ cytotoxic T cell therapy of cytomegalovirus and HIV infection. *Curr Opin Immunol* 1993;5: 484–491.
2. Ehtisham S, Sunil-Chandra NP, Nash AA. Pathogenesis of murine gamma-herpesvirus infection in mice deficient in CD4 and CD8 T cells. *J Virol* 1993;67:5247–5252.
3. Hou S, Doherty PC, Zijlstra M, Jaenisch R, Katz JM. Delayed clearance of Sendai virus in mice lacking class I MHC-restricted CD8⁺ T cells. *J Immunol* 1992;149:1319–1325.

4. Kast WM, Offringa R, Peters PJ, Melven RH, van der Eb AJ, Melief CJM. Eradication of adenovirus E1-induced tumors by E1a-specific cytotoxic T lymphocytes. *Cell* 1989;59:603–614.

5. Cox AL, Skipper J, Cehn Y, et al. Identification of a peptide recognized by five melanoma-specific human cytotoxic T cell lines. *Science* 1994; 264:716–719.

6. Klein J. *Natural history of the major histocompatibility complex*. New York: Wiley-Interscience, 1986.

7. Reddehase MJ, Mutter W, Much K, Buhring H-J, Koszinowski UH. CD8-positive T lymphocytes specific for murine cytomegalovirus immediate-early antigens mediate protective immunity. *J Virol* 1987; 61;3102–3108.

8. Larsen HS, Feng MF, Horohov DW, Moore RN, Rouse BT. Role of T-lymphocyte subsets in recovery from herpes simplex virus infection. *J Virol* 1984;50:56–59.

9. Lukacher AE, Braciale VL, Braciale TJ. *In vivo* effector function of influenza virus-specific cytotoxic T lymphocyte clones is highly specific. *J Exp Med* 1984;160:814–826.

10. Bender BS, Croghan T, Zhang L, Small PA Jr. Transgenic mice lacking class I major histocompatibility complex-restricted T cells have delayed viral clearance and increased mortality after influenza virus challenge. *J Exp Med* 1992;175;1143–1145.

11. Mackenzie CD, Taylor PM, Askonas BA. Rapid recovery of lung histology correlates with clearance of influenza virus by specific CD8+ cytotoxic T cells. *Immunology* 1989;67:375–381.

12. Doherty PC, Allan W, Eichelberger M, Carding SR. Role of αβ and γδ T cell subsets in viral immunity. *Annu Rev Immunol* 1992;10:123–151.

13. Buchmeier MJ, Welsh RM, Dutko FJ, Oldstone MBA. The virology and immunobiology of lymphocytic choriomeningitis virus infection. *Adv Immunol* 1980;30:275–331.

14. McMichael AJ, Gotch FM, Noble GR, Beare PAS. Cytotoxic T-cell immunity to influenza. *N Engl J Med* 1983;309:13–17.

15. Riddell SR, Watanabe KS, Goodrich JM, Li CR, Agha ME, Greenberg PD. Restoration of viral immunity in immunodeficient humans by the adoptive transfer of T cell clones. *Science* 1992;257:238–241.

16. Kagi D, Ledermann B, Burki K, Hengartner H, Zinkernagel RM. CD8+ T cell-mediated protection against an intracellular bacterium by perforin-dependent cytotoxicity. *Eur J Immunol* 1994;24:3068–3072.

17. Kaufmann SHE. CD8+ T lymphocytes in intracellular microbial infections. *Immunol Today* 1988;9:168–174.

18. Romero P, Maryanski JL, Corradin G, Nussenzweig RS, Nussenzweig V, Zavala F. Cloned cytotoxic T cells recognize an epitope in the circumsporozoite protein and protect against malaria. *Nature* 1989;341:323–326.

19. Tarleton RL, Koller BH, Latour A, Postan M. Susceptibility of beta 2-microglobulin-deficient mice to *Trypanosoma cruzi* infection. *Nature* 1992;356:338–340.

20. Herberman RB. Cell-mediated immunity to tumor cells. *Adv Cancer Res* 1974;19:207–263.

21. Velders MP, Nieland JD, Rudolf MP, et al. Identification of peptides for immunotherapy of cancer: it is still worth the effort. *Crit Rev Immunol* 1998;18:7–27.

22. Rosenberg SA, Packard BS, Aebersold PM, et al. Use of tumor-infiltrating lymphocytes and interleukin-2 in the immunotherapy of patients with metastatic melanoma: a preliminary report. *N Engl J Med* 1988; 319:1676–1680.

23. Melief CJM. Tumor eradication by adoptive transfer of cytotoxic T lymphocytes. *Adv Cancer Res* 1992;58:143–175.

24. Govaertz A. Cellular antibodies in kidney homotransplantation. *J Immunol* 1960;85:516–522.

25. Auchincloss H, Sachs DH. Transplantation and graft rejection. In: Paul WE, ed. *Fundamental immunology*, 3rd ed. New York: Raven Press, 1993;1099–1142.

26. Neefjes JJ, Momburg F. Cell biology of antigen presentation. *Curr Opin Immunol* 1993;5:27–34.

27. Rotzschke O, Falk K, Deres K, et al. Isolation and analysis of naturally processed viral peptides as recognized by cytotoxic T cells. *Nature* 1990;348:252–254.

28. Schumacher TN, De Bruijn ML, Vernie LN, et al. Peptide selection by MHC class I molecules. *Nature* 1991;350:703–706.

29. Goldberg AL, Rock KL. Proteolysis, proteasomes and antigen presentation. *Nature* 1992;357:375–379.

30. Sadasivan B, Lehner PJ, Ortmann B, Spies T, Cresswell P. Roles for calreticulin and a novel glycoprotein, tapasin, in the interaction of MHC class 1 molecules with TAP. *Immunity* 1996;5:103–114.

31. Townsend A, Bodmer H. Antigen recognition by class I-restricted T lymphocytes. *Annu Rev Immunol* 1989;7:601–624.

32. Ramshaw IA, Ramsay AJ, Karupiah G, Rolph MS, Mahalingam S, Ruby JC. Cytokines and immunity to viral infections. *Immunol Rev* 1997;159:119–135.

33. Harding F, Allison J. CD28-B7 interactions allow the induction of CD8+ cytotoxic T lymphocytes in the absence of exogenous help. *J Exp Med* 1993;177:1791–1796.

34. Berke G. The CTL's kiss of death. *Cell* 1995;81:9–12.

35. Clark WR, Walsh CM, Glass AA, Hayashi F, Matloubian M, Ahmed R. Molecular pathways of CTL-mediated cytotoxicity. *Immunol Rev* 1995; 146:33–44.

36. Henkart PA, Williams MS, Zacharchuk CM, Sarin A. Do CTL kill target cells by inducing apoptosis? *Semin Immunol* 1997;9:135–144.

37. Podack ER, Ding-E Young J, Cohn ZA. Isolation and biochemical and functional characterization of perforin 1 from cytolytic T-cell granules. *Proc Natl Acad SCI USA* 1985;82:8629–8633.

38. Smyth MJ, Trapani JA. Granzymes: exogenous proteinases that induce target cell apoptosis. *Immunol Today* 1995;16:202–206.

39. Duke RC, Persechini PM, Chang S, Liu C-C, Cohen JJ, Young JD-E. Purified perforin induces target cell lysis but not DNA fragmentation. *J Exp Med* 1989;170:1451–1456.

40. Shi L, Ka C-M, Powers JC, Aebersold R, Greenberg AH. Purification of three cytotoxic lymphocyte granule serine proteases that induce apoptosis through distinct substrate and target cell interactions. *J Exp Med* 1992;176:1521–1529.

41. Nakajima H, Park HL, Henkart PA. Synergistic roles of granzymes A and B in mediating target cell death by rat basophilic leukemia mast cell tumors also expressing cytolysin/perforin. *J Exp Med* 1995;181: 1037–1047.

42. Salvesen GS, Dixit VM. Caspases: intracellular signaling by proteolysis. *Cell* 1997;91:443–446.

43. Talanian RV, Yang XH, Turbov J, et al. Granule-mediated killing: pathways for granzyme B-initiated apoptosis. *J Exp Med* 1997;186: 1323–1331.

44. Froelich CJ, Dixit VM, Yang X. Lymphocyte granule-mediated apoptosis: matters of viral mimicry and deadly proteases. *Immunol Today* 1998;19:30–36.

45. Suda T, Okazaki T, Naito Y, et al. Expression of the Fas ligand in cells of T cell lineage. *J Immunol* 1995;154:3808–3813.

46. Rouvier E, Luciani M-F, Golstein P. Fas involvement in Ca(2+)-independent T cell-mediated cytotoxicity. *J Exp Med* 1993;177:195–200.

47. Los M, Van de Caen, Penning LC, et al. Requirement of an ICE/CED-3 protease for Fas/APO-1-mediated apoptosis. *Nature* 1995;375:81–83.

48. Enari M, Hug H, Nagata S. Involvement of an ICE-like protease in Fas-mediated apoptosis. *Nature* 1995;375:78–81.

49. Cocchi F, DeVico AL, Garzino-Demo A, Arya SK, Gallo RC, Lusso P. Identification of RANTES, MIP-1α, and MIP-1β as the major HIV-suppressive factors produced by CD8+ T cells. *Science* 1995;270:1811–1815.

50. Rollins BJ. Chemokines. *Blood* 1997;90:909–928.

51. Pircher H, Moskphidis A, Rohrer U, Burki K, Hengartner H, Zinkernagel RM. Viral escape by selection of cytotoxic T cell-resistant variants *in vivo*. *Nature* 1990;346:629–633.

52. Phillips RE, Rowland-Jones S, Nixon DF, et al. Human immunodeficiency virus genetic variation that can escape cytotoxic T cell recognition. *Nature* 1991;354:433–434.

53. Oldstone MB. How viruses escape from cytotoxic T lymphocytes: molecular parameters and players. *Virology* 1997;234:179–185.

54. Martz E. The 51Cr-release assay for CTL-mediated target cell lysis. In: Sitkovsky MV, Henkart PA, eds. *Cytotoxic cells: recognition, effector function, generation, and methods*. Boston: Birkhäuser, 1993:457–467.

55. Morris AG, Lin YL, Askonas BA. Immune interferon release when a cloned cytotoxic T-cell line meets its correct influenza-infected target cell. *Nature* 1982;295:150–152.

56. Doherty PC, Topham DJ, Tripp RA. Establishment and persistence of virus-specific CD4+ and CD8+ T cell memory. *Immunol Rev* 1996;150: 23–44.

57. Altman JD, Moss PAH, Goulder JR, et al. Phenotypic analysis of antigen-specific T lymphocytes. *Science* 1996;274:94–96.

58. Mescher MF. Molecular interactions in the activation of effector and precursor cytotoxic T lymphocytes. *Immunol Rev* 1995;146:177–210.

59. Roederer M, Dubs JG, Anderson MT, Raju PA, Herzenberg LA. CD8 naive T cell counts decrease progressively in HIV-infected adults. *J Clin Invest* 1995;95:2061–2066.

60. Morimoto C, Rudd CE, Letvin NL, Schlossman SF. A novel epitope of the LFA-1 antigen which can distinguish killer effector and suppressor cells in human CD8 cells. *Nature* 1987;330:479–482.

61. Okumura M, Fujii Y, Inada K, Nakahara K, Matsuda H. Both CD45RA$^+$ and CD45RA$^-$ subpopulations of CD8$^+$ T cells contain cells with high levels of lymphocyte function-associated antigen-1 expression, a phenotype of primed T cells. *J Immunol* 1993;150:429–437.

62. Figdor CG, van Kooyk Y, Keizer GD. On the mode of action of LFA-1. *Immunol Today* 1990;11:277–280.

63. Hourihan H, Allen TD, Ager A. Lymphocyte migration across high endothelium is associated with increases in alpha 4 beta 1 integrin (VLA-4) affinity. *J Cell Sci* 1993;104:1049–1059.

64. Kagi D, Ledermann B, Burki K, et al. Cytotoxicity mediated by T cells and natural killer cells is greatly impaired in perforin-deficient mice. *Nature* 1994;369:31–37.

65. Eddleston AL, Mondelli M. Immunopathological mechanisms of liver cell injury in chronic hepatitis B virus infection. *J Hepatol* 1986;3 [Suppl 2]:S17–23.

66. Plata F, Autran B, Pedroza-Martins L, et al. AIDS virus-specific cytotoxic T-lymphocytes in lung disorders. *Nature* 1987;328:348–351.

Inflammation: Basic Principles and Clinical Correlates,
3rd ed., edited by John I. Gallin and Ralph Snyderman.
Published by Lippincott Williams & Wilkins, Philadelphia 1999.

CHAPTER 14

Role of Co-Stimulation in the Host Response to Infection

Kelvin P. Lee, David M. Harlan, and Carl H. June

DEVELOPMENT OF THE THEORY OF CO-STIMULATION

For more than one-half century, immunologists have sought to understand how self-tolerance is induced and maintained. The concept of immunologic tolerance first arose from transplantation studies performed early in the 20th century. The studies by Ray Owen in the 1940s using freemartin cattle (i.e., dizygotic twins that are hematopoietic mixed chimeras) led to studies by Billingham, who made the dramatic observation that these animals were unable to reject each other's skin. It took several decades for immunologists to derive a satisfactory theoretical framework to understand these observations, and by the 1970s, tolerance was thought to be maintained at the cellular level by lymphocytes using thymic or postthymic mechanisms. Bretscher and Cohn first proposed a two-signal model of B lymphocyte activation (1), which was later modified by Lafferty and Cunningham (2) for T-cell activation and allograft rejection (Fig. 14-1).

The essential feature of these models was that activation of lymphocytes requires an antigen-specific signal 1 and a second antigen nonspecific event called signal 2. Moreover, the theories proposed that signal 1 in the absence of the co-stimulatory signal 2 led to tolerance. Antigen binding to the T-cell receptor (TCR) in the absence of co-stimulation fails to activate the cell and leads to a state called *anergy,* in which the T cell becomes refractory to subsequent activation. Although the original two-signal models

are now regarded as over simplified, they are supported by strong experimental evidence and continue to provide a basis for understanding the discrimination of self from nonself in the case of extrathymic antigens.

Because self-tolerance is critical for normal immune system function, years of evolutionary pressure have led to a great redundancy in mechanisms to bridle potential antiself immune responses. Experimental data support the existence of multiple mechanisms other than a lack of co-stimulation to account for tolerance, such as ignorance, indifference, and suppression (3–5). This chapter focuses on the role of co-stimulation in the maintenance of tolerance, with particular emphasis on infectious agents and vaccines.

CO-STIMULATORY SIGNAL TRANSDUCTION

Unlike B-cell immunoglobulin receptors that can bind native antigens directly, TCRs bind antigen fragments and major histocompatibility complex (MHC) molecules. Antigen recognition by the TCR requires accessory molecules, CD4 or CD8, to enhance the avidity of the TCR for the antigen–MHC complex. The signal 1 delivered to the T cell by the TCR depends on a complicated, multicomponent receptor complex involving the TCR binding to antigen-MHC and CD4 or CD8 binding directly to nonpolymorphic parts of class II or class I MHC molecules. Antigen receptor signal transduction is considered further in Chapter 42.

The antigen-specific clonal expansion of naive T cells requires a second, co-stimulatory signal (i.e., signal 2) that must be delivered by the same antigen-presenting cell (APC) on which the T cell recognizes its specific antigen. The nature of the co-stimulatory requirement varies as a function of the differentiation of the T cell. Naive T cells usually have the most stringent co-stimula-

*K. P. Lee, *D. M. Harlan, and †C. H. June: *Immune Cell Biology Program, Naval Medical Research Institute, Bethesda, Maryland 20889; †Henry M. Jackson Foundation for the Advancement of Military Medicine, U.S. Military HIV Research Program, Bethesda, Maryland 20889; and *†Department of Medicine, Uniformed Services University of the Health Sciences, Bethesda, Maryland 20814.

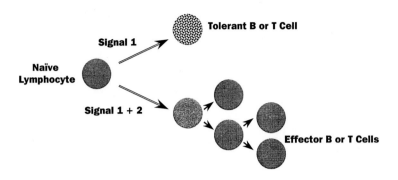

FIG. 14-1. The original two-signal theory of lymphocyte activation was proposed by Bretscher and Cohn in the 1960s and later modified by Lafferty and Cunningham in the 1970s. Bretscher and Cohn's model addressed B-cell activation and proposed that signal 2 was a carrier antibody, whereas Lafferty and Cunningham's model addressed T-cell activation and proposed that accessory cells delivered signal 2.

tory requirements. Effector T cells have far less stringent dependence on co-stimulation and, in many cases, function without co-stimulatory signals.

The mediators of co-stimulatory signaling are being investigated. It is thought that co-stimulation can be delivered by a variety of membrane-membrane interactions. The best characterized co-stimulatory molecules on APCs are the structurally related glycoproteins CD80 (B7-1) and CD86 (B7-2). The receptors for B7 molecules on the T cell are CD28 and CD152 (CTLA-4), structurally related members of the immunoglobulin superfamily. Ligation of CD28 by B7 molecules or by anti-CD28 antibodies co-stimulates the growth of naive T cells, whereas naive T-cell responses can be inhibited by anti-B7 antibodies that prevent binding of the B7 receptors to CD28 and CD152.

One feature of the two-signal theory is the requirement for simultaneous delivery of antigen-specific and co-stimulatory signals by one APC to activate the naive T cell. *In vivo*, it appears that only dendritic cells, so-called professional APCs, can initiate naive T-cell responses. Inappropriate T-cell activation is prevented by the two-signal requirement and by compartmentalization of the immune system (4). For example, naive T cells primarily traffic to lymph nodes, but dendritic cells provide surveillance in the periphery and only migrate to lymph nodes after encountering antigen and inflammatory signals. The requirement that the same cell must present the specific antigen and the co-stimulatory signal is important in preventing destructive immune responses to self tissues.

A second prediction of the two-signal theory is the existence of biochemically distinct forms of signal transduction after tolerance induction (signal 1 only) and productive antigen presentation (signals 1 and 2). A major roadblock to the investigation of anergic cells has been the lack of a suitable surface marker to permit identification of unresponsive cells. Despite this problem, substantial progress has been made in understanding the induction, maintenance, and *in vivo* relevance of the unresponsive state called anergy. T cells rendered anergic are characterized by their loss of an autocrine proliferative response to antigenic challenge because of a block in interleukin-2 (IL-2) production. Anergic CD4 cells are still able to produce IL-4, but they do not proliferate in response to IL-4. Anergic T cells also have a partial defect in their ability to express surface CD40L,

and in conjunction with impaired cytokine secretion, this may result in B-cell nonresponsiveness (6).

Signal transduction through CD28 is poorly understood. The cytosolic tail of CD28 binds several intracellular proteins, including phosphatidylinositol 3-kinase, growth factor receptor–bound protein-2 (GRB2), and the protein tyrosine kinase ITK (7). The SRC homology-2 (SH2) and -3 (SH3) domains of GRB2 also contribute to CD28 binding (8).

Anergy is associated with decreased activation of LCK, ZAP-70, RAS and defective activation of the IL-2 enhancer elements AP-1 and NF-AT (9,10). Anergic T cells display constitutive Cb1 phosphorylation and its association with the adapter protein Crkl and the guanine nucleotide-releasing factor C3G (11). Rap-1 GTP is constitutively detectable in anergic cells, whereas in productively activated T cells, the complex is only slightly and transiently induced after stimulation. In contrast, RAS is activated by conversion to the GTP bound form in control but not in anergic cells after antigen and B7 stimulation (Fig. 14-2).

After the T cells are activated, antigen-specific and antigen-nonspecific mechanisms have evolved to downregulate the response. Although the only counterreceptor for B7 molecules on naive T cells appears to be CD28, activated T cells express an additional receptor for B7 called CD152 (CTLA-4). CD152 has sequence homology to CD28, and the two molecules are encoded by closely linked genes. CD152 binds B7 molecules more avidly than CD28 and appears to deliver a dominant negative signal to the activated T cell (12). The activated progeny of a naive T cell are less sensitive to stimulation by the APC by virtue of their CD152 expression, which limits the amount of IL-2 produced (13). As a dramatic example of the important downregulatory role served by CD152, CD152 knock-out mice die from a fulminant polyclonal lymphoproliferative syndrome (14,15). The binding of CD152 to B7 molecules plays an essential role in limiting the proliferative response of activated T cells to antigen and B7 on the surface of APCs. Even though CD152 and CD28 share the same ligands, they appear to have potent and opposing roles in T-cell activation.

Clarification of CD152 function has resulted in the original two-signal model of T-cell activation being modified to a more complex three-signal model of activation (Fig. 14-3). For example, evidence indicates that

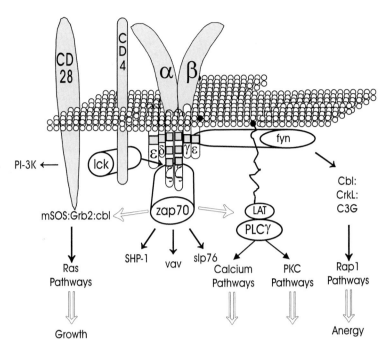

FIG. 14-2. Signaling complexes associated with antigen receptor and co-stimulatory signal transduction. Signaling complexes and pathways associated with the T-cell antigen receptor (TCR). The eight-chain TCR and the CD4 and CD28 coreceptors are shown with associated kinases LCK, FYN, and ZAP-70. Ten immunoreceptor tyrosine-based activation motifs (ITAM) are encoded in the TCR subunits *(shaded boxes)*. Tyrosine kinase activation results in the phosphorylation of several substrates, including phospholipase C (PLC). TCR-mediated activation of PLC results in increased calcium concentration and protein kinase C (PKC) activity in anergic and normal T cells. In normal cells, tyrosine kinase activation after TCR and CD28 stimulation also leads to activation of RAS through Cb1 binding through its SRC homology domain-3 (SH3) to growth factor receptor-bound protein-2 plus mammalian son of sevenless (GRB-2:SOS). In anergic cells, Cb1 binds to Crkl through its SRC homology domain-2 (SH2) domain and C3G, leading to Rap-1 activation and inhibition of RAS activation. SHP-1, SH2-containing tyrosine phosphatase-1; LAT, linker for activation of T cells.

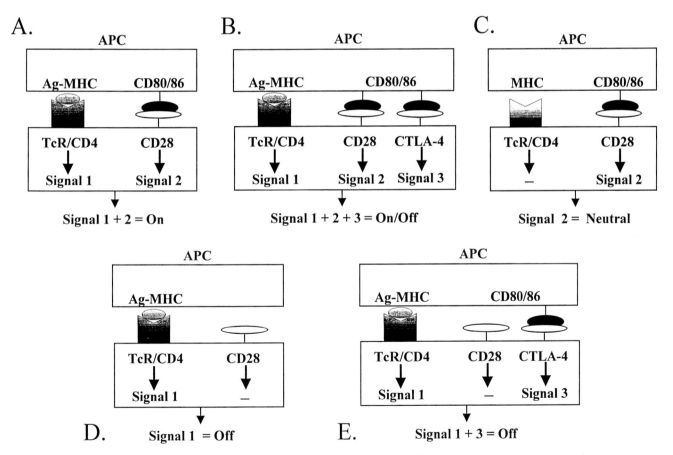

FIG. 14-3 A–E. The three-signal model of lymphocyte activation. Different types of antigen-presenting cells activate distinct forms of signal transduction in T cells, leading to differential signaling to CD28 and CTLA-4 (CD152), and the balance of signals determines the outcome of activation, anergy, or apoptosis.

an APC expressing antigen through appropriate MHC and B7 molecules presents a mixture of stimulating and inhibitory signals to a cognate T cell. If the T cell is resting and only expresses CD28, it is activated (see Fig. 14-3*A*). In contrast, depending on the level of B7 expression and on the activation state of the T cell (i.e., whether it is expressing CD152), the encounter can lead to activation or inhibition of the T cell (see Fig. 14-3*B*). Transgenic experiments testing the effect of ectopic B7 expression indicate that a B7-positive APC that does not express stimulatory peptide–MHC complexes presents a neutral signal and does not activate T cells (16) (see Fig. 14-3*C*).

There is controversy concerning the signals required to induce anergy. Some *in vitro* culture models indicate that signal 1 in the absence of co-stimulation leads to anergy (17), in agreement with the original two-signal model (see Fig. 14-3*D*). However, experiments using CD152 mutant mice bred onto mice expressing transgenic TCRs suggest that CD152 signaling (i.e., signals 1 through 3) is required for the induction of anergy *in vivo* (18) (see Fig. 14-3*E*).

OTHER CO-STIMULATORY RECEPTORS

Many receptors have been reported to enhance T-cell activation (Table 14-1). In some cases, activation is mediated by enhanced T-cell–APC adhesion. Lymphocyte function antigen-1 (LFA-1), an integrin with natural ligands intercellular adhesion molecules (ICAM)-1, -2, and -3, is the best described T-cell adhesion molecule. Although LFA-1 is critical for full T-cell activation and for the generation of signal 1, experiments with mutant mice indicate that CD28 is required to prevent the induction of anergy and that LFA-1 can not substitute for the signal provided by CD28 (19). However, some other molecules appear to have independent co-stimulatory functions. Activated T cells express CD40 ligand (CD40L, renamed CD154), a member of the tumor necrosis factor (TNF) ligand superfamily that includes TNF-α and ligands for CD27, CD30, 4-1BB, and OX40. For example, the binding of CD154 to CD40 strongly induces B7 expression on APCs, but CD40 can also mediate CD28-independent forms of co-stimulation (20). Other co-stimulatory molecules such as 4-1BB and OX40 appear to have important roles in T-cell activation and may provide co-stimulatory signals independent from CD28, particularly when CD28 is not expressed. Given the complexity of the CD28 and CD152 system, the task of uncovering the functions of these other receptor families is daunting.

CO-STIMULATION AND INFECTION

Infection and the Immune System

Because it is reasonable to believe that harmful invasion by exogenous organisms exerts negative selection pressure and that the immune system developed in response to these pressures, the most successful pathogens persist because they do not elicit an immune response or evade the response after it has occurred. Over millions of years of co-evolution with their hosts, pathogens have developed various strategies for avoiding destruction by the immune system. Although for colonial metazoans (i.e., animals) like Porifera (i.e., sponges) invasion may represent settlement by other colonists (21), in vertebrate metazoans immunity protects against infection by subcellular, unicellular, and multicellular pathogens.

Multiple interlocking layers of immune protection have evolved from passive barriers to innate immunity mediated by cells bearing nonclonal receptors to adaptive immunity mediated by antigen-specific lymphocytes. T-cell responses are a component of this latter protection system, which evolved approximately 300 million years ago. It is evident that T cells are not absolutely required for protection against infection, as the plant kingdom has not been overwhelmed by disease for lack of a thymus. For plants, resistance to new pathogens occurs as a result of selection pressure on the whole population, with significantly less adaptability at the individual level. Knockout mice lacking individual co-stimulatory ligands or receptors (e.g., CD28, CD80, CD86, CD152, CD154) are not particularly susceptible to common infectious agents and do not require germ-free isolation. Similarly, patients with loss of T-cell function because of acquired immunodeficiency syndrome (AIDS) are not more susceptible to most common bacterial infections. However, passive barriers and the innate immune system appear to be important lines of defense against bacterial sepsis, as evidenced by the heightened susceptibility of burn victims and neutropenic patients after chemotherapy.

However, the innate and adaptive responses should not be regarded as two separate entities. Receptor signaling involved in innate immune responses may also activate adaptive immunity. For example, the human homologue of Toll, a receptor that mediates potent antifungal responses in *Drosophila,* has been shown to upregulate CD80 (22,23). T-cell–mediated immunity, in addition to providing help for antibody responses, appears to be particularly important against "eukaryotic" pathogens, either discrete organisms such as protozoa or helminths or intracellular pathogens such as viruses and *Leishmania.* Even as cellular immunity has adapted to combat these infections, the infectious agents themselves have counteradapted to avoid or even subvert these immune responses.

Broadly then, what is the role for co-stimulation in T-cell responses to infection? From a beneficial standpoint, co-stimulation is the second signal required for T-cell activation on antigen presentation by professional APCs. Co-stimulation can qualitatively and quantitatively enhance T-cell effector function and appears to be particularly important in cases of low immunogenicity (i.e.,

TABLE 14-1. *Co-stimulatory receptors and ligands*

Molecule	Expression pattern	Gene family	Function	References
CD27	Medullary thymocytes, T cells, NK cells, some B cells	TNF receptor superfamily	Binds CD70; can function as a co-stimulator for T and B cells	136
CD28	T-cell subsets, NK cells, mast cells, plasma cells	Immunoglobulin superfamily	Receptor for co-stimulatory signal for activation of naive CD4 T cells; binds CD80 (B7-1) and CD86 (B7-2)	137–139
CD30	Activated T, B, and NK cells, monocytes	TNF receptor superfamily	Binds CD30L; cross-linking CD30 enhances proliferation of B and T cells, and induces NF-κB activation and HIV expression in chronically infected T lymphocytes	140–143
CD40	B cells, macrophages, dendritic cells, basal epithelial cells, and endothelial cells	TNF receptor superfamily	Binds CD40L; receptor for co-stimulatory signal for B cells, promotes growth, differentiation, and isotype switching of B cells, and cytokine production by macrophages and dendritic cells; required for cell-mediated immunity to *L. major* infection	20, 144
CD43	T cells, thymocytes, neutrophils, and platelets	Mucin-like	Co-stimulator in a CD28-independent fashion because anti-CD43 activates T cells from CD28-deficient mice and wild-type mice; altered in Wiscott-Aldrich syndrome	145, 146
CD70	Activated T and B cells, macrophages	TNF ligand superfamily	Ligand for CD27, may function in co-stimulation of B and T cells	147, 148
CD80 (B7-1)	Monocytes, activated B cells, dendritic cells	Immunoglobulin superfamily	Co-stimulator, ligand for CD28 and CD152	149
CD86 (B7-2)	Monocytes, activated B cells, dendritic cells	Immunoglobulin superfamily	Co-stimulator, ligand for CD28 and CD152	150
OX-2	Activated B and T cells, and brain	Immunoglobulin superfamily	Co-stimulator, ligand unknown	151–153
CD134 (OX40)	Activated T cells	TNF receptor superfamily	T-dependent antibody formation; co-stimulates T cells, OX40 and OX40L, which are induced by HTLV-I infection and directly mediate the adhesion between HTLV-I–infected T cells and vascular endothelial cells	154–156
CDw137 (4-1BB)	Activated T cells	TNF receptor superfamily	Co-stimulator of T-cell proliferation; can function on CD28-negative T cells	154, 157–159
CD152 (CTLA-4)	Activated T cells	Immunoglobulin superfamily	Receptor for CD80 (B7-1) and CD86 (B7-2); negative regulator of T-cell activation	12, 160
CD153 (CD30L)	Activated T cells, activated macrophages, neutrophils, B cells	TNF ligand superfamily	Ligand for CD30, may co-stimulate T cells; CD30 mutant mice have increased thymic size	141, 161
CD154 (CD40L)	Activated CD4 T cells	TNF ligand superfamily	Ligand for CD40	20, 144
CD134L (OX40L)	T cells, dendritic cells	TNF ligand superfamily	Ligand for CD134	162–164
CD137 (4-1BBL)	Activated B cells, macrophages and dendritic cells	TNF ligand superfamily	Ligand for CD137	159, 165

HIV, human immunodeficiency virus; HTLV-I, human T-cell lymphotropic virus type I; *L. major, Leishmania major*; TNF, tumor necrosis factor; NK, natural killer.

low signal 1 strength) in infection and after vaccination (24–26). Co-stimulatory ligand expression by infected cells may also allow for direct CD8+ cytotoxic T cell (CTL) and natural killer (NK) cell recognition and destruction of these cells, similar to host antitumor responses.

From a detrimental standpoint, some infectious agents have developed superantigens capable of crossbinding the nonvariant domains of whole Vβ TCR families and MHC class II molecules. This delivery of signal 1 in the presence of co-stimulation results in widespread T-cell activation and cytokine release, leading to toxic shock and immunosuppression (e.g., staphylococcal exotoxins) and spreading viral infection (e.g., murine mammary tumor virus). Other infectious agents downregulate co-stimulatory ligand expression, preventing CTL-mediated destruction of infected cells or even maintaining a state of immunosuppression. Some pathogens may subvert co-stimulation to qualitatively change the nature of the immune response from a protective (i.e., type 1 helper T cells [T_H1]) to a non-protective one (i.e., type 2 helper T cells [T_H2]). Such persistent infections often induce immune-mediated injury of uninfected tissue that becomes the major pathology of the disease.

The CD28 and CD40 receptor families are the best understood of the co-stimulatory pathways. As a paradigm for the co-stimulation required by the adaptive immune response, we explore the CD28 and CD154 receptor pathways, with the caveat that the other co-stimulatory pathways listed in Table 14-1 are also undoubtedly important in the responses to infection.

Infection and Autoimmunity

Clinical observations have long indicated that intercurrent infections can cause disease exacerbations in patients with autoimmune disorders. For example, some infections such as dysentery can trigger the onset of autoimmune illness (e.g., Reiter's syndrome) in genetically predisposed individuals. Infections can trigger graft-versus-host disease in recipients of allogeneic marrow transplants. Infectious agents may break potentially autoreactive CD4+ T-cell tolerance in some experimental models. For example, concomitant infection with the nematode *Nippostrongylus brasiliensis* breaks an established T-cell tolerance previously induced by injection of mice with *Staphylococcus* enterotoxin B (SEB) (27). Some systemic infections are also potent inducers of bystander T-cell proliferation, another potential means to break self-tolerance (28). Although the causes of autoimmune illness are undoubtedly multifactorial, activation of anergic, potentially autoreactive CD4+ T cells by infectious agents has long been suspected as a mechanism for the initiation of some autoimmune diseases.

Co-stimulation and Viral Infection

Protective Responses

The importance of T cells in antiviral immunity is underscored by the particular susceptibility of animals and patients with primary and secondary T-cell immunodeficiency (i.e., nude mice, human DiGeorge's syndrome and AIDS) or T- and B-cell immunodeficiency to viral infections. The nature of the T-cell responses is a reflection of the viral life cycle and where antigen can be found. The simplest synopsis of viral infection is the invasion of host cells, commandeering of the intracellular machinery, generation of more virus, departure from the host cell (often to that cell's detriment), and repetition of the cycle. T-cell responses can therefore be broadly characterized as directed against intracellular virus (i.e., infected cells) or as coordinating the humoral reaction against extracellular free virus.

In a naive host, the immune system is first alerted to a typical virus after it has infected host cells. Because intracellular virus and malignancy pose many of the same problems to the immune system, it is not surprising that mechanisms of antigen presentation, T-cell activation, and effector function involved in viral immune responses are often those found in antitumor responses. Antiviral and antitumor immunity are arguably essentially the same. Antigen presentation, directly by the infected or neoplastic cell or indirectly by APCs that have picked up shed antigen, results in activation of virus-specific CD8+ cytotoxic T cells early in the course of viral infection.

A requirement for CD28-mediated co-stimulation for the induction of an antiviral CTL response is not absolute but correlates with how immunogenic the infection is. Virulent viruses, such as vaccinia or lymphocytic choriomeningitis virus (LCMV), have prolonged and high levels of replication, and they induce vigorous CTL responses in the absence of CD28 activation, as has been demonstrated in the CD28 knock-out mouse (29,30) and a transgenic mouse strain that expresses blocking levels of soluble fusion protein CTLAIg (31). These data strongly suggest that robust infections with accompanying cell destruction and inflammatory cell infiltrates induce other ligands or cytokines that can substitute for CD28 co-stimulation. B7 expression can be induced by inflammatory cytokines, at least *in vitro*, on cells other than professional APCs, such as fibroblasts (32). Because CD28-independent CTL induction depends on sustained viral antigen presentation and signal 1 delivery, the nature of signal 1 appears to directly influence the requirement for co-stimulation.

Other viruses are more stealthy in their life cycle, and an effective immune response to those invaders appears to depend more on CD28 co-stimulation. For instance, in mice infected with vesicular stomatitis virus (VSV), CD28 activation is necessary for CTL induction, and infection with VSV in CD28 knock-out mice induces anergy in CD8$^+$ cells. These observations led to the notion that cell-mediated immune responses against infection with low-virulence viruses depend more on T-cell help and on CD28-mediated co-stimulation.

A central role for CD28 in the generation of T-cell help is even more evident in the humoral responses to viral infection. Whereas cell-mediated responses predominate in the early phases of infection and are critical for control of intracellular virus, development of neutralizing antibodies against free virus is generally crucial for resolution of the primary infection and for more durable protection against reinfection. Initial antibody responses are primarily of the IgM isotype, followed by affinity maturation and immunoglobulin class switching as independent but typically simultaneous events. The early IgM responses can be T cell dependent or independent, depending on the virus. Isotype switching from IgM to IgG, IgA, or IgE confers different physical and biologic properties on the antibody, which usually enhance efficacy. For example, dimeric IgG has a longer serum half-life and an increased ability to diffuse into tissue compared with the larger pentameric IgM, properties which may enhance protection against reinfection (33).

In contrast to some initial IgM responses, B cells are entirely dependent on CD4$^+$ T-cell help to switch immunoglobulin isotypes. Consistent with the lack of CTL induction, switching from IgM to IgG after VSV infection is significantly reduced in the absence of CD28 co-stimulation (29,31). And, even though induction of CTL is unaffected after LCMV infection, isotype class switching, particularly to neutralizing antibodies, is severely impaired by the lack of CD28. This difference probably reflects differential quantitative and qualitative requirements for co-stimulation by CD4$^+$ and CD8$^+$ cells. These observations underscore the importance of co-stimulation and T-cell help in the generation of a complete immune response to viral infection.

Pathogenic Responses and Viral Subversion

The rationale for MHC-restricted cytotoxic responses is that, although they are bad for the host in that cells are killed, they are worse for the virus. Given the downside of cellular fratricide, it is not surprising that, in contrast to long-lived antibody responses, measurable CTL activity disappears rapidly after infections have resolved. Unfortunately, in some instances after infection (typically with noncytopathic viruses) the virus is incompletely cleared, leading to chronic infection. These chronic immune responses cause the primary pathology of the infection, with persistent cytotoxicity and inflammation resulting in extensive destruction and fibrosis of the tissue harboring the invading virus. One example is chronic active viral hepatitis with progressive immune-mediated liver destruction and cirrhosis (34). Fibrotic changes may benefit the virus by disrupting vascular delivery of effector cells and by disrupting local components of immunity such as barriers or resident immune cells.

The virus also may subvert the immune response by fueling the cytotoxic responses through the direct or indirect induction of co-stimulatory ligands on host cells. For example, 7 of 7 cell lines derived from human hepatocellular carcinoma, a primary tumor of the liver highly associated with hepatitis B infection (35), were reported to express CD80 and CD86 (36). In patients with chronic active hepatitis C infection, CD80 is strongly expressed on hepatocytes (37). The degree of CD80 expression closely correlates with the activity of the hepatitis as determined by histologic measures of inflammation and necrosis and serologically determined by serum alanine transferase elevations. Whether the virus induces B7 expression to increase inflammation or increased inflammation induces B7 expression is not yet clear, but it is evident that protection and pathology are two outcomes of the same antiviral immune response.

Productive infection by many viruses, particularly retroviruses, is enhanced if the target cell is proliferating. If the target cells are T or B cells, co-stimulation may be an important component of the virus-induced cell proliferation that facilitates infection. One example is the mouse mammary tumor virus (MMTV). MMTV is a retrovirus that primarily infects B cells (38). B-cell proliferation is required for viral amplification and for completion of the viral infection cycle (i.e., vertical transmission through the mammary glands to produce milk-borne virus for nursing offspring) (39,40). MMTV induces B-cell proliferation through expression of a viral superantigen, which binds to MHC class II molecules on the B cell and the V region of a specific TCR chain family on the T cell. This T-B interaction triggers T-cell activation, cytokine secretion, and delivery of T-cell help, which supports the proliferation and differentiation of the infected B cell.

MMTV dependence on CD28 signaling can be demonstrated by parenterally infecting CD28 knock-out mice or CTLA-4Ig–producing transgenic mice. In either case, diminished T- and B-cell activation, reduced B-cell proliferation and differentiation, and decreased viral infection and dissemination are observed (41,42). However, oral milk-borne infection is not affected by the loss of CD28 co-stimulation (41), possibly because of CD40-mediated co-stimulation by the infected B cells in the Peyer's patches (43) or by other B7-binding receptors on gut-associated lymphatic tissue–associated T cells (44).

Murine acquired immunodeficiency syndrome (MAIDS) is a fatal disease induced by a mixture of retroviruses known as BM5. It is characterized by splenomegaly, lymphadenopathy, hypergammaglobulinemia, loss of T- and B-cell function, and development of B-cell lymphomas. As the disease progresses, the CD4$^+$ T-cell response to antigens and mitogens is blunted, and the CD4$^+$ T-cell population becomes anergic. Proliferation and cytokine production were restored in the early stages of infection by the addition of a co-stimulatory signal (anti-CD28) and a cytokine (IL-12) but not at later stages when anergy was well established (45). CTLA-4Ig administration substantially delays but does not prevent the onset of MAIDS (46). MAIDS' onset is accompanied by an increase in the level of B7 expression on B cells.

CD4$^+$ T cells from mice with MAIDS are unable to respond to TCR stimulation as measured by proliferation, IL-2 production, or IL-2R upregulation, although responsiveness was restored with pharmacologic receptor bypass activation with phorbol myristate acetate and ionomycin. The inability of MAIDS CD4$^+$ T cells to respond to CD3 stimulation was not associated with reduced surface expression of CD3, CD4, or CD28 and could not be overcome by co-stimulation with anti-CD28 antibody. MAIDS CD4$^+$ T cells have decreased antigen receptor signal transduction with diminished inositol 1,4,5-trisphosphate (IP$_3$) production and reduced Ca^{2+} mobilization compared with normal controls (47,48). Results of these studies indicate that after anergy has been established in MAIDS, unlike many other forms of anergy, it cannot be reversed by providing co-stimulation through CD28 and cytokines.

Human Immunodeficiency Virus Infection

As a consequence of the massive effort devoted to the human immunodeficiency virus (HIV) pandemic, the immune response against HIV-1 and HIV-2 is now the best characterized of all the human and nonhuman primate infections. Findings indicate that more than 30 million persons—approximately 1 of every 100 persons of reproductive age worldwide—are infected by HIV.

Perhaps the most characteristic immunologic abnormality in patients with untreated HIV infection is the lack of virus-specific CD4$^+$ helper T cell responses. The immune response to acute HIV-1 infection is characterized by the rapid development of an antigen-specific CTL response and a broadly directed serologic response. In early HIV-1 infection, the strength of the CTL response, particularly the CTL response with specificity for env, is associated with lower viral loads and with slower declines in CD4$^+$ cell counts (49). High CTL levels are also characteristically found in patients classified as long-term nonprogressors (LTNP). Increased secretion of the β-chemokines RANTES (regulated on activation, normally T-cell expressed and secreted), macrophage inflammatory proteins (MIP-1α and MIP-1β) (50), and other factors secreted by CD8$^+$ cells (51) correlates with delayed progression of HIV-1. Co-stimulation by triggering CD28 *in vitro* strongly enhances secretion of these factors (52–54).

With regard to the serologic response, high-titer and broadly cross-reactive neutralizing antibodies are associated with control of virus replication and low virus load

in LTNP (55,56). Curiously, although neutralizing antibody responses are slow to develop during primary infection, perhaps related to impaired CD4$^+$ helper T function, neutralizing antibody responses are uniquely broad in patients who are LTNPs.

The mechanism of the decline in CD4$^+$ cells during HIV infection remains unknown. Some evidence supports the idea of perturbed T-cell homeostasis, because the numbers of CD3$^+$ T cells remain constant for most of the course of infection, with a reciprocal increase in CD8$^+$ T cells compensating for the loss of CD4$^+$ cells (57). Initial studies based on the response to administration of potent antiretroviral agents proposed a high rate of CD4$^+$ cell turnover in HIV infection, but later studies suggested that the turnover rate is not markedly elevated, leading to the hypothesis that T-cell production is also impaired (58). Measurements of CD4$^+$ cell telomeric terminal restriction fragment length as a index of replicative history have been consistent with this notion (59,60). Although overall CD8$^+$ T-cell numbers are increased during the asymptomatic stage of the infection, studies indicate that CD4$^+$ and CD8$^+$ cells with a naive phenotype decline at similar rates during progressive HIV-1 infection (61). Other studies found that changes in the number of CD8$^+$CD28$^+$ cells closely paralleled those of the CD4$^+$CD28$^+$ T-cell subset, while the presence of CD8$^+$CD28$^-$ T cells correlated inversely with CD4$^+$ and CD8$^+$CD28$^+$ T cells (62). The simplest notion to explain these data is that there is a progressive loss of naive CD28$^+$ T cells in CD4$^+$ and CD8$^+$ subsets with a replacement with CD8$^+$CD28$^-$ T cells and that the CD4$^+$CD28$^+$ T cells die by apoptosis or as a result of viral infection.

Several findings indicate that co-stimulation may be impaired with HIV disease progression. First, a pathologic accumulation of CD28$^-$ T cells occurs in most patients with HIV infection (63–65). These T cells have limited replicative capacity and would be expected to be activated by CD28-independent forms of co-stimulation. Second, the induction of the T-cell anti-apoptotic gene *BCL$_X$* is impaired in patients with HIV-1 infection (66). Studies with mice have indicated that *BCL$_X$* induction depends on CD28 co-stimulation (67). Third, a low index of T-cell proliferation after anti-CD3/CD28 stimulation predicts progression to AIDS and was an independent predictor from CD4$^+$ cell counts (68). Fourth, the lymph node architecture is destroyed during progressive HIV infection (69). The loss of lymphoid mass, in conjunction with the fact that monocytes and dendritic cells are primary HIV-1 targets, suggests that co-stimulation by professional APCs may be decreased during HIV-1 infection. It is unknown whether this is related to the progression of disease that ultimately occurs in most patients.

Studies have evaluated the role of the spleen and of other secondary lymphoid organs for the induction of protective antiviral immune responses. Investigators have employed homeobox gene 11 knock-out mice

(Hox11–/–), which lack a spleen, and homozygous alymphoplastic mutant mice (aly/aly), which possess a structurally altered spleen but lack lymph nodes and Peyer's patches (70). In aly/aly mice, the thymus-independent IgM response against VSV was delayed and reduced, and the subsequent T-dependent switch to the protective IgG was absent. The aly/aly mice were highly susceptible to VSV infection. In contrast, absence of the spleen in the Hox11-/- mice had no major effects on the protective immune response. There is a critical role for organized secondary lymphoid organs for the activation of naive T cells where encounters with foreign antigens occur and a requirement for intact co-stimulatory pathways to avoid progressive anergy of T cells.

Lymph nodes from patients with HIV-1 infection have increased amounts of T cells secreting cytokines and other evidence of increased immune activation. One report indicated that infection of human peripheral blood lymphocytes with HIV-1 *in vitro* followed by T-cell activation through the CD3 and CD28 receptors resulted in enhanced IL-2 secretion. Evidence suggests that the *tat* gene may be responsible for the augmented IL-2 production *in vitro* (71). A T-cell co-stimulatory pathway abnormality induced by HIV-1 infection may play some role in the chronic state of immune hyperactivation observed in untreated patients and thereby abet the spread of virus by promoting bystander T-cell proliferation.

Infection of CD4$^+$ T lymphocytes by HIV-1 is initiated by the virion binding to the CD4 receptor on the cell surface. Fusion and cellular entry, however, depends on interactions between CD4, the viral envelope glycoprotein gp120, and the recently identified family of viral chemokine coreceptors expressed on the cell surface. It has been demonstrated that activation of CD4$^+$ T lymphocytes through the CD28 co-stimulatory pathway renders them resistant to infection with M-tropic HIV-1 (72). CD28 stimulation induces an HIV-1 resistance phenotype similar to that seen in some highly exposed and HIV-uninfected individuals who have homozygous Δ32 mutations of the *CCR5* gene by interrupting the viral life cycle at the level of viral entry (73,74). Further clarification is required to determine the role, if any, of signaling of the CD28 and CD152 (CTLA-4) receptors in the pathogenesis of HIV-1 infection.

Co-stimulation and Bacterial Infections

The primary defense against most bacterial infections is a combination of passive barriers, antigen-nonspecific effector cells such as polymorphonuclear cells or macrophage-monocytes, and antigen-specific antibodies and complement. Direct T-cell involvement is less critical. Indirect T-cell involvement in primary responses to bacterial infection is manifested by the delivery of help necessary for effective B-cell or antibody responses. Consistent with this function, bacterial products such as

lipopolysaccharide (LPS) (75–78) induce CD80 and CD86 on professional APCs. Neisserial porins (79) also induce CD86 on B cells. Although plasmacytoma cells express CD28, the role played by co-stimulatory receptor signaling in plasma cell function remains unknown (80, 81). Mast cells, which do not endogenously express antigen-specific receptors, can nonetheless elicit antigen-specific responses by binding antigen-specific antibody through FcεRI and Fcγ receptors and by upregulating functional CD28 expression on exposure to LPS (82). The role of co-stimulatory receptors on cells of the innate immune system is only beginning to be appreciated, and their role in host defense requires further study.

The nature of the CD4$^+$ T-cell helper or effector subset induced significantly affects the outcome of many infections. Although debate continues regarding the validity of the separation into T$_H$1 and T$_H$2 subsets, particularly in the human immune system, the basic paradigm is that different subsets of CD4$^+$ T cells provide qualitatively different T-cell help based primarily on the constellation of cytokines they secrete. T$_H$1 cells characteristically secrete interferon-γ (IFN-γ), IL-2, and TNF-α on activation, whereas T$_H$2 cells secrete IL-3, IL-4, IL-5, IL-6, and IL-10 (see Chapter 12). Because of these cytokine profiles, T$_H$1 cells are thought to induce macrophage activation, delayed-type hypersensitivity (DTH) responses, and immunoglobulin class switching to isotypes that fix complement and bind readily to macrophage Fc receptors— all responses involved in elimination of intracellular pathogens. T$_H$2 cells are thought to provide B-cell help, induce IgG1 and IgE class switching, and mast cell and eosinophil activation responses important in helminth infection. Each T$_H$ response reciprocally inhibits the other at several different levels as a means of focusing the immune response appropriately for the given challenge.

Some studies have addressed the role of co-stimulation and the T$_H$2 response in the genetic resistance to murine Lyme borreliosis. CTLA-4Ig or anti-CD80 and anti-CD86 monoclonal antibodies were used to investigate the contribution of CD80 and CD86 to the T$_H$2 cytokine profile and development of arthritis in BALB/c mice infected with *Borrelia burgdorferi*. Effective blockade of CD86-CD28 interaction was demonstrated by elimination of IL-4 and upregulation of IFN responses by *B. burgdorferi*-specific T cells and by reduction of *B. burgdorferi*-specific immunoglobulin G. Despite the shift toward a T$_H$1 cytokine pattern, which has been associated with disease susceptibility, the severity of arthritis was unchanged (83). Moreover, combined CD80 and CD86 blockade by using anti-CD80 and anti-CD86 monoclonal antibodies or CTLA-4Ig enhanced IFN production over that seen with CD86 blockade alone, but augmentation of this T$_H$1-associated cytokine did not enhance disease. The IL-4 production by T cells in *B. burgdorferi*-infected BALB/c mice depends on CD86/CD28 interaction, and this cytokine does not apparently contribute significantly to host resistance to the development of arthritis. Combined CD80 and CD86 blockade resulted in preferential expansion of IFN-producing T cells in *B. burgdorferi* infection, suggesting that co-stimulatory pathways other than B7/CD28 may contribute to T-cell activation during continuous antigen stimulation. Studies involving *Borrelia* and *Leishmania* indicate that the B7/CD28 pathway has some role in chronic infections in which deviation of T$_H$ cell immune responses occurs and antigen is persistently present.

Intracellular Bacteria

Intracellular bacteria cause a wide range of human disease, including tuberculosis *(Mycobacterium tuberculosis)*, leprosy *(M. leprae)*, typhoid fever *(Salmonella typhi)*, brucellosis (Brucella species) and listeriosis *(Listeria monocytogenes)*. The first three together have an estimated global prevalence of over 1 billion cases and cause 3.6 million deaths annually. A resurgence of tuberculosis among AIDS patients underscores the importance of T-cell–mediated immunity to these pathogens. The problems presented to the immune system by these intracellular bacteria are the same ones presented by viruses and all other intracellular pathogens. From a protective standpoint, T cells play a central role in responses to intracellular bacteria. Compared with antiviral responses, cell-mediated immunity to intracellular bacteria may be even more important, because it is central to controlling the primary infection and preventing disease recurrence. Sterilizing immunity is seldom achieved in these infections, and failure to contain residual organisms is the primary cause of relapse. For mycobacterial infections such as tuberculosis and leprosy, there is no substantial protection mediated by antibodies, and granuloma formation involving T cells and macrophage-monocytes is the primary mechanism by which residual organisms are held in check.

The interaction between most intracellular bacteria and effector T cells is complicated by the fact that the infected cells are primarily macrophages or monocytes as the bacteria induce their own phagocytosis and use a variety of approaches to avoid intracellular destruction. However, other cell types can also be infected and serve as reservoirs (e.g., hepatocytes for *L. monocytogenes,* Schwann cells for *M. leprae*). Because macrophages/monocytes are professional APCs, infected cells may induce or subvert T-cell activation. Activated macrophage-monocytes and cytotoxic T cells play the central role in effective antimicrobial immune responses (84). Macrophage-monocytes are primarily activated by IFN-γ, with synergy from TNF-α, both of which are secreted by activated T cells. The activated macrophages induce intracellular bactericidal or bacteriostatic effects targeting the infecting organisms (85). CD28-mediated co-stimulation sig-

nificantly enhances T-cell IFN-γ secretion by enhancing cytokine mRNA stability (86). After *L. monocytogenes* infection, CD80- or CD86-induced CD28 co-stimulation *in vivo* is required for IFN production by T cells (88). Consistent with these results, infection of human dendritic cells (but not monocytes) with *M. tuberculosis* induces substantial upregulation of CD40 and CD80 expression (87).

Leprosy is even more complex, because the causal bacterium, *M. leprae,* may suppress cell-mediated immunity or humoral immunity in a mutually exclusive way, leading to the two major forms of the disease: lepromatous and tuberculoid leprosy. In lepromatous leprosy, cell-mediated immunity is profoundly depressed, *M. leprae* organisms are present in abundance, and immune responses to many antigens are suppressed. This produces a clinical state in patients called *anergy,* meaning in this case the absence of delayed-type hypersensitivity to a wide range of antigens unrelated to *M. leprae*. In contrast, patients with tuberculoid leprosy display a potent cell-mediated immunity that controls but does not eradicate infection. Although few viable microorganisms are found in their tissues and the patients usually survive, most of the pathology is caused by the inflammatory response to the persistent microorganisms. Tuberculoid leprosy patients express high levels of CD80, CD86, and CD28 in their skin lesions. Cloned, class II–restricted helper T cells reactive against *M. leprae* antigens derived from leprosy patients have been inhibited by soluble anti-CD28 antibody *in vitro* (89). In contrast, a study of lesions from lepromatous leprosy patients has revealed low CD80, CD86, and CD28 expression but high CTLA-4 expression (90–92). In addition to macrophage-monocyte–mediated killing, cytotoxic effector cells (i.e., NK, CD4+, and CD8+ T cells) can target infected cells (93). Such cytotoxic responses also underlie some of the pathology seen in these diseases, such as the peripheral neuropathy in leprosy secondary to infected Schwann cell destruction (94) or hepatitis in murine listeriosis (95).

It is not surprising that one mechanism used by intracellular bacteria to avoid immune destruction is to down-regulate co-stimulatory receptors on the infected macrophage or monocyte. This would decrease T-cell activation and IFN-γ secretion, reduce susceptibility to cytotoxic T and NK cells, and potentially induce anergy. *M. tuberculosis* infection does not upregulate CD40 or CD80 expression on human monocytes as it does for dendritic cells. *M. tuberculosis* or *S. typhimurium* infection in mice results in downregulation of B7 expression on the infected macrophage (96,97). *M. tuberculosis*-infected macrophages were significantly less effective at inducing antigen-specific T cell-mediated DTH responses than uninfected or rifampin-treated (to kill the intracellular pathogens) macrophages, illustrating an escape mechanism resulting from co-stimulatory ligand downregulation.

Bacterial Toxins

Not all T-cell responses resulting from bacterial invasion are good for the host. This is particularly true in the case of certain staphylococcal toxins, such as staphylococcal enterotoxin A (SEA), SEB, SEC1, SEC2, SEC3, SED, and SEE; toxic shock syndrome toxin-1 (TSST-1); and streptococcal toxins, such as SPE-A and SPE-C. All of these toxins act as superantigens (98–100). Exposure to these toxins results in a wide spectrum of symptoms, including vomiting, diarrhea, high fever, erythroderma with skin desquamation, acute inflammatory lung injury, liver and kidney failure, shock, and even death. These toxins cause disease ranging from common food poisoning (25% of all cases in the United States are caused by staphylococcal enterotoxins) to toxic shock syndrome, with a case-fatality rate of 50% to 90% (101,102). These bacterial superantigens activate entire T-cell families by crossbinding MHC class II to specific TCR Vβ chains. The stimulated T cells proliferate and overproduce the inflammatory cytokines, which cause the syndrome, and the activated T cells then rapidly undergo apoptosis, leaving the victim with generalized immunosuppression and with the deletion of many T cell subsets.

In toxic shock syndrome for example, mass T-cell activation by TSST-1 results in the pathologic release of TNF-α, initiating a cytokine cascade that results in the clinical syndrome. *In vivo*, this immunopathology appears to depend on CD28-mediated co-stimulation. The administration of anti-CD28 antibody to normal mice prevents the septic shock syndrome and death otherwise induced by TSST-1 (103). The protection provided by anti-CD28 antibody was associated with decreased TNF-α levels in the circulation. Serum from anti-CD28 antibody–treated mice was capable of inhibiting the production of TNF-α by bone marrow–derived macrophages after treatment with LPS, perhaps through increased IL-10 secretion. Further, CD28 knock-out mice are completely resistant to the morbidity and mortality induced by TSST-1 (104). Development of toxic shock is also prevented by agents that block CD28 activation such as CTLA-4Ig (105) or anti-CD86 antibodies (106,107). *In vivo*, superantigen responses are augmented by anti-CD152 (CTLA-4) blockade (108) in accord with the three-signal model of T-cell activation (see Fig. 14-3).

CTLA-4Ig treatment prevents the acute sequelae of superantigen exposure, and it also results in long-term protection against rechallenge with TSST-1, even in the absence of further treatment with CTLA-4Ig. This protection was not solely the result of reactive T-cell tolerance (i.e., toxin-mediated signal 1 without co-stimulation), because adoptively transferred CD8+ cells from TSST-1/CTLA-4Ig–treated mice protected naive animals from toxin challenge (105) and further underscores the complexity of antigen-specific T-cell responses.

Co-stimulation and Protozoal Infections

Protozoal infections such as malaria (*Plasmodium* spp), Chagas disease (*Trypanosoma cruzi*), toxoplasmosis (*Toxoplasma gondii*), and leishmaniasis (*Leishmania* spp) represent an enormous health problem, infecting hundreds of millions of people worldwide. Infection of cattle with the protozoan *Theileria parva* caused a financial scourge in East Africa. Most protozoa have complex life cycles involving multiple hosts and the intracellular infection of host cells (see Chapter 62). Predictably, co-stimulatory signals play an important role in an effective immune response against these infections. In addition to the T-cell help required for the development of humoral immunity, the importance of direct T-cell responses in controlling disease is illustrated by the high incidence of *Pneumocystis carinii, T. gondii*, and *Cryptosporidium* infection in patients with AIDS. Similarly, many protozoal parasites (e.g, *T. cruzi, T. gondii, Leishmania major*) are phagocytosed by macrophages but somehow evade intracellular destruction and replicate inside the infected cell. Similarly, effective immunity against the primary infection and containment of residual organisms is mediated by activated macrophages and cell-mediated immunity involving co-stimulation through CD28.

Cytosolic infection of bovine T cells with *T. parva* results in T-cell transformation and clonal expansion of infected cells. Bovine T cells infected with the parasite *T. para* proliferate continuously and display autocrine constitutive secretion of IL-2 (109). Treatment of infected cultures with antitheilerial drugs results in growth arrest and reversion of the infected cells to a resting state. Several lines of evidence indicate that co-stimulation activates the NF-κB family of transcription factors, which may be responsible for the lymphoproliferative disorder induced by *T. parva* infection. Genetic studies show that the phenotype of the *Rel* knock-out mouse reveals immunodeficiencies consistent with decreased co-stimulation (110,111). Signal transduction studies indicate that stimulation of T cells with anti-CD28 increases the binding of the p50/Rel family of transcription factors to the IL-2 and IL-2Ra promoters (112,113). CD28 co-stimulation causes prolonged nuclear translocation of inhibitor IκBα in T cells (114). Findings indicate that the parasite mediates continuous phosphorylation and proteolysis of IκBα and IκBβ (115). This infection leads to persistent activation of NF-κB, suggesting that parasitic appropriation of co-stimulatory signal transduction pathways is important in the pathogenesis of this infection.

CD28-mediated co-stimulation substantially augments T-cell proliferation, secretion of proinflammatory cytokines (e.g., IL-2, granulocyte-macrophage colony-stimulating factor, TNF-α, IFN-γ) and induction of CD8+ CTL function. Activation of macrophages by T-cell IFN-γ secretion is critical for responses against *T. cruzi* (116).

Macrophages infected by *T. cruzi* strongly upregulate CD86 expression within 24 to 48 hours but not other co-stimulatory ligands such as CD80, ICAM-1, and LFA-3 (117). This upregulation markedly enhances the ability of infected macrophages to activate T cells. Patients chronically infected with *T. cruzi* have significantly lower numbers of circulating CD28+ (CD4+ and CD8+) T cells, than uninfected individuals (118). Whether this decrease in CD28+ T cells is caused by the organism itself or is a consequence of the ongoing immune response is unclear, but the similarity to patients with HIV infection described previously is striking.

NK cells are also an important component of immunity to many protozoa, functioning as a source of IFN-γ and as cytotoxic effectors. Infection by *T. gondii* induces macrophages to secrete IL-15 (119), which induces CD28 expression on NK cells (120). *T. gondii* induction of the CD28+ population of NK cells results in enhanced NK cell IFN-γ production and cytolytic activity. The importance of NK cell CD28 for *T. gondii* resistance is demonstrated by severe combined immunodeficiency mice that lack T and B cells but retain functional NK cells. Blockade of CD28 co-stimulation with CTLA-4Ig in these mice significantly increases the *T. gondii* parasite burden.

Co-stimulation is critical for control of infection by *Leishmania* species. After *L. major* infection, susceptible strains of mice (e.g., Balb/c) generate predominantly T_H2 responses that cannot control replication of the parasite, leading to the death of the animal. Conversely, resistant strains of mice that generate T_H1 responses (e.g., C57BL/6) contain the infection, in large part because of activation of macrophages by IFN-γ. CD28-mediated co-stimulation plays an important role in the generation of T_H1 or T_H2 responses. Early blockade of CD28 activation by CTLA-4Ig or antibody treatment with anti-CD86 monoclonal antibody abrogated progressive infection in normally susceptible Balb/c mice (121,122). This protection resulted from the loss of T_H2 responses, suggesting that T_H2 responses depend much more on CD28- and CD86-mediated co-stimulation than T_H1 responses. Whereas a single dose of CTLA-4Ig conferred protection, continued weekly administration abolished the ability of the mice to contain the infection, thus indicating the requirement of CD28 co-stimulation in the ongoing immune responses. Consistent with this is the observation that *Leishmania* infection interferes with the ability of the infected macrophage to upregulate co-stimulatory ligands.

Infection with *Leishmania donovani* has been reported to induce a dominant T_H1-type response in all strains of mice examined. Blockade of the co-stimulatory molecule CD86 (B7-2), but not CD80 (B7-1), significantly enhances disease severity, as measured by the day 28 parasite burden in the liver but not spleen (123). The effects of B7-2 blockade were associated with increased numbers of IFN-γ– and (surprisingly) IL-4–producing cells. Macrophages infected with *L. donovani* downregulate CD80 expression *in vivo* and *in vitro*, decreasing the ability of these cells to provide co-stimulation to CD4+ T cells (124) and inhibiting generation of DTH-mediated functions (125). Infected macrophages are also unable to upregulate CD80 expression in response to other stimuli, such as LPS or supernatants from Con A–treated T cells (124). The ability of infected macrophages to upregulate CD80 expression can be restored by prostaglandin inhibitors (125), and this results in recovery of antileishmanial immune responses. Similarly, studies at the London School of Hygiene and Tropical Medicine indicate that blockade of CTLA-4 with injections of anti-CTLA-4 antibody results in potent augmentation of leishmanial immunity.

However, Balb/c (susceptible) or C57BL/6 (resistant) mice bred onto a CD28 knock-out background unexpectedly retain their strain-related T_H bias and susceptibility to *L. major* infection, suggesting other factors are involved or can compensate for the loss of CD28 function (126). These studies did not examine the role of the other B7-binding receptor, CD152 (CTLA-4), on the generation of T_H2 responses. Anti-CD152 (CTLA-4) in CD28 knock-out mice affects the response and outcome of infection with *Leishmania* (B. Saha, unpublished observations).

Co-stimulation and Worms

Helminths differ from the previously examined organisms in that the infection is not intracellular and that immunity is primarily mediated by T_H2 responses. The role for CD28 in immunity to helminth infection is demonstrated by responses to *Schistosoma mansoni*. *S. mansoni* is a tissue-dwelling trematode parasite that elicits immediate hypersensitivity responses characterized by eosinophilia and elevated serum IgE levels, mediated in large part by T-cell IL-4 and IL-5 production (127). The ova of adult worms also elicit potent T_H2 responses (128), and it is these responses against ova lodged in tissues, primarily liver, that result in substantial pathology of the disease. Deviation to T_H2 responses is accompanied by downregulation of T_H1 responses, which may subvert responses that are potentially protective against reinfection by schistosomal larvae (129).

Blockade of CD28 activation with CTLA-4Ig significantly decreases production of the T_H2 cytokines IL-4 and IL-5 in response to schistosomal egg antigens while enhancing IFN-γ secretion (130). Likewise, CD28 knock-out mice have impaired T_H2 responses to egg antigens and schistosome infection, with the latter manifested by decreases in serum IgE and adult worm-specific IgG1 levels. Consequently, CD28 knock-out mice had significantly greater adult parasite loads than their wild-type counterparts. In further studies concerning the mechanism of granuloma formation, mice were injected with *S.*

mansoni eggs and followed for induction of pulmonary granulomas. Anti-B7-2 treatment inhibited pulmonary granuloma formation by 74% and decreased levels of lung IL-5 and IL-13 transcripts compared with those in animals given control immunoglobulin by 20- and 5-fold, respectively, and anti-B7-1 administration had no effect (131). Similarly, treatment with anti-CD86 antibody but not anti-CD80 inhibited T_H2 responses as assessed by IL-4, IgG1, and IgE to infection with *N. brasiliensis* (132).

T_H2 responses to mucosal infection with the gastrointestinal nematode *Heligmosomoides polygyrus* are also inhibited by treatment with CTLA-4Ig (133) or anti-CD80+ anti-CD86 antibodies, but not by either alone, suggesting that either CD80 or CD86 was sufficient to initiate the response (134). Increases in the number of IL-4– but not IL-5–secreting cells were also inhibited by CTLA-4Ig and *H. polygyrus*-induced elevations in serum IgE levels, but not blood eosinophils, were markedly inhibited by CTLA-4Ig. Surprisingly, whereas T_H2 responses to anti-IgD activation were lost in CD28 knock-out mice, the T_H2 responses to *H. polygyrus* were preserved (44). This observation suggests that compensatory co-stimulation pathways have developed in these mice or that a B7-dependent, CD28-independent mechanism such as CTLA-4 activation exists, as has been suggested for NK-mediated killing (135) and immunity to *M. leprae* (92).

In summary, many studies indicate that co-stimulation has a role in determination of self from nonself reactivity. It is possible that the necessity of this distinction has been evolutionarily driven, in part by the need to recognize intracellular eukaryotic pathogens. In some cases, pathogens appear to have counteradapted to avoid, interdict, or subvert immune responses at the level of co-stimulation.

ACKNOWLEDGMENTS

The views expressed in this article are those of the authors and do not reflect the official policy or position of the Department of the Army and Navy, Department of Defense, nor the United States Government. The work was supported in part by Naval Medical Research and Development Command Grant EW.0095.003.1412 and by Army contract #DAMD17-93-V-3004.

REFERENCES

1. Bretscher P, Cohn M. A theory of self-nonself discrimination. *Science* 1970;169:1042–1049.
2. Lafferty KJ, Cunningham AJ. A new analysis of allogeneic interactions. *Aust J Exp Biol Med Sci* 1975;53:27–42.
3. MacDonald HR. Mechanisms of immunological tolerance. *Science* 1989;246:982.
4. Zinkernagel RM. Immunology taught by viruses. *Science* 1996;271:173–178.
5. Groux H, O'Garra A, Bigler M, et al. A CD4- T-cell subset inhibits antigen-specific T-cell responses and prevents colitis. *Nature* 1997;389:737–742.
6. Telander DG, Mueller DL. Impaired lymphokine secretion in anergic CD4$^+$ T cells leads to defective help for B cell growth and differentiation. *J Immunol* 1997;158:4704–4713.
7. Ward SG, June CH, Olive D. PI 3-kinase: a pivotal pathway in T cell activation? *Immunol Today* 1996;17:187–197.
8. Kim HH, Tharayil M, Rudd CE. Growth factor receptor-bound protein 2 SH2/SH3 domain binding to CD28 and its role in co-signaling. *J Biol Chem* 1998;273:296–301.
9. Fields PE, Gajewski TF, Fitch FW. Blocked Ras activation in anergic CD4$^+$ T cells. *Science* 1996;271:1276–1278.
10. Li W, Whaley CD, Mondino A, Mueller DL. Blocked signal transduction to the ERK and JNK protein kinases in anergic CD4$^+$ T cells. *Science* 1996;271:1272–1276.
11. Boussiotis VA, Freeman GJ, Berezovskaya A, Barber DL, Nadler LM. Maintenance of human T cell anergy: blocking of IL-2 gene transcription by activated Rap1. *Science* 1997;278:124–128.
12. Bluestone JA. Is CTLA-4 a master switch for peripheral T cell tolerance? *J Immunol* 1997;158:1989–1993.
13. Blair PJ, Riley JL, Levine BL, et al. CTLA-4 ligation delivers a unique signal to human CD4 T cells that supports cell survival but not IL-2 secretion. *J Immunol* 1998;160:12–15.
14. Tivol EA, Borriello F, Schweitzer AN, Lynch WP, Bluestone JA, Sharpe AH. Loss of CTLA-4 leads to massive lymphoproliferation and fatal multiorgan tissue destruction, revealing a critical negative regulatory role of CTLA-4. *Immunity* 1995;3:541–547.
15. Waterhouse P, Penninger JM, Timms E, et al. CTLA-4 deficiency causes lymphoproliferative disorder with early lethality. *Science* 1995;270:985–988.
16. Harlan DM, Hengartner H, Huang ML, et al. Mice expressing both B7-1 and viral glycoprotein on pancreatic beta cells along with glycoprotein-specfic transgenic T cells develop diabetes due to a breakdown of T-lymphocyte unresponsiveness. *Proc Natl Acad Sci USA* 1994;91:3137–3141.
17. Johnson JG, Jenkins MK. Accessory cell-derived signals required for T cell. *Immunol Res* 1993;12:48–64.
18. Perez VL, Van Parijs L, Biuckians A, Zheng XX, Strom TB, Abbas AK. Induction of peripheral T cell tolerance *in vivo* requires CTLA-4 engagement. *Immunity* 1997;6:411–417.
19. Bachmann MF, McKall-Faienza K, Schmits R, et al. Distinct roles for LFA-1 and CD28 during activation of naive T cells: adhesion versus costimulation. *Immunity* 1997;7:549–557.
20. Larsen CP, Pearson TC. The CD40 pathway in allograft rejection, acceptance, and tolerance. *Curr Opin Immunol* 1997;9:641–647.
21. Smith LC, Hildemann WH. Allograft rejection, autograft fusion and inflammatory responses to injury in *Callyspongia diffusa* (Porifera; Demospongia). *Proc R Soc Lond B Biol Sci* 1986;226:445–464.
22. Lemaitre B, Nicolas E, Michaut L, Reichhart JM, Hoffmann JA. The dorsoventral regulatory gene cassette spatzle/Toll/cactus controls the potent antifungal response in *Drosophila* adults. *Cell* 1996;86:973–983.
23. Medzhitov R, Preston-Hurlburt P, Janeway CA. A human homologue of the *Drosophila* Toll protein signals activation of adaptive immunity. *Nature* 1997;388:394–397.
24. Kundig TM, Shahinian A, Kawai K, et al. Duration of TCR stimulation determines costimulatory requirement of T cells. *Immunity* 1996;5:41–52.
25. Reiser H, Stadecker MJ. Costimulatory B7 molecules in the pathogenesis of infectious and autoimmune diseases. *N Engl J Med* 1996;335:1369–1377.
26. Horspool JH, Perrin PJ, Woodcock JB, et al. Nucleic acid vaccine-induced immune responses require CD28 costimulation and are regulated by CTLA4. *J Immunol* 1998;160:3589.
27. Rocken M, Urban JF, Shevach EM. Infection breaks T-cell tolerance. *Nature* 1992;359:79–82.
28. Tough DF, Borrow P, Sprent J. Induction of bystander T cell proliferation by viruses and type I interferon *in vivo*. *Science* 1996;272:1947–1950.
29. Shahinian A, Pfeffer K, Lee KP, et al. Differential T cell costimulatory requirements in CD28-deficient mice. *Science* 1993;261:609–612.
30. Kundig TM, Shahinian A, Kawai K, et al. Duration of TCR stimulation determines costimulatory requirement of T cells. *Immunity* 1996;5:41–52.
31. Zimmermann C, Seiler P, Lane P, Zinkernagel RM. Antiviral immune responses in CTLA4 transgenic mice. *J Virol* 1997;71:1802–1807.
32. Pechhold K, Patterson NB, Craighead N, Lee KP, June CH, Harlan

DM. Inflammatory cytokines INF-gamma plus TNF-α induce regulated expression of CD80 (B7-1) but not CD86 (B7-2) on murine fibroblasts. *J Immunol* 1997;158:4921–4929.

33. Snapper C, Finkelman FD. Immunoglobulin class switching. In: Paul WE, ed. *Fundamental immunology.* New York: Raven Press, 1993: 837–864.

34. Koziel MJ, Dudley D, Wong JT, et al. Intrahepatic cytotoxic T lymphocytes specific for hepatitis C virus in persons with chronic hepatitis. *J Immunol* 1992;149:3339–3344.

35. Beasley RP, Hwang LY, Lin CC, Chien CS. Hepatocellular carcinoma and hepatitis B virus: a prospective study of 22,707 men in Taiwan. *Lancet* 1981;2:1129–1133.

36. Tatsumi T, Takehara T, Katayama K, et al. Expression of costimulatory molecules B7-1 (CD80) and B7-2 (CD86) on human hepatocellular carcinoma. *Hepatology* 1997;25:1108–1114.

37. Mochizuki K, Hayashi N, Katayama K, et al. B7/BB-1 expression and hepatitis activity in liver tissues of patients with chronic hepatitis C. *Hepatology* 1997;25:713–718.

38. Held W, Shakhov AN, Izui S, et al. Superantigen-reactive CD4+ T cells are required to stimulate B cells after infection with mouse mammary tumor virus. *J Exp Med* 1993;177:359–366.

39. Golovkina TV, Chervonsky A, Dudley JP, Ross SR. Transgenic mouse mammary tumor virus superantigen expression prevents viral infection. *Cell* 1992;69:637–645.

40. Held W, Waanders GA, Shakhov AN, Scarpellino L, Acha-Orbea H, MacDonald HR. Superantigen-induced immune stimulation amplifies mouse mammary tumor virus infection and allows virus transmission. *Cell* 1993;74:529–540.

41. Palmer LD, Saha B, Hodes RJ, Abe R. The role of CD28 costimulation in immune-mediated responses against mouse mammary tumor viruses. *J Immunol* 1996;156:2112–2118.

42. Champagne E, Scarpellino L, Lane P, Acha-Orbea H. CD28/CTLA4-B7 interaction is dispensable for T cell stimulation by mouse mammary tumor superantigen but not for B cell differentiation and virus dissemination. *Eur J Immunol* 1996;26:1595–1602.

43. Chervonsky AV, Xu J, Barlow AK, Khery M, Flavell RA, Janeway CA. Direct physical interaction involving CD40 ligand on T cells and CD40 on B cells is required to propagate MMTV. *Immunity* 1995;3:139–146.

44. Gause WC, Chen SJ, Greenwald RJ, et al. CD28-dependence of T cell differentiation to IL-4 production varies with the particular type 2 immune response. *J Immunol* 1997;158:4082–4087.

45. Andrews C, Swain SL, Muralidhar G. CD4 T cell anergy in murine AIDS: costimulation via CD28 and the addition of IL-12 are not sufficient to rescue anergic CD4 T cells. *J Immunol* 1997;159:2132–2138.

46. de Leval L. CTLA4 Ig treatment of MAIDS syndrome. *J Virol* 1998 (in press).

47. Fitzpatrick EA, Kaplan AM, Cohen DA. Defective CD4+ T cell signaling in murine AIDS: uncoupling of the T cell receptor complex from PIP2 hydrolysis. *Cell Immunol* 1996;167:176–187.

48. Selvey LA, Morse HC III, June CH, Hodes RJ. Analysis of antigen receptor signaling in B cells from mice with a retrovirus-induced acquired immunodeficiency syndrome. *J Immunol* 1995;154:171–179.

49. Musey L, Hughes J, Schacker T, Shea T, Corey L, McElrath MJ. Cytotoxic-T-cell responses, viral load, and disease progression in early human immunodeficiency virus type 1 infection. *N Engl J Med* 1997; 337:1267–1274.

50. Rosenberg ES, Billingsley JM, Caliendo AM, et al. Vigorous HIV-1–specific CD4+ T cell responses associated with control of viremia. *Science* 1997;278:1447–1450.

51. Walker CM, Moody DJ, Stites DP, Levy JA. CD8+ lymphocytes can control HIV infection *in vitro* by suppressing virus replication. *Science* 1986;234:1563–1566.

52. Riley JL, Carroll RG, Levine BL, et al. Intrinsic resistance to T cell infection with human immunodeficiency virus type 1 induced by CD28 costimulation. *J Immunol* 1997;158:5545–5553.

53. Greenfield EA, Howard E, Paradis T, et al. B7.2 expressed by T cells does not induce CD28-mediated costimulatory activity but retains CTLA4 binding: implications for induction of antitumor immunity to T cell tumors. *J Immunol* 1997;158:2025–2034.

54. Barker E, Bossart KN, Fujimura SH, Levy JA. CD28 costimulation increases CD8+ cell suppression of HIV replication. *J Immunol* 1997;159:5123–5131.

55. Zhang YJ, Fracasso C, Fiore JR, et al. Augmented serum neutralizing activity against primary human immunodeficiency virus type 1 (HIV-1) isolates in two groups of HIV-1–infected long-term nonprogressors. *J Infect Dis* 1997;176:1180–1187.

56. Pilgrim AK, Pantaleo G, Cohen OJ, et al. Neutralizing antibody responses to human immunodeficiency virus type 1 in primary infection and long-term-nonprogressive infection. *J Infect Dis* 1997;176: 924–932.

57. Margolick JB, Munoz A, Donnenberg AD, et al. Failure of T-cell homeostasis preceding AIDS in HIV-1 infection. *Nat Med* 1995;1: 674–680.

58. Hellerstein MK, McCune JM. T cell turnover in HIV-1 disease. *Immunity* 1997;7:583–589.

59. Wolthers KC, Otto SA, Lens SMA, et al. Increased expression of CD80, CD86 and CD70 on T cells from HIV-infected individuals upon activation *in vitro*: regulation by CD4+ T cells. *Eur J Immunol* 1996;26:1700–1706.

60. Palmer LD, Weng N-P, Levine BL, June CH, Lane HC, Hodes RJ. Telomere length, telomerase activity, and replicative potential in HIV infection: analysis of CD4+ and CD8+ T cells from HIV-discordant monozygotic twins. *J Exp Med* 1997;185:1381–1386.

61. Roederer M, Dubs JG, Anderson MT, Raju PA, Herzenberg LA. CD8 naive T cell counts decrease progressively in HIV-infected adults. *J Clin Invest* 1995;95:2061–2066.

62. Caruso A, Licenziati S, Canaris AD, et al. Contribution of CD4(+), CD8(+)CD28(+), and CD8(+)CD28(-) T cells to CD3(+) lymphocyte homeostasis during the natural course of HIV-1 infection. *J Clin Invest* 1998;101:137–144.

63. Caruso A, Cantalamessa A, Licenziati S, et al. Expression of CD28 on CD8+ and CD4+ lymphocytes during HIV infection. *Scand J Immunol* 1994;40:485–490.

64. Choremi-Papadopoulou H, Viglis V, Gargalianos P, Kordossis T, Iniotaki-Theodoraki A, Kosmidis J. Downregulation of CD28 surface antigen on CD4+ and CD8+ T lymphocytes during HIV-1 infection. *J Acquir Immune Defic Syndr* 1994;7:245–253.

65. Lewis DE, Tang DS, Adu-Oppong A, Schober W, Rodgers JR. Anergy and apoptosis in CD8+ T cells from HIV-infected persons. *J Immunol* 1994;153:412–420.

66. Blair PJ, Boise LH, Perfetto SP, et al. Impaired induction of the apoptosis-protective protein Bcl-XL in asymptomatic HIV-infected individuals. *J Clin Immunol* 1997;17:234–246.

67. Boise LH, Minn AJ, Accavitti MA, June CH, Lindsten T, Thompson CB. CD28 costimulation can promote T cell survival by inducing the expression of Bcl-XL. *Immunity* 1995;3:87–98.

68. Roos MT, Miedema F, Meinesz AP, et al. Low T cell reactivity to combined CD3 plus CD28 stimulation is predictive for progression to AIDS: correlation with decreased CD28 expression. *Clin Exp Immunol* 1996;105:409–415.

69. Fauci AS. Host factors and the pathogenesis of HIV-induced disease. *Nature* 1996;384:529–534.

70. Karrer U, Althage A, Odermatt B, et al. On the key role of secondary lymphoid organs in antiviral immune responses studied in alymphoplastic (aly/aly) and spleenless (Hox11(-)/-) mutant mice. *J Exp Med* 1997;185:2157–2170.

71. Ott M, Emiliani S, Van L C, et al. Immune hyperactivation of HIV-1–infected T cells mediated by tat and the CD28 pathway. *Science* 1997;275:1481–1485.

72. Levine BL, Mosca J, Riley JL, et al. Antiviral effect and *ex vivo* CD4+ T cell proliferation in HIV-positive patients as a result of CD28 costimulation. *Science* 1996;272:1939–1943.

73. Carroll RG, Riley JL, Levine BL, et al. Differential regulation of HIV-1 fusion cofactor expression by CD28 costimulation of CD4+ T cells. *Science* 1997;276:273–276.

74. Paxton WA, Martin SR, Tse D, et al. Relative resistance to HIV-1 infection of CD4 lymphocytes from persons who remain uninfected despite multiple high-risk sexual exposure. *Nat Med* 1996;2:412–417.

75. Razi-Wolf Z, Freeman GJ, Galvin F, Benacerraf B, Nadler L, Reiser H. Expression and function of the murine B7 antigen, the major costimulatory molecule expressed by peritoneal exudate. *Proc Natl Acad Sci USA* 1992;89:4210–4214.

76. Freeman GJ, Borriello F, Hodes RJ, et al. Uncovering of functional alternative CTLA-4 counter-receptor in B7-deficient mice. *Science* 1993;262:907–909.

77. Hathcock KS, Laszlo G, Dickler HB, Bradshaw J, Linsley P, Hodes RJ. Identification of an alternative CTLA-4 ligand costimulatory for T cell activation. *Science* 1993;262:905–907.

78. Schmittel A, Scheibenbogen C, Keilholz U. Lipopolysaccharide effectively up-regulates B7-1 (CD80) expression and costimulatory function of human monocytes. *Scand J Immunol* 1995;42:701–704.

79. Wetzler LW, Ho Y, Reiser H. Neisserial porins induce B lymphocytes to express costimulatory B7-2 molecules and to proliferate. *J Exp Med* 1996;183:1151–1159.

80. Kozbor D, Moretta A, Messner HA, Moretta L, Croce CM. Tp44 molecules involved in antigen-independent T cell activation are expressed on human plasma cells. *J Immunol* 1987;138:4128–4132.

81. Pellat Deceunynck C, Bataille R, Robillard N, et al. Expression of CD28 and CD40 in human myeloma cells: a comparative study with normal plasma cells. *Blood* 1994;84:2597–2603.

82. Marietta EV, Weis JJ, Weis JH. CD28 expression by mouse mast cells is modulated by lipopolysaccharide and outer surface protein A lipoprotein from *Borrelia burgdorferi*. *J Immunol* 1997;159:2840–2848.

83. Shanafelt MC, Kang I, Barthold SW, Bockenstedt LK. Modulation of murine Lyme borreliosis by interruption of the B7/CD28 T-cell co-stimulatory pathway. *Infect Immun* 1998;66:266–271.

84. Celada A, Nathan C. Macrophage activation revisited. *Immunol Today* 1994;15:100–102.

85. Kaufmann S. Immunity to intracellular bacteria. In: Paul WE, ed. *Fundamental immunology*. New York: Raven Press, 1993: 1151–1186.

86. Lindsten T, June CH, Ledbetter JA, Stella G, Thompson CB. Regulation of lymphokine messenger RNA stability by a surface-mediated T cell activation pathway. *Science* 1989;244:339–343.

87. Henderson RA, Watkins SC, Flynn JL. Activation of human dendritic cells following infection with Mycobacterium tuberculosis. *J Immunol* 1997;159:635–643.

88. Zhan Y, Cheers C. Either B7-1 or B7-2 is required for Listeria monocytogenes-specific production of gamma interferon and interleukin-2. *Infect Immun* 1996;64:5439–5441.

89. Lesslauer W, Koning F, Ottenhoff T, Giphart M, Goulmy E, van Rood JJ. T90/44 (9.3 antigen): a cell surface molecule with a function in human T cell activation. *Eur J Immunol* 1986;16:1289–1296.

90. Li SG, Ottenhoff TH, Van der Eisen P, et al. Human suppressor T cell clones lack CD28. *Eur J Immunol* 1990;20:1281–1288.

91. Mesret Y, Reed AH, Howe RC. Proliferative responses of T cells from the skin and nerve lesions of leprosy patients. *Clin Immunol Immunopathol* 1995;77:243–252.

92. Schlienger K, Uyemura K, Jullien D, et al. B7-1, but not CD28, is crucial for the maintenance of the CD4+ T cell responses in human leprosy. *J Immunol* 1998;161:2407.

93. Kaufmann SH. Immunity to intracellular bacteria. *Annu Rev Immunol* 1993;11:129–163.

94. Steinhoff U, Kaufmann SH. Specific lysis by CD8+ T cells of Schwann cells expressing *Mycobacterium leprae* antigens. *Eur J Immunol* 1988;18:969–972.

95. Sasaki T, Mieno M, Udono H, et al. Roles of CD4+ and CD8+ cells, and the effect of administration of recombinant murine interferon gamma in listerial infection. *J Exp Med* 1990;171:1141–1154.

96. Saha B, Das G, Vohra H, Ganguly NK, Mishra GC. Macrophage–T cell interaction in experimental mycobacterial infection: selective regulation of co-stimulatory molecules on *Mycobacterium*-infected macrophages and its implication in the suppression of cell-mediated immune response. *Eur J Immunol* 1994;24:2618–2624.

97. Gupta S, Vohra H, Saha B, Nain CK, Ganguly NK. Macrophage-T cell interaction in murine salmonellosis: selective down-regulation of ICAM-1 and B7 molecules in infected macrophages and its probable role in cell-mediated immunity. *Eur J Immunol* 1996;26:563–570.

98. Kotb M. Bacterial pyrogenic exotoxins as superantigens. *Clin Microbiol Rev* 1995;8:411–426.

99. Ulrich R, Sidell S, Taylor T, Wilhelmsen C, Franz D. Staphylococcal enteroxtoxin B and related pyrogenic toxins. In: Sidell F, Takafuji E, Franz D, eds. *Medical aspects of chemical and biological warfare*. Bethesda, MD: Department of the Army, 1997:621–630.

100. Reda K, Rich RR. Superantigens. In: Rich RR, ed. *Principles of clinical immunology*. St. Louis: Mosby–Year Book, 1998:132–148.

101. Freedman JD, Beer DJ. Expanding perspectives on the toxic shock syndrome. *Adv Intern Med* 1991;36:363–397.

102. Schlievert PM. Role of superantigens in human disease. *J Infect Dis* 1993;167:997–1002.

103. Wang R, Fang Q, Zhang L, et al. CD28 ligation prevents bacterial toxin-induced septic shock in mice by inducing IL-10 expression. *J Immunol* 1997;158:2856–2861.

104. Saha B, Harlan DM, Lee KP, June CH, Abe R. Protection against lethal toxic shock by targeted disruption of the CD28 gene. *J Exp Med* 1996;183:2675–2680.

105. Saha B, Jaklic E, Harlan DM, Gray GS, June CH, Abe R. Toxic shock syndrome toxin-1 (TSST-1) induced death is prevented by CTLA4-Ig. *J Immunol* 1996;157:3869–3875.

106. Muraille E, De Smedt T, Thielemans K, Urbain J, Moser M, Leo O. Activation of murine T cells by bacterial superantigens requires B7-mediated costimulation. *Cell Immunol* 1995;162:315–320.

107. Muraille E, De Smedt T, Urbain J, Moser M, Leo O. B7-2 provides costimulatory functions *in vivo* in response to staphylococcal enterotoxin B. *Eur J Immunol* 1995;25:2111–2114.

108. Krummel MF, Sullivan TJ, Allison JP. Superantigen responses and costimulation: CD28 and CTLA-4 have opposing effects on T cell expansion *in vitro* and *in vivo*. *Int Immunol* 1996;8:519–523.

109. Dobbelaere DA, Coquerelle TM, Roditi IJ, Eichhorn M, Williams RO. *Theileria parva* infection induces autocrine growth of bovine lymphocytes. *Proc Natl Acad Sci USA* 1988;85:4730–4734.

110. Kontgen F, Grumont RJ, Strasser A, et al. Mice lacking the c-rel proto-oncogene exhibit defects in lymphocyte proliferation, humoral immunity, and interleukin-2 expression. *Genes Dev* 1995;9:1965–1977.

111. Gerondakis S, Strasser A, Metcalf D, Grigoriadis G, Scheerlinck JY, Grumont RJ. Rel-deficient T cells exhibit defects in production of interleukin 3 and granulocyte-macrophage colony-stimulating factor. *Proc Natl Acad Sci USA* 1996;93:3405–3409.

112. Ghosh P, Tan TH, Rice NR, Sica A, Young HA. The interleukin-2 CD28-responsive complex contains at least three members of the NF kappa B family: c-Rel, p50, and p65. *Proc Natl Acad Sci USA* 1993;90:1696–1700.

113. Himes SR, Coles LS, Reeves R, Shannon MF. High mobility group protein I(Y) is required for function and for c-Rel binding to CD28 response elements within the GM-CSF and IL-2 promoters. *Immunity* 1996;5:479–489.

114. Lai JH, Tan TH. CD28 signaling causes a sustained down-regulation of I kappa B alpha which can be prevented by the immunosuppressant rapamycin. *J Biol Chem* 1994;269:30077–30080.

115. Palmer GH, Machado JJ, Fernandez P, Heussler V, Perinat T, Dobbelaere DA. Parasite-mediated nuclear factor kappa B regulation in lymphoproliferation caused by *Theileria parva* infection. *Proc Natl Acad Sci U S A* 1997;94:12527–12532.

116. Reed SG. *In vivo* administration of recombinant IFN-gamma induces macrophage activation, and prevents acute disease, immune suppression, and death in experimental *Trypanosoma cruzi* infections. *J Immunol* 1988;140:4342–4347.

117. Frosch S, Kuntzlin D, Fleischer B. Infection with *Trypanosoma cruzi* selectively upregulates B7-2 molecules on macrophages and enhances their costimulatory activity. *Infect Immun* 1997;65:971–977.

118. Dutra WO, Martins-Filho OA, Cancado JR, et al. Chagasic patients lack CD28 expression on many of their circulating T lymphocytes. *Scand J Immunol* 1996;43:88–93.

119. Doherty TM, Seder RA, Sher A. Induction and regulation of IL-15 expression in murine macrophages. *J Immunol* 1996;156:735–741.

120. Hunter CA, Ellis-Neyer L, Gabriel KE, et al. The role of the CD28/B7 interaction in the regulation of NK cell responses during infection with *Toxoplasma gondii*. *J Immunol* 1997;158:2285–2293.

121. Corry DB, Reiner SL, Linsley PS, Locksley RM. Differential effects of blockade of CD28-B7 on the development of Th1 or Th2 effector cells in experimental leishmaniasis. *J Immunol* 1994;153:4142–4148.

122. Brown JA, Titus RG, Nabavi N, Glimcher LH. Blockade of CD86 ameliorates *Leishmania major* infection by down-regulating the Th2 response. *J Infect Dis* 1996;174:1303–1308.

123. Murphy ML, Engwerda CR, Gorak PM, Kaye PM. B7-2 blockade enhances T cell responses to *Leishmania donovani*. *J Immunol* 1997;159:4460–4466.

124. Kaye PM, Rogers NJ, Curry AJ, Scott JC. Deficient expression of co-stimulatory molecules on *Leishmania*-infected macrophages. *Eur J Immunol* 1994;24:2850–2854.

125. Saha B, Das G, Vohra H, Ganguly NK, Mishra GC. Macrophage-T

cell interaction in experimental visceral leishmaniasis: failure to express costimulatory molecules on *Leishmania*-infected macrophages and its implication in the suppression of cell-mediated immunity. *Eur J Immunol* 1995;25:2492–2498.

126. Brown DR, Green JM, Moskowitz NH, Davis M, Thompson CB, Reiner SL. Limited role of CD28-mediated signals in T helper subset differentiation. *J Exp Med* 1996;184:803–810.

127. Sher A, Coffman RL. Regulation of immunity to parasites by T cells and T cell-derived cytokines. *Annu Rev Immunol* 1992;10:385–409.

128. Grzych JM, Pearce E, Cheever A, et al. Egg deposition is the major stimulus for the production of Th2 cytokines in murine *Schistosomiasis mansoni*. *J Immunol* 1991;146:1322–1327.

129. Pearce EJ, Caspar P, Grzych JM, Lewis FA, Sher A. Downregulation of Th1 cytokine production accompanies induction of Th2 responses by a parasitic helminth, *Schistosoma mansoni*. *J Exp Med* 1991;173:159–166.

130. King CL, Xianli J, June CH, Abe R, Lee KP. CD28-deficient mice generate an impaired Th2 response to *Schistosoma mansoni* infection. *Eur J Immunol* 1996;25:2448–2455.

131. Subramanian G, Kazura JW, Pearlman E, Jia X, Malhotra I, King CL. B7-2 requirement for helminth-induced granuloma formation and CD4 type 2 T helper cell cytokine expression. *J Immunol* 1997;158:5914–5920.

132. Nakajima A, Watanabe N, Yoshino S, Yagita H, Okumura K, Azuma M. Requirement of CD28-CD86 co-stimulation in the interaction between antigen-primed T helper type 2 and B cells. *Int Immunol* 1997;9:637–644.

133. Lu P, di Zhou X, Chen SJ, et al. CTLA-4 ligands are required to induce an *in vivo* interleukin 4 response to a gastrointestinal nematode parasite. *J Exp Med* 1994;180:693–698.

134. Greenwald R, Lu P, Halvorson M, et al. Effects of blocking B7-1 and B7-2 interactions during a type 2 *in vivo* immune response. *J Immunol* 1997;158:4088–4096.

135. Chambers BJ, Salcedo M, Ljunggren HG. Triggering of natural killer cells by the costimulatory molecule CD80 (B7-1). *Immunity* 1996;5:311–317.

136. Hintzen RQ, Lens SM, Lammers K, Kuiper H, Beckmann MP, van Lier RA. Engagement of CD27 with its ligand CD70 provides a second signal for T cell activation. *J Immunol* 1995;154:2612–2623.

137. June CH, Bluestone JA, Nadler LM, Thompson CB. The B7 and CD28 receptor families. *Immunol Today* 1994;15:321–331.

138. Lenschow DJ, Walunas TL, Bluestone JA. CD28/B7 system of T cell costimulation. *Annu Rev Immunol* 1996;14:233–258.

139. Levine BL, Bernstein W, Craighead N, Lindsten T, Thompson CB, June CH. Effects of CD28 costimulation on long term proliferation of CD4+ T cells in the absence of exogenous feeder cells. *J Immunol* 1997;159:5921–5930.

140. Tsitsikov EN, Wright DA, Geha RS. CD30 induction of human immunodeficiency virus gene transcription is mediated by TRAF2. *Proc Natl Acad Sci USA* 1997;94:1390–1395.

141. Amakawa R, Hakem A, Kundig TM, et al. Impaired negative selection of T cells in Hodgkin's disease antigen CD30-deficient mice. *Cell* 1996;84:551–562.

142. Ellis TM, Simms PE, Slivnick DJ, Jack HM, Fisher RI. CD30 is a signal-transducing molecule that defines a subset of human activated CD45RO+ T cells. *J Immunol* 1993;151:2380–2389.

143. Maggi E, Annunziato F, Manetti R, et al. Activation of HIV expression by CD30 triggering in CD4+ T cells from HIV-infected individuals. *Immunity* 1995;3:251–255.

144. Noelle RJ. CD40 and its ligand in host defense. *Immunity* 1996;4:415–419.

145. Sperling AI, Green JM, Mosley RL, et al. CD43 is a murine T cell cos-

146. Fanales-Belasio E, Zambruno G, Cavani A, Girolomoni G. Antibodies against sialophorin (CD43) enhance the capacity of dendritic cells to cluster and activate T lymphocytes. *J Immunol* 1997;159:2203–2211.

147. Agematsu K, Kobata T, Sugita K, Hirose T, Schlossman SF, Morimoto C. Direct cellular communications between CD45R0 and CD45RA T cell subsets via CD27/CD70. *J Immunol* 1995;154:3627–3635.

148. Bowman MR, Crimmins MA, Yetz-Aldape J, Kriz R, Kelleher K, Herrmann S. The cloning of CD70 and its identification as the ligand for CD27. *J Immunol* 1994;152:1756–1761.

149. Boussiotis VA, Freeman GJ, Gribben JG, Nadler LM. The role of B7-1/B7-2:CD28/CLTA-4 pathways in the prevention of anergy, induction of productive immunity and down-regulation of the immune response. *Immunol Rev* 1996;153:5–26.

150. Guinan EC, Gribben JG, Boussiotis VA, Freeman GJ, Nadler LM. Pivotal role of the B7:CD28 pathway in transplantation tolerance and tumor immunity. *Blood* 1994;84:3261–3282.

151. Borriello F, Lederer J, Scott S, Sharpe AH. MRC OX-2 defines a novel T cell costimulatory pathway. *J Immunol* 1997;158:4548–4554.

152. Preston S, Wright GJ, Starr K, Barclay AN, Brown MH. The leukocyte/neuron cell surface antigen OX2 binds to a ligand on macrophages. *Eur J Immunol* 1997;27:1911–1918.

153. McCaughan GW, Clark MJ, Barclay AN. Characterization of the human homolog of the rat MRC OX-2 membrane glycoprotein. *Immunogenetics* 1987;25:329–335.

154. Arch RH, Thompson CB. 4-1BB and Ox40 are members of a tumor necrosis factor (TNF)–nerve growth factor receptor subfamily that bind TNF receptor-associated factors and activate nuclear factor kappa B. *Mol Cell Biol* 1998;18:558–565.

155. Uchiyama T. Human T cell leukemia virus type I (HTLV-I) and human diseases. *Annu Rev Immunol* 1997;15:15–37.

156. Stuber E, Strober W. The T cell–B cell interaction via OX40-OX40L is necessary for the T cell-dependent humoral immune response. *J Exp Med* 1996;183:979–989.

157. Shuford WW, Klussman K, Tritchler DD, et al. 4-1BB costimulatory signals preferentially induce CD8+ T cell proliferation and lead to the amplification *in vivo* of cytotoxic T cell responses. *J Exp Med* 1997;186:47–55.

158. Melero I, Shuford WW, Newby SA, et al. Monoclonal antibodies against the 4-1BB T-cell activation molecule eradicate established tumors. *Nat Med* 1997;3:682–685.

159. DeBenedette MA, Shahinian A, Mak TW, Watts TH. Costimulation of CD28- T lymphocytes by 4-1BB ligand. *J Immunol* 1997;158:551–559.

160. Thompson CB, Allison JP. The emerging role of CTLA-4 as an immune attenuator. *Immunity* 1997;7:445–450.

161. Gruss HJ, Boiani N, Williams DE, Armitage RJ, Smith CA, Goodwin RG. Pleiotropic effects of the CD30 ligand on CD30-expressing cells and lymphoma cell lines. *Blood* 1994;83:2045–2056.

162. Baum PR, Gayle RB III, Ramsdell F, et al. Molecular characterization of murine and human OX40/OX40 ligand systems: identification of a human OX40 ligand as the HTLV-1–regulated protein gp34. *EMBO J* 1994;13:3992–4001.

163. Godfrey WR, Fagnoni FF, Harara MA, Buck D, Engleman EG. Identification of a human OX-40 ligand, a costimulator of CD4- T cells with homology to tumor necrosis factor. *J Exp Med* 1994;180:757–762.

164. Ohshima Y, Tanaka Y, Tozawa H, Takahashi Y, Maliszewski C, Delespesse G. Expression and function of OX40 ligand on human dendritic cells. *J Immunol* 1997;159:3838–3848.

165. Chu NR, DeBenedette MA, Stiernholm BJ, Barber BH, Watts TH. Role of IL-12 and 4-1BB ligand in cytokine production by CD28+ and CD28- T cells. *J Immunol* 1997;158:3081–3089.

timulatory receptor that functions independently of CD28. *J Exp Med* 1995;182:139–146.

Inflammation: Basic Principles and Clinical Correlates,
3rd ed., edited by John I. Gallin and Ralph Snyderman.
Lippincott Williams & Wilkins, Philadelphia © 1999.

CHAPTER 15

The Vascular Endothelium

Roy L. Silverstein

The vascular endothelium is a single-cell layer that forms a continuous lining for the large container that holds circulating blood. The area of this lining is estimated to be several thousand square meters, most of which is found in the microcirculation of the capillary beds, where the ratio of surface area to blood volume is highest and contact between endothelial cells and blood components is maximized. The endothelium is not merely a passive liner; it provides a dynamic interface between blood and tissue parenchyma. In the late 19th century, anatomists recognized the critical role of the endothelium in inflammation. During the 1860s, Metchnikoff described leukocyte "paving" on endothelium in inflamed tissue and considered endothelial cells to be second in importance only to leukocytes in the inflammatory response (1). With the development in 1973 by Jaffe et al. (2) and Gimbrone et al. (3) of straightforward methods to maintain, propagate, and identify mammalian endothelial cells in culture, interest in the biology of these cells blossomed. In addition to studies following Metchnikoff's legacy on the role of endothelium in inflammation, considerable insight into endothelial cell biology has come from study of the critical role of endothelium in disease states. Folkman's observations that growth of malignant tumors beyond a few millimeters in diameter required the development of new blood vessels and capillary beds (4), a process called angiogenesis, spawned intense study of the mechanisms of endothelial cell growth and differentiation. Similarly, Ross's hypothesis that atherosclerosis represents a "response" to vascular injury (5) has led to considerable study of the mechanisms and consequences by which endothelial cells react to their environment.

The vascular endothelium plays several critical roles in homeostasis, and endothelial dysfunction contributes to many pathologic processes (6). Maintenance of the normal fluid state of blood mostly is a function of the natural anticoagulant properties of the endothelial layer (7). Disruption of these properties is an important cause of pathologic thrombus formation. Similarly, disruption of the normal mechanisms by which endothelium regulates vascular tone may contribute to chronic hypertension and to circulatory collapse associated with shock states.

Perhaps the most obvious function of the endothelium is to provide a homeostatic barrier between blood and tissues. This barrier is exquisitely sensitive to environmental change. The endothelium is an organ with remarkable capacity to respond to a local "microenvironmental" stimulus with highly localized responses. Among the regulated barrier functions of the endothelium are permeability to fluid and macromolecules and the entry into tissues of inflammatory cells (i.e., polymorphonuclear cells [PMNs], monocytes, and eosinophils), immune effector cells (i.e., B and T lymphocytes and natural killer [NK] cells), and hematopoietic precursors.

DEVELOPMENTAL BIOLOGY OF VASCULAR ENDOTHELIUM

Vasculogenesis

The first organ to develop in the vertebrate embryo is the cardiovascular system, including heart and blood vessels. Primordial blood vessels develop from mesenchymal derived endothelial cell precursors, called angioblasts. These cells have the potential to differentiate into endothelial cells, but they express no characteristic endothelial markers and are not organized into lumen containing structures (8). They arise during the early primitive streak stage of development in extraembryonic sites, where they aggregate in the developing yolk sac to form the blood islands. Cells at the periphery of the blood islands become angioblasts, and the cells at the center become hematopoietic progenitors. This observation led

R. L. Silverstein: Division of Hematology and Medical Oncology, Department of Medicine, Weill Medical College of Cornell University, New York, New York 10021.

to the hypothesis of a common precursor cell, the hemangioblast (9), and may explain why endothelial cells share many common features with blood cells. In adults, a circulating pool of monocytic cells that express the hematopoietic precursor cell marker, CD34, may contain a subpopulation committed to endothelial cell differentiation (10,11).

Angioblasts are also found intraembryonically as solitary cells and as small clusters of cells along the wall of the aorta. Under the influence of specific growth factors, angioblasts migrate, proliferate, and eventually differentiate to form primary capillary plexuses, a process called vasculogenesis. The tyrosine kinase FLK-1 (fetal liver kinase-1, also known as KDR) is the first specific marker to appear on primitive endothelial cells, and as a receptor for the potent mitogen vascular endothelial growth factor (VEGF), it plays a key role in these early events (12). FLK-1 is a receptor tyrosine kinase related to the platelet-derived growth factor (PDGF) receptor. It is a type II transmembrane glycoprotein containing seven extracellular immunoglobulin-like domains and a split intracellular kinase domain (13,14). Its ligand, VEGF, is a highly conserved disulfide-bonded dimer of 34 to 45 kd, structurally related to the B chain of PDGF (15,16). Four isoforms of 121, 165, 185, and 206 amino acids are generated by differential splicing of a single gene product (17). VEGF is made by many embryonic cell types and is prominent in areas of blood vessel development. The key role of the VEGF/FLK-1 system in vasculogenesis is supported by murine genetic knock-out experiments in which FLK-1 nulls and VEGF nulls are early embryonic lethals (i.e., before day 10.5) (13,18,19). The FLK-1 null embryos do not form blood islands, and neither hematopoietic nor endothelial precursors appear. VEGF nulls also have severely abnormal blood vessel development. Heterozygous gene deletion of *VEGF* also leads to embryonic lethality, suggesting that threshold VEGF concentrations are critical for blood vessel development (18,19).

Cells within the developing primary capillary plexus differentiate further to form cords and then reorganize to form lumens. Lumen formation within the capillary sprout is thought to occur by the joining of an endothelial cell with itself or with another endothelial cell to form a ring. Although *in vitro* experiments have suggested a role for the endothelial cell adhesion molecules E-selectin (CD62E) and vascular endothelial cadherin (VE-cadherin) in lumen formation, the lack of phenotype of E-selectin null mice has left these data open to interpretation (20). Extensive regression and remodeling of these early vascular networks ensues to establish vascular connections and a continuous lumen, a process called network remodeling (8). Eventually, smooth muscle cell precursors are recruited into the developing blood vessel network as arteries and veins, and organ-specific capillary beds form. Within developing organs, blood vessels also form by invasive angiogenesis, as in the case of ecto-

dermal and mesenchymal organs such as brain and kidney, and *de novo* from resident mesenchymal precursors, as in the case of endodermal derived organs such as lung and spleen. The former involves sprouting of blood vessels from preexisting capillaries. These processes (i.e., lumen formation, network remodeling, large vessel formation, and embryonic angiogenesis) are presumably regulated by a network of growth factors and receptors and by cell-cell and cell-matrix interactions. Mice null for certain integrins, such as the fibronectin receptor components α_5 and β_1, have early lethal vascular defects, highlighting the importance of extracellular matrix interactions in vasculogenesis (21,22).

Several additional members of the VEGF family, including VEGF-B, VEGF-C, and placental growth factor, have been identified and shown to participate in vasculogenesis along with FLK-1 and the related receptor tyrosine kinases FLT-1 and FLT-4 (FMS-like kinase-1 and -4) (12,23,24). The latter functions as a receptor for VEGF-B, is expressed in early developing blood vessels, and then becomes restricted to lymphatic endothelium.

Two members of a second family of endothelial-specific tyrosine kinases that appear sightly later in development than FLK-1 (day 7.5 to 8 in the mouse) and are also highly expressed in blood vessels of developing organs such as brain, have been identified (25). They are novel receptors with extracellular regions consisting of an immunoglobulin-like domain, fibronectin-type III repeats, and an EGF repeat—hence the names TIE-1 and TIE-2 (*t*yrosine kinases with *i*mmunoglobulin and *E*GF homology domains). TIE ligands are mesenchymal produced and secreted glycoproteins called angiopoietins (26). Mice null for TIE receptors and angiopoietin-1 have severe vascular developmental defects, including absent angiogenesis in the neural tube (27–29). Mutations in the *TIE2* gene, in the region encoding the kinase domain of the receptor, have been associated with a familial syndrome of mucosal cavernous venous malformations (30). The disorganized endothelial cell–smooth muscle cell interactions in these malformations are similar to those in angiopoietin-1 null mice, suggesting an important role for the TIE-2 system in organizing endothelial-smooth muscle interactions. The functional role of other members of the angiopoietin family has not been determined.

Angiogenesis

In the adult organism, endothelial cells proliferate at an extremely slow rate; turnover times have been estimated as high as decades (4). Under certain physiologic and pathophysiologic conditions, including wound healing, inflammation, tumor growth, ovulation, diabetic retinopathy, and rheumatoid arthritis, new blood vessels can grow rapidly from preexisting capillaries by a sprouting process similar to embryonic angiogenesis (31). The cellular and molecular mechanisms of angiogenesis are complex and include at least three pivotal endothelial cell processes: proliferation, migration, and elaboration of proteases. Metalloproteases and serine proteases, such as collagenase and plasminogen activator, degrade extracellular matrix, facilitating cellular migration.

Based on *in vitro* assays using cultured capillary endothelial cell monolayers, heparin-binding growth factors have been identified that are capable of eliciting one or more of the activities associated with angiogenesis (16,32–34). These include acidic and basic fibroblast growth factor (aFGF and bFGF), VEGF, and hepatocyte growth factor, also known as scatter factor. These growth factors also stimulate angiogenesis in animal model systems such as in the rabbit or rodent cornea or the chick chorioallantoic membrane. VEGF is thought to be the most important physiologic regulator of angiogenesis, based on its expression in angiogenic tissues such as endometrium and corpus luteum, its broad pattern of inducible expression by angiogenic stimuli, and the endothelial cell–restricted expression of its receptors, FLT-1 and FLK-1 (8,16,34). An early response of endothelial cells to most angiogenic growth factors is upregulation of expression of the FLT-1 and FLK-1 kinases, further supporting the primacy of VEGF. Endothelial cells express other mitogenic receptors, including KIT, the interleukin-3 (IL-3) receptor, and the protease responsive receptor-2 (35–37), although their physiologic significance has not been documented.

CXC chemokines are small chemoattractants distinguished by the presence of cystein-x-cysteine motif. Several, including IL-8 and neutrophil-acitivating protein-2 (NAP-2), have angiogenic activity by virtue of their ability to stimulate endothelial cell migration (38). Other molecules shown to have *in vivo* angiogenic activity, such as PDGF, tumor necrosis factor-β (TGF-β), soluble E-selectin, and angiogenin (a copper-binding protein with high homology to pancreatic ribonuclease), do not stimulate the full range of endothelial cell angiogenic activities and may act indirectly, such as by stimulating production of VEGF (38).

The interaction of angiogenic endothelial cells with specific extracellular matrix components is also an essential component of the angiogenic response (21,39). Expression of the $\alpha_v\beta_3$ integrin is upregulated on angiogenic cells, and treatment of endothelial cells with inhibitory antibodies or peptides that block $\alpha_v\beta_3$-integrin interactions with specific matrix components blocks angiogenesis (40–42). Exposure of endothelial cells to VEGF also results in a rapid increase in vascular permeability (34) with extravasation of fibrinogen and formation of a provisional fibrin matrix, which is an excellent substrate to support endothelial cell migration and proliferation (43).

Angiogenesis is a tightly regulated process involving inhibitory and stimulatory influences (38). Some antiangiogenic molecules, including prostaglandin synthesis inhibitors and heparin (44), are probably not acting directly on endothelial cells, because they do not regulate the key endothelial angiogenic functions *in vitro*. Among the antiangiogenic molecules acting directly on endothelium are the cytokines interferon-γ and IL-12 and the CXC chemokine platelet factor-4 (8,38,45). Retinoids, including all-*trans*- and 13-*cis*-retinoic acids, block angiogenic effects of VEGF and FGF (46), presumably through interaction with retinoic acid receptor-α expressed in endothelial cells. Considerable attention has focused on matrix-associated molecules that function as antiangiogenesis factors. These include proteolytic fragments of collagen and plasminogen (i.e., endostatin [47] and angiostatin [48]) and thrombospondin-1 (49,50). Angiostatin and endostatin were originally identified as products of tumor cells, although they may also be generated by nonmalignant tissues. Thrombospondin-1 is a large-molecular-weight matrix glycoprotein secreted by endothelial and other vascular cells and is a highly regulated component of the extracellular matrix (51,52). Its secretion is regulated by many of the same agonists that control angiogenesis (53). Thrombospondin-1 and several proteolytic fragments of thrombospondin-1 inhibit endothelial cell migration to angiogenic stimuli and inhibit angiogenesis in animal models (54,55). Thrombospondin-1 peptides induce endothelial cell apoptosis, and mice null for thrombospondin-1 have increased blood vessel formation in granulation tissue (56). The antiangiogenic effects of thrombospondin-1 may be related to its binding to $\alpha_v\beta_3$ integrin and disruption of focal adhesions (57,58). However, a unique nonintegrin cellular receptor for thrombospondin-1, CD36, is preferentially expressed on capillary endothelial cells and is a likely mediator of the antiangiogenic effects of thrombospondin-1 (59). Blocking antibodies and peptides to CD36 inhibit the effect of thrombospondin-1 on endothelial cell migration, and other CD36 ligands, such as oxidized LDL, have similar antiangiogenic properties (55). Mice null for CD36, similar to the thrombospondin-1 null mice, have increased blood vessel formation and do not demonstrate an antiangiogenic response to thrombospondin-1 (60).

There is considerable interest in developing therapeutic agents based on the cell and molecular biology of angiogenesis for clinical use (31,38). For example, development of proangiogenic agents may be useful to promote revascularization of ischemic limbs and myocardium in patients with advanced atherosclerosis. Early preclinical and clinical studies delivering VEGF by gene transfer into ischemic tissues have shown enhanced formation of collateral vessels and increased blood flow, and delivery of VEGF onto diseased arteries after angioplasty has led to more rapid reendothelialization and less neointimal proliferation (61–63). The use of antiangiogenic agents to prevent tumor progression (64) and to slow progression of destructive angiogenesis such as seen in diabetic retinas and rheumatoid synovium is being developed. Angiostatin and endostatin, alone or in combination, show promise in cancer therapeutics.

Apoptosis

Endothelial cell apoptosis is an essential feature of vasculogenesis and angiogenesis, particularly during the remodeling phases. Capillary regression is also critical to the development of certain avascular tissues, such as cartilage and the vitreous of the eye, and to the terminal phases of wound healing (8). The molecular mechanisms that control endothelial cell apoptosis are not well understood, although endothelial cells have been shown to express receptors known to regulate apoptosis in other cells, including the tumor necrosis factor-α (TNF-α) receptor and CD40. Immunologic blockade of $\alpha_v\beta_3$ integrins on proliferating endothelial cells can induce apoptosis (65), consistent with study findings suggesting that ligation of this receptor by matrix proteins may provide an important survival signal to proliferating cells (41).

Blood flow is also important in maintaining endothelial cell survival. In embryonic tissues, absence of flow results in capillary regression (8). The finding that blood platelets contain significant amounts of VEGF may mean that platelets in flowing blood provide a tonic survival signal to endothelial cells, because blocking antibodies to VEGF in culture has been shown to induce endothelial cell apoptosis. Abnormal endothelial cell apoptosis may also have important pathophysiologic implications. Laurence et al. (66) showed that sera from patients with thrombotic thrombocytopenic purpura (TTP) and hemolytic uremic syndrome (HUS) induced apoptosis in certain types of cultured endothelial cells, suggesting that loss of survival signals or abnormal proapoptosis signals may provide a possible mechanism for pathologic conditions such as the severe microangiopathic vasculopathy seen in TTP and HUS.

ANATOMY OF VASCULAR ENDOTHELIUM

Ultrastructure of the Endothelium

Endothelial ultrastructure was initially described by Palade et al. in the 1960s. The cells contain numerous unique, electron-dense, membrane-bound organelles, called Weibel-Palade bodies (67), that contain a high concentration of high-molecular-weight multimers of von Willebrand factor (vWF). Their membranes express the leukocyte adhesion molecule P-selectin (68). When endothelial cells are exposed to certain agonists, including thrombin and histamine, these organelles "flow" to the surface, where their contents are secreted into the blood, and their membranes fuse with the cell surface membrane. This results in localized high concentration of the more active molecular form of vWF and in surface expression of P-selectin.

The presence of flask-shaped surface membrane invaginations (i.e., caveolae) and complex intracellular vesicles and channels suggests that considerable transport of macromolecules may occur directly through endothelial cells (69). Endothelial cell caveolae have been implicated in signal transduction, because many signaling molecules are localized in or around caveolae, including the PDGF receptor, protein kinase C, nonreceptor SRC-like tyrosine kinases, phospholipase C, sphingomyelin, and phosphatidyl inositol 3 kinase (70). PDGF exposure to endothelial cells increases phosphorylation of caveolae-associated proteins, and disruption of caveolae by cholesterol depletion blocks PDGF signaling (71).

Endothelial cells are in most cases flat and continuously attached to each other by numerous intercellular junctions. These junctions create a polarity with clear-cut differences between the apical surface facing the blood and the basal surface facing connective tissue. The most prevalent of the endothelial cell junctions are the adherens junctions, which are mainly localized at the basal side of endothelial cell intercellular contacts (72). These are formed by homophilic interaction of the extracellular domains of clusters of members of the cadherin family of transmembrane adhesion molecules. The major endothelial cadherin is VE-cadherin, also called cadherin-5. VE-cadherin is a single-chain phosphoglycoprotein consisting of five homologous repeats of a 110 amino acid calcium-binding cadherin domain (73). Cadherins interact in a dynamic fashion through their cytoplasmic domains with a network of cytoskeletal proteins, including β-catenin, plakoglobulin, and p120, all of which are members of the armadillo family of cytosolic signaling molecules (72). They link VE-cadherin to the actin cytoskeleton through interactions with α-catenin.

In addition to its role in cell adhesion and maintaining intercellular connections, the adherens junction is involved in mediating signal transduction (74). Signaling molecules, including RAS, SRC-like kinases, and phosphatases are localized at the intracellular face of the adherens junction. VE-cadherin associates with the adenomatosis polyposis coli (APC) gene product, a cell cycle inhibitor, and regulates cytoplasmic levels of catenins, which can cross the nuclear membrane and regulate gene transcription. Forced over expression of VE-cadherin results in inhibition of cellular proliferation, suggesting that VE-cadherin may play a role in mediating contact inhibition of growth (75). In confluent endothelial cell cultures, where junctions are stable, phosphorylation of VE-cadherin is low, and it is mainly linked to plakoglobulin and the actin cytoskeleton. In migrating cells or at early stages of confluence and where junctions are weak, VE-cadherin is heavily phosphorylated, and it is mostly linked to β-catenin and p120 (74).

The regulated and dynamic interactions of VE-cadherin with cytosolic components are probably important in mediating endothelial cell development and function. Exposure of endothelial cells in culture to VEGF, for example, increases VE-cadherin phosphorylation, changing intercellular interactions, increasing permeability, and possibly contributing to the proliferative and migratory phenotype of angiogenic cells. Similarly, exposure of endothelial cells to thrombin or attachment of neutrophils to the endothelial surface results in increased phosphorylation of VE-cadherin and disassembly of adherens junctions, leading to increased permeability and facilitating cellular transmigration (76,77).

Certain endothelial cell-cell contacts, as in the microcirculation of the brain, are marked by abundant tight junctions (78). These are usually localized near the apical side of the lateral cell-cell contact, where they create a high transcellular resistance and a barrier to unregulated transport. Tight junction proteins ZO-1 and occludin are heavily and specifically expressed at cell-cell contacts in the microcirculation of the brain (79).

Other transmembrane glycoproteins associate at sites of endothelial cell-cell contacts, including platelet/endothelial cell adhesion molecule-1 (PECAM-1, CD31), CD34, and endoglin (80). PECAM-1 is involved in leukocyte transmigration (81). CD34 may play a role in lymphocyte trafficking (82), and endoglin has been postulated to regulate latent TGF-β activation (83).

The basal surface of endothelial cells is attached to the extracellular matrix and is distinguished by the presence of focal adhesion plaques, β_1 and β_3 integrins, syndecan-1 and -4, and proteoglycans. Expression of β_3 integrins and syndecan is also regulated by angiogenic stimuli, perhaps related to the gain of a motile phenotype (22,84).

Endothelial Cell Heterogeneity

The endothelium exhibits considerable microheterogeneity and macroheterogeneity (85). Behavioral and structural differences distinguish arterial, venous, sinusoidal, lymphatic, and capillary endothelia; large vessel and small vessel endothelia; and endothelia from different organs. The most obvious examples of endothelial cell heterogeneity are found among the cells that form the microvasculature of different organs. Highly specialized endothelial cells have been described in certain tissues, such as the blood-brain barrier of brain microvasculature (78), the sinusoidal endothelium of the bone marrow (86), and the cuboidal "high endothelium" of postcapillary venules in lymphoid organs (87). Development of endothelial cell microheterogeneity is poorly understood (88), although studies of the developing brain suggest that local cues provided by parenchymal cells and by extracellular matrix direct the specific differentiation of endothelial cells (89,90). Similarly, in the absence of afferent lymph, the cuboidal endothelium of the high endothelial venules (HEV) becomes flattened. In general, plasticity of endothelial cells seems to decrease with age.

Microvascular endothelial cells can be described as discontinuous or continuous, depending on whether visible gaps are seen at the level of ultrastructure (85). In the central nervous system, muscles, and lymph nodes, where nutrient transport, barrier functions, and regulated immune cell homing are critical, the endothelium is mostly continuous. In the gastrointestinal tract, endocrine organs, choroid plexus, bone marrow, liver, and kidney, where absorption, secretion, filtration, and delivery of cells are paramount, the endothelium is mostly discontinuous. Discontinuous endothelial cells are described as being fenestrated, as in the peritubular capillaries of the kidney, or nonfenestrated.

Endothelial Cell Markers

Immunologic and biochemical markers for endothelial cells have been useful in studying vasculogenesis, angiogenesis, and other cellular functions, as well as in characterizing endothelial heterogeneity and in identifying endothelial cells and blood vessels in pathologic specimens. The first endothelial cell marker identified was the coagulation factor VIII–related antigen, later designated vWF (91). This factor is present mainly in the Weibel-Palade bodies (68). Other markers constitutively expressed include angiotensin-converting enzyme, PECAM-1 (CD31), binding sites for *Ulex europaens* lectin, a receptor for acetylated low-density lipoproteins (LDLs), thrombomodulin, endoglin (CD105), CD40, CD34, CD73, intercellular adhesion molecule-2 (ICAM-2, CD102), $\alpha_v\beta_3$ integrin (CD51/61), CD36, FLK-1, FLT-1, TIE-1, TIE-2, VE-cadherin, and numerous receptors for cytokines and growth factors, including those for IL-1, TNF-α, IL-3, IL-4, IL-6, IL-10, oncostatin-M, thrombin, TGF-β, FGF, PDGF, and stem cell factor (81,86,92). None of these is entirely specific for endothelial cells.

Certain adhesion molecules, such as glycosylation-dependent cell adhesion molecule 1 (GlyCAM-1), mucosal addressin cell adhesion molecule-1 (MadCAM-1), and vascular adhesion protein-1 (VAP-1), are expressed preferentially on high endothelial venules at areas of specific leukocyte trafficking, and others, such as intercellular adhesion molecule-1 (ICAM-1, CD54), E- and P-selectin (CD62E and CD62P), and vascular cell adhesion molecule-1 (VCAM-1, CD106) are expressed mainly in response to endothelial cell stimulation. FLK-1, FLT-1, TIE-1, and TIE-2 levels are increased on angiogenic endothelial cells, and CD36 is mainly restricted to capillary vessels. FLT-4 is mainly restricted to lymphatic vessels. The glucose transporter GLUT-1, the transferrin receptor (CD73), P-glycoprotein (i.e., product of the multidrug resistance-1a gene), ZO-1, and occludin are expressed mainly in brain microvasculature. This list is by no means complete, because many additional antigens less completely characterized have also been described.

ENDOTHELIAL CELL PHYSIOLOGY

Endothelial Cell Activation

Central to the critical role of endothelial cells in maintaining homeostasis is their ability to respond to myriad environmental signals with specific "programmed" responses (93). Included among these signals (Table 15-1) are biomechanical forces (94), cytokines (93), chemokines (95), lymphocyte surface co-stimulating molecules, growth factors (96), bioactive amines (68,97), retinoids (98), peptides, enzymes (76), complement components (99), eicosanoids (100,101), and nitric oxide (NO) (102). Pathologic conditions such as hypoxia (103) and infectious and pathologic agents such as bacterial endotoxin (93), viruses (104), viral proteins, oxidized lipoproteins (5), polar phospholipids (105,106), advanced glycation products (107), and certain antibodies (108) also can activate endothelial cells.

Endothelial Cell Inflammatory Response

Certain endothelial responses are rapid and do not require new gene transcription or protein synthesis. These include secretion of Weibel-Palade bodies with concomitant expression of surface P-selectin, activation of eicosanoid and NO metabolic pathways, and cytoskeletal or junctional reorganization resulting in increased vascular permeability (67,68,100,109). These responses are the hallmark of the early, non–leukocyte-dependent phase of inflammation. Agonists capable of eliciting this type of response include thrombin, histamine, neurogenic peptides, and complement components. Many endothelial responses, however, are the result of altered transcription of specific gene products (110), including the adhesion molecules E-selectin, ICAM-1 and -2, and VCAM, proinflammatory cytokines, growth factors, tissue factor procoagulant, and plasminogen activator inhibitor-1.

Perhaps the best described of these endothelial responses is that to the inflammatory mediators IL-1, TNF-α, or bacterial endotoxin (93). Within a few hours of exposure in culture, the cells begin to express E-selectin (111) and VCAM (112) and increase their expression of ICAM-1 (113). Expression peaks in 4 to 6 hours and then begins to fall, reaching baseline levels at 12 to 24 hours for E-selectin and somewhat later for the others. Tissue factor procoagulant is also expressed in this setting (114–116), along with plasminogen activator and plasminogen activator inhibitor-1 (PAI-1) (117–119), metalloproteinases and tissue inhibitors of metalloproteinases (98), platelet-activating factor (PAF) (120), a secreted sphingomyelinase, monocyte chemotactic protein-1 (MCP-1), PDGF, FGF, TGF-β, and IL-1 (121–123). The net result is leukocyte recruitment, adhesion, activation, and transmigration; platelet adhesion and activation; and fibrin deposition—all of which contribute to and amplify the inflammatory response.

Interferon-γ (IFN-γ), unlike TNF and IL-1, has little effect on expression of E-selectin, procoagulants, and cytokines, but it induces expression of major histocompatibility (MHC) class II antigens over a period measured in days (124). IFN-γ also induces formation of gaps in intercellular endothelial junctions, leading to increased transendothelial permeability (125). If IFN-γ is added to cells with TNF, expression of adhesion molecules is markedly prolonged. Similarly, IL-10 (126) and perhaps IL-3 (127) can stimulate endothelial cell adhesion molecule expression in a prolonged manner, suggesting that these cytokines may play a role in mediating more chronic inflammatory responses.

Oncostatin-M, an IL-6–related cytokine (128), has the dual capacity to induce rapid P-selectin expression and delayed expression of E-selectin. Oncostatin-M and IL-4 also increase transcription of the P-selectin gene and result in longer-term surface expression over several days (129).

Endothelial cells also express CD40 (130). Exposure of the cells to CD40 ligand, for example on the surface of activated T cells, may be another mechanism to recruit endothelial cells into an immune response.

The endothelial cell activation response can be blunted or blocked by other soluble agents. For example TGF-β (97), IL-4, or NO (102), when added to endothelial cells in the presence of TNF, blunts the typical activation response described earlier. Retinoids, including 13-cis- and all-trans-retinoic acids (98,131), also have potent endothelial cell antiinflammatory actions. This correlates

---

TABLE 15-1. *Endothelial cell agonists*

Biomechanical forces: shear stress, hydrostatic pressure, cyclic strain
Cytokines: IL-1, TNF-α, IL-3, IL-4, IL-6, IL-10, IL-12, oncostatin-M, IFN-γ, TGF-β
Chemokines: IL-8, NAP-2, platelet factor-4
Growth factors: bFGF, aFGF, VEGF, HGF, PDGF, stem cell factor (KIT ligand), angiopoietin-1
Vasoactive compounds: histamine, kinins, endothelin-1
Enzymes: thrombin, cathepsin G
Complement components: C5a, C5b-9 complex
Eicosanoids and lipoxins
Retinoids: 13-cis-retinoic acid, all-trans-retinoic acid
Nitric oxide
Viruses: DNA viruses (cytomegalovirus, herpes simplex), viral proteins (HIV tat)
Lipoproteins: oxidized LDL, lysophosphatidyl choline
Antibodies: antiphospholipid antibodies, anti-MHC, xenoreactive antibodies

aFGF, acidic fibroblast growth factor; bFGF, basic fibroblast growth factor; HGF, hepatocyte growth factor; HIV, human immunodeficiency virus; IFN, interferon; IL, interleukin; LDL, low-density lipoprotein; MHC, major histocompatibility complex; NAP, neutrophil-activating protein; PDGF, platelet-derived growth factor; TGF, transforming growth factor; TNF, tumor necrosis factor; VEGF, vascular endothelial growth factor.

well with the known antiinflammatory effects of retinoids in cutaneous disease. For example, if human dermal microvascular endothelial cells are pretreated with retinoids, subsequent exposure to TNF-α does not result in increased VCAM-1 gene transcription (132). ICAM-1 and E-selectin upregulation are not affected, providing some specificity for blockade of T-cell entry into inflammatory sites. Retinoids also modulate endothelial cell cytoskeletal changes and production of proteases in response to angiogenic and inflammatory stimuli while not affecting proliferation (46).

Specific nuclear transcription factors play an essential role in orchestrating the endothelial cell responses described earlier. In particular, the promotor regions of many of the genes activated by inflammatory mediators contain shear stress response elements (SSRE) and consensus sequences for activation by NF-κB (133). Complex interplay among intracellular signaling systems and among positive and negative transcriptional mediators probably accounts for the subtle differences in endothelial cell responses to different agonists and combinations of agonists. Pharmacologic and gene transfer approaches to limit NF-κB activity in endothelial cells are being developed as antiinflammatory therapies.

Endothelial Cell Response to Hypoxia

The endothelial response to hypoxia is complex. Immediately after exposure to hypoxic conditions, such as a PO_2 of 20 mm Hg, Weibel-Palade bodies are exocytosed, leading to vWF secretion and P-selectin expression, with concomitant recruitment of platelets and leukocytes (103). In a murine model system, P-selectin null animals exhibited a more than 10-fold decrement of neutrophil recruitment to a hypoxic region. Hypoxia results in a more delayed synthesis and secretion of endothelin-1, FGF, IL-1, IL-6, IL-8, and PAF, inducing local vasoconstriction, and in generating an angiogenic response and a leukocyte inflammatory reaction (134).

Endothelial Cell Response to Biomechanical Forces

Endothelial cells can respond to at least three types of biomechanical force: shear stress, cyclic strain, and hydrostatic pressure. Endothelial cells grown in culture under static conditions, when exposed to physiologic linear shear stress, exhibit marked morphologic changes and realignment of stress fibers in the direction of the flow (95,135). Associated with these morphologic changes are changes in intracellular calcium concentrations (136), tyrosine and serine-threonine phosphorylation of cytoplasmic components (137), changes in basolateral cell contacts (135), and changes in gene transcription (133,138–140). At 2.5 to 46 dynes/cm² of steady unidirectional linear shear stress, inducible nitric oxide synthase (NOS) and cyclooxygenase-2 genes are upregulated

(141), as is ICAM-1, but not VCAM-1 or E-selectin (142). VCAM-1 responses to cytokine stimulation are blunted at shear stresses of 0.7 to 7 dynes/cm². Turbulent flow does not increase cyclooxygenase-2 or inducible NOS levels. These studies suggest that endothelial cells possess sensors that can distinguish between uniform and turbulent flow and levels of linear shear stress. The role of these systems in pathologic entities such as atherosclerosis is under active study.

Endothelial Cell Responses to Pathologic Agents

Interaction of pathologic agents with endothelial cells may play important roles in multiple infectious and noninfectious disease states. Bacterial endotoxin is a potent endothelial cell inflammatory agonist and may be the major mediator of shock and disseminated intravascular coagulopathy states associated with gram-negative bacterial sepsis. Human immunodeficiency virus type 1 (HIV-1) tat protein has been shown to induce ICAM-1 and VCAM-1 expression on endothelial cells, suggesting a potential role in fostering extravasation of HIV infected cells (143). Infection of endothelial cells with herpesviruses, including herpes simplex (104) and cytomegalovirus (144), is associated with induction of adhesion molecules and a prothrombotic state, which may play a role in certain forms of atherosclerosis, such as the accelerated disease that follows cardiac transplantation. Herpesvirus DNA sequences have been found in the vessel wall in atheromatous vessels, supporting this hypothesis (145).

Endothelial cell activation by modified lipids and lipoproteins, such as oxidized LDL and lysophophatidyl choline (105,106), has been postulated to contribute to atherogenesis. The receptors that mediate this response are unknown, although endothelial cells have been shown to express type A and type B scavenger receptors (59). Endothelial cells also express receptors for advanced glycation protein adducts (107), such as are generated in patients with diabetes. A proinflammatory, proatherogenic response to these modified proteins has been hypothesized to contribute to the severe vasculopathy associated with diabetes.

Endothelial cell responses to circulating antibodies have been an area of considerable interest in disease pathogenesis. The presence of circulating autoantibodies directed against negatively charged phospholipids is associated with a clinical syndrome of arterial and venous thrombosis, repeated abortion, and thrombocytopenia. This syndrome, called antiphospholipid syndrome, is seen in patients with systemic lupus erythematosus and those with an idiopathic autoimmune disorder, and it may account for as much as 10% to 15% of so-called idiopathic thromboembolic disease. These autoantibodies react with vascular endothelial cells and can induce expression of chemokines, cytokines, and cell adhesion molecules, resulting in monocyte recruitment, activation, and a prothrombotic state (108). Antiphospholipid antibodies have also been associated with increased risk of coronary disease, which may be related to cross-reactivity of the antiphospholipid syndrome with oxidized LDL.

Anti-endothelial cell antibodies have also been described in patients with other autoimmune diseases. Their relationship to pathophysiology remains largely unknown, although disordered endothelial function has been implicated in vasculitic syndromes, systemic sclerosis, rheumatoid synovitis, and Kawasaki's disease. A clear-cut case where anti-endothelial cell antibodies contribute to pathogenesis is in transplant rejection. Anti-MHC class I antibodies have been shown to activate endothelial cells (146) and may contribute to allograft rejection. More dramatically, host xenoreactive antibodies, primarily complement-dependent IgMs with carbohydrate specificities, rapidly activate endothelial cells, inducing thrombin formation and leukocyte adhesion. Hyperacute rejection is the immediate consequence (147). Promising genetic engineering strategies to prevent hyperacute xenograft rejection have focused on donor-organ endothelial cell heterologous expression of natural anticoagulant and complement regulatory proteins.

Permeability Barrier and Transport Functions of Endothelium

Regulation of macromolecule and fluid flux between blood and the extravascular space is a critical function of endothelium. Endothelial cells express active transport systems for adenosine, serotonin, and LDL, and they may have the capacity to transfer some of these molecules or their metabolic products across the cell layer (85). Internalization and clearance of oxidized lipoproteins, advanced glycation adducts of proteins, and proteinase-proteinase inhibitor complexes are accomplished by specialized receptors expressed mainly on microvascular endothelial cells. These include the type I/II scavenger receptor, CD36, and LDL receptor–related protein. In certain regions, endothelial cells meet highly specialized transport needs, such as those of the blood-brain barrier, the glomerular filtration system, and the pulmonary gas exchange system.

Abnormal endothelial barrier function can have considerable untoward effects. For example, tissue edema induced by inflammatory reactions can compromise organ function, particularly in the lung, where large volumes of fluid can accumulate rapidly. A severe vascular leak syndrome commonly occurs in patients treated with high doses of IL-2 for malignancy. Because endothelial cells do not express receptors for IL-2, this reaction may be mediated by products of IL-2–activated T cells.

The structural correlate of "vascular leak" and tissue edema in inflammation is the appearance of gaps in intercellular endothelial cell connections (125). Cotran et al. have shown that such gaps can be induced by interferon-γ, other cytokines, PAF, kinins, histamine, neurogenic mediators, and thrombin, and they are associated with changes in endothelial cell shape, cytoskeletal organization, and junctions (15,34,76,93). This change may be related to agonist-mediated phosphorylation of VE-cadherin, a subsequent decreased association with cytoskeletal components such as plakoglobulin, and disassembly of adherens junctions (74).

Increased vascular permeability may also play an important role in the pathogenesis of atherosclerosis. Entry of lipoprotein particles, such as LDL and very-low-density lipoproteins (VLDLs), into the subendothelial space as a response to vascular injury (5) places them in a privileged compartment where they are susceptible to oxidative modification by endothelium and leukocyte-derived reactive oxygen metabolites. Oxidized lipoproteins can then be taken up by macrophages through "scavenger" pathways, leading to formation of foam cells and atheromatous plaque. Oxidized LDL and lysophosphatidic lipids can also interact with and activate endothelial cells, smooth muscle cells, leukocytes, and platelets, contributing to and augmenting the injury response.

The blood-brain barrier represents a highly specialized endothelial organization in the brain parenchymal microcirculation that is distinguished by abundant expression of intercellular tight junctions (78). Brain parenchymal transcellular resistance is as high as 5000 to 8000 ohm/cm^2, compared with 1000 to 1500 ohm/cm^2 in extraparenchymal vessels. The highly polarized endothelial cells of the blood-brain barrier express surface molecules specialized for bidirectional transport of small molecules between blood and brain (88). Examples include GLUT-1 (148), the LDL receptor, the transferrin receptor, and the product of the multidrug resistance-1a gene, P-glycoprotein (149,150). In rodents, ICAM and VCAM are absent from brain endothelial cells, although T cells and monocytes have been shown to enter the brain even with an intact blood-brain barrier (78). How leukocytes cross the tight junctions of the blood-brain barrier is not clear, although experiments suggest that inflammatory cytokines may downmodulate endothelial expression of tight junction components such as ZO-1 and thereby disassemble the junctions (149).

Hemostatic Functions of Endothelium

Under normal conditions, endothelial cells present a nonthrombogenic surface to flowing blood and play an active role in maintaining blood fluidity (7,151) (Fig. 15-1). Through the constitutive secretion of low levels of prostacyclin (100), a potent inhibitor of platelet activation, and expression of a surface ecto-ADPase (152), endothelial cells prevent inappropriate platelet activation and limit the degree of platelet response to an activating signal. The endothelial cell surface ecto-ADPase has been identified as CD39 (153), a single-chain transmembrane glycoprotein of 80 kd that was originally described as a B-cell marker and later shown to be expressed on NK cells, T-cell subsets, and endothelial cells. It is a calcium-magnesium–dependent E-type ATP diphosphohydrolase with specificity for ATP and ADP, but not AMP. It is antithrombotic by virtue of its ability to metabolize ATP and ADP, secreted from platelets, into AMP, which is not active as a platelet agonist.

The endothelial surface is also antithrombotic by virtue of constitutive expression of the natural regulators of thrombin generation and fibrin formation. These include tissue factor pathway inhibitor (TFPI) (154), a lipoprotein-associated, Kunitz-type protease inhibitor that is the major inhibitor of coagulation factor VIIa, and antithrombin III, a serine protease inhibitor with specificity for the major vitamin K–dependent proteases of the coagulation cascade, factors Xa, IXa, and thrombin. These are interesting inhibitors in that the inhibitory activity of TFPI requires complex formation with activated coagulation factor X, whereas that of antithrombin III requires complex formation with heparan sulfate proteoglycans (155). These inhibitory systems are activated by products of the activated coagulation cascade and localized in their action to the endothelial surface and subendothelial space.

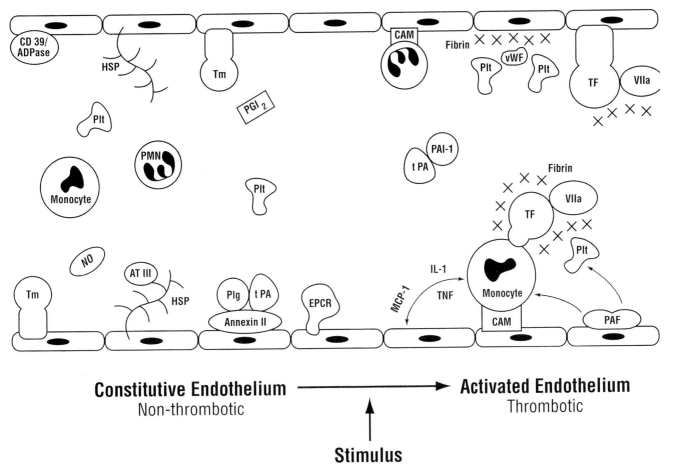

Constitutive Endothelium
Non-thrombotic

Activated Endothelium
Thrombotic

Stimulus

FIG. 15-1. Endothelial cell regulation of hemostasis. The resting endothelium normally expresses a nonthrombotic, noninflammatory phenotype marked by expression of thrombomodulin (Tm), heparan sulfate proteoglycan (HSP) species with high affinity for antithrombin III (ATIII), CD39/ectoADPase, endothelial protein C receptor (EPCR), prostacyclin (PGI₂), nitric oxide (NO), and receptors such as annexin II for plasminogen (Plg) and tissue plasminogen activator (tPA). On stimulation (arrow), the cells convert to a prothrombotic, proinflammatory phenotype marked by loss of Tm and HSP expression and by induction of expression of cytokines (including interleukin-1), chemokines (including monocyte chemotactic protein-1 [MCP-1]), growth factors (including platelet-derived growth factor [PDGF]), plasminogen activator inhibitor-1 (PAI-1), platelet-activating factor (PAF), von Willebrand factor (vWF), endothelin-1 (ET-1), and cell adhesion molecules (CAMS). Leukocytes bound to the CAMs can release cytokines and express tissue factor, amplifying the response.

The protein C system (156), a third critical regulator of thrombin generation, is itself also regulated in a complex manner. Activated protein C is a vitamin K–dependent serine protease that downregulates thrombin generation by proteolytic destruction of the major protein cofactors of the coagulation cascade, factors V and VIII. The zymogen protein C is converted to its active form by thrombin-mediated limited proteolytic cleavage (156,157). Thrombin gains specificity for protein C only when it is bound on the endothelial cell surface to a unique endothelial receptor, thrombomodulin (158), a transmembrane glycoprotein structurally related to the LDL receptor. An endothelial cell receptor for activated protein C (EPCR) has been identified and cloned (159,160). This transmembrane glycoprotein is related to CD1 and MHC class I, binds protein C, and facilitates its activation by thrombin. Endothelial cells also constitutively secrete tissue-type plasminogen activator (t-PA), single-chain urinary-type plasminogen activator (u-PA), and the GPI-linked cellular u-PA receptor (UPAR) (117–119,161). Annexin II expressed on the endothelial surface has been shown by Hajjar to function as a receptor for plasminogen and t-PA (162,163), localizing zymogen and activator to the vessel wall and altering the kinetics of activation to favor plasmin generation. Even though endothelial cells also express PAI-1, evidence suggests that under normal conditions the balance favors activators over inhibitors and that trace amounts of active plasmin are present on the endothelial surface (164).

Although the resting endothelial phenotype is antiplatelet, antithrombin, and profibrinolytic, endothelial cell activation, such as by TNF-α or lipopolysaccharide, results in a dramatic switch to a prothrombotic phenotype (7,151,155). The molecular basis of this change is complex (see Fig. 15-1) and includes loss of expression of thrombomodulin, EPCR, and heparan sulfate proteoglycans from the cell surface (155,165–168), downmodulating the ability to generate active protein C and functional antithrombin III. PAI-1 secretion also increases (117–119), resulting in a net antifibrinolytic state. Thrombin generation is directly promoted by induced surface expression of tissue factor procoagulant, the most important and efficient initiator of the coagulation cascade (114–116). Endothelial cells also express a cellular receptor for coagulation factor Xa (169–170). This novel 55-kd protein, called effector cell protease-1 (EPR-1), is also expressed on B and T cells, where it may participate in cell signaling (171). Its role on the endothelial surface is not yet established, although it has been shown to bind factor Xa, not the inactive zymogen, and therefore may play a role in generating a surface bound prothrombinase. Antiplatelet effects on the endothelial surface are also downmodulated by the resulting generation of thrombin, a potent platelet agonist, and the concomitant expression of PAF (120).

Generation of thrombin, fibrin, and activated platelets probably contributes to the "injury response" and facilitates inflammation and wound healing. Pathologic thrombus formation, however, could also result from such endothelial activation (7,151). Many acquired hypercoagulable states, including cancer, diabetes, the antiphospholipid syndrome, and disseminated intravascular coagulopathy associated with sepsis, may be the result of such inappropriate endothelial cell activation. Endothelial cell tissue factor expression and loss of thrombomodulin have been described in atheroma and in acute thrombosis associated with tumors and graft rejection.

Although a hallmark of the activated endothelial cell is expression of a prothrombotic phenotype, endothelial cell activation by cytokines and angiogenic stimuli also upregulates expression of plasminogen activators, t-PA and u-PA, and the u-PA receptor, UPAR (118,172,173). The latter localizes at focal adhesion points and at the leading edge of migratory cells, suggesting that highly localized plasmin generation is necessary for remodeling and angiogenesis. This may be related to the importance of plasmin in activating latent matrix-degrading metalloproteases.

Regulation of Vascular Tone by Endothelium

Vascular tone is provided primarily by arterial smooth muscle cells under the control of the autonomic nervous system, although large and medium vessel endothelium plays an important regulatory role. In studies using isolated aortic rings, Furchgott (174) first established that the vasodilatory effect of acetylcholine and histamine required an intact endothelium. The identity of this endothelium-dependent relaxing factor was eventually demonstrated independently by the laboratories of Moncada and Ignarro (175,176) to be indistinguishable from NO, consistent with other studies showing that the vasodilatory effect of nitroglycerin-related drugs resulted from their metabolism to NO. Perhaps one of the most significant scientific developments in vascular biology and immunology during the past decade has been the characterization of the cellular mechanisms for generating NO and the recognition of the pleiotropic role of NO in regulating many important cellular functions (177,178).

NO, by virtue of its ability to activate guanylyl cyclase and generate cGMP, is a potent vasodilator and inhibitor of platelet function. NO is an unstable gas that binds tightly to hemoglobin and therefore has an extraordinarily brief plasma lifespan, limiting its action to the microenvironment in which it is produced. NO is generated from L-arginine by the action of NOS, a family of tightly regulated enzymes found in many cells, including in brain, blood vessels, and macrophages. Endothelial cells express a constitutive NOS that can be activated rapidly by agonists that increase intracellular calcium concentrations. Endothelial cells may also synthesize a second, inducible form of NOS when exposed to inflammatory cytokines such as TNF. The inducible NOS generates NO in the absence of increases in intracellular calcium. It has been postulated that dysfunction of these systems may contribute to chronic hypertension, atherosclerosis, and shock (179).

Endothelial cells constitutively express eicosanoid-metabolizing enzymes, including cyclooxygenase-1 (COX-1) and prostacyclin synthase, producing prostacyclin as the major prostaglandin end product (100,109). Like NO, this is a potent vasodilator and antiplatelet agent with an extremely brief plasma half-life. On stimulation with thrombin, shear stress, and other agonists, phospholipase A_2 and other enzymes are activated, leading to prostacyclin generation (180). Whereas platelets and endothelial cells both express COX-1, endothelial cells metabolize its product to prostacyclin, and platelets instead form thromboxane as the major prostaglandin metabolite. Inhibition of COX-1 by aspirin or non-steroidal antiinflammatory agents blocks production of the vasoconstricting, platelet-activating thromboxane and the vasodilating, antiplatelet prostacyclin. Preferential platelet inhibition, however, can be accomplished with use of a single small daily aspirin dose (80 to 100 mg). Because aspirin inhibits COX-1 irreversibly and because platelets do not have the capacity to synthesize new proteins, a platelet exposed to aspirin, even at this low dose, is permanently paralyzed with respect to thromboxane synthesis. In contrast, endothelial cells have an intact RNA transcriptional and protein translational system and continue to synthesize new enzymes after a dose of aspirin is metabolized so that a single low daily dose has little effect on prostacyclin generation. Endothelial cells also express a second COX isoform (COX-2) that can be induced rapidly in response to TNF and other agonists, increasing the output of prostacyclin after exposure to appropriate stimuli.

Endothelial cells express vasoconstrictor systems (109), including angiotensin-converting enzyme, which generates the potent vasoconstrictor angiotensin II from its precursor, and endothelin-1 (ET-1), the most potent vasoconstricting substance described (181). ET-1 is a 21 amino acid peptide formed by enzymatic cleavage of a 200 amino acid pro-precursor protein to form a 40 amino acid precursor known as big ET (182). This is cleaved by a family of transmembrane ET-converting enzymes related to the enkephalin-converting enzymes of the brain. There are three known ETs, all members of a family of peptide hormones related to vasoconstrictor snake venoms (183). The biologic function of ET is mediated by a pair of seven transmembrane G-protein–coupled cellular receptors, ET receptors A and B. ETA is expressed on vascular smooth muscle and mediates the vasoconstrictor effects of ET-1. Endothelial cells express ETB, originally thought to be a clearance receptor but now known to control local vascular tone by mediating constitutive release of local vasodilators (184). In mice, specific pharmacologic inhibition of ETB leads to a significant rise in blood pressure that can be blocked by treatment with cyclooxygenase inhibitors, although not with inhibitors of NO production. Similarly, mice deficient in ET-1 are hypertensive (185).

Although the physiologic role of ET-1 in humans is not clear, its production and release by endothelial cells is slowly increased in response to epinephrine, thrombin, shear stress, and oxidized lipoproteins, suggesting a potential role in the endothelial cell injury response. High levels have been reported in hypoxic kidneys, perhaps indicating a role in shock-related acute renal failure.

Hematopoietic Functions of the Endothelium

During early embryonic development, hematopoietic precursors are found in direct contact with endothelial precursors within blood islands of the extraembryonic yolk sac and along the wall of the thoracic aorta (8,9). Close contact between hematopoietic precursors and differentiated endothelial cells is maintained throughout development in the fetal liver and then postnatally in the vascular sinusoids of the bone marrow. The endothelial cells that form these discontinuous, fenestrated sinusoids represent another example of a uniquely differentiated microvascular system (85). Endothelial cells isolated and propagated from bone marrow microvessels, unlike other cultured endothelial cells, constitutively secrete growth factors and cytokines critical for hematopoietic development, including stem cell factor, VEGF, leukemia inhibitory factor, IL-6, and macrophage, granulocyte, and granulocyte-macrophage colony-stimulating factors (186).

Coculture of CD34-positive hematopoietic precursors isolated from marrow or blood with bone marrow-derived endothelial cells supports long-term proliferation and differentiation of the hematopoietic cells in the absence of added cytokines (86,187). This coculture system also supports long-term maintenance of the endothelial cells in the absence of added endothelial growth factors, perhaps related to VEGF and angiopoietin produced by the CD34-positive precursors. Endothelial cells cultured from sites other than bone marrow also secrete hematopoietic cytokines and growth factors, although only in response to inflammatory cytokines, such as IL-1 (188–190). This distinction presumably reflects the proinflammatory and not hematopoietic functions of these cytokines.

The mechanisms that regulate release of differentiated hematopoietic cells from the bone marrow sinusoids and trafficking of hematopoietic precursors to and from the marrow are poorly understood, but they presumably are related to expression of specific adhesion molecules. Although the physiologic significance and molecular basis of hematopoietic precursor traffic are unknown, isolation of circulating progenitors by apheresis has become a standard method for preparing autologous stem cells for autotransplantation or gene therapy.

Endothelial Cell Role in Leukocyte Trafficking

Perhaps the most important function of the vascular endothelium with respect to inflammation is its role in orchestrating the complex trafficking of leukocytes from blood to tissues. For a circulating leukocyte to enter tissues, it must first encounter and cross the endothelium of the vessels in that tissue. At least three types of leukocyte traffic have been described:

1. Recruitment of inflammatory leukocytes (i.e., PMNs, monocytes, eosinophils, NK cells) into tissues in response to mediators of inflammation such as lipopolysaccharide, IL-1, and TNF-α
2. Constant recirculation of naive lymphocytes from blood to tissues and lymphoid organs as part of normal immune surveillance
3. Recruitment of memory lymphocytes into tissues and lymphoid organs as part of a secondary immune response (6,191,192)

In considering the large number of different cell types that traffic specifically to large numbers of different tissues (e.g., T cells to nodes, B cells to gut, memory cells to skin, PMNs to inflamed tissue), it is obvious that an elaborate system for leukocyte-endothelial cell recognition must exist and that scores of different and regulated cell-cell recognition events must occur. Unlike the case of embryologic development, this constant cell sorting must occur rapidly and under conditions of flow and shear stress (193).

The model for leukocyte trafficking that is supported by a large amount of elegant experimental cell and molecular biology from many laboratories involves a multistep cascade of adhesion steps (6,113,191,194). These are mediated by sequential interaction of specific leukocyte adhesion receptors with specific ligands or counterreceptors expressed on the surface of endothelial cells. These receptor-ligand interactions provide a specific "area code" (191), targeting the appropriate leukocyte subpopulation to its appropriate endothelial surface. The multistep adhesion cascade model is summarized in Figure 15-2 and consists of four major steps:

1. Attachment or tethering of the circulating leukocyte to the endothelial cell, which in certain vascular beds (e.g., small venules of the mesenteric circulation) is associated with rolling of the leukocyte down the blood vessel wall
2. Triggering or activation of additional adhesion molecules on the leukocyte surface

3. Firm attachment of leukocyte to endothelial cell, which is associated with arrest and spreading of the rolling leukocyte on the vessel wall
4. Migration or diapedesis of the leukocyte between adjacent endothelial cells into the subendothelial space

The initial attachment step is usually mediated by the selectin family of adhesion molecules (82). These are transmembrane glycoproteins consisting of an amino terminal C-type lectin (or carbohydrate recognition) domain, followed by an EGF-like domain, a variable number of short, repeating domains related to those in complement regulatory proteins, a transmembrane domain and a short carboxyl-terminal intracytoplasmic domain. Endothelial cells express two selectins, E and P (CD62E and CD62P), after stimulation by inflammatory mediators (68,111). Although *in vitro* cell culture experiments predicted a major role for E-selectin in acute inflammation, murine knock-out studies demonstrated that E-selectin null mice had little or no abnormalities (195). In contrast, P-selectin null mice showed partial inhibition of leukocyte rolling on inflamed mesenteric vessels, blunted delayed-type hypersensitivity, and decreased peritoneal recruitment of leukocytes (196,197). The double E- and P-selectin null mice demonstrated absent rolling, spontaneous skin infections, and poor wound healing, suggesting that the selectins may function cooperatively *in vivo* (198–201).

E-selectin and P-selectin interact with carbohydrate antigens expressed on the surface of PMNs, monocytes, eosinophils, and certain lymphocyte subpopulations (82). The major ligands are sialylated fucosylated tetrasaccharides, such as sialylated Lewis^X and sialylated Lewis^A, which are expressed in high concentration on the microvilli of PMNs and monocytes. P-selectin and the lymphocyte selectin, L-selectin, may also bind sulfatides and sulfated glycosoaminoglycans. Specific glycoprotein ligands for E- and P-selectin (ESL-1 and PSGL-1, respectively) have been identified and cloned. These presumably carry the necessary carbohydrate side chains and other recognition sites.

The firm attachment or arrest step of the cascade is mediated by the interaction of leukocyte integrins with endothelial cell immunoglobulin superfamily adhesion molecules (6,191). These include the interaction of the β_2 (CD11/CD18) integrins with ICAM-1 and ICAM-2, which are upregulated on the surface of cytokine-activated endothelial cells. Leukocyte $\alpha_4\beta_1$ integrin also interacts with endothelial VCAM-1. These integrin-mediated interactions are capable of transducing signals to the leukocyte (202) and lead to cytoskeletal reorganization and spreading. In general, the leukocyte integrins are functionally inactive on circulating cells; so while tethering of resting leukocytes occurs on activated endothelium, a leukocyte triggering or activation step must be

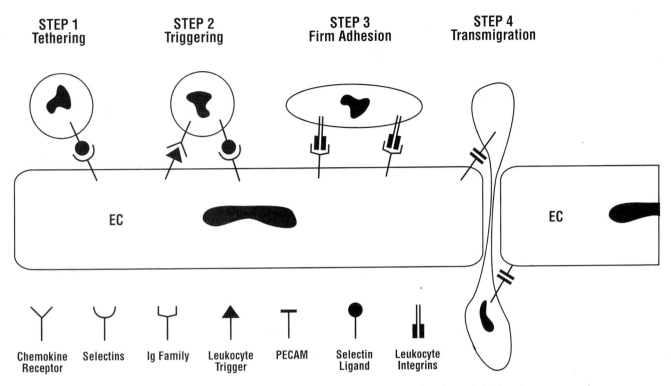

FIG. 15-2. Leukocyte adhesion cascade. Adhesion and transmigration of leukocytes across the endothelial cell layer is a multistep process involving sequential interaction of specific adhesion molecules on the endothelial surface with counterreceptors on the leukocyte surface. The first step is the tethering or rolling of the leukocyte to selectins expressed on the surface of activated endothelial cells. The second step is triggering of the tethered leukocyte that results in activation of leukocyte integrins. Triggering molecules include selectins themselves, platelet-activating factor, endothelial cell chemokines, and other inflammatory mediators. The third step is firm adhesion and spreading of the leukocyte on the endothelial surface, which is mediated by interactions of the activated leukocyte integrins with the immunoglobulin superfamily cell adhesion molecules on the endothelial surface. The final step is transmigration of the leukocyte through the endothelial barrier, which is mediated by platelet-endothelial cell adhesion molecule (PECAM)–dependent homophilic adhesive interactions.

interposed between attachment and firm adhesion. Multiple pathways of leukocyte triggering have been described. Some studies have shown that engagement of E-selectin, P-selectin, or both on the leukocyte surface can lead to triggering (203). In the latter case, PAF has been shown to play an important role (120). Soluble mediators, such as *N*-formyl-methionyl-leucyl-phenylalanine, leukotriene B$_4$, and C5a may also provide a signal.

Perhaps the most important activating signals are provided by chemokines produced locally at the site of vascular response (204). These are small, soluble mediators with potent leukocyte chemotactic properties that fall into two major families containing at least 25 members, the CXC family (e.g., IL-8) and the CC family (e.g., MCP-1, RANTES [regulated on activation, normally T-cell expressed and secreted]). Each has its own specificity, such as IL-8 for PMNs, MCP-1 for monocytes, and RANTES for memory T cells, determined by the specificity and expression pattern of a family of receptors (205). These are all seven transmembrane domain, G-protein–coupled signaling molecules and have variable

specificities. The IL-8 receptor is quite specific, but the receptor originally identified as the Duffy blood antigen is promiscuous. A subfamily of receptors with shared specificity, including one for MCP-1, has generated considerable interest as critical coreceptors for HIV cell entry. Chemokines such as MCP-1 and IL-8 are produced by activated endothelial cells and then presented to tethered leukocytes by surface presentation molecules such as proteoglycans. By providing precise sorting signals to subpopulations of tethered leukocytes, the chemokines and their receptors act as the traffic cops of the adhesion superhighway (191).

The final step of leukocyte trafficking is transmigration. This is accomplished by squeezing the cells between the intercellular junctions of adjacent endothelial cells. Work by Muller et al. (81) identified the immunoglobulin (Ig) superfamily molecule CD31 (i.e., PECAM-1) as necessary for this step. This protein, which probably functions as a homophilic adhesion molecule, is expressed on most leukocytes and occurs in high concentrations on the endothelial surface, localized to the lateral cell-cell junctions. Antibodies to CD31 or soluble CD31/Ig fusion proteins have been shown to block monocyte migration across endothelial cell monolayers in culture and to inhibit monocyte recruitment into inflamed peritoneum in animal models.

The cascade described earlier and summarized in Figure 15-2 is particularly relevant to the recruitment of PMNs, monocytes, eosinophils, NK cells, and certain lymphocyte subpopulations to inflammatory lesions. This is a specific, rapid, and efficient process; it has been estimated that up to 10^8 PMNs can enter a rheumatoid joint per hour, probably mainly through the flat endothelium of small postcapillary venules. Recirculation of naive lymphocytes, in contrast, occurs at a slower but more constant rate (192), occurring mainly through the high endothelial cells of postcapillary venules (i.e., HEVs) in lymphoid tissues. Pioneering studies of Stamper and Woodruff (87) demonstrated that lymphocyte subclasses bound with differing specificities to HEVs in thin sections cut from frozen lymphoid tissues. For example, T cells bound better to peripheral node HEVs, but B cells bound better to Peyer's patch HEVs. Lymphocyte L-selectin interactions with HEV mucin-like adhesion molecules GlyCAM-1, VAP-1, and CD34 determine attachment to peripheral nodes, and interactions with a different adhesion protein MadCAM-1 determine attachment to Peyer's patches (206–208). MadCAM-1 is an unusual Ig superfamily molecule that also has a mucin-like domain. MadCAM-1 also binds the lymphocyte integrin $\alpha_4\beta_7$, providing a specific firm adhesion pathway in Peyer's patch HEVs (208–210).

Recruitment of memory cells to lymphoid and cutaneous tissues is probably mediated by subtly different pathways. Skin T cells, for example, express a unique cutaneous lymphoid-associated antigen similar to Lewis^x that probably specifies initial tethering to flat cutaneous endothelial cells through E-selectin. Memory cells express different classes of integrins; gut-associated cells, for example, express high levels of β_7 integrins (α_E and α_4), and skin-associated cells express little or no β_7 but considerable $\alpha_4\beta_1$ (191,192,207,208). Studies also suggest that expression of certain L-selectin ligands by HEVs may require the presence of foreign antigen in the tissue.

Ongoing research is identifying the endothelial addressins and lymphocyte ligands that mediate the myriad and complex trafficking events. Table 15-2 summarizes some of the major adhesion pairs identified. The observation that tumor cells may also express specific ligands for endothelial cell adhesion molecules may explain the fairly specific and predictable metastatic patterns of certain cancers.

The vascular endothelium is a complex organ, precisely regulated to perform many crucial functions, most of which have direct relevance to the inflammatory response. These include regulation of vascular tone and

TABLE 15-2. *Families of endothelial cell adhesion molecules and their leukocyte ligands*

Endothelial cell adhesion molecules	Leukocyte ligands
Selectins	
E-selectin	sLe^x, sLe^a, CLA, ESL-1
P-selectin	sLe^x, sLe^a, PSGL-1
Ig family	
ICAM-1	$\alpha_M\beta_2$, $\alpha_L\beta_2$
ICAM-2	$\alpha_L\beta_2$
VCAM-1	$\alpha_4\beta_1$, $\alpha_4\beta_7$
MadCAM-1	$\alpha_4\beta_7$, L-selectin
PECAM	PECAM
Mucin-like molecules	
MadCAM-1	$\alpha_4\beta_7$, L-selectin
GlyCAM-1	L-selectin
CD34	L-selectin
Other sialoglycoprotein	
VAP-1	Unknown T-cell antigen

CLA, lymphoid-associated antigen; ESL, E-selectin–specific ligand; ICAM, intercellular adhesion molecule; MadCAM-1, mucosal addressin cell adhesion molecule-1; PECAM, platlet-endothelial cell adhesion molecule; PSGL, P-selectin–specific glycoprotein ligand; sLe, sialyl Lewis; VAP, vascular adhesion protein; VCAM, vascular cell adhesion molecule.

permeability, control of leukocyte traffic, wound repair, and hematopoiesis. Disordered endothelial function has been implicated in vasculitic syndromes, systemic sclerosis, thrombosis associated with lupus and antiphospholipid syndrome, and rheumatoid synovitis. Anti-endothelial cell autoantibodies have been described in many autoimmune diseases and may be pathogenic in some cases, such as Kawasaki's disease, systemic sclerosis, and antiphospholipid syndrome. Viral activation of endothelial cells has been described by several laboratories and may have particular relevance to the accelerated atherosclerosis seen after cardiac transplantation. New therapeutic approaches based on endothelial cell function are being developed for inflammatory disease, thrombotic disease, hypertension, atherosclerosis, cancer, myocardial infarction, and diabetic complications. Antibody-targeted therapy aimed at specific endothelial antigens is being developed for thrombosis and gene transfer.

REFERENCES

1. Metchnikoff E. Starling FA, Starling EH, translators. *Lectures on the comparative pathology of inflammation*. New York: Dover Publications, 1968:135–137.
2. Jaffe EA, Nachman RL, Becker CG. Culture of human endothelial cells derived from umbilical veins: identification by morphological and immunologic criteria. *J Clin Invest* 1973;52:2745–2758.
3. Gimbrone MA Jr, Cotran RS, Folkman J. Human vascular endothelial cells in culture: growth and DNA synthesis. *J Cell Biol* 1964;60: 673–682.
4. Folkman J, Cotran RS. Relation of vascular proliferation to tumor growth. *Int Rev Exp Pathol* 1976;16:207–248.
5. Ross R. The pathogenesis of atherosclerosis: a perspective for the 1990's. *Nature* 1993;362:801–809.

6. Luscinskas FW, Gimbrone MA Jr. Endothelial-dependent mechanisms in chronic inflammatory leukocyte recruitment. *Annu Rev Med* 1996;47:413–421.

7. Schafer AI. Vascular endothelium: in defense of blood fluidity. *J Clin Invest* 1997;99:1143–1144.

8. Risau W. Mechanisms of angiogenesis. *Nature* 1997;386:671–674.

9. Pardanaud L, Yassine F, Dieterlen-Lievre F. Relationship between vasculogenesis, angiogenesis and haemopoiesis during avian ontogeny. *Development* 1989;105:473–485.

10. Asahara T, Murohara T, Sullivan A, et al. Isolation of putative progenitor endothelial cells for angiogenesis. *Science* 1997;275:964–967.

11. Shi Q, Rafii S, Wu MH-D, et al. Evidence for circulating bone marrow-derived endothelial progenitor cells (personal communication, 1997).

12. Mustonen T, Alitalo K. Endothelial receptor tyrosine kinases involved in angiogenesis. *J Cell Biol* 1995;129:895–898.

13. Shalaby F, Rossant J, Yamaguchi TP, Gertsenstein M, Wu XF, Breitman ML, Schuh AC. Failure of blood-island formation and vasculogenesis in Flk-1–deficient mice. *Nature* 1995;376:62–66.

14. Shalaby F, Ho J, Stanford WL, et al. A requirement for Flk-1 in primitive and definitive hematopoiesis and vasculogenesis. *Cell* 1997;89:981–990.

15. Keck PJ, Hauser SD, Krivi G, et al. Vascular permeability factor, an endothelial cell mitogen related to PDGF. *Science* 1989;246:1309–1312.

16. Thomas KA. Vascular endothelial growth factor and potent and selective angiogenesis agent. *J Biol Chem* 1996;271:603–606.

17. Maglione D, Guerriero V, Viglietto G, Delli-Bovi P, Persico MG. Isolation of a human placenta cDNA coding for a protein related to the vascular permeability factor. *Proc Natl Acad Sci USA* 1991;88:9267–9271.

18. Ferra N, Carver-Moore K, Chen H, et al. Heterozygous embryonic lethality induced by targeted inactivation of the *VEGF* gene. *Nature* 1996;380:439–442.

19. Carmeliet P, Verreira V, Breier G, et al. Abnormal blood vessel development and lethality in embryos lacking a single *VEGF* allele. *Nature* 1996;380:435–439.

20. Gerritsen ME, Shen CP, Atkinson WJ, Padgett RC, Gimbrone MA Jr, Milstone DS. Microvascular endothelial cells from E-selectin–deficient mice form tubes *in vitro*. *Lab Invest* 1996;75:175–184.

21. Hynes RO, Bader BL. Targeted mutations in integrins and their ligands: their implications for vascular biology. *Thromb Haemost* 1997;78:83–87.

22. Brooks PC, Clark RA, Cheresh DA. Requirement of vascular integrin $\alpha_v\beta_3$ for angiogenesis. *Science* 1994;264:569–571.

23. Joukov V, Pajusola K, Kaipainen A, et al. A novel vascular endothelial growth factor, VEGF-C, is a ligand for the flt4 and (VEGFR-3) receptor tyrosine kinases. *EMBO J* 1996;15:290–298.

24. Kaipainen A, Korthonen J, Mustonen T, et al. Expression of the fms-like tyrosine kinase 4 gene becomes restricted to lymphatic endothelium during development. *Proc Natl Acad Sci USA* 1995;92:3566–3570.

25. Sato TN, Qin Y, Kozak CA, Audus KL. Tie-1 and Tie-2 define another class of putative receptor tyrosine kinase genes expressed in early embryonic vascular system. *Proc Natl Acad Sci USA* 1993;90:9355–9358.

26. Davis S, Aldrich TH, Jones PF, et al. Isolation of angiopoetin-1, a ligand for the Tie-2 receptor, by secretion-trap expression cloning. *Cell* 1996;87:1161–1169.

27. Sato TN, Tozawa Y, Deutsch U, et al. Distinct roles of the receptor tyrosine kinase Tie-1 and Tie-2 in blood vessel formation. *Nature* 1995;376:70–74.

28. Puri MC, Rossant J, Alitalo K. The receptor tyrosine kinase TIE is required for integrity and survival of vascular endothelial cells. *EMBO J* 1995;14:5884–5891.

29. Suri C, Jones P, Patan S, et al. Requisite role of angiopoietin-1, a ligand for the TIE2 receptor, during embryonic angiogenesis. *Cell* 1996;87:1171–1180.

30. Vikkula M, Boon LM, Carraway KL 3rd, et al. Vascular dysmorphogenesis caused by an activating mutation in the receptor tyrosine kinase TIE2. *Cell* 1996;87:1181–1190.

31. Folkman J. Clinical applications of research on angiogenesis. *N Engl J Med* 1995;333:1757–1763.

32. Folkman J, Klagsbrun M. Angiogenic factors. *Science* 1987;235:442–443.

33. Thomas KA, Gimenez-Gallego G. Fibroblast growth factors: broad spectrum mitogens with potent angiogenic activity. *Trends Biochem Sci* 1986;11:81–84.

34. Dvorak HF, Brown LF, Detmar M, Dvorak AM. Vascular permeability factor/vascular endothelial growth factor, microvascular hyperpermeability and angiogenesis. *Am J Pathol* 1995;146:1029–1039.

35. Konig A, Corbacioglu S, Ballmaier M, Welte K. Downregulation of c-kit expression in human endothelial cells by inflammatory stimuli. *Blood* 1997;90:148–155.

36. Brizzi MF, Garbarino G, Rossi PR, et al. Interleukin-3 stimulates proliferation and triggers endothelial-leukocyte adhesion molecule 1 gene activation of human endothelial cells. *J Clin Invest* 1993;91:2887–2892.

37. Mirza H, Yatsula V, Bahou WF. The proteinase activated receptor-2 (PAR-2) mediates mitogenic responses in human vascular endothelial cells. *J Clin Invest* 1996;97:1705–1714.

38. Mousa SA. Angiogenesis promoters and inhibitors: potential therapeutic implications. *Mol Med Today* 1996;2:140–142.

39. Meredith JE Jr, Fazeli B, Schwartz MA. The extracellular matrix as a cell survival factor. *Mol Biol Cell* 1993;4:953–961.

40. Stromblad S, Becker JC, Yebra M, Brooks PC, Cheresh DA. Suppression of p53 activity and p21WAF1/CIP1 expression by vascular cell integrin $\alpha_v\beta_3$ during angiogenesis. *J Clin Invest* 1996;98:426–433.

41. Brooks PC, Montgomery AM, Rosenfeld M, et al. Integrin $\alpha_v\beta_3$ antagonists promote tumor regression by inducing apoptosis of angiogenic blood vessels. *Cell* 1994;79:1157–1164.

42. Friedlander M, Brooks PC, Shaffer RW, Kincaid CM, Varner JA, Cheresh DA. Definition of two angiogenic pathways by distinct α_v integrins. *Science* 1995;270:1500–1502.

43. Dvorak HF, Harvey VS, Estella P, et al. Fibrin containing gels induce angiogenesis: implications for tumor stroma generation and wound healing. *Lab Invest* 1987;57:673–686.

44. Peterson HI. Tumor angiogenesis inhibition by prostaglandin synthetase inhibitors. *Anticancer Res* 1986;6:251–254.

45. Iruela-Arispe MF, Dvorak HF. Angiogenesis: a dynamic balance of stimulators and inhibitors. *Thromb Haemost* 1997;78:632–672.

46. Lingen MW, Polverini PJ, Bouck NP. Inhibition of squamous cell carcinoma angiogenesis by direct interaction of retinoic acid with endothelial cells. *Lab Invest* 1996;74:476–483.

47. O'Reilly MS, Boehm T, Shing Y, et al. Endostatin: an endogenous inhibitor of angiogenesis and tumor growth. *Cell* 1997;88:277–285.

48. O'Reilly MS, Holmgren L, Shing Y, et al. Angiostatin: a novel angiogenesis inhibitor that mediates the suppression of metastases by a Lewis lung carcinoma. *Cell* 1994;79:315–328.

49. Good DJ, Polverini PJ, Rastinejad F, et al. A tumor suppressor-dependent inhibitor of angiogenesis is immunologically and functionally indistinguishable from a fragment of thrombospondin. *Proc Natl Acad Sci USA* 1990;87:6624–6628.

50. Tolsma S, Volpert OV, Good DJ, Frazier WA, Polverini P, Bouck N. Peptides derived from two separate domains of the matrix protein thrombospondin-1 have anti-angiogenic activity. *J Cell Biol* 1993;122:497–511.

51. Frazier WA. Thrombospondins. *Curr Opin Cell Biol* 1991;3:792–799.

52. Bornstein P. The thrombospondins: structure and regulation of expression. *FASEB J* 1992;6:3290–3299.

53. Reed MJ, Iruela-Arispe ML, O'Brien ER, et al. Expression of thrombospondins by endothelial cells: injury is correlated with TSP-1. *Am J Pathol* 1995;147:1068–1080.

54. Irulea-Arispe ML, Bornstein P, Sage H. Thrombospondin exerts an antiangiogenic effect on tube formation by endothelial cells *in vitro*. *Proc Natl Acad Sci USA* 1991;88:5026–5030.

55. Dawson DW, Pearce SFA, Zhong R, Silverstein RL, Frazier WA, Bouck NP. CD36 mediates the inhibitory effects of thrombospondin-1 on endothelial cells. *J Cell Biol* 1997;138:707–717.

56. Polverini PJ, DiPietro LA, Dixit VM, Hynes RO, Lawler J. TSP-1 knockout mice showed delayed organization and prolonged vascularization of skin wounds. *FASEB J* 1995;9:272a(abst).

57. Lawler J, Weinstein R, Hynes RO. Cell attachment to thrombospondin: the role of ARG-GLY-ASP, calcium, and integrin receptors. *J Cell Biol* 1988;107:2351–2361.

58. Murphy-Ullrich JE, Hook M. Thrombospondin modulates focal adhesions in endothelial cells. *J Cell Biol* 1989;109:1309–1319.

59. Greenwalt DE, Lipsky RH, Ockenhouse CF, Ikeda H, Tandon NN, Jamieson GA. Membrane glycoprotein CD36: a review of its roles in

adherence, signal transduction, and transfusion medicine. *Blood* 1992; 80:1105–1115.

60. Febbraio M, Volpert O, Bouck NP, Silverstein RL. Absense of anti-angiogenic effect of TSP-1 in CD36 null mice [personal communication], 1998.

61. Isner JM, Pieczek A, Schainfeld R, et al. Clinical evidence of angiogenesis after arterial gene transfer of phVEGF165 in patient with ischaemic limb. *Lancet* 1996;348:370–374.

62. Asahara T, Chen D, Tsurumi Y, et al. Accelerated restitution of endothelial integrity and endothelium-dependent function after phVEGF165 gene transfer. *Circulation* 1996;94:3291–3302.

63. Asahara T, Bauters C, Pastore C, et al. Local delivery of vascular endothelial growth factor accelerates reendothelialization and attenuates intimal hyperplasia in balloon-injured rat carotid artery. *Circulation* 1995;91:2793–2801.

64. Kim KJ, Li B, Winer J, Armanini M, Gillett N, Phillips HS, Ferrara N. Inhibition of vascular endothelial growth factor-induced angiogenesis suppresses tumour growth *in vivo*. *Nature* 1993;362:841–844.

65. Brooks PC, Montgomeray AMP, Rosenfeld M, et al. Integrin $\alpha_v\beta_3$ antagonists promote further tumor regression by inducing apoptosis of angiogenic blood vessels. *Cell* 1994;79:1157–1164.

66. Laurence J, Mitra D, Steiner M, Staiano-Coico L, Jaffe E. Plasma from patients with idiopathic and human immunodeficiency virus-associated thrombotic thrombocytopenic purpura induces apoptosis in microvascular endothelial cells. *Blood* 1996;87:3245–3254.

67. Weibel ER, Palade GE. New cytoplasmic components in arterial endothelial. *J Cell Biol* 1964;23:101–112.

68. Wagner DD. The Weibel-Palade body: the storage granule for von Willebrand factor and P-selectin. *Thromb Haemost* 1993;70:105–110.

69. Liu J, Oh P, Horner T, Rogers RA, Schnitzer JE. Organized endothelial cell surface signal transduction in caveolae distinct from glycosylphosphatidylinositol-anchored protein microdomains. *J Biol Chem* 1997;272:7211–7222.

70. Schnitzer JE, Liu J, Oh P. Endothelial caveolae have the molecular transport machinery for vesicle budding, docking, and fusion including VAMP, NSF, SNAP, annexins, and GTPases. *J Biol Chem* 1995; 270:14399–14404.

71. Schnitzer JE, Oh P, Pinney E, Allard J. Filipin-sensitive caveolae-mediated transport in endothelium: reduced transcytosis, scavenger endocytosis, and capillary permeability of select macromolecules. *J Cell Biol* 1994;127:1217–1232.

72. Lampugnani MG, Corada M, Caveda L, et al. The molecular organization of endothelial cell to cell junctions: differential association of plakoglobin, beta-catenin, and alpha-catenin with vascular endothelial cadherin (VE-cadherin). *J Cell Biol* 1995;129:203–217.

73. Breier G, Breviario F, Caveda L, et al. Molecular cloning and expression of murine vascular endothelial-cadherin in early stage development of cardiovascular system. *Blood* 1996;87:630–641.

74. Dejana E. Endothelial adherens junctions: implications in the control of vascular permeability and angiogenesis. *J Clin Invest* 1996;98: 1949–1953.

75. Caveda L, Martin-Padura I, Navarro P, et al. Inhibition of cultured cell growth by vascular endothelial cadherin (cadherin-5/VE-cadherin). *J Clin Invest* 1996;98:886–893.

76. Rabiet MJ, Plantier JL, Rival Y, Genoux Y, Lampugnani MG, Dejana E. Thrombin-induced increase in endothelial permeability is associated with changes in cell-to-cell junction organization. *Arterioscler Thromb Vasc Biol* 1996;16:488–496.

77. Del Maschio A, Zanetti A, Corada M, et al. Polymorphonuclear leukocyte adhesion triggers the disorganization of endothelial cell-to-cell adherens junctions. *J Cell Biol* 1996;135:497–510.

78. Perry VH, Anthony DC, Bolton SJ, Brown HC. The blood-brain barrier and the inflammatory response. *Mol Med Today* 1997;3:335–341.

79. Risau W, Wolburg H. Development of the blood-brain barrier. *Trends Neurosci* 1990;13:174–178.

80. Ayalon O, Sabanai H, Lampugnani MG, Dejana E, Geiger B. Spatial and temporal relationships between cadherins and PECAM-1 in cell-cell junctions of human endothelial cells. *J Cell Biol* 1994;126: 247–258.

81. Muller WA, Weigl SA, Deng X, Phillips DM. PECAM-1 is required for transendothelial migration of leukocytes. *J Exp Med* 1993;178:449–460.

82. Kansas GS. Selectins and their ligands: current concepts and controversies. *Blood* 1996;88:3259–3287.

83. McAllister KA, Grogg KM, Johnson DW, et al. Endoglin, a TGF-beta binding protein of endothelial cells, is the gene for hereditary haemorrhagic telangiectasia type 1. *Nat Genet* 1994;8:345–351.

84. Couchman JR, Woods A. Syndecans, signaling, and cell adhesion. *J Cell Biochem* 1996;61:578–584.

85. Risau W. Differentiation of endothelium. *FASEB J* 1995;9:926–933.

86. Rafii S, Shapiro F, Rimarachin J, et al. Isolation and characterization of human bone marrow microvascular endothelial cells: hematopoietic progenitor cell adhesion. *Blood* 1994;84:10–19.

87. Stamper HB Jr, Woodruff JJ. Lymphocyte homing into lymph nodes: *in vitro* demonstration of the selective affinity of recirculating lymphocytes for high-endothelial venules. *J Exp Med* 1976;144: 828–834.

88. Risau W, Hallmann R, Albrecht U. Differentiation-dependent expression of proteins in brain endothelium during development of the blood-brain barrier. *Dev Biol* 1986;117:537–545.

89. Risau W, Hallmann R, Albrecht U, Henke-Fahle S. Brain induces the expression of an early cell surface marker for blood-brain barrier-specific endothelium. *EMBO J* 1986;5:3179–3183.

90. Kniesel U, Risau W, Wolburg H. Development of blood-brain barrier tight junctions in the rat cortex. *Brain Res Dev Brain Res* 1996;96: 229–240.

91. Jaffe EA. Synthesis of factor VIII by endothelial cells. *Ann N Y Acad Sci* 1982;401:163–170.

92. Jacobson BS, Stolz DB, Schnitzer JE. Identification of endothelial cell-surface proteins as targets for diagnosis and treatment of disease. *Nat Med* 1996;2:482–484.

93. Pober JS, Cotran RS. Cytokines and endothelial cell biology. *Physiol Rev* 1990;70:427–452.

94. Davies PF. Flow-mediated endothelial mechanotransduction. *Physiol Rev* 1995;75:519–560.

95. Gimbrone MA Jr, Obin MS, Brock AF, et al. Endothelial interleukin-8: a novel inhibitor of leukocyte-endothelial interactions. *Science* 1989;246:1601–63.

96. Brock TA, Brugnara C, Canessa M, Gimbrone MA Jr. Bradykinin and vasopressin stimulate Na^+-K^+-Cl^- cotransport in cultured endothelial cells. *Am J Physiol* 1986;250:888–895.

97. Smith WB, Noack L, Khew-Goodall Y, Isenmann S, Vadas MA, Gamble JR. Transforming growth factor-beta 1 inhibits the production of IL-8 and the transmigration of neutrophils through activated endothelium. *J Immunol* 1996;157:360–368.

98. Braunhut SJ, Moses MA. Retinoids modulate endothelial cell production of matrix-degrading proteases and tissue inhibitors of metalloproteinases (TIMP). *J Biol Chem* 1994;269:13472–13479.

99. Saadi S, Holzknecht RA, Patte CP, Stern DM, Platt JL. Complement-mediated regulation of tissue factor activity in endothelium. *J Exp Med* 1995;182:1807–1814.

100. Weksler BB, Marcus AJ, Jaffe EA. Synthesis of prostaglandin 12 (prostacyclin) by cultured human and bovine endothelial cells. *Proc Natl Acad Sci USA* 1977;74:3922–3928.

101. Brezinski ME, Gimbrone MA Jr, Nicolaou KC, Serhan CN. Lipoxins stimulate prostacyclin generation by human endothelial cells. *FEBS Lett* 1989;245:167–172.

102. De Caterina R, Libby P, Peng HB, et al. Nitric oxide decreases cytokine-induced endothelial activation. Nitric oxide selectively reduces endothelial expression of adhesion molecules and proinflammatory cytokines. *J Clin Invest* 1995;96:60–68.

103. Pinsky DJ, Naka Y, Liao H, et al. Hypoxia-induced exocytosis of endothelial cell Weibel-Palade bodies: a mechanism for rapid neutrophil recruitment after cardiac preservation. *J Clin Invest* 1996;97: 493–500.

104. Etingin OR, Silverstein RL, Friedman HM, Hajjar DP. Viral activation of the coagulation cascade: molecular interactions at the surface of infected endothelial cells. *Cell* 1990;61:657–662.

105. Kume N, Gimbrone MA Jr. Lysophosphatidylcholine transcriptionally induces growth factor gene expression in cultured human endothelial cells. *J Clin Invest* 1994;93:907–911.

106. Kume N, Cybulsky MI, Gimbrone MA Jr. Lysophosphatidylcholine, a component of atherogenic lipoproteins, induces mononuclear leukocyte adhesion molecules in cultured human and rabbit arterial endothelial cells. *J Clin Invest* 1992;90:1138–1144.

107. Greten J, Kreis I, Wiesel K, et al. Receptors for advance glycation end-products (AGE) expression by endothelial cells in non-diabetic uraemic patients. *Nephrol Dial Transplant* 1996;11:786–790.

108. Simantov R, LaSala JM, Lo SK, et al. Activation of cultured vascular

endothelium by antiphospholipid antibodies. *J Clin Invest* 1995;96: 2219–2221.

109. Vane R, Anggard E, Botting M. Regulatory functions of the vascular endothelium. *N Engl J Med* 1990;323:27–36.

110. Collins T, Palmer J, Whitley Z, Neish S, Williams J. A common theme in endothelial activation: insights from the structural analysis of the genes for E-selectin and VCAM-1. *Trends Cell Biol* 1993;3:92–97.

111. Bevilacqua MP, Stengelin S, Gimbrone MA Jr, Seed B. Endothelial leukocyte adhesion molecule 1: an inducible receptor for neutrophils related to complement regulatory proteins and lectins. *Science* 1989; 243:1160–1165.

112. Cybulsky MI, Gimbrone MA Jr. Endothelial expression of a mononuclear leukocyte adhesion molecule during atherogenesis. *Science* 1991;251:788–791.

113. Bevilacqua MP. Endothelial-leukocyte adhesion molecules. *Annu Rev Immunol* 1993;11:767–804.

114. Nawroth PP, Handley DA, Esmon CT, Stern DM. Interleukin-1 induces endothelial cell procoagulant while suppressing cell-surface anticoagulant activity. *Proc Natl Acad Sci USA* 1986;83:3460–3464.

115. Nawroth PP, Stern DM. Modulation of endothelial cell hemostatic properties by tumor necrosis factor. *J Exp Med* 1986;163:740–745.

116. Bevilacqua MP, Pober JS, Majeau GR, Cotran RS, Gimbrone MA Jr. Interleukin 1 (IL-1) induces biosynthesis and cell surface expression of procoagulant activity in human vascular endothelial cells. *J Exp Med* 1984;160:618–623.

117. Nachman RL, Hajjar KA, Silverstein RL, Dinarello C. Interleukin-1 induces endothelial cell synthesis of plasminogen activator inhibitor. *J Exp Med* 1986;163:1595–1600.

118. Bevilacqua MP, Schleef RR, Gimbrone MA Jr, Loskutoff DJ. Regulation of the fibrinolytic system of cultured human vascular endothelium by interleukin-1. *J Clin Invest* 1986;78:587–591.

119. Schleef RR, Bevilacqua MP, Sawdey M, Gimbrone MA Jr, Loskutoff DJ. Cytokine activation of vascular endothelium: effects on tissue-type plasminogen activator and type 1 plasminogen activator inhibitor. *J Biol Chem* 1988;263:5797–5803.

120. Lorant DE, Patel KD, McIntyre TM, McEver RP, Prescott SM, Zimmerman GA. Coexpression of GMP-140 and PAF by endothelium stimulated by histamine or thrombin: a juxtacrine system for adhesion and activation of neutrophils. *J Cell Biol* 1991;115:223–234.

121. Hajjar KA, Hajjar DP, Silverstein RL, Nachman RL. Tumor necrosis factor-mediated release of platelet-derived growth factor from cultured endothelial cells. *J Exp Med* 1987;166:235–245.

122. Collins T, Pober JS, Gimbrone MA Jr, et al. Cultured human endothelial cells express platelet-derived growth factor A chain. *Am J Pathol* 1987;126:7–12.

123. Hannan RL, Kourembanas S, Flanders KC, et al. Endothelial cells synthesize basic fibroblast growth factor and transforming growth factor beta. *Growth Factors* 1988;1:7–17.

124. Pober JS, Gimbrone MA Jr, Cotran RS, et al. Ia expression by vascular endothelium is inducible by activated T cells and by human gamma interferon. *J Exp Med* 1983;157:1339–1353.

125. Cotran RS. The delayed and prolonged vascular leakage in inflammation: II. An electron microscopic study of the vascular response after internal injury. *Am J Pathol* 1965;46:589–620.

126. Vora M, Romero LI, Karasek MA. Interleukin-10 induces E-selectin on small and large blood vessel endothelial cells. *J Exp Med* 1996; 184:821–829.

127. Khew-Goodall Y, Butcher CM, Litwin MS, et al. Chronic expression of P-selectin on endothelial cells stimulated by the T-cell cytokine, interleukin-3. *Blood* 1996;87:1432–1438.

128. Yao L, Pan J, Setiadi H, Patel KD, McEver RP. Interleukin 4 or oncostatin M induces a prolonged increase in P-selectin mRNA and protein in human endothelial cells. *J Exp Med* 1996;184:81–92.

129. Schleimer RP, Sterbinsky SA, Kaiser J, et al. IL-4 induces adherence of human eosinophils and basophils but not neutrophils to endothelium: association with expression of VCAM-1. *J Immunol* 1992;148: 1086–1092.

130. Mach F, Schonbeck U, Sukhova GK, et al. Functional CD40 ligand is expressed on human vascular endothelial cells, smooth muscle cells, and macrophages: implications for CD40-CD40 ligand signaling in atherosclerosis. *Proc Natl Acad Sci USA*. 1997;94:1931–1936.

131. Kojima S, Rifkin DB. Mechanism of retinoid-induced activation of latent transforming growth factor-beta in bovine endothelial cells. *J Cell Physiol* 1993;155:323–332.

132. Gille J, Paxton LLL, Lawley TJ, Caughman SW, Swerlick RA. Retinoic acid inhibits the regulated expression of vascular cell adhesion molecule by cultured dermal microvascular endothelial cells. *J Clin Invest* 1997;99:492–500.

133. Yan SF, Ogawa S, Stern DM, Pinsky DJ. Hypoxia-induced modulation of endothelial cell properties: regulation of barrier function and expression of interleukin-6. *Kidney Int* 1997;51:419–425.

134. Gimbrone MA Jr, Nagel T, Topper JN. Biomechanical activation: an emerging paradigm in endothelial adhesion biology. *J Clin Invest* 1997; 99:1809–1813.

135. Shen J, Luscinskas FW, Connolly A, Dewey CFJ, Gimbrone MA Jr. Fluid shear stress modulates cytosolic free calcium in vascular endothelial: spatial and temporal analysis. *Am J Physiol* 1992;262: C1411–C1417.

136. Tseng H, Peterson T, Berk BC. Fluid shear stress stimulates mitogen-activated protein kinases in bovine aortic endothelial cells. *Circ Res* 1995;77:869–878.

137. Resnick N, Gimbrone MA Jr. Hemodynamic forces are complex regulators of endothelial gene expression. *FASEB J* 1995;9:874–882.

138. Khachigian LM, Collins T. Inducible expression of Egr-1-dependent genes. A paradigm of transcriptional activation in vascular endothelium. *Circ Res* 1997;81:457–461.

139. Resnick N, Collins T, Atkinson W, Bonthron DT, Dewey CF Jr, Gimbrone MA Jr. Platelet-derived growth factor B chain promoter contains a cis-acting fluid shear-stress-responsive element. *Proc Natl Acad Sci USA* 1993;90:7908.

140. Khachigian LM, Resnick N, Gimbrone MA Jr, Collins T. Nuclear factor-kappa B interacts functionally with the platelet-derived growth factor B-chain shear-stress response element in vascular endothelial cells exposed to fluid shear stress. *J Clin Invest* 1995;96:1169–1175.

141. Topper JN, Cai J, Falb D, Gimbrone MA Jr. Identification of vascular endothelial genes differentially responsive to fluid mechanical stimuli: cyclooxygenase-2, manganese superoxide dismutase, and endothelial cell nitric oxide synthase are selectively up-regulated by steady laminar shear stress. *Proc Natl Acad Sci USA* 1996;93: 10417–10422.

142. Nagel T, Resnick N, Atkinson WJ, Dewey CF Jr, Gimbrone MA Jr. Shear stress selectively upregulates intercellular adhesion molecule-1 expression in cultured human vascular endothelial cells. *J Clin Invest* 1994;94:885–891.

143. Hofman FM, Dohadwala MM, Wright AD, Hinton DR, Walker SM. Exogenous tat protein activates central nervous system-derived endothelial cells. *J Neuroimmunol* 1994;54:19–28.

144. Zhou YF, Leon MB, Waclawiw MA, et al. Association between prior cytomegalovirus infection and the risk of restenosis after coronary atherectomy. *N Engl J Med* 1996;335:624–630.

145. Epstein SE, Speir E, Zhou YF, Guetta E, Leon M, Finkel T. The role of infection in restenosis and atherosclerosis: focus on cytomegalovirus. *Lancet* 1996;348[Suppl 1]:13–17.

146. Bian H, Harris PE, Mulder A, Reed EF. Anti-HLA antibody ligation to HLA class I molecules expressed by endothelial cells stimulates tyrosine phosphorylation, inositol phosphate generation, and proliferation. *Hum Immunol* 1997;53:90–97.

147. Bach FH, Ferran C, Soares M, et al. Modification of vascular responses in xenotransplantation: inflammation and apoptosis. *Nat Med* 1997;3:944–948.

148. Maher F, Vannucci SJ, Simpson IA. Glucose transporter proteins in brain. *FASEB J* 1994;8:1003–1011.

149. Schinkel AH, Smit JJ, van Tellingen O, et al. Disruption of the mouse *mdr1a* P-glycoprotein gene leads to a deficiency in the blood-brain barrier and to increased sensitivity to drugs. *Cell* 1994;77:491–502.

150. Qin Y, Sato TN. Mouse multidrug resistance 1a/3 gene is the earliest known endothelial cell differentiation marker during blood-brain barrier development. *Dev Dyn* 1995;202:172–180.

151. Nachman RL, Silverstein RL. Hypercoagulable states. *Ann Intern Med* 1993;119:819–827.

152. Marcus AJ, Safier LB, Hajjar KA, et al. Inhibition of platelet function by an aspirin-insensitive endothelial cell ADPase: thromboregulation by endothelial cells. *J Clin Invest* 1991;88:1690–1696.

153. Marcus AJ, Broekman MJ, Drosopoulos JH, et al. The endothelial cell ecto-ADPase responsible for inhibition of platelet function is CD39. *J Clin Invest* 1997;99:1351–1360.

154. Huang ZF, Wun TC, Broze GJ Jr. Kinetics of factor Xa inhibition by tissue factor pathway inhibitor. *J Biol Chem* 1993;268:26950–26955.

155. Shworak NW, Shirakawa M, Colliec-Jouault S, et al. Pathway-specific regulation of the synthesis of anticoagulantly active heparan sulfate. *J Biol Chem* 1994;269:24941–24952.

156. Esmon CT. The protein C anticoagulant pathway. *Arterioscler Thromb* 1992;12:135–145.

157. Esmon CT. The roles of protein C and thrombomodulin in the regulation of blood coagulation. *J Biol Chem* 1989;264:4743–4746.

158. Jackman RW, Beeler DL, Van De Water L, Rosenberg RD. Characterization of a thrombomodulin cDNA reveals structural similarity to the low density lipoprotein receptor. *Proc Natl Acad Sci USA* 1986;83: 8834–8838.

159. Stearns-Kurosawa DJ, Kurosawa S, Mollica JS, Ferrell GL, Esmon CT. The endothelial cell protein C receptor augments protein C activation by the thrombin-thrombomodulin complex. *Proc Natl Acad Sci USA* 1996;93:10212–10216.

160. Fukudome K, Esmon CT. Molecular cloning and expression of murine and bovine endothelial cell protein C/activated protein C receptor (EPCR): the structural and functional conservation in human, bovine, and murine EPCR. *J Biol Chem* 1995;270:5571–5577.

161. Mignatti P, Mazzieri R, Rifkin DB. Expression of the urokinase receptor in vascular endothelial cells is stimulated by basic fibroblast growth factor. *J Cell Biol* 1991;113:1193–1201.

162. Hajjar KA, Jacovina AT, Chacko J. An endothelial cell receptor for plasminogen/tissue plasminogen activator. I. Identity with annexin II. *J Biol Chem* 1994;269:21191–21197.

163. Cesarman GM, Guevara CA, Hajjar KA. An endothelial cell receptor for plasminogen/tissue plasminogen activator (t-PA). II. Annexin II–mediated enhancement of t-PA–dependent plasminogen activation. *J Biol Chem* 1994;269:21198–21203.

164. Hajjar KA, Nachman RL. Endothelial cell-mediated conversion of Glu-plasminogen to Lys-plasminogen. Further evidence for assembly of the fibrinolytic system on the endothelial cell surface. *J Clin Invest* 1988;82:1769–1778.

165. Antonov AS, Key NS, Smirnov MD, Jacob HS, Vercellotti GM, Smirnov VN. Prothrombotic phenotype diversity of human aortic endothelial cells in culture. *Thromb Res* 1992;67:135–145.

166. Moore KL, Esmon CT, Esmon NL. Tumor necrosis factor leads to the internalization and degradation of thrombomodulin from the surface of bovine aortic endothelial cells in culture. *Blood* 1989;73:159–165.

167. Malek AM, Jackman R, Rosenberg RD, Izumo S. Endothelial expression of thrombomodulin is reversibly regulated by fluid shear stress. *Circ Res* 1994;74:852–860.

168. Key NS, Vercellotti GM, Winkelmann JC, et al. Infection of vascular endothelial cells with herpes simplex virus enhances tissue factor activity and reduces thrombomodulin expression. *Proc Natl Acad Sci USA* 1990;87:7095–7099.

169. Tijburg PN, Ryan J, Stern DM, et al. Activation of the coagulation mechanism on tumor necrosis factor-stimulated cultured endothelial cells and their extracellular matrix: the role of flow and factor IX/IXa. *J Biol Chem* 1991;266:12067–12074.

170. Nicholson AC, Nachman RL, Altieri DC, et al. Effector cell protease receptor-1 is a vascular receptor for coagulation factor Xa. *J Biol Chem* 1996;271:28407–28413.

171. Altieri DC. Molecular cloning of effector cell protease receptor-1, a novel cell surface receptor for the protease factor Xa. *J Biol Chem* 1994;269:3139–3142.

172. Mandriota SJ, Seghezzi G, Vassalli JD, et al. Vascular endothelial growth factor increases urokinase receptor expression in vascular endothelial cells. *J Biol Chem* 1995;270:9709–9716.

173. Pepper MS, Sappino AP, Stocklin R, Montesano R, Orci L, Vassalli JD. Upregulation of urokinase receptor expression on migrating endothelial cells. *J Cell Biol* 1993;122:673–684.

174. Furchgott RF, Zawadzki JV. The obligatory role of endothelial cells in the relaxation of arterial smooth muscle by acetylcholine. *Nature* 1980;288:373–376.

175. Ignarro LJ, Byrns RE, Buga GM, Wood KS. Endothelium-derived relaxing factor (EDRF) released from artery and vein appears to be nitric oxide (NO) or a closely related radical species. *Fed Proc* 1987; 46:644.

176. Palmer RM, Ferrige AG, Moncada S. Nitric oxide release accounts for the biological activity of endothelium-derived relaxing factor. *Nature* 1987;327:524–526.

177. Nathan C. Inducible nitric oxide synthase: regulation subserves function. *Curr Top Microbiol Immunol* 1995;196:1–4.

178. Nathan C, Xie QW. Nitric oxide synthases: roles, tolls, and controls. *Cell* 1994;78:915–918.

179. Gross SS, Kilbourn RG, Griffith OW. NO in septic shock: good, bad or ugly? Learning from iNOS knockouts. *Trends Microbiol* 1996;4:47–49.

180. Weksler BB. Regulation of prostaglandin synthesis in human vascular cells. *Ann N Y Acad Sci* 1987;509:142–148.

181. Yanagisawa M, Kurihara H, Kimura S, et al. A novel potent vasoconstrictor peptide produced by vascular endothelial cells. *Nature* 1988; 332:411–415.

182. Xu D, Emoto N, Giaid A, et al. ECE-1: a membrane-bound metalloprotease that catalyzes the proteolytic activation of big endothelin-1. *Cell* 1994;78:473–485.

183. Yanagisawa M. The endothelin system: a new target for therapeutic intervention. *Circulation* 1994;89:1320–1322.

184. Tsukahara H, Ende H, Magazine HI, Bahou WF, Goligorsky MS. Molecular and functional characterization of the non-isopeptide-selective ETB receptor in endothelial cells: receptor coupling to nitric oxide synthase. *J Biol Chem* 1994;269:21778–21785.

185. Mizuguchi T, Nishiyama M, Moroi K, et al. Analysis of two pharmacologically predicted endothelin B receptor subtypes by using the endothelin B receptor gene knockout mouse. *Br J Pharmacol* 1997; 120:1427–1430.

186. Mohle R, Green D, Moore MA, Nachman RL, Rafii S. Constitutive production and thrombin-induced release of vascular endothelial growth factor by human megakaryocytes and platelets. *Proc Natl Acad Sci USA* 1997;94:663–668.

187. Rafii S, Shapiro F, Pettengell R, et al. Human bone marrow microvascular endothelial cells support long-term proliferation and differentiation of myeloid and megakaryocytic progenitors. *Blood* 1995;86: 3353–3363.

188. Zsebo KM, Yuschenkoff VN, Schiffer S, et al. Vascular endothelial cells and granulopoiesis: interleukin-1 stimulates release of G-CSF and GM-CSF. *Blood* 1988;71:99–103.

189. Seelentag WK, Mermod JJ, Montesano R, Vassalli P. Additive effects of interleukin 1 and tumour necrosis factor-alpha on the accumulation of the three granulocyte and macrophage colony-stimulating factor mRNAs in human endothelial cells. *EMBO J* 1987;6:2261–2265.

190. Sieff CA, Niemeyer CM, Mentzer SJ, Faller DV. Interleukin-1, tumor necrosis factor, and the production of colony-stimulating factors by cultured mesenchymal cells. *Blood* 1988;72:1316–1323.

191. Springer TA. Traffic signals for lymphocytes recirculation and leukocyte emigration: the multistep paradigm. *Cell* 1994;76:301–314.

192. Picker LJ, Butcher EC. Physiological and molecular mechanisms of lymphocyte homing. *Annu Rev Immunol* 1992;10:561–591.

194. Butcher EC. Leukocyte-endothelial cell recognition: three (or more) steps to specificity and diversity. *Cell* 1991;67:1033–1036.

195. Kontgen F, Stewart CL, McIntyre KW, Will PC, Burns DK, Wolitzky BA. Characterization of E-selectin-deficient mice: demonstration of overlapping function of the endothelial selectins. *Immunity* 1994;1: 709–720.

196. Mayadas TN, Johnson RC, Rayburn H, Hynes RO, Wagner DD. Leukocyte rolling and extravasation are severely compromised in P selectin--deficient mice. *Cell* 1993;74:541–554.

197. Yamada S, Mayadas TN, Yuan F, et al. Rolling in P-selectin-deficient mice is reduced but not eliminated in the dorsal skin. *Blood* 1995; 86:3487–3492.

198. Subramaniam M, Saffaripour S, Van De Water L, et al. Role of endothelial selectins in wound repair. *Am J Pathol* 1997;150: 1701–1709.

199. Frenette PS, Mayadas TN, Rayburn H, Hynes RO, Wagner DD. Double knockout highlights value of endothelial selectins. *Immunol Today* 1996;17:205.

200. Frenette PS, Mayadas TN, Rayburn H, Hynes RO, Wagner DD. Susceptibility to infection and altered hematopoiesis in mice deficient in both P- and E-selectins. *Cell* 1997;84:563–574.

201. Luscinskas FW, Kansas GS, Ding H, et al. Monocyte rolling, arrest and spreading on IL-4–activated vascular endothelium under flow is mediated via sequential action of L-selectin, beta 1-integrins, and beta 2-integrins. *J Cell Biol* 1994;125:1417–1427.

202. Zimmerman GA, Prescott SM, McIntyre TM. Endothelial cell interactions with granulocytes: tethering and signaling molecules. *Immunol Today* 1992;13:93–100.

203. Lo SK, Lee S, Ramos RA, Lobb R, Rosa M, Chi-Rosso G, Wright SD.

Endothelial-leukocyte adhesion molecule 1 stimulates the adhesive activity of leukocyte integrin CR3 (CD11b/CD18, Mac-1, $\alpha_m\beta_2$) on human neutrophils. *J Exp Med* 1991;173:1493–1500.

204. Miller MD, Krangel MS. Biology and biochemistry of the chemokines: a family of chemotactic and inflammatory cytokines. *Crit Rev Immunol* 1992;12:17–46.

205. Premack BA, Schall TJ. Chemokine receptors: gateways to inflammation and infection. *Nat Med* 1996;2:1174–1178.

206. Salmi M, Jalkanen S. A 90-kilodalton endothelial cell molecule mediating lymphocyte binding in humans. *Science* 1992;257:1407–1409.

207. Butcher EC, Picker LJ. Lymphocyte homing and homeostasis. *Science* 1996;272:60–66.

208. Rott LS, Briskin MJ, Andrew DP, Berg EL, Butcher EC. A fundamental subdivision of circulating lymphocytes defined by adhesion to mucosal addressin cell adhesion molecule-1: comparison with vascular cell adhesion molecule-1 and correlation with beta 7 integrins and memory differentiation. *J Immunol* 1996;156:3727–3736.

209. Briskin MJ, Rott L, Butcher EC. Structural requirements for mucosal vascular addressin binding to its lymphocyte receptor alpha₄ beta₇: common themes among integrin-Ig family interactions. *J Immunol* 1996;156:719–726.

210. Andrew DP, Berlin C, Honda S, et al. Distinct but overlapping epitopes are involved in alpha₄ beta₇-mediated adhesion to vascular cell adhesion molecule-1, mucosal addressin-1, fibronectin, and lymphocyte aggregation. *J Immunol* 1994;153:3847–3861.

Inflammation: Basic Principles and Clinical Correlates,
3rd ed., edited by John I. Gallin and Ralph Snyderman.
Published by Lippincott Williams & Wilkins, Philadelphia 1999.

CHAPTER 16

Fibroblasts and Matrix Proteins

Arnold E. Postlethwaite and Andrew H. Kang

Fibroblasts synthesize matrix constituents that comprise the various connective tissues of the body, and they are major players in immune and nonimmune inflammatory reactions. The matrix constituents (e.g., collagens, proteoglycans, noncollagenous structural glycoproteins), formerly regarded as having only structural support functions to provide the scaffolding and framework or an organizational structure for the various body organs and specialized tissues, also interact with somatic cells and cells of the immune system. This chapter describes the biology and function of fibroblasts and their matrix constituents, the nonstructural functions of matrix components, and the interaction of fibroblasts with the immune system. Fibroblast functions of adherence, proliferation, chemotaxis, and synthesis of matrix components and matrix-degrading enzymes are reviewed, as are the roles of fibroblasts in tissue repair and fibrosis.

FIBROBLAST FUNCTIONS

Fibroblasts are mesenchyme-derived cells. The term *fibroblast* often is used to describe several different cell types that share similar morphology determined by light microscopy but that have different functional roles. For example, the term is used to describe connective tissue stem cells, matrix- and protein-synthesizing cells (i.e., fibrocytes), contractile cells (i.e., myofibroblasts), and in some instances, tissue phagocytic cells (i.e., histiocytes) (1).

Myofibroblasts are present in increased numbers in wounds 3 to 10 days after injury occurs (1). Although they are identical in appearance to fibrocytes under light microscopy, electron microscopy reveals that myofibroblasts have abundant contractile actin-myosin filaments in their peripheral cytoplasm and synthetic organelles in

the perinuclear region (1). They express smooth muscle (SM) α-actin (2). Myofibroblasts have an indented nucleus and are usually surrounded by an incomplete basement membrane (1).

Fibrocytes are particularly suited for synthesis of matrix elements and have a prominent rough endoplasmic reticulum, a perinuclear Golgi complex, and an elaborate system of cell infoldings (1). Fibrocytes are present in increased numbers 6 to 12 days after injury at wound sites (1).

Fibroblasts play critical roles in the mature animal and during embryogenesis. In addition to synthesizing matrix, they determine the structure of the skeleton, location of muscle cells, routes taken by nerve fibers, and organization of the skin (3–5). They accomplish their organizational functions by attaching collagenous fibrils and cables to embryonic cells. The fibrils pull the cells into proper position and alignment to form parts of the developing organism (6).

In growing and mature animals, fibroblasts continue to synthesize and maintain constituents of the connective tissue matrix, which they constantly turn over and remodel by means of the degradative enzymes they produce. These synthetic and other functions of fibroblasts are controlled and regulated by signals from the matrix, growth factors, and cytokines.

The ability of fibroblasts to evoke a fibrotic reaction in response to a host of insults from the environment, including injury to tissue resulting from trauma inflicted by physical, chemical, or thermal forces, and from immunologic and infectious insults, has survival advantages for animals. Redundant systems have evolved to promote fibroblast adherence, chemotaxis, proliferation and synthesis of matrix constituents and enzymes. These are critical to the successful generation and remodeling of scar tissue, which repairs defects in the integument resulting from injury; walls off infections by pathogenic infectious agents; and repairs damage done to internal organs as a result of injury.

A. E. Postlethwaite and A. H. Kang: Department of Medicine, University of Tennessee, Memphis, Tennessee 38163.

SYNTHESIS OF MATRIX COMPONENTS

Connective tissue matrix is composed of various combinations of collagens (types I to XIX), elastins, hyaluronic acid, and a host of different proteoglycans and glycoproteins, and it can exhibit myriad structural and functional characteristics. As a result of their inherent tensile strength, fibrillar collagens with various contributions from elastin convey most of the mechanical properties of diverse connective tissue types such as tendons, ligaments, cartilage, cornea, and bone.

Collagens

Of all animal proteins, collagens are the most abundant and ubiquitous. In humans and most other vertebrates, they account for approximately one third of the total body proteins. They are the major structural proteins that hold cells together to give organs their characteristic architecture.

Nineteen distinct types of collagen have been identified in connective tissue or cultures of cells from mammals, and approximately 10 additional proteins also have collagen-like domains (Table 16-1). Collagens are composed of constituent polypeptide chains called α chains. Three α chains come together to form a single collagen molecule or monomer. A feature common to all of the collagens is that they contain triple-helical and globular domains (7,8) (Fig. 16-1). In each α chain, the triple-helical regions result from stretches of repeating triplet amino acid sequences, Gly-X-Y, in which X and Y can be any amino acid but are often proline and hydroxyproline, imino acids that accommodate close packing of the chains. The stereochemical configuration of the imino acids causes each α chain to assume a left-handed helical confirmation (i.e., minor helix), with a residue repeat distance of 0.291 nm and a relative twist of 110 degrees, a configuration that provides 3.27 residues per turn of the helix and 0.87 nm between each third glycine (9). To comply with the structural constraints of the helix, every third residue in the α chain must be glycine, which is the smallest amino acid. Because there are no bulky side chains on the α carbon atom of glycine, the three α chains can wind around a common axis to form a right-handed superhelix. A cross section of the triple-helical regions of a collagen molecule would reveal only

TABLE 16-1. *Collagens*

Type	Gene	Chromosome	Expression
I	COL1A2	17q21.3-p22	Most connective tissues
	COL1A2	7q21.3-q22	
II	COL2A1	12q13-q14	Cartilage, vitreous humor
III	COL3A1	2q24.3-q31	Extensible connective tissues (e.g., skin, lung, vascular system)
IV	COL4A1	13q34	Basement membranes
	COL4A2	13q34	
	COL4A3	2q35-q37	
	COL4A4	2q35-q37	
	COL4A5	Xq22	
	COL4A6	Xq22	
V	COL5A1	9q34.2-q34.3	Tissues containing collagen I, quantitatively minor component
	COL5A2	2q34.3-q31	
	COL5A3		
VI	COL6A1	21q22.3	Most connective tissues
	COL6A2	21q22.3	
	COL6A3	2q37	
VII	COL7A1	3p21	Anchoring fibrils
VIII	COL8A1	3q12-q13.1	Many tissues, especially endothelium
	COL8A2	1p32.3-p34.3	
IX	COL9A1	6q12-q14	Tissues containing collagen II
	COL9A2	1p32	
	COL9A3		
X	COL10A1	6q21-q22	Hypertrophic cartilage
XI	COL11A1	1p21	Tissues containing collagen II
	COL11A2	6p21.2	
	COL2A1	12q13-q14	
XII	COL12A1	6	Tissues containing collagen I
XIII	COL13A1	10q22	Many tissues
XIV	COL14A1		Tissues containing collagen I
XV	COL15A1	q21-22	Many tissues
XVI	COL16A1	1q34-35	Many tissues
XVII	COL17A1	10q24.3	Skin hemidesmosomes
XVIII	COL18A1	21q22.3	Many tissues, especially liver and kidney
XIV	COL19A1	6q12-q14	Rhabdomyosarcoma cells

From ref. 8, with permission.

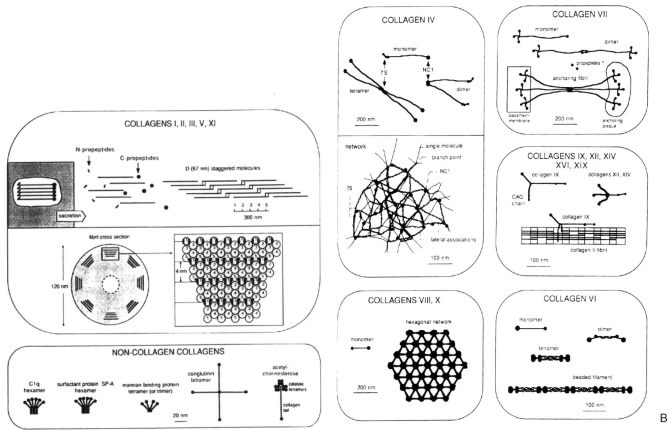

FIG. 16-1. (A) Diagrams of individual collagen molecules (shown with N termini to the left) are based on electron microscopic images of rotary shadowed preparations. Lines represent triple-helical regions, and non–triple-helical regions are shown as filled circles or tridentate structures. Notice the use of different scales. For collagens I, II, III, V, and XI, procollagen secretion, processing, D-staggered collagen assembly, and crosslinks *(short vertical lines)* are indicated. The rates and degrees of processing differ among the collagen types. The cross-sectional fibril shows crystalline domains, as observed (355) in the fibrils of collagen I. Within a crystalline domain, a likely molecular packing arrangement is shown in the enlarged view; each circle represents a molecule in cross section, and the numbers refer to relative axial locations (see the scale at the top). Crosslinks between adjacent molecules are shown by short, thick lines. There is evidence for a concentric, helical (356) organization around the fibril core *(lighter shading)*, which in the case of heterotypic fibrils may consist of collagen V or XI. Crystalline molecular packing has been observed only in the outer regions of large-diameter collagen I fibrils; in general, the lateral packing (i.e., perpendicular to the fibril axis) is likely to be much less regular. (From ref. 7, with permission). **(B)** For the structure of collagen IV, the lower part of the figure has a different scale. (From ref. 357, with permission.) For collagen VI, the beaded filaments can associate side by side to form 110-nm periodic fibrils. For collagen VII, propeptide processing appears to occur during maturation of dimers into anchoring fibrils. For collagens VIII and X, the nodes probably are connected by bundles of molecules, although the number of molecules in each bundle is unknown. For collagens IX, XII, XIV, XVI, and XIX, the location of a crosslink between collagens II and IX is shown by a short vertical line. For the noncollagen collagens, notice the relatively small scale. (From ref. 7, with permission.)

glycine in the central core with X and Y amino acid side chains radiating away from the core. Interchain hydrogen bonds, especially with the hydroxyl groups of hydroxyproline, stabilize the triple-helical structure.

Collagens make up a diverse superfamily and have been subdivided into 6 different classes (see Fig. 16-1) based on the characteristics of the polymeric structures they form or characteristic structural features of the collagens themselves (7,8). These collagens are not discussed in detail, but they have been reviewed elsewhere (7,8,10–13). As illustrated in Figure 16-1, *fibrillar colla-gens* consist of types I, II, III, V, and XI; *network-forming collagens* consist of types IV, VIII, and X; *FACIT collagens* have interrupted triple helices and include types IX, XII, XIV, XVI, and XIX; *bead-forming collagen* is type VI; *collagen type VII* forms anchoring fibrils for basement membranes; *transmembrane collagens* have a transmembrane domain (types XIII and XVII); *type XV and XVIII collagens* have not been well characterized in terms of structure or function; and *noncollagen collagens* are proteins that were belatedly found to have triple-helical collagenous domains (8).

Regulation of Type I Collagen Gene Expression

Regulation of the type I collagen-α1 gene *(COL1A1)* has received much attention. There are regulatory elements, including a TATA box at −23 bp and a CCAAT motif at −125 bp in the 5′ flanking region of the human *COL1A1* gene (14). The 5′ flanking region of *COL1A1* also contains additional upstream sequences that have homologies to consensus transcription factor binding sites (14). Basal expression of the human *COL1A1* gene depends on 129 bp 5′ from the transcription start site that contains binding sites for transcription factor SP1 and CCAAT box transcription factor/nuclear factor-1 (CTF/NF-1) (14).

Negative regulation of *COL1A1* expression may involve RAS- and RAF-modulated serine-threonine phosphorylation cascade, a complex element at −107 bp with overlapping binding sites for CTF/NF-1 and activator protein-2 (AP-2) that mediates repression of transcription by lipoxygenase inhibitors, and cKrox, which is a skin-specific zinc-finger transcription factor that binds regulatory elements in the promoter region of *COL1A1* and *COL1A2* (15–18).

Consequences of Mutations in Collagen Genes

Mutations in the *COL1A1* or *COL1A2* genes are associated with osteogenesis imperfecta, osteoporosis, and Ehlers-Danlos syndrome type VIIA and VIIB. Mutations in the *COL2A1* gene causes chondrodysplasias and severe osteoarthritis; mutations in *COL3A1* are associated with Ehlers-Danlos syndrome type IV and aortic aneurysms; and mutations in *COL4A3, COL3A4,* or *COL4A5* lead to Alport syndrome. Mutations in *COL4A5* and *COL4A6* cause X-linked Alport syndrome with diffuse esophageal leiomatosis. Mutations in *COL7A1* cause epidermolysis bullosa. Mutations in *COL9A1* cause osteoarthritis, and mutations in *COL9A2* cause multiple epiphyseal dysplasia. Mutations in *COL10A1* cause Schmid metaphyseal chondrodysplasia, and mutations in *COL11A2* cause nonocular Stickler syndrome. Mutations in lysyl hydroxylase cause type VI Ehlers-Danlos syndrome; mutations in type I *N*-proteinase cause type VIIC Ehlers-Danlos syndrome; and mutations in lysyl oxidase cause occipital horn syndrome and Menkes syndrome (8).

Elastin

Elastin is a unique fibrous protein constituent of the connective tissue matrix. It exists in two forms in elastic fibers as elastin and as microfibrils. It is found in high concentrations in specialized ligaments, lung fibrocartilage, and the media of large blood vessels. It is present in relatively small but important amounts in the skin, tendon, and bone. The elastic properties of tissue, ligaments, and tendons result from the elastin fibers in the extracellular matrix (ECM).

Elastin is the most insoluble protein in the body and is able to resist harsh chemical extraction procedures. Elastin is turned over very slowly, and in some tissue, it may last a lifetime. Elastin has an unusual amino acid composition. Approximately 33% of its amino acid residues are glycine and 10% to 13% are proline, similar to collagen (19,20). However, it contains little hydroxyproline and no hydroxylysine. Elastin is rich in the nonpolar amino acids alanine, valine, isoleucine, and leucine, but contains few polar amino acids (19,20). The lysyl residues are posttranslationally modified by lysyl oxidase to form α-amino-δ-semialdehyde (21).

Another difference between collagen and elastin is the extent to which there is crosslinking within and between polypeptide chains. Interstitial collagens contain 1 or 2 lysine- or hydroxylysine-derived crosslinks per 1000 residues, but elastin can have as many as 40 lysine-derived crosslinks per 1000 residues (22). The crosslinks of elastin are of four basic types: dehydrolysinonoerleucine (and its reduced form lysinonorleucine), desmosine, the product of aldol condensation of two allysines, and dehydromerodesmosine (22). The extensive crosslinking of elastin has retarded progress on the study of its primary amino acid sequence. Most of the structural data regarding elastin has been obtained by analyzing tropoelastin (67 kd), the precursor of elastin that can be obtained from aortas of piglets with copper deficiency, a condition that results in a general inhibition of crosslinking of elastin (23). Sequence analysis of purified tryptic peptides from porcine tropoelastin revealed long segments of hydrophobic amino acid residues that are interrupted with shorter segments of polyalanine sequences with clusters of lysines. These shorter segments are in α-helix conformation, and the larger hydrophobic sequences comprise a β-spiral structure with elastomeric properties (24). An interacting, repeating pentapeptide (Pro-Gly-Val-Gly-Val) in the hydrophobic regions apparently confers some unusual folding properties on elastin (24).

Cloning of the elastin gene from human fetal aorta has demonstrated that functionally distinct domains (i.e., hydrophobic, crosslinking) segregate into exons (25). The gene contains 34 exons in approximately 45 kb of genomic DNA. The elastin gene has some features of "housekeeping" genes in that the 5′-flanking region lacks a canonical TATA sequence, has several SP1 binding sites and an AP-2 site, and is G-C rich (25). Primer extension and S1 nuclease protection studies have revealed that transcription of elastin mRNA is initiated at multiple sites within the elastin gene (25). Alternative splicing of selected exons gives rise to nucleotide sequence heterogeneity in human and bovine elastin cDNAs that could give rise to isoforms of tropoelastin (26–29).

Binding of elastin to a 67-kd laminin receptor on fetal bovine articular chondroblasts and human A2058 melanoma cells has been demonstrated (30). The receptor, apparently not an integrin, recognizes a hydrophobic hexapeptide sequence in elastin, Val-Gly-Val-Ala-Pro-Gly (VGVAPG), which is a cell-recognition domain involved in the chemotactic response of fibroblasts to elastin (30).

Elastin mRNA and protein expression by chick embryonic skin fibroblasts and by rat neonatal lung fibroblasts are upregulated by retinoids (31,32). Latent transforming growth factor-β1 (TGF-β1) and its binding protein-1 (LTBP-1) are apparently stored in elastin microfibrils in human dermis *in vivo* (33). LTBP-1 is also released from cultured human skin fibroblasts by treatment with elastase *in vitro* (33). Release of latent TGF-β1 from the elastin microfibrils may be a mechanism by which TGF-β1 is regulated *in vivo*.

Keratinocytes synthesize fibrillin-1 and fibrillin-2 and assemble microfibrillar bundles containing elastin at the dermal-epidermal junction (34). TGF-β1 added to cultures of neonatal rat or human fetal lung fibroblasts increases synthesis of elastin *in vitro* to steady-state levels of elastin mRNA by increasing elastin mRNA stability (34–36).

Glucocorticoids upregulate fibroblast elastin synthesis by binding to three glucocorticoid response elements within the human elastin promoter (37). Fibroblasts from the upper layer of the dermis have higher basal and TGF-β1–stimulated mRNA levels than fibroblasts from the lower dermis (38). Basic fibroblast growth factor (bFGF) downregulates elastin mRNA in fibroblasts only from the upper dermis (38). The elastin gene bFGF responsive element has been localized to sequences spanning -900 to -200 bp (39).

Ascorbate reduces elastin mRNA levels but increases types I and III collagen mRNA levels in skin fibroblasts (40). Ascorbate reduces stability of elastin mRNA (40).

A 67-kd protein that resembles an enzymatically inactive, spliced variant of β-galactosidase is a major component of the elastin-laminin nonintegrin cell surface receptor on fibroblasts and other cells (41). This receptor recognizes several nonidentical hydrophobic domains on elastin, laminin, and type IV collagen (41). In fibroblasts and other elastin-producing cells, this 67-kd protein associates with tropoelastin and acts as a molecular chaperon for intracellular transport and extracellular assembly of tropoelastin (41). Fibroblasts, vascular smooth muscle cells, endothelial cells, monocytes, polymorphonuclear leukocytes, and T lymphocytes have an elastin-laminin receptor that, when activated, induces chemotactic migration to an elastin peptide gradient, release of lytic enzymes and oxygen-free radicals, and changes in ion fluxes (42).

Proteoglycans

Proteoglycans are a diverse group of complex macromolecules composed of sulfated polysaccharide chains that are linked covalently to a protein core. The long, linear carbohydrate chains called glycosaminoglycans are made up of repeating disaccharide subunits. More than 25 genes code for protein cores with at least one glycosaminoglycan chain. There are six different glycosaminoglycans: hyaluronic acid, chondroitin sulfate, dermatan sulfate, heparan sulfate, heparin, and keratan sulfate. The glycan backbone of each glycosaminoglycan is composed of one or two of the following disaccharide units: [HexA-Gal N]$_n$, [HexA-Glc N]$_n$, and [Gal-Glc N]$_n$ disaccharide. Dermatan sulfate and chondroitin sulfate contain [HexA-Gal N]$_n$, and hyaluronic acid heparan sulfate and heparin contain [Hex A-Glc N]$_n$ (43). The heparan sulfate and heparin structures are shown in Figure 16-2.

The disaccharides in hyaluronic acid are not sulfated, but those in the remaining glycosaminoglycans are sulfated to different degrees, giving rise to extensive sequence heterogeneity. The number of repeat disaccharides can vary but usually is on the order of 50. The protein core, which can vary from 11 to more than 400 kd, is also substituted with a number of *N*- or *O*-linked oligosaccharides similar to those found in glycoproteins (44,45). One or two different types of glycosaminoglycans are present in each proteoglycan molecule, and the total number of glycosaminoglycan chains may vary from one or two to more than 100, with a potential for as many as 10,000 negatively charged groups per proteoglycan molecule. The molecular mass of proteoglycans ranges from 50,000 to several million daltons, and some types of proteoglycans can form aggregates with molecular masses greater than 100 million daltons.

Although originally found in the ECM, proteoglycans are synthesized by most cells and play key roles in many cellular processes (e.g., motility, cell adhesion, proliferation, differentiation, morphogenesis) because of their inherent ability to bind to other molecules. They are found intracellularly in secretory granules (e.g., heparin) and on cell surface membranes, and they exist as transmembrane molecules (e.g., syndecans). Proteoglycans are listed in Table 16-2.

The extracellular small and large (i.e., modulator multidomain) proteoglycans provide mechanical support along with other matrix molecules and affect collagen fibrillogenesis, cell migration, and aggregation. Extracellular proteoglycans bind other matrix molecules (e.g., fibronectin, laminin, collagens) primarily through the interaction of glycosaminoglycan chains with specific binding sites on the matrix protein. Several observations suggest that proteoglycans may be important in modulating the proliferation and differentiation of cells. For example, chondrocytes synthesize aggrecan but the mesenchymal fibroblast-like precursor cells do not, and aggrecan may prevent chondrocyte dedifferentiation to fibroblasts by inhibiting cell adhesion (46). Aggrecan also fosters normal bone growth (46). The core protein

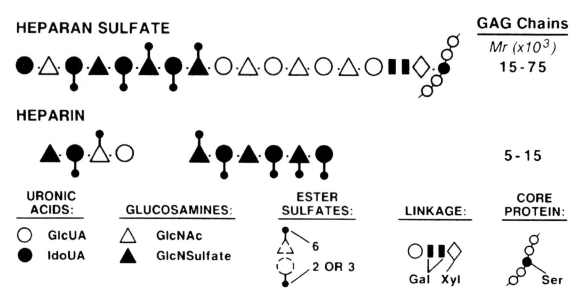

FIG. 16-2. Schematic structures of heparan sulfate (HS) and heparin. The HS chain contains a tetrasaccharide that links the core protein to a linear assembly of alternating uronic acid and N-substituted glucosamine residues. The chain is initially synthesized as a copolymer of D-glucuronic acid and N-acetyl glucosamine, which is then modified by sequential enzymatic deacetylation. N-sulfation and C5 epimerization of D-glucuronate to L-iduronate and O-sulfation at various positions yield chains with considerable sequence diversity, primarily the result of variable sulfation (358). This sequence heterogeneity, in which each chain is probably distinct, presumably arises because the product of each modification reaction is the substrate for the next and because the reactions do not go to completion. Commercial heparin, a pharmaceutical degradation product, contains fragments of chains with the same overall structure and heterogeneity as HS but that are rich in L-iduronate, N-sulfate, and O-sulfate. Heparan sulfate contains nonsulfated regions interspersed with these heparin-like highly sulfated regions. It is unclear how the size and distribution of these regions are regulated. (From ref. 52, with permission.)

portion of decorin also binds to collagen and fibronectin (47,48). *In vitro*, decorin has been shown to cause thinner collagen fibrils to form, and heparin added to collagen gels inhibits contraction of the gel induced by fibroblasts (49). Some extracellular proteoglycans, such as aggrecan and decorin-like dermatan sulfate proteoglycans, inhibit cell binding to collagen and fibronectin by attaching to the glycosaminoglycan binding domain of these proteins (49). Inhibition of cell migration by some proteoglycans may be effected by a similar mechanism (49,50).

Transmembrane and cell surface proteoglycans are largely of the heparan sulfate type and may be important in the attachment of fibroblasts to matrix structures that bind glycosaminoglycans (43,51,52). Syndecan-1 on fibroblasts and other cells binds types I, III, and V collagen fibrils; fibronectin; thrombospondin; and tenascin through its heparan sulfate chains (52). Syndecan-1 also binds precursor B cells to type I collagen (53). Syndecan-1 is cleaved from the plasma membrane of epithelial cells when they change shape and plays an important role in maintaining epithelial organization (52).

Expression of heparan sulfate on vascular endothelial cell surfaces is probably important in preventing thrombosis (54). Heparan sulfate on cell surfaces is essential for bFGF to bind to its high-affinity receptor (55). Syndecans

are coreceptors for binding several growth factors, matrix components, cell adhesion molecules, proteases, and protease inhibition (52). Cell surface glypican induces thrombin adhesive properties in plasmin-treated thrombin (56). Cell surface proteoglycans may also interact with matrix molecules to promote formation of adhesion plaques and organization of actin into stress fibers in attaching fibroblasts (57,58). The transferrin receptor on fibroblasts has a proteoglycan structure and regulates uptake of transferrin.

Extracellular Glycoproteins

Most extracellular proteins are glycosylated and are technically glycoproteins. There are four types of carbohydrate linkage to proteins among the vertebrates: proteoglycans, with polysaccharide (glycosaminoglycan) O-glycosidically linked through xylose to serine or threonine; the collagens, with glycose and galactose O-glycosidically linked to hydroxylysine; the mucins, with oligosaccharide o-glycosidically linked to serine or threonine; and the large body of glycoproteins in which oligosaccharide with a mannose core is N-glycosidically linked to asparagine. This section focuses on four glycoproteins synthesized by fibroblasts: fibronectin, laminin, tenascin, and vitronectin.

TABLE 16-2. *Transmembrane and secreted pericellular proteoglycans*

Designation	Protein core (kd)	GAG (No.)	Tissue distribution
Extracellular, small, leucine-rich proteoglycans			
Decorin	36	CS/DS (1)	Ubiquitous, collagenous matrices, bone, teeth, mesothelia, floor plate
Biglycan	38	CS/DS (1–2)	Interstitium, and cell surfaces
Fibromodulin	42	KS (4)	Collagenous matrices
Lumican	38	KS (2–3)	Cornea, intestine, liver, muscle, cartilage
Epiphycan	36	CS/DS (2)	Epiphyseal cartilage
Extracellular, modular, multidomain proteoglycans			
Versican	265–370	CS/DS (10–30)	Blood vessels, brain, skin, cartilage
Aggrecan	220	CS ($\approx$100)	Cartilage, brain, blood vessels
Neurocan	136	CS (3–7)	Brain, cartilage
Brevican	100	CS (1–3)	Brain
Perlecan	400–467	HS/CS (3–10)	Basement membranes, cell surfaces, sinusoidal spaces, cartilage
Agrin	200	HS (3–6)	Synaptic sites of neuromuscular junctions, renal basement membranes
Testican	44	HS/CS (1–2)	Seminal fluid
Transmembrane proteolgycans			
Syndecan-1	31	HS	Mammary epithelia fibroblasts, vascular endothelia
Syndecan-2	20	HS	Lung fibroblasts
Syndecan-3	38	HS	Chick embryo limb buds, rat newborn Schwann cells
Syndecan-4	20	HS	Chick embryo limb buds, rat microvascular endothelia
Betaglycan	100–200	CS/HS	
Transferrin receptor	2×90	HS	Fibroblasts and other cells
CD44		HS	Oligodendrocytes
Glypican		HS	Variety of cells
Cerebroglycan		HS	Brain
Intracellular proteoglycans			
Chromogranin A PG	48	CS (1)	Leukocytes
Serglycins	17–19	CS,DS,HS, heparin	Mast cells
Chromaffin granules	14	1–2 CS/DS	Leukocytes

PG, proteoglycan; CS, chondroitin sulfate; DS, dermatan sulfate; GAG, glycosaminoglycans; HS, heparan sulfate; KS, keratan sulfate.

Adapted from refs. 43, 52, and 358, with permission.

Fibronectin

The fibronectins are multifunctional, high-molecular-weight glycoproteins that are found on cell surfaces and in the pericellular and intercellular matrix, basement membranes, and a variety of body fluids. Fibronectin and other glycoproteins are intimately involved in the interactions of cells with one another and with their extracellular environment. Fibronectin is synthesized by a variety of cells and is closely associated with fibroblasts, endothelial cells, chondrocytes, glial cells, amniotic cells, myocytes, platelets, and monocytes (59). Its primary role is to attach cells to the ECM through integrin receptors.

Fibronectin is composed of two similar, 250-kd polypeptide chains. The polypeptides are joined near their C termini by disulfide bonds and have a series of tightly folded globular domains that have specialized binding characteristics formed by 10 residues that assume a coiled, antiparallel configuration (60) (Fig. 16-3). Fibronectin structure depends on its cell of origin. Plasma fibronectin from hepatocytes is smaller than the fibronectin synthesized by various cells in culture (61,62).

Each chain of fibronectin is made of four modular elements or domains called fibronectin type I (FnI), type II (FnII), and type III (FnIII), and the V domains (63). The domains in the major fibronectins are organized such that 6 type I domains are followed by 2 type II domains, 3 type I domains, 14 type III domains, the V domain, 1 type III domain, and 3 type I domains (see Fig. 16-3). Variation in structure by alternative gene splicing occurs so that additional type III domains can be inserted, one each after the 7th and after the 11th FnIII domain, or change the size of the V domain or delete it (64).

The cell adhesion function of fibronectin involves binding by integrins. Integrins interact with the synergy site in [9]FnIII and with an RGD sequence in [10]FnIII (see Fig. 16-3). The residues in the synergy site are important for discrimination by different classes of integrins. For example, Asp-1373 and Arg-1374 are necessary for

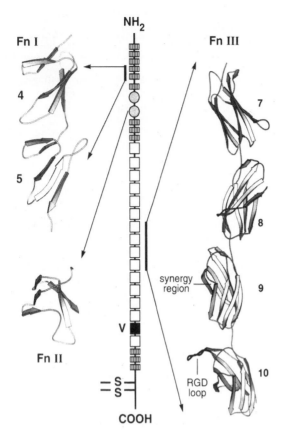

FIG. 16-3. The domain structure of fibronectin *(middle)* is shown schematically. The fibronectin type I (FnI) domains are represented by rectangles with bars; FnII domains are represented by shaded circles; and FnIII domains are represented by open squares. The structure of the fourth and fifth type I domains (359) *(top left)*, a type II domain from bovine seminal fluid protein (PDC-109) *(bottom left)*, and the structure of the segment of fibronectin formed by the seventh to tenth FnIII domains (360) *(right)* are shown. The integrin binding site involves the RGD tripeptide in [10]FnIII and the synergy region in [9]FnIII. (From ref. 63, with permission.)

recognition of $\alpha_{IIb}\beta_3$ integrin but not with $\alpha_5\beta_1$ integrin, and Arg-1379 is necessary for recognition of $\alpha_{IIb}\beta_3$ integrin (65,66). The heparin-binding region on [13]FnIII involves six arginines and one lysine on the A and B strands of the same sheet (63).

Fibronectin binds to most native and denatured (i.e., gelatin) collagens. The gelatin-type collagen binding domain resides in the two type II repeats (67,68). For type I collagen, the site of binding on the collagen molecule is near or at the mammalian collagenase cleavage site (69). The DNA-binding site is adjacent to the collagen binding domain, the significance of which is unknown (67,70).

Fibronectin has important biologic effects on a variety of target cells. It promotes anchorage and growth of fibroblasts and other normal cells in culture, establishment of polarity of basement membranes, migration of a variety of cells, and chemical attraction of fibroblasts

(67). Fibronectin is critical to migration of fibroblasts *in vitro* from a three-dimensional collagen matrix into a fibrin clot, suggesting that it may provide a conduit for migration from normal collagen-rich connective tissue into a fibrin clot at sites of wounds *in vivo* (71). Differentiation of a variety of cells is affected by fibronectin. For example, chondrocytes become fibroblastic, smooth muscle cells lose their contractile phenotype, formation of multicellular modules by aortic smooth muscle cells is inhibited, and malignant and virus-transformed cells revert to a normal-appearing phenotype in the presence of fibronectin (67).

Laminin

Laminin is a large, cross-shaped, 800-kd complex containing three (α, β, and γ) long polypeptide chains held together by disulfide bonds (72) (Fig. 16-4). There are five different α chains, three different β chains, and two different γ chains that form in different combination, and 11 laminin isoforms are recognized (73). Laminin-1, -2, and -4 can form quasihexagonal networks (72).

Laminin influences adhesion, morphology, growth differentiation, and migration of fibroblasts and other cells (72). Laminin promotes metastasis of tumors by inducing their attachment, migration, and production of collagenase IV (74,75). A variety of laminin receptors have been described, including integrins and nonintegrins. Integrins that bind laminin include $\alpha_1\beta_1$, $\alpha_2\beta_1$, $\alpha_3\beta_1$, $\alpha_v\beta_3$, $\alpha_6\beta_1$, $\alpha_6\beta_4$, and $\alpha_7\beta_1$ (75,76). Laminin stimulates DNA synthesis and growth in cells with epidermal growth factor (EGF) receptors and anti-laminin receptor antibodies inhibit EGF-mediated cell growth (77). This pattern indicates a relationship exists between laminin- and EGF receptor–mediated events (77). Expression of α_6 integrin in a murine fibroblast cell line unresponsive to EGF and laminin revealed that this integrin was largely responsible for laminin-mediated cell attachment and chemotactic migration of these α_6 integrin–expressing fibroblasts (77).

Tenascin

Tenascins are a family of extracellular glycoproteins: TN-C, TN-R, TN-X, and TN-Y (78,79). Tenascins contain four types of sequence motifs that fold independently into structural units (79) (Fig. 16-5). At the NH2 terminus, there are 3 to 3.5 hepad repeats, then 4.5 to 18.5 TN-type EGF-like repeats, followed by fibronectin type III–like (FNIII) domain (78,79). At the COOH terminus is a fibrinogen-like domain that is highly conserved (78). The FNIII domain is most variable and is subject to alternative splicing, giving rise to various splice forms of differing numbers (79). TN-R in chicken exhibits differential splicing in the cysteine-rich NH2 terminus (80). TN-Y has only been described in chickens and is produced by

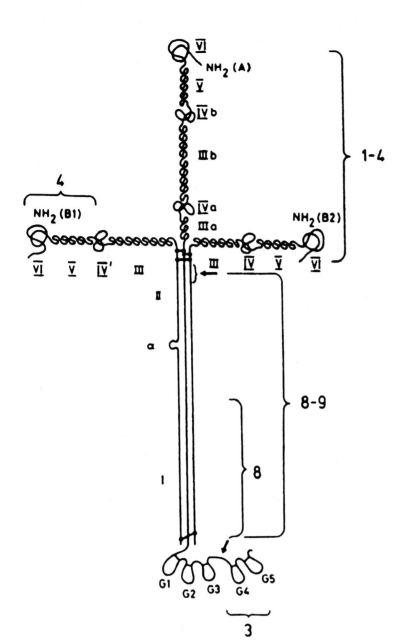

FIG. 16-4. Structural model of laminin. Domains are designated by roman numerals (361). Cys-rich rod domains in the short arms are designated by the symbol S and the triple coiled-coil region (domain I-II) of the long arm by parallel lines. In the B1 chain, the α-helical coiled domains are interrupted by a small, Cys-rich domain α. Interchain disulfide bridges *(thick bars)*; the primary cleavage sites of cathepsin G *(arrows)*, and regions of the molecule corresponding to fragments 1–4, 4, 8–9, 8, and 3 are indicated. (From ref. 72, with permission.)

fibroblasts of muscle tissue origin (79). It is unique among the tenascins in that the FNIII domains are interrupted by a new type of domain that is rich in serine-proline-X (X = any amino acid) repeats (79).

TN-C was originally called hexabrachion because its two subunit trimers formed a six-armed structure through disulfide linkage. TN-R usually forms trimers, dimers, and monomers (80,81). Because TN-X and TN-Y lack NH2-terminal cysteines, they probably only form dimers or timers (79,82).

TN-C is expressed in developing organs and some adult tissues (83). TN-R is only expressed in the central nervous system (84). TN-X is expressed in different embryonic and adult tissues (82,85). Tenascins are expressed redundantly in different tissues, and TN-C knock-out mice develop normally (85). In adult skin, TN-C is restricted to

a thin band in the papillary dermis (86). It is transiently expressed in wound healing preceding cell migration and collagen synthesis (87,88). Tenascin also has been described in some cancers, scleroderma fibrotic tissue, and rheumatoid synovium (89,90).

Interleukin-4 (IL-4) can induce higher levels of TN-C expression in dermal fibroblasts from normal adults and those with scleroderma (91). Platelet-derived growth factor (PDGF) and bFGF can induce TN-C expression in these same fibroblast lines (91). The cytokines (e.g., IL-1, IL-6, TGF-β, interferon-γ [IFN-γ], and tumor necrosis factor-α [TNF-α]) did not modulate TN-C synthesis by normal or scleroderma fibroblasts (91). IL-4 and TN-C are deposited in scleroderma fibrotic tissue in increased amounts, and these data support the concept that increased TN-C deposition may result from IL-4 upregulation.

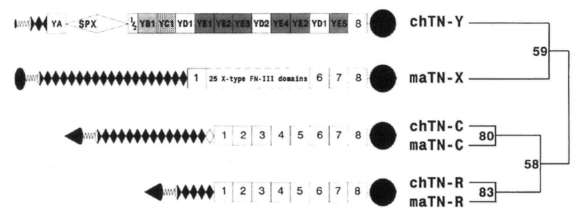

FIG. 16-5. The structures of the tenascins in chicken and mammals are compared. The dendrogram was created by the multiple alignment program pileup based on the amino acid sequence of the fibrinogen globe and the adjacent fibronectin type III (FnIII) domain 8 (362). Numbers in the dendrogram indicate sequence identifies in %. TN-Y and TN-X are similar (59%), as are TN-C and TN-R (58%). Only the smallest variant of each tenascin is shown *(left)*. Differences at the NH₂ termini of the tenascins are indicated *(black ellipses, pie segments)*; heptads *(wavy lines)* are followed by epidermal growth factor (EGF)–like repeats *(black diamonds)*. Chicken and mammalian TN-C differ in one EGF-like repeat *(white diamond)*. Constant FNIII domains 1 through 8 in TN-C and TN-R and the equivalent domains in TN-X (6 through 8) and in TN-Y (8) are shown *(white boxes)*. For TN-Y, distinct shading patterns for the repetitive FNIII domains were used to label the different types: YB, YC, YD, and YE. The SPX-containing domain, unique to TN-Y, that interrupts the FNIII domain series is shown as a rhomb, which is bisected by a dotted line that demarcates the part with repeated SPX motifs from the second part, which is joined in the one-half FNIII domain. The 25 X-type FNIII domains *(dotted box)* are not shown to scale. The NH₂-terminal fibrinogen globes *(black circles)* are indicated for all tenascins. (From ref. 79, with permission.)

TN-X and TN-Y share some functional properties but are structurally different. For example, they are both expressed in the skeletal muscle and heart tissues by fibroblasts between myocytes (85,92). In contrast, TN-C is expressed by tendon fibroblasts and by fibroblasts close to myotendinous junction (93). TN-C is strongly expressed in the tunica media of arteries, but TN-X and TN-Y are not (92). TN-X expression by fibroblasts is downregulated by glucocorticoids (94).

TN-C synthesis by chick embryo fibroblasts cultured on collagen matrix depends on the nature of the gel and whether it is floating or restrained (95). Cultures of the fibroblasts on floating gels does not result in upregulation of TN-C, whereas culture of the fibroblast on a restrained gel with resultant development of tenascin greatly upregulates TN-C synthesis (95). The TN-C gene is upregulated at the transcriptional level (95). Studies with reporter gene constructs suggest that different promoters probably are involved in fibroblast TN-C upregulation by mechanical stress and by serum (95). Alternative splicing of TN-C pre-mRNA in human lung and skin fibroblasts is modulated by small pH variations (7.2 to 6.9) (96).

Vitronectin

Vitronectin, also known as serum spreading factor, and fibronectin are the major cell-adhesive glycoproteins in plasma and serum (97–99). Vitronectin binds to specific integrins on fibroblasts and other cells through an RGD sequence, as discussed earlier (100–102). Vitronectin has been found in plasma, serum, urine, platelets, amniotic fluid, and connective tissue (103–105). It is synthesized by fibroblasts and hepatocytes, and like fibronectin, it affects cell differentiation, migration, proliferation, and spreading. Human vitronectin has a molecular mass of 75 kd and has a monomeric structure (106). The cDNA for human vitronectin has been identified and the deduced amino acid sequence determined (5,107). It is composed of 459 amino acids, with three asparagines that probably link to carbohydrates (106).

Several functional domains have been described for human vitronectin. The sequence of 44 amino acids in its N terminus is homologous to somatomedin B (108). A cell attachment site is located within a 5-kd fragment adjacent to the somatomedin domain. The 12-kd C terminus contains a glycosaminoglycan binding site that binds heparin and chondroitin sulfate (108). This domain has other properties, including the ability to bind to complement components C7, C8, and C9 and inhibit cell lysis of the membrane attack complex C5b, C6, C7, C8, and C9 (109). The glycosaminoglycan binding domain also binds to a pore-forming protein, perforin, from the cytoplasmic granules of cytotoxic T cells inhibiting lysis of these cells (109).

Human mast cells attach to artificial surfaces coated with vitronectin through αᵥ integrins (110). However, the

α_v integrins are not involved in attachment of mast cells to human fibroblast monolayers (110).

Vitronectin is removed from the matrix by receptor-mediated endocytosis and lyosomal degradation, and these processes involve heparan sulfate proteoglycans by undetermined mechanisms (110). Migration of fibroblasts on serum- or vitronectin-coated surfaces involves an autocrine loop with urokinase-urokinase receptors and is subject to downregulation by low-density-lipoprotein receptor-related protein (111). Fibroblasts and other cells undergoing active mitosis selectively adhere to vitronectin-coated surfaces and express high levels of vitronectin receptor, $\alpha_v\beta_3$, and lesser amounts of $\alpha_5\beta_1$ integrin (112).

SYNTHESIS OF MATRIX-DEGRADING ENZYMES

Matrix Metalloproteinases

Some of the enzymes capable of degrading all matrix components are synthesized by fibroblasts, and others are secreted by inflammatory or organ-specific cells. Enzymes capable of degrading the ECM are called matrix metalloproteinases (MMPs) (Table 16-3). These enzymes play a central role in remodeling wounds, embryonic development, pregnancy and parturition, malignant neoplasia, bone resorption, and mammary involution (113). The MMP family is able to degrade matrix constituents; is secreted in a proenzyme or latent form that requires activation; contains a zinc ion, rendering them suscepti-

ble to inhibition by chelation; shares common amino acid sequences; and is inhibited by tissue inhibitors of metalloproteinases (TIMPs) (113). Two new members of the MMP family (MMP-11 [stromelysin-3] and MMP-14 [MT1-MMP]) (see Table 16-3) do not directly degrade matrix constituents (113). The main substrate for MMP-11 is a serpin serine protease inhibitor (114). The main substrate for MMP-14 is inactive MMP-2 (gelatinase A). The expression of MMP activity is tightly regulated by mRNA transcription, activation of latent MMP, and inhibition by TIMPs.

The first event in degradation of collagen by collagenases (MMP-1, -8, and -13) is probably the depolymerization of the collagen fibrils. Polymorphonuclear leukocyte elastase (MMP-12) and cathepsin G depolymerize fibrillar collagen by degrading the nonhelical ends of collagen molecules (115). Mammalian collagenases can also degrade crosslinked collagen fibrils by attacking the collagen molecule at one specific locus one fourth of the distance from the C terminus (116). Collagen types I, II, and III are all cleaved in this manner (116). At temperatures higher than 33°C, the collagenase-cleaved collagen fibril spontaneously denatures and forms random coil fragments, which can be further degraded by a variety of tissue- and cell-secreted proteinases (116). Collagenases cleave at Gly-Leu or Gly-Ile bonds (117).

Degradation of tissue collagens involves MMPs (i.e., collagenases, stromelysins, and gelatinases), cysteine proteinases (i.e., cathepsin B and L), and serine proteinases (i.e., plasmin and plasminogen activator) (118).

TABLE 16-3. *Matrix metalloproteinases*

MMP	Proteinase	Main substrate or activity
Secreted matrix metalloproteinases		
MMP-1	Collagenase	Fibrillar collagens
MMP-2	Gelatinase A (72 kd)	Type IV and V collagens, fibronectin
MMP-3	Stromelysin	Laminin, fibronectin, nonfibrillar collagen
MMP-7	Matrilysin	Laminin, fibronectin, nonfibrillar collagen
MMP-8	Neutrophil collagenase	Fibrillar collagens
MMP-9	Gelatinase B (92 kd)	Fibrillar collagens
MMP-10	Stromelysin-2	Laminin, fibronectin, nonfibrillar collagen
MMP-11	Stromelysin-3	Serpin
MMP-12	Metalloelastase	Elastin
MMP-13	Collagenase-3	Fibrillar collagens
Membrane–type metalloproteinases[b]		
MMP-14	MT1-MMP	Pro-MMP-2 (gelatinase A)
	MT2-MMP	Pro-MMP-2 (gelatinase A)
	MT3-MMP	Pro-MMP-2 (gelatinase A)
Metalloproteinase-disintegrins[a]		
	Snake venom disintegrin	Platelet integrin $\alpha_{116}\beta_3$?
	Fertilin	Sperm-egg fusion
	Meltrin-α	Muscle fusion
	Kuzbanian (KUZ)	Cleaves *Drosophila* notch
	TNF-α convertase (TACE)	Releases membrane TNF-α
	MDC/ADAM 10	Activation of human notch receptors, neural development

MMP, matrix metalloproteinases; MT-MMP, membrane-type metalloproteinases.
[a]Partial list from more than 20 Adams family members.
Adapted from refs. 113 and 364, with permission.
[b]From ref. 363, with permission.

All MMPs can be activated *in vitro* by organomercurial agents such as 4-aminophenylmercuric acetate, and MMP-1 and -9 can be activated by some serine proteinases (119–121).

Several MMPs participate in a cascade to undergo activation from inactive proenzyme to active enzyme in preparation for matrix degradation. Pro-MMP-2 can be activated by MT-MMP, active MMP-7, and active MMP-1 (113,122). Pro-MMP-9 can be activated by active MMP-1 and MMP-2 and by active MMP-3, which can also activate pro-MMP-1 (113). Plasmin can activate pro-MMP-3, pro-MMP-1, and pro-MMP-9 (113).

Collagen types IV and V are resistant to degradation by mammalian collagenases that degrade type I, II, and III collagen (116). However, some enzymes can degrade type IV collagen (e.g., chymotrypsin-like enzyme from mast cells, neutrophil elastase, cathepsin G and B, metalloproteases from bone culture) and type V collagen (e.g., metalloprotease from bone culture, metalloproteases from macrophages) (116,123–125).

Fibroblasts from rheumatoid synovium express high levels of major histocompatibility complex (MHC) class II molecules. When these cells are stimulated with staphylococcal enterotoxin A (SEA) superantigen, which is a natural MHC class II ligand, they produce increased levels of MMP-1 and TIMP-1 through a prostaglandin E_2 (PGE_2)–dependent pathway that uses cyclooxygenase-2 (COX-2) and cytosolic phospholipase (cPLA) A_2 (126). IL-4 and dexamethasone added to cultures of SEA-stimulated rheumatoid synovial cells inhibited MMP-1 production but did not affect TIMP-1 production (126). TGF-β1 added to SEA-stimulated rheumatoid synovial fibroblast cultures inhibited MMP-1 production and increased TIMP-1 production. IL-4, TGF-β1, and dexamethasone inhibited phosphorylation of COX-2 and cPLA₂, suggesting that SEA superantigen stimulation of MHC class II on rheumatoid synovial fibroblasts and resultant MMP-1 upregulation uses COX-2– and PLA₂–dependent pathways (126). Stimulation of rheumatoid synovial fibroblasts with PDGF, EGF, or insulin also induces secretion of stromelysin-1 and MMP-1 (127).

Human keratinocytes and tumor cells contain a cell surface protein called extracellular matrix metalloproteinase inducer, which induces synthesis of collagenase-1, gelatinase A, and stromelysin-1 by dermal fibroblasts (128). Neonatal and fetal human fibroblasts in monolayer culture synthesize different basal levels of gelatinases and respond differently to growth factors (129). Although basal levels of gelatinase A (MMP-2) are similar in both cell types, basal levels of gelatinase B (MMP-9) are higher in fetal fibroblast cultures (129).

Collagenase gene expression is markedly increased when fibroblasts are cultured in a three-dimensional collagen gel compared with results when they are grown on artificial surfaces (130). Decorin, when added to surfaces coated with vitronectin or the 120-kd cell-binding domain of fibronectin, causes rabbit synovial fibroblasts to upregulate expression of MMP-1 (131).

MMPs can degrade other substrates. For example, IL-1β but not IL-1α is degraded by MMP-1 (interstitial collagenase), MMP-2 (gelatinase A), MMP-3 (stromelysin-1), and MMP-9 (gelatinase B) (132). The degradation of IL-1 is blocked by TIMP-1 (132).

Stromelysin-1 (MMP-3) is secreted by fibroblasts constitutively and in response to certain agents such as IL-1α and β, TNF-α, EGF, and phorbol myristate acetate (PMA) (133,134). β2-microglobulin is a component of amyloid fibrils in hemodialysis-associated amyloidosis (135). β2-microglobulin stimulates synovial fibroblasts to produce stromelysin-1 (MMP-3) but not TIMP-2 (MMP-2) (135). Stromelysin-3 (MMP-11) is associated only with stromal fibroblasts adjacent to cancer cells (136). Cancer cells (e.g., breast carcinoma cells) can activate a putative response element between 0.46 and 3.4 kb upstream of the transcription start site of MMP-11 (136). Retinoic acid stimulates human dermal fibroblast stromelysin-3 and represses interstitial collagenase (MMP-1) through transcriptional mechanisms (137).

Inhibitors of Metalloproteinases

Various inhibitors of collagenases and other MMPs (e.g., α_2-macroglobulin, β_1-anticollagenase) have been identified in plasma and cultured mammalian tissues such as rabbit bone, skin, and uterus; human tendon; bovine aorta; chick cartilage and bone; and cultured fibroblasts, synovial cells, smooth muscle cells, epithelial cells, gingival fibroblasts, and human amniotic fluid (e.g., TIMP) (116). Another metalloproteinase inhibitor (76 kd) from fibroblasts is called large inhibitor of metalloproteinases (LIMP) (138). LIMP inhibits MMP-1, -2, and -3 (138).

The degradation of collagen and other matrix components in normal and inflamed tissues probably depends on upsetting the balance between MMPs and their inhibitors (116). *TIMP1, TIMP2, TIMP3,* and *TIMP4* constitute a gene family whose products form complexes with MMPs to regulate their enzymatic activities (139). Imbalances between TIMPs and MMPs favoring excess TIMPs results in no degradation of matrix, whereas imbalances favoring excess MMPs results in matrix degradation. The right balance between MMPs and TIMPs is vital during physiologic ECM turnover during animal development and maturation. Imbalances between TIMPs and MMPs favoring excess MMPs or possibly mutations in *TIMP* genes are believed to be important in the pathogenesis of retinal degeneration, periodontal diseases, atherosclerotic plaque rupture, osteoarthritis, rheumatoid arthritis, and neoplastic cell invasion of normal tissues.

In addition to their ability to complex with MMPs to inhibit enzymatic degradation of matrix, they also have mitogenic effects on cells and have antimetastatic activities because of their ability to inhibit angiogenesis (140,141). TIMP-3 is a 21-kd, ECM-associated protein that has mitogenic effects on nontransformed cells and antiangiogenic properties (142–145).

TIMP-1's stromelysin-inhibiting activity is lost after incubation of TIMP-1 with neutrophil elastase (129), which destroys the Val^{69}-Cys^{70} bond. However, if the TIMP-1 and stromelysin complex is reacted with neutrophil elastase, the Val^{69}-Cys^{70} bond is protected, suggesting that this is a site of contact between TIMP-1 and the catalytic domain of stromelysin-1 (129).

Elastase

Elastin is degraded by only a few enzymes that, because of this property, are called elastases. Unlike mammalian collagenases, elastases lack specificity and are general and powerful proteases. Pancreatic and neutrophil elastases are serine proteases and are inhibited by α-1 antiprotease in plasma (146). Macrophage elastase is inhibited by α2-macroglobulin but not by α-1 antiprotease (146). Neutrophil elastase also degrades type IV collagen (147). These three elastases cleave elastin at different sites (146). The pancreatic elastase probably largely serves a digestive function, but in the presence of pancreatitis, it can contribute to tissue destruction. The neutrophil and macrophage elastases are probably important in degrading elastin and perhaps other proteins at sites of inflammatory reactions. Fibroblast elastase activity is the result of the concerted action of an endopeptidase and an aminopeptidase (148). IL-1 stimulates fibroblasts to synthesize elastase (147).

Leukocyte elastase also degrades fibrin and factor XIII–polymerized fibrin clots (149). MMP-9 and MMP-2 are elastolytic MMPs expressed and found in increased amounts in human aneurysmal tissues (150). Fibulin-1 and fibulin-2 are rodlike proteins in basement membranes and in interstitial fibrils (151). Fibulin-1 and fibulin-2 are readily cleaved by leukocyte elastase (151).

Peptides from the degradation of collagen and elastin stimulate human heart fibroblasts and upregulate elastase mRNA and protein *in vitro* (152). Elastase-treated human neutrophils undergo apoptosis *in vitro* (153). This suggests that elastase may be involved in neutrophil apoptosis, which may be responsible for the normal cessation of inflammation by eliminating toxic neutrophils (153).

Proteoglycanases and Glycosaminoglycanases

The core protein and link proteins of proteoglycans are partially degraded by proteases (154), allowing fragments to diffuse away or be further degraded in the pericellular area by proteases such as cathepsin B (155). Glycosaminoglycan peptides and free proteoglycans are pinocytosed by cells, where they are further degraded in the lysosomes by cathepsins with an acidic pH optimum of about 3, such as cathepsin D. The glycosaminoglycans are depolymerized by endoglycosidases and further degraded by several exoenzymes (156). Sulfate groups are removed first by sulfatases, each of which is specific for a given sulfate group. The next step is *N*-acetylation, and monosaccharides then are removed by the alternating action of specific iduronidases or glucuronidases and specific *N*-acetylglucosaminidases, which together degrade glycosaminoglycans to free sulfate and monosaccharide residues. IL-1α, IL-1β, and TNF-α induce synthesis of proteoglycanase by fibroblasts (157).

Glycoproteinases

Fibronectin and other extracellular glycoproteins are susceptible to degradation by a wide variety of tissue- and cell-associated proteases, including chymotrypsin, thrombin, pepsin, elastases, trypsin, plasmin, and cathepsin G and D (158). It appears that glycoproteins can be readily degraded at sites of inflammation by the concerted action of proteases from neutrophils, macrophages, and fibroblasts. Some intermediate fragments from fibronectin degradation may retain biologic activity, such as binding characteristics and the chemotactic property for fibroblasts, which promotes tissue repair.

Cytokine Regulation of Matrix-Degrading Enzymes and Inhibitors

Procollagenase (MMP-1) mRNA is stimulated by cytokines (e.g., IL-1α, β, TNFα) and by phorbol esters (159). The protooncogene *JUN* (formerly designated c-*jun*), which is part of the activator protein-1 (AP-1) complex, probably is an important *trans*-acting factor regulating transcription of the procollagenase gene (159). TNF-α and IL-1β induce rapid increases in *JUN*-encoded mRNA levels in fibroblasts, which precede increases in levels of procollagenase mRNA (159,160). EGF, bFGF, and PDGF also stimulate fibroblast collagenase synthesis (157,161).

TNF receptor p55 mediates TNF-α induction of collagenase expression by human dermal fibroblasts (162). A leukocyte chemotactic peptide fragment of TNF-α 36–62 also upregulates collagenase synthesis by human dermal fibroblasts (162).

During rat skin wound healing, stromelysin-1 and -3, collagenase-3, gelatinase A, gelatinase B, and membrane type 1 matrix metalloproteinase (MT1-MMP) are highly expressed (163). During wound healing, progelatinase A and progelatinase B are activated by MT1-MMP and stromelysin-1, respectively (163). TGF-β1 stimulates production of procollagenase B in fetal and neonatal fibroblast cultures and progelatinase A and activated gelatinase B only in fetal fibroblast cultures (129). PDGF stimulates gelatinase A and B more in fetal than in neonatal fibroblasts.

TIMP-1 is induced in a variety of cells (e.g., human lung and synovial fibroblasts, chondrocytes) by EGF, PDGF, bFGF, oncostatin M, IL-6, IL-11, and TGF-β1 (157,164–167). Retinoic acid added to cultures of human foreskin and synovial fibroblasts with EGF or bFGF synergistically increases production of TIMP-1 protein and inhibits MMP-1 (137).

Considerable attention has been focused on TGF-β regulation of *COL1A1* and *COL1A2* genes. The ACTF/NF-1 binding site between −346 and −300 bp upstream from the transcription start site is critical for TGF-β stimulation of murine *COL1A2* transcription (168). SP1 and AP-1 have also been implicated in activation of the *COL1A2* promoter by TGF-β (169). AP-2 and CTF/NF-1 binding motifs located in a negative response element at −1.6 kb appear to be important for transcription of rat *COL1A1* (170). A region between −1746 and −84 bp in human *COL1A1* containing potential binding sites for SP1, CTF/NF-1, and YB (i.e., type of tenascin domain) has been identified as a TGF-β–responsive element (168).

In cultured human dermal fibroblasts, type VII mRNA is strongly upregulated by IL-1α, IL-1 , TNF-α, and leukoregulin (LR), whereas IL-1 has less of a stimulatory effect on type I collagen gene expression, and TNF-α and LR reduce type I collagen gene expression (171,172). TGF-β acts in an additive manner with IL-1, TNF-α, and LR to stimulate type VII collagen gene expression, but these agents counteract TGF-β upregulation of type I collagen gene expression (171).

FIBROBLAST ADHESION

Fibroblasts *in vivo* adhere to and grow in a complex ECM. The adherence of fibroblasts to the matrix influences their morphology, migration, growth, and differentiation. In some tissues, especially the skin, fibroblasts attach to and pull on the surrounding matrix, causing it to contract and decrease the surface area of wounds. Just how fibroblast functions are influenced by matrix components *in vivo* remains a mystery, but adhesion of fibroblasts to substrate-coated surfaces has been studied *in vitro*. The pseudopodia of fibroblasts attach to substrates at loci called focal adhesions. Focal adhesions are composed of aggregated transmembrane ECM-integrin receptors that, on the outside of fibroblasts and other cells, bind to ECM components (e.g., collagens, fibronectin, elastin, vitronectin) and, on the inside, interact with actin filaments (173).

Most of the integrins comprising focal adhesions are β_1 or β_3 types (173). ECM protein receptors are found by pairing various α chains with the two β integrins, and the particular ECM protein next to the cell determines the type of integrins making up focal adhesions (173). Focal adhesions on fibroblasts grown on serum or vitronectin-coated surfaces express $\alpha_v\beta_3$, the vitronectin receptor, and fibroblasts grown on fibronectin-coated surfaces contain the fibronectin integrin receptor $\alpha_5\beta_1$ (173). RGD sequences in fibronectin and in vitronectin are recognized by $\alpha_5\beta_1$ and $\alpha_v\beta_3$, respectively (173). Cell adherence studies performed with surfaces coated with synthetic RGD peptides suggest that a high density of integrin ligands is needed for focal adhesion formation to occur (174).

The transmembrane proteoglycan, syndecan-4, and dystroglycan (laminin-binding protein-120 [cranin]) are components of focal adhesions on some cells (173). The cytoplasmic domains of the α and β subunits control targeting of integrins to focal adhesions, with the β subunit facilitating and the α subunit inhibiting the process (173). A host of cytoplasmic proteins participate in focal adhesion formation, some of which are illustrated in Figure 16-6 and reviewed by Burridge and Chrzanowska-Wodnicka (173).

Although many different focal adhesion proteins can bind to actin, many investigators believe that talin and vinculin are mostly involved in focal adhesion formation and that α-actin is probably critical in maintaining and stabilizing microfilament attachment in mature focal adhesions (173,175–178). Tensin, talin, and other focal adhesion proteins also have multiple actin-binding sites that may allow subunit addition as they remain bound to actin, or the multiple binding sites may cross-link actin filaments, stabilizing attachments to the membrane (173,179). Vinculin also binds acidic phospholipids (e.g., phosphatidylinositol 4,5-bisphosphate [PIP$_2$]), which brings about a change in its conformation, exposing binding sites for actin, talin, and potential phosphokinase C phosphorylation sites (173,180,181).

RHO, a RAS superfamily protein, is a small GTP-binding protein with regulatory effects on focal adhesion formation and generation of stress fibers (i.e., bundle of actin filaments adjacent to the site on the cell surface where tension is applied) (173). Other members of the RAS superfamily, RAC and CDC42, also affect cells. RAC participates in membrane ruffling (i.e., lamellipodia), and CDC42 generates filopodia formation (i.e., extensions of microspikes) (182,183). Activated RHO stimulates PIP$_2$ synthesis from PIP, and PIP$_2$ acts on cytoskeletal proteins that promote active polymerization and focal adhesion formation (173,184). RHO activates a complex kinase cascade and may increase binding of integrins to their ligands perhaps by inside-out signaling (173,185). The net result is cell contraction. In cells bound to a substrate, this generates isometric tension, bundling of actin filaments, and aggregation of integrins in the plane of the cell membrane (173). The aggregation of integrins leads to tyrosine phosphorylation, ion fluxes, and ligand metabolism that affects downstream pathways involved in cell-cycle progression, gene expression, and apoptosis (173,186,187).

Cultured dermal human fibroblasts express integrin receptors for fibronectin, vitronectin, and fibrinogen

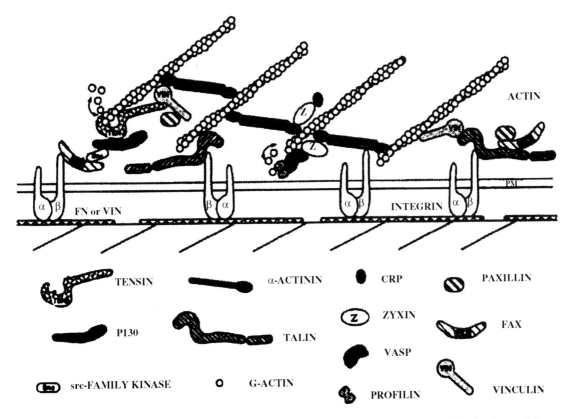

FIG. 16-6. A focal adhesion. The model shows some of the interactions determined *in vitro* for proteins within focal adhesions formed on a surface coated with fibronectin (FN) or vitronectin (VN). To allow linking proteins to be visualized, integrins are shown dispersed rather than clustered. They are linked to actin microfilaments by talin, vinculin, or α-actinin. Actin polymerization at these sites may involve tensin or profilin, which interacts with VASP, a zyxin-binding protein. A few of the signaling components (e.g., FAK, paxillin, p130cas, SRC family kinases) also have been included, but several focal adhesion proteins and many of the interactions have been omitted. The diagram misrepresents the stoichiometry of components in focal adhesions; some, such as vinculin and talin, appear to be many times more abundant than others, such as FAK, paxillin, tensin, and zyxin. (From ref. 173, with permission).

($\alpha_3\beta_1$, $\alpha_4\beta_1$, $\alpha_v\beta_1$, $\alpha_v\beta_3$, and $\alpha_5\beta_5$) (71). The integrin receptors $\alpha_4\beta_1$, $\alpha_5\beta_1$, and $\alpha_v\beta_1$ are used to attach to fibronectin, and $\alpha_v\beta_3$ and $\alpha_v\beta_5$ are used to attach to vitronectin (188). Fibroblasts adhere to substrates coated with fibrinogen, fibrin, or fibrinogen break-down product RGD through $\alpha_v\beta_3$ integrin and other unknown fibrinogen-binding surface proteins (189). The attachment and spreading of fibroblasts on fibrin monomer–coated surfaces also involves the integrin subunit (190).

FIBROBLAST MIGRATION AND CHEMOTAXIS

Fibroblasts are capable of extensive migration *in vivo* and *in vitro* (191–194). Studies of migrating fibroblasts on plastic or glass surfaces *in vitro* have shown that as they migrate they send out lamellipodia that adhere to the surface and allow the body of the fibroblast to be drawn up to the new adhesion site by activation of the contractile filaments within the cell (191,192,194). Neighboring

connective tissue fibroblasts can migrate to the site of corneal injury in rabbits and to sites of surgical wounds (193,195,196).

Studies demonstrating the migratory potential of fibroblasts *in vitro* and *in vivo* suggested that fibroblasts, like monocytes, T cells, and polymorphonuclear leukocytes, might be capable of directed migration toward specific chemoattractants. However, until development of an *in vitro* fibroblast chemotaxis assay, it was not possible to identify chemoattractants for fibroblasts. In 1976, the first description of a fibroblast chemotactic assay was published (197). It employed the Boyden technique and used gelatin-coated polycarbonate filters with 8-μm pores to separate the lower test compartment from the upper cell compartment (197). Fibroblasts from monolayer cultures were used as target cells (197). Since 1976, a host of different fibroblast chemoattractants have been described using this assay or slight variations on how the polycarbonate filter are coated.

Fibroblast Chemoattractants

Cytokines

The first fibroblast chemoattractant to be described was isolated from supernatants from cultures of antigen- or mitogen-stimulated human peripheral blood mononuclear leukocytes and was named LDCF-F (197). This factor was isolated from T cells and was produced as a latent molecule that could be converted to active form (22 kd) by limited trypsin digestion or extracts from sonicated macrophages (197,198). A larger guinea pig LDCF-F with a molecular size of 80 kd was identified (199). In light of data obtained with recombinant cytokines and growth factors, these fibroblast chemotactic factors probably were one or more of the known cytokines or growth factors.

Human recombinant (hr) TNF-α is a potent chemoattractant for human dermal fibroblasts *in vitro* (200). The chemotactic epitope in TNF-α is contained in residues 31–68 (200). TNF-α is synthesized predominantly by macrophages and related cell types and can be released at any inflammatory site where these cells are located.

HrIL-4 induces chemotaxis of human dermal fibroblasts in a dose-dependent manner (201). By using synthetic oligopeptides, two chemotactic epitopes were identified in residues 70–88 and 89–122 (201). IL-4, which is synthesized by T cells and mast cells, may attract fibroblasts to initiate repair at sites of immune reactions.

Growth Factors

The four growth factors—TGF-β, PDGF, bFGF, and EGF—are chemotactic factors for fibroblasts *in vitro* (161,202–204). These growth factors are synthesized by a variety of cells and should be a ready source of chemoattractants at sites of inflammation. The large stores of TGF-β1 and PDGF in platelets can be released at any location where platelets are aggregating (205). The production of TGF-β by many different tumor cell types may be responsible for the fibrotic reaction observed with some tumors (202). The mitogenic and chemotactic epitopes of PDGF-A and -B chains may be different, because elastase treatment of PDGF yields some peptides with only chemotactic or mitogenic activity (205). The PDGF-α receptor appears to be an essential regulatory receptor subtype for various PDGF isoforms to induce optimal chemotactic response of fibroblasts (206). A variety of oligopeptides spanning the 12.5-kd homodimer chain of human TGF-β1 were synthesized. Synthetic peptides contained in the 7-residue sequence of TGF-β1 368–374 (Val-Tyr-Tyr-Val-Gly-Arg-Lys) induce fibroblast, neutrophil, and monocyte chemotaxis (207).

Human gingival fibroblasts are chemically attracted to insulin-like growth factor (IGF) types I and II in a dose-dependent manner, with maximal migration occurring between 10^{-10} and 10^{-9} mmol/L (208). Endothelin (ET) types 1 and 3 (ET-1, ET-3) are chemoattractants for fibroblasts *in vitro* (209). ET-1 is produced by pulmonary artery endothelial cells in hypoxic states, and its chemotactic property may promote fibroblast accumulation in hypoxic pulmonary arteries, leading to pulmonary hypertension (210).

NIH 3T3 fibroblasts transfected with EGF receptor HER-1 or HER-4 are chemically attracted to heparin-binding epidermal growth factor (HB-EGF) (211). Chemotaxis is inhibited by wortmannin (i.e., P13-K inhibitor), implicating a P13-K–dependent signal transduction pathway in this effect of HB-EGF (211).

Neuropeptides

The neuropeptide neurokinin A (NKA) is chemotactic for human lung fibroblasts *in vitro*, and other neuropeptides (e.g., substance P, vasoactive intestinal peptide, calcitonin gene–related peptide) are not (212). NKA may contribute to the increased subepithelial fibroblasts observed in patients with asthma, because it is thought to be released from airway sensory nerves through a local axon reflex (212).

Secretoneurin is a 33 amino acid residue neuropeptide found with substance P in afferent C fibers and is widely distributed through the central and peripheral nervous systems (213). When tested *in vitro*, secretoneurin induced chemotaxis of human dermal fibroblasts at concentrations between 10^{-6} to 10^{-10} mmol/L. A 15-residue carboxyl-terminal fragment of secretoneurin also induces fibroblast chemotaxis (213). Secretoneurin does not stimulate fibroblast mitogenesis (213). Damage to peripheral nerves would be expected to cause release of secretoneurin, which could induce migration of neighboring connective tissue fibroblasts to the site of injury.

Human fibroblasts express the urokinase-type plasminogen activator (u-PA) receptor (UPAR), and *in vitro*, u-PA (5 to 500 ng/mL) triggers chemotaxis of these cells (214). Chemotaxis of fibroblasts to u-PA is inhibited by downregulation of protein kinase C with phorbol myristate acetate (214). Diacylglycerol is produced by engagement of the UPAR receptor by u-PA (214).

Chemokines

Chemokines are a family of small proteins with conserved cysteines at the amino terminal domain. The CC-chemokine subfamily includes RANTES (i.e., regulated on activation, normally T-cell expressed and secreted), macrophage chemotactic protein-3 (MCP-3), eotaxin, and MCP-4 (215). MCP-4 induces chemotaxis of eosinophils and releases Ca^{2+} and reactive oxygen species from these cells (215,216). Treatment of human dermal fibroblasts with rhIL-4, IFN-γ, and TNF-α upregulates MCP-4 mRNA and MCP-4 protein production (215). Production of MCP-4 by fibroblasts would lead to subsequent accumulation of eosinophils at the reaction site, which is typical of asthma, eosinophilic fasciitis, and eosinophilia myalgia syndrome.

The α-chemokine IL-8 induces chemotactic migration of rat embryo fibroblasts *in vitro* (208). Specific binding of IL-8 to human gingival fibroblasts has also been demonstrated (208).

Enzymes

Degranulation of mast cells results in the release of tryptase. Purified tryptase induces chemotaxis of dermal fibroblasts *in vitro* (217). Mast cells often infiltrate tissue that is undergoing fibrosis, and the release of tryptase may chemically attract fibroblasts to the area.

Complement

Activation of serum complement by the classic or alternative pathways generates an 80-kd, C5-derived fragment that is chemotactic for fibroblasts (218). Monocytes and neutrophils do not respond to this C5 fragment (218). It is doubtful that the larger 80,000 M_r, C5 fragment is related to C5a, because it is not chemotactic for neutrophils or monocytes, which do respond chemotactically to C5a (218). Purified human C5a has induced fibroblast chemotaxis (219).

Matrix

Types I, II, and III fibrillar collagens provide chemotactic signals for fibroblasts (220) and monocytes (221). Synthetic tripeptides containing the Gly-X-Y sequence, in which X or Y is proline or hydroxyproline, are also chemotactic for fibroblasts (220). The potency of various cyanogen bromide peptides of type I collagen correlated with their degree of binding to collagen receptors on fibroblasts (222).

Fibronectin isolated from human plasma is a potent fibroblast chemoattractant (223). It is active over a range of 0.8 to 1.6 µg/mL (223). The chemotactic epitope resides somewhere in the 140-kd, nongelatin binding fragment of fibronectin (203,223).

Tropoelastin and bovine elastin, when degraded by pancreatic elastase, induce chemotaxis of human skin fibroblasts *in vitro* (224). A synthetic peptide common to elastin, VGVAPG, is chemotactic for human fibroblasts at a concentration of 10^{-8} mmol/L (225).

Eicosanoids

Leukocytes are a major source of leukotriene B₄, which is generated in a variety of inflammatory reactions. This compound can induce chemotactic migration of fibroblasts, monocytes, neutrophils, and eosinophils (226).

Other Fibroblast Chemoattractants

SV40NIH 3T3–derived fibroblast chemotactic factor is produced by SV40 virus–transformed 3T3 cells (227). This factor is 20 to 30 kd (227) and may be TGF-β1 or other chemotactic cytokines or growth factors.

Breast cancer cell line–derived fibroblast chemotactic factor is a fibroblast chemotactic factor of about 100 kd. It has been isolated from a human breast carcinoma cell line (2R-75-1) (228). This chemotactic activity, unlike PDGF or fibronectin, is destroyed by pepsin, trypsin, and reduction and alkylation with 2-mercaptoethanol (228).

Modulators of Fibroblast Chemotaxis and Migration

Mannose 6-phosphate and IGF-II enhance PDGF-induced fibroblast chemotaxis *in vitro* (229). It has been suggested that lysosomal enzymes that bear mannose 6-phosphate molecules may be involved in chemotaxis of fibroblasts, because α-mannosidase and cathepsin D inhibitor, pepstatin, are potent inhibitors of fibroblast chemotaxis (229). Mannose 6-phosphate also stimulates fibroblast prolidase activity, the enzyme involved in the final step of collagen degradation (229).

Pretreatment of human skin fibroblasts for 24 hours with TGF-β1 or bFGF induces a twofold to threefold greater increase in the chemotactic response to PDGF than in control cells (230). These data support the concept that these growth factors may act synergistically with PDGF to attract fibroblasts to human wound sites.

PIP₂ binds to some actin-binding proteins and modulates phosphatidylinositol-specific phospholipase C (PLC) activity (231). Such actin-binding proteins may play a role in receptor signaling by restructuring the membrane cytoskeleton and modifying second messenger generation through the phosphoinositide cycle (232). Cap G is a member of the gelsolin family that binds Ca^{2+} and polyphosphoinositide, caps actin filaments without severing, and does not bind actin monomers (233–235). Overexpression of Cap G in NIH 3T3 fibroblasts leads to heightened proliferative and chemotactic responses to PDGF, more circular dorsal membrane ruffles, higher phosphoinositide turnover, and higher inositol 1,4,5-triphosphate (IP₃) generation and Ca^{2+} signaling responses consistent with enhanced PLC activity (232). These results suggest that Cap G and related proteins may link membrane signaling with actin filament changes related to cell stimulation (232).

Because so many chemoattractants exist for fibroblasts, it is reasonable to suspect that inhibitors may exist that could stop the chemotactic migration of fibroblasts. We found that serum from normal human donors contains a large-molecular-mass (about 210 kd) trypsin-sensitive protein, serum inhibitor of fibroblast migration (SIFM), that inhibits fibroblast migration to all known chemoattractants (236). This inhibitor is not cytotoxic to fibroblasts and does not alter collagen or protein synthesis (236). The serum inhibitor may function to control and modulate fibroblast chemotactic responses in general.

IFN-γ and IFN-α at relatively high doses (0.1 to 100 ng) have also been found to inhibit fibroblast chemotaxis to some agents (237).

The Clara cells of bronchiolar epithelium synthesizes Clara cell protein-16 (CC-16), which is the 15.8-kd human counterpart of rabbit uteroglobin (238). CC-16 is identical to human urinary protein-1 (hUP-1) (238). Although the biologic functions of CC-16 are not well known, it does inhibit phospholipase A₂ (PLA_2) and is related to lipocortins and antiflammins (239). CC-16 inhibits fibroblast migration to PDGF by 90% at a concentration of 30 μg/mL, and this inhibition is reversible by reducing CC-16 (238). Levels of CC-16 are reduced in alveolar fluids from patients with idiopathic pulmonary fibrosis and bleomycin-induced lung fibrosis (238). CC-16 deficiency may lead to increases in fibroblasts in these fibrosing lung diseases (238).

Cigarette smoke extract (CSE), an aqueous extract produced by bubbling, nonfiltered cigarette smoke through Hank's balanced salt solution, contains a non-volatile substance that dose-dependently inhibits chemotactic migration of human fetal lung fibroblasts to fibronectin when fibroblasts are precultured with CSE for 24 hours before assay (240). Cell viability is not affected by the CSE (240). Components in cigarette smoke may help tip the balance between injury and repair to favor emphysema (240).

FIBROBLAST PROLIFERATION

The mechanisms involved in the transmission of mitogenic signals to fibroblasts are not completely understood, and it is likely that they are different for different classes of growth factors. Specific receptors have been identified on fibroblasts for several growth factors (e.g., EGF; TGF-β, IL-1, PDGF) (241–250). The receptor on murine fibroblasts for PDGF has been cloned (241). The primary deduced structure for the PDGF receptor is similar to that of the *KIT* (formerly designated v-*kit*) oncogene product and the receptor for macrophage colony-stimulating factor (241). Its overall structure has properties consistent with a receptor and includes transmembrane and tyrosinase kinase domains (241). There is a potential site for *N*-linked glycosylation in the extracellular domain (241). The protein encoded by the cDNA clone would have an apparent mass of 120,000d after the signal sequence is removed (241). The molecular mass of the native receptor for PDGF is 180,000d, and the increase in molecular mass from the predicted figure may be explained by extensive glycosylation and the covalent linking of ubiquitin and phosphate groups (241).

Growth Factors

Addition of growth factors (e.g., EGF, PDGF, serum) to serum-starved, density-arrested 3T3 fibroblasts leads to rapid elevations in mRNA for vinculin and β₁ integrin by a protein kinase C–independent mechanism (242). This occurs after activation of genes encoding FOS, MYC, actin, and fibronectin (242). These observations suggest an important role for morphology in the control of fibroblast proliferative response to growth factors (242). EGF and PDGF binding to receptors appear to initiate increased Na^+/H^+ exchange and phosphorylation of tyrosine residues (243). EGF stimulates metabolism of arachidonic acid to produce oxygenated metabolites that are necessary for stimulation of MYC expression and DNA synthesis (244). Arachidonic acid and metabolites are not necessary for PDGF-induced mitogenesis in BALB/c3T3 cells (244). Binding of PDGF to fibroblast cell surface receptors generates inositol triphosphate and diacylglycerol, followed by increases in cytosolic calcium levels and stimulation of protein kinase C (245). EGF does not induce inositol triphosphate synthesis, except when cAMP is elevated by experimental manipulations of cells (244,245).

Some cytokines and growth factors exert their mitogenic effects on fibroblasts in part by indirectly inducing fibroblasts to synthesize their own growth factor in an autocrine-like or paracrine-like fashion. For example, IL-1α, IL-1β, TNF-α, EGF, and PDGF induce a transient increase in PDGF-A chain, but not PDGF-B chain, mRNA, with synthesis and release of a PDGF-like protein (probably a PDGF-AA dimer) (246–248). TGF-β induces synthesis of a PDGF-B chain mRNA (SIS) and release of PDGF-like protein but also may increase synthesis of fibroblast PDGF-A chain (249). TGF-β also induces expression of β-integrin, actin, fibronectin, MYC, and FOS (250–253).

PDGF and other growth factors stimulate cytoskeletal rearrangement, increase turnover of phosphatidylinositol, and enhance expression of a family of genes, including *MYC* and *FOS* proto-oncogenes. These effects probably are important in the eventual mitosis of fibroblasts and other targets of various growth factors, although exactly how these events are related to mitosis remains to be established.

Neuropeptides

Neuropeptides have been the focus of asthma research. NKA and substance P have been localized to different nerves of the airways and are thought to contribute to bronchoconstriction, airway microvascular leakage, and mucus secretion in patients with asthma (212). NKA stimulates proliferation of human lung fibroblasts when added to cultures *in vitro* (212). Substance P, like NKA, stimulates growth of normal human diploid lung fibroblasts *in vitro* (212). NKA and substance P may contribute to the increased accumulation of subepithelial myofibroblasts and fibrosis in patients with asthma (212).

ET-1 and ET-3 stimulate fibroblast mitogenesis and may play critical roles in expanding numbers of fibroblasts in the walls of hypoxic pulmonary arteries (209). Because ET-1 is also produced by pulmonary endothelial cells, it could expand fibroblast numbers in the lung parenchyma in conditions associated with pulmonary fibrosis, such as systemic sclerosis and crytogenic fibrosing alveolitis (210,254).

Human dermal fibroblasts are stimulated to undergo mitogenesis *in vitro* by native u-PA, although not by the amino terminal fragment of u-PA, u-PA-ATF (214). This suggests that UPARs on fibroblasts have to be fully engaged (i.e., receptor occupancy and activity of the u-PA catalytic site) to undergo mitogenesis by u-PA (214).

INTERPLAY OF FIBROBLASTS, EXTRACELLULAR MATRIX, AND THE IMMUNE SYSTEM

The association of lymphocyte infiltrates with fibrosis had long been observed but unexplained in human diseases such as pulmonary tuberculosis and pulmonary sarcoidosis. In 1976, two papers were published that shed light on this mystery. Johnson and Ziff reported that supernatants from cultures of activated peripheral blood lymphocyte-monocyte cultures stimulated synthesis of collagen when added to cultures of fibroblasts (255). Postlethwaite et al. reported that a 22-kd protein elaborated by antigen- and mitogen-stimulated human peripheral T cells induced chemotactic migration of fibroblasts *in vitro* (197). These papers offered the first tangible evidence that the immune system communicated with and modulated fibroblast matrix deposition and migration. That year, several other papers were published showing that peripheral blood T cells from patients with scleroderma and idiopathic pulmonary fibrosis elaborated lymphokines when cultured with collagen and other matrix components (256–258). Since 1976, there has been a tremendous expansion of research on and information about how fibroblasts, the ECM, and components of the immune and host defense systems communicate and interact.

Matrix and Leukocyte Interactions

T Cells

In addition to providing important structural functions, the ECM participates in important functions of cells of the immune system and virtually all other cells of the body. For T cells, the ECM provides regulatory signals and co-stimulatory messages that constantly modulate their activities as they migrate into tissues of various organs.

Fibronectin, laminin, and collagen types I, III, and IV can act as co-stimulators for activated CD4+ T cells (259,260). The receptors on T cells involved in interaction with collagen as a co-stimulator are CD26 and CD29 (260). For laminin, the T-cell receptor is VLA6 (261). For fibronectin, the T-cell receptors are VLA5 and CD29 (259,260). Peptides containing RGD or Gly-Pro-X amino acid sequences inhibit collagen co-stimulation of activated CD4+ T cells, suggesting that peptides containing these sequences contain important sites for interaction with CD4+ lymphocytes (260). Laminin, fibronectin, and collagen types I, III, and IV provide co-stimulatory signals to CD4+ T cells. This leads to expansion of CD4+ T cells and elaboration of cytokines. Addition of TN-C to cultures of human T cells inhibits T-cell proliferation, probably through TN-C's ability to compete with fibronectin binding to T cells (261). TN-C also inhibits anti-CD3/IL-2 or phorbol ester (in the absence of fibronectin) T-cell proliferation, suggesting that TN-C delivers a separate inhibitory signal to T cells (261). TN-C inhibits expression of IL-2 receptors and generation of functional NF-AT1 transcription factor complexes in nuclear extracts of T cells stimulated by phorbol ester or anti-CD3/IL-2 in the absence of fibronectin (261). TN-C may function *in vivo* to suppress T cell activation near certain tumors and at sites of tissue repair where TN-C is expressed.

In a normal resting state, neither T cells nor the ECM components possess all the necessary signals for T-cell activation and migration or homing to specific tissues (262). However, when an injury occurs to tissue or cellular components of tissue, T cells and the ECM can express cytokines, chemokines, matrix-degrading enzymes, and other inflammatory mediators that, collectively, can transduce co-stimulatory and modulatory signals involving T cells and other accompanying immune cells (262). For example, if vascular endothelium is damaged, as during allogeneic reactions in organ grafts, the underlying adjacent ECM can become "activated" or modified to facilitate recruitment and extravastion of T cells and other leukocytes.

The migration of T cells, other leukocytes, and platelets leads to secretion of heparanase and other matrix-degrading enzymes (263). After antigen activation, naive T cells synthesize heparanase, and memory CD4+ T cells release it from stores (263). Heparanase cleaves heparan sulfate proteoglycan and releases cytokines and growth factors bound to this type proteoglycan (262). By degrading heparan sulfate proteoglycans, T-cell migration is facilitated through tissue. The enzyme activity of heparanase is inhibited by heparin, and therefore migration of T cells is blocked (262). Because heparan sulfates are present on cell surfaces and form complex structural associations with collagens and other matrix molecules, their degradation by heparanase completely modifies properties of extracellular cell membranes and of the ECM, leading to exposure of an array of new determinants on cells and within the ECM for interaction with T cells (262). Heparan sulfate proteoglycans can regulate antigen-presenting functions of cells; bind growth factors, chemokines, and cytokines; and present mediators to leukocytes in biologically active forms (262).

Binding and storage of cytokines such as TNF-α to ECM components such as fibronectin or laminin facilitate their association with T cells and leukocytes responding to chemotactic signals, and this process restricts the activities of such bound cytokines (262). Low doses of TNF-α that would be available on the ECM molecules synergize with antigen, increasing the binding properties of ECM-specific $β_1$-integrins expressed on T cells (263,264). Chemokines (e.g., macrophage inflammatory protein-1β [MIP-1β], RANTES) interact with ECM glycosaminoglycans and may modulate migration, adhesion and haptotaxis of lymphocytes (e.g., $CD4^+$ T cells) within the ECM (262).

Extracellular Matrix Components as Autoantigens for T Cells

ECM components such as collagen types I, III, and III can act as autoantigens. Many patients with rheumatoid arthritis have T-cell immunity predominantly to the collagen type II present in joint cartilage (265). Patients with systemic sclerosis and those with idiopathic pulmonary fibrosis have T-cell immunity to collagen types I and III (256,258,266,267). T cells react to discrete epitopes on the collagen molecules (A. Postlethwaite, personal observation, 1998).

Monocytes and Macrophages

Monocytes and macrophages elaborate immunomodulatory cytokines when they adhere to matrix. For example, fibronectin adherence leads to synthesis of granulocyte-macrophage colony-stimulating factor (GM-CSF) and CSF-1, and collagen adherence leads to synthesis of IL-1 and TNF-α (268–270).

Modulation of Matrix Synthesis by Cytokines

A variety of cytokines modulate fibroblast matrix synthesis. IL-1α and IL-1β stimulate collagen synthesis in confluent skin fibroblast cultures (172) and stimulate synthesis of hyaluronic acid (271). TNF-α has stimulatory and inhibitory effects on fibroblast collagen synthesis, depending on the culture conditions and tissue of origin of the fibroblasts (272). TNF-α also stimulates glycosaminoglycan synthesis and decreases synthesis of fibronectin (272). IL-4 stimulates collagen, fibronectin, and hyaluronic acid by fibroblasts (273). IFN-γ inhibits collagen and fibronectin synthesis (272,274). PDGF has a modest stimulatory effect on collagen synthesis (272). FGF stimulates fibroblast synthesis of collagen, proteoglycan, and fibronectin (275). TGF-β stimulates synthesis of collagen, glycosaminoglycan and fibronectin (252,276–278).

Leukocyte and Fibroblast Interactions

Synovial T cells from rheumatoid arthritis and gout patients can be rescued from spontaneous apoptosis *in vitro* by IL-2R chain signaling cytokines that upregulate expression of BCL-2 and BCL-X or by exposure to synovial fibroblasts, which upregulates production of BCL-X but not BCL-2 (279). The rescue of rheumatoid T cells from apoptosis by fibroblasts involves RGD binding of integrins (279). This ability of synovial fibroblasts to inhibit T-cell apoptosis may be responsible for the blockade of T-cell death in rheumatoid synovium (280).

Fibroblast Interleukin-2 Receptors

Human embryonic skin fibroblasts express IL-2α chains but not β chains, bind [^{125}I]IL-2 in a specific manner and express two classes of receptors (280). The fibroblasts express 186±26 binding sites per cell with a K_d of 0.11±0.02 mmol/L and 659±48 binding sites per cell with a K_d of 32.1±1.8 nmol/L (280). They also express IL-2α and -2β chain mRNA (280). IL-2 (a T-cell derived cytokine) added to these fibroblasts stimulates JE gene expression that codes for MCP-1 and increased MCP-1 protein (280). Other fibroblast cytokines (e.g., IL-1, IL-5, IL-6, IL-7, IL-8, IL-9, GM-CSF, M-CSF, and TNF-α) are not upregulated by IL-2.

Fibroblast CD40

CD40 is a 50-kd receptor member of the TNF-α receptor superfamily. Although originally described on cells of bone marrow origin, it has been found on fibroblasts from human lung, orbit, thyroid, and gingiva. Engagement of the CD40 receptor by CD40 ligand results in upregulation of the transcription factor NF-κB, which results in synthesis and release of IL-6 and IL-8 (281). Activated T cells, eosinophils, and mast cells display gp39 (CD154), which is the CD40 ligand. These cells, when adjacent to fibroblasts, can engage CD40 on fibroblasts and upregulate the synthesis of IL-6, IL-8, intercellular adhesion molecule-1 (ICAM-1), and vascular cell adhesion molecule-1 (VCAM-1) (281). Fibroblasts from human lung massively upregulate COX-2 mRNA and protein synthesis and PGE_2 synthesis, especially in the presence of IFN-γ (282). PGE_2 is a potent mediator of inflammation, promoting vasodilation and pain.

Fibroblast CD80

Murine fibroblasts cultured from various tissues constitutively express CD80 (B7-1), which can be markedly increased by the addition of IFN-γ and TNF-α (283). These CD80-expressing fibroblasts are able to provide a co-stimulation signal to antigen specific T cells, suggesting that *in vivo* CD80 expressed on fibroblasts may deliver a co-stimulatory signal to T cells participating in inflammatory reactions (283).

β₂-*Integrins*

Human neutrophils use predominantly the β₂ integrin Mac-1 (i.e., α$_m$β₂ or CD 11b/CD18) to migrate through a barrier *in vitro* of human synovial or dermal fibroblasts (284). Neutrophils stimulated with platelet-activating factor (PAF) markedly adhere by CD11/CD18 (β₂) integrins to cultured fibroblasts but do not migrate (285). The addition of IL-8 to PAF-adherent neutrophils induces their migration, which is CD18 dependent along fibroblast monolayer surfaces (285).

Fibroblasts and other cell types express various heterophilic cell-cell adhesion molecules on their surfaces that mediate binding of cells of different types to each other. Many molecules are related structurally and belong to the immunoglobulin superfamily. Fibroblasts have several such cell adhesion molecules on their surface, including lymphocyte function-associated antigen-3 (LFA-3), HCAM (i.e., CD44 or Hermes antigen), and ICAM-1 (286). HCAM is expressed on fibroblasts, and this adhesion molecule belongs to the cartilage link protein family (287). LFA-3 is present on many different cell types and is a ligand for CD2, which is on all T cells (288). CD2 is also a member of the immunoglobulin superfamily (288). LFA-3–CD2 binding is important in T-cell adhesion to fibroblasts. ICAM-1 is also present on a wide variety of cell types and is a ligand for LFA-1 (CD11a), which is present on all leukocytes (287). ICAM-1–LFA-1 binding is important in leukocyte adhesion to fibroblasts. Fibroblasts from patients with scleroderma express higher degrees of ICAM-1 (289). Treatment of rheumatoid synovial fibroblasts with IL-1β, TNF-α, or IFN-γ leads to increased expression of ICAM-1 and class I MHC molecules on their surfaces (286). IFN-γ increases HLA class II antigen expression on fibroblasts (286). Fibroblast LFA-3 does not appear to be modulated by these cytokines (286).

Thy-1⁺ and Thy-1⁻ *Murine Fibroblasts*

Thy-1 antigen is a 25-kd cell surface glycoprotein originally described on thymocytes, T cells, and brain tissues in the mouse. Thy-1⁺ fibroblasts have been found in adult murine lungs, spleen, bone marrow and lymph nodes (287). Thy-1⁻ and Thy-1⁺ fibroblasts from murine spleens and lungs respond differently to IFN-γ and IL-4. Between 50% and 65% of murine spleen fibroblasts were Thy-1⁺ (287). Cloned Thy-1⁺ and Thy-1⁻ splenic fibroblast lines were established (287). Thy-1⁺ and Th-1⁻ splenic fibro-

blasts expressed class I MHC molecules, ICAM-1, VCAM-1, and CD44 without stimulation, but Thy-1⁺ fibroblasts produced more IL-6 (287). IFN-γ induced expression of class II MHC molecules that were capable of presenting antigen to an I-A^b-restricted T-cell line (287).

Cloned Thy-1⁺ and Thy-1⁻ murine lung fibroblasts were analyzed for their responses to IL-4 and IFN-γ (289). IL-4 caused significant increases in type I and type III collagen mRNAs and total collagen protein only in Thy-1⁺ cells, whereas IFN-γ decreased collagen production by 50% in Thy-1⁺ and Thy-1⁻ fibroblasts (289). Thy-1⁻ fibroblasts also proliferated to a greater extent than Thy-1⁺ fibroblasts when exposed to IL-1α, IL-4, and IL-6 (290).

Fibroblast-Derived Cytokines

Fibroblasts that have been activated by cytokines or that reside in connective tissue that has sustained an injury are a ready source of several cytokines and growth factors that play significant roles in modulating immune responses and affecting inflammatory and repair processes. IL-1α, IL-1β, double-stranded RNA, viruses, TNF-α, PDGF, and IFN-β stimulate fibroblasts to synthesize IL-6 (i.e., IFN-β₂/B-cell stimulatory factor 2) (291). IL-6 is the major cytokine involved in stimulation of acute-phase protein synthesis by hepatocytes. IL-6 also stimulates immunoglobulin synthesis and enhances B-cell growth (291). TNF-α induces IL-1α synthesis, but not IL-1β, by fibroblasts (292). IL-1β and TNF-α stimulate fibroblast synthesis of factor B, C3, and factor H (292). IL-1β and poly(rI).poly(rC) stimulate fibroblasts to synthesize granulocyte colony-stimulating factors (G-CSF), M-CSF and, GM-CSF (293). IL-1 induces synthesis of IFN-β and IL-8 by fibroblasts (294). IL-1 and TNF-α, but not lipopolysaccharide or IL-6, stimulate fibroblasts to synthesize monocyte chemotactic and activating protein (MCAF) (295,296). IL-1 induces synthesis of PDGF-AA by fibroblasts that act in an autocrine manner to effect fibroblast mitogenesis (246). Fibroblasts are also capable of synthesizing TGF-α and TGF-β (297). These fibroblast-derived cytokines and growth factors collectively exert multiple effects on leukocytes that include stimulation of their growth and release from bone marrow and the chemotaxis and accumulation of fibroblasts, neutrophils, monocytes, and T cells.

Epitaxin is a 35-kd motility factor for transformed epithelial cells. It is produced by transformed and normal human fibroblasts cultured *in vitro* (298). Although the function of this factor is not entirely understood, it may facilitate invasion and metastasis by epithelial tumors (298).

Keratinocyte growth factor (KGF), also known as fibroblast growth factor-7 (FGF-7), is produced by mesenchymal cells, including human dermal and lung fibroblasts (299). KGF production by fibroblasts is upregulated by IL-1α, PDGF-BB, and TGF-α but downregulated by glucocorticoids (299). KGF is thought to play a critical role in interactions between epithelial and mesenchymal cells during embryogenesis and in tissue repair in adults (299). Glucocorticoids downregulate KGF expression by reducing the rate of *FGF7* gene transcription and by causing destabilization of FGF-7 mRNA (299). This inhibitory effect of glucocorticoids on *FGF7* gene expression may be one mechanism by which they impair wound healing.

IL-11 is megakaryocyte progenitor colony-stimulating factor that acts synergistically with IL-3 to shorten the G_0 period of early progenitors (300). IL-11 mRNA is upregulated in adult human dermal and neonatal foreskin fibroblasts in culture and in lung fibroblasts by IL-1α, TGF-β1 , and TGF-β2 (301,302). Because the bone marrow stroma is particularly rich in fibroblasts (60% to 70%), fibroblasts probably are a major source of IL-11 to stimulate megakaryocyte formation (301).

Nerve growth factor (NGF) is involved in nerve growth and regeneration after injury. Several cytokines and growth factors, including TNF-α, IL-1α, IL-1β, EGF, bFGF, IFN-γ, and TGF-β stimulate in a dose-dependent fashion the production of NGF in mouse 3T3 fibroblasts *in vitro* (303). TNF-α synergistically increased NGF production in the presence of IL-1α, IL-1β, and IFN-γ, whereas TNF-α and IL-1β alone had modest effects on NGF production (303). Because Wallerian degeneration is necessary for peripheral sensory nerve regeneration to occur, it is likely that macrophages elaborate TNF-α, IL-1α, and IL-1β as they invade the nerve lesion site, and these cytokines together greatly increase NGF production by fibroblasts in the connective tissue in the area of the nerve injury.

Vascular endothelial growth factor (VEGF) is a major angiogenic factor involved in vascular growth in normal and pathologic conditions such as retinal neovascularization and rheumatoid pannus formation (304). When added to cultures of synovial fibroblasts from patients with rheumatoid arthritis, PGE_2, PGE_1, and IL-1α induced increased expression of VEGF mRNA (304). Further study revealed that EP2-type prostaglandin receptors probably are involved in PGE_1 and PGE_2-mediated induction of VEGF (304). These results suggest that VEGF, which is upregulated in synovial tissue of patients with rheumatoid arthritis, may be a major angiogenic factor in rheumatoid arthritis pannus formation (304).

IL-8 is an α-chemokine that is a potent chemoattractant for neutrophils (305). The early stages of periodontal disease is characterized by the influx of neutrophils and increases in IL-1β, TNF-α, and IFN-γ (306). Human gingival fibroblasts in culture increased levels of IL-8 mRNA and protein when stimulated with IL-1β or TNF-α (305). IL-1β and TNF-α added to human gingival fibroblasts synergistically increased IL-8 production, whereas IFN-γ inhibited IL-8 mRNA transcription induced by IL-1β or TNF-α (305). These results indicate that neutrophil accumulation in periodontal disease may be differentially regulated by a cytokine network consisting of IL-1β and TNF-α, which increase IL-8 production by human gingival fibroblasts, and by IFN-γ, which decreases IL-8 production (305). IL-8 production by human dermal fibroblasts is also downregulated by IFNγ (307).

KC is the product of an early response gene in mouse fibroblasts stimulated by PDGF. KC is a potent chemoattractant and upregulator of Mac-1 cell surface expression in murine neutrophils (308). KC has homology to human IL-8 and may be a major regulator of neutrophil trafficking to sites of inflammation in mice (308).

MCP-1 and MCP-2 are CXC or α-chemokines. MCP-1 and MCP-2 are upregulated in normal human diploid fibroblasts stimulated by IL-1β, IFN-γ, poly(rI), poly (rC), and measles virus (309). MCP-2 was induced in larger amounts than MCP-1 by all of these agents. MCP-1 and MCP-2 are equally potent chemoattractants for monocytes (309).

MIP-1β levels are higher in synovial fluid from patients with osteoarthritis than in synovial fluids from patients with rheumatoid arthritis (310). Cultured osteoarthritis synovial fibroblasts produced increased amounts of MIP-1β when stimulated with TNF-α, IL-1β, or lipopolysaccharide (LPS) from *Escherichia coli*. LPS from *Porphyromonas gingivalis* stimulates MCP-1 production through CD14 on human gingival fibroblasts (311). The mRNA for MCP-1 measured by in situ hybridization is prominently expressed in gingival fibroblasts in sites of gingival inflammation where there is fibrosis (312). These results suggest that MIP-1β may facilitate accumulation of monocytes in the joints exhibiting osteoarthritis. MIP-1β was responsible for 28% of the monocyte chemotactic activity in osteoarthritis synovial fluid (310).

Human dermal fibroblasts and rheumatoid synovial fibroblasts stimulated with TNF-α or IL-1β produce RANTES (313,314). Dermal fibroblasts produce a truncated form of RANTES lacking the first two N-terminal amino acids [Tyr-RANTES][66] instead of natural [Ser-RANTES][68] (313). This truncated RANTES is equally as potent as natural RANTES in inducing eosinophil chemotaxis *in vitro* (313). The same supernatants from cultures of dermal fibroblasts that contained truncated [Tyr-RANTES][66] contained another eosinophil chemoattractant, GM-CSF (313). These observations suggest that dermal fibroblasts are a rich source of eosinophil chemoattractants that are possibly released in affected tissues exhibiting atopic dermatitis or other allergic condition (313).

ET-1 stimulates synthesis of collagen (209,314). Because ET-1 is synthesized by pulmonary endothelial cells and probably by airway epithelium, it may contribute to collagen deposition in pulmonary artery walls and lung parenchyma in conditions associated with pulmonary hypertension and pulmonary fibrosis, respectively (314).

FIBROBLASTS IN WOUND HEALING

During healing of dermal wounds, a coordinated series of biologic events is set in motion. These events include platelet-induced hemostasis (with release of TGF-β1 and PDGF), followed by chemotaxis and accumulation of neutrophils, monocytes and fibroblasts and myofibroblasts, synthesis of new ECM, formation of new blood vessels to constitute new granulation tissue, and proliferation of fibroblasts to reconstitute the connective tissue (315). The growth factors and cytokines that signal cells to effect the healing process are primarily derived from platelets, neutrophils, monocytes, endothelial cells, lymphocytes, and fibroblasts (316).

At first, platelets are the major source of TGF-β1 and PDGF (316). Neutrophils migrate into the injury site 24 to 48 hours after wounding has occurred, and this is followed in 48 to 72 hours by macrophages, which become activated and are the major source for growth factors and cytokines that modulate tissue repair. These growth factors and cytokines include TGF-β1, PDGF, bFGF, TGF-α, IGF-I, IGF-II, TNF-α, and IL-1 (316–329). Angiogenesis and accumulation of fibroblasts is evident by 72 hours after wounding. A variety of chemoattractants may play a role in recruiting fibroblasts to the wound area, including TGF-β, PDGF, TNF-α, IL-4, fibronectin, collagen-derived peptides, tropoelastin and elastin peptides, leukotriene B₄, an 80-kd C5 fragment, and C5 (199–203, 207,218–220,223,224,226). The accumulation of fibroblasts is followed by increased synthesis of collagen, proteoglycans, laminin, and fibronectin. Wound strength is initially determined by the degree of new collagen synthesis, but after 7 to 14 days, collagen crosslinking appears to be the major predictor of wound strength (330).

A variety of growth factors and cytokines (e.g., TGF-β, PDGF, FGF, EGF, TGF-α, IL-1) have been added to wounds of different types in animal models and have been found to promote wound healing (331–342). TGF-β1 was shown in pigs to markedly enhance granulation tissue formation and to increase mRNAs for collagen types I and III, elastin, and TGF-β1 and to reduce expression of the matrix-degrading enzyme stromelysin (343). Similar results were shown earlier in a rat incisional wound model (340). A single intravenous dose (100 or 500 μg/kg) of TGF-β1 increased the wound-breaking strength in old and glucocorticoid-treated rats (344). TGF-β2 applied to an incisional wound in pigs significantly increased wound-breaking strength at day 8 after wounding and caused increased accumulation of connective tissue matrix (342). The role of TGF-β3 in the healing of adult wounds is less well defined, but it may diminish scar formation (345).

TNF-α is one of many different cytokines (e.g., TGF-β, IL-1α, IL-1β, IL-6, PDGF) produced by macrophages participating in inflammatory reactions (346). When hrTNF-α is injected subcutaneously into mice, it induces an acute inflammatory reaction that is followed by chronic inflammation, accumulation of fibroblasts, and fibrosis (347). TNF-α has fibrogenic and antifibrogenic effects on fibroblasts when tested in isolated cultures of these cells *in vitro*. TNF-α is a potent mitogen and chemoattractant for fibroblasts (200,348). However, it inhibits fibroblast synthesis of collagen and fibronectin and increases synthesis of collagenase and PGE₂ (349–351). TNF-α has been detected in significant quantities in wound fluid from healing wounds (346). Topical application of TNF-α to incisional wounds increased wound-breaking strength, and the addition of murine TNF-α to subcutaneously inserted polyvinyl alcohol sponges increased collagen deposition because of its mitogenic and chemotactic effects to expand the number of fibroblasts in wound sites (352,353).

After wounding of mouse skin, levels of IL-1β peak at 3 hours, and IL-1α levels peak at 6 hours; neutrophils are the major source of these cytokines (354). A second increase in IL-1α and IL-1β levels occurs 72 hours after wounding and is accompanied by an accumulation of fibroblasts and granulation tissue (354). Addition of exogenous IL-1β to mouse dermal incisional wounds promotes increased wound tensile strength in irradiated mice but not in normal mice.

ACKNOWLEDGMENTS

The authors acknowledge the excellent assistance of Phyllis Mikula in typing and preparing this chapter and the suggestions by Dr. Karen Hasty. The time and effort exerted by the authors in preparing this chapter were supported in part by research funds from the Department of Veterans Affairs and by PHS grant AR26034 and AR39166.

REFERENCES

1. Martinez-Hernandez A, Amenta PS. Basic concepts in wound healing. In: Leadbetter WB, Buckwalter JA, Gordon SL, eds. *Sports-induced inflammation.* Park Ridge, IL: American Academy of Orthopedic Surgeons, 1990:55–101.
2. Schmitt-Graff A, Desmouliere A, Gabbiani G. Heterogeneity of myofibroblast phenotype features: an example of fibroblastic cell plasticity. *Virchows Arch* 1994;425:3–24.
3. Lewis J, Chevallier A, Kieny M, et al. Muscle nerve branches do not develop in chick wings devoid of muscle. *J Embryol Exp Morphol* 1981;64:211–232.
4. Sengel P. *Morphogenesis of skin.* Cambridge, UK: Cambridge University Press, 1975.
5. Suzuki S, Oldberg A, Hayman EG, Pierschbacher MD, Ruoslahti E. Complete amino acid sequence of human vitronectin deduced from cDNA: similarity of cell attachment sites in vitronectin and fibronectin. *EMBO J* 1985;4:2519–2524.
6. Stopak D, Harris AK. Connective tissue morphogenesis by fibroblast traction. *Dev Biol* 1982;90:383–398.
7. Hulmes DJS. The collagen superfamily—diverse structures and assemblies. *Essays Biochem* 1992;27:49–67.
8. Prockop DJ. Collagens: molecular biology, diseases and potentials for therapy. *Annu Rev Biochem* 1995;64:403–434.
9. Ramachandran GN. Molecular structure. In: Ramachandran GN,

Reddi AH, eds. *Biochemistry of collagen*. New York: Plenum, 1976:45–84.

10. Engel J, Prockop DJ. The zipper-like folding of collagen triple helices and the effects of mutations that disrupt the zipper. *Ann Rev Biophys Chem* 1991;20:137–152.

11. Shaw LM, Olsen BR. FACIT collagens: diverse molecular bridges in extracellular matrices. *Trends Biochem Sci* 1991;16:191–194.

12. Mayne R, Brewton RG. New members of the collagen superfamily. *Curr Opin Cell Biol* 1993;5:883–890.

13. Van der Rest M, Garbone R. Collagen family proteins. *FASEB J* 1991;5:2814–2823.

14. Jimenez SA, Varga J, Olsen A, Li L, Diaz A, Herhal J, Koch J. Functional analysis of human α1(I) procollagen gene promoter. *J Biol Chem* 1994;269:12684–12691.

15. Slack JL, Parker MI, Bornstein P. Transcriptional repression of the α1(I) collagen gene by *ras* is mediated in part by an intronic AP1 site. *J Cell Biochem* 1995;58:380–392.

16. Chen A, Beno DWA, Davis BH. Suppression of stellate cell type I collagen gene expression involves AP-2 transmodulation of nuclear factor-1–dependent gene transcription. *J Biol Chem* 1996;271:25994–25998.

17. Galera P, Musso M, Ducy P, Karsenty G. c-Krox, a transcriptional regulator of type I collagen gene expression, is preferentially expressed in skin. *Proc Natl Acad Sci USA* 1994;91:9372–9376.

18. Galera P, Park R-W, Ducy P, Mattei M-G, Karsenty G. c-Krox binds to several sites in the promoter of both mouse type I collagen genes. *J Biol Chem* 1996;271:21331–21339.

19. Graves PN, Olsen BR, Fietzek PP, Dickson LA, Pesciotta DM, Hofmann H. Comparison of the NH$_2$-terminal sequence of chick type I preprocollagen chains synthesized in an mRNA-dependent reticulocyte lysate. *Eur J Biochem* 1981;118:363–372.

20. Sandberg LB, Gray WR, Franzblau C. *Elastin and elastic tissue*. New York: Plenum, 1977.

21. Kagan H, Mecham RP, eds. *Regulation of matrix accumulation*. New York: Academic Press, 1986:322–398.

22. Gallop PM, Blumenfeld OO, Seifter S. Structure and metabolism of connective tissue proteins. *Ann Rev Biochem* 1972;41:617–645.

23. Sandberg LB, Weissman N, Smith DW. The purification and partial characterization of a soluble elastin like protein from copper-deficient porcine aorta. *Biochemistry* 1969;8:2940–2949.

24. Sandberg LB, Soskel NJ, Walt MS. Structure of the elastic fiber: An overview. *J Invest Dermatol* 1982;79:128–140.

25. Bashir MM, Indik Z, Yeh H, et al. Characterization of the complete human elastic gene: delineation of unusual features in the 5′-flanking region. *J Biol Chem* 1989;264:8887–8891.

26. Indik Z, Yeh H, Ornstein-Goldstein N, et al. Alternative splicing of human elastin mRNA indicated by sequence analysis of cloned genomic and complementary DNA. *Proc Natl Acad Sci USA* 1987;84:5680–5684.

27. Raju K, Anwar RA. Primary structures of bovine elastin a, b, and c deduced from the sequences of cDNA clones. *J Biol Chem* 1987;262:5755–5762.

28. Yeh H, Ornstein-Goldstein N, Indik Z, et al. Sequence variation of bovine elastin mRNA due to alternative splicing. *Collagen Relat Res* 1987;7:235–247.

29. Zardi L, Carnemolla B, Siri A, et al. Transformed human cells produce a new fibronectin isoform by preferential alternative splicing of a previously unobserved exon. *EMBO J* 1987;6:2337–2342.

30. Mecham RP, Hinek A, Griffin GL, Senior RM, Liotta LA. The elastin receptor shows structural and functional similarities to the 67-kDa tumor cell laminin receptor. *J Biol Chem* 1989;264:16652–16657.

31. Tajima S, Hayashi A, Suzuki T. Elastin expression is upregulated by retinoic acid but not by retinol in chick embryonic skin fibroblasts. *J Dermatol Sci* 1997;15:166–172.

32. McGowan SE, Doro MM, Jackson SK. Endogenous retinoids increase perinatal elastin gene expression in rat lung fibroblasts and fetal explants. *Am J Physiol* 1997;273:L410–L416.

33. Karonen T, Jeskanen L, Keski-Oja J. Transforming growth factor beta 1 and its latent form binding protein-1 associate with elastic fibres in human dermis: accumulation in actinic damage and absence in anetoderma. *Br J Dermatol* 1997;137:51–58.

34. Haynes SL, Shuttleworth CA, Kielty CM. Keratinocytes express fibrillin and assemble microfibrils: implications for dermal matrix organization. *Br J Dermatol* 1997;137:17–23.

35. McGowan SE, Jackson SK, Olson PJ, Parekh T, Gold LI. Exogenous and endogenous transforming growth factors-beta influence elastin gene expression in cultured lung fibroblasts. *Am J Respir Cell Mol Biol* 1997;17:25–35.

36. Kucich U, Rosenbloom JC, Abrams WR, Bashir MM, Rosenbloom J. Stabilization of elastin mRNA by TGF-β: initial characterization of signaling pathway. *Am J Respir Cell Mol Biol* 1997;17:10–16.

37. Del Monaco M, Covello SP, Kennedy SH, Gilinger G, Litwack G, Uitto J. Identification of novel glucocorticoid-response elements in human elastin promoter and demonstration of nucleotide sequence specificity of the receptor binding. *J Invest Dermatol* 1997;108:938–942.

38. Tajima S, Izumi T. Differential *in vitro* responses of elastin expression to basic fibroblast growth factor and transforming growth factor beta 1 in upper, middle and lower dermal fibroblasts. *Arch Dermatol Res* 1996;288:753–756.

39. Rich CB, Nugent MA, Stone P, Foster JA. Elastase release of basic fibroblast growth factor in pulmonary fibroblast cultures results in down-regulation of elastin gene transcription: a role for basic fibroblast growth factor in regulating lung repair. *J Biol Chem* 1996;271:23043–23048.

40. Davidson JM, LuValle PA, Zoia O, Quaglino D Jr, Giro M. Ascorbate differentially regulates elastin and collagen biosynthesis in vascular smooth muscle cells and skin fibroblasts by pretranslational mechanisms. *J Biol Chem* 1997;272:345–352.

41. Hinek A. Biological roles of the non-integrin elastin/laminin receptor. *Biol Chem Hoppe Seyler* 1996;377:471–480.

42. Peterszegi G, Robert AM, Robert L. Presence of the elastin-laminin receptor on human activated lymphocytes. *Compts Rendus Acad Sci III* 1996;319:799–803.

43. Kjellen L, Lindahl U. Proteoglycans: structures and interactions. *Annu Rev Biochem* 1996;60:443–475.

44. Lohmander LS, De Luca S, Nilsson B. Oligosaccharides on proteoglycans from the swarm rat chondrosarcoma. *J Biol Chem* 1980;255:6084–6091.

45. Nilsson B, De Luca S, Lohmander S. Structures of *N*-linked and *O*-linked oligosaccharides on proteoglycans monomer isolated from the swarm rat chondrosarcoma. *J Biol Chem* 1982;257:10920–10927.

46. Stripe NS, Argraves WS, Goetinck PF. Chondrocytes from the cartilage proteoglycan deficient mutant, nanomelia, synthesize greatly reduced levels of the proteoglycan core protein transcript. *Dev Biol* 1987;124:77–81.

47. Vogel KG, Fisher LW. Comparisons of antibody reactivity and enzyme sensitivity between small proteoglycans from bovine tendon, bone and cartilage. *J Biol Chem* 1986;261:11334–11340.

48. Lewandoska K, Choi HU, Rosenberg LC, Zardi L, Culp LA. Fibronectin-mediated adhesion of fibroblasts: inhibition by dermatan sulfate proteoglycan and evidence for a cryptic glycosaminoglycan-binding domain. *J Cell Biol* 1987;105:1443–1454.

49. Ruoslahti E. Structure and biology of proteoglycans. *Ann Rev Cell Biol* 1988;4:229–255.

50. Ruoslahti E, Pierschbacher MD. New perspectives in cell adhesion: RGD and integrins. *Science* 1987;238:491–497.

51. Lark MW, Culp LA. Turnover of heparan sulfate proteoglycans from substratum adhesion sites of murine fibroblasts. *J Biol Chem* 1984;259:212–217.

52. Bernfield M, Kokenyesi R, Kato M, et al. Biology of the syndecans: a family of transmembrane heparan sulfate proteoglycans. *Annu Rev Cell Biol* 1992;8:365–393.

53. Lindahl U, Feingold DS, Roden L. Biosynthesis of heparin. *Trends Biochem Sci* 1986;11:221–225.

54. Kojima T, Leone CW, Marchildon GA, Marcum JA, Rosenberg RD. Isolation and characterization of heparan sulfate proteoglycans produced by cloned rat microvascular endothelial cells. *J Biol Chem* 1992;267:4859–4869.

55. Yayon A, Klgsbrun M, Esko JD, Leder P, Ornitz DM. Cell surface, heparin like molecules are required for binding of basic fibroblast growth factor to its high affinity receptor. *Cell* 1991;64:841–848.

56. Bar-Shavit R, Maoz M, Ginzburg Y, Vlodavsky I. Specific involvement of glypican in thrombin adhesive properties. *J Cell Biochem* 1996;61:278–291.

57. Oldberg A, Hayman EG, Ruoslahti E. Isolation of a chondroitin sulfate proteoglycan from a rat yolk sac tumor and immunochemical demonstration of its cell surface localization. *J Biol Chem* 1987;256:10847–10852.

58. Izzard CS, Radinsky R, Culp LA. Substratum contacts and cytoskeletal reorganization of BABL/c 3T3 cells on a cell-binding fragment and heparin-binding fragments of plasma fibronectin. *Exp Cell Res* 1986; 165:320–336.

59. Ruoslahti E, Engvall E, Hayman E. Fibronectin: current concepts of its structure and function. *Collagen Res* 1981;1:95–128.

60. Kar L, Lai C-S, Wolff CE, Nettesheim D, Sherman S, Johnson ME. ^{1}H NMR-based determination of the three-dimensional structure of the human plasma fibronectin fragment containing inter-chain disulfide bonds. *J Biol Chem* 1993;268:8580–8589.

61. Yamada KM, Kennedy DW. Fibroblast cellular and plasma fibronectin are similar but not identical. *J Cell Biol* 1979;80:492–498.

62. Tamkun JW, Schwarzbauer JE, Hynes RO. A single rat fibronectin gene generates three different mRNAs by alternative splicing of a complex exon. *Proc Natl Acad Sci USA* 1984;81:6140–5144.

63. Chothia C, Jones EY. The molecular structure of cell adhesion molecules. *Annu Rev Biochem* 1997;66:823–862.

64. Schwarzbauer JE. Alternative splicing of fibronectin: three variants, three functions. *Bioessays* 1991;13:527–533.

65. Aota S-I, Nomizu M, Yamada KM. The short amino acid sequence Pro-His-Ser-Arg-Asn in human fibronectin enhances cell-adhesive function. *J Biol Chem* 1994;269:24756–24761.

66. Bowditch RD, Hariharan M, Tominna EF, et al. Identification of a novel integrin binding site in fibronectin: differential utilization by beta 3 integrins. *J Biol Chem* 1994;269:10856–10863.

67. Ruoslahti E. Fibronectin and its receptors. *Annu Rev Biochem* 1988; 57:375–413.

68. Owens RJ, Baralle FE. Mapping the collagen-binding site of human fibronectin by expression in Escherichia coli. *EMBO J* 1986;5: 2825–2830.

69. Kleinman HK, McGoodwin EB, Martin GR. Localization of the binding site for cell attachment in the alpha (I) chain of collagen. *J Biol Chem* 1978;253:5642–5646.

70. Pande H, Calaycay J, Hawke D, Ben-Avram CM, Shively JE. Primary structure of a glycosylated DNA-binding domain in human plasma fibronectin. *J Biol Chem* 1985;260:2301–2306.

71. Greiling D, Clark RA. Fibronectin provides a conduit for fibroblast transmigration from collagenous stroma into fibrin clot provisional matrix. *J Cell Sci* 1997;110:861–870.

72. Beck K, Hunter I, Engel J. Structure and function of laminin: anatomy of a multidomain glycoprotein. *FASEB J* 1990;4:148–160.

73. Timpl R. Macromolecular organization of basement membranes. *Curr Opin Cell Biol* 1996;8:618–624.

74. Kleinman HK, Kibbey MC. Basement membrane regulation of tumor growth and metastasis. *J Natl Inst Health Res* 1991;3:54–55.

75. Hynes RO. Integrins: versatility, modulation and signaling in cell adhesion. *Cell* 1992;69:11–25.

76. Kramer RH, Cheng Y-F, Clyman R. Human microvascular endothelial cells use β1 and β3 integrin receptor complexes to attach to laminin. *J Cell Biol* 1990;111:1233–1243.

77. Lin M-L, Bertics PJ. Laminin responsiveness is associated with changes in fibroblast morphology, motility, and anchorage-independent growth: cell system for examining the interaction between laminin and EGF signaling pathways. *J Cell Physiol* 1995;164:593–604.

78. Erickson HP. Evolution of the tenascin family-implications for function of the C-terminal fibrinogen-like domain. *Perspect Dev Neurobiol* 1994;2:9–19.

79. Hagios C, Koch M, Spring J, Matthias C, Chiquet-Ehrismann R. Tenascin-Y. A protein of novel domain structure is secreted by differentiated fibroblasts of muscle connective tissue. *J Cell Biol* 1996;134: 1499–1512.

80. Norenberg U, Wille H, Wolff JM, Frank R, Rathjen FG. The chicken neural extracellular matrix molecule restrictin: similarity with EGF fibronectin type III and fibrinogen-like motifs. *Neuron* 1992;8: 849–863.

81. Pesheva P, Spiess E, Schachner M. J1-160 and J1-180 are oligodendrocyte-secreted nonpermissive substrates for cell adhesion. *J Cell Biol* 1989;109:1765–1778.

82. Bristow J, Kian M, Tee SE, Gitelman SE, Mellon SH, Miller WL. Tenascin-X: a novel extracellular matrix protein encoded by the human XB gene overlapping P450c21B. *J Cell Biol* 1993;122:265–278.

83. Chiquet-Ehrismann R. Tenascins: a growing family of extracellular matrix proteins. *Experientia* 1995;51:853–862.

84. Rathjen FG, Wolff JM, Chiquet-Ehrismann R. Restrictin: a chick neural extracellular matrix protein involved in cell attachment copurifies with the cell recognition molecules F11. *Development* 1991;113: 151–164.

85. Saga Y, Yagi T, Ikawa Y, Sakakura T, Aizawa S. Mice develop normally without tenascin. *Genes Dev* 1992;6:1821–1831.

86. Lightner VA, Gumkowski F, Bigner DD, Erickson HP. Tenascin/hexabrachion in human skin: biochemical identification and localization by light and electron microscopy. *J Cell Biol* 1989;108:2483–2493.

87. Koukoulis GK, Gould VE, Bhattacharyya A, Gould JE, Howeedy AA, Vitanen I. Tenascin in normal, reactive, hyperplastic and neoplastic tissue: biologic and pathologic implication. *Hum Pathol* 1991;22: 636–643.

88. Gailit J, Clark RA. Wound repair in the context of extracellular matrix. *Curr Opin Cell Biol* 1994;6:717–725.

89. Lacour JP, Vitetta A, Chiquet-Ehrismann R, Pisani A, Ortonne JP. Increased expression of tenascin in the dermis in scleroderma. *Br J Dermatol* 1992;127:328–334.

90. Salter DM. Tenascin is increased in cartilage and synovium from arthritic knees. *Br J Rheumatol* 1993;132:780–786.

91. Makhluf HA, Stepniakowska J, Hoffman S, Smith E, LeRoy C, Trojanowska M. IL-4 upregulates tenascin synthesis in scleroderma and healthy skin fibroblasts. *J Invest Dermatol* 1996;107:856–859.

92. Burch GH, Bedolli MA, McDonough S, Rosenthal SM, Bristow J. Embryonic expression of tenascin-X suggests a role in limb, muscle and heart development. *Dev Dyn* 1995;203:491–504.

93. Chiquet M, Fambrough DM. Chick myotendinous antigen. I. A monoclonal antibody as a marker for tendon and muscle morphogenesis. *J Cell Biol* 1984;98:1926–1936.

94. Sakai T, Furukawa Y, Chiquet-Ehrismann R, et al. Tenascin-X expression in tumor cells and fibroblasts: glucocorticoids as negative regulators in fibroblasts. *J Cell Sci* 1996;109:2069–2077.

95. Chiquet-Ehrismann R, Tannheimer M, Koch M, et al. Tenascin-C expression by fibroblasts is elevated in stressed collagen gels. *J Cell Biol* 1994;127:2093–2101.

96. Borsi L, Balza E, Gaggero B, Allemanni G, Zardi L. The alternative splicing pattern of the tenascin-C pre-mRNA is controlled by the extracellular pH. *J Biol Chem* 1995;270:6243–6245.

97. Holmes R. Preparation from human serum of an alpha-one protein which induces the immediate growth of unadapted cells *in vitro*. *J Cell Biol* 1967;32:297–308.

98. Yamada KM. Cell surface interactions with extracellular materials. *Annu Rev Biochem* 1983;52:761–799.

99. Ruoslahti E, Suzuki S, Hayman EG, Ill CR, Pierschbacher MD. Purification and characterization of vitronectin. *Methods Enzymol* 1987;144:430–437.

100. Urushihara H, Yamada KM. Evidence for involvement of more than one class of glycoprotein in cell interactions with fibronectin. *J Cell Physiol* 1986;126:323–332.

101. Ruoslahti E, Pierschbacher MD. Arg-Gly-Asp: a versatile cell recognition signal. *Cell* 1986;44:517–518.

102. Pytela R, Pierschbacher MD, Ginsberg MH, Plow EF, Ruoslahti E. Platelet membrane glycoprotein IIb/IIIa: member of a family of Arg-Gly-Asp-specific adhesion receptors. *Science* 1986;231:1559–1562.

103. Shaffer MC, Foley TP, Barnes DW. Quantitation of spreading factor in human biologic fluids. *J Lab Clin Med* 1984;103:783–791.

104. Barnes DW, Silnutzer J, See C, Shaffer M. Characterization of human serum spreading factor with monoclonal antibody. *Proc Natl Acad Sci USA* 1983;80:1362–1366.

105. Hayman EG, Pierschbacher MD, Ohgren Y, Ruoshlati E. Serum spreading factor (vitronectin) is present at the cell surface and in tissues. *Proc Natl Acad Sci USA* 1983;80:4003–4007.

106. Kitagaki-Ogawa H, Yatohgo T, Izumi M, et al. Diversities in animal vitronectins: differences in molecular weight, immunoreactivity and carbohydrate chains. *Biochim Biophys Acta* 1990;1033:49–56.

107. Jenne D, Stanley KK. Molecular cloning of S-protein: a link between complement, coagulation, and cell-substrate adhesion. *EMBO J* 1985; 4:3153–3157.

108. Suzuki S, Pierschbacher MD, Hayman EG, Nguyen K, Ohgren Y, Ruoslahti E. Domain structure of vitronectin: alignment of active sites. *J Biol Chem* 1984;259:15307–15314.

109. Tschopp J, Masson D, Schafer S, Peitsch M, Preissner KT. The heparin binding domain of S-protein/vitronectin binds to complement components C7, C8, C9 and performin from cytolytic T-cells and inhibits their lytic activities. *Biochemistry* 1988;27:4103–4109.

110. Trautmann A, Feuerstein B, Ernst N, Brocker EB, Klein CE. Heterotypic cell-cell adhesion of human mast cells to fibroblasts. *Arch Dermatol Res* 1997;289:194–203.

111. Weaver AM, Hussaini IM, Mazar A, Henkin J, Gonias SL. Embryonic fibroblasts that are genetically deficient in low density lipoprotein receptor-related protein demonstrate increased activity of the urokinase receptor system and accelerated migration on vitronectin. *J Biol Chem* 1997;272:14372–14379.

112. Anilkumar N, Bhattacharya AK, Manogaran PS, Pande G. Modulation of alpha 5 beta 1 and alpha V beta 3 integrins on the cell surface during mitosis. *J Cell Biochem* 1996;61:338–349.

113. Parsons SL, Watson SA, Brown PD, Collins HM, Steele RJC. Matrix metalloproteinases. *Br J Surg* 1997;84:160–166.

114. Basset P, Bellocq JP, Wolf C, et al. A novel metalloproteinase gene specifically expressed in stromal cells of breast carcinomas. *Nature* 1990;348:699–704.

115. Startex PM, Barratt AJ, Burleigh MC. The degradation of articular collagen by neutrophil proteinases. *Biochem Biophys Acta* 1977;183:386–397.

116. Woolley DE. Mammalian collagenases. In: Piez KA, Reddi AH, eds. *Extracellular matrix biochemistry*. New York: Elsevier, 1984;119–157.

117. Miller EJ, Harris ED Jr, Chung E. Cleavage of type II and III collagens with mammalian collagenase: site of cleavage and primary structure at the NH$_2$-terminal portion of the smaller fragment released from both collagens. *Biochemistry* 1976;15:787–792.

118. Everts V, van der Zee E, Creemers L, Beersten W. Phagocytosis and intracellular digestion of collagen: its role in turnover and remodelling. *Histochem J* 1996;28:229–245.

119. Okada Y, Gonoji Y, Naka K, et al. Matrix metalloproteinase 9 (92-kDa gelatinase/type IV collagenase) from HT1080 human fibrosarcoma cells. *J Biol Chem* 1992;267:21712–21719.

120. Okada Y, Tsuchiya H, Shimizu H, et al. Induction and stimulation of 92-kDa gelatinase/type IV collagenase production in osteosarcoma and fibrosarcoma cell lines by tumor necrosis factor alpha. *Biochem Biophys Res Commun* 1990;171:610–617.

121. Suzuki K, Enghild JJ, Morodomi T, Salvesen G, Nagase H. Mechanisms of activation of tissue procollagenase by matrix metalloproteinase 3 (stromelysin). *Biochemistry* 1990;29:10251–10270.

122. Sang QA, Bodden MK, Windsor LJ. Activation of human progelatinase A by collagenase and matrilysin: activation of procollagenase by matrilysin. *J Protein Chem* 1996;15:243–253.

123. Davies M, Barrett AJ, Travis J, et al. The degradation of human glomerular basement membrane with purified lysosomal proteinases. *Clin Sci Mol Med* 1977;54:233–240.

124. Mainardi CL, Seyer JM, Kang AH. Type specific collagenolysis: a type V collagen-degrading enzyme from macrophages. *Biochem Biophys Res Commun* 1980;97:1108–1115.

125. Mainardi CL, Dixit SN, Kang AH. Degradation of type IV (basement membrane) collagen by a proteinase isolated from human polymorphonuclear leukocyte granules. *J Biol Chem* 1980;255:5435–5441.

126. Mehindate K, Al-Daccak R, Aoudjit F, et al. Interleukin-4, transforming growth factor 1, and dexamethasone inhibit superantigen-induced prostaglandin E$_2$-dependent collagenase gene expression through their action on cyclooxygenase-2 and cytosolic phospholipase A$_2$. *Lab Invest* 1996;75:529–538.

127. Hiraoka K, Sasaguri Y, Kamiya S, Inoue A, Morimatsu M. Cell proliferation-related production of metalloproteinases 1 (tissue collagenase) and 3 (stromelysin) by cultured human rheumatoid synovial fibroblasts. *Biochem Int* 1992;27:1083–1091.

128. DeCastro R, Zhang Y, Guo H, et al. Human keratinocytes express EMMPRIN an extracellular matrix metalloproteinase inducer. *J Invest Dermatol* 1996;106:1260–1265.

129. Cullen B, Silcock D, Brown LJ, Gosiewska A, Geesin JC. The differential regulation and secretion of proteinases from fetal and neonatal fibroblasts by growth factors. *Int J Biochem Cell Biol* 1997;29:241–250.

130. Mauch C, Adelmann-Grill B, Hatamochi A, Krieg T. Collagenase gene expression in fibroblasts is regulated by a three dimensional contact with collagen. *FEBS Lett* 1989;250:301–305.

131. Huttenlocher A, Werb Z, Tremble P, Huhtala P, Rosenberg L, Damsky CH. Decorin regulates collagenase gene expression in fibroblasts adhering to vitronectin. *Matrix Biol* 1996;15:239–250.

132. Ito A, Mukaiyama A, Itoh Y, et al. Degradation of interleukin 1 beta by matrix metalloproteinases. *J Biol Chem* 1996;271:14657–14660.

133. MacNaul KL, Chartrain N, Lark M, Tocci MJ, Hutchinson NI. Discoordinate expression of stromelysin, collagenase, and tissue inhibitor of metalloproteinases-1 in rheumatoid human synovial fibroblasts. *J Biol Chem* 1990;265:17238–17245.

134. McDonnell SE, Kerr LD, Matrisian LM. Epidermal growth factor stimulation of stromelysin mRNA in rat fibroblasts requires induction of proto-oncogenes c-*fos* and c-*jun* and activation of protein kinase C. *Mol Cell Biol* 1990;10:4284–4293.

135. Migita K, Eguchi K, Tominaga M, Origuchi T, Kawabe Y, Nagataki S. Beta 2-microglobulin induces stromelysin production by human synovial fibroblasts. *Biochem Biophys Res Commun* 1997;239:621–625.

136. Ahmad A, Marshall JF, Bassett P, Anglard P, Hart IR. Modulation of human stromelysin 3 promoter activity and gene expression by human breast cancer cells. *Int J Cancer* 1997;73:290–296.

137. Guerin E, Ludwig MG, Basset P, Anglard P. Stromelysin-3 induction and interstitial collagenase repression by retinoic acid: therapeutical implication of receptor-selective retinoids dissociating transactivation and AP-1–mediated transrepression. *J Biol Chem* 1997;272:11088–11095.

138. Cawston TE, Curry VA, Clark IM, Hazelman BL. Identification of a new metalloproteinase inhibitor that forms tight-binding complexes with collagenase. *Biochem J* 1990;269:183–187.

139. Matrisian LM. The matrix-degrading metalloproteinases. *Bioessays* 1992;14:455–463.

140. Hayakawa T, Yamashita K, Ohuchi E, Shinagawa A. Cell growth-promoting activity of tissue inhibitor of metalloproteinases-2 (TIMP-2). *J Cell Sci* 1994;107:2373–2379.

141. Yamashita K, Suzuki M, Iwata H, et al. Tyrosine phosphorylation is crucial for growth signaling by tissue inhibitors of metalloproteinases (TIMP-1 and TIMP-2). *FEBS Lett* 1996;396:103–107.

142. Blenis J, Hawkes SP. Transformation-sensitive protein associated with the cell substratum of chicken embryo fibroblasts. *Proc Natl Acad Sci USA* 1983;80:770–774.

143. Pavloff NP, Staskus PW, Kishnani NS, Hawkes SP. A new inhibitor of metalloproteinases from chicken: ChIMP-3. A third member of the TIMP family. *J Biol Chem* 1992;267:17321–17326.

144. Yang TT, Hawkes SP. Role of the 21-kDa protein TIMP-3 in oncogenic transformation of cultured chicken embryo fibroblasts. *Proc Natl Acad Sci USA* 1992;89:10676–10680.

145. Anande-Apte B, Bao L, Smith R, Iwata K, Olsen BR, Zetter B, Apte SS. A review of tissue inhibitor of metalloproteinases-3 (TIMP-3) and experimental analysis of its effect on primary tumor growth. *Biochem Cell Biol* 1996;74:853–859.

146. Gosline JM, Rosenbloom J. Elastin. In: Piez KA, Reddi AH, eds. *Extracellular matrix biochemistry*. New York: Elsevier, 1984:191–227.

147. Briggaman RA, Schechter NM, Fraki J. Interleukin-1β stimulates fibroblast elastase activity. *Br J Dermatol* 1991;124:538–541.

148. Homsy R, Pelletier-Lebon P, Tixier JM. Characterization of human skin fibroblast elastase activity. *J Invest Dermatol* 1988;91:472–477.

149. Carmassi F, deNegri F, Morale M, Song KY, Chung SI. Fibrin degradation in the synovial fluid of rheumatoid arthritis patients: a model for extravascular fibrinolysis. *Semin Thromb Hemost* 1996;22:489–496.

150. Thompson RW, Parks WC. Role of matrix metalloproteinases in abdominal aortic aneurysms. *Ann N Y Acad Sci* 1996;800:157–174.

151. Sasaki T, Mann K, Murphy G, Chu ML, Timpl R. Different susceptibilities of fibulin-1 and fibulin-2 to cleavage by matrix metalloproteinases and other tissue proteases. *Eur J Biochem* 1996;240:427–434.

152. Tyagi SC, Kumar SG, Alla SR, Reddy HK, Voelker DJ, Janicki JS. Extracellular matrix regulation of metalloproteinase and antiproteinase in human heart fibroblast cells. *J Cell Physiol* 1996;167:137–147.

153. Trevani AS, Andonegui G, Giordano M, et al. Neutrophil apoptosis induced by proteolytic enzymes. *Lab Invest* 1996;74:711–721.

154. Sandy JD, Brown HLG, Lowther DA. Degradation of proteoglycan in articular cartilage. *Biochem Biophys Acta* 1978;543:536–544.

155. Truppe W, Kresse H. Uptake of proteoglycans and sulfated glycosaminoglycans by culture skin fibroblasts. *Eur J Biochem* 1978;85:351–356.

156. Wateson A, Amado R, Ingmar B, et al. Degradation of chondroitin sulphate by lysosomal enzymes from embryonic chick cartilage. *Protides Biol Fluids Proc Calloq Bruges* 1975;22:431–435.

157. Masure S, Opdenakker G. Cytokine-mediated proteolysis in tissue remodelling. *Experentia* 1989;45:542–549.

158. Hakomori S, Fukuda M, Sekiguchi K, et al. Fibronectin, laminin, and other extracellular glycoproteins. In: Piez KA, Reddi AH, eds. *Extracellular matrix biochemistry.* New York: Elsevier, 1984:229–275.

159. Conca W, Kaplan PB, Krane SM. Increases in levels of procollagenase messenger RNA in cultured fibroblast-induced by human recombinant interleukin 1b or serum follow c-*jun* expression and are dependent on new protein synthesis. *J Clin Invest* 1989;83:1753–1757.

160. Brenner DA, O Hara M, Angel P, Chojkier M, Karin M. Prolonged activation of c-*jun* and collagenase genes by tumor necrosis factor-α. *Nature* 1989;337:661–663.

161. Buckley-Sturrock A, Woodward SC, Senior RM, Griffin GL, Klagsbrun M, Davidson JM. Differential stimulation of collagenase and chemotactic activity in fibroblasts derived from rat wound repair tissue and human skin by growth factors. *J Cell Physiol* 1989;138: 70–78.

162. Rekdal O, Osterud B, Svendsen JS, Winberg JO. Evidence for exclusive role of the p55 tumor necrosis factor receptor in mediating the TNF-induced collagenase expression by human dermal fibroblasts. *J Invest Dermatol* 1996;107:565–568.

163. Okada A, Tomasetto C, Lutz Y, Bellocq JP, Rio MC, Basset P. Expression of matrix metalloproteinases during rat skin wound healing: evidence that membrane type-1 matrix metalloproteinase is a stromal activator of pro-gelatinase A. *J Cell Biol* 1997;137:67–77.

164. Zafarullah M, Su S, Martel-Pelletier J, et al. Tissue inhibitor of metalloproteinase-2 (TIMP-2) mRNA is constitutively expressed in bovine, human normal, and osteoarthritic articular chondrocytes. *J Cell Biochem* 1996;60:211–217.

165. Nemoto O, Yamada H, Mukaida M, Shimmei M. Stimulation of TIMP-1 production by oncostatin M in human articular cartilage. *Arthritis Rheum* 1996;39:560–566.

166. Maier R, Ganu V, Lotz M. Interleukin-11, an inducible cytokine in human articular chondrocytes and synoviocytes, stimulates the production of the tissue inhibitor of metalloproteinases. *J Biol Chem* 1993;268:21527–21532.

167. Guerne P-A, Carson DA, Lotz M. IL-6 production by human articular chondrocytes: modulation of its synthesis by cytokines, growth factors, and hormones *in vitro. J Immunol* 1990;144:499–505.

168. Rossi P, Karsenty G, Roberts AB, Roche NS, Sporn MB, Crombrugghe B. A nuclear factor 1 binding site mediates the transcriptional activation of a type I collagen promoter by transforming growth factor-β. *Cell* 1988;52:405–414.

169. Greenwel P, Inagaki Y, Hu W, Walsh M, Ramirez F. Sp1 is required for the early response of α2(I) collagen to transforming growth factor-β1. *J Biol Chem* 1997;272:19738–19745.

170. Ritzenthaler JB, Goldstein RH, Fine A, Lichtler AC, Rowe DW, Smith BD. Transforming growth factor β activation elements in the distal promoter region of the rate α1 type I collagen gene. *Biochem J* 1991;280:157–162.

171. Mauviel A, Lapiere JC, Halcin C, Evans CH, Uitto J. Differential cytokine regulation of type I and type VII collagen gene expression in cultured human dermal fibroblasts. *J Biol Chem* 1994;269:25–28.

172. Postlethwaite AE, Raghow R, Stricklin GP, Poppleton H, Seyer JM, Kang AH. Modulation of fibroblast functions by interleukin-1: increased steady-state accumulation of type I procollagen mRNAs and stimulation of other functions but not chemotaxis by human recombinant interleukin-1α and β. *J Cell Biol* 1988;106:311–318.

173. Burridge K, Chrzanowska-Wodnickam M. Focal adhesions, contractility and signaling. *Annu Rev Cell Dev Biol* 1996;12:463–519.

174. Massia SP, Hubbel JA. An RGC spacing of 440 nm is sufficient for integrin α$_v$β$_3$-mediated fibroblast spreading and 140 nm for focal contact and stress fiber formation. *J Cell Biol* 1991;114:1089–1100.

175. DePasquale JA, Izzard CS. Evidence for an actin-containing cytoplasmic precursor of the focal contact and the timing of incorporation of vinculin at the focal contact. *J Cell Biol* 1987;105:2803–2809.

176. DePasquale JA, Izzard CS. Accumulation of talin in nodes at the edge of the lamellipodium and separate incorporation into adhesion plaques at focal contacts in fibroblasts. *J Cell Biol* 1991;113: 1351–1359.

177. Pavalko FM, Burridge K. Disruption of the actin cytoskeleton after microinjection of proteolytic fragments of α-actinin. *J Cell Biol* 1991;114:481–491.

178. Nuckolls GH, Romer LH, Burridge K. Microinjection of antibodies against talin inhibits the spreading and migration of fibroblasts. *J Cell Sci* 1992;102:753–762.

179. Lo SH, Janmey PA, Hartwig JH, Chen LB. Interactions of tensin with actin and identification of its three distinct actin-binding domains. *J Cell Biol* 1994;125:1067–1075.

180. Weekes J, Barry ST, Critchley DR. Acidic phospholipids inhibit the intramolecular association between the N- and C-terminal regions of vinculin exposing actin-binding and protein kinase C phosphorylation sites. *Biochem J* 1996;314:827–832.

181. Gilmore AP, Burridge K. Regulation of vinculin binding to talin and actin by phosphatidylinistol-4-5-bisphosphate. *Nature* 1996;381: 531–535.

182. Ridley AJ, Hall A. The small GTP binding protein rho regulates the assembly of focal adhesions and actin stress fibers in response to growth factors. *Cell* 1992;70:389–399.

183. Nobes CD, Hawkins P, Stephens L, Hall A. Activation of the small GTP binding proteins rho and rac by growth factor receptors. *J Cell Sci* 1995;108:225–233.

184. Chong LD, Raynor-Kaplan A, Bokoch GM, Schwartz MA. The small GTP-binding protein Rho regulates a phosphatidylinositol 4-phosphate 5-kinase in mammalian cells. *Cell* 1994;79:507–513.

185. Ginsberg MH, Xiaoping D, O'Toole TE, Loftus JC, Plow EF. Platelet integrins. *Thromb Haemost* 1993;70:87–93.

186. Clark EA, Brugge JS. Integrins and signal transduction pathways: the road taken. *Science* 1995;268:233–239.

187. Schwartz MA, Schaller MD, Ginsberg MH. Integrins: emerging paradigms of signal transduction. *Annu Rev Cell Biol* 1995;11:549–599.

188. Gailit J, Clark RA. Studies *in vitro* on the role of alpha v and beta 1 integrins in the adhesion of human dermal fibroblasts to provisional matrix proteins fibronectin, vitronectin, and fibrinogen. *J Invest Dermatol* 1996;106:102–108.

189. Gailit J, Clarke C, Newman D, Tonnesen MG, Mosesson MW, Clark RA. Human fibroblasts bind directly to fibrinogen at RGD sites through integrin alpha(v)beta 3. *Exp Cell Res* 1997;232:118–126.

190. Asakura S, Niwa K, Tomozawa T, et al. Fibroblasts spread on immobilized fibrin monomer by mobilizing a beta 1-class integrin together with a vitronectin receptor alpha v beta 3 on their surface. *J Biol Chem* 1997;272:8824–8829.

191. Abercrombie M, Heaysman JEM, Pegrum SM. The locomotion of fibroblasts in culture. IV: Electron microscopy of the leading lamella. *Exp Cell Res* 1970;67:359–367.

192. Abercrombie M, Heaysman JEM, Pegrum SM. Locomotion of fibroblasts in culture. V: Surface marking with conconavalin A. *Exp Cell Res* 1972;73:536–539.

193. Baum JL. Source of the fibroblast in central corneal wound healing. *Arch Ophthalmol* 1972;85:473–477.

194. Harris A, Dunn G. Centripetal transport of attached particles on both surfaces of moving fibroblasts. *Exp Cell Res* 1972;73:519–523.

195. Cohen K, Moore CD, Diegelmann RF. Onset and localization of collagen synthesis during wound healing in open rat skin wounds. *Proc Soc Exp Biol* 1979;160:458–462.

196. Schilling JA. Wound healing. *Surg Clin North Am* 1976;56:859–874.

197. Postlethwaite AE, Snyderman R, Kang AH. The chemotactic attraction of human fibroblasts to a lymphocyte-derived factor. *J Exp Med* 1976;144:1188–1203.

198. Postlethwaite AE, Kang AH. Latent lymphokines: isolation of human latent lymphocyte-derived chemotactic factor for fibroblasts. In: Oppenheim JJ, Cohen S, eds. *Interleukin lymphokines and cytokines. Proceedings of the Third International Lymphokine Workshop.* New York: Academic Press, 1983:535–54l.

199. Postlethwaite AE, Kang AH. Characterization of guinea pig lymphocyte-derived chemotactic factor for fibroblasts. *J Immunol* 1980;124: 1462–1466.

200. Postlethwaite AE, Seyer JM. Stimulation of fibroblast chemotaxis by human recombinant tumor necrosis factor α (TNFα) and a synthetic TNFα 31-68 peptide. *J Exp Med* 1990;172:1749–1756.

201. Postlethwaite AE, Seyer JM. Fibroblast chemotaxis induction by human recombinant interleukin-4: identification by synthetic peptide analysis of two chemotactic domains residing in amino acid sequences 70–88 and 89–122. *J Clin Invest* 1991;87:2147–2152.

202. Postlethwaite AE, Keski-Oja J, Moses HL, Kang AH. Stimulation of the chemotactic migration of human fibroblasts by transforming growth factor β. *J Exp Med* 1987;165:251–256.

203. Seppa H, Seppa S, Yamada KM. The cell binding fragment of

fibronectin and platelet-derived growth factor are chemoattractants for fibroblasts. *J Cell Biol* 1980;87:323a(abst).

204. Senior RM, Huang JS, Griffin GL, Deuel TF. Dissociation of the chemotactic and mitogenic activities of PDGF by human neutrophil elastase. *J Cell Biol* 1985;100:351–356.

205. Senior RM, Huang JS, Griffin GL, Deuel TF. Dissociation of the chemotactic and mitogenic activities of platelet-derived growth factor by human neutrophil elastase. *J Cell Biol* 1985;100:351–356.

206. Osornio-Vargas AR, Lindroos PM, Coin PG, Budgett A, Hernandez-Rodriguez NA, Bonner JC. Maximal PDGF-induced lung fibroblast chemotaxis requires PDGF receptor α. *Am J Physiol* 1996;271:L93–L99.

207. Postlethwaite AE, Seyer JM. Identification of a chemotactic epitope in human TGF-β1 spanning amino acid residues 368–374. *J Cell Physiol* 1995;164:587–592.

208. Nishimura F, Terranova VP. Comparative study of the chemotactic responses of periodontal ligament cells and gingival fibroblasts to polypeptide growth factors. *J Dent Res* 1996;75:986–992.

209. Peacock AJ, Dawes KE, Shock A, Gray AJ, Reeves JT, Laurent GJ. Endothelin-1 and endothelin-3 induce chemotaxis and replication of pulmonary artery fibroblasts. *Am J Respir Cell Mol Biol* 1992;7:492–499.

210. Barnes PJ. Endothelins and pulmonary diseases. *J Appl Physiol* 1994;77:1051–1059.

211. Elenius K, Paul S, Allison G, Sun J, Klagsbrun M. Activation of HER4 by heparin-binding EGF-like growth factor stimulates chemotaxis but not proliferation. *EMBO J* 1997;16:1268–1278.

212. Harrison NK, Dawes KE, Kwon OJ, Barnes PJ, Laurent GJ, Chung KF. Effects of neuropeptides on human lung fibroblast proliferation and chemotaxis. *Am J Physiol* 1995;268:278–283.

213. Kahler CM, Bellmann R, Reinisch N, Schratzberger P, Gruber B, Wiedermann CJ. Stimulation of human skin fibroblast migration by the neuropeptide secreteurin. *Eur J Pharmacol* 1996;304:135–139.

214. Anichini E, Fibbi G, Pucci M, Caldini R, Chevanne M, Del Rosso M. Production of second messengers following chemotactic and mitogenic urokinase-receptor interaction in human fibroblasts and mouse fibroblasts transfected. *Exp Cell Res* 1994;213:438–448.

215. Petering H, Hochstetter R, Kimmig D, Smolarski R, Kapp A, Elsner J. Detection of MCP-4 in dermal fibroblasts and its activation of the respiratory burst in human eosinophils. *J Immunol* 1998;160:555–558.

216. Uguccioni M, Loetscher P, Forssmann U, et al. Monocyte chemotactic protein 4 (MCP-4) a novel structural and functional analogue of MCP-3 and eotaxin. *J Exp Med* 1996;183:2379–2384.

217. Gruber BL, Kew R, Jelaska A, et al. Human mast cells activate fibroblasts: tryptase is a fibrogenic factor stimulating collagen messenger ribonucleic acid synthesis and fibroblast chemotaxis. *J Immunol* 1997;158:2310–2317.

218. Postlethwaite AE, Snyderman R, Kang AH. Generation of a fibroblast chemotactic factor in serum by activation of complement. *J Clin Invest* 1979;64:1379–1385.

219. Senior RM, Griffin GL, Perez HD, et al. Human C5a and C5a des arg exhibit chemotactic activity for fibroblasts. *J Immunol* 1988;141:3570–3574.

220. Postlethwaite AE, Seyer JM, Kang AH. Chemotactic attraction of human fibroblasts to type I, II and III collagens and collagen-derived peptides. *Proc Natl Acad Sci USA* 1978;75:871–875.

221. Postlethwaite AE. Cell-cell interaction in collagen biosynthesis and fibroblast migration. In: Weissmann G, ed. *Advances in inflammation research*. New York: Raven Press, 1983:27–55.

222. Chiang TM, Postlethwaite AE, Beachey EH, Seyer JM, Kang AH. Binding of chemotactic collagen peptides to fibroblasts: the relationship to fibroblast chemotaxis. *J Clin Invest* 1978;62:916–922.

223. Postlethwaite AE, Keski-Oja J, Kang AH. Induction of fibroblast chemotaxis by fibronectin: localization of the chemotactic region to a 140,000 molecular weight. *J Exp Med* 1981;153:494–499.

224. Senior RM, Griffin GL, Mecham RP. Chemotactic responses of fibroblasts to tropoelastin and elastin-derived peptides. *J Clin Invest* 1982;70:614–618.

225. Senior RM, Griffin GL, Mecham RP, et al. Val-Gly-Val-Ala-Pro-Gly, a repeating peptide in elastin, is chemotactic for fibroblasts and monocytes. *J Cell Biol* 1984;99:870–874.

226. Mensing H, Czarnetozki BM. Leukotriene B4 induces *in vitro* fibroblast chemotaxis. *J Invest Dermatol* 1984;82:9–12.

227. Bleiberg I, Harvey AK, Smale G, Grotendorst GR. Identification of a PDGF-like mitoattractant produced by NIH/3T3 cells after transformation with SV40. *J Cell Biol* 1985;123:161–166.

228. Geiger B. A 130 K protein from chicken gizzard: its localization at the termini of microfilament bundles in cultured chicken cells. *Cell* 1979;18:193–205.

229. Palka JA, Karna E, Miltyk W. Fibroblast chemotaxis and prolidase activity modulation by insulin-like growth factor II and mannose 6-phosphate. *Mol Cell Biochem* 1997;168:177–183.

230. Soma Y, Takehara K, Ishibashi Y. Alteration of the chemotactic response of human skin fibroblasts to PDGF by growth factors. *Exp Cell Res* 1994;212:274–277.

231. Stossel TP. On the crawling of animal cells. *Science* 1993;260:1086–1094.

232. Sun H-Q, Kwaitkowska K, Wooten DC, Yin HL. Effects of CapG overexpression on agonist-induced motility and second messenger generation. *J Cell Biol* 1995;129:147–156.

233. Young CL, Southwick FS, Weber A. Kinetics of the interaction of a 41-kilodalton macrophage capping protein with actin: promotion of nucleation during prolongation of the lag period. *Biochemistry* 1990;29:2232–2240.

234. Yu F-X, Johnson PA, Sudhof TC, Yin HL. gCap39, a calcium ion- and polyphosphoinositide-regulated actin capping protein. *Biochemistry* 1990;29:2232–2240.

235. Yu F-X, Zhou D, Yin HL. Chimeric and truncated gCap39 elucidate the requirements for actin filament severing and end capping by the gelsolin family of proteins. *J Biol Chem* 1991;266:19269–19275.

236. Ochs ME, Postlethwaite AE, Kang AH. Identification of a protein in sera of normal individuals that inhibits fibroblast chemotactic and random migration *in vitro*. *J Invest Dermatol* 1987;88:183–190.

237. Adelmann-Grill BC, Hein R, Wach F, Krieg T. Inhibition of fibroblast chemotaxis by recombinant human interferon γ and interferon α. *J Cell Physiol* 1987;130:270–275.

238. Lesur O, Bernard A, Arsalane K, et al. Clara cell protein (CC-16) induces a phospholipase A2-mediated inhibition of fibroblast migration *in vitro*. *Am J Respir Crit Care Med* 1995;152:290–297.

239. Miele L, Cordella-Miel E, Facchiano A, Mukherjee AB. Novel anti-inflammatory peptides from the region of the highest similarity between uteroglobin and lipocortin I. *Nature* 1988;335:726–730.

240. Nakamura Y, Romberger DJ, Tate L, et al. Cigarette inhibits lung fibroblast and chemotaxis. *Am J Respir Crit Care Med* 1995;151:1497–1503.

241. Yarden Y, Escobedo JA, Kuang WJ, et al. Structure of the receptor for platelet-derived growth factor helps define a family of closely related growth factor receptors. *Nature* 1986;323:226–232.

242. Bellas RE, Bendori R, Farmer SR. Epidermal growth factor activation of vinculin and β1 integrin gene transcription in quiescent Swiss 3T3 cells. *J Biol Chem* 1991;266:12008–12014.

243. Rosengurt E. Early signals in the mitogenic response. *Science* 1986;234:161–166.

244. Handler JA, Danilowicz RM, Eling TE. Mitogenic signaling of epidermal growth factor (EGF) but not platelet-derived growth factor, requires arachidonic acid metabolism in BALB/c3T3 cells: modulation of EGF-dependent c-*myc* expression by prostaglandins. *J Biol Chem* 1990;265:3669–3673.

245. Besterman JM, Watson SP, Cuatrecasas P. Lack of association of epidermal growth factor-, insulin-, and serum-induced mitogenesis with stimulation of phosphoinositide degradation in BALB/c3T3 fibroblasts. *J Biol Chem* 1986;261:723–727.

246. Raines EW, Dower SK, Ross R. Interleukin-1 mitogenic activity for fibroblasts and smooth muscle cells is due to PDGF-AA. *Science* 1989;243:393–396.

247. Paulsson Y, Austgulen R, Hofsli E, Heldin CH, Westermark B, Nissen-Meyer J. Tumor necrosis factor-induced expression of platelet-derived growth factor A-chain messenger RNA in fibroblasts. *Exp Cell Res* 1989;180:490–496.

248. Paulsson Y, Hammacher A, Heldin C-H, Westermark B. Possible positive autocrine feedback in the prereplicate phase of human fibroblasts. *Nature* 1987;328:715–717.

249. Battegay EJ, Raines EW, Ross R. Biphasic modulation of proliferation of quiescent human arterial smooth muscle cells by TGF-β. *FASEB J* 1990;4:A889.

250. Carpenter G, Wahl MI. Peptide growth factors and their receptors. In: Sporn MB, Roberts AB, eds. *Handbook of experimental pharmacology*, vol 95. New York: Springer-Verlag, 1990:69–171.

251. Leof EB, Proper JA, Getz MJ, Moses HL. Transforming growth factor type beta regulation of actin mRNA. *J Cell Physiol* 1986;127:83–88.

252. Ignotz RA, Massague J. Transforming growth factor-beta stimulates the expression of fibronectin and collagen and their incorporation into the extracellular matrix. *J Biol Chem* 1986;261:4337–4345.

253. Massague J. The TGF-beta family of growth and differentiation factors. *Cell* 1987;49:437–438.

254. Giaid A, Michel RP, Steward DJ, Sheppard M, Corrin B, Hamid Q. Expression of endothelin-1 in lungs of patients with cryptogenic fibrosing alveolitis. *Lancet* 1993;341:1550–1554.

255. Johnson RL, Ziff M. Lymphokine stimulation of collagen accumulation. *J Clin Invest* 1976;58:240–248.

256. Kravis TC, Ahmed A, Brown TE, Fulmer JD, Crystal RG. Pathogenic mechanisms in pulmonary fibrosis. Collagen-induced migration inhibition factor production and cytotoxicity mediated by lymphocyte. *J Clin Invest* 1976;58:1233–1240.

257. Kondo H, Rabin BS, Rodnan GP. Cutaneous antigen stimulating lymphokine production by lymphocytes of patients with progressive systemic sclerosis (scleroderma). *J Clin Invest* 1976;58:1388–1412.

258. Stuart JM, Postlethwaite AE, Kang AH. Evidence for cell-mediated immunity to collagen in progressive systemic sclerosis. *J Lab Clin Med* 1976;88:601–607.

259. Matsuyama T, Yamada A, Kay J, et al. Activation of CD4 cells by fibronectin and anti-CD3 antibody: a synergistic effect mediated by the VLA-5 fibronectin receptor complex. *J Exp Med* 1989;170:1133–1148.

260. Dang NH, Torimoto Y, Schlossman SF, Morimoto C. Human CD4 helper T cell activation: functional involvement of two distinct collagen receptors, 1F7 and VLA integrin family. *J Exp Med* 1990;172:649–652.

261. Hemesath TJ, Marton LS, Stefansson K. Inhibition of T cell activation by the extracellular matrix protein tenascin. *J Immunol* 1994;152:5199–5207.

262. Gilat D, Cahalon L, Hershkoviz R, Lider O. Interplay of T cells and cytokines in the context of enzymatically modified extracellular matrix. *Immunol Today* 1996;17:16–20.

263. Fridman R, Lider O, Naparstek Y, Fuks Z, Vlodavsky I, Cohen IR. Soluble antigen induces T lymphocytes to secrete an endoglycosidase that degrades the heparan sulfate moiety of subendothelial extracellular matrix. *J Cell Physiol* 1987;130:85–92.

264. Hershkoviz R, Goldkorn I, Lider O. Tumour necrosis factor-alpha interacts with laminin and functions as a pro-adhesive cytokine. *Immunology* 1995;85:125–130.

265. Stuart JM, Postlethwaite AE, Townes AS, et al. Cell-mediated immunity to collagen α chains in rheumatoid arthritis and other rheumatic diseases. *Am J Med* 1980;69:13–18.

266. Gurram M, Pahwa S, Frieri M. Increased interleukin 6 production in peripheral blood mononuclear cells from patients with systemic sclerosis. *J Allergy Clin Immunol* 1992;89:291a.

267. Hawrylko E, Spertus A. Mele CA, Oster N, Frieri M. Increased interleukin-2 production in response to human type 1 collagen stimulation in patients with systemic sclerosis. *Arthritis Rheum* 1991;34:580–587.

268. Thorens B, Mermod J-J, Vassalli P. Phagocytosis and inflammatory stimuli induce GM-CSF mRNA in macrophages through posttranscriptional regulation. *Cell* 1987;48:671–679.

269. Eierman DF, Johnson CE, Haskill JS. Human monocyte inflammatory mediator gene expression is selectively regulated by adherence substrates. *J Immunol* 1989;142:1970–1976.

270. Dayer J-M, Ricard-Blum S, Kaufmann M-T, Herbage D. Type IX collagen is a potent inducer of PGE_2 and interleukin 1 production by human monocyte macrophages. *FEBS Lett* 1986;198:208–212.

271. Postlethwaite AE, Smith Jr GN, Lachman LB, et al. Stimulation of glycosaminoglycan synthesis in cultured human dermal fibroblasts by interleukin 1: induction of hyaluronic acid synthesis by natural and recombinant IL-1s and synthetic IL-1β peptide 163–171. *J Clin Invest* 1989;83:629–636.

272. Duncan MR, Berman B. Differential regulation of collagen, glycosaminoglycans, fibronectin, and collagenase activity production in cultured human adult dermal fibroblasts by interleukin-1-alpha and beta and tumor necrosis factor-alpha and beta. *J Invest Dermatol* 1989;92:699–706.

273. Postlethwaite AE, Katai H, Raghow R. Stimulation of extracellular matrix biosynthesis in fibroblasts by interleukin-4. *Arthritis Rheum* 1989;32[SupplB]:B167.

274. Jimenez SA, Freundlich B, Rosenbloom J. Selective inhibition of

275. Gospodarowicz D, Ferrara N, Schweigerer L, Neufeld G. Structural characterization and biological functions of fibroblast growth factor. *Endocr Rev* 1987;8:95–114.

276. Keski-Oja J, Raghow R, Sawdey M, et al. Regulation of mRNAs for type-1 plasminogen activator inhibitor, fibronectin, and type I procollagen by transforming growth factor-β: divergent responses in lung fibroblasts and carcinoma cells. *J Biol Chem* 1988;263:3111–3115.

277. Raghow R, Postlethwaite AE, Keski-Oja J, Moses HL, Kang AH. Transforming growth factor-β increases steady state levels of type I procollagen and fibronectin mRNAs posttranscriptionally in cultured human dermal fibroblasts. *J Clin Invest* 1987;79:1285–1288.

278. Cook JJ, Haynes KM, Werther GA. Mitogenic effects of growth hormone in cultured human fibroblasts: evidence for action via local insulin-like growth factor I production. *J Clin Invest* 1988;81:206–212.

279. Salmon M, Scheel-Toellner S, Huissoon AP, et al. Inhibition of T cell apoptosis in the rheumatoid synovium. *J Clin Invest* 1997;99:439–446.

280. Gruss HJ, Scott C, Rollins BJ, Brach MA, Herrmann F. Human fibroblasts express functional IL-2 receptors formed by the IL-2R α- and chain subunits. *J Immunol* 1996;157:851–857.

281. Sempowski GD, Chess PR, Phipps RP. CD40 is a functional activation antigen and B7-independent T cell costimulatory molecule on normal human lung fibroblasts. *J Immunol* 1997;158:4670–4677.

282. Zhang Y, Cao HJ, Braf B, Meekins H, Smith TJ, Phipps RP. CD40 engagement up-regulates cyclooxygenase-2 expression and prostaglandin E_2 production in human lung fibroblasts. *J Immunol* 1998;160:1053–1057.

283. Pechold K, Patterson NB, Craighead N, Lee KP, June CH, Harlan DM. Inflammatory cytokines IFN-γ plus TNF-α induce regulated expression of CD80 (B7-1) but not CD86 (B7-2) on murine fibroblasts. *J Immunol* 1997;158:4921–4929.

284. Gao J-X, Issekutz C. Mac-1 (CD11b/CD18) is the predominant β2 (CD18) integrin mediating human neutrophil migration through synovial and dermal fibroblast barriers. *Immunology* 1996;88:461–470.

285. Burns AR, Simon SI, Kukielka GL, et al. Chemotactic factors stimulate CD18-dependent canine neutrophil adherence and motility on lung fibroblasts. *J Immunol* 1996;156:3389–3401.

286. Chin JE, Wintervowd GE, Krzesicki RF, Sanders ME. Role of cytokines in inflammatory synovitis. *Arthritis Rheum* 1990;33:1776–1786.

287. Phipps RP, Penney DP, Keng P, et al. Characterization of two major populations of lung fibroblasts: distinguishing morphology and discordant display of Thy 1 and class II MHC. *Am J Respir Cell Mol Biol* 1989;1:65–74.

288. Springer TA, Dustin ML, Kishimoto TK, Marlin SD. The lymphocyte function-associated LFA-1, CD2 and LFA-3 molecules: cell adhesion receptors of the immune system. *Annu Rev Immunol* 1987;5:223–252.

289. Sempowski GD, Derdak S, Phipps R. Interleukin-4 and interferon-γ discordantly regulate collagen biosynthesis by functionally distinct lung fibroblast subsets. *J Cell Physiol* 1996;167:290–296.

290. Sempowski GD, Borrello MA, Brieden TM, Barth RK, Phipps RP. Fibroblast heterogeneity in the healing wound. *Wound Repair Regen* 1995;3:120–131.

291. Walther Z, May LT, Sehgal PB. Transcriptional regulation of the interferon-β2/B cell differentiation factor BSF-21 hepatocyte-stimulating factor gene in human fibroblasts by other cytokines. *J Immunol* 1988;140:974–977.

292. Le J, Weinstein D, Gubler U, Vilcek J. Induction of membrane-associated interleukin 1 by tumor necrosis factor in human fibroblasts. *J Immunol* 1987;138:2137–2142.

293. Fibbe WE, Van Damme JV, Billiau A, et al. Human fibroblasts produce granulocyte-CSF, macrophage-CSF, and granulocyte-macrophage-CSF following stimulation by interleukin-1 and poly(rI). poly(rC). *Blood* 1988;72:860–866.

294. Van Damme J, Opdenakker G. Interaction of interferons with skin reactive cytokines from interleukin-1 to interleukin-8. *J Invest Dermatol* 1990;95(6 Suppl):90S–93S.

295. Strieter RM, Wiggins R, Phan SH, et al. Monocyte chemotactic protein gene expression by cytokine-treated human fibroblasts and endothelial cells. *Biochem Biophys Res Commun* 1989;162:694–700.

296. Larsen CG, Zachariae COC, Oppenheim JJ, Matsushima K. Production of monocyte chemotactic and activating factor (MCAF) by

human dermal fibroblasts in response to interleukin 1 or tumor necrosis factor. *Biochem Biophys Res Commun* 1989;160:1403–1408.

297. Deuel TF. Polypeptide growth factors: roles in normal and abnormal cell growth. *Annu Rev Cell Biol* 1987;3:443–492.

298. Shimonaka M, Yamaguchi Y. Purification and biological characterization of epitaxin, a fibroblast-derived motility factor for epithelial cells. *J Biol Chem* 1994;269:14284–14289.

299. Chedid M, Hoyle JR, Csaky KG, Rubin JS. Glucocorticoids inhibit keratinocyte growth factor production in primary dermal fibroblasts. *Endocrinology* 1996;137:2232–2237.

300. Musashi M, Yang Y, Paul S, Clark S, Sudo T, Ogawa M. Direct and synergistic effects of interleukin-11 on murine hemopoiesis in culture. *Proc Natl Acad Sci USA* 1991;88:765–771.

301. Suen Y, Chang M, Min Lee S, Buzby JS, Cairo MS. Regulation of interleukin-11 protein and mRNA expression in neonatal and adult fibroblasts and endothelial cells. *Blood* 1994;84:4125–4134.

302. Elias J, Zheng T, Whiting N, et al. IL-1 and transforming growth factor-β regulation of fibroblast-derived IL-11. *J Immunol* 1994;15:2421–2429.

303. Hattori A, Iwasaki S, Murase K, et al. Tumor necrosis factor is markedly synergistic with interleukin 1 and interferon-γ in stimulating the production of nerve growth factor in fibroblasts. *FEBS Lett* 1994;340:177–180.

304. Ben-Av P, Crofford LJ, Wilder RL, Hla T. Induction of vascular endothelial growth factor expression in synovial fibroblasts by prostaglandin E and interleukin-1: a potential mechanism for inflammatory angiogenesis. *FEBS Lett* 1995;372:83–87.

305. Baggiolini M, Dewald B, Moser B. Interleukin-8 and related chemotactic cytokines—CXC and CC chemokines. *Adv Immunol* 1994;55:97–179.

306. Takigawa M, Takashiba S, Myokai F, et al. Cytokine-dependent synergistic regulation of interleukin-8 production from human gingival fibroblasts. *J Periodontol* 1994;65:1002–1007.

307. Friedland JS, Shattock RJ, Griffin GE. Phagocytosis of *Mycobacterium tuberculosis* on particulate stimuli by human fibroblasts: unique mechanism of transcriptional inhibition by interferon. *Proc Natl Acad Sci USA* 1993;89:9094–9098.

308. Bozic CR, Kolakowski LF, Gerard NP, et al. Expression and biologic characterization of the murine chemokine KC. *J Immunol* 1995;154:6048–6057.

309. VanDamme J, Proost P, Put W, et al. Induction of monocyte chemotactic proteins MCP-1 and MCP-2 in human fibroblasts and leukocytes by cytokines and cytokine inducers: chemical synthesis of MCP-2 and development of a specific RIA. *J Immunol* 1994;152:5495–5502.

310. Koch AE, Kunkel SL, Shah PMR, et al. Macrophage inflammatory protein-1: a C-C chemokine in osteoarthritis. *Clin Immunol Immunopathol* 1995;77:307–314.

311. Watanabe A, Takeshita A, Kitano S, Hanazawa S. CD14-mediated signal pathway of *Porphyromonas gingivalis* lipopolysaccharide in human gingival fibroblasts. *Infect Immun* 1996;64:4488–4494.

312. Yu X, Graves DT. Fibroblasts, mononuclear phagocytes, and endothelial cells express monocyte chemoattractant protein-1 (MCP-1) in inflamed human gingiva. *J Periodontal* 1995;66:80–88.

313. Noso N, Sticherling M, Bartels J, Mallet AI, Christophers E, Schroder J-M. Identification of an N-terminally truncated form of the chemokine RANTES and granulocyte-macrophage colony stimulating factor are major eosinophil attractants released by cytokine-stimulated dermal fibroblasts. *J Immunol* 1996;157:1946–1953.

314. Brewster CEP, Howarth PH, Djukanovic R, Wilson J, Holgate SJ, Roches WR. Myofibroblasts and subepithelial fibrosis in bronchial asthma. *Am J Respir Cell Mol Biol* 1990;3:507–551.

315. Davidson JM. Wound repair. In: Gallin JI, Goldstein IM, Snyderman R, eds. *Inflammation:* basic principles and clinical correlates, 2nd ed. New York: Raven Press, 1992:809–819.

316. Cromack DT, Porras-Reyes B, Mustoe TA. Current concepts in wound healing: growth factor and macrophage interaction. *J Trauma* 1990;30[Suppl S]:S129–S133.

317. Gibran NS, Isik FF, Heimbach DM, Gordon D. Basic FGF in the early human burn wound. *Proc Am Burn Assoc* 1992;24:30–36.

318. Gartner MH, Benson JD, Caldwell MD. Time course of EGF mRNA expression in healing wounds using polymerase chain reaction. *Surg Forum* 1991;42:643–649.

319. Gartner MH, Benson JD, Caldwell MD. Time course of TGF-beta 1 and 2 expression in the healing wound. *Proc Wound Healing Soc* 1992;2:3–10.

320. Howard M, Farrar J, Hilfiker M, et al. T cell-derived B cell growth factor distinct from IL-2. *J Exp Med* 1982;155:914–923.

321. Gartner MH, Richards JR, Caldwell MD. Interrelationships between growth factor messenger RNA and protein product in the healing wound. *Surg Forum* 1992;43:683–689.

322. Whitby DJ, Ferguson MWJ. Immunohistochemical localization of growth factors in fetal wound healing. *Dev Biol* 1991;147:207–215.

323. Wong DT, Donoff RB, Yang J, et al. Sequential expression of TGFα and β1 by eosinophils during cutaneous wound healing in the hamster. *Am J Pathol* 1993;143:130–142.

324. Appleton I, Tomlinson A, Colville-Nash PR, Willoughby DA. Temporal and spatial immunolocalization of cytokines in murine chronic granulomatous tissue: implications for their role in tissue development and repair processes. *Lab Invest* 1993;69:405–414.

325. Antoniades HN, Galanopoulos T, Neville-Golden J, Kiritsy CP, Lynch SE. Injury induces in vivo expression of PDGF and PDGF receptor mRNAs in skin epithelial cells and connective tissue fibroblasts. *Proc Natl Acad Sci USA* 1991;88:565–569.

326. Brasken P, Renvall S, Sandbert M. Expression of EGF and EGF receptor genes in healing colonic anastomoses in rats. *Eur J Surg* 1991;157:607–611.

327. Peus D, Jungtaubl H, Knaub S. Localization of PDGF receptor subunit expression in chronic venous leg ulcers. *Wound Repair Regen* 1995;3:265–270.

328. Wenczak B, Nanney L, Lynch JB. Evidence for a functional epidermal growth factor receptor in burn wounds. *Proc Am Burn Assoc* 1992;24:27–35.

329. Goretsky MJ, Greenhalgh DG. Delayed expression of IGF-II but not TGF- 1 in wounds of diabetic mice. *Proc Assoc Acad Surg* 1995;29:123–136.

330. Madden JW, Peacock EE. Studies on the biology of collagen during wound healing: rate of collagen synthesis and deposition in cutaneous wounds of the rat. *Surgery* 1988;64:288–296.

331. Barbul A, Hansen JK, Wasserkrug HL, Efron G. Interleukin 2 enhances wound healing in rats. *J Surg Res* 1986;40:315–319.

332. Mustoe TA, Purdy GF, Grumates P, Deuel TF, Thomason A, Pierce GF. Reversal of impaired wound healing in irradiated rats by PDGF-BB. *Ann J Surg* 1989;158:345–350.

333. Pierce GF, Mustoe TA, Lingelbach J, et al. PDGF and TGF induce in vivo and in vitro tissue repair. *J Cell Biol* 1989;109:429–440.

334. Pierce GF, Mustoe TA, Senior RM, et al. In vivo incisional wound healing augmented by PDGF and recombinant c-sis proteins. *J Exp Med* 1988;167:974–987.

335. Bitar MS, Labbad ZN. Transforming growth factor-β and insulin-like growth factor-1 is relative to diabetes-induced impairment of wound healing. *J Surg Res* 1996;61:113–119.

336. Bernstein EF, Harisiadis L, Salomon G, et al. Transforming growth factor-β improves healing and radiation-impaired wounds. *J Invest Dermatol* 1991;97:430–434.

337. Shah M, Foreman DM, Ferguson WJ. Neutralization of TGF-β1 and TGF-β2 on exogenous addition of TGF-β3 to cutaneous rat wounds reduces scarring. *J Cell Sci* 1995;108:985–1002.

338. Konig A, Bruckner-Tuberman L. Transforming growth factor-β promotes deposition of collagen VII in a modified organ-typic skin model. *Lab Invest* 1994;70:203–209.

339. Vegesna V, McBride WH, Taylor JMG, Withers HR. The effects of IL-1 on radiation-impaired murine skin wound healing. *J Surg Res* 1995;59:699–704.

340. Mustoe TA, Pierce GF, Thomason A, Gramates P, Sporn MB, Denel TF. Accelerated healing of incisional wounds induced by TGF-β. *Science* 1987;237:1335–1337.

341. Bernstein EF, Harisiadis L, Salomon G, et al. TGF-β improves healing of radiation impaired wounds. *J Invest Dermatol* 1991;97:430–434.

342. Ksander GA, Ogawa Y, Chu GH, McMullin H, Rosenblatt JS, McPherson JM. Exogenous transforming growth factor beta 2 enhances connective tissue formation and wound strength in guinea pig dermal wounds healing of secondary intent. *Ann Surg* 1990;211:288–294.

343. Quaglino D Jr, Nanney LB, Dietsheim JA, Davidson JM. TGF-β stimulates wound healing & modulates extracellular matrix gene expression in pig skin. *J Invest Dermatol* 1991;97:34–42.

344. Beck LS, DeGuzman L, Lee WP, Yu Y, Siegel MW, Amento EP. One administration of TGF-β1 reverses impaired wound healing. *J Clin Invest* 1993;92:2841–2849.

345. Levine JH, Moses HL, Gold LI, Nanney LB. Spatial and temporal patterns of immunoreactive transforming growth factor β1, β2, and β3 during excisional wound repair. *Am J Pathol* 1993;143:368–380.

346. Ford H, Hoffman RA, Wing EJ. Characterization of wound cytokines in the sponge matrix model. *Arch Surg* 1985;124:1422–1428.

347. Sharpe RJ, Margolis RJ, Askari M, Amento EP, Grandstein RD. Induction of dermal and subcutaneous inflammation TNFα in the mouse. *J Invest Dermatol* 1988;91:353–357.

348. Postlethwaite AE, Kang AH. Induction of fibroblast proliferation by human mononuclear leukocyte-derived proteins. *Arthritis Rheum* 1983;26:22–27.

349. Solis-Herrazo JA, Brenner DA, Chojkier M. TNF-α inhibits collagen gene transcription and collagen synthesis in cultured fibroblasts. *J Biol Chem* 1988;263:5841–5845.

350. Dayer JM, Beutler B, Cerami A. TNFα stimulates collagenase and prostaglandin E_2 production by human synovial cells and dermal fibroblasts. *J Exp Med* 1985;162:2163–2168.

351. Sugarman BJ, Aggarwal BB, Hass PE, Figari IS, Palladino MA, Shepard HM. TNF-α: effects on proliferation of normal and transformed cells *in vitro*. *Science* 1985;230:943–945.

352. Mooney DP, O'Reilly M, Gamelli RL. TNF and wound healing. *Ann Surg* 1990;211:124–129.

353. Regan MC, Kirk SJ, Hurson M, Sodeyama M, Wasserkrug HL, Barbul A. Tumor necrosis factor-α inhibits *in vivo* collagen synthesis. *Surgery* 1993;113:173–177.

354. Kondo T, Ohshima T. The dynamics of inflammatory cytokines in the healing process of mouse skin wounds. *Int J Legal Med* 1996;108:231–236.

355. Hulmes DJS, Holmes DF, Cummings C. Crystalline regions in collagen fibrils. *J Mol Biol 1985*;184:473–477.

356. Raspanti M, Ottani V, Ruggeri A. Different architectures of the collagen fibril: morphological aspects and functional implications. *Int J Biol Macromol* 1989;11:367–371.

357. Yurchenco PD, Schittny JC. Molecular architecture of basement membranes. *FASEB J* 1990;4:1577–1590.

358. Iozzo RV, Murdoch AD. Proteoglycans of the extracellular environment: clues from the gene and protein side offer novel perspectives in molecular diversity and function. *FASEB J* 1996;10:598–614.

359. Williams MJ, Phan I, Harvey TS, Rostagno A, Gold LI, Campbell ID. Solution structure of a pair of fibronectin type 1 modules with fibrin binding activity. *J Mol Biol* 1994;235:1302–1311.

360. Leahy DJ, Aukhil I, Erickson HP. 2.0 Å crystal structure of a four-domain segment of human fibronectin encompassing the RGD loop and synergy region. *Cell* 1996;84:155–164.

361. Sasaki M, Kleinman HK, Huber H, Deutzmann R, Yamada Y. Laminin, a multidomain protein: the A chain has a unique globular domain and homology with the basement membrane proteoglycan and the laminin B chains. *J Biol Chem* 1988;263:16536–16544.

362. Chiquet-Ehrismann R, Hagios C, Matsumoto K-I. The tenascin gene family. *Perspect Dev Neurobiol* 1994;2:3–7.

363. Sato H, Okada Y, Seiki M. Membrane-type matrix metalloproteinasaes (MT-MMPs) in cell invasion. *Thromb Haemost* 1997;78:497–500.

364. Biobel CP. Metalloprotease-disintegrins: links to cell adhesion and cleavage of TNFα and notch. *Cell* 1997;90:589–592.

Inflammation: Basic Principles and Clinical Correlates,
3rd ed., edited by John I. Gallin and Ralph Snyderman.
Lippincott Williams & Wilkins, Philadelphia © 1999.

CHAPTER 17

Extracellular Matrix Proteins and Proteoglycans

Erkki Ruoslahti

Extracellular matrices (ECMs) of our tissues consist primarily of adhesive glycoproteins, collagens, proteoglycans, and hyaluronic acid. By forming fibrils and by binding to one another, these ECM components form an insoluble network that fills the intercellular spaces. The matrix adheres to cells, and it binds various regulatory molecules such as growth factors, creating a network that guides the functions of the cells that come in contact with it.

STRUCTURAL COMPONENTS OF EXTRACELLULAR MATRICES

Glycoproteins and Collagens

The main adhesive ECM glycoproteins are fibronectin and laminin. Fibronectin is a characteristic component of ECM in connective tissues, whereas laminins are almost exclusively confined to basement membranes, the specialized ECM sheets that underlie epithelia and endothelia. Other ECM glycoproteins include vitronectin, tenascins, thrombospondins, fibrillin, fibulins, and von Willebrand factor (vWF). Among these ECM proteins, fibronectin, vitronectin, and vWF are also present in the blood as relatively abundant plasma proteins (1). The ECM glycoproteins are typically multimodular. They are composed of structurally and functionally autonomous domains.

The molecular ropes and straps that keep our tissues together are made of collagens (2). The amino acid sequences of these highly specialized proteins are characterized by the repeating triplet Gly-x-y; x and y can be any amino acid but are often proline or hydroxyproline. The Gly-x-y repeat makes it possible for three collagen chains to wind together into a triple helix that forms the trimeric collagen monomer. The monomers assemble into long polymers that are subsequently stabilized by crosslinking.

Proteoglycans

Members of this class of proteins are universally expressed at cell surfaces and in ECM (3–5). Proteoglycans serve structural functions and are regulators of various growth factor and cytokine activities.

Proteoglycans carry one or more glycosaminoglycan chains from a specialized class of glycoproteins. The glycosaminoglycans that characterize the proteoglycan structure are large carbohydrates composed of repeating disaccharide units. They exist in four main forms: heparan sulfate and heparin, chondroitin sulfate and dermatan sulfate, keratan sulfate, and hyaluronic acid. The first three are protein-bound glycosaminoglycans and contain sulfate; hyaluronic acid is made as a free glycosaminoglycan and lacks sulfate (5).

The glycosaminoglycans carry a strong negative charge. They bind many substances, including other ECM proteins and growth factors, through charge interactions. Heparin and heparan sulfate, which are the most highly sulfated of the glycosaminoglycans, are particularly effective in this regard. A typical binding site for heparin in a protein contains the sequence B-B-X-B, in which B is a basic amino acid (6). However, the charge is not the whole basis of the binding; a protein can bind specifically to a given type of glycosaminoglycan. Certain proteoglycans bind only to hyaluronic acid among the glycosaminoglycans. A protein also can differentiate among subtypes of a glycosaminoglycan; antithrombin, for example, binds to a specific hexasaccharide sequence in heparin, made unique by differential sulfation of the sugars that comprise the heparin chain (7).

Proteoglycans have many different types of core proteins and glycosaminoglycan substitutions (Fig. 17-1). The core proteins are as diverse as those of other types of glycoproteins, but there are far fewer proteoglycans than there of other kinds of proteoglycans (3,4).

Many proteoglycans are constituents of the ECM. Lecticans are a family of large chondroitin sulfate proteoglycans

E. Ruoslahti: La Jolla Cancer Research Center, The Burnham Institute, La Jolla, California 92037.

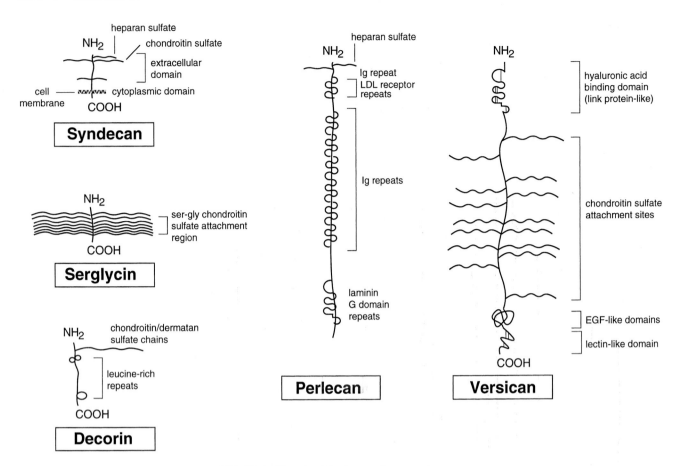

FIG. 17-1. Structural features of proteoglycans.

that includes aggrecan, versican, neurocan, and brevican (8). They are particularly abundant in the ECM of cartilage and brain. The small chondroitin sulfate proteoglycan family of decorin, fibromodulin, biglycan, and lumican is characterized by collagen-binding properties (9). The large heparan sulfate proteoglycan perlecan is a major component of basement membranes, thin sheets of ECM that underlie epithelia and endothelia and form sheaths around muscle fibers (10). Some proteoglycans have membrane-anchored core proteins. These include the heparan sulfate proteoglycans, syndecans, and glypicans (11,12). Serglycin resides in the secretory granules of various types of hematopoietic cells (13). CD44, which is a hyaluronic acid receptor important in lymphocyte homing, can also be a proteoglycan (14). The functions of proteoglycans are varied, but many of them play important roles in the regulation of growth factor and cytokine activities, as does the extracellular matrix in general.

GROWTH FACTOR–REGULATING ACTIVITIES OF MATRIX

Extracellular Matrix Can Localize Growth Factor Activity

Whereas hormones circulate in the blood and affect their target tissues from a distance, most growth factors,

cytokines, and chemokines appear to be designed to act over short distances. In the body, molecules with these activities bind to ECM components and to cell surface proteoglycans. Because both are ubiquitous, this prevents the active substance from traveling very far from its source and creates a reservoir of immobilized, potentially active substance that is ready to act on the cells in the immediate vicinity. An active factor can be generated by proteolysis of the proteoglycan core proteins or partial degradation of the glycosaminoglycan (usually heparan sulfate) component. The result of ECM and cell surface proteoglycan binding of growth factors and cytokines is a tight spatial control of the distribution of growth factors and cytokines and their growth-promoting and migration-enhancing activities. This mechanism probably is of major significance in the formation and maintenance of tissue architecture. It can localize certain inflammatory processes.

Heparan Sulfate in Growth Factor Binding to Extracellular Matrices and to Cell Surfaces

When fibroblast growth factor (FGF), which binds strongly to heparin and heparan sulfate, is applied as a small spot to a cell culture, it spreads only a short distance from the site of application (15). However, if it is mixed with heparin before adding the culture, it spreads much farther. The explanation is that the free FGF binds to the heparan sulfate proteoglycans in the culture, whereas the heparin-bound FGF cannot do this and consequently diffuses farther.

Serglycin is a chondroitin sulfate proteoglycan in the granules of hematopoietic cells. It has a very small core protein that contains essentially only glycosaminoglycan attachment sites to which the several chondroitin sulfate chains are linked (13). Platelet factor-4 (PF4), which is the prototype molecule in a family of a dozen or so growth factors and cytokines (16), binds to chondroitin sulfate, in addition to binding to heparin. PF4 exists in platelet α granules complexed with serglycin, suggesting that serglycin may, like heparin and heparan sulfate, serve as a carrier of cytokines.

Another example of the importance of the binding of growth factors to heparan sulfate in proteoglycans is the binding of the cytokine macrophage inflammatory protein-1β to heparan sulfate at the surface of endothelial cells (17). This cytokine binds to receptors on leukocytes that have been transiently slowed down at an inflammatory site, activating leukocyte integrins at these sites and causing the integrins to attach the leukocytes firmly to the endothelium, causing their migration into the tissue (18). Without the proteoglycan binding, the cytokine would be washed away in the bloodstream and would not be able to bind to the leukocyte receptors.

Heparan Sulfate as a Cofactor for Growth Factors

The binding of basic FGF (bFGF) to its receptor requires prior binding to the heparan sulfate side chains of a membrane heparan sulfate proteoglycan or to free heparan sulfate (heparin) chains (19,20). The glycosaminoglycan may change the conformation of bFGF so that it acquires an ability to bind to the receptor. However, evidence indicates that the glycosaminoglycan acts by effecting the oligomerization of bFGF; this makes it possible for the growth factor to cause dimerization of the receptors, which is a prerequisite for signal transmission by receptor tyrosine kinases such as the FGF receptors (21,22). Figure 17-2 depicts some of the effects of heparan sulfate proteoglycans on a growth factor such as FGF.

Other growth factors that bind to heparin and heparan sulfate include granulocyte-macrophage colony-stimulating factor, interleukin-3, and pleiotrophin or HB-CAM (23,24). The effects of ECM and cell surface proteoglycan binding on the activities of these growth factors are less well understood than those on FGF, but they are probably similar.

Transforming growth factor-β (TGF-β) binds to proteoglycans through the core protein of the proteoglycans. One of the three receptors for TGF-β, betaglycan, is a proteoglycan (25). The glycosaminoglycan component of betaglycan is not needed for the TGF-β binding. Betaglycan apparently does not function directly in signal transduction, but it is thought to play a supporting role by binding TGF-β for subsequent delivery to the signal transduction receptors.

TGF-β also binds to the extracellular matrix proteoglycan decorin. Like betaglycan, decorin binds TGF-β through its core protein (26). Decorin binds TGF-β, and it can neutralize the activity of the growth factor. The inhibition of TGF-β activity may result from competition between decorin and TGF-β receptors for the same or adjacent binding sites on TGF-β, or it may be caused by some indirect effect. As a result, decorin may function in a negative feedback loop that regulates TGF-β activity.

Decorin also inhibits cell proliferation. In fibroblastic cells, this effect may be secondary to counteracting TGF-β, which usually is a growth factor in fibroblasts (26,27). In epithelially derived tumor cells, inhibition of cell proliferation by decorin appears to be independent of TGF-β and is linked to increased expression of the cell cycle inhibitor, p21 Cip (28,29).

Other ECM components that have been reported to bind TGF-β include type IV collagen and trombospondin (30,31). TGF-β bound to ECM in tissue may form a reservoir of the growth factor, and thrombospondin accelerates the conversion of the inactive precursor to active TGF-β.

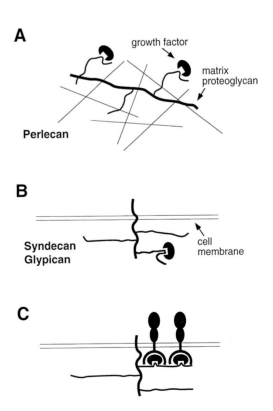

FIG. 17-2. Growth factor regulation by proteoglycans. Growth factors form a reservoir in the extracellular matrix **(A)** and at cell surfaces **(B)**. Dimerization of growth factors **(C)** facilitates receptor clustering and signaling.

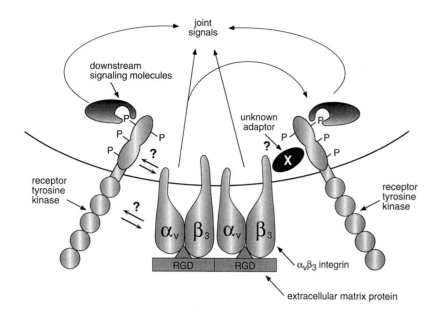

FIG. 17-3. Certain growth factor receptors associate with the $\alpha_v\beta_3$ integrin. When the integrin is bound to an extracellular matrix component (through the integrin-recognition sequence RGD), growth factor signaling is enhanced. The exact molecular pathways of these interactions and effects have not been determined.

Systemic administration of decorin suppresses kidney fibrosis in animal models of glomerulonephritis and some other fibrotic diseases that are caused by excessive TGF-β production and activity (32,33). Decorin may find use as an antifibrotic agent.

Extracellular Matrix Receptors Enhance Growth Factor Responses

ECMs also affect growth factors through the ECM receptors, integrins (see Chapter 37). The $\alpha_v\beta_3$ integrin physically associates with the receptors for insulin, insulin-like growth factor, and platelet-derived growth factor (34). When cells are bound to a matrix through this integrin, the mitogenic and cell migration–promoting activities of the growth factors are enhanced (Fig. 17-3). These responses may be important in angiogenesis, wound healing, and inflammatory responses (35–37).

In summary, components of the ECM through their receptors bind growth factors and cytokines and interact in various ways with their receptors. As a result, ECM-interacting growth factors and cytokines are concentrated in certain locations, and their activities can be suppressed or enhanced.

ACKNOWLEDGMENT

The author's research reviewed in this chapter was supported by grant CA60725 and Cancer Center Support Grant CA30199, both from the National Cancer Institute, Department of Health and Human Services.

REFERENCES

1. Hay E, ed. *Cell biology of extracellular matrix,* 2nd ed. New York: Plenum Press, 1991.
2. Prockop DJ, Kivirikko KI. Collagens: molecular biology, diseases, and potentials for therapy. *Annu Rev Biochem* 1995;64:403–434.
3. Ruoslahti E. Structure and biology of proteoglycans. *Annu Rev Cell Biol* 1988;4:229–255.
4. Iozzo R, Murdoch AD. Proteoglycans of the extracellular environment: clues from the gene and protein side offer novel perspectives in molecular diversity and function. *FASEB J* 1996;10:598–614.
5. Hascall VC, Calabro A, Midura RJ, Yanagishita M. Isolation and characterization of proteoglycans. *Methods Enzymol* 1994;230:390–417.
6. Cardin AD, Weintraub HJR. Molecular modeling of protein-glycosaminoglycan interactions. *Arteriosclerosis* 1989;9:21–32.
7. Bray B, Lane DA, Breyssinet J-M, Pejler G, Lindahl U. Anti-thrombin activities of heparin. *Biochem J* 1989;262:225–232.
8. Ruoslahti E. Brain extracellular matrix. *Glycobiology* 1996;6:489–492.
9. Hedbom E, Heinegård D. Binding of fibromodulin and decorin to separate sites on fibrillar collagens. *J Biol Chem* 1993;268:27307–27312.
10. Iozzo RV. Perlecan: a gem of a proteoglycan. *Matrix Biol* 1994;14:203–208.
11. Bernfield M. Developmental expression of the syndecans: possible function and regulation. *Development* 1993;xx[Suppl]:202–212.
12. Watanabe K, Yamada H, Yamaguchi Y. K-glypican: a novel heparan sulfate proteoglycan that is highly expressed in developing brain and kidney. *J Cell Biol* 1995;130:1207–1218.
13. Ruoslahti E. Proteoglycans in cell regulation: minireview. *J Biol Chem* 1989;264:13369–13372.
14. Jalkanen S, Jalkanen M. Lymphocyte CD44 binds to the COOH-terminal heparin-binding domain of fibronectin. *J Cell Biol* 1992;116:817–825.
15. Saksela O, Moscatelli D, Sommer A, Rifkin DB. Endothelial cell-derived heparan sulfate binds basic fibroblast growth factor and protects it from proteolytic degradation. *J Cell Biol* 1988;107:743–751.
16. Stoeckle MY, Barker KA. Two burgeoning families of platelet factor 4-related proteins: mediators of the inflammatory response. *New Biologist* 1990;2:313–323.
17. Tanaka Y, Adams DH, Hubscher S, Hirano H, Siebenlist U, Shaw S. T-cell adhesion induced by proteoglycan-immobilized cytokine MIP-1β. *Nature* 1993;361:79–82.
18. Springer TA. Traffic signals for lymphocyte recirculation and leukocyte emigration: the multistep paradigm. *Cell* 1994;76:301–314.
19. Yayon A, Klagsbrun M, Esko JD, Leder P, Ornitz DM. Cell surface, heparin-like molecules are required for binding of basic fibroblast growth factor to its high affinity receptor. *Cell* 1991;64:841–848.
20. Ruoslahti E, Yamaguchi Y. Proteoglycans as modulators of growth factor activities. *Cell* 1990;64:867–869.
21. Ornitz DM, Yayon A, Flanagan JG, Svahn CM, Levi E, Leder P. Heparin is required for cell-free binding of basic fibroblast growth factor to a soluble receptor and for mitogenesis in whole cells. *Mol Cell Biol* 1992;12:240–247.

22. Schlessinger J, Lax I, Lemmon M. Regulation of growth factor activation by proteoglycans: what is the role of the low affinity receptors. *Cell* 1995;83:357–360.

23. Roberts R, Gallagher J, Spooncer E, Allen TD, Bloomfield F, Dexter TM. Heparan sulfate bound growth factors: a mechanism for stromal cell mediated haemopoiesis. *Nature* 1988;332:376–378.

24. Merenmies J, Rauvala H. Molecular cloning of the 18-kDa growth-associated protein of developing brain. *J Biol Chem* 1990;265:16721–16724.

25. Massagué J. TGF beta signaling: receptors, transducers, and Mad proteins. *Cell* 1996;85:947–950.

26. Yamaguchi Y, Mann DM, Ruoslahti E. Negative regulation of transforming growth factor-β by the proteoglycan decorin. *Nature* 1990;346:281–284.

27. Yamaguchi Y, Ruoslahti E. Proteoglycans as modulators of growth factor activities. *Cell* 1991;64:867–869.

28. Santra M, Skorski T, Calabretta B, Lattime DC, Iozzo RV. De novo decorin gene expression suppresses the malignant phenotype in human colon cancer cells. *Proc Natl Acad Sci USA* 1995;92:7016–7020.

29. DeLuca A, Santra M, Baldi A, Giordano A, Iozzo RV. Decorin-induced growth suppression is associated with up-regulation of p21, an inhibitor of cyclin-dependent kinases. *J Biol Chem* 1996;271:18961–18965.

30. Paralkar VM, Vukicevic S, Reddi AH. Transforming growth factor beta type 1 binds to collagen IV of basement membrane matrix: implications for development. *Dev Biol* 1991;43:303–308.

31. Murphy-Ullrich JE, Schultz-Cherry S, Hook M. Transforming growth factor-beta complexes with thrombospondin. *Mol Biol Cell* 1992;3:181–188.

32. Border WA, Okuda S, Languino LR, Sporn M, Ruoslahti E. Suppression of experimental glomerulonephritis by antiserum against transforming growth factor β1. *Nature* 1990;346:371–374.

33. Border WA, Noble N. Targeting TGF-β for treatment of disease. *Nat Genet* 1995;1:1000–1001.

34. Schneller M, Vuori K, Ruoslahti E. $\alpha_v\beta_3$ Integrin associated with activated insulin and PDGFβ receptors and potentiates the biological activity of PDGF. *EMBO J* 1998 *(in press)*.

35. Varner JA, Brooks PC, Cheresh DA. Review: the integrin $\alpha_v\beta_3$: angiogenesis and apoptosis. *Cell Adhes Commun* 1995;3:367–374.

36. Gailit JO, Clark RAF. Integrins. *Adv Dermatol* 1993;8:129–153.

37. Sheppard D. Epithelial integrins. *Bioessays* 1996;18:655–660.

PART II

Mediators of Inflammation

Inflammation: Basic Principles and Clinical Correlates,
3rd ed., edited by John I. Gallin and Ralph Snyderman.
Lippincott Williams & Wilkins, Philadelphia © 1999.

CHAPTER 18

Immunoglobulins

Robyn L. Stanfield and Ian A. Wilson

The immune system has developed two main paths of response to foreign intruders. The humoral system uses antibodies to recognize and bind foreign materials, and in the cellular system the T-cell receptor interacts with molecules of the major histocompatibility complex (MHC) bound to foreign antigens digested from whole proteins, bacteria, and viruses. The two systems work together to protect against foreign invaders and tumors while being tolerant to self proteins (see Chapter 12 for overview). Since the first x-ray crystallographic structures of an antibody Fab fragment were determined (1,2), many more structural elucidations have provided detailed images of the multitude of components of both branches of the immune system. These x-ray structures have helped to answer many questions about antibody-antigen interactions and the structural basis of immune recognition.

ANTIBODY STRUCTURE AND DIVERSITY

Immunoglobulins typically are made of two copies each of two protein chains, called the light and heavy chains. Five different types of heavy chains (γ, μ, α, δ, and ε) and two different types of light chains (κ and λ) occur in humans. Five different classes of antibody (immunoglobulin G [IgG], IgM, IgA, IgD, and IgE) are determined by the nature of the constant region of the heavy chain. The basic structural unit for each antibody class is a Y-shaped molecule made up of two light and two heavy chains. Some classes exist as polymers of this basic unit; for example, IgM exists as a pentamer of five Y-shaped units. This chapter focuses on the IgG class (one Y-shaped unit), because structural information is largely confined to this class.

The IgG light and heavy chains have molecular masses of about 25,000 and 50,000 Da, respectively. The four

protein chains associate to form a molecule with three distinct regions. The two Fab arms each consist of one light chain and the N-terminal half of a heavy chain, whereas the Fc domain consists of a dimer of the C-terminal halves of the two heavy chains (Fig. 18-1). Each Fab region is attached to the Fc region by flexible polypeptides called the hinge region. The Fab domain can be further dissected into variable and constant regions (Fig. 18-2), and the Fc domain can be subdivided into C_H2 and C_H3 regions (Fig. 18-3). The variable region of the Fab is the portion of the antibody that interacts with

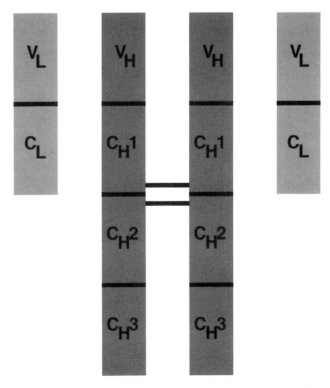

FIG. 18-1. Schematic drawing of the light and heavy chains making up an Fab fragment.

R. L. Stanfield and I. A. Wilson: Department of Molecular Biology, The Scripps Research Institute, La Jolla, California 92037.

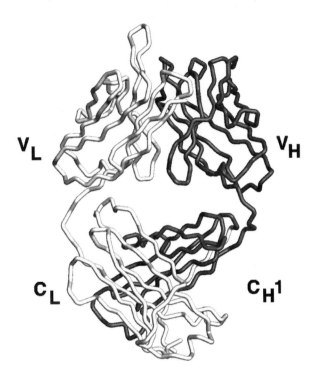

FIG. 18-2. Fab fragment. The x-ray crystallographic structure of the Fab fragment from antibody B13I2 (34) is shown. The light chain is on the left in light gray, and the heavy chain is on the right in darker gray, with the variable domain on the top and the constant domain on the bottom. This and all remaining figures were prepared with the use of the MIDAS display system (74).

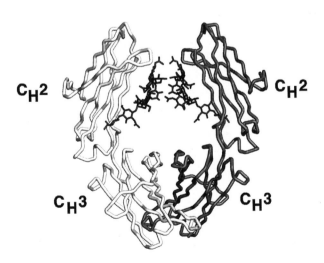

FIG. 18-3. Fc fragment. The x-ray crystallographic structure of a human immunoglobulin (IgG1) Fc fragment (75) is shown. The molecule is a dimer of two heavy chains, with the C_H2 domain on top and the C_H3 domain on the bottom. Note the carbohydrates found in the core of the molecule between the C_H2 domains.

antigen; it consists of the V_L and V_H chains. The constant region of the Fab is a dimer of the C_L and C_H1 domains. The Fc region consists of two dimers, one comprising the two C_H2 domains and the other two C_H3 domains.

Immunoglobulin Fold

Each antibody domain (V_L, V_H, C_L, C_H1, C_H2, and C_H3) is folded into a Greek key β-barrel, with either seven or nine strands forming the barrel; this is called the *immunoglobulin domain* or *immunoglobulin fold*. The constant domains have seven strands, four in one β-sheet and three in another (Fig. 18-4A). The domains in the variable region of the Fab fragment have nine β-strands, with the two extra strands (C' and C") forming a loop between strands C and D (3) (Fig. 18-4B). This domain topology has been found in Ig as well as some non-Ig proteins. In the Igs, a conserved disulfide bridge is found between the B and F strands on opposing β-sheets (4). However, this disulfide is not found in all of the Ig-like proteins; for example, it is not found in the first domain of CD2 (5) or in the third domain of CD4 (6).

Complementarity-Determining Regions

In 1965, the first analyses of amino acid sequences from Bence Jones proteins (dimers of IgG light chains found in urine of patients with multiple myeloma) revealed highly conserved sequences at the C-terminal half of the light chains but much more variable sequences throughout the N-terminal half (7). A few years later, with many more amino acid sequences available for analysis, several groups identified three regions in the N-terminal portion of the chain that were highly variable in their sequence (8–11). These "hypervariable" regions exist in both the light and heavy chains and are called the *complementarity-determining regions* (CDRs). Before any x-ray crystallographic structure of a Fab fragment was determined, these loops were postulated to be the primary recognition sites for antigen. The first Fab-antigen complex structure, determined in the early 1970s, verified this hypothesis (McPC603; 1). The CDR loops are referred to as L1, L2, and L3 (from the light chain) and H1, H2, and H3 (from the heavy chain) (Fig. 18-5). Several of the loops vary in length as well as in sequence (L1, H2, and especially H3). The remainder of the Fab variable region, referred to as the *framework region*, is highly conserved in sequence and in structure.

Immune Diversity

The immune system is able to produce antibodies that bind almost any cell, virus, protein, peptide, carbohydrate, or small-molecule antigen. The amazing diversity of this system is achieved by the genetic recombination of different gene segments to produce a staggering number

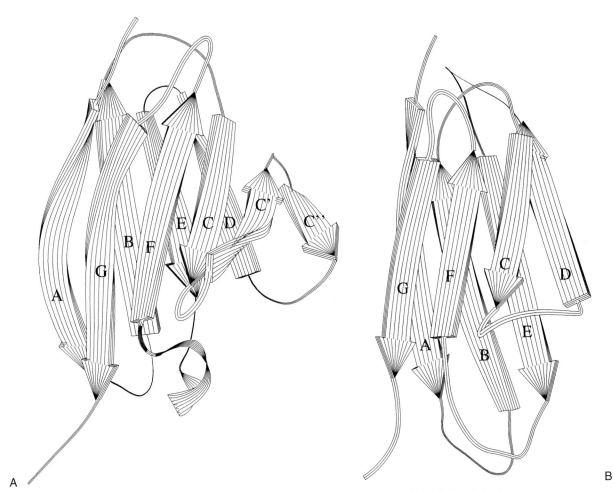

FIG. 18-4. Immunoglobulin domains. (**A**) The V$_L$ domain from antibody HyHEL-5 (76) is shown as a representative of the nine-stranded immunoglobulin domain family. Note especially the extra C'-C" loop inserted between strands C and D. (**B**) The C$_L$ domain from antibody HyHEL-5 is shown as a representative of the seven-stranded family. This figure was prepared with the RIBBON drawing program (77).

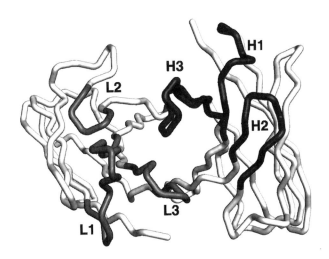

FIG. 18-5. Complementarity-determining region (CDR) loops. A view of antibody B13I2 is shown, looking down into the antibody-binding site. The light chain is on the left, and the heavy chain is on the right. The CDR loops are labeled.

of antibodies that can then be further modified by somatic mutations to achieve high affinity and specificity for almost any antigen. The antibody heavy-chain gene is generated by the recombination of three types of germline gene segments: the variable (V$_H$), diversity (D), and joining (J$_H$) segments (12). This event, called *V(D)J recombination*, involves joining of the D segment to the J segment, followed by joining of the V segment to the DJ segment. Additional nucleotides (N and P) can be added or removed at each site of recombination, further adding to the diversity of the system.

The human germ-line V$_H$, J$_H$, and D segments have now been completely mapped and sequenced. The human repertoire consists of 51 V$_H$ (13,14), 6 J$_H$ (15), and 27 D segments (16,17). The recombination of these three different types ($51 \times 6 \times 27$) can result in more than 8,000 different heavy-chain genes, which can be further modified by nucleotide additions at the junctions and then by somatic mutations throughout the variable region. Similarly, the light-chain gene is produced by recombination of a V_L and a J_L segment, sometimes with N additions (18,19). The gene segments for the human λ and κ chains have been mapped and sequenced. There are 40 $V_κ$ (20), 5 $J_κ$ (21), 30 $V_λ$ (17), and 4 $J_λ$ functional gene segments (22), allowing for at least 200 different possible κ chains and 120 different λ chains, without considering the further diversity from N additions and somatic mutation.

The most diverse region of the antibody is the heavy-chain CDR3, which occurs around the V_H-D-J_H junction (23). This CDR exhibits not only substantial sequence variation but also a large range in lengths: when the H3 loop is defined as occurring between heavy-chain residues 95 and 102, lengths have been seen to vary from 6 to 19 residues (24). Mutational studies have also suggested that this CDR loop is the most important for binding specificity (23,25).

STRUCTURAL ALTERATIONS

Canonical Conformations

Once a sufficient database of antibody structures had been generated, Chothia and Lesk and others (26–32) found that although the antibody CDR loops are highly variable in sequence, they are usually found in defined sets of conserved structures, called *canonical conformations*. These conformations depend on several "key" residues in and around each loop. Based on the antibody sequence, the canonical conformations for the L1, L2, L3, H1, and H2 loops can be predicted with a high degree of accuracy in most cases. The H3 loop, which is the most variable in sequence, length, and structure, has been difficult to classify, but it has been shown that this loop has at least two different conserved structural "stems" onto which the more structurally variable tip of the loop is mounted (31,33) (Fig. 18-6).

Conformational Changes

For years, the mechanism of antibody binding to antigen has been debated. Two main theories that describe the binding event are the "lock-and-key" and the "induced fit" theories. In the former, the antibody-binding surface has a rigid shape that is an exact fit with the antigen. In the latter theory, the antibody surface is capable of structural changes to more closely fit the antigen, or the antigen can change to better fit the antibody. In 1990, the first example of an x-ray structure for the same antibody in both the antigen-bound and antigen-free forms was determined for the anti-peptide antibody B13I2 (34). A comparison of the structures of the two forms showed that the H3 CDR moved as a rigid loop about 1 Å away from the binding site to allow the peptide to bind. Shortly thereafter, the structures of an anti-DNA antibody

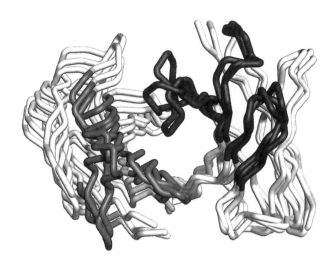

FIG. 18-6. Superposition of three different Fabs. Fabs B13I2, DB3, and HyHEL-5 are shown superimposed by framework residues in the heavy chain. The light chain is on the left. Notice the different lengths and conformations for the H3 loop. Note also that when the heavy chains are superimposed, the light chains show some variation in their packing with respect to the heavy chains.

(BV04-01; 35) and of another anti-peptide antibody (17/9; 36,37) were determined with and without antigen. Both of these complexes showed large rearrangements in the H3 CDR loop on binding of antigen. In addition, the BV04-01 structure showed a change of about 7 degrees in the relative disposition of the V_L and V_H domains, which added significantly to the changes in the nature and shape of the binding pocket.

By September 1997, coordinates were deposited in the Brookhaven Protein Data Bank for 17 antibodies in both their free and bound forms, some of these with multiple antigens. Just as the availability of multiple sequences led in 1970 to a description of hypervariable regions, these structures have permitted initial description of the types and ranges of conformational changes that occur in the antigen-binding process. Conformational changes have now been seen in all the CDR loops with the exception of the short L2 CDR loop. The types of conformational changes observed have included simple side-chain movements, segmental movements in which the CDR loop moves as a rigid unit by 1 to 2 Å, and main-chain rearrangements of CDR loops. In addition, quaternary V_L-V_H rearrangements as large as 16 degrees have been identified (38).

Not all antibodies use all of these types of conformational changes to maximize their fit with antigen. Free and bound forms of some antibody structures are virtually superimposable. Although the antibody-binding site can differ in antigen-bound and antigen-free states, it has been difficult to provide concrete proof of "induced fit," which implies that the antigen somehow causes the struc-

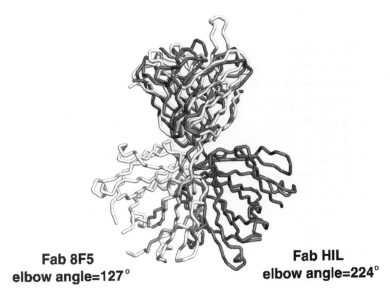

Fab 8F5
elbow angle=127°

Fab HIL
elbow angle=224°

FIG. 18-7. Elbow angles. The structures for the Fab fragments with the two most bent elbow angles known are shown. The Fab 8F5 (78) has an elbow angle of 127 degrees, and HIL (79) has an elbow angle of 224 degrees. The HIL crystal structure has two Fab fragments in the asymmetric unit, each with a different elbow angle. Other Fab structures show elbow angles distributed between these two extremes.

tural changes to take place. Another possible scenario that has been put forward is that the antibody can exist in a solution equilibrium population of two (or more) distinct conformations, one of which is more favorable for antigen binding (39). A third possibility is that the unliganded antibody is highly flexible and makes small adaptations to fit during binding of the antigen, thereby becoming more locked or fixed in conformation. By whatever means this event occurs, it is now obvious that, in addition to the tremendous sequence variability that can be used to bind a multitude of antigens, structural changes further extend the conformational range of binding-site structures to obtain fine specificity for the particular antigen.

Elbow Angle

Another area of flexibility in the antibody is at the connection or "elbow angle" between the variable and constant domains. This angle is defined as the angle between the pseudo-twofold rotation axis relating the V_L to the V_H domain and the axis relating the C_L to the C_H1 domain. These angles have been seen to vary between 127 and 224 degrees in different Fab fragments, as determined by x-ray crystallography (40) (Fig. 18-7). It was proposed early on that a change in this angle could signal the antigen-binding event to the constant region (41). The hypothesis was that open angles (elbow approximately 180 degrees) and closed angles (elbow much smaller than 180 degrees) would correlate

with free and bound forms of the antibody, respectively. However, this theory was disproved when the first example of an antibody-antigen complex (D1.3; 42) showed the bound form of the antibody to have an open elbow angle (43). Later, several examples were documented in which two molecules in the same crystallographic asymmetric unit had different elbow angles: Fab 50.1 with 164- and 177-degree angles (44) and an intact immunoglobulin monoclonal antibody (Mab231) with 144- and 160-degree angles (45). These findings argue against any hypothesis that the binding of antigen is signaled to the Fc region by changes in the elbow angle and, hence, in the relative disposition of the V and C domains.

ANTIBODY-ANTIGEN COMPLEXES

Since the first x-ray crystallographic determinations of the structure of an antibody-hapten complex in 1973 (McPC603; 1,46) and of an antibody-protein complex in 1985 (D1.3; 42,47), many more examples of such complexes have been deduced. These complexes have included Fab and Fv fragments with proteins, peptides, carbohydrates, DNA, steroids, and other small molecules. The Fv is the variable domain (V_H, V_L) of the Fab fragment, often genetically engineered to be covalently tethered by a short peptide linker. The detailed information gathered from these structures has greatly increased understanding of the antigen-binding process. As expected, the antigens bind to the CDR loops at the tip of the Fab fragment (Fig. 18-8). However, depending on the antigen, not all of the CDR loops make contact in any one complex, even for large protein antigens.

Currently, more than 20 structures of Fab-protein complexes have been deposited in the Brookhaven Protein Data Bank (48). The protein antigens have included lysozyme, neuraminidase, histidine-containing protein, influenza virus hemagglutinin, staphylococcal nuclease, human immunodeficiency virus reverse transcriptase, protein G, and tissue factor. Several examples of idiotope–anti-idiotope complexes are also available; in these complexes, one antibody is bound to another antibody (anti-idiotope) raised against it. Examination of these complex structures shows that, although each antibody-antigen interaction is unique, many shared features are present. Most protein antigens cover the entire antibody-binding surface, making contact with all six CDR loops (Table 18-1). Usually about 600 to 900 Å^2 of surface is buried on each molecule in these complexes, with a combined buried surface size ranging from 1,100 to 1,850 Å^2 (Table 18-2). The Fab-antigen interactions include van der Waals contacts, hydrogen bonds, and charged interactions, with usually 100 to 200 contacts and 6 to 17 hydrogen bonds and charged interactions. The protein antigens usually bind to a rather flat and undulating Fab surface (Fig. 18-9). Interestingly, analysis of the struc-

ture of a rheumatoid factor Fab in complex with Fc reveals that the antigen (Fc) binds to one side of the antibody-binding pocket, rather than directly on top of it (Fig. 18-10). Only the CDRs H1, H2, H3, and L2 make contact with the antigen. It has been proposed that a second, unknown antigen may bind to the remainder of the antibody-binding site, perhaps simultaneously with the Fc (49).

More than ten x-ray structures have been determined for Fab-peptide complexes. Many of the same features of Fab interactions with much larger protein antigens are seen in these peptide complexes, but with slightly smaller binding surfaces and correspondingly fewer contacts and hydrogen bonds between antigen and antibody (see Table 18-2). The surfaces on Fab or peptide that are buried on binding range from about 500 to 600 Å^2, with 100 to 150 van der Waals contacts and 5 to 14 hydrogen bonds and charged interactions. However, the peptides usually bind in grooves or pockets on the Fab surface, in contrast to the flatter, more undulating surfaces of anti-protein antibodies (see Fig. 18-9). The majority of the peptides form some type of β-turn when bound to antibody, although completely extended peptide conformations have also been observed (40,50).

Most of the antibody-antigen complexes that have been determined involve small haptenic antigens, including

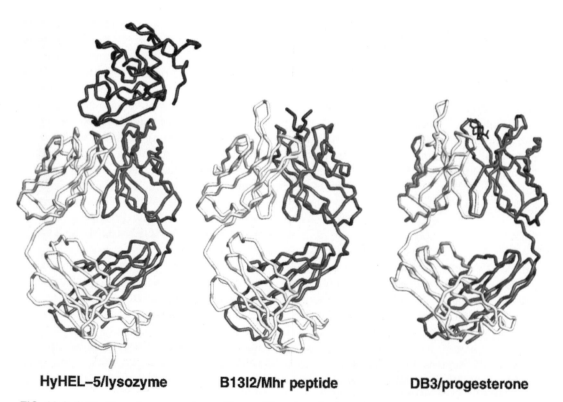

HyHEL–5/lysozyme   **B13I2/Mhr peptide**   **DB3/progesterone**

FIG. 18-8. Antibody-antigen complexes. Three different antibody-antigen complexes are shown to illustrate the variety of sizes found in antigens. On the left, is the complex of HyHEL-5 (77) with lysozyme, an example of an antibody-protein complex. In the middle, is the complex of B13I2 (34) with myohemerythrin peptide. On the right, is the complex between DB3 (80) and the small hapten progesterone.

TABLE 18-1. *Sizes of buried surface areas in antibody-antigen complexes[a]*

Fab	Fab buried surface area (Å²)	Antigen	Antigen mass (KDa)	Antigen buried surface area (Å²)	% antigen buried
McPC603	161	phosphocholine	182	137	81
DB3	286	progesterone	314	246	89
Se155-4	297	dodecasaccharide	472	248	66
4-4-20	308	fluorescein	332	266	94
AN02	350	DNP spin-label	392	232	67
17/9	468	HA peptide	929	436	59
59.1	469	GP120 peptide	975	429	49
BV04	515	d(pT)3	930	454	66
50.1	530	GP120 peptide	980	475	56
B13I2	560	Mhr peptide	836	462	66
D1.3	690	lysozyme	14,300	680	12
HyHEL-10	721	lysozyme	14,300	774	14
HyHEL-5	746	lysozyme	14,300	750	14
NC41	916	neuraminidase	45,300	899	6

[a]Listed here are a few representative examples of antibody-antigen complexes whose structures have been determined. The buried surface area is the size of the antibody and antigen surfaces involved in binding. Antigens shown here include small molecules, peptides, and proteins. Buried surface area calculated with MS[81] with a 1.7Å probe radius. Coordinates used are found in the Brookhaven Protein Databank[48] and are McPC603,[82] DB3,[80] Se155-4,[83] 4-4-20,[84] AN02,[85] 17/9,[36,37] 59.1,[86] BV04-01,[35] 50.1,[44] B13I2,[34] D1.3,[87] HyHEL-10,[88] HyHEL-5,[77] and NC41.[89]

TABLE 18-2. *Hypervariable loops used in antigen binding[a]*

Fab	PDB id	L1(%)	L2(%)	L3(%)	H1(%)	H2(%)	H3(%)	FW(%)
Haptens								
DB3	1dba	4	0	27	6	17	41	6
CHA255	1ind	13	0	28	8	31	20	0
AN02	1baf	14	6	38	0	5	32	5
1F7	1fig	0	0	10	24	4	61	1
26-10	1igj	0	0	21	16	2	35	6
4-4-20	4fab	30	0	12	20	6	32	0
NC6.8	2cgr	13	0	21	15	15	34	1
Peptides								
50.1	1ggi	9	8	18	1	27	23	14
17/9	1him	5	0	21	1	43	30	0
26/9	1frg	6	0	26	2	38	29	0
TE33	1tet	29	2	11	13	17	27	1
B13I2	2igf	8	0	14	10	34	32	2
59.1	1acy	19	0	26	5	20	30	0
BV04-01	1cbv	21	1	21	5	19	33	0
Se155-4	1mfb	23	0	25	17	20	15	0
Proteins								
NC41	1nca	1	22	17	11	13	28	8
D1.3	1fdl	9	14	17	10	19	26	5
D11.15	1jhl	7	3	23	18	22	24	3
HyHEL-5	2hfl	13	2	26	14	25	15	4
HyHEL-10	3hfm	12	12	17	18	25	9	7
Jel142	1jel	26	0	6	12	27	28	2
N10	1nsn	20	6	19	9	32	6	9
camelV$_H$	1mel	0	0	0	7	17	68	8

[a]This table lists the percentage each complementarity-determining region (CDR) loop contributes to the buried surface for the antibody when bound to antigen. The percentage contributed by framework residues is noted by "FW." Shown are antibodies bound to small antigens DB3,[80] CHA255,[90] AN02,[85] 1F7,[91] 26-10,[92] 4-4-20,[84] and NC6.8[93]; peptide, DNA, and carbohydrate antigens 50.1,[44] 17/9,[36,37] 26/9,[94] TE33,[95] B13I2,[34] 59.1,[86] BV04-01,[35] Se155-4[83]; and protein antigens (NC41,[89] D1.3,[87] D11.15,[96] HyHEL-5,[77] HyHEL-10,[88] Jel142,[97] camel VH,[66] and N10.[61] Most antibodies use the H3 CDR loop predominantly, but there are exceptions, such as antibody N10 in its complex with staphylococcal nuclease. L2 frequently is not used in binding, especially for the smaller antigens.

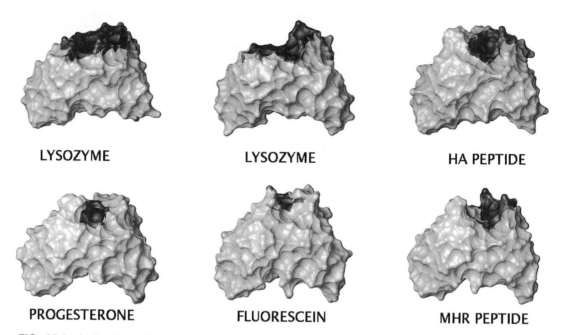

LYSOZYME   LYSOZYME   HA PEPTIDE

PROGESTERONE   FLUORESCEIN   MHR PEPTIDE

FIG. 18-9. Antibody-binding surfaces. Several representative surfaces of antibodies are shown. The region where antigen binds is highlighted in dark gray, and the antigen for the antibody is labeled under each. The anti-protein surfaces are usually more flat and undulating than the pockets and grooves found in anti-peptide and anti-hapten antibodies. This figure was created with the program MCS.

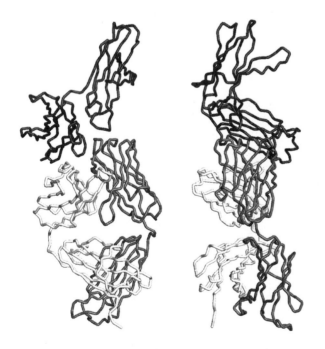

FIG. 18-10. The x-ray structure of antibody RF-AN and rheumatoid factor (49). The rheumatoid factor binds to one side of the Fab, contacting complementarity-determining regions (CDRs) H1, H2, H3, and L2. The light and heavy chains of the Fab are shown in light and dark gray, respectively. Two orthogonal views are shown for clarity.

progesterone, fluorescein, digoxin, ouabain, derivatives of ethylenediamine tetraacetic acid, sweet-tasting compounds, and transition-state analogues of chemical reactions. In these complexes, the small antigen usually is buried in a deep pocket in the antibody-combining site and usually makes many more interactions with the heavy chain than with the light chain. Again, van der Waals contacts, hydrogen bonds, and charged interactions are features of these binding sites (see Table 18-1), but no one type of interaction is predominant or even present in all complexes.

CATALYTIC ANTIBODIES

Since the first reports of monoclonal antibodies capable of catalyzing enzymatic reactions (51,52), many interesting catalytic antibodies have been produced. These antibodies are obtained by immunization with transition-state analogues of the desired reaction covalently linked to protein immunogens. Antibodies have now been obtained that catalyze reactions from all major enzyme classes (with the exception of nucleotide-dependent ligases) (53). Catalytic antibodies have also been produced that can catalyze reactions for which there are no natural enzyme catalysts. Many of these antibody catalysts have the highly desirable property of stereoselectivity; that is, they produce only one enantiomeric product of the desired reaction.

Another approach in immunogen design is that of "reactive immunization." Here, instead of being immunizing with an inert transition-state analogue of the desired reaction, the immunogen is a hybrid combining both a transition-state mimic and a portion that actually reacts with residues in the antibody-binding site. This method has been successful in producing potent hydrolytic antibodies (54) and an aldolase antibody with a broad range of substrate specificity (55). The x-ray structures for several catalytic antibodies and their transition-state analogues have now been determined, and these have resulted in a better understanding of how antibodies can be developed in a matter of weeks to catalyze reactions for which the natural enzyme (if one exists) evolved over millions of years. Additionally, the esterase catalytic antibody 48G7 has now been structurally compared with its germ-line precursor, with structures for both antibodies available in antigen-bound and antigen-free forms (56,57). The germ-line and mature antibodies differ by six and three amino acids in the heavy and light chains, respectively. These structures have demonstrated that there can also be large conformational changes in the germ-line antibody on binding of antigen; however, in this case no changes are seen between the bound and free forms for the mature 48G7. It has been hypothesized that this antibody uses conformational changes to optimize binding in the germ-line antibody and that these changes are later stabilized in the mature antibody through somatic mutations (56).

STRUCTURE OF INTACT IMMUNOGLOBULIN G

Until recently, there has been difficulty in obtaining a high-resolution x-ray crystallographic structure for an intact immunoglobulin because the high degree of flexibility between the Fab and Fc portions of the molecule has hampered efforts to obtain well-ordered crystals. This has resulted in the common practice of enzymatic cleavage of the immunoglobulin to prepare only Fab or Fab' fragments for crystallographic studies. Early work with intact immunoglobulins resulted in three structures, one in which the Fc region was disordered (Kol, 41), and two in which the hinge peptide was mutated to be abnormally short, thereby reducing the flexibility between Fab and Fc (McG, 58; DOB, 59). More recently, the structure of an intact antibody with a normal hinge region has been determined (45). These structures verify that the Fab arms are very flexible with respect to the Fc region, allowing the immunoglobulin to bind to two distinct antigenic sites. One of these structures is shown in Fig. 18-11.

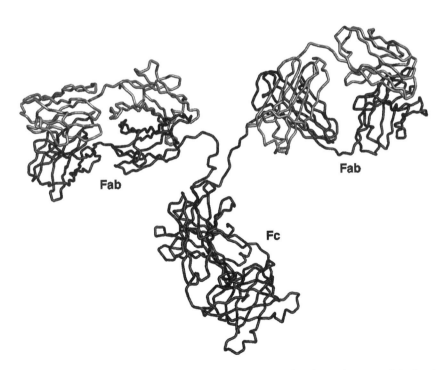

FIG. 18-11. Intact immunoglobulin. Shown is the structure for the first intact immunoglobulin visualized in its entirety by x-ray crystallography (antibody 231) (45). Note that each Fab fragment has a different elbow angle, and also note the flexible hinge peptides linking the Fab fragments to the Fc fragment. These flexible linkers allow the antibody a large degree of flexibility in binding bivalently to antigens.

ANTIBODY-VIRUS INTERACTIONS

In order to advance understanding of the mechanism of antibody neutralization of viruses, several structural studies with Fabs and viruses or viral antigens have been undertaken. Two viral surface antigens from influenza virus hemagglutinin have been studied in complex with antibody. One of these is influenza virus neuraminidase in complex with Fabs NC41 (60) and NC10 (61). The neuraminidase is a tetrameric glycoprotein, consisting of a head and a stalk region, which is responsible for destroying the cellular receptor for the virus by cleaving a sialic acid moiety. The NC41 and NC10 Fabs have been cocrystallized with native and mutant neuraminidase head regions. These structures show that the antibody may inhibit neuraminidase activity by blocking the active-site pocket. Although the two different antibodies bind to almost the same epitope on the neuraminidase, they bind in different orientations, showing that antibodies can evolve different ways to bind to the same epitope (60). The other influenza virus viral antigen studied in complex with antibody is the hemagglutinin. The hemagglutinin trimer is responsible for binding of the virus to the host cell and also for fusion and for transfer of the virus into the cell. The "top" region of the hemagglutinin molecule can be released by enzymatic digestion, and this portion has been crystallized and determined in complex with Fab HC19. The binding of the Fab may block access to the conserved sialic acid receptor-binding site.

Several structure determinations for Fabs bound to intact virus are also of special interest. The first of these is for cowpea mosaic virus (CPMV) complexed with monoclonal antibodies 5B2 (Fab and IgG) and 10B7 (Fab), which was determined by a combination of cryoelectron microscopy and x-ray crystallography to 23-Å resolution (62). The structures clearly showed the Fab fragments bound to the surface of the virus with icosahedral symmetry and revealed that the IgG bound with only one Fab arm. The two antibodies bound to virtually identical epitopes, related to the antigenic site 3B on poliovirus.

Another Fab-virus complex determined at about the same time was that of Fab 17-IA bound to human rhinovirus 14 (HRV 14) (63,64). This structure was determined by a combination of x-ray crystallography and cryoelectron microscopy to a resolution of 4.0 Å. In this complex, the Fab was unexpectedly found to bind deep into the viral "canyon," a depression located around each five-fold icosahedral axis in this virus (Fig. 18-12). The binding site for receptor is at the bottom of this canyon, so that binding of antibody can directly prevent binding of the virus to its receptor through competition for the binding site. This complex also shows that the Fab binds to virus not only with the CDR regions at the tip of the Fab fragment but also with the side of the V_H domain. The Fab buries about 550 Å^2 on the CDR region and an additional

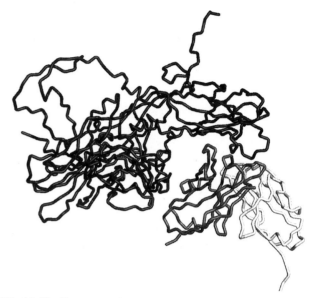

FIG. 18-12. Structure of Fab 17-IA with human rhinovirus 14 (HRV 14) (63,64). The Fv portion of the Fab is shown bound into a cleft on the viral surface. Only a small portion of the virus coat is depicted. The light and heavy chains of the Fv are shown in light and dark gray, respectively.

300 Å^2 along the side of the V_H domain, including residues from CDR H3 and framework residues in this region.

One other example is that of Fab SD6 bound to foot-and-mouth-disease virus (65). This structure has been determined to a resolution of 30 Å by a combination of cryoelectron microscopy and image reconstruction. The Fab binds to the surface of the virus and interacts with the major antigenic site on the virus. Again, the binding of this Fab blocks access to the receptor binding site. The structure has also been determined for this Fab in complex with the peptide corresponding to the continuous epitope on the virus.

CAMELID ANTIBODIES

A new class of antibodies, consisting only of heavy chains, has been found in camelid species (66). These antibodies have a normal Fc region, consisting of a dimer of the C_H2 and C_H3 regions of the heavy chain, but the Fab region consists of only the V_H domain. A structure determination of a camel V_H domain in complex with lysozyme showed that this solitary V_H domain can act much as a normal Fab V_L-V_H dimer in binding to antigen. The size of the interface buried between the camel V_H and lysozyme was 770 Å^2, comparable to the size buried in Fab-protein antigen interfaces (see Table 18-1). The domains differ from "normal" V_H domains primarily at framework residue positions, where the residues that would ordinarily be buried in the V_L-V_H

interface are instead changed to more hydrophilic amino acids to allow solvent exposure in the camel V_H domain. Another structure determined for a llama V_H domain in the unbound form showed similar solubility properties for this binding fragment (67). The discovery of these single-domain binding fragments is exciting for the field of antibody engineering, where smaller proteins are desirable because of their increased solubility, ease of production, longer lifetime *in vivo*, and better tissue penetration (68).

ANTIBODY ENGINEERING

As alluded to in the previous section, the field of antibody engineering has grown rapidly in the last few years (69). The ability to clone and express antibody genes has allowed the production of fragments and fusions of antibody domains not found in nature (70). In addition to the Fab fragment, there are the Fv (V_L-V_H dimer) fragment; the single-chain Fv, in which the V_L and V_H chains are expressed as one polypeptide; and the single-chain Fab, in which the light and heavy chains are expressed as one polypeptide. Diabodies and triabodies have also been formed. In diabodies (71,72), the V_L chain is linked to the V_H chain, and then dimers of these chains are formed, with V_L from one chain dimerizing with V_H from the other chain. In triabodies (73), the V_L domain is fused to the C terminus of the V_H domain, with no linking region. The combination of three of these units gives rise to three Fv fragments linked together, making up the triabody. The size of the linker region used to pair these segments appears to control the propensity for Fv, diabody, or triabody formation. With all of these antibody constructs, an attempt is made to maximize the number of binding sites per molecule and hence the effectiveness of the construct as a possible therapeutic agent. Additionally, as discussed previously, the discovery of the single-subunit V_H domain from camelid species has allowed antibody engineers to modify the solubility properties of similar single-domain molecules, so as to prepare very small binding domains suitable for human therapy.

CONCLUSION

Extensive sequencing and structural information about immunoglobulins has greatly increased the understanding of antibodies and how they participate in the immune response. Crystal structures of antibodies in complex with a wide array of antigens have shown how antibodies recognize these antigens and how conformational changes can assist in the binding process. Knowledge of the structure of immunoglobulin molecules has also helped in the development of immunoglobulin-based diagnostic tools and immunotherapeutic agents.

ACKNOWLEDGMENTS

The authors thank Dr. T. Smith for Fab 17-IA coordinates and Drs. A. Corper and B. Sutton for Fab RF-AN coordinates. This is manuscript #11208-MB from The Scripps Research Institute. Authors supported by NIH grants GM46192, GM49497, HL16411, CA27489.

REFERENCES

1. Padlan EA, Segal DM, Spande TF, Davies DR, Rudikoff S, Potter M. Structure at 4.5 Å resolution of a phosphorylcholine-binding fab. *Nat New Biol* 1973;245:165–167.
2. Poljak RJ, Amzel LM, Avey HP, Chen BL, Phizackerley RP, Saul F. Three-dimensional structure of the Fab' fragment of a human immunoglobulin at 2.8-Å resolution. *Proc Natl Acad Sci U S A* 1973;70:3305–3310.
3. Bork P, Holm L, Sander C. The immunoglobulin fold: structural classification, sequence patterns and common core. *J Mol Biol* 1994;242:309–320.
4. Lesk AM, Chothia C. Evolution of proteins formed by β-sheets: II. The core of the immunoglobulin domains. *J Mol Biol* 1982;160:325–342.
5. Jones EY, Davis SJ, Williams AF, Harlos K, Stuart DI. Crystal structure at 2.8 Å resolution of a soluble form of the cell adhesion molecule CD2. *Nature* 1992;360:232–239.
6. Brady RL, Dodson EJ, Dodson GG, et al. Crystal structure of domains 3 and 4 of rat CD4: Relation to the NH$_2$-terminal domains. *Science* 1993;260:979–983.
7. Hilschmann N, Craig LC. Amino acid sequence studies with Bence Jones proteins. *Proc Natl Acad Sci U S A* 1965;53:1403–1409.
8. Kabat EA. Unique features of the variable regions of Bence Jones proteins and their possible relation to antibody complementarity. *Proc Natl Acad Sci U S A* 1968;59:613–619.
9. Franêk F. *Symposium on developmental aspects of antibody formation and structure.* Prague, 1969.
10. Milstein C. Linked groups of residues in immunoglobulin κ chains. *Nature* 1967;216:330–332.
11. Wu TT, Kabat EA. An analysis of the sequences of the variable regions of Bence Jones proteins and myeloma light chains and their implications for antibody complementarity. *J Exp Med* 1970;132:211–250.
12. Tonegawa S. Somatic generation of antibody diversity. *Nature* 1983;302:575–581.
13. Tomlinson IM, Walter G, Marks JD, Llewelyn MB, Winter G. The repertoire of human germline V_H sequences reveals about fifty groups of V_H segments with different hypervariable loops. *J Mol Biol* 1992;227:776–798.
14. Cook GP, Tomlinson IM. The human immunoglobulin V_H repertoire. *Immunol Today* 1995;16:237–242.
15. Ravetch JV, Siebenlist U, Korsmeyer S, Waldmann T, Leder P. Structure of the human immunoglobulin mu locus: characterization of embryonic and rearranged J and D genes. *Cell* 1981;27:583–591.
16. Corbett SJ, Tomlinson IM, Sonnhammer ELL, Buck D, Winter G. Sequence of the human immunoglobulin diversity (D) segment locus: a systematic analysis provides no evidence for the use of DIR segments, inverted D segments, "minor" D segments or D-D recombination. *J Mol Biol* 1997;270:587–597.
17. Williams SC, Frippiat JP, Tomlinson IM, Ignatovich O, Lefranc MP, Winter G. Sequence and evolution of the human germline V_λ repertoire. *J Mol Biol* 1996;264:220–232.
18. Victor KD, Capra JD. An apparently common mechanism of generating antibody diversity: length variation of the V_L-J_L junction. *Mol Immunol* 1994;31:39–46.
19. Milstein C, Even J, Jarvis JM, Gonzales-Fernandez A, Gherardi E. Non-random features of the repertoire expressed by the members of one V_κ gene family and of the V-J recombination. *Eur J Immunol* 1992;22:1958.
20. Schable KF, Zachau HG. The variable genes of the human immunoglobulin kappa locus. *Biol Chem Hoppe-Seyler* 1993;374:1001–1022.
21. Hieter PA, Maizel JV Jr, Leder P. Evolution of human immunoglobulin κ J region genes. *J Biol Chem* 1982;257:1516–1522.

22. Vasicek TJ, Leder P. Structure and expression of the human immunoglobulin λ genes. *J Exp Med* 1990;172:609–620.

23. Kabat EA, Wu TT. Identical V region amino acid sequences and segments of sequences in antibodies of different specificities: relative contributions of V_H and V_L genes, minigenes, and complementarity-determining regions to binding of antibody-combining sites. *J Immunol* 1991;147:1709–1719.

24. Kabat EA, Wu TT, Perry HM, Gottesman KS, Foeller C. *Sequences of proteins of immunological interest*, 5th ed, vol 1. US Department of Health and Human Services, 1991.

25. Ohno S, Mori N, Matsunaga T. Antigen-binding specificities of antibodies are primarily determined by seven residues of V_H. *Proc Natl Acad Sci U S A* 1985;82:2945–2949.

26. Chothia C, Lesk AM, Levitt M, et al. The predicted structure of immunoglobulin D1.3 and its comparison with the crystal structure. *Science* 1986;233:755–758.

27. Chothia C, Lesk AM. Canonical structures for the hypervariable regions of immunoglobulins. *J Mol Biol* 1987;196:901–917.

28. Chothia C, Lesk AM, Tramontano A, et al. Conformations of immunoglobulin hypervariable regions. *Nature* 1989;342:877–883.

29. Chothia C, Lesk AM, Gherardi E, et al. Structural repertoire of the human V_H segments. *J Mol Biol* 1992;227:799–817.

30. Tramontano A, Chothia C, Lesk AM. Framework residue 71 is a major determinant of the position and conformation of the second hypervariable region in the V_H domains of immunoglobulins. *J Mol Biol* 1990;215:175–182.

31. Martin AC, Thornton JM. Structural families in loops of homologous proteins: automatic classification, modelling and application to antibodies. *J Mol Biol* 1996;263:800–815.

32. Al-Lazikani B, Lesk A, Chothia C. Standard conformations for the canonical structures of immunoglobulins. *J Mol Biol* (*in press*).

33. Shirai H, Kidera A, Nakamura H. Structural classification of CDR-H3 in antibodies. *FEBS Lett* 1996;399:1–8.

34. Stanfield RL, Fieser TM, Lerner RA, Wilson IA. Crystal structures of an antibody to a peptide and its complex with peptide antigen at 2.8 Å. *Science* 1990;248:712–719.

35. Herron JN, He XM, Ballard DW, et al. An autoantibody to single-stranded DNA: comparison of the three-dimensional structures of the unliganded Fab and a deoxynucleotide-Fab complex. *Proteins* 1991;11:159–175.

36. Rini JM, Schulze-Gahmen U, Wilson IA. Structural evidence for induced fit as a mechanism for antibody-antigen recognition. *Science* 1992;255:959–965.

37. Schulze-Gahmen U, Rini JM, Wilson IA. Detailed analysis of the free and bound conformations of an antibody: X-ray structures of Fab 17/9 and three different Fab-peptide complexes. *J Mol Biol* 1993;234:1098–1118.

38. Stanfield RL, Takimoto-Kamimura M, Rini JM, Profy AT, Wilson IA. Major antigen-induced domain rearrangements in an antibody. *Structure* 1993;1:83–93.

39. Foote J, Milstein C. Conformational isomerism and the diversity of antibodies. *Proc Natl Acad Sci U S A* 1994;91:10370–10374.

40. Stanfield RL, Wilson IA. X-ray crystallographic studies of antibody-peptide complexes. *Immunomethods* 1993;3:211–221.

41. Marquart M, Deisenhofer J, Huber R, Palm W. Crystallographic refinement and atomic models of the intact immunoglobulin molecule Kol and its antigen-binding fragment at 3.0 Å and 1.9 Å resolution. *J Mol Biol* 1980;141:369–391.

42. Amit AG, Mariuzza RA, Phillips SE, Poljak RJ. Three-dimensional structure of an antigen-antibody complex at 2.8 Å resolution. *Science* 1986;233:747–753.

43. Huber R. Structural basis for antigen-antibody recognition. *Science* 1986;233:702–703.

44. Rini JM, Stanfield RL, Stura EA, Salinas PA, Profy AT, Wilson IA. Crystal structure of a human immunodeficiency virus type 1 neutralizing antibody, 50.1, in complex with its V3 loop peptide antigen. *Proc Natl Acad Sci U S A* 1993;90:6325–6329.

45. Harris LJ, Larson SB, Hasel KW, McPherson A. Refined structure of an intact IgG2a monoclonal antibody. *Biochemistry* 1997;36:1581–1597.

46. Segal DM, Padlan EA, Cohen GH, Rudikoff S, Potter M, Davies DR. The three-dimensional structure of a phosphorylcholine-binding mouse immunoglobulin Fab and the nature of the antigen binding site. *Proc Natl Acad Sci U S A* 1974;71:4298–4302.

47. Amit AG, Mariuzza RA, Phillips SE, Poljak RJ. Three-dimensional structure of an antigen-antibody complex at 6 Å resolution. *Nature* 1985;313:156–158.

48. Bernstein FC, Koetzle TF, Williams GJ, et al. The Protein Data Bank: a computer-based archival file for macromolecular structures. *J Mol Biol* 1977;112:535–542.

49. Corper AL, Sohi MK, Bonagura VR, et al. Structure of human IgM rheumatoid factor Fab bound to its autoantigen IgG Fc reveals a novel topology of antibody-antigen interaction. *Nat Struct Biol* 1997;4:374–381.

50. Stanfield RL, Wilson IA. Protein-peptide interactions. *Curr Opin Struct Biol* 1995;5:103–113.

51. Tramontano A, Janda KD, Lerner RA. Catalytic antibodies. *Science* 1986;234:1566–1570.

52. Pollack SJ, Jacobs JW, Schultz PG. Selective chemical catalysis by an antibody. *Science* 1986;234:1570–1573.

53. Thomas NR. Catalytic antibodies: Reaching adolescence? *Nat Prod Rep* 1996;13:479–511.

54. Wirsching P, Ashley JA, Lo CH, Janda KD, Lerner RA. Reactive immunization. *Science* 1995;270:1775–1782.

55. Wagner J, Lerner RA, Barbas CF 3rd. Efficient aldolase catalytic antibodies that use the enamine mechanism of natural enzymes. *Science* 1995;270:1797–1800.

56. Wedemayer GJ, Patten PA, Wang LH, Schultz PG, Stevens RC. Structural insights into the evolution of an antibody combining site. *Science* 1997;276:1665–1669.

57. Wedemayer GJ, Wang LH, Patten PA, Schultz PG, Stevens RC. Crystal structures of the free and liganded form of an esterolytic catalytic antibody. *J Mol Biol* 1997;268:390–400.

58. Guddat LW, Herron JN, Edmundson AB. Three-dimensional structure of a human immunoglobulin with a hinge deletion. *Proc Natl Acad Sci U S A* 1993;90:4271–4275.

59. Silverton EW, Navia MA, Davies DR. Three-dimensional structure of an intact human immunoglobulin. *Proc Natl Acad Sci USA* 1977;74:5140–5144.

60. Tulip WR, Varghese JN, Webster RG, Air GM, Laver WG, Colman PM. Crystal structures of neuraminidase-antibody complexes. *Cold Spring Harb Symp Quant Biol* 1989;54:257–263.

61. Colman PM, Tulip WR, Varghese JN, et al. Three-dimensional structures of influenza virus neuraminidase-antibody complexes. *Philos Trans R Soc Lond B Biol Sci* 1989;323:511–518.

62. Porta C, Wang G, Cheng H, Chen Z, Baker TS, Johnson JE. Direct imaging of interactions between an icosahedral virus and conjugate F(ab) fragments by cryoelectron microscopy and X-ray crystallography. *Virology* 1994;204:777–788.

63. Liu H, Smith TJ, Lee WM, et al. Structure determination of an Fab fragment that neutralizes human rhinovirus 14 and analysis of the Fab-virus complex. *J Mol Biol* 1994;240:127–137.

64. Smith TJ, Chase ES, Schmidt TJ, Olson NH, Baker TS. Neutralizing antibody to human rhinovirus 14 penetrates the receptor-binding canyon. *Nature* 1996;383:350–354.

65. Hewat EA, Verdaguer N, Fita I, et al. Structure of the complex of an Fab fragment of a neutralizing antibody with foot-and-mouth disease virus: positioning of a highly mobile antigenic loop. *EMBO J* 1997;16:1492–1500.

66. Desmyter A, Transue TR, Ghahroudi MA, et al. Crystal structure of a camel single-domain V_H antibody fragment in complex with lysozyme. *Nat Struct Biol* 1996;3:803–811.

67. Spinelli S, Frenken L, Bourgeois D, et al. The crystal structure of a llama heavy chain variable domain. *Nat Struct Biol* 1996;3:752–757.

68. Sheriff S, Constantine KL. Redefining the minimal antigen-binding fragment. *Nat Struct Biol* 1996;3:733–736.

69. Carter P, Merchant AM. Engineering antibodies for imaging and therapy. *Curr Opin Biotechnol* 1997;8:449–454.

70. Pluckthun A, Pack P. New protein engineering approaches to multivalent and bispecific antibody fragments. *Immunotechnology* 1997;3:83–105.

71. Perisic O, Webb PA, Holliger P, Winter G, Williams RL. Crystal structure of a diabody, a bivalent antibody fragment. *Structure* 1994;2:1217–1226.

72. Poljak RJ. Production and structure of diabodies. *Structure* 1994;2:1121–1123.

73. Pei XY, Holliger P, Murzin AG, Williams RL. The 2.0-Å resolution crystal structure of a trimeric antibody fragment with noncognate V_H-V_L domain pairs shows a rearrangement of V_H CDR3. *Proc Natl Acad Sci U S A* 1997;94:9637–9642.

74. Ferrin TE, Huang CC, Jarvis LE, Langridge R. The MIDAS display system. *J Mol Graph* 1988;6:13–27.

75. Deisenhofer J. Crystallographic refinement and atomic models of a human Fc fragment and its complex with fragment B of protein A from *Staphylococcus aureus* at 2.9- and 2.8-Å resolution. *Biochemistry* 1981;20:2361–2370.

76. Sheriff S, Silverton EW, Padlan EA, et al. Three-dimensional structure of an antibody-antigen complex. *Proc Natl Acad Sci U S A* 1987;84:8075–8079.

77. Priestle JP. RIBBON: A stereo cartoon drawing program for proteins. *J Appl Crystallogr* 1988;21:572–576.

78. Tormo J, Stadler E, Skern T, et al. Three-dimensional structure of the Fab fragment of a neutralizing antibody to human rhinovirus serotype 2. *Protein Science* 1992;1:1154–1161.

79. Chiu YY, Lopez de Castro JA, Poljak RJ. Amino acid sequence of the V_H region of human myeloma cryoimmunoglobulin IgG Hil. *Biochemistry* 1979;18:553–560.

80. Arévalo JH, Stura EA, Taussig MJ, Wilson IA. Three-dimensional structure of an anti-steroid Fab′ and progesterone-Fab′ complex. *J Mol Biol* 1993;231:103–118.

81. Connolly ML. The molecular surface package. *J Mol Graph* 1993;11:139–141.

82. Satow Y, Cohen GH, Padlan EA, Davies DR. Phosphocholine binding immunoglobulin Fab McPC603: an x-ray diffraction study at 2.7 Å. *J Mol Biol* 1986;190:593–604.

83. Zdanov A, Li Y, Bundle DR, et al. Structure of a single-chain antibody variable domain (Fv) fragment complexed with a carbohydrate antigen at 1.7-Å resolution. *Proc Natl Acad Sci U S A* 1994;91:6423–6427.

84. Herron JN, Terry AH, Johnston S, et al. High resolution structures of the 4-4-20 Fab-fluorescein complex in two solvent systems: effects of solvent on structure and antigen-binding affinity. *Biophys J* 1994;67:2167–2183.

85. Brunger AT, Leahy DJ, Hynes TR, Fox RO. 2.9 Å resolution structure of an anti-dinitrophenyl-spin-label monoclonal antibody Fab fragment with bound hapten. *J Mol Biol* 1991;221:239–256.

86. Ghiara JB, Stura EA, Stanfield RL, Profy AT, Wilson IA. Crystal structure of the principal neutralization site of HIV-1. *Science* 1994;264:82–85.

87. Fischmann TO, Bentley GA, Bhat TN, et al. Crystallographic refinement of the three-dimensional structure of the Fab D1.3-lysozyme complex at 2.5-Å resolution. *J Biol Chem* 1991;266:12915–12920.

88. Padlan EA, Silverton EW, Sheriff S, Cohen GH, Smith-Gill SJ, Davies DR. Structure of an antibody-antigen complex: crystal structure of the HyHEL-10 Fab-lysozyme complex. *Proc Natl Acad Sci U S A* 1989;86:5938–5942.

89. Tulip WR, Varghese JN, Laver WG, Webster RG, Colman PM. Refined crystal structure of the influenza virus N9 neuraminidase-NC41 Fab complex. *J Mol Biol* 1992;227:122–148.

90. Love RA, Villafranca JE, Aust RM, et al. How the anti-(metal chelate) antibody CHA255 is specific for the metal ion of its antigen: X-ray structures for two Fab′/hapten complexes with different metals in the chelate. *Biochemistry* 1993;32:10950–10959.

91. Haynes MR, Stura EA, Hilvert D, Wilson IA. Routes to catalysis: structure of a catalytic antibody and comparison with its natural counterpart. *Science* 1994;263:646–652.

92. Jeffrey PD, Strong RK, Sieker LC, et al. 26-10 Fab-digoxin complex: affinity and specificity due to surface complementarity. *Proc Natl Acad Sci U S A* 1993;90:10310–10314.

93. Guddat LW, Shan L, Anchin JM, Linthicum DS, Edmundson AB. Local and transmitted conformational changes on complexation of an anti-sweetener Fab. *J Mol Biol* 1994;236:247–274.

94. Churchill ME, Stura EA, Pinilla C, et al. Crystal structure of a peptide complex of anti-influenza peptide antibody Fab 26/9: comparison of two different antibodies bound to the same peptide antigen. *J Mol Biol* 1994;241:534–556.

95. Shoham M. Crystal structure of an anticholera toxin peptide complex at 2.3 Å. *J Mol Biol* 1993;232:1169–1175.

96. Chitarra V, Alzari PM, Bentley GA, et al. Three-dimensional structure of a heteroclitic antigen-antibody cross-reaction complex. *Proc Natl Acad Sci U S A* 1993;90:7711–7715.

97. Prasad L, Sharma S, Vandonselaar M, et al. Evaluation of mutagenesis for epitope mapping: structure of an antibody-protein antigen complex. *J Biol Chem* 1993;268:10705–10708.

Inflammation: Basic Principles and Clinical Correlates,
3rd ed., edited by John I. Gallin and Ralph Snyderman.
Lippincott Williams & Wilkins, Philadelphia © 1999.

CHAPTER 19

Biology of the Complement System

Neil R. Cooper

Complement is a complex and highly regulated biologic effector system. Many of the functions of the complement system are concerned with the recognition and elimination of pathogens and altered host cells. In this context, complement is a major component of the innate immune system, with the ability to discriminate self from nonself and to facilitate the elimination of pathogens and nonself antigens (Ag) through multiple proinflammatory, opsonic, phagocytic, cytotoxic, and cytolytic actions. Entirely separate from these functions, the actions of the complement system are integrated with those of the adaptive immune system, and complement possesses a number of immunoregulatory actions concerned with Ag capture, Ag processing, and the regulation of antibody (Ab) responses.

The natural bactericidal action of blood, which is a result of Ab and complement, was discovered in 1888 by George Nuttall, who named it *alexin* (from the Greek, "protective substance"), and the next year by Hans Buchner (1). Jules Bordet used the same term to describe the ability of fresh, but not heated, serum to lyse erythrocytes in the presence of Ab (immune hemolysis), a phenomenon which he discovered in 1898. Paul Ehrlich named this activity *complement* (komplement), since its function in immune hemolysis appeared to complement that of the Ab. The crucial functions of Ab and complement in immune hemolysis and the bactericidal reaction were evaluated in numerous experimental studies and extensively discussed in theoretical treatises over the next few years by Bordet, Ehrlich, and other prominent microbiologists of the time, including Elie Metchnikoff, Julius Morgenroth, and Karl Landsteiner. Metchnikoff and Ehrlich (1908), and Bordet (1919) received Nobel prizes for these and related studies. Physicochemical and biologic approaches quickly showed that complement was

not a single substance, and by 1926 four of its components had been described. Although studies of complement continued during the next decades, rapid progress in molecular characterization of the complement proteins and elucidation of their reaction mechanisms, biologic functions, and genetics began with the advent of modern functional, biochemical, and biophysical techniques in the early 1960s and the development of molecular genetic approaches and monoclonal antibodies (MAbs) in the late 1970s.

This chapter reviews the many host defense and immunoregulatory functions of the complement system. The molecular characteristics of the complement proteins and their reaction mechanisms are not described in depth but are summarized to provide a background for understanding the biologic functions of the complement system. The reader is referred to the many comprehensive reviews of the complement proteins and their reaction mechanisms for detailed information and citations of the original papers (2–8). Other topics, including complement phylogeny, molecular genetics, and biosynthetic regulatory processes, are not considered here; these subjects have also been the focus of review articles (9–11).

COMPLEMENT ACTIVATION AND REGULATORY MECHANISMS

As a major component of the innate or natural immune system, the complement system possesses the ability to directly recognize and eliminate or destroy pathogens and damaged or malignant host cells in the absence of Ab or specific cellular immune mechanisms. However, these host defense functions are significantly augmented in the presence of specific or cross-reactive Ab. The mechanisms mediating these actions of the complement system are considered here.

The complement system, together with its regulatory factors and specific cellular receptors, consists of more

N.R. Cooper: Department of Immunology, The Scripps Research Institute, La Jolla, California 92037.

than 30 distinct plasma and cell-membrane proteins. Activation, a prerequisite for the manifestation of biologic activity by the system, initiates a precisely regulated series of interactions of the complement components with each other, with the activator, and with cell membranes. These reactions can be divided into three phases: recognition and initiation of one of the three complement activation pathways; C3 activation, binding, and amplification; and assembly of the C5b–9 membrane attack complex (MAC).

The complement system is triggered by binding of the recognition component of one of the three independent activation pathways to a bacterium or other complement activator. The three pathways are the classical complement pathway (CCP), the mannose-binding lectin (MBL) pathway, and the alternative complement pathway (ACP) (Fig. 19-1). Binding triggers the activation of complement proenzymes through limited proteolytic cleavage and the formation of protein-protein complexes with novel binding or enzymatic activities. The CCP comprises the reaction steps of C1q, which serves as the recognition unit; two proenzymes, C1r and C1s; and two proteins, C4 and C2, which interact to form a novel protease after proteolytic activation. The MBL pathway includes the reaction steps of MBL, which functions as the recognition unit; two enzymes, MBL-associated serine protease-1 and -2 (MASP-1 and MASP-2); and C4 and C2, which function as in the CCP. The ACP consists of reaction steps involving activated C3, which binds to the activator; and two enzymes, factors B and D.

Each of the complement activation pathways culminates with the formation of a C3 cleaving enzyme (C3 convertase). These indigenous complement enzymes mediate the cleavage and activation of large numbers of C3 molecules, thereby generating C3b and enormously amplifying complement activation at this crucial central stage of the reaction sequence.

The sequential enzyme-substrate and protein-protein complex interactions that characterize the three activation pathways and the C3 amplification step are negatively modulated by a number of complement regulatory molecules. These molecules function as enzyme inhibitors, specific enzymes, cofactors for these enzymes, or active site inhibitors. They include C1 inhibitor (C1In), C4-binding protein (C4bp), factor I for the CCP and the MBL; and factors H and I for the ACP and the C3 amplification step. All of these molecules prevent significant complement activation in plasma and thereby prevent potentially life-threatening systemic complement activation. On the surface of autologous cells, complement receptor type 1 (CR1, also called CD35); decay-accelerating factor (DAF, or CD55); and membrane cofactor protein (MCP, or CD46) block significant complement activation and amplification on the cell surface, thereby preventing cellular damage. ACP activation at the C3 step is positively regulated by properdin.

Mediation of the activation and C3 amplification phases of the complement reaction sequence by combinations of enzyme-substrate and protein-protein interactions has several implications for the biologic activities of the first two phases. First, these steps are associated with amplification of initially weak activation stimuli, since

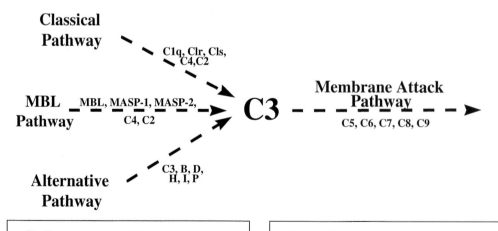

FIG. 19-1. Pathways and biology of the complement system.

each complement enzyme can cleave multiple complement substrate molecules. Second, limited proteolysis generates, in several instances, small complement peptides that are released from the parent molecule on the activator surface; these peptides bind to specific receptors on other cell types and initiate additional biologic reactions. Third, the larger complement cleavage fragments, which remain attached to the activator, acquire the ability to bind to specific complement receptors on various cell types, thereby mediating the attachment of the complement activator to such effector cells via a complement "bridge." These interactions trigger many additional reactions and specific biologic responses by the effector cells.

The terminal portion of the complement reaction sequence involves the assembly of a large multimolecular complex, the MAC. This portion of the reaction sequence is initiated by C5 cleavage into two fragments by the activator-bound C5 convertases generated by the activation pathways. The smaller fragment, C5a, which dissociates from C5, interacts with specific receptors on several cell types and elicits multiple biologic reactions. The larger fragment, C5b, initiates a self-assembly process involving C6, C7, C8, and C9 that leads to formation of the C5b–9 complex (MAC). Formation of this complex is associated with lytic disruption of cellular membranes. MAC formation and insertion into membranes is negatively regulated by several plasma proteins (S protein, SP40,40) and by cell membrane complement regulators (CD59 and homologous restriction factor [HRF]).

Complement Protein Families

Molecular cloning studies have shown that many of the complement proteins can be grouped into families on the basis of genetic, structural, or functional similarities. In addition, a number of the complement factors are mosaic proteins composed of multiple domains with characteristic structural features (7,11–13) (Table 19-1). This type of structure undoubtedly originated from exon shuffling of ancestral genes and gene segments. Some of these mosaic units are associated with enzymatic, binding, or other functional activities, and others serve unknown but probably structural purposes. Examples include C1r and C1s, which contain epidermal growth factor (EGF) and serine esterase domains as well as complement control protein short consensus repeats (SCR). Many different combinations of domains are found among the complement proteins. For example, C6 and C7 also contain EGF and SCR domains and, in addition, possess a low-density lipoprotein receptor, thrombospondin, and pore-forming protein domains, but lack a serine esterase domain. The extracellular domains of CR1 and CR2 are entirely composed of SCR domains. These combinations of domains and functions permit the grouping of the complement components into several families. In some cases, further gene duplication of ancestral proteins within a family has produced homologous proteins with similar, but not identical, functions or mechanisms of action. The genes encoding these homologous proteins may be linked, as with the genes for the regulators of complement activation (CR1, CR2, C4bp, factor H, DAF, MCP) on chromosome 1, or not linked, as with the C3, C4, and C5 genes. These classifications help to clarify the phylogeny of complement and the relation of complement to other effector systems. They also facilitate understanding of the mechanisms of activation and the biology of the system.

TABLE 19-1. *Complement protein families*

Family	Proteins	Thioester	Collagen	Ts	EGF	LDL	SCR	Perforin	vWF	Protease
Serine protease	C1r/C1s				+		+			+
	C2/B						+		+	+
	Factor I					+				+
RCA proteins	CR1, CR2						+			
	MCP, DAF						+			
	Factor H						+			
	C4bp						+			
Pore-forming proteins	C6/C7			+	+	+	+	+		
	C8			+	+	+		+		
	C9			+	+	+		+		
Membrane-binding proteins	C3/4	+								
	C5									
Collagen-like domain proteins	C1q		+							
	MBL		+							

Ts, thrombospondin; EGF, epidermal growth factor–like; LDL, low-density lipoprotein receptor–like; SCR, short consensus repeat; vWF, von Willebrand factor–like; RCA, regulators of complement activation.

The Classical Pathway

Initiation

The CCP is the primary mediator of adaptive humoral immunity, because it is activated by immune complexes containing immunoglobulins M (IgM) or G (IgG). IgG3 is a stronger activator than IgG1, which is much stronger than IgG2. Immune complexes containing IgG4, IgA, IgD, or IgE generally do not activate complement. In addition to its role as the primary effector system triggered by the binding of specific Ab to Ag, the CCP is efficiently activated by a large number of pathogens and other diverse and harmful agents in the absence of Ab (2,3,14). In this context, the CCP differentiates self from nonself. CCP activators comprise many gram-negative bacteria (e.g., *Salmonella* strains) and gram-positive bacteria (e.g., *Streptococcus* strains), as well as a number of viruses, including Sindbis virus (a togavirus), Newcastle disease virus (a paramyxovirus), and animal retroviruses such as the murine tumor viruses (15) and the human lentiviruses, which include the human immunodeficiency virus-1 (HIV-1) (16) and human T-cell lymphotrophic virus type I (HTLV-I). Other activators include parasites (e.g., *Schistosoma mansoni*, *Trypanosoma brucei*); mycoplasma; the Alzheimer's disease amyloid peptide (17,18); serum amyloid P component (19); myelin and myelin basic protein; certain carbohydrates (e.g., a polysaccharide from ant venom); C-reactive protein in complex with phosphoryl choline (20); cytoplasmic intermediate filaments; certain cellular membranes (e.g., mitochondrial membranes); polyanions (e.g., heparin, polynucleotides, DNA) (21); monosodium urate crystals; and others. All of the activators of the CCP either are aggregated or contain multiple subunits or other repeating structures, a required feature for CCP activation.

In all of these instances, the CCP is activated as a consequence of C1q binding to the activator. C1q binds to the heavy-chain constant-region C_H3 domain of IgM molecules and to the C_H2 domain of IgG molecules. In the case of the nonimmune activators, the precise molecular features responsible for activation are not known. However, for the nonprotein activators, and possibly also for the protein activators, clusters of highly charged species probably play an important role (22).

Structurally, C1q is a large (410 kd), unusual molecule that is composed of six copies of each of three, closely related polypeptide chains, designated A, B, and C (2,3). The amino-terminal residues 78 through 81 of each of these chains exhibit a collagen-like sequence. Electron microscopic images reveal a structure resembling a "bouquet of six tulips." The 18 polypeptide chains are arranged into 6 structural units, each containing a single copy of each of the three different polypeptide chains, with the relatively rigid, collagen-like portions of the polypeptide chains corresponding to the tulip "stems" and the carboxyl-terminal, noncollagen-like sequences representing the globular "heads" of the tulips.

C1q binds by means of its globular "heads" to immune complexes. However, in the case of the amyloid peptide, the amyloid P component, C-reactive protein, and DNA, binding is to a localized sequence (residues 14–26) in the collagen-like region of the A chain of C1q (18–21). Whether this is the case with other nonimmunoglobulin-containing activators remains to be determined. In any case, the presence of six identical binding sites facilitates multivalent attachment of C1q to the activator, a feature that is known to be important for CCP activation.

Activation, Formation of the CCP C3 Convertase, and Regulation

C1q is normally present in native C1 in plasma in a noncovalent complex with two molecules of C1r and two of C1s (2,3). C1r and C1s are homologous, genetically related proenzymes. In order for C1 activation to occur, at least two of the subunits of the C1q molecule must engage two sites on the activator. After binding, both of the C1r molecules are activated by means of an autocatalytic process involving cleavage of a single peptide bond in each identical C1r molecule. Because the $C1r_2C1s_2$ complex in a C1 molecule is intimately associated with the "stems" of the C1q molecule, autocatalytic cleavage is probably initiated by conformational changes in the C1r subunits induced by binding of two or more of the stems of the closely associated C1q molecule to the activator, although this has not been definitively demonstrated. The smaller subunits of cleaved, activated C1r possess serine protease activity and cleave a single peptide bond in each of the two C1s molecules in the complex. The smaller C1s subunits also possess serine protease activity. This process completes the activation of activator-bound C1.

Activated C1s in the macromolecular C1 complex hydrolyzes a single bond in C4, the next reacting component, thereby yielding small (C4a) and large (C4b) fragments (6–8). The susceptible bond is located in the largest (α) polypeptide chain of the three-chain C4 molecule. C4a possesses cytokine-like biologic activities (see later discussion). C4, like C3 (also discussed later), contains a thioester bond that is activated after C4 cleavage by C1s. The metastable activated acyl group of the glutamine residue of the cleaved thioester bond, which is located in the α chain of C4b, is able to form ester or amide bonds with appropriate hydroxyl or amino groups on the surface of the complement activator. These covalently bound C4b molecules form clusters around the bound activated C1 molecules. Only a proportion of the C4b molecules achieve binding, because the activated thioester of most C4b molecules reacts with water, with a resulting loss of binding potential. Despite the inefficiency of C4b binding, considerable amplification of complement activation occurs at this step, because it is enzymatically mediated. The next reacting component, C2, a single-chain zymogen, binds to C4b in a magnesium-dependent manner. Activated C1s in nearby C1 molecules cleave such C2 molecules at a single site, yielding two cleavage products. The larger (C2a) fragment remains bound to C4b and acquires serine protease activity, and the smaller (C2b) product diffuses away. The bound bimolecular C4b2a complex is the C3 convertase of the CCP. The C4b2a complex can be formed in plasma, but this process is inefficient because of the actions of control proteins (see later discussion). C4 and C2 can also be cleaved independently by activated C1s in plasma, but this reaction does not yield C3 convertase activity.

The C4b2a C3 convertase cleaves a single peptide bond in the larger (α) polypeptide chain of the two-chain C3 molecule, yielding 9.1-kd C3a and 184-kd C3b fragments. C3a has a number of biologic properties (see later discussion). Some C3b molecules may bind covalently to C4b or to the activator, but most are further degraded.

Further proteolytic processing of C3b in plasma and on cell and particle surfaces is mediated by factor I, a serine protease, in conjunction with a cofactor molecule (factor H, CR1, or MCP). Proteolytic processing of C3b is not random but occurs in orderly steps (6). First, with factor H acting as a cofactor, factor I cleaves the α chain of C3b at two closely spaced sites, yielding a major product (iC3b), which remains covalently bound to the activator, and a small 2-kd fragment (C3f), which is released. The product, iC3b, is unable to mediate C5b–9 assembly but possesses other potent biologic activities involving receptor interactions and phagocytosis (see later discussion). Bound iC3b undergoes cleavage of an additional bond in the α chain by factor I to yield a larger 140-kd fragment (C3c), which is released from the surface of the activator, and a single-chain 43-kd fragment (C3dg), which remains covalently bound to the activator. The cofactor for factor I in this second cleavage of C3b is CR1; neither factor H nor MCP can facilitate this cleavage. C3dg does not facilitate phagocytosis but has potent immunoregulatory properties (see later discussion); C3c is not known to possess biologic activities.

The CCP is regulated at each activation step. At the C1 step, spontaneous C1r activation is prevented by C1In. C1In also rapidly forms covalent complexes with activated C1r and C1s after C1 activation on the surface of an activator and thereby irreversibly inactivates both proteases. This process leads to the formation and release of two inactive C1rC1s(C1In)₂ complexes from each activated C1 molecule, leaving C1q bound to the complement activator. A second level of regulation occurs at the C4 step. The plasma control protein, C4bp, binds to C4b on the surface of a complement activator or in plasma and serves as a cofactor for the enzymatic degradation of C4b by factor I. C4bp also binds to C4b in C4b2a complexes,

thereby dissociating C2a and rendering C4b susceptible to degradation by factor I, which yields fragments comparable to those described previously for C3b. C4b2a complexes can form on the surface of autologous cells. However, further progression of the complement reaction sequence and cell damage on autologous cells is effectively prevented by the activity of three membrane-associated complement regulatory proteins—CR1, DAF, and MCP. CR1 and DAF inhibit the binding of C2 to C4b and promote the dissociation of C2a from C4b (decay acceleration). CR1 and MCP also serve as cofactors for the enzymatic degradation of C4b by factor I.

The MBL Pathway

Initiation

The MBL pathway is activated by pathogens but not by normal host components. This ability to discriminate self from nonself derives from the ability of MBL, the recognition component of the pathway, to recognize high-mannose-containing polysaccharides and several other neutral oligosaccharides in characteristic linkages that are not generally found on host cells and proteins (23,24). MBL has been shown to bind to a large number of infectious agents, including bacteria (strains of *Streptococcus, Escherichia, Neisseria, Haemophilus,* and *Salmonella*); viruses (HIV-1, HIV-2, influenza); fungi (*Candida albicans* and *Cryptococcus neoformans*); and parasites (*Leishmania*) (23–25). Many more examples undoubtedly will emerge with further study.

MBL is a member of the C-type lectin (collectin) family (23,24). MBL resembles C1q structurally. It consists of multiple copies of three related polypeptide chains, each containing a collagen-like sequence, assembled into subunits exhibiting a "tulip-like" structure. MBL molecules contain three, four, five, or six such trimeric subunits. MBL binds to carbohydrates in a calcium-dependent manner by means of the globular heads, which contain the carbohydrate recognition domain.

Activation, Formation of the MBL Pathway C3 Convertase, and Regulation

Several studies have indicated that MBL interacts with and mediates the activation of C1r and C1s, which in turn activate C4 and C2 (26,27). However, the cloning of MASP-1 and MASP-2 (28–30), two proteins that are structurally and functionally similar to C1r and C1s and also exist in complex with MBL, strongly implies that the earlier-reported activation of C1r and C1s by MBL represented MASP-1 and MASP-2 activation. Structurally, MASP-1 is more similar to C1r than to C1s, and MASP-2 is more similar to C1s than to C1r, findings in accord with the ability of activated MASP-2, but not MASP-1, to activate C4 (30). These data indicate that MBL–MASP-1

–MASP-2 and the C1 complex represent parallel and homologous, but distinct, complement activation pathways. The activation of C4 and C2 and the formation of the C4b2a C3 convertase by the MBL pathway appear to be the same as in the CCP (28–30).

The Alternative Pathway

Initiation

The ACP is a major mediator of innate immunity. Activators of the ACP include many pathogens, among which are gram-positive bacteria (*Streptococcus, Staphylococcus, Pneumococcus*); gram-negative bacteria (*Escherichia*); viruses (herpesvirus, paramyxovirus, togavirus, rhabdovirus, human lentiviruses); fungi (*Cryptococcus, Saccharomyces, Candida, Histoplasma*); and parasites (*Entamoeba, Acanthamoeba, Trichomonas, Leishmania, Schistosoma*) (4–6). The ACP also is activated by cells infected with various viruses (31); neutral sugars with a polymeric structure (various β glucans, inulin, zymosan); bacterial lipopolysaccharides (LPS); peptidoglycans; and some immune complexes (4–6).

In contrast to the targeted activation of the CCP and MBL pathways (i.e., binding of C1 or MBL to specific structures on pathogens and other complement activators), the ACP is activated in a different manner (4–6,32,33). The pathway is triggered by covalent binding of the C3b activation fragment to locations on the surface of cells or other activating particles where it is relatively protected from the actions of regulatory proteins. C3b is thus the recognition component for ACP activation. Clearly, pathogens and most other ACP-activating particles lack the mammalian cellular C3 regulatory proteins (CR1, DAF, and MCP).

However, the plasma C3 regulatory protein, factor H, also is largely prevented from binding to C3b on ACP activators, via mechanisms that are not entirely clear. For this reason, ACP activators are often described as protected surfaces.

The initial C3b molecules for ACP activation are produced by low-level C3 cleavage in plasma by a fluid-phase C3 convertase (5,6,32,33). C3 (like C4, as noted previously) possesses an unusual secondary thioester linkage located in the larger (α) polypeptide chain of the two-chain native molecule (Fig. 19-2). The thioester links the α-carboxyl group of a glutamine residue to the sulfhydryl group of a cysteine residue three amino acids away in the primary sequence (Gly-Cys-Gly-Glu-Gln-Asn). This bond is relatively metastable and is susceptible to very slow hydrolysis by water molecules in plasma; this hydrolysis generates an activated form of C3, variously designated C3(H_2O), C3*, or C3i, which possesses the ability to bind factor B in the presence of magnesium. Factor B in the C3(H_2O)B complex is cleaved by factor D (a circulating serine protease) at a single site, yielding a larger fragment (Bb), which remains bound to C3(H_2O) as a C3(H_2O)Bb complex, and a smaller fragment (Ba), which is released.

C3(H_2O)Bb is a C3 convertase able to cleave a peptide bond in native C3 to yield a small (C3a) and a large (C3b) fragment, exactly as described for the CCP C3 convertase. This process is accompanied by hydrolysis of the thioester bond in native C3. Although factor H binds to C3(H_2O) and to C3b, thereby rendering the molecules susceptible to further degradation by factor I, some C3b molecules achieve binding to the surface of the activator before being thus inactivated. This process of continuous low-level generation of C3(H_2O) and C3b, with binding

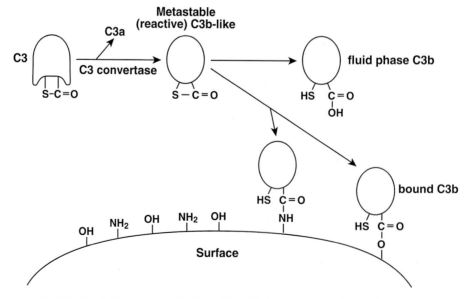

FIG. 19-2. Activation and binding of the third component of complement.

of C3b to surfaces, is frequently called C3 "tickover." The bound C3b molecules are for the most part protected from access by factor H, as described previously, and therefore are able to mediate the formation of additional C3 convertase molecules (see next section). Binding of C3b to surfaces is covalent, via ester or amide bonds formed between the reactive carbonyl group of the glutamic acid of the cleaved thioester bond and hydroxyl (ester) or amino (amide) groups on the surface of the activator. The continuous low-level attack on the thioester bond in C3 by water molecules in plasma ensures a constant supply of C3(H$_2$O) for ACP activation.

Formation and Regulation of the ACP C3 Convertase on ACP Activators

C3b on ACP activator surfaces is relatively protected from access by factor H and therefore is largely resistant to degradation and inactivation by plasma factor I. In addition, most ACP activators lack intrinsic membrane complement regulatory molecules, so C3b on such surfaces is not exposed to the regulatory activities of CR1, DAF, and MCP. The exception is human cells infected with any of a number of different viruses, including numerous members of the paramyxovirus, herpesvirus, togavirus, rhabdovirus, and human lentivirus families (14,31). Because such cells possess normal mammalian cell-membrane complement regulatory proteins, it is likely that viral proteins expressed on the cell surface or virus-induced alterations in the structure or composition of the membrane act to restrict access of complement control proteins to bound C3b.

C3 tickover and covalent C3b binding to surfaces is continuous and entirely random (see previous discussion). This process is not restricted to complement activators but also occurs with normal mammalian cells, which also possess numerous surface structures able to mediate covalent bond formation with C3b. However, on such surfaces, intrinsic (CR1, DAF, MCP) and extrinsic (factor H, factor I) complement regulatory proteins efficiently prevent the formation of C3 convertase molecules.

Protected C3b molecules on activator surfaces are capable of binding circulating factor B in the presence of magnesium, a process that renders factor B susceptible to cleavage at a single site by factor D. As a result, the C3bBb C3 convertase is formed on the surface of the activator. This process is identical to that which mediates the formation of the initial ACP C3 convertase, except for the involvement of bound C3b, rather than fluid-phase C3(H$_2$O), as a constituent of the convertase.

The C3b Amplification Feedback Loop

The C3b amplification feedback loop is mediated exclusively by the ACP components C3b, factor B, and

factor D. Bound C3 convertases on protected ACP surfaces cleave additional circulating C3 molecules, thereby generating more C3b molecules, some of which bind covalently to the activator surface and to covalently attached C3b molecules on the activator. These newly deposited C3b molecules serve as a nidus for the formation of more C3 convertase enzymes on the surface (5,6,32,33). This process markedly augments ACP-dependent complement activation at the C3 step. Another complement component, properdin, binds to and stabilizes cell-bound C3bBb complexes, thereby further augmenting amplification at the C3b step. Although the CCP does not mediate a comparable amplification loop, C3b molecules deposited on activators via CCP activation may sometimes trigger the ACP-dependent amplification loop. This apparently occurs because C3b molecules that become bound to Ab molecules, and perhaps to certain other sites via CCP activation, are on occasion relatively protected from the actions of factors H and I. Such C3b molecules can engage the ACP C3b amplification feedback loop. Some of the additional C3b molecules that become bound may also arrive in protected areas and continue the amplification process. The additional C3b molecules that deposit on complement activators through the activity of the amplification loop bind in clustered arrays around the initially bound C3b molecules.

The importance of amplification at the C3 stage is threefold. First, binding of additional C3b molecules to the initial C3b molecules is a requirement for the generation of a C5 convertase, and therefore for continued activation through the C5 step and formation of the MAC. Second, clusters of bound C3 activation fragments (C3b, iC3b, C3dg) on the surface of an activator are a requirement for high-affinity binding to the CR1 and CR3 receptors on phagocytic cells, and therefore for clearance of immune complexes from the circulation and for complement-mediated opsonization and phagocytosis. Third, it is probable that such clustered C3b molecules also are important for complement-mediated solubilization of immune complexes (these processes are described later).

C3b molecules generated in the fluid phase by the amplification loop, and C3b molecules that bind to nonprotected sites on the activator, interact with plasma factor H and CR1. Such C3b molecules undergo factor I–mediated further processing to iC3b and C3c plus C3dg, as described previously.

The Membrane Attack Pathway

Initiation

The membrane attack pathway is triggered by the C5 convertases of the CCP or the ACP (34,35). The CCP and ACP C5 convertases are formed by covalent addition of a single additional C3b molecule to the C3 convertases of the two pathways to form C4b2a3b and C3bBb3b, respectively. The binding of this C3b molecule to the C4b or C3b subunits of the CCP or ACP C3 convertases does not modify their enzymatic specificity but rather binds and modifies the substrate, C5 (6,36). A single peptide bond in the larger of the two polypeptide chains of C5 is cleaved by the C5 convertases of the two pathways, yielding C5a (11 kd), which has numerous potent biologic activities (see later discussion), and C5b (180 kd). Although highly homologous in structure to C3 and C4, C5 does not contain a thioester bond and therefore is unable to bind covalently to the C5 convertases or to surfaces.

Activation

The remaining portion of the complement reaction sequence is not enzymatically mediated; rather, C5 cleavage by the CCP or ACP C5 convertases initiates a series of protein-protein interactions involving C5, C6, C7, C8, and C9. The self-assembly process culminates with the formation of the multimolecular C5b–9 complex, or MAC (6,34,35). Activated C5b is metastable; it is able to bind C6 for a short time after generation and, thereby, to form a stable bimolecular C5b6 (C5b–6) complex. This complex possesses the ability to bind C7, a single-chain protein that is structurally related to C6, thus generating a C5b67 (C5b–7) complex. This second complex exhibits amphiphilic characteristics and possesses the ability to insert into the hydrocarbon core of lipid bilayer membranes. The insertion of C5b–7 into the external membrane of nearby host cells or pathogens does not lead to "leakiness" of the cells. The ability of C5b–7 to insert into membranes is extremely transient (milliseconds); failing such insertion, the complex self aggregates in solution and becomes functionally inactive.

Each membrane-inserted C5b–7 complex is able to bind a single C8 molecule to form a C5b–8 complex (34,35). C5b–7 complexes in plasma also can bind C8, but the resulting complexes are functionally inactive because they are not able to insert into membranes. On cell membranes, however, the binding of C8 to the C5b–7 complex further increases the hydrophobicity of the complex, which, as a result, inserts more deeply into the cellular membrane. This produces small pores with a functional diameter of 10 to 15 Å, sufficient to permit limited lysis of certain cell types (35,37). Under the electron microscope, the C5b–8 complex is an irregular, rod-like structure projecting out of lipid membranes (34). Functionally, it is a C9 acceptor. A single molecule of C9 binds first. The resulting complex initiates the nonenzymatic polymerization of additional C9 molecules, which bind to the initial C9 molecule bound to the C5b–8 complex and then laterally to each other, by mechanisms that are not completely understood (34,35,38). The fully assembled complex contains up to 16 C9 molecules. The characteristic complement-dependent circular cell-membrane lesions visualized on electron microscopy (39) largely represent polymerized C9 (poly-C9) (34,35,38). When viewed from the side, poly-C9 is tubular and projects approximately 120 Å above the outer surface of the lipid membrane (34,35,38). The central pore of a fully assembled, membrane-inserted C5b–8, $C9_{16}$ or $C5b–8C9_{16}$ complex is approximately 100 Å in diameter, and the tubular complex appears to penetrate both leaflets of the bilayer membrane (34,40). Although the membrane phospholipids surrounding the poly-C9 tubular structure are markedly disrupted by the presence of large numbers of inserted amphiphilic C5b–9 MACs, it is probably the unobstructed passage of ions and water through the central channels that initiates osmotically mediated cell lysis.

Regulation

The MAC and its assembly intermediates possess a number of potent biologic activities (see later discussion). These functional activities are membrane directed. It is therefore not surprising that membrane insertion and formation of the fully assembled complex is tightly controlled by a number of plasma and cell-membrane proteins. The primary plasma inhibitor of MAC action is S protein, a single-chain, 80-kd glycoprotein also known as vitronectin (35). S protein binds to the C5b–7 complex in plasma and prevents its membrane insertion, thereby abrogating assembly of the MAC on cell membranes (35). Although unable to bind to cell membranes, the SC5b–7 complex can bind C8 and two or three molecules of C9, forming functionally inactive fluid-phase SC5b–8 and SC5b–9 complexes (34,35). S protein prevents the polymerization of C9 into large tubular structures (34,35). Other plasma proteins, including SP40,40; apolipoprotein J; apolipoproteins (AI and AII) (41); and SGP-2 (clusterin) (42) also bind to the C5b–7 complex and prevent membrane insertion.

Assembly of MAC complexes that can evade control by plasma regulators and insert into host cell membranes is controlled by two mammalian membrane complement regulatory proteins (6,43). One of these proteins is CD59—also known as protectin, membrane inhibitor of reactive lysis (MIRL)—an 18- to 25-kd intrinsic membrane protein on many cell types that binds to C8 in membrane-inserted C5b–8 complexes (43,44). The resulting complexes in membranes bind a single molecule of C9, but binding of additional C9 molecules and subsequent C9 polymerization are prevented, and MAC-dependent cytolysis of autologous cells does not occur. The second intrinsic membrane protein is HRF, also known as C8-binding protein. HRF, which has not been cloned, is a 65-kd protein found on many cell types. HRF appears to function similarly to CD59; both proteins are attached to cell membranes by a glycosyl phosphatidylinositol (GPI) bond.

HOST DEFENSE FUNCTIONS OF THE COMPLEMENT SYSTEM

The mechanisms that enable the complement system to destroy pathogens and altered host cells (e.g., virus-infected cells, malignant cells, aged cells) are considered here (Table 19-2). They involve the multiple cytokine-like actions of C3a, C4a, and C5a, which, together with inter-leukin-1 (IL-1), IL-6, tumor necrosis factor-α (TNF-α), and other proinflammatory cytokines, chemokines, and other mediators, produce inflammation and trigger directed migration of leukocytes into the area of complement activation. These activities are integrated with the opsonic actions of C1q, MBL, C3b, iC3b, C4b, and iC4b and the interactions of these proteins with specific receptors on neutrophils, monocytes, and macrophages. Also involved are the cytotoxic and cell-signaling properties of the MAC. These various functions together account for the proinflammatory actions of the complement system.

Also considered here are the various mechanisms by which the complement system helps to reduce the deleterious effects of immune complexes on host cells and tissues. The formation of Ab is a central feature of the adaptive humoral response to pathogens and foreign substances. However, intrinsic to the reaction of Abs with Ags on pathogens, pathogen-derived Ags, and foreign soluble Ags is the formation of immune complexes and their subsequent removal by the reticuloendothelial system. Although these are largely beneficial actions, immune complexes of particular sizes can injure blood vessels and filtering organs. The complement system possesses the ability to regulate the size of immune complexes and can also solubilize immune complexes. The mechanisms involved in these actions of the complement system are distinct from those that mediate pathogen destruction.

Destruction of Pathogens and Altered Host Cells

The Inflammatory Response and Chemotaxis

Inflammation is a localized process characterized by redness, swelling, heat, and pain. This classic tetrad of symptoms, described in the first century by Celsius,

TABLE 19-2. *Host defense functions of the complement system*

Destruction of pathogens and altered host cells
  Inflammation and chemotoxis
  Cytotoxic and cytolytic actions of the C5b-9 complex
  Opsonization, complement receptor engagement, and
    phagocytosis
Regulation of immune complex processing
  CR1-mediated clearance of immune complexes
  Regulation of immune complex size
  Solubilization of immune complexes

CR1, complement receptor type 1.

occurs as a consequence of vasodilation, increased vascular permeability, transudation of fluids and cells, edema, and the actions of various cellular mediators that produce pain. These activities serve the physiologic function of preventing systemic dissemination of a localized infectious or injurious process. C3a, C4a, and C5a, termed anaphylatoxins because of their ability to induce anaphylactic-type reactions in animals, are able to produce the symptoms of inflammation. However, localized inflammation *in vivo* is a very complex process that involves the integrated and synergistic actions of multiple humoral and cellular effector systems (45,46).

C3a and C4a are 77-amino-acid activation fragments of C3 and C4, respectively, and C5a is a 74-residue fragment of C5 (47,48). C3a and C4a are not glycosylated, but C5a contains a single complex oligosaccharide moiety, which is important for the activities of the molecule (see later discussion). The three anaphylatoxins increase vascular permeability, contract smooth muscle, and trigger the release of histamine and other vasoactive substances from mast cells and basophils (47,48). C5a is 15 to 250 times more potent than C3a in these various activities, and C4a is two logs less active than C3a. These biologic actions are mediated not only by histamine but probably also by prostaglandins and leukotrienes released from cells as a consequence of the binding of the anaphylatoxins (46,48). Plasma contains a carboxypeptidase B–type enzyme, called the anaphylatoxin inactivator, that removes the carboxyl-terminal arginine residues of C3a, C4a, and C5a, thereby generating the "des Arg" forms of these peptides (49). Serum carboxypeptidase B differs in structure from pancreatic carboxypeptidase B. The permeability-increasing and spasmogenic activities of C3a and C4a are rapidly inactivated by the actions of this enzyme, as is the smooth muscle–contracting activity of C5a, although C5a des Arg possesses permeability-inducing and other capabilities (47,50) (see later discussion). In tissues, where localized inflammation occurs, the anaphylatoxins are likely to increase vascular permeability and contract smooth muscle before they are inactivated by plasma carboxypeptidase B.

C5a also has important and potent actions on neutrophils, monocytes, and macrophages (45,47,48,51). These actions include induced secretion of lysosomal enzymes and various mediators, including eicosanoids and platelet-activating factor (PAF); augmented oxidative metabolism; increased adherence to surfaces; induction of monocyte and neutrophil aggregation; augmented expression of C3 receptors, integrins, and other membrane proteins; induction of procoagulant activity; and triggering of directed migration (chemotaxis). In addition, C5a induces the synthesis and secretion of proinflammatory cytokines, including IL-1, TNF-α, and IL-6, from monocytes and macrophages (47,48). These various activities of C5a are reduced up to 10-fold, but not eliminated, by the action of plasma carboxypeptidase B (47,48). C5a activity is related, in a manner that is incompletely understood, to the single complex oligosaccharide moiety that the peptide bears. Removal of the oligosaccharide moiety by treatment with glycosidases largely restores anaphylatoxin activity to C5a des Arg (52). In addition, and further emphasizing the importance of the oligosaccharide, a 60-kd protein in normal human serum (cochemotaxin), binds to the oligosaccharide moiety on C5a des Arg, resulting in a marked increase in chemotactic activity (53). The 60-kd factor has been identified as Gc globulin (54,55).

The reactions that bind C5a and the other anaphylatoxins to cells exhibit the classic characteristics of receptor-mediated interactions: specificity, high affinity, saturability, and reversibility (47,48,56). Studies with radiolabeled C3a and C5a and with peptides duplicating portions of their primary amino acid sequences, coupled with various physicochemical approaches, provided much information on binding affinity, numbers of receptors on various cell types, and structural requirements for activity. They also revealed that C5a and C3a bind to different receptors (47,48,56–59). Although similar studies initially suggested that C3a and C4a use the same receptor (47), more recent experiments indicate that the C3a and C4a receptors also are distinct (60). Molecular cloning studies have revealed that the C3a and C5a receptors are structurally related and exhibit 37% identity at the nucleotide level; both have seven transmembrane spanning regions and are closely related to other G protein–coupled receptors (61–63), findings in accord with predictions.

Binding of C5a to cells triggers G protein–coupled intracellular processes including exchange of guanosine triphosphate (GTP) and guanosine diphosphate (GDP), activation of phospholipase C (PLC), activation of phosphatidylinositol 3-kinase, metabolism of arachidonic acid, and various intracellular signaling pathways (45–48). Similarly, binding of C3a to its receptor triggers intracellular signaling pathways that involve GTP-GDP exchange and lead to changes in intracellular calcium; however, C3a does not activate phosphatidylinositol 3-kinase, a finding which, together with other data (64–66), suggests that C3a and C5a activate overlapping but different intracellular pathways. Expression of the C3a and C5a receptors is regulated in part by interferon-γ and other cytokines; and, reciprocally, both anaphylatoxins induce the secretion of multiple cytokines, including TNF-α, IL-1, and IL-8 (67–71). These findings emphasize the multiple connections that exist among the anaphylatoxins and the proinflammatory cytokines. Interconnections among the chemokines and other mediators are also likely but have not been directly investigated. The relations of these various mediator systems and intracellular signaling pathways to the many different biologic activities manifested by the anaphylatoxins have yet to be addressed in depth.

C5a (but not C3a or C4a) is chemotactic for neutrophils, monocytes, and macrophages. It has been reported that C3a is a potent chemoattractant for human eosinophils and mast cells but not for neutrophils (72,73). Binding of C5a to the C5a receptor on neutrophils and monocytes triggers a complex sequence of events that induces the cell to migrate toward the complement-activating stimulus (46–48,74). C5a stimulates virtually instantaneous changes in cell shape and induces transient microtubule assembly and fusion of lysosomal granules with each other and with the plasma membrane (48,74). Studies with other chemotactic stimuli, the results of which probably also apply to C5a, have shown that chemotaxis involves a highly regulated sequence of events mediated by the actin-myosin system and related proteins, which provide the contractile force, together with microtubules and related proteins, which provide directionality (46,75,76). The intracellular events involved in chemotaxis and lysosomal enzyme release are related to those involved in phagocytosis, although they may occur independently of ingestion (48,74,77).

In addition to the anaphylatoxins, various other complement activation products have been implicated in the induction of inflammatory processes. These include C3e, a C3 activation/processing fragment that mobilizes leukocytes from bone marrow, increases vascular permeability, and induces the release of lysosomal enzymes (48,78,79). A 9-amino-acid peptide found in C3e, and also in a kallikrein-generated fragment of C3 called C3d-K, also induces leukocytosis (80). Fragments of factor B have been reported to possess chemotactic properties and to induce cell adherence and lysosomal enzyme secretion (81–83).

Also, sublytic concentrations of the MAC possess intracellular signaling properties. These include stimulation of arachidonic acid metabolism; production and release of reactive oxygen products; release of cytokines, including IL-8 and monocyte chemoattractant protein-1; release of procoagulant molecules such as von Willebrand's factor; and induced membrane expression of adhesion-related molecules including E-selectin, P-selectin, and intracellular adhesion molecule-1 (48,84–90). The biologic importance of these various activities has not been determined.

It should be kept in mind that a localized acute inflammatory response is multifactorial and extremely complex. Also simultaneously involved with complement are other mediator systems, each of which, like the anaphylatoxins, can produce many if not all of the various cellular reactions that comprise the local response to injury or infection. For example, leukotrienes and prostaglandins, bradykinin, and other activation products of the contact and kinogen systems have the ability to increase small blood vessel permeability and contract smooth muscle. Furthermore, various cytokines, including IL-1 and TNF-α and some of the leukotrienes and thromboxanes, can increase cellular adherence. Cytokines such as IL-8 and

TNF-α, PAF, and bacterial products such as formyl peptides can activate cells and produce mediator and lysosomal granule release. Numerous other agents, including some leukotrienes, cytokines (e.g., IL-8, chemokines), PAF, and formyl peptides are chemotactic. Interactions among the various mediation systems occur at multiple levels, including activation by the same agents, crossover between activation pathways, activation of other mediation systems by products from each, and cross-regulation. The anaphylatoxins are important, but they are seldom, if ever, the sole system involved in acute inflammatory processes.

Cytotoxic and Cytolytic Actions of the Membrane Attack Complex

Complement is activated through the C9 step by both gram-positive and gram-negative bacteria in the presence, and often in the absence, of Ab. However, gram-positive bacteria are resistant to MAC-mediated lytic destruction, presumably because the thick peptidoglycan layer restricts access of MAC to the cytoplasmic membrane. Serum-sensitive, rough strains of gram-negative bacteria are susceptible to complement-mediated lytic destruction, although complement-mediated opsonization and phagocytosis represent more important host defense mechanisms (91–93). *Neisseria* is an exception: complement-mediated lysis is the primary host defense mechanism for elimination of these gram-negative bacteria, as shown by the susceptibility of persons with C5, C6, C7, and C8 deficiencies to repeated meningococcal and gonococcal infections (see later discussion). Serum-resistant, smooth strains of gram-negative bacteria also activate complement through the C9 step, but they evade both complement-mediated lysis and phagocytic destruction by multiple different mechanisms (also discussed later).

Nonenveloped viral particles are not susceptible to complement-mediated lysis because of the absence of a lipid-containing envelope. Enveloped viral particles, which efficiently activate complement in the presence, and often in the absence, of Ab, can be lysed by the complement system, as demonstrated for numerous members of the alphavirus, arenavirus, coronavirus, herpesvirus, orthomyxovirus, paramyxovirus, and retrovirus families (14,31). These reactions, however, are not very efficient and are therefore unlikely to represent an important host defense mechanism. In addition, viruses have evolved many mechanisms by which to interfere with complement-dependent destructive processes (see later discussion).

Human cells infected with many RNA and DNA viruses, including herpesviruses, orthomyxovirus, paramyxoviruses, and members of the retrovirus families, also activate complement in the presence and in the absence of Ab, and such virus-infected cells may undergo complement-mediated lysis (14,31,94–96). However, in many cases such lysis is inefficient, and a very high concentration of Ab, or a very potent activation stimulus, is required to produce lysis, probably because of the presence of normal mammalian complement regulatory proteins on the cell membranes coupled with the existence of various virus-induced complement evasion mechanisms (discussed later). For these reasons, complement-mediated lytic destruction of virus-infected human cells is unlikely to represent an important host defense mechanism.

Some malignant human cells activate the complement system. This has been most clearly demonstrated with transformed and malignant human cells infected with Epstein-Barr virus (EBV), a human herpesvirus, which are efficiently lysed by the human complement system in the absence of Ab (31,96,97). Since complement activation by such host cells is mediated by a normal cell-membrane protein, it is possible that this represents a mechanism for dealing with altered normal host cells.

Complement Receptor Engagement and Phagocytosis

Several complement proteins, including C3b, iC3b, C1q, and MBL, target complement activators for ingestion and destruction by phagocytic cells. When bound to complement activators, these opsonic complement proteins engage specific complement receptors on the membranes of neutrophils, monocytes, and macrophages. C3 activation/processing fragments and bound C1q and MBL molecules have a clustered distribution on the surface of complement activators, as described earlier; this feature facilitates the simultaneous engagement of multiple cellular C3 or C1q/MBL receptors, increasing the binding affinity, which is otherwise very low. The binding activity of complement receptors is constitutive, and attachment does not require the expenditure of energy, although the presence of various cytokines and cellular activation may increase or decrease the binding affinity (45,98,99). Ingestion and degradation, in contrast to binding, is a highly complex, regulated activity that depends on cellular activation and energy.

CR1 (CD35), CR3 (CD11b/CD18), and CR4 (CD11c/CD18) bind C3 activation/processing fragments. The C1q-MBL receptor binds C1q or MBL after activation of C1 or the homologous MBL–MASP-1–MASP-2 complex. Complement activation is therefore a prerequisite for engagement of the complement receptors and for manifestation of the biologic activities of the receptors. These complement receptors, which are found on all phagocytic cells (neutrophils, monocytes, and macrophages), mediate or augment phagocytosis. CR2, another complement receptor, does not mediate phagocytosis but rather possesses immunoregulatory functions (see later discussion).

CR1, also known as the C3b receptor and the immune adherence receptor, binds both C3b and C4b (100–102). C3b binds to the first two SCRs of the first and second long homologous repeats (LHRs) of the amino terminus, whereas C4b binds to the first two SCRs of the third LHR. CR1 on erythrocytes primarily mediates immune complex binding and clearance (see later discussion) and also regulates activation, as discussed previously. The extracellular domain of CR1, a single-chain type 1 membrane glycoprotein, is composed of tandem 60- to 70-amino-acid SCRs assembled in LHRs, each of which contains seven SCRs. CR1 exists in four allelic forms, ranging in molecular weight from 160 to 250 kd.

CR3 and CR4 are members of the β_2 family of leukocyte integrins (98,103,104). CR3 (also known as the iC3b receptor) and CR4 (also called p150,95) are related membrane glycoproteins composed of two noncovalently linked polypeptide chains. The larger α chains of the CR3 and CR4 heterodimeric proteins have molecular weights of 185 kd and 150 kd, respectively, and the β chains, which are identical, have a molecular weight of 95 kd. CR3 and CR4 preferentially bind the iC3b activation/processing fragment of C3. In addition, both of these complement receptors mediate direct binding of a number of gram-positive and gram-negative organisms, parasites, and fungi in the absence of complement; these interactions may also be followed by phagocytosis (98).

After binding of C1 to a complement activator, the activated C1r and C1s subunits interact with C1In and the Clr-Cls-C1In complexes dissociate from C1q. This process enables C1q, which remains bound to the complement activator, to interact via its collagen-like region with a cellular C1q receptor on phagocytic cells (98,105). MBL and the structurally similar pulmonary surfactant protein (SP-A), which also contains a collagen-like region, bind to cell surface receptors on phagocytic cells (23,24,106). Because MBL is normally complexed to MASP-1 and MASP-2, a similar process to that described for C1q may expose the collagen-like portion of the molecule. C1q, MBL, and SP-A all bind to the same cell surface receptor, which has been cloned (107).

Although engagement of some cellular receptors on phagocytes (e.g., the Fc-γ receptors) leads directly to phagocytosis, this is not true of the binding of complement ligands to C3 receptors on phagocytic cells. Ingestion via CR1 and CR3 requires a second, cellular activation stimulus (45,98,99). A number of ligands can fulfill this function. Most important are IgG molecules (if they are also present on the target complement activator), which simultaneously engage cellular Fc receptors. Other identified stimuli include a unique T-cell cytokine, an incompletely characterized serum protein, PAF, amyloid P protein, phorbol esters, and components of the extracellular matrix including fibronectin, laminin, and type I collagen (98,99,108—111). The insoluble matrix-associated factors are likely to be important in facilitating phagocytosis of complement-coated pathogens in localized inflammatory sites. The mechanisms by which these various ligands activate cells to permit phagocytosis via C3b and iC3b complement receptors are not known. However, new protein synthesis is not required, and changes in the numbers of cellular C3 receptors do not occur.

The MBL/C1q receptor is unable to mediate phagocytosis directly and therefore is not an independent opsonic receptor (98,112). It does, however, enhance phagocytosis initiated by engagement of CR1 or the Fcγ receptor.

Phagocytosis is an active, energy-requiring process. It is initiated by the appearance of localized micropseudopodia at the region of the initial ligand-receptor contact (98,99,113). Spreading of the pseudopodia around the particle is facilitated by the progressive formation of additional ligand-receptor contacts, leading, as the pseudopodia meet and fuse, to engulfment of the particle into a single phagocytic vacuole. This "zipper" mechanism is well supported by experimental data. This process clearly involves a continuous series of positive interactions of membrane receptors with elements of the cytoskeleton, followed by the regulated disruption of such contacts. Although numerous studies have implicated components of the cytoskeleton and intracellular signaling pathways in phagocytosis, mechanistic details are not known. With specific regard to C3 receptors, neither CR1 nor CR3 ligation triggers an oxidative burst, release of reactive oxygen species, or arachidonic acid metabolism (114,115). Changes in intracellular calcium also do not appear to be involved, and this probably also applies to cyclic nucleotides and G proteins (98,99). Although IL-1 synthesis and secretion occur with complement receptor engagement (116), this is unlikely to be relevant to phagocytosis. The intracellular events that mediate ingestion are completely unknown.

Regulation of Immune Complex Processing and Solubility

The formation of immune complexes as a consequence of the binding of Ab to pathogens and pathogen-derived Ag is an important component of host defense mechanisms. However, immune complexes of certain sizes can be deposited in blood vessel walls and in filtering organs before clearance by the reticuloendothelial system, thus producing localized inflammation leading to vasculitis and acute and chronic immune complex disease. These potentially damaging processes are mainly restricted to large immune complexes. Three different complement-dependent mechanisms operate to regulate immune complex solubility and processing (see Table 19-2): CR1-mediated clearance of immune complexes; complement-dependent inhibition of the formation of large immune complexes; and complement-mediated solubilization of immune complexes.

CR1-Mediated Clearance of Immune Complexes

As described previously, immune complexes and other complement activators bearing covalently bound C3b molecules bind to CR1 on various cell types. Neutrophils, monocytes, macrophages, erythrocytes, and lymphocytes, among other cell types, possess CR1. In the case of phagocytic cells, adherence is an opsonic stimulus and may be followed by phagocytic ingestion of the complement activator, as described earlier.

Complement-mediated binding of immune complexes to erythrocytes has been known since the 1930s. This phenomenon, which can occur with any immune complex, is known as *immune adherence* (117,118). Immune adherence was demonstrated *in vivo* in Rhesus monkeys as the virtually instantaneous binding to erythrocytes of injected bacteria coated with Ab (118). Subsequently, the receptor that mediates C3b-dependent adherence to erythrocytes was shown to be CR1 (119). Although erythrocytes contain relatively few CR1 molecules per cell compared with neutrophils, monocytes, and lymphocytes, the enormous number of erythrocytes in relation to the various CR1-positive leukocytes suggested that most C3b-bearing immune complexes and other activators will bind to erythrocytes, a prediction that has been verified *in vitro* (120–124) and *in vivo* in nonhuman primates (125). Similar results were obtained in human volunteers (122,126–128). These studies showed that immune complex binding to CR1 represents a clearance mechanism in which erythrocytes bearing immune complexes are carried to the liver, where the complexes are removed, and the undamaged erythrocytes reenter the circulation (122,125–128). The reaction is efficient, and 9% to 15% of immune complexes are removed from the circulation each minute. This reaction sequence removes potentially harmful complement-bearing immune complexes from the circulation before they can be deposited in blood vessels or filtering organs to induce inflammation and subsequent tissue damage. Clearance probably is mediated by attachment of the erythrocyte-bound immune complexes to C3 and Fc receptors on fixed tissue macrophages in the liver, followed by stripping of the complexes from the surface of the erythrocytes and ingestion (125).

Regulation of the Size of Immune Complexes

Soluble Abs and Ags interact to form insoluble immune complexes both in conditions of Ab excess and at equivalence. Initial precipitation of immune complexes, which occurs *in vitro* and *in vivo*, is induced by Ab binding to Ag combined with Fc-Fc interactions (129). As immune complexes become larger, they acquire a lattice-like structure characterized by closely-spaced, alternating Ag and Ab molecules. Immune complexes that form in plasma, and therefore in the presence of complement, bind C1 and efficiently activate the CCP, leading to covalent attachment of C3b and C4b to the complexes. Despite this, it has been known since the 1940s that complement reduces the rate of precipitation of immune complexes and thereby helps to maintain the complexes in the soluble state (129,130). Studies have shown that inhibition of immune precipitation is absolutely dependent on C3 activation via the CCP (129,131,132). It is likely that covalent binding of large numbers of C3b molecules to Ab molecules in immune complexes, and possibly also to the Ag, interferes with the orderly molecular interactions required for the lattice-like arrangement of Ag and Ab molecules that characterizes insoluble immune complexes (129). Maintenance of the solubility of immune complexes is undoubtedly important in preventing their deposition in blood vessel walls and in filtering organs, and therefore it is important in inflammation and tissue damage *in vivo*.

Solubilization of Immune Complexes

Complement also has the ability to solubilize insoluble immune complexes (129,133). Solubilization is absolutely dependent on covalent binding of C3b to the immune complex, probably primarily to the Ab molecule, where it is largely protected from the degradative actions of factors H and I and can therefore effectively mediate activation and amplification of the ACP (134). Solubilization is an exclusive property of the ACP; the CCP has minimal complex-solubilizing properties (129,135,136). The mechanisms by which covalently bound C3b dissociates immune complexes are not understood but probably involve disruption of the lattice-like structure of the joined Ag and Ab molecules. Solubilization of immune complexes, in contrast to prevention of immune precipitation, is extremely inefficient; and marked complement activation by the insoluble complexes is required for solubilization to occur (129). For these reasons, complement-dependent solubilization is not likely to be biologically important.

IMMUNOREGULATORY ACTIONS OF THE COMPLEMENT SYSTEM

The studies that led to the discovery of complement a century ago suggested that the system functioned in host defense against infection. Numerous studies in the intervening years, and especially in the past 30 years, have documented many host defense–related effector functions of the complement system that are concerned with pathogen recognition, opsonization, phagocytosis, cytolysis, and inflammation. In the mid-1970s, experiments with cobra venom factor (CVF), which activates the ACP and leads to C3 depletion, suggested that complement also possesses functions related to the induction of immune responses. These experiments demonstrated that immune responses to thymus (T)–dependent and T-independent Ags were markedly reduced in C3-depleted mice (137,138). CVF-treated mice were also shown to be severely impaired in their ability to localize Ag on follicular dendritic cells (FDCs), form germinal centers, undergo isotype switching, and generate memory B cells (139,140). Subsequent studies in animals genetically deficient in various complement components, coupled with experiments with MAbs and studies in animals with targeted disruptions of complement and complement receptor genes, have clearly shown that complement possesses many immunoregulatory functions and that these depend on C3, CR2, and intracellular signaling molecules associated with CR2 and CD19 (Table 19-3).

Complement-Dependent Enhancement of Immune Responses

Until the experiments with CVF-treated mice, there was no evidence for an influence of complement on the induction of Ag-specific (adaptive) immune responses. However, it is now known that complement is intimately involved in the induction and regulation of primary and secondary Ab responses, including roles in Ag capture, processing, and presentation; generation of germinal centers; isotype switching; and induction of memory B cells. Complement augments and regulates the induction of specific T-dependent Ab responses to certain Ags. The findings suggest that complement may play a major and extremely important role when limited amounts of Ag interact with low-affinity Ag receptors. The mechanisms thus far identified are described here.

Role in Antigen Capture, Processing, and Presentation

Many pathogens, foreign Ags, and immune complexes activate complement; and this process leads to covalent binding of C3b and C4b activation fragments to the surface of the Ag, as discussed previously. Soluble and particulate Ags and immune complexes bearing C3 and C4 activation fragments were thought to possess the ability to simultaneously engage both the Ag receptor and complement receptors on the surface of Ag-specific B cells,

TABLE 19-3. *Immunoregulatory actions of the complement system*

Complement-dependent enhancement of immune responses
  Role in antigen capture and antigen processing
  Role in primary and secondary immune responses to T-dependent and T-independent antigens
  CR2-independent intracellular signaling
Regulation of B-cell development and function

CR2, complement receptor type 2.

thereby binding more firmly. In confirmation of this prediction, complexes of C3b covalently joined to tetanus toxin (TT) bound to Ag-specific B cells considerably better than TT alone, and such binding was largely inhibited by anti-CR2 (and anti-TT) Ab but not by anti-CR1 Ab (141). Ags bearing only C3 fragments (i.e., direct complement activators) were anticipated to bind to B cells via CR2; and this was also demonstrated, since TT-C3b complexes bound to nonspecific B cells via CR2. In another example, pneumococcal polysaccharide–C3d complexes bound via CR2 to B cells (142). In addition to increased Ag capture via CR2, evidence was obtained in the TT system for delayed intracellular proteolysis of the complexes containing C3b and consequently for more effective Ag processing of TT-C3b complexes, compared with TT (143).

With regard to Ag presentation, TT-C3b complexes were 100-fold more effective in stimulating the proliferation of TT-specific helper T cells; the presence of C3b also permitted TT to be presented by Ag-nonspecific B cells to TT-specific T cells (143,144). C3b covalently bound to MAb also enhanced T-cell responses to the immunoglobulin heavy chain (145). In a different example, complexes of soluble keyhole limpet hemocyanin, a T-dependent Ag, with natural IgM or IgG Abs activated complement and bound to Ag-specific and Ag-nonspecific B cells by means of their complement receptors; subsequent internalization and degradation depended on C3 and CR2 (146). The presence of C3 also endowed non–Ag-specific B cells with the ability to trigger the proliferation of Ag-specific helper T cells (146).

Role in Induction of Primary and Secondary Humoral Responses to T-Dependent and T-Independent Antigens

CVF stably interacts with factor B and thereby renders it susceptible to proteolytic activation by factor D, leading to formation of a fluid-phase ACP C3 convertase, which rapidly mediates complete activation and cleavage of plasma C3 (5,147). Experiments with CVF-treated mice in the 1970s revealed that they were virtually unable to generate primary immune responses to either T-dependent or T-independent Ag (137,138,148). Secondary immune responses also were reduced by CVF, but not as profoundly. CVF-treated mice also exhibited a defect in Ag localization to germinal centers (149,150).

Studies in the 1980s showed that C3-deficient guinea pigs were profoundly impaired in their ability to generate primary and secondary immune responses to limited concentrations of a T-dependent Ag and were unable to undergo isotype switching from IgM to IgG; these effects were dose dependent and were not evident at higher Ag concentrations (151–153). C3-deficient dogs also exhibited deficient Ab responses to T-independent Ag (154), as did C4-deficient humans and C2- and C4-deficient guinea pigs (151,155), but C5-deficient mice showed normal responses (156).

Cumulatively, these data strongly suggest that C3 activation via the CCP, but not the actions of C5a or MAC, are important for the formation of Ab in response to low concentrations of Ag. Complement activation fragments mediate their biologic reactions by binding to complement receptors. As noted, CR2 primarily binds C3dg, whereas CR1 has highest affinity for C3b. In the mouse, CR2 and CR1 are derived from the same gene by alternative splicing (157–159), whereas CR2 and CR1 in humans are separate proteins encoded by closely linked genes (102,160,161). Murine CR2 contains 15 SCRs, a transmembrane region, and a short cytoplasmic tail; the binding sites for C3dg are in the two amino-terminal SCRs (157–159,162,163). Murine CR1 contains the 15 SCRs of murine CR2, and therefore binds C3dg, but there are 6 additional, unique SCRs attached to the amino-terminal end of the molecule. The CR2 portion of murine CR1 was implicated in mediating the effects on Ab formation. In these experiments, *in vivo* administration of receptor-function–blocking MAb to the CR2 region of the protein markedly inhibited primary IgG and IgM Ab responses to low, but not to high concentrations of a variety of T-dependent and T-independent Ags (164–166). B-cell memory induction and secondary immune responses were either less susceptible (166,167) or unaffected (165) by *in vivo* administration of MAb to CR2. The fact that induction of helper T cells was not influenced by MAb to CR2 (167), implicated CR2 on either B cells or FDCs (the two murine cell types that possess CR2) in mediation of C3-dependent enhancement of immune responses. Direct evidence implicating murine CR2 came from studies showing that *in vivo* administration of a recombinant CR2 construct markedly reduced primary Ab formation to a soluble and to an insoluble T-dependent Ag and inhibited subsequent isotype switching (168).

The critical roles of CR2 and C3dg in induced immune responses were also demonstrated *in vivo* by a completely different approach. In these studies, mice were immunized with hen egg lysozyme (HEL) and with HEL fusion protein constructs bearing two or three copies of murine C3d (169). These fusion proteins mimic the covalent complexes that are formed between C3 activation fragments and complement activators. HEL constructs bearing two and three copies of C3d were 1000- and 10,000-fold more immunogenic, respectively, than HEL, as assessed by the formation of IgG1 Ab. Secondary immune responses also were comparably enhanced. These effects were completely blocked by an inhibitory MAb directed against murine CR2, demonstrating absolute dependence on this receptor.

The roles of C3, C4, and CR2 in the enhancement of primary and secondary immune responses to low doses of T-dependent Ags were confirmed and markedly extended by a series of experiments in mice that had been rendered selectively deficient in C3, C4, and CR2 by targeted gene disruption. Mice that were made completely deficient in either C3 or C4 by gene targeting in embryonic stem cells exhibited a profound defect in their ability to mount a primary IgM Ab response to low doses of a T-dependent Ag (170). Furthermore, the mice exhibited markedly reduced numbers of germinal centers and did not undergo isotype switching to IgG. The complement-deficient mice exhibited normal helper T-cell activity, and their B cells responded normally to other activation stimuli, indicating that the defect was entirely due to C3- or C4-dependent B-cell activation, leading to the formation of germinal centers. The defect was not absolute and could be partially overcome with 10-fold higher levels of Ag (170).

Similar results were obtained for CR2- and CR1-deficient mice generated by targeted disruption of the CR2/CR1 gene (171,172). These mice possessed normal levels of B cells (except for CD5$^+$ B-1a B cells, as described later) and exhibited normal intracellular activation responses to various noncomplement ligands (171). The receptor-deficient mice also had normal levels of IgM, IgG1, and IgA; but they showed modestly reduced levels of switched isotypes (IgG2a, IgG2b, and IgG3). After immunization, these mice were found to be markedly deficient in their ability to generate primary and secondary immune responses to T-dependent Ag, and this defect was only slightly overcome by 10-fold higher doses of Ag. The complement receptor–deficient mice and wild-type control mice had equivalent numbers of primary follicles (171). However, one study found that germinal centers formed in CR2/CR1-deficient mice after secondary challenge with Ag (172); whereas in the other study, a marked reduction in the number and size of germinal centers was found after secondary challenge with Ag (171). The reasons for this single major difference in findings between the studies are not known.

B-cell CR2 could potentially mediate the C3- and CR2-dependent effects on Ab formation and germinal center development, through the known ability of this receptor to modulate Ag-dependent immune responses. However, C3-dependent Ag retention by CR2 on FDC also could explain the results. Two different experimental approaches in the CR2/CR1 knock-out mice have definitively identified B-cell CR2 as mediating the modulating effects of C3 and CR2 on primary and secondary immune responses (171,173). First, CR2/CR1-deficient mice were reconstituted with normal bone marrow from major histocompatibility complex (MHC)-matched littermates (171). B cells from such mice expressed CR2 and CR1, but FDCs remained negative for these proteins. The reconstituted chimeric mice exhibited normal primary and secondary immune responses to a T-dependent Ag and formed normal numbers of germinal centers. These results indicate that the defect observed in the humoral response lies at the level of the B cell, not the FDC. In the second approach, blastocyst complementation in mice deficient in recombination-activating gene-2 (RAG-2) was used to generate mice with the reverse phenotype—that is, with B cells lacking CR2 and CR1 and FDCs exhibiting normal expression of CR2 and CR1 (173). RAG-2–deficient mice are unable to form lymphocytes but otherwise are normal (174). In these experiments, blastocysts from RAG-2–deficient mice were microinjected with embryonic stem cells from CR2/CR1-deficient mice before implantation into foster mothers for development. The resulting chimeric mice had B cells that were CR2- and CR1-deficient, because they were derived entirely from the injected CR2/CR1-deficient embryonic stem cells. Their FDCs, which were unaffected by the deletion of RAG-2, possessed these complement receptors. The chimeric mice were unable to generate an Ab response to a soluble T-dependent Ag. Both experimental approaches—the studies of mice with B cells lacking CR2 and CR1 and FDCs possessing them and the studies of mice with B cells possessing both complement receptors and FDCs lacking them—indicated that CR2 on B cells, and not on FDCs, is responsible for the C3-dependent effects on T-dependent Ab responses.

The mechanisms responsible for the B cell–specific enhancement of immune responses by C3 and CR2 are not yet clear. However, the well documented ability of CR2 ligands to synergistically enhance B-cell activation induced through the B-cell antigen receptor (BCR) and to augment Ag-nonspecific intracellular B-cell activation (175–178) provide a very likely explanation for a portion of these results. The demonstration that CD19-deficient mice, generated by targeted gene disruption, exhibit similar profound defects in the ability to form Abs to T-dependent Ags, in isotype switching, and in the ability to generate germinal centers (179,180) supports this conclusion, because CD19 is a major mediator of CR2-initiated intracellular activation (see later discussion). Complement-dependent enhancement of Ag-specific B-cell activation probably finds its *in vivo* counterpart in the activation of virgin B cells within the periarteriolar lymphoid sheath (140) by limited amounts of Ag binding to low-affinity B-cell Ag receptors (170,171,178). However, the dependence of germinal center development and/or maintenance on CR2 indicates that there is at least one additional site of action involved in the CR2-dependent effects on Ab formation. This has been postulated to be at the level of B-cell survival within the germinal center (171,178). Enhanced binding of B cells to Ag and to C3 fragments on FDCs could potentially mediate increased survival (173,178), a possibility rendered more likely by the demonstration that certain CR2 ligands reduce B-cell apoptosis (181,182). Complement-dependent enhanced Ag capture and more effective Ag processing (141,143, 144,146), discussed previously, could also be involved at both stages. A number of other possibilities exist. The

demonstration that CR2 on B cells has 15 SCRs but CR2 on FDCs has 16 SCRs (183) suggests that the additional SCR may impart a unique function to FDCs in germinal center development. Studies in the various lines of knock-out mice should elucidate the mechanisms involved.

CR2-Dependent Intracellular Signaling

B-cell CR2 is a member of an intracellular signaling pathway that modulates B-cell activation, growth, and differentiation (176–178,184,185). As indicated earlier, it is likely that the signal-transducing properties of CR2 play an important role in the C3-dependent enhancement of the humoral immune response to T-dependent Ag, although the mechanisms by which this is accomplished are not yet apparent.

Numerous studies have supported a role for CR2 in the modulation of Ag-dependent responses in B cells. These include the findings that CR2 associates with Igm in the B cell membrane, and that CR2 ligands, prime B cells for subsequent activation through the BCR, and synergize with Ab to the BCR in activating B cells, whether measured by changes in intracellular calcium, proliferation, or transcription of the *FOS* nuclear protooncogene (169,175,176,186–193). Co-ligation of CR2 with the BCR has also been reported to rescue B cells from apoptosis induced by Ab to the BCR (182). The ability of C3 and other CR2 ligands to modulate Ag-specific B-cell responses is conceptually appealing, because it provides the important element of Ag specificity, which C3 activation fragments lack. The concept is physiologically reasonable, because covalent Ag-C3dg complexes generated by complement activation would be expected to co-ligate CR2 and the BCR.

In addition, however, CR2 ligands trigger certain intracellular signaling responses in B cells independently of BCR ligation; such stimulation has generally been found to depend on the presence of T-cell–derived cytokines or to require an additional B-cell activation signal. CR2 ligands (including C3dg, some CR2 MAb, and EBV) are able to stimulate B-cell proliferation and differentiation in the presence of T cells, T-cell–derived growth factors, or a B-cell coactivator (194–202); to induce B-cell homotypic aggregation (186,193); to trigger IL-6 and CD23 transcription and protein synthesis (203,204); to activate the NF-κB transcription factor (184); to induce phosphorylation of certain intracellular proteins (205,206); and to maintain the growth of B-cell lines under suboptimal culture conditions (207,208). CD23 (which also binds CR2) and certain CR2 MAbs rescue germinal center B cells from apoptosis in the presence of IL-1 (181,209). Although the biologic significance of these various CR2-initiated reactions is unclear, they emphasize that CR2 ligands trigger one or more B-cell intracellular signaling pathways independently of BCR involvement.

Intracellular signaling reactions are initiated and driven by sequential interactions between proteins or other signal-transducing components that lead to activation of kinases, other enzymes, and signaling factors. Because CR2 has a 34-residue cytoplasmic tail that is devoid of known signaling motifs or enzymatic activity, CR2-initiated intracellular signaling undoubtedly depends on associations with other proteins. Immunoprecipitation and transfection approaches have shown that very little CR2 in the B-cell membrane is free; virtually all is physically associated with either CR1 (CD35) in a bimolecular complex or with CD19 and CD81 in a trimolecular complex (190,210,211). LEU-13 is occasionally also present in the latter complex. CR1 has not been shown to possess immunoregulatory functions (102). However, several lines of evidence indicate that CD19, which has a long cytoplasmic component, has signal-transducing properties (177,212). For example, CD19 is tyrosine phosphorylated after addition of Ab to CD19 (213), and it is one of the few proteins that is tyrosine phosphorylated after BCR ligation (213–216). This activity may be mediated by SRC-family kinases such as LYN or FYN, or by the SYK tyrosine kinase, all of which are associated with CD19 (214,217,218). Tyrosine phosphorylation occurs on multiple sites in CD19, including two YXXM motifs that interact with two SRC homology (SH2) domains in the p85 subunit of phosphatidylinositol 3-kinase and lead to activation of the enzymatic p110 subunit of the kinase (177,213). Other phosphorylated tyrosines in CD19 may interact with SH2 domains in other intracellular signaling molecules, as has been demonstrated for the SRC-family kinase, FYN, and the product of the *VAV* protooncogene (218,219). Crosslinking of CD19 also leads to increased intracellular calcium and to activation of PLC (177).

These findings strongly suggest that CD19 transduces intracellular signals triggered by binding of CR2 ligands. Other indirect evidence suggesting that CD19 is the intracellular signaling component includes the finding that crosslinking of CD19 with the BCR leads to the same synergistic activation of B cells as observed on crosslinking of CR2 with the BCR (220,221) and the demonstration that CD19 (and CD81) crosslinking, like CR2 ligation, induces comparable tyrosine kinase–dependent, homotypic B-cell activation, which is regulated by the CD45 cell-membrane phosphatase (211,222,223). In addition, CD19-null mice generated by homologous recombination exhibit a phenotype very similar to that of CR2 knock-out animals, since they exhibit profound defects in the ability to generate Ab to T-dependent Ag and in the ability to form germinal centers and also show impaired development of CD5+ B-1a B cells (179,180, 224). Mice lacking the protooncogene product VAV, which binds to CD19, also exhibit similar defects in Ag-dependent responses (225,226).

Although CD19 appears to transduce intracellular signals initiated by Ab to the BCR or by CR2 ligands, as

described, relatively few constituents of the signaling pathway have been identified. There are also suggestions of differences in the intracellular signaling pathways triggered by the BCR and by the CR2/CD19/CD81 complex. For example, BCR and CD19 ligation each lead to activation of PLC-γ, but this is associated with tyrosine phosphorylation of PLC-γ only in the former case (177). Also BCR ligation, but not CR2 or CD19 ligation, stimulates transcription of two cellular immediate early genes, *FOS* and *MYC* (193,227). B-cell activation triggered by BCR or CR2 ligation also exhibits a different pattern of inhibition by a panel of protein kinase C and protein-tyrosine kinase inhibitors (193,204). Isolation and characterization of the constituents of the signaling pathways are clearly needed.

It is critical to identify the downstream targets of the signaling pathways that modulate the expression of specific genes mediating the C3- and CR2-dependent effects on T-dependent Ab formation and germinal center development. These important goals can be most easily addressed by *in vivo* studies in mice bearing targeted disruptions of specific candidate genes, and combinations thereof, coupled with *in vitro* studies with cells from such mice.

Regulation of B-Cell Development and Function

As described previously, mice that lack CD19 have reduced numbers of peritoneal CD5+ B-1a B cells (CD5 B cells, LY-1 B cells) (179,180). B-1a B cells, a self-renewing subpopulation of B cells predominately found in the peritoneal cavity of adult mice, differ from conventional B cells (B2 B cells) in surface phenotype, Ag specificity, signaling, and growth properties (228). B-1a B cells represent the major source of plasma IgM and are closely associated with autoimmune responses. Normal adult mice treated with Ab to CD19 exhibited a progressive reduction in the numbers of B-1a B cells (229). Conversely, mice bearing a human CD19 transgene, and therefore exhibiting increased levels of CD19, showed a CD19-dependent dramatic increase in the numbers of B-1a B cells in the peritoneum and spleen, coupled with increased concentrations of circulating autoantibodies (Ab against single-stranded DNA and rheumatoid factor) and decreased numbers of mature conventional B cells (224,230,231). These data indicate that CD19 is required for normal maintenance of B-1a B cells, possibly because of its effects on stimulation via the BCR; BCR activation may be required for self-renewal of B-1a B cells (179,229–232). Further supporting a role for CD19 in maintenance of B-1a B cells is the finding that mice rendered deficient in the *Vav* protooncogene, which is associated with CD19 (219), also lack B-1a B cells (225,226). CD21-deficient mice generated by gene targeting also were found to lack peritoneal B-1a B cells in one of the two reports of such knock-outs (171). Possibly related, mice with a mutation in the BTK (Bruton's tyrosine kinase) protein-tyrosine kinase gene (*Btk*, formerly *Xid*), or engineered to lack this kinase, exhibited reduced numbers of B-1a B cells (233,234), whereas mice with mutations in the *Me* (moth-eaten) gene, which encodes a protein tyrosine phosphatase (SHP-1, PTP1c), exhibited greatly increased numbers of B-1a cells (235). In addition to their enzymatic activities, BTK and SHP1 contain SH2 domains that could mediate interactions with phosphorylated tyrosines either in CD19 or in other regulatory proteins associated with CD19, CD21, and the BCR, including CD22, FcγRIIB, CD40, SYK, other tyrosine kinases, protein phosphatases, and certain integrins (231, 236–238).

In addition to a role in B-1a B-cell maintenance and development, the 48% to 86% reduction in the various immunoglobulin classes and isotypes observed in nonimmunized CD19-deficient mice suggests additional functions for CD19 in B-cell development and activation (179,180,224,231,239). An expanded role is further supported by the demonstration that B cells from CD19-deficient mice exhibit moderate reductions in proliferative ability in response to LPS, to cross-linking of surface IgM, and to submitogenic doses of anti-IgM together with IL-4 (180). Conversely, mice overexpressing human CD19 showed increased mitogenic responses and immunoglobulin levels (180,239). Although CD19-deficient mice exhibited no major defects in the numbers of pro-B, pre-B, and immature or mature B cells (179,180), mice overexpressing this molecule showed markedly reduced numbers of immature and mature B cells (55% and 81%, respectively) in the bone marrow and severely reduced numbers of peripheral, splenic, and peritoneal B cells (95%, 82%, and 70%, respectively), indicative of a partial block in B-cell development at the pre-B-cell stage (230).

Possibly playing a role in these abnormalities in B-cell development is the finding that IL-7 enhanced the expression of CD19 in B-cell precursors (240,241). IL-7 binding also led to tyrosine phosphorylation of B-cell CD19 (214), an event that would be anticipated to enable CD19 to interact with intracellular signaling molecules. In addition, IL-7 downregulated mRNA levels for terminal deoxynucleotidyl transferase (TdT) and RAG-1 and RAG-2 in pro-B cells (240); RAG-1 and RAG-2 are essential for Ig gene rearrangement, and therefore for B-cell maturation. CD19 ligation with Ab did not influence TdT or RAG expression directly but completely blocked the downregulation of RAG expression by IL-7. The CD19 Ab effects did not occur in BTK-deficient pro-B cells, a finding that implicates this tyrosine kinase as an essential element in the IL-7/CD19 signaling pathway mediating RAG-1 and RAG-2 downregulation (240). Therefore, CD19, together with IL-7, regulates RAG expression and subsequent Ig gene rearrangement and B-cell maturation. Interference with these normal reciprocal relations could be responsible for the impairment of B-cell development at the pre-B-cell stage in mice that overexpress CD19.

On the basis of the studies in CD19-deficient and CD19-overexpressing mice cited in this and the preceding section, it has been postulated that CD19 is a major *in vivo* regulator of B-cell responses to Ag and other cell-surface receptors involved in B-cell development, negative selection, proliferation, differentiation, and clonal expansion. (180,224,231). Some of these CD19-dependent effects are undoubtedly initiated by an intracellular signaling pathway triggered by C3dg binding to CR2. However, it is difficult to visualize a role for C3 activation followed by C3dg binding to CR2 and signaling through CD19 in B-cell development and maturation in unimmunized animals. These roles of CD19 are probably initiated by binding of CD19 to an as yet unidentified ligand.

COMPLEMENT AND DISEASE

Genetic Complement Deficiencies

The first description of inherited total complement deficiency was in the early part of the 20th century. Several strains of complement-deficient guinea pigs were identified and used in a number of *in vitro* studies of the complement system in the 1920s (242). Although overtly healthy, they were more susceptible than other guinea pigs to infection with pathogenic bacterial strains. Autosomal recessive inheritance of the deficiency was shown, and complement activity was restored by trace amounts of heated normal guinea pig serum (243). These and other characteristics suggested that C3 was the deficient component, but the strains were lost before the deficiency could be definitively identified. Studies in the 1960s showed that almost half of the inbred strains of mice then available lacked complement activity, a trait shown to be inherited as a recessive characteristic (244). Since then mice, guinea pigs, rabbits, and dogs with deficiencies of C2, C3, C4, and C6 have been identified and studied (245). These various strains of complement-deficient animals have been extremely helpful in elucidating the role of complement in certain experimentally induced infections and disease models *in vivo* and the role of complement in numerous reactions *in vitro*. The complement-deficient animal strains have all been healthy, and their deficiencies have been discovered by chance. This is also true of the first identified humans with complement deficiencies, who lacked C2 (245). Subsequent studies have revealed that many persons who genetically lack various complement components are not entirely healthy but rather suffer from various diseases, as summarized in the following sections. In general, these disease complexes would not readily be detected in laboratory animals.

Patterns of Disease

Although they are quite rare, genetically determined deficiencies of most of the complement components and regulatory proteins have been described and carefully characterized over the last 30 years. Most of the deficiencies are inherited in an autosomal recessive manner. Studies of individuals and families with complement deficiencies have revealed previously unsuspected functions of the complement system *in vivo*, and certain characteristic disease complexes have been found to be highly associated with specific complement deficiencies (Table 19-4). Deficiencies of the CCP components (C1q, C1r, C1s, C2, and C4) are all associated with an increased frequency of systemic lupus erythematosus (SLE) and immune complex diseases, with more than half of affected persons manifesting these diseases. The absence of C1In, or the presence of a nonfunctional form of this regulatory protein, is associated with hereditary angioedema. MBL deficiency is associated with the symptoms of immunodeficiency and a markedly increased susceptibility to infection. Virtually all persons who lack C3 or its regulatory proteins, factors H and I, experience recurrent, life-threatening infections with pyogenic organisms, as well as immune complex disease. Those lacking the ACP components (factor D and properdin) or the terminal complement components (C5, C6, C7, and C8) have recurrent infections with *Neisseria* strains. The absence of GPI-linked proteins, which include DAF and CD59, is associated with paroxysmal nocturnal hemoglobinuria. Persons with a deficiency in the β_2-integrins (including CR3 and CR4) or LFA-1 have severe immunodeficiency and defective leukocyte functions.

Deficiencies of CCP Components and Regulatory Proteins

Two types of C1q deficiency have been described (246,247). Approximately 60% of the more than 40 persons reported to have C1q deficiency lacked C1q protein, while the remainder possessed antigenically normal but functionally defective C1q. All of these patients had severe SLE, and some also had recurrent pyogenic infections. Approximately ten cases of C1r deficiency have been reported, all in association with partial C1s deficiency; most of these individuals also had SLE (246,247). Complete deficiencies of the MHC-encoded CCP proteins C4, reported in more than 20 persons, and C2, observed in more than 100 patients, are strongly associated with SLE (129,247,248). More than 75% of the C4-deficient patients had severe SLE associated with immune complex disease of the kidney, and one third to one half of the C2-deficient patients had SLE of typical severity. Many of these patients also had recurrent pyogenic infections. The remaining C2- and C4-deficient persons were healthy.

Several hundred cases of C1In deficiency have been reported. C1In absence or dysfunction is associated with hereditary angioedema, a syndrome characterized by recurrent episodes of edema of the subcutaneous tissues of the skin and other organs. A cause of death of patients with hereditary angioedema is edema of the nasopharynx. In the more common type I deficiency, very low concentrations of C1In are present in the circulation; in the type II variant, various point mutations lead to relatively normal levels of nonfunctional protein (249,250). The disease is transmitted as an autosomal dominant trait.

A single case of partial C4bp deficiency has been reported (251). The patient had angioedema and exhibited symptoms of autoimmune disease.

Mannose-binding Lectin Deficiency

Three different inherited mutations in the collagen-like region of MBL have been described in various ethnic groups (24). Two of these are point mutations of the glycine residue of different Gly-X-Y triplets, alterations that apparently interfere with assembly of the MBL molecule, since homozygous persons have very low serum concentrations of MBL. Both of these mutations are common, with gene frequencies in certain populations of 0.11 to 0.16 (codon 54 mutation) and 0.23–0.29 (codon 57 mutation). The third mutation, which substitutes cysteine for an arginine in codon 52, does not disrupt the Gly-X-Y triplet and has less effect on serum MBL levels. This mutation occurs with a frequency of 0.05 or less. All of these mutations are associated with defective opsonization and phagocytosis of bacteria *in vitro* and a markedly increased risk of infection in both children and adults (24,252).

Deficiencies of ACP Components and Regulatory Proteins

One case of complete factor D deficiency has been reported in a patient who had repeated severe neisserial infections, including generalized infections (253). More

TABLE 19-4. *Patterns of disease associated with congenital complement deficiencies*

Deficient component	Disease association
C1q, C1r, C1s, C4, C2	SLE and other autoimmune diseases, immune complex disease, recurrent pyogenic infections
MBL	Recurrent pyogenic infections
Factor D, properdin	Recurrent neisserial infections
C3, factor H, factor I	Recurrent infections with pyogenic organisms, immune complex disease
C5, C6, C7, C8,	Recurrent neisserial infections
C1 inhibitor	Hereditary angioedema
CR3, CR4 (and LFA-1)	Severe immunodeficiency, recurrent infections, leukocyte dysfunction
DAF, CD59 (and GPI linked protein)	Paroxysmal nocturnal hemoglobinuria

MBL, mannose-binding lectin; LFA-1, lymphocyte function antigen-1; SLE, systemic lupus erythematosus.

than 70 cases of total properdin deficiency have been described; this deficiency is inherited as an X-linked trait (247,254). Most of those affected had repeated systemic, life-threatening *Neisseria* infections. No homozygous factor B–deficient persons have been found, although a single heterozygous case of factor B deficiency has been reported (255).

Deficiencies of C3 and the C3 Regulatory Proteins

Homozygous C3 deficiency has been described in approximately 25 persons. The defect is transmitted as an autosomal recessive trait. Most of those affected had recurrent life-threatening infections with encapsulated pyogenic bacteria, particularly *Neisseria*, and several also had SLE, glomerulonephritis, or syndromes reminiscent of autoimmune disease (247,256).

Inherited deficiencies of factor H and factor I have each been reported in 10 to 15 patients (257). These proteins, when present, mediate the rapid inactivation of C3b in plasma and on cells. In their absence, small amounts of C3b interact with factors B and D to form an uncontrolled C3 convertase, which rapidly cleaves and inactivates all of the C3 in plasma. Persons lacking these regulatory proteins exhibit acquired C3 deficiency. The diseases they manifest are the same as those that characterize inherited C3 deficiency: recurrent life-threatening pyogenic infections and manifestations of immune complex disease (257).

Deficiencies of the Terminal Complement Components

Complete C5 deficiency has been reported in approximately 30 persons, C6 deficiency in more than 100, C7 deficiency in approximately 80, C8 deficiency in about 80, and C9 deficiency in more than 500 persons (258). Striking differences in the frequencies of these homozygous deficiencies have been observed in various geographic and racial populations (255,258). Many of those with C5, C6, C7, or C8 deficiency were prone to neisserial infections, many had repeated episodes of meningococcal meningitis, and some had disseminated gonococcal infections. Most of the infections were not life-threatening. Individuals with C9 deficiency, in contrast, were generally healthy.

Deficiencies of the Membrane-Associated Complement Regulatory Proteins

Both DAF and CD59 are attached to cell membranes by means of a GPI bond. These proteins are not present on the membrane of cells in persons with paroxysmal nocturnal hemoglobinuria, an acquired hematopoietic stem cell disorder in which the cells are unable to synthesize the GPI linkage (259). In these persons, DAF, CD59, and the many other GPI-linked proteins are absent from cell membranes. The disease is characterized by recurrent complement-mediated hemolytic episodes. One person with a selective CD59 deficiency was reported to have paroxysmal nocturnal hemoglobinuria (260).

Deficiencies of Membrane Complement Receptors

Inherited deficiencies of CR1 and CR2 have not been reported. However, persons lacking the heterodimeric β_2 integrins—CD11a/CD18 (LFA-1), CD11b/CD18 (CR3), and CD11c/CD18 (CR4)—as a consequence of mutations in the CD18 β chain exhibit the syndrome called leukocyte adhesion deficiency (LAD) (104,261). They have increased susceptibility to infections with pyogenic bacteria; these infections may be mild, or they may be recurrent and life-threatening.

Implications of the Genetic Complement Deficiencies for the Biologic Significance of the Complement System

The mechanism responsible for the striking association of SLE and immune complex disease with genetic deficiencies of C1q, C1r, C1s, C4, and C2 is not known. Ascertainment artefacts (more complement tests on SLE patients than on other individuals) are not likely to explain this association, since large screening studies of Swiss army recruits and Japanese blood donors failed to identify any persons with complement deficiencies (255). Linkage with a disease susceptibility gene was initially thought to be responsible, because the association of SLE with C4 and C2 deficiency, both of which are MHC linked, was discovered and studied first. However, this explanation was ruled out by the finding that SLE is also strongly associated with C1q and C1r/C1s deficiencies, which are not linked to each other or to the MHC. Another early hypothesis was that the absence of CCP function permitted uncontrolled infection with a transforming retrovirus that provoked autoimmune responses, since the CCP exclusively mediated inactivation of all retroviruses studied (15). This theory was rendered unlikely by the finding that this phenomenon prevails only with animal retroviruses and is not observed with human lentiviruses.

The absence of any of the CCP components, rather than a particular complement component, is associated with the development of SLE. It follows, therefore, that the inability to activate the CCP through the C2 step, and probably the C3 step, predisposes to the development of SLE. Inability to activate the CCP would abrogate the various biologic activities that derive from CCP or C3 activation. C3-dependent opsonization and phagocytosis, the ability to regulate immune complex size, processing and clearance of immune complexes, and Ab formation to T-dependent Ags would be impaired. As a consequence, Abs generated in the absence of a functional CCP would be directed mainly to T-independent Ags. The Abs would form large immune complexes with the Ags which, in the absence of C3 activation, would not be cleared by the C3b/CR1–dependent immune complex clearing mechanism. These complexes probably would be deposited in the kidneys and in blood vessel walls in skin, muscle, and other tissues, leading to tissue damage that would be amplified by associated inflammatory processes. Tissue damage leading to enzymatic degradation of host components also would be anticipated to produce autoantigens, which, in turn, could generate autoantibodies and additional immune complexes. Furthermore, impaired Ab formation to T-dependent Ags would yield low-affinity Abs, probably directed primarily to bacterial Ags, because of the inability to opsonize and destroy pyogenic bacteria. These low-affinity Abs could generate additional immune complexes. Also, it is likely that some of these Abs would cross-react with normal cellular Ags. Such cyclic processes may be responsible for the continuous formation of immune complexes and the presence of the numerous autoantibodies, characteristics that typify SLE.

In addition to SLE, patients lacking CCP components (C3, factor H, factor I) are susceptible to repeated pyogenic infections by strains of *Staphylococcus, Streptococcus, Pneumococcus,* and other organisms. In the absence of CCP function, C3 activation by bacterial strains could occur only via the ACP. Many bacterial strains lack the ability to activate the ACP, or do so only inefficiently. C3-dependent opsonization and phagocytosis of those bacterial strains and of other pathogens that activate the CCP directly, and in the presence of Ab, would not occur in the absence of CCP function. This is undoubtedly the explanation for the increased susceptibility to infection with pyogenic organisms exhibited by persons with deficiencies in CCP components or in C3 or its regulatory factors. These findings emphasize the importance of C3 as a requirement for effective phagocytic destruction of bacteria (129).

Whereas impaired CCP activation is associated with autoimmune disease, immune complex disease, and repeated infections, increased and uncontrolled CCP activation occurs in the absence of the CCP regulatory protein, C1In. This member of the serine protease inhibitor (serpin) superfamily not only inhibits spontaneous C1 activation and the activity of activated C1r and C1s but also inhibits the activated proteases of the contact system (kallikrein), the clotting system (factors XII and XI), and the thrombolytic system (plasmin). The edema that is responsible for hereditary angioedema is probably caused by actions of peptides derived from C2 (C2 kinin) and high-molecular-weight kinogen (bradykinin), both of which enhance the permeability of postcapillary venules (249,262).

Appreciation of the existence of the MBL pathway of complement activation is relatively recent. This also applies to the realization that MBL mutations predispose to defects in opsonization and phagocytosis, frequent infections, and the symptoms of immunodeficiency.

Because mannose residues are uncommon on mammalian cells but are widely expressed on gram-positive and gram-negative bacteria, viruses, fungi, and other pathogens, the MBL pathway possesses the ability to differentiate self from nonself. Although the MBL pathway probably antedates the adaptive immune system in evolution, the persistence of the system after the development of specific immunity indicates that it provides a biologic advantage (263). This concept is reinforced by the susceptibility of patients with homozygous MBL deficiencies to various infections despite the integrity of the immune system, the CCP, and the ACP.

The association of ACP deficiencies (factor D and properdin) and membrane attack pathway deficiencies (C5, C6, C7, and C8) with recurrent *Neisseria* infections is striking. It is apparent that *Neisseria* must preferentially activate the ACP and that assembly of the MAC must be necessary for destruction of these organisms. The finding that most C9-deficient persons are not prone to repeated infections with *Neisseria* suggests that full MAC assembly is not required to kill *Neisseria*; however, virtually all of the cases of C9 deficiency occurred in Japan, where meninogococcal meningitis is rare. One study indicated that C9 deficiency does carry an increased risk for development of meningococcal disease (264).

In paroxysmal nocturnal hemoglobinuria, GPI-linked proteins are absent from the plasma membrane. The identification of a patient with a genetically determined CD59 deficiency but normal DAF expression who had paroxysmal nocturnal hemoglobinuria (260), coupled with the asymptomatic characteristics of several persons with inherited DAF deficiencies (265), suggests that CD59 plays a more important functional role in the regulation of complement-dependent cellular lysis than does DAF. Additional study of this point is needed, however, because DAF incorporated into cell membranes *in vitro* has profound effects on the amplification of the complement cascade and subsequent lysis of the cells (266).

Numerous defects in leukocyte adherence and function are evident in patients with LAD, who have impaired LFA-1, CR3, and CR4 function as a consequence of mutations in the β_2 integrin subunit. Persons with LAD are susceptible to pyogenic infections by the same organisms that infect patients with homozygous C3, factor H, or factor I deficiencies. Since CR3 and CR4 bind C3 activation/processing fragments and are largely expressed on monocytes and granulocytes, whereas LFA-1 primarily influences lymphocyte functions, the increased susceptibility to infection exhibited by LAD patients again emphasizes the critical roles of C3 activation, opsonization, and phagocytosis in host defense against many pyogenic bacteria.

Human Diseases and Complement Activation

Evidence for the physiologic functions and importance of the complement system in host defense comes from four sources: the disease susceptibility of individuals with homozygous complement deficiencies; the direct demonstration of complement activation in sites of tissue damage in a number of human diseases; insights gained from studies of the role of complement in animal models of human disease; and results of *in vitro* studies of the biologic activities of the complement system. Cumulatively, these data indicate that the important physiologic functions of the complement system are, first, the production of inflammatory responses, which serve the important function of preventing the dissemination of infectious and injurious processes; second, the destruction of infectious agents and altered host cells by lytic disruption or by opsonization and phagocytosis, or both; and third, immunoregulation (see Tables 19-2 and 19-3).

Complement activation has been demonstrated in many human bacterial, fungal, and protozoal infectious diseases; in autoimmune diseases such as SLE, Sjögren's syndrome, Behçet's syndrome, rheumatoid arthritis, dermatomyositis, and myasthenia gravis; in bullous pemphigoid and certain other dermatologic conditions; in immune complex deposition diseases; in Alzheimer's disease, multiple sclerosis, and other neurologic diseases; and in many other conditions (7,48,267–269). In these various pathologic processes, complement components (usually including C1q, C4, C3, and often MAC components) have been found in association with tissue damage in the skin, in filtering organs such as the kidney and choroid plexus, in blood vessel walls, or in muscles and other tissues, depending on the particular disease and sites of tissue injury.

Deposition of complement components, and in particular the MAC, is also seen near areas of ischemia in experimental models of tissue injury (7,48,269). This has been prominently shown in experimental myocardial infarction and reperfusion injury; extension of the initial cardiac damage has been shown to be complement mediated, since it is prevented by complement depletion or by infusion of soluble CR1. Similar findings have been made in experimental burns in animal model systems. Complement activation by damaged and ischemic tissues undoubtedly occurs in humans.

Systemic complement activation frequently occurs in cases of septicemia resulting from infection with gram-negative organisms, shock in association with disseminated intravascular coagulation, and the acute respiratory distress syndrome (7,48,269). A common feature of these life-threatening conditions is the generation of anaphylatoxins and the consequences of their actions on the various leukocyte populations in the circulation and adjacent tissues. Of these, the most damaging is C5a-dependent neutrophil aggregation and clumping in the circulation that is followed by embolization to the lung. In the lung, trapped and activated neutrophils cause extensive damage as a consequence of enzyme release from the cells, free radical generation, damage to small pulmonary blood vessels and alveoli, arterial hypoxemia, and interstitial edema.

Extensive studies have shown that complement activation by the membranes employed for renal dialysis and for cardiopulmonary bypass surgery is, in part, responsible for various symptoms in patients undergoing these techniques, including chest pain, dyspnea, hypotension, and organ dysfunction (270). These studies have led to considerable efforts to reduce the complement-activating potential of such membranes.

Xenotransplantation represents a viable approach to alleviate the shortage of human organs for transplantation. However, organs and tissues from most mammals (except humans and Old World monkeys) efficiently activate human complement *in vitro*, and porcine xenotransplants in rhesus monkeys undergo hyperacute rejection. These reactions are triggered by intense complement activation initiated by binding of natural Abs to an Ag (Gal[α_{1-3}]Gal) that is expressed on endothelial and other cells of most mammals—except humans and old world monkeys, which lack the necessary enzyme to generate this carbohydrate epitope (271–273). Depletion of the Ab, or *in vivo* complement depletion or inactivation, essentially abrogates hyperacute rejection (274). Expression of human complement control proteins (DAF and CD59) in porcine tissues as products of transgenes is being explored as an approach to obtain compatible porcine organs for transplantation in man (275).

Manipulation of the Complement System by Pathogens to Facilitate Infection

Many bacterial, viral, fungal, and protozoal pathogens are able to avoid inactivation or destruction by the complement system. Numerous different mechanisms by which they evade the recognition and effector functions of the complement system have been described. These include interference with the activation of specific complement components, prevention of complement component binding to the surface of the pathogen, blocking of C3-dependent effector functions, and interference with MAC assembly or action (14,31,92,93,276,277). Most striking are the findings that some pathogens have developed the ability to use the same mechanisms that enable normal mammalian cells to evade destruction by the complement system (14,31,276,277). A number of different types of pathogens also have evolved the ability to use the proteins of the complement system to increase infectivity, either by using cell surface complement proteins as receptors to initiate infection or by employing complement regulatory functions to augment infection (14,31,276,277).

Evasion of Complement-Mediated Inactivation and Destruction

Some pathogens have developed the ability to interfere with the initiation of complement activation or the deposition of C3b on their surface, or both (14,92,93,277). Capsules of gram-positive and gram-negative organisms activate the ACP poorly, in part because of the presence of sialic acid. The presence of sialic acid on *Treponema* strains also has an adverse effect on complement-activating potential. *Salmonella* strains exhibit striking differences in their ability to activate the ACP as a result of differences in the chemical structure of the O Ag side chains of their LPS molecules. Rickettsial strains have also been found to vary in complement-activating potential depending on the structure of their LPS molecules. Structures of certain *Streptococcus* and *Campylobacter* strains interfere with ACP C3 convertase assembly. In other cases, as with M protein–containing *Streptococcus* and some strains of *Escherichia, Pseudomonas,* and *Treponema,* degradation to iC3b is accelerated; as a consequence, further formation of a C3 convertase on the bacterial surface and additional C3b deposition are prevented, inhibiting efficient MAC formation and opsonization. LPS-rich *Escherichia* and *Salmonella* strains bind and activate C1, but such C1 is unduly susceptible to inactivation by C1In, and CCP activation does not occur. Paramyosins of some parasitic organisms such as *S. mansoni* and *Taenia solium* bind C1q and interfere with C1 activation by the organisms. Blocking proteins and C3-inactivating enzymes have been postulated to account for the inability of the vertebrate-host forms of *Trypanosoma* and *Leishmania* to activate complement. The presence of proteins that interfere with C3b binding to the surface of the pathogen or of C3-cleaving proteases (or both) is a common feature also exhibited by some *Escherichia, Streptococcus, Pseudomonas,* and *Serratia* strains, as well as by *Aspergillus fumigatus, Porphyromonas gingivalis, Entamoeba histolytica, Leishmania* strains, and *S. mansoni.* Some virulence factors, including the *Escherichia coli* TraT and Iss gene products, the *Salmonella typhimurium* Rsk gene product, the porins of *Neisseria* and *Salmonella,* the *Yersinia enterocolitica* YadA protein, and *Leishmania* gp63, among others, influence complement activation or C3-fragment deposition via unknown mechanisms.

Most bacteria are eliminated by phagocytosis. Bacteria have evolved several mechanisms to evade phagocytic destruction (14,92,93,276,277). C3b is deposited on the cell wall of encapsulated and nonencapsulated *Streptococcus, Staphylococcus, Escherichia,* and *Salmonella* strains, but access of phagocytic cells to opsonic C3b is restricted by the capsule. Another mechanism pertains to the presence of antiphagocytic proteins, including streptococcal M protein and staphylococcal protein A.

Bacteria and other pathogens have also evolved multiple mechanisms to interfere with MAC assembly or lytic activity (14,92,93,276,277). *Serratia marcescens* possesses an enzyme that cleaves C5, and this organism and *Streptococcus pyogenes* possess the ability to cleave and inactivate C5a. The *E. coli* TraT virulence gene product may interfere with C5b–6 assembly. The protein encoded

by the *rck* gene of *S. typhimurium* appears to retard C9 polymerization. The *Y. enterocolitica* Ail protein probably functions in a similar manner. This may also be true of the *Y. enterocolitica* YadA surface protein, which also acts at the C3 stage. Gram-positive bacteria mediate MAC activation but do not lyse, probably because the peptidoglycan layer prevents insertion of the MAC into the membrane. Gram-negative bacteria manifest several different mechanisms by which to evade MAC-mediated damage. One of these, exemplified by some serum-resistant *Salmonella* and *Escherichia* strains, is ineffective insertion of the MAC into the outer membrane, or accelerated shedding of the MAC. On serum-resistant strains bearing LPS molecules with long O Ag side chains, complement activation and MAC assembly occur far from the membrane, and, as a consequence, little MAC inserts into the outer membrane. The MAC is unable to bind to the surface membranes of some complement-sensitive *Salmonella* strains, exemplifying a second mechanism. Yet another process prevails with serum-resistant *Neisseria gonorrhoeae* strains. Serum-resistant and serum-sensitive strains bind similar amounts of MAC, but the complex binds to different sites; it does not insert into the lipid bilayer outer membrane of the resistant strain and, as a consequence, is rapidly shed from the surface.

Similar mechanisms may prevail with the vertebrate-host stages of *Trypanosoma cruzi* and *Leishmania major.* These protozoan parasites efficiently activate complement through the C9 step, but MAC fails to insert effectively into the lipid bilayer of *T. cruzi* amastigotes, and *L. major* noninfective promastigotes release MAC from the membrane. Furthermore, the presence of *Leishmania* gp63 appears to interfere with MAC binding to the organisms (278).

Use of Cellular Complement Receptors and Regulatory Molecules to Initiate Infection

A number of different pathogens have evolved the ability to initiate infection by binding directly to cellular complement receptors and complement regulatory molecules (14,31,92,276) (Table 19-5). This mechanism does not depend on complement activation by the microorganisms. As discussed previously, most pathogens also activate complement in the absence or presence of Ab and become coated with covalently bound C3 fragments. Although these pathogens are normally cleared via binding to complement receptors and subsequent ingestion by phagocytes, several groups have developed the ability to initiate infection in this manner via bound C3 activation fragments, as described in the following sections.

Bacteria

Bacteria that initiate infection by binding directly to complement regulatory molecules include *E. coli* strains

TABLE 19-5. *Cellular complement receptors and regulatory molecules used by pathogens to initiate infection*

Type of Pathogen	Microorganism	Cellular receptor	Complement-dependent	Ligand
Bacterial	*Escherichia coli*	DAF	—	Dr adhesin
	Mycobacterium leprae	CR1, CR3, CR4	—	Unknown
Viral	Measles virus	MCP	—	Hemagglutin
	Coxsackie group B viruses	DAF	—	Unknown
	Echoviruses	DAF	—	Unknown
	Enterovirus 70	DAF	—	Unknown
	EBV	CR2	—	C3-like sequence in gp350/220
Fungal	*Histoplasma capsulatum*	CR3, CR4	—	Unknown
Parasitic	*Leishmania major/Leishmania donovani*	CR3, CR4	—	Unknown, gp63
Bacterial	*Legionella pneumophila*	CR1/CR3	+	C3b or iC3b
	M. leprae	CR1, CR3	+	C3b or iC3b
	Mycobacterium tuberculosis	CR1, CR3, CR4	+	C3b or iC3b
Viral	HIV	CR3	+	C3b, iC3b
	HIV	CR2	+	C3b
	West Nile virus	CR3	+	iC3b
Parasitic	*Babesia rodhaini*	CR1	+	C3b
	L. major	CR1, CR3	+	C3b or iC3b

EBV, Epstein-Barr virus; HIV, human immunodeficiency virus; DAF, decay accelerating factor; CR1, complement receptor type 1; CR2, complement receptor type 2; CR3, complement receptor type 3; CR4, complement receptor type 4; MCP, membrane cofactor protein.

expressing Dr or related adhesins, which account for approximately 30% of clinical infections with this organism. By means of their Dr adhesions, these strains bind to SCR 3 of cell-surface DAF (279). *Mycobacterium leprae* binds directly to CR1 and CR3 on monocytes and macrophages, thereby initiating infection of these cell types (280). Mycobacteria also are capable of initiating infection via interactions of bound complement proteins with CR1, CR3, and CR4 on the surface of mononuclear phagocytes (281). *Legionella pneumophila* bearing C3 fragments is also able to bind to and infect cells via complement receptors (282).

Viruses

Measles virus initiates infection of various cells by binding directly to MCP *in vitro* (283–285). Measles virus is able to infect mice expressing human MCP as a transgene, a finding that also provides the first nonprimate model in which to study measles virus pathogenesis (286). The virus binds to the N-glycan of SCR 2 of MCP, via the viral hemagglutinin (287,288); measles virus has also been shown to bind independently to a site in SCR 1 (289).

A number of echovirus serotypes bind to and infect susceptible epithelial cells via DAF (290). A number of coxsackievirus group B strains, which are also picornaviruses, use DAF to infect cells (291,292). Studies with Abs suggest that DAF SCR 2 or SCR 3, or both, mediate binding of both picornaviruses. Another picornavirus, enterovirus 70, also has been shown to initiate infection through DAF (293).

Infection of human B cells by EBV is initiated by direct binding of the virus, via the viral glycoprotein gp350/220, to CR2 (186,294–297). The restricted distribution of CR2 is largely responsible for the selective tropism of this virus for B cells. The binding site for CR2 in gp350/220 is a nine-residue linear sequence epitope that is homologous in sequence to the CR2-binding epitope in C3dg (298).

HIV coated with C3 activation fragments as a result of complement activation binds to and infects B and T cells via CR2 (299–301) and monocytic cells via CR3 (301,302). West Nile virus, a flavivirus, activates complement and enters macrophages via CR3 (303).

Fungi

Histoplasma capsulatum has been reported to infect macrophages by binding to CR3 and CR4 (304).

Parasitic Organisms

Infectious metacyclic promastigotes of *Leishmania major* and *Leishmania donovani* bind directly to CR3 and CR4 (and LFA-1) via either of two parasite glycoproteins (305,306). One of these, gp63, contains a sequence reported to be cross-reactive with C3 (307). *Leishmania* promastigotes at various developmental stages also activate the CCP or the ACP and bind, via C3 activation fragments, to CR1 or CR3 on monocytes, a process followed by infection (305,308). This process is considerably augmented by the presence of gp63 (278). *Babesia rodhaini* activates complement and enters erythrocytes by binding to CR1 (309).

Use of Complement Regulatory Epitopes to Evade Complement-Mediated Destruction

A number of different types of pathogens have developed functional properties that are similar or identical to those used by normal mammalian cells to protect themselves from complement-mediated destruction (14,31, 276,277) (Table 19-6). The proteins that mediate these reactions are encoded by the genome of the pathogen and therefore differ structurally and functionally from their mammalian counterparts. However, some of the pathogen-encoded proteins that mediate complement-related functional activities are antigenically or genetically related to their mammalian homologues. In addition, several examples of the "capture" of mammalian complement regulatory proteins by microorganisms have been reported.

Bacteria

A single example of a bacterial protein with complement regulatory functions has been reported. The major virulence factor of β-hemolytic group A streptococci, M protein, has C3b-like properties and binds factor H (310). As a consequence, M protein retards assembly of the ACP C3 convertase on the streptococcal surface, a property that accounts for the ability of M protein to inhibit complement activation (311,312).

Viruses

There are a number of examples of virus-encoded proteins that possess complement regulatory functions. Vaccinia virus, a poxvirus, expresses a 35-kd protein that binds C4b; prevents formation of, and accelerates the decay of, the CCP and ACP C3 convertases; and serves as a cofactor for cleavage of C4b and C3b by factor I (313–316). The vaccinia virus protein contains four SCRs that are 38% identical to the four amino-terminal SCRs of human C4b (313,314). A vaccinia virus deletion mutant lacking the protein was found to be attenuated in vitro and in vivo (315). Proteins similar to the vaccinia virus complement control protein have been reported in cells infected with two other poxviruses, cowpox and ectromelia, but they have not been characterized (314). A 42-kd protein that expresses sequence similarity with the 35-kd vaccinia complement control protein and with factor H and C4bp has been described but has not been analyzed for complement regulatory properties (317,318). Vaccinia virus and rabbitpox virus also contain other uncharacterized genes that exhibit sequence homology to C3, C4, and C5 (319).

The other viral complement regulatory proteins that have been described occur in three different members of the herpesvirus family. Their presence is probably important, because herpesviruses persist indefinitely in latent form in host cells after infection, and continuing evasion of host defense mechanisms is a requirement for such persistence. The glycoprotein C (gC) envelope protein of herpes simplex virus types 1 and 2 (HSV-1, HSV-2) binds C3b (320–322). This glycoprotein lacks SCRs or obvious sequence similarity with CR1 or other C3b-binding proteins (322,323). Viral gC-1 accelerates decay of the ACP C3 convertase but lacks MCP activity and possesses no CCP inhibitory functions (324,325); this complex of properties differentiates gC-1 from known mammalian complement regulatory proteins. The presence of gC-1 protects HSV-1 from complement-mediated damage (321). HSV-1 strains expressing gC-1 mutants were found to be considerably less pathogenic, and the gC mutant strains and wild-type HSV-1 strains produced similar susceptibility to disease in C3-deficient guinea pigs (326). These findings suggest that gC contributes to HSV-1 pathogenesis in vivo by protecting the virus from complement-mediated destruction.

EBV possesses several complement regulatory proteins (327). The virus serves as a factor I–dependent cofactor for cleavage of C3b, iC3b, C4b, and iC4b, and it accelerates decay of the ACP C3 convertase. This unique combination of complement regulatory proteins is not shared by any known mammalian system. For example, EBV does not bind C3b, unlike CR1 and MCP; EBV serves as a cofactor for factor I–mediated cleavage of iC3b and iC4b, unlike MCP; and EBV does not accelerate decay of the CCP C3 convertase, unlike DAF. The viral proteins responsible for these activities have not been identified; the viral genome does not contain SCRs.

Herpesvirus saimiri (HVS) expresses two complement regulatory proteins. The first is an envelope protein composed of four SCRs that is 20% to 46% identical with human MCP or DAF, depending on the SCR that is compared (328). Cells transfected with this HVS gene exhibit resistance to complement-mediated damage, and the site of action is at the C3 step (329). HVS also contains a GPI-linked protein that is 48% identical in sequence to human CD59 (330,331). Cells expressing the CD59 homologue are resistant to the action of MAC (330,331).

Several viruses have been shown to acquire normal complement regulatory proteins during the process of viral maturation within host cells. Examples include three enveloped viruses—HIV-1, HTLV-I, and simian immunodeficiency virus (SIV)—which have been shown to acquire functionally active DAF and CD59 (332–335). Host cell–derived MCP has also been found to be associated with HIV-1 and SIV but has not yet been characterized for function (332). Human cytomegalovirus, an enveloped herpesvirus, has been shown to acquire DAF and CD59 from host cells, but functional activity has not been verified (31,333). Acquisition of functionally active host cell–derived MCP by human cytomegalovirus has been demonstrated (31).

TABLE 19-6. Complement binding and regulatory epitopes used by pathogens to evade the complement system or augment infection

Type of Pathogen	Pathogen	Pathogen protein	Source	Homologous complement protein(s)	Complement regulatory functions	Complement-like structural features
Bacterial	β hemolytic streptococci	M Protein	Pathogen	C3b	Binds factor H and blocks ACP C3 convertase assembly	Unknown
Viral	VV	35 kd	Pathogen	CR1, DAF, MCP	Binds C3b and C4b, factor I cofactor for C3 and C4 cleavage	Contains 4 SCRs
	VV	45 kd	Pathogen	C4bp, Factor H	Blocks CCP C3 convertase assembly and disassembles ACP and CCP C3 convertases	Contains SCRs
	HSV-1, HSV-2	gC-1, gC-2	Pathogen	CR1, DAF	Unknown	Unknown
	EBV	Unknown	Pathogen	CR1, DAF, MCP	Binds C3b and disassembles ACP C3 convertase	Unknown
	HVS	65–75 kd	Pathogen	CR1, DAF, MCP	Factor I cofactor for C3 and C4 cleavage and disassembles ACP C3 convertase	Contains 4 SCRs
	HVS	20 kd	Pathogen	CD59	Inhibits complement, acts at C3 step	Sequence homologous to CD59
	HIV-1	DAF	Host	DAF	Disassembles C3 convertases	Host SCRs
	HIV-1	MCP	Host	MCP	Unknown	Host SCRs
	HIV-1	CD59	Host	CD59	C5b-9 inhibition	Host CD59
	HTLV-1	DAF	Host	DAF	Disassembles C3 convertases	Host SCRs
	HTLV-1	CD59	Host	CD59	C5b-9 inhibition	Host CD59
	SIV	DAF	Host	DAF	Disassembles C3 convertases	Host SCRs
	SIV	MCP	Host	MCP	Unknown	Host SCRs
	SIV	CD59	Host	CD59	C5b-9 inhibition	Host CD59
	HCMV	DAF	Host	DAF	Unknown	Host SCRs
	HCMV	MCP	Host	MCP	Factor I cofactor for C3 and C4 cleavage	Host SCRs
	HCMV	CD59	Host	CD59	Unknown	Host CD59
Fungal	Candida albicans	130–165 kd	Pathogen	CR3	iC3b binding	Integrin
	C. albicans	60 kd	Pathogen	CR2	C3d binding	Unknown
	C. albicans	70 kd	Pathogen	Unknown	C3d binding	Unknown
Parasitic	Trypanosoma cruzi	160 kd	Pathogen	CR1, DAF	Binds C3b, and blocks ACP C3 convertase assembly	Contains SCRs
	T. cruzi	87–93 kd	Pathogen	CR1, DAF	Blocks assembly of and disassembles ACP and CCP C3 convertases	Unknown
	T. cruzi	58–68 kd	Pathogen	DAF	Blocks assembly of and disassembles ACP C3 convertase	Unknown
	T. cruzi	Unknown	Pathogen	C9	Induce lysis	C9 related
	Entamoeba histolytica	Adhesin	Pathogen	CD59	C5b-9 inhibition	Sequence homologous to CD59
	Schistosoma mansoni	130 kd	Pathogen	CR1	Binds C3	Unknown
	S. mansoni	70 kd	Pathogen	CR1	Binds C3b	Unknown
	S. mansoni	Unknown	Pathogen	CD59	C5b-9 inhibition	Sequence homologous to CD59
	S. mansoni	DAF	Host	DAF	Disassembles C3 convertase	Host SCRs

VV, vaccinia virus; VCP, virus complement control protein; HSV, herpes simplex virus; EBV, Epstein-Barr virus; HCMV, human cytomegalovirus; HVS, herpesvirus saimiri; SIV, simian immunodeficiency virus; HIV, human immunodeficiency virus; HTLV, human T-cell leukemia virus; CCP, classical pathway; ACP, alternative pathway; SCR, short consensus repeat; DAF, decay accelerating factor; CR1, complement receptor type 1; CR2, complement receptor type 2; MCP, membrane cofactor protein.

Fungi

C. albicans expresses various proteins that bind different C3 fragments. One of these, a 130- to 165-kd protein, is structurally and functionally related to the integrin complement receptor CR3, because it binds iC3b, reacts with some Abs to the α polypeptide chain of CR3, and exhibits integrin-like motifs in its primary nucleotide sequence (336–339). An MAb to human CR3 inhibited binding of *C. albicans* to iC3b and immunoprecipitated a 140-kd protein from solubilized organisms (338). The *Candida* CR3 homologue plays a role in pathogenesis, because it is involved in adherence to host tissues, a primary requirement for infection (340). Pathogenicity probably is also related in part to iC3b binding potential, since the more pathogenic strains bind iC3b more strongly than the less pathogenic strains (336,337,340); this could be related to adherence to iC3b on opsonized erythrocytes, a postulated bacterial mechanism for acquiring the iron needed for growth (341). *Candida* also possesses 60- and 70-kd glycoproteins that bind C3d (342). The 60-kd C3d-binding molecule, which is cross-reactive with CR2, has been purified but has not been characterized functionally (343–345).

Parasitic Organisms

The vertebrate-host forms of parasitic organisms are generally resistant to the actions of Ab and complement. In part, their resistance to such destruction is a result of complement regulatory properties that impede complement-mediated destruction. Several complement regulatory proteins have been described in the vertebrate bloodstream trypomastigote and amastigote forms of *T. cruzi*. These include a 87- to 93-kd molecule that possesses DAF-like activity for the C3 convertases of both pathways (346,347) and a 58- to 68-kd protein that possesses decay-accelerating activity for the ACP but not for the CCP C3 convertase (348). These proteins have been purified but not cloned. In addition, *T. cruzi* trypomastigotes contain a developmentally regulated 160-kd GPI-linked membrane glycoprotein that binds C3b and inhibits the ACP C3 convertase; the *T. cruzi* 160-kd gene hybridized with human DAF cDNA in Southern blotting studies under moderately stringent conditions, indicating genetic homology (349). Despite this, SCRs have not been identified in the complete cDNA sequence (350). *T. cruzi* also possesses a protein that is reactive with Abs against human C9 (351); this property may facilitate disruption of intracellular vacuolar membranes by the parasite, a requirement for entry into the cytoplasm. Finally, evidence for a *T. cruzi* epimastigote protein that regulates C9 binding has been obtained (352), a finding which suggests that the parasite possesses a CD59-like molecule.

Trophozoites of both pathogenic and nonpathogenic strains of *E. histolytica* activate the ACP during hematogenous spread throughout the body, but only the nonpathogenic strains are destroyed by MAC (353,354). The purified galactose-specific adhesin of *E. histolytica* binds C8 and C9 and confers MAC resistance to the complement-sensitive amoeba (355). Additionally, and further emphasizing the CD59-like properties, the adhesin is cross-reactive and exhibits some sequence similarity to CD59 (355).

S. mansoni, a parasitic helminth, possesses several complement regulatory properties. As with protozoan organisms, parasitic stages from vertebrate hosts are complement resistant. The organisms contain a 130-kd protein that binds C3 (356,357); however, its functional parameters have not yet been assessed. A 70-kd C3b-binding protein has also been isolated from *S. mansoni* (277), but it has not been determined whether the protein plays a role in complement resistance. *S. mansoni* also contains a GPI-linked CD59-like molecule that binds to C8 and C9 and inhibits the action of the MAC, probably by this mechanism (358). The protein is sufficiently similar to human CD59 to be purified with Ab to human CD59 (358). The *S. mansoni* CD59 homologue clearly plays a role in the complement resistance of the vertebrate-host form of the organism, because Ab to human CD59 renders the parasites vulnerable to complement-mediated destruction (358).

Adult *S. mansoni* worms use yet another mechanism to avoid destruction by the complement system (359,360). This mechanism involves the acquisition and insertion of human DAF into the parasite membrane in functionally active form.

ACKNOWLEDGMENTS

I wish to thank Catalina Hope and Joan Gausepohl for assistance with the manuscript. Studies from the author's laboratory were supported by USPHS grants CA14692, AI33244, CA52241 and NS34682. This is manuscript No. 11230-IMM at The Scripps Research Institute.

REFERENCES

1. Silverstein AM. *A history of immunology.* San Diego: Academic Press, 1989:1–422.
2. Cooper NR. The classical complement pathway: activation and regulation of the first complement component. *Adv Immunol* 1985;37:151–207.
3. Sim RB, Reid KBM. C1: molecular interactions with activating systems. *Immunol Today* 1991;12:307–311.
4. Atkinson JP, Farries T. Separation of self from non-self in the complement system. *Immunol Today* 1987;8:212–215.
5. Pangburn MK. The alternative pathway. In: Ross GD, ed. *Immunobiology of the complement system.* Orlando: Academic Press, 1986:45–62.
6. Müller-Eberhard HJ. Complement: chemistry and pathways. In: Gallin JI, Goldstein IM, Snyderman R, eds. *Inflammation: basic principles and clinical correlates,* 2nd ed. New York: Raven Press, 1992:33–61.
7. Roitt I, Brostoff J, Male D. Complement. In: Roitt I, Brostoff J, Male D, eds. *Immunology,* 3rd ed. St. Louis: Mosby, 1993:12.1–12.17.

8. Liszewski MK, Atkinson JP. The complement system. In: Paul WE, ed. *Fundamental immunology.* New York: Raven Press, 1993: 917–939.

9. Campbell RD, Law SKA, Reid KBM, Sim RB. Structure, organization, and regulation of the complement genes. *Annu Rev Immunol* 1988;6:161–195.

10. Volanakis JE. Transcriptional regulation of complement genes. *Annu Rev Immunol* 1995;13:277–305.

11. Farries TC, Atkinson JP. Evolution of the complement system. *Immunol Today* 1991;12:295–300.

12. Reid KBM, Day AJ. Structure-function relationships of the complement components. *Immunol Today* 1989;10:177–180.

13. Campbell ID, Baron M. The structure and function of protein modules. *Philos Trans R Soc Lond B Biol Sci* 1991;332:165–170.

14. Cooper NR. Interactions of the complement system with microorganisms. In: Erdei A, ed. *New aspects of complement structure and function.* Austin, TX: RG Landes, 1994:133–149.

15. Cooper NR, Jensen FC, Welsh RM Jr, Oldstone MBA. Lysis of RNA tumor viruses by human serum: direct antibody independent triggering of the classical complement pathway. *J Exp Med* 1976;144: 970–984.

16. Ebenbichler CF, Thielens NM, Vornhagen R, Marschang P, Arlaud GJ, Dierich MP. Human immunodeficiency virus type 1 activates the classical pathway of complement by direct C1 binding through specific sites in the transmembrane glycoprotein gp41. *J Exp Med* 1991;174: 1417–1424.

17. Rogers J, Cooper NR, Webster S, et al. Complement activation by β-amyloid in Alzheimer disease. *Proc Natl Acad Sci U S A* 1992;89: 10016–10020.

18. Jiang H, Burdick D, Glabe CG, Cotman CW, Tenner AJ. β-Amyloid activates complement by binding to a specific region of the collagen-like domain of the C1q A chain. *J Immunol* 1994;152:5050–5059.

19. Ying S-C, Gewurz AT, Jiang H, Gewurz H. Human serum amyloid P component oligomers bind and activate the classical complement pathway via residues 14–26 and 76–92 of the A chain collagen-like region of C1q. *J Immunol* 1993;150:169–176.

20. Jiang H, Robey FA, Gewurz H. Localization of sites through which CRP binds and activates complement to residues 14--26 and 76--92 of the human C1q A chain. *J Exp Med* 1992;175:1373–1379.

21. Jiang H, Cooper B, Robey FA, Gewurz H. DNA binds and activates complement via residues 14–26 of the human C1q A chain. *J Biol Chem* 1992;267:25597–25601.

22. Sim RB, Malhotra R. Interactions of carbohydrates and lectins with complement. *Biochem Soc Trans* 1993;22:106–111.

23. Holmskov U, Malhotra R, Sim RB, Jensenius JC. Collectins: collagenous C-type lectins of the innate immune defense system. *Immunol Today* 1994;15:67–73.

24. Turner MW. Mannose-binding lectin: the pluripotent molecule of the innate immune system. *Immunol Today* 1996;17:532–540.

25. Green PJ, Feizi T, Stoll MS, Thiel S, Prescott A, Mcconville M. Recognition of the major cell surface glycoconjugates of *Leishmania* parasites by the human serum mannan-binding protein. *Mol Biochem Parasitol* 1994;66:319–328.

26. Lu J, Thiel S, Wiedemann H. Binding of the pentamer/hexamer forms of mannan-binding protein to zymosan activates the proenzyme C1r₂C1s₂ complex, of the classical pathway of complement, without involvement of C1q. *J Immunol* 1990;144:2287–2294.

27. Ohta M, Okada M, Yamashina I. The mechanism of carbohydrate-mediated complement activation by the serum mannan-binding protein, *J Biol Chem* 1990;265:1980–1984.

28. Matsushita M, Fujita T. Activation of the classical complement pathway by mannose-binding protein in association with a novel C1s-like serine protease. *J Exp Med* 1992;176:1497–1502.

29. Takayama Y, Takada F, Takahashi A, Kawakami M. A 100-kDa protein in the C4-activating component of Ra-reactive factor is a new serine protease having module organization similar to C1r and C1s. *J Immunol* 1994;152:2308–2316.

30. Thiel S, Vorup-Jensen T, Stover CM, et al. A second serine protease associated with mannan-binding lectin that activates complement. *Nature* 1997;386:506–510.

31. Cooper NR. Complement and viruses. In: Frank M, Volanakis JE, eds. *The human complement system in health and disease.* New York: Marcel Dekker, 1997:393–407.

32. Fearon DT. Regulation of the amplification C3 convertase of human

33. Lachmann PJ, Hughes-Jones NC. Initiation of complement activation. In: Müller-Eberhard HJ, Miescher PA, eds. *Complement.* New York: Springer-Verlag, 1985:147–166.

34. Podack ER. Assembly and functions of the terminal components. In: Ross GD, ed. *Immunobiology of the complement system.* San Diego: Academic Press, 1986:115–137.

35. Müller-Eberhard HJ. The membrane attack complex of complement. *Annu Rev Immunol* 1986;4:503–528.

36. Isenman DE, Podack ER, Cooper NR. The interaction of C5 with C3b in free solution: a sufficient condition for cleavage by a fluid phase C3/C5 convertase. *J Immunol* 1980;124:326–331.

37. Zalman LS, Müller-Eberhard HJ. Comparison of channels formed by poly C9, C5b-8 and the membrane attack complex of complement. *Mol Immunol* 1990;27:533–537.

38. Tschopp J, Müller-Eberhard HJ, Podack ER. Formation of transmembrane tubules by spontaneous polymerization of hydrophilic complement protein C9. *Nature* 1982;298:534–538.

39. Humphrey JH, Dourmashkin RR. The lesions in cell membranes caused by complement. *Adv Immunol* 1969;11:75–115.

40. Peitsch MC, Amiguet P, Guy R, Brunner J, Maizel JV, Tschopp J. Localization and molecular modeling of the membrane-inserted domain of the ninth component of human complement and perforin. *Mol Immunol* 1990;27:589–602.

41. Hamilton KK, Zhao J, Sims PJ. Interaction between apolipoproteins A-I and A-II and the membrane attack complex of complement: affinity of the apolipoproteins for polymeric C9. *J Biol Chem* 1993;268: 3632–3638.

42. Tshopp J, Jenne D. Clusterin: the intriguing guises of a widely expressed glycoprotein. *Trends Biochem Sci* 1992;17:154–159.

43. Morgan BP, Meri S. Membrane proteins that protect against complement lysis. *Springer Semin Immunopathol* 1994;15:369–396.

44. Davies A, Lachmann PJ. Membrane defence against complement lysis: the structure and biological properties of CD59. *Immunol Res* 1993;12:258–275.

45. Frank MM, Fries LF. The role of complement in inflammation and phagocytosis. *Immunol Today* 1991;12:322–325.

46. Gallin JI. Inflammation. In: Paul WE, ed. *Fundamental immunology,* 3rd ed. New York: Raven Press, 1993:1015–1032.

47. Hugli TE. Structure and function of the anaphylatoxins. *Springer Semin Immunopathol* 1984;7:193–219.

48. Goldstein IM. Complement: biologically active products. In: Gallin JI, Goldstein IM, Snyderman R, eds. *Inflammation: basic principles and clinical correlates.* New York: Raven Press, 1992:63–80.

49. Bokisch VA, Müller-Eberhard HJ. Anaphylatoxin inactivator of human plasma: its isolation and characterization as a carboxypeptidase. *J Clin Invest* 1970;49:2427–2436.

50. Jose PJ, Forrest MJ, Williams TJ. Human C5a des Arg increases vascular permeability. *J Immunol* 1981;127:2376–2380.

51. Wetsel RA. Structure, function and cellular expression of complement anaphylatoxin receptors. *Curr Biol* 1995;7:48–53.

52. Gerard C, Hugli TE. Identification of classical anaphylatoxin as the des-Arg form of the C5a molecule: evidence for a modulator role for the oligosaccharide unit in human des-Arg74-C5a. *Proc Natl Acad Sci U S A* 1981;78:1833–1837.

53. Perez HD, Goldstein IM, Webster RO, Henson PM. Attachment of human C5a des Arg to its cochemotaxin is required for maximun expression of chemotactic activity. *J Clin Invest* 1986;78:1589–1895.

54. Kew RR, Webster RO. Gc-globulin (vitamin D–binding protein) enhances the neutrophil chemotactic activity of C5a and C5a des Arg. *J Clin Invest* 1988;82:364–369.

55. Perez HD, Kelly E, Chenoweth DE, Elfman F. Identification of the C5a des Arg cochemotaxin: homology with vitamin D–binding protein (group specific component globulin). *J Clin Invest* 1988; 82:360–363.

56. Chenoweth DE, Hugli TE. Demonstration of a specific C5a receptor on intact human polymorphonuclear leukocytes. *Proc Natl Acad Sci U S A* 1978;75:3943–3947.

57. Hugli TE. Human anaphylatoxin (C3a) from the third component of complement: primary structure. *J Biol Chem* 1975;250:8293–8301.

58. Caporale LH, Tippett PS, Erickson BW, Hugli TE. The active site of C3a anaphylatoxin. *J Biol Chem* 1980;255:10758–10763.

59. Gorski JP, Hugli TE, Müller-Eberhard HJ. C4a: the third anaphyla-

toxin of the human complement system. *Proc Natl Acad Sci U S A* 1979;76:5299–5302.

60. Murakami Y, Yamamoto T, Imamichi T, et al. Cellular responses of guinea-pig macrophages to C4a: inhibition of C3a-induced 0$_2$-generation by C4a. *Immunol Lett* 1993;36:301–304.

61. Gerard NP, Gerard C. The chemotactic receptor for human C5a anaphylatoxin. *Nature* 1991;349:614–617.

62. Ames RS, Li Y, Sarau HM, et al. Molecular cloning and characterization of the human anaphylatoxin C3a receptor. *J Biol Chem* 1996;271:20231–20234.

63. Crass T, Raffetseder U, Martin U, et al. Expression cloning of the human C3a anaphylatoxin receptor (C3aR) from differentiated U-937 cells. *Eur J Immunol* 1996;26:1944–1950.

64. Burg M, Martin U, Bock D, Rheinheimer C, Köhl J, Bautsch W, Klos A. Differential regulation of the C3a and C5a receptors (CD88) by IFN-gamma and PMA in U937 cells and related myeloblastic cell lines. *J Immunol* 1996;157:5574–5581.

65. Norgauer J, Dobos G, Kownatzki E, Dahinden C, Burger R, Kupper R, Gierschik P. Complement fragment C3a stimulates Ca^{2+} influx in neutrophils via a pertussis-toxin-sensitive G protein. *Eur J Biochem* 1993;217:289–294.

66. Murakami Y, Imamichi T, Nagasawa S. Characterization of C3a anaphylatoxin receptor on guinea-pig macrophages. *Immunology* 1993;79:633–638.

67. Okusawa S, Yancey KB, van der Meer JWM, et al. C5a stimulates secretion of tumor necrosis factor from human mononuclear cells *in vitro. J Exp Med* 1988;168:443–448.

68. Ember JA, Sanderson SD, Hugli TE, Morgan EL. Induction of interleukin-8 synthesis from monocytes by human C5a anaphylatoxin. *Am J Pathol* 1994;144:393–403.

69. McFarland HF. Complexities in the treatment of autoimmune disease. *Science* 1996;274:2037–2038.

70. Burg M, Martin U, Rheinheimer C, et al. IFN-gamma up-regulates the human C5a receptor (CD88) in myeloblastic U937 cells and related cell lines. *J Immunol* 1996;155:4419–4426.

71. Takabayashi T, Vannier E, Clark BD, et al. A new biologic role for C3a and C3a desArg: regulation of TNF-α and IL-1 synthesis. *J Immunol* 1996;156:3455–3460.

72. Daffern PJ, Pfeifer PH, Ember JA, Hugli TE. C3a is a chemotaxin for human eosinophils but not for neutrophils: I. C3a stimulation of neutrophils is secondary to eosinophil activation. *J Exp Med* 1995;181:2119–2127.

73. Nilsson G, Johnell M, Hammer CH, et al. C3a and C5a are chemotaxins for human mast cells and act through distinct receptors via a pertussis toxin-sensitive signal transduction pathway. *J Immunol* 1996;157:1693–1698.

74. Goldstein IM, Hoffstein S, Gallin J, Weissman G. Mechanisms of lysosomal enzyme release from human leukocytes: microtubule assembly and membrane fusion induced by a component of complement. *Proc Natl Acad Sci U S A* 1973;70:2916–2920.

75. Malech HL, Root RK, Gallin JI. Structural analysis of human neutrophil migration: centriole, microtubule and microfilament orientation and function during chemotaxis. *J Cell Biol* 1977;75:666–693.

76. Stossel TP. The mechanical responses of white blood cells. In: Gallin JI, Goldstein IM, Synderman R, eds. *Inflammation: basic principles and clinical correlates,* 2nd ed. New York: Raven Press, 1992:459–476.

77. Goldstein IM, Roos D, Weissmann G, Kaplan H. Complement and immunoglobulins stimulate superoxide production by human leukocytes independently of phagocytosis. *J Clin Invest* 1975;56:1155–1163.

78. Ghebrehiwet B, Müller-Eberhard HJ. C3e: an acidic fragment of human C3 with leukocytosis-inducing activity. *J Immunol* 1979;123:616–621.

79. Ghebrehiwet B. The release of lysosomal enzymes from human polymorphonuclear leukocytes by human C3e. *Clin Immunol Immunopathol* 1984;30:321–329.

80. Hugli TE. A synthetic nonapeptide corresponding to the NH$_2$ terminal sequence of C3d-K causes leukocytosis in rabbits. *J Biol Chem* 1978;120:438–444.

81. Hamuro J, Hadding U, Bitter-Suermann D. Fragments Ba and Bb derived from guinea pig factor B of the properdin system: purification, characterization, and biologic activities. *J Immunol* 1978;120:438–444.

82. Götze O, Bianco C, Cohn ZA. The induction of macrophage spreading by factor B of the properdin system. *J Exp Med* 1979;149:372–386.

83. Hirani S, Fair DS, Papin RA, Sundsmo JS. Leukocyte complement: interleukin-like properties of factor Bb. *Cell Immunol* 1985;92:235–246.

84. Wiedmer T, Esmon CT, Sims PJ. Complement proteins C5b-9 stimulate procoagulant activity through platelet prothrombinase. *Blood* 1986;68:875–880.

85. Lovett DH, Haensch G-M, Goppelt M, Resch K, Gemsa D. Activation of glomerular mesangial cells by the terminal membrane attack complex of complement. *J Immunol* 1987;138:2473–2480.

86. Hattori R, Hamilton KK, McEver RP, Sims PJ. Complement proteins C5b-9 induce secretion of high molecular weight multimers of endothelial von Willebrand factor and translocation of granule membrane protein GMP-140 to the cell surface. *J Biol Chem* 1989;264:9053–9060.

87. Biesecker G. The complement SC5b-9 complex mediates cell adhesion through a vitronectin receptor. *J Immunol* 1990;145:209–214.

88. Carney DF, Lang TJ, Shin ML. Multiple signal messengers generated by terminal complement complexes and their role in terminal complement complex elimination. *J Immunol* 1990;145:623–629.

89. Wang C, Gerard NP, Nicholson-Weller A. Signaling by hemolytically inactive C5b67, an agonist of polymorphonuclear leukocytes. *J Immunol* 1996;156:786–792.

90. Kilgore KS, Flory CM, Miller BF, Evans VM, Warren JS. The membrane attack complex of complement induces interleukin-8 and monocyte chemoattractant protein-1 secretion from human umbilical vein endothelial cells. *Am J Pathol* 1996;149:953–961.

91. Schreiber RD, Morrison DC, Podack ER, Müller-Eberhard HJ. Bactericidal activity of the alternative complement pathway generated from 11 isolated plasma proteins. *J Exp Med* 1979;149:870–882.

92. Joiner KA. Complement evasion by bacteria and parasites. *Annu Rev Microbiol* 1988;42:201–230.

93. Moffitt MC, Frank MM. Complement resistance in microbes. *Springer Semin Immunopathol* 1994;15:327–344.

94. Perrin LH, Joseph BS, Cooper NR, Oldstone MBA. Mechanism of injury of virus infected cells by antiviral antibody and complement: participation of IgG, Fab'$_2$ and the alternative complement pathway. *J Exp Med* 1976;143:1027–1041.

95. Sissons JGP, Schreiber RD, Perrin LH, Cooper NR, Müller-Eberhard HJ, Oldstone MBA. Lysis of measles virus infected cells by the purified cytolytic alternative complement pathway and antibody. *J Exp Med* 1979;150:445–454.

96. Cooper NR. Complement dependent virus neutralization. In: Rother K, Till G, Hansch GM, eds. *The complement system.* Ann Arbor: Springer-Verlag, 1997:302–309.

97. Mold C, Nemerow GR, Bradt BM, Cooper NR. CR2 is a complement activator and the covalent binding site for C3 during alternative pathway activation by Raji cells. *J Immunol* 1988;140:1923–1929.

98. Wright SD. Receptors for complement and the biology of phagocytosis. In: Gallin JI, Goldstein IM, Snyderman R, eds. *Inflammation: basic principles and clinical correlates.* New York: Raven Press, 1992:477–495.

99. Greenberg S, Silverstein SC. Phagocytosis. In: Paul WE, ed. *Fundamental immunology.* New York: Raven Press, 1993:941–964.

100. Schreiber RD. The chemistry and biology of complement receptors. In: Müller-Eberhard HJ, Miescher PA, eds. *Complement.* New York: Springer-Verlag, 1985:115–143.

101. Klickstein LB, Bartow TJ, Miletic V, Rabson LD, Smith JA, Fearon DT. Identification of distinct C3b and C4b recognition sites in the human C3b/C4b receptor (CR1,CD35) by deletion mutagenesis. *J Exp Med* 1988;168:1699–1717.

102. Ahearn JM, Fearon DT. Structure and function of the complement receptors, CR1 (CD35) and CR2 (CD21). *Adv Immunol* 1989;46:183–219.

103. Sanchez-Madrid F, Nagy JA, Robbins E, Simon P, Springer TA. Characterization of a human leukocyte differentiation antigen family with distinct α subunits and a common β subunit: the lymphocyte-function associated antigen (LFA-1), the C3bi complement receptor (OKM1/Mac1), and the p150,95 molecule. *J Exp Med* 1983;158:1785–1803.

104. Kishimoto TK, Larson R, Corbi AL, Dustin ML, Staunton DE, Springer TA. The leukocyte integrins. *Adv Immunol* 1989;46:149–182.

105. Tenner AJ, Cooper NR. Identification of types of cells in human peripheral blood that bind C1q. *J Immunol* 1981;126:1174–1179.

106. Malhotra R, Thiel S, Reid KBM, Sim RB. Human leukocyte C1q receptor binds other soluble proteins with collagen domains. *J Exp Med* 1990;172:955–959.

107. Nepomuceno RR, Henschen-Edman AH, Burgess WH, Tenner AJ. cDNA cloning and primary structure analysis of C1qRp, the human C1q/MBL/SPA receptor that mediates enhanced phagocytosis *in vitro*. *Immunity* 1997;6:119–129.

108. Griffin JA, Griffin FM Jr. Augmentation of macrophage complement receptor function *in vitro*: II. Characterization of the effects of a unique lymphokine upon the phagocytic capabilities of macrophages. *J Immunol* 1980;125:844–849.

109. Wright SD, Craigmyle LS, Silverstein SC. Fibronectin and serum amyloid P component stimulate C3b-and C3bi-mediated phagocytosis in cultured human monocytes. *J Exp Med* 1983;158:1338–1343.

110. Bohnsack JF, Kleinman HK, Takahashi T, O'Shea JJ, Brown EJ. Connective tissue proteins and phagocytic cell function: laminin enhances complement and Fc-mediated phagocytosis by cultured human phagocytes. *J Exp Med* 1985;161:912–923.

111. Skeel A, Yoshimura T, Showalter SD, Tanaka S, Appella E, Leonard EJ. Macrophage stimulating protein: purification, partial amino acid sequence, and cellular activity. *J Exp Med* 1991;173:1227–1234.

112. Tenner AJ, Robinson SL, Borchelt J, Wright JR. Human pulmonary surfactant protein (SP-A), a protein structurally homologous to C1q, can enhance FcR- and CR1-mediated phagocytosis. *J Biol Chem* 1989;264:13923–13928.

113. Griffin FM Jr, Griffin JA, Leider JE, Silverstein SC. Studies on the mechanism of phagocytosis: I. Requirements for circumferential attachment of particle-bound ligands to specific receptors on the macrophage plasma membrane. *J Exp Med* 1975;142:1263–1282.

114. Wright SD, Silverstein SC. Receptors for C3b and C3bi promote phagocytosis but not the release of toxic oxygen from human phagocytes. *J Exp Med* 1984;159:405–416.

115. Aderem AA, Wright SD, Silverstein SC, Cohn ZA. Ligated complement receptors do not activate the arachidonic acid cascade in resident peritoneal macrophages. *J Exp Med* 1985;161:617–622.

116. Bacle F, Haeffner-Cavaillon N, Laude M, Couturier C, Kazatchkine MD. Induction of IL-1 release through stimulation of the C3b/C4b complement receptor type one (CR1,CD35) on human monocytes. *J Immunol* 1990;144:147–152.

117. Nelson RA. The immune adherence phenomenon: an immunologically specific reaction between micro-organisms and erythrocytes leading to enhanced phagocytosis. *Science* 1953;118:733–737.

118. Nelson RA. The immune adherence phenomenon: a hypothetical role of erythrocytes in defence against bacteria and viruses. *Proc R Soc Med* 1956;49:55–69.

119. Fearon DT. Identification of the membrane glycoprotein that is the C3b receptor of the human erythrocyte, polymorphonuclear leukocyte, B lymphocyte, and monocyte. *J Exp Med* 1980;152:20–30.

120. Medof ME, Oger J. Competition for immune complexes by red cells in human blood. *J Clin Lab Immunol* 1982;7:7–13.

121. Schifferli JS, Ng YC, Peters DK. The role of complement and its receptor in the elimination of immune complexes. *N Engl J Med* 1986;315:488–495.

122. Davies KA, Hird V, Stewart S, et al. A study of *in vivo* immune complex formation and clearance in man. *J Immunol* 1990;144:4613–4620.

123. Beynon HLC, Davies KA, Haskard DO, Walport MJ. Erythrocyte complement receptor type 1 and interactions between immune complexes, neutrophils, and endothelium. *J Immunol* 1994;153:3160–3167.

124. Nielsen CH, Svehag S-E, Marquart HV, Leslie RGQ. Interactions of opsonized immune complexes with whole blood cells: binding to erythrocytes restricts complex uptake by leucocyte populations. *Scand J Immunol* 1994;40:228–236.

125. Cornacoff JB, Hebert LA, Smead WL, VanAman ME, Birmingham DJ, Waxman FJ. Primate erythrocyte-immune complex-clearing mechanism. *J Clin Invest* 1983;71:236–247.

126. Atkinson JP, Frank MM. Studies on the *in vivo* effects of antibody: interaction of IgM antibody and complement in the immune clearance and destruction of erythrocytes in man. *J Clin Invest* 1974;54:339–348.

127. Schifferli JA, Ng YC, Estreicher J, Walport MJ. The clearance of tetanus toxoid/anti-tetanus toxoid immune complexes from the circulation of humans: complement and erythrocyte complement receptor 1-dependent mechanisms. *J Immunol* 1988;140:899–904.

128. Schifferli JA, Ng YC, Estreicher J, Walport MJ. The clearance of tetanus toxoid/anti-tetanus toxoid immune complexes from the circulation of humans. *J Immunol* 1988;140:899–904.

129. Davies KA, Schifferli JA, Walport MJ. Complement deficiency and immune complex disease. *Springer Semin Immunopathol* 1994;15:397–416.

130. Moller NP, Steengaard J. Fc mediated immune precipitation: I. A new role of the Fc portion of IgG. *Immunology* 1979;38:631–640.

131. Schifferli JA, Woo P, Peters DK. Complement-mediated inhibition of immune precipitation: role of the classical and alternative pathways. *Clin Exp Immunol* 1982;47:555–562.

132. Naama JK, Hamilton AO, Yeung-Laiwah AC, Whaley K. Prevention of immune precipitation by puriified classical pathway components. *Clin Exp Immunol* 1984;58:486–492.

133. Miller GW, Nussenzweig V. A new complement function: solubilization of antigen-antibody aggregates. *Proc Natl Acad Sci U S A* 1975;72:418–422.

134. Fries LF, Gaither TA, Hammer CH, Frank MM. C3b covalently bound to IgG demonstrates a reduced rate of inactivation by factors H and I. *J Exp Med* 1984;160:1640–1655.

135. Späth PJ, Pascual M, Meyer-Hänni L, Schaad UB, Schifferli JA. Solubilization of immune precipitates by complement in the absence of properdin or factor D. *FEBS Lett* 1988;234:131–134.

136. Fujita T, Takata Y, Tamura N. Solubilization of immune precipitates by six isolated alternative pathway proteins. *J Exp Med* 1981;154:1743–1751.

137. Pepys MB. Role of complement in induction of antibody production *in vivo*: effect of cobra factor and other C3-reactive agents on thymus-dependent and thymus-independent antibody responses. *J Exp Med* 1974;140:126–145.

138. Pepys MB. Role of complement in the induction of immunological responses. *Transplant Rev* 1976;32:93–120.

139. Klaus GGB, Humphrey JH. A re-evaluation of the role of C3 in B-cell activation. *Immunol Today* 1986;7:163–165.

140. MacLennan ICM. Germinal centers. *Annu Rev Immunol* 1994;12:117–139.

141. Villiers M-B, Villiers CL, Jacquier-Sarlin MR, Gabert FM, Journet AM, Colomb MG. Covalent binding of C3b to tetanus toxin: influence on uptake/internalization of antigen by antigen-specific and non-specific B cells. *Immunology* 1996;89:348–355.

142. Griffioen AW, Rijkers GT, Janssens-Korpela P, Zegers BJM. Pneumococcal polysaccharides complexed with C3d bind to human B lymphocytes via complement receptor type 2. *Infect Immun* 1991;59:1839–1845.

143. Jacquier-Sarlin MR, Gabert FM, Villiers M-B, Colomb MG. Modulation of antigen processing and presentation by covalently linked complement C3b fragment. *Immunology* 1995;84:164–170.

144. Villiers M-B, Villiers CL, Wright JF, Maison CM, Colomb MG. Formation of covalent C3b-tetanus toxin complexes: a tool for the *in vitro* study of antigen presentation. *Scand J Immunol* 1991;34:585–595.

145. Santoro L, Drouet C, Reboul A, Mach JP, Colomb MG. Covalent binding of C3b to monoclonal antibodies selectively up-regulates heavy chain recognition by T cells. *Eur J Immunol* 1994;24:1620–1626.

146. Thornton BP, Vetvicka V, Ross GD. Natural antibody and complement-mediated antigen processing and presentation by B lymphocytes. *J Immunol* 1994;152:1727–1737.

147. Cochrane CG, Müller-Eberhard HJ, Aikin BS. Depletion of plasma complement *in vivo* by a protein of cobra venom: its effect on various immunologic reactions. *J Immunol* 1970;105:55–69.

148. Matsuda T, Martinelli GP, Osler AG. Studies on immunosuppression by cobra venom factor: II. On responses to DNP-Ficoll and DNP-Polyacrylamide. *J Immunol* 1978;121:2048–2051.

149. Papamichail M, Gutierrez C, Embling P, Johnson P, Holborow EJ, Pepys MB. Complement dependence of localization of aggregated IgG in germinal centers. *Scand J Immunol* 1975;4:343–347.

150. Klaus GGB, Humphrey JH, Kunkel A, Dongworth DW. The follicular dendritic cell: its role in antigen presentation in the generation of immunological memory. *Immunol Rev* 1997;53:3–28.

151. Böttger EC, Hoffmann T, Hadding U, Bitter-Suermann D. Influence of genetically inherited complement deficiencies on humoral immune response in guinea pigs. *J Immunol* 1985;135:4100–4107.

152. Böttger EC, Metzger S, Bitter-Suermann D, Stevenson S, Kleindienst S, Burger R. Impaired humoral immune response in complement C3-deficient guinea pigs: absence of a secondary antibody response. *Eur J Immunol* 1986;16:1231–1235.

153. Böttger EC, Bitter-Suermann D. Complement and the regulation of humoral immune responses. *Immunol Today* 1987;8:261–264.

154. O'Neil KM, Ochs HD, Heller SR, Cork LC, Morris JM, Winkelstein JA. Role of C3 in humoral immunity: defective antibody production in C3-deficient dogs. *J Immunol* 1988;140:1939–1945.

155. Jackson CG, Ochs HD, Wedgewood RJ. Immune response of a patient with deficiency of the fourth component of complement and systemic lupus erythematosus. *N Engl J Med* 1979;300:1124–1129.

156. Martinelli GP, Matsuda T, Waks HS. Studies on immunosuppression by cobra venom factor: III. On early responses to sheep erythrocytes in C5-deficient mice. *J Immunol* 1978;121:2052–2055.

157. Fingeroth JD, Benedict MA, Levy DN, Strominger JL. Identification of murine complement receptor type 2. *Proc Natl Acad Sci U S A* 1989;86:242–246.

158. Kurtz CB, O'Toole E, Christensen SM, Weis JH. The murine complement receptor gene family: IV. Alternative splicing of Cr2 gene transcripts predicts two distinct gene products that share homologous domains with both human CR2 and CR1. *J Immunol* 1990;144:3581–3591.

159. Molina H, Kinoshita T, Inque K, Carel J-C, Holers VM. A molecular and immunochemical characterization of mouse CR2: evidence for a single gene model of mouse complement receptors 1 and 2. *J Immunol* 1990;145:2974–2983.

160. Carroll MC, Alicot EM, Katzman PJ, Klickstein LB, Smith JA, Fearon DT. Organization of the genes encoding complement receptors type 1 and 2, decay-accelerating factor, and C4-binding protein in the RCA locus on human chromosome 1. *J Exp Med* 1988;167:1271–1280.

161. Rey-Campos JP, Rubinstein P, Cordoba RD. A physical map of the human regulator of complement activation gene cluster linking the complement genes. *J Exp Med* 1988;167:664–669.

162. Molina H, Kinoshita T, Webster CB, Holers VM. Analysis of C3b/C3d binding sites and factor I cofactor regions within mouse complement receptors 1 and 2. *J Immunol* 1994;153:789–795.

163. Kalli KR, Fearon DT. Binding of C3b and C4b by the CR1-like site in murine CR1. *J Immunol* 1994;152:2899–2903.

164. Heyman B, Wiersma EJ, Kinoshita T. *In vivo* inhibition of the antibody response by a complement receptor-specific monoclonal antibody. *J Exp Med* 1990;172:665–668.

165. Thyphronitis G, Kinoshita T, Inoue K, et al. Modulation of mouse complement receptors 1 and 2 suppresses antibody responses *in vivo*. *J Immunol* 1991;147:224–230.

166. Wiersma EJ, Kinoshita T, Heyman B. Inhibition of immunological memory and T-independent humoral responses by monoclonal antibodies specific for murine complement receptors. *Eur J Immunol* 1991;21:2501–2506.

167. Gustavsson S, Kinoshita T, Heyman B. Antibodies to murine complement receptor 1 and 2 can inhibit the antibody response *in vivo* without inhibiting T helper cell induction. *J Immunol* 1995;154:6524–6528.

168. Hebell T, Ahearn JM, Fearon DT. Suppression of the immune response by a soluble complement receptor of B lymphocytes. *Science* 1991;254:102–105.

169. Dempsey PW, Allison MED, Akkaraju S, Goodnow CC, Fearon DT. C3d of complement as a molecular adjuvant: bridging innate and acquired immunity. *Science* 1996;271:348–350.

170. Fischer MB, Ma M, Goerg S, et al. Regulation of the B cell response to T-dependent antigens by classical pathway complement. *J Immunol* 1996;157:549–556.

171. Ahearn JM, Fischer MB, Croix D, et al. Disruption of the Cr2 locus results in a reduction in B-1a cells and in an impaired B cell response to T-dependent antigen. *Immunity* 1996;4:251–262.

172. Molina H, Holers VM, Li B, et al. Markedly impaired humoral immune response in mice deficient in complement receptors 1 and 2. *Proc Natl Acad Sci U S A* 1996;95:3357–3361.

173. Croix DA, Ahearn JM, Rosengard AM, et al. Antibody response to a T-dependent antigen requires B cell expression of complement receptors. *J Exp Med* 1996;183:1857–1864.

174. Shinkai Y, Rathbun G, Lam K-P, et al. RAG-2-deficient mice lack mature lymphocytes owing to inability to initiate V(D)J rearrangement. *Cell* 1992;68:855–867.

175. Carter RH, Spycher MO, Ng YC, Hoffman R, Fearon DT. Synergistic interaction between complement receptor type 2 and membrane IgM on B lymphocytes. *J Immunol* 1988;141:457–463.

176. Nemerow G, Luxembourg A, Cooper N. CD21/CR2: its role in EBV infection and immune function. *Epstein Barr Rep* 1994;1:59–64.

177. Fearon DT, Carter RH. The CD19/CR2/TAPA-1 complex of B lymphocytes: linking natural to acquired immunity. *Ann Rev Immunol* 1995;13:127–149.

178. Carroll MC, Fischer MB. Complement and the immune response. *Curr Opin Immunol* 1997;9:64–69.

179. Rickert RC, Rajewsky K, Roes J. Impairment of T-cell-dependent B-cell responses and B-1 cell development in CD19-deficient mice. *Nature* 1995;376:352–355.

180. Engel P, Zhou L-J, Ord DC, Sato S, Koller B, Tedder TF. Abnormal B lymphocyte development, activation, and differentiation in mice that lack or overexpress the CD19 signal transduction molecule. *Immunity* 1995;3:39–50.

181. Bonnefoy J-Y, Henchoz S, Hardie D, Holder MJ, Gordon J. A subset of anti-CD21 antibodies promote the rescue of germinal center B cells from apoptosis. *Eur J Immunol* 1993;23:969–972.

182. Kozono Y, Duke RC, Schleicher MS, Holers VM. Co-ligation of mouse complement receptors 1 and 2 with surface IgM rescues splenic B cells and WEHI-231 cells from anti-surface IgM-induced apoptosis. *Eur J Immunol* 1995;25:1013–1017.

183. Liu Y-J, Xu J, de Bouteiller O, et al. Follicular dendritic cells specifically express the long CR2/CD21 isoform. *J Exp Med* 1997;185:165–170.

184. Sugano N, Chen W, Roberts ML, Cooper NR. Epstein-Barr virus binding to CD21 activates the initial viral promoter via NF-kappaB induction. *J Exp Med* 1997;186:731–737.

185. Cooper NR, Moore MD, Nemerow GR. Immunobiology of CR2, the B lymphocyte receptor for Epstein-Barr virus and the C3d complement fragment. *Ann Rev Immunol* 1988;6:85–113.

186. Tanner J, Weis J, Fearon D, Whang Y, Kieff E. Epstein-Barr virus gp350/220 binding to the B lymphocyte C3d receptor mediates adsorption, capping and endocytosis. *Cell* 1987;50:203–213.

187. Fingeroth JD, Heath ME, Ambrosino DM. Proliferation of resting B cells is modulated by CR2 and CR1. *Immunol Lett* 1989;21:291–302.

188. Carter RH, Fearon DT. Polymeric C3dg primes human B lymphocytes for proliferation induced by anti-IgM. *J Immunol* 1989;143:1755–1760.

189. Tsokos GC, Lambris JD, Finkelman FD, Anastassiou ED, June CH. Monovalent ligands of complement receptor 2 inhibit whereas polyvalent ligands enhance anti-Ig-induced human B cell intracytoplasmic free calcium concentration. *J Immunol* 1990;144:1640–1645.

190. Matsumoto AK, Kopicky-Burd J, Carter RH, Tuveson DA, Tedder TF, Fearon DT. Intersection of the complement and immune systems: a signal transduction complex of the B lymphocyte-containing complement receptor type 2 and CD19. *J Exp Med* 1991;173:55–64.

191. Hivroz C, Fischer E, Kazatchkine MD, Grillot-Courvalin C. Differential effects of the stimulation of complement receptors CR1 (CD35) and CR2 (CD21) on cell proliferation and intracellular Ca^{2+} mobilization of chronic lymphocytic leukemia B cells. *J Immunol* 1991;146:1766–1772.

192. Griffioen AW, Franklin SW, Zegers BJM, Rijkers GT. Expression and functional characteristics of the complement receptor type 2 on adult and neonatal B lymphocytes. *Clin Immunol Immunopathol* 1993;69:1–8.

193. Luxembourg AT, Cooper NR. Modulation of signaling via the B cell antigen receptor by CD21, the receptor for C3dg and Epstein-Barr virus. *J Immunol* 1994;153:4448–4457.

194. Wilson BS, Platt JL, Kay NE. Monoclonal antibodies to the 140,000 Mol Wt glycoprotein of B lymphocyte membranes (CR2 receptor) initiate proliferation of B cells *in vitro*. *Blood* 1985;66:824–829.

195. Nemerow GR, McNaughton ME, Cooper NR. Binding of monoclonal antibody to the Epstein-Barr virus (EBV)/CR2 receptor induces activation and differentiation of human B lymphocytes. *J Immunol* 1985;135:3068–3073.

196. Frade R, Crevon MC, Barel M, et al. Enhancement of human B cell proliferation by an antibody to the C3d receptor, the gp140 molecule. *Eur J Immunol* 1985;15:73–76.

197. Melchers F, Erdei A, Schulz T, Dierich MP. Growth control of activated, synchronized murine B cells by the C3d fragment of human complement. *Nature* 1985;317:264–267.

198. Erdei A, Melchers F, Schulz T, Dierich M. The action of human C3 in soluble or cross-linked form with resting and activated murine B lymphocytes. *Eur J Immunol* 1985;15:184–188.

199. Cheng-po H, Aman P, Masucci M-G, Klein E, Klein G. B cell activation by the nontransforming P3HR-1 substrain of the Epstein-Barr virus (EBV). *Eur J Immunol* 1986;16:841–845.

200. Hutt-Fletcher LM. Synergistic activation of cells by Epstein-Barr virus and B-cell growth factor. *J Virol* 1987;61:774–781.

201. Bohnsack JF, Cooper NR. CR2 ligands modulate human B cell activation. *J Immunol* 1988;141:2569–2576.

202. Griffioen AW, Toebes EAH, Zegers BJM, Rijkers GT. Role of CR2 in the human adult and neonatal *in vitro* antibody response to type 4 pneumococcal polysaccharide. *Cell Immunol* 1992;143:11–22.

203. Tanner JE, Alfieri C, Chatila TA, Diaz-Mitoma F. Induction of interleukin-6 after stimulation of human B-cell CD21 by Epstein-Barr adsorption to lymphocytes. *J Virol* 1996;70:570–575.

204. Roberts ML, Luxembourg AT, Cooper NR. Epstein-Barr virus binding to CD21, the virus receptor, activates resting B cells via an intracellular pathway that is linked to B cell infection. *J Gen Virol* 1996;77: 3077–3085.

205. Cheung RK, Dosch H-M. The tyrosine kinase *lck* is critically involved in the growth transformation of human B lymphocytes. *J Biol Chem* 1991;266:8667–8670.

206. Frade R, Hermann J, Barel M. A 16 amino acid synthetic peptide derived from human C3d triggers proliferation and specific tyrosine phosphorylation of transformed CR2-positive human lymphocytes and of normal resting B lymphocytes. *Biochem Biophys Res Commun* 1992;188:833–842.

207. Hatzfeld A, Fischer E, Levesque JP, Perrin R, Hatzfeld J, Kazatchkine MD. Binding of C3 and C3dg to the CR2 complement receptor induces growth of an Epstein-Barr virus positive human B cell line. *J Immunol* 1988;140:170–175.

208. Pernegger G, Schulz TF, Hosp M, et al. Cell cycle control of a Burkitt lymphoma cell line: responsiveness to growth signals engaging the C3d/EBV receptor. *Immunol* 1988;65:237–241.

209. Liu Y-J, Cairns JA, Holder MJ, et al. Recombinant 25-Da CD23 and interleukin 1 alpha promote the survival of germinal center B cells: evidence for bifurcation in the development of centrocytes rescued from apoptosis. *Eur J Immunol* 1991;21:1107–1114.

210. Tuveson DA, Ahearn JM, Matsumoto AK, Fearon DT. Molecular interactions of complement receptors on B lymphocytes: a CR1/CR2 complex distinct from the CR2/CD19 complex. *J Exp Med* 1991;173: 1083–1089.

211. Bradbury LE, Kansas GS, Levy S, Evans RL, Tedder TF. The CD19/CD21 signal transducing complex of human B lymphocytes includes the target of antiproliferative antibody-1 and Leu-13 molecules. *J Immunol* 1992;149:2841–2850.

212. Tedder TF, Zhou L-J, Engel P. The CD19/CD21 signal transduction complex of B lymphocytes. *Immunol Today* 1994;15:437–442.

213. Tuveson DA, Carter RH, Soltoff SP, Fearon DT. CD19 of B cells as a surrogate kinase insert region to bind phosphatidylinositol 3-kinase. *Science* 1993;260:986–989.

214. Uckun FM, Burkhardt AL, Jarvis L, et al. Signal transduction through the CD19 receptor during discrete development stages of human B-cell ontogeny. *J Biol Chem* 1993;268:21172–21184.

215. Roifman CM, Ke S. CD19 is a substrate of the antigen receptor-associated protein tyrosine kinase in human B cells. *Biochem Biophys Res Commun* 1993;194:222–225.

216. Chalupny NJ, Kanner SB, Schieven GL, et al. Tyrosine phosphorylation of CD19 in pre-B and mature B cells. *EMBO J* 1993;12: 2691–2696.

217. Van Noesel CJM, Lankester AC, Van Schijndel GMW, Van Lier RAW. The CR2/CD19 complex on human B cells contains the *src*-family kinase *lyn*. *Int Immunol* 1993;5:699–705.

218. Chalupny NJ, Aruffo A, Esselstyn JM, et al. Specific binding of fyn and phosphatidylinositol 3-kinase to the B cell surface glycoprotein CD19 through their src homology 2 domains. *Eur J Immunol* 1995; 25:2978–2984.

219. Weng W-K, Jarvis L, LeBien TW. Signaling through CD19 activates vav/mitogen-activated protein kinase pathway and induces formation of a CD19/Vav/phosphatidylinositol 3-kinase complex in human B cell precursors. *J Biol Chem* 1994;269:32514–32521.

220. Carter RH, Tuveson DA, Park DJ, Rhee SG, Fearon DT. The CD19 complex of B lymphocytes: activation of phospholipase C by a protein tyrosine kinase-dependent pathway that can be enhanced by the membrane IgM complex. *J Immunol* 1991;147:3663–3671.

221. Carter RH, Fearon DT. CD19: lowering the threshold for antigen receptor stimulation of B lymphocytes. *Science* 1992;256:105–107.

222. Kansas GS, Tedder TF. Transmembrane signals generated through MHC class II, CD19, CD20, CD39, and CD40 antigens induce LFA-1 dependent and independent adhesion in human B cells through a tyrosine kinase-dependent pathway. *J Immunol* 1991;147:4094–4102.

223. Wagner N, Engel P, Tedder TF. Regulation of the tyrosine kinase-dependent adhesion pathway in human lymphocytes through CD45. *J Immunol* 1993;150:4887–4899.

224. Sato S, Ono N, Steeber DA, Pisetsky DS, Tedder TF. CD19 regulates B lymphocyte signaling thresholds critical for the development of B-1 lineage cells and autoimmunity. *J Immunol* 1996;157:4371–4378.

225. Tarakhovsky A, Turner M, Schaal S, Mee PJ, Duddy LP, Rajewsky K, Tybulewicz VLJ. Defective antigen receptor-mediated proliferation of B and T cells in the absence of Vav. *Nature* 1995;374:467–470.

226. Zhang R, Alt FW, Davidson L, Orkin SH, Swat W. Defective signalling through the T- and B-cell antigen receptors in lymphoid cells lacking the vav proto-oncogene. *Nature* 1995;374:470–473.

227. Luxembourg AT, Cooper NR. T cell dependent B cell activating properties of antibody-coated small latex beads: a new model for B cell activation. *J Immunol* 1994;153:604–614.

228. Hardy RR, Hayakawa K. CD5 B cells, a fetal B cell lineage. *Adv Immunol* 1997;55:297–339.

229. Krop I, de Fougerolles AR, Hardy RR, Allison M, Schlissel MS, Fearon DT. Self-renewal of B-1 lymphocytes is dependent on CD19. *Eur J Immunol* 1996;26:238–242.

230. Zhou L, Smith HM, Waldschmidt TJ, Schwarting R, Daley J, Tedder TF. Tissue-specific expression of the human CD19 gene in transgenic mice inhibits antigen-independent B-lymphocyte development. *Mol Cell Biol* 1994;14:3884–3894.

231. Tedder TF, Inaoki M, Sato S. The CD19-CD21 complex regulates signal transduction thresholds governing humoral immunity and autoimmunity. *Immunity* 1997;6:107–118.

232. Doody GM, Dempsey PW, Fearon DT. Activation of B lymphocytes: integrating signals from CD19, CD22 and FcgammaRIIb1. *Curr Opin Immunol* 1996;8:378–382.

233. Hayakawa K, Hardy RR, Herzenberg LA. Peritoneal Ly-1 B cells: genetic control, autoantibody production, increased lambda light chain expression. *Eur J Immunol* 1986;16:450–456.

234. Khan WN, Alt FW, Gerstein RM, et al. Defective B cell development and function in *Btk*-deficient mice. *Immunity* 1995;3:283–299.

235. Kozlowski M, Mlinaric-Rascan I, Feng G-S, Shen R, Pawson T, Siminovitch KA. Expression and catalytic activity of the tyrosine phosphatase PTP1C is severely impaired in motheaten and viable motheaten mice. *J Exp Med* 1993;178:2157–2163.

236. O'Rourke L, Tooze R, Fearon DT. Co-receptors of B lymphocytes. *Curr Opin Immunol* 1997;9:324–329.

237. Carter RH, Doody GM, Bolen JB, Fearon DT. Membrane IgM-induced tyrosine phosphorylation of CD19 requires a CD19 domain that mediates association with components of the B cell antigen receptor complex. *J Immunol* 1997;158:3062–3069.

238. Xiao J, Messinger Y, Jin J, Myers DE, Bolen JB, Uckun FM. Signal transduction through the β 1 integrin family surface adhesion molecules VLA-4 and VLA-5 of human B-cell precursors activates CD19 receptor-associated protein-tyrosine kinases. *J Biol Chem* 1996;271: 7659–7664.

239. Sato S, Steeber DA, Tedder TF. The CD19 signal transduction molecule is a response regulator of B-lymphocyte differentiation. *Proc Natl Acad Sci U S A* 1995;92:11558–11562.

240. Billips LG, Nunez CA, Bertrand FE III, et al. Immunoglobulin recombinase gene activity is modulated reciprocally by interleukin 7 and CD19 in B cell progenitors. *J Exp Med* 1995;182:973–982.

241. Wolf ML, Weng W-K, Stieglbauer KT, Shah N, LeBien TW. Functional effect of IL-7-enhanced CD19 expression on human B cell precursors. *J Immunol* 1997;151:138–148.

242. Moore HD. Complementary and opsonic functions in their relation to immunity. *J Immunol* 1919;6:425–441.

243. Hyde RR. Complement-deficient guinea-pig serum. *J Immunol* 1923; 8:267–286.

244. Cinader B, Dubiski S, Wardlaw AC. Distribution, inheritance, and properties of an antigen, MUB1, and its relation to hemolytic complement. *J Exp Med* 1964;120:897–924.

245. Lachmann PJ, Walport MJ. Genetic deficiency diseases of the complement system. In: Ross GD, ed. *Immunobiology of the complement system.* San Diego: Harcourt Brace Jovanovich, 1986:237–261.

246. Reid KB. Deficiency of the first component of human complement. *Immunodefic Rev* 1989;1:247–260.

247. Colten HR. Complement deficiencies. *Annu Rev Immunol* 1992;10: 809–834.

248. Liszewski MK, Kahl LE, Atkinson JP. The functional role of complement genes in systemic lupus erythematosus and Sjögren's syndrome. *Curr Opin Rheumatol* 1989;1:347–352.

249. Davis AE III. C1 inhibitor and hereditary angioneurotic edema. *Annu Rev Immunol* 1988;6:595–628.

250. Oltvai ZN, Wong ECC, Atkinson JP, Tung KSK. C1 inhibitor deficiency: molecular and immunologic basis of hereditary and acquired angioedema. *Lab Invest* 1991;65:381–388.

251. Trapp RG, Fletcher M, Forristall J, West CD. C4 binding protein deficiency in a patient with atypical Behçet's disease. *J Rheumatol* 1987; 14:135–138.

252. Sumerfield JA, Ryder S, Sumiya M, et al. Mannose binding protein gene mutations associated with unusual and severe infections in adults. *Lancet* 1995;345:886–889.

253. Hiemstra PS, Langeler E, Compier B, et al. Complete and partial deficiencies of complement factor D in a Dutch family. *J Clin Invest* 1989;84:1957–1961.

254. Sjoholm AG, Krijper EJ, Tijssen CC, et al. Dysfunctional properdin in a Dutch family with meningococcal disease. *N Engl J Med* 1988; 319:33–77.

255. Morgan BP, Walport MJ. Complement deficiency and disease. *Immunology Today* 1991;12:301–306.

256. Botto M, Fong KY, So AK, Rudge A, Walport MJ. Molecular basis of hereditary C3 deficiency. *J Clin Invest* 1990;86:11581–11663.

257. Sim RB, Kölble K, McAleer MA, Dominguez O, Dee VM. Genetics and deficiencies of the soluble regulatory proteins of the complement system. *Int Rev Immunol* 1993;10:65–86.

258. Würzner R, Orren A, Lachmann PJ. Inherited deficiencies of the terminal components of human complement. *Immunodefic Rev* 1992;3: 123–147.

259. Rosse WF. Paroxysmal nocturnal hemoglobinuria. *Curr Top Microbiol Immunol* 1992;178:163–173.

260. Yamashina M, Ueda E, Kinoshita T, et al. Inherited complete deficiency of 20-kilodalton homologous restriction factor (CD59) as a cause of paroxysmal nocturnal hemoglobinuria. *N Engl J Med* 1990; 323:1184–1189.

261. Anderson DC, Springer TA. Leukocyte adhesion deficiency: an inherited defect in the Mac-1, LFA-1 and p150,95 glycoproteins. *Annu Rev Med* 1987;38:175–194.

262. Strang CJ, Cholin S, Spragg J, et al. Angioedema induced by a peptide derived from complement component C2. *J Exp Med* 1988;168: 1685–1698.

263. Reid KBM, Turner MW. Mammalian lectins in activation and clearance mechanisms involving the complement system. *Springer Semin Immunopathol* 1994;15:307–325.

264. Nagata M, Hara T, Aoki T. Inherited deficiency of ninth component of complement: an increased risk of meningococcal meningitis. *J Pediatr* 1989;114:260–264.

265. Telen MJ, Hall SE, Green A, Moulds AM, Moulds JJ, Rosse WF. Identification of human erythrocyte blood group antigens on decay accelerating factor (DAF) and an erythrocyte phenotype negative for DAF. *J Exp Med* 1988;167:1993–1998.

266. Medof ME, Kinoshita T, Nussenzweig V. Inhibition of complement activation on the surface of cells after incorporation of decay accelerating factor (DAF) into their membranes. *J Exp Med* 1984;160: 1558–1578.

267. Joiner KA. Role of complement in infectious diseases. In: Ross GD, ed. *Immunobiology of the complement system.* Orlando: Academic Press, 1986:183–195.

268. Atkinson JP, Kaine JL, Holers VM, Chan AC. Complement and rheumatic diseases. In: Ross GD, ed. *Immunobiology of the complement system.* Orlando: Academic Press, 1986:197–211.

269. Morgan BP. Intervention in the complement system: a therapeutic strategy in inflammation. *Biochem Soc Trans* 1996;24:224–229.

270. Videm V, Mollnes TE, Garred P, Svennevig JL, Thorac J. Biocompatibility of extracorporeal circulation: *in vitro* comparison of heparin-coated and uncoated oxygenator circuits. *J Thorac Cardiovasc Surg* 1991;101:654–660.

271. Platt JL, Fischel RJ, Matas AJ, Reif SA, Bolman RM, Bach FH. Immunopathology of hyperacute xenograft rejection in a swine-to-primate model. *Transplantation* 1991;52:214–220.

272. Galili U. Interaction of the natural anti-Gal antibody with α-galactosyl epitopes: a major obstacle for xenotransplantation in humans. *Immunol Today* 1993;14:480–482.

273. Takeuchi Y, Porter CD, Strahan KM, et al. Sensitization of cells and retroviruses to human serum by (α1-3) galactosyltransferase. *Nature* 1996;379:85–87.

274. Parker W, Saadi S, Lin SS, Holzknecht ZE, Bustos M, Platt JL. Transplantation of discordant xenografts: a challenge revisted. *Immunol Today* 1996;17:373–378.

275. McCurry KR, Kooyman DL, Alvarado CG. Human complement regulatory proteins protect swine-to-primate cardiac xenografts from humoral injury. *Nat Med* 1995;1:423–427.

276. Cooper NR. Complement evasion strategies of microorganisms. *Immunol Today* 1991;12:327–331.

277. Fishelson Z. Complement-related proteins in pathogenic organisms. *Springer Semin Immunopathol* 1994;15:345–368.

278. Brittingham A, Morrison CJ, McMaster WR, McGwire BS, Chang K-P, Mosser DM. Role of the *Leishmania* surface protease gp63 in complement fixation, cell adhesion, and resistance to complement-mediated lysis. *J Immunol* 1995;155:3102–3111.

279. Nowicki B, Hart A, Coyne KE, Lublin DM, Nowicki S. Short consensus repeat-3 domain of recombinant decay-accelerating factor is recognized by *Escherichia coli* recombinant Dr adhesin in a model of a cell-cell interaction. *J Exp Med* 1993;178:2115–2121.

280. Schlesinger LS, Horwitz MA. Phagocytosis of leprosy bacilli is mediated by complement receptors CR1 and CR3 on human monocytes and complement component C3 in serum. *J Clin Invest* 1990;85:1304–1314.

281. Schlesinger LS, Horwitz MA. Phagocytosis of *Mycobacterium leprae* by human monocyte-derived macrophages is mediated by complement receptors CR1 (CD35), CR3 (CD11b/CD18), and CR4 (CD11c/CD18) and IFN-gamma activation inhibits complement receptor function and phagocytosis of this bacterium. *J Immunol* 1991;147: 1983–1994.

282. Payne NR, Horwitz MA. Phagocytosis of *Legionella pneumophila* is mediated by human monocyte complement receptors. *J Exp Med* 1987;166:1377–1389.

283. Dörig RE, Marcil A, Chopra A, Richardson CD. The human CD46 molecule is a receptor for measles virus (Edmonston strain). *Cell* 1993;75:295–305.

284. Naniche D, Varior-Krishnan G, Cervoni F, et al. Human membrane cofactor protein (CD46) acts as a cellular receptor for measles virus. *J Virol* 1993;67:6025–6032.

285. Manchester M, Liszewski MK, Atkinson J-P, Oldstone MB. Multiple isoforms of CD46 (membrane cofactor protein) serve as receptors for measles virus. *Proc Natl Acad Sci U S A* 1994;91:2161–2165.

286. Rall GF, Manchester M, Daniels LR, Callahan EM, Belman AR, Oldstone MB. A transgenic mouse model for measles virus infection of the brain. *Proc Natl Acad Sci U S A* 1997;94:4659–4663.

287. Nussbaum O, Broder CC, Moss B, Bar-Lev Stern L, Rozenblatt S, Berger EA. Functional and structural interactions between measles virus hemagglutinin and CD46. *J Virol* 1995;69:3341–3349.

288. Maisner A, Alvarez J, Liszewski MK, Atkinson DJ, Atkinson JP, Herrler G. The N-glycan of the SCR 2 region is essential for membrane cofactor protein (CD46) to function as a measles virus receptor. *J Virol* 1996;70:4973–4977.

289. Manchester M, Gairin JE, Patterson JB, et al. Measles virus recognizes its receptor, CD46, via two distinct binding domains within SCR1-2. *Virology* 1997;233:174–184.

290. Bergelson JM, Chan M, Solomon KR, St John NF, Lin H, Finberg RW. Decay-accelerating factor (CD55), a glycosylphosphatidylinositol-anchored complement regulatory protein, is a receptor for several echoviruses. *Proc Natl Acad Sci U S A* 1994;91:6245–6248.

291. Shafren DR, Bates RC, Agrez MV, Herd RL, Burns GF, Barry RD. Coxsackieviruses B1, B3, and B5 use decay accelerating factor as a receptor for cell attachment. *J Virol* 1995;69:3873–3877.

292. Bergelson JM, Mohanty JG, Growell RL, St John NF, Lublin DM, Finberg RW. Coxsackievirus B3 adapted to growth in RD cells binds to decay-accelerating factor (CD55). *J Virol* 1995;69:1903–1906.

293. Karnauchow TM, Tolson DL, Harrison BA, Altman E, Lublin DM, Dimock K. The HeLa cell receptor for enterovirus 70 is decay-accelerating factor (CD55). *J Virol* 1996;70:5143–5152.

294. Fingeroth JD, Weis JJ, Tedder TF, Strominger JL, Biro PA, Fearon DT. Epstein-Barr virus receptor of human B lymphocytes is the C3d receptor CR2. *Proc Natl Acad Sci U S A* 1984;81:4510–4514.

295. Frade R, Barel M, Ehlin-Henriksson B, Klein G. gp140, the C3d

receptor of human B lymphocytes, is also the Epstein-Barr virus receptor. *Proc Natl Acad Sci U S A* 1985;82:1490–1493.

296. Nemerow GR, Wolfert R, McNaughton ME, Cooper NR. Identification and characterization of the Epstein-Barr virus receptor on human B lymphocytes and its relationship to the C3d complement receptor. *J Virol* 1985;55:347–351.

297. Nemerow GR, Mold C, Keivens-Schwend V, Tollefson V, Cooper NR. Identification of gp350 as the viral glycoprotein mediating attachment of Epstein-Barr virus (EBV) to the EBV/C3d receptor of B cells: sequence homology of gp350 and C3 complement fragment C3d. *J Virol* 1987;61:1416–1420.

298. Nemerow GR, Houghten RA, Moore MD, Cooper NR. Identification of the epitope in the major envelope protein of Epstein-Barr virus that mediates viral binding to the B lymphocyte EBV receptor (CR2). *Cell* 1989;56:369–377.

299. Boyer V, Desgranges C, Trabaud M-A, Fischer E, Kazatchkine MD. Complement mediates human immunodeficiency virus type 1 infection of a human T cell line in a CD4- and antibody-independent fashion. *J Exp Med* 1991;173:1151–1158.

300. Gras GS, Dormont D. Antibody-dependent and antibody-independent complement-mediated enhancement of human immunodeficiency virus type 1 infection in a human, Epstein-Barr virus–transformed B-lymphocytic cell line. *J Virol* 1991;65:541–545.

301. Dierich MP, Ebenbichler CF, Marschang P, Füst G, Thielens NM, Arlaud GJ. HIV and human complement: mechanisms of interaction and biological implication. *Immunol Today* 1993;14:435–439.

302. Soelder BM, Reisinger EC, Koeffler D. Complement receptors and HIV entry into cells. *Lancet* 1989;2:271–272.

303. Cardosa MJ, Peterfield JS, Gordon S. Complement receptors mediate enhanced flavivirus replication in macrophages. *J Exp Med* 1983;158:258–263.

304. Bullock WE, Wright SD. Role of the adherence-promoting receptors, CR3, LFA-1, and p150-95, in binding of *Histoplasma capsulatum* by human macrophages. *J Exp Med* 1987;165:195–210.

305. Da Silva RP, Hall BF, Joiner KA, Sacks DL. CR1, the C3b receptor, mediates binding of infective *Leishmania major* metacyclic promastigotes to human macrophages. *J Immunol* 1989;143:617–622.

306. Russell DG, Talamas-Rohana P. *Leishmania* and the macrophage: a marriage of inconvenience. *Immunol Today* 1989;10:328–333.

307. Russell DG, Talamas-Rohana P, Zelechowski J. Antibodies raised against synthetic peptides from the Arg-Gly-Asp–containing region of the *Leishmania* surface protein gp63 cross-react with human C3 and interfere with gp63-mediated binding to macrophages. *Infect Immun* 1989;57:630–639.

308. Puentes SM, Sacks DL, Da Silva RP, Joiner KA. Complement binding by two developmental stages of *Leishmania major* promastigotes varying in expression of a surface lipophosphoglycan. *J Exp Med* 1988;167:887–902.

309. Jack RM, Ward PA. *Babesia rodhaini* interactions with complement: relationship to parasitic entry into red cells. *J Immunol* 1980;124:1566–1573.

310. Horstmann RD, Sievertsen HJ, Leippe M, Fischetti VA. Role of fibrinogen in complement inhibition by streptococcal M protein. *Infect Immun* 1992;60:5036–5041.

311. Horstmann RD, Sievertsen HJ, Knobloch J, Fischetti VA. Antiphagocytic activity of streptococcal M protein: selective binding of complement control protein factor H. *Proc Nat Acad Sci U S A* 1988;85:1657–1661.

312. Hong K, Kinoshita T, Takeda J, et al. Inhibition of the alternative C3 convertase and classical C5 convertase of complement by group A streptococcal M protein. *Proc Natl Acad Sci U S A* 1990;58:2535–2541.

313. Kotwal GJ, Moss B. Vaccinia virus encodes a secretory polypeptide structurally related to complement control proteins. *Nature* 1988;335:176–178.

314. Kotwal GJ, Isaacs SN, McKenzie R, Frank MM, Moss B. Inhibition of the complement cascade by the major secretory protein of vaccinia virus. *Science* 1990;250:827–829.

315. Isaacs SN, Kotwal GJ, Moss B. Vaccinia virus complement-control protein prevents antibody-dependent complement-enhanced neutralization of infectivity and contributes to virulence. *Proc Natl Acad Sci U S A* 1992;89:628–632.

316. McKenzie R, Kotwal GJ. Regulation of complement activity by vaccinia virus complement-control protein. *J Infect Dis* 1992;166:1245–1250.

317. Takahashi-Nishimaki F, Funahashi S-I, Miki K, Hashizume S, Sugimoto M. Regulation of plaque size and host range by a vaccinia virus gene related to complement system proteins. *Virology* 1991;181:158–164.

318. Engelstad M, Howard ST, Smith GL. A constitutively expressed vaccinia gene encodes a 42-kDa glycoprotein related to complement control factors that forms part of the extracellular virus envelope. *Virology* 1992;188:801–810.

319. Bloom DC, Edwards KM, Hager C, Moyer RW. Identification and characterization of two nonessential regions of the rabbitpox virus genome involved in virulence. *J Virol* 1991;65:1530–1542.

320. Friedman HM, Cohen GH, Eisenberg RJ, Seidel CA, Cines DB. Glycoprotein C of herpes simplex virus 1 acts as a receptor for the C3b complement component on infected cells. *Nature* 1984;309:633–635.

321. McNearney TA, O'Dell C, Holers VM, Spear PG, Atkinson JP. Herpes simplex virus glycoproteins gC-1 and gC-2 bind to the third component of complement and provide protection against complement mediated neutralization of viral infectivity. *J Exp Med* 1987;166:1525–1535.

322. Seidel-Dugan C, Ponce de Leon M, Friedman HM, Eisenberg RJ, Cohen GH. Identification of C3b-binding regions on herpes simplex virus type 2 glycoprotein C. *J Virol* 1990;64:1897–1906.

323. Hung S-L, Peng C, Kostavasili I, et al. The interaction of glycoprotein C of herpes simplex virus types 1 and 2 with the alternative complement pathway. *Virology* 1994;203:299–312.

324. Fries LF, Friedman HM, Cohen GH, Eisenberg RJ, Hammer CH, Frank MM. Glycoprotein C of herpes simplex virus 1 is an inhibitor of the complement cascade. *J Immunol* 1986;137:1636–1641.

325. Kostavasili J, Sahu A, Friedman HM, Eisenberg RJ, Cohen GH, Lambris JD. Mechanism of complement inactivation by glycoprotein C of herpes simplex virus. *J Immunol* 1997;158:1763–1771.

326. Friedman HM, Wang L, Fishman NO, et al. Immune evasion properties of herpes simplex virus type 1 glycoprotein gC. *J Virol* 1996;70:4253–4260.

327. Mold C, Bradt BM, Nemerow GR, Cooper NR. Epstein-Barr virus regulates activation and processing of the third component of complement. *J Exp Med* 1988;168:949–969.

328. Albrecht J-C, Fleckenstein B. New member of the multigene family of complement control proteins in herpesvirus saimiri. *J Virol* 1992;66:3937–3940.

329. Fodor WL, Rollins SA, Bianco-Caron S, et al. The complement control protein homolog of herpesvirus saimiri regulates serum complement by inhibiting C3 convertase activity. *J Virol* 1995;69:3889–3896.

330. Albrecht J-C, Nicholas J, Cameron KR, Newman C, Fleckenstein B, Honess RW. Herpesvirus saimiri has a gene specifying a homologue of the cellular membrane glycoprotein CD59. *Virology* 1992;190:527–530.

331. Rother RP, Rollins SA, Fodor WL, et al. Inhibition of complement-mediated cytolysis by the terminal complement inhibitor of herpesvirus saimiri. *J Virol* 1994;68:730–737.

332. Montefiori DC, Cornell RJ, Zhou Y, Zhou T, Hirsch VM, Johnson PR. Complement control proteins, CD46, CD55, and CD59, as common surface constituents of human and simian immunodeficiency viruses and possible targets for vaccine protection. *Virology* 1994;205:82–92.

333. Spear GT, Lurain NS, Parker CJ, Ghassemi M, Payne GH, Saifuddin M. Host cell-derived complement control proteins CD55 and CD59 are incorporated into the virions of two unrelated enveloped viruses. *J Immunol* 1995;155:4376–4381.

334. Schmitz J, Zimmer JP, Kluxen B, et al. Antibody-dependent complement-mediated cytotoxicity in sera from patients with HIV-1 infection is controlled by CD55 and CD59. *J Clin Invest* 1995;96:1520–1526.

335. Stoiber H, Pinter C, Siccardi AG, Clivio A, Dierich MP. Efficient destruction of human immunodeficiency virus in human serum by inhibiting the protective action of complement factor H and decay accelerating factor (DAF,CD55). *J Exp Med* 1996;183:307–310.

336. Edwards JE Jr, Gaither TA, O'Shea JJ. Expression of specific binding sites on *candida* with functional and antigenic characteristics of human complement receptors. *J Immunol* 1986;137:3577–3583.

337. Gilmore BJ, Retsinas EM, Lorenz JS, Hostetter MK. An iC3b receptor on *Candida albicans*: structure, function, and correlates for pathogenicity. *J Infect Dis* 1988;157:38–46.

338. Eigentler A, Schulz TF, Larcher C, et al. C3bi-binding protein on *Candida albicans*: temperature-dependent expression and relationship to human complement receptor type 3. *Infect Immun* 1989;57:616–622.

339. Gale C, Finkel D, Tao N, et al. Cloning and expression of a gene

encoding an integrin-like protein in *Candida albicans*. *Proc Natl Acad Sci U S A* 1996;93:357–361.

340. Gustafson KS, Vercellotti GM, Bendel CM, Hostetter MK. Molecular mimicry in *Candida albicans*. *J Clin Invest* 1991;87:1896–1902.

341. Moors MA, Stull TL, Blank KJ, Buckley HR, Mosser DM. A role for complement receptor-like molecules in iron acquisition by *Candida albicans*. *J Exp Med* 1992;175:1643–1651.

342. Calderone RA, Linehan L, Wadsworth E, Sandberg AL. Identification of C3d receptors on *Candida albicans*. *Infect Immun* 1988;56:252–258.

343. Linehan L, Wadsworth E, Calderone R. *Candida albicans* C3d receptor, isolated by using a monoclonal antibody. *Infect Immun* 1986;56:1981–1986.

344. Saxena A, Calderone R. Purification and characterization of the extracellular C3d-binding protein of *Candida albicans*. *Infect Immun* 1990;58:309–314.

345. Fukayama M, Wadsworth E, Calderone R. Expression of the C3d-binding protein (CR2) from *Candida albicans* during experimental candidiasis as measured by lymphoblastogenesis. *Infect Immun* 1992;8–12.

346. Joiner KA, Dias daSilva W, Rimoldi MT, Hammer CH, Sher A, Kipnis TL. Biochemical characterization of a factor produced by trypomastigotes of *Trypanosoma cruzi* that accelerates the decay of complement C3 convertases. *J Biol Chem* 1988;263:11327–11335.

347. Rimoldi MT, Sher A, Heiny S, Lituchy A, Hammer CH, Joiner K. Developmentally regulated expression by *Trypanosoma cruzi* of molecules that accelerate the decay of complement C3 convertases. *Proc Natl Acad Sci U S A* 1988;85:193–197.

348. Fischer E, Quaissi MA, Velge P, Cornette J, Kazatchkine MD. gp 58/68, a parasite component that contributes to the escape of the trypomastigote form of *T. cruzi* from damage by the human alternative complement pathway. *Immunology* 1988;65:299–303.

349. Norris KA, Bradt B, Cooper NR, So M. Characterization of a *Trypanosoma cruzi* C3 binding protein with functional and genetic similarities to the human complement regulatory protein, decay-accelerating factor. *J Immunol* 1991;147:2240–2247.

350. Norris KA, Schrimpf JE, Szabo MJ. Identification of the gene family encoding the 160-kilodalton *Trypanosoma cruzi* complement regulatory protein. *Infect Immunol* 1997;65:349–357.

351. Andrews NW, Abrams CK, Slatin SL, Griffits G. A *T. cruzi*-secreted protein immunologically related to the complement component C9: evidence for membrane pore-forming activity at low pH. *Cell* 1990;61:1277–1287.

352. Iida K, Whitlow MB, Nussenzweig V. Amastigotes of *Trypanosoma cruzi* escape destruction by the terminal complement components. *J Exp Med* 1989;169:881–891.

353. Reed SL, Curd JG, Gigli I, Gillin FD, Braude AI. Activation of complement by pathogenic and nonpathogenic *Entamoeba histolytica*. *J Immunol* 1986;136:2265–2270.

354. Reed SL, Gigli I. Lysis of complement-sensitive *Entamoeba histolytica* by activated terminal complement components. *J Clin Invest* 1990;86:1815–1822.

355. Braga LL, Ninomiya H, McCoy JJ, et al. Inhibition of the complement membrane attack complex by the galactose-specific adhesin of *Entamoeba histolytica*. *J Clin Invest* 1992;90:1131–1137.

356. Tarleton RL, Kemp WM. Demonstration of IgG-Fc and C3 receptors on adult *Schistosoma mansoni*. *J Immunol* 1981;126:379–386.

357. Silva EE, Clarke MW, Posesta RB. Characterization of a C3 receptor on the envelope of *Schistosoma mansoni*. *J Immunol* 1993;151:7057–7066.

358. Parizade M, Arnon R, Lachmann PJ, Fishelson Z. Functional and antigenic similarities between a 94-kD protein of *Schistosoma mansoni* (SCIP-1) and human CD59. *J Exp Med* 1994;179:1625–1636.

359. Pearce EJ, Hall BF, Sher A. Host-specific evasion of the alternative complement pathway by schistosomes correlates with the presence of a phospholipase C-sensitive surface molecule resembling human decay accelerating factor. *J Immunol* 1990;144:2751–2756.

360. Fátima M, Horta M, Ramalho-Pinto FJ. Role of human decay-accelerating factor in the evasion of *Schistosoma mansoni* from complement-mediated killing *in vitro*. *J Exp Med* 1991;174:1399–1406.

Inflammation: Basic Principles and Clinical Correlates,
3rd ed., edited by John I. Gallin and Ralph Snyderman.
Lippincott Williams & Wilkins, Philadelphia © 1999.

CHAPTER 20

Acute Phase Response

Irving Kushner and Debra Rzewnicki

Avery never discussed the C-reactive protein without turning the conversation to what he was wont to call the chemistry of the host. Although he never spelled out what he meant by that expression, he clearly had in mind all the unidentified body substances and mechanisms of a non-immunological nature, both protective and destructive, that come into play in the course of infectious processes.

Rene J. Dubos (1)

HISTORICAL AND SEMANTIC CONSIDERATIONS

The term *inflammation* refers to the complex, localized responses elicited by a variety of noxious stimuli. In addition to these localized responses, a vast number of distant systemic changes may also occur if the stimulus is severe enough. These changes are referred to collectively as the acute phase response (APR) (2), because attention was first focused on them by the discovery of C-reactive protein (CRP) in the serum of patients in the acute phase of pneumococcal pneumonia (3). Oswald Avery, in whose laboratory this observation was made in 1930, was excited by this discovery, which he regarded as an important lead to understanding what he termed "the chemistry of the host"—the host response to disease. Maclyn McCarty noted that the Avery laboratory, whose core interest was the study of pneumonia, made two major contributions to unrelated areas of biology and medicine: the discoveries that genes are made of DNA and that polysaccharides have antigenic specificity. He suggested that the discovery of CRP may well represent a third major contribution (4).

Since we now know that the APR occurs during a wide variety of inflammatory states, not just gram-positive infections as was originally thought, the term *host response* is not entirely appropriate, but it is acceptable if we think of the host more broadly as the subject of an inflammatory rather than an infectious process. An unfortunate consequence of the use of the term *acute phase* is that many physicians incorrectly believe that acute phase changes are limited to acute inflammatory states and are not found in chronic inflammation. In fact, the APR persists in many chronic diseases, resulting in what might seem to be an oxymoron, a chronic APR. An APR comparable to that in humans is seen in all vertebrates, whereas lower species manifest lesser responses.

Many components of the APR have attracted the interest of highly focused biomedical investigators whose interests encompass only limited aspects of the broad APR. Two such examples are worthy of note. First, clinicians whose major concerns are the deleterious consequences of the APR have employed the terms *systemic inflammatory response syndrome* and *sepsis* to refer to the hemodynamic changes, diffuse alterations in capillary permeability, coagulation defects, and organ failure that may accompany severe infection (5). Second, investigators whose major focus is on the neuroendocrine aspects of the APR (6) have employed the term *stress response*, originated by Hans Selye in the 1940s. They define stress as a state of disharmony or threatened homeostasis (7). Many of these investigators have been particularly interested in the changes that are induced by psychological and emotional stimuli (8) and that are mediated by corticotropin-releasing hormone (CRH) and the autonomic nervous system. As indicated later, these types of stimuli may also influence other, nonneuroendocrine components of the APR.

THE PHENOMENON OF THE ACUTE PHASE RESPONSE

A large number of changes, distant from inflammatory sites and involving many organ systems, accompany inflammatory states (Fig. 20-1). New APR phe-

I. Kushner and D. Rzewnicki: Case Western Reserve University at MetroHealth Medical Center, Cleveland, Ohio 44109.

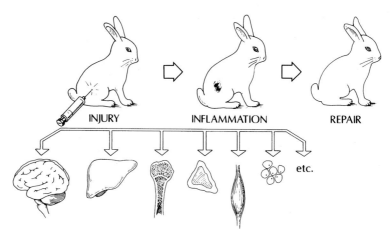

FIG. 20-1. Some of the organs participating in the systemic acute phase response are pictured here. Involvement of the BRAIN may result in fever, anorexia, somnolence, and increased synthesis of corticotropin-releasing hormone (CRH), corticotropin (ACTH), and other neuroendocrine products. The LIVER orchestrates synthesis of plasma proteins and synthesizes increased amounts of metallothionein and several antioxidants. In BONE, marrow erythropoiesis is suppressed, thrombocytosis is induced, and loss of bone substance occurs. The ADRENAL GLAND is the site of enhanced production of cortisol and norepinephrine. In MUSCLE, proteolysis and decreased protein synthesis may occur. FAT CELLS represent alterations in lipid metabolism. (From Kushner I. Regulation of the acute phase response by cytokines. In: Oppenheim J, Rossio J, Gearing A [eds]. *Clinical applications of cytokines: role in pathogenesis, diagnosis and therapy.* New York: Oxford University Press, 1993, with permission.)

nomena continue to be recognized, year after year. In general, these represent the substitution of new "set points" for the homeostatic mechanisms that normally maintain a constant internal environment during good health. These changes can be categorized as affecting plasma protein synthesis, the neuroendocrine and hematologic systems, metabolic processes, intrahepatic constituents, and nonprotein plasma components. All of these phenomena investigated thus far are induced by members of the same group of inflammation-associated cytokines.

Acute Phase Proteins

The term APR is frequently employed in a narrow sense to refer only to changes in concentration of a large number of plasma proteins, the *acute phase proteins.* These changes largely reflect reprogramming of plasma protein gene expression in hepatocytes. There probably are few plasma proteins whose production is not altered to some degree during the APR; a change of 25% has been suggested arbitrarily as the definition of an acute phase protein. Both increases (positive acute phase proteins) and decreases (negative acute phase proteins) are seen; changes in different proteins occur at different rates and to different degrees (Fig. 20-2). The rapidity of change of plasma protein concentrations generally parallels the magnitude of change. In the presence of severe liver disease, synthesis of some acute phase proteins is not affected and synthesis of others is inhibited (9).

A few plasma proteins have long been recognized as positive acute phase proteins. Ceruloplasmin and the complement components C3 and C4 exhibit relatively modest positive acute phase behavior (typically an increase of about 50%). Concentrations of haptoglobin, α_1-acid glycoprotein (α1-AGP), α_1-protease inhibitor, α_1-antichymotrypsin, and fibrinogen ordinarily increase about twofold to fivefold. The two major human acute phase proteins, however, are CRP and serum amyloid A (SAA). Both are normally present in plasma in only trace amounts but can manifest dramatic increases in rates of synthesis and plasma concentration after stimulation, achieving levels more than 1,000 times normal in some severely infected persons. The long-recognized negative acute phase reactants in humans are albumin and transferrin.

In addition, newly recognized positive and negative acute phase proteins continue to be reported. Among the positive acute phase proteins are other members of the *complement* system, including factor B, C1 inhibitor, C4b-binding protein, and mannose-binding lectin (10–13), and members of the *fibrinolytic and anticoagulant* systems, including plasminogen, tissue plasminogen activator, urokinase, protein S, and plasminogen activator inhibitor-1 (PAI-1) (14–16). Positive acute phase *antiproteases* include pancreatic secretory trypsin inhibitor (17) and members of the interalpha-protease inhibitor family members (18). Putative participants in the *inflammatory process* include secreted phospholipase A_2, interleukin-1 receptor antagonist (IL-1Ra), and lipopolysaccharide

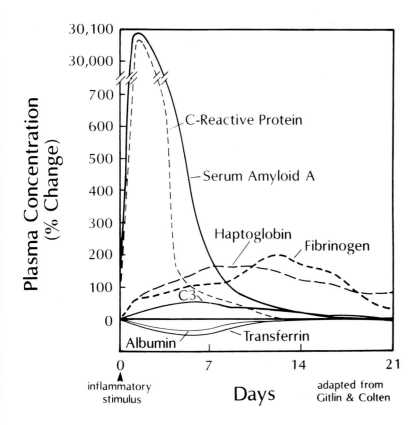

FIG. 20-2. Characteristic patterns of change in concentrations of some plasma proteins after a moderate inflammatory stimulus. (From Kushner I. Regulation of the acute phase response by cytokines. In: Oppenheim J, Rossio J, Gearing A [eds]. *Clinical applications of cytokines: role in pathogenesis, diagnosis and therapy.* New York: Oxford University Press, 1993, with permission.)

(LPS)-binding protein (19–21). Other miscellaneous acute phase reactants include fibronectin, hemopexin, and ferritin (22,23). Recently recognized negative human acute phase proteins include transthyretin, α_2-HS glycoprotein, α-fetoprotein, T4-binding globulin, and insulin-like growth factor-I (IGF-I) (24–26). Altered production of some acute phase proteins occurs at both extrahepatic and hepatic sites (10,27–30).

There are significant differences among species in acute phase protein expression. A notable example is CRP. Massively induced in humans and rabbits, it is only minimally induced by inflammatory stimuli in mice; in rats, it is constitutively expressed at high levels, with only a several-fold increase after stimulation. Another example is α_2-macroglobulin, which is a major acute phase protein in the rat but not ordinarily in humans. Haptoglobin is only a modest acute phase reactant in humans; in ruminants, it is normally undetectable but behaves as a major acute phase reactant (31).

Other Acute Phase Phenomena

Among the *neuroendocrine* changes are fever (literally a resetting of the thermostat), somnolence, anorexia, the "sick euthyroid syndrome" (32), and altered synthesis of many endocrine hormones including CRH, glucagon, insulin, corticotropin (ACTH), cortisol, adrenal catecholamines, growth hormone, thyroid-stimulating hormone, thyroxin, aldosterone, and arginine vasopressin

(6). Involvement of the *hematopoietic* system includes leukocytosis, thrombocytosis, and the "anemia of chronic disease" (better designated the "anemia of chronic inflammation") (33), which is seen in most patients with chronic inflammatory states. Erythropoietin levels are reported to rise greatly in nonsurviving patients with septic shock (34). *Metabolic* changes include decreased gluconeogenesis, negative nitrogen balance, and substantial alterations in lipid metabolism (35). An extreme consequence of the latter two conditions is the cachexia seen in persons with severe chronic infection or advanced malignancy. Osteoporosis appears to belong in this category also, as does the reported increase in blood leptin levels in inflammatory states (36).

A very large number of enzymatic, morphologic, and chemical changes occur in the *liver* (2), including increases in metallothionein, inducible nitric oxide synthase (iNOS), heme oxygenase, manganese superoxide dismutase, hepatocyte growth factor activator (37), and glutathione (38). Markedly decreased expression of the gap junction subunit connexin 32 (39) and a decrease in catalase and phosphoenolpyruvate carboxykinase (PEPCK) activity occur (40). Decreased expression of many members of the cytochrome P450 family is seen, but several others are induced (41). Finally, changes in nonprotein *plasma constituents* include hypozincemia, hypoferremia, hypercupremia, increased retinol (42), and increased glutathione secondary to increased hepatic levels (38).

Stimuli That Elicit an Acute Phase Response

Recognition of an acute phase phenomenon requires *in vivo* induction by any of a variety of inflammatory stimuli. In humans, stimuli that commonly give rise to the APR include bacterial and, to a lesser extent, viral infection; surgical or other trauma; neoplasm; burn injury; tissue infarction; various immunologically mediated and crystal-induced inflammatory states; strenuous exercise (43); heatstroke; and childbirth. Several psychiatric illnesses (44,45) and psychological stress (46) are associated with acute phase changes, as is chronic fatigue syndrome (47), a condition of unknown pathogenesis. The most commonly employed animal models are injection of bacterial endotoxin (LPS) or turpentine. Studies in knock-out mice indicate that these two animal models are not equivalent, however. Many acute phase changes induced by the localized tissue damage of sterile turpentine injection are blocked in both IL-1β and IL-6 knock-out mice but are not inhibited when LPS is administered to these same mice (48).

REGULATION OF ACUTE PHASE PROTEINS

Extracellular Signals

Most of the data bearing on acute phase protein regulation are derived from studies in hepatoma-derived cell lines, which may not accurately reflect processes in normal hepatocytes. Nonetheless, they cast considerable light on what may occur *in vivo*. A number of inflammation-associated cytokines play central roles in regulation of the acute phase protein response. The cytokine effects are influenced by a variety of circulating molecules, notably cytokine modulators (e.g., cytokine receptors, receptor antagonists, antibodies to cytokines) and some endocrine hormones. Although it was initially believed that the APR was a uniform, coordinately regulated response, it is now clear that the acute phase protein genes are independently regulated by differing combinations and subsets of cytokines and their modulators.

Inflammation-associated Cytokines

A number of different cytokines, alone or in a network, may influence acute phase protein synthesis (see Chapter 29). These cytokines are elicited during, and participate in, the inflammatory process. They include IL-6, IL-1, tumor necrosis factor-α (TNF-α), interferon-γ (IFN-γ), and transforming growth factor-β (TGF-β). Some of these cytokines are regarded as proinflammatory, while others are regarded as antiinflammatory. Inflammation-associated cytokines may be produced by many different cells, including monocytes, macrophages, fibroblasts, endothelial cells, T lymphocytes, and epithelial cells, but macrophages and monocytes at inflammatory sites clearly play major roles. Mechanisms by which LPS induces cytokines are well described, and effects of non-LPS stimuli continue to be reported (49–51). TGF-β, released at sites of tissue injury by degranulating platelets, may stimulate local cells to secrete cytokines (52), and phagocytosis of particulate stimuli by macrophages may itself set the inflammatory process in motion (53). Psychological stresses may stimulate IL-6 production through release of catecholamines (6).

IL-6 serves as the major acute phase protein inducer. This conclusion is based on the large number and magnitude of changes in plasma proteins induced by this cytokine in model systems, the strong correlation often found clinically between serum IL-6 levels and acute phase protein changes, and the ability of antibodies to IL-6 to block production of a number of acute phase proteins when administered to humans. Effects comparable to those induced by IL-6 are also produced in model systems by IL-11, leukemia inhibitor factor, oncostatin M, ciliary neurotrophic factor, and cardiotropin (54), all of which share a signal transducing unit with IL-6. However, it is unlikely that all of these cytokines contribute to the APR *in vivo*. Neither IL-11 nor leukemia inhibitor factor appears to participate significantly in acute phase protein induction (55). Although IL-6 was found to be significantly elevated in sera of rheumatoid arthritis patients, IL-11, oncostatin M, and leukemia inhibitor factor were not (56).

Observations in both IL-1β and IL-6 knock-out mice indicate that the importance of IL-6 in acute phase protein induction depends on the nature or site of the inflammatory stimulus (48). The acute phase protein response was largely inhibited in IL-6 knockout mice when turpentine injection was the inflammatory stimulus. In contrast, a virtually intact APR was observed in these animals when LPS was the inflammatory stimulus, indicating that LPS injection causes production of unidentified, non–IL-6 cytokines capable of inducing acute phase proteins that are IL-6 dependent when turpentine is the stimulus. The same differences in acute phase protein responses to these stimuli were observed in IL-1β knockout mice. The decreased APR to turpentine injection in this group of mice was accompanied by inhibition of IL-6 production, indicating that IL-6 production after turpentine injection is induced by IL-1β and that IL-6 is required to induce the APR after local injection of turpentine. These studies demonstrate that patterns of cytokine production differ in different inflammatory conditions, a generalization that is undoubtedly true in human pathophysiology as well.

In addition to IL-6–related cytokines, IL-1 and TNF-α both affect the synthesis of a large number of acute phase proteins, including CRP, SAA, α1-AGP, C3, factor B, and haptoglobin. Both of these cytokines inhibit induction of fibrinogen by IL-6. When the important role of IL-6 in acute phase protein production was initially appreciated, it was proposed that the acute phase proteins be divided into two classes: those whose maximal induction is achieved by the combination of IL-6 and IL-1 (class 1) and those whose responses to IL-6 are not enhanced by IL-1 (class 2) (57). However, it is increasingly difficult to fit newly acquired knowledge into this system, now that the influences of cytokines other than IL-6 and IL-1 are better appreciated and more acute phase proteins are recognized. The following discussion outlines examples not consistent with this classification. IL-6 alone had no or minimal effects on induction of PAI-1 but greatly enhanced the inducing effect of IL-1 (58). Similar findings were reported for IL-1Ra: its induction by IL-1β was greatly enhanced by IL-6, which alone had little effect (20). Human C1 inhibitor was strongly induced by IFN-γ and, to a lesser extent, by IL-6; although IL-1β enhanced induction by IFN-γ, it inhibited induction by IL-6 (11). C4b-binding protein could be induced in a rat hepatoma cell line by TNF-α; addition of either IL-1α or IL-6 alone had little effect, but synergistic induction was observed when all three cytokines were used (59). TGF-β appears to be the major inducer of human urokinase and both human (16) and mouse PAI-1 (60). Both IL-1β and TNF-α depressed levels of IGF-I, whereas IL-6 had no effect (61). Taken together, these findings cast doubt on the utility of a classification based largely on whether a gene is responsive to IL-1 in a single model system.

Finally, TGF-β and IFN-γ each influence production of subsets of acute phase proteins. IFN-γ is noteworthy for its ability to induce a number of complement components (10,11). TGF-β, whose net effects in vivo are antiinflammatory, induces several antiproteases (62) and negative acute phase proteins (24), as well as urokinase and PAI-1.

Cytokine Modulators and Other Intercellular Signaling Molecules

The effects of cytokines may be influenced by other cytokines and hormones, particularly by cytokine modulators such as IL-1Ra; by soluble receptors, some of which are upregulatory (e.g., the gp54 IL-6 receptor) and some downregulatory (e.g., TNF-α receptors); and by autoantibodies to cytokines (63–65). Hormones—the term employed here in the original sense of intercellular chemical mediators (66)—also participate in acute phase protein regulation. Corticosteroids potentiate the effects of cytokines on induction of many human acute phase proteins but do not themselves substantially alter their synthesis (67). Insulin can modulate acute phase protein production in a complex fashion (68), and thrombin has a synergistic effect on induction of PAI-1 by TGF-β in HepG2 cells (16). In addition, histamine and retinoic acid modulate the APR (69,70), and in vivo studies suggest that CRH may mediate acute phase protein induction (71). Finally, studies indicate that TNF-α serves as a major mediator of LPS induction of parathyroid hor-

mone-related protein (PTHrP) in multiple organs, that PTHrP behaves like a member of the inflammatory cytokine cascade, and that it may participate in acute phase protein induction (72).

Target cells such as hepatocytes are not usually exposed to individual cytokines alone but rather to complex mixtures of intercellular signaling molecules. Combinations of cytokines may produce additive, inhibitory, and synergistic effects. Synthesis of individual plasma proteins is regulated differentially by various combinations of cytokines, with proteins exhibiting distinct responses to different combinations of cytokines (73). These observations indicate that the acute phase plasma protein response is not a single, coordinate, global phenomenon but rather that it represents the integrated sum of multiple, separately regulated changes in gene expression. Thus far, combinations of more than two cytokines have rarely been studied. It is likely that a very complex scenario of combinations of large numbers of cytokines, modulators, and hormones, in varying sequences and concentrations, most accurately reflects the in vivo pathophysiologic environment.

Intracellular Events

In all instances studied thus far, except apoferritin (discussed later), increased transcription has played a substantial if not the only role in enhancing acute phase protein expression. Crosstalk between signal transducing factors and transcription factors, by pathways which are partly parallel and partly interconnecting, plays an important role in regulation of gene transcription by cytokines. Binding of IL-6 to its receptor causes activation of members of the JAK family of signal transducers, with subsequent phosphorylation of STAT3, an important transcriptional enhancer of most IL-6–responsive genes. Members C/EBP transcription factor family that are activated by mitogen-activated protein kinase also mediate IL-6 effects. It is likely that various combinations of STAT3, C/EBP, and perhaps other IL-6 response factors, in their unique promoter contexts, enhance transcription of each IL-6–responsive acute phase gene (74). Both C/EBP and NF-κB play significant roles in mediating effects of IL-1 on gene expression, and interactions between C/EBP and NF-κB transcription factors are well described (75). In addition, posttranscriptional regulation also participates in the APR (76,77). Processing or stabilization of mRNAs for various acute phase proteins may play a role in some acute phase changes (77), and apoferritin induction by IL-1β is regulated at the level of translation in HepG2 cells (78).

Three types of change in glycosylation of plasma proteins are observed during the APR. Best studied are the changes in binding of some acute phase proteins to concanavalin A, which reflect differences in the number of branches in the antennary structures of the glycan side chains of these glycoproteins. Glycan branching has been found to be regulated by inflammation-associated cytokines independently of effects on protein production (79). Binding of plasma glycoproteins to concanavalin A is increased in several acute inflammatory states and decreased in a number of chronic diseases, suggesting that the cytokines or other extracellular signals operative during acute and chronic inflammatory states may differ. Second, increased α1,3-fucosylation and sialyl Lewis[x] expression of α1-AGP, induced by inflammation-associated cytokines, is observed in acute inflammatory states (80). Finally, decreased galactosylation of immunoglobulin G is observed in a number of chronic inflammatory diseases (81). The possible participation of cytokines in this process has not been clarified.

Secretion of CRP, a process distinct from synthesis, is separately regulated during the course of the APR. Studies of intracellular transport of newly synthesized rabbit CRP showed that the intracellular transit time for CRP was decreased dramatically in hepatocytes from inflamed rabbits compared with those from controls (82). Subsequent radioligand binding studies indicated that CRP is retained within the endoplasmic reticulum of the resting hepatocyte by specific interaction with an endoplasmic reticulum–restricted 60-kd serine carboxylesterase (82). During the APR, more efficient secretion of CRP is associated with a decrease in the binding affinity of this esterase for CRP, probably as a result of secondary modification of the esterase.

REGULATION OF OTHER ACUTE PHASE PHENOMENA

Acute phase phenomena other than plasma protein changes, although not as well studied, are also primarily induced by the same group of inflammation-associated cytokines that induce acute phase protein changes. In addition, IL-4 and IL-13 have been implicated in induction of hypoferremia (83). Studies have indicated that vagal afferent fibers also mediate some of the effects of inflammatory stimuli on brain-controlled functions (84,85).

Intrahepatic Changes

Many intracellular hepatic constituents are altered during the APR. The intracellular heavy metal–binding protein metallothionein is induced by IL-6, but not by IL-1α, with concomitant increase in cellular zinc content (86) and secondary hypozincemia. IL-6 induces transglutaminase activity (87). Cytokines increase synthesis of two physiologically important hepatic antioxidants: manganese superoxide dismutase, which is synergistically induced in hepatocytes by IL-6, IL-1, and TNF-α (88), and microsomal heme oxygenase, which is induced by IL-6 in Hep3B cells (89).

A tissue inhibitor of metalloproteinase (TIMP-1) is induced in HepG2 cells by both IL-6 and TGF-β (90). IL-1β, IL-6, and interferons are capable of altering the expression of a number of hepatic P450 cytochromes during inflammatory states (91,92). IL-1β and TNF-α can each induce iNOS in cultured rat hepatocytes (93). Low IGF-I blood levels may be caused by reduced hepatocyte responsiveness to growth hormone, secondary to downregulation of growth hormone receptor in hepatocytes in response to IL-1β or TNF-α (26).

Fever

The mechanisms by which cytokines lead to fever have been clarified considerably by studies in knock-out mice (94). In brief, these studies suggest that the final step in induction of fever requires that IL-6, derived from the endothelium of the hypothalamic circumventricular organs, access the thermoregulatory center in the preoptic region. Induction of IL-6 in this endothelial site could result from stimulation by circulating IL-1β or TNF-α arising peripherally or, conceivably, from a direct stimulus such as LPS itself. Alternatively, circulating IL-6 could cross the blood-brain barrier to stimulate the thermoregulatory center. A different scenario has also been proposed, in which IL-1β produced in the central nervous system serves as the ultimate stimulus for the development of fever (95). The finding that subdiaphragmatic vagotomy blocks the febrile response to intraperitoneal but not to intramuscular injection of LPS (84) indicates that induction of the febrile response may be even more complex than previously thought.

Other Neuroendocrine Changes

Changes in the neuroendocrine system that occur as a result of both inflammatory stimuli and "stress" unrelated to inflammation reflect complex interactions between inflammation-associated cytokines on the one hand and the hypothalamic-pituitary-adrenal axis and other components of the neuroendocrine system on the other (6). IL-6, IL-1, and TNF-α are induced by inflammatory stimuli (or, in noninflammatory states, apparently by catecholamines) and activate the hypothalamic-pituitary-adrenal axis by stimulating the corticotropin secretagogues CRH and arginine vasopressin, with consequent increased production of ACTH and cortisol. A direct stimulatory effect of IL-6 on adrenal cells has been reported (96), and nitric oxide was found to inhibit the ACTH response to IL-1β (97). In addition, the adrenomedullary and sympathetic systems respond with production of a variety of neurotransmitters whose effects are governed by both positive and negative feedback loops. IL-6 induction of arginine vasopressin may be responsible for the inappropriate secretion of antidiuretic hormone seen during the APR. The paraventricular hypothalamic nucleus appears to play a key role in integrating diverse stimuli to generate the cerebral component of the APR (98).

As with fever, studies of molecular mechanisms inducing somnolence, lethargy, and anorexia are often difficult to interpret because of the requirement for *in vivo* models. IL-1 and TNF-α are both *somnogenic* on injection into the lateral cerebral ventricle of rabbits, enhancing non–rapid eye movement (non-REM) sleep while inhibiting REM sleep, and presumably directly affecting the anterior hypothalamic preoptic area. Brain-derived IL-1 may be central to this process (99), and nitric oxide seems to mediate cytokine-induced sleep (100). IL-6, which is required for several types of sickness behavior after turpentine injection, is not required for development of *lethargy* (101), suggesting that other cytokines mediate the latter phenomenon. Mice deficient in the type I receptor for IL-1 do not demonstrate lethargy after turpentine injection, suggesting that IL-1 mediates the response to this stimulus (102).

Several cytokines are implicated in the pathogenesis of *anorexia*. Anorexia is blocked in both IL-6 knock-out mice and IL-1 receptor type I knock-out mice after turpentine injection, but not after LPS injection (102,103). These findings are consistent with data indicating that IL-1 induces IL-6 production after turpentine (but not LPS) injection and that IL-6 is required for anorexia after turpentine injection. Older data suggest that local TNF-α production in the brain may also participate in the development of anorexia (104). In addition, the observation that leptin is an acute phase reactant suggests that leptin may also contribute to inflammation-associated anorexia. Existing data suggest that IL-1β is the major contributor to leptin induction (36). Finally, vagal nerve afferents appear to be required for intraperitoneal IL-1β and LPS to induce anorexia in mice (85).

Hematopoietic System

The mechanisms responsible for the *anemia* of chronic inflammation, although somewhat poorly understood, include decreased proliferation of red cell progenitors and inadequate erythropoietin production, both caused at least in part by inflammation-associated cytokines (105). Some of these cytokines cause erythrocyte precursors to be relatively refractory to erythropoietin, and others suppress erythropoietin production (106). The importance of both the decreased iron utilization in marrow and the somewhat increased hemolysis found in many patients with this type of anemia is questionable, because clinical observations demonstrate that the anemia of chronic inflammation can usually be overcome by erythropoietin administration alone. Another acute phase phenomenon, *thrombocytosis,* also appears to be caused by IL-6 (107).

Hypoferremia seen during the APR is largely caused by iron sequestration in the reticuloendothelial system. This sequestration appears to result from increased apoferritin translation in macrophages induced by IL-4 and IL-13, with consequent inhibition of iron release (83). As indicated previously, it is not clear that hypoferremia contributes significantly to the anemia of chronic inflammation, although it may contribute to the microcytosis that usually is seen with that condition.

Metabolic Changes

Cachexia, the loss of body mass that accompanies chronic inflammatory states and cancer, results from decreases in skeletal muscle, fat tissue, and bone mass. There is considerable evidence that IL-1, IL-6, TNF-α, and IFN-γ all contribute to these processes (108,109). Loss of skeletal muscle is caused by the combination of decreased protein synthesis and increased *proteolysis*. Both IL-1 and TNF-α seem to be involved in these processes, and the effects of both are reversed by administration of IL-1Ra (110). IL-6 is also implicated; transgenic mice overexpressing IL-6 demonstrate gastrocnemius muscle atrophy and increased lysosomal cathepsin activity (111). Muscle wasting caused by injection of TNF-α–transfected Chinese hamster ovary (CHO) cells can be prevented by iNOS inhibitors (112), suggesting that nitric oxide may mediate this cytokine-induced process. *Osteoporosis* is also a consequence of chronic inflammation. Several inflammation-associated cytokines stimulate bone resorption (113) and suppress osteocalcin expression (114).

Lipid metabolism is markedly altered during the APR. Loss of fat tissue results, at least in part, from inhibition of lipoprotein lipase production by cytokines (115). Increases in serum triglycerides, very-low-density lipoproteins, and low-density lipoproteins are seen (116). Effects on high-density lipoproteins (HDLs) are particularly striking. HDL levels fall during inflammatory states, and SAA may largely displace apolipoprotein I (apo A-I) in HDL (117), with accompanying increase in HDL size and density and in HDL triglyceride concentration. Effects of cytokines on hepatic production of apolipoproteins and lecithin-cholesterol acyltransferase have been reported, but differences among species and among results from different laboratories make it difficult to arrive at firm conclusions about the effects of specific cytokines (118–120). Cytokines induce both lipolysis and *de novo* fatty acid synthesis, thus providing fatty acids for increased production of triglycerides (121). Chronic IL-6 administration can cause hypocholesterolemia in rhesus monkeys (122). The complexity of regulation of lipid metabolism during inflammatory states was emphasized by Grunfeld et al. (35), who concluded that "multiple cytokines . . . influence lipid metabolism at multiple sites by multiple mechanisms."

IL-10, regarded as an antiinflammatory cytokine, has been implicated in the pathogenesis of *postoperative immunosuppression*, which is probably also an acute phase phenomenon (123). Inflammation-associated cytokines play a major role in the pathogenesis of septic shock (124) and are believed to play a role in the "sick euthyroid syndrome" (32).

FUNCTION OF THE ACUTE PHASE RESPONSE

Discussion of the function of the APR must be tempered by two caveats. First, we presume that acute phase changes play a major role in adaptation and defense because we are inclined to believe that nature tries to accomplish useful purposes. This is not necessarily true. The host response may be either protective or destructive; sepsis is a specific example of the latter case. Second, our presumptions about the functions of the acute phase proteins are largely based on their known functional capabilities *in vitro* and on logical speculation as to how these may serve useful purposes. We are not always certain that these presumptions are valid in *in vivo* situations.

The term *inflammation* describes a group of complex, highly orchestrated processes that are initiated in response to various noxious stimuli and then amplified and sustained. Although the function of inflammation appears to be primarily defensive, an uncontrolled inflammatory response clearly has the potential of causing harm to the host; therefore, the mechanisms that keep inflammation under control (modulate it) and ultimately cause it to resolve are critically important. Many cell types and molecules participate in the evolution of these complex processes, as demonstrated by the table of contents of this volume. Acute phase proteins may be expected to influence any of these.

The characterization of molecules as either "proinflammatory" or "antiinflammatory" introduces three problems. First, it is often forgotten that even purely antiinflammatory molecules are intrinsic components of the inflammatory process, as indicated previously. Second, although some cytokines may only initiate and sustain inflammation and others may only modulate it, many cytokines are multifunctional and play different roles at different points in the process. Finally, as with hepatocytes, it is likely that cells participating in the localized inflammatory response are rarely exposed to only a single cytokine, arachidonic acid metabolite, neuropeptide, or other molecule capable of influencing inflammation. Accordingly, the effect of a cytokine on a target cell probably depends on other molecules capable of influencing cell behavior that are present at that point in the evolution of inflammation.

Illuminating data about the differing roles that cytokines may play at various points in the inflammatory process continue to accumulate. It has long been recognized that TGF-β is both an extremely potent monocyte chemoattractant and activator and an important contributor to wound healing (125). We now know that the net effects of TGF-β are antiinflammatory (126). Studies also have indicated that both IL-12 and IFN-γ play stimulatory roles in early collagen-induced arthritis but suppress inflammation in late disease (127,128); likewise, IFN-α is both proinflammatory and antiinflammatory (129). In addition, some "proinflammatory" cytokines (IL-1 and TNF-α) have been implicated in wound healing (130). The "antiinflammatory" cytokines IL-4 and IL-13 upregulate adhesion molecules, and IL-13 can recruit inflammatory cells (131). Finally, IL-6 is commonly regarded as proinflammatory, but the argument has been advanced that it is actually antiinflammatory (132). It is likely that both viewpoints are correct.

Acute Phase Proteins

Although a simple classification of acute phase proteins as either proinflammatory or antiinflammatory has been suggested (132), it is not clear that such a classification is helpful in understanding *in vivo* molecular mechanisms because, as indicated previously, many exceptions to these broad characterizations are being recognized. A number of acute phase proteins have the potential to influence the inflammatory and tissue repair processes (133). CRP, for example, can be regarded as a component of the primitive innate, or natural, immune system. A very large number of binding specificities and biologic effects of CRP are reported (134), and a major function of CRP is presumed to be "proinflammatory," related to its ability to specifically bind to phosphocholine and some nuclear components. Through such binding, CRP could recognize some foreign pathogens, as well as both phospholipid and nuclear constituents of damaged or necrotic cells. Further, CRP can activate the complement system when bound to one of its ligands and can also bind to phagocytic cells, suggesting that it can initiate elimination of targeted cells by interaction with humoral and cellular effector systems of inflammation (133). This argument is supported by the observation that CRP can induce production of inflammatory cytokines (135) and tissue factor (136), the main initiator of blood coagulation, by monocytes. In contrast, studies of the effects of CRP on chemotaxis, phagocytosis, and respiratory burst activity of phagocytic cells suggest a significant antiinflammatory role. For example, CRP has been reported to inhibit neutrophil chemotaxis, to inhibit superoxide generation by neutrophils (137–139), and to induce particularly large amounts of IL-1Ra in peripheral blood mononuclear cells (140). Finally, studies in transgenic mice suggest that the net effect of CRP *in vivo* is antiinflammatory (141–143). In sum, it is likely that CRP plays multiple roles in the course of the inflammatory process.

SAA, the other major human acute phase protein, has been shown to induce adhesion and chemotaxis of phagocytic cells and lymphocytes (144). In addition, the findings that macrophages bear specific binding sites for SAA and that SAA-rich HDLs display increased ability to transfer cholesterol to macrophages at inflammatory sites (145) suggest a role of SAA in the transfer of cholesterol to inflammatory cells. SAA also has been reported to enhance low-density lipoprotein oxidation in arterial cell walls (146). The complement components, many of which are acute phase reactants, are recognized as being central to innate immunity. They can affect chemotaxis, opsonization, vascular permeability, and vascular dilatation when activated, and they may lead to cytotoxicity as well. The important role of the acute phase protein mannose-binding lectin in the innate immune system was reviewed by Turner (147).

Proinflammatory functions of acute phase proteins can be ascribed to the findings that transthyretin, a negative acute phase reactant, inhibits IL-1 production by monocytes and endothelial cells (148); that α1-AGP increases tissue factor expression and TNF-α secretion by monocytes (149); and that ceruloplasmin enhances oxidation of low-density lipoproteins (150). In contrast, haptoglobin, hemopexin, and ceruloplasmin play antioxidant roles and can be presumed to modulate the inflammatory process, as can the antiproteases α1-AGP, α_1-antichymotrypsin, and C1 inhibitor (133). Mice are protected from the lethal effect of TNF-α by α_1-protease inhibitor (151), and both this serpin and α1-AGP protect against TNF-α–induced liver failure (152). Superoxide anion generation is suppressed by α_1-antichymotrypsin (153), and α1-AGP modulates neutrophil function (154), both reflecting antiinflammatory effects. Finally, fibrinogen, in addition to its participation in the clotting process, can lead to endothelial cell adhesion, spreading, and proliferation, all critical to wound repair. Haptoglobin can aid in wound repair by stimulating angiogenesis (155), but the dependence of chronic inflammation on angiogenesis (156) raises the possibility that the ultimate effect of haptoglobin may not be entirely benign.

Other Acute Phase Phenomena

The functions of many acute phase phenomena seem self-evident. The value of increasing the number of available granulocytes to provide additional bacterial killing power in infection is obvious. Platelets are significant participants in the inflammatory process (see Chapter 6) and may also be useful in promoting wound healing. Increased hepatic heme oxygenase, TIMP-1 (90), and manganese superoxide dismutase are presumed to play protective roles against oxidant-mediated injury. Overexpression of manganese superoxide dismutase has also been shown to modulate IL-1α levels (157). Somnolence clearly leads to reduced energy demands. Decreases in serum levels of iron and zinc may have beneficial effects in defense against bacterial infection and in tissue repair.

It has been hypothesized that decreased zinc concentrations benefit the host by influencing the production of cytokines (158). Increased sialyl Lewis^X expression on α1-AGP might block the binding of leukocytes to endothelial selectin molecules (80).

Several acute phase changes such as fever and hypercortisolemia are presumed to provide a systemic environment appropriate for the adaptive requirements of coping with significant tissue injury or infection. The influence of fever on host defenses was reviewed by Hasday (159), and arguments supporting its adaptive value were presented by Kluger et al. (160). It is presumed that fever is beneficial during infections, on the basis of its effects on survival in some *in vivo* models, but the cellular or molecular bases for such a phenomenon are still ill-defined. Although temperature can influence a number of inflammatory and immunologic processes, including chemotaxis, cytokine production and function, complement-mediated opsonization, and T-cell function, a coherent picture is yet to emerge.

Finally, the functional usefulness of some acute phase changes must be questioned. Not only may some changes actually have harmful effects (e.g., sepsis), but some changes may be stereotyped, occurring in inflammatory states other than the ones in which they serve a useful purpose. For example, although fever may be useful in certain infectious states, it does not seem useful after a surgical procedure or acute myocardial infarction.

SUMMARY

Many metabolic, physiologic, behavioral, and nutritional changes distant from the inflammatory site accompany inflammatory states. In a given patient, the APR represents the integrated sum of multiple, separately regulated changes induced primarily by inflammation-associated cytokines and influenced by modulators of cytokine function (cytokine inhibitors, soluble receptors, autoantibodies), some endocrine hormones, and other circulating molecules. Although many of these changes commonly occur together, clinical experience teaches that not all of them occur in all patients, indicating that they must be individually regulated. For example, febrile patients may have normal blood levels of CRP and vice versa, leukocytosis does not always accompany other acute phase phenomena, and instances of discordance between levels of the various acute phase proteins are regularly encountered. These variations may be explained by differences in patterns of specific cytokines or cytokine modulators in the various pathophysiologic states.

Cytokines function as part of a complex regulatory network, a signaling language in which information is conveyed to cells by combinations, and perhaps sequences, of a variety of hormones. In the original sense of the word, a cytokine is just another hormone, as is a cytokine modulator. The effects of combinations of hormones are complex.

Using the simile of human communication, individual hormones can be thought of as *words* that bear informational content. Although on occasion a single hormone, like a single word, may communicate a complete message, more commonly the complete messages received by cells probably resemble *sentences*, in which combinations and sequences of words convey information.

The plasma protein response to inflammatory stimuli seen in hepatocytes can serve as a paradigm for the APR in other organs. Currently available data suggest that hepatocytes receive a complex mixture of humoral or paracrine signals during the APR, which are then integrated by multiple interacting signal transducing mechanisms to cause finely regulated changes in plasma protein gene expression. Regulation occurs mainly by transcriptional control, but posttranscriptional mechanisms, including translational regulation, may also participate. Both the extracellular and the intracellular mechanisms that mediate the response of the hepatocyte to inflammatory stimuli are highly complex and involve multiple overlapping and parallel pathways. IL-6 is a major participant in many of these plasma protein changes. Regulation of nonhepatocyte acute phase phenomena has not been delineated as thoroughly, but they clearly also involve some of the same group of inflammation-associated cytokines.

It is widely held that components of the APR influence the inflammatory response or enhance adaptation to noxious stimuli. Although this probably is true most of the time, it is not invariably true. The host response may be either protective or destructive; an example of the latter is septic shock. It is possible to adduce the putative usefulness of a number of acute phase changes, based on the known functional capabilities of acute phase proteins and on logical speculation as to how these may serve useful purposes. There is reason to believe that some acute phase proteins participate in initiation, amplification, modulation, or resolution of the inflammatory process, and a number of acute phase changes are presumed to play protective roles, contributing to a systemic environment required for coping with significant tissue injury or infection. Finally, it is likely that some changes occur in inflammatory states other than the ones in which they do serve a useful purpose.

ACKNOWLEDGMENT

This work was supported in part by NIH grant #AG-02467. We express our gratitude to John Harris and David Samols for review of the manuscript.

REFERENCES

1. Dubos RJ. *The professor, the institute and DNA.* New York: The Rockefeller University Press, 1976.
2. Kushner I. The phenomenon of the acute phase response. *Ann N Y Acad Sci* 1982;389:39–48.
3. Tillet WS, Francis TJ. Serological reactions in pneumonia with a non-protein somatic fraction of pneumococcus. *J Exp Med* 1930;52:561–585.
4. McCarty M. Historical perspective on C-reactive protein. *Ann N Y Acad Sci* 1982;389:1–10.
5. Members of the American College of Chest Physicians/Society of Critical Care Medicine Consensus Conference Committee. American College of Chest Physicians/Society of Critical Care Medicine Consensus Conference: Definitions for sepsis and organ failure and guidelines for the use of innovative therapies in sepsis. *Crit Care Med* 1992;20:864–874.
6. Chrousos GP. The hypothalamic-pituitary-adrenal axis and immune-mediated inflammation. *N Engl J Med* 1995;332:1351–1362.
7. Chrousos GP, Gold PW. The concepts of stress system disorders: overview of behavioral and physical homeostasis. *JAMA* 1992;267:1244–1252.
8. Sternberg EM. Emotions and disease: from balance of humors to balance of molecules. *Nat Med* 1997;3:264–267.
9. Izumi S, Hughes RD, Langley PG, Pernambuco JRB, Williams R. Extent of the acute phase response in fulminant hepatic failure. *Gut* 1994;35:982–986.
10. Colten H. Tissue-specific regulation of inflammation. *J Appl Physiol* 1992;72:1–7.
11. Zuraw BL, Lotz M. Regulation of the hepatic synthesis of C1 inhibitor by the hepatocyte stimulating factors interleukin-6 and interferon gamma. *J Biol Chem* 1990;265:12664–12670.
12. de Frutos P, Alim RIM, Härdig Y, Zöller B, Dahlbäck B. Differential regulation of α and β chains of C4b-binding protein during acute-phase response resulting in stable plasma levels of free anticoagulant protein S. *Blood* 1994;84:815–822.
13. Ezekowitz RAB, Day LE, Herman GA. A human mannose-binding protein is an acute-phase reactant that shares sequence homology with other vertebrate lectins. *J Exp Med* 1988;167:1034–1046.
14. Jenkins G, Seiffert D, Parmer RJ, Miles LA. Regulation of plasminogen gene expression by interleukin-6. *Blood* 1997;89:2394–2403.
15. Hooper WC, Phillips DJ, Ribeiro M, Benson J, Evatt BL. IL-6 upregulates protein S expression in the HepG-2 hepatoma cells. *Thromb Haemost* 1995;73:819–824.
16. Hopkins WE, Fujii S, Sobel BE. Synergistic induction of plasminogen activator inhibitor type-1 in HEP G2 cells by thrombin and transforming growth factor-β. *Blood* 1992;79:75–81.
17. Omachi Y, Murata A, Yasuda T, et al. Expression of the pancreatic secretory trypsin inhibitor gene in the liver infected with hepatitis B virus. *J Hepatol* 1994;21:1012–1016.
18. Sarafan N, Martin JP, Bourguignon J, et al. The human inter-alpha-trypsin inhibitor genes respond differently to interleukin-6 in HepG2 cells. *Eur J Biochem* 1995;227:808–815.
19. Crowl RM, Stoller TJ, Conroy RR, Stoner CR. Induction of phospholipase A2 gene expression in human hepatoma cells by mediators of the acute phase response. *J Biol Chem* 1991;266:2647–2651.
20. Gabay C, Smith M Jr, Eidlen D, Arend WP. Interleukin 1 receptor antagonist (IL-1Ra) is an acute-phase protein. *J Clin Invest* 1997;99:2930–2940.
21. Schumann RR, Kirschning CJ, Unbehaun A, et al. The lipopolysaccharide-binding protein is a secretory class 1 acute-phase protein whose gene is transcriptionally activated by APRF/STAT-3 and other cytokine-inducible nuclear proteins. *Mol Cell Biol* 1996;16:3490–3503.
22. Thompson PN, Cho E, Blumenstock FA, Shah DM, Saba TM. Rebound elevation of fibronectin after tissue injury and ischemia: role of fibronectin synthesis. *Am J Physiol* 1992;263:G437–G445.
23. Lee MH, Means RT. Extremely elevated serum ferritin levels in a university hospital: associated diseases and clinical significance. *Am J Med* 1995;98:566–571.
24. Beauchamp RD, Sheng H, Alam T, Townsend CM Jr, Papaconstantinou J. Posttranscriptional regulation of albumin and α-fetoprotein messenger RNA by transforming growth factor-β1 requires de novo RNA and protein synthesis. *Mol Endocrinol* 1992;6:1789–1796.
25. Bartalena L, Faresetti A, Flink IL, Robbins J. Effects of interleukin-6 on the expression of thyroid hormone-binding protein genes in cultured human hepatoblastoma-derived (HepG2) cells. *Mol Endocrinol* 1992;6:935–942.
26. Wolf M, Bohm S, Brand M, Kreymann G. Proinflammatory cytokines interleukin 1 beta and tumor necrosis factor α inhibit growth hormone

stimulation of insulin-like growth factor I synthesis and growth hormone receptor mRNA levels in cultured rat liver cells. *Eur J Endocrinol* 1996;135:729–737.

27. Haidaris PJS. Induction of fibrinogen biosynthesis and secretion from cultured pulmonary epithelial cells. *Blood* 1997;89:873–882.

28. Ramadori G, Sipe J, Colten HR. Expression and regulation of the murine serum amyloid A (SAA) gene in extrahepatic sites. *J Immunol* 1985;135:3645–3647.

29. Cichy J, Potempa J, Travis J. Biosynthesis of alpha (1)-proteinase inhibitor by human lung-derived epithelial cells. *J Biol Chem* 1997;272:8250–8255.

30. Hardardottir I, Sipe J, Moser AH, Fielding CJ, Feingold KR, Grunfeld C. LPS and cytokines regulate extra hepatic mRNA levels of apolipoproteins during the acute phase response in Syrian hamsters. *Biochim Biophys Acta* 1997;1334:210–220.

31. Sheffield CL, Kamps-Holtzapple C, DeLoach JR, Stanker LH. Production and characterization of a monoclonal antibody against bovine haptoglobin and its use in an ELISA. *Vet Immunol Immunopathol* 1994;42:171–183.

32. Boelen A, Platvoetterschiphorst MC, Wiersinga WM. Immunoneutralization of interleukin-1, tumor necrosis factor interleukin-6 or interferon does not prevent the LPS-induced sick euthyroid syndrome in mice. *J Endocrinol* 1997;153:115–122.

33. Schilling RF. Anemia of chronic disease: a misnomer. *Ann Intern Med* 1991;115:572–573.

34. Abel J, Spannbrucker N, Fandrey J, Jelkmann W. Serum erythropoietin levels in patients with sepsis and septic shock. *Eur J Haematol* 1996;57:359–363.

35. Grunfeld C, Soued M, Adi S, et al. Interleukin 4 inhibits stimulation of hepatic lipogenesis by tumor necrosis factor, interleukin 1, and interleukin 6 but not by interferon-α1. *Cancer Res* 1991;51:2803–2807.

36. Sarraf P, Frederich RC, Turner EM, et al. Multiple cytokines and acute inflammation raise mouse leptin levels: potential role in inflammatory anorexia. *J Exp Med* 1997;185:171–175.

37. Okajima A, Miyazawa K, Naitoh Y, Inoue K, Kitamura N. Induction of hepatocyte growth factor activator messenger RNA in the liver following tissue injury and acute inflammation. *Hepatology* 1997;25:97–102.

38. Portoles MT, Catala M, Anton A, Pagani R. Hepatic response to the oxidative stress induced by *E. coli* endotoxin: glutathione as an index of the acute phase during the endotoxic shock. *Mol Cell Biochem* 1996;159:115–121.

39. Gingalewski C, Wang K, Clemens MG, De Maio A. Posttranscriptional regulation of connexin 32 expression in liver during acute inflammation. *J Cell Physiol* 1996;166:461–467.

40. Deutschman CS, DeMaio A, Clemens MG. Sepsis-induced attenuation of glucagon and 8-BrcAMP modulation of the phosphoenolpyruvate carboxykinase gene. *Am J Physiol* 1995;269:R584–R591.

41. Sewer MB, Koop DR, Morgan ET. Differential inductive and suppressive effects of endotoxin and particulate irritants on hepatic and renal cytochrome P-450 expression. *J Pharmacol Exp Ther* 1997;280:1445–1454.

42. Duggan C, Colin AA, Agil A, Higgins L, Rifai N. Vitamin A status in acute exacerbations of cystic fibrosis. *Am J Clin Nutr* 1996;64:635–639.

43. Castell LM, Poortmans JR, Leclercq R, Brasseur M, Duchateau J, Newsholme EA. Some aspects of the acute phase response after a marathon race, and the effects of glutamine supplementation. *Eur J Appl Physiol* 1997;75:47–53.

44. Joyce PR, Hawes CR, Mulder RT, Sellman JD, Wilson DA, Boswell DR. Elevated levels of acute phase plasma proteins in major depression. *Biol Psychiatry* 1992;32:1035–1041.

45. Maes M, Delange J, Ranjan R, et al. Acute phase proteins in schizophrenia, mania and major depression: modulation by psychotropic drugs. *Psychiatry Research* 1997;66:1–11.

46. LeMay LG, Vander AJ, Kluger MJ. The effects of psychological stress on plasma interleukin-6 activity in rats. *Physiol Behav* 1990;47:957–961.

47. Buchwald D, Wener MH, Pearlman T, Kith P. Markers of inflammation and immune activation in chronic fatigue and chronic fatigue syndrome. *J Rheumatol* 1997;24:372–376.

48. Fantuzzi G, Dinarello CA. The inflammatory response in interleukin-1β-deficient mice: comparison with other cytokine-related knock-out mice. *J Leukoc Biol* 1996;59:489–493.

49. Sterpetti AV, Cucina A, Morena AR, et al. Shear stress increases the release of interleukin-1 and interleukin-6 by aortic endothelial cells. *Surgery* 1993;114:911–914.

50. Kurdowska A, Travis J. Acute phase protein stimulation by α1-antichymotrypsin-cathepsin G complexes. *J Biol Chem* 1990;265:21023–21026.

51. Henderson B, Wilson M. Cytokine induction by bacteria: beyond lipopolysaccharide. *Cytokine* 1996;8:269–282.

52. Wahl SM, Costa GL, Mizel DE, Allen JB, Skaleric U, Mangan DF. Role of transforming growth factor beta in the pathophysiology of chronic inflammation. *J Periodontol* 1993;64:450–455.

53. Kobzik L, Huang S, Paulauskis JD, Godleski JJ. Particle opsonization and lung macrophage cytokine response. *J Immunol* 1993;151:2753–2759.

54. Richards CD, Langdon C, Pennica D, Gauldie J. Murine cardiotrophin-1 stimulates the acute-phase response in rat hepatocytes and H35 hepatoma cells. *J Interferon Cytokine Res* 1996;16:69–76.

55. Gabay C, Singwe M, Genin B, et al. Circulating levels of IL-11 and leukaemia inhibitory factor (LIF) do not significantly participate in the production of acute-phase proteins by the liver. *Clin Exp Immunol* 1996;105:260–265.

56. Okamoto H, Yamamura M, Morita Y, Harada S, Makino H, Ota Z. The synovial expression and serum levels of interleukin-6, interleukin-11, leukemia inhibitory factor, and oncostatin M in rheumatoid arthritis. *Arthritis Rheum* 1997;40:1096–1105.

57. Gauldie J, Richards C, Northemann W, Fey G, Baumann H. IFNβ2/BSF2/IL-6 is the monocyte-derived HSF that regulates receptor-specific acute phase gene regulation in hepatocytes. *Ann N Y Acad Sci* 1988;557:46–59.

58. Healy AM, Gelehrter TD. Induction of plasminogen activator inhibitor-1 in HepG2 human hepatoma cells by mediators of the acute phase response. *J Biol Chem* 1994;269:19095–19100.

59. Moffat GJ, Tack BF. Regulation of C4b-binding protein gene expression by the acute-phase mediators tumor necrosis factor-alpha, interleukin-6, and interleukin-1. *Biochemistry* 1992;31:12376–12384.

60. Seki T, Gelehrter TD. Interleukin-1 induction of type-1 plasminogen activator inhibitor (PAI-1) gene expression in the mouse hepatocyte line, AML 12. *J Cell Physiol* 1996;168:648–656.

61. Thissen JP, Verniers J. Inhibition by interleukin-1 beta and tumor necrosis factor-alpha of the insulin-like growth factor I messenger ribonucleic acid response to growth hormone in rat hepatocyte primary culture. *Endocrinology* 1997;138:1078–1084.

62. Mackiewicz A, Ganapathi MK, Schultz D, et al. Transforming growth factor β1 regulates production of acute phase proteins. *Proc Natl Acad Sci U S A* 1990;87:1491–1495.

63. Damtew B, Rzewnicki D, Lozanski G, Kushner I. IL-1 receptor antagonist affects the plasma protein response of Hep 3B cells to conditioned medium from LPS-stimulated monocytes. *J Immunol* 1993;150:4001–4007.

64. Mackiewicz A, Schooltink H, Heinrich PC, Rose-John S. Soluble human interleukin-6-receptor upregulates synthesis of acute-phase proteins. *J Immunol* 1992;306:257–261.

65. May LT, Neta R, Moldawer LL, Kenney JS, Patel K, Sehgal PB. Antibodies chaperone circulating IL-6. Paradoxical effects of anti-IL-6 "neutralizing" antibodies in vivo. *J Immunol* 1993;151:3225–3236.

66. Van Wyk JJ. Remembrances of our founders: will growth factors, oncogenes, cytokines and gastrointestinal hormones return us to our beginnings? *Endocrinology* 1992;130:3–5.

67. Baumann H, Richards C, Gauldie J. Interaction among hepatocyte-stimulating factors, interleukin 1, and glucocorticoids for regulation of acute phase plasma proteins in human hepatoma (Hep G2) cells. *J Immunol* 1987;139:4122–4128.

68. Campos SP, Wang Y, Koj A, Baumann H. Insulin cooperates with IL-1 in regulating expression of α1-acid glycoprotein gene in rat hepatoma cells. *Cytokine* 1994;6:485–492.

69. Falus A. Histamine modulates the acute phase response at multiple points. *Immunol Today* 1994;15:59.

70. Pierzchalski P, Rokita H, Koj A, Fries E, Åkerström B. Synthesis of α1-microglobulin in cultured rat hapatocytes is stimulated by interleukin-6, leukemia inhibitory factor, dexamethasone and retinoic acid. *FEBS Lett* 1992;198:165–168.

71. Hagan PM, Poole S, Bristow AF. Corticotrophin-releasing factor as a mediator of the acute-phase response in rats, mice and rabbits. *J Endocrinol* 1993;136:207–216.

72. Funk JL, Moser AH, Grunfeld C, Feingold KR. Parathyroid hormone-related protein is induced in the adult liver during endotoxemia and stimulates the hepatic acute phase response. *Endocrinology* 1997;138:2665–2673.

73. Mackiewicz A, Speroff T, Ganapathi MK, Kushner I. Effects of cytokine combinations on acute phase protein production in two human hepatoma cell lines. *J Immunol* 1991;146:3032–3037.

74. Sun M, Zhang D, Evans J, Samols D, Kushner I. Roles of STAT3 and C/EBP binding sites in C-reactive protein (CRP) transcription induced by IL-6 in Hep3B cells. *J Investig Med* 1997;45:271A.

75. Matsusaka T, Fujikawa K, Nishio Y, et al. Transcription factors NF-IL6 and NF-κB synergistically activate transcription of the inflammatory cytokines, interleukin 6 and interleukin 8. *Proc Natl Acad Sci U S A* 1993;90:10193–10197.

76. Jiang S, Samols D, Rzewnicki D, et al. Kinetic modeling and mathematical analysis indicate that acute phase gene expression in Hep 3B cells is regulated by both transcriptional and post-transcriptional mechanisms. *J Clin Invest* 1995;95:1253–1261.

77. Mitchell TJ, Naughton M, Norsworthy P, Davies KA, Walport MJ, Morley BJ. IFN-gamma up-regulates expression of the complement components C3 and C4 by stabilization of mRNA. *J Immunol* 1996;156:4429–4434.

78. Rogers JT, Bridges KR, Durmowicz GP, Glass J, Auron PE, Munro HN. Translational control during the acute phase response: ferritin synthesis in response to interleukin 1. *J Biol Chem* 1990;265:14572–14578.

79. van Dijk W, Mackiewicz A. Interleukin-6-type cytokine-induced changes in acute phase protein glycosylation. *Ann N Y Acad Sci* 1995;762:319–330.

80. de Graaf TW, Van der Stelt ME, Anberge MG, van Dijk W. Inflammation-induced expression of sialyl Lewis X-containing glycan structures on alpha 1-acid glycoprotein (orosomucoid) in human serum. *J Exp Med* 1993;177:657–666.

81. Dubé R, Rook GAW, Steele J, et al. Agalactosyl IgG in inflammatory bowel disease: correlation with C-reactive protein. *Gut* 1990;31:431–434.

82. Macintyre S, Samols D, Dailey P. Two carboxylesterases bind C-reactive protein within the endoplasmic reticulum and regulate its secretion during the acute phase response. *J Biol Chem* 1994;269:24496–24503.

83. Weiss G, Bogdan C, Hentze MW. Pathways for the regulation of macrophage iron metabolism by the anti-inflammatory cytokines IL-4 and IL-13. *J Immunol* 1997;158:420–425.

84. Goldbach JM, Roth J, Zeisberger E. Fever suppression by subdiaphragmatic vagotomy in guinea pigs depends on the route of pyrogen administration. *Am J Physiol* 1997;272:R675–R681.

85. Bret-Dibat JL, Bluthe RM, Kent S, Kelley KW, Dantzer R. Lipopolysaccharide and interleukin-1 depress food-motivated behavior in mice by a vagal-mediated mechanism. *Brain Behav Immun* 1995;9:242–246.

86. Schroeder JJ, Cousins RJ. Interleukin 6 regulates metallothionein gene expression and zinc metabolism in hepatocyte monolayer cultures. *Proc Natl Acad Sci U S A* 1990;87:3137–3141.

87. Suto N, Ikura K, Sasaki R. Expression induced by interleukin-6 of tissue-type transglutaminase in human hepatoblastoma HepG2 cells. *J Biol Chem* 1993;268:7469–7473.

88. Ono M, Kohda H, Kawaguchi T, et al. Induction of Mn-superoxide dismutase by tumor necrosis factor, interleukin-1 and interleukin-6 in human hepatoma cells. *Biochem Biophys Res Commun* 1992;182:1100–1107.

89. Mitani K, Fujita H, Kappas A, Sassa S. Heme oxygenase is a positive acute-phase reactant in human Hep 3B hepatoma cells. *Blood* 1992;79:1255–1259.

90. Kordula T, Guttgemann I, Rose-John S, et al. Synthesis of tissue inhibitor of metalloproteinase-1 (TIMP-1) in human hepatoma cells (HepG2). *FEBS Lett* 1992;313:143–147.

91. Chen JQ, Nikolova-Karakashian M, Merrill AH, Morgan ET. Regulation of cytochrome P450 2C11 (CYP2C11) gene expression by interleukin-1, sphingomyelin hydrolysis, and ceramides in rat hepatocytes. *J Biol Chem* 1995;270:25233–25238.

92. Delaporte E, Renton KW. Cytochrome P4501A1 and cytochrome P4501A2 are downregulated at both transcriptional and post-transcriptional levels by conditions resulting in interferon-alpha/beta induction. *Life Sci* 1997;60:687–696.

93. Geller DA, Freeswick PD, Nguyen D, et al. Differential induction of nitric oxide synthase in hepatocytes during endotoxemia and the acute-phase response. *Arch Surg* 1994;129:165–171.

94. Dinarello CA. Cytokines as endogenous pyrogens. In: Mackowiak PA (ed). *Fever: basic mechanisms and management* 2nd ed. Philadelphia: Lippincott-Raven, 1997:87–116.

95. Lucino J, Wong M. Interleukin 1b and fever. *Nat Med* 1996;2:1314–1315.

96. Path G, Bornstein SR, Spathschwalbe E, Scherbaum WA. Direct effects of interleukin-6 on human adrenal cells. *Endocr Res* 1996;22:867–873.

97. Turnbull AV, Rivier C. Cytokine effects on neuroendocrine axes: influence of nitric oxide and carbon monoxide. In: Rothwell NJ (ed). *Cytokines in the nervous system.* Austin, TX: RG Landes, 1996:93.

98. Elmquist JK, Saper CB. Activation of neurons projecting to the paraventricular hypothalamic nucleus by intravenous lipopolysaccharide. *J Comp Neurol* 1996;374:315–331.

99. Takahashi S, Kapas L, Fang JD, Seyer JM, Wang Y, Krueger JM. An interleukin-1 receptor fragment inhibits spontaneous sleep and muramyl dipeptide-induced sleep in rabbits. *Am J Physiol* 1996;271:R101–R108.

100. Krueger JM. Cytokine involvement in sleep responses to infection and physiological sleep. In: Rothwell NJ (ed). *Cytokines in the nervous system.* Austin, TX: RG Landes, 1996:41.

101. Leon LR, Kozak W, Peschon J, Kluger MJ. Exacerbated febrile responses to LPS, but not turpentine, in TNF double receptor-knockout mice. *Am J Physiol* 1997;272:R563–R569.

102. Leon LR, Conn CA, Glaccum M, Kluger MJ. IL-1 type I receptor mediates acute phase response to turpentine, but not lipopolysaccharide, in mice. *Am J Physiol* 1996;40:R1668–R1675.

103. Fattori E, Cappelletti M, Costa P, et al. Defective inflammatory response in interleukin 6–deficient mice. *J Exp Med* 1994;180:1243–1250.

104. Tracey KJ, Morgello S, Koplin B, et al. Metabolic effects of cachectin/tumor necrosis factor are modified by site of production. *J Clin Invest* 1990;86:2014–2024.

105. Means RT. Pathogenesis of the anemia of chronic disease: a cytokine-mediated anemia. *Stem Cells* 1995;13:32–37.

106. Faquin WC, Schneider TJ, Goldberg MA. Effect of inflammatory cytokines on hypoxia-induced erythropoietin production. *Blood* 1992;79:1987–1994.

107. Zeidler C, Kanz L, Hurkuck F, et al. *In vivo* effects of interleukin-6 on thrombopoiesis in healthy and irradiated primates. *Blood* 1992;80:2740–2745.

108. Espat NJ, Moldawer LL, Copeland EM III. Cytokine-mediated alterations in host metabolism prevent nutritional repletion in cachectic cancer patients. *J Surg Oncol* 1995;58:77–82.

109. Tisdale MJ. Cancer cachexia: metabolic alterations and clinical manifestations. *Nutrition* 1997;13:1–7.

110. Cannon JG. Cytokines in aging and muscle homeostasis. *J Gerontol A Biol Sci Med Sci* 1995;50:120–123.

111. Fujita J, Tsujinaka T, Ebisui C, et al. Role of interleukin-6 in skeletal muscle protein breakdown and cathepsin activity *in vivo*. *Eur Surg Res* 1996;28:361–366.

112. Buck M, Chojkier M. Muscle wasting and dedifferentiation induced by oxidative stress in a murine model of cachexia is prevented by inhibitors of nitric oxide synthesis and antioxidants. *EMBO J* 1996;15:1753–1765.

113. Mundy GR. Role of cytokines in bone resorption. *J Cell Biochem* 1993;53:296–300.

114. Li Y, Stashenko P. Proinflammatory cytokines tumor necrosis factor-α and IL-6, but not IL-1, down-regulate the osteocalcin gene promotor. *J Immunol* 1992;148:788–794.

115. Feingold KR, Marshall M, Gulli R, Moser AH, Grunfeld C. Effect of endotoxin and cytokines on lipoprotein lipase activity in mice. *Arterioscler Thromb* 1994;14:1866–1872.

116. Liao W, Florén C. Hyperlipidemic response to endotoxin: a part of the host-defense mechanism. *Scand J Infect Dis* 1993;25:675–682.

117. Banka CL, Yuan T, de Beer MC, Kindy M, Curtiss LK, de Beer FC. Serum amyloid A (SAA): influence on HDL-mediated cellular cholesterol efflux. *J Lipid Res* 1995;36:1058–1065.

118. Skretting G, Gjernes E, Prydz H. Regulation of lecithin : cholesterol acyltransferase by TGF-beta and interleukin-6. *Biochim Biophys Acta* 1995;1255:267–272.

119. Ettinger WHJ, Varma VK, Sorci-Thomas M, et al. Cytokines decrease

apolipoprotein accumulation in medium from Hep G2 cells. *Arterioscler Thromb* 1994;14:8–13.

120. Delers F, Mangeney M, Raffa D, et al. Changes in rat liver mRNA for alpha-1-acid-glycoprotein, apolipoprotein E, apolipoprotein B and beta-actin after mouse recombinant tumor necrosis factor injection. *Biochem Biophys Res Commun* 1989;161:81–89.

121. Nonogaki K, Pan XM, Moser AH, et al. LIF and CNTF, which share the gp130 transduction system, stimulate hepatic lipid metabolism in rats. *Am J Physiol* 1996;271:E521–E528.

122. Ettinger WHJ, Sun WH, Binkley N, Kouba E, Ershler W. Interleukin-6 causes hypocholesterolemia in middle-aged and old rhesus monkeys. *J Gerontol* 1995;50:M137–M140.

123. Klava A, Woodhouse LF, Ramsen C, Farmery SM, Guillou PJ. IL-10: a candidate for the immunosuppressive effects of surgical injury? *Cytokine* 1995;7:620.

124. Bone RC. Toward a theory regarding the pathogenesis of the systemic inflammatory response syndrome: what we do and do not know about cytokine regulation. *Crit Care Med* 1996;24:163–172.

125. Wahl SM, McCartney-Francis N, Mergenhagen SE. Inflammatory and immunomodulatory roles of TGFβ. *Immunol Today* 1989;10:258–261.

126. Kulkarni AB, Karlsson S. Transforming growth factor-β₁ knockout mice. *Am J Pathol* 1993;143:3–9.

127. van den Berg WB. Cytokines *in vivo* in animal models of arthritis. *Eur Cytokine Netw* 1996;7:434.

128. Boissier MC, Chiocchia G, Bessis N, et al. Biphasic effect of interferon-gamma in murine collagen-induced arthritis. *Eur J Immunol* 1995;25:1184–1190.

129. Tilg H, Peschel C. Interferon-alpha and its effects on the cytokine cascade: a pro- and anti-inflammatory cytokine. *Leuk Lymphoma* 1996; 23:55–60.

130. Hubner G, Brauchle M, Smola H, Madlener M, Fassler R, Werner S. Differential regulation of pro-inflammatory cytokines during wound healing in normal and glucocorticoid-treated mice. *Cytokine* 1996;8: 548–556.

131. Ying S, Meng Q, Barata LT, Robinson DS, Durham SR, Kay AB. Associations between IL-13 and IL-4 (mRNA and protein), vascular cell adhesion molecule-1 expression, and the infiltration of eosinophils, macrophages, and T cells in allergen-induced late-phase cutaneous reactions in atopic subjects. *J Immunol* 1997;158: 5050–5057.

132. Tilg H, Dinarello CA. Interleukin-6 and acute phase proteins: antiinflammatory and immunsuppressive mediators. *Immunol Today* 1997; 18:428–432.

133. Volanakis JE. Acute phase proteins in rheumatic disease. In: Koopman WJ (ed). *Arthritis and allied conditions: a textbook of rheumatology.* Baltimore: Williams & Wilkins, 1997:505–514.

134. Schultz DR, Arnold PI. Properties of four acute phase proteins: C-reactive protein, serum amyloid A, α1-acid glycoprotein, and fibrinogen. *Semin Arthritis Rheum* 1990;20:129–147.

135. Ballou SP, Lozanski G. Induction of inflammatory cytokines release from cultured human monocytes by C-reactive protein. *Cytokine* 1992;4:361–368.

136. Cermak J, Key NS, Bach RR, Jacob HS, Vercellotti GM. C-reactive protein induces human peripheral blood monocytes to synthesize tissue factor. *Blood* 1993;82:513–520.

137. Shephard EG, Anderson R, Rosen O, Fridkin M. C-reactive protein (CRP) peptides inactivate enolase in human neutrophils leading to depletion of intracellular ATP and inhibition of superoxide generation. *Immunology* 1992;76:79–85.

138. Földes-Filep É, Filep JG, Sirois P. C-reactive protein inhibits intracellular calcium mobilization and superoxide production by guinea pig alveolar macrophages. *J Leukoc Biol* 1992;51:13–18.

139. Dobrinich R, Spagnuolo PJ. Binding of C-reactive protein to human neutrophils: inhibition of respiratory burst activity. *Arthritis Rheum* 1991;34:1031–1038.

140. Tilg H, Vannier E, Vachine G, Dinarello CA, Mier JW. Antiinflammatory properties of hepatic acute phase proteins: preferential induction of interleukin 1 (IL-1) receptor antagonist over IL-1β synthesis by human peripheral blood mononuclear cells. *J Exp Med* 1993;178: 1629–1636.

141. Ahmed N, Thorley R, Xia D, Samols D, Webster RO. Transgenic mice expressing rabbit C-reactive protein exhibit diminished chemotactic factor-induced alveolitis. *Am J Respir Crit Care Med* 1996;153: 1141–1147.

142. Xia D, Samols D. Transgenic mice expressing rabbit C-reactive protein are resistant to endotoxemia. *Proc Natl Acad Sci U S A* 1997;94: 2575–2580.

143. Heuertz RM, Xia D, Samols D, Webster RO. Inhibition of C5a des Arg–induced neutrophil alveolitis in transgenic mice expressing C-reactive protein. *Am J Physiol* 1994;266:L649–L654.

144. Xu L, Badolato R, Murphy WJ, et al. A novel biologic function of serum amyloid A: induction of T lymphocyte migration and adhesion. *J Immunol* 1995;155:1184–1190.

145. Kisilevsky R, Subrahmanyan L. Serum amyloid A changes high density lipoprotein's cellular affinity. *Lab Invest* 1992;66:778–785.

146. Berliner JA, Navab M, Fogelman AM, et al. Atherosclerosis: basic mechanisms—oxidation, inflammation, and genetics. *Circulation* 1995;91:2488–2496.

147. Turner MW. Mannose-binding lectin: the pluripotent molecule of the innate immune system. *Immunol Today* 1996;17:532–540.

148. Borish L, King MS, Mascali JJ, Johnson S, Coll B, Rosenwasser LJ. Transthyretin is an inhibitor of monocyte and endothelial cell interleukin-1 production. *Inflammation* 1992;16:471–476.

149. Su SJ, Yeh TM. Effects of alpha 1-acid glycoprotein on tissue factor expression and tumor necrosis factor secretion in human monocytes. *Immunopharmacology* 1996;34:139–145.

150. Ehrenwald E, Chisolm GM, Fox PL. Intact human ceruloplasmin oxidatively modifies low density lipoprotein. *J Clin Invest* 1994;93: 1493–1501.

151. Libert C, Van Molle W, Brouckaert P, Fiers W. α1-Antitrypsin inhibits the lethal response to TNF in mice. *J Immunol* 1996;157:5126–5129.

152. Brouckaert P, Libert C, Cauwels A, et al. Inhibition of and sensitization to the lethal effects of tumor necrosis factor. *J Inflamm* 1996;47: 18–26.

153. Kilpatrick L, McCawley L, Nachiappan V, et al. α-1-Antichymotrypsin inhibits the NADPH oxidase-enzyme complex in phorbol ester-stimulated neutrophil membranes. *J Immunol* 1992;149: 3059–3065.

154. Lainé E, Couderc R, Roch-Arveiller M, Vasson MP, Giroud JP, Raichvarg D. Modulation of human polymorphonuclear neutrophil functions by α₁-acid glycoprotein. *Inflammation* 1990;14:1–9.

155. Cid MC, Grant DS, Hoffman GS, Fauci AS, Kleinman HK. Identification of haptoglobin as an angiogenic factor in sera from patients with systemic vasculitis. *J Clin Invest* 1993;91:977–985.

156. Jackson JR, Seed MP, Kircher CH, Willoughby DA, Winkler JD. The codependence of angiogenesis and chronic inflammation. *FASEB J* 1997;11:457–465.

157. Melendez JA, Davies KJA. Manganese superoxide dismutase modulates interleukin-1 alpha levels in HT-1080 fibrosarcoma cells. *J Biol Chem* 1996;271:18898–18903.

158. Braunschweig CL, Sowers M, Kovacevich DS, Hill GM, August DA. Parenteral zinc supplementation in adult humans during the acute phase response increases the febrile response. *J Nutr* 1997;127:70–74.

159. Hasday JD. The influence of fever on host defenses. In: Mackowiak PA (ed). *Fever: basic mechanisms and management* 2nd edition. Philadelphia: Lippincott-Raven, 1997:177–196.

160. Kluger MJ, Kozak W, Conn CA, Leon LR, Soszynski D. The adaptive value of fever. In: Mackowiak PA (ed). *Fever: basic mechanisms and management* 2nd edition. Philadelphia: Lippincott-Raven, 1997: 255–266.

Inflammation: Basic Principles and Clinical Correlates,
3rd ed., edited by John I. Gallin and Ralph Snyderman.
Lippincott Williams & Wilkins, Philadelphia © 1999.

CHAPTER 21

Bradykinin Formation:

Plasma and Tissue Pathways and Cellular Interactions

Allen P. Kaplan, Kusumam Joseph, Yoji Shibayama, Yoshitaka Nakazawa, Berhane Ghebrehiwet, Sesha Reddigari, and Michael Silverberg

The plasma kinin-forming system consists of three essential plasma proteins that interact in a complex fashion once they are bound to certain negatively charged inorganic surfaces, macromolecular complexes formed during an inflammation response, or proteins along cell surfaces. These plasma proteins are coagulation factor XII (Hageman factor), prekallikrein, and high-molecular-weight kininogen (HK). Factor XII, once it is activated to factor XIIa, converts plasma prekallikrein to kallikrein; kallikrein then digests HK to liberate bradykinin. Factor XIIa has a second substrate in plasma, coagulation factor XI. Activation of surface-bound factor XI by factor XIIa initiates the intrinsic coagulation cascade. The interactions of all four of these proteins are known collectively as *contact activation*, and bradykinin is formed as a cleavage product of the initiating step of this cascade (Fig. 21-1).

Bradykinin is also generated by a *tissue pathway*. Intracellular conversion of a prokallikrein to tissue kallikrein occurs by means of enzymes that are not well characterized, and tissue kallikrein is secreted into the local milieu. There, it digests low-molecular-weight kininogen (LK) to generate lysyl-bradykinin (kallidin), and a plasma aminopeptidase converts kallidin to bradykinin.

These various pathways and their related cell interactions and contributions to human disease are discussed

A. P. Kaplan, K. Joseph, M. Silverberg, Y. Nakazawa: Division of Pulmonary and Critical Care Medicine, Allergy and Clinical Immunology, Medical University of South Carolina, Charleston, South Carolina 29425.

B. Ghebrehiwet: Department of Medicine, State University of New York, Health Science Center, Stony Brook, New York 11794.

Y. Shibayama: Nippon Zoki Pharmaceuticals, Osaka, Japan.

S. Reddigari: Enzyme Research Laboratories, South Bend, Indiana 46601.

in this chapter. Data suggest that the constituents of the plasma kinin-forming cascade are bound along the surfaces of cells such as endothelial cells, platelets, and neutrophils and that activation may occur along the cell surface.

PROTEIN CONSTITUENTS

Factor XII

Factor XII circulates as a single-chain zymogen with no detectable enzymatic activity (1). It has a molecular weight of 80,000 d on sodium dodecyl sulfate (SDS) gel electrophoresis (2) (Table 21-1). It is synthesized in the liver and circulates in plasma at a concentration of 30 to 35 μg/mL. Its primary sequence has been deduced from cDNA analysis (3,4) and from direct protein sequence data (5,6). The 596 amino acids present account for a molecular weight of 66,915 d; the remainder (16.8%) is carbohydrate. The protein has distinct domains homologous to fibronectin, plasminogen, and plasminogen activators (3,7) at its N-terminal end, and the COOH terminus has the catalytic domain. This latter portion is homologous to serine proteases such as pancreatic trypsin and even more so to the catalytic domain of plasminogen activators.

Factor XII is unusual because it is capable of autoactivating once it is bound to initiating surfaces (8,9). Factor XII that is bound undergoes a conformational change that renders it a substrate for factor XIIa (10). Gradually, all of the bound factor XII can be converted to factor XIIa. Whether plasma normally contains a trace amount of factor XIIa is unknown, but, if so, its concentration is less than 0.01% that of factor XII. The alternative is that the first molecule of factor XIIa is formed by interaction of two factor XII zymogens. In this case, any activity that

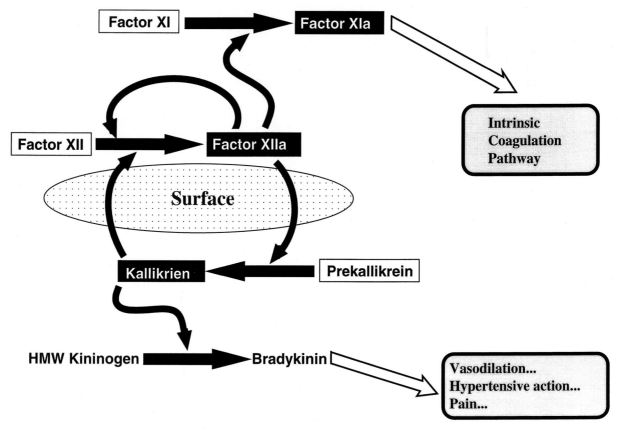

FIG. 21-1. The pathways of contact activation. *Open boxes,* zymogens; *black boxes,* proteases; *graded arrows,* activation reactions; *solid arrows,* catalytic activation.

the factor XII zymogen might possess is below the limits of detection (11). However, observations regarding activation along cell surfaces suggest possibilities for the generation of minute amounts of active enzymes that escape inhibition.

Activation of factor XII is caused by cleavage of the molecule at a critical Arg-Val bond (5). This bond is contained within a disulfide bridge, so that the resultant factor XIIa is a two-chain, disulfide-linked, 80-kd enzyme consisting of a heavy chain of 50 kd and a light chain of 28 kd (12). The light chain contains the enzymatic-active site (13) and is at the carboxyl-terminal end, whereas the heavy chain contains the binding site for the surface and

is at the amino-terminal end (14). Further cleavage can occur at the C-terminal end of the heavy chain to produce a series of fragments of activated factor XII that retain enzymatic activity (15,16). The most prominent of these is a 30-kd species termed factor XIIf. Careful examination of factor XIIf on SDS gels under nonreducing conditions has revealed a doublet in which the higher band, at 30 kd, is gradually converted to the lower band, at 28.5 kd (14). Reduced gels demonstrate that these species are comprised of the light chain of factor XIIa and a very small piece of the original heavy chain. These fragments lack the surface-binding site; they have lost much of the ability of factor XIIa to convert factor XI to factor XIa,

TABLE 21-1. *Physicochemical properties of proteins of the contact activation cascade*

Protein	Factor XII	Prekallikrein	Factor XI	HMW kininogen
Mass, calculated (daltons)	80,427	79,545	140,000	116,643
Carbohydrate (w/w)	16.8%	15%	5%	40%
Isoelectric point	6.3	8.7	8.6	4.7
Extinction coefficient ($E^{1\%}$ 280/nm)	14.2	11.7	13.4	7.0
Plasma concentration				
μg/mL	30–45	35–50	4–6	70–90
nmol/L (average)	400	534	36	686

HMW, high-molecular-weight.

and they do not participate in factor XII autoactivation. Nonetheless, these fragments remain potent activators of prekallikrein (15). Formation of factor XIIf allows bradykinin production to continue until the enzyme is inactivated. Thus the reactions can proceed at sites distant from the initiating surface. A diagrammatic representation of the cleavages in factor XII that generate factor XIIa and factor XIIf is shown in Figure 21-2.

Once factor XIIa interacts with prekallikrein, rapid conversion to kallikrein ensues. This is followed by an important positive feedback in which kallikrein digests surface-bound factor XII to form factor XIIa and then factor XIIf (13,18,19). This reaction is far more rapid than the autoactivation reaction (9,19), and the reciprocal reaction in which factor XII and prekallikrein interact to generate both factor XIIa and kallikrein is augmented by many thousands of times (9). Quantitatively, therefore, most of the factor XIIa or factor XIIf activity generated when plasma is activated results from kallikrein activation of factor XII. Yet, autoactivation can be demonstrated in plasma that is congenitally deficient in prekallikrein (Fletcher trait) and can-

not therefore generate any bradykinin (20-22). Clotting (i.e., conversion of factor XI to factor XIa by factor XIIa) does proceed, albeit at a much slower rate, and the partial thromboplastin time (PTT) progressively shortens as the time of incubation of the plasma with the surface is increased before recalcification. This is probably a result of factor XII autoactivation on the surface. As more and more factor XIIa forms, the rate of factor XI activation increases and the PTT approaches normal.

Prekallikrein

Prekallikrein is a zymogen without detectable proteolytic activity that is converted to kallikrein by cleavage during contact activation (23). On SDS gels, it has two bands, at 88 and 85 kd. The entire amino acid sequence of the protein has been determined by a combination of direct protein sequencing and amino acid sequence prediction from cDNAs isolated from a λgt-11 phage expression library (24). A signal peptide of 19 residues (which is cleaved off before secretion) is followed by the sequence

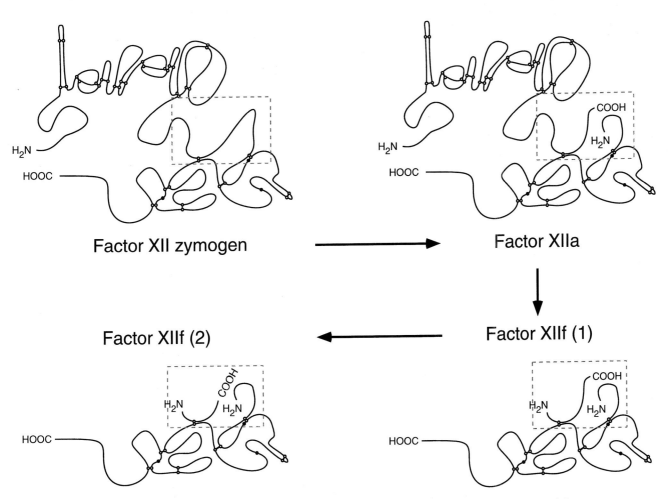

FIG. 21-2. Diagram of the activation of factor XII to factor XIIa and the sequential production of the two forms of factor XIIf.

of the mature plasma prekallikrein, which has 619 amino acids and a calculated molecular weight of 69,710 d. There is 15% carbohydrate as well. The heterogeneity observed by SDS gel electrophoresis is not reflected in the amino acid sequence, so it may be a result of two variant glycosylation forms. Activation of prekallikrein by factor XIIa or factor XIIf results from cleavage of a single Arg-Ile band within a disulfide bridge, so that a heavy chain of 56 kd is disulfide-linked to a light chain of either 33 or 36 kd, each of which has a DFP-inhibitable active site (16,25). This light chain heterogeneity reflects the two forms of the zymogen.

The amino acid sequence of the kallikrein heavy chain is unusual and is homologous only to the corresponding portion of factor XI. It has four tandem repeats, each of which contains approximately 90 to 91 amino acids. The presence of six cysteines per repeat suggests a repeating structure with three disulfide loops. It is postulated that a gene coding for the ancestor of this repeat sequence duplicated and that the entire segment duplicated again to give the present structure. The light chain, containing the active site, is homologous to many of the catalytic domains of other enzymes of the coagulation cascade.

In contrast to factor XII, prekallikrein does not circulate as a separate protein. It is bound to HK in a 1:1 bimolecular complex through a site on its heavy chain. The binding is firm, with a dissociation constant (K_d) of 12 to 15 nmol/L (26,27), a value that does not change on conversion of prekallikrein to kallikrein. About 80% to 90% of prekallikrein is normally complexed to HK in plasma. It is the prekallikrein-HK complex that binds to surfaces during contact activation, and the binding is primarily through HK (28), although some interaction of prekallikrein with the surface can be inferred (29). The dissociation of 10% to 20% of the kallikrein that forms along the surface may serve to propagate the formation of bradykinin in the fluid phase and at sites distant from the initiating reaction (8,30).

Prokallikrein and Tissue Kallikreins

Tissue kallikrein is a single-chain, acidic glycoprotein that is physicochemically and immunologically distinct from plasma kallikrein. The reported molecular weight ranges from 25 to 43 kd, and considerable heterogeneity is observed, primarily as a result of proteolysis after secretion. It is produced in abundance by organs such as the pancreas, salivary glands, and kidney (31), but it is actually widespread and can be found in colon (32), prostate, pituitary gland (33,34), and brain (35), as well as in neutrophils (33).

Within a given species, tissue kallikreins derived from all organs are immunologically identical (36), and cDNA cloning and subsequent analysis reveals the same amino acid sequence of 238 residues (37,38). In rodents, tissue kallikrein is a member of a large multigene family of more than 20 members; in humans, it is encoded by no more than two or three closely related genes, only one of which yields *bona fide* tissue kallikrein (37,39). Tissue kallikrein is synthesized within tissue cells as a preproenzyme that is converted intracellularly to tissue kallikrein. This reaction may be only partial. Urine, for example, contains a mixture of prokallikrein and tissue kallikrein (40). A multitude of isoelectric forms can be found, reflecting microheterogeneity caused by variable glycosylation. Intracellular conversion of prokallikrein to kallikrein occurs by means of enzymes that are not well characterized. Secreted prokallikrein can be converted to tissue kallikrein extracellularly by either plasmin or plasma kallikrein (40,41).

Factor XI

Coagulation factor XI is the second substrate of factor XIIa (see Fig. 21-1), but it has no role in bradykinin formation. Factor XI is unique among the clotting factors because the circulating zymogen consists of two identical chains linked by disulfide bonds (42,43). The dimer has an apparent molecular weight of 160 kd on SDS gel electrophoresis but reveals a single 80-kd protein on reduction. Factor XI activation follows the familiar pattern of cleavage of a single peptide band (Arg-Ile) within a disulfide bridge to yield an amino-terminal heavy chain of 50 kd and a disulfide-linked light chain of 33 kd. Since both subunits can be cleaved by factor XIIa and each resultant light chain bears a functional active site, factor XIa is a four-chain protein with two active sites. The concentration in plasma is only 4 to 8 µg/mL, the lowest among the contact proteins. Its heavy chain, like that of kallikrein, binds to the light chain of HK. Therefore, factor XI and HK also circulate as a complex (44). The K_d is 70 nmol/L (45), which is high enough to ensure that virtually all the factor XI is complexed. The molar ratio of the complex can consist of 1 or 2 molecules of HK per molecule of factor XI because of the dimeric nature of factor XI (46). The binding site of HK on factor XI has been localized to the first (N-terminal) tandem repeat (47). The factor XI–HK complex binds to the surface, and conversion to XIa by factor XIIf is only 2% to 4% that of surface-bound factor XIIa (16). The primary function of factor XIa is to activate factor IX to IXa, which is the first calcium-dependent reaction in the intrinsic coagulation cascade.

The amino acid sequence of human factor XI has been determined by cDNA analysis and is closely homologous to that of prekallikrein. It has a 19-amino-acid leader peptide followed by a 607-amino-acid sequence for each of the two chains of the mature protein. The amino acid sequence of the heavy chain of factor XIa, like that of kallikrein, has four tandem repeats of about 90 amino acids with six cysteines per repeat, implying three disulfide bands. Unpaired cysteines in the first and fourth repeats are postulated to form the interchain disulfide bridges between monomers that produce the homodimer.

High-Molecular-Weight Kininogen

HK circulates in plasma as a 115-kd, nonenzymatic glycoprotein at a concentration of 70 to 90 µg/mL (48-52). Its apparent molecular weight by gel filtration is aberrant at about 200,000 d, indicative of a large partial specific volume owing to its conformation in solution (27). It forms noncovalent complexes with both prekallikrein and factor XI, with a K_d of 15 nmol/L (26,53) and 70 nmol/L (45,54), respectively. There is sufficient HK in plasma to theoretically bind both factor XII substrates, and the excess HK (about 10% to 20%) circulates uncomplexed. The complexes of HK with prekallikrein or factor XI are formed with the light-chain region of HK; the isolated light chain (after reduction and alkylation) possesses the same binding characteristics as the whole molecule (54,55). HK functions as a coagulation cofactor, and this activity resides in the light chain (55). The light chain consists of a basic (histidine-rich) amino-terminal domain that binds to initiating surfaces (56) and a carboxyl-terminal domain that binds prekallikrein or factor XI (57). The one cysteine in the light chain links it to the heavy chain. The kallikrein binding site maps to residues 194–224 (45,57), and the factor XI site to residues 185–252 (45). Since these sites overlap, one molecule of HK can interact with only one molecule of prekallikrein or factor XI at a time.

During contact activation, kallikrein cleaves HK at two positions within a disulfide bridge, first at the C-terminal Arg-Ser (58,59) and then at the N-terminal Lys-Arg, to release the nonapeptide bradykinin (Arg-Pro-Pro-Gly-Phe-Ser-Pro-Phe-Arg). The two-chain, disulfide-linked, kinin-free HK that results from this activity consists of a heavy chain of 65,000 d and a light chain, variously reported at molecular weights of 46,000 to 49,000 d (53,58-61), that retains all light-chain functions. Tissue kallikrein can also digest HK to liberate kallidin, leaving the heavy chain disulfide-linked to a 56- to 62-kd light chain; the additional cleavage of the light chain to 46 to 49 kd is made by plasma kallikrein but not by tissue kallikrein (60). Tissue kallikrein is immunologically and structurally unrelated to plasma kallikrein. It is secreted by various organs or cells such as salivary glands, kidney, pancreas, prostate, pituitary gland, and neutrophils and is found in high concentrations in saliva, urine, and prostatic fluid. Its primary substrate is LK, but it can release kallidin from either HK or LK. Kallidin is functionally very similar to bradykinin, albeit slightly less potent. A plasma aminopeptidase (62) removes the N-terminal lysine to convert it to bradykinin.

The very unusual domain structure of HK is shown in Figure 21-3. Domain 5, the histidine-rich region at the N-terminal end of the light chain, binds to initiating surfaces. The binding of prekallikrein or factor XI at the C-terminal domain 6 of the light chain accounts for the cofactor function of HK in intrinsic coagulation and kinin generation. The complete amino acid sequence of HK has been determined as translated from the cDNA and by direct sequence analysis of the purified protein (63-66). HK has 626 amino acids, with a calculated molecular weight of 69,896 d. An unusually high content of carbohydrate accounts for 40% of the observed molecular

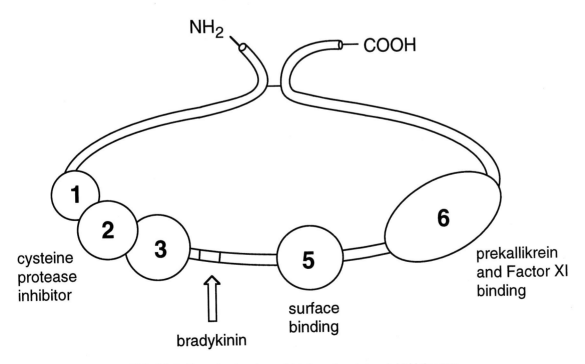

FIG. 21-3. Domain structure of high-molecular-weight kininogen.

weight of 115 kd. The heavy chain of 362 residues is derived from the amino terminus. This is followed by the 9-residue bradykinin (domain 4) sequence and then the light chain of 265 residues. The N-terminal end is blocked with pyroglutamic acid (cyclic glutamate). The carbohydrate is distributed via three N-linked glycosidic linkages on the heavy chain and nine O-linked glycosidic linkages on the light chain. The heavy chain has three contiguous and homologous apple-type domains consisting of residues 1–116, 117–238, and 239–360 (see Fig. 21-3). There are 17 cysteines; one of them is disulfide-linked to the light chain, and the others form eight disulfide loops within these domains (63). The three domains on the heavy chain are homologous to the cystatin family of protease inhibitors (e.g., sulfhydryl proteases such as cathepsins). Domains 2 and 3 (but not domain 1) retain this inhibitory function; for example, native HK can bind and inactivate 2 molecules of papain (67-70). Limited proteolysis of the heavy chain can occur at susceptible bonds that separate the domains; in this manner, individ-

ual domains can be isolated. Cleavage at these sites may occur under certain pathologic conditions.

Low-Molecular-Weight Kininogen and Kininogen Genes

Another precursor of bradykinin in plasma is LK. Its digestion by tissue kallikrein yields kallidin and a kinin-free two-chain molecule consisting of a 65-kd heavy chain disulfide-linked to a light chain of only 4 kd (63,65,71-73). LK is not cleaved by plasma kallikrein. The amino acid sequences of HK and LK are identical from the amino terminus through the bradykinin sequence plus the next 12 residues (73), after which the two sequences diverge. LK does not bind to surfaces or to prekallikrein or factor XI. The kininogens are produced from a single gene that is thought to have originated from two successive duplications of a primordial cystatin-like gene (64). As represented in Figure 21-4, there are 11 exons. The first nine code for the heavy chain, with each of the three domains in

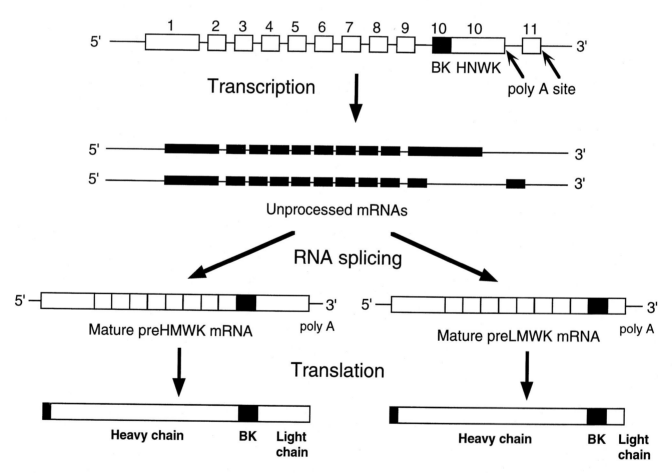

FIG. 21-4. The gene for high-molecular-weight kininogen (HMWK). The boxes labeled 1 through 9 represent the exon coding for the heavy chain of both HMWK and low-molecular-weight kininogen (LMWK). Exon 10 codes for the bradykinin (BK) sequence and the light chain of HMWK. The mature mRNAs are assembled by alternative splicing events in which the light-chain sequences are attached to the 3′ end of the 12-amino-acid common-sequence C-terminal to BK.

this portion of the protein being represented by three exons. The tenth exon codes for bradykinin and the light chain of HK, and exon 11 encodes the light chain of LK. The mRNAs for HK and LK are produced by alternative splicing at a point 12 amino acids beyond the bradykinin sequence, thus enabling the two proteins to have different light chains (see Fig. 21-4).

BRADYKININ FORMATION BY CONTACT ACTIVATION

Contact activation was initially observed in the interaction of blood with glass surfaces (74); subsequently, finely derived kaolin was used extensively as an experimental surface and for coagulation assays such as the PTT (75). Ellagic acid (76), a tannin-like substance used as a component of many commercial assay systems, was purported to be a soluble initiator but was later shown to form large sedimentable aggregates catalyzed by trace heavy metal ions, so it too is particulate (77). Somewhat later, dextran sulfate (78,79) and sulfatide (78) were used to study contact activation. Although sulfatide, a galactose sulfate sphingolipid found in nerve tissue, is an activator, it occurs in quantities too small to be an effective one. However, when purified, it can form highly charged micelles that are very efficient initiators (80,81). Dextran sulfate is a truly soluble activator and a close homologue of naturally occurring sulfated mucopolysaccharides. High-molecular-weight preparations of 500 kd are typically used (9,11,78), but in a study of factor XII autoactivation (82) much smaller fractions were effective, down to as low as 5 kd. The rate of factor XII activation increased markedly with dextran sulfate at 10 kd (or more), a level at which the theoretical number of factor XII molecules capable of binding per particle increased from 1 to 2; similar results were seen with heparin. This presumably provides a critical intermolecular interaction required for optimal autoactivation.

Naturally occurring polysaccharides are effective if they are highly sulfated, and these include heparin and chondroitin sulfate E (described in rodent mucosal mast cells) (83). Other mucopolysaccharides known to catalyze factor XII autoactivation are dermatan sulfate, keratin polysulfate, and chondroitin sulfate C (84). The basement membrane of endothelial cell matrix may support contact activation, but this has not been demonstrated *in vivo*. Collagen, long thought to be an initiator, was proved to be ineffective, and the activity reported was possibly caused by contaminating matrix proteins. One pathophysiologic substance very likely to initiate contact activation *in vivo* is endotoxin (85-87). There is good reason to believe that the contact cascade is activated in septic shock and that the observed symptoms result, in part, from the generation of bradykinin (88,89). Crystals of uric acid and pyrophosphate also can initiate kinin formation by this pathway (90,91).

The various interactions of these constituents are shown in Fig. 21-5, which also includes the steps inhibited by C1 inhibitor (C1In). The autoactivation of factor XII as shown is very slow. However, the reciprocal reactions involving kallikrein contribute to a tremendously fast activation of factor XII, as illustrated by the finding that if one molecule each of factor XIIa and kallikrein per milliliter were present in a mixture of factor XII and prekallikrein at their plasma concentrations, 50% of factor XII would be activated in 13 seconds (9). This corresponds to a 5×10^{-13}% solution of active enzyme in the preparations. The source of the active enzyme is unknown, but it may be formed by other plasma proteases (e.g., plasmin) or by endogenous activation along cell surfaces. In fact, very slow turnover of the cascade may be ongoing (92-95) and controlled by plasma inhibitors (96). Introduction of a surface or other polyanionic substances could accelerate by many thousand-fold the baseline turnover of factor XII and prekallikrein to ignite the cascade. The addition of the cofactor HK (which was not included in the aforementioned kinetic analysis) accelerates these reactions even further, but a surface must be present.

The surface appears to create a local milieu in the contiguous fluid phase (1,80,97); there, the local concentrations of reactants are greatly increased, which increases the rates of the reciprocal interactions. In addition, surface-bound factor XII undergoes a conformational change that renders it more susceptible to cleavage (10). The alternative idea (29,98,99), that binding of factor XII induces a conformational change that exposes an active site, has essentially been disproved. Inhibitors such as C1In are not bound to the surface, so the balance between activation and inactivation is upset. Dilution of plasma diminishes the effect of inhibitors, far more than any slowing of enzymatic reaction rates. The net effect is, therefore, a marked augmentation of reaction rate.

When dextran sulfate was used, the effect of the surface on the rate of factor XIIa conversion of prekallikrein to kallikrein was increased 70-fold (9), and digestion of factor XII by kallikrein was increased by as much as 3,000- to 12,000-fold (9,100). This latter reaction is about 2,000-fold more rapid than the rate of factor XII autoactivation, and this kinetic dominance means that prekallikrein must be considered to be a coagulation factor. As indicated earlier, the PTT of prekallikrein-deficient plasma is much prolonged, but it does autocorrect as factor XII autoactivates on the surface. On the other hand, factor XII-deficient plasma has a markedly abnormal PTT, does not autocorrect, and is essentially devoid of intrinsic clotting or kinin formation. Alternatively, purified factor XII preparations activate when tested with a surface or polyanion under physiologic conditions (9,101,102), whereas prekallikrein does not. Hence, factor XII is considered to be absolutely requisite for intrinsic coagulation, whereas prekallikrein acts as an accelerator.

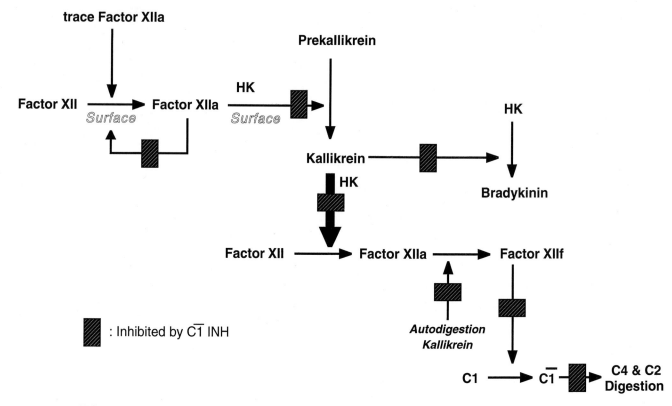

FIG. 21-5. The plasma kinin-forming cascade. The initiating autoactivation step, the positive feedback involving kallikrein, and a linkage to the complement cascade are depicted. All steps inhibitable by C1 inhibitor (C1 INH) are shown.

In plasma, the involvement of HK was indicated by the discovery of persons whose plasma had a very prolonged PTT and generated no bradykinin on incubation with kaolin, but who were not deficient in factor XII or prekallikrein (103-105). This phenomenon was explained by the identification of HK as a nonenzymatic cofactor in contact activation. It appeared to accelerate activation of both factor XII and prekallikrein, as well as factor XI (12,13,28,97). The discovery that prekallikrein and factor XII circulate, bound to HK, provided the mechanistic key to the explanation (49). One function of HK is to present the substrates of factor XIIa in a conformation that facilitates their activation. Prekallikrein that is bound to a surface in the absence of HK is not readily cleaved and cannot dissociate from the surface. A synthetic peptide containing the HK binding site for prekallikrein disrupts contact activation by competitively interfering with the binding of prekallikrein to the HK light chain (45); similarly, a monoclonal antibody to this binding site inhibits coagulation and kinin formation in plasma (106).

Factor XI activation depends almost totally on the formation of a surface-binding complex with HK. HK also augments the rate of factor XII activation in plasma (12,28), although it does not augment the activity of kallikrein against synthetic substrates. The effect seems to be largely indirect. First, it is required for efficient for-

mation of kallikrein in surface-activated plasma. Second, since kallikrein is able to dissociate from surface-bound HK, it can interact with surface-bound factor XII on an adjacent particle, thereby disseminating the reaction (8,28,30). As a result, the effective ratio of kallikrein to factor XII is increased in the presence of HK. Finally, in plasma, HK can displace other adhesive glycoproteins, such as fibrinogen, in binding to the surface (107). These data indicate that HK must also be considered to be a coagulation cofactor, because it is required for the generation of kallikrein (a factor XII activator) and for the activation of factor XI. HK-deficient plasma has a profoundly prolonged activated PTT that is almost as abnormal as that seen in patients with factor XII deficiency (103-105), although persons with congenital HK deficiency have no bleeding diathesis.

REGULATION OF THE KININ-FORMING PATHWAYS

Contact Activation

Regulation of contact activation occurs by means of plasma protease inhibitors. A summary of the major control proteins of this pathway is given in Table 21-2. The C1In is a major inhibitor of factor XIIa or XIIf (108-111),

TABLE 21-2. *Plasma inhibitors of enzymes of contact activation: relative contributions to inhibition in normal plasma*

Inhibitor	Enzyme			
	Factors		Kallikrein	Factor XIa
	XIIa	XIIf		
C1 Inhibitor	91.3	93	52 (84[a])	47
Antithrombin III[b]	1.5	4	n d	5
α_2-Macrogloblin	4.3	—	35 (16[a])	—
α_2-Protease inhibitor	—	—	nd	25
α_1-Antiplasmin	3.0	3	nd	8
α_1-Antitrypsin	—	—	5 (0)	23

nd, not determined separately
[a]Data obtained from generation of kallikrein *in situ*
[b]Data are for results obtained in the absence of added heparin

and it is not active against other coagulation enzymes except factor XIa. The inhibitor is cleaved by the protease and then binds at the active site of the protease in a 1 : 1 molar covalent complex that completely inactivates the enzyme (112). Antithrombin III, which is a critical control protein for much of the coagulation cascade, makes a minor contribution to factor XIIa(f) inactivation (108,110,113,114). Heparin can augment the inhibition by antithrombin III, although reports as to the magnitude of augmentation vary. Heparin can also function as an activating polyanion for contact activation (82,83). Curiously, α_2-macroglobulin, which is an inhibitor of broad reactivity with enzymes, does not significantly inhibit any of the forms of activated factor XII.

Kallikrein is inhibited by both C1In and α_2-macroglobulin (115-117), which together account for more than 90% of the inhibitory activity of plasma (118,119). α_2-macroglobulin does not bind to the active site; rather, it traps the protease within its structure so as to sterically interfere with its ability to cleave large protein substrates (120). About one third of the enzyme's activity on small synthetic substrates is retained by the complex, whereas the activity on its natural substrates is less than 1%. Although these two inhibitors contribute roughly equally when kallikrein is added to plasma (118,119,121), when a surface such as kaolin is added, 70% to 80% of the kallikrein formed is bound to C1In (121). The reason for this difference is unknown. Conversely, at low temperatures, C1In is less effective, and much of the kallikrein inhibition is mediated by α_2-macroglobulin (121).

Factor XIa is inhibited to a great extent by C1In (122,123). When purified factor XIa was added to plasma and its distribution among various inhibitors was determined, most of the added factor XIa was found complexed to C1In, even in the presence of heparin; complexes of factor XIa with α_1-antitrypsin were next most common, followed by factor XIa with α_2-antiplasmin. However α_1-antitrypsin was found to be the major inhibitor when chromatographic plasma fractions were tested for factor XIa inhibitory activity (124,125).

Antithrombin III has also been reported previously to inhibit factor XIa (122,125).

Activation on a surface occurs very quickly, whereas inhibition has a slower reaction rate. In plasma of patients with hereditary angioedema, in whom C1In is absent or dysfunctional, the amount of surface needed to produce maximal activation is 10- to 20-fold less than that needed to activate normal plasma (113).

Tissue Kallikrein

The tissue pathway for bradykinin formation is far simpler, because only tissue kallikrein is involved, regardless of which cell or tissue produces it. Tissue kallikrein (126) digests HK or LK to kallidin, and a plasma aminopeptidase rapidly converts kallidin to bradykinin (127). Kallidin and bradykinin possess similar biologic activities (see later discussion) and act on the same receptor, but in most assays, kallidin has 80% to 90% of the potency of bradykinin. Because the concentration of LK is much greater than that of HK, LK is preferentially cleaved. By contrast, plasma kallikrein is quite specific in utilizing HK as substrate.

The regulatory mechanisms of the tissue kallikrein pathway of bradykinin formation are not well known, and it was believed in the past that none of the inhibitors of the contact pathway were involved in controlling tissue kallikrein. However, Rahman et al. (128) detected tissue kallikrein–α_1-antitrypsin complexes in synovial fluid from rheumatoid arthritis patients. In porcine plasma, exogenously added tissue kallikrein was found, to some extent, to form complexes with α_2-macroglobulin and α_1-antitrypsin (129). However, tissue kallikrein activity was still present some 12 hours after the addition, suggesting that these macromolecular inhibitors may not provide significant regulation of tissue kallikrein in plasma. Since tissue kallikrein is not relevant to plasma kinin generation, the significance of these studies is unclear. Other kallikrein-binding proteins, such as kallistatin, which specifically binds and inhibits tissue kallikrein but not plasma kallikrein, have been identified in rat and human tissues (130). However the functional significance of this binding protein is still unclear. Peptide sequences analogous to the C-terminal sequence of kinins (Ac-Ser-Pro-Phe-Arg-Ser-Val-Gln-NH$_2$) have been reported to be potent synthetic inhibitors of tissue kallikrein (131).

Bradykinin Function and Control Mechanisms

The functions of bradykinin include venular dilatation, increased vascular permeability (132), constriction of uterine and gastrointestinal smooth muscle, constriction of coronary and pulmonary vasculature, bronchoconstriction, and activation of phospholipase A$_2$ to augment arachidonic acid metabolism. Bradykinin acts on most tissues by means of B2 receptors, and selective B2 receptor antagonists have been synthesized. In plasma, bradykinin is first digested by carboxypeptidase N (also known as anaphylatoxin inactivator) (133), which removes the C-terminal Arg, leaving des-Arg^9-bradykinin (134). This peptide lacks the inflammatory function of bradykinin (i.e., vasodilatation, increased permeability) that is evident in skin or smooth muscle, but it can interact with B1 receptors in the vasculature to cause hypotension. The major agonist for the B1 receptor is, however, des-Arg^{10}-kallidin. It has been reported that B1 receptors are induced during inflammatory conditions (132), whereas B2 receptors are synthesized constitutively. However, in cultured bovine pulmonary artery endothelial cells, Smith et al. showed that both B1 and B2 receptors are made constitutively (135).

When serum is examined, the rate of removal of the C-terminal Arg is more rapid than can be attributed to carboxypeptidase N (95). This may be a result of secretion (from cells) or activation of carboxypeptidase U, an exopeptidase (136). The next cleavage is by angiotensin-converting enzyme (ACE), which digests des-Arg^9-bradykinin (Arg-Pro-Pro-Gly-Phe-Ser-Pro-Phe) by its tripeptidase activity (137) (in contrast to the dipeptidase activity that converts angiotensin I to angiotensin II) to yield Arg-Pro-Pro-Gly-Phe plus Ser-Pro-Phe. These products are inactive on both B1 and B2 receptors. Further slow digestion leads to the final products of Arg-Pro-Pro, plus 1 mole each of the amino acids Gly, Ser, Pro, and Arg, and 2 moles of Phe (127).

In vivo, kinin degradation occurs rapidly along endothelial cells of the pulmonary vasculature. Here, however, the predominant enzyme is ACE, which acts as a dipeptidase if the C-terminal Arg is present to remove Phe-Arg. The resultant heptapeptide is cleaved once again at the C-terminal end to liberate Ser-Pro, leaving the pentapeptide Arg-Pro-Pro-Gly-Phe (137). These peptides are further metabolized to Arg-Pro-Pro and free amino acids, as indicated earlier. The cough and angioedema associated with the use of ACE inhibitors may be caused by the accumulation of bradykinin.

CELL SURFACE ASSEMBLY OF THE PLASMA KININ-FORMING CASCADE

All the components of the contact activation cascade have been demonstrated to bind to endothelial cells. Schmaier et al. (138) and van Iwaarden et al. (139) first described binding of HK to human umbilical vein endothelial cells in a zinc-dependent reaction. This binding subsequently was demonstrated *in situ* by immunochemical staining of umbilical cord segments after incubation with HK (140). The interaction of HK with the human umbilical vein endothelial cells is saturable, is reversible, depends on the presence of 25 to 50 µmol/L zinc (normal plasma concentration), and fulfills the characteristics of a receptor-mediated interaction. There are $1-3\times10^6$ binding sites with a high affinity (K$_d$, 40 to 50 nmol/L). Binding is seen with either the heavy or the light chain of HK, so a complex interaction with subsites within the receptor seems likely (141). A similar complex interaction has been observed with platelets, although the number of binding sites is far fewer. Since prekallikrein and factor XI circulate bound to HK, they are brought to the endothelial cell surface by HK (142). There are no separate receptor sites for either prekallikrein or factor XI. When we examined binding of factor XII, we found receptor binding characteristics strikingly similar to those seen with HK, including a requirement for zinc (141). We then demonstrated that HK and factor XII can compete for binding at a comparable molar basis, suggesting that they bind to the same receptor (94).

We also demonstrated that factor XII can slowly autoactivate when bound to endothelial cells (94) and that addition of kallikrein can digest bound HK to liberate bradykinin at a rate proportional to the kallikrein concentration and with a final bradykinin level dependent on the amount of bound HK. Therefore, activation of the cascade may occur along the endothelial cell surface, as illustrated in Figure 21-6; bradykinin is liberated and then interacts with the B2 receptor to increase permeability. Bradykinin also can stimulate cultured endothelial cells to secrete tissue plasminogen activator (143), prostaglandin I$_2$ (prostacyclin), and thromboxane A$_2$ (144,145) and can thereby modulate platelet function and stimulate local fibrinolysis.

Endothelial cell binding proteins have been isolated from cell membrane preparations, and a major binding protein for both HK and factor XII appears to be gC1qR, the receptor for the globular heads of C1q (146,147). Binding of factor XII and HK to gC1qR is zinc dependent; HK and factor XII compete with each other for binding; and use of site-specific monoclonal antisera localized the binding site to the C-terminal domain of gC1qR. The isolated heavy and light chains derived from kinin-free kininogen can each interact with endothelial cells (141); this binding has been shown to depend on domains 3 and 5, respectively (148,149), although bradykinin may link

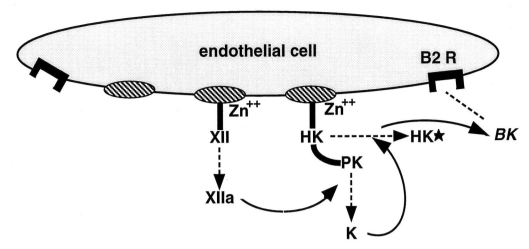

FIG. 21-6. Assembly of the proteins involved in bradykinin formation along the endothelial cell surface. A common receptor (gC1qR) binds factor XII and HK, an action that requires zinc ion. Bradykinin, once liberated, acts on the B2 receptor to activate endothelial cells and increase vascular permeability. (HK, HMW kininogen; PK, prekallikrein; K, kallikrein; HK*, cleaved HK; BK, bradykinin.)

the two sites and contribute to binding in the intact protein (150). The interaction with gC1qR appears to depend on the light chain (i.e., domain 5) (146). C1q itself binds to an N-terminal site and therefore does not compete with either HK or factor XII for binding, and the reaction of C1q with gC1qR is not zinc dependent. Finally, antisera to the relevant gC1qR domain inhibits HK binding to intact endothelial cells (147).

The interaction of the kinin-forming cascade with endothelial cells is yet more complex. Additional cell-derived proteins are involved, and observations may vary with the state of activation of the cell. Cleaved HK (a two-chain, disulfide-linked molecule with bradykinin removed) was found to bind to the receptor for urokinase (urokinase plasminogen activator receptor, or UPAR) in an analogous zinc-dependent reaction (151), and anti-receptor antibody also inhibited binding. It is not clear whether this occurs via the heavy chain (domain 3) or the light chain (domain 5). Others have described binding of HK to a cytokeratin on the endothelial cell surface (152,153), a case in which antibody to cytokeratin also inhibits HK binding. Finally, gC1qR expression at the endothelial cell surface has been questioned (154,155), because its concentration within the cell is far greater than at the surface and it lacks a transmembrane domain. However, other data confirm surface expression (156), and the calculated binding sites for C1q (157) are the same as the number of HK binding sites (94,139). HK and C1q do not, however, compete for binding to gC1qR, because C1q interacts with an N-terminal domain of gC1qR, whereas HK and factor XII bind to a C-terminal site (147).

Other observations suggest an additional level of interaction of the kinin cascade with fibrinolysis. For example, kallikrein converts prourokinase to urokinase (158), and prourokinase bound to UPAR is activated more readily. Therefore, if kallikrein is generated along the cell surface via HK interaction with UPAR, fibrinolysis can occur along the cell surface. There is also evidence that endothelial cells can secrete a cysteine-protease that converts prekallikrein to kallikrein (with prekallikrein bound to HK, which in turn is bound to the cell surface) in the absence of factor XII (159). We have confirmed this observation; however, the addition of factor XII markedly augments the rate of prekallikrein activation. Factor XII can be converted to factor XIIa by either autoactivation through binding to gC1qR (160); digestion by kallikrein formed by cysteine-protease activation of prekallikrein; or enzymatic activation of factor XII by a cell enzyme, as was suggested many years ago (161).

The interaction of HK (but not factor XII) with platelets has been studied extensively; it resembles that observed with endothelial cells qualitatively, but the quantitation is vastly different. Vascular endothelial cells have approximately 3×10^6 binding sites per cell, whereas platelets possess 1,000 times fewer sites. Binding of HK to platelets is zinc dependent; the heavy and light chains of HK can each bind (162), and the binding depends on domains 3 and 5, respectively (163). HK (domain 3) also inhibits the ability of thrombin to activate platelets, an activity not shared by factor XII (164). Because there appears to be no interaction of HK with thrombin, an interaction with the thrombin receptor or with a thrombin-binding protein is suggested. We have purified an HK-binding protein from platelet membranes that is indistinguishable from the α chain of glycoprotein 1b (glycocalicin) by affinity chromatography of platelet membranes and HK sepharose as ligand. Binding requires zinc, and the same protein binds factor XII and thrombin (165). The thrombin receptor copurifies with it, but it does not bind HK and may be linked within the membrane to glycoprotein 1b. Thrombospondin is an additional HK-binding protein derived from platelets that may participate in these reactions (166).

Other observations with regard to platelet interactions with proteins of the kinin-forming cascade are of interest. Bradford et al. reported that the HK inhibition of platelet aggregation is not observed in platelets that are congenitally deficient in the glycoprotein 1b–factor IX–factor V complex and that antisera to the complex also prevents the HK inhibition (167). These data indirectly support our observation that a key platelet membrane protein that binds HK domain 3 is in fact glycoprotein 1b (165).

Neutrophils also bind HK via the iC3b receptor (CR3) (168), which is absent on endothelial cells, and all components of the kinin-forming cascade can interact at the cell surface (169).

THE KININ SYSTEM AND DISEASE

Endotoxic Shock

Early studies of endotoxic shock suggested activation of the plasma kinin-forming cascade based on depletion of prekallikrein, formation of kallikrein complexes with C1In or α_2-macroglobulin, and HK depletion of cleavage (170,171). Direct activation of factor XII by endotoxic shock is also readily demonstrable (85). In a baboon model of endotoxic shock, activation of the plasma kinin-forming cascade was observed (172). In addition, infusion of a monoclonal antibody to factor XII inhibited the resultant hypotension, and mortality was significantly decreased (173). Any possible contribution of tissue kallikrein to HK cleavage or to kallidin or bradykinin formation was not assessed. The disseminated intravascular coagulation associated with endotoxic shock was not inhibited, indicating that it is independent of contact activation and is probably mediated by tissue factor.

Pancreatitis

Among the enzymes liberated from the pancreas in the course of acute hemorrhagic pancreatitis is tissue kallikrein; tissue kallikrein levels in peritoneal fluid are markedly increased. It is hypothesized that kinin formation contributes to the severe pooling of fluid in the abdominal cavity. Hypotension can be caused by hypovolemia as well as peripheral vasodilatation, and the mortality rate is high.

Alzheimer's Disease

The protein associated with Alzheimer's disease (Aβ) has been shown to bind HK and factor XII in a zinc-dependent reaction that requires aggregation of Aβ (174). Aggregation of Aβ is similarly zinc dependent, or at least zinc accelerated (175). Binding of factor XII to Aβ leads to gradual autoactivation, and prominent conversion of prekallikrein to kallikrein is observed on incubation of aggregated Aβ with factor XII, prekallikrein, and HK in the presence of 50 μmol/L zinc. The reaction is strictly factor XII dependent. Factor XII has also been found bound to the plaques of patients with Alzheimer's disease. Together, the data suggest activation of the plasma kinin-forming cascade in the brains of patients with Alzheimer's disease, and the likely initiator is aggregated Aβ, which is present in senile plaques.

Hereditary Angioedema

Although absence of C1In or presence of a dysfunctional C1In is clearly the cause of the swelling that characterizes hereditary angioedema and the various forms of acquired C1In deficiency, the identity of the vasoactive peptide responsible for the increased vascular permeability is uncertain. The bulk of evidence favors bradykinin. Incubation of plasma from patients with hereditary angioedema leads to evolution of bradykinin as the sole identifiable vasoactive substance (176,177). During attacks of angioedema, depletion of prekallikrein and HK occurs (178), and blisters induced on the skin of such patients contain increased levels of plasma kallikrein (179). Because complement is activated in this disorder, with diminished levels of C4 and C2 during attacks, an alternative consideration, for which there is some evidence, is that a vasoactive peptide may be cleaved from C2 or C2b by enzymes such as plasmin (180), which has bradykinin-like properties. It has not been possible, however, to demonstrate this peptide by direct cleavage of C2 or C2b (176,177), however, such a peptide seems to be present within the C2b amino acid sequence, as identified by testing of synthetic peptides for permeability-increasing capability (181). Nevertheless, the proponents of this alternative have very recently isolated a vasoactive factor from normal plasma or from C2-deficient plasma from which C1In was depleted, and identified the peptide as bradykinin (182). An atypical C1In mutation, which inhibits C1 but not enzymes of the kinin-forming cascade, has been described, which also points to bradykinin as the most likely pathogenic peptide.

Allergic Disease

Activation of the plasma and tissue kinin-forming systems has been observed in allergic reactions in the nose, lungs, and skin. This activation includes both the immediate reaction and the late phase reaction, although the contributions of the plasma and tissue kallikrein pathways to each aspect of allergic inflammation are probably different. Antigen challenge of the nose, followed by nasal lavage, has revealed an increase in tosyl arginine methyl ester (TAME) esterase activity that is largely attributable to kallikreins (183). The activation has been seen during both the immediate response and the late phase reaction (184). Both LK and HK have been shown to be present in nasal lavage fluids (185), and fractionation of nasal washings has demonstrated evidence of both tissue kallikrein (186) and plasma kallikrein (187). Tissue kallikrein can be secreted by glandular tissue or by infiltrating cells such as neutrophils, and it digests HK to yield kallidin. Plasma kallikrein digests HK to yield bradykinin directly. High-performance liquid chromatographic analysis of kinins in nasal washings have revealed both kallidin and bradykinin. Although the latter can be formed from kallidin by aminopeptidase action, a portion of the bradykinin is likely to be the direct result of plasma kallikrein activity. Tissue kallikrein also has been found in bronchoalveolar lavage fluids of asthmatics (188), and bradykinin can be a stimulus for neuropeptide release from sensory nerve endings.

Studies of allergen-induced late phase reaction in the skin (189) have demonstrated the presence of kallikrein-C1In and activated factor XIIa–C1In complexes in induced blisters observed for an 8-hour period. Increased levels of those complexes were seen at 3 to 6 hours, coincident with the late phase response, and were specific for the allergen to which the patient was sensitive.

Hypertension

Bradykinin has been considered to be a counterbalance to the renin-angiotensin system in the control of blood pressure. Therefore, it is possible that diminished generation of bradykinin could be a cause or a contributor to the pathogenesis of essential hypertension. There are no primary data in humans, but in rodent models of hypertension there is an association of essential hypertension with diminished levels of tissue kallikrein in urine, and presumably with diminished tissue kinin levels. Of particular interest is a study of the efficacy of ACE inhibitors in the treatment of hypertension. Although levels of angiotensin II are diminished, it is possible that increased bradykinin levels contribute to the lowering of blood pressure. Consistent with that possibility is the observation that administration of B2-receptor antagonists can reverse the therapeutic effect of the ACE inhibitor. This observation also lends support to the idea that increased bradykinin levels are responsible for ACE-induced angioedema or cough (190).

REFERENCES

1. Silverberg M, Diehl SV. The activation of the contact system of human plasma by polysaccharide sulfates. *Ann N Y Acad Sci* 1987;516: 268–279.
2. Revak SD, Cochrane CG, Griffin JH. The binding and cleavage characteristics of human Hageman factor during contact activation: a comparison of normal plasma with plasma deficient in factor XI, prekallikrein, or high molecular weight kininogen. *J Clin Invest* 1977; 58:1167.
3. Cool DE, Edgell CS, Louie GV, Zoller MJ, Brayer GD, MacGillivray RTA. Characterization of human blood coagulation factor XII cDNA. *J Biol Chem* 1985;25:13666–13676.
4. Que BG, Davie EW. Characterization of a cDNA coding for human factor XII (Hageman factor). *Biochemistry* 1986;8:1525–1528.
5. Fujikawa K, McMullen BA. Amino acid sequence of human β-factor XIIa. *J Biol Chem* 1983;258:10924–10933.
5. Proctor RR, Rapaport SI. The partial thromboplastin time with kaolin: a simple screening test for first stage clotting deficiencies. *Am J Clin Pathol* 1961;35:212.
6. McMullen BA, Fujikawa K. Amino acid sequence of the heavy chain of human α-factor XIIa (activated Hageman factor). *J Biol Chem* 1985;260:5328–5341.
7. Castellino FJ, Beals JM. The genetic relationships between the kringle domains of human plasminogen, prothrombin, tissue plasminogen activator, urokinase, and coagulation factor XII. *J Mol Evol* 1987;26: 358–369.
8. Silverberg M, Nicoll JE, Kaplan AP. The mechanism by which the light chain of cleaved HMW-kininogen augments the activation of prekallikrein, factor XI, and Hageman factor. *Thromb Res* 1980;20: 173–189.
9. Tankersley DL, Finlayson JS. Kinetics of activation and autoactivation of human factor XII. *Biochemistry* 1984;23:273–279.
10. Griffin JH. Role of surface in surface-dependent activation of Hageman factor (blood coagulation factor XII). *Proc Natl Acad Sci U S A* 1978;75:1998–2002.
11. Silverberg M, Kaplan AP. Enzymatic activities of activated and zymogen forms of human Hageman factor (factor XII). *Blood* 1982;60: 64–70.
12. Revak SD, Cochrane CG, Johnston AR, Hugli TE. Structural changes accompanying enzymatic activation of human Hageman factor. *J Clin Invest* 1974;54:619–627.
13. Meier HL, Pierce JV, Colman RW, Kaplan AP. Activation and function of human Hageman factor: the role of high molecular kininogen and prekallikrein. *J Clin Invest* 1977;60:18–31.
14. Pixley RA, Stumpo LG, Birkmeyer K, Silver L, Colman RW. A monoclonal antibody recognizing an icosapeptide sequence in the heavy chain of human factor XII inhibits surface-catalyzed activation. *J Biol Chem* 1987;262:10140–10145.
15. Kaplan AP, Austen KF. A prealbumin activator of prekallikrein. *J Immunol* 1970;105:802–811.
16. Kaplan AP, Austen KF. A prealbumin activator of prekallikrein II: derivation of activators of prekallikrein from active Hageman factor by digestion with plasmin. *J Exp Med* 1971;133:696–712.
17. Dunn JT, Kaplan AP. Formation and structure of human Hageman factor fragments. *J Clin Invest* 1982;70:627.
18. Cochrane CG, Revak SD, Wuepper KD. Activation of Hageman factor in solid and fluid phases: a critical role of kallikrein. *J Exp Med* 1973;138:1564.
19. Dunn JT, Silverberg M, Kaplan AP. The cleavage and formation of activated human Hageman factor by autodigestion and by kallikrein. *J Biol Chem* 1982;257:1779–1784.
20. Saito H, Ratnoff OD, Donaldson VH. Defective activation of clotting, fibrinolytic, and permeability-enhancing systems in human Fletcher trait. *Circ Res* 1974;34:641–651.
21. Weiss AS, Gallin JI, Kaplan AP. Fletcher factor deficiency: a diminished rate of Hageman factor activation caused by absence of prekallikrein with abnormalities of coagulation, fibrinolysis, chemotactic activity and kinin generation. *J Clin Invest* 1974;53:622–633.
22. Wuepper KD. Prekallikrein deficiency in man. *J Exp Med* 1973;138: 1345–1355.
23. Mandle RJ, Kaplan AP. Hageman factor substrates: II. Human plasma prekallikrein: mechanism of activation by Hageman factor and participation in Hageman factor-dependent fibrinolysis. *J Biol Chem* 1977; 252:6097.
24. Chung DW, Fujikawa K, McMullen BA, Davie EW. Human plasma prekallikrein, a zymogen to a serine protease that contains four tandem repeats. *Biochemistry* 1986;25:2410–2417.
25. Bouma BN, Miles LA, Barretta G, Griffin JH. Human plasma prekallikrein: studies of its activated factor XII and of its inactivation by diisopropyl phosphofluoridate. *Biochemistry* 1980;19:1151.
26. Bock PE, Shore JD, Tans G, Griffin JH. Protein-protein interactions in contact activation of blood coagulation: binding of high molecular weight kininogen and the 5-(iodoacetamido) fluorescein-labeled kinino-

gen light chain to prekallikrein, kallikrein, and the separated kallikrein heavy and light chains. *J Biol Chem* 1985;260:12434–12443.

27. Mandle RJ, Colman RW, Kaplan AP. Identification of prekallikrein and high molecular weight kininogen as a complex in human plasma. *Proc Natl Acad Sci U S A* 1976;73:4179–4183.

28. Wiggins RC, Bouma BN, Cochrane CG, Griffin JH. Role of high molecular weight kininogen in surface binding and activation of coagulation factor XI and prekallikrein. *Proc Natl Acad Sci U S A* 1977;77:4636.

29. McMillin CR, Saito H, Ratnoff OD, Walton AG. The secondary structure of human Hageman factor (factor XII) and its alteration by activating agents. *J Clin Invest* 1974;54:1312.

30. Cochrane CG, Revak SD. Dissemination of contact activation in plasma by plasma kallikrein. *J Exp Med* 1980;152:608–619.

31. Ole-Moiyoi O, Spragg J, Helbert SP. Immunologic reactivity of purified human urinary kallikrein (urokallikrein) with anti-serum directed against human pancreas. *J Immunol* 1977;118:667.

32. Schachter M, Peret MW, Billing AG. Immunolocalization of protease kallikrein in the color. *J Histochem Cytochem* 1983;31:1255.

33. Figueroa C, Maciver AG, Bhoola KD. Identification of tissue kallikrein in human polymorphonuclear leukocytes. *Br J Haematol* 1989;72:321.

34. Powers CA, Nasjletti A. A novel kinin generating protease (kininogenase) in the porcine anterior pituitary. *J Biol Chem* 1982;257:5594.

35. Chao J, Woodley-Miller C, Chao L. Identification of tissue kallikrein in brain and in the cell-free translation product encoded by brain mRNA. *J Biol Chem* 1983;258:15173.

36. Fritz H, Fiedler F, Dietl T. On the relationship between porcine pancreatic, submandibular and urinary kallikrein. In: Haberland GL, Rohen JW, Suzuki T, eds. *Kininogenases: kallikrein.* New York: Schattauer-Verlag, 1977:15.

37. Baker AR, Shine J. Human kidney kallikrein: cDNA cloning and sequence analysis. *DNA* 1985;4:445.

38. Fukushima D, Kitamura N, Nakanishi S. Nucleotide sequence of cloned cDNA for human pancreatic kallikrein. *Biochemistry* 1985;24:8037.

39. Wines DR, Brady JM, Pritchett DB. Organization and expression of the rat kallikrein gene family. *J Biol Chem* 1989;264:7653.

40. Takada Y, Skidgel RA, Erdos EG. Purification of human urinary prokallikrein: identification of the site of activation by the metalloproteinase thermolysin. *Biochem J* 1985;232:851.

41. Takahaski S, Irie A, Katayama Y, Ito K, Miyake Y. N-terminal amino acid sequence of human urinary prokallikrein. *J Biochem (Tokyo)* 1986;99:989–992.

42. Bouma BN, Griffin JH. Human blood coagulation factor XI: purification, properties, and mechanism of activation by factor XII. *J Biol Chem* 1977;252:6432.

43. Kurachi K, Davie EW. Activation of human factor XI (plasma thromboplastin antecedent) by factor XII (activated Hageman factor). *Biochemistry* 1977;16:5831.

44. Thompson RE, Mandle RJ, Kaplan AP. Association of factor XI and high molecular weight kininogen in human plasma. *J Clin Invest* 1977;60:1376–1380.

45. Tait J, Fujikawa K. Primary structure requirements for the binding of human high molecular weight kininogen to plasma prekallikrein and factor XI. *J Biol Chem* 1987;262:11651–11656.

46. Warn-Cramer BJ, Bajaj SP. Stoichiometry of binding of high molecular weight kininogen to factor XI/XIA. *Biochem Biophys Res Commun* 1985;133:417.

47. Baglia FA, Sinha D, Walsh PN. Functional domains in the heavy-chain region of factor XI: a high molecular weight kininogen-binding site and a substrate binding site for factor IX. *Blood* 1989;74:244–251.

48. Adam A, Albert A, Calay G, Closset J, Damas J, Franchimont P. Human kininogens of low and high molecular mass: quantification by radioimmunoassay and determination of reference values. *Clin Chem* 1985;31:423–426.

49. Berrettini M, Lammle B, White T, et al. Detection of *in vitro* and *in vivo* cleavage of high molecular weight kininogen in human plasma by immunoblotting with monoclonal antibodies. *Blood* 1986;68:455–462.

50. Colman RW, Müller-Esterl W. Nomenclature of kininogens. *Thromb Haemost* 1988;60:340–341.

51. Proud D, Pierce JV, Pisano JJ. Radioimmunoassay of human high molecular weight kininogen in normal and deficient plasma. *J Lab Clin Med* 1980;95:563.

52. Reddigari SR, Kaplan AP. Quantification of human high molecular weight kininogen by immunoblotting with a monoclonal anti-light chain antibody. *J Immunol Methods* 1989:19–25.

53. Bock PE, Shore JD. Protein-protein interactions in contact activation of blood coagulation: characterization of fluorescein-labeled human high molecular weight kininogen-light chain as a probe. *J Biol Chem* 1983;258:15079–15086.

54. Thompson RE, Mandle RJ, Kaplan AP. Studies of the binding of prekallikrein and factor XI to high molecular weight kininogen and its light chain. *Proc Natl Acad Sci U S A* 1979;79:4862.

55. Thompson RE, Mandle RJ, Kaplan AP. Characterization of human high molecular weight kininogens: procoagulant activity associated with the light chain of kinin-free molecular weight kininogen. *J Exp Med* 1978;147:488.

56. Ikari N, Sugo T, Fujii S, Kato H, Iwanaga S. The role of bovine high molecular weight kininogen in contact-mediated activation of bovine factor XII: interaction of HMW kininogen with kaolin and plasma prekallikrein. *J Biochem (Tokyo)* 1981;89:1699–1701.

57. Tait J, Fujikawa K. Identification of the binding site plasma prekallikrein in human high molecular weight kininogen. *J Biol Chem* 1986;261:15396–15401.

58. Mori K, Nagasawa S. Studies on human high molecular weight (HMW) kininogen: II. Structural change in HMW kininogen by the action of human plasma kallikrein. *J Biochem (Tokyo)* 1981;89:1465–1473.

59. Mori K, Sakamoto W, Nagasawa S. Studies on human high molecular weight (HMW) kininogen: III. Cleavage of HMW kininogen by the action human salivary kallikrein. *J Biochem (Tokyo)* 1981;90:503–509.

60. Reddigari SR, Kaplan AP. Cleavage of high molecular weight kininogen by purified kallikreins and upon contact activation of plasma. *Blood* 1988;71:1334–1340.

61. Schiffman S, Mannhalter C, Tynerk D. Human high molecular weight kininogen: effects of cleavage by kallikrein on protein structure and procoagulant activity. *J Biol Chem* 1980;255:6433.

62. Guimaraes JA, Borges DR, Prado ES, Prado JL. Kinin converting aminopeptidase from human serum. *Biochem Pharmacol* 1973;22:403.

63. Kellermann J, Lottspeich F, Henschen A, Müller-Esterl W. Completion of the primary structure of human high molecular weight kininogen: the amino acid sequence of the entire heavy chain and evidence for its evolution by gene triplication. *Eur J Biochem* 1986;154:471–478.

64. Kitamura N, Kitagawa H, Fukushima D, Takagaki Y, Miyata T, Nakanishi S. Structural organization of the human kininogen gene and a model for its evolution. *J Biol Chem* 1985;260:8610–8617.

65. Lottspeich F, Kellermann J, Henschen A, Foertsch B, Müller-Esterl W. The amino acid sequence of the light chain of human high molecular mass kininogen. *Eur J Biochem* 1985;152:307–314.

66. Takagaki Y, Kitamura N, Nakanishi S. Cloning and sequence analysis of cDNAs for high molecular weight and low molecular weight prekininogens. *J Biol Chem* 1985;260:8601–8609.

67. Gounaris AD, Brown MA, Barrett AJ. Human plasma α1-cysteine proteinase inhibitor: purification by affinity chromatography, characterization, and isolation of an active fragment. *Biochem J* 1984;221:445.

68. Higashiyama S, Ohkubo I, Ishiguro H, Kunimatsu M, Sawaki K, Sasaki M. Human high molecular weight kininogen as a thiol protease inhibitor: presence of the entire inhibition capacity in the native form of heavy chain. *Biochemistry* 1986;25:1669–1675.

69. Ishiguro H, Higashiyama S, Ohkubo I, Sasaki M. Mapping of functional domains of human high molecular weight and low molecular weight kininogens using murine monoclonal antibodies. *Biochemistry* 1987;26:7021–7029.

70. Müller-Esterl W, Fritz H, Machleidt IW, et al. Human plasma kininogens are identical with α2-cysteine protease inhibitors: evidence from immunological, enzymological, and sequence data. *FEBS Lett* 1985;182:310–314.

71. Jacobsen S, Kritz M. Some data on two purified kininogens from human plasma. *Br J Pharmacol* 1967;29:25.

72. Johnson DA, Salveson G, Brown M, Barrett AJ. Rapid isolation of human kininogens. *Thromb Res* 1987;48:187–193.

73. Müller-Esterl W, Rauth G, Lottspeich F, Kellermann J, Henschen A. Limited proteolysis of human low-molecular mass kininogen by tissue kallikrein: isolation and characterization of the heavy and light chains. *Eur J Biochem* 1985;149:15.

74. Margolis J. Activation of plasma by contact with glass: evidence for a common reaction which releases plasma kinin and initiates coagulation. *J Physiol* 1958;144:1.

76. Ratnoff OD, Crum JD. Activation of Hageman factor by solutions of ellagic acid. *J Lab Clin Med* 1964;63:359–377.

77. Bock PE, Srinivasan KR, Shore JD. Activation of intrinsic blood coagulation by ellagic acid: insoluble ellagic acid metal ion complexes are the activating species. *Biochemistry* 1981;20:7258–7271.

78. Fujikawa K, Heimark RL, Kurachi K, Davie EW. Activation of bovine factor XII (Hageman factor) by plasma kallikrein. *Biochemistry* 1980; 19:1322–1330.

79. Kluft C. Determination of prekallikrein in human plasma: optimal conditions for activating prekallikrein. *J Lab Clin Med* 1978;91:83–93.

80. Griep MA, Fujikawa K, Nelsestuen GL. Binding and activation properties of human factor XII, prekallikrein and derived peptides with acidic lipid vesicles. *Biochemistry* 1985;24:4124–4130.

81. Tans G, Griffin JH. Properties of sulfatides in factor XII dependent contact activation. *Blood* 1982;59:69.

82. Silverberg M, Diehl SV. The autoactivation of factor XII (Hageman factor) induced by low-Mr heparin and dextran sulphate: the effect of the Mr of the activating polyanion. *Biochem J* 1987;248:715–720.

83. Hojima Y, Cochrane CG, Wiggins RC, Austen KF, Stevens RL. *In vitro* activation of the contact (Hageman factor) system of plasma by heparin and chondroitin sulfate E. *Blood* 1984;63:1453–1459.

84. Brunnée T, Reddigari SR, Shibayama Y, Salerno V, Kaplan AP, Silverberg M. Activation of the contact system by glycosaminoglycan derived from mast cell proteoglycan. *Clin Exp Allergy* 1997;27:653–663.

85. Morrison DC, Cochrane CG. Direct evidence for Hageman factor (factor XII) activation by bacterial lipopolysaccharides (endotoxins). *J Exp Med* 1974;140:787.

86. Pettinger MA, Young R. Endotoxin-induced kinin (bradykinin) formation: activation of Hageman factor and plasma kallikrein in human plasma. *Life Sci* 1970;9:313.

87. Roeise O, Bouma BN, Stadaas JO, Aasen AO. Dose dependence of endotoxin-induced activation of the plasma contact system: an *in vitro* study. *Circ Shock* 1988;26:419–430.

88. Kaufman N, Page JD, Pixley RA, Schein R, Schmaier AH, Colman RW. α2-Macroglobulin-kallikrein complexes detect contact system activation in hereditary angioedema and human sepsis. *Blood* 1991;77:2660–2667.

89. Mason JW, Kleeberg UR, Dolan P, Colman RW. Plasma kallikrein and Hageman factor in gram-negative bacteremia. *Ann Intern Med* 1970; 73:545.

90. Ginsberg M, Jaques B, Cochrane CG, Griffin JH. Urate crystal dependent cleavage of Hageman factor in human plasma and synovial fluid. *J Lab Clin Med* 1980;95:497.

91. Kellermeyer RW, Breckenridge RT. The inflammatory process in acute gouty arthritis, I: activation of Hageman factor by sodium urate crystals. *J Lab Clin Med* 1965;63:307.

92. Bernardo MM, Day DF, Halvarson HR, Olson ST, Shore JD. Surface-independent acceleration of factor XII activation by zinc ions: II. Direct binding and fluorescence studies. *J Biol Chem* 1993;268: 12477.

93. Bernardo MM, Day DF, Olson ST, Shore JD. Surface-independent acceleration of factor XII activation by zinc ions: I. Kinetic characterization of the metal ion rate enhancement. *J Biol Chem* 1993;268: 12468–12476.

94. Reddigari SR, Shibayama Y, Brunnée T, Kaplan AP. Human Hageman factor (factor XII) and high molecular weight kininogen compete for the same binding site on human umbilical vein endothelial cells. *J Biol Chem* 1993;268:11982–11987.

95. Shibayama Y, Brunnée T, Kaplan AP. Activation of human Hageman factor (factor XII) in the presence of zinc and phosphate ions. *Braz J Med Biol Res* 1994;27:1817.

96. Weiss R, Silverberg M, Kaplan AP. The effect of C1 inhibitor upon Hageman factor autoactivation. *Blood* 1986;68:239–243.

97. Griffin JH, Cochrane CG. Mechanisms for the involvement of high molecular weight kininogen in surface-dependent reactions of Hageman factor. *Proc Natl Acad Sci U S A* 1976;73:2554.

98. Kurachi K, Fujikawa K, Davie EW. Mechanism of activation of bovine factor XI by factor XII and factor XIIa. *Biochemistry* 1980:19: 1330–1338.

99. Ratnoff OD, Saito H. Amidolytic properties of single chain activated Hageman factor. *Proc Natl Acad Sci U S A* 1979;76:1411.

100. Rosing J, Tans G, Griffin JH. Surface-dependent activation of human factor XII by kallikrein, and its light chain. *Eur J Biochem* 1985;151: 531–538.

101. Silverberg M, Dunn JT, Garen L, Kaplan AP. Autoactivation of human Hageman factor: demonstration utilizing a synthetic substrate. *J Biol Chem* 1980;255:7281–7286.

102. Tans G, Rosing J, Griffin JD. Sulfatide dependent autoactivation of human blood coagulation factor XII (Hageman factor). *J Biol Chem* 1983;258:8215.

103. Colman RW, Bagdasarian A, Talamo RC, et al. Williams trait: human kininogen deficiency with diminished levels of plasminogen proactivator and prekallikrein associated with abnormalities of the Hageman factor-dependent pathways. *J Clin Invest* 1975;56:1650–1662.

104. Donaldson VH, Glueck HI, Miller MA. Kininogen deficiency in Fitzgerald trait: role of high molecular weight kininogen in clotting and fibrinolysis. *J Lab Clin Med* 1976;89:327.

105. Wuepper KD, Miller DR, LaCombe MJ. Flaujeac trait: deficiency of human plasma kininogen. *J Clin Invest* 1975;56:1663.

106. Reddigari SR, Kaplan AP. Monoclonal antibody to human high molecular weight kininogen recognizes its prekallikrein binding site and inhibits its coagulant activity. *Blood* 1989;72:695–702.

107. Schmaier AH, Silver L, Adams AL, et al. The effect of high molecular weight kininogen on surface-adsorbed fibrinogen. *Thromb Res* 1984;33:51–67.

108. de Agostini A, Lijnen HR, Pixley RA, Colman RW, Schapira M. Inactivation of factor XII active fragment in normal plasma: predominant role of C1-inhibitor. *J Clin Invest* 1984;73:1542.

109. Forbes CO, Pensky J, Ratnoff OD. Inhibition of activated Hageman factor and activated plasma thromboplastin antecedent by purified C1 inactivator. *J Lab Clin Med* 1970;76:809.

110. Pixley RA, Schapira M, Colman RW. The regulation of human factor XII by plasma proteinase inhibitors. *J Biol Chem* 1985;260:1723–1729.

111. Schreiber AD, Kaplan AP, Austen KF. Inhibition by C1 INH of Hageman factor fragment activation of coagulation, fibrinolysis, and kinin generation. *J Clin Invest* 1973;52:1402.

112. Travis J, Salvesen GS. Human plasma proteinase inhibitors. *Ann Rev Biochem* 1983;52:655–709.

113. Cameron CL, Fisslthaler B, Sherman A, Reddigari S, Silverberg M. Studies on contact activation: effects of surface and inhibitors. *Med Prog Technol* 1989;15:53–62.

114. Stead N, Kaplan AP, Rosenberg RD. Inhibition of activated factor XII by antithrombin-heparin cofactor. *J Biol Chem* 1976;251:6481–6488.

115. Gigli I, Mason JW, Colman RW, Austen KF. Interaction of plasma kallikrein with C1 inhibitor. *J Immunol* 1970;104:574.

116. Harpel PC. Circulatory inhibitors of human plasma kallikrein. In: *Chemistry and biology of the kallikrein-kinin system in health and disease.* Fogerty International Center Proceedings. No. 27 1974;27:169.

117. McConnell DJ. Inhibitors of kallikrein in human plasma. *J Clin Invest* 1972;51:1611.

118. Schapira M, Scott CF, Colman RW. Contribution of plasma protease inhibitors to the inactivation of kallikrein in plasma. *J Clin Invest* 1982;69:462–468.

119. Van der Graaf F, Koedam JA, Bouma BN. Inactivation of kallikrein in human plasma. *J Clin Invest* 1983;71:149–158.

120. Barrett AJ, Starkey PM. The interaction of α2-macroglobulin with proteinases. *Biochem J* 1973;133:709–724.

121. Harpel PC, Lewin MF, Kaplan AP. Distribution of plasma kallikrein between C1 inactivator and α2-macroglobulin-kallikrein complexes. *J Biol Chem* 1985;4257–4263.

122. Meijers JC, Vlooswijk RAA, Bouma BN. Inhibition of human blood coagulation factor XIa by C1 Inhibitor. *Biochemistry* 1988;27: 959–963.

123. Wuillemin WA, Minnema M, Meijers JC. Inactivation of factor XIA in human plasma assessed by measuring factor XIA-protease inhibitor complexes: major role for C1-inhibitor. *Blood* 1995;85:1517.

124. Heck LW, Kaplan AP. Substrates of Hageman factor: I. Isolation and characterization of human factor XI (PTA) and inhibition of the activated enzyme by α1-antitrypsin. *J Exp Med* 1974;140:1615.

125. Scott CF, Schapira M, James HL, Cohen AG, Colman RW. Inactivation of factor XIA by plasma protease inhibitors: predominant role of α1-protease inhibitor and protective effect of high molecular weight kininogen. *J Clin Invest* 1982;69:844.

126. Nustad K, Orstavik TB, Bautvik KM. Glandular kallikreins. *Gen Pharmacol* 1978;9:1.

127. Sheikh IA, Kaplan AP. The mechanism of digestion of bradykinin and lysylbradykinin (kallidin) in human serum: the role of carboxy-peptidase, angiotensin converting enzyme, and determination of final degradation products. *Biochem Pharmacol* 1989;38:993–1000.

128. Rahman MM, Worthy K, Elson CJ. Inhibitor regulation of tissue kallikrein activity in the synovial fluid of patients with rheumatoid arthritis. *Br J Rheumatol* 1994;33:215.

129. Blackberg M. Interactions *in vitro* and *in vivo* between porcine tissue kallikrein and porcine plasma proteinase inhibitors. *J Clin Lab Invest* 1994;54:643.

130. Bhoola KD, Figueroa CD, Worthy K. Bioregulation of kinins: kallikrein, kininogen, and kininases. *Pharmacol Rev* 1992;44:1.

131. Burton J, Benetos A. The design of specific inhibitors of tissue kallikrein and their effect on the blood pressure of rat. *Adv Exp Med Biol* 1989;247B:9.

132. Regoli D, Barabe J. Pharmacology of bradykinin and related kinins. *Pharmacol Rev* 1980;32:1.

133. Erdos EG, Sloane GM. An enzyme in human plasma that inactivates bradykinin and kallidins. *Biochem Pharmacol* 1962;11:585.

134. Sheikh IA, Kaplan AP. Studies of the digestion of bradykinin, lysylbradykinin and kinin degradation products by carboxypeptidases A, B, N. *Biochem Pharmacol* 1986;35:1957.

135. Smith AMJ, Webb C, Holford J. Signal transduction pathways for B1 and B2 bradykinin receptors in bovine pulmonary artery endothelial cells. *Mol Pharmacol* 1995;47:525.

136. Wang W, Hendriks DK, Scharpe SS. Carboxypeptidase U, a plasma carboxypeptidase with high affinity for plasminogen. *J Biol Chem* 1994;269:15937.

137. Sheikh IA, Kaplan AP. Studies of the digestion of bradykinin, lysylbradykinin and des-arg^9 bradykinin by angiotensin converting enzyme. *Biochem Pharmacol* 1986;35:1951.

138. Schmaier AH, Kuo A, Lundberg D, Murray S, Cines DB. The expression of high molecular weight kininogen on human umbilical vein endothelial cells. *J Biol Chem* 1988;263:16327–16333.

139. Van Iwaarden F, de Groot PG, Bouma BN. The binding of high molecular weight kininogen to cultured human endothelial cells. *J Biol Chem* 1988;263:4698–4703.

140. Nishikawa K, Shibayama Y, Kuna P, Calcaterra E, Kaplan AP, Reddigari SR. Generation of the vasoactive peptide bradykinin from human umbilical vein endothelium-bound high molecular weight kininogen by plasma kallikrein. *Blood* 1992;80:1980–1988.

141. Reddigari SR, Kuna P, Miragliotta G, Shibayama Y, Nishikawa K, Kaplan AP. Human high molecular weight kininogen binds to human umbilical vein endothelial cells via its heavy and light chains. *Blood* 1993;81:1306–1311.

142. Berrettini M, Schleef RR, Heeb MJ, Hopmeier P, Griffin JH. Assembly and expression of an intrinsic factor IX activator complex on the surface of cultured human endothelial cells. *J Biol Chem* 1992;267:19833–19839.

143. Smith D, Gilbert M, Owen WG. Tissue plasminogen activator release *in vivo* in response to vasoactive agents. *Blood* 1985;66:835–839.

144. Crutchly DJ, Ryan JW, Ryan US, Fisher GH. Bradykinin induced release of prostacyclin and thromboxanes from bovine pulmonary artery endothelial cells. *Biochem Biophys Acta* 1983;751:99.

145. Hong SL. Effect of bradykinin and thrombin on prostacyclin synthesis in endothelial cells from calf and pig aorta and human umbilical cord vein. *Thromb Res* 1980;18:787.

146. Herwald H, Dedio J, Kellner R, Loos M, Müller-Esterl W. Isolation and characterization of the kininogen-binding protein p33 from endothelial cells. *J Biol Chem* 1996;271:13040–13047.

147. Joseph K, Ghebrehiwet B, Peerschke EIB, Reid KB, Kaplan AP. Identification of the zinc-dependent endothelial cell binding protein for high molecular weight kininogen and factor XII: identity with the receptor that binds to the globular "heads" of C1q (gC1qR). *Proc Natl Acad Sci U S A* 1996;14:36.

148. Hasan AA, Cines DB, Herwald H, Schmaier AH, Müller-Esterl W. Mapping the cell binding site on high molecular weight kininogen domain 5. *J Biol Chem* 1995;270:19256–19261.

149. Herwald H, Hasan AA, Godovac-Zimmermann J, Schmaier AH, Müller-Esterl W. Identification of an endothelial cell binding site on kininogen domain D3. *J Biol Chem* 1995;270:14634–14642.

150. Hasan AA, Cines DB, Zhang J, Schmaier AH. The carboxyl terminus of bradykinin and amino terminus of the light chain of kininogens comprise an endothelial cell binding domain. *J Biol Chem* 1994;269:31822–31830.

151. Colman RW, Pixley RA, Najamunnisa S, et al. Binding of high molecular weight kininogen to human endothelial cells is mediated via a site within domains 2 and 3 of the urokinase receptor. *J Clin Invest* 1997;100:1481–1487.

152. Hasan AAK, Zisman T, Schmaier AH. Cytokeratin 1 is the major cell receptor for kininogens [abstract]. *Thromb Haemost* 1997;77(Suppl):141.

153. Shariat-Mador Z, Mahdi F, Rojkjaer R, Schmaier AH. Mapping of the kininogen binding domain on its endothelial cell receptor, cytokeratin 1. *Blood* 1997;90(Suppl 1):79b.

154. Dedio J, Müller-Esterl W. Kininogen binding protein p331gC1qR is localized in the vesicular fraction of endothelial cells. *FEBS Lett* 1996;399:255–258.

155. Vandenberg RH, Prins F, Faber-Krol MC, et al. Intracellular localization of the human receptor for the globular domains of C1q. *J Immunol* 1997;158:3909–3916.

156. Ghebrehiwet B, Lu PD, Zhang W, et al. Evidence that the two C1q binding membrane proteins gC1qR and cC1qR associate to form a complex. *J Immunol* 1997;159:1429–1436.

157. Peerschke EIB, Smyth SS, Tang EI, Dalzell M, Ghebrehiwet B. Human umbilical vein endothelial cells possess binding sites for the globular domain of C1q. *J Immunol* 1996;157:4154–4158.

158. Ichinose A, Fujikawa K, Suyama T. The activation of pro-urokinase by plasma kallikrein and its inhibition by thrombin. *J Biol Chem* 1986;261:3486–3489.

159. Motta G, Hasan AAK, Cines DB, Schmaier AH. High molecular weight kininogen and prekallikrein assembly on endothelial cells produce plasminogen activation independent of factor XII. *Blood* 1995;86(Suppl 1):374a.

160. Shibayama Y, Joseph K, Ghebrehiwet B, Peerschke EIB, Reid KBM, Kaplan AP. Evidence that the receptor for the globular heads of C1q (gC1qR) can serve as a naturally occurring initiator of the plasma kinin-generating pathway. *J Clin Invest* (submitted).

161. Wiggins RC, Loskatoff DJ, Cochrane CG, Griffin JH, Edgington TS. Activation of the rabbit Hageman factor by homogenates cultured rabbit endothelial cells. *J Clin Invest* 1980;65:197–206.

162. Meloni FJ, Gustafson EJ, Schmaier AH. High molecular weight kininogen binds to platelets by its heavy and light chains and when bound has altered susceptibility to kallikrein cleavage. *Blood* 1992;79:1233–1244.

163. Jiang YP, Müller-Esterl W, Schmaier AH. Domain 3 of kininogens contains a cell-binding site and a site that modifies thrombin activation of platelets. *J Biol Chem* 1992;267:3712–3717.

164. Puri RN, Zhou F, Hu CJ, Colman RW. High molecular weight kininogen inhibits thrombin-induced platelet aggregation and cleavage of aggregin by inhibiting binding of thrombin to platelets. *Blood* 1991;77:500.

165. Joseph K, Bahou W, Kaplan AP. Evidence that the zinc-dependent platelet binding protein of factor XII and high molecular weight kininogen is glycoprotein Ib. *J Invest Med* 1997;45:267A.

166. De La Cadena RA, Wyshock EG, Kunapuri SP, et al. Platelet thrombospondin interacts with human high and low molecular weight kininogens. *Thromb Haemost* 1994;72:125–131.

167. Bradford HN, De la Cadena RA, Kunapuli SP, Dong JF, Lopez JA, Colman RW. Human kininogens regulate thrombin binding to platelets through the glycoprotein 1b-IX-V complex. *Blood* 1997;90:1508–1515.

168. Wachtfogel YT, De la Cadena RA, Kunapuli SP, et al. High molecular weight kininogen binds to Mac-1 on neutrophils by its heavy chain (domain 3) and its light chain (domain 5). *J Biol Chem* 1994;269:19307–19312.

169. Henderson LM, Figueroa CD, Müller-Esterl W. Assembly of contact phase factors on the surface of the human neutrophil membrane. *Blood* 1994;84:474.

170. De la Cadena RA, Suffredini AF, Page JD, et al. Activation of the kallikrein-kinin system after endotoxin administration to normal volunteers. *Blood* 1993;81:3313.

171. Martinez-Brotóns F, Oncins JR, Mestres J, Amargós V, Reynaldo C. Plasma kallikrein-kinin system in patients with uncomplicated sepsis and septic shock: comparison with cardiogenic shock. *Thromb Haemost* 1987;4:709–713.

172. Pixley RA, De la Cadena RA, Page JD, et al. Activation of the contact system in lethal hypotensive bacteremic in a baboon model. *Am J Pathol* 1992;140:897.

173. Pixley RA, De La Cadena R, Page JD, et al. The contact system con-

tributes to hypotension but not disseminated intravascular coagulation in lethal bacteremia: *in vivo* use of a monoclonal anti-factor XII antibody to block contact activation in baboons. *J Clin Invest* 1993;91: 61–68.

174. Shibayama Y, Joseph K, Ghebrehiwet B, Peerschke EIB, Kaplan AP. Zinc-dependent activation of the plasma kinin formation cascade by aggregated amyloid protein. *Clinical Immunology and Immunopathology* (*in press*).

175. Bush AI, Pettingell WH Jr, Paradis MD, Tanzi RE. Modulation of A beta adhesiveness and secretase site cleavage by zinc. *J Biol Chem* 1994;269:12152–12158.

176. Curd JG, Yelvington M, Burridge N, et al. Generation of bradykinin during incubation of hereditary angioedema plasma. *Mol Immunol* 1983;19:1365.

177. Fields T, Ghebrehiwet B, Kaplan AP. Kinin formation in hereditary angioedema plasma: evidence against kinin derivation from C2 and in support of "spontaneous" formation of bradykinin. *J Allergy Clin Immunol* 1983;72:54–60.

178. Schapira M, Silver LD, Scott CF, et al. Prekallikrein activation and high molecular weight kininogen consumption in hereditary angioedema. *N Engl J Med* 1985;3:1050–1054.

179. Curd JG, Prograis LJJ, Cochrane CG. Detection of active kallikrein in induced blister fluids of hereditary angioedema patients. *J Exp Med* 1980;152:242.

180. Donaldson VH, Rosen FS, Bing DH. Role of the second component of complement (C2) and plasmin in kinin release in hereditary angioneurotic edema (HANE) plasma. *Trans Assoc Am Physicians* 1977;40:174.

181. Strang CJ, Cholin S, Spragg J, et al. Angioedema induced by a peptide derived from complement component C2. *J Exp Med* 1988;166:1685.

182. Shoemuker LR, Schurmeen SJ, Donaldson VH, Davis AEI. Hereditary angioneurotic oedema: characterization of plasma kinin and vascular permeability-enhancing activities. *Clin Exp Immunol* 1994;95:22.

183. Proud D, Togias A, Naclerio RM, Crush SB, Norman PS, Lichtenstein LM. Kinins are generated *in vivo* following nasal airway challenge of allergic individuals with allergen. *J Clin Invest* 1983;72:1678.

184. Creticos PS, Van Metre TE, Mardiney MR, Rosenberg GL, Norman PS, Adkinson NF Jr. Dose response of IgE and IgG antibodies during ragweed immunotherapy. *J Allergy Clin Immunol* 1984;73:94–104.

185. Baumgarten CR, Togias AG, Naclerio RM, Lichtenstein LM, Norman PS, Proud D. Influx of kininogens into nasal secretions after antigen challenge of allergic individuals. *J Clin Invest* 1985;76:191.

186. Baumgarten CR, Nichols RC, Naclerio RM, Lichtenstein LM, Norman PS, Proud D. Plasma kallikrein during experimentally-induced allergic rhinitis: role in kinin formation and contribution to TAME-esterase activity in nasal secretions. *J Immunol* 1986;137:977.

187. Baumgarten CR, Nichols RC, Naclerio RM, Proud D. Concentrations of glandular kallikrein in human nasal secretions increase during experimentally-induced allergic rhinitis. *J Immunol* 1986;137:1323.

188. Christiansen SC, Proud D, Cochrane CG. Detection of tissue kallikrein in the bronchoalveolar lavage fluids of asthmatic subjects. *J Clin Invest* 1987;79;188.

189. Atkins PC, Miragliotta G, Talbot SF, Zweiman B, Kaplan AP. Activation of plasma Hageman factor and kallikrein in ongoing allergic reactions in the skin. *J Immunol*. 1987;139:2744–2748.

190. Israili ZH, Hall WD. Cough and angioneurotic edema associated with angiotensin-converting enzyme inhibitor therapy. *Annals Int Med* 1992;117:234–242.

Inflammation: Basic Principles and Clinical Correlates,
3rd ed., edited by John I. Gallin and Ralph Snyderman.
Lippincott Williams & Wilkins, Philadelphia © 1999.

CHAPTER 22

Prostaglandins and Inflammation

Richard J. Griffiths

Prostaglandins have been one of the most intensively studied group of mediators of the inflammatory response, and insights into their production and biologic mode of action continue to be revealed. Historically, the origins of prostaglandin research are in a different area of physiology altogether. The biologic activity of the group of substances now called prostaglandins was first detected in seminal fluid and extracts of the accessory genital glands. The ability of seminal fluid to affect the tone of the human uterus was first reported in 1931 (1). Independent work demonstrated that human seminal fluid contained a smooth muscle–stimulating, vasodepressor substance that could be distinguished by pharmacologic and chemical means from other biologically active substances (2–4). This work led to the introduction of the term *prostaglandin,* because the prostate gland was assumed to be the source of the biologic activity. However, we now know that prostaglandins are secretions of the seminal vesicles.

It was not until the development of more refined chemical techniques that the active substance responsible for the biologic activity could be isolated (5) and separated into two fractions that had smooth muscle–stimulating activity (prostaglandin F [PGF]) (6) and smooth muscle–stimulating activity and vasodepressor activity (prostaglandin E [PGE]) (7). The structural elucidation of PGE and PGF rapidly followed, and the basic structure of both compounds was shown to be an unsaturated 20-carbon-chain acidic lipid, with one, two, or three double bonds. The structure of the prostaglandins bears a striking resemblance to the essential fatty acids, a group of substances necessary for maintenance of life but the exact function of which had remained an enigma.

Independent work by two groups demonstrated that the essential fatty acid, arachidonic acid, was converted by means of an enzyme, cyclooxygenase, in sheep vesicular

gland to PGE_2 (8,9) and that dihomo-γ-linolenic acid and eicosapentaenoic acid were precursors for PGE_1 and PGE_3, respectively. Because of the potent biologic effects of prostaglandins, it was suggested that the function of the essential fatty acids was to serve as precursors for prostaglandin synthesis. Arachidonic acid is the most abundant precursor fatty acid for prostaglandin synthesis in mammalian cells; therefore, prostaglandins with two double bonds are found in higher concentrations than those with one or three double bonds. Arachidonic acid also serves as the precursor for the production of leukotrienes (see Chapter 23).

All prostaglandins have 20 carbon atoms, which are numbered from the carbon attached to the carboxyl group (C1). The five-membered cyclopentane ring spans carbons 8 through 12. The hydroxyl group at position C15 is required for biologic activity (Fig. 22-1).

Early studies on the conversion of arachidonic acid into prostaglandins suggested that an intermediate compound existed. Further evidence for the existence of this intermediate came with the demonstration of the release of an unstable substance, rabbit aorta–contracting substance (RCS), from antigen-challenged guinea-pig lungs (10). The release of RCS was increased by arachidonic acid. RCS rapidly decomposed nonenzymatically at room temperature, and this change was associated with increased production of a PGE_2-like substance (11). Studies on the metabolism of arachidonic acid by microsomal fractions of sheep vesicular gland also demonstrated the presence of an unstable intermediate that contracted the rabbit aorta and spontaneously decomposed to form classic prostaglandins (12,13). Later work showed the presence of two unstable intermediates, a 15-hydroperoxy derivative and a 15-hydroxyl derivative of arachidonic acid. These endoperoxide intermediates are called PGG_2 and PGH_2. Both endoperoxides contracted the rabbit aorta and induced platelet aggregation. Although the prostaglandin endoperoxides have potent biologic activity in their own right, the amounts released from antigen-challenged guinea-pig

R. J. Griffiths: Department of Respiratory, Allergy, Immunology, Inflammation, Infectious Diseases, Central Research Division, Pfizer, Inc., Groton, Connecticut 06340.

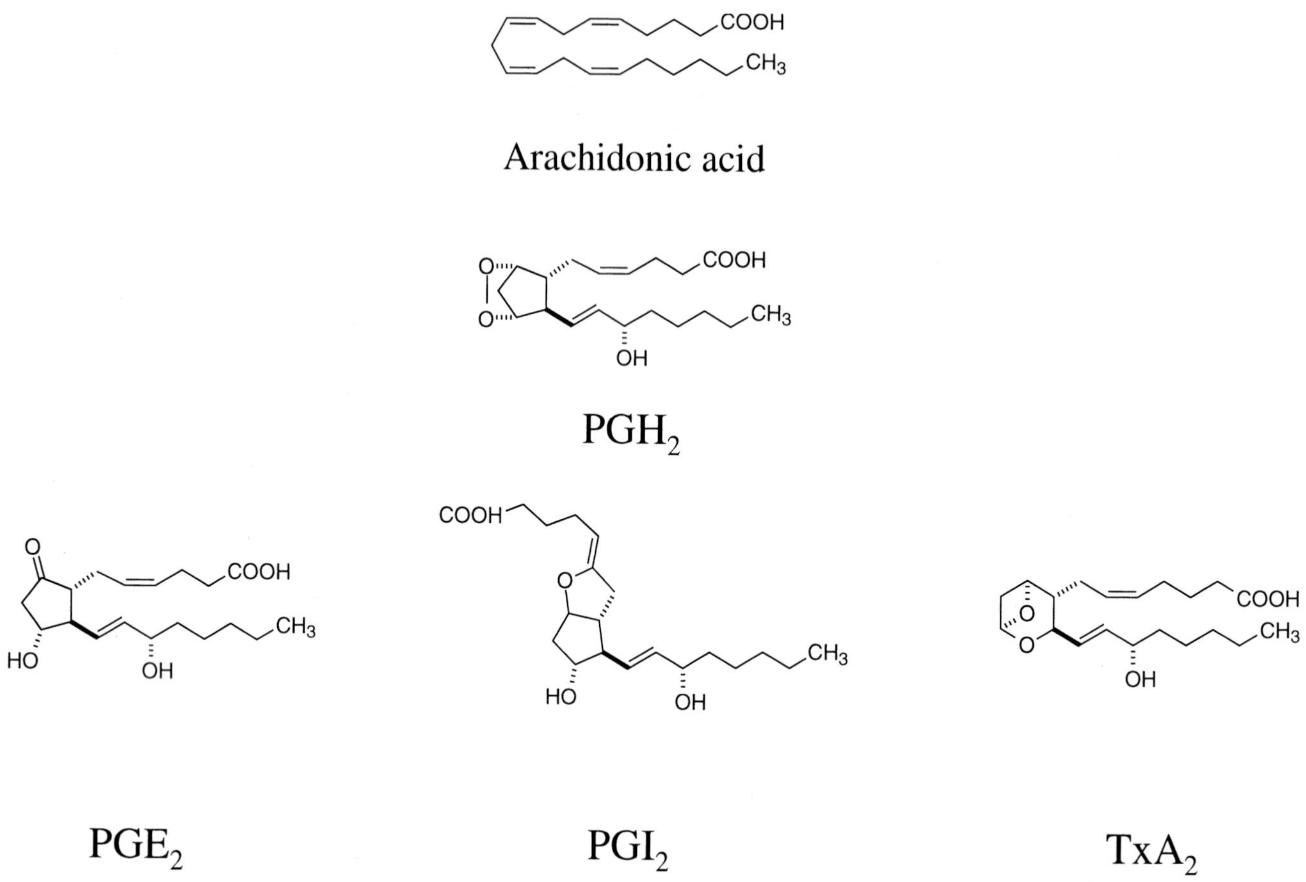

Arachidonic acid

PGH$_2$

PGE$_2$ **PGI$_2$**   **TxA$_2$**

FIG. 22-1. The structure of arachidonic acid and related prostanoids.

lungs or platelets and their stability ($T_{1/2}$ = 4 to 5 minutes at 37°C, pH 7.4) were not sufficient to account for the biologic activity and stability of RCS ($T_{1/2}$ = 30 to 40 seconds at 37°C, pH 7.4).

A study of arachidonic acid metabolism by platelets demonstrated that a stable nonprostaglandin, the hemiacetal derivative of 8-(1-hydroxy-3-oxopropyl)-9-12-L-dihydroxy-5,10-heptadecadienoic acid (thromboxane B$_2$ [TxB$_2$]) was formed (14). The experimental data suggested that TxB$_2$ was formed from PGG$_2$ by rearrangement and subsequent incorporation of one molecule of H$_2$O. The addition of nucleophilic reagents to incubations of radiolabeled PGG$_2$ with platelets trapped an intermediate in the formation of TxB$_2$. The new substance, TxA$_2$ was unstable ($T_{1/2}$ = 30 to 40 seconds, pH 7.4, 37°C), contracted the rabbit aorta, and induced platelet aggregation. TxA$_2$ is the major component of RCS from aggregating platelets and guinea-pig lungs (15). The ring structure of thromboxanes (i.e., oxetane) is different from the cyclopentane ring in the classic prostaglandins (see Fig. 22-1). The term *prostanoids* is used to refer collectively to prostaglandins and thromboxanes.

The discovery of the structure of TxA$_2$ prompted the search for other tissues that were capable of producing it. Studies of the biologic transformation of prostaglandin

endoperoxides by microsomal fractions of various tissues using the superfusion bioassay technique led to the discovery that blood vessels converted endoperoxides to a novel substance that had the opposite biologic effects to TXA$_2$; it relaxed vascular smooth muscle and inhibited platelet aggregation (16). This new prostaglandin was unstable and spontaneously hydrolyzed in neutral and acidic aqueous media to form 6-oxo-PGF$_{1\alpha}$, a stable compound first isolated from rat stomach homogenates. The structure of the new prostaglandin was elucidated and called PGI$_2$, with the trivial name prostacyclin (17). The history of the discovery of prostaglandins illustrates the value of bioassays in identifying interesting biologic activities that can then be subjected to careful chemical analysis.

BIOSYNTHESIS OF PROSTAGLANDINS

Stimuli for Prostaglandin Production

There are many ways of inducing prostaglandin synthesis, and these may be cell type specific. Immunologic stimuli, such as phagocytosis of particles mediated by the CD11b receptor and immune complexes mediated by Fcγ receptors on monocytes-macrophages, leads to PGE$_2$ and TxA$_2$ synthesis (18), as does stimulation of the CD14 receptor for lipopolysaccharide (LPS) (19). Activation of the Fc receptor or certain cytokine receptors on mast cells leads to PGD_2 production (20). Stimulation of fibroblasts, epithelial cells, and chondrocytes with cytokines such as interleukin-1 (IL-1) and tumor necrosis factor-α (TNF-α) (21,22) leads to PGE_2 production. Activation of endothelial cells with IL-1, bradykinin, or thrombin stimulates predominantly PGI_2 formation (23). Several of these cell types exist throughout the body and may contribute to the prostaglandins measured at sites of inflammation *in vivo*.

Prostaglandins have been detected in almost all experimental models of inflammation studied (24,25) and in the synovial fluid of patients with arthritis (26). In most cases, the major prostaglandins found are PGE_2 and PGI_2. In experimental forms of arthritis, the production of PGE_2 is prevented by suppressing leukocyte influx into the joint (24,27). It is not clear whether the infiltrating leukocytes produce PGE_2 or they provide a stimulus required to initiate prostaglandin production by resident joint tissues. In contrast, injection of zymosan or immune complexes into the peritoneal cavity initiates a rapid (minutes) phase of PGE_2 and PGI_2 production, but in this case, resident peritoneal macrophages are the most likely source of prostanoids because these cells respond *in vitro* to these stimuli by producing PGE_2 and PGI_2 (24,28,29).

Role of Phospholipase A_2 in Prostaglandin Synthesis

Although it had been proved that prostaglandins were formed from essential fatty acids, it was not clear how the substrate was made available for enzymatic conversion to prostaglandins, because only free fatty acids could serve as precursors for prostaglandin synthesis. Concentrations of free fatty acids in cells are extremely low, and prostaglandins are synthesized on demand rather than being stored in cells. Perfusion of organs with phospholipase or arachidonic acid greatly increases the release of prostaglandins from the organ (30). This observation suggested that, although the organ had a high biosynthetic capacity, it was limited by the rate of release of the precursor fatty acid.

Evidence for the role of phospholipase in prostaglandin synthesis came from studies that followed the fate of radiolabeled arachidonic acid. The radiolabel was accumulated in phospholipid and neutral lipid pools, could be selectively released from the phospholipid pool by chemical or mechanical stimulation, and was subsequently converted to prostaglandins (31,32). The arachidonic acid was incorporated exclusively into the sn-2 position of the glycerol backbone of the phospholipid, and a phospholipase A_2 (PLA$_2$) enzyme therefore was presumed to be responsible for this rate-limiting step in prostanoid biosynthesis (Fig. 22-2).

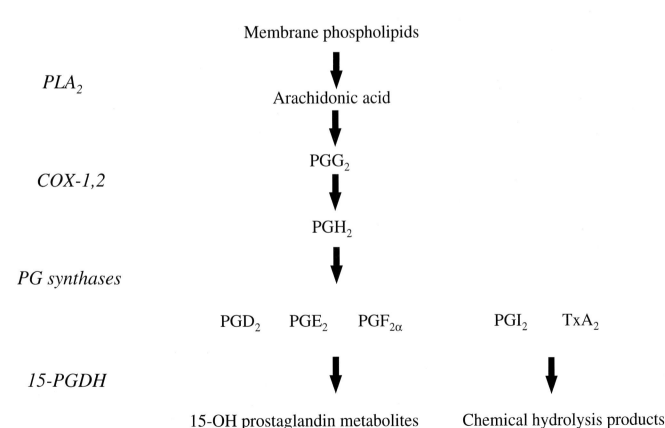

FIG. 22-2. The prostanoid biosynthetic pathway.

Much work has been conducted in the past 20 years to establish the identity of the phospholipase A_2 responsible for liberating arachidonic acid. The phospholipase A_2 family of enzymes is large and growing in number (33,34). Most work has been focused on two types of PLA_2, the secreted 14-kd form (35) and the type IV cytosolic 85-kd enzyme (36,37). There is evidence that a 14-kd PLA_2 and the 85-kd PLA_2 are involved in prostaglandin generation and that the relative importance of each may depend on the cell type and the activating stimulus (38). The 85-kd cytosolic enzyme selectively cleaves fatty acids at the sn-2 position of phospholipids and is regulated by phosphorylation through a mitogen-activated protein kinase pathway and by calcium-dependent translocation to membranes, where substrate is located (36). The nuclear envelope and the endoplasmic reticulum are the major sites within the cell that this form of PLA_2 translocates to on cell activation, rather than the plasma membrane (39,40). In monocytes and mast cells, the 85-kd PLA_2 appears to be involved in prostaglandin generation induced by a variety of stimuli (41). The secreted 14-kd enzyme does not specifically cleave fatty acids at the sn-2 position, and unlike the type IV cytosolic enzyme, it cleaves fatty acid from the external surface of the plasma membrane. This form of the enzyme is transcriptionally upregulated in certain cell types such as fibroblasts and chondrocytes by cytokines such as IL-1 and TNF-α (42), whereas in other cells, it exists preformed.

Several forms of the 14-kd enzyme represent the products of different genes. Until recently, it was assumed that the type IIA enzyme, originally described in synovial fluid and platelets, was probably involved in release of arachidonic acid. However, recent evidence cast doubt on this idea, and instead, another member of this family, the type V enzyme, probably is involved (43). Mast cells isolated from mice with a genetic deficiency of the type IIA enzyme secrete equivalent amounts of PLA_2 activity, compared with that of cells isolated from wild-type mice, and synthesize PGD_2 normally (38,44). In mouse macrophages, the type IIA enzyme is not responsible for arachidonic acid release, as determined by work with antisense probes (45). It seems likely that a type V 14-kd enzyme is involved in these cells. This new form of PLA_2 has been characterized in several species, including humans (46), and although similar to the type IIA enzyme in many respects, it is a different enzyme. However, inhibitors of the type IIA enzyme also inhibit the type V and many of the immunologic methods used to detect the type IIA form may also measure the type V (43). Further work is needed to clarify the roles of these two enzymes in prostanoid biosynthesis.

Role of Cyclooxygenase

Arachidonic acid is converted to the prostaglandin endoperoxides PGG_2 and PGH_2 by two enzymes, cyclooxygenase-1 and cyclooxygenase-2 (47). Both enzymes catalyze the insertion of molecular oxygen into arachidonic acid at C11, resulting in a bicyclic cyclopentenyl endoperoxide in which the oxygen bridges C9 and C11. The subsequent insertion of oxygen at C15 results in the formation of PGG_2. A peroxidase activity, also catalyzed by cyclooxygenase-1 and cyclooxygenase-2, reduces the 15-hydroperoxy to a 15-hydroxy group to form PGH_2. Discovery of the two forms of the cyclooxygenase enzyme is the most significant finding in this area since 1971, when Sir John Vane discovered that cyclooxygenase was the molecular target for aspirin-like drugs (48) (see Chapter 74). For many years, it was assumed that cyclooxygenase was constitutively expressed in cells and that the main regulator of its activity was the phospholipase A_2, which supplied substrate by mediating the release of arachidonic acid. However, studies of the mechanism of enhanced prostaglandin synthesis by the hydronephrotic rabbit kidney indicated that cyclooxygenase levels were regulated by new protein synthesis as a result of tissue injury (49,50).

During the 1980s, it became clear that the regulation of cyclooxygenase activity was more complex than at first thought. Several reports demonstrated that cyclooxygenase activity showed a time-dependent increase in many cell types when exposed to inflammatory agents. For example, Needleman and coworkers showed that glucocorticoids and inhibitors of protein synthesis could suppress the increase in cyclooxygenase activity observed when fibroblasts or monocytes were exposed to cytokines, but that they had no effect on the basal level of cyclooxygenase activity (19,51).

Cyclooxygenase-1 was cloned from sheep, mouse, and human sources in 1988 through 1990. The proteins from these species are approximately 90% homologous (52–57). However, studies in cell-based systems in which cyclooxygenase activity increased did not reveal an increase in mRNA for cyclooxygenase-1. Coincident with these observations was the discovery of an inducible form of cyclooxygenase (i.e., cyclooxygenase-2) as a serum- and phorbol ester–inducible gene in chicken and mouse fibroblasts (58–60). The human (61–63) and rat (64) genes have also been cloned. Many studies have shown that the increase in cyclooxygenase activity observed on exposure of cells to inflammatory stimuli is caused by increased expression of cyclooxygenase-2 (65–67). Glucocorticoids suppress the induction of cyclooxygenase-2 but do not affect expression of cyclooxygenase-1, explaining the selective effect of these agents on cyclooxygenase activity observed by Needleman (68,69).

The tissue distribution of cyclooxygenase-1 and cyclooxygenase-2 *in vivo* are different. Cyclooxygenase-1 is constitutively expressed in many tissues, whereas cyclooxygenase-2 is mainly induced at sites of inflammation and injury. This is somewhat oversimplified, because cyclooxygenase-2 is constitutively expressed in brain and kidney, and cyclooxygenase-1 levels change during development (70,71). Little is known about the regulation of cyclooxygenase-1, but induction of cycloxygenase-2 by cytokines appears to be regulated by the transcription factor NF-κB (72,73) and the p38 mitogen–activated kinase pathway (18,74). The discovery of cyclooxygenase-2 has led to the search for isozyme selective inhibitors to maintain the desired therapeutic effects of cyclooxygenase inhibitors without the gastrointestinal and renal side effects that plague the use of the current generation of drugs (see Chapter 74).

Cyclooxygenase-1 and cyclooxygenase-2 share approximately 60% homology at the amino acid level, and both catalyze the formation of PGH_2 from arachidonic acid with similar kinetic properties. X-ray structures for both enzymes indicate that the enzymes contain a unique membrane-binding domain that is used to anchor the proteins in the membrane of the endoplasmic reticulum and nuclear envelope (75). The larger active site of cyclooxygenase-2 compared with cyclooxygenase-1 helps to explain the mechanism for the selective inhibition of this enzyme by certain cyclooxygenase inhibitors (76,77). In addition to different patterns of expression of the two isozymes, the enzymes are activated by different stimuli, use different pools of substrate, and may couple to different phospholipase A_2 enzymes. These patterns have been elegantly demonstrated in murine cells; when the activity of cyclooxygenase-2 is blocked, arachidonic acid released by certain stimuli cannot be converted to prostaglandins even though functional cyclooxygenase-1 is present in the cell (20,78,79).

Mice with genetic deletions of cyclooxygenase-1 or -2 have been created by homologous recombination in embryonic stem cells. Mice deficient in cyclooxygenase-2 develop a renal pathology because of a reduction in the number of nephrons (80,81). Cyclooxygenase-1–deficient mice have normal kidney function and none of the gastrointestinal abnormalities that would have been predicted based on the ability of cyclooxygenase inhibitors to produce gastric ulceration (82).

Role of Prostaglandin Synthases

PGH_2 spontaneously decomposes in aqueous solution to form a mixture of PGD_2, PGE_2, and PGF_{2*}. However, distinct enzymes catalyze the formation of each of these prostaglandins plus TXA_2 and PGI_2. The cellular expression pattern of each of these synthases may profoundly influence the type of prostaglandin produced by a particular cell. For example, platelets produce predominantly thromboxane A_2, endothelial cells PGI_2, and mast cells PGD_2. Genes for PGD synthase (83), PGF synthase (84), PGI synthase (85–87), and thromboxane A_2 synthase (88) have been cloned. PGD synthase is identical to β-trace protein, a major constituent of cerebrospinal fluid. This may reflect the role of PGD_2 as a sleep-promoting substance. In

addition to catalyzing the conversion of PGH_2 to $PGF_{2\alpha}$, PGF synthase also converts PGD_2 to $9\alpha11\beta$ PGF, an isomer of $PGF_{2\alpha}$, and is a member of the aldoketo reductase superfamily (89). A second form of PGD synthase that depends on reduced glutathione (GSH) for activity has been purified, but its gene has not been cloned. This form of the enzyme has been found to occur in mast cells (89). The most closely studied synthase is thromboxane synthase because of the interest in producing inhibitors of this enzyme as antithrombotic drugs. This enzyme is homologous to members of the cytochrome P450 family, as is PGI synthase, but there is only 16% homology between PGI synthase and thromboxane synthase. The genes for the prostanoid synthases are regulated, as evidenced by the changes in their pattern of expression during leukocyte activation and differentiation (90–92).

METABOLISM OF PROSTAGLANDINS

The biologic activity of prostaglandins is regulated by rates of synthesis and by an active degradative process. Once formed, prostaglandins of the E and F series are rapidly inactivated by a two-stage process that involves uptake into the cell cytosol followed by a series of enzymatic reactions. As charged organic anions at physiologic pH, prostanoids traverse biologic membranes poorly. An energy-requiring transport system that carries prostaglandins to the site of inactivation has been demonstrated in a variety of organs but has been most intensively studied in the lung. PGE_2 and $PGF_{2\alpha}$ are inactivated 80% to 95% during transit across the pulmonary circulation and therefore do not reach the arterial side of the circulation (93). The transport protein responsible for this first step in prostaglandin metabolism has been cloned and belongs to a family of 12 transmembrane-spanning carrier proteins (94,95).

The enzymes responsible for metabolism of prostaglandins are located in the cytosolic fractions of cellular homogenates (96), and the initial, rate-limiting step is the oxidation of the hydroxyl group at C15 to an oxo group catalyzed by the enzyme 15-hydroxyprostaglandin dehydrogenase (15-PGDH) (97). 15-PGDH is an NAD^+-dependent enzyme that has been cloned from mouse (98), rat (99), and human tissue (100). The primary structure indicates that it falls into the family of short-chain alcohol dehydrogenase enzymes. At least three different splice variants of the enzyme exist, but the biologic significance of this is not clear (101). The second step in prostaglandin metabolism is reduction of the 13,14 double bond catalyzed by the enzyme prostaglandin delta-13 reductase. The 15-oxo-13,14-dihydro prostaglandin products of these reactions have a greatly reduced biologic activity compared with that of the parent compounds, and this represents an efficient inactivation pathway. The products of these reactions may be further metabolized by β and ω oxidation before excretion in the urine.

In vitro, PGE$_2$, PGF$_{2\alpha}$, and PGI$_2$ are all good substrates for 15-PGDH, whereas TXB$_2$ and PGD$_2$ are poor substrates (102). PGI$_2$ is a poor substrate for the transporter protein that takes prostaglandins into cells, and exogenously administered PGI$_2$ therefore is not inactivated during passage across the lungs (103). However, endogenously produced PGI$_2$ is extensively metabolized by 15-PGDH in certain tissues (104). It appears that PGI$_2$ and TXA$_2$ catabolism proceeds through two competing pathways: spontaneous hydrolysis to form 6-oxo-PGF$_{1\alpha}$ and TXB$_2$, respectively, and enzymatic catabolism by 15-PGDH.

PROSTAGLANDIN RECEPTORS

Prostaglandins are liberated from cells and exert their biologic effects by binding to a family of high-affinity cell surface receptors. These receptors were originally classified using classic pharmacologic techniques, such as comparing the rank order of potency of a variety of prostanoid analogues on a panel of bioassay tissues (105). These studies, together with the discovery of antagonists for certain receptor subtypes, set the stage for a working classification based on the recognition that there was at least one receptor subtype for each of the five naturally occurring prostanoids. At each of these receptors, one of the naturally occurring prostanoids was at least one order of magnitude more potent than any of the others. The prefix P (prostanoid) is used to designate each receptor subtype; the FP receptor is preferentially activated by PGF$_{2\alpha}$, and the IP receptor is preferentially activated by PGI$_2$ (106). There appears to be only one receptor for PGD$_2$, PGF$_{2\alpha}$, and PGI$_2$; two for TxA$_2$; and four subtypes for PGE$_2$ (EP1 through EP4) (Table 22-1). The pharmacologic evidence for multiple prostanoid receptors proved to be extremely accurate when clones for the individual receptors were eventually isolated.

In 1991, the thromboxane receptor was the first member of this family to be cloned (107), and since then, the remaining family members have been identified. The prostanoid receptors belong to the superfamily of seven-transmembrane-spanning G-protein–coupled receptors (108–119). The only real surprise from the cloning exercise was the discovery of multiple isoforms of the TP (120) and EP3 receptors generated by alternative splicing of a single gene. In the case of the EP3 receptor, at least three isoforms are known in all species from which they have been cloned, including humans (121). All of the isoforms have very similar ligand-binding properties but differ in their cytoplasmic domain. This results in differences in coupling to intracellular effector molecules (122) and differential rates of desensitization (123). The two forms of the TP receptor, the platelet TP-α and the endothelial TP-β, are identical in their extracellular domains but differ in their cytoplasmic tails. Unlike the EP3 isoforms, pharmacologic and biochemical studies had predicted at least two forms of the TP receptor.

The signal transduction pathways activated by prostanoid receptors vary (see Table 22-1). For example, the EP2 and EP4 receptors couple to adenylate cyclase and stimulate cAMP formation, whereas the EP1 receptor triggers increases in intracellular calcium. EP3 isoforms can couple to several signal transduction pathways, including inhibition of adenylate cyclase and stimulation of phosphoinositide production. The transduction pathway in the case of all members of the family is initiated by the recruitment and activation of a trimeric G protein.

Genetic deletion of individual prostanoid receptors helps to clarify the role of each subtype. This process has been reported only for the prostacyclin receptor (124). Despite the fact that prostacyclin is a potent vasodilator, there is no effect on resting blood pressure in mice lacking this receptor, though the animals are more susceptible to arterial thrombosis.

TABLE 22-1. *Characterization of prostanoid receptors*

Receptor	Isoforms	Signal transduction	Selective agonist	Selective antagonist	Human cloning reference
EP1		↑Intracellular Ca^{2+}	17-phenyl PGE$_2$	SC19220	113
EP2		↑cAMP	Butaprost		116
EP3	Several—generated by alternate splicing	↓cAMP ↑PI turnover	Enprostil		121
EP4		↑cAMP		AH23848	109
DP		↑cAMP	BW245C	BW866C	112
FP		↑PI turnover	Fluprostonol		108
IP		↑cAMP	Cicaprost		111
TP	α, β—generated by alternate splicing	↑PI turnover	U44069	GR32191	107

EP1–EP4, receptors preferentially activated by PGE$_2$; FP, receptor preferentially activated by PGF$_{2\alpha}$; IP, receptor preferentially activated by PGI$_2$ PGE$_2$, prostaglandin E$_2$; TP, receptor preferentially activated by thromboxane; ↑, increased; ↓, decreased.

ROLE OF PROSTAGLANDINS IN REGULATING THE INFLAMMATORY RESPONSE

The role of prostaglandins in regulating the inflammatory response has been investigated by studying the effects of injections of these substances into animals and humans and by studying the effects of nonsteroidal anti-inflammatory drugs that inhibit cyclooxygenase and, therefore, prostaglandin production. The biologic effects of prostaglandins are extremely wide ranging, suggesting they may play a role in many aspects of physiology and pathology. However, four areas are particularly pertinent to the regulation of the inflammatory response: fever, pain, edema, and regulation of leukocyte function.

Fever

Fever is a complex neuroendocrine response to injury and infection, and there is still considerable debate about whether it is beneficial to the host (125). Despite this uncertainty, it is clear that prostanoids are key mediators of this response. Prostaglandins of the E series cause an increase in body temperature in many species (126,127), and the levels of PGE_2 are increased in cerebrospinal fluid from febrile animals (128). The increased prostaglandin production probably occurs within the central nervous system and is mediated by cytokines released in response to bacterial products. Body temperature is normally regulated within strict limits (i.e., the set point), and it seems likely that PGE_2 acts on neurons in the thermoregulatory network of the hypothalamus and elevates the set point, resulting in an increase in body temperature (129). The receptors by which PGE_2 exerts this effect have not been characterized.

Cyclooxygenase inhibitors are used clinically as antipyretic agents, adding weight to the hypothesis that prostaglandins are key mediators of pyrexia. In rodents, selective cyclooxygenase-2 inhibitors are equally as effective as nonselective cyclooxygenase inhibitors in reducing fever (130,131). The level of the mRNA for cyclooxygenase-2 in the brain is increased after administration of bacterial LPS (64,132), suggesting that production of the prostaglandins involved in the pyretic response depends on cyclooxygenase-2 rather than cyclooxygenase-1.

Pain

Prostaglandins usually do not induce a painful response when injected alone. However, they do produce a condition known as hyperalgesia, i.e., the response to a chemical, mechanical, or thermal stimulus that does induce pain, which is greatly increased in the presence of a prostaglandin. Hyperalgesia does induce pain and is greatly increased in the presence of a prostaglandin. PGE_2 and PGI_2 are the most potent prostaglandins in this respect (133), but it is not clear which EP receptor subtype mediates this response. Prostaglandins are important for the processing of pain by sensitizing the peripheral terminals of primary afferent nociceptors and by augmenting processing of pain information at the spinal level. Cyclooxygenase inhibitors are used clinically as analgesic agents, lending support to the concept that prostaglandins play a key role in pain perception. In experimental models that demonstrate pharmacologic sensitivity to cyclooxygenase inhibitors, prostaglandin production has been directly measured at the site of injury (29,134,135).

Until recently, it was unclear whether PGI_2 or PGE_2 is the most important mediator of the pain response. Development of a monoclonal antibody to PGE_2 that is effective at neutralizing the biologic activity of this prostanoid and the generation of mice with genetic deficiencies in prostaglandin receptors helped to clarify this question. In the phenylbenzoquinone mouse-writhing model, anti-PGE_2 treatment inhibits the response by 80% (135). Nonselective cyclooxygenase inhibitors cause complete suppression in this model. In contrast, in the rat paw, thermal hypersensitivity model anti-PGE_2 was equally effective as a cyclooxygenase inhibitor (136). In the rat paw thermal hypersensitivity model, selective cyclooxygenase-2 inhibitors are equally effective as nonselective agents, indicating that the inducible form of cyclooxygenase is responsible for the production of PGE_2 that contributes to this response (130,137). In contrast, in IP receptor–deficient mice, the writhing responses to intraperitoneal injection of acetic acid is reduced to an extent similar to that observed with a cyclooxygenase inhibitor (124). The EP and IP receptors therefore are involved in pain perception, and their relative importance depends on the experimental system used.

Edema

Edema, like pain, is not produced by injection of prostaglandins alone. However, PGE_2 and PGI_2 do have a profound influence on the edema associated with inflammation by virtue of their ability to increase blood flow to the inflamed site (138,139). This is brought about by arteriolar dilation. The increased blood flow alone cannot promote edema, but in the presence of an agent that increases the permeability of venules to plasma proteins, a synergistic increase in the extent of plasma leakage is observed (140,141). This process has been most closely studied experimentally in the rabbit and guinea-pig. Application of PGE_2 or PGI_2 alone increases blood flow but does not promote edema. However, coinjection of either agent with substances such as the chemotactic factors LTB_4 and IL-8 or mediators that directly act on the endothelial cells such as platelet-activating factor and bradykinin causes profound plasma protein leakage (142). The increased blood flow can enhance delivery of leukocytes to the inflamed site and thereby contribute to an enhancement of the inflammatory response (143–145). The EP receptor subtypes involved in increased arteriolar dilation are unknown, but because binding to the EP2 and EP4 subtypes has resulted in relaxation of the smooth muscle of large blood vessels, they appear to be the most likely candidates (106).

Cyclooxygenase inhibitors are used clinically to reduce the swelling of joints affected by rheumatoid arthritis, suggesting that prostanoids contribute to the regulation of microvascular permeability in this disease. Historically, the clinical effects of the prototypes of this class of drug (i.e., aspirin) were observed in humans many years before the mechanism of action had been elucidated. To find drugs with improved efficacy compared with aspirin, models such as the guinea-pig ultraviolet light–induced erythema model (146) and carrageenan-induced paw swelling in the rat were used (147). Both models are sensitive to aspirin, and the erythema in the skin is a direct reflection of increased blood flow, whereas the edema response to carrageenan is an example of the synergy between prostaglandin-induced vasodilation and the promotion of increased vessel permeability by other inflammatory mediators. Similar to findings in models of inflammatory pain, anti-PGE_2 antibody treatment is as effective as a cyclooxygenase inhibitor in reducing the edema induced by carrageenan injection into the rat paw and that associated with adjuvant-induced arthritis in the rat (136). Studies on the form of cyclooxygenase present at sites of inflammation and the use of selective cyclooxygenase-2 inhibitors have shown that the inducible form of cyclooxygenase is the major source of PGE_2 during inflammatory responses in rats.

Cyclooxygenase-2–selective agents are equally as effective antiinflammatory agents when compared with nonselective cyclooxygenase inhibitors (69,131,134,137,148). Early clinical studies with these agents suggest that selective inhibition of cyclooxygenase-2 also is antiinflammatory and analgesic in humans (149).

Regulation of Leukocyte Function

Prostaglandins also modulate leukocyte function, suggesting they may also downregulate the inflammatory response. This seems paradoxical given that drugs that inhibit prostaglandin synthesis are widely used as antiinflammatory agents. However, evidence indicates that prostaglandin-induced suppression of the inflammatory response can occur *in vivo* (150,151). PGE_2, PGD_2, and PGI_2 all inhibit neutrophil activation *in vitro*, as measured by chemotaxis or superoxide production (152). The inhibitory effect is associated with increased cAMP formation. Intravenous infusions of PGI_2 (at doses that do not affect systemic blood pressure) can also inhibit neutrophil-dependent plasma protein extravasation in the rabbit *in vivo* (153). The effects of PGI_2 in this model therefore depend on the route of administration; the effects of local administration are proinflammatory, whereas those of systemic administration are antiinflammatory.

PGE_2 is also a potent inhibitor of monocyte activation; the most notable effect is inhibition of TNF production (154). The TNF gene is regulated by cAMP concentrations within the cell, and it seems likely that the effect of PGE_2 is mediated through the EP2 or EP4 receptor, which increases cAMP levels. This effect also occurs *in vivo*, because administration of cyclooxygenase inhibitors to animals and humans enhances the release of TNF in response to administration of LPS (155,156). In mice, this enhanced release of TNF is associated with an increase in the sensitivity of the animals to the lethal effects of LPS (155). There is also evidence that administration of cyclooxygenase inhibitors to animals at doses that produce an antiinflammatory effect may exacerbate cartilage degradation, perhaps also linked to enhanced TNF production (157,158).

In addition to affecting the function of myeloid cells, PGE_2 inhibits lymphocyte function. T-cell proliferation (159), cytokine production (160,161), and T-cell migration (162) are inhibited by PGE_2 through a cAMP-mediated mechanism, suggesting the involvement of the EP2 or EP4 receptor. It appears that the inhibitory effects of PGE_2 on cytokine production are more evident in T cells having the helper T cell type 1 (T_H1) phenotype rather than those with the T_H2 phenotype (163). These findings suggest that prostaglandins may influence the type of immune response mounted to an antigen and perhaps favor the induction of an allergic phenotype.

CONCLUSIONS

Since the last edition of this book was published, tremendous advances have been made in our understanding at the molecular level of the enzymes by which prostanoids are synthesized and of the receptors by which they exert their biological activities. The ability to selectively delete genes from the mouse genome has aided our understanding of the physiological roles of prostaglandins which had been hampered by the lack of selective and potent pharmacological antagonists. In addition, these studies have allowed the development of a new generation of drugs, the selective cyclooxygenase-2 inhibitors, which retain the beneficial therapeutic effects of earlier drugs without the GI problems that were associated with the class as a whole.

REFERENCES

1. Kurzrok R, Lieb C. Biochemical studies of human semen: action of semen on the human uterus. *Proc Soc Exp Biol* 1931;28:268–272.
2. von Euler US. Uber die spezifische blutdrucksenkende Substanz des menschlichen Prostata—und Samenblasensekretes. *Klin Wochenschr* 1935;14:1182–1183.
3. Von Euler US. Zur Kenntnis der pharmakologishen Wirkungen von Nativsekreten und Extrakten mannlicher accessorischer Geschlechtsdrusen. *Naunyn Schmiedebergs Arch Exp Pathol* 1934;175:78–84.
4. Goldblatt MW. A depressor substance in seminal fluid. *J Soc Chem Ind* 1933;52:1056–1057.
5. Bergstrom S, Sjoval J. The isolation of prostaglandin. *Acta Chem Scand* 1957;11:1086–1087.

6. Bergstrom S, Sjoval J. The isolation of prostaglandin F from sheep prostate glands. *Acta Chem Scand* 1960;14:1693–1701.

7. Bergstrom S, Sjoval J. The isolation of prostaglandin E from sheep prostate glands. *Acta Chem Scand* 1960;14:1701–1708.

8. Bergstrom S, Danielsson H, Samuelsson B. The enzymatic formation of prostaglandin E_2 from arachidonic acid. Prostaglandins and related factors. *Biochim Biophys Acta* 1964;90:207–210.

9. Van Dorp DA, Beerthius RK, Nugteren DH, et al. Enzymatic conversion of all-*cis*-polyunsaturated fatty acids into prostaglandins. *Nature* 1964;203:839–841.

10. Piper PJ, Vane JR. Release of additional factors in anaphylaxis and its antagonism by anti-inflammatory drugs. *Nature* 1969;223:29–35.

11. Gryglewski R, Vane JR. The generation from arachidonic acid of rabbit aorta contracting substance (RCS) by a microsomal enzyme preparation which also generates prostaglandins. *Br J Pharmacol* 1972;46:449–457.

12. Hamberg M, Samuelsson B. Detection and isolation of an endoperoxide intermediate in prostaglandin biosynthesis. *Proc Natl Acad Sci USA* 1973;70:899–903.

13. Nugteren DH, Hazelhof E. Isolation and properties of intermediates in prostaglandin biosynthesis. *Biochim Biophys Acta* 1973;326:448–461.

14. Hamberg M, Samuelsson B. Prostaglandin endoperoxides. Novel transformations of arachidonic acid in human platelets. *Proc Natl Acad Sci USA* 1974;71:3400–3404.

15. Hamberg M, Svensson J, Samuelsson B. Thromboxanes: a new group of biologically active compounds derived from prostaglandin endoperoxides. *Proc Natl Acad Sci USA* 1975;72:2994–2998.

16. Moncada S, Gryglewski R, Bunting S, et al. An enzyme isolated from arteries transforms prostaglandin endoperoxides to an unstable substance that inhibits platelet aggregation. *Nature* 1976;263:663–665.

17. Whittaker N, Bunting S, Salmon J, et al. The chemical structure of prostaglandin X (prostacyclin). *Prostaglandins* 1976;12:915–928.

18. Pouliot M, Baillargeon J, Lee JC, et al. Inhibition of prostaglandin endoperoxide synthase-2 expression in stimulated human monocytes by inhibitors of p38 mitogen-activated protein kinase. *J Immunol* 1997;158:4930–4937.

19. Fu J, Masferrer JL, Siebert K, et al. The induction and suppression of prostaglandin H2 synthase (cyclooxygenase) in human monocytes. *J Biol Chem* 1990;265:1–4.

20. Murakami M, Matsumoto R, Austen KF, et al. Prostaglandin endoperoxide synthase-1 and -2 couple to different transmembrane stimuli to generate prostaglandin D_2 in mouse bone marrow-derived mast cells. *J Biol Chem* 1994;269:22269–22275.

21. Dayer J-M, Beutler B, Cerami A. Cachectin/tumor necrosis factor stimulates collagenase and prostaglandin E_2 production by human synovial cells and dermal fibroblasts. *J Exp Med* 1985;162:2163–2168.

22. Dayer J-M, de Rochemonteix B, Burrus B, et al. Human recombinant interleukin 1 stimulates collagenase and prostaglandin E_2 production by human synovial cells. *J Clin Invest* 1986;77:645–648.

23. Albrightson CR, Baenzinger NL, Needleman P. Exaggerated human vascular cell prostaglandin biosynthesis mediated by monocytes: role of monokines and interleukin 1. *J Immunol* 1985;135:1872–1877.

24. Griffiths RJ, Li SW, Wood BE, et al. A comparison of the anti-inflammatory activity of selective 5-lipoxygenase inhibitors with dexamethasone and colchicine in a model of zymosan induced inflammation in the rat knee joint and peritoneal cavity. *Agents Actions* 1991;32:313–320.

25. Henderson B, Higgs GA. Synthesis of arachidonate oxidation products by synovial joint tissues during the development of chronic erosive arthritis. *Arthritis Rheum* 1987;30:1149–1156.

26. Day RO, Francis H, Vial J, et al. Naproxen concentrations in plasma and synovial fluid and effects on prostanoid concentrations. *J Rheumatol* 1995;22:2295–2303.

27. Pettipher ER, Henderson B, Moncada S, et al. Leukocyte infiltration and cartilage proteoglycan loss in immune arthritis in the rabbit. *Br J Pharmacol* 1988;95:169–176.

28. Bonney RJ, Naruns P, Davies P, et al. Antigen-antibody complexes stimulate synthesis and release of prostaglandins by mouse peritoneal macrophages. *Prostaglandins* 1979;18:605–616.

29. Doherty NS, Poubelle P, Borgeat P, et al. Intraperitoneal injection of zymosan in mice induces pain, inflammation and the synthesis of peptidoleukotrienes and prostaglandin E_2. *Prostaglandins* 1985;30:769–789.

30. Bartels JH, Kunze H, Vogt W, et al. Prostaglandin: liberation from and formation in perfused frog intestine. *Naunyn Schmiedebergs Arch Pharmacol* 1970;266:199–207.

31. Hong S, Levine L. Inhibition of arachidonic acid release from cells as the biochemical action of anti-inflammatory corticosteroids. *Proc Natl Acad Sci USA* 1976;73:1730–1734.

32. Flower RJ, Blackwell GJ. The importance of phospholipase A_2 in prostaglandin biosynthesis. *Biochem Pharmacol* 1976;25:285–291.

33. Dennis EA. The growing phospholipase A_2 superfamily of signal transduction enzymes. *Trends Biochem Sci* 1997;22:1–2.

34. Leslie CC. Properties and regulation of cytosolic phospholipase A_2. *J Biol Chem* 1997;272:16709–16712.

35. Seilhamer JJ, Pruzanski W, Vadas P, et ai. Cloning and recombinant expression of phospholipase A_2 present in rheumatoid arthritic synovial fluid. *J Biol Chem* 1989;264:5335–5338.

36. Clark JD, Lin L-L, Kriz RW. A novel arachidonic acid-selective cytosolic PLA_2 contains a Ca^{2+}-dependent translocation domain with homology to PKC and GAP. *Cell* 1991;65:1043–1051.

37. Sharp JD, White DL, Chiou XG, et al. Molecular cloning and expression of human Ca^{++}-sensitive cytosolic phospholipase A_2. *J Biol Chem* 1991;266:14850–14853.

38. Bingham CO III, Murakami M, Fujishima H, et al. A heparin-sensitive phospholipase A_2 and prostaglandin endoperoxide synthase-2 are functionally linked in the delayed phase of prostaglandin D_2 generation in mouse bone marrow-derived mast cells. *J Biol Chem* 1996;271:25936–25944.

39. Peters-Golden M, Song K, Marshall T, et al. Translocation of cytosolic phospholipase A_2 to the nuclear envelope elicits topographically localized phospholipid hydrolysis. *Biochem J* 1996;318:797–803.

40. Schievella AR, Regier MK, Smith WL, et al. Calcium-mediated translocation of cytosolic phospholipase A_2 to the nuclear envelope and endoplasmic reticulum. *J Biol Chem* 1995;270:30749–30754.

41. Marshall LA, Bolognese B, Winkler JD, et al. Depletion of human monocyte 85-kDa phospholipase A_2 does not alter leukotriene formation. *J Biol Chem* 1997;272:759–765.

42. Lyons-Giordano B, Davis GL, Galbraith W, et al. Interleukin-1 beta stimulates phospholipase A_2 mRNA synthesis in rabbit articular chondrocytes. *Biochem Biophys Res Commun* 1989;164:488–495.

43. Tischfield JA. A reassessment of the low molecular weight phospholipase A_2 gene family in mammals. *J Biol Chem* 1997;272:17247–17250.

44. Reddy ST, Winstead MV, Tischfield JA, et al. Analysis of the secretory phospholipase A_2 that mediates prostaglandin production in mast cells. *J Biol Chem* 1997;272:13591–13596.

45. Balboa MA, Balsinde J, Winstead MV, et al. Novel group V phospholipase A_2 involved in arachidonic acid mobilization in murine P388D1 macrophages. *J Biol Chem* 1996;271:32381–32384.

46. Chen J, Engle SJ, Seilhamer JJ, et al. Cloning and recombinant expression of a novel human low molecular weight Ca^{++}-dependent phospholipase A_2. *J Biol Chem* 1994;269:2365–2368.

47. Smith WL, Garavito RM, DeWitt DL. Prostaglandin endoperoxide H synthases (cyclooxygenases)-1 and -2. *J Biol Chem* 1996;271:33157–33160.

48. Vane JR. Inhibition of prostaglandin synthesis as a mechanism of action for aspirin-like drugs. *Nat New Biol* 1971;231:232–235.

49. Morrison AR, Nishikawa K, Needleman P. Thromboxane A_2 biosynthesis in the ureter obstructed isolated perfused kidney of the rabbit. *J Pharmacol Exp Ther* 1978;205:1–8.

50. Seibert K, Masferrer JL, Needleman P, et al. Pharmacological manipulation of cyclo-oxygenase-2 in the inflamed hydronephrotic kidney. *Br J Pharmacol* 1996;117:1016–1020.

51. Raz A, Wyche A, Siegal N, et al. Regulation of fibroblast cyclooxygenase synthesis by interleukin-1. *J Biol Chem* 1988;263:3022–3028.

52. DeWitt DL, Smith WL. Primary structure of prostaglandin G/H synthase from sheep vesicular gland determined from the complementary DNA sequence. *Proc Natl Acad Sci USA* 1988;85:1412–1416.

53. DeWitt DL, El-Harith EA, Kraemer SA, et al. The aspirin and heme-binding sites of ovine and murine prostaglandin endoperoxide synthases. *J Biol Chem* 1990;265:5192–5198.

54. Funk CD, Funk LB, Kennedy ME, et al. Human platelet/erythroleukemia cell prostaglandin G/H synthase cDNA cloning, expression and gene chromosomal assignment. *FASEB J* 1991;1991:2304–2312.

55. Merlie JP, Fagan D, Mudd J, et al. Isolation and characterization of the complementary DNA for sheep seminal vesicle prostaglandin endoperoxide synthase (cyclooxygenase). *J Biol Chem* 1988;263:3550–3553.

56. Yokoyama C, Tanabe T. Cloning of human gene encoding prostaglandin endoperoxide synthase and primary structure of the enzyme. *Biochem Biophys Res Commun* 1989;165:888–894.

57. Yokayama C, Takai T, Tanabe T, et al. Primary structure of sheep

prostaglandin endoperoxide synthase deduced from cDNA sequence. *FEBS Lett* 1988;231:347–351.

58. Kujubu DA, Fletcher BS, Varnum BC, et al. TIS10, a phorbol ester tumor promoter-inducible mRNA from Swiss 3T3 cells encodes a novel prostaglandin synthase/cyclooxygenase homologue. *J Biol Chem* 1991;266:12866–12872.

59. Xie W, Chipman JG, Robertson DL, et al. Expression of a mitogen-responsive gene encoding prostaglandin synthase is regulated by mRNA splicing. *Proc Natl Acad Sci USA* 1991;88:2692–2696.

60. Fletcher BS, Kujuba DA, Perrin DM, et al. Structure of the mitogen-inducible TIS10 gene and demonstration that the TIS10-encoded protein is a functional prostaglandin G/H synthase. *J Biol Chem* 1992; 267:4338–4344.

61. O'Bannion MK, Winn VD, Young DA. cDNA cloning and functional activity of a glucocorticoid regulated inflammatory cyclooxygenase. *Proc Natl Acad Sci USA* 1992;89:4888–4892.

62. Jones DA, Carlton DP, McIntyre TM, et al. Molecular cloning of human prostaglandin endoperoxide synthase type II and demonstration of expression in response to cytokines. *J Biol Chem* 1993;268: 9049–9054.

63. Hla T, Neilson K. Human cyclooxygenase-2 cDNA. *Proc Natl Acad Sci USA* 1992;89:7384–7388.

64. Kennedy BP, Chan C-C, Culp SA, et al. Cloning and expression of rat prostaglandin endoperoxide synthase (cyclooxygenase)-2 cDNA. *Biochem Biophys Res Commun* 1993;197:494–500.

65. Crofford LJ, Wilder RL, Ristimaki AP, et al. Cyclooxygenase-1 and -2 expression in rheumatoid synovial tissues: effects of interleukin-1β, phorbol ester, and corticosteroids. *J Clin Invest* 1994;93:1095–1101.

66. Sano H, Hla T, Maier JAM, et al. *In vivo* cyclooxygenase expression in synovial tissue of patients with rheumatoid arthritis and osteoarthritis and rats with adjuvant and streptococcal cell wall arthritis. *J Clin Invest* 1992;89:97–108.

67. O'Sullivan MG, Chilton FH, Huggins EMJ, et al. Lipopolysaccharide priming of alveolar macrophages for enhanced synthesis of prostanoids involves induction of a novel prostaglandin H synthase. *J Biol Chem* 1992;267:14547–14550.

68. Masferrer JL, Zweifel BS, Seibert K, et al. Endogenous glucocorticoids regulate an inducible cyclooxygenase enzyme. *Proc Natl Acad Sci USA* 1992;89:3917–3921.

69. Masferrer JL, Zweifel BS, Seibert K, et al. Selective inhibition of inducible cyclooxygenase 2 *in vivo* is antiinflammatory and nonulcerogenic. *Proc Natl Acad Sci USA* 1994;91:3228–3232.

70. Harris RC, McKanna JA, Akai Y, et al. Cyclooxygenase-2 is associated with the macula densa of rat kidney and increases with salt restriction. *J Clin Invest* 1994;93:2504–2510.

71. O'Neill G, Ford-Hutchinson A. Expression of mRNA for cyclooxygenase-1 and cyclooxygenase-2 in human tissues. *FEBS Lett* 1993; 330:156–160.

72. Crofford LJ, Tan B, McCarthy CJ, et al. Involvement of nuclear factor kappa-B in the regulation of cyclooxygenase-2 expression by interleukin-1 in rheumatoid synoviocytes. *Arthritis Rheum* 1997;40: 226–236.

73. Schmedtje JF, Ji YS, Liu WL, et al. Hypoxia induces cyclooxygenase-2 via the NF-kappa-B p65 transcription factor in human vascular endothelial cells. *J Biol Chem* 1997;272:601–608.

74. Ridley SH, Sarsfield SJ, Lee JC, et al. Actions of IL-1 are selectively controlled by p38 mitogen-activated protein kinase. *J Immunol* 1997; 158:3165–3173.

75. Morita I, Schindler M, Regier MK, et al. Different intracellular locations for prostaglandin endoperoxide H synthase-1 and -2. *J Biol Chem* 1995;270:10902–10908.

76. Kurumball RG, Stevens AM, Gierse JK, et al. Structural basis for selective inhibition of cyclooxygenase-2 by antiinflammatory agents. *Nature* 1996;384:644–648.

77. Luong C, Miller A, Barnett J, et al. Flexibility of the NSAID binding site in the structure of human cyclooxygenase-2. *Nature Structural Biology* 1996;3:927–933.

78. Reddy ST, Herschman HR. Ligand-induced prostaglandin synthesis requires expression of the TIS10/PGHS-2 prostaglandin synthase gene in murine fibroblasts and macrophages. *J Biol Chem* 1994;269: 15473–15480.

79. Reddy ST. Prostaglandin synthase-1 and prostaglandin synthase-2 are coupled to distinct phospholipases for the generation of prostaglandin D2 in activated mast cells. *J Biol Chem* 1997;272:3231–3237.

80. Dinchuk JE, Car BD, Focht RJ, et al. Renal abnormalities and an altered inflammatory response in mice lacking cyclooxygenase II. *Nature* 1995;378:406–409.

81. Morham SG, Langenbach R, Loftin CD, et al. Prostaglandin synthase 2 gene disruption causes severe renal pathology in the mouse. *Cell* 1995;83:473–482.

82. Langenbach R, Morham SG, Tiano HF, et al. Prostaglandin synthase 1 gene disruption in mice reduces arachidonic acid-induced inflammation and indomethacin-induced gastric ulceration. *Cell* 1995;83:483–490.

83. Nagata A, Susuki Y, Igarashi M, et al. Human brain prostaglandin D synthase has been evolutionarily differentiated from lipophilic-ligand carrier proteins. *Proc Natl Acad Sci USA* 1991;88:4020–4024.

84. Watanabe K, Yutaka F, Nakayama K, et al. Structural similarity of bovine lung prostaglandin F synthase to lens ε-crystallin of the European common frog. *Proc Natl Acad Sci USA* 1988;85:11–15.

85. Hara S, Miyata A, Yokoyama C, et al. Isolation and molecular cloning of prostacyclin synthase from bovine endothelial cells. *J Biol Chem* 1994;269:19897–19903.

86. Miyata A, Hara S, Yokoyama C, et al. Molecular cloning and expression of human prostacyclin synthase. *Biochem Biophys Res Commun* 1994;200:1728–1734.

87. Pereira B, Wu KK, Wang LH. Molecular cloning and characterization of bovine prostacyclin synthase. *Biochem Biophys Res Commun* 1994; 203:59–66.

88. Yokayama C, Miyata A, Ihara H, et al. Molecular cloning of human platelet thromboxane A synthase. *Biochem Biophys Res Commun* 1991;178:1479–1444.

89. Urade Y, Watanabe K, Hayaishi O. Prostaglandin D, E, and F synthases. *J Lipid Mediat Cell Signal* 1995;12:257–273.

90. Kuwamoto S, Inoue H, Tone Y, et al. Inverse gene expression of prostacyclin and thromboxane synthases in resident and activated peritoneal macrophages. *FEBS Lett* 1997;409:242–246.

91. Matsumoto H, Naraba H, Murakami M, et al. Concordant induction of prostaglandin E synthase with cyclooxygenase-2 leads to preferred production of prostaglandin E2 over thromboxane and prostaglandin D2 in lipopolysaccharide-stimulated rat peritoneal macrophages. *Biochem Biophys Res Commun* 1997;230:110–114.

92. Nusing R, Goerig M, Habenicht AJ, et al. Selective eicosanoid formation during HL-60 macrophage differentiation: regulation of thromboxane synthase. *Eur J Biochem* 1993;212:371–376.

93. Ferreira SH, Vane JR. Prostaglandins: their disappearance from and release into the circulation. *Nature* 1967;216:868–873.

94. Kanai N, Lu R, Satriano JA, et al. Identification and characterization of a prostaglandin transporter. *Science* 1995;268:866–869.

95. Lu R, Kanai N, Bao Y, et al. Cloning, *in vitro* expression, and tissue distribution of a human prostaglandin transporter cDNA (hPGT). *J Clin Invest* 1996;98:1142–1149.

96. Anggard E, Samuelsson B. Metabolism of prostaglandin E1 in guinea pig lung: the structure of two metabolites. *J Biol Chem* 1964;239: 4097–4102.

97. Tai H-H, Ensor CM. 15-Hydroxyprostaglandin dehydrogenase. *J Lipid Mediat Cell Signal* 1995;12:313–319.

98. Matsuo M, Ensor CM, Tai H-H. Cloning and expression of the cDNA for mouse NAD+-dependent 15-hydroxyprostaglandin dehydrogenase. *Biochim Biophys Acta* 1996;1309:21–24.

99. Zhang H, Matsuo M, Zhou H, et al. Cloning and expression of the cDNA for rat NAD+-dependent 15-hydroxyprostaglandin dehydrogenase. *Gene* 1997;188:41–44.

100. Ensor CM, Yang YY, Okita RT, et al. Cloning and sequence analysis of the cDNA for human placental NAD+-dependent 15-hydroxyprostaglandin dehydrogenase. *J Biol Chem* 1990;265:14888–14891.

101. Delage-Mourroux R, Pichaud F, Frendo JL, et al. Cloning and sequencing of a new 15-hydroxyprostaglandin dehydrogenase related mRNA. *Gene* 1997;188:143–148.

102. McGuire JC, Sun FF. Metabolism of prostacyclin: oxidation by rhesus monkey lung 15-hydroxyl prostaglandin dehydrogenase. *Arch Biochem Biophys* 1978;189:92–96.

103. Armstrong JM, Lattimer N, Moncada S, et al. Comparison of the vasodepressor effects of prostacyclin and 6-oxo-prostaglandin F1α with those of prostaglandin E2 in rats and rabbits. *Br J Pharmacol* 1978;62:125–130.

104. Machleidt C, Forstermann U, Anhut H, et al. Formation and elimination of prostacyclin metabolites in the cat *in vivo* as determined by radioimmunoassay of unextracted plasma. *Eur J Pharmacol* 1981;74:19–26.

105. Kennedy I, Coleman RA, Humphrey PPA, et al. Studies on the characterization of prostanoid receptors: a proposed classification. *Prostaglandins* 1982;24:667–689.

106. Coleman RA, Smith WL, Narumiya S. Classification of prostanoid receptors: properties, distribution, and structure of the receptors and their subtypes. *Pharmacol Rev* 1994;46:205–229.

107. Hirata M, Hayashi Y, Ushikubi F, et al. Cloning and expression of the cDNA for a human thromboxane A_2 receptor gene. *Nature* 1991;349:617–620.

108. Abramovitz M, Boie Y, Nguyen T, et al. Cloning and expression of a cDNA for the human prostanoid FP receptor. *J Biol Chem* 1994;269:2632–2636.

109. Bastien L, Sawyer N, Grygorczyk R, et al. Cloning, functional expression, and characterization of the human prostaglandin E_2 receptor EP2 subtype. *J Biol Chem* 1994;269:11873–11877.

110. An S, Yang J, Xia M, et al. Cloning and expression of the EP2 subtype of human receptors for prostaglandin E_2. *Biochem Biophys Res Commun* 1993;197:263–270.

111. Boie Y, Rushmore TH, Darmon-Goodwin A, et al. Cloning and expression of a cDNA for the human prostanoid IP receptor. *J Biol Chem* 1994;269:12173–12178.

112. Boie Y, Sawyer N, Slipetz DM, et al. Molecular cloning and characterization of the human prostanoid DP receptor. *J Biol Chem* 1995;270:18910–18916.

113. Funk CD, Furci L, FitzGerald GA, et al. Cloning and expression of a cDNA for the human prostaglandin E receptor EP1 subtype. *J Biol Chem* 1993;268:26767–26772.

114. Honda A, Sugimoto Y, Namba T, et al. Cloning and expression of a cDNA for mouse prostaglandin E receptor EP2 subtype. *J Biol Chem* 1993;268:7759–7762.

115. Nishigaki N, Negishi M, Honda A, et al. Identification of prostaglandin E receptor "EP2" cloned from mastocytoma cells as EP4 subtype. *FEBS Lett* 1995;364:339–341.

116. Regan JW, Bailey TJ, Pepperl DJ, et al. Cloning of a novel human prostaglandin receptor with characteristics of the pharmacologically defined EP2 subtype. *Mol Pharmacol* 1994;46:213–220.

117. Sando T, Usui T, Tanaka I, et al. Molecular cloning and expression of rat prostaglandin E receptor EP2 subtype. *Biochem Biophys Res Commun* 1994;200:1329–1333.

118. Sugimoto Y, Namba T, Honda A, et al. Cloning and expression of a cDNA for mouse prostaglandin E receptor EP3 subtype. *J Biol Chem* 1992;267:6463–6466.

119. Watabe A, Sugimoto Y, Honda A, et al. Cloning and expression of cDNA for a mouse EP1 subtype of prostaglandin E receptor. *J Biol Chem* 1993;268:20175–20178.

120. Raychowdhury MK, Yukawa M, Collins LJ, et al. Alternative splicing produces a divergent cytoplasmic tail in the human endothelial thromboxane A_2 receptor. *J Biol Chem* 1994;269:19256–19261.

121. Regan JW, Bailey TJ, Donello JE, et al. Molecular cloning and expression of human EP3 receptors: evidence of three variants with differing carboxyl termini. *Br J Pharmacol* 1994;112:377–385.

122. An S, Yang J, So SW, et al. Isoforms of the EP3 subtype of human prostaglandin E_2 receptor transduce both intracellular calcium and cAMP. *Biochemistry* 1994;33:14496–14502.

123. Namba T, Sugimoto Y, Negishi M, et al. Alternative splicing of C-terminal tail of prostaglandin E receptor subtype determines G-protein specificity. *Nature* 1993;365:166–170.

124. Murata T, Ushikubi F, Matsuoka T, et al. Altered pain perception and inflammatory response in mice lacking prostacyclin receptor. *Nature* 1997;388:678–682.

125. Kluger MJ. Fever: role of pyrogens and cryogens. *Physiol Rev* 1991;71:93–127.

126. Feldberg W, Saxena PN. Fever produced by prostaglandin E_1. *J Physiol* 1971;217:547–556.

127. Milton AS, Wendlandt S. Effects on body temperature of prostaglandins of the A, E and F series on injection into the third ventricle of unanaesthetized cats and rabbits. *J Physiol* 1971;218:325–336.

128. Feldberg W, Gupta KP. Pyrogen fever and prostaglandin-like activity in cerebrospinal fluid. *J Physiol* 1973;228:41–53.

129. Stitt JT. Prostaglandin E as the neural mediator of the febrile response. *Yale J Biol Med* 1986;59:137–149.

130. Boyce S, Chan C-C, Gordon R, et al. L-745,337: a selective inhibitor of cyclooxygenase-2 elicits antinociception but not gastric ulceration in rats. *Neuropharmacology* 1994;33:1609–1611.

131. Riendeau R, Percival MD, Boyce S, et al. Biochemical and pharmacological profile of a tetrasubstituted furanone as a highly selective COX-2 inhibitor. *Br J Pharmacol* 1997;121:105–117.

132. Cao CY, Matsumura K, Yamagata K, et al. Involvement of cyclooxygenase-2 in LPS-induced fever and regulation of its mRNA by LPS in the rat brain. *Am J Physiol* 1997;41:R1712–R1725.

133. Ferreira SH, Nakamura M, Abreu Castro MS. The hyperalgesic effects of prostacyclin and PGE2. *Prostaglandins* 1978;16:31–38.

134. Chan C-C, Boyce S, Brideau C, et al. Pharmacology of a selective cyclooxygenase-2 inhibitor, L-745,337: a novel nonsteroidal anti-inflammatory agent with an ulcerogenic sparing effect in rat and non-human primate. *J Pharmacol Exp Ther* 1995;274:1531–1537.

135. Mnich SJ, Veenhuizen AW, Monahan JB, et al. Characterization of a monoclonal antibody that neutralizes the activity of prostaglandin E_2. *J Immunol* 1995;155:4437–4444.

136. Portanova JP, Zhang Y, Anderson GD. Selective neutralization of prostaglandin E_2 blocks inflammation, hyperalgesia, and interleukin 6 production *in vivo. J Exp Med* 1996;184:883–891.

137. Seibert K, Zhang Y, Leahy K, et al. Pharmacological and biochemical demonstration of the role of cyclooxygenase 2 in inflammation and pain. *Proc Natl Acad Sci USA* 1994;91:12013–12017.

138. Moncada S, Vane J, Ferreira SH. Prostaglandins, aspirin-like drugs and the odema of inflammation. *Nature* 1973;246:217–219.

139. Williams TJ, Morley J. Prostaglandins as potentiators of increased vascular permeability in inflammation. *Nature* 1973;246:215–217.

140. Williams TJ, Peck MJ. Role of prostaglandin-mediated vasodilatation in inflammation. *Nature* 1977;270:530–532.

141. Williams TJ. Prostaglandin E_2, prostaglandin I_2 and the vascular changes of inflammation. *Br J Pharmacol* 1979;65:517–524.

142. Wedmore CV, Williams TJ. Control of vascular permeability by polymorphonuclear leukocytes in inflammation. *Nature* 1981;289:646–650.

143. Issekutz AC. Effect of vasoactive agents on polymorphonuclear leukocyte emigration *in vivo. Lab Invest* 1981;45:234–240.

144. Issekutz AC, Movat HZ. The effect of vasodilator prostaglandins on polymorphonuclear leukocyte infiltration and vascular injury. *Am J Pathol* 1982;107:300–309.

145. Teixeira MM, Williams TJ, Hellewell PG. E-type prostaglandins enhance local oedema formation and neutrophil accumulation but suppress eosinophil accumulation in guinea-pig skin. *Br J Pharmacol* 1993;110:416–422.

146. Wilhelmi G. Ueber die pharmakologischen Eigenschaften von irgapyrin, einem neuen Praparat aus der Pyrazolreihe. *Schweiz Med Wochenschr* 1949;79:577–582.

147. Winter CA, Risley EA, Nuss GW. Carrageenan-induced edema in the hind paw of the rat as an assay for antiinflammatory drugs. *Proc Soc Exp Biol Med* 1962;111:544–547.

148. Anderson GD, Hauser SD, McGarity KL, et al. Selective inhibition of cyclooxygenase (COX)-2 reverses inflammation and expression of COX-2 and interleukin 6 in rat adjuvant arthritis. *J Clin Invest* 1996;97:2672–2679.

149. Lipsky PE, Isakson PC. Outcome of specific COX-2 inhibition in rheumatoid arthritis. *J Rheumatol* 1997;24[Suppl 49]:9–14.

150. Fantone JC, Kunkel SL, Ward PA, et al. Suppression by prostaglandin E_1 of vascular permeability by vasoactive inflammatory mediators. *J immunol* 1980;125:2591–2596.

151. Kunkel SL, Thrall RS, Kunkel RG, et al. Suppression of immune complex vasculitis in rats by prostaglandin. *J Clin Invest* 1979;64:1525–1529.

152. Wheeldon A, Vardey CJ. Characterization of the inhibitory prostanoid receptors on human neutrophils. *Br J Pharmacol* 1993;108:1051–1054.

153. Rampart M, Williams TJ. Polymorphonuclear leukocyte-dependent plasma leakage in the rabbit skin enhanced or inhibited by prostacyclin, depending on the route of administration. *Am J Pathol* 1986;124:285–296.

154. Kunkel SL, Wiggings RC, Chensue SW, et al. Regulation of macrophage tumor necrosis factor production by prostaglandin E_2. *Biochem Biophys Res Commun* 1986;137:404–409.

155. Pettipher ER, Wimberley DJ. Cyclooxygenase inhibitors enhance tumor necrosis factor production and mortality in murine endotoxic shock. *Cytokine* 1994;6:500–503.

156. Martich GD, Danner RL, Ceska M, et al. Detection of interleukin 8 and tumor necrosis factor in normal humans after intravenous endotoxin: the effect of antiinflammatory agents. *J Exp Med* 1991;173:1021–1024.

157. Bottomley KMK, Griffiths RJ, Rising TJ, et al. A modified mouse air pouch model for evaluating the effects of compounds on granuloma-induced cartilage degradation. *Br J Pharmacol* 1988;93: 627–635.

158. Pettipher ER, Henderson B, Edwards JCW, et al. Effect of indomethacin on swelling, lymphocyte influx and cartilage proteoglycan depletion in experimental arthritis. *Ann Rheum Dis* 1989;48:623–627.

159. Goodwin JS, Bankhurst AD, Messner RP. Suppression of human T-cell mitogenesis by prostaglandin. *J Exp Med* 1977;146:1719–1725.

160. Snijdewint FGM. Prostaglandin E_2 differentially modulates cytokine secretion profiles of human T helper lymphocytes. *J Immunol* 1993; 150:5321–5329.

161. van der Pouw Kraan TCTM, Boeije LCM, Smeenk RJT, et al. Prostaglandin E_2 is a potent inhibitor of human interleukin 12 production. *J Exp Med* 1995;181:775–779.

162. Oppenheimer-Marks N, Kavanaugh AF, Lipsky PE. Inhibition of the transendothelial migration of human T lymphocytes by prostaglandin E_2. *J Immunol* 1994;152:5703–5713.

163. Betz M, Fox BS. Prostaglandin E_2 inhibits production of Th1 lymphokines but not of Th2 lymphokines. *J Immunol* 1991;146:108–113.

Inflammation: Basic Principles and Clinical Correlates,
3rd ed., edited by John I. Gallin and Ralph Snyderman.
Lippincott Williams & Wilkins, Philadelphia © 1999.

CHAPTER 23

Leukotrienes:

Biosynthetic Pathways, Release, and Receptor-Mediated Actions With Relevance to Disease States

John F. Penrose, K. Frank Austen, and Bing K. Lam

Leukotrienes are one of the three major families of arachidonic acid-based lipid mediators of inflammation, which also include prostaglandins and lipoxins. Leukotrienes are formed from the catalytic oxygenation of 20-carbon polyunsaturated fatty acids, most notably arachidonic acid. The term *leukotriene* describes leukocyte-derived molecules with three conjugated double bonds (i.e., trienes) (1) (Fig. 23-1). The potent biologic activities of these molecules have been implicated in the pathobiology of immediate-type hypersensitivity reactions and inflammation (2). Although initially discovered in the 1940s and described as the slow-reacting substance of anaphylaxis (3,4), the cysteinyl leukotrienes and the dihydroxy-leukotrienes were not defined chemically for more than 3 decades (5,6). Leukotrienes have been implicated in a broad array of functions and disease processes, and therapeutic agents that inhibit leukotriene biosynthesis and that antagonize leukotriene receptor-mediated effects have been developed.

This chapter reviews the biochemistry of leukotriene biosynthesis and release and the cDNAs or genes that encode the proteins involved in these pathways. Leukotriene effects, mediated through leukotriene receptors, are described at the cellular level in clinical disease states, and therapeutic modalities directed to the attenuation of these effects are reviewed.

LEUKOTRIENE BIOSYNTHESIS: BIOCHEMICAL AND MOLECULAR CHARACTERIZATION OF THE ACTIVE PROTEINS

The initial step in the generation of leukotrienes is the enzymatic release of arachidonic acid from cell *membrane phospholipids* (Fig. 23-2A). This reaction is catalyzed by phospholipase A_2, of which multiple isoforms have been identified with different physicochemical properties, molecular masses, and subcellular localizations (7). The first committed step in leukotriene formation from arachidonic acid is through the enzymatic action of 5-lipoxygenase (5-LO).

5-Lipoxygenase

Human 5-LO is a 78-kd enzyme, which acts as a stereospecific dioxygenase that catalyzes the insertion of molecular oxygen into arachidonic acid, leading to the formation of 5-hydroperoxyeicosatetraenoic acid (5-HPETE) (8). 5-HPETE then undergoes enzymatic dehydration by 5-LO to form leukotriene A_4 (LTA$_4$) (9,10) (see Fig. 23-2A).

5-LO has been identified in several cell types of myelomonocytic origin; they include neutrophils, eosinophils, basophils, monocytes, macrophages, and mast cells (10). Detailed kinetic studies of 5-LO have been difficult to perform because of rapid turnover inactivation (10); however, purified 5-LO from human leukocytes has an apparent K_m of 10 to 20 μmol/L for arachidonic acid and a V_{max} value of 5 μmol/min/mg for HPETE (9,11) (Table 23-1).

In resting cells, 5-LO is localized mainly to the cytosol or nucleoplasm. In neutrophils, cellular activa-

J. F. Penrose, K. F. Austen, and B. K. Lam: Department of Medicine, Harvard Medical School, and Division of Rheumatology, Immunology, and Allergy, Brigham and Women's Hospital, Boston, Massachusetts 02115.

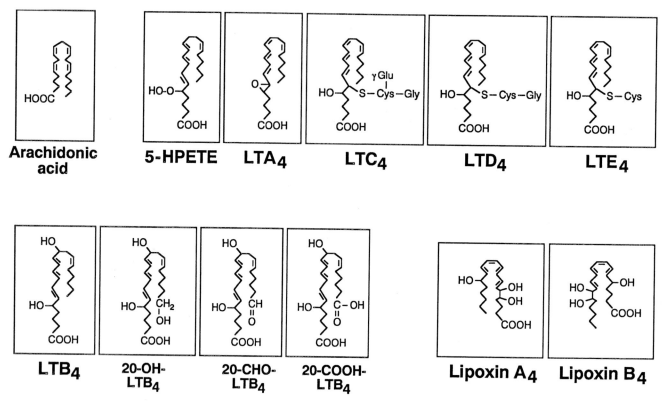

FIG. 23-1. Chemical structures of the arachidonic acid products of the 5-lipoxygenase pathway. The chemical structures of arachidonic acid, 5-hydroperoxyeicosatetraenoic acid (5-HPETE), the hydroxy and cysteinyl leukotrienes, and the lipoxins are shown.

tion causes the calcium-dependent translocation of 5-LO from the cytosol to the nuclear membrane; whereas in mast cells and basophils, the movement occurs from the nucleoplasm to the nuclear membrane (12–15). A portion of 5-LO colocalizes with 5-LO–activating protein (FLAP) after cellular activation. 5-LO contains a proline rich region in the carboxyl terminus, with an amino acid consensus sequence for an SRC homologous (SH3) domain (16). That such a domain interacts with cytoskeletal proteins such as growth factor receptor-bound protein-2, actin, and α-actinin may explain the effect of 5-LO in cell remodeling, an effect that probably is distinct from the known catalytic function of the enzyme (16).

The cDNA for 5-LO predicts a protein of 674 amino acids, with a molecular mass of 78 kd (17). The deduced amino acid sequence does not contain easily identifiable sequences for the binding domains of adenosine triphosphate (ATP) or Ca^{2+}, despite their apparent augmentation of subcellular 5-LO function (10). Homology between human 5-LO and other lipoxygenases and across species occurs in the carboxyl tail, suggesting that this highly conserved region may contain the active site (17). Site-directed mutagenesis studies reveal that histidine residues 368 and 373 are involved in coordination of the iron atom and are essential for enzyme activity (18–20).

The human 5-LO gene is more than 82 kilobases (kb), composed of 14 exons and 13 introns, and is localized on human chromosome 10 (21,22). The 5′-untranslated region of the 5-LO gene contains a GC-rich promoter region and lacks TATA or CCAAT regions, consistent with the features of a housekeeping gene (Table 23-2). The 5-LO gene has been subjected to targeted disruption in mice, and this process has revealed selective involvement of lipoxygenase products in a variety of induced inflammatory states (23,24). The absence of leukotrienes was associated with a reduced cellular inflammatory response in glycogen- and zymosan-induced peritonitis. An edematous inflammatory response mediated by the application of arachidonic acid was impaired. The endotoxin-induced shock response was intact; however, the 5-LO–deficient mice were resistant to platelet-activating factor–induced hypotension (23,24). 5-LO–deficient mice incurred increased lethality from *Klebsiella*-induced pneumonia. There was no defect in neutrophil recruitment, although macrophages were impaired in phagocytosis and killing; this defect could be restored with the administration of LTB₄ (25).

The function of 5-LO in leukotriene formation is pivotal, because LTA₄ is the common precursor of the two major bioactive classes of leukotrienes: the dihydroxy leukotriene, LTB₄, and the cysteinyl leukotrienes (see Figs. 23-1 and 23-2*C*). The synthesis of the leukotrienes appears to be differentially regulated so that few cell types produce both classes. LTA$_4$ may be exported for transcellular metabolism as in neutrophils, in which a portion of the abundantly produced LTA$_4$ is exported for potential transcellular metabolism. Smooth muscle cells and endothelial cells possess a bifunctional microsomal glutathione-*S*-transferase (mGST-II) (26) that catalyzes the formation of LTC$_4$ from LTA$_4$ (27,28). The transcellular conversion of LTA$_4$ to LTC$_4$ by platelets, however, occurs by the action of authentic LTC$_4$ synthase (29) (Fig. 23-2*C*). LTA$_4$ has an additional potential fate in the platelet, which through the action of 12-lipoxygenase can form the biologically active trihydroxytetraenes or lipoxins (30,31) (see Figs. 23-1 and 23-2*C*), which act as distinct mediators (32).

5-Lipoxygenase–Activating Protein

In activated neutrophils, 5-LO is translocated to the perinuclear membrane (33) from the cytoplasm as a result of a rise in intracellular calcium (10,12); there, it associates with an 18-kd integral perinuclear membrane protein known as 5-LO–activating protein (FLAP) (34). FLAP appears to present arachidonic acid to 5-LO (35). The secondary structure prediction for FLAP suggests three hydrophobic domains with two interspersed hydrophilic loops (36). The carboxyl-terminal end of the first loop contains amino acid residues responsible for the binding of drugs, called FLAP inhibitors, which attenuate cellular leukotriene biosynthesis but not subcellular 5-LO function, implying an effect on intracellular arachidonic acid presentation (37). FLAP has been shown by amino acid sequencing and genomic organization to be similar to another 18-kd integral membrane protein in the biosynthetic pathway of cysteinyl leukotrienes, LTC$_4$ synthase (36). The 161–amino acid protein is 31% identical to LTC$_4$ synthase, with 44% homology within the N-terminal two thirds of the molecule, including the FLAP inhibitor–binding domain. Genomic cloning reveals that the human FLAP gene contains 5 exons and 4 introns, which span more than 31 kb, and is located on chromosome 13q12 (10,38) (see Table 23-2). When the FLAP gene is subjected to targeted disruption, results are similar to those obtained in the 5-LO gene-disrupted mice. The mice develop normally and have normal delayed-type hypersensitivity reactions and IgE-mediated passive anaphylaxis; however, they have a blunted inflammatory response to topical arachidonic acid, increased resistance to platelet-activating factor–induced shock, and reduced edema in a zymosan-induced model of peritonitis (39). Collagen-induced arthritis is also significantly reduced in FLAP gene-disrupted mice (40).

Leukotriene A$_4$ Hydrolase

5*S*,12*R*-(dihydroxy)-6,8,10,14 (Z,E,E,Z)-eicosatetraenoic acid (LTB$_4$) is generated by the action of LTA$_4$ hydrolase,

a 70-kd cytosolic metalloenzyme with specific substrate requirements, that is distinct from liver epoxide hydrolase (41,42). This zinc-requiring enzyme contains two overlapping active sites with separate functions (43). The epoxide hydrolase activity acts only on LTA$_4$ with a stereospecific structure of a 5,6-epoxide with 7,9,11,14 (E,E,Z,Z) double bonds and converts it to LTB$_4$ (44). The epoxide hydrolase activity is activated by chloride ions and is suicide inactivated by the covalent binding of the enzyme to the substrate, LTA$_4$ (41,42). LTA$_4$ hydrolase has a K$_m$ value for LTA$_4$ of 5.8 µmol/L and a V$_{max}$ value of 692 nmol/min/mg for epoxide hydrolase activity (45,46). A separate catalytic site of the enzyme exhibits an aminopeptidase activity, for which a natural substrate has not been defined (41,46).

The cDNA of LTA$_4$ hydrolase predicts an encoded protein of 610 amino acids, and the deduced amino acid sequence shares no significant homology with liver epoxide hydrolase (47). Site-directed mutagenesis studies have revealed that histidine 295, histidine 299, and glutamic acid 318 are zinc-binding residues; that glutamic acid 296 and tyrosine 383 are catalytic residues for the peptidase function; and that enzyme inactivation by the substrate LTA$_4$ depends on a tyrosine residue in position 378 (48–51). In contrast to 5-LO, which is expressed in limited numbers of cells, LTA$_4$ hydrolase is widely distributed. The human gene for LTA$_4$ hydrolase is larger than 35 kb, has 19 exons, and is localized on chromosome 12q22 (52) (see Table 23-2).

Leukotriene C$_4$ Synthase

LTA$_4$, as the pivotal compound of leukotriene formation, is also a substrate for LTC$_4$ synthase. This 18-kd integral membrane protein conjugates reduced glutathione (GSH) to LTA$_4$ to form the parent cysteinyl leukotriene, 5*S*-hydroxy-6*R*-*S*-glutathionyl-7,9,11,14 (E,E,Z,Z)-eicosatetraenoic acid (LTC$_4$) (53,54) (see Figs. 23-1 and 23-2*C*). In contrast, mGST-II, which forms a homologous gene family with LTC$_4$ synthase and FLAP, is bifunctional in conjugating GSH to LTA$_4$ or the xenobiotic 1-chloro-2,4-dinitrobenzene (55). mGST-II is widely distributed in cells, including those cells lacking 5-LO expression, such as in the liver; this finding implies that the primary function of mGST-II is detoxification rather than serving as a central source of proinflammatory cysteinyl leukotrienes. LTC$_4$ synthase conjugates only LTA$_4$ and its analogues to GSH and has no ability to conjugate xenobiotics to GSH. LTC$_4$ synthase is expressed in a restricted population of hematopoietic cells, including eosinophils, basophils, mast cells, and monocytes-macrophages (56–59). Purified recombinant LTC$_4$ synthase exhibits K$_m$ values for LTA$_4$ and GSH of 3.6 µmol/L and 1.6 mmol/L, respectively, with V$_{max}$ values of 1.3 and 2.7 µmol/min/mg, respectively (60) (see Table 23-1).

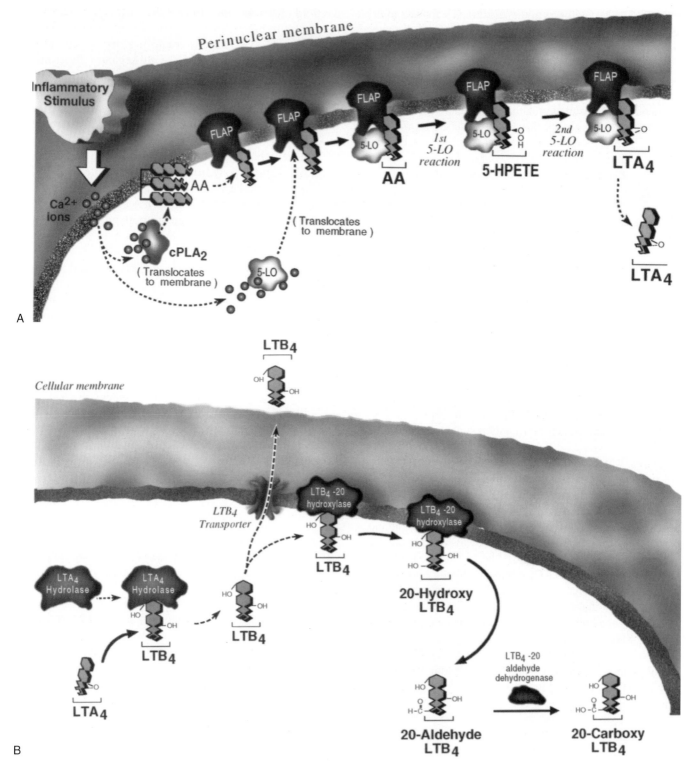

FIG. 23-2. (A) The 5-lipoxygenase pathway for the biosynthesis of the pivotal leukotriene, LTA$_4$, shows the enzymes and proteins for each of the biosynthetic steps in the formation of LTA$_4$, which acts as the common precursor to the dihydroxy and cysteinyl leukotrienes. **(B)** The leukotriene B$_4$ metabolism pathway shows the biosynthetic enzymes responsible for LTB$_4$ generation and 20-carbon oxidative inactivation in human neutrophils.

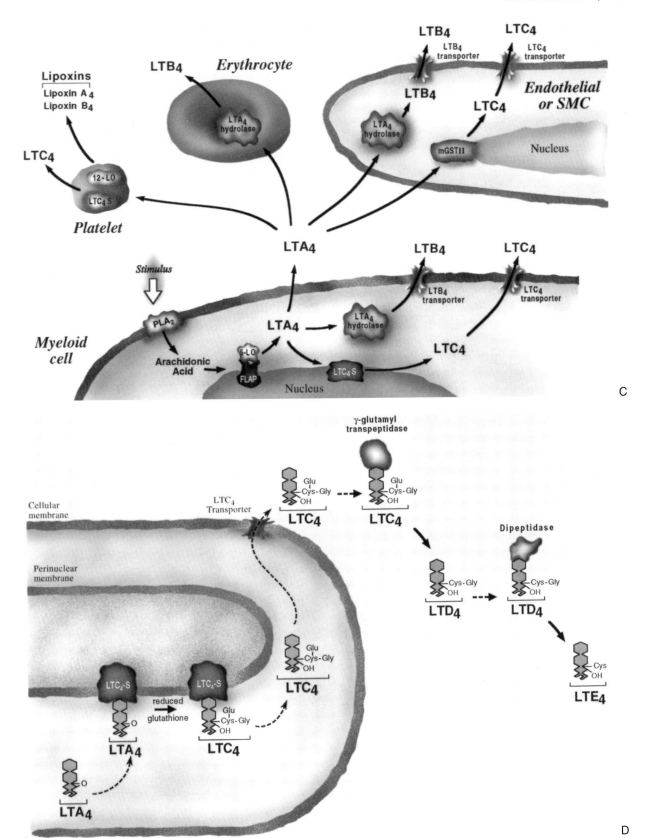

FIG. 23-2. *(continued)* **(C)** The pathway of LTA$_4$ metabolism in myeloid cells and the transcellular metabolism of LTA$_4$ in nonmyeloid cells are compared. The full complement of enzymes and other proteins is present for LTB$_4$ and LTC$_4$ generation in myeloid cells, whereas only terminal enzymes are present in nonmyeloid and nonhematopoietic cells. **(D)** Cysteinyl leukotriene metabolism. The intracellular generation of LTC$_4$ in the perinuclear location is depicted with its subsequent carrier-mediated export and extracellular conversion to LTD$_4$ and LTE$_4$. AA, arachidonic acid; cPLA$_2$, cytosolic phospholipase A$_2$; smc, smooth muscle cell.

TABLE 23-1. *Biochemical properties of the major enzymes and proteins of the 5-lipoxygenase biosynthetic pathway in humans*

Enzyme/protein	Size	K_m	V_{max}	pH optimum	Cofactors	Subcellular location	Reference
5-Lipoxygenase	78-kd, 674-amino-acid residues	10–20 µmol/L for arachidonic acid	5 µmol/min/mg protein for HPETE	7.5	Ca^{2+}, ATP	Cytosol or nucleoplasm; (translocates with cellular activation)	8,10,12–15
5-Lipoxygenase activating protein	18-kd, 161-amino-acid residues	—	—	—	—	Perinuclear integral membrane protein	15,34,35
Leukotriene A_4 hydrolase	70-kd, 610-amino-acid residues	5.8 µmol/L for LTA_4	0.6 µmol/min/mg protein for epoxide hydrolase activity	8.0	—	Cytosol	42–45
Leukotriene C_4 synthase	18-kd, 150-amino-acid residues	3.6 µmol/L for 1.6 LTA_4, 1.6mmol/L for GSH	1.3 µmol/min/mg for LTA_4 protein, 2.7 µmol/min/mg for GSH	8.5	—	Perinuclear integral membrane protein	29,53,54,60

GSH, reduced glutathione; HPETE, hydroperoxyeicosatetraenoic acid; LTA_4, leukotriene A_4.

TABLE 23-2. *Properties of the human genes for the major enzymes and proteins of the 5-lipoxygenase biosynthetic pathway*

Enzyme/protein	Gene size and structure	Promoter	Chromosomal localization	Reference
5-Lipoxygenase	<82 kb; 14 exons, 13 introns	5 tandem SP-1 sites	10	17,21
5-Lipoxygenase activating protein	>31 kb; 5 exons, 4 introns	Modified TATA box	13q12	38
Leukotriene A_4 hydrolase	>35 kb; 19 exons, 18 introns	No TATA, CAAT, or SP-1 promoter	12q22	52
Leukotriene C_4 synthase	2.5 kb; 5 exons, 4 introns	SP-1 site; no TATA or CAAT	5q35	62

The cDNAs for human and mouse LTC_4 synthases are 88% homologous at the nucleotide level and 87% homologous in amino acid sequence (60). The cDNAs encode for a 150–amino acid protein with three hydrophobic domains interspersed by two hydrophilic loops (36). Site-directed mutagenesis has suggested that arginine 51 is required to open the epoxide ring by acid catalysis of LTA_4, whereas tyrosine 93 provides the thiolate ion by base catalysis of GSH, resulting in conjugation to form LTC_4 (61). The gene for LTC_4 synthase is 2.5 kb and has an identical intron/exon alignment to that of FLAP; however, its chromosomal location of 5q35 is in proximity to the genes for helper T cell type 2 (T_H2) cytokines, which are implicated in allergic and asthmatic inflammation (62) (see Table 23-2).

LEUKOTRIENE TRANSPORT

After biosynthesis, leukotrienes are transported from human granulocytic cells in a carrier-mediated process that is temperature dependent and substrate specific and that exhibits saturation kinetics. Distinct and specific transporters export LTB_4 and LTC_4, respectively (63, 64).

The export of LTB_4 from neutrophils, the major cell type that generates this mediator, has a Q_{10} value of 3.0 and an energy of activation value of 19.9 kcal/mol (63). The transport of LTB_4 is significantly more rapid than that of its 20-OH metabolite and is inhibited by its structural analogue, LTB_5. The transport of LTB_4 is concentration dependent and exhibits saturation kinetics, with a calculated K_m of 80 pmol/10^6 cells and a V_{max} of 115 pmol/min/10^6 cells (63). The K_m and V_{max} values of LTC_4 export from the myelocytic cell line KG-1 are 80 pmol/10^6 cells and 38.5 pmol/min/10^6 cells/min, respectively (64). LTC_4 export from human eosinophils has a Q_{10} value of 3.7 and an energy of activation value of 28 kcal/mol (64), and these characteristics also hold for the KG-1 and dimethylsulfoxide-differentiated HL-60 cell lines. LTC_4 transport is inhibited in a dose-dependent fashion by competition with LTC_5 and by an intracellular glutathione conjugate of 1-chloro-2,4-dinitrobenzene (64). Probenecid inhibits the transport of LTC_4, but not that of LTB_4.

The observation that the export of LTC_4 competes with other GSH conjugates is compatible with a possible role of the ATP-dependent, multidrug-resistant associated protein (MRP) as a leukotriene transport protein (65).

The transfection of the cDNA for the MRP into HeLa cells increased the ATP-dependent uptake of LTC$_4$ by inside-out vesicles of the transfected cells. That cyclosporin, probenecid, and the leukotriene receptor antagonist, MK-571, all inhibit the uptake of LTC$_4$ by the inside-out vesicles suggests that the 190-kd MRP may be a LTC$_4$ carrier protein (66).

LEUKOTRIENE METABOLISM

LTB$_4$ may be exported from the cell by a carrier-mediated transport system to exert its biologic activity, or it may be retained intracellularly with attenuation of activity. In human neutrophils, the biologic activity of LTB$_4$ is attenuated by a series of oxidations of the terminal (C20) carbon (67) (see Fig. 23-2B). A microsomal P450 enzyme, LTB$_4$ 20-hydroxylase, sequentially catalyzes the formation of partially active 20-hydroxy LTB$_4$ (20-OH LTB$_4$) and the unstable intermediate, 20-aldehyde LTB$_4$ (20-CHO LTB$_4$) (68). The LTB$_4$ 20-hydroxylase cDNA encodes a 60-kd deduced protein of 520 amino acids (69). A 20-aldehyde dehydrogenase converts 20-aldehyde LTB$_4$ to 20-carboxyl LTB$_4$ (20-COOH LTB$_4$) (70), which is inactive in functional assays of chemotaxis or smooth muscle contractile responses. Other cells such as monocytes, macrophages, and mesangial cells metabolize LTB$_4$ by oxidation of C12, and keratinocytes adduct GSH to LTB$_4$ (71).

In animal models of systemic metabolism in which LTB$_4$ was infused, β oxidation metabolites appeared in the urine (72). The parent compound of the cysteinyl leukotrienes, LTC$_4$, is metabolized to receptor-active products or is inactivated after export. Gamma-glutamyl transpeptidase removes glutamic acid to form the cysteinylglycyl derivative, LTD$_4$ (73). LTD$_4$ is converted to the final bioactive cysteinyl leukotriene derivative, LTE$_4$, by dipeptidase cleav-

age of the glycine residue (74) (Fig. 23-2D). LTE$_4$ is excreted in the urine directly or after N-acetylation. In the microenvironment of an inflammatory reaction, cysteinyl leukotrienes may be inactivated by hypochlorous acid formed from myeloperoxidase-dependent hydrogen peroxidase and chloride ions. Hypochlorous acid can attack the sulfur bridge to generate inactive sulfoxides and the 6-trans-diastereoisomers of LTB$_4$ (75).

LEUKOTRIENE RECEPTORS

The receptors for LTB$_4$ are characterized by their ability to bind and transduce the effects of LTB$_4$ and by their selective blockade by several potent and selective antagonists (76,77) (Table 23-3). In neutrophils, the LTB$_4$ receptor appears to have two different affinity states. The high-affinity receptor state, with a K$_d$ of 0.3 nmol/L, transduces the functions of chemotaxis and adhesion, and the low-affinity receptor state, with a K$_d$ of 200 nmol/L, mediates the secretion of granule contents and superoxide generation when activated by LTB$_4$ (78). A cell-surface G-protein–coupled receptor for LTB$_4$ has been cloned and predicts a seven-transmembrane-spanning protein of 352 amino acids, with homology to receptors for rat somatostatin, human interleukin-8, lipoxin A$_4$, and the formylated tripeptide, methionine-leucine-phenylanine (79). This receptor is highly expressed in human leukocytes, transduces leukocyte chemotaxis and chemokinesis, and has a K$_d$ for LTB$_4$ of 0.15 nmol/L that corresponds to the high-affinity receptor that has been biochemically characterized. This receptor increases intracellular calcium and inositol triphosphate accumulation with adenylyl cyclase inhibition through pertussis-sensitive and -insensitive G proteins (79).

LTD$_4$ binds to high- and low-affinity receptor states in human lung and transduces signals through G-protein–

TABLE 23-3. *Characteristics of the leukotriene receptors*

Receptor	K$_d$	Protein size	Signal transduction	Distribution	Specific antagonists	Selected references
LTB$_4$ (OH-LTR)	0.15 nmol/L (high affinity) for [^{3}H]LTB$_4$ 53–80 nmol/L (low affinity) for [^{3}H]LTB$_4$	60-kd	G-protein–coupled; activates phospholipase C, increases Ca^{2+}, increases IP$_3$ turnover	Neutrophils, spleen, lung	LY223982 ONO-4057 SC 41930 RP 69698 SB 201993	76–79
LTC$_4$ (Cys-LTR$_2$)	Unknown	Unknown	G-protein–coupled; increases PI turnover, increases Ca^{2+}	Pulmonary vein	—	76,77,80, 81
LTD$_4$ (Cys-LTR$_1$)	0.4 nmol/L for [^{3}H]LTD$_4$	45-kd (guinea pig lung)	G-protein–coupled; increases PI turnover, increases Ca^{2+}	Bronchial smooth muscle, lung, GI tissues (animals)	MK-571 ICI 204,219 ICI 198,615 SK&F 104353 FPL 55712	76,77,80, 81

GI, gastrointestinal; IP$_3$, inositol 1,4,5-triphosphate; LTB$_4$, leukotriene B$_4$; LTC$_4$, leukotriene C$_4$; LTD$_4$, leukotriene D$_4$; PI, phosphatidyl inositol.

linked phospholipase C (80) (see Table 23-3). This receptor apparently is heterogeneous in guinea-pig lungs, as shown by the greater potency of LTE_4 relative to LTD_4 in contracting tracheal smooth muscle preparations, whereas the ratio is reversed in the contraction of parenchymal strips (81). LTC_4 binds cytosolic and membrane-bound GSTs, although no specific signal transduction has been shown by these interactions (82,83).

A classification system has been proposed in which the cysteinyl leukotriene receptors are divided into two categories. The receptors in the category of Cys-LTR1 interact with LTD_4/LTE_4 and are capable of being blocked by available receptor antagonists. The receptors in the category of Cys-LTR2 interact with LTC_4, are narrowly distributed, and are resistant to agonists that act on Cys-LTR1. Neither Cys-LTR1 nor Cys-LTR2 represents a homogeneous population of receptors based on affinity values determined for a range of antagonists (76,77) (see Table 23-3).

ROLE OF LEUKOTRIENES IN THE BIOLOGY OF INFLAMMATION

Pathophysiologic Effects of Leukotrienes

LTB_4 promotes neutrophil-induced inflammation by causing cell degranulation and release of lysosomal enzymes; it then provides autoamplification for these inflammatory effects by mediating adhesion, migration, and further accumulation of activated neutrophils (84,85). B lymphocytes respond to LTB_4 with enhanced activation and immunoglobulin production (86). Apart from these cell-surface receptor-mediated effects, LTB_4 acts as an intracellular messenger. LTB_4 is a ligand for the peroxisome proliferator-activated receptor-α (PPAR-α) (87), an orphan nuclear receptor that acts as a transcription factor to induce the expression of enzymes involved in fatty acid oxidation and adipogenesis. LTB_4 initiates and amplifies the inflammatory response, and through the actions of PPAR-α activation, it putatively initiates and controls its own metabolism (87).

Cysteinyl leukotrienes systemically administered to rats decrease glomerular filtration because of renovascular constriction with glomeruloconstriction (88) and have negative inotropic effects on myocardium because of coronary vasoconstriction (89). In bronchial asthma, the pathobiologic changes mediated by the cysteinyl leukotrienes result from their effects on smooth muscle: constriction of bronchial tissue and edema mediated by augmented venular permeability (90,91). This allergic pulmonary inflammation results from the activation of bone marrow–derived cells with a full 5-LO/LTC_4 synthase pathway, including monocytes, eosinophils, basophils, and mast cells (59,92–95). Of these cells, only monocytes generate LTB_4 and LTC_4 when stimulated with an appropriate stimulus, and the ratio of these leukotrienes varies with the stimulus (92).

Identification of Leukotrienes at Lesional Sites

Leukotrienes are present in the biologic fluids of inflammatory lesions in several disease states. Target organ allergen challenge induces the formation of cysteinyl leukotrienes which appear in the serum, bronchial lavage fluid, and urine of patients with bronchial asthma (96–98), in the nasal secretions of those with allergic rhinitis, and in the tears of patients with conjunctivitis (99). In other pulmonary conditions such as adult respiratory distress syndrome (100), neonatal pulmonary hypertension (101), and chronic obstructive pulmonary disease, cysteinyl leukotrienes are present in bronchial fluids or sputum (Table 23-4) (102). Cysteinyl leukotriene generation is markedly increased in patients with juvenile chronic arthritis, and there is an association between increased LTE_4 excretion and the number of affected joints (103).

LTB_4 is found in the rectal fluid of patients with inflammatory bowel disease (104), the skin lesions of patients with psoriasis (105), and the synovial fluid of patients with gout (106). In patients with rheumatoid arthritis, the elevated levels of LTB_4 in the synovial fluid (107) correlate with the increases in synovial fluid leukocytes, immune complexes, and rheumatoid factor (108). Synovial tissues from patients with rheumatoid arthritis, osteoarthritis, and pseudogout produce prostanoids and leukotrienes *in vitro* in response to calcium ionophore (109).

Therapeutic Interventions with Agents Active Against 5-Lipoxygenase Products

In clinical studies of patients with moderate asthma, agents active against leukotriene biosynthesis or cysteinyl leukotriene receptors produced relief within 30 minutes of administration through reduction of the basal level of airway tone produced by chronic overproduction of the cysteinyl leukotrienes in this population (110). Patients with cold air- and exercise-induced asthma exhibit only partial responses to agents active against 5-LO biosynthesis or cysteinyl leukotriene receptor antagonists, suggesting that these pulmonary function abnormalities are mediated through additional mechanisms (111–113). Episodes of experimentally initiated asthma, induced by the administration of antigens, are attenuated with increasingly more effective inhibitors of 5-LO (114–118), and aspirin-induced asthma appears to be a subset mediated almost exclusively by the cysteinyl leukotrienes (119–121). In patients with chronic stable asthma, increased airflow, as measured by the forced expiratory volume in 1 second (FEV_1), and a reduction of concomitant medication use were effected by administration of an LTD_4 receptor antagonist (121) and a 5-LO inhibitor, respectively (110) (see Table 23-4).

In two clinical studies of patients with ulcerative colitis, an orally administered specific 5-LO inhibitor modestly decreased the symptoms of the disease (122,123). In

TABLE 23-4. *Evidence linking leukotrienes to inflammatory diseases*

Disease	5-Lipoxygenase products involved	Supporting therapeutic intervention	Selected references
Allergic and airways diseases			
Asthma	LTD_4, LTE_4, and 20-OH LTB_4 in the serum and/or urine of patients with asthma and bronchial hyperreactivity	Zileuton, a 5-lipoxygenase inhibitor; MK-886, a FLAP inhibitor; ICI 204,219 (Zafirlukast) and MK-571, MK-0476 (Montelukast), MK-0679, LTD_4 receptor antagonists that relieve various forms of asthma	96–98, 110–121
Adult respiratory distress syndrome	LTC_4 in bronchial fluids/sputum	—	100
Chronic obstructive pulmonary disease	LTB_4, cysteinyl leukotrienes in sputum	—	102
Allergic rhinitis and conjunctivitis	LTC_4 and LTB_4 in nasal fluid	Zileuton reduces leukotriene formation and decreases symptoms.	98,99
Skin disease			
Psoriasis	LTB_4, LTC_4, and LTD_4 in skin lesion fluid	Methotrexate reduces 5-lipoxygenase products and reduces symptoms. R68151 and RA43179 improve erythema and scaling of psoriasis.	105,125–127
Inflammatory bowel disease			
Ulcerative colitis, Crohn's disease	LTB_4 in rectal secretions	Zileuton reduces the symptoms of colitis. R68151 and RA43179 reduce signs and symptoms of colitis and improve gross appearance of mucosa.	104,122–124
Arthritides			
Rheumatoid arthritis	LTB_4, LTD_4, and LTE_4 in synovial fluid	Methotrexate reduces LTB_4 formation and improves disease signs and symptoms. Zileuton demonstrates a trend toward reduced symptoms.	107–109, 128
Juvenile rheumatoid arthritis	LTE_4 in urine	—	103
Gout	LTB_4 in synovial fluid	—	106

FLAP, 5-lipoxygenase–activating protein; LTB_4, leukotriene B_4; LTC_4, leukotriene C_4; LTD_4, leukotriene D_4; LTE_4, leukotriene E_4.

a multicenter trial of another 5-LO inhibitor, the level of LTB_4 was reduced, but there was no correlation with remission (124).

In clinical trials of patients with psoriasis, the administration of topical 5-LO inhibitors resulted in decreased symptom scores, scaling, and erythema (125,126). A short trial of an oral FLAP-inhibitor demonstrated reduced leukotriene levels but no clinical improvement (127).

In a 4-week, placebo-controlled trial of a 5-LO inhibitor in patients with rheumatoid arthritis who did not receive nonsteroidal antiinflammatory drug therapy, the trend toward fewer painful and swollen joints and better scores in the joint swelling index did not reach statistical significance. The amount of LTB_4 synthesis with calcium ionophore stimulation of whole blood was reduced by 70% (128).

REFERENCES

1. Samuelsson B, Borgeat P, Hammarström S, Murphy RC. Introduction of a nomenclature: leukotrienes. *Prostaglandins* 1979;17:785–787.
2. Samuelsson B. Leukotrienes: mediators of immediate hypersensitivity reactions and inflammation. *Science* 1983;220:568–575.
3. Kellaway CH, Trethewie WR. The liberation of a slow reacting smooth muscle-stimulating substance in anaphylaxis. *Q J Exp Physiol* 1940;30:121–145.
4. Brocklehurst WE. Occurrence of an unidentified substance during anaphylactic shock in cavy lung. *J Physiol* 1953;120:16–17.
5. Murphy RC, Hammarström S, Samuelsson B. Leukotriene C: a slow reacting substance for murine mastocytoma cells. *Proc Natl Acad Sci USA* 1979;76:4275–4279.
6. Lewis RA, Drazen JM, Austen KF, Clark DA, Corey EJ. Identification of the c(6)-*S*-conjugate of leukotriene A with cysteine as naturally occurring slow reacting substance of anaphylaxis (SRS-A): importance of the 11-*cis*-geometry for biological activity. *Biochem Biophys Res Commun* 1980;96:271–277.
7. Dennis EA. Diversity of group types, regulation, and function of phospholipase A_2. *J Biol Chem* 1994;269:13057–13060.
8. Rouzer CA, Matsumoto T, Samuelsson B. Single protein from human leukocytes possesses 5-lipoxygenase and leukotriene A_4 synthase activities. *Proc Natl Acad Sci USA* 1986;83:857–861.
9. Ueda N, Kaneko S, Yoshimoto T, Yamamoto S. Purification of arachidonate 5-lipoxygenase from porcine leukocytes and its reactivity with hydroperoxy-eicosatetraenoic acids. *J Biol Chem* 1986;261:7982–7988.
10. Ford-Hutchinson AW, Gresser M, Young RN. 5-Lipoxygenase. *Ann Rev Biochem* 1994;63:383–417.
11. Percival MD. Human 5-lipoxygenase contains an essential iron. *J Biol Chem* 1991;261:10058–10061.
12. Brock TG, Paine R, Peters-Golden M. Localization of 5-lipoxygenase to the nucleus of unstimulated rat basophilic leukemia cells. *J Biol Chem* 1994;269:22059–22066.
13. Reid GK, Kargman S, Vickers PJ, et al. Correlation between expression of 5-lipoxygenase-activating protein, 5-lipoxygenase, and cellular leukotriene biosynthesis. *J Biol Chem* 1990;265:19818–19823.
14. Woods JW, Coffey MJ, Brock TG, Singer II, Peters-Golden M. 5-Lipoxygenase is located in the euchromatin of the nucleus in resting

human alveolar macrophages and translocates to the nuclear envelope on cell activation. *J Clin Invest* 1995;95:2035–2046.

15. Woods JW, Evans JF, Ethier D, et al. 5-Lipoxygenase and 5-lipoxygenase activating protein are localized in the nuclear envelope of activated human leukocytes. *J Exp Med* 1993;178:1935–1946.

16. Lepley RA, Fitzpatrick FA. 5-Lipoxygenase contains a functional Src homology 3-binding motif that interacts with the Src homology 3 domain of Grb2 and cytoskeletal proteins. *J Biol Chem* 1994;269:24163–24168.

17. Dixon RAF, Jones RE, Diehl RE, Bennet CD, Kargman S, Rouzer CA. Cloning of the cDNA for human 5-lipoxygenase. *Proc Natl Acad Sci USA* 1988;85:416–420.

18. Nguyen T, Falguryret J-P, Abramovitz M, Riendeau D. Evaluation of the role of conserved His and Met residues among lipoxygenases by site-directed mutagenesis of recombinant 5-lipoxygenase. *J Biol Chem* 1991;266:22057–22062.

19. Zhang YY, Rådmark O, Samuelsson B. Mutagenesis of some conserved residues in human 5-lipoxygenase. *Proc Natl Acad Sci USA* 1992;89:485–489.

20. Ishii S, Noguchi M, Miyano M, Matsumoto T, Noma M. Mutagenesis studies on the amino acid residues involved in the iron-binding and the activity of human 5-lipoxygenase. *Biochem Biophys Res Commun* 1992;182:1482–1490.

21. Funk CD, Hoshiko S, Matsumoto T, Rådmark O, Samuelsson B. Characterization of the human 5-lipoxygenase gene. *Proc Natl Acad Sci USA* 1989;86:2587–2591.

22. Chen X-S, Naumann TA, Kurre U, Jenkins NA, Copeland NG, Funk CD. cDNA cloning, expression, mutagenesis, intracellular localization, and gene chromosomal assignment of mouse 5-lipoxygenase. *J Biol Chem* 1995;270:17993–17999.

23. Chen X-S, Sheller JR, Johnson EN, Funk CD. Role of leukotrienes revealed by targeted disruption of the 5-lipoxygenase gene. *Nature* 1994;372:179–182.

24. Goulet JL, Snouwaert JN, Latour AM, Coffman TM, Koller BH. Altered inflammatory responses in leukotriene-deficient mice. *Proc Natl Acad Sci USA* 1994;91:12852–12856.

25. Bailie MB, Standiford J, Aaichalk LL, Coffey MJ, Stieter D, Peters-Golden M. Leukotriene-deficient mice manifest enhanced lethality from *Klebsiella* pneumonia in association with decreased alveolar macrophage phagocytic and bactericidal activities. *J Immunol* 1996;157:5221–5224.

26. Scoggan KA, Jakobsson P-J, Ford-Hutchinson AW. Production of leukotriene C4 in different human tissues is attributable to distinct membrane-bound biosynthetic enzymes. *J Biol Chem* 1997;272:10182–10187.

27. Feinmark SJ, Cannon J. Vascular smooth muscle cell leukotriene C4 synthesis: requirement for transcellular leukotriene A4 metabolism. *Biochim Biophys Acta* 1987;922:125–132.

28. Feinmark SJ. The role of the endothelial cell in leukotriene biosynthesis. *Am Rev Respir Dis* 1992;146:S51–S55.

29. Penrose JF, Spector J, Lam BK, Friend DS, Xu K, Jack RM, Austen KF. Purification of human lung leukotriene C4 synthase and preparation of a polyclonal antibody. *Am J Respir Crit Care Med* 1995;152:283–289.

30. Serhan CN, Sheppard KA, Fiore S. Lipoxin formation: evaluation of the role and actions of leukotriene A4. *Adv Prostaglandin Thromboxane Leukot Res* 1990;20:54–62.

31. Lindgren JA, Edenius C. Platelet-granulocyte interactions and the production of leukotrienes and lipoxins. *Adv Prostaglandin Thromboxane Leukot Res* 1990;20:63–70.

32. Serhan CN. Lipoxins: eicosanoids carrying intra- and intercellular messages. *J Bioenerg Biomembr* 1991;23:105–122.

33. Rouzer CA, Kargman S. Translocation of 5-lipoxygenase to the membrane in human leukocytes challenged with ionophore A23187. *J Biol Chem* 1990;263:10980–10988.

34. Dixon RAF, Diehl RE, Opas E, et al. Requirement of a 5-lipoxygenase activating protein for leukotriene synthesis. *Nature* 1990;343:282–284.

35. Miller DK, Gillard JW, Vickers PJ, et al. Identification and isolation of a membrane protein necessary for leukotriene production. *Nature* 1990;343:278–281.

36. Lam BK, Penrose JF, Freeman G, Austen KF. Expression cloning of a cDNA for human leukotriene C4 synthase, an integral membrane protein conjugating reduced glutathione to leukotriene A4. *Proc Natl Acad Sci USA* 1994;91:7663.

37. Vickers PJ, Adam M, Charleson S, Coppolino MG, Evans JF, Mancini JA. Identification of amino acid residues of 5-lipoxygenase activating protein essential for the binding of leukotriene biosynthesis inhibitors. *Mol Pharmacol* 1992;42:94–102.

38. Kennedy BP, Diehl RE, Boie Y, Adam M, Dixon RAF. Gene characterization and promotor analysis of the human 5-lipoxygenase-activating protein (FLAP). *J Biol Chem* 1991;266:8511–8516.

39. Byrum RS, Goulet JL, Griffiths RJ, Koller BH. Role of the 5-lipoxygenase-activating protein (FLAP) in murine acute inflammatory responses. *J Exp Med* 1997;185:1065–1075.

40. Griffiths RJ, Smith M, Roach ML, et al. Collagen-induced arthritis is reduced in 5-lipoxygenase-activating protein-deficient mice. *J Exp Med* 1997;185:1123–1129.

41. McGee J, Fitzpatrick F. Enzymatic hydration of leukotriene A4: purification and characterization of a novel epoxide hydrolase from human erythrocytes. *J Biol Chem* 1985;260:12832–12837.

42. Rådmark O, Shimizu T, Jornvall H, Sameulsson B. Leukotriene A4 hydrolase in human leukocytes: purification and properties. *J Biol Chem* 1984;259:12339–12345.

43. Haeggström JZ, Wetterholm A, Vallee BL, Samuelsson B. Leukotriene A4 hydrolase: an epoxide hydrolase with peptidase activity. *Biochem Biophys Res Commun* 1990;173:620–626.

44. Ohishi N, Izumi T, Minami M, et al. Leukotriene A4 hydrolase in human lung: interaction of the enzyme with leukotriene A4 hydrolase isomers. *J Biol Chem* 1987;262:10200–10205.

45. Haeggström JZ, Wetterholm A, Medina J, et al. Novel structural and functional properties of leukotriene A4 hydrolase: implications for the development of enzyme inhibitors. *Adv Prostaglandin Thromboxane Leukot Res* 1994;22:3.

46. Örning L, Krivi G, Bild G, Gierse J, Aykent S, Fitzpatrick FA. Inhibition of leukotriene A4 hydrolase/aminopeptidase by captopril. *J Biol Chem* 1991;26:16507–16511.

47. Funk CD, Rådmark O, Fu JY, et al. Molecular cloning and amino acid sequence of leukotriene A4 hydrolase. *Proc Natl Acad Sci USA* 1987;84:6677–6681.

48. Mueller MJ, Blomster M, Opperman UCT, Jornvall H, Samuelsson B, Haeggström JZ. Leukotriene A4 hydrolase: protection from mechanism-based inactivation by mutation of tyrosine-378. *Proc Natl Acad Sci USA* 1996;93:5931–5935.

49. Medina JF, Wetterholm A, Rådmark O, et al. Leukotriene A4 hydrolase: determination of the three zinc-binding ligands by site-directed mutagenesis and zinc analysis. *Proc Natl Acad Sci USA* 1991;88:7620–7624.

50. Wetterholm A, Medina JF, Rådmark O, et al. Leukotriene A4 hydrolase: abrogation of the peptidase activity by mutation of glutamic acid-296. *Proc Natl Acad Sci USA* 1992;89:9141–9145.

51. Blomster M, Wetterholm A, Mueller MJ, Haeggström. Evidence for a catalytic role of tyrosine 383 in the peptidase reaction of leukotriene A4 hydrolase. *Eur J Biochem* 1995;231:528–534.

52. Mancini JA, Evans JF. Cloning and characterization of the human leukotriene A4 hydrolase gene. *Eur J Biochem* 1995;231:65–71.

53. Penrose JF, Gagnon L, Goppelt-Struebe M, et al. Purification of human leukotriene C4 synthase. *Proc Natl Acad Sci USA* 1992;89:11603–11606.

54. Nicholson DW, Ali A, Vaillancourt JP, et al. Purification to homogeneity and the N-terminal sequence of human leukotriene C4 synthase: a homodimeric glutathione S-transferase composed of 18-kDa subunits. *Proc Natl Acad Sci USA* 1993;90:2015–2019.

55. Jakobsson P-J, Mancini JA, Ford-Hutchinson AW. Identification and characterization of a novel human microsomal glutathione S-transferase with leukotriene C4 synthase activity and significant sequence identity to 5-lipoxygenase activating protein and leukotriene C4 synthase. *J Biol Chem* 1996;271:22203–22210.

56. Weller PF, Lee CW, Foster DW, Corey EF, Austen KF, Lewis RA. Generation and metabolism of 5-lipoxygenase pathway leukotrienes by human eosinophils: predominant production of leukotriene C4. *Proc Natl Acad Sci USA* 1983;80:7626–7630.

57. MacGlashan DW Jr, Schleimer RP, Peters SP, et al. Generation of leukotrienes by purified human lung mast cells. *J Clin Invest* 1982;70:747–751.

58. Soderström M, Mannervik B, Garkov V, Hammarström S. On the nature of LTC4 synthase in human platelets. *Arch Biochim Biophys* 1992;294:70–74.

59. Williams JD, Czop JK, Austen KF. Release of leukotrienes by human monocytes on stimulation of their phagocytic receptor for particulate activators. *J Immunol* 1984;132:3034–3040.

60. Lam BK, Penrose JF, Rokach J, Xu K, Baldasaro MH, Austen KF. Molecular cloning, expression and characterization of mouse leukotriene C$_4$ synthase. *Eur J Biochem* 1996;238:606–612.

61. Lam BK, Penrose JF, Xu K, Baldasaro M, Austen KF. Site directed mutagenesis of leukotriene C$_4$ synthase. *J Biol Chem* 1997;273:13923–13928.

62. Penrose JF, Spector JS, Baldasaro M, et al. Molecular cloning of the gene for human leukotriene C$_4$ synthase: organization, nucleotide sequence, and chromosomal localization to 5q35. *J Biol Chem* 1996;271:11356–11361.

63. Lam BK, Gagnon L, Austen KF, Soberman RJ. The mechanism of leukotriene B$_4$ export from human polymorphonuclear leukocytes. *J Biol Chem* 1990;265:13438–13441.

64. Lam BK, Owen WF Jr, Austen KF, Soberman RJ. The identification of a distinct export step following the biosynthesis of leukotriene C$_4$ by human eosinophils. *J Biol Chem* 1989;264:12885–12889.

65. Leier I, Muller M, Jedlitschky G, Keppler D. Leukotriene uptake by hepatocytes and hepatoma cells. *Eur J Biochem* 1992;209:281–289.

66. Leier I, Kedlitschky G, Buchholz U, Coles SPC, Deeley RG, Keppler D. The MRP gene encodes an ATP-dependent export pump for leukotriene C$_4$ and structurally related conjugates. *J Biol Chem* 1994;269:27807–27810.

67. Soberman RJ, Harper TW, Murphy RC, Austen KF. Identification and functional characterization of leukotriene B$_4$ 20-hydroxylase of human polymorphonuclear leukocytes. *Proc Natl Acad Sci USA* 1985;82:2292–2295.

68. Soberman RJ, Sutyak JP, Okita RT, et al. The identification and formation of 20-aldehyde leukotriene B$_4$. *J Biol Chem* 1988;263:7996–8002.

69. Kikuta Y, Kusunose E, Endo K, et al. A novel form of cytochrome P-450 family 4 in human polymorphonuclear leukocytes. cDNA cloning and expression of leukotriene B$_4$ omega hydroxylase. *J Biol Chem* 1993;268:9376–9380.

70. Sutyak J, Austen KF, Soberman RJ. Identification of an aldehyde dehydrogenase in the microsomes of human polymorphonuclear leukocytes that metabolizes 20-aldehyde leukotriene B$_4$. *J Biol Chem* 1989;264:14818–14823.

71. Wheelan P, Zirrolli JA, Morelli JG, Murphy RC. Metabolism of leukotriene B$_4$ (LTB$_4$) by cultured human keratinocytes. Formation of glutathione conjugates and dihydro metabolites. *J Biol Chem* 1993;268:25439–25448.

72. Serafin WE, Oates JA, Jubbard WC. Metabolism of leukotriene B$_4$ in the monkey: identification of the principal nonvolatile metabolite in the urine. *Prostaglandins* 1984;27:899.

73. Anderson ME, Allison RD, Meister A. Interconversion of leukotrienes catalyzed by purified gamma-glutamyl transpeptidase: concomitant formation of leukotriene D$_4$ gamma-glutamyl amino acid. *Proc Natl Acad Sci USA* 1982;79:1088–1091.

74. Lee CW, Lewis RA, Corey EJ, Austen KF. Conversion of leukotriene D$_4$ to leukotriene E$_4$ by a dipeptidase released from the specific granules of human polymorphonuclear leukocytes. *Immunology* 1983;48:27–35.

75. Lee CW, Lewis RA, Tauber AI, Mehrotra M, Corey EJ, Austen KF. The myeloperoxidase-dependent metabolism of leukotrienes C$_4$, D$_4$ and E$_4$ to 6-*trans*-leukotriene B$_4$ diastereoisomers and the subclass-specific *S*-diastereoisomeric sulfoxides. *J Biol Chem* 1983;258:15004–15009.

76. Coleman RA, Dahlen SE, Drazen JM, et al. Classification of leukotriene receptors. In: Proceedings of the 9th International Conference on Prostaglandins and Related Compounds, Florence, Italy, June 6–10, 1994;1–7.

77. Metters KM. Leukotriene receptors. *J Lipid Mediat* 1995;12:413–427.

78. Goldman DW, Goetzl EJ. Heterogeneity of human polymorphonuclear leukocyte receptors for leukotriene B$_4$: identification of a subset of high affinity receptors that transduce the chemotactic response. *J Exp Med* 1984;159:1027–1041.

79. Yokomizo T, Izumi T, Chang K, Takuwa Y, Shimizu T. A G-protein–coupled receptor for leukotriene B$_4$ that mediates chemotaxis. *Nature* 1997;387:620–624.

80. Rovati GE, Fiovanazzi S, Mezzetti M, et al. Heterogeneity of binding sites for ICI 198,615 in human lung parenchyma. *Biochem Pharmacol* 1992;44:1411–1415.

81. Lee TH, Austen KF, Corey EJ, et al. Leukotriene E$_4$-induced airway hyperresponsiveness of guinea pig tracheal smooth muscle to histamine and evidence for three separate sulfidopeptide leukotriene receptors. *Proc Natl Acad Sci USA* 1984;81:4922–4925.

82. Sun FF, Chau L-Y, Spur B, Corey EJ, Lewis RA, Austen KF. Identification of a high affinity leukotriene C$_4$-binding protein in rat liver cytosol as glutathione S-transferase. *J Biol Chem* 1986;261:8540–8546.

83. Metter KM, Sawyer N, Nicholson DW. Microsomal glutathione-S-transferase is the predominant leukotriene C$_4$ binding site in cellular membranes. *J Biol Chem* 1994;269:12816–12823.

84. Ford-Hutchinson AW, Bray MA, Doig MV, Shipley ME, Smith MJH. Leukotriene B, a potent chemokinetic and aggregating substance released from polymorphonuclear leukocytes. *Nature* 1980;286:264–265.

85. Palmblad J, Malmsten CL, Uden AM, Rådmark O, Engstrot L, Samuelsson B. Leukotriene B$_4$ is a potent stereospecific stimulator of neutrophil chemotaxis and adherence. *Blood* 1981;58:658–661.

86. Samuelsson B, Claesson H-E. Leukotriene B$_4$: biosynthesis and role in lymphocytes. *Adv Prostaglandin Thromboxane Leukot Res* 1990;20:1–13.

87. Devchand PR, Keller H, Peters JM, Vasquez M, Gonzalez FJ, Wahli W. The PPARα-leukotriene B$_4$ pathway to inflammation control. *Nature* 1996;384:39–43.

88. Badr KF, Baylis C, Pfeffer JM, et al. Renal and systemic hemodynamic responses to intravenous infusion of leukotriene C$_4$ in the rat. *Circ Res* 1984;54:492–499.

89. Bittl JA, Pfeffer MA, Lewis RA, Hegrotra MM, Corey EJ, Austen KF. Mechanism of the negative inotropic action of leukotrienes C$_4$ and D$_4$ on isolated rat heart. *Cardiovasc Res* 1985;119:426–432.

90. Dahlén S-E, Björk J, Hedqvist P, et al. Leukotrienes promote plasma leakage and leukocyte adherence in post capillary venules: *in vivo* effects with relevance to the acute inflammatory response. *Proc Natl Acad Sci USA* 1981;78:3887–3891.

91. Dahlén S-E, Hedqvist P, Hammarström S, Samuelsson B. Leukotrienes are potent constrictors of human bronchi. *Nature* 1981;268:484–486.

92. Boyce JA, Lam BK, Penrose JF, et al. Expression of LTC$_4$ synthase during the development of eosinophils *in vitro* from cord blood progenitors. *Blood* 1996;11:4338–4347.

93. Shaw RJ, Walsh GM, Cromwell O, Moqbel R, Spry CJF, Kay AB. Activated human eosinophils generated SRS-A leukotrienes following IgG-dependent stimulation. *Nature* 1985;316:150–152.

94. Levi-Shaffer F, Austen KF, Caulfield JP, Hein A, Gravallese PM, Steven RL. Co-culture of human lung-derived mast cells with mouse 3T3 fibroblasts: morphology and IgE-mediated release of histamine, prostaglandin D$_2$, and leukotrienes. *J Immunol* 1987;139:494–500.

95. McGlashan DW Jr, Peters SP, Warner J, Lichtenstein LM. Characteristics of human basophil sulfidopeptide leukotriene release: releasability defined as the ability of the basophil to respond to dimeric cross-links. *J Immunol* 1986;136:2231–2239.

96. Okubo T, Takahashi H, Sumitomo M, Shindoh K, Suzuki S. Plasma levels of leukotrienes C$_4$ and D$_4$ during wheezing attack in asthmatic patients. *Int Arch Allergy Appl Immunol* 1987;84:149–155.

97. Wardlaw AJ, Hay H, Cromwell O, Collins JV, Kay AB. Leukotrienes, LTC$_4$ and LTB$_4$, in bronchoalveolar lavage in bronchial asthma and other respiratory disease. *J Allergy Clin Immunol* 1989;84:19–26.

98. Creticos PS, Peters SP, Adkinson NF Jr, et al. Peptide leukotriene release after antigen challenge in patients sensitive to ragweed. *N Engl J Med* 1984;310:1626–1630.

99. Bisgaard H, Ford-Hutchinson AW, Charleson S, Taudorf E. Production of leukotrienes in human skin and conjunctival mucosa after specific allergen challenge. *Allergy* 1985;40:417–423.

100. Matthay MA, Eschenbacher WL, Goetzl EJ. Elevated concentrations of leukotriene D$_4$ in pulmonary edema fluid of patients with adult respiratory distress syndrome. *J Clin Immunol* 1984;4:479–483.

101. Stenmark KR, James SL, Voelkel NF, Toews WH, Reeves JT, Murphy RC. Leukotriene C$_4$ and D$_4$ in neonates with hypoxemia and pulmonary hypertension. *N Engl J Med* 1983;309:77–80.

102. O'Driscoll BR, Cromwell O, Kay AB. Sputum leukotrienes in obstructive airways diseases. *Clin Exp Immunol* 1984;55:397–404.

103. Fauler J, Thon A, Tsikas D, von der Hardt H, Frolich J. Enhanced synthesis of cysteinyl leukotrienes in juvenile rheumatoid arthritis. *Arthritis Rheum* 1994;37:93–99.

104. Sharon P, Stenson WF. Enhanced synthesis of leukotriene B$_4$ by colonic mucosa in inflammatory bowel disease. *Gastroenterology* 1984;86:453–460.

105. Brain S, Camp R, Dowd P, Black AK, Greaves M. The release of leukotriene B$_4$-like material in biologically active amounts from the lesional skin of patients with psoriasis. *J Invest Dermatol* 1984;83:70–73.

106. Rae SA, Davidson EM, Smith MJH. Leukotriene B₄, an inflammatory mediator in gout. *Lancet* 1982;2:1122–1124.

107. Davidson EM, Rae SA, Smith MJH. Leukotriene B₄, a mediator of inflammation present in synovial fluid in rheumatoid arthritis. *Ann Rheum Dis* 1983;43:677–679.

108. Ahmadzadeh N, Shingu M, Nobunaga M, et al. Relationship between leukotriene B₄ and immunological parameters in rheumatoid synovial fluids. *Inflammation* 1991;15:497–501.

109. Wittenberg RH, Willburger RE, Kleemeyer K, Peskar BA. *In vitro* release of prostaglandins and leukotrienes from synovial tissue, cartilage, and bone in degenerative joint diseases. *Arthritis Rheum* 1993;10:1444–1450.

110. Israel EJ, Rubin P, Kemp JP, et al. The effect of inhibition of 5-lipoxygenase by Zileuton in mild-to-moderate asthma. *Ann Intern Med* 1993;119:1059–1066.

111. Manning PJ, Watson RM, Margolskee DJ, Williams VC, Schwartz JI, O'Byrne PM. Inhibition of exercise-induced asthma. *N Engl J Med* 1990;232:1736–1739.

112. Finnerty JP, Wood-Baker R, Thomson H, Holgate ST. Role of leukotrienes in exercise-induced asthma; inhibitory effect of ICI 204,219, a potent leukotriene D₄ receptor antagonist. *Am Rev Respir Dis* 1992;145:746–749.

113. Israel E, Dermarkarian R, Rosenberg M, et al. The effects of a 5-lipoxygenase inhibitor on asthma induced by cold, dry air. *N Engl J Med* 1990;323:1740–1744.

114. Rasmussen JB, Margolskee DJ, Eriksson LO, Williams VC, Andersson KE. Leukotriene (LT) D₄ is involved in antigen-induced asthma: a study with the LTD₄ receptor antagonist, MK-571. *Ann N Y Acad Sci* 1991;629:436.

115. Gaddy JN, Margolskee DJ, Bush RK, Williams VC, Busse WW. Bronchodilatation with a potent and selective leukotriene D₄ (LTD₄) antagonist (MK-571) in patients with asthma. *Am Rev Respir Dis* 1992;146:358–363.

116. O'Shaughnessy KM, Taylor IK, O'Connor B, O'Connell F, Thomson H, Dollery CT. Potent leukotriene D(4) receptor antagonist ICI-204,219 given by the inhaled route inhibits the early but not the late phase of allergen-induced bronchoconstriction. *Am Rev Respir Dis* 1993;146:1431–1435.

117. Friedman BS, Gel EH, Buntinx A, et al. Oral leukotriene inhibitor (MK-886) blocks allergen-induced airway responses. *Am Rev Respir Dis* 1993;147:839–844.

118. Taylor IK, O'Shaughnessy KM, Fuller RW, Dollery CT. Effect of cysteinyl leukotriene receptor antagonist ICI 204,219 on allergen-induced bronchoconstriction and airway hyperreactivity in atopic subjects. *Lancet* 1991;337:690–694.

119. Christie PE, Smith CM, Lee TH. The potent and selective sulfidopeptide leukotriene antagonist, SK&F 104353, inhibits aspirin-induced asthma. *Am Rev Respir Dis* 1991;144:957–958.

120. Israel E, Fischer AR, Rosenberg MA, et al. The pivotal role of 5-lipoxygenase products in the reaction of aspirin-sensitive asthmatics to aspirin. *Am Rev Respir Dis* 1993;148:1447–1451.

121. Cloud ML, Enas GC, Kemp J, et al. A specific LTD₄/LTE₄ receptor antagonist improves pulmonary function in patients with mild, chronic asthma. *Am Rev Respir Dis* 1989;140:1336–1339.

122. Collawn C, Rubin P, Perez N, et al. Phase II study of the safety and efficacy of a 5-lipoxygenase inhibitor in patients with ulcerative colitis. *Am J Gastroenterol* 1992;87:342–346.

123. Rask-Madsen J, Bukhave K, Laursen LS, et al. 5-Lipoxygenase inhibitors for the treatment of inflammatory bowel disease. *Agents Actions* 1992;C37–C46.

124. Roberts WG, Simon TJ, Berlin RG, et al. Leukotrienes in ulcerative colitis: results of a multicenter trial of a leukotriene biosynthesis inhibitor, MK-591. *Gastroenterology* 1997;112:725–732.

125. Degreef H, Dockx P, DeDoncker P, DeBeule K, Cauwenbergh G. A double-blind vehicle-controlled study of R68151 in psoriasis: a topical 5-lipoxygenase inhibitor. *J Am Acad Dermatol* 1990;22:751–755.

126. Black AK, Camp RD, Mallet AI, Cunningham FM, Hofbauer N, Greaves MW. Pharmacologic and clinical effects of Ionapalene (RA43179), a 5-lipoxygenase inhibitor, in psoriasis. *J Invest Dermatol* 1990;95:50–54.

127. DeJong EM, van Vlijmen IM, Scholte JC, et al. Clinical and biochemical effects of an oral leukotriene biosynthesis inhibitor (MK886) in psoriasis. *Skin Pharmacol* 1991;4:278–285.

128. Weinblatt ME, Kremer JM, Coblyn JS, et al. Zileuton, a 5-lipoxygenase inhibitor in rheumatoid arthritis. *J Rheumatol* 1992;19:1537–1541.

Inflammation: Basic Principles and Clinical Correlates,
3rd ed., edited by John I. Gallin and Ralph Snyderman.
Lippincott Williams & Wilkins, Philadelphia © 1999.

CHAPTER 24

Lipoxins and Aspirin-Triggered 15-epi-Lipoxins

Charles N. Serhan

Lipid-derived mediators play critical roles within their cells of origin and function as local extracellular signals in inflammation and other multicellular processes, including vascular disease, atherosclerosis, thrombosis, and asthma (1). Two classes of eicosanoids, leukotrienes and prostaglandins (see Chapters 22 and 23), are mediators of human airway inflammation and vascular events, and they may regulate human myelopoiesis (2,3). Administration of pharmacologic agents that inhibit leukotriene biosynthesis or leukotriene receptor antagonist appear to have a salutary effect on asthma (4). Although the evidence for proinflammatory roles of leukotriene is established, there is also evidence that other eicosanoids such as lipoxins and aspirin-triggered lipoxins (ATLs), such as 15-epi-lipoxin (5) (Fig. 24-1), possess potent counterregulatory actions (6–8). The integrated response of the host, recognized as human diseases such as vasculitis and arthritis, in part may reflect an overall balance and temporal orchestration between proinflammatory and antiinflammatory signals. Among such signals, the role of lipid-derived mediators has remained unclear, probably because these products are rapidly generated, often through transcellular biosynthesis; exist ephemerally; and act within the local microenvironment. Lipoxin and the aspirin-triggered 15-epi-lipoxins are of particular interest.

Lipid mediators are derived from lipid precursors through sequential action of two lipoxygenases (see Fig. 24-1). Because of the requirement for two lipoxygenation steps, it seemed likely that these molecules were formed through transcellular biosynthesis. The potential requirement for transcellular biosynthesis originally led to questions about whether lipoxins could be formed *in vivo*. The enzymatic lipoxin formation that involves two main steps

and subsequent reactions is similar to that of prostaglandins, which also require the insertion of molecular oxygen at two sites within the prostanoid structure, at carbon 9 (C9) and C11 of arachidonate. Because of the requirement for two lipoxygenation steps in lipoxin biosynthesis to generate two of the alcohol groups and the third from water (C6 position in lipoxin A4 [LXA4] and C14 position alcohol in lipoxin B4 [LXB4] are derived from H_2O), these molecules probably were formed by transcellular biosynthesis (Figs. 24-2 and 24-3). Numerous studies have shown that lipoxins are formed *in vitro* from endogenous sources of arachidonate in isolated cells and are formed *in vivo* and across many species, from fish to humans (9). This chapter addresses the major routes and bioactions of lipoxins and whether their formation and actions can have therapeutic value in regulating inflammation.

LIPOXIN BIOSYNTHESIS

Biosynthesis of mediators by *transcellular* and *cell-cell interactions* is recognized as an important means of amplifying and generating lipid-derived mediators, particularly those produced by lipoxygenases (6,10,11). In humans, lipoxin biosynthesis is an example of lipoxygenase-lipoxygenase interactions through transcellular routes (see Figs. 24-2 and 24-3) (6–8). Lipoxins can be generated by two lipoxygenase routes; the first described involves initial lipoxygenation by 15-lipoxygenase (inserting O_2 in predominantly the *S* configuration), followed by 5-lipoxygenase and generation of a 5,6-epoxytetraene (see Fig. 24-2). My colleagues and I also established another, initiated by 5-lipoxygenase from leukocytes with formation of leukotriene A4 (LTA4), which unexpectedly is converted by platelet 12-lipoxygenase (see Fig. 24-3). This platelet-polymorphonuclear cell (PMN) model exemplifies the pivotal role of LTA4 released by activated PMN that can be converted to leu-

C. N. Serhan: Center for Experimental Therapeutics and Reperfusion Injury, Brigham and Women's Hospital and Harvard Medical School, Boston, Massachusetts 02115.

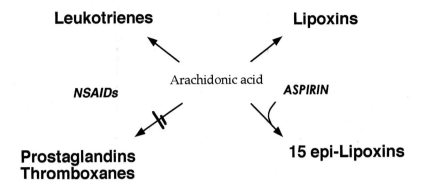

FIG. 24-1. Novel concepts in eicosanoid formation.

kotriene C4 (LTC4) or lipoxin by platelets (7,11,12). Results with recombinant platelet 12-lipoxygenase confirmed this and revealed that it also serves as a lipoxin synthase, producing LXA4 and LXB4 (13).

A third and unexpected pathway was uncovered (Fig. 24-4). It is triggered by acetylsalicylic acid (ASA) acetylation of prostaglandin H synthase-2 (PGHS-2), which is also designated cyclooxygenase-2, in endothelial cells and generates (15R)-hydroxyeicosatetraenoic acid ([15R]-HETE) from arachidonic acid, which is rapidly transformed by leukocytes in a transcellular biosynthetic route involving leukocytes and vascular endothelial cells or epithelial cells (5,14). These 15-epi-lipoxins can also be initiated by cytochrome P450 oxygenation of arachidonate and 5-lipoxygenase oxygenation in leukocytes (14). The ATLs or 15-epi-lipoxins display intriguing bioactions, including antiinflammatory and antiproliferative effects *in vitro* (14–16), which may be linked to ASA's reduction of vascular disease and protection against certain malignancies, including breast, lung, and colon cancers (17,18). This novel action of ASA and generation of 15-epi-lipoxin as potential endogenous mediators (see Fig. 24-1) are considered along with results from my laboratory that indicate that the bioavailability and biologic half-life of ATL can be increased and exploited for pharmacologic use in *in vivo* models of inflammation (15,16).

15-Lipoxygenase–Initiated Pathway

The first lipoxin biosynthetic pathway described in 1984 rationalized the generation of lipoxins by routes involving insertion of molecular oxygen into the C15 position of arachidonic acid, predominantly in the *S* configuration (see Fig. 24-2). This pathway implicated involvement of a 15-lipoxygenase in the generation of bioactive molecules (19) and was of interest because the role of 15-lipoxygenase was unknown (20). Human 15-lipoxygenase, subsequently found to be abundant in human eosinophils, alveolar macrophages, monocytes, and epithelial cells, is controlled by cytokines and regulated primarily by interleukin-4 (IL-4) and IL-13 (21–24). These two cytokines are implicated as negative regulators of the inflammatory response or antiinflammatory

cytokines (25). Studies on the actions of lipoxin implicate LXA4 and LXB4 as potential antiinflammatory compounds.

Oxygenation of arachidonic acid at the C15 position generates hydroperoxyeicosatetraenoic acids (HPETEs). The (15S)-hydroperoxy form and (15S)-HETE, the reduced alcohol form, can each serve as a substrate for 5-lipoxygenase in leukocytes. These transformations occur within the cell type of origin or through transcellular routes in humans. The product of the 5-lipoxygenase's action on 15-HPETE is a (5S)-hydroperoxy form, (15S)-hydroperoxy-diHPETE, which is then rapidly converted to a 5(6)epoxytetraene. The 5-lipoxygenase is also regulated by cytokines such as granulocyte-macrophage colony-stimulating factor (GM-CSF) and IL-3 (26—28), and 5-lipoxygenase is highly expressed in human neutrophils and monocytes. Once formed, as illustrated in Figure 24-2, the 5(6)epoxytetraene is rapidly converted by hydrolases to (5S,6R,15S)-trihydroxy-7,9,13-*trans*-11-*cis*-eicosatetraenoic acid, also called lipoxin A4 (LXA4), or transformed through lipoxin B4 hydrolase to (5S, 14R,15S)-trihydroxy-6,10,12-*trans*-8-*cis*-eicosatetrenoic acid, also called lipoxin B4 (LXB4). LXA4 and LXB4 are each vasoactive, primarily vasodilatory in most isolated organs and *in vivo* models tested (29,30), and they both regulate leukocyte functions (16,31,32), perhaps serving as downregulatory molecules.

Temporally concomitant with the biosynthesis of lipoxins by the 15-lipoxygenase–initiated route, leukotriene biosynthesis is blocked at the 5-lipoxygenase level (8,14), resulting in an inverse relationship between leukotriene and lipoxin biosynthesis. When lipoxins are generated by neutrophils from conversion of 15-HETE carrying its alcohol in the *R* or *S* configuration, leukotriene formation is dramatically reduced, and lipoxins and 15-epi-lipoxin are formed and released. Lipoxins also functionally block the actions of LTB4 and the peptidoleukotriene LTD4 (31–33).

Evidence indicates that primed leukocytes from individuals with inflammatory disorders such as asthma that are exposed to various cytokines and other inflammatory stimuli *in vivo* generate lipoxins entirely from endogenous sources of arachidonic acid from a single cell type. The finding that primed cells (12,34–36) and cells from periph-

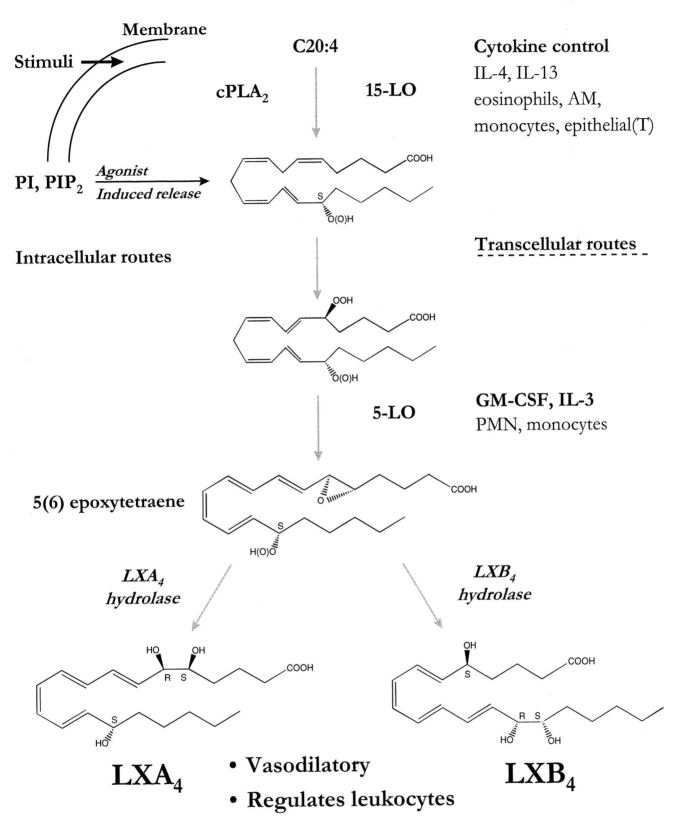

FIG. 24-2. 15-Lipoxygenase–initiated lipoxin biosynthesis on mucosal surfaces. (From Serhan CN. Lipoxins and novel aspirin-triggered 15-epi-lipoxins (ATL): a jungle of cell-cell interactions or a thera-peutic opportunity? *Prostaglandins* 1997;53:107–137, with permission.)

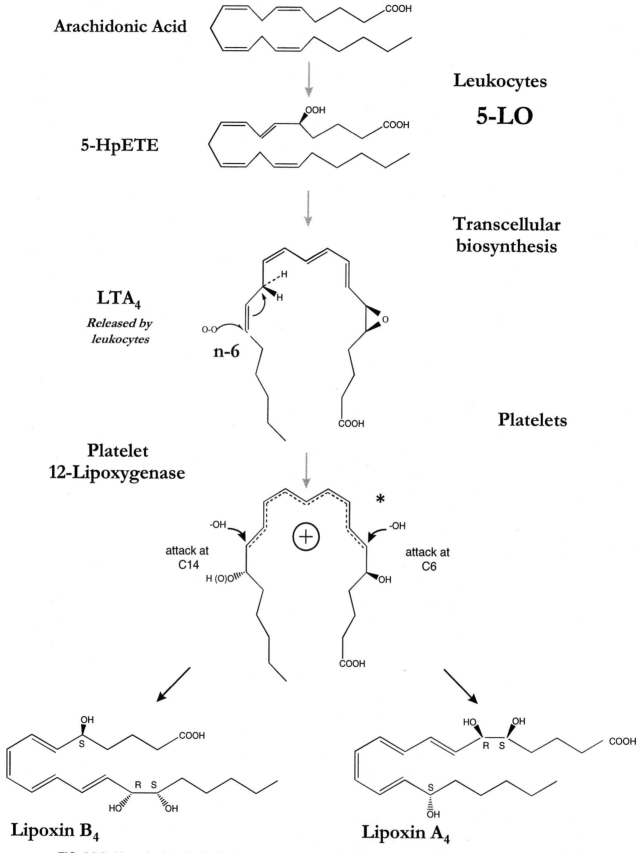

FIG. 24-3. Vascular intraluminal 5-lipoxygenase and 12-lipoxygenase interactions in lipoxin biosynthesis. (From Serhan CN. Lipoxins and novel aspirin-triggered 15-epi-lipoxins (ATL): a jungle of cell-cell interactions or a therapeutic opportunity? *Prostaglandins* 1997;53:107–137, with permission.)

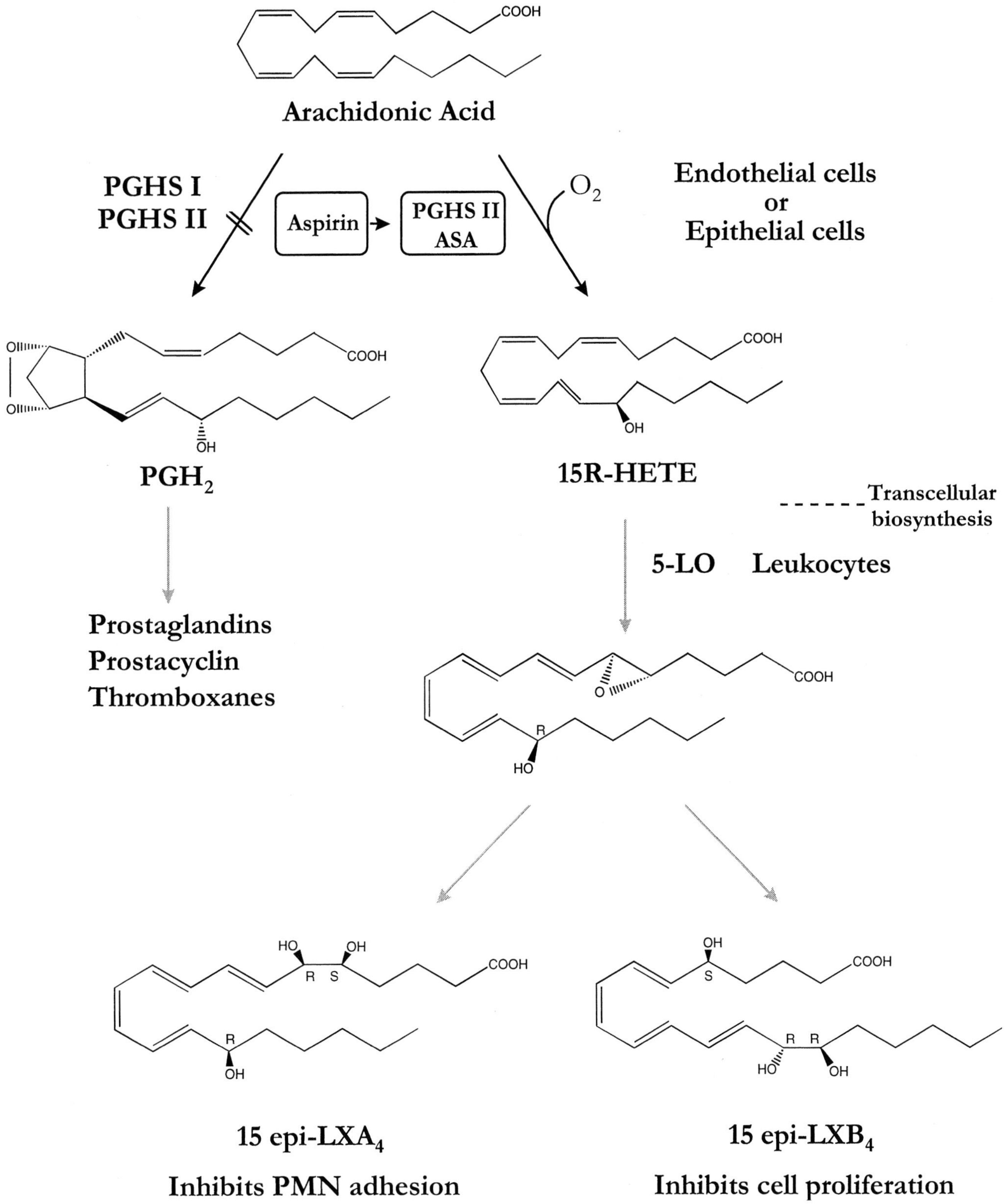

FIG. 24-4. Aspirin-triggered 15-epi-lipoxin biosynthesis. (From Serhan CN. Lipoxins and novel aspirin-triggered 15-epi-lipoxins (ATL): a jungle of cell-cell interactions or a therapeutic opportunity? *Prostaglandins* 1997;53:107–137, with permission.)

eral blood of individuals with various diseases can generate lipoxins from endogenous sources of arachidonic acid raises questions about our current understanding of the generation of eicosanoids in inflammatory diseases. What is the temporal relationship between the eicosanoid classes during the progression of an inflammatory response from acute to chronic status (see Fig. 24-1)? Does diet affect the temporal relationships between classes? Information along these lines can help in understanding the biologic impact of each class of compound, because in experimental models, they regulate key responses during multicellular events. This is particularly evident in view of findings with transgenic rabbits that express 15-lipoxygenase in a macrophage-specific fashion (37). When the 15-lipoxygenase–overexpressing rabbits were fed an atherogenic diet, the expression of 15-lipoxygenase was found to have a protective effect on the development of atherosclerosis. This action of 15-lipoxygenase probably is causally related to biosynthesis of local antiinflammatory mediators such as lipoxin.

5-Lipoxygenase–Initiated Pathway

The second route recognized for lipoxin biosynthesis, the LTA_4-dependent lipoxin biosynthetic route, occurs between cell types of the vasculature. These intraluminal sources of lipoxygenase products show a sharp contrast between interstitial or mucosal origins. This pathway is best studied with the interaction of human neutrophils with platelets (see Fig. 24-3). The key insertion of molecular oxygen in this biosynthetic scheme involves 5-lipoxygenase within human neutrophils and 12-lipoxygenase in high levels in human platelets (7,11,12,38). The platelet-leukocyte interactions in the biosynthesis of lipoxins and other eicosanoids serve as a model of cell-cell interactions in other tissues and cell types because of the ease with which we can obtain sufficient numbers of neutrophils and platelets to carry out experiments in vitro. Unprimed neutrophils apparently do not generate appreciable quantities of lipoxins on their own (11,12), and more than 50% of their LTA_4, formed from the 5-lipoxygenase, is released into the extracellular milieu (39).

Platelets that adhere to PMN pick up LTA_4 and convert it by means of 12-lipoxygenase to a carbonium cation intermediate in a reaction mechanism that is similar to the 15-lipoxygenase mechanism (11,40). The platelet 12-lipoxygenase abstracts hydrogen at the C13 position and inserts molecular oxygen into the C15 position of LTA_4 (see Fig. 24-3), converting it to a cation intermediate that opens to lipoxin B_4 when attacked by water at the C14 position or LXA_4 when attacked by water at the C6 position (13,41,42). The formation of LXB_4 and LXA_4 is unique to the 12-lipoxygenase; 15-lipoxygenase does convert LTA_4 to the 5(6)epoxytetraene and then nonenzymatically opens to LXA_4 and its isomers without a high-yield generation of LXB_4.

This new activity of 12-lipoxygenase, for which a functional role of the enzyme in platelets had remained elusive, indicates that the 12-lipoxygenase serves as a lipoxin synthase in platelets (11). Observations of isolated, intact platelets from human peripheral blood were confirmed with studies using recombinant 12-lipoxygenase. The 12-lipoxygenase converts LTA_4 to LXA_4 and LXB_4 (13). The enzyme undergoes suicide inactivation with LTA_4 as substrate for LXB_4 but continues to produce LXA_4. This catalytic regulatory mechanism has implications for the separate biologic actions of lipoxin A_4 and B_4 when generated within the vasculature, which probably is the place for platelets and leukocytes to adhere and interact (43,44). Cell-cell interactions, exemplified here with platelets and leukocytes, result in the formation of new molecules by transcellular communication that regulates cell function (see Chapter 6).

Aspirin-Triggered 15-epi-Lipoxin Circuit

A third major route to tetraene-containing eicosanoids (5,14) was uncovered (see Figs. 24-1 and 24-4). In this transcellular biosynthetic scheme (see Fig. 24-4), PGHS-2, expressed in endothelial cells or epithelial cells after exposure to proinflammatory cytokines such as IL-1β, lipopolysaccharide, or tumor necrosis factor, switches its catalytic activity in the presence of aspirin, generating 15(R)HETE instead of prostaglandin intermediates. In this setting, aspirin inhibits prostaglandin biosynthesis by PGHS-1 and PGHS-2 (45). PGHS-2, when acetylated in endothelial or epithelial cells, is not enzymatically inactive. Instead, this isozyme converts endogenous arachidonic acid to 15(R)HETE, which is released and transformed through transcellular routes to form 15-epi-lipoxins by leukocytes in proximity. The activated and, in most instances, adherent leukocytes in this scenario possess 5-lipoxygenase and transform 15(R)HETE to a 5,6-epoxytetraene within leukocytes, which carries its C15-position alcohol in the R configuration. This proposed common intermediate leads to the formation of 15-epi-lipoxin A_4 (15-epi-LXA_4) and 15-epi-lipoxin B_4, which each carry the R configuration at C15. The 15-epi-LXA_4 proves to be more potent than native LXA_4 in inhibiting neutrophil adhesion (5,16), and 15-epi-LXB_4 inhibits cell proliferation (14). The R configuration increases the bioactivity of both molecules.

Recombinant PGHS-2, when acetylated by ASA, switches its substrate binding to an altered conformer that favors the generation of 15(R)HETE (46). The well-known in vivo inhibition of prostaglandin H_2 by ASA is readily demonstrable by means of recombinant enzymes, with the appearance of lipoxygenase activity or 15(R)generating activity within minutes that reduces sharply with time. The interest in the pathway outlined in Figure 24-4 is that PGHS-2 is present in abundance in inflammatory reactions and in disease states, including colon cancer

(45,47), and is in place when individuals take aspirin for its therapeutic benefit. PGHS-2 is likely to be in place *in vivo* when ASA is taken, and it is more than likely that inflammatory cell types are adhering and in appropriate proximity in these scenarios (see Chapter 6).

We are accustomed to thinking of aspirin as an inhibitor of eicosanoid biosynthesis, and these new results establish that aspirin can trigger the biosynthesis of novel compounds, such as the ATLs, which can serve as potential endogenous antiinflammatory signals or mediators of some of aspirin's beneficial actions. These benefits include prevention of myocardial infarction (48,49) and protection from colorectal adenoma and other forms of cancer (47,50). The mechanism of ASA's beneficial actions probably includes the biosynthesis of 15-epi-lipoxin and related compounds and may represent a novel mechanism for this old drug for which a wealth of toxicology data is available worldwide. Because of ASA's widespread use and absence of a clear mechanism to explain its newly appreciated actions, it is important to gain a more complete understanding of its cellular impact and the sites of its therapeutic actions.

CELL-CELL INTERFACING TO LIPOXIN CIRCUITS AND LOCAL BIOLOGIC IMPACT

The three major routes that lead to the formation of tri-hydroxytetraene-containing eicosanoids can operate independently or simultaneously within the vasculature. For example, GM-CSF–primed neutrophils recruited to an inflammatory site can interact with platelets. After the platelets adhere to the neutrophil surface (11,43,44,51), activated PMNs generate LTA4 that is released and transformed by means of 12-lipoxygenase in platelets to generate lipoxins (see Fig. 24-3). These routes are not inhibited by ASA or other nonsteroidal antiinflammatory drugs, and leukotriene and lipoxin biosynthesis persist with these drugs on board (42). Within the vasculature, the aspirin-triggered lipoxin pathway can be operative with activated endothelial cells interacting with adherent neutrophils generating 15-epi-lipoxin. Leukocytes interacting with epithelial surfaces, as in the case of respiratory, renal, or gastrointestinal inflammation, can also generate lipoxins through bidirectional routes, in which (15S)-HETE and (15R)-HETE are released by the epithelial cell and converted to lipoxin by neutrophils.

The other component of this bidirectional interaction can involve neutrophil-released LTA4 (52) that is converted by the abundant 15-lipoxygenase in epithelial cells (53), particularly tracheal epithelial cells, to generate lipoxins through a LTA4-dependent mechanism. LTA4 is also a substrate for the 15-lipoxygenase and can be converted to lipoxin (11,53). A less prominent route to their formation involves 5,6-dihydroxyeicosanoids, which are also substrates for lipoxin production (54). These reactions can include 15-lipoxygenase conversion or 12-lipoxygenase conversion of 5,6-dihydroxyeicosanoid substrates to lipoxin (54), which are enhanced by cell-cell adhesion interactions (55).

Impact of Cytokines and Priming

Individual cytokines enhance the appearance of the required enzymes and prime for lipoxin formation, suggesting that there is a close association between the local cytokines within the site of generation of lipoxins and the site of lipoxin action.

Another recognized source of lipoxin biosynthesis involves a form of priming that involves esterification of 15-HETE (see Fig. 24-2) in inositol-containing phospholipids within the membranes of human neutrophils (56). Cells rapidly esterify 15-HETE into their inositol-containing lipids, which on subsequent agonist stimulation, release 15-HETE from this source, which is further transformed (see Fig. 24-2). The deacylated mono-HETEs are released and transformed, in this case, to lipoxin or perhaps to other eicosanoids that have yet to be discovered. This pathway, illustrated in Figure 24-2, suggests that precursors of lipoxin biosynthesis can be stored within membranes of inflammatory cells and then released by stimuli activating phospholipase A2 (56). This form of membrane priming to generate bioactive lipid mediators has implications in the second messengers generated, such as 15-hydroxy-phosphatidylinositol-4-phosphate and diglyceride, which contain 15-HETE that may alter their intracellular signaling activities. As is the case with (15S)-HETE, (15R)-HETE is rapidly esterified into membrane phospholipids and probably serves as a reservoir for 15-epi-lipoxin formation (14).

GM-CSF and IL-3 regulate expression of 5-lipoxygenase, and IL-4 and IL-13 specifically regulate the gene expression of 15-lipoxygenase (21–23,26,27). Specific cytokine regulators of 12-lipoxygenase expression in human megakaryocytes have not been observed (41).

Functional integration of these pathways and their regulation by cytokines provides cells and tissues with diverse routes to generate lipoxin. The redundant biosynthetic capacity for producing lipoxins in human tissues is orchestrated by cell-cell interactions of diverse cell types and probably reflects the basic functional requirements for these compounds in regulating essential tissue responses.

PMN-platelet microaggregates form in vivo (43,44), and key eicosanoid biosynthetic enzymes are regulated by specific cytokines (22,23). This understanding of cell-cell interactions provides new concepts for appreciating the signaling networks involved in lipoxin formation (55) and actions. GM-CSF enhances lipoxin generation during receptor-mediated PMN and platelet interactions (12), and helper T cells type 2 (TH2 cells) can produce the 15-lipoxygenase, regulating cytokines IL-4 and IL-13, which are in the microenvironment (21,22,25). *In vivo* microenvironments, particularly for specific disease states, probably contain specific cytokines that can enhance production of lipoxins and other novel bioactive lipid mediators.

Role for Cell Adhesion and Transcellular Biosynthesis *In Vivo*

This type of cellular lipoxin circuit is demonstrated in an animal model of glomerular nephritis in which platelet-leukocyte interactions lead to the generation of lipoxins *in vivo* (51). Antibodies against P-selectin, a mediator of platelet-leukocyte adhesion, block transcellular lipoxin biosynthesis *in vitro* and in glomerular nephritis *in vivo* (57). Neutrophil infiltration was unexpectedly more pronounced during acute nephrotoxic serum nephritis in P-selectin knock-out mice than in wild-type mice, because it was anticipated that infiltration of PMNs in the P-selectin–deficient mouse would be reduced, not enhanced, as was observed. Consistent with this notion, P-selectin deficient mice show a reduced efficiency of transcellular lipoxin generation (51). LXA$_4$ levels are restored, and the difference in neutrophil infiltration is eliminated when the P-selectin–deficient mice are infused with wild-type platelets. These observations raise the possibility that platelet-neutrophil adherence and transcellular biosynthesis are important inflammatory events that regulate neutrophil recruitment by initiating the formation of lipid mediators that suppress proinflammatory responses. Lipoxin generation by platelets may help regulate the entry of recruiting and infiltrating neutrophils.

Transcellular biosynthetic circuits and networks such as those illustrated by the model of platelet-neutrophil interactions can yield lipoxins (see Fig. 24-3) and leukotrienes. If lipoxins act as a braking signal or as an endogenous stop signal for the recruitment of leukocytes, it is likely that molecular switches are thrown that direct eicosanoid product profiles from a proinflammatory to an antiinflammatory phenotype. In this regard, cytokines and the local redox potential of the inflammatory microenvironment play important roles in the generation of lipoxins, particularly in platelets. Agents that reduce the intracellular platelet level of glutathione, such as nitroprusside, enhance lipoxin generation by platelets and block the formation of cysteinyl-containing leukotrienes (12).

Conserved Structures

Lipoxins are evolutionarily conserved molecules in that they are generated in large quantities (i.e., microgram amounts during incubation) by a variety of fish tissues, including leukocytes and brain (9). The levels generated by isolated fish cells are approximately 10 to 100 times greater than the amount generated by human cells in coincubation, suggesting that they possess important roles in fish. Their role in fish brain is unknown, but lipoxins inhibit proliferation of fish lymphocytes (9). Phylogenetic analysis shows that lipoxins are also generated by frog leukocytes and thrombocytes (58). LXA$_4$ stimulates chemotaxis of trout macrophages (9), a response that is shared by human monocytes (59) but not by human neutrophils (15). Produced in human marrow, lipoxins are implicated in regulating myelopoiesis (3). It appears that lipoxins have a primitive physiologic function that has evolved and changed in humans but has held the lipoxin structure conserved.

LIPOXINS IN TISSUES AND DISEASES

Lipoxin Generation *In Vivo*

Lipoxins are generated in human organs and are associated with a variety of inflammatory events; the first demonstration was made by bronchial lavage (60). LXA$_4$ and LXB$_4$ are formed in nasal polyps (53), and LXA$_4$ is generated in nasal lavage from ASA-sensitive asthmatics (61) and in experimental nephritis (57). Along these lines, Chavis et al. (34) proposed that lipoxin are useful biomarkers of asthma, and Thomas et al. (36) proposed that lipoxins are biomarkers of long-term clinical improvement in arthritic patients.

The list of diseases and tissues in Table 24-1 is not exhaustive, and it is likely to represent examples of *in vivo* scenarios in which cell-cell interaction is accelerated and the generation of lipoxins is detected because of the abundance of cytokines and cell-cell interactions in these settings. Rupture of the atherosclerotic plaque leads to rapid generation of lipoxin A$_4$ in the intracoronary artery (62). Lipoxins are also generated by normal human bone marrow (3,63). During chronic myelocytic leukemia, platelets lose 12-lipoxygenase. They also lose their ability to generate lipoxins, and this finding may be related to the blast crisis observed in chronic myelocytic leukemia (3).

Vasoactive and Antiinflammatory Lipoxin Bioactions

Lipoxins display vasodilatory and counterregulatory roles in *in vivo* and *in vitro* models (8,30). LXA$_4$ and LXB$_4$ promote vasorelaxation and relax aorta and pul-

TABLE 24-1. *Lipoxins in tissues and diseases*

Asthma
Aspirin-sensitive asthma
Angioplasty-induced plaque rupture
Bone marrow generation
Lipoxin biosynthesis—defect in chronic myeloid leukemia
Glomerulonephritis
Sarcoidosis
Pneumonia
Nasal polyps
Rheumatoid arthritis

TABLE 24-2. *Vascular and smooth muscle actions of lipoxins*

Vasodilatory
Relax aorta and pulmonary artery
Reverse $PGF_{2\alpha}$ and endothelin (ET-1) contraction
Stimulate nitric oxide generation
Stimulate endothelial prostacyclin formation
Stimulate $cPLA_2$-dependent arachidonate release and conversion

PGF, prostaglandin F; $cPLA_2$, cytosolic phospholipase A_2.

monary arteries (Table 24-2). LXA_4 reverses precontraction of the pulmonary artery induced by prostaglandin $F_{2\alpha}$ and the potent vasoconstrictor enzyme endothelin-1. The mechanisms of LXA_4- and LXB_4-induced vasodilation involve endothelium-dependent vasorelaxation and involve prostaglandin-dependent and independent pathways (30). In certain tissues, lipoxins can stimulate the formation of, for example, prostacyclin by endothelial cells (64), which can contribute to vasodilation. These prostanoid-dependent actions of lipoxins are inhibited by cyclooxygenase inhibitors (30) and indicate that lipoxins can stimulate the biosynthesis of a second set of mediators. These also include lipoxin-stimulated generation of nitric oxide (65), which may mediate a component of lipoxin-regulated vascular tone. LXA_4 stimulation of nitric oxide also regulates cholinergic neurotransmission and reduces vagal nerve-mediated contraction of airway smooth muscle (66).

The actions of lipoxins contrast with those of most other lipid mediators that are primarily proinflammatory, such as leukotriene, platelet-activating factor, and thromboxane. LXA_4 displays human leukocyte-selective actions (Table 24-3). Lipoxins in the nanomolar range inhibit neutrophil and eosinophil chemotaxis (33,67). LXA_4 inhibits PMN transmigration across endothelial and epithelial cells (68), blocks PMN diapedesis from postcapillary venules (69), and inhibits PMN entry into inflamed tissues in animal models (57).

TABLE 24-3. *Human leukocyte selective actions*

Cell type	Lipoxin	Action
PMN	LXA_4 and LXB_4	Block emigration, transmigration, and chemotaxis; downregulate CD11/18 and intracellular IP_3, Ca^{2+}; inhibit PMN-endothelial cell and epithelial cell interactions
Eosinophils	LXA_4	Inhibit chemotaxis to PAF and FMLP
Monocytes	LXA_4 and LXB_4	Stimulate chemotaxis and adherence; stimulate myeloid bone marrow-derived progenitors

LX, lipoxins; PMN, polymorphonuclear cell.

At nanomolar concentrations in human PMNs, LXA_4 and LXB_4 block transmigration and chemotaxis by a mechanism that regulates CD11/CD18 (70,71) and blocks agonist-induced generation of inositol 1,4,5-trisphosphate (72). Unlike PMNs and eosinophils (67,72), lipoxins are potent chemoattractants for monocytes (73). LXA_4 and LXB_4 stimulate monocyte chemotaxis and adherence, which may be related to the recruitment of monocytes to sites of wound injury. However, monocytes do not generate superoxide anions or degranulate in response to lipoxins, suggesting that their actions on these cells are selective and are related to locomotion. Lipoxins in the subnanomolar concentration range stimulate myeloid progenitors (3). The selective actions of lipoxins on leukocytes are of interest because of the finding that lipoxins are not further transformed by PMN but are rapidly converted through dehydrogenation to inactive compounds by human monocytes (16). The biologic half-life of lipoxin is regulated by peripheral blood mononuclear cells; like other autacoids, lipoxins are rapidly formed and inactivated by specific metabolic routes.

In humans, a potentially important role for LXA_4 is underscored by the finding that inhalation of LXA_4 blocks airway constriction in asthmatic patients (74). *In vivo*, lipoxins inhibit diapedesis of PMNs from postcapillary venules (69) and inhibit the entry of leukocytes into inflamed tissues (71). LXA_4 downregulates LTB_4-mediated delayed-type hypersensitive reactions (75), and it antagonizes the actions of LTD_4 in renal hemodynamics and competes at the receptor for LTD_4 (32). LXB_4, which has not yet been studied extensively *in vivo*, induces sleep, much like the effect of prostaglandin D_2. In this respect, LXB_4 is less potent than prostaglandin D_2 (76). Lipoxins serve counterregulatory roles in the physiologic events of interest in inflammation, and enantiomerically modified lipoxins, as generated by aspirin (see Fig. 24-4), may also be effectors of well-established antiinflammatory therapies.

LIPOXIN INACTIVATION PATHWAYS

Aspirin-Triggered Lipoxins as Endogenous Lipoxin Stable Analogues

Eicosanoids and other bioactive lipids are rapidly generated within seconds, act locally, and are rapidly inactivated. Most lipoxygenase-derived products are rapidly inactivated by ω oxidation at the C20 position (8). Prostaglandins and other cyclooxygenase products usually are rapidly inactivated by dehydrogenation at C15 by an enzyme called prostaglandin dehydrogenase. Lipoxins undergo ω oxidation at C20 and then undergo dehydrogenation (16,73). Dehydrogenation or ω oxidation of lipoxins is organ and cell type specific. The major route of lipoxin inactivation is through dehydrogenation by monocytes that convert LXA_4 to 15-oxo-LXA_4 and LXB_4 to 5-oxo-LXB_4, followed by specific reduction of the double bond adjacent to the ketone. The enzymatic steps of dehydrogenation followed by reduction of lipoxin-derived intermediates resemble the inactivation of prostaglandins (73). Because the lipoxin and ATL appear to serve as downregulating autacoids, a series of analogues were designed and prepared by total organic synthesis to increase the biologic half-life of the lipoxins and enhance their bioavailability. The goal was to further test the notion that these lipoxin pathways and bioactions are antiinflammatory *in vivo*.

LXA$_4$ analogues were constructed with bulky groups placed at the C15 and the omega or C20 end (see Fig. 24-2). LXB$_4$ analogues were designed with bulky groups at C5 to disrupt the dehydrogenation step at this site. Placement of these specific groups within the LXA$_4$ structure template prevents oxidation and lipoxin inactivation, and it proved to be a modest enough change to retain their native bioactivities. In some cases, the analogues proved to be equal or more potent than the native lipoxin structures. Their potencies depend on the tissues and routes of inactivation effected. For example, LXA$_4$ stable analogues are potent inhibitors of PMN adherence to endothelial cells and PMN transmigration across endothelial cell surfaces (16). During coincubations of PMN with endothelial cells, native LXA$_4$ is not further metabolized in appreciable quantities or inactivated. LXA$_4$ and its analogues are essentially equipotent, with a rank order of LXA$_4$ ≈ (15R/S)-methyl-LXA$_4$-ME ≈ 15-cyclohexyl-LXA$_4$-ME ≈ 16-phenoxy-LXA$_4$-ME, with an apparent 50% effective concentration (EC$_{50}$) of approximately 1 nmol/L. In contrast, PMN coincubations of epithelial cells show sharp differences in rank order and potency of the lipoxin analogues, because epithelial cells can degrade lipoxin *in vitro*. In these cell-cell interactions, (15R/S)-methyl-LXA$_4$-ME and 16-phenoxy-LXA$_4$-ME proved to be more potent than native LXA$_4$, with inhibition of PMN transmigration observed at concentrations of the lipoxin analogues as low as picomolar levels.

The ATL 15-epi-LXA$_4$ is less effectively converted *in vitro* to its 15-oxo-metabolite than LXA$_4$ is converted by recombinant prostaglandin dehydrogenase (16). This indicates that the dehydrogenation step is highly stereospecific and suggests that, when ATLs are generated *in vivo*, their biologic half-life is increased by about twofold greater than that of native LXA$_4$, thereby enhancing their ability to evoke bioactions. These LXA$_4$ stable analogues proved to inhibit PMN adhesion and transmigration, and they were as potent stimuli for monocyte migration as the native LXA$_4$ (59). Biologically stable analogues of lipoxin and ATL can be engineered to enhance the bioactions, which suggests that they are useful tools and offer leads for developing therapeutic modalities.

Antiinflammatory Signaling and Lipoxin-Specific Receptors

Lipoxin actions are cell type, species, and organ specific. These actions can be assigned to one or a combination of three mechanisms:

1. Lipoxins act at their own specific cell surface receptors (i.e., LXA$_4$ specific and separate LXB$_4$ receptor) (77).
2. LXA$_4$ interacts with a subclass of LTD$_4$ receptors (pharmacologically defined) that also binds LXA$_4$ (30,32).
3. Lipoxins can act at *intracellular targets* after lipoxin transport and uptake or within its cell of origin (77,78).

LXA$_4$ and LXB$_4$ act at two distinct sites, and in some cell types, they evoke similar actions, but their actions are distinct in others. The profile of LXA$_4$ actions in responses relevant to inflammation (see Table 24-2) suggested that its actions as an autacoid are mediated by a cell surface receptor and that lipoxin could evoke responses in its cell of origin by acting on specific enzyme systems (8,77). Labeled LXA$_4$ facilitates identification of specific LXA$_4$ receptors on leukocytes (15,77). These receptors are inducible in HL-60 cells (i.e., human acute promyelocytic leukemic line), and specific binding of the ^{3}H-labeled LXA$_4$ correlates with the appearance of function in these cells. The temporal appearance of surface binding and functional responses led to identification of orphan cDNA clones of a seven-transmembrane-spanning, G-protein–coupled receptor that specifically binds LXA$_4$ and transmits its signal in transfected cells. The LXA$_4$ receptor is expressed on PMNs, monocytes, and endothelial cells, and it evokes actions in each cell type (79).

To further explore LXA$_4$ action *in vivo*, the mouse LXA$_4$ receptor was cloned (15). The mRNA distribution of this receptor is most abundant in neutrophils, followed by spleen and lung tissue, and this pattern is similar in humans and mice. The mouse receptor is 76% homologous at the nucleotide level to the human receptor, with 100% homology of the second intracellular loop, suggesting important roles for these regions in intracellular signaling. Each of the LXA$_4$ analogues that evokes actions on PMNs and monocytes acts at this receptor (15,70,73), as demonstrated by competitive binding and by receptor desensitization. The postreceptor events that lead to inhibition of PMNs and activation of monocyte migration have not been elucidated. Nevertheless, it is clear that G-protein activation is critical in both cell types. Although it appeared possible that cAMP levels could be the intracellular effector for LXA$_4$, later evidence indicated that LXA$_4$ did not stimulate adenylate cyclase activity in leukocytes, excluding a role for G$_s$ in lipoxin signaling.

ATL 15-epi-LXA$_4$ acts at the same receptor as LXA$_4$ and its bioactive analogue (15,59). To explore the possible links between aspirin and 15-epi-LXA$_4$ generation and actions, some of the lipoxin stable synthetic analogues previously mentioned were designed to carry 15R configurations: (15R/S)-methyl-LXA$_4$ and (15R)-16-phenoxy-17,18,19,20-tetranor-LXA$_4$. When added topically to the mouse ear model of acute inflammation, these analogues proved to be potent pharmacologic inhibitors of neutrophil infiltration, with actions rivaling those of the well-established antiinflammatory dexamethasone (15). These findings have therapeutic implications for the development of lipoxin- and ATL-like analogues as pharmacologic tools and drugs, and they provide direct evidence for the endogenous antiinflammatory action of LXA_4 and 15-epi-LXA_4. Because the active LXA_4 analogues act at the LXA_4 receptor, their ability to inhibit PMN infiltration *in vivo* provides evidence for antiinflammatory seven-transmembrane receptors and pathways. Although the LXB_4 receptor has not yet been identified, it is likely to be a member of the class. Because inflammation and wound healing are normally self-limited events in healthy individuals, it is not surprising that endogenous pathways and receptors exist to counteract the sequelae of severe or potentially overwhelming levels of proinflammatory mediators.

CONCLUSIONS

Lipoxins are trihydroxytetraene-containing eicosanoids that are generated primarily through cell-cell interactions and transcellular biosynthesis to regulate inflammatory events. LXA_4 and LXB_4 are positional isomers that are vasodilators; they also inhibit neutrophil transmigration and adhesion and stimulate monocyte recruitment. Lipoxins are generated within blood vessels by platelet-leukocyte interactions and on mucosal surfaces by leukocyte interactions with epithelial cells. These biosynthetic routes are distinct—one involves mainly initial oxygenation of arachidonate at C5 by 5-lipoxygenase (platelet-PMN) and the other by 15-lipoxygenase (mucosal). These lipoxin biosynthetic routes are controlled by cytokines such as IL-4 and IL-13, which specifically stimulate expression of 15-lipoxygenase, and GM-CSF and IL-3, which regulate 5-lipoxygenase in leukocytes. The importance of these events is heightened by the finding that aspirin triggers the biosynthesis of 15-epi-lipoxin during PMN-endothelial cell and PMN–adenocarcinoma-derived epithelial cell interactions (see Fig. 24-4). ATLs also inhibit PMN adhesion to endothelium and block proliferation of airway epithelial adenocarcinoma cells (14).

Stop signals in the process of inflammation may be involved in switching the cellular response from additional recruitment of PMNs toward monocytes that could assist in wound healing. This hypothesis places lipoxin and ATL as pivotal mediators in tissue-level protection events whose function could peak after initial leukotriene and prostaglandin generation. Lipoxin's ability to inhibit key events in asthma in humans (74), in renal inflammation in rodents (57), and in acute inflammation in mouse ear (15) lends support to this hypothesis. Lipoxin and lipoxin stable analogue responses appear to be evoked, at least in part, by specific lipoxin receptors.

Availability of LXA_4 receptor cDNA enables dissection of the postreceptor ligand interactions and the identification of lipoxin mimetics and antagonists. Lipoxin and ATL stable analogues represent useful tools to evaluate the potential of pharmacologic manipulation of the lipoxin and ATL system *in vivo* (15) as means to developing new and selective therapies. This approach may yield agents that can selectively focus on the beneficial actions of aspirin and related drugs in a variety of clinical settings.

ACKNOWLEDGMENTS

The author thanks Mary Halm Small for expert assistance in the preparation of this chapter. Studies from the author's laboratory were supported in part by National Institutes of Health grants GM-38765 and P01-HL-36028.

REFERENCES

1. Serhan CN, Haeggström JZ, Leslie CC. Lipid mediator networks in cell signaling: update and impact of cytokines. *FASEB J* 1996;10:1147–1158.
2. Dahlén S-E, Dahlén B, Kumlin M, Björck T, Ihre E, Zetterström O. Clinical and experimental studies of leukotrienes as mediators of airway obstruction in humans. *Adv Prostaglandin Thromboxane Leukot Res* 1994;22:155–166.
3. Stenke L, Reizenstein P, Lindgren JA. Leukotrienes and lipoxins—new potential performers in the regulation of human myelopoiesis. *Leuk Res* 1994;18:727–732.
4. Israel E, Dermarkarian R, Rosenberg M, et al. The effects of a 5-lipoxygenase inhibitor on asthma induced by cold, dry air. *N Engl J Med* 1990;323:1740–1744.
5. Clària J, Serhan CN. Aspirin triggers previously undescribed bioactive eicosanoids by human endothelial cell-leukocyte interactions. *Proc Natl Acad Sci USA* 1995;92:9475–9479.
6. Samuelsson B, Dahlén SE, Lindgren JÅ, Rouzer CA, Serhan CN. Leukotrienes and lipoxins: structures, biosynthesis, and biological effects. *Science* 1987;237:1171–1176.
7. Lindgren JA, Edenius C. Transcellular biosynthesis of leukotrienes and lipoxins via leukotriene A_4 transfer. *Trends Pharmacol Sci* 1993;14: 351–354.
8. Serhan CN. Lipoxin biosynthesis and its impact in inflammatory and vascular events. *Biochim Biophys Acta* 1994;1212:1–25.
9. Rowley AF, Hill DJ, Ray CE, Munro R. Haemostasis in fish—an evolutionary perspective. *Thromb Haemost* 1997;77:227–233.
10. Marcus AJ, Broekman MJ, Safier LB, et al. Formation of leukotrienes and other hydroxy acids during platelet-neutrophil interactions *in vitro*. *Biochem Biophys Res Commun* 1982;109:130–137.
11. Serhan CN, Sheppard KA. Lipoxin formation during human neutrophil-platelet interactions: evidence for the transformation of leukotriene A_4 by platelet 12-lipoxygenase *in vitro*. *J Clin Invest* 1990;85:772–780.
12. Fiore S, Serhan CN. Formation of lipoxins and leukotrienes during receptor-mediated interactions of human platelets and recombinant human granulocyte/macrophage colony-stimulating factor-primed neutrophils. *J Exp Med* 1990;172:1451–1457.
13. Romano M, Chen XS, Takahashi Y, Yamamoto S, Funk CD, Serhan CN. Lipoxin synthase activity of human platelet 12-lipoxygenase. *Biochem J* 1993;296:127–133.
14. Clària J, Lee MH, Serhan CN. Aspirin-triggered lipoxins (15-epi-LX) are generated by the human lung adenocarcinoma cell line (A549)-neutrophil interactions and are potent inhibitors of cell proliferation. *Mol Med* 1996;2:583–596.
15. Takano T, Fiore S, Maddox JF, Brady HR, Petasis NA, Serhan CN. Aspirin-triggered 15-epi-lipoxin A_4 and LXA_4 stable analogs are potent inhibitors of acute inflammation: evidence for anti-inflammatory receptors. *J Exp Med* 1997;185:1693–1704.
16. Serhan CN, Maddox JF, Petasis NA, et al. Design of lipoxin A_4 stable analogs that block transmigration and adhesion of human neutrophils. *Biochemistry* 1995;34:14609–14615.

17. Marcus AJ. Aspirin as prophylaxis against colorectal cancer. *N Engl J Med* 1995;333:656–658.

18. Giovannucci E, Rimm EB, Stampfer MJ, Colditz GA, Ascherio A, Willett WC. Aspirin use and the risk for colorectal cancer and adenoma in male health professionals. *Ann Intern Med* 1994;121:241–246.

19. Serhan CN, Hamberg M, Samuelsson B. Lipoxins: novel series of biologically active compounds formed from arachidonic acid in human leukocytes. *Proc Natl Acad Sci USA* 1984;81:5335–5339.

20. Ford-Hutchinson AW. Arachidonate 15-lipoxygenase: characteristics and potential biological significance. *Eicosanoids* 1991;4:65–74.

21. Levy BD, Romano M, Chapman HA, Reilly JJ, Drazen J, Serhan CN. Human alveolar macrophages have 15-lipoxygenase and generate (15S)-hydroxy-5,8,11-*cis*-13-transeicosatetraenoic acid and lipoxins. *J Clin Invest* 1993;92:1572–1579.

22. Nassar GM, Morrow JD, Roberts LJ II, Lakkis FG, Badr KF. Induction of 15-lipoxygenase by interleukin-13 in human blood monocytes. *J Biol Chem* 1994;269:27631–27634.

23. Sigal E, Conrad DJ. Human 15-lipoxygenase: a potential effector molecule for interleukin-4. *Adv Prostaglandin Thromboxane Leukot Res* 1994;22:309–316.

24. Katoh T, Lakkis FG, Makita N, Badr KF. Co-regulated expression of glomerular 12/15-lipoxygenase and interleukin-4 mRNA in rat nephrotoxic nephritis. *Kidney Int* 1994;46:341–349.

25. Anderson GP, Coyle AJ. TH2 and "TH2-like" cells in allergy and asthma: pharmacological perspectives. *Trends Pharmacol Sci* 1994;15:324.

26. Pouliot M, McDonald PP, Borgeat P, McColl SR. Granulocyte/macrophage colony-stimulating factor stimulates the expression of the 5-lipoxygenase-activating protein (FLAP) in human neutrophils. *J Exp Med* 1994;179:1225–1232.

27. Ring WL, Riddick CA, Baker JR, Munafo DA, Bigby TD. Lymphocytes stimulate expression of 5-lipoxygenase and its activating protein in monocytes *in vitro* via granulocyte-macrophage colony stimulating factor and interleukin-3. *J Clin Invest* 1996;97:1293–1301.

28. L'Heureux GP, Bourgoin S, Jean N, McColl SR, Naccache PH. Diverging signal transduction pathways activated by interleukin-8 and related chemokines in human neutrophils: interleukin-8, but not NAP-2 or GROAα, stimulates phospholipase D activity. *Blood* 1995;85:522–531.

29. Lefer AM, Stahl GL, Lefer DJ, et al. Lipoxins A4 and B4: comparison of icosanoids having bronchoconstrictor and vasodilator actions but lacking platelet aggregatory activity. *Proc Natl Acad Sci USA* 1988;85:8340–8344.

30. Dahlén S-E, Serhan CN. Lipoxins: bioactive lipoxygenase interaction products. In: Wong A, Crooke ST, eds. *Lipoxygenases and their products.* San Diego: Academic Press, 1991:235–276.

31. Lee TH, Lympany P, Crea AE, Spur BW. Inhibition of leukotriene B4-induced neutrophil migration by lipoxin A4: structure-function relationships. *Biochem Biophys Res Commun* 1991;180:1416–1421.

32. Badr KF, DeBoer DK, Schwartzberg M, Serhan CN. Lipoxin A4 antagonizes cellular and *in vivo* actions of leukotriene D4 in rat glomerular mesangial cells: evidence for competition at a common receptor. *Proc Natl Acad Sci USA* 1989;86:3438–3442.

33. Lee TH, Horton CE, Kyan-Aung U, Haskard D, Crea AE, Spur BW. Lipoxin A4 and lipoxin B4 inhibit chemotactic responses of human neutrophils stimulated by leukotriene B4 and *N*-formyl-L-methionyl-L-leucyl-L-phenylalanine. *Clin Sci* 1989;77:195–203.

34. Chavis C, Chanez P, Vachier I, Bousquet J, Michel FB, Godard P. 5-15-diHETE and lipoxins generated by neutrophils from endogenous arachidonic acid as asthma biomarkers. *Biochem Biophys Res Commun* 1995;207:273–279.

35. Chavis C, Vachier I, Chanez P, Bousquet J, Godard P. (5S,15S)-Dihydroxyeicosatetraenoic acid and lipoxin generation in human polymorphonuclear cells: dual specificity of 5-lipoxygenase towards endogenous and exogenous precursors. *J Exp Med* 1996;183:1633–1643.

36. Thomas E, Leroux JL, Blotman F, Chavis C. Conversion of endogenous arachidonic acid to 5,15-diHETE and lipoxins by polymorphonuclear cells from patients with rheumatoid arthritis. *Inflamm Res* 1995;44:121–124.

37. Shen J, Herderick E, Cornhill JF, et al. Macrophage-mediated 15-lipoxygenase expression protects against atherosclerosis development. *J Clin Invest* 1996;98:2201–2208.

38. Edenius C, Haeggström J, Lindgren JA. Transcellular conversion of endogenous arachidonic acid to lipoxins in mixed human platelet-granulocyte suspensions [published erratum appears in *Biochem Biophys*

39. Fiore S, Serhan CN. Phospholipid bilayers enhance the stability of leukotriene A4 and epoxytetraenes: stabilization of eicosanoids by liposomes. *Biochem Biophys Res Commun* 1989;159:477–481.

40. Corey EJ, Mehrotra MM. A stereoselective and practical synthesis of 5,6(5,5)-epoxy-15(s)-hydroxyl-7(E), 9(E), 11(2), 13(E)-eicosatetraenoic acid (4), possible precursor of the lipoxins. *Tetrahedron Lett* 1986;27:5173–5176.

41. Sheppard KA, Greenberg SM, Funk CD, Romano M, Serhan CN. Lipoxin generation by human megakaryocyte-induced 12-lipoxygenase. *Biochim Biophys Acta* 1992;1133:223–234.

42. Romano M, Serhan CN. Lipoxin generation by permeabilized human platelets. *Biochemistry* 1992;31:8269–8277.

43. Lehr H-A, Olofsson AM, Carew TE, et al. P-selectin mediates the interaction of circulating leukocytes with platelets and microvascular endothelium in response to oxidized lipoprotein *in vivo*. *Lab Invest* 1994;71:380–386.

44. Lehr H-A, Frei B, Arfors K-E. Vitamin C prevents cigarette smoke-induced leukocyte aggregation and adhesion to endothelium *in vivo*. *Proc Natl Acad Sci USA* 1994;91:7688–7692.

45. Herschman HR. Prostaglandin synthase 2. *Biochim Biophys Acta* 1996;1299:125–140.

46. Xiao G, Tsai A-L, Palmer G, Boyar WC, Marshall PJ, Kulmacz RJ. Analysis of hydroperoxide-induced tyrosyl radicals and lipoxygenase activity in aspirin-treated human prostaglandin H synthase-2. *Biochemistry* 1997;36:1836–1845.

47. Levy GN. Prostaglandin H synthases, nonsteroidal anti-inflammatory drugs, and colon cancer. *FASEB J* 1997;11:234–247.

48. Savage MP, Goldberg S, Bove AA, et al. Effect of thromboxane A2 blockade on clinical outcome and restenosis after successful coronary angioplasty. *Circulation* 1995;92:3194–3200.

49. Hennekens C, Jonas M, Buring J. The benefits of aspirin in acute myocardial infarction. Still a well-kept secret in the United States. *Arch Intern Med* 1994;154:37–39.

50. Giovannucci E, Egan KM, Hunter DJ, et al. Aspirin and the risk of colorectal cancer in women. *N Engl J Med* 1995;333:609–614.

51. Mayadas TN, Mendrick DL, Brady HR, et al. Acute passive anti-glomerular basement membrane nephritis in P-selectin-deficient mice. *Kidney Int* 1996;49:1342–1349.

52. Garrick R, Wong PY. Enzymatic formation and regulatory function of lipoxins and leukotriene B4 in rat kidney mesangial cells. *Adv Exp Med Biol* 1991;314:361–369.

53. Edenius C, Kumlin M, Björk T, Anggard A, Lindgren JA. Lipoxin formation in human nasal polyps and bronchial tissue. *FEBS Lett* 1990;272:25–28.

54. Tornhamre S, Gigou A, Edenius C, Lellouche JP, Lindgren JA. Conversion of 5,6-dihydroxyeicosatetraenoic acids: a novel pathway for lipoxin formation by human platelets. *FEBS Lett* 1992;304:78–82.

55. Brady HR, Serhan CN. Adhesion promotes transcellular leukotriene biosynthesis during neutrophil-glomerular endothelial cell interactions: inhibition by antibodies against CD18 and L-selectin. *Biochem Biophys Res Commun* 1992;186:1307–1314.

56. Brezinski ME, Serhan CN. Selective incorporation of (15S)-hydroxyeicosatetraenoic acid in phosphatidylinositol of human neutrophils: agonist-induced deacylation and transformation of stored hydroxyeicosanoids. *Proc Natl Acad Sci USA* 1990;87:6248–6252.

57. Papayianni A, Serhan CN, Phillips ML, Rennke HG, Brady HR. Transcellular biosynthesis of lipoxin A4 during adhesion of platelets and neutrophils in experimental immune complex glomerulonephritis. *Kidney Int* 1995;47:1295–1302.

58. Gronert K, Virk SM, Herman CA. Thrombocytes are the predominant source of endogenous sulfidopeptide leukotrienes in the bullfrog (*Rana catesbeiana*). *Biochim Biophys Acta* 1995;1255:311–319.

59. Maddox JF, Hachicha M, Takano T, Petasis NA, Fokin VV, Serhan CN. Lipoxin A4 stable analogs are potent mimetics that stimulate human monocytes and THP-1 cells via a G-protein linked lipoxin A4 receptor. *J Biol Chem* 1997;272:6972–6978.

60. Lee TH, Crea AE, Gant V, et al. Identification of lipoxin A4 and its relationship to the sulfidopeptide leukotrienes C4, D4, and E4 in the bronchoalveolar lavage fluids obtained from patients with selected pulmonary diseases. *Am Rev Respir Dis* 1990;141:1453–1458.

61. Levy BD, Bertram S, Tai HH, et al. Agonist-induced lipoxin A4 gener-

Res Commun 1989;159:370]. *Biochem Biophys Res Commun* 1988;157:801–807.

ation: detection by a novel lipoxin A4-ELISA. *Lipids* 1993;28: 1047–1053.

62. Brezinski DA, Nesto RW, Serhan CN. Angioplasty triggers intracoronary leukotrienes and lipoxin A4. Impact of aspirin therapy. *Circulation* 1992;86:56–63.

63. Stenke L, Näsman-Glaser B, Edenius C, Samuelsson J, Palmblad J, Lindgren JÅ. Lipoxygenase products in myeloproliferative disorders: increased leukotriene C4 and decreased lipoxin formation in chronic myeloid leukemia. *Adv Prostaglandin Thromboxane Leukot Res* 1990; 21B:883–886.

64. Leszczynski D, Ustinov J. Protein kinase C-regulated production of prostacyclin by rat endothelium is increased in the presence of lipoxin A4. *FEBS Lett* 1990;263:117–120.

65. Bratt J, Gyllenhammar H. The role of nitric oxide in lipoxin A4-induced polymorphonuclear neutrophil-dependent cytotoxicity to human vascular endothelium *in vitro*. *Arthritis Rheum* 1995;38:768–776.

66. Tamaoki J, Tagaya E, Yamawaki I, Konno K. Lipoxin A4 inhibits cholinergic neurotransmission through nitric oxide generation in the rabbit trachea. *Eur J Pharmacol* 1995;287:233–238.

67. Soyombo O, Spur BW, Lee TH. Effects of lipoxin A4 on chemotaxis and degranulation of human eosinophils stimulated by platelet-activating factor and *N*-formyl-L-methionyl-L-leucyl-L-phenylalanine. *Allergy* 1994;49:230–234.

68. Colgan SP, Serhan CN, Parkos CA, Delp-Archer C, Madara JL. Lipoxin A4 modulates transmigration of human neutrophils across intestinal epithelial monolayers. *J Clin Invest* 1993;92:75–82.

69. Raud J, Palmertz U, Dahlén SE, Hedqvist P. Lipoxins inhibit microvascular inflammatory actions of leukotriene B4. *Adv Exp Med Biol* 1991; 314:185–192.

70. Fiore S, Serhan CN. Lipoxin A4 receptor activation is distinct from that of the formyl peptide receptor in myeloid cells: inhibition of CD11/18 expression by lipoxin A4-lipoxin A4 receptor interaction. *Biochemistry* 1995;34:16678–16686.

71. Papayianni A, Serhan CN, Brady HR. Lipoxin A4 and B4 inhibit leukotriene-stimulated interactions of human neutrophils and endothelial cells. *J Immunol* 1996;156:2264–2272.

72. Grandordy BM, Lacroix H, Mavoungou E, et al. Lipoxin A4 inhibits phosphoinositide hydrolysis in human neutrophils. *Biochem Biophys Res Commun* 1990;167:1022–1029.

73. Maddox JF, Serhan CN. Lipoxin A4 and B4 are potent stimuli for human monocyte migration and adhesion: selective inactivation by dehydrogenation and reduction. *J Exp Med* 1996;183:137–146.

74. Christie PE, Spur BW, Lee TH. The effects of lipoxin A4 on airway responses in asthmatic subjects. *Am Rev Respir Dis* 1992;145:1281–1284.

75. Feng Z, Godfrey HP, Mandy S, et al. Leukotriene B4 modulates in vivo expression of delayed-type hypersensitivity by a receptor-mediated mechanism: regulation by lipoxin A4. *J Pharmacol Exp Ther* 1996;278: 950–956.

76. Kantha SS, Matsumura H, Kubo E, et al. Effect of prostaglandin D2, lipoxins and leukotrienes on sleep and brain temperature of rats. *Prostaglandins Leukot Essent Fatty Acids* 1994;51:87–93.

77. Fiore S, Ryeom SW, Weller PF, Serhan CN. Lipoxin recognition sites. Specific binding of labeled lipoxin A4 with human neutrophils. *J Biol Chem* 1992;267:16168–16176.

78. Simchowitz L, Fiore S, Serhan CN. Carrier-mediated transport of lipoxin A4 in human neutrophils. *Am J Physiol* 1994;267:C1525–1534.

79. Fiore S, Romano M, Reardon EM, Serhan CN. Induction of functional lipoxin A4 receptors in HL-60 cells. *Blood* 1993;81:3395–3403.

Inflammation: Basic Principles and Clinical Correlates,
3rd ed., edited by John I. Gallin and Ralph Snyderman.
Lippincott Williams & Wilkins, Philadelphia © 1999.

CHAPTER 25

Platelet-Activating Factor:

A Phospholipid Mediator of Inflammation

Stephen M. Prescott, Thomas M. McIntyre, and Guy A. Zimmerman

Platelet-activating factor (PAF, 1-*O*-alkyl-2-acetyl-*sn*-glycero-3-phosphocholine) is a potent mediator with diverse effects in a variety of cells and tissues. It was discovered during separate investigations of a platelet-activating factor in the plasma of rabbits undergoing anaphylaxis and an endogenous polar lipid from kidney that caused hypotension. When the structures of the active compounds were identified, they were identical. The trivial name, PAF, has achieved widespread acceptance, even though it describes only one of the compound's many effects; PAF's predominant role is in inflammation. It exerts its actions through a cell surface receptor—the first one identified for a phospholipid mediator—and receptor antagonists have been tested in inflammatory disorders.

As with eicosanoids, PAF is synthesized when inflammatory cells are activated, and its synthesis and subsequent secretion are closely regulated. In pathologic states, the regulation of the synthesis can be bypassed, or related compounds are made through unregulated mechanisms. In such circumstances, control of the proinflammatory actions is achieved by the rate of removal of PAF, which is accomplished by PAF acetylhydrolases. This chapter summarizes key aspects of the role of PAF in inflammation; more detailed discussions of specific points can be found in other reviews (1–3).

PLATELET-ACTIVATING FACTOR IN THE EARLY STEPS OF PHYSIOLOGIC INFLAMMATION

Inflammation can be a homeostatic response, as in protecting against infection and participating in wound

repair. In physiologic inflammation, an initial, rapid step is activation of endothelial cells, which change their surface properties to become adhesive for leukocytes (4). In the first few minutes after activation of the endothelial cells, they express an adhesion protein, P-selectin, on their surface (Fig. 25-1), and polymorphonuclear (PMNs) leukocytes and monocytes bind to it. This step, called tethering, accounts for leukocyte rolling *in vivo* (5). The activated endothelial cells also synthesize PAF and its acyl analogue, with the same time course (a few minutes). PAF is directed to the cell surface but is not secreted. The leukocytes that have been tethered by P-selectin are then activated by PAF (6). This step, called signaling, induces tight (integrin-dependent) binding of leukocytes to the vascular wall and their subsequent emigration and priming for secretion of their granular contents.

The spatial specificity of this response is crucial. The tethering protein and the activating phospholipid PAF are both retained at the surface of the endothelial cell. This ensures that the leukocytes are attracted to the site where they are needed but not at uninflamed areas of the vasculature or at downstream locations. The two-step process has additional safety features—the initial tethering step does not fully activate the leukocyte, although it primes the leukocyte for activation responses, and the adhesion is relatively low affinity. If the leukocyte does not receive an additional activating signal (from the PAF on the endothelial surface), it can be released and return to the bloodstream without damaging the tissue there or downstream.

The *in vitro* demonstration that P-selectin and PAF cooperatively mediate the adhesion of PMNs to activated endothelial cells is supported by *in vivo* studies in which antibodies to P-selectin (7,8) and PAF receptor antagonists (7) suppressed inflammation. Mice that had P-selectin specifically deleted (5) also had depressed

S. M. Prescott, T. M. McIntyre, and G. A. Zimmerman: Huntsman Cancer Institute, Nora Eccles Harrison Cardiovascular Research and Training Institute, and Department of Internal Medicine, University of Utah, Salt Lake City, Utah 84112.

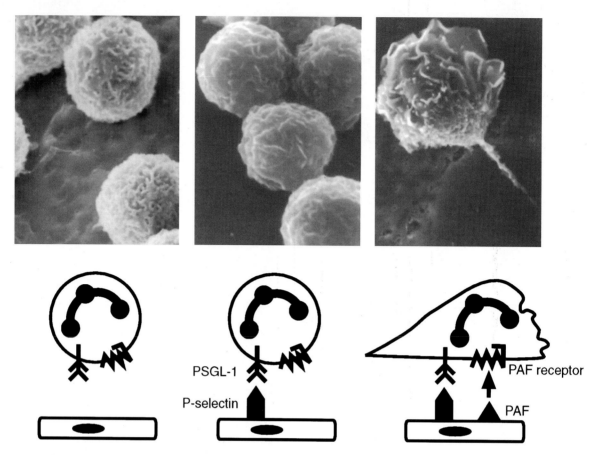

FIG. 25-1. Platelet-activating factor provides the activation signal for leukocytes adhering to endothelium that expresses P-selectin.

inflammatory responses. A similar mechanism has been described for the adhesion of platelets to neutrophils, with PAF on the surface of the latter activating the platelets (9). PAF serves an early function in inflammation; however, analogous effects have been described by other pairs of tethering and signaling molecules in the rapid and slower forms of leukocyte recruitment (4), indicating that this step, as with others in inflammation, has intrinsic redundancy.

In contrast to regulated leukocyte attraction and activation, the inappropriate activation of leukocytes can be devastating. Experimental evidence supports the idea that this as an essential feature of acute lung injury, ischemia-reperfusion, and multiorgan failure after sepsis. Bacterial toxins (10–12) and oxidants (13) circumvent the usual controls to activate endothelial cells. In some cases, P-selectin is expressed, and PAF is synthesized through the usual biochemical pathways, although in response to an inappropriate and persistent stimulus. This process can contribute to excessive inflammation, although in a localized environment. In other cases, pathologic stimuli cause the synthesis of PAF or generation of analogues through free-radical–mediated processes, and the lipid mediators escape into the circulation (14,15). This causes leukocyte activation in the circulating blood, which results in systemic responses, often with devastating outcomes. PAF and related compounds can play diametrically opposing roles, such as a regulated signal for physiologic inflammation or as a potent, pleiotropic mediator of disseminated inflammation.

PLATELET-ACTIVATING FACTOR SYNTHESIS

Two pathways have been described for PAF synthesis: *remodeling* and *de novo* (Fig. 25-2). The remodeling pathway was described first and probably is the more important in inflammation. PAF is not produced by this pathway in resting cells; they must be activated to initiate the synthesis. The synthesis is initiated by a phospholipase A_2 (PLA$_2$), and arachidonate release and PAF synthesis are closely coupled (16). The arachidonic acid is converted to eicosanoids, which also have diverse, potent actions (see Chapters 22 and 23). The lyso-PAF is converted to PAF by a specific acetyltransferase, which is activated by phosphorylation on cell stimulation (17–20).

The identity of the PLA$_2$ that initiates PAF synthesis has been addressed using multiple approaches, but one of the most compelling comes from a study of cells derived from mice genetically engineered to lack the cytoplasmic form (cPLA$_2$). This 110-kd enzyme requires calcium and

Remodeling   **De Novo**

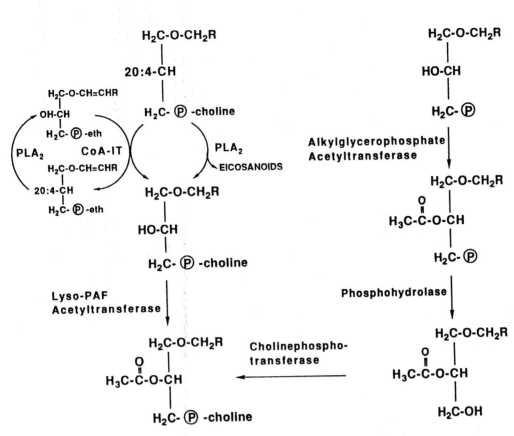

FIG. 25-2. Pathways for platelet-activating factor synthesis.

is activated through a G-protein–coupled pathway that includes activation of protein kinase C (PKC) and then phosphorylation of cPLA₂ by mitogen-activated protein (MAP) kinase. All of these properties are features of the remodeling pathway as assessed in whole-cell experiments. Another connection is that cPLA₂ selectively hydrolyzes arachidonate-containing phospholipids, which could explain the association of PAF and eicosanoid synthesis. cPLA₂ was a likely candidate for the initiation of PAF synthesis, and two groups reported that cells from animals that lacked the cPLA2 could not synthesize PAF (21,22). However, what is apparently the initial step in PAF synthesis may not be as simple as the hydrolysis of arachidonate from a common precursor, because a coenzyme A–independent transacylase also is involved in the production of PAF (2). Although a PLA₂ is still required for the initiation of PAF synthesis in this scenario, it may not act directly on 1-*O*-alkyl-2-arachidonoyl-*sn*-glycero-3-phosphocholine, a direct PAF precursor (see Fig. 25-2).

The second step of PAF synthesis (see Fig. 25-2) also is regulated in that lyso-PAF acetyltransferase is activated by phosphorylation. Whole-cell experiments have implicated the involvement of PKC in the regulation of the acetyltransferase, although the effect observed may have

been primarily at the PLA₂ step. Direct support for this regulation has been obtained in cell-free experiments in which several protein kinases were shown to activate the acetyltransferase (17,19,20). Using information from the various studies of this pathway, we have proposed that activation of cPLA₂ is a conditional step (i.e., absolutely required for the synthesis of PAF) and that activation of the lyso-PAF acetyltransferase modulates the amount of PAF produced from the lyso-PAF precursor (18).

PAF can also be synthesized by a *de novo* pathway (see Fig. 25-2) in which the enzymes are constitutively active and regulated by the availability of substrate (2). It has been proposed that this pathway produces a small amount of PAF to support some basal physiologic role, but definitive studies using whole cells or animals have not been reported.

PLATELET-ACTIVING FACTOR RECEPTOR

Virtually all of the effects of PAF are mediated through a specific receptor that was cloned independently by expression cloning and homology to other G-protein–linked receptors (23–26). Although the guinea-pig cDNA showed hybridization with 2.2-, 3.0-, and 4.0-

kb mRNAs (23), subsequent studies of human tissues showed a single message of approximately 4 kb (25,26). The human gene encodes a protein of 39 kd (342 amino acids) that is more than 80% identical to the guinea-pig protein. Since characterization of the cDNA encoding the PAF receptor, there has been rapid progress in defining the basis for signaling downstream of it. This resulted from the opportunity to transfect cells that lack the PAF receptor with a cDNA that encodes it, thereby conferring responsiveness to PAF in a cell that previously was unresponsive. In such studies, Ali et al. found that the signal generated by the PAF receptor led to a rise in the intracellular calcium level that was not blocked by pertussis toxin but, in contrast, that phosphatidylinositol turnover was partially inhibited (27). Both responses were blocked by analogues of GTP, indicating that signaling required a G protein. This work suggested that the signaling through the PAF receptor used two different G proteins.

Honda et al. used a similar protocol—stably transfected cells—to study signaling through MAP kinases (28). They found that the 42- and 44-kd forms of ERK were activated and phosphorylated on tyrosine residues in response to stimulation of the cells with PAF. Likewise, they found signals that increased the turnover of phosphatidylinositol and inhibited cyclic AMP (cAMP). They also found that there were G-protein pathways that were sensitive and insensitive to pertussis toxin. They were unable to detect activation of RAS under identical conditions, indicating that MAP kinase activation occurred through a different mechanism (28). Findings of many of these studies were consistent with the previous work on platelets and leukocytes that demonstrated that PAF receptor functions through G proteins to induce the turnover of phosphatidylinositol, inhibit cAMP, release arachidonic acid, activate phospholipase D, and stimulate protein tyrosine kinases (29).

Several groups have investigated the structure-function relationships of the PAF receptor by mutating various portions of the receptor, transfecting cells, and carrying out binding or signaling assays. One goal has been to define the area of the receptor responsible for binding PAF; this still has not been established unequivocally, but one group proposed that histidine residues 188, 248, and 249 may form a binding pocket for PAF (30). Mutation of these residues (Fig. 25-3) provided supporting evidence for this conclusion. These workers and others have shown that zinc can inhibit the binding of PAF to its receptor, which also implicates the histidine residues. Such a site would be consistent with findings for other G-protein–coupled receptors, for which the ligand binding site is composed of residues from several of the transmembrane-spanning regions.

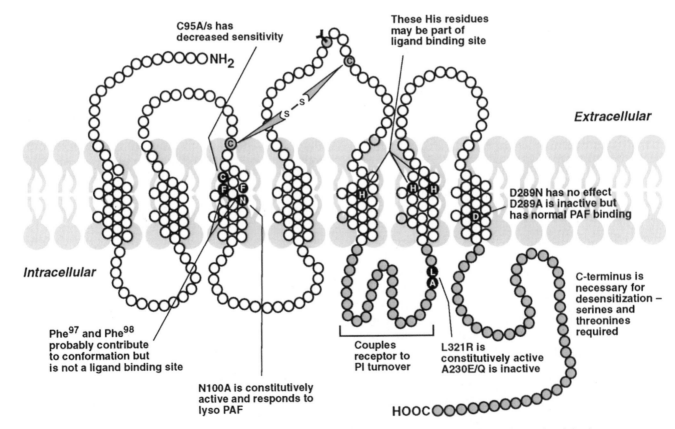

FIG. 25-3. Structure-function studies of the platelet-activating factor receptor have determined the key regions responsible for ligand binding, intracellular signaling, and desensitization.

Another important issue has been to define the regions of the receptor that are responsible for transducing the intracellular signals in response to the binding of the ligand. Experiments carried out in multiple laboratories have implicated the third intracellular loop in this function. For example, Carlson et al. showed that artificial constructs with the sequence from this region inhibited the response by other receptors (essentially a "dominant negative" strategy to saturate the downstream signaling pathways) (31). Moreover, by establishing chimeric receptors that included or lacked this region, they could shift the signaling response, consistent with this conclusion. From these experiments, it seemed clear that the third intracellular loop of the receptor is critically important for signaling phosphatidylinositol turnover.

Ishii et al. examined these issues further by systematically mutating all of the polar amino acids in the transmembrane domains of the guinea-pig receptor (see Fig. 25-3). They found that mutations in domains II, III, and VII had higher affinities for PAF than did the wild-type receptor and that mutants in transmembrane segments V, VI, and VII had lower affinities (30). The binding studies correlated well with functional responses in that representative mutations that had higher affinities were more responsive to PAF and those with lower affinities had a decreased or absent response. A mutation in the third transmembrane domain was constitutively active and had lost some of the substrate specificity; the mutant receptor responded well to lyso-PAF, which normally gives no response.

Parent et al. examined the role of various amino acids in the transmembrane domains. They found that two adjacent phenylalanine residues (see Fig. 25-3) appeared to be important for structural stability of the receptor but had no substantial effect on ligand binding (32). They also examined the role of an aspartic acid at position 289, which at the corresponding position is an asparagine in most of the G-protein–coupled receptors that have been examined. In their experiments, there was no substantial change by making this substitution (32). The same researchers examined the role of several cysteine residues in the receptor. Their experiments showed that there probably is a disulfide bond between the conserved residues at positions 90 and 173 (33). They also found that the nearby cysteine at position 95 was required for function—at least at an optimal level—and proposed that it might be involved in binding to another cysteine. In addition to the mutation (N100A) described by Ishii et al., which results in constitutive activation of the PAF receptor, work by Parent et al. showed that mutation of alanine 230 to glutamic acid also led to constitutive activity and an increased affinity for binding of PAF (34). Mutation of the adjacent residue led to a marked decrease in activity. The central portion of the receptor appears to function in ligand binding and downstream signaling.

The PAF receptor, as with other G-protein–coupled receptors, undergoes a desensitization response. Ali et al. studied this phenomenon and found that desensitization was accompanied by phosphorylation of the PAF receptor and that this was partially blocked by inhibitors of PKC. Because PKC was known to be activated by PAF, the finding indicated that a negative feedback mechanism could desensitize it, at least partially (27). In contrast, manipulations that activated cAMP-dependent kinase caused a low-level phosphorylation of the receptor but did not desensitize the receptor (27). Takano et al. examined this issue by creating a PAF receptor that lacked the C-terminal intracellular "tail" and another in which several serine and one threonine residues were replaced with alanine (35). They found that the tail and the phosphorylation sites were required for desensitization to occur. However, pretreatment with phorbol esters or PKC inhibitors had no effect, indicating that PKC was not the responsible kinase. They also found that a peptide representing the carboxyl-terminal 18 amino acids of the receptor was an excellent substrate for the G-protein–coupled receptor kinase-1 (GRK) (35). The carboxyl terminus of the PAF receptor is the target for phosphorylation, which functionally downregulates the receptor. The responsible kinase has not been established unequivocally, but it is likely to be a member of the GRK family.

Additional mechanisms for desensitization of cellular responses to PAF have been elucidated by taking advantage of the phenomena of homologous and heterologous desensitization. In the former, receptors are desensitized only by their own ligand (or family members), whereas in the latter case, receptors of one type can be downregulated after stimulation of a receptor from a different class. Previous studies had shown that the PAF receptor underwent heterologous desensitization when some peptide receptors were activated, and other work has shown that this results from PKC-mediated phosphorylation of the carboxyl terminus (36). In the same report, additional findings demonstrated that the converse can be true—that signals through the PAF receptor can downregulate peptide receptors through an effect on downstream enzymes (37). Homologous desensitization to PAF is accomplished by a combination of two mechanisms: phosphorylation of the receptor (probably a GRK) and inactivation of the key downstream effector PLC-β3 by PKC. Heterologous desensitization of the PAF receptor uses a third mechanism: phosphorylation of the receptor by PKC.

In addition to conveying signals, the PAF receptor has the unusual property of participating in the uptake and degradation of the ligand (38). In these studies, COS-7 cells were transfected with the PAF receptor, and the binding of PAF and its internalization were studied at 4°C and 37°C. There was a dramatic increase in the amount of PAF associated with the cells at 37°C, which resulted from increased internalization. Cells that did not express the receptor did not internalize PAF, and all of the uptake in the transfected cells could be blocked by including an antagonist of the receptor. The utility of this aspect of

PAF receptor function is not apparent, but it may be a mechanism to remove and degrade PAF or other receptor ligands under some circumstances.

The coding sequence of the human PAF receptor gene does not contain introns, and the gene has been localized to human chromosome 1p35-p34.3 (39,40). Expression of the receptor is regulated strongly by a variety of inflammatory agonists, including PAF itself (41–45). Two different transcripts have been described in different tissues, and the transcriptional start sites for each of them have been determined. Transcript 1 was found to be uniquely expressed in peripheral leukocytes and in a human eosinophilic cell line. This transcript, which has consensus sequences for NFκB, SP-1, and INR, is the one that responds to stimulation with PAF. Transcript 1, also referred to as the leukocyte-type, is induced by PAF and by phorbol esters in cells that contain both transcripts or those that express it selectively. The response to PAF and phorbol esters requires sequences that contain the NFκB consensus binding sites (41). Phorbol esters, but not PAF, also increased the expression of transcript 2, which required a functional AP-1 site for the response (41). Transcript 2 responded to stimulation with retinoic acid or thyroid hormone, but transcript 1 did not (46). The *cis*-acting elements responsible for this effect were mapped to three hexamer repeats located between -67 to -44 of the transcription start site. The transcriptional regulation seems to be specific—the 5′ sequence of transcript 1 responds to inflammatory stimuli, and transcript 2 is regulated by signals involved in differentiation. For example, exposure of a B lymphocyte cell line to transforming growth factor-β resulted in increased transcription of the receptor gene, and the response element was mapped to -44 to -17 of the transcript 1 sequence (44). Monocytes exposed to tumor necrosis factor-α (TNF-α) or a rat intestinal injury model induced by PAF or endotoxin showed increased expression of PAF receptor (43). In the intestinal injury model, a key component of the signaling was endogenous TNF-α.

Another form of regulation of the receptor was described in studies in which it was observed that the mRNA levels for the PAF receptor in human monocytes fell in response to activation of PKC. Under these circumstances, the $T_{1/2}$ for the mRNA was markedly decreased, and the investigators concluded that decreased stability of the messenger RNA was another potential regulatory mechanism (42).

PLATELET-ACTIVATING FACTOR RECEPTOR LIGANDS

Activated inflammatory cells can produce an analogue of PAF (acyl-PAF) that has a fatty acid rather than a fatty alcohol ligated at the *sn*-1 position of the glycerol backbone. This is the major acetylated lipid synthesized by stimulated mast cells, basophils, and endothelial cells (47). The relative production of PAF compared with that of acyl-PAF does not derive from specificity of the enzymes in the synthetic pathway, but rather reflects the abundance of the respective phospholipid precursors (47–49). Acyl-PAF is 100- to 1,000-fold less potent than PAF, but it still has actions at low concentrations (<0.1 μmol/L) and has been implicated as a priming agent in neutrophils (50). In another type of experimental protocol, pretreatment with acyl-PAF diminished a subsequent response to PAF (51), a result that may have reflected desensitization of the receptor by the pretreatment. Because it is the major product in endothelial cells, acyl-PAF, like PAF, may regulate neutrophil adhesion to endothelial cells.

The PAF receptor can bind lysophosphatidylcholine and send downstream signals, which can be blocked by receptor antagonists (52). This function is important, because lysophosphatidylcholine has been identified in a variety of pathologic circumstances and is known to activate inflammatory responses in the vascular wall. A criticism of the previous reports on the effects of lysophosphatidylcholine has been that the responses usually occur only at very high concentrations, levels at which detergent effects are also seen. It was not clear whether the response was a specific one or represented a generic response of the cell to damage. This issue was addressed in the studies by Ogita et al. (52). They found that manipulations that markedly decrease the detergent effects of lysophosphatidylcholine on cells did not abolish the signaling through the PAF receptor. Even so, the concentrations required were still very high, at least a 1,000-fold higher than required for PAF.

Oxidation of phospholipids that have a polyunsaturated fatty acid, particularly arachidonic acid, at the *sn*-2 position is another source of compounds that bind to the receptor and elicit the same responses as PAF (53,54). Tokumura et al. found such compounds in brain and identified them as phosphatidylcholines with oxidatively fragmented residues at the *sn*-2 position (55–57). Watson et al. reported the structure of two compounds from low-density lipoproteins (LDLs) that had been oxidized *in vitro* (58). One was the *sn*-2 butyroyl compound, and the other had a 5-oxovaleroyl residue at the *sn*-2 position—a PAF mimetic that we had described (53).

Oxidative attack on cellular and LDL-associated lipids may be an important mechanism for tissue injury. For example, oxidized phospholipids have been implicated in inflammation provoked by cigarette smoking. Imaizumi had subjects smoke cigarettes and found transient accumulation of a lipid with PAF bioactivity in the blood (59). He did not determine whether the active compound was authentic PAF or an oxidized phospholipid, but our results from an animal model of cigarette smoking definitively showed that smoking generates a phospholipid with PAF bioactivity through an oxidation mechanism (15). There are no definitive reports of these oxidatively modified compounds in human inflammation, but there are some suggestive observations. For multiple syndromes, including ischemia-reperfusion (60), stroke (61,62), acute asthmatic attacks (63), and sepsis, investigators have described PAF-like bioactivity or immunoreactivity but did not have proof of the structure. It is plausible that some or all of the bioactivity resulted from oxidized phospholipids, because all of these situations have had oxidation implicated as an important mechanism. This has a significant corollary: PAF is synthesized through tightly regulated enzymatic pathways (see Fig. 25-2), and oxidatively modified phospholipids are generated in an uncontrolled, possibly exponential, reaction, which could result in large quantities of a bioactive lipid.

Bacteria and bacterial toxins can activate the PAF receptor, and *Streptococcus pneumoniae* can bind to thrombin-stimulated endothelial cells through the PAF receptor (64). Experiments were expanded using a variety of strategies, including transfected cell lines in which it was shown that this type of binding depended on the presence of the PAF receptor and that the binding could be blocked by an antagonist of the receptor. Nakumara et al. showed that *Escherichia coli* endotoxin binds to the PAF receptor (65). These experiments demonstrated that the key portion of the molecule was the lipid backbone, because a precursor, lipid A, activated the PAF receptor as well as endotoxin did. The investigators demonstrated specific binding and activation as evidenced by a calcium flux. Antagonists of the receptor blocked the response to endotoxin and lipid A. These results are particularly interesting because antagonists of the PAF receptor have been shown to block a variety of shock syndromes induced by bacteria or their toxins. The traditional interpretation for this effect was that the bacteria or toxins stimulated the synthesis of PAF by cells in the host and that this PAF then induced pathophysiologic responses that resulted in shock. The antagonist interrupted this sequence by blocking the binding of the synthesized PAF to its receptor (PAF analogues such as oxidized phospholipids could fit in the sequence equally well). However, the findings that certain bacteria and endotoxin can bind directly to the PAF receptor and activate it suggest another possibility—they could directly stimulate the sepsis syndrome without PAF being generated. This seems less likely but should be considered during future studies and clinical trials.

The observations reviewed in this section indicate that the PAF receptor may be important in conveying signals from a variety of potential pathologic ligands. This mechanism would fit with the diversity of chemical structures of receptor antagonists, which range from structural analogues of PAF to completely unrelated natural products. We speculate that the phospholipids derived from oxidation of membranes and lipoproteins are particularly important endogenous ligands for the PAF receptor and account for many of the pathologic actions attributed to PAF.

REMOVING INFLAMMATORY LIPIDS BY PLATELET-ACTIVATING FACTOR ACETYLHYDROLASE

Inflammatory responses are regulated in a variety of ways, but a key mechanism is to turn off the signal by degrading PAF or oxidized phospholipids. This is the function of PAF acetylhydrolase, which is also called a "signal terminator" (66). The enzyme responsible for the degradation of PAF in blood and presumably in the extracellular space of tissues is plasma PAF acetylhydrolase; there are intracellular forms that regulate PAF signaling inside cells (1), but they do not influence the $T_{1/2}$ of PAF in blood (67).

PAF acetylhydrolase is a phospholipase that is specific for PAF and other lipids with short acyl chains at the sn-2 position. This specificity allows the enzyme to circulate in the plasma in its active form without continuously degrading cell membranes or lipoproteins. The precise role of PAF acetylhydrolase in inflammation is incompletely defined, but studies suggest that acquired deficiency is common and detrimental. Graham et al. compared the plasma PAF acetylhydrolase activity in 13 patients with clinical sepsis with the activity in 10 normal subjects. They found that the activity in the septic patients was decreased by about 50% and that the half-life of PAF in plasma was prolonged in the patients with the worst outcomes (68). This finding was supported by a report of the plasma PAF acetylhydrolase activity in 26 seriously injured patients who were at high risk for multiple organ failure syndrome (69). Eight of the subjects developed the syndrome, and their PAF acetylhydrolase activity was substantially lower than the patients who had a more successful course. The differences were seen at the earliest time after injury (12 hours) and persisted for at least 6 days. Likewise, Nakos et al. found that PAF acetylhydrolase activity in bronchoalveolar lavage (BAL) fluid was decreased in patients with adult respiratory distress syndrome (ARDS) compared with the activity in normal subjects. The researchers found a strong inverse correlation between the amount of PAF bioactivity in the BAL fluid and the PAF acetylhydrolase activity, which suggests that the enzyme is an important determinant of the concentration of PAF (or PAF-like lipids) in critically ill patients (70).

Results of these studies suggest that there may not be much functional excess in the amount of circulating PAF acetylhydrolase and that acquired deficiency may leave the patient without a key mechanism for regulating inflammation (66). If so, "replacement" therapy should provide protection, and animal studies of acute inflammation support this approach (71). Resolution of this issue will be particularly relevant in Japan and perhaps for other Asian populations, because they have a high prevalence of inherited deficiency of the plasma PAF acetylhydrolase (72,73).

Extensive studies *in vivo* have shown that PAF acetylhydrolase activity is regulated by estrogen and dexamethasone (74,75), and hormonal regulation has been examined in cultured macrophages and hepatocytes. We showed that HepG2 cells and primary cultures of hepatocytes secreted PAF acetylhydrolase (although at relatively low levels compared with macrophages) and that estradiol inhibited the secretion (76); similar findings were reported by Satoh et al. (77). We found no substantial effect of dexamethasone in hepatocytes, but Narahara et al. showed that it increased secretion from HL-60 cells that had differentiated to macrophages (78). Estrogen had no effect on the macrophage secretion in their experiments, and we observed the same in monocyte-derived macrophages. Lipopolysaccharide, interleukin-1α and -1β, and TNF-α reduced the secretion from decidual macrophages (78).

Another regulator of PAF acetylhydrolase expression is its substrate. Satoh et al. showed that PAF—but not the product of the reaction, lyso-PAF—stimulated the secretion of PAF acetylhydrolase from HepG2 cells (77), and we found a similar effect on transcription of the gene in macrophages. One of the most dramatic examples of regulation of PAF acetylhydrolase synthesis is during the differentiation from monocytes to macrophages. We showed previously that monocytes do not secrete PAF acetylhydrolase but that it increases dramatically during spontaneous differentiation to macrophages (71,79,80).

PLATELET-ACTIVATING FACTOR IN ANIMAL MODELS AND HUMAN INFLAMMATORY DISORDERS

Work from a variety of sources has suggested that PAF is a mediator of sepsis. For example, receptor antagonists blocked endotoxin-induced recruitment of platelets to the lung (81), and PAF infusion caused platelet accumulation (82). PAF was shown to enhance endotoxin's effects, including systemic hypotension, accumulation of PMNs and platelets in the lung, and pulmonary edema (83). A PAF receptor antagonist blocked IL-2–induced accumulation of PMNs and elevated lung water content (84), endotoxin-induced systemic hypotension, pulmonary vasoconstriction, and capillary leak (85). One important observation was that PAF bioactivity was present in the plasma of septic patients and that their platelets had decreased PAF binding sites compared with controls, indicating that the receptor had been downregulated after exposure to PAF *in vivo* (86). Subsequently, Szabo et al. showed that a substantial part of the hypotension in endotoxic animals resulted from the synthesis of nitric oxide, the induction of which is mediated by PAF; antagonists of the PAF receptor blocked the induction of nitric oxide synthase and hypotension (87).

Other investigators found PAF in BAL fluid from ARDS patients (88). Immunoassay results showed there was no measurable PAF in the lavage fluid of eight normal subjects; however, it was detected in 14 of the 19 patients with ARDS, with values ranging from about 80 to 1,800 pg/mL (mean, 237.5±86 pg/mL). Others found that BAL samples from ARDS patients had 406±96 pg of PAF bioactivity in a 9-mL sample; patients with pulmonary edema from other causes had somewhat lower levels (196±83 pg), and normal subjects had little or none ($P<0.001$ for ARDS patients compared with controls) (70). PAF bioactivity was detected in the BAL fluid from infants with bronchopulmonary dysplasia after hyaline membrane disease (89) and in a baboon model of hyaline membrane disease (90). In this model, which examined barotrauma, PAF bioactivity was found in the BAL fluid of seven of the eight animals that developed the syndrome, in contrast to the four that did not.

A role for PAF in systemic inflammation was supported in experiments using transgenic mice that overexpress the PAF receptor (91) and that were more sensitive to endotoxin than normal animals. The essential role of the PAF receptor was confirmed when an antagonist reversed the increased sensitivity of the transgenics. There is extensive evidence that PAF and related compounds are important inflammatory mediators in sepsis and probably are factors in other severe systemic inflammatory disorders such as ARDS. The responses PAF evokes are consistent with this role, appropriate bioactivity has been found in plasma during sepsis and in BAL fluid after acute lung injury, and receptor antagonists have a beneficial effect in animal models of sepsis. Two clinical trials have suggested that PAF receptor antagonists may be beneficial in treating sepsis (92) and pancreatitis (93). Both studies showed a favorable trend in phase II or III trials, supporting a role for PAF in systemic inflammation and suggesting that therapies that target PAF may have a beneficial action.

ACKNOWLEDGMENTS

We are grateful for the contributions of many dedicated and creative students, postdoctoral fellows, and technical associates for the past 15 years. We are particularly indebted to Dr. Diana Stafforini, who also provided a critical review of this chapter, and to our collaborators here and at other institutions. Our work has been supported by grants from the National Institutes of Health, The American Heart Association, and the Nora Eccles Treadwell Foundation.

REFERENCES

1. Stafforini DM, McIntyre TM, Zimmerman GA, Prescott SM. Platelet-activating factor acetylhydrolases. *J Biol Chem* 1997:272:17895–17898.
2. Venable ME, Zimmerman GA, McIntyre TM, Prescott SM. Platelet-activating factor: a phospholipid autacoid with diverse actions. *J Lipid Res* 1993;34:691–702.

3. Imaizumi T-A, Stafforini DM, Yamada Y, McIntyre TM, Prescott SM, Zimmerman GA. Platelet-activating factor: a mediator for clinicians. *J Intern Med* 1995;238:5–20.

4. Zimmerman GA, McIntyre TM, Prescott SM. Adhesion and signaling in vascular cell-cell interactions. *J Clin Invest* 1996;98:1699–1702.

5. Mayadas TN, Johnson RC, Rayburn H, Hynes RO, Wagner DD. Leukocyte rolling and extravasation are severely compromised in P selectin-deficient mice. *Cell* 1993;74:541–554.

6. Zimmerman GA, Prescott SM, McIntyre TM. Endothelial cell interactions with granulocytes: tethering and signaling molecules. *Immunol Today* 1992;13:93–100.

7. Coughlan AF, Hau H, Dunlop LC, Berndt MC, Hancock WW. P-selectin and platelet-activating factor mediate initial endotoxin-induced neutropenia. *J Exp Med* 1994;179:329–334.

8. Weyrich AS, Ma X-L, Lefer DJ, Albertine KH, Lefer AM. In vivo neutralization of P-selectin protects feline heart and endothelium in myocardial ischemia and reperfusion injury. *J Clin Invest* 1993;91:2620–2629.

9. Zhou W, Javors MA, Olson MS. Platelet-activating factor as an intercellular signal in neutrophil-dependent platelet activation. *J Immunol* 1992;149:1763–1769.

10. Bunting M, Lorant DE, Bryant AE, et al. *C. Perfringens* alpha toxin induces proinflammatory changes in endothelial cells. *J Clin Invest* 1997;99:565–574.

11. Modur V, Zimmerman GA, Prescott SM, McIntyre TM. Endothelial cell inflammatory responses to TNFα: ceramide-dependent and independent MAP kinase cascades. *J Biol Chem* 1996;271:13094–13102.

12. Whatley RE, Nelson P, Zimmerman GA, et al. The regulation of platelet-activating factor production in endothelial cells. *J Biol Chem* 1989;264:6325–6333.

13. Patel KD, Zimmerman GA, Prescott SM, McEver RP, McIntyre TM. Oxygen radicals induce human endothelial cells to express GMP-140 and bind neutrophils. *J Cell Biol* 1991;112:749–759.

14. Patel KD, Zimmerman GA, Prescott SM, McIntyre TM. Novel leukocyte agonists are released by endothelial cells exposed to peroxide. *J Biol Chem* 1992;267:15168–15175.

15. Lehr H-A, Weyrich AS, Saetzler RK, et al. Vitamin C blocks inflammatory platelet-activating factor mimetics created by cigarette smoking. *J Clin Invest* 1997;99:2358–2364.

16. Chilton FH, Ellis JM, Olson SC, Wykle RL. 1-*O*-alkyl-2-arachidonoyl-*sn*-glycero-3-phosphocholine: a common source of platelet-activating factor and arachidonate in human polymorphonuclear leukocytes. *J Biol Chem* 1984;259:12014–12019.

17. Domenech C, Domenech EM-D, Soling H-D. Regulation of acetyl-CoA:1-alkyl-*sn*-glycero-3-phosphocholine O₂-acetyltransferase (lyso-PAF-acetyltransferase) in exocrine glands: evidence for an activation via phosphorylation by calcium/calmodulin-dependent protein kinase. *J Biol Chem* 1987;262:5671–5676.

18. Holland MR, Venable ME, Whatley RE, Zimmerman GA, McIntyre TM, Prescott SM. Activation of the acetyl-coenzyme A: lysoplatelet-activating factor acetyltransferase regulates platelet-activating factor synthesis in human endothelial cells. *J Biol Chem* 1992;267:22883–22890.

19. Lenihan DJ, Lee T-C. Regulation of platelet-activating factor synthesis: modulation of 1-alkyl-2-lyso-*sn*-glycero-3-phosphocholine: acetyl-CoA acetyltransferase by phosphorylation and dephosphorylation in rat spleen microsomes. *Biochem Biophys Res Commun* 1984;120:834–839.

20. Nieto ML, Velasco S, Crespo MS. Modulation of acetyl-CoA:1-alkyl-2-lyso-*sn*-glycero-3-phosphocholine (lyso-PAF) acetyltransferase in human polymorphonuclear cells: the role of cyclic AMP-dependent and phospholipid sensitive, calcium-dependent protein kinases. *J Biol Chem* 1988;263:4607–4611.

21. Bonventre JV, Huang Z, Taheri MR, et al. Reduced fertility and postischaemic brain injury in mice deficient in cytosolic phospholipase A2. *Nature* 1997;390:622–625.

22. Uozumi N, Kume K, Nagase T, et al. Role of cytosolic phospholipase A2 in allergic response and parturition. *Nature* 1997;390:618–622.

23. Honda Z, Nakamura M, Miki I, et al. Cloning by functional expression of platelet-activating factor receptor from guinea-pig lung. *Nature* 1991;349:342–346.

24. Nakamura M, Honda Z-i, Izumi T, et al. Molecular cloning and expression of platelet-activating factor receptor from human leukocytes. *J Biol Chem* 1991;266:20400–20405.

25. Kunz D, Gerard NP, Gerard C. The human leukocyte platelet-activating factor receptor. *J Biol Chem* 1992;267:9101–9106.

26. Ye RD, Prossnitz ER, Zou A, Cochrane CG. Characterization of a human cDNA that encodes a functional receptor for platelet activating factor. *Biochem Biophys Res Commun* 1991;180:105–111.

27. Ali H, Richardson RM, Tomhave ED, DuBose RA, Haribabu B, Snyderman R. Regulation of stably transfected platelet activating factor receptor in RBL-2H3 cells. *J Biol Chem* 1994;269:24557–24563.

28. Honda Z-i, Takano T, Gotoh Y, Nishida E, Ito K, Shimizu T. Transfected platelet-activating factor receptor activates mitogen-activated protein (MAP) kinase and MAP kinase in Chinese hamster ovary cells. *J Biol Chem* 1994;269:2307–2315.

29. Shukla SD. Platelet-activating factor receptor and signal transduction mechanisms. *FASEB J* 1992;6:2296–2301.

30. Ishii I, Izumi T, Tsukamoto H, Umeyama H, Ui M, Shimizu T. Alanine exchanges of polar amino acids in the transmembrane domains of a platelet-activating factor receptor generate both constitutively active and inactive mutants. *J Biol Chem* 1997;272:7846–7854.

31. Carlson SA, Chatterjee TK, Fisher RA. The third intracellular domain of the platelet-activating factor receptor is a critical determinant in receptor coupling to phosphoinositide phospholipase C-activating G proteins. *J Biol Chem* 1996;271:23146–23153.

32. Parent J, Gouill C, Escher E, Rola-Pleszczynsji M, Stankova J. Identification of transmembrane domain residues determinant in the structure-function relationship of the human platelet-activating factor receptor by site-directed mutagenesis. *J Biol Chem* 1996;271:23298–23303.

33. Gouill CL, Parent J, Rola-Pleszczynski M, Stankova J. Role of the Cys⁹⁰, Cys⁹⁵ and Cys¹⁷³ residues in the structure and function of the human platelet-activating factor receptor. *FEBS Lett* 1997;402:203–208.

34. Parent J, Gouill CL, Brum-Fernandes AJD, Rola-Pleszczynski M, Stankova J. Mutations of two adjacent amino acids generate inactive and constitutively active forms of the human platelet-activating factor receptor. *J Biol Chem* 1996;271:7949–7955.

35. Takano T, Honda Z-i, Sakanaka C, et al. Role of cytoplasmic tail phosphorylation sites of platelet-activating factor receptor in agonist-induced desensitization. *J Biol Chem* 1994;269:22453–22458.

36. Richardson RM, Haribabu B, Ali H, Snyderman R. Cross-desensitization among receptors for platelet activating factor and peptide chemoattractants. *J Biol Chem* 1996;271:28717–28724.

37. Ali H, Fisher I, Haribabu B, Richardson RM, Snyderman R. Role of phospholipase CB3 phosphorylation in the desensitization of cellular responses to platelet-activating factor. *J Biol Chem* 1997;272:11706–11709.

38. Gerard NP, Gerard C. Receptor-dependent internalization of platelet-activating factor. *J Immunol* 1994;152:793–800.

39. Chase PB, Yang J-M, Thompson FH, Halonen M, Regan JW. Regional mapping of the human platelet-activating factor receptor gene (PTAFR) to 1p35-p34.3 by fluorescence in situ hybridization. *Cytogenet Cell Genet* 1996;72:205–207.

40. Seyfried CE, Schweickart VL, Godiska R, Gray PW. The human platelet activating factor receptor gene (PTAFR) contains no introns and maps to chromosome 1. *Genomics* 1992;13:832–834.

41. Mutoh H, Ishii S, Izumi T, Kato S, Shimizu T. Platelet-activating factor (PAF) positively auto-regulates the expression of human PAF receptor transcript 1 (leukocyte-type) through NF-κB. *Biochem Biophys Res Commun* 1994;205:1137–1142.

42. Thivierge M, Parent J-L, Stankova J, Rola-Pleszczynski M. Modulation of human platelet-activating factor receptor gene expression by protein kinase C activation. *J Immunol* 1996;157:4681–4687.

43. Wang H, Tan X-D, Chang H, Gonzalez-Crussi F, Remick DG, Hsueh W. Regulation of platelet-activating factor receptor gene expression *in vivo* by endotoxin, platelet-activating factor and endogenous tumour necrosis factor. *Biochem J* 1997;322:603–608.

44. Yang H-H, Pang J-HS, Hung R-Y, Chau L-Y. Transcriptional regulation of platelet-activating factor receptor gene in B lymphoblastoid ramos cells TGF-β1. *J Immunol* 1997;158:2771–2778.

45. Dagenais P, Thivierge M, Parent J-L, Stankova J, Rola-Pleszczynski M. Augmented expression of platelet-activating factor receptor gene by TNF-x through transcriptional activation in human monocytes. *J Leukoc Biol* 1997;61:106–112.

46. Mutoh H, Fukuda T, Kitamoto T, et al. Tissue-specific response of the human platelet-activating factor receptor gene to retinoic acid and thyroid hormone by alternative promoter usage. *Proc Natl Acad Sci USA* 1996;93:774–779.

47. Triggiani M, Schleimer RP, Warner JA, Chilton FH. Differential synthesis of 1-acyl-2-acetyl-*sn*-glycero-3-phosphocholine and platelet-activating factor by human inflammatory cells. *J Immunol* 1991;147:660–666.

48. Whatley RE, Clay KL, Chilton FH, et al. Relative amounts of 1-*O*-alkyl- and 1-acyl-2-acetyl-*sn*-glycero-3-phosphocholine in stimulated endothelial cells. *Prostaglandins* 1992;43:21–29.

49. Takamura H, Kasai H, Arita H, Kito M. Phospholipid molecular species in human umbilical artery and vein endothelial cells. *J Lipid Res* 1990; 31:709–717.

50. Pinckard RN, Showell HJ, Castillo R, et al. Differential responsiveness of human neutrophils to the autocrine actions of 1-*O*-alkyl homologs and 1-acyl analogs of platelet-activating factor. *J Immunol* 1992;148: 3528–3535.

51. Triggiani M, Goldman DW, Chilton FH. Biological effects of 1-acyl-2-acetyl-*sn*-glycero-3-phosphocholine in the human neutrophil. *Biochim Biophys Acta* 1991;1084:41–47.

52. Ogita T, Tanaka Y, Nakaoka T, et al. Lysophosphatidylcholine transduces Ca^{2+} signaling via the platelet-activating factor receptor in macrophages. *Am J Physiol* 1997;272:H17–H24.

53. Smiley PL, Stremler KE, Prescott SM, Zimmerman GA, McIntyre TM. Oxidatively fragmented phosphatidylcholines activate human neutrophils through the receptor for platelet-activating factor. *J Biol Chem* 1991;266:11104–11110.

54. Heery JM, Kozak M, Stafforini DM, et al. Oxidatively modified LDL contains phospholipids with PAF-like activity and stimulates the growth of smooth muscle cells. *J Clin Invest* 1995;96:2322–2330.

55. Tokumura A, Takauchi K, Asai T, Kamiyasu K, Ogawa T, Tsukatani H. Novel molecular analogues of phosphatidylcholines in a lipid extract from bovine brain: 1-long-chain acyl-2-short-chain acyl-*sn*-glycero-3-phosphocholines. *J Lipid Res* 1989;30:219–224.

56. Tokumura A, Tanaka T, Yotsumoto T, Tsukatani H. Identification of *sn*-2-omega-hydroxycarboxylate-containing phospholipids in a lipid extract from bovine brain. *Biochem Biophys Res Commun* 1991;177:466–473.

57. Tanaka T, Minamino H, Unezaki S, Tsukatani H, Tokumura A. Formation of platelet-activating factor-like phospholipids by Fe^{2+}/ascorbate/EDTA-induced lipid peroxidation. *Biochim Biophys Acta* 1993; 1166:264–274.

58. Watson AD, Leitinger N, Navab M, et al. Structural identification by mass spectrometry of oxidized phospholipids in minimally oxidized low density lipoprotein that induce monocyte/endothelial interactions and evidence for their presence *in vivo*. *J Biol Chem* 1997;272:13597–13607.

59. Imaizumi T-A. Intravascular release of a platelet-activating factor-like lipid (PAF-LL) induced by cigarette smoking. *Lipids* 1991;26:1269–1273.

60. Kubes P, Ibbotson G, Russell J, Wallace JL, Granger DN. Role of platelet-activating factor in ischemia/reperfusion-induced leukocyte adherence. *Am J Physiol* 1990;259:G300–G305.

61. Hirashima Y, Endo S, Ohmori T, Kato R, Takaku A. Platelet-activating factor (PAF) concentration and PAF acetylhydrolase activity in cerebrospinal fluid of patients with subarachnoid hemorrhage. *J Neurosurg* 1994;80:31–36.

62. Satoh K, Imaizumi T-A, Yoshida H, Hiramoto M, Takamatsu S. Increased levels of blood platelet-activating factor (PAF) and PAF-like lipids in patients with ischemic stroke. *Acta Neurol Scand* 1992;85: 122–127.

63. Hsieh K-H, Ng C-K. Increased plasma platelet-activating factor in children with acute asthmatic attacks and decreased *in vivo* and *in vitro* production of platelet-activating factor after immunotherapy. *J Allergy Clin Immunol* 1993;91:650–657.

64. Cundell D, Gerard NP, Gerard C, Idanpaan-Heikkila I, Tuomanen EI. Streptococcus pneumoniae anchor to activated human cells by the receptor for platelet-activating factor. *Nature* 1995;377:435–438.

65. Nakamura M, Honda Z, Waga I, Matsumoto T, Noma M, Shimizu T. Endotoxin transduces Ca^{2+} signaling via platelet-activating factor receptor. *FEBS Lett* 1992;314:125–129.

66. Bazan NG. A signal terminator. *Nature* 1995;374:501–502.

67. Stafforini DM, McIntyre TM, Carter ME, Prescott SM. Human plasma platelet-activating factor acetylhydrolase: association with lipoprotein particles and role in the degradation of platelet-activating factor. *J Biol Chem* 1987;262:4215–4222.

68. Graham RM, Stephens CJ, Silvester W, Leong LLL, Strurm MJ, Taylor RR. Plasma degradation of platelet-activating factor in severely ill patients with clinical sepsis. *Crit Care Med* 1994;22:204–212.

69. Partrick DA, Moore EE, Moore FA, Biffl WL, Barnett CC. Reduced PAF-acetylhydrolase activity is associated with postinjury multiple organ failure. *Shock* 1997;7:170–174.

70. Nakos G, Pneumatikos J, Tsangaris I, Tellis C, Lekka M. Proteins and phospholipids in BAL from patients with hydrostatic pulmonary edema. *Am J Respir Crit Care Med* 1997;155:945–951.

71. Tjoelker LW, Wilder C, Eberhardt C, et al. Anti-inflammatory properties of a platelet-activating factor acetylhydrolase. *Nature* 1995;374:549–553.

72. Miwa M, Miyake T, Yamanaka T, et al. Characterization of serum platelet-activating factor (PAF) acetylhydrolase: correlation between deficiency of serum PAF acetylhydrolase and respiratory symptoms in asthmatic children. *J Clin Invest* 1988;82:1983–1991.

73. Stafforini DM, Satoh K, Atkinson DL, et al. Platelet-activating factor acetylhydrolase deficiency. *J Clin Invest* 1996;97:2784–2791.

74. Contador M, Moya FR, Zhao B, et al. Effect of dexamethasone on rat plasma platelet activating factor acetylhydrolase during the perinatal period. *Early Hum Dev* 1997;47:167–176.

75. Yasuda K, Johnston JM. The hormonal regulation of platelet-activating factor acetylhydrolase in the rat. *Endocrinology* 1992;130:708–716.

76. Tarbet EB, Stafforini DM, Elstad MR, Zimmerman GA, McIntyre TM, Prescott SM. Liver cells secrete the plasma form of platelet-activating factor acetylhydrolase. *J Biol Chem* 1991;266:16667–16673.

77. Satoh K, Imaizumi T-A, Kawamura Y, et al. Platelet-activating factor (PAF) stimulates the production of PAF acetylhydrolase by the human hepatoma cell line, HepG2. *J Clin Invest* 1991;87:476–481.

78. Narahara H, Frenkel RA, Johnston JM. Secretion of platelet-activating factor acetylhydrolase following phorbol ester-stimulated differentiation of HL-60 cells. *Arch Biochem Biophys* 1993;301:275–281.

79. Elstad MR, Stafforini DM, McIntyre TM, Prescott SM, Zimmerman GA. Platelet-activating factor acetylhydrolase increases during macrophage differentiation: a novel mechanism that regulates accumulation of platelet-activating factor. *J Biol Chem* 1989;264:8467–8470.

80. Stafforini DM, Elstad MR, McIntyre TM, Zimmerman GA, Prescott SM. Human macrophages secrete platelet-activating factor acetylhydrolase. *J Biol Chem* 1990;265:9682–9687.

81. Beijer L, Botting J, Oyckan AO, Page CP, Rylander R. The involvement of platelet activating factor in endotoxin-induced pulmonary platelet recruitment in the guinea-pig. *Br J Pharmacol* 1987;92:803–808.

82. Christman BW, Lefferts PL, King GA, Snapper JR. Role of circulating platelets and granulocytes in PAF-induced pulmonary dysfunction in awake sheep. *J Appl Physiol* 1988;64:2033–2041.

83. Rabinovici R, Esser KM, Lysko PG, et al. Priming by platelet-activating factor of endotoxin-induced lung injury and cardiovascular shock. *Circ Res* 1991;69:12–25.

84. Rabinovici R, Sofronski MD, Renz JF, et al. Platelet activating factor mediates interleukin-2-induced lung injury in the rat. *J Clin Invest* 1992; 89:1669–1673.

85. Chang S-W, Feddersen CO, Henson PM, Voelkel NF. Platelet-activating factor mediates hemodynamic changes and lung injury in endotoxin-treated rats. *J Clin Invest* 1987;79:1498–1509.

86. Diez FL, Nieto MI, Fernandez-Gallardo S, Gijon MA, Crespo MS. Occupancy of platelet receptors for platelet-activating factor in patients with septicemia. *J Clin Invest* 1989;83:1733–1740.

87. Szabo C, Wu C-C, Mitchell JA, Gross SS, Thiemermann C, Vane JR. Platelet-activating factor contributes to the induction of nitric oxide synthase by bacterial lipopolysaccharide. *Circ Res* 1993;73:991–999.

88. Matsumoto K, Taki F, Kondoh Y, Taniguchi H, Takagi K. Platelet-activating factor in bronchoalveolar lavage fluid of patients with adult respiratory distress syndrome. *Clin Exp Pharmacol Physiol* 1992;19: 509–515.

89. Stenmark KR, Eyzaguirre M, Westcott JY, Henson PM, Murphy RC. Potential role of eicosanoids and PAF in the pathophysiology of bronchopulmonary dysplasia. *Am Rev Respir Dis* 1987;136:770–772.

90. Meredith KS, deLemos RA, Coalson JJ, et al. Role of lung injury in the pathogenesis of hyaline membrane disease in premature baboons. *J Appl Physiol* 1989;66:2150–2158.

91. Ishii S, Nagase T, Tashiro F, et al. Bronchial hyperreactivity, increased endotoxin lethality and melanocytic tumorigenesis in transgenic mice overexpressing platelet-activating factor receptor. *EMBO J* 1997;16: 133–142.

92. Dhainaut J-FA, Tenaillon A, Tulzo YL, et al. Platelet-activating factor receptor antagonist BN 52021 in the treatment of severe sepsis: a randomized, double-blind, placebo-controlled, multicenter clinical trial. *Crit Care Med* 1994;22:1720–1728.

93. Kingsnorth AN, Galloway SW, Formela LJ. Randomized, double-blind phase II trail of Lexipafant, a platelet-activating factor antagonist, in human acute pancreatitis. *Br J Surg* 1995;82:1414–1420.

Inflammation: Basic Principles and Clinical Correlates,
3rd ed., edited by John I. Gallin and Ralph Snyderman.
Lippincott Williams & Wilkins, Philadelphia © 1999.

CHAPTER **26**

Neuropeptides in Inflammation and Immunity

Richard D. Granstein

The concept that the nervous system may be involved with immunity and inflammation is supported by a number of observations and considerable data. Certain inflammatory diseases, such as psoriasis, atopic dermatitis, and inflammatory bowel disease, appear to worsen with anxiety (1–3). Much experimental evidence indicates that certain aspects of immune responses are suppressed during periods of psychologic stress, and some data suggest that this effect is mediated in part through neuroendocrine pathways (4–6).

A direct role for nerves in cutaneous inflammation has been recognized for more than a century. Researchers observed that antidromic stimulation of the peripheral stumps of transected sensory nerves induced vasodilation and other signs of inflammation in the skin, suggesting that afferent neurons have a sensory role and take part in effector functions (7). When irritants are applied directly to the skin, the flare component of the triple response (i.e., vasodilation) spreads far beyond the point of the initial stimulus. This phenomenon depends on sensory innervation and involves nerve conduction. It is referred to as an *axon reflex*, a term that presupposes that sensory nerves branch in the periphery, with one or some branches forming a sensory ending for reception of the stimulus and the other branches innervating a blood vessel. After activation of the sensory ending, nerve conduction travels centrally at the branch and antidromically to the blood vessel. These observations provided important support for the concept of neurologic inflammation. A neurogenic component of IgE-mediated cutaneous inflammation has been identified in an experimental model; decreased inflammation was associated with denervation (8).

Anatomic evidence also suggests a role for nerve-derived factors in inflammation and immunity. For example, the lymphoid organs are innervated (9–13), and an anatomic association of nerves with mast cells (14) and

Langerhans cells (15) in the skin is recognized. T cells and mast cells also are associated in the gut (16).

This chapter discusses evidence that certain peptide products of nerves have functions that directly or indirectly play a role in inflammation and immunologic responses. The inflammatory and immunologic effects of substance P (SP), vasoactive intestinal polypeptide (VIP), calcitonin gene-related peptide (CGRP), and somatostatin (SOM) have been well studied. SP is an 11 amino acid peptide that is part of the tachykinin family along with neurokinin A (NKA) and neurokinin B (NKB) (17,18). These three peptides share a common C-terminal amino acid sequence and produce their activity through specific receptors on target cells. Three distinct tachykinin receptors, called NK-1, NK-2, and NK-3, have been found. Although these receptors differ in their affinities for the various tachykinins, each receptor can be activated by any tachykinin, and there is cross-reactivity between these factors. VIP is a 28 amino acid peptide (17,19). It is distributed throughout the central and peripheral nervous system. The family of VIP-related peptides is large and includes glycocin, corticotropin-releasing factor, and secretin. CGRP is a 37 amino acid peptide that results from alternative splicing of a calcitonin gene transcript (17). It exists in two forms, called α and β or I and II. Expression of CGRP is widespread throughout the central and peripheral nervous systems, and it is a potent vasodilator thought to play an important role in regulating vascular tone. SOM exists as a 28 amino acid peptide and as a 14 amino acid cleavage product of the 28 amino acid molecule, both of which are biologically active (17,20). It frequently colocalizes with SP in sensory nerves. SOM may function as a neurotransmitter in the central and peripheral nervous systems (21,22).

NEUROPEPTIDES AND INFLAMMATION

The possibility that neuropeptides can play a role in inflammation is suggested by several observations. Cuta-

R. D. Granstein: Department of Dermatology, Weill College of Medicine of Cornell University, New York, New York 10021.

neous mast cells release histamine in culture in response to several neuropeptides, including SP, VIP, and SOM (23). The specificity of this observation is demonstrated by the fact that NKA, NKB, CGRP, and neurotensin induce only negligible histamine release *in vitro* (23). However, one report indicates that intradermal CGRP can induce cerebrovascular mast cell degranulation (24). In support of the concept that these neuropeptides induce mast cell degranulation *in situ,* it has been shown that treatment of human skin with capsaicin, a substance that stimulates peptide release from sensory neurons, results in degranulation of mast cells (25). Capsaicin does not release histamine from mast cells *in vitro*, demonstrating that degranulation probably results from the release of neuropeptides from sensory nerves.

SP, VIP, and CGRP induce neutrophil influx after intradermal injection, along with rapid induction of E-selectin expression by endothelial cells (26). Neuropeptide Y and SP prime neutrophil oxidative metabolism, but CGRP fails to do so (27). There are reports that SP is chemotactic for neutrophils and monocytes (28) and that VIP is chemotactic for macrophages and T cells (29). SP and CGRP are involved in vasodilatation and edema formation. SP can stimulate chemotaxis and lysosomal enzyme secretion by neutrophils (at least in rabbit cells) (30) and stimulate neutrophil phagocytosis (31). In rat skin, CGRP potentiates SP-induced erythema (32). VIP also induces vasodilatation (33). Further support for a functional role for neuropeptides in inflammation comes from the study demonstrating that pretreatment of mice with capsaicin to deplete sensory neuropeptides greatly reduces the subsequent influx of polymorphonuclear leukocytes in response to injection of interleukin-1 (IL-1) (34). Topical application of SP, CGRP, and SOM increases irritant inflammation in the skin (35).

The proinflammatory effects may, at least for some factors, depend on the experimental protocol. For example, CGRP can have antiinflammatory effects (36). When administered along with croton oil or acetic acid, CGRP inhibits the degree of inflammation induced by these agents alone.

Neuropeptides may also influence inflammation in the skin through induction of proinflammatory cytokines. SP induces tumor necrosis factor-α (TNF-α) mRNA expression in mast cells (37) and stimulates IL-1 production by monocytes (38), IL-1 and IL-6 production by bone marrow cells (39), IL-6 production by astrocytes (40), and IL-2 production by murine lymphocytes (41). This peptide induces IL-1α, IL-1β, and IL-1 receptor antagonist expression in keratinocytes and causes human microvascular and endothelial cells to produce IL-8 (42). It also stimulates IL-3 and granulocyte-macrophage colony-stimulating factor (GM-CSF) production by bone marrow cells, partially through IL-1 and IL-6 mediation (39).

Cytokines may induce neuropeptide expression. For example, IL-1 induces SP production by cultured sympathetic ganglia (43). α-Melanocyte stimulating hormone (α-MSH) inhibits acute inflammation in several models, including irritation of the skin, and may help regulate cutaneous inflammation (44,45). This effect of α-MSH appears to result from processes mediated through the central nervous system (CNS) and processes not mediated through the CNS. Topical administration of α-MSH can also inhibit the induction and elicitation of contact hypersensitivity in mice (46). *In vitro*, α-MSH inhibits interferon-γ (IFN-γ) production by antigen-stimulated lymph node cells (47) and by lymphocytes stimulated by α-MSH–treated antigen-presenting cells in some circumstances (47). Keratinocytes are capable of producing α-MSH and corticotropin (48).

NEUROPEPTIDES AND IMMUNITY

Anatomic associations exist between nerve fibers and cellular components of the immune system, suggesting a functional relationship between these elements. In support of this concept, several products of neurons regulate the function of lymphocytes, macrophages, and dendritic cells.

Several lines of evidence implicate CGRP as an important modulator of immune functions. CGRP has effects on the functioning of T cells, macrophages, and Langerhans cells (15,49–52). CGRP inhibits T-cell proliferation and IL-2 production *in vitro* (49). *In vitro* treatment of macrophages inhibits several functions, including oxidative metabolism and antigen-presenting ability (50). The presence of CGRP-containing nerves in the thymus led to speculation that CGRP plays a role in positive and negative selection of the T-cell repertoire (53). Most significantly, CGRP inhibits the ability of macrophages and Langerhans cells to present antigen in several systems (15,50,51). The mechanisms by which CGRP exerts these effects have been partially elucidated. Treatment of macrophages or a Langerhans cell–like line (used as a surrogate for Langerhans cells) with CGRP inhibits upregulation of the co-stimulatory molecule B7-2 (51). It also augments expression of IL-10 induced by lipopolysaccharide (LPS) and inhibits the LPS-induced expression of IL-1β and IL-12 (52). Experiments using neutralizing antisera to IL-10 indicate that the effects of CGRP on B7-2 expression, IL-12 expression, and at least in one assay, antigen presentation, may be mediated by IL-10 induction (52).

There is now direct anatomic evidence for a mechanism by which Langerhans cells encounter CGRP. Experiments using laser confocal scanning microscopy and double immunofluorescence staining demonstrated apparent apposition of CGRP-containing nerves with Langerhans cells within human epidermis (15). This anatomic association was confirmed with transmission electron microscopy. A small number of Langerhans cells in normal skin were found to have immunoreactive

CGRP at or on their surfaces, as if a nerve had deposited CGRP in the vicinity of the cell where it then bound to CGRP receptors on the cell. Administration of CGRP intradermally into naive mice followed by immunization epicutaneously with haptens at the site of injection leads to a lesser contact hypersensitivity response compared with control mice injected with diluent alone, further supporting a role for CGRP as an endogenous modulator of immune responses (54). One report provided convincing evidence that CGRP plays a role in the cascade of events that result in impaired contact hypersensitivity responses after exposure of mice to ultraviolet radiation (55).

VIP has several inhibitory effects on immunocompetent cells (56). It inhibits T-cell mitogen-induced proliferation but fails to affect proliferation induced by the B-cell mitogen LPS (57). These observations are consistent with a report that T cells have high-affinity receptors for VIP but that B cells do not (57). VIP has also been shown to inhibit IL-2 and IFN-γ production by lymphocytes (59). Effects of VIP on immunoglobulin production depend on the site from which the B cells were obtained (56). IgA production by concanavalin A–stimulated cells derived from spleen and mesenteric lymph nodes was increased somewhat by exposure to VIP, but production by cells from Peyer's patches much more potently increased (60). Cells derived from Peyer's patches also produced more IgM after exposure to VIP, but VIP had no effect on IgM production by cells from the spleen or lymph nodes (60). Whether these effects result entirely from interactions of VIP with B cells or from effects derived from T cells is unknown (56). However, B and T cells have VIP receptors, although B cells appear to have lower binding affinity (61). VIP also can inhibit human natural killer cell activity (61).

In addition to the proinflammatory effects of SP previously described, SP has direct effects on immunocompetent cells. SP enhances T-cell proliferation (64) and stimulates IgA and IgM production, although apparently not IgG (60).

SOM receptors have been found on some lymphoid cell lines, including a human myeloma line and a line of leukemic human T cells (65). SOM inhibits T-cell proliferation under several different conditions, although at high concentrations, it can stimulate lymphocyte proliferation (17). SOM can inhibit natural killer cell activity (66). Staphylococcal enterotoxin A–stimulated IFN-γ secretion and endotoxin-induced leukocytosis are inhibited by SOM (63,67). The effects of SOM on immunoglobulin synthesis appear to be complex. IgE production is decreased by SOM, but SOM enhances IgG2 production (68,69). IgA production can be inhibited or enhanced, depending on the experimental protocol (70,71).

The neurotoxin capsaicin causes release of sensory neuropeptides locally in the skin when it is applied epicutaneously (72). When administered systemically in sufficient amounts, it can largely deplete sensory nerves of neuropeptides throughout an animal (72). Systemic treatment of mice and rats with capsaicin results in augmented contact and delayed-type hypersensitivity responses (73,74). Topical treatment of human skin with capsaicin results in an enhanced contact hypersensitivity response on challenge at capsaicin-treated sites with relevant allergens in sensitive individuals (75). Although these experiments do not identify the neuropeptides responsible for inhibiting hypersensitivity reactions, they do suggest strongly that the net effect of sensory nerves is to inhibit these responses. Nonsensitized irritant responses in these capsaicin-treated animals are reduced, consistent with the role of sensory neuropeptides in neurogenic inflammation.

NEUROPEPTIDES AND INFLAMMATORY DISEASES

The role of neuropeptides as mediators of inflammatory and immune reactivity suggests that they must also play some role in inflammatory disease states. This is an evolving area, and much of the information is incomplete. The following sections review some of the data available on the role of neuropeptides in specific inflammatory disorders.

Psoriasis

The role of neuropeptides in psoriasis is suggested most strongly by reports that psoriasis clears in areas of skin that have become denervated (76,77). In support of this are other reports stating psoriasis improves after administration of agents that block nerve impulses (78). Several studies have addressed the question of whether cutaneous innervation is abnormal in psoriatic lesions, but these studies provide contradictory data. Immunohistochemistry with an antibody directed against protein gene product 9.5 showed a reduction of epidermal nerve fiber density in psoriatic skin. Another study using immunocytochemical analysis of SP and VIP showed no difference between psoriatic and normal skin, while a study looking at protein gene product 9.5 showed an increase in nerve fibers and the dermal epidermal junction, in the papillary dermis, and at the eccrine sweat glands in lesional psoriatic skin (79–82). An additional study looked at psoriatic lesions induced by the Koebner phenomenon (i.e., trauma) in a serial manner, and the investigators found an increase in SP- and VIP-positive fibers in the dermal papillae of mature psoriatic plaques and in nerve–mast cell contacts (82). Because each of these studies used different techniques and examined different endpoints, it is hard to draw conclusions.

The SP and VIP content of skin was found by radioimmunoassay to be significantly elevated in psoriatic plaques (83). No difference between the plasma levels of these neuropeptides in psoriatic patients compared with control subjects was found in that study. This was confirmed by other investigators who examined plasma levels of α-MSH, β-endorphin, met-enkephalin, and SP (84). No significant differences between the plasma levels of any of these neuropeptides were observed among active psoriatic patients, stable psoriatic patients, and control subjects. However, other studies found an increased plasma concentration of β-endorphin in patients with psoriasis (85) and in those with systemic sclerosis or atopic dermatitis (86).

Atopic Dermatitis

Skin reactivity to intradermally injected neuropeptides, including CGRP, VIP, SP, neurotensin, and neurokinin A, is less in patients with atopic dermatitis than in controls (87). The concentration of SP is lower and that of VIP higher in lesional skin of atopic dermatitis patients compared with control subjects (88). These findings may suggest a role for neuropeptides in atopic dermatitis. Langerhans cells express IgE receptors, and in atopic dermatitis, these cells often have IgE on their surfaces (89,90). Hypothetically, such IgE, if directed against specific antigens, may play a role in atopic dermatitis by providing for more efficient trapping and subsequent internalization of relevant antigens. IgE-induced inflammation appears to be regulated in part by nerves (8). After allergen challenge in patients with allergic rhinitis, there is an immediate increase in VIP, CGRP, and SP content in nasal secretions (91), a pattern that may correlate with the role of neuropeptides in atopic dermatitis.

Inflammatory Bowel Disease

The two major clinical entities comprising chronic inflammatory bowel disease are ulcerative colitis and Crohn's disease (92). The cause and pathogenesis of these disorders remain unclear. A host of mediators of inflammation have been identified as candidate mediators in inflammatory bowel disease (93,94). Among these are several neuropeptides.

Polymodal nociceptor activation yields axon reflexes involving primary afferent neurons and that result in the release of SP (92). In support of a role for SP in inflammation in inflammatory bowel disease, it has been demonstrated that intestinal inflammation decreased the level of neutral endopeptidase (94), resulting in an increase in the availability of SP in the gut. Other observations support the possibility that nervous influences contribute to inflammation and inflammatory bowel disease. Surgical denervation of the pelvis or vagotomy has been used successfully to treat refractory inflammatory bowel disease (95–97). Clonidine, nicotine, and lidocaine are beneficial in treating inflammatory bowel disease (99–100), and their effects may result from influencing

nerve function, although direct antiinflammatory effects of these agents may also be possible. Using immunoperoxidase staining, SP immunoactivity was found to be increased in ulcerative colitis and Crohn's disease, while vasoactive intestinal polypeptide staining was decreased (101).

Other studies reported that the number of VIP- and SP-containing nerves are decreased in severe inflammatory lesions in Crohn's disease and ulcerative colitis (102,103); they are almost completely absent around crypt abscesses. Decreased levels of VIP protein have been detected in the mucosal or submucosal layer of ulcerative colitis (104). By Northern blot analysis, mRNA levels were increased 260% in ulcerative colitis (104). The decreased level observed at the protein level did not appear to result from deceased transcription. These data could be interpreted to suggest that axonal degeneration in ulcerative colitis leads to increased VIP gene expression.

Inflammatory Joint Disease

Circumstantial evidence implicates neuropeptides in inflammatory joint disease, particularly rheumatoid arthritis (105). Synovial joints are innervated by myelinated and unmyelinated afferent nerve fibers (106–111). Small-diameter nerve fibers have been found in the fibrous capsule, ligaments, tendons, and synovium of joints (105,111). Immunostaining shows these fibers contain SP and CGRP (105,110,111). SP- and CGRP-reactive fibers are frequently found in perivascular locations, but many also extend freely through the synovium. These anatomic findings suggest a possible role for neuropeptides in joint inflammation, especially since the role of C fibers in neurogenic inflammation is so well documented. Consistent with this idea, pretreatment of rats with capsaicin to destroy unmyelinated nerves attenuates adjuvant arthritis (112). Synovial tissue has been reported to have free stromal nerves frequently failing to stain for neuropeptides in the setting of rheumatoid arthritis, as if neuropeptides had been released (111,113). Administration of SP into the joints of animals with adjuvant arthritis leads to enhanced bone and cartilage damage (114).

Farrell et al. performed a series of experiments that suggest a role for neuropeptides in joint inflammation (105). They demonstrated that there is a neurogenic component, mediated by SP and possibly by other neuropeptides, to carrageenan-induced joint inflammation. They demonstrated that antidromic electrical stimulation of C fibers in the joints leads to vasodilatation. Because neuropeptides mediate mast cell degranulation, secretion of prostaglandins, and collagenase from synovial cells and secretion of IL-1 from macrophages, it is surmised that they would have inflammatory effects in joints (105). Although it has been reported that neuropeptides, including VIP (115), SP (116), CGRP (117), and SOM (118), are present in the synovial fluid of

TABLE 26-1. *Effects of selected neuropeptides*

Neuropeptide	Vasodilates or induces erythema in skin	Releases histamine from mast cells *in vitro*	Induces neutrophil influx *in vivo*	Inhibits antigen presentation	Inhibits inflammation	Inhibits contact hypersensitivity	T-cell effects
SP	+	+	+	—	—	—	Enhances proliferation
VIP	+	+	+	—	—	—	Inhibits proliferation Inhibits IFN-γ production
CGRP	+	—	+	+	+ (some models)	+	Inhibits proliferation
SOM	—	+	—	—	—	—	Inhibits proliferation Inhibits IFN-γ production
αMSH	—	—	—	—	+	+	Inhibits IFN-γ production

CGRP, calcitonin gene-related peptide; IFN, interferon; MSH, melanocyte-stimulating hormone; SOM, somatostatin; SP, substance P; VIP, vasoactive intestinal polypeptide; +, positive effect.

patients with rheumatoid arthritis, a conflicting report stated that SP is not present and that NKA was present in levels below that in controls (119). However, the failure to find SP may mean that it has been released and degraded. A specific inhibitor of the NK-1 receptor can block SP-induced vasodilatation in a rat knee joint (120). Induction of adjuvant arthritis in rats is associated with increased CGRP and SP concentrations in ankle joints and corresponding dorsal root ganglia (121). Immunocytochemical analysis of this model showed increased CGRP- and SP-containing fibers in synovium, with the increase more pronounced for CGRP. Although largely circumstantial, there is abundant evidence implicating neuropeptides as mediators in inflammatory joint disease.

CONCLUSIONS

A large body of evidence supports a role for neuropeptides in inflammation and immunity. Neuropeptides can directly cause vasodilation, induction of other inflammatory mediators, and recruitment of inflammatory cells (Table 26-1). Evidence for a regulatory role for products of nerves in immunity comes from anatomic and functional observations, including the apparent apposition of Langerhans cells, mast cells and lymphocytes to nerves and the functional effects of neuropeptides on antigen presentation and macrophage effector functions. Several neuropeptides affect lymphocyte proliferation, production of cytokines, and other cellular responses.

A role for neuropeptides in disease can be inferred from the functions previously described. A more direct role for neuropeptides in the pathogenesis of inflammatory disease is suggested by the observations that destruction of neural pathways can ameliorate experimental models of inflammatory joint disease, that inflammatory bowel disease clinically improves with interruption of nerves, and that interruption of nerve pathways leads to improvement in psoriasis.

Neuropeptides can be thought of in many ways as being similar to cytokines. Many have pleiotrophic effects on a wide variety of cells and tissues, and some

have been shown to be produced by extraneural cells and tissues, suggesting that they may be involved in signaling from a variety of cell types. The study of nervous system influences on immunity and inflammation is in its infancy, and developments in this area of research promise to be exciting and useful.

REFERENCES

1. Winchell SA, Watts RA. Relaxation therapies in the treatment of psoriasis and possible pathophysiologic mechanisms. *J Am Acad Dermatol* 1988;18:101–104.
2. Ostlere LS, Cowen T, Rustin MH. Neuropeptides in the skin of patients with atopic dermatitis. *Clin Exp Dermatol* 1995;20:462–467.
3. Talal AH, Drossman DA. Psychosocial factors in inflammatory bowel disease. *Gastroenterol Clin North Am* 1995;24:699–716.
4. Hassig A, Wen XL, Stampfi K. Stress-induced suppression of the cellular immune reactions: on the neuroendocrine control of the immune system. *Med Hypotheses* 1996;46:551–555.
5. Birmaher B, Rabin BS, Garcia MR, et al. Cellular immunity in depressed, conduct disorder, and normal adolescents: role of adverse life events. *J Am Acad Child Adolesc Psychiatry* 1994;33:671–678.
6. Peters LJ, Kelly H. The influence of stress and stress hormones on the transplantability of a non-immunogenic syngeneic murine tumor. *Cancer* 1977;39:1482–1488.
7. Lynn B. Neurogenic inflammation. *Skin Pharmacol* 1988;1:217–224.
8. Miller GW, Liuzzi FJ, Ratzlaff RE. Involvement of an axonal reflex in IgE-mediated inflammation in mouse skin. *J Neuroimmunol* 1995;57:137–141.
9. Bulloch K. Neuroanatomy of lymphoid tissue: a review. In: Guillemin R, Cohn M, Melnechuk T, eds. *Neural modulation of immunity.* New York: Raven Press, 1985:111.
10. Felten DL, Ackerman KD, Wiegand SJ, Felten SY. Noradrenergic sympathetic innervation of the spleen: I. Nerve fibers associated with lymphocytes and macrophages in specific compartments of the splenic white pulp. *J Neurosci Res* 1987;18:28–36.
11. Stead RH, Bienenstock J, Stanisz M. Neuropeptide regulation of mucosal immunity. *Immunol Rev* 1987;100:333–359.
12. Walker RF, Codd EE. Neuroimmunomodulatory interactions of norepinephrine and serotonin. *J Neuroimmunol* 1985;10:41–58.
13. Lorton D, Bellinger DL, Felten SY, Felten DL. Substance P innervation of spleen in rats: nerve fibers associate with lymphocytes and macrophages in specific compartments of the spleen. *Brain Behav Immunol* 1991;5:29–40.
14. Naukkarinen A, Harvima I, Paukkonen K, Aalto ML, Horsmanheimo M. Immunohistochemical analysis of sensory nerves and neuropeptides, and their contacts with mast cells in developing and mature psoriatic lesions. *Arch Dermatol Res* 1993;285:341-346.
15. Hosoi J, Murphy GF, Egan CL, et al. Regulation of Langerhans cell function by nerves containing calcitonin gene-related peptide. *Nature* 1993;363:159–163.
16. Arizono N, Matsuda S, Hattori T, Kojima Y, Maeda T, Galli SJ.

Anatomical variation in mast cells nerve associations in the rat small intestine, heart, lung, and skin: similarities of distance between neural processes and mast cells, eosinophils, or plasma cells in the jejunal lamina propria. *Lab Invest* 1990;62:626–634.

17. Stanisz AM. Neuronal factors modulating immunity. *Neuroimmunomodulation* 1994;1:217–230.

18. McGill JP, Mitsuhashi M, Payan DG. Immunomodulation by tachykinin neuropeptides. *Ann N Y Acad Sci* 1990;594:85–94.

19. Said SI. Vasoactive intestinal polypeptide (VIP): current status. *Peptides* 1984;5:143–150.

20. Wass JAH. Somatostatin. In: DeGroot LJ, Besser GM, Cahill GF, eds. *Endocrinology.* Philadelphia: WB Saunders, 1990:152–153.

21. Funekes CL, Minth CD, Deschenes R, et al. Cloning and characterization of a mRNA encoding rat preprosomatostatin. *J Biol Chem* 1981; 30:127–131.

22. Schultzberg M, Hokfelt T, Nilsson G, et al. Distribution of peptide and catecholamine-containing neurons in the gastrointestinal tract of rat and guinea pig: immunohistochemical studies with antisera to substance P, vasoactive intestinal polypeptide, enkephalins, somatostatin, gastrin/cholecystokinin, neurotensin, and dopamine β-hydroxylase. *Neuroscience* 1980;5:689–744.

23. Lowman MA, Benyon RC, Church MK. Characterization of neuropeptide-induced histamine release from human dispersed skin mast cells. *Br J Pharmacol* 1988;95:121–130.

24. Raynier-Rebuffel AM, Mathiau P, Callebert J, et al. Substance P, calcitonin gene-related peptide, and capsaicin release serotonin from cerebrovascular mast cells. *Am J Physiol* 1994;267:R1421–1429.

25. Bunker CB, Cerio R, Bull HA, Evans J, Dowd PM, Foreman JC. The effect of capsaicin application on mast cells in normal human skin. *Agents Actions* 1991;33:195–196.

26. Smith HC, Barker JN, Morris RW, MacDonald DM, Lee TH. Neuropeptides induce rapid expression of endothelial cell adhesion molecules and elicit granulocytic infiltration in human skin. *J Immunol* 1993;151:3274–3282.

27. Hafstrom I, Ringhertz B, Lundeberg T, Palmblad J. The effect of endothelin, neuropeptide Y, calcitonin gene-related peptide and substance P on neutrophil functions. *Acta Physiol Scand* 1993;148: 341–346.

28. Locatelli L, Sacerdote P, Mantegazza P, Panerai AE. Effect of ibuprofen and diclofenac on the chemotaxis induced by substance P and transforming growth factor-beta on human monocytes and polymorphonuclear cells. *Int J Immunopharmacol* 1993;15:833–838.

29. Johnston JA, Taub DD, Lloyd AR, Conlon K, Oppenheim JJ, Kevlin DJ. Human T lymphocyte chemotaxis and adhesion induced by vasoactive intestinal peptide. *J Immunol* 1994;153:1762–1768.

30. Marasco WA, Showell HJ, Becker EL. Substance P binds to the formylpeptide chemotaxis receptor on the rabbit neutrophil. *Biochem Biophys Res Commun* 1982;99:1065–1072.

31. Bar-shavit Z, Goldman R, Stabinsky R, et al. Enhancement of phagocytosis-A newly found activity of substance P in its N-terminal tetrapeptide sequence. *Biochem Biophys Res Commun* 1980;94: 1445–1451.

32. Hartung HP, Wolters K, Toyka KV. Substance P binding properties and studies on cellular responses in guinea-pig macrophages. *J Immunol* 1986;136:3856–3863.

33. Cooper JR, Bloom FE, Roth RH. *The biochemical basis of neuropharmacology,* 5th ed. New York: Oxford University Press, 1986:352–393.

34. Pewrretti M, Ahluwalia A, Flower RJ, Manzini S. Endogenous tachykinins play a role in IL-1-induced neutrophil accumulation: involvement of NK-1 receptors. *Immunology* 1993;80:73–77.

35. Gutwald J, Goebeler M, Sorg C. Neuropeptides enhance irritant and allergic contact dermatitis. *J Invest Dermatol* 1991;96:695–698.

36. Clementi G, Caruso A, Cutuli VM, et al. Anti-inflammatory activity of amylin and CGRP in different experimental models of inflammation. *Life Sci* 1995;57:PL193–197.

37. Ansel JC, Brown JR, Payan DG, Brown MA. Substance P selectively activates TNF-alpha gene expression in murine mast cells. *J Immunol* 1993;150:4478–4485.

38. Laurenzi MA, Persson MA, Dalsgaard CJ, Haegerstrand A. The neuropeptide substance P stimulates production of interleukin 1 in human blood monocytes: activated cells are preferentially influenced by the neuropeptide. *Scand J Immunol* 1990;31:529–533.

39. Rameshwar P, Ganea D, Gascon P. Induction of IL-3 and granulocyte-macrophage colony-stimulating factor by substance P in bone marrow cells is partially mediated through the release of IL-1 and IL-6. *J Immunology* 1994;152:4044–4054.

40. Gitter BD, Regoli D, Howbert JJ, Glasebrook AL, Waters DC. Interleukin-6 secretion from human astrocytoma cells induced by substance P. *J Neuroimmunol* 1994;51:101–108.

41. Rameshwar P, Gascon P, Ganea D. Stimulation of IL-2 production in murine lymphocytes by substance P and related tachykinins. *J Immunol* 1993;151:2484–2496.

42. Ansel JC, Kaynard AH, Armstrong CA, Olerud J, Bunnett N, Payan D. Skin–nervous system interactions. *J Invest Dermatol* 1996;106: 198–204.

43. Hart RP, Shadiack AM, Jonakait GM. Substance P gene expression is regulated by interleukin-1 in cultured sympathetic ganglia. *J Neurosci Res* 1991;29:282–291.

44. Rheins LA, Cotleur AL, Kleier RS, Hoppenjans WB, Sauder DN, Nordlund JJ. Alpha-melanocyte stimulating hormone modulates contact hypersensitivity responses in C57BL/6 mice. *J Invest Dermatol* 1989;93:511–517.

45. Ceriani G, Macaluso A, Catania A, Lipton JM. Central neurogenic antiinflammatory action of alpha-MSH: modulation of peripheral inflammation induced by cytokines and other mediators of inflammation. *Neuroendocrinology* 1994;59:138–143.

46. Macaluso A, McCoy D, Ceriani G, et al. Antiinflammatory influences of alpha-MSH molecules: central neurogenic and peripheral actions. *J Neurosci* 1994;14:2377–2382.

47. Taylor AW, Streilen JW, Cousins SW. Alpha melanocyte-stimulatng hormone suppresses antigen-stimulated T cell production of gamma interferon. *Neuroimmunomodulation* 1994;1:188–194.

48. Schauer E, Trautinger F, Kock A, et al. Proopiomelanocortin-derived peptides are synthesized and released by human keratinocytes. *J Clin Invest* 1994;93:2258–2262.

49. Wang F, Millet I, Bottomly K, Vignery A. Calcitonin gene-related peptide inhibits interleukin 2 production by murine T lymphocytes. *J Biol Chem* 1992;267:21052–21057.

50. Nong YH, Titus RG, Ribeiro JM, Remold HG. Peptides encoded by the calcitonin gene inhibit macrophage function. *J Immunol* 1989; 143:45–49.

51. Asahina A, Moro O, Hosoi J, et al. Specific induction of cyclic AMP in Langerhans cells by calcitonin gene-related peptide: relevance to functional effects. *Proc Natl Acad Sci USA* 1995;92:8323–8327.

52. Torii H, Hosoi J, Beissert S, et al. Regulation of cytokine expression in macrophages and the Langerhans cell-like line XS52 by calcitonin gene-related peptide. *J Leukoc Biol* 1997;61:216–223.

53. Bulloch K, McEwen BS, Diwa A, Radojcic T, Hausman J, Baird S. The role of calcitonin gene-related peptide in the mouse thymus revisited. *Ann N Y Acad Sci* 1994;741:129–136.

54. Asahina A, Hosoi J, Beissert S, Stratigos A, Granstein RD. Inhibition of the induction of delayed-type and contact hypersensitivity by calcitonin gene-related peptide. *J Immunol* 1995;154:3056–3061.

55. Gillardon F, Moll I, Michel S, Benrath J, Weihe E, Zimmermann M. Calcitonin gene-related peptide and nitric oxide are involved in ultraviolet radiation-induced immunosuppression. *Eur J Pharmacol* 1995; 293:395–400.

56. Johnson HM, Downs MO, Pontzer CH. Neuroendocrine peptide hormone regulation of immunity. *Chem Immunol* 1992;52:49–83.

57. Ottaway CA, Greenberg GR. Interaction of vasoactive intestinal peptide with mouse lymphocytes: specific binding and the modulation of mitogen responses. *J Immunol* 1984;132:417–423.

58. Ottaway CA, Bernaerts C, Chan B, Greenberg GR. Specific binding of VIP to human circulating mononuclear cells. *Can J Physiol Pharmacol* 1983;61:664–671.

59. Ottaway CA. Selective effects of vasoactive intestinal peptide in the mitogenic responses of murine T cells. *Immunology* 1987;62:291–297.

60. Stanisz AM, Befus D, Bienenstock J. Differential effects of vasoactive intestinal peptide, substance P, and somatostatin on immunoglobulin synthesis and proliferation by lymphocytes from Peyer's patches, mesenteric lymph nodes, and spleen. *J Immunol* 1986;136:152–156.

61. Ottaway CA, Lay TE, Greenberg GR. High affinity specific binding of vasoactive intestinal peptide to human circulating T cells, B cells and large granular lymphocytes. *J Neuroimmunol* 1990;29:149–155.

62. Rola-Pleszczynski M, Bolduc D, St Pierre S. The effects of vasoactive

intestinal peptide on human natural killer cell function. *J Immunol* 1985;135:2569–2573.

63. Muscettola M, Grasso G. Somatostatin and vasoactive intestinal peptide reduce interferon-gamma production by human peripheral blood mononuclear cells. *Immunobiology* 1990;180:419–430.

64. Payan DG, Brewster DR, Goetzl EJ. Specific stimulation of human T lymphocytes by substance P. *J Immunol* 1983;13:1613–1615.

65. Sreedharan SP, Kodama KT, Peterson KE, Goetzl EJ. Distinct subsets of somatostatin receptors on cultured human lymphocytes. *J Biol Chem* 1989;264:949–952.

66. Agro A, Padol I, Stanisz AM. Immunomodulatory activities of the somatostatin analogue RIM 23014c: effects on murine lymphocyte proliferation and natural killer activity. *Regul Pept* 1991;32:129–139.

67. Wagner M, Hengst K, Zierden E, Gerlach U. Investigations of the antiproliferative effect of somatostatin in man and rats. *Metab Clin Exp* 1979;27:1381–1386.

68. Kimata H, Yoshida A, Ishioka C, Mikawa H. Differential effect of vasoactive intestinal peptide, somatostatin and substance P on human IgE and IgG subclass production. *Cell Immunol* 1992;144:429–442.

69. Kimata H, Yoshida A, Fujimoto M, Mikawa H. Effect of vasoactive intestinal peptide, somatostatin and substance P on spontaneous IgE and IgC4 production in atopic patients. *J Immunol* 1993;150:4630–4640.

70. Serechitano R, Dazin P, Bienenstock J, Payan PG, Stanisz AM. The murine IgA-secreting plasmacytoma MOPC-315 expresses somatostatin receptors. *J Immunol* 1988;141:937–941.

71. Fais S, Annibale B, Boirivant M, Santoro F, Pallone F, DeleFave G. Effect of somatostatin on human intestinal lamina propria lymphocytes. *J Neuroimmunol* 1991;31:211–219.

72. Rains C, Bryson HM. Topical capsaicin: a review of its pharmacological properties and therapeutic potential in post-herpetic neuralgia, diabetic neuropathy and osteoarthritis. *Drugs Aging* 1995;7:317–328.

73. Nilsson G, Ahlstedt S. Increased delayed-type hypersensitivity reaction in rats neuromanipulated with capsaicin. *Int Arch Allergy Appl Immunol* 1989;90:256–260.

74. Wallengren J, Ekman R, Moller H. Capsaicin enhances allergic contact dermatitis in the guinea pig. *Contact Dermatitis* 1991;24:30–34.

75. Wallengren J, Moller H. The effect of capsaicin on som experimental inflammations in human skin. *Acta Derm Venereol* 1986;66:375–380.

76. Raychaudhuri SP, Farber EM. Are sensory nerves essential for the development of psoriatic lesions? *J Am Acad Dermatol* 1993;28:488–489.

77. Dewing SB. Remission of psoriasis associated with cutaneous nerve section. *Arch Dermatol* 1971;104:220–221

78. Perlman HH. Remission of psoriasis vulgaris from the use of nerve-blocking agents. *Arch Dermatol* 1972;105:128–129.

79. Johansson O, Han SW, Enhamre A. Altered cutaneous innervation in psoriatic skin as revealed by PGP 9.5 immunohistochemistry. *Arch Dermatol Res* 1991;283:519–523.

80. Naukkarinen A, Harvima IT, Aalto ML, Harvima RJ, Horsmanheimo M. Quantitative analysis of contact sites between mast cells and sensory nerves in cutaneous psoriasis and lichen planus based on a histochemical double staining technique. *Arch Dermatol Res* 1991;283:433–437.

81. Al'Abadie MS, Senior HJ, Bleehen SS, Gawkrodger DJ. Neuropeptides and general neuronal marker in psoriasis—an immunohistochemical study. *Clin Exp Dermatol* 1995;20:384–389.

82. Naukkarinen A, Harvima I, Paukkonen K, Aalto ML, Horsmanheimo M. Immunohistochemical analysis of sensory nerves and neuropeptides, and their contacts with mast cells in developing and mature psoriatic lesions. *Arch Dermatol Res* 1993;285:341–346.

83. Eedy DJ, Johnston CF, Shaw C, Buchanan KD. Neuropeptides in psoriasis: an immunocytochemical and radioimmunoassay study. *J Invest Dermatol* 1991;96:434–438.

84. Mozzanica N, Cattaneo A, Vignati G, Finzi A. Plasma neuropeptide levels in psoriasis. *Acta Derm Venereol Suppl* 1994;186:67–68.

85. Glinski W, Brodecka H, Glinska-Ferenz M, Kowalski D. Neuropeptides in psoriasis: possible role of beta-endorphin in the pathomechanism of the disease. *Int J Dermatol* 1994;33:356–360.

86. Glinski W, Brodecka H, Glinska-Ferenz M, Kowalski D. Increased concentration of beta-endorphin in sera of patients with psoriasis and other inflammatory dermatoses. *Br J Dermatol* 1994;131:260–264.

87. Gianetti A, Girolomoni G. Skin reactivity to neuropeptides in atopic dermatitis. *Br J Dermatol* 1989;121:681–688.

88. Gianetti A, Fantini F, Cimitan A, Pincelli C. Vasoactive intestinal polypeptide and substance P in the pathogenesis of atopic dermatitis. *Acta Derm Venereol* 1992;176:90–92.

89. Cooper KD. Atopic dermatitis: recent trends in pathogenesis and therapy. *J Invest Dermatol* 1994;102:128–137.

90. Bieber T. Fc epsilon RI on human Langerhans cells: a receptor in search of new functions. *Immunol Today* 1994;15:52–53.

91. Mosimann BL, White MV, Hohman RJ, Goldrich MS, Kaulbach HC, Kaliner MA. Substance P, calcitonin gene-related peptide, and vasoactive intestinal peptide increase in nasal secretions after allergen challenge in atopic patients. *J Allergy Clin Immunol* 1993;92:95–104.

92. Nielsen OH, Rask-Madsen J. Mediators of inflammation in chronic inflammatory bowel disease. *Scand J Gastroenterol* 1996;31[Suppl 216]:146–159.

93. Collins SM. The immunomodulation of enteric neuromuscular function: implications for motility and inflammatory disorders. *Gastroenterology* 1996;111:1683–1699.

94. Hwang L, Leichter R, Okamoto A, Payan D, Collins SM, Bunnett NW. Downregulation of neutral endopeptidase (EC 3.4.24.11) in the inflamed rat intestine. *Am J Physiol* 1993;264:G735–G743.

95. Shafiroff GP, Hinton J. Denervation of the pelvic colon for ulcerative colitis. *Surg Forum* 1950;134–139.

96. Thorek P. Vagotomy for idiopathic ulcerative colitis and regional enteritis. *JAMA* 1951;145:140–146.

97. Dennis C, Eddy FD, Frykman MH, McCarthy AM, Westover D. The response to vagotomy in idiopathic ulcerative colitis and regional enteritis. *Ann Surg* 1946;128:479–496.

98. Lechin F, van der Dijs B, Insausti CL. Treatment of ulcerative colitis with clonidine. *J Clin Pharmacol* 1985;25:255–262.

99. Lashner BA, Hanauer SB, Siverstein MD. Testing nicotine gum for ulcerative colitis patients: experience with single patient trials. *Dig Dis Sci* 1990;35:827–832.

100. Bjorck S, Dahlstrom A, Johansson L, Ahlman H. Treatment of the mucosa with local anaesthetics in ulcerative colitis. *Agents Actions* 1992;10:C61–72.

101. Mazumdar S, Moy Das K. Immunocytochemical localization of vasoactive intestinal peptide and substance P in the colon from normal subjects and patients with inflammatory bowel disease. *Am J Gastroenterol* 1992;87:176–181.

102. Kubota Y, Petras RE, Ottaway CA, Tubbs RR, Farmer RG, Fiocchi C. Colonic vasoactive intestinal peptide nerves in inflammatory bowel disease. *Gastroenterology* 1992;102:1242–1251.

103. Kimura M, Masuda T, Hiwatashi N, Toyota T, Nagura H. Changes in neuropeptide-containing nerves in human colonic mucosa with inflammatory bowel disease. *Pathol Int* 1994;44:624–634.

104. Schulte-Bockholt A, Fink JG, Meier DA, et al. Expression of mRNA for vasoactive intestinal peptide in human colon and during inflammation. *Mol Cell Biochem* 1995;142:1–7.

105. Scott DT, Lam FY, Ferrell WR. Acute joint inflammation—mechanisms and mediators. *Gen Pharmacol* 1994;25:1285–1296.

106. Samuel EP. The autonomic and somatic innervation of the articular capsule. *Anat Rec* 1952;168:161–172.

107. Skoglund S. Anatomical and physiological studies of knee joint innervation in the cat. *Acta Physiol Scand* 1956;36[Suppl 124]:1–101.

108. Ferrell WR, Lam FY, Montgomery I. Differences in the axon composition of nerves supplying the rat knee joint following intraarticular injection of capsaicin. *Neurosci Lett* 1992;141:259–261.

109. Langford LA, Schmidt RF. Afferent and efferent axons in the medical and posterior articular nerves of the cat. *Anat Rec* 1983;206:71–78.

110. Freeman MAR, Wyke B. The innervation of the knee joint: an anatomical and histological study in the cat. *J Anat* 1967;101:505–532.

111. Mapp PI, Kidd BL, Gison SJ, et al. Substance P, calcitonin gene-related peptide, and C-flanking peptide of neuropeptide Y-immunoreactive nerve fibres are present in normal synovium but depleted in patients with rheumatoid arthritis. *Neuroscience* 1990;37:143–153.

112. Colpaer FC, Donnere J, Lembeck F. Effects of capsaicin on inflammation and on the substance P content of nervous tissue in rats with adjuvant arthritis. *Life Sci* 1983;32:1827–1934.

113. Grondblad M, Konntinen YT, Korkala O, Liesi P, Hukkanen M, Polak J. Neuropeptides in the synovium of patients with rheumatoid arthritis and osteoarthritis. *J Rheum* 1988;15:1807–1810.

114. Levine JD, Clark R, Devor M, Helms C, Moskowitz MA, Basbaum AI. Intraneuronal substance P contributes to the severity of experimental arthritis. *Science* 1984;226:547–549.

115. Lygren I, Ostensen M, Burhol PG, Husby G. Gastrointestinal peptides in serum and synovial fluid from patients with inflammatory joint disease. *Ann Rheum* Dis 1986;45:637–640.

116. Sacerdote P, Carrabba M, Galante A, Pisat R, Manfredi I, Pancrai AE. Plasma and synovial fluid interleukin-1, interleukin-6, and substance P concentrations in rheumatoid arthritis patients: effect of the nonsteroidal antiinflammatory drugs indomethacin, diclofenac, and naproxen. *Inflamm Res* 1995;44:486—490.

117. Arnalich F, de Miguel E, Peroz-Ayala C, et al. Neuropeptides and interleukin-6 in human joint inflammation: relationship between intraarticular substance P and interleukin-6 concentrations. *Neurosci Lett* 1994;170:251–254.

118. Marabini S, Matucci-Cerinic M, Geppetti P, et al. Substance P and somatostatin levels in rheumatoid arthritis, osteoarthritis and psoriatic arthritis synovial fluid. *Ann N Y Acad Sci* 1991;632:435–436.

119. Larsson LA, Ekbom A, Henrikson K, Lundeberg T, Theodorsson E. Concentration of substance P, neurokinin A, calcitonin gene-related peptide, neuropeptide Y and vasoactive intestinal polypeptide in synovial fluid from knee joints in patients suffering from rheumatoid arthritis. *Scand J Rheum* 1991;20:326–335.

120. Lam FY, Ferrell WR. Effects of interactions of naturally occurring neuropeptides on blood flow in the rat knee joint. *Br J Pharmacol* 1993;108:694–699.

121. Ahmed M, Bjurholm A, Schultzberg M, Theodorsson E. Kreiebergs A. Increased levels of substance P and calcitonin gene-related peptide in rat adjuvant arthritis: a combined immunohistochemical and radioimmunoassay analysis. *Arthritis Rheum* 1995;38:699–709.

Inflammation: Basic Principles and Clinical Correlates,
3rd ed., edited by John I. Gallin and Ralph Snyderman.
Lippincott Williams & Wilkins, Philadelphia © 1999.

CHAPTER 27

Myeloid Growth Factors

Donald Metcalf

The mature neutrophils, monocytes, eosinophils, and mast cells involved in inflammatory responses are short-lived cells that must be replaced continuously, even under basal conditions. This cell production is part of the complex hematopoietic process in which cells of eight functionally distinct lineages are generated from a small population of self-renewing multipotential hematopoietic stem cells (1). Cellular production in each lineage occurs in distinct steps, with cells of each succeeding step being more numerous than those of the preceding step (2) (Fig. 27-1).

Multipotential stem cells first generate progenitor cell progeny that are restricted in their lineage potential, in most cases ultimately to a single lineage (3–5). Such progenitor cells have no capacity for self-renewal, but each can generate up to 10,000 maturing progeny (6). In a simple lineage, such as that of the neutrophil (granulocytic) series, the progeny of progenitors pass through successive maturation stages until mature, postmitotic neutrophils result. This sequence is potentially more complex for monocytes and eosinophils, because under some circumstances, apparently mature cells of these types may exhibit some limited mitotic activity. Although mitotic activity in monocyte-macrophages or eosinophils is not prominent in inflammatory foci, some local proliferation of these cells may occur.

Mature monocytes can transform to a variety of macrophages after seeding from the circulation into appropriate tissue sites. Although all tissue macrophages are originally marrow derived, local production of cells can occur and, in the case of peritoneal macrophages, seems likely to be able to sustain basal numbers of macrophages (7,8). Under inflammatory conditions, most of the greatly increased population of macrophages are of recent bone marrow origin (9).

All neutrophilic granulocytes are regarded as equivalent, with no evidence for the existence of specialized subsets, although this question warrants further exploration. A similar comment can be made regarding eosinophils. Macrophages in different tissues vary greatly in size, shape, surface markers, and biologic activity (10). It remains unclear whether these are merely tissue-dictated phenotypic changes or distinct sublineages of macrophages exist, each with their own progenitor cells and tissue-homing characteristics.

The heterogeneous macrophage populations include one subpopulation of major importance for inflammatory responses. Dendritic cells capture antigens and present them in modified form to induce the T-cell activation that initiates immune responses. There are two general classes of dendritic cells, one lymphoid in origin (11) and the other (including dendritic cells in the skin, lymph nodes, gut and lungs) derived from macrophage progenitor cells (12). The role of macrophage precursors in inflammatory responses is therefore twofold. They provide the variety of macrophages available for local responses and a major subset of dendritic cells needed for the initiation of classic immune responses.

In mice and humans, bipotential granulocyte-macrophage progenitors can form granulocytic and macrophage progeny (13,14). It is unclear whether such progeny are essentially identical to those produced from unipotential progenitor cells.

Immature cells cannot revert to progenitor cells, progenitor cells cannot switch their differentiation lineage to another, and progenitor cells cannot revert to stem cells. Because progenitor cells cannot self-renew, they expend themselves by forming more mature progeny. The increased production of mature cells to engage in a sustained inflammatory response therefore requires the coordinated regulation of two cellular processes: the formation by stem cells of committed progenitor cells and the formation of mature progeny by committed progenitor cells.

D. Metcalf: The Walter and Eliza Hall Institute of Medical Research, The Royal Melbourne Hospital, 3050, Victoria, Australia.

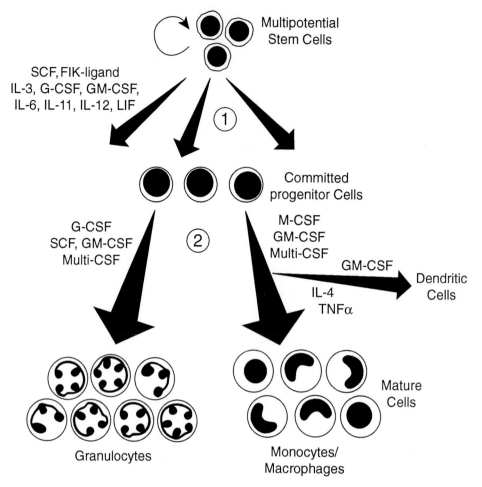

FIG. 27-1. Sequential cellular events in the formation of mature neutrophils, macrophages, and dendritic cells and the hematopoietic regulators controlling this cell production.

PRINCIPLES OF REGULATORY CONTROL

The formation of neutrophils, monocytes, and eosinophils occurs in only two organs—the bone marrow and, to a lesser extent, the spleen. Under conditions of stress, such as infections or acute inflammation, cell production in the marrow can increase in humans because not all of the marrow space is usually occupied by hematopoietic tissue. In the mouse, the capacity of the marrow to expand cell production is limited, but the spleen can then dramatically increase its size and ability to contain additional hematopoietic cells.

Hematopoiesis restricted to the marrow and spleen suggests that this cellular activity probably depends on special microenvironmental cells in these organs that can sustain or stimulate cell formation (15). This conclusion has been supported by tissue culture studies indicating that a complex mixture of stromal cells exists in marrow and spleen tissue and that contact of immature hematopoietic cells with these stromal cells is essential for sustained hematopoiesis (16,17). The precise mechanisms involved have not been fully characterized, nor has

it been established whether subsets of stromal cells have specific roles in supporting or stimulating hematopoiesis of one type or another. Various adhesion molecules appear to be important in permitting responsiveness of hematopoietic cells or in modulating their response to specific regulatory factors (18). The glycocalyx of stromal cells is capable of loosely binding some regulatory factors and possibly then releases these for action on adjacent hematopoietic cells (19). Stromal cells can produce many hematopoietic regulatory factors by secreting them into the local microenvironment or displaying them on their cell membranes (as is the case with macrophage colony-stimulating factor (M-CSF) or stem cell factor (SCF) (20–25).

There are at least 25 identified growth factors, or cytokines, with proliferative actions on various hematopoietic cells. Certain generalizations can be made about these regulators. They are almost all glycoproteins. The carbohydrate moiety of these molecules is not necessary for their biologic action *in vitro* but can be important *in vivo* by modulating the half-life of the factors. These factors have high biologic activity, are active on target cells at picogram to nanogram per milliliter concentrations, and can be produced as secreted molecules or, less often, in the form of membrane-displayed molecules. For some, local production and action are dominant (i.e., paracrine action), whereas others behave as typical humoral factors and are transported in the blood to their target cells. The combination of humoral and paracrine aspects makes it difficult to establish the concentrations of a particular factor available locally, either at sites of cell production or in an inflammatory focus.

A further complexity exists in that none of these factors is absolutely lineage specific in its actions (2). Although many have a dominant action on cells of one particular lineage, all have additional actions on cells of at least some other lineages (Table 27-1). This situation is made possible by the simultaneous display on immature and mature hematopoietic cells of specific receptors for multiple regulatory factors. This arrangement allows the combined actions on individual cells of two or more factors that are usually synergistic in nature and allows subtle alterations to be achieved in the number of mature cells of different lineages being produced in any inflammatory situation (26).

The regulatory factors are products of multiple cell types located in multiple organs in the body (2,27,28). Cell types typically able to produce regulatory factors are stromal cells, fibroblasts, endothelial cells, T lymphocytes, mast cells, and various epithelial cell types. Studies with T lymphocytes have documented that individual cells can produce multiple regulatory factors, often simultaneously (29). In general, the level of production of regulatory factors is very low under basal conditions. In response to inductive signals, cells can, within minutes to hours, greatly increase their levels of transcription or production of regulators (21,23,30). This ability coupled with the relatively short plasma half-lives of many of these regulators (typically a few hours) gives the control system a high degree of lability in response to changing demands.

Regulators active in the formation of progenitor cells by stem cells are SCF, multi-CSF (i.e., interleukin-3 [IL-3]), IL-6, IL-1, fetal liver kinase (FLK) ligand, IL-11, IL-12, granulocyte-macrophage colony-stimulating factor (GM-CSF), granulocyte colony-stimulating factor (G-CSF), and leukemia inhibitory factor (LIF) (see Fig. 27-1) (31-37). Of these, the most active are SCF and FLK ligand, but cellular production is characterized by the need for multiple regulators to act simultaneously (38,39), unlike the situation with progenitor cell proliferation, in which individual regulators acting alone can stimulate unequivocal cell proliferation. Stem cells tend to generate various progenitor cells in a stochastic fashion (3–5), but the use of combinations of different regulators with SCF can skew the relative rates of production of particular types of progenitor cells (40,41) and thereby modulate the formation of neutrophils, monocytes, and eosinophils during an inflammatory response.

Analysis of the regulatory control of cell production *in vitro* by progenitors of neutrophils, monocytes, and eosinophils has identified a number of positive regulators of cell proliferation (see Fig. 27-1). The relative importance of these regulators for cell production can be assessed *in vitro* from the concentrations required, the numbers of colonies generated from marrow cells in clonal cultures, and the cell numbers in such colonies. *In vivo*, the situation depends on the relative production rates and concentrations of these factors, and a valid assessment requires the use of mice with selective inactivation of the genes encoding the various regulatory factors or their receptors. Such studies are not complete for all these factors, but they have identified G-CSF (42) and SCF (43,44) as major regulators of granulocyte production, M-CSF as a major regulator of macrophage production (45,46), and IL-5 as a regulator of eosinophil production (47,48). In each case, it is clear from current gene inactivation data that other regulators, not yet characterized, must exist and play a role in these processes (49).

The *in vivo* response to injected regulatory factors does not wholly agree with the assessment of which regulators are the most important, based on studies on basal hematopoiesis in mice with gene inactivation. Injection of G-CSF is outstanding in stimulating granulocyte production (50,51), but the action of injected SCF is weak (52). Similarly, only at high doses does injected M-CSF produce a selective monocytosis, and this is a relatively weak response (53). These findings suggest that the vari-

TABLE 27-1. *Major human myeloid regulators controlling formation of neutrophilic granulocytes, monocyte-macrophages, and eosinophils*

Factor	M$_r$ polypeptide	Gene location	Strong actions	Weaker or accessory actions
G-CSF	18,600	17q21-22	G	M, Stem
GM-CSF	14,700	5q21-32	G,M.Eo	Meg, E, Stem
M-CSF	41,000–63,000	1p13-21	M	G, Stem (?)
Multi-CSF (IL-3)	15,400	5q21-32	G, M, Eo, Meg, E, Stem, Mast	B-lymphocytes
Stem cell factor	18,400	12q22-24	Stem, G	M, E, Meg, Mast
Interleukin-5	24,000	5q31	Eo	

CSF, colony-stimulating factor; G, neutrophilic granulocytes; M, macrophage; Eo, eosinophils; Meg, megakaryocytes; E, erythroid cells; Mast, mast cells; Stem, stem cells (blast colony-forming cells).

ous regulatory factors may change their importance under emergency conditions, distinct from their role in basal hematopoiesis.

COLONY-STIMULATING FACTORS

Some regulators were named colony-stimulating factors (CSFs) because of their ability to stimulate individual progenitor cells *in vitro* to form colonies of maturing progeny.

Granulocyte Cololony-Stimulating Factor

G-CSF was first recognized as a distinct CSF produced by human placenta (54) and was purified to homogeneity from mouse lung conditioned medium (55). Human G-CSF was subsequently purified from medium conditioned by two human tumor cell lines (56,57).

Murine and human G-CSF are synthesized with a 30 amino acid leader sequence typical of secreted proteins. The mature proteins contain 178 amino acids (M_r 19,061) in mice and 174 amino acids (M_r 18,627) in humans (56–58). The larger apparent molecular mass (22,000 to 25,000) of the secreted proteins is the result of the addition of O-linked carbohydrate. G-CSF contains two cysteine-cysteine disulfide bonds necessary for maintaining the three-dimensional morphology and functional activity of the molecule in its 4α-helical configuration (59,60).

The gene encoding G-CSF contains 5 exons and spans about 2.3 kbp on chromosome 17q11-22 in humans (61) and on the syntenic region of chromosome 11 D-E2 in mice (62). The two genes are highly homologous, with 69% nucleic acid identity in coding and noncoding regions. The cross-species conservation of G-CSF is the highest of the four CSFs, allowing a wide range of cross-species biologic activity.

G-CSF can be produced by a wide range of cell types, including endothelial cells, fibroblasts, stromal cells, and macrophages (21,30,63,64)—cells that are well located to make early contact with invading microorganisms or their products. Low levels of G-CSF (25±20 pg/mL) (65,66) are detectable in normal human sera and in mice. G-CSF in low concentrations is extractable from most major organs.

Production of G-CSF is highly responsive to agents such as bacterial lipopolysaccharide (LPS), IL-1, tumor necrosis factor (TNF), or GM-CSF in a process involving stabilization of G-CSF mRNA (67) and increased rates of transcription regulated by regions upstream of the transcription initiation site—regions homologous to the cytokine (CK)-1, CK-2, and nucleus factor (NF)-IL-6 elements (68). These regulatory elements appear to differ in relative importance in different types of producer cells and with the inducing agent (68,69).

Of considerable interest is the absence of G-CSF mRNA from extracts of human or murine marrow cells (28,70), although after induction *in vitro*, various marrow cell types can produce G-CSF. This ability implies that, under normal conditions, G-CSF acts as a humoral agent when it regulates granulocyte formation in marrow populations.

Model studies in mice and rats confirm the ability of cells to rapidly increase G-CSF production within hours in inflammatory peritoneal exudates (71) or in the lungs of animals with induced infections (72), and circulating levels of G-CSF rise to as high as 2 µg/mL 3 hours after the intravenous injection of endotoxin in mice (73).

During infections, G-CSF levels can be elevated in mice up to 180 ng/mL (74) and in humans up to 10,000 pg/mL (65,66,75), but this response was not observed in all nonneutropenic patients with infections (66). Similar elevations, and possibly infections, are observed in the more complex clinical situations of chemotherapy-induced neutropenia.

G-CSF exerts its actions on responding cells by interacting with a membrane-displayed unique receptor. This receptor belongs to the cytokine receptor superfamily and in its high-affinity form is a homodimer of two identical glycoprotein chains (76,77). The cytoplasmic domain of the receptor includes a juxtamembrane region (box 1 and 2), initiating mitotic signaling through interaction with JAK kinases and a more C-terminal domain required for initiation of maturation in responding cells (78).

Actions In Vitro

In clonal cultures of marrow cells, the characteristic action of G-CSF is to stimulate the formation of neutrophilic granulocytic colonies, with maximum numbers of colonies developing at a concentration of 2 to 10 ng/mL. Typically, these colonies are of relatively small size, and by 7 days of incubation, they contain mainly mature neutrophils (79,80), suggesting that G-CSF preferentially stimulates the proliferation of relatively mature neutrophilic progenitor cells. G-CSF possesses a much weaker capacity to stimulate macrophage colony formation and no capacity to stimulate the proliferation of eosinophils, mast cells, erythroid cells, or megakaryocytic cells (79).

When acting with SCF, G-CSF can enhance progenitor cell formation by stem cells (40), with the production of neutrophilic progenitors and also progenitors for macrophages, eosinophils, megakaryocytes, and erythroid cells (41). These actions on stem cells appear to be the basis for the broader responses to G-CSF observable *in vivo*.

As is true for all the CSFs, G-CSF can enhance the functional activity of mature cells. G-CSF can stimulate neutrophilic granulocytes to exhibit enhanced superoxide production and antibody-dependent cytotoxicity (2).

In Vivo *Actions*

When injected into mice or humans, G-CSF exhibits a dose-dependent capacity to elevate blood neutrophil levels, with responses peaking after 3 to 5 days of administration and the height of the plateau depending on the dose used (50,51,81). After G-CSF administration stops, blood neutrophil levels return to preinjection levels within a few days. The G-CSF–induced elevations of blood neutrophils are sustainable indefinitely, with no indication that responsiveness is lost or that the neutrophil precursor population becomes depleted.

The magnitude of the neutrophil responses observed to a given dose of G-CSF vary from one human to another over a tenfold range (82). The only disease state in which responsiveness to G-CSF is decreased is congenital neutropenia (83), and some of these patients have defective G-CSF receptors (84).

The initial events after injection of G-CSF are complex, but the ultimate basis for the sustained increase in blood neutrophil levels is an increase in neutrophil production by increased numbers of progenitor cells. Analysis has shown a transient initial decrease in total marrow granulocytic progenitor cells in mice, which is corrected within a few days, and the numbers thereafter are slightly higher than normal (2). In parallel, the number of granulocytic progenitor cells in the spleen rises progressively and exceeds in total the number in the entire bone marrow after 5 days. G-CSF also induces a major increase in progenitor cells of other lineages, probably because of increased progenitor production by stem cells under the combined actions of SCF and G-CSF.

A feature of clinical importance is the G-CSF–induced rise in stem and progenitor cells in the peripheral blood, a response that becomes evident after 3 to 5 days and peaks in humans at day 8 (85,86). The regulatory basis for this rise is likely to be the combined action of SCF and G-CSF, because responses are diminished in mice lacking SCF receptors (W^v mice) or lacking the ability to produce SCF (Sl^d mice) (87). Stem and progenitor cell populations released to the blood are capable of repopulating recipients more rapidly and efficiently than marrow populations, even those from G-CSF–treated donors (88).

Studies with engrafted or genetically manipulated mice extend these observations on G-CSF action *in vivo*. Mice transplanted with marrow cells overproducing G-CSF exhibited extensive granulocytic hyperplasia, with extreme elevations of neutrophils in the blood, marrow, spleen, liver, and lymph nodes (89). Conversely, in mice with inactivation of the G-CSF gene, blood neutrophil levels fall to 30% of normal levels, and there is a 50% reduction in marrow neutrophil numbers and in the number of progenitor cells of all types in the bone marrow (42).

For inflammatory responses, the G-CSF–dependent production of neutrophils is important because it provides the effector cells required. However, although G-CSF has been claimed to be a chemotactic agent *in vitro* (90), it is unlikely that G-CSF plays a major role in accelerating neutrophil release from the marrow during an inflammatory response or in attracting neutrophils to the inflammatory site. Mice with inactivated G-CSF genes or mice injected with G-CSF exhibited an unaltered capacity to accumulate neutrophils in an inflammatory site (71), and other studies suggest that such trafficking is regulated by chemokines such as IL-8 (91).

Granulocyte-Macrophage Colony-Stimulating Factor

GM-CSF was first recognized as a distinct CSF produced by mouse lung-conditioned medium (92) and was purified to homogeneity from that source (93). A corresponding human GM-CSF was purified to homogeneity from the Mo human T-lymphocyte leukemic cell line (94). Human and murine GM-CSFs are glycosylated with *N*- and *O*-linked carbohydrate and have an apparent molecular mass of 18,000 to 33,000.

GM-CSF has a 4α-helical configuration. Human and murine GM-CSF are synthesized with a 17 amino acid hydrophobic leader sequence that is cleaved during secretion (95,96). The mature protein consists of 127 amino acids (human) and 124 amino acids (murine), with core polypeptide molecular masses of 14,700 and 14,400, respectively. There is only 52% amino acid identity between the two species and no biologic cross-reactivity. Although both contain two cysteine-cysteine disulfide bonds, only one of these is required for biologic activity (97).

The gene encoding GM-CSF is on chromosome 5q21-32 in humans (98) and on chromosome 11A5-B1 in the mouse (99). Both genes contain 4 exons and produce a single transcript. The GM-CSF mRNA is highly labile because of AT-rich sequences in the 3'-untranslated region of the mRNA (100).

GM-CSF can be produced by a wide range of cell types, including stromal cells, fibroblasts, endothelial cells, T lymphocytes, macrophages, osteoblasts, mast cells (20,101–105), and probably a number of epithelial cell types—a range of cells well suited to make early contact with the products of invading microorganisms.

The transcription and production of GM-CSF are highly labile and can be induced by agents such as TNF, IL-1, LPS, and T-cell mitogens (106). Some of these agents initially increase GM-CSF production by inducing increased stability in GM-CSF mRNA, but initiating agents also activate transcription by inducing binding of nuclear factors to several regulatory upstream elements of the gene (107-109).

GM-CSF is undetectable in normal sera or present at low concentrations (<20 pg/mL) (66,110). Serum GM-CSF levels can be elevated in mice by the injection of endotoxin or by model infections, although the levels are usually low (<500 pg/mL) (74), and in patients with infections, GM-CSF often remains undetectable (66). Based on these data, GM-CSF is commonly regarded as acting as a humoral factor only under exceptional circumstances and normally being produced in significant concentrations locally at sites of cell proliferation or in inflammatory foci.

GM-CSF exerts its action through a specific low-affinity α chain that is also a member of the hemopoietin class of receptors (111). In high-affinity signaling form, the specific α chain becomes associated with a signaling β chain that is shared by the specific α chains of IL-3 and IL-5 (112–114). The β chain contains two distinct signaling domains, a juxtamembrane box 1 and box 2 region signaling proliferation and a more C-terminal domain influencing maturation and differentiation induction (115).

Actions In Vitro

In clonal cultures of murine or human marrow cells, the most prominent action of GM-CSF is to stimulate the formation of colonies of granulocytes, macrophages, or both cell types. However, it is also an effective stimulus for eosinophil colony formation and, at higher concentrations, can stimulate the formation of megakaryocyte and some early erythroid colonies (116,117). GM-CSF can enhance SCF-stimulated proliferation of stem cells to form progenitor cells in various lineages (40).

GM-CSF has a unique role in stimulating the formation or functional activity of dendritic cells originating from myeloid precursors. This action is more evident when GM-CSF acts in association with TNF-α or IL-4 (12). GM-CSF can enhance the in vitro survival of cells expressing GM-CSF receptors, regardless of maturation stage (118,119); can initiate differentiation commitment and maturation in granulocyte-macrophage precursor cells (13); and can activate a variety of functions of mature neutrophils, macrophages, and eosinophils (2,120).

In Vivo Actions

When injected into humans, GM-CSF can induce elevations in blood neutrophils, monocytes, and sometimes, eosinophils with kinetics that are similar to those for G-CSF, although at comparable dose levels, the elevation of neutrophil numbers is lower than that achievable by G-CSF (121,122). Similarly, in mice, GM-CSF also stimulates increased hemopoiesis in the spleen but not to the levels achieved by G-CSF (123).

When injected intraperitoneally into mice, GM-CSF has the most potent action of all the four CSFs in inducing a major rise in local macrophage cell numbers, partially because of the induction of mitotic activity in local cells (123). This more potent action of GM-CSF has supported the notion that GM-CSF may be designed to function more as a locally acting agent. Like G-CSF, GM-CSF has the capacity increase blood levels of stem and progenitor cells, although not to the high levels achievable by G-CSF (124,125).

In local inflammatory models in mice, GM-CSF levels rise even earlier than levels of G-CSF. However, evidence from mice with inactivation of the GM-CSF gene or its receptor indicates that GM-CSF is not essential for the accumulation of neutrophils or eosinophils, and injected GM-CSF did not induce the acute (within 3 hours) migration of inflammatory cells into the local site (71).

In transgenic mice with constitutively elevated (80- to 100-fold) levels of serum GM-CSF, no effects were observed on blood, marrow, or spleen cellularity (126). However, these mice develop massive accumulations of macrophages in the peritoneal and pleural cavities and evidence of selective functional activation of these cells (127,128). Such animals die prematurely with a variety of chronic inflammatory lesions in the eye, skeletal muscle, and pleural and peritoneal cavities and can also exhibit wasting, hind limb paralysis, and gut damage, possibly the consequence of overstimulation of macrophages by GM-CSF with the production of toxic agents such as TNF and plasminogen activator.

Mice repopulated by marrow cells overexpressing GM-CSF exhibited elevated numbers of neutrophils, macrophages, and eosinophils and had marked hyperplasia of hemopoietic tissues (129). Such mice died prematurely with massive macrophage and granulocyte infiltrations of the liver and lung.

In mice with inactivation of the GM-CSF gene or its receptor, no decrease was observed in neutrophil, monocyte, or eosinophil levels in the blood, marrow, or spleen, but the mice consistently developed surfactant accumulation in the lung with associated proteinaceous exudates— a disease state identical to alveolar proteinosis (130,131). The basis for these changes is a failure of alveolar macrophages to turn over surfactant. It has also been observed that type II alveolar cells depend on GM-CSF for proliferative activity. GM-CSF therefore plays a unique role in maintaining the functional integrity of alveolar macrophages and alveolar cells and is likely to play a vital role in lung inflammatory states and their proper resolution.

Macrophage Colony-Stimulating Factor

M-CSF was first purified as the major CSF in human urine (132) and was later purified from mouse L-cell fibroblast–conditioned medium (133). Unlike the other CSFs, M-CSF is a homodimer of two 4α-helical polypeptide chains linked end to end (134). A wide variety of M-CSF molecules has been described, based on the existence of alternate spliced forms of M-CSF mRNA and a widely varying carbohydrate content (135,136). These variants have mature M-CSF molecular masses that can range from 45,000 to more than 200,000. Unlike the other CSFs, M-CSF can be produced in a membrane-displayed form, which is able to stimulate the proliferation of hematopoietic cells making contact with such cells (24).

The gene encoding M-CSF is located on chromosome 1p13-21 (137) in humans and on chromosome 3F3 (also the osteopetrosis, op/op locus) in the mouse (45,138). In op/op mice, a single base insertion leads to a frameshift in the M-CSF coding sequence and to a failure of M-CSF production.

M-CSF is produced by a wide range of cell types, including fibroblasts, macrophages, endothelial cells, stromal cells, uterine decidual cells, and in humans, by T lymphocytes (22,133,139-142). M-CSF has a unique role during pregnancy (142), with CSF production in uterine tissue switching from GM-CSF and G-CSF in the non-pregnant state to a massive overproduction of M-CSF (27,28). A mouse lacking M-CSF cannot sustain pregnancy, but the cellular mechanisms responsible have not been determined. No other CSF fluctuates in this manner in response to sex steroids or pregnancy.

An unusual aspect of the biology of M-CSF is that, despite its ability to be produced in a fixed membrane-displayed form, serum levels of M-CSF are far higher in normal health than those of other CSFs, with normal levels in mice and humans of 1,000 to 8,000 pg/mL (66,143). These levels can increase after the injection of endotoxin in mice (73) or during infections in humans (66), and elevations have also been observed in patients with lymphoid malignancies (144).

M-CSF interacts with a specific membrane receptor on macrophages, macrophage precursors, and, in lower numbers, on neutrophils. The M-CSF receptor is the pro-tooncogene *FMS* (c-*fms*) (145); the transforming version (v-*fms*) is constitutively activated and capable of ligand-independent proliferative signaling. The high-affinity M-CSF receptor is a homodimer of two transmembrane glycoprotein chains with classic tyrosine kinase cytoplasmic domains; ligand binding results in transphosphorylation of these domains and initiation of proliferative and other signaling (146).

Actions In Vitro

In clonal cultures of human marrow cells, M-CSF has little or no capacity to stimulate colony formation. However, when combined with low concentrations of GM-CSF, a striking enhancement of colony-stimulating activity is observed (147). In cultures of murine marrow cells, M-CSF is a strong stimulus for macrophage colony formation, with maximum colony numbers developing at a concentration of 5 to 10 ng/mL. M-CSF also stimulates the formation of some granulocyte-macrophage and granulocytic colonies but not eosinophil, megakaryocytic, or erythroid colonies (2).

Little enhancing action has been observed for M-CSF in combination with SCF when acting on stem cells (40), although combination of IL-1 with M-CSF can enhance the formation of very large macrophage colonies that are likely to be formed by less mature cells than conventional macrophage progenitor cells (33). M-CSF can enhance progenitor cell survival *in vitro* and can commit bipotential granulocyte-macrophage progenitors to the exclusive formation of macrophage progeny (13). M-CSF has a range of actions on mature macrophages, including enhancement of phagocytosis and cytotoxicity for *Candida* or tumor cells, enhanced respiratory burst responses, and increased production of G-CSF, interferon, plasminogin activator-1 and -2, thromboplastin, and superoxide (148,149).

Actions In Vivo

Injection of mice with up to 10 µg of M-CSF induces a selective rise in blood monocytes (53), and a similar selective monocytosis has been observed in humans, although the absolute elevations are relatively minor in magnitude (150). On continued injection of M-CSF, some reduction in platelet levels has been observed, probably resulting from excess destruction of platelets in the spleen (151). When injected into the peritoneal cavity of mice, M-CSF induced only a minor increase in macrophage cell numbers (2).

These relatively minor responses to injected M-CSF suggest that M-CSF is not a major regulator of cell production *in vivo*. However, studies in op/op mice lacking the capacity to produce M-CSF have indicated that M-CSF is a major regulator of macrophage cell numbers. The op/op mice have a profound defect in osteoclasts, a derivative of macrophages, and this is the basis for the bone overgrowth and osteopetrotic state in these mice (46,152). This defect can be reversed by the injection of M-CSF. The op/op mice also exhibit failure of teeth eruption and major deficiencies in tissue macrophages in some organs. Mice lacking M-CSF and GM-CSF have a more severe depletion of macrophages, but some tissue macrophages are still present (153), suggesting the existence of other, as yet uncharacterized, macrophage-stimulating factors.

Multipotential Colony-Stimulating Factor: Interleukin-3

Multi-CSF, or IL-3, was first identified as a product of the murine myelomonocytic leukemic cell line WEHI-3B and was purified to homogeneity from this source and from activated T-lymphocyte–conditioned media (154,155). Murine multi-CSF is synthesized with a 26 amino acid hydrophobic leader sequence that is cleaved before secretion. The mature murine protein contains 140 amino acids, with four cysteine residues forming two intramolecular disulfide bonds and a protein core M_r of 16,200 (156,157). The molecule is variably glycosylated, giving an apparent size ranging from 22 to 34 kd. Human IL-3 is synthesized with a 19 amino acid leader sequence and is secreted as a mature protein of 133 amino acids (protein core M_r 15,400). It contains only one disulfide bond, which is homologous with one of the murine bonds (158).

The gene encoding multi-CSF is on chromosome 5q21-32 (159) in humans and on chromosome 11A5 B1 in mice (99). In both species, the IL-3 gene is closely linked to the GM-CSF gene, separated by only 9 kbp in humans and 14 kbp in mice, and both may respond to common control elements, at least in T lymphocytes.

The multi-CSF receptor is composed of a specific α chain of low affinity that, in its high-affinity form, is complexed as a heterodimer with the same β common chain used by the specific receptors for GM-CSF and IL-5 (113-115). On murine cells, a second multi-CSF–specific β chain is coexpressed and is the preferred partner in associating with the specific α chain (160).

Cells capable of producing multi-CSF *in vitro* are more restricted in range than cells able to produce the other CSFs. The dominant producer is the mitogen-activated T-lymphocyte (161), but mast cells have also been reported to produce multi-CSF (162), and there have been isolated reports of multi-CSF production by keratinocytes, eosinophils, and stromal cells (2).

The most puzzling aspect of the biology of multi-CSF is the failure to detect multi-CSF in normal serum, tissue extracts, or organ-conditioned media from such tissues (28). This deficiency is in stark contrast to the ease of producing multi-CSF *in vitro*. Because T-cell activation must be occurring even in normal animals, the failure to obtain evidence of multi-CSF production or transcription, even with polymerase chain reaction methods, is difficult to explain. However, under conditions of extreme T-cell activation, such as graft-versus-host responses, small numbers of lymphocytes produce multi-CSF (163).

Actions In Vitro

Multi-CSF is the most broadly acting of all the CSFs, and in clonal cultures of murine marrow cells, it can stimulate development of neutrophil, macrophage, eosinophil, megakaryocyte, erythroid, and blast cell colonies (164). It is also a proliferative stimulus for mast cells (165) and has a potent potentiating action when combined with SCF on the formation of progenitor cells by stem cells (40,41).

Multi-CSF also has a proliferative action on some B lymphocytes (166) and can stimulate the functional activity of macrophages and eosinophils (165,167). Multi-CSF has no action on mature human neutrophils because, unlike the situation in the mouse, the human neutrophil does not express receptors for multi-CSF.

Actions In Vivo

When injected into mice or humans, multi-CSF (IL-3) weakly elevates granulocyte or monocyte levels (164, 168,169) and elevates peripheral blood levels of progenitor cells (170). It also increases hematopoiesis in the mouse spleen and strongly elevates mast cell numbers in this organ and elsewhere (168).

More extreme changes in these populations have been observed in mice transplanted with bone marrow cells overexpressing multi-CSF (171). The likely absence of multi-CSF in the normal body is in accord with observations that mice with inactivation of the multi-CSF gene *(IL3)* show no perturbations in hematopoiesis (172).

STEM CELL FACTOR

SCF is a glycoprotein of M_r 28,000 that functions most effectively in a membrane-displayed form, although it is also produced in a secreted form. Most SCF studies have been concerned with its action on hematopoietic stem cells (31), but it also has a strong direct proliferative effect on granulocyte precursors (40). Its role in inflammatory responses has not been studied adequately.

When injected, the secreted form of SCF produces only minor elevations of granulocyte numbers (52). However, in mutant W^v or Sl^d mice lacking the ability to produce, respectively, effective SCF receptors or SCF, the animals have a moderate deficit in granulocytes (43,44) and respond relatively poorly to injected G-CSF (87).

Because of its actions on progenitor cell formation and direct actions on granulocyte formation, SCF is an important regulator of myeloid cell production and probably plays a significant role in inflammatory responses needing to be sustained.

INTERLEUKIN-5

From *in vitro* studies, only three regulatory factors are known to stimulate eosinophil formation: GM-CSF, multi-CSF, and IL-5. The action of IL-5 differs in failing to stimulate neutrophil, granulocyte, or macrophage formation (2).

IL-5 is a homodimeric glycoprotein of M_r 45,000 that may be an exclusive product of activated T lymphocytes (173).

Mice lacking the capacity to produce IL-5 or the β chain of the IL-5 receptor (shared with the GM-CSF and IL-3 α receptor chains [114]) exhibit a profound reduction in circulating eosinophils and an inability to mount effective eosinophilic inflammatory responses to helminth infestations (47,48,131). IL-5 appears not to be chemotactic for eosinophils; the active agent attracting eosinophils to inflammatory sites appears to be eotaxin (174).

ROLE OF MYELOID GROWTH FACTORS IN INFLAMMATION

Myeloid regulatory factors such as the CSFs are polyfunctional (2). They control cell proliferation, differentiation commitment, maturation, and the functional activity of the mature cells. In inflammation or infection, the myeloid regulatory factors play two distinct roles: ensuring production of the mature cells needed to take part in the inflammatory response and activating or enhancing the cellular responses made at the inflammatory site.

As determined from gene-inactivation data, G-CSF and SCF are major determinants in sustaining or elevating the production of neutrophils. The sequence of events during inflammation may be that products of microorganisms induce the local production of CSFs and chemotactic agents by direct action on producing cells or through a simple cytokine network, such as microbial products → IL-1 → G-CSF induction. Attraction of existing mature cells to the infection site, with functional activation of these cells, would in most cases terminate the infection (Fig. 27-2) in a process requiring only minutes or hours. When the magnitude of a local infection becomes sufficient to allow microbial products to enter the circulation, the resulting systemic elevation of CSF levels stimulates increased granulocyte and macrophage production in the marrow and the spleen, resulting in leukocytosis and localization of increased numbers of inflammatory cells at the infection site to resolve the infection (Fig. 27-3).

Because germ-free animals fail to develop elevated CSF levels in response to irradiation or cytotoxic drugs (2), it is less likely that products of damaged cells are a sufficient or particularly effective stimulus for eliciting CSF production. Sterile inflammatory responses are therefore less likely to result in enhanced production of CSF.

As determined in gene-inactivation studies, GM-CSF may not play an important role in controlling the production of mature granulocytes and macrophages, but it clearly plays a major role in controlling macrophage function in the lung and possibly other sites. GM-CSF has a unique role in controlling the formation of dendritic cells needed to initiate T-lymphocyte responses.

Gene-inactivation studies have established M-CSF as a major regulator of macrophage production. Enhanced levels of M-CSF production, first local and then systemic, can be expected to play a generally similar role in inflammatory responses to that outlined for G-CSF. No evidence links multi-CSF to inflammatory responses, but in principle, enhanced multi-CSF production could occur in situations involving significant T-lymphocyte activation.

Administration of CSFs protects animals against experimental infections (72,175–180). CSFs are most effective if given before an infectious challenge, possibly because this allows increased numbers of effector cells to be produced and to be available for inflammatory responses. A similar protective effect of CSF administration is observed in patients with cyclic or congenital neutropenia (181,182) and less clearly in cancer patients, in whom chemotherapy has reduced white blood cell levels (88,183,184).

ETIOLOGIC ROLE OF COLONY-STIMULATING FACTORS IN INFLAMMATION

The CSFs have a protective role in infections, but they also can cause tissue damage and chronic inflammatory

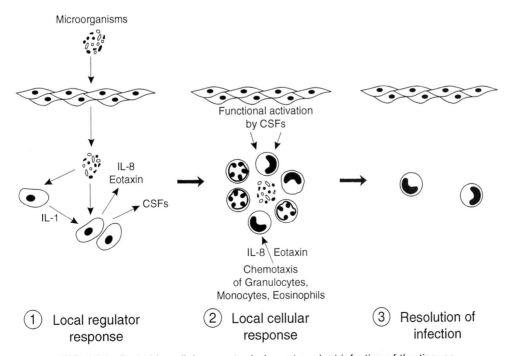

FIG. 27-2. Probable cellular events during a transient infection of the tissues.

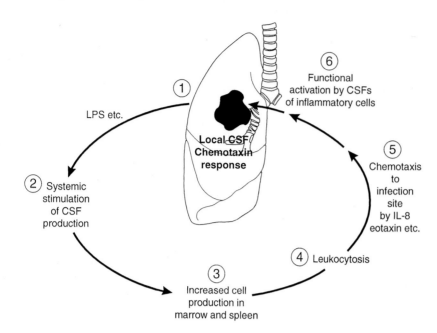

FIG. 27-3. Sequence of events occurring in response to a major microbial infection, when resolution of the infection requires production of increased numbers of mature effector cells.

states—particularly CSFs active in stimulating macrophage function. The local production of GM-CSF or M-CSF may be a proinflammatory event in certain situations in which CSF-stimulated macrophage products cause tissue damage. This appears to be the situation in GM-CSF transgenic mice (126,185), and it is conceivable that a similar series of events may occur in several inflammatory states in humans. More evidence is needed on local production of GM-CSF and M-CSF in such lesions to evaluate whether this is a significant process in initiating or sustaining an inflammatory state.

REFERENCES

1. Metcalf D, Moore MAS. *Haemopoietic cells.* Amsterdam: North-Holland, 1971.
2. Metcalf D, Nicola NA. *The hemopoietic colony stimulating factors.* Cambridge, UK: Cambridge University Press, 1995.
3. Johnson GR, Metcalf D. The commitment of multipotential hemopoietic stem cells: studies *in vivo* and *in vitro.* In: Le Douarin N, ed. *Cell lineage, stem cells and cell determination.* INSERM Symposium No. 10. The Netherlands: Elsevier/North-Holland Biomedical Press, 1979; 199–213.
4. Nakahata T, Gross AJ, Ogawa M. A stochastic model of self-renewal and commitment to differentiation of the primitive hemopoietic stem cells in culture. *J Cell Physiol* 1982;113:455–458.
5. Ogawa M, Porter PN, Nakahata T. Renewal and commitment of differentiation of hemopoietic stem cells (an interpretive review). *Blood* 1983;61: 823–829.
6. Metcalf D. *The hemopoietic colony stimulating factors.* Amsterdam: Elsevier, 1984.
7. Parwaresch MR, Wacker H-H. Origin and kinetics of resident tissue macrophages. *Cell Tissue Kinet* 1984;17:25–39.
8. Volkman A. Disparity in origin of mononuclear phagocyte populations. *J Reticuloendothel Soc* 1976;19:249–268.
9. Volkman A. The origin and turnover of mononuclear cells in peritoneal exudates in rats. *J Exp Med* 1966;124:241–254.
10. Gordon S, Perry VH, Rabinowitz S, Chung LP, Rosen H. Plasma membrane receptors of the mononuclear phagocyte system. *J Cell Sci Suppl* 1988;9:1–26.
11. Ardavin C, Wu L, Li CL, Shortman K. Thymic dendritic cells and T cells develop simultaneously in the thymus from a common precursor population. *Nature* 1993;362:761–763.
12. Young JW, Steinman RM. The hematopoietic development of dendritic cells: a distinct pathway for myeloid differentiation. *Stem Cells* 1996;14:376–387.
13. Metcalf D, Burgess AW. Clonal analysis of progenitor cell commitment to granulocyte or macrophage production. *J Cell Physiol* 1982; 111:275–283.
14. Dao C, Metcalf D, Zittoun R, Bilski-Pasquier G. Normal human bone marrow cultures *in vitro*: cellular composition and maturation of granulocytic colonies. *Br J Haematol* 1977;37:127–136.
15. Trentin JJ. Hemopoietic microenvironments. In: Tavassoli M, ed. *Handbook of the hemopoietic microenvironment.* Clifton: Humana Press, 1989:1–86.
16. Dexter TM, Spooncer E, Simons P, Allen TD. Long-term marrow culture: an overview of techniques and experience. In: Wright DG, Greenberger JS, eds. *Long-term bone marrow culture.* New York: Alan R Liss, 1984:57–96.
17. Cashman J, Eaves AC, Eaves CJ. Regulated proliferation of primitive hematopoietic progenitor cells in long-term human marrow cultures. *Blood* 1985;66:1002–1005.
18. Clark BR, Gallagher JT, Dexter TM. Cell adhesion in the stromal regulation of haemopoiesis. *Baillieres Clin Haematol* 1992;5:619–652.
19. Gordon MY, Riley GP, Watt SM, Greaves MF. Compartmentalization of a haematopoietic growth factor (GM-CSF) by a glycosaminoglycans in the bone marrow microenvironment. *Nature* 1987;326:403–405.
20. Broudy VC, Zuckerman KS, Jetmalani S, Fitchan JH, Bagby GC Jr. Monocytes stimulate fibroblastoid bone marrow stromal cells to produce multilineage hematopoietic growth factors. *Blood* 1986;68:530–534.
21. Rennick D, Yang G, Gemmell L, Lee F. Control of hemopoiesis by a bone marrow stromal cell clone: lipopolysaccharide- and interleukin-1–inducible production of colony stimulating factors. *Blood* 1987;69: 682–691.
22. Lanotte M, Metcalf D, Dexter TM. Production of monocyte/macrophage colony-stimulating factor by preadipocyte cell lines derived from murine marrow stroma. *J Cell Physiol* 1982;112:123–127.
23. Migliaccio AR, Migliaccio G, Adamson JW, Torok-Storb B. Production of granulocyte colony-stimulating factor and granulocyte/macrophage colony-stimulating factor after interleukin-1 stimulation of marrow stromal cell cultures from normal or aplastic anemia donors. *J Cell Physiol* 1992;152:199–206.
24. Stein J, Borzillo GV, Rettenmier CW. Direct stimulation of cells expressing receptors for macrophage colony-stimulating factor (CSF-1) by a plasma membrane-bound precursor of human CSF-1. *Blood* 1990;76:1308–1314.

25. Toksoz D, Zsebo KM, Smith KA, et al. Support of human hematopoiesis in long-term bone marrow cultures by murine stromal cells selectively expressing the membrane-bound and secreted forms of the human homolog of the Steel gene product, stem cell factor. *Proc Natl Acad Sci USA* 1992;89:7350–7354.

26. Metcalf D. Hemopoietic regulators: redundancy or subtlety? *Blood* 1993;82:3515–3523.

27. Bartocci A, Pollard JW, Stanley ER. Regulation of colony-stimulating factor 1 during pregnancy. *J Exp Med* 1986;164: 956–961.

28. Metcalf D, Willson TA, Hilton DJ, Di Rago L, Mifsud S. Production of hematopoietic regulatory factors in cultures of adult and fetal mouse organs: measurement by specific bioassays. *Leukemia* 1995;9: 1556–1564.

29. Kelso A, Gough NM. Coexpression of granulocyte-macrophage colony-stimulating factor, γ-interferon, and interleukins 3 and 4 is random in murine alloreactive T-lymphocyte clones. *Proc Natl Acad Sci USA* 1988;85:9189–9983.

30. Broudy VC, Kaushansky K, Harlan JM, Adamson JW. Interleukin 1 stimulates human endothelial cells to produce granulocyte-macrophage colony-stimulating factor and granulocyte colony-stimulating factor. *J Immunol* 1987;139:464–468.

31. Galli SJ, Zsebo KM, Geissler EN. The kit ligand, stem cell factor. *Adv Immunol* 1994;55:1–96.

32. Ikebuchi K, Wong GG, Clark SC, Ihle JN, Hirai Y, Ogawa M. Interleukin-6 enhancement of interleukin-3-dependent proliferation of multipotential hemopoietic progenitors. *Proc Natl Acad Sci USA* 1987;84:9035–9039.

33. Bradley TR, Hodgson GS, Bertoncello I. Characterization of macrophage progenitor cells with high proliferative potential: their relationships to cells with marrow repopulating ability in 5-fluorouracil treated mouse bone marrow. In: Baum SJ, Ledney GD, Van Bekkum DW, eds. *Experimental hematology today.* New York: Karger, 1980:285–297.

34. Hudak S, Hunte B, Culpepper J, et al. FLT3/FLK2 ligand promotes the growth and expansion of colony-forming cells and spleen colony-forming units. *Blood* 1995;85:2747–2755.

35. Jacobsen SE, Okkenhaug C, Myklebust J, Veiby OP, Lyman SD. The FLT3 ligand potently and directly stimulates the growth and expansion of primitive murine bone marrow progenitor cells *in vitro*: synergistic interactions with interleukin (IL) 11, IL-12, and other hematopoietic growth factors. *J Exp Med* 1995;181:1357–1363.

36. Jacobsen SEW, Veiby OP, Smeland EB. Cytotoxic lymphocyte maturation factor (interleukin-12) is a synergistic growth factor for hematopoietic stem cells. *J Exp Med* 1993; 178:413–418.

37. Keller JR. Gooya JM, Ruscetti FW. Direct synergistic effects of leukemia inhibitory factor on hematopoietic progenitor cell growth: comparison with other hematopoietins that use the gp130 receptor subunit. *Blood* 1996;88:863–869.

38. Li CL, Johnson GR. Rhodamine 123 reveals heterogeneity within murine Lin⁻, Sca-1⁺ hemopoietic stem cells. *J Exp Med* 1992;175: 1443–1447.

39. Meunch MD, Schneider JG, Moore MAS. Interaction amongst colony stimulating factors, IL-1β, IL-6 and kit-ligand in the regulation of primitive murine hematopoietic cells. *Exp Hematol* 1992;20:339–349.

40. Metcalf D, Nicola NA. Direct proliferative actions of stem cell factor on murine bone marrow cells *in vitro*: effects of combination with colony-stimulating factors. *Proc Natl Acad Sci USA* 1991;88: 6239–6243.

41. Metcalf D. The cellular basis for enhancement interactions between stem cell factor and the colony stimulating factors. *Stem Cells* 1993;11[Suppl 2]:1–11.

42. Lieschke GJ, Grail D, Hodgson G, et al. Mice lacking granulocyte colony-stimulating factor have chronic neutropenia, granulocyte and macrophage progenitor cell deficiency, and impaired neutrophil mobilization. *Blood* 1994;84:1737–1746.

43. Chervenick PA, Boggs DR. Decreased neutrophils and megakaryocytes in anemic mice of genotype W/Wᵛ. *J Cell Physiol* 1969;73: 25–30.

44. Ruscetti FW, Boggs DR, Torok BJ, Boggs SS. Reduced blood and marrow neutrophils and granulocytic colony-forming cells in Sl/Slᵈ mice. *Proc Soc Exp Biol Med* 1976;152:398–402.

45. Yoshida H, Hayashi S, Kunisada T, et al. The murine mutation osteopetrosis is in the coding region of the macrophage colony stimulating factor gene. *Nature* 1990;345:442–444.

46. Wiktor-Jedrzejczak W, Ratajczak MZ, Ptasznik A, Sell KW, Ahmed-Ansari A, Ostertag W. CSF-1 deficiency in the op/op mouse has differential effects on macrophage populations and differentiation stages. *Exp Hematol* 1992;20:1004–1010.

47. Kopf M, Brombacher F, Hodgkin PD, et al. IL-5–deficient mice have a developmental defect in CD5⁺ B-1 cells and lack eosinophilia but have normal antibody and cytotoxic T cell responses. *Immunity* 1996; 4:15–24.

48. Yoshida T, Ikuta K, Sugaya H, et al. Defective B-1 cell development and impaired immunity against *Angiostrongylus cantonensis* in IL-5Rα-deficient mice. *Immunity* 1996;4:483–494.

49. Metcalf D. The granulocyte-macrophage regulators: reappraisal by gene inactivation. *Exp Hematol* 1995;23:569–572.

50. Morstyn G, Campbell L, Souza LM, et al. Effect of granulocyte colony-stimulating factor on neutropenia induced by cytotoxic chemotherapy. *Lancet* 1988;1:667–672.

51. Anderlini P, Przepiorka D, Champlin R, Korbling M. Biologic and clinical effects of granulocyte colony-stimulating factor in normal individuals. *Blood* 1996;88:2819–2825.

52. Briddell RA, Hartley CA, Smith KA, McNiece IK. Recombinant rat stem cell factor synergizes with recombinant human granulocyte colony-stimulating factor *in vivo* in mice to mobilize peripheral blood progenitor cells that have enhanced repopulating potential. *Blood* 1993;82:1720–1723.

53. Hume DA, Pavli P, Donahue RE, Fidler IJ. The effect of human recombinant macrophage colony-stimulating factor (CSF-1) on the murine mononuclear phagocyte system *in vivo*. *J Immunol* 1988;141: 3405–3409.

54. Nicola NA, Metcalf D, Johnson GR, Burgess AW. Preparation of colony stimulating factors from human placental conditioned medium. *Leuk Res* 1978;2:313–322.

55. Nicola NA, Metcalf D, Matsumoto M, Johnson GR. Purification of a factor inducing differentiation in murine myelomonocytic leukemia cells: identification as granulocyte colony-stimulating factor. *J Biol Chem* 1983;258:9017–9023.

56. Souza LM, Boone TC, Gabrilove J, et al. Recombinant human granulocyte colony-stimulating factor: effects on normal and leukemic myeloid cells. *Science* 1986;232:61–65.

57. Nagata S, Tsuchiya M, Asano S, et al. Molecular cloning and expression of cDNA for human granulocyte colony-stimulating factor. *Nature* 1986;319:415–418.

58. Tsuchiya M, Asano S, Kaziro Y, Nagata S. Isolation and characterization of the cDNA for murine granulocyte colony-stimulating factor. *Proc Natl Acad Sci USA* 1986;83:7633–7637.

59. Hill CP, Osslund TD, Eisenberg D. The structure of granulocyte colony-stimulating factor and its relationship to other growth factors. *Proc Natl Acad Sci USA* 1993;90:5167–5171.

60. Lovejoy B, Cascio D, Eisenberg D. Crystal structure of canine and bovine granulocyte colony-stimulating factor (G-CSF). *J Mol Biol* 1993;234:640–653.

61. Kanda N, Fukushige S, Murotsu T, et al. Human gene coding for granulocyte colony-stimulating factor is assigned to the q21-q22 region of chromosome 17. *Somat Cell Mol Genet* 1987;13:679–684.

62. Tsuchiya M, Kaziro Y, Nagata S. The chromosomal gene structure for murine granulocyte colony-stimulating factor. *Eur J Biochem* 1987; 165:7–12.

63. Metcalf D, Nicola NA. Synthesis by mouse peritoneal cells of G-CSF, the differentiation inducer for myeloid leukemia cells: stimulation by endotoxin, M-CSF and multi-CSF. *Leuk Res* 1985;1:35–50.

64. Koeffler HP, Gasson J, Ranyard J, Souza L, Shepard M, Munker R. Recombinant human TNFα stimulates production of granulocyte colony-stimulating factor. *Blood* 1987;70:55–59.

65. Kawakami M, Tsutsumi H, Kumakawa T, et al. Levels of serum granulocyte colony-stimulating factor in patients with infections. *Blood* 1990;76:1962–1964.

66. Cebon J, Layton JE, Maher D, Morstyn G. Endogenous haemopoietic growth factors in neutropenia and infection. *Br J Haematol* 1994; 86:265–274.

67. Koeffler HP, Gasson J, Tobler A. Transcriptional and posttranscriptional modulation of myeloid colony-stimulating factor expression by tumor necrosis factor and other agents. *Mol Cell Biol* 1988;8: 3432–3438.

68. Shannon MF, Coles LS, Fielke RK, Goodall GJ, Lagnado CA, Vadas MA. Three essential promoter elements mediate tumour necrosis fac-

tor and interleukin-1 activation of the granulocyte colony-stimulating factor gene. *Growth Factors* 1992;7:181–193.

69. Nishizawa M, Nagata G. Regulatory elements responsible for inducible expression of the granulocyte colony-stimulating factor gene in macrophages. *Mol Cell Biol* 1990;10:2002–2011.

70. Cluitmans FHM, Esendam BHJ, Landegent JE, Willemze R, Falkenberg JHF. Constitutive *in vivo* cytokine and hematopoietic growth factor gene expression in the bone marrow and peripheral blood of healthy individuals. *Blood* 1995;85:2038–2044.

71. Metcalf D, Robb L, Dunn AR, Mifsud S, Di Rago L. Role of granulocyte-macrophage colony-stimulating factor and granulocyte colony-stimulating factor in the development of an acute neutrophil inflammatory response in mice. *Blood* 1996;88:3755–3764.

72. Nelson S, Daifuku R, Andresen J. Use of filgrastim (r-metHuG-CSF) in infectious diseases. In: Morstyn G, Dexter TM. eds. *Filgrastim in clinical practice.* New York: Marcel Dekker, 1994:253–266.

73. Metcalf D, Roberts AW, Willson TA. The regulation of hematopoiesis in *max 41* transgenic mice with sustained excess granulopoiesis. Leukemia 1996;10:311–320.

74. Cheers C, Haigh AM, Kelso A, Metcalf D, Stanley ER, Young AM. Production of colony-stimulating factors (CSFs) during infection: separate determinations of macrophage-, granulocyte-, granulocyte-macrophage and multi-CSFs. *Infect Immun* 1988;56: 247–251.

75. Watari S, Asano S, Shirafuji N, et al. Serum granulocyte colony-stimulating factor levels in healthy volunteers and patients with various disorders as estimated by enzyme immunoassay. *Blood* 1989;73:117–122.

76. Fukunaga R, Ishizaka-Ikeda E, Seto Y, Nagata S. Expression cloning of a receptor for murine granulocyte colony-stimulating factor. *Cell* 1990;61:341–350.

77. Larsen A, Davis T, Curtis BM, et al. Expression cloning of a human granulocyte colony-stimulating factor receptor: a structural mosaic of hematopoietin receptor, immunoglobulin, and fibronectin domains. *J Exp Med* 1990;172:1559–1570.

78. Avalos BR. Molecular analysis of the granulocyte colony-stimulating factor receptor. *Blood* 1996;88:761–777.

79. Metcalf D, Nicola NA. Proliferative effects of purified granulocyte colony-stimulating factor (G-CSF) on normal mouse hematopoietic cells. *J Cell Physiol* 1983;116:198–206.

80. Begley CG, Metcalf D, Lopez AF, Nicola NA. Fractionated populations of normal human marrow cells respond to both human colony-stimulating factors with granulocyte-macrophage activity. *Exp Hematol* 1985;13: 956–962.

81. Molineux G, Pojda Z, Dexter TM. A comparison of hematopoiesis in normal and splenectomized mice treated with granulocyte colony-stimulating factor. *Blood* 1990;75:563–569.

82. Grigg AP, Roberts AW, Raunow H, et al. Optimising dose and scheduling of filgrastim (granulocyte colony-stimulating factor) for mobilization and collection of peripheral blood progenitor cells in normal volunteers. *Blood* 1995;86:4437–4445.

83. Bonilla MA, Gillio AP, Ruggeiro M, et al. Effects of recombinant human granulocyte colony stimulating factor on neutropenia in patients with congenital agranulocytosis. *N Engl J Med* 1989;320: 1574–1580.

84. Dong F, Hoefsloot LH, Schelen AM, et al. Identification of nonsense mutation in the granulocyte colony-stimulating factor receptor in severe congenital neutropenia. *Proc Natl Acad Sci USA* 1994;91: 4480–4484.

85. Dührsen U, Villeval J-L, Boyd J, Kannourakis G, Morstyn G, Metcalf D. Effects of recombinant human granulocyte colony-stimulating factor on hemopoietic progenitor cells in cancer patients. *Blood* 1988;72: 2074–2081.

86. DeLuca E, Sheridan WP, Watson D, Szer J, Begley CG. Prior chemotherapy does not prevent effective mobilisation by G-CSF of peripheral blood progenitor cells. *Br J Cancer* 1992;66:893–899.

87. Cynshi O, Satoh K, Shimonaka Y, et al. Reduced response to granulocyte colony-stimulating factor in W/Wᵛ and Sl/Slᵈ mice. *Leukemia* 1991;5:75–77.

88. Welte K, Gabrilove J, Bronchud MH, Platzer E, Morstyn G. Filgrastim (r-metHuG-CSF): the first 10 years. *Blood* 1996;88:1907–1929.

89. Chang JM, Metcalf D, Gonda TJ, Johnson GR. Long-term exposure to retrovirally expressed G-CSF induces a non-neoplastic granulocytic and progenitor cell hyperplasia without tissue damage in mice. *J Lab Clin Invest* 1989;84:1488–1496.

90. Wang JM, Colella S, Allavena P, Mantovani A. Chemotactic activity

91. Cacalano G, Lee J, Kikly K, et al. Neutrophil and B cell expansion in mice that lack the murine IL-8 receptor homolog. *Science* 1994; 265:682–684.

92. Sheridan JW, Metcalf D. A low molecular weight factor in lung-conditioned medium stimulating granulocyte and monocyte colony formation *in vitro. J Cell Physiol* 1973;81:11–24.

93. Burgess AW, Camakaris J, Metcalf D. Purification and properties of colony-stimulating factor from mouse lung conditioned medium. *J Biol Chem* 1977;252:1998–2003.

94. Gasson JC, Weisbart RH, Kauffman SE, Clark SC, Hewick RM, Wong GG. Purified human granulocyte-macrophage colony-stimulating factor: direct action on neutrophils. *Science* 1984;226:1339–1342.

95. Gough NM, Gough J, Metcalf D, et al. Molecular cloning of cDNA encoding a murine haematopoietic growth regulator, granulocyte-macrophage colony stimulating factor. *Nature* 1984;309:763–767.

96. Wong GG, Witek JS, Temple PA, et al. Human GM-CSF: molecular cloning of the complementary DNA and purification of the natural and recombinant proteins. *Science* 1985;228:810–815.

97. Shanafelt AB, Kastelein RA. Identification of critical regions in mouse granulocyte-macrophage colony-stimulating factor by scanning-deletion analysis. *Proc Natl Acad Sci USA* 1989;86:4872–4876.

98. Huebner K, Isobe M, Croce CM, Golde DW, Kaufman SE, Gasson JC. The human gene encoding GM-CSF is at 5q21-q32, the chromosome region deleted in the 5q- anomaly. *Science* 1985;230:1282–1285.

99. Barlow DP, Bucan M, Lehrach H, Hogan BL, Gough NM. Close genetic and physical linkage between the murine haemopoietic growth factor genes GM-CSF and multi-CSF (IL3). *EMBO J* 1987;6: 617–623.

100. Shaw G, Kamen R. A conserved AU sequence from the 3′ untranslated region of GM-CSF mRNA mediates selective mRNA degradation. *Cell* 1986;46:659–667.

101. Burgess AW, Metcalf D, Russell SHM, Nicola NA. Granulocyte/macrophage-, megakaryocyte-, eosinophil- and erythroid colony-stimulating factors produced by mouse spleen cells. *Biochem J* 1980; 185:301–314.

102. Quesenberry PJ, Gimbrone MA. Vascular endothelium as a regulator of granulopoiesis: production of colony-stimulating activity by cultured human endothelial cells. *Blood* 1980;56:1060–1067.

103. Rich IN. A role for the macrophage in normal hemopoiesis. I. Functional capacity of bone-marrow–derived macrophages to release hemopoietic growth factors. *Exp Hematol* 1986;14:738–745.

104. Horowitz MC, Coleman DL, Flood PM, Kupper TS, Jilka RL. Parathyroid hormone and lipopolysaccharide induce murine osteoblast-like cells to secrete a cytokine indistinguishable from granulocyte-macrophage colony-stimulating factor. *J Clin Invest* 1989; 83:149–157.

105. Plaut M, Pierce JH, Watson CJ, Hanley-Hyde J, Nordan RP, Paul WE. Mast cell lines produce lymphokines in response to cross-linkage of FcεRI or to calcium ionophores. *Nature* 1989;339:64–67.

106. Gasson JC. Molecular physiology of granulocyte-macrophage colony-stimulating factor. *Blood* 1991;77:1131–1145.

107. Arai N, Naito Y, Watanabe M, et al. Activation of lymphokine genes in T cells: role of *cis*-acting DNA elements that respond to T cell activation signals. *Pharmacol Ther* 1992;55:303–318.

108. Shannon MF, Gamble JR, Vadas MA. Nuclear proteins interacting with the promoter region of the human granulocyte/macrophage colony-stimulating factor gene. *Proc Natl Acad Sci USA* 1988;85:674–678.

109. Cockerill PN, Shannon MF, Bert AG, Ryan GR, Vadas MA. The granulocyte-macrophage colony-stimulating factor/interleukin 3 locus is regulated by an inducible cyclosporin A–sensitive enhancer. *Proc Natl Acad Sci USA* 1993;90:2466–2470.

110. Baiocchi G, Scambia G, Benedetti P, et al. Autologous stem cell transplantation: sequential production of hematopoietic cytokines underlying granulocytic recovery. *Cancer Res* 1993;53:1297–1303.

111. Gearing DP, King JA, Gough NM, Nicola NA. Expression cloning of a receptor for human granulocyte-macrophage colony-stimulating factor. *EMBO J* 1989;8:3667–3676.

112. Hayashida K, Kitamura T, Gorman DM, Arai K, Yokota T, Miyajima A. Molecular cloning of a second subunit of the receptor for human granulocyte-macrophage colony-stimulating factor (GM-CSF): reconstitution of a high-affinity GM-CSF receptor. *Proc Natl Acad Sci USA* 1990;87:9655–9659.

113. Kitamura T, Hayashida K, Sakamaki K, Yokota T, Arai K, Miyajima A. Reconstitution of functional receptors for human granulocyte/macrophage colony-stimulating factor (GM-CSF): evidence that the protein encoded by the AIC2B cDNA is a subunit of the murine GM-CSF receptor. *Proc Natl Acad Sci USA* 1991;88:5082–5086.

114. Tavernier J, Devos R, Cornelis S, et al. A human high affinity interleukin-5 receptor (IL5R) is composed of an IL5-specific alpha chain and a beta chain shared with the receptor for GM-CSF. *Cell* 1991;66:1175–1184.

115. Smith A, Metcalf D, Nicola NA. Cytoplasmic domains of the common β-chain of the GM-CSF/IL-3/IL-5 receptors that are required for inducing differentiation or clonal suppression in myeloid leukaemic cell lines. *EMBO J* 1997;16:451–464.

116. Metcalf D, Burgess AW, Johnson GR, et al. *In vitro* actions on hemopoietic cells of recombinant murine GM-CSF purified after production in *Escherichia coli:* comparison with purified native GM-CSF. *J Cell Physiol* 1986;128:421–431.

117. Metcalf D, Begley CG, Johnson GR, et al. Biologic properties *in vitro* of a recombinant human granulocyte-macrophage colony-stimulating factor. *Blood* 1986;67:37–45.

118. Metcalf D, Merchav S. Effects of GM-CSF deprivation on precursors of granulocytes and macrophages. *J Cell Physiol* 1982;112:411–418.

119. Begley CG, Lopez AF, Nicola NA, et al. Purified colony stimulating factors enhance the survival of human neutrophils and eosinophils *in vitro*: a rapid and sensitive microassay for colony stimulating factors. *Blood* 1986;68:162–166.

120. Grant SM, Heel RC. Recombinant granulocyte-macrophage colony-stimulating factor (rGM-CSF). A review of its pharmacological properties and prospective role in the management of myelosuppression. *Drugs* 1992;43:516–560.

121. Lieschke GJ, Maher D, Cebon J, et al. Effects of bacterially synthesized recombinant human granulocyte-macrophage colony-stimulating factor in patients with advanced malignancy. *Ann Intern Med* 1989;110:357–364.

122. Ganser A, Völkers B, Greher J, et al. Recombinant human granulocyte-macrophage colony-stimulating factor in patients with myelodysplastic syndromes: a phase I/II trial. *Blood* 1989;73:31–37.

123. Metcalf D, Begley CG, Williamson D, et al. Hemopoietic responses in mice injected with purified recombinant murine GM-CSF. *Exp Hematol* 1987;15:1–9.

124. Socinski MA, Cannistra SA, Elias A, Antman KH, Schnipper L, Griffin JD. Granulocyte-macrophage colony-stimulating factor expands the circulating haemopoietic progenitor cell compartment in man. *Lancet* 1988;1:1194–1198.

125. Villeval J-L, Dührsen U, Morstyn G, Metcalf D. Effect of recombinant human granulocyte-macrophage colony-stimulating factor on progenitor cells in patients with advanced malignancies. *Br J Haematol* 1990;74:36–44.

126. Lang RA, Metcalf D, Cuthbertson RA, et al. Transgenic mice expressing a hemopoietic growth factor gene (GM-CSF) develop accumulations of macrophages, blindness and a fatal syndrome of tissue damage. *Cell* 1987;51:675–686.

127. Metcalf D, Elliott MJ, Nicola NA. The excess numbers of peritoneal macrophages in granulocyte-macrophage colony-stimulating factor transgenic mice are generated by local proliferation. *J Exp Med* 1992;175:877–884.

128. Elliott MJ, Strasser A, Metcalf D. Selective up-regulation of macrophage function in granulocyte-macrophage colony-stimulating factor transgenic mice. *J Immunol* 1991;147:2957–2963.

129. Johnson GR, Gonda TJ, Metcalf D, Hariharan IK, Cory S. A lethal myeloproliferative syndrome in mice transplanted with bone marrow cells infected with a retrovirus expressing granulocyte-macrophage colony-stimulating factor. *EMBO J* 1989;8:441–448.

130. Dranoff G, Crawford AD, Sadelain M, et al. Involvement of granulocyte-macrophage colony-stimulating factor in pulmonary homeostasis. *Science* 1994;264:713–716.

131. Robb L, Drinkwater CC, Metcalf D, et al. Hematopoietic and lung abnormalities in mice with a null mutation of the common β subunit of the receptors for granulocyte-macrophage colony-stimulating factor and interleukins 3 and 5. *Proc Natl Acad Sci USA* 1995;92:9565–9569.

132. Stanley ER, Hansen G, Woodcock J, Metcalf D. Colony stimulating factor and the regulation of granulopoiesis and macrophage production. *Fed Proc* 1975;34:2272–2278.

133. Stanley ER, Heard PM. Factors regulating macrophage production and growth. Purification and some properties of the colony stimulating factor from medium conditioned by mouse L cells. *J Biol Chem* 1977;252:4305–4312.

134. Pandit J, Bohm A, Jancarik J, Halenbeck R, Koths K, Kim SH. Three-dimensional structure of dimeric human recombinant macrophage colony-stimulating factor. *Science* 1992;258:1358–1362.

135. Cerretti DP, Wignall J, Anderson D, et al. Human macrophage colony-stimulating factor: alternative RNA and protein processing from a single gene. *Mol Immunol* 1988;25:761–770.

136. Baccarini M, Stanley ER. Colony stimulating factor-1. In: Habenicht A, ed. *Growth factors, differentiation factors, and cytokines*. Berlin: Springer-Verlag, 1990:189–200.

137. Morris SW, Valentine MB, Shapiro DN, et al. Reassignment of the human CSF1 gene to chromosome 1p13-p21. *Blood* 1991;78:2013–2020.

138. Wiktor-Jedrzejczak W, Bartocci A, Ferrante AW Jr, et al. Total absence of colony-stimulating factor 1 in the macrophage-deficient osteopetrotic (op/op) mouse. *Proc Natl Acad Sci USA* 1990;87:4828–4832.

139. Horiguchi J, Warren MK, Ralph P, Kufe D. Expression of the macrophage specific colony-stimulating factor (CSF-1) during monocytic differentiation. *Biochem Biophys Res Commun* 1986;141:924–930.

140. Seelentag WK, Mermod J-J, Montesano R, Vassalli P. Additive effects of interleukin 1 and tumour necrosis factor-alpha on the accumulation of the three granulocyte and macrophage colony-stimulating factor mRNAs in human endothelial cells. *EMBO J* 1987;6:2261–2265.

141. Wong GG, Temple PA, Leary AC, et al. Human CSF-1: molecular cloning and expression of 4 kb encoding the human urinary protein. *Science* 1987;235:1504–1508.

142. Bartocci A, Pollard JW, Stanley ER. Regulation of colony-stimulating factor 1 during pregnancy. *J Exp Med* 1986;164:956–961.

143. Aihara T, Misago M, Hanamura T, et al. Within-day and day-to-day variations of serum M-CSF levels in healthy volunteers. *Rinsho Byori* 1993;41:268–272.

144. Janowska-Wieczorek A, Belch AR, Jacobs A, et al. Increased circulating colony-stimulating factor-1 in patients with preleukemia, leukemia, and lymphoid malignancies. Blood 1991;77:1796–1803.

145. Sherr CJ, Rettenmier CW, Sacca R, Roussel MF, Look AT, Stanley ER. The c-fms proto-oncogene product is related to the receptor for the mononuclear phagocyte growth factor, CSF-1. *Cell* 1985;41:665–676.

146. Sherr CJ. Colony-stimulating factor-1 receptor. *Blood* 1990;75:1–12.

147. Caracciolo D, Shirsat N, Wong GG, Lange B, Clark S, Rovera G. Recombinant human macrophage colony-stimulating factor (M-CSF) requires subliminal concentrations of granulocyte/macrophage (GM)-CSF for optimal stimulation of human macrophage colony formation *in vitro*. *J Exp Med* 1987;166:1851–1860.

148. Nemunaitis J. Macrophage function activating cytokines: potential clinical application. *Crit Rev Oncol Hematol* 1993;14:152–171.

149. Van de Pol CJ, Garnick MB. Clinical applications of recombinant macrophage colony-stimulating factor (rhM-CSF). *Biotechnol Ther* 1991;2:231–239.

150. Redman BC, Flaherty L, Chan TH, et al. Phase I trial of recombinant macrophage colony-stimulating factor by rapid intravenous infusion in patients with cancer. *J Immunother* 1992;12:50–54.

151. Garnick MB, Stoudemire JB. Preclinical and clinical evaluation of recombinant human macrophage colony-stimulating factor (rhM-CSF). *Int J Cell Cloning* 1990;8:356–371.

152. Witmer-Pack MD, Hughes DA, Schuler G, Lawson L, McWilliam A, Inaba K, Steinman RM, Gordon S. Identification of macrophages and dendritic cells in the osteopetrotic (op/op) mouse. *J Cell Sci* 1993;104:1021–1029.

153. Lieschke GJ, Stanley E, Grail D, et al. Mice lacking both macrophage- and granulocyte-macrophage colony-stimulating factor have macrophages and co-existent osteopetrosis and severe lung disease. *Blood* 1994;84:27–35.

154. Ihle JN, Keller J, Henderson L, Klein F, Palaszynski E. Procedures for the purification of interleukin 3 to homogeneity. *J Immunol* 1982;129:2431–2436.

155. Cutler RL, Metcalf D, Nicola NA, Johnson GR. Purification of a multipotential colony stimulating factor from pokeweed mitogen-stimulated mouse spleen cell conditioned medium. *J Biol Chem* 1985;260:6579–6587.

156. Fung M-C, Hapel AJ, Ymer S, et al. Molecular cloning of cDNA for murine interleukin-3. *Nature* 1984;307:233–237.

157. Clark-Lewis I, Hood LE, Kent SB. Role of disulfide bridges in determining the biological activity of interleukin 3. *Proc Natl Acad Sci USA* 1988;85:7897–7901.

158. Yang Y-C, Ciarletta AB, Temple PA, et al. Human IL-3 (multi-CSF): identification by expression cloning of a novel hematopoietic growth factor related to murine IL-3. *Cell* 1986;47:3–10.

159. Yang YC, Kovacic S, Kriz R, et al. The human genes for GM-CSF and IL3 are closely linked in tandem in chromosome 5. *Blood* 1988;71:958–961.

160. Nicola NA, Robb L, Metcalf D, Cary D, Drinkwater CC, Begley CG. Functional inactivation in mice of the gene for the interleukin-3 (IL-3)-specific receptor β-chain: implications for IL-3 function and the mechanism of receptor transmodulation in hematopoietic cells. *Blood* 1996;87:2665–2674.

161. Kelso A, Metcalf D. T lymphocyte-derived colony-stimulating factors. *Adv Immunol* 1990;48:69–105.

162. Wodnar-Filipowicz A, Heusser CH, Moroni C. Production of the haemopoietic growth factors GM-CSF and interleukin-3 by mast cells in response to IgE receptor-mediated activation. *Nature* 1989; 339:150–152.

163. Troutt AB, Kelso A. Enumeration of lymphokine mRNA-containing cells *in vivo* in a murine graft-versus-host reaction using the PCR. *Proc Natl Acad Sci USA* 1992;89:5276–5280.

164. Metcalf D, Begley CG, Nicola NA, Johnson GR. Quantitative responsiveness of murine hemopoietic populations *in vitro* and *in vivo* to recombinant multi-CSF (IL-3). *Exp Hematol* 1987;15:288–295.

165. Clark-Lewis I, Schrader JW. Molecular structure and biological activities of P cell-stimulating factor (interleukin 3). *Lymphokines* 1988;15:1–37.

166. Xia X, Li L, Choi YS. Human recombinant IL-3 is a growth factor for normal B cells. *J Immunol* 1992;148:491–497.

167. Yang YC, Clark SC. Interleukin-3: molecular biology and biologic activities. *Hematol Clin North Am* 1989;3:441–452.

168. Metcalf D, Begley CG, Johnson GR, Nicola NA, Lopez AF, Williamson DJ. Effects of purified bacterially synthesized murine multi-CSF (IL-3) on hematopoiesis in normal adult mice. *Blood* 1986;68:46–57.

169. Ganser A, Lindemann A, Seipelt G, et al. Effects of recombinant human interleukin-3 in patients with normal hematopoiesis and in patients with bone marrow failure. *Blood* 1990;76:666–676.

170. Ottmann OG, Ganser A, Seipelt IG, Eder M, Schulz G, Hoelzer D. Effects of recombinant human interleukin-3 on human hematopoietic progenitor and precursor cells *in vivo*. *Blood* 1990;76:1494–1502.

171. Chang JM, Metcalf D, Lang RA, Gonda TJ, Johnson GR. Non-neoplastic hematopoietic myeloproliferative syndrome induced by dysregulated multi-CSF (IL-3) expression. *Blood* 1989;73:1487–1497.

172. Nishinakamura R, Miyajima A, Mee PJ, Tybulewicz VLJ, Murray R. Hematopoiesis in mice lacking the entire granulocyte-macrophage colony-stimulating factor/interleukin-3/interleukin-5 functions. *Blood* 1996;88:2458–2464.

173. Sanderson C. Interleukin-5, eosinophils and disease. *Blood* 1992;79:3101–3109.

174. Collins PD, Marleau S, Griffiths-Johnson DA, Jose PJ, Williams TJ. Cooperation between interleukin-5 and chemokine eotaxin to induce eosinophil accumulation *in vivo*. *J Exp Med* 1995;182:1169–1174.

175. Matsumoto M, Matsubara S, Matsuno T, et al. Protective effect of human granulocyte colony-stimulating factor on microbial infection in neutropenic mice. *Infect Immun* 1987;55:2715–2720.

176. Yasuda H, Ajiki Y, Shimozato T, et al. Therapeutic efficacy of granulocyte colony-stimulating factor alone and in combination with antibiotics against *Pseudomonas aeruginosa* infections in mice. *Infect Immun* 1990;58:2502–2509.

177. Cairo MS, Mauss D, Kommareddy S, Norris K, Van de Ven C, Modanlou H. Prophylactic or simultaneous administration of recombinant human granulocyte colony stimulating factor in the treatment of group B streptococcal sepsis in neonatal rats. *Pediatr Res* 1990;27:612–616.

178. Toda H, Murata A, Matsuura N, et al. Therapeutic efficacy of granulocyte colony stimulating factor against rat cecal ligation and puncture model. *Stem Cells* 1993;11:228–234.

179. Talmadge JF, Tribble H, Pennington R, et al. Protective, restorative and therapeutic properties of recombinant colony stimulating factors. *Blood* 1989;73:2093–2103.

180. Tanikawa S, Nose M, Aoki Y, Tsuneoka K, Shikita M, Nara N. Effects of recombinant human granulocyte colony-stimulating factor on the hematologic recovery and survival of irradiated mice. *Blood* 1990;76:445–449.

181. Welte K, Zeidler C, Reiter A, et al. Differential effects of granulocyte-macrophage colony-stimulating factor and granulocyte colony-stimulating factor in children with severe congenital neutropenia. *Blood* 1990;75:1056–1063.

182. Dale DC, Bonilla MA, Davis MW, et al. Randomized controlled phase III trial of recombinant human granulocyte colony-stimulating factor (filgrastim) for treatment of severe chronic neutropenia. *Blood* 1993;81:2496–2502.

183. Crawford J, Ozer H, Stoller R, et al. Reduction by granulocyte colony-stimulating factor of fever and neutropenia induced by chemotherapy in patients with small-cell lung cancer. *N Engl J Med* 1991;325:164–170.

184. Nemunaitis J, Shannon-Dorey K, Appelbaum FR, et al. Long-term follow-up of patients with invasive fungal disease who received adjunctive therapy with recombinant human macrophage colony-stimulating factor. *Blood* 1993;82:1422–1427.

185. Metcalf D, Moore JG. Divergent disease patterns in GM-CSF transgenic mice associated with differing transgene insertion sites. *Proc Natl Acad Sci USA* 1988;85:7767–7771.

Inflammation: Basic Principles and Clinical Correlates,
3rd ed., edited by John I. Gallin and Ralph Snyderman.
Lippincott Williams & Wilkins, Philadelphia © 1999.

CHAPTER 28

Chemokines

Marco Baggiolini, Beatrice Dewald, and Bernhard Moser

In 1991, when we submitted the manuscript for the second edition of this book, only few chemokines had been reported (1,2), and no publication on chemokine receptors had yet appeared. Today, nearly 40 human chemokines and 12 chemokine receptors are known. Chemokines are by far the largest family of cytokines and form a complex system for the chemotactic activation of all types of leukocytes. The expression of chemokine receptors differs with the type of leukocyte, and in some cells (T lymphocytes in particular), it depends on the degree of activation. Receptor expression and generation of different chemokines are the basis for the selective recruitment of leukocytes and the composition of the inflammatory infiltrate as observed in different inflammation pathologies. Chemokines are studied mainly because of their effects on leukocytes and their roles in inflammation and immunity. Additional interest arose from the discovery that chemokine receptors function as cellular recognition sites for human immunodeficiency virus (HIV) and that chemokines have HIV-suppressive activity.

In this chapter, we present the essential properties of human chemokines and chemokine receptors and describe their main functions. No references are given for well-established facts, which can be traced in our two comprehensive reviews (3,4). Additional reviews may be consulted for special aspects of the field (5–9). The systematic nomenclature for chemokine receptors, which was elaborated at the 1996 Gordon Research Conference on Chemotactic Cytokines, is used. Depending on their selectivity for CXC or CC chemokines, receptors are designated as CXCR or CCR followed by a number (Table 28-1).

CHEMOKINE STRUCTURES

Chemokines have four conserved cysteines that form two disulfide bonds (Cys1 → Cys3 and Cys2 → Cys4). Two subfamilies, CXC and CC chemokines or α and β chemokines, are distinguished according to the position of the first two cysteines that are adjacent (CC) or separated by one amino acid (CXC). Most chemokine cDNAs encode proteins of 92 to 125 amino acids with leader sequences of 20 to 25 amino acids. Interleukin-8 (IL-8) may be regarded as the prototype for CXC chemokines and monocyte chemotactic protein-1 (MCP-1) as the prototype for CC chemokines (3).

Three-Dimensional Structure

In concentrated solution and on crystallization, IL-8 is present as a dimer, as shown by nuclear magnetic resonance (NMR) spectroscopy and x-ray crystallography (10,11). The monomer has a short, conformationally flexible NH_2-terminal domain followed by three antiparallel β strands connected by loops and a prominent COOH-terminal α helix. The dimer is stabilized by hydrogen bonds between the first β strands of the monomers and by amino acid side chain interactions. The structures of growth-related oncogene-α (GRO-α) and neutrophil-activating protein-2 (NAP-2) are similar to that of IL-8 at the monomer and dimer level (4). The monomer structure of CC chemokines is analogous to that of CXC chemokines. As shown for macrophage inflammatory protein-1β (MIP-1β) and RANTES (regulated on activation, normally T-cell expressed and secreted), CC chemokines also form dimers in solution, but the site of interaction between the monomers is in the NH_2-terminal region, and the dimer has an elongated, cylindrical shape (12,13,14). The different mode of dimerization of CXC and CC chemokines presumably reflects the different distribution of hydrophobicity regions on the surface of the monomers (15,16). In contrast, the core hydrophobicity

M. Baggiolini, B. Dewald, and B. Moser: Theodor-Kocher Institute, University of Bern, Bern, Switzerland CH-3012.

TABLE 28-1. *Human chemokine receptors and their ligands*

| Receptors | Nomenclature | | Ligands[a] |
	New	Old	
CXC chemokine receptors	CXCR1	IL-8R1 (type A)	IL-8, GCP-2
	CXCR2	IL-8R2 (type B)	IL-8, GROα,β,γ, NAP-2, ENA78, GCP-2
	CXCR3	IP10/MigR	IP10, Mig, I-TAC
	CXCR4	LESTR, HUMSTR, fusin, etc.	SDF-1
CC chemokine receptors	CCR1	RANTES/MIP-1αR	RANTES, MIP-1α, MCP-2, MCP-3
	CCR2	MCP-1R	MCP-1, MCP-2, MCP-3, MCP-4
	CCR3	EotaxinR	Eotaxin, Eotaxin-2, RANTES, MCP-2, MCP-3, MCP-4
	CCR4		TARC
	CCR5		RANTES, MIP-1α, MIP-1β
	CCR6	CKR-L3, STRL22	LARC (MIP-3α)
	CCR7	EBI1, BLR2	ELC (MIP-3β)
	CCR8	TER1, ChemR1, CKR-L1	I-309

[a]Shown by high-affinity binding or induction of Ca^{2+}-mobilization.

clusters have a similar distribution in chemokines of both subfamilies, and this explains why the three-dimensional structures of the monomers are comparable.

Monomers and Dimers

Because several chemokines form dimers in solution, it was proposed that the dimer is the biologically relevant structure (4). However, chemokines exert their biologic effects at nanomolar concentrations, far below the dissociation constant of the dimers (17,18). To show that IL-8 can function as a monomer, an analogue was synthesized with N-methyl-Leu instead of Leu at position 25 of the 72 amino acid form. The methyl group disturbs hydrogen bond formation and prevents dimerization, but the analogue is as active as wild-type IL-8 (19). Monomeric forms of MIP-1α are also biologically active (20), and NMR structure studies have shown that macrophage chemotactic protein-3 (MCP-3) does not dimerize (21).

CHEMOKINE EXPRESSION

Numerous publications document the expression of CXC and CC chemokines at sites of inflammation, infection, and immune reactions. The main sources are immigrant leukocytes, resident macrophages, mast cells, and tissue cells such as fibroblasts, endothelial cells, and epithelial cells. The most common inducers are inflammatory cytokines (e.g., IL-1, tumor necrosis factor [TNF], interferon-γ [IFN-γ]), endotoxins, hematopoietic growth factors, and phagocytosis (3). Most chemokines are products of inducible genes responding to local stimulation, but some, such as stromal cell–derived factor-1 (SDF-1) (22) and HCC-1 (23), appear to be produced constitutively. Studies with cultured leukocytes or cell lines and *in situ* analysis of inflamed tissues show that chemokines of different kinds are often generated concomitantly.

BIOLOGIC ACTIVITIES

The dendrogram in Figure 28-1 presents all human chemokines for which receptors or at least clear activities on leukocytes have been reported. Chemokines act mainly on leukocytes and induce chemotaxis that may be assessed *in vitro* or *in vivo*. In granulocytes, chemokine activities are similar to those of the classic chemoattractants, C5a, N-formyl-L-methionyl-L-leucyl-L-phenylalanine (fMLP), platelet-activating factor, and leukotriene B$_4$. Like these, the chemokines elicit migration and a characteristic pattern of functions that are required for host defense in infection and inflammation, including activation of the cytoskeleton, enhanced adhesion, granule exocytosis, formation of bioactive lipids, and a respiratory burst (3).

CXC Chemokines

In the past, CXC chemokines were thought to act through IL-8 receptors exclusively on neutrophils. This simple concept had to be revised when two new CXC chemokine receptors, CXCR3 and CXCR4, were characterized and shown to mediate lymphocyte and monocyte chemotaxis (24–26).

Interleukin-8 and Other Neutrophil-Activating Chemokines

IL-8 has been studied much more extensively than any other chemokine. It was identified as an agonist for neutrophils on the basis of two *in vitro* effects—chemotaxis and the release of granule enzymes (27–29)—and was subsequently shown to bind to two receptors that are abundantly expressed on neutrophils, CXCR1 and CXCR2 (3). In our laboratory, the study of IL-8 at the level of the receptors, signaling, and functional responses became the basis of comparison for the characterization of many other chemokines (3,30).

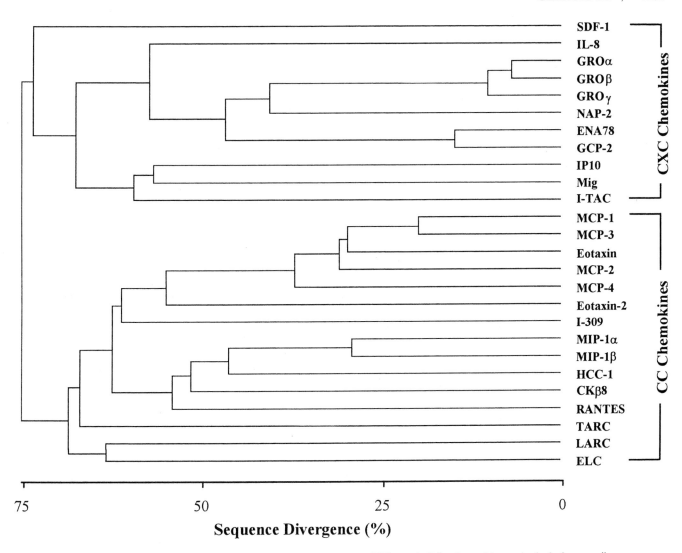

FIG. 28-1. Structure similarity is shown for human CXC and CC chemokines. Included are all chemokines with defined function and receptor selectivity. The distance to the branching points indicates the percentage (%) of sequence divergence. The overall similarity of the two subfamilies of chemokines is 24.5%.

The *shape change* reflects the activation of the cytoskeleton and the transient assembly of filamentous actin, a prerequisite for adherence to endothelial cells and migration. *Exocytosis* leads to the release of enzymes and other contents from subcellular storage granules. The granules fuse with the plasma membrane and partly change its properties, such as by upregulating the expression of integrins. The *formation of bioactive lipids,* prostanoids, leukotrienes, and platelet-activating factor, is a complex and important proinflammatory process that is initiated by activation of phospholipase A_2 (31,32). The *respiratory burst* is a characteristic feature of stimulated phagocytes. It is induced by the assembly and activation of a membrane-bound electron transport chain that oxidizes cytosolic NADPH and reduces extracellular oxygen to superoxide (33). All these receptor-mediated responses are preceded by a characteristic, rapid rise of the intracellular free Ca^{2+}

concentration ($[Ca^{2+}]_i$), which can be taken as a correlate of chemokine activity in all types of leukocytes.

Six other CXC chemokines, NAP-2, GRO-α, GRO-β, GRO-γ, epithelial cell–derived neutrophil-activating peptide-78 (ENA-78), and granulocyte chemotactic protein-2 (GCP-2), are also selective chemoattractants for neutrophils and elicit responses similar to those of IL-8 (3). They share with IL-8 the short sequence motif Glu-Leu-Arg (ELR) preceding the first cysteine that is required for receptor triggering. Unlike IL-8, which binds with high affinity to CXCR1 and CXCR2, all other ELR chemokines have high affinity for CXCR2 but only low affinity for CXCR1.

The responses elicited by single IL-8 receptors were analyzed in Jurkat cells stably transfected with the cDNA coding for CXCR1 or CXCR2. Both receptors mediate chemotaxis in response to IL-8, GRO-α, and NAP-2.

Cells expressing CXCR2 are equally responsive to IL-8 and the related chemokines, but cells expressing CXCR1 are 300- to 1000-fold less sensitive to GRO-α or NAP-2 than to IL-8, in agreement with the differences in binding affinity (34). Monoclonal antibodies that selectively block one or the other receptor reveal functional differences between CXCR1 and CXCR2 in neutrophils. Whereas $[Ca^{2+}]_i$ changes, chemotaxis, and granule enzyme release are mediated by both receptors, the respiratory burst and the activation of phospholipase D depend exclusively on CXCR1 (35,36). IL-8 also acts on basophils, eosinophils, and monocytes (3); natural killer (NK) cells (37); and subsets of naive T lymphocytes (38). The responses observed, however, are very weak in comparison with those of neutrophils.

Interferon-γ–Inducible Protein-10 and Monokine Induced by Interferon-γ

IFN-γ–inducible protein-10 (IP-10) and monokine induced by IFN-γ (MIG) are CXC chemokines (39,40). IP-10 was found in delayed-type hypersensitivity reactions of the skin, which are characterized by a lymphocytic infiltration (41), but its function remained unclear for many years. IP-10 was reported to attract human monocytes, T lymphocytes, and NK cells (42,43), and MIG was shown to attract tumor-infiltrating T lymphocytes (44). The riddle of the two interferon-inducible chemokines was solved with the cloning of a novel CXC chemokine receptor, CXCR3, which is selective for IP-10 and MIG and is expressed exclusively on activated T lymphocytes (24). The restricted expression and selectivity of CXCR3 and the fact that IP-10 and MIG are induced by IFN-γ suggest that these chemokines mediate the characteristic accumulation of lymphocytes that is observed in viral infections, autoimmune inflammation, and delayed-type hypersensitivity where IFN-γ is upregulated. In a survey of chemokine levels in cerebrospinal fluid, IP-10 was detected in 80% of the patients with viral meningitis, but not in patients with Guillian-Barré syndrome (44a). Interferon-inducible T cell alpha chemoattractant (I-TAC) is another IFN-γ–induced chemokine that selectively binds CXCR3 (44b).

Stromal Cell–Derived Factor-1

SDF-1 corresponds to pre-B-cell growth-stimulating factor (22,45,46). It was originally described as a product of bone marrow stromal cells that acts in synergy with IL-7 as a stimulus of progenitor B-cell proliferation. SDF-1 has all the structural features of a CXC chemokine. Human SDF-1 consists of 67 amino acids and differs from its murine homologue by a single substitution (Val[18] instead of Ile[18]) and the deletion of the COOH-terminal lysine. Such a high degree of sequence identity between human and murine chemokines is unique.

SDF-1 was characterized as a chemoattractant for lymphocytes, monocytes, and neutrophils and qualified as a chemokine in terms of function (25,26). It acts through CXCR4, a chemokine receptor that was cloned in several laboratories and is expressed in different types of leukocytes (4). Work has established that SDF-1 attracts CD34+ B precursor cells at early stages of maturation (47,48). Disruption of the SDF-1 gene in mice results in a marked reduction of B-lymphocyte and myeloid cell progenitors in the bone marrow and developmental disturbances, including a septal defect of the heart, that lead to perinatal death. SDF-1 is an unusual chemokine that may display functions that go beyond chemotaxis and leukocyte activation (24). It became prominent as HIV-1 suppressive factor (25,26) when CXCR4 was recognized as HIV-1 coreceptor (49).

CC Chemokines

Monocyte Chemotactic Proteins

MCP-1 was the first CC chemokine to be characterized. It was shown to attract monocytes but not neutrophils, and it was initially viewed as the counterpart of IL-8, which has the opposite properties (3). Two related proteins, MCP-2 and MCP-3, were subsequently identified (50), and MCP-4 was described later (51). The MCPs are closely related to each other and to eotaxin (56% to 71% amino acid sequence identity). All MCPs have a 10-residue NH₂-terminal domain preceding the first cysteine, which starts with pyroglutamic acid followed by proline.

All MCPs act on monocytes, T lymphocytes, and basophils. MCP-2, MCP-3, and MCP-4 are also active on eosinophils, whereas MCP-1 is not (4). At least three receptors mediate these responses: CCR2, which recognizes all the MCPs, and CCR1 and CCR3, which recognize MCP-2, MCP-3, and MCP-4. In basophils, MCP-1 is a strong stimulus of histamine and leukotriene release but only a moderate chemoattractant, whereas RANTES is a strong chemoattractant and a weak inducer of release. This suggests that CCR1 (receptor for RANTES) and CCR2 (receptor for MCP-1) are functionally different; MCP-3, which binds equally well to both receptors, is highly effective as stimulus of migration and release (5).

The effects of the MCPs on lymphocytes are of particular interest. Studies on human CD4 or CD8+ T-cell clones and blood mononuclear cells demonstrate that all four MCPs are potent attractants for activated T lymphocytes (51–53). MCP-1, MCP-3, and MCP-4 induce $[Ca^{2+}]_i$ changes that are inhibited by pretreatment with pertussis toxin and attract more T cells than RANTES, MIP-1α, and MIP-1β across bare or endothelial cell–coated filters (51,53). Similar migration responses were observed with dendritic cells (54) and NK cells (55), in which the MCPs induce $[Ca^{2+}]_i$ changes and exocytosis of granzyme A and *N*-acetyl-β-D-glucosamini-dase (56).

RANTES and Macrophage Inflammatory Proteins

RANTES was originally presented as a chemoattractant for T lymphocytes (57) that were subsequently shown to respond to the macrophage inflammatory proteins MIP-1α and MIP-1β as well (58). T cells express CCR1, a receptor for RANTES and MIP-1α, and CCR5, which is the only receptor that binds RANTES, MIP-1α, and MIP-1β (see Table 28-1). RANTES is a powerful chemoattractant for basophils (through CCR1 and CCR3) and eosinophils (through CCR3), and these effects are probably more important than those on T lymphocytes, which respond more readily to the MCPs and some chemokines, such as IP-10 and MIG, that are selective for these cells.

Murine MIP-1α and MIP-1β enhance the proliferation of granulocyte-macrophage progenitor cells in the presence of granulocyte-macrophage colony-stimulating factor (GM-CSF) or colony-stimulating factor-1 (59). In contrast, the proliferation of earlier progenitor cells that depend on IL-3 is suppressed by MIP-1α (60). The stem cell–inhibiting effect of MIP-1α (61) is prevented by MIP-1β (62). The effects of MIP-1α on hematopoietic precursors were reviewed by Cook (63). Disruption of the MIP-1α gene in mice did not yield overt abnormalities of blood or bone marrow cells, indicating that MIP-1α is not necessary for normal hematopoiesis. These mice, however, have a reduced inflammatory response to influenza virus and are resistant to coxsackievirus-induced myocarditis (63,64). Several other chemokines affected colony formation in bone marrow cultures, but despite intensive research, the roles of chemokines in hematopoiesis and their mechanisms of action remain unclear (65).

Eotaxin

Eotaxin was originally isolated from the bronchoalveolar fluid of guinea pigs with allergic lung inflammation (66) and the murine (67) and human homologues (68) were subsequently cloned. Its sequence is closely related to that of the MCPs, but eotaxin has only 7 instead of 10 amino acids before the first cysteine and lacks the pyroglutamate-proline motif that is conserved among the MCPs (4). Human eotaxin is selective for the chemokine receptor CCR3, whereas other chemokines (especially MCP-3, MCP-4, and RANTES) recognize CCR3 in addition to other receptors. CCR3 is highly expressed on eosinophils (69,70) and basophils (71,72), and it is found on subsets of T lymphocytes (73). All these cells readily respond to eotaxin, which is inactive on neutrophils and monocytes (51,68). Eotaxin attracts eosinophils when applied *in vivo*, and its expression is enhanced in tissue cells at sites of eosinophil accumulation (68).

Eotaxin-2 is a functional homologue of eotaxin that acts exclusively through CCR3 (74). It is chemotactic for eosinophils and basophils, and it induces the release of histamine and leukotriene C_4 from basophils. When applied intradermally in a monkey, eotaxin-2 induced a marked local infiltration of eosinophils (74). The functional similarity is surprising because eotaxin and eotaxin-2 share only 39% identical amino acids and differ almost completely in the NH_2-terminal region.

Other New CC Chemokines

Several other human chemokines have been identified and at least partially characterized. HCC-1 has 46% sequence identity with MIP-1α and MIP-1β and was reported to enhance the proliferation of $CD34^+$ myeloid progenitor cells (23). A peculiar feature is the constitutive expression of this chemokine in several tissues, including spleen, liver, skeletal and heart muscle, gut, and bone marrow, as well as its presence at high concentration in plasma (23).

CK-β8 (75) is a CC chemokine with six cysteines. It is expressed in liver, in the gastrointestinal tract, and by monocytes activated with IL-1β or IFN-γ. It is chemotactic for monocytes but not for T lymphocytes, eosinophils, or neutrophils. Cross-desensitization experiments suggest that CK-β8 acts by means of a receptor that is recognized by all MCPs, MIP-1α, MIP-1β, and RANTES, and it therefore appears to differ from the chemokine receptors previously described.

TARC (thymus and activation-regulated chemokine) (76) is expressed constitutively in the thymus but also in phytohemagglutinin antigen–stimulated blood mononuclear cells. TARC is a specific ligand for CCR4 and was reported to be chemotactic for T cell lines.

LARC (liver and activation-regulated chemokine) (77), which is also called MIP-3α (78), is expressed mainly in the liver, but also in lymph nodes, appendix, fetal lung, blood mononuclear cells, activated monocytes, and several tumor cell lines. LARC is a selective chemoattractant for lymphocytes and is a specific ligand for CCR6 (77).

Another chemokine, Epstein-Barr virus–induced-1-ligand chemokine (ELC) (79), also called MIP-3β (78), is expressed in the thymus, lymph nodes, appendix, and activated monocytes (79). ELC binds to CCR7 and was shown to be chemotactic for HUT78 cells. Its gene was mapped to chromosome 9p13, which is unusual for CC chemokines, which are clustered on chromosome 17q11.2.

C and CXXXC Chemokines

A protein called lymphotactin with two instead of four cysteines and some sequence similarity to chemokines was reported to attract T lymphocytes (80) and NK cells (81). There is still no agreement, however, on the biologic effects of human lymphotactin. In CD4$^+$ and CD8$^+$ T cells, a chemotactic response could not be demonstrated, but chemokinesis was observed with purified and chemically synthesized lymphotactin (82). Chemotaxis assays with human NK cell clones yielded ambiguous results (83). A membrane protein carrying a chemokine-like structure on top of a mucin domain was cloned, and a soluble fragment was reported to be chemotactic for leukocytes (84,85). The first two cysteines of the chemokine-like region are separated by three amino acids (CXXXC motif). It was proposed that lymphotactin constitutes the third and the CXXXC protein the fourth subfamily of chemokines. It takes at least two to make a family, and it will therefore be important to find the relatives.

CHEMOKINE RECEPTORS

Chemokines act through seven-transmembrane-domain receptors (4,6) that signal through heterotrimeric GTP-binding proteins. Four CXC chemokine receptors (36% to 77% identity) and eight CC chemokine receptors (33% to 74% identity) have been identified. Most chemokine receptors recognize more than one chemokine, and several chemokines bind to more than one receptor (see Table 28-1). The occurrence of chemokine receptors on leukocytes is summarized in Table 28-2.

CXC Chemokine Receptors

Neutrophils express two receptors for IL-8: CXCR1 and CXCR2. They are similar, especially in the transmembrane regions and the connecting loops, but they differ considerably in the NH$_2$-terminal and COOH-terminal regions. CXCR1 has high affinity for IL-8 and low affinity for the other ELR chemokines, whereas CXCR2 has high affinity for all ELR chemokines (3). Both receptors recognize the ELR motif.

The regions that determine selectivity for different ELR chemokines were studied with mutant and chimeric receptors. Recognition is complex and involves several, partly overlapping binding epitopes (8). IL-8 receptors are also found on monocytes, basophils, and eosinophils, but their functional role is unclear, because the responses of these cells depend largely on CC chemokine receptors (3,4). Flow cytometry showed that CXCR1 and CXCR2 can be detected on natural killer cells and CD8$^+$ T lymphocytes (38,86). Low levels of both receptors were detected in melanocytes, fibroblasts, smooth muscle cells, and skin epithelial cells by immunocytochemistry or reverse transcriptase–polymerase chain reaction methods (4).

Two additional CXC chemokine receptors, CXCR3 and CXCR4, have been identified. CXCR3 is selective for IP-10 and MIG (24). It consists of 368 amino acids and shares 41% sequence identity with the two IL-8 receptors. CXCR3 is highly expressed in IL-2–activated CD4$^+$ and CD8$^+$ T lymphocytes, but is not detectable or not functional in resting T lymphocytes, B lymphocytes, monocytes, or granulocytes. Because of its ligand selectivity and its restriction to activated T lymphocytes, CXCR3 is considered important for lymphocyte recruitment (24).

A putative chemokine receptor, CXCR4, was cloned some years ago in several laboratories (4). It was then found to function as the coreceptor for the entry of lymphocyte-tropic, syncytium-inducing HIV-1 strains (49). The only known ligand for CXCR4 is SDF-1, which was shown to act as HIV-1 suppressive factor (25,26). CXCR4 is relatively distant from the other chemokine receptors (33% to 36% identical amino acids). Its gene, however, is localized on chromosome 2q21 in proximity to the genes for CXCR1 and CXCR2 (4). As a chemokine receptor, CXCR4 has an unusually wide distribution. It is highly expressed in leukocytes, lymphocytes, hematopoietic precursor cells, and in a variety of tissues, including heart, brain, liver, and colon (4,87).

TABLE 28-2. *Expression of human CXC and CC chemokine receptors*

Receptor	Main cellular expression	Minor cellular expression
CXCR1	Neutrophils	Monocytes, NK cells
CXCR2	Neutrophils	Monocytes, basophils, eosinophils, NK cells
CXCR3	Activated T lymphocytes	
CXCR4	T and B lymphocytes, monocytes, macrophages, granulocytes, precursor B lymphocytes, dendritic cells, tissue cells	
CCR1	Monocytes, basophils, activated T lymphocytes	Eosinophils
CCR2	Monocytes, basophils, activated T lymphocytes	
CCR3	Eosinophils, basophils, activated T lymphocytes	
CCR4	Freshly isolated CD4$^+$ T lymphocytes	
CCR5	Activated monocytes, activated T lymphocytes, dendritic cells	
CCR6	Activated T lymphocytes, B lymphocytes	
CCR7	EBV-B cell lines, T cell lines	
CCR8	NK cell lines, activated T lymphocytes	

EBV, Epstein-Barr virus; NK, natural killer.

CC Chemokine Receptors

Eight different CC chemokine receptors have been identified during the past 4 years. CCR1 and CCR2 were originally designated as RANTES/MIP-1α and MCP-1 receptors, respectively, based on the ligands they were first shown to recognize (4). Both receptors are widely expressed and are functional in monocytes, granulocytes, IL-2–activated T lymphocytes, and related cell lines (4,8). CCR1 transcripts were also found in neutrophils, but the receptor does not appear to be fully functional, because RANTES and MIP-1α induce $[Ca^{2+}]_i$ changes but not other responses (88,89). CCR2 occurs in two RNA splicing variants, CCR2a and CCR2b, with differences in the COOH-terminal region that affect their selectivity for G proteins (90). The term MCP receptor remains appropriate, because CCR2 is the only chemokine receptor that binds all MCPs.

CCR3 is the only receptor that binds eotaxin and eotaxin-2 (70,74,91). It has, however, some functional similarity with CCR1 and recognizes RANTES, MCP-2, MCP-3, and MCP-4. CCR3 was thought to be exclusively expressed by eosinophils, but studies have shown that it also occurs in basophils (71,72) and in a subset of T lymphocytes that associate with eosinophils at sites of allergic inflammation (73).

CCR4 was cloned from a basophilic cell line cDNA library (92) and was reported to bind RANTES and MIP-1α when expressed in HL-60 cells (93). However, studies using transfected K562 cells showed that CCR4 has high affinity for the CC chemokine TARC, which was not displaced by RANTES or MIP-1α (94). CCR4 transcripts are found in blood $CD4^+$ T lymphocytes but not in B lymphocytes, NK cells, monocytes, or granulocytes. These observations suggest that CCR4 may be involved in the selective recruitment of T lymphocytes.

CCR5 was cloned from human mononuclear phagocyte cDNA and genomic DNA libraries (95,96), and it remains the only known receptor with high affinity for MIP-1β. CCR5 also binds RANTES and MIP-1α. Although its role in leukocyte recruitment is unexplored, this receptor gained considerable attention from studies demonstrating its function as HIV-1 coreceptor with selectivity for monocyte-macrophage–tropic strains. CCR5 is highly expressed in phytohemagglutinin antigen–treated blood mononuclear cells, macrophages, and IL-2–activated T lymphocytes, but it is only weakly expressed in unstimulated leukocytes (97,98).

Three additional CC chemokine receptors were identified or characterized. CCR6 was known as an orphan receptor called STRL22 (99) or CKR-L3 (100) and was found to selectively bind LARC (77), a chemokine that was also called MIP-3α (78). CCR6 is expressed in T and B lymphocytes but not in NK cells, monocytes, or granulocytes (101). CCR7 corresponds to the former orphan receptor EBI1 that was cloned from Epstein-Barr

virus–infected Burkitt's lymphoma cells (102). It binds the novel CC chemokine ELC (MIP-3β) and is selectively expressed in B and T lymphocyte lines (79). CCR8 is the receptor for I-309 (103,104) and was previously described as an orphan receptor called TER-1 (105) or CKR-L1 (100). CCR8 is weakly expressed in cultured NK cells and monocytes. No cell bearing high numbers of this receptor has been found, and the target for its ligand, I-309, remains elusive.

Orphan and Viral Receptors

Several cDNAs encoding putative chemokine receptors with unknown ligands have been reported. Of particular interest are Burkitt's lymphoma–derived receptor-1 (BLR-1) and its NH_2-terminal splicing variant, monocyte-derived receptor-15 (MDR-15), which are highly expressed in mature B and T lymphocytes (106,107). Mice lacking the *BLR1* gene have defective formation of spleen follicles and germinal centers, indicating that the product of *BLR1* may be involved in directing the migration of B lymphocytes into lymphoid areas (108). Another orphan receptor, CMKBRL-1 (109) or V28 (110), has 39% to 44% sequence identity with CC chemokine receptors and is expressed in neutrophils, monocytes, and blood lymphocytes and in lymphoid and neuronal tissues. Its gene and the gene of another orphan receptor, GPR5 (111), is localized on chromosome 3 together with the genes of chemokine receptors CCR1 to CCR5 (112).

Some receptors that bind chemokines are encoded by viruses. US28 from human cytomegalovirus recognizes several CC chemokines, including MCP-1, RANTES, MIP-1α, and MIP-1β (113,114). ECRF-3 is encoded by herpesvirus saimiri and binds IL-8, GRO-α, and NAP-2 but not CC chemokines (115). In human fibroblasts, cytomegalovirus has been shown to induce the expression of IL-8 receptors and to replicate more rapidly when the cells are exposed to IL-8 (116). Genes for putative chemokine receptors are also found in herpesvirus strains associated with Kaposi's sarcoma (117–119). The viral strain HHV8 encodes a receptor that causes enhanced cell proliferation when transfected into rat kidney fibroblasts (120), suggesting that virally encoded chemokine receptors may favor viral replication.

Receptor Function and Signal Transduction

Most studies on signaling were performed with neutrophils and cell lines transfected with one or the other IL-8 receptor. Signal transduction in IL-8–stimulated neutrophils depends on *Bordetella pertussis* toxin–sensitive, GTP-binding proteins and the activation of a phosphatidylinositol-specific phospholipase C, which delivers two second messengers, inositol 1,4,5-trisphosphate (IP_3) and diacylglycerol. IP_3 induces a rise in the cytosolic-free calcium level, and diacylglycerol activates protein kinase C (3). The mechanisms that mediate responses to IL-8 appear similar to those observed after stimulation with the classic chemotactic agonists such as fMLP and C5a (121).

Using Jurkat cells stably transfected with CXCR1 or CXCR2 cDNA, we showed that both receptors respond equally well to IL-8, as judged by the activation of p42/p44 mitogen-activated protein kinase (122), Ca^{2+} mobilization, and chemotaxis (34) and that they function independently of each other. By blocking one or the other receptor in neutrophils using monoclonal antibodies, it was found that phospholipase D activation and the respiratory burst are mediated by CXCR1 only (35). In agreement with these observations, it was reported that phospholipase D is activated by stimulation with IL-8, although not with GRO-α or NAP-2 (36).

There is strong evidence for a role of phosphatidylinositol 3-kinase (PI3K) in chemokine-mediated signal transduction (123,124). PI3K may become activated by interaction with the $\beta\gamma$ subunit of G proteins or by small GTPases, SRC-related tyrosine kinases, or phosphotyrosines that bind to the SRC homology-2 (SH2) domain of PI3K. In murine pre-B cells transfected with CXCR1, RHO was implicated in IL-8–mediated adhesion to fibrinogen (125), suggesting that ligation of IL-8 leads to activation of small GTPases, which are involved in cytoskeletal rearrangement, phospholipase D activation, and assembly of the respiratory burst oxidase (126). Leukocyte responses to chemokines are characteristically transient, and the receptors become rapidly desensitized. Phosphorylation of serines and threonines in the COOH-terminal region of CXCR1 and CXCR2 correlates with homologous desensitization after stimulation with IL-8 or GRO-α, respectively (3,127,128). In rat basophilic leukemia cells expressing CXCR1 and the C5a receptor, heterologous desensitization correlated with COOH-terminal receptor phosphorylation (129).

Regulation of CC Chemokine Receptor Expression in Lymphocytes

The expression of CC chemokine receptors in T lymphocytes depends on the state of activation. Using blood T cells of the memory type (CD45RO$^+$), we observed that chemotaxis in response to RANTES, MCP-1, and other CC chemokines depended on pretreatment with IL-2, which markedly enhanced the expression of CCR1 and CCR2 (89). This effect is reversible; receptor numbers and responsiveness are rapidly lost when IL-2 is withdrawn and fully restored when it is added again. IL-4, IL-10, and IL-12 have similar effects but are less potent, whereas other cytokines known to act on T lymphocytes, such as IL-13, IFN-γ, IL-1β, and TNF-α, are inactive. Other stimulatory conditions, such as treatment with anti-CD3 or anti-CD28 (or both), lead to rapid receptor down-

regulation and loss of chemotactic migration. These observations show that T lymphocyte responses to chemokines are strictly regulated. The cells appear to respond after IL-2–mediated expansion but not after antigen-dependent activation, suggesting that antigen recognition may lead to transient immobilization of the T cells. The IL-2 effect is also observed for expression of CCR5 (97,98) and CXCR3 (24). Understanding receptor upregulation in lymphocytes became more important after recognition of the role of chemokine receptors in HIV infection (130).

In contrast to most CC chemokine receptors, CXCR4 and presumably CCR4 are expressed in nonactivated T lymphocytes and are not upregulated by IL-2 (25,26,94). CCR4 is apparently restricted to T cells, whereas CXCR4 is widely distributed in leukocytes. Because their respective ligands, SDF-1 and TARC, are constitutively produced in primary lymphoid tissues, CXCR4 and CCR4 may be involved in the physiologic, disease-unrelated lymphocyte traffic.

Human Immunodeficiency Virus Coreceptor Function

Some chemokine receptors are recognition sites for HIV-1 infection, and some chemokines have HIV-1–suppressive properties (131–134). In a search for suppressive factors, Cocchi et al. (135) found that RANTES, MIP-1α, and MIP-1β inhibited infection by monocyte-macrophage–tropic HIV-1 strains. Shortly thereafter, Feng et al. (49) showed that a chemokine receptor, CXCR4, functioned together with CD4 as binding site for HIV-1 entry into cells. SDF-1, the ligand for CXCR4, was then found to be a potent inhibitor of infection by T-cell–tropic HIV-1 strains (25,26). CCR5, a receptor for RANTES, MIP-1α, and MIP-1β, was identified by several groups as the main coreceptor for entry of monocyte-macrophage–tropic HIV-1 strains (131–133).

Coreceptor function has also been reported for CCR2 and CCR3. CCR5 is expressed in activated but not resting T cells, adherent monocytes, and dendritic cells (98,136). The HIV-1 glycoprotein gp120, which determines viral tropism through variations in the V3 loop, is a poor ligand for CCR5. Binding, however, is markedly enhanced in the presence of CD4, which is thought to induce a conformational change of gp120 that confers high affinity for CCR5 (137,138). The role of CCR5 is further documented by the discovery of a mutation of the CCR5 gene. A 32-bp deletion resulting in a nonfunctional receptor was shown to confer resistance to infection by monocyte-macrophage–tropic HIV isolates, whereas infection by T-cell–tropic viruses was not affected (134,139–141).

CXCR4 is the only coreceptor that is selective for syncytium-inducing T-cell–tropic HIV-1. These viruses are believed to emerge at later stages in HIV-positive individuals when the CD4$^+$ T cell count is low and symptoms of the disease become apparent (142). In contrast to CCR5, CXCR4 is expressed by all types of white blood cells and many different tissue cells. This pattern may contribute to disease progression.

Chemokines and their receptors represent promising new targets for therapeutic intervention. Novel strategies for the prevention of HIV proliferation and dissemination may include gene therapy aiming at deleting the CCR5 gene in blood cells, vaccination for the generation of antibodies that block coreceptor function, modulation of coreceptor and chemokine expression, and the generation of modified chemokines as antagonists for HIV coreceptors. Structural variation of chemokines has already yielded several potent receptor antagonists, and variants with NH$_2$-terminal truncation or modification of RANTES blocked infection by monocyte-macrophage–tropic HIV-1 (143,144).

STRUCTURE-ACTIVITY RELATIONSHIPS

All chemokines have a short NH$_2$-terminal sequence, a core made of the β strands and loops extending between the first and fourth cysteine, and a COOH-terminal domain, which usually comprises 20 to 30 amino acids but can exceed 50. The disulfide bonds and hydrophobic interactions confer a well-ordered structure to the core, whereas the NH$_2$- and COOH-terminal domains are disordered, especially at their extremities. Structural studies, which have been performed for several chemokines, indicate that receptor recognition and triggering depends on interaction with a few NH$_2$-terminal residues and discrete regions of the core structure.

Role of the NH$_2$-Terminus

The first evidence for the importance of the NH$_2$-terminus came from studies with IL-8. It was found that the Glu-Leu-Arg (ELR motif) preceding the first cysteine is required for recognition and triggering of both IL-8 receptors, CXCR1 and CXCR2. This binding site, however, is not sufficient, because oligopeptides containing the ELR motif are inactive, and the introduction of the ELR motif into unrelated chemokines such as IP-10 or MCP-1 does not result in activity on neutrophils. The second binding site depends on proper folding, as suggested by the finding that IL-8 activity is lost when the disulfide bonds are reduced (3). The length of the NH$_2$-terminus is also critical, and maximum activity is obtained when the ELR chemokines are NH$_2$-terminally truncated to optimally expose the ELR motif (3). The secondary binding domain is not fully identified, but extensive mutation analysis and studies with hybrid chemokines indicate that the region between residues 10 and 17 of the 72 amino acid form of IL-8 and Gly^{31}-Pro^{32} before the third cysteine are of primary importance (4). The secondary bind-

ing site determines the affinity for binding to CXCR1 and CXCR2 (which recognize the ELR motif equally well). Significant structural differences are observed between IL-8 and GRO-α or NAP-2 in the region between residue 10 and 17 (145).

Truncation studies demonstrate that the NH$_2$-terminal region is also essential for receptor recognition and activation by CC chemokines. However, as shown for MCP-1, the structural requirements are more strict, because the entire sequence of 10 amino acids preceding the first cysteine is necessary for full activity (18). Considerable loss of activity was observed after NH$_2$-terminal truncation or elongation, but replacement of the NH$_2$-terminal pyroglutamate by several noncyclic residues was tolerated. The effect of truncation of MCP-1 was studied in monocytes, basophils, and eosinophils. The most dramatic effect was obtained by deletion of the pyroglutamate, which leads to a 50-fold decrease in activity on monocytes (146) and basophils (147). Surprisingly, this deletion confers MCP-1 activity on eosinophils, which do not respond to the full-length chemokine (147).

Receptor Antagonists

IL-8 receptor antagonists are generated by deletions and substitutions within the ELR motif. The two antagonists, (R)IL-8 and (AAR)IL-8 (with the NH$_2$-terminal sequences Arg-Cys and Ala-Ala-Arg-Cys, respectively), that were studied most extensively are potent inhibitors of IL-8 binding and of exocytosis and chemotaxis induced in neutrophils by IL-8, GRO-α, or NAP-2 (148). We studied the receptor selectivity of antagonists with an Arg-Cys NH$_2$-terminal sequence using transfected cells expressing CXCR1 or CXCR2. Whereas (R)IL-8 had similar affinity for CXCR1 and CXCR2 and blocked responses mediated by both receptors, the corresponding analogues of GRO-α and platelet factor-4, (R)GRO-α and (R)PF4, were selective for CXCR2, as shown by binding competition and inhibition of functional responses (149).

NH$_2$-terminally truncated CC chemokines are also potent antagonists. MCP-1 derivatives obtained by deletion of 8 or 9 NH$_2$-terminal residues, MCP-1(9–76) and MCP-1(10–76), block CCR2 and prevent the responses elicited by MCP-1, MCP-2, and MCP-3, although not by RANTES, MIP-1α, or MIP-1β (146). In contrast, the corresponding truncation analogues of RANTES, RANTES(9-68), and of MCP-3, MCP-3(10-76), block several CC chemokine receptors and inhibit the responses induced by MCP-1, MCP-3, and RANTES (150). The loss of selectivity suggests that receptor specificity of these chemokines depends on determinants within the NH$_2$-terminal domain while other domains ensure the interaction with multiple receptors. Antagonists were obtained by NH$_2$-terminal extension of MCP-3 with Arg-Glu-Phe (151) or RANTES with a methionine (152) and by chemical modification of the NH₂-terminus of RANTES (144).

ACKNOWLEDGMENTS

This work was supported by Grant 31-039744.93 to Marco Baggiolini and Bernhard Moser from the Swiss National Science Foundation. Bernhard Moser also is a recipient of a career development award from the Professor Max Cloëtta Foundation.

REFERENCES

1. Stoeckle MY, Barker KA. Two burgeoning families of platelet factor 4-related proteins: mediators of the inflammatory response. *New Biologist* 1990;2:313–323.
2. Schall TJ. Biology of the RANTES/SIS cytokine family. *Cytokine* 1991;3:165–183.
3. Baggiolini M, Dewald B, Moser B. Interleukin-8 and related chemotactic cytokines—CXC and CC chemokines. *Adv Immunol* 1994;55: 97–179.
4. Baggiolini M, Dewald B, Moser B. Human chemokines: an update. *Annu Rev Immunol* 1997;15:675–705.
5. Baggiolini M, Dahinden CA. CC chemokines in allergic inflammation. *Immunol Today* 1994;15:127–133.
6. Murphy PM. The molecular biology of leukocyte chemoattractant receptors. *Annu Rev Immunol* 1994;12:593–633.
7. Schall TJ, Bacon KB. Chemokines, leukocyte trafficking, and inflammation. *Curr Opin Immunol* 1994;6:865–873.
8. Murphy PM. Chemokine receptors: structure, function and role in microbial pathogenesis. *Cytokine Growth Factor Rev* 1996;7:47–64.
9. Moser B, Loetscher M, Piali L, Loetscher P. Lymphocyte responses to chemokines. *Int Rev Immunol* 1998;16:323–344.
10. Clore GM, Appella E, Yamada M, Matsushima K, Gronenborn AM. Three-dimensional structure of interleukin 8 in solution. *Biochemistry* 1990;29:1689–1696.
11. Baldwin ET, Weber IT, St. Charles R, et al. Crystal structure of interleukin 8: symbiosis of NMR and crystallography. *Proc Natl Acad Sci USA* 1991;88:502–506.
12. Lodi PJ, Garrett DS, Kuszewski J, et al. High-resolution solution structure of the β chemokine hMIP-1β by multidimensional NMR. *Science* 1994;263:1762–1767.
13. Skelton NJ, Aspiras F, Ogez J, Schall TJ. Proton NMR assignments and solution conformation of RANTES, a chemokine of the C-C type. *Biochemistry* 1995;34:5329–5342.
14. Chung C, Cooke RM, Proudfoot AEI, Wells TNC. The three-dimensional solution structure of RANTES. *Biochemistry* 1995;34: 9307–9314.
15. Covell DG, Smythers GW, Gronenborn AM, Clore GM. Analysis of hydrophobicity in the α and β chemokine families and its relevance to dimerization. *Protein Sci* 1994;3:2064–2072.
16. Clore GM, Gronenborn AM. Three-dimensional structures of α and β chemokines. *FASEB J* 1995;9:57–62.
17. Burrows SD, Doyle ML, Murphy KP, et al. Determination of the monomer-dimer equilibrium of interleukin-8 reveals it is a monomer at physiological concentrations. *Biochemistry* 1994;33:12741–12745.
18. Clark-Lewis I, Kim K-S, Rajarathnam K, et al. Structure-activity relationships of chemokines. *J Leukoc Biol* 1995;57:703–711.
19. Rajarathnam K, Sykes BD, Kay CM, et al. Neutrophil activation by monomeric interleukin-8. *Science* 1994;264:90–92.
20. Graham GJ, MacKenzie J, Lowe S, et al. Aggregation of the chemokine MIP-1α is a dynamic and reversible phenomenon. Biochemical and biological analyses. *J Biol Chem* 1994;269:4974–4978.
21. Kim KS, Rajarathnam K, Clark-Lewis I, Sykes BD. Structural characterization of a monomeric chemokine: monocyte chemoattractant protein-3. *FEBS Lett* 1996;395:277–282.
22. Shirozu M, Nakano T, Inazawa J, et al. Structure and chromosomal localization of the human stromal cell-derived factor 1 (SDF1) gene. *Genomics* 1995;28:495–500.
23. Schulz-Knappe P, Mägert HJ, Dewald B, et al. HCC-1, a novel chemokine from human plasma. *J Exp Med* 1996;183:295–299.
24. Loetscher M, Gerber B, Loetscher P, et al. Chemokine receptor specific for IP10 and Mig: structure, function, and expression in activated T-lymphocytes. *J Exp Med* 1996;184:963–969.
25. Oberlin E, Amara A, Bachelerie F, et al. The CXC chemokine SDF-1 is the ligand for LESTR/fusin and prevents infection by T-cell-line–adapted HIV-1. *Nature* 1996;382:833–835.
26. Bleul CC, Farzan M, Choe H, et al. The lymphocyte chemoattractant SDF-1 is a ligand for LESTR/fusin and blocks HIV-1 entry. *Nature* 1996;382:829–833.
27. Walz A, Peveri P, Aschauer H, Baggiolini M. Purification and amino acid sequencing of NAF, a novel neutrophil-activating factor produced by monocytes. *Biochem Biophys Res Commun* 1987;149:755–761.
28. Yoshimura T, Matsushima K, Tanaka S, et al. Purification of a human monocyte-derived neutrophil chemotactic factor that has peptide sequence similarity to other host defense cytokines. *Proc Natl Acad Sci USA* 1987;84:9233–9237.
29. Schröder J-M, Mrowietz U, Morita E, Christophers E. Purification and partial biochemical characterization of a human monocyte-derived, neutrophil-activating peptide that lacks interleukin 1 activity. *J Immunol* 1987;139:3474–3483.
30. Baggiolini M, Imboden P, Detmers P. Neutrophil activation and the effects of interleukin-8/neutrophil-activating peptide 1 (IL-8/NAP-1). In: Baggiolini M, Sorg C, eds. *Cytokines,* vol 4. *Interleukin-8 (NAP-1) and related chemotactic cytokines.* Basel: Karger, 1992:1–17.
31. McDonald PP, Pouliot M, Borgeat P, McColl SR. Induction by chemokines of lipid mediator synthesis in granulocyte-macrophage colony-stimulating factor-treated human neutrophils. *J Immunol* 1993;151:6399–6409.
32. Serhan CN, Haeggström JZ, Leslie CC. Lipid mediator networks in cell signaling: update and impact of cytokines. *FASEB J* 1996;10: 1147–1158.
33. Thelen M, Dewald B, Baggiolini M. Neutrophil signal transduction and activation of the respiratory burst. *Physiol Rev* 1993;73:797–821.
34. Loetscher P, Seitz M, Clark-Lewis I, Baggiolini M, Moser B. Both interleukin-8 receptors independently mediate chemotaxis. Jurkat cells transfected with IL-8R1 or IL-8R2 migrate in response to IL-8, GRO-α and NAP-2. *FEBS Lett* 1994;341:187–192.
35. Jones SA, Wolf M, Qin SX, Mackay CR, Baggiolini M. Different functions for the interleukin 8 receptors (IL-8R) of human neutrophil leukocytes: NADPH oxidase and phospholipase D are activated through IL-8R1 but not IL-8R2. *Proc Natl Acad Sci USA* 1996;93:6682–6686.
36. L'Heureux GP, Bourgoin S, Jean N, McColl SR, Naccache PH. Diverging signal transduction pathways activated by interleukin-8 and related chemokines in human neutrophils: interleukin-8, but not NAP-2 or GRO-α, stimulates phospholipase D activity. *Blood* 1995;85: 522–531.
37. Sebok K, Woodside D, Al-Aoukaty A, Ho AD, Gluck S, Maghazachi AA. IL-8 induces the locomotion of human IL-2–activated natural killer cells: involvement of a guanine nucleotide binding (Gₒ) protein. *J Immunol* 1993;150:1524–1534.
38. Qin SX, LaRosa G, Campbell JJ, et al. Expression of monocyte chemoattractant protein-1 and interleukin-8 receptors on subsets of T cells: correlation with transendothelial chemotactic potential. *Eur J Immunol* 1996;26:640–647.
39. Luster AD, Ravetch JV. Biochemical characterization of a gamma interferon-inducible cytokine (IP-10). *J Exp Med* 1987;166: 1084–1097.
40. Farber JM. HuMIG: a new human member of the chemokine family of cytokines. *Biochem Biophys Res Commun* 1993;192:223–230.
41. Kaplan G, Luster AD, Hancock G, Cohn ZA. The expression of a gamma interferon-induced protein (IP-10) in delayed immune responses in human skin. *J Exp Med* 1987;166:1098–1108.
42. Taub DD, Lloyd AR, Conlon K, et al. Recombinant human interferon-inducible protein 10 is a chemoattractant for human monocytes and T lymphocytes and promotes T cell adhesion to endothelial cells. *J Exp Med* 1993;177:1809–1814.
43. Taub DD, Sayers TJ, Carter CRD, Ortaldo JR. α and β chemokines induce NK cell migration and enhance NK-mediated cytolysis. *J Immunol* 1995;155:3877–3888.
44. Liao F, Rabin RL, Yannelli JR, Koniaris LG, Vanguri P, Farber JM. Human MIG chemokine: biochemical and functional characterization. *J Exp Med* 1995;182:1301–1314.

44a. Lahrtz F, Piali L, Nadal D, et al. Chemotactic activity on mononuclear cells in the cerebrospinal fluid of patients with viral meningitis is mediated by interferon-gamma inducible protein-10 and monocyte chemotactic protein-1. *Eur J Immunol* 1997;27:2484–2489.

44b. Cole KE, Strick CA, Paradis TJ, et al. Interferon-inducible T cell alpha chemoattractant (I-TAC): A novel non-ELRCXC chemokine with potent activity on activated T cells through selective high affinity binding to CXCR3. *J Exp Med* 1998;187:2009–2021.

45. Tashiro K, Tada H, Heilker R, Shirozu M, Nakano T, Honjo T. Signal sequence trap: a cloning strategy for secreted proteins and type I membrane proteins. *Science* 1993;261:600–603.

46. Nagasawa T, Kikutani H, Kishimoto T. Molecular cloning and structure of a pre-B-cell growth-stimulating factor. *Proc Natl Acad Sci USA* 1994;91:2305–2309.

47. Aiuti A, Webb IJ, Bleul C, Springer T, Gutierrez-Ramos JC. The chemokine SDF-1 is a chemoattractant for human CD34$^+$ hematopoietic progenitor cells and provides a new mechanism to explain the mobilization of CD34$^+$ progenitors to peripheral blood. *J Exp Med* 1997;185:111–120.

48. D'Apuzzo M, Rolink A, Loetscher M, et al. The chemokine SDF-1, stromal cell-derived factor 1, attracts early stage B cell precursors via the chemokine receptor CXCR4. *Eur J Immunol* 1997;27:1788–1793.

49. Feng Y, Broder CC, Kennedy PE, Berger EA. HIV-1 entry cofactor: functional cDNA cloning of a seven-transmembrane, G protein–coupled receptor. *Science* 1996;272:872–877.

50. Van Damme J, Proost P, Lenaerts J-P, Opdenakker G. Structural and functional identification of two human, tumor-derived monocyte chemotactic proteins (MCP-2 and MCP-3) belonging to the chemokine family. *J Exp Med* 1992;176:59–65.

51. Uguccioni M, Loetscher P, Forssmann U, et al. Monocyte chemotactic protein 4 (MCP-4), a novel structural and functional analogue of MCP-3 and eotaxin. *J Exp Med* 1996;183:2379–2384.

52. Carr MW, Roth SJ, Luther E, Rose SS, Springer TA. Monocyte chemoattractant protein 1 acts as a T-lymphocyte chemoattractant. *Proc Natl Acad Sci USA* 1994;91:3652–3656.

53. Loetscher P, Seitz M, Clark-Lewis I, Baggiolini M, Moser B. The monocyte chemotactic proteins, MCP-1, MCP-2 and MCP-3, are major attractants for human CD4$^+$ and CD8$^+$ T lymphocytes. *FASEB J* 1994;8:1055–1060.

54. Sozzani S, Sallusto F, Luini W, et al. Migration of dendritic cells in response to formyl peptides, C5a, and a distinct set of chemokines. *J Immunol* 1995;155:3292–3295.

55. Allavena P, Bianchi G, Zhou D, et al. Induction of natural killer cell migration by monocyte chemotactic protein-1, -2 and -3. *Eur J Immunol* 1994;24:3233–3236.

56. Loetscher P, Seitz M, Clark-Lewis I, Baggiolini M, Moser B. Activation of NK cells by CC chemokines—chemotaxis, Ca^{2+} mobilization, and enzyme release. *J Immunol* 1996;156:322–327.

57. Schall TJ, Bacon K, Toy KJ, Goeddel DV. Selective attraction of monocytes and T lymphocytes of the memory phenotype by cytokine RANTES. *Nature* 1990;347:669–671.

58. Taub DD, Conlon K, Lloyd AR, Oppenheim JJ, Kelvin DJ. Preferential migration of activated CD4$^+$ and CD8$^+$ T cells in response to MIP-1α and MIP-1β. *Science* 1993;260:355–358.

59. Broxmeyer HE, Sherry B, Lu L, et al. Myelopoietic enhancing effects of murine macrophage inflammatory proteins 1 and 2 on colony formation *in vitro* by murine and human bone marrow granulocyte/macrophage progenitor cells. *J Exp Med* 1989;170:1583–1594.

60. Broxmeyer HE, Sherry B, Lu L, et al. Enhancing and suppressing effects of recombinant murine macrophage inflammatory proteins on colony formation *in vitro* by bone marrow myeloid progenitor cells. *Blood* 1990;76:1110–1116.

61. Graham GJ, Wright EG, Hewick R, et al. Identification and characterization of an inhibitor of haemopoietic stem cell proliferation. *Nature* 1990;344:442–444.

62. Broxmeyer HE, Sherry B, Cooper S, et al. Macrophage inflammatory protein (MIP)-1β abrogates the capacity of MIP-1α to suppress myeloid progenitor cell growth. *J Immunol* 1991;147:2586–2594.

63. Cook DN. The role of MIP-1α in inflammation and hematopoiesis. *J Leukocyte Biol* 1996;59:61–66.

64. Cook DN, Beck MA, Coffman TM, et al. Requirement of MIP-1α for an inflammatory response to viral infection. *Science* 1995;269:1583–1585.

65. Verfaillie CM. Chemokines as inhibitors of hematopoietic progenitors. *J Lab Clin Med* 1996;127:148–150.

66. Jose PJ, Griffiths-Johnson DA, Collins PD, et al. Eotaxin: a potent eosinophil chemoattractant cytokine detected in a guinea pig model of allergic airways inflammation. *J Exp Med* 1994;179:881–887.

67. Rothenberg ME, Luster AD, Leder P. Murine eotaxin: an eosinophil chemoattractant inducible in endothelial cells and in interleukin 4-induced tumor suppression. *Proc Natl Acad Sci USA* 1995;92:8960–8964.

68. Ponath PD, Qin SX, Ringler DJ, et al. Cloning of the human eosinophil chemoattractant, eotaxin: expression, receptor binding, and functional properties suggest a mechanism for the selective recruitment of eosinophils. *J Clin Invest* 1996;97:604–612.

69. Combadiere C, Ahuja SK, Murphy PM. Cloning and functional expression of a human eosinophil CC chemokine receptor. *J Biol Chem* 1995;270:16491–16494 [correction *J Biol Chem* 1995;270:30235].

70. Daugherty BL, Siciliano SJ, DeMartino JA, Malkowitz L, Sirotina A, Springer MS. Cloning, expression, and characterization of the human eosinophil eotaxin receptor. *J Exp Med* 1996;183:2349–2354.

71. Uguccioni M, Mackay C, Ochensberger B, et al. High expression of the chemokine receptor CCR3 in human blood basophils. Role in activation by eotaxin MCP-4 and other chemokines. *J Clin Invest* 1997;(in press).

72. Yamada H, Hirai K, Miyamasu M, et al. Eotaxin is a potent chemotaxin for human basophils. *Biochem Biophys Res Commun* 1997;231:365–368.

73. Gerber BO, Zanni MP, Uguccioni M, et al. Functional expression of the eotaxin receptor CCR3, in T lymphocytes co-localizing with eosinophils. *Curr Biol* 1997;7:836–843.

74. Forssmann U, Uguccioni M, Loetscher P, et al. Eotaxin-2, a novel CC chemokine that is selective for the chemokine receptor CCR3, and acts like eotaxin on human eosinophil and basophil leukocytes. *J Exp Med* 1997;185:2171–2176.

75. Forssmann U, Delgado MB, Uguccioni M, Loetscher P, Garotta G, Baggiolini M. CKβ8, a novel CC chemokine that predominantly acts on monocytes. *FEBS Lett* 1997;408:211–216.

76. Imai T, Yoshida T, Baba M, Nishimura M, Kakizaki M, Yoshie O. Molecular cloning of a novel T cell–directed CC chemokine expressed in thymus by signal sequence trap using Epstein-Barr virus vector. *J Biol Chem* 1996;271:21514–21521.

77. Hieshima K, Imai T, Opdenakker G, et al. Molecular cloning of a novel human CC chemokine liver and activation-regulated chemokine (LARC) expressed in liver: chemotactic activity for lymphocytes and gene localization on chromosome. *J Biol Chem* 1997;272:5846–5853.

78. Rossi DL, Vicari AP, Franz-Bacon K, McClanahan TK, Zlotnik A. Identification through bioinformatics of two new macrophage proinflammatory human chemokines MIP-3α and MIP-3β. *J Immunol* 1997;158:1033–1036.

79. Yoshida R, Imai T, Hieshima K, et al. Molecular cloning of a novel human CC chemokine EBI1-ligand chemokine that is a specific functional ligand for EBI1, CCR7. *J Biol Chem* 1997;272:13803–13809.

80. Kennedy J, Kelner GS, Kleyensteuber S, et al. Molecular cloning and functional characterization of human lymphotactin. *J Immunol* 1995;155:203–209.

81. Bianchi G, Sozzani S, Zlotnik A, Mantovani A, Allavena P. Migratory response of human natural killer cells to lymphotactin. *Eur J Immunol* 1996;26:3238–3241.

82. Dorner B, Müller S, Entschladen F, et al. Purification, structural analysis, and function of natural ATAC, a cytokine secreted by CD8$^+$ T cells. *J Biol Chem* 1997;272:8817–8823.

83. Hedrick JA, Saylor V, Figueroa D, et al. Lymphotactin is produced by NK cells and attracts both NK cells and T cells *in vivo*. *J Immunol* 1997;158:1533–1540.

84. Bazan JF, Bacon KB, Hardiman G, et al. A new class of membrane-bound chemokine with a CX$_3$C motif. *Nature* 1997;385:640–644.

85. Pan Y, Lloyd C, Zhou H, et al. Neurotactin, a membrane-anchored chemokine upregulated in brain inflammation. *Nature* 1997;387:611–617.

86. Chuntharapai A, Lee J, Hébert CA, Kim KJ. Monoclonal antibodies detect different distribution patterns of IL-8 receptor A and IL-8 receptor B on human peripheral blood leukocytes. *J Immunol* 1994;153:5682–5688.

87. Federsppiel B, Melhado IG, Duncan AMV, et al. Molecular cloning of

the cDNA and chromosomal localization of the gene for a putative seven-transmembrane segment (7-TMS) receptor isolated from human spleen. *Genomics* 1993;16:707–712.

88. McColl SR, Hachicha M, Levasseur S, Neote K, Schall TJ. Uncoupling of early signal transduction events from effector function in human peripheral blood neutrophils in response to recombinant macrophage inflammatory proteins-1α and -1β. *J Immunol* 1993;150: 4550–4560.

89. Loetscher P, Seitz M, Baggiolini M, Moser B. Interleukin-2 regulates CC chemokine receptor expression and chemotactic responsiveness in T lymphocytes. *J Exp Med* 1996;184:569–577.

90. Kuang YN, Wu YP, Jiang HP, Wu DQ. Selective G protein coupling by C-C chemokine receptors. *J Biol Chem* 1996;271:3975–3978.

91. Ponath PD, Qin SX, Post TW, et al. Molecular cloning and characterization of a human eotaxin receptor expressed selectively on eosinophils. *J Exp Med* 1996;183:2437–2448.

92. Power CA, Meyer A, Nemeth K, et al. Molecular cloning and functional expression of a novel CC chemokine receptor cDNA from a human basophilic cell line. *J Biol Chem* 1995;270:19495–19500.

93. Hoogewerf AJ, Black D, Proudfoot AEI, Wells TNC, Power CA. Molecular cloning of murine CC CKR-4 and high affinity binding of chemokines to murine and human CC CKR-4. *Biochem Biophys Res Commun* 1996;218:337–343.

94. Imai T, Baba M, Nishimura M, Kakizaki M, Takagi S, Yoshie O. The T cell–directed CC chemokine TARC is a highly specific biological ligand for CC chemokine receptor 4. *J Biol Chem* 1997;272: 15036–15042.

95. Samson M, Labbe O, Mollereau C, Vassart G, Parmentier M. Molecular cloning and functional expression of a new human CC-chemokine receptor gene. *Biochemistry* 1996;35:3362–3367.

96. Raport CJ, Gosling J, Schweickart VL, Gray PW, Charo IF. Molecular cloning and functional characterization of a novel human CC chemokine receptor (CCR5) for RANTES, MIP-1β, and MIP-1α. *J Biol Chem* 1996;271:17161–17166.

97. Bleul CC, Wu LJ, Hoxie JA, Springer TA, Mackay CR. The HIV coreceptors CXCR4 and CCR5 are differentially expressed and regulated on human T lymphocytes. *Proc Natl Acad Sci USA* 1997;94:1925–1930.

98. Wu LJ, Paxton WA, Kassam N, et al. CCR5 levels and expression pattern correlate with infectability by macrophage-tropic HIV-1, *in vitro*. *J Exp Med* 1997;185:1681–1691.

99. Liao F, Lee HH, Farber JM. Cloning of STRL22, a new human gene encoding a G-protein–coupled receptor related to chemokine receptors and located on chromosome 6q27. *Genomics* 1997;40:175–180.

100. Zaballos A, Varona R, Gutiérrez J, Lind P, Márquez G. Molecular cloning and RNA expression of two new human chemokine receptor-like genes. *Biochem Biophys Res Commun* 1996;227:846–853.

101. Baba M, Imai T, Nishimura M, et al. Identification of CCR6, the specific receptor for a novel lymphocyte-directed CC chemokine LARC. *J Biol Chem* 1997;272:14893–14898.

102. Birkenbach M, Josefsen K, Yalamanchili R, Lenoir G, Kieff E. Epstein-Barr virus-induced genes: first lymphocyte-specific G protein–coupled peptide receptors. *J Virol* 1993;67:2209–2220.

103. Roos RS, Loetscher M, Legler DF, Clark-Lewis I, Baggiolini M, Moser B. Identification of CCR8, the receptor for the human CC chemokine I-309. *J Biol Chem* 1997;272:17251–17254.

104. Tiffany HL, Lautens LL, Gao J-L, et al. Identification of CCR8: a human monocyte and thymus receptor for the CC chemokine I-309. *J Exp Med* 1997;186:165–170.

105. Napolitano M, Zingoni A, Bernardini G, et al. Molecular cloning of *TER1*, a chemokine receptor-like gene expressed by lymphoid tissues. *J Immunol* 1996;157:2759–2763.

106. Dobner T, Wolf I, Emrich T, Lipp M. Differentiation-specific expression of a novel G protein–coupled receptor from Burkitt's lymphoma. *Eur J Immunol* 1992;22:2795–2799.

107. Barella L, Loetscher M, Tobler A, Baggiolini M, Moser B. Sequence variation of a novel heptahelical leucocyte receptor through alternative transcript formation. *Biochem J* 1995;309:773–779.

108. Förster R, Mattis AE, Kremmer E, Wolf E, Brem G, Lipp M. A putative chemokine receptor, BLR1, directs B cell migration to defined lymphoid organs and specific anatomic compartments of the spleen. *Cell* 1996;87:1037–1047.

109. Combadiere C, Ahuja SK, Murphy PM. Cloning, chromosomal localization, and RNA expression of a human β chemokine receptor-like gene. *DNA Cell Biol* 1995;14:673–680.

110. Raport CJ, Schweickart VL, Chantry D, et al. New members of the chemokine receptor gene family. *J Leukoc Biol* 1996;59:18–23.

111. Heiber M, Docherty JM, Shah G, et al. Isolation of three novel human genes encoding G protein–coupled receptors. *DNA Cell Biol* 1995;14: 25–35.

112. Samson M, Soularue P, Vassart G, Parmentier M. The genes encoding the human CC-chemokine receptors CC-CKR1 to CC-CKR5 (CMKBR1-CMKBR5) are clustered in the p21.3-p24 region of chromosome 3. *Genomics* 1996;36:522–526.

113. Neote K, DiGregorio D, Mak JY, Horuk R, Schall TJ. Molecular cloning, functional expression, and signaling characteristics of a C-C chemokine receptor. *Cell* 1993;72:415–425.

114. Gao J-L, Murphy PM. Human cytomegalovirus open reading frame US28 encodes a functional β chemokine receptor. *J Biol Chem* 1994;269:28539–28542.

115. Ahuja SK, Murphy PM. Molecular piracy of mammalian interleukin-8 receptor type B by herpesvirus saimiri. *J Biol Chem* 1993;268: 20691–20694.

116. Murayama T, Kuno K, Jisaki F, et al. Enhancement of human cytomegalovirus replication in a human lung fibroblast cell line by interleukin-8. *J Virol* 1994;68:7582–7585.

117. Nicholas J, Cameron KR, Honess RW. Herpesvirus saimiri encodes homologues of G protein–coupled receptors and cyclins. *Nature* 1992; 355:362–365.

118. Gompels UA, Nicholas J, Lawrence G, et al. The DNA sequence of human herpesvirus-6: structure, coding content, and genome evolution. *Virology* 1995;209:29–51.

119. Nicholas J. Determination and analysis of the complete nucleotide sequence of human herpesvirus 7. *J Virol* 1996;70:5975–5989.

120. Arvanitakis L, Geras-Raaka E, Varma A, Gershengorn MC, Cesarman E. Human herpesvirus KSHV encodes a constitutively active G-protein–coupled receptor linked to cell proliferation. *Nature* 1997;385: 347–350.

121. Baggiolini M, Kernen P. Neutrophil activation: control of shape change, exocytosis, and respiratory burst. *News Physiol Sci* 1992;7: 215–219.

122. Jones SA, Moser B, Thelen M. A comparison of post-receptor signal transduction events in Jurkat cells transfected with either IL-8R1 or IL-8R2: chemokine mediated activation of p42/p44 MAP-kinase (ERK-2). *FEBS Lett* 1995;364:211–214.

123. Thelen M, Uguccioni M, Bösiger J. PI 3-kinase-dependent and independent chemotaxis of human neutrophil leukocytes. *Biochem Biophys Res Commun* 1995;217:1255–1262.

124. Turner L, Ward SG, Westwick J. RANTES-activated human T lymphocytes: a role for phosphoinositide 3-kinase. *J Immunol* 1995;155: 2437–2444.

125. Laudanna C, Campbell JJ, Butcher EC. Role of Rho in chemoattractant-activated leukocyte adhesion through integrins. *Science* 1996; 271:981–983.

126. Bokoch GM. Chemoattractant signaling and leukocyte activation. *Blood* 1995;86:1649–1660.

127. Mueller SG, Schraw WP, Richmond A. Melanoma growth stimulatory activity enhances the phosphorylation of the class II interleukin-8 receptor in non-hematopoietic cells. *J Biol Chem* 1994;269: 1973–1980.

128. Richardson RM, DuBose RA, Ali H, Tomhave ED, Haribabu B, Snyderman R. Regulation of human interleukin-8 receptor A: identification of a phosphorylation site involved in modulating receptor functions. *Biochemistry* 1995;34:14193–14201.

129. Richardon RM, Ali H, Tomhave ED, Haribabu B, Snyderman R. Cross-desensitization of chemoattractant receptors occurs at multiple levels: evidence for a role for inhibition of phospholipase C activity. *J Biol Chem* 1995;270:27829–27833.

130. Moore JP, Koup RA. Chemoattractants attract HIV researchers. *J Exp Med* 1996;184:311–313.

131. Moser B. Chemokines and HIV: a remarkable synergism. *Trends Microbiol* 1997;5:88–90.

132. D'Souza MP, Harden VA. Chemokines and HIV-1 second receptors: confluence of two fields generates optimism in AIDS research. *Nature Med* 1996;2:1293–1300.

133. Fauci AS. Host factors and the pathogenesis of HIV-induced disease. *Nature* 1996;384:529–534.

134. Moore JP. Coreceptors: implications for HIV pathogenesis and therapy. *Science* 1997;276:51–52.

135. Cocchi F, DeVico AL, Garzino-Demo A, Arya SK, Gallo RC, Lusso P. Identification of RANTES, MIP-1α, and MIP-1β as the major HIV-suppressive factors produced by CD8⁺ T cells. *Science* 1995;270: 1811–1815.

136. Granelli-Piperno A, Moser B, Pope M, et al. Efficient interaction of HIV-1 with purified dendritic cells via multiple chemokine coreceptors. *J Exp Med* 1996;184:2433–2438.

137. Wu LJ, Gerard NP, Wyatt R, et al. CD4-induced interaction of primary HIV-1 gp120 glycoproteins with the chemokine receptor CCR-5. *Nature* 1996;384:179–183.

138. Trkola A, Dragic T, Arthos J, et al. CD4-dependent, antibody-sensitive interactions between HIV-1 and its co-receptor CCR-5. *Nature* 1996; 384:184–187.

139. Dean M, Carrington M, Winkler C, et al. Genetic restriction of HIV-1 infection and progression to AIDS by a deletion allele of the CKR5 structural gene. *Science* 1996;273:1856–1862.

140. Liu R, Paxton WA, Choe S, et al. Homozygous defect in HIV-1 coreceptor accounts for resistance of some multiply-exposed individuals to HIV-1 infection. *Cell* 1996;86:367–377.

141. Samson M, Libert F, Doranz BJ, et al. Resistance to HIV-1 infection in Caucasian individuals bearing mutant alleles of the CCR-5 chemokine receptor gene. *Nature* 1996;382:722–725.

142. Connor RI, Sheridan KE, Ceradini D, Choe S, Landau NR. Change in coreceptor use correlates with disease progression in HIV-1–infected individuals. *J Exp Med* 1997;185:621–628.

143. Arenzana-Seisdedos F, Virelizier JL, Rousset D, et al. HIV blocked by chemokine antagonist. *Nature* 1996;383:400.

144. Simmons G, Clapham PR, Picard L, et al. Potent inhibition of HIV-1 infectivity in macrophages and lymphocytes by a novel CCR5 antagonist. *Science* 1997;276:276–279.

145. Kim K-S, Clark-Lewis I, Sykes BD. Solution structure of GRO/melanoma growth stimulatory activity determined by ¹H NMR spectroscopy. *J Biol Chem* 1994;269:32909–32915.

146. Gong J-H, Clark-Lewis I. Antagonists of monocyte chemoattractant protein 1 identified by modification of functionally critical NH₂-terminal residues. *J Exp Med* 1995;181:631–640.

147. Weber M, Uguccioni M, Baggiolini M, Clark-Lewis I, Dahinden CA. Deletion of the NH₂-terminal residue converts monocyte chemotactic protein 1 from an activator of basophil mediator release to an eosinophil chemoattractant. *J Exp Med* 1996;183:681–685.

148. Moser B, Dewald B, Barella L, Schumacher C, Baggiolini M, Clark-Lewis I. Interleukin-8 antagonists generated by N-terminal modification. *J Biol Chem* 1993;268:7125–7128.

149. Jones SA, Dewald B, Clark-Lewis I, Baggiolini M. Chemokine antagonists that discriminate between interleukin-8 receptors. *J Biol Chem* 1997;272:16166–16169.

150. Gong JH, Uguccioni M, Dewald B, Baggiolini M, Clark-Lewis I. RANTES and MCP-3 antagonists bind multiple chemokine receptors. *J Biol Chem* 1996;271:10521–10527.

151. Masure S, Paemen L, Proost P, Van Damme J, Opdenakker G. Expression of a human mutant monocyte chemotactic protein 3 in *Pichia pastoris* and characterization as an MCP-3 receptor antagonist. *J Interferon Cytokine Res* 1995;15:955–963.

152. Proudfoot AEI, Power CA, Hoogewerf AJ, et al. Extension of recombinant human RANTES by the retention of the initiating methionine produces a potent antagonist. *J Biol Chem* 1996;271:2599–2603.

Inflammation: Basic Principles and Clinical Correlates, 3rd ed., edited by John I. Gallin and Ralph Snyderman. Lippincott Williams & Wilkins, Philadelphia © 1999.

CHAPTER 29

Cytokines in Normal and Pathogenic Inflammatory Responses

John S. Sundy, Dhavalkumar D. Patel, and Barton F. Haynes

The term *cytokine* refers to a myriad of cellular proteins that mediate pleiotropic proinflammatory and antiinflammatory modulatory effects (Table 29-1). The biologic responses to cytokines result from cytokine ligation of specific cytokine receptors on target cells. Although cytokines regulate many functions in a variety of cell types, the scope of this chapter is limited to the general roles that cytokines play in mediating normal and pathologic inflammatory and immune responses. This chapter provides an overview of the general concepts of cytokine and cytokine receptor classification and function, illustrated with examples of selected cytokines. More information regarding specific cytokines and their functions can be found in Appendix B and in many other chapters in this book.

NOMENCLATURE

The terminology used to describe cytokines can be confusing, because an individual cytokine often has multiple names based on its cell of origin, biologic effect, or molecular size. However, conventions have been established, and formalized nomenclatures have been adopted for the naming of many cytokines (see Appendix B) (1). When considered as classes of molecules, cytokines produced by cells of the monocyte lineage have been called *monokines,* and lymphocyte-derived cytokines have been called *lymphokines.* However, monokines and lymphokines may be produced by a variety of cell types, including endothelial cells, fibroblasts, and epithelial cells, and it is therefore more accurate to use the term

J. S. Sundy, D. D. Patel, and B. F. Haynes: Department of Medicine, Duke University Medical Center, Durham, North Carolina 27710.

cytokine. The term *interleukin* was originally used to describe cytokines that were produced by leukocytes and acted on leukocytes. This term has been adopted as part of the recognized general nomenclature of cytokines and does not necessarily imply that any given *interleukin* is produced by or acts on leukocytes (1). The term *chemokine* describes a subset of cytokines that share structural characteristics and induce the movement of leukocytes (2). Chemokines are designated CC or CXC based on the presence or absence of an amino acid between the two amino-terminal cysteine (C) residues.

PROINFLAMMATORY CYTOKINE PLEIOTROPY, REDUNDANCY, AND CASCADES

Cytokines often exhibit *pleiotropic* activity; they act on many types of cells to stimulate numerous cell functions. At the same time, more than one cytokine may induce a particular biologic activity; functions of individual cytokines can be *redundant.*

Interleukin-1 (IL-1) is a pleiotropic cytokine. IL-1 acts on virtually all leukocytes and leukocyte precursors, as well as on endothelial cells, hepatocytes, myocytes, adipose tissue, and certain neurons in the central and peripheral nervous systems (3). The biologic effects of IL-1 include upregulated expression of adhesion molecules, cytokines, and arachidonic acid metabolites; enhanced neutrophil accumulation, fibroblast proliferation, and angiogenesis; hepatic acute phase protein synthesis; and induction of fever (3). Similar pleiotropic activity has been observed with tumor necrosis factor-α (TNF-α), IL-6, IL-4, IL-10, transforming growth factor-β (TGF-β), and members of the interferon (IFN) cytokine family (4–9).

The functions of IL-1 and TNF-α are excellent examples of cytokine functional redundancy. Among the over-

TABLE 29-1. *Characteristic features of cytokines*

Most cytokines are simple polypeptides or glycoproteins with molecular weight ≤ 30 kd.
Constitutive production of cytokines is uncommon; production is regulated by inducing stimuli at the level of transcription and translation.
Cytokine production is transient and the action radius is usually short.
Cytokines act by binding to high-affinity cell-surface receptors ($K_d = 10^{-9}$–10^{-12} M).
Most cytokine actions are attributed to altered gene expression in the target cells.

From ref. 1, with permission.

lapping functions of IL-1 and TNF-α are adhesion molecule upregulation, accumulation of leukocytes in sites of inflammation, acute phase protein synthesis, and angiogenesis (3,10). Another example includes members of the IL-6 cytokine family, oncostatin-M, leukemia inhibitory factor, IL-11, and IL-6; cytokines that share redundant functions of acute phase protein induction; growth promotion of myeloma cells; and growth of hematopoietic progenitors (11).

Cytokine gene disruption experiments in mice have highlighted the concept of cytokine redundancy. Mice deficient in IL-2 have normal immune system ontogeny (12). IL-2 deficient mice had only partially reduced cytotoxic T-cell responses and surprisingly were capable of rejecting allografts (13,14). Deficiency of IL-2 and IL-4 in "double knock-out" mice also resulted in normal lymphocyte subset development, with mice demonstrating increased lymphocyte proliferative responses (15). Mice deficient in key cytokines that regulate T-cell proliferation are able to function relatively normally, presumably on the basis of compensatory and redundant function of other T-cell trophic cytokines. The redundancy of function in the IL-2 system can be explained in part by the observation that IL-2 shares a common receptor component with IL-4, IL-7, IL-9, and IL-15 that can transduce identical signals into the cell, regardless of the specific cytokine ligating the cytokine receptor (16).

Cytokines often induce the production of additional cytokines, resulting in a cytokine *cascade*. Lipopolysaccharide (LPS)–induced sepsis in animals provides a well-characterized example of a cytokine cascade (17). Injection of LPS is followed by a progression of systemic cytokine production that is initiated by TNF-α and followed by successive waves of IL-1 and IL-6 production. This process is driven by TNF-α; exogenous TNF-α administration triggers the same cascade in the absence of LPS (17).

The proinflammatory effects of the cell surface receptor for hyaluronan, CD44, include regulation of other adhesion molecule functions, induction of monocyte and T-cell cytokine production, leukocyte rolling on endothelial cells, and migration into inflammatory sites (18).

Although IL-3, IL-2, granulocyte-macrophage colony-stimulating factor (GM-CSF), IL-1α, IL-1β, IL-15, and IL-10 induce CD44 to bind hyaluronan on monocytes, in each case, the effect is achieved through secondarily induced TNF-α (19).

Mediation of Normal and Pathologic Inflammatory and Immune Responses

Cytokines appear to be critical for mediating normal and abnormal states of inflammation and immune responses. For example, the ability to normally produce IFN-γ is critical for generating normal cytotoxic T-cell responses and controlling infections such as those of *Listeria monocytogenes,* cytomegalovirus, and herpes simplex (20,21). Overproduction of TNF-α is associated with the occurrence of life-threatening malaria (22), and overproduction of IL-5 is associated with the occurrence of the hypereosinophilic syndrome (23).

Regulation of Proinflammatory Cytokine Function

The biologic activity of cytokines depends on binding to specific cytokine receptors. Several mechanisms of cytokine-receptor interactions have been identified, most of which involve soluble cytokines (Fig. 29-1). The most

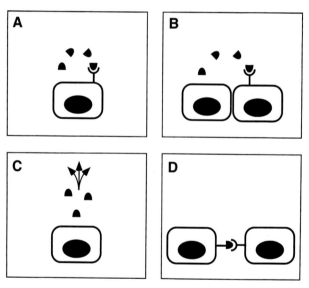

FIG. 29-1. Cytokine-receptor interactions. Most cytokines have a short action radius, and after being secreted, they interact with cytokine receptors in an autocrine manner (i.e., bind receptors on cell of origin) **(A)** or paracrine manner (i.e., bind receptors on adjacent cells) **(B)**. Some cytokines, such as tumor necrosis factor, interleukin-1, and interleukin-6, bind receptors expressed on distant cells and may therefore function in an endocrine manner **(C)**. Juxtacrine cytokine-receptor interactions **(D)** occur when a membrane-anchored cytokine binds its receptor on the same cell or an adjacent cell.

common mechanisms by which a cytokine interacts with its receptor are through *paracrine* and *autocrine* pathways; cytokines generally have a short action radius (24). Paracrine pathways allow cytokines to signal cells in the local microenvironment, leading to inflammatory cell accumulation and activation. Most cytokines function in a paracrine manner. Autocrine pathways are important in cytokine-induced inflammatory and immune responses, because autocrine cytokine stimulation enables amplification of inflammatory responses. For example, activation of T lymphocytes results in upregulation of IL-2 and IL-2 receptor expression, creating a positive feedback loop that stimulates proliferation of activated T cells and the clonal expansion of antigen-specific T cells.

Cytokines released into the peripheral circulation may also function in an *endocrine* manner. IL-1, IL-6, and TNF-α function in an endocrine manner, inducing hepatic cell acute phase protein production and induction of generalized septic shock syndrome (3,7,17). *Juxtacrine* signaling occurs when a membrane-bound cytokine binds its receptor on an adjacent cell (25). Several cytokines are expressed on the cell surface in membrane-bound form and have biologic activity; the best characterized are members of the IL-1 and TNF families of cytokines (26,27).

Cytokines are potent biologic response modifiers, and numerous cellular and molecular mechanisms have therefore evolved to regulate cytokine function. The primary mechanism of regulating cytokine production occurs at the level of gene transcription. In most cases, cytokines are not stored in the cell but are produced *de novo* after cell activation. Cytokine gene transcription is transitory, and the resulting mRNAs are generally short lived. For example, resting T cells contain no IL-2 mRNA (28,29). However, antigen stimulation of T cells leads to IL-2 gene transcription within 30 minutes, with steady-state levels that peak after 4 to 8 hours and return to baseline within 24 hours (28–31). Rapid degradation of IL-2 mRNA is in part caused by an inducible selective mechanism for cytokine mRNA degradation in the cell (31–33). Co-stimulation of T cells through the surface molecule, CD28, prolongs the half-life of IL-2 mRNA by inhibiting IL-2 mRNA degradation (31,32). In general, transcription of most cytokine genes is tightly regulated.

Regulation of the function of several cytokines occurs through the regulation of conversion of inactive procytokines to their active form. Among the cytokines that undergo activation from inactive forms are IL-1α, IL-1β, TNF-α, TGF-α, and TGF-β. For example, IL-1β is synthesized as a procytokine that remains in the cytosol and is essentially inactive until it is cleaved by the intracellular cysteine protease, IL-1–converting enzyme (34–36). In contrast, TNF-α is produced as a biologically active membrane protein. Secretion takes place only after proteolytic cleavage by TNF-α–converting enzyme, a member of the metalloproteinase family (37–39). TGF-β is expressed as a latent molecule in association with two proteins that target the latent cytokine to the extracellular matrix (40). TGF-β becomes activated after cleavage by proteases, predominantly plasmin (40).

Regulation of cytokine function also occurs through control of expression of the cytokine receptor, in that receptor expression determines responsiveness to secreted cytokines. The IL-2 receptor (IL-2R) is not expressed on resting T cells; it is an early marker of T-cell activation and allows expansion of activated T cells (41). Similarly, IL-6 and IL-6R are not normally expressed in normal neuronal tissue of mice. However, after tissue injury, IL-6 is expressed by neuronal Schwann cells, and IL-6R is expressed on injured nerve cell bodies, with subsequent IL-6–mediated nerve regeneration (42).

Novel cytokine receptor characteristics can also regulate cytokine functional activity. For example, IL-1 has two receptors, designated type I and type II IL-1Rs (3). The type I IL-1R is capable of transducing signals in response to IL-1α and IL-1β binding, whereas the type II IL-1R does not. The type II IL-1R instead functions as a decoy that adsorbs IL-1α and IL-1β, limiting IL-1 bioactivity (43). An analogue of IL-1β, known as the IL-1 receptor antagonist (IL-1Ra), binds to the IL-1R without transducing a signal (3). When expressed in sufficient levels, IL-1Ra prevents IL-1β binding to the type I IL-1R, decreasing the biologic activity of IL-1β. Recombinant human IL-1Ra has been studied with various degrees of success in therapeutic trials in patients with leukemia, rheumatoid arthritis, and graft-versus-host disease (3).

The release of soluble cytokine receptors is another mechanism for regulating cytokine activity. Soluble TNF receptors (TNFRs) are detected in the serum of patients with inflammatory diseases and downregulate TNF-α activity *in vitro*. The importance of intrinsic soluble TNFR in modulating TNF-α activity *in vivo* is unknown. However, recombinant soluble TNFR has been used in pharmacologic doses to successfully treat human rheumatoid arthritis (44). Soluble IL-6Rs have also been detected in human serum at concentrations that are biologically significant *in vitro* (45). The IL-6/IL-6R complex maintains bioactivity and can associate with the common gp130 IL-6 receptor family signaling subunit on cell surfaces, conferring IL-6 responsiveness to cells that do not express the IL-6 receptor (11). Soluble cytokine receptors may have complex effects on the biologic activities of their respective cytokines, with the abilities to inhibit or possibly stimulate cytokine activity on target cells.

ANTIINFLAMMATORY ACTIVITIES OF CYTOKINES

Downregulating inflammation is equally as important in the host's inflammatory response as initiating inflammation. Failure to control inflammatory responses can lead to extensive tissue damage; for example, defective regulation of inflammation may contribute to the pathogenesis of many autoimmune diseases. Among the mechanisms for downregulating inflammatory responses are apoptosis of inflammatory cells, production of inhibitors of activated complement components, and production of cytokine receptor antagonists. Certain cytokines, such as IL-4, IL-10, IL-13, and TGF-β, have intrinsic antiinflammatory activities.

The cytokines IL-4, IL-10, and IL-13 are produced predominantly by T cells. When considering their antiinflammatory actions, it is important to appreciate the functional dichotomy of $CD4^+$ helper T cells. Helper T cells may be divided into functional types, T_H1 and T_H2, based on their patterns of cytokine expression (see Chapter 12). T_H1 cells produce IFN-γ, IL-2, and lymphotoxin, and they stimulate cellular immune responses such as cytotoxic T-cell formation and drive IgG1 (murine IgG2a/b) antibody responses. T_H2 cells produce IL-4, IL-5, IL-10, and IL-13 and drive IgG4 (murine IgG1) and IgE antibody responses (46–48). Some of the cytokines produced by helper T cells mediate complex regulatory roles; for example, IFN-γ stimulates T_H1 and inhibits T_H2 formation, and IL-4 and IL-10 stimulate T_H2 and inhibit T_H1 responses (49,50). Some of the antiinflammatory actions of IL-4 and IL-10 may result from downregulation of T_H1 immune responses. In support of this notion, interleukin-10 deficient mice spontaneously develop severe $CD4^+$ T_H1-mediated enterocolitis, presumably on the basis of unopposed stimulation of T_H1 T cells by enteric antigens (51).

IL-4 and IL-10 share similar activities in the induction of immunity and in the induction of antiinflammatory activities. IL-4 is produced by activated T cells, mast cells, and basophils, and it binds to receptors expressed on T and B lymphocytes, mast cells, endothelial cells, macrophages, keratinocytes, fibroblasts, hepatocytes, stromal cells, and neuroblasts (4). IL-10 is produced by activated T and B lymphocytes, macrophages, mast cells, and keratinocytes, and it binds to receptors expressed on T and B lymphocytes, natural killer cells, macrophages, and mast cells (48).

Alone or in combination, IL-4 and IL-10 decrease LPS-induced macrophage production of proinflammatory cytokines IL-1, IL-6, IL-8, IL-12, and TNF-α (4,52,53). Other effects of IL-4 or IL-10 on macrophages include decreased major histocompatibility complex class II antigen expression, decreased expression of the T-cell co-stimulatory molecule B7, decreased nitric oxide production, and reduced expression of hydrogen peroxide (4,52). IL-10 and IL-4 decrease in vitro prostaglandin E_2 (PGE_2) production in LPS-stimulated neutrophils. The reduction in PGE_2 correlated with decreased levels of the synthetic enzyme cyclooxygenase-2 mRNA (54). IL-4 decreases the expression of intercellular adhesion molecule-1 and endothelial leukocyte adhesion molecule-1 (also called E-selectin or CD62E) on endothelial cells (4).

Evidence for antiinflammatory effects of IL-4 and IL-10 has been found in animal models of disease and in human diseases. Exogenous administration of IL-4 prevents mice from developing type I diabetes mellitus (55). Similarly, decreased IL-4 mRNA expression is seen in in vitro activated peripheral blood mononuclear cells and T cells from patients with newly diagnosed type I diabetes mellitus (56). IL-4 and IL-10 appear to be important in downregulating proinflammatory responses in the placenta. CBA × DBA/2 mouse placentas have defects in production of IL-4 and IL-10 that result in excessive fetal wastage. This defect is corrected by administration of IL-10 and is exacerbated by administration of anti-IL-10 (57). IL-4 inhibits production of the proinflammatory cytokine leukemia inhibitory factor by cultured human synovium obtained from rheumatoid arthritis patients (58). Recombinant IL-10 reduced the severity of collagen-induced arthritis in DBA1/J mice (59). These observations have provided the rationale for administering recombinant human IL-4 and IL-10 to treat patients with inflammatory diseases such as rheumatoid arthritis.

IL-13 shares structural and functional characteristics with IL-4 (60). It is produced by T cells, mast cells, and basophils and exerts biologic effects similar to IL-4 on macrophages, B cells, mast cells, basophils, and natural killer cells, but not on T cells (60–62). IL-4 and IL-13 share receptor components on monocytes, accounting for some of these interleukins' common functions (63). IL-13 inhibits LPS-stimulated monocyte production of IL-1, IL-6, IL-8, macrophage inflammatory protein-1α, TNF-α, IL-10, IL-12, GM-CSF, and granulocyte colony-stimulating factor, but it upregulates IL-1Ra expression (60). IL-4 and IL-13 are potent downregulators of a wide variety of proinflammatory events, including the induction by TNF-α of the ability of monocyte-macrophage CD44 to bind hyaluronan (19). IL-13 increases the ability of macrophages to present antigen, resulting in increased T-cell proliferative responses. This pattern suggests that IL-13 does not globally inhibit macrophage function, but that it instead selectively inhibits cytotoxic and proinflammatory macrophage functions (60). In vivo, IL-13 protects against lethal endotoxemia in mice, a finding that was correlated with decreased production of IL-12, TNF-α, and IFN-γ (64). In summary, IL-13 has antiinflammatory activities similar to IL-4 and IL-10 but does not have the ability to directly act on T lymphocytes.

TGF-β exists in three isoforms, TGF-β1, TGF-β2, and TGF-β3 (65). At least one or more isoforms are produced by virtually all cells, and all cells have TGF-β receptors (65). TGF-β stimulates a variety of responses that are antiinflammatory and others that may lead to tissue injury. TGF-β induces fibroblast proliferation and increased extracellular matrix production. Consequently, TGF-β has been implicated in the pathogenesis of fibrosing diseases such as glomerulosclerosis and scleroderma (66,67). However, TGF-β also inhibits T-cell proliferative responses to mitogens, inhibits macrophage activation, and antagonizes proinflammatory actions on endothelial cells and fibroblasts (68). TGF-β1–deficient mice have uncontrolled inflammatory responses, a process that reflects reciprocal regulation of immune function between IFN-γ and TGF-β (69,70). Susceptibility to experimental autoimmune myasthenia gravis in rats correlated with decreased T-cell expression of TGF-β relative to IFN-γ (71). Recombinant TGF-β decreases T-cell proliferative responses and IL-2 production in a rat model of bacterial sepsis (72). Disease activity of patients with sarcoid correlated inversely with TGF-β production in the supernatants of cultured bronchoalveolar lavage cells, suggesting that increased production of TGF-β may play a role in reducing sarcoid disease activity (73). Taken together, these data suggest antiinflammatory and immunosuppressive effects of TGF-β, but the biologic activities of TGF-β are complex and incompletely characterized.

CYTOKINE RECEPTORS

Cytokines bind specific cell-surface receptors that transduce signals across the cell membrane into the cell. Cytokine receptors are transmembrane proteins and have been divided into receptor families based on structural similarities (Fig. 29-2). With few exceptions, cytokine receptors are heterodimers with one receptor subunit binding cytokine and the other transducing signals into the cell (74). Type I cytokine receptors share a conserved amino acid sequence (WSXWS) with four paired cysteines (CCCC) in their extracellular domain.

Type II cytokine receptors share sequence homology with type I receptors but have an additional cysteine pair and have conserved proline and tyrosine residues (74). Interferons are the ligands for this receptor family.

A third type of cytokine receptor family contains immunoglobulin domains. Ligands of the immunoglobu-lin family of receptors include IL-1α and IL-1β and many of the hematopoietic growth factor cytokines, such as IL-3 and GM-CSF.

The TNF receptor family is characterized by type I membrane proteins that contain a cysteine-rich region in the extracellular domain. The prototype receptors in this family are TNF receptors type I and II, each of which binds both TNF-α and lymphotoxin (6). Other members of this family include receptor molecules whose ligands are membrane proteins instead of soluble cytokines. Examples include CD40, whose ligand is gp39 (CD40L), and FAS (CD95), which binds the FAS ligand (6).

The fifth family of cytokine receptors is among the larger superfamily of seven-transmembrane-spanning receptors. They have as their ligands the CC or the CXC chemokines (75).

Cytokine receptors frequently function as a complex of two or three molecules. The receptors for several different cytokines often share a common receptor subunit (see Appendix B). For example, the high affinity IL-2 receptor is a heterotrimer composed of α, β, and γ subunits (16). However, the γ subunit has been shown to be the critical signaling subunit in this receptor, and it also is a member of the receptor complex for IL-4, IL-7, IL-9, and IL-15 (16). Mutation of the common γ chain results in X-linked severe combined immunodeficiency disease (SCID) in humans, canines, and mice (16). The IL-6R has similar characteristics; it is composed of an IL-6–binding subunit that is associated with a signal transducing subunit, gp130 (11). Gp130 is also the signaling subunit in the receptors for the cytokines oncostatin-M, leukemia inhibitory factor, ciliary neurotrophic factor, IL-11, and cardiotrophin-1 (11). Targeted disruption of gp130 is a lethal mutation, with embryos exhibiting hypoplastic myocardium, decreased primordial germ cells, hematopoietic abnormalities, and altered placental development (11). A common β subunit (gp150) comprises part of the receptors for the cytokines IL-3, IL-5, and GM-CSF (76).

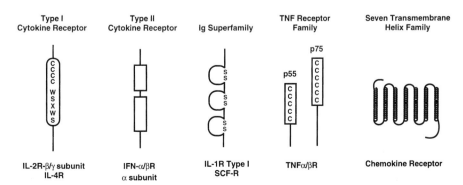

FIG. 29-2. Cytokine receptors are grouped into families on the basis of shared structural motifs. (From ref. 85, with permission.)

OTHER MOLECULES THAT BIND CYTOKINES

The manner in which cytokines are presented to receptor-expressing cells is another level at which regulation can occur. Cells can encounter cytokines in soluble form, bound to the extracellular matrix or on other cell surfaces as transmembrane proteins (i.e., TNF and fractalkine), or soluble cytokines that are bound to the cell surface (i.e., growth factors and chemokines). The ability of fibroblast growth factors (FGFs) to bind to and transduce signals through FGF receptors is enhanced by the binding of FGFs to glycosaminoglycans (77,78). Chemokines binding to cell-surface glycosaminoglycans can increase local chemokine concentrations to induce chemokine oligomerization—a step that may be necessary for the function of specific chemokines at physiologic nanomolar concentrations (79). Macrophage chemotactic protein-1 (MCP-1), for example, functions as a dimer (80,81). Chemokine binding to glycosaminoglycans, such as the CD44 molecule, on endothelial cells may also be necessary to present chemokines to rolling leukocytes for leukocyte migration.

SIGNALING BY CYTOKINE RECEPTORS

Interaction of cytokines with specific receptors initiates signals that modify cell functions in the cytoplasm and the nucleus. The rapid induction of new gene transcription is a common outcome of cytokine signaling. Darnell et al. (74) elucidated a new mechanism of cytokine signal transduction known as the JAK-STAT pathway. Although cytokine-receptor interactions initiate a variety of biologic responses, the JAK-STAT pathway has emerged as a major pathway by which transcriptional activation signals are transmitted to the nucleus by many cytokines.

A schematic representation of the JAK-STAT pathway is shown in Figure 29-3. The Janus kinases (i.e., JAKs) are a family of four tyrosine kinases: TYK-2, JAK-1, JAK-2, and JAK-3. The JAKs are soluble proteins that are associated in inactive forms with cytoplasmic components of cytokine receptors. Binding of a cytokine to its receptor dimerizes the receptor chains, allowing the JAKs to transphosphorylate each other. JAK phosphorylation allows association of STATs (i.e., signal transducers and activators of transcription), a family of six proteins (STAT-1 through STAT-6) that possess a SRC homology-2 (SH2) phosphotyrosine binding domain and a conserved tyrosine residue at amino acid 700. Subsequent phosphorylation of STATs results in homodimerization or heterodimerization, which permits STAT translocation into the nucleus, where the activated STAT dimers bind DNA and regulate the transcription of cytokine-responsive genes. Examples of

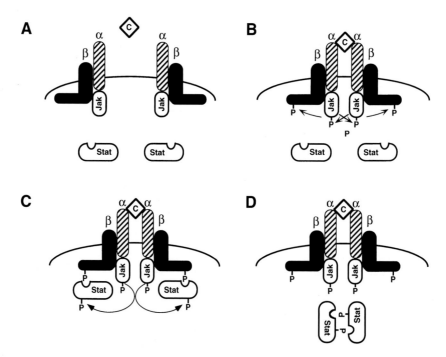

FIG. 29-3. JAK-STAT signaling pathway. **(A)** JAK components are associated in an inactive form with the cytoplasmic portion of cytokine receptors. **(B)** Cytokine binding leads to cytokine receptor aggregation. Adjacent JAKs become activated and phosphorylate each other and phosphorylate tyrosine residues on the cytoplasmic region of the cytokine receptor. **(C)** Through the SH2 domain, STATs bind phosphotyrosine residues on the cytoplasmic portion of cytokine receptors. Bound STAT proteins are phosphorylated by bound JAK proteins and subsequently dissociate. **(D)** Phosphorylated STAT proteins dimerize and then move to the nucleus, where they activate transcription by binding to specific sequences known as interferon-stimulated response elements (ISREs). (From ref. 74, with permission.)

JAK and STAT proteins known to be associated with specific cytokine signaling pathways are shown in Table 29-2.

The tissue distribution of JAK-STAT proteins is broad. All JAKs are expressed in most tissues, with the exception of JAK-3, which is limited to the myelocytic and lymphocytic cell types (74). STAT-1 through STAT-3 are expressed in most tissues, and STAT-4 is expressed primarily in testis and thymus. STAT-5 occurs in myeloid cells and in mammary tissue (74).

An important area of research is aimed at defining the mechanisms by which the specificity of cytokine functions are maintained despite signaling through a limited array of JAK and STAT proteins. The notion has emerged that specificity is maintained at multiple levels through differences in the ability of STATs to associate with particular cytokine receptors. Differences in the DNA binding properties of STAT homodimers and heterodimers also enable a measure of specificity. Other transcriptional regulators undoubtedly influence the signaling functions of the JAK-STAT pathway and help to maintain tissue-specific and cytokine-specific responses to cytokine-receptor interactions.

The JAK-STAT pathway is important in disease pathogenesis. Mutations in the JAK-3 protein lead to an autosomal recessive form of SCID (82). SCID related to JAK-3 deficiency is autosomally transmitted but is phenotypically similar to X-linked SCID, which is caused by mutations in the common γ chain of the IL-2 receptor family. JAK-3 is a critical member of the signaling cascade through the IL-2 receptor family, explaining the phenotypic similarities of SCID in the setting of IL-2Rγ or JAK-3 mutations, despite different modes of inheritance of the genes encoding these proteins. A fusion protein between TEL, a member of the ETS transcription factor family, and JAK-2 was described in a patient with a T-cell leukemia characterized by a t(9;12)(p24;p13) chromosomal translocation (83). The fusion protein contained the catalytic domain of JAK-2 and exhibited constitutive kinase activity. Similarly, the *BCR-ABL* oncogene, present in chronic myelogenous leukemia, results in constitutive activation of STAT-5, providing a mechanism for malignant transformation of leukocyte precursors in leukemia (84).

CONCLUSIONS

From the data reviewed in this chapter and in Appendix B, it is clear that cytokines are central and critical mediators of normal host defenses and are key mediators of abnormal pathogenic host inflammatory responses. Although redundancy in cytokine function results in effective antiinfective agent host immune responses, redundancy in cytokine function also results in systems that are difficult to inhibit for antiinflammatory therapy. Understanding how to modulate host pathologic cytokine production while leaving normal host defense intact is a major challenge for future research in the development of novel therapies for diseases of pathologic inflammation.

TABLE 29-2. *Jak-STAT components of cytokine signaling pathways*

Cytokine	Jak	STAT
IFN α/β	Jak-1, Tyk-2	STAT1, STAT2
IFNγ	Jak-1, Jak-2	STAT1a
IL-2	Jak-1, Jak-3	STAT5, STAT3
IL-3	Jak-1, Jak-2	STAT5
IL-4	Jak-1, Jak-3, Jak-2	STAT6
IL-5	Jak-1, Jak-2	STAT5
IL-6	Jak-1, Jak-2, Jak-3	STAT1, STAT3
IL-7	Jak-1, Jak-3	STAT5
IL-10	Unknown	STAT1, STAT3
IL-12	Jak-1, Tyk-2	STAT3, STAT4
IL-13	Jak-2	STAT6
IL-15	Jak-1, Jak-3	STAT5, STAT3
GM-CSF	Jak-1, Jak-2	STAT5
G-CSF	Jak-1, Jak-2	STAT3

Jak and Tyk, Janus kinases; STAT, signal transducer and activator of transcription.
From ref. 85, with permission.

REFERENCES

1. Vilcek J, Le J. Immunology of cytokines. In: Thomson A, ed. *The cytokine handbook,* 2nd ed. New York: Academic Press, 1994.
2. Schall TJ. The chemokines. In: Thomson A, ed. *The cytokine handbook,* 2nd ed. New York: Academic Press, 1994.
3. Dinarello CA. Biologic basis for interleukin-1 in disease. *Blood* 1996; 87:2095–2147.
4. Ryan JJ. Interleukin 4 and its receptor: essential mediators of the allergic response. *J Allergy Clin Immunol* 1997;99:1–5.
5. Mossman TR. Properties and functions of interleukin-10. *Adv Immunol* 1994;56:1–26.
6. Bazzoni F, Beutler B. The tumor necrosis factor ligand and receptor families. *N Engl J Med* 1996;26:1717–1725.
7. Akira S, Taga T, Kishimoto T. Interleukin-6 in biology and medicine. *Adv Immunol* 1993;54:1–78.
8. Letterio JJ, Roberts AB. TGF-beta: a critical modulator of immune cell function. *Clin Immunol Immunopathol* 1997;84:244–50.
9. Gresser I. Wherefore interferon? *J Leukoc Biol* 1997;61:567–574.
10. Bemelmans MHA, van Tits LJH, Buuman WA. Tumor necrosis factor: function, release and clearance. *Crit Rev Immunol* 1996;16:1–11.
11. Taga T, Kishimoto T. Gp130 and the interleukin-6 family of cytokines. *Annu Rev Immunol* 1997;15:797–819.
12. Schorle H, Holtschke T, Hinig T, Schimpl A, Horak I. Development and function of T cells in mice rendered interleukin-2 deficient by gene targeting. *Nature* 1991;352:621–624.
13. Kindig TM, Schorle H, Bachmann M, Hengartner H, Zinkernagel RM, Horak I. Immune responses in interleukin-2 deficient mice. *Science* 1993;262:1059–1061.
14. Steiger J, Nickerson PW, Steurer W, Moscovitch-Lopatin M, Strom TB. IL-2 knockout recipient mice reject islet cell allografts. *J Immunol* 1995;155:489–498.
15. Sadlack B, Lohler J, Schorle H, Rajewsky K, Miller W, Horak I. Development and function of lymphocytes in mice deficient for both interleukins 2 and 4. *Eur J Immunol* 1995;24:281–284.
16. Sugamura K, Asao H, Kondo M, et al. The interleukin-2 receptor gamma chain: its role in the multiple cytokine receptor complexes and T cell development in XSCID. *Annu Rev Immunol* 1996;14:179–205.
17. Beutler B, Cerami A. The endogenous mediator of endotoxic shock. *Clin Res* 1987;35:192–197.
18. Haynes BF, Telen MJ, Hale LP, Denning SM. CD44: a molecule

involved in leukocyte adherence and T cell activation. *Immunol Today* 1989;10:423.

19. Levesque MC, Haynes BF. Cytokine induction of the ability of human monocyte CD44 to bind hyaluronan is mediated primarily by TNF-alpha and is inhibited by IL-4 and IL-13. *J Immunol* 1997;159: 6184–6194.

20. Young HA, Hardy KJ. Role of interferon-gamma in immune cell regulation. *J Leukoc Biol* 1995;58:373–381.

21. Boehm U, Klamp T, Groot M, Howard JC. Cellular responses to interferon-gamma. *Annu Rev Immunol* 1997;15:749–795.

22. Shaffer N, Grau GE, Hedberg K, et al. Tumor necrosis factor and severe malaria. *J Infect Dis* 1991;163:96–101.

23. Brugnoni D, Airo P, Rossi G, et al. A case of hypereosinophilic syndrome is associated with the expansion of a CD3-CD4$^+$ T-cell population able to secrete large amounts of interleukin-5. *Blood* 1996;87: 1416–1422.

24. Kaplan D. Autocrine secretion and the physiologic concentration of cytokines. *Immunol Today* 1996;17:303–304.

25. Bosenberg MW, Massague J. Juxtacrine cell signaling molecules. *Curr Opin Cell Biol* 1993;5:832–838.

26. Kaplanski G, Farnarier C, Kaplanski S, et al. Interleukin-1 induces interleukin-8 secretion from endothelial cells by a juxtacrine mechanism. *Blood* 1994;84:4242–4248.

27. Schmid EF, Binder K, Grell M, Scheurich P, Pfizenmaier K. Both tumor necrosis factor receptors, TNFR60 and TNFR80, are involved in signaling endothelial tissue factor expression by juxtacrine tumor necrosis factor alpha. *Blood* 1995;86:1836–1841.

28. Jain J, Loh C, Rao A. Transcriptional regulation of the IL-2 gene. *Curr Opin Immunol* 1995;7:333–342.

29. Lacour M, Arrighi J-F, Muller KM, Carlberg C, Saurat J-H, Hause C. cAMP up-regulates IL-4 and IL-5 production from activated CD4$^+$ T cells while decreasing IL-2 release and NF-AT induction. *Int Immunol* 1994;6:1333–1343.

30. Shaw J, Meerovitch K, Bleackley RC, Paetkau V. Mechanisms regulating the level of IL-2 mRNA in T lymphocytes. *J Immunol* 1988;140: 2243–2248.

31. Umlauf SW, Beverly B, Lantz O, Schwartz RH. Regulation of IL-2 gene expression by CD28 costimulation in mouse T cell clones. Both nuclear and cytoplasmic RNA are regulated with complex kinetics. *Mol Cell Biol* 1995;15:3197–3205.

32. Lindsten T, June CH, Ledbetter JA, Stella G, Thompson CB. Regulation of lymphokine messenger RNA stability by a surface-mediated T cell activation pathway. *Science* 1989;244:339–343.

33. Bohjanen PR, Petryniak B, June CH, Thompson CB, Lindsten T. An inducible cytoplasmic factor (AU-B) binds selectively to AUUUA multimers in the 3′ untranslated region of lymphokine mRNA. *Mol Cell Biol* 1991;11:3288–3295.

34. Hazuda DJ, Strickler J, Kueppers F, Simon PL, Young PR. Processing of precursor interleukin-1 beta and inflammatory disease. *J Biol Chem* 1990;265:6318–6322.

35. Cerretti DP, Kozlosky CJ, Mosley B, et al. Molecular cloning of the IL-1β processing enzyme. *Science* 1992;256:97–100.

36. Thornberry NA, Bull HG, Calaycay JR, et al. A novel heterodimeric cysteine protease is required for interleukin-1 beta processing in monocytes. *Nature* 1992;356:768–774.

37. Perez C, Albert I, DeFay K, Zachariades N, Gooding L, Kriegler M. A nonsecretable cell surface mutant of tumor necrosis factor (TNF) kills by cell-to-cell contact. *Cell* 1990;63(2):251–258.

38. Utsumi T, Levitan A, Hung MC, Klostergaard J. Effects of truncation of human pro-tumor necrosis factor transmembrane domain on cellular targeting. *J Biol Chem* 1993;268:9511–9516.

39. Moss ML, Jin SL, Milla ME, et al. Cloning of a disintegrin metalloproteinase that processes precursor tumor-necrosis factor alpha. *Nature* 1997;385:733–736.

40. Munger JS, Harpel JG, Gleizes PE, Mazzieri R, Nunes I, Rifkin DB. Latent transforming growth factor-beta: structural features and mechanisms of activation. *Kidney Int* 1997;51:1376–1382.

41. Karnitz LM, Abraham RT. Interleukin-2 receptor signaling mechanisms. *Adv Immunol* 1996;61:147–199.

42. Hirota H, Kiyama H, Kishimoto T, Taga T. Accelerated nerve regeneration in mice by upregulated expression of interleukin (IL) 6 and IL-6 receptor after trauma. *J Exp Med* 1996;183:2627–2634.

43. Colotta F, Dower SK, Sims JE, Mantovani A. The type II decoy receptor: a novel regulatory pathway for interleukin-1. *Immunol Today* 1994; 15:562–566.

44. Moreland LW, Baumgartner SW, Schiff MH. Treatment of rheumatoid arthritis with a recombinant human tumor necrosis factor receptor (p75)-Fc fusion protein. *N Engl J Med* 1997;337:141–147.

45. Narazaki M, Yasukawa K, Saito T, et al. Soluble forms of the interleukin-6 signal-transducing receptor component gp130 in human serum possessing a potential to inhibit signals through membrane-anchored gp130. *Blood* 1993;82:1220–1226.

46. Cherwinski HM, Schumaker JH, Brown KD, Mosmann TR. Two types of mouse helper T cell clone. III. Further differences in lymphokine synthesis between Th1 and Th2 clones revealed by RNA hybridization, functionally monospecific bioassays, and monoclonal antibodies. *J Exp Med* 1987;166:1229–1244.

47. Mosmann TR, Cherwinski H, Bond MW, Giedlin MA, Coffman RL. Two types of murine helper T cell clones. I. Definition according to profiles of lymphokine activities and secreted proteins. *J Immunol* 1987;136:2348–2357.

48. Mosmann TR, Li L, Hengartner H, Kagi D, Fu W, Sad S. Differentiation and functions of T cell subsets. *Ciba Found Symp* 1997;204: 148–154.

49. Mosmann TR, Coffman RL. Heterogeneity of cytokine secretion patterns and functions of helper T cells. *Adv Immunol* 1989;46:111–147.

50. Swain SL, Weinberg AD, English M, Huston G. IL-4 directs the development of Th2-like helper effectors. *J Immunol* 1990;145:3796–3806.

51. Rennick DM, Fort MM, Davidson NJ. Studies with IL-10 −/− mice: an overview. *J Leukoc Biol* 1997;61:389–396.

52. Mosmann TR. Properties and functions of interleukin-10. *Adv Immunol* 1994;56:1–26.

53. Chernoff AE, Granowitz EV, Shapiro L, et al. A randomized controlled trial of interleukin-10 in humans: inhibition of inflammatory cytokine production and immune responses. *J Immunol* 1995;154:5492.

54. Niiro H, Otsuka T, Izuhara K, et al. Regulation by interleukin 10 and interleukin 4 of cyclooxygenase-2 expression in human neutrophils. *Blood* 1997;89:1621–1628.

55. Rabinovitch A. Immunoregulatory and cytokine imbalances in the pathogenesis of IDDM: therapeutic intervention by immunostimulation. *Diabetes* 1994;43:613.

56. Berman MA, Sandborg CI, Wang Z, et al. Decreased IL-4 production in new onset type I insulin-dependent diabetes mellitus. *J Immunol* 1996;157:4690–4696.

57. Chaouat G, Assal Meliani A, et al. IL-10 prevents naturally occurring fetal loss in the CBA × DBA/2 mating combination, and local defect in IL-10 production in this abortion-prone combination is corrected by *in vivo* injection of IFN-tau. *J Immunol* 1996;154:4261–4268.

58. Dechanet J, Taupin JL, Chomarat P, et al. Interleukin-4 but not interleukin-10 inhibits the production of leukemia inhibitory factor by rheumatoid synovium and synoviocytes. *Eur J Immunol* 1994;24: 3222–3228.

59. Tanaka Y, Otsuka T, Hotokebuchi T, et al. Effect of IL-10 on collagen-induced arthritis in mice. *Inflamm Res* 1996;45:283–288.

60. Zurawski G, de Vries JE. Interleukin 13, an interleukin 4-like cytokine that acts on monocytes and B cells, but not on T cells. *Immunol Today* 1994;15:19–26.

61. Li H, Sim TC, Alam R. IL-13 released by and localized in human basophils. *J Immunol* 1996;156:4833–4838.

62. Burd PR, Thompson CR, Max EE, Mills FC. Activated mast cells produce interleukin 13. *J Exp Med* 1995;181:1373–1380.

63. Keegan AD, Ryan JJ, Paul WE. IL-4 regulates growth and differentiation by distinct mechanisms. *Immunologist* 1996;4:194.

64. Muchamuel T, Menon S, Pisacane P, Howard MC, Cockayne DA. IL-13 protects mice from lipopolysaccharide-induced lethal endotoxemia: correlation with down-modulation of TNF-alpha, IFN-gamma, and IL-12 production. *J Immunol* 1997;158:2898–2903.

65. Lawrence DA. Transforming growth factor-β: an overview. *Kidney Int* 1995;49:S19–S23.

66. Kitamura M, Suto TS. TGF-beta and glomerulonephritis: anti-inflammatory versus prosclerotic actions. *Nephrol Dial Transplant* 1997;12: 669–679.

67. Rudnicka L, Varga J, Christiano AM, Iozzo RV, Jimenez SA, Uitto J. Elevated expression of type VII collagen in the skin of patients with systemic sclerosis: regulation by transforming growth factor-beta. *J Clin Invest* 1994;93:1709–1715.

68. Letterio JJ, Roberts AB. TGF-beta: a critical modulator of immune cell function. *Clin Immunol Immunopathol* 1997;84:244–250.

69. Bottinger EP, Letterio JJ, Roberts AB. Biology of TGF-beta in knockout and transgenic mouse models. *Kidney Int* 1997;51:1355–1360.

70. Strober W, Kelsall B, Fuss I, et al. Reciprocal IFN-gamma and TGF-beta responses regulate the occurrence of mucosal inflammation. *Immunol Today* 1997;18:61–64.

71. Zhang GX, Ma CG, Xiao BG, van de Meide PH, Link H. Autoreactive T cell responses and cytokine patterns reflect resistance to experimental autoimmune myasthenia gravis in Wistar Furth rats. *Eur J Immunol* 1996;26:2552–2558.

72. Ahmad S, Choudry MA, Shanker R, Sayeed MM. Transforming growth factor-beta negatively modulates responses in sepsis. *FEBS Lett* 1997; 402:213–218.

73. Zissel G, Homolka J, Schlaak J, Schlaak M, Muller-Quernheim J. Anti-inflammatory cytokine release by alveolar macrophages in pulmonary sarcoidosis. *Am J Respir Crit Care Med* 1996;154:713–719.

74. Schindler C, Darnell JE. Transcriptional responses to polypeptide ligands: the JAK-STAT pathway. *Annu Rev Biochem* 1995;64:621–651.

75. Baggiolini M, Dewald B, Moser B. Human chemokines: an update. *Annu Rev Immunol* 1997;15:675–705.

76. Bagley CJ, Woodcock JM, Stomski FC, Lopez AF. The structural and functional basis of cytokine receptor activation: lessons from the common beta subunit of the granulocyte-macrophage colony-stimulating factor, interleukin-3 (IL-3), and IL-5 receptors. *Blood* 1997;89: 1471–1482.

77. Vlodavsky I, Miao HQ, Medalion B, Danagher P, Ron D. Involvement of heparan sulfate and related molecules in sequestration and growth promoting activity of fibroblast growth factor. *Cancer Metastasis Rev* 1996;15:177–186.

78. Rusnati M, Presta M. Interaction of angiogenic basic fibroblast growth factor with endothelial cell heparan sulfate proteoglycans: biological implications in neovascularization. *Int J Clin Lab Res* 1996;26:15–23.

79. Hoogewerf AJ, Kuschert GSV, Proudfoot AEI, et al. Glycosaminoglycans mediate cell surface oligomerization of chemokines. *Biochemistry* 1997;36:13570–13578.

80. Paolini JF, Willard D, Consler T, Luther M, Krangel MS. The chemokines IL-8, monocyte chemoattractant protein-1, and I-309 are monomers at physiologically relevant concentrations. *J Immunol* 1994;153:2704–2717.

81. Zhang Y, Rollins BJ. A dominant negative inhibitor indicates that monocyte chemoattractant protein 1 functions as a dimer. *Mol Cell Biol* 1995;15(9):4851–4855.

82. Macchi P, Villa A, Gillani S, et al. Mutations of JAK-3 gene in patients with autosomal severe combined immune deficiency (SCID). *Nature* 1995;377:65–68.

83. Lacronique V, Boureux A, Valle VD, et al. A TEL-JAK2 fusion protein with constitutive kinase activity in human leukemia. *Science* 1997;278: 1309–1312.

84. Shuai K, Halpern J, ten Hoeve J, Rao X, Sawyers CL. Constitutive activation of STAT5 by the *BCR-ABL* oncogene in chronic myelogenous leukemia. *Oncogene* 1996;13:247–254.

85. Abbas A, Lichtman AH, Pober JS. *Cellular and molecular immunology,* 3rd ed. Philadelphia: WB Saunders, 1997:250–277.

Inflammation: Basic Principles and Clinical Correlates,
3rd ed., edited by John I. Gallin and Ralph Snyderman.
Lippincott Williams & Wilkins, Philadelphia © 1999.

CHAPTER 30

Interleukin-1:

A Proinflammatory Cytokine

Charles A. Dinarello

Interleukin-1 (IL-1) is the prototypic "multifunctional" cytokine. The two forms of IL-1 are IL-1α and IL-1β, and in most studies, their effects in terms of biologic activity are indistinguishable. Unlike the lymphocyte and colony-stimulating growth factors, IL-1 affects nearly every cell type, often in concert with another proinflammatory cytokine, tumor necrosis factor (TNF). Although IL-1 can upregulate host defenses and be an immunoadjuvant, IL-1 is a highly inflammatory cytokine. The margin between clinical benefit and unacceptable toxicity in humans is exceedingly narrow. In contrast, agents that reduce the production or activity of IL-1 are likely to have an impact on clinical medicine. In support of this concept, there is growing evidence that the production and activity of IL-1, particularly IL-1β, are tightly regulated events that appear destined to reduce the response to IL-1 during disease. In addition to controlling gene expression, synthesis, and secretion, this regulation extends to surface receptors, soluble receptors, and a receptor antagonist.

Investigators have studied how production of the different members of the IL-1 family is controlled, the various biologic activities of IL-1, the distinct and various functions of the IL-1 receptor (IL-1R) family, and the complexity of intracellular signaling. Mice deficient in IL-1β, IL-1β–converting enzyme (ICE), and IL-1R type I have also been studied. Humans have been injected with IL-1 (IL-1α or IL-1β) to enhance bone marrow recovery and for cancer treatment. The IL-1–specific receptor antagonist (IL-1Ra) has also been tested in clinical trials.

There are three members of the IL-1 gene family: genes for IL-1α *(IL1A)*, IL-1β *(IL1B)*, and IL-1Ra *(IL1RN)*. IL-

1α and IL-1β are agonists, and IL-1Ra is a specific receptor antagonist. The naturally occurring IL-1Ra appears to be a unique situation in cytokine biology. The intron-exon organization of the three IL-1 genes suggests duplication of a common gene about 350 million years ago. Before this common IL-1 gene, there may have been an ancestral gene from which fibroblast growth factor (FGF) evolved, because IL-1 and FGF share significant amino acid homologies, lack a signal peptide, and form an all β-pleated sheet tertiary structure. IL-1α and IL-1β are synthesized as precursors without leader sequences. The molecular mass of each precursor is 31 kd. Processing of IL-1α or IL-1β to "mature" forms of 17 kd requires specific cellular proteases. In contrast, IL-1Ra evolved with a signal peptide and is readily transported out of the cells and called secreted IL-1Ra (sIL-1Ra).

There are two primary cell surface binding proteins (IL-1Rs) for IL-1. IL-1 type I receptor (IL-1RI) transduces a signal, whereas the type II receptor (IL-1RII) binds IL-1 but does not transduce a signal. IL-1RII acts as a sink for IL-1β and has been called a decoy receptor, which is somewhat unique to cytokine biology (1). When IL-1 binds to IL-1RI, a complex is formed that then binds to the IL-1R accessory protein (IL-1R-AcP), resulting in high-affinity binding (2). The IL-1R-AcP itself does not bind IL-1. It is likely that the heterodimerization of the cytosolic domains of IL-1RI and IL-1R-AcP triggers IL-1 signal transduction.

As with other cytokines, IL-1's importance in development and health has been revealed using targeted gene disruption in mice. Gene expression and synthesis of IL-1α, IL-1β, or IL-1Ra have been demonstrated in ovarian granulosa and theca cells and in the dividing embryo. Although IL-1 is found in placental trophoblasts and appears to play a role in embryonic development, the implantation, birth, and neonatal development of mice deficient in IL-1β, ICE,

---

C. A. Dinarello: Department of Medicine, Division of Infectious Diseases, University of Colorado Health Science Center, Denver, Colorado 80262.

or IL-1RI suggest that ovulation, fertilization, implantation, and parturition do not require IL-1R signaling or that compensatory cytokines are used by these mice. Mice deficient in IL-1β, ICE, or IL-1RI are not susceptible to infection in a standard animal facility, in sharp contrast to mice deficient in IL-10 or transforming growth factor-β.

INTERLEUKIN-1 ADMINISTERED TO HUMANS

Although the systemic effects of IL-1 have been studied in animals, there also are data on the effects and sensitivity to IL-1 in humans. IL-1α or IL-1β has been injected into patients with various solid tumors or as part of a reconstitution strategy in bone marrow transplantation. The acute toxicities of IL-1α or IL-1β were greater after intravenous than subcutaneous injection; subcutaneous injection was associated with significant local pain, erythema, and swelling (3,4). Chills and fever are observed in nearly all patients, even in the group receiving a dose of 1 ng/kg (5). The febrile response increased in magnitude with increasing doses (6–8), and chills and fever were abated with indomethacin treatment (9). Almost all patients receiving IL-1α (7) or IL-1β (6,8) experienced significant hypotension at doses of 100 ng/kg or greater. Systolic blood pressure fell steadily and reached a nadir of 90 mm Hg or less 3 to 5 hours after the infusion of IL-1 (6,7,10). At doses of 300 ng/kg, most patients required intravenous pressors. By comparison, in a trial of 16 patients given IL-1β subcutaneously in doses of 4 to 32 ng/kg, there was only one episode of hypotension at the highest dose level (4). These results suggest that the hypotension probably is caused by induction of nitric oxide and elevated levels of serum nitrate that have been measured in patients with IL-1–induced hypotension (7).

At 30 to 100 ng/kg, IL-1β produced a sharp increase in cortisol levels 2 to 3 hours after the injection (6,11). Similar increases were observed in patients given IL-1α (7). In 13 of 17 patients given IL-1β, the serum glucose levels fell within the first hour of administration, and in 11 patients, the glucose level fell to 70 mg/100 mL or lower (6). Levels of corticotropin and thyroid-stimulating hormone increased, but the testosterone level decreased (7). No changes were observed in coagulation parameters such as prothrombin time, partial thromboplastin, or fibrinogen degradation products (7). This latter finding contrasts with TNF-α infusion into healthy humans, which results in a distinct coagulopathy syndrome (12).

Not unexpectedly, IL-1 infusion into humans significantly increased circulating IL-6 levels in a dose-dependent fashion (7). At a dose of 30 ng/kg, mean IL-6 levels were 500 pg/mL 4 hours after IL-1 (baseline <50 pg/mL) and 8,000 pg/mL after a dose of 300 ng/kg. In another study, infusion of 30 ng/kg of IL-1α elevated IL-6 levels within 2 hours (13). These elevations in IL-6 are associated with a rise in C-reactive protein concentrations and a decrease in albumin levels (7). The serum concentra-

tions of granulocyte-macrophage colony-stimulating factor (GM-CSF) were less than 50 pg/mL. In two studies, one with IL-1α (14) and one with IL-1β (15), rapid increases in the levels of circulating IL-1Ra and TNF soluble receptors (p55 and p75) were observed after a 30-minute intravenous infusion. The rise in the circulating levels of both naturally occurring antagonists was greater than the levels measured in human volunteers injected with lipopolysaccharide (LPS) (16,17).

INTERLEUKIN-1α

The 31-kd IL-1α precursor (proIL-1α) is not synthesized in the endoplasmic reticulum but rather in association with cytoskeletal microtubules (18). ProIL-1α is fully active as a precursor (19) but remains mostly intracellularly (Fig. 30-1). The opposite is true for the IL-1β precursor (proIL-1β) which is not fully active, and a considerable amount of which is secreted after cleavage by a specific, intracellular protease. When cells die, proIL-1α is released and can be cleaved by extracellular proteases (20). ProIL-1α can also be cleaved by activation of the calcium-dependent, membrane-associated cysteine proteases called calpains (21,22). In transformed cell lines constitutively synthesizing proIL-1α, the addition of a calcium ionophore stimulates calpain, which cleaves the precursor. The release of the 17-kd IL-1α can take place without cell death (23).

Because of the lack of a leader peptide, proIIL-1α remains in the cytosol soon after translation, and there is no appreciable accumulation of IL-1 in any specific organelle. Immunohistochemical studies of IL-1α in endotoxin-stimulated human blood monocytes reveal a diffuse staining pattern, but by comparison in the same cell, IL-1Ra is localized to the Golgi (24). There is a better correlation of disease severity with tissue levels of IL-1α than with those of IL-1β, presumably because of the cell-associated nature of IL-1α. IL-1α is not commonly found in the circulation or in body fluids except during severe disease, in which case the cytokine may be released from dying cells or by proteolysis after calpain-mediated cleavage (23).

Initially, Mizel and et al. (25) reported that radiolabeled, 17-kd, recombinant IL-1α bound to the cell surface receptors was rapidly internalized and that, after 2 to 3 hours, was associated with the nucleus. It was unclear whether the nuclear binding comprised the IL-1α/IL-1R complex or just the ligand. Using truncated mutants of the cytoplasmic domain of IL-1RI, rapid internalization and nuclear localization of IL-1β were observed with several mutants not capable of transducing a biologic signal (26). It was later shown that the IL-1α/IL-1R complex, but not 17-kd IL-1α, bound to immobilized DNA, could be eluted under the same salt conditions as that of the estrogen receptor (27).

The cytoplasmic domain of IL-1RI is highly conserved and contains a consensus sequence (residues 517 through 529) similar to those that transport viral proteins (26). If

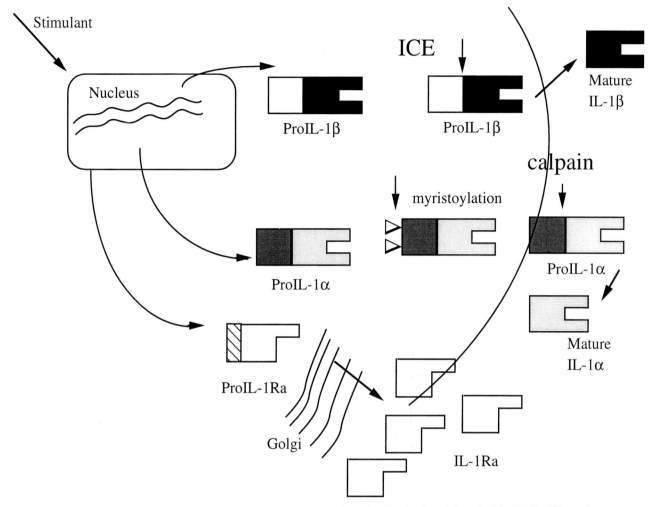

FIG. 30-1. Scheme for the synthesis and secretion of interleukin-1α (IL-α), interleukin-1β (IL-1β), and interleukin-1 receptor agonist (IL-1Ra).

proIL-1α plays an essential role in cellular differentiation (28,29), it is not in conjunction with the type I IL-1R, because mice deficient in this receptor appear to have a normal phenotype, including gross examination of skin and fur (M. Labow, personal communication,). The IL-1RI–deficient mouse has no response to IL-1 signaling.

Using antibodies directed specifically to proIL-1α (18) and transfection with plasmids containing the first 115 amino acids of proIL-1α, also called the IL-1α propiece, it appears that the propiece rather than the carboxyl-terminal, mature segment of IL-1α localizes to the nucleus (30). This concept is supported by the observation that a specific peptide in the propiece of IL-1α binds to DNA (31). Phosphorylation (32) and myristoylation (33) of the IL-1α propiece may facilitate nuclear localization. Myristoylation takes place on lysine residues 82 and 83 of the IL-1α propiece that is found in the nuclear localization sequence KVLKKRR (31). Transfecting endothelial cells with a plasmid containing this sequence revealed nuclear localization (30). Transfecting cells with

the propiece of IL-1α results in slower rate of proliferation (30), consistent with a role for IL-1α in early endothelial senescence (34). Transfection of an intracellular IL-1–producing plasmid increases IL-2 production in thymoma cells, and this biologic effect is prevented by antisense IL-1 (35), suggesting that IL-1α without its receptor is functional as an intracellular molecule.

ProIL-1α can be found on the surface of several cells, particularly on monocytes and B lymphocytes after stimulation *in vitro*. Approximately 10% to 15% of the IL-1α is myristoylated (33), and this form is thought to be transported to the cell surface, where it is called membrane IL-1 (36). Myristoylation on specific lysines facilitates passage to the cell membrane (33). This membrane IL-1α is biologically active; its biologic activities are neutralized by anti-IL-1α but not anti-IL-1β antibodies, and it appears to be anchored through a lectin interaction involving mannose residues (37). Using high concentrations of IL-1Ra to prevent IL-1α binding to the cell surface IL-1R during fixation, the biologic activity of membrane IL-1α was unaffected. In contrast, a mannose-like receptor appears to bind membrane IL-1α (38). Although IL-1α has glycosylation sites, recombinant forms of mature IL-1 are biologically active when expressed in *Escherichia coli,* which lacks the ability to glycosylate proteins. Because membrane IL-1α probably is a glycosylated or myristoylated form of the cytokine, it accounts for no more than 5% of the total proIL-1α synthesized by the cell. There has been some dispute about whether membrane IL-1α represents a "leak" of intracellular IL-1 (39), but with prolonged fixation, leakage does not account for the activity of membrane IL-1 (38,40).

INTERLEUKIN-1β

Depending on the stimulant, IL-1β mRNA levels rise rapidly within 15 minutes but start to fall after 4 hours. This decrease probably is caused by synthesis of a transcriptional repressor, decrease in the mRNA half-life, or both (41,42). Using IL-1 as a stimulant of its own gene expression, IL-1β mRNA levels were sustained for more than 24 hours (43,44). Raising cAMP levels in these same cells with histamine enhances IL-1α–induced IL-1β gene expression and protein synthesis (45). In human peripheral blood mononuclear cells (PBMCs), retinoic acid induces IL-1β gene expression, but the primary precursor transcripts fail to yield mature mRNA (42). Inhibition of translation by cycloheximide results in enhanced splicing of exons, excision of introns, and increased levels of mature mRNA (superinduction) by two orders of magnitude. Synthesis of mature IL-1β mRNA requires an activation step to overcome an apparently intrinsic inhibition to process precursor mRNA.

Dissociation between transcription and translation is characteristic of IL-1β and TNF-α (46). It appears that the stimuli are not sufficient to provide a signal for translation despite a vigorous signal for transcription. Without translation, most of the IL-1β mRNA is degraded, and this situation has been observed in humans undergoing hemodialysis with complement-activating membranes (47). Although the IL-1β mRNA assembles into large polyribosomes, there is little significant elongation of the peptide (48). However, adding bacterial endotoxin or IL-1 itself to cells with high levels of steady-state IL-1β mRNA results in augmented translation (46,49) in somewhat the same manner as the removal of cycloheximide after superinduction. One explanation is that stabilization of the AU-rich 3'-untranslated region takes place in cells stimulated with LPS. These AU-rich sequences suppress normal hemoglobin synthesis. The stabilization of mRNA by microbial products may explain why low concentrations of LPS or a few bacteria or *Borrelia* organisms per cell induce the translation of large amounts of IL-1β (50).

Another explanation is that IL-1 stabilizes its own mRNA (43) by preventing deadenylation, as it does for the chemokine growth-related peptide-α (GRO-α) (51).

Removal of IL-1 from cells after 2 hours increases the shortening of poly (A) segment, and IL-1 apparently is an important regulator of GRO synthesis because it prevents deadenylation. Of the several cytokines induced by IL-1, large amounts of the chemokine family are produced in response to low concentrations of IL-1. For example, 1 pmol/L of IL-1 stimulates fibroblasts to synthesize 10 nmol/L of IL-8 (52).

After synthesis, proIL-1β remains primarily cytosolic until it is cleaved and transported out of the cell (see Fig. 30-1). The IL-1β propiece (amino acids 1 through 116) is also myristoylated on lysine residues (33), but unlike IL-1α, proIL-1β has no known membrane form, and proIL-1β is only marginally active (53). Some IL-1β is found in lysosomes (54) or associated with microtubules (18,55), and either localization may play a role in the secretion of IL-1β. In mononuclear phagocytes, a small amount of proIL-1β is secreted from intact cells (56,57), but the pathway for this secretion remains unknown. However, release of mature IL-1β appears to be linked to processing at the aspartic acid–alanine (116–117) peptide cleavage by ICE (58).

Although well controlled in the setting of laboratory cell culture, death and rupture of inflammatory cells are not unusual occurrences *in vivo.* Several sites in the N-terminal, 16-kd part of proIL-1β are vulnerable to cleavage by enzymes in the vicinity of alanine 117: trypsin (20), elastase (59), chymotrypsin (60), a mast cell chymase (61), and a variety of proteases (62,63) that are commonly found in inflammatory fluids. The extent that these proteases play in the *in vivo* conversion of proIL-1β to mature forms is uncertain, but in each case, a biologically active IL-1β species is produced. The affinity of proIL-1β for IL-1R type II, a constitutively produced soluble receptor, is high and may prevent haphazard cleavage of the precursor by these enzymes in inflammatory fluids.

INTERLEUKIN-1β–CONVERTING ENZYME

Structure and Function

ProIL-1β requires cleavage before the mature form is secreted (see Fig. 30-1). The cDNA encoding ICE has been reported (64,65). The 45-kd precursor of ICE requires two internal cleavages before becoming the enzymatically active heterodimer composed of 10- and 20-kd chains. The active site cysteine is located on the 20-kd chain. ICE itself contributes to autoprocessing of the ICE precursor by undergoing oligomerization with itself or homologues of ICE (66,67). ICE is the first member of a family of intracellular cysteine proteases called caspases. The term *caspase* is used to connote the activity of the cysteine proteases cleaving after an aspartic acid residue. ICE is caspase-1.

The tertiary structure of the active site has been reported (66,68). Two molecules of the ICE heterodimer form a tetramer with two molecules of proIL-1β for cleavage (66,68). The aspartic acid at position 116 of the proIL-1β is the recognition amino acid for ICE cleavage. ICE does not cleave the IL-1α precursor. Enzymes such as elastase (59) and granzyme A (69) cleave proIL-1β at amino acids 112 and 120, respectively, yielding biologically active IL-1β. The propiece of IL-1β can be found inside and outside the cell (70). The propiece exhibits biologic activity as a chemoattractant for fibroblasts through an IL-1R–mediated event (71).

In the presence of a tetrapeptide competitive substrate inhibitor of ICE, the generation and secretion of mature IL-1β is reduced, and proIL-1β accumulates mostly inside but also outside the cell (65). This latter finding supports the concept that proIL-1β can be released from a cell independent of processing by ICE. Similar to the situation for thioredoxin (72) and basic FGF (73), exocytosis has been proposed as a possible mechanism of proIL-1β release. A putative membrane "channel" where active ICE is localized has also been proposed. In this model, mature IL-1β is released through this channel (74). When ICE activity is blocked by a reversible competitive substrate inhibitor, greater amounts of proIL-1β are found in the supernatants (65,74), and the putative channel may provide a passive secretory pathway for proIL-1β and mature IL-1β.

Macrophages from ICE-deficient mice do not release mature IL-1β on stimulation *in vitro* (75,76). Although neutrophil enzymes such as elastase and granzyme A (69) can cleave proIL-1β at sites close to alanine 117, proIL-1β accumulates in cells from ICE-deficient mice (75,76). IL-1α production in macrophages from ICE-deficient mice is reduced, a finding consistent with self-induction of IL-1 gene expression and synthesis (77). ICE-deficient mice can be resistant (75) or susceptible (76) to lethal endotoxemia. Studies suggest that mice deficient in ICE fail to develop collagen-induced arthritis.

Interleukin-1β–Converting Enzyme and Interferon-γ–Inducing Factor

Endotoxin-induced serum activity that stimulated production of interferon-γ (IFN-γ) from mouse spleen cells was described in 1989 (78). This serum activity functioned not as a direct inducer of IFN-γ but rather as a co-stimulant with IL-2 or mitogens. An attempt to purify the activity from endotoxin-treated mouse serum revealed an apparently homogeneous 50- to 55-kd protein (79). Because other cytokines can act as co-stimulants for IFN-γ production, the failure of neutralizing antibodies to IL-1, IL-4, IL-5, IL-6, or TNF to neutralize the serum activity suggested it was a distinct factor.

In 1995, a third report from the same scientists demonstrated that the endotoxin-induced co-stimulant for IFN-γ production was present in extracts of livers from mice preconditioned with *Propionibacterium acnes* (80). In this model, the hepatic macrophage population (i.e., Kupffer cells) expands, and in these mice, a low dose of bacterial LPS, which in nonpreconditioned mice is not lethal, becomes lethal. The factor, named IFN-γ–inducing factor (IGIF), was purified to homogeneity from 1,200 g of *P.acnes*-treated mouse livers. Its molecular weight was 18 to 19 kd, and an N-terminal amino acid sequence was reported (80). Similar to the endotoxin-induced serum activity, IGIF did not induce IFN-γ by itself but functioned primarily as a co-stimulant with mitogens or IL-2. Degenerate oligonucleotides derived from amino acid sequences of purified IGIF were used to clone a murine IGIF cDNA (81). Recombinant IGIF did not induce IFN-γ by itself but only in the presence of a mitogen or IL-2. However, the co-induction of IFN-γ was independent of IL-12 induction of IFN-γ.

Neutralizing antibodies to mouse IGIF can prevent the lethality of low-dose LPS in *P. acnes*–preconditioned mice (81). Others had reported the importance of IFN-γ as a mediator of LPS lethality in preconditioned mice. For example, neutralizing anti-IFN-γ antibodies protected mice against Shwartzman-like shock (82), and galactosamine-treated mice deficient in the IFN-γ receptor were resistant to LPS-induced death (83). It was not unexpected that neutralizing antibodies to murine IGIF protected *P. acnes*–preconditioned mice against lethal LPS (81). Anti-murine IGIF treatment also protected surviving mice against severe hepatic cytotoxicty. After the murine form was cloned (81), the human cDNA sequence for IGIF was reported in 1996 (84). Recombinant human IGIF exhibited natural IGIF activity (84). Human recombinant IGIF did not have direct IFN-γ–inducing activity on human T cells but acted as a co-stimulant for production of IFN-γ and other helper T-cell type 1 (T$_H$1) cytokines (84). IGIF induced T-cell and NK-cell IFN-γ production independently of IL-12 and *vice versa* (81). IGIF is thought of as primarily a co-stimulant for T$_H$1 cytokine production (i.e., IFN-γ, IL-2, and GM-CSF) (85) and as a co-stimulant for FAS ligand–mediated cytotoxicity of murine NK cell clones (86). *In vivo*, endogenous IGIF activity appears to account for IFN-γ production in *P. acnes*– and LPS-mediated lethality (81).

Scientists working on other IFN-γ–inducing cytokines analyzed the computer-generated protein folding pattern of murine IGIF and compared its pattern with those of others in the data bank. Using a validated compatibility relatedness program, the mature murine IGIF had the highest score when compared with mature human IL-1β; the IGIF amino acid sequence matched best with amino acids that form the all-β–pleated-sheet folding pattern of human IL-1β (87). A high degree of alignment was present in the sequences that comprise the 12 β-sheets of the mature IL-1β structure. Using this alignment of conserved amino acids, there is a 19% positional identity of mature murine IGIF with mature human IL-1β and a 12% identity with human IL-1α. Using this same positional alignment, the identity of IL-1β compared with IL-1α is 23%. It has been suggested that the name IGIF be changed to interleukin-1γ (IL-1γ) (87). Does IGIF bind to IL-1 type I receptors? This would be an essential criterion for assigning the name IL-1γ, because the type I IL-1R is the signaling receptor for the biologic activity of IL-1. In the absence of evidence that IGIF binds to IL-1RI (unpublished data,), IL-18 rather than IL-1γ is a more appropriate name (84). Little is known about the spectrum of its activities.

Similar to proIL-1β, precursor IL-18 (proIL-18) does not contain a signal peptide required for the removal of the precursor amino acids with subsequent secretion. The N-terminal amino acid sequence of the secreted form of murine IL-18 (80) was consistent with the sequence following cleavage after an aspartic acid residue, a typical cleavage site for ICE. This analysis alerted investigators that the cleavage of proIL-18 at the aspartic acid site probably requires ICE (87), and it was not surprising that ICE cleaved proIL-18 (after the aspartic acid 19) and resulted in the mature and active protein (88).

INTERLEUKIN-1 RECEPTOR ANTAGONIST

ProIL-1Ra, which possesses a leader sequence, is synthesized, processed, and secreted from the cell (see Fig. 30-1). On stimulation with LPS, human blood monocytes initially express the gene for sIL-1Ra (89). During the first 4 to 6 hours, sIL-1Ra protein can be visualized in the Golgi (24). After 24 hours, the primary transcript in these cells is intracellular IL-1Ra (icIL-1Ra), which, lacking a leader peptide, stains diffusely in the cytosol and remains intracellular (24). It has been proposed that icIL-1Ra constitutively produced in keratinocytes and epithelial cells may block the binding of IL-1α to nuclear DNA (89,90).

The primary amino acid homology of mature human IL-1β to IL-1Ra is 26%, which is greater than that between IL-1α and IL-1β. Each member of the human IL-1 family is composed of an all-β–strand molecule that forms an open barrel-like structure (91–93) closely related to structure of FGF (94). Because each member of the IL-1 family binds to the IL-1RI, it is not surprising that IL-1α, IL-1β, and IL-1Ra share structural similarities. How does IL-1Ra bind to IL-1RI with nearly the same affinity as IL-1α or IL-1β but not trigger a response? Crystal structural analysis of the IL-1R/IL-1Ra complex reveals that IL-1Ra contacts all three domains of IL-1RI (95).

IL-1β has two sites of binding to IL-1RI. There is a primary binding site located at the open top of its barrel shape (96), which is similar but not identical to that of IL-1α (97). A second site is on the back side of the IL-1β molecule (96). IL-1Ra also has two binding sites similar to those of IL-1β (93,98). However, the backside site in IL-1Ra is more homologous to that of IL-1β than the primary binding site (98). The backside site of IL-1Ra prob-

ably binds to IL-1RI and occupies the receptor. Lacking the second binding site, IL-1Ra does not trigger a signal. After IL-1Ra binds to IL-1RI–bearing cells, there is no phosphorylation of the epidermal growth factor receptor (99), a well-established and sensitive assessment of IL-1 signal transduction (100). Moreover, when injected intravenously into humans at doses 1,000,000-fold greater than that of IL-1α or IL-1β (6,101), IL-1Ra has no agonist activity (102).

The formation of the heterodimer consisting of the IL-1RI and IL-1R-AcP (2) probably explains the failure of IL-1Ra to trigger a signal. Judging from the structural differences previously described between IL-1β and IL-1Ra, the second binding site missing from the IL-1Ra probably is the site that binds the accessory protein. The cross-linked complex of radiolabeled IL-1Ra to the type I receptor was not precipitated by a specific antibody to the accessory protein (2). As shown in Figure 30-2, IL-1Ra binds to the type I receptor with the same affinity as that of IL-1, but lacking the second binding site, the IL-1R-AcP does not dock to the IL-1Ra, and the heterodimer is not formed. The binding of IL-1Ra to the type I receptor probably prevents or disrupts the complex between IL-1 and the type I receptor. This model implies that signal transduction takes place only when the heterodimer is formed. A triple mutation in IL-1Ra (103) may have partially reconstituted the second binding domain so that a degree of dimerization takes place between the cytosolic domains of IL-1RI and IL-1R-AcP, resulting in increased agonist activity of the mutated IL-1Ra (103).

IL-1β have resulted in molecules with greater than a 100-fold loss in biologic activity but only a small decrease in IL-1RI binding (104,105). Healthy humans are the most sensitive indicators of IL-1 agonist activity; 1 ng/kg of intravenous IL-1β produces symptoms (5). In contrast, the intravenous infusion of 10 mg/kg of IL-1Ra in healthy humans, a 10 million-fold molar excess, has no effects (102). What are the structural requirements of the respective molecules that account for this dramatic difference? The ability of IL-1β to optimally trigger cell signaling requires stability of the overall tertiary structure of the cytokine so that mutations in one amino acid may unfold the molecule, resulting in a several hundred-fold loss in activity but no loss in receptor binding. This suggests that biologic activity requires binding of IL-1β to a relatively broad area on the receptor. The tertiary structure of IL-1Ra, which is closely related to that of IL-1β, allows tight binding to the IL-1RI, but IL-1Ra lacks the second binding site that allows docking of the IL-1R-AcP to form the heterodimer. Without dimerization, no signal is transduced, but occupancy of the IL-1RI by IL-1Ra results in effective prevention of IL-1 signal transduction. Small molecules may mimic the near-perfect receptor antagonism of IL-1Ra, but none have been reported.

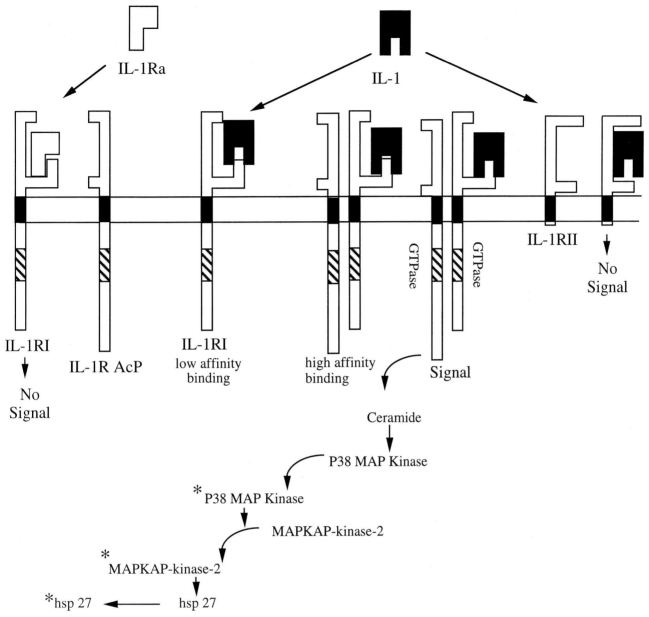

FIG. 30-2. Interleukin-β (IL-1β) is used to demonstrate interleukin-1 receptors and cell signaling.

INTERLEUKIN-1 RECEPTORS

Two primary IL-1 binding proteins (i.e., receptors) and one receptor accessory protein (IL-1R-AcP) have been identified. The extracellular domains of the two receptors and the IL-1R-AcP are members of the immunoglobulin (Ig) superfamily. Each comprises three IgG-like domains and shares significant homology to the others (2,106, 107). The two IL-1Rs are distinct gene products, and in humans, the genes for IL-1RI and IL-1RII are located on the long arm of chromosome 2 (108).

IL-1RI is an 80-kd glycoprotein found prominently on endothelial cells, smooth muscle cells, epithelial cells, hepatocytes, fibroblasts, keratinocytes, epidermal dendritic cells, and T lymphocytes. IL-1RI is heavily glycosylated, and blocking the glycosylation sites reduces the binding of IL-1 (109). Surface expression of this receptor probably occurs on most IL-1–responsive cells, because biologic activity of IL-1 is a better assessment of receptor expression than ligand binding to cell surfaces (110). Failure to show specific and saturable IL-1 binding often results from the low numbers of surface IL-1RI on primary cells. In cell lines, the number of IL-1RI can reach 5,000 per cell, but primary cells usually express fewer that 200 receptors per cell. In some primary cells, there are fewer than 50 per cell (111), and IL-1 signal transduction has been observed in cells expressing fewer than 10 type I receptors per cell (112). The low number of IL-1RI on cells and the discrepancy between binding affinities and biologic activities can be explained by the increased binding affinity of IL-1 in the complex with the IL-1R-AcP (2).

IL-1RI has a single transmembrane segment and a cytoplasmic domain (see Fig. 30-2). Using specific neutralizing antibodies, IL-1RI, but not IL-1RII, is the primary signal transducing receptor (112–115). Antisense oligonucleotides directed against IL-1RI block IL-1 activities *in vitro* and *in vivo* (116). The cytoplasmic domain of IL-1RI has no apparent intrinsic tyrosine kinase activity, but when IL-1 binds to only a few receptors, the remaining unoccupied receptors appear to undergo phosphorylation (117), probably by a member of the mitogen-activated protein (MAP) kinase family. The cytosolic domain of IL-1RI has a 45% amino acid homology with the cytosolic domain of the *Drosophila* gene for Toll (118). Toll is a transmembrane protein that acts like a receptor, although the ligand for the Toll protein is unknown. Gene organization and amino acid homology suggest that the IL-1RI and the cytosolic Toll are derived from a common ancestor and trigger similar signals (119,120).

Like other models of two chain receptors, IL-1 binds first to the IL-1RI with a low affinity (see Fig. 30-2). Although there is no direct evidence, a structural change may take place in IL-1, allowing docking of IL-1R-AcP to the IL-1RI/IL-1 complex. After IL-1RI/IL-1 binds to IL-1R-AcP, high-affinity binding is observed. Antibodies to the type I receptor and to the IL-1R-AcP block IL-1 binding and activity (2). The IL-1R-AcP is essential to IL-1 signaling; in cells deficient of the IL-1R-AcP, no IL-1–induced activation of the stress kinases takes place, but this response is restored on transfection with a construct expressing the IL-1R-AcP (121). IL-1 may therefore bind to the type I receptor with a low affinity, causing a structural change in the ligand followed by recognition by the IL-1R-AcP. Alternatively, cells express IL-1RI/IL-1R-AcP already complexed, and the high-affinity binding takes place on the preformed complexes.

Similar to IL-1RI and IL-1RII, a soluble form of the IL-1R-AcP exists. Unlike the soluble forms of the IL-1RI and IL-1RII, the soluble IL-1R-AcP is not formed by proteolytic cleavage of the full-length accessory protein. Because the IL-1R-AcP does not bind IL-1 (2), the effect of the soluble IL-1R-AcP on the binding of IL-1 remains unclear. IL-1Ra does not form a complex with the IL-1RI, which probably explains how the IL-1Ra can bind so tightly to the IL-1RI but not exhibit agonist activity (see Fig. 30-2). The IL-1RI/IL-1/IL-1R-AcP complex triggers the cell, and without the IL-1R-AcP participation, the IL-1 signal by means of IL-1RI is weak or nonexistent.

IL-1RII has a short cytosolic domain consisting of 29 amino acids. The type II receptor appears to act as a decoy molecule, particularly for IL-1β. The receptor binds IL-1β tightly, preventing binding to the signal transducing type I receptor (122). It is the lack of a signal transducing cytosolic domain that makes the type II receptor a functionally negative receptor. For example, when the extracellular portion of the type II receptor is fused to the cytoplasmic domain of the type I receptor, a biologic signal occurs (123). The extracellular portion of the type II receptor is found in body fluids, where it is called IL-1 soluble receptor type II (IL-1sRII). It is assumed that a proteolytic cleavage of the extracellular domain of the IL-1RII from the cell surface is the source of the IL-1sRII.

As cell-bound IL-1RII increases, a comparable increase in soluble forms probably occurs (124). Similar to soluble receptors for TNF, the extracellular domain of the type I and type II IL-1R are found as "soluble" molecules in the circulation and urine of healthy subjects and in inflammatory synovial and other pathologic body fluids (115,125–128). In healthy humans, the circulating levels of IL-1sRII are 100 to 200 pmol/L (127–130), whereas levels of IL-1sRI are 10-fold less (115,128,130). The rank of affinities for the two soluble receptors are remarkably different for each of the three IL-1 molecules. The rank for the three IL-1 ligands binding to IL-1sRI is IL-1Ra > IL-1α > IL-1β, whereas for IL-1sRII, the rank is IL-1β > IL-1α > IL-1Ra. Elevated levels of IL-1sRII are found in the circulation of patients with sepsis (129) and in the synovial fluid of patients with active rheumatoid arthritis (128), whereas the elevations of soluble type I receptor in these fluids are 10-fold lower (128). High-dose IL-2 therapy induces IL-1sRI and IL-1sRII (130).

Unlike other cytokine receptors, in cells expressing IL-1 type I and type II receptors, there is competition to bind IL-1 first. This competition between signaling and nonsignaling receptors for the same ligand appears unique to cytokine receptors, although it exists for atrial natriuretic factor receptors (131). The type II receptor is more likely to bind to IL-1β than IL-1α, a pattern that can result in a diminished response to IL-1β. The soluble form of IL-1sRII circulates in healthy humans at molar concentrations that are 10-fold greater than those of IL-1β measured in septic patients and 100-fold greater than the concentration of IL-1β after intravenous administration (6). Why do humans have a systemic response to an infusion of IL-1β? Binding of IL-1β to the soluble form of IL-1R type II exhibits a slow on rate compared with the cell IL-1RI.

In addition to naturally occurring conditions that reduce a biologic response to IL-1β, neutralizing antibodies to IL-1α are present in many subjects and probably reduce the activity of IL-1α. Vaccinia and cowpox virus genes encode for a protein with a high amino acid homology to the type II receptor, and this protein binds IL-1β (132,133). Despite the portfolio of soluble receptors and naturally occurring antibodies, IL-1 produced during disease does trigger the type I receptor, because blocking receptors or neutralizing IL-1 ameliorates disease in animals and humans. These findings underscore the high functional level of only a few IL-1 type I receptors. They also imply that the postreceptor triggering events are greatly amplified. It seems reasonable to conclude that treating disease based on blocking IL-1R needs to take into account the efficiency of so few type I receptors initiating a biologic event.

SIGNAL TRANSDUCTION

Early Events in Interleukin-1 Signal Transduction

Within a few minutes after binding to cells, IL-1 induces several biochemical events (134–137). It remains unclear which is the most upstream triggering event or whether several occur at the same time. No sequential order or cascade has been identified, but several signaling events appear to be taking place during the first 2 to 5 minutes. Some of the biochemical changes associated with signal transduction probably are cell specific. Within 2 minutes, hydrolysis of GTP (138), phosphatidylcholine, phosphatidylserine, or phosphatidylethanolamine (110,139) and release of ceramide by neutral (140), not acidic, sphingomyelinase (141) have been reported. In general, multiple protein phosphorylations and activation of phosphatases can be observed with 5 minutes (142), and some are thought to be initiated by the release of lipid mediators. The release of ceramide has attracted attention as a possible early signaling event (143). Phosphorylation of phospholipase A_2 (PLA_2) activating protein also occurs in the first few minutes (144), leading to a rapid release of arachidonic acid. Multiple and similar signaling events have also been reported for TNF.

Of special consideration for IL-1 signal transduction is the unusual discrepancy between the low number of receptors (<10 in some cells) and the low concentrations of IL-1, which can induce a biologic response (145). This latter observation, however, may be clarified in studies on high-affinity binding with the IL-1R-AcP complex (2). A rather extensive "amplification" step takes place after the initial postreceptor binding event. The most likely mechanism for signal amplification is multiple and sequential phosphorylations (or dephosphorylations) of kinases that result in nuclear translocation of transcription factors and activation of proteins participating in translation of mRNA. IL-1RI is phosphorylated after IL-1 binding (117). It is unknown whether the IL-1R-AcP is phosphorylated during receptor complex formation. In primary cells, the number of IL-1RI type I is very low (<100/cell), and a biologic response occurs when only as few as 2% to 3% of IL-1RI receptors are occupied (117,146). IL-1–responsive cells probably have constitutive expression of the IL-1R-AcP.

There is general agreement that IL-1 does not stimulate hydrolysis of phosphatidylinositol nor increase intracellular calcium. Without a clear increase in intracellular calcium, early postreceptor binding events nevertheless include hydrolysis of a GTP with no associated increase in adenyl cyclase (137,138), activation of adenyl cyclase (147,148), hydrolysis of phospholipids (110,149), release of ceramide (150), and release of arachidonic acid from phospholipids through cytosolic PLA_2 after its activation by PLA_2-activating protein (144,151). Tyrosine phosphorylations have been reported (152). Each of these mechanisms occurs within the first few minutes after the addition of IL-1 to cultured cells.

Although few comparative studies have been reported, it appears that some IL-1 signaling events are prominent in different cells. Postreceptor signaling mechanisms may therefore provide cellular specificity. For example, in some cells, IL-1 is a growth factor, and signaling is associated with serine or threonine phosphorylation of the p42/44 MAP kinase in mesangial cells (153). The p38 MAP kinase, another member of the MAP kinase family, is phosphorylated in fibroblasts (154), as is the p54a MAP kinase in hepatocytes (155). These somewhat different phosphorylations may distinguish the phenotypic response in various cells stimulated with IL-1.

Characteristics of the Cytoplasmic Domain of Interleukin-1 Type I Receptor

The cytoplasmic domain of the IL-1RI does not contain a consensus sequence for intrinsic tyrosine phosphorylation, but deletion mutants of the receptor reveal specific functions of some domains. Four nuclear localization sequences share homology with the glucocorticoid receptor. Three amino acids (Arg^{518}, Lys^{515}, Arg^{518}), also found in the Toll protein, are essential for IL-1–induced IL-2 production (120). However, deletion of a segment containing these amino acids did not affect IL-1–induced IL-8 (156). If this discrepancy results from different signaling pathways for IL-1–induced IL-2 or for induction of IL-8, the cytoplasmic domain of IL-1RI can induce more than one biochemical event. There are also two cytoplasmic domains in the IL-1RI that share homology with the IL-6–signaling gp130 receptor. When these regions are deleted, IL-1–induced IL-8 production is lost (156).

The C-terminal 30 amino acids of the IL-1RI can be deleted without affecting biologic activity (157). Two independent studies have focused on the area between amino acids 513 and 529. Amino acids 508 through 521 contain sites required for the activation of nuclear factor NF-κB. In one study, deletion of this segment abolished IL-1–induced IL-8 expression (156), and in another study, specific mutations of amino acids 513 and 520 to alanine prevented IL-1–driven E-selectin promoter activity (157). This area is also present in the Toll protein domain associated with NF-κB translocation and previously shown to be part of the IL-1 signaling mechanism

452 / CHAPTER 30

(120). The 513–520 area is also responsible for activating a kinase that associates with the receptor. This kinase, called IL-1RI–associated kinase, phosphorylates a 100-kd substrate (157). Others have reported a serine/threonine kinase that coprecipitates with the IL-1RI (158). Amino acid sequence comparisons of the cytosolic domain of the IL-1RI have revealed similarities with a protein kinase C (PKC) acceptor site. Because PKC activators usually do not mimic IL-1–induced responses, the significance of this observation is unclear.

GTPase

Hopp (159) reported a detailed sequence and structural comparison of the cytosolic segment of IL-1RI with the RAS family of GTPases. In this analysis, the known amino acid residues for GTP binding and hydrolysis by the GTPase family were found to align with residues in the cytoplasmic domain of the IL-1RI. RAC, a member of the RHO family of GTPases, were also present in the binding and hydrolytic domains of the IL-1RI cytosolic domains. These observations are consistent with the observations that GTP analogues undergo a rapid hydrolysis when membrane preparations of IL-1RI are incubated with IL-1 (135,137). Amino acid sequences in the cytosolic domain of the IL-1R-AcP also align with the same binding and hydrolytic regions of the GTPases (T. P. Hopp, personal communication,). A protein similar to G-protein–activating protein associates with the cytosolic domain of the IL-1RI (160). This finding is consistent with the hypothesis that an early event in IL-1R signaling involves dimerization of the two cytosolic domains, activation of putative GTP binding sites on the cytosolic domains, binding of a G protein, hydrolysis of GTP, and activation of a phospholipase. Hydrolysis of phospholipids generates diacylglycerol or phosphatidic acids.

Activation of MAP Kinases After Interleukin-1 Receptor Binding

Multiple phosphorylations take place during the first 15 minutes after IL-1R binding. A comparison of IL-1–induced phosphorylations with those induced by phorbol esters through PKC reveals some similarities. However, unique, non-PKC–activated kinases are also stimulated by IL-1, possibly through release of diacylglycerol (110) with activation on non-PKC kinases (140). Most consistently, IL-1 activates protein kinases that phosphorylate serine and threonine residues, which are the targets of the MAP kinase family. An early study reported an IL-1–induced serine/threonine phosphorylation of a 65-kd protein that was unrelated to those phosphorylated by PKC (161). Other studies have implicated a role for PKC (148). As reviewed by O'Neill (137), before IL-1 activation of serine/threonine kinases, IL-1R binding results in the phosphorylation of tyrosine residues (154,155). Tyrosine phosphorylation induced by IL-1 probably is caused by activation of MAP kinase, which then phosphorylates tyrosine and threonine on MAP kinases.

After activation of MAP kinases, there are phosphorylations on serine and threonine residues of the epidermal growth factor receptor, heat-shock protein p27 (HSP-27), myelin basic protein, and serines 56 and 156 of β-casein, each of which has been observed in IL-1–stimulated cells (162,163). TNF also activates these kinases. There are at least three families of MAP kinases. The p42/44 MAP kinase family is associated with signal transduction by growth factors, including RAS–RAF-1 signal pathways. In rat mesangial cells, IL-1 activates the p42/44 MAP kinase within 10 minutes and increases *de novo* synthesis of p42 (153).

In addition to p42/44, two members of the MAP kinase family (p38 and p54) have been identified as part of an IL-1 phosphorylation pathway and are responsible for phosphorylating HSP-27 (154,155). These MAP kinases are highly conserved proteins homologous to the *HOG1* stress gene in yeasts. When *HOG1* is deleted, yeasts fail to grow in hyperosmotic conditions; however, the mammalian gene coding for the IL-1–inducible p38 MAP kinase (155) can reconstitute the ability of the yeast to grow in hyperosmotic conditions (164). In cells stimulated with hyperosmolar NaCl, LPS, IL-1, or TNF, indistinguishable phosphorylation of the p38 MAP kinase takes place (165). In human monocytes exposed to hyperosmolar NaCl (375 to 425 mOsm/L), IL-8 gene expression and synthesis takes place, which is indistinguishable from that induced by LPS or IL-1 (166). The MAP p38 kinase pathways involved in IL-1, TNF, and LPS signal transductions share certain elements that are related to the primitive stress-induced pathway. The dependency of RHO members of the GTPase family for IL-1–induced activation of p38 MAP kinases has been demonstrated (167), an observation that links the intrinsic GTPase domains of IL-1RI and IL-1R-AcP with activation of the p38 MAP kinase.

Drugs of the pyridinyl imidazole class primarily inhibit translation rather than transcription of LPS- and IL-1–induced cytokines (168). The target for these drugs has been identified as a homologue of the *HOG1* gene family (168); its sequence is identical to that of the p38 MAP kinase activating protein-2 (168,169). As expected, this class of imidazoles also prevents the downstream phosphorylation of HSP-27 (170). Compounds of this class appear to be highly specific for inhibition of the p38 MAP kinase in that there was no inhibition of 12 other kinases (170). Using one of these compounds, hyperosmotic NaCl- and IL-1α–induced IL-8 synthesis was inhibited (166).

Transcription Factors

The cytosolic domain of IL-1RI shares significant homology with the receptor-like *Toll* gene and suggests that both molecules signal similar events. After IL-1 stimulation, phosphorylation of inhibitory κB (I-κB) takes place, and this molecule is rapidly degraded within the proteosome (171). NF-κB is then translocated to the nucleus (112,172). A substrate for the β-casein kinase in IL-1– and TNF-activated cells (173) has been identified as the p65 subunit of NF-κB (174). Most of the biologic effects of IL-1 take place in cells after nuclear translocation of NF-κB and activating protein-1 (AP-1), two nuclear factors common to many IL-1–induced genes. Addition of IL-1 to T lymphocytes and cultured hepatocytes increases nuclear binding of JUN and FOS, the two components of AP-1 (175). Similar to NF-κB, AP-1 sites are present in the promoter regions of many IL-1–inducible genes. IL-1 also increases the transcription of *JUN* (formerly designated *c-jun*) by activating two novel nuclear factors (JUN-1 and JUN-2) that bind to the promoter of the *JUN* gene and stimulate *JUN* transcription (176).

Because so few IL-1RI are expressed on primary cells and because so few of these receptors need to be triggered to initiate a biologic response to IL-1, one concludes that the signaling mechanism is highly efficient and greatly amplified. Dimerization of the cytosolic domains of type I receptor with the IL-1R-AcP likely initiates the signal. The best explanation for the potency of IL-1–induced signaling is postreceptor amplification through multiple phosphorylations of protein kinases. Phosphorylation and dephosphorylation of transcription factors enable the cell to transcribe genes controlled by the IL-1 activation of these transcription factors. The multiple postreceptor phosphorylations may explain why IL-1 induces several genes in the same cell at the same time. LPS and TNF share with IL-1 many of these same MAP kinase pathways, most of them related to the *HOG1* stress gene family of MAP kinases. These observations support the concept that IL-1 signal transducing events mimic the evolutionary benefit of cell stress.

INTERLEUKIN-1 RECEPTOR ANTAGONIST AND AMELIORATION OF DISEASE

Determining the Biologic Response

Blocking IL-1Rs with IL-1Ra has increased our understanding of IL-1 as a mediator of disease. Numerous animal studies have employed IL-1Ra to demonstrate a role for IL-1 in disease processes. Table 30-1 lists several studies in which administration of IL-1Ra has reduced the severity of disease. In addition to administration of IL-1Ra, rat synoviocytes have been transfected with IL-1Ra, and when expressed in the joint, a decrease in arthritis has been observed (177). Findings of these studies form the basis for gene therapy with IL-1Ra. Mice with a null mutation for the IL-1Ra gene have increased rates of death caused by lethal endotoxemia (178). Transgenic

mice overproducing IL-1Ra have increased protection against lethal endotoxemia (178). Methods such as neutralizing anti-IL-1 antibodies, antibodies to IL-1RI, and soluble IL-1Rs are equally effective, although limited by their animal specificity. In most disease models, other cytokines are produced in addition to IL-1. The data depicted in Table 30-1 reveal that IL-1 plays an important role in the pathogenesis of inflammatory and immunologically mediated disease. In these studies, a reduction of at least 50% is observed, but in many, the amelioration of pathologic changes can be complete. One consistent observation is the reduction in the number of infiltrating neutrophils associated with local inflammation, and this effect of IL-1Ra may result from preventing IL-1–induced synthesis of IL-8 and related chemokines (179).

However, in most studies, IL-1Ra has been administered just before the challenging event. This has been the case in models of infection in which injecting IL-1Ra before a lethal challenge has significantly reduced mortality; however, when IL-1Ra was injected shortly after the challenge, it had little or no effect on reducing death rates. On the other hand, in acute pancreatitis, a dose-dependent administration of IL-1Ra later in the disease reduced the severity of tissue damage (180,181). In some models of chronic disease, administration of IL-1Ra after the onset of disease can dramatically reduce severity (182,183).

It is not uncommon to inject a high dose of IL-1Ra (10 mg/kg) to observe an ameliorating effect in acute models of infection or inflammation despite the relatively low concentrations of circulating IL-1 in these animals. Why is so much IL-1Ra required? The plasma half-life of IL-1Ra is only 6 minutes, and these models are usually severe. For example, in the bacteremic model, the number of organisms injected intravenously is 10^9 to 10^{11} per kilogram of body weight. Although systemic levels of IL-1 can be low, tissue production of IL-1 can be high (184) because of membrane IL-1α (38) and IL-1 from activated platelets (185). In addition to these sources of IL-1, there is rapid excretion of IL-1Ra, a slow receptor "on" rate, increased IL-1RI expression, IL-1Ra binding to the soluble type I receptor, and poor tissue penetration of IL-1Ra. The binding of IL-1Ra to the cell-bound type I receptor is decreased as the pH falls. The acidic environment of inflammation can reduce the effectiveness of IL-1Ra, requiring large amounts.

Because triggering so few IL-1Rs results in a biologic response, it is necessary to sustain a high level of IL-1Ra to block unoccupied receptors. When exogenous IL-1 is injected intravenously into animals, pretreatment with a 100-fold molar excess of IL-1Ra prevents the response to IL-1. For example, injecting rabbits with 100 ng/kg of IL-1β produces fever; preinjection of 10 μg/kg of IL-1Ra prevents the fever. However, under natural conditions in which endogenous IL-1 and other cytokines are released,

TABLE 30-1. *Effects of the interleukin-1 receptor antagonist (IL-1Ra)*

Models of infection

Improved survival in endotoxin shock in mice, rats, and rabbits

Improved survival in *Klebsiella pneumoniae* infection in newborn rats

Reduction in shock and mortality in rabbits and baboons from *Escherichia coli* or *Staphylococcus epidermidis* bacteremia

Amelioration of shock and reduction in death after cecal ligation and puncture

Attenuation of LPS-induced lung nitric oxide activity

Decreased hypoglycemia, production of CSF, and early tolerance in mice after administration of endotoxin

Reduction in LPS-induced hyperalgesia

Protection against TNF-induced lethality in D-galactosamine–treated mice

Reduction in nematode-induced intestinal nerve dysfunction

Decreased circulating or cellular TNF production in models of sepsis

Decreased IL-6 production after LPS

Protection from *Bacillus anthracis* toxin-induced lethality in mice

Decreased intestinal inflammation and bacterial invasion in shigellosis

Models of local inflammation

Decreased neutrophil accumulation in inflammatory peritonitis in mice

Reduction in immune complex–induced neutrophil infiltration, eicosanoid production, and tissue necrosis in rabbit colitis

Reduction in acid-induced neutrophil infiltration and enterocolitis in rats

Decreased endotoxin-induced intestinal secretory diarrhea in mice

Reduction in ischemia and excitotoxic-induced brain damage in rats

Decrease in number of necrotic neurons in cerebral artery occlusion

Inhibition of permanganate-induced granulomas in rats

Inhibition of LPS-induced intraarticular neutrophil infiltration

Decreased IL-1–induced synovitis and loss of cartilage proteoglycan

Reduced myocardial neutrophil accumulation after coronary occlusions in dogs

Reduced inflammation and mortality in acute pancreatitis

Decreased hepatic inflammation after hemorrhagic shock

Models of acute or chronic lung injury

Decreased local LPS-induced neutrophil infiltration in rats

Inhibition of antigen-induced pulmonary eosinophil accumulation and airway hyperactivity in guinea pigs

Prevention of bleomycin or silica-induced pulmonary fibrosis

Reduction in hypoxia-induced pulmonary hypertension

Reduction in carrageenan-induced pleurisy in rats

Decreased intratracheal IL-1–induced fluid leak (systemic administration)

Decreased albumin leak after systemic LPS

Inhibition of antigen-induced eosinophil accumulation in guinea pigs

Models of metabolic dysfunction

Reduction in hepatocellular damage after ischemia-reperfusion

Improved survival after hemorrhagic shock in mice

Inhibition of SAA gene expression and synthesis in high-dose IL-2 toxicity

Decreased muscle protein breakdown in rats with peritonitis due to cecal ligation

Reduced muscle protein breakdown in rats with chronic septic peritonitis

Inhibition of weight loss after muscle tissue injury

Decrease in bone loss in ovariectomized rats

Reversal of LPS-induced CRF gene expression in the hypothalamus

Prevention of LPS-induced corticotropin release

Models of autoimmune disease

Diminution of *Streptococcus* wall-induced arthritis in rats

Reduction in collagen arthritis in mice

Suppression of anti–basement membrane glomerulonephritis

Delayed hyperglycemia in the diabetic BB rat

Reduction in streptozotocin-induced diabetes

Models of immune-mediated disease

Prevention of graft-versus-host disease in mice

Prolongation of islet allograft survival

Reduction in autoimmune encephalomyelitis

Reduction in skin contact hypersensitivity

Decrease in coronary artery fibronectin deposition in heterotopic cardiac transplantation

Models of malignant disease

Reduction in the number and size of metastatic melanoma

Reduction in growth of subcutaneous melanoma tumors

Reduced LPS-induced augmentation of metastatic melanoma

Reduction in tumor-mediated cachexia (intratumoral injection)

Miscellaneous

Inhibition of TNF-induced social depression in mice

Prevention of stress-induced hypothalamic monoamine release

Reduction in LPS-induced sickness behavior in rats

Suppression of crescentic glomerulonephritis in rats

Attenuation of muramyl dipeptide-induced sleep in rabbits

Impairment of host responses

Decreased sciatic nerve regeneration in mice

Increased mortality to *K. pneumoniae* in newborn rats (high dose)

Increased mortality to *Listeria* infection

Enhanced growth of *Mycobacterium avium* in organs

Worsening of infectious arthritis (late administration)

Increased vascular leak in mice given high-dose IL-2

Studies without an effect of IL-1Ra

Antigen-induced arthritis in rabbits

LPS-and *S. epidermidis* bacteremia–induced fever in rabbits

Fever after LPS injection into the brain

Leukopenia in rats after LPS

Hypertriglyceridemia after LPS in mice

LPS-induced increase in skin blood flow

LPS, lipopolysaccharide; CSF, colony-stimulating factor; TNF, tumor necrosis factor.

an IL-1Ra plasma level of 20 to 30 µg/mL is needed before observing a reduction in disease severity (186). In humans, similar levels of IL-1Ra are needed to block the hematologic response to LPS. *In vitro*, considerably lower concentrations of IL-1Ra are needed (187). For example, a 1 : 1 molar ratio of IL-1Ra to IL-1 blocks 50% of the IL-1–induced response in blood monocytes (188), and a concentration of 100 ng/mL of IL-1Ra reduces the spontaneous proliferation, colony formation, and cytokine production of acute myelogenous leukemia (AML) or chronic myelogenous leukemia (CML) cells (189–191).

The molar "ratio" of endogenous IL-1Ra to IL-1β levels in body fluids from patients with infectious, inflammatory, or autoimmune disease is often 10-fold to 1000-fold more IL-1Ra than IL-1β. In some selected clinical conditions, the ratio is far less. If the molar ratio of endogenous IL-1Ra to IL-1 falls, does it affect disease outcome? Some data provide important findings. In AML cells in which IL-1β is spontaneously expressed, IL-1Ra gene expression is suppressed even when stimulated with GM-CSF (190). In 81 patients with CML, cell lysates contained more IL-1β than cells from healthy subjects, whereas the levels of IL-1Ra were the same for both groups (192). The survival rate of 44 patients with elevated IL-1β was lower than that of patients with low IL-1β levels. During accelerated blast crisis, IL-1Ra levels were lower compared with levels of patients in a chronic phase (192). Stromal cultures established from bone marrow of patients with aplastic anemia produced less spontaneous and induced IL-1Ra compared with stromal cells established from normal bone marrow (193). We measured high circulating levels of IL-1sII (127) in 25 patients with hairy cell leukemia that correlated with high levels of IL-1β (194); however, there was no increase in IL-1Ra levels in these patients.

In patients with acute Lyme arthritis, the duration of joint inflammation is shortest in those with the highest joint fluid levels of IL-1Ra, whereas it is prolonged in patients with low levels of IL-1Ra (195). The reciprocal relationship was found for synovial fluid levels of IL-1β in the same patients. Similar findings were found in the relative production of IL-1Ra and IL-1β in synovial tissue explants of patients with rheumatoid or osteoarthritis (196–198). In normal skin, icIL-1Ra is present in higher concentrations than IL-1α (29), but in psoriatic lesions, the balance is in favor of IL-1α (29,199).

Does endogenous production of IL-1Ra affect disease outcome? Elevated production of IL-1Ra is an excellent marker of disease and certainly a better indicator than IL-1 itself. In some clinical conditions, the elevation in IL-1Ra rather than IL-1 may indicate the presence of a pathologic condition. Elevated IL-1Ra production may indicate a natural compensatory mechanism to counter the activity of IL-1, as in persons with rheumatoid arthritis (200) or human immunodeficiency virus type 1 infection (201). Is the amount of IL-1Ra produced in disease

sufficient to dampen the response to IL-1? Using specific, neutralizing antibodies to mouse IL-1Ra, an increase in the formation of schistosome egg granulomas was observed when endogenous IL-1Ra was neutralized (202). In rabbits with immune complex colitis, infusion of a neutralizing antibody to rabbit IL-1Ra resulted in exacerbation and prolongation of the colitis (203). The phenotype of an IL-1Ra–deficient mouse is unknown, but neutralizing endogenous IL-1Ra appears to worsen inflammation.

Interleukin-1 Receptor Agonist Administered to Humans

Effect on Healthy Subjects

IL-1Ra given intravenously to healthy volunteers produces no side effects or changes in biochemical, hematologic, or endocrinologic parameters, even when peak blood levels reach 30 µg/mL and are sustained above 10 µg/mL for several hours (102). These studies support the concept that there is no role for IL-1 in the regulation of body temperature, blood pressure, or hematopoiesis in health. PBMCs taken from these volunteers after receiving IL-1Ra failed to produce IL-6 when stimulated *ex vivo* with LPS (102). A role for IL-1R on PBMCs in LPS-stimulated IL-6 *in vitro* has been reported (188).

To evaluate the effect of IL-1R blockade in clinical disease under controlled experimental conditions, healthy volunteers were challenged with intravenous endotoxin and administered an infusion of IL-1Ra at the same time. Even at 10 mg of IL-1Ra/kg, there was no effect on endotoxin-induced fever, although blood levels of IL-1Ra were not significantly elevated until 1 hour after the bolus injection of endotoxin. Humans injected with antibodies to TNF before endotoxin also did not have a reduction in fever (H. Michie, personal communication,). In animal studies, peripheral endotoxin induces fever by triggering IL-1 induction of IL-6 synthesis in the central nervous system (204). Because IL-1Ra does not cross the blood-brain barrier, this may account for the inability of IL-1Ra to diminish endotoxin fever (205). However, IL-1R blockade was accomplished, because there was a 50% reduction in the endotoxin-induced neutrophilia and a reduction in the circulating levels of granulocyte colony-stimulating factor compared with subjects injected with endotoxin plus saline (206).

Endotoxin injection suppresses the mitogen-induced proliferative response of PBMCs *in vitro*. However, in volunteers injected with endotoxin plus IL-1Ra, there was no suppression of the response (206). Mitogen- and antigen-induced proliferation is a well-established parameter of immunocompetence and is associated with decreased production of IL-2. Similar to results for experimental endotoxin injection, this suppression is observed in patients with multiple trauma, sepsis, and cardiopulmonary bypass. In experimental endotoxemia and the previously described clinical conditions, treatment with cyclooxygenase inhibitors restores these cell-mediated immune responses (207). This effect of cyclooxygenase inhibitors is consistent with the well-known suppressive effects of prostaglandin E_2 (PGE_2) on IL-2 production and T-cell proliferation. Because IL-1 is a potent inducer of cyclooxygenase-2, it is not surprising that blocking IL-1Rs during endotoxemia reduces IL-1–induced PGE_2 production during endotoxemia. These studies establish that, under conditions of low-dose endotoxemia, it is possible to block IL-1–mediated responses with IL-1Ra. The host response parameters that were unaffected by IL-1Ra probably result from other cytokines such as TNF or IL-6 or the combination of these cytokines with IL-1.

Effect as a Therapeutic Agent

IL-1Ra has been in given to patients with septic shock, rheumatoid arthritis, steroid resistant graft-versus-host disease, AML, and CML. The initial (phase II) trial was a randomized, placebo-controlled, open-label study that recruited 99 patients. Patients received placebo or a loading bolus of 100 mg followed by a 3-day infusion of 17, 67, or 133 mg of IL-1Ra per hour (208). A dose-dependent improvement in the 28-day mortality rate was observed; it was reduced from 44% in the placebo group to 16% in the group receiving the highest dose of IL-1Ra ($P = 0.015$). In that study, there was a dose-related fall in the circulating levels of IL-6 24 hours after the initiation of IL-1Ra infusion. This fall in IL-6 levels is consistent with the well-established control of circulating IL-6 levels by IL-1 (209,210) and the correlation of disease severity and outcome with IL-6 levels (211). A large phase III trial with 893 patients revealed a trend but without a statistically significant reduction in the 28-day mortality rate (212). However, a retrospective analysis of 563 patients with a predicted risk of mortality of 24% or greater (213) revealed a significant reduction in 28-day mortality (45% in the placebo group and 35% in patients receiving 2 mg/kg/h for 72 hours, $P = 0.005$) (212). A second phase III trial using 10 g of IL-1Ra infused over 3 days was undertaken but terminated during an interim analysis because a reduction in the overall 28-day mortality rate would not likely reach statistical significance. Patient heterogeneity is thought to contribute to a failure to bridge the gap between animal and clinical data in sepsis.

IL-1Ra was initially tested in a trial with 25 patients with rheumatoid arthritis. In the group receiving a single subcutaneous dose of 6 mg/kg, there was a fall in the mean number of tender joints ($P < 0.05$) (214). In patients receiving 4 mg/kg per day for 7 days, there was a reduction in the number of tender joints from 24 to 10, the erythrocyte sedimentation rate fell from 48 to 31 and C-reactive protein decreased from 2.9 to 1.9 mg/mL. In this group, the mean plasma concentration of IL-1Ra was 660 ± 240 ng/mL (214). In an expanded trial, IL-1Ra was given to 175 patients (215). Patients were enrolled into the study with active disease and while taking nonsteroidal antiinflammatory drugs, up to 10 mg/day of prednisone, or both. There was an initial phase of 3 weeks of 20, 70, or 200 mg administered one, three, or seven times per week. Thereafter, patients received the same dose once weekly for 4 weeks. Placebo was given to patients once weekly for the entire 7-week study period. Four measurements of efficacy were used: number of swollen joints, number of painful joints, and patient and physician assessments of disease severity. A reduction of 50% or more in these scores from baseline was considered significant in the analysis. A statistically significant reduction in the total number of parameters was observed with the optimal improvement in patients receiving 70 mg/d.

A large, double-blind, placebo-controlled trial of IL-1Ra with 472 patients with rheumatoid arthritis used three doses: 30, 75, and 150 mg/day for 24 weeks. There was a dose-dependent reduction in the number of swollen joints and the overall assessment of patient scores ($P = 0.048$) (216). There was a fall in C-reactive protein and sedimentation rate. In this trial, there was a reduction in new bone erosions (217).

A phase I/II trial of escalating doses of IL-1Ra in 17 patients with steroid-resistant graft-versus-host disease has been completed (218). IL-1Ra (400 to 3,400 mg/d) was given as a continuous intravenous infusion every 24 hours for 7 days. Using an organ-specific, acute disease scale, there was improvement in 16 of the 17 patients. Moreover, a decrease in the steady state mRNA for TNF-α in peripheral blood mononuclear cells correlated with improvement ($P = 0.001$) (218). These studies in humans are similar to the use of IL-1Ra in animal models of graft-versus-host disease (219).

For clinical efficacy, IL-1Ra in patients with rheumatoid arthritis exhibits a dose-dependent response. Even the reduction of endotoxin-induced neutrophilia in healthy subjects is dose dependent. Animal studies support these clinical observations. The requirement for such high plasma levels of IL-1Ra is not completely understood, because IL-1Ra levels are already several logs higher than measurable IL-1 levels in the most severe cases of septic shock (211). Rapid renal clearance, binding to the soluble form of the type I receptor, and the effect of acidosis locally or systemically may explain a need for these high levels.

ACKNOWLEDGMENTS

The studies of Dr. Dinarello are supported by NIH grant AI-15614.

REFERENCES

1. Colotta F, Dower SK, Sims JE, Mantovani A. The type II "decoy" receptor: a novel regulatory pathway for interleukin-1. *Immunol Today* 1994;15:562–566.

2. Greenfeder SA, Nunes P, Kwee L, Labow M, Chizzonite RA, Ju G. Molecular cloning and characterization of a second subunit of the interleukin-1 receptor complex. *J Biol Chem* 1995;270:13757–13765.

3. Kitamura T, Takaku F. A preclinical and phase I clinical trial of IL-1. *Exp Med* 1989;7:170–177.

4. Laughlin MJ, Kirkpatrick G, Sabiston N, Peters W, Kurtzberg J. Hematopoietic recovery following high-dose combined alkylating-agent chemotherapy and autologous bone marrow support in patients in phase I clinical trials of colony stimulating factors: G-CSF, GM-CSF, IL-1, IL-2 and M-CSF. *Ann Hematol* 1993;67:267–276.

5. Tewari A, Buhles WC Jr, Starnes HF Jr. Preliminary report: effects of interleukin-1 on platelet counts. *Lancet* 1990;336:712–714.

6. Crown J, Jakubowski A, Kemeny N, et al. A phase I trial of recombinant human interleukin-1β alone and in combination with myelosuppressive doses of 5-fluorouracil in patients with gastrointestinal cancer. *Blood* 1991;78:1420–1427.

7. Smith JW, Urba WJ, Curti BD, et al. The toxic and hematologic effects of interleukin-1 alpha administered in a phase I trial to patients with advanced malignancies. *J Clin Oncol* 1992;10:1141–1152.

8. Nemunaitis J, Appelbaum FR, Lilleby K, et al. Phase I study of recombinant interleukin-1β in patients undergoing autologous bone marrow transplantation for acute myelogenous leukemia. *Blood* 1994;83:3473–3479.

9. Iizumi T, Sato S, Iiyama T, et al. Recombinant human interleukin-1 beta analogue as a regulator of hematopoiesis in patients receiving chemotherapy for urogenital cancers. *Cancer* 1991;68:1520–1523.

10. Smith JW, Longo D, Alford WG, et al. The effects of treatment with interleukin-1α on platelet recovery after high-dose carboplatin. *N Engl J Med* 1993;328:756–761.

11. Starnes HF. Biological effects and possible clinical applications of interleukin-1. *Semin Hematol* 1991;28:43–41.

12. van der Poll T, Bueller HR, ten Cate H, et al. Activation of coagulation after administration of tumor necrosis factor to normal subjects. *N Engl J Med* 1990;322:1622–1627.

13. Tilg H, Trehu E, Atkins MB, Dinarello CA, Mier JW. Interleukin-6 (IL-6) as an anti-inflammatory cytokine: induction of circulating IL-1 receptor antagonist and soluble tumor necrosis factor receptor p55. *Blood* 1994;83:113–118.

14. Tilg H, Trehu E, Shapiro L, et al. Induction of circulating soluble tumour necrosis factor receptor and interleukin 1 receptor antagonist following interleukin-1α infusion in humans. *Cytokine* 1994;6:215–219.

15. Bargetzi MJ, Lantz M, Smith CG, et al. Interleukin-1 beta induces interleukin-1 receptor antagonist and tumor necrosis factor binding proteins. *Cancer Res* 1993;53:4010–4013.

16. Granowitz EV, Santos A, Poutsiaka DD, et al. Circulating interleukin-1 receptor antagonist levels during experimental endotoxemia in humans. *Lancet* 1991;338:1423–1424.

17. Shapiro L, Clark BD, Orencole SF, Poutsiaka DD, Granowitz EV, Dinarello CA. Detection of tumor necrosis factor soluble receptor p55 in blood samples from healthy and endotoxemic humans. *J Infect Dis* 1993;167:1344–1350.

18. Stevenson FT, Torrano F, Locksley RM, Lovett DH. Interleukin-1: the patterns of translation and intracellular distribution support alternative secretory mechanisms. *J Cell Physiol* 1992;152:223–231.

19. Mosley B, Urdal DL, Prickett KS, et al. The interleukin-1 receptor binds the human interleukin-1α precursor but not the interleukin-1β precursor. *J Biol Chem* 1987;262:2941–2944.

20. Kobayashi Y, Oppenheim JJ, Matsushima K. Human pre-interleukin-1α and β: structural features revealed by limited proteolysis. *Chem Pharm Bull (Tokyo)* 1991;39:1513–1517.

21. Kobayashi Y, Yamamoto K, Saido T, Kawasaki H, Oppenheim JJ, Matsushima K. Identification of calcium-activated neutral protease as a processing enzyme of human interleukin 1 alpha. *Proc Natl Acad Sci USA* 1990;87:5548–5552.

22. Miller AC, Schattenberg DG, Malkinson AM, Ross D. Decreased content of the IL-1α processing enzyme calpain in murine bone marrow-derived macrophages after treatment with the benzene metabolite hydroquinone. *Toxicol Lett* 1994;74:177–184.

23. Watanabe N, Kobayashi Y. Selective release of a processed form of interleukin-1α. *Cytokine* 1994;6:597–601.

24. Andersson J, Björk L, Dinarello CA, Towbin H, Andersson U. Lipopolysaccharide induces human interleukin-1 receptor antagonist and interleukin-1 production in the same cell. *Eur J Immunol* 1992;22:2617–2623.

25. Mizel SB, Kilian PL, Lewis JC, Paganelli KA, Chizzonite RA. The interleukin 1 receptor: dynamics of interleukin 1 binding and internalization in T cells and fibroblasts. *J Immunol* 1987;138:2906–2912.

26. Heguy A, Baldari C, Bush K, et al. Internalization and nuclear localization of interleukin 1 are not sufficient for function. *Cell Growth Differ* 1991;2:311–315.

27. Weizmann MN, Savage N. Nuclear internalization and DNA binding activities of interleukin-1, interleukin-1 receptor complexes. *Biochem Biophys Res Commun* 1992;187:1166–1171.

28. Hauser C, Saurat J-H, Schmitt A, Jaunin F, Dayer J-M. Interleukin-1 is present in normal epidermis. *J Immunol* 1986;136:3317–3222.

29. Hammerberg C, Arend WP, Fisher GJ, et al. Interleukin-1 receptor antagonist in normal and psoriatic epidermis. *J Clin Invest* 1992;90:571–583.

30. Maier JAM, Statuto M, Ragnotti G. Endogenous interleukin-1 alpha must be transported to the nucleus to exert its activity in human endothelial cells. *Mol Cell Biol* 1994;14:1845–1851.

31. Wessendorf JHM, Garfinkel S, Zhan X, Brown S, Maciag T. Identification of a nuclear localization sequence within the structure of the human interleukin-1α precursor. *J Biol Chem* 1993;268:22100–22104.

32. Beuscher HU, Nickells MW, Colten HR. The precursor of interleukin-1α is phosphorylated at residue serine 90. *J Biol Chem* 1988;263:4023–4028.

33. Stevenson FT, Bursten SL, Fanton C, Locksley RM, Lovett DH. The 31-kDa precursor of interleukin-1α is myristoylated on specific lysines within the 16-kDa N-terminal propiece. *Proc Natl Acad Sci USA* 1993;90:7245–7249.

34. Maier JAM, Voulalas P, Roeder D, Maciag T. Extension of the life span of human endothelial cells by an interleukin-1α antisense oligomer. *Science* 1990;249:1570–1574.

35. Falk W, Hofmeister R. Intracellular IL-1 replaces signaling by the membrane IL-1 type I receptor. *Cytokine* 1994;6:558.

36. Kurt-Jones EA, Beller DI, Mizel SB, Unanue ER. Identification of a membrane-associated interleukin-1 in macrophages. *Proc Natl Acad Sci USA* 1985;82:1204–1208.

37. Brody DT, Durum SK. Membrane IL-1: IL-1α precursor binds to the plasma membrane via a lectin-like interaction. *J Immunol* 1989;143:1183.

38. Kaplanski G, Farnarier C, Kaplanski S, et al. Interleukin-1 induces interleukin-8 from endothelial cells by a juxacrine mechanism. *Blood* 1994;84:4242–4248.

39. Minnich-Carruth LL, Suttles J, Mizel SB. Evidence against the existence of a membrane form of murine IL-1α. *J Immunol* 1989;142:526.

40. Bailly S, Ferrua B, Fay M, Gougerot-Pocidalo M-A. Paraformaldehyde fixation of LPS-stimulated human monocytes: technical parameters permitting the study of membrane IL-1 activity. *Eur Cytokine Netw* 1990;1:47–51.

41. Fenton MJ, Vermeulen MW, Clark BD, Webb AC, Auron PE. Human pro-IL-1 beta gene expression in monocytic cells is regulated by two distinct pathways. *J Immunol* 1988;140:2267–2273.

42. Jarrous N, Kaempfer R. Induction of human interleukin-1 gene expression by retinoic acid and its regulation at processing of precursor transcripts. *J Biol Chem* 1994;269:23141–23149.

43. Schindler R, Ghezzi P, Dinarello CA. IL-1 induces IL-1. IV. IFN-γ suppresses IL-1 but not lipopolysaccharide-induced transcription of IL-1. *J Immunol* 1990;144:2216–2222.

44. Serkkola E, Hurme M. Synergism between protein-kinase C and cAMP-dependent pathways in the expression of the interleukin-1β gene is mediated via the activator-protein-1 (AP-1) enhancer activity. *Eur J Biochem* 1993;213:243–249.

45. Vannier E, Dinarello CA. Histamine enhances interleukin (IL)-1–induced IL-1 gene expression and protein synthesis via H2 receptors in peripheral blood mononuclear cells: comparison with IL-1 receptor antagonist. *J Clin Invest* 1993;92:281–287.

46. Schindler R, Clark BD, Dinarello CA. Dissociation between interleukin-1β mRNA and protein synthesis in human peripheral blood mononuclear cells. *J Biol Chem* 1990;265:10232–10237.

47. Schindler R, Linnenweber S, Schulze M, et al. Gene expression of interleukin-1β during hemodialysis. *Kidney Int* 1993;43:712–721.

48. Kaspar RL, Gehrke L. Peripheral blood mononuclear cells stimulated with C5a or lipopolysaccharide to synthesize equivalent levels of IL-1β mRNA show unequal IL-1β protein accumulation but similar polyribosome profiles. *J Immunol* 1994;153:277–286.

49. Schindler R, Gelfand JA, Dinarello CA. Recombinant C5a stimulates transcription rather than translation of IL-1 and TNF; cytokine synthesis induced by LPS, IL-1 or PMA. *Blood* 1990;76:1631–1638.

50. Miller LC, Isa S, Vannier E, Georgilis K, Steere AC, Dinarello CA. Live *Borrelia burgdorferi* preferentially activate IL-1β gene expression and protein synthesis over the interleukin-1 receptor antagonist. *J Clin Invest* 1992;90:906–912.

51. Stoeckle MY, Guan L. High-resolution analysis of gro-α mRNA poly (A) shortening: regulation by interleukin-1β. *Nucl Acid Res* 1993;21:1613–1617.

52. Shapiro L, Panayotatos N, Meydani SN, Wu D, Dinarello CA. Ciliary neurotrophic factor combined with soluble receptor inhibits synthesis of pro-inflammatory cytokines and prostaglandin-E2 *in vitro*. *Exp Cell Res* 1994;215:51–56.

53. Jobling SA, Auron PE, Gurka G, Webb AC, McDonald B, Rosenwasser LJ, Gehrke L. Biological activity and receptor binding of human prointerleukin-1β and subpeptides. *J Biol Chem* 1988;263:16372.

54. Bakouche O, Brown DC, Lachman LB. Subcellular localization of human monocyte interleukin 1: evidence for an inactive precursor molecule and a possible mechanism for IL-1 release. *J Immunol* 1987;138:4249–4255.

55. Rubartelli A, Cozzolino F, Talio M, Sitia R. A novel secretory pathway for interleukin-1 beta, a protein lacking a signal sequence. *EMBO J* 1990;9:1503–1510.

56. Auron PE, Warner SJ, Webb AC, et al. Studies on the molecular nature of human interleukin 1. *J Immunol* 1987;138:1447–1456.

57. Beuscher HU, Guenther C, Roellinghoff M. IL-1β is secreted by activated murine macrophages as biologically inactive precursor. *J Immunol* 1990;144:2179–2183.

58. Black RA, Kronheim SR, Cantrell M, et al. Generation of biologically active interleukin-1 beta by proteolytic cleavage of the inactive precursor. *J Biol Chem* 1988;263:9437–9442.

59. Dinarello CA, Cannon JG, Mier JW, et al. Multiple biological activities of human recombinant interleukin 1. *J Clin Invest* 1986;77:1734–1739.

60. Mizutani H, Black RA, Kupper TS. Human keratinocytes produce but do not process pro-interleukin-1β. *J Clin Invest* 1991;87:1066–1071.

61. Mizutani H, Schecter N, Zazarus G, Black RA, Kupper TS. Rapid and specific conversion of precursor interleukin-1β to an active IL-1 species by human mast cell chymase. *J Exp Med* 1991;174:821–825.

62. Hazuda DJ, Strickler J, Kueppers F, Simon PL, Young PR. Processing of precursor interleukin-1 beta and inflammatory disease. *J Biol Chem* 1990;265:6318–6322.

63. Hazuda DJ, Strickler J, Simon P, Young PR. Structure-function mapping of interleukin 1 precursors: cleavage leads to a conformational change in the mature protein. *J Biol Chem* 1991;266:7081–7086.

64. Cerretti DP, Kozlosky CJ, Mosley B, et al. Molecular cloning of the IL-1β processing enzyme. *Science* 1992;256:97–100.

65. Thornberry NA, Bull HG, Calaycay JR, et al. A novel heterodimeric cysteine protease is required for interleukin-1 beta processing in monocytes. *Nature* 1992;356:768–774.

66. Wilson KP, Black JA, Thomson JA, et al. Structure and mechanism of interleukin-1β converting enzyme. *Nature* 1994;370:270–275.

67. Gu Y, Wu J, Faucheu C, Lalanne J-L, Diu A, Livingston DL, Su MS-S. Interleukin-1β converting enzyme requires oligomerization for activity of processed forms *in vivo*. *EMBO J* 1995;14:1923–1931.

68. Walker NP, Talanian RV, Brady KD, et al. Crystal structure of the cysteine protease interleukin-1 beta-converting enzyme: a (p20/p10)2 homodimer. *Cell* 1994;78:343–352.

69. Irmler M, Hertig S, MacDonald HR, et al. Granzyme A is an interleukin-1β-converting enzyme. *J Exp Med* 1995;181:1917–1922.

70. Higgins GC, Foster JL, Postlethwaite AE. Interleukin-1 beta propeptide is detected intracellularly and extracellularly when human monocytes are stimulated with LPS *in vitro*. *J Exp Med* 1994;180:607–614.

71. Higgins GC, Foster JL, Postlethwaite AE. Synthesis and biological activity of human interleukin-1β propiece *in vitro*. *Arthritis Rheum* 1993;39:S153.

72. Rubartelli A, Bajetto A, Allavena G, Wollman E, Sitia R. Secretion of thioredoxin by normal and neoplastic cells through a leaderless secretory pathway. *J Biol Chem* 1992;267:24161–24164.

73. Mignatti P, Rifkin DB. Release of basic fibroblast growth factor, an angiogenic factor devoid of secretory signal sequence: a trivial phenomenon or a novel secretion mechanism? *J Cell Biochem* 1991;47:201–217.

74. Singer II, Scott S, Chin J, Kostura MJ, Miller DK, Chapman K, Bayne EK. Interleukin-1β converting enzyme is localized on the external cell-surface membranes and in the cytoplasmic ground substance of activated human monocytes by immuno-electronmicroscopy. *Lymphokine Cytokine Res* 1993;12:340(abst).

75. Li P, Allen H, Banerjee S, et al. Mice deficient in interleukin-1 converting enzyme (ICE) are defective in production of mature interleukin-1β and resistant to endotoxic shock. *Cell* 1995;80:401–411.

76. Kuida K, Lippke JA, Ku G, et al. Altered cytokine export and apoptosis in mice deficient in interleukin-1β converting enzyme. *Science* 1995;267:2000–2003.

77. Dinarello CA, Ikejima T, Warner SJ, et al. Interleukin 1 induces interleukin 1. I. Induction of circulating interleukin 1 in rabbits *in vivo* and in human mononuclear cells *in vitro*. *J Immunol* 1987;139:1902–1910.

78. Nakamura K, Okamura H, Wada M, Nagata K, Tamura T. Endotoxin-induced serum factor that stimulates gamma interferon production. *Infect Immun* 1989;57:590–595.

79. Nakamura K, Okamura H, Nagata K, Komatsu T, Tamura T. Purification of a factor which provides a costimulatory signal for gamma interferon production. *Infect Immun* 1993;61:64–70.

80. Okamura H, Nagata K, Komatsu T, et al. A novel costimulatory factor for gamma interferon induction found in the livers of mice causes endotoxic shock. *Infect Immun* 1995;63:3966–3972.

81. Okamura H, Tsutsui H, Komatsu T, et al. Cloning of a new cytokine that induces interferon-γ. *Nature* 1995;378:88–91.

82. Heremans H, van Damme J, Dillen C, Dikman R, Billiau A. Interferon-γ, a mediator of lethal lipopolysaccharide-induced Shwartzman-like shock in mice. *J Exp Med* 1990;171:1853–1861.

83. Car BD, Eng VM, Schnyder B, et al. Interferon γ receptor deficient mice are resistant to endotoxic shock. *J Exp Med* 1994;179:1437–1444.

84. Ushio S, Namba M, Okura T, et al. Cloning of the cDNA for human IFN-γ-inducing factor, expression in *Escherichia coli*, and studies on the biologic activities of the protein. *J Immunol* 1996;156:4274–4279.

85. Kohno K, Kataoka J, Ohtsuki T, et al. IFN-γ-inducing factor (IGIF) is a co-stimulatory factor on the activation of Th1 but not Th2 cells and exerts its effect independently of IL-12. *J Immunol* 158:1541–1550.

86. Tsutsui H, Nakanishi K, Matsui K, et al. IFN-γ-inducing factor up-regulates Fas ligand-mediated cytotoxic activity of murine natural killer cell clones. *J Immunol* 1996;157:3967–3973.

87. Bazan JF, Timans JC, Kaselein RA. A newly defined interleukin-1? *Nature* 1996;379:591.

88. Gu Y, Kuida K, Tsutsui H, et al. Activation of interferon-γ inducing factor mediated by interleukin-1β converting enzyme. *Science* 1997;275:206–209.

89. Arend WP. Interleukin-1 receptor antagonist. *Adv Immunol* 1993;54:167–227.

90. Haskill S, Martin M, VanLe L, et al. cDNA cloning of a novel form of the interleukin-1 receptor antagonist associated with epithelium. *Proc Natl Acad Sci USA* 1991;88:3681–3685.

91. Preistle JP, Schar HP, Grutter MG. Crystallographic refinement of interleukin 1 beta at 2.0 Å resolution. *Proc Natl Acad Sci USA* 1989;86:9667–9671.

92. Graves BJ, Hatada MH, Hendrickson WA, Miller JK, Madison VS, Satow Y. Structure of interleukin-1α at 2.7 Å resolution. *Biochem* 1990;29:2679–2684.

93. Vigers GP, Caffes P, Evans RJ, Thompson RC, Eisenberg SP, Brandhuber BJ. X-ray structure of interleukin-1 receptor antagonist at 2.0-Å resolution. *J Biol Chem* 1994;269:12874–12879.

94. Murzin AG, Lesk AM, Chothia C. β-Trefoil fold: patterns of structure and sequence in the Kunitz inhibitors interleukins-1β and 1α and fibroblast growth factors. *J Mol Biol* 1992;223:531–543.

95. Schreuder H. Crystal structure of the interleukin-1 receptor antagonist complex. *Cytokine* 1995;7:599.

96. Gruetter MG, van Oostrum J, Priestle JP, et al. A mutational analysis of receptor binding sites of interleukin-1β: differences in binding of

human interleukin-1β mureins to human and mouse receptors. *Protein Eng* 1994;7:663–671.

97. Lambriola-Tomkins E, Chandran C, Varnell TA, Madison VS, Ju G. Structure-function analysis of human IL-1α: identification of residues required for binding to the human type I IL-1 receptor. *Protein Eng* 1993;6:535–539.

98. Evans RJ, Bray J, Childs JD, et al. Mapping receptor binding sites in the IL-1 receptor antagonist and IL-1β by site-directed mutagenesis: identification of a single site in IL-1ra and two sites in IL-1β. *J Biol Chem* 1994;270:11477–11483.

99. Dripps DJ, Brandhuber BJ, Thompson RC, Eisenberg SP. Effect of IL-1ra on IL-1 signal transduction. *J Biol Chem* 1991;266:10331–10336.

100. Bird TA, Saklatvala J. IL-1 and TNF transmodulate epidermal growth factor receptors by a protein kinase C-independent mechanism. *J Immunol* 1989;142:126–133.

101. Smith JW, Urba WJ, Curti BD, et al. Phase II trial of interleukin-1 alpha in combination with indomethacin in melanoma patients. *Proc Am Soc Clin Oncol* 1991;10:293(abst).

102. Granowitz EV, Porat R, Mier JW, et al. Pharmacokinetics, safety, and immunomodulatory effects of human recombinant interleukin-1 receptor antagonist in healthy humans. *Cytokine* 1992;4:353–360.

103. Greenfeder SA, Varnell T, Powers G, et al. Insertion of a structural domain of interleukin-1β confers agonist activity to the IL-1 receptor antagonist. *J Biol Chem* 1995;270:22460–22465.

104. Gehrke L, Jobling SA, Paik LS, McDonald B, Rosenwasser LJ, Auron PE. A point mutation uncouples human interleukin-1β biological activity and receptor binding. *J Biol Chem* 1990;265:5922–5925.

105. Simoncsits A, Bristulf J, Tjornhammar ML, et al. Deletion mutants of human IL-1β with significantly reduced agonist properties: search for the agonist/antgonist switch in ligands to the interleukin-1 receptors. *Cytokine* 1994;6:206–214.

106. Sims JE, March CJ, Cosman D, et al. cDNA expression cloning of the IL-1 receptor, a member of the immunoglobulin superfamily. *Science* 1988;241:585–589.

107. McMahon CJ, Slack JL, Mosley B, et al. A novel IL-1 receptor cloned form B cells by mammalian expression is expressed in many cell types. *EMBO J* 1991;10:2821–2832.

108. Sims JE, Painter SL, Gow IR. Genomic organization of the type I and type II IL-1 receptors. *Cytokine* 1995;7:483–490.

109. Mancilla J, Ikejima I, Dinarello CA. Glycosylation of the interleukin-1 receptor type I is required for optimal binding of interleukin-1. *Lymphokine Cytokine Res* 1992;11:197–205.

110. Rosoff PM, Savage N, Dinarello CA. Interleukin-1 stimulates diacylglycerol production in T lymphocytes by a novel mechanism. *Cell* 1988;54:73–81.

111. Shirakawa F, Tanaka Y, Ota T, Suzuki H, Eto S, Yamashita U. Expression of interleukin-1 receptors on human peripheral T-cells. *J Immunol* 1987;138:4243–4248.

112. Stylianou E, O'Neill LAJ, Rawlinson L, Edbrooke MR, Woo P, Saklatvala J. Interleukin-1 induces NFκB through its type I but not type II receptor in lymphocytes. *J Biol Chem* 1992;267:15836–15841.

113. Sims JE, Gayle MA, Slack JL, et al. Interleukin-1 signaling occurs exclusively via the type I receptor. *Proc Natl Acad Sci USA* 1993;90:6155–6159.

114. Dower SK, Fanslow W, Jacobs C, Waugh S, Sims JE, Widmer MB. Interleukin-1 antagonists. *Ther Immunol* 1994;1:113–122.

115. Sims JE, Giri JG, Dower SK. The two interleukin-1 receptors play different roles in IL-1 activities. *Clin Immunol Immunopathol* 1994;72:9–14.

116. Burch RM, Mahan LC. Oligonucleotides antisense to the interleukin-1 receptor mRNA block the effects of interleukin-1 in cultured murine and human fibroblasts and in mice. *J Clin Invest* 1991;88:1190–1196.

117. Gallis B, Prickett KS, Jackson J, Slack J, Schooley K, Sims JE, Dower SK. IL-1 induces rapid phosphorylation of the IL-1 receptor. *J Immunol* 1989;143:3235–3240.

118. Gay NJ, Keith FJ. *Drosophila* Toll and IL-1 receptor. *Nature* 1991;351:355–356.

119. Guida S, Heguy A, Melli M. The chicken IL-1 receptor: differential evolution of the cytoplasmic and extracellular domains. *Gene* 1992;111:239–243.

120. Heguy A, Baldari CT, Macchia G, Telford JL, Melli M. Amino acids conserved in interleukin-1 receptors and the *Drosophila* Toll protein are essential for IL-1R signal transduction. *J Biol Chem* 1992;267:2605–2609.

121. Wesche H, Korherr C, Kracht M, Falk W, Resch K, Martin MU. The interleukin-1 receptor accessory protein is essential for IL-1–induced activation of interleukin-1 receptor–associated kinase (IRAK) and stress-activated protein kinases (SAP kinases). *J Biol Chem* 1997;272:7727–7731.

122. Colotta F, Re F, Muzio M, et al. Interleukin-1 type II receptor: a decoy target for IL-1 that is regulated by IL-4. *Science* 1993;261:472–475.

123. Heguy A, Baldari CT, Censini S, Ghiara P, Telford JL. A chimeric type II/I interleukin-1 receptor can mediate interleukin-1 induction of gene expression in T cells. *J Biol Chem* 1993;268:10490–10494.

124. Giri J, Newton RC, Horuk R. Identification of soluble interleukin-1 binding protein in cell-free supernatants. *J Biol Chem* 1990;265:17416–17419.

125. Symons JA, Eastgate JA, Duff GW. Purification and characterization of a novel soluble receptor for interleukin-1. *J Exp Med* 1991;174:1251–1254.

126. Symons JA, Young PA, Duff GW. The soluble interleukin-1 receptor: ligand binding properties and mechanisms of release. *Lymphokine Cytokine Res* 1993;12:381.

127. Orencole SF, Vannier E, Dinarello CA. Detection of soluble IL-1 receptor type II (IL-1sRII) in sera and plasma from healthy volunteers. *Cytokine* 1994;6:554(abst).

128. Arend WP, Malyak M, Smith MF, et al. Binding of IL-1α, IL-1β, and IL-1 receptor antagonist by soluble IL-1 receptors and levels of soluble IL-1 receptors in synovial fluids. *J Immunol* 1994;153:4766–4774.

129. Giri JG, Wells J, Dower SK, et al. Elevated levels of shed type II IL-1 receptor in sepsis. *J Immunol* 1994;153:5802–5813.

130. Orencole SF, Fantuzzi G, Vannier E, Dinarello CA. Circulating levels of IL-1 soluble receptors in health and after endotoxin or IL-2. *Cytokine* 1995;7:642.

131. Leitman DC, Andersen JW, Kuno T, Kamisaki Y, Chang J, Murad F. Identification of multiple binding sites for atrial natriuretic factor by affinity cross—linking in cultured endothelial cells. *J Biol Chem* 1986;261:11650–11656.

132. Alcami A, Smith GL. A soluble receptor for interleukin-1β encoded by vaccinia virus: a novel mechanism of virus modulation of the host response to infection. *Cell* 1992;71:153–167.

133. Spriggs MK, Hruby DE, Maliszewski CR, et al. Vaccinia and cowpox viruses encode a novel secreted interleukin-1 binding protein. *Cell* 1992;71:145–152.

134. Rossi B. IL-1 transduction signals. *Eur Cytokine Netw* 1993;4:181–187.

135. Mizel SB. IL-1 signal transduction. *Eur Cytokine Netw* 1994;5:xxx-xxx.

136. Kuno K, Matsushima K. The IL-1 receptor signaling pathway. *J Leukoc Biol* 1994;56:542–547.

137. O'Neill LAJ. Towards an understanding of the signal transduction pathways for interleukin-1. *Biochim Biophys Acta* 1995;1266:31–44.

138. O'Neill LAJ, Bird TA, Saklatvala J. Interleukin-1 signal transduction. *Immunol Today* 1990;11:392–394.

139. Rosoff PM. Characterization of the interleukin-1–stimulated phospholipase C activity in human T lymphocytes. *Lymphokine Res* 1989;8:407–413.

140. Schutze S, Machleidt T, Kronke M. The role of diacylglycerol and ceramide in tumor necrosis factor and interleukin-1 signal transduction. *J Leukoc Biol* 1994;56:533–541.

141. Andrieu N, Salvayre R, Levade T. Evidence against involvement of the acid lysosomal shingomyelinase in the tumor necrosis factor and interleukin-1–induced sphigomyelin cycle and cell proliferation in human fibroblasts. *Biochem J* 1994;303:341–345.

142. Bomalaski JS, Steiner MR, Simon PL, Clark MA. IL-1 increases phospholipase A_2 activity, expression of phospholipase A_2–activating protein, and release of linoleic acid from the murine T helper cell line EL-4. *J Immunol* 1992;148:155–160.

143. Kolesnick R, Golde DW. The sphingomyelin pathway in tumor necrosis factor and interleukin-1 signalling. *Cell* 1994;77:325–328.

144. Gronich J, Konieczkowski M, Gelb MH, Nemenoff RA, Sedor JR. Interleukin-1α causes a rapid activation of cytosolic phospholipase A_2 by phosphorylation in rat mesangial cells. *J Clin Invest* 1994;93:1224–1233.

145. Orencole SF, Dinarello CA. Characterization of a subclone (D10S) of the D10.G4.1 helper T-cell line which proliferates to attomolar concentrations of interleukin-1 in the absence of mitogens. *Cytokine* 1989;1:14–22.

146. Ye K, Koch K-C, Clark BD, Dinarello CA. Interleukin-1 down regulates gene and surface expression of interleukin-1 receptor type I by destabilizing its mRNA whereas interleukin-2 increases its expression. *Immunology* 1992;75:427–434.

147. Mizel SB. Cyclic AMP and interleukin-1 signal transduction. *Immunol Today* 1990;11:390–391.

148. Munoz E, Beutner U, Zubiaga A, Huber BT. IL-1 activates two separate signal transduction pathways in T helper type II cells. *J Immunol* 1990;144:964–969.

149. Kester M, Siomonson MS, Mene P, Sedor JR. Interleukin-1 generates transmembrane signals from phospholipids through novel pathways in cultured rat mesangial cells. *J Clin Invest* 1989;83:718–723.

150. Mathias S, Younes A, Kan C-C, Orlow I, Joseph C, Kolesnick RN. Activation of the sphingomyelin signaling pathway in intact EL4 cells and in a cell-free system by IL-1β. *Science* 1993;259:519–522.

151. Clark MA, Özgür LE, Conway TM, Dispoto J, Crooke ST, Bomalaski JS. Cloning of a phospholipase A₂-activating protein. *Proc Natl Acad Sci USA* 1991;88:5418–5422.

152. Rzymkiewicz DM, DuMaine J, Morrison AR. IL-1β regulates rat mesangial cyclooxygenase II gene expression by tyrosine phosphorylation. *Kidney Int* 1995;47:1354–1363.

153. Huwiler A, Pfeilschifter J. Interleukin-1 stimulates de novo synthesis of mitogen-activated protein kinase in glomerular mesangial cells. *FEBS Lett* 1994;350:135–138.

154. Freshney NW, Rawlinson L, Guesdon F, et al. Interleukin-1 activates a novel protein cascade that results in the phosphorylation of hsp27. *Cell* 1994;78:1039–1049.

155. Kracht M, Truong O, Totty NF, Shiroo M, Saklatvala J. Interleukin-1α activates two forms of p54a mitogen-activated protein kinase in rabbit liver. *J Exp Med* 1994;180:2017–2027.

156. Kuno K, Okamoto S, Hirose K, Murakami S, Matsushima K. Structure and function of the intracellular portion of the mouse interleukin-1 receptor (type I). *J Biol Chem* 1993;268:13510–13518.

157. Croston GE, Cao Z, Goeddel DV. NFκB activation by interleukin-1 requires an IL-1 receptor-associated protein kinase activity. *J Biol Chem* 1995;270:16514–16517.

158. Martin M, Bol GF, Eriksson A, Resch K, Brigelius-Flohe R. Interleukin-1–induced activation of a protein kinase co-precipitating with the type I interleukin-1 receptor in T-cells. *Eur J Immunol* 1994;24:1566–1571.

159. Hopp TP. Evidence from sequence information that the interleukin-1 receptor is a transmembrane GTPase. *Protein Sci* 1995;4:1851–1859.

160. Mitchum JL, Sims JE. IIP1: a novel human protein that interacts with the IL-1 receptor. *Cytokine* 1995;7:595(abst).

161. Matsushima K, Kobayashi Y, Copeland TD, Akahoshi T, Oppenheim JJ. Phosphorylation of a cytosolic 65-kDa protein induced by interleukin-1 in glucocorticoid pretreated normal human peripheral blood mononuclear leukocytes. *J Immunol* 1987;139:3367–3374.

162. Bird TA, Sleath PR, de Roos PC, Dower SK, Virca GD. Interleukin-1 represents a new modality for the activation of extracellular signal-related kinases/microtubule-associated protein-2 kinases. *J Biol Chem* 1991;266:22661–22670.

163. Guesdon F, Freshney N, Waller RJ, Rawlinson L, Saklatvala J. Interleukin 1 and tumor necrosis factor stimulate two novel protein kinases that phosphorylate the heat shock protein hsp27 and beta-casein. *J Biol Chem* 1993;268:4236–4243.

164. Galcheva-Gargova Z, Dérijard B, Wu I-H, Davis RJ. An osmosensing signal transduction pathway in mammalian cells. *Science* 1994;265:806–809.

165. Han J, Lee J-D, Bibbs L, Ulevitch RJ. A MAP kinase targeted by endotoxin and hyperosmolarity in mammalian cells. *Science* 1994;265:808–811.

166. Shapiro L, Dinarello CA. Osmotic regulation of cytokine synthesis *in vitro*. *Proc Natl Acad Sci USA* 1995;92:12230–12234.

167. Zhang S, Han J, Sells MA, Chernoff J, Knaus UG, Ulevitch RJ, Bokoch GM. Rho family GTPases regulate p38 mitogen-activated protein kinase through the downstream mediator Pak1. *J Biol Chem* 1995;270:23934–23936.

168. Lee JC, Laydon JT, McDonnell PC, et al. A protein kinase involved in the regulation of inflammatory cytokine biosynthesis. *Nature* 1994;372:739–747.

169. Han J, Richter B, Li Z, Kravchenko VV, Ulevitch RJ. Molecular cloning of human p38 MAP kinase. *Biochim Biophys Acta* 1995;1265:224–227.

170. Cuenda A, Rouse J, Doza YN, et al. SB 203580 is a specific inhibitor of a MAP kinase homologue which is stimulated by stresses and interleukin-1. *FEBS Lett* 1995;364:229–233.

171. DiDonato JA, Mercurio F, Karin M. Phosphorylation of IκBa precedes but is not sufficient for its dissociation from NFκB. *Mol Cell Biol* 1995;15:1302–1311.

172. Shirakawa F, Mizel SB. *In vitro* activation and nuclear translocation of NF-kappa B catalyzed by cyclic AMP-derived protein kinase and protein kinase C. *Mol Cell Biol* 1989;9:2424–2430.

173. Guesdon F, Waller RJ, Saklatvala J. Specific activation of β-casein kinase by the inflammatory cytokines interleukin-1 and tumour necrosis factor. *Biochem J* 1994;304:761–768.

174. Bird TA, Downey H, Virca GD. Interleukin-1 regulates casein kinase II-mediated phosphorylation of the p65 subunit of NGκB. *Cytokine* 1995;7:603(abst).

175. Muegge K, Williams TM, Kant J, et al. Interleukin-1 costimulatory activity on the interleukin-2 promoter via AP-1. *Science* 1989;246:249–251.

176. Muegge K, Vila M, Gusella GL, Musso T, Herrlich P, Stein B, Durum SK. IL-1 induction of the c-jun promoter. *Proc Natl Acad Sci USA* 1993;90:7054–7058.

177. Makarov SS, Olsen JC, Johnston WN, et al. Suppression of experimental arthritis by gene transfer of interleukin-1 receptor antagonist cDNA. *Proc Natl Acad Sci USA* 1995;92:11301–11315.

178. Hirsch E, Irikura VM, Paul SM, Hirsh D. Functions of interleukin-1 receptor antagonist in gene knockout and overproducing mice. *Proc Natl Acad Sci USA* 1996;93:11008–11013.

179. Porat R, Poutsiaka DD, Miller LC, Granowitz EV, Dinarello CA. Interleukin-1 (IL-1) receptor blockade reduces endotoxin and *Borrelia burgdorferi*-stimulated IL-8 synthesis in human mononuclear cells. *FASEB J* 1992;6:2482–2486.

180. Norman JG, Franz MG, Messina J, et al. Interleukin-1 receptor antagonist decreases severity of experimental acute pancreatitis. *Surgery* 1995;117:648–655.

181. Norman JG, Franz MG, Fink GS, et al. Decreased mortality of severe acute pancreatitis after proximal cytokine blockade. *Ann Surg* 1995;221:625–634.

182. Dayer-Metroz MD, Duhamel D, Rufer N, et al. IL-1ra delays the spontaneous autoimmune diabetes in the BB rat. *Eur J Clin Invest* 1992;22:A50(abst).

183. Vidal-Vanaclocha F, Amézaga C, Asumendi A, Kaplanski G, Dinarello CA. Interleukin-1 receptor blockade reduces the number and size of murine B16 melanoma hepatic metastases. *Cancer Res* 1994;54:2667–2672.

184. Cominelli F, Nast CC, Clark BD, et al. Interleukin-1 gene expression, synthesis and effect of specific IL-1 receptor blockade in rabbit immune complex colitis. *J Clin Invest* 1990;86:972–980.

185. Kaplanski G, Porat R, Aiura K, Erban JK, Gelfand JA, Dinarello CA. Activated platelets induce endothelial secretion of interleukin-8 *in vitro* via an interleukin-1–mediated event. *Blood* 1993;81:2492–2495.

186. Aiura K, Gelfand JA, Wakabayashi G, Burke JF, Thompson RC, Dinarello CA. Interleukin-1 (IL-1) receptor antagonist prevents *Staphylococcus epidermidis*-induced hypotension and reduces circulating levels of tumor necrosis factor and IL-1β in rabbits. *Infect Immun* 1993;61:3342–3350.

187. Arend WP, Welgus HG, Thompson RC, Eisenberg SP. Biological properties of recombinant human monocyte-derived interleukin-1 receptor antagonist. *J Clin Invest* 1990;85:1694–1697.

188. Granowitz EV, Clark BD, Vannier E, Callahan MV, Dinarello CA. Effect of interleukin-1 (IL-1) blockade on cytokine synthesis: I. IL-1 receptor antagonist inhibits IL-1–induced cytokine synthesis and blocks the binding of IL-1 to its type II receptor on human monocytes. *Blood* 1992;79:2356–2363.

189. Estrov Z, Kurzrock R, Wetzler M, et al. Suppression of chronic myelogenous leukemia colony growth by IL-1 receptor antagonist and soluble IL-1 receptors: a novel application for inhibitors of IL-1 activity. *Blood* 1991;78:1476–1484.

190. Rambaldi A, Torcia M, Bettoni S, et al. Modulation of cell proliferation and cytokine production in acute myeloblastic leukemia by interleukin-1 receptor antagonist and lack of its expression by leukemic cells. *Blood* 1991;78:3248–3253.

191. Schirò R, Longoni D, Rossi V, et al. Suppression of juvenile chronic myelogenous leukemia colony growth by interleukin-1 receptor antagonist. *Blood* 1993;83:460–465.

192. Wetzler M, Kurrzock R, Estrov Z, et al. Altered levels of interleukin-1β and interleukin-1 receptor antagonist in chronic myelogenous leukemia: clinical and prognostic correlates. *Blood* 1994;84:3142–3147.

193. Holmberg LA, Seidel K, Leisenring W, Torok-Storb B. Aplastic anemia analysis of stromal cell-function in long-term marrow cultures. *Blood* 1994;84:3685–3690.

194. Barak V, Nisman B, Dann EJ, et al. Serum interleukin-1β levels as a marker in hairy cell leukemia: correlation with disease status and sIL-2R levels. *Leuk Lymphoma* 1994;14:33–39.

195. Miller LC, Lynch EA, Isa S, Logan JW, Dinarello CA, Steere AC. Balance of synovial fluid IL-1β and IL-1 receptor antagonist and recovery from Lyme arthritis. *Lancet* 1993;341:146–148.

196. Firestein GS, Berger AE, Tracey DE, et al. IL-1 receptor antagonist protein production and gene expression in rheumatoid arthritis and osteoarthritis synovium. *J Immunol* 1992;149:1054–1062.

197. Roux-Lombard P, Modoux C, Vischer T, Grassi J, Dayer J-M. Inhibitors of interleukin 1 activity in synovial fluids and in cultured synovial fluid mononuclear cells. *J Rheumatol* 1992;19:517–523.

198. Firestein GS, Boyle DL, Yu C, et al. Synovial IL-1 receptor antagonist and interleukin-1 balance in rheumatoid arthritis. *Arthritis Rheum* 1994;37:644–652.

199. Kristensen M, Deleuran B, Eedy DJ, Feldmann M, Breathnach SM, Brennan FM. Distribution of interleukin-1 receptor antagonist protein (IRAP), interleukin-1 receptor, and interleukin-1 alpha in normal and psoriatic skin. *Br J Dermatol* 1992;127:305–311.

200. Chomarat P, Vannier E, Dechanet J, et al. The balance of IL-1 receptor antagonist/IL-1β in rheumatoid synovium and its regulation by IL-4 and IL-10. *J Immunol* 1995;154:1432–1439.

201. Thea DM, Porat R, Nagimbi K, et al. Plasma cytokines, plasma cytokine antagonists, and disease progression in African women infected with HIV-1. *Ann Intern Med* 1996;124:757–762.

202. Chensue SW, Bienkowski M, Eessalu TE, et al. Endogenous IL-1 receptor antagonist protein (IRAP) regulates schistosome egg granuloma formation and the regional lymphoid response. *J Immunol* 1993;151:3654–3662.

203. Ferretti M, Casini-Raggi V, Pizarro TT, Eisenberg SP, Nast CC, Cominelli F. Neutralization of endogenous IL-1 receptor antagonist exacerbates and prolongs inflammation in rabbit immune colitis. *J Clin Invest* 1994;94:449–453.

204. LeMay LG, Otterness IG, Vander AJ, Kluger MJ. *In vivo* evidence that the rise in plasma IL-6 following injection of a fever-inducing dose of LPS is mediated by IL-1 beta. *Cytokine* 1990;2:199–204.

205. Dinarello CA, Zhang XX, Wen HD, Wolff SM, Ikejima T. The effect of interleukin-1 receptor antagonist on IL-1, LPS, *Staphylococcus epidermidis* and tumor necrosis factor fever. In: Bartfai T, Ottoson D, eds. *Neuro-immunology of fever.* Oxford: Pergamon Press, 1992:11–18.

206. Granowitz EV, Porat R, Mier JW, et al. Hematological and immunomodulatory effects of an interleukin-1 receptor antagonist coinfusion during low-dose endotoxemia in healthy humans. *Blood* 1993;82:2985–2990.

207. Markewitz A, Faist E, Lang S, Endres S, Fuchs B, Reichart B. Successful restoration of cell-mediated immune response after cardiopulmonary bypass by immunomodulation. *J Thorac Cardiovasc Surg* 1993;105:15–24.

208. Fisher CJJ, Slotman GJ, Opal SM, et al. Initial evaluation of human recombinant interleukin-1 receptor antagonist in the treatment of sepsis syndrome: a randomized, open-label, placebo-controlled multicenter trial. *Crit Care Med* 1994;22:12–21.

209. Gershenwald JE, Fong YM, Fahey TJ, Calvano SE, Chizzonite R, Kilian PL, Lowry SF, Moldawer LL. Interleukin 1 receptor blockade attenuates the host inflammatory response. *Proc Natl Acad Sci USA* 1990;87:4966–4970.

210. Fischer E, Marano MA, Barber AE, et al. A comparison between the effects of interleukin-1α administration and sublethal endotoxemia in primates. *Am J Physiol* 1991;261:R442–R449.

211. Casey LC, Balk RA, Bone RC. Plasma cytokines and endotoxin levels correlate with survival in patients with the sepsis syndrome. *Ann Intern Med* 1993;119:771–778.

212. Fisher CJJ, Dhainaut JF, Opal SM, et al. Recombinant human interleukin-1 receptor antagonist in the treatment of patients with sepsis syndrome: results from a randomized, double blind, placebo-controlled trial. *JAMA* 1994;271:1836–1843.

213. Knaus WA, Harrell FE, Fisher CJ, et al. The clinical evaluation of new drugs for sepsis. *JAMA* 1993;270:1233–1241.

214. Lebsack ME, Paul CC, Bloedow DC, et al. Subcutaneous IL-1 receptor antagonist in patients with rheumatoid arthritis. *Arthritis Rheum* 1991;34[Suppl]:S67.

215. Lebsack ME, Paul CC, Martindale JJ, Catalano MA. A dose- and regimen-ranging study of IL-1 receptor antagonist in patients with rheumatoid arthritis. *Arthritis Rheum* 1993;36:S39.

216. Bresnihan B, Lookabaugh J, Witt K, Musikic P. Treatment with recombinant human interleukin-1 receptor antagonist in rheumatoid arthritis: results of a randomized, double-blind, placebo-controlled multicenter trial. *Arthritis Rheum* 1996;39:S73(abst).

217. Watt I, Cobby M. Recombinant human interleukin-1 receptor antagonist reduces the rate of joint erosion in rheumatoid arthritis. *Arthritis Rheum* 1996;39:S123.

218. Antin JH, Weinstein HJ, Guinan EC, et al. Recombinant human interleukin-1 receptor antagonist in the treatment of steroid-resistant graft-versus-host disease. *Blood* 1994;84:1342–1348.

219. McCarthy PL, Abhyankar S, Neben S, et al. Inhibition of interleukin-1 by interleukin-1 receptor antagonist prevents graft versus host disease. *Blood* 1991;78:1915–1918.

Inflammation: Basic Principles and Clinical Correlates,
3rd ed., edited by John I. Gallin and Ralph Snyderman.
Lippincott Williams & Wilkins, Philadelphia © 1999.

CHAPTER 31

Interleukin-2

Kendall A. Smith, Carol Beadling, and Elizabeth Leef Jacobson

INTERLEUKIN-2 HISTORY

The history of IL-2 can be traced to the beginning of lymphocyte cultures, first described by Nowell in 1960 (1). Nowell astutely observed that lymphocytes stimulated to proliferate by phytohemagglutinin (PHA) underwent a "long latent period," in that he "consistently failed to observe mitosis in cultures of normal leukocytes before the 3rd day *in vitro*." He postulated "the possibility that some such essential factor, perhaps a cell product, does exist in our cultures, although the fact remains that it alone, in the absence of PHA does not initiate mitosis." In 1965, Kasakura and Lowenstein (2) and Gordon and MacLean (3) simultaneously reported in *Nature* that medium conditioned by mixed leukocyte cultures contained a mitogenic factor they called *blastogenic factor*, which promoted the proliferation of freshly isolated leukocytes. During the ensuing decade, numerous lymphocyte mitogenic factors were reported by various names, including *potentiating factor* (4), *autostimulating factor* (5), *immune response restorer activity* (6), and *lymphocyte-activating factor* (7). However, the activities of all of these factors found in lymphocyte-conditioned medium were only tested for their effects on short-term cell growth assays of a few days' duration.

In the mid-1970s, there were several reports of extending the culture of lymphocytes by repetitive stimulation with the initial antigenic stimulus. In 1973, a successful secondary alloantigen stimulation was reported (8), and as many as four sequential alloantigen stimulations of the same initial cell population over 64 days was attained (9). It was shown that lymphocytes could be re-stimulated with allogenic lymphocytes every second week and could be maintained for up to 4 months (10), and in 1976, T

cells sensitized *in vitro* to alloantigens were propagated for more than 9 months by repetitive alloantigen stimulation (11).

These early attempts to promote long-term lymphocyte growth by repetitive alloantigen stimulation reflected the prevailing dogma at the time that the primary mitogenic stimulus was delivered by the antigen, as originally suggested by Nowell. Soluble factors were thought to merely amplify the proliferative reaction that had already been initiated by antigen. In 1976, the accidental discovery by Doris Morgan that PHA-stimulated lymphocyte-conditioned medium selected for and maintained the growth of normal human T cells was a major breakthrough. While trying to promote and sustain the growth of myeloid leukemic cells, Morgan et al. (12) found that PHA-stimulated lymphocyte-conditioned medium consistently selected for T-cell growth that could be sustained for as long as 13 months.

The Morgan results prompted our laboratory to use a similar approach to try to generate long-term antigen-specific T-cell lines, first by stimulating with antigen to select only for antigen reactive cells, followed by long-term growth in conditioned medium. Contrary to the belief that antigen was the only mitogenic stimulus necessary, concanavalin A (Con A)–stimulated murine spleen cell–conditioned medium (but not fresh medium containing Con A) supported the long-term growth of cytolytic T-lymphocyte lines (CTLLs) (13). Subsequently, the conditioned medium was used to obtain the first clones of T cells (14).

Even though antigen-specific T-cell clones could be generated, it was not clear initially whether one or several molecules in the conditioned media promoted the long-term T-cell growth. Moreover, the role of the mitogenic lectins (i.e., PHA or Con A) in relation to any "factors" in the conditioned medium was not understood. To elucidate the nature of the molecules that were responsible for the mitogenic activity, CTLL clones were used to create a rapid, sensitive, and quantitative bioassay for the T-cell

K. A. Smith, C. Beadling, and E. L. Jacobson: The Immunology Program, Cornell University Graduate School of Medical Sciences, and the Department of Medicine, Division of Immunology, Cornell University Medical College, New York, New York 10021.

growth factor (TCGF) activity (15). Patterned after an assay created for erythropoietin (16), the TCGF assay was instrumental in experiments directed toward characterizing TCGF. The TCGF activity was only produced by mitogen- or antigen-stimulated T cells, and it promoted the growth solely of mitogen or antigen-activated T cells, with resting T cells remaining unresponsive (15,17).

To characterize and purify the molecule responsible for TCGF activity, many liters of conditioned medium were produced from PHA-stimulated human tonsil lymphocytes. Biochemical analysis indicated that all of the activity detectable by the TCGF assay could be ascribed to a single molecule that migrated as a peak of 15.5 kd on SDS-PAGE gels and had an isoelectric point (pI) of 8.2 (18). To facilitate identification and purification of the molecule, TCGF-neutralizing monoclonal antibodies were generated and the molecule was purified by antibody affinity adsorption (19). The antibody-purified TCGF molecules were homogeneous as assessed by amino acid sequence analysis, and for the first time, the precise molecular characteristics of the molecule that came to be known as interleukin-2 (IL-2) were defined (18,19).

The bioassay was then used by Taniguchi et al. (20) to detect and isolate a cDNA encoding IL-2 activity. Analysis of the amino acid sequence predicted from the cDNA confirmed all of the molecular characteristics that we had defined from purified natural IL-2, including the molecular size, pI, and N-terminal amino acid sequence. In just 5 years, the molecule responsible for the TCGF activity had been identified, characterized biologically and biochemically, and purified to homogeneity, and the gene encoding the molecule was cloned.

INTERLEUKIN-2 RECEPTOR HISTORY

Like the TCGF bioassay, the discovery and definition of the IL-2 receptor (IL-2R) can be traced to experiments on the biologic activity of erythropoietin (16). In the late 1960s and early 1970s, receptors had been identified for only a few classic hormones, such as insulin. One of the approaches used to discern whether the ligand bound to the target cells was to perform adsorption experiments. Fetal liver cells, which are rich in erythroblasts, were searched for erythropoietin adsorptive capacity. Monitored by the erythropoietin assay, these target cells removed erythropoietin activity in a time-, temperature-, and cell concentration–dependent manner, suggesting the presence of a cellular receptor for this hormone (16).

After the TCGF bioassay had been developed, the same kind of adsorptive assays were performed, with similar results. Only mitogen- or antigen-activated T cells had absorptive capacity; resting T cells and B cells activated by lipopolysaccharide (LPS) did not (21). These findings were consistent with the observation that conditioned medium containing TCGF activity only maintained the growth of mitogen- or antigen-activated T cells, thereby pointing to the antigen-induced expression of receptors only by T cells.

The discovery of IL-2Rs and their characterization had to await the purification of IL-2 to homogeneity so that the molecule could be radiolabeled and classic radiolabeled ligand binding experiments could be performed (22). Initially, biosynthetically radiolabeled TCGF was purified painstakingly by gel filtration and isoelectric focusing. Subsequently, immunoaffinity purification using TCGF-reactive monoclonal antibodies greatly facilitated the experiments (19).

IL-2 binding sites were saturable at very low IL-2 concentrations (about 100 pmol/L), which were identical to the IL-2 concentrations that promoted T-cell proliferation (22). Moreover, IL-2–specific binding sites were detectable only on antigen-activated T cells, resting T cells, and LPS-activated B cells remaining negative. The IL-2 binding sites satisfied all of the criteria to be called true receptors, as defined by classic endocrinology.

The discovery of IL-2Rs and their characterization as classic hormone receptors opened a new era in immunology. Before the molecular identification of the nature of IL-2 and the mechanism whereby it interacted with antigen-activated T cells, the lymphokine (cytokine) field suffered from phenomenology, because experiments dealt with biologic "activities." After these discoveries, classic biochemical and pharmacologic principles were found to underlie the most fundamental of immunologic responses of lymphocytes to antigenic stimulation: proliferation and differentiation.

INTERLEUKIN-2 AND ITS RECEPTOR: STRUCTURE-ACTIVITY RELATIONSHIPS

Although the primary structure of IL-2 was known by 1983, a decade of further research was necessary before the full three-dimensional structure became known (23). Similarly, even though high-affinity binding of IL-2 by IL-2Rs was first observed in 1981, a decade of additional research was necessary before the primary structures of the three chains making up this receptor became fully realized (24–27). The complete picture of IL-2 bound to its receptor still remains to be elucidated.

The structure of IL-2 is prototypic for many of the members of the interleukin hematopoietic growth factor family. IL-2 is comprised of 133 amino acid residues that are organized into four main antiparallel amphipathic α helices. The molecule is stable to extremes of pH and heat, with a strong hydrophobic core and a hydrophilic exterior. The original biochemical analysis of IL-2 (18) revealed that the molecule is variably glycosylated, but the carbohydrates are not involved in mediating its biologic activity, because nonglycosylated IL-2 is just as active as fully glycosylated IL-2.

The three identifiable classes of IL-2Rs are shown in Table 31-1. High-affinity ($K_d=10^{-11}$ mol/L) receptors are

TABLE 31-1. *Interleukin-2*

Property	Affinity class		
	High	Intermediate	Low
Binding affinity (K_d)	10^{-11} M	10^{-9} M	10^{-8} M
Chains	α, β, γ	β, γ	α
Cells	Activated T and B lymphocytes, 10% NK	90% NK	—
[IL-2]	10^{-12}–10^{-10}	10^{-10}–10^{-8}	10^{-9}–10^{-7}
No. cells	10^8	10^9	—

NK, natural killer cells; [IL-2], concentration of interleukin-2.

heterotrimers of distinct chains designated α (p55), β (p75), and γ (p65). Detailed kinetic binding studies revealed how the three different chains cooperate to create a very-high-affinity IL-2 binding site (28). The α chain contributes a very rapid association rate ($k=10^7$ mol/L^{-1}s^{-1}), and a combination of the βγ dimer contributes a slow rate of dissociation ($k^{-1}=10^{-4}$ s^{-1}). Because the equilibrium dissociation constant (K_d) is made up of the ratio of the two rate constants, the $K_d=k^1/k=10^{-4}$ s^{-1}/10^7 mol/L^{-1}s^{-1}=10^{-11} M. Of utmost significance and importance for the biologic activity of IL-2 and for the pharmacologic use of IL-2, the expression of high affinity heterotrimeric IL-2Rs is restricted to antigen-activated T cells and B cells (29) and a minor proportion (about 10%) of natural killer (NK) cells (30) (see Table 31-1). Normal individuals have up to 10^8 circulating cells with these high-affinity IL-2Rs among the 10^{10} total circulating lymphocytes.

By comparison, intermediate affinity IL-2Rs ($K_d=10^{-9}$ mol/L) lack an α chain, so that they are composed of βγ heterodimers. The missing α chain results in a much slower association rate ($k=10^5$ mol/L^{-1}s^{-1}) and, consequently, a 100-fold lower affinity for binding than the heterotrimeric, high-affinity receptor. The importance of this class of receptors resides in the finding that 90% of NK cells express this receptor constitutively (30). Consequently, 100-fold higher IL-2 concentrations are necessary to saturate the intermediate affinity IL-2Rs expressed by most NK cells, compared with the much lower IL-2 concentrations that can saturate the high-affinity IL-2Rs expressed by antigen-activated T cells and B cells (29,30).

These findings explained Nowell's 1960 observation that PHA was necessary to activate lymphocyte proliferation (1). Moreover, they explained how blastogenic factor (2,3) had mitogenic activity for freshly isolated lymphocytes that had not been activated by lectin or antigen (e.g., NK cells). They also elucidated how Morgan's PHA-stimulated lymphocyte-conditioned medium selected for T-cell growth: it contained the mitogenic lectin that stimulated expression of IL-2Rs on T cells and stimulated production

of the growth factor IL-2 that is necessary to bind to these receptors and promote cell cycle progression.

Interleukin-2 Signaling

Endocrinologists and pharmacologists make a distinction between a binding site and a receptor. In addition to binding the ligand with high affinity and specificity, a true receptor is capable of delivering a signal to the cell (29). A true receptor has two functions, that of an on-off switch and that of a timer. How long a receptor signals often dictates the type of biologic response obtained. For the IL-2R, it is evident that only the β chain and γ chain are involved in creating the signal that is delivered to the interior of the cells (31,32). Binding of IL-2 to the receptor functions to stabilize a complex of the IL-2 β chain with the γ chain. This stabilization is thought to provide the on switch (31,32). The timer function of the receptor is determined by the rate of dissociation of IL-2 from the βγ dimer (t$^{1/2}$=45 minutes) compared with the rate of internalization of the IL-2–receptor complex (t$^{1/2}$=15 minutes). After it is internalized, acidification of the receptors promotes dissociation of IL-2 from its binding site, the receptor is switched off, and signaling ceases (33).

The biochemical reactions responsible for generating the signals that invade the interior of the cell are still being unraveled. Soon after the discovery of the β chain of the IL-2R, it was demonstrated that IL-2R triggering led to rapid tyrosine-specific phosphorylation of several cytoplasmic proteins, most notably the β chain of the receptor itself (34). The kinases responsible for these events remained obscure until the discovery of the Janus family of intracellular kinases (JAK), which originally was found to be involved in interferon receptor signaling, but is now known to be responsible for the tyrosine-specific phosphorylation triggered by many of the receptors in the interleukin-hematopoietic growth factor family (35). It remains controversial whether members of the SRC family of tyrosine-specific kinases are also involved early in the IL-2R triggering events (36).

The close approximation of the β chain and the γ chain of the receptor mediated by IL-2 binding brings together the JAK-1 kinase, which is associated with the most membrane-proximal segments of the β chain, and JAK-3, which is associated with a similar region of the chain. Almost instantaneously, the JAKs begin to phosphorylate one another and specific tyrosine residues on the β and γ chains (37,38), initiating signaling by at least three distinct biochemical pathways.

Phosphorylation of the most membrane-proximal tyrosine of the β chain, Y-338, eventually leads to activation of the RAS-RAF-MEK-MAP/ERK pathway (39). When phosphorylated, Y-338 binds the phosphotyrosine binding domain of the adapter protein SHC, and SHC itself becomes phosphorylated (40,41). The P-Tyr in SHC serves as a docking site for the SRC homology-2 (SH2) region of the adapter protein growth factor receptor-bound protein-2 (GRB-2). GRB-2 binds to proline-rich sequences of the nucleotide exchange factor Son of Sevenders (SOS). The net effect of these associations is to bring SOS into proximity with membrane-associated RAS, thereby favoring the accumulation of RAS in the active, GTP-bound state, rather than the inactive GDP-bound state (42,43). As in other signaling pathways, active RAS binds to downstream effectors, including RAF-1 (44,45), contributing to activation of the RAF-MEK-MAP kinase cascade.

A second signaling pathway, which involves activation of phosphatidylinositol 3-kinase (PI3K), has been traced to Y-392 of the IL-2Rβ chain (46). The 85-kd regulatory subunit of PI3K is tyrosine phosphorylated itself within a minute of IL-2 binding, and the association of PI3K with the IL-2Rβ chain is blocked by a Tyr phosphopeptide containing Y-392. Once activated, PI3K activates downstream effectors, including p70S6 kinase (47) and the serine/threonine kinase encoded by the *AKT* protooncogene (48), also called protein kinase B (PKB). PI3K activates a lipid intermediate, phosphatidylinositol 3,4,5-triphosphate, which is instrumental in facilitating the activation of PKB, probably through intermediate upstream serine/threonine kinases (49).

A third IL-2R–triggered signaling pathway involves the signal transducer and activator of transcription (STAT) proteins (35). IL-2R triggering has been reported to activate STAT-3 and STAT-5 (50,51). These proteins are activated by tyrosine-specific phosphorylation, thought to be mediated by the JAKs, which subsequently is necessary for dimerization of the STATs through their SH2 domains, a prerequisite before the STAT homodimers or heterodimers can translocate to the nucleus, where they bind to STAT-specific response elements and activate transcription. Like the activation of the other two signaling pathways, phosphorylation of Tyr residues of the IL-2R β chain (Tyr 392 and 510) has been implicated in activation of the STAT proteins (39). When phosphorylated, these IL-2R Tyr residues bind the STAT proteins through their SH2 domains. Recruitment into the receptor complex is required for STAT activation, presumably for bringing the STATs into proximity of the JAKs so they can be phosphorylated. STATs also must be serine phosphorylated, which is necessary for maximal transactivation capability (52). In the case of IL-2–induced STAT-5 serine phosphorylation, the kinase responsible appears to be independent of RAF-MAPK/ERK or p70S6K (53) and is possibly PKB.

Interleukin-2–Induced Gene Expression

The signal transduction pathways culminate in the activation of transcriptional initiation factors, which stimulate the expression of specific genes. The STATs are the only IL-2–induced transcription factors identified conclusively, although the search for additional factors continues. Even more obscure are the genes activated by these factors. We and others identified a number of cellular protooncogenes expressed soon after IL-2 stimulation, including *MYB* (54), *MYC, FOS* (55), *PIM* (56), and *BCL2* (57). Because these genes encode products known to be involved in cell growth, they remain important candidates that are thought to function by carrying on the effects initiated by IL-2R triggering.

Of the genes known to specify products important for cell cycle progression, the G_1 cyclins D2 and D3 are noteworthy. It is still obscure whether cyclin D2 gene expression is directly activated by an IL-2R signaling pathway or is expressed as a consequence of cell cycle progression. However, cyclin D2 mRNA expression, which is first evident in early G_1 and then disappears in late G_1 just as cyclin D3 mRNA transcripts appear, establishes a landmark of gene expression during the G_1 phase of the cell cycle (58). The kinetics of the expression of cyclin D3 are similar to those of PCNA, an auxiliary factor of DNA polymerase delta, which is expressed at the G_1 to S phase transition (59). Other genes under the coordinate control of the E2F family of transcription factors also are expressed at the G_1 to S phase boundary in IL-2–stimulated lymphocytes (60,61), and their gene products are required for optimal DNA synthesis and DNA replication.

Although the genes expressed in the second half of G_1 that promote G_1 to S phase transition have become better defined, the events occurring in the first half of G_1 responsible for stimulating the later events have remained obscure. To identify genes expressed in an immediate or early fashion as a result of IL-2R signaling, we developed a method to enrich for and isolate genes transcribed within the first 2 hours of receptor activation (62). By stimulating the cells in the presence of cycloheximide to block intermediate gene expression, we could focus on immediate or early genes. Cycloheximide often superinduces transiently expressed genes. Newly transcribed mRNA transcripts were labeled by including thiol-derivatized uridine during the culture interval. Subsequently, the IL-2–induced thiol-labeled transcripts could be selected by phenyl mercury affinity adsorption. Together, these methods enable a 10,000-fold increase in the efficiency of identifying ligand-induced gene expression.

We have identified 7 novel genes activated by IL-2. The mechanisms responsible for activating their expression and their functional roles in promoting IL-2–initiated events are being investigated. It should be possible to connect the most immediate biochemical reactions activated by the IL-2R to the immediate genes activated and then to the intermediate and late events that occur as a consequence of IL-2R activation.

Biologic and Immunologic Effects

The only normal cells known to express IL-2Rs are antigen-activated T cells, B cells, and NK cells. IL-2 stimulates these target cells to undergo two fundamental changes: proliferation and differentiation (63). Even though much is known about the immediate signaling events activated by the IL-2R within the first few minutes of IL-2R binding, exactly how these reactions dictate the subsequent events that eventually lead to cell cycle progression remain unknown. However, it is clear that there is a threshold of IL-2/IL-2R interactions that must be surpassed before the cell can move beyond the G_1 restriction point and progress to the S phase (33). An estimate of these interactions indicates that at least 5 hours of exposure and 10,000 IL-2/IL-2R interactions are necessary. Because most T cells only express 1,000 high-affinity IL-2Rs, there must be ongoing synthesis of new receptors to replace those that are internalized and degraded during this interval (33).

The progressive degradation of the cell cycle inhibitor p27 is a critical event that occurs during early G_1 downstream from the biochemical signaling pathways (64). The exact connection of the signaling pathways with the protein degradation mechanisms has yet to be determined. However, the stoichiometric relationship between the concentration of p27 and the concentration of the cyclin-cyclin–dependent kinases is thought to determine the G_1 restriction point (65).

After these conditions have been satisfied, an IL-2–stimulated cell progresses completely through G_1 to S, G_2, and M phase. Simultaneously, the cells differentiate, such that their appropriate differentiated effector functions are expressed. Helper T cells stimulated by IL-2 secrete cytokines, especially interferon-γ (IFN-γ) (66), and cytolytic T cells secrete even more IFN-γ than helper T cells, and they also express cytolytic molecules, such as perforin and proteases, that make up the contents of the cytolytic granules (66,67). NK cells stimulated by IL-2 also proliferate and secrete a specific subset of cytokines that preferentially activate monocytes and macrophages, including IFN-γ, granulocyte-macrophage colony-stimulating factor (GM-CSF), and tumor necrosis factor-α (TNF-α). Moreover, IL-2 potentiates the capacity of NK cells to effect cytolysis, presumably by promoting the expression of the cytolytic molecules (68).

The end result of these IL-2 activities is to promote innate host defenses mediated by NK cells and macrophages and antigen-specific acquired immune responses mediated by T cells and B cells. In particular, the stimulation of NK cells sets into motion an intercellular cytokine communication system that favors a strong cell-mediated response. IFN-γ released by IL-2–activated NK cells activates macrophages to release IL-12, which further stimulates NK cells and improves their functional capacity. Complementing these effects, the IL-2 promoted clonal expansion of antigen-selected helper and cytolytic T cells furthers host defenses through their cytokine secretion and cytolytic effector mechanisms.

Given the biologic effects of IL-2, it is not surprising that, when injected, IL-2 produces all of the classic signs of inflammation: rubor, calor, tumor, and dolor (69). Cytokines rather than microbial products can be responsible for promoting the macroscopic and microscopic changes that are classically associated with the inflammatory response to infection, and the injection of IL-2 intradermally produces a classic delayed-type hypersensitivity reaction in the complete absence of antigen or microbial products (69). Moreover, if high doses of IL-2 are injected intravenously, a systemic inflammatory response syndrome (SIRS) results, with all of the classic signs and symptoms of this syndrome, including high fever, rigor, severe myalgia, and vascular collapse (70).

THERAPEUTIC POTENTIAL OF INTERLEUKIN-2

Soon after recombinant IL-2 was made available in sufficient quantities for clinical trials, it was tried as a form of antitumor therapy in severely ill patients with metastatic cancers. Using the principles of cytotoxic chemotherapy of dose intensification, Rosenberg et al. (70) dramatically reported in 1985 that patients with cancers refractory to standard therapy had a 44% response rate to very high IL-2 doses given along with peripheral blood mononuclear cells that had been cultured *ex vivo* for 3 days in IL-2, the so-called lymphokine-activated killer (LAK) cells. IL-2 was given as an intravenous bolus injection every 8 hours at 50 million IU for 5 days. Subsequent studies showed that the LAK cells were unnecessary, and that the response rate was not 44%, but rather 20%, with a 10% complete response in patients with metastatic renal cell carcinoma. With 10 years of follow-up, those fortunate patients who achieved complete remission appear to have been cured (71).

Impressive as these results are, the mechanisms responsible for the complete responses remain unknown. Moreover, the reasons for the lack of a response in 80% of the patients are obscure. It has been maintained by Rosenberg and other oncologists that the therapeutic effect is associated with the toxicities generated by the very high doses. World Health Organization grade III and IV toxic reactions, with high fevers, severe myalgia, and vascular collapse, occur in all patients treated with high-dose IL-2, usually necessitating hospitalization in an intensive care unit (70). Most of these toxicities result from the release of secondary cytokines, primarily from NK cells and monocytes-macrophages. IL-2 promotes the release of IFN-γ, GM-CSF, and TNF-α from NK cells, which promote the release of the proinflammatory cytokines TNF-α, IL-1, and IL-6 from monocytes and macrophages (69). The end result is the SIRS.

Several years ago, in collaboration with Ritz and Caligiuri from the Dana-Farber Cancer Institute, dose-finding, safety-toxicity studies were initiated to establish

TABLE 31-2. *Interleukin-2 equivalents[a]*

Doses		Plasma [IL-2][b]			% of receptors occupied[c]	
IU (×10⁶)	μg	IU/mL	ng/mL	pM	High Affinity	Intermediate Affinity
150.0	10,000	10,714	714	47,000	99	98
15.0	1,000	1,071	71	4,700	99	82
1.5	100	107	7	470	98	32
0.1	10	11	1	47	82	2

[a]Based on a specific activity of 15 million IU/mg IL-2 protein and a molecular size of 15 kD.
[b]Assuming V_D = 14 L of total extracellular fluid.
[c]Based on the formula $\%R_{occ} = [IL\text{-}2]/([IL\text{-}2] + K_d) \times 100$

doses of IL-2 that could be administered continuously with few or no side effects (72). Studying ambulatory cancer patients, doses of IL-2 in the range of 600,000 IU/m²/d were found to be tolerable for 3 months when administered as a 24-hour continuous intravenous infusion. The biologic response to this therapy was readily detectable as a progressive increase in circulating NK cells (73).

In New York, this approach was extended to individuals who had human immunodeficiency virus (HIV) infections but were asymptomatic, and the route of administration was changed to a daily subcutaneous injection (74). A dose of 250,000 IU/m²/d is the maximum dose that can be administered to these patients daily for 6 months with no side effects. This dose is safe, causing no change in circulating HIV RNA, even though there are readily detectable stimulatory effects on the immune system. For example, there are progressive increases in circulating NK cells, eosinophils, and monocytes. There is a progressive, rapid increase in circulating CD4⁺ T cells (28 cells/mm³ per month), and the delayed-type hypersensitivity responses to common environmental antigens double after 6 months of therapy. This immunotherapy approach has been extended to additional patients and combined with the most effective antiviral chemotherapy. Moreover, this approach is being extended to other infectious diseases and is used as an adjuvant for vaccines and as adjuvant therapy in cancer patients to boost immune responses in those with minimal residual tumor burdens after primary therapy.

Others have used IL-2 in HIV-positive individuals in approximately 50-fold higher doses (12 million IU/m²/d) than used in our studies, but for only 5 days every 2 months (75). At these doses, a progressive increase in circulating CD4⁺ T cells has been observed, but just as in the high-dose regimens used in cancer therapy, patients experience severe, grade III and IV toxicities. Moreover, the safety of this approach is questionable, because during and immediately after the IL-2 injections, HIV plasma levels increase by as much as 50-fold.

Comparisons of the IL-2 doses that have been used in various clinical trials, their equivalents, the peak plasma concentrations attained, and the percentage of IL-2Rs

occupied at each of these concentrations are shown in Table 31-2. The expression of IL-2 doses only in international units of biologic activity as defined by the CTLL bioassay can be misleading unless the specific activity is given as international units per milligram of protein. The dose used in cancer therapy of 150 million IU is equivalent to 10 mg, at a specific activity of 15 million IU/mg IL-2 protein. Because IL-2 is a small, globular protein, it freely passes through capillaries and lymphatics, distributing into total extracellular fluid, which in a normal adult of 70 kg is about 14 L. The plasma concentration of IL-2 after distribution of 10 mg into total extracellular fluid is 47 nmol/L. Such a high concentration saturates 99% of high-affinity IL-2Rs expressed by antigen-activated T cells and B cells and 98% of the intermediate-affinity IL-2Rs expressed by most NK cells. There are about 1 billion circulating NK cells, and IL-2 activation of all of these cells simultaneously leads to massive production of secondary cytokines, which produces the SIRS. Based on these calculations, even a 10-fold reduction in dose to 15 million IU (1 mg), the dose used by Kovacs et al. (75) in treating HIV-positive individuals, yields a plasma concentration of 4.7 nmol/L, which can saturate 99% of the high-affinity IL-2Rs, and 82% of the intermediate-affinity IL2 receptors expressed by NK cells. It is understandable why this dose causes such severe grade III and IV toxicities.

From the data shown in Table 31-2, it is apparent that doses in the range of 0.15 to 1.5 million IU (i.e., 10 to 100 μg), would yield plasma IL-2 concentrations sufficient to saturate most high-affinity IL-2Rs but only a small fraction of intermediate affinity IL-2Rs. The end result is a therapeutic agent and regimen that can be used for a broad range of indications when enhancement of the function of the immune system is desirable.

REFERENCES

1. Nowell PC. Phytohemagglutinin: an initiator of mitosis in cultures of normal human leukocytes. *Cancer Res* 1960;20:462–466.
2. Kasakura S, Lowenstein L. A factor stimulating DNA synthesis derived from the medium of leucocyte cultures. *Nature* 1965;208:794–795.
3. Gordon J, MacLean LD. A lymphocyte-stimulating factor produced *in vitro. Nature* 1965;208:795–796.

4. Janis M, Bach FH. Potentiation of *in vitro* lymphocyte reactivity. *Nature* 1970;225:238–239.

5. Powles R, Balchin L, Currie GA, Alexander P. Specific autostimulating factor released by lymphocytes. *Nature* 1971;231:161–164.

6. Hoffman M, Dutton RW. Immune response restoration with macrophage culture supernatants. *Science* 1971;172:1047–1048.

7. Gery I, Gershon RK, Waksman BH. Potentiation of the T-lymphocyte response to mitogens. *J Exp Med* 1972;136:128–142.

8. Andersson LC, Hayry P. Specific priming of mouse thymus-dependent lymphocytes to allogeneic cells *in vitro*. *Eur J Immunol* 1973;3:595–599.

9. MacDonald HR, Engers HD, Cerottini J-C, Brunner KT. Generation of cytotoxic T lymphocytes *in vitro*. *J Exp Med* 1974;140:718–730.

10. Svedmyr E. Long-term maintenance *in vitro* of human T cells by repeated exposure to the same stimulator cells. *Scand J Immunol* 1975;4:421–427.

11. Dennert G, De Rose M. Continuously proliferating T killer cells specific for H-2^b targets: selection and characterization. *J Immunol* 1976;116:1601–1606.

12. Morgan DA, Ruscetti FW, Gallo R. Selective *in vitro* growth of T lymphocytes from normal human bone marrows. *Science* 1976;193:1007–1008.

13. Gillis S, Smith KA. Long-term culture of cytotoxic T-lymphocytes. *Nature* 1977;268:154–156.

14. Baker PE, Gillis S, Smith KA. Monoclonal cytolytic T-cell lines. *J Exp Med* 1979;149:273–278.

15. Gillis S, Ferm MM, Ou W, Smith KA. T-cell growth factor: parameters of production and a quantitative microassay for activity. *J Immunol* 1978;120:2027–2032.

16. Fredrickson TN, Smith KA, Cornell CJ, Jasmin C, McIntyre OR. The interaction of erythropoietin with fetal liver cells. I. Measurement of proliferation by tritiated thymidine incorporation. *Exp Hem* 1977;5:254–265.

17. Baker PE, Gillis S, Smith KA. The effect of T-cell growth factor on the generation of cytolytic T-cells. *J Immunol* 1978;121:2168–2173.

18. Robb RJ, Smith KA. Heterogeneity of human T-cell growth factor due to glycosylation. *Mol Immunol* 1981;18:1087–1094.

19. Smith KA, Favata MF, Oroszlan S. Production and characterization of monoclonal antibodies to human interleukin-2: strategy and tactics. *J Immunol* 1983;131:1808–1815.

20. Taniguchi T, Matsui H, Fujita T, et al. Structure and expression of a cloned cDNA for human interleukin 2. *Nature* 1983;302:305–310.

21. Smith KA, Gillis S, Baker PE, McKenzie D, Ruscetti FW. T-cell growth factor-mediated T-cell proliferation. *Ann NY Acad Sci* 1979;332:423–432.

22. Robb RJ, Munck A, Smith KA. T-cell growth factor receptors: quantitation, specificity and biological relevance. *J Exp Med* 1981;154:1455–1474.

23. Bazan JF. Unraveling the structure of IL-2. *Science* 1992;257:410–413.

24. Leonard WJ, Depper JM, Crabtree GR, et al. Molecular cloning and expression of cDNAs for the human interleukin-2 receptor. *Nature* 1984;311:626–631.

25. Nikaido T, Shimizu A, Ishida N, et al. Molecular cloning of cDNA encoding human interleukin-2 receptor. *Nature* 1984;311:631–635.

26. Hatakeyama M, Tsudo M, Minamoto S, et al. Interleukin-2 receptor chain gene: generation of three receptor forms by cloned human α and β chain cDNAs. *Science* 1989;244:551–556.

27. Takeshita T, Asao H, Ohtani K, et al. Cloning of the chain of the human IL-2 receptor. *Science* 1992;257:379–382.

28. Wang H, Smith KA. The interleukin 2 receptor: functional consequences of its bimolecular structure. *J Exp Med* 1987;166:1055–1069.

29. Smith KA. The interleukin 2 receptor. In: Palade GE, ed. *Annual review of cell biology*. California: Annual Reviews, 1989:397–425.

30. Caligiuri MA, Zmuidzinas A, Manley TJ, Levin H, Smith KA, Ritz J. Functional consequences of IL-2 receptor expression on resting human lymphocytes: identification of a novel NK cell subset with high affinity receptors. *J Exp Med* 1990;171:1509–1526.

31. Nakamura Y, Russell SM, Mess SA, et al. Heterodimerization of the IL-2 receptor β- and γ-chain cytoplasmic domains is required for signaling. *Nature* 1994;369:330–333.

32. Nelson BH, Lord JD, Greenberg PD. Cytoplasmic domains of the interleukin-2 receptor β- and γ-chains mediate the signal for T-cell proliferation. *Nature* 1994;369:333–336.

33. Smith KA. Cell growth signal transduction is quantal. *Ann N Y Acad Sci* 1995;766:263–271.

34. Kumaki S, Asao H, Takeshita T, et al. Cell type-specific tyrosine phosphorylation of IL-2 receptor chain in response to IL-2. *FEBS Lett* 1992;310:22–26.

35. Schindler C, Darnell JE Jr. Transcriptional responses to polypeptide ligands: the JAK-STAT pathway. *Annu Rev Biochem* 1995;64:621–651.

36. Hatakeyama M, Kono T, Kobayashi N, et al. Interaction of the IL-2 receptor with the src-family kinase p56^lck: identification of novel intermolecular association. *Science* 1991;252:1523–1528.

37. Johnston JA, Kawamura M, Kirken RA, et al. Phosphorylation and activation of the Jak-3 Janus kinase in response to interleukin-2. *Nature* 1994;370:151–153.

38. Witthuhn BA, Silvennoinen O, Miura O, et al. Involvement of the Jak-3 Janus kinase in signaling by interleukins 2 and 4 in lymphoid and myeloid cells. *Nature* 1994;370:153–157.

39. Friedmann MC, Migone T, Rusell SM, Leonard WJ. Different interleukin 2 receptor β-chain tyrosines couple to at least two signaling pathways and synergistically mediate interleukin 2–induced proliferation. *Proc Natl Acad Sci USA* 1996;93:2077–2082.

40. Ravichandran KS, Burakoff SJ. The adapter protein Shc interacts with the interleukin-2 (IL-2) receptor upon IL-2 stimulation. *J Biol Chem* 1994;269:1599–1602.

41. Ravichandran KS, Igras V, Shoelson SE, Fesik SW, Burakoff SJ. Evidence for a role for the phosphotyrosine-binding domain of Shc in interleukin 2 signaling. *Proc Natl Acad Sci USA* 1996;93:5275–5280.

42. Satoh T, Nakafuku M, Miyajima A, Kaziro Y. Involvement of ras p21 protein in signal-transduction pathways from interleukin 2, interleukin 3, and granulocyte/macrophage colony-stimulating factor, but not from interleukin 4. *Proc Natl Acad Sci USA* 1991;88:3314–3318.

43. Graves JD, Downward J, Izquierdo-Pastor M, Rayter S, Warne PH, Cantrell DA. The growth factor IL-2 activates p21 ras proteins in normal human T lymphocytes. *J Immunol* 1992;148:2417–2422.

44. Turner B, Rapp U, App H, Greene M, Dobashi K, Reed J. Interleukin 2 induces tyrosine phosphorylation and activation of p72-74 Raf-1 kinase in a T-cell line. *Proc Natl Acad Sci USA* 1991;88:1227–1231.

45. Zmuidzinas A, Mamon H, Roberts TM, Smith KA. Interleukin-2–triggered Raf-1 expression, phosphorylation, and associated kinase activity increase through G$_1$ and S in CD3-stimulated primary human T cells. *Mol Cell Biol* 1991;11:2794–2803.

46. Truitt KE, Millis GB, Turck CW, Imboden JB. SH2-dependent association of phosphatidylinositol 3′-kinase 85-kDa regulatory subunit with the interleukin-2 receptor beta chain. *J Biol Chem* 1994;269:5937–5943.

47. Monfar M, Lemon K, Grammar TC, et al. Activation of pp70/85 S6 kinases in interleukin-2–responsive lymphoid cells is mediated by phosphatidylinositol 3-kinase and inhibited by cyclic AMP. *Mol Cell Biol* 1995;15:326–337.

48. Ahmed NN, Grimes HL, Bellacosa A, Chan TO, Tsichlis PN. Transduction of interleukin-2 antiapoptotic and proliferative signals via Akt protein kinase. *Proc Natl Acad Sci USA* 1997;94:3627–3632.

49. Stokoe D, Stephens LR, Copeland T, et al. Dual role of phosphatidylinositol-3,4,5-trisphosphate in the activation of protein kinase B. *Science* 1997;277:567–570.

50. Hou J, Schindler U, Henzel WJ, Wong SC, McKnight SL. Identification and purification of human STAT proteins activated in response to interleukin-2. *Immunity* 1995;2:321–329.

51. Lin J, Migone T, Tsang M, et al. The role of shared receptor motifs and common STAT proteins in the generation of cytokine pleiotropy and redundancy by IL-2, IL-4, IL-7, IL-13, and IL-15. *Immunity* 1995;2:331–339.

52. Wen Z, Zhong Z, Darnell JE Jr. Maximal activation of transcription by STAT1 and STAT3 requires both tyrosine and serine phosphorylation. *Cell* 1995;82:241–250.

53. Beadling C, Ng J, Babbage JW, Cantrell DA. Interleukin-2 activation of STAT5 requires the convergent action of tyrosine kinases and a serine/threonine kinase pathway distinct from the Raf1/ERK2 MAP kinase pathway. *Embo J* 1996;15:1902–1913.

54. Stern JB, Smith KA. Interleukin-2 induction of T-cell G$_1$ progression and c-*myb* expression. *Science* 1986;233:203–206.

55. Reed JC, Alpers JD, Scherle PA, Hoover RG, Nowell PC, Prystowsky MB. Proto-oncogene expression in cloned T lymphocytes: mitogens and growth factors induce different patterns of expression. *Oncogene* 1987;1:223–228.

56. Dautry F, Weil D, Yu J, Dautry-Varsat A. Regulation of pim and myb mRNA accumulation by interleukin 2 and interleukin 3 in murine hematopoietic cell lines. *J Biol Chem* 1988;263:17615–17620.

57. Reed JC, Tsujimoto Y, Alphers JD, Croce CM, Nowell PC. Regulation of bcl-2 proto-oncogene expression during normal human lymphocyte proliferation. *Science* 1987;236:1295–1299.

58. Turner JM. IL-2–dependent induction of G_1 cyclins in primary T cells is not blocked by rapamycin or cyclosporin A. *Int Immunol* 1993;5: 1199–1209.

59. Shipman-Appasamy P, Cohen KS, Prystowsky MB. Interleukin 2–induced expression of proliferating cell nuclear antigen is regulated by transcriptional and post-transcriptional mechanisms. *J Biol Chem* 1990;265:19180–19184.

60. Furukawa Y, Piwnica-Worms H, Ernst TJ, Kanakura Y, Griffen JD. *Cdc2* gene expression at the G_1 to S transition in human T lymphocytes. *Science* 1990;250:805–808.

61. Neckers LM, Cossman J. Transferrin receptor induction in mitogen-stimulated human T lymphocytes is required for DNA synthesis and cell division and is regulated by interleukin 2. *Proc Natl Acad Sci USA* 1983;80:3494–3498.

62. Beadling C, Johnson KW, Smith KA. Isolation of interleukin-2–stimulated immediate-early genes. *Proc Natl Acad Sci USA* 1993;90:2719–2723.

63. Smith KA. Interleukin 2: inception, impact, and implications. *Science* 1988;240:1169–1176.

64. Nourse J, Firpo E, Flanagan WM, et al. Interleukin-2–mediated elimination of the p27^{Kip1} cyclin-dependent kinase inhibitor prevented by rapamycin. *Nature* 1994;372:570–573.

65. Sherr CJ. Mammalian G_1 cyclins. *Cell* 1993;73:1059–1065.

66. Weil D, Dautry F. Induction of tumor necrosis factor-α and -β and interferon-γ mRNA by interleukin 2 in murine lymphocytic cell lines. *Oncol Res* 1988;3:409–414.

67. Liu CC, Granelli-Piperno A, Trapani JA, Young JD. Perforin and serine esterase gene expression in stimulated human T cells. Kinetics, mitogen requirements, and effects of cyclosporin A. *J Exp Med* 1989;170: 2105–2118.

68. Manyak CL, Norton GP, Lobe CG, et al. IL-2 induces expression of serine protease enzymes and genes in natural killer and nonspecific T killer cells. *J Immunol* 1989;142:3707–3713.

69. Smith KA. Lowest dose interleukin 2 immunotherapy. *Blood* 1993;18: 1414–1423.

70. Rosenberg SA, Lotze MT, Muul LM, et al. Observations on the systemic administration of autologous lymphokine-activated killer cells and recombinant interleukin-2 to patients with metastatic cancer. *N Engl J Med* 1985;313:1485–1492.

71. Rosenberg SA. Keynote address: Perspectives on the use of interleukin 2 in cancer treatment. *The Cancer Journal* 1997;3SI;82–86.

72. Caligiuri MA, Murray C, Soiffer RJ, et al. Extended continuous infusion low-dose recombinant interleukin-2 in advanced cancer: prolonged immunomodulation without significant toxicity. *J Clin Oncol* 1991;9:2110–2119.

73. Caligiuri MA, Murray C, Robertson MJ, et al. Selective modulation of human natural killer cells *in vivo* following prolonged infusion of low-dose recombinant interleukin 2. *J Clin Invest* 1993;91:123–132.

74. Jacobson EL, Pilaro F, Smith KA. Rational interleukin 2 therapy for HIV$^+$ individuals: daily low doses enhance immune function without toxicity. *Proc Natl Acad Sci USA* 1996;93:10405–10410.

75. Kovacs JA, Vogel S, Albert JM, et al. Controlled trial of interleukin-2 infusions in patients infected with the human immunodeficiency virus. *N Engl J Med* 1996;335:1350–1356.

Inflammation: Basic Principles and Clinical Correlates,
3rd ed., edited by John I. Gallin and Ralph Snyderman.
Lippincott Williams & Wilkins, Philadelphia © 1999.

CHAPTER 32

Tumor Necrosis Factor, Interleukin-6, Macrophage Migration Inhibitory Factor, and Macrophage Inflammatory Protein-1 in Inflammation

Haichao Wang and Kevin J. Tracey

Excessive or dysregulated inflammation contributes to the pathogenesis of infection, trauma, and autoimmune diseases. Monocyte-macrophages play an important role in the host recognition of microbial products, which trigger the release of endogenous proinflammatory mediators in this process. Prominent among the proinflammatory mediators released by these cells are tumor necrosis factor (TNF), interleukin-6 (IL-6), macrophage inflammatory protein-1 (MIP-1), and macrophage migration inhibitory factor (MIF). In this chapter, we review the spectrum of inflammatory responses, beneficial and injurious, mediated by these factors, and discuss their participation in the host response to infection and tissue invasion (Fig. 32-1). These cytokines link activities between a variety of cells and tissues, providing common threads between physiologic and pathologic states. TNF, which is among the very first cytokines produced by various cells, induces the release of many other cytokines including IL-6, MIF (1,2), and MIP-1 (3). Once released, MIF, MIP-1, and other components of the cytokine cascade may restimulate the production of TNF, thereby amplifying the inflammatory response to infection or tissue invasion.

TUMOR NECROSIS FACTOR

TNF, one of the earliest cytokines produced by activated macrophage-monocytes, occupies a pivotal role in

H. Wang and K. J. Tracey: Departments of Emergency Medicine and Surgery, North Shore University Hospital–New York University School of Medicine and The Picower Institute for Medical Research, Manhasset, New York 11030.

the pathogenesis of inflammation, septic shock, and tissue injury (4–8). Although TNF shares with other cytokines (e.g., interleukin-6 [IL-6]) a pleiotropic range of beneficial and injurious effects, it is the only cytokine identified capable of triggering the complete physiologic, humoral, and tissue injury responses that define septic shock syndrome.

Regulation of TNF Expression

The TNF gene *(TNF)* is located on the short arm of chromosome 6 and encodes a 233–amino acid precursor (pro-TNF). This 26-kd precursor is anchored to the cytoplasmic membrane and subsequently cleaved into a 17-kd mature, soluble TNF. Three 17-kd, soluble TNFs associate as a homotrimer that is responsible for the major bioactivity, although the 26-kd transmembrane pro-TNF can also interact with TNF receptors (9). TNF responses in target cells are mediated by receptor aggregation. To mediate cytotoxicity through cell-cell interactions (10, 11), the mature TNF domains of pro-TNF are arranged as a compact, bell-shaped trimer, similar to the arrangement in the mature TNF crystal (12).

TNF synthesis can be stimulated in various cell types by a wide range of stimuli. Although TNF is produced predominantly in monocyte-macrophages, it is also made by numerous other cells (Table 32-1). The principal source of serum TNF during endotoxemia is the liver (13). Exogenous and endogenous factors produced by bacteria, viruses, parasites, and tumors are capable of inducing cells to produce TNF (see Table 32-1). Under

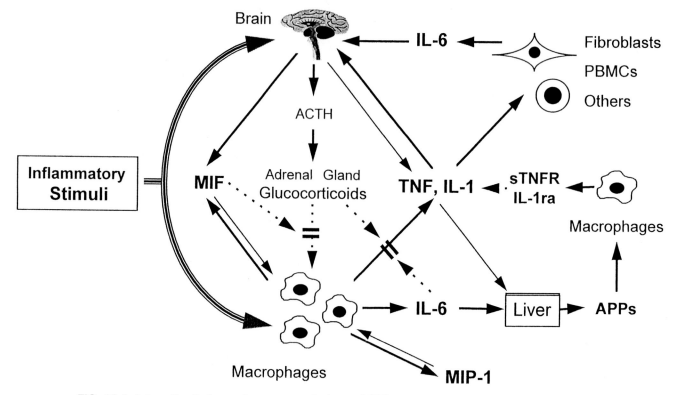

FIG. 32-1. Interaction between tumor necrosis factor (TNF), macrophage migration inhibitory factor (MIF), interleukin-6 (IL-6), macrophage inflammatory protein-1 (MIP-1), and glucocorticoid hormone. TNF and IL-6 from activated macrophages or produced locally in brain stimulate the release of corticotropin (ACTH) from the pituitary gland and subsequently stimulate the release of glucocorticoids from the adrenal gland. Glucocorticoids and IL-6 suppress TNF and IL-1 synthesis. The production of IL-6 is further amplified by TNF and IL-1. IL-6 from activated macrophages, in combination with IL-1 and TNF, induces hepatic acute phase protein (APP) synthesis, and in combination with IL-6, APP induces interleukin-1 receptor agonist (IL-1Ra) synthesis and the shedding of soluble TNF receptors (sTNFRs). The release of MIF from macrophages is stimulated by low concentrations of glucocorticoids (10 to 16 mol/L). MIF from activated macrophages or the pituitary gland overrides the suppressive effect of glucocorticoids on macrophages. MIP-1 from activated macrophages induces the release of several inflammatory cytokines such as TNF, IL-1, and IL-6. PBMC, peripheral blood mononuclear cells.

normal conditions, the synthesis of TNF is tightly controlled to ensure the production of vanishingly small amounts of TNF in quiescent cells. On stimulation by a variety of stimuli, the transcription and translation of the TNF gene are rapidly upregulated, enabling the release of large quantities of soluble TNF. Regulation of TNF expression is controlled by many factors at multiple levels, and cell activation *in vivo* ultimately results in a characteristic rise of serum TNF within 90 minutes of stimulation, followed by an abrupt fall to baseline (undetectable) levels within 4 hours.

Several regulatory sequences are found upstream of the TNF gene, including NF-κB sites, NF-AT–binding sites (14), "Y" box, cAMP-responsive elements for ATF-2/JUN (15), SP-1 sites (16), AP-1 and AP-2 sites for FOS/JUN (17), and EGR-1 binding sites (18). These regulatory sequences can bind to various transcriptional factors such as NF-κB, FOS/JUN, and NFAT. For instance, TNF induction in lipopolysaccharide (LPS)–activated macrophages is associated with activation of the tran-

scription factor NF-κB. Increases of TNF mRNA levels are observed within 15 to 30 minutes, even in the absence of *de novo* protein synthesis, indicating that factors necessary for induction of TNF mRNA expression preexist in unstimulated normal cells. These transcriptional mechanisms enable the rapid mobilization of TNF synthesis during the early response to host invasion.

The expression of TNF is further regulated at the translational level, which enforces efficient regulation of TNF production during an acute response, and protects the host from the harmful effects of uncontrolled overproduction. A key element for translational regulation of TNF has been identified in the 3′ untranslated region (UTR) of TNF mRNA (19). It is an AU-rich sequence (UUAUUUAU), which can decrease the stability of TNF mRNA (20,21), and it may also inhibit the process of translation. It has been suggested that translational regulation by the AU-rich sequence occurs through a physical interaction with the poly (A) tail to prevent polysome formation (22). The minimal motif that confers mRNA

TABLE 32-1. *Sources and roles of tumor necrosis factor during inflammation*

Cell sources	Macrophages, monocytes, astrocytes, B cells, basophils, cardiac myocytes, eosinophils, fibroblasts, glial cells, granulosa cells, keratinocytes, mast cells, neurons, neutrophils, NK cells, T cells, osteoblasts, retinal pigment epithelial cells, smooth muscle cells, spermatogenic cells, tumor cells
Stimuli	Bacterial endotoxin (LPS), antibodies to LFA-3, calcium ionophores, C5a, CD44, CD45, enterotoxin, GM-CSF, hypoxia, IL-1, irradiation, leukotrienes, mellitin, MIP-1α, mycobacterial lipoarabinomannan, nitric oxide, oxygen radicals, parasites, phorbol esters, synthetic lipid A, TNF, toxic shock toxin-1, viruses
Biologic roles	
Central nervous system	Fever
	Anorexia
	Altered pituitary hormone secretion
Inflammation	Activation of cell cytotoxicity
	Enhanced NK cell function
	Mediation of IL-2 tumor toxicity
	Stimulation of neutrophil respiratory burst activation of macrophages
Cardiovascular	Shock
	Capillary leakage syndrome
	Tissue injury

GM-CSF, granulocyte-macrophage colony-stimulating factor; IFN, interferon; IL, interleukin; LFA-3, lymphocyte function antigen-3; LPS, lipopolysaccharide; MIP, macrophage inflammatory protein; NK, natural killer; TNF, tumor necrosis factor.

instability is the UUAUUUAUU sequence (23,24), and the presence of a single octanucleotide UUAUUUAU in the 3′UTR is sufficient to significantly inhibit translation. A complete understanding of these mechanisms is lacking, because the AU-rich sequence has no significant effect on TNF mRNA stability in RAW 264.7 macrophages (25,26). Moreover, evidence suggests a possible regulatory role for the p38 mitogen-activated protein (MAP) kinase family in the regulation of TNF translation (27), but it remains unclear whether the effects of p38 MAP kinase on TNF translation depend on direct interaction with the AU-rich sequence of TNF mRNA.

Newly synthesized, 233–amino acid pro-TNF is processed by myristylation (28), which targets its insertion into the plasma membrane through the N-terminal hydrophobic domain. Pro-TNF possesses activity in the standard cell cytotoxicity bioassay and may function as a nondiffusible mediator of cell-cell interaction in B-cell activation by T cells (29–31). In macrophage and other cells that release TNF, pro-TNF is processed by proteolytic cleavage to a bioactive 157–amino acid TNF peptide. The TNF-converting enzyme (TCE) has been identified as a matrix metalloproteinase (MMP)–like enzyme (32,33). Metalloproteinase inhibitors that inhibit TCE effectively block the release of soluble TNF in animal models of endotoxemia (34).

Inhibition of TNF Synthesis

The relative overproduction of TNF has been implicated in the pathogenesis of numerous diseases and heightened interest in the development of therapeutic strategies to inhibit TNF synthesis (35,36). Several potential targets have been identified based on an understanding of each level of TNF synthesis (37–39). For instance, glucocorticoids and pentoxifylline inhibit the activation of NF-κB to suppress TNF expression at the transcriptional level (Table 32-2). Two separate strategies have exploited the role of p38 MAP kinase. In one approach, a class of cytokine synthesis inhibitors called cytokine-suppressing antiinflammatory drugs (40) act to directly inhibit the activity of p38 MAP kinase. Another approach uses a newly identified class of multivalent guanylhydrazones that inhibit the upstream phosphorylation of p38 MAP kinase, thereby preventing its activation. These approaches exert their major suppressive effects on TNF at the translational level (41–44) (see Table 32-2). Strategies to directly inhibit TNF activity with antibodies or soluble TNF receptors (sTNFRs) are effective in animal models (45) (see Table 32-2) and are being used in clinical trials (46–49).

TABLE 32-2. *Strategies for preventing tumor necrosis factor toxicity*

Suppression of TNF synthesis	
Transcriptional level (NF-κB)	Glucocorticoids
	Pentoxifyline
Translational level (p38 MAP kinase)	CSAIDs
	CNI-1493
	Spermine
	Thalidomide
Posttranslational level (TACE)	BB-94
Neutralization of TNF activity	Antibodies
	Soluble TNF receptor
	Soluble TNF receptor fusion protein

CSAIDs, cytokine-suppressing antiinflammatory drugs; MAP, mitogen-activated protein; NF-κB, nuclear transcription factor κB; TNF, tumor necrosis factor.

TNF Receptors

The activities of TNF are mediated through at least two types of membrane-associated receptors called type I (TNFR1, p55) and type II (TNFR2, p75) receptors (Table 32-3). Each of the TNF receptors is present on virtually all cell types, except for red blood cells (50). TNFR1 is responsible for the major TNF bioactivity, including cytotoxicity, cytostasis, and activation of neutrophils and endothelial cells. TNFR2 alone is not sufficient to stimulate these functions and appears to be mainly confined to cells of the immune system, where it contributes to stimulation of proliferation of T and B cells (51), induction of NF-κB, and cytotoxicity (52). One important role of TNFR2 may be to potentiate the effects of TNFR1, because TNF-TNFR2 complexes rapidly disassociate, which enables TNF to be passed to TNFR1.

TNFR1 has at least three functional intracellular domains, the C-terminal death domain, the neutral sphingomyelinase (N-SMase)–activating domain (NSD), and the acidic sphingomyelinase (A-SMase)–activating domain (ASD). The death domain of TNFR1 is associated with activation of phosphatidylcholine-phospholipase e (PC-PLC) (53), which transmits a signal to the apoptosis pathway associated with interleukin-1β–converting enzyme and NF-κB. The N-SMase mediates a number of cellular TNF responses, including cell growth and inflammation through MAP kinase (ERK) and phospholipase A₂, whereas A-SMase can activate NF-κB, a factor involved in induction (54) or inhibition of apopto-

sis (55). TNFR2, however, lacks the intracellular death domain and may inhibit apoptosis through downregulation of an anti-apoptotic protein, BCL-XL (56).

Both types of TNF receptors can be proteolytically processed, can be released from the membrane, and can appear in the extracellular space and circulation. These soluble receptors (sTNFRs) bind to TNF and function as TNF-binding proteins (TNFBPs) that neutralize TNF activity (57). The proteases responsible for receptor release are still unknown, but metalloprotease inhibitors have been observed to block the shedding of the two TNFRs (58,59). The TNFBPs function as inflammatory regulators that are released in response to a number of stimuli that activate immune responses, including phorbol myristate acetate, LPS, and cytokines such as TNF and IL-1. Increased levels of sTNFRs are found in clinical samples from patients with rheumatoid arthritis, sepsis, chronic infection, and other illnesses (60–63). The biologic role of sTNFRs may be dose dependent, because higher concentrations reduce the bioactivity of TNF by competing for TNF binding with cell-associated receptors, whereas lower concentrations can stabilize the trimeric structure of TNF, thereby slowing spontaneous decay of its bioactivity (63). Low amounts of sTNFRs may augment the long-term effects of TNF by providing a reservoir of bioactive TNF that is slowly released.

TNF Role in Infection

After intravenous endotoxemia, serum TNF reaches a peak level in 90 to 120 minutes, subsequently declines, and becomes undetectable within 4 to 6 hours. TNF disappears from the serum by binding to TNF receptors and soluble TNF-binding proteins, which are then cleared through the kidney. Interpretation of the serum TNF concentration during infection may be confounded by its stereotypical pattern of transient appearance and by the contemporaneous release of sTNFRs that remove bioactivity but may not block detection in immunoassays. Moreover, TNF may be produced and act locally in vital tissues without reaching the bloodstream (64). Compartmentalized production of TNF in the central nervous system (CNS) has been studied in meningitis and multiple sclerosis, and serum levels usually do not correlate with the levels in cerebrospinal fluid. The overproduction of TNF in this central body compartment has been implicated in the development of tissue necrosis in meningitis, anorexia, inflammation, and demyelination in multiple sclerosis (7,8).

The role of TNF has been exhaustively studied in septic shock, which is characterized by the development of hypotension, dehydration, myocardial suppression, diffuse capillary leakage, hemorrhagic necrosis of tissues, and multiple organ failure after infections. At least three lines of evidence indicate that TNF plays a critical role in septic shock. First, TNF is acutely overproduced system-

TABLE 32-3. *Receptors for tumor necrosis factor, interleukin-1, macrophage inflammatory protein, and macrophage migration inhibitory protein*

TNF receptors	
Type I (TNFR1, or P55)	C-terminal death domain
	N-SMase-activating domain (NSD)
	A-SMase-activating domain (ASD)
Type II (TNF R2, or P75)	Lacking C-terminal death domain
IL-6 receptor complex	Ligand-binding subunit (IL-6R) (60 kd)
	Lacking tyrosine kinase activity, relying on gp130 subunit to transmit the signal
MIF receptor	Not identified
MIP-1 receptors	CCR1 (for MIP-1α, RANTES, MCP-3)
	CCR4 (for MIP-1α, RANTES, MCP-1)
	CCR5 (for RANTES, MIP-1α, MIP-1β)

CCR, CC chemokine receptors; IL, interleukin; MIF, macrophage migration inhibitory protein; MIP, macrophage inflammatory protein; RANTES, regulated on activation, normally T-cell expressed and secreted; TNF, tumor necrosis factor.

ically during overwhelming sepsis, and persistent increases are associated with mortality and multiple organ failure (65). Second, direct injection of recombinant TNF causes hypotension, metabolic acidosis, hemoconcentration, and death, a pattern indistinguishable from the cardiovascular response in endotoxin-induced septic shock (4). Third, neutralization of TNF using antibodies prevents septic shock syndrome during lethal bacteremia in baboons (8). Initial transgenic mouse models supported a critical role for TNF in mediating lethal endotoxemia, because TNF receptor knock-out (TNFRp55-/-) mice are protected against lethal dosages of LPS (66). Moreover, these animals exhibited increased sensitivity to infection with *Listeria monocytogenes,* indicating that the effects of TNF on intracellular infection are predominantly beneficial.

Antibodies to TNF prevent the activation of a cytokine cascade in lethal bacteremia (8). The availability of TNF knock-out (TNF–/–) mice has enabled this role to be studied during lethal endotoxemia. These studies revealed delayed activation of the cytokine cascade during lethal endotoxemia and delayed lethality (67,68). Although interpretation of these transgenic studies is confounded by the absence of TNF during development, results do suggest that other complementary death mechanisms can be activated in the absence of TNF. These studies therefore have confirmed a role for TNF as a mediator of early lethality and established that, in the absence of the earlier cytokine response, other mediators take over. Translation of these mechanisms into clinical use for septic shock syndrome has been hampered by the difficulties and expense of large-scale trials with critically ill patients with sepsis, but Abraham et al. (69) observed a trend toward mortality reduction in patients with early septic shock during a phase II study of p55-IgG. The role of the compensatory cytokine response in human sepsis is unknown.

TNF Role in the Central Nervous System

TNF can be produced by various cells in the CNS, including microglia, astrocytes, and neurons (70). In the normal brain, TNF expression is low and localized to specific neuron cell population in the hypothalamus (71,72). TNF expression is dramatically increased after pathologic stimuli such as injury, ischemia, or infection (73). Elevated levels of TNF are implicated in the pathogenesis of several human CNS disorders, notably bacterial meningitis (74,75), Alzheimer's disease (76), and multiple sclerosis (77). The inflammatory effects of TNF are pivotal to the pathogenesis of cerebral inflammation and edema during meningitis. During cerebral ischemia, the expression of TNF and its receptors (TNFRs) are significantly upregulated within the ischemic cortex (73). The cells that are abundantly stained by anti-TNF antibodies include neurons, astrocytes, microglia, and infiltrating polymorphonuclear neutrophils (PMNs) (73,78).

Two contrasting roles, beneficial or injurious, have been proposed for TNF in the pathogenesis of cerebral ischemia. The beneficial role of TNF in cerebral ischemia is supported by observations that administration of neutralizing anti-TNF antibodies into the brain cortex significantly reduced ischemic brain damage (79,80). Moreover, systemic administration of a tetravalent guanylhydrazone compound, CNI-1493, effectively inhibited endogenous brain TNF synthesis and conferred significant protection against the development of cerebral infarction (79).

TNF Genetics and Disease Risk

Ultimately, the variability of TNF production between individuals appears to be critical in determining susceptibility to diseases such as multiple sclerosis, rheumatoid arthritis, and infections with parasites, bacteria, or viruses (81). The TNF locus is located in the class II region of the major histocompatibility complex (MHC) on the short arm of human chromosome 6, where there is a high degree of gene polymorphism. At least five polymorphisms described in the TNF locus have been linked to variable TNF production rates between individuals. For instance, *TNF2* homozygosity is associated with high TNF levels in children who are at increased risk for cerebral malaria (81). The *LTA2* allele has also been associated with higher levels of TNF production in patients with lower survival with multiple organ failure secondary to severe sepsis (82,83). As the understanding of allelic regulatory differences improves, it should be possible to more effectively translate our basic research advances in TNF mechanisms into clinically useful methods to prevent the sequelae of excessive TNF and to improve the potential benefits of its controlled local production, as in cancer.

INTERLEUKIN-6

IL-6 is a pleiotropic cytokine that occupies an important role in regulating the immune response. It plays a prominent role in the coordinated systemic host defense response to injury by regulating inflammatory responses and hepatic acute phase protein synthesis.

Regulation of Expression

IL-6 was discovered and characterized independently in several laboratories. Weissenbach et al. (84) identified IL-6 during an effort to clone human fibroblast interferon-β (IFN-β). Because this new mRNA did not crosshybridize with IFN-β mRNA, the resultant protein was called IFN-β_2. Content et al. (85) cloned the same species from fibroblasts and designated it 26-kd protein. In 1986, the purification of a human B-cell differentiation factor, called B-cell stimulatory factor-2 (BSF-2) was reported by Hirano et al. (86), which was subsequently pointed out by Billiau (87) to be identical to IFN-β_2 and the 26-kd protein. Gauldie et al. (88) discovered a cytokine regulating the hepatic acute phase protein (APP) response, called hepatocyte-stimulating factor, that was identical to IFN-β_2 (88).

The human IL-6 gene, located on human chromosome 7p15-21, is organized within five exons spanning approximately 5 kb of genomic sequence (89). The IL-6 cDNA contains a single, large open-reading frame encoding a protein of 184 amino acids plus a 28–amino acid signal sequence (90). Human IL-6 protein has two potential N-glycosylation sites (at amino acids 45 and 144) and is variably glycosylated (91). As a result, IL-6 is secreted by mammalian cells as a heterogeneous set of proteins with molecular masses ranging from 19 to 30 kd (92). Nonglycosylated bacteria-derived recombinant IL-6 is biologically active, and there are no apparent qualitative differences in biologic activity from the glycosylated forms.

IL-6 mRNA is constitutively expressed at low levels in numerous cell types, including peripheral blood leukocytes, spleen, liver, kidney, and intestine of healthy individuals. Its expression is induced during infection, trauma, or immunologic challenge in nearly every human tissue and cell type (93–95) (Table 32-4). Among bone marrow–derived cells, mononuclear phagocytes are an important source of IL-6, but lymphocytes, neutrophils, eosinophils, and mast cells can also be induced to express this cytokine (96). The expression of IL-6 is activated by numerous factors, including other cytokines, growth factors, hormones, neuropeptides, leukotrienes, and microbial and viral products (see Table 32-4). *In vivo*, systemic administration of TNF, IL-1, or LPS causes rapid induction of circulating IL-6. The stimulation of IL-6 synthesis is regulated in part by a 23-bp multiple response element on the promoter of IL-6 gene (97) that contains binding sites for transcription factors such as NF-IL-6 and NF-κB. Transcription factor NF-IL-6 is also induced transcriptionally by LPS, IL-1, and IL-6 (98). In contrast, IL-6 expression can be downregulated by glucocorticoids (99,100) and certain cytokines (101–103) (see Table 32-4).

Receptors

The pleiotropic effects of IL-6 are mediated through the interaction of IL-6 with its receptor complex on the target cells. The IL-6 receptor (IL-6R) complex is composed of a 60-kd, ligand-binding subunit (IL-6R) and a 130-kd, signal-transducing subunit (gp130) (see Table 32-3). The gp130 molecule is ubiquitously expressed and is the principal signal-transducing component of receptors for other cytokines such as IL-6 and IL-11 (104,105). The IL-6R contains 468 amino acids, consisting of a 19–amino acid signal peptide and two functional domains, one belonging to the immunoglobulin superfamily and the other belonging to the cytokine receptor family (106). Although the significance of the immunoglobulin-like domain is unclear, the cytokine receptor-like domain contains specific binding sites for IL-6. Two types of IL-6R complex have been characterized based on their affinity to IL-6. The high-affinity human IL-6R complex consists of two molecules each of IL-6, IL-6R, and gp130 (β-subunit) (107), which interact

---

TABLE 32-4. *Sources and roles of interleukin-6 during inflammation*

Cell sources	Monocytes, macrophages, amnion, astrocytes, B cells, bone marrow stromal cells, chondrocytes, endothelial cells, eosinophils, epithelial cells, fibroblasts, glial cells, hepatoma cells, keratinocytes, Kupffer cells, mast cells, mesangial cells, neutrophils, osteoblasts, osteoclasts, smooth muscle cells, synoviovytes, T cells
Stimuli	IL-1, TNF, bacterial endotoxin (LPS), calcium ionophore A23187, cAMP, diacylglycerols, GM-CSF, IFN, leukotrienes, platelet-activating factor, platelet-derived growth factor, reactive oxygen metabolites, TGF-β, viruses
Factors suppressing IL-6 expression	Glucocorticoids
	Retinoic acid
	Cytokines (IL-4, IL-10, IL-13)
	Nitric oxide
	Prostaglandin E_2
Biologic roles	
Immune response	B-cell maturation/differentiation
	T-cell/thymocyte activation
Acute-phase response	Stimulates acute-phase protein synthesis
Hematopoiesis	Hemopoietic stem cell growth
	Granulocyte-macrophage colony-stimulating factor induction
Nervous system	Induces fever through PGE_2-dependent mechanism
	Alters release of pituitary hormone (corticotropin)

GM-CSF, granulocyte-macrophage colony-stimulating factor; IFN, interferon; IL, interleukin; LPS, lipopolysaccharide; PGE_2, prostaglandin E_2; TGF, transforming growth factor; TNF, tumor necrosis factor.

to mediate intracellular signaling. The low-affinity receptor complex consists of one molecule each of IL-6 and IL-6R. Because the intracellular domain of IL-6R lacks tyrosine kinase activity, the IL-6/IL-6R complex probably requires the gp130 subunit for signal transduction. After IL-6 binding and homodimerization of gp130, the protein tyrosine kinase JAK (Janus kinase) is activated by phosphorylation, which activates a latent cytoplasmic transcription factor, a signal transducer and activator of transcription (STAT) (108). Dimeric, activated STAT translocates to the nucleus, binds to nuclear transcription factors, such as the nuclear factor (NF)-IL-6 and the acute phase response factor, and stimulates transcription of specific acute-phase protein genes.

Expression of specific IL-6Rs is subject to regulatory control. For instance, the IL-6R subunit is upregulated by dexamethasone and downregulated by granulocyte-macrophage colony-stimulating factor and IL-6 (109,110). As with some other cytokine receptor families, the IL-6R can be shed from the cell surface through proteolytic cleavage. The function of shed (soluble) IL-6Rs is not completely understood, but they may compete with membrane-bound receptors for circulating IL-6 and attenuate the activity of IL-6 on the cell. They may also enhance IL-6 activity by transporting IL-6, protecting it from proteolysis, creating a reservoir of active IL-6, and facilitating presentation of IL-6 to a broader distribution of cell types (111,112). Circulating IL-6 can also be protected from protease digestion by binding to serum carrier proteins such as α_2-macroglobulin, complement factors C3b and C4b, C-reactive protein, and albumin. These circulating complexes may serve as additional reservoirs for IL-6.

Roles of IL-6 in Inflammation

IL-6 is a multifunctional cytokine involved in the induction of B-cell terminal differentiation, induction of acute phase protein synthesis in hepatocytes, stimulation of hemopoietic progenitors, and activation of T cells and thymocytes (see Table 32-4).

Immune Response

Serum IL-6 levels are elevated in patients who develop an acute phase response, such as in sepsis, and this increase of circulating IL-6 may be a marker for outcome in septic shock (113–116). Ultimately, the biologic role of IL-6 may depend on the level in serum and tissue compartments. Relatively low levels may be beneficial, whereas very high levels may contribute to organ dysfunction. For instance, in systemic autoimmune diseases, IL-6 has been implicated in stimulating differentiation of B lymphocytes into antibody-secreting cells (117,118). Intraperitoneal administration of recombinant IL-6 to mice potentiated the antibody response to foreign antigens (119). Further overexpression of IL-6 in transgenic

mice is associated with hypergammaglobulinemia, enhanced production of autoantibodies, and induction of IL-6–responsive genes. Although these animals give no evidence of inflammatory and immunologic disturbance before 18 months of age (120), later in life, some of the IL-6–transgenic mice develop lymphomas of B-cell origin. This may reflect IL-6–induced B-cell proliferation or an immunosuppressive mechanism of IL-6. IL-6 infusion in humans and animals results in fever but does not cause shock or a capillary-leakage–like syndrome, as observed with proinflammatory cytokines such as TNF (121).

Acute Phase Response

The liver occupies a central role in limiting the local and systemic response to inflammation. Acute inflammation is accompanied by changes in the concentrations of a family of hepatocyte-derived plasma proteins known as acute phase proteins (122), such as C-reactive protein, serum amyloid A, fibrinogen, and many others. These proteins can inactivate serine proteases, support wound healing, and scavenge oxygen radicals. IL-1 and TNF stimulate the generation of only a limited subset of the acute phase proteins (123–126) (Table 32-5). IL-6, however, induces a broad spectrum of acute phase proteins in hepatoma cells and hepatocytes (127–129) (see Table 32-5). Administration of IL-6 to experimental animals activates the production of a complete set of acute phase protein responses that is similar to the response to a number of experimental models of inflammation. IL-6–deficient (IL-6-/-) mice are unable to mount a physiologic APP response to tissue injury or infection (130).

Maximal expression of the complete acute phase response requires the presence of IL-6, glucocorticoids, IL-1, and TNF. The interactions among IL-1, TNF, and IL-6 occur at two levels. IL-1 and TNF promote IL-6 production, and all three cytokines cooperate in inducing the acute phase reactants. IL-6 can suppress LPS-induced synthesis of TNF (131) in human monocytic cell line U937 and in intact mice. When considered together, it appears that IL-6 mediates an important counterregula-

TABLE 32-5. *Acute-phase proteins regulated by inflammatory cytokines*

Induced by IL-1 and TNF	Induced by IL-6 only
α_1-acid glycoprotein	α_1-acid glycoprotein
C-reactive protein	α_1-cysteine proteinase inhibitor
Complement C3	α_2-macroglobulin
Factor B	Complement C3
Hemopexin	β-fibrinogen
Haptoglobin (rat)	α_1-proteinase inhibitor
	Haptoglobin (human)
	α_1-antitrypsin
	C1 esterase inhibitor

IL, interleukin; TNF, tumor necrosis factor.

tory function that balances or limits the inflammatory sequelae of TNF and other mediators.

Hematopoiesis

Hematopoiesis is a complex process by which a small number of stem cells give rise to the enormous number of mature blood cells, including T and B lymphocytes, neutrophils, eosinophils, basophils, monocytes, platelets, and erythrocytes. Decreased red blood cell production, anemia, thrombocytosis, and granulocytosis are the hematologic changes classically associated with the acute phase response (132). Production of cytokines by activated PMNs, macrophages, and fibroblasts in the bone marrow plays a major role in the genesis of postinjury inflammation and tissue injury. Proliferation of PMN progenitors in the bone marrow favors the persistence of a hyperinflammatory state. Although IL-6 alone is not sufficient, a combination of hematopoietic growth factors, including stem cell factor, erythropoietin, IL-1, IL-3, and IL-6, triggers maximal *ex vivo* expansion of total nucleated cells and CD34$^+$ clonogenic progenitor cells (133).

Role in the Central Nervous System

IL-6 is produced in the nervous system in response to trauma, infection, and autoimmune disease. Intracerebral IL-6 activates the hypothalamic-pituitary-adrenal axis and induces fever through a prostaglandin E$_2$–dependent mechanism (134). Intravenous administration of IL-6 induces the release of corticotropin (135–138), which increases synthesis of glucocorticoids in the adrenal gland. Glucocorticoids can suppress the synthesis of proinflammatory cytokines IL-1 and TNF, upregulate the high-affinity IL-6R and gp130 on hepatocytes, and thereby augment the hepatic response to IL-6, particularly the synthesis of APPs. The activities of IL-6 in the nervous and the immune systems coordinate the two systems, in which IL-6 can activate a central inflammatory response and a peripheral, protective negative feedback response that can be considered antiinflammatory or counterregulatory.

MACROPHAGE MIGRATION INHIBITORY FACTOR

MIF was first described more than 30 years ago as an antigen- or mitogen-induced T-lymphocyte–derived lymphokine that inhibited the random migration of macrophages (139,140). MIF was rediscovered as a pituitary and macrophage-derived cytokine that is secreted after stimulation by bacterial endotoxin or glucocorticoids. Once released, MIF can override the inhibitory effects of glucocorticoids on TNF, IL-1, IL-6, and IL-8 production by LPS-stimulated monocytes *in vitro* and suppress the protective effects of steroids against lethal endotoxemia *in vivo*.

Although human MIF cDNA was cloned in 1989, the discovery of its central physiologic role in inflammation has emerged only recently from studies addressing inflammation-induced pituitary factors. When the secretory profile of an LPS-stimulated murine pituitary cell line (AtT-20) was analyzed, a 12.5-kd protein was found. N-terminal amino acid sequencing analysis demonstrated this 12.5-kd protein to be highly homologous to a human MIF (90% identity over 115 amino acids) (141). Cloning of the genes confirmed the identity of the pituitary protein as MIF (142).

Nonstimulated pituitary cells were found to contain significant amounts of preformed, intracellular MIF, which is released in response to LPS (143). *In vivo* studies demonstrated that the amount of preformed MIF protein in the pituitary gland was decreased 16 to 24 hours after endotoxin administration while the serum levels increased (143). The pituitary appears to be an important source of the MIF, because the gradual increase in serum MIF over 20 hours was not observed in hypophysectomized mice. Instead, an earlier serum MIF peak (<3 hours after injection of LPS) was observed, attributable to MIF release from other LPS-sensitive cells, such as monocytes and macrophages. Significant amounts of preformed MIF protein were found in resting monocyte-macrophages and in various murine and human monocyte cell lines (143). Moreover, proinflammatory stimuli (e.g., LPS, TNF, IFN-γ) stimulated the secretion of MIF by macrophages (Table 32-6). In contrast to other proinflammatory cytokines such as TNF and IL-1, secretion of MIF occurred at much lower LPS concentrations (10 to 100 pg/mL). The appearance of serum MIF was also examined in T-cell–deficient mice, revealing a dramatic delay in the accumulation of serum MIF in these mutant mice. These data suggest that T cells can contribute directly to the early rise of serum MIF and act indirectly by releasing cytokines such as TNF or IFN-γ that promote the release of additional macrophage MIF (144). The

TABLE 32-6. *Sources and roles of macrophage migration inhibitory factor*

Cell sources	Macrophages, monocytes
	Pituitary cells
	T cells
Stimuli	Bacterial endotoxins (LPS, TSST-1)
	Malarial pigment
	IFN-γ
	TNF
	Glucocorticoids (at low concentration)
Biologic roles	Inflammatory response: stimulates macrophage TNF and NO production
	Counterregulates the antiinflammatory and immunosuppressive effects of glucocorticoids on immune cells (macrophages, T cells)

IFN, interferon; LPS, lipopolysaccharide; NO, nitric oxide; TNF, tumor necrosis factor; TSST-1, toxic shock syndrome toxin-1.

(K_d) of 1.6 nmol
1β, and RANT
human immunoc
in human periph
ies revealed tha
tropic) HIV-1 int
the primary viru:
tor CCR5 (180,
major entry cof:
the observations
uninfected indi
chemokines (18.

Roles of MIP-1

The biologic r
extensive, inclu(
tion, regulation
modulation of in
producing these
macrophages, ly
epithelial cells,

Chemotaxis

The recruitm(
cells to sites of
inflammation ai
ment of an imm
ulated in part by
including chem
32-7). Intradern
a marked infla
nantly of neutr(
matory change
brospinal fluid
changes inclu(
increases of se
opment of bra
murine MIP-1(
when administe
tration of neutr
subsequent *in*
material have
(186). Althoug
chemokinetic f
vitro, it did trig
centrations, as
peroxide (187)

MIP-1s also
CD8+ T lymph
in vivo, presum
such as RANT
pressive activit
blocked by a
against RANT

mouse MIF gene has been cloned (145,146) and located on chromosome 10. It spans approximately 1 kb and contains three exons and two short introns of 201 and 145 nucleotides. Various consensus sequences for transcription factors were identified upstream of the transcription start site, which include a FOS binding site, an SP-1 site, a cAMP-responsive element, an AP-1 site, and a negative glucocorticoid responsive element (147). Northern blotting analysis of mouse tissue showed MIF mRNA is expressed as a single 0.6-kb transcript in most tissues examined. Moreover, whole-tissue analyses demonstrated significant amounts of MIF protein in organs that have a high content of macrophages including liver, spleen, kidney, and brain (148–151). Mouse and human MIF proteins lack a typical N-terminal signal sequence and appear to be released from cells by a nonconventional protein secretion pathway (148).

The crystal structure of human MIF has been solved and reveals a homotrimer that forms a barrel-like structure containing a solvent-accessible channel (149–151). This MIF homotrimer displays three-dimensional structural (but not primary sequence) homology with the bacterial enzymes 4-oxalocrotonate tautomerase and 5-carboxymethyl-2-hydroxymuconate isomerase (152).

Role in Inflammation

Initial evidence for the proinflammatory activities of MIF was derived from observations that MIF significantly potentiated the lethality of endotoxin (i.e., LPS) and that neutralizing anti-MIF antibodies conferred protection against endotoxic shock (153). *In vitro*, MIF possesses several macrophage-activating properties, such as the ability to induce the release of TNF by macrophages, to act together with IFN-γ to promote the release of nitric oxide, and to augment killing of intracellular pathogens (154,155) (see Table 32-6). Unlike the inhibition produced by other proinflammatory mediators, low concentrations of glucocorticoids induce MIF production from monocyte-macrophages and T cells. The release of MIF was triggered by dexamethasone at concentrations as low as 10^{-16} mol/L, peaked at 10^{-14} to 10^{-12} mol/L, and decreased at higher concentrations (10^{-8} to 10^{-6} mol/L). This observation led to identification of a mechanism by which MIF acts to counterregulate the antiinflammatory activities of glucocorticoids (156–158). The addition of exogenous rMIF overrides glucocorticoid-mediated inhibition of cytokine production *in vitro*. Similar effects are observed by administering rMIF to endotoxemic mice. MIF functions as a counterregulatory mediator that enables immune cells to produce cytokines even in the presence of glucocorticoids (159).

Role in the Central Nervous System

MIF plays an important role in the integration of central and peripheral inflammatory responses. The release of MIF by the pituitary provides a basis for a direct, neurohu-

moral cytokine response to infection and tissue invasion. MIF is also released by peripheral macrophages, indicating that the macrophage is a target and an important source of MIF *in vivo* (143). Once released, macrophage-derived MIF may act in concert with TNF to initiate local responses to infection or tissue invasion. Pituitary-derived MIF may prime systemic immune responses after a localized inflammatory site fails to contain an invasive agent or act as a cell-derived stress signal to activate the immune system in anticipation of an impending, invasive stimulus (156–158). MIF and corticotropin occupy balancing, antagonistic roles in regulating the influence of glucocorticoids on the development of inflammation.

MACROPHAGE INFLAMMATORY PROTEIN-1

During early stages of infection or tissue injury, leukocytes emigrate outward into tissues and move toward the provocator of the inflammation response (e.g., clump of bacteria, group of damaged cells). This process of directional locomotion, called *chemotaxis*, is partially mediated by members of the chemokine superfamily. The chemokine superfamily is divided into two subfamilies based on arrangement of the first two cysteines, which are separated by one amino acid (i.e., CXC chemokines such as MIP-2) or are adjacent (i.e., CC chemokines, such as MIP-1). Whereas the CXC chemokines predominantly activate neutrophils, the CC chemokines generally activate monocytes, lymphocytes, basophils, and eosinophils. This large family of chemokines is reviewed in detail elsewhere (160,161), but for the purpose of this abridged discussion, we focus on a prototypic example of one cytokine, MIP-1, in inflammation.

Regulation of Expression

Whereas many of the CXC chemokines were identified by protein chemistry, most of the CC chemokines were characterized by molecular cloning. MIP-1 proteins were originally identified as secretory products of endotoxin-stimulated murine macrophages (162,163), which migrated as a doublet of two peptides with molecular masses of about 8000 daltons on SDS-PAGE gels (164). Further biochemical separation of the doublet yielded two distinct molecules, MIP-1α and MIP-1β. The name is derived from the cell source and from the fact that this protein preparation elicited an inflammatory response on injection into mice foot pads (165). N-terminal amino acid sequence analysis of these two peptides revealed a high degree of homology to members of the CC chemokine subfamily. The cDNAs for MIP-1α and MIP-1β in mice and humans are about 70% identical to each other in their mature secreted forms (68 or 69 amino acids).

One hallmark of the controlled expression of the MIP-1 peptides is their inducibility by inflammatory stimuli (Table 32-7). The purification of MIP-1 as a doublet of mouse bone marrow and spleen and decreased the number of circulating neutrophils by 50%.

RESEARCH PERSPECTIVES

Identification of cytokine mechanisms in inflammation has been hampered by the complexity and redundancy of the host inflammatory responses and by the pleiotropism and synergy that are essential features of cytokine biology. The discovery and characterization of new cytokines and activities remain important to the development of therapies for inflammation. For instance, there is widespread interest in developing strategies to suppress the proinflammatory activities of TNF, IL-6, MIP-1α, and MIP-1β. The tetravalent guanylhydrazone compound CNI-1493 blocks synthesis of these cytokines and suppresses inflammatory responses in animal models of septic shock (203), cerebral ischemia (76), and pancreatitis (204). Recently, it was shown that the negative acute phase protein fetuin is required for the inhibition of cytokine synthesis by CNI-1493 (205). Fetuin also functions at the local cellular level to inactivate cytokine synthesis in the presence of spermine (206,207). Thus, under conditions in which fetuin levels are decreased (e.g., trauma patients), the suppression of macrophages by endogenous polyamines may be impaired, contributing to the uncontrolled, aberrant overproduction of proinflammatory cytokines. In contrast, under conditions in which spermine and fetuin levels are very high (e.g., in the fetus), they may be ideally poised to counterregulate the cytokine production in pregnancy (207). This scenario is analogous to other diseases in which the levels of cytokine activity determine whether the host helped or harmed.

REFERENCES

1. Hirokawa J, Sakaue S, Tagami S, et al. Identification of macrophage migration inhibitory factor in adipose tissue and its induction by tumor necrosis factor-alpha. *Biochem Biophys Res Commun* 1997; 235:94–98.
2. Lan HY, Yang N, Metz C, et al. TNF-alpha up-regulates renal MIF expression in rat crescentic glomerulonephritis. *Mol Med* 1997;3: 136–144.
3. Dudley DJ, Spencer S, Edwin S, Mitchell MD. Regulation of human decidual cell macrophage inflammatory protein-1 alpha (MIP-1 alpha) production by inflammatory cytokines. *Am J Reprod Immunol* 1995;34:231–235.
4. Tracey KJ, Beutler B, Lowry SF, et al. Shock and tissue injury induced by recombinant human cachectin. *Science* 1986;234:470–474.
5. Tracey KJ, Beutler B, Lowry SF, et al. Anti-cachectin/TNF monoclonal antibodies prevent septic shock during lethal bacteraemia. *Nature* 1987;330:662–664.
6. Tracey KJ, Wei H, Manogue KR, et al. Cachectin/tumor necrosis factor induces cachexia, anemia, and inflammation. *J Exp Med* 1988;167: 1211–1227.
7. Tracey KJ, Lowry SF. The role of cytokine mediators in septic shock. *Adv Surg* 1990;23:21–56.
8. Tracey KJ. Tumor necrosis factor (cachectin) in the biology of septic shock syndrome. *Circ Shock* 1991;35:123–128.
9. Grell M, Krammer PH, Scheurich P. TNF receptors TR60 and TR80 can mediate apoptosis via induction of distinct signal pathways. *J Immunol* 1994;153:1963–1972.
10. Kriegler M, Perez C, De Fay K, Albert I, Lu SD. A nonsecretable cell surface mutant of tumor necrosis factor (TNF) kills by cell-to-cell contact. *Cell* 1990;63:251–258.
11. Perez C, Albert I, De Fay K, Zachariades N, Gooding L, Kriegler M. The structure of tumor necrosis factor-alpha at 2.6 A resolution: implications for receptor binding. *J Biol Chem* 1989;264:17595–17605.
12. Eck MJ, Beutler B, Kuo G, Merryweather JP, Sprang SR. Structure of tumour necrosis factor. *Nature* 1989;338:225–228.
13. Kumins NH, Hunt J, Gamelli RL, Filkins JP. Partial hepatectomy reduces the endotoxin-induced peak circulating level of tumor necrosis factor in rats. *Shock* 1996;5:385–388.
14. Goldfeld AE, Flemington EK, Boussiotis VA, et al. Tumor necrosis factor alpha gene regulation in activated T cells involves ATF-2/Jun and NFATp. *Mol Cell Biol* 1996;16:459–467.
15. Tsai EY, Jain J, Pesavento PA, Rao A, Goldfeld AE. Cell-type-specific regulation of the human tumor necrosis factor alpha gene in B cells and T cells by NFATp and ATF-2/JUN. *Mol Cell Biol* 1996;16: 5232–5244.
16. Kramer B, Meichle A, Hensel G, Charnay P, Kronke M. Regulation of the human TNF promoter by the transcription factor Ets. *J Biol Chem* 1995;270:6577–6583.
17. Leitman DC, Ribeiro RC, Mackow ER, Baxter JD, West BL. The core promoter region of the tumor necrosis factor alpha gene confers phorbol ester responsiveness to upstream transcriptional activators. *Mol Cell Biol* 1992;12:1352–1356.
18. Kramer B, Wiegmann K, Kronke M. Identification of a tumor necrosis factor-responsive element in the tumor necrosis factor alpha gene. *J Biol Chem* 1991;266:9343–9346.
19. Wang E, Ma WJ, Aghajanian C, Spriggs DR. Posttranscriptional regulation of protein expression in human epithelial carcinoma cells by adenine-uridine–rich elements in the 3′-untranslated region of tumor necrosis factor-alpha messenger RNA. *Cancer Res* 1997;57:5426–5433.
20. Aharon T, Schneider RJ. Selective destabilization of short-lived mRNAs with the granulocyte-macrophage colony-stimulating factor AU-rich 3′ noncoding region is mediated by a cotranslational mechanism. *Mol Cell Biol* 1993;13:1971–1980.
21. Shaw G, Kamen R. A conserved AU sequence from the 3′ untranslated region of GM-CSF mRNA mediates selective mRNA degradation. *Cell* 1986;46:659–667.
22. Grafi G, Sela I, Galili G. The nonamer UUAUUUAUU is the key AU-rich sequence motif that mediates mRNA degradation. *Mol Cell Biol* 1995;15:2219–2230.
23. Zubiaga AM, Belasco JG, Greenberg ME. AUUUA is not sufficient to promote poly (A) shortening and degradation of an mRNA: the functional sequence within AU-rich elements may be UUAUUUA (U/A)(U/A). *Mol Cell Biol* 1994;14:7984–7995.
24. Lagnado CA, Brown CY, Goodall GJ. Translational blockade imposed by cytokine-derived UA-rich sequences. *Science* 1989;245:852–855.
25. Han JH, Beutler B, Huez G. Complex regulation of tumor necrosis factor mRNA turnover in lipopolysaccharide-activated macrophages. *Biochim Biophys Acta* 1991;1090:22–28.
26. Han J, Huez G, Beutler B. Interactive effects of the tumor necrosis factor promoter and 3′-untranslated regions. *J Immunol* 1991;146: 1843–1848.
27. Nahas N, Molski TF, Fernandez GA, Sha'afi RI. Tyrosine phosphorylation and activation of a new mitogen-activated protein (MAP) kinase cascade in human neutrophils stimulated with various agonists. *Biochem J* 1996;318:247–253.
28. Stevenson FT, Bursten SL, Locksley RM, Lovett DH. Myristyl acylation of the tumor necrosis factor alpha precursor on specific lysine residues. *J Exp Med* 1992;176:1053–1062.
29. Ware CF, Van Arsdale S, Van Arsdale TL. Expression of surface lymphotoxin and tumor necrosis factor on activated T, B, and natural killer cells. *J Immunol* 1992;149:3881–3888.
30. Ware CF, Crowe PD, Grayson MH, Androlewicz MJ, Browning JL. The 26-kD transmembrane form of tumor necrosis factor alpha on activated CD4$^+$ T cell clones provides a costimulatory signal for human B cell activation. *J Exp Med* 1993;177:1575–1585.
31. Aversa G, Punnonen J, de Vries JE. A metalloproteinase disintegrin that releases tumour-necrosis factor-alpha from cells. *Nature* 1997; 385:729–733.
32. Black RA, Rauch CT, Kozlosky CJ, et al. Cloning of a disintegrin metalloproteinase that processes precursor tumour-necrosis factor-alpha. *Nature* 1997;385:733–736.

33. Moss ML, Jin SL, Milla ME, et al. *In vitro* processing of human tumor necrosis factor-alpha. *J Biol Chem* 1995;270:23688–23692.

34. Gearing AJ, Beckett P, Christodoulou M, et al. Processing of tumour necrosis factor-alpha precursor by metalloproteinases. *Nature* 1994; 370:555–557.

35. Tracey KJ, Cerami A. Tumor necrosis factor: a pleiotropic cytokine and therapeutic target. *Annu Rev Med* 1994;45:491–503.

36. Gearing AJ, Beckett P, Christodoulou M, et al. TNF inhibitors: a new therapeutic perspective in chronic inflammatory diseases in rheumatology? [Translated from German]. *Z Rheumatol* 1995;54:158–164.

37. Han J, Huez G, Beutler B. Dexamethasone and pentoxifylline inhibit endotoxin-induced cachectin/tumor necrosis factor synthesis at separate points in the signaling pathway. *J Exp Med* 1990;172:391–394.

38. Waage A, Halstensen A, Shalaby R, Brandtzaeg P, Kierulf P, Espevik T. Glucocorticoids suppress the production of tumour necrosis factor by lipopolysaccharide-stimulated human monocytes. *Immunology* 1988;63:299–302.

39. Lauterbach R, Zembala M. Pentoxifylline reduces plasma tumour necrosis factor-alpha concentration in premature infants with sepsis. *Eur J Pediatr* 1996;155:404–409.

40. Griswold DE, Hillegass LM, Breton JJ, Esser KM, Adams JL. Differentiation *in vivo* of classical non-steroidal antiinflammatory drugs from cytokine suppressive antiinflammatory drugs and other pharmacological classes using mouse tumour necrosis factor alpha production. *Drugs Exp Clin Res* 1993;19:243–248.

41. Cohen PS, Nakshatri H, Dennis J, Caragine T, Bianchi M, Cerami A, Tracey KJ. Cni-1493 inhibits monocyte/macrophage tumor necrosis factor by suppression of translation efficiency. *Proc Natl Acad Sci USA* 1996;93:3967–3971.

42. Cohen PS, Schmidtmayerova H, Dennis J, et al. The critical role of p38 MAP kinase in T cell HIV-1 replication. *Mol Med* 1997;3: 339–346.

43. Bianchi M, Ulrich P, Bloom O, et al. An inhibitor of macrophage arginine transport and nitric oxide production (CNI-1493) prevents acute inflammation and endotoxin lethality. *Mol Med* 1995;1:254–266.

44. Bianchi M, Bloom O, Raabe T, et al. Suppression of proinflammatory cytokines in monocytes by a tetravalent guanylhydrazone. *J Exp Med* 1996;183:927–936.

45. Peppel K, Crawford D, Beutler B. Shock and tissue injury induced by recombinant human cachectin. *Science* 1986;234:470–474.

46. Fisher CJ Jr, Opal SM, Dhainaut JF, et al. Influence of an anti-tumor necrosis factor monoclonal antibody on cytokine levels in patients with sepsis: the CB0006 Sepsis Syndrome Study Group [see comments]. *Crit Care Med* 1993;21:318–327.

47. Abraham E, Glauser MP, Butler T, et al. P55 tumor necrosis factor receptor fusion protein in the treatment of patients with severe sepsis and septic shock—a randomized controlled multicenter trial: Ro 45-2081 Study Group. *JAMA* 1997;277:1531–1538.

48. Schattner A, el-Hador I, Hahn T, Landau Z. Triple anti-TNF-alpha therapy in early sepsis: a preliminary report. *J Int Med Res* 1997;25: 112–116.

49. Reinhart K, Wiegand-Lohnert C, Grimminger F, et al. Assessment of the safety and efficacy of the monoclonal anti-tumor necrosis factor antibody-fragment, MAK 195F, in patients with sepsis and septic shock: a multicenter, randomized, placebo-controlled, dose-ranging study. *Crit Care Med* 1996;24:733–742.

50. Hohmann HP, Remy R, Brockhaus M, van Loon AP. Tumor necrosis factors-alpha and -beta bind to the same two types of tumor necrosis factor receptors and maximally activate the transcription factor NF-kappa B at low receptor occupancy and within minutes after receptor binding. *J Biol Chem* 1990;265:15183–15188.

51. Barbara JA, Smith WB, Gamble JR, et al. Function of the p55 tumor necrosis factor receptor "death domain" mediated by phosphatidylcholine-specific phospholipase C. *J Exp Med* 1996;184:725–733.

52. Hohmann HP, Remy R, Poschl B, van Loon AP. Expression of the types A and B tumor necrosis factor (TNF) receptors is independently regulated, and both receptors mediate activation of the transcription factor NF-kappa B. TNF alpha is not needed for induction of a biological effect via TNF receptors. *J Biol Chem* 1990;265:22409–22417.

53. Machleidt T, Kramer B, Adam D, et al. Stress-induced apoptosis and the sphingomyelin pathway. *Biochem Pharmacol* 1997;53:615–621.

54. Pena LA, Fuks Z, Kolesnick R. TNF- and cancer therapy-induced apoptosis: potentiation by inhibition of NF-kappaB [see comments]. *Science* 1996;274:784–787.

55. Wang CY, Mayo MW, Baldwin AS Jr. Bcl-x(L) can inhibit apoptosis in cells that have undergone Fas-induced protease activation. *Proc Natl Acad Sci USA* 1997;94:3759–3764.

56. Boise LH, Thompson CB. Antibodies to a soluble form of a tumor necrosis factor (TNF) receptor have TNF-like activity. *J Biol Chem* 1990;265:14497–14504.

57. Engelmann H, Holtmann H, Brakebusch C, et al. Two tumor necrosis factor-binding proteins purified from human urine: evidence for immunological cross-reactivity with cell surface tumor necrosis factor receptors. *J Biol Chem* 1990;265:1531–1536.

58. Engelmann H, Novick D, Wallach D. A metalloprotease inhibitor blocks shedding of the 80-kD TNF receptor and TNF processing in T lymphocytes. *J Exp Med* 1995;181:1205–1210.

59. Crowe PD, Walter BN, Mohler KM, Otten-Evans C, Black RA, Ware CF. A metalloprotease inhibitor blocks shedding of the IL-6 receptor and the p60 TNF receptor. *J Immunol* 1995;155:5198–5205.

60. Mullberg J, Durie FH, Otten-Evans C, et al. The potential biological and clinical significance of the soluble tumor necrosis factor receptors. *Cytokine Growth Factor Rev* 1996;7:231–240.

61. Aderka D. Protection against endotoxic shock by a tumor necrosis factor receptor immunoadhesin. *Proc Natl Acad Sci USA* 1991;88: 10535–10539.

62. Aderka D, Engelmann H, Maor Y, Brakebusch C, Wallach D. Tumor necrosis factor in sepsis: mediator of multiple organ failure or essential part of host defense? [Editorial]. *Shock* 1995;3:1–12.

63. Ashkenazi A, Marsters SA, Capon DJ, et al. Stabilization of the bioactivity of tumor necrosis factor by its soluble receptors. *J Exp Med* 1992;175:323–329.

64. Tracey KJ, Morgello S, Koplin B, et al. Metabolic effects of cachectin/tumor necrosis factor are modified by site of production. Cachectin/tumor necrosis factor-secreting tumor in skeletal muscle induces chronic cachexia, while implantation in brain induces predominantly acute anorexia. *J Clin Invest* 1990;86:2014–2024.

65. Van der Poll T, Lowry SF. Tumor necrosis factor in sepsis: mediator of multiple organ failure or essential part of host defense? [Editorial]. *Shock* 1995;3:1–12.

66. Pfeffer K, Matsuyama T, Kundig TM, et al. Mice deficient for the 55 kd tumor necrosis factor receptor are resistant to endotoxic shock, yet succumb to *L. monocytogenes* infection. *Cell* 1993;73:457–467.

67. Amiot F, Fitting C, Tracey KJ, Cavallion JM, Dautry F. Lipopolysaccharide-induced cytokine cascade and lethality in LT alpha/TNF alpha-deficient mice. *Mol Med* 1997;3:864–875.

68. Marino MW, Dunn A, Grail D, et al. Characterization of tumor necrosis factor-deficient mice. *Proc Natl Acad Sci USA* 1997;94: 8093–8098.

69. Abraham E, Wunderink R, Silverman H, et al. Efficacy and safety of monoclonal antibody to human tumor necrosis factor alpha in patients with sepsis syndrome: a randomized, controlled, double-blind, multicenter clinical trial. TNF-alpha MAb Sepsis Study Group. *JAMA* 1995;273:934–941.

70. Cheng B, Christakos S, Mattson MP. Tumor necrosis factors protect neurons against metabolic-excitotoxic insults and promote maintenance of calcium homeostasis. *Neuron* 1994;12:139–153.

71. Breder CD, Hazuka C, Ghayur T, et al. Regional induction of tumor necrosis factor alpha expression in the mouse brain after systemic lipopolysaccharide administration. *Proc Natl Acad Sci USA* 1994;91: 11393–11397.

72. Breder CD, Tsujimoto M, Terano Y, Scott DW, Saper CB. Distribution and characterization of tumor necrosis factor-alpha–like immunoreactivity in the murine central nervous system. *J Comp Neurol* 1993;337: 543–567.

73. Botchkina GI, Meistrell ME 3rd, Botchkina IL, Tracey KJ. Expression of TNF and TNF receptors (p55 and p75) in the rat brain after focal cerebral ischemia [In Process Citation]. *Mol Med* 1997;3:765–781.

74. Waage A, Slupphaug G, Shalaby R. Local production of tumor necrosis factor alpha, interleukin 1, and interleukin 6 in meningococcal meningitis: relation to the inflammatory response. *J Exp Med* 1989; 170:1859–1867.

75. Waage A, Bakke O. *In vivo* relationship of tumor necrosis factor-alpha to blood-brain barrier damage in patients with active multiple sclerosis. *J Neuroimmunol* 1992;38:27–33.

76. Sharief MK, Thompson EJ. Elevated circulating tumor necrosis factor levels in Alzheimer's disease. *Neurosci Lett* 1991;129:318–320.

77. Sarchielli P, Orlacchio A, Vicinanza F, et al. Cytokine secretion and

nitric oxide production by mononuclear cells of patients with multiple sclerosis. *J Neuroimmunol* 1997;80:76–86.

78. Barone FC, Arvin B, White RF, et al. Tumor necrosis factor-alpha: a mediator of focal ischemic brain injury. *Stroke* 1997;28:1233–1244.

79. Meistrell ME, 3rd, Botchkina GI, Wang H, et al. Tumor necrosis factor is a brain damaging cytokine in cerebral ischemia. *Shock* 1997;8: 341–348.

80. Dawson DA, Martin D, Hallenbeck JM. Inhibition of tumor necrosis factor-alpha reduces focal cerebral ischemic injury in the spontaneously hypertensive rat. *Neurosci Lett* 1996;218:41–44.

81. McGuire W, Hill AV, Allsopp CE, et al. Variation in the TNF-alpha promoter region associated with susceptibility to cerebral malaria. *Nature* 1994;371:508–510.

82. Stuber F, Petersen M, Bokelmann F, Schade U. A genomic polymorphism within the tumor necrosis factor locus influences plasma tumor necrosis factor-alpha concentrations and outcome of patients with severe sepsis [see comments]. *Crit Care Med* 1996;24:381–384.

83. Stuber F, Udalova IA, Book M, et al. -308 Tumor necrosis factor (TNF) polymorphism is not associated with survival in severe sepsis and is unrelated to lipopolysaccharide inducibility of the human TNF promoter [see comments]. *J Inflamm* 1995;46:42–50.

84. Weissenbach J, Chernajovsky Y, Zeevi M, et al. Two interferon mRNAs in human fibroblasts: *in vitro* translation and *Escherichia coli* cloning studies. *Proc Natl Acad Sci USA* 1980;77:7152–7156.

85. Content J, De Wit L, Pierard D, Derynck R, De Clercq E, Fiers W. Secretory proteins induced in human fibroblasts under conditions used for the production of interferon beta. *Proc Natl Acad Sci USA* 1982;79:2768–2772.

86. Hirano T, Yasukawa K, Harada H, et al. Complementary DNA for a novel human interleukin (BSF-2) that induces B lymphocytes to produce immunoglobulin. *Nature* 1986;324:73–76.

87. Scholz W. Human beta 2 interferon and B-cell differentiation factor BSF-2 are identical. *Science* 1987;235:731–732.

88. Gauldie J, Richards C, Harnish D, Lansdorp P, Baumann H. Interferon beta 2/B-cell stimulatory factor type 2 shares identity with monocyte-derived hepatocyte-stimulating factor and regulates the major acute phase protein response in liver cells. *Proc Natl Acad Sci USA* 1987;84:7251–7255.

89. Sehgal PB, Zilberstein A, Ruggieri RM, et al. Complementary DNA for a novel human interleukin (BSF-2) that induces B lymphocytes to produce immunoglobulin. *Nature* 1986;324:73–76.

90. Hirano T, Yasukawa K, Harada H, et al. Post-translational modifications of human interleukin-6. *Arch Biochem Biophys* 1989;274: 161–170.

91. Santhanam U, Ghrayeb J, Sehgal PB, May LT. Synthesis and secretion of multiple forms of beta 2–interferon/B-cell differentiation factor 2/hepatocyte-stimulating factor by human fibroblasts and monocytes. *J Biol Chem* 1988;263:7760–7766.

92. May LT, Ghrayeb J, Santhanam U, et al. Human eosinophils synthesize and secrete interleukin-6, *in vitro*. *Blood* 1992;80:1496–1501.

93. Barton BE. IL-6: insights into novel biological activities. *Clin Immunol Immunopathol* 1997;85:16–20.

94. Hirano T. The biology of interleukin-6. *Chem Immunol* 1992;51: 153–180.

95. Hamid Q, Barkans J, Meng Q, et al. Interleukin-6: an overview. *Annu Rev Immunol* 1990;8:253–278.

96. Lotz M. Interleukin-6: a comprehensive review. *Cancer Treat Res* 1995;80:209–233.

97. Sehgal PB. A nuclear factor for the IL-6 gene (NF-IL6). *Chem Immunol* 1992;51:299–322.

98. Akira S, Isshiki H, Nakajima T, et al. Cytokine serum level during severe sepsis in human IL-6 as a marker of severity. *Ann Surg* 1992; 215:356–362.

99. Van Snick J. Inhibition by glucocorticoids of the formation of interleukin-1 alpha, interleukin-1 beta, and interleukin-6: mediation by decreased mRNA stability. *Mol Pharmacol* 1993;43:176–182.

100. Cheng B, Christakos S, Mattson MP. Glucocorticoids inhibit the production of IL6 from monocytes, endothelial cells and fibroblasts. *Eur J Immunol* 1990;20:2439–2443.

101. de Waal Malefyt R, Abrams J, Bennett B, Figdor CG, de Vries JE. Recombinant IL-4 inhibits IL-6 synthesis by adherent peripheral blood cells *in vitro*. *Lymphokine Res* 1990;9:283–293.

102. de Waal Malefyt R, Abrams J, Bennett B, Figdor CG, de Vries JE. Interleukin 10 (IL-10) inhibits cytokine synthesis by human mono-

cytes: an autoregulatory role of IL-10 produced by monocytes. *J Exp Med* 1991;174:1209–1220.

103. de Waal Malefyt R, Haanen J, Spits H, et al. Interleukin 10 (IL-10) and viral IL-10 strongly reduce antigen-specific human T cell proliferation by diminishing the antigen-presenting capacity of monocytes via downregulation of class II major histocompatibility complex expression. *J Exp Med* 1991;174:915–924.

104. Taga T. The signal transducer gp130 is shared by interleukin-6 family of haematopoietic and neurotrophic cytokines. *Ann Med* 1997;29: 63–72 .

105. Taga T, Kishimoto T. Gp130 and the interleukin-6 family of cytokines. *Annu Rev Immunol* 1997;15:797–819.

106. Kishimoto T, Tanaka T, Yoshida K, Akira S, Taga T. The molecular biology of interleukin 6 and its receptor. *Ciba Found Symp* 1992;167: 5–16.

107. Kishimoto T, Hibi M, Murakami M, Narazaki M, Saito M, Taga T. High affinity interleukin-6 receptor is a hexameric complex consisting of two molecules each of interleukin-6, interleukin-6 receptor, and gp-130. *J Biol Chem* 1994;269:23286–23289.

108. Zhong Z, Wen Z, Darnell JE Jr. Stat3: a STAT family member activated by tyrosine phosphorylation in response to epidermal growth factor and interleukin-6. *Science* 1994;264:95–98.

109. Nesbitt JE, Fuller GM. The hepatic interleukin-6 receptor. Studies on its structure and regulation by phorbol 12-myristate 13-acetate-dexamethasone. *J Biol Chem* 1993;268:4250–4258.

110. Zohlnhofer D, Graeve L, Rose-John S, Schooltink H, Dittrich E, Heinrich PC. The hepatic interleukin-6 receptor: down-regulation of the interleukin-6 binding subunit (gp80) by its ligand. *FEBS Lett* 1992; 306:219–222.

111. Biffl WL, Moore EE, Moore FA, Peterson VM. Interleukin 6 in diseases: cause or cure? *Immunopharmacology* 1996;31:131–150.

112. Peters M, Meyer zum Buschenfelde KH, Rose-John S. The function of the soluble IL-6 receptor *in vivo*. *Immunol Lett* 1996;54:177–184.

113. Damas P, Ledoux D, Nys M, et al. Increased plasma levels of interleukin-6 in sepsis [see comments]. *Blood* 1989;74:1704–1710.

114. Hack CE, De Groot ER, Felt-Bersma RJ, et al. Limited involvement of interleukin-6 in the pathogenesis of lethal septic shock as revealed by the effect of monoclonal antibodies against interleukin-6 or its receptor in various murine models. *Eur J Immunol* 1992;22:2625–2630.

115. Biffl WL, Moore EE, Moore FA, Peterson VM. Interleukin-6 in the injured patient: marker of injury or mediator of inflammation? *Ann Surg* 1996;224:647–664.

116. Ryffel B, Mihatsch MJ, Woerly G. Pathology induced by interleukin-6. *Int Rev Exp Pathol* 1993;34[Pt A]:79–89.

117. Chen-Kiang S. Regulation of terminal differentiation of human B-cells by IL-6. *Curr Top Microbiol Immunol* 1995;194:189–198.

118. Yoshizaki K, Kuritani T, Kishimoto T. Interleukin-6 in autoimmune disorders. *Semin Immunol* 1992;4:155–166.

119. Waage A, Kaufmann C, Espevik T, Husby G. Human recombinant IL-6/B cell stimulatory factor 2 augments murine antigen-specific antibody responses *in vitro* and *in vivo*. *J Immunol* 1988;141:3072–3077.

120. Woodroofe C, Muller W, Ruther U. Long-term consequences of interleukin-6 overexpression in transgenic mice. *DNA Cell Biol* 1992;11: 587–592.

121. Mastorakos G, Chrousos GP, Weber JS. Recombinant interleukin-6 activates the hypothalamic-pituitary-adrenal axis in humans. *J Clin Endocrinol Metab* 1993;77:1690–1694.

122. Geng Y, Zhang B, Lotz M. Interleukin-6: a regulator of plasma protein gene expression in hepatic and non-hepatic tissues. *Mol Biol Med* 1990;7:117–130.

123. Mastorakos G, Chrousos GP, Weber JS. Cachectin/tumor necrosis factor regulates hepatic acute-phase gene expression. *J Clin Invest* 1986; 78:1349–1354.

124. Perlmutter DH, Dinarello CA, Punsal PI, Colten HR. Distinct sets of acute phase plasma proteins are stimulated by separate human hepatocyte-stimulating factors and monokines in rat hepatoma cells. *J Biol Chem* 1987;262:9756–9768.

125. Baumann H, Onorato V, Gauldie J, Jahreis GP. Interferon beta 2/B-cell stimulatory factor type 2 shares identity with monocyte-derived hepatocyte-stimulating factor and regulates the major acute phase protein response in liver cells. *Proc Natl Acad Sci USA* 1987;84:7251–7255.

126. Gauldie J, Richards C. Induction of rat acute-phase proteins by interleukin 6 *in vivo*. *Eur J Immunol* 1988;18:717–721.

127. Gauldie J, Richards C, Harnish D, Lansdorp P, Baumann H. Effects of

interleukin-6 and leukemia inhibitory factor on the acute phase response and DNA synthesis in cultured rat hepatocytes. *Lymphokine Cytokine Res* 1991;10:23–26.

128. Kordula T, Rokita H, Koj A, Fiers W, Gauldie J, Baumann H. The relationship of serum IL-6 levels to acute graft-versus-host disease and hepatorenal disease after human bone marrow transplantation. *Transplantation* 1992;54:457–462.

129. Tilg H, Dinarello CA, Mier JW. IL-6 and APPs: anti-inflammatory and immunosuppressive mediators. *Immunol Today* 1997;18:428–432.

130. Kopf M, Baumann H, Freer G, et al. Impaired immune and acute-phase responses in interleukin-6–deficient mice. *Nature* 1994;368:339–342.

131. Kopf M, Baumann H, Freer G, et al. IL-6 inhibits lipopolysaccharide-induced tumor necrosis factor production in cultured human monocytes, U937 cells, and in mice. *J Immunol* 1989;143:3517–3523.

132. Van Snick J. Interleukin-6: an overview. *Annu Rev Immunol* 1990;8:253–278.

133. Bermudez LE, Wu M, Petrofsky M, Young LS. Ex vivo expansion of enriched peripheral blood CD34- progenitor cells by stem cell factor, interleukin-1 beta (IL-1 beta), IL-6, IL-3, interferon-gamma, and erythropoietin. *Blood* 1993;81:2579–2584.

134. Brugger W, Mocklin W, Heimfeld S, Berenson RJ, Mertelsmann R, Kanz L. Interleukin-6 as an endogenous pyrogen: induction of prostaglandin E2 in brain but not in peripheral blood mononuclear cells. *Brain Res* 1991;562:199–206.

135. Dinarello CA, Cannon JG, Mancilla J, Bishai I, Lees J, Coceani F. Corticotropin-releasing activity of monokines. *Science* 1985;230:1035–1037.

136. Dinarello CA, Bunn PA Jr. Fever. *Semin Oncol* 1997;24:288–298.

137. Raber J, O'Shea RD, Bloom FE, Campbell IL. Modulation of hypothalamic-pituitary-adrenal function by transgenic expression of interleukin-6 in the CNS of mice. *J Neurosci* 1997;17:9473–9480.

138. Lenczowski MJ, Van Dam AM, Poole S, Larrick JW, Tilders FJ. Role of circulating endotoxin and interleukin-6 in the ACTH and corticosterone response to intraperitoneal LPS. *Am J Physiol* 1997;273:R1870–1877.

139. Bloom BR, Bennett B. Mechanism of a reaction *in vitro* associated with delayed-type hypersensitivity. *Science* 1966;153:80–82.

140. David JR. Dual immunological unresponsiveness induced by cell membrane coupled hapten or antigen. *Nature* 1966;212:156–157.

141. Bernhagen J, Mitchell RA, Calandra T, Voelter W, Cerami A, Bucala R. Purification, bioactivity, and secondary structure analysis of mouse and human macrophage migration inhibitory factor (MIF). *Biochemistry* 1994;33:14144–14155.

142. Weiser WY, Temple PA, Witek-Giannotti JS, Remold HG, Clark SC, David JR. Molecular cloning of a cDNA encoding a human macrophage migration inhibitory factor. *Proc Natl Acad Sci USA* 1989;86:7522–7526.

143. Calandra T, Bernhagen J, Mitchell RA, Bucala R. The macrophage is an important and previously unrecognized source of macrophage migration inhibitory factor. *J Exp Med* 1994;179:1895–1902.

144. Calandra T, Bernhagen J, Metz CN, et al. Macrophage migration inhibitory factor is a neuroendocrine mediator of endotoxaemia. *Trends Microbiol* 1994;2:198–201.

145. Kozak CA, Adamson MC, Buckler CE, Segovia L, Paralkar V, Wistow G. Cloning and characterization of the gene for mouse macrophage migration inhibitory factor (MIF). *J Immunol* 1995;154:3863–3870.

146. Kozak CA, Adamson MC, Buckler CE, Segovia L, Paralkar V, Wistow G. Genomic cloning of mouse MIF (macrophage inhibitory factor) and genetic mapping of the human and mouse expressed gene and nine mouse pseudogenes. *Genomics* 1995;27:405–411.

147. Calandra T, Bucala R. MIF rediscovered: cytokine, pituitary hormone, and glucocorticoid-induced regulator of the immune response. *FASEB J* 1996;10:1607–1613.

148. Bernhagen J, Bacher M, Calandra T, et al. Localization of macrophage migration inhibitory factor (MIF) to secretory granules within the corticotrophic and thyrotrophic cells of the pituitary gland. *Mol Med* 1995;1:781–788.

149. Lan HY, Mu W, Yang N, et al. NMR characterization of structure, backbone dynamics, and glutathione binding of the human macrophage migration inhibitory factor (MIF). *Protein Sci* 1996;5:2095–2103.

150. Muhlhahn P, Bernhagen J, Czisch M, et al. The subunit structure of human macrophage migration inhibitory factor: evidence for a trimer. *Protein Eng* 1996;9:631–635.

151. Bucala R. Purification, bioactivity, and secondary structure analysis of mouse and human macrophage migration inhibitory factor (MIF). *Biochemistry* 1994;33:14144–14155.

152. Sugimoto H, Taniguchi M, Nakagawa A, Tanaka I, Suzuki M, Nishihira J. Crystallization and preliminary X-ray analysis of human D-dopachrome tautomerase. *J Struct Biol* 1997;120:105–108.

153. Bernhagen J, Calandra T, Mitchell RA, et al. MIF is a pituitary-derived cytokine that potentiates lethal endotoxaemia. *Nature* 1993;365:756–759.

154. Bucala R. MIF rediscovered: cytokine, pituitary hormone, and glucocorticoid-induced regulator of the immune response. *FASEB J* 1996;10:1607–1613.

155. Metz CN, Bucala R. Role of macrophage migration inhibitory factor in the regulation of the immune response. *Adv Immunol* 1997;66:197–223.

156. Calandra T, Bernhagen J, Metz CN, et al. MIF as a glucocorticoid-induced modulator of cytokine production. *Nature* 1995;377:68–71.

157. Calandra T, Bucala R. Macrophage migration inhibitory factor: a counter-regulator of glucocorticoid action and critical mediator of septic shock. *J Inflamm* 1995;47:39–51.

158. Calandra T, Bucala R. Macrophage migration inhibitory factor (MIF): a glucocorticoid counter-regulator within the immune system. *Crit Rev Immunol* 1997;17:77–88.

159. Donnelly SC, Bucala R. Macrophage migration inhibitory factor: a regulator of glucocorticoid activity with a critical role in inflammatory disease. *Mol Med Today* 1997;3:502–507.

160. Baggiolini M, Dewald B, Moser B. Human chemokines: an update. *Annu Rev Immunol* 1997;15:675–705.

161. Baggiolini M, Loetscher P, Moser B. Interleukin-8 and the chemokine family. *Int J Immunopharmacol* 1995;17:103–108.

162. Davatelis G, Wolpe SD, Sherry B, Dayer JM, Chicheportiche R, Cerami A. Cloning and characterization of a cDNA for murine macrophage inflammatory protein (MIP), a novel monokine with inflammatory and chemokinetic properties [published erratum appears in *J Exp Med* 1989;170:2189]. *J Exp Med* 1988;167:1939–1944.

163. Davatelis G, Tekamp-Olson P, Wolpe SD, et al. Macrophages secrete a novel heparin-binding protein with inflammatory and neutrophil chemokinetic properties. *J Exp Med* 1988;167:570–581.

164. Sherry B, Tekamp-Olson P, Gallegos C, et al. Resolution of the two components of macrophage inflammatory protein 1, and cloning and characterization of one of those components, macrophage inflammatory protein 1 beta. *J Exp Med* 1988;168:2251–2259.

165. Sherry BA, Alava G, Tracey KJ, Martinez J, Cerami A, Slater AF. Malaria-specific metabolite hemozoin mediates the release of several potent endogenous pyrogens (TNF, MIP-1 alpha, and MIP-1 beta) *in vitro*, and altered thermoregulation *in vivo*. *J Inflamm* 1995;45:85–96.

166. Broxmeyer HE, Sherry B, Lu L, et al. Two inflammatory mediator cytokine genes are closely linked and variably amplified on chromosome 17q. *Nucleic Acids Res* 1990;18:3261–3270.

167. Tekamp-Olson P, Gallegos C, Bauer D, et al. Cloning and characterization of cDNAs for murine macrophage inflammatory protein 2 and its human homologues. *J Exp Med* 1990;172:911–919.

168. Combadiere C, Ahuja SK, Murphy PM. Genomic cloning and promoter analysis of macrophage inflammatory protein (MIP)-2, MIP-1 alpha, and MIP-1 beta, members of the chemokine superfamily of proinflammatory cytokines. *J Immunol* 1993;150:4996–5012.

169. Venkatesan S, Moss B. Cell-type specific protein binding to the enhancer of simian virus 40 in nuclear extracts. *Nature* 1986;323:544–548.

170. Widmer U, Yang Z, van Deventer S, Manogue KR, Sherry B, Cerami A. Genomic structure of murine macrophage inflammatory protein-1 alpha and conservation of potential regulatory sequences with a human homolog, LD78. *J Immunol* 1991;146:4031–4040.

171. Davidson I, Fromental C, Augereau P, Wildeman A, Zenke M, Chambon P. Cell-type specific protein binding to the enhancer of simian virus 40 in nuclear extracts. *Nature* 1986;323:544–548.

172. Kelvin DJ, Michiel DF, Johnston JA, et al. Chemokines and serpentines: the molecular biology of chemokine receptors. *J Leukoc Biol* 1993;54:604–612.

173. Irving SG, Zipfel PF, Balke J, et al. Identification of cell surface receptors for murine macrophage inflammatory protein-1 alpha. *J Immunol* 1991;147:2978–2983.

174. Wang JM, Sherry B, Fivash MJ, Kelvin DJ, Oppenheim JJ. Human recombinant macrophage inflammatory protein-1 alpha and -beta and

monocyte chemotactic and activating factor use common and unique receptors on human monocytes. *J Immunol* 1993;150:3022–3029.

175. Wang JM, McVicar DW, Oppenheim JJ, Kelvin DJ. Identification of RANTES receptors on human monocytic cells: competition for binding and desensitization by homologous chemotactic cytokines. *J Exp Med* 1993;177:699–705.

176. Nibbs RJB, Wylie SM, Pragnell IB, Graham GJ. Molecular cloning, functional expression, and signaling characteristics of a C-C chemokine receptor. *Cell* 1993;72:415–425.

177. Ahuja SK, Gao JL, Murphy PM. Chemokine receptors and molecular mimicry. *Immunol Today* 1994;15:281–287.

178. Raport CJ, Gosling J, Schweickart VL, Gray PW, Charo IF. Molecular cloning and functional characterization of a novel human CC chemokine receptor (CCR5) for RANTES, MIP-1beta, and MIP-1alpha. *J Biol Chem* 1996;271:17161–17166.

179. Alkhatib G, Combadiere C, Broder CC, et al. CC CKR5: a RANTES, MIP-1alpha, MIP-1beta receptor as a fusion cofactor for macrophage-tropic HIV-1. *Science* 1996;272:1955–1958.

180. Rucker J, Samson M, Doranz BJ, et al. Regions in beta-chemokine receptors CCR5 and CCR2b that determine HIV-1 cofactor specificity. *Cell* 1996;87:437–446.

181. Moore JP, Trkola A, Dragic T. Co-receptors for HIV-1 entry [see comments]. *Curr Opin Immunol* 1997;9:551–562.

182. Dragic T, Litwin V, Allaway GP, et al. HIV-1 entry into CD4- cells is mediated by the chemokine receptor CC-CKR-5 [see comments]. *Nature* 1996;381:667–673.

183. Cook DN. The role of MIP-1 alpha in inflammation and hematopoiesis. *J Leukoc Biol* 1996;59:61–66.

184. Broxmeyer HE, Sherry B, Cooper S, et al. Macrophage inflammatory protein 1 modulates macrophage function. *J Immunol* 1992;148:2764–2769.

185. Wolpe SD, Davatelis G, Sherry B, et al. Macrophages secrete a novel heparin-binding protein with inflammatory and neutrophil chemokinetic properties. *J Exp Med* 1988;167:570–581.

186. McColl SR, Hachicha M, Levasseur S, Neote K, Schall TJ. Uncoupling of early signal transduction events from effector function in human peripheral blood neutrophils in response to recombinant macrophage inflammatory proteins-1 alpha and -1 beta. *J Immunol* 1993;150:4550–4560.

187. Schall TJ, Bacon K, Camp RD, Kaspari JW, Goeddel DV. Human macrophage inflammatory protein alpha (MIP-1 alpha) and MIP-1 beta chemokines attract distinct populations of lymphocytes. *J Exp Med* 1993;177:1821–1826.

188. Fahey TJ 3rd, Tracey KJ, Tekamp-Olson P, et al. Macrophage inflammatory protein (MIP)-1 beta abrogates the capacity of MIP-1 alpha to suppress myeloid progenitor cell growth. *J Immunol* 1991;147:2586–2594.

189. Myers RD, Lopez-Valpuesta FJ, Minano FJ, Wooten MH, Barwick VS, Wolpe SD. Macrophage inflammatory protein-1: a prostaglandin-independent endogenous pyrogen. *Science* 1989;243:1066–1068.

190. Saukkonen K, Sande S, Cioffe C, Wolpe S, Sherry B, Cerami A, Tuomanen E. Fever and feeding: differential actions of macrophage inflammatory protein-1 (MIP-1), MIP-1 alpha and MIP-1 beta on rat hypothalamus. *Neurochem Res* 1993;18:667–673.

191. Oh KO, Zhou Z, Kim KK, et al. Hypothalamic indomethacin fails to block fever induced in rats by central macrophage inflammatory protein-1 (MIP-1). *Pharmacol Biochem Behav* 1991;39:535–539.

192. Minano FJ, Sancibrian M, Vizcaino M, et al. Macrophage inflammatory protein-1: unique action on the hypothalamus to evoke fever. *Brain Res Bull* 1990;24:849–852.

193. Minano FJ, Vizcaino M, Myers RD. Fever induced by macrophage inflammatory protein-1 (MIP-1) in rats: hypothalamic sites of action. *Brain Res Bull* 1991;27:701–706.

194. Myers RD, Lopez-Valpuesta FJ, Minano FJ, Wooten MH, Barwick VS, Wolpe SD. Fever and feeding in the rat: actions of intrahypothalamic interleukin-6 compared to macrophage inflammatory protein-1 beta (MIP-1 beta). *J Neurosci Res* 1994;39:31–37.

195. Fahey TJ 3d, Sherry B, Tracey KJ, et al. Cytokine production in a model of wound healing: the appearance of MIP-1, MIP-2, cachectin/TNF and IL-1. *Cytokine* 1990;2:92–99.

196. Smith RS, Smith TJ, Blieden TM, Phipps RP. Fibroblasts as sentinel cells: synthesis of chemokines and regulation of inflammation. *Am J Pathol* 1997;151:317–322.

197. Myers RD, Paez X, Roscoe AK, Sherry B, Cerami A. Comparative analysis of the human macrophage inflammatory protein family of cytokines (chemokines) on proliferation of human myeloid progenitor cells. Interacting effects involving suppression, synergistic suppression, and blocking of suppression. *J Immunol* 1993;150:3448–3458.

198. Tilg H, Dinarello CA, Mier JW. The role of MIP-1 alpha in inflammation and hematopoiesis. *J Leukoc Biol* 1996;59:61–66.

199. Fahey TJ 3d, Sherry B, Tracey KJ, et al. Myelopoietic enhancing effects of murine macrophage inflammatory proteins 1 and 2 on colony formation *in vitro* by murine and human bone marrow granulocyte/macrophage progenitor cells. *J Exp Med* 1989;170:1583–1594.

200. Broxmeyer HE, Sherry B, Lu L, et al. Myelopoietic enhancing effects of murine macrophage inflammatory proteins 1 and 2 on colony formation *in vitro* by murine and human bone marrow granulocyte/macrophage progenitor cells. *J Exp Med* 1989;170:1583–1594.

201. Broxmeyer HE, Sherry B, Lu L, et al. Enhancing and suppressing effects of recombinant murine macrophage inflammatory proteins on colony formation *in vitro* by bone marrow myeloid progenitor cells. *Blood* 1990;76:1110–1116.

202. Broxmeyer HE, Sherry B, Cooper S, et al. Comparative analysis of the human macrophage inflammatory protein family of cytokines (chemokines) on proliferation of human myeloid progenitor cells: interacting effects involving suppression, synergistic suppression, and blocking of suppression. *J Immunol* 1993;150:3448–3458.

203. Villa P, Meazza C, Sironi M, et al. A low molecular weight TNF inhibitor (CNI-1493) protects mice from sepsis and sepsis-associated pulmonary infiltration. *Eur Cytokine Network* 1997;7:506.

204. Denham W, Fink G, Yang J, Ulrich P, Tracey K, Norman J. Small molecule inhibition of tumor necrosis factor gene processing during acute pancreatitis prevents cytokine cascade progression and attenuates pancreatitis severity. *Am Surg* 1997;63:1045–1049.

205. Wang H, Zhang M, Bianchi M, et al. Fetuin (α_2-HS-glycoprotein) opsonizes cationic macrophage-deactivating molecules. *Proc Natl Acad Sci USA* 1998;95:(in press).

206. Zhang M, Caragine T, Wang H, et al. Spermine inhibits proinflammatory cytokine synthesis in human mononuclear cells: a counterregulatory mechanism that restrains the immune response. *J Exp Med* 1997;185:1759–1768.

207. Wang H, Zhang M, Soda K, Sama A, Tracey KJ. Fetuin protects the fetus from TNF [Letter]. *Lancet* 1997;350:861–862.

Inflammation: Basic Principles and Clinical Correlates,
3rd ed., edited by John I. Gallin and Ralph Snyderman.
Lippincott Williams & Wilkins, Philadelphia © 1999.

CHAPTER 33

Biochemistry, Mechanism of Action, and Biology of the Interferons

Erika A. Bach, Daniel H. Kaplan, and Robert D. Schreiber

Our understanding of interferon (IFN) biology has grown exponentially during the last 20 years. During this period, the genes encoding the IFNs and their cognate receptors have been cloned and expressed, and the corresponding polypeptides have been extensively characterized. The ability to produce large quantities of highly purified, recombinant IFN proteins has facilitated the molecular definition of IFN receptors and the elucidation of their mechanism of action. IFN-specific monoclonal antibodies have been generated and used to study IFN biosynthesis and structure, and they have helped establish many of the *in vivo* functions of this family of proteins. Mice lacking IFN family members, IFN receptor components, or IFN signaling components have been generated and used to further define the physiologic roles of the IFNs *in vivo*. Human patients with inactivating mutations in the IFN-γ signaling pathway have been discovered, and the characterization of their immunocompromised state has unequivocally established the important functions of the IFN proteins in preventing human disease.

The combination of basic and clinical research has established a relatively clear view of the biochemistry and biology of the IFN system. In this chapter, key aspects of IFN biochemistry and biology are discussed, and special attention is paid to the important role of IFN-γ in promoting inflammatory processes, host resistance to microbial pathogens and tumors, and in modulating immune system activity.

STRUCTURE OF THE INTERFERON GENES AND PROTEINS

The IFNs were originally described as agents capable of protecting cells from viral infection (1,2). Based on several criteria such as their cellular source, gene and protein structures, and functional activity, IFN family members have been divided into two groups (Table 33-1). Type I IFNs are primarily induced in response to viral infection of cells and have been further subdivided into two classes (IFN-α and IFN-β) based on their cell of origin (3). The IFN-α family consists of more than 22 structurally related polypeptides encoded by distinct genes that are produced largely by leukocytes (4,5). There is only one form of IFN-β. It is encoded by a single, distinct gene that is expressed largely in fibroblasts (3). Type II IFN, now designated IFN-γ, is a product of a single gene and is synthesized by T lymphocytes and natural killer (NK) cells after activation with immune and inflammatory stimuli (6,7).

Interferon-α and Interferon-β Genes and Proteins

Twenty-six IFN-α genes, at least five of which are pseudogenes, have been identified (4). These genes reside in a gene cluster on human chromosome 9 and mouse chromosome 4 (8). IFN-α genes are organized in an identical manner and lack introns. It is believed that this gene family evolved from a common ancestral gene 100 million years ago. In humans and mice, the single IFN-β gene is located next to the IFN-α gene cluster. Because the organization of the IFN-β gene is closely related to that of the IFN-α genes, IFN-β and IFN-α genes probably evolved from the same common ancestral gene.

IFN-α proteins are single-chained polypeptides that contain 165 to 167 amino acids in their mature form. At

E. A. Bach, D. H. Kaplan, and R. D. Schreiber: Center for Immunology and Department of Pathology, Washington University School of Medicine, St. Louis, Missouri 63110.

TABLE 33-1. *Properties of interferons*

Property	Interferon-α	Interferon-β	Interferon-γ
Nomenclature	Type I, leukocyte	Type I, fibroblast	Type II, immune
Major inducers	Virus	Virus, LPS, ds-poly RNA	Antigens, mitogens, TNF-α + IL-12
Physical properties			
Molecular mass (kd), predicted/mature	20/20	20/20–25	17/34–50
Amino acids	165–166	166	143
N-linked glycosylation	Some species	Yes	2 sites
Subunit composition	Single polypeptide	Single polypeptide	Noncovalent homodimer
pH stability	Stable	Stable	Labile
Gene structure			
Number of genes	26	1	1
Chromosomal location			
Human	9	9	12
Murine	4	4	10
Presence of introns	None	None	3
Cellular source	T cells, B cells, macrophages	Fibroblasts, epithelial cells	T cells, natural killer cells

LPS, lipopolysaccharide; ds, double stranded; TNF-α, tumor necrosis factor-α.

least 25 distinct forms of mature human IFN-α have been identified with molecular masses that range from 16 to 27.5 kd (5). However, some of these represent differentially glycosylated forms of the same gene product. The human IFN-α polypeptides display 68% sequence identity with one another and approximately 40% homology with their murine IFN-α counterparts. Most forms of IFN-α are heat and pH stable. Whereas some types of IFN-α proteins display species specificity in their ability to bind cell surface receptors and activate cellular responses, others do not. Mature human and murine IFN-β are glycoproteins that consist of 166 and 161 amino acids and have molecular masses of 20 and 26 kd, respectively. Despite the overall similarity in the organization of the IFN-α and IFN-β genes, the proteins they encode share only 15% to 30% identity at the amino acid level. However, sufficient similarity exists between the key functional domains of the proteins that they bind to the same cell surface receptor and induce a highly overlapping array of biologic responses (9).

Interferon-γ Genes and Proteins

IFN-γ is not related to IFN-α or IFN-β at the gene or polypeptide levels. IFN-γ is encoded by a single 6-kb gene that resides on human chromosome 12 and murine chromosome 10 (10,11). The gene in humans and mice is organized in an identical fashion and contains 4 exons and 3 introns. The human IFN-γ gene encodes a 1.2-kb mRNA that gives rise to a 166–amino acid polypeptide. After cleavage of a 23–amino acid signal sequence, the mature human IFN-γ polypeptide contains 143 amino acids and displays a molecular mass of 17 kd. However, because of differential glycosylation at the 2 N-linked glycosylation sites, mature human IFN-γ polypeptides have molecular masses of 17, 20, and 25 kd (12). The

murine IFN-γ gene produces a 1.2-kb mRNA that gives rise to a 134–amino acid mature polypeptide that, depending on its glycosylation state, has a molecular mass of 15.4, 20, or 25 kd. In both species, the fully glycosylated form of IFN-γ predominates. Human and murine IFN-γ coding sequences display 60% identity, but the polypeptides share only 40% identity. This primary amino acid sequence diversity is the basis for the strict species specificity that human and murine IFN-γ display in binding to and inducing responses from human and murine cells, respectively (6).

Under physiologic conditions two IFN-γ polypeptides self-associate to form a noncovalently bonded homodimer with a molecular mass of 50 kd (13,14). The IFN-γ homodimer is a labile molecule that can be denatured by extremes of temperature (>65°C) or pH (<4 or >9). Only the homodimeric form of IFN-γ is fully capable of binding to the IFN-γ receptor on cells and inducing biologic responses. The crystal structure of the IFN-γ dimer has been solved and indicates that two IFN-γ monomers associate in an antiparallel fashion to form a symmetrical dimer (15). Subsequent crystallographic studies of the complex of IFN-γ bound to the ligand-binding chain of the IFN-γ receptor indicate that the IFN-γ homodimer contains two identical receptor binding sites and interacts with two receptor molecules (16).

BIOSYNTHESIS OF THE INTERFERONS

Interferon-α and Interferon-β Production

Biosynthesis of Type I IFNs is not a specialized cellular function, because most cells are capable of producing at least one form of Type I IFN after exposure to the appropriate inducing stimuli (17–20). The most important physiologic inducer of IFN-α and IFN-β is viral infection. However, Type I IFN family members can also be induced by double-stranded RNA, inflammatory stimuli such as bacterial endotoxin, interleukin-1 (IL-1), tumor necrosis factor (TNF), and even IFN itself. Analysis of the regulatory elements of the Type I IFN genes reveals the presence of binding sites for NF-κB and IFN regulatory factor-1 (IRF-1) transcription factors that are activated by the known IFN inducers. Type I IFN induction is rapid, and IFN-α and IFN-β can be detected in the extracellular environment within 6 hours after cellular stimulation.

Interferon-γ Production

In contrast to the production of Type I IFNs, IFN-γ biosynthesis is highly regulated in that it occurs only in a few specialized cell types stimulated with specific stimuli (6,7). T cells are one of the two major cellular sources of IFN-γ in the normal host. All CD8$^+$ T cells and the T$_H$0 and T$_H$1 subsets of CD4$^+$ helper T cells secrete IFN-γ in response to peptide antigen bound to a major histocompatibility (MHC) protein and the appropriate co-stimulatory signal. Synthesis can also be induced through antibody-dependent cross-linking of the T-cell receptor, mitogens, or pharmacologic stimuli. In resting T cells, the IFN-γ gene is transcriptionally silent. However, after T-cell activation, IFN-γ transcripts can be detected within 6 to 8 hours, reach maximum levels by 12 to 24 hours, and then subsequently decline to baseline values. IFN-γ proteins are secreted immediately after synthesis and reach maximal extracellular levels 18 to 24 hr after T-cell stimulation (6).

Although the molecular events that underlie IFN-γ production in T cells have not been fully elucidated, it is clear that interleukin-12 (IL-12) and interleukin-18 (IL-18) play important roles in regulating IFN-γ synthesis (21–24) through mechanisms involving the transcription factors STAT-4 and NF-κB (25,26). However, more work is needed to define whether these transcription factors act directly on the IFN-γ promoter or act in an indirect manner through the induction of other transcription factors that regulate IFN-γ production.

The other major cellular source of IFN-γ is activated NK cells, which, in contrast to T cells, produce the cytokine in a rapid and MHC-unrestricted manner. Studies of severe combined immunodeficiency mice infected with the gram-positive bacteria *Listeria monocytogenes* defined a positive amplification system involving NK cells and IFN-γ and two other cytokines: IL-12 and TNF-α (27,28). These studies revealed that, on interaction with bacterial products, tissue macrophages produce low amounts of TNF-α and IL-12. These two cytokines then stimulate NK cells to secrete low levels of IFN-γ. NK cell–derived IFN-γ then activates macrophages in the vicinity of the infectious focus such that they produce greater quantities of TNF-α and IL-12 when they encounter the infectious agent. The increased levels of IL-12 and TNF-α that accumulate in the environment stimulate NK cells to produce enhanced quantities of IFN-γ, which induce more IL-12 and TNF-α production from macrophages. This type of reciprocal stimulation forms a positive amplification loop that results in the rapid production of substantial quantities of IFN-γ early during the course of infection and that facilitates the generation of large numbers of activated macrophages with antimicrobial activity. The mutual synergistic effects that IFN-γ, IL-12, and TNF-α have on macrophages and NK cells provide the host with an innate mechanism for IFN-γ production and macrophage activation that facilitates early control of infection (29).

IL-10 is one of the major negative regulators of IFN-γ production in NK cells and T cells (26,28,30). IL-10 exerts its effects on either cell type in an indirect manner. In the case of NK cells, IL-10 prevents macrophage secretion of TNF-α and IL-12 and thereby inhibits NK cell activation for IFN-γ production. In the case of T cells, the action of this cytokine remains somewhat less clear. Because IL-10 limits the ability of antigen-presenting cells to produce IL-12, it exerts its inhibitory effects on T cells in a manner that is similar to that for NK cells. However, IL-10 also has been shown to downregulate expression of MHC class II proteins in human mononuclear phagocytes (31) and may block T-cell activation and cytokine production inhibiting the process of antigen presentation.

INTERFERON RECEPTORS

Interferonα/β Receptor

All Type I IFNs bind to a single, high-affinity, cell surface IFN-α/β receptor (9,32). Functionally active IFN-α/β receptors are composed of two distinct subunits: a 110-kd IFNAR1 polypeptide (also known as IFNaR1) and a 102-kd IFNAR2 polypeptide (also called IFNaR2) (Table 33-2 and Fig. 33-1). The IFNAR1 and IFNAR2 polypeptides are members of the class 2 cytokine receptor family, which also includes the subunits of the IFN-γ receptor, the IL-10 receptor, and tissue factor (33). Like all class 2 cytokine receptor family members, the intracellular domains of the IFN-α/β receptor subunits are devoid of intrinsic kinase or phosphatase activities. The genes encoding IFNAR1 and IFNAR2 are located in a gene cluster on human chromosome 21 and murine chromosome 16. These syntenic chromosomal regions also contain the genes of many of the other class 2 cytokine receptor family members, including the α subunit of the IFN-γ receptor and CRF-2-4, which functions as the β chain of the IL-10 receptor (34,35).

The human *IFNAR1* gene encodes a 557-amino acid polypeptide that contains a 27–amino acid signal sequence (9). The mature 530–amino acid IFNAR1 polypeptide contains a 409–amino acid extracellular domain, a 21–amino

TABLE 33-2. *Properties of interferon receptors*

Property	Interferon-α/β receptor		Interferon-γ receptor	
	IFNAR1[a]	IFNAR2[a]	α Chain (IFNGR1)[a]	β Chain (IFNGR2)[a]
Molecular mass (kd) predicted/mature	60.5/95–100	34.7/102	52.6/85–95	34.8/62
Amino acids (aa)	530	315	472	316
Domain structure				
Extracellular (aa)	409	217	228	226
Transmembrane (aa)	21	21	23	24
Intracellular (aa)	100	251	221	66
Glycosylation sites	12	3	5	5
Chromosomal location				
Murine	16	16	10	16
Human	21	21	6	21

[a]Polypeptide receptor subunits.

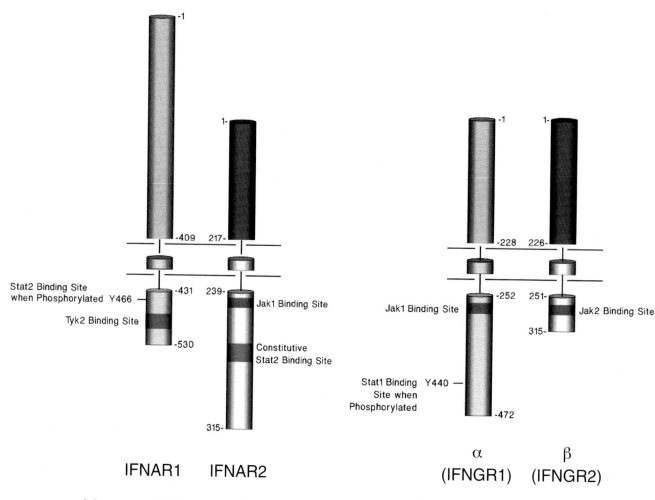

A

B

FIG. 33-1. Schematic representation of the human interferon (IFN)-α/β and IFN-γ receptors. **(A)** The IFNAR1 and IFNAR2 subunits of the IFN-α/β receptor. **(B)** The α (IFNGR1) and β (IFNGR2) subunits of the IFN-γ receptor. The positions of the amino acids are shown, and the functionally important intracellular domain sequences are identified.

acid transmembrane domain, and a 100–amino acid cytoplasmic domain. The human *IFNAR2* gene encodes a mature polypeptide of 489 amino acids and consists of a 217–amino acid extracellular domain, a 21–amino acid transmembrane domain, and a 251–amino acid intracellular domain. Although expression of human IFNAR1 is sufficient to confer on cells the ability to bind and respond to one IFN-α family member (IFN-α8), binding of *all* IFN-α family members requires the coexpression of both IFN-α/β receptor subunits (9,36). Although a distinct receptor for IFN-β has been proposed, no data are available to unequivocally support the existence of such a protein.

Interferon-γ Receptor

IFN-γ exerts its pleiotropic effects on cells by interacting with a high-affinity (K_d=10–100pM) specific receptor that is expressed on nearly all cell surfaces (16,37). IFN-γ receptors consist of two species-matched polypeptides (see Table 33-2 and Fig. 33-1). The IFN-γ receptor α chain (i.e., IFNGR1, IFN-γR1, or CDw119) is a 90-kd protein that is encoded by a gene on human chromosome 6 and murine chromosome 10. The receptor α chain is responsible for ligand binding and ligand trafficking through the cell, and it is necessary but not sufficient for signal transduction. The IFN-γ receptor β chain (i.e., IFNGR2, IFN-γR2, or accessory factor-1 [AF-1]) is a 62-kd protein encoded by a gene on human chromosome 21 and murine chromosome 16. The IFN-γ receptor β chain plays only a minor role in ligand binding but is absolutely required for IFN-γ signaling. Expression of the two IFN-γ receptor subunits differs significantly. The IFN-γ receptor α chain is constitutively expressed at moderate levels on the surface of nearly all cells (200 to 25,000 sites/cell), and its expression does not appear to be modulated by external stimuli. In contrast, the IFN-γ receptor β chain is constitutively expressed on cells at extremely low levels, but expression is regulated in certain cell types, such as T lymphocytes, by external stimuli (38,39). In some cells, the expression of the IFN-γ receptor β chain gene becomes a critical factor in determining whether they can respond to IFN-γ.

The cDNA encoding the human IFN-γ receptor α chain encodes a 489–amino acid precursor that contains a 17–amino acid signal sequence (40). The murine receptor α subunit gene encodes a 477–amino acid polypeptide containing a 26–amino acid signal peptide (41–45). The murine and human proteins are organized in a similar manner as both contain identically sized extracellular and transmembrane domains of 228 and 23 amino acids, respectively, and relatively large, serine- and threonine-rich intracellular domains. Despite this organizational similarity, the two polypeptides exhibit only 52.5% overall sequence identity, which extends throughout the extracellular and intracellular domains of the polypeptides. Mature human IFN-γ receptor α subunits from different

cells display molecular masses that vary between 80 and 95 kd because of cell-specific differences in glycosylation (46–48).

The human and murine IFN-γ receptor β subunits are also structurally similar to one another. The human IFN-γ receptor β subunit is a 337–amino acid type I transmembrane polypeptide, which contains a 21–amino acid signal sequence, an extracellular domain of 226 amino acids, a single 24–amino acid transmembrane domain, and a relatively short intracellular domain of only 66 amino acids (49). The murine receptor β chain consists of an 18–amino acid signal sequence, a 224–amino acid extracellular domain, a 24–amino acid transmembrane domain, and a 64–amino acid intracellular domain (50). Although human and murine receptor β chains exhibit 58% identity overall, this value increases to 73% when their cytoplasmic domains are compared. The human and murine cDNAs encode polypeptides of 38 kd. However, mature forms of human and murine receptor β chains have molecular masses of 62 kd (39). This difference is most likely explained by postsynthetic glycosylation of the polypeptides, although the composition and location of β-chain–associated carbohydrates has not yet been established.

SIGNAL TRANSDUCTION THROUGH INTERFERON RECEPTORS

JAK-STAT Pathway: Janus Kinases and Signal Transducers and Activators of Transcription

During the past 6 years, our understanding of signal transduction through the IFN-α/β receptor and IFN-γ receptors has been greatly advanced. Both IFN receptor systems function as a result of the ligand-induced coupling of the cognate cell surface receptor to a cytosolic signal transduction pathway known as the JAK-STAT pathway (16,32,51–54). The JAK-STAT pathway uniquely represents a mechanism capable of rapidly transferring signals directly from the cell surface to the nucleus. This pathway is responsible for mediating the effects of a large number of cytokine and growth factor receptors.

To achieve the biologic diversity needed to promote the specific biologic actions of such a wide range of ligand and receptor systems, two families of signaling proteins have evolved that play distinct roles in the signal transduction process. One is a family of related protein tyrosine kinases known as Janus kinases (JAKs). The second is a family of latent cytosolic transcription factors known as signal transducers and activators of transcription (STATs).

The Janus kinase family contains four members: JAK-1, JAK-2, JAK-3, and TYK-2 (51,54,55). These enzymes are responsible for phosphorylating activated cytokine receptors and STAT proteins. Structurally, the members of the Janus kinase family are unusual compared with other protein tyrosine kinases because they contain two carboxyl-terminal, kinase-like domains, with only the domain at the extreme COOH terminus having documented kinase activity. Although the JAKs associate with receptor subunits in a specific manner (56–58), their catalytic domains are interchangeable (59). This observation has led to the suggestion that JAKs participate in cytokine signaling by activating the STATs and by recruiting other signaling pathways to the activated cytokine receptor complex. It is possible to envisage a mechanism in which cytokines that address different receptors that activate the same STAT protein can induce distinct biologic responses in cells.

The STAT protein family consists of seven distinct gene products: STAT-1, STAT-2, STAT-3, STAT-4, STAT-5A, STAT-5B, and STAT-6 (52,54). Based on studies using cells and mice engineered to lack particular STAT proteins, it has been possible to establish that the STATs are the major components that determine cytokine receptor signaling specificity (51,60,61). The STATs are unique among transcription factors in that they possess SRC homology-2 (SH2) domains capable of binding to phosphotyrosine-containing sequences. The sequence differences within the SH2 domains of the STAT proteins are responsible for effecting the selective recruitment of distinct STATs to activated, tyrosine-phosphorylated cytokine receptor subunits and the subsequent specific pairing that occurs between two tyrosine-phosphorylated STAT proteins that form the functionally active transcription factor complex.

Interferon-γ Receptor Signaling

Based on a large body of data concerning the structure and function of the IFN-γ receptor, the JAKs, and the STATs, it has been possible to construct a relatively comprehensive model of IFN-γ signal transduction through the JAK-STAT pathway (Fig. 33-2). This model serves as the signaling paradigm for many cytokine receptors that belong to the type I cytokine receptor family.

In unstimulated cells, the IFN-γ receptor subunits are not preassociated with one another (62), but rather constitutively, and specifically associate through their intracellular domains with inactive JAK family members (62–65). JAK-1 binds to a ^{266}LPKS^{269} sequence in the membrane proximal portion of the intracellular domain of the IFN-γ receptor α chain, and JAK-2 associates with a 12–amino acid sequence (^{263}PPSIPLQIEEYL^{274}) in the intracellular domain of the IFN-γ receptor β chain. Signal transduction is initiated when a homodimeric IFN-γ molecule binds to two IFN-γ receptor α subunits, leading to the formation of a complex to which two receptor β subunits subsequently bind. Within the ligand assembled receptor complex, the inactive subunit-associated kinases are brought into juxtaposition with one another and are activated by mechanisms involving autophosphorylation and transphosphorylation. The activated kinases then phosphorylate a key tyrosine residue within a ^{440}YDKPH^{444} sequence residing near the COOH terminus of the receptor α chain, thereby forming the phosphorylated sequence that is specifically recognized by the SH2 domain of STAT-1 (66,67). Two STAT-1 molecules then bind to the paired docking sites on the activated receptor complex; are brought into proximity with the receptor-associated, activated tyrosine kinases; and are phosphorylated at a specific tyrosine residue (Y701) that resides near the COOH terminus of the transcription factor (68,69).

The two phosphorylated STAT-1 proteins, which have also become serine phosphorylated in an undefined step in the pathway, then dissociate from their receptor tether, form reciprocal homodimers, and translocate to the nucleus. In the nucleus, the STAT-1 homodimers bind to specific promoter elements (i.e., IFN-γ–activated sites or GAS elements) and thereby effect transcription of IFN-γ–induced genes (16,51).

Using cells and mice with induced genetic deficiencies of different JAKs and STATs, most IFN-γ–induced biologic responses have been shown to require the participation of STAT-1, JAK-1, and JAK-2 (56–58,60,61). These studies have unequivocally established the validity and physiologic relevance of this signaling model.

Interferon-α/β Receptor Signaling

Signaling through the IFN-α/β receptor is similar to that of the IFN-γ receptor, but there are some important differences (see Fig. 33-2). Like IFN-γ receptor signaling, the IFN-α/β receptor subunits constitutively and specifically associate with inactive JAKs in unstimulated cells. TYK-2 binds to the membrane-proximal region of the IFNAR1 intracellular domain (70), and JAK-1 associates with a ^{274}LPKV^{277} sequence in the intracellular domain of IFNAR2 (71,72). However, unlike IFN-γ receptor signaling, latent forms of STAT-1 and STAT-2 preassociate with the membrane-proximal region of the intracellular domain of IFNAR2 in unstimulated cells (73). The molecular basis for the association of STAT-1 and STAT-2 with IFNAR2 is not well understood but is not mediated through the interaction of phosphotyrosine containing receptor sequences and the SH2 domains of the STATs. When IFN-α/β receptor–bearing cells are exposed to Type I IFN, the subunits oligomerize, the JAKs become activated, and the activated kinases then phosphorylate a ^{466}YVFFP^{470} sequence in the IFNAR1 intracellular domain (74). The tyrosine-phosphorylated IFNAR1 sequence functions as a receptor docking site for the SH2 domain of STAT-2, leading to the establishment of a high-affinity association between STAT-2 and the activated IFN-α/β receptor (75). STAT-2 is tyrosine phosphorylated by the receptor-associated JAKs and then functions as an adapter that is recognized by the SH2 domain of STAT-1. When STAT-1 binds to IFNAR1-associated STAT-2, it is also tyrosine phosphorylated.

On the activated receptor, the STAT-1/STAT-2 complex has two fates (32). First, some of the activated STAT-1 proteins dissociate from their STAT-2 tethers and form

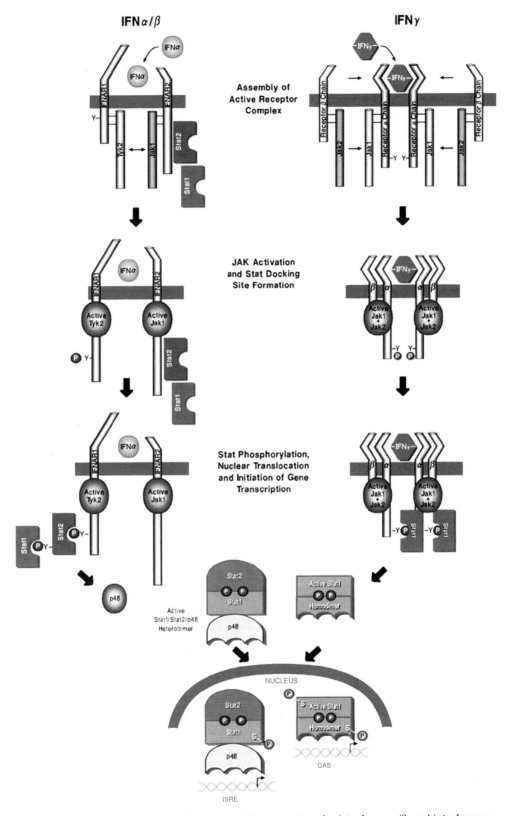

FIG. 33-2. Comparison of signaling through the receptors for interferon-α/β and interferon-γ.

STAT-1 homodimers. These homodimers translocate to the nucleus, bind to GAS elements, and activate transcription of IFN-γ–inducible genes. To some extent, this mechanism explains the overlapping pattern of genes induced by IFN-α/β and IFN-γ. Second, the STAT-1/STAT-2 dimer (i.e., ISGF-3α) can dissociate as an intact heterocomplex from the IFN-α/β receptor. The heterodimer can neither translocate to the nucleus nor bind DNA. However, it can associate with a cytosolic DNA binding protein, called p48 or ISGF-3γ, to form the trimolecular complex known as ISGF-3 that is competent for nuclear translocation and transcriptional activation. In the nucleus, ISGF-3 interacts with a promoter element, known as the IFN-stimulated response element (ISRE), which is distinct from the GAS element and thereby promotes transcription of IFN-α/β–inducible genes. In this manner, type I IFNs can effect activation of a set of genes that are not induced by IFN-γ (51,74).

Regulation of Interferon Receptor Signaling

At least four distinct mechanisms have been proposed that may control IFN-dependent JAK-STAT pathway signaling. One is a mechanism involving protein tyrosine phosphatases. Because the signaling pathway is driven by tyrosine kinases, it was predicted that phosphatases should play an important regulatory role. Evidence for the participation of phosphatases in the IFN signaling pathway has been obtained and largely comes from experiments showing that phosphorylation of the receptor subunits and the STATs is extremely transient. Moreover, a phosphatase activity has been coprecipitated with the activated IFN-α/β receptor complex (76). However, no specific phosphatase has been identified that plays an obligatory role in pathway regulation, and no phosphatase activity that associates with the activated IFN-γ receptor has been reported yet. More work is needed to clarify this issue.

The work from three laboratories has defined a family of proteins known as SOCS proteins, JABs, or SSI proteins, whose production is stimulated by cytokines and which function as JAK inhibitors (77–79). At least six closely related members of the family have been found, and another 14 members have been identified that are more distantly related (80). The proteins are rapidly induced (about 20 minutes) after cytokine stimulation of cells and then rapidly disappear (about 2 hours). Using overexpression approaches in intact cells and cell-free systems, these proteins were found to be capable of significantly reducing the catalytic activity of all JAKs but not other tyrosine kinases. However, the specificity of induction and action of these proteins and their cellular distribution have yet to be determined. It remains unclear whether, under physiologic conditions, the SOCS/JAB/SSI proteins serve as specific regulators of distinct cytokine signaling responses or represent a generalized mechanism to effect the return of an activated cytokine signaling pathway to its homeostatic baseline.

Another family of proteins known as proteins that inhibit activated STATs (PIAS) has been discovered (81). Each of the two related proteins identified shows a high degree of specificity for a particular activated STAT complex. PIAS-1 binds selectively to activated STAT-1 homodimers while PIAS-3 binds selectively activated STAT-3 homodimers. These components are zinc finger proteins that form complexes with activated STAT dimers and block the STATs from binding to DNA. However, more work is needed to define the other members of the PIAS family and to determine their mechanism of action.

IFN signaling can be regulated by a mechanism involving expression of particular receptor subunits. The IFN-γ receptor β chain is downregulated in T cells as they differentiate to the T_H1 CD4$^+$ subset (38,39). Downregulation appears to occur at the transcriptional level. In newly developing T-cell clones, exposure of the cells to IFN-γ leads to a loss of IFN-γ receptor β chain, message, and protein. In long-term T_H1 cell clones, IFN-γ receptor β chain expression is permanently suppressed. The generality and molecular basis of the mechanism underlying this unusual type of homologous desensitization remain poorly understood.

INTERFERON-INDUCIBLE GENES

The rapid signaling action of the JAK-STAT pathway makes it an ideal system to regulate the activation of immediate-early genes that could provide the host with a rapid mechanism to respond to an infectious agent. Over the years, it has been possible to identify a large number of IFN-stimulated genes (ISGs) that are induced rapidly (15 to 30 minutes) in IFN-treated cells and whose transcription does not depend on new protein synthesis (82,83). The promoter regions of these ISGs harbor two classes of conserved nucleotide sequences that direct their rapid transcriptional activation (51,52) (Table 33-3). One is the ISRE mentioned previously. It is a 12- to 15-nucleotide sequence that displays a consensus motif of AGTTTCNNTTTCNC/T and is responsible for driving expression of IFN-α/β–inducible genes. This site is recognized by the trimolecular ISGF-3 signaling complex induced by IFN-α/β. The other is the GAS element which

TABLE 33-3. *DNA binding specificities exhibited by different STAT complexes*

STAT protein	DNA sequence recognized
STAT-1	TTCC(G>C)GGAA
STAT-2	not defined
STAT-3	TTCC(G=C)GGAA
STAT-4	TTCC(G>C)GGAA
STAT-5	TTCC(A>T)GGAA
STAT-6	TTCC(A>T,N)GGAA
Consensus	TTNCNNNAA
ISGF3 (STAT-1, STAT-2, P48)	TTTCNNTTTC

From ref. 55, with permission.

TABLE 33-4. *Representative IFN-γ–regulated genes involved in inflammation*

Category	Examples
LPS response	CD14 (membrane and soluble)↓
	RAF-1 kinase↓
Acute-phase reactants	α1-antichymotrypsin↓[a]
	HNF-3β↑
	Fibrinogen↓[a]
	Serine protease inhibitor↑
	Haptoglobin↓[a]
Nitric oxide and respiratory burst	iNOS↑[a]
	MPO↓
	Mn-SOD↑
	gp91-phox↑, p47-phox↑↓[a], p67-phox↑[a] (components of NADPH oxidase)
Cytokines and cytokine receptors	IL-12↑
	TNF-α↑[a], TNFR1↑, TNFR2↑↓[a]
	IL-6↑[a]
	IL-6R↑
	CSF-1↑
	CD40↑
Chemokines	
C-C family	MCP-1↑
	MCP-2↑
	MCP-3↑
	MIP-1α↑↓[a]
	MIP-1β↑↓[a]
C-X-C family	RANTES↑[a]
	IP-10↑
	MIG↑
	MGSA (GROα, GRO1, GRO)↓[a]
Classic chemoattractants	PAF↑[a]
	PAFR↑
	fMLP-R↑
	HGF↑
	C5aR↑↓
Transcription factors	IRF-1↑
	IRF-2↑
	ICSBP↑
	ISGF3γ(p48)↑
	CIITA↑
Lymphocyte-activation markers	Ly-6A/E↑
	B7/BB-1↑
	CD80↑↓
	1–8 gene family↑
Fc receptors	CD23↓
	FcγRI↑
	pIgR↑
Complement system	C1q↑
	C2↑
	C3↑↓
	C4↑
	Factor B↑
	Factor H↑
	Factor I↑
Selectins	L-selectin (CD62L)↑
	E-selectin (CD62E)↑[a]
Selectin ligands	CD34↓
	CD15↓
	MadCAM-1↓[a]↑
	PNAd↑
Integrins	VLA-1↑, -2↑, -3↑, -4↑↓, -5↓, -6↑
	CD11a, b, c↑
	CD18↑

TABLE 33-4. *(Continued)*

Category	Examples
Cellular adhesion molecules	ICAM-1↑
	VCAM-1↑
	LFA-3↓[a]
	CD56↑
	CD44 (CD44)↑
Extracellular matrix and cytoskeleton-associated proteins	collagen type I↓, III↑, IV (α1-chain)↓
	Keratin↑
	Fibronectin↑↓
Lipids and steroids	15-lipoxygenase↓[a]
	Glucocorticoid receptor↑
	Phospholipase A$_2$ (PLA$_2$)↑
	Cytosolic PLA$_2$↑

CIITA, MHC Class II transactivating factor; CSF, colony-stimulating factor; fMLP, *N*-formylmethionyl-leucyl-phenylalanine; GRO, oncogenes with growth-stimulating activity; HGF, human growth factor; HNF, hepatocyte nuclear factor; ICAM, intercellular adhesion molecule; ICSBP, interferon consensus sequence-binding factor; IL, interleukin; iNOS, inducible form of nitric oxide synthase; IP-10, interferon-gamma–inducible 10-kd protein; IRF, interferon regulatory factor; LFA, lymphocyte function antigen; LPS, lipopolysaccharide; MadCAM-1, mucosal addressin cell adhesion molecule-1; MCP, monocyte chemotactic protein; MGSA, melanoma growth stimulatory activity; MIG, monokine induced by interferon-γ; MIP, macrophage inflammatory protein; MPO, myeloperoxidase; PAF, platlet-activating factor; PNAd, peripheral lymph node addressin; RANTES, regulated on activation, normally T-cell expressed and secreted; SOD, superoxide dismutase; TNF, tumor necrosis factor; VCAM, vascular cell adhesion molecule; VLA, very late activation antigen; ↑, denotes genes that are upregulated by IFN-γ; ↓, denotes genes that are downregulated by IFN-γ.

[a]Genes require a second cytokine or stimulus to effect upregulation or downregulation.

From ref. 7, with permission.

functions to promote transcriptional activation of IFN-γ–induced genes. The GAS site is a 9-nucleotide sequence that contains the consensus sequence of TTNCNNNAA. STAT-1 homodimers bind to this site and thereby promote transcription of IFN-γ–inducible genes.

Activated dimeric forms of STAT-3, STAT-4, STAT-5, and STAT-6 recognize nucleotide elements that resemble the GAS element but are subtly different (54) (see Table 33-3). This observation indicates that activated STAT proteins bind to short, palindromic sequences. The specific ability of each activated STAT dimer to effect the activation of a particular array of cytokine-induced genes is based in part on the nucleotide specificity displayed by the DNA binding domain that is formed on dimerization of tyrosine phosphorylated STAT proteins.

Table 33-4 presents a sampling of genes regulated by IFN-γ. This list contains several examples of IFN-γ–regulated immediate-early genes such as IFN regulatory factor-1 (IRF-1), guanylate binding protein-1 and the type I Fcγ receptor (IFN-γRI) that participate in inflammatory and immune responses. The list also contains several IFN-γ–regulated intermediate genes, which are induced within 6 to 8 hours of stimulation but which require additional protein synthesis for transcriptional activation to occur. Examples of these genes include those that encode class I and class II MHC proteins. The characterization of STAT-1–deficient mice has shown that STAT-1 plays an obligate and early role in the activation of most IFN-γ– and IFN-α/β–inducible genes (60,61). A more complete discussion of IFN-γ–inducible genes is provided by the excellent reviews from Kerr and Stark (82,83) and Howard (7).

BIOLOGIC ACTIVITIES OF INTERFERONS

Antiviral and Antiproliferative Activities

Type I and Type II IFNs can protect cells from viral infection and exert profound antiproliferative actions on normal and neoplastic cells. The molecular basis of the antiviral effects of the IFNs has been extensively studied during the past 15 years. The IFNs promote antiviral responses that are intrinsic to the infected cell itself or extrinsic in that they effect recognition and destruction of infected cells by components of the innate or specific limbs of the host immune response.

IFN induces several proteins in cells that promote intrinsic mechanisms of cellular resistance to viral infection (84). Three mechanisms have been identified. The first is the result of the induction and actions of a family of enzymes known as 2'-5'-oligoadenylate synthetases (85). These enzymes are induced by Type I and Type II IFNs and are activated in the presence of double-stranded RNA (which are intermediates or byproducts of viral RNA replication). The activated enzymes polymerize ATP into 2'-5'-linked oligomers that activate RNAse L, a latent, constitutively expressed endoribonuclease. Activated RNAse L degrades single-stranded RNA and thereby inhibits protein synthesis in cells. The second mechanism is based on the protein PKR (i.e., double-stranded RNA-dependent kinase, P1 kinase, p68 kinase, or eIF-2 kinase), which is a serine/threonine kinase that is also induced by IFN and activated by double-stranded RNA (86,87). PKR phosphorylates and inactivates the eukaryotic protein synthesis initiation factor (eIF-2), thereby blocking protein synthesis in cells. These two mechanisms produce their antiviral effects by inhibiting cellular protein synthesis. The third mechanism depends on the Mx protein, which is induced only by Type I IFNs (88). The mechanism of action of this protein is poorly understood but is directed primarily at inhibiting replication of orthomyxoviruses such as influenza virus.

Extrinsic antiviral mechanisms induced by the IFNs are largely those that direct the development of innate and specific immune responses. Type I IFNs induce enhanced cytolytic activity in NK cells and thereby promote the capacity of these cells to lyse virally infected target cells. Type I and Type II IFNs promote antigen processing and presentation and thereby play a key role in the induction of antiviral cellular and humoral immune responses.

Both classes of IFNs manifest antiproliferative effects on cells. Although these biologic effects are well documented, their molecular bases are not well defined. At least some of the antiproliferative actions of the IFNs are caused by the induction of proteins that inhibit the enzymes involved in cell cycle progression. For example, IFN can induce, through the JAK-STAT pathway, expression of the protein p21$^{WAF1/CIP1/CAP1}$, which is an inhibitor of CDK2 (89). However, this process occurs in a relatively cell specific manner, and it is uncertain whether other cell cycle inhibitors may also be involved in the process. Nevertheless, this negative biologic response can still be attributed to a positive induction of a particular gene product.

Macrophage Activation and Innate Immunity

Of the IFN family members, IFN-γ is clearly distinct in its ability to function as the major macrophage-activating factor (90–92). It is crucial in promoting nonspecific host defense mechanisms against a number of pathogens. Data supporting this concept come from *in vitro* and *in vivo* studies demonstrating that IFN-γ can induce in macrophages the capacity to nonspecifically kill a variety of intracellular and extracellular parasites and kill neoplastic cells (6,93). IFN-γ reduces the susceptibility of macrophages to microbial infection and enhances recognition of targets during the early innate phase of immunity through regulation of macrophage cell surface proteins that remain undefined (94). The physiologic role played by IFN-γ in macrophage activation and host defense against microbial pathogens has been demonstrated in several *in vivo* murine infection models. Mice pretreated with neutralizing antibodies to IFN-γ lose the ability to resist a sublethal challenge of a variety of microbial pathogens, such as *L. monocytogenes* (27,91), *Toxoplasma gondii* (95) or *Leishmania major* (96). Mice with

disrupted genes for IFN-γ, the IFN-γ receptor α chain, or the IFN signaling protein STAT-1 die when challenged with sublethal doses of microbial pathogens such as *Mycobacterium bovis, L. monocytogenes,* or *L. major* (60,97,98).

Activated macrophages kill microbial targets using a variety of toxic substances, such as reactive oxygen and nitrogen intermediates that are induced by IFN-γ. Much of the antimicrobial function of IFN-γ–activated macrophages can be attributed to the actions of nitric oxide (NO) or reactive oxygen intermediates (99,100). Nitric oxide is produced in activated macrophages by the inducible form of nitric oxide synthase (iNOS). The gene encoding iNOS is transcriptionally activated after treatment of cells with IFN-γ plus a variety of second signals that activate the transcription factor NF-κB such as TNF-α, IL-1, or bacterial endotoxin. The enzyme catalyzes the conversion of L-arginine to L-citrulline, giving rise to large amounts of the toxic gas NO.

NO is thought to kill target cells by one of two mechanisms. It can form an iron-nitrosyl complex with Fe-S groups of aconitase and complex I or complex II, causing the inactivation of the mitochondrial electron transport chain. Alternatively, NO may react with superoxide anion (a reactive oxygen intermediate formed by the IFN-γ–induced enzyme NADPH oxidase) to form peroxynitrite, which decays rapidly after protonation to form the highly toxic compound hydroxyl radical. Evidence that NO is responsible for macrophage killing of intracellular parasites comes from a number of studies with *Listeria* and *Leishmania*. Mice pretreated with the L-arginine analogue iNOS inhibitor *N*-monomethyl-L-arginine (NMMA) were unable to resolve footpad infection with *Leishmania* parasites. Similarly, mice treated with another iNOS inhibitor (aminoguanidine) succumbed to sublethal *Listeria* infection (101). Mice lacking the iNOS gene are highly susceptible to infection with microbial pathogens (99,100).

Antigen Processing and Presentation

One of the major immunoregulatory roles of the IFNs is their ability to promote the inductive phase of immune responses. These cytokines significantly influence the generation and presentation of antigenic peptides on cell surfaces (6,7). Among the IFN family members, IFN-γ is uniquely capable of regulating expression of MHC class II proteins, thereby promoting enhanced CD4$^+$ T-cell responses (7,102). IFN-γ induces MHC class II protein expression on many cells, such as mononuclear phagocytes, endothelial cells and epithelial cells. IFN-γ inhibits IL-4–dependent class II expression on B cells (103), although the molecular basis for this apparently discordant effect is unknown. Type I IFN cannot induce MHC class II proteins on cells by itself. However, it can inhibit or enhance IFN-γ's ability to induce MHC class II. In the case of mononuclear phagocytes, preexposure of cells to Type I IFNs induces a state of unresponsiveness to IFN-γ. In contrast, treatment of cells with IFN-α/β concomitant with or after IFN-γ treatment leads to enhanced class II expression. A similar type of modulation of IFN-γ's MHC class II inducing activity is observed with other stimuli such as TNF, bacterial endotoxin, and immune complexes. A cell's ability to express MHC class II in response to IFN-γ is thus influenced by the composition of the microenvironment (6).

One function all IFN family members share is the ability to regulate expression of molecules involved in the MHC class I antigen presentation pathway (7). Some of these effects are at the level of regulating cell surface molecules. Type I IFN and IFN-γ enhance expression of MHC class I proteins and β2-microglobulin on a wide variety of cell types, thereby increasing cell surface levels of functional MHC class I molecules. The proteins also enhance expression of several cell surface proteins, such as intercellular adhesion molecule-1 and B-7, responsible for increasing target cell–T-cell contact and T-cell co-stimulation, respectively (104,105).

The IFNs also promote antigen processing by regulating expression of many intracellular proteins required for antigenic peptide generation (7,105). IFN-γ plays a key role in modifying the activity of the proteasome, a multisubunit enzyme complex that is responsible for generating the peptides that bind to MHC class I proteins. To some extent, IFN-γ mediates its effects by modulating the expression of the enzymatic proteasome subunits. It induces increased expression of LMP-2, LMP-7 (low molecular weight polypeptide proteasome subunit), and MECL-1 and decreased expression of subunits x, y, and z, thereby altering proteasome composition and specificity (105–107). However, IFN-γ also induces expression of nonenzymatic proteasome components, such as the α and β subunits of PA-28 (i.e., the 11S regulator of the proteasome) that function to regulate proteasome enzymatic activity (108). Purified 20S and 26S proteasomes from IFN-γ–treated cells have an increased capacity to generate the types of 9–amino acid peptides that most commonly bind to MHC class I (106).

IFN-γ increases expression of the peptide transporters TAP-1 and TAP-2 (transporters associated with antigen presentation), which transfer peptides that have been generated in the cytoplasm by the proteasome into the endoplasmic reticulum where they can bind to nascently produced MHC class I proteins (104,105). Moreover, IFN-γ increases expression of the heat shock protein gp96, which may play a role in transferring peptide within the cell from the TAPs to MHC class I and between cells from nonprofessional antigen presenting cells to a subset of macrophages (109). Taken together, these observations show that IFN-γ plays an important role in enhancing immunogenicity by increasing the quantity and the repertoire of peptides displayed on MHC class I proteins.

Helper T-Cell Phenotype Development

Human and murine CD4+ T cells can be divided into two subsets defined by their pattern of cytokine secretion after stimulation (26,110). Type 1 helper T cells (T$_H$1) promote cell-mediated immunity and delayed-type hypersensitivity responses through their production of IFN-γ, lymphotoxin, and IL-2. T$_H$2 cells predominantly produce IL-4, IL-5, and IL-10 and thereby provide help for humoral immune responses. IFN-γ plays an important role in T$_H$1 development. In vitro, antibody neutralization of IFN-γ greatly reduces the development of T$_H$1 cells and augments the development of T$_H$2 cells. Administration of exogenous IFN-γ in vitro or in vivo does not drive a T$_H$1 response. Thus, IFN-γ is necessary but is not sufficient for T$_H$1 development.

The single-most important cytokine that drives T cells to the T$_H$1 pole is IL-12, as shown in in vitro and in vivo studies (111,112). Bacterial products promote T$_H$1 cell development by inducing IL-12 production from antigen-presenting cells such as macrophages. Mice deficient in the gene for IL-12 or the IL-12 signaling protein STAT-4 are unable to generate T$_H$1 cells and display reduced delayed-type hypersensitivity responses.

The role of IFN-γ in this process results from its effects at the level of the macrophage and the CD4+ T cell. The effects of IFN-γ on macrophages were elucidated in studies that used transgenic mice lacking IFN-γ sensitivity specifically in the macrophage compartment. IFN-γ–insensitive macrophages were unable to support efficient T$_H$1 development because of a severely reduced capacity to produce IL-12 (113). IFN-γ also directly affects the developing T$_H$ cells. IFN-γ maintains expression of the β2 subunit of the IL-12 receptor on developing T cells, thereby preserving sensitivity of these cells to IL-12 and promoting their development into a T$_H$1 phenotype (114). IFN-γ also blocks development of T$_H$2 phenotype through two mechanisms. First, IFN-γ inhibits synthesis of IL-4 from undifferentiated, antigen-stimulated T cells, thereby inhibiting production of the cytokine that is absolutely required for T$_H$2 development (115). Second, IFN-γ inhibits T$_H$2 cell expansion by directly inhibiting proliferation of T$_H$2 cells (116). The antiproliferative effects of IFN-γ are not observed on T$_H$1 cells, because these cells do not express the IFN-γ receptor β subunit (38,39). IFN-γ simultaneously promotes cell-mediated immunity through facilitating T$_H$1 cell formation and inhibits development of humoral immunity through blockade of T$_H$2 cell expansion.

Humoral Immunity

The IFNs play complex and conflicting roles in regulating humoral immunity. Most analyses have been directed at defining the influence of IFN-γ in the process, although later observations suggest that the Type I IFNs may cause many of the same biologic effects. The IFNs exert their effects indirectly by regulating the development of specific helper T-cell subsets or directly at the level of the B cell. In the latter case, the IFNs are predominantly responsible for regulating three specialized B-cell functions: B-cell development and proliferation, immunoglobulin secretion, and immunoglobulin heavy chain switching.

In the case of murine B-cell differentiation and proliferation, IFN-γ inhibits IL-4–dependent induction of MHC class II protein expression and proliferation of B cells stimulated with anti-immunoglobulin (anti-Ig) and IL-4. In contrast, IFN-γ enhances proliferative responses in human B cells activated with anti-Ig. IFN-γ can also enhance or inhibit Ig secretion by murine or human B cells. However, in this process, IFN-γ's effects depend on the differentiation state of the B cell, the timing of IFN-γ stimulation, and the nature of the activating stimulus.

The best-characterized B-cell–directed actions of the IFNs are their ability to influence Ig heavy chain switching. Immunoglobulin class switching is significant because the different Ig isotypes promote distinct effector functions in the host. IgE is the only isotype that can bind to Fcε receptors on mast cells and basophils and thereby promotes immediate-type hypersensitivity and allergic reactions. IgG2a fixes complement and can, in monomeric form, bind to FcγRI on murine macrophages, a high-affinity Fc receptor that is upregulated during IFN-γ–induced macrophage activation. Activated macrophages can efficiently use antibodies of the IgG2a isotype to mediate antibody-dependent cellular cytotoxicity (ADCC). IgG3 can self-aggregate, which may enhance its opsonic activity and, with IgG2a, can bind to the NK cell IgG receptor CD16 and effect NK-mediated ADCC. By favoring the production of IgG2a and IgG3 while inhibiting the production of IgE isotypes, the IFNs can facilitate the interaction between the humoral and cellular effector limbs of the immune response and increase host defense against certain bacteria and viruses.

In vitro, IFN-γ is able to direct immunoglobulin class switching from IgM to the IgG2a subtype in lipopolysaccharide-stimulated murine B cells and to IgG2a and IgG3 in murine B cells that have been stimulated with activated T cells (117,118). Moreover, IFN-γ blocks IL-4–induced Ig class switching in murine B cells to IgG1 or IgE (119). The validity of these observations has been stringently tested in experiments in which immunoglobulin subclass production was monitored in mice that were injected with IgD-specific antiserum to achieve polyclonal activation of B cells. Mice treated in this manner produced large quantities of IgG1 and IgE. However, when IFN-γ was administered to the mice before anti-IgD treatment, they produced high levels of IgG2a and decreased levels of IgG1. Thus, IFN-γ is an important regulator of immunoglobulin class switching *in vivo* (120).

A role for Type I IFNs in this process has been identified (121). Mice deficient in the receptors for IFN-γ,

IFN-α/β, or both Type I and Type II IFNs were infected with live lymphocytic choriomeningitis virus (LCMV), and the profile of the LCMV-specific antibodies generated was determined. Comparable levels of LCMV-specific IgG2a antibodies were observed in the sera of normal mice and of mice that were unresponsive to IFN-γ or IFN-α/β. In contrast, IgG2a antibodies were not produced in mice with combined unresponsiveness to both types of IFN. These results demonstrate that, when induced during the immune response, Type I IFNs can function in a redundant manner to IFN-γ in effecting immunoglobulin class switching.

Tumor Immunity

An accumulating body of evidence suggests that IFN family members play important roles in promoting host defense to tumors. The IFNs can exert profound antiproliferative effects on a variety of tumor cells. IFN-α/β is, in general, more active in promoting this response than IFN-γ. The IFNs may also inhibit tumor generation by directly increasing expression of several tumor suppressor genes such as those for IRF-1 and PKR.

However, several antitumor activities are unique to IFN-γ. *In vitro*, IFN-γ is able to activate macrophages to nonspecifically lyse certain tumor cells (93,122). IFN-γ is required for robust IL-12 secretion by macrophages. IL-12 has been shown in several studies to possess potent antitumor activities, even in mice with preestablished tumors (112). Injection of recombinant IL-12 into tumor bearing mice reduces the rate of metastasis, slows tumor growth, and in some cases, effects complete tumor regression. IFN-γ is required for IL-12 mediated antitumor effects. This conclusion is based on the observation that neutralizing IFN-γ–specific monoclonal antibodies ablate the effects of IL-12 on tumors *in vivo* (123,124).

Other data support the concept that IFN-γ itself is able to effect antitumor responses under physiologic conditions. Direct injection of IFN-γ *in vivo* reduces the frequency of spontaneous melanoma and hepatic metastasis and reduces tumor growth in several murine tumor models. The actions of IFN-γ in these models appear to be mediated through an augmentation of tumor immunity. For example, lymphocytes harvested from draining lymph nodes of mice harboring the fibrosarcoma MCA105 were able to adoptively transfer immunity to naive mice. This effect was abrogated by *in vivo* administration of neutralizing IFN-γ antibodies to recipient mice.

Work with ultraviolet light–induced murine sarcomas has elegantly demonstrated that CD8+ cytotoxic T lymphocytes can recognize tumor-specific rejection antigens and effect antitumor responses (125–127). For a tumor to grow progressively in an immunocompetent host, it must evade lysis by CD8+ cytotoxic T lymphocytes. Several examples of tumors with specific deficits in many sites along the MHC class I peptide presentation pathway have been identified. Some successfully established tumors have lost expression of antigenic epitopes, MHC molecules, or proteins involved in MHC class I peptide loading. Because IFN-γ increases expression of many of these proteins, it is likely that a major effect of IFN-γ in this process is to increase antigenicity of transformed cells, thereby enhancing tumor specific immunity. There are examples in which IFN-γ treatment was able to restore immunogenicity to nonantigenic, aggressively growing tumors *in vitro* and *in vivo*. In the B16 murine melanoma model, IFN-γ treatment of the tumor cells enhanced *in vitro* lysis of the cells by CD8+ cytotoxic T lymphocytes. IFN-γ–treated B16 melanoma cells when injected into syngeneic mice demonstrated a decreased rate of metastasis and a subsequent increase in host survival compared with untreated cells.

A clear demonstration of a role for IFN-γ in immune-mediated tumor rejection comes from studies that used a variety of transplantable murine fibrosarcomas (128). Overexpression of a mutant nonfunctional IFN-γ receptor α chain in these tumor cells rendered them insensitive to IFN-γ and enhanced their tumorigenicity *in vivo*. IFN-γ–insensitive fibrosarcomas grew more rapidly in naive syngeneic mice than did control tumors and were not rejected when the tumor-bearing mice were treated with lipopolysaccharide. The IFN-γ–insensitive tumors neither primed naive mice for induction of tumor specific immunity nor were rejected in mice with preestablished immunity to the wild-type, IFN-γ–sensitive tumor cell counterpart. This effect was not caused by the antiproliferative actions of IFN-γ. Thus, the ability of the immune system to recognize and reject certain tumors depends on the tumor's ability to respond to IFN-γ.

This conclusion is supported by findings of studies that evaluated whether endogenously produced IFN-γ plays an important role in controlling growth of nascently transformed cells (i.e., whether it controls the formation of primary tumors) (129). For this purpose, IFN-γ receptor knock-out mice, STAT-1 knock-out mice, and wild-type mice, all of which had a pure inbred 129/Sv/Ev background, were treated with different doses of the chemical carcinogen methylcholanthrene, and tumor development was followed through 160 days. At every methylcholanthrene dose examined, IFN-γ–insensitive mice developed tumors significantly more rapidly and with greater frequency compared with wild-type mice. Tumor cells derived from IFN-γ–insensitive mice grew progressively with identical kinetics when transplanted into wild-type mice or the corresponding IFN-γ–insensitive mouse strain. Moreover, introduction of the missing IFN-γ signaling protein into these cells by gene transfer reconstituted their capacity to respond to IFN-γ and converted them into immunogenic tumors that were rejected in wild-type 129/Sv/Ev mice but not mice devoid of lymphocytes. Similar observations were made in a second model in which spontaneous tumor formation was moni-

tored in IFN-γ–sensitive and –insensitive mice that lacked the *P53* tumor suppressor gene.

These results demonstrate that the interplay between IFN-γ and the specific immune system forms the basis of an effective tumor surveillance system in the host. These observations also indicate that the major target of IFN-γ's surveillance functions is the tumor cell itself.

IN VIVO DYSFUNCTION OF INTERFERON-γ SIGNALING

Mice with Disrupted Genes of Interferon-γ Signaling Proteins

The physiologic consequences of global *in vivo* inactivation of the IFN-γ signaling pathway in mice were originally uncovered using neutralizing monoclonal antibodies specific for IFN-γ (91). However, the physiologic roles of IFN-γ were more broadly defined subsequently using mice with disrupted forms of the IFN-γ structural gene (97), the genes encoding the IFN-γ receptor α subunit (98,130), or the genes encoding the three signaling proteins required by IFN-γ for biologic response induction: STAT-1 (60,61), JAK-1 (56), and JAK-2 (57,58). As a group, these mice display a greatly impaired ability to resist infection by a variety of microbial pathogens including *L. monocytogenes*, *L. major*, and several mycobacterial species, including *M. bovis* and *Mycobacterium avium*. Mice lacking the IFN-γ receptor α chain are able to mount a curative response to many viruses, and mice lacking the IFN-α/β receptor or STAT-1 and cells of mice deficient in JAK-1 or JAK-2 are not. These results demonstrate that the antiviral effects of the IFN system are largely mediated through Type I IFNs (131).

Human Patients Who Lack the Interferon-γ Receptor α Chain

Results obtained from IFN-γ receptor–deficient mice suggested that individuals with inactivating mutations in the human IFN-γ receptor α chain gene might suffer from recurrent microbial but not viral infections. Two research groups have identified children with such mutations who manifest a severe susceptibility to weakly pathogenic mycobacterial species (132,133). Four unrelated sets of patients have been identified with inactivating mutations in the IFN-γ receptor α chain gene. One study identified a group of related Maltese children who showed extreme susceptibility to infection with *Mycobacterium fortuitum*, *M. avium*, and *Mycobacterium chelonei* (132). In the other study, a Tunisian child was identified with disseminated *M. bovis* infection after bacillus Calmette-Guérin (BCG) vaccination (133). A third study identified a child of distinct ancestry who had a similar immunocompromised phenotype (134).

Genetic analysis of the families of these patients revealed that the mutations are inherited in an autosomal recessive manner. These patients only showed enhanced susceptibility to mycobacteria and not typical bacteria or other common microbial pathogens or fungi. Moreover, in all three kindred, the patients were able to mount antibody or curative responses to several different viruses. It is important to determine why IFN-γ receptor defects in humans lead exclusively to enhanced susceptibility to mycobacterial infection.

RESEARCH PROSPECTS

In this chapter, we reviewed the basic biochemical and biologic aspects of the IFN family, concentrating on the unique characteristics that differentiate IFN-γ from IFN-α/β. Advances in the field have led to a dramatic increase in our understanding of the molecular mechanisms that underlie IFN receptor signal transduction and in the physiologic roles played by the IFNs in promoting host defense. It is likely that future IFN research will continue to reveal new insights into the physiologic functions of these cytokines and may help in the development of novel therapeutic strategies aimed at regulating the actions of the IFNs in a manner that will promote host defense or dampen immunopathologic processes.

ACKNOWLEDGMENTS

Work performed in the authors' laboratory that was included in this chapter was supported by NIH grant number CA43059 and by grants from Genentech, Inc., and Abbot Laboratories, Inc. The authors are also grateful to past and present members of the Schreiber laboratory for their participation in these studies. This chapter is dedicated to the memory of Dr. Hans Müller-Eberhard, who contributed greatly to our understanding of the innate and specific molecular mechanisms that promote inflammation and with whom Robert D. Schreiber had the privilege of working.

REFERENCES

1. Isaacs A, Lindenmann J. Virus interference. I. The interferon. *Proc R Soc Lond B Biol Sci* 1957;147:258.
2. Wheelock EF. Interferon-like virus-inhibitor induced in human leukocytes by phytohemagglutinin. *Science* 1965;149:310–311.
3. Pestka S, Langer JA, Zoon KC, Samuel CE. Interferons and their actions. *Annu Rev Biochem* 1987;56:727–777.
4. Henco K, Brosius J, Fujisawa A, et al. Structural relationships of human interferon alpha genes and pseudogenes. *J Mol Biol* 1985;185:227–260.
5. Zoon KC, Miller D, Bekisz J, et al. Purification and characterization of multiple components of human lymphoblastoid interferon alpha. *J Biol Chem* 1992;267:15210–15216.
6. Farrar MA, Schreiber RD. The molecular cell biology of interferon-γ and its receptor. *Annu Rev Immunol* 1993;11:571–611.
7. Boehm U, Klamp T, Groot M, Howard JC. Cellular responses to interferon-γ. *Annu Rev Immunol* 1997;15:749–795.
8. Trent JM, Olson S, Lawn RM. Chromosomal localization of human leukocyte, fibroblast, and immune interferon genes by means of *in situ* hybridization. *Proc Natl Acad Sci USA* 1982;79:7809–7813.
9. Uzé G, Lutfalla G, Mogensen KE. Alpha and beta interferon and their receptor and their friends and relations. *J Interferon Res* 1995;15:3–26.
10. Naylor SL, Sakaguchi AY, Shows TB, Law ML, Goeddel DV, Gray PW. Human immune interferon gene is located on chromosome 12. *J Exp Med* 1983;157:1020–1027.
11. Naylor SL, Gray PW, Lalley PA. Mouse immune interferon (IFN-γ) gene is on human chromosome 10. *Somat Cell Mol Genet* 1984;10:531–534.
12. Kelker HC, Le J, Rubin BY, Yip YK, Nagler C, Vilcek J. Three molecular weight forms of natural human interferon-gamma revealed by immunoprecipitation with monoclonal antibody. *J Biol Chem* 1984;259:4301–4304.
13. Scahill SJ, Devos R, Van der Heyden J, Fiers W. Expression and characterization of the product of a human immune interferon cDNA gene in Chinese hamster ovary cells. *Proc Natl Acad Sci USA* 1983;80:4654–4658.
14. Chang TW, McKinney S, Liu V, Kung PC, Vilcek J, Le J. Use of monoclonal antibodies as sensitive and specific probes for biologically active human gamma-interferon. *Proc Natl Acad Sci USA* 1984;81:5219–5222.
15. Ealick SE, Cook WJ, Vijay-Kumar S, et al. Three-dimensional structure of recombinant human interferon-γ. *Science* 1991;252:698–702.
16. Bach EA, Aguet M, Schreiber RD. The IFN-γ receptor: a paradigm for cytokine receptor signaling. *Annu Rev Immunol* 1997;15:563–591.
17. Maniatis T. Mechanisms of human β-interferon gene regulation. *Harvey Lect* 1988;82:71–104.
18. Taniguchi T. Regulation of interferon-β gene: structure and function of *cis*-elements and *trans*-acting factors. *J Interferon Res* 1989;9:633–640.
19. Pitha PM, Au W-C. Induction of interferon alpha genes expression. *Virology* 1995;6:151–159.
20. Tanaka N, Taniguchi T. Cytokine gene regulation: regulatory *cis*-elements and DNA binding factors involved in the interferon system. *Adv Immunol* 1992;52:263–281.
21. Wolf SF, Temple PA, Kobayashi M, et al. Cloning of cDNA for natural killer cell stimulatory factor, a heterodimeric cytokine with multiple biologic effects on T and natural killer cells. *J Immunol* 1991;146:3074–3080.
22. Stern AS, Podlaski FJ, Hulmes JD, et al. Purification to homogeneity and partial characterization of cytotoxic lymphocyte maturation factor from human B-lymphoblastoid cells. *Proc Natl Acad Sci USA* 1990;87:6808–6812.
23. Jacobson NG, Szabo SJ, Weber-Nordt RM, et al. Interleukin 12 signaling in T helper type 1 (Th1) cells involves tyrosine phosphorylation of signal transducer and activator of transcription (Stat) 3 and Stat4. *J Exp Med* 1995;181:1755–1762.
24. Okamura H, Tsutsui H, Komatsu T, et al. Cloning of a new cytokine that induces IFN-γ production by T cells. *Nature* 1995;378:88–91.
25. Robinson D, Shibuya K, Mui A, et al. IGIG does not drive Th1 development, but synergizes with IL-12 for IFN-γ production, and activates IRAK and NF-κB. *Immunity* 1997;7:571–581.
26. O'Garra A. Cytokines induce the development of functionally heterogeneous T helper cell subsets. *Immunity* 1998;8:275–283.
27. Bancroft GJ, Schreiber RD, Unanue ER. Natural immunity, a T-cell–independent pathway of macrophage activation, defined in the scid mouse. *Immunol Rev* 1991;124:5–24.
28. Tripp CS, Wolf SF, Unanue ER. Interleukin-12 and tumor necrosis factor alpha are costimulators of interferon-gamma production by natural killer cells in severe combined immunodeficiency mice with listeriosis, and interleukin-10 is a physiologic antagonist. *Proc Natl Acad Sci USA* 1993;90:3725–3729.
29. Unanue ER. Interrelationship among macrophages, NK cells and neutrophils in early stages of Listeria resistance. *Curr Opin Immunol* 1997;9:35–43.
30. Fiorentino DF, Zlotnik A, Mosmann TR, Howard M, O'Garra A. IL-10 inhibits cytokine production by activated macrophages. *J Immunol* 1991;147:3815–3822.
31. Koppelman B, Neefjes JJ, De Vries JE, de Waal Malefyt R. Interleukin-10 down-regulates MHC class II αβ peptide complexes at the plasma membrane of monocytes by affecting arrival and recycling. *Immunity* 1997;7:861–871.
32. Stark GR, Kerr IM, Williams BRG, Silverman RH, Schreiber RD. How cells respond to interferons. *Annu Rev Biochem* 1998;67:227–264.
33. Bazan JF. Structural design and molecular evolution of a cytokine receptor superfamily. *Proc Natl Acad Sci USA* 1990;87:6934–6938.
34. Cook JR, Emanuel SL, Donnelly RJ, et al. Sublocalization of the human interferon-gamma receptor accessory factor gene and charac-

terization of accessory factor activity by yeast artificial chromosomal fragmentation. *J Biol Chem* 1994;269:7013–7018.

35. Spencer SD, Di Marco F, Hooley J, et al. The orphan receptor CRF2-4 is an essential subunit of the interleukin 10 receptor. *J Exp Med* 1998;187:571–578.

36. Uzé G, Lutfalla G, Gresser I. Genetic transfer of a functional human interferon alpha receptor into mouse cells: cloning and expression of its cDNA. *Cell* 1990;60:225–234.

37. Pestka S, Kotenko SV, Muthukumaran G, Izotova LS, Cook JR, Garotta G. The interferon gamma (IFN-γ) receptor: a paradigm for the multi-chain cytokine receptor. *Cytokine Growth Factor Rev* 1997;8:189–206.

38. Pernis A, Gupta S, Gollob KJ, et al. Lack of interferon-γ receptor β chain and the prevention of interferon-γ signaling in T$_H$1 cells. *Science* 1995;269:245–247.

39. Bach EA, Szabo SJ, Dighe AS, et al. Ligand-induced autoregulation of IFN-γ receptor β chain expression in T helper cell subsets. *Science* 1995;270:1215–1218.

40. Aguet M, Dembic Z, Merlin G. Molecular cloning and expression of the human interferon-γ receptor. *Cell* 1988;55:273–280.

41. Gray PW, Leong S, Fennie EH, et al. Cloning and expression of the cDNA for the murine interferon gamma receptor. *Proc Natl Acad Sci USA* 1989;86:8497–8501.

42. Kumar CS, Muthukumaran G, Frost LJ, et al. Molecular characterization of the murine interferon-γ receptor cDNA. *J Biol Chem* 1989;264: 17939–17946.

43. Munro S, Maniatis T. Expression and cloning of the murine interferon-γ receptor cDNA. *Proc Natl Acad Sci USA* 1989;86:9248–9252.

44. Hemmi S, Peghini P, Metzler M, Merlin G, Dembic Z, Aguet M. Cloning of murine interferon gamma receptor cDNA: expression in human cells mediates high-affinity binding but is not sufficient to confer sensitivity to murine interferon gamma. *Proc Natl Acad Sci USA* 1989;86:9901–9905.

45. Cofano F, Moore SK, Tanaka S, Yuhki N, Landolfo S, Applella E. Affinity purification, peptide analysis, and cDNA sequence of the mouse interferon-γ receptor. *J Biol Chem* 1990;265:4064–4071.

46. Hershey GK, Schreiber RD. Biosynthetic analysis of the human interferon-gamma receptor. Identification of *N*-linked glycosylation intermediates. *J Biol Chem* 1989;264:11981–11988.

47. Mao C, Aguet M, Merlin G. Molecular characterization of the human interferon-gamma receptor: analysis of polymorphism and glycosylation. *J Interferon Res* 1989;9:659–669.

48. Fischer T, Thoma B, Scheurich P, Pfizenmaier K. Glycosylation of the human interferon-gamma receptor: *N*-linked carbohydrates contribute to structural heterogeneity and are required for ligand binding. *J Biol Chem* 1990;265:1710–1717.

49. Soh J, Donnelly RO, Kotenko S, et al. Identification and sequence of an accessory factor required for activation of the human interferon-γ receptor. *Cell* 1994;76:793–802.

50. Hemmi S, Bohni R, Stark G, DiMarco F, Aguet M. A novel member of the interferon receptor family complements functionality of the murine interferon γ receptor in human cells. *Cell* 1994;76:803–810.

51. Darnell JE Jr, Kerr IM, Stark GR. Jak-STAT pathways and transcriptional activation in response to IFNs and other extracellular signaling proteins. *Science* 1994;264:1415–1421.

52. Schindler C, Darnell JE Jr. Transcriptional responses to polypeptide ligands: the JAK-STAT pathway. *Annu Rev Biochem* 1995;64:621–651.

53. Darnell JE Jr. STATs and gene regulation. *Science* 1997;277: 1630–1635.

54. O'Shea JJ. Jaks, STATs, cytokine signal transduction, and immunoregulation: are we there yet? *Immunity* 1997;7:1–11.

55. Ihle JN, Witthuhn BA, Quelle FW, Yamamoto K, Silvennoinen O. Signaling through the hematopoietic cytokine receptors. *Annu Rev Immunol* 1995;13:369–398.

56. Rodig SJ, Meraz MA, White JM, et al. Disruption of the Jak1 gene demonstrates obligatory and nonredundant roles of the Jaks in cytokine-induced biologic responses. *Cell* 1998;93:373–383.

57. Paraganas E, Wang D, Stravopodis D, et al. Jak2 is essential for signaling through a variety of cytokine receptors. *Cell* 1998;93:385–395.

58. Neubauer H, Cumano A, Muller M, Wu H, Huffstadt U, Pfeffer K. Jak2 deficiency defines an essential developmental checkpoint in definitive hematopoiesis. *Cell* 1998;93:397–409.

59. Kotenko SV, Izotova LS, Pollack BP, et al. Other kinases can substitute for Jak2 in signal transduction by interferon-γ. *J Biol Chem* 1996; 271:17174–17182.

60. Meraz MA, White JM, Sheehan KCF, et al. Targeted disruption of the STAT1 gene in mice reveals unexpected physiologic specificity in the Jak-STAT signaling pathway. *Cell* 1996;84:431–442.

61. Durbin JE, Hackenmiller R, Simon MC, Levy DE. Targeted disruption of the mouse Stat1 gene results in compromised innate immunity to viral infection. *Cell* 1996;84:443–450.

62. Bach EA, Tanner JW, Marsters SA, et al. Ligand-induced assembly and activation of the gamma interferon receptor in intact cells. *Mol Cell Biol* 1996;16:3214–3221.

63. Kaplan DH, Greenlund AC, Tanner JW, Shaw AS, Schreiber RD. Identification of an interferon-γ receptor α chain sequence required for JAK-1 binding. *J Biol Chem* 1996;271:9–12.

64. Kotenko S, Izotova L, Pollack B, et al. Interaction between the components of the interferon gamma receptor complex. *J Biol Chem* 1995; 270:20915–20921.

65. Sakatsume M, Igarashi K, Winestock KD, Garotta G, Larner AC, Finbloom DS. The Jak kinases differentially associate with the α and β (accessory factor) chains of the interferon-γ receptor to form a functional receptor unit capable of activating STAT transcription factors. *J Biol Chem* 1995;270:17528–17534.

66. Greenlund AC, Farrar MA, Viviano BL, Schreiber RD. Ligand induced IFN-γ receptor phosphorylation couples the receptor to its signal transduction system (p91). *EMBO J* 1994;13:1591–1600.

67. Greenlund AC, Morales MO, Viviano BL, Yan H, Krolewski J, Schreiber RD. STAT recruitment by tyrosine-phosphorylated cytokine receptors: an ordered reversible affinity-driven process. *Immunity* 1995;2:677–687.

68. Schindler C, Shuai K, Prezioso VR, Darnell JE Jr. Interferon-dependent tyrosine phosphorylation of a latent cytoplasmic transcription factor. *Science* 1992;257:809–813.

69. Shuai K, Stark GR, Kerr IM, Darnell JE Jr. A single phosphotyrosine residue of Stat 91 required for gene activation by interferon-γ. *Science* 1993;261:1744–1746.

70. Colamonici O, Yan H, Domanski P, et al. Direct binding to and tyrosine phosphorylation of the α subunit of the type 1 interferon receptor by p135tyk2 tyrosine kinase. *Mol Cell Biol* 1994;14:8133–8142.

71. Gauzzi MC, Velazquez L, McKendry R, Mogensen KE, Fellous M, Pellegrini S. Interferon-α–dependent activation of Tyk2 requires phosphorylation of positive regulatory tyrosines by another kinase. *J Biol Chem* 1996;271:20494–20500.

72. Novick D, Cohen B, Rubinstein M. The human interferon α/β receptor: characterization and molecular cloning. *Cell* 1994;77:391–400.

73. Li X, Leung S, Kerr IM, Stark GR. Functional subdomains of STAT2 required for preassociation with the α interferon receptor and for signaling. *Mol Cell Biol* 1997;17:2048–2056.

74. Yan H, Krishnan K, Greenlund AC, et al. Phosphorylated interferon-α receptor 1 subunit (IFNaR1) acts as a docking site for the latent form of the 113 kDa STAT2 protein. *EMBO J* 1996;15:1064–1074.

75. Leung S, Qureshi SA, Kerr IM, Darnell JE Jr, Stark GR. Role of STAT2 in alpha interferon signaling pathway. *Mol Cell Biol* 1995;15: 1312–1317.

76. David M, Zhou G, Pine R, Dixon JE, Larner AC. The SH2 domain-containing tyrosine phosphatase PTP1D is required for interferon α/β–induced gene expression. *J Biol Chem* 1996;271:15862–15865.

77. Starr R, Wilson TA, Viney EM, et al. A family of cytokine-inducible inhibitors of signalling. *Nature* 1997;387:917–920.

78. Endo TA, Masuhara M, Yokouchi M, et al. A new protein containing an SH2 domain that inhibits JAK kinases. *Nature* 1997;387:921–924.

79. Naka T, Narazaki M, Hirata M, et al. Structure and function of a new STAT-induced STAT inhibitor. *Nature* 1997;387:924–928.

80. Hilton DJ, Richardson RT, Alexander WS, et al. Twenty proteins containing a C-terminal SOCS box form five structural classes. *Proc Natl Acad Sci USA* 1998;95:114–119.

81. Chung CD, Liao JY, Liu B, et al. Specific inhibition of Stat3 signal transduction by PIAS3. *Science* 1997;278:1803–1805.

82. Kerr IM, Stark GR. The control of interferon-inducible gene expression. *FEBS Lett* 1991;285:194–198.

83. Lewin AR, Reid LE, McMahon M, Stark GR, Kerr IM. Molecular analysis of a human interferon-inducible gene family. *Eur J Biochem* 1991;199:417–423.

84. Vilcek J, Sen GC. Interferons and other cytokines. In: Fields BN, Knipe DM, Howley PM, eds. *Fields virology.* Philadelphia: Lippincott-Raven Publishers, 1996:375–400.

85. Silverman RH, Cirino NM. RNA decay by the Interferon-regulated 2-

5A system as a host defense against viruses. In: Morris DR, Harford JB, eds. *mRNA metabolism and post-transcriptional gene regulation.* New York: John Wiley & Sons, 1997:295–309.

86. Meurs E, Chong K, Galabru J, et al. Molecular cloning and characterization of the human double-stranded RNA-activated protein kinase induced by interferon. *Cell* 1990;62:379–390.

87. McMillan NAJ, Williams BRG. Structure and function of the interferon-induced protein kinase, PKR, and related enzymes. In: Clemens MJ, ed. *Protein phosphorylation in cell growth regulation.* London: Harwood Academic Publishers, 1996:225–254.

88. Arnheiter H, Frese M, Kambadur R, Meier E, Haller O. Mx transgenic mice—animal models of health. *Curr Top Microbiol Immunol* 1996; 206:119–147.

89. Chin YE, Kitagawa M, Su WS, You Z, Iwamoto Y, Fu X. Cell growth arrest and induction of cyclin-dependent kinase inhibitor p21 mediated by Stat1. *Science* 1996;272:719–722.

90. Schreiber RD, Pace JL, Russell SW, Altman A, Katz DH. Macrophage-activating factor produced by a T cell hybridoma: physiochemical and biosynthetic resemblance to gamma-interferon. *J Immunol* 1983;131:826–832.

91. Buchmeier NA, Schreiber RD. Requirement of endogenous interferon-gamma production for resolution of *Listeria monocytogenes* infection. *Proc Natl Acad Sci USA* 1985;82:7404–7408.

92. Nathan CF, Murray HW, Wiebe ME, Rubin BY. Identification of interferon-gamma as the lymphokine that activates human macrophage oxidative metabolism and antimicrobial activity. *J Exp Med* 1983; 158:670–689.

93. Schreiber RD, Celada A. Molecular characterization of interferon gamma as a macrophage activating factor. *Lymphokines* 1985;11: 87–118.

94. Belosevic M, Davis CE, Meltzer MS, Nacy CA. Regulation of activated macrophage antimicrobial activities: identification of lymphokines that cooperate with IFN-gamma for induction of resistance to infection. *J Immunol* 1988;141:890–896.

95. Suzuki Y, Orellana MA, Schreiber RD, Remington JS. Interferon-gamma: the major mediator of resistance against *Toxoplasma gondii.* *Science* 1988;240:516–518.

96. Nacy CA, Fortier AH, Meltzer MS, Buchmeier NA, Schreiber RD. Macrophage activation to kill *Leishmania major*: activation of macrophages for intracellular destruction of amastigotes can be induced by both recombinant interferon-gamma and non-interferon lymphokines. *J Immunol* 1985;135:3505–3511.

97. Dalton DK, Pitts-Meek S, Keshav S, Figari IS, Bradley A, Stewart TA. Multiple defects of immune function in mice with disrupted interferon-γ genes. *Science* 1993;259:1739–1742.

98. Huang S, Hendriks W, Althage A, et al. Immune response in mice that lack the interferon-γ receptor. *Science* 1993;259:1742–1745.

99. Nathan C. Natural resistance and nitric oxide. *Cell* 1995;82:873–876.

100. MacMicking J, Xie Q-W, Nathan C. Nitric oxide and macrophage function. *Annu Rev Immunol* 1997;15:323–350.

101. Beckerman KP, Rogers HW, Corbett JA, Schreiber RD, McDaniel ML, Unanue ER. Release of nitric oxide during the T cell–independent pathway of macrophage activation: its role in resistance to *Listeria monocytogenes.* *J Immunol* 1993;150:888–895.

102. Mach B, Steimle V, Martinez-Soria E, Reith W. Regulation of MHC class II genes: lessons from a disease. *Annu Rev Immunol* 1996;14: 301–331.

103. Mond JJ, Carman J, Sarma C, Ohara J, Finkelman FD. Interferon-gamma suppresses B-cell stimulation factor (BSF-1) induction of class II MHC determinants on B cells. *J Immunol* 1986;137: 3534–3537.

104. Germain RN. Antigen processing and presentation. In: Paul WE, ed. *Fundamental immunology.* New York: Raven Press, 1993:629–676.

105. Pamer E, Cresswell P. Mechanisms of MHC class I restricted antigen processing. *Annu Rev Immunol* 1998;16:323–358.

106. Gaczynska M, Rock KL, Spies T, Goldberg AL. Peptidase activities of proteasomes are differentially regulated by the major histocompatibility complex-encoded genes for LMP2 and LMP7. *Proc Natl Acad Sci USA* 1994;91:9213–9217.

107. York IA, Rock KL. Antigen processing and presentation by the class I major histocompatibility complex. *Annu Rev Immunol* 1996;14: 369–396.

108. Groettrup M, Soza A, Eggers M, et al. A role for the proteasome regulator PA28α in antigen presentation. *Nature* 1996;381:166–168.

109. Suto R, Srivastava PK. A mechanism for the specific immunogenicity of heat shock proteins-chaperoned peptides. *Science* 1995;269: 1585–1588.

110. Abbas AK, Murphy KM, Sher A. Functional diversity of helper T lymphocytes. *Nature* 1997;383:787–793.

111. Hsieh C-S, Macatonia S, Tripp CS, Wolf SF, O'Garra A, Murphy KM. Development of Th1 CD4+ T cells through IL-12 produced by *Listeria*-induced macrophages. *Science* 1993;260:547–549.

112. Gately MK, Renzetti LM, Magram J, et al. Interleukin-12/interleukin-12-receptor system: role in normal and pathologic immune responses. *Annu Rev Immunol* 1998;16:495–521.

113. Dighe AS, Campbell D, Hsieh C-S, et al. Tissue specific targeting of cytokine unresponsiveness in transgenic mice. *Immunity* 1995;3: 657–666.

114. Szabo SJ, Dighe AS, Gubler U, Murphy KM. Regulation of the interleukin (IL)-12R B2 subunit expression in developing T helper 1 (Th1) and Th2 cells. *J Exp Med* 1997;185:817–824.

115. Szabo SJ, Jacobson NG, Dighe AS, Gubler U, Murphy KM. Developmental commitment to the Th2 lineage by extinction of IL-12 signaling. *Immunity* 1995;2:665–675.

116. Gajewski TF, Fitch FW. Anti-proliferative effect of IFN-gamma in immune regulation. IV. Murine CTL clones produce IL-3 and GM-CSF, the activity of which is masked by the inhibitory action of secreted IFN-gamma. *J Immunol* 1990;144:548–556.

117. Snapper CM, Peschel C, Paul WE. IFN-gamma stimulates IgG2a secretion by murine B cells stimulated with bacterial lipopolysaccharide. *J Immunol* 1988;140:2121–2127.

118. Snapper CM, McIntyre TM, Mandler R, et al. Induction of IgG3 secretion by interferon gamma: a model for T cell–independent class switching in response to T cell–independent type 2 antigens. *J Exp Med* 1992;175:1367–1371.

119. Snapper CM, Paul WE. Interferon-gamma and B cell stimulatory factor-1 reciprocally regulate Ig isotype production. *Science* 1987;236: 944–947.

120. Snapper CM. Interferon-gamma. In: Snapper CM, ed. *Cytokine regulation of humoral immunity.* West Sussex: John Wiley & Sons, 1996: 325–346.

121. van den Broek MF, Muller U, Huang S, Aguet M, Zinkernagel RM. Antiviral defense in mice lacking both alpha/beta and gamma interferon receptors. *J Virol* 1995;69:4792–4796.

122. Adams DO, Hamilton TA. The cell biology of macrophage activation. *Annu Rev Immunol* 1984;2:283–318.

123. Nastala CL, Edington HD, McKinney TG, et al. Recombinant IL-12 administration induces tumor regression in association with IFN-γ production. *J Immunol* 1994;153:1697–1706.

124. Brunda MJ. Interleukin-12. *J Leukoc Biol* 1994;55:280–288.

125. Kripke ML. Immunologic mechanisms in UV radiation carcinogenesis. *Adv Cancer Res* 1981;34:69–106.

126. Schreiber H, Ward PL, Rowley DA, Strauss HJ. Unique tumor-specific antigens. *Annu Rev Immunol* 1988;6:465–483.

127. Schreiber H. Tumor immunology. In: Paul WE, ed. *Fundamental immunology.* New York: Raven Press, 1993:1143–1178.

128. Dighe AS, Richards E, Old LJ, Schreiber RD. Enhanced *in vivo* growth and resistance to rejection of tumor cells expressing dominant negative IFNγ receptors. *Immunity* 1994;1:447–456.

129. Kaplan DH, Shankaran V, Dighe AS, et al. Demonstration of an IFNγ dependent tumor surveillance system in immunocompetent mice. *Proc Natl Acad Sci USA* 1998;95:7556–7561.

130. Kamijo R, Le J, Shapiro D, Havell EA, et al. Mice that lack the interferon-γ receptor have profoundly altered responses to infection with bacillus Calmette-Guérin and subsequent challenge with lipopolysaccharide. *J Exp Med* 1993;178:1435–1440.

131. Müller U, Steinhoff U, Reis LFL, et al. Functional role of type I and type II interferons in antiviral defense. *Science* 1994;264: 1918–1921.

132. Newport MJ, Huxley CM, Huston S, et al. A mutation in the interferon-γ-receptor gene and susceptibility to mycobacterial infection. *N Engl J Med* 1996;335:1941–1949.

133. Jouanguy E, Altare F, Lamhamedi S, et al. Interferon-γ-receptor deficiency in an infant with fatal bacille Calmette-Guérin infection. *N Engl J Med* 1996;335:1956–1961.

134. Pierre-Audigier C, Jouanguy E, Lamhamedi S, et al. Fatal disseminated *Mycobacterium smegmatis* infection in a child with inherited interferon γ receptor deficiency. *Clin Infect Dis* 1997;24:982–984.

Inflammation: Basic Principles and Clinical Correlates,
3rd ed., edited by John I. Gallin and Ralph Snyderman.
Lippincott Williams & Wilkins, Philadelphia © 1999.

CHAPTER 34

Interleukin-12

Giorgio Trinchieri

Interleukin-12 (IL-12) is a heterodimeric cytokine, composed of a heavy chain of 40 kd (p40) and a light chain of 35 kd (p35), originally described with the names of natural killer stimulatory factor (1) or cytotoxic lymphocyte maturation factor (2). IL-12 is produced within a few hours of infection, particularly in the case of bacteria and intracellular parasites (3), and it acts as a proinflammatory cytokine, activating natural killer (NK) cells (1) and, through its ability to induce IFN-γ production (1,4,5), enhancing the phagocytic and bacteriocidal activity of phagocytic cells and their ability to release proinflammatory cytokines, including IL-12 itself (6). IL-12 produced during the early phases of infection and inflammation sets the stage for the ensuing antigen-specific immune response, favoring differentiation and function of helper T cells type 1 (T$_H$1) T cells while inhibiting the differentiation of T$_H$2 T cells (7–9). IL-12, in addition to being a potent proinflammatory cytokine, is a key immunoregulator molecule in T$_H$1 responses.

INTERLEUKIN-12 GENES AND RECEPTOR

The two genes encoding the two chains of IL-12 are separate and unrelated (10,11); the gene encoding the p35 light chain has limited homology with other single-chain cytokines (12), whereas the gene encoding the p40 heavy chain is homologous to the extracellular domain of genes of the hemopoietic cytokine receptor family (13). The p35 and the p40 chains are covalently linked to form a biologically active heterodimer (p70). The IL-12 heterodimer resembles a cytokine linked to a soluble form of its receptor; an analogous situation is observed for IL-6, IL-11, and ciliary neurotropic factor (CNTF), three cytokines that can bind in solution to the soluble form of one chain of their receptor to create complexes that bind to other transmembrane chains of their receptor, including the shared gp130 chain, inducing signal transduction and biologic functions.

The p40 heavy chain of IL-12 is most homologous to the CNTF receptor and to the IL-6 receptor (α chain) (13,14), whereas the p35 light chain has some homology with IL-6 itself (12). IL-12 probably is evolutionarily derived from a primordial cytokine similar to IL-6/CNTF and from a chain of its original receptor.

The p35 subunit has seven cysteine residues, six of which are involved in intrachain disulfide bonds or form the intersubunit disulfide pairing (15). The p40 subunit possesses 10 cysteine residues, 8 of which are involved in intrachain disulfide bonds (15). All the intramolecular pairs support the homology of IL-12 p35 and p40 to IL-6 and IL-6 receptor, respectively. The p35 gene is located on human chromosome 3p12-q13.2 (16). The Cys^{252} of the p40 chain does not have a corresponding residue in the IL-6 receptor, and it is not paired with any other cysteine in IL-12 but is cysteinylated or contains thioglycolate paired with sulfur (15). The gene encoding the p40 heavy chain of IL-12 is located on human chromosome 5q31-q33 within or close to a cluster of genes encoding other cytokines and cytokine receptors, including IL-4 (16).

Two or more IL-12 binding affinities are observed on IL-12–responsive cells, and the receptors with the highest affinity, in the picomolar range, are probably responsible for IL-12 biologic activity (17,18). Two chains of the IL-12 receptor, IL-12Rβ1 and IL-12Rβ2, have been cloned and are members of the cytokine receptor superfamily and within that family are most closely related to gp130 (18–20). IL-12Rβ1 and IL-12Rβ2 have cytoplasmic regions that contain the characteristic box I and II motifs found in other cytokine receptors (18,19). However, conserved cytoplasmic tyrosine residues are missing from the β1 subunit, whereas the IL-12R β2 subunit contains three cytoplasmic tyrosine residues that probably are involved in signaling processes. Each subunit alone binds IL-12 with only low affinity (K$_d$=2 to 5 nmol/L). Coexpression of both receptor subunits results in high-affinity (K$_d$=50 pmol/L) and low-affinity (K$_d$=5 nmol/L) IL-12 binding sites (18). IL-12 p40 interacts mostly with IL-

G. Trinchieri: The Wistar Institute, Philadelphia, Pennsylvania 19104.

12Rβ1, whereas IL-12 p35, or possibly an epitope on IL-12 composed of both ligand subunits, appears to interact mostly with the IL-12Rβ2 of the receptor complex (18).

The cells producing IL-12 secrete a large excess of the free p40 chain over the biologically active heterodimer, from a few-fold, as observed in activated phagocytic cells, to 100- to 1,000-fold (3,21). Human and murine recombinant p40 IL-12 is secreted by transfected cells as a disulfide-bonded homodimer and as a monomer. Homodimer p40 production has been observed in vivo in the mouse, although not in humans (22). Murine p40 homodimers bind to the IL-12Rβ1 chain with an affinity similar to that of the heterodimers and compete with the heterodimers for binding to the IL-12 receptor, effectively blocking the biologic functions of IL-12 on murine cells (23,24). On human cells, the homodimers bind to the IL-12R with a much lower affinity than the heterodimers and act as antagonists only at much higher concentrations than on murine cells (25). In the mouse, but probably not in humans, the IL-12 p40 homodimer may represent a physiologic antagonist of IL-12.

Resting T and NK cells do not express or express only at very low levels the IL-12R (26); however, resting peripheral blood T and NK cells rapidly respond to IL-12 with IFN-γ production and enhancement of cytotoxic functions, suggesting that the receptor is present at least in a proportion of the cells or that it can be rapidly activated in culture (1). Activation of T and NK cells induces upregulation of IL-12R, as identified by low- and high-affinity binding and upregulation at least of the IL-12Rβ1 gene (26,27). Certain cell types, such as human B-lymphoblastoid cell lines and normal B cells, also express the IL-12Rβ1 mRNA, usually without expressing IL-12 binding sites (28,29), suggesting that IL-12Rβ1 is essential but not sufficient for expression of functional, high-affinity IL-12R and that the IL-12Rβ2 subunit may be more restricted in its expression than IL-12Rβ1.

Signal transduction through the IL-12R induces tyrosine phosphorylation of the Janus family kinases JAK-2 and TYK-2 (30) and of the transcription factors STAT-3 and STAT-4 (31,32); the induction of STAT-4 is rather selective for IL-12, although one study has suggested that another cytokine, IFN-α, may share this ability with IL-12 (33). STAT-4 activation appears to mediate many or most of the activity of IL-12, because mice genetically deficient in STAT-4 appear to have a phenotype equivalent to that of IL-12 p40-deficient mice (34–36). Phosphorylation and activation of the 44-kd mitogen-activated protein (MAP) kinase may be responsible for the serine phosphorylation also observed in STAT-4 on stimulation of T cells with IL-12 (37).

CELL TYPES PRODUCING INTERLEUKIN-12

IL-12 was originally discovered as a product of Epstein-Barr virus (EBV)–transformed B-cell lines,

which all constitutively produce at least low levels of IL-12 p40 (1,2,28). Although malignant or EBV-transformed B-cell lines produce IL-12, the physiologic relevance of IL-12 production from normal B cells remains to be established, and subsequent studies suggested that phagocytic cells are the major physiologic producers of IL-12 (38), a conclusion supported by many in vitro and in vivo studies. Monocytes produce high levels of IL-12 p40 and p70 when stimulated by bacteria, such as heat-fixed Staphylococcus aureus or bacterial products such as lipopolysaccharide (LPS) or Streptococcus extracts (38). In addition to monocytes, polymorphonuclear cells (PMNs) also respond to LPS stimulation with production of IL-12 (39).

On monocytes and PMNs, IFN-γ has a powerful enhancing effect on IL-12 production (6,40), probably potentiating it within inflammatory tissues. The ability of IFN-γ to enhance the production of IL-12 by phagocytic cells is of particular interest because IL-12 is a potent inducer of IFN-γ production by T and NK cells (1,4,5). IL-12–induced IFN-γ exerts positive feedback in inflammation by enhancing IL-12 production. Because IL-12 is the major cytokine responsible for the differentiation of type 1 helper T cells (T$_H$1), which are producers of IFN-γ (7–9), the enhancing effect of IFN-γ on IL-12 production may represent a mechanism by which T$_H$1 responses are maintained in vivo. The ability of IFN-γ to enhance IL-12 production is particularly evident and required for IL-12 production in response to certain infectious agents, such as mycobacteria, which are rather poor inducers of IL-12 production (41). However, with many other inducers, such as LPS, Toxoplasma gondii, and S. aureus, IL-12 production in vivo and in vitro precedes and is required for IFN-γ production (42–44).

The positive feedback amplification of IL-12 production mediated by IFN-γ represents a potentially dangerous mechanism leading to uncontrolled cytokine production. There are, however, potent mechanisms of downregulation of IL-12 production and of the ability of T and NK cells to respond to IL-12. IL-10 is a potent inhibitor of IL-12 production by phagocytic cells (45). The ability of IL-10 to suppress production of IFN-γ and other T$_H$1 cytokines primarily results from its inhibition of IL-12 production from antigen-presenting cells (APCs) and inhibition of expression of co-stimulatory surface molecules (e.g., B-7) and soluble cytokines (e.g., TNF-α, IL-1β) (45–47). Another powerful inhibitor of IL-12 production is TGF-β (38). IL-4 and IL-13 also partially inhibit IL-12 production (38), suggesting that T$_H$2 cells, by producing cytokines such as IL-10, IL-4, and IL-13, suppress IL-12 production and prevent the emergence of a T$_H$1 response (48).

Another cell type reported to express IL-12 mRNAs and possibly secrete minute levels of IL-12 protein is the keratinocyte (49,50). However, the physiologic significance of this production is doubtful because, when used as APCs, keratinocytes induce no stimulation of IFN-γ production unless exogenous IL-12 is added to the cultures (51). Analysis of IL-12 production by skin cells suggests that Langerhans cells rather than keratinocytes are the major producers (52).

The production of IL-12 by Langerhans cells raises the issue of the ability of professional APCs, such as dendritic cells, to produce IL-12 and their role during antigen-presentation and T-cell activation. Definitive evidence that dendritic cells are producers of IL-12 came from studies demonstrating that, when endogenous IL-4 production is blocked, these cells induce a T_H1 response, which is prevented by neutralizing anti-IL-12 antibodies (53). Extensive studies with human and mouse dendritic cells have confirmed that dendritic cells are efficient producers of the IL-12 that acts in inducing T_H1 responses on antigen presentation by these APCs (54–56).

In addition to the induction of IL-12 observed in response to infectious agents, activated T cells stimulate production of IL-12 by macrophages and dendritic cells (53,57). The mechanism of this T-cell–dependent induction of IL-12 is based on the interaction of CD40 ligand (CD40L) on the surface of activated T cells with CD40 on the APCs and can be mimicked by crosslinking CD40 on the surface of IL-12 producing cells with anti-CD40 antibodies or recombinant CD40L (56,58–60). The induction of IL-12 by bacterial or other infectious agents and by activated T cells represents two independent pathways of APC activation, as shown by the observation that spleen cells from CD40 knock-out mice are completely unable to produce IL-12 in response to activated T cells but produce normal levels of IL-12 in response to endotoxin or *S. aureus* (61). However, during an infection or an immune response *in vivo*, it is probable that both pathways are activated, the T-cell–independent path during the inflammatory phase of innate resistance and the T-cell–dependent one during the subsequent adaptive immune response. The inflammatory pathway may be responsible for the initiation of the T_H1 response and the T-cell–dependent pathway for its maintenance.

MOLECULAR CONTROL OF INTERLEUKIN-12 PRODUCTION

On activation of phagocytic cells with LPS or *S. aureus,* accumulation of IL-12 p40 mRNA is observed within 2 to 4 hours, slightly delayed compared with that of other proinflammatory cytokines such as tumor necrosis factor-α (TNF-α), and then it subsides after several hours (45). The induction of p40 expression is largely controlled at the transcriptional level, and the enhancing effect of IFN-γ and the inhibitory effect of IL-10 are reflected in changes in the rate of IL-12 gene transcription (40,62). The promoter of the p40 gene is constitutively active in EBV-transformed cell lines and inducible in myeloid cell lines, but not in T-cell lines; IFN-γ priming of the myeloid cells greatly enhances the activation of the promoter by LPS (40). A region responsible for promoter induction and activity is between nucleotides -196 and -224, and it binds a series of IFN-γ– and LPS-induced nuclear proteins, including ETS-2 and ETS-related factors (63). Promoter constructs with deletion or mutations in this region display a reduced but still detectable IFN-γ/LPS inducible promoter activity, contributed in part by a site between -123 and -99, to which the transcriptional factor NF-κB binds (64).

Gene expression for p35 is also upregulated on activation of phagocytic cells, although its ubiquitous constitutive expression has complicated analysis of its expression using nonpurified cell preparations (3,65,66). P35 upregulation is inhibited by IL-10, whereas IFN-γ enhances transcription and mRNA accumulation of the p35 gene (40,62). In activated phagocytic cells and in B-cell lines, p40 mRNA is approximately 10-fold more abundant than p35 mRNA, consistent with the overproduction and secretion of the free p40 chain over the p35-containing heterodimer.

BIOLOGIC ACTIVITIES

IL-12 synergizes with other hematopoietic factors in enhancing survival and proliferation of early multipotent hematopoietic progenitor cells and lineage-committed precursor cells (40,67,68). Although *in vitro* IL-12 has prevalently stimulatory effects on hematopoiesis, *in vivo* IL-12 treatment results in decreased bone marrow hematopoiesis and in transient anemia and neutropenia (69,70). The toxic effects of IL-12 on hematopoiesis are mostly mediated by IFN-γ, and in its absence, treatment with IL-12 results only in stimulation of hematopoiesis (71).

IL-12 induces T and NK cells to produce several cytokines, particularly IFN-γ (4,72). IL-12–induced IFN-γ production requires the presence of low levels of TNF and IL-1 (45). The importance of IL-12 as an IFN-γ inducer consists of its high efficiency at low concentrations and its synergy with many other activating stimuli (4,5,46). IL-12 is required for optimal IFN-γ production *in vivo* during immune responses, especially in bacterial or parasitic infections (36). In response to macrophage-produced IL-12, NK cells readily produce IFN-γ, which activates macrophages and enhances their bacteriocidal activity, providing a mechanism of T-cell–independent macrophage activation during the early phases of innate resistance (73–75).

IL-12 does not induce proliferation of resting peripheral blood T cells or NK cells, although it potentiates the proliferation of T cells induced by various mitogens and has a direct proliferative effect on preactivated T and NK cells (1,76,77). IL-12 is effective at lower concentrations than IL-2, although the levels of proliferation obtained with IL-12 are much lower than those observed with IL-2 (77). However, co-stimulation through the CD28 receptor by the B-7 ligand or anti-CD28 antibodies strongly synergizes with IL-12 in inducing efficient T-cell proliferation and cytokine production (46,47). Because B-7 is a surface molecule and IL-12 is a secreted product of APCs, their synergistic effect on T cells plays an important role in inducing T-cell proliferation and IFN-γ production on antigen presentation to T cells.

IL-12 also enhances the generation of cytotoxic T lymphocytes (CTLs) and lymphokine activated killer (LAK) cells, and potentiates the cytotoxic activity of CTLs and NK cells (1,78). Some of the effects of IL-12 on cell-mediated cytotoxicity result from increased formation of cytoplasmic granules and induction of transcription of genes encoding cytotoxic granule-associated molecules, such as perforin and granzymes (72,79). The ability of IL-12 to induce expression of adhesion molecules on T and NK cells also may affect their cytotoxic activity and their ability to migrate to tissues (80,81).

Induction of T_H1 Responses

IL-12 is required for T_H1 cell development during the immune response to pathogens, and the type of T_H cell differentiation is most likely determined early after infection by the balance between IL-12 and IL-4, which favors T_H1 and T_H2 development, respectively (7–9). IL-12 is produced by phagocytic cells, other APCs, and possibly B cells, whereas IL-4 is produced by subsets of T cells and by mast cells.

The defining characteristic of the T_H1 and T_H2 cells is that they stably express the ability to produce certain cytokines but not others. IL-12 is particularly powerful, when present early in clonal expansion, in priming CD4$^+$ and CD8$^+$ T cells to produce high levels of IFN-γ on restimulation (82–84). IL-12, produced during the inflammatory phase of infections or immune responses, induces NK cells and T cells to produce IFN-γ; IL-12, in cooperation with IFN-γ, then induces the T-cell clones expanding in response to the specific antigens to differentiate into T_H1 cells by priming them for expression of cytokines such as IFN-γ and by exerting other positive or negative selective mechanisms, including, for example, deletion of IL-4 producing cells or preferential expansion of cells with T_H1-like phenotype (84).

During developmental commitment of BALB/c CD4$^+$ T cells to the T_H2 lineage, the ability of T cells to signal in response to IL-12 is extinguished because of downregulation of IL-12Rβ2 expression (85,86). Similarly, human T_H2 clones lose expression of the IL-12Rβ2 chain (87). However, T_H2 cells are not completely unresponsive to IL-12, at least in the human (82), and IL-12Rβ2 may be upregulated on T_H2 cells by IFN-γ in mice (86) and IFN-α/β in the human (87). After a T_H1 response is induced in vivo, IL-12 is, in most cases, unnecessary for maintaining it (88–90). However, differentiated T_H1 cells maintain IL-12 responsiveness, and IL-12, produced by APCs during cognate antigen presentation to T cells, appears to be important, at least in autoimmune diseases,

for optimal proliferation and cytokine production of the T_H1 cells in response to antigens (47,91,92).

Many of the effects of IL-12 on B-cell activation and immunoglobulin isotype production could be interpreted as mediated by either subset of the helper T cells or by their products, IFN-γ in particular (93). However, evidence has been provided that IL-12 may directly affect B-cell proliferation and differentiation (94).

Role in Infections

The proinflammatory functions of IL-12 and its ability to stimulate innate resistance and to generate a T_H1-type immune response are essential for resistance to infection, particularly by bacteria, fungi, and intracellular parasites (95,96). The most acute instance of IL-12 production resulting in IFN-γ induction is observed in models of endotoxic-induced shock (42,97). Similar pathogenetic mechanisms mediated by IL-12 are involved in the toxic shock–like syndromes induced by superantigenic exotoxins produced by gram-positive bacteria, such as Streptococcus pyogenes and S. aureus (98). The role of endogenous IL-12 in resistance to infection or the possibility of using IL-12 in therapy of infections has been analyzed in many studies (95,96). In helminthic infections, T_H2 responses are most effective in the elimination of the pathogen and their eggs, while IL-12 treatment decreases the resistance of the host (99).

Unlike what is observed in bacterial and intracellular parasite infections, IL-12 has a relatively minor role in resistance to virus infection, where IL-12–independent mechanisms of IFN-γ production are operative (100,101). Even if IL-12 has a modest role in viral resistance, its immunoregulatory activity can be used by including IL-12 as an adjuvant in vaccines composed of inactivated viruses or isolated viral proteins (102,103).

The ability of peripheral blood mononuclear cells from patients infected with human immunodeficiency virus (HIV) to produce IL-12 in vitro is profoundly and selectively depressed (104,105). However, NK and T cells from HIV-infected patients respond normally to exogenous IL-12 (106,107). IL-12 can prevent apoptosis in T cells of HIV-infected patients and correct in vitro their defective proliferative response to recall antigens, alloantigens, and mitogens (107,108). Because IL-12 has immunoregulatory effects favoring generation of T_H1 cells and cell-mediated cytotoxicity and because in vivo treatment of animals with neutralizing anti-IL-12 antibodies results in a loss of delayed-type hypersensitivity responses similar to that observed in HIV-infected patients, a deficient in vivo production of IL-12 may be in part responsible for HIV-induced immunodeficiency.

A transient loss of delayed-type hypersensitivity and immunodeficiency is observed in patients infected or vaccinated with measles virus; in vitro measles virus selectively inhibits production of IL-12 and transcription of the two genes encoding IL-12, without significantly affecting the production of other proinflammatory cytokines (109). This inhibition is also observed using other ligands of the measles receptor (CD46 or membrane cofactor protein) such as anti-CD46 monoclonal antibodies or polymerized complement (109).

POSSIBLE CLINICAL APPLICATIONS

The immunoregulatory role of IL-12 is of central importance in the immunity against invaders such as bacteria, intracellular parasites, and tumors, which require immunity based on cell-mediated mechanisms and phagocytic cell activation supported by T_H1 cells. Administration of IL-12 early in infection enhances the efficiency of an immune response and can convert an inefficient T_H2 response to intracellular pathogens to a protective T_H1 response, as exemplified by the studies of cutaneous leishmaniasis and other infectious pathogens in mice (110,111). In a clinical situation, it is usually impossible to treat a patient at the time of infection, and after the immune response to an infectious pathogen is established, the administration of IL-12 is relatively inefficient in modifying it (110,112), making its direct use in infections problematic. However, it has been shown that when used in combination with other drugs directly affecting pathogen replication and load, IL-12 may convert an established T_H2 response to a protective T_H1, reflecting a possible clinical use (113). In mice susceptible to *Mycobacterium avium* infection and with inadequate production of endogenous IL-12, replacement therapy with IL-12 ameliorates an established infection (114).

The ability of IL-12 to facilitate T_H1 immune responses is at the basis of its successful use as an adjuvant in vaccination in combination with soluble antigens or killed pathogens, usually poor vaccines, to induce a T_H1-biased memory response able to maintain protective immunity (102,103,111). As an adjuvant in vaccination, IL-12 has a potentiating effect on antibody formation of all isotypes (115,116); these results suggest that IL-12 may have more complex immunoregulatory effects than those previously characterized and suggest its potential use in vaccination against a variety of infections against which cellular or humoral immunity is required. Although these potential uses of IL-12 in therapy, particularly its use as an adjuvant in vaccination, are strongly supported by preclinical data, no clinical trials in infectious disease have been started, with the exception of limited phase I trials enrolling patients with HIV infections, with the hope of boosting their compromised immune system in responding to infection with HIV itself or opportunistic pathogens, and those with chronic hepatitis, in an attempt to use the *in vivo* antiviral activity of IL-12.

Although IL-12 as a powerful proinflammatory cytokine plays a crucial role in the first line of defense against infec-

tion, it is also responsible for some of the negative side effects of inflammation. These include hematologic alterations, damage to the liver and gastrointestinal tract, and sensitization to the lethal effects of endotoxin (71,117). These pathogenic effects of IL-12 resulted in considerable toxicity in phase I and II clinical trials with cancer patients and limited the tolerated dosage (118).

The remarkable antitumor activity of IL-12 observed in preclinical studies (69,119) has still to be transformed into clinical utility. The antitumor effect of IL-12 is indirect and based on several mechanisms: activation of innate and antigen-specific adaptive immunity against the tumor cells and ability through IFN-γ to inhibit tumor angiogenesis (119–121). The preclinical studies suggest that appropriate schedules of administration and the combination of IL-12 with other cytokines, such as IL-2 (122), or with a co-stimulator factor, such as the B-7 ligand for the CD28 receptor on T cells, may be used clinically to reduce the toxicity of IL-12 treatment and maximize its antitumor effect.

Based on its ability to block T_H2 cell differentiation, particularly IL-4 production, IL-12 also has an antiallergic activity, demonstrated by its ability to prevent airway hyperresponsiveness and asthma, even in already sensitized animals, which reflects the stage of disease in patients (123). Because of the role of IL-12 in inducing and maintaining T_H1 response, overexpression of this cytokine is likely to play a role in organ-specific autoimmunity, as confirmed by emerging evidence in many of these syndromes (91,124). Antagonists of IL-12 production or action could find a therapeutic use in these syndromes.

CONCLUSIONS

IL-12 is a proinflammatory cytokine and a potent immunoregulatory molecule. It provides an important functional bridge between innate resistance and adaptive immunity. It plays a central and necessary role in the resistance to many intracellular pathogens. Because its potent activity may result in severe systemic and tissue toxicity, its production is strictly regulated, even more than that of other proinflammatory cytokines. Its activities suggest great therapeutic potential for this cytokine in infectious diseases and cancer, but its serious toxicity presents a challenge.

ACKNOWLEDGMENTS

The experimental work of the author described in this chapter was in part supported by NIH grants CA10815, CA20833, CA32898, and AI34412.

REFERENCES

1. Kobayashi M, Fitz L, Ryan M, et al. Identification and purification of natural killer cell stimulatory factor (NKSF), a cytokine with multiple biologic effects on human lymphocytes. *J Exp Med* 1989;170: 827–846.

2. Stern AS, Podlaski FJ, Hulmes JD, et al. Purification to homogeneity and partial characterization of cytotoxic lymphocyte maturation factor from human B-lymphoblastoid cells. *Proc Natl Acad Sci USA* 1990; 87:6808–6812.

3. D'Andrea A, Rengaraju M, Valiante NM, et al. Production of natural killer cell stimulatory factor (NKSF/IL-12) by peripheral blood mononuclear cells. *J Exp Med* 1992;176:1387–1398.

4. Chan SH, Perussia B, Gupta JW, et al. Induction of IFN-γ production by NK cell stimulatory factor (NKSF): characterization of the responder cells and synergy with other inducers. *J Exp Med* 1991;173: 869–879.

5. Chan SH, Kobayashi M, Santoli D, Perussia B, Trinchieri G. Mechanisms of IFN-γ induction by natural killer cell stimulatory factor (NKSF/IL-12): role of transcription and mRNA stability in the synergistic interaction between NKSF and IL-2. *J Immunol* 1992;148: 92–98.

6. Kubin M, Chow JM, Trinchieri G. Differential regulation of interleukin-12 (IL-12), tumor necrosis factor-α, and IL-1β production in human myeloid leukemia cell lines and peripheral blood mononuclear cells. *Blood* 1994;83:1847–1855.

7. Manetti R, Parronchi P, Giudizi MG, et al. Natural killer cell stimulatory factor (NKSF/IL-12) induces Th1-type specific immune responses and inhibits the development of IL-4 producing Th cells. *J Exp Med* 1993;177:1199–1204.

8. Hsieh C, Macatonia SE, Tripp CS, Wolf SF, O'Garra A, Murphy KM. *Listeria*-induced Th1 development in α-TCR transgenic CD4⁺ T cells occurs through macrophage production of IL-12. *Science* 1993;260: 547–549.

9. Trinchieri G. Interleukin-12 and its role in the generation of T$_H$1 cells. *Immunol Today* 1993;14:335–338.

10. Wolf SF, Temple PA, Kobayashi M, et al. Cloning of cDNA for natural killer cell stimulatory factor, a heterodimeric cytokine with multiple biologic effects on T and natural killer cells. *J Immunol* 1991;146: 3074–3081.

11. Gubler U, Chua AO, Schoenhaut DS, et al. Coexpression of two distinct genes is required to generate secreted bioactive cytotoxic lymphocyte maturation factor. *Proc Natl Acad Sci USA* 1991;88:4143–4147.

12. Merberg DM, Wolf SF, Clark SC. Sequence similarity between NKSF and the IL-6/G-CSF family. *Immunol Today* 1992;13:77–78.

13. Gearing DP, Cosman D. Homology of the p40 subunit of natural killer cell stimulatory factor (NKSF) with the extracellular domain of the interleukin-6 receptor. *Cell* 1991;66:9–10.

14. Schoenhaut DS, Chua AO, Wolitzky AG, et al. Cloning and expression of murine IL-12. *J Immunol* 1992;148:3433–3440.

15. Tangarone BS, Vath JE, Nickbarg EB, Yu W, Harris AS, Scoble HA. The disulfide bond structure of recombinant human interleukin-12. In: Marshak DR, ed. *Techniques in protein chemistry. VII: Abstracts of the 9th Symposium of the Protein Society;* July 1995. Boston: Academic Press, 1996:150.

16. Sieburth D, Jabs EW, Warrington JA, et al. Assignment of genes encoding a unique cytokine (IL12) composed of two unrelated subunits to chromosomes 3 and 5. *Genomics* 1992;14:59–62.

17. Chizzonite R, Truitt T, Desai BB, et al. IL-12 receptor. I. Characterization of the receptor on PHA-activated human lymphoblasts. *J Immunol* 1992;148:3117–3124.

18. Presky DH, Yang H, Minetti LJ, et al. A functional interleukin 12 receptor complex is composed of two beta-type cytokine receptor subunits. *Proc Natl Acad Sci USA* 1996;93:14002–14007.

19. Chua AO, Chizzonite R, Desai BB, et al. Expression cloning of a human IL-12 receptor component: a new member of the cytokine receptor superfamily with strong homology to gp130. *J Immunol* 1994;153:128–136.

20. Chua AO, Wilkinson VL, Presky DH, Gubler U. Cloning and characterization of a mouse IL-12 receptor-β component. *J Immunol* 1995; 155:4286–4294.

21. Gray PW, Goeddel DV. Structure of the human immune interferon gene. *Nature* 1982;298:859–863.

22. Gately MK, Carvajal DM, Connaughton SE, et al. Interleukin-12 antagonist activity of mouse interleukin-12 p40 homodimer *in vitro* and *in vivo*. *Ann N Y Acad Sci* 1996;795:1–12.

23. Mattner F, Fischer S, Guckes S, et al. The interleukin-12 subunit p40 specifically inhibits effects of the interleukin-12 heterodimer. *Eur J Immunol* 1993;23:2202–2208.

24. Gillessen S, Carvajal D, Ling P, et al. Mouse interleukin-12 (IL-12)

25. Ling P, Gately MK, Gubler U, et al. Human IL-12 p40 homodimer binds to the IL-12 receptor but does not mediate biologic activity. *J Immunol* 1995;154:116–127.

26. Desai BB, Quinn PM, Wolitzky AG, Mongini PKA, Chizzonite R, Gately MK. The IL-12 receptor. II. Distribution and regulation of receptor expression. *J Immunol* 1992;148:3125–3132.

27. Wu C, Warrier RR, Wang X, Presky DH, Gately MK. Regulation of interleukin-12 receptor beta 1 chain expression and interleukin-12 binding by human peripheral blood mononuclear cells. *Eur J Immunol* 1997;27:147–154.

28. Benjamin D, Sharma V, Kubin M, et al. IL-12 expression in AIDS-related lymphoma B cell lines. *J Immunol* 1996;156:1626–1637.

29. Vogel LA, Showe LC, Lester TL, McNutt RM, Van Cleave VH, Metzger DW. Direct binding of IL-12 to human and murine B lymphocytes. *Int Immunol* 1996;8:1955–1962.

30. Bacon CM, McVicar DW, Ortaldo JR, Rees RC, O'Shea JJ, Johnston JA. Interleukin 12 (IL-12) induces tyrosine phosphorylation of JAK2 and TYK2: differential use of Janus family tyrosine kinases by IL-2 and IL-12. *J Exp Med* 1995;181:399–404.

31. Jacobson NG, Szabo SJ, Weber-Nordt RM, et al. Interleukin 12 signaling in T helper type 1 (Th1) cells involves tyrosine phosphorylation of signal transducer and activator of transcription (Stat)3 and Stat4. *J Exp Med* 1995;181:1755–1762.

32. Bacon CM, Petricoin EF III, Ortaldo JR, et al. IL-12 induces tyrosine phosphorylation and activation of STAT4 in human lymphocytes. *Proc Natl Acad Sci USA* 1995;92:7307–7311.

33. Cho SS, Bacon CM, Sudarshan C, et al. Activation of STAT4 by IL-12 and IFN-α: evidence for the involvement of ligand-induced tyrosine and serine phosphorylation. *J Immunol* 1996;157:4781–4789.

34. Thierfelder WE, van Deursen JM, Yamamoto K, et al. Requirement for Stat4 in interleukin-12–mediated responses of natural killer and T cells. *Nature* 1996;382:171–174.

35. Kaplan MH, Sun Y, Hoey T, Grusby MJ. Impaired IL-12 responses and enhanced development of Th2 cells in Stat4-deficient mice. *Nature* 1996;382:174–177.

36. Magram J, Connaughton SE, Warrier RR, et al. IL-12–deficient mice are defective in IFN gamma production and type 1 cytokine responses. *Immunity* 1996;4:471–481.

37. Pignata C, Sanghera JS, Cossette L, Pelech S, Ritz J. Interleukin-12 induces tyrosine phosphorylation and activation of 44-kD mitogen-activated protein kinase in human T cells. *Blood* 1994;83:184–190.

38. D'Andrea A, Ma X, Aste-Amezaga M, Paganin C, Trinchieri G. Stimulatory and inhibitory effects of IL-4 and IL-13 on production of cytokines by human peripheral blood mononuclear cells: priming for IL-12 and TNF-α production. *J Exp Med* 1995;181:537–546.

39. Cassatella MA, Meda L, Gasperini S, D'Andrea A, Ma X, Trinchieri G. Interleukin-12 production by human polymorphonuclear leukocytes. *Eur J Immunol* 1995;25:1–5.

40. Ma X, Chow JM, Gri G, et al. The interleukin-12 p40 gene promoter is primed by interferon-γ in monocytic cells. *J Exp Med* 1996;183: 147–157.

41. Flesch IEA, Hess JH, Huang S, et al. Early interleukin 12 production by macrophages in response to mycobacterial infection depends on interferon and tumor necrosis factor α. *J Exp Med* 1995;181:1615–1621.

42. Wysocka M, Kubin M, Vieira LQ, et al. Interleukin-12 is required for interferon-γ production and lethality in lipopolysaccharide-induced shock in mice. *Eur J Immunol* 1995;25:672–676.

43. Heinzel FP, Rerko RM, Ahmed F, Hujer AM. IFN—independent production of IL-12 during murine endotoxemia. *J Immunol* 1996;157: 4521–4528.

44. Scharton-Kersten TM, Wynn TA, Denkers EY, et al. In the absence of endogenous IFN-γ, mice develop unimpaired IL-12 responses to *Toxoplasma gondii* while failing to control acute infection. *J Immunol* 1996;157:4045–4054.

45. D'Andrea A, Aste-Amezaga M, Valiante NM, Ma X, Kubin M, Trinchieri G. Interleukin-10 inhibits human lymphocyte IFN-γ production by suppressing natural killer cell stimulatory factor/interleukin-12 synthesis in accessory cells. *J Exp Med* 1993;178:1041–1048.

46. Kubin M, Kamoun M, Trinchieri G. Interleukin-12 synergizes with B7/CD28 interaction in inducing efficient proliferation and cytokine production of human T cells. *J Exp Med* 1994;180:211–222.

47. Murphy EE, Terres G, Macatonia SE, et al. B7 and IL-12 cooperate

p40 homodimer: a potent IL-12 antagonist. *Eur J Immunol* 1995;25: 200–206.

for proliferation and IFN-γ production by mouse T helper clones that are unresponsive to B7 costimulation. *J Exp Med* 1994;180:223–231.

48. Hino A, Nariuchi H. Negative feedback mechanism suppresses interleukin-12 production by antigen-presenting cells interacting with T helper 2 cells. *Eur J Immunol* 1996;26:623–628.

49. Aragane Y, Riemann H, Barhdwaj RS, et al. IL-12 is expressed and released by human keratinocytes and epidermoid carcinoma cell lines. *J Immunol* 1994;153:5366–5372.

50. Muller G, Saloga J, Germann T, et al. Identification and induction of human keratinocyte-derived IL-12. *J Clin Invest* 1994;94:1799–1805.

51. Goodman RE, Nestle F, Naidu YM, et al. Keratinocyte-derived T cell costimulation induces preferential production of IL-2 and IL-4 but not IFN-γ. *J Immunol* 1994;152:5189–5198.

52. Kang K, Kubin M, Cooper KD, Lessin SR, Trinchieri G, Rook AH. IL-12 synthesis by human Langerhans cells. *J Immunol* 1996;156: 1402–1407.

53. Macatonia SE, Hosken NA, Litton M, et al. Dendritic cells produce IL-12 and direct the development of Th1 cells from naive CD4+ T cells. *J Immunol* 1995;154:5071–5079.

54. Heufler C, Koch F, Stanzl U, et al. Interleukin-12 is produced by dendritic cells and mediates Th1 development as well as IFN-γ production by Th1 cells. *Eur J Immunol* 1996;26:659–668.

55. Koch F, Stanzl U, Jennewein P, et al. High level IL-12 production by murine dendritic cells: upregulation via MHC class II and CD40 molecules and downregulation by IL-4 and IL-10. *J Exp Med* 1996;184: 741–746.

56. Cella M, Scheidegger D, Plamer-Lehmann K, Lane P, Lanzavecchia A, Alber G. Ligation of CD40 on dendritic cells triggers production of high levels of interleukin-12 and enhances T cell stimulatory capacity: T-T help via APC activation. *J Exp Med* 1996;184:747–752.

57. Germann T, Gately MK, Schoenhaut DS, et al. Interleukin-12/T cell stimulating factor, a cytokine with multiple effects on T helper type 1 (T$_H$1) but not on T$_H$2 cells. *Eur J Immunol* 1993;23:1762–1770.

58. Shu U, Kiniwa M, Wu CY, et al. Activated T cells induce interleukin-12 production by monocytes via CD40-CD40 ligand interaction. *Eur J Immunol* 1995;25:1125–1128.

59. Stüber E, Strober W, Neurath M. Blocking the CD40L-CD40 interaction *in vivo* specifically prevents the priming of T helper 1 cells through the inhibition of interleukin 12 secretion. *J Exp Med* 1996; 183:693–698.

60. Kennedy MK, Picha KS, Fanslow WC, et al. CD40/CD40 ligand interactions are required for T cell-dependent production of interleukin-12 by mouse macrophages. *Eur J Immunol* 1996;26:370–378.

61. Maruo S, Oh-Hora M, Ahn H, et al. B cells regulate CD40 ligand-induced IL-12 production in antigen-presenting cells (APC) during T cell/APC interactions. *J Immunol* 1997;158:120–126.

62. Aste-Amezaga M, Ma X, Trinchieri G. Regulation by interleukin-10 of *Staphylococcus aureus*- and lipopolysaccharide-induced interleukin-12 gene expression in human peripheral blood mononuclear cells. *Ann N Y Acad Sci* 1996;795:319–320.

63. Ma X, Neurath M, Gri G, Trinchieri G. Identification and characterization of a novel ets-2–related nuclear complex implicated in the activation of the human IL-12 p40 gene promoter. *J Biol Chem* 1997;272: 10389–10401.

64. Murphy TL, Cleveland MG, Kulesza P, Magram J, Murphy KM. Regulation of interleukin 12 p40 expression through an NF-κB half-site. *Mol Cell Biol* 1995;15:5258–5267.

65. Yoshimoto T, Kojima K, Funakoshi T, Endo Y, Fujita T, Nariuchi H. Molecular cloning and characterization of murine IL-12 genes. *J Immunol* 1996;156:1082–1088.

66. Tone Y, Thompson SA, Babik JM, et al. Structure and chromosomal location of the mouse interleukin-12 p35 and p40 subunit genes. *Eur J Immunol* 1996;26:1222–1227.

67. Jacobsen SE, Okkenhaug C, Myklebust J, Veiby OP, Lyman SD. The FLT3 ligand potently and directly stimulates the growth and expansion of primitive murine bone marrow progenitor cells *in vitro*: synergistic interactions with interleukin (IL) 11, IL-12, and other hematopoietic growth factors. *J Exp Med* 1995;181:1357–1363.

68. Bellone G, Trinchieri G. Dual stimulatory and inhibitory effect of NK cell stimulatory factor/IL-12 on human hematopoiesis. *J Immunol* 1994;153:930–937.

69. Brunda MJ, Luistro L, Warrier RR, et al. Antitumor and antimetastatic activity of interleukin 12 against murine tumors. *J Exp Med* 1993; 178:1223–1230.

70. Sarmiento UM, Riley JH, Knaack PA, et al. Biologic effects of recombinant human interleukin-12 in squirrel monkeys *(Sciureus saimiri)*. *Lab Invest* 1994;71:862–873.

71. Eng VM, Car BD, Schnyder B, et al. The stimulatory effects of interleukin (IL)-12 on hematopoiesis are antagonized by IL-12–induced interferon gamma *in vivo*. *J Exp Med* 1995;181:1893–1898.

72. Aste-Amezaga M, D'Andrea A, Kubin M, Trinchieri G. Cooperation of natural killer cell stimulatory factor/interleukin-12 with other stimuli in the induction of cytokines and cytotoxic cell-associated molecules in human T and NK cells. *Cell Immunol* 1994;156:480–492.

73. Gazzinelli RT, Wysocka M, Hayashi S, et al. Parasite induced IL-12 stimulates early IFN-γ synthesis and resistance during acute infection with *Toxoplasma gondii*. *J Immunol* 1994;153:2533–2543.

74. Tripp CS, Wolf SF, Unanue ER. Interleukin 12 and tumor necrosis factor alpha are costimulators of interferon gamma production by natural killer cells in severe combined immunodeficiency mice with listeriosis, and interleukin 10 is a physiologic antagonist. *Proc Natl Acad Sci USA* 1993;90:3725–3729.

75. Scharton-Kersten T, Afonso LCC, Wysocka M, Trinchieri G, Scott P. IL-12 is required for NK cell activation and subsequent Th1 cell development in experimental leishmaniasis. *J Immunol* 1995;154: 5320–5330.

76. Gately MK, Desai BB, Wolitzky AG, et al. Regulation of human lymphocyte proliferation by a heterodimeric cytokine, IL-12 (cytotoxic lymphocyte maturation factor). *J Immunol* 1991;147:874–882.

77. Perussia B, Chan S, D'Andrea A, et al. Natural killer cell stimulatory factor or IL-12 has differential effects on the proliferation of TCRαβ+, TCRγδ+ T lymphocytes and NK cells. *J Immunol* 1992;149:3495–3502.

78. Gately MK, Wolitzky AG, Quinn PM, Chizzonite R. Regulation of human cytolytic lymphocyte responses by interleukin-12. *Cell Immunol* 1992;143:127–142.

79. Salcedo TW, Azzoni L, Wolf SF, Perussia B. Modulation of perforin and granzyme messenger RNA expression in human natural killer cells. *J Immunol* 1993;151:2511–2520.

80. Rabinowich H, Herberman RB, Whiteside TL. Differential effects of IL-12 and IL-2 on expression and function of cellular adhesion molecules on purified human natural killer cells. *Cell Immunol* 1993;152: 481–498.

81. Robertson MJ, Soiffer RJ, Wolf SF, et al. Response of human natural killer (NK) cells to NK cell stimulatory factor (NKSF): cytolytic activity and proliferation of NK cells are differentially regulated by NKSF. *J Exp Med* 1992;175:779–788.

82. Manetti R, Gerosa F, Giudizi MG, et al. Interleukin-12 induces stable priming for interferon-γ (IFN)-γ production during differentiation of human T helper (Th) cells and transient IFN-γ production in established Th2 cell clones. *J Exp Med* 1994;179:1273–1283.

83. Gerosa F, Paganin C, Peritt D, et al. Interleukin-12 primes human CD4 and CD8 T cell clones for high production of both interferon-γ and interleukin-10. *J Exp Med* 1996;183:2559–2569.

84. Seder RA, Gazzinelli R, Sher A, Paul WE. IL-12 acts directly on CD4+ T cells to enhance priming for IFN production and diminishes IL-4 inhibition of such priming. *Proc Natl Acad Sci USA* 1993;90: 10188–10192.

85. Szabo SJ, Jacobson NG, Dighe AS, Gubler U, Murphy KM. Developmental commitment to the Th2 lineage by extinction of IL-12 signaling. *Immunity* 1995;2:665–675.

86. Szabo SJ, Dighe AS, Gubler U, Murphy KM. Regulation of the interleukin (IL)-12R 2 subunit expression in developing T helper (Th1) and Th2 cells. *J Exp Med* 1997;185:817–824.

87. Rogge L, Barberis-Maino L, Biffi M, et al. Selective expression of an interleukin-12 receptor component by human T helper 1 cells. *J Exp Med* 1997;185:825–831.

88. Gazzinelli RT, Wysocka M, Hieny S, et al. In the absence of endogenous IL-10, mice acutely infected with *Toxoplasma gondii* succumb to a lethal immune response dependent on CD4+ T cells and accompanied by overproduction of IL-12, IFN-γ, and TNF-α. *J Immunol* 1996; 157:798–805.

89. Tripp CS, Kanagawa O, Unanue ER. Secondary response to Listeria infection requires IFN-gamma but is partially independent of IL-12. *J Immunol* 1995;155:3427–3432.

90. Heinzel FP, Rerko RM, Ahmed F, Pearlman E. Endogenous IL-12 is required for control of Th2 cytokine responses capable of exacerbating leishmaniasis in normally resistant mice. *J Immunol* 1995;155: 730–739.

91. Seder RA, Kelsall BL, Jankovic D. Differential roles for IL-12 in the maintenance of immune responses in infectious versus autoimmune disease. *J Immunol* 1996;157:2745–2748.

92. Neurath MF, Fuss I, Kelsall BL, Stüber E, Strober W. Antibodies to interleukin 12 abrogate established experimental colitis in mice. *J Exp Med* 1995;182:1281–1290.

93. Metzger DW, Buchanan JM, Collins JT, et al. Enhancement of humoral immunity by interleukin-12. *Ann N Y Acad Sci* 1996;795:100–115.

94. Jelinek DF, Braaten JK. Role of IL-12 in human B lymphocyte proliferation and differentiation. *J Immunol* 1995;154:1606–1613.

95. Biron CA, Gazzinelli RT. Effects of IL-12 on immune responses to microbial infections: a key mediator in regulating disease outcome. *Curr Opin Immunol* 1995;7:485–496.

96. Trinchieri G. Proinflammatory and immunoregulatory functions of interleukin-12. *Int Rev Immunol* 1998;16:365–396.

97. Heinzel FP, Rerko RM, Ling P, Hakimi J, Schoenhaut DS. Interleukin 12 is produced *in vivo* during endotoxemia and stimulates synthesis of gamma interferon. *Infect Immun* 1994;62:4244–4249.

98. Leung DYM, Gately M, Trumble A, Ferguson-Darnell B, Schlievert PM, Picker LJ. Bacterial superantigens induce T cell expression of the skin-selective homing receptor, the cutaneous lymphocyte-associated antigen, via stimulation of interleukin 12 production. *J Exp Med* 1995;181:747–753.

99. Finkelman FD, Madden KB, Cheever AW, et al. Effects of interleukin 12 on immune responses and host protection in mice infected with intestinal nematode parasites. *J Exp Med* 1994;179:1563–1572.

100. Orange JS, Biron CA. An absolute and restricted requirement for IL-12 in natural killer cell IFN-gamma production and antiviral defense: studies of natural killer and T cell responses in contrasting viral infections. *J Immunol* 1996;156:1138–1142.

101. Biron CA. Cytokines in the generation of immune responses to, and resolution of, virus infection. *Curr Opin Immunol* 1994;6:530–538.

102. Tang YW, Graham BS. Interleukin-12 treatment during immunization elicits a T helper cell type 1–like immune response in mice challenged with respiratory syncytial virus and improves vaccine immunogenicity. *J Infect Dis* 1995;172:734–738.

103. Schijns VE, Haagmans BL, Horzinek MC. IL-12 stimulates an antiviral type 1 cytokine response but lacks adjuvant activity in IFN—receptor-deficient mice. *J Immunol* 1995;155:2525–2532.

104. Chehimi J, Starr S, Frank I, et al. Impaired interleukin-12 production in human immunodeficiency virus-infected patients. *J Exp Med* 1994;179:1361–1366.

105. Gazzinelli RT, Bala S, Stevens R, et al. HIV infection suppresses type 1 lymphokine and IL-12 responses to *Toxoplasma gondii* but fails to inhibit the synthesis of other parasite-induced monokines. *J Immunol* 1995;155:1565–1574.

106. Chehimi J, Starr S, Frank I, et al. Natural killer cell stimulatory factor (NKSF) increases the cytotoxic activity of NK cells from both healthy donors and HIV-infected patients. *J Exp Med* 1992;175:789–796.

107. Clerici M, Lucey DR, Berzofsky JA, et al. Restoration of HIV-specific cell-mediated immune responses by interleukin-12 *in vitro*. *Science* 1993;262:1721–1724.

108. Clerici M, Sarin A, Coffman RL, et al. Type 1/type 2 cytokine modulation of T cell programmed cell death as a model for HIV pathogenesis. *Proc Natl Acad Sci USA* 1994;91:11811–11815.

109. Karp CL, Wysocka M, Wahl LM, et al. Mechanism of suppression of cell-mediated immunity by measles virus. *Science* 1996;273:228–231.

110. Heinzel FP, Schoenhaut DS, Rerko RM, Rosser LE, Gately MK. Recombinant interleukin 12 cures mice infected with *Leishmania major*. *J Exp Med* 1993;177:1505–1509.

111. Afonso LCC, Scharton TM, Vieira LQ, Wysocka M, Trinchieri G, Scott P. The adjuvant effect of interleukin-12 in a vaccine against *Leishmania major*. *Science* 1994;263:235–237.

112. Sypek JP, Chung CL, Mayor SEH, et al. Resolution of cutaneous leishmaniasis: interleukin-12 initiates a protective T helper type 1 immune response. *J Exp Med* 1993;177:1797–1802.

113. Nabors GS, Afonso LC, Farrell JP, Scott P. Switch from a type 2 to a type 1 T helper cell response and cure of established *Leishmania major* infection in mice is induced by combined therapy with interleukin 12 and Pentostam. *Proc Natl Acad Sci USA* 1995;92:3142–3146.

114. Kobayashi K, Yamazaki J, Kasama T, et al. Interleukin (IL)-12 deficiency in susceptible mice infected with *Mycobacterium avium* and amelioration of established infection by IL-12 replacement therapy. *J Infect Dis* 1996;174:564–573.

115. Bliss J, Van Cleave V, Murray K, et al. IL-12, as an adjuvant, promotes a T helper 1 cell, but does not suppress a T helper 2 cell recall response. *J Immunol* 1996;156:887–894.

116. Germann T, Bongartz M, Dlugonska H, et al. Interleukin-12 profoundly up-regulates the synthesis of antigen-specific complement-fixing IgG2a, IgG2b and IgG3 antibody subclasses *in vivo*. *Eur J Immunol* 1995;25:823–829.

117. Car BD, Eng VM, Schnyder B, et al. Role of interferon-γ in IL-12–induced pathology in mice. *Am J Pathol* 1995;147:1693–1707.

118. Cohen J. IL-12 deaths: explanation and a puzzle. *Science* 1995;270:908.

119. Nastala CL, Edington HD, McKinney TG, et al. Recombinant IL-12 administration induces tumor regression in association with IFN-γ production. *J Immunol* 1994;153:1697–1706.

120. Yu WG, Yamamoto N, Takenaka H, et al. Molecular mechanisms underlying IFN-gamma-mediated tumor growth inhibition induced during tumor immunotherapy with rIL-12. *Int Immunol* 1996;8:855–865.

121. Voest EE, Kenyon BM, O'Reilly MS, Truitt G, D'Amato RJ, Folkman J. Inhibition of angiogenesis *in vivo* by interleukin 12. *J Natl Cancer Inst* 1995;87:581–586.

122. Wigginton JM, Komschlies KL, Back TC, Franco JL, Brunda MJ, Wiltrout RH. Administration of interleukin 12 with pulse interleukin 2 and the rapid and complete eradication of murine renal carcinoma. *J Natl Cancer Inst* 1996;88:38–43.

123. Gavett SH, O'Hearn DJ, Li X, Huang SK, Finkelman FD, Wills-Karp M. Interleukin 12 inhibits antigen-induced airway hyperresponsiveness, inflammation, and Th2 cytokine expression in mice. *J Exp Med* 1995;182:1527–1536.

124. Adorini L, Gregori S, Magram J, Trembleau S. The role of IL-12 in the pathogenesis of Th1 cell-mediated autoimmune diseases. *Ann N Y Acad Sci* 1996;795:208–215.

PART III

Cellular Mechanisms

Inflammation: Basic Principles and Clinical Correlates,
3rd ed., edited by John I. Gallin and Ralph Snyderman.
Lippincott Williams & Wilkins, Philadelphia © 1999.

CHAPTER 35

Receptors for Microbial Products:

Carbohydrates

Iain P. Fraser and R. Alan B. Ezekowitz

Multicellular organisms have evolved mechanisms to protect themselves from noxious stimuli. These external challenges often are microbial pathogens. The ability of host receptors to recognize conserved, shared motifs on the surfaces of pathogens has led to the concept of pattern recognition as a cornerstone of the innate immune system (1). Pathogen-associated molecular patterns (PAMPs) are the invariant motifs shared by many different groups of microorganisms (2). PAMPs are recognized by a variety of host-encoded pattern recognition receptors (PRRs), which couple recognition to effector functions (2).

PRRs may exist as soluble proteins or as endocytic-phagocytic receptors. It is likely that the primary function of PRRs in primitive organisms was initially in development and that they evolved to play a role in host defense. This paradigm is likely to apply to PRRs that recognize molecular patterns on diverse targets such as apoptotic cells. Accordingly, recognition systems of primitive organisms are less specialized and are likely to recognize general features such as charge or geometry of their ligands. It appears that these primitive recognition systems have persisted in and adapted to the wider needs of more complex hosts and have formed the template of innate immunity in vertebrates.

There appears to be a link between innate and adaptive immunity. Macrophages play a dual role. They are an essential part of innate or first-line host defense, and their versatile properties have been coopted by the adaptive immune response, in which they play a role as accessory cells. Macrophages recognize a wide array of different antigens and in an extension of the concept of pattern recognition, we consider all macrophage cell surface receptors as PRRs. We hypothesize that among these receptors there is a hierarchy of recognition. The scavenger receptors (SRs) represent the most primitive, recognizing the most general patterns, and the Fc receptors represent the most specialized. Macrophages can therefore recognize PAMPs directly through SRs or lectin-like molecules like the mannose receptor. Alternatively, the recognition pattern may be provided by opsonins such as antibody (i.e., the pattern is the Fc portion of immunoglobulin), complement components, or collectins such as the mannose-binding protein (Table 35-1).

Glycoconjugates on the surfaces of pathogenic microorganisms serve as a class of PAMP that has been selected for by the innate immune system. The PRRs that interact specifically with these PAMPs are the subject of this review. Although we have focused on the host recognition of carbohydrate PAMPs in pathogens, microorganisms themselves express a range of lectins that recognize specific carbohydrate residues on host cells and that are used in microbial pathogenesis and virulence (3).

LESSONS LEARNED FROM PRIMITIVE RECOGNITION SYSTEMS

Studies using relatively simple organisms such as *Drosophila, Periplanta, Sarcophaga,* and *Limulus* have yielded important information about primitive host defense mechanisms and provided insights into the ways in which more sophisticated systems may have evolved.

The blood of the horseshoe crab *Limulus* contains a coagulation cascade that is activated on detection of pathogens or foreign invaders (4). This cascade may be triggered specifically by carbohydrates or lipids present

I. P. Fraser and R. A. B. Ezekowitz: Laboratory of Developmental Immunology and Department of Pediatrics, Massachusetts General Hospital, Boston, Massachusetts 02114.

TABLE 35-1. *Hierarchy of recognition*

Receptor	Pattern recognition
1. Scavenger receptors (classes A, B, and C)	Modified proteins, specific polyanions, apoptotic cells, LPS
2. CD14	LPS/LBP
3. Lectins (types C–, S–, I–, P–)	Specific carbohydrate conformations
4. Integrins	RGD sequence; other ligands
5. Collectin receptors	Collagen stalks of collectins
6. Complement receptors	Cleaved C3
7. Fc receptors	Fc portion of immunoglobulin

LPS, lipopolysaccharide; LBP, LPS-binding protein; RGD, arginine-glycine-aspartate.

on microorganisms and results in the formation of an insoluble gel that immobilizes and localizes the invading microbes. This facilitates killing of the trapped microbes by antimicrobial substances released by host hemocytes. Lipid-dependent activation of this cascade results from an interaction between the crab factor C and lipopolysaccharide (LPS) located on the surfaces of invading microorganisms. This system is so sensitive to trace amounts of LPS that it is used as the standard laboratory assay for LPS contamination of reagents (5).

An independent, carbohydrate-dependent activation pathway is triggered by a specific interaction between (1,3)-β-glucan (present on fungal surfaces) and the *Limulus* serine protease zymogen, factor G. Binding of the β-glucan to the heterodimeric factor G complex results in autocatalytic activation to an active serine protease that then triggers the remainder of the coagulation cascade. This action ultimately results in the conversion of a soluble coagulogen precursor to an insoluble coagulin gel (6). In this case, pathogen recognition by a soluble PRR is coupled to a humoral effector response.

The hemolymph of the freshwater crayfish *(Pacifastacus leniusculus)* also contains a (1,3)-β-glucan binding protein (BGBP). This BGBP is structurally unrelated to the *Limulus* factor G molecule and contains no serine protease domain (7). On ligation, the BGBP-ligand complex binds to a membrane receptor on the surface of hemocytes. In addition to enhancing phagocytosis through an opsonic mechanism, binding to the receptor triggers hemocyte degranulation and spreading, further enhancing host defense mechanisms. In this case, a soluble PRR is coupled to a cellular effector response through a hemocyte cell surface receptor.

These simple yet elegant systems indicate how a single PAMP may generate different effector responses, depending on the nature of the PRR encountered. They also illustrate how these molecules contribute to effective host defense, even in the absence of a clonal immune system.

The hemolymph of the American cockroach *(Periplanta americana)* contains a protein with affinity for some forms of LPS (8). Unlike other LPS-binding proteins that have been described, this lectin recognizes tetrasaccharides present at the proximal ends of LPS chains but not the lipid A component. Because the glycosylation patterns of LPS vary among bacteria, not all forms of LPS are recognized. The cDNA of this lectin predicts a C-terminal carbohydrate recognition domain (CRD) similar to that found in animal lectins. It also behaves as an acute phase reactant, in that its expression is transiently upregulated on injection of *Escherichia coli* into adult cockroaches. Although the downstream effector mechanisms and biologic significance of this carbohydrate-binding protein have not been determined, it nonetheless provides another example of primitive pattern recognition that may have been coopted in the evolutionary development of higher organisms.

Larvae of the flesh-fly *(Sarcophaga peregrina)* can be induced to express a galactose-binding lectin (9). This lectin is absent from normal larvae, but its expression is rapidly upregulated by direct injury to the body wall, such as that induced experimentally by a hypodermic needle. After induction, this lectin appears to upregulate the phagocytic and killing capacity of hemocytes, illustrating another link between pattern recognition and host defense function. In this case, interaction between a carbohydrate PAMP and a PRR leads to enhancement of effector cell function, rather than to a direct antimicrobial effect.

PRIMITIVE RECOGNITION SYSTEMS: SCAVENGER RECEPTOR SUPERFAMILY

These cell surface PRRs are expressed in a wide range of organisms, from flies to humans, and are categorized as class A, B, or C based on protein sequence similarities. The class A SRs were the first to be described (10) and include the AI, AII (11), and MARCO (macrophage receptor with collagenous structure) (12) molecules. Although originally described for their ability to recognize chemically modified (but not native) low-density lipoprotein (LDL) particles, subsequent studies demonstrated an impressive promiscuity of ligand recognition, suggesting a role more fundamental than one confined to lipid metabolism. These receptors are largely macrophage-restricted and have a broad polyanionic pattern recognition specificity. Their known ligands include acetylated or oxidized LDL, polyinosinic acid, polyguanylic acid, maleylated bovine serum albumin, fucoidan, dextran sulfate, carrageenan, phosphatidylserine, and polyvinyl sulfate. All known ligands are polyanionic, but only those polyanions with appropriately spaced negative charges bind to these receptors (13). The PAMP of this class of PRR therefore appears to be charge based. Microbial ligands described for the class A receptors include the lipid A component of LPS (14) and lipoteichoic acid (as expressed on the surface of many gram-positive bacteria) (15).

The binding and uptake of LPS through the SR appears to be a mechanism of LPS clearance, because no release of tumor necrosis factor (TNF) or interleukin-6 (IL-6) results from the interaction. This contrasts with the interaction between LPS and the CD14 receptor. The MARCO receptor binds gram-positive *(Staphylococcus aureus)* and gram-negative *(E. coli)* bacteria, but not yeast *(Saccharomyces cerevisiae)*, in a specific fashion (12). Availability of SR-A–null mice has made it possible to start to address the physiologic functioning of these receptors *in vivo*. Targeted disruption of the gene encoding murine AI and AII receptors resulted in increased susceptibility to infection *in vivo* with *Listeria monocytogenes* and herpes simplex virus type 1, implicating these SRs directly in host defense mechanisms (16). It is not clear whether these receptors are scavenging microbes from the bloodstream and thereby reducing pathogen load or if a more subtle interplay with other immune mechanisms is operational. A later report indicates that these SR knock-out mice have increased mortality in response to *in vivo* challenge with endotoxin (17), confirming earlier observations of the class A receptors as nonsignaling LPS scavengers (14). The extent to which MARCO may be compensating for the lack of these receptors in the knock-out animals remains undetermined but is potentially testable after MARCO-deficient mice become available.

The class B SRs constitute the CD36 family. Their pattern recognition repertoire includes modified proteins (e.g., thrombospondin, collagen, long-chain fatty acids, oxidatively modified LDL), but identified ligands do not have the broad polyanionic pattern characteristic of class A ligands.

It is likely that primitive organisms would employ cell surface PRRs to facilitate phagocytosis and signal transduction on encountering nonself or apoptotic particles or cells. Using a dual candidate gene or sequence homology strategy based on this premise, Franc et al. (18) identified just such a molecule in the fruit fly. Croquemort (from the French for "catcher of death") is a CD36-like molecule expressed on the surface of *Drosophila melanogaster* hemocytes-macrophages, which mediates the recognition and uptake of apoptotic cells *in vitro* and *in vivo* in embryogenesis. The molecular specificity of this interaction and a role in fly immunity have yet to be established.

Recognition of apoptotic cells appears to be a highly conserved function of the class B SRs, as manifested in flies (18) and mammals (19,20). CD36 itself has been implicated in the binding and uptake of apoptotic inflammatory human leukocytes. This process may be important in limiting inflammatory responses *in vivo*, particularly because phagocytosis through this mechanism does not appear to be coupled to a proinflammatory cytokine response (21). The only pathogen–class B SR interaction described is that between CD36 and malaria-parasitized erythrocytes (22). In this case, the PAMP recognized is contained in the knobs on the surface of the parasitized erythrocyte and not directly on the pathogen itself (23). Murine SR-BI (which shares 30% homology with CD36) was originally identified for its SR-like ability to bind modified lipoproteins (24). This receptor has since been shown to function primarily as a receptor for high-density lipoprotein (25,26), calling into question its function as a true SR (27).

The only class C SR described was cloned from a *Drosophila*-derived cell line. The receptor (dSR-CI) was first identified for its ability to mediate endocytosis of classic class A SR ligands in fruit fly embryo macrophages and in a *Drosophila*-derived cell line (28). Expression cloning of the dSR-CI cDNA revealed a predicted primary structure that is unrelated to that of the other SRs (29). The presence of two complement control protein motifs (which are found in a number of complement proteins and clotting factors, including the *Limulus* coagulation factor C [30]), suggests a possible role in protein-protein interactions. In *Drosophila* embryos, dSR-CI appears to be macrophage-restricted, consistent with its function as a SR, but a physiologic PAMP ligand has yet to be described.

LECTINS IN HIGHER ORGANISMS

Animal lectins are classified according to the primary structure and function of their CRDs: C- (i.e., calcium-dependent, extracellular, wide range of carbohydrate specificity), S- (i.e., thiol-containing, calcium-independent, intracellular and extracellular, β-galactoside specificity), I- (i.e., immunoglobulin domain-containing, sialoadhesin family), and P- (i.e., mannose-6-phosphate specificity) lectins.

The C-type lectins have been strongly implicated in host-pathogen interactions. This is a family of extracellular, calcium-dependent molecules with different carbohydrate specificities. They are found in a variety of proteins, including endocytic-phagocytic receptors, homing-adhesion receptors, soluble lectins, and proteoglycans. The C-type CRD is a compact domain with a hydrophobic core, oriented with the N and C termini adjacent to each other. Two intrachain disulfide bonds and two calcium binding sites are present in each CRD. The pH-dependent uncoupling of ligands that is characteristic of this domain is probably mediated by decreased calcium binding at low pH. The carbohydrate specificities of CRD-containing receptors may be altered *in vitro* by site-directed mutagenesis of critical amino acids within the CRDs (31), suggesting that different carbohydrate specificities may have arisen in evolution by mutation within a primordial CRD framework structure. By combining CRDs with other protein domains (soluble or cell associated), specific carbohydrate recognition may be coupled with different effector functions. In this fashion, a single PAMP may give rise to a variety of host effects, depending on the nature of the PRR to which it binds.

Mammalian Asialoglycoprotein Receptor

The asialoglycoprotein receptor (ASGP-R) was the first model system to describe the carbohydrate-discriminating capacity of animal lectins (32). Two separate genes encode two proteins that associate to form the functional receptor at the hepatocyte cell surface (33,34). Each subunit is a type II transmembrane protein with a single C-terminal CRD in the extracellular domain. The lectin possesses a Gal/GalNAc specificity and mediates the calcium-dependent binding and endocytosis of galactose-terminated glycoproteins (35). When the terminal sialic acid residues on N-linked oligosaccharides of glycoproteins are removed, terminal galactose residues are displayed, and the proteins become effective ligands for this receptor. Its primary function appears to be the clearance of senescent erythrocytes and glycoproteins from the circulation, but it can recognize appropriate carbohydrates on pathogens such as Neisseria gonorrhoeae (36), Marburg virus (37), and hepatitis B virus (38). In the case of the ASGP-R, the pattern recognized by the receptor is present on some self-glycoproteins, but only on those that have been modified to earmark them for destruction.

Collectins, Including Mannose-Binding Protein

The collectins are soluble C-type lectins that appear to function in first-line host defense (39) (Table 35-2). Their ligand-recognition ability is contained in a globular, C-terminal, carbohydrate recognition domain (CRD), and their effector functions are mediated by their conserved collagenous tails. In vivo, these lectins multimerize, increasing their avidity for their cognate ligands and, by virtue of the resultant spatial orientation of their CRDs, conferring a specificity for the carbohydrate residues present on the surfaces of microorganisms (as opposed to those residues located on the surfaces of self-glycoproteins). These PRRs are able to perform their function in first-line host defense by virtue of their broad range of ligand recognition, their ability to distinguish self from nonself, their appropriate effector mechanisms, and their wide distribution in bodily fluids and cavities.

The mannose-binding protein (MBP) has the broadest range of pathogen recognition of all the collectins. Microbes recognized include bacteria (gram-positive and gram-negative forms), yeast, viruses (including influenza A and human immunodeficiency virus), and parasites (see Table 35-2). The structural basis of carbohydrate recognition has been well described (40,41). The CRD

contains five sheets, two α-helices, and four extended loops. A calcium ion in the CRD binding site coordinates with equatorial 3-OH and 4-OH groups in the terminal mannose residue of the carbohydrate ligand. The carbohydrate specificity of the MBP CRD is precisely defined by this requirement for adjacent pairs of hydroxyl groups. So finely tuned is this carbohydrate recognition that simply switching an amide group between two amino acids in the binding site by in vitro mutagenesis alters the specificity of recognition from mannose to galactose (42). Some specificity for nonself carbohydrates is obtained by virtue of the orientation of adjacent CRDs during multimerization. The MBP trimerization domain (i.e., neck region connecting the CRD head to the collagen tail) orients the CRD carbohydrate binding sites exactly 4.5 nanometers (human) or 5.3 nanometers (rat) apart, thereby favorably orienting the binding sites to carbohydrate repeats on pathogen surfaces (43–45).

On ligation of MBP, the bound ligand may be cleared through an opsonic interaction with specific cell surface receptors expressed on the surfaces of phagocytes, or other effector functions may be activated. MBP, lung surfactant protein-A (SP-A), and C1q (the recognition component of the classic complement pathway) enhance macrophage FcR-mediated phagocytosis by binding to a 126-kd cell surface receptor (46). This illustrates how a soluble PRR may act as a signaling molecule to enhance host cellular immune function. In addition to enhancing FcR activity, this cell surface receptor is thought to play a role in the clearance of particles opsonized by MBP, SP-A, or C1q. Cloning of the cDNA of this receptor (designated C1qRp) has shown it to be a novel type I membrane protein, containing a C-type CRD, five epidermal growth factor–like domains, a transmembrane domain, and a short cytoplasmic tail (47). Although other receptors have been described for C1q (48), and SP-A (49), this is the only receptor described for MBP.

Other effector functions of MBP include activation of the classic and alternative complement pathways directly or through activation of associated proteases such as the MBP-associated protease (MASP), which is able to amplify the generation of the third component of complement (50). Human MBP is able to substitute for C1q in its interaction with the C1r and C1s serine proteases and is thereby able to activate the C3 convertase of the classic complement pathway (51,52). Binding of MBP to mannose-rich pathogens has also been shown to directly activate the alternative pathway of complement (53). MASP was identified as a serine protease with similarities to C1r and C1s that co-purified with MBP. Ligation of MBP activates MASP, which then cleaves C3 directly or activates the classic pathway C3 convertase (50). The elucidation of the multi-exon MASP gene structure has suggested that it may have been the evolutionary prototype for other serine proteases such as C1r and C1s (54). By activating complement, MBP illustrates the interac-

TABLE 35-2. *Collectins and their characteristics*

Collectin	MBP	SP-A	SP-D	Conglutin	CL-43
Species	Mouse, rat, rabbit, chicken, bovine, human	Mouse, rat, rabbit, dog, bovine, human	Mouse, rat, bovine, human	Bovine	Bovine
Human gene	7 kb, 4 exons	4.5 kb, 5 exons	11 kb, 8 exons	—	—
Chromosomal localization (human)	10q11.2-q21	10q22.2-q23.1	10q22.2-q23.1	—	—
Carbohydrate specificity	Mannose, fucose, glucose, GlcNAc	ManNAc, fucose	Maltose, glucose	GlcNAc	Mannose, ManNAc
Complement activation	Yes	No	No	Binds to iC3b	No
Organisms bound					
Bacteria					
Gram negative	Klebsiella pneumoniae, Pseudomonas aeruginosa, Salmonella typhimurium, Salmonella montevideo, E. coli	Escherichia coli	K. pneumoniae, E. coli	—	—
Gram positive	S. aureus, viridans streptococci, Streptococcus pneumoniae, group B streptococci	S. aureus	—	—	—
Yeast	Cryptococcus neoformans, Saecharomyces cerevisiae, Candida albicans	C. neoformans	C. neoformans,	C. neoformans S. cerevisiae	C. neoformans
Viruses	HIV, IAV, HSV	IAV, HSV	IAV	HIV, IAV, HSV	
Mycobacteria	Mycobacterium tuberculosis, M. avium, M. leprae				
Protozoa	Trypanosoma cruzi, Pneumocystis carinii	P. carinii	P. carinii		

MBP, mannose-binding protein; SP-A, lung surfactant protein-A; SP-D, lung surfactant protein-D; CL-43, serum bovine collectin-43; GlcNAc, *N*-acetyl glucosamine; ManNAc, *N*-acetyl mannosamine; IAV, influenza A virus; HSV, herpes simplex virus; HIV, human immunodeficiency virus

(Reproduced from ref. 39, with permission of the editors.)

tion between a soluble PRR and other soluble immune effector mechanisms.

The similarities of function of MBP with those of immunoglobulin led to the concept of collectins as antibodies. The wide range of carbohydrate ligands recognized by the collectin CRDs enables interaction with pathogens during the time lag when specific immune responses (immunoglobulin and T cell receptor repertoires) are being generated (55). This hypothesis is supported by the observation that children with genetically determined low levels of MBP are predisposed to recurrent bacterial infections. This susceptibility is particularly marked for children younger than 2 years of age, a time when anti-carbohydrate immunoglobulin production is markedly diminished (56,57).

Mannose Receptor and Related Transmembrane Lectins

The macrophage mannose receptor (MR) is an approximately 180-kd transmembrane receptor expressed on resident macrophage subpopulations, dendritic cells, and subsets of endothelial cells. Ligands bearing terminal mannose, fucose, or *N*-acetylglucosamine are bound in a calcium-dependent fashion and then internalized by this lectin. Although the MR has been extensively studied as a classic recycling endocytic receptor (58), it is also able to mediate phagocytic uptake of particles bearing mannose-rich residues, including pathogens such as *Pneumocystis carinii* (59). The carbohydrate specificity of pattern recognition is the same as that of the MBP and a wide range of pathogens has been reported to bind to the MR. Cellular expression of the MR is tightly regulated (60). Regulation by lymphocyte-derived cytokines (e.g., the dramatic upregulation of MR expression by prototypical T_H2 cytokines (61,62)), strongly implicates this receptor in inflammatory conditions; however, *in vivo* data describing a physiologic role are lacking.

Molecular cloning of the cDNA for this receptor has revealed the predicted primary structure of a type I transmembrane molecule: an N-terminal, cysteine-rich domain, followed by a fibronectin type II–like domain, eight CRDs in tandem, a single transmembrane domain, and a 45 residue cytoplasmic tail at the C terminus (63–65). Since the cloning of the MR, a number of molecules with significant primary structure homology have been identified (Table 35-3), thereby defining a family of MR-like type C lectins, characterized by the presence of multiple tandem CRD repeats within a single polypeptide chain. Not all members of this family function as lectins, however, suggesting that their CRD domains have been used as a structural or framework motif, rather than as a specific carbohydrate-binding domain.

Analysis of truncated forms of the MR expressed in fibroblasts showed that neither the cysteine-rich nor fibronectin type II–like domains were involved in carbohydrate binding (66). Most of the carbohydrate-binding activity of the intact receptor was mediated by CRDs 4 through 8: CRD-4 was the only CRD able to bind monosaccharides, and CRDs-4, -5, and -7 were required in combination to mediate high-affinity binding of complex ligands such as glycoproteins (66). The clustering of CRDs to achieve high-affinity binding is reminiscent of that seen in the soluble MBP, in which clustering is achieved through multimerization of single CRD-bearing monomers, rather than through tandem positioning in a single polypeptide chain.

Although playing no discernible role in carbohydrate binding, the cysteine-rich and fibronectin type II–like domains of the MR are highly conserved across species. This prompted Gordon et al. (67) to seek alternative ligands for these domains. By means of chimeric proteins consisting of these two MR domains fused to the Fc portion of immunoglobulin, putative ligands for the cysteine-rich domain of MR were identified (67). These ligands were associated with subsets of macrophages and B lymphocytes in the spleen and lymph nodes of mice. Upregulation and migration of these putative ligands were observed on antigenic stimulation of the mice, hinting at a role for MR in cell-cell interaction, antigen transport, or transfer to regions where humoral responses are generated. Further investigation of the nature of these newly recognized MR ligands is underway.

It has been postulated that MR may be acting as a bifunctional molecule, using its CRDs to capture carbohydrate-bearing ligands and its cysteine-rich region to direct these bound antigens to appropriate effector cells.

Additional evidence for a role in cell-cell interactions has come from studies in which inhibitors of MR were able to prevent IL-4–induced macrophage fusion in an *in vitro* model (68). IL-13 and IL-4 induced macrophage fusion and foreign body–type giant cell formation *in vitro*, while upregulating MR expression on these cells (69). The MR domains mediating these events and the role of other molecules in this process have yet to be determined.

Dendritic cells, as the most significant and potent stimulators of primary immune responses (70), would be expected to be capable of effectively sampling body interfaces, recognizing nonself molecules or pathogens and rapidly processing them for evaluation by the immune system. Evidence is accumulating that immature dendritic cells express high levels of the MR and that this receptor is a major pathway for the uptake of antigens and their subsequent delivery to major histocompatibility complex class II (MHC II) compartments within the dendritic cells (71,72). In addition to this MHC II pathway, MR plays a critical role in the presentation of lipoglycan antigens (in pathogens such as mycobacteria and fungi) to T cells by delivering these antigens to intracellular CD1b molecules in antigen presenting cells (73). It appears that MR is expressed at high levels on immature dendritic cells (i.e., those in antigen-capturing mode) and is then downregulated by the same inflammatory stimuli that cause migration and maturation of the dendritic cells into their antigen-presenting mode (74,75). In this fashion, the broad ligand specificity of a PRR, the mannose receptor, is coupled with the finely tuned recognition capabilities of the specific, clonal immune system. This may be an important mechanism to ensure that nonself molecules are preferentially presented to stimulate host T lymphocytes.

Although MR-mediated ligation and uptake leads to enhanced macrophage microbicidal activity (76) and cytokine secretion (77), the downstream signaling pathway has not been defined. Likewise, while the intracellular mechanisms of Fc receptor-mediated phagocytosis are becoming well defined (78,79), those of MR remain unelucidated. In a series of experiments using chimeric receptors, it was demonstrated that the cytoplasmic and transmembrane domains from the MR were required to mediate optimal phagocytosis *in vitro* (80). Studies directed toward molecules that may interact with the MR cytoplasmic tail may help to further refine these observations.

Other members of the endocytic mannose receptor C-type lectin family are indicated in Table 35-3. All are type I transmembrane proteins containing a cysteine-rich domain, fibronectin type II–like domain, and 8 or 10 tandem CRD repeats. The DEC-205 molecule is expressed on dendritic cells and thymic epithelium and has 10 CRDs. Although its carbohydrate recognition pattern has not been reported, antigens that bind DEC-205 are presented to T lymphocytes more efficiently than are similar

TABLE 35-3. *Endocytic mannose receptor type C lectin family*

Receptor	Number of CRDs	References
Mannose receptor	8	63, 64
DEC-205	10	81
PLA$_2$ receptor	8	82
"Novel lectin"	8	85

CRD, carbohydrate recognition domain; PLA$_2$, phospholipase A$_2$.

antigens that are not DEC-205 ligands (81). Molecular cloning of the mammalian receptors for phospholipase A_2 (a secretory enzyme) revealed a similar primary structure to that of the MR (82,83). High-affinity binding of phospholipase enzymes, which contain no carbohydrate residues, to these receptors is mediated by the CRDs, but is calcium and carbohydrate independent (82), suggesting that the CRD framework has been coopted in evolution to provide different pattern recognition abilities. The CRDs in the phospholipase A_2 receptor are still capable of binding some carbohydrate ligands with high affinity, even though carbohydrates are not involved in binding of physiologic ligands (84).

Recently, another member of this family was identified by its homology with the CRD from E-selectin (85). This novel lectin is expressed in highly endothelialized sites (e.g., lung, choroid plexus, renal glomeruli) and in chondrocytes in cartilaginous regions of the embryo, but no ligand specificity or physiologic functions have been reported.

CONCLUSIONS

The carbohydrate residues that decorate the surfaces of pathogens provide PAMPs that are recognized by host-encoded PRRs. The information conveyed by these interactions enables the host to distinguish self from nonself and to initiate an appropriately targeted immune response. Although much is known about key PRRs, many questions remain to be addressed. Further analysis of the downstream signaling pathways of PRRs will enable a greater understanding of the role of PRRs in cellular activation and other immune responses. The relative contributions of different PRRs that recognize the same PAMPs (e.g., soluble MBP, cell surface MR) to effector responses *in vivo* remain to be determined. Further delineation of the cooperation and interplay between the innate and clonal immune systems may lead to novel therapeutic interventions. Stimulating or augmenting innate immune responses in the setting of a failing, depleted, or suppressed clonal immune system may be one way of preventing or treating infections in this setting.

Studies of naturally occurring polymorphisms and mutations (as described for MBP) shed some light on the functions of PRRs *in vivo*. These experiments of nature are difficult to interpret however, chiefly because of a multiplicity of confounding variables. The use of simpler organisms with the attendant ability to perform mass genetic screens on large populations has proved useful in the past and is likely to continue to do so. This approach may yield new PRRs and is also likely to provide insight into PRR-mediated signal transduction. The experience with human MBP mutations suggests that the loss or diminution of function of a single PRR may not give rise to a readily appreciated phenotype.

The increasing availability of a range of knock-out mice and the ability to breed double and triple gene knock-outs will help to circumvent this problem in at least two ways. First, the effects of the loss of multiple PRRs in a single animal can be studied, and redundancy and cooperativity of PRRs can be defined. Second, PRR-deficient mice can be crossed with mice deficient in other components of the immune system (e.g., complement, B lymphocytes, T lymphocytes), and the interplay and cross-talk between the innate and clonal immune systems can be further dissected.

REFERENCES

1. Janeway CAJ. The immune system evolved to discriminate infectious nonself from noninfectious self. *Immunol Today* 1992;13:11–16.
2. Medzhitov R, Janeway CAJ. Innate immunity: the virtues of a nonclonal system of recognition. *Cell* 1997;91:295–298.
3. Ofek I, Goldhar J, Keisari Y, Sharon N. Nonopsonic phagocytosis of microorganisms. *Annu Rev Microbiol* 1995;49:239–276.
4. Muta T, Iwanaga S. The role of hemolymph coagulation in innate immunity. *Curr Opin Immunol* 1996;8:41–47.
5. Tanaka S, Iwanaga S. *Limulus* test for detecting bacterial endotoxins. *Metab Enzymol* 1993;223:358–364.
6. Seki N, Muta T, Oda T, et al. Horseshoe crab (1,3)-beta-D-glucan-sensitive coagulation factor G: a serine protease zymogen heterodimer with similarities to beta-glucan-binding proteins. *J Biol Chem* 1994;269:1370–1374.
7. Cerenius L, Liang Z, Duvic B, et al. Structure and biological activity of a 1,3-beta-D-glucan-binding protein in crustacean blood. *J Biol Chem* 1994;269:29462–29467.
8. Jomori T, Natori S. Molecular cloning of cDNA for lipopolysaccharide-binding protein from the hemolymph of the American cockroach, *Periplanta americana*: similarity of the protein with animal lectins and its acute phase expression. *J Biol Chem* 1991;266:13318–13323.
9. Takahashi H, Komano H, Kawaguchi N, Kitamura N, Nakanishi S, Natori S. Cloning and sequencing of cDNA of Sarcophaga peregrina humoral lectin induced on injury of the body wall. *J Biol Chem* 1985;260:12228–12233.
10. Goldstein JL, Ho YK, Basu SK, Brown MS. Binding site on macrophages that mediates uptake and degradation of acetylated low density lipoprotein producing massive cholesterol deposition. *Proc Natl Acad Sci USA* 1979;76:333–337.
11. Krieger M, Acton S, Ashkenas J, Pearson A, Penman M, Resnick D. Molecular flypaper, host defense, and atherosclerosis. *J Biol Chem* 1993;268:4569–4572.
12. Elomaa O, Kangas M, Sahlberg C, et al. Cloning of a novel bacteria-binding receptor structurally related to scavenger receptors and expressed in a subset of macrophages. *Cell* 1995;80:603–609.
13. Emi M, Asaoka H, Matsumoto A, et al. Structure, organization, and chromosomal mapping of the human macrophage scavenger receptor gene. *J Biol Chem* 1993;268:2120–2125.
14. Hampton RY, Golenbock DT, Penman M, Krieger M, Raetz CRH. Recognition and plasma clearance of endotoxin by scavenger receptors. *Nature* 1991;352:342–344.
15. Dunne DW, Resnick D, Greenberg J, Krieger M, Joiner KA. The type I macrophage scavenger receptor binds to gram-positive bacteria and recognizes lipoteichoic acid. *Proc Natl Acad Sci USA* 1994;91:1863–1867.
16. Suzuki H, Kurihara Y, Takeya M, et al. A role for macrophage scavenger receptors in atherosclerosis and susceptibility to infection. *Nature* 1997;386:292–296.
17. Haworth R, Platt N, Keshav S, et al. The macrophage scavenger receptor type A is expressed by activated macrophages and protects the host against lethal endotoxic shock. *J Exp Med* 1997;186:1431–1439.
18. Franc NC, Dimarcq J-L, Lagueux M, Hoffmann J, Ezekowitz RAB. Croquemort, a novel *Drosophila* hemocyte/macrophage receptor that recognizes apoptotic cells. *Immunity* 1996;4:431–443.
19. Savill J, Hogg N, Ren Y, Haslett C. Thrombospondin cooperates with

CD36 and the vitronectin receptor in macrophage recognition of neutrophils undergoing apoptosis. *J Clin Invest* 1992;90:1513–1522.

20. Savill J. Macrophage recognition of senescent neutrophils. *Clin Sci* 1992;83:649–655.

21. Stern M, Savill J, Haslett C. Human monocyte-derived macrophage phagocytosis of senescent eosinophils undergoing apoptosis. Mediation by alpha V beta 3/CD36/thrombospondin recognition mechanism and lack of phlogistic response. *Am J Pathol* 1996;149:911–921.

22. Oquendo P, Hundt E, Lawler J, Seed B. CD36 directly mediates cytoadherence of *Plasmodium falciparum* parasitized erythrocytes. *Cell* 1989; 58:95–101.

23. Crabb BS, Cooke BM, Reeder JC, et al. Targeted gene disruption shows that knobs enable malaria-infected red cells to cytoadhere under physiological shear stress. *Cell* 1997;89:287–296.

24. Acton SL, Scherer PE, Lodish HF, Krieger M. Expression cloning of SR-BI, a CD36-related class B scavenger receptor. *J Biol Chem* 1994; 269:21003–21009.

25. Acton S, Rigotti S, Landschulz KT, Hobbs HH, Krieger M. Identification of scavenger receptor SR-BI as a high density lipoprotein receptor. *Science* 1996;271:518–520.

26. Kozarsky KF, Donahee MH, Rigotti A, Iqbal SN, Edelman ER, Krieger M. Overexpression of the HDL receptor SR-BI alters plasma HDL and bile cholesterol levels. *Nature* 1997;387:414–417.

27. Steinberg D. A docking receptor for HDL cholesterol esters. *Science* 1996;271:460–461.

28. Abrams JM, Lux A, Steller H, Krieger M. Macrophages in Drosophila embryos and L2 cells exhibit scavenger receptor-mediated endocytosis. *Proc Natl Acad Sci USA* 1992;89:10375–10379.

29. Pearson A, Lux A, Krieger M. Expression cloning of dSR-CI, a class C macrophage-specific scavenger receptor from *Drosophila melanogaster*. *Proc Natl Acad Sci USA* 1995;92:4056–4060.

30. Reid KBM, Day AJ. Structure-function relationships of the complement components. *Immunol Today* 1989;10:177–180.

31. Iobst ST, Drickamer K. Binding of sugar ligands to Ca(2+)-dependent animal lectins. II. Generation of high-affinity galactose binding by site-directed mutagenesis. *J Biol Chem* 1994;269:15512–15519.

32. Spiess M. The asialoglycoprotein receptor: a model for endocytic transport receptors. *Biochemistry* 1990;29:10009–10018.

33. Holland EC, Leung JO, Drickamer K. Rat liver asialoglycoprotein receptor lacks a cleavable NH$_2$-terminal signal sequence. *Proc Natl Acad Sci USA* 1984;81:7338–7342.

34. Spiess M, Lodish HF. Sequence of a second human asialoglycoprotein receptor: conservation of two receptor genes during evolution. *Proc Natl Acad Sci USA* 1985;82:6465–6469.

35. Ii M, Kurata H, Itoh N, Yamashira I, Kawasaki T. Molecular cloning and sequence analysis of cDNA encoding the macrophage lectin specific for galactose and *N*-acetylgalactosamine. *J Biol Chem* 1990;265: 11295–11298.

36. Porat N, Apicella MA, Blake MS. *Neisseria gonorrhoeae* utilizes and enhances the biosynthesis of the asialoglycoprotein receptor expressed on the surface of the hepatic HepG2 cell line. *Infect Immun* 1995;63: 1498–1506.

37. Becker S, Spiess M, Klenk HD. The asialoglycoprotein receptor is a potential liver-specific receptor for Marburg virus. *J Gen Virol* 1995; 76:393–399.

38. Treichel U, Meyer zum Buschenfelde KH, Stockert RJ, Poralla T, Gerken G. The asialoglycoprotein receptor mediates hepatic binding and uptake of natural hepatitis B virus particles derived from viraemic carriers. *J Gen Virol* 1994;75:3021–3029.

39. Epstein J, Eichbaum Q, Sheriff S, Ezekowitz RAB. The collectins in innate immunity. *Curr Opin Immunol* 1996;8:29–35.

40. Weis WI, Kahn R, Fourme R, Drickamer K, Hendrickson WA. Structure of the calcium-dependent lectin domain from a rat mannose-binding protein determined by MAD phasing. *Science* 1991;254:1608–1615.

41. Weis WI, Drickamer K, Hendrickson WA. Structure of a C-type mannose-binding protein complexed with an oligosaccharide. *Nature* 1992; 360:127–134.

42. Drickamer K. Engineering galactose-binding activity into a C-type mannose-binding protein. *Nature* 1992;360:183–186.

43. Hoppe HJ, Barlow PN, Reid KB. A parallel three stranded alpha-helical bundle at the nucleation site of collagen triple-helix formation. *FEBS Lett* 1994;344:191–195.

44. Sheriff S, Chang CY, Ezekowitz RAB. Human mannose-binding protein carbohydrate recognition domain trimerizes through a triple alpha-helical coiled-coil. *Nat Struct Biol* 1994;1:789–794.

45. Weis WI, Drickamer K. Trimeric structure of a C-type mannose binding protein. *Structure* 1994;2:1227–1240.

46. Tenner AJ, Robinson SL, Ezekowitz RAB. Mannose binding protein (MBP) enhances mononuclear phagocyte function via a receptor that contains the 126,000 M(r) component of the C1q receptor. *Immunity* 1995;3:485–493.

47. Nepomuceno RR, Henschen-Edman AH, Burgess WH, Tenner AJ. cDNA cloning and primary structure analysis of C1qR(P), the human C1q/MBL/SPA receptor that mediates enhanced phagocytosis *in vitro*. *Immunity* 1997;6:119–129.

48. Malhotra R, Willis AC, Jensenius JC, Jackson J, Sim RB. Structure and homology of human C1q receptor (collectin receptor). *Immunology* 1993;78:341–348.

49. Pison U, Wright JR, Hawgood S. Specific binding of surfactant apoprotein SP-A to rat alveolar macrophages. *Am J Physiol* 1992;262: L412–L417.

50. Matsushita M, Fujita T. Activation of the classical complement pathway by mannose-binding protein in association with a novel C1s-like serine protease. *J Exp Med* 1992;176:1497–1502.

51. Ikeda K, Sannoh T, Kawasaki N, Kawasaki T, Yamashina I. Serum lectin with known structure activates complement through the classical pathway. *J Biol Chem* 1987;262:7451–7454.

52. Lu JH, Thiel S, Wiedmann H, Timpl R, Reid KB. Binding of the pentamer/hexamer forms of mannan-binding protein to zymosan activates the proenzyme C1r2C1s2 complex of the classical pathway of complement, without involvement of C1q. *J Immunol* 1990;144:2287–2294.

53. Schweinle J, Ezekowitz RAB, Tenner A, Joiner K. Human mannose-binding protein activates the alternative pathway and enhances serum bactericidal activity on a mannose-rich isolate of Salmonella. *J Clin Invest* 1989;84:1821–1829.

54. Endo Y, Sato T, Matsushita M, Fujita T. Exon structure of the gene encoding the human mannose-binding protein-associated serine protease light chain: comparison with complement C1r and C1s genes. *Int Immunol* 1996;8:1355–1358.

55. Ezekowitz RAB. Ante-antibody immunity. *Curr Biol* 1991;1:60–62.

56. Super M, Thiel S, Lu J, Levindsky RJ, Turner MW. Association of low levels of mannan-binding protein with a common defect of opsonization. *Lancet* 1989;2:1236–1238.

57. Summerfield JA, Sumiya M, Levin M, Turner MW. Association of mutations in mannose binding protein gene with childhood infection in consecutive hospital series. *BMJ* 1997;314:1229–1232.

58. Stahl P, Schlesinger PH, Sigardson E, Rodman JS, Lee YC. Receptor-mediated pinocytosis of mannose glycoconjugates by macrophages: characterization and evidence for receptor recycling. *Cell* 1980;19: 207–215.

59. Ezekowitz RAB, Williams DJ, Koziel H, et al. Uptake of *Pneumocystis carinii* mediated by the macrophage mannose receptor. *Nature* 1991; 351:155–158.

60. Mokoena T, Gordon S. Modulation of mannosyl-fucosyl receptor activity *in vitro* by lymphokines, γ and α interferons and dexamethasone. *J Clin Invest* 1985;75:624–631.

61. Stein M, Keshav S, Harris N, Gordon S. Interleukin 4 potently enhances murine macrophage mannose receptor activity: a marker of alternative immunologic macrophage activation. *J Exp Med* 1992;176: 287–292.

62. Doyle AG, Herbein G, Montaner LJ, et al. Interleukin-13 alters the activation state of murine macrophages *in vitro*: comparison with interleukin-4 and interferon-gamma. *Eur J Immunol* 1994;24:1441–1445.

63. Ezekowitz RAB, Sastry K, Bailly P, Warner A. Molecular characterization of the human macrophage mannose receptor: demonstration of multiple carbohydrate recognition-like domains and phagocytosis of yeasts in COS-1 cells. *J Exp Med* 1990;172:1785–1794.

64. Taylor ME, Conary JT, Lennartz MR, Stahl PD, Drickamer K. Primary structure of the mannose receptor contains multiple motifs resembling carbohydrate recognition domains. *J Biol Chem* 1990;265:12156–12162.

65. Harris N, Super M, Rits M, Chang G, Ezekowitz RAB. Characterization of the murine macrophage mannose receptor: demonstration that the downregulation of receptor expression mediated by interferon-γ occurs at the level of transcription. *Blood* 1992;80:2363–2373.

66. Taylor ME, Bezouska K, Drickamer K. Contribution to ligand binding by multiple carbohydrate-recognition domains in the macrophage mannose receptor. *J Biol Chem* 1992;267:1719–1726.

67. Martinez-Pomares L, Kosco-Vilbois M, Darley E, et al. Fc chimeric protein containing the cysteine-rich domain of the murine mannose receptor binds to macrophages from splenic marginal zone and lymph

node subcapsular sinus and to germinal centers. *J Exp Med* 1996;184: 1927–1937.

68. McNally AK, DeFife KM, Anderson JM. Interleukin-4–induced macrophage fusion is prevented by inhibitors of mannose receptor activity. *Am J Pathol* 1996;149:975–985.

69. DeFife KM, Jenney CR, McNally AK, Colton E, Anderson JM. Interleukin-13 induces human monocyte/macrophage fusion and macrophage mannose receptor expression. *J Immunol* 1997;158:3385–3390.

70. Hart DNJ. Dendritic cells: unique leukocyte populations which control the primary immune response. *Blood* 1997;90:3245–3287.

71. Sallusto F, Cella M, Danieli C, Lanzavecchia A. Dendritic cells use macropinocytosis and the mannose receptor to concentrate macromolecules in the major histocompatibility complex class II compartment: downregulation by cytokines and bacterial products. *J Exp Med* 1995; 182:389–400.

72. Lanzavecchia A. Mechanisms of antigen uptake for presentation. *Curr Opin Immunol* 1996;8:348–354.

73. Prigozy TI, Sieling PA, Clemens D, et al. The mannose receptor delivers lipoglycan antigens to endosomes for presentation to T cells by CD1b molecules. *Immunity* 1997;6:187–197.

74. Cella M, Engering A, Pinet V, Pieters J, Lanzavecchia A. Inflammatory stimuli induce accumulation of MHC class II complexes on dendritic cells. *Nature* 1997;388:782–787.

75. Pierre P, Turley SJ, Gatti E, et al. Developmental regulation of MHC class II transport in mouse dendritic cells. *Nature* 1997;388:787–792.

76. Lefkowitz DL, Lincoln JA, Lefkowitz SS, Bollen A, Moguilevsky N. Enhancement of macrophage-mediated bactericidal activity by macrophage mannose receptor–ligand interaction. *Immunol Cell Biol* 1997; 75:136–141.

77. Yamamoto Y, Klein TW, Friedman H. Involvement of mannose receptor in cytokine interleukin-1 beta (IL-1 beta), IL-6, and granulocyte-macrophage colony-stimulating factor responses, but not in chemokine macrophage inflammatory protein 1 beta (MIP-1 beta), MIP-2, and KC responses, caused by attachment of *Candida albicans* to macrophages. *Infect Immun* 1997;65:1077–1082.

78. Crowley MT, Costello PS, Fitzer-Attas CJ, et al. A critical role for Syk in signal transduction and phagocytosis mediated by Fcγ receptors on macrophages. *J Exp Med* 1997;186:1027–1039.

79. Hackam DJ, Rotstein OD, Schreiber A, Zhang W-J, Grinstein S. Rho is required for the initiation of calcium signalling and phagocytosis by Fcγ receptors in macrophages. *J Exp Med* 1997;186:955–966.

80. Kruskal BA, Sastry K, Warner AB, Mathieu CE, Ezekowitz RAB. Phagocytic chimeric receptors require both transmembrane and cytoplasmic domains from the mannose receptor. *J Exp Med* 1992;176:1673–1680.

81. Jiang W, Swiggard WJ, Heufler C, et al. The receptor DEC-205 expressed by dendritic cells and thymic epithelial cells is involved in antigen processing. *Nature* 1995;375:151–155.

82. Ishizaki J, Hanasaki K, Higashino K-I, et al. Molecular cloning of pancreatic group I phospholipase A2 receptor. *J Biol Chem* 1994;269: 5897–5904.

83. Ancian P, Lambeau G, Mattei M-G, Lazdunski M. The human 180-kDa receptor for secretory phospholipase A_2: molecular cloning, identification of a secreted soluble form, expression, and chromosomal localization. *J Biol Chem* 1995;270:8963–8970.

84. Lambeau G, Ancian P, Barhanin J, Lazdunski M. Cloning and expression of a membrane receptor for secretory phospholipase A_2. *J Biol Chem* 1994;269:1575–1578.

85. Wu K, Yuan J, Lasky LA. Characterization of a novel member of the macrophage mannose receptor type C lectin family. *J Biol Chem* 1996; 271:21323–21330.

Inflammation: Basic Principles and Clinical Correlates,
3rd ed., edited by John I. Gallin and Ralph Snyderman.
Lippincott Williams & Wilkins, Philadelphia © 1999.

CHAPTER 36

Innate Recognition of Microbial Lipids

Samuel D. Wright

Bacteria express lipids that have structures and colligative properties different from those of their mammalian counterparts, and certain of these lipids provoke dramatic responses in inflammatory cells. Gram-negative lipopolysaccharide (LPS, endotoxin) is by far the most potent bacterial stimulator of inflammation, with picogram per milliliter concentrations yielding strong responses *in vitro* and *in vivo*. This chapter first concentrates on LPS as a paradigm for understanding innate responses to microbial lipids and then discusses other microbial lipids.

A large body of work suggests that LPS is necessary and sufficient for sensitive innate responses to gram-negative bacteria. Injection of animals with purified LPS replicates the full spectrum of inflammatory responses observed with whole bacteria (1), and systemic responses to bacteria can be blocked by anti-LPS antibodies or LPS-neutralizing proteins (2,3). A mutation in the bacterial enzyme that attaches myristic acid to LPS (Fig. 36-1) yields an LPS molecule that has lost the ability to stimulate mammalian cells, and whole bacteria with this mutation have a 1,000-fold depressed ability to stimulate cellular responses (4). The responses to LPS are innate and do not depend on an adaptive immune response. Immunologically virgin piglets, delivered by aseptic hysterectomy from sows raised in a germ-free environment, have no passive immunity or anamnestic response but exhibit a full range of responses to LPS (5). Moreover, monocytes, neutrophils, and endothelial cells each respond to bacteria in vitro with no requirement for IgG, and LPS strongly stimulates lower phyla (e.g., mollusks, arthropods), which do not even possess an adaptive immune system. These studies make it clear that recognition of LPS serves as a cornerstone of the innate response to gram-negative bacteria.

LPS induces a very wide range of effects in mammals, including fever, nausea, increased leptin levels, anorexia, hypertriglyceridemia, hypotension, tachycardia, and diarrhea (6–8). It is evident that LPS causes these complex physiologic changes in a largely indirect fashion by triggering cascades of secondary mediators. In this review, we concentrate on responses that are directly caused by the interaction of LPS with cells. Some of the direct cellular effects of LPS are listed in Table 36-1.

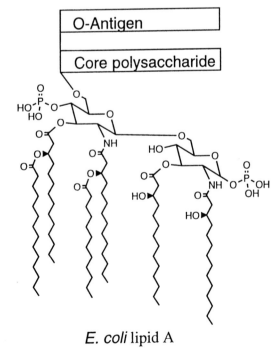

E. coli lipid A

FIG. 36-1. The structure of gram-negative lipopolysaccharide details a representative lipid A region and the placement of core polysaccharides and O-antigen.

S. D. Wright: Department of Lipid Biochemistry, Merck Research Laboratories, Rahway, New Jersey 07065.

TABLE 36-1. *Direct effects of lipopolysaccharide on cells*

Response	Cell type	References
Synthesis of cytokines (TNF, IL-1, IL-8, IL-6)	Monocytes, macrophages, PMN, astrocytes	Many
Synthesis of adhesion molecules (ICAM-1, E-selectin, VCAM-1)	Endothelial cells	9, 117
Activation of leukocyte integrins	PMN	118
Synthesis of tissue factor	Endothelial cells, monocytes	119, 120
Priming for arachidonic acid release	Macrophages, PMN	121, 122
Priming for superoxide anion release	Macrophages, PMN	123, 124
Synthesis of iNOS	Monocytes, macrophages	125
Synthesis of PGHS-II (COXII)	Monocytes, macrophages	126
Synthesis of plasminogen activator inhibitor I	Hepatocyte, endothelial cells	127
Synthesis of antibiotic peptides	Epithelial cells	128

ICAM, intercellular adhesion molecule; IL, interleukin; iNOS, inducible form of nitric oxide synthase; PGHS-II, prostaglandin H synthase-2; PMN, polymorphonuclear cell; VCAM, vascular cell adhesion molecule.

INFLAMMATORY REACTIONS TO LIPOPOLYSACCHARIDE

Beneficial Localized Responses

The integrated functions of the responses to LPS are best seen in localized bacterial infections. Bacterial products act on nearby cells to induce molecules that participate in cell-to-cell adhesion, including intercellular adhesion molecule-1 (ICAM-1) and E-selectin (ELAM-1, CD62E) on endothelial cells (9–11) and leukocyte integrins on polymorphonuclear cells (PMNs) (11–13,118) and monocytes (14). LPS also induces nearby cells to secrete proinflammatory cytokines and chemoattractants for leukocytes such as tumor necrosis factor (TNF), interleukin-1 (IL-1), IL-6, and IL-8 and to produce procoagulant molecules such as tissue factor (see Table 36-1). These processes lead to the well-known cardinal signs of inflammation, swelling, redness, heat, and pain. They bring leukocytes and other bactericidal effectors to the infectious focus and promote resolution of the infection. The beneficial nature of the response to LPS is confirmed by studies on mice with the *Lps^d* trait. Leukocytes from animals with this genetic defect require 10-fold to 1,000-fold more LPS to initiate a response than cells from normal mice, and animals with this defect are extremely susceptible to infectious challenge with *Salmonella typhimurium* (15). A prompt inflammatory response is clearly an evolutionary advantage conferred by the well-conserved recognition of LPS.

Septic Shock Response

In septic shock, the normally beneficial responses to LPS are detrimental because they occur systemically. In response to systemic endotoxemia, phagocytes move to the site of infection and into uninfected tissues and may provoke tissue damage and multi-organ failure. The procoagulant activity that may limit bacterial spread locally may cause disastrous disseminated intravascular coagulation systemically. The enhanced blood flow that is beneficial locally cannot be sustained throughout the body, and hypotension (shock) results; this has been called the systemic inflammatory response syndrome and should be thought of as a misdirected inflammatory response. Unfortunately, septic shock is one of the leading causes of death in the United States (16,17). Approximately 400,000 cases occur annually, with a mortality rate of nearly 40%. Septic shock is the leading cause of death in intensive care units, and the annual medical costs are estimated to be $5 to $10 billion. Approximately 50% of all septic shock-related deaths are of gram-negative origin. The absence of a specific treatment for septic shock makes it an object of active research. Because LPS can be separated from the bacterium that produced it and can be transported far from the site of infection, it is the prime suspect in misdirecting the inflammatory response in septic shock.

STRUCTURE OF LIPOPOLYSACCHARIDE

LPS is the predominant lipid in the outer leaflet of the outer membrane of nearly all gram-negative bacteria. The structure of LPS from a variety of strains has been determined, and excellent reviews have described LPS structure and biosynthesis (18,19). A prototypic LPS molecule is diagrammed in Figure 36-1 and may be divided into three regions.

O-antigen is a portion of LPS that is composed of a variable number of repeats of a unit comprising three to six sugar residues. Bacterial strains show tremendous variation in the nature and length of these repeats, and more than a thousand immunochemically distinct variants exist. The O-antigen is not necessary for bacterial growth, and "rough" strains lack the O-antigen entirely. The O-antigen is also unnecessary for the inflammatory activity of LPS.

The *core polysaccharide* region contains 10 or more sugars and a variable number of phosphate and ethanolamine residues. It is often divided into an "inner core" containing sugars unique to LPS such as 3-deoxy-D-manno-octulosonic acid (KDO) and L-glycero-D-manno-heptose and an "outer core" containing hexoses. Only the KDO residues are necessary for bacterial growth. The core polysaccharides are also not necessary for the inflammatory activity of LPS.

The *lipid A* region is composed of two acylated glucosamine phosphate residues joined by a β1–6 bond. The lipid A structure and the enzymes involved in its biosynthesis are highly conserved throughout the enterobacteriaceae (19). Lipid A is necessary for growth of bacteria, and mutations in most of the lipid A biosynthetic genes are lethal. Lipid A biosynthetic enzymes may be favorable targets for novel antibiotics (20). Unlike the core and O-antigen, lipid A is necessary and sufficient for initiating inflammatory responses and may be thought of as the "endotoxic" portion of LPS. Many studies on responses to LPS have used synthetic lipid A or lipid A derived by chemical cleavage of the core polysaccharides. Because lipid A and LPS have the same active principle, we refer to both as endotoxins.

As expected of a membrane-forming lipid, LPS is amphiphilic, with the six or more hydrocarbon chains forming the hydrophobe and sugars and phosphates forming the hydrophile. LPS may serve as a constituent of bacterial outer membranes, phospholipid liposomes, lipoproteins, and cell membranes. Further in keeping with these properties, LPS has a vanishingly low solubility as a monomer, existing rather as membranes or micelles (21), and it does not spontaneously diffuse from one membrane to another without the assistance of lipid transfer proteins (22).

LIPOPOLYSACCHARIDE-BINDING PROTEIN AND CD14 IN RESPONSES TO LIPOPOLYSACCHARIDE *IN VITRO*

Studies have defined two plasma proteins, CD14 and lipopolysaccharide-binding protein (LBP), that are necessary for systemic responses to LPS in the range of picograms to nanograms per milliliter. These two proteins transfer lipids from membrane to membrane in a two-step reaction. In the first step, LBP transfers an LPS monomer to a binding site on CD14. The resulting lipid-CD14 complex diffuses freely, and in a second reaction, the bound lipid is unloaded into a target membrane or lipoprotein. In this way, LBP and CD14 can hasten the movement of LPS from bacteria or shed fragments of bacteria to leukocytes and thereby enhance the inflammatory response. The actions of these proteins are considered in detail.

Lipopolysaccharide-Binding Protein

Role as a Lipid-Transfer Protein

LBP was discovered as an acute phase reactant that binds LPS (23). As its name implies, LBP was once thought to function as a "binding protein" that might stably recognize LPS in the same way that IgG recognizes foreign proteins. This view is mistaken; LBP is a relatively promiscuous lipid transfer protein that overcomes diffusion limits of an amphiphile such as LPS.

LBP is a member of a family of lipid transfer proteins that includes phospholipid transfer protein (PLTP), cholesterol ester transfer protein (CETP), and bactericidal permeability increasing protein (BPI) (24–28). Each of these glycoproteins has a molecular weight of approximately 50 kd and shows sequence identity of about 24% with the other members throughout its length. PLTP is carried on high-density lipoprotein (HDL) and exchanges phospholipids between lipoproteins (26). CETP, also carried on HDL, exchanges triglyceride in one lipoprotein particle with cholesterol ester in a second particle (27). Transfer activity for BPI has not been formally demonstrated, but x-ray crystalographic data show that the protein contains two moles of tightly bound phospholipid in separate binding sites (28). In keeping with the properties of the class, LBP is also carried on HDL particles (25,29) and mediates the exchange of phospholipids and LPS between lipoprotein particles, phospholipid vesicles, and CD14 (22,25,30).

LBP moves LPS monomers between aggregates and a binding site on CD14. The lipid transfer activity of LBP was first demonstrated by the finding that it dramatically accelerates movement of LPS from aggregates to a monomer binding site on CD14 (11). Under the conditions employed, each LBP molecule mediates the movement of over 100 LPS molecules, indicating a catalytic mechanism. Additional studies using real time measurements of the movement of fluorescently labeled LPS have revealed the Km for LPS (31), Km for CD14 (31), the first order reaction rate (32), the Vmax (31), and the "ternary complex" reaction mechanism employed by this bisubstrate catalyst (31). As expected of a catalyst, LBP enhances the forward and the reverse reactions; it accelerates the movement of LPS into CD14 and the movement of bound, radioactive LPS out of CD14 and into aggregates of unlabeled LPS (unpublished observations, 1996), lipoproteins (25) or phospholipid vesicles (22). The binding site for LPS aggregates has been mapped to the amino-terminal half of LBP, and transfer of LPS to CD14 requires the carboxyl-terminal half of the molecule (33,34).

LBP transfers not only LPS but also other phospholipids. One study documented LBP-catalyzed transfer of phosphatidyl inositol, phosphatidyl ethanolamine, and phosphatidyl choline to CD14 (30). Additional evidence suggests that LBP catalyzes a reciprocal transfer of lipids into and out of CD14 (30). The movement of each LPS molecule from CD14 to a phospholipid vesicle is accompanied by the reverse movement of one or two molecules of phospholipid from that vesicle into CD14. In this respect, LBP acts like CETP, which catalyzes an obligate exchange of triglyceride for cholesterol ester (27).

Roles of LBP in Inflammatory Responses to Lipopolysaccharide

LBP may both enhance and inhibit inflammatory responses to LPS. The broad specificity of LBP suggests that it may not be a pivotal recognition point in generating a response to bacterial infection. Additional observations show that LBP has activities that may work to enhance and to blunt inflammatory responses, further complicating its role in innate immunity.

LBP enhances responses of CD14-bearing cells to LPS in vitro. LBP may enhance responses of cells to LPS by speeding the transfer of LPS to CD14. LPS-CD14 complexes are key intermediates in sensitive responses to LPS, and by accelerating this transfer, LBP may speed and enhance a cellular response. The importance of this function of LBP is seen in studies with PMN in which addition of LBP may cause a >1000-fold enhancement in sensitivity to LPS. In this setting, the function of LBP is only to transfer LPS into membrane-associated CD14 because the requirement for LBP can be obviated by stimulating cells with preformed LPS-sCD14 complexes rather than LPS aggregates (11,35). LBP is not absolutely essential for responses to LPS, and in some settings it does not even stimulate them (10,24,36–38). The increase in sensitivity observed on addition of LBP varies from more than 1,000-fold for the rapid responses of PMN to essentially zero in assays that employ long incubations (24 to 48 hours) with LPS. It appears likely that with sufficient time for spontaneous diffusion into CD14, a catalyst may not be necessary.

LBP mediates the neutralization of LPS by lipoproteins. LBP hastens the movement of LPS out of LPS-CD14 complexes into lipoprotein particles (39). Incorporation of LPS into lipoproteins has long been known to "neutralize" the ability of LPS to stimulate biologic responses (39–42), and this action of LBP counteracts the stimulatory effect of LPS transfer to CD14. LBP can also accelerate transfer of lipids to HDL particles in the absence of CD14, though this reaction proceeds at a slower rate than the transfer from CD14 (22,25,39). The ability of LBP to transfer LPS to lipoproteins provides a countervailing force that may retard the spread of inflammation from a site of infection. Transgenic mice that overexpress high-density lipoproteins show reduced systemic responses to LPS (43).

LBP may act as an opsonin. LBP binds to LPS-coated particles (23), and these particles can be bound by CD14-bearing cells such as macrophages (44). Binding of LBP-coated bacteria to the surface of leukocytes is followed by phagocytosis (44,45), and LBP-coated LPS aggregates may also be endocytosed (46,47). In this way, LBP may serve in clearance of bacteria and shed LPS. LPS-LBP complexes bind to CD14 on the surface of cells (47,48) and this binding may be the first step in the transfer of LPS monomers to CD14. However, in some cases the binding of LPS-LBP complexes may cause endocytosis of large LPS aggregates or bacteria in such a way that an inflammatory response is not initiated. Certain monoclonal antibodies to LBP block transfer of LPS to CD14 (47). These antibodies inhibit cellular responses to LPS but do not block binding of LPS-LBP complexes to cell surface CD14. Further, site-directed mutagenesis of LBP has yielded a form that fails to transfer LPS monomers from aggregates to CD14 (49). This form still binds LPS and mediates binding of LBP-LPS complexes to cell surface CD14, but it does not enhance cellular responses to LPS. These studies highlight the lipid transfer activity of LBP as a key to its ability to provoke cellular responses and suggest that endocytosis of LPS-LBP complexes, in contrast, acts to remove LPS without cellular responses. The precise role of the opsonic function of LBP and the balance between cell stimulation and LPS clearance remains to be determined.

LBP knock-out mice respond to LPS. The gene encoding LBP was deleted from mice by homologous recombination (38). As expected from the *in vitro* findings, whole blood taken from these animals showed a striking deficiency in the ability to produce TNF in response to LPS. However, injection of LPS into LBP knock-out animals produced a cytokine response that was indistinguishable from that of wild type mice. These data further highlight the multifunctional nature of LBP. They also suggest the existence of an additional protein or factor that may substitute for LBP in the transfer of LPS to CD14 that underlies the systemic response to endotoxin.

CD14

Structure and Expression

CD14 is a 55-kd glycoprotein expressed on the surfaces of monocytes, macrophages, and PMN. A potential role for CD14 in recognition of LPS was discovered by experiments in which depletion of mCD14 from the surface of macrophages prevented binding of particles coated with LPS and LBP (50). Although LPS-LBP complexes do bind to CD14, the binding is transient and occurs during LBP-catalyzed transfer of an LPS monomer to a binding site on CD14. CD14 binds LPS in the absence of LBP and should be thought of as a lipid-binding protein.

The two types of CD14 are membrane CD14 (mCD14) and soluble CD14 (sCD14). Though CD14 was first discovered as a cell surface differentiation antigen, the majority (>99%) of CD14 in the blood exists as a soluble protein present at about 3 µg/mL (51,52). This is possible because CD14 is held at the cell surface by a GPI anchor and, like many GPI anchored proteins, it may be readily shed (53). It was originally proposed that the sCD14 would act as a competitive inhibitor of the action of mCD14 (54). However, sCD14 acts like mCD14 to enhance responses of cells to LPS. This was first shown in studies of the responses of endothelial cells to LPS (10). These cells exhibit a strong, CD14-dependent response to LPS despite the fact that they do not express mCD14. Endothelial cells employ sCD14 from plasma in place of mCD14. These findings have been confirmed and extended with many cell types that do not express mCD14 (10,55–57). The ability of sCD14 to enhance rather than block responses to LPS suggests that CD14 does not act as a typical receptor. It is instead most consistent with a role for CD14 in the shuttling of lipid monomers.

Role of CD14 in Cellular Responses to Lipopolysaccharide

A wide variety of studies have documented that CD14 is necessary for cells to respond to low concentrations of LPS. Anti-CD14 antibodies block responses of cells (50) and animals (58) to LPS, transfection of CD14 enhances sensitivity of cells to LPS (59,60), addition of sCD14 to cells that do not express mCD14 enables responses to LPS (10), and deletion of the CD14 gene from mice yields animals that fail to respond to doses of LPS that kill CD14-sufficient animals (61). How does CD14 enable responses to LPS? CD14 clearly hastens the association of LPS with responsive cells (47,48,62,63), and this function is undoubtedly important for cell stimulation. It is equally clear that simple proximity of LPS to the cells or even endocytosis of LPS aggregates is not sufficient for cell stimulation. Anti-LPS IgG causes macrophages to bind and endocytose LPS without cell stimulation (64), and LPS-LBP complexes can be bound and endocytosed without cell stimulation if the transfer of LPS to the binding site on CD14 is inhibited (47,49).

CD14 can insert LPS into phospholipid bilayers (22,25,30), and several lines of evidence suggest that LPS must be inserted into the plasma membrane of cells to initiate responses and that CD14 hastens this precise step. A requirement for membrane insertion of LPS was elegantly shown by studies of LPS incorporated into viral membranes. Binding of these membranes to cells did not lead to stimulation, but fusion of the viral membranes with leukocyte membranes caused cell stimulation (65). Like viral envelopes, CD14 delivers LPS into the cell membrane with each mCD14 shuttling 15 or more LPS molecules into the monocyte membrane in 30 minutes (63). Delivery of LPS from CD14 into the membrane appears necessary for cell stimulation because perturbations that halt lipid delivery to the membrane halt cellular responses to LPS. Anti-CD14 antibodies that block binding and shuttling of LPS block cellular responses while certain antibodies that do not block binding or shuttling do not affect responses (35,50,63,66). Moreover, mutations in CD14 that block LPS binding and lipid shuttling also block the ability of CD14 to mediate cell stim-

ulation (66–68). LPS-sCD14 complexes appear incapable of stimulating cells if the LPS cannot be transferred out of the CD14 and into cells. Cell stimulation by LPS-sCD14 complexes is blocked by excess "empty" sCD14 (35). Under these conditions, mass action retains LPS in the sCD14 pool. Cell stimulation by LPS-sCD14 complexes is also blocked by protease treatment of cells that prevents uptake of the LPS (63). These experiments make it clear that CD14 mediates sensitive responses to cells by a mechanism that differs from that of any classic "receptor" and is most consistent with the function of a transport protein. The mechanism by which CD14 transports LPS into cell membranes is described in the next section.

CD14 binds LPS monomers. CD14 does not bind to LPS aggregates or the surface of bacteria. Rather, soluble, monomeric sCD14 binds with a 1:1 stoichiometry to LPS monomers. This was established using native gel electrophoresis to separate sCD14 and LPS-sCD14 complexes from LPS aggregates (11) and has been confirmed by measurements of the spectroscopic change of fluorescently labeled LPS on binding to CD14 (31,32). LPS has a large hydrophobic region but is kept in solution as a monomer upon interaction with sCD14. It is thus likely that the hydrophobe of LPS interacts extensively with CD14 and is hidden from the solvent.

The affinity of CD14 for LPS has not been rigorously established. In fact, because of the physical properties of LPS and CD14, it is not clear which of several binding reactions are most relevant to the function of CD14. It is energetically favorable for LPS to move from aggregates in aqueous solution to the binding site on recombinant sCD14 (11,31), suggesting that a high affinity could be measured under these conditions. It is also energetically favorable for LPS to depart sCD14 and bind to phospholipid vesicles (22,25,30), suggesting a low affinity may be measured under these conditions. An explanation of these findings comes from work showing that CD14 also binds phospholipids and that the binding of LPS to CD14 may be coupled with the exit of a phospholipid (30). Because the energetics of LPS binding probably are dictated both by the binding properties of LPS and by the identity and the fate of the displaced lipid, affinity measurements are relevant only for certain well-defined, *in vitro* conditions that may not be mimicked at any place in the body.

The binding site for LPS has been partially mapped using protease protection, site-directed mutagenesis, and epitope mapped antibodies (66–68). The carboxyl-terminal four-fifths of the protein is composed of 10 tandem copies of the so called "leucine-rich" repeat that is common in a variety of proteins (69). These repeats do not appear essential for LPS binding or the function of CD14, because 7 of the 10 repeats can be deleted without substantially altering the function of CD14 (67). In contrast, the amino terminus bears no homology to any protein known and residues 57 through 64 appear essential for

LPS binding (66). Although the data demonstrating a role for residues 57 through 64 are strong, it is equally clear that these do not comprise the entire binding site. Eight residues are insufficient to interact with the large LPS molecule and are not exceptionally well conserved in the four species of CD14 sequenced, and several studies have described other mutations in the amino-terminal region that affect LPS binding (70,71).

LPS spontaneously exchanges between CD14 molecules. As expected from its physical properties, LPS monomers seldom enter or "sample" the aqueous environment. Because of this, movement of LPS monomers to the binding site on CD14 requires catalysis by LBP. In contrast, LPS monomers bound to CD14 readily exchange between CD14 molecules (35), and LBP does not appear to accelerate this exchange. The exchange of LPS between CD14 molecules may allow mCD14 and sCD14 to work together in transporting and responding to LPS. Addition of sCD14 has been shown to enhance the responses of mCD14-bearing cells to some forms of LPS (35,72), and expression of functional mCD14 enhances the responses of cells to LPS-sCD14 complexes. Moreover, mCD14 strongly enhances the cellular uptake of radioactive LPS from LPS-sCD14 complexes (63). Because of its privileged position near the plasma membrane, mCD14 may be more likely to participate in lipid exchange reactions with the plasma membrane. Most CD14 in blood is the soluble form, and this sCD14 is the most likely to first receive LPS from bacteria or shed fragments of bacteria.

Role of CD14 in Shuttling Lipids Between Membranes

LBP efficiently "loads" sCD14 with LPS monomers. The resulting approximately 60-kd LPS-sCD14 complexes may then diffuse through the aqueous medium and, in the reverse reaction, the LPS can be unloaded into a different membrane. This "shuttle" activity of sCD14 was first described for the transport of LPS to lipoprotein particles (39). Movement of LPS to HDL occurs slowly but is dramatically accelerated by the addition of LBP and sCD14. During this transfer, LPS-sCD14 complexes can be observed as an intermediate in the process. Additional studies have shown that LBP and sCD14 can shuttle LPS into phospholipid vesicles (22,30) and can shuttle phospholipids between vesicles in a similar fashion (30). CD14 acts as a carrier protein, akin to serum albumin, to transfer large hydrophobic molecules. This function of CD14 is clearly established and should be considered a major if not the major role of CD14.

CD14 shuttles lipids into HDL and phospholipid vesicles and into the membranes of cells. A large number of studies have documented that CD14 promotes the association of LPS with cells; binding of radioactive or fluorescent LPS is enhanced by the addition of CD14, and uptake of LPS into CD14-bearing cells is blocked by

anti-CD14 antibodies (48,50,59,62,63,73,74). Studies strongly suggest that in the uptake process, LPS is unloaded from CD14 into the plasma membrane (63). During uptake of LPS into monocytes from LPS-sCD14 complexes, the LPS binds first to mCD14, because anti-mCD14 blocks uptake. Under these conditions, monocytes clearly take up more than 15 LPS molecules per mCD14 molecule. Because mCD14 cannot simultaneously bind 15 LPS molecules, transfer to the membrane appears likely. Further support for the transfer of LPS from CD14 to cell membranes comes from the observation that endothelial cells take up LPS from LPS-sCD14 complexes, but CD14 cannot be found associated with the cell under these conditions (75 and unpublished observations).

Role of CD14 in Innate Immunity

Because CD14 binds LPS, it has been proposed that CD14 is a "pattern recognition receptor" that binds and recognizes foreign molecules (76). Several observations suggest that this is not the case. For example Delude et al. (77) observed that certain LPS precursors are LPS antagonists in human cells but agonists in murine cells. These authors then transfected murine cells with human CD14 and human cells with murine CD14. Human cells recognized the analogue as an antagonist, regardless of the species of CD14 at the surface, and murine cells recognized the analogue as an agonist, regardless of the species of CD14 at the cell surface. These experiments make it clear that discrimination of lipid species occurs in cells but not at the level of CD14. It is also clear that CD14 does not have appropriate binding specificity to serve as a pattern recognition receptor. CD14 binds not only LPS, but also phosphatidyl inositol, phosphatidyl ethanol, phosphatidyl choline (30), and lipoteichoic acid (78), and this broad specificity is not consistent with discrimination of host from pathogen.

If CD14 does not cleanly discriminate inflammatory microbial lipids from benign host lipids, what is its role in innate immunity? Two alternatives may be envisioned. In the first, CD14 may represent one step in a multistep recognition process (79). For example, LBP may recognize one subset of lipids in the broad array available in the environment. Among these, CD14 may recognize a smaller subset, and after transport of the selected lipids to cells, further discrimination may occur. In this way inflammatory lipids may be winnowed and selected by the serial action of several proteins in the absence of any single master recognition protein.

An alternative view is that neither CD14 nor LBP has any beneficial role in the local inflammatory responses to bacteria. Rather, the ability of LBP and CD14 to spread LPS to distant tissues may be an unwanted and dangerous consequence of their function in lipid transport. Seen in this light, LBP and CD14 may play a critical role in generating septic shock but not in generating protection from infectious agents. Several arguments favor this view. First, LBP and CD14 transport lipids in a catalytic fashion, moving hundreds of molecules per LBP per hour, but LBP and CD14 are found in 3- to 4-log molar excess of LPS, even in patients with fatal septic shock. This observation suggests a principal function other than recognition of bacterial products. Second, the two-step mode of action of LBP and CD14 leads to an LPS-CD14 complex with a half-life of >10 minutes in whole plasma (39). This time allows LPS in the vasculature to travel in the bloodstream far from the source of the infection. Although monocytes and PMNs do express CD14 at the cell surface and this CD14 can target LPS to these cells, most of the CD14 in blood is soluble and capable of carrying LPS away from sites of infection. Third, in keeping with a role in lipid transport, the highest levels of CD14 mRNA in stimulated mice are found in adipose tissue (80). Fourth, CD14 certainly is involved in promoting the systemic response to LPS; anti-CD14 antibodies block production of TNF, IL-1, IL-6, IL-8 and hypotension in a monkey model of endotoxemia (58), and CD14 knock-out mice have strongly attenuated systemic cytokine responses to endotoxin challenge (61). Fifth, the most important observation suggesting that CD14 is not needed for beneficial inflammation is that CD14 knock-out mice survive and recover completely from live bacterial challenge that is fatal in wild type control animals. After intraperitoneal challenge, bacteremia in CD14 knock-out animals is actually reduced in comparison with wild type control animals (61). Additional studies are needed to clarify whether CD14 and LBP are actually beneficial participants in the recognition or response to infection.

CELLULAR RECOGNITION OF LIPOPOLYSACCHARIDE

Cells recognize microbial lipids after they are transferred to the plasma membrane. How do cells discriminate microbial lipids such as LPS from endogenous phospholipids? It is well known that cells recognize and sort lipids with subtle chemical differences, segregating sphingomyelin, for example, from the closely similar phosphatidyl choline (81). It is possible that similar types of lipid sorting might serve in innate recognition of microbial products. In keeping with this notion, it was observed that the introduction of fluorescent LPS monomers into the plasma membranes of cells was followed by rapid transport of LPS to a perinuclear site (82). This transport appears to discriminate biologically active from inactive LPS species because inactive chemical homologues of LPS were not transported in this way (83). The transport to the perinuclear site also appears necessary for cell stimulation because blocking of transport with inhibitors of vesicular transport prevented responses to LPS (82). Moreover; this transport was greatly attenu-

ated in cells from mice with a genetic deficiency in responsiveness to LPS (84). The mechanism for selective recognition and transport of LPS (or any membrane lipid) is not known at this time and is an area of active research.

Innate Responses to Microbial Lipids Other Than Lipopolysaccharide

Lipoteichoic Acid

Gram-positive bacteria express macroamphophiles, the best characterized of which is lipoteichoic acid (LTA) (85). The hydrophile of this molecule is composed of a variable number of repeats of glycerol phosphate and the hydrophobe is a glycerol esterified with two fatty acids. The hydrophobe and hydrophile of LTA are connected through a variable carbohydrate linkage. LTA binds to CD14 (78) and certain LTA species cause stimulation of inflammatory cells in a CD14-dependent fashion (78,86,87). Gram-positive bacteria stimulate inflammatory cells, and LTA is a good candidate for the inflammatory principle. However, the precise contribution of LTA to inflammatory responses to gram-positive bacteria has not been defined.

Peptidoglycan

The cell wall peptidoglycan of gram-positive bacteria is exposed to the medium, and several studies have shown that peptidoglycan preparations activate cells in a CD14-dependent fashion (76,87–89). Although it is clear that CD14 enhances responses of leukocytes to gram-positive cell wall preparations, the nature of the CD14-binding entity in these preparations is controversial. A direct interaction of peptidoglycan with CD14 has been proposed by some authors (88,89), while others suggest that a lipid contaminant of peptidoglycan is the CD14-binding, cell-stimulating agent (87).

Sphingolipids

The soil bacterium *Sphingomonas* is a gram-negative bacterium that does not express LPS. Instead, it expresses a glycosylated sphingolipid (90), and this lipid has been shown to stimulate cells (91), albeit with less potency than LPS. These findings are consistent with the observation that sphingolipids and LPS show striking structural similarity (92) and that ceramides stimulate many cells in a fashion similar to LPS (93).

Lipoarabinomannan

Mycobacteria express lipoglycans composed of branched carbohydrate polymers joined to a phosphatidylinositol (41). Lipoarabinomannan is the major antigenic lipoglycan of *Mycobacterium tuberculosis* and

Mycobacterium leprae. LAM stimulates inflammatory cells and anti-CD14 antibodies have been shown to block response to this complex ligand (76,95,96).

Acylated Bacterial Proteins

The spirochete, *Borrelia burgdorferi,* expresses surface proteins (i.e., OspA, OspB) that are implicated in the inflammatory response to the bacterium (97). Each of these proteins bears covalently attached lipid; a cysteine residue at the N terminus bears an amide-linked palmitate and a thioether linked diglyceride yielding three moles of palmitate per mole of protein (98). Several lines of evidence indicate that the covalently attached lipid is essential for these proteins to initiate responses in inflammatory cells. Recombinant proteins without the N-terminal cysteine fail to stimulate leukocytes (99,100), and short, lipidated peptides made synthetically (99) or by protease digestion of the mature bacterial protein (101) are capable of stimulating cells.

CD14 plays a facilitating role in mediating responses of cells to acylated proteins from *Borrelia.* The acylated proteins bind to sCD14 *in vitro*, and this binding requires acylation and the well-characterized LPS binding site on CD14 (101). Addition of CD14 enhances the responses of endothelial cells to the proteins, and the blockade of CD14 on monocytes inhibits responses. The requirement for CD14, however, is not complete and can be overcome by raising the amount of acylated protein by a factor of 10 to 100. It appears that, by acting as a nonspecific lipid transfer protein, CD14 may hasten the interaction of these proteins with cells and thereby enhance responses.

Responses to Mammalian Lipids

Macrophages bind and phagocytose apoptotic cells and cellular debris, and at least a portion of this recognition is mediated by lipids (102). The plasma membrane of living cells is asymmetric, with aminophospholipids disposed almost exclusively on the cytoplasmic leaflet. On cell death, the asymmetry is lost and aminophospholipids, such as phosphatidyl serine (PS), appear at the cell surface. Work from several laboratories has shown that recognition of apoptotic cells by macrophages occurs on exposure of PS at the plasma membrane and that blockade of the PS with a binding protein or occupation of PS receptors on macrophages with PS liposomes can block recognition (102–104). The "PS receptor" on macrophages has not been defined, but the ability of CD14 to interact with purified PS (22) suggests an additional potential role for this protein.

Other Receptors for Lipopolysaccharide

LPS has been reported to bind a relatively large number of different cell surface proteins (105). We focus below on known, cloned proteins shown to bind LPS, and proteins identified only as a binding site or a band on a gel are not discussed.

Scavenger Receptor A

SRA was first recognized for its binding to modified lipoprotein particles and is thought to serve in the clearance of oxidized or damaged lipoproteins (106). Hampton et al. (107) have shown that this molecule also binds a metabolic precursor of LPS known as lipid IVa, and Dunne et al. suggested an interaction with LTA (108). Blockade of SRA slows hepatic uptake of LPS (107), suggesting a role for SRA in clearance of LPS. However, blockade of SRA does not prevent responses to LPS (107), and the broad binding specificity of SRA makes it an unlikely candidate for directing innate immune recognition.

Leukocyte Integrins

Leukocytes express three heterodimeric adhesion proteins known as β2 integrins or leukocyte integrins (CD antigens). The individual members are better known by the names LFA-1, CR3 (also known as Mac-1), and p150,95. Each of these integrins has been shown to bind gram-negative bacteria and LPS-coated particles (109) and may play a role in clearance of whole bacteria or shed fragments of LPS. A potential role for these receptors in mediating responses to LPS has been suggested by the finding that transfection of CHO cells with DNA for p150,95 (110) or CR3 (111) enhances the responsiveness of cells to LPS. On the other hand, monocytes from patients with a genetic deficiency in all three leukocyte integrins show normal synthesis of cytokines to LPS *in vitro* (112), and a strong febrile response to infection is a hallmark of patients with this disease (see Chapter 37). If leukocyte integrins make a contribution to recognition of LPS, it is minor.

AREAS OF FUTURE RESEARCH

Recognition of microbial lipids clearly plays an important role in innate immune responses. Nevertheless, the lipids of many pathogens are poorly characterized with respect to structure and proinflammatory capabilities. Further study of these molecules is likely to be a fruitful pursuit.

The greatest single intellectual problem for understanding innate responses to microbial lipids is understanding how cells sense, sort, and initiate responses to small molecules that become incorporated into the plasma membrane. This is particularly challenging because the mechanisms for sorting endogenous phospholipids are currently obscure. Studies have identified proteins involved in vesicular transport (113), flipping lipids from leaflet to leaflet (114), and transport of cholesterol into mitochondria (115) and out of lysosomes (116). These proteins or homologues of these proteins may play important roles in handling and responding to microbial lipids. Conversely, it is also likely that studies using microbial lipids may lead to identification of proteins that have broader roles in cellular lipid homeostasis.

ACKNOWLEDGMENT

I wish to thank Drs. P. A. Detmers, R. Thieringer, C. T. Park, N. Thieblemont, and T. Vasselon for critically reading the manuscript.

REFERENCES

1. Morrison DC, Ulevitch RJ. The effects of bacterial endotoxins on host mediation systems. *Am J Pathol* 1978;93:526–617.
2. Baumgartner JD, Heumann D, Gerain J, Weinbrech P, Grau GE, Glauser MP. Association between protective efficacy of anti-lipopolysaccharide (LPS) antibodies and suppression of LPS-induced tumor necrosis factor α and interleukin 6. *J Exp Med* 1990;171:889–896.
3. Kohn FR, Kung AHC. Role of endotoxin in acute inflammation induced by gram-negative bacteria: specific inhibition of lipopolysaccharide-mediated responses with an amino-terminal fragment of bactericidal/permeability-increasing protein. *Infect Immun* 1995;63:333–339.
4. Somerville JE Jr, Cassiano L, Bainbridge B, Cunningham MD, Darveau RP. A novel *Escherichia coli* lipid A mutant that produces an antiinflammatory lipopolysaccharide. *J Clin Invest* 1996;97:359–365.
5. Kim YB, Watson DW. Role of antibodies in reactions to gram-negative bacterial endotoxins. *Ann N Y Acad Sci* 1996;133:727–745.
6. Hardardottir I, Grunfeld C, Feingold KR. Effects of endotoxin and cytokines on lipid metabolism. *Curr Opin Lipidol* 1994;5:207–215.
7. Fong Y, Marano MA, Moldawer LL, et al. The acute splanchnic and peripheral tissue metabolic response to endotoxin in human. *J Clin Invest* 1990;85:1896–1904.
8. Sarraf P, Frederich RC, Turner EM, et al. Multiple cytokines and acute inflammation raise mouse leptin levels: potential role in inflammatory anorexia. *J Exp Med* 1997;185:171–175.
9. Bevilacqua MP. Endothelial-leukocyte adhesion molecules. *Ann Rev Immunol* 1993;11:767–804.
10. Frey EA, Miller DS, Jahr TG, et al. Soluble CD14 participates in the response of cells to LPS. *J Exp Med* 1992;176:1665–1671.
11. Hailman E, Lichenstein HS, Wurfel MM, et al. Lipopolysaccharide (LPS)-binding protein accelerates the binding of LPS to CD14. *J Exp Med* 1994;179:269–277.
12. Wright SD, Ramos RA, Patel M, Miller DS. Septin: a factor in plasma that opsonizes lipopolysaccharide-bearing particles for recognition by CD14 on phagocytes. *J Exp Med* 1992;176:719–727.
13. Detmers PA, Zhou D, Powell DE. Different signaling pathways for CD18-mediated adhesion and Fc-mediated phagocytosis. *J Immunol* 1994;153:2137–2145.
14. Maio M, Tessitori G, Pinto A, Temponi M, Colombatti A, Ferrone S. Differential role of distinct determinants of intercellular adhesion molecule-1 in immunologic phenomena. *J Immunol* 1989;143:181–188.
15. Rosenstreich DL. Genetic control of endotoxin response: C3H/HeJ mice. In: Berry LJ, ed. *Handbook of endotoxin: cellular biology of endotoxin,* vol 3. New York: Elsevier Science Publishers, 1995.
16. Bone RC. The pathogenesis of sepsis. *Ann Intern Med* 1991;115:457.
17. Stone R. Search for sepsis drugs goes on despite past failures. *Science* 1994;264:365.
18. Raetz CRH. Biochemistry of endotoxins. *Annu Rev Biochem* 1990;59:129–170.
19. Raetz CRH. In: Neidhardt FC, ed. *Escherichia coli and Salmonella: cellular and molecular biology,* vol 1, 2nd ed. Washington, DC: American Society for Microbiology, 1996:1035–1063.
20. Onishi HR, Pelak BA, Gerckens LS, et al. Antibacterial agents that inhibit lipid A biosynthesis. *Science* 1996;274:980–982.
21. Din ZZ, Mukerjee P, Kastowsky M, Takayama K. Effect of pH on solubility and ionic state of lipopolysaccharide obtained from the deep rough mutant of *Escherichia coli*. *Biochemistry* 1993;32:4579–4586.
22. Wurfel MM, Wright SD. Lipopolysaccharide-binding protein and soluble CD14 transfer lipopolysaccharide to phospholipid bilayers. *J Immunol* 1997;158:3925–3934.
23. Tobias PS, Soldau K, Ulevitch RJ. Isolation of a lipopolysaccharide-binding acute phase reactant from rabbit serum. *J Exp Med* 1986;164:777–793.
24. Schumann RR, Leong SR, Flaggs GW, Gray, et al. Structure and function of lipopolysaccharide binding protein. *Science* 1990;249:1429–1431.
25. Wurfel MM, Kunitake ST, Lichenstein H, Kane JP, Wright SD. Lipopolysaccharide (LPS)-binding protein is carried on lipoproteins and acts as a cofactor in the neutralization of LPS. *J Exp Med* 1994;180:1025–1035.
26. Albers JJ, Tu A-T, Wolfbauer G, Cheung MC, Marcovina SM. Molecular biology of phospholipid transfer protein. *Curr Opin Lipidol* 1996;7:86–93.
27. Bruce C, Tall AR. Cholesteryl ester transfer proteins, reverse cholesterol transport, and atherosclerosis. *Curr Opin Lipidol* 1995;6:306–311.
28. Beamer LJ, Carroll SF, Eisenberg D. Crystal structure of human BPI and two bound phospholipids at 2.4 angstrom resolution. *Science* 1997;276:1861–1864.
29. Park CT, Wright SD. Plasma lipopolysaccharide-binding protein is found associated with a particle containing apolipoprotein A-I, phospholipid, and factor H-related proteins. *J Biol Chem* 1996;271:18054–18060.
30. Yu B, Hailman E, Wright SD. LPS binding protein (LBP) and sCD14 catalyze exchange of phospholipids. *J Clin Invest* 1997;99:315–324.
31. Yu B, Wright SD. Catalytic properties of lipopolysaccharide (LPS)-binding protein (LBP): I. Transfer of LPS to soluble CD14. *J Biol Chem* 1996;271:4100–4105.
32. Tobias PS, Soldau K, Gegner JA, Mintz D, Ulevitch RJ. Lipopolysaccharide binding protein–mediated complexation of lipopolysaccharide with soluble CD14. *J Biol Chem* 1995;270:10482–10488.
33. Han J, Mathison JC, Ulevitch RJ, Tobias PS. Lipopolysaccharide (LPS) binding protein, truncated at Ile-197, binds LPS but does not transfer LPS to CD14. *J Biol Chem* 1994;269:8172–8175.
34. Theofan G, Horwitz AH, Williams RE, et al. An amino-terminal fragment of human lipopolysaccharide-binding protein retains lipid A binding but not CD14-stimulatory activity. *J Immunol* 1994;152:3623–3629.
35. Hailman E, Vasselon T, Kelley M, et al. Stimulation of macrophages and neutrophils by complexes of lipopolysaccharides and soluble CD14. *J Immunol* 1996;56:4384–4390.
36. Mathison JC, Tobias PS, Wolfson E, Ulevitch RJ. Plasma lipopolysaccharide (LPS)-binding protein. A key component in macrophage recognition of gram-negative LPS. *J Immunol* 1992;149:200–206.
37. Lynn WA, Liu Y, Golenbock DT. Neither CD14 nor serum is absolutely necessary for activation of mononuclear phagocytes by bacterial lipopolysaccharide. *Infect Immun* 1993;61:4452–4461.
38. Wurfel MM, Monks BG, Ingalls RR, et al. Targeted deletion of the LBP gene leads to profound suppression of LPS responses ex vivo while *in vivo* responses remain intact. *J Exp Med* 1997;186:2051–2056.
39. Wurfel MM, Hailman E, Wright SD. Soluble CD14 acts as a shuttle in the neutralization of LPS by LPS-binding protein and reconstituted high-density lipoprotein. *J Exp Med* 1995;181:1743–1754.
40. Skarnes RC. *In vivo* interaction of endotoxin with a lipoprotein having esterase activity. *J Bacteriol* 1968;95:2031–2034.
41. Ulevitch RJ, Johnston AR, Weinstein DB. New function for high density lipoproteins. *J Clin Invest* 1979;64:1516–1524.
42. Munford RS, Hall CL, Lipton JM, Dietschy JM. Biological activity, lipoprotein-binding behavior, and *in vivo* disposition of extracted and native forms of *Salmonella typhimurium* lipopolysaccharides. *J Clin Invest* 1982;70:877–888.
43. Levine DM, Parker TS, Donnelly TM, Walsh A, Rubin AL. *In vivo* protection against endotoxin by plasma high density lipoprotein. *Proc Natl Acad Sci USA* 1993;90:12040–12044.
44. Wright SD, Tobias PS, Ulevitch RJ, Ramos R. Lipopolysaccharide binding protein opsonizes LPS-bearing particles for recognition by a novel receptor on macrophages. *J Exp Med* 1989;170:1231–1241.
45. Grunwald U, Fan X, Jack RS, et al. Monocytes can phagocytose gram-negative bacteria by a CD14-dependent mechanism. *J Immunol* 1996;157:4119–4125.

46. Luchi M, Munford RS. Binding, internalization, and deacylation of bacterial lipopolysaccharide by human neutrophils. *J Immunol* 1993; 151:959–969.

47. Gegner JA, Ulevitch RJ, Tobias PS. Lipopolysaccharide (LPS) signal transduction and clearance: dual roles for LPS binding protein and membrane CD14. *J Biol Chem* 1995;270:5320–5325.

48. Troelstra A, Antal-Szalmas P, DeGraaf-Miltenburg AM, et al. Saturable CD14-dependent binding of fluorescein-labeled lipopolysaccharide to human monocytes. *Infect Immun* 1997;65:2272–2277.

49. Lamping N, Hoess A, Yu B, et al. Effects of site-directed mutagenesis of basic residues (Arg 94, Lys 95, Lys 99) of lipopolysaccharide (LPS)-binding protein on binding and transfer of LPS and subsequent immune cell activation. *J Immunol* 1996;157:4648–4656.

50. Wright SD, Ramos RA, Tobias PS, Ulevitch RJ, Mathison JC. CD14, a receptor for complexes of lipopolysaccharide (LPS) and LPS binding protein. *Science* 1990;249:1431–1433.

51. Goyert SM, Ferrero E, Rettig WJ, Yenamandra AK, Obata D, LeBeau MM. The CD14 monocyte differentiation antigen maps to a region encoding growth factors and receptors. *Science* 1988;239:497–500.

52. Bazil V, Baudys M, Hilgert I, et al. Structural relationship between the soluble and membrane-bound forms of human monocyte surface glycoprotein CD14. *Mol Immunol* 1989;26:657–662.

53. Bazil V, Strominger JL. Shedding as a mechanism of down-modulation of CD14 on stimulated human monocytes. *J Immunol* 1991;147: 1567–1574.

54. Maliszewski CR. CD14 and immune response to lipopolysaccharide. *Science* 1991;252:1321–1322.

55. Pugin J, Schurer-Maly C-C, Leturcq D, Moriarty A, Ulevitch RJ, Tobias PS. Lipopolysaccharide activation of human endothelial and epithelial cells is mediated by lipopolysaccharide-binding protein and soluble CD14. *Proc Natl Acad Sci USA* 1993;90:2744–2748.

56. Haziot A, Rong G-W, Silver J, Goyert SM. Recombinant soluble CD14 mediates the activation of endothelial cells by lipopolysaccharide. *J Immunol* 1993;151:1500–1507.

57. Arditi M, Zhou J, Dorio R, Rong GW, Goyert SM, Kim KS. Endotoxin-mediated endothelial cell injury and activation: role of soluble CD14. *Infect Immun* 1993;61:3149–3156.

58. Leturcq DJ, Moriarty AM, Talbott G, Winn RK, Martin TR, Ulevitch RJ. Antibodies against CD14 protect primates from endotoxin-induced shock. *J Clin Invest* 1996;98:1533–1538.

59. Lee J-D, Kato K, Tobias PS, Kirkland TN, Ulevitch RJ. Transfection of CD14 into 70Z/3 cells dramatically enhances the sensitivity to complexes of lipopolysaccharide (LPS) and LPS binding protein. *J Exp Med* 1992;175:1697–1705.

60. Golenbock DT, Liu Y, Millham FH, Freeman MW, Zoeller RA. Surface expression of human CD14 in Chinese hamster ovary fibroblasts imparts macrophage-like responsiveness to bacterial endotoxin. *J Biol Chem* 1993;268:22055–22059.

61. Haziot A, Ferrero E, Kontgen F, et al. Resistance to endotoxin shock and reduced dissemination of gram-negative bacteria in CD14-deficient mice. *Immunity* 1996;4:407–414.

62. Couturier C, Haeffner-Cavaillon N, Caroff M, Kazatchkine MD. Binding sites for endotoxins (lipopolysaccharides) on human monocytes. *J Immunol* 1991;147:1899–1904.

63. Vasselon T, Pironkova R, Detmers PA. Sensitive responses of leukocytes to LPS require a protein distinct from CD14 at the cell surface. *J Immunol* 1997;159:4498–4505.

64. Burd RS, Battafarano RJ, Cody CS, Farber MS, Ratz CA, Dum DL. Anti-endotoxin monoclonal antibodies inhibit secretion of tumor necrosis factor-alpha by two distinct mechanisms. *Ann Surg* 1993; 218:250–259.

65. Dijkstra J, Bron R, Wilschut J, deHaan A, Ryan JL. Activation of murine lymphocytes by lipopolysaccharide incorporated in fusogenic, reconstituted influenza virus envelopes (virosomes). *J Immunol* 1996; 157:1028–1036.

66. Juan TS, Hailman E, Kelley MJ, et al. Identification of a lipopolysaccharide (LPS)-binding domain in CD14 between amino acids 57 and 64. *J Biol Chem* 1995;270:5219–5224.

67. Juan TS, Kelley MJ, Johnson DA, et al. Soluble CD14 truncated at amino acid 152 binds lipopolysaccharide (LPS) and enables cellular response to LPS. *J Biol Chem* 1995;270:1382–1387.

68. Juan TS, Hailman E, Kelley MJ, Wright SD, Lichenstein HS. Identification of a domain in CD14 essential for lipopolysaccharide (LPS) signaling but not LPS binding. *J Biol Chem* 1995;270:17237–17242.

69. Setoguchi M, Nasu N, Yoshida S, Higuchi Y, Akizuki S, Yamamoto S. Mouse and human CD14 (myeloid cell-specific leucine-rich glycoprotein) primary structure deduced from cDNA clones. *Biochim Biophys Acta* 1989;1008:213–222.

70. Viriyakosol S, Kirkland TN. A region of human CD14 required for lipopolysaccharide binding. *J Biol Chem* 1995;270:361–368.

71. Stelter F, Bernheiden M, Menzel R, et al. Mutation of amino acids 39–44 of human CD14 abrogates binding of lipopolysaccharide and *Escherichia coli. Eur J Biochem* 1997;243:100–109.

72. Troelstra A, Giepmans BN, Van Kessel KP, Lichenstein HS, Verhoef J, Van Strijp JA. Dual effects of soluble CD14 on LPS priming of neutrophils. *J Leukoc Biol* 1997;61:173–178.

73. Troelstra A, Antal-Szalmas P, de Graaf-Miltenburg LA, et al. Saturable CD14-dependent binding of fluorescein-labeled lipopolysaccharide to human monocytes. *Infect Immun* 1997;65:2272–2277.

74. Kitchens RL, Ulevitch RJ, Munford RS. Lipopolysaccharide (LPS) partial structures inhibit responses to LPS in a human macrophage cell line without inhibiting LPS uptake by a CD14-mediated pathway. *J Exp Med* 1992;176:485–494.

75. Tapping RI, Tobias PS. Cellular binding of soluble CD14 requires lipopolysaccharide (LPS) and LPS-binding protein. *J Biol Chem* 1997;272:23157–23164.

76. Pugin J, Heumann ID, Tomasz A, et al. CD14 is a pattern recognition receptor. *Immunity* 1994;1:509–516.

77. Delude RL, Savedra R Jr, Zhao H, et al. CD14 enhances cellular responses to endotoxin without imparting ligand-specific recognition. *Proc Natl Acad Sci USA* 1995;92:9288–9292.

78. Kusunoki T, Hailman E, Juan TS-C, Lichenstein H, Wright SD. Molecules from *Staphylococcus aureus* that bind CD14 and stimulate innate immune responses. *J Exp Med* 182:1673.

79. Wright SD. CD14 and innate recognition of bacteria. *J Immunol* 1995; 155:6–8.

80. Fearns C, Kravchenko VV, Ulevitch RJ, Loskutoff DJ. Murine CD14 gene expression *in vivo*: extramyeloid synthesis and regulation by lipopolysaccharide. *J Exp Med* 1995;181:857–866.

81. van Meer G. Lipid traffic in animal cells. *Annu Rev Cell Biol* 1989; 5:247–275.

82. Detmers PA, Thieblemont N, Vasselon T, Pironkova R, Miller D, Wright SD. Potential role of membrane internalization and vesicle fusion in adhesion of neutrophils response to lipopolysaccharide and TNF. *J Immunol* 1996;157:5589–5596.

83. Thieblemont T, Thieringer R, Wright SD. Innate immune recognition of bacterial lipopolysaccharide: dependence on interactions with membrane lipids and endocytic movement. *Immunity* 1998;8:771–777.

84. Thieblemont N, Wright SD. Mice genetically hyporesponsive to LPS exhibit a defect in endocytic uptake of LPS and ceramide. *J Exp Med* 1997;185:2095–2100.

85. Fischer W. Bacterial phosphoglycolipids and lipoteichoic acids. In: Hannah DJ, eds. *Handbook of lipid research,* vol 6. New York: Plenum Press, 1989;123–234.

86. Suda Y, Tochio H, Kawano K, Takada H, et al. Cytokine-inducing glycolipids in the lipoteichoic acid fraction from *Enterococcus hirae* ATCC 9790. *FEMS Immunol Med Microbiol* 1995;12:97–112.

87. Kusunoki T, Wright SD. Chemical characterization of *Staphylococcus aureus* molecules that have CD14-dependent cell stimulatory activity. *J Immunol* 1996;157:5112–5117.

88. Gupta D, Kirkland TN, Viriyakosol S, Dziarski R. CD14 is a cell-activating receptor for bacterial peptidoglycan. *J Biol Chem* 1996;271: 23310–23316.

89. Weidemann B, Schletter J, Dziarski R, et al. Specific binding of soluble peptidoglycan and muramyldipeptide to CD14 on human monocytes. *Infect Immun* 1997;65:858–864.

90. Kawahara K, Seydel U, Matsuura M, Danbara H, Reitschel ETH, Zahringer U. Chemical structure of glycosphingolipids isolated from *Sphingomonas paucimobilis. FEBS Lett* 1991;292:107–110.

91. Krziwon C, Zahringer U, Kawahara K, et al. Glycosphingolipids from *Sphingomonas paucimobilis* induce monokine production in human mononuclear cells. *Infect Immun* 1995;63:2899–2905.

92. Joseph CK, Wright SD, Bornmann WG, et al. Bacterial lipopolysaccharide has structural similarity to ceramide and stimulates ceramide-activated protein kinase in myeloid cells. *J Biol Chem* 1994;269: 17606–17610.

93. Wright SD, Kolesnick RM. Does endotoxin stimulate cells by mimicking ceramide? *Immunol Today* 1995;16:297–302.

94. Hunter SD, Gaylord H, Brennan PJ. Structure and antigenicity of the phosphorylated lipopolysaccharide antigens from the leprosy and tubercle bacilli. *J Biol Chem* 1986;261:12345–12351.

95. Zhang Y, Doerfler M, Lee TC, Guillemin B, Rom WN. Mechanisms of stimulation of interleukin-1β and tumor necrosis factor-α by *Mycobacterium tuberculosis* components. *J Clin Invest* 1993;91:2076–2083.

96. Savedra R, Delude RL, Ingalls RR, Fenton MJ, Golenbock DT. Mycobacterial lipoarabinomannan recognition requires a receptor that shares components of the endotoxin signaling system. *J Immunol* 1996;157:2549–2554.

97. Radolf JD, Norgard MC, Brandt ME, Isaacs RD, Thompson PA, Beutler B. Lipoproteins of *Borrelia burgdorferi* and *Treponema pallidum* activate cachectin/tumor necrosis factor synthesis. *J Immunol* 1991;147:1968–1974.

98. Brandt ME, Riley BS, Radolf JD, Norgard MV. Immunogenic integral membrane proteins of *Borrelia burgdorferi* are lipoproteins. *Infect Immun* 1990;58:983–991.

99. Radolf JD, Arndt LL, Akins DR, et al. *Treponema pallidum* and *Borrelia burgdorferi* lipoproteins and synthetic lipopeptides activate monocytes/macrophages. *J Immunol* 1995;154:2866–2877.

100. Weis JJ, Ma Y, Erdile LF. Biological activities of native and recombinant *Borrelia burgdorferi* outer surface protein A: dependence on lipid modification. *Infect Immun* 1994;62:4632–4636.

101. Wooten RM, Morrison TB, Weis JH, Wright SD, Thieringer R, Weis JJ. The role of CD14 in signaling mediated by outer membrane lipoproteins of *Borrelia burgdorferi*. *J Immunol* 1998;160:5485–5492.

102. Bruckheimer EM, Schroit AJ. Membrane phospholipid asymmetry: host response to the externalization of phosphatidylserine. *J Leukoc Biol* 1996;59:784–788.

103. McEvoy L, Williamson P, Schlegel RA. Membrane phospholipid asymmetry as a determinant of erythrocyte recognition by macrophages. *Proc Natl Acad Sci USA* 1986;83:3311–3315.

104. Fadok VA, Voelker DR, Campbell PA, Cohen JJ, Bratton DL, Henson PM. Exposure of phosphatidylserine on the surface of apoptotic lymphocytes triggers specific recognition and removal by macrophages. *J Immunol* 1992;148:2207–2216.

105. Wright SD. Multiple receptors for endotoxin. *Curr Opin Immunol* 1991;3:83–90.

106. Pearson AM. Scavenger receptors in innate immunity. *Curr Opin Immunol* 1996;8:20–28.

107. Hampton RY, Golenbock DT, Penman M, Krieger M, Raetz CRH. Recognition and plasma clearance of endotoxin by scavenger receptors. *Nature* 1991;352:342–344.

108. Dunne DW, Resnick D, Greenberg J, Krieger M, Joiner KA. The type I macrophage scavenger receptor binds to gram-positive bacteria and recognizes lipoteichoic acid. *Proc Natl Acad Sci USA* 1994;91:1863–1867.

109. Wright SD, Jong MTC. Adhesion-promoting receptors on human macrophages recognize *E. coli* by binding to lipopolysaccharide. *J Exp Med* 1986;164:1876–1888.

110. Ingalls RR, Golenbock DT. CD11c/CD18, a transmembrane signaling receptor for lipopolysaccharide. *J Exp Med* 1995;181:14733–1479.

111. Ingalls RR, Arnaout MA, Golenbock DT. Outside-in signaling by lipopolysaccharide through a tailless integrin. *J Immunol* 1997;159:433–438.

112. Wright SD, Detmers PA, Aida Y, et al. CD18-deficient cells respond to lipopolysaccharide *in vitro*. *J Immunol* 1990;144:2566–2571.

113. Rothman JE, Weiland FT. Protein sorting by transport vesicles. *Science* 1996;272:227–234.

114. van Helvoort A, Smith AJ, Sprong H, et al. MDR1 P-glycoprotein is a lipid translocase of broad specificity, while MDR3 P-glycoprotein specifically translocates phosphatidylcholine. *Cell* 1996;87:507–517.

115. Stocco DM, Clark BJ. Role of the steroidogenic acute regulatory protein (StAR) in steroidogenesis. *Biochem Pharmacol* 1996;51:197–205.

116. Carstea ED, Morris JA, Coleman KG, et al. Niemann-Pick C1 disease gene: homology to mediators of cholesterol homeostasis. *Science* 1997;277:228–231.

117. Haraldsen G, Kvale D, Lien B, Farstad IN, Brandtzaeg P. Cytokine-regulated expression of E-selectin, intercellular adhesion molecule-1 (ICAM-1), and vascular cell adhesion molecule-1 (VCAM-1) in human microvascular endothelial cells. *J Immunol* 1996;156:2558–2565.

118. Wright SD, Ramos R, Hermanowski-Vosatka A, Rockwell P, Detmers PA. Activation of the adhesive capacity of CR3 on neutrophils by endotoxin: dependence on lipopolysaccharide binding protein and CD14. *J Exp Med* 1991;173:1281–1286.

119. Maier RV, Ulevitch RJ. The induction of a unique procoagulant activity in rabbit hepatic macrophages by bacterial lipopolysaccharides. *J Immunol* 1981;127:1596–1600.

120. Colucci M, Balconi G, Lorenzet R, et al. Cultured human endothelial cells generate tissue factor in response to endotoxin. *J Clin Invest* 1983;71:1893–1896.

121. Surette ME, Palmantier R, Gosselin J, Borgeat P. Lipopolysaccharides prime whole human blood and isolated neutrophils for the increased synthesis of 5-lipoxygenase products by enhancing arachidonic acid availability: involvement of the CD14 antigen. *J Exp Med* 1993;178:1347–1355.

122. Surette ME, Nadeau M, Borgeat P, Gosselin J. Priming of human peripheral blood mononuclear cells with lipopolysaccharides for enhanced arachidonic acid release and leukotriene synthesis. *J Leukoc Biol* 1996;59:709–715.

123. Pabst MJ, Johnston RB Jr. Increased production of superoxide anion by macrophages exposed *in vitro* to muramyl dipeptide or lipopolysaccharide. *J Exp Med* 1980;151:101–114.

124. Guthrie LA, McPhail LC, Henson PM, Johnston RB Jr. Priming of neutrophils for enhanced release of oxygen metabolites by bacterial lipopolysaccharide: evidence for increased activity of the superoxide-producing enzyme. *J Exp Med* 1984;160:1656–1671.

125. Ding AH, Nathan CF, Stuehr DJ. Release of reactive nitrogen intermediates and reactive oxygen intermediates from mouse peritoneal macrophages. *J Immunol* 1988;141:2407–2412.

126. Hempel SL, Monick MM, Hunninghake GW. Lipopolysaccharide induces prostaglandin H synthase-2 protein and mRNA in human alveolar macrophages and blood monocytes. *J Clin Invest* 1994;93:391–396.

127. Fearns C, Loskutoff DJ. Induction of plasminogen activator inhibitor 1 gene expression in murine liver by lipopolysaccharide: cellular localization and role of endogenous tumor factor-alpha. *Am J Pathol* 1997;150:579–590.

128. Diamond G, Russell JP, Bevins CL. Inducible expression of an antibiotic peptide gene in lipopolysaccharide-challenged tracheal epithelial cells. *Proc Natl Acad Sci USA* 1996;93:5156–5160.

Inflammation: Basic Principles and Clinical Correlates,
3rd ed., edited by John I. Gallin and Ralph Snyderman.
Lippincott Williams & Wilkins, Philadelphia © 1999.

CHAPTER 37

The Role of β₂ Integrins in Inflammation

Takashi Kei Kishimoto, Eric T. Baldwin, and Donald C. Anderson

THE INTEGRIN FAMILY: DEFINITION AND HISTORICAL PERSPECTIVE

The integrins are a large family of cell adhesion molecules that influence or directly regulate diverse cellular functions including growth, differentiation, motility, and polarity. As a consequence, the integrins have played a fundamental role in the evolution of multicellular organisms. Cellular migration and rearrangements during embryogenesis as well as cellular differentiation and organization during organogenesis involve specific and highly regulated adherence interactions of cells with their environment. Leukocytes are by necessity mobile cells that circulate through the vascular and lymphatic compartments and survey the body for potential pathogenic microorganisms. The nature of the immune system puts extraordinary demands on the mechanisms that regulate the temporal and spatial specificities of leukocyte adhesive interactions. Leukocyte adhesion is critical for regulation of the immune response, trafficking of leukocytes, and cell-mediated effector functions. While leukocytes are capable of expressing a wide array of adhesion receptors, the β₂ integrins play a central role in many leukocyte functions.

The term *integrin* was originally suggested to describe membrane receptors that integrate the extracellular environment (matrix or other cells) with the intracellular cytoskeleton (1). All integrins are cell membrane heterodimeric glycoproteins consisting of noncovalently associated α and β subunits. The integrins were originally divided into three subfamilies based on distinct β subunits that shared multiple α subunits (Fig. 37-1A). The β₁ subfamily encompasses many extracellular matrix receptors,

including the classic fibronectin receptor. Some of the β₁ integrins also mediate cell-cell interactions, notably the α₄β₁ integrin, which plays an important role in lymphocyte, monocyte, and eosinophil adhesion. The β₂ family includes the leukocyte integrins lymphocyte function antigen-1 (LFA-1), Mac-1, p150,95, and α_dβ₂. This subfamily of integrins is expressed exclusively by leukocytes. The β₃ family is composed of gpIIbIIIa and the vitronectin receptor. This subclassification of integrins has been complicated by the discovery of novel β subunits and the recognition that some α subunits can pair with multiple β subunits. Currently, there are 16 known α subunits and 8 known β subunits, which can pair to form at least 22 unique αβ heterodimers (Fig. 37-1A).

The β₂ integrin family plays an integral role in the inflammatory response. A hallmark feature of inflammation is the massive migration and infiltration of leukocytes into the affected tissue. Three major developments over the past decade underscore the importance of the β₂ or "leukocyte" integrins (also termed the CD11/CD18 complex) as adhesion receptors fundamental to specific immunity and inflammation: (a) Retrospectively, it was recognized that these proteins were evolutionary related to other previously recognized integrins known to play a major role in guiding cell migration during embryogenesis, organogenesis, and wound healing. By analogy, it is perhaps not surprising that the β₂ integrins would be later demonstrated to provide a somewhat similar means for guiding leukocyte localization in inflamed tissues. (b) The recognition of molecular ligands for LFA-1 or other β₂ integrins further defined and underscored the specificity and versatility of the leukocyte integrin complex. Of particular importance was the identification of intracellular adhesion molecule-1 (ICAM-1), which was shown to be inducible by several inflammatory mediators and to regulate leukocyte localization in inflamed tissue. (c) The biologic importance of the β₂ integrins was dramatically demonstrated by the identification and characterization of its genetic deficiency in humans,

T. K. Kishimoto: Section of Cell Adhesion, Department of Biology, Boehringer Ingelheim Pharmaceuticals, Ridgefield, Connecticut 06877.

E. T. Baldwin and D. C. Anderson: Discovery Research, Pharmacia and Upjohn, Kalamazoo, Michigan 49007.

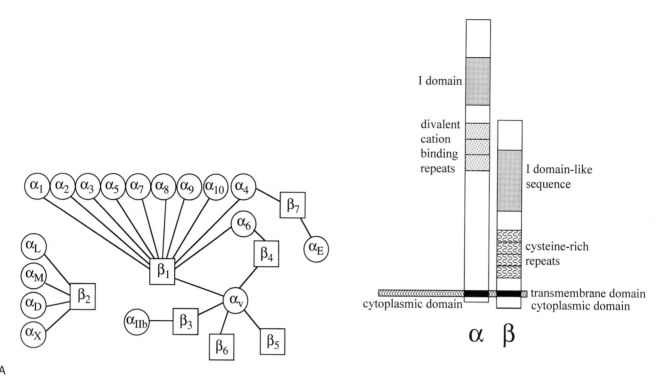

FIG. 37-1. The integrin family of adhesion receptors. **A:** The integrin adhesion molecules consist of $\alpha\beta$ heterodimers in a 1:1 stoichiometry. The subfamilies of integrin receptors are defined by the β subunit *(squares)*, of which there are eight known; these can associate with one or more α subunits *(circles)* to form at least 22 distinct $\alpha\beta$ heterodimers, as indicated by the connecting lines. The β_2 subfamily is composed of the $\alpha_L\beta_2$, $\alpha_M\beta_2$, $\alpha_d\beta_2$, and $\alpha_x\beta_2$ heterodimers. **B:** Structural features of the β_2 integrins.

canine, and bovine. Severe and often fatal infectious complications and impaired would healing in patients with this disorder [now termed leukocyte adhesion deficiency (LAD)] underscored the physiologic requirements for β_2 integrin in a wide spectrum of adhesion-dependent inflammatory functions of myeloid and lymphoid cells. Characterizations of LAD together with studies exploiting subunit-specific monoclonal antibodies to β_2 integrins have allowed for rich insights into our present understanding of the role of leukocyte adhesion determinants in immunologic host defense. The β_2 integrins, in concert with other integrins (notably $\alpha_4\beta_1$ and $\alpha_4\beta_7$) and with adhesion receptors of the immunoglobulin, selectin, and CD44 adhesion families, contribute to the development of immunocompetence and guide leukocyte localization during inflammation. This chapter focuses on the β_2 integrins and their role in inflammation.

THE β_2 INTEGRINS AND THEIR LIGANDS

Basic Features of CD11/CD18 Subunits

Basic Structure and Nomenclature of β_2 Integrins

The β_2 integrin subfamily consists of four heterodimeric integral membrane proteins including LFA-1

($\alpha_L\beta_2$), Mac-1 ($\alpha_M\beta_2$), p150,95 ($\alpha_x\beta_2$), and $\alpha_d\beta_2$. The nomenclature, structure, cell distribution, and functions of these proteins are summarized in Table 37-1, and a schematic representation of their primary structure is shown in Fig. 1B. Each of these prototype integrin glycoproteins consists of noncovalently associated α and β subunits with $\alpha_1\beta_1$ stoichiometry. They share an identical β subunit ($M_r = 95,000$) and are distinguished immunologically by α subunits whose molecular weights are as follows: $M_r = 165,000$ for Mac-1α (α_M); $M_r = 177,000$ for LFA-1α (α_L); $M_r = 150,000$ for p150,95α (α_x); and $M_r = 160,000$ for α_d. The World Health Organization designation for these glycoproteins is CD18 for β_2; CD11a for α_L; CD11b for α_M; and CD11c for α_x. The recently identified α_d subunit will likely receive the designation CD11d at the next International Leukocyte Typing Workshop. The entire complex is termed CD11/CD18 or the β_2 integrin subfamily.

Distribution

LFA-1, Mac-1, and p150,95 have different and yet overlapping roles in adhesion in part due to their characteristics of expression on immune cells. LFA-1 is expressed on virtually all immune cells, with the excep-

TABLE 37-1. *Cellular distribution and functional activities of β_2-integrin heterodimers*[a]

Property	LFA-1 (CD11a/CD18)	Mac-1 (CD11b/CD18)	P150, 95 (CD11c/CD18)	$\alpha_d\beta_2$ (CD11d/CD18)
Leukocyte distribution	T and B lymphocytes; large granular lymphocytes; monocytes; and granulocytes	Granulocytes; monocytes; macrophages; large granular lymphocytes	Macrophages; monocytes; granulocytes	Specialized tissue macrophages > monocytes, granulocytes, and lymphocytes. The predominant expression on specialized cells in tissues (e.g., foam cells in atherosclerotic lesions) suggests that αD may contribute to phagocytic functions. α_d is expressed at low levels on blood granulocytes, T cells, and monocytes; functional contribution on these cells is uncertain. $\alpha_d\beta_2$ CHO transfectants bind with soluble and immobilized ICAM-3, but not ICAM-1.
Myeloid cell functions	Natural killing; Antibody-dependent cellular cytotoxicity; Adhesion to endothelium or other mesenchymal or epithelial cells expressing ICAM-1, ICAM-2, ICAM-3	Complement receptor type 3 functions; iC3b binding; Phagocytosis and intracellular killing or cytolysis of complement-opsonized targets; Binding of microbial determinants (*Leishmania* GP63, *Bordetella* FHA); Homotypic aggregation; Adhesion to endothelium or protein substrates (fibrinogen, ICAM-1); Adhesion-dependent potentiation of oxidative burst and degranulation; Chemotaxis, random migration; Antibody-dependent cellular cytotoxicity; Cytotoxicity by large granular lymphocytes	iC3b binding (complement receptor type 4 activity?); Adhesion to endothelium or protein substrates; Chemotaxis, phagocytosis and aggregation (?)	
Lymphoid cell functions	Cytolytic T-lymphocyte-mediated killing; Natural killing; Antigen-, mitogen-, or alloantigen-induced proliferation; Phorbol-ester-elicited T- and B-lymphocyte aggregation; T-helper-cell responses		Cytolytic-T-cell, target-cell conjugation?	

ICAM, intercellular adhesion molecule 1; FHA, filamentous hemagglutinin; CHO, Chinese hamster ovary cells; LAD, leukocyte adhesion deficiency.
[a]Determined by subunit-specific MAb inhibition studies and/or observations of LAD leukocyte functions *in vitro.*

tion of some tissue macrophages (2,3). The distribution of Mac-1 is somewhat more limited. It is expressed predominantly in myeloid cells including blood monocytes, macrophages, and granulocytes (neutrophils, eosinophils, and basophils) (4–6), but it is also expressed on large granular lymphocytes and subsets of CD5$^+$ B cells (7) and CD8$^+$ T cells (8,9). A similar distribution exists for p150,95 as for Mac-1, although it is more highly expressed on tissue macrophages than on blood monocytes (10–12). p150,95 is also expressed on some activated lymphocytes and is a marker for hairy cell leukemia (7,13). The recently characterized $\alpha_d\beta_2$ is also expressed primarily on cells of the myeloid lineage, in particular tissue macrophages (14). Expression of $\alpha_d\beta_2$ has been found on foam cells in atherosclerotic plaques (14).

Biosynthesis

The β subunits of LFA-1, Mac-1, and p150,95 and their common β_2 subunit are synthesized as distinct precursors that are cotranslationally glycosylated with N-linked high mannose carbohydrate groups (15–17). An association of α subunit and β subunit precursors, which occurs 1 to 2 hours after synthesis, is required for further conversion to complex-type N-linked carbohydrates in the Golgi apparatus. Mature $\alpha\beta$ complexes are then transported to the cell surface or to intracellular secretory vesicles (18–22).

In unstimulated blood granulocytes and monocytes, Mac-1 and p150,95 are present in intracellular, vesicular compartments as well as on the cell surface (18–21). Electron microscopy studies reveal that β_2 integrins are associated with peroxidase negative (secondary and tertiary) granules in neutrophils or monocytes (19,20). In studies of fractionated neutrophils, it has been demonstrated that Mac-1 co-sediments with secondary granules (rich in vitamin B_{12} transport protein or lactoferrin) as well as higher density gelatinase-rich granules (22,23). Inflammatory mediators including chemotactic factors [(C5a, f-Met-Leu-Phe, and leukotriene B_4 (LTB$_4$)] and certain cytokines [tumor necrosis factor-α (TNF-α) and interleukin-8 (IL-8)] stimulate a three- to tenfold increase of Mac-1 and p150,95 on the surface of granulocytes and monocytes through translocation of intracellular stores to the cell surface (18,19,22).

Primary Structure

β Subunit Structure

The deduced amino acid sequence of the β_2 cDNA shows the characteristic features of an integral membrane protein with an N-terminal 677 amino acid extracellular domain containing 6 N-linked glycosylation sites, a 23 amino acid membrane spanning domain, and a 46 amino acid cytoplasmic tail (24,25). As observed for other β integrins, β_2 is rich in cystine residues (7.4% overall) and contains a fourfold repeat of an unusual cystine motif. This high cysteine content may provide for a rigid tertiary structure of the β subunit. Northern blot and Southern blot analyses employing the β_2 cDNA as a probe confirmed immunochemical evidence that a single gene encodes β_2 (24). The CD18 gene has been localized to chromosome 21 band q22 by in situ hybridization techniques (26). The genomic sequence encoding the β_2 integrin gene includes 16 exons spanning over 40 kb of genomic DNA (27).

The β_2 subunit shares 37% to 45% amino acid identity with the β_1 and β_3 subunits; especially high conservation among these three β subunits is evident within a 241 amino acid region in the extracellular domain (64%) (1,24,25,28). This region has been implicated as a potential site for divalent cation binding and for α subunit association (see below). All 56 cystine residues are conserved in each of β_1, β_2, and β_3 (and most other β integrins), including the fourfold cystine motif repeat. In contrast to β_1 and β_3, which contain a consensus tyrosine phosphorylation sequence in their cytoplasmic domains, no such sequence is found in the β_2 subunit.

α Subunit Structure

The α subunits of LFA-1 (29), Mac-1 (30–32), p150,95 (33), and $\alpha_d\beta_2$ (14) are structurally related integral membrane proteins with long extracellular domains, single hydrophobic membrane spanning domains, and short cytoplasmic tails (α_L, 53 amino acids; α_M, 19 amino acids: α_X, 29 amino acids; α_d, 38 amino acids). The α subunits of the β_2 integrins are more similar to each other (~47% identity) than to those of matrix receptors of the β_1 and β_3 subfamilies (~27% identity). The Mac-1 α subunit, p150,95 α subunit, and α_d subunit share 60% to 66% amino acid identity with one another, but only 35% identity with the LFA-1α subunit. Each subunit contains three homologous repeats that have putative divalent cation-binding sites that are similar to the Ca^{2+} binding E-F handloop sequences for calmodulin, troponin C, and parvalbumin. These metal-binding repeats are among the most highly conserved regions of these integrin α subunits. They may account in part for the divalent cation-dependency of β_2 integrin adherence functions. Divalent cations appear to stabilize $\alpha\beta$ chain association during immunopurification of LFA-1 in a functional form (34).

The divalent cation-binding motifs in the E-F handloops of the integrin α subunits have only five of six predicted metal coordination sites. Therefore, it has been suggested that "in integrin binding to RGD [arginine–glycine–aspartic acid] containing ligands, the Asp residue (D) in RGD binds to the metal held in the divalent cation-binding pocket of the α subunit, thereby forming a sixth coordination site" (30). The role of RGD recognition in ligand binding by β_2 as compared to several β_1- or β_3-ligand interactions is unclear. The primary structure of ICAM-1, a natural ligand for both LFA-1 and Mac-1, lacks an RGD motif, and detailed site-directed mutation studies indicate complex, probably noncontiguous, recognition sites within the immunoglobulin (Ig) domain 1 and domain 2 of this counterreceptor (35).

All four α subunits of the β_2 family contain a ~200 amino acid segment in their extracellular domains that is not found in α subunits of other integrins with the exception of $\alpha_1\beta_1$, $\alpha_2\beta_1$, and $\alpha_E\beta_7$. This unique domain, designated the "I" domain (for inserted or interactive domain), is highly homologous to the A domains of von Willebrand factor, to a domain in the complement proteins C2 and factor B, and to two domains in the cartilage matrix protein (30–32). Since the I domain structure is related to ligand-binding repeats in other nonintegrin proteins, it has been proposed that it confers modes of ligand recognition to the leukocyte integrins in addition to those common to all integrins. Antibodies that block integrin function often map to the I domain (36,37). Recently, the I domain of LFA-1 and Mac-1 have been expressed as an independent domain and extensively analyzed by binding studies and by x-ray crystallography (see below).

The genomic structure of the Mac-1 and p150,95 α subunit genes consists of 30 exons (38,39). The I domain is defined by four separate exons (exons 6–9) and its 5' and 3' boundaries correspond precisely with the intron between exon 4 and 5 of the αIIb gene, which lacks an I domain. The gene structure supports the idea that the I domain was inserted during evolution of this subfamily. Each of the E-F handloops is encoded by a separate exon. *In situ* hybridization data showed that the LFA-1, Mac-1, and p150,95 α subunit genes map between band p11 and p13.1 on chromosome 16 (26). These findings define a gene cluster of cell adhesion molecules and support the concept that the α subunit genes evolved by gene duplication. Chromosomal inversions and translocations in this region of chromosome 16 have been identified in patients with acute myelomonocytic leukemia (40).

Functional Characteristics of β_2 Integrins; *In Vitro* Applications of Monoclonal Antibodies

LFA-1 Function

LFA-1 participates in a broad spectrum of adhesive interactions of immune cells including the intercellular interactions among lymphoid and myeloid cells with other cell types (41–47). As shown in early studies with anti–LFA-1 monoclonal antibody (MAb), LFA-1 participates in antigen-independent adhesion of lymphocytes and monocytes to a variety of targets. LFA-1 is required for cytotoxic T-lymphocyte (CTL)-antigen-dependent adhesion to and killing of some target cells (48,49). Similarly, LFA-1 has been demonstrated to be important in

natural killing and antibody-dependent killing by NK cells and granulocytes, and in T-lymphocyte helper cell interactions (41,50,51). Not unexpectedly, abnormalities of many of these cellular functions were later recognized in studies of leukocytes of patients with genetic deficiency of the β_2 integrins (discussed in detail below).

Homotypic aggregation of T lymphocytes and lymphoid cell lines in response to phorbol ester stimulation *in vitro* is both inhibitable and reversible by anti–LFA-1 MAb (52–54). The requirements for aggregation are similar to those for the adhesion phase of CTL conjugate formation to target cells. Both processes are Mg^{2+}, energy, and temperature dependent, and both appear to involve interactions with an intact cytoskeleton (52). As shown in recent studies, LFA-1 purified from cell membranes in the presence of Mg^{2+} remains associated in an $\alpha\beta$ complex and mediates adhesion of several human cell lines when incorporated into planar membranes. Cell binding is inhibited by the pretreatment of the monolayer with LFA-1 MAb or the removal of Mg^{2+} and is energy independent.

The recognition of ICAM-1, a ligand for LFA-1 widely distributed on vascular endothelial cells, fibroblasts, epidermal keratinocytes, synovial cells, hepatocytes, and other cell types, led to studies defining the important role of LFA-1 in lymphocyte localization in lymphoid organs and inflamed tissues and its participation in the process of allograft rejection. These are discussed below. T-lymphocyte adhesion to endothelial cells (42,43,45), epidermal keratinocytes (44), synovial cells (46), hepatocytes (47), or other cell types is at least partially inhibited by LFA-1 MAb. Enhanced LFA-1–dependent adhesion to these cell types is facilitated by their exposure to cytokines (e.g., TNF-α, TNF-γ, IL-1) or lipopolysaccharides (LPSs) as a result of the upregulation of ICAM-1. Lymphocyte binding to high endothelial venules (HEV) of uninflamed lymphocyte organs appears to involve LFA-1 as an adhesion determinant accessory to organ-specific homing receptors (55). Lymphoid hypoplasia has been reported in pathologic studies of patients with leukocyte adhesion (β_2) deficiency (56).

Mac-1 Function

A functional role for Mac-1 was initially shown by the ability of anti–Mac-1α (CD11b) MAb to inhibit monocyte and granulocyte binding of iC3b-coated erythrocytes, findings indicating the identity of the Mac-1 protein and the complement receptor type 3 (CR-3) (57). Monoclonal antibodies to Mac-1 inhibit binding and phagocytosis of iC3b-opsonized particles by granulocytes and macrophages (57–59) as well as the heightened activity of natural killer (NK) cells against iC3b-coated target cells (60). Mac-1–dependent binding to microbial ligands has been implicated as a mechanism for the phagocytosis of *Leishmania promastigotes* (61,62), bordetella organisms (63), and histoplasma organisms (64) as well as ingestion of complement-opsonized bacteria by human granulocytes (59).

In addition to CR3 mediated functions, Mac-1 plays a more general role in adhesive interactions with a variety of protein substrates or cell types (59,65–68). Neutrophil aggregation elicited by chemotactic factors, phorbol esters, or calcium ionophores is inhibitable by some anti–Mac-1 MAb, but not by anti–LFA-1 MAb. Chemotaxis of neutrophils and monocytes (when assessed in adhesion-dependent assays) is also inhibitable by selected anti–Mac-1 MAb (59), as is adhesion of neutrophils to plastic or glass coated with certain proteins including serum, albumin, fibrinogen, and keyhole limpet hemocyanin (KLH) (59). Similarly, anti–Mac-1, but not anti–LFA-1, MAb inhibit adhesion of eosinophils to immune complex–coated plastic (69). The important role of Mac-1 in neutrophil, monocyte, or eosinophil adhesion to endothelial cell ligands is discussed below.

Mac-1–dependent adhesion to matrix proteins or endothelial cells contributes to a massive secretion of H_2O_2 by neutrophils activated by chemotactic factors or cytokines (68,70). Generation of reactive oxygen by neutrophils/mononuclear phagocytes not only is essential for intracellular microbicidal activities of these cells, but it also contributes to inflammatory tissue injury in a variety of pathophysiologic conditions. Chemotactic factors and other physiologic agonists generally elicit minimal levels of reactive oxygen release by neutrophil suspensions in vitro. However, these stimuli elicit a massive release of H_2O_2 by neutrophils adherent to matrix or endothelial substrates, a process inhibitable by anti-CD11b or CD18 MAb (70). Furthermore, essentially no H_2O_2 production by LAD neutrophils (which fail to normally adhere to these substrates) is detectable in this experimental system. The mechanism by which Mac-1–dependent adhesion potentiates the respiratory burst by adherent stimulated neutrophils is unclear, but these observations suggest that Mac-1 plays a fundamental role in transducing extracellular signals that influence the effector functions of the neutrophil oxidase and other secretory functions. Furthermore, this process would appear to be of considerable physiologic and possibly pathologic importance in vivo, as inflammatory cells interact with vascular endothelial or other biologic substrates in the presence of inflammatory mediators.

A role for Mac-1 in the regulation of phagocytosis independent of its ligand-binding function has been demonstrated by Brown et al. (71). In a series of studies, these investigators showed that the phagocytosis of Ig-opsonized targets is inhibited by a monoclonal antibody directed at an immobile subset of membrane Mac-1, which may be linked to the cytoskeleton (72). These studies are consistent with the earlier report of Arnaout et al. (73), who also demonstrated the inhibition of phagocytosis of C3 or IgG-coated particles by anti–Mac-1 MAb.

Collectively, these findings suggest that Mac-1 indirectly contributes to phagocytic function by its association with Fc receptors.

Mac-1 may also play an important role in regulating apoptosis of neutrophils. Accumulation of large numbers of neutrophils into inflammatory sites may exacerbate the tissue damage associated with inflammatory diseases. Normally, neutrophils undergo apoptosis and are then cleared by macrophages. Coxon et al. (74) made the unexpected finding that mice deficient in Mac-1 expression showed increased accumulation of neutrophils into thioglycollate-inflamed peritoneum. The increased accumulation was associated with delayed apoptosis of the recruited neutrophils. In vitro analysis showed that neutrophils undergo apoptosis following phagocytosis of opsonized particles. Apoptosis can be blocked with anti–Mac-1 MAbs. Thus, Mac-1–dependent adhesion, associated with activation may signal programmed cell death, an important mechanism for eliminating activated neutrophils.

p150,95 and $\alpha_d\beta_2$ Function

The function of these integrins is less well defined. A role for p150,95 as a complement receptor was initially demonstrated by the finding that this glycoprotein (as well as Mac-1) can be eluted from iC3b affinity columns (75,76). The contributions of p150,95 to iC3b binding by neutrophils and monocytes has been demonstrated in studies designed to exclude the contributions of the complement receptor 1 (CR-1) and CR-3 (which is expressed in tenfold excess of p150,95 on these cell types) (77). This activity has been designated CR-4, but its overall physiologic significance is unknown. As is also true for Mac-1, p150,95 appears to play a role in adhesion to substrates other than iC3b. Anti-CD11c MAb inhibits neutrophil adhesion to protein-coated glass or plastic but does not inhibit aggregation or chemotaxis (59). Studies by Figdor's team (78,79) and Arnaout et al. (80) indicate that p150,95 contributes to monocyte adhesion functions including adherence to protein substrates and endothelial cells, phagocytosis of latex spheres, and chemotaxis.

There is little known at this time about the physiologic function of the $\alpha_d\beta_2$ integrin. The distribution of $\alpha_d\beta_2$ integrin on macrophages and its high affinity interaction with ICAM-3 suggest that the $\alpha_d\beta_2$ integrin may be involved in antigen presentation (14). Both $\alpha_d\beta_2$ and p150,95 are expressed at higher levels on tissue macrophages than on blood monocytes.

Regulation of Expression and Functional Activity

The β_2 integrins are exquisitely regulated at several levels, a characteristic feature contributing to their functional and biologic diversity. Regulatory mechanisms include those at a biosynthetic level, which are largely linked to hematopoietic cell differentiation, and others that influence the expression or function of cell surface receptors or intracellular pools of receptors.

Biosynthesis Regulation

Studies of hematopoietic cell differentiation indicate that LFA-1 is first expressed in cytoplasmic μ chain–positive pre-B cells and late myeloblasts (81), and that Mac-1 expression is associated with committed granulocyte or monocyte precursors in bone marrow (82). These observations are in agreement with findings of β_2 expression on the promyeloblastic cell line HL-60. Whereas undifferentiated HL-60 cells express only LFA-1, differentiation promoted by phorbol esters (to a monocytoid lineage) or retinoic acid (to a granulocytic lineage) results in the expression of both Mac-1 and p150,95 (83). Blood monocytes express low amounts of p150,95 and high amounts of Mac-1, but this pattern of expression is reversed on further differentiated tissue macrophages (10). A downregulation of LFA-1 on murine blood monocytes during differentiation to tissue macrophages has also been reported (84). The underlying mechanisms and physiologic significance of variable levels of expression of β_2 integrins on hematopoietic cells during differentiation in bone marrow or other tissues remains to be determined.

Receptor Mobilization of Intracellular Preformed Pools (Quantitative Upregulation)

Following their biosynthesis, a proportion of Mac-1 and p150,95 (but not LFA-1) heterodimers are targeted for secondary and tertiary granules in granulocytes and in peroxidase negative granules in monocytes as well as the cell membrane (18–23). Upon cell activation by chemotactic factors, phorbol esters and certain cytokines [for example, TNF-α and granulocyte-macrophage colony-stimulating factor (GM-CSF)], the surface expression of Mac-1 and p150,95 increases severalfold. This occurs, in part, as a result of the translocation of granule-associated intracellular pools to the cell surface. This process of upregulation occurs within minutes after agonist exposure, is not impeded by protein synthesis inhibitors, and appears to involve the fusion of granule and cell membranes accompanying degranulation. The finding that blood granulocytes and monocytes upregulate the surface expression of these receptors when emigrating into inflammatory sites further suggests a physiologic role for this process (85). Moreover, impaired upregulation has been proposed to underlie the diminished granulocyte adhesive functions in patients with β_2 integrin deficiency (86), neutrophil specific granule deficiency (87), and human neonates (23,88).

Functional Regulation

On resting leukocytes, the β_2 integrins are expressed in an inactive state. Phorbol esters stimulate LFA-1–dependent homotypic aggregation of lymphocytes without altering the surface expression of LFA-1 (or its ligand ICAM-1) on these cells (52,89). In T lymphocytes, crosslinking of the T-cell receptor complex (90,91) results in increased LFA-1 adhesiveness, which peaks at 5 to 10 minutes and returns to baseline by 30 minutes. Neutrophil β_2 integrins have been shown to be transiently modulated by a variety of chemoattractants, including f-Met-Leu-Phe, C5a, LTB₄, IL-8, and platelet-activating factor (PAF). Extracellular nucleotides, such as adenosine diphosphate (ADP) and adenosine triphosphate (ATP), induce neutrophil aggregation (92) and appear to increase avidity of Mac-1 for factor X and fibrinogen (93–95). The capacity of inflammatory mediators to induce β_2-mediated adhesion has been termed inside-out signaling, as intracellular signals must be processed to somehow alter the adhesive interactions of the leukocyte with its extracellular environment. Chemokine activation of β_2 integrins occurs via a rho-dependent mechanism (96).

Regulation of β_2 integrin function is complex and involves multiple mechanisms including high affinity states of β_2 integrins, receptor clustering, and cell spreading (97–99). Two affinity states of LFA-1 have been described on intact cells—a low-affinity state with a K_d of approximately 100 μM and a high-affinity form that is 200-fold higher in affinity (100). The structural basis of β_2 integrin affinity modulation is not clear, although divalent cations appear to play a role. High concentrations of exogenous Mg^{2+} induce a high-affinity state of LFA-1, as evidenced by the MAb 24 activation epitope and by binding of soluble ICAM-1 (99,101,102).

In contrast, phorbol esters do not induce MAb 24 epitope or soluble ICAM-1 binding, but appear to mediate adhesion to ICAM-1–bearing cells in a cytoskeleton-dependent manner. Single particle tracking techniques show that diffusion of LFA-1 within the plasma membrane greatly increases upon activation with phorbol esters (103). Similar results are seen with the use of cytochalasin D, a microfilament-disrupting agent (103). The interpretation is that the nonadhesive state of LFA-1 in unactivated cells is maintained by cytoskeletal interactions, and that activation allows LFA-1 to diffuse and possibly cluster at the site of cell-cell contact. Clustering of LFA-1 requires calcium (97,104) and is evidenced by the calcium-dependent L16 MAb epitope. The Jurkat T-cell line, which is unable to mediate adhesion to ICAM-1 even with phorbol ester activation, lacks the L16 epitope (105,106). Ultrastructural studies (107) have demonstrated that PMA induces the formation of Mac-1 clusters on neutrophil surfaces, which correlates with their capacity to bind iC3b.

The cytoplasmic domains of integrins are critical to the regulation of integrin function. All integrin α subunits contain a conserved motif, GlyPhePheLysArg, proximal to the membrane. Deletion of this motif results in the expression of constitutively active integrins capable of ligand binding. The β_2 subunit contains a ThrThrThr motif that is necessary for β_2 function (108,109), possibly through cytoskeletal binding (110). Cells expressing the α subunit truncated in the GFFK motif and a β_2 subunit mutated in the ThrThrThr motif show defective adhesion, despite the fact that the receptors are locked in a high-affinity state. These double mutants show impaired cell spreading and decreased ability to organize cytoskeleton. The β_2 integrins have been shown to be associated with cytoskeletal components such as α-actinin (111), talin (112), filamin (113), and vinculin (114).

Recently, Kolanus et al. (115) used the yeast two-hybrid system to identify cytoadhesin-1 as an adapter protein that binds to the cytoplasmic tail of the β_2 integrin. Cytoadhesin-1 contains a pleckstrin homology (PH) domain, which may bind phospholipids and act as a guanosine diphosphate (GDP)–guanosine triphosphate (GTP) exchange factor, and a sec 7 homology domain, which binds directly to the cytoplasmic domain of the β_2 subunit. Overexpression of the PH domain of cytoadhesin-1 in T lymphocytes inhibited T-cell adhesion.

Receptor phosphorylation among other intracellular mechanisms may serve to regulate β_2 integrin function and activation (116). All α subunits of the β_2 integrin family are intrinsically phosphorylated (on serine and threonine residues) in isolated human mononuclear cells, whereas little or no phosphorylation is detected on the β_2 subunit itself (116). Phorbol esters, known to stimulate protein kinase C, elicit phosphorylation of β_2 in lymphocytes undergoing homotypic aggregation (117). However, phorbol ester–induced aggregation differs significantly from aggregation induced by chemotactic agents, in that the former is characterized by stable aggregates while the latter is a more physiologic event and involves a transient response followed by dis-aggregation. The phosphorylation pattern of the β subunit differs in phorbol ester–stimulated and f-Met-Leu-Phe–stimulated neutrophils. Phorbol esters induce a sustained and intense phosphorylation of the β subunit, while activation with f-Met-Leu-Phe results in little (116) or no (118) phosphorylation of the β subunit. Staurosporine, an inhibitor of protein kinase C, inhibited both PMA-induced aggregation and β subunit phosphorylation. However, staurosporine reduced the small amount of phosphorylation induced with f-Met-Leu-Phe, but actually enhanced the f-Met-Leu-Phe–induced aggregation response. These results suggest that phosphorylation of the β subunit is not required for activation of Mac-1 by a chemoattractant.

Signaling by Leukocyte Integrins

LFA-1 has been cast as an accessory cell molecule that mediates adhesive interactions necessary for immune cell function. Recently, there have been a number of reports suggesting that the leukocyte integrins can also transmit signals to within the cell (119). Crosslinking of the T-cell receptor complex is known to induce a Ca^{2+} flux resulting in T-cell activation and proliferation. This activation event, whether measured by Ca^{2+} flux or by proliferation, is markedly enhanced by co-crosslinking of LFA-1 (120,121). Crosslinking of LFA-1 can also synergize with phorbol esters to cause lymphocyte proliferation. Binding through LFA-1 also enhances biosynthesis of TNF-α and IL-2 by activated T cells (122). Other groups report that crosslinking of LFA-1, in the absence of any other stimulus, can induce a Ca^{2+} flux (123) and reorganization of the cytoskeleton (124) (Fig. 37-2).

Mac-1 has also been implicated in transmitting signals to myeloid cells. An early report showed that prolonged exposure of murine macrophages to soluble anti–Mac-1 MAb induces increased expression of major histocompatibility complex (MHC) class II, decreased phagocytosis, decreased secretion of proteins, and increased superoxide response triggered by PMA (125). These changes resemble macrophage activation with interferon-γ. More recent studies indicate that crosslinking of LFA-1 or Mac-1 induces production of cell-associated IL-1, but not release of this cytokine (126). This response may be important during antigen presentation. Crosslinking Mac-1 also synergizes with LPS or T-cell cytokines to induce increased expression of tissue factor and an enhanced TNF-α response (127), and to induce tyrosine phosphorylation of paxillin (128). Ligation of Mac-1 also induces the adhesion-dependent respiratory burst by neutrophils stimulated with chemoattractants (68). Similarly, superoxide production in response to concanavalin A has been suggested to be due to crosslinking of p150,95 (129).

Adhesion through LFA-1 has been implicated in a number of signal transducing events, including tyrosine phosphorylation of p130cas and the subsequent binding of p130cas to c-CrkII (130). Crosslinking of Mac-1 on neutrophils induces tyrosine phosphorylation of the *vav* protooncogene and activation of the GTP-binding protein, p21ras (131). Crosslinking of β_2 on neutrophils induces tyrosine phosphorylation of phospholipase C-γ_2 (PLC-γ_2), which parallels an increase in inositol 1,4,5-trisphosphate (IP_3) and may regulate the release of Ca^{2+} from intracellular stores (132).

Association with Other Cell Surface Receptors

The β_2 integrins appear to be functionally associated with a number of other cell surface receptors. LFA-1 has been physically linked to the T-cell receptor and the CD2 antigen on the surfaces of T lymphocytes. On neutrophils, Mac-1 interacts with the FcγRIII receptor and the uroki-

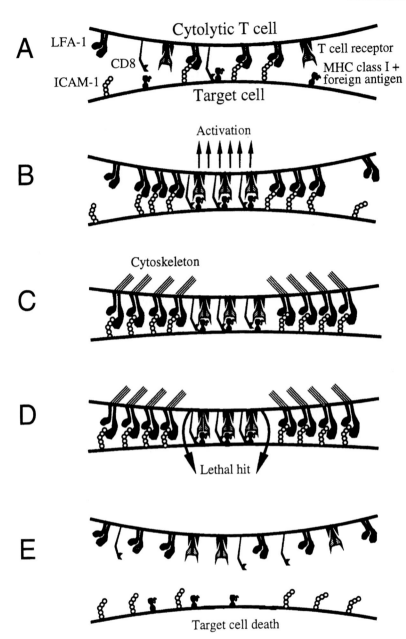

FIG. 37-2. A hypothetical model for cytolytic T-lymphocyte (CTL)–target cell interaction. The role of lymphocyte function antigen-1 (LFA-1) in CTL-mediated killing is depicted in five steps. **A:** Antigen-independent adhesion. Nonproductive antigen-independent interactions must be weak and freely reversible, as CTLs sample potential targets. **B:** Antigen-specific T-cell activation. CTL activation occurs if the T-cell receptor complex (TCR) engages the appropriate foreign antigen in context of major histocompatibility complex (MHC) class I antigen. Crosslinking of the TCR complex results in a rapid Ca²⁺ flux. Crosslinking of LFA-1 provides a co-stimulatory signal. **C:** Adhesion strengthening. Crosslinking of the TCR complex results in a transient, high-avidity state of LFA-1, which stabilizes the conjugate. The cytoskeleton is reorganized, resulting in clustering of LFA-1 at the contact site. **D:** Delivery of the lethal hit. The close contact between the CTL and the target cell, mediated in part by LFA-1, ensures that only the target cell is killed and that bystander cells are not harmed. **E:** Conjugate dissociation. Once the CTL has delivered the lethal hit, it is able to release the target cell and engage new target cells. LFA-1 returns to its low-avidity state.

nase-type plasminogen activator receptor (uPAR) (133). The interaction of Mac-1 with FcγRIII is critical for FcγRIII-mediated phagocytosis (71,72,134–136) and for efficient signal transduction leading to Ca²⁺ flux and oxidative burst (137). As FcγRIII is a glycosyl phosphotidyl inositol (GPI)-linked protein, lacking classical transmembrane and cytoplasmic domains, it has been proposed that FcγRIII transduces signal through its association with Mac-1. A similar situation occurs for the interaction of Mac-1 with the uPA receptor (uPAR) (138,139). The uPAR is a GPI-linked protein that binds and activates uPA, leading to conversion of plasminogen to plasmin. Signaling through uPAR requires association with Mac-1 (138–142). Thus, Mac-1 serves as a versatile signaling molecule in addition to its role in cell adhesion.

Ligands for β₂ Integrins

Ligands for LFA-1

Intercellular Adhesion Molecule-1 (ICAM-1)

This β₂ integrin counterreceptor was initially identified with a novel MAb (RR1/1) capable of inhibiting LFA-1–dependent homotypic aggregation of lymphoblasts (89). The strategy used to prepare this MAb was based on the observation that lymphocytes (as well as granulocytes) of patients with LAD are incapable of homotypic aggregation in response to phorbol esters or chemotactic factor stimulation, but are capable of forming heterotypic aggregates with normal leukocytes (52,89). These results suggested the presence on LAD cells of an adhesion determinant interactive with, but distinct from LFA-1 (or Mac-1). Thus, LAD lymphoblasts were employed in immunization protocols, and hybridoma supernatants were screened for the ability to inhibit LFA-1–dependent lymphocyte aggregation. Immunoprecipitation studies with this MAb defined a 76,000 to 114,000 dalton heavily glycosylated molecule, termed intercellular adhesion molecule-1 (ICAM-1), which was expressed on both normal and LAD lymphoblasts (89,143).

That ICAM-1 represents a ligand for LFA-1 was more formally proven in LFA-1–dependent lymphocyte or myeloid cell adhesion assays incorporating purified ICAM-1 in planar membranes or ICAM-1 cDNA transfected into mammalian cells (144–147). In each of these assay systems, lymphocyte binding is inhibitable by pretreatment of ICAM-1 substrates with RR1/1 or other anti–ICAM-1 MAb or by preincubation of cells with anti–LFA-1 MAb. Consistent with the above findings, LAD lymphoblasts or neutrophils fail to adhere to ICAM-1 substrates (67). Reciprocal studies using purified LFA-1 protein substrates further confirm the receptor-ligand interactions of LFA-1 and ICAM-1 (90). Binding of ICAM-1–bearing cells to purified LFA-1 substrates is inhibited by anti–ICAM-1 MAb, and purified LFA-1 binds to ICAM-1 incorporated in planar membranes (90). Purified LFA-1 binds to purified ICAM-1 with a K_d of ~130 nM (148), which is consistent with the high-affinity state of LFA-1 described on intact cells (100).

In striking contrast to the cellular distribution of β_2 integrins, ICAM-1 is widely distributed in non-hematopoietic cells including endothelial cells, fibroblasts, dendritic cells, keratinocytes, other mesenchymal cells, or cell lines in certain epithelial cells (143). Basal expression of ICAM-1 on nonhematopoietic cells is low, but surface expression is markedly upregulated by a variety of inflammatory mediators including LPS and cytokines such as IL-1, TNF-α, and interferon-γ (INF-γ) (44,45,143,149–151). ICAM-1 expression is markedly elevated on endothelial cells, other mesenchymal cells, and certain epithelial cells at sites of inflammation in vivo (69,143). Cytokine-elicited expression on cultured cells is inhibitable by protein or DNA synthesis inhibitors, achieves maximal levels following 18 to 24 hours of stimulation (143), and accounts for increased levels of LFA-1–dependent adhesion by T lymphocytes to endothelial cells (45), fibroblasts (143), epidermal keratinocytes (44), synovial cells (46), or hepatocytes (47). Upregulation of ICAM-1 by cytokines or LPS also facilitates enhanced neutrophil binding to and migration through cultured endothelial cell monolayers in vitro, a process involving the interactions of Mac-1 and LFA-1 with ICAM-1 (67) (see below). Immunofluorescence studies have shown a punctate distribution of ICAM-1 when expressed in COS cells or on microvillous structures of endothelial cells. A localized distribution of ICAM-1 on

these cells may facilitate its interaction with LFA-1 and Mac-1. ICAM-1 is presented on the cell surface as a homodimer (152,153), which may facilitate high-affinity interactions with LFA-1.

ICAM-1 is a member of the immunoglobulin gene superfamily (145,146), which includes other adhesion molecules such as neural crest adhesion molecule-1 (NCAM-1) and myelin adhesion glycoprotein. It contains five extracellular Ig domains, a transmembrane domain, and a short cytoplasmic tail at its C terminus. Alternatively spliced forms of ICAM-1 that lack one or more Ig domains are expressed in low levels in normal mice (154). Recently reported amino acid substitution and deletion mutation studies indicate that LFA-1 binding to transfected COS cells is mediated via recognition sites in domain 1, and to a lesser extent domain 2 (155). Comparison of the binding sites of ICAM-1, ICAM-2, and ICAM-3 led to a proposed sequence binding motif Ile/Leu-Glu-Thr-Pro/Ser-Leu (156). A similar motif has been described for VCAM-1 and the CS-1 domain of fibronectin (ligands for $\alpha_4\beta_1$) (157) and for MAdCAM-1, a ligand for $\alpha_4\beta_7$ (158). This critical motif is common to these integrin ligands even though the $\alpha_4\beta_1$ and $\alpha_4\beta_7$ integrins lack the I domain insertion.

A soluble form of ICAM-1 has been identified in normal human plasma at levels of 100 to 200 ng/ml (159). The levels of circulating ICAM-1 increase markedly in a number of clinical settings, providing a useful diagnostic marker for various inflammatory and immunologic diseases, including transplantation, stroke, insulin-dependent diabetes, arthritis, and cancer (160–166). The physiologic function of circulating ICAM-1 is unknown.

ICAM-1 has also been shown to function as a ligand for Mac-1 (see below), fibrinogen (167,168), and as receptor for the major group rhinovirus (169,170) and Plasmodium falciparum–infected red blood cells (171, 172). The major group rhinoviruses bind to the same two N-terminal domains interacting with LFA-1, and this binding to ICAM-1 is inhibited with the same MAb that blocks LFA-1–ICAM-1 interactions (155).

Intracellular Adhesion Molecule-2 (ICAM-2)

Early studies of LFA-1–dependent lymphocyte adhesion provided indirect evidence that ICAM-1 was not the only ligand for LFA-1. For example, phorbol ester–induced homotypic aggregation of the SKW3 T-cell line was inhibitable by LFA-1 MAb but not by ICAM-1 MAb (89). Moreover, in studies of LFA-1–dependent T-cell adhesion to endothelial cells, both ICAM-1–dependent and ICAM-1–independent pathways were evident; an ICAM-1–dependent pathway was elicited by cytokines, whereas ICAM-1–independent adhesion was not (44,45). These findings of differential LFA-1 binding prompted the development of a novel strategy to identify alternative ligands for LFA-1 (173). A cDNA library derived from LPS-elicited endothelial cells was expressed in COS cells and screened for clones mediating binding to LFA-1 substrates in the presence of ICAM-1 MAb. Sequence analysis of one isolated clone conferring this type of differential adhesion revealed a novel integral membrane protein, termed ICAM-2 (173).

ICAM-2 is an integral membrane protein of 28 to 46 kD with two as opposed to five N-terminal extracellular Ig-like domains sharing 35% sequence identity with domains 1 and 2 of ICAM-1 (173). Based on these characteristics, ICAM-1 and ICAM-2 represent a subfamily within the immunoglobulin gene family of molecules. ICAM-2 is constitutively expressed on endothelial cells, lymphocytes (174), and platelets (175), but unlike ICAM-1, it is not elicited by inflammatory mediators. The relative role and importance of ICAM-2 in inflammatory reactions *in vivo* remain to be determined.

Recently, the crystal structure of ICAM-2 has been described (176) and provides the first x-ray view of a β₂ integrin ligand. The general structure is similar to that described for domains 1 and 2 of VCAM-1 (177). The two independently folded Ig-like domains of ICAM-2 present a critical glutamic acid, E37, that projects from the edge of the C strand rather than the tip of the CD turn as in VCAM-1. Thus, the binding feature recognized by LFA-1 is a flat surface that includes the CD edge and the GFC-β sheet. Residues Y54, Q30, and Q75 have also been shown by mutagenesis to be important for ICAM binding to LFA-1 (see Fig. 37-2), and they define a surface that extends on either side of E37. Docking of the LFA-1 I domain and the ICAM-2 crystal structures can be accomplished without substantial protein adjustment.

Intracellular Adhesion Molecule-3 (ICAM-3)

ICAM-3, like ICAM-1, has five Ig-like domains (178–180). Unlike other ICAM molecules, ICAM-3 is restricted primarily to leukocytes (181), although some expression on vascular endothelium has been detected in some disease states (182). In contrast to ICAM-1, ICAM-3 is expressed constitutively and is not greatly altered by proinflammatory cytokines. ICAM-3 is highly expressed on resting leukocytes, including neutrophils, blood dendritic cells, and epidermal Langerhans cells (181,183). The pattern of distribution and expression has led to the suggestion that ICAM-3 may be involved in the initiation of primary immune responses, while ICAM-1 may be more involved in the interactions of activated lymphocytes. ICAM-3 is a major co-stimulatory ligand for LFA-1 on blood dendritic cells (183,184). ICAM-3 binds with a higher apparent affinity to $\alpha_d\beta_2$ than to LFA-1 (14).

Other ICAM-Related Ligands

Homology searches of recently cloned genes have revealed two novel ICAM-like ligands for LFA-1. The LW blood group antigen, recently termed ICAM-4, is a red blood cell antigen with significant homology to ICAM-1 (185). Subsequent binding studies revealed that ICAM-4 can bind directly to both LFA-1 and Mac-1 (186). The physiologic function of this interaction is not yet known, but may be involved in red blood cell homeostasis. Senescent red blood cells may be retained in the spleen by splenic macrophages via LFA-1 or Mac-1 binding to ICAM-4.

Another antigen, telecephalin, was originally cloned as a telecephalon-specific marker of rabbit brains (187). Telecephalin has nine Ig-like domains, of which the N-terminal five domains show significant homology to ICAM-1. ICAM-1, -3, -4, and telecephalin are all clustered on chromosome 19p13.2 (188). Again, subsequent ligand-binding studies showed that telecephalin can bind LFA-1 (189), although binding was divalent cation-independent and did not increase with phorbol ester activation (188). Telecephalin is constitutively expressed on neurons, while LFA-1 is constitutively expressed on microglial cells in the brain. In central nervous system (CNS) neurodegenerative diseases or in brain trauma, microglial cells become activated and migrate to damaged neurons. The physiologic role of telecephalin in normal brain function or in neurodegenerative diseases remains to be investigated.

Mac-1 Ligands

ICAM-1

ICAM-1 can also serve as a functional ligand for Mac-1 (66–68). Smith et al. (67) showed that adhesion of f-Met-Leu-Phe–stimulated neutrophils to endothelial cells is largely Mac-1 (and to a lesser extent LFA-1) dependent. In contrast, adhesion of unstimulated neutrophils is exclusively LFA-1 dependent. Since anti–ICAM-1 MAb inhibited adhesion of both unstimulated and stimulated neutrophils to endothelial cells or purified ICAM-1 in planar membranes in these studies, it was concluded that both LFA-1 and Mac-1 interact with ICAM-1.

Diamond et al. (66) employed immunoaffinity purified Mac-1 and ICAM-1 and cell lines transfected with Mac-1 and ICAM-1 cDNAs to more directly explore the possible interactions of ICAM-1 and Mac-1. They showed that cytokine-stimulated endothelial cells bound to purified Mac-1 absorbed to artificial substrates, a process inhibited by both anti–ICAM-1 and Mac-1 MAb. Murine L cells or monkey COS cells transfected with ICAM-1 cDNA bound to purified Mac-1 in a specific and dose-dependent manner; this attachment was of lower avidity, was more temperature sensitive, and was inhibited by different anti–ICAM-1 MAb when compared to LFA-1–binding characteristics. In reciprocal studies, COS cells cotransfected with the α and β subunits of Mac-1 or LFA-1 attached avidly to purified ICAM-1 substrates; this binding was inhibited by MAb to ICAM-1, LFA-1, and Mac-1. Parallel cell conjugation experiments showed that f-Met-Leu-Phe–stimulated (but not –unstimulated) neutrophils bind human endothelial cells stimulated with LPS for 24 hours to induce high levels of ICAM-1. Binding among these cell suspensions was significantly inhibited by anti–Mac-1 but not anti–LFA-1 MAb, and a combination of anti–LFA-1 and Mac-1 MAb demonstrated additive and almost total inhibition of cell binding. A mixture of anti–ICAM-1 MAbs only partially inhibited cell binding, findings suggesting that Mac-1 and/or LFA-1 may be interacting with non–ICAM-1 ligands on LPS-elicited endothelium as previously suggested by Lo et al. (190). ICAM-2 does not appear to represent one of these ligands, since anti–ICAM-2 MAb was not inhibitory of adhesion in this system. Of a panel of nine ICAM-1 MAb tested, only the R6.5 MAb used by Smith et al. (67) was capable of inhibiting both Mac-1–ICAM-1 and LFA-1–ICAM-1 interactions. Other ICAM-1 MAbs block LFA-1–ICAM-1 interactions but not Mac-1–ICAM-1 interactions. These results are consistent with mapping studies showing that LFA-1 binds domain 1 of ICAM-1 while Mac-1 binds domain-3. The ICAM-1 domain 3 sequence reveals a critical leucine–aspartic acid–valine (LDV)-like motif.

iC3b

The iC3b fragment of complement was the first ligand to be demonstrated for Mac-1 (57,191), thus defining Mac-1 as the complement receptor type three (CR-3). The C3b fragment is generated during the complement cascade and is covalently bound to target surfaces. The iC3b binding activity of Mac-1 has been shown to be sufficient in promoting neutrophil phagocytosis and lysis of iC3b-coated erythrocytes in an Fc receptor–independent fashion (58). In contrast to Fc receptor–mediated phagocytosis, phagocytosis of iC3b-coated targets does not promote release of oxygen radicals (191) or arachidonic acid metabolites (192). Mac-1–positive NK cells show elevated cytolytic activity against C3bi-coated targets (60). In addition, the deposition of iC3b on endothelial cells provides a rapid means of inducing neutrophil adhesion in a Mac-1–dependent, LFA-1/p150,95–independent fashion (193). Various MAbs directed at CD11b appear to recognize specific CR-3 epitopes capable of inhibiting iC3b rosetting or iC3b-dependent cytotoxicity but not other Mac-1–dependent functions such as homotypic aggregation or adhesion of endothelial cells (59).

Polysaccharides

The existence of binding sites for polysaccharides on Mac-1 has been suggested by the finding that certain MAbs inhibit neutrophil adhesion to substrates such as zymosan (194) or polysaccharide determinants of bacter-ial capsules (195). Binding of Mac-1 to zymosan is inhibited by N-acetyl-D-glycocyamine and is mediated by a site in Mac-1 distinct from the iC3b-binding site (194). Cells transfected with Mac-1 gain the ability to bind β-glucan, supporting the view that Mac-1 has a lectin-like activity (196). Recent studies suggest that iC3b-opsonin, in addition to incompletely defined constituents of group B Streptococcus capsular polysaccharide, mediates Mac-1–dependent ingestion and killing by neutrophils (195).

Other Ligands

Coagulation factor X and fibrinogen α bind to Mac-1 on activated but not basal myeloid cells (93–95,197). Binding of factor X to "activated" Mac-1 is specific for the zymogen but not the activated form of factor X, and it requires the Ca^{2+} ion but not the Mg^{2+} ion. Fibrinogen α and factor X compete with each other and with iC3b for binding to Mac-1 of activated cells, suggesting that a common activation epitope of Mac-1 mediates binding of all three ligands. Mac-1–dependent binding of factor X and fibrinogen α to activated macrophages or neutrophils may play a role in the initiation of coagulation and thrombosis at inflammatory sites.

A wide range of diverse proteins has been identified or proposed as ligands for Mac-1. Mac-1 has also been shown to bind to haptoglobin, an acute-phase protein (198); high molecular weight kininogen (199); collagen (200); fibronectin (200,201); heparin (65); CD23 (202); and ICAM-4 (185). Thus, Mac-1 is unusually promiscuous in its binding specificity. One interesting hypothesis is that Mac-1 may bind to determinants on denatured proteins (203), an activity that may enable neutrophils and monocytes to clear antigens that have been damaged by infectious agents or by superoxide and proteases generated during the course of an inflammatory event.

p150,95 and $\alpha_d\beta_2$ Ligands

The p150,95 integrin exhibits some of the promiscuous binding activity of Mac-1. Various ligands have been proposed for p150,95, including ICAM-1, iC3b, heparin, CD23, fibrinogen, and a yet-unidentified ligand on activated endothelial cells. Typically, antibodies against p150,95 are much less potent in inhibiting leukocyte adhesion than anti–Mac-1 MAbs, making it difficult to assess the physiologic contribution of p150,95 to leukocyte function.

The $\alpha_d\beta_2$ integrin has only been recently identified and is not fully characterized in ligand-binding specificity. However, it has been shown to bind ICAM-3 preferentially over ICAM-1 (14). Chinese hamster ovary (CHO) cells expressing $\alpha_d\beta_2$ bind to ICAM-3 but not ICAM-1. Furthermore, $\alpha_d\beta_2$ transfectants, but not LFA-1 transfectants, bind soluble ICAM-3–Ig chimeras, suggesting that the affinity of $\alpha_d\beta_2$ for ICAM-3 is greater than that of LFA-1. The preferential binding of $\alpha_d\beta_2$ for ICAM-3 suggests some specialized function for this interaction. One interesting proposal is that $\alpha_d\beta_2$–ICAM-3 interaction may be more involved in the initiation of the primary immune response.

Structural Definitions of Putative Ligand-Binding Sites in LFA-1 and Mac-1 I Domains

LFA-1 and Mac-1 I Domain Structure/Function Relationships

One of the most significant recent advances has been the elucidation of the x-ray crystal structure of the I domain from Mac-1 and LFA-1 (204–207; Baldwin, unpublished data). The domain comprises about 180 amino acids and adopts a familiar structural topology, the Rossmann or nucleotide-binding fold. The I domain has a six-stranded β sheet, with strand C being anti-parallel, and seven α helices. Helix 5 is slightly shorter in LFA-1 due to a seven amino acid deletion (Fig. 37-3B). The crystal structures support the idea that the I domain was "inserted" into a preexisting α subunit as a structural appendage. The N and C termini of the domain are in close proximity, and the compact, globular I domain is

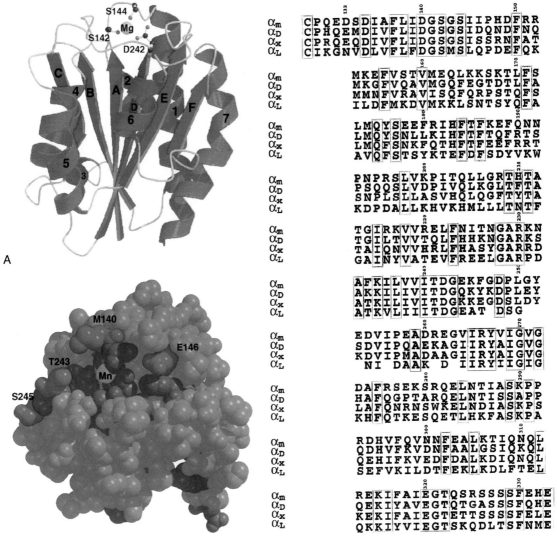

FIG. 37-3. Structural features of the I domain. **A:** Ribbon diagram of the Mac-1 I domain with Mn ion bound at the COOH-terminal end of the mostly parallel β sheet *(green)*. The seven α helices are shown *(red)*. The Mg ion is coordinated by the conserved residues S142, S144, and D242. The NH₂- and COOH-termini are in close proximity to each other and denoted as N and C, respectively. **B:** Structural alignment of the human protein sequences of the I domains from the α subunits of LFA-1, Mac-1, p150,95, and $\alpha_d\beta_2$. The sequences were aligned using the Mac-1 (Baldwin, unpublished data) and LFA-1 I domain (1zon.pdb) x-ray structures. The α_D and α_x I domains could be aligned to Mac-1 without gaps. The I domain spans approximately 200 amino acids, while the entire α subunit is nearly 1,200 amino acids in length. The invariant amino acids among the I domains are boxed. **C:** Space-filling model of the Mac-1 I domain. The invariant residues *(blue)* (see above) cluster around the Mn ion in a shallow groove across the surface of the I domain.

stable in solution, independent of the rest of the α subunit, and does not require the β subunit for folding (208).

The C-terminal end of the β sheet (Fig. 3A, top) is the general location of ligand-binding function for this structural class of proteins. For example, in subtilisin the protease active site is found there; in proteins with nucleotide cofactors, the flavin-adenine dinucleotide (FAD) or nicotinamide-adenine dinucleotide (NAD) is bound in the crevice at the C-terminus of the sheet; and several sugar-binding proteins like arabinose-binding protein also use this motif for ligand binding. In the I domain, the crevice is the location of a group of conserved amino acids, S142, S144, and D242 (Mac-1, sequence numbering), which coordinate a metal ion, Mg^{2+} or Mn^{2+}. This motif, termed MIDAS (metal ion dependent adhesion site), is critical for the interaction of the I domain with β2 ligands.

Ueda et al. (209) demonstrated that recombinant I domain required either Mn^{2+}, Mg^{2+}, or Mg^{2+} and Ca^{2+} for binding to iC3b, while Ca^{2+} alone was ineffective. Metal-binding studies (210) have shown that Mn^{2+} binds with a low micromolar affinity constant, while Mg^{2+} binds with a tenfold lower affinity. Calcium ion binds with a 500- to 1000-fold lower affinity than Mn^{2+}. Crystal structures of both LFA-1 and Mac-1 I domain confirmed that either Mg^{2+} or Mn^{2+} can bind in the MIDAS metal ion–binding site (204–207). While Mn and Mg ions could be easily soaked into metal free I domain crystals, Ca ion was not observed in electron density maps even when the crystals were soaked at 100 mM $CaCl_2$ (Baldwin, unpublished data). The crystal structure of LFA-1 and Mac-1 I domains without metal ions (1zon.pdb) adopt a protein conformation that is unaffected by the addition of either Mn or Mg ion (207; Baldwin, unpublished data). Mutagenesis studies showed that mutation of D140A/S142A or D242A blocked metal binding and iC3b binding when the mutant α chain was coexpressed with β2 on whole cells (210). The crystal structure definitively proved that Mn or Mg ion is directly coordinated by D242, S142, and S144. The remaining three coordination sites are occupied by three waters or two waters and a chloride ion. The relatively open coordination geometry of the metal ion binding site in the I domain and the observation that β2 ligands like ICAM-1 have critical acidic residues suggest the possibility that an ICAM acidic side chain may directly (or indirectly through water) coordinate with the metal ion during ICAM-integrin binding. This attractive hypothesis has yet to be proven.

A comparison of the β2 I domains shows that the most highly conserved region is near the metal-binding site (Fig. 37-3C, blue residues). Most of these residues directly coordinate with the metal (D242, etc.) or makeup residues in the floor of the shallow ligand-binding crevice found on either side of the metal. A number of recent studies have investigated site-directed mutations in the I domain in the context of full-length α chain coexpressed with wild-type β2 chain. These studies have shown that metal coordinating residues in the I domain, as well as residues located in or along the crevice where the metal binds on I domain, are needed for binding of protein ligands like ICAM or iC3b.

In Mac-1, mutation of D140A, S142A, S144A, T209A, D248A, or Y252A or a deletion of F246-Y252 eliminated or reduced binding to iC3b (210-212). Zhang and Plow (213) also showed that deletion of D248-Y252 blocked iC3b and ICAM binding to Mac-1. Similarly for LFA-1, mutation of T206A, D137A, D239A, D239K, or D137K prevented LFA-1 from binding to ICAM (211,214,215). Proline-192A also prevented binding of ICAM (214), but T208A still bound ICAM-1 (211). Huang and Springer (216) prepared a series of LFA-1 I domain mutants with diminished binding of ICAM-1 to LFA-1. Since mouse LFA-1 does not bind to human ICAM-1, a series of chimeric I domains were prepared to delineate the general location of sequences important for ICAM-1 binding. When specific mutants were introduced into LFA-1 I domain, and the relative binding to ICAM-1 evaluated, four mutants seemed to be the most important: M140Q, 35% WT; E146D, 50% WT; T243S, 40% wild type (WT); and S245K, 30% WT. These mutants have been mapped in red upon the LFA-1 surface in Fig. 3C. These mutations fall along the edge of the metal binding crevice and overlap with the general location of the Mac-1 iC3b mutants of McGuire and Bajt (212). Taken together, these data underscore the importance of the metal coordinating residues and crevice for Mac-1 and LFA-1 function. Another residue in the crevice T206 (LFA)/T209 (Mac-1) forms a water-mediated hydrogen bond to the metal ion in many crystal structures. This residue may play additional roles in ligand interaction (204).

The deletion of residues at the beginning of helix 5 (212,213) was prepared to mimic the LFA-1 I domain deletion relative to the Mac-1 I domain. Such insertion/deletions often occur in β turns and result in the lengthening or shortening of a surface loop. For the Mac-1/LFA-1 I domains, this was clearly not the case. The deletion converts part of helix 5 into a β meander and results in a dispersed structural alignment (Fig. 37-3B). The deletion of contiguous residues of Mac-1 I domain clearly diminishes function, but the necessary structural rearrangements could perturb ligand recognition in a variety of ways. Mac-1 residues D248 and Y252 do not project from the surface of I domain in a manner suggestive of residues involved in critical protein-protein interactions. Rather, important structural roles are played by D248 and Y252. Conversion of these residues to alanine (212) would result in the loss of side chain to main chain hydrogen bonds and bulk, which would likely destabilize the conformation of helix 5 (Baldwin, unpublished data). Huang and Springer (216) have also noted topologically related mutations that affect ICAM-1 binding to LFA-1 I domain (see above and Fig. 3C; S245K and T243S).

The mutation of P195A of Mac-1 (210) and P192A of LFA-1 (214) is found on the opposite face of the I domain from the metal-binding site. This proline is the first residue of α helix 3. Michishita et al. (210) reported that the proline mutant did not affect binding of whole Mac-1 to iC3b, but did increase the apparent K_d for Mn ion. Edwards et al. (214) examined the corresponding mutation in LFA-1 I domain and found a complete loss of ICAM-1 binding. Zhang and Plow (213) found that replacement of Mac-1 I domain residues around this proline with the corresponding residues from LFA-1 could convert Mac-1 to spontaneously adhere to fibrinogen without activation. While these data suggest that residues including P195 may be important for some ligand-binding interactions for both LFA-1 and Mac-1, the exact structural manifestation of these mutations is unclear.

An I-Domain–Like MIDAS Motif of the β_2 Subunit

The β subunits of the integrin family contain a highly conserved 200 amino acid segment that has been implicated in $\alpha\beta$ association and in ligand binding. While the primary sequence of this region of the β_2 subunit has no obvious homology to the I domain of the integrin α subunits, secondary structure predictions of these regions show remarkably similar hydropathic profiles, which are indicative of β strands and α helices (204). Even more striking, the N-terminus of this region of the β_2 subunit contains a conserved metal-binding motif, DXSXS, like that found in the α subunit I domains. Based on these observations, Lee et al. (204) proposed that the β_2 subunit contains an I-domain–like MIDAS motif. Initial site-directed mutagenesis experiments demonstrated that the residues in the β_2 subunit DXSXS motif were required for ligand recognition. The analogue of D140 of Mac-1 I domain in the β_2 subunit has been mutated with loss of ligand-binding function: D134, β_2 (217). Additionally, mutation of the S142 analogue (217) also affects ligand-binding function. Taken together, these results indicate that the MIDAS motifs of the α subunit, the β subunit, metal ions, and ligand are intimately associated during integrin-mediated adhesion.

β-Propeller Model for Folding of the Integrin α Subunit

Springer (218) has proposed a model for the N-terminal third of the α subunit of integrins (approximately 440 amino acids, exclusive of the I domain). The sevenfold repeated FG...GAP motif (33) is threaded through a seven-bladed β-propeller. Each blade of the propeller is composed of a four-stranded antiparallel β sheet. The "FG" would begin the first strand of each blade, and "GAP" ends the second strand. The seventh blade is composed of strand 4 from the N-terminus and strands 1 to 3 from the C-terminus, a common feature of the motif,

which helps to stabilize the protein torus. Strand 1 of the blade is found near the center of the donut-shaped protein and strand 4 is at the perimeter. The loops that connect strands 2 to 3 and 4 to 1 are proposed to project to form part of the ligand-binding surface, at the top, while loops 1 to 2 and 3 to 4, which coordinate some of the calcium ions required for integrin function, are found on the bottom surface of the torus. The upper surface loop or central cavity of β-propellers often bind metals. In the α subunit model, an Mg ion is modeled in the center of the cavity. Springer notes that in galactose oxidase a polypeptide finger fills the central cavity from below and provides an acidic residue for metal coordination. He speculates that perhaps some of the important α-β subunit interactions required for integrin function provide just such an acidic finger from the β subunit. Finally, the insertion of the I domain into to the α subunit in some of the integrins is found in loop 4 to 1 (top surface) between blades 2 and 3 of the α subunit β-propeller. The I domain folds independently and is perhaps free to adopt a limited number of orientations relative to the β-propeller domain (208). This hinge motion could be important for integrin activation or modulation of adhesive function.

β_2 INTEGRINS IN HOST-DEFENSE AND INFLAMMATORY INJURY

Leukocyte Adhesion Deficiency (LAD)

Early Characterizations

Prior to 1990, several reports documented a group of human patients with widespread bacterial and fungal infections, defective polymorphonuclear (PMN) leukocyte mobility and phagocytosis, impaired wound healing, or delayed umbilical cord severance (219). Crowley et al. (220) were the first to propose that defects in neutrophil chemotaxis and phagocytosis and associated susceptibility to recurrent infection were secondary to an abnormality in leukocyte adhesion. Neutrophils of one of their patients showed impaired adhesion and spreading on plastic substrates. Moreover, lysates of whole-blood neutrophils from this patient lacked a cell surface protein (M_r = 110,000) termed gp110. Subsequently, other similar patients were shown to lack surface glycoproteins ranging in M_r from 130,000 to 180,000 daltons (221,222). Patient cells studied by Bowen et al. (222) failed to adhere and spread to a variety of artificial substrates, while those studied by Arnaout et al. (221) demonstrated defective neutrophil receptor–mediated phagocytosis of complement-opsonized particles.

The M_r range of 110,000 to 180,000 daltons for the missing surface glycoproteins was consistent with that of the 165,000 M_r α subunit of Mac-1. Studies in 1984 revealed that both the α and β subunits of Mac-1 (223–226) and LFA-1 (224,226,227) were deficient on patient leukocytes. Thus, it was proposed that the primary defect in this disorder was related to the β_2 subunit and that the β_2 subunit was necessary for cell surface expression of α subunits (reviewed in ref. 219). This group of patients sharing similar clinical features and the same molecular defect defined a novel pathologic disorder, designated as leukocyte adhesion deficiency (LAD). Very similar clinical disorders in Irish setters (228) and Holstein cattle (229) have been described and shown to be due to deficiency of β_2 integrins. Bovine LAD, prevalent among Holstein cattle in the United States, Europe, and Japan in the early 1990s, resulted from highly regulated breeding practices of the U.S. Department of Agriculture. All recognized cases are related to a single β_2 integrin mutant allele transmitted via artificial insemination from a single bull carrier.

Clinical Characteristics and Histopathologic Features

Clinical and histopathologic features of LAD are remarkably similar among affected human, canine, and bovine subjects (Fig. 37- 4) (86,226,228–232). Recurrent necrotic and indolent infections of soft tissues primarily involving skin, mucous membranes, and intestinal tract are clinical hallmarks of this autosomal/recessive trait now recognized in over 100 patients worldwide (Fig. 37-4). Superficial infections on body surfaces may invade locally or systemically. Typical small, erythematous, non-pustular skin lesions often progress to large, well-demarcated ulcerative craters or pyoderma gangrenosa, which heal slowly or with dysplastic eschars (86). Staphylococcal or gram-negative enteric bacterial organisms may be cultured from such lesions for up to several weeks despite antimicrobial therapy. Fulminant progression of gangrene of soft tissues of a distal extremity in one case prompted surgical amputation as a lifesaving measure (222). Septicemia progressing from omphalitis associated with delayed severance of the umbilical cord is a common and unique feature of LAD (226). Perirectal abscess or cellulitis leading to peritonitis and/or septicemia has been reported in multiple patients, and facial or deep neck cellulitis has been observed to progress from ulcerative mucous membrane lesions of the oral cavity (86,221, 222). Recurrent invasive candidal or nonspecific esophagitis, erosive gastritis, acute appendicidal or ileal perforation, and necrotizing enterocolitis represent common and often fatal complications of LAD. Recurrent otitis media occurs commonly, and may progress to mastoiditis and/or facial nerve paralysis. Other reported respiratory infections include severe (bacterial) laryngotracheitis with airway compromise, recurrent or necrotizing pneumonitis, and sinusitis (86).

Severe gingivitis and/or periodontitis is a major feature among all patients who survive infancy (Fig. 37-4) (233). Acute gingivitis has appeared in all cases with eruption of the primary dentition. Subsequently, these patients developed characteristic features of progressive generalized prepubescent periodontitis, including gingival proliferation, defective recession, mobility, and advanced alveolar bone loss associated with periodontal pocket formation and partial or total loss of both the deciduous and permanent dentitions (233).

Recurrent infections and poor wound healing reflect a profound impairment of blood leukocyte mobilization into extravascular inflammatory sites of LAD patients (Fig. 4). Artificial inflammatory "skin windows" as well as biopsies of infected tissues demonstrate inflammatory infiltrates almost totally devoid of neutrophils (86,222,234). This histopathologic feature is observed in all tissues with the exception of lung and is particularly striking considering that marked peripheral blood leukocytosis and neutrophilia (4- to 24-fold normal values) are constant features of LAD (Table 37-2). Transfusions of leukocytes results in the appearance of donor neutrophils and monocytes in skin windows or chambers and in inflamed tissues (222,235). Impaired healing of traumatic or surgical wounds commonly observed in LAD represents a clinical feature not commonly reported in patients with neutropenia or other neutrophil dysfunction disorders. Unusual paper-thin or dysplastic cutaneous scars found in some patients (86) may reflect the lack of monocyte infiltration and lack of elaboration of inflammatory mediators contributing to healing such as angiogenesis factors. The wide spectrum of gram-positive and gram-negative bacterial and fungal microorganisms afflicting LAD patients is also characteristic of patients with primary neutropenia syndromes (236,237) and individuals with primary neutrophil-specific granule deficiency (238). These clinical models also demonstrate insufficient tissue leukocyte infiltration. However, deep-seated granulomatous infections typical of phagocyte oxidative killing defects (e.g., chronic granulomatous disease) have not been observed in LAD.

Limited evidence suggests increased susceptibility to viral infection in LAD (86,230,239), which might be expected considering the important role of LFA-1 in cytotoxic and other functions of lymphocytes and myeloid cells *in vitro*. Most LAD patients demonstrate apparently normal and self-limited courses of varicella or other viral respiratory infections. Five of 10 patients in one report demonstrated no untoward reactions to live viral vaccine administration (219). However, one patient died of an overwhelming infection with picornavirus involving the oral pharynx, glottis, trachea, and lungs, and three patients of the same series had one or more episodes of aseptic (presumably viral) meningitis (86).

The severity of clinical features among LAD patients appears to be directly related to the degree of glycoprotein deficiency on leukocyte surfaces (86). Two general phenotypes, designated severe and moderate (or partial) deficiency, have been identified (Table 37-2) (86,219). As assessed by immunofluorescence flow cytometry and verified by radioimmunoassay and immunoprecipitation

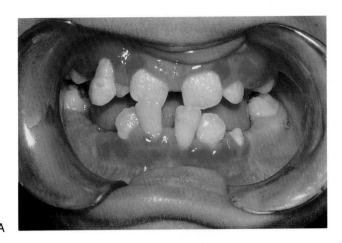
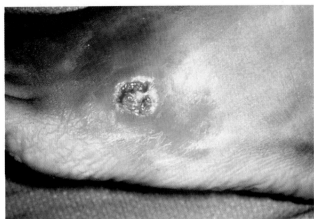

A

B

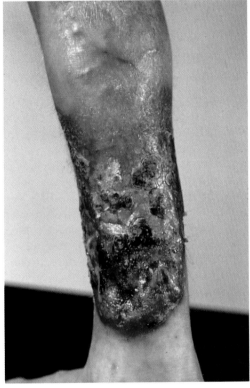
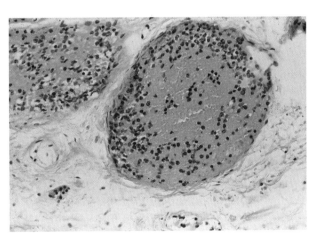

C

D

FIG. 37-4. Clinical pathologic characteristics of leukocyte adhesion deficiency. **A:** Severe gingivitis and periodontitis involving the permanent dentition of a 9-year-old. Gingivae exhibit acute inflammation, proliferation, recession, and periodontal pocket formation. Of teeth remaining, all exhibit severe mobility. Radiographs of this area demonstrate greater than 60% loss of alveolar bone. **B:** A typical necrotic (i.e., nonpustular) cutaneous ulcer of the dorsal foot. *Pseudomonas maltophilia* was isolated from this lesion, which failed to heal despite several weeks of antibiotic therapy. **C:** Dysplastic eschar resulting from a chronic superficial infection and delayed healing of lower-extremity lesion. **D:** Submucosal vessels in an ulcerated and infected region of the ilium, which was surgically resected at 18 months of age. Although numerous neutrophils are present in the dilated veins, only a mild polymorphonuclear (PMN) infiltrate is evident in the extravascular connective tissues (H&E; ×300).

techniques, four severely deficient patients in one series had essentially undetectable expression (≤0.3% of normal) of all three αβ complexes on their neutrophils. Six moderately deficient patients in the same series expressed 2.5% to 6% of all three αβ complexes. Patients of this series with severe phenotype LAD either died in infancy or demonstrated susceptibility to severe, life-threatening systemic infections. In contrast, among the six moderate patients (mean age 27 years, range 18–49 years), life-threatening infections have been infrequently observed. These relationships have been generally observed among recognized LAD kindreds as illustrated

TABLE 37-2. *Clinical features of patients with leukocyte adhesion deficiency among Texas kindreds*

Clinical features	Severe[a]	Moderate[b]
Delayed umbilical cord severance	3/4	0/6
Persistent granulocytosis (15,000–161,000/mm^3)	4/4	6/6
Recurrent infections		
Cutaneous abscess or cellulitis	4/4	6/6
Perirectal cellulitis with sepsis	4/4	0/6
Stomatitis and facial cellulitis	4/4	3/6
Gingivitis and periodontitis	4/4	6/6
Pneumonitis	4/4	2/6
Necrotizing enterocolitis, peritonitis	2/4	0/6
Impaired wound healing	3/4	2/6
Parenteral consanguinity	2/4	3/6
Age range (y)	1–6	11–38

[a]Leukocytes from these four patients had less than 0.3% of the normal amount of Mac-1 on their surfaces.

[b]Leukocytes from these six patients had 2.5–6% of the normal amount of Mac-1 on their surfaces.

by the actuarial survival among 22 severe and 24 moderate LAD patients, respectively, summarized by Fischer et al. (232) (Fig. 37-5). While a precise definition of moderate versus severe phenotype based on clinical features and leukocyte protein expression is not always possible (239,240), this classification has proven generally useful for prognostic purposes and for guiding therapeutic intervention among individual cases (86). Importantly, allogeneic bone marrow transplantation represents a lifesaving and viable option for severe phenotype patients even without the availability of human leukocyte antigen (HLA)-matched donor cells (241,242), whereas the relative longevity of moderately affected patients does not justify this high-risk intervention. As predicted for an autosomal recessive trait, heterozygous carriers of CD18 mutations among all reported LAD kindreds demonstrate intermediate (approximately half normal) levels of β$_2$ protein subunits on their leukocyte surfaces and do not show any distinctive clinical features (86,219,230,232).

Definition of the Molecular Basis of LAD

Biosynthesis and Somatic Cell Hybrid Studies

Early studies showing that all recognized LAD patients were deficient in the expression of all three leukocyte integrins (219) suggested that a primary defect in the common β subunit of Mac-1, LFA-1, and p150,95 accounted for this disease. This possibility was supported by initial biosynthesis studies using available LFA-1α and β MAb. As shown using Epstein-Barr virus transformed B lymphocytes and mitogen-stimulated T-lymphocyte cell lines, healthy individuals synthesize the LFA-1α subunit and the common β subunit and express the LFA-1αβ complex on the cell surface. In contrast, cell lines from patients synthesized an apparently normal LFA-1α subunit precursor, but this precursor did not undergo carbohydrate processing, did not associate in an αβ complex, and was not expressed on the cell surface (226,243). These findings indicate that the LFA-1α sub-

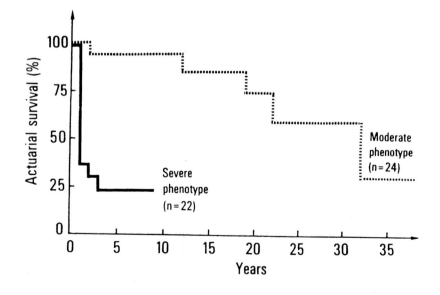

FIG. 37-5. Actuarial survival of patients of leukocyte adhesion deficiency (LAD). Patients who have undergone bone marrow transplantation are not included. Patients were classified as severe or moderate phenotype based on surface expression of LFA-1 (<1% and 5–10% of normal, respectively).

unit precursor is apparently degraded in the absence of a normal β subunit (226). The underlying pathologic role of the β subunit was further implicated in somatic cell complementation studies (244). In hybrids of human and mouse lymphocytes, human LFA-1α and β subunits from healthy controls associate with mouse LFA-1α and β subunits to form interspecies hybrid αβ complexes. In hybrids of patient and mouse lymphocytes, the α_L but not the β₂ subunit was rescued by the formation of interspecies complexes that were expressed on the hybrid cell surfaces. These findings indicate that the LFA-1α subunit in genetically deficient cells is competent for surface expression in the presence of an appropriate mouse β₂ subunit. These complementation protocols also facilitated mapping of the β₂ subunit to chromosome 21, findings in agreement with several lines of evidence that LAD is an autosomal recessive trait (86).

The Molecular Basis of Heterogeneity Among Severe and Moderate Deficiency LAD Kindreds

Heterogeneity among LAD patients was first observed in the extent of β₂ integrin deficiency on leukocyte surfaces, and, as previously discussed, the severity of clinical features and magnitude of functional deficits in vitro are directly related to the degree of protein deficiency (Table 37-2) (86,232). Early observations of the extent of β₂ precursor or mRNA deficiency in some patients correlated to some extent with the severe or moderate clinical phenotype. However, among a large population of reported LAD patients demonstrating apparently normal levels of β₂ subunit mRNA and protein precursors, it was later unclear why some are of the moderate and some of the severe phenotype (243,245–249). An elucidation of diverse mutant CD18 alleles is comprehensively described elsewhere (250).

In molecular analyses of one extended kindred, which included four related patients with moderate phenotype, an aberrantly small β₂ precursor of identical size was identified in each case. Of ten relatives within this kindred, nine were typed as heterozygote carriers and one as a noncarrier on the basis of cell surface expression of LFA-1 (86). All nine heterozygotes showed both a normal and an abnormally small β₂ precursor, and the noncarrier showed only the normal β₂ precursor. Detailed studies of this kindred confirmed that a predominant aberrantly small β₂ precursor is biosynthesized and then degraded in patient cells, prior to transport to the Golgi apparatus (251). However, ¹²⁵I surface labeling of large numbers of patient cells revealed that small amounts of a normally sized LFA-1αβ complex are biosynthesized and transported to the cell surface, findings consistent with a moderate phenotype (86). S1 nuclease protection studies revealed a 90-nucleotide deletion in the β₂ subunit mRNA, and sequence analysis indicated a 90-nt deletion within the I-domain–like region of the β₂ gene.

Analysis of genomic DNA revealed that this 90-bp region is encoded by a single exon in both the patient and normal. However, sequence analysis of patient genomic DNA revealed a single G to C substitution in the sequence of the 5′ splice site, suggesting aberrant RNA splicing. A small amount of normally spliced message, as detected by polymerase chain reaction (PCR) amplification, appears to encode a normal β₂ subunit, which accounts for the low but detectable levels (3–6% of normal) of β₂ integrin expression in these affected patients.

Functional Properties of LAD Leukocytes

Some of the heterogeneity in functional abnormalities among reported LAD patients or kindreds may reflect methodologic differences. However, abnormalities of adherence to substrates and adhesion-dependent functions including chemotaxis, phagocytosis, and aggregation have been observed among all patients studied (86,220,224, 230,231). Chemotaxis appears to be affected because it requires adhesion (224). CR3-dependent binding and phagocytosis of iC3b-opsonized particles are deficient, in agreement with the identity of the CR3 with Mac-1 (57). In addition, since particles opsonized with iC3b are phagocytosed poorly by LAD cells, they fail to trigger the respiratory burst (221,224,234,241,252–255). Abnormalities of antibody-dependent cellular cytotoxicity have also been observed in several patients (50,51,86). In contrast, some adherence-independent cellular functions including f-Met-Leu-Phe receptor-ligand binding and oxidative metabolism or degranulation when mediated by soluble stimuli are generally normal (86,222,224,241,256,257). Intracellular microbicidal activity (e.g., the ability to kill *Staphylococcus aureus*) in most reported patients is relatively normal (86,222,224,225), indicating that receptors other than CR-3 (e.g., FcRγ or CR-1) are sufficient to promote a normal level of phagocytosis and intracellular microbial killing in most instances (73,86,87,224,226). Overall, more profound functional abnormalities have been observed among severely deficient as compared with moderately deficient patients (86).

The predominance of bacterial (as opposed to viral or fungal) infections in patients with LAD implies that the functions of neutrophils or monocytes are more profoundly affected than those of lymphocytes. However, deficits of the LFA-1–dependent functions of lymphocytes have been observed in many patients. Furthermore, in cases where LFA-1–dependent functions are nearly normal, they are inhibited by much lower concentrations of monoclonal antibodies to LFA-1 than for normal cells. T-lymphocyte–mediated killing, proliferative responses, natural killing, and antibody-dependent killing by patients' lymphocytes are deficient compared with that in adult controls (50,51,234,238,241,257–260). In primary mixed lymphocyte cultures, LAD lymphocytes have demonstrated profoundly diminished cytotoxic and proliferative responses and interferon production in several studies (258–261). However, after further stimulation, these responses increase to nearly normal levels (259). This may be due to compensatory mechanisms, perhaps involving an increase in the affinity of the T-lymphocyte antigen receptor, and may account for the relatively normal functions of B and T lymphocytes observed in many cases. Delayed cutaneous hypersensitivity reactions are normal in most patients tested, and most individuals demonstrate normal specific antibody synthesis (86,222,232,256). However, T-lymphocyte–dependent antibody responses *in vivo* (for example, to repeated vaccination with tetanus, diphtheria toxoids, and polio virus) are impaired, and antibody production *in vivo* or *in vitro* in response to influenza virus was found to be abnormal in one patient (262). Thus, responses of lymphocytes *in vivo* may be found deficient in only some of the patients whose β_2 subunit mutation is particularly deleterious to the expression of LFA-1.

Functional deficits of LAD neutrophils and monocytes (and other leukocyte cell types) are related in part to impaired mobilization of Mac-1 and p150,95 from intracellular granular pools to the cell surface and/or impaired qualitative activation of these surface receptors (as well as LFA-1 and $\alpha_d\beta_2$) in response to inflammatory mediators (86). A three- to tenfold increase in Mac-1 and p150,95 surface expression accompanies the hyperadherence, aggregation, and/or chemotactic responses of normal granulocytes to f-Met-Leu-Phe and/or phorbol esters (18,21,22). In contrast, little or no increase of these surface molecules and no enhancement of adhesion or motility on artificial substrates as well as impaired homotypic aggregation or heterotypic adhesion to platelets (263) are characteristic of LAD neutrophils exposed to these chemotactic factors (18,86,226). In contrast to these findings, several adhesion or ligand-independent functions of LAD cells are normally elicited by chemotactic factors or phorbol esters, including cell bipolarization (224), complement receptor type-1 (CR-1) upregulation (86,224), L-selectin downregulation (264), specific granule release (86,224), superoxide production (86), and actin polymerization (265).

As illustrated by *in vitro* studies of LAD cells, β_2 integrins potentiate leukocyte effector functions in the presence of inflammatory mediators, especially under conditions of CD18-dependent adhesion or ligand engagement. For example, whereas stimulation of normal PMNs with inflammatory mediators markedly recruits or augments Fc and CR-1 receptor-mediated ingestion, LAD neutrophils fail to recruit phagocytic functions in response to phorbol esters, cytokines, or RGD-containing ligands (134). Studies by Nathan et al. (70) demonstrated that LAD cells, unlike normal cells, failed to elaborate hydrogen peroxide in response to

TNF-α exposure while incubated on extracellular matrix protein substrates (fibronectin, vitronectin, fibrinogen, thrombospondin); similar results (i.e., an attenuated respiratory burst) were observed with normal neutrophils preincubated with anti-CD18 MAb when studied under the same conditions. Shappell et al. (68) extended these observations to show that chemotactically stimulated LAD neutrophils fail to secrete hydrogen peroxide (unlike that of normal neutrophils) when incubated on human umbilical vein endothelial cells or the artificial Mac-1–dependent adherence substrate KLH. Such results indicate that Mac-1 or other β_2 integrins can potentiate the neutrophil (or monocyte) respiratory burst under conditions of inflammatory mediator-driven and β_2 integrin–dependent hyperadherence. As stimulated surface expression of Mac-1 and enhanced adherence of neutrophils to endothelium or extracellular matrix proteins are likely a general response of activated neutrophils (and other leukocytes) *in vivo,* these observations are relevant to pathologic inflammatory events in which cytotoxic leukocyte effector functions are presumably amplified via CD11/CD18-dependent adhesion to biologic substrates.

Further studies of LAD PMNs by Graham et al. (128) demonstrated the capacity of Mac-1 (CR-3) to transduce signals related to cytoskeletal reorganization, a general requirement for diverse functions of phagocytic cells. These involved comparative evaluations of the tyrosine phosphorylation of paxillin, a microfilament-associated vinculin-binding protein previously shown to be tyrosine phosphorylated in fibroblasts at sites of focal contacts with integrin substrates. Upon exposure to inflammatory mediators (PMA, f-Met-Leu-Phe, TNF-α) in suspension, or in response to adhesion to immune complexes or extracellular matrix proteins induced by phorbal esters, LAD neutrophils failed to demonstrate paxillin tyrosine phosphorylation, as was consistently demonstrated with normal leukocytes under these experimental conditions. Collectively, these studies imply that normal granulocyte hyperadherence, aggregation, and adhesion-primed cytotoxic functions *in vivo* are facilitated by an increased surface expression and/or functional activation of Mac-1 and p150,95 in response to inflammatory mediators. The profound inability of LAD granulocytes to localize and function normally in inflamed tissues appears to reflect (a) impaired hyperadherence to and emigration through vascular endothelium and/or extravascular substrates normally mediated by upregulated or activated Mac-1 and p150,95 (and probably other β_2 integrins), and (b) impaired signal transduction events promoting or regulating diverse extracellular functions including those contributing to cytotoxicity. Studies documenting deficient CD18-dependent adhesion of LAD granulocytes and monocytes to endothelial cells *in vitro* and *in vivo* are described below.

Applications of LAD Cells to Validate a Multistep Dynamic Model of Leukocyte-Endothelial Adherence Interactions

Leukocyte–Endothelial Cell Interactions

Three families of adhesion molecules appear to be involved in neutrophil or monocyte–endothelial cell adhesion including the β_2 integrins, members of the immunoglobulin gene family, and the selectin gene family (266–268) (Fig. 37-6). The physiologic interactions of blood leukocytes with vascular endothelium involves a division of labor with respect to families of adhesion molecules and their counterreceptors. L-selectin and P-selectin may be involved in the process of neutrophil margination (or vascular rolling equivalent) rather than emigration. In contrast, the leukocyte integrins (LFA-1 and Mac-1) and ICAM-1 would appear to be critical to extravasation at inflammatory sites. Histopathologic and clinical observations in LAD patients are totally consistent with these possibilities. LAD neutrophils fail to emigrate into most inflamed tissues despite their capacity to mediate normal adherence to endothelium *in vitro* via L-selectin and E-selectin (264). Moreover, they demonstrate normal endothelial margination or vascular rolling under conditions of sheer stress *in vitro* (269), and they demarginate normally in response to the systemic administration of epinephrine, a process apparently not dependent on β_2 integrins (86,219,270). The capacity of LAD lymphocytes and monocytes (as opposed to neutrophils) to migrate into inflamed tissues appears to reflect in part the expression of very late activation antigen-4 (VLA-4) on the former and not the latter cell type, in turn facilitating adhesive interactions of lymphocytes and eosinophils with VCAM-1. Further confirmation of these emerging concepts of leukocyte-endothelial interactions is provided by studies in other clinical models characterized by defective expression or function of neutrophil adherence molecules and associated inflammatory deficits and by experimental applications of monoclonal antibodies directed at leukocyte or endothelial adherence proteins in animal models of acute or chronic inflammation (discussed below).

An important role of the CD11/CD18 complex of glycoproteins in leukocyte-endothelial adhesion interactions *in vivo* was initially suggested by observations that LAD neutrophils and monocytes fail to infiltrate inflamed tissues despite the occurrence of profound blood granulocytosis in affected patients (86,219). Experimental applications of β_2 integrin subunit MAb in *in vitro* assays of neutrophil or monocyte adhesion to endothelial cell monolayers and in animal models of inflammation *in vivo* have convincingly confirmed this hypothesis. These findings and concepts based on the LAD model have facilitated a variety of investigations revealing several distinct, and yet integrated, adhesion receptor–ligand pairs involved in the process of transendothelial migration *in vitro* or emigration by peripheral blood leukocytes *in vivo* (231,271).

Transendothelial migration of neutrophils can be induced *in vitro* under two general conditions: the establishment of a chemotactic gradient across the endothelial monolayer (272) and the stimulation of the endothelial monolayer with LPS or cytokines such as IL-1 or TNF-α (67,151,271,273,274). Under both conditions, migration requires β_2 integrins since anti-CD18 MAbs almost completely block migration, and, more convincingly, LAD

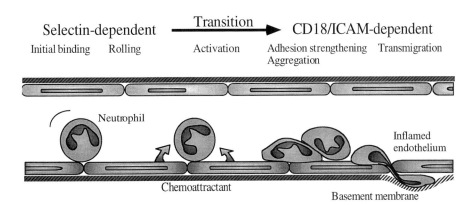

FIG. 37-6. A dynamic model for neutrophil interaction with inflamed endothelium. Endothelial cells adjacent to a site of inflammation are stimulated by cytokines, such as tumor necrosis factor (TNF) and interleukin-1 (IL-1), to synthesize intracellular adhesion molecule-1 (ICAM-1) and E-selectin adhesion molecules. These inducible adhesion molecules provide position-specific information for the circulating neutrophils. L-selectin on the neutrophil and E-selectin on the endothelium mediate initial capture and rolling of neutrophils. The transiently bound neutrophil is exposed to chemotactic factors generated by the endothelial cells or at the site of inflammation, inducing a rapid transition in neutrophil morphology and adhesiveness. Neutrophil crawling and transendothelial migration are largely mediated by the β_2 integrins.

neutrophils fail to demonstrate transendothelial migration when assessed in the absence of shear stress (67,151,271). Additional studies using monoclonal antibodies to LFA-1 and Mac-1 indicate that these heterodimers cooperate in this process via adhesion interactions with ICAM-1 (67,271). ICAM-1 appears to be obligatory for transendothelial migration *in vitro,* as anti–ICAM-1 MAbs are almost completely inhibitory in the presence or absence of shear stress conditions (271). In contrast, adhesion receptor–ligand pairs other than β_2 integrins and ICAM-1 do not appear to induce transendothelial migration independently. MAbs against neutrophil L-selectin produce little inhibition of migration (264).

β_2 Integrins and ICAM-1 in Pharmacologic and Genetic Mouse Models of Inflammation

Rationale for Antiadhesion Strategies in Inflammatory Disorders

The localization and function of neutrophils and mononuclear leukocytes normally provide for immunologic host defense and repair of tissues. However, as evidenced by a large body of experimental data, these cells can mediate microvascular and tissue injury in response to a variety of inflammatory mediators generated by diverse pathogenic mechanisms (275–279). Intercellular adhesion is critical to these proinflammatory injurious events, not only because the localization and infiltration of leukocytes in inflamed tissues is determined by specific interactions of adhesion molecules and their counterreceptors, but also because leukocyte adhesion to biologic substrates (i.e., other cells or matrix proteins) appears to amplify cytotoxic functions (e.g., oxidative or secretory processes) in the presence of proinflammatory mediators (68,280–282) via molecular mechanisms described above. Leukocyte-mediated vascular and tissue injury has been defined in a number of clinical entities in which the induction of leukocyte or endothelial adhesion mechanisms has been directly demonstrated (275–277, 283–290) or inferred (see ref. 277 for a review). Among these entities are adult respiratory distress syndrome (ARDS); asthma; immune complex or complement-mediated lung injury; diverse ischemia-reperfusion or reoxygenation states (including hypovolemic shock, with multiple organ injury); allograft rejection; chronic inflammatory states such as rheumatoid arthritis, systemic lupus erythematosus (SLE), or inflammatory skin disorders; and acute suppurative meningitis. The rationale for antiadhesion strategies in the clinical management of these disorders is based on observations of the inhibitory effects of anti-β_2 integrin MAb with respect to several adhesion functions of leukocytes *in vitro*, which are proposed to facilitate multiple pathogenic mechanisms contributing to inflammatory injury *in vivo*. These functions include heterotypic interactions with endothelial cells, antigen presenting cells, or other cells expressing ligands for β_2 integrins, which are thought to mediate the localization, cytotoxic and/or co-stimulatory functions of neutrophils, monocytes, and lymphocytes, as well as homotypic interactions of these cells, which may in turn facilitate leukocyte emboli and vascular occlusion (discussed above).

In Vivo β_2 or ICAM-1 Monoclonal Antibody Protection Protocols

Applications of monoclonal antibodies recognizing leukocyte integrins or their ligands in experimental animals have emphasized the physiologic importance of these adhesion receptors and have provided some insights concerning their mechanisms of action *in vivo*. While they convincingly support the concept that transendothelial migration is CD18- and ICAM-1–dependent (as suggested by *in vitro* studies discussed above), they also indicate that β_2 integrins cooperate with other leukocyte adhesion proteins (e.g., VLA-4, L-selectin, etc.) in this process. Moreover, these studies also indicate that adherence-independent mechanisms play an important role in inflammatory cell sequestration in selected tissues and/or in response to specific inflammatory stimuli.

Several monoclonal antibodies capable of binding to functional epitopes of β_2 integrin subunits have been shown to be potent inhibitors of neutrophil or monocyte localization or emigration in response to experimental inflammatory stimuli (see refs. 250,277,291 for reviews). Systemically administered anti-CD18 MAbs profoundly inhibit (>90%) neutrophil emigration elicited by chemotactic factors (292) or endotoxin (293) in rabbit skin. In a similar fashion, the intravenous administration of anti-CD11b MAb in mice profoundly inhibits the recruitment of PMNs and monocytes into thioglycolate-elicited peritoneal exudate (294) or the T-lymphocyte–dependent recruitment of myelomonocytic cells at cutaneous sites of antigen challenge in sensitized animals (295). Anti-CD18 MAbs have been reported to reduce PMN/monocyte emigration and inflammatory injury associated with experimental bacterial meningitis in rabbits (296). In one additional study, MAbs directed at CD18 as well as CD11a and ICAM-1 significantly (but not totally) inhibited the accumulation of PMNs in a lapine model of acute lung injury (297). These findings are consistent with histopathologic observations in LAD patients (56,86) and support the concept based on the LAD model that transendothelial migration is CD11/CD18 and ICAM-1 dependent.

MAbs directed at β_2 integrin subunits in animal models of ischemia-reperfusion injury substantially reduce neutrophil localization, microvascular permeability, and tissue injury. Protective effects in such models were anticipated, since inflammatory mediators capable of upregulating Mac-1 on neutrophils/monocytes and ICAM-1 on vascular endothelial cells are elaborated in ischemic tissues (298). As shown in several independent studies, anti-CD11/CD18 MAbs (a) diminish leukocyte sequestration and vascular permeability in models of intestinal ischemia (299), (b) attenuate leukocyte sequestration and/or infarct size and myocardial dysfunction in dog (300,301) or rabbit (302,303), (c) prevent or limit tissue injury and edema in transected rabbit ear (304), and (d) diminish hepatic and gastrointestinal or other organ injury and mortality in lapine or primate models of hemorrhagic shock and resuscitation (305,306).

More recent studies in lapine models of lung injury or infection emphasize a role for CD18-independent mechanisms of neutrophil emigration into pulmonary air spaces (307). Pulmonary recruitment by *Streptococcus pneumoniae* organisms, in contrast to LPS or *Escherichia coli* organisms or PMA, is only minimally influenced by anti-CD18 MAb (60.3), even though recruitment into inflamed peritoneum is almost totally abolished by this MAb in the same experimental animals. Consistent with these findings, autopsy studies in a LAD patient who died with gram-negative pneumonia demonstrated vigorous neutrophil recruitment into pulmonary air spaces as opposed to impaired localization in several other inflamed tissues (56). These observations suggest that neutrophil emigration into inflamed lung (and possibly other tissues) may be stimulus specific and that mechanisms of inflammatory emigration may be tissue specific. The relative participation of adhesion receptor–ligand pairs in various tissues as well as influences of locally elaborated cytokines may play a role in determining these specificities.

Results of still other studies employing monoclonal antibodies suggest that CD18-independent and possibly adhesion-independent mechanisms account for pulmonary localization of neutrophils (308). For example, systemic administration of chemotactic factors in rabbits promotes a rapid (<30 minutes) sequestration of neutrophils in the pulmonary vasculature and, as a consequence, neutropenia. This localization was not influenced by pretreatment of experimental animals with the anti-CD11b MAb 60.3, a reagent previously shown to totally inhibit neutrophil emigration elicited by intradermal administration of chemotactic factors (292). Evidence exists that this CD18-independent phenomenon is related to mechanical trapping. The average size of circulating neutrophils is >7.5 µM in diameter as compared to the average of 5.5 µM in capillaries in vascular beds such as in lungs (309). Thus, neutrophils must deform to pass through capillaries, a process influenced by rheologic factors as well as intrinsic properties of neutrophils. Worthen et al. (309) have shown that passage of neutrophils through 5-µM-diameter micropore filters is markedly reduced by chemotactic factors, a process independent of cell adhesiveness but directly related to the

stiffness of the cells (i.e., a lack of deformability). These findings suggest that the rapid pulmonary localization of neutrophils in response to intravenously administered chemotactic factors results from mechanical trapping of nondeformable neutrophils rather than CD18-dependent adhesion. This appears to be true even though Mac-1 on circulating blood neutrophils is significantly upregulated in this experimental setting (308).

As also observed for cytokine- and LPS-stimulated endothelial cells *in vitro,* endothelial cells and other mesenchymal or epithelial cells of inflamed tissues demonstrate high levels of expression of ICAM-1 as compared to low but detectable levels on cells of uninflamed tissues or unstimulated cells in culture (44,69,143,284,290, 310–313). Vejlsgaard et al. (310) documented induction of ICAM-1 on vascular endothelial cells and keratinocytes in skin biopsy specimens of sensitive individuals in whom haptens were applied for allergic contact dermatitis testing. ICAM-1 expression on keratinocytes was induced as early as 4 to 24 hours, concurrent with a heavy mononuclear cell dermal infiltrate, findings suggesting that ICAM-1 plays a role in facilitating either antigen presentation or leukocyte infiltration (44). Adams et al. (311) further demonstrated that ICAM-1 is markedly induced on bile ducts, endothelium, and perivenular hepatocytes in liver allografts of patients during acute rejection. Patients with stable grafts demonstrated the same low levels of ICAM-1 on these cells as seen on donor grafts, and among patients with resolving rejection, ICAM-1 expression was greatly reduced after high-dose corticosteroid therapy. These investigators proposed that induction of ICAM-1 on hepatic tissues may play an important role in the initiation of the inflammatory response of rejection and in determining which cells are targets of LFA-1–dependent immune damage by lymphocytes and neutrophils (311).

These clinicopathologic findings in human patients have potentially important therapeutic implications. They suggest that MAb or other reagents such as antisense oligonucleotides (314) designed to inhibit ICAM-1–dependent adhesion reactions may prevent or attenuate inflammatory injury in a number of clinical disorders. Evidence for this possibility has been demonstrated in recent studies employing systemically administered ICAM-1 MAb in animal models (69,297,315). In a primate model of allergic asthma, Wegner et al. (69) demonstrated that the anti–ICAM-1 MAb R6.5 significantly diminishes eosinophil recruitment, bronchial mucosal injury, and airway hyperresponsiveness to inhaled ascaris antigen. These inhibitory results were consistent with additional findings that ICAM-1 MAb partially inhibits (and anti-CD18 MAb totally inhibits) eosinophil adherence to endothelial cells *in vitro,* and that ICAM-1 is markedly upregulated by IL-1β, TNF-α, and TNF-α on bronchial epithelial cells *in vitro,* and is expressed on inflamed but not normal bronchial epithelium *in vivo.*

Similar findings have been reported by Richards et al. (313) in a rodent model of antigen-induced lung injury.

The potential efficacy of anti–ICAM-1 MAb in preventing or therapeutically reversing renal allograft rejection has been studied by Cosimi et al. (315) in cynomolgous monkeys. "Prophylactic" ICAM-1 MAb (0.5–2.0 mg/kg IV for 12 days beginning 48 hours prior to allograft procedures) preserved normal renal function and markedly prolonged survival in test as compared to untreated control animals. "Therapeutic" ICAM-1 MAb given for 10 days after the onset of rejection normalized renal function in most animals and also prolonged survival. Intense R6.5 MAb deposition was evident on grafts (but not other tissues), especially on arterioles, capillaries, and glomeruli of untreated animals. Notable in the R6.5 MAb "prophylactic" group was the almost complete lack of vascular rejection during treatment and the lack of progression of vascular rejection in the therapeutic group. In the latter group, recovery of renal function was accompanied by decreased interstitial edema and hemorrhage (evidence of peritubular injury) but little or no decrease in mononuclear infiltrates in grafts. These findings suggest that blockade of T-lymphocyte–mediated vascular injury may be a major mechanism of action of the R6.5 MAb and emphasize that ICAM-1 is a critical molecule in the pathogenesis of allograft rejection.

Genetic Models of β₂ Integrins or ICAM-1 Deficiency

The emergence of gene targeting technologies has facilitated the creation of mutant mouse models to test diverse hypotheses concerning the physiologic and pathologic roles of β_2 integrins and ICAM-1 (316–318). By preparing an insertion mutation in the murine CD18 gene, Wilson et al. (316) produced a hypomorphic rather than null allele due to low expression from a cryptic promoter. Resulting homozygous mutant mice demonstrated mild granulocytosis, 2% to 16% of normal levels of CD18 on blood leukocytes, impaired inflammatory responses to chemical peritonitis, and delayed rejection of cardiac transplants. Genetically ICAM-1–deficient mice prepared by gene targeting demonstrate abnormalities of neutrophil inflammatory responses, diminished contact hypersensitivity, and defective allogenic T-cell responses (317–319). These mutant mice are resistant to lethal effects of endotoxin, an observation that appears causally related to a diminution in critical leukocyte-endothelial interactions (317). Overall, the inflammatory and immunologic defects observed in these murine models are consistent with findings in studies of the human LAD model.

Recently, mice with targeted selected deficiency of LFA-1 alone (320,321) or of Mac-1 alone (74,322) have been generated. Surprisingly, neutrophil trafficking to thioglycollate-inflamed peritoneum was not deficient in the Mac-1–deficient animals (74,322). On the contrary, at late time points (5–10 hours), the number of neutrophils in the inflamed peritoneum was markedly enhanced in the Mac-1–deficient mice (74). This enhancement was shown to be due to a defect in neutrophil apoptosis, suggesting that Mac-1 plays a critical role in eliminating extravasated neutrophils (74). The Mac-1–deficient neutrophils showed a severe defect in oxidative burst, phagocytosis, degranulation, and adhesion to fibrinogen-coated disks (74,322). Trafficking of the Mac-1 deficient neutrophils into the inflamed peritoneum could be blocked with an anti–LFA-1 MAb (322). In agreement with these findings, neutrophils from LFA-1–deficient mice showed impaired migration into the inflamed peritoneum (320), although migration into an LPS-inflamed skin site was unimpaired (321). Not surprisingly, the LFA-1–deficient mice showed more defects in lymphocyte-mediated functions, including proliferation in mixed lymphocyte response and in response to mitogen (320,321). The LFA-1–deficient mice were defective in rejecting immunogenic tumors (320,321). However, there were some discrepancies reported for CTL activity, NK activity, and delayed-type hypersensitivity response in independently derived LFA-1–deficient mouse lines (320,321). Unexpectedly, mice deficient in either Mac-1 or in ICAM-1 are prone to spontaneous obesity, compared to wild-type mice (323). These observations suggest that leukocytes may play a role in regulating excess body fat deposition.

Applications of CD18 and ICAM-1–deficient mice in specific disease models have provided further evidence for the role of β_2 integrins in inflammatory pathology. Results of these studies are largely consistent with those employing anti–β_2 integrin or ICAM-1 blocking MAb in animal models of inflammation (discussed above). ICAM-1– and/or CD18-deficient mice are less susceptible to ischemia-reperfusion injury in models of cerebral vascular occlusion (324,325), acute tubular necrosis (326), or hepatic leukostasis and hypoxic stress (327). ICAM-1–deficient mice also demonstrate reduced susceptibility to collagen-induced arthritis (328). A reduced incidence of arthritis in heterozygous or homozygous mutant mice is not due to a lack of immunity to type II collagen, since these mice demonstrate similar levels of anti–type II collagen IgG compared to wild-type mice, and positive delayed-type hypersensitivity reactions to type II collagen. These results suggest that naturally occurring genetic variations in the expression of ICAM-1 or related inflammatory cell adhesion molecules may influence susceptibility to rheumatoid arthritis disease in humans, and they support the concept that pharmacologic antagonists of ICAM-1 expression may be of therapeutic value. ICAM-1 deficiency also protects against a rapidly fatal form of autoimmune disease (vasculitis and glomerulonephritis) similar to severe SLE in humans, as observed in MRL/MpJ-Fas^{lpr} mice (329). Crossed ICAM-1–deficient MRL/MpJ-Fas^{lpr} (ICAM-1/Fas^{lpr}) mice demonstrate increased survival associated with delayed elevations of blood urea nitrogen, a reduction of glomerular pathology, and a significant reduction in vasculitis in kidney, lung, skin, and salivary glands when compared to *Fas*^lpr animals.

Based on considerable evidence for an inflammatory component in atherosclerosis, including the enhanced expression of endothelial cell adhesion molecules, cytokines, and growth factors, Nageh et al. (330) applied CD18, ICAM-1, or double CD18/ICAM-1 mutant mice to test the hypothesis that deficient expression of these inflammatory cell adhesion determinants would reduce susceptibility to atherosclerosis. Among C57BL/6 mice fed a high-fat diet, a 50% to 70% reduction in atherosclerotic fatty streaks was observed in each mutant strain compared to background. These findings suggest that genetic variation at these foci could influence susceptibility to atherosclerosis in humans and that pharmacologic reduction of the expression or function of these cell adhesion molecules may be protective.

Further applications of these mutant mice in models of lung inflammation have demonstrated somewhat disparate findings concerning the role of β₂ integrins/ICAM-1. In a model of ovalbumin-induced pulmonary eosinophilia, Gonzalo et al. (331) showed that mice deficient in ICAM-1 and VCAM-1 failed to develop pulmonary eosinophilic infiltrates. In a model of endotoxin-induced lung injury, Kumasaka et al. (314) examined neutrophil pulmonary emigration in ICAM-1–deficient mice and wild-type mice administered antisense ICAM-1 oligonucleotides or anti–ICAM-1 MAb. Neutrophil emigration into alveolar air spaces was significantly inhibited by ICAM-1–directed MAb or antisense probes, but no attenuation was observed in the ICAM-1 mutant animals. These findings suggest that mutant mice use ICAM-1–independent mechanisms including alternative adhesion pathways for recruiting neutrophils into endotoxin injured lungs. In another study, neutrophil accumulation in lungs of ICAM-1 versus wild-type mice administered intrapulmonary *Pseudomonas aeruginosa* showed similar results (332). Whereas anti-CD11a, anti-CD11b, or anti–ICAM-1 MAb potently inhibited neutrophil accumulation after infection, pulmonary neutrophilia was normal in infected mutant animals. In still another report, Bullard et al. (333) showed that P-selectin/ICAM-1 double mutant mice demonstrate completely absent neutrophil emigration into peritoneum of animals experimentally infected with *S. pneumoniae*, but normal neutrophil accumulation in pulmonary alveoli following *S. pneumoniae*–induced pneumonitis. These findings provide evidence for ICAM-1 and P-selectin–independent mechanisms in the inflammatory response of lung.

FUTURE DIRECTIONS

The field of leukocyte adhesion molecules has reached a mature phase, where many (but certainly not all) of the adhesion receptors and their ligand interactions have been defined. Over the last several years, there have been significant advances in elucidating the specific roles of adhesion receptors through the generation of gene-targeted knockout animals. The first glimpse into the structural basis of adhesion interactions has been provided by x-ray crystallography of ICAM-2 and of the I domains of LFA-1 and Mac-1. It is also appreciated that the adhesion molecules, and not just cellular Velcro, can provide signals to the cell that can influence cell activation, migration, and even life and death through the process of apoptosis. The advances in these and other areas will certainly continue, as adhesion receptor–deficient animals are tested in a wider range of disease-relevant models, as structural data for other receptors and perhaps even for an integrin αβ heterodimer become available, as signal cascades become elucidated, and as new insights and discoveries are made that direct the field into unexpected and unexplored territory. The ultimate question for the future is whether this wealth of knowledge can be harnessed to develop therapeutics that can be used to safely and effectively treat a wide range of inflammatory and immunologic diseases. Monoclonal antibody-based therapeutics may lead the way into the clinic, but a vast array of recombinant biologics, antisense oligonucleotides, and small molecule compounds that inhibit or influence leukocyte adhesion are not far behind. The next 5 years should be an exciting period for the field of leukocyte cell adhesion.

REFERENCES

1. Tamkun JW, DeSimone DW, Fonda D, et al. Structure of integrin, a glycoprotein involved in the transmembrane linkage between fibronectin and actin. *Cell* 1986;46:271–282.
2. Krensky AM, Sanchez-Madrid F, Robbins E, Nagy J, Springer TA, Burakoff SJ. The functional significance, distribution, and structure of LFA-1, LFA-2, and LFA-3: cell surface antigens associated with CTL-target interactions. *J Immunol* 1983;131:611–616.
3. Kurzinger K, Reynolds T, Germain RN, Davignon D, Martz E, Springer TA. A novel lymphocyte function-associated antigen (LFA-1): cellular distribution, quantitative expression, and structure. *J Immunol* 1981;127:596–602.
4. Eddy A, Newman SL, Cosio F, LeBien T, Michael A. The distribution of the CR3 receptor on human cells and tissue as revealed by a monoclonal antibody. *Clin Immunol Immunopathol* 1984;31:371–389.
5. Ho MK, Springer TA. Mac-1 antigen: quantitative expression in macrophage populations and tissues, and immunofluorescent localization in spleen. *J Immunol* 1982;128:2281–2286.
6. Todd RF III, Nadler LM, Schlossman SF. Antigens on human monocytes identified by monoclonal antibodies. *J Immunol* 1981;126:1435–1442.
7. de la Hera A, Alvarez-Mon M, Sanchez-Madrid F, Martinez AC, Durantez A. Co-expression of MAC-1 and p150,95 on CD5⁺ B cells. Structural and functional characterization in a human chronic lymphocytic leukemia. *Eur J Immunol* 1988;18:1131–1134.
8. McFarland HI, Nahill SR, Maciaszek JW, Welsh RM. CD11b (Mac-1): a marker for CD8⁺ cytotoxic T cell activation and memory in virus infection. *J Immunol* 1992;149:1326–1333.
9. Hoshino T, Yamada A, Honda J, et al. Tissue-specific distribution and age-dependent increase of human CD11b⁺ T cells. *J Immunol* 1993;151:2237–2246.
10. Hogg N, Takacs L, Palmer DG, Selvendran Y, Allen C. The p150,95 molecule is a marker of human mononuclear phagocytes: comparison

with expression of class II molecules. *Eur J Immunol* 1986;16: 240–248.

11. Postigo AA, Corbí AL, Sánchez-Madrid F, De Landázuri MO. Regulated expression and function of CD11c/CD18 integrin on human B lymphocytes. Relation between attachment to fibrinogen and triggering of proliferation through CD11c/CD18. *J Exp Med* 1991;174: 1313–1322.

12. MacDonald SM, Pulford K, Falini B, Micklem K, Mason DY. A monoclonal antibody recognizing the p150/95 leucocyte differentiation antigen. *Immunology* 1986;59:427–431.

13. Schwarting R, Stein H, Wang CY. The monoclonal antibodies anti S-HCL 1 (anti Leu 14) and anti S-HCL 3 (anti Leu M5) allow the diagnosis of hairy cell leukemia. *Blood* 1985;65:974–983.

14. Van der Vieren M, Le Trong H, Wood CL, et al. A novel leukointegrin, alpha d beta 2, binds preferentially to ICAM-3. *Immunity* 1995;3: 683–690.

15. Sanchez-Madrid F, Nagy J, Robbins E, Simon P, Springer TA. A human leukocyte differentiation antigen family with distinct alpha subunits and a common beta subunit: the lymphocyte function-associated antigen (LFA-1), the C3bi complement receptor (OKM1/Mac-1), and the p150,95 molecule. *J Exp Med* 1983;158:1785–1803.

16. Miller LJ, Springer TA. Biosynthesis and glycosylation of p150,95 and related leukocyte adhesion proteins. *J Immunol* 1987;139: 842–847.

17. Sastre L, Kishimoto TK, Gee C, Roberts T, Springer TA. The mouse leukocyte adhesion proteins Mac-1 and LFA-1: studies on mRNA translation and protein glycosylation with emphasis on Mac-1. *J Immunol* 1986;137:1060–1065.

18. Todd RFI, Arnaout MA, Rosin RE, Crowley CA, Peters WA, Babior BM. Subcellular localization of the large subunit of Mo1 (Mo1 alpha; formerly gp 110), a surface glycoprotein associated with neutrophil adhesion. *J Clin Invest* 1984;74:1280–1290.

19. Miller LJ, Bainton DF, Borregaard N, Springer TA. Stimulated mobilization of monocyte Mac-1 and p150,95 adhesion proteins from an intracellular vesicular compartment to the cell surface. *J Clin Invest* 1987;80:535–544.

20. Bainton DF, Miller LJ, Kishimoto TK, Springer TA. Leukocyte adhesion receptors are stored in peroxidase-negative granules of human neutrophils. *J Exp Med* 1987;166:1641–1653.

21. Borregaard N, Miller LJ, Springer TA. Chemoattractant-regulated fusion of a novel, mobilizable intracellular compartment with the plasma membrane in human neutrophils. *Science* 1987;237: 1204–1206.

22. Jones DH, Anderson DC, Burr BL, et al. Quantitation of intracellular Mac-1 (CD11b/CD18) pools in human neutrophils. *J Leukoc Biol* 1988;44:535–544.

23. Jones DH, Schmalstieg FC, Dempsey K, et al. Subcellular distribution and mobilization of MAC-1 (CD11b/CD18) in neonatal neutrophils. *Blood* 1990;75:488–498.

24. Kishimoto TK, O'Connor K, Lee A, Roberts TM, Springer TA. Cloning of the beta subunit of the leukocyte adhesion proteins: homology to an extracellular matrix receptor defines a novel supergene family. *Cell* 1987;48:681–690.

25. Law SKA, Gagnon J, Hildreth JEK, Wells CE, Willis AC, Wong AJ. The primary structure of the beta subunit of the cell surface adhesion glycoproteins LFA-1, CR3 and p150,95 and its relationship to the fibronectin receptor. *EMBO J* 1987;6:915–919.

26. Corbi AL, Larson RS, Kishimoto TK, Springer TA, Morton CC. Chromosomal location of the genes encoding the leukocyte adhesion receptors LFA-1, Mac-1 and p150,95. Identification of a gene cluster involved in cell adhesion. *J Exp Med* 1988;167:1597–1607.

27. Weitzman JB, Wells CE, Wright AH, Clark PA, Law SKA. The gene organisation of the human β2 integrin subunit (CD18). *FEBS Lett* 1991;294:97–103.

28. Fitzgerald LA, Steiner B, Rall SC Jr, Lo S, Phillips DR. Protein sequence of endothelial glycoprotein IIIa derived from a cDNA clone. Identity with platelet glycoprotein IIIa and similarity to "integrin." *J Biol Chem* 1987;262:3936–3939.

29. Larson RS, Corbi AL, Berman L, Springer TA. Primary structure of the LFA-1 alpha subunit: an integrin with an embedded domain defining a protein superfamily. *J Cell Biol* 1989;108:703–712.

30. Corbi AL, Kishimoto TK, Miller LJ, Springer TA. The human leukocyte adhesion glycoprotein Mac-1 (Complement receptor type 3, CD11b) alpha subunit: cloning, primary structure, and relation to the integrins, von Willebrand factor and factor B. *J Biol Chem* 1988;263: 12403–12411.

31. Pytela R. Amino acid sequence of the murine Mac-1 alpha chain reveals homology with the integrin family and an additional domain related to von Willebrand factor. *EMBO J* 1988;7:1371–1378.

32. Arnaout MA, Gupta SK, Pierce MW, Tenen DG. Amino acid sequence of the alpha subunit of human leukocyte adhesion receptor Mo1 (complement receptor type 3). *J Cell Biol* 1988;106:2153–2158.

33. Corbi AL, Miller LJ, O'Connor K, Larson RS, Springer TA. cDNA cloning and complete primary structure of the alpha subunit of a leukocyte adhesion glycoprotein, p150,95. *EMBO J* 1987;6: 4023–4028.

34. Dustin ML, Springer TA. Role of lymphocyte adhesion receptors in transient interactions and cell locomotion. *Annu Rev Immunol* 1991;9: 27–66.

35. Staunton DE, Dustin ML, Erickson HP, Springer TA. The LFA-1 and rhinovirus binding sites of ICAM-1 and arrangement of its Ig-like domains. *Cell* 1990;61:243–253.

36. Diamond MS, Garcia-Aguilar J, Bickford JK, Corbi AL, Springer TA. The I domain is a major recognition site on the leukocyte integrin Mac-1 (CD11b/CD18) for four distinct adhesion ligands. *J Cell Biol* 1993;120:1031–1043.

37. Landis RC, McDowall A, Holness CL, Littler AJ, Simmons DL, Hogg N. Involvement of the "I" domain of LFA-1 in selective binding to ligands ICAM-1 and ICAM-3. *J Cell Biol* 1994;126:529–537.

38. Corbi AL, Garcia-Aguilar J, Springer TA. Genomic structure of an integrin alpha subunit, the leukocyte p150,95 molecule. *J Biol Chem* 1990;265:2782–2788.

39. Fleming JC, Pahl HL, Gonzalez DA, Smith TF, Tenen DG. Structural analysis of the CD11b gene and phylogenetic analysis of the alpha-integrin gene family demonstrate remarkable conservation of genomic organization and suggest early diversification during evolution. *J Immunol* 1993;150:480–490.

40. Le Beau MM, Diaz MO, Karin M, Rowley JD. Metallothionein gene cluster is split by chromosome 16 rearrangements in myelomonocytic leukaemia. *Nature* 1985;313:709–711.

41. Springer TA, Dustin ML, Kishimoto TK, Marlin SD. The lymphocyte function-associated LFA-1, CD2, and LFA-3 molecules: cell adhesion receptors of the immune system. *Annu Rev Immunol* 1987;5:223–252.

42. Mentzer SJ, Burakoff SJ, Faller DV. Adhesion of T lymphocytes to human endothelial cells is regulated by the LFA-1 membrane molecule. *J Cell Physiol* 1986;126:285–290.

43. Haskard D, Cavender D, Beatty P, Springer T, Ziff M. T lymphocyte adhesion to endothelial cells: mechanisms demonstrated by anti–LFA-1 monoclonal antibodies. *J Immunol* 1986;137:2901–2906.

44. Dustin ML, Singer KH, Tuck DT, Springer TA. Adhesion of T lymphoblasts to epidermal keratinocytes is regulated by interferon gamma and is mediated by intercellular adhesion molecule-1 (ICAM-1). *J Exp Med* 1988;167:1323–1340.

45. Dustin ML, Springer TA. Lymphocyte function associated antigen-1 (LFA-1) interaction with intercellular adhesion molecule-1 (ICAM-1) is one of at least three mechanisms for lymphocyte adhesion to cultured endothelial cells. *J Cell Biol* 1988;107:321–331.

46. Mentzer SJ, Rothlein R, Springer TA, Faller DV. Intercellular adhesion molecule-1 (ICAM-1) is involved in the cytolytic T lymphocyte interaction with human synovial cells. *J Cell Physiol* 1988;137:173–178.

47. Roos E, Roossien FF. Involvement of leukocyte function-associated antigen-1 (LFA-1) in the invasion of hepatocyte cultures by lymphoma and T-cell hybridoma cells. *J Cell Biol* 1987;105:553–559.

48. Davignon D, Martz E, Reynolds T, Kurzinger K, Springer TA. Monoclonal antibody to a novel lymphocyte function-associated antigen (LFA-1): mechanism of blocking of T lymphocyte-mediated killing and effects on other T and B lymphocyte functions. *J Immunol* 1981; 127:590–595.

49. Sanchez-Madrid F, Krensky AM, Ware CF, et al. Three distinct antigens associated with human T lymphocyte-mediated cytolysis: LFA-1, LFA-2, and LFA-3. *Proc Natl Acad Sci USA* 1982;79:7489–7493.

50. Kohl S, Springer TA, Schmalstieg FC, Loo LS, Anderson DC. Defective natural killer cytotoxicity and polymorphonuclear leukocyte antibody-dependent cellular cytotoxicity in patients with LFA-1/OKM-1 deficiency. *J Immunol* 1984;133:2972–2978.

51. Kohl S, Loo LS, Schmalstieg FS, Anderson DC. The genetic deficiency of leukocyte surface glycoproteins Mac-1, LFA-1, p150,95 in humans is associated with defective antibody dependent cellular cyto-

toxicity *in vitro* and defective protection against herpes simplex virus infection *in vivo*. *J Immunol* 1986;137:1688–1694.

52. Rothlein R, Springer TA. The requirement for lymphocyte function-associated antigen 1 in homotypic leukocyte adhesion stimulated by phorbol ester. *J Exp Med* 1986;163:1132–1149.

53. Patarroyo M, Beatty PG, Fabre JW, Gahmberg CG. Identification of a cell surface protein complex mediating phorbol ester-induced adhesion (binding) among human mononuclear leukocytes. *Scand J Immunol* 1985;22:171–182.

54. Mentzer SJ, Gromkowski SH, Krensky AM, Burakoff SJ, Martz E. LFA-1 membrane molecule in the regulation of homotypic adhesions of human B lymphocytes. *J Immunol* 1985;135:9–11.

55. Hamann A, Westrich DJ, Duijevstijn A, et al. Evidence for an accessory role of LFA-1 in lymphocyte-high endothelium interaction during homing. *J Immunol* 1988;140:693–699.

56. Hawkins HK, Heffelfinger SC, Anderson DC. Leukocyte adhesion deficiency: clinical and postmortem observations. *Pediatr Pathol* 1992;12:119–130.

57. Beller DI, Springer TA, Schreiber RD. Anti–Mac-1 selectively inhibits the mouse and human type three complement receptor. *J Exp Med* 1982;156:1000–1009.

58. Rothlein R, Springer TA. Complement receptor type three-dependent degradation of opsonized erythrocytes by mouse macrophages. *J Immunol* 1985;135:2668–2672.

59. Anderson DC, Miller LJ, Schmalstieg FC, Rothlein R, Springer TA. Contributions of the Mac-1 glycoprotein family to adherence-dependent granulocyte functions: structure-function assessments employing subunit-specific monoclonal antibodies. *J Immunol* 1986;137:15–27.

60. Ramos OF, Kai C, Yefenof E, Klein E. The elevated natural killer sensitivity of targets carrying surface-attached C3 fragments require the availability of the iC3b receptor (CR3) on the effectors. *J Immunol* 1988;140:1239–1243.

61. Mosser DM, Edelson PJ. The mouse macrophage receptor for C3bi (CR3) is a major mechanism in the phagocytosis of *Leishmania promastigotes*. *J Immunol* 1985;135:2785–2789.

62. Mosser DM, Springer TA, Diamond MS. *Leishmania promastigotes* require opsonic complement to bind to the human leukocyte integrin Mac-1 (CD11b/CD18). *J Cell Biol* 1992;116:511–520.

63. Relman D, Tuomanen E, Falkow S, Golenbock DT, Saukkonen K, Wright SD. Recognition of a bacterial adhesion by an integrin: macrophage CR3 (alpha M beta 2, CD11b/CD18) binds filamentous hemagglutinin of *Bordetella pertussis*. *Cell* 1990;61:1375–1382.

64. Bullock WE, Wright SD. Role of the adherence-promoting receptors, CR3, LFA-1 and p150,95, in binding of *Histoplasma capsulatum* by human macrophages. *J Exp Med* 1987;165:195–210.

65. Diamond MS, Alon R, Parkos CA, Quinn MT, Springer TA. Heparin is an adhesive ligand for the leukocyte integrin Mac-1 (CD11b/CD1). *J Cell Biol* 1995;130:1473–1482.

66. Diamond MS, Staunton DE, De Fougerolles AR, et al. ICAM-1 (CD54): a counter-receptor for Mac-1 (CD11b/CD18). *J Cell Biol* 1990;111:3129–3139.

67. Smith CW, Marlin SD, Rothlein R, Toman C, Anderson DC. Cooperative interactions of LFA-1 and Mac-1 with intercellular adhesion molecule-1 in facilitating adherence and transendothelial migration of human neutrophils *in vitro*. *J Clin Invest* 1989;83:2008–2017.

68. Shappell SB, Toman C, Anderson DC, Taylor AA, Entman ML, Smith CW. Mac-1 (CD11b/CD18) mediates adherence-dependent hydrogen peroxide production by human and canine neutrophils. *J Immunol* 1990;144:2702–2711.

69. Wegner CD, Gundel RH, Reilly P, Haynes N, Letts LG, Rothlein R. Intercellular adhesion molecule-1 (ICAM-1) in the pathogenesis of asthma. *Science* 1990;247:456–459.

70. Nathan C, Srimal S, Farber C, et al. Cytokine-induced respiratory burst of human neutrophils: dependence on extracellular matrix proteins and CD11/CD18 integrins. *J Cell Biol* 1989;109:1341–1349.

71. Brown EJ, Bohnsack JF, Gresham HD. Mechanism of inhibition of immunoglobulin G-mediated phagocytosis by monoclonal antibodies that recognize the Mac-1 antigen. *J Clin Invest* 1988;81:365–375.

72. Graham IL, Gresham HD, Brown EJ. An immobile subset of plasma membrane CD11b/CD18 (Mac-1) is involved in phagocytosis of targets recognized by multiple receptors. *J Immunol* 1989;142:2352–2358.

73. Arnaout MA, Todd RF III, Dana N, Melamed J, Schlossman SF, Colten HR. Inhibition of phagocytosis of complement C3- or immunoglobulin G-coated particles and of C3bi binding by monoclonal antibodies to a monocyte-granulocyte membrane glycoprotein (Mo1). *J Clin Invest* 1983;72:171–179.

74. Coxon A, Rieu P, Barkalow FJ, Askari S, et al. A novel role for the beta-2 integrin CD11b/CD18 in neutrophil apoptosis—a homeostatic mechanism in inflammation. *Immunity* 1996;5:653–666.

75. Micklem KJ, Sim RB. Isolation of complement-fragment-iC3b-binding proteins by affinity chromatography. *Biochem J* 1985;231:233–236.

76. Malhotra V, Hogg N, Sim RB. Ligand binding by the p150,95 antigen of U937 monocytic cells: properties in common with complement receptor type 3 (CR3). *Eur J Immunol* 1986;16:1117–1123.

77. Myones BL, Dalzell JG, Hogg N, Ross GD. Neutrophil and monocyte cell surface p150,95 has iC3b-receptor (CR4) activity resembling CR3. *J Clin Invest* 1988;82:640–651.

78. Keizer GD, te Velde AA, Schwarting R, Figdor CG, de Vries JE. Role of p150,95 in adhesion, migration, chemotaxis and phagocytosis of human monocytes. *Eur J Immunol* 1987;17:1317–1322.

79. te Velde AA, Keizer GD, Figdor CG. Differential function of LFA-1 family molecules (CD11 and CD18) in adhesion of human monocytes to melanoma and endothelial cells. *Immunology* 1987;61:261–267.

80. Arnaout MA, Lanier LL, Faller D. Relative contribution of the leukocyte molecules Mo1, LFA-1, and p150,95 (leuM5) in adhesion of granulocytes and monocytes to vascular endothelium is tissue- and stimulus-specific. *J Cell Physiol* 1989;137:305–309.

81. Campana D, Sheridan B, Tidman N, Hoffbrand AV, Janossy G. Human leukocyte function-associated antigens on lympho-hemopoietic precursor cells. *Eur J Immunol* 1986;16:537–542.

82. Miller BA, Antognetti G, Springer T. Identification of cell surface antigens present on murine hematopoietic stem cells. *J Immunol* 1985;134:3286–3290.

83. Miller LJ, Schwarting R, Springer TA. Regulated expression of the Mac-1, LFA-1, p150,95 glycoprotein family during leukocyte differentiation. *J Immunol* 1986;137:2891–2900.

84. Strassmann G, Springer TA, Haskill SJ, Miraglia CC, Lanier LL, Adams DO. Antigens associated with the activation of murine mononuclear phagocytes *in vivo*: differential expression of lymphocyte function-associated antigen in the several stages of development. *Cell Immunol* 1985;94:265–275.

85. Jutila MA, Rott L, Berg EL, Butcher EC. Function and regulation of the neutrophil MEL-14 antigen *in vivo*: comparison with LFA-1 and Mac-1. *J Immunol* 1989;143:3318–3324.

86. Anderson DC, Schmalstieg FC, Finegold MJ, et al. The severe and moderate phenotypes of heritable Mac-1, LFA-1 deficiency: their quantitative definition and relation to leukocyte dysfunction and clinical features. *J Infect Dis* 1985;152:668–689.

87. O'Shea JJ, Brown EJ, Seligmann BE, Metcalf JA, Frank MM, Gallin JI. Evidence for distinct intracellular pools of receptors for C3b and C3bi in human neutrophils. *J Immunol* 1985;134:2580–2587.

88. Anderson DC, Rothlein R, Marlin SD, Krater SS, Smith CW. Impaired transendothelial migration by neonatal neutrophils: abnormalities of Mac-1 (CD11b/CD18)-dependent adherence reactions. *Blood* 1990;76:2613–2621.

89. Rothlein R, Dustin ML, Marlin SD, Springer TA. A human intercellular adhesion molecule (ICAM-1) distinct from LFA-1. *J Immunol* 1986;137:1270–1274.

90. Dustin ML, Springer TA. T cell receptor cross-linking transiently stimulates adhesiveness through LFA-1. *Nature* 1989;341:619–624.

91. Van Kooyk Y, Van de Wiel-van Kemenade P, Weder P, Kuijpers TW, Figdor CG. Enhancement of LFA-1–mediated cell adhesion by triggering through CD2 or CD3 on T lymphocytes. *Nature* 1989;342:811–813.

92. Freyer DR, Boxer LA, Axtell RA, Todd RF. Stimulation of human netrophil adhesive properties by adenine nucleotides. *J Immunol* 1988;141:580–586.

93. Altieri DC, Bader R, Mannucci PM, Edgington TS. Oligospecificity of the cellular adhesion receptor Mac-1 encompasses an inducible recognition specificity for fibrinogen. *J Cell Biol* 1988;107:1893–1900.

94. Altieri DC, Edgington TS. The saturable high affinity association of factor X to ADP-stimulated monocytes defines a novel function of the Mac-1 receptor. *J Biol Chem* 1988;263:7007–7015.

95. Altieri DC, Morrissey JH, Edgington TS. Adhesive receptor Mac-1 coordinates the activation of factor X on stimulated cells of monocytic

and myeloid differentiation: an alternative initiation of the coagulation protease cascade. *Proc Nat Acad Sci USA* 1988;85:7462–7466.

96. Laudanna C, Campbell JJ, Butcher EC. Role of Rho in chemoattractant-activated leukocyte adhesion through integrins. *Science* 1996; 271:981–983.

97. Lub M, Van Kooyk Y, Figdor CG. Ins and outs of LFA-1. *Immunol Today* 1995;16:479–483.

98. Stewart M, Hogg N. Regulation of leukocyte integrin function: affinity vs. avidity [Review]. *J Cell Biochem* 1996;61:554–561.

99. Stewart MP, Cabanas C, Hogg N. T cell adhesion to intercellular adhesion molecule-1 (ICAM-1) is controlled by cell spreading and the activation of integrin LFA-1. *J Immunol* 1996;156:1810–1817.

100. Lollo BA, Chan KW, Hanson EM, Moy VT, Brian AA. Direct evidence for two affinity states for lymphocyte function-associated antigen 1 on activated T cells [published erratum appears in *J Biol Chem* 1994;269(13):10184]. *J Biol Chem* 1993;268:21693–21700.

101. Dransfield I, Hogg N. Regulated expression of Mg^{2+} binding epitope on leukocyte integrin alpha subunits. *EMBO J* 1989;8:3759–3765.

102. Dransfield I, Cabanas C, Craig A, Hogg N. Divalent cation regulation of the function of the leukocyte integrin LFA-1. *J Cell Biol* 1992;116: 219–226.

103. Kucik DF, Dustin ML, Miller JM, Brown EJ. Adhesion-activating phorbol ester increases the mobility of leukocyte integrin LFA-1 in cultured lymphocytes. *J Clin Invest* 1996;97:2139–2144.

104. Van Kooyk Y, Weder P, Heije K, Figdor CG. Extracellular Ca^{2+} modulates leukocyte function-associated antigen-1 cell surface distribution on T lymphocytes and consequently affects cell adhesion. *J Cell Biol* 1994;124:1061–1070.

105. Mobley JL, Ennis E, Shimizu Y. Differential activation-dependent regulation of integrin function in cultured human T-leukemic cell lines. *Blood* 1994;83:1039–1050.

106. Van Kooyk Y, Van de Wiel-van Kemenade E, Weder P, Huijbens RJF, Figdor CG. Lymphocyte function-associated antigen 1 dominates very late antigen 4 in binding of activated T cells to endothelium. *J Exp Med* 1993;177:185–190.

107. Detmers PA, Wright SD, Olsen E, Kimball B, Cohn ZA. Aggregation of complement receptors on human neutrophils in the absence of ligand. *J Cell Biol* 1987;105:1137–1145.

108. Hibbs ML, Xu H, Stacker SA, Springer TA. Regulation of adhesion to ICAM-1 by the cytoplasmic domain of LFA-1 integrin β subunit. *Science* 1991;251:1611–1613.

109. Hibbs ML, Jakes S, Stacker SA, Wallace RW, Springer TA. The cytoplasmic domain of the integrin lymphocyte function-associated antigen-1 β subunit: sites required for binding to intercellular adhesion molecule 1 and the phorbol ester–stimulated phosphorylation site. *J Exp Med* 1991;174:1227–1238.

110. Peter K, O'Toole TE. Modulation of cell adhesion by changes in $\alpha_L \beta_2$ (LFA-1, CD11a/CD18) cytoplasmic domain/cytoskeleton interaction. *J Exp Med* 1995;181:315–326.

111. Pavalko FM, LaRoche SM. Activation of human neutrophils induces an interaction between the integrin $β_2$-subunit (CD18) and the actin binding protein α-actinin. *J Immunol* 1993;151:3795–3807.

112. Burn P, Kupfer A, Singer SJ. Dynamic membrane-cytoskeleton interactions: specific association of integrin and talin arises *in vivo* after phorbol ester treatment of peripheral blood lymphocytes. *Proc Natl Acad Sci USA* 1988;85:497–501.

113. Sharma CP, Ezzell RM, Arnaout MA. Direct interaction of filamin (ABP-280) with the $β_2$-integrin subunit CD18. *J Immunol* 1995;154: 3461–3470.

114. Pardi R, Inverardi L, Rugarli C, Bender JR. Antigen-receptor complex stimulation triggers protein kinase C-dependent CD11a/CD18–cytoskeleton association in T lymphocytes. *J Cell Biol* 1992;116: 1211–1220.

115. Kolanus W, Nagel W, Schiller B, et al. Alpha L beta 2 integrin/LFA-1 binding to ICAM-1 induced by cytohesin-1, a cytoplasmic regulatory molecule. *Cell* 1996;86:233–242.

116. Chatila TA, Geha RS, Arnaout MA. Constitutive and stimulus-induced phosphorylation of CD11/CD18 leukocyte adhesion molecules. *J Cell Biol* 1989;109:3435–3444.

117. Hara T, Fu SM. Phosphorylation of alpha,beta subunits of 180/100-Kd polypeptides (LFA-1) and related antigens. In: Reinherz EL, Haynes BF, Nadler LM, et al., eds. *Leukocyte typing II. Vol. 3: Human myeloid and hematopoietic cells.* New York: Springer-Verlag, 1986:77–84.

118. Merrill JT, Slade SG, Weissmann G, Winchester R, Buyon JP. Two

119. pathways of CD11b/CD18-mediated neutrophil aggregation with different involvement of protein kinase C-dependent phosphorylation. *J Immunol* 1990;145:2608–2615.

119. Dustin ML. Two-way signalling through the LFA-1 lymphocyte adhesion receptor. *Bioessays* 1990;12:421–427.

120. Wacholtz MC, Patel SS, Lipsky PE. Leukocyte function-associated antigen 1 is an activation molecule for human T cells. *J Exp Med* 1989;170:431–448.

121. Carrera AC, Rincon M, Sanchez-Madrid F, Lopez-Botet M, De Landazuri MO. Triggering of co-mitogenic signals in T cell proliferation by anti–LFA-1 (CD18, CD11a), LFA-3, and CD7 monoclonal antibodies. *J Immunol* 1988;141:1919–1924.

122. Fan ST, Brian AA, Lollo BA, Mackman N, Shen NL, Edgington TS. CD11a/CD18 (LFA-1) integrin engagement enhances biosynthesis of early cytokines by activated T cells. *Cell Immunol* 1993;148:48–59.

123. Pardi R, Bender JR, Dettori C, Giannazza E, Engleman EG. Heterogeneous distribution and transmembrane signaling properties of lymphocyte function-associated antigen (LFA-1) in human lymphocyte subsets. *J Immunol* 1989;143:3157–3166.

124. Kelleher D, Murphy A, Cullen D. Leukocyte function-associated antigen 1 (LFA-1) is a signaling molecule for cytoskeletal changes in a human T cell line. *Eur J Immunol* 1990;20:2351–2354.

125. Ding A, Wright SD, Nathan C. Activation of mouse peritoneal macrophages by monoclonal antibodies to Mac-1 (complement receptor type 3). *J Exp Med* 1987;165:733–749.

126. Couturier C, Haeffner-Cavaillon N, Weiss L, Fischer E, Kazatchkine MD. Induction of cell-associated interleukin 1 through stimulation of the adhesion-promoting proteins LFA-1 (CD11a/CD18) and CR3 (CD11b/CD18) of human monocytes. *Eur J Immunol* 1990;20: 999–1005.

127. Fan S-T, Edgington TS. Integrin regulation of leukocyte inflammatory functions: CD11b/CD18 enhancement of the tumor necrosis factor-a responses of monocytes. *J Immunol* 1993;150:2972–2980.

128. Graham IL, Anderson DC, Holers VM, Brown EJ. Complement receptor 3 (CR3, Mac-1, integrin $\alpha_M\beta_2$, CD11b/CD18) is required for tyrosine phosphorylation of paxillin in adherent and nonadherent neutrophils. *J Cell Biol* 1994;127:1139–1147.

129. Lacal PM, Balsinde J, Cabañas C, Bernabeu C, Sánchez-Madrid F, Mollinedo F. The CD11c antigen couples concanavalin A binding to generation of superoxide anion in human phagocytes. *Biochem J* 1990;268:707–712.

130. Petruzzelli L, Takami M, Herrera R. Adhesion through the interaction of lymphocyte function-associated antigen-1 with intracellular adhesion molecule-1 induces tyrosine phosphorylation of p130cas and its association with c-CrkII. *J Biol Chem* 1996;271:7796–7801.

131. Zheng L, Sjolander A, Eckerdal J, Andersson T. Antibody-induced engagement of beta 2 integrins on adherent human neutrophils triggers activation of p21ras through tyrosine phosphorylation of the protooncogene product Vav. *Proc Natl Acad Sci USA* 1996;93: 8431–8436.

132. Hellberg C, Molony L, Zheng L, Andersson T. Ca^{2+} signalling mechanisms of the beta 2 integrin on neutrophils: involvement of phospholipase C gamma 2 and Ins(1,4,5)P_3. *Biochem J* 1996;317:403–409.

133. Sitrin RG, Todd RF3, Albrecht E, Gyetko MR. The urokinase receptor (CD87) facilitates CD11b/CD18-mediated adhesion of human monocytes. *J Clin Invest* 1996;97:1942–1951.

134. Gresham HD, Graham IL, Anderson DC, Brown EJ. Leukocyte adhesion-deficient neutrophils fail to amplify phagocytic function in response to stimulation. Evidence for CD11b/CD18-dependent and-independent mechanisms of phagocytosis. *J Clin Invest* 1991;88: 588–597.

135. Krauss JC, PooH, Xue W, Mayo-Bond L, Todd RF 3rd, Petty HR. Reconstitution of antibody-dependent phagocytosis in fibroblasts expressing Fc gamma receptor IIIB and the complement receptor type 3. *J Immunol* 1994;153:1769–1777.

136. Zhou MJ, Brown EJ. CR3 (Mac-1, alpha M beta 2, CD11b/CD18) and Fc gamma RIII cooperate in generation of a neutrophil respiratory burst: requirement for Fc gamma RIII and tyrosine phosphorylation. *J Cell Biol* 1994;125:1407–1416.

137. Sehgal G, Zhang K, Todd RF 3rd, Boxer LA, Petty HR. Lectin-like inhibition of immune complex receptor-mediated stimulation of neutrophils. Effects on cytosolic calcium release and superoxide production. *J Immunol* 1993;150:4571–4580.

138. Xue W, Kindzelskii AL, Todd RF 3rd, Petty HR. Physical association

of complement receptor type 3 and urokinase-type plasminogen activator receptor in neutrophil membranes. *J Immunol* 1994;152: 4630–4640.

139. Cao D, Mizukami IF, Garni-Wagner BA, et al. Human urokinase-type plasminogen activator primes neutrophils for superoxide anion release. Possible roles of complement receptor type 3 and calcium. *J Immunol* 1995;154:1817–1829.

140. Wong WS, Simon DI, Rosoff PM, Rao NK, Chapman HA. Mechanisms of pertussis toxin-induced myelomonocytic cell adhesion: role of Mac-1(CD11b/CD18) and urokinase receptor (CD87). *Immunology* 1996;88:90–97.

141. Wei Y, Lukashev M, Simon DI, et al. Regulation of integrin function by the urokinase receptor. *Science* 1996;273:1551–1555.

142. Waltz DA, Sailor LZ, Chapman HA. Cytokines induce urokinase-dependent adhesion of human myeloid cells. A regulatory role for plasminogen activator inhibitors. *J Clin Invest* 1993;91:1541–1552.

143. Dustin ML, Rothlein R, Bhan AK, Dinarello CA, Springer TA. Induction by IL-1 and interferon, tissue distribution, biochemistry, and function of a natural adherence molecule (ICAM-1). *J Immunol* 1986; 137:245–254.

144. Marlin SD, Springer TA. Purified intercellular adhesion molecule-1 (ICAM-1) is a ligand for lymphocyte function-associated antigen 1 (LFA-1). *Cell* 1987;51:813–819.

145. Makgoba MW, Sanders ME, Luce GEG, et al. ICAM-1: definition by multiple antibodies of a ligand for LFA-1 dependent adhesion of B, T and myeloid cell. *Nature* 1988;331:86–88.

146. Simmons D, Makgoba MW, Seed B. ICAM, an adhesion ligand of LFA-1, is homologous to the neural cell adhesion molecule NCAM. *Nature* 1988;331:624–627.

147. Staunton DE, Marlin SD, Stratowa C, Dustin ML, Springer TA. Primary structure of intercellular adhesion molecule 1 (ICAM-1) demonstrates interaction between members of the immunoglobulin and integrin supergene families. *Cell* 1988;52:925–933.

148. Woska JR Jr, Morelock MM, Jeanfavre DD, Bormann BJ. Characterization of molecular interactions between intercellular adhesion molecule-1 and leukocyte function-associated antigen-1. *J Immunol* 1996; 156:4680–4685.

149. Pober JS, Gimbrone MA Jr, Lapierre LA, et al. Overlapping patterns of activation of human endothelial cells by interleukin 1, tumor necrosis factor and immune interferon. *J Immunol* 1986;137:1893–1896.

150. Pober JS, Lapierre LA, Stolpen AH, et al. Activation of cultured human endothelial cells by recombinant lymphotoxin: comparison with tumor necrosis factor and interleukin 1 species. *J Immunol* 1987; 138:3319–3324.

151. Smith CW, Rothlein R, Hughes BJ, Mariscalco MM, Schmalstieg FC, Anderson DC. Recognition of an endothelial determinant for CD18-dependent neutrophil adherence and transendothelial migration. *J Clin Invest* 1988;82:1746–1756.

152. Miller J, Knorr R, Ferrone M, Houdei R, Carron CP, Dustin ML. Intercellular adhesion molecule-1 dimerization and its consequences for adhesion mediated by lymphocyte function associated-1. *J Exp Med* 1995;182:1231–1241.

153. Reilly PL, Woska JR Jr, Jeanfavre DD, McNally E, Rothlein R, Bormann BJ. The native structure of intercellular adhesion molecule-1 (ICAM-1) is a dimer. Correlation with binding to LFA-1. *J Immunol* 1995;155:529–532.

154. King PD, Sandberg ET, Selvakumar A, Fang P, Beaudet AL, Dupont B. Novel isoforms of murine intercellular adhesion molecule-1 generated by alternative RNA splicing. *J Immunol* 1995;154:6080–6093.

155. Staunton DE, Dustin ML, Erickson HP, Springer TA. The arrangement of the immunoglobulin-like domains of ICAM-1 and the binding sites for LFA-1 and rhinovirus. *Cell* 1990;61:243–254.

156. Holness CL, Simmons DL. Structural motifs for recognition and adhesion in members of the immunoglobulin superfamily. *J Cell Sci* 1994;107:2065–2070.

157. Vonderheide RH, Tedder TF, Springer TA, Staunton DE. Residues within a conserved amino acid motif of domains 1 and 4 of VCAM-1 are required for binding to VLA-4. *J Cell Biol* 1994;125:215–222.

158. Briskin MJ, Rott L, Butcher EC. Structural requirements for mucosal vascular addressin binding to its lymphocyte receptor alpha 4 beta 7. Common themes among integrin-Ig family interactions. *J Immunol* 1996;156:719–726.

159. Rothlein R, Mainolfi EA, Czajkowski M, Marlin SD. A form of circulating ICAM-1 in human serum. *J Immunol* 1991;147:3788–3793.

160. Haught WH, Mansour M, Rothlein R, et al. Alterations in circulating intercellular adhesion molecule-1 and L-selectin: further evidence for chronic inflammation in ischemic heart disease. *Am Heart J* 1996; 132:1–8.

161. Dore-Duffy P, Newman W, Balabanov R, et al. Circulating, soluble adhesion proteins in cerebrospinal fluid and serum of patients with multiple sclerosis: correlation with clinical activity. *Ann Neurol* 1995; 37:55–62.

162. Ballantyne CM, Mainolfi EA, Young JB, et al. Relationship of increased levels of circulating intercellular adhesion molecule 1 after heart transplantation to rejection: human leukocyte antigen mismatch and survival. *J Heart Lung Transplant* 1994;13:597–603.

163. Adams DH, Mainolfi E, Elias E, Neuberger JM, Rothlein R. Detection of circulating intercellular adhesion molecule-1 after liver transplantation—evidence of local release within the liver during graft rejection. *Transplantation* 1993;55:83–87.

164. Clark WM, Coull BM, Briley DP, Mainolfi E, Rothlein R. Circulating intercellular adhesion molecule-1 levels and neutrophil adhesion in stroke. *J Neuroimmunol* 1993;44:123–126.

165. Cush JJ, Rothlein R, Lindsley HB, Mainolfi EA, Lipsky PE. Increased levels of circulating intercellular adhesion molecule 1 in the sera of patients with rheumatoid arthritis. *Arthritis Rheum* 1993;36: 1098–1102.

166. Lampeter ER, Kishimoto TK, Rothlein R, et al. Elevated levels of circulating adhesion molecules in IDDM patients and in subjects at risk for IDDM. *Diabetes* 1992;41:1668–1671.

167. Languino LR, Plescia J, Duperray A, et al. Fibrinogen mediates leukocyte adhesion to vascular endothelium through an ICAM-1–dependent pathway. *Cell* 1993;73:1423–1434.

168. Languino LR, Duperray A, Joganic KJ, Fornaro M, Thornton GB, Altieri DC. Regulation of leukocyte-endothelium interaction and leukocyte transendothelial migration by intercellular adhesion molecule-1 fibrinogen recognition. *Proc Natl Acad Sci USA* 1995;92: 1505–1509.

169. Staunton DE, Merluzzi VJ, Rothlein R, Barton R, Marlin SD, Springer TA. A cell adhesion molecule, ICAM-1, is the major surface receptor for rhinoviruses. *Cell* 1989;56:849–853.

170. Greve JM, Davis G, Meyer AM, et al. The major human rhinovirus receptor is ICAM-1. *Cell* 1989;56:839–847.

171. Ockenhouse CF, Betageri R, Springer TA, Staunton DE. Plasmodium falciparum-infected erythrocytes bind ICAM-1 at a site distinct from LFA-1, Mac-1, and human rhinovirus [published erratum appears in *Cell* 1992;68(5):following 994]. *Cell* 1992;68:63–69.

172. Berendt AR, Simmons DL, Tansey J, Newbold CI, Marsh K. Intercellular adhesion molecule-1 is an endothelial cell adhesion receptor for *Plasmodium falciparum*. *Nature* 1989;341:57–59.

173. Staunton DE, Dustin ML, Springer TA. Functional cloning of ICAM-2, a cell adhesion ligand for LFA-1 homologous to ICAM-1. *Nature* 1989;339:61–64.

174. De Fougerolles AR, Stacker SA, Schwarting R, Springer TA. Characterization of ICAM-2 and evidence for a third counterreceptor for LFA-1. *J Exp Med* 1991;174:253–267.

175. Diacovo TG, DeFougerolles AR, Bainton DF, Springer TA. A functional integrin ligand on the surface of platelets: intercellular adhesion molecule-2. *J Clin Invest* 1994;94:1243–1251.

176. Casasnovas JM, Springer TA, Liu JH, Harrison SC, Wang JH. Crystal structure of ICAM-2 reveals a distinctive integrin recognition surface. *Nature* 1997;387:312–315.

177. Jones EY, Harlos K, Bottomley MJ, et al. Crystal structure of an integrin-binding fragment of vascular cell adhesion molecule-1 at 1.8 A resolution. *Nature* 1995;373:539–544.

178. Vazeux R, Hoffman PA, Tomita JK, et al. Cloning and characterization of a new intercellular adhesion molecule ICAM-R. *Nature* 1992;360: 485–488.

179. Fawcett J, Holness CLL, Needham LA, et al. Molecular cloning of ICAM-3, a third ligand for LFA-1, constitutively expressed on resting leukocytes. *Nature* 1992;360:481–484.

180. De Fougerolles AR, Klickstein LB, Springer TA. Cloning and expression of intercellular adhesion molecule 3 reveals strong homology to other immunoglobulin family counter-receptors for lymphocyte function-associated antigen 1. *J Exp Med* 1993;177:1187–1192.

181. De Fougerolles AR, Springer TA. Intercellular adhesion molecule 3, a third adhesion counter-receptor for lymphocyte function-associated molecule 1 on resting lymphocytes. *J Exp Med* 1992;175:185–190.

182. Doussis-Anagnostopoulou I, Kaklamanis L, Cordell J, et al. ICAM-3 expression on endothelium in lymphoid malignancy. *Am J Pathol* 1993;143:1040–1043.

183. Teunissen MB, Koomen CW, Bos JD. Intercellular adhesion molecule-3 (CD50) on human epidermal Langerhans cells participates in T-cell activation. *J Invest Dermatol* 1995;104:995–998.

184. Starling GC, McLellan AD, Egner W, et al. Intercellular adhesion molecule-3 is the predominant co-stimulatory ligand for leukocyte function antigen-1 on human blood dendritic cells. *Eur J Immunol* 1995;25:2528–2532.

185. Bailly P, Hermand P, Callebaut I, et al. The LW blood group glycoprotein is homologous to intercellular adhesion molecules. *Proc Natl Acad Sci USA* 1994;91:5306–5310.

186. Bailly P, Tontti E, Hermand P, Cartron JP, Gahmberg CG. The red cell LW blood group protein is an intercellular adhesion molecule which binds to CD11/CD18 leukocyte integrins. *Eur J Immunol* 1995;25:3316–3320.

187. Yoshihara Y, Oka S, Nemoto Y, et al. An ICAM-related neuronal glycoprotein, telencephalin, with brain segment-specific expression. *Neuron* 1994;12:541–553.

188. Mizuno T, Yoshihara Y, Inazawa J, Kagamiyama H, Mori K. cDNA cloning and chromosomal localization of the human telencephalin and its distinctive interaction with lymphocyte function-associated antigen-1. *J Biol Chem* 1997;272:1156–1163.

189. Tian L, Yoshihara Y, Mizuno T, Mori K, Gahmberg CG. The neuronal glycoprotein telencephalin is a cellular ligand for the CD11a/CD18 leukocyte integrin. *J Immunol* 1997;158:928–936.

190. Lo SK, Van Seventer GA, Levin SM, Wright SD. Two leukocyte receptors (CD11a/CD18 and CD11b/CD18) mediate transient adhesion to endothelium by binding to different ligands. *J Immunol* 1989;143:3325–3329.

191. Wright SD, Rao PE, Van Voorhis WC, et al. Identification of the C3bi receptor of human monocytes and macrophages with monoclonal antibodies. *Proc Natl Acad Sci USA* 1983;80:5699–5703.

192. Aderem AA, Wright SD, Silverstein SC, Cohn ZA. Ligated complement receptors do not activate the arachidonic acid cascade in resident peritoneal macrophages. *J Exp Med* 1985;161:617–622.

193. Marks RM, Todd RF, Ward PA. Rapid induction of neutrophil-endothelial adhesion by endothelial complement fixation. *Nature* 1989;339:314–317.

194. Ross GD, Cain JA, Lachmann PJ. Membrane complement receptor type three (CR3) has lectin-like properties analogous to bovine conglutinin and functions as a receptor for zymosan and rabbit erythrocytes as well as a receptor for iC3b. *J Immunol* 1985;134:3307–3315.

195. Smith CL, Baker CJ, Anderson DC, Edwards MS. Role of complement receptors in opsonophagocytosis of group B streptococci by adult and neonatal neutrophils. *J Infect Dis* 1990;162:489–495.

196. Thornton BP, Vetvicka V, Pitman M, Goldman RC, Ross GD. Analysis of the sugar specificity and molecular location of the beta-glucan-binding lectin site of complement receptor type 3 (CD11b/CD18). *J Immunol* 1996;156:1235–1246.

197. Wright SD, Weitz JI, Huang AJ, Levin SM, Silverstein SC, Loike JD. Complement receptor type three (CD11b/CD18) of human polymorphonuclear leukocytes recognizes firinogen. *Proc Natl Acad Sci USA* 1988;85:7734–7738.

198. El Ghmati SM, Van Hoeyveld EM, Van Strijp JG, Ceuppens JL, Stevens EA. Identification of haptoglobin as an alternative ligand for CD11b/CD18. *J Immunol* 1996;156:2542–2552.

199. Wachtfogel YT, DeLa Cadena RA, Kunapuli SP, et al. High molecular weight kininogen binds to Mac-1 on neutrophils by its heavy chain (domain 3) and its light chain (domain 5). *J Biol Chem* 1994;269:19307–19312.

200. Monboisse J-C, Garnotel R, Randoux A, Dufer J, Borel J-P. Adhesion of human neutrophils to and activation by type I collagen involving a β_2 integrin. *J Leukoc Biol* 1991;50:373–380.

201. Thompson HL, Matsushima K. Human polymorphonuclear leucocytes stimulated by tumour necrosis factor-alpha show increased adherence to extracellular matrix proteins which is mediated via the CD11b/18 complex. *Clin Exp Immunol* 1992;90:280–285.

202. Lecoanet-Henchoz S, Gauchat JF, Aubry JP, et al. CD23 regulates monocyte activation through a novel interaction with the adhesion molecules CD11b-CD18 and CD11c-CD18. *Immunity* 1995;3:119–125.

203. Davis GE. The Mac-1 and p150,95 beta 2 integrins bind denatured proteins to mediate leukocyte cell-substrate adhesion. *Exp Cell Res* 1992;200:242–252.

204. Lee JO, Rieu P, Arnaout MA, Liddington R. Crystal structure of the A domain from the alpha subunit of integrin CR3 (CD11b/CD18). *Cell* 1995;80:631–638.

205. Lee JO, Bankston LA, Arnaout MA, Liddington RC. Two conformations of the integrin A-domain (I-domain): a pathway for activation? *Structure* 1995;3:1333–1340.

206. Qu A, Leahy DJ. Crystal structure of the I-domain from the CD11a/CD18 (LFA-1, alpha L beta 2) integrin. *Proc Natl Acad Sci USA* 1995;92:10277–10281.

207. Qu A, Leahy DJ. The role of the divalent cation in the structure of the I domain from the CD11a/CD18 integrin. *Structure* 1996;4:931–942.

208. Huang C, Springer TA. Folding of the beta-propeller domain of the integrin alphaL subunit is independent of the I domain and dependent on the beta2 subunit. *Proc Natl Acad Sci USA* 1997;94:3162–3167.

209. Ueda T, Rieu P, Brayer J, Arnaout MA. Identification of the complement iC3b binding site in the β_2 integrin CR3 (CD11b/CD18). *Proc Natl Acad Sci USA* 1994;91:10680–10684.

210. Michishita M, Videm V, Arnaout MA. A novel divalent cation-binding site in the A domain of the β_2 integrin CR3 (CD11b/CD18) is essential for ligand binding. *Cell* 1993;72:857–867.

211. Kamata T, Wright R, Takada Y. Critical threonine and aspartic acid residues within the I domains of beta 2 integrins for interactions with intercellular adhesion molecule 1 (ICAM-1) and C3bi. *J Biol Chem* 1995;270:12531–12535.

212. McGuire SL, Bajt ML. Distinct ligand binding sites in the I domain of integrin alpha M beta 2 that differentially affect a divalent cation-dependent conformation. *J Biol Chem* 1995;270:25866–25871.

213. Zhang L, Plow EF. Overlapping, but not identical, sites are involved in the recognition of C3bi, neutrophil inhibitory factor, and adhesive ligands by the alphaMbeta2 integrin. *J Biol Chem* 1996;271:18211–18216.

214. Edwards CP, Champe M, Gonzalez T, et al. Identification of amino acids in the CD11a I-domain important for binding of the leukocyte function-associated antigen-1 (LFA-1) to intercellular adhesion molecule-1 (ICAM-1). *J Biol Chem* 1995;270:12635–12640.

215. Binnerts ME, Van Kooyk Y, Edwards CP, et al. Antibodies that selectively inhibit leukocyte function-associated antigen 1 binding to intercellular adhesion molecule-3 recognize a unique epitope within the CD11a I domain. *J Biol Chem* 1996;271:9962–9968.

216. Huang C, Springer TA. A binding interface on the I domain of lymphocyte function-associated antigen-1 (LFA-1) required for specific interaction with intercellular adhesion molecule 1 (ICAM-1). *J Biol Chem* 1995;270:19008–19016.

217. Bajt ML, Goodman T, McGuire SL. Beta 2 (CD18) mutations abolish ligand recognition by I domain integrins LFA-1 (alpha L beta 2, CD11a/CD18) and MAC-1 (alpha M beta 2, CD11b/CD18). *J Biol Chem* 1995;270:94–98.

218. Springer TA. Folding of the N-terminal, ligand-binding region of integrin alpha-subunits into a beta-propeller domain. *Proc Natl Acad Sci USA* 1997;94:65–72.

219. Anderson DC, Springer TA. Leukocyte adhesion deficiency: an inherited defect in the Mac-1, LFA-1, and p150,95 glycoproteins. *Annu Rev Med* 1987;38:175–194.

220. Crowley CA, Curnutte JT, Rosin RE, et al. An inherited abnormality of neutrophil adhesion: its genetic transmission and its association with a missing protein. *N Engl J Med* 1980;302:1163–1168.

221. Arnaout MA, Pitt J, Cohen HJ, Melamed J, Rosen FS, Colten HR. Deficiency of a granulocyte-membrane glycoprotein (gpl50) in a boy with recurrent bacterial infections. *N Engl J Med* 1982;306:693–699.

222. Bowen TJ, Ochs HD, Altman LC, et al. Severe recurrent bacterial infections associated with defective adherence and chemotaxis in two patients with neutrophils deficient in a cell-associated glycoprotein. *J Pediatr* 1982;101:932–940.

223. Dana N, Todd RF III, Pitt J, Springer TA, Arnaout MA. Deficiency of a surface membrane glycoprotein (Mo1) in man. *J Clin Invest* 1984;73:153–159.

224. Anderson DC, Schmalstieg FC, Arnaout MA, et al. Abnormalities of polymorphonuclear leukocyte function associated with a heritable deficiency of high molecular weight surface glycoproteins (GP138): common relationship to diminished cell adherence. *J Clin Invest* 1984;74:536–551.

225. Diener AM, Beatty PG, Ochs HD, Harlan JM. The role of neutrophil membrane glycoprotein 150 (GP-150) in neutrophil-mediated endothelial cell injury in vitro. J Immunol 1985;135:537–543.

226. Springer TA, Thompson WS, Miller LJ, Schmalstieg FC, Anderson DC. Inherited deficiency of the Mac-1, LFA-1, p150,95 glycoprotein family and its molecular basis. J Exp Med 1984;160:1901–1918.

227. Arnaout MA, Spits H, Terhorst C, Pitt J, Todd RFI. Deficiency of a leukocyte surface glycoprotein (LFA-1) in two patients with Mo1 deficiency. J Clin Invest 1984;74:1291–1300.

228. Giger U, Boxer LA, Simpson PJ, Lucchesi BR, Todd RFI. Deficiency of leukocyte surface glycoproteins Mo1, LFA-1, and Leu M5 in a dog with recurrent bacterial infections: an animal model. Blood 1987;69:1622–1630.

229. Kehrli ME Jr, Schmalstieg FC, Anderson DC, et al. Molecular definition of the bovine granulocytopathy syndrome: identification of deficiency of the Mac-1 (CD11b/CD18) glycoprotein. Am J Vet Res 1990; 51:1826–1836.

230. Arnaout MA. Leukocyte adhesion molecules deficiency: its structural basis, pathophysiology and implications for modulating the inflammatory response [Review]. Immunol Rev 1990;114:145–180.

231. Harlan JM. Leukocyte adhesion deficiency syndrome: insights into the molecular basis of leukocyte emigration [Review]. Clin Immunol Immunopathol 1993;67:S16–24.

232. Fischer A, Lisowska-Grospierre B, Anderson DC, Springer TA. The leukocyte adhesion deficiency: molecular basis and functional consequences. Immunodef Rev 1988;1:39–54.

233. Waldrop TC, Anderson DC, Hallmon WW, Schmalstieg FC, Jacobs RL. Periodontal manifestations of the heritable Mac-1, LFA-1 deficiency syndrome—clinical, histopathologic and molecular characteristics. J Periodont 1986;137:400–416.

234. Weisman SJ, Berkow RL, Plautz G, et al. Glycoprotein-180 deficiency: genetics and abnormal neutrophil activation. Blood 1985;65: 696–704.

235. Boxer LA, Hedley-Whyte ET, Stossel TP. Neutrophil actin dysfunction and abnormal neutrophil behavior. N Engl J Med 1974;291: 1093–1099.

236. Wright DG, Dale DC, Fauci AS, Wolff SM. Human cyclic neutropenia: clinical review and long-term follow-up of patients. Medicine 1981;60:1–13.

237. Greenberg PL, Mara B, Steed S, Boxer L. The chronic idiopathic neutropenia syndrome: correlation of clinical features with in vitro parameters of granulocytopoiesis. Blood 1980;55:915–921.

238. Boxer LA, Coates TD, Haak RA, Wolach JB, Hoffstein S, Baehner RL. Lactoferrin deficiency associated with altered granulocyte function. N Engl J Med 1982;307:404–410.

239. Lau YL, Low LCK, Jones BM, Lawton JWM. Defective neutrophil and lymphocyte function in leucocyte adhesion deficiency. Clin Exp Immunol 1991;85:202–208.

240. Wright AH, Douglass WA, Taylor GM, et al. Molecular characterization of leukocyte adhesion deficiency in six patients. Eur J Immunol 1995;25:717–722.

241. Fischer A, Descamps-Latscha B, Gerota I, et al. Bone-marrow transplantation for inborn error of phagocytic cells associated with defective adherence, chemotaxis, and oxidative response during opsonised particle phagocytosis. Lancet 1983;2:473–476.

242. Fischer A, Blanche S, Veber F, et al. Correction of immune disorders by HLA matched and mismatched bone marrow transplantation. In: Gale RP, ed. Recent advances in bone marrow transplantation. New York: Alan R. Liss, 1986:37–49.

243. Kishimoto TK, Hollander N, Roberts TM, Anderson DC, Springer TA. Heterogenous mutations in the beta subunit common to the LFA-1, Mac-1, and p150,95 glycoproteins cause leukocyte adhesion deficiency. Cell 1987;50:193–202.

244. Marlin SD, Morton CC, Anderson DC, Springer TA. LFA-1 immunodeficiency disease: definition of the genetic defect and chromosomal mapping of alpha and beta subunits of the lymphocyte function-associated antigen 1 (LFA-1) by complementation in hybrid cells. J Exp Med 1986;164:855–867.

245. Wardlaw AJ, Hibbs ML, Stacker SA, Springer TA. Distinct mutations in two patients with leukocyte adhesion deficiency and their functional correlates. J Exp Med 1990;172:335–345.

246. Dana N, Clayton LK, Tennen DG, et al. Leukocytes from four patients with complete or partial Leu-CAM deficiency contain the common

247. Dimanche MT, Le Deist F, Fischer A, Arnaout MA, Griscelli C, Lisowska-Grospierre B. LFA-1 beta-chain synthesis and degradation in patients with leukocyte adhesive protein deficiency. Eur J Immunol 1987;17:417–419.

248. Arnaout MA, Dana N, Gupta SK, Tenen DG, Fathallah DM. Point mutations impairing cell surface expression of the common β subunit (CD18) in a patient with leukocyte adhesion molecule (Leu-CAM) deficiency. J Clin Invest 1990;85:977–981.

249. Sligh JE Jr, Hurwitz MY, Zhu C, Anderson DC, Beaudet AL. An initiation codon mutation in CD18 in association with the moderate phenotype of leukocyte adhesion deficiency. J Biol Chem 1992;267: 714–718.

250. Anderson DC, Kishimoto TK, Smith CW. Leukocyte adhesion deficiency and other disorders of leukocyte adherence and motility. In: Scrivner CR, Beaudet AL, Sly WS, et al., eds. The metabolic and molecular basis of inherited disease. New York: McGraw-Hill, 1995: 3955–3994.

251. Kishimoto TK, O'Connor K, Springer TA. Leukocyte adhesion deficiency: aberrant splicing of a conserved integrin sequence causes a moderate deficiency phenotype. J Biol Chem 1989;264:3588–3595.

252. Abramson JS, Mills EL, Sawyer MK, Regelmann WR, Nelson JD, Quie PG. Recurrent infections and delayed separation of the umbilical cord in an infant with abnormal phagocytic cell locomotion and oxidative response during particle phagocytosis. J Pediatr 1981;99: 887–894.

253. Harvath L, Andersen BR. Defective initiation of oxidative metabolism in polymorphonuclear leukocytes. N Engl J Med 1979;300: 1130–1135.

254. Thompson RA, Candy DCA, McNeish AS. Familial defect of polymorph neutrophil phagocytosis associated with absence of a surface glycoprotein antigen (OKMI). Clin Exp Immunol 1984;58:229–236.

255. Weening RS, Roos D, Weemaes CMR, Homan-Muller JWT, van Schaik MLJ. Defective initiation of the metabolic stimulation in phagocytizing granulocytes: a new congenital defect. J Lab Clin Med 1976;88:757–768.

256. Buescher ES, Gaither T, Nath J, Gallin JI. Abnormal adherence-related functions of neutrophils, monocytes, and Epstein-Barr virus-transformed B cells in a patient with C3bi receptor deficiency. Blood 1985;65:1382–1390.

257. Ross GD, Thompson RA, Walport MJ, et al. Characterization of patients with an increased susceptibility to bacterial infections and a genetic deficiency of leukocyte membrane complement receptor type 3 and the related membrane antigen LFA-1. Blood 1985;66: 882–890.

258. Davies EG, Isaacs D, Levinsky RJ. Defective immune interferon production and natural killer activity associated with poor neutrophil mobility and delayed umbilical cord separation. Clin Exp Immunol 1982;50:454–460.

259. Krensky AM, Mentzer SJ, Clayberger C, et al. Heritable lymphocyte function-associated antigen-1 deficiency: abnormalities of cytotoxicity and proliferation associated with abnormal expression of LFA-1. J Immunol 1985;135:3102–3108.

260. Fischer A, Seger R, Durandy A, et al. Deficiency of the adhesive protein complex lymphocyte function antigen 1, complement receptor type 3, glycoprotein p150,95 in a girl with recurrent bacterial infections. J Clin Invest 1985;76:2385–2392.

261. Beatty PG, Harlan JM, Rosen H, et al. Absence of monoclonal-antibody-defined protein complex in boy with abnormal leukocyte function. Lancet 1984;1:535–537.

262. Fischer A, Durandy A, Sterkers G, Griscelli C. Role of the LFA-1 molecule in cellular interactions required for antibody production in humans. J Immunol 1986;136:3198–3203.

263. Diacovo TG, Roth SJ, Buccola JM, Bainton DF, Springer TA. Neutrophil rolling, arrest, and transmigration across activated, surface-adherent platelets via sequential action of P-selectin and the beta 2-integrin CD11b/CD18. Blood 1996;88:146–157.

264. Smith CW, Kishimoto TK, Abbassi O, et al. Chemotactic factors regulate lectin adhesion molecule-1 (LECAM-1)-dependent neutrophil adhesion to cytokine-stimulated endothelial cells in vitro. J Clin Invest 1991;87:609–618.

265. Southwick FS, Holbrook T, Howard T, Springer T, Stossel TP, Arnaout

beta-subunit precursor and beta-subunit messenger RNA. J Clin Invest 1987;79:1010–1015.

MA. Neutrophil actin dysfunction is associated with a deficiency of Mo1. *Clin Res* 1986;34:533A.

266. Kishimoto TK. A dynamic model for neutrophil localization to inflammatory sites. *J NIH Res* 1991;3:75–77.

267. Butcher EC. Leukocyte-endothelial cell recognition: three (or more) steps to specificity and diversity. *Cell* 1991;67:1033–1036.

268. Springer TA. Traffic signals for lymphocyte recirculation and leukocyte emigration: the multistep paradigm. *Cell* 1994;76:301–314.

269. Lawrence MB, Smith CW, Eskin SG, McIntire LV. Effect of venous shear stress on CD18-mediated neutrophil adhesion to cultured endothelium. *Blood* 1990;75:227–237.

270. Buchanan MR, Crowley CA, Rosin RE, Gimbrone MA, Babior BM. Studies on the interaction between GP-180–deficient neutrophils and vascular endothelium. *Blood* 1982;60:160–165.

271. Smith CW, Marlin SD, Rothlein R, et al. Role of ICAM-1 in the adherence of human neutrophils to human endothelial cells *in vitro*. In: Springer TA, Anderson DC, Rosenthal AS, et al., eds. *Leukocyte adhesion molecules*. New York: Springer-Verlag, 1989:170–189.

272. Furie MB, Tancinco MCA, Smith CW. Monoclonal antibodies to leukocyte integrins CD11a/CD18 and CD11b/CD18 or intercellular adhesion molecule-1 inhibit chemoattractant-stimulated neutrophil transendothelial migration *in vitro*. *Blood* 1991;78:2089–2097.

273. Furie MB, McHugh DD. Migration of neutrophils across endothelial monolayers is stimulated by treatment of the monolayers with interleukin-1 or tumor necrosis factor-alpha. *J Immunol* 1989;143:3309–3317.

274. Moser R, Schleiffenbaum B, Groscurth P, Fehr J. Interleukin 1 and tumor necrosis factor stimulate human vascular endothelial cells to promote transendothelial neutrophil passage. *J Clin Invest* 1989;83:444–455.

275. Thiagarajan RR, Winn RK, Harlan JM. The role of leukocyte and endothelial adhesion molecules in ischemia-reperfusion injury [Review]. *Thromb Haemost* 1997;78:310–314.

276. Cornejo CJ, Winn RK, Harlan JM. Anti-adhesion therapy [Review]. *Adv Pharmacol* 1997;39:99–142.

277. Harlan JM, Winn RK, Vedder NB, et al. *In vivo* models of leukocyte adherence to endothelium. In: Harlan JM, Liu DY, eds. *Adhesion: its role in inflammatory disease*. New York: W.H. Freeman, 1992:117–150.

278. Smith CW, Anderson DC, Taylor AA, Rossen RD, Entman ML. Leukocyte adhesion molecules and myocardial ischemia. *Trends Cardiovasc Med* 1991;1:167–170.

279. Weiss SJ. Tissue destruction by neutrophils [see comments] [Review]. *N Engl J Med* 1989;320:365–376.

280. Nathan CF. Neutrophil activation on biological surfaces. Massive secretion of hydrogen peroxide in response to products of macrophages and lymphocytes. *J Clin Invest* 1987;80:1550–1560.

281. Nathan CF. Respiratory burst in adherent human neutrophils: triggering by colony-stimulating factors CSF-GM and CSF-G. *Blood* 1989;73:301–306.

282. Nathan C, Srimal S, Farber C, et al. Cytokine-induced respiratory burst of human neutrophils: dependence on extracellular matrix proteins and CD11/CD18 integrins. *J Cell Biol* 1989;109:1341–1349.

283. Corbi AL. *Leukocyte integrins: structure, expression, and function.* Austin, TX: R.G. Landes, 1996.

284. Panes J, Perry MA, Anderson DC, et al. Regional differences in constitutive and induced ICAM-1 expression *in vivo*. *Am J Physiol* 1995;269:H1955–H1964.

285. Manning AM, Bell FP, Rosenbloom CL, et al. NF-kappa B is activated during acute inflammation *in vivo* in association with elevated endothelial cell adhesion molecule gene expression and leukocyte recruitment. *J Inflamm* 1995;45:283–296.

286. Kukielka GL, Hawkins HK, Michael L, et al. Regulation of intercellular adhesion molecule-1 (ICAM-1) in ischemic and reperfused canine myocardium. *J Clin Invest* 1993;92:1504–1516.

287. Mulligan MS, Smith CW, Anderson DC, et al. Role of leukocyte adhesion molecules in complement-induced lung injury. *J Immunol* 1993;150:2401–2406.

288. Mulligan MS, Wilson GP, Todd RF, et al. Role of β_1, β_2 integrins and ICAM-1 in lung injury after deposition of IgG and IgA immune complexes. *J Immunol* 1993;150:2407–2417.

289. Panes J, Perry MA, Anderson DC, et al. Portal hypertension enhances endotoxin-induced intercellular adhesion molecule 1 up-regulation in the rat. *Gastroenterology* 1996;110:866–874.

290. Komatsu S, Flores S, Gerritsen ME, Anderson DC, Granger DN. Differential up-regulation of circulating soluble and endothelial cell intercellular adhesion molecule-1 in mice. *Am J Pathol* 1997;151:205–214.

291. Korthuis RJ, Anderson DC, Granger DN. Role of neutrophil-endothelial cell adhesion in inflammatory disorders [Review]. *J Crit Care* 1994;9:47–71.

292. Arfors K-E, Lundberg C, Lindborm L, Lundberg K, Beatty PG, Harlan JM. A monoclonal antibody to the membrane glycoprotein complex CD18 inhibits polymorphonuclear leukocyte accumulation and plasma leakage *in vivo*. *Blood* 1987;69:338–340.

293. Price TH, Beatty PG, Corpuz SR. *In vivo* inhibition of neutrophil function in the rabbit using monoclonal antibody to CD18. *J Immunol* 1987;139:4174–4177.

294. Rosen H, Gordon S. Monoclonal antibody to the murine type 3 complement receptor inhibits adhesion of myelomonocytic cells *in vitro* and inflammatory cell recruitment *in vivo*. *J Exp Med* 1987;166:1685–1701.

295. Rosen H, Milon G, Gordon S. Antibody to the murine type 3 complement receptor inhibits T lymphocyte-dependent recruitment of myelomonocytic cells *in vivo*. *J Exp Med* 1989;169:535–548.

296. Tuomanen EI, Saukkonen K, Sande S, Cioffe C, Wright SD. Reduction of inflammation, tissue damage, and mortality in bacterial meningitis in rabbits treated with monoclonal antibodies against adhesion-promoting receptors of leukocytes. *J Exp Med* 1989;170:959–968.

297. Barton RW, Rothlein R, Ksiazek J, Kennedy C. The effect of anti-intercellular adhesion molecule-1 on phorbol-ester-induced rabbit lund inflammation. *J Immunol* 1989;143:1278–1282.

298. Dreyer WJ, Smith CW, Michael LH, et al. Canine neutrophil activation by cardiac lymph obtained during reperfusion of ischemic myocardium. *Circ Res* 1989;65:1751–1762.

299. Kurose I, Anderson DC, Miyasaka M, et al. Molecular determinants of reperfusion-induced leukocyte adhesion and vascular protein leakage. *Circ Res* 1994;74:336–343.

300. Simpson PJ, Todd RFI, Fantone JC, et al. Reduction of experimental canine myocardial reperfusion injury by a monoclonal antibody (anti-Mo1, anti-CD11b) that inhibits leukocyte adhesion. *J Clin Invest* 1988;81:624–629.

301. Dreyer WJ, Micheal LH, West MS, et al. Neutrophil accumulation in ischemic canine myocardium: insights into the time course, distribution, and mechanism of localization during early reperfusion. *Circulation* 1991;84:400–411.

302. Seewaldt-Becker E, Rothlein R, Dammgen J. CDw18 dependent adhesion of leukocytes to endothelium and its relevance for cardiac reperfusion. In: Springer TA, Anderson DC, Rosenthal AS, et al., eds. *Leukocyte adhesion molecules: structure, function, and regulation.* New York: Springer-Verlag, 1990:138–148.

303. Williams FM, Collins PD, Tanniere-Zeller M, Williams TJ. The relationship between neutrophils and increased microvascular permeability in a model of myocardial ischaemia and reperfusion in the rabbit. *Br J Pharmacol* 1990;100:729–734.

304. Vedder NB, Winn RK, Rice CL, Chi EY, Arfors K-E, Harlan JM. Inhibition of leukocyte adherence by anti-CD18 monoclonal antibody attenuates reperfusion injury in the rabbit ear. *Proc Natl Acad Sci USA* 1990;87:2643–2646.

305. Vedder NB, Winn RK, Rice CL, Chi EY, Artors K-E, Harlan JM. A monoclonal antibody to the adherence-promoting leukocyte glycoprotein, CD18, reduces organ injury and improves survival from hemorrhagic shock and resuscitation in rabbits. *J Clin Invest* 1988;81:939–944.

306. Mileski WJ, Winn RJ, Vedder NB, Pohlman TH, Harlan JM, Rice CL. Inhibition of CD18–dependent neutrophil adherence reduces organ injury after hemorrhagic shock in primates. *Surgery* 1990;108:206–212.

307. Berke G, Fishelson Z, Schick B. Hyperthermia and formaldehyde can dissociate the binding and killing activities of cytolytic T lymphocytes. *Transplant Proc* 1979;11:804–806.

308. Lundberg C, Wright SD. Relation of the CD11/CD18 family of leukocyte antigens to the transient neutropenia caused by chemoattractants. *Blood* 1990;76:1240–1245.

309. Worthen GS, Schwab B 3rd, Elson EL, Downey GP. Mechanics of stimulated neutrophils: cell stiffening induces retention in capillaries. *Science* 1989;245:183–186.

310. Vejlsgaard GL, Ralfkiaer E, Avnstorp C, Czajkowski M, Marlin SD, Rothlein R. Kinetics and characterization of intercellular adhesion molecule-1 (ICAM-1) expression on keratinocytes in various inflam-

matory skin lesions and malignant cutaneous lymphomas. *J Am Acad Dermatol* 1989;20:782–790.

311. Adams DH, Hubscher SG, Shaw J, Rothlein R, Neuberger JM. Intercellular adhesion molecule 1 on liver allografts during rejection. *Lancet* 1989;2:1122–1125.

312. Zhang RL, Chopp M, Zaloga C, et al. The temporal profiles of ICAM-1 protein and mRNA expression after transient MCA occlusion in the rat. *Brain Res* 1995;682:182–188.

313. Richards IM, Kolbasa KP, Winterrowd GE, et al. Role of intercellular adhesion molecule-1 in antigen-induced lung inflammation in brown Norway rats. *Am J Physiol* 1996;271:L267–L276.

314. Kumasaka T, Quinlan WM, Doyle NA, et al. Role of the intercellular adhesion molecule-1(ICAM-1) in endotoxin-induced pneumonia evaluated using ICAM-1 antisense oligonucleotides, anti–ICAM-1 monoclonal antibodies, and ICAM-1 mutant mice. *J Clin Invest* 1996;97: 2362–2369.

315. Cosimi AB, Conti D, Delmonico FL, et al. *In vivo* effects of monoclonal antibody to ICAM-1 (CD54) in nonhuman primates with renal allografts. *J Immunol* 1990;144:4604–4612.

316. Wilson RW, Ballantyne CM, Smith CW, et al. Gene targeting yields a CD18–mutant mouse for study of inflammation. *J Immunol* 1993;151: 1571–1578.

317. Xu H, Gonzalo JA, St. Pierre Y, et al. Leukocytosis and resistance to septic shock in intercellular adhesion molecule 1–deficient mice. *J Exp Med* 1994;180:95–109.

318. Sligh JE Jr, Ballantyne CM, Rich SS, et al. Inflammatory and immune responses are impaired in mice deficient in intercellular adhesion molecule 1. *Proc Natl Acad Sci USA* 1993;90:8529–8533.

319. Christensen JP, Marker O, Thomsen AR. T-cell-mediated immunity to lymphocytic choriomeningitis virus in beta2-integrin (CD18)- and ICAM-1 (CD54)-deficient mice. *J Virol* 1996;70:8997–9002.

320. Schmits R, Kundig TM, Baker DM, et al. LFA-1–deficient mice show normal CTL responses to virus but fail to reject immunogenic tumor. *J Exp Med* 1996;183:1415–1426.

321. Shier P, Otulakowski G, Ngo K, et al. Impaired immune responses toward alloantigens and tumor cells but normal thymic selection in mice deficient in the beta2 integrin leukocyte function-associated antigen-1. *J Immunol* 1996;157:5375–5386.

322. Lu H, Smith CW, Perrard J, et al. LFA-1 is sufficient in mediating neutrophil emigration in Mac-1–deficient mice. *J Clin Invest* 1997;99: 1340–1350.

323. Dong ZM, Gutierrez-Ramos JC, Coxon A, Mayadas TN, Wagner DD. A new class of obesity genes encodes leukocyte adhesion receptors. *Proc Natl Acad Sci USA* 1997;94:7526–7530.

324. Soriano SG, Lipton SA, Wang YF, et al. Intercellular adhesion molecule-1–deficient mice are less susceptible to cerebral ischemia-reperfusion injury. *Ann Neurol* 1996;39:618–624.

325. Connolly ES Jr, Winfree CJ, Springer TA, et al. Cerebral protection in homozygous null ICAM-1 mice after middle cerebral artery occlusion. Role of neutrophil adhesion in the pathogenesis of stroke. *J Clin Invest* 1996;97:209–216.

326. Kelly KJ, Williams WW Jr, Colvin RB, et al. Intercellular adhesion molecule-1–deficient mice are protected against ischemic renal injury. *J Clin Invest* 1996;97:1056–1063.

327. Horie Y, Wolf R, Anderson DC, Granger DN. Hepatic leukostasis and hypoxic stress in adhesion molecule-deficient mice after gut ischemia/reperfusion. *J Clin Invest* 1997;99:781–788.

328. Bullard DC, Hurley LA, Lorenzo I, Sly LM, Beaudet AL, Staite ND. Reduced susceptibility to collagen-induced arthritis in mice deficient in intercellular adhesion molecule-1. *J Immunol* 1996;157:3153–3158.

329. Bullard DC, King PD, Hicks MJ, Dupont B, Beaudet AL, Elkon KB. Intercellular adhesion molecule-1 deficiency protects MRL/MpJ-Fas(lpr) mice from early lethality. *J Immunol* 1997;159:2058–2067.

330. Nageh MF, Sandberg ET, Marotti KR, et al. Deficiency of inflammatory cell adhesion molecules protects against atherosclerosis in mice. *Arterioscler Thromb Vasc Biol* 1997;17:1517–1520.

331. Gonzalo JA, Lloyd CM, Kremer L, et al. Eosinophil recruitment to the lung in a murine model of allergic inflammation. The role of T cells, chemokines, and adhesion receptors. *J Clin Invest* 1996;98:2332–2345.

332. Qin L, Quinlan WM, Doyle NA, et al. The roles of CD11/CD18 and ICAM-1 in acute *Pseudomonas aeruginosa*–induced pneumonia in mice. *J Immunol* 1996;157:5016–5021.

333. Bullard DC, Qin L, Lorenzo I, et al. P-selectin/ICAM-1 double mutant mice: acute emigration of neutrophils into the peritoneum is completely absent but is normal into pulmonary alveoli. *J Clin Invest* 1995;95:1782–1788.

Inflammation: Basic Principles and Clinical Correlates,
3rd ed., edited by John I. Gallin and Ralph Snyderman.
Lippincott Williams & Wilkins, Philadelphia © 1999.

CHAPTER 38

The Selectins in Inflammation

Lisa A. Robinson, Douglas A. Steeber, and Thomas F. Tedder

One of the hallmarks of inflammation is the recruitment of circulating leukocytes into tissue sites of injury or disease. This emigration involves a series of interdependent and closely regulated adhesive interactions between leukocytes and the vascular endothelium (Fig. 38-1) (1). The first of these interactions is mediated predominantly by the selectin family of adhesion molecules, which are specialized at capturing free-flowing leukocytes from the blood (2). Once captured, leukocytes roll along the venular endothelium via interactions among multiple members of the selectin, integrin, and immunoglobulin families (3). Transition from rolling to firm arrest depends on the presence of appropriate activation signals primarily provided by chemoattractants. Chemoattractant-induced upregulation of leukocyte β_2 [lymphocyte function antigen-1 (LFA-1), CD11a/CD18; Mac-1, CD11b/CD18] and β_1 [very late activation antigen-4 (VLA-4), CD49d/CD29] integrins arrests the rolling cell via specific interactions with their immunoglobulin family counterreceptors expressed on the vascular endothelium (4). Expression of immunoglobulin family members such as intercellular adhesion molecule-1 (ICAM-1, CD54) and vascular cell adhesion molecule-1 (VCAM-1, CD106) increases dramatically following activation with proinflammatory cytokines, while others such as ICAM-2 (CD102) are constitutively expressed. Subsequent to firm adhesion, diapedesis of the leukocyte at endothelial cell junctions occurs in a CD31 [platelet endothelial cell adhesion molecule-1 (PECAM-1)]-dependent manner.

The three members of the selectin family, L-selectin [MEL-14 antigen, leukocyte adhesion molecule-1 (LAM-1), CD62L], P-selectin [platelet activation-dependent granule external membrane protein (PADGEM), granule membrane protein-140 (GMP-140), CD62P] and E-selectin [endothelial leukocyte adhesion molecule-1 (ELAM-1), CD62E], although closely related in structure, have very different patterns of expression (2). L-selectin is expressed by the majority of leukocytes and mediates binding to an inducible vascular ligand(s) at sites of inflammation. In addition, the recirculation of lymphocytes through the peripheral lymphoid tissues is largely mediated through the interaction of L-selectin with constitutively expressed ligands present on specialized venules, called high endothelial venules (HEVs), within these tissues. In contrast, P-selectin is rapidly mobilized to the surface of activated platelets and endothelial cells from preformed intracellular stores. E-selectin surface expression on cytokine-activated endothelial cells requires de novo protein synthesis and is therefore slower than that of P-selectin. Both P- and E-selectin bind to cell surface ligands expressed by myeloid cells and subpopulations of lymphocytes. In this way, the selective expression of the selectins and selectin ligands provides a key regulatory mechanism for leukocyte emigration from the vasculature.

SELECTIN STRUCTURE

L-, E-, and P-selectin share a unique extracellular region composed of an amino-terminal calcium-dependent lectin domain, an epidermal growth factor (EGF)-like domain, and short consensus repeat (SCR) units homologous to domains found in complement regulatory proteins (Figure 38-2). L-selectin contains two SCR domains, while E- and P-selectin contain six and nine SCR domains, respectively. Human L-, E-, and P-selectin are closely related in amino acid sequence, ranging from ~65% identity in the lectin and EGF domains to ~40% identity in the SCR domains. This high degree of sequence conservation among the lectin domains results in the recognition of similar, if not identical, carbohydrate epitopes decorating various protein scaffolds. In contrast

L. A. Robinson, D. A. Steeber, and T. F. Tedder: Department of Immunology, Duke University Medical Center, Durham, North Carolina 27710.

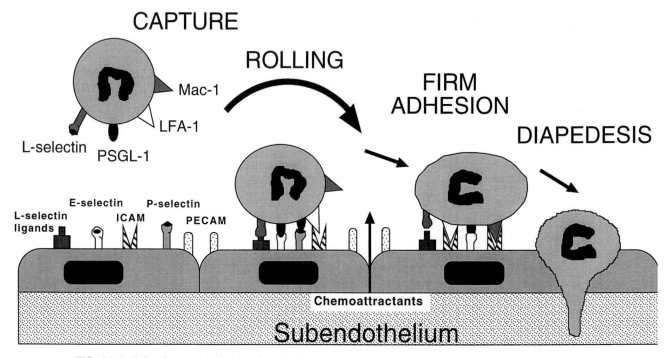

FIG. 38-1. Adhesion molecules involved in leukocyte interactions with vascular endothelium at sites of inflammation. Vascular expression of P-selectin and ligands for L-selectin predominantly mediate the initial capture of leukocytes from the flowing blood. L-selectin and P-selectin glycoprotein ligand-1 (PSGL-1) are concentrated on microvilli of unstimulated neutrophils, a location that may facilitate cell-cell contacts. Optimal leukocyte rolling is mediated by two or all of the selectins functioning in concert. In addition, leukocyte integrins interacting with their vascular ligands function synergistically with the selectins to slow rolling velocities prior to mediating firm adhesion. Subsequent to firm adhesion, leukocytes migrate between endothelial cells in a platelet endothelial cell adhesion molecule (PECAM)-dependent process.

to the extracellular domains, the cytoplasmic tails are highly diverse.

Ligand-binding ability of the selectins is predominantly conferred by the lectin domain, with some function also attributed to the EGF and SCR domains. This is demonstrated by the finding that the most effective L-selectin function-blocking monoclonal antibodies (MAbs) bind epitopes localized within the lectin domain (5–8), although a few have been mapped to regions within the EGF domain (5,6,9). In addition, functional studies using chimeric selectins also demonstrate that both the lectin and EGF domains are directly involved in cell adhesion (8,10,11). Despite lower levels of homology between selectin SCR domains, these domains are critical for optimal selectin function. Extending the lectin and EGF domains of E- and P-selectin from the cell surface appears to be important in promoting interactions that would be spatially unfavorable for a more membrane proximal receptor such as L-selectin (12,13). Thus, cooperative interactions among the individual extracellular domains of the selectins promote ligand binding.

L-Selectin

L-selectin has an ~74,000 M_r when expressed by human lymphocytes but has an apparent 90 to 110,000 M_r

when expressed by neutrophils (14,15). These size differences reflect changes in glycosylation rather than differences in the protein core (16). The membrane proximal region of L-selectin contains a site that is susceptible to endoproteolytic cleavage by an endogenous membrane-bound protease following cell activation (Fig. 38-2) (17). The cleavage product has a 69,000 M_r, is functionally active, and is present at high levels (1.6 ± 0.8 µg/ml) in normal serum where it may downregulate inflammatory responses (18). Although it has been proposed that L-selectin cleavage from the cell surface is prerequisite to diapedesis, recent findings do not support this idea (19). The cytoplasmic domain of L-selectin is very short, consisting of only 17 amino acid residues including two serine and one tyrosine residue as potential targets for phosphorylation. Although not critical for ligand binding, the cytoplasmic domain is required for optimal cell surface receptor function (20). This latter observation may relate to the finding that the ligand-binding activity of L-selectin is rapidly upregulated by exposing leukocytes to a variety of proinflammatory agents that activate protein kinase C (PKC), including chemoattractants (21). Within seconds of chemoattractant receptor activation, L-selectin is phosphorylated on cytoplasmic serine residues through a PKC-dependent pathway (22). Moreover, inhibitors of PKC prevent the upregulation of L-

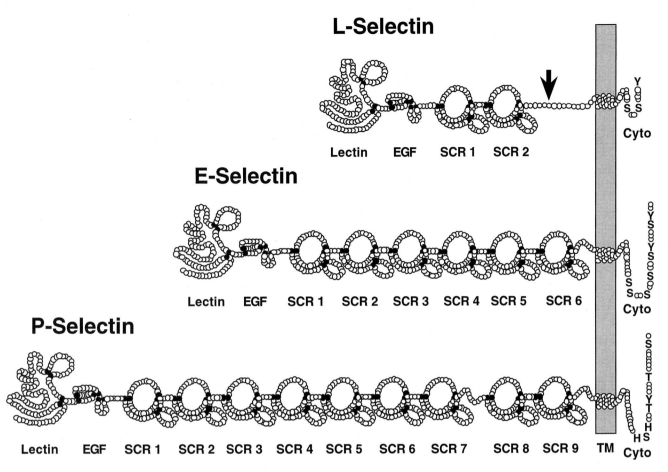

FIG. 38-2. Selectin structure. The lectin, epidermal growth factor (EGF)-like, short consensus repeat (SCR), transmembrane (TM), and cytoplasmic (Cyto) domains of each selectin are shown. Serine (S), threonine (T), tyrosine (Y), and histidine (H) residues located within the cytoplasmic domain are indicated. *Open circles* represent amino acid residues; *filled circles* indicate conserved cysteines. *Arrow* indicates primary site of endoproteolytic cleavage of L-selectin from the cell surface.

selectin–dependent lymphocyte binding to HEV following activation. Thus, phosphorylation of the L-selectin cytoplasmic domain may be a physiologically relevant mechanism for the synergistic regulation of adhesion molecules during leukocyte migration.

P-Selectin

P-selectin is a 140,000 M_r protein in humans of which almost 30% of its apparent mass represents complex *N*-linked oligosaccharides (23). Three species of P-selectin have been described. Two differ in the number of SCR domains (Fig. 38-2; major species, nine; minor species, eight), while a third form lacks a transmembrane domain (24). Soluble P-selectin is functionally active and is found in normal plasma at concentrations in the range of ~40 to ~200 ng/ml (25,26). The cytoplasmic domain of P-selectin consists of 35 amino acid residues including two serine, two threonine, and one tyrosine residue, which are rapidly phosphorylated following activation (Fig. 38-2) (27,28). In addition, rapid and

selective dephosphorylation occurs on the threonine and tyrosine residues (28). Interestingly, histidine phosphorylation of P-selectin in activated platelets has also been demonstrated (29). In contrast to L-selectin, the cytoplasmic domain of P-selectin is not essential for leukocyte adhesion (30).

E-Selectin

Human cytokine-activated endothelial cells predominantly express E-selectin as a 115,000 M_r glycoprotein (31). The short cytoplasmic tail consists of 32 amino acid residues including six serine and two tyrosine residues as potential sites for phosphorylation (Fig. 38-2). E-selectin expressed by tumor necrosis factor-α (TNF-α)–activated human umbilical vein endothelial cells (HUVECs) is constitutively serine phosphorylated (32) with time-dependent dephosphorylation following leukocyte adhesion or E-selectin crosslinking (33). Activated endothelial cells release a truncated form of E-selectin (~94,000 M_r) that lacks an intact cytoplasmic domain (34,35). Normal plasma levels of soluble E-selectin have been reported in the range of 0.1 to ~3 ng/ml (34). Similar to P-selectin, the cytoplasmic domain of E-selectin is not essential for leukocyte adhesion (30).

SELECTIN EXPRESSION AND LIGAND BINDING

Expression

L-selectin is expressed by all classes of leukocytes at most stages of differentiation (36,37). Among lymphocytes, the majority of circulating virgin/naive T cells express L-selectin and enter peripheral lymphoid tissues, although distinct subpopulations of both CD4$^+$ and CD8$^+$ memory cells that lack L-selectin are present (37,38). Recently activated helper T cells with a memory phenotype generally lack L-selectin expression but reacquire surface receptor expression during further maturation into fully competent helper cells (14,39). In addition, intrinsic differences in expression levels of L-selectin among lymphocyte subsets regulate in part, their differential migration patterns (38). Thus, both naive and mature memory lymphocytes utilize L-selectin to enter lymphoid tissues where effective helper function is provided.

P-selectin is constitutively found in the membranes of Weibel-Palade bodies within endothelial cells and in the α-granules of platelets (40). Within minutes following activation by thrombogenic or inflammatory mediators, granules containing P-selectin fuse with the plasma membrane, thereby expressing P-selectin on the cell surface. Activating agents include thrombin, histamine, complement fragments, oxygen-derived free radicals, lipopolysaccharide (LPS), and cytokines. In vivo, LPS and TNF-α treatment increase expression of P-selectin on endothelial cells. P-selectin expression is generally short-lived (minutes), which is consistent with its role in mediating early leukocyte-endothelial cell interactions (41). However, in vivo studies of P-selectin function suggest that it may also be important at later time points as a cytokine-induced adhesion molecule.

E-selectin is expressed by activated but not resting endothelial cells (31). E-selectin protein production is strongly induced by a variety of inflammatory mediators, including interleukin-1β (IL-1β), TNF-α, interferon-γ, substance P, and LPS. E-selectin expression on HUVEC peaks at 4 to 6 hours following activation and declines to basal levels by 24 to 48 hours (31,42). However, E-selectin expression in HUVEC may not be generalized to reflect its expression in other tissues in vivo since sustained expression has been observed in endothelial cells isolated from different vascular beds (43–45). Therefore, the kinetics of E-selectin expression are variable, likely reflecting differences in both the microvascular bed and the type of inflammatory insult.

Ligands

The molecular basis of selectin adhesion involves carbohydrate recognition by the lectin domain (46). The selectins recognize a variety of complex carbohydrates in vitro, although it is likely that each selectin only binds to a very restricted number of high-affinity ligands in vivo (Table 38-1). The tetrasaccharide sialyl Lewis^x (sLe^x, CD15s) binds to each of the selectins and therefore has been identified as a prototype selectin ligand. In vitro, murine L-selectin has been shown to recognize at least four different heavily glycosylated mucin-like proteins constitutively expressed by HEV: glycosylation-dependent cell adhesion molecule-1 (GlyCAM-1, CD34, MAd-CAM-1 (mucosal addressin that primarily mediates α$_4$β$_7$ integrin-dependent binding) (47), and a 200,000-M$_r$ HEV ligand (sgp200). Each of these molecules is decorated with sulfated, sialylated, and fucosylated O-linked carbohydrate side chains which appear to be essential for L-selectin recognition (48). At present it remains unclear which, if any, of the above molecules functions as the dominant physiologic ligand for L-selectin. Ligands for L-selectin expressed on HEV have previously been identified by the MECA-79 MAb (49–51). MECA-79 reactivity is also found on venules at sites of chronic inflammation (52,53). However, HEVs from fucosyltransferase VII–deficient mice that lack selectin ligands express normal levels of the MECA-79 epitope (54). Recent studies have shown that L-selectin also binds to P-selectin glycoprotein ligand-1 (PSGL-1, see below) expressed by leukocytes (8,55,56), although much less efficiently than does P-selectin (8). An unidentified cytokine-inducible ligand for L-selectin has been described for cultured HUVEC and microvascular endothelial cells (57–59). Both HEV and endothelial cells of skin venules express a carbohydrate sLe^x-like epitope defined by the 2H5 MAb (60–62). The 2H5 determinant is induced on vascular endothelial cells at sites of inflammation, and, importantly, this MAb blocks L-selectin–dependent leukocyte binding and migration. Therefore, it is likely that the 2H5 MAb recognizes a physiologically relevant L-selectin ligand.

P-selectin glycoprotein ligand-1 has been shown to be the dominant physiologic ligand for P-selectin (Table 38-1) (63,64). In fact, all P-selectin–dependent leukocyte rolling in vivo has been shown to be mediated by PSGL-1 (64). PSGL-1 was originally identified as a P- and E-selectin ligand and is decorated by N-linked glycans and numerous sialylated O-linked glycans, including O-linked polylactosamine determinants that carry sLe^x. O-linked glycans are required for P-selectin recognition, whereas the N-linked glycans are not. P-selectin binding through the amino-terminal region of PSGL-1 is blocked by a specific anti–PSGL-1 MAb (PL1) and by O-sialoglycoprotein endopeptidase (OSGE)-mediated cleavage of PSGL-1 from the cell surface.

TABLE 38-1. *Selectin ligands*

Selectin	Name	Size (kd)	Location	Comments
			Ligand	
L-selectin	GlyCAM-1	50,000	PLN HEV Lung Mammary epithelium	Constitutively expressed. Secreted protein.
	sgp200	200,000	PLN HEV	Both cell membrane–associated and secreted forms.
	CD34	90,000	Endothelial cells Hematopoietic stem cells	Constitutively expressed. Type 1 transmembrane glycoprotein. Proposed regulation by tissue- specific O-glycosylation.
	MadCAM-1	58,000–66,000	PP HEV MLN HEV Intestinal lamina propria vessels	Mucin-like domain binds L-selectin. Ig-like domain binds $\alpha_4\beta_7$ integrin. Tissue-specific glycosylation. Increased expression in IBD. Pancreatic expression in NOD mice. CNS expression in relapsing EAE.
	PSGL-1	220,000 M_r homodimer	Myeloid cells, eosinophils, thymocytes, lymphocytes, NK cells, dendritic cells	Binds L- and P-selectin through identical overlapping regions.
P-selectin	PSGL-1		As above	Requires modification by sialylated $\alpha(1,3)$fucosylated O-linked glycans for P-selectin recognition. Amino-terminal sulfated tyrosine residues required for P-selectin binding. Mediates all P-selectin-dependent leukocyte rolling *in vivo*.
E-selectin	PSGL-1		As above	Requires appropriate glycosylation and fucosylation.
	ESL-1	150,000	Murine neutrophils	Variant of a chicken FGF receptor. Requires fucosylation for binding activity.

GlyCAM-1, glycosylation-dependent cell adhesion molecule-1; PLN, peripheral lymph node; HEV, high endothelial venules; MLN, mesenteric lymph node; PP, Peyer's patches; MAdCAM-1, mucosal addressin cell adhesion molecule-1; Ig, immunoglobulin; CNS, central nervous system; PSGL-1, P-selectin glycoprotein ligand-1; NK, natural killer; ESL-1, E-selectin ligand-1; NOD, nonobese diabetic; EAE, experimental allergic encephalomyelitis; IBD, inflammatory bowel disease; FGF, fibroblast growth factor.

Although E- and P-selectin can bind identical carbohydrate moieties, glycoprotein ligands unique to P- and E-selectin have been identified (Table 38-1). E-selectin binds to appropriately glycosylated PSGL-1 on myeloid cells (65). E-selectin also binds to the cutaneous lymphocyte-associated antigen (CLA), a carbohydrate determinant that is recognized by the HECA-452 MAb and is associated with tissue-selective homing of T cells to sites of chronic cutaneous inflammation (66). Lymphocyte CLA has been recently identified as a modified form of PSGL-1 (67). E-selectin also binds a 260,000 M_r glycoprotein on bovine $\gamma\delta$ T cells (68) and a predominant 150,000 M_r glycoprotein and minor 250,000 M_r protein on mouse neutrophils (69). The 150,000 M_r glycoprotein, termed the E-selectin ligand-1 (ESL-1), is a variant of a chicken fibroblast growth factor receptor (70). The above observations have led to the suggestion that E- and P-selectin recognize two types of glycoprotein ligands, one being monospecific and the second common for both endothelial selectins (71).

INFLAMMATION IN SELECTIN-DEFICIENT MOUSE MODELS

The generation of selectin-deficient mice has done much to elucidate the role of the selectins in inflammation, as well as their interplay with other adhesion receptors (72–74). Selectin-deficient mice develop normally and are generally healthy.

L-Selectin–Deficient Mice

L-selectin–deficient mice initially have normal levels of leukocyte rolling along inflamed venules but show a marked decline in rolling thereafter (41,73,75). This initial rolling has been shown to be mediated by P-selectin (41). The decreased rolling observed in L-selectin–deficient mice results in a pronounced reduction in the ability of leukocytes to migrate into inflamed tissues. Specifically, L-selectin–deficient mice demonstrate decreased leukocyte recruitment into the inflamed peritoneal cavity at early (<4 hours) and late (4–72 hours) time points (73,76). Significant reductions in delayed contact hypersensitivity responses and in susceptibility to LPS-induced septic shock are also characteristic of these mice (76). L-selectin is involved in lymphocyte migration to cutaneous sites of inflammation since rejection of skin allografts is significantly delayed in L-selectin–deficient mice despite the generation of a normal cytotoxic T lymphocyte response (77). Taken together, these findings demonstrate that L-selectin plays a major role in mediating leukocyte rolling and thereby entry into tissue sites during inflammation.

P-Selectin–Deficient Mice

P-selectin–deficient mice have two- to threefold more circulating neutrophils compared to wild-type mice (72). In contrast to L-selectin–deficient mice, these mice show a complete absence of leukocyte rolling along venules at the onset of inflammation, but rolling is observed at time points beyond an hour (41,72,75,78). As a result, leukocyte entry into the peritoneal cavity of P-selectin–deficient mice is significantly reduced at early time points following induction of peritonitis (72). At later time points, these mice have fewer infiltrating monocytes but near-normal numbers of neutrophils and lymphocytes (78). Although delayed contact hypersensitivity responses are not reduced by P-selectin MAb treatment (74), these responses are variable in P-selectin–deficient mice (79,80). In addition, rejection of allogeneic skin grafts is not altered in P-selectin–deficient mice (77). Therefore, P-selectin predominantly mediates leukocyte interactions during the early phases of inflammatory responses, but is not strictly required later during inflammation.

E-Selectin–Deficient Mice

Inflammatory responses are remarkably normal in E-selectin–deficient mice (74). These findings are in contrast to reports showing decreased leukocyte migration into sites of inflammation following treatment with E-selectin neutralizing MAbs (81,82). However, in E-selectin–deficient mice, both the number of rolling leukocytes and rolling velocities are increased in TNF-α–treated venules (75). Moreover, the normal increase in leukocyte stable adhesion to TNF-α–treated microvascular endothelium is significantly reduced in E-selectin–deficient mice (83). Interestingly, treatment with P-selectin blocking antibodies significantly reduces inflammation and neutrophil influx during delayed-contact hypersensitivity responses in E-selectin–deficient mice, but has no effect in wild-type mice (74). Similarly, E-selectin antibodies block cytokine-induced leukocyte rolling in P-selectin–deficient mice, but have little effect in wild-type mice (75). These results suggest that E-selectin has subtle effects on leukocyte influx into sites of inflammation and that E- and P-selectin are at least partially redundant *in vivo*.

Fucosyltransferase-Deficient Mice

Congenital deficiencies in leukocyte adhesion resulting from reduced or absent expression of β_2 integrins [leukocyte adhesion deficiency-I (LAD-I)] or from a defect in endogenous fucose metabolism (LAD-II) have been described. Neutrophils from LAD-II patients are able to bind endothelium under static conditions but roll poorly along inflamed venules (84). This is consistent with the finding that ligands for each of the selectins require appropriate fucosylation. This has been confirmed experimentally by generation of a mouse deficient in $\alpha(1,3)$fucosyltransferase VII (54). These mice demonstrate leukocytosis, decreased leukocyte rolling along inflamed venules, decreased neutrophil emigration during peritonitis, and severely reduced lymphocyte migration into peripheral lymph nodes. Therefore, fucosyltransferase VII plays an essential role in the generation of physiologic ligands for each of the selectins.

THE SELECTINS IN DISEASE

Leukocyte infiltration is central to the pathogenesis of diverse inflammatory processes associated with human disease. Therefore, it is not surprising that much attention has focused on elucidating the role of adhesion molecules in the initiation and maintenance of inflammatory disease. An increasing number of reports have identified crucial roles for the selectins in both local and systemic disease settings. Consequently, novel therapeutic approaches aimed at disrupting selectin function hold great promise for alleviating the pathology associated with inflammation.

Localized Inflammation

End-organ ischemia is associated with a number of disease states including myocardial ischemia/infarction, cerebrovascular accident, solid organ transplantation, and hypotension. The ensuing injury associated with tissue reperfusion is initiated by neutrophil interactions with damaged endothelium. Several *in vivo* models have suggested a crucial role for the selectins in promoting these interactions. P-selectin expression is enhanced on the coronary vasculature following ligation-induced myocardial ischemia and subsequent reperfusion in cats (85). Similar P-selectin staining has been found in a model of rabbit ear reperfusion injury (86). Upregulated E-selectin mRNA expression, with a corresponding increase in neutrophilic infiltration, has recently been observed in ischemic rat kidney, peaking within 6 hours (87). Ischemic injury in striatal muscle appears to be L-selectin–dependent, as evidenced by the ability of anti–L-selectin MAb to alleviate tissue damage (88). Thus, it is highly likely that selectin-mediated neutrophil recruitment contributes to postischemic injury.

In acute rejection of a transplanted allogeneic organ, progressive organ dysfunction occurs in conjunction with interstitial infiltration of leukocytes, most notably lymphocytes, macrophages, and neutrophils. Despite improved short-term survival due to more efficacious clinical therapies, many grafts succumb in the long-term to chronic rejection. The histopathologic hallmarks of this type of rejection are progressive interstitial mononuclear infiltration and fibrosis, as well as vessel sclerosis. Therefore, it is likely that selectin-mediated leukocyte recruitment may contribute to both acute and chronic allograft rejection. E-selectin staining has been variably demonstrated in the normal kidney, ranging from no staining to intertubular capillary endothelial staining (89,90). In acute rejection, however, cell surface E-selectin is upregulated on peritubular capillaries and large vessels (90,91). Similarly, endothelial E-selectin expression is upregulated on human cardiac allografts that have been subjected to perioperative ischemia (92). More importantly, enhanced E-selectin expression was predictive of an imminent rejection episode. In addition, during renal allograft rejection, peritubular capillaries develop a plump endothelial lining, a morphologic characteristic of HEV, and bind both an L-selectin/immunoglobulin G (IgG) fusion protein and an antibody to sLe^x (93). Therefore, both E- and L-selectin mediate leukocyte migration into transplanted organs and may thereby contribute to their ultimate destruction.

Several studies also support a role for the selectins in xenograft rejection. Both E- and P-selectin are upregulated on vascularized guinea pig hearts placed into rats (94,95). Our recent studies show that TNF-α–activated porcine aortic endothelial cells express a vascular ligand that recognizes human L-selectin (96). Moreover, monoclonal antibodies directed against porcine E-selectin, human L-selectin, or human PSGL-1 can inhibit attachment of human neutrophils to activated porcine vascular endothelial monolayers under physiologic flow conditions. Similarly, pretreatment with anti–L-selectin antibody inhibits lymphocyte adhesion under nonstatic conditions. These studies suggest that interrupting the selectin-mediated arm of the adhesion cascade would impair the ability of human leukocytes to infiltrate a transplanted porcine organ.

In asthmatics, the bronchial epithelial mucosa becomes extensively infiltrated by eosinophils, monocytes, lymphocytes, and neutrophils in response to allergen challenge. Several studies have demonstrated constitutive E-selectin expression in the bronchial vasculature, which is upregulated in antigen-induced reactive airways disease (97–99). In a primate model of extrinsic allergic asthma, E-selectin expression and corresponding neutrophil infiltration of the bronchial mucosa occurred within 6 hours

of inhalational antigen challenge (97). In addition, L-selectin expression is significantly lower on eosinophils recovered from bronchoalveolar lavage fluid compared to those recovered from blood in challenged allergic asthmatics (100), likely reflecting local cellular activation. Soluble E-selectin levels rise acutely in the blood during exacerbations of asthma (101,102), and in bronchoalveolar lavage fluid following segmental antigen challenge (103), indicating endothelial cell activation. These reports suggest that E-selectin is instrumental in recruiting circulating leukocytes to inflamed airways.

Numerous studies suggest a role for the selectins in targeting neutrophils to the lung in acute pulmonary injury. The development of an animal model of cobra venom factor–induced acute lung injury, which is neutrophil dependent, has provided considerable insight. In this model, P-selectin is rapidly expressed in the pulmonary vasculature within minutes of cobra venom factor administration (104). In similar studies, E-selectin expression on pulmonary venules and interstitial capillaries was dramatically upregulated following induction of immune-complex–mediated injury (82). Both P- and E-selectin in the lung are induced de novo during staphylococcal enterotoxin B–induced acute lung injury (105). In addition, L-selectin plays an important role in the recruitment of neutrophils to inflamed lung at later time points (>5 minutes) (106). Specifically, L-selectin–deficient mice have reduced pulmonary neutrophil accumulation in response to either complement-induced injury or bacterial pneumonia. Examination of soluble selectin levels in patients with acute respiratory distress syndrome (ARDS) has provided a convincing human clinical correlate (107). Neutrophils have been shown to mediate the pathogenesis of ARDS, and the acute lung injury seen is characterized by profound neutrophilic invasion as well as widespread endothelial activation and damage. This process results in loss of integrity of the alveolar-capillary barrier, and culminates in extensive fluid extravasation into alveoli. In a study involving at-risk human patients, low plasma levels of soluble L-selectin predicted subsequent development of ARDS (107). Moreover, low circulating L-selectin levels correlated with the severity of pulmonary injury, and predicted progression to multiorgan failure. Thus, soluble L-selectin levels may be of both diagnostic and prognostic importance.

Both allergic and atopic forms of cutaneous inflammation are associated with intraepidermal edema and leukocytic infiltrates. In uninflamed skin, E-selectin is minimally expressed on dermal vascular endothelial cells, but is intensely upregulated in allergic contact dermatitis and, to a lesser extent, in atopic dermatitis (108). In allergic contact dermatitis, vessels staining positive for E-selectin are marked by perivascular lymphohistiocytic infiltration. In contrast, in atopic dermatitis, E-selectin staining does not necessarily correlate with cellular infiltration. E-selectin expression is also enhanced following intradermal allergen challenge in atopic subjects, and is associated with an inflammatory infiltrate consisting of eosinophils, neutrophils, and mononuclear cells (109). Serum levels of soluble E-selectin are also significantly increased in atopic dermatitis, but return toward baseline with disease remission (110). Thus, soluble E-selectin may provide a useful marker of disease activity and response to treatment in various types of cutaneous inflammation.

Multisystem Disease

Rheumatoid arthritis (RA) is an autoimmune disease with a broad spectrum of clinical activity, including symmetric polyarthritis, vasculitis, and serositis. Central to the development of arthritis is the infiltration of leukocytes into inflamed synovial tissues, and much evidence exists that this process is adhesion molecule dependent. Rheumatoid synovium contains HEV-like vessels, similar to those found in peripheral lymph nodes, which support leukocyte binding and migration (111–113). Increased E-selectin expression has been consistently demonstrated on RA synovial endothelium, both in vitro and in situ (114–117). Antiinflammatory therapies, such as anti–TNF-α antibody, pulse intravenous methylprednisolone, and intramuscular gold, decrease vascular endothelial E-selectin expression in synovial biopsy specimens (116,118,119). In addition, intense, diffuse synovial P-selectin expression and/or P-selectin–mediated monocyte adhesion has been described in some (113), but not other (115), patients with RA. Although serum levels of L- and P-selectin are elevated in RA patients, only P-selectin levels correlate with disease activity (120,121). Serum E-selectin levels are increased in patients with active disease, but fall in response to antiinflammatory therapy (122). Thus, in RA, each of the selectins appears to play a role in recruiting leukocytes into the inflamed synovium. Furthermore, both soluble P- and E-selectin may serve as markers of disease activity and may potentially be used to gauge response to therapy.

Systemic lupus erythematosus (SLE) is a multisystem autoimmune disease marked by arthritis, glomerulonephritis, mucositis, serositis, vasculitis, cutaneous lesions, and immune complex deposition. SLE is associated with high titers of antinuclear antibodies whose binding to vascular endothelial cells may upregulate E-selectin expression (123). Increased E-selectin expression has also been demonstrated in quadriceps muscle and nonlesional, non–sun-exposed skin in patients with SLE (124,125). E-selectin expression is also enhanced on glomerular and interstitial venular endothelial cells, and on glomerular parietal epithelium in patients with lupus nephritis (126). Levels of soluble P-selectin are elevated, particularly in the presence of nephropathy, but do not correlate with most other laboratory markers (120).

Therefore, tissue-specific E-selectin expression in SLE reflects localized endothelial activation at diverse sites, thereby contributing to the constellation of symptoms seen in these patients.

The hallmark of insulin-dependent diabetes mellitus is T-cell–mediated destruction of pancreatic islet cells, resulting in the clinical syndrome of hyperglycemia, nephropathy, neuropathy, retinopathy, and micro- and macroangiopathy. Much is unknown about the mechanisms by which lymphocytic infiltration of the pancreas occurs. However, use of a murine model of spontaneous insulin-dependent diabetes, the nonobese diabetic (NOD) mouse, has provided significant new insights (127). In NOD mice, vascular endothelium associated with inflamed islets expresses the MECA-79 antigen and MAdCAM-1 (52). Correspondingly, both L-selectin and $\alpha_4\beta_7$ integrin-dependent lymphocyte migration have been shown to be involved in the generation of disease in these mice (128,129). These studies highlight the important role of adhesion molecules, notably L-selectin, in the pathogenesis of diabetes.

Multiorgan failure is a near-certain consequence of the profound systemic hypotension associated with septic shock, and is characterized histopathologically by disseminated intravascular coagulation and end-organ leukocyte infiltration. Widespread E-selectin expression has been described within 6 hours of induction of septic shock in a baboon model (130). In human patients, soluble E-selectin levels were markedly elevated in the serum of bacteremic patients with hypotension, as compared to normotensive controls (34). These findings likely represent generalized organ hypoperfusion with consequent endothelial activation. In addition, a prominent role for L-selectin in the development of lethal septic shock is demonstrated by the extreme resistance of L-selectin–deficient mice to high-dose LPS treatment (76). This protection is likely the result of impaired leukocyte migration into multiple tissue sites, thereby preventing associated end-organ damage. Thus, L-selectin function, and possibly that of E-selectin, may influence mortality in septic shock.

Selectin-Directed Therapies

The inappropriate recruitment of leukocytes to specific sites is central to the pathogenesis of numerous inflammatory diseases. In view of this, therapies designed to disrupt leukocyte-endothelial interactions would be anticipated to slow the progression of inflammatory responses. A variety of selectin-targeted therapies have been developed and examined for their ability to reduce pathology in a number of in vivo models of inflammation.

Monoclonal antibody blockade of selectin function has proven to be an effective method of reducing leukocyte migration into sites of inflammation. Specifically, blocking leukocyte L-selectin function with antibodies alleviates the severity of injury and the degree of leukocyte infiltration in numerous models of ischemic and thermal injury (88,131–136) and attenuates insulitis in the NOD murine model of diabetes mellitus (128). Anti–P-selectin therapy has also been shown to attenuate ischemia/reperfusion injury associated with both localized ischemia and systemic shock (85,86,137), and to protect against complement-associated acute lung injury in a rat model (104). P-selectin function blockade also improves xenograft graft survival in a guinea pig–to-rat cardiac transplant model (95). Lastly, anti–E-selectin MAb treatment has been demonstrated to decrease bronchial neutrophil infiltration in a primate model of extrinsic allergic asthma (97).

As selectin-mediated leukocyte recruitment is central to the propagation of inflammation, it would follow that competitive inhibition of selectin-receptor binding would present therapeutic benefit. Several studies support this hypothesis. A soluble form of P-selectin has been shown to inhibit adhesion of cytokine-activated neutrophils to human vascular endothelial cells (138). In contrast, recombinant soluble E-selectin only weakly inhibits in vitro adhesion of myeloid cells to vascular endothelium (139). Chimeric selectin-IgG proteins have been effective in reducing inflammatory responses in several models. Specifically, an L-selectin/IgG fusion protein decreased neutrophil influx in response to peritoneal instillation of thioglycollate (140), and diminished both complement- and immune complex–associated acute lung injury in a dose-dependent manner (141). Similarly, P-selectin– and E-selectin–fusion proteins lessen cobra venom factor–induced and immune complex–mediated lung injury, respectively (141). Further studies to examine the therapeutic efficacy of such agents are warranted.

Therapies using oligosaccharide analogues of selectin ligands effectively attenuate inflammation. However, the pharmacokinetics of these agents remains unclear. The agents currently available bind the selectins with only modest affinity, dictating a need for high doses of the drug. Moreover, the in vivo half-lives of these agents are short, promoting speculation that their observed protective effects occur via mechanisms other than inhibition of selectin-mediated adhesion. Nonetheless, blocking L-selectin function with soluble carbohydrates has significant protective effects in tissues following ischemia and reperfusion in rats (88). An sLe^x-containing oligosaccharide reduces feline myocardial reperfusion injury (142), and sialylated oligosaccharides attenuate immune complex–mediated acute pulmonary injury in rats (143). In addition, heparin oligosaccharides that bind both L- and P-selectin in vitro as well as inositol polyanions effectively block neutrophil entry into the inflamed peritoneal cavity in mice (144,145). More recent work suggests that soluble PSGL-1 effectively prevents leukocyte infiltration and accompanying renal dysfunction in uninephrectomized rats subjected to renal ischemia, and thus may

have antiinflammatory properties (87). Although selectin ligand analogues represent promising antiinflammatory agents, further studies are needed to evaluate their efficacy and mode of action. Moreover, modification of existing oligosaccharide ligands may produce higher affinity reagents (146).

In response to inflammatory mediators, vascular endothelial cells upregulate adhesion receptor expression, thereby increasing their capacity to bind circulating leukocytes and thus promoting a more effective immune response. Upregulated E-selectin cell surface expression and, to some extent, that of P-selectin reflect enhanced transcription of the corresponding genes. Therefore, interfering with transcription of these genes may alleviate inflammation. This has been tested using antisense oligonucleotides. These molecules are synthetic oligonucleotides that hybridize to the mRNA of interest and subsequently inhibit protein expression. Although few reports exist concerning the application of this method to selectin expression, an antisense oligonucleotide that selectively recognizes E-selectin mRNA has been shown to decrease E-selectin expression in human vascular endothelial cells, resulting in a decreased ability to bind myeloid cells (147). Future work is required to determine the applicability of this approach to the other selectins and/or their ligands.

CONCLUSIONS

Leukocyte recruitment from the circulation into inflamed tissues is a dynamic process involving cooperative interactions among multiple families of adhesion receptors. Selectin interactions with their ligands are crucial for initial leukocyte capture from the bloodstream. Subsequently, selectin and integrin functions synergistically promote leukocyte rolling and firm adhesion to the venular endothelium. The entire process culminates in transmigration of the leukocyte across the endothelial layer, and entry into the injured tissue. Early events are regulated by multiple mechanisms, including rapid translocation of preformed P-selectin to the cell surface, increased selectin protein synthesis, expression of vascular ligands for L-selectin, activation-dependent changes in the avidity of L-selectin for its ligands, and rapid endoproteolytic release of L-selectin from the cell surface. Regulation of selectin ligand function occurs at the level of protein synthesis and differential carbohydrate decoration. The selectins and/or their ligands have been implicated in the pathogenesis of a myriad of clinical syndromes, both localized and systemic. Furthermore, selectin-neutralizing therapies have proven effective in a number of these diseases and disease models, including ischemia/reperfusion injury, diabetes mellitus, acute lung injury, graft rejection, and asthma. It is hoped that the rapid expansion of knowledge regarding selectin function, coupled with the identification of physiologically relevant ligands, will allow the development of specifically targeted therapeutics aimed at abrogating the leukocyte influx central to the pathogenesis of so many diseases.

ACKNOWLEDGMENTS

This work was supported by grants HL-50985, AI-26872, and CA-54464 from the National Institutes of Health. We thank members of our laboratory for review of the manuscript.

REFERENCES

1. Ley K, Tedder TF. Leukocyte interactions with vascular endothelium: new insights into selectin-mediated attachment and rolling. *J Immunol* 1995;155:525–528.
2. Tedder TF, Steeber DA, Chen A, Engel P. The selectins: vascular adhesion molecules. *FASEB J* 1995;9:866–873.
3. Steeber DA, Campbell MA, Basit A, Ley K, Tedder TF. Optimal selectin-mediated rolling of leukocytes during inflammation *in vivo* requires intercellular adhesion molecule-1 expression. *Proc Natl Acad Sci USA* 1998;95:7562–7567.
4. Springer TA. Traffic signals on endothelium for lymphocyte recirculation and leukocyte emigration. *Annu Rev Physiol* 1995;57:827–872.
5. Kansas GS, Spertini O, Stoolman LM, Tedder TF. Molecular mapping of functional domains of the leukocyte receptor for endothelium, LAM-1. *J Cell Biol* 1991;114:351–358.
6. Spertini O, Kansas GS, Reimann KA, Mackay CR, Tedder TF. Functional and evolutionary conservation of distinct epitopes on the leukocyte adhesion molecule-1 (LAM-1) that regulate leukocyte migration. *J Immunol* 1991;147:942–949.
7. Steeber DA, Engel P, Miller AS, Sheetz MP, Tedder TF. Ligation of L-selectin through conserved regions within the lectin domain activates signal transduction pathways and integrin function in human, mouse and rat leukocytes. *J Immunol* 1997;159:952–963.
8. Tu L, Chen A, Delahunty MD, et al. L-selectin binds to P-selectin glycoprotein ligand-1 on leukocytes. Interactions between the lectin, EGF and consensus repeat domains of the selectins determine ligand binding specificity. *J Immunol* 1996;156:3995–4004.
9. Siegelman MH, Cheng IC, Weissman IL, Wakeland EK. The mouse lymph node homing receptor is identical with the lymphocyte cell surface marker Ly-22: role of the EGF domain in endothelial binding. *Cell* 1990;61:611–622.
10. Kansas GS, Saunders KB, Ley K, et al. A role for the epidermal growth factor-like domain of P-selectin in ligand recognition and cell adhesion. *J Cell Biol* 1994;124:609–618.
11. Gibson RM, Kansas GS, Tedder TF, Furie B, Furie BC. Lectin and epidermal growth factor domains of P-selectin at physiological density are the recognition unit for leukocyte binding. *Blood* 1995;85:151–158.
12. Patel KD, Nollert MU, McEver RP. P-selectin must extend a sufficient length from the plasma membrane to mediate rolling of neutrophils. *J Cell Biol* 1995;131:8193–1902.
13. Li SH, Burns DK, Rumberger JM, et al. Consensus repeat domains of E-selectin enhance ligand binding. *J Biol Chem* 1994;269:4431–4437.
14. Tedder TF, Matsuyama T, Rothstein DM, Schlossman SF, Morimoto C. Human antigen-specific memory T cells express the homing receptor necessary for lymphocyte recirculation. *Eur J Immunol* 1990;20:1351–1355.
15. Griffin JD, Spertini O, Ernst TJ, et al. GM-CSF and other cytokines regulate surface expression of the leukocyte adhesion molecule-1 on human neutrophils, monocytes, and their precursors. *J Immunol* 1990;145:576–584.
16. Ord DC, Ernst TJ, Zhou LJ, et al. Structure of the gene encoding the human leukocyte adhesion molecule-1 (TQ1, Leu-8) of lymphocytes and neutrophils. *J Biol Chem* 1990;265:7760–7767.
17. Chen A, Engel P, Tedder TF. Structural requirements regulate endoproteolytic release of the L-selectin (CD62L) adhesion receptor from the cell surface of leukocytes. *J Exp Med* 1995;182:519–530.
18. Schleiffenbaum BE, Spertini O, Tedder TF. Soluble L-selectin is present in human plasma at high levels and retains functional activity. *J Cell Biol* 1992;119:229–238.
19. Allport JR, Ding HT, Ager A, Steeber DA, Tedder TF, Luscinskas FW. L-selectin shedding does not regulate human neutrophil attachment, rolling or transmigration across human vascular endothelium *in vitro*. *J Immunol* 1997;158:4365–4372.
20. Kansas GS, Ley K, Munro JM, Tedder TF. Regulation of leukocyte rolling and adhesion to HEV through the cytoplasm domain of L-selectin. *J Exp Med* 1993;177:833–838.
21. Spertini O, Kansas GS, Munro JM, Griffin JD, Tedder TF. Regulation of leukocyte migration by activation of the leukocyte adhesion molecule-1 (LAM-1) selectin. *Nature* 1991;349:691–694.
22. Haribabu B, Steeber DA, Ali H, Richardson RM, Snyderman R, Tedder TF. Chemoattractant receptor-induced phosphorylation of L-selectin. *J Biol Chem* 1997;272:13961–13965.
23. Johnston GI, Kurosky A, McEver RP. Structural and biosynthetic studies of the granule membrane protein, GMP-140, from human platelets and endothelial cells. *J Biol Chem* 1989;264:1816–1823.
24. Johnston GI, Cook RG, McEver RP. Cloning of GMP-140, a granule membrane protein of platelets and endothelium: sequence similarity to proteins involved in cell adhesion and inflammation. *Cell* 1989;56:1033–1044.
25. Ushiyama S, Laue TM, Moore KL, Erickson HP, McEver RP. Structural and functional characterization of monomeric soluble P-selectin and comparison with membrane P-selectin. *J Biol Chem* 1993;268:15229–15237.
26. Dunlop LC, Skinner MP, Bendall LJ, et al. Characterization of GMP-140 (P-selectin) as a circulating plasma protein. *J Exp Med* 1992;175:1147–1150.
27. Fujimoto T, McEver RP. The cytoplasmic domain of P-selectin is phosphorylated on serine and threonine residues. *Blood* 1993;82:1758–1766.
28. Crovello CS, Furie BC, Furie B. Rapid phosphorylation and selective dephosphorylation of P-selectin accompanies platelet activation. *J Biol Chem* 1993;268:14590–14593.
29. Crovello CS, Furie BC, Furie B. Histidine phosphorylation of P-selectin upon stimulation of human platelets: a novel pathway for activation-dependent signal transduction. *Cell* 1995;82:279–286.
30. Kansas GS, Pavalko FM. The cytoplasmic domain of E- and P-selectin do not constitutively interact with α-actinin and are not essential for leukocyte adhesion. *J Immunol* 1996;157:321–325.
31. Bevilacqua MP, Pober JS, Mendrick DL, Cotran RS, Gimbrone MA Jr. Identification of an inducible endothelial-leukocyte adhesion molecule. *Proc Natl Acad Sci USA* 1987;84:9238–9243.
32. Smeets EF, de Vries T, Leeuwenberg JFM, van den Eijnden DH, Buurman WA, Neefjes JJ. Phosphorylation of surface E-selectin and the effect of soluble ligand (sialyl Lewis^x) on the half-life of E-selectin. *Eur J Immunol* 1993;23:147–151.
33. Yoshida M, Szente BE, Kiely J-M, Rosenzweig A, Gimbrone MA Jr. Phosphorylation of the cytoplasmic domain of E-selectin is regulated during leukocyte-endothelial adhesion. *J Immunol* 1998;16:933–941.
34. Newman W, Beall LD, Carson CW, et al. Soluble E-selectin is found in supernatants of activated endothelial cells and is elevated in the serum of patients with septic shock. *J Immunol* 1993;150:644–654.
35. Leeuwenberg JFM, Smeets EF, Neefjes JJ, et al. E-selectin and intercellular adhesion molecule-1 are released by activated human endothelial cells *in vitro*. *Immunology* 1992;77:543–549.
36. Gallatin WM, Weissman IL, Butcher EC. A cell-surface molecule involved in organ-specific homing of lymphocytes. *Nature* 1983;304:30–34.
37. Tedder TF, Penta AC, Levine HB, Freedman AS. Expression of the human leukocyte adhesion molecule, LAM1. Identity with the TQ1 and Leu-8 differentiation antigens. *J Immunol* 1990;144:532–540.
38. Tang MLK, Steeber DA, Zhang XQ, Tedder TF. Intrinsic differences in L-selectin expression levels affect T and B lymphocyte subset-specific recirculation pathways. *J Immunol* 1998;160:5113–5121.
39. Steeber DA, Green NE, Sato S, Tedder TF. Lymphocyte migration in L-selectin–deficient mice: altered subset migration and aging of the immune system. *J Immunol* 1996;157:1096–1106.
40. McEver RP, Beckstead JH, Moore KL, Marshal-Carlson L, Bainton DF. GMP-140, a platelet alpha granule membrane protein, is also synthesized by vascular endothelial cells and is localized in Weibel-Palade bodies. *J Clin Invest* 1989;84:92–99.

41. Ley KE, Bullard D, Arbones ML, et al. Sequential contribution of L- and P-selectin to leukocyte rolling *in vivo*. *J Exp Med* 1995;181:669–675.

42. Bevilacqua MP, Stengelin S, Gimbrone MA Jr, Seed B. Endothelial leukocyte adhesion molecule 1: an inducible receptor for neutrophils related to complement regulatory proteins and lectins. *Science* 1989;243:1160–1164.

43. Keelan ET, Licence ST, Peters AM, Binns RM, Haskard DO. Characterization of E-selectin expression *in vivo* with use of a radiolabeled monoclonal antibody. *Am J Physiol* 1994;266:H278–290.

44. Silber A, Newman W, Reimann KA, Hendricks E, Walsh D, Ringler DJ. Kinetic expression of endothelial adhesion molecules and relationship to leukocyte recruitment in two cutaneous models of inflammation. *Lab Invest* 1994;70:163–175.

45. Petzelbauer P, Bender JR, Wilson J, Pober JS. Heterogeneity of dermal microvascular endothelial cell antigen expression and cytokine responsiveness *in situ* and in cell culture. *J Immunol* 1993;151:5062–5072.

46. Rosen SD, Bertozzi CR. The selectins and their ligands. *Curr Opin Cell Biol* 1994;6:663–673.

47. Streeter PR, Berg EL, Rouse BN, Bargatze RF, Butcher EC. A tissue-specific endothelial cell molecule involved in lymphocyte homing. *Nature* 1988;331:41–46.

48. Lowe JB. Selectin ligands, leukocyte trafficking, and fucosyltransferase genes. *Kidney Int* 1997;51:1418–1426.

49. Streeter PR, Rouse BTN, Butcher EC. Immunologic and functional characterization of a vascular addressin involved in lymphocyte homing into peripheral lymph nodes. *J Cell Biol* 1988;107:1853–1862.

50. Hemmerich S, Butcher EC, Rosen SD. Sulfation-dependent recognition of HEV-ligands by L-selectin and MECA 79, an adhesion-blocking mAb. *J Exp Med* 1994;180:2219–2226.

51. Berg EL, Robinson MK, Warnock RA, Butcher EC. The human peripheral lymph node vascular addressin is a ligand for LECAM-1, the peripheral lymph node homing receptor. *J Cell Biol* 1991;114:343–349.

52. Hanninen A, Taylor C, Streeter PR, et al. Vascular addressins are induced on islet vessels during insulitis in nonobese diabetic mice and are involved in lymphoid binding to islet endothelium. *J Clin Invest* 1993;92:2509–2515.

53. Michie SA, Streeter PR, Bolt PA, Butcher EC, Picker LJ. The human peripheral lymph node vascular addressin. An inducible endothelial antigen involved in lymphocyte homing. *Am J Pathol* 1993;143:1688–1698.

54. Maly P, Thall AD, Petryniak B, et al. The α(1,3) fucosyltransferase Fuc-TVII controls leukocyte trafficking through an essential role in L-, E-, and P-selectin ligand biosynthesis. *Cell* 1996;86:643–653.

55. Guyer DA, Moore KL, Lynam EB, et al. P-selectin glycoprotein ligand-1 (PSGL-1) is a ligand for L-selectin in neutrophil aggregation. *Blood* 1996;88:2415–2421.

56. Walcheck B, Moore KL, McEver RP, Kishimoto TK. Neutrophil-neutrophil interactions under hydrodynamic shear stress involve L-selectin and PSGL-1. A mechanism that amplifies initial leukocyte accumulation on P-selectin *in vitro*. *J Clin Invest* 1996;98:1081–1087.

57. Spertini O, Luscinskas FW, Kansas GS, et al. Leukocyte adhesion molecule-1 (LAM-1, L-selectin) interacts with an inducible endothelial cell ligand to support leukocyte adhesion. *J Immunol* 1991;147:2565–2573.

58. Spertini O, Luscinskas FW, Gimbrone MA Jr, Tedder TF. Monocyte attachment to activated human vascular endothelium *in vitro* is mediated by Leukocyte Adhesion Molecule-1 (L-selectin) under non-static conditions. *J Exp Med* 1992;175:1789–1792.

59. Brady HR, Spertini O, Jimenez W, Brenner BM, Marsden PA, Tedder TF. Neutrophils, monocytes and lymphocytes bind to cytokine-activated kidney glomerular endothelial cells through L-selectin (LAM-1) *in vitro*. *J Immunol* 1992;149:2437–2444.

60. Sawada M, Takada A, Ohwaki I, et al. Specific expression of a complex sialyl Lewis X antigen on high endothelial venules of human lymph nodes: possible candidate for L-selectin ligand. *Biochem Biophys Res Commun* 1993;193:337–347.

61. Mitsuoka C, Kawakami-Kimura N, Kasugai-Sawada M, et al. Sulfated sialyl Lewis X, the putative L-selectin ligand, detected on endothelial cells of high endothelial venules by a distinct set of anti-sialyl Lewis X antibodies. *Biochem Biophys Res Commun* 1997;230:546–551.

62. Akahori T, Yuzawa Y, Nishikawa K, et al. Role of a sialyl Lewis[x]-like epitope selectively expressed on vascular endothelial cells in local skin inflammation of the rat. *J Immunol* 1997;158:5384–5392.

63. Moore KL, Patel KD, Breuhl RE, et al. P-selectin glycoprotein ligand-1 mediates rolling of human neutrophils on P-selectin. *J Cell Biol* 1995;128:661–671.

64. Norman KE, Moore KL, McEver RP, Ley K. Leukocyte rolling *in vivo* is mediated by P-selectin glycoprotein ligand-1. *Blood* 1996;86:4417–4421.

65. Asa D, Raycroft L, Ma L, et al. The P-selectin glycoprotein ligand functions as a common human leukocyte ligand for P- and E-selectins. *J Biol Chem* 1995;270:11662–11672.

66. Picker LJ, Treer JR, Ferguson DB, Collins PA, Bergstresser PR, Terstappen LWNN. Control of lymphocyte recirculation in man. Differential regulation of the cutaneous lymphocyte-associated antigen, a tissue-selective homing receptor for skin-homing T cells. *J Immunol* 1993;150:1122–1136.

67. Fuhlbrigge RC, Kieffer JD, Armerding D, Kupper TS. Cutaneous lymphocyte antigen is a specialized form of PSGL-1 expressed on skin-homing T cells. *Nature* 1997;389:978–981.

68. Walcheck B, Watts G, Jutila MA. Bovine γδ T cells bind E-selectin via a novel glycoprotein receptor: first characterization of a lymphocyte/E-selectin interaction in an animal model. *J Exp Med* 1993;178:853–863.

69. Levinovitz A, Muhlhoff J, Isenmann S, Vestweber D. Identification of a glycoprotein ligand for E-selectin on mouse myeloid cells. *J Cell Biol* 1993;121:449–459.

70. Steegmaler M, Levinovitz A, Isenmann S, et al. The E-selectin-ligand ESL-1 is a variant of a receptor for fibroblast growth factor. *Nature* 1995;373:615–620.

71. Lenter M, Levinovitz S, Isenmann S, Vestweber D. Monospecific and common glycoprotein ligands for E- and P-selectin on myeloid cells. *J Cell Biol* 1994;125:471–481.

72. Mayadas TN, Johnson RC, Rayburn H, Hynes RO, Wagner DD. Leukocyte rolling and extravasation are severely compromised in P selectin–deficient mice. *Cell* 1993;74:541–554.

73. Arbones ML, Ord DC, Ley K, et al. Lymphocyte homing and leukocyte rolling and migration are impaired in L-selectin (CD62L) deficient mice. *Immunity* 1994;1:247–260.

74. Labow MA, Norton CR, Rumberger JM, et al. Characterization of E-selectin–deficient mice: demonstration of overlapping function of the endothelial selectins. *Immunity* 1994;1:709–720.

75. Kunkel EJ, Ley K. Distinct phenotype of E-selectin–deficient mice. E-selectin is required for slow leukocyte rolling *in vivo*. *Circ Res* 1996;79:1196–1204.

76. Tedder TF, Steeber DA, Pizcueta P. L-selectin deficient mice have impaired leukocyte recruitment into inflammatory sites. *J Exp Med* 1995;181:2259–2264.

77. Tang MLK, Hale LP, Steeber DA, Tedder TF. L-selectin is involved in lymphocyte migration to sites of inflammation in the skin: delayed rejection of allografts in L-selectin–deficient mice. *J Immunol* 1997;158:5191–5199.

78. Johnson RC, Mayadas TN, Frenette PS, et al. Blood cell dynamics in P-selectin–deficient mice. *Blood* 1995;86:1106–1114.

79. Subramaniam M, Saffaripour S, Watson SR, Mayadas TN, Hynes RO, Wagner DD. Reduced recruitment of inflammatory cells in a contact hypersensitivity response in P-selectin–deficient mice. *J Exp Med* 1995;181:2277–2282.

80. Staite ND, Justen JM, Sly LM, Beaudet AL, Bullard DC. Inhibition of delayed-type contact hypersensitivity in mice deficient in both E-selectin and P-selectin. *Blood* 1996;88:2973–2979.

81. Silber A, Newman W, Sasseville VG, et al. Recruitment of lymphocytes during cutaneous delayed hypersensitivity in nonhuman primates is dependent on E-selectin and vascular cell adhesion molecule 1. *J Clin Invest* 1994;93:1554–1563.

82. Mulligan MS, Varani J, Dame MK, et al. Role of endothelial-leukocyte adhesion molecule (ELAM-1) in neutrophil-mediated lung injury in rats. *J Clin Invest* 1991;88:1396–1406.

83. Milstone DS, Fukumura D, Padgett RC, et al. Mice lacking E-selectin show normal numbers of rolling leukocytes but reduced leukocyte stable arrest on cytokine-activated microvascular endothelium. (Submitted).

84. von Andrian UH, Berger EM, Ramezani L, et al. *In vivo* behavior of neutrophils from two patients with distinct inherited leukocyte adhesion deficiency syndromes. *J Clin Invest* 1993;91:2893–2897.

85. Weyrich AS, Ma X-L, Lefer DJ, Albertine KH, Lefer AM. *In vivo* neutralization of P-selectin protects feline heart and endothelium in

myocardial ischemia and reperfusion injury. *J Clin Invest* 1993;91: 2620–2629.

86. Winn RK, Liggitt D, Vedder NB, Paulson JC, Harlan JM. Anti-P-selectin monoclonal antibody attenuates reperfusion injury to the rabbit ear. *J Clin Invest* 1993;92:2042–2047.

87. Takada M, Nadeau KC, Shaw GD, Marquette KA, Tilney NL. The cytokine-adhesion molecule cascade in ischemia/reperfusion injury of the rat kidney. Inhibition by a soluble P-selectin ligand. *J Clin Invest* 1997;99:2682–2690.

88. Seekamp A, Till GO, Mulligan MS, et al. Role of selectins in local and remote tissue injury following ischemia and reperfusion. *Am J Pathol* 1994;144:592–598.

89. Fuggle SV, Sanderson JB, Gray DWR, Richardson A, Morris PJ. Variation in expression of endothelial adhesion molecules in pretransplant and transplanted kidneys—correlation with intragraft events. *Transplantation* 1993;55:117–123.

90. Brockmeyer C, Ulbrecht M, Schendel DJ, et al. Distribution of cell adhesion molecules (ICAM-1, VCAM-1, ELAM-1) in renal tissue during allograft rejection. *Transplantation* 1993;55:610–615.

91. Brady HR. Leukocyte adhesion molecules and kidney diseases. *Kidney Int* 1994;45:1285–1300.

92. Briscoe DM, Yeung AC, Schoen EL, et al. Predictive value of inducible endothelial cell adhesion molecule expression for acute rejection of human cardiac allografts. *Transplantation* 1995;59: 204–211.

93. Turunen JP, Paavonen T, Majuri M-L, et al. Sialyl Lewis(x) and L-selectin–dependent site-specific lymphocyte extravasation into renal transplants during acute rejection. *Eur J Immunol* 1994;24: 1130–1136.

94. Blakely ML, Van der Werf WJ, Berndt MC, Dalmasso AP, Bach FH, Hancock WW. Activation of intragraft endothelial and mononuclear cells during discordant xenograft rejection. *Transplantation* 1994;58: 1059–1066.

95. Coughlan AF, Berndt MC, Dunlop LC, Hancock WW. *In vivo* studies of P-selectin and platelet activating factor during endotoxemia, accelerated allograft rejection, and discordant xenograft rejection. *Transplant Proc* 1993;25:2930–2931.

96. Robinson LA, Tu LL, Steeber DA, Preis O, Platt JL, Tedder TF. The role of adhesion molecules in human leukocyte attachment to porcine vascular endothelium: implications for xenotransplantation. *J Immunol* 1998 (in press).

97. Gundel RH, Wegner CD, Torcellini C, et al. Endothelial leukocyte adhesion molecule-1 mediates antigen-induced acute airway inflammation and late-phase airway obstruction in monkeys. *J Clin Invest* 1991;88:1407–1411.

98. Gosset P, Tillie-Leblond I, Janin A, et al. Expression of E-selectin, ICAM-1 and VCAM-1 on bronchial biopsies from allergic and non-allergic asthmatic patients. *Int Arch Allergy Immunol* 1995;106:69–77.

99. Montefort S, Gratziou C, Goulding D, et al. Bronchial biopsy evidence for leukocyte infiltration and upregulation of leukocyte-endothelial cell adhesion molecules 6 hours after local allergen challenge of sensitized asthmatic airways. *J Clin Invest* 1994;93: 1411–1421.

100. Mengelers HJ, Maikoe T, Brinkman L, Hooibrink B, Lammers JW, Koenderman L. Immunophenotyping of eosinophils recovered from blood and BAL of allergic asthmatics. *Am J Respir Crit Care Med* 1994;149:345–351.

101. Montefort S, Lai CK, Kapahi P, et al. Circulating adhesion molecules in asthma. *Am J Respir Crit Care Med* 1994;149:1149–1152.

102. Kobayashi T, Hashimoto S, Imai K, et al. Elevation of serum soluble intercellular adhesion molecule-1 (sICAM-1) and sE-selectin levels in bronchial asthma. *Clin Exp Immunol* 1994;96:110–115.

103. Georas SN, Liu MC, Newman W, Beall LD, Stealey BA, Bochner BS. Altered adhesion molecule expression and endothelial cell activation accompany the recruitment of human granulocytes to the lung after segmental antigen challenge. *Am J Respir Cell Mol Biol* 1992;7: 261–269.

104. Mulligan MS, Polley MJ, Bayer RJ, Nunn MF, Paulson JC, Ward PA. Neutrophil dependent acute lung injury. Requirement for P-selectin. *J Clin Invest* 1992;90:1600–1607.

105. Neumann B, Engelhardt B, Wagner H, Holzmann B. Induction of acute inflammatory lung injury by staphylococcal enterotoxin B. *J Immunol* 1997;158:1862–1871.

106. Doyle NA, Bhagwan SD, Meek BB, et al. Neutrophil margination, sequestration, and emigration in the lungs of L-selectin–deficient mice. *J Clin Invest* 1997;99:526–533.

107. Donnelly SC, Haslett C, Dransfield I, et al. Role of selectins in development of adult respiratory distress syndrome. *Lancet* 1994;344: 215–219.

108. Groves RW, Allen MH, Barker JN, Haskard DO, MacDonald DM. Endothelial leukocyte adhesion molecule-1 (ELAM-1) expression in cutaneous inflammation. *Br J Dermatol* 1991;124:117–123.

109. Kyan-Aung U, Haskard DO, Poston RN, Thornhill MT, Lee TH. Endothelial leukocyte adhesion molecule-1 and intercellular adhesion molecule-1 mediate the adhesion of eosinophils to endothelial cells *in vitro* and are expressed by endothelium in allergic cutaneous inflammation *in vivo*. *J Immunol* 1991;146:521–528.

110. Czech W, Schopf E, Kapp A. Soluble E-selectin in sera of patients with atopic dermatitis and psoriasis- correlation with disease activity. *Br J Dermatol* 1996;134:17–21.

111. Cronstein BN. Adhesion molecules in the pathogenesis of rheumatoid arthritis. *Curr Opin Rheumatol* 1994;6:300–304.

112. Szekanecz Z, Szegedi G, Koch AE. Cellular adhesion molecules in rheumatoid arthritis: regulation by cytokines and possible clinical importance. *J Invest Med* 1996;44:124–135.

113. Grober JS, Bowen BL, Ebling H, et al. Monocyte-endothelial adhesion in chronic rheumatoid arthritis. *In situ* detection of selectin and integrin-dependent interactions. *J Clin Invest* 1993;91:2609–2619.

114. McMurray RW. Adhesion molecules in autoimmune disease. *Semin Arthritis Rheum* 1996;25:215–233.

115. To SS, Newman PM, Hyland VJ, Robinson BG, Schrieber L. Regulation of adhesion molecule expression by human synovial microvascular endothelial cells *in vitro*. *Arthritis Rheum* 1996;39:467–477.

116. Tak PP, Taylor PC, Breedveld FC, et al. Decrease in cellularity and expression of adhesion molecules by anti-tumor necrosis factor alpha monoclonal antibody treatment in patients with rheumatoid arthritis. *Arthritis Rheum* 1996;39:1077–1081.

117. Kriegsman J, Keyszer GM, Geiler T, et al. Expression of E-selectin messenger RNA and protein in rheumatoid arthritis. *Arthritis Rheum* 1995;38:750–754.

118. Youssef PP, Triantafillou S, Parker A, et al. Effects of pulse methylprednisolone on cell adhesion molecules in the synovial membrane in rheumatoid arthritis. *Arthritis Rheum* 1996;39:1970–1979.

119. Corkill MM, Kirkham BW, Haskard DO, Barbatis C, Gibson T, Panayi GS. Gold treatment of rheumatoid arthritis decreases synovial expression of the endothelial leukocyte adhesion receptor ELAM-1. *J Rheumatol* 1991;18:1453–1460.

120. Takeda I, Kaise S, Nishimaki T, Kasukawa R. Soluble P-selectin in the plasma of patients with connective tissue diseases. *Int Arch Allergy Immunol* 1994;105:128–134.

121. Littler AJ, Buckley CD, Wordsworth P, Collins I, Martinson J, Simmons DL. A distinct profile of six soluble adhesion molecules (ICAM-1, ICAM-3, VCAM-1, E-selectin, L-selectin and P-selectin) in rheumatoid arthritis. *Br J Rheumatol* 1997;36:164–169.

122. Paleolog EM, Hunt M, Elliott MJ, Feldmann M, Maini RN, Woody JN. Deactivation of vascular endothelium by monoclonal anti-tumor necrosis factor α antibody in rheumatoid arthritis. *Arthritis Rheum* 1996;39:1082–1091.

123. Chan TM, Yu PM, Cheng IK. Endothelial cell binding by human polyclonal anti-DNA antibodies: relationship to disease activity and endothelial functional alterations. *Clin Exp Immunol* 1995;100:506–513.

124. Pallis M, Robson DK, Haskard DO, Powell RJ. Distribution of cell adhesion molecules in skeletal muscle from patients with systemic lupus erythematosus. *Ann Rheum Dis* 1993;52:667–671.

125. Belmont HM, Buyon J, Giorno R, Abramson S. Up-regulation of endothelial cell adhesion molecules characterizes disease activity in systemic lupus erythematosus. The Shwartzman phenomenon revisited. *Arthritis Rheum* 1994;37:376–383.

126. Bruijn JA, Dinklo NJCM. Distinct patterns of expression of intercellular adhesion molecule-1, vascular cell adhesion molecule-1, and endothelial-leukocyte adhesion molecule-1 in renal disease. *Lab Invest* 1993;69:329–335.

127. Tisch R, McDevitt H. Insulin-dependent diabetes mellitus. *Cell* 1996; 85:291–297.

128. Yang X-D, Karin N, Tisch R, Steinman L, McDevitt HO. Inhibition of insulitis and prevention of diabetes in nonobese diabetic mice by blocking L-selectin and very late antigen 4 adhesion receptors. *Proc Natl Acad Sci USA* 1993;90:10494–10498.

129. Yang X-D, Michie SA, Tisch R, Karin N, Steinman L, McDevitt HO. A predominant role of integrin α4 in the spontaneous development of autoimmune diabetes in nonobese diabetic mice. *Proc Natl Acad Sci USA* 1994;91:12604–12608.

130. Drake TA, Cheng J, Chang A, Taylor FB Jr. Expression of tissue factor, thrombomodulin, and E-selectin in baboons with lethal *Escherichia coli* sepsis. *Am J Pathol* 1993;142:1458–1470.

131. Ramamoorthy C, Sharar SR, Harlan JM, Tedder TF, Winn RK. Blocking L-selectin function attenuates reperfusion injury following hemorrhagic shock in rabbits. *Am J Physiol* 1996;271:H1871–H1877.

132. Mihelcic D, Schleiffenbaum B, Tedder TF, Harlan JM, Winn RK. Inhibition of leukocyte L-selectin function with a monoclonal antibody attenuates reperfusion injury to the rabbit ear. *Blood* 1994;84:2322–2328.

133. Kurose I, Anderson DC, Miyasaka M, et al. Molecular determinants of reperfusion-induced leukocyte adhesion and vascular protein leakage. *Circ Res* 1994;74:336–343.

134. Ma X-L, Weyrich AS, Lefer DJ, Buerke M, Albertine KH, Kishimoto TK, Lefer AM. Monoclonal antibody to L-selectin attenuates neutrophil accumulation and protects ischemic reperfused cat myocardium. *Circulation* 1993;88:649–658.

135. Buerke M, Weyrich AS, Murohara T, et al. Humanized monoclonal antibody DREG-200 directed against L-selectin protects in feline myocardial reperfusion injury. *J Pharmacol Exp Ther* 1994;271:134–142.

136. Mulligan MS, Till GO, Smith CW, et al. Role of leukocyte adhesion molecules in lung and dermal vascular injury after thermal trauma of skin. *Am J Pathol* 1994;144:1008–1015.

137. Winn RK, Paulson JC, Harlan JM. A monoclonal antibody to P-selectin ameliorates injury associated with hemorrhagic shock in rabbits. *Am J Physiol* 1994;267:H2391–H2397.

138. Gamble JR, Skinner MP, Berndt MC, Vadas MA. Prevention of activated neutrophil adhesion to endothelium by soluble adhesion protein GMP-140. *Science* 1990;249:414–417.

139. Lobb RR, Chi-Rosso G, Leone DR, et al. Expression and functional characterization of a soluble form of endothelial-leukocyte adhesion molecule 1. *J Immunol* 1991;147:124–129.

140. Watson SR, Fennie C, Lasky LA. Neutrophil influx into an inflammatory site inhibited by a soluble homing receptor-IgG chimera. *Nature* 1991;349:164–167.

141. Mulligan MS, Watson SR, Fennie C, Ward PA. Protective effects of selectin chimeras in neutrophil-mediated lung injury. *J Immunol* 1993;151:6410–6417.

142. Buerke M, Weyrich AS, Zheng Z, Gaeta FCA, Forrest MJ, Lefer AM. Sialyl Lewis^x-containing oligosaccharide attenuates myocardial reperfusion injury in cats. *J Clin Invest* 1994;93:1140–1148.

143. Mulligan MS, Paulson JC, De Frees S, Zheng Z-L, Lowe JB, Ward PA. Protective effects of oligosaccharides in P-selectin–dependent lung injury. *Nature* 1993;364:149–151.

144. Nelson RM, Ceccioni O, Roberts WG, Aruffo A, Linhardt RJ, Bevilacqua MP. Heparin oligosaccharides bind L- and P-selectin and inhibit acute inflammation. *Blood* 1993;82:3253–3258.

145. Cecconi O, Nelson RM, Roberts WG, et al. Inositol polyanions. Noncarbohydrate inhibitors of L- and P-selectin that block inflammation. *J Biol Chem* 1994;269:15060–15066.

146. Nelson RM, Dolich S, Aruffo A, Cecconi O, Bevilacqua MP. Higher-affinity oligosaccharide ligands for E-selectin. *J Clin Invest* 1993;91:1157–1166.

147. Bennett CF, Condon TP, Grimm S, Chan H, Chiang M. Inhibition of endothelial adhesion molecule expression with antisense oligonucleotides. *J Immunol* 1993;152:3530–3540.

Inflammation: Basic Principles and Clinical Correlates,
3rd ed., edited by John I. Gallin and Ralph Snyderman.
Lippincott Williams & Wilkins, Philadelphia © 1999.

CHAPTER 39

Leukocyte-Endothelial Cell Adhesion Molecules in Transendothelial Migration

William A. Muller

LEUKOCYTE EMIGRATION INVOLVES A COORDINATED SERIES OF ADHESIVE EVENTS

When leukocytes are recruited to a site of inflammation, a stereotyped series of adhesion events appears to mediate their emigration from blood to tissues. These sequential events—rolling, activation, adhesion, and transendothelial migration—occur regardless of the inflammatory stimulus and the type of leukocyte being recruited. However, the stereotyped behavior belies a highly selective and specific process. In humans, neutrophils [polymorphonuclear cells (PMNs)] appear within hours at sites of acute inflammation such as bacterial infection and tissue necrosis, but are conspicuously absent from the infiltrate in a delayed-type hypersensitivity reaction. Eosinophils are selectively recruited into the bronchial soft tissue in asthmatics, despite the fact that eosinophils make up a minor population of the circulating leukocytes.

The actual adhesion molecules that carry out the adhesion may differ according to the inflammatory stimulus, the type of leukocyte being recruited, and perhaps the location in the body, but in general those mediating each separate step are members of a common cell adhesion molecule (CAM) family. This sequence of events is completed within seconds *in vivo* as well as in some *in vitro* models.

The process of leukocyte emigration has been dissected into a series of sequential adhesion events in the following working model (Fig. 39-1): In the first step, some of the leukocytes entering a postcapillary venule in an area of inflammation leave the circulatory stream, and adhere loosely, tentatively, and reversibly to the endothelial cell surfaces in a process aptly named "rolling." The selectin family of adhesion molecules and their sialylated-Lewis[x]–decorated ligands appear to be primarily responsible for this initial interaction (reviewed in refs. 1,2; see Chapter 38). Rolling leukocytes come into direct contact with the endothelium, exposing them to a variety of signals capable of promoting the next step—activating the leukocyte-specific integrins (see Chapter 37). The binding of leukocytes to E-selectin itself may be a sufficient signal (3). Alternatively or additionally, the leukocytes tethered by selectins are now in a position to be activated by platelet-activating factor (4) or other lipid modulators (5), chemokines bound to endothelial surface glycosaminoglycans (6), soluble chemoattractants (7), or ligands that cross-link leukocyte CD31 (8–10).

Upon activation of their integrins to the high-affinity binding state, leukocytes cease rolling and adhere tightly to the endothelial surface. For monocytes and lymphocytes, which express integrins of both the β_1 and β_2 families, engagement by either integrin may suffice to promote attachment for subsequent transmigration (11). The identified counterreceptors for β_1 and β_2 integrin-mediated adhesion include intracellular adhesion molecule-1 (ICAM-1), ICAM-2, and vascular cell adhesion molecule-1 (VCAM-1), members of the immunoglobulin gene superfamily. Leukocytes bound tightly to the luminal surface of the endothelial cell crawl rapidly to an intercellular junction, a process that requires successive cycles of adhesion and disadhesion, as the leukocytes attach at their forward ends and release at their rear. Upon reaching the junction, they insert pseudopods between tightly apposed endothelial cells and crawl through, in ameboid fashion, while retaining tight contacts with the endothelial cell. This step is referred to as transendothelial migration, or transmigration. Platelet endothelial cell adhesion

W. A. Muller: Department of Pathology and the Center for Vascular Biology, Weill Medical College of Cornell University, New York, New York 10021.

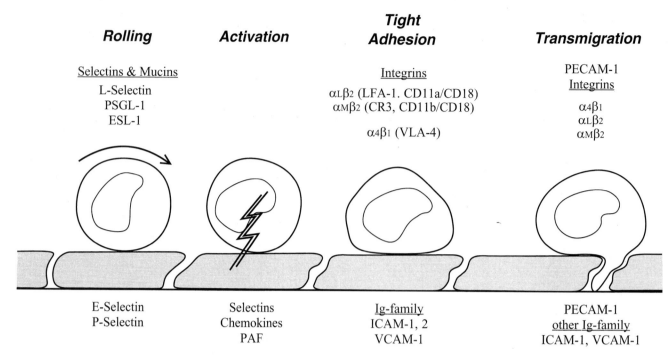

FIG. 39-1. Leukocyte emigration is molecularly dissectable into distinct steps involving sequential interactions of different families of adhesion molecules on the leukocyte and endothelial cell. Some of the leukocyte adhesion molecules implicated in these steps are printed above the leukocytes, while those involved on the endothelial side are printed below the endothelial cells (shaded). The rolling step involves interaction between members of the selectin family of adhesion molecules and their sialylated Lewis^x-bearing ligands, some of which are on defined proteins that have been identified [P-selectin glycoprotein ligand-1 (PSGL-1), E-selectin ligand-1 (ESL-1)]. Leukocytes rolling along the endothelium are in a position to have their integrins activated by a variety of stimuli presented by the endothelial cell. Activation of integrins is followed rapidly by tight adhesion to the apical surface of the endothelial cell. This adhesion depends on leukocyte integrins of the β_2 family as well as $\alpha_4\beta_1$. Where the counterreceptors for this adhesion have been identified, they are members of the immunoglobulin gene superfamily. Adhesion must be reversible, as the leukocytes crawl over the endothelium to an intercellular border. Transmigration involves the squeezing of leukocytes in ameboid fashion between tightly apposed endothelial cells. This step is sometimes referred to as diapedesis. Platelet endothelial cell adhesion molecule-1 (PECAM-1) on both leukocytes and endothelium plays a crucial role in this process. There is evidence that the leukocyte integrins and their counterreceptors are involved, as well. (From ref. 65, with permission.)

molecule-1 (PECAM, also known as CD31), a CAM of the immunoglobulin superfamily, expressed on the surfaces of leukocytes and platelets and concentrated in the borders between endothelial cells is involved in this step. Contact between leukocyte PECAM and endothelial PECAM is crucial for the transmigration of the vast majority of neutrophils and monocytes *in vitro* (12) and *in vivo* (13,14). There is experimental evidence that leukocyte integrins and their endothelial cell counterreceptors are involved in this process as well.

We can divide leukocyte emigration into these steps because we have reagents that can block each one of these steps. There may be additional adhesion molecules awaiting discovery that interact at steps intermediate to or distal to these. Several investigators can block monocyte adhesion/transmigration almost completely with antibodies against CD11/CD18 and $\alpha_4\beta_1$, but incompletely even

with combinations of antibodies against the endothelial cell ICAMs and VCAM-1 (15,16). This suggests that there is at least one additional counterreceptor for leukocyte integrins on the endothelial cell.

The scenario above is compelling and in general has been borne out by *in vivo* studies in several species. However, leukocyte emigration is unlikely to be so simply regulated. In fact, several exceptions and additions have already been identified. For example, under some conditions *in vitro*, the leukocyte $\alpha_4\beta_1$ can mediate rolling (17). When monocyte CD11/CD18 is blocked, $\alpha_4\beta_1$ allows arrest of monocytes on the surface of interleukin-4 (IL-4)–activated endothelial cells, but does not promote spreading and migration of the monocytes (18). As will be discussed in detail below, there is evidence that molecules other than PECAM may be involved in transendothelial migration.

There are numerous *in vivo* examples of exceptions to these rules. Although the vast majority of transmigration appears to involve leukocytes passing through the interendothelial junctions (19), there may be situations in which leukocytes enter the inflamed tissues by moving *through* the endothelial cells rather than *between* them (20–22).

Migration of leukocytes to sites of inflammation in the lung may use alternative molecules. One oft-cited example is a patient with leukocyte adhesion deficiency (LAD) type I syndrome who died with overwhelming bacterial infections (23). Despite a massive granulocytosis, the patient's neutrophils, which lacked β_2 (CD18) integrins, could not emigrate to sites of infection. At autopsy, overwhelming bacterial growth was found in his skin and most other organs. However, his lungs showed typical bronchopneumonia—an appropriate neutrophil response.

Doerschuk et al. (24) have demonstrated in several animal models that although CD18-dependent migration in response to bacterial infection is the rule in many/most vascular beds, response to *Streptococcus pneumoniae* in the lung is CD18 independent. This may be because in contrast to other sites of inflammation where diapedesis takes place across postcapillary venules, in the lung PMNs cross capillaries. Not only are the vessels of a different phenotype, but the rheologic characteristics of the lung may be very different. The pulmonary capillaries are narrow and poorly deformable. These physical barriers may serve to slow and stop leukocytes, making them less dependent on cell adhesion molecules to mediate these processes.

There may be other factors at work here, however. LAD patients and adhesion molecule knock-out mice have demonstrated the redundancy of adhesion molecules that mediate the various steps in leukocyte migration. While it comes now as no surprise that leukocytes bearing $\alpha_4\beta_1$ [CD49d/CD29, very late activation antigen-4 (VLA-4)], such as monocytes, lymphocytes, and eosinophils, can migrate independently of CD18 by virtue of VLA-4/VCAM-1 interactions, neutrophils, which are characteristically much more dependent on CD18 for their function, may "learn" ways around this if given the proper environment or enough time. Mileski et al. (25) showed that transfer of inflammatory cells from one rabbit to another could render the response of the recipient to *S. pneumoniae* CD18 independent in the mesenteric vascular bed, normally a site of CD18-dependent migration.

Mice rendered genetically deficient in CD18 (equivalent to the human LAD type I syndrome) mount a very poor acute inflammatory response to challenge by cutaneous irritant, but respond as well as wild-type littermates to intraperitoneal challenge by thioglycollate broth or *S. pneumoniae* (26). It is not known why these mice develop a CD18-independent inflammatory response in the peritoneum. Possibilities include the following: (a) A chronic low-grade inflammation in the peritoneal cavity induced the same factor(s) as in the inflammatory cell transfer experiment described above (25). (b) These mice developed in the absence of β_2 integrins, and so vital functions of the β_2 integrins may have been taken over by other families of cell adhesion molecules or other leukocyte integrins that either do not normally subserve those functions, or that are not normally present in sufficient numbers on the neutrophil surface. One obvious candidate would be VLA-4. (c) A CD18-independent pathway(s) normally exists, but is relatively insignificant and therefore not noticed in acute experiments. In the absence of CD18, this pathway expands in importance by upregulation of the appropriate adhesion molecules and/or signaling pathways.

Transendothelial Migration

The molecules involved in transmigration may vary depending on the leukocyte type, the situation, and the location in the vascular system. Monocytes and natural killer (NK) cells emigrate constitutively at low levels. T lymphocytes constitutively "home" selectively to their appropriate lymph nodes, binding to and crossing the high endothelial venules to enter the lymph node parenchyma. On the other hand, there can be rapid recruitment of neutrophils, eosinophils, and mononuclear cells to sites of acute or chronic inflammation. To a large extent, differences in adhesion molecules used for the rolling and adhesion phases of emigration in these circumstances may be responsible for this variability.

Diapedesis is the process by which the leukocyte squeezes in ameboid fashion across the endothelial cell barrier. While in most instances this passage is believed to occur along the junctions between tightly apposed endothelial cells (19,27,28), there is at least one experimental model in which migration of neutrophils directly through endothelial cells has been documented by serial electron micrographs (22). The molecular mechanisms underlying the latter type of migration are not known. We will therefore confine this discussion to the intercellular pathway.

Leukocyte rolling and firm adhesion are prerequisites for transmigration. Blockade of these adhesion molecules blocks transmigration in an assay of transmigration. However, it is not clear whether there is a role for these adhesion molecules in transmigration apart from their role in adhesion to the apical surface of the endothelial cell. Diapedesis appears to be an independent step in the process of leukocyte emigration because it can be dissected from the preceding steps of rolling and adhesion.

Table 39-1 summarizes a number of *in vitro* studies reporting the roles of adhesion molecules in transendothelial migration. In almost all cases the role of these adhesion molecules on the transendothelial migration or

TABLE 39-1. *Adhesion molecules involved in transendothelial migration of leukocytes*[a]

Assay[b]	Activation leukocyte	Activation endothelium	Adhesion molecule involvement		Comment[d]	Reference No.
			Leukocyte[c]	Endothelium		
Neutrophils						
Collagen gel	—	TNF-α	PECAM-1	PECAM-1	1	12
Collagen gel	fMLP	—	CD18			53
	—	IL-1	CD18			
Collagen gel	—	IL-1	CD11a/CD18	ICAM-1		54
			CD11b/CD18	E-selectin		
Collagen gel	—	IL-1	CD18			55
Filter chamb.	IL-8	—	IAP			
	—	TNF-α	IAP	IAP		56
Coverslip	—	IL-1, LPS	CD18	ICAM-1	2	57
Coverslip	—	IL-1	CD11a>CD11b		3	58
Coverslip	—	IL-1	CD11b			59
Monocytes						
Collagen gel	—	Unstimulated	PECAM-1	PECAM-1	1	12
		TNF-α	PECAM-1	PECAM-1	1	12
Amnion	—	Unstimulated	CD18			11
		IL-1	CD18 + VLA-4	VCAM-1	4	
Filter chamb.	C5a	—	CD18>VLA-4			15
	—	IL-1, TNF-α	VLA-4	VCAM-1		
T Cells						
Coverslip	—	IL-1	CD11a/CD18		3	60
Filter chamb.	PDB, Iono.	—	CD11a/CD18			29
	—	IL-1	CD11a/CD18			
		IL-1	CD44			
Filter chamb.	—	IL-1		ICAM-1		30
Eosinophils						
ECM	—	IL-4	CD11a/CD18			61
			CD11b/CD18			
			VLA-4			
Filter chamb.	—	IL-1, TNF-α	CD11b/CD18	ICAM-1	5	62
			CD11a/CD18			
Filter chamb.	C5a, PAF	—	CD29			63
Natural Killer Cells						
Filter chamb.	—	Unstimulated	CD11a/CD18			64
	—	IL-1	VLA-4	VCAM-1		
			CD11a/CD18			

fMLP, formyl-methionyl-leucyl-phenylalanine; IL-1, interleukin-1; LPS, bacterial lipopolysaccharide; IL-4, interleukin-4; IL-8, interleukin-8; TNF-α tumor necrosis factor-α; PAF, platelet-activating factor; C5a, activated form of the fifth component of complement, IAP, integrin-associated protein (CD47).

[a]This table lists representative studies on transendothelial migration *in vitro* by cell type. All studies used cultured human umbilical vein endothelial cells and human leukocytes. Adhesion molecules are identified as important for transmigration by virtue of significant block of transmigration by monoclonal antibodies against those antigens. Negative results are not listed. The caveats discussed in the text regarding whether the block is at the adhesion, diapedesis, or migration step of transendothelial migration apply here. Endothelial and leukocyte adhesion molecules listed on the same line are presumed to be interacting with each other. Adhesion molecules listed on consecutive lines of the same entry are shown that way to save space. Common names are generally used, except for the leukocyte integrins where monoclonal antibodies against the separate α and β chains have been used. Therefore, the CD nomenclature is given in the chart.

[b]The *in vitro* assay system used in the studies (see text). Filter chamb; filter chamber, similar to Transwell system; PDB, Iono, phorbol dibutyrate and ionomycin added to T-cell cultures for 1 to 2 days to activate T cells; ECM, extracellular matrix from fibroblast cultures used as a substratum for growing human endothelial cells.

[c]Cluster designation nomenclature: PECAM-1 (CD31), LFA-1 (CD11a/CD18), Mac-1 (CD11b/CD18), ICAM-1 (CD54), E-selectin (CD62E), integrin associated protein (CD47), VLA-4 (CD49d/CD29), VCAM-1 (CD106).

[d]Comments:

1. Homophilic interaction between PECAM on the leukocyte and PECAM at the endothelial junction is presumed to occur.

2. Endothelial cells were cultured on glass coverslips. Phase-contrast microscopy was used to assess which leukocytes had migrated beneath the endothelial monolayer in this and all similar "coverslip" entries.

3. No effect was seen with anti-CD11b mAb alone, but synergy was observed when it was mixed with anti-CD11a mAb.

4. No block was observed unless anti-CD18 and anti-VLA-4 mAb were added together, implying that either adhesion molecule was sufficient to mediate transmigration in this system.

5. Anti-CD11b blocked better than anti-CD11a.

From ref. 65 by permission of RG Landes Co.

diapedesis step itself cannot be distinguished from a role in the earlier or subsequent steps as summarized above. The prime exception to this is PECAM-1.

One thought to bear in mind when examining this literature is what percentage of leukocytes added to a culture system bind and/or transmigrate. Most investigators find that the vast majority of monocytes will bind and transmigrate, whereas only about half of the PMNs added to a system will adhere tightly to the endothelium. T cells are a major interpretative problem: Only a small percentage of the added cells transmigrate endothelium even after 4 hours at 37°C (29,30), making the significance of this migration and any blockade using antibodies against adhesion molecules open to question. However, the small percentage of T cells that transmigrate may in fact be physiologically relevant. As subsets of T cells with different surface antigens and correspondingly different functional phenotypes have been discovered, the observation that certain subsets of T cells are particularly prone to transmigration (31,32) sheds new light on these experiments. *In vivo,* the constant emigration of a small defined T-cell subset would produce a substantial inflammatory infiltrate.

Platelet Endothelial Cell Adhesion Molecule-1 and Diapedesis

Platelet endothelial cell adhesion molecule-1 (PECAM-1/CD31) is a cell adhesion molecule of the immunoglobulin (Ig) superfamily (33) that has a unique role in diapedesis (12). This molecule is expressed abundantly by endothelial cells (10^6 molecules/cell), which concentrate it in the junctions between adjacent cells (34). It is also diffusely expressed on the surfaces of most leukocyte classes as well as platelets (33,35). Blockade of PECAM-1 can block diapedesis of PMNs, monocytes (Mo), and NK cells *in vitro* and *in vivo* without affecting the ability of these leukocytes to adhere to the endothelial surface (12–14,36–39).

During diapedesis, leukocyte PECAM interacts in a homophilic manner with PECAM in the endothelial junctions. The amino-terminal domains of both leukocyte and endothelial PECAM are involved in this interaction, since it can be blocked either by monoclonal antibodies directed against domains 1 and/or 2 on the leukocyte (36,40), or by soluble recombinant domain 1 mimicking endothelial PECAM (37). These same domains have been shown to be involved in the binding of soluble recombinant PECAM to PECAM on endothelial cells (37,41) and purified PECAM in liposomes (41). However, efficient interaction of leukocyte and endothelial PECAM during diapedesis requires more than just the presence of the amino-terminal domains. While domains 1 and 2 of PECAM are the only domains necessary for homophilic adhesion, presentation of these domains on a molecular stalk of appropriate length is also a prerequisite for binding to PECAM presented on cells. Full-length (domains 1–6) soluble recombinant PECAM binds avidly to endothelial cell PECAM (37,41), yet a construct lacking one or more of the distal domains will not bind (Liao and Muller, unpublished observations). Murine PECAM will not bind to human PECAM when both are expressed on transfected L cells; however, a construct in which human PECAM domains 1 and 2 are ligated to murine domains 3 to 6 will bind as well as the complete human molecule to human PECAM (42).

Blockade of PECAM function on either the endothelial cell or leukocyte by reagents that bind to or mimic PECAM domains 1 and/or 2 selectively blocks diapedesis. *In vitro* leukocytes are arrested on the apical surface of endothelial monolayers just above the intercellular junctions (12). These leukocytes are tightly adherent to the underlying endothelium and resist dislodgment by inverted centrifugation in low concentrations of ethyleneglycoltetraacetic acid (EGTA). However, the block is reversible. When excess reagent is washed away, bound anti-PECAM MAb or soluble PECAM is metabolized and full transendothelial migration is complete within 1 to 2 hours (12). Transmigration appears to be blocked at the same step *in vivo* as well. Monoclonal antibodies against domain 1 of murine PECAM (13) or soluble domain 1 of murine PECAM (37) block neutrophil and monocyte recruitment to the peritoneal cavity of mice in response to thioglycollate broth. Histologic sections of the mesenteric microvasculature of these mice show intravascular leukocytes arrested on the luminal surface of postcapillary venules (13,37). In the *scid*-hu chimeric mouse, a similar picture is seen when PMNs are attracted to a site of dermal inflammation: blocking MAb to either murine neutrophils' or human endothelial cells' PECAM blocked emigration. The local vasculature showed abundant intravascular leukocytes, but little emigration (39).

In addition to the examples cited above, PECAM blockade has been shown to block emigration in a number of other acute inflammatory models in different tissues and species. These include myocardial ischemia-reperfusion injuries in both cat (43) and rat (44), and infiltration into the rat lung in response to immune complexes (14). In all published studies, both *in vitro* and *in vivo,* the inhibition of migration ranged from about 70% to 90%, suggesting that PECAM-independent pathways of leukocyte emigration exist and account for the residual transmigration.

Transendothelial migration involves an obligatory increase in intracytoplasmic-free calcium in the endothelial cells. Huang et al. (45) demonstrated that buffering intracellular calcium with the chelator bis(2-amino-5-methylphenoxy)ethane-N,N,N',N'-tetraacetic acid tetraacetoxymethyl ester (MAPTAM) blocked diapedesis of PMNs without interfering with their ability to adhere to the apical surface of the endothelial monolayer. The rise in intracellular calcium has been linked to phosphorylation of myosin light chain kinase (46). This in turn activates the regulatory light chain associated with myosin II of non-muscle cells, leading to enhanced actin-myosin interaction and tension generation. It is hypothesized that this tension is responsible for retraction of the endothelial cells from each other at their borders, allowing the leukocyte to pass through (46). Whether PECAM-1 (or any other CAM) is involved in generating this calcium signal is currently a focus of investigation.

Migration Across Basal Lamina

Once the leukocyte has traversed the intercellular junction, it encounters the subendothelial basal lamina, the next barrier on its way into the site of inflammation. The basal lamina is a dense meshwork of extracellular matrix proteins, including type IV collagen, laminin, fibronectin, and heparan sulfate–containing glycosaminoglycans.

There has been considerable controversy over whether breaching the basal lamina requires digestion by leukocyte proteases, or whether the leukocytes can push the strands of matrix apart as they squeeze through. Studies by Weiss and colleagues (47) indicated that neutrophil proteases are capable of degrading subendothelial basal lamina. However, migration was reported to alter the retentive properties of the matrix without causing detectable structural alterations (48). In vivo transmigration occurs in the presence of plasma, which is replete with protease inhibitors. On the other hand, leukocytes can secrete into "protected compartments" (49,50), tight appositions of cell membrane to the substratum from which molecules larger than 40,000 daltons are excluded. In vitro, protease inhibitors are excluded from these compartments. In addition, neutrophils are able to inactivate some of the naturally occurring protease inhibitors (51). Thus, a role for proteolysis in the passage of leukocytes across basal lamina has not been ruled out.

Leukocyte PECAM-1 also plays a role in migration across the basal lamina. Since there is no PECAM in the basal lamina, this must be a heterophilic interaction in which leukocyte PECAM is interacting with a different molecule. In fact, this interaction involves a different part of the PECAM molecule than is involved in transendothelial migration (TEM). While transmigration involves domains 1 and/or 2 of leukocyte PECAM interacting with domains 1 and/or 2 of endothelial cell PECAM, it is domain 6 (the most membrane proximal) that appears to interact with the basal lamina (36). In a study by Liao et al. (36), monoclonal antibodies to PECAM domain 6 had no effect on TEM, but arrested monocytes between the basal surface of the endothelium and the subendothelial basal lamina. Conversely, MAb against domains 1 and 2 that blocked passage across the endothelial monolayer had no effect on this step. The important epitopes appeared to be localized to or near domain 6, since two MAbs to domain 6 blocked, but a MAb whose epitope mapped to domain 5 did not. This was the first demonstration that migration across the basal lamina could be inhibited distinctly from other steps in transmigration (36). Further experiments (Muller, unpublished data) demonstrated that the role of PECAM-1 in migration across basal lamina was independent of its role in transmigration: When confluent monolayers of human umbilical vein endothelial cells (HUVECs) were nonenzymatically removed from atop collagen gel cultures, monocyte migration across the remaining basal lamina into the collagen gel in response to chemoattractant was selectively blocked by MAbs against PECAM domain 6.

The role for PECAM-1 in migration across basal lamina has been demonstrated in vivo as well. Wakelin et al. (52) treated rats with a cross-reacting rabbit antihuman PECAM antibody prior to intraperitoneal stimulation with IL-1β. Four hours later, there was a striking reduction in extravasated leukocytes, as expected. When they examined the affected mesenteric microvessels ultrastructurally at 4 hours, they found that in the rats treated with anti-PECAM antibody, almost twice as many leukocytes were seen between the basal surface of the endothelium and the basement membrane as in mice treated with control antibody (52). The relatively large effect of this polyclonal antibody on the passage of leukocytes across the basal lamina relative to the effect on transendothelial migration in this model is probably due to species differences. That is, the antibody may cross-react with epitopes on rat domain 6 more extensively than against epitopes on the amino terminal portions of rat PECAM. The same antibody used in the scid-hu mice clearly blocked the ability of leukocytes to transmigrate the endothelial cells (14).

It is clear that transendothelial migration of leukocytes involves a coordinated series of adhesive and disadhesive events that involve transduced signals leading to cytoskeletal rearrangements, membrane deformations, and further adhesive interactions. There is likely to be a molecular signaling dialogue between the leukocytes and endothelium that is both instructional (facilitating the next step in emigration) and regulatory (providing feedback augmentation or inhibition of inflammation). Leukocytes pass through the endothelial lining without permanent disruption of its integrity or that of the basal lamina. This complex choreography takes place in a matter of seconds, so that signal transduction and response mechanisms must be rapid and precise. A better understanding of the molecules involved in transendothelial migration and their regulation will undoubtedly lead to more rational antiinflammatory therapies. It may also provide many new paradigms for the study of coordinated transient cell-cell interactions.

ACKNOWLEDGMENTS

Supported by National Institutes of Health grant HL46849. W.A.M. is an Established Investigator of the American Heart Association.

REFERENCES

1. Lasky LA. Selectins: interpreters of cell-specific carbohydrate information during inflammation. *Science* 1992;258:964–969.
2. Springer TA. Traffic signals for lymphocyte recirculation and leukocyte emigration: the multistep paradigm. *Cell* 1994;76:301–314.
3. Lo SK, Lee S, Ramos RA, et al. Endothelial-leukocyte adhesion molecule 1 stimulates the adhesive activity of leukocyte integrin CD3 (CD11B/CD18, Mac-1, alpha m beta 2) on human neutrophils. *J Exp Med* 1991;173:1493–1500.
4. Lorant DE, Patel KD, McIntyre TM, McEver RP, Prescott SM, Zimmerman GA. Coexpression of GMP-140 and PAF by endothelium stimulated by histamine or thrombin: a juxtacrine system for adhesion and activation of neutrophils. *J Cell Biol* 1991;115:223–234.
5. Hermanowski-Vosatka A, Van Strijp JAG, Swiggard WJ, Wright SD. Integrin modulating factor-1: a lipid that alters the function of leukocyte integrins. *Cell* 1992;68:341–352.
6. Tanaka Y, Adams DH, Hubscher S, Hirano H, Siebenlist U, Shaw S. T-cell adhesion induced by proteoglycan-immobilized cytokine MIP-1 beta. *Nature* 1993;361:79–82.
7. Huber AR, Kunkel SL, Todd RF III, Weiss SJ. Regulation of transendothelial neurophil migration by endogenous interleukin-8. *Science* 1991;254:99–102.
8. Tanaka Y, Albelda SM, Horgan KJ, et al. CD31 expressed on distinctive T cell subsets is a preferential amplifier of beta1 integrin-mediated adhesion. *J Exp Med* 1992;176:245–253.
9. Piali L, Albelda SM, Baldwin HS, Hammel P, Gisler RH, Imhof BA. Murine platelet endothelial cell adhesion molecule (PECAM-1/CD31) modulates beta2 integrins on lymphokine-activated killer cells. *Eur J Immunol* 1993;23:2464–2471.
10. Berman ME, Muller WA. Ligation of platelet/endothelial cell adhesion molecule 1 (PECAM-1/CD31) on monocytes and neutrophils increases binding capacity of leukocyte CR3(CD11b/CD18). *J Immunol* 1995;154:299–307.
11. Meerschaert J, Furie MB. Monocytes use either CD11/CD18 or VLA-4 to migrate across human endothelium *in vitro*. *J Immunol* 1994;152:1915–1926.
12. Muller WA, Weigl SA, Deng X, Phillips DM. PECAM-1 is required for transendothelial migration of leukocytes. *J Exp Med* 1993;178:449–460.
13. Bogen S, Pak J, Garifallou M, Deng X, Muller WA. Monoclonal antibody to murine PECAM-1 (CD31) blocks acute inflammation *in vivo*. *J Exp Med* 1994;179:1059–1064.
14. Vaporciyan AA, Delisser HM, Yan H-C, et al. Involvement of platelet-endothelial cell adhesion molecule-1 in neutrophil recruitment *in vivo*. *Science* 1993;262:1580–1582.
15. Luscinskas FW, Ding H, Lichtman AH. P-selectin and vascular cell adhesion molecule 1 mediate rolling and arrest, respectively, of CD4⁺ T lymphocytes on tumor necrosis factor alpha-activated vascular endothelium under flow. *J Exp Med* 1995;181:1179–1186.
16. Meerschaert J, Furie MB. The adhesion molecules used by monocytes for migration across endothelium include CD11a/CD18, CD11b/CD18, and VLA-4 on monocytes and ICAM-1, VCAM-1, and other ligands on endothelium. *J Immunol* 1995;154:4099–4112.
17. Berlin C, Bargatze RF, Campbell JJ, et al. Alpha 4 integrins mediate lymphocyte attachment and rolling under physiologic flow. *Cell* 1995;80:413–422.
18. Luscinskas FW, Kansas GS, Ding H, et al. Monocyte rolling, arrest and spreading on IL-4-activated vascular endothelium under flow is mediated via sequential action of L-selectin, β1-integrins, and β2-integrins. *J Cell Biol* 1994;125:1417–1427.
19. Muller WA. Migration of leukocytes across the vascular intima. Molecules and mechanisms. *Trends Cardiovasc Med* 1995;5:15–20.
20. Marchesi VT, Gowans JL. The migration of lymphocytes through the endothelium of venules in lymph nodes: an electron microscope study. *Proc R Soc B* 1964;159:283–290.
21. Walker DC, Chu F, MacKenzie A. Pathway of leukocyte emigration from the pulmonary vasculature during pneumonia in rabbits. *Am Rev Respir Dis* 1991;143:A541.
22. Feng D, Nagy JA, Pyne K, Dvorak HF, Dvorak AM. Neutrophils emigrate from venules by a transendothelial cell pathway in response to fMLP. *J Exp Med* 1998;187:903–915.
23. Hawkins HK, Heffelfinger SC, Anderson DC. Leukocyte adhesion deficiency: clinical and postmortem observations. *Pediatr Pathol* 1992;12:119–130.
24. Doerschuk CM, Winn RK, Coxson HO, Harlan JM. CD18-dependent and -independent mechanisms of neutrophil emigration in the pulmonary and systemic microcirculation of rabbits. *J Immunol* 1990;144:2327–2333.
25. Mileski W, Harlan J, Rice C, Winn R. *Streptococcus pneumoniae*–stimulated macrophages induce neutrophils to emigrate by a CD18-independent mechanism of adherence. *Circ Shock* 1990;31:259–267.
26. Mizgerd JP, Kubo H, Kutkoski GJ, et al. Neutrophil emigration in the skin, lungs, and peritoneum: different requirements for CD11/CD18 revealed by CD18-deficient mice. *J Exp Med* 1997;186:1357–1364.
27. Furie MB, Naprstek BL, Silverstein SC. Migration of neutrophils across monolayers of cultured microvascular endothelial cells: an *in vitro* model of leukocyte extravasation. *J Cell Sci* 1987;88:161–175.
28. Marchesi VT, Florey HW. Electron micrographic observations on the emigration of leukocytes. *J Exp Physiol* 1960;45:343–347.
29. Oppenheimer-Marks N, Davis LS, Lipsky PE. Human T lymphocyte adhesion to endothelial cells and transendothelial migration. Alteration of receptor use relates to the activation status of both the T cell and the transendothelial cell. *J Immunol* 1990;145:140–148.
30. Oppenheimer-Marks N, Davis LS, Bogue DT, Ramberg J, Lipsky PE. Differential utilization of ICAM-1 and VCAM-1 during the adhesion and transendothelial migration of human T lymphocytes. *J Immunol* 1991;147:2913–2921.
31. Pietschmann P, Cush JJ, Lipsky PE, Oppenheimer-Marks N. Identification of subsets of human T cells capable of enhanced transendothelial migration. *J Immunol* 1992;149:1170–1178.
32. Brezinschek RI, Lipsky PE, Galea P, Vita R, Oppenheimer-Marks N. Phenotypic characterization of CD4⁺ T cells that exhibit a transendothelial migratory capacity. *J Immunol* 1995;154:3062–3077.
33. Newman PJ, Berndt MC, Gorski J, et al. PECAM-1 (CD31) cloning and relation to adhesion molecules of the immunoglobulin gene superfamily. *Science* 1990;247:1219–1222.
34. Muller WA, Ratti CM, McDonnell SL, Cohn ZA. A human endothelial cell-restricted, externally disposed plasmalemmal protein enriched in intercellular junctions. *J Exp Med* 1989;170:399–414.
35. Newman PJ. The biology of PECAM-1. *J Clin Invest* 1997;99:3–8.
36. Liao F, Huynh HK, Eiroa A, Greene T, Polizzi E, Muller WA. Migration of monocytes across endothelium and passage through extracellular matrix involve separate molecular domains of PECAM-1. *J Exp Med* 1995;182:1337–1343.
37. Liao F, Ali J, Greene T, Muller WA. Soluble domain 1 of platelet-endothelial cell adhesion molecule (PECAM) is sufficient to block transendothelial migration *in vitro* and *in vivo*. *J Exp Med* 1997;185:1349–1357.
38. Berman ME, Xie Y, Muller WA. Roles of platelet/endothelial cell adhesion molecule-1 (PECAM-1, CD31) in natural killer cell transendothelial migration and beta 2 integrin activation. *J Immunol* 1996;156:1515–1524.
39. Christofidou-Solomidou M, Nakada MT, Williams J, Muller WA, Delisser HM. Neutrophil platelet endothelial cell adhesion molecule-1 participates in neutrophil recruitment at inflammatory sites and is down-regulated after leukocyte extravasation. *J Immunol* 1997;158:4872–4878.
40. Muller WA, Greene T, Liao F. CD31 Workshop: Transendothelial migration and interstitial migration of monocytes are mediated by separate domains of monocyte CD31. In: Kishimoto et al., eds. *Leukocyte typing VI. White cell differentiation antigens.* London: Garland, 1996.
41. Sun Q-H, Delisser HM, Zukowski MM, Paddock C, Albelda SM, Newman PJ. Individually distinct Ig homology domains in PECAM-1 regulate homophilic binding and modulate receptor affinity. *J Biol Chem* 1996;271:11090–11098.
42. Sun J, Williams J, Yan H, Amin KM, Albelda SM, Delisser HM. Platelet/endothelial cell adhesion molecule-1 (PECAM-1) homophilic adhesion is mediated by immunoglobulin-like domains 1 and 2 and depends on the cytoplasmic domain and the level of surface expression. *J Biol Chem* 1996;271:18561–18570.
43. Murohara T, Delyani JA, Albelda SM, Lefer AM. Blockade of platelet endothelial cell adhesion molecule-1 protects against myocardial ischemia and reperfusion injury in cats. *J Immunol* 1996;156:3550–3557.
44. Gumina RJ, Schultz JE, Yao Z, et al. Antibody to platelet/endothelial cell adhesion molecule-1 reduces myocardial infarct size in a rat model of ischemia-reperfusion injury. *Circulation* 1996;94:3327–3333.
45. Huang AJ, Manning JE, Bandak TM, Ratau MC, Hanser KR, Silver-

stein SC. Endothelial cell cytosolic free calcium regulates neutrophil migration across monolayers of endothelial cells. *J Cell Biol* 1993;120: 1371–1380.

46. Hixenbaugh EA, Goeckeler ZM, Papaiya NN, Wysolmerski RB, Silverstein SC, Huang AJ. Chemoattractant-stimulated neutrophils induce regulatory myosin light chain phosphorylation and isometric tension development in endothelial cells. *Am J Physiol* 1997;273:H981–H988.

47. Weiss SJ, Curnutte JT, Regiani S. Neutrophil-mediated solubilization of the subendothelial matrix: oxidative and nonoxidative mechanisms of proteolysis used by normal and chronic granulomatous disease phagocytes. *J Immunol* 1986;136:636–641.

48. Huber AR, Weiss SJ. Disruption of subendothelial basement membrane during neutrophil diapedesis in an *in vitro* construct of a blood vessel wall. *J Clin Invest* 1989;83:1122–1136.

49. Wright SD, Silverstein SC. Phagocytosing macrophages exclude proteins from the zones of contact with opsonized targets. *Nature* 1984; 309:359–361.

50. Loike JD, Silverstein R, Wright SD, Weitz JI, Huang AJ, Silverstein SC. The role of protected extracellular compartments in interactions between leukocytes, and platelets, and fibrin/fibrinogen matrices. *Ann NY Acad Sci* 1992;667:163–172.

51. Weiss SJ, Regiani S. Neutrophils degrade subendothelial matrices in the presence of alpha-1-proteinase inhibitor. Cooperative use of lysosomal proteinases and oxygen metabolites. *J Clin Invest* 1984;73:1297–1303.

52. Wakelin MW, Sanz M-J, Dewar A, et al. An anti-platelet/endothelial cell adhesion molecule-1 antibody inhibits leukocyte extravasation from mesenteric microvessels *in vivo* by blocking the passage through basement membrane. *J Exp Med* 1996;184:229–239.

53. Hakkert BC, Rentenaar JM, Van Aken WG, Roos D, van Mourik JA. A three-dimensional model system to study the interactions between human leukocytes and endothelial cells. *Eur J Immunol* 1990;20:2775–2781.

54. Luscinskas FW, Cybulsky MI, Kiely JM, Peckins CS, Davis VM, Gimbrone MA Jr. Cytokine-activated human endothelial monolayers support enhanced neutrophil transmigration via a mechanism involving both endothelial-leukocyte adhesion molecule-1 and intercellular adhesion molecule-1. *J Immunol* 1991;146:1617–1625.

55. Rice GE, Munro JM, Bevilacqua MP. Inducible cell adhesion molecule 110 (INCAM-110) is an endothelial receptor for lymphocytes. *J Exp Med* 1990;171:1369–1374.

56. Ley K, Bullard DC, Arbones ML, et al. Sequential contribution of L-and P-selectin to leukocyte rolling *in vivo*. *J Exp Med* 1995;181:669–675.

57. Smith CW, Rothlein R, Hughes BJ, et al. Recognition of an endothelial determinant for CD18-dependent human neutrophil adherence and transendothelial migration. *J Clin Invest* 1988;82:1746–1756.

58. Smith CW, Marlin SD, Rothlein R, Toman C, Anderson DC. Cooperative interactions of LFA-1 and Mac-1 with intercellular adhesion molecule-1 in facilitating adherence and transendothelial migration of human neutrophils *in vitro*. *J Clin Invest* 1989;83:2008.

59. Anderson DC, Rothlein R, Marlin SD, Krater SS, Smith CW. Impaired transendothelial migration by neonatal neutrophils: abnormalities of Mac-1 (CD11b/CD18)-dependent adherence reactions. *Blood* 1990;76: 2613–2621.

60. van Epps DE, Potter J, Vachula M, Smith CW, Anderson DC. Suppression of human lymphocyte chemotaxis and transendothelial migration by anti-LFA-1 antibody. *J Immunol* 1989;143:3207–3210.

61. Moser R, Fehr J, Bruijnzeel PLB. IL-4 controls the selective endothelium-driven transmigration of eosinophils from allergic individuals. *J Immunol* 1992;149:1432–1438.

62. Ebisawa M, Bochner BS, Georas SN, Schleimer RP. Eosinophil transendothelial migration induced by cytokines. I. Role of endothelial and eosinophil adhesion molecules in IL-1b-induced transendothelial migration. *J Immunol* 1992;149:4021–4028.

63. Pinola M, Saksela E, Tiisala S, Renkomen R. Human NK cells expressing $\alpha_4\beta_1/\beta_7$ adhere to VCAM-1 without preactivation. *Scand J Immunol* 1994;39:131–136.

64. Lastres P, Almendro N, Bellon T, Lopez-Guerrero JA, Eritja R, Bernabeu C. Functional regulation of platelet /endothelial cell adhesion molecule-1 by TGF-1 in promonocytic U-937 cells. *J Immunol* 1995; 153:4206–4218.

65. Muller WA. Transendothelial migration of leukocytes. In: G. Peltz, ed. *Leukocyte recruitment in inflammatory disease. Section I. Molecular and cellular components.* Austin, TX: R.G. Landes, 1996:3–18.

Inflammation: Basic Principles and Clinical Correlates,
3rd ed., edited by John I. Gallin and Ralph Snyderman.
Lippincott Williams & Wilkins, Philadelphia © 1999.

CHAPTER 40

Molecular Basis of Lymphocyte Migration

Douglas A. Steeber and Thomas F. Tedder

The immune system is composed of functionally diverse tissues spread throughout the body that must remain functionally integrated to provide optimal immune responses. Lymphocyte migration into lymphoid and nonlymphoid tissues and their recirculation between tissues are important aspects of immune surveillance that allow maximal interactions between lymphocytes and foreign antigens and enable the dissemination of effector lymphocytes (1). Lymphocytes migrate continuously between lymphoid and nonlymphoid tissues using the blood and lymph vessels as traffic routes (2–4). Lymphocyte migration is tightly regulated during normal homeostasis and is rapidly modified and magnified during immune responses and inflammation.

The first step in lymphocyte recirculation is selective migration from the blood across specialized vascular endothelium within postcapillary venules located in nonlymphoid and lymphoid organs (5). This process depends on selective interactions between adhesion molecules on lymphocytes and tissue-specific determinants expressed by vascular endothelial cells (6). Chemokines are an integral part of this process when expressed by or displayed on vascular endothelium (see Chapter 28). After entering lymphoid tissues, B and T lymphocytes segregate into distinct zones and compartments, where they are retained or exit the tissue. Lymphocytes leave most lymphoid tissues by migrating through interstitial and lymphatic channels to eventually return to the blood. Although more lymphocytes pass through the spleen than recirculate through all other lymphoid tissues, little is known about the molecular mechanisms involved in lymphocyte migration to and entry into this organ (7). Similarly, the molecular basis for lymphocyte migration into nonlymphoid tissues remains poorly understood. However, studies suggest that many of the molecular mechanisms that contribute to lymphocyte migration into lymphoid tissues

such as peripheral lymph nodes also function at sites of inflammation.

This review focuses primarily on the molecular basis of lymphocyte migration into lymphoid tissues, because many molecular events are common to lymphocyte migration into sites of inflammation. Because many of the advances in our understanding of leukocyte migration are derived from studies performed in mice, this chapter primarily focuses on mouse studies, although identical mechanisms probably operate in other species. Reviews of lymphocyte migration in other species are available and can be divided into those examining the general physiology of migration (8,9) and those examining the cell surface molecules involved in lymphocyte interactions with specialized high endothelial venules (HEVs) that line postcapillary venules of some lymphoid organs (10,11).

GENERAL LEUKOCYTE-ENDOTHELIAL CELL INTERACTIONS

Lymphocyte migration represents a complex process with multiple adhesion molecules operating cooperatively and in parallel to facilitate leukocyte and endothelial cell interactions. The selectin family of adhesion molecules mediates the initial capture and attachment of leukocytes to vascular endothelial cells, which initiates the rolling of leukocytes along the venular wall (12). The selectin family consists of three closely related cell-surface molecules: L-selectin, E-selectin, and P-selectin.

In addition to the selectins, leukocyte integrins interact with their immunoglobulin superfamily ligands to stabilize leukocyte rolling and regulate leukocyte rolling velocities (13). Only intercellular adhesion molecule-1 (ICAM-1, CD54) and α_4 integrins are critically involved in leukocyte rolling. However, multiple leukocyte integrins are likely to be involved in this process, including lymphocyte function antigen-1 (LFA-1, CD11a/CD18) and HML-1 ($\alpha_E\beta_7$). These integrins bind to members of the immunoglobulin superfamily expressed by vascular

D. A. Steeber and T. F. Tedder: Department of Immunology, Duke University Medical Center, Durham, North Carolina 27710.

endothelium such as vascular cell adhesion molecule-1 (VCAM-1, CD106), ICAM-1, and ICAM-2 (CD102). Upregulation of L-selectin and integrin avidity during rolling contribute to the arrest of rolling leukocytes, which initiates firm adhesion with vascular endothelium (14).

Most adhesion pathways appear to operate through common mechanisms with overlapping use of independently regulated selectin, integrin, and immunoglobulin superfamily members. The differential usage of adhesion molecules by different leukocyte subclasses allows for diversity and specificity in leukocyte migration as these cells pass through different vascular beds throughout the body.

MIGRATION ACROSS HIGH ENDOTHELIAL VENULES OF LYMPHOID TISSUES

Specific patterns of lymphocyte migration were suspected when lymph nodes were found to be the preferred site of lymphocyte emigration among lymphoid tissues after their intravenous infusion into rats (4). It was also observed that lymph draining lymphoid tissues contained many more lymphocytes than lymph draining nonlymphoid tissues (15–17). Lymphocytes exited the blood in lymph nodes by passing between the specialized "high" endothelial cells of HEVs (18), a process controlled by specific molecular interactions between lymphocytes and endothelial cells (19). HEVs are found in peripheral lymph nodes (PLNs), mesenteric lymph nodes (MLNs), Peyer's patches, tonsils, and some inflamed nonlymphoid tissues. Lymphocyte entry into Peyer's patches and tonsils entirely depends on lymphocyte-HEV interactions (20). HEVs represent the major site for lymphocytes entering a resting lymph node, because about 95% of the lymphocytes within efferent lymph are derived from the blood rather than from lymphocyte proliferation within the node (21) or from afferent lymph (17,22,23). In sheep, approximately one of every three or four lymphocytes passing through HEV of lymph nodes is extracted from the blood (24,25). In rats, one of four blood lymphocytes passing through Peyer's patches migrates across HEVs (26). However, only about 2% of lymphocytes are found within the circulation, and fewer than 10% of all recirculating lymphocytes migrate across HEVs into peripheral lymphoid tissues. Most migrating lymphocytes enter organs such as spleen, liver, and lung through normal venules or sinuses (8).

ADHESION MOLECULES MEDIATING ORGAN-SPECIFIC MIGRATION

L-selectin Regulates Lymphocyte Migration Into Peripheral Lymphoid Tissues

In 1976, Stamper and Woodruff demonstrated that lymphocyte binding to lymph node HEVs was a specific event (19). Binding was mediated by L-selectin, as later identified by the MEL-14 monoclonal antibody (MAb) that blocks mouse lymphocyte binding to HEVs of PLNs *in vitro* and inhibits lymphocyte migration into PLNs *in vivo* (27). L-selectin is expressed by all classes of leukocytes at most stages of differentiation and serves a functional role in the migration of all leukocyte lineages (28). L-selectin is expressed by most circulating T and B lymphocytes (29,30) and a subpopulation of circulating NK cells (29). Blood lymphocytes express L-selectin at higher frequencies and levels than most tissue lymphocytes (29,31,32). Distinct subpopulations of $CD4^+$ and $CD8^+$ cells that lack L-selectin are found in the circulation of humans and mice (29,33–35). Functional analysis of these cells reveals that activated or memory helper T cells generally lack L-selectin expression, but they appear to reacquire surface receptor expression during their further maturation into fully competent helper cells (33). This suggests that fully mature memory cells use L-selectin to reenter lymphoid tissues, where effective helper function is actually performed. The positive and negative modulation of L-selectin expression by lymphocytes significantly influences the localization of leukocyte subsets to various lymphoid tissues.

Mice deficient in L-selectin expression are viable, have no developmental defects, and do not succumb to multifocal infections (36–38). These mice have a significant reduction (70% to 90%) in the number of resident lymphocytes within their PLNs, and lymphocytes from these mice cannot attach to HEVs of PLNs during *in vitro* binding assays (36,39). Consistent with these findings, lymphocytes from L-selectin–deficient mice are unable to migrate into PLNs of normal mice during short-term (1 hour) and long-term (48 hours) *in vivo* migration experiments (Fig. 40-1). Lymphocyte entry into PLNs during inflammatory responses is completely blocked by the absence of L-selectin, even when lymph node size increases dramatically. Infused wild-type lymphocytes migrate to PLNs of L-selectin–deficient mice at a normal rate despite a reduction in the number of histologically distinct HEVs observed in these tissues (39).

The localization of $CD4^+$ T cells and memory T cells is more severely affected by the loss of L-selectin than that of other cell populations. Among circulating lymphocyte populations, the loss of L-selectin results in a gradual increase in the frequency of $CD4^+$ T cells and the accelerated accumulation of memory T cells in the blood and spleen (39). The frequency of circulating monocytes is also increased in L-selectin–deficient mice. These studies demonstrate an essential role for L-selectin in lymphocyte binding to HEVs and subsequent entry into peripheral and mucosal lymphoid tissues.

In contrast to PLNs, the spleens of L-selectin–deficient mice contain 30% to 50% more lymphocytes compared with spleens of wild-type mice (36,39), and L-selectin–deficient lymphocytes preferentially enter the spleen during *in vivo* migration assays (see Fig. 40-1).

1 Hour

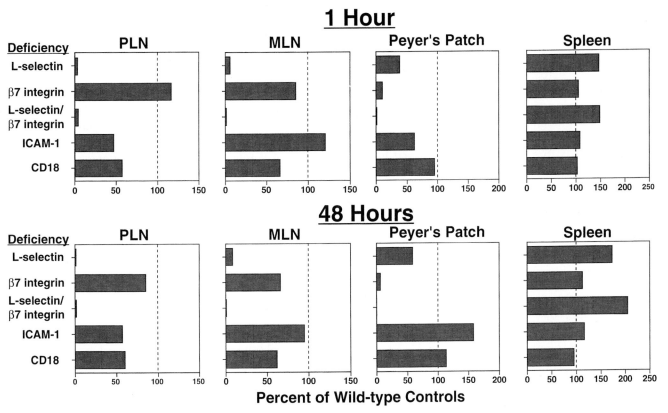

FIG. 40-1. Adhesion molecules involved in lymphocyte migration into secondary lymphoid tissues. Bars represent the relative ability of lymphocytes from adhesion molecule–deficient mice to migrate into the indicated tissues compared with lymphocytes from wild-type littermates. These migration assays were performed using isolated splenocytes deficient in one or more of the indicated adhesion molecules that were labeled with fluorochrome and injected intravenously into recipient wild-type mice, as previously described (32,36). In the case of intercellular adhesion molecule-1 (ICAM-1), the deficiency was in the recipient mice. Immigrant cells were detected and analyzed by fluorescence-based flow cytometry after 1 or 48 hours of migration. The dashed lines are placed for reference and indicate the migration of wild-type lymphocytes (100%).

These findings demonstrate that lymphocyte migration is also regulated by the specific loss of L-selectin, rather than only by the expression or acquisition of adhesion receptors specific for particular lymphoid tissues. Adhesion molecules or ligands specific to the spleen have not been defined, but they clearly are different from those that regulate lymphocyte migration into lymph nodes, Peyer's patches, or tonsils (7). The spleen may serve as a natural reservoir for cells that are not specifically recruited into other secondary lymphoid tissues. The rapid downregulation of L-selectin from the cell surface by endoproteolytic release (40), as occurs after cell activation (29,41), may therefore be an effective mechanism for increasing the number of lymphocytes entering the spleen or other tissues.

L-selectin Ligands on High Endothelial Venules and Leukocytes

The lectin domain of each of the selectins can recognize multiple complex carbohydrates *in vitro* (42). Of these, sia-lyl Lewis[X] (sLe[X], CD15s) serves as the prototypic selectin carbohydrate ligand. However, L-selectin binds with a higher avidity to carbohydrate determinants displayed in the proper context on a limited number of glycoproteins or proteoglycans (42,43). Mouse L-selectin binds to at least five heavily glycosylated mucin-like proteins expressed by HEVs: glycosylation-dependent cell adhesion molecule-1 (GlyCAM-1) (44,45), CD34 (45,46), mucosal addressin cell adhesion molecule-1 (MAdCAM-1) (47), and a ligand with a molecular mass of 200,000 (48). Podocalyxin supports L-selectin–dependent binding and is expressed on HEVs (49). Although there is considerable *in vitro* evidence that L-selectin interacts with multiple sialomucins, a direct physiologic role for any of these molecules in the mediation of lymphocyte adhesion to HEVs *in vivo* has not been proven. L-selectin binds the P-selectin glycoprotein ligand (PSGL-1) expressed by leukocytes (50–52). Thereby, L-selectin may also contribute to leukocyte rolling on adherent leukocytes (53), although this process contributes minimally to leukocyte accumulation at sites of inflammation or migration *in vivo* (54).

Each of these mucins bear sulfated, sialylated, and fucosylated *O*-linked carbohydrate side chains that appear essential for L-selectin binding activity. These ligands are also identified by the MECA-79 MAb (55) that identifies a sulfated sLe^X-like carbohydrate determinant (48). This MAb blocks lymphocyte binding to murine peripheral lymph node HEV by 95% (56) and inhibits lymphocyte migration into PLNs by about 80% *in vivo* (56,57). In humans, the MECA-79 MAb only partially inhibits (by 30% to 50%) lymphocyte binding to PLN HEV, and other L-selectin ligands that do not express the MECA-79 antigen have been described (58,59). The presence of MECA-79 antigen–independent L-selectin ligands is further supported by the finding that the HEVs of PLNs from $\alpha(1,3)$fucosyltransferase VII–deficient mice are unable to support L-selectin–mediated lymphocyte binding despite expressing the MECA-79 antigen at normal levels (60). Moreover, 6-sulfo sLe^X, which does not react with the MECA-79 MAb, is a major carbohydrate capping group of L-selectin ligands expressed on HEVs of human lymph nodes (61–63). The precise nature and identity of the L-selectin ligands on all HEVs remain unresolved, although this is an active area of research.

β_7 Integrins Influence Lymphocyte Migration Into Gut-Associated Lymphoid Tissues

The integrin β_7 chain associates with two α chains to generate the integrins $\alpha_4\beta_7$ and $\alpha_E\beta_7$ (64). Most lymphocytes express the $\alpha_4\beta_7$ integrin, which interacts with mucosal HEV determinants to mediate lymphocyte migration into Peyer's patches and MLNs (57). The $\alpha_E\beta_7$ integrin has a much more restricted distribution on lymphocyte populations than the $\alpha_4\beta_7$ integrin and is primarily expressed on intraepithelial lymphocytes and lymphocytes migrating to the mucosa (65,66). Early studies suggested that lymphocyte attachment to Peyer's patch HEVs was primarily controlled by the $\alpha_4\beta_7$ integrin, because the MEL-14 MAb did not block lymphocyte binding to Peyer's patch HEVs or inhibit lymphocyte migration into Peyer's patches (27,67,68). Lymphocyte attachment to Peyer's patch HEVs is also specifically and completely blocked by antibodies against α_4 or β_7 integrin chains (69). Treatment of peripheral lymph node HEV with sialidase inactivated adhesive ligands for L-selectin but had no apparent effect on lymphocyte attachment to Peyer's patch HEV (70,71). In most instances, L-selectin–IgG fusion proteins do not stain or block lymphocyte binding to Peyer's patch HEVs (72). These studies suggested that L-selectin mediated lymphocyte migration to PLNs and MLNs, while β_7 integrins mediated migration to Peyer's patches and MLNs.

The dominant physiologic ligand for the $\alpha_4\beta_7$ integrin is MAdCAM-1 (57,73). MAdCAM-1 is an immunoglobulin superfamily member with a high degree of homology with ICAM-1 and VCAM-1 (74). MAdCAM-1 is expressed on HEVs located within Peyer's patches and MLNs, on vessels within the lamina propria, and on follicular dendritic cells within Peyer's patches and chronically inflamed PLNs and spleen (56,75). In addition to its three immunoglobulin-like domains, mouse MAdCAM-1 expressed on HEVs contains a mucin-like domain that is decorated with carbohydrates recognized by the MECA-79 MAb (47,76). In this way, MAdCAM-1 is proposed to mediate L-selectin- and $\alpha_4\beta_7$ integrin–dependent adhesion (77).

Mice deficient in β_7 integrin expression are healthy, viable, and develop normally (78). The major phenotype of these mice is a dramatic reduction in the size of their Peyer's patches, which are hypocellular and contain only rudimentary follicles. The numbers of lamina propria and intraepithelial lymphocytes are significantly reduced relative to wild-type mice. Consistent with these findings, β_7 integrin–deficient lymphocytes are severely impaired in their ability to enter Peyer's patches of wild-type mice during short-term *in vivo* migration assays (see Fig. 40-1) (78). Migration into MLNs is also reduced with β_7 integrin loss, although not as severely as for Peyer's patches. Intravital microscopic analysis of exteriorized Peyer's patches showed that, although the number of leukocytes rolling along the HEVs was not different from that observed in wild-type mice, the number that arrested and firmly adhered was dramatically reduced (78,79). Leukocyte rolling in Peyer's patch HEVs occurs at faster characteristic velocities in β_7 integrin–deficient mice (79), which may in part explain why fewer leukocytes arrest and firmly adhere to Peyer's patch HEVs.

L-selectin and β_7 Integrins Regulate All Lymphocyte Migration Across High Endothelial Venules

In addition to the β_7 integrins, L-selectin is critically involved in lymphocyte migration to the gut and Peyer's patches (32,36,39). L-selectin–deficient lymphocytes are significantly reduced (about 60%) in their ability to migrate into Peyer's patches during short-term *in vivo* migration experiments (see Fig. 40-1). Lymphocyte migration into mouse Peyer's patches is also partially inhibited by Fab fragments of the MEL-14 MAb (80). However, L-selectin–deficient lymphocytes do accumulate in Peyer's patches in long-term migration assays (32,36,39). This suggests that $\alpha_4\beta_7$ integrins mediate a low level of selectin-independent cell capture from the blood. This idea is supported by intravital microscopic analysis of isolated Peyer's patches, demonstrating that L-selectin and, to a lesser degree, $\alpha_4\beta_7$ integrins participate in the initial interaction between lymphocytes and HEVs and in subsequent rolling (77,79). Although β_7 integrins are less efficient than L-selectin in mediating lymphocyte interactions with Peyer's patch HEVs, they can contribute significantly to lymphocyte entry into this tissue.

Lymphocyte migration into MLNs of normal mice is also significantly inhibited (>90%; see Fig. 40-1) by the loss of L-selectin, although not as completely as with PLNs (32,36). In this case, a dual migratory specificity for MLNs involving L-selectin and $\alpha_4\beta_7$ integrins confirms previous *in vitro* studies (57,70,81). HEVs of mesenteric lymph nodes express high levels of the MECA-79 antigen (76) and MAdCAM-1 (57). The presence of MAdCAM-1 and presumably $\alpha_4\beta_7$ integrin/ MAdCAM-1 interactions in MLNs may explain why lymphocyte migration to these tissues in L-selectin–deficient mice is less severely inhibited than migration to PLNs, which lack this ligand.

Because lymphocyte migration across HEVs within some lymphoid tissues occurs in the L-selectin– and the β_7 integrin–deficient mice, it could not be concluded that other adhesion molecules were not involved in initiating lymphocyte-HEV interactions. The generation of mice deficient in expression of L-selectin and β_7 integrins confirmed this hypothesis. Initial characterization of these double-deficient mice demonstrated that peripheral and mucosal lymphoid tissues are dramatically reduced while concurrent increases are found in splenic and circulating lymphocyte populations (81a, 81b). Consistent with this, lymphocytes isolated from these mice are essentially excluded from entering PLNs, MLNs, or Peyer's patches during short- and long-term *in vivo* migration assays (see Fig. 40-1). These cells show increased localization in the spleen, similar to that observed with L-selectin–deficient lymphocytes and an increased number remaining in the circulation. These mice therefore confirm a major role for L-selectin in mediating lymphocyte rolling within Peyer's patches, with the β_7 integrins regulating lymphocyte adhesion within gut-associated lymphoid tissues. L-selectin and β_7 integrins regulate most normal lymphocyte migration across HEVs within secondary lymphoid tissues.

CD18 Integrins and Intercellular Adhesion Molecule-1

The CD18 integrins consist of four members: CD11a/ CD18 (LFA-1, $\alpha_L\beta_2$), CD11b/CD18 (Mac-1, $\alpha_M\beta_2$), CD11c/CD18 (p150,95, $\alpha_X\beta_2$), and α_d/CD18 (82,83). Of these, LFA-1 has the widest distribution among leukocyte populations, is the most well-characterized, and clearly facilitates leukocyte firm adhesion to vascular endothelium at sites of inflammation (84). Ligands for LFA-1 are ICAM-1, -2, and -3, of which only ICAM-1 and -2 are expressed on vascular endothelium. ICAM-1 is typically expressed at low levels on resting endothelium and is dramatically upregulated during inflammation. In contrast, ICAM-2 is constitutively expressed on resting endothelium at higher levels than ICAM-1, but expression is not increased on activation. The increased expression of ICAM-1 is critical in mediating the greatly enhanced leukocyte adherence to the endothelium during inflammatory responses (85). The critical role of CD18 integrins in

mediating leukocyte migration is illustrated in leukocyte adhesion deficiency type I patients, who are unable to produce functional β_2 integrin chains as a result of mutations within the CD18 gene (86). These patients suffer from recurrent, life-threatening bacterial and fungal infections as a result of markedly deficient leukocyte adhesion and migration at sites of infection.

An accessory role for LFA-1 in mediating lymphocyte migration through peripheral lymphoid tissues has been suggested based on studies using function-blocking MAbs. The adhesion of lymphocytes to HEVs *in vitro* (87) and the *in vivo* migration of lymphocytes to peripheral lymphoid tissues can be partially blocked with anti-LFA-1 MAbs (87–89). Anti-ICAM-1 MAb treatment *in vivo* results in a modest reduction in numbers of lymphocytes within PLNs (90). However, studies using mice deficient in expression of either of these molecules have not unequivocally confirmed this accessory role. Peripheral lymphoid tissues of CD18-deficient mice are of normal size and contain a normal distribution of lymphocyte populations (91). Similarly, LFA-1–deficient mice have lymphoid organs within a normal size range, although PLN size tends to be reduced, and they have a normal distribution of leukocyte subsets (92). In contrast, a twofold increase in spleen size and a 75% reduction in PLN size were reported in a second line of LFA-1–deficient mice (93). ICAM-1–deficient mice have normal lymphoid tissues, including PLNs, and have normal distributions of lymphocyte populations within these tissues (94,95). Our studies indicate that lymphocytes isolated from CD18-deficient mice have a reduced ability to migrate to PLNs and MLNs of wild-type mice during short- and long-term *in vivo* migration assays (see Fig. 40-1). The short-term *in vivo* migration of wild-type lymphocytes into PLNs and, to a lesser degree, into Peyer's patches of ICAM-1–deficient mice is reduced (see Fig. 40-1). Migration into PLNs remains reduced by about 50% after long-term migration assays. These findings support a role for ICAM-2 in mediating lymphocyte-HEV interactions. However, the findings with the CD18- and the LFA-1–deficient mice are surprising given that lymphocytes in these mice lack ICAM-1 and ICAM-2–mediated interactions. *In vivo* treatment with anti-VCAM-1 MAb does not inhibit the migration of wild-type lymphocytes into PLNs, MLNs, or Peyer's patches in short-term migration assays (1998). These results suggest that other receptor-ligand pairs important in mediating lymphocyte-HEV adhesion within peripheral lymphoid tissues remain to be defined.

How Adhesion Molecules Work Together

Leukocyte interactions with vascular endothelial cells involve multiple steps, including the capture of flowing leukocytes with their subsequent rolling, firm adhesion, and diapedesis (96). For migration, multiple adhesion molecules function synergistically to mediate the interrelated steps of this cascade and to mediate optimal lymphocyte entry into tissues. L-selectin predominantly mediates leukocyte capture from the blood for migration into PLNs, MLNs, and Peyer's patches. L-selectin and the β_7 integrins contribute cooperatively to lymphocyte rolling when their appropriate ligands are expressed by HEVs. However, the β_7 integrins can mediate this process with low efficiency in the absence of L-selectin expression. Studies using intravital microscopy of exteriorized cremaster muscle vasculature have shown that L-selectin and ICAM-1 function synergistically to mediate optimal leukocyte–endothelial cell interactions at sites of inflammation (13). Leukocytes in ICAM-1–deficient mice exhibit significantly increased rolling velocities compared with those in wild-type mice. Increased rolling velocities cause a reduction in the frequency of leukocytes rolling along the endothelium, which results in fewer leukocytes entering sites of inflammation. Similarly, leukocyte rolling in Peyer's patch HEVs occurs at slower and faster characteristic velocities in L-selectin- and β_7 integrin–deficient mice, respectively (79), which suggests that these receptors function cooperatively to retard lymphocyte rolling and facilitate firm adhesion. This interrelated function among members from different families of adhesion molecules probably regulates the normal migration of lymphocytes into lymphoid tissues. Lymphocyte migration probably is significantly influenced by the relative expression levels of the different adhesion molecules on lymphocytes and endothelium.

SUBSET-SPECIFIC LYMPHOCYTE MIGRATION

In addition to organ-specific molecular mechanisms, the nonrandom, hierarchical migration of CD4$^+$ helper T cells, CD8$^+$ cytotoxic T cells, B cells, and naive or memory lymphocytes suggests the existence of subset-specific lymphocyte–endothelial cell recognition systems. For example, marked differences exist in the distribution of CD4$^+$ T cells, CD8$^+$ T cells and B cells between the blood and afferent and efferent lymph of lymph nodes in sheep (22,97). In sheep, CD4$^+$ T cells are extracted by the HEVs of PLNs at a faster rate than CD8$^+$ T cells or B cells (24,98,99), and CD4$^+$ T cells recirculate more efficiently than CD8$^+$ T cells (97,100). In humans, T cells bind preferentially to PLNs compared with B cells during Stamper-Woodruff *in vitro* binding assays (101). CD4$^+$ T cells bind preferentially to PLN endothelium compared with CD8$^+$ T cells, and CD8$^+$ T cells bind to gut-associated lymphoid tissues more efficiently than CD4$^+$ T cells. In rats, twice as many T cells as B cells enter MLNs and PLNs after intravenous injection (102,103), and approximately equal numbers of B and T cells enter Peyer's patches and spleen (103). B lymphocytes from MLNs bind about three times better to HEVs of Peyer's patches compared with HEVs of PLNs (104). However, the proportional binding of CD4$^+$ cells, CD8$^+$ cells, and B cells isolated from thoracic duct to PLNs, MLNs, or Peyer's patch HEVs is similar to their relative proportions within lymph (104). Despite these results, however, the existence of subset-specific lymphocyte–endothelial cell recognition systems remains controversial (104–106).

During *in vivo* migration assays in mice, more T cells migrate into PLNs, MLNs, and Peyer's patches than B cells (32). Seventeen times more T cells than B cells migrate into PLNs by 1 hour, nine times more T cells enter MLNs, and four times more T cells than B cells enter Peyer's patches (Fig. 40-2). After 48 hours, almost nine and six times more T cells than B cells localize in PLNs and MLNs, respectively (32). Twice as many immigrant B cells accumulate within Peyer's patches relative to T cells, because most entering B cells are retained, whereas T cells constantly enter and exit this tissue. In all cases, CD4$^+$ and CD8$^+$ T cells demonstrate similar migration patterns. These results contrast markedly with those of early studies demonstrating that two to five times more T cells bind to PLNs compared with B cells during *in vitro* frozen-section binding assays, two to three times more B cells bind to Peyer's patch HEVs compared with T cells, and equal numbers of T and B cells bind to HEVs of MLNs (107). Although a similar proportion of CD4$^+$ and CD8$^+$ cells bind to PLN endothelium *in vitro*, CD4$^+$ cells bind to frozen sections of Peyer's patch more efficiently than CD8$^+$ cells (108). The different binding properties of T and B cells are evident regardless of their tissue source (e.g., spleen, PLNs, MLNs, Peyer's patches) (107) or whether they are binding to HEVs of resting or antigen-stimulated PLNs (102). From these studies, it is apparent that T cells are the principal recirculating lymphocyte subpopulation and that B cells do not recirculate as efficiently in mice. Although *in vitro* binding assays suggest differences in expression of adhesion molecules, they do not predict migratory behavior (106).

Because most T and B cells derived from rat blood express L-selectin and $\alpha_4\beta_7$ integrins, it has been argued that tissue-specific lymphocyte–endothelial cell adhesive interactions do not regulate the selective migration of lymphocyte subsets through secondary lymphoid tissues (105). Similarly, most mouse lymphocytes simultaneously express L-selectin and $\alpha_4\beta_7$ integrins (32). However, T cells have intrinsic twofold higher levels of L-selectin expression than B cells (32), and B cells have intrinsically higher levels of $\alpha_4\beta_7$ integrin expression (32,109). Higher levels of L-selectin expression by lymphocytes directly translates into a greater ability to migrate into lymphoid tissues (32). High levels of L-selectin expression by T cells may explain their preferential migration into PLNs, MLNs, and Peyer's patches through interactions with HEVs. Whether higher levels of $\alpha_4\beta_7$ integrin expression by B cells allows these cells to preferentially interact with Peyer's patch HEVs has not been demonstrated. B cell migration into Peyer's

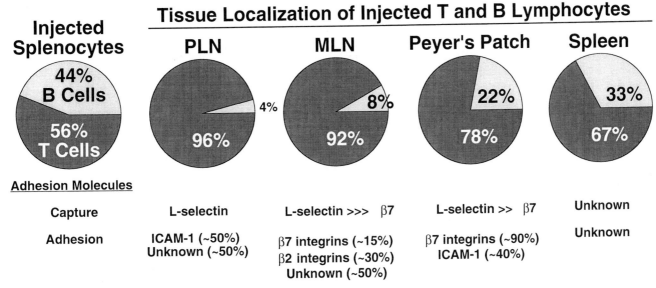

FIG. 40-2. Tissue localization of B cells and T cells during short-term (1-hour) *in vivo* migration assays carried out in mice. Pie graphs represent the average relative proportion of migrated T-cell and B-cell subsets into the indicated secondary lymphoid tissues compared with the proportion within the injected splenocyte population. Data were obtained using two-color *in vivo* migration assays, as previously described (32). The contributions of individual adhesion molecules to the capture and subsequent firm adhesion of the lymphocyte populations in each tissue are indicated below the graphs.

patches can occur independently of L-selectin expression, whereas CD4+ and CD8+ T cell migration into this tissue is predominantly L-selectin dependent. Alternatively, higher $\alpha_4\beta_7$ integrin expression by B cells may explain why B cells are retained in Peyer's patches while most T cells transit through this tissue. T cell use of $\alpha_4\beta_7$ integrins for entry into lymphoid tissues must be relatively inefficient, because T cells do not accumulate within Peyer's patches of L-selectin–deficient mice but rather localize in the spleen (36,39). Subset-specific migration of lymphocytes into secondary lymphoid tissues may be predominantly regulated by the endogenous levels of L-selectin and perhaps $\alpha_4\beta_7$ integrin expression (see Fig. 40-2).

The regulation of L-selectin expression levels is a complex and dynamic process, because L-selectin expression levels change rapidly in response to numerous stimuli, including cellular activation (110,111). This paradigm probably applies to other adhesion molecules as well. The differential migration of T and B lymphocyte subsets is regulated in part by differences in expression levels of cell surface adhesion receptors, and receptor density contributes to the efficiency of interactions between organ-specific receptors on lymphocytes and organ-specific determinants on HEVs.

Lymphocyte Homing

Homing is a term used to describe the increased propensity for previously activated lymphocytes to recirculate back into the tissues where they were initially acti-

vated (112). For example, lymphocytes obtained from efferent intestinal lymph recirculate preferentially through intestinal lymph nodes of sheep, whereas lymphocytes derived from efferent subcutaneous lymph recirculate preferentially through "peripheral" subcutaneous lymph nodes (113). The identification of specific pools of recirculating nodal and intestinal T lymphocytes with different migratory characteristics led to the hypothesis that these migration patterns might be mediated by tissue-specific lymphocyte–endothelial cell recognition mechanisms (114). These findings were extended when a third migration pathway was identified using dermal granulomas as a model tissue (115,116). Similar findings have been described for mice (81). All of these studies point to the fact that different lymphocyte populations have a tendency to migrate preferentially into specific lymphoid organs.

The molecular basis for lymphocyte homing probably can be explained by many factors. First, T cells have a tendency to preferentially localize in PLNs relative to B cells, and B cells tend to accumulate within mucosal lymphoid tissues. Studies using lymphocytes derived from tissues that contained relatively higher proportions of T cells therefore would expect to find more of these cells return to peripheral lymphoid tissues. Similarly, because Peyer's patches contain a higher percentage of B cells relative to PLNs, Peyer's patch lymphocytes would be expected to reaccumulate in Peyer's patches. Lymphocytes entering specific tissues display the appropriate receptors that facilitated their preferential accumulation within that tissue. The cells leaving that tissue should have an advantage for reentering their tissue of origin. The differential expression and use of adhesion molecules probably account for many of these differences, rather than the cells becoming specifically imprinted with a display of adhesion molecules that depend on the site at which they encountered antigen.

Lymphocyte activation within a site of inflammation or immune response probably alters the display of adhesion receptors expressed, which may also facilitate the retention of specific lymphocyte subpopulations within certain tissues. For example, the mucosal $\alpha_E\beta_7$ integrin is expressed on 95% of intraepithelial lymphocytes but on only 1% to 2% of peripheral blood lymphocytes (66,117). Expression of $\alpha_E\beta_7$ integrin is induced in the presence of transforming growth factor-β1, but expression of LFA-1 is reduced (65). Because the β_7 integrins play a specialized role in mucosal localization and adhesion, expression of β_7 integrins can facilitate increased migration to or retention within gut-associated lymphoid tissues. This is particularly true for activated lymphocytes that may express these integrins in an active binding state.

Naive and Memory T-Cell Migration

The migratory pathways of naive and memory lymphocytes have long been thought to be different based in part on the number of adhesion molecule changes that occur during the transition from a naive to memory phenotype (118). Naive lymphocytes are relatively uniform in expressing high levels of L-selectin and moderate to low levels of CD18, $\alpha_4\beta_7$ and $\alpha_4\beta_1$ integrins, and CD44. In contrast, lymphocyte activation induces significant alterations in surface receptor expression, including L-selectin downregulation (29,119,120) and the upregulation of CD18 and $\alpha_4\beta_1$ integrins and CD44 (121). Although numerous reports conclude that mouse memory CD4$^+$ T cells are L-selectin negative (120,122), other studies have demonstrated L-selectin expression on substantial proportions of memory CD4$^+$ T cells isolated from human blood (33,123) and mouse tissues (39,109,124,125). Expression levels of $\alpha_4\beta_7$ integrin are highly variable on mouse and human CD4$^+$ memory T cells (109,126). These complications, in addition to the complexity in defining memory lymphocyte phenotypes, indicate that the expression levels of adhesion molecules involved in lymphocyte migration are extremely heterogeneous among memory lymphocyte subpopulations.

The differential expression of L-selectin and other adhesion molecules by naive and memory lymphocytes suggests the existence of specific functional roles and migratory capabilities of cells with a defined phenotype during immune responses. It has been suggested that naive lymphocytes migrate directly from blood through an L-selectin–dependent interaction with HEVs in PLNs. Memory lymphocytes are proposed to use different adhesion receptors to migrate selectively to other tissues,

including the gut and skin, and then enter lymph nodes through the afferent lymphatics (22,127–129). Support for this concept has predominantly been obtained indirectly by determining the frequencies of naive and memory T lymphocytes in the afferent and efferent lymph of sheep (22,127–129). However, other studies have questioned whether it is appropriate to place naive and memory populations into such exclusive migratory pathways. It has been shown that naive T lymphocytes can migrate into lymph nodes and skin in other animal models (9,130). Rat thoracic duct lymphocytes with a memory phenotype migrate from the blood into the efferent lymph through lymph nodes at similar levels and during similar periods as naive lymphocytes (131). These memory cells also localize to HEVs of PLNs (9).

A characteristic feature in L-selectin–deficient mice is the accumulation of memory lymphocytes within the circulation and spleen, suggesting that the loss of L-selectin on a subset of these cells blocks their migration into peripheral lymphoid tissues (39). Lymphocyte migration is significantly affected by the array and density of adhesion molecules expressed by individual cells at any time. For example, large numbers of T cells enter Peyer's patches. For most lymphocytes, L-selectin is required for their initial capture and rolling on Peyer's patch HEVs (77,78). However, significant numbers of T cells enter Peyer's patches in the absence of L-selectin expression, possibly including $\alpha_4\beta_7$ integrin high-memory cells (39). Given these caveats, the difficulty in defining memory cells, and the considerable heterogeneity among memory cells, it is not appropriate to generalize and predict the tissue localization of broad populations of cells based on phenotype alone, because many factors influence this process (132).

LYMPHOCYTE MIGRATION TO THE SKIN

Specific migration of lymphocytes into inflamed skin is thought to be largely mediated by endothelial E-selectin. E-selectin is not normally expressed by resting endothelial cells and is not present in other cell types, but it is expressed by cytokine-activated endothelial cells *in vitro* by 4 to 6 hours, with sustained expression *in vivo* during inflammation (133–135). E-selectin binds to a carbohydrate determinant on leukocytes called the *cutaneous lymphocyte antigen* (CLA) during leukocyte–endothelial cell interactions (136–140). LFA-1 interacting with ICAM-1 and very late activation antigen-4 (VLA-4) interacting with VCAM-1 are thought to mediate subsequent firm adhesion (121,124). Consistent with this idea, ICAM-1–deficient mice have decreased contact hypersensitivity responses in the skin (94,95). However, E-selectin–deficient mice generate normal delayed-type hypersensitivity (DTH) responses in the skin, suggesting that other adhesion receptor pairs are also important in this process (141). P-selectin plays an important role in leukocyte migration to cutaneous sites, because P-selectin–deficient mice have reduced leukocyte recruitment into sites of contact hypersensitivity (142) and reduced leukocyte rolling in skin (143). However, allogeneic skin grafts are rejected normally in P-selectin–deficient mice (144).

L-selectin is also an important adhesion molecule for mediating leukocyte migration into inflamed skin. L-selectin–deficient mice have significantly impaired DTH responses because of decreased leukocyte recruitment into sites of cutaneous inflammation (37,145). Cutaneous lesions from a variety of disease states display increased expression of potential L-selectin ligands identified by the MECA-79 MAb (58,127) and the 2H5 MAb (61). The absence of L-selectin on lymphocytes recruited into the skin or draining lymph nodes during a cutaneous inflammatory response was previously used to argue against any involvement of L-selectin in lymphocyte homing to inflamed skin (121,124). However, several studies have demonstrated L-selectin surface expression on 80% to 90% of lymphocytes recruited into cutaneous suction blisters during DTH responses (138,146). Because cellular activation results in the endoproteolytic release of L-selectin from the cell surface, L-selectin expression may change rapidly during the recruitment process (40,41,119). L-selectin also plays a functionally significant role in allogeneic skin graft rejection (144). L-selectin–deficient mice reject primary and secondary allogeneic skin grafts significantly slower than wild-type littermates and have reduced numbers of $CD4^+$ and $CD8^+$ T cells present within the graft bed and dermis. Multiple adhesion molecule pairs, including L-selectin and its ligands, P-selectin and PSGL-1, E-selectin and CLA, VLA-4 and VCAM-1, and LFA-1 and ICAM-1, probably regulate leukocyte migration into cutaneous sites of inflammation.

LYMPHOCYTE MIGRATION TO SITES OF INFLAMMATION

L-selectin is the principal selectin operable for lymphocyte migration to sites of vascular inflammation. For example, lymphocyte migration into the peritoneal cavity of L-selectin–deficient mice is severely impaired subsequent to thioglycolate instillation (145). L-selectin ligands are induced on cytokine activated human umbilical vein endothelial cells, microvascular endothelial cells, and aortic endothelial cells (147–152). The L-selectin ligands expressed on vascular endothelium are carbohydrate determinants displayed by specific cell surface molecules, which are distinct from the MECA-79 MAb-defined ligands present on HEVs. Moreover, interactions between L-selectin and its vascular ligands are completely blocked by the HECA-452 MAb (152) that identifies CLA. CLA is similar to the 6-sulfo sLe^X and 6,6'-bis-sulfo sLe^X determinants, which can serve as L-selectin ligands on HEVs (62,153) and rat endothelium

at sites of inflammation (61). Because HEV-like vessels that support lymphocyte migration are observed in chronically inflamed nonlymphoid tissues (154), findings suggest that CLA induction on vascular endothelial cells generates a functional L-selectin ligand that may be related to the 6-sulfo sLe^X determinants, which can serve as HEV ligands for L-selectin. Subsequent to L-selectin–mediated capture of lymphocytes from the blood, LFA-1 and VLA-4 probably facilitate rolling and firm adhesion of lymphocytes before they adhere and enter sites of inflammation.

CONCLUSIONS

Whereas the migration of lymphocytes through lymphoid tissues is an essential component of the immune system, the inappropriate or abnormal sequestration of lymphocytes at specific sites is a central component in the development of a variety of autoimmune diseases and pathologic inflammatory disorders. Blocking the function of adhesion molecules involved in lymphocyte–endothelial cell attachment may have dramatic effects on inflammatory reactions. Blocking adhesion molecule function in a number of animal models has had beneficial effects on the progression of inflammatory responses in a variety of tissues (155,156). Therapeutic agents that specifically block adhesion molecule function will be advantageous in inflammatory situations but may also influence lymphocyte migration because common adhesion pathways appear to mediate both processes.

ACKNOWLEDGMENTS

This work was supported by grants HL-50985, AI-26872, and CA-54464 from the National Institutes of Health.

REFERENCES

1. Ford WL, Gowans JL. The role of lymphocytes in antibody formation. II. The influence of lymphocyte migration on the initiation of antibody formation in the isolated, perfused spleen. *Proc R Soc Lond B* 1967; 168:244–262.
2. Gowans JL. The recirculation of lymphocytes from blood to lymph in rat. *J Physiol* 1959;146:54–69.
3. Gowans JL. The effect of the continuous reinfusion of lymph and lymphocytes on the output of lymphocytes from the thoracic duct of unanaesthetized rats. *Br J Exp Pathol* 1957;38:67–78.
4. Gowans JL, Knight EJ. The route of recirculation of lymphocytes in the rat. *Proc R Soc Lond B* 1964;159:257–282.
5. Fossum S, Smith ME, Ford WL. The migration of lymphocytes across specialized vascular endothelium. VII. The migration of T and B lymphocytes from the blood of the athymic, nude rat. *Scand J Immunol* 1983;17:539–550.
6. Butcher EC. Specificity of leukocyte-endothelial interactions and diapedesis: physiologic and therapeutic implications of an active decision making process. *Res Immunol* 1993;144:695–698.
7. Pabst R. The spleen in lymphocyte migration. *Immunol Today* 1988;9: 43–45.
8. Pabst R, Binns RM. Heterogeneity of lymphocyte homing physiology: several mechanisms operate in the control of migration to lymphoid and non-lymphoid organs *in vivo*. *Immunol Rev* 1989;108:83–109.

9. Westermann J, Pabst R. How organ-specific is the migration of "naive" and "memory" T lymphocytes? *Immunol Today* 1996;17: 278–282.

10. Picker LJ, Butcher EC. Physiological and molecular mechanisms of lymphocyte homing. *Annu Rev Immunol* 1992;10:561–591.

11. Springer TA. Traffic signals on endothelium for lymphocyte recirculation and leukocyte emigration. *Annu Rev Physiol* 1995;57:827–872.

12. Tedder TF, Steeber DA, Chen A, Engel P. The selectins: vascular adhesion molecules. *FASEB J* 1995;9:866–873.

13. Steeber DA, Campbell MA, Basit A, Ley K, Tedder TF. Optimal selectin-mediated rolling of leukocytes during inflammation *in vivo* requires intercellular adhesion molecule-1 expression. *Proc Natl Acad Sci USA* 1998;95:7562–7567.

14. Spertini O, Kansas GS, Munro JM, Griffin JD, Tedder TF. Regulation of leukocyte migration by activation of the leukocyte adhesion molecule-1 (LAM-1) selectin. *Nature* 1991;349:691–694.

15. Hall JG. Quantitative aspects of the recirculation of lymphocytes: an analysis of data from experiments on sheep. *Q J Exp Physiol* 1967; 52:76.

16. Hall JG, Morris B. The output of cells in the efferent lymph from a single lymph node. *Q J Exp Physiol* 1962;47:360.

17. Smith JB, McIntosh GH, Morris B. The traffic of cells through tissues: a study of peripheral lymph in sheep. *J Anat* 1970;107:87–100.

18. Schoefl GI. The migration of lymphocytes across the vascular endothelium in lymphoid tissue: a reexamination. *J Exp Med* 1972;136: 568–588.

19. Stamper HB Jr, Woodruff JJ. Lymphocyte homing into lymph nodes: *in vitro* demonstration of the selective affinity of recirculating lymphocytes for high-endothelial venules. *J Exp Med* 1976;144:828–833.

20. Croitoru K, Bienenstock J. Characteristics and function of mucosa-associated lymphoid tissue. In: Ogra PL, Strober W, Mestecky J, McGhee JR, Lamm ME, Bienenstock J, eds. *Handbook of mucosal immunology.* San Diego: Academic Press, 1994:141.

21. Hall JG, Morris B. The origin of the cells in the efferent lymph from a single lymph node. *J Exp Med* 1965;121:901–910.

22. Mackay CR, Kimpton WG, Brandon MR, Cahill RNP. Lymphocyte subsets show marked differences in their distribution between blood and the afferent and efferent lymph of peripheral lymph nodes. *J Exp Med* 1988;167:1755–1765.

23. Hall JG, Morris B. The immediate effect of antigens on the cell output of a lymph node. *Br J Exp Pathol* 1965;46:450–454.

24. Washington EA, Kimpton WG, Cahill RNP. CD4+ lymphocytes are extracted from blood by peripheral lymph nodes at different rates than other T cell subsets and B cells. *Eur J Immunol* 1988;18:2093–2096.

25. Hay JB, Hobbs BB. The flow of blood to lymph nodes and its relation to lymphocyte traffic and the immune response. *J Exp Med* 1977; 145:31–44.

26. Bjerknes M, Cheng H, Ottaway CA. Dynamics of lymphocyte-endothelial interactions *in vivo. Science* 1986;231:402–405.

27. Gallatin WM, Weissman IL, Butcher EC. A cell-surface molecule involved in organ-specific homing of lymphocytes. *Nature* 1983;304: 30–34.

28. Robinson LA, Steeber DA, Tedder TF. The selectins in inflammation. In: Gallin JI, Snyderman R, eds. *Inflammation:* basic principles and clinical correlates. Philadelphia: Lippincott Williams & Wilkins, 1999.

29. Tedder TF, Penta AC, Levine HB, Freedman AS. Expression of the human leukocyte adhesion molecule, LAM1. Identity with the TQ1 and Leu-8 differentiation antigens. *J Immunol* 1990;144:532–540.

30. Kansas GS, Dailey MO. Expression of adhesion structures during B cell development in man. *J Immunol* 1989;142:3058–3062.

31. Wallace DL, Beverley PC. Characterization of a novel subset of T cells from human spleen that lacks L-selectin. *Immunology* 1993;78: 623–628.

32. Tang MLK, Steeber DA, Zhang X-Q, Tedder TF. Intrinsic differences in L-selectin expression levels affect T and B lymphocyte subset-specific recirculation pathways. *J Immunol* 1998;160:5113–5121.

33. Tedder TF, Matsuyama T, Rothstein DM, Schlossman SF, Morimoto C. Human antigen-specific memory T cells express the homing receptor necessary for lymphocyte recirculation. *Eur J Immunol* 1990;20:1351–1355.

34. Zola H, Flego L, Macardle PJ, Donohoe PJ, Ranford J, Roberton D. The CD45RO (p180, UCHL1) marker: complexity of expression in peripheral blood. *Cell Immunol* 1992;145:175–186.

35. Lee WT, Vitetta ES. The differential expression of homing and adhesion molecules on virgin and memory T cells in the mouse. *Cell Immunol* 1991;132:215–222.

36. Arbones ML, Ord DC, Ley K, et al. Lymphocyte homing and leukocyte rolling and migration are impaired in L-selectin (CD62L) deficient mice. *Immunity* 1994;1:247–260.

37. Xu J, Grewal IS, Geba GP, Flavell RA. Impaired primary T cell responses in L-selectin–deficient mice. *J Exp Med* 1996;183:589–598.

38. Catalina MD, Carroll MC, Arizpe H, Takashima A, Estess P, Siegelman MH. The route of antigen entry determines the requirement for L-selectin during immune responses. *J Exp Med* 1996;184:2341–2351.

39. Steeber DA, Green NE, Sato S, Tedder TF. Lymphocyte migration in L-selectin–deficient mice: altered subset migration and aging of the immune system. *J Immunol* 1996;157:1096–1106.

40. Chen A, Engel P, Tedder TF. Structural requirements regulate endoproteolytic release of the L-selectin (CD62L) adhesion receptor from the cell surface of leukocytes. *J Exp Med* 1995;182:519–530.

41. Griffin JD, Spertini O, Ernst TJ, et al. GM-CSF and other cytokines regulate surface expression of the leukocyte adhesion molecule-1 on human neutrophils, monocytes, and their precursors. *J Immunol* 1990;145:576–584.

42. Rosen SD, Bertozzi CR. The selectins and their ligands. *Curr Opin Cell Biol* 1994;6:663–673.

43. Shimizu Y, Shaw S. Cell adhesion: mucins in the mainstream. *Nature* 1993;366:630–631.

44. Lasky LA, Singer MS, Dowbenko D, et al. An endothelial ligand for L-selectin is a novel mucin-like molecule. *Cell* 1992;69:927–938.

45. Imai Y, Singer MS, Fennie C, Lasky LA, Rosen SD. Identification of a carbohydrate-based endothelial ligand for a lymphocyte homing receptor. *J Cell Biol* 1991;113:1213–1221.

46. Baumhueter S, Singer MS, Henzel W, et al. Binding of L-selectin to the vascular sialomucin CD34. *Science* 1993;262:436–438.

47. Berg EL, McEvoy LM, Berlin C, Bargatze RF, Butcher EC. L-selectin–mediated lymphocyte rolling on MAdCAM-1. *Nature* 1993; 366:695–698.

48. Hemmerich S, Butcher EC, Rosen SD. Sulfation-dependent recognition of HEV-ligands by L-selectin and MECA 79, an adhesion-blocking mAb. *J Exp Med* 1994;180:2219–2226.

49. Sassetti C, Tangemann K, Singer MS, Kershaw DB, Rosen SD. Identification of podocalyxin-like protein as a high endothelial venule ligand for L-selectin: parallels to CD34. *J Exp Med* 1998;187: 1965–1975.

50. Tu L, Chen A, Delahunty MD, Moore KL, Watson S, McEver RP, Tedder TF. L-selectin binds to P-selectin glycoprotein ligand-1 on leukocytes. Interactions between the lectin, EGF and consensus repeat domains of the selectins determine ligand binding specificity. *J Immunol* 1996;156:3995–4004.

51. Spertini O, Cordey A-S, Monai N, Giuffrè L, Schapira M. P-selectin glycoprotein ligand 1 is a ligand for L-selectin on neutrophils, monocytes, and CD34+ hematopoietic progenitor cells. *J Cell Biol* 1996; 135:523–531.

52. Laszik Z, Jansen PJ, Cummings RD, Tedder TF, McEver RP, Moore KL. P-selectin glycoprotein ligand-1 is broadly expressed in cells of myeloid, lymphoid, and dendritic lineage and in some non-hematopoietic cells. *Blood* 1996;88:3010–3021.

53. Bargatze RF, Kurk S, Butcher EC, Jutila MA. Neutrophils roll on adherent neutrophils bound to cytokine-induced endothelial cells via L-selectin on the rolling cells. *J Exp Med* 1994;180:1785–1792.

54. Kunkel EJ, Chomas JE, Ley K. Role of primary and secondary capture for leukocyte accumulation *in vivo. Circ Res* 1998;82:30–38.

55. Berg EL, Robinson MK, Warnock RA, Butcher EC. The human peripheral lymph node vascular addressin is a ligand for LECAM-1, the peripheral lymph node homing receptor. *J Cell Biol* 1991;114:343–349.

56. Streeter PR, Rouse BTN, Butcher EC. Immunologic and functional characterization of a vascular addressin involved in lymphocyte homing into peripheral lymph nodes. *J Cell Biol* 1988;107:1853–1862.

57. Streeter PR, Berg EL, Rouse BN, Bargatze RF, Butcher EC. A tissue-specific endothelial cell molecule involved in lymphocyte homing. *Nature* 1988;331:41–46.

58. Michie SA, Streeter PR, Bolt PA, Butcher EC, Picker LJ. The human peripheral lymph node vascular addressin: an inducible endothelial antigen involved in lymphocyte homing. *Am J Pathol* 1993;143:1688–1698.

59. Clark RA, Fuhlbrigge RC, Springer TA. L-selectin ligands that are *O*-glycoprotease resistant and distinct from MECA-79 antigen are suffi-

cient for tethering and rolling of lymphocytes on human high endothelial venules. *J Cell Biol* 1998;140:721–731.

60. Maly P, Thall AD, Petryniak B, et al. The α(1,3) fucosyltransferase Fuc-TVII controls leukocyte trafficking through an essential role in L-, E-, and P-selectin ligand biosynthesis. *Cell* 1996;86:643–653.

61. Akahori T, Yuzawa Y, Nishikawa K, et al. Role of a sialyl Lewis^X-like epitope selectively expressed on vascular endothelial cells in local skin inflammation of the rat. *J Immunol* 1997;158:5384–5392.

62. Mitsuoka C, Kawakami-Kimura N, Kasugai-Sawada M, et al. Sulfated sialyl Lewis X, the putative L-selectin ligand, detected on endothelial cells of high endothelial venules by a distinct set of anti-sialyl Lewis X antibodies. *Biochem Biophys Res Commun* 1997;230:546–551.

63. Seko Y, Enokawa Y, Tamatani T, et al. Expression of sialyl Lewis^X in rat heart with ischemia/reperfusion and reduction of myocardial reperfusion injury by a monoclonal antibody against sialyl Lewis^X. *J Pathol* 1996;180:305–310.

64. Parker CM, Cepek KL, Russell GJ, et al. A family of beta-7 integrins on human mucosal lymphocytes. *Proc Natl Acad Sci USA* 1992;89:1924–1928.

65. Cepek KL, Parker CM, Madara JL, Brenner MB. Integrin α$_E$β$_7$ mediates adhesion of T lymphocytes to epithelial cells. *J Immunol* 1993;150:3459–3470.

66. Cerf-Bensussan N, Jarry A, Brousse N, Lisowska-Grospierre B, Guy-Grand D, Griscelli C. A monoclonal antibody (HML-1) defining a novel membrane molecule present on human intestinal lymphocytes. *Eur J Immunol* 1987;17:1279–1285.

67. Geoffroy JS, Rosen S. Demonstration that a lectin-like receptor (gp90^{mel}) directly mediates adhesion of lymphocytes to high endothelial venules of lymph nodes. *J Cell Biol* 1989;109:2463–2469.

68. Holzmann B, McIntyre BW, Weissman IL. Identification of a murine Peyer's patch-specific lymphocyte homing receptor as an integrin molecule with an α chain homologous to human VLA-4α. *Cell* 1989;56:37–46.

69. Hu MC, Crowe DT, Weissman IL, Holzmann B. Cloning and expression of mouse integrin β$_p$(β$_7$): a functional role in Peyer's patch-specific lymphocyte homing. *Proc Natl Acad Sci USA* 1992;89:8254–8258.

70. Rosen SD, Singer MS, Yednock YA, Stoolman LM. Involvement of sialic acid on endothelial cells in organ-specific lymphocyte recirculation. *Science* 1985;228:1005–1007.

71. Rosen SD, Chi SI, True DD, Singer MS, Yednock TA. Intravenously injected sialidase inactivates attachment sites for lymphocytes on high endothelial venules. *J Immunol* 1989;142:1895–1902.

72. Watson SR, Imai Y, Fennie C, Geoffrey JS, Rosen SD, Lasky LA. A homing receptor-IgG chimera as a probe for adhesive ligands of lymph node high endothelial venules. *J Cell Biol* 1990;110:2221–2229.

73. Nakache M, Berg E, Streeter P, Butcher E. The mucosal vascular addressin is a tissue-specific endothelial cell adhesion molecule for circulating lymphocytes. *Nature* 1989;337:179–181.

74. Briskin MJ, McEvoy LM, Butcher EC. MAdCAM-1 has homology to immunoglobulin and mucin-like adhesion receptors and to IgA1. *Nature* 1993;363:461–464.

75. Szabo MC, Butcher EC, McEvoy LM. Specialization of mucosal follicular dendritic cells revealed by mucosal addressin-cell adhesion molecule-1 display. *J Immunol* 1997;158:5584–5588.

76. Bargatze RF, Streeter PR, Butcher EC. Expression of low levels of peripheral lymph node-associated vascular addressin in mucosal lymphoid tissues: possible relevance to the dissemination of passaged AKR lymphomas. *J Cell Biochem* 1990;42:219–227.

77. Bargatze RF, Jutila MA, Butcher EC. Distinct roles of L-selectin and integrins α$_4$β$_7$ and LFA-1 in lymphocyte homing to Peyer's patch-HEV *in situ*: the multistep hypothesis confirmed and refined. *Immunity* 1995;3:99–108.

78. Wagner N, Lohler J, Kunkel EJ, et al. Critical role for β7 integrins in formation of the gut-associated lymphoid tissue. *Nature* 1996;382:366–370.

79. Kunkel EJ, Ramos CL, Steeber DA, et al. The roles of L-selectin, B$_7$ integrins, and P-selectin in leukocyte rolling and adhesion in high endothelial venules of Peyer's patches. *J Immunol* 1998;161:2449–2456.

80. Hamann A, Jablonski-Westrich D, Jonas P, Thiele H. Homing receptors reexamined: mouse LECAM-1 (MEL-14 antigen) is involved in lymphocyte migration into gut-associated lymphoid tissue. *Eur J Immunol* 1991;21:2925–2929.

81. Butcher EC, Scollay RG, Weissman IL. Organ specificity of lymphocyte migration: mediation by highly selective lymphocyte interaction with organ-specific determinants on high endothelial venules. *Eur J Immunol* 1980;10:556–561.

81a. Steeber DA, Tang MLK, Zhang X-A, Müller W, Wagner N, Tedder TF. Efficient lymphocyte migration across high endothelial venules of mouse Peyer's patches requires overlapping expression of L-selectin and B$_7$ integrin. *J Immunol* 1998;161:(*in press*).

81b. Wagner N, Löhler J, Tedder TF, Rajewsky K, Müller W, Steeber DA. L-selectin and B$_7$ integrin synergistically mediate lymphocyte migration to mesenteric lymph nodes. *Eur J Immunol* 1998;(*in press*).

82. Larson RS, Springer TA. Structure and function of leukocyte integrins. *Immunol Rev* 1990;114:181–217.

83. Danilenko DM, Rossitto PV, Van der Vieren M, et al. A novel canine leukointegrin, α$_d$β$_2$, is expressed by specific macrophage subpopulations in tissue and a minor CD8$^+$ lymphocyte subpopulation in peripheral blood. *J Immunol* 1995;155:35–44.

84. Springer TA. Adhesion receptors of the immune system. *Nature* 1990;346:425–434.

85. Dustin ML, Springer TA. Lymphocyte function-associated antigen-1 (LFA-1) interaction with intercellular adhesion molecule-1 (ICAM-1) is one of at least three mechanisms for lymphocyte adhesion to cultured endothelial cells. *J Cell Biol* 1988;107:321–331.

86. Anderson DC, Springer TA. Leukocyte adhesion deficiency: an inherited defect in the Mac-1, LFA-1 and p150,95 glycoproteins. *Annu Rev Med* 1987;38:175–194.

87. Hamann A, Jablonski-Westrich D, Duijvestijn A, et al. Evidence for an accessory role of LFA-1 in lymphocyte-high endothelium interaction during homing. *J Immunol* 1988;140:693–699.

88. Camp RL, Scheynius A, Hohansson C, Pure E. CD44 is necessary for optimal contact allergic responses but is not required for normal leukocyte extravasation. *J Exp Med* 1993;178:497–507.

89. Issekutz TB. Inhibition of lymphocyte endothelial adhesion and *in vivo* lymphocyte migration to cutaneous inflammation by TA-3, a new monoclonal antibody to rat LFA-1. *J Immunol* 1992;149:3394–3402.

90. Scheynius A, Camp RL, Pure E. Reduced contact sensitivity reactions in mice treated with monoclonal antibodies to leukocyte function-associated molecule-1 and intercellular adhesion molecule-1. *J Immunol* 1993;150:655–663.

91. Wilson RW, Ballantyne CM, Smith CW, et al. Gene targeting yields a CD18-mutant mouse for study of inflammation. *J Immunol* 1993;151:1571–1578.

92. Shier P, Otulakowski G, Ngo K, et al. Impaired immune responses toward alloantigens and tumor cells but normal thymic selection in mice deficient in the β2 integrin leukocyte function-associated antigen-1. *J Immunol* 1996;157:5375–5386.

93. Schmits R, Kundig TM, Baker DM, et al. LFA-1–deficient mice show normal CTL responses to virus but fail to reject immunogenic tumor. *J Exp Med* 1996;183:1415–1426.

94. Xu H, Gonzalo JA, St Pierre Y, et al. Leukocytosis and resistance to septic shock in intercellular adhesion molecule 1–deficient mice. *J Exp Med* 1994;180:95–109.

95. Sligh JE Jr, Ballantyne CM, Rich SS, et al. Inflammatory and immune responses are impaired in mice deficient in intercellular adhesion molecule 1. *Proc Natl Acad Sci USA* 1993;90:8529–8533.

96. Ley K, Tedder TF. Leukocyte interactions with vascular endothelium: new insights into selectin-mediated attachment and rolling. *J Immunol* 1995;155:525–528.

97. Abernethy NJ, Hay JB, Kimpton WG, Washington E, Cahill RNP. Lymphocyte subset-specific and tissue-specific lymphocyte-endothelial cell recognition mechanisms independently direct the recirculation of lymphocytes from the blood to lymph in sheep. *Immunology* 1991;72:239–245.

98. Witherden DA, Kimpton WG, Washington EA, Cahill RNP. Non-random migration of CD4$^+$, CD8$^+$ and γ/δT19$^+$ lymphocytes through peripheral lymph nodes. *Immunology* 1990;70:235–240.

99. Reynolds JD, Chin W, Shmoorkoff J. T and B cells have similar recirculation kinetics in sheep. *Eur J Immunol* 1988;18:835–840.

100. Abernethy NJ, Hay JB, Kimpton WG, Washington EA, Cahill RNP. Nonrandom recirculation of small, CD4$^+$ and CD8$^+$ T lymphocytes in sheep: evidence for lymphocyte subset-specific endothelial cell recognition. *Int Immunol* 1990;2:231–238.

101. Pals ST, Kraal G, Horst E, de Groot A, Scheper RJ, Meijer CJLM. Human lymphocyte-high endothelial venule interaction: organ-selec-

tive binding of T and B lymphocyte populations to high endothelium. *J Immunol* 1986;137:760–763.

102. Kimpton WG, Poskitt DC, Ruby J, Petersons A, Muller HK. The entry of T and B lymphocytes into rat popliteal lymph nodes undergoing a graft-versus-host reaction. *Cell Immunol* 1983;80:143–150.

103. Fossum S, Smith ME, Ford WL. The recirculation of T and B lymphocytes in the athymic, nude rat. *Scand J Immunol* 1983;17:551–557.

104. Westermann J, Blaschke V, Zimmermann G, Hirschfeld U, Pabst R. Random entry of circulating lymphocyte subsets into peripheral lymph nodes and Peyer's patches: no evidence *in vivo* of a tissue-specific migration of B and T lymphocytes at the level of high endothelial venules. *Eur J Immunol* 1992;22:2219–2223.

105. Westermann J, Nagahori Y, Walter S, Heerwagen C, Miyasaka M, Pabst R. B and T lymphocyte subsets enter peripheral lymph nodes and Peyer's patches without preference *in vivo*: no correlation occurs between their localization in different types of high endothelial venules and the expression of CD44, VLA-4, LFA-1, ICAM-1, CD2 or L-selectin. *Eur J Immunol* 1994;24:2312–2316.

106. Walter S, Micheel B, Pabst R, Westermann J. Interaction of B and T lymphocyte subsets with high endothelial venules in the rat: binding *in vitro* does not reflect homing *in vivo*. *Eur J Immunol* 1995;25:1199–1205.

107. Stevens SK, Weissman IL, Butcher EC. Differences in the migration of B and T lymphocytes: organ-selective localization *in vivo* and the role of lymphocyte-endothelial cell recognition. *J Immunol* 1982;128: 844–851.

108. Kraal G, Weissman IL, Butcher EC. Differences in *in vivo* distribution and homing of T cell subsets to mucosal vs nonmucosal lymphoid organs. *J Immunol* 1983;130:1097–1102.

109. Andrew DP, Rott LS, Kilshaw PJ, Butcher EC. Distribution of $\alpha_4\beta_7$ and $\alpha_E\beta_7$ integrins on thymocytes, intestinal epithelial lymphocytes and peripheral lymphocytes. *Eur J Immunol* 1996;26:897–905.

110. Tedder TF. Regulation of L-selectin function: a leukocyte receptor for endothelium. In: Navarro J, ed. *Molecular basis of inflammation.* Rome: Ares-Serono Symposia Publications, 1994:185–200.

111. Munro JM, Briscoe DM, Tedder TF. Differential regulation of leukocyte L-selectin (CD62L) expression in normal lymphoid and inflamed extralymphoid tissues. *J Clin Pathol* 1996;49:721–727.

112. Butcher EC. The regulation of lymphocyte traffic. *Curr Top Microbiol Immunol* 1986;128:86–122.

113. Scollay R, Hopkins J, Hall JG. Possible role of surface Ig in non-random recirculation of small lymphocytes. *Nature* 1976;260:528–529.

114. Cahill RNP, Poskitt DC, Frost M, Trnka Z. Two distinct pools of recirculating T lymphocytes: migratory characteristics of nodal and intestinal T lymphocytes. *J Exp Med* 1977;145:420–428.

115. Chin W, Hay JB. A comparison of lymphocyte migration through intestinal lymph nodes, subcutaneous lymph nodes, and chronic inflammatory sites of sheep. *Gastroenterology* 1980;79:1231–1242.

116. Issekutz TB, Chin W, Hay JB. Lymphocyte traffic through granulomas: difference in the recovery of indium-111–labeled lymphocytes in afferent and efferent lymph. *Cell Immunol* 1980;54:79–86.

117. Cerf-Bensussan N, Begue B, Gagnon J, Meo T. The human intraepithelial lymphocyte marker HML-1 is an integrin consisting of a B-7 subunit associated with a distinctive α chain. *Eur J Immunol* 1992;22:273–277.

118. Mackay CR. T-cell memory: the connection between function, phenotype and migration pathways. *Immunol Today* 1991;12:189–192.

119. Jung TM, Gallatin WM, Weissman IL, Dailey MO. Down-regulation of homing receptors after T cell activation. *J Immunol* 1988;141: 4110–4117.

120. Bradley LM, Atkins GG, Swain SS. Long-term memory CD4+ T cells from spleen lack MEL-14, the lymph node homing receptor. *J Immunol* 1992;148:324–331.

121. Mobley JL, Dailey MO. Regulation of adhesion molecule expression by CD8 T cells *in vivo*. I. Differential regulation of gp90^MEL14 (LECAM-1), Pgp-1, LFA-1, and VLA-4α during the differentiation of CTL induced by allografts. *J Immunol* 1992;148:2348–2356.

122. Swain SL, Bradley LM, Croft M, et al. Helper T cell subsets: phenotype, function, and the role of lymphokines in regulating their development. *Immunol Rev* 1991;123:115–144.

123. Tsuji T, Nibu R, Iwai K, et al. Efficient induction of immunoglobulin production in neonatal naive B cells by memory CD4+ T cell subset expressing homing receptor L-selectin. *J Immunol* 1994;152: 4417–4424.

124. Mobley JL, Rigby SM, Dailey MO. Regulation of adhesion molecule

125. expression by CD8 T cells *in vivo*. II. Expression of L-selectin (CD62L) by memory cytolytic T cells responding to minor histocompatibility antigens. *J Immunol* 1994;153:5443–5452.

125. Tripp RA, Hou S, Doherty PC. Temporal loss of the activated L-selectin low phenotype for virus-specific CD8+ memory T cells. *J Immunol* 1995;154:5870–5875.

126. Schweighoffer T, Tanaka Y, Tidswell M, et al. Selective expression of integrin $\alpha_4\beta_7$ on a subset of human CD4+ memory T cells with hallmarks of gut-trophism. *J Immunol* 1993;151:717–729.

127. Mackay CR, Marston W, Dudler L. Altered patterns of T cell migration through lymph nodes and skin following antigen challenge. *Eur J Immunol* 1992;22:2205–2210.

128. Mackay CR, Marston WL, Dudler L, Spertini O, Tedder TF, Hein WR. Tissue-specific migration pathways by phenotypically distinct subpopulations of memory T cells. *Eur J Immunol* 1992;22:887–895.

129. Mackay CR, Marston WL, Dudler L. Naive and memory T cells show distinct pathways of lymphocyte recirculation. *J Exp Med* 1990;171: 801–817.

130. Washington EA, Kimpton WG, Holder JE, Cahill RN. Role of the thymus in the generation of skin-homing alpha beta and gamma delta virgin T cells. *Eur J Immunol* 1995;25:723–727.

131. Westermann J, Persin S, Matyas J, van der Meide P, Pabst R. Migration of so-called naive and memory T lymphocytes from blood to lymph in the rat. The influence of IFN-γ on the circulation pattern. *J Immunol* 1994;152:1744–1750.

132. Snider D. Memory T cell entry into Peyer's patches directed by $\alpha_4\beta_7$ integrin, *in vivo* evidence or selective interpretation. *Mucosal Immunol* 1998;6:11–14.

133. Bevilacqua MP, Pober JS, Mendrick DL, Cotran RS, Gimbrone MA Jr. Identification of an inducible endothelial-leukocyte adhesion molecule. *Proc Natl Acad Sci USA* 1987;84:9238–9243.

134. Keelan ET, Licence ST, Peters AM, Binns RM, Haskard DO. Characterization of E-selectin expression *in vivo* with use of a radiolabeled monoclonal antibody. *Am J Physiol* 1994;266:H278–290.

135. Silber A, Newman W, Reimann KA, Hendricks E, Walsh D, Ringler DJ. Kinetic expression of endothelial adhesion molecules and relationship to leukocyte recruitment in two cutaneous models of inflammation. *Lab Invest* 1994;70:163–175.

136. Munro JM, Pober JS, Cotran RS. Recruitment of neutrophils in the local endotoxin response: association with *de novo* endothelial expression of endothelial leukocyte adhesion molecule-1. *Lab Invest* 1991; 64:265–299.

137. Picker LJ, Kishimoto TK, Smith CW, Warnock RA, Butcher EC. ELAM-1 is an adhesion molecule for skin-homing T cells. *Nature* 1991;349:796–799.

138. Picker LJ, Treer JR, Ferguson DB, Collins PA, Bergstresser PR, Terstappen LWNN. Control of lymphocyte recirculation in man. Differential regulation of the cutaneous lymphocyte-associated antigen, a tissue-selective homing receptor for skin-homing T cells. *J Immunol* 1993;150:1122–1136.

139. Shimizu Y, Shaw S, Graber N, et al. Activation-independent binding of human memory T cells to adhesion molecule ELAM-1. *Nature* 1991;349:799–802.

140. Berg EL, Yoshino T, Rott LS, et al. The cutaneous lymphocyte antigen is a skin lymphocyte homing receptor for the vascular lectin endothelial cell-leukocyte adhesion molecule 1. *J Exp Med* 1991;174:1461–1466.

141. Labow MA, Norton CR, Rumberger JM, et al. Characterization of E-selectin–deficient mice: demonstration of overlapping function of the endothelial selectins. *Immunity* 1994;1:709–720.

142. Subramaniam M, Saffaripour S, Watson SR, Mayadas TN, Hynes RO, Wagner DD. Reduced recruitment of inflammatory cells in a contact hypersensitivity response in P-selectin–deficient mice. *J Exp Med* 1995;181:2277–2282.

143. Yamada S, Mayadas TN, Yuan F, et al. Rolling in P-selectin–deficient mice is reduced but not eliminated in the dorsal skin. *Blood* 1995;86:3487–3492.

144. Tang MLK, Hale LP, Steeber DA, Tedder TF. L-selectin is involved in lymphocyte migration to sites of inflammation in the skin: delayed rejection of allografts in L-selectin–deficient mice. *J Immunol* 1997;158:5191–5199.

145. Tedder TF, Steeber DA, Pizcueta P. L-selectin deficient mice have impaired leukocyte recruitment into inflammatory sites. *J Exp Med* 1995;181:2259–2264.

146. Picker LJ, Martin RJ, Trumble A, et al. Differential expression of lymphocyte homing receptors by human memory/effector T cells in pulmonary versus cutaneous immune effector sites. *Eur J Immunol* 1994;24:1269–1277.

147. Spertini O, Luscinskas FW, Kansas GS, et al. Leukocyte adhesion molecule-1 (LAM-1, L-selectin) interacts with an inducible endothelial cell ligand to support leukocyte adhesion. *J Immunol* 1991;147:2565–2573.

148. Spertini O, Luscinskas FW, Gimbrone MA Jr, Tedder TF. Monocyte attachment to activated human vascular endothelium *in vitro* is mediated by leukocyte adhesion molecule-1 (L-selectin) under non-static conditions. *J Exp Med* 1992;175:1789–1792.

149. Brady HR, Spertini O, Jimenez W, Brenner BM, Marsden PA, Tedder TF. Neutrophils, monocytes and lymphocytes bind to cytokine-activated kidney glomerular endothelial cells through L-selectin (LAM-1) *in vitro*. *J Immunol* 1992;149:2437–2444.

150. Giuffè L, Cordey A-S, Monai N, Tardy Y, Schapira M, Spertini O. Monocyte adhesion to activated aortic endothelium: role of L-selectin and heparan sulfate proteoglycans. *J Cell Biol* 1997;136:945–956.

151. Saunders KB, Munro M, Luscinskas FW, Mellors A, Tedder TF. Investigation of a role for CD34, a sialomucin expressed by human endothelial cells, in L-selectin-mediated adhesion. In: Schlossman SF, Boumsell L, Gilks W, Harlan J, Kishimoto T, Morimoto C, Ritz J, Shaw S, Silverstein R, Springer T, Tedder TF, Todd R, eds. *Leukocyte typing V: white cell differentiation antigens.* Oxford: Oxford University Press, 1994;2:1520–1521.

152. Tu L, Delahunty MD, Ding H, Luscinskas FW, Tedder TF. The cutaneous lymphocyte antigen (CLA) is an essential component of the L-selectin ligand induced in human vascular endothelial cells. *J Exp Med (in press).*

153. Sawada M, Takada A, Ohwaki I, et al. Specific expression of a complex sialyl Lewis X antigen on high endothelial venules of human lymph nodes: possible candidate for L-selectin ligand. *Biochem Biophys Res Commun* 1993;193:337–347.

154. Freemont AJ, Ford WL. Functional and morphological changes in post-capillary venules in relation to lymphocytic infiltration into BCG-induced granulomata in rat skin. *J Pathol* 1985;147:1–12.

155. Winn RK, Vedder NB, Mihelcic D, Flaherty LC, Langdale L, Harlan JM. The role of adhesion molecules in reperfusion injury. *Agents Actions Suppl* 1993;41:113–126.

156. Tedder TF, Green NE, Miller A, Steeber DA. L-selectin function and inflammatory disease. In: Peltz G, eds. *Leukocyte recruitment in inflammatory disease.* Austin: RG Landes, 1995:165–210.

Inflammation: Basic Principles and Clinical Correlates,
3rd ed., edited by John I. Gallin and Ralph Snyderman.
Lippincott Williams & Wilkins, Philadelphia © 1999.

CHAPTER 41

Chemoattractant Stimulus-Response Coupling

Ronald J. Uhing and Ralph Snyderman

Phagocytes migrate from the circulation to accumulate at sites of inflammation in response to proinflammatory mediators. At sites of inflammation, phagocytic leukocytes can become activated to enhance their ability to endocytize particles, produce toxic radicals, and secrete cytotoxic substances. The local accumulation of phagocytes is preceded by the binding of circulating leukocytes to the endothelium of postcapillary venules, followed by the emigration of the cells through gaps in the endothelium. A large group of mediators can cause accumulation of phagocytic leukocytes at sites of inflammation. Chemotactic factors bind to cell surface receptors and stimulate discrete biologic responses by leukocytes. Migratory responses of leukocytes are induced by chemoattractant doses that are at least 10-fold lower than those required to stimulate cytotoxic responses. At high concentrations, chemoattractants provoke potentially cytotoxic or microbicidal responses by leukocytes through the degranulation of storage vesicles and the production of toxic products, including oxygen radicals and nitric oxide. The differential natures of migratory and cytotoxic responses are evident in their pharmacologic manipulation and the specific biochemical mechanisms involved.

The molecular mechanisms of signal transduction involved in the actions of chemoattractants are better understood than those of any other group of leukocyte stimuli. Chemoattractants initiate their responses after binding to members of the general family of GTP-binding protein (G protein)–coupled receptors. Cloning and sequencing of chemoattractant receptors have shown that they form a separate group within this family with close similarities to other peptide receptors. The receptors for chemoattractants primarily couple to pertussis toxin–sensitive G proteins, although signaling by, for example, platelet-activating factor (PAF, 1-*O*-alkyl-2-acetyl-*sn*-glycero-3-phosphocholine), can involve other heterotrimeric G proteins.

Subunits of the heterotrimeric G protein initiate multiple signaling cascades, and βγ-mediated activation of phosphoinositide-specific phospholipase C is the best characterized. After the rapid (≤5 seconds) hydrolysis of phosphatidylinositol 4,5-bisphosphate, additional biochemical processes are observed under conditions in which cytotoxic responses are initiated. These include a sustained calcium influx and activation of additional signaling components, including low-molecular-weight (LMW) G proteins, phospholipases, and the tyrosine and serine/threonine protein kinases. Activation of phospholipase D with subsequent production of diacylglycerol probably is a prerequisite for cytotoxic activation.

Chemoattractant stimulation of leukocyte responses is tightly regulated and affected by other inflammatory mediators that potentiate or inhibit the observed response. The production of several prostanoids or histamine by immune cells results in elevation of intracellular cAMP levels in phagocytic leukocytes, with resultant attenuation of chemoattractant-induced activation. In contrast, lipopolysaccharide, thrombin, and several cytokines potentiate the ability of chemoattractants to induce cellular responses. The transient responses initiated by chemoattractants are terminated by the actions of several signal-regulated protein kinases acting on the receptor or associated downstream signaling components.

TYPES OF CHEMOATTRACTANTS

Identification of molecules that are capable of inducing the directed migration of leukocytes continues to expand. For the most part, chemoattractants use related G-protein–coupled receptors to mediate their actions, although other molecules with chemotactic activity (e.g., platelet-derived growth factor, transforming growth factor-β) have

R. J. Uhing: COVANCE Biotechnology Services Inc., Research Triangle Park, North Carolina 27709.
R. Snyderman: Duke University Medical Center, Duke University Health System, Durham, North Carolina 27710.

been described. Chemoattractants (Table 41-1) include bacterial products (e.g., formylpeptides), a product of the complement cascade (C5a), secreted products of stimulated phospholipid metabolism (e.g., PAF, leukotriene B_4 [LTB$_4$]), and large numbers of chemotactic cytokines or chemokines. The sequences of the chemoattractants are known, and in many cases, their three-dimensional structures have been determined. Receptors have been identified for the major classes of chemoattractants.

Chemoattractants stimulate phagocytic leukocytes in a dose-dependent manner to initiate chemotactic or cytotoxic responses including exocytosis and stimulation of the respiratory burst in neutrophils and mononuclear phagocytes. By definition, all stimulate chemotaxis through a mechanism involving activation of a phosphoinositide-specific phospholipase C and the release of calcium from intracellular stores. Chemoattractants are different with regard to their ability to stimulate secretory responses and activate signaling events (e.g., phospholipase D). Certain chemoattractants (i.e., LTB$_4$, interleukin-8 [IL-8], PAF), although equally potent and active as chemotactic agents, are less effective secretagogues. These differences are reflected in the signaling pathways.

N-formylmethionylpeptides were identified as chemoattractants produced by bacteria and were the first synthetic chemoattractants for leukocytes (1). Amino-terminal formylation occurs for bacterial and mitochondrial proteins, and the *N*-formylpeptide chemoattractant receptor may direct leukocytes after bacterial infection or cell destruction. Early structure-function studies using neutrophils indicated that formylation of the α-amino group on the amino terminal methionine was essential for biologic activity (2). The presence of alternative amino-terminal modifications (e.g., N-tert-butoxycarbonyl) was reported to give rise to potent antagonists. A later study (3) suggested that acetylation or no amino-terminal modification may be tolerated for certain agonist sequences. Additional studies have suggested that the hydrophobic nature of the peptide is important for binding to leukocyte receptors. Binding of the most active tripeptide, *N*-formyl-L-methionyl-L-leucyl-L-phenylalanine (fMLP), is further increased by the presence of additional hydrophobic residues on the carboxyl end (4).

C5a was the initial chemoattractant identified (5,6). It is a 74–amino acid protein with three disulfide bonds and is glycosylated on an asparagine at position 64 (7). Deletion of the caboxyl-terminal 5 amino acids abolishes the

TABLE 41-1. *Types of chemoattractants*

Chemoattractant	Structure or sequence
fMLP	formyl-MLF
PAF (C$_{16}$)	
LTB$_4$	
C5a	TLQKKIEEIAAKYKHSVVKKCCYDGACVNNDETCEQRAAR ISLGPRCIKAFTDCCVVASQLRANISHKDMQLGR
IL-8(CXC)	SAKELRCQCIKTYSKPFHPKFIKELRVIESGPHCANTEIIVK LSDGRELCLDPKENWVQRVVEKFLKRAENS
MCP-1 (CC)	QPDAINAPVTCCYNFTNRKISVQRLASYRRITSSKCPKEA VIFKTIVAKEICADPKQKWVQDSMDHLDKQTQTPKT

fMLP, *N*-formylmethionyl-leucyl-phenylalanine; IL, interleukin; LTB$_4$, leukotriene B$_4$; MCP-1, monocyte chemotactic protein-1; PAF, platelet-activating factor.

chemotactic activity of the molecule, although it still binds to the receptor (8,9). The amino-terminal portion is essential for activity (7,10). Two-dimensional nuclear magnetic resonance has been used to determine the solution structure of the molecule (11). These results confirmed the presence of significant helical content and the importance of positively charged residues in the putative receptor binding portion.

PAF and LTB$_4$ are generated from leukocytes and other cells as a consequence of stimulated phospholipase A$_2$ (PLA$_2$) activity. PAF is formed by transacetylase-mediated acetylation of lysophosphatidylcholine, which is generated by PLA$_2$. Its actions are normally transient due to the presence of acetylhydrolase activity in blood. PAF exerts effects on a variety of cell types through the actions of a calcium-mobilizing receptor (12). LTB$_4$ is a product of calcium-activated 5-lipoxygenase action on arachidonic acid, which occurs primarily in leukocytes. The primary cell mediating the proinflammatory actions of LTB$_4$ appears to be the neutrophil (13).

A large group of related chemokines have been identified that act on leukocytes, lymphocytes, and other cells (14) (see Chapter 28). These chemokines are approximately 8- to 10-kd proteins that can be separated into families based on the positions of cysteines forming disulfide bonds. For CC chemokines, the first two cysteines are adjacent, whereas for CXC chemokines, they are separated by a single amino acid. The three-dimensional structure of representative members of both these families have been determined (15). The monomeric structures of members of both families are similar with a triple-stranded antiparallel β sheet that has the carboxyl-terminal portion in an α helix on top. The amino terminus is an irregular strand. However, the formation of dimers involves different portions of the molecule between the two families. Evidence indicates that the chemokine monomer constitutes the active form. The amino-terminal portion of the chemokine contains most of the receptor-binding determinants.

CHEMOATTRACTANT RECEPTORS

Receptors for chemoattractants were initially identified through the use of radiolabeled ligands. Before the cloning of chemoattractant receptors, radioligand binding studies had demonstrated their relative abundance, affinity, specificity, and molecular mass. Data obtained using radiolabeled fMLP and intact human neutrophils demonstrated the presence of a single population of 50,000 binding sites per cell with a K$_d$ of about 20 nmol/L (16). Crosslinking studies had shown that the endogenous receptor for formylpeptides is glycosylated, with an approximately 32-kd protein core (17).

A variety of data have indicated that the formylpeptide receptor was coupled to a heterotrimeric G protein. Similar data have been obtained for most other types of

chemoattractant receptors before their cloning. Sequencing of chemoattractant receptors showed they belong to the large group of G-protein–coupled receptors, which are characterized by possessing an extracellular amino terminus, seven putative transmembrane domains, and an intracellular carboxyl terminus. The α-helical transmembrane segments of G-protein–coupled receptors are thought to be arranged in a counterclockwise orientation within the plasma membrane, with the extracellular portions of the segments participating in the binding of hydrophobic ligands. The amino terminus and the extracellular loops are indicated to participate in the binding of protein ligands. The carboxyl terminus contains multiple potential phosphorylation sites that are involved in the termination of receptor signaling and receptor internalization.

Expression cloning using COS cells and a cDNA library derived from differentiated HL60 cells was used to obtain the sequence for a human formylpeptide receptor (18). The guinea-pig receptor for PAF (19) and the human CXCR1 (IL-8) chemokine receptor (20) were also obtained by expression cloning. Random sequencing of cDNAs obtained from a subtraction library of retinoic acid–differentiated HL60 cells yielded a receptor identified as that for LTB$_4$ (21). The receptors for C5a (22) and a variety of receptors for CXC and CC chemokines (Table 41-2) were cloned based on sequence homologies (14,23).

Chemoattractant receptors usually have shorter than normal sequences (about 350 to 370 amino acids), with

TABLE 41-2. *Chemokine receptors*

Receptor	Preferred ligands
CXC receptors	
CXCR1	IL-8
CXCR2	IL-8, GRO-α, NAP-2, ENA78
CXCR3	IP10, MIG
CXCR4	SDF-1
CC receptors	
CCR1	RANTES, MIP-1α, MCP-2, MCP-3
CCR2(a/b)	MCP-1, MCP-2, MCP-3, MCP-4
CCR3	RANTES, MCP-3, MCRP-4, eotaxin
CCR4	RANTES, MIP-1α, MCP-1, TARC
CCR5	RANTES, MIP-1α, MIP-1β
CCR6	LARC
CCR7	ELC
CCR8	I-309

IL-8, interleukin-8; GRO-α, growth-related peptide-α; NAP-2, neutrophil-activating protein-2; ENA-78, epithelial-derived neutrophil-activating peptide-78; IP10, interferon-γ–inducible 10-kd protein; MIG, monokine induced by interferon-γ; SDF-1, stromal cell-derived factor-1; RANTES, regulated on activation, normally T-cell expressed and secreted; MIP, macrophage inflammatory protein; MCP, monocyte chemotactic protein; TARC, thymus and activation-regulated chemokine; LARC, liver and activation-regulated chemokine; ELC, EBI1-ligand chemokine; EBI, Epstein-Barr virus-induced gene; I-309, human homologue of murine TCA3, T-cell activation protein-3.

very short third intracellular loops. Most have extracellular N-linked glycosylation sites. They contain cysteine residues in the first and second extracellular loops that probably are disulfide linked. Chemokine receptors contain additional conserved cysteine residues in the amino terminus and third extracellular loop that may form an additional disulfide bond. Receptors for the lipid chemoattractants contain very short extracellular amino termini. Amino terminal regions of chemokine and C5a receptors are longer with an abundance of negatively charged amino acids consistent with an involvement in the binding of positively charged areas of the ligand.

As shown in Table 41-2, most chemokine receptors are used by multiple ligands. The number of chemokine receptors identified is expanding at nearly the rate of identification of chemokines, and a number of orphan receptors with significant homology have been found (see Chapter 28). In addition to specific CXC and CC chemokine receptors, the Duffy antigen of erythrocytes binds both types of chemokines and is the cellular recognition site for the malarial parasite. Certain chemokine receptors are not limited to leukocytes but regulate the migration of other cell types (14,23).

Chimeric chemoattractant receptors have been extensively used for the analyses of ligand binding determinants. The high degree of interspecies sequence variability for peptide chemoattractant receptors has provided useful information on the importance of specific residues. A murine fMLP receptor exhibits an affinity for the chemoattractant approximately 100-fold lower than the human receptor based on functional properties of the expressed receptors (24). Most of the nonconservative differences between the receptors occur in the extracellular regions. Similarly, sequence divergence between species is mainly evident in extracellular portions of the receptors for C5a and the chemokines. In many cases, this divergence results in species-specific ligand binding.

Replacement of the extracellular amino terminus of the fMLP receptor, such as with the amino terminus of the C5a receptor (25) or a low-affinity fMLP receptor (26), does not alter fMLP binding affinity. Extension of the substitution into the first transmembrane domain resulted in a 10-fold decrease in ligand affinity (27). Chimeras composed of altered extracellular loops displayed reduced ligand affinity, with the largest effects observed with changes in the first extracellular loop (25—27).

Receptors for C5a and chemokines use a two-stage mechanism for ligand recognition and signal generation. The amino terminus of the receptor contains most of the determinants for high-affinity binding of the peptide ligand. Subsequent signal generation requires additional ligand recognition sites on other extracellular or transmembrane portions of the receptor. In the case of C5a, antibodies to the amino terminus, but not other extracellular domains of the human C5a receptor, inhibit ligand binding (28,29). However, studies comparing the effects

of C5a and an active C-terminal fragment of C5a have concluded that the amino terminus and an additional part of the receptor are necessary for signaling (30). Similarly, the amino-terminal domain of the CCR2b receptor when expressed as a fusion protein is sufficient for high-affinity binding of monocyte chemotactic protein-1 (MCP-1) (31). When the fusion protein is coexpressed with a chimeric CCR2b receptor incapable of detectable high-affinity binding, signaling occurs in response to MCP-1.

Chemokine binding selectivity of the CXCR1 and CXCR2 receptors also is mediated by their amino terminus (14). A chimera composed of the amino terminus of CXCR2 on the CXCR1 receptor is capable of high-affinity binding of IL-8, growth-related peptide-α, and neutrophil-activating protein-2 (32). Activation of phospholipase C at similar ligand concentrations is observed only when additional portions of the CXCR2 receptor are included in the chimera. The amino terminus of chemokine receptors has also been suggested as the primary site for selectivity of CXC or CC chemokines (33). A single mutation in IL-8 allows the chemokine to bind to and activate CCR1 receptors or bind to a peptide composed of the amino-terminal sequence of the CCR1 receptor.

Similar regions of selected chemokine receptors appear to be involved in their coreceptor function for cell infection by human immunodeficiency virus (HIV). Cell entry by the virus requires CD4 binding to viral gp120, followed by recognition of this complex by strain-selective chemokine receptors. For the most part, T-tropic viruses use CXCR4, whereas M-tropic viruses use CCR5 as coreceptors, although there is some overlap of cell receptor expression and selected viral strains can also use CCR2b or CCR3 (34). RANTES (regulated on activation, normally T-cell expressed and secreted) and macrophage inflammatory proteins (MIP-1α and MIP-1β) inhibit binding of the virus to CCR5, whereas stromal cell—derived factor-1 (SDF-1) inhibits binding to CXCR4, indicating similar binding determinants for HIV and the natural ligands. The amino-terminal regions of these receptors appear to be important for recognition of some viral strains based on mutagenesis studies (34,35). Neither receptor signaling nor receptor internalization appear to be important for coreceptor function (36,37), suggesting that HIV may bind without inducing activation of chemokine receptors.

Signaling by a single dose of chemoattractant is rapidly initiated but does not persist for more than several minutes. The transient nature of chemoattractant responses can be explained, at least in part, by receptor phosphorylation with a resultant desensitization. Sequences from the third cytoplasmic loops and carboxyl termini of representative chemoattractant receptors are presented in Table 41-3. Potential serine and threonine phosphorylation sites have been highlighted. Each chemoattractant receptor contains multiple potential phosphorylation sites consistent with the stringent regu-

TABLE 41-3. *Potential phosphorylation sites for representative chemoattractant receptors*

Receptor	Third loop	Carboxyl terminus
fMLP	KQGLIKSSRPLR	QDFRERLIHALPASLERALTEDSTQTSDTATNSTLPSAEVALQAK
C5a	RRATRSTKTLK	QGFQGRLRKSLPSLLRNVLTEESVVRESKSFTRSTVDTMAQKTQAV
PAF	QPVQQQRNAEVKRR	KKFRKHLIEKFVSMRESSRKCSRASSDTVTEVVVPFNQIPGNSLKN
LTB₄	RRFRRSRRTGR	VGFVAKLLEGTGSEASSTRRGGSLGQTARSGPAALEPGPSESLTASSPLKLNELN
CXCR1	KAHMGQKHRAMR	QKFRHGFLKILAMHGLVSKEFLARHRVTSYTSSSVNVSSNL
CXCR2	KAHMGQKHRAMR	QKFRHGLLKILAIHGLISKDSLPKDSRPSFVGSSSGHTSTTL
CCR1	RRPNEKKSKAVR	ERFRKYLRQLFHRRVAVHLVKWLPFLSVDRERVSSTSPSTGEHELSAGF
CCR2B	RCRNEKKRHRAVR	EKFRRYLSVFFRKHITKRFCKQCPVFYRETVDGVTSTNTPSTGEQEVSAGL

CCR, receptor of chemokines with first two cysteines separated by one amino acid; CXCR, receptor of chemokines with adjacent first two cysteines; fMLP, *N*-formylmethionyl-leucyl-phenylalanine; LTB₄, leukotriene B₄; PAF, platelet-activating factor.

lation of responses. However, distinct differences exist between the receptors with regard to the sites present, and these differences are reflected in the nature of the desensitization observed. Desensitization can be affected by second messenger–induced phosphorylation of phospholipase C (see below).

HETEROTRIMERIC G PROTEINS AND RAPID ACTIVATION OF EFFECTOR PROTEINS

Chemoattractant receptors form a separate group of the large family of seven-transmembrane G-protein–coupled receptors. Like other seven-transmembrane receptors, chemoattractant receptors are physically associated with heterotrimeric GTP-binding proteins (G proteins) in the cell plasma membrane. Before receptor sequence determination, this G-protein coupling had been demonstrated. In the case of the endogenous formylpeptide receptor, data were obtained using membrane preparations demonstrating guanine nucleotide effects on ligand binding affinity (38,39), while formylpeptide binding was shown to stimulate guanine nucleotide binding (40) and GTPase activity (41,42). These studies provided early evidence that chemoattractant receptors were directly coupled to a GTP-binding protein.

Pertussis toxin, which causes the ADP ribosylation and inactivation of G proteins of the G_i/G_o and transducin families has been a valuable tool in the examination of G-protein–mediated events. Pretreatment of leukocytes with pertussis toxin results in an attenuation of signaling events initiated by endogenous receptors for formylpeptides, C5a, LTB₄, PAF, and CXC and CC chemokines, indicating that these endogenous receptors can all couple to pertussis toxin–sensitive G proteins. High concentrations of pertussis toxin substrates are present in leukocyte membranes (>20 pmol/mg protein) (43). Based on immunologic data, G_o and transducin are absent, whereas $G_i\alpha_2$ and $G_i\alpha_3$ are detected (43,44). Purification of receptor and G-protein complexes has demonstrated that $G_i\alpha_2$ copurifies with the endogenous formylpeptide receptor (45) and the endogenous C5a receptor (46), whereas immunologic methods have similarly detected an associ-

ation between $G_i\alpha_2$ and endogenous IL-8 receptors (47). These results indicate that activation of $G_i\alpha_2$ is a general event involved in signaling by a number of chemoattractant receptors.

Transfection studies have demonstrated that expressed chemoattractant receptors use a pertussis-sensitive G protein for signaling in a variety of cell types. The formylpeptide receptor, when expressed on HEK293 (48,49), COS-7 (50), or RBL-2H3 (51,52) cells, stimulates calcium mobilization or inhibits cAMP accumulation in a pertussis toxin–sensitive manner, indicating that the receptor couples to members of the G_i family in these cells. Signaling through the phosphatidylinositol/Ca^{2+} pathway has also been reported using expressed receptors for C5a, PAF, and CXC and CC chemokines on the same cell types. The responses of those examined were generally pertussis toxin sensitive. Coexpression studies using chemoattractant receptors and various G proteins demonstrated that coupling to pertussis toxin–insensitive G proteins can occur. Expressed receptors for fMLP, C5a, PAF, IL-8, MIP-1α, and MCP-1 can couple to expressed pertussis toxin–insensitive G proteins in COS-7 and HEK293 cells (50,53-58). The receptors exhibit different selectivities with regard to coupling to $G\alpha_q$, $G\alpha_{11}$, and $G\alpha_{16}$. Differences are also observed between the two cell types. The ability of many of the receptors to couple to $G\alpha_{16}$, a G protein found in hematopoietic cells (59), has led to suggestions that pertussis toxin–insensitive G proteins may participate in chemoattractant signaling through endogenous receptors. However, expressed $G\alpha_{16}$ has been shown to couple to a variety of G-protein–coupled receptors (60,61). The best evidence for the participation of pertussis toxin–insensitive G proteins in chemoattractant signaling is that which has been obtained for the PAF receptor. An examination of the pertussis toxin sensitivity of chemoattractant responses revealed a partial attenuation of PAF-induced calcium mobilization and secretion in neutrophils under conditions where the same responses induced by peptide chemoattractants were completely inhibited (62). In COS-7 cells, an expressed PAF receptor is capable of using endogenous pertussis toxin–insensitive G proteins to stimulate phosphoinositide metabolism (53), whereas other expressed chemoattractant receptors require coexpression of pertussis toxin–insensitive G proteins to stimulate endogenous phospholipase C (50,53–58) or expressed phospholipase Cβ₂ to use endogenous pertussis toxin–sensitive G proteins (50,56,57). In RBL-2H3 cells, stably transfected PAF receptor stimulates inositide metabolism with pertussis toxin–sensitive and –insensitive components, whereas signaling through fMLP and C5a receptors was completely abolished by the toxin (51,52). PAF receptor signaling through phospholipase Cβ₃ is indicated for RBL cells (63).

These results demonstrate that there are differences between the various chemoattractant receptors with regard to G-protein coupling preference. The receptor sequences determining specific G-protein recognition have not been determined. The determination of three-dimensional structures for some heterotrimeric G proteins (64) should facilitate the study of specific interactions with receptors. Generally, seven-transmembrane receptors mutated in the second or third cytoplasmic loop or the C-terminus can exhibit alterations in G-protein coupling (65). A study examining the affinity of peptides corresponding to intracellular regions of the fMLP receptor for Giα concluded that the third intracellular loop was not a major determi-

nant of G-protein coupling (66). Peptides corresponding to the second intracellular loop or regions of the carboxyl terminus were shown to bind to the G protein. Studies examining fMLP signaling by receptors with mutations in the third intracellular loop also indicated that it was not a major determinant for G-protein coupling (67). The third intracellular loop (58) and C-terminus (56) of MCP-1 receptors have been reported to be involved in receptor coupling to pertussis toxin–insensitive G proteins in cotransfected COS-7 cells. Future studies should provide additional information on receptor sequence-specific determination of G-protein coupling.

Evidence for direct G-protein regulation of a phosphoinositide-specific phospholipase C in leukocytes was initially obtained in membrane preparations (68,69). Heterotrimeric G proteins have been demonstrated to activate members of the phospholipase Cβ family (70,71). Members of this family are characterized as approximately 150-kd proteins with an N-terminal PH domain, a calcium-dependent phospholipid binding domain, two adjacent domains comprising a catalytic region, and a large C-terminal region that interacts with G-protein α subunits (Fig. 41-1). The α subunits of pertussis toxin–insen-

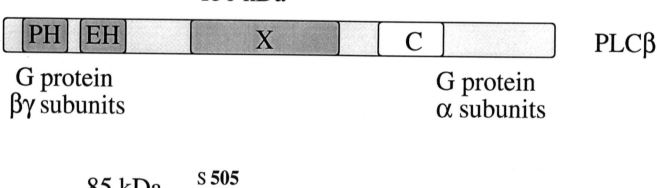

150 kDa

PLCβ

G protein βγ subunits

G protein α subunits

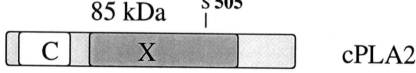

85 kDa

S 505

cPLA2

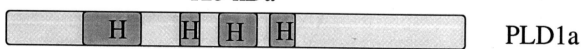

125 kDa

PLD1a

FIG. 41-1. Signal-regulated phospholipases in leukocytes. Depicted are models for phospholipase Cβ, phospholipase A₂, and a phospholipase D isozyme, with various regulatory regions indicated. X, the catalytic region; C, calcium-binding domain; PH, PH domain; EH, EH domain. Regions of homology between the isozymes of phospholipase D are indicated by H. The approximate regions of phospholipase Cβ interacting with either α or βγ subunits of heterotrimeric G proteins are shown, as is the position of the mitogen-activated protein (MAP) kinase phosphorylation site (S505) in phospholipase A₂.

sitive G proteins have been shown to activate phospholipase Cβs in transfected cells using the purified proteins. Pertussis toxin–sensitive α subunits are inactive in assays using purified phospholipase Cs. In contrast, βγ subunits derived from G_i have been demonstrated to activate phospholipase Cβ2 and phospholipase Cβ3. This activation is attenuated by the addition of $α_i$, presumably by binding the free βγ subunits.

Different regions of phospholipase C interact with α or βγ subunits (72). The α and γ subunits of heterotrimeric G proteins are multimember families (73). Differences exist in the ability of individual members of each family to associate with each other and with individual receptors and to activate phospholipase C. Phospholipase Cβ2 is abundant in leukocytes. Expressed chemoattractant receptors activate expressed phospholipase Cβ2 in COS-7 cells in a pertussis toxin–sensitive manner. Data indicate that at least in COS-7 cells phospholipase Cβ2 mediates pertussis toxin–sensitive chemoattractant activation of phosphoinositide metabolism. In contrast, chemoattractant receptors transfected into RBL-2H3 cells use phospholipase Cβ3 to activate phosphoinositide metabolism. Phospholipase Cβ usage by chemoattractant receptors may depend on isozyme availability. One study examined fMLP-mediated functions in mice lacking phospholipase Cβ2 (74). Loss of the enzyme resulted in decreases in fMLP-induced calcium fluxes and superoxide production but potentiated fMLP-mediated chemotaxis of certain cell populations.

In addition to the activation of phosphoinositide-specific phospholipase C, G_i-derived βγ probably regulates other intracellular signaling pathways (73). The earliest described effector of βγ subunits was adenylate cyclase, for which activity was attenuated and several members of the adenylate cyclase family are negatively regulated *in vitro*. Chemoattractant receptors attenuate cAMP accumulation through G_i in transfected cells. However, in leukocytes, chemoattractant receptors elevate cAMP levels through a calcium-dependent mechanism (75). In membrane preparations from neutrophils, fMLP was reported to not affect adenylate cyclase activity (75). Elevation of intracellular cAMP in neutrophils appears to be caused by the release of adenosine after chemoattractant stimulation, with subsequent activation of adenylate cyclase through A_2 receptors (76). The elevation of cAMP serves to dampen chemoattractant-induced responses through the phosphorylation of chemoattractant receptors and phospholipase C (see below).

The βγ subunits can directly activate a phosphoinositide 3-kinase and G-protein–coupled receptor kinases (GRKs) and are involved (independent of phospholipase C) in the ability of G_i–coupled receptors to activate RAS (a GTP-binding protein) and mitogen-activated protein (MAP) kinase. Activation of GRKs involves interaction of βγ subunits with the pleckstrin homology (PH) domain. Activation of Bruton tyrosine kinase family members by βγ also

occurs in a PH domain, although not all PH domain–containing proteins are regulated by βγ subunits. Based on current information, it is reasonable to assume that chemoattractant receptor-activated heterotrimeric G proteins directly affect multiple signaling cascades.

ROLES FOR PHOSPHOLIPID METABOLISM IN SIGNALING

Extensive phospholipid remodeling of leukocyte membranes is rapidly initiated in response to chemoattractants. Enzymatic activities that are stimulated include a phosphoinositide-specific phospholipase C, phosphoinositide kinases, a phospholipase D with preference for phosphatidylcholine, and PLA2. Downstream consequences of these stimulated activities include the elevation of intracellular calcium, the translocation and activation of protein kinase C and other signaling molecules, and the actions of newly synthesized eicosanoids and PAF. The stimulation of phospholipid metabolism is a general response to chemoattractants, although differences are observed for the stimulation of individual enzymes.

A significant increase in inositol phosphates is observed within seconds after the exposure of leukocytes to chemoattractants. Inositol 1,4,5-triphosphate is the initial aqueous product detected coincident with a decrease of the membrane phospholipid phosphatidylinositol 4,5-bisphosphate. Measurement of the intracellular concentration of inositol 1,4,5-triphosphate produced in response to fMLP (about 1 μmol/L of inositol 1,4,5-triphosphate [IP3] at 10^{-8} mol/L of fMLP) suggests sufficient quantities to maximally release calcium from the IP3-sensitive organelle (77). Increases in a variety of other inositol phosphates are observed at subsequent times because of the actions of phosphatases. These observations are consistent with stimulation of a phospholipase C with a preference for polyphosphoinositides. In addition to inositol phosphates formed because of phosphatase action on inositol 1,4,5-triphosphate, other metabolites phosphorylated at the 3 position are simultaneously observed (78).

Prior exposure of leukocytes to pertussis toxin attenuates phosphoinositide metabolism, indicating the involvement of G_i. Evidence suggests that βγ subunits of G_i directly stimulate phospholipases Cβ2 or Cβ3 as a result of chemoattractants binding to their receptors. In the case of PAF, α subunits of pertussis toxin–insensitive G proteins also are involved in signaling to phospholipase C. Using leukocyte membrane preparations, Smith et al. (69) reported that guanine nucleotide stimulation of phospholipase C required submicromolar calcium concentrations. Studies using purified recombinant phospholipase C have demonstrated a calcium-dependent phospholipid binding domain and the involvement of a calcium molecule at the active site (71). Phospholipase

C also contain a PH domain that binds phosphatidylinositol 4,5-bisphosphate and is likely involved in membrane targeting of the enzyme. The enzyme is sensitive to product inhibition, and this may contribute to the transient nature of chemoattractant activation.

Phosphatidylinositol 3-kinase (PI3K) activity was initially described in chemoattractant-stimulated leukocytes based on the formation of lipid products (79). PI3K activity is stimulated in neutrophils within seconds by formylpeptides (79,80), IL-8 (81), C5a (81), and PAF (80). Activation of PI3K activity is attenuated by prior treatment of the cells with pertussis toxin and does not appear to be because of changes in cytosolic calcium concentrations or stimulation of protein kinase C. An increase in the cellular products of the enzyme (primarily phosphatidylinositol 3,4,5-triphosphate and phosphatidylinositol 3,4-bisphosphate) is observed in response to a variety of extracellular stimuli (82). Two receptor-activated forms of the enzyme have been identified. The initial enzyme that was isolated is composed of a p85 regulatory subunit containing two SRC homology-2 (SH2) domains, a SRC homology-3 (SH3) domain, two proline-rich regions, and a p110 catalytic subunit, and it has been shown to be recruited by several tyrosine-phosphorylated growth factor receptors (82). A second enzyme form was initially identified in myeloid cells as being activated by G-protein $\beta\gamma$ subunits (83) and shown to have a p110γ catalytic subunit (with a PH domain) that is activated by $G_i\alpha$ ($G_t\alpha$ at higher concentrations) and $\beta\gamma$ (84). Both types of PI3K are inhibited by wortmannin at nanomolar concentrations, and inhibition of cellular functions by the fungal product is often used as evidence for PI3K involvement.

Chemoattractant-mediated stimulation of PI3K activity is unaffected by inhibitors of tyrosine kinases (85). However, p110 is associated with LYN (a tyrosine kinase) in immunoprecipitates from chemoattractant-stimulated cells. Wortmannin had no effect on chemoattractant-induced RAS activation, consistent with a potential role of RAS as an upstream regulator of PI3K (81). Inhibition of PI3K by wortmannin resulted in the attenuation of RAF and MAP kinase activation by chemoattractants suggesting a role in this signaling cascade. Similar concentrations of wortmannin attenuate the ability of chemoattractants to stimulate a respiratory burst (86) and granule secretion (87). Activation of PI3K by chemoattractants is therefore suggested to be an important signaling component for leukocyte activation although much of the signaling mechanism remains unclear.

Signaling by means of 3-phosphoinositides is caused by their interaction with selected SH2 and PH domains and results in membrane localization or activation (88–91). Interactions with PH domains of proteins is observed with the phospholipid and the corresponding aqueous inositol phosphates. Interactions with 3-phosphoinositides have been implicated in signal transmission to the LMW G-protein ADP-ribosylation factor (ARF, through ARF guanine nucleotide exchange factors [GEFs] containing PH domains) and RAC (through RAC GEF) and other signaling molecules. Selected PH domains have also been demonstrated to bind phosphatidylinositol 4,5-bisphosphate (PIP$_2$), and this lipid can directly regulate certain proteins (90,91). Both 3-phosphoinositides and PIP$_2$ interact with profilin and gelsolin, and these actions may be involved in cytoskeletal rearrangement and cell motility. The activity of phosphatidylinositol 4-phosphate 5-kinase is stimulated in response to a variety of agonists, including chemoattractants. The mechanism of stimulation appears to be through the direct interaction with RHO/RAC family members (92).

The hydrolysis of polyphosphoinositides by phospholipase C results in an increase of membrane diacylglycerol. This lipid synergizes with cytosolic calcium for the activation of the conventional members of the protein kinase C family. A variety of techniques has been used over the years to indicate an involvement of protein kinase C in the activation of the respiratory burst and exocytosis of specific granules. The formation of diacylglycerol in response to chemoattractants exhibits biphasic kinetics (93–95). The initial accumulation has been demonstrated to result from phosphatidylinositol metabolism, whereas the later phase is derived from phosphatidylcholine by the action of phospholipase D (96,97). In addition to diacylglycerol, approximately an equal amount of other diradylglycerols (alkyl and alkenyl containing) accumulate after chemoattractant stimulation, consistent with the composition of phosphatidylcholine in leukocytes. Lipid chemoattractants are poor stimuli for phospholipase D activation compared with peptide chemoattractants (94,98); they are weaker stimuli for secretory responses (62).

Data obtained using leukocytes indicate the involvement of LMW G proteins for the activation of phospholipase D. PLD activity has been associated with plasma membranes, cytosol, Golgi, and nuclei (99). A 120-kd human phospholipase D that is stimulated by LMW G proteins and localized to membranes has been cloned (100) together with a smaller splice variant (101) (see Fig. 41-1). Based on purification results and data from other species, additional human isozymes exist (99). In addition to the indicated roles for LMW G proteins, PIP$_2$ and PIP$_3$ also activate certain preparations of the enzyme. Roles for calcium and protein kinase C have also been suggested from cellular studies and results using purified proteins. Inhibition of calcium influx eliminates the second phase of chemoattractant-stimulated diacylglycerol accumulation (94). Evidence for an ATP-independent protein-protein interaction or a phosphorylation-dependent stimulation by protein kinase C have been presented (97,99). Which of these events is required for the delayed activation of phospholipase D by chemoattractants is unknown.

Multiple roles for the lipid products resulting from phospholipase D activation are possible, including a signaling role for phosphatidate (102), regulation of vesicular transport (103), and the recruitment and activation of protein kinase C isozymes. A role for protein kinase C in chemoattractant signaling has been indicated for the oxidative burst and exocytosis based on the actions of pharmacologic stimuli. Inhibitors of phospholipase D–stimulated diacylglycerol accumulation attenuate fMLP-activated superoxide production with similar potencies (104). Protein kinase C phosphorylates p47^{phox} *in vitro* at sites that are also phosphorylated in stimulated cells. fMLP, at doses that stimulate a respiratory burst and in the presence of cytochalasin, increases membrane-associated protein kinase C activity threefold (105). Pharmacologic agents that inhibit chemoattractant-stimulated respiratory burst activity also inhibit the translocation of protein kinase C (105).

The protein kinase C family of structurally related enzymes can be divided into three groups based on whether activity is stimulated by calcium and diacylglycerol (conventional), stimulated by diacylglycerol but not calcium (novel), or is stimulated by neither (atypical) (106). Members of all three groups have been immunologically detected in leukocytes (107–109). In the presence of cytochalasin, fMLP stimulates the translocation of some members of all three groups (107–109). Future research should determine the subcellular sites and signaling roles for the different protein kinase C isoforms.

In addition to the roles previously described for phosphatidylinositol and phosphatidylcholine, together with phosphatidylethanolamine, these phospholipids serve as precursors for eicosanoid synthesis in response to chemoattractants. Mononuclear phagocytes readily produce eicosanoids in response to chemoattractants, whereas chemoattractants are poor stimuli of eicosanoid synthesis when examined using unprimed human neutrophils. However, a variety of neutrophil stimuli prime for chemoattractant-induced activation of PLA$_2$.

As with many other chemoattractant signaling mechanisms, fMLP is the most studied chemoattractant stimulus of arachidonate metabolism. Pertussis toxin inhibits fMLP-induced formation of free arachidonate and cyclooxygenase and lipoxygenase products. An increase in cytosolic calcium is required for the activation of PLA$_2$. A stimulated influx of extracellular calcium with a resultant prolonged elevation of cytosolic calcium concentrations is required for the activation of 5-lipoxygenase by fMLP (110). Calcium is not required for cyclooxygenase activity. The translocation and phosphorylation of cytosolic PLA$_2$ (cPLA$_2$) in response to a variety of cellular stimuli suggests that this is the primary enzyme that initiates eicosanoid formation. The calcium-sensitive cPLA$_2$ is a 85-kd protein that is enriched in leukocytes but also present in a variety of cell types (111). The enzyme contains an amino-terminal calcium-binding (C2) domain that is required for association of the protein with membranes (see Fig. 41-1). Elevation of intracellular calcium cPLA$_2$ levels is associated with the translocation of cPLA$_2$ to the nuclear membrane and the plasma membrane. A number of phosphorylation sites have been identified, although only phosphorylation of serine 505 by proline-directed kinases has been demonstrated to result in activation. Extracellular signal regulated kinases (ERK-1 and ERK-2) and p38 kinase are capable of phosphorylating this site and activating the enzyme in response to stimuli. Full activation of the cPLA$_2$ is thought to require phosphorylation and elevation of cytosolic calcium. Phosphorylation of cPLA$_2$ occurs in response to chemoattractants and in response to several well-characterized priming agents.

CYTOSOLIC CALCIUM LEVEL ELEVATION IN LEUKOCYTE ACTIVATION

An immediate consequence of chemoattractant-induced activation of phospholipase C (i.e., production of inositol 1,4,5-triphosphate) is the transient elevation of intracellular calcium. Within 5 seconds, cytosolic calcium concentrations are maximally elevated (<100 nmol/L to >1 μmol/L) and exhibit a biphasic decline to return to resting levels within 5 minutes. This biphasic calcium response is caused by the ability of chemoattractants to stimulate the release of calcium from IP$_3$-sensitive intracellular stores and to enhance calcium influx. Lipid chemoattractants are less potent stimuli of the second phase of calcium elevation (62,94).

IP$_3$-sensitive calcium release has been localized to an intracellular organelle in leukocytes distinct from the endoplasmic reticulum called the calciosome (112). The IP$_3$ receptor (IP$_3$-activated calcium channel) has been sequenced and has significant homology with the ryanodine receptor from sarcoplasmic reticulum of striated muscle (113). It contains several transmembrane domains, two nucleotide binding sites, and potential phosphorylation sites for several protein kinases. The depletion of IP$_3$-sensitive calcium stores as a consequence of chemoattractant stimulation serves as the stimulus for calcium influx into neutrophils (114). This temporally coincides with the second phase of cytosolic calcium elevation.

The elevation of intracellular calcium appears to be essential for the stimulation of secretory responses by chemoattractants. Elevation of cytosolic calcium with calcium ionophores in the presence of extracellular calcium stimulates superoxide production and degranulation (115,116). Removal of extracellular calcium attenuates stimulation of the same responses by chemoattractants. However, evidence suggests that elevated calcium synergizes with additional signals induced by chemoattractants. When intracellular calcium was buffered at various concentrations using QUIN-2 and degranulation was examined, fMLP stimulation reduced the apparent EC$_{50}$

for calcium approximately 10-fold (115,116). Because no further changes in cytosolic calcium occurred under these conditions, the results demonstrated the involvement of an additional signaling component for chemoattractant stimulation. Similar data were obtained when thapsigargin was used to manipulate cytosolic calcium levels and the respiratory burst was examined (117). The fMLP and receptor interactions resulted in the generation of an unidentified signal that synergized with the pharmacologic elevation of cytosolic calcium for activation of the respiratory burst. These data demonstrate that calcium elevation is a required signal for secretory responses but that it also requires the participation of other signals for maximal stimulation.

The involvement of specific signals in cytoskeletal rearrangement and cell motility is less clear. Depletion of cell calcium has been reported to inhibit chemotaxis, whereas removal of extracellular calcium had only a small effect on directed migration (118). Buffering of intracellular calcium at various concentrations did not modify the ability of fMLP to stimulate actin polymerization or membrane ruffling (119). The absence of a clear role for chemoattractant-induced elevation of cytosolic calcium in these responses suggests that there may be a need for the involvement of other signaling pathways.

The nature of the second signals that synergize with calcium for stimulation of degranulation and activation of the respiratory burst remains to be clarified. PLA_2- and phospholipase D–derived lipid products and protein kinase C have each been indicated to participate in these processes. However, data obtained studying respiratory burst activation (117) suggested that the necessary second signal could be generated in the absence of chemoattractant-induced elevation of cytosolic calcium. All of these enzymes require the elevation of cytosolic calcium by chemoattractants for their activation.

LOW-MOLECULAR-WEIGHT G PROTEINS AND REGULATION OF DOWNSTREAM EFFECTORS

It has become apparent that chemoattractant signaling pathways that regulate the respiratory burst, chemotaxis, secretion of granules, and phospholipid metabolism involve LMW G proteins. Observations that pertussis toxin treatment of leukocytes attenuates chemoattractant stimulation of these processes indicate that these RAS-related G proteins act downstream of G_i. LMW G proteins are a large group of related GTP-binding proteins (about 18 to 26 kd) that have a specific subcellular localization and act as molecular switches in cellular processes (120,121). Based on sequence homology, they can be divided into families, including those of RAS, RHO/RAC, ARF, RAB, RAN, and RAD. LMW G proteins are monomeric and most are prenylated on the carboxyl-terminal end facilitating a membrane localization.

In general, they have a low intrinsic GTPase activity compared with their heterotrimeric counterparts. As is the case with other G proteins, the GTP-bound protein constitutes the active form. Regulation of GTPase activity and G-protein signaling ability is a consequence of interactions with GTPase-activating proteins (GAPs), GDP dissociation inhibitors (GDIs), and GEFs. With regard to signaling cascades, GEFs usually are the immediate upstream activator of the G protein, whereas downstream effectors are often GAPs.

Chemoattractant receptors activate an oxidative burst in neutrophils. The LMW G-protein RAC-2 is required for the stimulated activity. Activation of the respiratory burst involves translocation of the major components to the plasma membrane region of the cell (see Chapter 48). Phosphorylation of p47^{phox} is also required for activation. RAC is present as a complex with RHO GDI in the cytosol of unstimulated cells. On stimulation, RAC is translocated to the membrane fraction, whereas RHO GDI remains in the cytosol. RAC and CDC42, but not RHO, have been demonstrated to bind to p67^{phox} (122–124), although CDC42 does not activate the oxidative burst *in vitro*. The proximal signaling events regulating RAC involvement in this pathway are unclear, although PI3K-mediated activation of a RAC GEF has been reported (125) (Fig. 41-2). Phosphorylation of p47^{phox} by protein kinase C and an additional, unidentified protein kinase is required for activation of the oxidative burst by chemoattractants (126).

The RHO/RAC family of LMW G proteins, which includes RHO, RAC, and CDC42, has been implicated in other chemoattractant-stimulated leukocyte functions. Studies examining signaling through RHO proteins have been facilitated by the observation that they are ADP ribosylated by botulinum toxin C3 ADP-ribosyltransferase, with resultant inactivation of the proteins (127). Treatment of neutrophils with C3 ADP-ribosyltransferase inhibits chemoattractant-induced chemotaxis without similar effects on secretion or the oxidative burst (128). Lymphocytes containing transfected formylpeptide or IL-8 receptors exhibit chemoattractant-stimulated GTP loading of RHO, while inhibition of chemoattractant-stimulated integrin-mediated adherence by C3 ADP-ribosyltransferase is observed in transfected lymphocytes and normal neutrophils (129). RHO signaling probably is mediated by protein kinases. GTP-bound RHO directly activates protein kinases, including a p160 RHO kinase that can associate with membranes and phosphorylate myosin light chain (130–132) and protein kinase N (133, 134), which is phosphorylated in a botulinum toxin–sensitive manner in fibroblasts exposed to lysophosphatidic acid (134).

In fibroblasts, the RHO/RAC family of proteins has been demonstrated to be involved in the stimulated reorganization of the cytoskeleton (135). The formation of stress fibers involves RHO. Lamellipodia formation

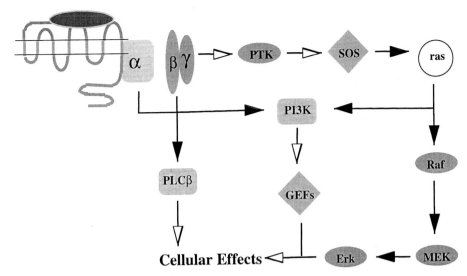

FIG. 41-2. Low-molecular-weight (LMW) G-protein activation pathways. The model summarizes chemoattractant signaling to LMW G proteins, including the proposed role of phosphatidylinositol 3-kinase (PI3K) in the regulation of guanine nucleotide exchange factors (GEFs) for several LMW proteins. In some steps, the two components directly interact *(closed arrows)*, and in some pathways *(open arrows)* multiple steps may occur. Diamond-shaped symbols represent GEFs; horizontal ellipses represent protein kinases (e.g., protein tyrosine kinase [PTK]); and rounded squares represent phospholipid-metabolizing enzymes.

requires RAC and filipodia extensions are mediated by CDC42. Based on microinjection studies using constitutively active or dominant negative forms of the proteins (constructed by single amino acid substitutions in the GTP-binding domain), it was suggested that these proteins act downstream of RAS in these processes. Data indicating that this family of proteins may also be involved in cytoskeletal rearrangement in stimulated leukocytes are summarized elsewhere (136).

The RAC proteins (RAC-1 and RAC-2) were identified initially in leukocytes, and RAC-2 was expressed preferentially in myeloid cells (137). RAC is translocated to the plasma membrane region of the cell in response to chemoattractants. Its association with and activation of oxidative burst components occurs within a submembranous cytoskeletal compartment (138). The proposed effects of RAC and CDC42 on the leukocyte cytoskeleton may involve the actions of a protein kinase. Members of the p21-activated protein kinase (PAK) family bind RAC and CDC42 in a GTP-dependent manner, are activated by RAC and CDC42, and constitutively active PAK can mimic downstream effects of RAC and CDC42 in transfection studies (139). In fibroblasts, PAKs have been demonstrated to be associated with cytoskeletal elements and the activation of PAKs results in actin reorganization (139). In leukocytes, PAKs are activated by exposure of cells to fMLP (140) and represent the previously described renaturable kinases that are rapidly activated in response to chemoattractants (141). A common feature of PAKs and several other signaling proteins that have been demonstrated to bind RAC or CDC42 is a motif for

CDC42/RAC *i*nteractive *b*inding (CRIB) (142). This motif has been useful in the identification of additional kinases that appear to be regulated similarly to PAKs (143).

LMW G proteins also mediate activation of phospholipase D by chemoattractants. Phospholipase D–mediated hydrolysis of phosphatidylcholine is a major mechanism for protein kinase C activation in response to chemoattractants. Initial experiments using subcellular fractions or permeabilized cells (neutrophils or HL60 cells) and endogenously labeled or exogenous phosphatidylcholine demonstrated guanine nucleotide stimulation of phospholipase D activity (144–147). Purification of a cytosolic component capable of reconstituting activity in cytosol-depleted assays resulted in the identification of ARF as the major active G protein (148,149). Prior research had identified ARF as a cytosolic component necessary for cholera toxin–mediated ADP-ribosylation of $G_s\alpha$ and subsequently as a family of proteins involved in vesicular trafficking. Effects on phospholipid metabolism may mediate ARF's involvement for vesicle movement (103). In addition to the effects of ARF on phospholipase D, RHO has been identified as a membrane component capable of stimulating phospholipase D activity (150). A subsequent study in HL60 cells presented evidence for cytosolic and membrane phospholipase D activities with different sensitivities to ARF and RHO family proteins (151). The cloning of phospholipases D should allow for the further delineation of signaling mechanisms involved in chemoattractant-mediated activation of the enzyme.

RAS was the initial LMW G protein identified and its role in intracellular signaling is the best understood. It is involved as an upstream component in the activation of MAP kinases in response to growth factors and other mitogens, including G-protein–coupled receptors (152). The activation of individual MAP kinases results in the subsequent phosphorylation and activation of specific transcription factors (153) and other proteins involved in cellular signaling, such as PLA₂. The signaling events involving RAS are most clear for the regulation of the MAP kinases ERK-1 and ERK-2. These serine/threonine kinases of 44 and 42 kd, respectively, are activated by phosporylation of threonine and tyrosine residues by MEK-1 and MEK-2. Several chemoattractant receptors have been demonstrated to mediate ERK-1 and ERK-2 activation, including endogenous receptors for formylpeptides (154,155), IL-8 (81), and C5a (81,156) and the PAF receptor after transfection into CHO cells (157) but not the endogenous neutrophil PAF receptor (158). Activation of ERK by chemoattractants is pertussis toxin sensitive and does not appear to involve calcium. Conflicting data concerning a potential role for protein kinase C have been obtained (155,159). Chemoattractant signaling involves an increase in GTP-bound RAS (81,155) and the subsequent activation of RAF and MEK-1 (159) (see Fig. 41-2), although an alternative pathway involving a different MEK kinase may also contribute to ERK activation (160).

RAS activation by chemoattractants occurs after the activation of nonreceptor tyrosine kinases. Tyrosine kinase inhibitors block chemoattractant-induced ERK activation (155,159). Exposure of neutrophils to fMLP results in the activation of the SRC-related kinase, Lyn (161). After immunoprecipitation of relevant proteins from activated neutrophils, complexes are observed of Lyn and Shc that also contain phosphatidylinositol 3-kinase. The ability of chemoattractants to activate RAS-mediated signaling is similar to that observed for other Gi-coupled receptors (162). The βγ portion of the receptor-associated G protein is involved in signaling for RAS activation based on the ability of transfected protein sequestrants of βγ to specifically inhibit stimulation. Sequestration of βγ by these proteins is caused by the presence of pleckstrin homology (PH) domains, a structural motif found in a variety of signaling molecules (163). The role of βγ for MAP kinase activation is distinct from its effects on adenylate cyclase or phospholipase C. As described for chemoattractant receptors, Shc phosphorylation, stimulation of phosphatidylinositol 3-kinase, and the activation of SRC-related tyrosine kinases are all observed for other Gi-coupled receptors. The molecular target for βγ and the identity of the initial tyrosine kinase, which is activated, remain to be elucidated.

FMLP also activates p38 MAP kinase (158,164,165) but does not activate JUN N-terminal kinase; stress activated protein kinase (JNK/SAPK) (158). Although PAF is a poor stimulus for ERK activation, it is comparable to fMLP as a stimulus for the activation of p38 MAP kinase

(158). Activation of p38 and JNK/SAPK MAP kinases also involves LMW G proteins. Constitutively active RAC and CDC42 activate JNK/SAPK and p38 kinase in transfected cells (166–169). As with the RAS/ERK pathway, the immediate effector of RAC and CDC42 in these pathways appears to be a protein kinase because constitutively active PAK activates JNK/SAPK in transfection studies (139).

In addition to the ability of GTP-bound RAS to bind to and activate RAF, the same effector domain of the active protein binds to and activates other signaling molecules, including the p110 subunit of a growth factor-regulated phosphatidylinositol 3-kinase (PI3K), ral GEF and a variety of other proteins with less clear signaling roles (170,171). Because of the similarity of LMW G proteins in the effector region, the specificity of these observations is unclear (170). Members of the RHO/RAC family of LMW G proteins, under certain conditions, also bind to and activate growth factor-regulated PI3K in a GTP-dependent manner *in vitro* (172,173). In contrast to RAS, these proteins bind to the p85 subunit. Chemoattractants stimulate PI3K activity and this stimulated activity has been indicated to participate in signaling.

The next several years should clarify chemoattractant signaling mechanisms regulating LMW G-protein function in leukocytes. Functions for individual rab family members in vesicular trafficking have been described and it is likely that this family of proteins is involved in phagocytosis and secretory mechanisms (174). RAN family members have been ascribed a role in directional nuclear transport of RNA and proteins (175) and may serve a regulated function during chemoattractant-induced activation of immediate early genes (176,177).

PRIMING OF CHEMOATTRACTANT RESPONSES

The ability of chemoattractants to induce secretory or respiratory burst responses in leukocytes is potentiated by prior exposure of the cells to a variety of agents. In the case of human neutrophils, these priming stimuli include tumor necrosis factor-α (TNF-α), granulocyte-macrophage colony-stimulating factor (GM-CSF), lipopolysaccharide (LPS), and low doses of chemoattractants themselves. The neutrophil responses where priming is best understood are the oxidative burst and eicosanoid synthesis. Potentiation of these chemoattractant-induced responses by prior exposure to the agents previously described has been demonstrated for isolated neutrophils, in whole blood, and *in vivo*. Priming by lipopolysaccharide and the cytokines occurs within minutes to hours, whereas priming by chemoattractants is evident within seconds. Although these cytokines can increase the number of cell surface receptors for several chemoattractants, these responses happen slower than priming. GM-CSF and TNF-α prime for sodium fluoride-induced superoxide production, indicating regulation at a postreceptor step (178). LPS (179), GM-CSF (180), and TNF-α (181) all rapidly increase plasma membrane $G_i\alpha$ levels and this effect has been suggested to explain their priming for oxidative burst activation. Priming of an early event in the signaling pathway is consistent with the reported inability of TNF-α and GM-CSF to prime for phorbol ester-induced superoxide production (178).

Priming for stimulated eicosanoid production also is evident at an early step in the signaling process. Priming for enhanced PLA_2 activity has been reported for GM-CSF (182) and LPS (183). GM-CSF was shown to stimulate the phosphorylation of $cPLA_2$, an effect that was blocked by tyrosine kinase inhibitors (182). The results suggested that MAP kinase–mediated phosphorylation of $cPLA_2$ enhanced the subsequent calcium-mediated activation of the enzyme by chemoattractants. In support of this idea, prior exposure to GM-CSF also enhances calcium ionophore-stimulated PLA_2 activation (184).

Low doses of chemoattractants prime for activation of secretory responses, whereas high concentrations desensitize for a second dose. Whereas lipid chemoattractants are poor stimuli for superoxide production, they are effective in priming for an fMLP-stimulated response (185,186). Priming by cytokines and LPS is long-lasting, whereas priming by PAF is maximal at ten minutes and reversed within two hours (187). Mechanisms involved in chemoattractant-induced priming are unclear. Priming is rapidly observed in response to low doses of phorbol esters or calcium ionophores (188). The same report demonstrated that influx of extracellular calcium was not required for priming by fMLP. However, depletion of intracellular calcium does attenuate priming by PAF (185,186). Current data indicate that chemoattractant-induced priming regulates protein kinase C because an increase in phorbol ester binding is observed after stimulation of primed cells compared with unprimed cells (186).

Exposure of RBL-2H3 cells to thrombin primes for chemoattractant-induced secretion, calcium mobilization, and phospholipase C activation by transfected pertussis toxin–sensitive chemoattractant receptors (189). This effect is observed within minutes of thrombin exposure and is apparently not mediated by the well-characterized G-protein–coupled thrombin receptor. Whether the mechanisms involved in thrombin priming are the same as those involved in the actions of other priming agents requires further study.

TERMINATION OF CHEMOATTRACTANT SIGNALING

Overview

Phagocytic leukocytes are capable of potent microbiocidal and host destructive activities that are tightly regulated. Moreover, these cells have receptors for many chemoattractants and other proinflammatory agents that are simultaneously present at inflammatory sites. Receptor regulation and cross-regulation play important roles in leukocyte physiology. Desensitization of leukocyte chemoattractant receptors can be defined as whether the down regulation is confined to ligand occupied receptors or is a consequence of processes not requiring receptor occupancy (i.e., homologous vs heterologous). These phenomena have been studied in detail, with a great deal of information resulting from studies of the visual and adrenergic systems. Based on this work, it has been determined that desensitization of G-protein–coupled receptors can be mediated by receptor phosphorylation involving at least three different types of kinases. Ligand-induced phosphorylation, presumably initiated by steric changes associated with receptor occupancy, leads to phosphorylation of a site on the receptor's cytoplasmic domain. This phosphorylation by GRKs is not mediated by additional second messengers but presumably is initiated by changes in receptor conformation associated with the active state. Activation of second messenger systems can lead to protein kinase A– or protein kinase C–mediated phosphorylation of receptors at other cytoplasmic sites. This type of phosphorylation can occur during receptor activation but can also lead to the phosphorylation of other receptors that contain the appropriate phosphorylation sites. Phosphorylation of G-protein–coupled receptors is associated with a reduced affinity for G proteins and an increased affinity for members of the arrestin family of proteins. The association of the receptor with arrestin targets the receptor for internalization presumably through clathrin-coated vesicles. A reduction of pH in the internalized vesicles results in the dissociation of the ligand and the dephosphorylation of the receptor before its eventual recycling to the cell surface.

The availability of cell lines capable of expressing functional, genetically modified chemoattractant receptors has allowed for a rapid expansion in our understanding of the role of receptor phosphorylation versus downstream events during chemoattractant desensitization. It has led to the determination that, for chemoattractant receptors, desensitization occurs at multiple levels. Similar to other G-protein–coupled receptors, chemoattractant receptors are desensitized by phosphorylation through GRKs and protein kinase C. A second site for desensitization has been identified at the level of phospholipase C (β_3 and presumably β_2). Selectivity for classes of chemoattractant receptors have been identified with regard to their ability to cross desensitize each other. This appears to be associated with the specific G protein to which the receptor normally couples. These observations, described in detail later, may explain a phenomenon originally observed in human neutrophils. Certain chemoattractant receptors, when activated, desensitize themselves as well as selected additional chemoattractant receptors.

For example, stimulation of the formylpeptide receptor on neutrophils not only desensitizes for further formylpeptide-stimulated calcium responses, but also those for C5a, IL-8, PAF, and LTB$_4$. In contrast, activation of the PAF receptor desensitizes for further PAF stimulation but not for formylpeptides, C5a, or IL-8. This phenomenon was called receptor class desensitization. The availability of cellular models to study chemoattractant activation has allowed for a better understanding of the molecular mechanisms of desensitization at the level of the receptor and at the level of activation of phospholipase C.

Desensitization at the Level of Chemoattractant Receptors

Chemoattractant activation results in the rapid phosphorylation of the corresponding chemoattractant receptor. Agonist-dependent phosphorylation and desensitization has been demonstrated using expressed receptors for fMLP (51,190,191), C5a (51,190,191), PAF (52,191), MCP-1 (192), and IL-8 (190,191,193–195). Specific residues that are phosphorylated have been determined for some chemoattractant receptors. Agonist-induced desensitization of CXCR1 and CXCR2 is caused by the phosphorylation within a short sequence containing multiple serines/threonines near the carboxyl terminus (193,194). Truncation of the PAF receptor (191) or mutation of the CCR2b receptor (192) have also demonstrated that desensitization is caused by phosphorylation of serine/threonine residues in the carboxyl terminus. The phosphorylation-deficient PAF receptor mutant stimulates phospholipase C and exocytosis to a greater and more prolonged degree than the corresponding wild type receptor consistent with a lack of desensitization of G-protein coupling and internalization after agonist exposure. The more intense signaling is also evidenced in the ability of the truncated, but not native, PAF receptor to cross-desensitize C5a and Il-8 receptors in RBL-2H3 cells (191).

Homologous desensitization of G-protein–coupled receptors has been demonstrated to be mediated by a family of GRKs that phosphorylate agonist-occupied receptors (196). These kinases are characterized by a central catalytic domain and a carboxyl-terminal domain that is necessary for membrane localization. The individual members exhibit differences in receptor specificity and mechanism of membrane binding (farnesylation, palmitoylation, or PH domains). GRKs 2, 3, 5, and 6 were shown to be expressed in human neutrophils (197). The roles of the individual isozymes for desensitization of chemoattractant receptors is unclear at the present time.

Most chemoattractant receptors are also phosphorylated in response to second messenger-regulated protein kinases. Activation of protein kinase C and the calcium-dependent increase in cAMP observed in response to chemoattractants have been indicated to inhibit early signaling events. Active phorbol esters stimulate the phosphorylation of expressed C5a (51), IL-8 (193), and PAF (52) receptors but not fMLP receptors (51) in stably transfected RBL-2H3 cells consistent with the absence of a putative protein kinase C phosphorylation site in the fMLP receptor. Similarly, a cell-permeable cAMP analog increased the phosphorylation of the expressed PAF receptor but not of the expressed receptors for C5a and fMLP (52), again consistent with the presence or absence, respectively, of putative phosphorylation sites in the third cytoplasmic loop and carboxyl tail. The examination of relative roles for phosphorylation by GRKs versus second messenger-regulated protein kinases has revealed that low doses of agonist stimulate receptor phosphorylation by protein kinase A and protein kinase C, whereas high concentrations of agonist are required for phosphorylation by GRKs.

Desensitization at the Level of Phospholipase C

In addition to the homologous and heterologous desensitization mechanisms described earlier, additional complexity is observed when examining cross-desensitization by chemoattractant receptors. Didsbury et al. (198) reported that expressed receptors for fMLP and C5a were capable of cross-desensitizing in HEK293 cells, whereas cross-desensitization with endogenous calcium-mobilizing purinergic receptors was not observed. This was called receptor class desensitization. Similarly, endogenous receptors for peptide chemoattractants in leukocytes are capable of cross-desensitizing but do not desensitize responses to a purinergic ligand (199). The peptide chemoattractants C5a, fMLP, and IL-8 are able to desensitize subsequent calcium mobilization in response to PAF and LTB$_4$ in neutrophils, whereas the reverse is not observed (199). In RBL-2H3 cells, expressed receptors for PAF do not mediate desensitization of expressed receptors for fMLP, C5a, or IL-8, whereas desensitization of PAF-mediated responses occur as a result of prior exposure to the peptide ligands (191).

Differences in signaling mechanisms are likely to result in the desensitization patterns described. Differences exist among chemoattractant receptors with regard to their ability to couple to pertussis toxin–insensitive and pertussis toxin–sensitive G proteins. The effectiveness of peptide chemoattractants for cross-desensitization of calcium mobilization suggests that they share a common mechanism through the activation of phospholipase C. Because α and $\beta\gamma$ subunits activate phospholipase Cβ through interactions with different regions of the molecule (72), phosphorylation of the enzyme could serve to differentially desensitize different classes of chemoattractants. Phosphorylation of phospholipase Cβ_2 by protein kinase A results in a decreased activation of the enzyme by $\beta\gamma$ but not α subunits (200). Furthermore, phosphorylation of phospholipase Cβ_3 in RBL cells is

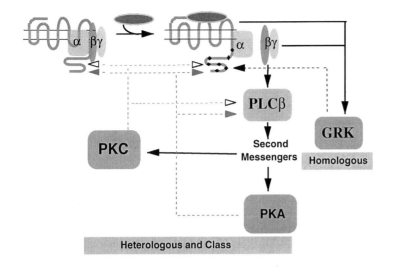

FIG. 41-3. Model for chemoattractant receptor phosphorylation. Depicted are the proposed routes for homologous desensitization in which a G-protein–coupled receptor kinase (GRK) phosphorylates an agonist-occupied receptor; heterologous desensitization whereby protein kinase C (PKC) or protein kinase A (PKA) activated by second messengers resulting from PLC activation phosphorylate all receptors containing the appropriate sequences; or class desensitization in which the same signal-regulated protein kinases phosphorylate phospholipase Cβ isozymes at sites that inhibit activation by α or βγ subunits of specific heterotrimeric G proteins. Solid lines refer to stimulatory events, and dashed lines refer to phosphorylation events involved in desensitization.

indicated to be involved in desensitization of PAF receptor signaling (63). A similar downstream locus for desensitization of fMLP responses is indicated from results demonstrating a lack of phosphorylation of the fMLP receptor during cross-desensitization (190). Current results indicate that termination of chemoattractant signaling involves the regulation of multiple components in the signaling cascade, including the phosphorylation and inactivation of chemoattractant receptors and phospholipase C (Fig. 41-3). An increased understanding of desensitization mechanisms should provide further information of signaling mechanisms used by the different chemoattractant receptors.

CONCLUSIONS

Chemoattractants use common and divergent mechanisms for the stimulation of chemotaxis and secretory functions. They bind to related G-protein–coupled receptors and activate a polyphosphoinositide-specific phospholipase C with a resultant increase in cytosolic calcium concentrations. This pathway is indicated to be essential for the initiation of downstream signaling events that are involved in specific secretory responses. Different efficacies are observed between the various types of chemoattractants with regard to specific downstream signaling events (e.g., calcium influx, phospholipase D, LMW G-protein activation) and the corresponding secretory events. By contrast, all chemoattractants exhibit similar potencies for the stimulation of chemotaxis and the biochemical mechanisms involved appear to differ from those described for secretion.

The ability of chemoattractants to stimulate various leukocyte functions can be primed or desensitized through multiple mechanisms. Cytokines and LPS prime leukocytes by regulating G protein and receptor availability, whereas low doses of chemoattractants prime downstream signaling events. High doses of chemoattractants

themselves or a variety of other leukocyte stimuli can desensitize signaling events. This desensitization is mediated by protein phosphorylation of the chemoattractant receptor or of other signaling molecules (e.g., phospholipase C).

The identification and sequence determination of proteins that are potentially involved in chemoattractant signaling is accumulating at a rapid pace. These proteins include not only additional chemokines and chemokine receptors but also lipid-metabolizing enzymes (phospholipases D and phosphatidylinositol 3-kinases), cytoskeletal-associated protein kinases, and lipid binding proteins with potential signaling roles. The near future should more clearly delineate the involvement of these molecules in signaling pathways controlling chemotactic and secretory functions of leukocytes.

REFERENCES

1. Schiffmann E, Corcoran BA, Wahl SM. *N*-formylmethionyl peptides as chemoattractants for leukocytes. *Proc Natl Acad Sci USA* 1975;72:1059–1063.
2. Showell HJ, Freer RJ, Zigmond SH, Schiffman E, Aswanikumar S, Corcoran B, Becker EL. The structure-activity relations of synthetic peptides as chemotactic factors and inducers of lysozymal enzyme secretion for neutrophils. *J Exp Med* 1976;143:1154–1169.
3. Gao J-L, Becker EL, Freer RJ, Muthukumaraswamy N, Murphy PM. A high potency nonformylated peptide agonist for the phagocyte *N*-formylpeptide chemotactic receptor. *J Exp Med* 1994;180:2191–2197.
4. Niedel J, Wilkinson S, Cuatrecasas P. Receptor-mediated uptake and degradation of ^{125}I-chemotactic peptide by human neutrophils. *J Biol Chem* 1979;254:10700–10706.
5. Snyderman R, Gewurz H, Mergenhagen SE. Interactions of the complement system with endotoxic lipopolysaccharide: generation of a factor chemotactic for polymorphonuclear leukocytes. *J Exp Med* 1968;128:259–275.
6. Shin HS, Snyderman R, Friedman E, Mellors A, Mayer MM. Chemotactic and anaphylactic fragment cleaved from the fifth component of guinea pig complement. *Science* 1968;162:361–363.
7. Gerard C, Gerard NP. C5a anaphylatoxin and its seven transmembrane-segment receptor. *Annu Rev Immunol* 1994;12:775–808.
8. Chenoweth DE, Erickson BW, Hugli TE. Human C5a-related synthetic peptides as neutrophil chemotactic factors. *Biochem Biophys Res Commun* 1979;68:227–231.

9. Chenoweth DE, Hugli TE. Human C5a and C5a analogs as probes of the neutrophil C5a receptor. *Mol Immunol* 1980;17:151–161.

10. Gerard C, Showell HJ, Hoeprich PD Jr, Hugli TE, Stimler NP. Evidence for a role of the amino-terminal region in the biological activity of the classical anaphylatoxin, porcine C5a des-Arg-74. *J Biol Chem* 1985;260:2613–2616.

11. Zuiderweg RP, Henkin J, Mollison KW, Carter GW, Greer J. Comparison of model and nuclear magnetic resonance structures for the human inflammatory protein C5a. *Proteins Struct Function Genet* 1988;3:139–145.

12. Chao W, Olson MS. Platelet-activating factor: receptors and signal transduction. *Biochem J* 1993;292:617–629.

13. Henderson WR Jr. The role of leukotrienes in inflammation. *Ann Intern Med* 1994;121:684–697.

14. Baggiolini M, Dewald B, Moser B. Human chemokines: an update. *Annu Rev Immunol* 1997;15:675–705.

15. Clore GM, Gronenborn AM. Three-dimensional structures of α and β chemokines. *FASEB J* 1995;9:57–62.

16. Williams LT, Snyderman R, Pike MC, Lefkowitz RJ. Specific receptor sites for chemotactic peptides on human polymorphonuclear leukocytes. *Proc Natl Acad Sci USA* 1977;74:1204–1208.

17. Malech HL, Gardner JP, Heiman DF, Rosenzweig SA. Asparagine-linked oligosaccharides on formyl peptide chemotactic receptors of human phagocytic cells. *J Biol Chem* 1985;260:2509–2514.

18. Boulay F, Tardif M, Brouchon L, Vignais P. Synthesis and use of a novel *N*-formyl peptide derivative to isolate a human *N*-formyl peptide receptor cDNA. *Biochem Biophys Res Commun* 1990;168:1103–1109.

19. Honda Z, Nakamura M, Miki I, et al. Cloning by functional expression of platelet-activating factor receptor from guinea-pig lung. *Nature* 1991;349:342–346.

20. Holmes WE, Lee J, Kuang W-J, Rice GC, Wood WI. Structure and functional expression of a human interleukin-8 receptor. *Science* 1991;253:1278–1280.

21. Yokomizo T, Izumi T, Chang K, Takuwa Y, Shimizu T. A G-protein–coupled receptor for leukotriene B₄ that mediates chemotaxis. *Nature* 1997;387:620–624.

22. Gerard NP, Gerard C. The chemotactic receptor for human C5a anaphylatoxin. *Nature* 1991;349:614–617.

23. Murphy PM. Chemokine receptors: structure, function and role in microbial pathogenesis. *Cytokine Growth Factor Rev* 1996;7:47–64.

24. Gao J-L, Murphy PM. Species and subtype variants of the *N*-formyl peptide chemotactic receptor reveal multiple important functional domains. *J Biol Chem* 1993;268:25395–25401.

25. Mery L, Boulay F. The NH₂-terminal region of C5aR but not that of FPR is critical for both protein transport and ligand binding. *J Biol Chem* 1994;269:3457–3463.

26. Queheuberger O, Prossnitz ER, Cavanagh SL, Cochrane CG, Ye RD. Multiple domains of the *N*-formyl peptide receptor are required for high-affinity ligand binding: construction and analysis of chimeric *N*-formyl peptide receptors. *J Biol Chem* 1993;268:18167–18175.

27. Perez HD, Holmes R, Vilander LR, Adams RR, Manzana W, Jolley D, Andrews WH. Formyl peptide receptor chimeras define domains involved in ligand binding. *J Biol Chem* 1993;268:2292–2295.

28. Morgan E, Ember JA, Sanderson SD, et al. Anti-C5a receptor antibodies: characterization of neutralizing antibodies specific for a peptide, C5ar-(9-29), derived from the predicted amino-terminal sequence of the human C5a receptor. *J Immunol* 1993;151:377–388.

29. Oppermann M, Raedt U, Hebell T, Schmidt B, Zimmerman B, Gotze O. Probing the human receptor for C5a anaphylatoxin with site-directed antibodies. Identification of a potential ligand binding site on the NH₂-terminal domain. *J Immunol* 1993;151:3785–3794.

30. Siciliano SJ, Rollins TE, DeMartino J, et al. Two-site binding of C5a by its receptor: an alternative binding paradigm for G protein-coupled receptors. *Proc Natl Acad Sci USA* 1994;91:1214–1218.

31. Monteclaro FS, Charo IF. The amino-terminal domain of CCR2 is both necessary and sufficient for high affinity binding of monocyte chemoattractant protein 1: receptor activation by a pseudo-tethered ligand. *J Biol Chem* 1997;272:23186–23190.

32. Ahuja SK, Lee JC, Murphy PM. CXC chemokines bind to unique sets of selectivity determinants that can function independently and are broadly distributed on multiple domains of human interleukin-8 receptor B: determinants of high affinity binding and receptor activation are distinct. *J Biol Chem* 1996;271:225–232.

33. Wells TNC, Power CA, Lusti-Narasimhan M, et al. Selectivity and antagonism of chemokine receptors. *J Leukoc Biol* 1996;59:53–60.

34. Clapham PR. HIV and chemokines: ligands sharing cell-surface receptors. *Trends Cell Biol* 1997;7:264–268.

35. Rucker J, Samson M, Doranz BJ, et al. Regions in β-chemokine receptors CCR5 and CCR2b that determine HIV-1 cofactor specificity. *Cell* 1996;87:437–446.

36. Oravezc T, Pall M, Norcross MA. β-Chemokine inhibition of a monocytotropic HIV-1 infection. Interference with a postbinding fusion step. *J Immunol* 1996;157:1329–1332.

37. Aramori I, Zhang J, Ferguson SSG, Bieniasz PD, Cullen BR, Caron MG. Molecular mechanism of desensitization of the chemokine receptor CCR-5: receptor signaling and internalization are dissociable from its role as an HIV-1 co-receptor. *EMBO J* 1997;16:4606–4616.

38. Koo C, Lefkowitz RJ, Snyderman R. Guanine nucleotides modulate the binding affinity of the oligopeptide chemoattractant receptor on human polymorphonuclear leukocytes. *J Clin Invest* 1983;72:748–753.

39. Snyderman R, Pike MC, Edge S, Lane B. A chemoattractant receptor on macrophages exists in two affinity states regulated by guanine nucleotides. *J Cell Biol* 1984;98:444–448.

40. Smith CD, Uhing RJ, Snyderman R. Nucleotide regulatory protein-mediated activation of phospholipase C in human polymorphonuclear leukocytes is disrupted by phorbol esters. *J Biol Chem* 1987;262:6121–6127.

41. Okajima F, Katada T, Ui M. Coupling of the guanine nucleotide regulatory protein to chemotactic peptide receptors in neutrophil membranes and its uncoupling by islet-activating protein, pertussis toxin: a possible role of the toxin substrate in Ca²⁺-mobilizing receptor-mediated signal transduction. *J Biol Chem* 1985;260:6761–6768.

42. Feltner DE, Smith RH, Marasco WA. Characterization of the plasma membrane GTPase from rabbit neutrophils. I. Evidence for an Nᵢ-like protein coupled to the formyl peptide, C5a, and leukotriene B₄ chemotaxis receptors. *J Immunol* 1986;137:1961–1970.

43. Giershik P, Falloon J, Milligan G, Pines M, Gallin JI, Spiegel A. Immunochemical evidence for a novel pertussis toxin substrate in human neutrophils. *J Biol Chem* 1986;261:8058–8062.

44. Goldsmith P, Rossiter K, Carter A, et al. Identification of the GTP-binding protein encoded by the Gᵢ3 complementary DNA. *J Biol Chem* 1988;263:6476–6479.

45. Polakis PG, Uhing RJ, Snyderman R. The formylpeptide chemoattractant receptor copurifies with a GTP-binding protein containing a distinct 40 kDa pertussis toxin substrate. *J Biol Chem* 1988;263:4969–4976.

46. Rollins TE, Siciliano S, Kobayashi S, et al. Purification of the active C5a receptor from human polymorphonuclear leukocytes as a receptor-Gᵢ complex. *Proc Natl Acad Sci USA* 1991;88:971–975.

47. Damaj BB, McColl SR, Mahana W, Crouch MF, Naccache PH. Physical association of Gᵢ2α with interleukin-8 receptors. *J Biol Chem* 1996;271:12783–12789.

48. Didsbury JR, Uhing RJ, Tomhave E, Gerard C, Gerard NP, Snyderman R. Functional high efficiency expression of cloned leukocyte chemoattractant receptor cDNAs. *FEBS Lett* 1992;297:275–279.

49. Uhing RJ, Gettys TW, Tomhave E, Snyderman R, Didsbury JR. Differential regulation of cAMP by endogenous versus transfected formylpeptide chemoattractant receptors: implications for Gᵢ-coupled receptor signaling. *Biochem Biophys Res Commun* 1992;183:1033–1039.

50. Jiang H, Kuang Y, Wu Y, Smrcka A, Simon MI, Wu D. Pertussis toxin-sensitive activation of phospholipase C by the C5a and fMet-Leu-Phe receptors. *J Biol Chem* 1996;271:13430–13434.

51. Ali H, Richardson RM, Tomhave ED, Didsbury JR, Snyderman R. Differences in phosphorylation of formylpeptide and C5a chemoattractant receptors correlate with differences in desensitization. *J Biol Chem* 1993;268:24247–24254.

52. Ali H, Richardson RM, Tomhave ED, DuBose RA, Haribabu B, Snyderman R. Regulation of stably transfected platelet activating factor receptor in RBL-2H3 cells: role of multiple G proteins and receptor phosphorylation. *J Biol Chem* 1994;269:24557–24563.

53. Amatruda TT III, Gerard NP, Gerard C, Simon MI. Specific interactions of chemoattractant factor receptors with G-proteins. *J Biol Chem* 1993;268:10139–10144.

54. Lee CH, Katz A, Simon MI. Multiple regions of Gα₁₆ contribute to the specificity of activation by the C5a receptor. *Mol Pharmacol* 1995;47:218–223.

55. Amatruda TT III, Dragas-Graonic S, Holmes R, Perez HD. Signal transduction by the formyl peptide receptor: studies using chimeric receptors and site-directed mutagenesis define a novel domain for interaction with G-proteins. *J Biol Chem* 1995;270:28010–28013.

56. Kuang Y, Wu Y, Jiang H, Wu D. Selective G protein coupling by C-C chemokine receptors. *J Biol Chem* 1996;271:3975–3978.

57. Wu D, LaRosa GJ, Simon MI. G protein-coupled signal transduction pathways for interleukin-8. *Science* 1993;261:101–103.

58. Arai H, Charo IF. Differential regulation of G-protein—mediated signaling by chemokine receptors. *J Biol Chem* 1996;271:21814–21819.

59. Amatruda TT III, Steele DA, Slepak VZ, Simon MI. $G\alpha_{16}$, a G protein α subunit specifically expressed in hematopoietic cells. *Proc Natl Acad Sci USA* 1991;88:5587–5591.

60. Offermanns S, Simon MI. $G\alpha_{15}$ and $G\alpha_{16}$ couple a wide variety of receptors to phospholipase C. *J Biol Chem* 1995;270:15175–15180.

61. Zhu X, Birnbaumer L. G protein subunits and the stimulation of phospholipase C by G_s- and G_i-coupled receptors: lack of receptor selectivity of $G\alpha_{16}$ and evidence for a synergic interaction between $G\beta\gamma$ and the α subunit of a receptor-activated G protein. *Proc Natl Acad Sci USA* 1996;93:2827–2831.

62. Verghese MW, Charles L, Jakoi L, Dillon SB, Snyderman R. Role of a guanine nucleotide regulatory protein in the activation of phospholipase C by different chemoattractants. *J Immunol* 1987;138:4374–4380.

63. Ali H, Fisher I, Haribabu B, Richardson RM, Snyderman R. Role of phospholipase Cβ3 phosphorylation in the desensitization of cellular responses to platelet-activating factor. *J Biol Chem* 1997;272:11706–11709.

64. Sprang SR. G protein mechanisms: insights from structural analysis. *Annu Rev Biochem* 1997;66:639–678.

65. Dohlman HG, Thorner J, Caron MG, Lefkowitz RJ. Model systems for the study of seven-transmembrane-segment receptors. *Annu Rev Biochem* 1991;60:653–688.

66. Schreiber RE, Prossnitz ER, Ye RD, Cochrane CG, Bokoch GM. Domains of the human neutrophil *N*-formyl peptide receptor involved in G protein coupling: mapping with receptor-derived peptides. *J Biol Chem* 1994;269:326–331.

67. Prossnitz ER, Quehenberger O, Cochrane CG, Ye RD. The role of the third intracellular loop of the neutrophil *N*-formyl peptide receptor in G protein coupling. *Biochem J* 1993;294:581–587.

68. Smith CD, Lane BC, Kusaka I, Verghese MW, Snyderman R. Chemoattractant receptor-induced hydrolysis of phosphatidylinositol 4,5-bis-phosphate in human polymorphonuclear leukocyte membranes: requirement of a guanine nucleotide regulatory protein. *J Biol Chem* 1985;260:5875–5878.

69. Smith CD, Cox CC, Snyderman R. Receptor-coupled activation of phosphoinositide-specific phospholipase C by an N protein. *Science* 1986;232:97–100.

70. Exton JH. Regulation of phosphoinositide phospholipases by hormones, neurotransmitters, and other agonists linked to G proteins. *Annu Rev Pharmacol Toxicol* 1996;36:481–509.

71. Rhee SG, Bae YS. Regulation of phosphoinositide-specific phospholipase C isozymes. *J Biol Chem* 1997;272:15045–15048.

72. Wu D, Katz A, Simon MI. Activation of phospholipase Cβ2 by the α and βγ subunits of trimeric GTP-binding protein. *Proc Natl Acad Sci USA* 1993;90:5297–5301.

73. Clapham DE, Neer EJ. G protein βγ subunits. *Annu Rev Pharmacol Toxicol* 1997;37:167–203.

74. Jiang H, Kuang Y, Wu Y, Xie W, Simon MI, Wu D. Roles of phospholipase Cβ2 in chemoattractant-elicited responses. *Proc Natl Acad Sci USA* 1997;94:7971–7975.

75. Verghese MW, Fox K, McPhail LC, Snyderman R. Chemoattractant-elicited alterations of cAMP levels in human polymorphonuclear leukocytes require a Ca⁺⁺-dependent mechanism which is independent of transmembrane activation of adenylate cyclase. *J Biol Chem* 1985;260:6769–6775.

76. Iannone MA, Wolberg G, Zimmerman TP. Chemotactic peptide induces cAMP elevation in human neutrophils by amplification of the adenylate cyclase response to endogenously produced adenosine. *J Biol Chem* 1989;264:20177–20180.

77. Bradford PG, Rubin RP. Quantitative changes in inositol 1,4,5-triphosphate in chemoattractant-stimulated neutrophils. *J Biol Chem* 1986;261:15644–15647.

78. Dillon SB, Murray JJ, Verghese MW, Snyderman R. Regulation of inositol phosphate metabolism in chemoattractant-stimulated human polymorphonuclear leukocytes: definition of distinct dephosphorylation pathways for IP₃ isomers. *J Biol Chem* 1987;262:11546–11552.

79. Traynor-Kaplan AE, Harris A, Thompson B, Taylor P, Sklar LA. An inositol tetrakisphosphate-containing phospholipid in activated neutrophils. *Nature* 1988;334:353–356.

80. Stephens L, Jackson T, Hawkins PT. Synthesis of phosphatidylinositol 3,4,5-trisphosphate in permeabilized neutrophils regulated by receptors and G-proteins. *J Biol Chem* 1993;268:17162–17172.

81. Knall C, Young S, Nick JA, Buhl AM, Worthen GS, Johnson GL. Interleukin-8 regulation of the Ras/Raf/mitogen-activated protein kinase pathway in human neutrophils. *J Biol Chem* 1996;271:2832–2838.

82. Kapeller R, Cantley LC. Phosphatidylinositol 3-kinase. *Bioessays* 1994;16:565–576.

83. Stephens L, Hawkins PT, Eguinoa A, Cooke F. A heterotrimeric GTPase-regulated isoform of PI3K and the regulation of its potential effectors. *Philos Trans R Soc Lond B* 1996;351:211–215.

84. Stoyanov B, Volinia S, Hanck T, et al. Cloning and characterization of a G protein-activated human phosphoinositide 3-kinase. *Science* 1995;269:690–693.

85. Stephens L, Eguinoa A, Corey S, Jackson T, Hawkins PT. Receptor stimulated accumulation of phosphatidylinositol (3,4,5)-trisphosphate by G-protein–mediated pathways in human myeloid derived cells. *EMBO J* 1993;12:2265–2273.

86. Baggiolini M, Dewald B, Schnyder J, Ruch W, Cooper PH, Payne TG. Inhibition of the phagocytosis-induced respiratory burst by the fungal metabolite wortmannin and some analogues. *Exp Cell Res* 1987;169:408–418.

87. Dewald B, Thelen M, Baggiolini M. Two transduction sequences are necessary for neutrophil activation by receptor agonists. *J Biol Chem* 1988;263:16179–16184.

88. Rameh LE, Chen C-S, Cantley LC. Phosphatidylinositol (3,4,5)P₃ interacts with SH2 domains and modulates PI 3-kinase association with tyrosine-phosphorylated proteins. *Cell* 1995;83:821–830.

89. Klarlund JK, Guilherme A, Holik JJ, Virbasius JV, Chawla A, Czech MP. Signaling by phosphoinositide-3,4,5-trisphosphate through proteins containing pleckstrin and Sec7 homology domains. *Science* 1997;275:1927–1930.

90. Lemmon MA, Falasca M, Ferguson KM, Schlessinger J. Regulatory recruitment of signalling molecules to the cell membrane by pleckstrin-homology domains. *Trends Cell Biol* 1997;7:237–242.

91. Toker A, Cantley LC. Signalling through the lipid products of phosphoinositide-3-OH kinase. *Nature* 1997;387:673–676.

92. Tapon N, Hall A. Rho, rac and cdc42 GTPases regulate the organization of the actin cytoskeleton. *Curr Opin Cell Biol* 1997;9:86–92.

93. Honeycutt PJ, Niedel JE. Cytochalasin B enhancement of the diacylglycerol response in formyl peptide-stimulated neutrophils. *J Biol Chem* 1986;261:15900–15905.

94. Truett AP III, Verghese MW, Dillon SB, Snyderman R. Calcium influx stimulates a second pathway for sustained diacylglycerol production in leukocytes activated by chemoattractants. *Proc Natl Acad Sci USA* 1988;85:1549–1553.

95. Uhing RJ, Prpic V, Hollenbach PW, Adams DO. Involvement of protein kinase C in platelet-activating factor-stimulated diacylglycerol accumulation in murine peritoneal macrophages. *J Biol Chem* 1989;264:9224–9230.

96. Exton JH. Phosphatidylcholine breakdown and signal transduction. *Biochim Biophys Acta* 1994;1212:26–42.

97. Olson SC, Lambeth JD. Biochemistry and cell biology of phospholipase D in human neutrophils. *Chem Phys Lipids* 1996;80:3–19.

98. Kanaho Y, Kanoh H, Saitoh K, Nozawa Y. Phospholipase D activation by platelet-activating factor, leukotriene B₄ and formyl-methionyl-leucyl-phenylalanine in rabbit neutrophils. Phospholipase D activation is involved in enzyme release. *J Immunol* 1991;146:3536–3541.

99. Exton JH. New developments in phospholipase D. *J Biol Chem* 1997;272:15579–15582.

100. Hammond SM, Altshuller YM, Sung TC, et al. Human ADP-ribosylation factor-activated phosphatidylcholine-specific phospholipase D defines a new and highly conserved gene family. *J Biol Chem* 1995;270:29640–29643.

101. Hammond SM, Jenco JM, Nakashima S, et al. Characterization of two alternatively spliced forms of phospholipase D1: activation of the purified enzymes by phosphatidylinositol 4,5-bisphosphate, ADP-

ribosylation factor, and rho family monomeric GTP-binding proteins and protein kinase C-α. *J Biol Chem* 1997;272:3860–3868.

102. English D. Phosphatidic acid: a lipid messenger involved in intracellular and extracellular signalling. *Cell Signal* 1996;8:341–347.

103. Morris AJ, Engebrecht J, Frohman MA. Structure and regulation of phospholipase D. *Trends Pharmacol Sci* 1996;17:182–185.

104. Bonser RW, Thompson NT, Randall RW, Garland LG. Phospholipase D activation is functionally linked to superoxide generation in the human neutrophil. *Biochem J* 1989;264:617–620.

105. Pike MC, Jakoi L, McPhail LC, Snyderman R. Chemoattractant-mediated stimulation of the respiratory burst in human polymorphonuclear leukocytes may require appearance of protein kinase activity in the cells' particulate fraction. *Blood* 1986;67:909–913.

106. Dekker LV, Parker PJ. Protein kinase C: a question of specificity. *Trends Biochem Sci* 1994;19:73–77.

107. Dang PM-C, Rais S, Hakim J, Perianin A. Redistribution of protein kinase C isoforms in human neutrophils stimulated by formyl peptides and phorbol myristate acetate. *Biochem Biophys Res Commun* 1995; 212:664–672.

108. Kent JD, Sergeant S, Burns DJ, McPhail LC. Identification and regulation of protein kinase C-δ in human neutrophils. *J Immunol* 1996; 157:4641–4647.

109. Tsao L-T, Wang J-P. Translocation of protein kinase C isoforms in rat neutrophils. *Biochem Biophys Res Commun* 1997;234:412–418.

110. Krump E, Pouliot M, Naccache PH, Borgeat P. Leukotriene synthesis in calcium-depleted human neutrophils: arachidonic acid release correlates with calcium influx. *Biochem J* 1995;310:681–688.

111. Leslie CC. Properties and regulation of cytosolic phospholipase A_2. *J Biol Chem* 1997;272:16709–16712.

112. Krause K-H, Pittet D, Volpe P, Pozzan T, Meldolesi J, Lew DP. Calciosome, a sarcoplasmic reticulum-like organelle involved in intracellular $[Ca^{2+}]$ handling by non-muscle cells: studies in human neutrophils and HL-60 cells. *Cell Calcium* 1989;10:351–361.

113. Ferris CD, Snyder SH. Inositol 1,4,5-trisphosphate-activated calcium channels. *Annu Rev Physiol* 1992;54:469–488.

114. Demaurex N, Monod A, Lew DP, Krause K-H. Characterization of receptor-mediated and store-regulated Ca^{2+} influx in human neutrophils. *Biochem J* 1994;297:595–601.

115. Lew PD, Wollheim CB, Waldvogel FA, Pozzan T. Modulation of cytosolic free calcium transients by changes in intracellular calcium-buffering capacity: correlation with exocytosis and O_2^- production in human neutrophils. *J Cell Biol* 1984;99:1212–1220.

116. Lew PD, Monod A, Waldvogel FA, Dewald B, Baggiolini M, Pozzan T. Quantitative analysis of the cytosolic free calcium dependency of exocytosis from three subcellular compartments in intact neutrophils. *J Cell Biol* 1986;102:2197–2204.

117. Foyouzi-Youssefi R, Petersson F, Lew DP, Krause K-H, Nusse O. Chemoattractant-induced respiratory burst: increases in cytosolic Ca^{2+} concentrations are essential and synergize with a kinetically distinct second signal. *Biochem J* 1997;322:709–718.

118. Elferink JGR, Deierkauf M. The effect of quin2 on chemotaxis by polymorphonuclear leukocytes. *Biochim Biophys Acta* 1985;846: 364–369.

119. Zaffran Y, Lepidi H, Bongrand P, Mege JL, Capo C. F-actin content and spatial distribution in resting and chemoattractant-stimulated human polymorphonuclear leukocytes: which role for intracellular free calcium? *J Cell Sci* 1993;105:675–684.

120. Bourne HR, Sanders DA, McCormick F. The GTPase superfamily: conserved structure and molecular mechanism. *Nature* 1991;349: 117–127.

121. Bockoch GM, Der CJ. Emerging concepts in the Ras superfamily of GTP-binding proteins. *FASEB J* 1993;7:750–759.

122. Diekmann D, Abo A, Johnston C, Segal AW, Hall A. Interaction of rac with p67phox and regulation of phagocytic NADPH oxidase activity. *Science* 1994;265:531–532.

123. Prigmore E, Ahmed S, Best A, et al. A 68-kDa kinase and NADPH oxidase component p67 are targets for cdc42Hs and rac1 in neutrophils. *J Biol Chem* 1995;270:10717–10722.

124. Dorseuil O, Reibel L, Bokoch GM, Camonis J, Gacon G. The rac target NADPH oxidase p67phox interacts preferentially with rac 2 rather than rac 1. *J Biol Chem* 1996;271:83–88.

125. Michiels F, Habets GGM, Stam JC, van der Kammen R, Collard J. A role for rac in Tiam-1–induced membrane ruffling and invasion. *Nature* 1995;375:338–340.

126. Park J-W, Hoyal CR, El Benna J, Babior BM. Kinase-dependent activation of the leukocyte NADPH oxidase in a cell free system. Phosphorylation of membranes and p47phox during oxidase activation. *J Biol Chem* 1997;11035–11043.

127. Quilliam LA, Lacal JC, Bokoch GM. Identification of rho as a substrate for botulinum toxin C3-catalyzed ADP-ribosylation. *FEBS Lett* 1989;247:221–226.

128. Stasia M, Jouan A, Bourmeyster N, Boquet P, Vignais PV. ADP-ribosylation of a small size GTP-binding protein in bovine neutrophils by the C3 exoenzyme of Clostridium botulinum and effect on the cell motility. *Biochem Biophys Res Commun* 1991;180:615–622.

129. Laudanna C, Campbell JJ, Butcher EC. Role of rho in chemoattractant-activated leukocyte adhesion through integrins. *Science* 1996; 271:981–983.

130. Leung T, Manser E, Tan L, Lim L. A novel serine/threonine kinase binding the ras-related rhoA GTPase which translocates the kinase to peripheral membranes. *J Biol Chem* 1995;270:29051–29054.

131. Matsui T, Amano M, Yamamoto T, et al. Rho-associated kinase, a novel serine/threonine kinase, as a putative target for the small GTP binding protein rho. *EMBO J* 1996;15:2208–2216.

132. Kureishi Y, Kobayashi S, Amano M, et al. Rho-associated kinase directly induces smooth muscle contraction through myosin light chain phosphorylation. *J Biol Chem* 1997;272:12257–12260.

133. Watanabe G, Saito Y, Madaule P, et al. Protein kinase N (PKN) and PKN-related rhophilin as targets of small GTPase rho. *Science* 1996; 271:645–648.

134. Amano M, Mukai H, Ono Y, et al. Identification of a putative target for rho as the serine-threonine kinase protein kinase N. *Science* 1996; 271:648–650.

135. Symons M. Rho GTPases: the cytoskeleton and beyond. *Trends Biochem Sci* 1996;21:178–181.

136. Dharmawardhane S, Bokoch GM. Rho GTPases and leukocyte cytoskeletal regulation. *Curr Opin Hematol* 1997;4:12–18.

137. Didsbury JR, Weber RF, Bokoch GM, Evans T, Snyderman R. Rac, a novel ras-related family of proteins that are botulinum toxin substrates. *J Biol Chem* 1989;264:16378–16382.

138. El Benna J, Ruedi JM, Babior BM. Cytosolic guanine nucleotide-binding protein Rac 2 operates *in vivo* as a component of the neutrophil respiratory burst oxidase. Transfer of Rac 2 and the cytosolic oxidase components p47phox and p67phox to the submembranous actin cytoskeleton during oxidase activation. *J Biol Chem* 1994;269: 6729–6734.

139. Sells MA, Chernoff J. Emerging from the Pak: the p21-activated protein kinase family. *Trends Cell Biol* 1997;7:162–167.

140. Knaus UG, Morris S, Dong H, Chernoff J, Bokoch GM. Regulation of human leukocyte p21-activated kinases through G protein–coupled receptors. *Science* 1995:269:221–223.

141. Ding J, Knaus UG, Lian JP, Bokoch GM, Badwey JA. The renaturable 69- and 63-kDa protein kinases that undergo rapid activation in chemoattractant-stimulated guinea pig neutrophils are p21-activated kinases. *J Biol Chem* 1996;271:24869–24873.

142. Burbelo PD, Drechsel D, Hall A. A conserved binding motif defines numerous candidate target proteins for both cdc42 and rac GTPases. *J Biol Chem* 1995:270:29071–29074.

143. Teramoto H, Coso OA, Miyata H, Igishi T, Miki T, Gutkind JS. Signaling from the small GTP-binding proteins rac1 and cdc42 to the c-Jun N-terminal kinase/stress-activated protein kinase pathway: a role for mixed lineage kinase 3/protein-tyrosine kinase 1, a novel member of the mixed lineage kinase family. *J Biol Chem* 1996;271: 27225–27228.

144. Anthes JC, Wang P, Siegel MI, Egan RW, Billah MM. Granulocyte phospholipase D is activated by a guanine nucleotide dependent protein factor. *Biochem Biophys Res Commun* 1991;175:236–243.

145. Xie M, Dubyak GR. Guanine-nucleotide– and adenine-nucleotide–dependent regulation of phospholipase D in electropermeabilized HL-60 granulocytes. *Biochem J* 1992;278:81–89.

146. Geny B, Fensome A, Cockcroft S. Rat brain cytosol contains a factor which reconstitutes guanine-nucleotide-binding-protein-regulated phospholipase-D activation in HL60 cells previously permeabilized with streptolysin O. *Eur J Biochem* 1992;215:389–396.

147. Geny B, Cockcroft S. Synergistic activation of phospholipase D by protein kinase C- and G-protein-mediated pathways in streptolysin O-permeabilized HL60 cells. *Biochem J* 1992;284:531–538.

148. Brown HA, Gutowski S, Moomaw CR, Slaughter C, Sternweus PC.

ADP-ribosylation factor, a small GTP-dependent regulatory protein, stimulates phospholipase D activity. *Cell* 1993;75:1137–1144.

149. Cockcroft S, Thomas GMH, Fensome A, et al. Phospholipase D: a downstream effector of ARF in granulocytes. *Science* 1994;263: 523–526.

150. Bowman EP, Uhlinger DJ, Lambeth JD. Neutrophil phospholipase D is activated by a membrane-associated rho family small molecular weight GTP-binding protein. *J Biol Chem* 1993;268:21509–21512.

151. Siddiqi AR, Smith JL, Ross AH, Qui R-G, Symons M, Exton JH. Regulation of phospholipase D in HL60 cells: evidence for a cytosolic phospholipase D. *J Biol Chem* 1995;270:8466–8473.

152. Marshall CJ. Specificity of receptor tyrosine kinase signaling: transient versus sustained extracellular signal-regulated kinase activation. *Cell* 1995;80:179–185.

153. Hill CS, Treisman R. Transcriptional regulation by extracellular signals: mechanisms and specificity. *Cell* 1995;80:199–211.

154. Grinstein S, Furuya W. Chemoattractant-induced tyrosine phosphorylation and activation of microtubule-associated protein kinase in human neutrophils. *J Biol Chem* 1992;267:18122–18125.

155. Worthen GS, Avdi N, Buhl AM, Suzuki N, Johnson GL. FMLP activates Ras and Raf in human neutrophils. *J Clin Invest* 1994;94: 815–823.

156. Buhl AM, Avdi N, Worthen GS, Johnson GL. Mapping of the C5a receptor signal transduction network in human neutrophils. *Proc Natl Acad Sci USA* 1994;91:9190–9194.

157. Honda Z, Takano T, Gotoh Y, Nishida E, Ito K, Shimizu T. Transfected platelet-activating receptor activates mitogen-activated protein (MAP) kinase and MAP kinase in Chinese hamster ovary cells. *J Biol Chem* 1994;269:2307–2315.

158. Nick JA, Avdi NJ, Young SK, et al. Common and distinct intracellular signaling pathways in human neutrophils utilized by platelet activating factor and FMLP. *J Clin Invest* 1997;99:975–986.

159. Grinstein S, Butler JR, Furuya W, L'Allemain G, Downey GP. Chemotactic peptides induce phosphorylation and activation of MEK-1 in human neutrophils. *J Biol Chem* 1994;269:19313–19320.

160. Avdi NJ, Winston BW, Russel M, Young SK, Johnson GL, Worthen GS. Activation of MEKK by formyl-methionyl-leucyl-phenylalanine in human neutrophils: mapping pathways for mitogen-activated protein kinase activation. *J Biol Chem* 1996;271:33598–33606.

161. Ptasznik A, Traynor-Kaplan A, Bokoch GM. G protein-coupled chemoattractant receptors regulate Lyn tyrosine kinase-Shc adapter protein signaling complexes. *J Biol Chem* 1995;270:19969–19973.

162. van Biesen T, Luttrell LM, Hawes BE, Lefkowitz RJ. Mitogenic signaling via G protein-coupled receptors. *Endocr Rev* 1996;17: 698–714.

163. Shaw G. The pleckstrin homology domain: an intriguing multifunctional protein module. *Bioessays* 1996;18:35–46.

164. El Benna J, Han J, Park JW, Schmid E, Ulevitch RJ, Babior BM. Activation of p38 in stimulated human neutrophils: phosphorylation of the oxidase component p47phox by p38 and ERK but not by JNK. *Arch Biochem Biophys* 1996;334:395–400.

165. Krump E, Sanghera JS, Pelech SL, Furuya W, Grinstein S. Chemotactic peptide *N*-formyl-Met-Leu-Phe activation of p38 mitogen-activated protein kinase (MAPK) and MAPK-activated protein kinase-2 in human neutrophils. *J Biol Chem* 1997;272:937–944.

166. Coso OA, Chiariello M, Yu J-C, et al. The small GTP-binding proteins rac1 and cdc42 regulate the activity of the JNK/SAPK signaling pathway. *Cell* 1995;81:1137–1146.

167. Minden A, Lin A, Claret F-X, Abo A, Karin M. Selective activation of the JNK signaling cascade and c-Jun transcriptional activity by the small GTPases rac and cdc42Hs. *Cell* 1995;81:1147–1157.

168. Zhang S, Han J, Sella MA, et al. Rho family GTPases regulate p38 mitogen-activated protein kinases through the downstream mediator Pak 1. *J Biol Chem* 1995;270:23934–23936.

169. Bagrodia S, Derijard B, Davis RJ, Cerione RA. Cdc42 and PAK-mediated signaling leads to Jun kinase and p38 mitogen-activated protein kinase activation. *J Biol Chem* 1995;270:27995–27998.

170. Wittinghofer A, Hermann C. Ras-effector interactions, the problem of specificity. *FEBS Lett* 1995;369:52–56.

171. Wittinghofer A, Nassar N. How ras-related proteins talk to their effectors. *Trends Biochem Sci* 1996;21;488–491.

172. Zheng Y, Bagrodia S, Cerione RA. Activation of phosphoinositide 3-kinase activity by CDC42Hs binding to p85. *J Biol Chem* 1994;269: 18727–18730.

173. Bokoch GM, Vlahos CJ, Wang Y, Knaus UG, Traynor-Kaplan AE. Rac GTPase interacts specifically with phosphatidylinositol 3-kinase. *Biochem J* 1996;315:775–779.

174. Bokoch GM. Chemoattractant signaling and leukocyte activation. *Blood* 1995;86:1649–1660.

175. Koepp DM, Silver PA. A GTPase controlling nuclear trafficking: running the right way or walking randomly. *Cell* 1996;87:1–4.

176. Ho Y-S, Lee WMF, Snyderman R. Chemoattractant-induced c-*fos* gene expression in human monocytes. *J Exp Med* 1987;165:1524–1538.

177. Ye RD, Pan Z, Kravchenko VV, Browning DD, Prossnitz ER. Gene transcription through activation of G-protein–coupled chemoattractant receptors. *Gene Expr* 1996;5:205–215.

178. McColl SR, Beauseigle D, Gilbert C, Naccache PH. Priming of the human neutrophil respiratory burst by granulocyte-macrophage colony-stimulating factor and tumor necrosis factor-α involves regulation at a post-cell surface receptor level: enhancement of the effect of agents which directly activate G proteins. *J Immunol* 1990;145: 3047–3053.

179. Yasui K, Becker EL, Sha'afi RI. Lipopolysaccharide and serum cause the translocation of G-protein to the membrane and prime neutrophils via CD14. *Biochem Biophys Res Commun* 1992;183:1280.

180. Durstin M, McColl SR, Gomez-Cambronero J, Naccache PH, Sha'afi RI. Up-regulation of the amount of $G_{\alpha i2}$ associated with the plasma membrane in human neutrophils stimulated by granulocyte-macrophage colony-stimulating factor. *Biochem J* 1993;292:183.

181. Klein JB, Scherzer JA, Harding G, Jacobs AA, McLeish KR. TNF-α stimulates increased plasma membrane guanine nucleotide binding protein activity in polymorphonuclear leukocytes. *J Leukoc Biol* 1995;57:500–506.

182. Nahas N, Waterman WH, Sha'afi RI. Granulocyte-macrophage colony-stimulating factor (GM-CSF) promotes phosphorylation and an increase in the activity of cytosolic phospholipase A_2 in human neutrophils. *Biochem J* 1996;313:503–508.

183. Surette ME, Palmantier R, Gosselin J, Borgeat P. Lipopolysaccharides prime whole human blood and isolated neutrophils for the increased synthesis of 5-lipoxygenase products by enhancing arachidonic acid availability-involvement of the CD14 antigen. *J Exp Med* 1993;178: 1347–1355.

184. Schatz-Munding M, Ullrich V. Priming of human polymorphonuclear leukocytes with granulocyte-macrophage colony-stimulating factor involves protein kinase C rather than enhanced calcium mobilisation. *Eur J Biochem* 1992;204:705–712.

185. Koenderman L, Yazdanbakhsh M, Roos D, Yehoeven AJ. Dual mechanisms in priming of the chemoattractant-induced respiratory burst in human granulocytes: a Ca^{2+}-dependent and a Ca^{2+}-independent route. *J Immunol* 1989;142:623–628.

186. O'Flaherty JT, Redman JF, Jacobson DP, Rossi AG. Stimulation and priming of protein kinase C translocation by a Ca^{2+} transient-independent mechanism: studies in human neutrophils challenged with platelet-activating factor and other receptor agonists. *J Biol Chem* 1990;265:21619–21623.

187. Kitchen E, Rossi AG, Condliffe AM, Haslett C, Chilvers ER. Demonstration of reversible priming of human neutrophils using platelet-activating factor. *Blood* 1996;88:4330–4337.

188. McPhail LC, Clayton CC, Snyderman R. The NADPH oxidase of human leukocytes: evidence for regulation by multiple signals. *J Biol Chem* 1984;259:5768–5775.

189. Ali H, Tomhave ED, Richardson RM, Haribabu B, Snyderman R. Thrombin primes responsiveness of selective chemoattractant receptors at a site distal to G protein activation. *J Biol Chem* 1996;271:3200–3206.

190. Richardson RM, Ali H, Tomhave ED, Haribabu B, Snyderman R. Cross-desensitization of chemoattractant receptors occurs at multiple levels: evidence for a role for inhibition of phospholipase C activity. *J Biol Chem* 1995;270:27829–27833.

191. Richardson RM, Haribabu B, Ali H, Snyderman R. Cross-desensitization among receptors for platelet activating factor and peptide chemoattractants: evidence for independent regulatory pathways. *J Biol Chem* 1996; 271:28717–28724.

192. Franci C, Gosling J, Tsou CL, Coughlin SR, Charo IF. Phosphorylation by a G protein–coupled kinase inhibits signaling and promotes internalization of the monocyte chemoattractant protein-1 receptor. Critical role of carboxyl-tail serines/threonines in receptor function. *J Immunol* 1996;157:5606–5612.

193. Richardson RM, DuBose RA, Ali H, Tomhave ED, Haribabu B, Sny-

derman R. Regulation of human interleukin-8 receptor A: identification of a phosphorylation site involved in modulating receptor functions. *Biochemistry* 1995;34:14193–14201.

194. Mueller SG, White JR, Schraw WP, Lam V, Richmond A. Ligand-induced desensitization of the human CXC chemokine receptor-2 is modulated by multiple serine residues in the carboxyl-terminal domain of the receptor. *J Biol Chem* 1997;272:8207–8214.

195. Mueller SG, Schraw WP, Richmond A. Melanoma growth stimulatory activity enhances the phosphorylation of the class II interleukin-8 receptor in non-hematopoietic cells. *J Biol Chem* 1994;269:1973–1980.

196. Premont RT, Inglese J, Lefkowitz RJ. Protein kinases that phosphorylate activated G protein-coupled receptors. *FASEB J* 1995;9:175–182.

197. Haribabu B, Snyderman R. Identification of additional members of human G-protein-coupled receptor kinase multigene family. *Proc Natl Acad Sci USA* 1993;90:9398–9402.

198. Didsbury JR, Uhing RJ, Tomhave ED, Gerard C, Gerard NP, Snyderman R. Receptor class-specific desensitization of leukocyte chemoattractant receptors. *Proc Natl Acad Sci USA* 1991;88:11564–11568.

199. Tomhave ED, Richardson RM, Didsbury JR, Menard L, Snyderman R, Ali H. Cross-desensitization of receptors for peptide chemoattractants: characterization of a new form of leukocyte regulation. *J Immunol* 1994;153:3267–3275.

200. Liu M, Simon MI. Regulation by cAMP-dependent protein kinase of a G-protein–mediated phospholipase C. *Nature* 1996;382:83–87.

Inflammation: Basic Principles and Clinical Correlates,
3rd ed., edited by John I. Gallin and Ralph Snyderman.
Lippincott Williams & Wilkins, Philadelphia © 1999.

CHAPTER 42

Signal Transduction in Lymphocytes

Gary A. Koretzky

Much has been learned about the molecular biology and biochemical events associated with lymphocyte activation. Many of the second messengers produced after engagement of numerous cell surface receptors on lymphocytes have been elucidated, but how these various signaling pathways are regulated and integrated to produce the appropriate biologic response remains largely unexplored. This chapter addresses some of what is known about signaling pathways initiated by ligation of antigen-specific and antigen-nonspecific receptors on T cells, B cells, and natural killer (NK) cells. Several examples illustrate how pathologic states may result from mutations in molecules that play critical roles in lymphocyte signal transduction.

ANTIGEN-SPECIFIC STIMULATION

Structures of the B-cell and T-cell Antigen Receptors

Because they must respond to a vast universe of potential antigens, B and T cells have evolved receptors that, through genetic recombination, are extremely diverse (see Chapters 9 and 10). The antigen-binding component of the B-cell antigen receptor (BCR) is the immunoglobulin molecule itself (1). The antigen-binding component of the T-cell antigen receptor (TCR) is similarly composed of two proteins (i.e., $\alpha\beta$ or $\gamma\delta$ heterodimer) that arise by rearranging gene segments (2). All of the information required for antigen (antigen plus major histocompatibility complex [MHC] molecule for T cells) binding resides in these clonotypically expressed receptors. However, these molecules cannot be transported to the lymphocyte cell surface in isolation. They are coexpressed with a series of dimers that are responsible for

signal transduction: Igα and Igβ for the BCR (3) and the CD3 complex for the TCR (4) (Fig. 42-1).

Igα, Igβ, and the CD3 proteins are capable of transducing signals, because each of these molecules contains at least one copy of an amino acid stretch called an immunoreceptor tyrosine-based activation motif (ITAM) (5–7). The ITAM sequence is characterized by two critical tyrosine residues spaced by a stretch of 9 to 11 amino acids. Phosphorylation of the ITAM tyrosines is a crucial step in lymphocyte activation.

Signals Delivered After Engagement of B-cell and T-cell Antigen Receptors

Engagement of the BCR and TCR results in activation of numerous second messenger cascades. The most proximal signaling event known to occur is stimulation of cytosolic protein tyrosine kinases (PTKs) of the SRC family (4,7). Among the substrates of these PTKs are the tyrosine residues within the ITAMs of the BCR and TCR (8,9). Phosphorylation of the ITAMs enables associations with other cellular proteins that contain SRC homology-2 (SH2) domains. SH2 domains are discreet, modular regions that allow proteins to bind other proteins that are phosphorylated on tyrosine residues (10). Several SH2 domain–containing proteins associate with the phosphorylated CD3 chains or with phosphorylated Igα or Igβ. Among these recruited proteins are PTKs (SYK in B cells [11] and ζ-associated protein-70 [ZAP-70] in T cells [12]). Activation of the BCR and TCR with subsequent recruitment of ZAP-70 or SYK converts cell surface receptors with no intrinsic enzymatic activity to complexes with PTK function (see Fig. 42-1).

After association of SYK with the BCR and ZAP-70 with the TCR, multiple cytosolic substrates are phosphorylated. Experiments using B and T cells have shown that activity of the PTKs is critical for downstream signaling events, because pharmacologic inhibitors of PTK

G. A. Koretzky: Department of Internal Medicine, University of Iowa College of Medicine, Iowa City, Iowa 52242.

function abrogate signals leading to cellular activation (13,14). Genetic studies using cell lines and mice made deficient in the PTKs by homologous recombination support the central role of this signaling pathway for all subsequent activation events (15–17). With this knowledge, the focus of many laboratories has turned to iden-

tification and characterization of substrates of the BCR- and TCR-stimulated PTKs to understand better the molecular and biochemical events that occur during lymphocyte activation.

Among the first of these substrates to be identified were members of the phospholipase C (PLC) γ family

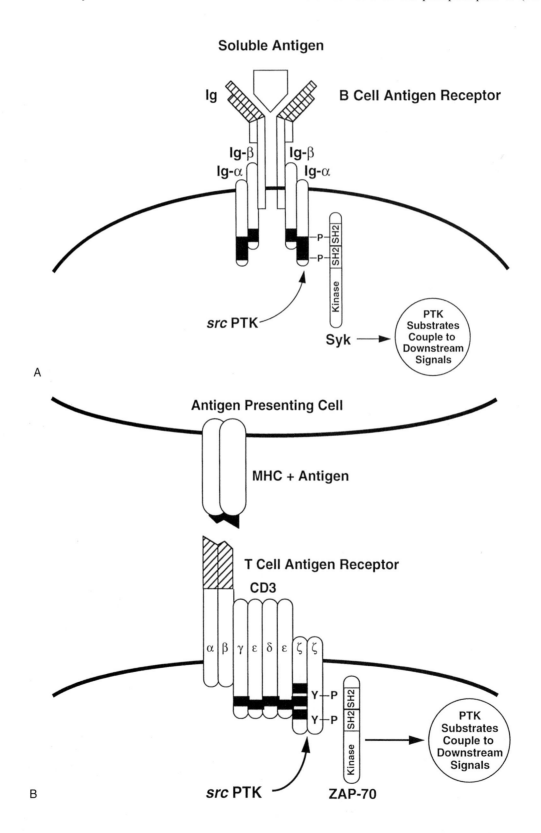

(18,19) (Fig. 42-2). These enzymes are responsible for initiating the phosphatidylinositol signaling cascade by hydrolyzing the membrane phospholipid phosphatidylinositol 4,5-bisphosphate into diacylglycerol (DAG) and inositol 1,4,5-trisphosphate (IP$_3$). DAG serves as a second messenger as an activator of some isoforms of protein kinase C (PKC) (20). IP$_3$ is a soluble sugar that interacts with specific receptors on the endoplasmic reticulum, resulting in its release of calcium (21). The importance of these signaling events for lymphocyte stimulation is supported by the observation that a combination of pharmacologic agents that activate PKC and increase cytosolic free calcium can bypass the BCR or TCR and lead to important cellular activation events. Although phosphorylation of PLC-γ is clearly critical for activation of this enzyme (22), it appears that other substrates of the antigen receptor-stimulated PTKs may also be important for the regulation of PLC-γ activity (23).

Some of the roles played by the second messengers generated by PLC-γ activity are understood. Increases in intracellular free calcium are required to activate calcineurin, a serine/threonine phosphatase (24), which is important in the regulation of transcription factors such as nuclear factor of activated T cells (NF-AT) (25). Similarly, activation of members of the PKC family probably serves important roles in transcriptional activation of new genes and in modifying other proteins important for cellular activation.

In addition to stimulation of phosphatidylinositol-derived second messengers, engagement of the BCR and TCR lead to activation of the RAS signaling pathway in a PTK-dependent fashion (26,27) (see Fig. 42-2). RAS, a small-molecular-mass guanine nucleotide–binding protein found at the plasma membrane, is bound to GDP in its inactive state and is associated with GTP when activated (28). RAS activation stimulates a series of serine/threonine kinases and kinases with serine/threonine and tyrosine specificity (28). This cascade of kinases leads ultimately to activation of transcription factors that initiate expression of other important activation genes.

Evidence suggests that, in addition to these signaling pathways, engagement of the specific antigen receptors on B and T lymphocytes leads to activation of other second messenger systems. Exactly how these signaling cascades are integrated, resulting in the appropriate distal activation events, remains unclear, but it is an area of intense research. One strategy being employed by numerous laboratories is to identify additional substrates of the antigen receptor–stimulated PTKs. This has led to the characterization of several novel molecules, some of which are expressed only in hematopoietic cells and others that are present in multiple tissues, which are thought to mediate protein-protein interactions important for linking signaling pathways (29–31).

Regulation of Proximal Signals by Protein Tyrosine Phosphatases

Protein tyrosine phosphatases (PTPs) are enzymes that remove phosphates from tyrosine residues. Two major classes of PTPs have been described: those that are restricted to the cytosol and those that traverse the plasma membrane (32). The first transmembrane PTP to be identified was CD45, a glycoprotein that is abundantly expressed on all nucleated hematopoietic cells (33). Because the most proximal consequence of engagement of the BCR and TCR is activation of several PTKs, after CD45 was identified as a PTP, it was assumed that this enzyme would serve a negative feedback role in lymphocyte activation by dephosphorylating substrates of the receptor-stimulated PTKs. It was surprising to discover that CD45 serves a critical stimulatory role in B- and T-cell activation (34–36). In one model, CD45 controls phosphorylation of a negative-regulatory tyrosine present in SRC family PTKs (37). Only after CD45 dephosphorylates these key tyrosines can receptor engagement couple with PTK activation (see Fig. 42-2).

Other PTPs function as negative regulators of lymphocyte signal transduction. Two PTPs interfere with lymphocyte activation; SHP-1 (38) and SHP-2 (39) are both

---

FIG. 42-1. (A) The B-cell antigen receptor (BCR) is composed of immunoglobulin to confer antigen specificity associated with Igα and Igβ, two proteins with signal transduction capability. The variable regions of the immunoglobulin molecule *(hatched region)* arise from rearranging gene segments and are extremely diverse; the constant regions *(open region)* are nonpolymorphic. Igα and Igβ are invariant, and each contains an immunoreceptor tyrosine-based activation motif (ITAM) *(filled region)*. Tyrosine residues within the ITAMs become phosphorylated by SRC family protein tyrosine kinases (PTK) after BCR engagement and recruit the SYK PTK through its SRC homology-2 (SH2) domains. All subsequent signaling events depend on the initial phosphorylation of the ITAMs and association with SYK. **(B)** Like the BCR, the T-cell antigen receptor (TCR) is composed of variable, antigen-binding proteins (α and β) associated with nonpolymorphic peptides (γ, δ, ϵ, and ζ) that transduce signals. Instead of binding soluble antigen, the TCR is triggered by a peptide antigen presented within the groove of major histocompatibility complex (MHC) molecules expressed on antigen-presenting cells. Engagement of the TCR leads to phosphorylation of the ITAMs by SRC family PTKs and subsequent recruitment of the ζ-associated protein-70 (ZAP-70) PTK. All subsequent signaling events depend on the initial phosphorylation of the ITAMs and association with ZAP-70.

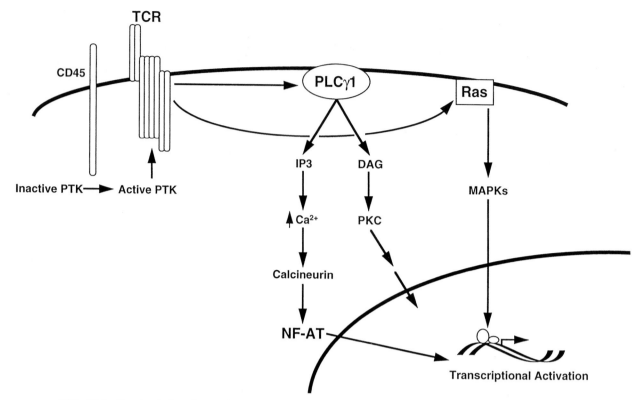

FIG. 42-2. Proximal signaling pathways stimulated by engagement of the T-cell antigen receptor (TCR). Surface expression of the CD45 tyrosine phosphatase is required for the TCR to couple with its signal transduction machinery. CD45 dephosphorylates several key protein tyrosine kinases (PTKs) on "negative-regulatory" tyrosines, enabling the PTKs to respond to TCR engagement by phosphorylating the TCR immunoreceptor tyrosine-based activation motifs (ITAMs) on tyrosine residues. ITAM phosphorylation leads to the recruitment of ζ-associated protein-70 (ZAP-70) and phosphorylation of numerous substrates, leading to other second messenger cascades such as activation of phospholipase Cγ1 (PLCγ1), which hydrolyzes a membrane phospholipid to form two second messengers, diacylglycerol (DAG) and inositol trisphosphate (IP₃). DAG is an activator of protein kinase C (PKC), which is important for stimulating transcription factors. IP₃ interacts with receptors on the endoplasmic reticulum, leading to the release of calcium into the cytosol. The increased calcium concentration is important for activation of calcineurin, a serine/threonine phosphatase that dephosphorylates the nuclear factor of activated T cells (NF-AT) and results in translocation of this transcription factor into the nucleus. PTK activation after TCR engagement also leads to activation of RAS. Active RAS stimulates a cascade of mitogen-activated protein (MAP) kinases, which are important activators of transcription factors.

cytosolic PTPs that can associate with tyrosine phosphorylated proteins through SH2 domains. The SH2 domains of these molecules are critical for their function. Work from several laboratories has provided insight into the identity of some of the physiologically relevant substrates for these enzymes (39a).

Downstream Activation Events of B and T Cells

After engagement of the BCR and TCR and subsequent stimulation of various signaling cascades, B and T cells perform several functions. Under appropriate conditions, B and T cells respond to antigenic challenge by clonal expansion, increasing the number of cells able to combat a specific pathogen. Activated B cells produce large quantities of immunoglobulin, leading to opsinization and subsequent elimination of a pathogen. T cells have direct effector function (e.g., killing cells that express the antigen that triggered the TCR) or helper function (e.g., producing various cytokines that stimulate other immune cells to act). Different helper T-cell subsets (i.e., T$_H$1 and T$_H$2 cells) produce a different spectrum of cytokines (40). Data suggest that the various patterns of cytokine production may be related to differences in proximal signals transduced by engagement of cell surface receptors and to cell subset–specific expression of unique transcription factors (41,42).

Stimulation of the specific antigen receptor is not sufficient for optimal cellular activation. For T cells, stimulation of the TCR alone results in long-lived unresponsiveness (i.e., anergy) or cellular death (i.e., apoptosis) instead of a proliferative response (43). The requirement for an "accessory signal" to prevent these outcomes has led to experiments designed to identify other cell surface receptors on lymphocytes that transduce signals important for antigen-specific responses.

Accessory Receptors That Transduce Signals

In addition to the BCR and TCR, many cell surface receptors present on B and T cells are capable of transducing signals that modulate cellular responsiveness. These "accessory" receptors are not antigen specific. Some are uniquely expressed on lymphocytes or lymphocyte subsets, and others are expressed on a wider spectrum of tissues. Engagement of some of these receptors leads to further activation events, while ligation of other accessory receptors leads to downregulation of cellular responses. Under some circumstances, the receptors modulate signals delivered by the BCR or TCR, and under other circumstances, engagement of these receptors leads to activation of new second messenger cascades.

CD28 is a homodimer expressed on most CD4$^+$ and approximately 50% of CD8$^+$ T cells (44). The natural ligands for CD28 are two molecules, B7-1 and B7-2, expressed in an inducible fashion on antigen presenting cells (45). Early studies indicated that when CD28 is engaged at the same time as the TCR, production of cytokines such as interleukin-2 is markedly augmented (46), which may result from increased cytokine gene transcription (47) and stabilization of existing cytokine mRNA (48). Even more striking was the observation that, although stimulation of cells through the TCR alone eventually leads to cell death, co-stimulation of these same cells through the TCR plus CD28 promotes cellular survival (49). Ligation of CD28 leads to overlapping, although not identical, signaling cascades stimulated by the TCR (44). Triggering both receptors leads to stimulation of cytosolic PTKs, but the particular kinases activated may differ.

In addition to the PTK pathway, CD28 is a potent activator of phosphatidylinositol 3-kinase (50), a lipid kinase that plays a key role in driving numerous downstream events (51). Work has shown that, although engagement of the TCR stimulates extracellularly regulated kinases (ERKs), members of the mitogen-activated protein (MAP) kinase family, ligation of the TCR plus CD28 results in activation of other MAP kinase family members (52). It remains unclear exactly how the different second messengers initiated by engagement of the TCR and CD28 are integrated and translated into biologic outcomes.

After activation, T cells inducibly express CTLA-4, another cell surface receptor that binds to B7-1 and B7-2 (53). CTLA-4 has a much higher affinity for its ligands than CD28 and is thought to compete effectively for binding to B7-1 and B7-2. Instead of signaling activation events, engagement of CTLA-4 stimulates signals that appear to turn off T-cell responses (54,55). Although the mechanism for this negative signaling is not fully understood, some experimental evidence has implicated the PTP SHP-2 in this process.

Nonantigen specific receptors on B cells play critical roles in cellular activation and modulation of specific antigen responses. For example, although ligation of the BCR with antigen results in activation of B cells, engagement of the same receptor with an antigen-antibody immune complex fails to result in cellular stimulation (56). Although the molecular basis for this inhibition of BCR signaling was not clear, it was appreciated that cross-linking FcγRIIB, a cell surface receptor that binds the constant region of IgG, with the BCR downregulates signals initiated by BCR binding (57). At least one mechanism by which FcγRIIB interferes with B-cell activation has been elucidated. When the BCR and FcγRIIB are co-ligated, the PTKs initiated by BCR engagement phosphorylate key tyrosines within the cytoplasmic tail of FcγRIIB (58). These tyrosines are found within an immunoreceptor tyrosine-based inhibitory motif (ITIM) sequence that is similar to the ITAM described previously (59). Phosphorylation of the tyrosine residues within the FcγRIIB ITIM allows for recruitment of SHP-1 through the SHP-1 SH2 domain (60). SHP-1 can then dephosphorylate the ITAMs of the BCR-associated molecules Igα and Igβ. Once dephosphorylated, these components of the BCR release the associated PTKs, terminating responses.

Numerous other cell surface receptors expressed on B and T cells modulate signaling by means of either the BCR, the TCR, or both receptors. Some of these molecules are expressed on both cell types, and others are expressed in a lineage-specific fashion. Some of these other receptors function by modulating (positively or negatively) signals delivered by the BCR or TCR, and others function by initiating unique signals of their own. A complete understanding of the process of lymphocyte activation requires full characterization of each of these receptors and how their signals are integrated to produce the appropriate downstream response.

Cytokine Receptor Signaling

One class of important antigen-nonspecific receptors expressed on B and T cells are those that respond to cytokines. Cytokines play a critical role initiating lymphocyte proliferation, producing other soluble mediators, and inducing immunoglobulin production and class switching. Work from a number of laboratories has established that cytokine receptors can be segregated into several distinct families based on common usage of signal transducing components (61). Although specificity for the cytokine is imparted by a unique chain or, in some circumstances, a combination of chains, the signals that are transduced after receptor engagement are dictated by use of associated common components. Similar to the signaling molecules associated with the BCR and TCR, the various common chains of the cytokine receptors do not have intrinsic enzymatic activity but associate with effector molecules after they are triggered by ligand binding (61).

Another similarity between signal transduction initiated by the TCR and BCR and through cytokine receptors is the importance of PTK activation. In the case of cytokine receptors, the most important PTKs that are stimulated belong to the Janus family of intracellular kinases (JAKs) (62). After ligand binding, these kinases become active and phosphorylate a series of proteins known as signal transducers and activators of transcription (STATs) (63). STAT phosphorylation results in formation of homodimers or heterodimers involving different members of this family. The STAT dimers then enter the nucleus to drive transcription of new genes connecting signals from the membrane to a downstream cellular response.

TERMINATION OF SPECIFIC IMMUNE RESPONSES

The appropriate response of the immune system to an antigenic challenge is clonal expansion of cells reactive against the inciting antigen. However, some receptors on B cells and T cells can transduce signals to downregulate activation events. After antigen has been cleared, there

must be a mechanism by which most of responding lymphocytes can be eliminated to avoid excessive accumulation of these cells. More is known about this process in T cells, but similar mechanisms probably occur in B cells.

In addition to providing signals leading to production of cytokines or activation of effector functions, stimulation of the TCR results in upregulation of CD95 (FAS), a surface receptor that binds specifically to a ligand (CD95 ligand), whose expression is also upregulated after TCR engagement (64,65) (Fig. 42-3). After binding its ligand, CD95 oligomerizes and associates with other cytosolic proteins through interactions with a motif within the CD95 cytoplasmic tail known as the "death domain" (66). The resulting protein complex includes molecules with protease activity that initiate a cascade of enzymatic events resulting in death of the cell (67), a process known as apoptosis. When T cells are co-stimulated through the TCR and other receptors (e.g., CD28), although they are protected from apoptosis, they upregulate expression of CD95 and CD95 ligand (68,69). It is not clear exactly how these cells avoid entering the death pathway, but data emerging from a number of laboratories suggest that co-

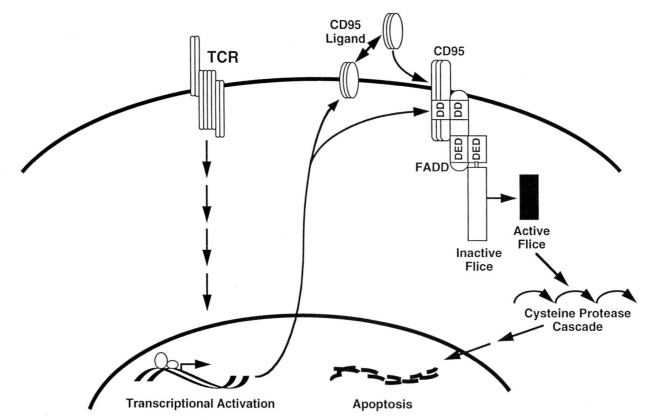

FIG. 42-3. T-cell antigen receptor (TCR) stimulation can lead to programmed cell death (i.e., apoptosis). Engagement of the TCR results in transcriptional activation of the genes encoding CD95 and CD95 ligand. In the absence of protective factors that may be induced by co-stimulating the T cell, the interaction between CD95 and its ligand leads to apoptosis. Ligation of CD95 induces its oligomerization and recruitment of FADD (FAS associated death domain containing protein) through the death domains (DD) of both molecules. The CD95/FADD complex then recruits an inactive form of FLICE, a novel FADD-homologous interleukin-1β–converting enzyme/CED-3–like protease, through the death effector domains (DEDs) of both molecules. FLICE is then activated and initiates a cascade of cysteine-directed proteases that lead eventually to death of the cell.

stimulation results in expression of protective proteins (e.g., members of the BCL2 family) that interfere with CD95-mediated initiation of apoptosis (70). The mechanism by which these proteins block programmed cell death is an area of intense investigation.

Appreciation for the role of CD95 and its ligand in stimulating apoptosis in T cells has shed light on an observation made many years ago. It was recognized that various tissues in the body are resistant to T-cell infiltration, even when infected with pathogens known to elicit T-cell responses in other tissues. These "immunologically privileged" sites constitutively express CD95 ligand (71,72). When inflammatory cells that express CD95 on their surface enter these areas, the invading cells undergo apoptosis, preventing accumulation of antigen-specific effector cells.

The interaction between CD95 and its ligand is not the only mechanism by which antigen specific lymphocytes are induced to undergo apoptosis. For example, in the developing thymus, T cells that express a TCR potentially reactive with self-antigens are eliminated by a process known as negative selection. Although this occurs also by apoptosis, experiments using mice deficient in expression of CD95 or its ligand demonstrate that negative selection occurs normally in the absence of this receptor and ligand system (73,74). Several other candidate receptors have been implicated as potentially important for apoptosis in B and T cells and in cells of other lineages.

NATURAL KILLER CELLS: NONANTIGEN-SPECIFIC LYMPHOCYTE RESPONSES

In addition to B cells and T cells, a third class of lymphocytes, NK cells, is delineated by a lack of specific antigen receptors. These cells spontaneously kill various tumor cell lines (75) (see Chapter 11). In contrast to cytolytic CD8+ T cells that only lyse targets that express specific peptide antigen within the groove of an appro-

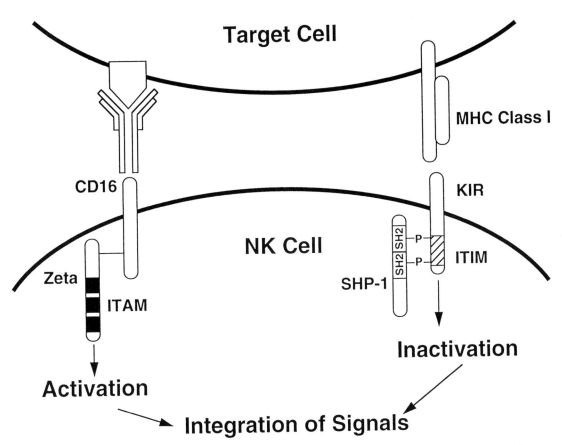

FIG. 42-4. Natural killer (NK) cells express activating and inhibitory receptors. NK cells interact with target cells that have been coated with antibody directed against surface molecules. The antibody Fc portion binds to the CD16/ζ complex on the NK cell, leading to phosphorylation of the ζ immunoreceptor tyrosine-based activation motif (ITAM) and subsequent activation signals. However, if the target cell expresses the appropriate class I major histocompatibility (MHC) molecule, a killer inhibitory receptor (KIR) on the NK cell also binds, leading to phosphorylation of its immunoreceptor tyrosine-based inhibitory motif (ITIM). The phosphorylated ITIM recruits the SHP-1 tyrosine phosphatase through its SRC homology-2 (SH2) domains, leading to dephosphorylation of key substrates and an inhibitory signal. The ultimate activation status of the NK cell depends on integration of these and other signals delivered by cell surface receptors.

priate MHC class I molecule, class I alleles of MHC molecules interfere with the ability of NK cells to lyse target cells (76). Several families of polymorphic NK cell receptors that bind to MHC class I molecules and deliver inhibitory signals have been identified. These include members of the Ly-49 family found on murine NK cells (77) and killer cell inhibitory receptors (KIR) on human cells (78). Considerable progress, based on the structures and proteins with which the cytoplasmic domains of these receptors interact, has been made in the understanding of the molecular events that occur after their engagement. Similar to FcγRIIB, which interferes with BCR-mediated signaling, Ly-49 receptors and KIRs contain ITIMs within their cytoplasmic domains (77,78). Stimulation of these receptors by engagement of particular MHC class I alleles results in phosphorylation of tyrosine residues within the ITIMs and subsequent recruitment of the PTP SHP-1 to the activated receptor. The relevant substrates of SHP-1 that lead to inhibition of NK cell function are unknown, but they probably include molecules bearing ITAMs. A greater understanding of the biology of NK cell inhibition will develop as more is learned about the Ly-49 and KIR families and other NK receptors that bind MHC class I alleles.

The ability of an NK cell to lyse a target appears to be based on a balance of activating and inhibitory signals delivered by its cell surface receptors (Fig. 42-4). Although a single, critical activating receptor has not been characterized (79), numerous candidate molecules have been identified. These include receptors for adhesion molecules and receptors for other co-stimulatory ligands that are expressed on B cells, T cells, and macrophages. Perhaps the best characterized activating receptor on NK cells is CD16, a low-affinity receptor for IgG (80). CD16 associates in NK cells with members of the TCR-ζ family (81). Ligation of CD16 induces phosphorylation of the ζ chain ITAMs and subsequent activation events similar to those seen after engagement of the TCR. Signals that are induced include PTK activation, generation of phosphatidylinositol-derived second messengers, increases in the concentration of cytosolic free calcium, and activation of phosphatidylinositol 3-kinase (82,83). It is likely, however, that to induce NK cell lytic activity, other activating receptors must also be engaged. Evidence for this has come from studies demonstrating that interfering with the interaction between the cell surface antigen CD58 present on target cells and the CD2 receptor on NK cells blocks target cell lysis (79), suggesting that, similar to T cells, co-stimulation of NK cells is required for their optimal function.

DISEASE STATES ARISING FROM MUTATIONS WITHIN SIGNALING MOLECULES

Many disorders are characterized by abnormalities in lymphocyte activation. Advances in mapping techniques

to locate disease genes coupled with improved understanding of the molecular events associated with lymphocyte activation have identified the genetic defects underlying a number of these disease states. In the following sections are examples of mutations in a cell surface receptor, a PTK, and a PTP that cause distinct immunodeficiency disorders described in human and/or murine hosts.

Immunodeficiency Associated With Mutation of the Common γ Chain Cytokine Receptor

Human X-linked severe combined immunodeficiency disease (XSCID) accounts for approximately one half of patients with primary SCID (84). This disorder, characterized by defects in humoral and cell-mediated immunity, was mapped to the q13 region of the X chromosome. Chromosomal mapping also demonstrated that the common γ chain of the receptor complexes for several critical cytokines (i.e., interleukin-2, -4, -7, -9, and -15) is found on Xq13 (85). Subsequent studies of affected individuals found nonsense, frame shift, deletion, and truncation mutations in the gene encoding the γ chain (86). Defects in the γ chain remain the most common identified causal mutations in XSCID. Some patients express no functional protein at all, but others express aberrant versions of the receptor. A mutation in a gene important for the function of multiple cytokines is consistent with the observation that XSCID patients have defects in lymphocyte development and lymphocyte function. As expected, the phenotype of patients with XSCID does not match exactly that of known patients with defects in any single cytokine that interacts with a receptor that uses the common γ chain. Although γ-chain–deficient mice have been generated (87,88), they do not share the exact phenotype of XSCID patients. Further molecular studies on the function of cytokines that bind receptors using the γ chain will provide additional insights into the pathogenesis of XSCID.

Immunodeficiency Associated with Mutation of ZAP-70

Shortly after the identification of ZAP-70 as a critical proximal mediator of TCR signaling, several patients were identified who had evidence for severe combined immunodeficiency but did not fit criteria for previously described disorders (89,90). Although these patients had normal levels of CD3+ cells, subset analysis revealed a near complete absence of CD8+ cells. The CD4+ cells failed to proliferate *in vitro* in response to engagement of the TCR, and *in vitro* studies revealed normal function of B cells and NK cells. These findings suggested that the defect in these patients was because of a molecule important for TCR-mediated signal transduction, although not for signaling through the BCR or NK cell receptors. Subsequent analysis demonstrated mutations within the gene encoding the ZAP-70 PTK resulting in production of an unstable protein that is degraded rapidly in the cell (91). The ZAP-70 abnormalities found in these patients explain why the CD4$^+$ T cells that are present fail to respond appropriately to stimulation. It remains unknown why these patients also demonstrate a skewed T-cell subset distribution. These patients have shown us that ZAP-70 probably plays a differential role in the thymic development of CD4$^+$ and CD8$^+$ cells, a finding that was not expected based on earlier studies in the laboratory. Further work investigating the role of ZAP-70 in T-cell development and function should help in understanding further the underlying mechanism of this immune disorder.

Immunodeficiency Associated with Mutation of SHP-1

Several decades ago, an inbred murine strain was developed that was characterized by the rapid onset of a fatal infiltrative pulmonary disorder. Designated *moth-eaten* because of its disheveled appearance, this strain was found to suffer from multiple immune cell abnormalities including hypergammaglobulinemia, autoantibody production, and proliferation of an unusual subset of B cells (92). Although the underlying molecular disorder that gave rise to its complex phenotype was unknown, it was clear that many cell types were involved. For example, mononuclear cells grow *in vitro* independently of growth factors that are required for maintaining such cultures from normal mice (92). Similarly, thymocytes from moth-eaten mice proliferate more robustly in culture than thymocytes from normal littermates (94). Collectively, data from numerous *in vitro* studies suggested that the moth-eaten defect led to a failure to downregulate activation events in lymphocytes and other mononuclear cells.

Insight into the molecular mechanism behind these abnormalities was provided by genetic mapping studies that placed the location of the gene encoding the PTP SHP-1 close to the site previously shown to harbor the moth-eaten mutation (95). Subsequent analysis of the mice demonstrated a single base change in the SHP-1 gene resulting in a premature stop codon eliminating its enzymatic activity (92,96). These findings corroborated other ongoing studies indicating that a major role of SHP-1 is to interfere with activation events initiated by engagement of PTK-associated cell surface receptors.

These are but three examples of many immune disorders resulting from mutations in molecules that play important roles in regulating lymphocyte function. Understanding the basic biology of lymphocyte activation has been important in our appreciation of how mutations in these molecules may lead to immune cell dysfunction. Similarly, identification and characterization of patients or murine strains with defined immunologic defects have taught us much about the biology of lymphocyte activation. Further studies investigating normal lymphocyte biology, together with studies of pathologic immune conditions, will provide important insights into the mechanism of disease and suggest novel therapeutic interventions.

REFERENCES

1. Cambier JC, Ransom JT. Molecular mechanisms of transmembrane signaling in B lymphocytes. *Annu Rev Immunol* 1987;5:175–199.
2. Clevers H, Alarcon B, Wileman T, Terhorst C. The T cell receptor/CD3 complex: a dynamic protein ensemble. *Annu Rev Immunol* 1988;6:629–662.
3. Hombach J, Tsubata T, Leciercq L, Stappert H, Reth M. Molecular components of the B-cell antigen receptor complex of the IgM class. *Nature* 1990;343:760–762.
4. Weiss A, Stobo JD. Requirement for the coexpression of T3 and the T cell antigen receptor on a malignant human T cell line. *J Exp Med* 1984;160:1284–1299.
5. Reth M. Antigen receptor tail clue. *Nature* 1989;338:383–384.
6. Weiss A. T cell antigen receptor signal transduction: a tale of tails and cytoplasmic protein-tyrosine kinases. *Cell* 1993;73:209–212.
7. DeFranco AL. Transmembrane signaling by antigen receptors of B and T lymphocytes. *Curr Opin Cell Biol* 1995;7:163–175.
8. Clark MR, Campbell KS, Kazlauskas A, et al. The B cell antigen receptor complex: association of Ig-a and Ig-b with distinct cytoplasmic effectors. *Science* 1992;258:123–126.
9. Weiss A, Littman DR. Signal transduction by lymphocyte antigen receptors. *Cell* 1994;76:263–274.
10. Pawson T. Protein modules and signalling networks. *Nature* 1995;373:573–580.
11. Bolen JB. Protein tyrosine kinases in the initiation of antigen receptor signaling. *Curr Opin Immunol* 1995;7:306–311.
12. Isakov N, Wange RL, Burgess WH, Watts JD, Aebersold R, Samelson LE. ZAP-70 binding specificity to T cell receptor tyrosine-based activation motifs: the tandem SH2 domain of ZAP-70 bind tyrosine based activation motifs with varying affinity. *J Exp Med* 1995;181:375–380.
13. Lane PJ, Ledbetter JA, McConnell FM, et al. The role of tyrosine phosphorylation in signal transduction through surface Ig in human B cells. *J Immunol* 1991;146:715–722.
14. June CH, Fletcher MC, Ledbetter JA, et al. Inhibition of tyrosine phosphorylation prevents T cell receptor-mediated signal transduction. *Proc Natl Acad Sci USA* 1990;87:7722–7726.
15. Cheng AM, Rowley B, Pao W, Hayday A, Bolen JB, Pawson T. Syk tyrosine kinase required for mouse viability and B-cell development. *Nature* 1995;378:303–306.
16. Straus DB, Weiss A. Genetic evidence for the involvement of the lck tyrosine kinase in signal transduction through the T cell antigen receptor. *Cell* 1992;70:585–593.
17. Levin SD, Anderson SJ, Forbush KA, Perlmutter RM. A dominant-negative transgene defines a role for p56^{lck} in thymopoiesis. *EMBO J* 1993;12:1671–1680.
18. Carter RH, Park DJ, Rhee SG, Fearon DT. Tyrosine phosphorylation of phospholipase C induced by membrane immunoglobulin in B lymphocytes. *Proc Natl Acad Sci USA* 1991;88:2745–2749.
19. Secrist JP, Karnitz L, Abraham RT. T-cell antigen receptor ligation induces tyrosine phosphorylation of phospholipase C-γl. *J Biol Chem* 1991;266:12135–12139.
20. Spiegel S, Foster D, Kolesnick R. Signal transduction through lipid second messengers. *Curr Opin Cell Biol* 1996;8:159–167.
21. Berridge MJ, Irvine RF. Inositol phosphates and cell signalling. *Nature* 1989;341:197–205.
22. Wahl MI, Daniel TO, Carpenter G. Antiphosphotyrosine recovery of phospholipase C activity after EGF treatment of A-431 cells. *Science* 1988;241:968–970.
23. Motto D, Musci M, Ross SE, Koretzky GA. Tyrosine phosphorylation of Grb2-associated proteins correlates with phospholipase Cγl activation in T cells. *Mol Cell Biol* 1996;16:2823–2829.
24. Schreiber SL, Crabtree GR. The mechanism of action of cyclosporin A and FK506. *Immunol Today* 1992;13:136–142.

25. Rao A. NF-Atp: a transcription factor required for the co-ordinate induction of several cytokine genes. *Immunol Today* 1994;15:274–281.

26. Tordai A, Franklin RA, Patel H, Gardner AM, Johnson GL, Gelfand EW. Cross-linking of surface IgM stimulates the Ras/Raf-1/MEK/MAPK cascade in human B lymphocytes. *J Biol Chem* 1994;269:7538–7543.

27. Woodrow M, Clipstone NA, Cantrell D. P21ras and calcineurin synergize to regulate the nuclear factor of activated T cells. *J Exp Med* 1993;178:1517–1522.

28. Downward J. Control of ras activation. *Cancer Surv* 1996;27:87–100.

29. Nel AE, Gupta S, Lee L, Ledbetter JA, Kanner SB. Ligation of the T-cell antigen receptor (TCR) induces association of Sos1, ZAP-70, phospholipase C-γ1, and other phosphoproteins with Grb2 and the zeta-chain of the TCR. *J Biol Chem* 1995;270:18428–18436.

30. Donovan JA, Wange RL, Langdon WY, Samelson LE. The protein product of the c-cbl protooncogene is the 120-kDa tyrosine-phosphorylated protein in Jurkat cells activated via the T cell antigen receptor. *J Biol Chem* 1994;269:22921–22924.

31. Jackman JK, Motto DG, Sun Q, et al. Molecular cloning of SLP-76, a 76 kDa tyrosine phosphoprotein associated with Grb2 in T cells. *J Biol Chem* 1995;270:7029–7032.

32. Dixon JE. Structure and catalytic properties of protein tyrosine phosphatases. *Ann N Y Acad Sci* 1995;766:18–22.

33. Koretzky GA. Role of the CD45 tyrosine phosphatase in signal transduction in the immune system. *FASEB J* 1993;7:420.

34. Pingel JT, Thomas ML. Evidence that the leukocyte-common antigen is required for antigen-induced T lymphocyte proliferation. *Cell* 1989;58:1055–1065.

35. Koretzky GA, Picus J, Thomas ML, Weiss A. Tyrosine phosphatase CD45 is essential for coupling T cell antigen receptor to the phosphatidylinositol pathway. *Nature* 1990;346:66–68.

36. Justement LB, Campbell KS, Chien NC, Cambier JC. Regulation of B cell antigen receptor signal transduction and phosphorylation by CD45. *Science* 1991;252:1839–1842.

37. Hurley TR, Hyman R, Sefton BM. Differential effects of expression of the CD45 tyrosine protein phosphatase on the tyrosine phosphorylation of the lck, fyn, and c-src tyrosine protein kinases. *Mol Cell Biol* 1993;13:1651–1656.

38. Plutzky J, Neel BG, Rosenberg RD. Isolation of a src homology 2–containing tyrosine phosphatase. *Proc Natl Acad Sci USA* 1992;89:1123.

39. Vogel W, Lammers R, Huang J, Ullrich A. Activation of a phosphotyrosine phosphatase by tyrosine phosphorylation. *Science* 1993;259:1611.

39a. Pani G, Siminovitch KA. Protein tyrosine phosphatase roles in the regulation of lymphocyte signaling. *Clinical Immunology & Immunopathology* 1997;84(1):1–16.

40. Mossmann TR, Sad S. The expanding universe of T-cell subsets: Th1, Th2 and more. *Immunol Today* 1996;17:138–146.

41. Ranger AM, Das MP, Kuchroo VK, Glimcher LH. B7-2 (CD86) is essential for the development of IL-4–producing T cells. *Int Immunol* 1996;8:1549–1560.

42. Hodge MR, Chun HJ, Rengarajan J, Alt A, Lieberson R, Glimcher LH. NF-AT-driven interleukin-4 transcription potentiated by NIP45. *Science* 1996;274:1903–1905.

43. Abbas AK. Die and let live: eliminating dangerous lymphocytes. *Cell* 1996;84:655–657.

44. Rudd, CE. Upstream-downstream: CD28 cosignaling pathways and T cell function. *Immunity* 1996;4:527–534.

45. Truneh A, Reddy M, Ryan P, et al. Differential recognition by CD28 of its cognate counter receptors CD80 (B7.1) and B70 (B7.2): analysis by site directed mutagenesis. *Mol Immunol* 1996;33:321–334.

46. Bjorndahl JM, Sung SS, Hansen JA, Fu SM. Human T cell activation: differential response to anti-CD28 as compared to anti-CD3 monoclonal antibodies. *Eur J Immunol* 1989;19:881–887.

47. Fraser JD, Irving BA, Crabtree G, Weiss A. Regulation of interleukin-2 gene enhancer activity by the T cell accessory molecule CD28. *Science* 1991;251:313–316.

48. Lindsten T, June CH, Ledbetter JA, Stella G, Thompson CB. Regulation of lymphokine messenger RNA stability by a surface-mediated T cell activation pathway. *Science* 1989;244:339–342.

49. Boise LH, Noel PJ, Thompson CB. CD28 and apoptosis. *Curr Opin Immunol* 1995;7:620–625.

50. Cai YC, Cefai D, Schneider H, Raab M, Nabavi N, Rudd CE. Selective CD28pYMNM mutations implicate phosphatidylinositol 3-kinase in CD86-CD28–mediated costimulation. *Immunity* 1995;3:417–426.

51. Fry MJ, Waterfield MD. Structure and function of phosphatidylinositol 3-kinase: a potential second messenger system involved in growth control. *Philos Trans R Soc Lond B Biol Sci* 1993;340:337–344.

52. Su B, Jacinto E, Hibi M, Kallunki T, Karin M, Ben-Neriah Y. JNK is involved in signal integration during costimulation of T lymphocytes. *Cell* 1994;77:727–736.

53. Linsley PS, Ledbetter JA. The role of the CD28 receptor during T cell responses to antigen. *Annu Rev Immunol* 1993;11:191–212.

54. Chambers CA, Allison JP. The role of tyrosine phosphorylation and PTP-1C in CTLA-4 signal transduction. *Eur J Immunol* 1996;26:3224–3229.

55. Marengere LE, Waterhouse P, Duncan GS, Mittrucker HW, Feng GS. Regulation of T cell receptor signaling by tyrosine phosphatase SYP association with CTLA-4. *Science* 1996;272:1170–1173.

56. Chan PL, Sinclair NR. Regulation of the immune response. V. An analysis of the function of the Fc portion of antibody in suppression of an immune response with respect to interaction with components of the lymphoid system. *Immunology* 1971;21:967–981.

57. Unkeless JC. Human Fc-γ receptors. *Curr Opin Immunol* 1989;2:63–67.

58. Muta T, Kurosaki T, Misulovin Z, Sanchez M, Nussenzweig MC, Ravetch JV. A 13-amino-acid motif in the cytoplasmic domain of FcγRIIB modulates B-cell receptor signalling. *Nature* 1994;369:340.

59. Daeron M, Latour S, Malbec O, et al. The same tyrosine-based inhibition motif, in the intracytoplasmic domain of FcγRIIB, regulates negatively BCR-, TCR-, and FcR-dependent cell activation. *Immunity* 1995;3:635–646.

60. D'Ambrosio D, Hippen KL, Minskoff SA, et al. Recruitment and activation of PTP1C in negative regulation of antigen receptor signaling by FcγRIIB1. *Science* 1995;268:293–255.

61. Taniguchi T. Cytokine signaling through nonreceptor protein tyrosine kinases. *Science* 1995;268:251–255.

62. Ihle JN. Janus kinases in cytokine signalling. *Philos Trans R Soc Lond B Biol Sci* 1996;351:159–166.

63. Darnell JE Jr, Kerr IM, Stark GR. Jak-STAT pathways and transcriptional activation in response to IFNs and other extracellular signaling proteins. *Science* 1994;264:1415–1421.

64. Brunner T, Mogil RJ, LaFace D, et al. Cell-autonomous Fas (CD95)/Fas-ligand interaction mediates activation-induced apoptosis in T-cell hybridomas. *Nature* 1995;373:441–444.

65. Alderson MR, Tough TW, Davis-Smith T, et al. Fas ligand mediates activation-induced cell death in human T lymphocytes. *J Exp Med* 1995;181:71–77.

66. Nagata S, Golstein P. The Fas death factor. *Science* 1995;267:1449–1456.

67. Muzio M, Chinnaiyan AM, Kischkel FC, et al. FLICE, a novel FADD-homologous ICE/CED-3–like protease, is recruited to the CD95 (Fas/APO-1) death-inducing signaling complex. *Cell* 1996;85:817–827.

68. van Parijs L, Ibraghimov A, Abbas AK. The roles of costimulation and fas in T cell apoptosis and peripheral tolerance. *Immunity* 1996;4:321–328.

69. Boise LH, Minn AJ, Noel PJ, et al. CD28 costimulation can promote T cell survival by enhancing the expression of Bcl-xL. *Immunity* 1995;3:87.

70. Yang E, Korsmeyer SJ. Molecular thanatopsis: a discourse on the BCL2 family and cell death. *Blood* 1996;88:386–401.

71. Bellgrau D, Gold D, Selawry H, Moore J, Franzusoff A, Duke RC. A role for CD95 ligand in preventing graft rejection. *Nature* 1995;377:630–632.

72. Griffith TS, Brunner T, Fletcher SM, Green DR, Ferguson TA. Fas ligand-induced apoptosis as a mechanism of immune privilege. *Science* 1995;270:1189–1192.

73. Cohen PL, Eisenberg RA. Lpr and gld: single gene models of systemic autoimmunity and lymphoproliferative disease. *Annu Rev Immunol* 1991;9:243–269.

74. Adachi M, Suematsu S, Suda T, et al. Enhanced and accelerated lymphoproliferation in Fas-null mice. *Proc Natl Acad Sci USA* 1996;93:2131–2136.

75. Kiessling R, Klein E, Wigzell H. "Natural" killer cells in the mouse.

I. Cytotoxic cells with specificity for mouse Moloney leukemia cell: specificity and distribution according to genotype. *Eur J Immunol* 1975;5:112–117.

76. Storkus WJ, Alexander J, Payne JA, Dawson JR, Cresswell P. Reversal of natural killing susceptibility in target cells expressing transfected class I genes. *Proc Natl Acad Sci USA* 1988;86:2361–2364.

77. Takei F, Brennan J, Mager DL. The Ly-49 family: genes, proteins, and recognition of class I MHC. *Immunol Rev* 1997;155:67–78.

78. Long EO, Burshtyn DN, Clark WP, et al. Killer cell inhibitory receptors: diversity, specificity, and function. *Immunol Rev* 1997;155:135–144.

78. Wagtmann N, Biassoni R, Cantoni C, et al. Molecular clones of the p58 NK cell receptor reveal immunoglobulin-related molecules with diversity in both the extra- and intracellular domains. *Immunity* 1995;2:439–449.

79. Lanier L, Corliss B, Phillips JH. Arousal and inhibition of human NK cells. *Immunol Rev* 1997;155:145–154.

80. Trinchieri G, Valiante N. Receptor for the Fc fragment of IgG on natural killer cells. *Nat Immun* 1993;12:218–234.

81. Anderson P, Caliguiri M, O'Brien C, Manley T, Ritz J, Schlossman SF. Fcγ receptor type III (Cd16) is included in the zeta NK receptor complex expressed by human natural killer cells. *Proc Natl Acad Sci USA* 1990;87:2274–2278.

82. Galandrini R, Palmieri G, Piccoli M, Frati L, Santoni A. CD16-mediated p21 ras activation is associated with Shc and p36 tyrosine phosphorylation and their binding with Grb2 in human natural killer cells. *J Exp Med* 1996;183:179–186.

83. Kanakaraj P, Duckworth B, Azzoni L, Kamoun M, Cantley LC, Perussia B. Phosphatidylinositol 3-kinase activation induced upon FcγRIIIA interaction. *J Exp Med* 1994;179:551–558.

84. Sagamura K, Asao H, Kondo M, et al. The interleukin-2 receptor γ chain: its role in the multiple cytokine receptor complexes and T cell development in XSCID. *Annu Rev Immunol* 1996;14:179–205.

85. Ishida N, Kanamorisd H, Noma T, et al. Molecular cloning and structure of the human interleukin 2 receptor gene. *Nucleic Acids Res* 1985;13:7579–7589.

86. Sugamura K, Asao H, Kondo M, et al. The common γ-chain for multiple cytokine receptors. *Adv Immunol* 1995;59:225–277.

87. DiSanto JP, Muller W, Guy-Grand D, Fischer A, Rajewsky K. Lymphoid development in mice with a targeted deletion of the interleukin 2 receptor γ chain. *Proc Natl Acad Sci USA* 1995;92:377–381.

88. Peschon JJ, Morrissey PJ, Grabstein KH, et al. Early lymphocyte expansion is severely impaired in interleukin 7 receptor-deficient mice. *J Exp Med* 1994;180:1955–1960.

89. Elder MD, Lin D, Clever J, et al. Human severe combined immunodeficiency due to a defect in ZAP-70, a T cell tyrosine kinase. *Science* 1994;264:1596–1599.

90. Arpaia E, Shahar M, Dadi H, Cohen A, Roifman CM. Defective T cell receptor signaling and CD8+ thymic selection in humans lacking Zap-70 kinase. *Cell* 1994;76:947–958.

91. Elder ME. Severe combined immunodeficiency due to a defect in the tyrosine kinase ZAP-70. *Pediatr Res* 1996;39:743–748.

92. Shultz LD, Schweitzer PA, Rajan TV, et al. Mutations at the murine motheaten locus are within the hematopoietic cell protein-tyrosine phosphatase (HCPh) gene. *Cell* 1993;73:1445–1454.

93. Shultz LD. Hematopoiesis and models of immunodeficiency. *Semin Immunol* 1991;3:397–408.

94. Lorenz U, Ravichandran KS, Burakoff SJ, Neel BG. Lack of SHPT1 results in src-family kinase hyperactivation and thymocyte hyperresponsiveness. *Proc Natl Acad Sci USA* 1996;93:9624–9629.

95. Yi T, Cleveland JL, Ihle JN. Protein tyrosine phosphatase containing SH2 domains: characterization, preferential expression in hematopoietic cells, and localization to human chromosome 12p12-p13. *Mol Cell Biol* 1992;12:836–846.

96. Kozlowski M, Mlinaric-Rascan I, Feng G-S, Shen R, Pawson T, Siminovitch KA. Expression and catalytic activity of the tyrosine phosphatase PTP1C is severely impaired in motheaten and viable motheaten mice. *J Exp Med* 1993;178:2157–2163.

Inflammation: Basic Principles and Clinical Correlates,
3rd ed., edited by John I. Gallin and Ralph Snyderman.
Lippincott Williams & Wilkins, Philadelphia © 1999.

CHAPTER **43**

Ion Channels and Carriers in Leukocytes:

Distribution and Functional Roles

Thomas E. DeCoursey and Sergio Grinstein

Leukocytes receive and respond to a variety of stimuli as part of their role in host defenses and immune function. As in other cells, information processing and signal transduction in leukocytes involves ion transport. The phospholipid bilayer membrane surrounding every cell constitutes a tight barrier against the permeation of ions. Ion channels and carriers are mechanisms that allow cells to regulate the entry or exit of ions across the membrane. This chapter reviews ion channels and carriers in leukocytes, and more detailed reviews of specific topics are mentioned.

ION CHANNELS

Ion channels were discovered in nerve and muscle and are best known for their role in the excitability of these tissues. Hodgkin and Huxley (1) showed that ion channels are responsible for the action potential, or nerve impulse. Ion channels also underlie synaptic transmission and initiate muscular contraction. In the past dozen years, we have learned that nonexcitable cells and most other cells have ion channels in their membranes. The ubiquity of these channels suggests widespread roles in cellular homeostasis. The ability of ion channels to respond rapidly (within milliseconds) and to change the membrane potential or intracellular ion concentrations facilitates their central roles in cellular signaling, such as in triggering secretion.

Increasing numbers of genetic diseases have been found to be caused by mutations of ion channels (e.g., Cl⁻ channels in cystic fibrosis and myotonia congenita).

Abnormal ion channel expression in autoimmune disease has been documented, but its relationship with the disease process has eluded us (2). As the functions of channels in healthy and diseased cells are elucidated, the possibilities of using ion channels as targets for therapeutic intervention expand. Their variety, rapid response, superficial cellular location, and pharmacologic sensitivity make ion channels ideally suited to extrinsic manipulation. Substantial research on ion channels as targets for modulating lymphocyte function is already underway.

What Are Ion Channels?

An ion channel is an integral membrane glycoprotein that forms a pathway by which ions can permeate the cell membrane. The original German word *Kanal* (3) means canal, channel, or conduit. Ion channels connect extracellular and intracellular solutions, usually by forming a water-filled pore spanning the cell membrane. Ion channels are usually composed of several (typically four or five) subunits or subunit-like domains, each with four to six membrane-spanning regions.

A fundamental characteristic of ion channels is that they can exist in two distinct states, open and closed. The opening and closing of channels is called gating. Without gating, the cell would have no way to regulate ionic fluxes, and channels would be pernicious holes. When a channel is open, ions rapidly pass through the pore down their electrochemical gradient; ionic current is driven by the transmembrane electrical potential and the concentration gradient. Ion channels conduct ions passively; they do not use energy (e.g., ATP), nor do they couple ion transport with the movement of other ions. Most ion channels are selectively permeable; they allow only certain ions to pass through them. For example, sodium

T. E. DeCoursey and *S. Grinstein: Department of Molecular Biophysics and Physiology, Rush Presbyterian St. Luke's Medical Center, Chicago, Illinois 60612; *Division of Cell Biology, Hospital for Sick Children at Toronto, Toronto, Ontario M5G 1X8, Canada.

channels pass Na⁺, and potassium channels pass K⁺. Usually, the selectivity is not perfect. Na⁺ channels usually conduct Li⁺ and Na⁺ but can also conduct K⁺ at about 8% as well. Most K⁺ channels are more selective, conducting K⁺ 100 times better than Na⁺. Ion selectivity results from a combination of steric and electrostatic interactions between the channel pore and permeating ions, including the ability of the channel to substitute for waters of hydration that normally surround ions in solution. Extremely high selectivity is observed for H⁺ channels, leading to speculation that permeation occurs by a distinct mechanism.

Ion channels have common names that express key features such as their selectivity (e.g., K⁺, Na⁺, H⁺, Ca²⁺, Cl⁻), their size (i.e., conductance, or the rate that ions pass through them, such as maxi-K), the things that cause them to open (e.g., Ca²⁺-activated K⁺ channels, acetylcholine receptor channels, voltage-gated channels), or their distinctive properties (e.g., inward rectifier K⁺ channels, inactivating delayed rectifier K⁺ channels). Current flow through ion channels can be blocked by drugs or ions. Sensitivity to specific blockers helps to identify ion

channels, and pharmacologic lesion experiments help to elucidate functional roles of ion channels. In the past decade, many ion channels have been cloned and sequenced, and relatively unambiguous molecular biologic terminology is often used (e.g., Kv1.3, Kv4.2, IRK1). Unfortunately, there is no consensus on this terminology; there are various degrees of nonhomology among similar channels in different tissues or species, and the process of renaming channels severs them from their historical context. Table 43-1 lists common and known genetic names of the main ion channels found in leukocytes.

Functions of Ion Channels

Membrane Potential Changes

When an ion channel is open, permeant ions pass through it down their electrochemical gradient. Ionic current has two main effects on cells, changing the ionic concentrations and membrane potential, V_m. Because ions are charged, ionic current changes the electrical potential

TABLE 43-1. *Ion channels in leukocytes and related cell lines*

Common name[a]	Genetic designation	Gating	Inhibitors[b]	Distribution: species	Distribution: cells	References
K⁺ channels						
Delayed rectifier (*n*-type)	Kv1.3	+V	ChTX, NxTX	H,M,R,G,L,X	L$_{T,B,NK}$, Mφ, μg, P	2,8,23,35,60,61, 69,72,84,113, 214–221,244
Delayed rectifier (*l*-type)	Kv3.1	+V	TEA	M,X	L$_T$ (mouse)	7–10,12,89
Delayed rectifier (*n'*-type)	?	+V	ChTX	M	L$_T$ (CD8⁺), μg	9,113
Inward rectifier	IRK1	-V, K⁺	Cs⁺, Ba²⁺	H, M, R, X	Mφ, μg, B	20,21,96,111,222, 223
Ca²⁺-activated (maxi-K)	*slo?*	+V, Ca²⁺	ChTX, TEA	H, B, X	Mφ, μg	20,97,100,224
Ca²⁺-activated (medium)	?	Ca²⁺	ChTX	H, R, M, X	L$_{T,B}$, Mφ, μg, P	25,27,28,98,114, 216,225,226
Ca²⁺-activated (small)	Kca1?	Ca²⁺	Apamin	H, R, X	L$_{T,B}$ (rare)	77,214,216
G-protein activated	?	G proteins	Nitrend, quin	M, R, X	Mφ, μg, B	29–31,227
Na⁺ channels	?	+V	TTX	H, M, X	L$_{T,B}$, μg	11,61,116,228
H⁺ channels	?	+V, pH	Zn²⁺, Cd²⁺	H, M, R, X	Mφ, μg, N, E	35–37,104,106, 132,229
Ca²⁺ channels (CRAC)	?	Ca²⁺ release	Cd²⁺, Ni²⁺	H, R, X	L$_T$, Mφ, N, B, N	42,146,151, 230–232
Cl⁻ channels						
Ca²⁺-activated	?	Ca²⁺	DIDS	H, R	Mφ, N, B, P	35,51,233–236
Stretch-activated	?	Osm	DIDS, SITS	H, M, X	L$_{T,B}$, Mφ, μg, N	28,52,53,83,237, 238
Voltage-gated	?	+V, -V	SITS, Zn²⁺	H, M, R, B, X	L$_{T,B}$, Mφ, μg, B	223,224,239–241

+V, depolarization; −V, hyperpolarization; B, basophil or mast cell; B, bovine; Ca²⁺, rise [Ca²⁺]ᵢ; ChTX, charybdotoxin; E, eosinophil; G, guinea pig; μg, microglia; H, human; L, leporine (rabbit); L$_B$, B lymphocyte; L$_{NK}$, natural killer; L$_T$, T lymphocyte; M, mouse; Mφ, macrophage; N, neutrophil; Nitrend, nitrendipine; NxTX, noxioustoxin; Osm, osmotic stress; P, platelet or megakaryocyte; quin, quinidine; R, rat; TEA, tetraethyl ammonium; TTX, tetrodotoxin; X, cell line.

[a]This table lists the most common ion channels in native leukocytes. Many channels have also been described in cell lines of leukocytic lineage; channels that have been described only in cell lines are not included. The expression of many of these channels varies dramatically with activation or differentiation.

[b]Potent, selective, or characteristic inhibitors are listed; many other inhibitors exist.

across the membrane. Ionic current always drives the V_m of a cell toward the Nernst potential for the permeating ion. The Nernst potential, or equilibrium potential, depends on the concentration of ions outside and inside the cell. The Nernst potential for K^+ is given by the following equation:

$$E_K = \frac{RT}{zF} \ln \frac{[K^+]_o}{[K^+]_i} \approx 61.5 \log_{10} \frac{[K^+]_o}{[K^+]_i} \text{ (mV at 37°C).}$$

For normal ionic conditions, E_K is roughly −90 mV, E_{Cl} is −35 mV, E_H is −20 mV, and E_{Na} and E_{Ca} are positive to 0 mV. Typical resting membrane potentials for leukocytes are not easy to measure and probably vary substantially, but they are roughly −30 to −70 mV. Opening K^+ channels therefore tends to hyperpolarize the cell membrane (i.e., make the intracellular potential more negative), whereas opening any other channel would tend to depolarize the membrane (i.e., make it more positive). The opening of Na^+ channels in excitable cells leads to the rapid transient depolarization that constitutes the action potential or nerve impulse, the fundamental response of all excitable cells (1).

Ionic current is governed by Ohm's Law, which dictates a simple, linear current-voltage relationship (e.g., doubling the voltage doubles the current). However, current through ion channels rarely obeys Ohm's Law. Violation of Ohm's Law is called rectification (like rectifiers in electronic circuits), which means more current flows in one direction than the other for the same driving voltage. Two mechanisms are responsible. First, many channels tend to open at certain V_m levels; this is voltage-dependent gating. A nearly ubiquitous group of K^+ channels were named *delayed rectifier channels* by Hodgkin, Huxley, and Katz (4), because they open with a sigmoid time course during a depolarizing pulse (i.e., delayed opening), and they conduct outward currents but not inward currents (i.e., rectification). The outward rectification of these channels is caused entirely by voltage-dependent gating, because when the channels are open, they conduct inward and outward currents about equally. When electrophysiologists speak of rectification, they usually mean that the current-voltage relationship of a single open channel is not linear. Most channels have nonlinear current-voltage relationships as a result of interactions between the permeating ion and the walls of the pore through which the ions pass. If the potential profile the ion experiences inside the pore is not symmetric, rectification occurs.

Concentration Changes

The second major effect of opening ion channels is to change the concentration of ions in the cell. This occurs most readily for ions such as Ca^{2+} or H^+, which normally are present at very low concentrations. Even very small inward Ca^{2+} currents increase the intracellular free Ca^{2+} concentration, $[Ca^{2+}]_i$, significantly above its low resting value of less than 200 nmol/L. However, although opening K^+ and Cl^- channels changes the intracellular concentrations of K^+ and Cl^-, $[K^+]_i$ and $[Cl^-]_i$, respectively, only very slowly, efflux of K^+ and Cl^- across the cell membrane can still have osmotic effects, effectively dragging water out of the cell in response to hypotonic stress-induced swelling.

Studies of Ion Channels

Ion channels are usually studied using voltage-clamp methods, in which V_m is clamped at an arbitrary command potential (i.e., voltage steps or ramps are common commands), and the resulting membrane current is observed. Studied under voltage-clamp, voltage-gated ion channels tend to open at some potentials and close at others. When several hundred ion channels in a whole-cell membrane are studied by voltage-clamp, the current typically increases with time during a depolarizing voltage pulse (+V channels in Table 43-1), as more and more channels open in a stochastic, or probabilistic, manner. If the channels inactivate, the current reaches a peak and then decreases as more channels become inactivated, after which they neither conduct nor reopen. If many channels are open and the voltage is stepped to a potential at which the channels tend to close, they do not close instantly but with a characteristic time course that depends on the channel and the potential, resulting in a tail current that decays away as the channels close. Although the voltage-clamp technique is a powerful experimental tool, the V_m of living cells is not fixed at any particular potential but fluctuates continuously as a result of electrogenic ion transport through channels and carriers.

The voltage-clamp technique of choice for studying ion channels in leukocytes is the patch-clamp technique. The widespread use of this powerful technique resulted in a Nobel Prize for its developers, Neher and Sakmann (5). The electrically tight seal that forms between the tip of a glass microelectrode and the cell membrane represented a great advance over conventional recording techniques. A small cell like phagocyte has such a small membrane area that the leak current flowing through the damaged site of a conventional microelectrode puncture may be orders of magnitude larger than the current flowing through the several dozen or few hundred ion channels in the entire cell membrane. It is possible to record from a few channels in the patch of membrane spanning the pipette tip (i.e., cell-attached patch and inside-out or outside-out excised patch configurations), or to rupture the patch and record from the whole cell membrane (whole-cell configuration). The patch-clamp technique is sensitive enough to allow measurement of current flowing through a single ion channel in real time and to detect conformational changes in this molecule as the channel opens and closes. The patch-clamp technique revolutionized the field of electrophysiology of nonexcitable cells by making these small but important cells accessible to exhaustive and detailed study.

Ion channels have been described in essentially all cells, but elucidation of their functional roles has been more difficult. This review summarizes the properties of the main ion channels in leukocytes and reviews the progress made in determining their functions.

ION CHANNELS IN LEUKOCYTES

Table 43-1 lists the main types of ion channels that have been found in leukocytes. There are many varieties of K^+ channels, and most cells have at least one type. K^+ channels appear to be a universal mechanism for maintaining a large negative V_m, which among other things acts as a battery to drive myriad cellular transport processes (e.g., Ca^{2+} influx, amino acid transport into cells). Inward rectifier and maxi-K channels are found characteristically in macrophages, type l K^+ channels are found only in lymphocytes. Microglia, specialized macrophage-like cells in the brain, express a panoply of ion channels similar to those of macrophages. The general properties of each type of channel are described, because a given channel behaves similarly in any cell. The evidence for involvement of specific ion channels in the functions of each type of leukocyte is summarized.

Voltage-Activated Potassium Channels

Voltage-gated K^+ channels are perhaps the most widely distributed ion channels. They are strongly voltage dependent; their probability of opening increases from 0 to about 1 within an approximately 20-mV range of V_m. Studied using voltage-clamp methods, delayed rectifier K^+ channels in leukocytes open rapidly on depolarization with a sigmoid time course, conduct outward K^+ current, and then slowly close into an inactivated state in which they are refractory to another stimulus.

Three types of delayed rectifier K^+ channels have been identified in leukocytes, distinguished by their gating kinetics and pharmacologic sensitivity. The most common is type n (so-called because it is found in normal lymphocytes), also called Kv1.3 (see Table 43-1). Type n K^+ channels open rapidly at potentials more positive than -50 mV (just positive to the resting potential of human T cells, -59 mV) (6), inactivate slowly but are very slow to recover from inactivation, and are blocked potently by several scorpion toxins such as charybdotoxin. Type l K^+ channels, named because of their discovery in mutant lpr (lymphoproliferation) mice, are blocked potently by tetraethylammonium (TEA^+) but not by charybdotoxin, recover rapidly from inactivation, and open at a more positive range of V_m (7–10). Although the gating of leukocyte delayed rectifier channels is influenced by the

species and concentration of permeant ions (11,12), divalent cations (13–15), and by cyclic AMP (14), their fundamental response is to V_m.

Inward Rectifier Potassium Channels

Inward rectifier (or anomalous rectifier) K^+ channels are unusual in several respects. They open preferentially during hyperpolarizing voltage pulses and are closed by depolarization. Their opening strongly depends on the extracellular K^+ concentration, such that they open at potentials near or negative to the Nernst potential for K^+, E_K. Inward rectifier channels open rapidly during hyperpolarizing voltage pulses and do not inactivate. The mechanism of the gating of inward rectifier channels has been investigated intensely. Part of the rectification results from rapid block of outward current by intracellular Mg^{2+} (16,17). The time-dependent gating mechanism does not result from Mg^{2+} block (18) and largely reflects voltage-dependent removal of the intracellular tetravalent cation spermine from the channel (19). Inward rectifier channels have no potent inhibitors but exhibit characteristic voltage-dependent block by extracellular Na^+, Cs^+, and Ba^{2+} (20,21).

The inward rectifier and delayed rectifier K^+ channels are capable of setting the resting potential of cells. Some macrophages express delayed rectifier K^+ channels or inward rectifier K^+ channels reciprocally, and they always have at least one type of K^+ channel capable of maintaining a large negative V_m (20–22).

Calcium-Activated Potassium Channels

Two main classes of K^+ channels are stimulated to open by increases in $[Ca^{2+}]_i$. Maxi-K channels are among the largest ion channels, with a single channel conductance of approximately 250 pS. The large conductance results in characteristically noisy whole-cell currents in small cells as single channels open and close stochastically. Maxi-K channels are voltage gated, opening with depolarization of V_m. However, elevating $[Ca^{2+}]_i$ shifts the voltage dependence of gating to more negative potentials, increasing the probability of channel opening at any given V_m. They are opened by depolarization or increases in $[Ca^{2+}]_i$ or both. Maxi-K channels do not inactivate and are blocked potently by charybdotoxin and TEA^+. Their large single-channel current amplitude and lack of inactivation make them favorites for elaborate studies of channel gating kinetics.

Other Ca^{2+}-activated K^+ channels with lower conductance are voltage independent, opening at any potential when $[Ca^{2+}]_i$ is increased. Their $[Ca^{2+}]_i$ sensitivity is quite steep, suggesting that several Ca^{2+} ions must bind to activate each channel. The channels are closed at the normal resting $[Ca^{2+}]_i$ of less than 200 nmol/L but are maximally activated at 1 μmol/L of $[Ca^{2+}]_i$ (24–27). Any intervention that increases $[Ca^{2+}]_i$ opens voltage-independent Ca^{2+}-activated K^+ channels. Subcategories of these channels (see Table 43-1) have different single-channel conductance and differential sensitivity to charybdotoxin and the bee venom apamin. These Ca^{2+}-activated K^+ channels exhibit voltage-dependent block by Cs^+ and Ba^{2+}, although at much higher concentrations than for inward rectifier channels (25,28).

G-Protein–Activated Potassium Channels

One component in the signaling pathway activated by chemoattractants involves G-protein activation. Intracellular application of G-protein activators such as GTPγS or AlF_4^- induces a non–voltage-gated, outwardly rectifying, K^+-selective conductance in macrophages (29) and mast cells (30). This conductance appears to be enhanced by local $[Ca^{2+}]_i$ elevation (31). Induction is prevented by preexposure to pertussis toxin (29,32), but the specific class of G proteins to which the channel is coupled has not been identified.

Sodium Channels

Voltage-gated Na^+ channels are best known for their involvement in initiating action potentials in excitable cells. Na^+ channels open rapidly during depolarizing pulses, and they rapidly inactivate. They are blocked selectively by tetrodotoxin from puffer fish.

Hydrogen Ion Channels

Voltage-gated H^+ channels are unique in several respects. H^+ currents are activated by depolarization of the membrane, but their threshold for activation is sensitive to internal and external pH, pH_i and pH_o, respectively. Lowering pH_i or increasing pH_o by one unit shifts the threshold by 40 mV to more negative potentials (33,34). Thus, the H^+ conductance is activated by intracellular acidification or extracellular alkalinization. Because pH_i and pH_o are equally effective, the voltage dependence is established by the pH gradient. H^+ channels open only at potentials positive to the Nernst potential, E_H, and their activation leads to acid extrusion from the cell. In phagocytes, H^+ channels open very slowly, taking several seconds or even minutes to reach a steady-state level of activation under some conditions (35–37). H^+ channels are inhibited by polyvalent metal cations, such as Cd^{2+}, Zn^{2+}, and La^{3+}.

Single H^+-channel currents are very small (35,38), only a few femtoamperes (1fA = 10^{-15} A), 1,000 times smaller than K^+ channels, but comparable with Ca^{2+} release–activated Ca^{2+} (CRAC) channels. The unitary current corresponds with efflux of several thousand H^+ per second, in the range of carriers. Several lines of evidence indicate that H^+ channels are not water-filled pores like other channels. Their selectivity is extremely high, with a relative permeability more than 10^6 higher for H^+ than for other cations, and there is no evidence that any other ion can permeate detectably (34,37,39). The rate-determining step in permeation is not diffusion of H^+ or protonated buffer to the channel but occurs in the pore itself (40). Deuterium permeates H^+ channels only about one half as well as protons, suggesting specific interaction with the pore during permeation (34). These observations suggest that protons permeate by a Grotthuss-like mechanism, hopping across a membrane-spanning hydrogen-bonded chain of side groups of amino acids (41).

Calcium Release–Activated Calcium Channels

Binding of antigens or mitogens to the T-cell antigen receptor results in a rapid rise in $[Ca^{2+}]i$. This Ca^{2+} influx is mediated by a novel Ca^{2+}-selective channel that is activated by depletion of Ca^{2+} from the endoplasmic reticulum (42,43), hence the name CRAC channels. The single-channel conductance is very small, 10 to 24 fS, consistent with carrier or channel mechanisms (43) and quite similar to H^+ channels. CRAC currents have an unusually high temperature sensitivity (44) compared with other channels. CRAC channels differ from the familiar Ca^{2+} channels of excitable cells in lacking a distinct voltage-gating mechanism, but they share the property that in the absence of Ca^{2+} they become permeable to monovalent cations (45,46). Ca^{2+} influx through CRAC channels is enhanced by membrane hyperpolarization (47), presumably because of the increased driving force. Evidence suggests that hyperpolarization may potentiate CRAC current also through a calcium-dependent mechanism (48). CRAC channel activity is controlled by a self-inhibitory feedback mechanism in which the channels are inactivated by Ca^{2+} binding to an internally accessible site (49). This feedback results in oscillations in $[Ca^{2+}]_i$ after activation of lymphocytes (42,50). CRAC channels appear to mediate Ca^{2+} signaling in many leukocytes (see Table 43-1).

Chloride Channels

A variety of Cl^--permeable channels have been reported, but most have not been characterized well enough to permit generalizations among different cells. Subtypes of Cl^- channels seem to be harder to distinguish than other channels, because they lack distinctive voltage-dependent gating. Several types of Cl^- channels are listed in Table 43-1 somewhat arbitrarily according to their mode of activation: by increased $[Ca^{2+}]_i$, osmotic stress, or V_m. However, the regulation of Cl^- channels is often complex, as in mast cells in which cAMP, inositol 1,4,5-trisphosphate (IP$_3$), elevated $[Ca^{2+}]_i$, and the nonhydrolysable GTP analog GTPγS in various combinations all stimulate the Cl^- conductance (51).

Cl⁻ channels are activated by hypotonic stress in many cells. The mechanism of activation is the actual stretching of the membrane, because hydrostatic pressure, osmotic pressure, or mechanical deformation can be sensed. These channels run down spontaneously in whole-cell experiments, becoming uninducible within a few minutes (52–54). Rundown is retarded by intracellular ATP in mouse lymphocytes and Jurkat cells (52,53) but not in human T cells (54). These mini-Cl⁻ channels (i.e., single-channel conductance of 0.6 to 2.4 pS) are weakly selective among anions (53), but they do not conduct cations. The current-voltage relation exhibits outward rectification. These channels are blocked by traditional Cl⁻ flux inhibitors DIDS (4,4′-diisothiocyanatostilbene-2,2′-disulfonic acid) and SITS (4-acetamido-4′-isothiocyanatostilbene-2,2′-disulfonic acid) (53,54) and by 2-(aminomethyl)phenols (55).

EXPRESSION AND PROPOSED FUNCTIONS OF LEUKOCYTE ION CHANNELS

Identifying the functions of ion channels in leukocytes has proven to be far more difficult than characterizing their properties. Despite the voluminous and expanding literature on the subject, there is little agreement on the functions of many of the ion channels that have been identified. Several types of evidence have been used to support proposed roles of ion channels, each of which has various pitfalls. The most direct is the pharmacologic lesion experiment, in which the functional effects of completely blocking a specific channel are evaluated. A modern version of this strategy is the gene knock-out technique, which generates transgenic animals (often mice) in which a specific gene has been mutated to be dysfunctional or nonexpressing. Indirect evidence for functions of ion channels arises when patterns of ion channel expression change in cells at various stages of differentiation or during responses to various physiologic interventions (20,56–58). These changes are quite dramatic in some cases, leading investigators to conclude that the cells alter their ion channel expression patterns for a reason. Acute effects of biologically active substances on ion channel behavior are often taken to indicate that part of the biologic activity of the substance is mediated by the observed changes in ion channel properties. The most satisfying proposed functions are those that can be explained in the context of a mechanism that lends itself to testable hypotheses.

Functions of Ion Channels in Lymphocytes

Calcium and Potassium Channels Facilitate Lymphocyte Proliferation

Interleukin-2 in Lymphocyte Proliferation

Functional delayed rectifier K⁺ channels appear to play a role during activation of human T lymphocytes (11,59–61) and B lymphocytes (62) to proliferate in response to mitogens and antigenic stimuli. The strongest evidence comes from pharmacologic lesion experiments showing that a chemically diverse group of compounds blocks K⁺ current and inhibits lymphocyte proliferation at comparable concentrations (56,58,63). All blockers of lymphocyte type n K⁺ channels inhibit lymphocyte proliferation, but certain selective and potent peptides may inhibit proliferation only partially (64–67). This result suggests that K⁺ channels perform some function that facilitates proliferation but are not in a direct signaling pathway.

K⁺ channel blockers inhibit interleukin-2 (IL-2) release without affecting the appearance of the IL-2 receptor (59), and the inhibition of proliferation can be overcome by exogenous IL-2 (65), suggesting that suppression of IL-2 release is the mechanism of the inhibition of proliferation. Blocking K⁺ channels in lymphocytes depolarizes V_m (66,68,69), and depolarization by a high extracellular K⁺ concentration, $[K^+]_o$, inhibits IL-2 release and proliferation (69–71). These results lend strong support to the idea that the main function of K⁺ channels during lymphocyte activation is to maintain a large negative V_m. Lymphocytes are small cells with electrically tight membranes, and opening a single K⁺ channel changes V_m by many millivolts (11,72). The resting potential of T lymphocytes fluctuates over a 20-mV range centered at -59 mV (6,27).

Maintaining the Resting Membrane Potential

Why is a large V_m important? An early signaling event in the response to mitogens is a rapid increase in $[Ca^{2+}]_i$ (71,73,74). This rise in $[Ca^{2+}]_i$ is required for IL-2 production (74). Ca^{2+} influx occurs through CRAC channels, and continuous monitoring reveals that $[Ca^{2+}]_i$ oscillates in parallel with CRAC channel activity (42,50). Because CRAC channels are not voltage gated, they conduct more Ca^{2+} at more negative potentials because of the increased driving force. Depolarization, by K⁺ channel blockade or by elevation of $[K^+]_o$, attenuates the Ca^{2+} signal (64,66,71,75,242) and thereby inhibits the mitogen response. Block of type n K⁺ channels by charybdotoxin does not inhibit production of mRNA for IL-2 in response to phorbol myristate acetate if the need for Ca^{2+} influx through CRAC channels is bypassed by adding a Ca^{2+} ionophore, A23187 (76). Evidence suggests that activation of voltage-independent Ca^{2+}-activated K⁺ channels by the mitogen-induced $[Ca^{2+}]_i$ rise may contribute to keeping V_m sufficiently negative to optimize the proliferative response (66,77). However, new nonpeptide compounds inhibit lymphocyte activation at concentrations that block voltage-gated but not Ca^{2+}-activated K⁺ channels (78).

The type n K⁺ channel has become a target for potential immunosuppressant drugs (63). In a dramatic demonstration of the importance of CRAC channels in lymphocyte proliferation, Partiseti et al. (79) reported that CRAC current was absent in lymphocytes from a patient with primary immunodeficiency, apparently causing defective T-cell proliferation. The type *n* K$^+$ channels, and perhaps the Ca^{2+}-activated K$^+$ channels, facilitate the proliferation of lymphocytes, most likely by maintaining a large negative V$_m$.

General Role of Potassium Channels

It is not clear how general is the requirement for K$^+$ channels during cellular proliferation. Blocking K$^+$ channels in a wide variety of cells inhibits proliferation (56,58,80). However, not all cells express type *n* K$^+$ channels or any K$^+$ channels, and the specific mechanism described earlier therefore can apply only in certain cells. Reduction of glial proliferation by nonselective K$^+$ channel blockers has been attributed to increased pH$_i$ (81). In an intriguing attempt to generalize the role of K$^+$ channels in proliferation of many cells, Dubois and Rouzaire-Dubois (56) proposed that proliferation is a consequence of K$^+$ efflux and attendant cell volume changes. The well-established involvement of K$^+$ and Cl$^-$ channels in lymphocyte volume regulation is discussed in the following section. Cl$^-$ channel blockers inhibit lymphocyte proliferation (82). That peptide blockers of delayed rectifier do not inhibit proliferation of cells lacking these channels (83) suggests that their effects in lymphocytes are caused by K$^+$ channel block.

Type n Potassium Channels in Natural Killer Cells

Natural killer cells, a subtype of lymphocytes, recognize and kill tumor cells. Several nonselective blockers of type *n* K$^+$ channels inhibit target cell lysis at concentrations comparable to those that block K$^+$ channels (84).

Type n Potassium and Chloride Ion Channels in Lymphocyte Volume Regulation

When cells are exposed to hypotonic solutions, they swell rapidly as water enters the cell, after which they more slowly regulate their volume back toward its original value. Various cells have adopted different strategies to deal with anisotonic conditions. Lymphocytes extrude water by efflux of Cl$^-$ and K$^+$ (85,86). The Cl$^-$ channel responsible for Cl$^-$ efflux is activated by hypotonic stress (52), and K$^+$ efflux is mediated by the type *n* K$^+$ channel (72,87). Membrane stretch activates the Cl$^-$ conductance, which depolarizes the membrane toward E$_{Cl}$, opening depolarization-activated delayed rectifier K$^+$ channels. The ability of type *n*, but not type *l*, K$^+$ channels to effect

volume regulation was demonstrated in elegant experiments by Deutsch and Chen (88). They showed that heterologous expression of type *n* K$^+$ channels enabled volume regulation in response to hypotonic stress in a T-lymphocytic cell line originally lacking K$^+$ channels and the ability to regulate its volume.

Type l Potassium Channels as Markers for Murine Autoimmune Disease

With the exception of a human lymphoma cell line (89), type *l* K$^+$ channels have been observed only in murine thymocytes and peripheral T lymphocytes of the cytotoxic or suppressor phenotype (52). Type *l* channels are expressed abundantly in CD4$^-$CD8$^-$ lymphocytes in several murine models of autoimmune diseases: systemic lupus erythematosus, generalized lymphoproliferative disease, diabetes mellitus, experimental allergic encephalomyelitis, and collagen arthritis (7,243,90,91). The correlation with autoimmunity is intriguing, but no mechanism relating these channels with disease has been proposed (2).

Ion Channels in Macrophages

Inward Rectifier Channels in Determining the Resting Potential of Macrophages

The inward rectifier K$^+$ channel is widely distributed among macrophages and related cells (57). Blocking inward rectifier channels with Ba^{2+} depolarizes V$_m$ (23,92,93). During adherence of J774.1 cells (a macrophage cell line) plated onto glass, V$_m$ hyperpolarizes in parallel with increases in the density of inward rectifier K$^+$ channels (23,94). Blocking inward rectifier channels does not impair chemotaxis, phagocytosis, or the respiratory burst (21). However, inhibition of the inward rectifier by blockers or antisense oligodeoxynucleotides inhibited the generation of hemopoietic progenitor cells (95).

Activation of G-protein signaling pathways appears to inhibit inward rectifier K$^+$ currents and activates G-protein–activated K$^+$ channels (29,30). The G-protein–activated K$^+$ current may assume responsibility for maintaining V$_m$ under these conditions.

Calcium-Activated Potassium Channels in Macrophage Responses

Among the earliest electrophysiologic investigations of leukocytes were pioneering studies showing that human macrophages exposed to chemotactic factors or mechanical stimuli responded by hyperpolarization of V$_m$ (57,96–101). As was proposed in these studies, the hyperpolarization was caused by activation of Ca^{2+}-activated

K$^+$ channels (98,102). Many physiologically active substances increase [Ca^{2+}]$_i$ in macrophages, opening voltage-independent Ca^{2+}-activated K$^+$ channels, preventing depolarization of V$_m$. Stimulation of the Fc receptor for immunoglobulin G does not directly open ion channels (93,103), but it leads to an increase in [Ca^{2+}]$_i$, which activates nonselective cation and K$^+$ channels (103).

Voltage-Gated Hydrogen Ion Channels in the Respiratory Burst

The nearly ubiquitous presence of H$^+$ channels in macrophages, other phagocytes (104,105), and related cells such as microglia (106,107) and osteoclasts (108) lends support to the idea that these channels help to sustain the respiratory burst in all phagocytes. This role is discussed in the section on neutrophils, in which it has been studied most intensively.

Ion Channel Expression Changes During Activation or Ramification of Microglia

Brain macrophages, or microglia, may play a role in Alzheimer's disease (109) and in more conventional host defense mechanisms. Microglia reside quietly in the brain in a highly ramified state and adopt a more compact ameboid shape when activated by bacteria or local neurologic injury. Unstimulated microglia and microglia in situ in brain slices express inward rectifier K$^+$ channels but not delayed rectifier (110,111). Stimulation by lipopolysaccharide results in the appearance of delayed rectifier (Kv1.3) channels in addition to inward rectifier channels (107,112). Differentiation with granulocyte-macrophage colony-stimulating factor (GM-CSF), but not with macrophage colony-stimulating factor (M-CSF), induces microglia to express delayed rectifier currents and to present antigen (106,113–115). Paradoxically, delayed rectifier currents also appear when ameboid microglia are transformed into ramified cells by co-culturing with astrocytes (116,117) or by addition of astrocyte-conditioned media (118), even though the cells appear morphologically to resemble quiescent microglia in the brain. However, the expression of delayed rectifier channels can be dissociated from the morphologic change, suggesting that different control mechanisms exist (118).

Voltage-gated H$^+$ currents are somewhat reduced in ramified microglia (C. Eder and R. Klee, personal communication, 1997), perhaps reflecting the less activated condition of the cells or possibly reflecting the appearance of other depolarization-activated (delayed rectifier) channels capable of repolarizing the membrane. Intriguingly, microglial ramification is inhibited by several chloride channel blockers but not by K$^+$ channel blockers or the Na$^+$ channel blocker tetrodotoxin (118).

Ion Channels in Neutrophils

Chloride Channels in Neutrophil Volume Regulation

Osmotic stress-activated Cl$^-$ channels similar to those in lymphocytes are responsible for the Cl$^-$ efflux that occurs during volume regulation in human neutrophils (55). Although K$^+$ efflux is also thought to occur, the channel responsible has not been identified.

Voltage-Gated Hydrogen Ion Channels in the Respiratory Burst

Phagocytes kill bacteria by engulfing them into a phagocytic vacuole and then secreting cytotoxic reactive oxygen species, as illustrated in Fig. 43-1. During this burst of metabolic activity, the respiratory burst, O^2, is consumed by the enzyme NADPH oxidase, which releases superoxide anion into the phagosome and at the same time stoichiometrically releases H$_+$ into the cell (119,120). This metabolically produced acid must be extruded to avoid lowering pH$_i$ and depolarizing V$_m$.

Several lines of evidence suggest that voltage-gated H$^+$ channels are activated during the respiratory burst in human neutrophils and extrude at least part of the acid produced. In functional studies, pH and V$_m$ changes have been explored using pH- and voltage-sensitive fluorescent dyes; properties deduced from these studies can be compared with the results of voltage-clamp studies of the H$^+$ channel. The respiratory burst can be elicited by a variety of stimuli including N-formyl-L-methionyl-L-leucyl-L-phenylalanine (fMLP, a chemotactic peptide), phorbol esters, arachidonic acid, and opsonized zymosan (121). NADPH oxidase is electrogenic (122,123), and its activity is limited by a requirement for compensating charge movement (124). H$^+$ efflux through channels is electrogenic, and opening only a small fraction of the H$^+$ channels in a human neutrophil is sufficient to extrude all the acid produced during the respiratory burst (35). H$^+$ extrusion can be inhibited by Cd^{2+} or Zn^{2+} (122,125), both of which inhibit voltage-gated H$^+$ channels in phagocytes (35–37,126). H$^+$ efflux and H$^+$ channels can be activated by lowering pH$_i$ (35,37,127). Arachidonic acid, an unsaturated fatty acid released by activated neutrophils, stimulates NADPH oxidase activity (121, 128–130), H$^+$ efflux (127,131), and the voltage-gated H$^+$ channel (35,126,132).

Blocking H$^+$ channels with Cd^{2+} or Zn^{2+} attenuates superoxide production (124). Several different mechanisms may contribute. Low pH$_i$ inhibits superoxide release (133,134). The pH optimum of NADPH oxidase is 7.0 to 7.5 (135), and H$^+$ current may serve to maintain pH$_i$ in this range. Membrane depolarization depresses the respiratory burst (136–138). H$^+$ current tends to raise pH$_i$ and to hyperpolarize V$_m$, with both actions helping to sustain and optimize superoxide release. By lowering local

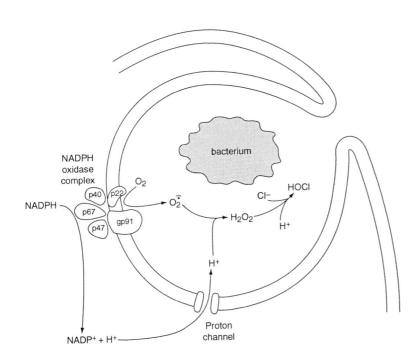

FIG. 43-1. Role of H$^+$ channels in the respiratory burst of phagocytes. After engulfing a bacterium into the phagocytic vacuole, the normally quiescent enzyme NADPH oxidase assembles in the phagosome membrane from five or more components from the membrane and cytosol. Reactive oxygen species generated by this enzyme contribute to the killing process. The superoxide anion (O$_2^-$) dismutates spontaneously to form hydrogen peroxide (H$_2$O$_2$). Myeloperoxidase then combines H$_2$O$_2$ with Cl$^-$ and H$^+$ to form hypochlorous acid (HOCl), the active ingredient in Chlorox bleach and a major bactericidal compound in phagocytes. The stoichiometries of the reactions shown are simplified. During O$_2^-$ production, protons (H$^+$) are released into the cell. To prevent accumulation of H$^+$ in the cell, which would lower pH$_i$ and depolarize V$_m$, H$^+$-selective ion channels open in the cell membrane, allowing passive H$^+$ extrusion. There is evidence for (211,212) and against (142,143) the idea that the gp91 subunit of the NADPH oxidase complex constitutes the H$^+$ channel. (Cartoon of the NADPH oxidase complex from ref. 135, redrawn with permission, with the addition of a 40-kd cytoplasmic subunit (213) and omission of small regulatory G proteins.)

pH$_o$, proton extrusion may facilitate the bactericidal action of acid proteases released by phagocytes (139).

The precursor cell line HL60 expresses small H$^+$ currents, but after induction, to differentiate into granulocyte-like cells, the H$^+$ channel density increases substantially, concurrently with the appearance of NADPH oxidase activity and the ability to mount a respiratory burst (140).

In chronic granulomatous disease (CGD), the NADPH oxidase of neutrophils is dysfunctional and as a result the patients suffer from recurrent infections. Nanda et al. (141) demonstrated that of three major acid-compensating systems of neutrophils, Na$^+$/H$^+$-antiport and H$^+$-ATPase responded normally to phorbol esters, but activation of H$^+$ efflux was only 12% to 15% normal in CGD. Most evidence indicates that the H$^+$ efflux elicited in CGD neutrophils is reduced because the oxidase is dysfunctional and does not generate the metabolic acid that normally activates the H$^+$ conductance (142,143).

How are H$^+$ channels activated during the respiratory burst? NADPH oxidase tends to lower pH$_i$ and to depolarize V$_m$, both of which tend to activate H$^+$ channels. Arachidonic acid enhances the H$^+$ conductance and shifts the threshold potential negatively (35,126,132), with both effects increasing the H$^+$ current at any given V$_m$. Extrusion of H$^+$ through channels costs the cell no metabolic energy. In contrast, H$^+$ pumps consume ATP directly, and the Na$^+$/H$^+$-antiporter extrudes H$^+$ at the expense of ATP required to pump Na$^+$ out of the cell. The Na$^+$/H$^+$-antiporter is electroneutral and therefore cannot dissipate excess positive charge from the cell. Although their relative contributions are unknown, all three mechanisms of

acid extrusion appear to be activated during the respiratory burst (120,144,145).

Ion Channels in Eosinophils

The only ion channels described in human eosinophils are voltage-activated H$^+$ channels (132), which are thought to serve the same role of acid extrusion during the respiratory burst in these cells as in neutrophils and other phagocytes (see Fig. 43-1). The H$^+$ current in eosinophils was enhanced by arachidonic acid and by elevation of [Ca^{2+}]$_i$ (132).

Ion Channels in Basophils or Mast Cells

Histamine secretion requires CRAC and K$^+$ channels. Mast cells secrete histamine in response to antigenic stimuli. Secretagogues activate three types of ion channels: CRAC channels, nonselective cation channels (146), and Cl$^-$ channels (51). Although the nonselective cation channels are permeable to Ca^{2+}, most of the Ca^{2+} signal enters mast cells through CRAC channels, which are highly Ca^{2+} selective (146). Binding of antigen to IgE receptors also activates G proteins, which activate an outwardly rectifying K$^+$ conductance (30,147). This K$^+$ conductance appears to facilitate secretion by maintaining a negative V$_m$ to drive Ca^{2+} entry through CRAC channels: blocking the K$^+$ conductance inhibits secretion (32). Blocking Cl$^-$ channels in mast cells only partially inhibits secretion (148,149), suggesting an ancillary role for Cl$^-$ channels. However, blocking CRAC channels by La^{3+} or by several

Cl⁻ channel blockers completely inhibits secretion, supporting a requirement for Ca^{2+} influx (149).

Ion Channels in Platelets and Megakaryocytes

Platelets or their Brobdingnagian precursors, megakaryocytes, express several of the familiar leukocyte ion channels, although for the most part their functions have not been elucidated. Platelets are anuclear, and their ion channels probably are synthesized during the megakaryocyte stage. Blocking type *n* delayed rectifier K^+ channels with charybdotoxin depolarizes the platelet V_m by 25 mV, demonstrating that this channel helps maintain the resting potential (150). An IP_3-dependent monovalent cation channel has been reported in the plasma membranes of rat megakaryocytes (151,152), which primarily conduct Na^+ under physiologic conditions. Further work is required to determine whether this pathway underlies the Na^+-dependent morphologic responses reported by Leven et al. (153). Thrombin activates platelets through a rise in $[Ca^{2+}]_i$ resulting from Ca^{2+} influx through CRAC channels (154).

ION CARRIERS

Terminology

Facilitated or carrier-mediated ion transport differs from that occurring through channels in that translocation of the ion is coupled to the displacement of all or part of the carrier molecule across the membrane. In biologic membranes, in which carriers usually are proteins or glycoproteins, transport is envisaged to require a conformational change of the polypeptide backbone of the transporter. As a result, the transport rates attained by carriers are considerably slower than those reported for channels.

In general, single inorganic cations or anions are not transported independently by plasma membrane carriers. Their translocation is stringently coupled to the concomitant displacement of other ionic species. Two types of coupling are recognized. One or more ions can be exchanged for ions traveling in the opposite direction. This process is called antiport or countertransport exchange. Alternatively, transmembrane movement of an ion may require the simultaneous translocation of other ions in the same direction. This form of coupled transport is known as cotransport or symport. The properties and distribution of the principal symports and antiports present in the plasma membranes of leukocytes (Table 43-2) are described in the following sections.

Sodium/Hydrogen Antiport

General Properties

Functional Characterization

A transporter that exchanges Na^+ for H^+ has been described in the plasma membranes of most mammalian cells, including leukocytes (155,156). The antiport is exquisitely cation-selective, transporting Na^+ and, to a lesser extent, Li^+, but not K^+, Rb^+, Cs^+, monovalent organic cations, or divalent cations. The stoichiometry of the exchange reaction is one Na^+ for one H^+. As a result, the transport cycle is electroneutral and insensitive to changes in transmembrane potential, V_m. The rate of Na^+/H^+ exchange (NHE) is a saturable function of the external Na^+ concentration and follows Michaelis-Menten kinetics. This behavior is consistent with the translocation of a single Na^+ ion per transport cycle. In view of the one-to-one stoichiometry of the exchange process, a single proton equivalent must be ejected per cycle (157).

The antiport function is reversible, and the predominant direction of the exchange process is dictated by the combined chemical (concentration) gradients of Na^+ and H^+. Under physiologic conditions, the antiport catalyzes the net uptake of external Na^+, coupled to the efflux of intracellular H^+. This results from the prevailing inward Na^+ gradient generated by the Na^+/K^+ pump. Although the antiport itself does not hydrolyze ATP, the energy for the continued extrusion of H^+ from the cells is indirectly provided by the Na^+/K^+ pump, through the formation and maintenance of the Na^+ gradient.

TABLE 43-2. *Inorganic ion carriers in leukocytes: inhibitor sensitivity and distribution*

Carrier	Stoichiometry	Inhibitors	Distribution
Na^+/H^+ exchange	1 to 1	Amiloride	Lymphocytes, neutrophils, monocytes, macrophages, myeloid cell lines (e.g., HL60, U937)
Cl^-/HCO_3^- exchange	1 to 1	Disulfonic stilbenes	Lymphocytes
Na^+-dependent anion exchange (with HCO_3^-)	1 Cl^- + 1 H^+ or 1 Cl^-	Disulfonic stilbenes	Lymphocytes
		Picrylsulfonate	Myeloid cell lines (U937,HL60?)
Na^+/Ca^{2+} exchange	3 to 1	Lanthanides	Lymphocytes
		Amiloride analogues	Neutrophils
Na^+-K^+-Cl^- cotransport	1 to 1 to 2	Bumetanide	Unfractionated mononuclear cells

One of the hallmarks of NHE is its susceptibility to inhibition by amiloride and a group of related pyrazine derivatives. In general, amiloride and its analogues are believed to inhibit the antiport competitively by interacting externally with the Na^+ binding site. Forward exchange (i.e., Na^+ influx for H^+ efflux) is inhibited by extracellular acidification, probably by competition between Na^+ and H^+ at the same external site. In contrast, a pronounced stimulation of NHE is observed when the cytoplasm is acidified. The steep relationship between the internal H^+ concentration and the rate of exchange suggests a cooperative process. This effect has been attributed to the existence of an inward-facing allosteric site that, when protonated, stimulates the rate of cation exchange (157). This putative "modifier" site is thought to be different from the site that binds the protons to be transported across the membrane.

The NHE functions primarily in the regulation of the intracellular (cytosolic) pH (pH_i). Through its ability to mediate the net extrusion of H^+, the antiport can counteract the spontaneous tendency of cells to become acidic because of passive (electrophoretic) H^+ influx and metabolic acid production. If unopposed, the latter can severely compromise pH_i homeostasis, particularly in activated cells. The allosteric modifier site is thought to confer on the antiport its pH_i regulatory properties. NHE takes place at significant rates only if the cytoplasm is acidified, when the allosteric controlling site is protonated. Conversely, transport essentially ceases after the normal resting pH_i is attained, because of deprotonation of this site.

Under certain conditions, the "set point" of the modifier site of the antiport can be adjusted upward, rendering the cytoplasm more alkaline. This occurs in osmotically shrunken cells, in which the resulting activation of NHE leads to a net osmotic gain and accompanying increases in cell water and volume. For this reason, the antiport is also thought to participate in the regulation of cellular volume. The set point of the allosteric modifier can be reset upward by a number of ligands through receptor-mediated processes. In leukocytes, the molecular mechanism underlying this shift has not been defined, but experiments with other cell types suggest that phosphorylation of the cytosolic moiety of the antiport is involved (158).

Molecular Characterization

The molecules responsible for NHE have been cloned and sequenced (245). Five NHE isoforms (NHE1 through NHE5), derived from distinct genes, have been described. Overall, NHE1 through NHE5 share approximately 34% to 60% amino acid identity, with predicted molecular masses of about 81 to 93 kD. Based on their primary structure, a similar membrane topology can be predicted for all isoforms, with 10 to 12 membrane-spanning domains at the N terminus and a large cytoplasmic region at the C terminus. The entire C-terminal domain is seemingly oriented toward the cytosol, because it is inaccessible to antibodies or proteases added extracellularly. Evidence suggests that the NHEs exist in the membrane as homodimers and can be glycosylated.

Only NHE1 has been detected in blood cells. Lymphocytes (159), neutrophils (160), and macrophages (161) were shown to express this isoform, and NHE2 through NHE4 have not been detected. The detailed distribution of NHE5 has not been reported, but this isoform may be present in leukocytes, because it is abundant in the spleen.

Sodium/Hydrogen Exchange in Lymphocytes

Na^+/H^+ antiport activity has been detected in the plasma membrane of rodent thymic lymphocytes (162), human (163) and porcine (164) peripheral blood lymphocytes, and several lymphoid cell lines derived from human or murine T or B cells (165). Although not studied in detail in every case, the properties of the antiport in these cells generally fit the typical pattern. A role for Na^+/H^+ exchange in the regulation of pH_i and of cellular volume has been well documented in lymphocytes (166). The antiport is activated by a variety of growth-promoting agents. In T cells, exchange has been shown to be stimulated by lectins (163), by monoclonal antibodies against the T3–T-cell receptor complex (167), by interleukins (168), and by co-mitogenic doses of phorbol esters and calcium ionophores (165). Interleukin-1 also stimulates the antiport in B cells, as does bacterial lipopolysaccharide (169,170).

Activation of NHE by these mitogens consistently precedes proliferation, suggesting that these events are causally related. The correlation was further stressed by the finding that proliferation induced by a variety of agents can be blocked by amiloride. Conversely, inhibition of NHE was suggested to be essential for the initiation of apoptosis in T cells (171). However, caution must be exercised in interpreting these results, because high concentrations of amiloride inhibit the antiport and a variety of protein kinases, protein synthesis, and other processes that are central to cell growth. Experiments using more potent and specific analogues of amiloride were able to dissociate the activation of the antiport from the initiation of lymphoproliferation (172). Stimulation of Na^+/H^+ exchange therefore does not appear to be an essential requirement for cell growth, and the significance of the activation by mitogens remains unclear.

Agents that promote B lymphocyte differentiation are able to stimulate Na^+/H^+ countertransport (169,170). As in the case of mitogens, stimulation of ion exchange precedes differentiation and the latter can be blocked by amiloride. A causal relationship between these events was further suggested by the observation that artificially elevating the cytoplasmic Na$^+$ content, thereby mimicking one of the effects of the antiport, sufficed to induce differentiation. However, subsequent experiments using more specific amiloride analogues questioned the validity of this hypothesis (169).

It appears unlikely that stimulation of Na$^+$/H$^+$ exchange by mitogens and differentiating agents is required for the expression of their biologic effects. More likely, the antiport is activated as a safeguard in anticipation of the increase in metabolic rate (and therefore acid generation) that occurs during proliferation and differentiation. Alternatively, the purpose of the elevated rate of cation exchange may be to increase the osmotic content of the cells. The associated water and volume gain may be an important prelude to the synthesis of macromolecules that follows mitogenic stimulation.

Sodium/Hydrogen Exchange in Phagocytic Leukocytes

The presence of an active Na$^+$/H$^+$ exchanger has been described in neutrophils from several species and in HL60 cells, a promyelocytic leukemia line (173,174). HL60 cells proliferate in culture in an undifferentiated state, but they can be induced to differentiate into granulocyte-like cells by agents such as dimethylsulfoxide. Undifferentiated and granulocytic HL60 cells display Na$^+$/H$^+$ antiport activity, although with somewhat different properties.

As in other cells, the antiport in neutrophils is thought to participate in pH$_i$ regulation, because it is greatly activated on cytosolic acidification. This role becomes particularly important during the respiratory burst, which is associated with a surge in intracellular acid generation. Whereas pH$_i$ normally remains above neutrality during activation, a pronounced intracellular acidification is observed in the absence of Na$^+$ or in the presence of amiloride (175). During neutrophil activation, the antiport is stimulated in part by the accumulation of intracellular H$^+$ but also directly by a shift in the pH$_i$ dependence of the modifier site. As a result, pH$_i$ is maintained in the face of increased metabolic H$^+$ generation and usually becomes more alkaline. Receptor-mediated activation of Na$^+$/H$^+$ exchange is induced in neutrophils by chemoattractants, phorbol esters, zymosan, lectins, and leukotrienes (119).

Maintenance of pH$_i$ by the antiport is essential for the bactericidal function of neutrophils. The NADPH oxidase is markedly pH$_i$ dependent, showing an alkaline optimum and rapid inactivation at acidic levels. Similarly, chemotaxis and chemokinesis are enhanced by alkalosis and depressed at low pH$_i$. As a result, neutrophil migration and the respiratory burst are inhibited by omission of external Na$^+$ and by amiloride and its analogues, ostensibly through inhibition of the antiport (134,176). The generation of eicosanoids is similarly impaired when antiport activity is precluded (119). The

swelling induced by Na$^+$/H$^+$ exchange may contribute to the migration of neutrophils (177). However, the ionic changes produced by the antiport do not by themselves generate any of the responses observed in cells activated by physiologic ligands. Activation of Na$^+$/H$^+$ exchange is necessary but not sufficient for normal neutrophil responsiveness.

Active Na$^+$/H$^+$ exchange has been verified in monocytes and macrophages from a variety of sources (178,179) and in several transformed myeloid cell lines, including AML-193, U-937, and HL60 (180,181). Because stimulated macrophages undergo a respiratory and metabolic burst like that of neutrophils, Na$^+$/H$^+$ exchange probably is important to the maintenance of pH$_i$ during activation (182,183). Increased countertransport has been reported when these cells are stimulated by phorbol esters. A variety of other stimuli also activate the exchanger, including zymosan, interferon-γ, platelet-activating factor, and GM-CSF (119,179). Several of the responses elicited by these ligands are impaired when amiloride or its analogues are present or when Na$^+$ is omitted. Although suggesting a direct linkage between responsiveness and Na$^+$/H$^+$ exchange, the findings merely reflect the pH$_i$ sensitivity of different facets of the activation process.

As in the case of lymphoid cells, monocyte and macrophage proliferation is associated with stimulation of the antiport. Blood monocytes and bone marrow–derived macrophages respond to colony-stimulating factor-1, a mitogenic agent, with increased Na$^+$/H$^+$ exchange activity. It has been proposed that the enhanced cycling of Na$^+$ into and out of the cells is important for their progression through the S phase of the growth cycle (179). This conclusion should be viewed as tentative, because it was reached solely on the basis of the inhibitory effects of amiloride analogues.

Chloride/Bicarbonate Exchange

General Properties

Functional Characterization

The Cl$^-$/HCO$_3^-$ exchanger is a tightly coupled carrier that translocates anions across the plasma membrane with a one-to-one stoichiometry. Like the Na$^+$/H$^+$ antiport, it is electroneutral, and its rate of transport is insensitive to variations in V_m the transmembrane potential. The Cl$^-$/HCO$_3^-$ exchanger is extremely anion specific: Cl$^-$ is transported over a million times faster than K$^+$, a cation of similar size. In contrast, its selectivity toward anions is comparatively limited; in addition to its main physiologic substrates, Cl$^-$ and HCO$_3^-$, it can transport a number of halides and larger, polyvalent anions such as sulfate and phosphate. In contrast to the cation-dependent anion exchanger, Na$^+$ is not transported by this system, nor is it required for the transport of anions.

As is true for the cation antiport, the anion exchanger is reversible but asymmetric. The rate and direction of transport are dictated by the concentration gradients of the substrate ions, and metabolic energy is not expended during the translocation event. Cl^-/HCO_3^- exchange is typically inhibited by externally added stilbene derivatives such as DIDS and SITS.

The primary role of anion exchange in nucleated cells is thought to be as a regulator of pH_i. When cells become excessively alkaline, HCO_3^-, a base equivalent, can be readily extruded from the cytoplasm in exchange for incoming Cl^-, preserving electroneutrality. In most cell types, the combined Cl^- and HCO_3^- gradients are poised to drive net base efflux from the cells even at the resting, physiologic pH_i. This phenomenon would seem to be deleterious to the cells, because it would compound the spontaneous tendency of the cells to acidify. However, evidence indicates that Cl^-/HCO_3^- exchange in nucleated cells, unlike that in red blood cells, is greatly inhibited at pH_i below about 7.2, the resting pH of most cells. A pronounced activation is observed at more alkaline levels (184). Cl^-/HCO_3^- exchange can function effectively in the defense of intracellular pH in the alkaline range, without contributing significantly to spontaneous acidification under physiologic conditions.

Molecular Characterization

Three isoforms of the anion exchanger (AE) have been identified and sequenced. The AE of red blood cells, called AE1, is a glycoprotein of molecular mass of about 95,000 and is also known as capnophorin or band 3 (185). It encompasses a hydrophobic C-terminal domain, has 10 to 14 transmembrane segments, and has a hydrophilic N-terminal tail. This bipartite topology is shared by two other distinct but closely related gene products in nucleated cells (184). AE2 is a rather ubiquitous isoform, which differs from AE1 in its sharper pH dependence, with acute inhibition at acidic pH. This is the isoform likely to prevail in white blood cells. A third isoform, AE3, is present in specialized regions of the brain and heart (186).

Chloride/Bicarbonate Exchange in Lymphocytes

The presence of a robust anion exchanger in lymphoid cells was initially inferred from the apparent discrepancy between electrical and isotopic measurements of Cl^- permeability. While the plasma membrane appeared very permeable to the anion, the measured conductance was minute (187). These observations can be explained by the presence of nonconductive (electroneutral) Cl^- transporters. A large fraction of the measured flux was later found to strictly depend on the availability of contralateral exchangeable anions and to be susceptible to inhibition by disulfonic stilbenes (188). These features are diagnostic of electroneutral anion exchange.

As found in several other nucleated cell types, anion exchange in lymphocytes is acutely sensitive to the cytosolic pH; the rate of exchange increases over 10-fold within 0.4 pH units. The cells are thereby endowed with a means to counteract cytosolic alkalosis by extrusion of HCO_3^-. However, pH_i rarely increases beyond the resting level. Moderate alkalosis tends to occur when the Na^+/H^+ antiport is activated. Under these conditions, Cl^-/HCO_3^- exchange also is stimulated, leading to a net uptake of NaCl and water. Such coupling between the cation and anion exchangers may be of significance in the control of cellular volume.

Anion exchange also plays a central role in the establishment of the steady state concentration of cytoplasmic Cl^-. Because Cl^- conductance is low in lymphoid cells, Cl^-/HCO_3^- exchange is the predominant pathway for Cl^- permeation. As a result, the transmembrane HCO_3^- gradient is the primary determinant of the distribution of Cl^-. This is evidenced by the changes in intracellular Cl^- concentration that follow alterations in the concentration of HCO_3^- (188). Because at constant P_{CO2} the concentration of HCO_3^- is a function of the pH, it follows that the transmembrane pH is the primary determinant of the Cl^- gradient in lymphocytes.

Chloride/Bicarbonate Exchange in Phagocytic Leukocytes

Anion exchange activity has been reported in the plasma membranes of human neutrophils and undifferentiated HL60 cells (189,190). In general, Cl^-/HCO_3^- exchange in these cells conforms to the typical pattern described previously; it shows broad anion selectivity, is asymmetric, has a one-to-one stoichiometry, and is consequently electroneutral. However, the exchanger in granulocytes displays certain unique features. It is comparatively insensitive to disulfonic stilbenes and is instead susceptible to inhibition by hydroxycinnamate derivatives (190).

The exquisite dependence of Cl^-/HCO_3^- exchange activity on pH_i described for lymphocytes and other cells is also evident in neutrophils (191). It is reasonable to assume that the exchanger also plays a role in the control of cytosolic pH in these cells. The exchanger may be an important determinant of the resting intracellular Cl^- concentration, which is reported to be much higher than expected for a passive (electrochemically driven) distribution (190). It is not clear whether the exchanger is involved in the large drop in Cl^- content reported to occur on neutrophil stimulation (192). It has been speculated that anion exchange may be essential to granule secretion, which is blocked by disulfonic stilbenes. However, inhibition of secretion by an effect of the stilbenes on processes other than anion exchange has not been ruled out.

There is minimal information concerning the existence and properties of Cl^-/HCO_3^- exchange in monocytes and macrophages. Because the exchanger is present in undifferentiated HL60 cells, it is reasonable to assume that it is preserved after monocytic differentiation, but no direct data are available. The promonocytic leukemia line U937 displays stilbene disulfonate-sensitive Cl^- uptake. In nominally bicarbonate-free medium, this uptake is dependent on the presence of contralateral (intracellular) Cl^-. These observations are consistent with the presence of anion exchange. However, the researchers (181) attributed the fluxes to the Na^+-dependent anion exchange system. Suggestive but inconclusive evidence was presented against the existence of cation-independent Cl^-/HCO_3^- exchange (181). The identification and characterization of anion exchange in mononuclear phagocytes awaits further study.

Sodium–Dependent Anion Exchange

General Properties

A distinct form of anion exchange, which strictly depends on the presence of Na^+, was identified in several mammalian cell types. In its forward (physiologic) mode, this transporter mediates the coupled entry of one Na^+ and the exit of one Cl^-, while removing from the cell two acid equivalents. This process is electroneutral and requires the presence of HCO_3^- (or CO_3^{2-}). Two possible coupling modes have been considered. First, Na^+ could be transported inward along with HCO_3^- in exchange for one Cl^- and one H^+. Second, Na^+ and CO_3^{2-} could combine at the external transport site to form a monovalent ion pair ($NaCO_3^-$) that would be exchanged for internal Cl^-. These two transport modes are functionally equivalent and thermodynamically indistinguishable; both are electrically neutral and result in the elimination of two intracellular acid equivalents. In the former case, one H^+ is extruded, and one cytosolic acid equivalent is eliminated by internal protonation of HCO_3^-. In the second mechanism, two cytosolic acid equivalents are used up by the protonation of CO_3^{2-}.

Under normal circumstances, the Na^+-dependent anion exchanger is thermodynamically poised to extrude acid from the cells. This extrusion is driven chiefly by the large inward Na^+ gradient and in part by the smaller inward HCO_3^- (or CO_3^{2-}) gradient, despite the net tendency of Cl^- to move inward through the exchanger (because $[Cl^-]_o > [Cl^-]_i$). Like the Na^+/H^+ antiport, the Na^+-dependent anion exchange system is virtually quiescent in the alkaline range but becomes activated as pH_i falls below a certain threshold, which is close to the physiologic pH_i. This peculiar pH sensitivity, together with its ability to eliminate acid equivalents from the cytoplasm,

led investigators to believe that the Na^+-dependent anion exchanger is important in the maintenance of the resting pH_i and in the prevention of acidosis during metabolic activation. In the few instances in which both systems have been measured, the Na^+-dependent anion exchanger is more active near the physiologic pH_i than the cation antiport. Under conditions in which Na^+/H^+ exchange is impaired (e.g., addition of amiloride or its analogues), most cells, including some leukocytes (189,193), maintain pH_i within the physiologic range, provided HCO_3^- is present. This in all likelihood reflects the operation of the Na^+-dependent anion exchanger.

As for the cation-insensitive Cl^-/HCO_3^- exchange system, the Na^+-dependent anion exchanger is also blocked by disulfonic stilbenes such as SITS and DIDS. Despite their similar pharmacology and anion selectivity, the Na^+-dependent and independent modes of anion exchange are believed to be mediated by separate and distinct molecular entities. This mechanism is suggested in part by the fact that some cell types display only one of the transport modalities. Moreover, in cells possessing both transport systems, differential sensitivity to certain inhibitors has been demonstrated. Ethacrynic acid preferentially inhibits cation-independent Cl^-/HCO_3^- exchange, with little effect on the Na^+-dependent system, but picrylsulfonate has the opposite effect (194).

Distribution

There is only one report of Na^+-dependent anion exchange in lymphoid cells. In rat thymic lymphocytes, pH_i was found to recover from an acid load under conditions in which Na^+/H^+ exchange was totally inhibited. The observed recovery was found to depend on the presence of extracellular Na^+ and was promoted by addition of HCO_3^-. Although the requirement for intracellular Cl^- was not analyzed, the observations are consistent with activation of Na^+-dependent anion exchange. The pH_i recovery was obliterated by stilbene disulfonates (195).

Information regarding N^+-dependent anion exchange in phagocytes is also scarce. In HL60 cells, the presence of the cation-dependent exchanger was suggested by pH_i determinations and Na^+ uptake measurements (196). As in the case of thymocytes, the Cl^- dependence and electrical correlates of the transport process were not defined. For this reason, ambiguity remains about whether the observations are attributable to Na^+-dependent anion exchange or to the Cl^--independent, electrogenic sodium bicarbonate ion cotransporter described in other cells. In HL60 cells, the Na^+ and bicarbonate-dependent pH_i recovery was observed in undifferentiated and retinoic acid-differentiated (granulocytic) cells. Unlike Na^+/H^+ exchange, which is activated after treatment with retinoic acid, the putative Na^+-dependent anion exchanger was unaffected during differentiation.

A *bona fide* Na$^+$-dependent anion exchanger was described in promonocytic U937 cells (181). These cells display a Na$^+$- and HCO$_3^-$-dependent pH$_i$ recovery process after acid loading. The recovery, indicative of HCO$_3^-$ (or CO$_3^{2-}$) entry, was accompanied by Na$^+$ uptake and by efflux of Cl$^-$, and all of these events were comparably inhibited by stilbene derivatives. The HCO$_3^-$-dependent entry of Na$^+$ was depressed by depletion of intracellular Cl$^-$, suggesting a tight coupling between the cation and anion fluxes. Based on the marked pH dependence of its transport rate, the Na$^+$-dependent anion exchanger was proposed to be an important pH$_i$ regulatory mechanism in myeloid cells.

Sodium/Calcium Exchange

General Properties

Functional Characterization

An antiport capable of exchanging Na$^+$ for Ca^{2+} exists in the plasma membranes of many cells, including leukocytes. Ca^{2+} is a substrate of the Na$^+$/Ca^{2+} exchanger and plays a regulatory role. At physiologic levels, cytosolic Ca^{2+} allosterically enhance the rate of transport. The stoichiometry of Na$^+$/Ca^{2+} exchange has been the subject of intense study (197). In most cells, three Na$^+$ ions are exchanged for one Ca^{2+} ion in each cycle. As a result of the dissimilar number of charges transported, the exchange process is electrogenic, with one net charge transported per cycle. For this reason, the activity of the Na$^+$/Ca^{2+} antiport varies with the transmembrane potential (V_m). The direction of net exchange is determined by the difference (ΔV) between V_m and the reversal potential of the exchanger ($E_{Na^+/Ca^{2+}}$), which is defined as

$$E_{Na^+/Ca^{2+}} = 3\ E_{Na^+} - 2\ E_{Ca^{2+}}$$

where E_{Na^+} and $E_{Ca^{2+}}$ are the equilibrium potentials for Na$^+$ and Ca^{2+}, respectively. Based on the V_m and the Na$^+$ and Ca^{2+} gradients prevailing in resting leukocytes, the exchanger can be calculated to be near equilibrium, slightly favoring net Ca^{2+} entry into the cells. At constant concentrations of Na$^+$ and Ca^{2+}, entry of Ca^{2+} through the antiport is enhanced by depolarization of V_m. Such influx may be of importance in inflammatory cells, some of which are known to depolarize abruptly on activation. When the cytosolic Ca^{2+} concentration rises, as is the case during stimulation of some leukocytes, the Na$^+$/Ca^{2+} antiport can catalyze net Ca^{2+} efflux from the cells. In this capacity, the exchanger probably functions as an effective Ca^{2+} extrusion system, complementing the plasmalemmal Ca^{2+} pump. The latter is thought to be a high-affinity, low-capacity system, but the exchanger has a much larger capacity, although with lower affinity for Ca^{2+} (198).

There are no potent and specific inhibitors of Na$^+$/Ca^{2+} exchange. Several agents have inhibitory action, including analogues of doxorubicin and amiloride and some local anesthetics, but comparatively high concentrations are required and side effects are observed. Divalent (e.g., Cd^{2+}, Sr^{2+}) and trivalent cations (e.g., La^{3+}, Nd^{3+}) inhibit competitively, binding to the Ca^{2+} site.

Molecular Characterization

Three proteins catalyzing Na$^+$/Ca^{2+} exchange, called NCX1 through NCX3, have been identified and cloned. The deduced sequence predicts a protein of between 921 and 970 residues, with a molecular mass of approximately 105 kD. The larger apparent molecular size (160 kD) detected by electrophoresis is attributable to glycosylation of an asparagine residue. The best studied of the exchangers, NCX1, is believed to span the membrane 11 times and to have a large cytosolic loop of about 520 residues between transmembrane segments 5 and 6. It is not clear which one of the isoforms is expressed in inflammatory cells.

Distribution

The evidence for the presence of Na$^+$/Ca^{2+} exchange in leukocytes is scant and often controversial. Several approaches failed to demonstrate exchange activity in intact lymphocytes (187). However, one report documented calcium entry mediated by this exchanger in human lymphocytes (199). The information in neutrophils is more abundant but is also inconsistent. No exchange activity was detectable through Ca^{2+} efflux measurements from intact cells or by monitoring free cytosolic [Ca^{2+}] while performing ionic substitutions (200,201). Ca^{2+} uptake determinations into inverted plasma membrane vesicles also failed to demonstrate Na$^+$/Ca^{2+} exchange (201). In contrast, convincing evidence was provided by Ca^{2+} uptake determinations into resting and stimulated cells (202). The influx of Ca^{2+} was found to be proportional to the intracellular Na$^+$ concentration and enhanced by depolarization. The flux was blocked by divalent and trivalent cations and by amiloride analogues. These features are hallmarks of the Na$^+$/Ca^{2+} antiport. The apparent inconsistency of the available results could be explained by assuming that an important fraction of Ca^{2+} uptake is mediated by Na$^+$/Ca^{2+} exchange, whereas most of the efflux occurs through the Ca^{2+} pump.

It has also been claimed that in neutrophils Na$^+$/Ca^{2+} exchange is stimulated by chemoattractants, underlying a major fraction of the activated Ca^{2+} influx and associated increase in cytosolic [Ca^{2+}]. This conclusion was based mainly on the susceptibility of the stimulated influx to inhibition by polyvalent inorganic cations and by analogues of amiloride (203). These agents were also found to block stimulation of the NADPH oxidase by chemotactic peptide, presumably by precluding the rise in [Ca^{2+}]. However, the inhibitors also affected the oxidase by means other than blocking Ca^{2+} uptake, inasmuch as they inhibited the Ca^{2+}-independent part of the respiratory response and the Ca^{2+}-dependent component.

Sr^{2+}, a Ca^{2+} surrogate, was used to detect Na^+/Ca^{2+} exchange in macrophages (204). Uptake of the divalent cation was stimulated by intracellular Na^+ loading and blocked by amiloride analogues, consistent with the presence of the antiport. The functional role of the Na^+/Ca^{2+} exchanger in mononuclear phagocytes has not been investigated.

Sodium, Potassium, and Chloride Cotransport

General Properties

Functional Characterization

A system that mediates the coupled transport of Na^+, K^+, and Cl^- across the plasma membrane has been described in a wide variety of cell types, including blood cells (205). In the mammalian tissues studied, the stoichiometry of the cotransport process is 1 Na^+, 1 K^+, and 2 Cl^- ions per cycle. Because equal numbers of cations and anions are translocated, the process is electrically neutral and potentially insensitive. Na^+-K^+-2 Cl^- cotransport is reversible and is driven by the concentration gradients of the substrate ions. Metabolic energy is not expended during the transport cycle. Nevertheless, the presence of intracellular ATP seems to be required for effective cotransport, at least in some cell types (205). These observations suggest that Na^+-K^+-2 Cl^- cotransport may be controlled by phosphorylation of the symporter itself or of a regulatory protein. Data obtained with phosphoprotein phosphatase inhibitors support this notion. The decay of cotransport activity after ATP depletion was found to be markedly delayed when dephosphorylation was inhibited (206).

A distinctive property of Na^+-K^+-2 Cl^- cotransport is its sensitivity to inhibition by loop diuretics, such as furosemide, piretanide and bumetanide. The most potent of these inhibitors are effective in the low micromolar range. Because of their potency and selectivity, radiolabeled diuretics can be used to quantify the number of cotransporters. Based on the number of active transporters determined by binding studies, and on the magnitude of the fluxes, the turnover number of the Na^+-K^+-2 Cl^- cotransporter has been reported to range between 50 and 4000 per second.

Na^+-K^+-2 Cl^- cotransport is thought to function in the maintenance and regulation of the cellular volume. Cotransport is greatly activated when cells shrink, promoting influx of Na^+, K^+, Cl^-, and osmotically obliged water. The cells swell, tending to restore their original volume. The cotransporter is also central to the establishment of the intracellular Cl^- concentration, particularly in cells with low anion conductance and poor anion exchange activity. In this instance, the inward Na^+ gradient drives Cl^- into the cytosol through the cotransporter,

attaining concentrations that surpass the levels predicted from electrochemical equilibrium.

Molecular Characterization

Molecular studies have identified two isoforms of the Na^+-K^+-2 Cl^- cotransporter, NKCC1 and NKCC2. The latter appears to be restricted to apical membranes of epithelia, whereas NKCC1 has a wide tissue distribution and is likely the isoform present in leukocytes. NKCC1 comprises about 1200 amino acids (molecular mass of about 130 kD) and is predicted to span the membrane 12 times. The protein has comparatively large hydrophilic N- and C-terminal domains, both of which are believed to be oriented toward the cytosol. A putative *N*-glycosylation site has been identified in the loop between transmembrane segments 7 and 8 (207).

Distribution

Na^+-K^+-2 Cl^- cotransport is expressed very poorly in most types of leukocytes studied. In thymic lymphocytes, addition of bumetanide or omission of extracellular K^+ or Cl^- had little effect on the rate of Na^+ uptake. Similarly, uptake of Cl^- was essentially unaffected by bumetanide or by removal of Na^+ or K^+ (188,208). In neutrophils, Cl^- uptake can be partially inhibited by furosemide, but this likely reflects a nonspecific effect of the inhibitor, because omission of external Na^+ or K^+ had no effect (196). In alveolar macrophages, only a minute component of the uptake of Rb^+ (used as a K^+ surrogate) was blocked by furosemide (209). Only one study reported a substantial inhibition of Na^+ transport by bumetanide in leukocytes (210). Because this report analyzed unfractionated human mononuclear cells, it is not possible to attribute the cotransport activity to a particular type of leukocyte. All of these measurements were carried out using unstimulated cells. It is conceivable that the cotransporter exists in a quiescent form, capable of being activated by changes in cell volume, by cyclic nucleotides or other stimuli known to stimulate Na^+-K^+-2 Cl^- cotransport in other cells.

CONCLUSIONS

Ion channels and carriers are important for the survival and activation of inflammatory cells. For these reasons, they are potential targets for therapeutic intervention. Their variety, specific distribution, rapid response, superficial cellular location, and sensitivity to exogenous agents make these transporters well suited to pharmacologic manipulation. Substantial research is already underway, and a productive outcome is anticipated in the near future.

ACKNOWLEDGMENTS

This work was supported in part by research grant HL52671 from the National Institutes of Health. The authors thank colleagues who provided preprints of their work and who commented on the manuscript.

REFERENCES

1. Hodgkin AL, Huxley AF. A quantitative description of membrane current and its application to conduction and excitation in nerve. *J Physiol* 1952;117:500–544.
2. DeCoursey TE. Type *l* (Kv3.1) K$^+$ channels in lymphocytes. *Cell Physiol Biochem* 1997;7:172–178.
3. Brücke E. Beiträge zur Lehre von der Diffusion tropfbarflüssiger Körper durch poröse Scheidenwände. *Ann Phys Chem* 1843;58:77–94.
4. Hodgkin AL, Huxley AF, Katz B. Ionic currents underlying activity in the giant axon of the squid. *Arch Sci Physiol* 1949;3:129–150.
5. Hamill OP, Marty A, Neher E, Sakmann B, Sigworth FJ. Improved patch-clamp techniques for high-resolution current recording from cells and cell-free membrane patches. *Pflügers Arch* 1981;391:85–100.
6. Verheugen JAH, Vijverberg HPM. Intracellular Ca^{2+} oscillations and membrane potential fluctuations in intact human T lymphocytes: role of K+ channels in Ca^{2+} signalling. *Cell Calcium* 1995;17:287–300.
7. Chandy KG, DeCoursey TE, Fischbach M, Talal N, Cahalan MD, Gupta S. Altered K$^+$ channel expression in abnormal T lymphocytes from mice with the l*pr* gene mutation. *Science* 1986;233:1197–1200.
8. DeCoursey TE, Chandy KG, Gupta S, Cahalan MD. Two types of potassium channels in murine T lymphocytes. *J Gen Physiol* 1987;89:379–404.
9. Lewis RS, Cahalan MD. Subset-specific expression of potassium channels in developing murine T lymphocytes. *Science* 1988;239:771–775.
10. Shapiro MS, DeCoursey TE. Selectivity and gating of the type L potassium channel in mouse lymphocytes. *J Gen Physiol* 1991;97:1227–1250.
11. Cahalan MD, Chandy KG, DeCoursey TE, Gupta S. A voltage-gated potassium channel in human T lymphocytes. *J Physiol* 1985;358:197–237.
12. Shapiro MS, DeCoursey TE. Permeant ion effects on the gating kinetics of the type L potassium channel in mouse lymphocytes. *J Gen Physiol* 1991;97:1251–1278.
13. Bregestovski P, Redkozubov A, Alexeev A. Elevation of intracellular calcium reduces voltage-dependent potassium conductance in human T cells. *Nature* 1986;319:776–778.
14. Choquet D, Sarthou P, Primi D, Cazenave PA, Korn H. Cyclic AMP-modulated potassium channels in murine B cells and their precursors. *Science* 1987;235:1211–1214.
15. Grissmer S, Cahalan MD. Divalent ion trapping inside potassium channels of human T lymphocytes. *J Gen Physiol* 1989;93:609–630.
16. Matsuda H, Saigusa A, Irisawa H. Ohmic conductance through the inwardly rectifying K channel and blocking by internal Mg^{2+}. *Nature* 1987;325:156–159.
17. Vandenberg CA. Inward rectification of a potassium channel in cardiac ventricular cells depends on internal magnesium ions. *Proc Natl Acad Sci USA* 1987;84:2560–2564.
18. Silver MR, DeCoursey TE. Intrinsic gating of inward rectifier in bovine pulmonary artery endothelial cells in the presence or absence of internal Mg^{2+}. *J Gen Physiol* 1990;96:109–133.
19. Lopatin AN, Nichols CG. [K$^+$] dependence of polyamine-induced rectification in inward rectifier potassium channels (IRK1, Kir2.1). *J Gen Physiol* 1996;108:105–113.
20. DeCoursey TE, Kim SY, Silver MR, Quandt FN. III. Ion channel expression in PMA-differentiated human THP-1 macrophages. *J Membr Biol* 1996;152:141–157.
21. McKinney LC, Gallin EK. Inwardly rectifying whole-cell and single-channel K currents in the murine macrophage cell line J774.1. *J Membr Biol* 1988;103:41–53.
22. Eder C. *Charakterisierung der spannungsabhängigen Ionenströme zytokinbehandelter kultivierter Mikrogliazellen.* Doctoral dissertation, University of Cologne, 1994.
23. Gallin EK, Sheehy PA. Differential expression of inward and outward potassium currents in the macrophage-like cell line J774.1. *J Physiol* 1985;369:475–499.
24. Grissmer S, Lewis RS, Cahalan MD. Ca^{2+}-activated K$^+$ channels in human leukemic T cells. *J Gen Physiol* 1992;99:63–84.
25. Grissmer S, Nguyen AN, Cahalan MD. Calcium-activated potassium channels in resting and activated human T lymphocytes: expression levels, calcium dependence, ion selectivity, and pharmacology. *J Gen Physiol* 1993;102:601–630.
26. Varnai P, Demaurex N, Jaconi M, Schlegel W, Lew DP, Krause KH. Highly co-operative Ca^{2+} activation of intermediate-conductance K$^+$ channels in granulocytes from a human cell line. *J Physiol* 1993;472:373–390.
27. Verheugen JAH, Vijverberg HPM, Oortgiesen M, Cahalan MD. Voltage-gated and Ca^{2+}-activated K$^+$ channels in intact human T lymphocytes: noninvasive measurements of membrane currents, membrane potential, and intracellular calcium. *J Gen Physiol* 1995;105:765–794.
28. Kim SY, Silver MR, DeCoursey TE. I. Ion channels in human THP-1 monocytes. *J Membr Biol* 1996;152:117–130.
29. McKinney LC, Gallin EK. G-protein activators induce a potassium conductance in murine macrophages. *J Membr Biol* 1992;130:265–276.
30. McCloskey MA, Cahalan MD. G protein control of potassium channel activity in a mast cell line. *J Gen Physiol* 1990;95:205–227.
31. Fan Y, McCloskey MA. Dual pathways for GTP-dependent regulation of chemoattractant-activated K$^+$ conductance in murine J774 macrophages. *J Biol Chem* 1994;269:31533–31543.
32. Qian YX, McCloskey MA. Activation of mast cell K$^+$ channels through multiple G protein–linked receptors. *Proc Natl Acad Sci USA* 1993;90:7844–7848.
33. Cherny VV, Markin VS, DeCoursey TE. The voltage-activated hydrogen ion conductance in rat alveolar epithelial cells is determined by the pH gradient. *J Gen Physiol* 1995;105:861–896.
34. DeCoursey TE, Cherny VV. Deuterium isotope effects on voltage-activated proton channels in rat alveolar epithelium. *J Gen Physiol* 1997;109:415–434.
35. DeCoursey TE, Cherny VV. Potential, pH, and arachidonate gate hydrogen ion currents in human neutrophils. *Biophys J* 1993;65:1590–1598.
36. DeCoursey TE, Cherny VV. II. Voltage-activated proton currents in human THP-1 monocytes. *J Membr Biol* 1996;152:131–140.
37. Kapus A, Romanek R, Qu AY, Rotstein OD, Grinstein S. A pH-sensitive and voltage-dependent proton conductance in the plasma membrane of macrophages. *J Gen Physiol* 1993;102:729–760.
38. Byerly L, Suen Y. Characterization of proton currents in neurones of the snail, *Lymnaea stagnalis*. *J Physiol* 1989;413:75–89.
39. DeCoursey TE, Cherny VV. Na$^+$/H$^+$-antiport detected through hydrogen ion currents in rat alveolar epithelial cells and human neutrophils. *J Gen Physiol* 1994;103:755–785.
40. DeCoursey TE, Cherny VV. Effects of buffer concentration on voltage-gated H$^+$ currents: does diffusion limit the conductance? *Biophys J* 1996;71:182–193.
41. Nagle JF, Morowitz HJ. Molecular mechanisms for proton transport in membranes. *Proc Natl Acad Sci USA* 1978;75:298–302.
42. Lewis RS, Cahalan MD. Mitogen-induced oscillations of cytosolic Ca^{2+} and transmembrane Ca^{2+} current in human leukemic T cells. *Cell Regul* 1989;1:99–112.
43. Zweifach A, Lewis RS. Mitogen-regulated Ca^{2+} current of T lymphocytes is activated by depletion of intracellular Ca^{2+} stores. *Proc Natl Acad Sci USA* 1993;90:6295–6299.
44. Somasundaram B, Mahaut-Smith MP, Floto RA. Temperature-dependent block of capacitative Ca^{2+} influx in the human leukemic cell line KU-812. *J Biol Chem* 1996;271:26096–26104.
45. Lepple-Wienhues A, Cahalan MD. Conductance and permeation of monovalent cations through depletion-activated Ca^{2+} channels (I$_{CRAC}$) in Jurkat cells. *Biophys J* 1996;71:787–794.
46. Premack BA, McDonald TV, Gardner P. Activation of Ca^{2+} current in Jurkat T cells following the depletion of Ca^{2+} stores by microsomal Ca^{2+}-ATPase inhibitors. *J Immunol* 1994;152:5226–5240.
47. Neher E. The influence of intracellular calcium concentration on degranulation of dialysed mast cells from rat peritoneum. *J Physiol* 1988;395:193–214.
48. Zweifach A, Lewis RS. Calcium-dependent potentiation of store-oper-

ated calcium channels in T lymphocytes. *J Gen Physiol* 1996;107: 597–610.

49. Zweifach A, Lewis RS. Slow calcium-dependent inactivation of depletion-activated calcium current: store-dependent and-independent mechanisms. *J Biol Chem* 1995;270:14445–14451.

50. Dolmetsch RE, Lewis RS. Signaling between intracellular Ca^{2+} stores and depletion-activated Ca^{2+} channels generates $[Ca^{2+}]_i$ oscillations in T lymphocytes. *J Gen Physiol* 1994;103:365–388.

51. Matthews G, Neher E, Penner R. Chloride conductance activated by external agonists and internal messengers in rat peritoneal mast cells. *J Physiol* 1989;418:131–144.

52. Cahalan MD, Lewis RS. Role of potassium and chloride channels in volume regulation by T lymphocytes. In: Gunn RB, Parker JC, eds. *Cell physiology of blood*. New York: Rockefeller University Press, 1988:281–301.

53. Lewis RS, Ross PE, Cahalan MD. Chloride channels activated by osmotic stress in T lymphocytes. *J Gen Physiol* 1993;101:801–826.

54. Schumacher PA, Sakellaropoulos G, Phipps DJ, Schlichter LC. Small-conductance chloride channels in human peripheral T lymphocytes. *J Membr Biol* 1995;145:217–232.

55. Simchowitz L, Textor JA, Cragoe ED. Cell volume regulation in human neutrophils: 2-(aminomethyl)phenols as Cl^- channel inhibitors. *Am J Physiol* 1993;265:C143–C155.

56. Dubois JM, Rouzaire-Dubois B. Role of potassium channels in mitogenesis. *Prog Biophys Mol Biol* 1993;59:1–21.

57. Gallin EK. Ion channels in leukocytes. *Physiol Rev* 1991;71:775–811.

58. Lewis RS, Cahalan MD. Potassium and calcium channels in lymphocytes. *Annu Rev Immunol* 1995;13:623–653.

59. Chandy KG, DeCoursey TE, Cahalan MD, McLaughlin C, Gupta S. Voltage-gated potassium channels are required for human T lymphocyte activation. *J Exp Med* 1984;160:369–385.

60. DeCoursey TE, Chandy KG, Gupta S, Cahalan MD. Voltage-gated K^+ channels in human T lymphocytes: a role in mitogenesis? *Nature* 1984;307:465–468.

61. DeCoursey TE, Chandy KG, Gupta S, Cahalan MD. Mitogenic induction of ion channels in murine T lymphocytes. *J Gen Physiol* 1987;89: 405–420.

62. Amigorena S, Choquet D, Teillaud JL, Korn H, Fridman WH. Ion channel blockers inhibit B cell activation at a precise stage of the G1 phase of the cell cycle. *J Immunol* 1990;144:2038–2045.

63. Slaughter RS, Garcia ML, Kaczorowski GJ. Ion channels as drug targets in the immune system. *Curr Pharm Design* 1996;2:610–623.

64. Lin CS, Boltz RC, Blake JT, et al. Voltage-gated potassium channels regulate calcium-dependent pathways involved in human T lymphocyte activation. *J Exp Med* 1993;177:637–645.

65. Price M, Lee SC, Deutsch C. Charybdotoxin inhibits proliferation and interleukin 2 production in human peripheral blood lymphocytes. *Proc Natl Acad Sci USA* 1989;86:10171–10175.

66. Rader RK, Kahn LE, Anderson GD, Martin CL, Chinn KS, Gregory SA. T cell activation is regulated by voltage-dependent and Ca^{2+}-activated K^+ channels. *J Immunol* 1996;156:1425–1430.

67. Verheugen JAH, Le Deist F, Devignot V, Korn H. Enhancement of calcium signaling and proliferation responses in activated human T lymphocytes: inhibitory effects of K^+ channel block by charybdotoxin depend on the T cell activation state. *Cell Calcium* 1997;21:1–17.

68. Grinstein S, Smith JD. Calcium-independent cell volume regulation in human lymphocytes. *J Gen Physiol* 1990;95:97–120.

69. Leonard RJ, Garcia ML, Slaughter RS, Reuben JP. Selective blockers of voltage-gated K^+ channels depolarize human T lymphocytes: mechanism of the antiproliferative effect of charybdotoxin. *Proc Natl Acad Sci USA* 1992;89:10094–10098.

70. Freedman BD, Price MA, Deutsch CJ. Evidence for voltage modulation of IL-2 production in mitogen-stimulated human peripheral blood lymphocytes. *J Immunol* 1992;149:3784–3794.

71. Gelfand EW, Cheung RK, Grinstein S. Role of membrane potential in the regulation of lectin-induced calcium uptake. *J Cell Physiol* 1984; 121:533–539.

72. DeCoursey TE, Chandy KG, Gupta S, Cahalan MD. Voltage-dependent ion channels in T-lymphocytes. *J Neuroimmunol* 1985;10:71–95.

73. Metcalf JC, Pozzan T, Smith GA, Hesketh TR. A calcium hypothesis for the control of cell growth. *Biochem Soc Symp* 1980;45:1–26.

74. Tsien RY, Pozzan T, Rink TJ. T-cell mitogens cause early changes in cytoplasmic free Ca^{2+} and membrane potential in lymphocytes. *Nature* 1982;295:68–71.

75. Oettgen HC, Terhorst C, Cantley LC, Rosoff PM. Stimulation of the T3-T cell receptor complex induces a membrane-potential-sensitive calcium influx. *Cell* 1985;40:583–590.

76. Attali B, Romey G, Honore E, et al. Cloning, functional expression, and regulation of two K^+ channels in human T lymphocytes. *J Biol Chem* 1992;267:8650–8657.

77. Mahaut-Smith MP, Mason MJ. Ca^{2+}-activated K^+ channels in rat thymic lymphocytes: activation by concanavalin A. *J Physiol* 1991; 439:513–528.

78. Nguyen A, Kath JC, Hanson DC, et al. Novel nonpeptide agents potently block the C-type inactivated conformation of Kv1.3 and suppress T cell activation. *Mol Pharmacol* 1996;50:1672–1679.

79. Partiseti M, Le Deist F, Hivroz C, Fischer A, Korn H, Choquet D. The calcium current activated by T cell receptor and store depletion in human lymphocytes is absent in a primary immunodeficiency. *J Biol Chem* 1994;69:32327–32335.

80. Wonderlin WF, Strobl JS. Potassium channels, proliferation and G1 progression. *J Membr Biol* 1996;154:91–107.

81. Pappas CA, Ullrich N, Sontheimer H. Reduction of glial proliferation by K^+ channel blockers is mediated by changes in pH$_i$. *Neuroreports* 1994;6:193–196.

82. Phipps DJ, Branch DR, Schlichter LC. Chloride-channel block inhibits T lymphocyte activation and signalling. *Cell Signal* 1996;8: 141–149.

83. Schlichter LC, Sakellaropoulos G, Ballyk B, Pennefather PS, Phipps DJ. Properties of K^+ and Cl^- channels and their involvement in proliferation of rat microglial cells. *Glia* 1996;17:225–236.

84. Schlichter LC, Sidell N, Hagiwara S. Potassium channels mediate killing by human natural killer cells. *Proc Natl Acad Sci USA* 1986;83: 451–455.

85. Deutsch C, Lee SC. Cell volume regulation in lymphocytes. *Ren Physiol Biochem* 1988;35:260–276.

86. Grinstein S, Foskett JK. Ionic mechanisms of cell volume regulation in leukocytes. *Annu Rev Physiol* 1990;52:399–414.

87. Lee SC, Price M, Prystowsky MB, Deutsch C. Volume response of quiescent and interleukin 2–stimulated T-lymphocytes to hypotonicity. *Am J Physiol* 1988;254:C286–C296.

88. Deutsch C, Chen LQ. Heterologous expression of specific K^+ channels in T lymphocytes: functional consequences for volume regulation. *Proc Natl Acad Sci USA* 1993;90:10036–10040.

89. Shapiro MS, DeCoursey TE. Two types of potassium channels in a lymphoma cell line. *Biophys J* 1988;53:550a.

90. Grissmer S, Cahalan MD, Chandy KG. Abundant expression of type *l* K^+ channels. *J Immunol* 1988;141:1137–1142.

91. Grissmer S, Hanson DC, Natoli EJ, Cahalan MD, Chandy KG. CD4⁻CD8⁻ T cells from mice with collagen arthritis display aberrant expression of type *l* K^+ channels. *J Immunol* 1990;145:2105–2109.

92. Gallin EK, Livengood DR. Inward rectification in mouse macrophages: evidence for a negative resistance region. *Am J Physiol* 1981; 241:C9–C17.

93. Randriamampita C, Trautmann A. Ionic channels in murine macrophages. *J Cell Biol* 1987;105:761–769.

94. McKinney LC, Gallin EK. Effect of adherence, cell morphology, and lipopolysaccharide on potassium conductance and passive membrane properties of murine macrophage J774.1 cells. *J Membr Biol* 1990; 116:47–56.

95. Shirihai O, Merchav S, Attali B, Dagan D. K^+ channel antisense oligodeoxynucleotides inhibit cytokine-induced expansion of human hemopoietic progenitors. *Pflügers Arch* 1996;431:632–638.

96. Gallin EK. Voltage clamp studies in macrophages from mouse spleen cultures. *Science* 1981;214:458–460.

97. Gallin EK. Calcium and voltage activated potassium channels in human macrophages. *Biophys J* 1984;46:821–825.

98. Gallin EK. Evidence for a Ca-activated inwardly rectifying K channel in human macrophages. *Am J Physiol* 1989;257:C77–C85.

99. Gallin EK, Gallin JI. Interaction of chemotactic factors with human macrophages: induction of transmembrane potential changes. *J Cell Biol* 1977;75:277–289.

100. Gallin EK, McKinney LC. Patch-clamp studies in human macrophages: single-channel and whole-cell characterization of two K^+ conductances. *J Membr Biol* 1988;103:55–66.

101. Gallin EK, Wiederhold ML, Lipsky PE, Rosenthal AS. Spontaneous and induced membrane hyperpolarizations in macrophages. *J Cell Physiol* 1975;86:653–662.

102. Ince C, Van Duijn B, Ypey DL, Van Bavel E, Weidema F, Leijh PCJ. Ionic channels and membrane hyperpolarization in human macrophages. *J Membr Biol* 1987;97:251–258.

103. Floto RA, Somasundaram B, Allen JM, Mahaut-Smith MP. Fcγ receptor I activation triggers a novel Ca^{2+}-activated current selective for monovalent cations in the human monocytic cell line, U937. *J Biol Chem* 1997;272:4753–4758.

104. DeCoursey TE, Cherny VV. Voltage-activated hydrogen ion currents. *J Membr Biol* 1994;141:203–223.

105. Lukacs GL, Kapus A, Nanda A, Romanek R, Grinstein S. Proton conductance of the plasma membrane: properties, regulation, and functional role. *Am J Physiol* 1993;265:C3–C14.

106. Eder C, Fischer HG, Hadding U, Heinemann U. Properties of voltage-gated currents of microglia developed using macrophage colony-stimulating factor. *Pflügers Arch* 1995;430:526–533.

107. Visentin S, Agresti C, Patrizio M, Levi G. Ion channels in rat microglia and their different sensitivity to lipopolysaccharide and interferon-γ. *J Neurosci Res* 1995;42:439–451.

108. Nordström T, Rotstein OD, Romanek R, et al. Regulation of cytoplasmic pH in osteoclasts: contribution of proton pumps and a proton-selective conductance. *J Biol Chem* 1995;270:2203–2212.

109. Streit WJ, Kincaid-Colton CA. The brain's immune system. *Sci Am* 1995;273:54–61.

110. Brockhaus J, Ilschner S, Banati RB, Kettenmann H. Membrane properties of ameboid microglial cells in the corpus callosum slice from early postnatal mice. *J Neurosci* 1993;13:4412–4421.

111. Kettenmann H, Hoppe D, Gottmann K, Banati R, Kreutzberg G. Cultured microglial cells have a distinct pattern of membrane channels different from peritoneal macrophages. *J Neurosci Res* 1990;26:278–287.

112. Nörenberg W, Gebicke-Haerter PJ, Illes P. Inflammatory stimuli induce a new K$^+$ outward current in cultured rat microglia. *Neurosci Lett* 1992;147:171–174.

113. Eder C, Fischer HG, Hadding U, Heinemann U. Properties of voltage-gated potassium currents of microglia differentiated with granulocyte/macrophage colony-stimulating factor. *J Membr Biol* 1995;147:137–147.

114. Eder C, Klee R, Heinemann U. Pharmacological properties of Ca^{2+}-activated K$^+$ currents of ramified murine brain macrophages. *Naunyn Schmiedebergs Arch Pharmacol* 1997;356:233–239.

115. Fischer HG, Eder C, Hadding U, Heinemann U. Cytokine-dependent K$^+$ channel profile of microglia at immunologically defined functional states. *Neuroscience* 1995;64:183–191.

116. Korotzer AR, Cotman CW. Voltage-gated currents expressed by rat microglia in culture. Glia 1992;6:81–88.

117. Sievers J, Schmidtmayer J, Parwaresch R. Blood monocytes and spleen macrophages differentiate into microglia-like cells when cultured on astrocytes. *Ann Anat* 1994;176:45–51.

118. Eder C, Klee R, Heinemann U. Distinct soluble astrocytic factors induce expression of outward K$^+$ currents and ramification of brain macrophages. *Neurosci Lett* 1997;226:147–150.

119. Decker K, Dieter P. The stimulus-activated Na$^+$/H$^+$ exchange in macrophages, neutrophils and platelets. In: Häussinger D, ed. *pH homeostasis: mechanisms and control.* San Diego: Academic Press, 1988:79–96.

120. Grinstein S, Furuya W. Cytoplasmic pH regulation in phorbol ester-activated human neutrophils. *Am J Physiol* 1986;251:C55–C65.

121. Badwey JA, Karnovsky ML. Production of superoxide by phagocytic leukocytes: a paradigm for stimulus-response phenomena. *Curr Top Cell Regul* 1986;28:183–208.

122. Henderson LM, Chappell JB, Jones OTG. The superoxide-generating NADPH oxidase of human neutrophils is electrogenic and associated with an H$^+$ channel. *Biochem J* 1987;246:325–329.

123. Nanda A, Grinstein S. Protein kinase C activates an H$^+$ (equivalent) conductance in the plasma membrane of human neutrophils. *Proc Natl Acad Sci USA* 1991;88:10816–10820.

124. Henderson LM, Chappell JB, Jones OTG. Superoxide generation by the electrogenic NADPH oxidase of human neutrophils is limited by the movement of a compensating charge. *Biochem J* 1988;255:285–290.

125. Henderson LM, Chappell JB, Jones OTG. Internal pH changes associated with the activity of NADPH oxidase of human neutrophils: further evidence for the presence of an H$^+$ conducting channel. *Biochem J* 1988;251:563–567.

126. Kapus A, Romanek R, Grinstein S. Arachidonic acid stimulates the plasma membrane H$^+$ conductance of macrophages. *J Biol Chem* 1994;269:4736–4745.

127. Kapus A, Susztak K, Ligeti E. Regulation of the electrogenic H$^+$ channel in the plasma membrane of neutrophils: possible role of phospholipase A$_2$, internal and external protons. *Biochem J* 1993;292:445–450.

128. Badwey JA, Curnutte JT, Karnovsky ML. *Cis*-polyunsaturated fatty acids induce high levels of superoxide production by human neutrophils. *J Biol Chem* 1981;256:12640–12643.

129. Bromberg Y, Pick E. Unsaturated fatty acids as second messengers of superoxide generation by macrophages. *Cell Immunol* 1983;79:240–252.

130. Kakinuma K. Effects of fatty acids on the oxidative metabolism of leukocytes. *Biochim Biophys Acta* 1974;348:76–85.

131. Henderson LM, Chappell JB. The NADPH-oxidase-associated H$^+$ channel is opened by arachidonate. *Biochem J* 1992;283:171–175.

132. Gordienko DV, Tare M, Parveen S, Fenech CJ, Robinson C, Bolton TB. Voltage-activated proton current in eosinophils from human blood. *J Physiol* 1996;496:299–316.

133. Nasmith PE, Grinstein S. Impairment of Na$^+$/H$^+$-exchange underlies inhibitory effects of Na$^+$-free media on leukocyte function. *FEBS Lett* 1986;202:79–85.

134. Simchowitz L. Intracellular pH modulates the generation of superoxide radicals by human neutrophils. *J Clin Invest* 1985;76:1079–1089.

135. Clark RA. The human neutrophil respiratory burst oxidase. *J Infect Dis* 1990;161:1140–1147.

136. Forman HJ, Kim E. Inhibition by linoleic acid hydroperoxide of alveolar macrophage superoxide production: effects upon mitochondrial and plasma membrane potentials. *Arch Biochem Biophys* 1989;274:443–452.

137. Martin MA, Nauseef WM, Clark RA. Depolarization blunts the oxidative burst of human neutrophils: parallel effects of monoclonal antibodies, depolarizing buffers, and glycolytic inhibitors. *J Immunol* 1988;140:3928–3935.

138. Novak MJ, Cohen HJ. Depolarization of polymorphonuclear leukocytes by *Porphyromonas (Bacteroides) gingivalis* 381 in the absence of respiratory burst activation. *Infect Immun* 1991;59:3134–3142.

139. Swallow CJ, Grinstein S, Rotstein OD. Regulation and functional significance of cytoplasmic pH in phagocytic leukocytes. *Curr Top Membr Transp* 1990;35:227–247.

140. Qu AY, Nanda A, Curnutte JT, Grinstein S. Development of a H$^+$-selective conductance during granulocytic differentiation of HL-60 cells. *Am J Physiol* 1994;266:C1263–C1270.

141. Nanda A, Grinstein S, Curnutte JT. Abnormal activation of H$^+$ conductance in NADPH oxidase-defective neutrophils. *Proc Natl Acad Sci USA* 1993;908:760–764.

142. Nanda A, Curnutte JT, Grinstein S. Activation of H$^+$ conductance in neutrophils requires assembly of components of the respiratory burst oxidase but not its redox function. *J Clin Invest* 1994;93:1770–1775.

143. Nanda A, Romanek R, Curnutte JT, Grinstein S. Assessment of the contribution of the cytochrome b moiety of the NADPH oxidase to the transmembrane H$^+$ conductance of leukocytes. *J Biol Chem* 1994;269:27280–27285.

144. Molski TFP, Naccache PH, Volpi M, Wolpert LM, Sha'afi RI. Specific modulation of the intracellular pH of rabbit neutrophils by chemotactic factors. *Biochem Biophys Res Commun* 1980;94:508–514.

145. Nanda A, Grinstein S. Chemoattractant-induced activation of vacuolar H$^+$ pumps and of an H$^+$-selective conductance in neutrophils. *J Cell Physiol* 1995;165:588–599.

146. Matthews G, Neher E, Penner R. Second messenger-activated calcium influx in rat peritoneal mast cells. *J Physiol* 1989;418:105–130.

147. Zhang L, McCloskey MA. Immunoglobulin E receptor-activated calcium conductance in rat mast cells. *J Physiol* 1995;483:59–66.

148. Dietrich J, Lindau M. Chloride channels in mast cells: block by DIDS and role in exocytosis. *J Gen Physiol* 1994;104:1099–1111.

149. Reinsprecht M, Rohn MH, Spadinger RJ, Pecht I, Schindler H, Romanin C. Blockade of capacitive Ca^{2+} influx by Cl$^-$ channel blockers inhibits secretion from rat mucosal-type mast cells. *Mol Pharmacol* 1995;47:1014–1020.

150. Mahaut-Smith MP, Rink TJ, Collins SC, Sage SO. Voltage-gated potassium channels and the control of membrane potential in human platelets. *J Physiol* 1990;428:723–735.

151. Somasundaram B, Mahaut-Smith MP. Three cation influx currents

activated by purinergic receptor stimulation in rat megakaryocytes. *J Physiol* 1994;480:225–231.

152. Somasundaram B, Mahaut-Smith MP. A novel monovalent cation channel activated by inositol triphosphate in the plasma membrane of rat megakaryocytes. *J Biol Chem* 1995;270:16638–16644.

153. Leven RM, Mullikin WH, Nachmias VT. Role of sodium in ADP- and thrombin-induced megakaryocyte spreading. *J Cell Biol* 1983;96:1234–1240.

154. Somasundaram B, Mason MJ, Mahaut-Smith MP. Thrombin-dependent calcium signalling in single human erythroleukaemia cells. *J Physiol* 1997;503:485–495.

155. Orlowski J, Grinstein S. Na/H exchangers of mammalian cells. *J Biol Chem* 1997;272:22373–22376.

156. Wakabayashi S, Shikegawa M, Pouyssegur J. Molecular physiology of vertebrate Na/H exchangers. *Physiol Rev* 1997;77:51–78.

157. Aronson PS. Kinetic properties of the plasma membrane Na/H exchanger. *Annu Rev Physiol* 1985;47:545–560.

158. Sardet C, Counillon L, Franchi A, Pouyssegur J. Growth factors induce phosphorylation of the Na/H antiporter. *Science* 1990;247:723–726.

159. Siffert W, Duesing R. Sodium-proton exchange and primary hypertension: an update. *Hypertension* 1995;27:649–655.

160. Fukushima T, Waddell TK, Grinstein S, Orlowski J, Downey GP. Na/H exchange activity during phagocytosis in human neutrophils. *J Cell Biol* 1996;132:1037.

161. Demaurex N, Orlowski J, Woodside M, Grinstein S. The mammalian Na^+/H^+ antiporters NHE1, NHE2 and NHE3 are electroneutral and voltage-independent but can couple to an H^+ conductance. *J Gen Physiol* 1995;106:85–111.

162. Grinstein S, Cohen S, Rothstein A. Cytoplasmic pH regulation in thymic lymphocytes by an amiloride-sensitive Na/H antiport. *J Gen Physiol* 1984;83:341–369.

163. Mills GB, Cheung RK, Grinstein S, Gelfand EW. Activation of Na/H antiport is not required for lectin-induced proliferation of human T lymphocytes. *J Immunol* 1986;136:1150–1154.

164. Prasad KV, Severini A, Kaplan JG. Sodium ion influx in proliferating lymphocytes: an early component of the mitogenic signal. *Arch Biochem Biophys* 1987;252:515–525.

165. Rosoff PM, Stein LF, Cantley LC. Phorbol esters induce differentiation in pre-B lymphocytes by enhancing Na/H exchange. *J Biol Chem* 1984;259:7056–7060.

166. Grinstein S, Rotin D, Mason MJ. Na/H exchange and growth factor induced cytosolic pH changes. Role in cellular proliferation. *Biochim Biophys Acta* 1989;988:73–97.

167. Rosoff PM, Cantley LC. Stimulation of the T3-T cell receptor associated Ca influx enhances the activity of the Na/H exchanger in a leukemic T cell line. *J Biol Chem* 1985;260:14053–14059.

168. Mills GB, Cragoe EJ, Gelfand EW, Grinstein S. Interleukin-2 induces a rapid increase in intracellular pH through activation of the Na/H antiport. *J Biol Chem* 1985;260:12500–12507.

169. Calalb MB, Stanton TH, Smith L, Cragoe EJ, Bomsztyk K. Recombinant human interleukin 1 stimulated Na/H exchange is not required for differentiation in pre-B lymphocytes. *J Biol Chem* 1987;262:3680–3684.

170. Rosoff PM, Cantley LC. Increasing the intracellular Na concentration induces differentiation in a pre-B lymphocyte cell line. *Proc Natl Acad Sci USA* 1983;80:7547–7550.

171. Li J, Eastman A. Apoptosis in an IL-2–dependent cytotoxic T cell line is associated with intracellular acidification. Role of the Na/H exchanger. *J Biol Chem* 1995;270:3203–3211.

172. Mills GB, Lee JWW, Cheung RK, Gelfand EW. Characterization of the requirements for human T cell mitogenesis by using suboptimal concentrations of phytohemagglutinin. *J Immunol* 1985;135:3087–3093.

173. Costa-Casnellie MR, Segel G, Cragoe EJ, Lichtman MA. Characterization of the Na/H exchanger during maturation of HL-60 cells induced by dimethylsulfoxide. *J Biol Chem* 1987;262:9093–9097.

174. Simchowitz L, Cragoe EJ. Intracellular acidification-induced alkali metal/H exchange in human neutrophils. *J Gen Physiol* 1987;90:737–762.

175. Grinstein S, Elder B, Furuya W. Phorbol ester-induced changes in cytoplasmic pH in neutrophils. *Am J Physiol* 1985;248:C379–C386.

176. Simchowitz L, Cragoe EJ. Regulation of human neutrophil chemotaxis by intracellular pH. *J Biol Chem* 1986;261:6492–6500.

177. Rosengren S, Henson PM, Worthen GS. Migration-associated volume changes in neutrophils facilitate the migratory process *in vitro*. *Am J Physiol* 1994;267:C1623–C1632.

178. Rotstein OD, Houston K, Grinstein S. Control of cytoplasmic pH by Na/H exchange in rat peritoneal macrophages activated with phorbol ester. *FEBS Lett* 1987;215:223–227.

179. Vairo G, Argyriou S, Bordun M, Gonda TJ, Cragoe EJ, Hamilton JH. Na/H exchange involvement in colony-stimulating factor 1–stimulated macrophage proliferation. *J Biol Chem* 1990;265:16929–16939.

180. Alvarez J, Garcia-Sancho J, Mollinedo F, Sanchez A. Intracellular Ca potentiates Na/H exchange and cell differentiation induced by phorbol esters in U937 cells. *Eur J Biochem* 1989;183:709–714.

181. Ladoux A, Krawice I, Cragoe EJ, Abita JP, Frelin C. Properties of the Na-dependent chloride-bicarbonate exchange system in U937 human leukemic cells. *Eur J Biochem* 1987;170:43–39.

182. Bidani A, Brown SES, Heming TH. pHi regulation in alveolar macrophages: relative roles of Na^+-H^+-antiport and H^+-ATPase. *Am J Physiol* 1994;259:C586–C598.

183. Murphy JK, Forman HJ. Effects of sodium and proton pump activity on respiratory burst and pH regulation of rat alveolar macrophages. *Am J Physiol* 1993;264:L523–L532.

184. Alper SL. The band 3–related anion exchanger (AE) gene family. *Annu Rev Physiol* 1992;53:549–564.

185. Jennings ML. Structure and function of the red cell anion transport protein. *Annu Rev Biophys Chem* 1989;18:397–430.

186. Reutz S, Lindsey AE, Kopito RR. Function and biosynthesis of erythroid and noneurythroid anion exchangers. In: Reuss L, Russell J, Jennings ML, eds. *Molecular biology of carrier proteins.* New York: Rockefeller University Press, 1992.

187. Grinstein S, Dixon SJ. Ion transport, membrane potential and cytoplasmic pH in lymphocytes: changes during activation. *Physiol Rev* 1989;69:417–481.

188. Garcia-Soto JJ, Grinstein S. Determinants of the transmembrane distribution of chloride in rat lymphocytes: role of chloride-bicarbonate exchange. *Am J Physiol* 1990;258:C1108–C1116.

189. Restrepo D, Kozody DJ, Spinelli LJ, Knauf PA. pH homeostasis in promyelocytic leukemic HL60 cells. *J Gen Physiol* 1988;92:489–507.

190. Simchowitz L, de Weer P. Chloride movements in human neutrophils: diffusion, exchange and active transport. *J Gen Physiol* 1986;88:167–194.

191. Simchowitz L, Davies AO. Internal alkalinization by reversal of anion exchange in human neutrophils: regulation of transport by pH. *Am J Physiol* 1991;260:C132–C142.

192. Shimizu Y, Daniels RH, Finnen MJ, Hill M, Lackie JM. Agonist stimulated Cl efflux from human neutrophils. *Biochem Pharmacol* 1993;45:1743–1751.

193. Vallance SJ, Downes CP, Cragoe EJ, Whetton AD. Granulocyte-macrophage colony-stimulating factor can stimulate macrophage proliferation via persistent activation of Na/H antiport. *Biochem J* 1990;265:359–364.

194. Madshus IH, Olsnes S. Selective inhibition of sodium-linked and sodium independent bicarbonate-chloride exchange. *J Biol Chem* 1987;262:7486–7491.

195. Grinstein S, Garcia-Soto JJ, Mason M. Differential role of cation and anion exchange in lymphocyte pH regulation. CIBA Symposium 139: *Proton passage across cell membranes.* London: John Wiley & Sons, 1988:70–79.

196. Ladoux A, Cragoe EJ, Geny B, Abita JP, Frelin C. Differentiation of human promyelocytic HL60 cells by retinoic acid is accompanied by an increase in the intracellular pH. *J Biol Chem* 1987;262:811–816.

197. Blaustein MP. Calcium transport and buffering in neurons. *Trends Neurosci* 1988;11:438–443.

198. Carafoli E. Intracellular calcium homeostasis. *Annu Rev Biochem* 1987;56:395–433.

199. Balasubramanyam M, Reeves JP, Gardner JP. Na/Ca exchange-mediated calcium entry in human lymphocytes. *J Clin Invest* 1994;94:2002–2008.

200. Nasmith PE, Grinstein S. Phorbol ester-induced changes in cytoplasmic calcium in human neutrophils. *J Biol Chem* 1987;262:13558–13566.

201. Volpi M, Naccache PH, Sha'afi RI. Calcium transport in inside-out membrane vesicles prepared from rabbit neutrophils. *J Biol Chem* 1983;258:4153–4158.

202. Simchowitz L, Cragoe EJ. Na-Ca exchange in human neutrophils. *Am J Physiol* 1988;254:C150–C164.

203. Simchowitz L, Foy MA, Cragoe EL. A role for Na/Ca exchange in the generation of superoxide radicals by human neutrophils. *J Biol Chem* 1990;265:13449–13456.

204. Galli C, Hannaert P, Soler A, Garay R. A study of the interaction between the Na-K pump and Na-Ca exchange in macrophages and vascular smooth muscle cells. *Am J Hypertens* 1988;1:64S-70S.

205. Haas M. Properties and diversity of Na-K-Cl cotransporters. *Annu Rev Physiol* 1989;51:443–457.

206. Altamirano AA, Breitweiser GE, Russell JM. Vanadate and fluoride effects on Na-K-Cl cotransport. *Am J Physiol* 1988;254:C582–C586.

207. Payne JA, Forbush B. Molecular characterization of the epithelial Na-K-Cl cotransporter isoforms. *Curr Opinion Cell Biol* 1995;7:493–503.

208. Senn N, Garay R. Regulation of Na and K contents in rat thymocytes. *Am J Physiol* 1989;257:C12–C18.

209. Bland RD, Boyd CAR. Cation transport in lung epithelial cells derived from fetal, newborn, and adult rabbits. *Am J Physiol* 1986;61:507–515.

210. Brossard M, Dagher G. Na fluxes in human mononuclear leucocytes. *Experientia* 1986;42:1262–1264.

211. Henderson LM, Banting G, Chappell JB. The arachidonate-activatable, NADPH oxidase-associated H^+ channel: evidence that gp91-*phox* functions as an essential part of the channel. *J Biol Chem* 1995;270:5909–5916.

212. Henderson LM, Chappell JB. NADPH oxidase of neutrophils. *Biochim Biophys Acta* 1996;1273:87–107.

213. Wientjes FB, Hsuan JJ, Totty NF, Segal AW. p40phox, a third cytosolic component of the activation complex of the NADPH oxidase to contain *src* homology 3 domains. *Biochem J* 1993;296:557–561.

214. Grissmer S, Dethlefs B, Wasmuth JJ, et al. Expression and chromosomal localization of a lymphocyte K^+ channel gene. *Proc Natl Acad Sci USA* 1990;87:9411–9415.

215. Kawa K. Voltage-gated calcium and potassium currents in megakaryocytes dissociated from guinea-pig bone marrow. *J Physiol* 1990;431:187–206.

216. Mahaut-Smith MP, Schlichter LC. Ca^{2+}-activated K^+ channels in human B lymphocytes and rat thymocytes. *J Physiol* 1989;415:69–83.

217. Maruyama Y. A patch-clamp study of mammalian platelets and their voltage-gated potassium current. *J Physiol* 1987;391:467–485.

218. Matteson DR, Deutsch C. K channels in T lymphocytes: a patch clamp study using monoclonal antibody adhesion. *Nature* 1984;307:468–471.

219. Nörenberg W, Gebicke-Haerter PJ, Illes P. Voltage-dependent potassium channels in activated rat microglia. *J Physiol* 1994;475:15–32.

220. Sands SB, Lewis RS, Cahalan MD. Charybdotoxin blocks voltage-gated K^+ channels in human and murine T lymphocytes. *J Gen Physiol* 1989;93:1061–1074.

221. Ypey DL, Clapham DE. Development of a delayed outward-rectifying K conductance in cultured mouse peritoneal macrophages. *Proc Natl Acad Sci USA* 1984;81:3083–3087.

222. Kubo Y, Baldwin TJ, Jan YN, Jan LY. Primary structure and functional expression of a mouse inward rectifier potassium channel. *Nature* 1993;362:127–133.

223. Lindau M, Fernandez JM. A patch-clamp study of histamine-secreting cells. *J Gen Physiol* 1986;88:349–368.

224. McLarnon JG, Sawyer D, Kim SU. Cation and anion unitary ion channel currents in cultured bovine microglia. *Brain Res* 1995;693:8–20.

225. Mahaut-Smith MP. Calcium-activated potassium channels in human platelets. *J Physiol* 1995;484:15–24.

226. Partiseti M, Choquet D, Diu A, Korn H. Differential regulation of voltage- and calcium-activated potassium channels in human B lymphocytes. *J Immunol* 1992;148:3361–3368.

227. Ilschner S, Nolte C, Kettenmann H. Complement factor C5a and epidermal growth factor trigger the activation of outward potassium currents in cultured murine microglia. *Neuroscience* 1996;73:1109–1120.

228. Sutro JB, Vayuvegula BS, Gupta S, Cahalan MD. Voltage-sensitive ion channels in human B lymphocytes. *Adv Exp Med Biol* 1989;254:113–122.

229. Demaurex N, Grinstein S, Jaconi M, Schlegel W, Lew DP, Krause KH. Proton currents in human granulocytes: regulation by membrane potential and intracellular pH. *J Physiol* 1993;466:329–344.

230. Demaurex N, Monod A, Lew DP, Krause KH. Characterization of receptor-mediated and store-regulated Ca^{2+} influx in human neutrophils. *Biochem J* 1994;297:595–601.

231. Hoth M, Penner R. Depletion of intracellular calcium stores activates a calcium current in mast cells. *Nature* 1992;355:353–356.

232. Maleyev A, Nelson DJ. Extracellular pH modulates the Ca^{2+} current activated by depletion of intracellular Ca^{2+} stores in human macrophages. *J Membr Biol* 1995;146:101–111.

233. Holevinsky KO, Jow F, Nelson DJ. Elevation in intracellular calcium activates both chloride and proton currents in human macrophages. *J Membr Biol* 1994;140:13–30.

234. Krause KH, Welsh MJ. Voltage-dependent and Ca^{2+}-activated ion channels in human neutrophils. *J Clin Invest* 1990;85:491–498.

235. MacKenzie AB, Mahaut-Smith MP. Chloride channels in excised membrane patches from human platelets: effect of intracellular calcium. *Biochim Biophys Acta* 1996;1278:131–136.

236. Mahaut-Smith MP. Chloride channels in human platelets: evidence for activation by internal calcium. *J Membr Biol* 1990;118:69–75.

237. Levitan I, Almonte C, Mollard P, Garber SS. Modulation of a volume-regulated chloride current by F-actin. *J Membr Biol* 1995;147:283–294.

238. Stoddard JS, Steinbach JH, Simchowitz L. Whole cell Cl^- currents in human neutrophils induced by cell swelling. *Am J Physiol* 1993;265:C156–C165.

239. McCann FV, McCarthy DC, Noelle RJ. Patch-clamp profile of ion channels in resting murine B lymphocytes. *J Membr Biol* 1990;114:175–188.

240. Pahapill PA, Schlichter LC. Cl^- channels in intact human T lymphocytes. *J Membr Biol* 1992;125:171–183.

241. Schwarze W, Kolb HA. Voltage-dependent kinetics of an anionic channel of large unit conductance in macrophages and myotube membranes. *Pflügers Arch* 1984;402:281–291.

242. Hess SD, Oortgiesen M, Cahalan MD. Calcium oscillations in human T and natural killer cells depend upon membrane potential and calcium influx. *J Immunol* 1993;150:2620–2633.

243. Chandy KG, Cahalan MD, Grissmer S. Autoimmune diseases linked to abnormal K^+ channel expression in double-negative $CD4^-CD8^-$ T cells. *Eur J Immunol* 1990;20:747–751.

244. Douglass J, Osborne PB, Cai YC, Wilkinson M, Christie MJ, Adelman JP. Characterization and functional expression of a rat genomic DNA clone encoding a lymphocyte potassium channel. *J Immunol* 1990;144:4841–4850.

245. Sardet C, Franchi A, Pouyssegur J. Molecular cloning, primary structure and expression of human growth factor-activatable Na/H antiporter. *Cell* 1989;56:271–280.

Inflammation: Basic Principles and Clinical Correlates,
3rd ed., edited by John I. Gallin and Ralph Snyderman.
Lippincott Williams & Wilkins, Philadelphia © 1999.

CHAPTER 44

Mechanical Responses of White Blood Cells

Thomas P. Stossel

CORTICAL CYTOPLASM AND LEUKOCYTE MECHANICAL RESPONSES

Locomotion, pinocytosis (endocytosis), phagocytosis, and exocytosis are mechanical responses of leukocytes because they involve movements of the plasma membrane caused by changes in the shape, resistance, or flow of the cytoplasm. Phagocytosis, locomotion, and granule movements were the first mechanical activities of leukocytes to be recognized. The descriptions of these events observed with the light microscope still form an important basis for understanding the mechanisms of these aspects of leukocyte behavior. This chapter describes the fundamental morphologic elements of leukocyte mechanics and reviews current opinions about the molecular basis of these mechanics. Many of the descriptions and molecular events germane to leukocytes are applicable to other cell types, such as amoebas, fibroblasts, epithelial cells, neuronal cells, tumor cells, and even yeasts; conversely, molecular information about other cell types, especially blood platelets, can be inferred to apply to leukocyte behavior. This area of knowledge therefore contains certain universal aspects as well as particulars which define the individuality of white blood cells. Readers are directed to review articles that address the comparative mechanical behaviors of different cell types (1–5).

Locomotion and Cortical Flow

The earliest descriptions of leukocyte movements reveal an appreciation that the leukocyte crawls rather than swims and that from its periphery extend organelle-excluding hyaline pseudopodia (often called lamellipodia) that determine direction and locomotion (Fig. 44-1).

The lamellipodia become briefly adherent to the substrate to provide the frictional force for movement. The cell body from which the pseudopod extends becomes elongated in the axis defined by the lamellar protrusion. Although adherence of the membrane to the substrate, mediated by a variety of externally disposed membrane receptors (see Chapters 41 and 45), is essential for translational locomotion, this motion requires that the adhesion be reversible, and the balance between protrusion and adhesion may determine the speed of movement of a cell (6). Sometimes the rear of the cell, which can acquire a knob-like protuberance called the uropod or simply the tail, adheres to the surface. This tail is the site where molecules on the cell membrane that have become cross-linked by various ligands migrate (cap) and are subsequently shed or internalized. Undulating waves move with the surface molecules, and this phenomenon has been called *cortical flow.*

Occasionally, as the cell moves forward, the attached tail stretches to form one or more thin strings; either motion is totally retarded by the tethered tail or else the strings (sometimes called retraction fibers) break. Most large organelles within the moving cell (e.g., the nucleus and hydrolase-containing granules) are relatively immobile, although they sometimes move anteriorly in concert with streaming of the internal cytoplasm from the rear to the front of the cell. On the other hand, relatively rapid granule movements take place just proximal to the lamellipodia (7).

With better optics it became apparent that the moving leukocyte's anterior pseudopodia are composed of a relatively broad and somewhat flattened region from which extend blebs and little spikes at the leading edge. As long as the lamellae advance, granules never come close to this leading edge. Two separate lamellipodia can transiently be splayed into different directions separated by as much as 180 degrees, as if they were in competition for pulling the cell; this situation does not persist, however,

T. P. Stossel: Hematology Division, Brigham and Women's Hospital, Boston, Massachusetts 02115.

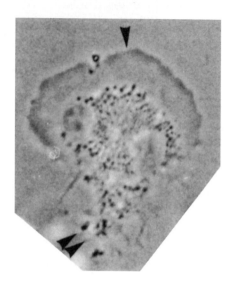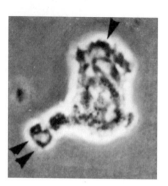

FIG. 44-1. Appearance of two crawling neutrophils photographed by phase-contrast microscopy, showing the anterior lamellae (*single arrowhead*) and the tail or uropod (*double arrowheads*) (original magnification, ×1200).

and one lamellipod or group of lamellipodia takes precedence. At this point the granules pour into the nondominant lamellipodia, which retract back to the cell body. Frequent reference has been made to a "contractile ring," a circumferential puckering of the cell surface located immediately behind the lamellipodia that forms from time to time and persists as cytoplasm moves forward through it (8).

The morphologic properties just summarized have been most frequently described in neutrophils, because of their propensity to polarize and move rapidly. Mononuclear phagocytes, especially macrophages, have a tendency to spread a completely circumferential hyaline lamella that folds upward at the edge, a process called *ruffling* (Fig. 44-2); the ruffles migrate to the cell body in a centripetal variation of the unidirectional cortical flow observed in locomoting neutrophils and lymphocytes. Macrophages also form pleats on, and extend spikes from, the nonadherent surface of the cell (9).

The dominance of the peripheral cytoplasm in light-microscopic descriptions of leukocyte movement implies, but does not prove, that this region is of primary importance to the mechanism of motility. A critical observation made by Keller and Bessis (10) and confirmed by Malawista and Boisfleury-Chevance (11) is that neutrophils heated to 40°C release lamellipodia from their cell bodies, and that these "cytokineplasts" persist in a rudimentary form of movement and even exhibit chemotaxis and phagocytosis of small particles. This discovery comes close to proving that the "motor" of leukocytes resides in the cell periphery and that events at the front of the cell are adequate for locomotion, at least under these experimental conditions. Nevertheless, as mentioned, observations of moving intact neutrophils clearly give the impression that some kind of peripheral contractile activity is squeezing the internal contents of the cell body (or of the rear of the cytokineplast) toward the leading lamella (12).

Phagocytosis, Pinocytosis (Endocytosis), Exocytosis, and Intracellular Parasitism

The peripheral cytoplasm is also of great importance in phagocytosis. This fact is particularly clear when the observer watches polymorphonuclear leukocytes migrate on a glass slide in the presence of objects they ingest (e.g., bacteria, yeast particles). The effects of molecules that

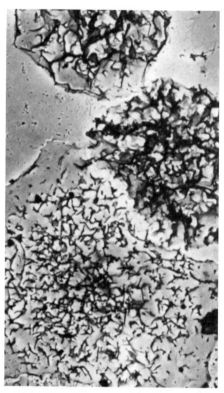

FIG. 44-2. Appearance of three spread macrophages that were rapidly frozen, rotary-shadowed with carbon-platinum, and photographed by electron microscopy, showing the peripheral spread lamellae and projecting veils on the dorsal surface of the cells (original magnification, ×3500). (Courtesy of John Hartwig.)

induce chemotaxis of leukocytes in orienting the direction of leukocyte movement, and the interactions of these molecules with receptors on phagocyte membranes, are discussed in Chapter 45. The leukocytes move toward the target particles guided by a gradient of chemotactic molecules emanating from them. The act of engulfment appears to be a variant of locomotion. The organelle-excluding, leading lamellipod surrounds an appropriately opsonized object and fuses at its distal end (8). For leukocytes in suspension or macrophages spread on a surface, the phagocytic act is more difficult to visualize by light microscopy because it is not limited to any one focal plane. However, scanning electron microscope images of leukocytes suspended with ingestible particles or of adherent macrophages ingesting particles on their free surfaces reveal the extension of a thin lamella around the object (13) although increasingly other morphological patterns of phagocytosis are being recognized (see Chapter 45). The region of the ruffled membrane of macrophages is the point of origin of "pinocytic" vesicles visible with the light microscope, and these vesicles move centripetally to the perinuclear region. In recent years the descriptive word for "cell drinking," pinocytosis, has tended to be supplanted by the more general term, *endocytosis*.

In the past, phagocytosis and endocytosis in leukocytes were thought to involve mainly the sequestration of pathogenic microorganisms and body microparts destined for destruction. It is now recognized that a subset of microorganisms, bacterial and viral, not only fail to be destroyed by leukocytes after engulfment but also use the mechanical machinery of the host leukocyte to mediate transit to other cells. By this mechanism these parasites spread while avoiding attacks from the immune system (14).

In polymorphonuclear leukocytes, granule movements become prominent at the base of the forming phagocytic vacuole, and the disappearance (degranulation) of the granules corresponds to a secretory act in which there is exocytosis of granule contents into the phagosomal vacuole (15). Because leukocytes release granule-associated enzymes into the medium during locomotion, it is possible that the movement of granules behind the advancing lamella during locomotion also represents an exocytic event. Balancing the internalization of membrane associated with endocytosis is a countertraffic of membrane vesicles; collectively, these processes account for enormous membrane turnover. This largely constitutive behavior within the cell is believed to differ mechanistically from the induced exocytosis of large granules described previously.

Agonal Events: Necrosis and Apoptosis

Under the light microscope, leukocytes that have exhibited the morphology described for a time may, especially in serum-free (i.e., growth factor–free) medium, begin to display extensive blebbing of the surface. The blebs are initially spherical and about 1 μm in diameter. Later they can become confluent and extend like sausages for impressive distances from the cell body, from which they are easily separated by minimal mechanical agitation. For the most part, the blebs continue to exclude granules, but when a granule enters the bleb it may demonstrate extensive movement that may be either saltatory or apparently Brownian in form. In such cells, which are evidently dying, internal granules may become much more mobile than in more viable leukocytes. Eventually all movements cease (9). Nowadays, the term *apoptosis* encompasses these morphologic elements of leukocyte death, which are accompanied by the sequential breakdown of DNA. Under physiologic conditions, the deteriorating leukocytes are engulfed by mononuclear phagocytes (16).

THE CYTOSKELETON, ESPECIALLY ACTIN, IN LEUKOCYTE MECHANICS

Consistency of Peripheral Cytoplasm

Aspiration (with micropipettes) of a piece of membrane with underlying cytoplasm reveals that the peripheral cytoplasm of a resting polymorphonuclear leukocyte resists initial deformation in a manner expected for an elastic or gel-like material, but on prolonged aspiration it flows. This kind of mechanical behavior is called *viscoelastic behavior*. Because the plasma membrane of the leukocyte in isotonic media has numerous folds and is believed to be a relatively delicate and fluid lipid bilayer, it is presumed to be passively deformed in such experiments and does not contribute to the measurement. Similar determinations on pseudopodia extended from activated leukocytes show them to resist deformation in a manner characteristic of a solid or a gel; however, they do not flow in response to relatively prolonged stress, suggesting that the pseudopod is more gelled than the peripheral cytoplasm of the resting cell. Similarly, the overall deformability of both phagocytes and lymphocytes diminishes (i.e., they become more rigid) when the cells are activated by chemotactic factors or mitogens, respectively (17–19). It is now accepted that the cytoskeleton, and in particular actin, accounts for the mechanical properties of leukocyte cortical cytoplasm.

Cytoskeleton

Actin filaments are the principal structures of leukocyte peripheral cytoplasm, and the total actin concentration in this region is estimated to be as high as 20 mg/mL (on the order of millimolar). Purified monomeric (G) actin forms double-helical filaments (F-actin), which morphologically appear as relatively straight rods. Actin filaments have a polarity first recognized by Hugh Huxley, who observed that proteolytically derived actin-binding fragments of myosin bind to actin filaments at an angle that produces arrowhead-like structures that are visible in the electron microscope. In muscle sarcomeres, actin filaments move against myosin filaments from the barbed to the pointed direction. As described later, the polarity of actin filaments is also manifested in actin assembly kinetics; the barbed filament ends are thought to be most important for assembly, the pointed ends for depolymerization.

About half of the total actin in leukocytes is in the form of filaments. Because of the high concentration of this protein in a filamentous form, the filaments, if sufficiently long, overlap and hinder one another's rotational movements. This impedance to filament rotational motion translates into viscoelastic behavior (20). Empiric measurements of solutions containing long, interpenetrated actin filaments (21), or else shorter actin filaments connected by agents that cross-link them (22), reveal a high rigidity, consistent with important mechanical strength imparted to the leukocyte periphery by filamentous actin.

A number of toxins that powerfully inhibit leukocyte locomotion and phagocytosis, enhance exocytosis, and cause retraction of the leukocyte cortical cytoplasm have the common biochemical effect of inhibiting actin filament assembly by a variety of mechanisms. It follows that remodeling of actin filaments, often referred to as *actin dynamics*, underlies the changes in cortical consistency and shape that are characteristic of the leukocyte functions described at the beginning of this chapter.

In contrast to the functional importance of actin and actin-associated proteins in the leukocyte peripheral cytoplasm, immunofluorescence microscopy suggests that the other known cytoskeletal protein systems, the tubulin polymers (microtubules) and the intermediate filaments (assemblies of the protein vimentin in leukocytes), are relatively few in number and are restricted to the cell body, although they penetrate the actin-rich peripheral cytoplasm to some extent (23,24). Chemicals that affect tubulin assembly (i.e., colchicine, vinblastine, or vincristine) inhibit tubulin's polymerization and cause net depolymerization of microtubules in leukocytes but do not have the profound inhibitory effects on leukocyte mechanical functions that are caused by the actin-related toxins (25). On the other hand, the centriole of leukocytes tends to orient itself on the side of the nucleus in the direction of cell migration, and it has been argued that a centriole–Golgi apparatus complex may be important for recycling of plasma membrane (26). In macrophages, microtubules and associated motor proteins influence the positioning of actin-based surface movements (27) as well as the distribution of intracellular structures called tubular lysosomes (28).

Leukocyte Actin Networks: Morphology

Almost all of the available data on the structure of filamentous actin in leukocytes is based on examinations of surface protrusions, the lamellae and finger-like extensions called filopodia (29). Almost nothing is known about the structure of actin investing the cell body of leukocytes. Based on ultrastructural morphologic findings in blood platelets, it is possible that some kind of membrane skeleton, resembling the two-dimensional lamina that invests the inner surface of erythrocytes, may be present. Biochemical studies have documented the existence of membrane skeletal proteins such as spectrin in leukocytes (where it is also designated nonerythroid spectrin or fodrin) (30,31). However, spectrin localizes to the centriole rather than to the plasma membrane in lymphocytes that have been studied (32,33). The cell body of neutrophils contains a stable population of filamentous actin, in contrast with the dynamic actin filaments in cellular protrusions (34), but its ultrastructure has not been examined. A detailed investigation of actin ultrastructure in the cell bodies of fibroblasts revealed a variety of filament bundle conformations, including bundles with filaments interdigitating with opposite polarities resembling sarcomeres and characteristic of extensively studied stress fibers. The most abundant class of bundles lies close to the cell's ventral surface and contains very long filaments oriented axially with barbed ends facing the plasma membrane, but more barbed ends extending in the direction of locomotion, a phenomenon described by the authors as "graded polarity." This system of bundles was postulated to be part of a motor system involved in cell body translocation (35).

Hartwig and Shevlin (36) examined the architecture of the lamellar cytoplasm of rabbit pulmonary macrophages that were fixed and detergent-extracted while spreading on a surface (Fig. 44-3). Both rapid freezing and critical point drying were employed in preparing the specimens for electron microscopy, to provide better reassurance that the three-dimensional structure observed was not affected by shrinkage artifacts. The authors confirmed with immunohistochemical techniques that most of the filaments in the cell cortex are actin. Using a computer-assisted morphometric technique to analyze stereo-pair electron micrographs, they determined that the actin filament concentration in the macrophage periphery was about 15 mg/mL (approximately 200 mmol/L), that the average spacing between filament overlaps was about 120 nm with a narrow distribution, and that the branch angle at filament overlaps was strongly biased toward the perpendicular. The polarity of branching was determined by decorating the actin filaments with myosin fragments. In the T-shaped branches that were predominant, the barbed ends of the actin filaments extended from the intersections where the pointed end inserted on the side of its partner. Relatively few free filament ends could be seen in these images; most were observed either attaching to the adherent surface of the lamellipod or extending upward from the free surface. Both barbed and pointed filament ends inserted into the plasma membrane.

Using a different technique, in which cells are first permeabilized and extracted and then negatively stained for viewing in the electron microscope, Small et al. saw pre-

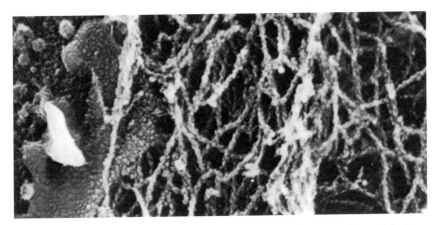

FIG. 44-3. Cortical actin gel of a rabbit lung macrophage. The membrane–actin gel interface was visualized with the use of a polylysine-coated coverslip to tear parts of the dorsal membrane from a macrophage adherent to glass. The ripped cell was incubated in a solution containing heavy meromyosin to elute intracellular soluble components and to allow the myosin fragments to bind actin filaments. Then the specimen was rapidly frozen, rotary-shadowed with tantalum-tungsten, and photographed in the electron microscope. The image reveals an orthogonal network of actin filaments, identified by the binding of heavy meromyosin to show an arrowhead configuration. Some of the actin filaments interact with the plasmalemma. The network's pores are small enough to exclude most organelles. (Photomicrograph courtesy of John Hartwig.)

dominantly long actin filaments that appeared to insert by their barbed ends into the plasma membrane at the leading edge of mouse peritoneal macrophages (37). The images agree with Hartwig and Shevlin's insofar as the filaments overlap more or less orthogonally. The two methodologic approaches may be somewhat selective, and both types of actin filament architecture may coexist. A detailed analysis of neutrophil lamellar cytoplasm has not been performed.

The ultrastructural examinations of the peripheral cytoplasm of these mononuclear leukocytes provide plausible explanations for the apparent rigidity and the organelle exclusion of the lamellipod. An orthogonal network of actin filaments with the dimensions observed could provide maximal extension of the lamellipod with an economy of mass, permitting solutes, water, and small vesicles to percolate through the network. On the other hand, the pore size of the network is sufficiently small to account for the exclusion of large organelles.

In contrast to the relatively isotropic organization of actin filaments in lamellae, actin filaments in filopodia align in parallel as bundles. Actin filament bundles have been analyzed extensively in microvilli of epithelial cells and in hairlike protrusions of many other cell types, but detailed descriptions of actin bundles in such extensions of normal leukocytes are lacking.

Leukocyte Actin Networks: Molecular Composition

Actin filaments have a marked propensity to align spontaneously into parallel bundles, especially at the high concentrations of actin in the cell. Both thermodynamic and ionic forces mediate this bundling tendency (38–41).

If actin filaments entangle sufficiently as they elongate, they can form isotropic networks because the entanglement impedes the filament rotation required for the chains to align in parallel (42). Prevention of bundle formation in short filaments, however, requires some kind of intervention by actin filament crossbridging proteins. Because actin filaments line up spontaneously, such proteins are not needed to produce alignment. Rather, they modify the way in which the filaments align or, possibly, they provide binding sites for other cellular components to associate with the actin filament system.

The high-angle branching of actin filaments observed in replicas of leukocyte cortical cytoplasm represents an extreme of crossbridging intervention. Thus far the only agent shown *in vitro* to produce the perpendicular branching of actin documented in leukocyte cortical cytoplasm is filamin-1 (ABP-280), a 540-kd homodimer composed of 280-kd subunits (43–45). The ability of this protein to effect the right-angle branching of actin is based on its large size and filamentous shape and explains its efficiency in causing a sol-to-gel transition of actin filaments of a given length. High-angle junctions minimize the opportunity for redundant crosslinks to accumulate between adjacent filaments. The actin gel composed of actin and filamin-1 could be rigid at the concentrations of these reagents that are estimated to exist in cortical cytoplasm, and experimental studies of the mechanical properties of reconstituted filamin-1–actin gels support this prediction (22). A molecule closely related to filamin-1, first isolated from smooth muscle, is filamin-2. Filamin is almost identical to filamin-1 in its amino acid sequence except that it lacks an insert known as a hinge near the carboxyl terminus (43,46). This difference may be sufficient to render filamin less efficient than filamin-1 in actin gelation (47). In addition, whereas filamin-1 is encoded by a gene on the X chromosome in humans, the filamin-2 gene resides on chromosome 7 (48–50). Although filamin has a more restricted tissue distribution than filamin-1, it is possible that these molecules coexist in the same cell types.

Strong evidence for the role of filamin-1 in creating the orthogonal actin network of leukocyte peripheral cytoplasm emerges from the identification of human malignant melanoma cell lines that fail to express filamin-1 mRNA or protein. These cells are very defective in translational locomotion, and they have unstable cortices that bleb constitutively in response to growth factors; their actin filaments form loose bundles but not orthogonal networks. Restoration of filamin-1 expression by genetic transfection yielded cell lines with stable membranes and repaired chemotactic responsiveness (51).

Another actin filament crosslinking agent identified in leukocytes, α-actinin, binds to F-actin with an affinity equivalent to that of filamin-1 (about 10^7 mol/L^{-1}) and joins the actin filaments side-to-side as loose bundles. α-Actinin is a short (100 nm) rod that, based on electron micrograph findings, binds to the sides of adjacent actin filaments to cross-link them. α-Actinin is inefficient in producing a sol-to-gel transformation of actin filaments *in vitro* compared with ABP at 37°C, as would be expected for low-angle cross-linking (52). There is as much α-actinin as filamin-1 in the leukocyte (about 1% of the total cell protein), and it is reasonable to conclude that α-actinin may stabilize points where actin filaments are observed to align in parallel in the cortical cytoplasm. An interesting feature of leukocyte and some other nonmuscle-cell α-actinins is that micromolar calcium concentrations decrease their ability to bind F-actin by about 2 orders of magnitude (52).

A third class of actin filament crosslinking protein identified in leukocytes is another rodlike protein variously named fimbrin and L-plastin—the "L" designating an isoform of this protein found in leukocytes as opposed to epithelial or tumor cells. L-plastin promotes stabilization of actin filament bundles, and calcium reportedly inhibits this bundle formation (53–55). L-plastin becomes phosphorylated within cells, although the functional consequences of this phosphorylation are unknown. Plastin phosphorylation takes place during Fc-mediated phagocytosis implying a role for this protein in that mechanical function (56).

REMODELING OF LEUKOCYTE ACTIN NETWORKS

Assembly of Actin *In Vitro*

To discuss the assembly of actin, it is first necessary to summarize briefly some information concerning its poly-merization into linear filaments which then are organized into different types of three-dimensional structures by actin filament bridging proteins. Actin is a highly conserved molecule. Although vertebrates possess several genes encoding actin, the proteins produced differ only slightly in primary structure, principally at the level of a few charged amino acids at the amino terminus of the molecule. Leukocytes contain two of these gene products, typical for nonmuscle cells, which are designated β and γ based on their isoelectric points and are present in cytoplasm in molar ratios of about 5:1 respectively (57). Although the reasons are not currently known, cell-specific isoforms appear not to be replaceable by other isoforms, despite the limited differences between them (58).

Pure monomeric actin is a slightly asymmetric, globular protein of relative molecular mass (M_r) 42,500 which, in the presence of neutral salts, spontaneously assembles to form the double-helical actin filament. A rate-limiting step in this assembly, first observed by Fumio Oosawa, is the formation of a nucleus composed of two or three monomers. The presence of preexisting actin nuclei, filaments, or other agents that substitute as nuclei can have an important effect on the kinetics of actin assembly. At the completion of polymerization from monomers, the monomers continue to exchange with the ends of filaments that have a large and exponential length distribution, ranging from a few that are many microns long to many that comprise only a few monomers (59).

The concentration of actin monomers is one important determinant of the assembly process. As in any bimolecular reaction, the rate of assembly is influenced by the concentration of the reactants and by the association and dissociation rate constants. In the case of actin, these constants are different for the opposite ends of actin nuclei or filaments. This difference in rate constants is one of several examples of the polarity of the actin filament.

In the case of actin assembly, the barbed filament end (with respect to the actin-decorating myosin arrowheads) has association and dissociation rate constants that are about 30 times faster than those of the pointed ends. Therefore, under steady-state conditions, actin monomers exchange with the two ends of filaments at different rates. In addition, the concentration of G actin in dynamic equilibrium with actin filaments (called the critical monomer concentration) is about 15 times lower for the barbed filament end than for the pointed filament end. Because exchange is so much faster at the barbed end, the critical concentration of pure actins is essentially that of the barbed end. Under ionic conditions believed to be reasonably physiologic, this concentration is about 0.1 μmol/L. In this circumstance the rate of addition of actin monomers to the barbed filament end is about 20 monomers per micromolar actin monomer concentration per second, and the off-rate is about 2 per second. Because one of the most prominent effects of the cytochalasins and of *Clostridium botulinum* iota and C toxins on actin *in vitro* is to bind the barbed filament ends and block exchange of actin monomers with that end (cytochalasins do this directly, whereas the bacterial toxins convert monomeric actin into an end-blocking species), it is apparent why these agents have the effect of inhibiting actin assembly from monomers and reducing the steady-state F-actin concentration.

The absolute values for these rate constants and critical concentrations vary depending on the temperature, the salt conditions, and the concentrations of other ambient metabolites. For example, as first inferred by Albrecht Wegner in the early 1970s, monomeric actin has a different conformation depending on whether it binds an adenosine triphosphate (ATP) molecule (G-ATP actin) or an adenosine diphosphate (ADP) molecule (G-ADP actin). ATP in G-ATP actin becomes hydrolyzed to ADP during assembly (F-ADP actin). When a monomer dissociates from F-actin, it exchanges its ADP for ATP, provided that ATP is present in the medium. Actin, therefore, may account for a high fraction of cellular ATP turnover. Depending on the rates of assembly and depolymerization, ATP hydrolysis and ATP-ADP exchange may or may not be kinetically coupled to the assembly. Therefore G-ATP actin may coexist with F-ATP actin or with F-ADP actin, depending on the conditions. The affinity of G-ATP actin for F-ATP actin is lower than that of G-ATP actin for F-ADP actin and much lower than that of G-ADP actin for F-ADP actin. It is therefore apparent that adenine nucleotides can play an important role in regulating the polarity of assembly of actin, and it is ATP binding, hydrolysis, and ADP-ATP exchange that account for the different assembly kinetic properties of the opposite ends of actin filaments (59).

Remodeling of Actin in Leukocytes

In the resting leukocyte, about half of the total actin is in the form of filaments, which remain in a cellular "cytoskeleton" when leukocytes are subjected to detergent solubilization of their membranes. The rest is in the form of monomers or small oligomers that are extracted along with other "soluble" proteins by detergent treatment. The fraction of polymerized actin in a cell can also be detected by reacting fixed and permeabilized cells with fluorescently labeled phallotoxin, a mushroom alkaloid that binds polymeric, but not monomeric, actin (60,61). When neutrophils are stimulated by addition of a number of other agonists that induce morphologic changes in the cell, the fraction of cytoskeletal actin, measured by either technique, transiently rises, the kinetics of the change depending on the nature of the stimulus. When leukocytes undergo active locomotion or other motile functions, the net amount of polymerized actin may not be different from at baseline; however, because of active remodeling, the turnover of actin between network and diffusible states, between linear polymers and monomers, may be increased over the basal rate (62).

Because the total actin concentration in the peripheral cytoplasm is on the order of 400 μmol/L, all but a tiny fraction (0.1 μmol/L) ought to be polymerized based on the critical concentration of pure actin under ionic, thermal, and metabolic conditions thought to exist in the cytoplasm of a resting leukocyte. Furthermore, the length distribution of actin filaments in cytoplasm is not the broad exponential range characteristic of actin filaments assembled from pure monomers. The assembly of actin in the leukocyte therefore must be regulated to keep so much of the actin unpolymerized in resting cells, to maintain a relatively uniform actin filament length distribution, and to allow for rapid polymerization and depolymerization of actin in response to stimulation. There are two theoretical approaches to describing this regulation. In one, a molecule alters actin monomers to prevent their nucleation or exchange onto filaments. In the other, molecules bind the ends of filaments to prevent monomer addition or loss. Both mechanisms seem to be active in leukocytes.

LEUKOCYTE PROTEINS REGULATING ACTIN POLYMERIZATION

Protein controls on actin polymerization are depicted in Figure 44-4).

Monomer Sequestration

A very basic protein (isoelectric point, 9.2; M_r, 20,000), originally isolated from spleen by Lindberg et al. and named profilin, was reported to bind actin monomers tightly and render them unpolymerizable, accounting for the large amount of unpolymerized actin in nonmuscle cells. Profilins have subsequently been purified from many cell types, including leukocytes, and two isoforms encoded

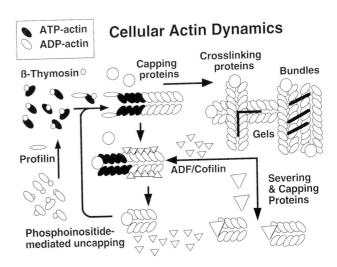

FIG. 44-4. Control of leukocyte actin assembly by proteins affecting actin monomer sequestration, actin barbed-end filament exchange, severing, and accelerated depolymerization of actin filaments in relation to transmembrane signaling.

by different genes have been identified. Nachmias identified a polymorphic set of heat-stable small polypeptides, the β thymosins (M_r, 5,000) with monomeric actin-binding properties. Thymosins are present in cells at concentrations of 0.4 μmol/L and are therefore considered most relevant for actin monomer sequestration *in vivo* (59).

The original concept of sequestration considered that actin subunits tightly complexed to profilin would not be competent to assemble until some form of cellular regulation dissociated the complexes. Experiments designed to understand this regulation led Lindberg to another important principle concerning cellular actin remodeling, namely that D_4 phosphoinositides (ppIs), a class of membrane lipids implicated in various aspects of cellular signal transduction, might control actin assembly (D_4 indicates a phosphate atom on the 4-position of the inositol ring). Phosphatidylinositol-4-phosphate (PIP) and phosphatidylinositol 4,5-bisphosphate (PIP$_2$) lower the affinity of both profilin isoforms for actin (59,63). Lindberg's notion was that ppIs could desequester actin from profilin, enabling its nucleation and its elongation onto the barbed ends of actin filaments.

Current views about control of cellular actin remodeling, although by no means unanimous, are somewhat different from these early ideas about profilin (64–66). Most researchers agree that the β thymosins prevent the spontaneous nucleation of monomeric actin and that control of this sequestration resides in other molecules. However, the affinity of the major thymosin isoform, β$_4$, for G-ATP actin is higher than for G-ADP actin, although neither state of G actin spontaneously nucleates well in the presence of β$_4$ thymosin. Neither G-ADP actin nor G-ATP actin remains sequestered by thymosins in the presence of actin filament barbed ends, which have higher affinities for the monomers than the sequestering agent. Because half of the actin in cells is polymerized, there should be plenty of barbed filament ends to soak up actin monomers. If, on the other hand, the barbed actin filament ends were blockaded, thymosin could inhibit spontaneous nucleation, and regulated uncapping of actin filament barbed ends could determine sites and times of actin filament assembly in the cell (67). As discussed later, there is considerable evidence that actin filament assembly is controlled at the level of capping of actin filament barbed ends. A prevalent view, moreover, is that profilin's principal role in the cell is not to sequester monomeric actin but to catalyze exchange between ADP- and ATP-monomeric actin, and to deliver ATP-monomers to the barbed ends of actin filaments. In the presence of free actin filament barbed ends, profilin reportedly accelerates actin filament assembly (67).

The ability of leukocytes to keep actin unpolymerized has several important implications. First, the monomeric actin can diffuse throughout the peripheral cytoplasm to serve as a reservoir for assembly on demand. Second, by keeping actin unpolymerized far above the critical concentration, assembly after modification by regulatory factors could occur rapidly on demand. However, this characteristic has the possible disadvantage that nucleation of actin could occur randomly in space. One way to gain spatial control is to couple changes in the polymerizability of actin monomers with regulation at the rapidly growing, barbed end of actin filaments. Much support for this mechanism for control of actin remodeling has come from extensive research on actin filament barbed end capping proteins.

Actin Filament End-Blockade and Its Regulation

The first cytoplasmic molecule recognized to confer this kind of regulation, and the prototype of the most powerful type of actin filament length-controlling factor known, is gelsolin, a protein (M_r, 82,000) purified from leukocytes in 1979 (68). This protein binds the fast-growing end of actin filaments and prevents exchange of monomers with that end. In addition to blocking the ends of actin filaments, gelsolin severs the noncovalent actin-actin bonds in filaments, thereby rupturing the filaments. This severing action efficiently dissolves an actin network gel (as described previously) and explains why the protein is named gelsolin. Because gelsolin binds to the barbed end of actin filaments, only the pointed filament ends exchange monomers. Therefore the critical concentration of gelsolin-blocked actin filaments rises to that of the pointed end, and it follows that gelsolin produces partial depolymerization as well as fragmentation of F-actin. The severing and blocking action of gelsolin *in vitro* is activated by micromolar calcium concentrations and independently by protons. In the presence of micromolar calcium concentrations or at pH less than 7.0, gelsolin first binds one actin molecule. This binding exposes a cryptic actin-binding site that binds a second actin with even higher affinity. This second binding is required for gelsolin to sever an actin filament. The severing site is at the amino terminus of the molecule, whereas the calcium-sensitive binding site resides in the carboxyl-terminal half of gelsolin.

Once gelsolin has interacted with actin in the presence of calcium, only the first-bound actin can be removed by chelation of calcium with ethyleneglycoltetraacetic acid (EGTA); the actin bound to the severing site is EGTA resistant. The EGTA-resistant gelsolin-actin complex can block the fast ends of actin filaments, but it neither severs actin filaments nor nucleates actin monomer assembly. In the presence of calcium, nucleating activity (but not severing activity) is regained. The EGTA-resistant actin monomer can, however, be dissociated from gelsolin by PIP or PIP$_2$, the phospholipids previously shown to dissociate profilin-actin complexes. As discussed later, the EGTA-resistant gelsolin-actin complex is useful for monitoring actin-gelsolin interactions in cells.

PIP or PIP$_2$ also inhibits the severing of actin filaments by gelsolin, even in the presence of protons or of calcium. The observations that gelsolin binds to ppIs and associates reversibly with membranes of leukocytes suggest that gelsolin operates in both cytosolic and membrane domains of the cell. Hence gelsolin is under dual regulation: Calcium or protons promote its binding to actin, its severing of actin filaments, and its blocking of monomer addition at the fast-growing filament end—all effects that lead to actin depolymerization and to the solution of a cross-linked actin gel. It follows that the reversal of gelsolin's tight binding to actin is necessary for actin assembly. Phosphoinositides could be responsible for this reversal, with the implication that gelsolin, in being regulated by the two known intracellular messengers—calcium and an intermediate of the ppI cycle—is positioned centrally in the transduction of surface stimulation into mechanical events in the cell (69). This reversal process may be sufficiently effective to keep gelsolin from forming tight complexes with actin even in the presence of micromolar calcium concentrations (70).

Although gelsolin is the most extensively studied actin filament barbed end capping protein and its atomic structure is partially known (71), cells (including leukocytes) contain other proteins that have similar functions. Some of these proteins are structurally related to gelsolin (e.g., CAPG in humans and Flightless in *Drosophila*) (72,73), but they do not all sever actin filaments and they differ from one another in details of regulation by ions. Nevertheless, all of these proteins have in common with one another and with a structurally different protein called capping protein (74) the fact that ppIs reduce their affinity for actin filament barbed ends (75,76).

There is accumulating evidence that control of actin filament barbed end capping is at least one important mechanism for the regulation of cellular actin assembly in general and in leukocytes in particular. The first recognition of this seemingly complex method for regulation arose from studies with *Dictyostelium* amoebas stimulated with the chemoattractant cyclic adenosine monophosphate. After cell perturbation, actin filament barbed end capping activity appeared in the soluble fraction of cell extracts and correlated with the simultaneous emergence of actin nucleation activity in the cytoskeletal fraction; and these events preceded net actin filament assembly (77). *N*-formyl-methionyl-leucyl-phenylalanine (fMLP)–stimulated and permeabilized neutrophils were then shown to have actin nucleating activity, and investigation of this system pointed to membrane-associated sites of nucleation that have characteristics consistent with actin filaments. This nucleation activity is directed to the barbed end, as evidenced by its inhibition with cytochalasin B (78,79). Neutrophil extracts also have considerable actin filament barbed end capping activity, predominantly mediated by capping protein (80). As described further in a later section, studies with other cell types, particularly blood platelets, are consistent with actin filament barbed end uncapping, with or without severing, as an important mechanism for cellular actin assembly. On the other hand, the possibility that stimuli leading to actin assembly in the cell initiate molecular interactions that create some kind

of nucleation site other than the barbed end of a filament has not been ruled out. Recently much interest has focused on the possible role of Arp2/3 (Actin-related proteins 2 and 3) as agents that bind to the pointed ends of actin filaments. In addition, they nucleate actin filament assembly in the barbed direction. It is possible that some of the actin nucleating activity in neutrophils results from an interaction involving Cdc42 and Arp2/3 independent of phosphoinositides. (80a,80b).

Actin Disassembly

Blockade of the actin filament barbed end inhibits assembly and shortens the average length of actin filaments *in vitro*. However, the rapid actin disassembly that accompanies actin remodeling during cell movements requires additional mechanisms to account for rapid filament shortening. As discussed previously, actin filament severing by gelsolin could account for this shortening. Studies of gelsolin-null knockout mice showing that a number of cell migration and cell migration–related activities are impaired by about half also indicate that gelsolin plays a role in cellular actin remodeling. Nevertheless, the viability of gelsolin knockout mice also attests to the importance of other actin regulatory proteins (81). Representing these other proteins, in addition to severing members of the gelsolin family, is a class of essential abundant low-molecular-weight proteins (M_r, 15,000 to 17,000) variously named actin depolymerizing factor, cofilin, and actophorin. These proteins promote actin disassembly, either by a weak severing activity or by promotion of dissociation of actin subunits from the pointed ends of actin filaments (82). This family of proteins is regulated by serine phosphorylation, and it is the dephosphorylated forms of the proteins that depolymerize actin filaments (83). The enzymes that phosphorylate and dephosphorylate these proteins have not been characterized. The cofilin family of proteins are also regulated by ppIs, in that ppIs inhibit their interaction with actin (84). The existence of numerous proteins of overlapping structures and functions regulating actin remodeling is hardly surprising, given the complexity of cell mechanics, the multiple mechanical functions of cells, and the need for cells to have alternative and backup systems to compensate for genetic, toxic, or other impairments of such vital functions.

Signaling Linkages between Cell Surface Stimulation and Actin Remodeling

The issues to be resolved in stimulus-response coupling concerning actin remodeling are the signals that lead to remodeling and the coordination of particular actin-remodeling proteins responding to these signals. In examining the problem, it is logical to investigate what happens to factors that regulate proteins thought to be involved in actin remodeling during cellular stimulation. Many agonists eliciting motile responses in leukocytes and net actin assembly act through heterotrimeric G protein–coupled sevenfold membrane spanning receptors (see Chapter 42). Others, such as cytokines or phagocytosable particles opsonized with immunoglobulin G (IgG), dimerize single spanning transmembrane receptors, leading to the phosphorylation of the cytoplasmic domains of the receptors and recruitment of adapter proteins that bring in additional phosphorylation reactions (85–87). Both types of cell surface perturbation can induce transient rises in intracellular calcium concentration (Ca^{2+}_i) and in intracellular pH (pH_i) and activate turnover of ppIs, consistent with the involvement of profilin as well as gelsolin- and cofilin-related proteins in actin remodeling.

The evidence for this involvement based on correlations with changes in signaling intermediates is inconsistent. Manipulation of neutrophil Ca^{2+}_i in electropermeabilized cells showed an inverse correlation between Ca^{2+}_i and cellular F-actin, consistent with promotion of actin depolymerization by calcium, possibly via its actions on gelsolin-related proteins (88). Studies by the late Fred Fay and colleagues with large newt eosinophils amenable to visualization of localized calcium concentrations consistently showed an inverse correlation between cell protrusion and localized free calcium (89). The persistence and speed of migration in neutrophils correlates with the Ca^{2+}_i level (90). However, protrusive surface activity and net actin assembly can occur in the absence of Ca^{2+}_i or pH_i transients and even at very low basal (nanomolar) Ca^{2+}_i levels (91,92). By the same token, in stimulated neutrophils levels of D_4 ppIs initially diminish at a time when net actin assembly occurs. In contrast, D_3 ppIs (ppIs with phosphate atoms in the 3 position of the inositol ring, either alone or with phosphates in the 4 and/or 5 positions) are present in much smaller quantities than D_4 ppIs but increase in mass and remain elevated after actin has assembled and returned to baseline (93,94). Diacylglycerol analogues that activate protein kinase C (e.g., tumor-promoting phorbol esters) cause flattening of leukocytes on a substrate in association with net actin assembly, although the kinetics of polymerization are slower than (and the extent is less than) what is observed with other agonists. These stimuli do not induce calcium transients, although they can increase ppI levels.

The problem with looking for correlations in messenger levels and actin remodeling in cells such as leukocytes is that actin remodeling occurs in space rather than in sequential time: net assembly takes place at the leading edge, with components disassembled elsewhere cycling to the site of assembly. As a result, bulk cellular concentrations of ions and lipids may not correlate with actin changes, measured biochemically, and the spatial resolution of microscopic localization is not able to detect local levels with sufficient precision. A further complication is the fact that D_3 and D_4 ppIs are increasingly being implicated in cellular reactions other than actin assembly, and changes in specific lipid types, specific structures, and particular cell locations may be more important than overall levels.

Several new lines of information, although mainly directed at cell types other than leukocytes, have begun to unravel this problem. One important advance was the discovery by Hall et al. that activated small GTPases, specifically RAC, RHO, and CDC42, induce particular actin-rich structures in cultured fibroblasts (95). These GTPases are active when bound to GTP, which they hydrolyze to GDP, thereby becoming inactive. Additional factors control the activity of the GTPases: GTPase activating proteins promote GTP degradation, other proteins promote exchange of bound GDP for GTP, and still others (guanine nucleotide exchange inhibitors) lock guanine nucleotides in the GTPases (see Chapter 41). Activated RAC elicits actin-based ruffling lamellae; activated RHO produces adhesion foci and actin-containing stress fiber bundles; and activated CDC42 leads to filopodia (95). The relevance of these findings to leukocytes is supported by the fact that in a macrophage cell line RAC induced ruffling, a dominant-negative form of RAC inhibited growth factor–mediated ruffling, and CDC42 elicited filopodia. These cells do not ordinarily produce stress fibers, and activated RHO causes the cells to round up (96). Bacterial toxins that inhibit activation of some of these GTPases inhibit actin assembly in neutrophils (97). The Wiskott-Aldrich syndrome, an inherited disorder associated with immunodeficiency and absence of surface projections on T lymphocytes, is caused by mutations affecting a gene, designated *WAS*, that interacts with CDC42, and overexpression of WAS causes cells to accumulate actin aggregates (98).

Initially no linkages between the GTPases and the known controls for actin assembly were apparent, but more recent information, particularly gleaned from platelets, indicates that ppIs interact both upstream and downstream of GTPases to produce various types of actin assembly. An advantage of the platelet as a research tool is that its actin remodeling takes place in time, as a distinct sequence throughout the platelet substance. Therefore it is possible to examine this sequence of events biochemically and quantitively as well as morphologically. The thrombin receptor of discoid resting platelets is a heterotrimeric G protein–coupled transmembrane protein. Its perturbation leads to heterotrimeric G protein–mediated activation of phospholipase C_β and transient hydrolysis of D_4 ppIs (99). The inositol trisphosphate generated by this hydrolysis mediates release of calcium from intracellular stores (see Chapter 41). The resultant increase in Ca^{2+}_i is obligatory for a documented severing of actin filaments that maintain the discoid shape of the resting platelet, and this severing facilitates transformation of the discoid platelet into a sphere (100). The severing correlates with the time course established for formation of gelsolin-actin complexes in the platelet (101).

Intracellular actin-gelsolin complexing in platelets has been monitored by immunoprecipitation experiments using high-affinity monoclonal anti-gelsolin antibodies conjugated to Sepharose beads to recover gelsolin quantitatively from cell extracts made from resting or stimulated cells. The cells are extracted in EGTA (low calcium) to prevent further complex formation between gelsolin and actin. The anti-gelsolin beads are included with the extract, and gelsolin—with or without actin bound to it—binds to the antibody. The beads are centrifuged and washed with EGTA-containing solutions, and the proteins associated with the beads are analyzed electrophoretically. Reversible actin-gelsolin associations have also been documented in leukocytes. In contrast to platelets, neutrophils or macrophages have complexes before activation (possibly owing to partial stimulation during harvesting). A chemotactic peptide, fMLP, or surface-induced spreading of the cells rapidly dissociates all actin-gelsolin complexes present (102–104). In contrast to leukocytes and other cells that remodel actin spatially as well as temporally, actin assembly off the barbed ends of the severed filaments correlates perfectly with the resynthesis of D_4 ppIs. In permeabilized platelets, ppIs uncap actin filament barbed ends. Moreover, coupling of thrombin receptor stimulation to such uncapping is preserved in the permeabilized platelets, and uncapping is blocked by peptides, derived from gelsolin, that bind ppIs. Activated RAC induces ppI synthesis and actin filament barbed end uncapping in the permeabilized platelets, and again the uncapping is blocked by ppI-binding peptides. These results provide compelling evidence that ppI-mediated actin filament barbed end uncapping is the terminal step in stimulated actin assembly in a pathway involving small GTPases (105). Furthermore, RAC associates directly with phosphoinositide kinases (106). The relevance of the thrombin pathway in platelets to leukocyte actin assembly is supported by the following considerations. First, both leukocytes and platelets are hematopoietic cells, derived from a common precursor. Second, both thrombin- and fMLP-mediated actin assembly, in platelets and leukocytes respectively, are inhibited by pertussis toxin, which inactivates the heterotrimeric GTPase linked to seven transmembrane spanning receptors.

Work with platelets has also begun to identify specific pathways involving D_3 and D_4 ppIs. D_3 ppIs are more effective in dissociating capping protein from actin filament barbed ends in permeabilized platelets, whereas D_4 ppIs are more effective for dissociation of gelsolin (107). Inhibition of D_3 ppI biosynthesis had no effect on thrombin-mediated platelet shape changes and resulted in massive actin assembly associated with actin filament remodeling leading to the formation of circumferential lamella (108). D_3 ppI synthesis inhibition also failed to impair fMLP-induced actin assembly in neutrophils (109) and fMLP-directed chemotaxis (110). However, such inhibi-tion prevented the modest burst of net actin assembly caused by phorbol myristate acetate. This actin assembly leads to extension of filopodia, and the principal role of the phorbol ester appears to be to phosphorylate plekstrin, which in turn stimulates protein kinase C activity (111).

Inhibition of D_3 ppI synthesis did limit growth factor–induced actin assembly and chemotaxis by fibroblasts and neutrophils (110,112,113); however, the concentrations of inhibitor used to effect complete chemotaxis inhibition were at levels at which intracellular reactions, such as myosin phosphorylation, might also be affected. It is unclear whether this inhibition is at the level of actin filament barbed end uncapping or at the upstream series of reactions leading to this event, beginning with dimerization of growth factor receptors. In fibroblasts, RAS stimulates D_3 ppI synthesis, which induces actin-based ruffling, and this ruffling requires active RAC, suggesting that in this case ppIs are working upstream of actin assembly (114).

Further evidence implicating D_4 ppIs in actin assembly includes the observations that forced genetic expression in cultured cells of phosphatidylinositol 4-phosphate 5-kinase, the enzyme that converts phosphatidylinositol 4-phosphate to PIP_2, induces abundant net actin assembly (115) and that micelles of D_3 ppIs induce cellular ruffling and migration (116).

D_3 and D_4 ppIs are increasingly recognized as important signaling molecules, and they may function upstream as well as at the end of actin assembly pathways and in other reactions important for leukocyte mechanical responses. For example, inhibition of synthesis of D_3 ppIs prevents the closure of phagosomes forming around objects by macrophages, implicating these lipids in a membrane fusion event (117). A role for ppIs in membrane fusion makes sense, because these lipids affect membrane curvature in artificial bilayers and are implicated in a growing number of intracellular vesicular trafficking pathways (118). The small GTPases and their regulatory proteins involved in signaling to actin assembly are also influenced by ppIs, as are many of the cytoplasmic molecules involved in cell-cell and cell-substrate adhesion, as discussed later in this chapter.

ACTIN-MEMBRANE ASSOCIATIONS

Attachments between the peripheral actin gel and the membrane bilayer must exist for retraction of pseudopodia and stabilization of the membrane against external forces to occur (Table 44–1). In some cases molecular information exists regarding the actin-membrane connections. For example, ABP-280 binds the submembrane actin gel of myeloid cells to the high-affinity IgG receptor, FcγRI (CD64) (119) and reportedly also binds to the β₂ leukocyte integrin, CD11b/CD18 (120). Another protein implicated in bridging cytoplasmic actin filaments

TABLE 44-1. *Proteins proposed to mediate actin membrane association in leukocytes*

Components of integrin-related adhesion complexes
  Talin
  Vinculin
  Paxillin
  α-Actinin
  Zyxin
  CRP
  Tensin
  FAK[125]
  Cortactin
  SRC, FYN, LCK
Other components
  Filamin-1
  MARCKS
  Unconventional myosins
  Fodrin (nonerythroid spectrin)
  Ezrin/moesin/p205

with the membrane is Myristoylated Arginine Rich Protein Kinase C Substrate (MARCKS). The binding of this protein to actin is regulated by calcium and through serine phosphorylation by protein kinase C (121).

The most extensively studied connection between the cell exterior and cytoplasmic actin is that between integrins and peripheral actin, which is mediated by a complex consisting of α-actinin, vinculin, paxillin, tensin, zyxin, talin, and members of a protein kinase cascade associated with focal adhesions (122). Because cells must generate a firm attachment and yet detach in coordination with events occurring outside and inside the cell, a system involving multiple regulated components, each contributing a small part of the strength of the complex, seems reasonable. The regulation of associations between components is in part mediated by phosphorylation reactions. Protein kinases found in adhesion complexes include the product of the *SRC* protooncogene and a variety of other tyrosine kinases as well as kinases associated with SRC, such as focal adhesion kinase (FAK[125]) (123,124). Vinculin, paxillin, tensin, and the focal adhesion kinases are targets of tyrosine phosphorylation (125,126). Control of adhesion by membrane ppIs has also been documented. Enzymes mediating ppI synthesis associate with components of adhesion complexes (127), and D₄ ppIs alter the conformation of vinculin, causing it to unfold and increase its avidity for talin and actin (128,129). This regulation is consistent with the observation that perturbation of cellular integrins leads to D₄ ppI synthesis (130). The ppI-binding protein gelsolin migrates transiently to integrin-rich adhesion complexes in neutrophils adhering to a matrix (131). Integrin-mediated adhesion is also an important source of signaling traffic moving both from outside to inside and from inside to outside the cell. Such integrin-associated signaling appears to be important in the process of complement-mediated phagocytosis (see Chapter 45).

CONTRACTILITY AND LEUKOCYTE MYOSINS

As described in the beginning of this chapter, observation of live leukocytes leads to the impression that contractility in the cell periphery may account for some of the intracellular movements of organelles and the puckering of membrane that forms occasionally during locomotion and phagocytosis. Since the discovery of actin and myosin in nonmuscle cells in the 1960s by Hatano and Oosawa, it has been assumed that actin-myosin interactions, reminiscent of muscle contraction, mediate such contractile events in nonmuscle cells (e.g., leukocytes). There has been relatively little recent work with leukocyte myosins, so the following comments depend primarily on research with other types of cells (Fig. 44-5).

Generically, myosins are complex molecules that ratchet vectorially along actin filaments by binding sequentially to serial subunits. "Conventional" myosins form bipolar filaments that can pull actin filaments of opposite polarity in an antiparallel direction, the classic example of this interaction being the generation of contractility in striated and smooth muscle (132). "Unconventional" myosins, of which numerous isoforms exist, may or may not form filaments and in some cases move membrane-bound cargos along actin filaments. Conventional leukocyte myosin molecules resemble muscle and most other nonmuscle myosins in having two sets of heavy chains (Mᵣ, 200,000) and two sets of light chains (Mᵣ, 20,000 and 15,000). Gene ablation experiments with amoebas indicate that conventional myosin is important for optimal cell motility, cell division, and capping, but unconventional myosins can contribute to intracellular organelle movements and rudimentary cell locomotion (133).

Leukocyte myosins, like muscle and other nonmuscle myosins, have low magnesium-dependent ATPase activity. Purified striated muscle myosin shows a marked increase in this activity in the presence of actin, and the actin-activated Mg^{2+}-ATPase activity of the myosin is an integral feature of the cyclic myosin head–actin monomer interaction that generates the contraction of muscle. The Mg^{2+}-ATPase activity of leukocyte myosin, unlike that of

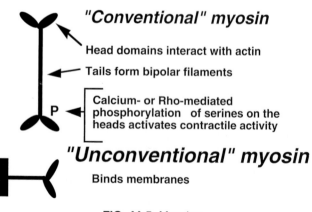

FIG. 44-5. Myosins.

striated muscle myosin, is not increased directly by the addition of F-actin. The actin-activated Mg^{2+}-ATPase activity of macrophage myosin correlates with the extent to which the 15-kd light chains of the myosin are phosphorylated. This suggests that the mechanism of regulation of leukocyte myosin is similar to what is thought to obtain in smooth muscle and in nonmuscle cells examined: a calcium-calmodulin complex activates a myosin light-chain kinase, which in turn phosphorylates the 15-kd myosin chain. A type 1 protein phosphatase in the cell reverses this activation. In addition, the ability of thymocyte myosin to form bipolar filaments is influenced positively by the extent of phosphorylation of the molecule. Therefore, the available information concerning regulation of the oligomeric state of myosin and its interactive properties with actin suggests that calcium can control filament formation and the interaction of myosin with actin (see Fig. 44-5).

The RHO family of GTPases have also been implicated as mediators of myosin activation and contractility in nonmuscle cells. The GTPase RHO activates a serine-threonine kinase (RHO-kinase) that phosphorylates myosin light chains and inhibits the dephosphorylating enzyme (134,135). This regulation works independently of calcium. Therefore, as with control of actin remodeling, calcium-dependent and -independent forms of oversight prevail, possibly protecting cells from toxins that inactivate one or the other signaling pathways.

For myosin to contract the cell cortex by working with actin, the actin network must be sufficiently intact to provide a continuous structure. Because calcium activates not only myosin but also gelsolin-related proteins (an effect expected to disrupt the network), cross-purposes would seem to be operating. It has been shown, however, that some of the cortical filamentous actin in leukocytes is relatively stable, suggesting that it is this population of filaments on which myosin operates. The biochemical basis for this stability is unclear. Two molecules that protect actin filaments from severing by gelsolin and inhibit depolymerization are tropomyosin and caldesmon, and both have been identified in leukocytes.

ACTIN REMODELING IN LEUKOCYTE FUNCTIONS

Mechanics of Membrane Protrusion in Locomotion

It is not immediately obvious how actin assembly from subunits induces protrusion of pseudopodia during spreading, locomotion, and other functions. Several, mutually nonexclusive ideas are plausible, and it is likely that cells use various means depending on the circumstances to effect membrane protrusion.

Actin assembly inside artificial lipid bilayers can cause distortion of these structures, suggesting that actin assembly per se can generate forces (136). In such model systems, however, actin is presumably not attached to the membrane; another problem is to explain how actin monomers in a cell attach to the end of a filament once it is pushed up against the planar surface of a membrane or against a fulcrum point elsewhere. Mogliner and Oster addressed this problem with the idea that actin subunits can intercalate between the membrane and the barbed filament end because of thermal fluctuations in the bilayer. This "Brownian ratchet" model in effect implies that actin polymerization is the initial driving force for protrusion (137).

The Brownian ratchet model supplanted an earlier idea of Oster's that the driving force for protrusion is osmotic rather than mechanical. According to this view, osmotic swelling of an actin gel takes place when it and its association with the plasmalemma are disrupted. Polymer gels have a swelling tendency that is balanced by mechanical restraints imposed by the crosslinks between filaments in the gel, and the release of these restraints allows the gel to swell further. Osmotic swelling would cause the plasma membrane to lift away from the underlying actin matrix and permit monomers to add onto barbed ends of actin filaments. As this assembly occurred, filamin-1 molecules could cross-link the incipient filaments into an orthogonal gel, thereby stabilizing the osmotically extruded pseudopod. Hydrostatic force generated by actin-myosin contraction of the cell body or parts of an extending lamella could also generate the protrusive force (138).

For local osmotic changes to be responsible for protrusive activity, the cell must be able to prevent rapid osmotic equilibrium throughout the cell, and it has been shown that actin networks cross-linked by filamin-1 in particular are capable of resisting osmotic forces (139).

Also consistent with this formulation to explain cell protrusive activity is the behavior of the filamin-1–deficient melanoma cell lines described previously. Despite lacking an important actin cross-linking protein, these cells extend blebs in response to stimulation (serum growth factors). The rate of bleb extension is too fast to be caused by actin polymerization, and cytochalasins do not inhibit bleb formation, but they completely prevent the recovery of these protrusions back to the cell body, suggesting that this latter step requires actin assembly. Monomeric actin enters expanding blebs, and only as the blebs stabilize and contract does filamentous actin appear. All of these results suggest that filamin-1, by cross-linking the assembling network, counteracts hydrostatically-induced or osmotic swelling, leading to the formation of pleats and pseudopodia rather than blebs. The extent to which the filamin-1–deficient cells can retract blebs presumably reflects the presence of other cross-linking proteins, or it may simply reflect the effects of long actin filaments' becoming interpenetrated, thereby accomplishing in a rudimentary fashion what filamin-1 does with greater efficiency (140). In either of these models, the initial stimulus for protrusion would be dissipative, namely a local breakdown of the cortical actin network and its attachments to the plasma membrane.

Another mechanism for cell protrusion involves myosins, which ratchet actin filaments centripetally on actin filaments left behind when a cell has contracted (141). Such a system can extend membrane only as far as it went before with its accompanying actin filaments, although a case has been made for unconventional myosins' actually driving membrane forward to accommodate new actin monomers on an extending filament (142). However, sperm cells of the nematode *Ascaris* undergo locomotion with a morphology highly reminiscent of migrating leukocytes, yet contain little actin. The movement of these cells derives from the polymerization and cross-linking of a protein completely unrelated to actin, called major sperm protein (MSP). MSP polymerization is regulated by pH_i, and it has been proposed that the compression of MSP filaments drives fluid forward, providing a hydrostatic force for movement (143). Most important is the fact that MSP has no motor proteins associated with it, so a myosin-related mechanism is at least not required for locomotion. Why MSP has been selected for motility in a biomass dominated by actin is unclear, but it is notable that the *Ascaris* sperm has no cellular role other than to migrate, and it is possible that MSP lacks the versatility of actin to mediate other mechanical functions.

Advancement of the actin network at the leading edge of leukocytes requires an adequate supply of component subunits. If the mechanisms for dissociation of monomer sequestering and barbed end filament capping proteins are at the leading edge of the cell, the concentrations of free forms of these regulatory proteins would become higher at this front than elsewhere. This concentration differential would create a bidirectional gradient in which unligated actin control proteins diffuse toward the rear of the pseudopodial network and complexed regulatory proteins diffuse forward. These gradients would provide both a continuous source of monomers and oligomers for actin assembly at the front of the network and a supply of free regulatory components to depolymerize actin from the rear of the network. The observation that filamin-1–deficient melanoma cells (in contrast to motile filamin-1–containing tumor cells) are unable to focus protrusive activity in one part of the cell suggests that filamin-1's ability to cross-link many actin filaments, thereby concentrating the target of actin-binding proteins in a region of the cell where actin assembly initially occurs, is responsible for establishing and maintaining the gradient of ingredients required to maintain protrusive activity.

Whereas the primary role of actin assembly and gelation in protrusive activity of leukocytes and the absolute requirement for this activity for locomotion appear well established, the actual mechanism of translational locomotion remains uncertain. Sequential episodes of protrusion, associated with transient adhesion of the extended part of the cell while contraction of the cell body brings it forward, could account for locomotion. The contractility of the cell body, mediated by myosin, can serve both to generate hydrostatic forces for protrusion and to draw the cell body in the direction of the extending lamella. The mechanism of cortical flow is even more mysterious. Most students of this phenomenon favor the idea that myosin-like motor molecules are somehow involved (144).

Actin Remodeling and Phagocytosis, Secretion, and Intracellular Parasitism

Most evidence indicates that the actin system does not play a primary role in the constitutive processes of membrane trafficking involving small vesicles (i.e., <0.1 nm). Rather, other protein skeletal elements (e.g., clathrin) mediate receptor-mediated endocytosis, and another protein, caveolin, determines the internalization of specialized vesicles called caveolae. In contrast, the actin system does appear to be important for endocytosis of large amounts of fluid mediated by the ruffling activity at the leading edge, in which folds of extruded membrane fuse to enclose external medium. The fluid-containing vesicles then migrate to the center of the cell. This fluid uptake method has sometimes been called macropinocytosis.

Actin also appears to be important for secretory activities mediated by larger organelles. For example, in order for exocytosis to take place at the base of a forming phagocytic vacuole, attenuation of the pseudopodial actin network is required to permit granule approach to, and fusion with, the plasmalemma. From the biochemical data presented, one mechanism to account for these findings would be for the calcium concentration to be sufficiently high at that region to keep gelsolin-related proteins active and the network dissolved. The remodeling of network components proposed to be associated with advancement of pseudopodia could also account for the network attenuation at the base of a phagocytic vacuole. The network decomposes at the base of the advancing pseudopod, during either phagocytosis or locomotion, and this degradation facilitates the fusion of granules with the plasma membrane at that location. Consistent with the role of calcium-activated actin disassembly in facilitating secretion are studies showing that, whereas phagocytosis can proceed in leukocytes with Ca^{2+}_i fixed at nanomolar levels, degranulation and exocytosis are markedly inhibited (145). Biosynthesis of ppIs also appears to be involved in exocytosis. In rat basophilic leukemia cells, IgE antibodies trigger secretion in sensitized cells, and the exocytic event is associated with actin assembly temporally correlated with D_4 ppI accumulation (146).

Also consonant with the actin barrier depletion hypothesis of secretion is the repeated observation that cytochalasins enhance exocytosis by agonist-stimulated phagocytes, provided that the cytochalasin is present before stimulation. This phenomenon has been taken as evidence that cortical actin filaments keep cytoplasmic granules away from the plasma membrane, because cytochalasins inhibit actin assembly and predictably inhibit the formation of intact actin networks. These findings are consistent with the model for agonist-activated actin assembly described here, because actin assembly after unblocking of fast-growing ends by signals resulting from stimulation would be blocked by cytochalasins, the peripheral actin gel would not assemble, and granule access to the plasmalemma would not be impaired. Once actin assembly was well established, however, its blockade by cytochalasins would not be expected to impair network formation, and, despite the activation of processes that permit granule fusion with the plasma membrane, granules would be separated from that site by the growing actin network.

When virulent *Listeria monocytogenes, Shigella flexnerii, Rickettsia prowazeckii,* and vaccinia viruses enter cells by endocytosis, they lyse the phagosome enclosing them and then migrate around the cell center. Eventually they move to the periphery, induce a filopodium, migrate to its tip, bud off, then lyse the double membrane and enter an adjacent cell (147). Neutrophils can kill these organisms, but macrophages, especially bone marrow macrophages and macrophage cell lines, accommodate parasite motility. In these migratory efforts the parasites subordinate the actin remodeling machinery of the host cell. The most striking findings are the rapidity with which the microbes move (0.05 to as much as 1.4 μm/s) and the trailing mass of actin filaments that follows the moving microorganism. The actin filaments are generally thought to be short (<1 μm) and crosslinked in random orientations by many of the actin filament bridging proteins found in cells, although there is also evidence for long axial filaments in the filopodia from which the parasites exit (148). Intense research has been directed at the remodeling of these filaments, which is required for microbial movement (149).

The actin tails, often called "rockets" or "comet tails," form at the interface of the bacterium with the tail, and they dissolve at the rear of the moving tail. The rate of actin turnover and the length of the tail are proportional to the rate of microbial movement (150,151). The microorganisms do not nucleate assembly of purified actin *in vitro* but can do so in various cell extracts, and in such media they can move at rates approximating migration in the living cell. The consensus therefore is that microbial components recruit cellular elements that lead to actin assembly (152,153). *Listeria* expresses a protein called ActA, which binds a host cellular protein called vasodilator-stimulated phosphoprotein (VASP). VASP is a phosphoprotein first identified in platelets that has multiple profilin-binding sites. Another protein, MENA, a mammalian homolog of a Drosophile gene product

enabled, is bound by ActA and in turn binds profilin. *Shigella* uses a protein called IcsA, which has been proposed to recruit cellular vinculin; proteolytic cleavage of vinculin exposes binding sites for VASP, which in turn brings profilin into the complex (154). The collection of high concentrations of profilin on VASP or MENA somehow eventuates in actin assembly, although none of these proteins directly nucleates actin assembly *in vitro*. Using platelet extracts and protein fractions derived from such extracts, a case has been made that actin-related proteins, previously shown to associate with profilin, may nucleate actin assembly (155). Most of the interpretations of how microorganisms assemble host actin assume that actin nucleates *de novo* from monomeric subunits (156), although a role for uncapping of actin filament barbed ends has also been proposed (157). Cofilin has been implicated as the major cellular factor required for disassembly of the actin tails (82,158).

Explaining the actual movement of the microorganisms again presents the problem of how the cell's leading edge membrane protrusion occurs. The Brownian ratchet model has been proposed to account for it, but the observation that the smaller *Shigella* organisms move faster than the larger *Listeria* ones is opposite of what Brownian motion would predict. Localized hydrostatic forces emanating from compaction of the actin filaments in the tail behind the microorganism, as proposed for the locomotion of *Ascaris* sperm, might apply.

Actin Remodeling and Apoptosis

The increase in peripheral granule movements and the generalized blebbing of the cell that occur during apoptosis in leukocytes after prolonged incubation, exposure to sonication, or exposure to various toxic substances could result from a pathologic disruption of the peripheral actin network. Because the plasma membrane is mechanically weak, even partial destruction of the underlying actin matrix might predispose the membrane to rupture, and it is common for membrane blebs to break away from the cell. Sonic waves close to the dimensions of the network can be predicted to disrupt it mechanically. Some of the cysteinyl proteinases (caspases) involved in apoptosis cleave actin and actin-binding proteins. One caspase that hydrolyzes interleukin-1β, interleukin 1-converting enzyme (ICE), degrades actin (13) as well as a cell growth–related intermediate protooncogene called GAS2, and the GAS2 derivative leads to actin filament rearrangements in cells (159). Metabolic toxicity to the cell might cause the intracellular calcium concentration to increase, thereby activating calpain, which has been shown to degrade fodrin during apoptosis (160). Cytosolic acidification during neutrophil apoptosis has been reported (161). Elevated calcium ions or protons are predicted to activate gelsolin-related proteins, resulting in widespread severing of the actin network.

Supporting this idea, gelsolin has been implicated as a substrate in metabolic pathways leading to apoptosis. Overexpression of gelsolin inhibited apoptosis in lymphoid cells exposed to a variety of treatments normally leading to apoptosis (162). On the other hand, gelsolin has been shown to be a substrate for caspace 3 in neutrophils, and the cleaved amino-terminal half of gelsolin mediates actin filament severing in apoptotic neutrophils. Gelsolin-null mouse neutrophils have markedly delayed apoptotic reactions (162a). Downregulation of actin biosynthesis during apoptosis has also been reported (163).

The metabolic functions of the cell may be optimal when energy-producing enzyme cascades are organized in association with the cortical actin network. For example, there is evidence that the activity of glycolytic enzymes is influenced by association with actin filaments (164). Therefore, better understanding of the changes in actin and actin-associated proteins accompanying cell injury and metabolic deprivation may be useful in devising strategies for protecting cells against irreversible damage.

Cytoskeletal Components and Leukocyte Dysfunction

Chronic granulomatous disease, the best-characterized functional deficiency of phagocytic leukocytes, results from failure of activation of the superoxide-generating, nicotinamide-adenine dinucleotide phosphate (NADPH)–linked oxidase in stimulated phagocytic leukocytes. This activation process has long been recognized to involve some association with the actin cytoskeleton, but the specific molecular events are unclear. The GTPases involved in leukocyte protrusion and oxidase activation seem to be shared (165). The identification of mutant WAS and its relation to CDC42 as a factor in the pathogenesis of the Wiskott-Aldrich syndrome and lymphoid dysregulation were discussed in the section on signal transduction. In the early 1970s the term "neutrophil actin dysfunction" described neutrophils in an apparently genetically transmitted condition that were morphologically abnormal, were defective in translocational migration, and had aberrant actin polymerization. This disorder may be the result of accumulation of a protein first identified in lymphocytes. This protein, called lymphocyte-specific protein-1 (LSP-1), is also expressed in neutrophils and other myeloid cells, and increased amounts of it are found in leukocytes of Tongan families with neutrophil dysfunction. LSP-1 is an actin-bundling protein *in vitro*, and when overexpressed in cultured cells it induces the formation of long branched filopodia, also seen in the affected patients (166). The function of LSP-1 in normal leukocytes is under investigation.

REFERENCES

1. Ayscough K, Drubin D. Actin: general principles from studies in yeast. *Annu Rev Cell Dev Biol* 1996;12:129–160.
2. Lauffenburger D, Horwitz A. Cell migration: a physically integrated molecular process. *Cell* 1996;84:359–369.
3. Mitchison T, Cramer L. Actin-based cell motility and cell locomotion. *Cell* 1996;84:371–379.
4. Noegel A, Luna J. The *Dictyostelium* cytoskeleton. *Experientia* 1995; 51:1135–1143.
5. Stossel T. On the crawling of animal cells. *Science* 1993;260: 1086–1094.
6. Palacek S, Loftus J, Ginsberg M, Lauffenburger D, Horwitz A. Integrin-ligand binding properties govern cell migration speed through cell-substratum adhesiveness. *Nature* 1997;385:537–540.
7. Schultze M. Ein heizbarer objekttisch und seine verwendung bei untersuchung des blutes. *Arch Mikrosk Anat* 1865;1:1–42.
8. Fukushima K, Senda N, Miura S, Ishigami S, Murakami Y. Dynamic pattern in the movement of leukocyte I and II. *Med J Osaka Univ* 1954;5:1–56.
9. Bessis M. *Living blood cells and their ultrastructure.* Heidelberg: Springer-Verlag, 1971.
10. Keller H, Bessis M. Migration and chemotaxis of anucleate cytoplasmic fragments. *Nature* 1975;258:723–724.
11. Malawista S, Boisfleury-Chevance A. The cytokineplast: purified, stable, and functional motile machinery from human blood polymorphonuclear leukocytes: possible formative role of heat-induced centrosomal dysfunction. *J Cell Biol* 1982;95:960–973.
12. Mizuno T, Kagami O, Sakai T, Kawasaki K. Locomotion of neutrophil fragments occurs by graded radial extension. *Cell Motil Cytoskeleton* 1996;35:289–297.
13. Mashima T, Naito M, Fujita N, Noguchi K, Tsuruo T. Identification of actin as a substrate of ICE and an ICE-like protease and involvement of an ICE-like protease but not ICE in VP-16-induced apoptosis. *Biochem Biophys Res Commun* 1995;217:1185–1192.
14. Weinhofer E, Zhao L, Cohan C. Actin dynamics and organization during growth cone morphogenesis in *Heliosoma* neurons. *Cell Motil Cytoskeleton* 1997;37:54–71.
15. Hirsch J. Cinemicrophotraphic observations on granule lysis in polymorphonuclear leukocytes during phagocytosis. *J Exp Med* 1962;116: 827–833.
16. Sullivan G, Gelrud A, Carper H, Mandell G. Interaction of tumor necrosis factor-α and granulocyte colony-stimulating factor on neutrophil apoptosis, receptor expression, and bactericidal function. *Proc Assoc Am Physicians* 1996;108:455–466.
17. Evans E. New physical concepts for cell amoeboid motion. *Biophys J* 1993;64:1306–1322.
18. Usami S, Wung S-L, Skiercyznski B, Skalak R, Chien S. Locomotion forces generated by a polymorphonuclear leukocyte. *Biophys J* 1992; 63:1663–1666.
19. Zhelev D, Hochmuth R. Mechanically stimulated cytoskeleton rearrangement and cortical contraction in human neutrophils. *Biophys J* 1995;68:2004–2014.
20. MacKintosh F, Käs J, Janmey P. Elasticity of semiflexible biopolymer networks. *Phys Rev Lett* 1995;75:4425–4428.
21. Janmey P, Hvidt S, Käs J, et al. The mechanical properties of actin gels. Elastic modulus and filament motions. *J Biol Chem* 1994;269: 32503–32513.
22. Janmey P, Hvidt S, Lamb J, Stossel TP. Resemblance of actin-binding protein/actin gels to covalently crosslinked networks. *Nature* 1990; 345:89–92.
23. Anderson D, Wible L, Hughes B, Smith CW, Brinkley B. Cytoplasmic microtubules in polymorphonuclear leukocytes: effects of chemotactic stimulation and colchicine. *Cell* 1982;31:719–729.
24. Cassimeris L, Wadsworth P, Salmond E. Dynamics of microtubule depolymerization in monocytes. *J Cell Biol* 1986;102:2023–2032.
25. Keller H, Niggli V. Colchicine-induced stimulation of PMN motility related to cytoskeletal changes in actin, α-actinin, and myosin. *Cell Motil Cytoskeleton* 1993;25:10–18.
26. Singer S, Kupfer A. The directed migration of eukaryotic cells. *Annu Rev Cell Biol* 1986;2:337–365.
27. Rosania G, Swanson J. Microtubules can modulate pseudopod activity from a distance inside macrophages. *Cell Motil Cytoskeleton* 1996; 34:230–245.
28. Hollenbeck P, Swanson J. Radial extension of macrophage tubular lysosomes supported by kinesin. *Nature* 1990;346:864–866.
29. Matsudaira P. Actin crosslinking proteins at the leading edge. *Semin Cell Biol* 1994;5:165–174.

30. Pestonjamasp K, Amieva M, Strassel C, Nauseef W, Furthmayr H, Luna E. Moesin, ezrin, and p205 are actin-binding proteins associated with neutophil plasma membranes. *Mol Biol Cell* 1995;6:247–259.

31. Stevenson KB, Clark RA, Nauseef WM. Fodrin and band 4.1 in a plasma membrane-associated fraction of human neutrophils. *Blood* 1989;74:2136–2143.

32. Gregorio C, Kubo R, Bankert R, Repasky E. Translocation of spectrin and protein kinase C to a cytoplasmic aggregate upon lymphocyte activation. *Proc Natl Acad Sci U S A* 1992;89:4947–4951.

33. Gregorio C, Repasky E, Fowler V, Black J. Dynamic properties of ankyrin in T lymphocytes: colocalization with spectrin and protein kinase Cβ. *J Cell Biol* 1994;125:345–358.

34. Cassimeris L, McNeill H, Zigmond S. Chemoattractant-stimulated polymorphonuclear leukocytes contain two populations of actin filaments that differ in their spatial distributions and relative stabilities. *J Cell Biol* 1990;110:1067–1075.

35. Cramer L, Siebert M, Mitchison T. Identification of novel graded polarity actin filament bundles in locomoting heart fibroblasts: implications for the generation of motile force. *J Cell Biol* 1997;136:1287–1305.

36. Hartwig JH, Shevlin P. The architecture of actin filaments and the ultrastructural location of actin-binding protein in the periphery of lung macrophages. *J Cell Biol* 1986;103:1007–1020.

37. Small J. Lamellipodia architecture: actin filament turnover and the lateral flow of actin filaments during motility. *Semin Cell Biol* 1994;5:157–163.

38. Furukawa R, Kundra R, Fechheimer M. Formation of liquid crystals from actin filaments. *Biochemistry* 1993;32:12346–12352.

39. Käs J, Strey H, Tang J, et al. F-actin, a model polymer for semiflexible chains in dilute, semidilute, and liquid crystalline solutions. *Biophys J* 1996;70:609–625.

40. Suzuki A, Yamazaki M, Ito T. Polymorphism of F-actin assembly: 1. A quantitative phase diagram of F-actin. *Biochemistry* 1996;35:5238–5244.

41. Tang J, Janmey P. The polyelectrolyte nature of F-actin and the mechanism of actin bundle formation. *J Biol Chem* 1996;271:8556–8583.

42. Käs J, Strey M, Sackmann E. Direct imaging of reptation for semiflexible actin filaments. *Nature* 1994;368:226–229.

43. Gorlin J, Yamin R, Egan S, et al. Human endothelial actin-binding protein (ABP, nonmuscle filamin): a molecular leaf spring. *J Cell Biol* 1990;111:1089–1105.

44. Hartwig J. Actin-binding proteins 1: spectrin superfamily. In: Sheterline P, ed. *Protein profile*. London: Academic Press, 1994:711–778.

45. Hartwig J, Kwiatkowski D. Actin-binding proteins. *Curr Opin Cell Biol* 1991;3:87–97.

46. Barry C, Xie J, Lemmon V, Young A. Molecular characterization of a multipromoter gene encoding a chicken filamin protein. *J Biol Chem* 1993;268:25577–25586.

47. Brotschi EA, Hartwig JH, Stossel TP. The gelation of actin by actin-binding protein. *J Biol Chem* 1978;253:8988–8993.

48. Gorlin J, Henske E, Warren S, et al. Actin-binding protein (ABP-280) filamin gene (FLN) maps telomeric to the color vision locus (R/CGP) and centromeric to G6PD in Xq28. *Genomics* 1993;17:496–498.

49. Maestrini E, Patrosso C, Mancini M, et al. Mapping of two genes encoding isoforms of the actin-binding protein ABP-280, a dystrophin like protein, to Xq28 and to chromosome 7. *Hum Mol Genet* 1993;2:761–766.

50. Patrosso M, Repetto M, Villa A, et al. The exon-intron organization of the human X-linked gene (FLN1) encoding actin-binding protein 280. *Genomics* 1994;21:71–76.

51. Cunningham C, Gorlin J, Kwiatkowski D, et al. Actin-binding protein requirement for cortical stability and efficient locomotion. *Science* 1992;255:325–327.

52. Bennett J, Zaner K, Stossel T. Isolation and some properties of macrophage δ-actinin. Evidence that it is not an actin gelling protein. *Biochemistry* 1984;23:5081–5086.

53. Arpin M, Friederich E, Algrain M, Vernel F, Louvard D. Functional differences between L- and T-plastin isoforms. *J Cell Biol* 1994;127:1995–2008.

54. Namba Y, Ito M, Zu Y, Shigesada K, Maruyama K. Human T cell L-plastin bundles actin filaments in a calcium-dependent manner. *J Biochem* 1992;112:503–507.

55. Pacaud M, Derancourt J. Purification and further characterization of macrophage 70-kDa protein, a calcium-regulated, actin-binding protein identical to L-plastin. *Biochemistry* 1993;32:3448–3455.

56. Jones S, Brown E. FcγRII-mediated adhesion and phagocytosis induced L-plastin phosphorylation in human neutrophils. *J Biol Chem* 1996;271:14623–14630.

57. P, Clayton J, Sparrow J. Actins. In: Sheterline P, ed, *Protein profile*. London, Academic Press, 1996.

58. Kumar A, Crawford K, Close L, et al. Rescue of cardiac α-actin-deficient mice by enteric smooth muscle γ-actin. *Proc Natl Acad Sci U S A* 1997;94:4406–4411.

59. Carlier M-F. Dynamic actin. *Curr Biol.* 1993;3:321–323.

60. Allen P, Janmey P. Gelsolin displaces phalloidin from actin filaments: a new fluorescence method shows that both Ca^{2+} and Mg^{2+} affect the rate at which gelsolin severs F-actin. *J Biol Chem* 1994;269:32916–32923.

61. De La Cruz E, Pollard T. Transient kinetic analysis of rhodamine phalloidin binding to actin filaments. *Biochemistry* 1994;33:14387–14392.

62. Howard T, Watts R. Actin polymerization and leukocyte function. *Curr Opin Hematol* 1994;1:61–68.

63. Gieselmann R, Kwiatkowski D, Janmey P, Witke W. Distinct biochemical characteristics of the two human profilin isoforms. *Eur J Biochem* 1995;229:621–628.

64. Fechheimer M, Zigmond S. Focusing on unpolymerized actin. *J Cell Biol* 1993;123:1–5.

65. Stossel T. The machinery of blood cell movements. *Blood* 1994;84:367–379.

66. Sun H-Q, Kwiatkowska K, Yin H. Actin monomer binding proteins. *Curr Opin Cell Biol* 1995;7:102–110.

67. Pantaloni D, Carlier M-F. How profilin promotes actin filament assembly in the presence of thymosin β4. *Cell* 1993;75:1007–1014.

68. Stossel T. From signal to pseudopod: how cells control cytoplasmic actin assembly. *J Biol Chem* 1989;264:18261–18264.

69. Janmey P. Protein regulation by phosphatidylinositol lipids. *Chem Biol* 1995;2:61–65.

70. Janmey P. Phosphoinositides and calcium as regulators of cellular actin assembly and disassembly. *Annu Rev Physiol* 1994;56:169–191.

71. McLaughlin P, Weeds A. Actin-binding protein complexes at atomic resolution. *Annu Rev Biophys Biomol Struct* 1995;24:643–675.

72. de Couet H, Fong K, Weeds A, McLaughlin P, Miklos G. Molecular and mutational analysis of a gelsolin-family member encoded by the flightless I gene of *Drosophila melanogaster*. *Genetics* 1995;141:1049–1059.

73. Southwick F. Gain-of-function mutations conferring actin-severing activity to human macrophage Cap G. *J Biol Chem* 1995;270:45–48.

74. Naum N, Speicher D, DiNubile M, Southwick F. Purification and properties of a Ca^{2+}-independent barbed-end actin filament capping protein, CapZ, from human polymorphonuclear leukocytes. *Biochemistry* 1996;35:3518–3524.

75. Onoda K, Yin H. gCap39 is phosphorylated: stimulation by okadaic acid and preferential association with nuclei. *J Biol Chem* 1993;268:4106–4112.

76. Schafer D, Jennings P, Cooper J. Dynamics of capping protein and actin assembly *in vitro*: uncapping barbed ends by polyphosphoinositides. *J Cell Biol* 1996;135:169–179.

77. Condeelis J. Life at the leading edge: the formation of cell protrusions. *Annu Rev Cell Biol* 1994;9:411–444.

78. Redmond T, Tardif M, Zigmond S. Induction of actin polymerization in permeabilized neutrophils. *J Biol Chem* 1994;269:21657–21663.

79. Redmond T, Zigmond S. Distribution of F-actin elongation sites in lysed polymorphonuclear leukocytes parallels the distribution of endogenous F-actin. *Cell Motil Cytoskeleton* 1993;26:7–18.

80. DiNubile M, Cassimeris L, Joyce M, Zigmond S. Actin filament barbed-end capping activity in neutrophil lysates: the role of capping protein-β2. *Mol Biol Cell* 1995;6:1659–1671.

80a. Zigmond SH, Joyce M, Yang C, Brown K, Huang M, Pring M. Mechanism of Cdc42-induced actin polymerization in neutrophil extracts. *J Cell Biol* 1998;142L:1001–1012.

80b. Zigmond SH. Actin cytoskeleton: the Arp 2/3 complex gets to the point. *Curr Biol* 1998;8:R654–R657.

81. Witke W, Sharpe A, Hartwig J, Azuma T, Stossel T, Kwiatkowski D. Hemostatic, inflammatory and fibroblast responses are blunted in mice lacking gelsolin. *Cell* 1995;81:41–51.

82. Carlier M-F, Laurent V, Santolini J, et al. Actin depolymerizing factor (ADF/cofilin) enhances the rate of filament turnover: implication in actin-based motility. *J Cell Biol* 1997;136:1307–1323.

83. Nagaokoa R, Abe H, Obinata T. Site-directed mutagenesis of the phosphorylation site of cofilin: its role in cofilin-actin interaction and cytoplasmic localization. *Cell Motil Cytoskeleton* 1996;35:200–209.

84. Hatanaka H, Ogura K, Moriyama K, Ichikawa S, Yahara I, Inagaki F. Tertiary structure of destrin and structural similarity between two actin-regulating protein families. *Cell* 1996;85:1047–1055.

85. Greenberg S, Chang P, Silverstein S. Tyrosine phosphorylation of the γ subunit of Fcγ receptors, p72^syk, and paxillin during Fc receptor-mediated phagocytosis in macrophges. *J Biol Chem* 1994;269:3897–3902.

86. Greenberg S, Chang P, Wang D-C, Xavier R, Seed B. Clustered syk tyrosine kinase domains trigger phagocytosis. *Proc Natl Acad Sci U S A* 1996;93:1103–1107.

87. Huang M-M, Indik Z, Brass L, Hoxie J, Schreiber A, Brugge J. Activation of FcγRII induces tyrosine phosphorylation of multiple proteins including FcγRII. *J Biol Chem* 1992;267:5467–5473.

88. Downey G, Chan C, Trudel S, Grinstein S. Actin assembly in electropermeabilized neutrophils: role of intracellular calcium. *J Cell Biol* 1990;110:1975–1982.

89. Gilbert S, Perry K, Fay F. Mediation of chemoattractant-induced changes in [Ca²⁺]ᵢ and cell shape, polarity and locomotion by InsP₃, DAG, and protein kinase C in newt eosinophils. *J Cell Biol* 1994;127:489–503.

90. Mandeville J, Ghosh R, Maxfield F. Intracellular calcium levels correlate with speed and persistent forward motion in migrating neutrophils. *Biophys J* 1995;68:1207–1217.

91. Laffafian I, Hallett M. Does cytosolic free Ca²⁺ signal neutrophil chemotaxis in response to formylated chemotactic peptide? *J Cell Sci* 1995;108:3199–3205.

92. Maxfield F. Regulation of leukocyte locomotion by Ca²⁺. *Trends Biol Sci* 1993;3:386–391.

93. Dobos G, Norgauer J, Eberle M, Schollmeyer P, Traynor-Kaplan A. C5a reduces formyl peptide-induced actin polymerization and phosphatidylinositol(3,4,5)trisphosphate formation, but not phosphatidylinositol(4,5) bisphosphate hydrolysis and superoxide production, in human neutrophils. *J Immunol* 1992;149:609–614.

94. Eberle M, Traynor-Kaplan A, Sklar L, Norgauer J. Is there a relationship between phosphatidylinositol trisphosphate and F-actin polymerization in human neutrophils? *J Biol Chem* 1990;265:16725–16728.

95. Hall A. Rho GTPases and the actin cytoskeleton. *Science* 1998;279:509–514.

96. Allen W, Jones G, Pollard J, Ridley A. Rho, Rac and Cdc42 regulate actin organization and cell adhesion in macrophages. *J Cell Sci* 1997;110:707–720.

97. Aktories K. Bacterial toxins that target rho proteins. *J Clin Invest* 1997;99:827–829.

98. Kirchhausen T, Rosen F. Unravelling Wiskott-Aldrich syndrome. *Curr Biol* 1996;6:676–678.

99. Grand R, Turnell A, Grabham P. Cellular consequences of thrombin-receptor activation. *Biochem J* 1996;313:353–368.

100. Hartwig J. Mechanisms of actin rearrangements mediating platelet activation. *J Cell Biol* 1992;118:1421–1442.

101. Lind SE, Janmey PA, Chaponnier C, Herbert T, Stossel TP. Reversible binding of actin to gelsolin and profilin in human platelet extracts. *J Cell Biol* 1987;105:833–842.

102. Deaton J, Guerrero T, Howard T. Role of gelsolin interaction with actin in regulation and creation of actin nuclei in chemotactic peptide activated polymorphonuclear neutrophils. *Mol Biol Cell* 1992;3:1427–1435.

103. Howard T, Chaponnier C, Yin H, Stossel T. Gelsolin-actin interaction and actin polymerization in human neutrophils. *J Cell Biol* 1990;110:1983–1991.

104. Watts R, Howard T. Evidence for a gelsolin-rich, labile F-actin pool in human polymorphonuclear leukocytes. *Cell Motil Cytoskeleton* 1992;21:25–37.

105. Hartwig J, Bokoch G, Carpenter C, et al. Thrombin receptor ligation and activated rac uncap actin filament barbed ends through phosphoinositide synthesis in permeabilized platelets. *Cell* 1995;82:643–653.

106. Tolias K, Cantley L, Carpenter C. Rho family GTPases bind to phosphoinositide kinases. *J Biol Chem* 1995;270:17656–17659.

107. Barkalow K, Witke W, Kwiatkowski D, Hartwig J. Coordinated regulation of platelet actin filament barbed ends by gelsolin and capping protein. *J Cell Biol* 1996;134:389–399.

108. Kovacsovics T, Bachelot C, Toker A, et al. Phosphoinositide 3-kinase inhibition spares actin assembly in activating platelets, but reverses platelet activation. *J Biol Chem* 1995;270:11358–11366.

109. Arcaro A, Wymann M. Wortmannin is a potent phosphatidylinositol 3-kinase inhibitor: the role of phosphatidylinositol 3,4,5-trisphosphate in neutrophil responses. *Biochem J* 1993;296:297–301.

110. Thelen M, Uguccioni M, Bösiger J. PI 3-kinase-dependent and independent chemotaxis of human neutrophil leukocytes. *Biochem Biophys Res Commun* 1995;217:1255–1262.

111. Hartwig J, Kung S, Kovacsovics T, et al. D3 phosphoinositides and outside-in integrin signaling by GPIIb/IIIa mediate platelet actin assembly and filopodial extension induced by phorbol 12-myristate acetate. *J Biol Chem* 1996;271:32986–32993.

112. Knall C, Worthen G, Johnson G. Interleukin 8-stimulated phosphatidylinositol-3-kinase activity regulates the migration of human neutrophils independent of mitogen-activated protein kinases. *Proc Natl Acad Sci U S A* 1997;94:3052–3057.

113. Wennström S, Siegbahn A, Yokote K, et al. Membrane ruffling and chemotaxis transduced by the PDGF β-receptor require the binding site for phosphatidylinositol 3′ kinase. *Oncogene* 1994;9:651–660.

114. Rodriguez-Viciana P, Warne P, Khwaja A, et al. Role of phosphoinositide 3-OH kinase in cell transformation and control of the actin cytoskeleton by Ras. *Cell* 1997;89:457–467.

115. Shibasaki Y, Ishihara H, Kizuki N, Asano T, Oka Y, Yazaki Y. Massive actin polymerization induced by phosphatylinositol-4-phosphate 5-kinase *in vivo*. *J Biol Chem* 1997;272:7578–7581.

116. Derman M, Toker A, Hartwig J, et al. The lipid products of phophoinositide 3-kinase increase cell motility through protein kinase C. *J Biol Chem* 1997;272:6465–6470.

117. Araki N, Johnson M, Swanson J. A role for phosphoinositide 3-kinase in the completion of macropinocytosis and phagocytosis by macrophages. *J Cell Biol* 1996;135:1249–1260.

118. De Camilli P, Emr S, McPherson P, Novick P. Phosphoinositides as regulators in membrane traffic. *Science* 1996;271:1533–1539.

119. Ohta Y, Stossel T, Hartwig J. Ligand-sensitive binding of actin-binding protein (ABP) to immunoglobulin G Fc receptor I(FcγR1, CD64). *Cell* 1991;67:275–282.

120. Sharma C, Ezzell R, Arnaout M. Direct interaction of filamin (ABP-280) with the β2-integrin subunit CD18. *J Immunol* 1995;154:3461–3470.

121. Allen L-A, Aderem A. A role for MARCKS, the α isozyme of protein kinase C and myosin I in zymosan phagocytosis by macrophages. *J Exp Med* 1995;182:829–840.

122. Burridge K, Chrzanowska-Wodnicka M. Focal adhesions, contractility and signaling. *Annu Rev Cell Dev Biol* 1996;12:463–519.

123. Hartley D, Corvera S. Formation of c-Cbl phosphatidylinositol 3-kinase complexes on lymphocyte membranes by a p56lck-independent mechanism. *J Biol Chem* 1996;271:21939–21943.

124. Manié S, Beck A, Astier A, et al. Involvement of p130^Cas and p105^HEF1, a novel Cas-like docking protein, in a cytoskeleton-dependent signaling pathway initated by ligation of integrin or antigen receptor on human B cells. *J Biol Chem* 1997;272:4230–4236.

125. Chen H-C, Appeddu P, Parsons J, Hildebrand J, Schaller M, Guan J-L. Interaction of focal adhesion kinase with cytoskeletal protein talin. *J Biol Chem* 1995;270:16995–16899.

126. Schaller M, Otey C, Hildebrand J, Parsons J. Focal adhesion kinase and paxillin bind to peptides mimicking β integrin cytoplasmic domains. *J Cell Biol* 1995;130:1181–1187.

127. Auger K, Songyang Z, Ho S, Roberts T, Chen L. Platelet-derived growth factor-induced formation of tensin and phosphoinositide 3-kinase complexes. *J Biol Chem* 1996;271:23452–23457.

128. Craig S, Johnson R. Assembly of focal adhesions: progress, paradigms, and portents. *Curr Opin Cell Biol* 1996;8:74–85.

129. Gilmore A, Burridge K. Regulation of vinculin binding to talin and actin by phoshatidylinositol-4,5-bisphosphate. *Nature* 1996;381:531–535.

130. Schwartz M, Schaller M, Ginsberg M. Integrins: emerging paradigms of signal transduction. *Annu Rev Cell Dev Biol* 1995;11:549–599.

131. Wang J-S, Coburn J, Tauber A, Zaner K. Role of gelsolin in actin depolymerization of adherent human neutrophils. *Mol Biol Cell* 1997;8:121–128.

132. Hasson T, Mooseker M. Vertebrate unconventional myosins. *J Biol Chem* 1996;271:16431–16434.

133. Spudich A. Myosin reorganization in activated RBL cells correlates temporally with stimulated secretion. *Cell Motil Cytoskeleton* 1995;29:345–353.

134. Amano M, Ito M, Kimura K, et al. Phosphorylation and activation of myosin by Rho-associated kinase (Rho-kinase). *J Biol Chem* 1996;271:20246–20249.

135. Kimura K, Ito M, Amano M, et al. Regulation of myosin phosphatase by Rho and Rho-associated kinase (Rho-kinase). *Science* 1996;273:245–248.

136. Cortese JD, Schwab B, Frieden C, Elson EL. Actin polymerization induces a shape change in actin-containing vesicles. *Proc Natl Acad Sci U S A* 1989;86:5773–5777.

137. Mogliner A, Oster G. Cell motility driven by actin polymerization. *Biophys J* 1996;71:3030–3045.

138. Keller H, Babie H. Protrusive activity quantitatively determines the rate and direction of cell locomotion. *Cell Motil Cytoskeleton* 1996;33:241–251.

139. Ito T, Suzuki A, Stossel R. Regulation of water flow by actin-binding protein-induced actin gelation. *Biophys J* 1992;61:1301–1305.

140. Cunningham C. Actin polymerization and intracellular solvent flow in cell surface blebbing. *J Cell Biol* 1995;129:1589–1599.

141. Cramer L, Mitchison T. Myosin is involved in postmitotic cell spreading. *J Cell Biol* 1995;131:179–189.

142. Sheetz M. Cell migration by graded attachment to substrates and contraction. *Semin Cell Biol* 1994;5:149–155.

143. Italiano J Jr, Roberts T, Stewart M, Fontana C. Reconstitution *in vitro* of the motile apparatus from the amoeboid sperm of *Ascaris* shows that filament assembly and bundling move membranes. *Cell* 1996;84:105–114.

144. Bretscher M. Getting membrane flow and the cytoskeleton to cooperate in moving cells. *Cell* 1996;87:601–606.

145. Jaconi M, Lew D, Carpentier J-L, Magnusson K. Cytosolic free calcium elevation mediates phagosome-lysosome fusion during phagocytosis in human neutrophils. *J Cell Biol* 1990;110:1555–1564.

146. Apgar J. Activation of protein kinase C in rat basophilic leukemia cells stimulates increased production of phosphatidylinositol 4-phosphate and phosphatidylinositol 4,5-bisphosphate: correlation with actin polymerization. *Mol Biol Cell* 1995;6:97–108.

147. Higley S, Way M. Actin and cell pathogenesis. *Curr Opin Cell Biol* 1997;9:62–69.

148. Sechi A, Wehland J, Small J. The isolated comet tail pseudopodium of *Listeria monocytogenes:* a tail of two filament populations, long and axial and short and random. *J Cell Biol* 1997;137:155–167.

149. Southwick F, Purich D. Intracellular pathogenesis of Listeriosis. *N Engl J Med.* 1996;334:770–776.

150. Dabiri G, Sanger J, Portnoy D, Southwick F. *Listeria monocytogenes* moves rapidly through the host cell cytoplasm by inducing directional actin assembly. *Proc Natl Acad Sci U S A* 1990;87:6068–6072.

151. Theriot J, Mitchison T, Tilney L, Portnoy D. The rate of actin-based motility of intracellular *Listeria monocytogenes* equals the rate of actin polymerization. *Nature* 1992;357:257–259.

152. Coso O, Teramoto H, Simonds W, Gutkind J. Signaling from G protein-coupled receptors to c-Jun kinase involves βγ subunits of heterotrimeric G proteins acting on a Ras and Rac1-dependent pathway. *J Biol Chem* 1996;271:3963–3966.

153. Cossart P, Boquet P, Normark S, Rappuoli R. Cellular microbiology emerging. *Science* 1996;271:315–316.

154. Zeile W, Purich D, Southwick F. Recognition of two classes of oligoproline sequences in profilin-mediated acceleration of actin-based *Shigella* motility. *J Cell Biol* 1996;133:49–59.

155. Welch M, Iwamatsu A, Mitchison T. Actin polymerization is induced by Arp2/3 protein complex at the surface of *Listeria monocytogenes.* *Nature* 1997;385:265–269.

156. Theriot J. The cell biology of infection by intracellular bacterial pathogens. *Annu Rev Cell Dev Biol* 1995;11:213–239.

157. Marchand J-B, Moreau P, Paoletti A, et al. Actin-based movement of *Listeria monocytogenes:* actin assembly results from the local maintenance of uncapped filament barbed ends at the bacterium surface. *J Cell Biol* 1995;130:331–343.

158. Rosenblatt J, Agnew B, Abe H, Bamburg J, Mitchison T. *Xenopus* actin depolymerizing factor/cofilin (XAC) is responsible for the turnover of actin filaments in *Listeria monocytogenes* tails. *J Cell Biol* 1997;136:1323–1332.

159. Brancolini C, Menedetti M, Schneider C. Microfilament reorganization during apoptosis: the role of Gas2, a possible substrate for ICE-like proteases. *EMBO J* 1995;14:5179–5190.

160. Martin S, O'Brien G, Nishioka W, et al. Proteolysis of fodrin (non-erythroid spectrin) during apoptosis. *J Biol Chem* 1995;270:6425–6428.

161. Meisenholder G, Martin S, Green D, Nordberg J, Babior B, Gottlieb R. Events in apoptosis: acidification is downstream of protease activation and BCL-2 protection. *J Biol Chem* 1996;271:16260–16262.

162. Ohtsu M, Sakai M, Fujita H, et al. Inhibition of apoptosis by the actin-regulatory protein gelsolin. *EMBO J* 1997;16:4650–4656.

162a. Kothakota S, Azuma T, Reinhard C, et al. Caspace-3–generated fragment of gelsolin: effector of morphological changes in apoptosis. *Science* 1997;278:294–296.

163. Guénal I, Risler Y, Mignotte B. Down-regulation of actin genes precedes microfilament network disruption and actin cleavage during p53-mediated apoptosis. *J Cell Sci* 1997;110:489–495.

164. Pagliaro L, Taylor D. 2-Deoxyglucose and cytochalasin D modulate aldolase mobility in living 3T3 cells. *J Cell Biol* 1992;118:859–963.

165. Bokoch G. Chemoattractant signaling and leukocyte activation. *Blood* 1995;86:1649–1660.

166. Howard T, Li Y, Torres M, Guerrero A, Coates T. The 47-kD protein increased in neutrophil actin dysfunction with 47- and 89-kD protein abnormalities is lymphocyte-specific protein. *Blood* 1994;83:231–241.

Inflammation: Basic Principles and Clinical Correlates,
3rd ed., edited by John I. Gallin and Ralph Snyderman.
Lippincott Williams & Wilkins, Philadelphia © 1999.

CHAPTER **45**

Biology of Phagocytosis

Steven Greenberg

"There is at bottom only one scientific therapy for all diseases, and that is to stimulate the phagocytes."
—George Bernard Shaw, *The Doctor's Dilemma*

Phagocytosis is a phylogenetically ancient response to
particulate stimuli adapted by specialized cells of the
immune system. These cells—primarily granulocytes and
mononuclear phagocytes—utilize highly conserved programs of signaling and motility to engulf foreign
pathogens. The remarkable similarity in the phagocytic
response of simple organisms such as *Dictyostelium* and
of higher-order eukaryotes suggests that phagocytosis
serves basic functions in amoeboid cells. Perhaps it is the
most efficient mechanism for extremely motile single-
cell organisms with high metabolic rates to acquire
energy sources. Alternatively, phagocytosis provides a
means of sequestering potentially harmful particulate
substances and microbial pathogens, thereby limiting
their toxic effects.

DISTINGUISHING FEATURES OF
PHAGOCYTOSIS

It was not appreciated until fairly recently that many
cells, including sessile ones, are capable of mediating
phagocytosis. Recent progress has revealed the multitude
and diversity of the phagocytic response. Three features
distinguish phagocytosis from other forms of endocytic
events: First, phagocytosis requires the specific recognition of insoluble ligands whose size exceeds about 0.5 μm
(the size of *Mycoplasma,* the smallest microbe known to
stimulate phagocytosis (reviewed in ref. 1). The next
smallest microbe, *Chlamydia,* enters cells by a poorly
understood but nonphagocytic mechanism (2). Similarly,
viruses do not engage the host cell phagocytic machinery,
but rather are internalized either by the host's endocytic

apparatus or, if the virus bears an envelope, by direct penetration. Second, participation of the host cell actin-based
cytoskeleton is required in nearly all cases of phagocytosis. Particles that engage the phagocytic machinery of the
host stimulate the formation of pseudopods rich in filamentous, or F-actin (Fig. 45-1). Furthermore, addition of
cytochalasins, toxins that block actin assembly at the
rapidly growing, or barbed end, of actin filaments, blocks
phagocytosis (3,4). Third, phagocytosis does not occur at
low temperatures, which are permissive for endocytosis.
Although the lowest temperature that supports phagocytosis is variable depending on the cell type and culture
conditions, it ranges between 13 and 18°C (5; S. Greenberg, unpublished data). It is not known why a temperature requirement for phagocytosis exists, since many biochemical events that are critical in phagocytosis, such as
actin assembly and protein phosphorylation, occur at
reduced temperatures *in vitro.*

CELLS THAT MEDIATE PHAGOCYTOSIS

To gain insight into the mechanisms underlying phagocytosis, it is useful to consider which pathways and
cytoskeletal elements are conserved among the various
cells capable of mediating phagocytosis. Until fairly
recently, this seemed like a straightforward task; polymorphonuclear leukocytes and mononuclear phagocytes,
both avidly phagocytic, share many morphologic features
in common, including an abundant cortical cytoplasm
with many pseudopodial projections. However, it is now
apparent that the spectrum of phagocytic cells is broad.
Some have scant cytoplasm, such as lymphocytes. Others
are sessile and polarized, such as epithelia. This diversity
suggests at least two models for phagocytosis: (a) cells
have evolved multiple pathways leading to phagocytosis
with only a paucity of features in common, or (2) the signal transduction pathways underlying phagocytosis are so
essential for cell survival that they are conserved. It is too
early to tell which of these models pertains.

S. Greenberg: Departments of Medicine and Pharmacology,
Columbia University, New York, New York 10032.

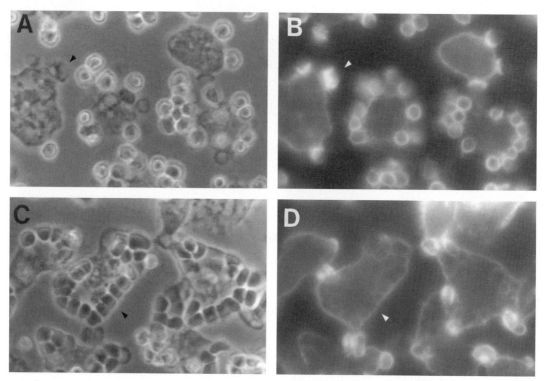

FIG. 45-1. Fc$_\gamma$R-mediated phagocytosis is accompanied by a transient accumulation of F-actin. Adherent mouse inflammatory peritoneal macrophages were challenged with immunoglobulin G (IgG)-coated erythrocytes for 2 minutes **(A,B)** or 10 minutes **(C,D),** and were fixed and stained with rhodamine-phalloidin to detect F-actin. Phase contrast **(A,C)** and fluorescence micrographs **(B,D)** depict phagocytic cups rich in F-actin. Note accumulation of F-actin in pseudopods within 2 minutes after the onset of phagocytosis (*arrowheads* in **A** and **C**) and disappearance of most of the F-actin following complete internalization of the particles (*arrowheads* in **B** and **D**). Magnification = 800×.

RECEPTORS THAT PROMOTE PHAGOCYTOSIS

Opsonic and Nonopsonic Recognition

Multiple cell surface receptors mediate phagocytosis (Table 45-1). Some of these function by binding unmodified epitopes on the surfaces of bacteria. Many of these interactions involve recognition of carbohydrate residues on bacteria by lectins on phagocyte cell surfaces (reviewed in ref. 6). This form of phagocytosis, termed "nonopsonic phagocytosis," is an important function of the innate immune system, whose development predated the acquired immune system characteristic of reptiles and higher organisms. Many substances bind either to microorganisms (termed "opsonins") or to host cells to further enhance phagocytosis (Table 45-2). These substances are found in the serum and in the lining fluid of body cavities, and are even secreted by the phagocytic cells themselves (7). However, the distinction between opsonin-dependent and opsonin-independent phagocytosis has become somewhat blurred by the realization that several receptors, such as complement receptor 3 (CR3), bear multiple recognition sites for opsonic and nonopsonic residues (8–14). What distinguishes phagocytosis mediated by different receptors is the nature of the sig-

naling pathways involved and postphagocytic events, such as phagosome-lysosome fusion, generation of microbicidal products, and activation of gene expression.

Fc$_\gamma$ Receptor-mediated Phagocytosis

The best studied class of phagocytic receptors is the Fc$_\gamma$ receptors (Fc$_\gamma$R), which recognize the Fc portion of IgG (reviewed in refs. 15–18). There are three principal types of human Fc$_\gamma$ receptors (Table 45-1). All three types are members of the Ig superfamily and all are capable of triggering phagocytosis independently (19). Although a detailed discussion of the structures of the various Fc$_\gamma$R gene products is beyond the scope of this chapter, certain structural features of Fc$_\gamma$Rs will be emphasized here that are relevant to their phagocytic functions. Fc$_\gamma$RI binds monomeric immunoglobulin G (IgG) with a K_a of 10^8 to 10^9 (15). In contrast, both Fc$_\gamma$RII and III are low-affinity receptors, and can effectively bind only multimeric IgG. This indicates that receptor affinity is not an important determinant of phagocytic competence. Fc$_\gamma$RI and IIIA are noncovalently associated with a small homodimer, the γ subunit, which confers signaling capabilities by virtue of its encoding an immunoreceptor tyrosine activation

TABLE 45-1. *Examples of phagocytosis-competent cells and phagocytosis-promoting receptors*[a]

Cell types	Receptor	Target	Ligand	References
PMN[b], Mo, MΦ	FcγRI (CD64)	IgG-opsonized bacteria	Fc portion of IgG	19
Leuk, Plts	FcγRIIA (CD32)	IgG-opsonized bacteria	Fc portion of IgG	19,305
MΦ, Mo[c]	FcγRIIIA (CD16)	IgG-opsonized bacteria	Fc portion of IgG	19,306,307
PMN	FcγRIIIB (CD16)[d]	IgG-opsonized bacteria	Fc portion of IgG	308
Mast, Eo	FcεRI	IgE-opsonized particles	Fc portion of IgE	309,310
PMN, Mo	FcαR (CD89)	IgA-opsonized particles	Fc portion of IgA	311,312
PMN, Mo, MΦ	CR1 (CD35)	Complement-opsonized bacteria	C3b, C4b	313,314
PMN, Mo, MΦ	CR3 (CD11b/CD18; $\alpha_M\beta_2$; Mac-1)	Complement-opsonized bacteria	C3b	315,316
		Gram-negative bacteria	Lipopolysaccharide	13,317
		Bordatella pertussis	Filamentous hemagglutinin	14
		Yeast	β-Glucan	8,318
MΦ	CR4 (CD11c/ CD18; p150,95)	Complement-opsonized bacteria	C3b, C4	319
MΦ	Mannose receptor	*Pneumocystis carinii, Candida albicans*	Mannosyl/fucosyl residues	320–322
MΦ	Scavenger receptor AI/II	Apoptotic lymphocytes	?	323
		Gram-positive cocci	Leipoteichoic acid	324
MΦ	CD36	Apoptotic cells	?Phosphatidylserine	325,326
Many	β_1 integrins	*Yersinia*	Invasin	121
MΦ	$\alpha_V\beta_3$ integrin	Vitronectin-coated apoptotic cells	Vitronectin	327,328
Epithelial	E-cadherin	*Listeria*	Internalin	204

Mo, monocytes; MΦ, macrophages; Leuk, leukocytes; PMN, polymorphonuclear leukocytes; Plts, platelets; Eo, eosinophils; Mast, mast cells; Ig, immunoglobulin.

[a]Specific inhibition of binding by these receptors correlates with inhibition of phagocytosis. However, with some notable exceptions (e.g, FcγRIIA, FcεRI, and the macrophage mannose receptor), it is possible that the indicated receptor serves to enhance ligand binding, rather than to participate directly in the ingestion process.

[b]FcγRI is present only on IFN-γ-stimulated PMNs.

[c]A subset of circulating monocytes (~13%) express FcγRIIIA (329).

[d]FcγRIIIB on PMNs is GPI-linked. Its function is somewhat controversial; one report claims it is independently capable of mediating phagocytosis (308), while another claims that it cannot trigger phagocytosis (19). FcγRIIIB is capable of triggering $[Ca^{2+}]_i$ fluxes (330) and actin polymerization (331).

TABLE 45-2. *Secreted proteins that enhance the efficiency of phagocytosis*[a]

Protein	Opsonin	Phagocytic receptor[b]	Reference
IgG, IgE, IgA	+	FcγR,FcεR,FcαR	332
C3b, C4b	+	CR1	333
C3bi, C4b, C3d	+	CR3	333
Surfactant Protein A (SP-A)	+[c]	FcγR,CR1	173
Mannan-binding protein (MBP)	+	FcγR,CR1	334,335
C1q	+	FcγR,CR1	336,337
LPS-binding protein (LBP)	+	?	338
Laminin		FcγR,CR1,CR3	138
Fibronectin		FcγR,CR1,CR3	136,137
Serum amyloid P		FcγR,CR1,CR3	136
P-selectin		?	339
IL-10[d]		Fcγ,CR	340
IL-1		FcγR	341,342
IL-4		FcγR,CR1,CR3	343
GM-CSF		FcγR	344,345
M-CSF		FcγR,CR1	343
TNF-α		FcγR	346,347

Ig, immunoglobulin; IL, interleukin; GM-CSF, granulocyte-macrophage-colony-stimulating factor; M-CSF, macrophage colony-stimulating factor; TNF-α, tumor necrosis factor-α.

[a]Some of these proteins bind directly to microorganisms and stimulate binding and/or ingestion; these are denoted as opsonins. Others stimulate phagocytosis indirectly by binding to phagocytic cells and enhancing ingestion of a variety of pathogens by other receptors.

[b]Indicates which phagocytic receptor is involved or upregulated. In some cases, the specific receptor mediating phagocytosis is not known.

[c]There is evidence that SP-A may act as an opsonin (348), and evidence that it upregulates phagocytosis indirectly (349).

[d]The effect of IL-10 and other cytokines on phagocytosis requires a prolonged incubation with the cells, probably reflecting a requirement for protein synthesis.

motif (ITAM; see below). $Fc_\gamma RIIA$, which is the most widely expressed human $Fc_\gamma R$ and which has no mouse homologue, contains an ITAM in its cytosolic domain.

$Fc_\gamma R$ Signal Transduction—ITAMs and Tyrosine Kinases

First recognized by Reth (20), the ITAM consensus sequence, $YxxLx_{5-12}Yx_{2-3}L/I$, is present in multiple subunits of the T-cell antigen receptor complex, the B-cell antigen receptor complex, and various Fc receptor families. Mutation of either of the tyrosine residues within this sequence markedly impairs receptor signaling (reviewed in ref. 21). $Fc_\gamma R$-mediated phagocytosis in the mouse requires expression of the γ subunit (22) and participation of one or more tyrosine kinases (23–27). Upon clustering of $Fc_\gamma Rs$ and their associated γ subunits by clustered Fc residues, the tyrosine residues within the γ subunit ITAMs become phosphorylated (28,29). These residues serve as high-affinity binding sites for members of the Syk family of tyrosine kinases (30–33). This family, of which only two members are known, contain tandem SH2 domains, each of which interact with tyrosine phosphorylated ITAMs.

The identity of the "initiating" kinase that phosphorylates tyrosine residues within the ITAM is unknown. There is evidence in T cells that the Src family members Lck and Fyn promote this function (reviewed in ref. 34). Indeed, several workers have co-precipitated multiple Src family members and various $Fc_\gamma Rs$ (35–41). On the other hand, there is no convincing evidence that Src family members are required for ITAM phosphorylation during phagocytosis, and it is possible that other tyrosine kinases fulfill this role. In fact, studies using Src family knock-out mice demonstrated that murine macrophages were capable of undergoing $Fc_\gamma R$-mediated phagocytosis in the absence of Lyn, Fgr, and Hck, the Src family members normally expressed in these cells (Clifford Lowell and Anthony DeFranco, personal communication). The constitutive association of Syk with subunits of the antigen receptor in resting B cells (30) and with $Fc_\gamma RIIA$ in THP-1 cells, a human monocyte-like cell line (42), suggests that Syk itself may serve as the "initiating" kinase. According to this view, a small percentage of Syk molecules or other cytosolic tyrosine kinases promote tyrosine phosphorylation of ITAM-bearing subunits in the absence of receptor ligation. This creates a limited number of Syk/ITAM complexes in resting cells. Following engagement of Fc_γ receptors by IgG, further recruitment of unphosphorylated ITAMs occurs; these become phosphorylated by nearby Syk/ITAM complexes, leading to further Syk recruitment from the cytosolic pool (Fig. 45-2). Thus, Syk activation may result from at least three interrelated events: (a) binding to phosphorylated ITAMs and localized submembranous recruitment; (b) activation of intrinsic Syk kinase activity by binding phosphory-

lated ITAMs (43–45); and (c) Syk phosphorylation, both by neighboring Syk molecules ["autophosphorylation" (46)] and by other recruited kinases. Indeed, several Src family members have the capacity to bind and activate Syk (47–50). All three mechanisms of Syk activation are likely to occur *in vivo*.

Downstream Signals Following SYK Activation—Phosphatidylinositol 3-Kinase and Other Tyrosine Kinase Substrates

Syk is required for ITAM-dependent actin assembly in a transfected cell model (51) and for $Fc_\gamma R$-mediated phagocytosis in human monocytes (52). What are the key events that are triggered by Syk recruitment that result in phagocytosis? One likely candidate is the activation of one or more members of the phosphatidylinositol (PI) 3-kinase family. The p85/p110 isoform of PI 3-kinase is a heterodimeric enzyme that phosphorylates the 3' hydroxyl group within the *myo*-inositol ring of phosphatidylinositol and its phosphorylated derivatives. Activation of $Fc_\gamma RIIA$ in platelets induces its association with PI 3-kinase (53) and $Fc_\gamma R$ activation in myeloid cells is accompanied by enhanced PI 3-kinase activity associated with phosphotyrosine residues (54,55). The demonstration of a requirement for this enzyme in phagocytosis is largely pharmacologic (54,56). In contrast to growth factor-mediated signaling, PI 3-kinase is not responsible for triggered actin assembly during $Fc_\gamma R$-mediated phagocytosis (56; S. Greenberg, unpublished observations). Since PI 3-kinase and/or one or more of its isoforms have been implicated in vesicular trafficking of multiple subcellular compartments (reviewed in ref. 57), one possibility is that PI 3-kinase is required for membrane trafficking necessary to support phagocytosis. Perhaps optimal pseudopod extension requires new membrane insertion from an intracellular pool. An alternative explanation is that PI 3-kinase is required for phagosomal closure (56).

Enhanced phosphorylation of other tyrosine kinase substrates has been reported following $Fc_\gamma R$ ligation. These include phospholipase C (PLC) γ-1 and γ-2 (58–60) (see below), paxillin (28), HS1 (61), Raf-1 (62), Vav (63,64) (see below), the adapter proteins Shc (58,62) and Nck (65), and Cbl (66–68). Cbl is a prominent tyrosine kinase substrate that interacts with multiple proteins implicated in $Fc_\gamma R$ signaling, including Lyn (69), Syk (70), PI 3-kinase (67,71,72), and Grb2 (73,74). Recent evidence suggests that Cbl acts as a negative regulator of Syk activation (75).

Activation of Phospholipases

$Fc_\gamma R$ ligation leads to the activation of one or more isoforms of phospholipase A_2 (PLA_2) (76–78). In human monocytes, a variety of PLA_2 inhibitors inhibited phago-

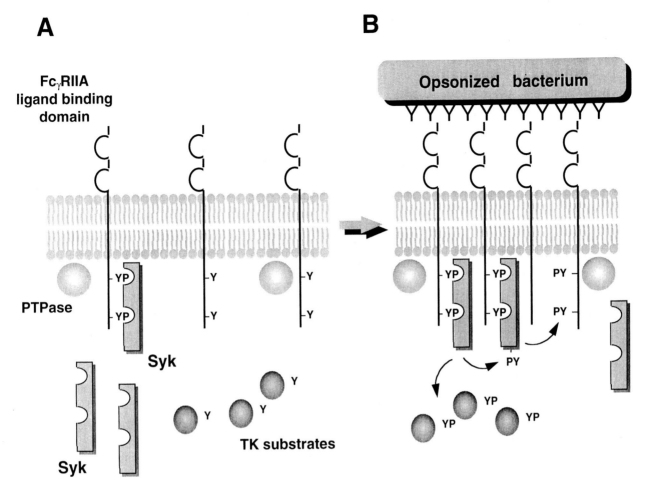

FIG. 45-2. Model for early signal transduction events during phagocytosis by Fc$_\gamma$RIIA. **A:** Fc$_\gamma$Rs are normally freely diffusible within the plane of the plasma membrane. Associated with the membrane are various protein tyrosine phosphatases (PTPase) that oppose the activity of plasma membrane-associated tyrosine kinases, creating a dynamic balance between the two. Syk is present predominantly in the cytosol; a small fraction is constitutively associated with freely mobile Fc$_\gamma$RIIA molecules via SH2 domain-phosphotyrosine interactions. **B:** Following engagement of Fc$_\gamma$Rs with IgG-opsonized bacterium, Fc$_\gamma$Rs cluster to conform with the distribution of IgG molecules bound to the surface of the bacterium. This causes apposition of Fc$_\gamma$Rs, some of which are already associated with Syk. This allows Syk to phosphorylate immunoreceptor tyrosine activation motifs (ITAMs) of neighboring Fc$_\gamma$RIIA, which serve to recruit additional Syk molecules to phosphorylated ITAMs. A localized imbalance of tyrosine kinase activity over basal PTPase activity occurs, which results in enhanced tyrosine phosphorylation of Syk (autophosphorylation) and Syk substrate *(arrows)*. Not depicted are additional tyrosine kinases, such as Lyn, which are recruited to Fc$_\gamma$Rs and which phosphorylate and further activate Syk.

cytosis, which was partially restored by addition of arachidonic acid (78). Partial purification of the Fc$_\gamma$R-activated PLA$_2$ activity revealed it to be Ca^{2+}-insensitive, utilizing phosphatidylethanolamine as a preferred substrate (79). The requirement for PLA$_2$ in regulating endosomal trafficking (80) raises the possibility that PLA$_2$, like PI 3-kinase, may be required for upregulating a vesicular compartment necessary for phagocytosis to occur. Treatment of macrophages and HeLa cells with inhibitors of PLA$_2$ inhibited cell spreading (81,82), and macrophages derived from mice with essential fatty acid deficiency displayed defects in cell spreading (81), suggesting that PLA$_2$ may be required for adhesive (e.g.,

binding to matrix) or protrusive (e.g., extension of pseudopods) events in general.

Other phospholipases are activated following Fc$_\gamma$R ligation. These include phospholipase C (58,60,83–87) and phospholipase D (88,89). Neither enzyme is likely to be required for Fc$_\gamma$R-mediated phagocytosis since neutrophils can ingest IgG-opsonized particles under conditions that block detectable rises of inositol phosphates (83), and several inhibitors of phospholipase D had no effect on Fc$_\gamma$R-mediated phagocytosis (S. Greenberg, unpublished results). Sphingomyelin hydrolysis has been reported in Fc$_\gamma$R-activated HL60 cells (90) and neutrophils (91). Since exogenous ceramide inhibits Fc$_\gamma$R-mediated phagocytosis (91), this suggests that sphingomyelinase activation may act as a negative regulator of phagocytosis.

Other Early Signals Sent by Ligated Fc$_\gamma$ Receptors

Many investigators have shown that Fc$_\gamma$R ligation triggers elevations in cytosolic free calcium concentrations ($[Ca^{2+}]_i$) in a variety of leukocytes (92–96). Peak $[Ca^{2+}]_i$ is observed in periphagosomal regions (94) and corresponds to a redistribution of several markers of intracellular Ca^{2+} stores (97). Are alterations in $[Ca^{2+}]_i$ required for phagocytosis? Use of intracellular Ca^{2+} chelators has produced disparate results, depending on the cell type, the nature of the Ca^{2+} chelator, and the type of particle (83,93,95,96,98–101). The ability of mouse peritoneal macrophages to undergo Fc$_\gamma$R-mediated phagocytosis and actin polymerization without detectable alterations in $[Ca^{2+}]_i$ indicates that $[Ca^{2+}]_i$ fluxes are unlikely to play a central role in the ingestion process in these cells (100,101). Since Fc$_\gamma$R-mediated phagocytosis in murine macrophages is dependent on expression of the γ subunit (22), these findings suggest that γ subunit–dependent cytoskeletal alterations are independent of fluxes of $[Ca^{2+}]_i$. In contrast, mutations in the cytosolic domain of human Fc$_\gamma$RIIA that inhibited $[Ca^{2+}]_i$ fluxes also inhibited phagocytosis (102), suggesting that alterations in $[Ca^{2+}]_i$ may play a role in phagocytosis mediated by this Fc$_\gamma$R isoform. It is also possible that these residues are important for recruitment of other signaling modules.

Cytosolic transients may be involved in other aspects of phagocytic function, such as chemotactic peptide enhancement of Fc$_\gamma$R-mediated phagocytosis in neutrophils (98), arachidonic acid production (103), and phagosome-lysosome fusion (104). However, here too, others have reported Fc$_\gamma$R-mediated, $[Ca^{2+}]_i$-independent enhanced PLA$_2$ activity (79) and $[Ca^{2+}]_i$-independent phagosome-lysosome fusion (105).

Other cation fluxes that accompany Fc$_\gamma$R ligation include those due to activation of plasma membrane channels (106,107) and a Na$^+$/H$^+$ exchanger (108). Alterations in cation fluxes are unlikely to play a role in promoting phagocytosis since Fc$_\gamma$R-mediated phagocytosis is insensitive to the cationic species in the extracellular medium (109).

Activation of many protein serine/threonine kinases has been reported following Fc$_\gamma$R ligation. These include protein kinase C (110,111), protein kinase A (112,113), casein kinase II (114), calcium/calmodulin-dependent protein kinase II (115), histone H4 protein kinase (115), and multiple isoforms of MAP kinases (40,62,115–117). The specific roles of these kinases in Fc$_\gamma$R-mediated signaling pathways are largely unknown. There is evidence that protein kinase C activity is required for Fc$_\gamma$R-mediated phagocytosis (26,111), but a requirement for this family of enzymes in phagocytosis may not be universal (24,118).

Fc$_\gamma$ Receptors and Cytoskeletal Coupling

Likely candidates to mediate actin assembly during phagocytosis are members of the Rho family of guanosine triphosphatases (GTPases). Experiments using dominant-negative constructs of Rho family members indicate that Rac1 and Cdc42 participate in the actin assembly that occurs during phagocytosis. Precisely how these proteins become activated during phagocytosis is unknown. Vav, a protooncogene with guanine nucleotide exchange factor activity toward Rac and Cdc42, becomes tyrosine phosphorylated upon Fc$_\gamma$R ligation (63,64), suggesting one plausible scenario. Vav directly associates with, and is phosphorylated by, Syk (119) and tyrosine phosphorylation of Vav activates guanine nucleotide exchange activity of Rac1 (120).

Integrin-Mediated Phagocytosis

Multiple classes of integrins share the capacity to mediate phagocytosis (Table 2). Despite the widespread recognition of integrin-mediated phagocytosis, the precise signals generated by ligated integrins that result in phagocytosis are largely unknown. Lack of progress in the field is partly due to the multiplicity and diversity of integrins expressed on mammalian cells. In addition, unlike Fc$_\gamma$Rs, integrins exist in several states of activation (a reflection of "inside-out" signaling) that influence their binding affinities for various ligands. This complicates interpretation of experiments designed to test whether a given cellular perturbation (e.g., the addition of an enzyme inhibitor) affects signaling events that occur downstream of receptor ligation, or whether inhibition is at the level of receptor binding.

β$_1$ Integrins

This family of integrins is responsible for the binding and ingestion of invasin-bearing bacteria, such as *Yersinia pseudotuberculosis,* by cultured epithelial cells (121). In studies of internalization efficiency, Isberg's team (122) found that receptor density and ligand affinity were important determinants of binding and ingestion efficiency, whereas the specific binding site within the integrin was less important. Using beads coated with mAbs of various affinities, they found a correlation between bead uptake and binding affinities for the individual mAbs. However, mAbs with 350- to 450-fold lower affinities than the highest affinity mAb used were still able to support phagocytosis at about half the extent of the high-affinity mAbs. These studies indicate that receptor affinity alone is not the sole determinant of the fate of a particle. In contrast, high-affinity interactions between bacteria and specific host cell surface receptors may prevent the microorganisms from interacting with other, competing receptors that may not trigger phagocytosis, such as those located at the basolateral surfaces (122).

What biochemical events are required to trigger β_1 integrin-dependent phagocytosis? Since beads coated with nonblocking mAbs are capable of triggering ingestion (122), it is unlikely that receptor occupancy is necessary. These data are consistent with earlier findings by Sheetz's team (123) that 1-μm beads coated with noncompetitive anti-β_1 integrin mAbs are transported centripetally on the dorsal surface of adherent cells, most likely by engaging the cytoskeleton (123). In contrast, these results are at variance with a requirement for receptor occupancy in integrin-mediated targeting to focal contacts and accumulation of a subset of cytoskeletal proteins, including F-actin (124). The source of this discrepancy is not clear, especially since actin assembly is required for invasin-dependent bacterial uptake (125). Perhaps receptor occupancy is required for integrin-cytoskeletal coupling when ligand density is low, as suggested in a recent study (126).

The above data indicate that, similar to FcγR-mediated phagocytosis, clustering is a major signal for phagocytic signaling via β_1 integrins. The ability of inhibitors of tyrosine kinases to block ingestion, but not binding, of invasin-bearing bacteria (127), suggests that β_1 integrin-mediated phagocytosis requires the participation of tyrosine kinases, as does FcγR-mediated phagocytosis. It is not clear which specific tyrosine kinase(s) are required for phagocytosis mediated by β_1 integrins, nor is it clear what steps beyond tyrosine phosphorylation are essential for this response. Pharmacologic blockade of PLA$_2$ or protein kinase C inhibits β_1 integrin–mediated spreading (82,128), suggesting these families of enzymes as possible candidates for mediating integrin-mediated phagocytosis.

Studies using site-directed mutagenesis indicate that an NPIY sequence in the cytosolic domain of the β_1 subunit is required for phagocytosis (129). This sequence, which is predicted to encode a tight β turn, is highly conserved among most β subunits. The specific role of this motif in promoting phagocytosis is unknown. One suggestion is that it is responsible for binding adapter complexes (reviewed in ref. 130). In fact, microinjection of anticlathrin or anti-AP2 antibodies inhibited bacterial internalization by 60% (129), and depletion of intracellular K$^+$, which blocks accumulation of clathrin, prevented internalization of *Shigella* (131) and invasin-bearing *Escherichia coli* (129). However, other consequences of deletions or mutations within this region include impaired attachment to, and spreading on, immobilized ligand (β_3 integrins; 132) and decreased ligand binding affinity (β_1 integrins; 133). Thus, assigning a role for this motif in signal transduction is complicated by its importance in supporting ligand binding.

β_2 Integrins

This family of integrins, which includes CR3, is expressed exclusively on hematopoetic cells. Analysis of leukocytes derived from patients with leukocyte adhesion deficiency, an inherited disorder of β_2 integrin expression, indicates that these integrins are important in leukocyte adhesion, diapedesis, and phagocytosis (reviewed in ref. 134). Unlike phagocytosis mediated by Fcγ receptors and most phagocytically competent receptors, CR3-mediated phagocytosis is regulated by the "activation state" of the receptor. On resting human neutrophils and monocytes, CR3 is capable of binding C3bi-coated erythrocytes (E-C3bi), but not ingesting them. Addition of several agents, including phorbol esters (135) and extracellular matrix proteins (136–138), capacitates CR3 for phagocytosis. In contrast, murine inflammatory macrophages derived from the peritoneal cavity are capable of ingesting E-C3bi without further stimulation (139). The constitutive activity of β_2 integrins on these cells probably reflects prior activation by one or more inflammatory components. Despite recognition of this phenomenon since 1982, there is no consensus as to the mechanism of CR3 activation. It is not likely to be solely a consequence of alteration in the affinity state of CR3, since addition of substances that increase receptor affinity, such as integrin modulating factor-1 (IMF-1), a lipid that is produced by phorbol myristate acetate (PMA)-stimulated neutrophils (140), and E-selectin (141), does not support phagocytic function. PMA-stimulated CD18 phosphorylation has been demonstrated (142,143), although it is not known whether this is required for phagocytosis. Integrin clustering may be required to promote phagocytosis. Indeed, addition of PMA to human neutrophils induced the appearance of CR3 heterodimers in a clustered configuration at the cells' surfaces (144), probably reflecting stimulus-induced protein-protein interactions. Perhaps a protein recruited to the cytoplasmic domain of either CD11b or CD18 is required to relay the phagocytic signal from ligated CR3 heterodimers. Since neutrophils contain intracellular pools of CR3 that colocalize with specific granule markers (145,146), it is possible that PMA upregulates surface expression of preclustered CR3 aggregates from this pool, rather than induces clustering of surface-bound CR3 (147).

Binding of ligand or MAbs to CR3 triggers multiple signal transduction events, including elevation of $[Ca^{2+}]_i$ (148–151), increases in F-actin content (150,152), activation of phospholipases C and D (153–155), enhanced protein tyrosine phosphorylation (156,157), and activation of Ras (158). Addition of a phorbol ester to HL60 cells abrogated both β_2 integrin-mediated $[Ca^{2+}]_i$ fluxes and enhanced protein tyrosine phosphorylation (159), raising the possibility that CR3-mediated phagocytosis is independent of these signaling events.

RECEPTOR COOPERATIVITY AND PHAGOCYTOSIS

While many studies of phagocytosis involve the use of artificial particles, such as erythrocytes opsonized with mono-specific ligands, it is apparent that bacteria and fungi bear multiple adhesins on their surfaces (reviewed in refs. 160 and 161). For example, phagocytosis of *Leishmania* or *Mycobacterium tuberculosis* by various macrophages is mediated by multiple complement receptors, scavenger receptors, and receptor(s) that recognize mannose residues (162–166). Recognition of unopsonized *Pseudomonas aeruginosa* by human macrophages is mediated by multiple receptors including, apparently, $Fc_\gamma Rs$ (167); another unusual feature of the phagocytosis of this organism is a requirement for glucose, probably by the macrophage (168). The simultaneous engagement of multiple receptors of the host cell increases the likelihood that cross-talk occurs downstream of receptor binding.

Activation of One Receptor Enhances Phagocytic Activity of Another

Examples of receptor cross-talk include activation of CR3 as described above, and activation of $Fc_\gamma Rs$ on human neutrophils by the chemotactic peptide formylmethionyl-leucyl-phenylalanine (fMLP). The molecular events that underlie receptor activation are unknown. Work by Brown et al. (169) has shown that the RGD-dependent activation of both $Fc_\gamma R$- and complement receptor-mediated phagocytosis occurs via ligation of a "leukocyte response integrin" immunologically related to a β_3 integrin. This integrin was found to be associated with a 50-kd associated protein [integrin-associated protein (IAP)] (169), later shown to be CD47 (170). IAP is a 50-kd protein with three or five membrane-spanning segments whose precise function is unknown (171). Mice rendered deficient in IAP demonstrated defects in phagocytosis and increased susceptibility to bacterial infection (172).

Receptor cooperativity is likely to be important in the alveolar lining of the lung. Surfactant protein A (SP-A) is the most abundant protein constituent of surfactant, the surface lining material of the lung. SP-A enhanced phagocytosis mediated by $Fc_\gamma Rs$ and CR1 (173). SP-A is a member of a family of proteins containing collagen-like regions contiguous with globular domains. Other members of the family include the complement protein C1q and mannose-binding lectin. The cDNA cloning of a receptor for this family of proteins was recently reported (174).

Phagocytic Receptors Associate in Multi-Subunit Complexes

Addition of mAbs to CR3 inhibited not only CR3-dependent phagocytosis, but $Fc_\gamma R$-mediated phagocytosis as well (175). Some MAbs that recognize CR3 also blocked binding of IgG-coated targets (176), raising the possibility that $Fc_\gamma Rs$ and CR3 are physically associated with each other. Many cell surface receptors, including

CR3 and $Fc_\gamma RIIIB$ (177), occupy microdomains on cell surfaces. Since $Fc_\gamma RIIIB$ is a GPI-linked protein, its association with CR3 most likely involves their extracellular domains perhaps in lectin-like interactions (178). Indeed, soluble $Fc_\gamma RIIIB$ interacted with both CD11b/CD18 and CD11c/CD18 and triggered release of interleukin (IL)-6 and IL-8 (179). The ability to trigger cell responses when present in soluble form suggests that $Fc_\gamma RIIIB$ might retain its function when shed from cell surfaces.

THE CYTOSKELETON AND PHAGOCYTOSIS

Light and electron microscopic micrographs of cells undergoing phagocytosis reveal certain characteristic features. One is the elaboration of pseudopods that extend from the perimeter of the cells and conform to the circumference of the test particles. The classic observation that ligands needed to be present around the entire circumference of the phagocytic particle for phagocytosis to be completed inspired the "zipper hypothesis" (180,181). Recently, alternative morphologies of phagocytosis have been demonstrated. *Salmonella* stimulates localized membrane ruffling resembling macropinocytosis (182). Pseudopods stimulated by contact with *Legionella* appear as coils that "wrap" around the bacteria (183). A similar morpology was seen during the ingestion of *Borrelia burgdorferi* (184) (Fig. 45-3).

Actin and Phagocytosis

Phagocytosis is accompanied by a net polymerization of actin (101,185,186). One to two micromolar cytochalasin Ds are sufficient to block by greater than 90% the ingestion of the vast majority of phagocytic particles. To the degree that cytochalasin D acts solely to disrupt actin polymerization, this indicates that actin assembly plays an essential role in phagocytosis. What proteins and pathways influence the turnover of actin filaments during phagocytosis? Immunofluorescence studies have provided candidate signal transduction intermediates and cytoskeletal proteins that are involved in phagocytosis (Table 45-3). Vinculin, an F-actin and talin-binding protein that localizes to focal adhesions, is recruited to phagosomes formed by *Shigella* (187) but not, apparently, by IgG-coated ligands (188,189). The most compelling evidence for a requirement for any of these proteins in cell motility is for ABP-280. Melanoma cell lines lacking this protein displayed gross defects in their cortical cytoplasm and were incapable of extending pseudopods (190). Another actin-binding protein, coronin, is required for efficient phagocytosis in *Dictyostelium*. Deletion of this protein reduced yeast uptake by 70% (191). Coronin or coronin-like proteins are probably expressed in mammalian cells, since a protein that shares 40% homology with coronin was cloned from an HL60

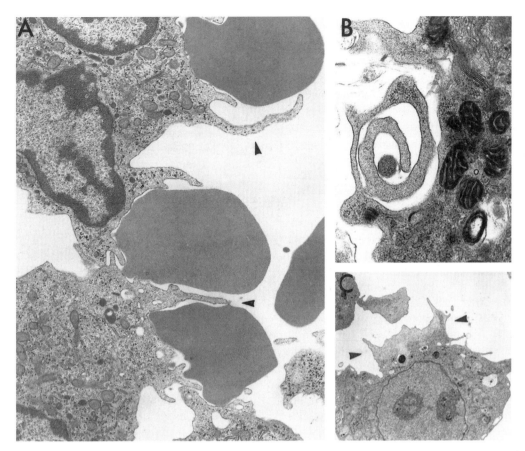

FIG. 45-3. The diversity of phagosomes. **A:** Electron micrograph of human monocyte challenged with IgG-coated erythrocytes. Note extension of pseudopod from the surface of the monocyte, which closely conforms to the topology of the particle. This is an example of the "zipper" mechanism of phagocytosis. **B:** Electron micrograph of *Salmonella enteriditis* invading an epithelial cell. Note localized membrane ruffling response. (Courtesy of Bärbel Raupach, Max-Planck-Intitut für Infektionsbiologie, Berlin, Germany.) **C:** Human monocyte challenged with unopsonized *Borrelia burgdorferi*. A "coiling phagosome" is seen enveloping the bacterium. (Courtesy of Michael Rittig, University of Erlangen-Nurnberg, Erlangen-Nurnberg, Germany.) × 42,000.

library (192). While it was suggested that MacMARCKS is required for phagocytosis of zymosan particles (193), studies using knock-out mice did not demonstrate a requirement for either MARCKS or MacMARCKS in phagocytosis (Alan Aderem, personal communication).

TABLE 45-3. *Cytoskeletal-associated proteins that accumulate in the periphagosomal region*

Protein	Reference
Paxillin	24,28
Ezrin	350
Talin	26,351,352
α-Actinin	26
Gelsolin	353
ABP-280	352,354
Cortactin	355
Coronin	191
T- and L-plastin	356
Myosin I	189,357
Tropomyosin	188
MARCKS	26,189
MacMARCKS	193

However, there is at least one well-documented example in which actin polymerization by host cells is not required for microbial invasion. Host cells expressing cytochalasin-resistant mutant β'-actin failed to ingest *Toxoplasma* in the presence of cytochalasin D, while cytochalasin-resistant mutants of *Toxoplasma* invaded wild-type host cells in the presence of cytochalasin, thus implicating parasitic F-actin in the ingestion process (194).

Mechanisms for Pseudopod Extension

Models for cell motility that account for the leading edge generally fall into two categories: those in which the force required for protrusion is provided by the growing actin meshwork itself, and those in which protrusive forces require the participation of motor proteins, such as members of the myosin superfamily (reviewed in refs. 195–201). There is no consensus as to which model best explains pseudopod extension. Two models are discussed below (see also chapter by Stossel).

Actin Polymerization Alone Powers Pseudopod Extension—The Case of Listeria

While induction of actin polymerization within lipid vesicles is capable of deforming the vesicles (202), evidence supporting this model *in vivo* is indirect. The best evidence for such a model comes from studies of *Listeria* motility (reviewed in refs. 196 and 203). *Listeria* enters host cells via a classic "zipper mechanism" of phagocytosis. In epithelial cells, E-cadherin serves as a receptor for internalin, a *Listeria* cell surface protein (204). Like Fc$_\gamma$R-mediated phagocytosis, ingestion is blocked by PI 3-kinase inhibitors, implicating one or more isoforms of PI 3-kinase in bacterial ingestion (205). Once ingested, viable bacteria exit the phagosomal membrane and, after a short lag period, "swim" within the host cell cytoplasm. The bacteria themselves are associated with bundles of actin filaments and other actin-binding proteins that appear as "comet tails" trailing the motile bacteria (206, 207). Since *Listeria* movement is correlated with the length of F-actin–rich "comet tails" and occurs in the apparent absence of associated host cell membrane, it has been suggested that actin polymerization alone powers movement (208). Studies using *Listeria* mutants indicate that ActA, a 610-amino acid surface protein, is required for motility. The amino terminus of ActA is required for inducing actin assembly, which is further enhanced by the proline-rich central region of the protein, possibly by recruiting VASP, a profilin-binding protein (209,210). Earlier studies suggest that profilin is crucial in supporting actin filament assembly by *Listeria* (211), possibly by donating actin monomers to uncapped barbed ends in the presence of the actin monomer capping protein, thymosin-β_4 (212,213). Recent studies have implicated isoforms of Arps, small proteins that associate with actin, in promoting *Listeria*-directed actin assembly (214).

Myosin Motors Power Pseudopod Extension— The Case of Neuronal Growth Cones

An alternative view of cell motility is provided by studies of neuronal growth cone extension. This type of motility, which superficially resembles pseudopod extension, requires the participation of one or more isoforms of myosin. Butanedione monoxime, a nonselective inhibitor of myosin adenosine triphosphatase (ATPase), inhibits growth cone extension, an effect mimicked by the addition of inactivated S1 fragments of myosin (215). Reinforcing the concept that the motility of intracellular *Listeria* differs from that occurring in neuronal growth cones, butanedione monoxime had no effect on the rate of *Listeria* movement (216).

The now-classic studies by De Lozanne and Spudich (217) and Knecht and Loomis (218) indicate that conventional myosin II is not required for phagocytosis in *Dictyostelium*. Using similar genetic methods and *Dictyostelium* as a model system, results from several groups indicate that several isoforms of myosin I (myoB and myoC) are important for optimal phagocytosis, whereas others (myoA and myoD) are not (reviewed in ref. 201). There are fewer studies of unconventional myosins in higher-order cells. One study implicates myosin-V in filopodial extension (219). Butanedione monoxime also inhibits Fc$_\gamma$R-mediated phagocytosis in mouse macrophages (S. Greenberg, unpublished data). Together with a lack of requirement for myosin II in phagocytosis of yeast by macrophages (220), this suggests that one or more unconventional myosins are required for phagocytosis in mammalian cells.

Rho Family Guanosine Triphosphatases

Analogous to their role in promoting membrane ruffling, filopodia, and stress fibers, several GTPases of the Rho family have been implicated in phagocytosis. Dominant-negative versions of Cdc42 (221) block ingestion of *Salmonella*. Both Rac1 and Cdc42 are required for Fc$_\gamma$R-mediated phagocytosis in macrophages. In contrast, Rho isoforms have been proposed to mediate entry of *Shigella* (187,222) but not *Salmonella* (187,223). Impairment of Rho function by C3 exotoxin abolished *Shigella*-induced membrane folding, but not the appearance of actin nucleation sites (222), suggesting an additional protein for this activity. Treatment of Chinese hamster ovary (CHO) cells with C3 exotoxin blocked early signaling events associated with phagocytosis, including enhanced protein tyrosine phosphorylation and bacterial association with the cells (187). This suggests that inhibition of Rho function adversely affected attachment of the bacteria to the cells, possibly by altering receptor affinity or mobility. Constitutively active forms of Rho enhanced bacterial association and phagocytosis (187), implying that Rho signals enhanced adhesive function of receptor(s) that bind *Shigella*. These findings are consistent with the finding that Rho is required for cell adhesion via β_1 and β_2 integrins (224).

Although the mechanism by which Rho family members trigger actin assembly is not known, Hartwig and Stossel's team (225) have demonstrated that addition of constitutively active versions of Rac1 to permeabilized platelets induces uncapping at the barbed ends of actin filaments. Together with the ability of Rho to stimulate phosphatidylinositol-5-kinase (226), these data suggest a model by which activation of Rho family GTPases leads to alterations in phosphoinositide levels and uncapping of actin filaments. The challenge for the future lies in determining how ligation of a diverse array of phagocytically competent receptors results in activation of these GTPases, and how these GTPases signal cytoskeletal assembly.

Receptor-Cytoskeletal Coupling—A Model for Cytoskeletal Alterations that Accompany Phagocytosis

Inhibitors of tyrosine kinases block phagocytosis of IgG-coated particles (23–27), invasin-bearing bacteria

(127), *Leishmania donovani* (227), and enteropathogenic *E. coli* (228). However, the same inhibitors did not block phagocytosis of complement-coated particles (26) or of *Salmonella typhimurium* (229). What are the minimal requirements for phagocytic signaling? A reductionist view would hold that the receptor must recognize a specific ligand on the phagocytic particle and transmit a signal that culminates in cytoskeletal alterations and actin assembly. These criteria do not require that the ligated receptors themselves either directly activate a signaling pathway or couple to the cytoskeleton. In fact, it is possible that it is freely mobile receptors, rather than those that are associated with the cytoskeleton, that are responsible for phagocytosis. Several lines of evidence support this: First, plating macrophages on immobilized immune complexes decreased the attachment of IgG-coated erythrocytes by 68% but decreased their ingestion by 98%. This suggests that the freely mobile fraction of $Fc_\gamma Rs$ was important for phagocytosis (230). Second, mutations in β_1 integrins that disrupted association with focal contacts (and presumably, the cytoskeleton) actually enhanced their phagocytic efficacy (129). Third, addition of IgG to cells expressing $Fc_\gamma RI$ reduced, rather than increased, association of $Fc_\gamma RI$ with the actin cross-linking protein ABP-280 (231). Finally, addition of phorbol ester or cytochalasin D led to an increase in the lateral mobility of LFA-1, a β_2 integrin, in human lymphocytes. Either treatment led to enhanced adhesion to intercellular adhesion molecule-1 (ICAM-1)–coated substrates (232).

Collectively, these data suggest that freely mobile receptors are a prerequisite for stimulating adhesion and uptake of phagocytic particles. Following diffusion of this mobile fraction of receptors to regions of cell-particle contact, the ligated receptors initiate a program of cytoskeletal rearrangement. A different set of proteins, such as members of the ERM (ezrin/radixin/moesin) family (reviewed in ref. 233) or actin cross-linking proteins may serve to provide a physical link between the growing actin meshwork and the plasma membrane. Alternatively, a fraction of cell surface integrins that bind directly to cytoskeletal proteins may serve this "anchoring function." For example, peptides derived from the cytosolic tails of β_1 and β_2 subunits bound α-actinin (234–236), ABP-280 (236), and talin (236) *in vitro*. This model of phagocytosis assigns a dual role to cell surface proteins that participate in phagocytosis: binding and transmission of the "phagocytic signal" by a freely mobile receptor pool, and anchoring to the cytoskeleton by a different subset.

MEMBRANE REMODELING AND PHAGOCYTOSIS

The phagocytic capacity of macrophages is prodigious. Single adherent macrophages can ingest scores of bacteria, yet the macrophages neither burst nor exhibit an obvious decline in membrane surface area. This is indicative of ongoing recruitment and remodeling of plasma membrane. As particle size increases, the capacity for phagocytosis is not limited by the number of phagocytic receptors (237), consistent with an upper limitation in membrane surface area. However, there is no clear picture as to the source of this membrane. Studies of macrophages spreading on immune complex-coated substrates showed that the Golgi apparatus fragmented and redistributed to areas beneath the plasma membrane adjacent to the substrate (238). More recent studies have indicated that a plasma membrane–derived endosomal compartment is recruited locally during phagocytosis. Inhibitors of PLA_2 blocked ingestion of IgG-coated particles by human monocytes and induced the accumulation of plasma membrane–derived, electron-lucent vesicles beneath the particles (239). This raises the possibility that $Fc_\gamma R$-directed PLA_2 activation precedes, and is required for, the insertion of endosomal membrane into the nascent phagosome. However, this does not address the proximate source of additional membrane needed for replenishment of the pool that is internalized during the engulfment process. Perhaps an endosomal pool that normally recycles at remote areas of the plasma membrane is recruited to forming phagosomes, and the endosomal pool itself is replenished from other intracellular stores.

Fusion of Phagosomes with Lysosomes and Endosomes

Most engulfed bacteria enjoy only a short-lived respite; within minutes to hours, lysosomes rich in hydrolytic enzymes fuse with phagosomes and contribute to bacterial killing and/or digestion. Phagosome-lysosome (P-L) fusion is enhanced in activated macrophages, and occurs in the presence of cytochalasins, indicating that the actin-based cytoskeleton plays little or no role (240). More recent studies indicate that phagosomes engage in sequential interactions with various endocytic compartments (241,242), and that microtubules play a role in the fusion of endosomes with phagosomes (242). Transfer between phagocytic vacuoles containing different microorganisms has been reported (243).

The signals required to effect P-L fusion are poorly understood. In a study of the structural requirements for lysosomal targeting, sequences within the cytosolic domain of murine $Fc_\gamma RII$ ($mFc_\gamma RII$) were required for PL fusion of IgG-coated *Toxoplasma gondii*. Isoforms of $mFc_\gamma RII$ that do not confer localization to clathrin-coated pits (244) were effective in mediating P-L fusion, arguing against a role for clathrin and related proteins in mediating P-L fusion (245). A Ca^{2+} requirement for P-L fusion was shown in one study (104) but not another (105). Given the widespread involvement of members of the Rab GTPase family in vesicular trafficking (reviewed in ref. 246), involvement of one or more members of this family in phagosomal fusion events is likely. Localization of early (Rab5) and late (Rab7) endosomal markers to isolated phagosomes has been demonstrated (242). Using an *in vitro* fusion assay, Stahl's team (247) showed that antibodies to Rab5 inhibited fusion of endosomes with phagosomes containing nonhemolytic mutants of *Listeria* (247). In a similar assay of P-L fusion, addition of Rab-GDI or of anti-NSF antibodies inhibited P-L fusion, further arguing for the importance of Rab proteins in phagosomal fusion events (248). Analysis of phagosomal proteins by two-dimensional gel analysis and immunocytochemistry indicated that multiple annexins associate with phagosomes (249,250); however, the role of these proteins in supporting fusion events during phagocytosis is unknown.

SUBVERSION OF PHAGOCYTOSIS BY PATHOGENS

Evasion of Phagosome-Endo/Lysosome Fusion

Several microorganisms have the capacity to subvert P-L fusion. These include *M. tuberculosis* (251), *T. gondii* (252), *Legionella pneumophila* (253), and *Listeria monocytogenes* (254). Inhibition of P-L fusion requires the presence of viable microorganisms, and is partially reversed by opsonization of the bacteria. The degree of inhibition of P-L fusion is relative and depends on the microorganism and the type of phagocytic cell. The P-L fusion inhibitory activity of *M. tuberculosis* has been attributed to the production of ammonium by the microorganism (255) and the presence of sulfatides in the cell wall (256). *L. donovani* promastigotes evade phagosome-endosome fusion by production of cell surface lipophosphoglycan (257).

Replication Within, or Escape From, the Phagocytic Vacuole

Rather than evade P-L fusion, several microorganisms persist and replicate within the host cell phagolysosomes. Pathogens such as *M. tuberculosis* and *Leishmania* have evolved multiple mechanisms for intracellular survival (reviewed in ref. 258). For example, *M. tuberculosis* survives in a compartment that lacks vesicular proton-ATPases, suggesting that the viable bacteria either exclude or remove it from the phagosomal membrane (259). Other organisms that block phagosomal acidification include *L. pneumophila* (260) and *T. gondii* (261). In contrast, organisms such as *Coxiella burnetti* (262) and *Leishmania* (263) replicate within the phagolysosome despite the ambient acidic pH. *S. typhimurium* may actually require an acidic pH for optimal intracellular replication (264).

An additional survival strategy is employed by *Leishmania* promastigotes. These parasites have the capacity to fix complement, probably via a lipophosphoglycan (265) and gp63, a protein expressed at the surface of the parasite (266). Complement deposition enhances intracellular survival of *Leishmania,* probably by diverting the parasite to phagosomes containing complement receptors that do not trigger the respiratory burst efficiently (267).

L. monocytogenes (206,207), *Rickettsia* spp. (268,269), *Trypanosome cruzi* (261), and *Shigella* (270,271) have evolved a remarkable mechanism for survival. Within 10 to 30 minutes of entry, they lyse the phagosomal membrane, escape into the host cytoplasm, and ultimately infect neighboring cells. For *L. monocytogenes,* pore-forming lysins, such as listeriolysin O, and several phospholipases are virulence factors that mediate escape from the phagosomal vacuole (272–274).

PHAGOCYTOSIS OF PATHOGENIC BACTERIA BY EPITHELIAL CELLS

There has been much progress in the past 5 years in the field of bacterial pathogenesis. What is strikingly apparent from the work of many laboratories is the diversity of receptors and signaling pathways used by host cells to ingest pathogenic microbes. Perhaps this diversity reflects multiple strategies used by different classes of bacteria to subvert the immune system, and the evolutionary pressures they exert on the host. Although it is beyond the scope of this chapter to discuss each microorganism in detail, the reader is referred elsewhere for several excellent reviews (275–278).

Ingestion of Salmonella

Addition of *Salmonella* to epithelial cells leads to a localized formation of membrane ruffles that resembles the process of macropinocytosis (182). This contrasts with the "zipper" mechanisms of phagocytosis characteristic of ingestion of most other bacteria and fungi. *Salmonella* expresses a type III secretion system including several proteins (SipA and SipD) that are required for invasiveness and that are homologous to similar proteins in *Shigella* (see below). Incubation of epithelial cells with *Salmonella* induces several signal transducing events, including phosphoinositide hydrolysis (279), elevations in $[Ca^{2+}]_i$ (280), and enhanced protein tyrosine phosphorylation (229). Inhibitor studies suggest that host cell fluxes of $[Ca^{2+}]_i$ are required for bacterial invasion, as are production of leukotrienes (280). A role of Cdc42 in phagocytosis of *Salmonella* was demonstrated (221). Once ingested, *Salmonella* resides in "spacious phagosomes" whose presence correlates with bacterial survival (281).

Ingestion of Shigella

Similar to *Salmonella, Shigella* induces a "trigger" mechanism of phagocytosis. Entry into mammalian cells is mediated by the IpA proteins, a complex of at least three subunits that is secreted by the bacteria (276). In CHO cells, IpA proteins interact with the $\alpha_5\beta_1$ integrin and trigger enhanced tyrosine phosphorylation of paxillin and focal adhesion kinase (282). The exact composition of the IpA complex is not known, but two constitutents, IpB and IpC, appear to be necessary for bacterial entry. Like phagocytosis of IgG-coated particles in mouse macrophages, ingestion of *Shigella* is independent of $[Ca^{2+}]_i$ (283). SRC is localized to *Shigella*-induced membrane ruffles and is activated during bacterial entry, suggesting a role for this kinase in phagocytosis (276). As discussed above, ingestion of *Shigella* is mediated by Rho (187,222). Compared to the "zipper" mechanism of phagocytosis, the "trigger" mechanism of *Shigella* phagocytosis is characterized by a less spatially localized rearrangement of cytoskeletal proteins. Perhaps this reflects the secretion and localized diffusion of the IpA complex.

Ingestion of Enteropathogenic *E. Coli*

Enteropathogenic *E. coli* (EPEC), another causative agent of diarrheal illness, binds to and invades the gut epithelia. EPEC expresses bundle-forming pili that create a network of fibers that bind together individual organisms (284). Tight adherence of the bacteria to epithelial cells requires the expression of the *eae* gene product. This gene encodes intimin, a 94-kd outer membrane protein homologous to the invasin of *Y. pseudotuberculosis* (285). EPEC induces host cell phosphoinositide hydrolysis (286) and enhanced protein tyrosine phosphorylation, particularly of a 90-kd protein (Hp90) (228). Another gene locus, *cfm,* is required to signal enhanced protein tyrosine phosphorylation of Hp90. Mutants of this locus neither induce enhanced tyrosine phosphorylation of Hp90 nor enter cells (228), and tyrosine kinase inhibitors block invasion of wild-type EPEC (127). Hp90 itself may bind directly to intimin (287). Finlay's team (287) suggested a model by which both intimin and the *cfm* gene product cooperate to induce ingestion of EPEC by epithelial cells. EPEC induces finger-like projections on epithelial cells that extend outward from the epithelial cells and bind additional bacteria (287).

PHAGOCYTOSIS AND THE IMMUNE SYSTEM

Phagocytosis by macrophages and other professional phagocytes results in ingestion and killing of a wide spectrum of microorganisms. What is the fate of the cells that have successfully ingested pathogens? Some of the cells migrate to regional lymph nodes (288). Others, particularly monocytes, undergo apoptosis (289,290), which may limit their capacity to present antigen (291). The fate of the macrophages, once in the lymph node, is unknown, but it is likely that they participate in antigen presentation. Dendritic cells (DCs) (reviewed in ref. 292) are par-

ticularly potent antigen-presenting cells whose immature forms are capable of ingesting a wide variety of particles *in vitro* (293) or *in vivo* (294). In a study of the role of phagocytosis and antigen presentation, granulocyte-macrophage colony-stimulating factor (GM-CSF)–treated bone marrow cultures were incubated with BCG *in vitro.* Following phagocytosis, the immature dendritic cells underwent further differentiation in culture, lost their ability to mediate phagocytosis, but became potent antigen-presenting cells (295). This led Steinman's team (295) to suggest that phagocytosis by immature dendritic cells accelerated or enhanced the development of a more mature phenotype with greater antigen-presenting ability.

The mechanism by which phagocytosis enhances antigen presentation is unknown, but may involve elaboration of a spectrum of cytokines in an autocrine fashion leading to a distinct "antigen-presenting" phenotype. For example, addition of tumor necrosis factor-α (TNF-α) or IL-1 to dendritic cells upregulated the expression of co-stimulatory molecules while downregulating expression of FcγRII (296). Alternatively, phagocytosis may enhance proteolytic processing of antigens and/or loading of antigen onto major histocompatibility complex (MHC) class II. This may explain the observation that targeting of antigen to FcγRs enhances antigen presentation by 100-fold or more (297,298).

There is clear evidence that phagocytosis *per se* enhances antigen presentation by MHC class I (MHC-I). Several studies have shown that a subset of macrophages have the capacity to load antigen onto MHC-I, but only when the antigen is introduced in an insoluble form. Antigen presentation was greatly attenuated by addition of cytochalasins (23,293,299–301). Several explanations have been offered to account for these results, including direct transfer of phagosomal material to the cytosol via a distinct pathway (23,302,303), peptide "regurgitation" from the phagosomes to cell surface MHC-I molecules (300,302), and an "indigestion model" invoking particle overloading of the phagosomal compartment with disruption of phagosomal membrane integrity (304).

ACKNOWLEDGMENTS

Work from this laboratory was supported by grant HL04164 from the National Institutes of Health and grant CB-170 from the American Cancer Society. S. Greenberg is an Established Investigator of the American Heart Association.

REFERENCES

1. Marshall AJ, Miles RJ, Richards L. The phagocytosis of mycoplasmas. *J Med Microbiol* 1995;43:239–250.
2. Gregory WW, Byrne GI, Gardner M, Moulder JW. Cytochalasin B does not inhibit ingestion of *Chlamydia psittaci* by mouse fibroblasts (L cells) and mouse peritoneal macrophages. *Infect Immun* 1979;25:463–466.
3. Zigmond SH, Hirsch JG. Effects of cytochalasin B on polymor-

phonuclear leukocyte locomotion, phagocytosis and glycolysis. *Exp Cell Res* 1972;73:383–393.

4. Axline SG, Reaven EP. Inhibition of phagocytosis and plasma membrane mobility of the cultivated macrophage by cytochalasin B. Role of subplasmalemmal microfilaments. *J Cell Biol* 1974;62:647–569.

5. Mahoney EM, Hamill AL, Scott WA, Cohn ZA. Response of endocytosis to altered fatty acyl composition of macrophage phospholipids. *Proc Natl Acad Sci USA* 1977;74:4895–4899.

6. Ofek I, Goldhar J, Keisari Y, Sharon N. Nonopsonic phagocytosis of microorganisms. *Annu Rev Microbiol* 1995;49:239–276.

7. Ezekowitz RAB, Sim RB, Hill M, Gordon S. Local opsonization by secreted macrophage complement components. *J Exp Med* 1983;159:244–260.

8. Ross GD, Cain JA, Lachmann PJ. Membrane complement receptor type three (CR₃) has lectin-like properties analogous to bovine conglutinin and functions as a receptor for zymosan and rabbit erythrocytes as well as a receptor for iC3b. *J Immunol* 1985;134:3307–3315.

9. Altieri DC, Edgington TS. The saturable high affinity association of factor X to ADP-stimulated monocytes defines a novel function of the Mac-1 receptor. *J Biol Chem* 1988;263:7007–7015.

10. Altieri MC, Bader R, Mannucci PM, Edgington TS. Oligospecificity of the cellular adhesion receptor MAC-1 encompasses an inducible recognition specificity for fibrinogen. *J Cell Biol* 1988;107:1893–1900.

11. Diamond MS, Alon R, Parkos CA, Quinn MT, Springer TA. Heparin is an adhesive ligand for the leukocyte integrin Mac-1 (CD11b/CD18). *J Cell Biol* 1995;130:1473–1482.

12. Wright SD, Weitz JI, Huang AJ, Levin SM, Silverstein SC, Loike JD. Complement receptor type three (CD11b/CD18) of human polymorphonuclear leukocytes recognizes fibrinogen. *Proc Natl Acad Sci USA* 1988;85:7734–7738.

13. Wright SD, Levin SM, Jong MTC, Chad Z, Kabbash LG. CR3 (CD11b/CD18) expresses one binding site for Arg-Gly-Asp-containing peptides and a second site for bacterial lipopolysaccharide. *J Exp Med* 1989;169:175–183.

14. Relman D, Tuomanen E, Falkow S, Golenbock DT, Saukkonen K, Wright SD. Recognition of a bacterial adhesion by an integrin: macrophage CR3($\alpha_M\beta_2$, CD11b/CD18) binds filamentous hemagglutinin of Bordetella pertussis. *Cell* 1990;61:1375–1382.

15. Hulett MD, Hogarth PM. Molecular basis of Fc receptor function. In: Dixon FJ, ed. *Advances in immunology,* vol 57. New York: Academic Press, 1994:1–127.

16. Ravetch JV. Fc receptors: rubor redux. *Cell* 1994;78:553–560.

17. Unkeless JC, Shen Z, Lin C-W, DeBeus E. Function of human FcγRIIA and FcγRIIIB. *Semin Immunol* 1995;7:37–44.

18. Indik ZK, Park J-G, Hunter S, Schreiber AD. Structure/function relationships of Fcγ receptors in phagoctyosis. *Semin Immunol* 1995;7:45–54.

19. Anderson CL, Shen L, Eicher DM, Wewers MD, Gill JK. Phagocytosis mediated by three distinct Fcγ receptor classes on human leukocytes. *J Exp Med* 1990;171:1333–1345.

20. Reth M. Antigen receptor tail clue. *Nature* 1989;338:384.

21. Cambier JC. Antigen and Fc receptor signaling: the awesome power of the immunoreceptor tyrosine-based activation motif (ITAM). *J Immunol* 1995;155:3281–3285.

22. Takai T, Li M, Sylvestre D, Clynes R, Ravetch JV. FcR γ chain deletion results in pleiotropic effector cell defects. *Cell* 1994;76:519–529.

23. Ghazizadeh S, Fleit HB. Tyrosine phosphorylation provides an obligatory early signal for Fcγ RII-mediated endocytosis in the monocytic cell line THP-1. *J Immunol* 1994;152:30–41.

24. Greenberg S, Chang P, Silverstein SC. Tyrosine phosphorylation is required for Fc receptor-mediated phagocytosis in mouse macrophages. *J Exp Med* 1993;177:529–534.

25. Davis W, Harrison PT, Hutchinson MJ, Allen JM. Two distinct regions of Fcγ RI initiate separate signalling pathways involved in endocytosis and phagocytosis. *EMBO J* 1995;14:432–441.

26. Allen LAH, Aderem A. Molecular definition of distinct cytoskeletal structures involved in complement- and Fc receptor-mediated phagocytosis in macrophages. *J Exp Med* 1996;184:627–637.

27. Fallman M, Andersson K, Hakansson S, Magnusson K-E, Stendahl O, Wolf-Watz H. *Yersinia pseudotuberculosis* inhibits Fc receptor-mediated phagocytosis in J774 cells. *Infect Immun* 1995;63:3117–3124.

28. Greenberg S, Chang P, Silverstein SC. Tyrosine phosphorylation of the γ subunit of Fcγ receptors, p72^{syk}, and paxillin during Fc receptor-mediated phagocytosis in macrophages. *J Biol Chem* 1994;269:3897–3902.

29. Duchemin AM, Ernst LK, Anderson CL. Clustering of the high affinity Fc receptor for immunoglobulin G (FcγRI) results in phosphorylation of its associated γ-chain. *J Biol Chem* 1994;269:12111–12117.

30. Law DA, Chan VWF, Datta SK, DeFranco AL. B-cell antigen receptor motifs have redundant signalling capabilities and bind the tyrosine kinases PTK72, Lyn and Fyn. *Curr Biol* 1993;3:645–657.

31. Agarwal A, Salem P, Robbins KC. Involvement of p72^{syk}, a protein-tyrosine kinase, in Fcγ receptor signaling. *J Biol Chem* 1993;268:15900–15905.

32. Kiener PA, Rankin BM, Burkhardt AL, et al. Cross-linking of Fcγ receptor I (Fcγ RI) and receptor II (Fcγ RII) on monocytic cells activates a signal transduction pathway common to both Fc receptors that involves the stimulation of p72^{Syk} protein tyrosine kinase. *J Biol Chem* 1993;268:24442–24448.

33. Benhamou M, Ryba NJ, Kihara H, Nishikata H, Siraganian RP. Protein-tyrosine kinase p72^{syk} in high affinity IgE receptor signaling. Identification as a component of pp72 and association with the receptor γ chain after receptor aggregation. *J Biol Chem* 1993;268:23318–23324.

34. Qian DP, Weiss A. T cell antigen receptor signal transduction. *Curr Opin Cell Biol* 1997;9:205–212.

35. Hamada F, Aoki M, Akiyama T, Toyoshima K. Association of immunoglobulin G Fc receptor II with SRC-like protein-tyrosine kinase Fgr in neutrophils. *Proc Natl Acad Sci USA* 1993;90:6305–6309.

36. Salcedo TW, Kurosaki T, Kanakaraj P, Ravetch JV, Perussia B. Physical and functional association of p56^{lck} with Fcγ RIIIA (CD16) in natural killer cells. *J Exp Med* 1993;177:1475–1480.

37. Ghazizadeh S, Bolen JB, Fleit HB. Physical and functional association of SRC-related protein tyrosine kinases with Fcγ RII in monocytic THP-1 cells. *J Biol Chem* 1994;269:8878–8884.

38. Sarmay G, Pecht I, Gergely J. Protein-tyrosine kinase activity tightly associated with human type II Fcγ receptors. *Proc Natl Acad Sci USA* 1994;91:4140–4144.

39. Wang AVT, Scholl PR, Geha RS. Physical and functional association of the high affinity immunoglobulin G receptor (FcγRI) with the kinases hck and lyn. *J Exp Med* 1994;180:1165–1170.

40. Durden DL, Kim HM, Calore B, Liu YB. The FcγRI receptor signals through the activation of *hck* and MAP kinase. *J Immunol* 1995;154:4039–4047.

41. Duchemin A-M, Anderson CL. Association of non-receptor protein tyrosine kinases with the FcγRI/γ-chain complex in monocytic cells. *J Immunol* 1997;158:865–871.

42. Ghazizadeh S, Bolen JB, Fleit HB. Tyrosine phosphorylation and association of SYK with Fcγ RII in monocytic THP-1 cells. *Biochem J* 1995;305:669–674.

43. Rowley RB, Burkhardt AL, Chao HG, Matsueda GR, Bolen JB. SYK protein-tyrosine kinase is regulated by tyrosine-phosphorylated Igα/Igβ immunoreceptor tyrosine activation motif binding and autophosphorylation. *J Biol Chem* 1995;270:11590–11594.

44. Shiue L, Zoller MJ, Brugge JS. SYK is activated by phosphotyrosine-containing peptides representing the tyrosine-based activation motifs of the high affinity receptor for IgE. *J Biol Chem* 1995;270:10498–10502.

45. Kimura T, Sakamoto H, Appella E, Siraganian RP. Conformational changes induced in the protein tyrosine kinase p72^{syk} by tyrosine phosphorylation or by binding of phosphorylated immunoreceptor tyrosine-based activation motif peptides. *Mol Cell Biol* 1996;16:1471–1478.

46. Kurosaki T, Johnson SA, Pao L, Sada K, Yamamura H, Cambier JC. Role of the SYK autophosphorylation site and SH2 domains in B cell antigen receptor signaling. *J Exp Med* 1995;182:1815–1823.

47. Kurosaki T, Takata M, Yamanashi Y, et al. SYK activation by the SRC-family tyrosine kinase in the B cell receptor signaling. *J Exp Med* 1994;179:1725–1729.

48. Sidorenko SP, Law CL, Chandran KA, Clark EA. Human spleen tyrosine kinase p72SYK associates with the SRC-family kinase p53/56Lyn and a 120-kDa phosphoprotein. *Proc Natl Acad Sci USA* 1995;92:359–363.

49. Ting AT, Dick CJ, Schoon RA, Karnitz LR, Abraham RT, Leibson PJ. Interaction between lck and SYK family tyrosine kinases in Fcγ receptor-initiated activation of natural killer cells. *J Biol Chem* 1995;270:16415–16421.

50. Amoui M, Draberova L, Tolar P, Draber P. Direct interaction of SYK and lyn protein tyrosine kinases in rat basophilic leukemia cells activated via type I Fcϵ receptors. *Eur J Immunol* 1997;27:321–328.

51. Cox D, Chang P, Kurosaki T, Greenberg S. SYK tyrosine kinase is required for immunoreceptor tyrosine activation motif-dependent actin assembly. *J Biol Chem* 1996;271:16597–16602.

52. Matsuda M, Park JG, Wang DC, Hunter S, Chien P, Schreiber AD. Abrogation of the Fc$_\gamma$ receptor IIA-mediated phagocytic signal by stem-loop SYK antisense oligonucleotides. *Mol Biol Cell* 1996;7:1095–1106.

53. Chacko GW, Brandt JT, Coggeshall KM, Anderson CL. Phosphoinositide 3-kinase and p72^{SYK} noncovalently associate with the low affinity Fc$_\gamma$ receptor on human platelets through an immunoreceptor tyrosine-based activation motif: reconstitution with synthetic phosphopeptides. *J Biol Chem* 1996;271:10775–10781.

54. Ninomiya N, Hazeki K, Fukui Y, Seya T, Okada T, Hazeki O, Ui M. Involvement of phosphatidylinositol 3-kinase in Fc$_\gamma$ receptor signaling. *J Biol Chem* 1994;269:22732–22737.

55. Kanakaraj P, Duckworth B, Azzoni L, Kamoun M, Cantley LC, Perussia B. Phosphatidylinsoitol-3 kinase activation induced upon Fc$_\gamma$RI-IIA-ligand interaction. *J Exp Med* 1994;179:551–558.

56. Arai N, Johnson MT, Swanson JA. A role for phosphoinositide 3-kinase in the completion of macropinocytosis and phagocytosis by macrophages. *J Cell Biol* 1997;135:1249–1260.

57. Shepherd PR, Reaves BJ, Davidson HW. Phosphoinositide 3-kinases and membrane traffic. *Trends Cell Biol* 1996;6:92–97.

58. Shen Z, Lin CT, Unkeless JC. Correlations among tyrosine phosphorylation of Shc, p72^{SYK}, PLCγ1, and [Ca^{2+}]$_i$ flux in Fc$_\gamma$ RIIA signaling. *J Immunol* 1994;152:3017–3023.

59. Ting AT, Einspahr KJ, Abraham RT, Leibson PJ. Fc$_\gamma$ receptor signal transduction in natural killer cells-coupling to phospholipase C via a G protein-independent, but tyrosine kinase-dependent pathway. *J Immunol* 1991;147:3122–3127.

60. Liao F, Shin HS, Rhee SG. Cross-linking of Fc$_\gamma$RIIIA on natural killer cells results in tyrosine phosphorylation of PLC-γ1 and PLC-γ2. *J Immunol* 1993;150:2668–2674.

61. Zeng H, Yoshida T, Kurosaki T, et al. Phosphorylation of HS1, GAP-associated p190 and a novel GAP-associated p60 protein by cross-linking of Fc$_\gamma$RIIIA. *J Biochem Tokyo* 1995;118:1166–1174.

62. Park RK, Liu YB, Durden DL. A role for Shc, Grb2, and Raf-1 in Fc$_\gamma$RI signal relay. *J Biol Chem* 1996;271:13342–13348.

63. Darby C, Geahlen RL, Schreiber AD. Stimulation of macrophage Fc$_\gamma$RIIIA activates the receptor-associated protein tyrosine kinase SYK and induces phosphorylation of multiple proteins including p95Vav and p62/GAP-associated protein. *J Immunol* 1994;152:5429–5437.

64. Xu XL, Chong SF. Vav in natural killer cells is tyrosine phosphorylated upon cross-linking of Fc$_\gamma$RIIIA and is constitutively associated with a serine/threonine kinase. *Biochem J* 1996;318:527–532.

65. Park D, Rhee SG. Phosphorylation of Nck in response to a variety of receptors, phorbol myristate acetate, and cyclic AMP. *Mol Cell Biol* 1992;12:5816–5823.

66. Li W, Hu P, Skolnik EY, Ullrich A, Schlessinger J. The SH2 and SH3 domain-containing Nck protein is oncogenic and a common target for phosphorylation by different surface receptors. *Mol Cell Biol* 1992;12:5824–5833.

67. Matsuo T, Hazeki K, Hazeki O, Katada T, Ui M. Specific association of phosphatidylinositol 3-kinase with the protooncogene product Cbl in Fc$_\gamma$ receptor signaling. *FEBS Lett* 1996;382:11–14.

68. Tanaka S, Neff L, Baron R, Levy JB. Tyrosine phosphorylation and translocation of the c-Cbl protein after activation of tyrosine kinase signaling pathways. *J Biol Chem* 1995;270:14347–14351.

69. Tezuka T, Umemori H, Fusaki N, et al. Physical and functional association of the cbl protooncogene product with an SRC-family protein tyrosine kinase, p53/56^{lyn}, in the B cell antigen receptor-mediated signaling. *J Exp Med* 1996;183:675–680.

70. Panchamoorthy G, Fukazawa T, Miyake S, et al. p120^{cbl} is a major substrate of tyrosine phosphorylation upon B cell antigen receptor stimulation and interacts *in vivo* with Fyn and SYK tyrosine kinases, Grb2 and Shc adaptors, and the p85 subunit of phosphatidylinositol 3-kinase. *J Biol Chem* 1996;271:3187–3194.

71. Kim TJ, Kim YT, Pillai S. Association of activated phosphatidylinositol 3-kinase with p120^{cbl} in antigen receptor-ligated B cells. *J Biol Chem* 1995;270:27504–27509.

72. Hartley D, Meisner H, Corvera S. Specific association of the beta isoform of the p85 subunit of phosphatidylinositol-3 kinase with the proto-oncogene c-cbl. *J Biol Chem* 1995;270:18260–18263.

73. Donovan JA, Ota Y, Langdon WY, Samelson LE. Regulation of the association of p120^{cbl} with Grb2 in Jurkat T cells. *J Biol Chem* 1996;271:26369–26374.

74. Khwaja A, Hallberg B, Warne PH, Downward J. Networks of interaction of p120*cbl* and p130^{cas} with Crk and Grb2 adaptor proteins. *Oncogene* 1996;12:2491–2498.

75. Ota Y, Samelson LE. The product of the proto-oncogene c-cbl: a negative regulator of the SYK tyrosine kinase. *Science* 1997;276:418–420.

76. Suzuki T, Saito-Taki T, Sadasivan R, Nitta T. Biochemical signal transmitted by Fc$_\gamma$ receptors: phospholipase A$_2$ activity of Fc$_\gamma$2b receptor of murine macrophage cell line P388D$_1$. *Proc Natl Acad Sci USA* 1982;79:591–595.

77. Aderem AA, Wright SD, Silverstein SC, Cohn ZA. Ligated complement receptors do not activate the arachidonic acid cascade in resident peritoneal macrophages. *J Exp Med* 1985;161:617–622.

78. Lennartz MR, Brown EJ. Arachidonic acid is essential for IgG Fc receptor-mediated phagocytosis by human monocytes. *J Immunol* 1991;147:621–626.

79. Lennartz MR, Lefkowith JB, Bromley FA, Brown EJ. Immunoglobulin G-mediated phagocytosis activates a calcium-independent, phosphatidylethanolamine-specific phospholipase. *J Leukoc Biol* 1993;54:389–398.

80. Mayorga LS, Colombo MI, Lennartz M, et al. Inhibition of endosome fusion by phospholipase A$_2$ (PLA2) inhibitors points to a role for PLA$_2$ in endocytosis. *Proc Natl Acad Sci USA* 1993;90:10255–10259.

81. Lefkowith JB, Rogers M, Lennartz MR, Brown EJ. Essential fatty acid deficiency impairs macrophage spreading and adherence. Role of arachidonate in cell adhesion. *J Biol Chem* 1991;266:1071–1076.

82. Auer KL, Jacobson BS. β_1 integrins signal lipid second messengers required during cell adhesion. *Mol Biol Cell* 1995;6:1305–1313.

83. Della Bianca V, Grzeskowiak M, Rossi F. Studies on molecular regulation of phagocytosis and activation of the NADPH oxidase in neutrophils-IgG- and C3b-mediated ingestion and associated respiratory burst independent of phospholipid turnover and Ca^{2+} transients. *J Immunol* 1990;144:1411–1417.

84. Ting AT, Karnitz LM, Schoon RA, Abraham RT, Leibson PJ. Fc$_\gamma$ receptor activation induces the tyrosine phosphorylation of both phospholipase C (PLC)-γ1 and PLC-γ2 in natural killer cells. *J Exp Med* 1992;176:1751–1755.

85. Scholl PR, Ahern D, Geha RS. Protein tyrosine phosphorylation induced via the IgG receptors Fc$_\gamma$RI and Fc$_\gamma$RII in the human monocytic cell line THP-1. *J Immunol* 1992;149:1751–1757.

86. Dusi S, Donini M, Della BV, Rossi F. Tyrosine phosphorylation of phospholipase C-γ2 is involved in the activation of phosphoinositide hydrolysis by Fc receptors in human neutrophils. *Biochim Biophys Acta* 1994;201:1100–1108.

87. Della Bianca V, Grzeskowiak M, Dusi S, Rossi F. Formation of inositol (1,4,5) trisphosphate and increase of cytosolic Ca^{2+} mediated by Fc receptors in human neutrophils. *Biochem Biophys Res Commun* 1993;196:1233–1239.

88. Della Bianca V, Grzeskowiak M, Dusi S, Rossi F. Transmembrane signaling pathways involved in phagocytosis and associated activation of NADPH oxidase mediated by Fc$_\gamma$Rs in human neutrophils. *J Leukoc Biol* 1993;53:427–438.

89. Gewirtz AT, Simons ER. Phospholipase D mediates Fc$_\gamma$ receptor activation of neutrophils and provides specificity between high-valency immune complexes and fMLP signaling pathways. *J Leukoc Biol* 1997;61:522–528.

90. Glick D, Barenholz Y. IgG immunoglobulins induce activation of the sphingomyelin cycle in HL-60 cells. *FEBS Lett* 1996;394:237–240.

91. Suchard SJ, Hinkovska-Galcheva V, Mansfield PJ, Boxer LA, Shayman JA. Ceramide inhibits IgG-dependent phagocytosis in human polymorphonuclear leukocytes. *Blood* 1997;89:2139–2147.

92. Young JD, Ko SS, Cohn ZA. The increase in intracellular free calcium associated with IgG γ2b/γ1 Fc receptor-ligand interactions: role in phagocytosis. *Proc Natl Acad Sci USA* 1984;81:5430–5434.

93. Lew DP, Andersson T, Hed J, Di Virgilio F, Pozzan T, Stendahl O. Ca^{2+}-dependent and Ca^{2+}-independent phagocytosis in human neutrophils. *Nature* 1985;315:509–511.

94. Sawyer DW, Sullivan JA, Mandell GL. Intracellular free calcium localization in neutrophils during phagocytosis. *Science* 1985;230:663–666.

95. Di Virgilio F, Meyer BC, Greenberg S, Silverstein SC. Fc receptor-mediated phagocytosis occurs in macrophages at exceedingly low cytosolic Ca^{2+} levels. *J Cell Biol* 1988;106:657–666.

96. Hishikawa T, Cheung JY, Yelamarty RV, Knutson DW. Calcium transients during Fc receptor-mediated and nonspecific phagocytosis by murine peritoneal macrophages. *J Cell Biol* 1991;115:59–66.

97. Stendahl O, Krause K-H, Krischer J, et al. Redistribution of intracellular Ca²⁺ stores during phagocytosis in human neutrophils. *Science* 1994;265:1439–1441.

98. Rosales C, Brown EJ. Two mechanisms for IgG Fc-receptor-mediated phagocytosis by human neutrophils. *J Immunol* 1991;146:3937–3944.

99. Odin JA, Edberg JC, Painter CJ, Kimberly RP, Unkeless JC. Regulation of phagocytosis and [Ca²⁺]ᵢ flux by distinct regions of an Fc receptor. *Science* 1991;254:1785–1788.

100. McNeil PL, Swanson JA, Wright SD, Silverstein SC, Taylor DL. Fc-receptor-mediated phagocytosis occurs in macrophages without an increase in average [Ca⁺⁺]ᵢ. *J Cell Biol* 1986;102:1586–1592.

101. Greenberg S, El Khoury J, Di Virgilio F, Kaplan EM, Silverstein SC. Ca²⁺-independent F-actin assembly and disassembly during Fc receptor-mediated phagocytosis in mouse macrophages. *J Cell Biol* 1991; 113:757–767.

102. Edberg JC, Lin CT, Lau D, Unkeless JC, Kimberly RP. The Ca²⁺ dependence of human Fc gamma receptor-initiated phagocytosis. *J Biol Chem* 1995;270:22301–22307.

103. Aderem AA, Scott WA, Cohn ZA. Evidence for sequential signals in the induction of the arachidonic acid cascade in macrophages. *J Exp Med* 1986;163:139–154.

104. Jaconi MEE, Lew DP, Carpentier J-L, Magnusson KE, Sjogren M, Stendahl O. Cytosolic free calcium elevation mediates the phago-some-lysosome fusion during phagocytosis in human neutrophils. *J Cell Biol* 1990;110:1555–1564.

105. Zimmerli S, Majeed M, Gustavsson M, Stendahl O, Sanan DA, Ernst JD. Phagosome-lysosome fusion is a calcium-independent event in macrophages. *J Cell Biol* 1996;132:49–61.

106. Nelson DJ, Jacobs ER, Tang JM, Zeller JM, Bone RC. Immunoglobu-lin-G-induced single ionic channels in human alveolar macrophage membranes. *J Clin Invest* 1985;76:500–507.

107. Ince C, Coremans JMCC, Ypey DL, Leijh PCJ, Verveen AA, van Furth R. Phagocytosis by human macrophages is accompanied by changes in ionic channel currents. *J Cell Biol* 1988;106:1873–1878.

108. Fukushima T, Waddell TK, Grinstein S, Goss GG, Orlowski J, Downey GP. Na⁺/H⁺ exchange activity during phagocytosis in human neutrophils: role of Fcγ receptors and tyrosine kinases. *J Cell Biol* 1996;132:1037–1052.

109. Pfefferkorn LC. Transmembrane signaling: anion flux-independent model for signal transduction by complexed Fc receptors. *J Cell Biol* 1984;99:2231–2240.

110. Brozna JP, Hauff NF, Phillips WA, Johnston JRB. Activation of the respiratory burst in macrophages. Phosphorylation specifically associated with Fc receptor-mediated stimulation. *J Immunol* 1988;141: 1642–1647.

111. Zheleznyak A, Brown EJ. Immunoglobulin-mediated phagocytosis by human monocytes requires protein kinase C activation. Evidence for protein kinase C translocation to phagosomes. *J Biol Chem* 1992;267: 12042–12048.

112. Nitta T, Suzuki T. Fcγ2b receptor-mediated prostaglandin synthesis by a murine macrophage cell line P388D₁. *J Immunol* 1982;128:2527–2532.

113. Smolen JE, Korchak HM, Weissmann G. Increased levels of cyclic adenosine-3′, 5′-monophosphate in human polymorphonuclear leuko-cytes after surface stimulation. *J Clin Invest* 1980;65:1077–1085.

114. Hirata Y, Suzuki T. Protein kinase activity associated with Fcγ2a receptor of a murine macrophage like cell line, P388D₁. *Biochem* 1987;26: 8189–8195.

115. Liang L, Huang C-K. Activation of multiple protein kinase induced by cross-linking of FcγRII in human neutrophils. *J Leukoc Biol* 1995;57: 326–331.

116. Rose DM, Winston BW, Chan ED, et al. Fcγ receptor cross-linking activates p42, p38, and JNK/SAPK mitogen-activated protein kinases in murine macrophages—Role for p42^MAPK in Fcγ receptor-stimulated TNF-α synthesis. *J Immunol* 1997;158:3433–3438.

117. Trotta R, Kanakaraj P, Perussia B. FcγR-dependent mitogen-activated protein kinase activation in leukocytes: a common signal transduction event necessary for expression of TNF-α and early activation genes. *J Exp Med* 1996;184:1027–1035.

118. Newman SL, Mikus LK, Tucci MA. Differential requirements for cellular cytoskeleton in human macrophage complement receptor- and Fc receptor-mediated phagocytosis. *J Immunol* 1991;146:967–974.

119. Deckert M, Tartaredeckert S, Couture C, Mustelin T, Altman A. Functional and physical interactions of SYK family kinases with the Vav proto-oncogene product. *Immunity* 1996;5:591–604.

120. Crespo P, Schuebel KE, Ostrom AA, Gutkind JS, Bustelo XR. Phosphotyrosine-dependent activation of Rac-1 GDP/GTP exchange by the *vav* proto-oncogene product. *Nature* 1997;385:169–172.

121. Isberg RR, Leong JM. Multiple β₁ chain integrins are receptors for invasin, a protein that promotes bacterial penetration into mammalian cells. *Cell* 1990;60:861–871.

122. Tran Van Nhieu G, Isberg RR. Bacterial internalization mediated by β₁ chain integrins is determined by ligand affinity and receptor density. *EMBO J* 1993;12:1887–1895.

123. Schmidt CE, Horwitz AF, Lauffenburger DA, Sheetz MP. Integrin-cytoskeletal interactions in migrating fibroblasts are dynamic, asymmetric, and regulated. *J Cell Biol* 1993;123:977–991.

124. Miyamoto S, Akiyama SK, Yamada KM. Synergistic roles for receptor occupancy and aggregation in integrin transmembrane function. *Science* 1995;267:883–885.

125. Finlay BB, Falkow S. Comparison of the invasion strategies used by *Salmonella cholerae-suis, Shigella flexneri* and *Yersinia enterocolitica* to enter cultured animal cells: endosome acidification is not required for bacterial invasion or intracellular replication. *Biochimie* 1988;70: 1089–1099.

126. Felsenfeld DP, Choquet D, Sheetz MP. Ligand binding regulates the directed movement of beta1 integrins on fibroblasts. *Nature* 1996; 383:438–440.

127. Rosenshine I, Duronio V, Finlay BB. Tyrosine protein kinase inhibitors block invasin-promoted bacterial uptake by epithelial cells. *Infect Immun* 1992;60:2211—2217.

128. Vuori K, Ruoslahti E. Activation of protein kinase C precedes α₅β₁ integrin-mediated cell spreading on fibronectin. *J Biol Chem* 1993; 268:21459–21462.

129. Tran Van Nhieu G, Krukonis ES, Reszka AA, Horwitz AF, Isberg RR. Mutations in the cytoplasmic domain of the integrin β₁ chain indicate a role for endocytosis factors in bacterial internalization. *J Biol Chem* 1996;271:7665–7672.

130. Marks MS, Ohno H, Kirchasusen T, Bonifacino JS. Protein sorting by tyrosine-based signals: adapting to the Ys and wherefors. *Trends Cell Biol* 1997;7:124–128.

131. Clerc PL, Sansonetti PJ. Evidence for clathrin mobilization during directed phagocytosis of *Shigella flexneri* by HEp2 cells. *Microbial Pathol* 1989;7:329–336.

132. Filardo EJ, Brooks PC, Deming SL, Damsky C, Cheresh DA. Requirement of the NPXY motif in the integrin β₃ subunit cytoplasmic tail for melanoma cell migration *in vitro* and *in vivo*. *J Cell Biol* 1995;130: 441–450.

133. O'Toole TE, Ylanne J, Culley BM. Regulation of integrin affinity states through an NPXY motif in the β subunit cytoplasmic domain. *J Biol Chem* 1995;270:8553–8558.

134. Harlan JM. Leukocyte adhesion deficiency syndrome: insights into the molecular basis of leukocyte emigration. *Clin Immunol Immuno-pathol* 1993;67:S16–S24.

135. Wright SD, Silverstein SC. Tumor-promoting phorbol esters stimulate C3b and C3bi receptor-mediated phagocytosis in cultured human monocytes. *J Exp Med* 1982;156:1149–1164.

136. Wright SD, Craigmyle LS, Silverstein SC. Fibronectin and serum amyloid P component stimulate C3b- and C3bi-mediated phagocytosis in cultured human monocytes. *J Exp Med* 1983;158: 1338–1343.

137. Pommier CG, Inada S, Fries LF, Takahashi T, Frank MM, Brown EJ. Plasma fibronectin enhances phagocytosis of opsonized particles by human peripheral blood monocytes. *J Exp Med* 1983;157:1844–1854.

138. Bohnsack JF, Kleinman HK, Takahashi T, Oshea JJ, Brown EJ. Connective tissue proteins and phagocytic cell function. Laminin enhances complement and Fc-mediated phagocytosis by cultured human phagocytes. *J Exp Med* 1985;161:912–923.

139. Bianco C, Griffin FM Jr, Silverstein SC. Studies of the macrophage complement receptor. Alteration of receptor function upon macrophage activation. *J Exp Med* 1975;141:1278–1290.

140. Hermanowski-Vosatka A, Van Strijp J, Swiggard WJ, Wright SD. Integrin modulating factor-1: a lipid that alters the function of leukocyte integrins. *Cell* 1992;68:341–352.

141. Lo SK, Lee S, Ramos RA, Lobb R, Rosa M, Chi-Rosso G, Wright SD. Endothelial-leukocyte adhesion molecule 1 stimulates the adhesive

activity of leukocyte integrin CR3(CD11b/CD18, Mac-1) on human neutrophils. *J Exp Med* 1991;173:1493–1500.

142. Buyon JP, Slade SG, Reibman J, et al. Constitutive and induced phosphorylation of the α- and β-chains of the CD11/CD18 leukocyte integrin family. Relationship to adhesion-dependent functions. *J Immunol* 1990;144:191–197.

143. Chatila TA, Geha RS, Arnaout MA. Constitutive and stimulus-induced phosphorylation of CD11/CD18 leukocyte adhesion molecules. *J Cell Biol* 1989;109:3435–3444.

144. Detmers PA, Wright SD, Olsen E, Kimball B, Cohn ZA. Aggregation of complement receptors on human neutrophils in the absence of ligand. *J Cell Biol* 1987;105:1137–1145.

145. Pryzwansky KB, Wyatt T, Reed W, Ross GD. Phorbol ester induces transient focal concentrations of functional, newly expressed CR3 in neutrophils at sites of specific granule exocytosis. *Eur J Cell Biol* 1991;54:61–75.

146. Miller LJ, Bainton DF, Borregaard N, Springer TA. Stimulated mobilization of monocyte Mac-1 and p150,95 adhesion proteins from an intracellular vesicular compartment to the cell surface. *J Clin Invest* 1987;80:535–544.

147. Petty HR, Francis JW, Todd RF III, Petrequin P, Boxer LA. Neutrophil C3bi receptors: formation of membrane clusters during cell triggering requires intracellular granules. *J Cell Physiol* 1987;133:235–242.

148. Jaconi ME, Theler JM, Schlegel W, Appel RD, Wright SD, Lew PD. Multiple elevations of cytosolic-free Ca^{2+} in human neutrophils: initiation by adherence receptors of the integrin family. *J Cell Biol* 1991;112:1249–1257.

149. Fuortes M, Jin WW, Nathan C. Adhesion-dependent protein tyrosine phosphorylation in neutrophils treated with tumor necrosis factor. *J Cell Biol* 1993;120:777–784.

150. Walzog B, Seifert R, Zakrzewicz A, Gaehtgens P, Ley K. Cross-linking of CD18 in human neutrophils induces an increase of intracellular free Ca^{2+}, exocytosis of azurophilic granules, quantitative up-regulation of CD18, shedding of L-selectin, and actin polymerization. *J Leukoc Biol* 1994;56:625–635.

151. Ng-Sikorski J, Andersson R, Patarroyo M, Andersson T. Calcium signaling capacity of the CD11b/CD18 integrin on human neutrophils. *Exp Cell Res* 1991;195:504–508.

152. Lofgren R, Ng SJ, Sjolander A, Andersson T. β2 integrin engagement triggers actin polymerization and phosphatidylinositol trisphosphate formation in non-adherent human neutrophils. *J Cell Biol* 1993;123:1597–1605.

153. Hellberg C, Molony L, Zheng L, Andersson T. Ca^{2+} signalling mechanisms of the β2 integrin on neutrophils: involvement of phospholipase Cγ2 and Ins(1,4,5)P3. *Biochem J* 1996;317:403–409.

154. Fallman M, Gullberg M, Hellberg C, Andersson T. Complement receptor-mediated phagocytosis is associated with accumulation of phosphatidylcholine-derived diglyceride in human neutrophils. Involvement of phospholipase D and direct evidence for a positive feedback signal of protein kinase. *J Biol Chem* 1992;267:2656–2663.

155. Serrander L, Fallman M, Stendahl O. Activation of phospholipase D is an early event in integrin-mediated signalling leading to phagocytosis in human neutrophils. *Inflammation* 1996;20:439–450.

156. Berton G, Fumagalli L, Laudanna C, Sorio C. β2 integrin-dependent protein tyrosine phosphorylation and activation of the FGR protein tyrosine kinase in human neutrophils. *J Cell Biol* 1994;126:1111–1121.

157. Walzog B, Offermanns S, Zakrzewicz A, Gaehtgens P, Ley K. β2 integrins mediate protein tyrosine phosphorylation in human neutrophils. *J Leukoc Biol* 1996;59:747–753.

158. Zheng L, Sjolander A, Eckerdal J, Andersson T. Antibody-induced engagement of β2 integrins on adherent human neutrophils triggers activation of p21ras through tyrosine phosphorylation of the protooncogene product Vav. *Proc Natl Acad Sci USA* 1996;93:8431–8436.

159. Hellberg C, Eierman D, Sjolander A, Andersson T. The Ca^{2+} signaling capacity of the β2-integrin on HL60-granulocytic cells is abrogated following phosphorylation of its CD18-chain: relation to impaired protein tyrosine phosphorylation. *Exp Cell Res* 1995;217:140–148.

160. Ofek I, Goldhar J, Keisari Y, Sharon N. Nonopsonic phagocytosis of microorganisms [Review]. *Annu Rev Microbiol* 1995;49:239–276.

161. Hauschildt S, Kleine B. Bacterial stimulators of macrophages. *Int Rev Cytol Surv Cell Biol* 1995;161:263–331.

162. Rosenthal LA, Sutterwala FS, Kehrli ME, Mosser DM. *Leishmania major*-human macrophage interactions: cooperation between Mac-1

163. Wilson ME, Pearson RD. Roles of CR3 and mannose receptors in the attachment and ingestion of *Leishmania donovani* by human mononuclear phagocytes. *Infect Immun* 1988;56:363–369.

164. Mosser DM, Springer TA, Diamond MS. *Leishmania* promastigotes require opsonic complement to bind to the human leukocyte integrin Mac-1(CD11b/CD18). *J Cell Biol* 1992;116:511–520.

165. Schlesinger LS. Role of mononuclear phagocytes in *M tuberculosis* pathogenesis. *J Invest Med* 1996;44:312–323.

166. Zimmerli S, Edwards S, Ernst JD. Selective receptor blockade during phagocytosis does not alter the survival and growth of *Mycobacterium tuberculosis* in human macrophages. *Am J Respir Cell Mol Biol* 1996;15:760–770.

167. Speert DP, Wright SD, Silverstein SC, Mah B. Functional characterization of macrophage receptors for *in vitro* phagocytosis of unopsonized *Pseudomonas aeruginosa*. *J Clin Invest* 1988;82:872–879.

168. Speert DP, Gordon S. Phagocytosis of unopsonized *Pseudomonas aeruginosa* by murine macrophages is a two-step process requiring glucose. *J Clin Invest* 1992;90:1085–1092.

169. Brown E, Hooper L, Ho T, Gresham H. Integrin-associated protein: a 50 kD plasma membrane antigen physically and functionally associated with integrins. *J Cell Biol* 1990;111:2785–2794.

170. Lindberg FP, Lublin DM, Telen MJ, et al. Rh-related antigen CD47 is the signal-transducer integrin-associated protein. *J Biol Chem* 1994;269:1567–1570.

171. Lindberg FP, Gresham HD, Schwarz E, Brown EJ. Molecular cloning of integrin-associated protein: an immunoglobulin family member with multiple membrane-spanning domains implicated in $\alpha_v\beta_3$-dependent ligand binding. *J Cell Biol* 1993;123:485–496.

172. Lindberg FP, Bullard DC, Caver TE, Gresham HD, Beaudet AL, Brown EJ. Decreased resistance to bacterial infection and granulocyte defects in IAP-deficient mice. *Science* 1996;274:795–798.

173. Tenner AJ, Robinson SL, Borchelt J, Wright JR. Human pulmonary surfactant protein (SP-A), a protein structurally homologous to C1q, can enhance FcR- and CR1-mediated phagocytosis. *J Biol Chem* 1989;264:13923–13928.

174. Nepomuceno RR, Henschen-Edman AH, Burgess WH, Tenner AJ. cDNA cloning and primary structure analysis of C1qRp, the human C1q/MBL/SPA receptor that mediates enhanced phagocytosis *in vitro*. *Immunity* 1997;6:119–129.

175. Arnaout MA, Todd RF, Dana N, Melamed J, Schlossman SF, Colten HR. Inhibition of phagocytosis of complement C3 or immunoglobulin G coated particles and of C3bi binding by monoclonal antibodies to the monocyte-granulocyte membrane glycoprotein (Mo1). *J Clin Invest* 1983;72:171–179.

176. Brown EJ, Bohnsack JF, Gresham HD. Mechanism of inhibition of immunoglobulin G-mediated phagocytosis by monoclonal antibodies that recognizes the Mac-1 antigen. *J Clin Invest* 1988;81:365–375.

177. Poo H, Krauss JC, Mayo BL, Todd RR, Petty HR. Interaction of Fcγ receptor type IIIB with complement receptor type 3 in fibroblast transfectants: evidence from lateral diffusion and resonance energy transfer studies. *J Mol Biol* 1995;247:597–603.

178. Zhou M-j, Todd RFd, van de Winkel JGJ, Petty HR. Cocapping of the leukoadhesin molecules complement receptor type 3 and lymphocyte function-associated antigen-1 with Fcγ receptor III on human neutrophils. Possible role of lectin-like interactions. *J Immunol* 1993;150:3030–3041.

179. Galon J, Gauchat JF, Mazieres N, et al. Soluble Fcγ receptor type III (FcγRIII, CD16) triggers cell activation through interaction with complement receptors. *J Immunol* 1996;157:1184–1192.

180. Griffin FMJ, Griffin JA, Leider JE, Silverstein SC. Studies on the mechanism of phagocytosis. I. Requirements for circumferential attachment of particle-bound ligands to specific receptors on the macrophage plasma membrane. *J Exp Med* 1975;142:1263–1282.

181. Griffin FMJ, Griffin JA, Silverstein SC. Studies on the mechanism of phagocytosis. II. The interaction of macrophages with anti-immunoglobulin IgG-coated bone marrow-derived lymphocytes. *J Exp Med* 1976;144:788–809.

182. Francis CL, Ryan TA, Jones BD, Smith SJ, Falkow S. Ruffles induced by *Salmonella* and other stimuli direct macropinocytosis of bacteria. *Nature* 1993;364:639–642.

183. Horwitz M. Phagocytosis of the Legionnaires' disease bacterium

(*Legionella pneumophila*) occurs by a novel mechanism: engulfment within a pseudopod coil. *Cell* 1984;36:27–33.

184. Rittig M, Krause A, Haupl T, et al. Coiling phagocytosis is the preferential phagocytic mechanism for *Borrelia burgdorferi*. *Infect Immun* 1992;60:4205–4212.

185. Bailey GB, Day DB, Gasque JW. Rapid polymerization of *Entamoeba histolytica* actin induced by interaction with target cells. *J Exp Med* 1985;162:546–558.

186. Sheterline P, Rickard JE, Richards RC. Fc receptor-directed phagocytic stimuli induce transient actin assembly at an early stage of phagocytosis in neutrophil leukocytes. *Eur J Cell Biol* 1984;34:80–87.

187. Watarai M, Kamata Y, Kozaki S, Sasakawa C. Rho, a small GTP-binding protein, is essential for *Shigella* invasion of epithelial cells. *J Exp Med* 1997;185:281–292.

188. Finlay BB, Ruschkowski S, Dedhar S. Cytoskeletal rearrangements accompanying salmonella entry into epithelial cells. *J Cell Sci* 1991; 99:283–296.

189. Allen LAH, Aderem A. A role for MARCKS, the α isozyme of protein kinase C and myosin I in zymosan phagocytosis by macrophages. *J Exp Med* 1995;182:829–840.

190. Cunningham CC, Gorlin JB, Kwiatkowski DJ, et al. Actin-binding protein requirement for cortical stability and efficient locomotion. *Science* 1992;255:325–327.

191. Maniak M, Rauchenberger R, Albrecht R, Murphy J, Gerisch G. Coronin involved in phagocytosis: dynamics of particle-induced relocalization visualized by a green fluorescent protein tag. *Cell* 1995;83: 915–924.

192. Suzuki K, Nishihata J, Arai Y, et al. Molecular cloning of a novel actin-binding protein, p57, with a WD repeat and a leucine zipper motif. *FEBS Lett* 1995;364:283–288.

193. Zhu ZX, Bao ZH, Li JX. MacMARCKS mutation blocks macrophage phagocytosis of zymosan. *J Biol Chem* 1995;270:17652–17655.

194. Dobrowolski JM, Sibley LD. Toxoplasma invasion of mammalian cells is powered by the actin cytoskeleton of the parasite. *Cell* 1996; 84:933–939.

195. Cooper J. The role of actin polymerization in cell motility. *Annu Rev Physiol* 1991;53:585–605.

196. Lasa I, Cossart P. Actin-based bacterial motility: towards a definition of the minimal requirements. *Trends Cell Biol* 1996;6:109–114.

197. Welch MD, Mallavarapu A, Rosenblatt J, Mitchison TJ. Actin dynamics *in vivo*. *Curr Opin Cell Biol* 1997;9:54–61.

198. Lauffenburger DA, Horwitz AF. Cell migration: a physically integrated molecular process. *Cell* 1996;84:359–369.

199. Titus MA. Unconventional myosins: new frontiers in actin-based motors. *Trends Cell Biol* 1997;7:119–123.

200. Bahler M. Myosins on the move to signal transduction. *Curr Opin Cell Biol* 1996;8:18–22.

201. Ostap EM, Pollard TD. Overlapping functions of myosin-I isoforms? *J Cell Biol* 1996;133:221–224.

202. Cortese JD, Schwab B, Frieden C, Elson EL. Actin polymerization induces a shape change in actin-containing vesicles. *Proc Natl Acad Sci USA* 1989;86:5773–5777.

203. Southwick FS, Purich DL. Mechanisms of disease: intracellular pathogenesis of listeriosis. *N Engl J Med* 1996;334:770–776.

204. Mengaud J, Ohayon H, Gounon P, Mege RM, Cossart P. E-cadherin is the receptor for internalin, a surface protein required for entry of L. monocytogenes into epithelial cells. *Cell* 1996;84:923–932.

205. Ireton K, Payrastre B, Chap H, et al. A role for phosphoinositide 3-kinase in bacterial invasion. *Science* 1996;274:780–782.

206. Tilney L, Portnoy D. Actin filaments and the growth, movement, and spread of the intracellular bacterial parasite, *Listeria monocytogenes*. *J Cell Biol* 1989;109:1597–1608.

207. Dabiri GA, Sanger JM, Portnoy DA, Southwick FS. *Listeria monocytogenes* moves rapidly through the host-cell cytoplasm by inducing directional actin assembly. *Proc Natl Acad Sci USA* 1990;87:6068–6072.

208. Theriot JA, Mitchison TJ, Tilney LG, Portnoy DA. The rate of actin-based motility of intracellular *Listeria monocytogenes* equals the rate of actin polymerization. *Nature* 1992;357:257–260.

209. Kocks C, Gouin E, Tabouret M, Berche P, Ohayon H, Cossart P. *Listeria monocytogenes* induced actin assembly requires the ActA gene product, a surface protein. *Cell* 1992;68:521–531.

210. Domann E, Wehland J, Rohde M, et al. A novel bacterial virulence gene in *Listeria monocytogenes* required for host cell microfilament interaction with homology to the proline-rich region of vinculinme. *EMBO J* 1992;11:1981–1990.

211. Theriot JA, Rosenblatt J, Portnoy DA, Goldschmidt-Clermont PJ, Mitchison TJ. Involvement of profilin in the actin-based motility of *L. monocytogenes* in cells and in cell-free extracts. *Cell* 1994;76:505–517.

212. Marchand JB, Moreau P, Paoletti A, Cossart P, Carlier MF, Pantaloni D. Actin-based movement of Listeria monocytogenes: actin assembly results from the local maintenance of uncapped filament barbed ends at the bacterium surface. *J Cell Biol* 1995;130:331–343.

213. Pantaloni D, Carlier MF. How profilin promotes actin filament assembly in the presence of thymosin β_4. *Cell* 1993;75:1007–1014.

214. Welch MD, Iwamatsu A, Mitchison TJ. Actin polymerization is induced by Arp2/3 protein complex at the surface of *Listeria monocytogenes*. *Nature* 1997;385:265–269.

215. Lin CH, Espreafico EM, Mooseker MS, Forscher P. Myosin drives retrograde F-actin flow in neuronal growth cones. *Neuron* 1996;16: 769–782.

216. Cramer LP, Mitchison TJ. Myosin is involved in postmitotic cell spreading. *J Cell Biol* 1995;131:179–189.

217. De Lozanne A, Spudich JA. Disruption of the *Dictyostelium* myosin heavy chain gene by homologous recombination. *Science* 1987;236: 1086–1091.

218. Knecht DA, Loomis WF. Antisense RNA inactivation of myosin heavy chain gene expression in *Dictyostelium discoideum*. *Science* 1987; 236:1081–1085.

219. Wang FS, Wolenski JS, Cheney RE, Mooseker MS, Jay DG. Function of myosin-V in filopodial extension of neuronal growth cones. *Science* 1996;273:660–663.

220. de Lanerolle P, Gorgas G, Li X, Schluns K. Myosin light chain phosphorylation does not increase during yeast phagocytosis by macrophages. *J Biol Chem* 1993;268:16883–16886.

221. Chen L-M, Hobbie S, Galan JE. Requirement of CDC42 for *Salmonella*-induced cytoskeletal and nuclear responses. *Nature* 1996;274: 2115–2118.

222. Adam T, Giry M, Boquet P, Sansonetti P. Rho-dependent membrane folding causes *Shigella* entry into epithelial cells. *EMBO J* 1996;15: 3315–3321.

223. Jones BD, Paterson HF, Hall A, Falkow S. *Salmonella typhimurium* induces membrane ruffling by a growth factor-receptor-independent mechanism. *Proc Natl Acad Sci USA* 1993;90:10390–10394.

224. Laudanna C, Campbell JJ, Butcher EC. Role of Rho in chemoattractant-activated leukocyte adhesion through integrins. *Science* 1996; 271:981–983.

225. Hartwig JH, Bokoch GM, Carpenter CL, et al. Thrombin receptor ligation and activated Rac uncap actin filament barbed ends through phosphoinositide synthesis in permeabilized human platelets. *Cell* 1995;82:643–653.

226. Chong LD, Traynorkaplan A, Bokoch GM, Schwartz MA. The small GTP-binding protein Rho regulates a phosphatidylinositol 4-phosphate 5-kinase in mammalian cells. *Cell* 1994;79:507–513.

227. Martiny A, Vannier-Santos MA, Borges VM, et al. Leishmania-induced tyrosine phosphorylation in the host macrophage and its implication to infection. *Eur J Cell Biol* 1996;71:206–215.

228. Rosenshine I, Donnenberg MS, Kaper JB, Finlay BB. Signal transduction between enteropathogenic *Escherichia coli* (EPEC) and epithelial cells: EPEC induces tyrosine phosphorylation of host cell proteins to initiate cytoskeletal rearrangement and bacterial uptake. *EMBO J* 1992;11:3551–3560.

229. Rosenshine I, Ruschkowski S, Foubister V, Finlay BB. *Salmonella typhimurium* invasion of epithelial cells: role of induced host cell tyrosine protein phosphorylation. *Infect Immun* 1994;62:4969–4974.

230. Michl J, Pieczonka MM, Unkeless JC, Silverstein SC. Effects of immobilized immune complexes on Fc- and complement-receptor function in resident and thioglycollate-elicited mouse peritoneal macrophages. *J Exp Med* 1979;150:607–621.

231. Ohta Y, Stossel TP, Hartwig JH. Ligand-sensitive binding of actin-binding proteins to immunoglobulin G Fc receptor I (Fc$_\gamma$RI). *Cell* 1991;67:275–282.

232. Kucik DF, Dustin ML, Miller JM, Brown EJ. Adhesion-activating phorbol ester increases the mobility of leukocyte integrin LFA-1 in cultured lymphocytes. *J Clin Invest* 1996;97:2139–2144.

233. Tsukita S, Yonemura S, Tsukita S. ERM proteins: head-to-tail regulation of actin-plasma membrane interaction. *Trends Biochem Sci* 1997; 22:53–58.

234. Pavalko FM, LaRoche SM. Activation of human neutrophils induces an interaction between the integrin β_2-subunit (CD18) and the actin binding protein α-actinin. *J Immunol* 1993;151:3795–3807.

235. Otey CA, Pavalko FM, Burridge K. An interaction between α-actinin and the β1 integrin subunit in vitro. J Cell Biol 1990;111:721–729.

236. Sharma CP, Ezzell RM, Arnaout MA. Direct interaction of filamin (ABP-280) with the β2 integrin subunit CD18. J Immunol 1995;154: 3461–3470.

237. Cannon GJ, Swanson JA. The macrophage capacity for phagocytosis. J Cell Sci 1992;101:907–913.

238. Bainton DF, Takemura R, Stenberg PE, Werb Z. Rapid fragmentation and reorganization of Golgi membranes during frustrated phagocytosis of immobile immune complexes by macrophages. Am J Pathol 1987;134:15–26.

239. Lennartz MR, Yuen AFC, Masi SM, Russell DG, Buttle KF, Smith JJ. Phospholipase A2 inhibition results in sequestration of plasma membrane into electron-lucent vesicles during IgG-mediated phagocytosis. J Cell Sci 1997;In press.

240. Kielian MC, Cohn ZA. Modulation of phagosome-lysosome fusion in mouse macrophages. J Exp Med 1981;153:1015–1020.

241. Mayorga LS, Bertini F, Stahl GC. Fusion of newly formed phagosomes with endosomes in intact cells and in a cell-free system. J Cell Biol 1993;266:6511–6517.

242. Desjardins M, Huber LA, Parton RG, Griffiths G. Biogenesis of phagolysosomes proceeds through a sequential series of interactions with the endocytic apparatus. J Cell Biol 1994;124:677–688.

243. Veras PST, de Chastellier D, Rabinovitch M. Transfer of zymosan (yeast cell walls) to the parasitophorous vacuoles of macrophage infected with Leishmania amazonensis. J Exp Med 1992;176:639–646.

244. Mietinen HM, Rose JK, Mellman I. Fc receptor isoforms exhibit distinct abilities for coated pit localization as a result of cytoplasmic domain heterogeneity. Cell 1989;58:317–327.

245. Joiner KA, Fuhrman SA, Miettinen HM, Kasper LH, Mellman I. Toxoplasma gondii: Fusion competence of parasitophorous vacuoles in Fc receptor-transfected fibroblasts. Science 1990;249:641–646.

246. Mellman I. Endocytosis and molecular sorting. Annu Rev Cell Dev Biol 1996;12:575–625.

247. Alvarez-Dominguez C, Barbieri AM, Beron W, Wandinger NA, Stahl PD. Phagocytosed live Listeria monocytogenes influences Rab5-regulated in vitro phagosome-endosome fusion. J Biol Chem 1996;271: 13834–13843.

248. Funato K, Beron W, Yang CZ, Mukhopadhyay A, Stahl PD. Reconstitution of phagosome-lysosome fusion in striptolyhsin O-permeabilized cells. J Biol Chem 1997;272:16147–16151.

249. Desjardins M, Celis JE, van Meer G, et al. Molecular characterization of phagosomes. J Biol Chem 1994;269:32194–32200.

250. Diakonova M, Gerke V, Ernst J, Liautard J-P, van der Vusse G, Griffiths G. Localization of five annexins in J774 macrophages and on isolated phagosomes. J Cell Sci 1997;110:1199–1213.

251. Armstrong JA, D'Arcy Hart P. Response of cultured macrophages to Mycobacterium tuberculosis, with observations of fusion of lysosomes with phagosomes. J Exp Med 1971;134:713–740.

252. Jones TC, Hirsch JG. The interaction between Toxoplasma gondii and mammalian cells. II. The absence of lysosomal fusion with phagocytic vacuoles containing living parasites. J Exp Med 1972;136:1173–1194.

253. Horwitz MA. The Legionnaires' disease bacterium (Legionella pneumophila) inhibits phagosome-lysosome fusion in human monocytes. J Exp Med 1983;158:2108–2126.

254. Alvarez-Dominguez C, Roberts R, Stahl PD. Internalized Listeria monocytogenes modulates intracellular trafficking and delays maturation of the phagosome. J Cell Sci 1997;110:731–743.

255. Gordon AH, D'Arcy Hart P, Young MR. Ammonia inhibits phagosome-lysosome fusion in macrophages. Nature 1980;286:79–80.

256. Goren MB, D'Arcy-Hart P, Young MR, Armstrong JA. Prevention of phagosome-lysosome fusion in cultured macrophage by sulfatides of Mycobacterium tuberculosis. J Exp Med 1976;73:2510–2514.

257. Desjardins M, Descoteaux A. Inhibition of phagosomal biogenesis by the Leishmania lipophosphoglycan. J Exp Med 1997;185:2061–2068.

258. Reiner SL, Locksley RM. The regulation of immunity to Leishmania major. Annu Rev Immunol 1995;13:151–177.

259. Sturgill-Koszycki S, Schlesinger PH, Chakraborty P, et al. Lack of acidification in Mycobacterium phagosomes produced by exclusion of the vesicular proton-ATPase. Science 1994;263:678–681.

260. Horwitz MA, Maxfield FR. Legionella pneumophila inhibits acidification of its phagosome in human monocytes. J Cell Biol 1984;99: 1936–1943.

261. Sibley LD, Weidner E, Krahenbuhl JL. Phagosome acidification blocked by intracellular Toxoplasma gondii. Nature 1985;315:416–419.

262. Maurin M, Benoliel AM, Bongrand P, Raoult D. Phagolysosomes of Coxiella burnetti-infected cells maintain an acidic pH during persistent infection. Infect Immun 1992;60:5013–5016.

263. Russell DG, Xu S, Chakraborty P. Intracellular trafficking and the parasitophorous vacuole of Leishmani mexicana-infected macrophages. J Cell Sci 1992;103:1193–1210.

264. Rathman M, Sjaastad MD, Falkow S. Acidification of phagosomes containing Salmonella typhimurium in murine macrophages. Infect Immun 1996;64:2765–2773.

265. Puentes SM, Sacks DL, Da SRP, Joiner KA. Complement binding by two developmental stages of Leishmania major promastigotes varying in expression of a surface lipophosphoglycan. J Exp Med 1988;167: 887–902.

266. Brittinhham A, Morrison CJ, McMaster WR, McGwire BS, Chang KP, Mosser DM. Role of the Leishmania surface protease gp63 in complement fixation, cell adhesion, and resistance to complement-mediated lysis. J Immunol 1995;155:3102–3111.

267. Mosser DM, Edelson PJ. The third component of complement (C3) is responsible for the intracellular survival of Leishmania major. Nature 1987;327:329–331.

268. Teysseire N, Chiche PC, Raoult D. Intracellular movements of Rickettsia conorii and R. typhi based on actin polymerization. Res Microbiol 1992;143:821–829.

269. Heinzen RA, Hayes SF, Peacock MG, Hackstadt T. Directional actin polymerization associated with spotted fever group Rikettsia infection of Vero cells. Infect Immun 1993;61:1926–1935.

270. Clerc P, Sansonetti PJ. Entry of Shigella flexneri into HeLa cells: evidence for directed phagocytosis involving actin polymerization and muosin accumulation. Infect Immun 1987;55:2681–2688.

271. Bernardini ML, Mounier J, D'Hauteville H, Coquis-Rondon M, Sansonetti PJ. Identification of icsA, a plasmid locus of Shigella flexneri that governs bacterial intra- and intercellular spread through interaction with F-actin. Proc Natl Acad Sci USA 1989;86:3867–3871.

272. Gaillard JL, Berche P, Mounier J, Richard S, Sansonetti P. In vitro model of penetration and intracellular growth of Listeria monocytogenes in the human enterocyte-like cell Caco-2. Infect Immun 1987;55: 2822–2829.

273. Bielecki J, Youngman P, Connelly P, Portnoy DA. Bacillus subtilis expressing a haemolysin gene from Listeria monocytogenes can grow in mammalian cells. Nature 1990;345:175–176.

274. Smith GA, Marquis H, Jones S, Johnston NC, Portnoy DA, Goldfine H. The two distinct phospholipases C of Listeria monocytogenes have overlapping roles in escape from a vacuole and cell-to-cell spread. Infect Immun 1995;63:4231–4237.

275. Parsot C, Sansonetti PJ. Invasion and the pathogenesis of Shigella infections. Curr Top Microbiol Immunol 1996;209:25–42.

276. Finlay BB, Cossart P. Exploitation of mammalian host cell functions by bacterial pathogens. Science 1997;276:718–725.

277. Cossart P. Subversion of the mammalian cell cytoskeleton by invasive bacteria. J Clin Invest 1997;99:2307–2311.

278. Galan JE, Bliska JB. Cross-talk between bacterial pathogens and their host cells. Annu Rev Cell Dev Biol 1996;12:221–255.

279. Ruschkowski S, Rosenshine I, Finlay BB. Salmonella typhimurium induces an inositol phosphate flux in infected epithelial cells. FEMS Microbiol Lett 1992;74:121–126.

280. Pace J, Hayman MJ, Galan JE. Signal transduction and invasion of epithelial cells by S. typhimurium. Cell 1993;72:505–514.

281. Alpuche-Aranda CM, Berthiaume EP, Mock B, Swanson JA, Miller SI. Spacious phagosome formation within mouse macrophages correlates with Salmonella serotype pathogenicity and host susceptibility. Infect Immun 1995;63:4456–4462.

282. Watarai M, Funato S, Sasakawa C. Interaction of Ipa proteins of Shigella flexneri with α5β1 integrin promotes entry of the bacteria into mammalian cells. J Exp Med 1996;183:991–999.

283. Clerc PL, Berthon B, Claret M, Sansonetti PJ. Internalization of Shigella flexneri into HeLa cells occurs without an increase in cytosolic Ca2+ concentration. Infect Immun 1989;57:2919–2922.

284. Giron JA, Suk Yue Ho A, Schoolnik GK. An inducible bundle-forming pilus of enteropathogenic Escherichia coli. Science 1991;254: 710–713.

285. Jerse AE, Yu J, Tall BD, Kaper JB. A genetic locus of enteropathogenic Escherichia coli necessary for the production of attaching and effacing lesions on tissue culture cells. Proc Natl Acad Sci USA 1990;87: 7839–7843.

286. Foubister V, Rosenshine I, Finlay BB. A diarrheal pathogen,

enteropathogenic *Escherichia coli* (EPEC), triggers a flux of inositol phosphates in infected epithelial cells. *J Exp Med* 1994;179:993–998.

287. Rosenshine I, Ruschkowski S, Stein M, Reinscheid DJ, Mills SD, Finlay BB. A pathogenic bacterium triggers epithelial signals to form a functional bacterial receptor that mediates actin pseudopod formation. *EMBO J* 1996;15:2613–2624.

288. Bellingan GJ, Caldwell H, Howie SE, Dransfield I, Haslett C. *In vivo* fate of the inflammatory macrophage during the resolution of inflammation: inflammatory macrophages do not die locally, but emigrate to the draining lymph nodes. *J Immunol* 1996;157:2577–2585.

289. Zychlinsky A, Prevost MC, Sansonetti PJ. *Shigella flexneri* induces apoptosis in infected macrophages. *Nature* 1992;358:167–169.

290. Baran J, Guzik K, Hryniewicz W, Ernst M, Flad HD, Pryjma J. Apoptosis of monocytes and prolonged survival of granulocytes as a result of phagocytosis of bacteria. *Infect Immun* 1996;64:4242–4248.

291. Pryjma J, Baran J, Ernst M, Woloszyn M, Flad HD. Altered antigen-presenting capacity of human monocytes after phagocytosis of bacteria. *Infect Immun* 1994;62:1961–1967.

292. Cella M, Sallusto F, Lanzavecchia A. Origin, maturation and antigen presenting function of dendritic cells. *Curr Opin Immunol* 1997;9:10–16.

293. Reis e Sousa C, Stahl PD, Austyn JM. Phagocytosis of antigens by Langerhans cells *in vitro. J Exp Med* 1993;178:509–519.

294. Matsuno K, Ezaki T, Kudo S, Uehara Y. A life stage of particle-laden rat dendritic cells *in vivo:* their terminal division, active phagocytosis, and translocation from the liver to the draining lymph. *J Exp Med* 1996;183:1865–1878.

295. Inaba K, Inaba M, Naito M, Steinman RM. Dendritic cell progenitors phagocytose particulates, including Bacillus Calmette-Guerin organisms, and sensitize mice to mycobacterial antigens *in vivo. J Exp Med* 1993;178:479–488.

296. Sallusto F, Cella M, Danieli C, Lanzavecchia A. Dendritic cells use macropinocytosis and the mannose receptor to concentrate macromolecules in the major histocompatibility complex class II compartment: downregulation by cytokines and bacterial products. *J Exp Med* 1995;182:389–400.

297. Snider DP, Kaubisch A, Segal DM. Enhanced antigen immunogenicity induced by bispecific antibodies. *J Exp Med* 1990;171:1957–1963.

298. Gosselin EJ, Wardwell K, Gosselin DR, Alter N, Fisher JL, Guyre PM. Enhanced antigen presentation using human Fc$_\gamma$ receptor (monocyte/macrophage)-specific immunogens. *J Immunol* 1992;149:3477–3481.

299. Kovacsovics-Bankowski M, Clark K, Benacerraf B, Rock KL. Efficient major histocompatibility complex class I presentation of exogenous antigen upon phagocytosis by macrophages. *Proc Natl Acad Sci USA* 1993;90:4942–4946.

300. Pfeifer JD, Wick MJ, Roberts RL, Findlay K, Normark SJ, Harding CV. Phagocytic processing of bacterial antigens for class I MHC presentation to T cells. *Nature* 1993;361:359–362.

301. Kovacsovics-Bankowski M, Rock KL. A phagosome-to-cytosol pathway for exogenous antigens presented on MHC class I molecules. *Science* 1995;267:243–246.

302. Harding CV, Song R. Phagocytic processing of exogenous particulate antigens by macrophages for presentation by class I MHC molecules. *J Immunol* 1994;153:4925–4933.

303. Norbury CC, Hewlett LJ, Prescott AR, Shastri N, Watts C. Class I MHC presentation of exogenous soluble antigen via macropinocytosis in bone marrow macrophages. *Immunity* 1995;3:783–791.

304. Reis e Sousa C, Germain RN. Major histocompatibility complex class I presentation of peptides derived from soluble exogenous antigen by a subset of cells engaged in phagocytosis. *J Exp Med* 1995;182:841–851.

305. Looney RJ, Ryan DH, Takahashi K, et al. Identification of a second class of IgG Fc receptors on human neutrophils. *J Exp Med* 1986;163:826–836.

306. Huizinga TWJ, van Kemenade F, Koenderman L, et al. The 40-kDa Fc$_\gamma$ receptor (FcγRII) on human neutrophils is essential for the IgG-induced respiratory burst and IgG-induced phagocytosis. *J Immunol* 1989;142:2365–2369.

307. Clarkson SB, Ory PA. Developmentally regulated IgG Fc receptors on cultured human monocytes. *J Exp Med* 1988;167:408–417.

308. Salmon JE, Kapur S, Kimberly RP. Opsonin-independent ligation of Fc gamma receptors. The 3G8-bearing receptors on neutrophils mediate the phagocytosis of concanavalin A-treated erythrocytes and nonopsonized *Escherichia coli. J Exp Med* 1987;166:1798–1813.

309. Daeron M, Malbec O, Bonnerot C, Latour S, Segal DM, Fridman WH. Tyrosine-containing activation motif-dependent phagocytosis in mast cells. *J Immunol* 1994;152:783–792.

310. Pierini L, Holowka D, Baird B. Fc$_\varepsilon$RI-mediated association of 6-μm beads with RBL-2H3 mast cells results in exclusion of signaling proteins from the forming phagosome and abrogation of normal downstream signaling. *J Cell Biol* 1996;134:1427–1439.

311. Shen L, Lasser R, Fanger MW. My43, a monoclonal antibody that reacts with human myeloid cells inhibits monocyte IgA binding and triggers function. *J Immunol* 1989;143:4117–4122.

312. Weisbart RH, Kacena A, Schuh A, Golde DW. GM-CSF induces human neutrophil IgA-mediated phagocytosis by an IgA Fc receptor activation mechanism. *Nature* 1988;332:647–648.

313. Ross GD, Lambris JD. Identification of a C3bi-specific membrane complement receptor that is expressed on lymphocytes, monocytes, neutrophils, and erythrocytes. *J Exp Med* 1982;155:96–110.

314. Newman SL, Devery-Pocius JE, Ross GD, Henson PM. Phagocytosis by human monocyte-derived macrophages. Independent function of receptors for C3b (CR$_1$) and iC3b (CR$_3$). *Complement* 1984;1:213–227.

315. Wright SD, Rao PE, Van Voorhis WC, et al. Identification of the C3bi receptor of human monocytes and macrophages by using monoclonal antibodies. *Proc Natl Acad Sci USA* 1983;80:5699–5703.

316. Beller DI, Springer TA, Schreiber RD. Anti-Mac-1 selectively inhibits the mouse and human type three complement receptor. *J Exp Med* 1982;156:1000–1009.

317. Wright SD, Jong MT. Adhesion-promoting receptors on human macrophages recognize *Escherichia coli* by binding to lipopolysaccharide. *J Exp Med* 1986;164:1876–1888.

318. Vetvicka V, Thornton BP, Ross GD. Soluble β-glucan polysaccharide binding to the lectin site of neutrophil or natural killer cell complement receptor type 3 (CD11b/CD18) generates a primed state of the receptor capable of mediating cytotoxicity of iC3b-opsonized target cells. *J Clin Invest* 1996;98:50–61.

319. Myones BL, Dalzell JG, Hogg N, Ross GD. Neutrophil and monocyte cell surface p150,95 has iC3b-receptor (CR4) activity resembling CR3. *J Clin Invest* 1988;82:640–651.

320. Kruskal BA, Sastry K, Warner AB, Mathieu CE, Ezekowitz RA. Phagocytic chimeric receptors require both transmembrane and cytoplasmic domains from the mannose receptor. *J Exp Med* 1992;176:1673–1680.

321. Ezekowitz RAB, Williams DJ, Koziel H, et al. Uptake of *Pneumocystis carinii* mediated by the macrophage mannose receptor. *Nature* 1991;351:155–158.

322. Ezekowitz RAB, Sastry K, Bailly P, Warner A. Molecular characterization of the human macrophage mannose receptor: demonstration of multiple carbohydrate recognition-like domains and phagocytosis of yeasts in Cos-1 cells. *J Exp Med* 1990;172:1785–1794.

323. Platt N, Suzuki H, Kurihara Y, Kodama T, Gordon S. Role for the class A macrophage scavenger receptor in the phagocytosis of apoptotic thymocytes *in vitro. Proc Natl Acad Sci USA* 1996;93:12456–12460.

324. Dunne DW, Resnick D, Greenberg J, Krieger M, Joiner KA. The type I macrophage scavenger receptor binds to gram-positive bacteria and recognizes lipoteichoic acid. *Proc Natl Acad Sci USA* 1994;91:1863–1867.

325. Ren Y, Silverstein RL, Allen J, Savill J. CD36 gene transfer confers capacity for phagocytosis of cells undergoing apoptosis. *J Exp Med* 1995;181:1857–1862.

326. Rigotti A, Acton SL, Krieger M. The class B scavenger receptors SR-BI and CD36 are receptors for anionic phospholipids. *J Biol Chem* 1995;270:16221–16224.

327. Fadok VA, Savill JS, Haslett C, et al. Different populations of macrophages use either the vitronectin receptor or the phosphatidylserine receptor to recognize and remove apoptotic cells. *J Immunol* 1992;149:4029–4036.

328. Savill J, Dransfield I, Hogg N, Haslett C. Vitronectin receptor-mediated phagocytosis of cells undergoing apoptosis. *Nature* 1990;343:170–173.

329. Passlick B, Flieger D, Ziegler-Heitbrock HWL. Identification and characterization of a novel monocyte subpopulation in human peripheral blood. *Blood* 1989;74:2527–2534.

330. Kimberly RP, Ahlstrom JW, Click ME, Edberg JC. The glycosyl phosphatidylinositol-linked FcγRIII$_{PMN}$ mediates transmembrane signaling events distinct from FcγRII. *J Exp Med* 1990;171:1239–1255.

331. Salmon JE, Brogle NL, Edberg JC, Kimberly RP. Fcγ receptor III induces actin polymerization in human neutrophils and primes phagocytosis mediated by Fcγ receptor II. *J Immunol* 1991;146:997–1004.

332. Greenberg S, Silverstein SC. Phagocytosis. In: Paul WE, ed. *Fundamental immunology*, 3rd ed. New York: Raven Press, 1993:941–964.

333. Liszewski MK, Atkinson JP. The complement system. In: Paul WE, ed. *Fundamental immunology*, 3rd ed. New York: Raven Press, 1993:917–939.

334. Kuhlman M, Joiner K, Ezekowitz RAB. The human mannose-binding protein functions as an opsonin. *J Exp Med* 1989;169:1733–1745.

335. Tenner AJ, Robinson SL, Ezekowitz RA. Mannose binding protein (MBP) enhances mononuclear phagocyte function via a receptor that contains the 126,000 M_r component of the C1q receptor. *Immunity* 1995;3:485–493.

336. Bobak DA, Gaither TA, Frank MM, Tenner AJ. Modulation of FcR function by complement: subcomponent C1q enhances the phagocytosis of IgG-opsonized targets by human monocytes and culture-derived macrophages. *J Immunol* 1987;138:1150–1156.

337. Bobak DA, Frank MM, Tenner AJ. C1q acts synergistically with phorbol dibutyrate to activate CR1-mediated phagocytosis by human mononuclear phagocytes. *Eur J Immunol* 1988;18:2001–2007.

338. Wright SD, Tobias PS, Ulevitch RJ, Ramos RA. Lipopolysaccharide (LPS) binding protein opsonizes LPS-bearing particles for recognition by a novel receptor on macrophages. *J Exp Med* 1989;170:1231–1241.

339. Cooper D, Butcher CM, Berndt MC, Vadas MA. P-selectin interacts with a β2-integrin to enhance phagocytosis. *J Immunol* 1994;153:3199–3209.

340. Capsoni F, Minonzio F, Ongari AM, Carbonelli V, Galli A, Zanussi C. IL-10 up-regulates human monocyte phagocytosis in the presence of IL-4 and IFN-γ. *J Leukoc Biol* 1995;58:351–358.

341. Simms HH, Gaither TA, Fries LF, Frank MM. Monokines released during short-term Fcγ receptor phagocytosis up-regulate polymorphonuclear leukocytes and monocyte-phagocytic function. *J Immunol* 1991;147:265–272.

342. Moxey-Mims MM, Simms HH, Frnak MM, Lin EY, Gaither TA. The effects of IL-1, IL-2, and tumor necrosis factor on polymorphonuclear leukocyte Fcγ receptor-mediated phagocytosis. *J Immunol* 1991;147:1823–1830.

343. Sampson LL, Heuser J, Brown EJ. Cytokine regulation of complement receptor-mediated ingestion by mouse peritoneal macrophages. M-CSF and IL-4 activate phagocytosis by a common mechanism requiring autostimulation by IFN-β. *J Immunol* 1991;146:1005–1013.

344. Collins HL, Bancroft GJ. Cytokine enhancement of complement-dependent phagocytosis by macrophages: synergy of tumor necrosis factor-α and granulocyte-macrophage colony-stimulating factor for phagocytosis of *Cryptococcus neoformans*. *Eur J Immunol* 1992;22:1447–1454.

345. Capsoni F, Bonara P, Minonzio F, et al. The effect of cytokines on human neutrophil Fc receptor-mediated phagocytosis. *J Clin Lab Immunol* 1991;34:115–124.

346. Klebanoff SJ, Vadas MA, Harlan JM, et al. Stimulation of neutrophils by tumor necrosis factor. *J Immunol* 1986;136:4220–4225.

347. Gresham HD, Zheleznyak A, Mormol JS, Brown EJ. Studies on the molecular mechanisms of human neutrophil Fc receptor-mediated phagocytosis. Evidence that a distinct pathway for activation of the respiratory burst results in reactive oxygen metabolite-dependent amplification of ingestion. *J Biol Chem* 1990;265:7819–7826.

348. Kabha K, Schmegner J, Keisari Y, Parolis H, Schlepper-Schaefer J, Ofek I. SP-A enhances phagocytosis of *Klebsiella* by interaction with capsular polysaccharides and alveolar macrophages. *Am J Physiol* 1997;272:L344–L352.

349. Gaynor CD, Mccormack FX, Voelker DR, Mcgowan SE, Schlesinger LS. Pulmonary surfactant protein A mediates enhanced phagocytosis of *Mycobacterium tuberculosis* by a direct interaction with human macrophages. *J Immunol* 1995;155:5343–5351.

350. Finlay BB, Rosenshine I, Donnenberg MS, Kaper JB. Cytoskeletal composition of attaching and effacing lesions associated with enteropathogenic *Escherichia coli* adherence to HeLa cells. *Infect Immun* 1992;60:2541–2543.

351. Greenberg S, Burridge K, Silverstein SC. Colocalization of F-actin and talin during Fc receptor-mediated phagocytosis in mouse macrophages. *J Exp Med* 1990;172:1853–1856.

352. Young VB, Falkow S, Schoolnik GK. The invasin protein of *Yersinia enterocolitica*: internalization of invasin-bearing bacteria by eukaryotic cells is associated with reorganization of the cytoskeleton. *J Cell Biol* 1992;116:197–207.

353. Yin HL, Albrecht JH, Fattoum A. Identification of gelsolin, a Ca^{2+}-dependent regulatory protein of actin gel-sol transformation, and its intracellular distribution in a variety of cells and tissues. *J Cell Biol* 1981;91:901–906.

354. Valerius NH, Stendahl OI, Hartwig JH, Stossel TP. Distribution of actin-binding protein and myosin in neutrophils during chemotaxis and phagocytosis. *Adv Exp Med Biol* 1982;141:19–28.

355. Dehio C, Prevost MC, Sansonetti PJ. Invasion of epithelial cells by Shigella flexneri induces tyrosine phosphorylation of cortactin by a pp60[c-src]-mediated signalling pathway. *EMBO J* 1995;14:2471–2482.

356. Adam T, Arpin M, Prevost MC, Gounon P, Sansonetti PJ. Cytoskeletal rearrangements and the functional role of T-plastin during entry of *Shigella flexneri* into HeLa cells. *J Cell Biol* 1995;129:367–381.

357. Fukui Y, Lynch TJ, Brzeska H, Korn ED. Myosin I is located at the leading edges of locomoting *Dictyostelium* amoebae. *Nature* 1989;341:328–331.

Inflammation: Basic Principles and Clinical Correlates,
3rd ed., edited by John I. Gallin and Ralph Snyderman.
Lippincott Williams & Wilkins, Philadelphia © 1999.

CHAPTER 46

Degranulation

Giorgio Berton

Neutrophils are secretory cells that, on interaction with a wide array of stimuli, release microbicidal and proinflammatory agents in the extracellular milieu. At least three distinct pathways of secretion, differing in terms of regulation and time of occurrence, have been identified in phagocytic cells. Agonists of neutrophil responses elicit a rapid (within seconds) release of newly synthesized compounds such as reactive oxygen intermediates and phospholipid-derived mediators. Soon afterward (within seconds or minutes), preformed enzymes and proteins stored in intracellular granules are discharged (degranulation). Finally, activation of gene transcription results (within a few hours) in synthesis and secretion of proinflammatory cytokines (1).

The first two pathways of secretion are indistinguishable as far as the eliciting stimuli and signals involved. In addition, these secretory pathways are coordinated rather than independent events. For example, phospholipid turnover influences degranulation, and mobilization of intracellular compartments regulates assembly of components of nicotinamide-adenine dinucleotide phosphate (NADPH) oxidase, the superoxide anion–generating enzymatic system.

Degranulation has significance in the context of several important aspects of phagocyte biology, including killing of pathogens, transmigration into inflamed tissues, and tissue damage and remodeling. This chapter deals with only some of the more recent developments in the field of degranulation. In particular, the significance of degranulation in the context of leukocyte-endothelial cell interaction, the mechanisms of granule–plasma membrane fusion, and the signaling mechanisms for degranulation are addressed.

HETEROGENEITY OF NEUTROPHIL GRANULES AND THEIR CONTENT

The traditional classification of neutrophil granules is based on the order of appearance of different granule subsets during myelopoiesis and the presence or absence of the enzyme myeloperoxidase. This classification distinguishes two main granule populations: *primary* (or *azurophil*), peroxidase-positive granules and *secondary* (or *specific*), peroxidase-negative granules. Early, pivotal studies on biogenesis of neutrophil granules were reviewed in detail by Klebanoff and Clark (2) and by Bainton (3,4). Later studies showed that specific granules could be distinguished on the basis of their content of lactoferrin and gelatinase. This finding led to classification of a lactoferrin-negative, gelatinase-containing specific granule subset as *tertiary* (or *gelatinase*) granules (5). Borregaard et al. (6,7) described a fourth mobilizable intracellular compartment, of endocytic origin (7), named *secretory vesicles*. The distinction among azurophil granules (primary), specific granules (secondary), gelatinase granules (tertiary) and secretory vesicles has meaning also in the context of the degranulation process. In fact, the four compartments are mobilized (i.e., fuse with the plasma membrane) according to a well defined hierarchy. Both *in vitro* and *in vivo* studies (8–10) demonstrated that the speed of mobilization from highest to lowest is as follows: secretory vesicles, gelatinase granules, specific granules, azurophil granules.

The content of neutrophil granule subsets has been extensively characterized (2–5,11–13; see Chapter 2). Recent findings have shed light on mechanisms underlying the segregation of different proteins in distinct granule subsets. These findings led Borregaard to propose an hypothesis based on "targeting by timing of biosynthesis" (14,15). According to this hypothesis (Fig. 46-1), the characteristic protein profile of the different granule populations is explained by the profile of granule proteins synthesized at a given stage during neutrophil maturation. This hypothesis well explains the finding that some granule constituents are contained in more than one granule subset.

Major constituents of neutrophil granules and their compartmental localization are reported in Table 46-1. In

G. Berton: Institute of General Pathology, University of Verona, Verona, Italy.

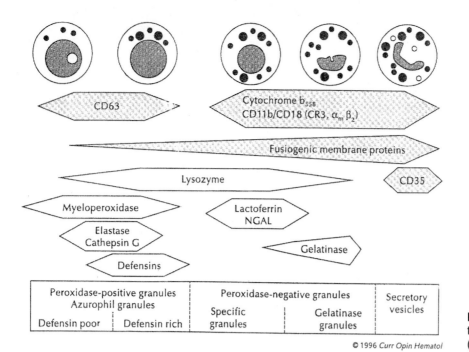

FIG. 46-1. Borregaard's "targeting by timing of biosynthesis" hypothesis. (From ref. 14, with permission.)

© 1996 Curr Opin Hematol

TABLE 46-1. Constituents of neutrophil granules[a]

Class of constituent	Example	Compartment
Microbicidal enzymes	Myeloperoxidase	Azurophil granules
	Lysozyme	Azurophil and specific granules
	Phospholipase A_2 (group II)	Specific granules
Acid hydrolases	Cathepsins	Azurophil granules
	β-glucuronidase	
	N-acetyl-β-glucosaminidase	
	Phosphatases	
Neutral proteinases	Serprocidins	Azurophil granules
	Elastase	
	Proteinase 3	
	Cathepsin G	
	Azurocidin (CAP-37)	
	Gelatinase	Specific granules
	Collagenase	Specific granules
Antimicrobial peptides	Bactericidal/permeability-increasing protein	Azurophil granules
	Defensins	Azurophil granules
	Lactoferrin	Specific granules
	Cathelicidins	Specific granules
Receptors	Transmembrane	Specific granules and/or secretory vesicles
	CR1 (CD35)	
	TNF-R (type I)	
	fMLP-R	
	IL-8R	
	GPI-linked	Specific granules and/or secretory vesicles
	Fcγ-RIII	
	uPAR	
	CD14 (LPS-receptor)	
Adhesion receptors	CR3 (CD11b/CD18; Mac-1)	Specific granules and/or secretory vesicles
	CR4 (CD11c/CD18; gp150,95)	
Effector molecules	NADPH oxidase components	Specific granules and/or secretory vesicles
	(gp91-phox, p22-phox)	
Cytoplasmic proteins	iNOS	Azurophil granules
	Fgr (Src family tyrosine kinase)	Specific granules
	Hck (Src family tyrosine kinase)	Azurophil granules

CAP-37, cationic antimicrobial protein-37; TNF-R, tumor necrosis factor receptor; fMLP-R, N-formyl-methionyl-leucyl-phenylalanine receptor; IL-8R, interleukin-8 receptor; LPS, lipopolysaccharide; NADPH, nicotinamide-adenine dinucleotide phosphate; iNOS, inducible nitric oxide synthese; uPAR, urokinase-type plasminogen activator receptor.

[a]References are reported in the text. Note that expression of Fcγ-RIII is initially enhanced by cell stimulation but then the molecule is shed from the neutrophil surface (27,29,39,49).

addition to microbicidal enzymes (lysozyme, acid hydrolases, proteases), neutrophil granules contain peptides with broad-spectrum bactericidal activity (i.e., defensins, cathelicidins, and bactericidal/permeability-increasing protein), which belong to a wide group of antimicrobial peptides in cell types of both mammalian and nonmammalian species. Excellent reviews addressing the structure and function of these peptides have been published (16–18; see Chapter 50). The 14-kd (group II) secreted phospholipase A_2 (19) is included within the group of human leukocyte microbicidal peptides (18) because of its identification as a constituent of neutrophil specific granules that is secreted in response to cell stimulation (20) and accounts for most of the bactericidal activity of ascitic fluid against *Staphylococcus aureus* (21).

As reported in Table 46-1, in addition to their constituents implicated in microbial killing, neutrophil granules store molecules that are destined to be inserted in the plasma membrane as true transmembrane proteins or as proteins linked to the external leaflet by a glycosyl phosphatidylinositol (GPI) anchor. Some of these components have been identified both in specific granules and in secretory vesicles, another finding supporting the "targeting by timing of biosynthesis" hypothesis (14). The recognition of translocation to the plasma membrane of proteins with a clearly identified function from neutrophil intracellular compartments was pioneered by studies demonstrating activation-dependent translocation of cytochrome b_{558} (22). Subsequently, several transmembrane and GPI-linked proteins were shown to be translocated from secretory vesicles or specific granules, or both, to the plasma membrane (5). The former group included CR1 (CD35), CR3 (CD11b/CD18), CR4 (CD11c/CD18), tumor necrosis factor receptor (TNF-R) type I, *N*-formyl-methionyl-leucyl-phenylalanine receptor (fMLP-R), interleukin-8 receptor (IL-8R), gp91-phox, and p22-phox (23–38); the latter group included the low-affinity immunoglobulin G receptor FcγRIII (CD16), urokinase-type plasminogen activator receptor (uPAR), and CD14 (39–41). These findings assigned to degranulation a significance far beyond its established role in microbial killing and tissue damage (see later discussion). GPI-linked molecules interact functionally with CR3 and CR4 (42). GPI-linked and signaling proteins colocalize, together with the marker protein caveolin, in submembranous vesicles named *caveolae*, in various cell types (43,44). The possible relation between secretory vesicles and caveolae has not been investigated because it was assumed that these organelles are not present in neutrophils (42). However, the evidence that neutrophils express caveolin (45) suggests caution in excluding the presence of caveola-like structures in neutrophils.

Neutrophil granules have been also reported to bind cytoplasmic molecules (46–48) (see Table 46-1). This finding suggests that degranulation may also redistribute effector or signaling proteins, thus dictating their site of action within the cell.

DEGRANULATION IN THE CONTEXT OF NEUTROPHIL-ENDOTHELIAL CELL INTERACTION

Degranulation can be induced by a wide variety of stimuli that interact with distinct surface receptors and are able to elicit other neutrophil responses. Stimuli inducing degranulation include chemotactic factors and chemokines, FcγR ligands, and cytokines (granulocyte colony-stimulating factor, granulocyte-macrophage colony-stimulating factor, TNF). In addition, adhesion receptors have been implicated as inducers of degranulation (see later discussion). Such forms of control indicate that neutrophils interacting with endothelial cells (ECs) in vessels of inflamed tissues may be stimulated to degranulate, and degranulation may regulate neutrophil adhesion and transmigration at different levels.

Migration of neutrophils into inflamed tissues is now viewed as a phenomenon occurring in distinct steps (50–53): (a) at first, neutrophils adhere to and roll along inflamed endothelium as a result of adhesive interactions mediated by selectins; (b) tethering to the ECs favors the interaction of neutrophils with chemotactic substances or chemokines that trigger signals activating integrin avidity for endothelial counterreceptors; (c) activation of integrin avidity for ligands belonging to the immunoglobulin supergene family expressed by ECs promotes firm adhesion of neutrophils and arrest on the EC surface; (d) after arrest, neutrophils migrate into the subendothelial space.

During the first step of neutrophil-EC interaction (i.e., selectin-mediated tethering), neutrophils may be stimulated to degranulate. L-selectin engagement triggers an increase in cytosolic free Ca^{2+} (54,55), and small increases of cytosolic Ca^{2+} mobilize secretory vesicles (9). L-selectin engagement upregulates expression of CD11b/CD18 (56), which is stored in secretory vesicles and specific granules (Table 46-1), indicating mobilization of at least these two compartments during L-selectin–mediated neutrophil-EC interaction. In addition, selectin-mediated tethering of neutrophils to the EC surface favors interaction with surface-bound chemotactic factors and chemokines, which promotes the generation of signals by chemoattractant receptors (juxtacrine signaling) (57).

The significance of degranulation in the context of neutrophil-EC interaction probably goes beyond increased expression of β_2 integrins. Neutrophil adhesiveness is enhanced by stimuli that induce degranulation (58,59). The release of sialidases (60,61), which by acting on surface sialoproteins reduce the neutrophil negative charge, and elastase (61–63) or other proteases (64,65), which cause shedding of the sialoprotein CD43, has been implicated in regulation of neutrophil spreading. Elastase-induced shedding of CD43 was required for neutrophil spreading (61) in assay conditions in which spreading was demonstrated to be strictly β_2 integrin dependent (66,67).

Neutrophil activation by agonists of degranulation is also accompanied by shedding of L-selectin (68,69). The significance of L-selectin shedding in regulation of neutrophil adhesiveness is unclear. It may be that once L-selectin has tethered neutrophils to the EC surface, thus favoring juxtacrine signaling from surface-bound chemoattractants, removal of the molecule facilitates integrin-dependent adhesion and spreading, analogously to CD43 removal. L-selectin "sheddases" have been identified as metalloproteinases (68,69) that probably are associated with membranes rather than secreted (69). However, it must be considered that gelatinase also sheds L-selectin (69), suggesting a possible role of degranulation in L-selectin shedding.

The third of the sequential steps regulating neutrophil-EC interaction (i.e., integrin-dependent adhesion and spreading), also can induce degranulation. Integrin ligation triggers cytosolic Ca^{2+} transients (70–74). Integrin-dependent neutrophil spreading is accompanied by release of lactoferrin (75), and antibody engagement of the β_2 integrin subunit induces elastase release from neutrophils (72). Degranulation in the context of neutrophil-EC interaction has been demonstrated by analysis of neutrophils that migrated into skin window chambers and the chamber fluid (10).

The evidence summarized here—indicating that selectin-mediated tethering of neutrophils to the EC surface, interaction with surface-bound chemoattractants, and integrin-dependent adhesion and spreading can elicit degranulation—raises the issue of the significance of degranulation in the context of neutrophil adhesion to the EC surface and transmigration into the inflammatory site. This significance can be summarized as follows. First, as mentioned, mobilization of secretory vesicles may be required to increase expression of adhesion receptors (CR3 and CR4) and of chemoattractant receptors (fMLP, IL-8, TNF). In addition, secretory vesicles also store uPAR (see Table 46–1), which is involved in regulation of neutrophil chemotaxis by way of its capability to interact with CR3 (76). The mechanisms and significance of the interactions of uPAR, FcγRIII, and CD14 with CR3 are reviewed by Petty and Todd (42). Second, translocation of cytochrome b_{558} (gp91-phox and p22-phox) from secretory vesicles and specific granules to the plasma membrane favors assembly of NADPH oxidase and release of oxidants in response to surface-bound or soluble stimuli. Oxidants can regulate EC functions such as expression of P-selectin (77), intercellular adhesion molecule-1 (78), and vascular cell adhesion molecule type-1 (79), and they induce release from ECs of phosphatidylcholine-derived platelet-activating factor–like phospholipids, which bind to leukocyte platelet-activating factor receptors (80).

Third, secretion of granule constituents induces shedding of surface molecules (i.e., CD43 and possibly L-selectin), which favors leukocyte-EC interaction and cell spreading. Moreover, cathepsin G and elastase have been reported to inhibit integrin-dependent spreading (81,82), an effect that can be viewed in the context of the detachment of neutrophils after integrin-mediated arrest on the EC surface that precedes cell movement and transmigration. Finally, granule constituents can affect functions of other bystander inflammatory cells. For example, cathepsin G activates platelets (83), and azurocidin/CAP-37 acts as a T-cell chemoattractant (84).

Release of granule constituents on interaction with ECs probably plays a major role in the pathogenesis of the vasculitis induced by anti-neutrophil cytoplasmic autoantibodies (85,86).

MECHANISMS OF GRANULE–PLASMA MEMBRANE FUSION

Transport of proteins within the cell, their delivery to various compartments, and their eventual secretion in the extracellular milieu require formation of vesicles in the endoplasmic reticulum and the Golgi stack that move away from their site of origin, dock with a target membrane, and eventually fuse with it (87–92). With the exception of secretory vesicles, which have an endocytic origin (7), fusion of neutrophil granules with the plasma membrane represents a heterotypic fusion event (89) involving two distinct membrane compartments. Fusion between two different membrane compartments involves protein-protein interactions that dock a vesicle to its final destination and proteins that favor the interaction between the phospholipid bilayer of the vesicle and its target membrane. In addition, membrane lipids participate in regulation of membrane traffic and degranulation.

Role of SNAREs and the Small GTP-binding Proteins ARF and RAB

SNAREs (*SNAP receptors*) are membrane proteins that bind a complex formed by the soluble proteins NSF (*N-ethylmaleimide-sensitive fusion protein*) and SNAP (*soluble NSF-attachment protein*). According to the "SNARE hypothesis" (88,91,92), vesicle docking results from the interaction between a vesicular SNARE (v-SNARE) and a SNARE present in the target membrane (t-SNARE) in complex with SNAPs and NSF. In mammalian cells, SNAREs involved in synaptic vesicle secretion have been characterized in detail (93) and include two v-SNAREs—synaptotagmin and synaptobrevin/VAMP (*vesicle-associated membrane protein*)—and two t-SNAREs—syntaxin and SNAP-25 (*synaptosome-associated protein*).

In addition to SNAREs and their associated proteins, other components involved in vesicle transport include members of two distinct subfamilies of small guanosine triphosphate (GTP)–binding proteins, ARF and RAB. ARF (*a*denosine diphosphate-*r*ibosylation *f*actor) was initially characterized for its role in regulation of the budding of COP (*co*at *p*rotein)-coated vesicles from the Golgi stack (88). More recent findings have assigned an important role to ARF in degranulation. The current knowledge explains this role in light of the ability of ARF to activate phospholipase D and to promote synthesis of phosphatidylinositol 4,5-bisphosphate (PIP_2), as discussed later. RAB proteins are thought to regulate v-SNARE–t-SNARE interactions as well as other events implicated in membrane traffic. The roles played by ARF and RAB in regulation of membrane traffic have been reviewed (88, 90,94–96).

Investigation of the roles of SNAREs and RAB in the regulation of neutrophil degranulation has just begun. Brumel et al. identified a v-SNARE (VAMP-2) and a t-SNARE (syntaxin-4) in human neutrophils (97). VAMP-2 was found to be concentrated in gelatinase-containing specific granules and secretory vesicles and to be translocated to the plasma membrane in response to an increase in cytosolic Ca^{2+}. Syntaxin-4 was found almost exclusively in the plasma membrane. The finding that syntaxin-1, two other v-SNAREs (VAMP-1 and cellubrevin), SNAP-25, and synaptophysin are absent from neutrophils led the authors to suggest that syntaxin-4 and VAMP-2 are the SNAREs involved in fusion of the plasma membrane with secretory vesicles and gelatinase-containing granules. This same study identified SCAMP (*s*ecretory *ca*rrier *m*embrane *p*rotein), an integral vesicular membrane protein (93), in specific granules and secretory vesicles in neutrophils. Evidence also has been presented for a role of RAB proteins in phagocyte degranulation. Early studies demonstrated that RAB-5 expression increases during differentiation of myelomonocytic cell lines to monocytes or granulocytes (98). RAB-5 was detected in human neutrophils and found to be translocated from the cytosol to a membrane fraction on cell stimulation (99). RAB-5 was shown to regulate fusion of endosomal membranes with phagosomes containing *Listeria monocytogenes* and to be enriched in the phagosomal membrane in a macrophage cell line (100).

Annexins and Degranulation

Besides SNAREs and associated proteins, heterotypic fusion also implicates a group of proteins, the annexins, that mediate interactions between negatively charged phospholipids of the granule and the plasma membrane (101,102). Annexins are encoded by at least ten distinct genes in mammalian cells and display the ability to bind membrane lipids in a Ca^{2+}-dependent manner. Members of this protein family are classified I to XIII, including non-mammalian annexins (102). Annexins have a common structure (101,102) that usually consists of four 70-amino-acid domains containing the so-called endonexin-fold

sequence at the C-terminus ("core"), and a unique N-terminal domain ("tail") containing phosphorylation sites and probably dictating specialized functions. In the presence of Ca^{2+}, annexins bind acidic phospholipids (phosphatidic acid, phosphatidylserine, phosphatidylinositol) with high affinity (102). This property makes them good candidates for promotors of membrane fusion. Besides exocytosis and membrane transport, annexins have been reported to regulate ion channel activity, inflammation, proliferation, and other cell functions (102,103). Crystallographic studies have offered new clues for understanding mechanisms of annexin association with membranes (104).

Annexins expressed by neutrophils include annexin I (lipocortin I), II (calpactin I heavy chain), III (lipocortin III), IV (endonexin I), VI (p68), VII (synexin), and a fragment of annexin XI (CAP-50) (105–113). Evidence for a role of annexins in neutrophil degranulation derives from two sets of observations. First, in the presence of Ca^{2+}, annexins induce aggregation of neutrophil granules and their fusion with liposomes (105,106,108,109). Second, some annexins are redistributed from the cytosol to plasma or granule membranes in response to agonists of degranulation or as a consequence of increase in cytosolic Ca^{2+} (110–113). Annexins I and III can be detected in contact with the phagosomal membrane in phagocytosing neutrophils (107,112). Redistribution of annexins to different granule subsets displays some selectivity. For example, annexin III (111), an annexin XI fragment (111), and other annexin-like proteins (110) associate primarily with specific granules. In addition, binding of annexin II to secretory vesicles and specific granules displays a Ca^{2+}-dependency different from that associated with binding to azurophil granules (110). The variation in Ca^{2+} dependency for secretion of distinct granule subsets (8,9) may depend on different Ca^{2+} requirements for the binding of annexins to each granule population.

Lipids as Regulators of Degranulation

Besides docking proteins and annexins, the lipid compositions of the granule and the plasma membrane also regulate granule-membrane fusion. Modifications of membrane phospholipids by phospholipase A_2, with generation of *cis*-unsaturated fatty acids, is known to facilitate membrane fusion (101). Arachidonic acid lowers to physiologic levels the concentrations of Ca^{2+} required for fusion of neutrophil granules with complex liposomes and triggers degranulation (114,115). In addition, accumulating evidence indicates that inositol lipids phosphorylated at the D_4/D_5 and D_3 positions regulate different pathways of membrane transport, including degranulation.

PIP_2 has been shown to play a critical role in the regulation of vesicles budding from the trans-Golgi network and other steps of membrane traffic in yeast and mammalian cells, independently of its being a source of classic intracellular messengers such as inositol 1,4,5-trisphosphate

(IP$_3$) and diacylglycerol (116,117). PIP$_2$ synthesis is required for Ca^{2+}-dependent neurotransmitter secretion in PC12 cells (118). Work by Cockcroft et al. demonstrated that PIP$_2$ also regulates degranulation in permeabilized granulocytic cells (119).

The mechanisms by which PIP$_2$ regulates membrane transport are a subject of speculation. It has been suggested that generation of a high local concentration of PIP$_2$ may be sufficient to induce vesicle budding from intracellular membranes (116,117). As far as degranulation is concerned, PIP$_2$ may be involved because of its ability to bind annexins (102). However, PIP$_2$ synthesis is the point of convergence of signaling pathways that result in generation of other intracellular messengers, and PIP$_2$ also affects downstream targets.

PIP$_2$ synthesis in neutrophils is activated by agonists of degranulation that interact with distinct receptors (120). ARF activates PIP$_2$ synthesis, an effect that probably is mediated by activation of phospholipase D, whose product, phosphatidic acid, activates enzymes involved in PIP$_2$ synthesis, such as phosphatidylinositol 4-phosphate 5-kinase (116,117,119,120–129). Therefore, the role played by ARF in degranulation is probably related to its ability to increase PIP$_2$ synthesis (119,120). ARF-dependent activation of phospholipase D might facilitate membrane fusion by mechanisms alternative to PIP$_2$ synthesis. Phosphatidic acid, the product of phospholipase D, binds with high affinity to annexins (102). In addition, phosphatidic acid can be dephosphorylated to form diacylglycerol (130,131), thus inducing activation of protein kinase C (PKC).

Another mechanism for the generation of PIP$_2$ relies on the action of phosphatidylinositol transfer protein (PITP). PITP induces neurotransmitter release by PC12 cells (118) and granulocytic cell degranulation (119). In permeabilized HL60 cells, recombinant PITP restores GTPγS–dependent secretion and PIP$_2$ synthesis without modulating phospholipase D activity, suggesting that PIP$_2$ per se facilitates degranulation (119).

The relation between ARF, phospholipase D, and PIP$_2$ is further complicated by evidence that PIP$_2$ increases phospholipase D activity (120,127,128,132,133) and may activate ARF by increasing the exchange between guanosine diphosphate (GDP) and GTP (134). Taken together, these findings point to the existence of a positive feedback loop involving ARF, phospholipase D, and PIP$_2$ and leading to a high local production of PIP$_2$ (116) as well as other lipids (phosphatidic acid, diacylglycerol, and possibly arachidonic acid; see later discussion) that may favor degranulation. Neutrophil agonists that elicit degranulation also activate phospholipase D and formation of phosphatidic acid and diacylglycerol (135–147). Diversion of production of phosphatidic acid to phosphatidylethanol with the use of ethanol inhibits neutrophil degranulation (119,146,148,149).

In addition to ARF, proteins belonging to the RHO subfamily of GTP-binding proteins have been implicated in the synthesis of PIP$_2$. RHO proteins (RHO, RAC, CDC42) activate phospholipase D in different cell types (120,127,128,150–153), although in HL60 cells ARF seems to play a major role (126). In addition, RAC activates phosphatidylinositol 4-phosphate 5-kinase directly (154–158). RHO proteins seem to be involved in a positive feedback loop sustained by the RHO proteins themselves, phospholipase D, and PIP$_2$. RHO-stimulated phospholipase D activity is increased by PIP$_2$ (127,128); and, in analogy with ARF (as previously described), PIP$_2$ has been reported to activate CDC42 and RHO, increasing dissociation of GDP (159). Evidence has been also presented that phosphatidic acid generation by phospholipase D may be upstream of RHO activation (160). RAC has been reported to activate phospholipase A$_2$, forming arachidonic acid, another lipid implicated in membrane fusion (161). RHO proteins regulate secretion in mast cells and basophilic leukemia cells (162–164).

Another mechanism of regulation of membrane traffic and degranulation by PIP$_2$ may be represented by its role as a precursor of phosphatidylinositol 3,4,5-trisphosphate (PIP$_3$). PIP$_2$ is one of the substrates of phosphoinositide 3-kinases, enzymes that phosphorylate phosphatidylinositol lipids at the D$_3$ position (165). Genetic studies in yeast (117) provided formal proof for a role of phosphoinositide 3-kinase in regulation of transport from Golgi membranes to vacuoles. The role of phosphoinositide 3-kinase in the regulation of membrane traffic in mammalian cells has been investigated with the use of selective inhibitors of the enzyme. Inhibition of phosphoinositide 3-kinase with the fungal metabolite wortmannin or the compound LY294002 blocks transport to lysosomes in mammalian cells (166,167). In addition, wortmannin inhibits translocation of glucose transporters to the adipocyte plasma membrane (168,169), as well as degranulation in mast cells, basophils, and natural killer cells (170–175). Both degranulation and production of reactive oxygen intermediates by neutrophils are effectively inhibited by phosphoinositide 3-kinase inhibitors (176–180).

By analogy with PIP$_2$, PIP$_3$ per se may favor vesicle budding and vesicle–plasma membrane fusion. Alternatively, it may affect downstream targets. For example, PIP$_3$ activates some PKC isoforms (see later discussion) and at least one component of the fusion apparatus, RAB-5 (181). In addition, phosphoinositide 3-kinase is linked in a complex manner to both RAS (182–189) and RHO (190–196) proteins, because it may be either upstream and downstream of each of them. These findings suggest that PIP$_3$ also may be a component of a positive feedback loop consisting of ARF, RHO proteins, phospholipase D, phosphatidylinositol-kinases, PITP, PIP$_2$, and PIP$_3$ itself (Fig. 46-2).

Although mechanisms of degranulation in neutrophils are still poorly understood, the demonstration that certain components involved in membrane traffic and fusion

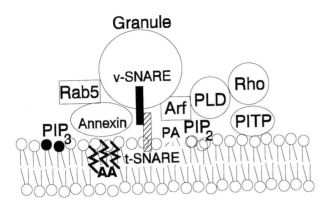

FIG. 46-2. Components possibly implicated in granule–plasma membrane fusion in neutrophils. Granule-membrane interaction requires docking proteins (SNAREs), phospholipid-binding proteins (annexins), and regulatory proteins (RAB-5) (see text). Reconstitution studies in permeabilized cells established that phosphatidylinositol 4,5-bisphosphate [PtdIns(4,5)P$_2$ or PIP$_2$] synthesis stimulated by ARF(RHO?)-dependent phospholipase D (PLD) activity or by phosphatidylinositol transfer protein (PITP) is essential for degranulation (119). PIP$_2$ and its product phosphatidylinositol 3,4,5-trisphosphate [PtdIns(3,4,5)P$_3$ or PIP$_3$], together with arachidonic acid (AA) and phosphatidic acid (PA), may favor granule–plasma membrane fusion through unidentified mechanisms.

(SNAREs, RAB-5, annexins) are expressed in phagocytic cells makes it possible to put neutrophil degranulation in the context of processes that are conserved from yeast to mammals. Studies with inhibitors have provided important clues for the identification of some essential components (phospholipase D, phosphoinositide 3-kinase). Finally, reconstitution of functions in cytosol-depleted myelomonocytic cell lines with recombinant ARF proteins and PITP (119) has opened new perspectives. However, much remains to be done to elucidate a process that is further complicated by the fact that neutrophils contain at least three distinct mobilizable organelles whose fusion with the plasma membrane is differentially regulated (8–10).

SIGNALING FOR DEGRANULATION

Fig. 46–3 summarizes current knowledge of some key aspects of signal transduction by receptors eliciting neutrophil responses and highlights signaling pathways implicated in degranulation. Signaling pathways involved in degranulation in other cell types and possibly playing a role in neutrophils are also depicted. Signals regulating degranulation include: (a) increase in cytosolic free Ca^{2+} and activation of PKC as a consequence of PIP$_2$ breakdown by phosphoinositidase C and the formation of IP$_3$ and diacylglycerol; (b) activation of phospholipase A$_2$ and phospholipase D and the consequent modification of membrane phospholipids with formation of arachidonic acid, phosphatidic acid, and PIP$_2$; (c) activation of phos-

phoinositide 3-kinase with formation of PIP$_3$; (d) activation of cytoplasmic protein-tyrosine kinases (PTKs); and (e) activation of members of the RHO family of small GTP-binding proteins.

The role of Ca^{2+} as a regulator of degranulation in neutrophils was recognized more than 20 years ago on the basis that ionophores that increase cytosolic free Ca^{2+} induce degranulation (2,260–263). A hierarchy in mobilization of different granule subsets depending on the level of intracellular free Ca^{2+} has been demonstrated (8,9); from highest to lowest, these are secretory vesicles, gelatinase-containing granules, specific granules, azurophil granules. Although Ca^{2+} alone can induce degranulation, a receptor agonist such as fMLP lowers the Ca^{2+} requirement of the process (8,9). Together with the evidence that blunting the increase of cytosolic free Ca^{2+} with intracellular Ca^{2+} chelators does not totally inhibit fMLP-induced degranulation of specific granules (9), this finding points to the requirement for additional signals to induce degranulation. The role of Ca^{2+} in regulating mobilization of secretory vesicles is of particular interest. Small increases in cytosolic free Ca^{2+} mobilize secretory vesicles completely, but elimination of fMLP-induced Ca^{2+} transients with intracellular Ca^{2+} chelators inhibits them negligibly (9). Therefore, at least as far as secretory vesicles are concerned, cytosolic Ca^{2+} does not need to be increased, provided additional signals are generated by fMLP receptors. Receptor agonists inducing an increase of cytosolic free Ca^{2+} also lead to activation of PKC (see Fig. 46-3). Phorbol esters, which stimulate PKC directly, are powerful elicitors of degranulation. Regulation of degranulation by Ca^{2+} and PKC might depend on their ability to modulate phospholipase A$_2$ and phospholipase D activities (see Fig. 46-3). In addition, Ca^{2+} is required for binding of annexin to phospholipids (see previous discussion). Ca^{2+} regulates the actin-filament-severing activity of gelsolin (258), and cytochalasins, fungal metabolites that disassemble actin filaments, have long been used to enhance degranulation (2). Evidence discussed later suggests that the relation between cytoskeleton dynamics and degranulation may be more complex than expected.

The role of phospholipase A$_2$ and phospholipase D in regulating degranulation has already been discussed. Phospholipase A$_2$ and phospholipase D activation can modify membrane phospholipids and form lipid domains enriched in arachidonic acid and phosphatidic acid. PIP$_2$ synthesis, regulated by ARF, PITP, and phospholipase D, is currently viewed as a critical step in degranulation. As anticipated, inhibition of phosphatidic acid formation with alcohols blocks neutrophil degranulation (119,146, 148,149), and ARF and PITP reconstitute GTPγS-dependent degranulation in permeabilized granulocytic cells (119). Ca^{2+}, PKC, phosphoinositide 3-kinase, RAS, and RHO protein signals can all converge in activation of phospholipase A$_2$ or phospholipase D (see Fig. 46–3).

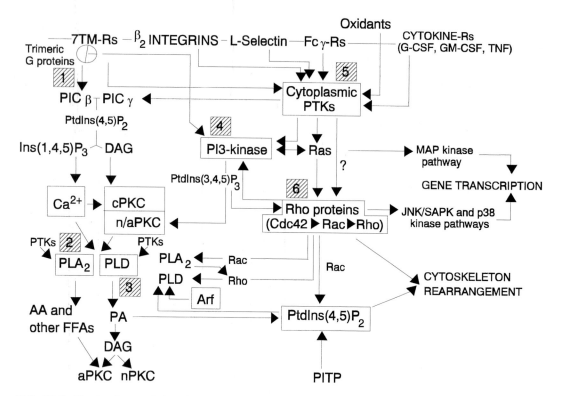

FIG. 46-3. Mechanisms of signal transduction by receptors triggering degranulation. The main pathways of transmembrane signaling by receptors expressed by phagocytes and possibly involved in stimulation of degranulation are shown. Crosstalk between some of the illustrated signaling pathways has not been demonstrated in phagocytic cells but is well characterized in other cell types and is included to put signaling for degranulation in phagocytic cells in perspective. Components that have been clearly implicated in degranulation, either in neutrophils or in other cell types, are framed in rectangles. Major pathways are indicated by numbers and are briefly described in the following paragraphs, along with references to a limited number of original papers or reviews.

Pathway #1: Generation of messengers via hydrolysis of phosphatidylinositol 4,5-bisphosphate [$PtdIns(4,5)P_2$ or PIP_2] *by trimeric G protein–coupled receptors.* Mechanisms of transmembrane signaling by heterotrimeric G protein–coupled receptors, which include the wide family of structurally related seven-transmembrane spanning chemotactic receptors (7TM-Rs), were the first to be characterized in detail (197–201). The nomenclature used here is that proposed by Divecha and Irvine (202). Activation of β isoforms of phosphoinositidase C (PIC) results in the breakdown of $PtdIns(4,5)P_2$ and formation of inositol 1,4,5-trisphosphate [$Ins(1,4,5)P_3$ or IP_3] and diacylglycerol (DAG). Ca^{2+} mobilized from intracellular stores by $Ins(1,4,5)P_3$ and DAG activates "classic"—or "conventional"—protein kinase C isoforms (cPKC) (203–205). PKC activation can be sustained by a second wave of formation of DAG deriving from the hydrolysis of phosphatidylcholine by phospholipase D (PLD) acting in concert with arachidonic acid (AA) and other *cis*-unsaturated fatty acids (FFAs). Both "new" (nPKC) and "atypical" PKC (aPKC) isoforms can be regulated by DAG and fatty acids (203).

Pathway #2: Activation of phospholipase A_2 (PLA$_2$) *and generation of AA.* Activation of the cytosolic, 85-kd (group IV) PLA$_2$ (19) probably plays a major role in AA generation in neutrophils and other phagocytic cells (131,198). Ca^{2+} regulates activity of this PLA$_2$ mainly by inducing redistribution of the protein from the cytosol to the plasma membrane (19). Additional mechanisms of regulation that have been described include phosphorylation of the protein by serine-threonine or tyrosine kinases (19,131,206). 7TM-Rs activate PLA$_2$, possibly via release of Ca^{2+} and activation of PKC. Also extracellular regulated kinase phosphorylates and activates PLA$_2$ (19,131,198). This finding is of interest because agonists of 7TM-Rs activate the mitogen-activated protein (MAP) kinase pathways in neutrophils (described in a later paragraph). The RHO protein RAC has been shown to mediate growth factor–induced release of AA in fibroblasts (161). Because different signaling pathways can converge in activation of RHO proteins (see later paragraph), this finding suggests the existence of an additional mechanism leading to PLA$_2$ activation.

Pathway #3: Activation of PLD. Several different signaling pathways lead to PLD activation. First, stimulation of PKC by phorbol esters activates PLD in various cell types, including neutrophils (127,131, 136,138,139,141). Neutrophil stimulation with chemotactic agonists also results in PLD activation, a finding that can be explained as a consequence of an increase in cytosolic Ca2+ (131,142) as well as PKC activation. Second, studies have implicated the small guanoside triphosphate (GTP)—binding proteins ARF and RHO members in regulation of PLD activity in various cell types, including myelomonocytic cells (116,117,119,120–129,150–153). $PtdIns(4,5)P_2$, whose synthesis is increased by PLD, is also a regulator of PLD activity (120,127,128,132,133). Finally, PLD can be activated by either receptor or cytoplasmic protein-tyrosine kinases (PTKs) (131). Tyrosine phosphorylation can activate PLD in neutrophils and in HL60 cells (207–209). *SRC*-induced activation of PLD in fibroblasts depends on RAS (210), suggesting that a possible alternative pathway involves activation of PLD by RAS, either through activation of phosphoinositide 3-kinase (PI3-kinase) and phosphatidylinositol 3,4,5-trisphosphate [PtdIns(3,4,5)P_3 or PIP$_3$]–dependent activation of some PKC isoforms or through RHO proteins (see later paragraph). Because the RAS pathway can be activated by receptors as well as by oxidants in neutrophils (see later paragraph), it may lead to PLD activation. Alternatively, activation of cytoplasmic PTKs by different receptors can lead to activation of PI3-kinase (see next paragraph) and hence PtdIns(3,4,5)P_3-dependent activation of some PKC isoforms.

Pathway #4: Activation of PI3-kinase. Activation of PI3-kinase and the consequent formation of D_3-phosphorylated inositol lipids is an important signaling pathway in leukocytes (165,211), and biochemically distinct PI3-kinases have been identified (165,212). 7TM-Rs can trigger formation of PtdIns(3,4,5)P_3 in neutrophils, and a PI3-kinase isoform present in myelomonocytic cells is activated by trimeric G-protein subunits (213). Alternatively, signaling by receptor and cytoplasmic PTKs results in activation of a PI3-kinase (165). SRC-family tyrosine kinases activate PI3-kinase in lymphocytes (211) and in neutrophils (214,215). Moreover, PI3-kinase has been identified as a target of RAS (184,185,187,188) and RHO family members (154–158). Because signaling by tyrosine kinases activates RAS and possibly RHO members in various cell types, including neutrophils (see later paragraph), activation of PI3-kinase by tyrosine kinases may be mediated by these entities. PI3-kinase also can be upstream of RAS (182,183, 186,187) and RHO members (192–196). Placing of PI3-kinase both upstream and downstream of RAS has been suggested to depend on its ability to compete with GTPase activating protein for binding to the RAS effector domain, thus increasing the GTP-bound form of RAS (187). PtdIns(3,4,5)P_3 can activate some PKC isoforms (203), suggesting that signaling pathways originating from PtdIns(4,5)P_2 hydrolysis by PIC and the PTKs/RAS/RHO/PI3-kinase pathways converge in PKC activation.

Pathway #5: Activation of cytoplasmic PTKs. Cytoplasmic PTKs play an important role in signal transduction by different surface receptors in numerous cell types, including hematopoietic cells. Agonists of 7TM-Rs activate tyrosine kinases in various cell types, leading to activation of the MAP kinase pathway (216,217). Cytoplasmic PTKs implicated in signaling by 7TM-Rs include the SRC-family kinases SRC (218–222) and LYN (214,215,223), SYK (223), FAK (224), and the recently cloned FAK-family member PYK2 (221,225). Mechanisms of activation of cytoplasmic PTKs by 7TM-Rs are unknown. "Classic" signals such as Ca^{2+} and PKC induce phosphorylation of FAK (224) and PYK2 (225), and PKC activation with phorbol myristate acetate (PMA) enhances the activity of the SRC-family kinases FGR and LYN in neutrophils (45). Therefore, involvement of cytoplasmic PTKs by 7TM-Rs may be secondary to PtdIns(4,5)P_2 hydrolysis by PIC. PKC activation triggers actin polymerization, and the association of PTKs with cytoskeletal protein complexes may activate cytoplasmic PTKs (226). Some of the effects of 7TM-R agonists thus may be mediated by their ability to activate integrin adhesiveness and integrin-mediated reorganization of the cytoskeleton (74). Activation of FGR by *N*-formyl-methionyl-leucyl-phenylalanine (fMLP) and PMA in adherent neutrophils depends on β_2 integrins (227). Both SRC-family kinases and SYK are implicated in β_2-integrin signaling in neutrophils (226–229), and integrin signaling is defective in neutrophils from *fgr*/-hck-/- double-knockout mice (230). Integrin signaling leads to activation of the MAP kinase pathway in various cell types (231–234), including neutrophils (235). Chemotactic peptides (236–240), chemokines (241), L-selectin (242), and cytokines (243,244) activate this pathway in neutrophils. In addition, oxidants may activate the MAP kinase pathway in neutrophils (245), an effect that conceivably results from their ability to trigger protein tyrosine phosphorylation and to activate SRC-family kinases (246,247). Besides activating RAS and the MAP kinase pathway, tyrosine kinases have been placed upstream of PI3-kinase in various cell types, including neutrophils (see previous paragraph), pointing to a possible mechanism of activation of some PKC isoforms via PTK-mediated formation of PtdIns(3,4,5)P_3. Other possible downstream targets of cytoplasmic PTKs include PLD (see earlier paragraph) and, by analogy with RAS, RHO family members. The immunoglobulin G receptors (FcγRs) and some cytokines, such as granulocyte colony-stimulating factor (G-CSF), granulocyte-macrophage colony-stimulating factor (GM-CSF), and tumor necrosis factor (TNF), may activate neutrophil functions, including degranulation, by activating cytoplasmic PTKs (248–251).

Pathway #6: Activation of RHO proteins. RHO proteins can be involved in signaling for gene transcription, cytoskeleton rearrangements, and activation of other signaling pathways (154–158,252). Mechanisms of activation of RHO proteins are poorly understood. In fibroblasts, RAS can activate RAC, and activation of CDC42 leads to the sequential activation of RAC and RHO (252,253). The ability of RAS to activate RAC may be, in part, indirect. RAS may activate PI3-kinase, and formation of PtdIns(3,4,5)P_3 may then lead to RHO activation (see earlier paragraph). By analogy with RAS, cytoplasmic PTKs could activate RHO members either directly or via activation of PtdIns(3,4,5)P_3 formation. Stimulation of RHO-mediated stress fiber formation by 7TM-Rs in fibroblasts requires a tyrosine kinase activity (254). Several downstream targets of RHO proteins have been identified (154–158). By analogy with RAS, RHO proteins can be either downstream or upstream of PI3-kinase (see previous paragraph and the text). RHO proteins can activate PLA$_2$, PLD, and PtdIns(4,5)P_2 synthesis (see text), as well as the JNK/SAPK and p38 kinase pathway (255–257). PtdIns(4,5)P_2 synthesis can mediate actin polymerization (154-156,258,259). Moreover, regulation of the assembly of the cytoskeleton by RHO proteins can also occur independently of PtdIns(4,5)P_2 synthesis (154,156,157).

Evidence for the implication of phosphoinositide 3-kinase and PIP$_3$ in the regulation of degranulation derives from studies on the effects of selective phosphoinositide 3-kinase inhibitors and was addressed earlier. Phosphoinositide 3-kinase can be activated directly by trimeric G-protein subunits or cytoplasmic PTKs or, alternatively, by RAS and RHO proteins (see Fig. 46-3). PIP$_3$ can act on downstream targets (some PKC isoforms, RAS, and RHO) (see Fig. 46-3), or it can play a direct role in degranulation (see previous discussion).

Accumulating data point to an important role of cytoplasmic PTKs in signal transduction (see Fig. 46-3). An increase in phosphorylation of proteins in tyrosine residues has been reported to occur in response to different agonists of degranulation, such as chemotactic agents and chemokines, ligands for Fc receptors, cytokines, inflammatory microcrystals, and phorbol myristate acetate (45,264–278). Engagement of β_2 integrins (227,228, 249–251) or L-selectin (242) also stimulates protein tyrosine phosphorylation. Tyrosine phosphorylated proteins and the SRC-family tyrosine kinase LYN were found to localize in the periphagosomal membrane in macrophages (279,280). Studies with PTK inhibitors indicated that mobilization of secretory vesicles requires tyrosine phosphorylation (281). Degranulation in response to monosodium urate crystals (282,283) or concanavalin A (284), but not chemotactic agents (285), is inhibited by PTK inhibitors. Degranulation was shown to be sensitive to tyrosine kinase inhibitors also in eosinophils, mast cells, basophils, and cytotoxic T lymphocytes (286–293). In neutrophils, the SRC-family kinases FGR, HCK, and LYN and the tyrosine kinase SYK may be involved in signal transduction by seven transmembrane spanning receptors (7-TMRs) (214,215,294), β_2 integrins (227–230,295), FcγRs (296–301), and other stimuli (302,303). Mechanisms of activation of tyrosine kinase in neutrophils are poorly understood (74). Some agonists of neutrophil responses may activate PTKs indirectly, via activation of integrin adhesiveness (74).

The RHO family member RAC is essential for regulation of NADPH oxidase activity in neutrophils (304). So far, its possible role in mediation of neutrophil degranulation has not been investigated. RHO proteins can act on downstream targets that regulate degranulation (e.g., phospholipase A$_2$, phospholipase D, phosphoinositide 3-kinase; see Fig. 46-3). RHO proteins are now viewed as essential components in the regulation of cytoskeleton assembly (154–158,258,259). Their possible regulatory role in degranulation is in apparent contradiction with the old knowledge that disruption of actin filaments with cytochalasins enhances degranulation (2). However, it must be considered that degranulation occurs coincident with phagocytosis, a process that has been defined as "regurgitation during feeding" (2), and cytoskeletal proteins, including F-actin, are detected adjacent to the phagosome surface (280). Moreover, more than 25 years

has passed since adhesion to surfaces was observed to induce neutrophil degranulation, a process referred to as "reverse endocytosis" or "frustrated phagocytosis" (2). More recent studies with surfaces coated with integrin ligands showed that neutrophil adhesion may also result in cell spreading, a process requiring an extensive rearrangement of the cytoskeleton (66,249). Nonetheless, neutrophils induced to spread with TNF release lactoferrin extracellularly (75). Cytoskeleton rearrangement is a highly dynamic process, and this property is required to perform specialized functions such as chemotaxis (258). Localized rearrangements of the cytoskeleton can result in severing of actin filaments between adjacent granule and surface membranes, but, at the same time, polymerization of actin filaments at the periphery of the apposed membranes can provide a driving force for fusion. In disassembling the cytoskeleton, cytochalasins may simply redistribute granules to the cell periphery, thereby artificially enhancing granule plasma membrane fusion. However, it is tempting to anticipate that one of the possible mechanisms of action of RHO proteins in regulating degranulation may derive from their capacity to induce localized rearrangements of the cytoskeleton.

ACKNOWLEDGMENTS

The author wishes to thank Professors Filippo Rossi, Siamon Gordon, and Domenico Romeo, who guided him into the complexity of phagocyte biology; the many colleagues of the Institute of General Pathology of the University of Verona with whom he has collaborated and exchanged ideas in the last 15 years; and Professor Niels Borregaard, who kindly gave permission to include one of his figures in this chapter. Special thanks to Paola and Beatrice for the joy they bring my life.

REFERENCES

1. Cassatella MA. *Cytokines produced by polymorphonuclear neutrophils: molecular and biological aspects.* Austin, TX: RG Landes, 1996.
2. Klebanoff SJ, Clark RA. *The neutrophil: function and clinical disorders.* Amsterdam: North-Holland Publishing Company, 1978.
3. Bainton DF. Phagocytic cells: developmental biology of neutrophils and eosinophils. In: Gallin JI, Goldstein IM, Snyderman R (eds). *Inflammation: basic principles and clinical correlates.* New York: Raven Press, 1988:265–280.
4. Bainton DF. Developmental biology of neutrophils and eosinophils. In: Gallin JI, Goldstein IM, Snyderman R (eds). *Inflammation: basic principles and clinical correlates,* 2nd ed. New York: Raven Press, 1992:303–324.
5. Borregaard N, Lollike K, Kjeldsen L, et al. Human neutrophil granules and secretory vesicles. *Eur J Haematol* 1993;51:187–198.
6. Borregaard N, Miller LJ, Springer TA. Chemoattractant regulated mobilization of a novel intracellular compartment in human neutrophils. *Science* 1987; 237:1204–1206.
7. Borregaard N, Kjeldsen L, Rygaard K, et al. Stimulus-dependent secretion of plasma proteins from human neutrophils. *J Clin Invest* 1992;90:86–96.
8. Lew PD, Monod A, Waldvogel FA, Dewald B, Baggiolini M, Pozzan T. Quantitative analysis of the cytosolic free calcium dependency of exocytosis from three subcellular compartments in intact human neutrophils. *J Cell Biol* 1986;102:2197–2204.

9. Sengelov H, Kjeldsen L, Borregaard N. Control of exocytosis in early neutrophil activation. *J Immunol* 1993;150:1535–1543.

10. Sengelov H, Follin P, Kjeldsen L, Lollike K, Dahlgren C, Borregaard N. Mobilization of granules and secretory vesicles during *in vivo* exudation of human neutrophils. *J Immunol* 1995;154:4157–4165.

11. Baggiolini M. The neutrophil. In: Weissmann G (ed). *Handbook of inflammation, vol 2: the cell biology of inflammation*. Amsterdam: North-Holland Biomedical Press, 1980:163–187.

12. Henson PM, Henson JE, Fittschen C, Kimani G, Bratton DL, Riches DWH. Phagocytic cells: degranulation and secretion. In: Gallin JI, Goldstein IM, Snyderman R (eds). *Inflammation: basic principles and clinical correlates*. New York: Raven Press, 1988:363–390.

13. Henson PM, Henson JE, Fittschen C, Bratton DL, Riches DWH. Degranulation and secretion in phagocytic cells. In: Gallin JI, Goldstein IM, Snyderman R (eds). *Inflammation: basic principles and clinical correlates, 2nd ed.* New York: Raven Press, 1992:511–539.

14. Borregaard N. Current concepts about neutrophil granule physiology. *Curr Opin Hematol* 1996;3:11–18.

15. Le Cabec V, Cowland JB, Calafat J, Borregaard N. Targeting of proteins to granule subsets is determined by timing and not by sorting: the specific granule protein NGAL is localized to azurophil granules when expressed in HL 60 cells. *Proc Natl Acad Sci U S A* 1996;93:6454–6457.

16. Martin E, Ganz T, Lehrer RI. Defensins and other endogenous peptide antibiotics of vertebrates. *J Leukoc Biol* 1995;58:128–136.

17. Zanetti M, Gennaro R, Romeo D. Cathelicidins: a novel protein family with a common proregion and a variable C terminal antimicrobial domain. *FEBS Lett* 1995;374:1–5.

18. Ganz T, Lehrer RI. Antimicrobial peptides of leukocytes. *Curr Opin Hematol* 1997;4:53–58.

19. Dennis EA. Diversity of group types, regulation, and function of phospholipase A_2. *J Biol Chem* 1994;269:13057–13060.

20. Rosenthal MD, Gordon MN, Buescher ES, Slusser JH, Harris LK, Franson RC. Human neutrophils store type II 14 kDa phospholipase A_2 in granules and secrete active enzyme in response to soluble stimuli. *Biochem Biophys Res Commun* 1995;208:650–656.

21. Weinrauch Y, Elsbach P, Madsen LM, Foreman A, Weiss J. The potent anti-*Staphylococcus aureus* activity of a sterile rabbit inflammatory fluid is due to a 14 kD phospholipase A_2. *J Clin Invest* 1996;97:250–257.

22. Borregaard N, Heiple JM, Simons ER, Clark RA. Subcellular localization of the b-cytochrome component of the human neutrophil microbicidal oxidase: translocation during activation. *J Cell Biol* 1983;97:52–61.

23. Todd RF III, Arnaout MA, Rosin RE, Crowley CA, Peters WA, Babior BA. Subcellular localization of the large subunit of Mo1 (Mo1 alpha; formerly gp110), a surface glycoprotein associated with neutrophil adhesion. *J Clin Invest* 1984;74:1280–1290.

24. Berger M, O'Shea J, Cross AS, et al. Human neutrophils increase expression of C3bi as well as C3b receptors upon activation. *J Clin Invest* 1984;74:1566–1571.

25. Miller LJ, Bainton DF, Borregaard N, Springer TA. Stimulated mobilization of monocyte Mac 1 and p150,95 adhesion proteins from an intracellular vesicular compartment to the cell surface. *J Clin Invest* 1987;80:535–544.

26. Bainton DF, Miller LJ, Kishimoto TK, Springer TA. Leukocyte adhesion receptors are stored in peroxidase negative granules of human neutrophils. *J Exp Med* 1987;166:1641–1653.

27. Kuijpers TW, Tool AT, van der Schoot CE, et al. Membrane surface antigen expression on neutrophils: a reappraisal of the use of surface markers for neutrophil activation. *Blood* 1991;78:1105–1111.

28. Porteu P, Nathan CF. Mobilizable intracellular pool of p55 (type I) tumor necrosis factor receptors in human neutrophils. *J Leukoc Biol* 1992;52:122–124.

29. Tosi MF, Zakem H. Surface expression of Fcγ receptor III (CD16) on chemoattractant-stimulated neutrophils is determined by both surface shedding and translocation from storage compartments. *J Clin Invest* 1992;90:462–470.

30. Sengelov H, Kjeldsen L, Diamond MS, Springer TA, Borregaard N. Subcellular localization and dynamics of Mac 1 ($\alpha_M\beta_2$) in human neutrophils. *J Clin Invest* 1993;92:1467–1476.

31. Calafat J, Kuijpers TW, Janssen H, Borregaard N, Verhoeven AJ, Roos D. Evidence for small intracellular vesicles in human blood phagocytes containing cytochrome b558 and the adhesion molecule CD11b/CD18. *Blood* 1993;81:3122–3129.

32. Borregaard N, Kjeldsen L, Sengelov H, et al. Changes in subcellular localization and surface expression of L selectin, alkaline phosphatase, and Mac 1 in human neutrophils during stimulation with inflammatory mediators. *J Leukoc Biol* 1994;56: 80–87.

33. Kjeldsen L, Sengelov H, Lollike K, Nielsen MH, Borregaard N. Isolation and characterization of gelatinase granules from human neutrophils. *Blood* 1994;83:1640–1649.

34. Sengelov H, Boulay F, Kjeldsen L, Borregaard N. Subcellular localization and translocation of the receptor for N formylmethionyl leucyl phenylalanine in human neutrophils. *Biochem J* 1994;299:473–479.

35. Sengelov H, Kjeldsen L, Kroeze W, Berger M, Borregaard N. Secretory vesicles are the intracellular reservoir of complement receptor 1 in human neutrophils. *J Immunol* 1994;153:804–810.

36. Simms HH, D'Amico R. Subcellular location of neutrophil opsonic receptors is altered by exogenous reactive oxygen species. *Cell Immunol* 1995;166:71–82.

37. Sengelov H. Complement receptors in neutrophils. *Crit Rev Immunol* 1995:107–131.

38. Manna SK, Samanta AK. Upregulation of interleukin 8 receptor in human polymorphonuclear neutrophils by formyl peptide and lipopolysaccharide. *FEBS Lett* 1995;367:117–121.

39. de Haas M, Kerst JM, van der Schoot CE, et al. Granulocyte colony stimulating factor administration to healthy volunteers: analysis of the immediate activating effects on circulating neutrophils. *Blood* 1994; 84:3885–3894.

40. Plesner T, Ploug M, Ellis V, et al. The receptor for urokinase type plasminogen activator and urokinase is translocated from two distinct intracellular compartments to the plasma membrane on stimulation of human neutrophils. *Blood* 1994;83:808–815.

41. Detmers PA, Zhou D, Powell D, Lichenstein H, Kelley M, Pironkova R. Endotoxin receptors (CD14) are found with CD16 (Fc gamma RIII) in an intracellular compartment of neutrophils that contains alkaline phosphatase. *J Immunol* 1995;155:2085–2095.

42. Petty HR, Todd RF III. Integrins as promiscuous signal transduction devices. *Immunol Today* 1996;17:209–212.

43. Lisanti MP, Scherer PE, Tang ZL, Sargiacomo M. Caveolae, caveolin and caveolin-rich membrane domains: a signalling hypothesis. *Trends Cell Biol* 1994;4:231–235.

44. Parton RG. Caveolae and caveolins. *Curr Opin Cell Biol* 1996;8: 542–548.

45. Yan SR, Fumagalli L, Berton G. Activation of SRC family kinases in human neutrophils: evidence that p58C FGR and p53/56 LYN redistributed to a Triton X 100 insoluble cytoskeletal fraction, also enriched in the caveolar protein caveolin, display an enhanced kinase activity. *FEBS Lett* 1996;380:198–203.

46. Gutkind JS, Robbins KC. Translocation of the FGR protein tyrosine kinase as a consequence of neutrophil activation. *Proc Natl Acad Sci U S A* 1989;86 8783–8787.

47. Mohn H, Le Cabec V, Fischer S, Maridonneau-Parini I. The src family protein tyrosine kinase p59^{hck} is located on the secretory granules in human neutrophils and translocates towards the phagosome during cell activation. *Biochem J* 1995;309:657–665.

48. Evans TJ, Buttery LD, Carpenter A, Springall DR, Polak JM, Cohen J. Cytokine treated human neutrophils contain inducible nitric oxide synthase that produces nitration of ingested bacteria. *Proc Natl Acad Sci U S A* 1996;93:9553–9558.

49. Huizinga TW, van der Schoot CE, Jost C, et al. The PI linked receptor FcRIII is released on stimulation of neutrophils. *Nature* 1988;333: 667–669.

50. Butcher EC. Leukocyte-endothelial cell recognition: three (or more) steps to specificity and diversity. *Cell* 1991;67:1033–1036.

51. McEver RP. Leukocyte-endothelial cell interactions. *Curr Opin Cell Biol* 1992:4:840–849.

52. Springer TA. Traffic signals for lymphocyte recirculation and leukocyte emigration: the multistep paradigm. *Cell* 1994;76:301–304.

53. Carlos TM, Harlan JM. Leukocyte-endothelial adhesion molecules. *Blood* 1994;84:2068–2101

54. Laudanna C, Constantin G, Baron P, et al. Sulfatides trigger increase of cytosolic free calcium and enhanced expression of tumor necrosis factor-alpha and interleukin 8 mRNA in human neutrophils. Evidence for a role of L-selectin as a signaling molecule. *J Biol Chem* 1994; 269:4021–4026.

55. Waddell TK, Fialkow L, Chan CK, Kishimoto TK, Downey GP. Potentiation of the oxidative burst of human neutrophils: a signaling role for L selectin. *J Biol Chem* 1994;269:18485–18491.

56. Simon SI, Burns AR, Taylor AD, et al. L selectin (CD62L) cross link-ing signals neutrophil adhesive functions via the Mac 1 (CD11b/CD18) beta 2 integrin. *J Immunol* 1995;155:1502–1514.

57. Zimmerman GA, McIntyre TM, Prescott SM. Adhesion and signaling in vascular cell-cell interactions. *J Clin Invest* 1996;98:1699–1702.

58. Hoover RL, Briggs RT, Karnovsky MJ. The adhesive interactions between polymorphonuclear leukocytes and endothelial cells *in vitro*. *Cell* 1978;14:423–428.

59. Gallin JI. Degranulating stimuli decrease the negative surface charge and increase the adhesiveness of human neutrophils. *J Clin Invest* 1980;65:298–306.

60. Cross AS, Wright DG. Mobilization of sialidase from intracellular stores to the surface of human neutrophils and its role in stimulated adhesion responses of these cells. *J Clin Invest* 1991;88:2067–2076.

61. Nathan C, Xie QW, Halbwachs-Mecarelli L, Jin WW. Albumin inhibits neutrophil spreading and hydrogen peroxide release by block-ing the shedding of CD43 (sialophorin, leukosialin). *J Cell Biol* 1993; 122:243–256.

62. Remold O'Donnell E, Parent D. Specific sensitivity of CD43 to neu-trophil elastase. *Blood* 1995;86:2395–2402.

63. Halbwachs-Mecarelli L, Bessou G, Lesavre P, Renesto P, Chignard M. Neutrophil serine proteases are most probably involved in the release of CD43 (leukosialin, sialophorin) from the neutrophil membrane during cell activation *Blood* 1996;87:1200–1202.

64. Bazil V, Strominger JL. CD43, the major sialoglycoprotein of human leukocytes, is proteolytically cleaved from the surface of stimulated lymphocytes and granulocytes. *Proc Natl Acad Sci U S A* 1993;90: 3792–3796.

65. Remold O'Donnell E, Parent D. Two proteolytic pathways for down-regulation of the barrier molecule CD43 of human neutrophils. *J Immunol* 1994;152:3595–3605.

66. Nathan C, Sanchez E. Tumor necrosis factor and CD11/CD18 (β2) integrins act synergistically to lower cAMP in human neutrophils. *J Cell Biol* 1990;111:2171–2181.

67. Nathan C, Srimal S, Farber C, et al. Cytokine induced respiratory burst of human neutrophils: dependence on extracellular matrix pro-teins and CD11/CD18 integrins. *J Cell Biol* 1989;109:1341–1349.

68. Bennett TA, Lynam EB, Sklar LA, Rogelj S. Hydroxamate based met-alloprotease inhibitor blocks shedding of L selectin adhesion mole-cule from leukocytes: functional consequences for neutrophil aggre-gation. *J Immunol* 1996;156:3093–3097.

69. Preece G, Murphy G, Ager A. Metalloproteinase mediated regulation of L-selectin levels on leucocytes. *J Biol Chem* 1996;271:11634–11640.

70. Ng-Sikorski J, Andersson R, Patarroyo M, Andersson T. Calcium sig-naling capacity of the CD11b/CD18 integrin on human neutrophils. *Exp Cell Res* 1991;195:504–508.

71. Jaconi MEE, Theler JM, Schlegel W, Appel RD, Wright SD, Lew PD. Multiple elevations of cytosolic-free Ca^{2+} in human neutrophils: initi-ation by adherence receptors of the integrin family. *J Cell Biol* 1991;112:1249–1257.

72. Walzog B, Seifert R, Zakrzewicz A, Gaehtgens P, Ley K. Cross-link-ing of CD18 in human neutrophils induces an increase of intracellular free Ca2+, exocytosis of azurophilic granules, quantitative up regula-tion of CD18, shedding of L selectin, and actin polymerization. *J Leukoc Biol* 1994;56:625–635.

73. Pettit EJ, Hallett MB. Localised and global cytosolic Ca2+ changes in neutrophils during engagement of CD11b/CD18 integrin visu-alised using confocal laser scanning reconstruction. *J Cell Sci* 1996; 1689–1694.

74. Berton G, Yan SR, Fumagalli L, Lowell CA. Neutrophil activation by adhesion: mechanisms and pathophysiological implications. *Int J Clin Lab Res* 1996;26:160–177.

75. Suchard SJ, Boxer LA. Exocytosis of a subpopulation of specific granules coincides with H_2O_2 production in adherent human neu-trophils. *J Immunol* 1994;152:290–300.

76. Gyetko MR, Sitrin RG, Fuller JA, Todd RF III, Petty H, Standiford TJ. Function of the urokinase receptor (CD87) in neutrophil chemotaxis. *J Leukoc Biol* 1995;58:533–538.

77. Patel KD, Zimmermann GA, Prescott SM, McEver RP, McIntyre TM. Oxygen radicals induce human endothelial cells to express GMP-140 and bind neutrophils. *J Cell Biol* 1991;112:749–759.

78. Roebuck KA, Rahman A, Lakshminarayanan V, Janakidevi K, Malik AB. H2O2 and tumor necrosis factor-α activate intercellular adhesion molecule-1 (ICAM-1) gene transcription through distinct *cis*-regula-

79. tory elements within the ICAM-1 promoter. *J Biol Chem* 1995;270: 18966–18974.

79. Marui N, Offermann MK, Swerlick R, et al. Vascular cell adhesion molecule-1 (VCAM-1) gene transcription and expression are regu-lated through an antioxidant-sensitive mechanism in human vascular endothelial cells. *J Clin Invest* 1993;92:1866–1874.

80. Patel KD, Zimmermann GA, Prescott SM, McIntyre TM. Novel leukocyte agonists are released by endothelial cells exposed to perox-ide. *J Biol Chem* 1992;267:15168–15175.

81. Renesto P, Halbwachs-Mecarelli L, Bessou G, Balloy V, Chignard M. Inhibition of neutrophil endothelial cell adhesion by a neutrophil product, cathepsin G. *J Leukoc Biol* 1996;59:855–863.

82. Cai TQ, Wright SD. Human leukocyte elastase is an endogenous ligand for the integrin CR3 (CD11b/CD18, Mac 1, $\alpha_M\beta_2$) and modulates poly-morphonuclear leukocyte adhesion. *J Exp Med* 1996;184:1213–1223.

83. Si-Tahar M, Renesto P, Falet H, Rendu F, Chignard M. The phospho-lipase C/protein kinase C pathway is involved in cathepsin G-induced human platelet aggregation: comparison with thrombin. *Biochem J* 1996;313:401–408.

84. Chertov O, Michiel DF, Xu L, et al. Identification of defensin 1, defensin 2, and CAP37/azurocidin as T cell chemoattractant proteins released from interleukin 8 stimulated neutrophils. *J Biol Chem* 1996;271:2935–2940.

85. Zhao MH, Short AK, Lockwood CM. Antineutrophil cytoplasm autoantibodies and vasculitis. *Curr Opin Hematol* 1995;2:96–102.

86. Grimminger F, Hattar K, Papavassilis C, et al. Neutrophil activation by anti-protease 3 antibodies in Wegener's granulomatosis: role of exoge-nous arachidonic acid and leukotriene B4 generation. *J Exp Med* 1996;184:1567–1572.

87. Ferro-Novick S, Jahn R. Vesicle fusion from yeast to man. *Nature* 1994;370:191–193.

88. Rothman JE. Mechanisms of intracellular protein transport. *Nature* 1994;372:55–63.

89. Mellman I. Enigma variations: protein mediators of membrane fusion. *Cell* 1995;82: 869–872.

90. Denesvre C, Malhotra V. Membrane fusion in organelle biogenesis. *Curr Opin Cell Biol* 1996;8:519–523.

91. Rothman JE, Wieland FT. Protein sorting by transport vesicles. *Sci-ence* 1996;272:227–234.

92. Pfeffer SR. Transport vesicle docking: SNAREs and associates. *Annu Rev Cell Dev Biol* 1996;12:441–461.

93. Sudhof TC. The synaptic vesicle cycle: a cascade of protein protein interactions. *Nature* 1995;375:645–653.

94. Gruenberg J, Clague MJ. Regulation of intracellular membrane trans-port. *Curr Opin Cell Biol* 1992;4:593–599.

95. Zerial M, Stenk H. Rab GTPases in vesicular transport. *Curr Opin Cell Biol* 1993;5:613–620.

96. Boman AL, Kahn RA. Arf proteins: the membrane traffic police? *Trends Biochem Sci* 1995;20:147–150.

97. Brumell JH, Volchuk A, Sengelov H, et al. Subcellular distribution of docking/fusion proteins in neutrophils, secretory cells with multiple exocytic compartments. *J Immunol* 1995;155:5750–5759.

98. Maridonneau-Parini I, Yang CZ, Bornens M, Goud B. Increase in the expression of a family of small guanosine triphosphate binding pro-teins, rab proteins, during induced phagocyte differentiation. *J Clin Invest* 1991;87:901–907.

99. Vita F, Soranzo MR, Borelli V, Bertoncin P, Zabucchi G. Subcellular localization of the small GTPase Rab5a in resting and stimulated human neutrophils. *Exp Cell Res* 1996;227:367–373

100. Alvarez-Dominguez C, Barbieri AM, Beron W, Wandinger-Ness A, Stahl PD. Phagocytosed live *Listeria monocytogenes* influences Rab5 regulated *in vitro* phagosome endosome fusion. *J Biol Chem* 1996; 271:13834–13843.

101. Creutz CE. The annexins and exocytosis. *Science* 1992;258:924–931.

102. Raynal P, Pollard HB. Annexins: the problem of assessing the biolog-ical role for a gene family of multifunctional calcium and phospho-lipid binding proteins. *Biochim Biophys Acta* 1994;1197:63–93.

103. Moss SE. Ion channels: annexins taken to task. *Nature* 1995;378: 446–447.

104. Luecke H, Chang BT, Mailliard WS, Schlaepfer DD, Haigler HT. Crystal structure of the annexin XII hexamer and implications for bilayer insertion. *Nature* 1995;378:512–515.

105. Meers P, Ernst JD, Duzgunes N, et al. Synexin like proteins from human polymorphonuclear leukocytes: identification and characteri-

zation of granule aggregating and membrane fusing activities. *J Biol Chem* 1987;262:7850–7858.

106. Ernst JD, Hoye E, Blackwood RA, Jaye D. Purification and characterization of an abundant cytosolic protein from human neutrophils that promotes Ca(2+) dependent aggregation of isolated specific granules. *J Clin Invest* 1990;85:1065–1071.

107. Ernst JD. Annexin III translocates to the periphagosomal region when neutrophils ingest opsonized yeast. *J Immunol* 1991;146:3110–3114.

108. Francis JW, Balazovich KJ, Smolen JE, Margolis DI, Boxer LA. Human neutrophil annexin I promotes granule aggregation and modulates Ca(2+) dependent membrane fusion. *J Clin Invest* 1992;90:537–544.

109. Meers P, Mealy T, Tauber AI. Annexin I interactions with human neutrophil specific granules: fusogenicity and coaggregation with plasma membrane vesicles. *Biochim Biophys Acta* 1993;1147:177–184.

110. Sjolin C, Stendahl O, Dahlgren C. Calcium-induced translocation of annexins to subcellular organelles of human neutrophils. *Biochem J* 1994;300:325–330.

111. Le Cabec V, Maridonneau-Parini I. Annexin 3 is associated with cytoplasmic granules in neutrophils and monocytes and translocates to the plasma membrane in activated cells. *Biochem J* 1994;303:481–487.

112. Kaufman M, Leto T, Levy R. Translocation of annexin I to plasma membranes and phagosomes in human neutrophils upon stimulation with opsonized zymosan: possible role in phagosome function. *Biochem J* 1996;316:35–42.

113. Sjolin C, Dahlgren C. Isolation by calcium dependent translation to neutrophil specific granules of a 42 kD cytosolic protein, identified as being a fragment of annexin XI. *Blood* 1996;87:4817–4823.

114. Blackwood RA, Transue AT, Harsh DM, et al. PLA2 promotes fusion between PMN specific granules and complex liposomes. *J Leukoc Biol* 1996;59:663–670.

115. Takasaki J, Kawauchi Y, Yasunaga T, Masuho Y. Human type II phospholipase A2-induced Mac-1 expression on human neutrophils. *J Leukoc Biol* 1996;60:174–180.

116. Liscovitch M, Cantley LC. Signal transduction and membrane traffic: the PITP/phosphoinositide connection. *Cell* 1995;81:659–662.

117. De Camilli P, Emr SD, McPherson PS, Novick P. Phosphoinositide regulators in membrane traffic. *Science* 1996;271:1533–1539.

118. Hay JC, Fisette PL, Jenkins GH, et al. ATP dependent inositide phosphorylation required for Ca(2+) activated secretion. *Nature* 1995;374:173–177.

119. Fensome A, Cunningham E, Prosser S, et al. Arf and PITP restore GTPγS-stimulated protein secretion from cytosol-depleted HL60 cells by promoting PIP2 synthesis. *Curr Biol* 1996;6:730–738.

120. Cockcroft S. Phospholipid signaling in leukocytes. *Curr Opin Hematol* 1996;3:48–54.

121. Brown HA, Gutowski S, Moomaw CR, Slaughter C, Sternweis PC. ADP ribosylation factor, a small GTP dependent regulatory protein, stimulates phospholipase D activity. *Cell* 1993;75:1137–1144.

122. Cockcroft S, Thomas GM, Fensome A, et al. Phospholipase D: a downstream effector of ARF in granulocytes. *Science* 1994;263:523–526.

123. Siddiqi AR, Smith JL, Ross AH, Qiu RG, Symons M, Exton JH. Regulation of phospholipase D in HL60 cells: evidence for a cytosolic phospholipase D. *J Biol Chem* 1995;270:8466–8473.

124. Jenkins GH, Fisette PL, Anderson RA. Type I phosphatidylinositol 4 phosphate 5 kinase isoforms are specifically stimulated by phosphatidic acid. *J Biol Chem* 1994;269:11547–11554.

125. Hammond SM, Altshuller YM, Sung TC, et al. Human ADP ribosylation factor activated phosphatidylcholine specific phospholipase D defines a new and highly conserved gene family. *J Biol Chem* 1995;270:29640–29643.

126. Martin A, Brown FD, Hodgkin MN, et al. Activation of phospholipase D and phosphatidylinositol 4 phosphate 5 kinase in HL60 membranes is mediated by endogenous Arf but not Rho. *J Biol Chem* 1996;271:17397–17403.

127. Morris AJ, Engebrecht J, Frohman MA. Structure and regulation of phospholipase D. *Trends Pharmacol Sci* 1996;17:182–185.

128. Frohman MA, Morris AJ. Phospholipid signalling: Rho is only ARF the story. *Curr Biol* 1996;6:945–947.

129. Cockcroft S. ARF regulated phospholipase D: a potential role in membrane traffic. *Chem Phys Lipids* 1996;80:59–80.

130. Billah MM, Anthes JC. The regulation and cellular functions of phosphatidylcholine hydrolysis. *Biochem J* 1990;269:281–291.

131. Exton JH. Phosphatidylcholine breakdown and signal transduction. *Biochim Biophys Acta* 1994;1212:26–42.

132. Liscovitch M, Chalifa V, Pertile P, Chen CS, Cantley LC. Novel function of phosphatidylinositol 4,5 bisphosphate as a cofactor for brain membrane phospholipase D. *J Biol Chem* 1994;269:21403–21406.

133. Pertile P, Liscovitch M, Chalifa V, Cantley LC. Phosphatidylinositol 4,5 bisphosphate synthesis is required for activation of phospholipase D in U937 cells. *J Biol Chem* 1995;270:5130–5135.

134. Terui T, Kahn RA, Randazzo PA. Effects of acid phospholipids on nucleotide exchange properties of ADP ribosylation factor 1: evidence for specific interaction with phosphatidylinositol 4,5 bisphosphate. *J Biol Chem* 1994;269:28130–28135.

135. Pai JK, Siegel MI, Egan RW, Billah MM. Phospholipase D catalyzes phospholipid metabolism in chemotactic peptide stimulated HL 60 granulocytes. *J Biol Chem* 1988;263:12472–12477.

136. Gelas P, Ribbes G, Record M, Terce F, Chap H. Differential activation by fMet-Leu-Phe and phorbol ester of a plasma membrane phosphatidylcholine specific phospholipase D in human neutrophil. *FEBS Lett* 1989;251:213–218.

137. Bonser RW, Thompson NT, Randall RW, Garland LG. Phospholipase D activation is functionally linked to superoxide generation in the human neutrophil. *Biochem J* 1989;264:617–620.

138. Agwu DE, McPhail LC, Chabot MC, Daniel LW, Wykle RL, McCall CE. Choline-linked phosphoglycerides: a source of phosphatidic acid and diglycerides in stimulated neutrophils. *J Biol Chem* 1989;264:1405–1413.

139. Fallman M, Stendahl O, Andersson T. Phorbol ester induced activation of protein kinase C leads to increased formation of diacylglycerol in human neutrophils. *Exp Cell Res* 1989;181:217–225.

140. Mullmann TJ, Siegel MI, Egan RW, Billah MM. Phorbol-12 myristate-13-acetate activation of phospholipase D in human neutrophils leads to the production of phosphatides and diglycerides. *Biochem Biophys Res Commun* 1990;170:1197–1202.

141. Mullmann TJ, Siegel MI, Egan RW, Billah MM. Complement C5a activation of phospholipase D in human neutrophils: a major route to the production of phosphatidates and diglycerides. *J Immunol* 1990;144:1901–1908.

142. Reinhold SL, Prescott SM, Zimmerman GA, McIntyre TM. Activation of human neutrophil phospholipase D by three separable mechanisms. *FASEB J* 1990;4:208–214.

143. Rossi F, Grzeskowiak M, Della Bianca V, Calzetti F, Gandini G. Phosphatidic acid and not diacylglycerol generated by phospholipase D is functionally linked to the activation of the NADPH oxidase by FMLP in human neutrophils. *Biochem Biophys Res Commun* 1990;168:320–327.

144. Della Bianca V, Grzeskowiak M, Lissandrini D, Rossi F. Source and role of diacylglycerol formed during phagocytosis of opsonized yeast particles and associated respiratory burst in human neutrophils. *Biochem Biophys Res Commun* 1991;177:948–955.

145. Kanaho Y, Nishida A, Nozawa Y. Calcium rather than protein kinase C is the major factor to activate phospholipase D in FMLP-stimulated rabbit peritoneal neutrophils: possible involvement of calmodulin/myosin L chain kinase pathway. *J Immunol* 1992;149:622–628.

146. Suchard SJ, Nakamura T, Abe A, Shayman JA, Boxer LA. Phospholipase D mediated diradylglycerol formation coincides with H2O2 and lactoferrin release in adherent human neutrophils. *J Biol Chem* 1994;269:8063–8068.

147. Nakamura T, Suchard SJ, Abe A, Shayman JA, Boxer LA. Role of diradylglycerol formation in H2O2 and lactoferrin release in adherent human polymorphonuclear leukocytes. *J Leukoc Biol* 1994;56:105–109.

148. Stutchfield J, Cockcroft S. Correlation between secretion and phospholipase D activation in differentiated HL60 cells. *Biochem J* 1993;293:649–655.

149. Zhou HL, Chabot-Fletcher M, Foley JJ, et al. Association between leukotriene B4 induced phospholipase D activation and degranulation of human neutrophils. *Biochem Pharmacol* 1993;46:139–148.

150. Bowman EP, Uhlinger DJ, Lambeth JD. Neutrophil phospholipase D is activated by a membrane-associated Rho family small molecular weight GTP-binding protein. *J Biol Chem* 1993;268:21509–21512.

151. Singer WD, Brown HA, Bokoch GM, Sternweis PC. Resolved phospholipase D activity is modulated by cytosolic factors other than Arf. *J Biol Chem* 1995;270:14944–14950.

152. Kuribara H, Tago K, Yokozeki T, et al. Synergistic activation of rat brain phospholipase D by ADP ribosylation factor and rhoA p21, and its inhibition by *Clostridium botulinum* C3 exoenzyme. *J Biol Chem* 1995;270:25667–25671.

153. Schmidt M, Rumenapp U, Bienek C, Keller J, von Eichel-Streiber C, Jakobs KH. Inhibition of receptor signaling to phospholipase D by *Clostridium difficile* toxin B: role of Rho proteins. *J Biol Chem* 1996; 271:2422–2426.

154. Machesky LM, Hall A. Rho: a connection between membrane receptor signalling and the cytoskeleton. *Trends Cell Biol* 1996;6:304–310.

155. Symons M. Rho family GTPases: the cytoskeleton and beyond. *Trends Biochem Sci* 1996;21:178–181.

156. Zigmond SH. Signal transduction and actin filament organization. *Curr Opin Cell Biol* 1996;8:66–73.

157. Ridley AJ. Rho: theme and variations. *Curr Biol* 1996;10:1256–1264.

158. Dharmawardhane S, Bokoch GM. Rho GTPases and leukocyte cytoskeletal regulation. *Curr Opin Hematol* 1997;4:12–18.

159. Zheng Y, Glaven JA, Wu WJ, Cerione RA. Phosphatidylinositol 4,5-bisphosphate provides an alternative to guanine nucleotide exchange factors by stimulating the dissociation of GDP from Cdc42Hs. *J Biol Chem* 1996;27:23815–23819.

160. Cross MJ, Roberts S, Ridley AJ, et al. Stimulation of actin stress fibre formation mediated by activation of phospholipase D. *Curr Biol* 1996;6:588–597.

161. Peppelenbosch MP, Qiu RG, de Vries-Smits, et al. Rac mediates growth factor induced arachidonic acid release. *Cell* 1995;81:849–856.

162. Price LS, Norman JC, Ridley AJ, Koffer A. The small GTPases Rac and Rho as regulators of secretion in mast cells. *Curr Biol* 1995;5: 68–73.

163. Mariot P, O'Sullivan AJ, Brown AM, Tatham PER. Rho guanine nucleotide dissociation inhibitor protein (RhoGDI) inhibits exocytosis in mast cells. *EMBO J* 1996;15:6476–6482.

164. Prepens U, Just I, von Eichel-Streiber C, Aktories K. Inhibition of FcεRI mediated activation of rat basophilic leukemia cells by *Clostridium difficile* toxin B (monoglucosyltransferase). *J Biol Chem* 1996;271:7324–7329.

165. Carpenter CL, Cantley LC. Phosphoinositide kinases. *Curr Opin Cell Biol* 1996;8:153–158.

166. Brown WJ, DeWald DB, Emr SD, Plutner H, Balch WE. Role for phosphatidylinositol 3-kinase in the sorting and transport of newly synthesized lysosomal enzymes in mammalian cells. *J Cell Biol* 1995;130:781–796.

167. Davidson HW. Wortmannin causes mistargeting of procathepsin D: evidence for the involvement of a phosphatidylinositol 3-kinase in vesicular transport to lysosomes. *J Cell Biol* 1995;130:797–805.

168. Martin SS, Haruta T, Morris AJ, Klippel A, Williams LT, Olefsky JM. Activated phosphatidylinositol 3-kinase is sufficient to mediate actin rearrangement and GLUT4 translocation in 3T3 L1 adipocytes. *J Biol Chem* 1996;271:17605–17608.

169. Yang J, Clarke JF, Ester CJ, Young PW, Kasuga M, Holman GD. Phosphatidylinositol 3-kinase acts at an intracellular membrane site to enhance GLUT4 exocytosis in 3T3 L1 cells. *Biochem J* 1996;313: 125–131.

170. Yano H, Nakanishi S, Kimura K, et al. Inhibition of histamine secretion by wortmannin through the blockade of phosphatidylinositol 3-kinase in RBL 2H3 cells. *J Biol Chem* 1993;268:25846–25856.

171. Ozawa K, Masujima T, Ikeda K, Kodama Y, Nonomura Y. Different pathways of inhibitory effects of wortmannin on exocytosis are revealed by video enhanced light microscope. *Biochem Biophys Res Commun* 1996;222:243–248.

172. Marquardt DL, Alongi JL, Walker LL. The phosphatidylinositol 3-kinase inhibitor wortmannin blocks mast cell exocytosis but not IL 6 production. *J Immunol* 1996;156:1942–1945.

173. Teng JM, Liu XR, Mills GB, Dupont B. CD28 mediated cytotoxicity by the human leukemic NK cell line YT involves tyrosine phosphorylation, activation of phosphatidylinositol 3-kinase, and protein kinase C. *J Immunol* 1996;156:3222–3232.

174. Bonnema JD, Karnitz LM, Schoon RA, Abraham RT, Leibson PJ. Fc receptor stimulation of phosphatidylinositol 3-kinase in natural killer cells is associated with protein kinase C independent granule release and cell mediated cytotoxicity. *J Exp Med* 1994;80:1427–1435.

175. Nakanishi S, Yano H, Matsuda Y. Novel functions of phosphatidylinositol 3-kinase in terminally differentiated cells. *Cell Signal* 1995; 7:545–557.

176. Dewald B, Thelen M, Baggiolini M. Two transduction sequences are necessary for neutrophil activation by receptor agonists. *J Biol Chem* 1988;263:16179–16184.

177. Arcaro A, Wymann MP. Wortmannin is a potent phosphatidylinositol 3-kinase inhibitor: the role of phosphatidylinositol 3,4,5 trisphosphate in neutrophil responses. *Biochem J* 1993;296:297–301.

178. Thelen M, Wymann MP, Langen H. Wortmannin binds specifically to 1 phosphatidylinositol 3-kinase while inhibiting guanine nucleotide binding protein-coupled receptor signaling in neutrophil leukocytes. *Proc Natl Acad Sci U S A* 1994;91:4960–4964.

179. Okada T, Sakuma L, Fukui Y, Hazeki O, Ui M. Blockage of chemotactic peptide-induced stimulation of neutrophils by wortmannin as a result of selective inhibition of phosphatidylinositol 3-kinase. *J Biol Chem* 1994;269:3563–3567.

180. Vlahos CJ, Matter WF, Brown RF, et al. Investigation of neutrophil signal transduction using a specific inhibitor of phosphatidylinositol 3 kinase. *J Immunol* 1995;154:2413–2422.

181. Li G, D'Souza-Schorey C, Barbieri MA, et al. Evidence for phosphatidylinositol 3 kinase as a regulator of endocytosis via activation of Rab5. *Proc Natl Acad Sci U S A* 1995;92:10207–10211.

182. Valius M, Kazlauskas A. Phospholipase C-γ1 and phosphatidylinositol 3-kinase are the downstream mediators of the PDGF receptor's mitogenic signal. *Cell* 1993;73:321–334.

183. Yamauchi K, Holt K, Pessin JE. Phosphatidylinositol 3-kinase functions upstream of Ras and Raf in mediating insulin stimulation of c-fos transcription. *J Biol Chem* 1993;268:14597–14600.

184. Rodriguez-Viciana P, Warne PH, Dhand R, et al. Phosphatidylinositol 3-OH-kinase as a direct target of Ras. *Nature* 1994;370:527–532.

185. Kodaki T, Woscholski R, Hallberg B, Rodriguez Viciana P, Downward J, Parker PJ. The activation of phosphatidylinositol 3-kinase by Ras. *Curr Biol* 1994;4:798–806.

186. Hu Q, Klippel A, Muslin AJ, Fanti WJ, Williams WT. Ras-dependent induction of cellular responses by constitutively active phosphatidylinositol 3-kinase. *Science* 1995;268:100–102.

187. Feig LA, Schaffhausen B. Signal transduction: the hunt for Ras targets. *Nature* 1994;370:508–509.

188. Marshall MS. Ras target proteins in eukaryotic cells. *FASEB J* 1995; 9:1311–1318.

189. Marshall CJ. Ras effectors. *Curr Opin Cell Biol* 1996;8:197–204.

190. Zhang J, King WG, Dillon S, Hall A, Feig L, Rittenhouse SE. Activation of platelet phosphatidylinositide 3-kinase requires the small GTP-binding protein Rho. *J Biol Chem* 1993;268:22251–22254.

191. Zheng Y, Bagrodia S, Cerione RA. Activation of phosphoinositide 3-kinase activity by Cdc42Hs binding to p85. *J Biol Chem* 1994;269: 18727–18730.

192. Hawkins PT, Eguinoa A, Qiu RG, et al. PDGF stimulates an increase in GTP-Rac via activation of phosphoinositide 3-kinase. *Curr Biol* 1995;5:393–403.

193. Parker PJ. Intracellular signalling: PI 3-kinase puts GTP on the Rac. *Curr Biol* 1995;5:577–579.

194. Tolias KF, Cantley LC, Carpenter CL. Rho family GTPases bind to phosphoinositide kinases. *J Biol Chem* 1995;270:17656–17659.

195. Bokoch GM, Vlahos CJ, Wang Y, Knaus UG, Traynor-Kaplan AE. Rac GTPase interacts specifically with phosphatidylinositol 3-kinase. *Biochem J* 1996;315:775–779.

196. Reif K, Nobes CD, Thomas G, Hall A, Cantrell DA. Phosphatidylinositol 3-kinase signals activate a selective subset of Rac/Rho-dependent effector pathways. *Curr Biol* 1996;11:1445–1455.

197. Gerard C, Gerard NP. The pro-inflammatory seven-transmembrane segment receptors of the leukocyte. *Curr Opin Immunol* 1994;6: 140–145.

198. Thelen M, Wirthmueller U. Phospholipases and protein kinases during phagocyte activation. *Curr Opin Immunol* 1994;6:106–112.

199. Bokoch GM. Chemoattractant signaling and leukocyte activation. *Blood* 1995;86:1649–1660.

200. Downey GP, Fukushima T, Fialkow L. Signaling mechanisms in human neutrophils. *Curr Opin Hematol* 1995;2:76–88.

201. Premack BA, Schall TJ. Chemokine receptors: gateways to inflammation and infection. *Nat Med* 1996;2:1174–1178.

202. Divecha N, Irvine RF. Phospholipid signaling. *Cell* 1995;80:269–278.

203. Nishizuka Y. Protein kinase C and lipid signaling for sustained cellular responses. *FASEB J* 1995;9:484–496.

204. Jaken S. Protein kinase C isozymes and substrates. *Curr Opin Cell Biol* 1996;8:168–173.

205. Spiegel S, Foster D, Kolesnick R. Signal transduction through lipid second messengers. *Curr Opin Cell Biol* 1996;8:159–167.

206. Zor U, Ferber E, Gergely P, Szucs K, Dombradi V, Goldman R. Reactive oxygen species mediate phorbol ester regulated tyrosine phos-

phorylation and phospholipase A_2 activation: potentiation by vanadate. *Biochem J* 1993;295:879–888

207. Bourgoin S, Grinstein S. Peroxides of vanadate induce activation of phospholipase D in HL 60 cells: role of tyrosine phosphorylation. *J Biol Chem* 1992;267:11908–11916.

208. Uings IJ, Thompson NT, Randall RW, et al. Tyrosine phosphorylation is involved in receptor coupling to phospholipase D but not phospholipase C in the human neutrophil. *Biochem J* 1992;281:597–600.

209. Dubyak GR, Schomisch SJ, Kusner DJ, Xie M. Phospholipase D activity in phagocytic leucocytes is synergistically regulated by G protein and tyrosine kinase based mechanisms. *Biochem J* 1993,292:121–128.

210. Jiang H, Lu Z, Luo JQ, Wolfman A, Foster DA. Ras mediates the activation of phospholipase D by v-Src. *J Biol Chem* 1995;270:6006–6009.

211. Ward SG, June CH, Olive D. PI 3 kinase: a pivotal pathway in T cell activation? *Immunol Today* 1996;17:187–197.

212. Stoyanov B, Volinia S, Hanck T, et al. Cloning and characterization of a G protein activated human phosphoinositide 3-kinase. *Science* 1995;269:690–693.

213. Stephens L, Smrcka A, Cooke FT, Jackson TR, Sternweis PC, Hawkins PT. A novel phosphoinositide 3-kinase activity in myeloid derived cells is activated by G protein $\beta\gamma$ subunits. *Cell* 1994;77:83–93.

214. Ptasznik A, Traynor-Kaplan A, Bokoch GM. G protein-coupled chemoattractant receptors regulate Lyn tyrosine kinase·Shc adapter protein signaling complexes. *J Biol Chem* 1995;270:19969–19973.

215. Ptasznik A, Prossnitz ER, Yoshikawa D, et al. A tyrosine kinase signaling pathway accounts for the majority of phosphatidylinositol 3,4,5 trisphosphate formation in chemoattractant stimulated human neutrophils. *J Biol Chem* 1996;271:25204–25207.

216. Bourne HR. Signal transduction: team blue sees red. *Nature* 1995;376:727–729.

217. Bokoch GM. Interplay between Ras related and heterotrimeric GTP-binding proteins: lifestyles of the BIG and little. *FASEB J* 1996;10:1290–1295.

218. Clark EA, Brugge JS. Redistribution of activated pp60[c-src] to integrin-dependent cytoskeletal complexes in thrombin stimulated platelets. *Mol Cell Biol* 1993;13:1863–1871.

219. Erpel T, Courtneidge SA. Src family protein tyrosine kinases and cellular signal transduction pathways. *Curr Opin Cell Biol* 1995;7:176–182.

220. Luttrell LM, Hawes BE, van Biesen T, Luttrell DK, Lansing TJ, Lefkowitz RJ. Role of c-Src tyrosine kinase in G protein-coupled receptor and G$\beta\gamma$ subunit-mediated activation of mitogen activated protein kinases. *J Biol Chem* 1996;271:19443–19550.

221. Dikic I, Tokiwa G, Lev S, Courtneidge SA, Schlessinger J. A role for Pyk2 and Src in linking G-protein-coupled receptors with MAP kinase activation. *Nature* 1996;383:547–550.

222. Rodriguez-Fernandez JL, Rozengurt E. Bombesin, bradykinin, vasopressin, and phorbol esters rapidly and transiently activate Src family tyrosine kinases in Swiss 3T3 cells: dissociation from tyrosine phosphorylation of p125 focal adhesion kinase. *J Biol Chem* 1996;271:27895–27901.

223. Wan Y, Kurosaki T, Huang XY. Tyrosine kinases in activation of the MAP kinase cascade by G protein coupled receptors. *Nature* 1996;380:541–544.

224. Schaller MD, Parsons JT. Focal adhesion kinase and associated proteins. *Curr Opin Cell Biol* 1994;6:705–710.

225. Lev S, Moreno H, Martinez R, et al. Protein tyrosine kinase PYK2 involved in Ca(2+) induced regulation of ion channel and MAP kinase functions. *Nature* 1995;376:737–745.

226. Clark EA, Brugge JS. Integrins and signal transduction pathways: the road taken. *Science* 1995;268:233–239.

227. Berton G, Fumagalli L, Laudanna C, Sorio C. β2 integrin-dependent protein tyrosine phosphorylation and activation of the FGR protein tyrosine kinase in human neutrophils. *J Cell Biol* 1994;126:1111–1121.

228. Yan SR, Fumagalli L, Berton G. Activation of p58[c-fgr] and p53/56[lyn] in adherent human neutrophils: evidence for a role of divalent cations in regulating neutrophil adhesion and protein tyrosine kinase activities. *J Inflammation* 1995;45:297–311.

229. Yan SR, Huang M, Berton G. Signaling by adhesion in human neutrophils. Activation of the p72[syk] tyrosine kinase and formation of protein complexes containing p72[syk] and Src family tyrosine kinases in neutrophils spreading over fibrinogen. *J Immunol* 1997;158:1902–1910.

230. Lowell CA, Fumagalli L, Berton G. Deficiency of Src family kinases p59/61[hck] and p58[c-fgr] results in defective adhesion dependent neutrophil functions. *J Cell Biol* 1996;133:895–910.

231. Kapron-Bras C, Fitz-Gibbon L, Jeevaratnam P, Wilkins J, Dedhar S. Stimulation of tyrosine phosphorylation and accumulation of GTP-bound p21[ras] upon antibody mediated $\alpha2\beta1$ integrin activation in T-lymphoblastic cells. *J Biol Chem* 1993;268:20701–20704.

232. Clark EA, Hynes RO. Ras activation is necessary for integrin mediated activation of extracellular signal-regulated kinase 2 and cytosolic phospholipase A_2 but not for cytoskeletal organization. *J Biol Chem* 1996;271:14814–14818.

233. Chen Q, Lin TH, Der CJ, Juliano RL. Integrin mediated activation of MEK and mitogen-activated protein (MAP) kinase is independent of Ras. *J Biol Chem* 1996;271:18122–18127.

234. Miyamoto S, Teramoto H, Gutkind JS, Yamada KM. Integrins can collaborate with growth factors for phosphorylation of receptor tyrosine kinases and MAP kinase activation: roles of integrin aggregation and occupancy of receptors. *J Cell Biol* 1996;135:1633–1642.

235. Zheng L, Sjolander A, Eckerdal J, Andersson T. Antibody induced engagement of β_2 integrins on adherent human neutrophils triggers activation of p21[ras] through tyrosine phosphorylation of the protooncogene product Vav. *Proc Natl Acad Sci U S A* 1996;93:8431–8436.

236. Grinstein S, Furuya W. Chemoattractant-induced tyrosine phosphorylation and activation of microtubule-associated protein kinase in human neutrophils. *J Biol Chem* 1992;267:18122–18125.

237. Torres M, Hall FL, O'Neill K. Stimulation of human neutrophils with formyl-methionyl-leucyl-phenylalanine induces tyrosine phosphorylation and activation of two distinct mitogen-activated protein kinases. *J Immunol* 1993;150:1563–1577.

238. Worthen GS, Avdi N, Buhl AM, Suzuki N, Johnson GL. FMLP activates Ras and Raf in human neutrophils: potential role in activation of MAP kinase. *J Clin Invest* 1994;94:815–823.

239. Pillinger MH, Feoktistov AS, Capodici C, et al. Mitogen-activated protein kinase in neutrophils and enucleate neutrophil cytoplasts: evidence for regulation of cell-cell adhesion. *J Biol Chem* 1996;271:12049–12056.

240. Downey GP, Butler JR, Brumell J, et al. Chemotactic peptide induced activation of MEK-2, the predominant isoform in human neutrophils: inhibition by wortmannin. *J Biol Chem* 1996;271:21005–21011.

241. Knall C, Young S, Nick JA, Buhl AM, Worthen GS, Johnson GL. Interleukin-8 regulation of the Ras/Raf/mitogen activated protein kinase pathway in human neutrophils. *J Biol Chem* 1996;271:2832–2838.

242. Waddell TK, Fialkow L, Chan CK, Kishimoto TK, Downey GP. Signaling functions of L-selectin: enhancement of tyrosine phosphorylation and activation of MAP kinase. *J Biol Chem* 1995;270:15403–15411.

243. Gomez-Cambronero J, Colasanto JM, Huang CK, Sha'afi RI. Direct stimulation by tyrosine phosphorylation of microtubule-associated protein (MAP) kinase activity by granulocyte-macrophage colony-stimulating factor in human neutrophils. *Biochem J* 1993;291:211–217.

244. Rafiee P, Lee JK, Leung CC, Raffin TA. TNF alpha induces tyrosine phosphorylation of mitogen activated protein kinase in adherent human neutrophils. *J Immunol* 1995;154:4785–4792.

245. Fialkow L, Chan CK, Rotin D, Grinstein S, Downey GP. Activation of the mitogen activated protein kinase signaling pathway in neutrophils: role of oxidants. *J Biol Chem* 1994;269:31234–31242.

246. Brumell JH, Burkhardt AL, Bolen JB, Grinstein S. Endogenous reactive oxygen intermediates activate tyrosine kinases in human neutrophils. *J Biol Chem* 1996;271:1455–1461.

247. Yan SR, Berton G. Regulation of Src family tyrosine kinase activities in adherent human neutrophils: evidence that reactive oxygen intermediates produced by adherent neutrophils increase the activity of the p58[c-fgr] and p53/56[lyn] tyrosine kinases. *J Biol Chem* 1996;271:23464–23471.

248. Santana C, Noris G, Espinoza B, Ortega E. Protein tyrosine phosphorylation in leukocyte activation through receptors for IgG. *J Leukoc Biol* 1996;60:433–440.

249. Fuortes M, Jin WW, Nathan C. Adhesion-dependent protein tyrosine phosphorylation in neutrophils treated with tumor necrosis factor. *J Cell Biol* 1993;120:777–784.

250. Graham IL, Anderson DC, Holers VM, Brown EJ. Complement receptor 3 (CR3, Mac-1, integrin $\alpha_M\beta_2$, CD11b/CD18) is required for tyrosine phosphorylation of paxillin in adherent and nonadherent neutrophils. *J Cell Biol* 1994;127:1139–1147.

251. Fuortes M, Jin WW, Nathan C. β₂ integrin dependent tyrosine phosphorylation of paxillin in human neutrophils treated with tumor necrosis factor. *J Cell Biol* 1994;127:1477–1483.

252. Hall A. Small GTP binding proteins and the regulation of the actin cytoskeleton. *Annu Rev Cell Biol* 1994;10:31–54.

253. Nobes CD, Hall A. Rho, rac, and cdc42 GTPases regulate the assembly of multimolecular focal complexes associated with actin stress fibers, lamellipodia, and filopodia. *Cell* 1995;81:53–62.

254. Ridley AJ, Hall A. Signal transduction pathways regulating Rho mediated stress fibre formation: requirement for a tyrosine kinase. *EMBO J* 1994;13:2600–2610.

255. Vojtek AB, Cooper JA. Rho family members: activators of MAP kinase cascades. *Cell* 1995;82:527–529.

256. Kyriakis JM, Avruch J. Sounding the alarm: protein kinase cascades activated by stress and inflammation. *J Biol Chem* 1996;271:24313–24316.

257. Canman CE, Kastan MB. Signal transduction: three paths to stress relief. *Nature* 1996;384:213–214.

258. Stossel TP. On the crawling of animal cells. *Science* 1993;260:1086–1094.

259. Hartwig JH, Bokoch GM, Carpenter CL, et al. Thrombin receptor ligation and activated Rac uncap actin filament barbed ends through phosphoinositide synthesis in permeabilized human platelets. *Cell* 1995;82:643–653.

260. Goldstein IM, Horn JK, Kaplan HB, Weissmann G. Calcium-induced lysozyme secretion from human polymorphonuclear leukocytes. *Biochem Biophys Res Commun* 1974;60:807–812.

261. Koza EP, Wright TE, Becker EL. Lysosomal enzyme secretion and volume contraction induced in neutrophils by cytochalasin B, chemotactic factor and A23187. *Proc Soc Exp Biol* 1975;149:476–479.

262. Zabucchi G, Soranzo MR, Rossi F, Romeo D. Exocytosis in human polymorphonuclear leukocytes induced by A23187 and calcium. *FEBS Lett* 1975;54:44–48.

263. Smith C, Ignarro LJ. Bioregulation of lysosomal enzyme secretion from human neutrophils: roles of guanosine 3,5-monophosphate and calcium in stimulus-secretion coupling. *Proc Natl Acad Sci U S A* 1975;72:108–112.

264. Huang CK, Laramee GR, Casnellie JE. Chemotactic factor-induced tyrosine phosphorylation of membrane-associated proteins in rabbit peritoneal neutrophils. *Biochem Biophys Res Commun* 1988;151:794–801.

265. Gomez-Cambronero J, Huang CK, Bonak VA, et al. Tyrosine phosphorylation in human neutrophil. *Biochem Biophys Res Commun* 1989;162:1478–1485.

266. Huang CK, Bonak V, Laramee GR, Casnellie JE. Protein tyrosine phosphorylation in rabbit peritoneal neutrophils. *Biochem J* 1990;269:431–436.

267. Gomez-Cambronero J, Wang E, Johnson G, Huang CK, Sha'afi RI. Platelet activating factor induces tyrosine phosphorylation in human neutrophils. *J Biol Chem* 1991;266:6240–6245.

268. Berkow RL, Dodson RW. Tyrosine specific protein phosphorylation during activation of human neutrophils. *Blood* 1990;75:2445–2452.

269. McColl SR, DiPersio JF, Caon AC, Ho P, Naccache PH. Involvement of tyrosine kinases in the activation of human peripheral blood neutrophils by granulocyte-macrophage colony-stimulating factor. *Blood* 1991;78:1842–1852.

270. Connelly PA, Farrell CA, Merenda JM, Conklyn MJ, Showell HJ. Tyrosine phosphorylation is an early signaling event common to Fc receptor crosslinking in human neutrophils and rat basophilic leukemia cells (RBL 2H3). *Biochem Biophys Res Commun* 1991;177:192–201.

271. Gomez-Cambronero J, Huang CK, Gomez-Cambronero TM, Waterman WH, Becker EL, Sha'afi RI. Granulocyte macrophage colony stimulating factor induced protein tyrosine phosphorylation of microtubule associated protein kinase in human neutrophils. *Proc Natl Acad Sci U S A* 1992;89:7551–7555.

272. Ohta S, Inazu T, Taniguchi T, Nakagawara G, Yamamura H. Protein-tyrosine phosphorylation induced by concanavalin A and N-formyl-methionyl-leucyl-phenylalanine in human neutrophils. *Eur J Biochem* 1992;206:895–900.

273. Gaudry M, Roberge CJ, de Medicis R, Lussier A, Poubelle PE, Naccache PH. Crystal induced neutrophil activation: III. Inflammatory microcrystals induce a distinct pattern of tyrosine phosphorylation in human neutrophils. *J Clin Invest* 1993;91:1649–1655.

274. Richard S, Shaw AS, Showell HJ, Connelly PA. The role of individual Fcγ receptors in aggregated IgG-stimulated protein tyrosine phosphorylation in the human neutrophil. *Biochem Biophys Res Commun* 1994;199:653–661.

275. Dusi S, Donini M, Rossi F. Tyrosine phosphorylation and activation of NADPH oxidase in human neutrophils: a possible role for MAP kinases and for a 75 kDa protein. *Biochem J* 1994;304:243–250.

276. Dusi S, Donini M, Della Bianca V, Rossi F. Tyrosine phosphorylation of phospholipase Cγ-2 is involved in the activation of phosphoinositide hydrolysis by Fc receptors in human neutrophils. *Biochem Biophys Res Commun* 1994;201:1100–1108.

277. Richard S, Farrell CA, Shaw AS, Showell HJ, Connelly PA. C5a as a model for chemotactic factor stimulated tyrosine phosphorylation in the human neutrophil. *J Immunol* 1994;152:2479–2487.

278. Liang L, Huang CK. Tyrosine phosphorylation induced by cross-linking of Fcγ receptor type II in human neutrophils. *Biochem J* 1995;306:489–495.

279. Zaffran Y, Escallier JC, Ruta S, Capo C, Mege JL. Zymosan-triggered association of tyrosine phosphoproteins and lyn kinase with cytoskeleton in human monocytes. *J Immunol* 1995;154:3488–3497.

280. Allen LA, Aderem A. Molecular definition of distinct cytoskeletal structures involved in complement and Fc receptor-mediated phagocytosis in macrophages. *J Exp Med* 1996;184:627–637.

281. Naccache PH, Jean N, Liao NW, Bator JM, McColl SR, Kubes P. Regulation of stimulated integrin surface expression in human neutrophils by tyrosine phosphorylation. *Blood* 1994;84:616–624.

282. Burt HM, Jackson JK, Dryden P, Salari H. Crystal-induced protein tyrosine phosphorylation in neutrophils and the effect of a tyrosine kinase inhibitor on neutrophil responses. *Mol Pharmacol* 1993;43:30–38.

283. Burt HM, Jackson JK, Salari H. Inhibition of crystal-induced neutrophil activation by a protein tyrosine kinase inhibitor. *J Leukoc Biol* 1994;55:112–119.

284. Asahi M, Taniguchi T, Hashimoto E, Inazu T, Maeda H, Yamamura H. Activation of protein tyrosine kinase p72^syk with concanavalin A in polymorphonuclear neutrophils. *J Biol Chem* 1993;268:23334–23338.

285. Naccache PH, Gilbert C, Caon AC, et al. Selective inhibition of human neutrophil functional responsiveness by erbstatin, an inhibitor of tyrosine protein kinase. *Blood* 1990;76:2098–2104.

286. Oliver JM, Burg DL, Wilson BS, McLaughlin JL, Geahlen RL. Inhibition of mast cell FcεRI-mediated signaling and effector function by the Syk-selective inhibitor, piceatannol. *J Biol Chem* 1994;269:29697–29703.

287. Rivera VM, Brugge JS. Clustering of Syk is sufficient to induce tyrosine phosphorylation and release of allergic mediators from rat basophilic leukemia cells. *Mol Cell Biol* 1995;15:1582–1590.

288. Zhang J, Berenstein EH, Evans RL, Siraganian RP. Transfection of Syk protein tyrosine kinase reconstitutes high affinity IgE receptor-mediated degranulation in a Syk negative variant of rat basophilic leukemia RBL 2H3 cells. *J Exp Med* 1996;184:71–79.

289. Lavens SE, Goldring K, Thomas LH, Warner JA. Effects of integrin clustering on human lung mast cells and basophils. *Am J Respir Cell Mol Biol* 1996;14:95–103.

290. Taylor JA, Karas JL, Ram MK, Green OM, Seidel-Dugan C. Activation of the high-affinity immunoglobulin E receptor FcεRI in RBL-2H3 cells is inhibited by Syk SH2 domains. *Mol Cell Biol* 1995;15:4149–4157.

291. Kato M, Abraham RT, Kita H. Tyrosine phosphorylation is required for eosinophil degranulation induced by immobilized immunoglobulins. *J Immunol* 1995;155:357–366.

292. Anel A, Richieri GV, Kleinfeld AM. A tyrosine phosphorylation requirement for cytotoxic T lymphocyte degranulation. *J Biol Chem* 1994;269:9506–9513.

293. O'Rourke AM, Mescher MF. Signals for activation of CD8-dependent adhesion and costimulation in CTLs. *J Immunol* 1994;152:4358–4367.

294. Gaudry M, Gilbert C, Barabe F, Poubelle PE, Naccache PH. Activation of Lyn is a common element of the stimulation of human neutrophils by soluble and particulate stimuli. *Blood* 1995;86:3567–3574.

295. Lin TH, Rosales C, Mondal K, Bolen JB, Haskill S, Jiano RL. Integrin-mediated tyrosine phosphorylation and cytokine message induction in monocytic cells: a possible signaling role for the Syk tyrosine kinase. *J Biol Chem* 1995;270:16189–16197.

296. Hamada F, Aoki M, Akiyama T, Toyoshima K. Association of immunoglobulin G Fc receptor II with Src-like protein tyrosine kinase Fgr in neutrophils. *Proc Natl Acad Sci U S A* 1993;90:6305–6309.

297. Kiener PA, Rankin BM, Burkhardt AL, Schieven GL, Gilliland LK, Rowley RB, Bolen JB, Ledbetter JA. Cross-linking of Fcγ receptor I (FcγRI) and receptor II (FcγRII) on monocytic cells activates a signal transduction pathway common to both Fc receptors that involves the stimulation of p72 Syk protein tyrosine kinase. *J Biol Chem* 1993;268: 24442–24448.

298. Greenberg S, Chang P, Silverstein SC. Tyrosine phosphorylation of the γ subunit of Fcγ receptors, p72^{syk}, and paxillin during Fc receptor-mediated phagocytosis in macrophages. *J Biol Chem* 1994;269:3897–3902.

299. Darby C, Geahlen RL, Schreiber AD. Stimulation of macrophage FcγRIIIA activates the receptor-associated protein tyrosine kinase Syk and induces phosphorylation of multiple proteins including p95Vav and p62/GAP associated protein. *J Immunol* 1994;152:5429–5437.

300. Durden DL, Kim HM, Calore B, Liu Y. The FcγRI receptor signals through the activation of hck and MAP kinase. *J Immunol* 1995;154: 4039–4047.

301. Zhou MJ, Lublin DM, Link DC, Brown EJ. Distinct tyrosine kinase activation and Triton X-100 insolubility upon FcγRII or FcγRIIIB ligation in human polymorphonuclear leukocytes: implications for immune complex activation of the respiratory burst. *J Biol Chem* 1995; 270:13553–13560.

302. Corey SJ, Burkhardt AL, Bolen JB, Geahlen RL, Tkatch LS, Tweardy DJ. Granulocyte colony-stimulating factor receptor signaling involves the formation of a three-component complex with Lyn and Syk protein-tyrosine kinases. *Proc Natl Acad Sci U S A* 1994;91: 4683–4687.

303. Welch H, Maridonneau-Parini I. Hck is activated by opsonized zymosan and A23187 in distinct subcellular fractions of human granulocytes. *J Biol Chem* 1997;272:102–109.

304. Bokoch GM. Regulation of the human neutrophil NADPH oxidase by the Rac GTP binding proteins. *Curr Opin Cell Biol* 1994;6: 212–218.

Inflammation: Basic Principles and Clinical Correlates,
3rd ed., edited by John I. Gallin and Ralph Snyderman.
Lippincott Williams & Wilkins, Philadelphia © 1999.

CHAPTER 47

Oxygen Metabolites from Phagocytes

Seymour J. Klebanoff

Professional phagocytes (neutrophils, eosinophils, monocytes/macrophages) have among their functions the phagocytosis and destruction of microorganisms. These cells, when appropriately stimulated, also can release toxic agents to the outside of the cell, with the potential for attack on adjacent normal tissue, malignant cells, invading organisms too large to be ingested, and certain soluble mediators. They perform these functions through a variety of mechanisms (1) that can be conveniently divided into those that are dependent on oxygen and those that are not. This chapter discusses the microbicidal and cytotoxic systems that are oxygen dependent. The oxygen-independent toxic systems of phagocytes are considered in the chapter by Elsbach et al.

Oxygen is a very reactive molecule thermodynamically and thus can react with most elements and many organic molecules. However, from a kinetic standpoint, oxygen is rather inert and, in most instances, requires a catalyst to overcome this kinetic barrier. This is a necessary property, since without the kinetic barrier, the high reactivity of oxygen would result in its depletion from the environment and the loss of aerobic life as we know it. The basis for the kinetic inertness of oxygen is its electronic configuration. In most instances, electrons occur in pairs stabilized by spins in the opposite direction. When this is not the case, i.e., an electron is unpaired, the molecule is a highly reactive free radical. Molecular oxygen is a diradical in which two of its valence electrons, located in different orbitals, are unpaired and have parallel spins (Fig. 47-1). In oxidation reactions, oxygen accepts electrons from the molecule that it oxidizes and in the process is reduced. In reactions with a nonradical, this transfer of electrons

occurs from an electron pair with opposite spins, and thus inversion of spin is necessary if both of the vacant spaces in the unfilled orbitals of oxygen are to be filled. This restriction to electron transfer accounts for the sluggishness of oxygen reactivity.

The reactivity of O_2 can be increased by either reduction or excitation. Oxygen is reduced ultimately to water by the acceptance of four electrons; however, partial reduction can occur with the formation of highly reactive intermediates, namely the superoxide anion (O_2^-), hydrogen peroxide (H_2O_2), and the hydroxyl radical ($\cdot OH$) (Fig. 47-1). Excitation occurs when an absorption of energy shifts one of the unpaired electrons of oxygen to an orbital of higher energy with an inversion of spin. The product (singlet oxygen, $^1O_2$) can occur in two forms: delta singlet oxygen ($^1\Delta_g O_2$), in which the newly paired electrons occupy the same orbital (with the other orbital empty); and sigma singlet oxygen ($^1\Sigma_g^+ O_2$), in which the two electrons now with opposite spins occupy different orbitals. The formation of these toxic oxygen products and their involvement in the activity of phagocytes are considered here (reviewed in refs. 2,3).

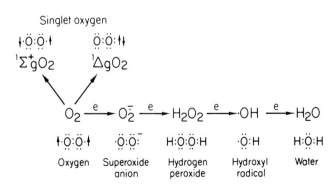

FIG. 47-1. The reduction and excitation of oxygen.

S.J. Klebanoff: Department of Medicine, University of Washington, Seattle, Washington 98195.

NEUTROPHILS

A striking feature of neutrophils is their response to stimulation with a marked increase in oxygen consumption. Early findings indicated that the respiratory burst of neutrophils was not needed for the generation of the metabolic energy required for phagocytosis; rather, the respiratory burst appeared to be required for optimum microbicidal activity as indicated by the decrease (but not loss) of microbicidal activity on exposure of neutrophils to hypoxic conditions (4,5) and by the association of a microbicidal defect (6) with the absence of the respiratory burst (7) in the leukocytes of patients with chronic granulomatous disease (CGD). The nature of the oxidase responsible for the respiratory burst is considered in the chapter by Leto. This chapter focuses on the nature and mode of action of the toxic products formed.

Superoxide Anion (O_2^-)

The initial product of the respiratory burst formed when oxygen accepts a single electron is O_2^- (8):

$$O_2 + e \rightarrow O_2^-$$

Reports of the redox potential of the O_2/O_2^- couple have ranged from +0.5 to −590 mV; a value of −330 mV has been proposed by several investigators (9,10). O_2^- is in equilibrium with its protonated form, the perhydroxyl radical (HO_2^-):

$$HO_2^- \rightleftharpoons O_2^- : + H^+$$

The pKa of the dissociation is 4.88 (11,12). Thus, the radical exists almost entirely as O_2^- at neutral or alkaline pH. O_2^- is predominantly a reductant, as, for example, in the reduction of ferricytochrome C, where it loses an electron and is converted back to oxygen. It can, however, also act as an oxidant, as, for example, in the oxidation of epinephrine, where it gains an electron and is converted to H_2O_2. When two molecules interact, one is oxidized and the other is reduced in a dismutation reaction with the formation of oxygen and H_2O_2:

$$O_2^- + O_2^- + 2H^+ \rightarrow O_2 + H_2O_2$$

This reaction can occur spontaneously or be catalyzed by the enzyme superoxide dismutase (SOD). Three distinct SODs exist, which vary in their metal component (copper-zinc SOD, manganese SOD, iron SOD) and in their distribution in cells (13).

Spontaneous dismutation occurs optimally at pH 4.8, where O_2^- and HO_2^- are present in equal concentrations. At this pH, the rate constant for spontaneous dismutation [$8.5 \times 10^7 M^{-1}sec^{-1}$ (11)] approaches that of SOD-catalyzed dismutation [$1.9 \times 10^9 M^{-1}sec^{-1}$ (14)]. The rate constant for spontaneous dismutation falls when the pH is lowered and HO_2^- predominates and is particularly low at alkaline pH where O_2^- predominates (11,12). Indeed, it is probable that spontaneous dismutation does not occur when O_2^- is the sole species. The rate constant for SOD-catalyzed dismutation is little affected by pH over the range 5.0 to 10.0 (14) and is thus a particularly effective catalyst at neutral or alkaline pH where spontaneous dismutation is relatively low. Although SOD is present in neutrophils (15), its release into the phagosome has not been demonstrated. SOD, however, can be introduced there as a component of the ingested organism. Most studies have indicated a fall in pH in the phagosome to a level where spontaneous dismutation is rapid (1,16); however, an early rise in pH has been reported (17,18).

The direct toxicity of O_2^- has been the subject of some controversy. O_2^- reacts rather sluggishly with many biologically important compounds, leading to the suggestion by some (19,20) that O_2^- does not have the necessary reactivity to be directly toxic to cells. However, a few words of caution. The chemical reactivity of O_2^- is considerably increased in a nonpolar environment as may exist in the hydrophobic region of a membrane where its reactions are not in competition with the proton-requiring dismutation reaction. Under these conditions, O_2^- is a powerful base with considerable nucleophilicity and reducing activity. Further, the protonated form, HO_2^-, is a considerably stronger oxidant than is O_2^- (21,22), raising the possibility that a local fall in pH as might occur within a phagosome or at a membrane surface may cause a shift in the $HO_2^- \rightleftharpoons O_2^-$ equilibrium toward the more reactive protonated form with localized damage. The low steady-state concentration of O_2^- would limit its dissipation by spontaneous dismutation, and this, together with its relatively low reactivity, may allow it to diffuse over significant distances, where it can be toxic through a local fall in pH or the formation of more reactive oxidants. In this regard, O_2^- can penetrate some cell membranes, including those of granulocytes (23), by passage through anion channels (24–27).

A direct toxic effect of O_2^- is suggested when the toxicity of an O_2^--generating system is inhibited by SOD but not by catalase or by ·OH scavengers. O_2^--generating systems are toxic to a variety of cells and compounds, and the inhibitory effect of SOD has implicated O_2^- either as a direct toxin or in the generation of a more distal oxidant. In some studies SOD was the only inhibitor tested, in other instances toxicity was also inhibited by catalase and ·OH scavengers, implicating ·OH and, in yet other studies catalase or ·OH scavengers were inhibitory but not both. However, in some cases only SOD was inhibitory (13,28).

Hydrogen Peroxide (H_2O_2)

H_2O_2 is formed in large amounts by stimulated phagocytes (29). Its formation is predominantly by dismutation of O_2^-, which occurs rapidly and efficiently (30). However, under some conditions H_2O_2 may be formed, in part, directly from oxygen by divalent reduction without an apparent O_2^- intermediate (31–35).

H_2O_2 is a well-known germicidal agent and its involvement in the microbicidal activity of phagocytes was therefore proposed (29). The reactivity of H_2O_2, however, is relatively low as compared to some of the other toxic products of the respiratory burst (e.g., ·OH, hypohalous acids). This allows H_2O_2 to pass intact through cell membranes (36) and through complex biologic fluids, rebounding intact from collisions to be toxic at a distance under conditions in which the more reactive oxygen products are readily scavenged. Organisms vary widely in their susceptibility to H_2O_2 and in general this correlates with the level of H_2O_2-scavenging enzymes in the target cell. These include catalase, which breaks down H_2O_2 to oxygen and water, and the glutathione cycle (Fig. 47-2). The glutathione cycle is a sequence of reactions by which the degradation of H_2O_2 is coupled to the increased activity of the hexose monophosphate shunt (HMS). The first two enzymes of the HMS, glucose 6-phosphate dehydrogenase and 6-phosphogluconate dehydrogenase, reduce the oxidized form of nicotinamide adenine dinucleotide phosphate ($NADP^+$) to the reduced form (NADPH), and the continued activity of the shunt is dependent on the reoxidation of NADPH. This can be accomplished by the glutathione cycle, which is initiated by the oxidation of reduced glutathione (GSH) by H_2O_2 catalyzed by glutathione peroxidase. The oxidized glutathione (GSSG) formed is reduced by NADPH in the presence of glutathione reductase with the formation of $NADP^+$. The HMS is thus a sink for excess H_2O_2, with the increased oxidation of glucose carbon-1 to CO_2 as evidence of its use.

H_2O_2 released by phagocytes can be toxic nonenzymatically to a number of targets *in vitro*. Indeed, when toxicity occurs at a distance through a fluid rich in proteins and other scavengers of the more reactive oxidants, H_2O_2 may be the chief, perhaps only, product of the respiratory burst that is toxic. Further, H_2O_2 has been impli-

cated in the autotoxicity of stimulated neutrophils (37,38), although in this (39) and other systems, H_2O_2 may not act alone but in conjunction with some other component of the reaction mixture or cell, such as iron. Neutrophils are protected from the toxic effects of exogenous or endogenous H_2O_2 by their content of catalase (40,41) and the components of the glutathione cycle (42,43) (Fig. 47-2).

The toxicity of H_2O_2 can be increased many orders of magnitude by a number of mechanisms. Three mechanisms, reaction with peroxidase and a halide to form hypohalous acids, synergism with proteinases, and reaction with ferrous iron to form ·OH, are considered in detail below.

Peroxidase-H_2O_2-Halide System

A number of distinct peroxidases exist in mammalian tissues that differ in primary structure and in their heme prosthetic group, but have in common the ability to increase the rate of H_2O_2-dependent reactions many orders of magnitude. Peroxidases alone have not been shown to exert an antimicrobial effect, although the strongly basic nature of some peroxidases, for example, eosinophil peroxidase (EPO) and, to a lesser degree, myeloperoxidase (MPO), suggests that, like other basic proteins, they may be antimicrobial at high concentrations. However, peroxidase can exert an antimicrobial effect indirectly by catalyzing the conversion of a substance, such as a halide, with little or no antimicrobial activity to one that is strongly toxic. The myeloperoxidase-H_2O_2-halide system (Fig. 47-3) appears to be operative in neutrophils (reviewed in ref. 44).

Myeloperoxidase

A peroxidase first appears in the developing human granulocyte in the promyelocyte stage, where it is synthesized and packaged into the azurophil (primary) granules (45). This process ceases at the end of the promyelocyte stage and the peroxidase-positive azurophil granules

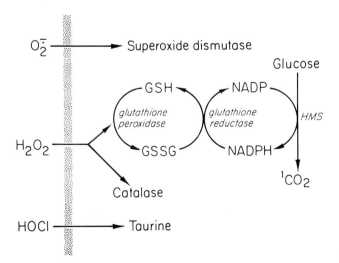

FIG. 47-2. Scavengers of reactive oxygen species.

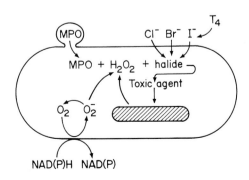

FIG. 47-3. The myeloperoxidase-H_2O_2-halide antimicrobial system in the phagosome.

are distributed to daughter cells and intermingled with the newly formed peroxidase-negative specific (secondary) granules during the myelocyte stage of granulocyte development. Mature neutrophils contain their total complement of MPO in azurophil granules. In human cells, these granules are morphologically heterogenous, varying in shape from spherical to ellipsoid (45), and can be separated into two peroxidase-positive populations on the basis of density (46–48). Following phagocytosis, degranulation occurs with the release of MPO into the phagosome, and leakage or secretion of MPO to the outside of the cell can occur either during phagocytosis or following exposure of neutrophils to an antibody-coated surface or to a soluble stimulus. In addition, MPO can be released by cell lysis. Following release, MPO is inactivated by products of the respiratory burst (49–51), with loss of the visible absorption spectrum. It also can be cleared from the extracellular fluid by reaction with the mannose receptor of macrophages with internalization (52).

MPO is present in human neutrophils in exceptionally high concentrations, with estimates varying from 1% to 2% of the dry weight of the cell (53) to greater than 5% (54,55); it is an intense green color, and the green color of pus is due to its presence. The MPO gene has been cloned by a number of laboratories (56–62). It is a single gene of approximately 11 kb, composed of 11 introns and 12 exons (63). It has been localized on the long arm of chromosome 17 in segment q12-24 (60,64–66) and has been reported to be in close proximity to the translocation breakpoint in acute promyelocytic leukemia (64). The initial translation product (pre-MPO) is approximately 84 kd (67) (Fig. 47-4). The 41 amino acid leader sequence of pre-MPO is cleaved in the endoplasmic reticulum and N-linked glycosylation occurs with incorporation of high mannose side chains into the heavy (α) subunit (68,69) to form an 89- to 90-kd heme-free apopro-MPO (63). The Ca^{2+}-binding protein calreticulin associates with the fully glycosylated heme-free apopro-MPO in the endoplasmic reticulum and acts as a molecular chaperone for the developing MPO molecule (70). Phosphorylation of the oligosaccharide side chains may occur (68). Heme is inserted to produce an enzymatically active pro-MPO, and this insertion is required for the further processing of MPO (71–73). The 125 amino acid prosequence is cleaved, probably in lysosomes, and the remainder of the molecule is cleaved into an 112 amino acid small (β) subunit (12 kd) and a 467 amino acid large (α) subunit (57 kd). The final product is a complex protein with a molecular weight that ranges in different estimates from 120 to 160 kd (1,74). An 89-kd precursor of MPO is released extracellularly by HL-60 cells (75,76). A human recombinant, single chain, enzymatically active MPO precursor of ~84 kd has been expressed (77–79).

The native enzyme consists of two heavy (α) (55–63 kd) and two light (β) (10–15 kd) subunits (80–82), with both the heme and carbohydrate bound to the heavy subunit (81–83; see, however, ref. 82). It has been proposed that the two heavy-light protomers are linked by a single disulfide bond between the two heavy subunits along their long axis (80) (Fig. 47-4). Conversion of the monomeric to dimeric form occurs relatively late in maturation, probably in mature azurophil granules (84). Reduction and alkylation separated the two protomers into hemi-myeloperoxidase consisting of a heavy and light subunit, which retained enzymatic and bactericidal activity (80,85). The two heavy subunits of MPO appear to be structurally different (86,87). Studies of the x-ray crystal structure of canine (88–91) and human (92) MPO have appeared.

MPO has been resolved by ion exchange chromatography into three distinct isoforms (MPO I, MPO II, MPO III) in the same individual, which vary in solubility, enzymatic activity, sensitivity to inhibition by aminotriazole, subunit structure, distribution in azurophil granule subpopulations, and release on neutrophil stimulation (87,93–97). Structural heterogeneity in the same isoform has also been reported (87).

MPO contains two iron-containing prosthetic groups per molecule (98) which are covalently linked to the heavy subunits (81,99–101), by a methionyl sulfonium bond with Met^{409} (91,102,103). The iron is normally in the ferric form. Magnetic circular dichroism (104) and resonance Raman spectroscopy (105,106) suggested that the prosthetic groups are iron chlorins (107), whereas other studies suggested that the prosthetic group was an

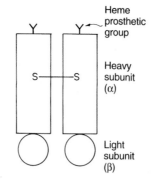

FIG. 47-4. Primary translation product of human MPO.

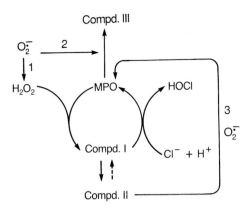

FIG. 47-5. MPO-complex formation. MPO forms three complexes: compound I, II and III. O_2^- can influence the reactivity of MPO by (1) forming H_2O_2 by dismutation, which reacts with MPO to form compound I; (2) reacting with MPO to form compound III; (3) converting the inactive compound II to native MPO.

iron porphyrin related to protoporphyrin IX (91,103, 108). There has been some controversy as to whether the two iron centers are identical in structure and function, with some studies indicating equivalence (105,106) and others inequivalence (98,109,110). It has been proposed that at low concentrations, H_2O_2 reacts with only one of the two iron atoms, whereas at high concentrations, H_2O_2 binds to both and is degraded catalatically to O_2 and H_2O with associated inactivation of the enzyme (111). This latter reaction would serve to modulate the activity of the peroxidase system by both the degradation of H_2O_2 and the inactivation of MPO. MPO has been reported to contain two tightly bound calcium ions (112). Although MPO may have effects on biologic systems unrelated to its enzyme activity, but based on its strong positive charge or its high mannose content leading to reaction with mannose receptors on macrophages (113), most of its effects are believed to be a consequence of its enzymatic reaction with H_2O_2 and a halide.

H_2O_2

The respiratory burst of phagocytes serves as the primary source of H_2O_2 for MPO-catalyzed reactions. In addition, certain ingested microorganisms can generate H_2O_2, and thus contribute to their own destruction by the peroxidase system. Lactic acid bacteria (e.g., pneumococci, streptococci, lactobacilli) lack heme and as a result do not utilize the cytochrome system (which reduces oxygen to water) for terminal oxidations. Rather, flavoproteins are employed, which reduce oxygen to H_2O_2, which, in the absence of the heme-protein catalase, is released into the medium (114). H_2O_2 also is produced by certain mycoplasmal strains (115–118) and by *Candida albicans* (119).

MPO forms three different complexes on reaction with products of the respiratory burst—compounds I, II and

III—with distinct spectral properties (Fig. 47-5). H_2O_2 at relatively low (equimolar) concentrations reacts with the iron of MPO to form compound I (120). It is the primary catalytic peroxide compound of MPO, is highly unstable, and is at an oxidized level equivalent to that of ferric MPO. Compound I reacts with chloride to form hypochlorous acid (HOCl) with regeneration of the native Fe^{3+}-MPO. When an excess of H_2O_2 is added, compound I is converted to compound II, which is at an oxidized level one equivalent above that of the ferric enzyme (120). Compound II is an inactive form of MPO in respect to the oxidation of chloride (121). Compound II can be reduced to Fe^{3+}-MPO by O_2^- (122–124), ascorbic acid (125,126), urate (122), as well as certain other reducing agents with restoration of chlorinating activity. Thus, O_2^- may function in part to maintain MPO in a catalytically active form, thus potentiating its toxic activity. The formation of O_2^- during the reaction of MPO and H_2O_2 has also been reported (127).

Compound III is an oxyperoxidase that, like oxyhemoglobin or oxymyoglobin, has oxygen attached to the heme iron (128,129). It is at the three-equivalent oxidized level above ferric MPO and is formed by reaction of compound II with H_2O_2 (120), by the aerobic oxidation of NADH (120), by the reaction of ferrous MPO with oxygen (120), or by the reaction of ferric MPO with O_2^- (120,130–132). The reaction of MPO with O_2^- to form compound III is an order of magnitude slower than the reaction of MPO with H_2O_2 (133). Compound III is unstable, decaying to ferric peroxidase with a half-decay time of several minutes at room temperature (128,134). It can react with a number of electron donors (128,135–137) and with certain electron acceptors (137), raising the possibility that MPO compound III formed by reaction with O_2^- may be a catalytically active form of MPO in neutrophils. The conversion of compound III to the native enzyme by reducing agents such as ascorbic acid leads to a return in compound I–dependent HOCl production (138). Spectral changes suggestive of MPO compound III formation have been detected in intact stimulated neutrophils, or on incubation of purified MPO with either phorbol myristate acetate (PMA)-stimulated neutrophils or the xanthine oxidase system (131).

Peroxidases also can use molecular oxygen for oxidative reactions. The number of substances that can be oxidized by peroxidase and oxygen in the absence of added H_2O_2 are limited. They include NADH and NADPH (139) in a reaction that is strongly stimulated by Mn^{2+} and by certain phenolic compounds such as the thyroid hormones (140) and estrogens (140,141). H_2O_2 is formed in the reaction and used either for the oxidation of the reduced pyridine nucleotides or for coupled oxidations of other substances (142). O_2^- is formed when peroxidase acts as an oxidase (136,143) and may serve as an intermediate in H_2O_2 formation or react directly with peroxidase to form compound III (120,130).

Halides

Iodide, bromide, chloride (144,145), or the pseudo-halide thiocyanate (146,147) can serve as the halide component of the MPO-mediated antimicrobial system. Of the halides, iodide is the most effective on a molar basis (145). The concentration of inorganic iodide in serum, however, is very low (<1 mg%) and its contribution to the peroxidase system may therefore be small. Iodide also can be provided by deiodination of the thyroid hormones (144). Bromide is intermediate in effectiveness between iodide and chloride (145); however, its concentration in biologic fluids is considerably higher than that of iodide (148), raising the possibility that bromide may serve as a physiologic halide. Thiocyanate is oxidized by intact neutrophils to the antimicrobial agent hypothiocyanite when the concentration of thiocyanate is high relative to that of chloride as occurs in saliva; but under conditions similar to those in plasma, where the thiocyanate concentration is low relative to chloride, chloride is preferentially oxidized (149). The concentration of chloride in biologic fluids is considerably greater than that required for the isolated MPO-mediated antimicrobial system, suggesting that it is the primary halide used by the MPO system *in situ*.

The halides at high concentration can inhibit the MPO-mediated antimicrobial system. Thus, bromide was consistently less effective as the halide component of the MPO system at a high, as opposed to low, concentration (145), and an inhibitory effect of thiocyanate on the MPO-H_2O_2-halide system has been described (1,144, 145,149,150). Two distinct binding sites for chloride on MPO have been proposed: one, the substrate binding site, is unaffected by pH and leads to the production of HOCl, and the second, the inhibitor binding site, requires prior protonation (acid pH) and leads to the competitive inhibition of H_2O_2 binding to MPO (121,151–153). The substrate binding site for chloride appears to be at or close to the iron of MPO (154–157).

Toxic Products Formed

The halides are oxidized by compound I and possibly also by compound III (131) to form toxic agents that vary with the halide, its concentration, pH and other factors (reviewed in ref. 158); the products include hypohalous acids, halogens, long-lived oxidants such as chloramines or aldehydes, and possibly hydroxyl radicals and singlet oxygen.

Hypohalous Acids

Chloride is oxidized to HOCl by MPO and H_2O_2 (159–161) and by intact neutrophils (162–164) (Fig. 47-6). Since HOCl has a pK$_a$ of 7.53, it exists as a mixture of the undissociated acid and the hypochlorite ion at physi-

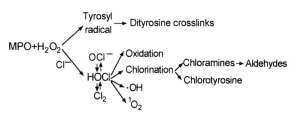

FIG. 47-6. Products of the MPO system.

ologic pH levels. When the pH is lowered, as may occur within the phagosome, HOCl would predominate. Hypobromous acid (HOBr) and hypothiocyanous acid (HOSCN) and the corresponding hypohalite ions appear to be the primary products formed by the peroxidase catalyzed oxidation of bromide and thiocyanate, and, although hypoiodous acid (HOI) may be formed by iodide oxidation by peroxidases, it is not clear whether it or iodine is the predominant species formed.

Halogens

The halogens chlorine (Cl_2), bromine (Br_2), iodine (I_2), and the pseudohalogen thiocyanogen [$(SCN)_2$] may be formed by halide oxidation, although the initial species, at least with chloride, bromide, and thiocyanate, appears to be the hypohalous acid. The hypohalous acid can react with excess halide at acid pH to form the corresponding halogen as follows (for chloride):

$$HOCl + Cl^- \rightarrow Cl_2 + H_2O$$

The generation of chlorine gas by the MPO-H_2O_2-chloride system has been demonstrated by gas chromatography–mass spectrometry and its formation by intact phagocytosing neutrophils has been proposed based on the conversion of L-tyrosine to 3-chlorotyrosine, a reaction mediated by Cl_2 and not by HOCl/OCl- (165). Iodine is a major product of iodide oxidation by peroxidase and H_2O_2. The MPO-H_2O_2-iodide antimicrobial system is effective at an iodide concentration that is considerably lower than that of the reagent iodine needed to produce a comparable antimicrobial effect (144). However, this discrepancy has been explained by the catalytic activity of iodide, in which iodide is oxidized by peroxidase and H_2O_2 to iodine, and the iodine is then reduced by reaction with a surface sulfhydryl or other oxidizable group and reutilized by the peroxidase system (166,167). Reactions of this sort with other halogens may amplify their contribution to the antimicrobial effect.

Chloramines

HOCl formed by neutrophils can react with nitrogen-containing compounds to form nitrogen-chlorine derivatives with retention of oxidizing activity (Fig. 47-6) (158,168–171). Some of these compounds are relatively long-lived, thus providing a mechanism for the prolongation of the oxidant activity of the peroxidase system. The toxicity of the chloramine can occur in a number of ways:

1. The nitrogen-chloride derivative may be directly toxic. Taurine, which is present in neutrophils in high concentration (172,173), forms a relatively stable chloramine, and it was proposed that taurine chloramine formed by the MPO-H_2O_2-chloride system may serve a microbicidal function (174). Taurine, however, inhibits the bactericidal activity of the MPO-H_2O_2-chloride system (175,176), suggesting that the formation of taurine chloramine is competitive with, rather than required for, microbicidal activity. *N*-chlorotaurine, however, can oxidize sulfhydryl or sulfur-ether groups (170) and thus may have sufficient oxidant activity to inactivate soluble mediators dependent on an intact sulfur-ether group (171), but have insufficient activity to induce a microbicidal effect (177). The limited cytotoxicity has been attributed to the hydrophilic nature of the organic chloramines. In contrast, reaction of HOCl with ammonium ions forms a lipophilic oxidizing agent monochloramine (NH_2Cl) with considerably increased toxic activity (168,176,178). It has been concluded that taurine and other organic amines protect certain targets including neutrophils by scavenging HOCl in a form that is relatively nontoxic (Fig. 47-2).

2. Chloramines are generally unstable, hydrolyzing to continuously release their available chlorine in an activated form such as HOCl (179) or NH_2Cl (168).

3. Degradation of unstable chloramines may result in the formation of a non–chloride-containing derivative with toxic properties. The formation of toxic aldehydes by the deamination and decarboxylation of amino acids by MPO, H_2O_2, and chloride (174,180, 181) was proposed to be a microbicidal mechanism (175,181). Although certain aldehydes are toxic to microorganisms in high concentrations, the involvement of free aldehydes in the toxicity of the peroxidase system *in situ* remains to be established. Chlorination of glycine or glycylpeptides can yield hydrogen cyanide (HCN), which can be chlorinated to cyanogen chloride (ClCN) (182–184). It is not known whether these agents are produced in sufficient quantities to contribute to the toxic effect.

4. The long-lived *N*-chloramines can react with iodide to form a highly toxic species that may be free iodine or some other oxidized product (177).

5. The organic monochloramine (RNHCl) can undergo dismutation to form the more powerful dichloramine ($RNCl_2$) (185).

6. The amine chlorinated by the MPO-H_2O_2-chloride system can be covalently bound to protein (186). However, this reaction is slow, is quantitatively minor, and requires a high pH, suggesting that it does not contribute significantly to the antimicrobial activity of the MPO system. Glucosamine is incorporated into protein by stimulated neutrophils by an MPO-dependent process (187) and, although the mechanism of incorporation was not established, a chlorinated intermediate may be involved.

Hydroxyl Radicals

The formation of ·OH by the MPO system is considered under Hydroxyl Radical (·OH), below.

Singlet Oxygen

The formation of $^1O_2$ by the MPO system is considered under Singlet Oxygen($^1O_2$), below.

Nature of the Destructive Lesion

The products of halide oxidation are powerful toxins that can attack the target at a variety of chemical sites. There are two main modes of attack: halogenation, in which the halide is covalently bound to cellular constituents; and oxidation, in which exposed groups are oxidized.

Halogenation

MPO and H_2O_2 oxidize the halide to a form that binds in covalent linkage to components on the ingested organism. With iodide as the halide, iodination is indicated by the conversion of radioiodide to a trichloroacetic acid precipitable form and by the radioautographic localization of the fixed iodide on the organism (144). Tyrosine residues of protein are readily iodinated to form mono- and diiodotyrosine, and the exposed tyrosine residues of the organism appear to be the primary site of iodination by the peroxidase system (167). In addition, unsaturated fatty acids (188), sulfhydryl groups (167), as well as a number of other compounds may be iodinated. Bromination of cell surface constituents also occurs. Chlorination of microorganisms by purified MPO, H_2O_2, and chloride, and by granulocytes that have ingested bacteria, is indicated by ^{36}Cl incorporation (189). This, together with the formation of chlorinated derivatives on the addition of taurine or 1,3,5-trimethoxybenzene to stimulated neutrophils (162–164), suggests that chlorination of components of the ingested organism occurs. The chlorinated derivatives include monochloramines and dichloramines [preferentially involving the N-terminal amino group of peptides or proteins (183)], chlorhydrins (190,191), and chlorotyrosine (192). The glycine residues of bacterial peptidoglycan (182), reduced pyridine nucleotides (193), and adenine nucleotides (194) are also chlorinated. Chlorinated NAD(P)H is no longer catalytically active. The substitution of a bulky halide atom for a hydrogen at a crucial location on the cell surface or the subsequent degradative changes initiated by the halogenation reaction may contribute to the toxicity.

Oxidation

It is probable that toxicity results primarily from the oxidation of essential cell constituents. HOCl, as well as the other products of halide oxidation, are powerful oxidants capable of the oxidation of a number of biologically important substances (195,196) through reaction with a variety of chemical groups, some of which are considered below.

1. Sulfhydryl groups. A number of enzymes and other biologically important compounds require a free sulfhydryl group for optimum activity, and the oxidation of essential sulfhydryl groups by the peroxidase system may contribute to its toxicity. The sulfhydryl groups of *Escherichia coli* are readily oxidized by peroxidase, H_2O_2, and iodide, and by one of the products of that system, I_2 (167), and by MPO, H_2O_2, and chloride and its major product, HOCl (176). Only a portion of the oxidizing equivalents consumed could be accounted for by sulfhydryl oxidation, although there was a close correlation between the oxidation of bacterial sulfhydryl groups and cell death.

 The MPO-H_2O_2-halide system oxidizes GSH to GSSG, with the effectiveness of the halides being on the order I>Br>Cl (197). GSH is also oxidized by stimulated neutrophils through the formation of a product of the MPO system (198). It is not known, however, whether GSH is oxidized within intact organisms and, if so, whether this would contribute to cell death or serve a protective function.

2. Iron-sulfur centers. The iron-sulfur centers of ferredoxin are very rapidly oxidized by the MPO-H_2O_2-chloride system and by its product HOCl (195,199), raising the possibility that proteins with iron-sulfur centers (which are important constituents of the electron transport system of the microbial cytoplasmic membrane) may be a site of attack by the peroxidase system. The microbicidal effect of the MPO-H_2O_2-halide system on *E. coli* is associated with the loss of iron into the medium as measured by the release of ^{59}Fe from prelabeled organisms (200). Iron loss, which reached levels in excess of 70% of the total microbial iron, was observed with chloride or bromide but not with iodide as the halide. That a portion of the iron loss was due to the oxidation of *E. coli* iron-sulfur centers by the peroxidase system was suggested by the loss of labile sulfide content (199). In contrast to iron loss, the effectiveness of the halides, on a molar basis, in inducing labile sulfide oxidation was in the order I>Br>Cl. Thus, iodide-derived oxidants appeared to oxidize microbial iron-sulfur centers without the release of iron into the medium. The amount of oxidant required to destroy iron-sulfur centers in the respiratory chain exceeded the amount required to inhibit respiration or kill the organism by a factor of 4 to 5, with the loss of respiration being due to a lesion between the iron sulfur center and ubiquinone reductase in the respiratory chain (201).

3. Heme-proteins. Porphyrins, hemes, and heme-proteins are rapidly oxidized by HOCl and by the peroxidase-H_2O_2-halide system (195,196,200). The oxidation of cytochrome C by the MPO-H_2O_2-halide system was associated with the release of the heme iron and, as with iron release from the intact organism, chloride or bromide but not iodide could meet the halide requirement (200). MPO, which is a heme-protein, is inactivated by H_2O_2 and a halide (202).

4. Sulfur-ether groups. The MPO-H_2O_2-Cl- system oxidizes the sulfur-ether group of free (203) and peptide-bound methionine (204–207) and of the sulfidopeptide leukotrienes (208,209) to the corresponding sulfoxide, and thus the oxidation of sulfur-ether groups in the target organism may contribute to cell death.

5. Oxidative decarboxylation, deamination, and peptide cleavage of proteins. The oxidative decarboxylation and deamination of free and peptide-linked amino acids (174,175,180,181,210–212) occurs with the formation of the corresponding aldehyde. Associated peptide cleavage may occur (211). The amino acids of particulate proteins are decarboxylated in the phagosome by the peroxidase system, whereas free soluble amino acids pass into the cytoplasm, where they are decarboxylated predominantly after transamination, by the normal, nonperoxidase, cellular amino acid oxidative pathway (210). It is not clear whether peptide cleavage is a direct consequence of the action of the peroxidase system in intact cells, or whether decarboxylation of amino acids or peptides follows cleavage of the protein by proteases released into the phagosome.

6. Lipid peroxidation. Lipid peroxidation, that is the oxidation of polyunsaturated fatty acids, has been implicated in membrane damage. It can be initiated by a variety of oxygen species and is maintained in a chain reaction (propagation) by radical species formed. Lipid peroxidation occurs in phagocytes following particle ingestion (213,214) and its relationship to the respiratory burst is indicated by its absence in CGD leukocytes (213,214) unless an H_2O_2-generating organism is ingested (213). The peroxidase-H_2O_2-halide system can initiate lipid peroxidation (215,216), raising the possibility that this effect may contribute to its toxicity.

Primary Lesion

The nature of the chemical lesion in the target cell that causes death is not known. The primary lesion may differ in different cell types, and perhaps death is a consequence of multiple hits at a variety of chemical sites rather than to a single lesion. The attack on the microorganism is very rapid. In one study (217), HOCl prevented *E. coli* replication, as measured by colony formation, in milliseconds. The highly reactive nature of the oxidants formed suggests that the attack is at, or close to, the surface of the organism, i.e., at the cell membrane. Intracellular biomolecules are attacked only when concentrations of HOCl are employed that are considerably higher than those that are lethal (195,218,219). An early effect of the MPO system and its product HOCl on microorganisms is the loss of membrane transport function with associated leakage of small molecules (1,220–222), an effect that correlated closely to the loss of viability as measured by replication (220,221). The loss of transport function is not due to membrane lysis, since some membrane functions, e.g., transmembrane proton conductance and glycerol permeability, are unaffected by HOCl (220), but may be due to a direct oxidative attack on transport proteins, to the dissipation of adenylate energy reserves (223), or to inactivation of adenosine triphosphate (ATP) synthetase (222). The loss of adenine nucleotides from the target cell by the formation of adenine nucleotide chloramines that bind to proteins and nucleic acids has been proposed (194). Other proposed mechanisms of toxicity include disruption of the membrane electron transport chain (201,224–226) through inactivation of dehydrogenases (224,226), inactivation of the enzymes involved in the remodeling of peptidoglycan cell wall (penicillin-binding proteins) (226a,226b), and inhibition of DNA replication through disruption of the interaction between the cell membrane and chromosomal DNA (227,228). An early attack on tumor cell membrane sulfhydryl groups has been proposed (229).

Halide-Independent Effects of MPO and H₂O₂

Although MPO and H_2O_2 are believed to produce their toxic effects predominantly by reaction with a halide, particularly chloride, to form a potent oxidant such as HOCl or Cl_2, direct oxidation of a tissue component other than a halide also may occur. For example free or peptide-linked tyrosine can be oxidized by isolated or phagocyte-associated MPO and H_2O_2 to form the tyrosyl radical that can initiate lipid peroxidation in low-density lipoproteins (230) and form dityrosine, trityrosine, pulcherosine, and isotyrosine from free tyrosine (231,232), or stably cross-linked protein dityrosine linkages (233).

Targets for the Inhibitory Activity of the MPO System

Two lines of evidence have been employed in support of a role for the MPO system in the toxic effect of neutrophils on a particular target.

First, toxicity is produced by a purified preparation of MPO when combined with H_2O_2 (or an H_2O_2-generating enzyme system) and a halide. This toxicity requires each component of the MPO system and is inhibited by peroxidase inhibitors such as azide and cyanide, and by catalase. Protein and low molecular weight components of complex biologic fluids inhibit the peroxidase-H_2O_2-halide system by scavenging its toxic products, and when maintenance of target cell viability requires the presence of protein in the medium, the toxicity of the peroxidase system may not be demonstrable (234,235). Indeed, in complex biologic fluids, the toxicity of H_2O_2 can be reduced by peroxidase and a halide (236,237), presumably due to the utilization of H_2O_2 for the formation of more powerful oxidants that are scavenged by the components of the reaction mixture prior to their reaching the target cells. Preincubation of the target cell with the peroxidase for a short period allows the demonstration of toxicity of the peroxidase system, even in the presence of large amounts of protein. MPO, and particularly EPO, are strongly basic proteins that bind firmly to anionic surfaces, including those of target cells. Thus, following preincubation, the toxic products are directed to the target cell surface by the bound peroxidase (234,235). The peroxidase system can be targeted to a particular cell type by conjugation of either an H_2O_2-generating enzyme such as glucose oxidase or xanthine oxidase (238–240), or both an H_2O_2-generating enzyme and peroxidase (241–245) to specific antibody.

Second, toxicity is produced by intact phagocytes that have the following properties:

1. Toxicity is dependent on stimulation of the phagocytes, either by a particulate or soluble stimulus.
2. A halide is required for optimum activity. If possible, an incubation medium should be employed that lacks chloride, unless it is added as a component of the MPO system, in order to be able to detect a chloride requirement. When intact cells are employed, isotonic solutions in which chloride is replaced by sulfate or nitrate can generally be used, since incubations are usually short. If chloride is an absolute requirement for maintenance of the viability of the cells, then a halide requirement can be inferred from the inhibitory effect of agents, such as methionine and taurine, that react with HOCl, although the specificity of this reaction is not absolute. Further, the addition of a second halide, i.e., iodide or bromide, may increase the toxicity of the peroxidase system. Iodination of the target is compatible with halide involvement, since it demonstrates an interaction between a product of halide oxidation by the MPO system and the target. However, it should be emphasized that iodination per se is not the mechanism of toxicity.
3. Toxicity is decreased by peroxidase inhibitors such as azide or cyanide and by catalase (but not by heated

catalase). When the target cell is sensitive both to H_2O_2 alone and to the peroxidase-H_2O_2-halide system (at lower H_2O_2 concentrations), the addition of a heme-enzyme inhibitor such as azide may not inhibit toxicity and may even increase it. Azide, by inhibiting the degradation of H_2O_2 by the peroxidase (and catalase) of the phagocyte, results in the buildup of H_2O_2 to relatively high levels, which can be toxic in the absence of peroxidase. Further, inhibition of the catalase of the target cell by the heme-enzyme inhibitor may increase the sensitivity of the cell to H_2O_2 toxicity. This paradoxical effect of heme enzyme inhibitors has been observed with the release of platelet constituents by neutrophils activated by phagocytosis (246) and the inactivation of granule enzymes by phagocytosing neutrophils (247). An additional problem with the use of inhibitors, particularly those of large molecular weight, is the possible exclusion of the inhibitor from the site of action of the peroxidase (or other) antimicrobial system.

4. Toxicity is decreased when CGD leukocytes are employed, and this decrease in toxicity is not observed when H_2O_2 or an H_2O_2-generating enzyme system is added. This indicates a requirement for H_2O_2 in the toxicity.

5. Toxicity is decreased when MPO-deficient leukocytes are employed, and this decrease in toxicity is prevented by the addition of MPO. As described below, MPO-deficient leukocytes may substitute an MPO-independent system for the normally operative MPO-dependent one, and it is sometimes possible through the use of inhibitors to determine the nature of the toxic system.

The MPO-mediated antimicrobial system has been implicated in the effects of neutrophils on a variety of targets through studies of this kind (Table 47-1). The peroxidase system is generally inhibitory in its activity, but in some instances it can be stimulatory.

Microorganisms

Using some or all of the procedures described above, the MPO-H_2O_2-halide system has been shown to be toxic to a variety of bacteria (144,145,248) including mycoplasma (249), chlamydia (250), *Mycobacterium leprae* (251), *Actinobacillus actinomycetemcomitans* (252), and *Legionella pneumophila* (253). The MPO system also is toxic to fungi (254–259); viruses (260), including human immunodeficiency virus-1 (HIV-1) (261–263); protozoa such as *Trypanosoma dionisii* (264), *Trypanosoma cruzi* (265), and *Leishmania donovani* (266,267); amoebae, such as *Neigleria fowleri* (268); and helminths such as the schistosomula of *Schistosoma mansoni* (269,270) and the newborn larvae of *Trichinella spiralis* (271). In most instances, the microorganisms are

TABLE 47-1. *Effects of the myeloperoxidase system*

In vitro inhibitory effects
  Microorganisms: bacteria, fungi, viruses, protozoa, amoebae, helminths
  Mammalian cells: spermatozoa, blood cells (e.g., granulocytes, lymphocytes, erythrocytes, platelets), tumor cells
  Soluble agents: chemotactic factors (C5a, fMLP), α_1-proteinase inhibitor, bacterial toxins (e.g., diphtheria toxin, pneumolysin, clostridial toxins), neutrophil granule components (e.g., lysosomal enzymes, vitamin B_{12}–binding protein), arachidonic acid metabolites (e.g., prostaglandins, leukotrienes), elastin, transferrin, fluorescent probes

In vitro stimulatory effects
  Cell secretion (e.g., platelets, mast cells), enzyme activation (e.g., collagenase, gelatinase), complement acivation

In vivo effects
  Pulmonary injury, renal injury, tumor cell destruction, atherosclerosis

ingested and toxicity occurs in the phagosome; however, the toxic effect of the MPO system on all of these organisms may be extracellular, and on some, e.g., helminths, it is generally extracellular.

Bacterial Toxins

Many microorganisms form and release potent exotoxins either into the phagosome, where they can affect the viability of the phagocyte, or into the extracellular fluid, where they can have profound local and systemic effects. The first demonstration of the inactivation of a biologic product by MPO was that of Agner (272–274), who observed that diphtheria toxin was detoxified by MPO, H_2O_2, and a dialyzable cofactor found in casein hydrolysates, urine, and other materials. Although partially purified, the nature of the dialyzable cofactor was not established at that time. More recently, other bacterial toxins such as the cytotoxin of *Clostridium difficile* (275), the pneumolysin of *Streptococcus pneumoniae* (276), the leukotoxin of *A. actinomycetemcomitans* (277), and aflotoxin (278) have been shown to be rapidly inactivated by the MPO-H_2O_2-halide system.

Tumor Cells

Tumor cells are readily inhibited or killed by the cell-free peroxidase-H_2O_2-halide system (239,279,280) and by the MPO system released by intact neutrophils stimulated by phagocytosis (281), concanavalin A (282), or PMA (283–287). The antibody-dependent tumor cell cytotoxic activity of neutrophils, however, does not appear to be dependent on MPO (288,289). Although neutrophils can be present adjacent to tumor cells *in situ,* it is not known whether neutrophil-derived reactive oxygen species play an important role in the host defense against malignancy. Patients with CGD are not noted to have an increased incidence of malignancy, even though their neutrophils lack a respiratory burst and thus do not generate reactive oxygen species. Although this may be due in part to the short life expectancy of CGD patients, if neutrophil respiratory burst activity was required for the destruction of tumor cells, childhood malignancies would have been expected. A high incidence of malignancy has been reported in patients with MPO deficiency (290), although most patients with this condition have not been noted to have tumors.

Granulocytes

The MPO-H_2O_2-halide system is toxic to neutrophils as well as to blood mononuclear cells (291), raising the possibility that this system may be autoinhibitory when released by stimulated phagocytes. Self-destruction of neutrophils during stimulation has been reported and, although H_2O_2 has been implicated (37–39), the involvement of the peroxidase system has not been described.

The MPO system can inhibit phagocytosis by human neutrophils under conditions in which the respiratory burst and chemotactic response are unaffected (292). Preincubation of the opsonized particles with the MPO-H_2O_2-halide system also inhibited their phagocytic uptake (293), suggesting that the MPO system can affect both the cell and the opsonized particle. The binding of fluorescein isothiocyanate (FITC)-labeled anti–immunoglobulin G (IgG) or anti-C3b to the yeast particles was decreased following exposure of the opsonized particles to the peroxidase system (293), suggesting either the loss of the ligand from the particle surface or its modification to a form unreactive with specific antibody. IgG exposed to MPO, H_2O_2, and catechol form large amounts of heavy IgG aggregates that behave like immune complexes in that they consume complement, precipitate with monoclonal rheumatoid factor, and are detected by the Raji cell and solid-phase C1q assays (294). Crosslinking of immune complexes by the MPO system of intact leukocytes has been reported (295).

Stimulated neutrophils can also inactivate some of their own granule components (lysosomal enzymes, vitamin B_{12}–binding protein) in part or totally through the action of the MPO-H_2O_2-halide system (247,296–300). These components are released by the degranulation process and thus their action may be modulated by the peroxidase system either in the phagosome or the extracellular fluid.

MPO can also be inactivated by the strong oxidants formed. A characteristic of peroxidases is their susceptibility to inactivation by excess H_2O_2, and MPO is particularly sensitive in this regard (53,111). Inactivation of MPO by H_2O_2 is potentiated by chloride (180,202,207, 301,302), presumably due to autoxidation by products of chloride oxidation. Disappearance of the Soret band (180,207,301) and oxidation of methionine and tyrosine residues (207) of MPO have been reported. MPO loses activity following release from stimulated neutrophils (49–51).

Lymphocytes

Natural killer (NK) cell activity, lymphocyte proliferation in response to mitogens, and generation of immunoglobulin-secreting cells were suppressed on exposure of human mononuclear leukocytes to the MPO-H_2O_2-halide system or HOCl (303–305). Stimulated neutrophils also suppressed lymphocyte function through the release of the MPO system (306). When the H_2O_2 flux was raised or the number of mononuclear leukocytes decreased, lymphocyte suppression could be mediated by H_2O_2 alone. The various lymphocyte functions tested were affected to a different degree by the MPO system, and removal of the monocytes from the mononuclear cell preparation increased the susceptibility of the lymphocytes to oxidant injury. The toxic nature of the MPO system raises the possibility that the effect on function is secondary to a loss of viability of lymphocytes. Normal trypan blue exclusion, fluorescein diacetate uptake, target cell binding frequency by the treated mononuclear leukocytes, and the reversibility of the lesion would argue against this as the mechanism for loss of function and thus point to an immunoregulatory role for the MPO system.

Erythrocytes

Erythrocytes can be lysed by exposure to the MPO-H_2O_2-halide system (307) and by reactive oxygen species formed by stimulated neutrophils (308–313). The nature of the oxygen species responsible for erythrocyte lysis by intact neutrophils has varied in these studies (314). In general, the MPO-H_2O_2-halide system was not implicated, although in one study (309) an inhibition of the lysis of chicken erythrocytes by azide, catalase, and the substitution of CGD for normal neutrophils suggested that the MPO system may be involved.

Oxidant injury to erythrocytes that does not progress to lysis can also be induced by stimulated neutrophils. Thus, the GSH level of glucose-6-phosphate dehydrogenase deficient (but not normal) erythrocytes was depressed by phagocytosing neutrophils with associated rapid removal of the cells from the circulation; H_2O_2 was implicated as the toxic species (315). When erythrocytes are exposed to stimulated neutrophils, some hydrophilic products of the peroxidase system, e.g., taurine chloramine, can enter the cell through anion channels and be trapped intracellularly as taurine following reduction by GSH (185), whereas lipophilic oxidants, e.g., NH_2Cl, penetrate the lipid bilayer and produce oxidant damage (168).

Platelets

The granule marker serotonin and the cytoplasmic marker adenine were released by platelets exposed either to the cell-free MPO-H_2O_2-halide system (316) or to intact neutrophils stimulated by phagocytosis (246). The considerably greater serotonin than adenine release by the cell-free system suggested in part a nonlytic secretory process (see below), whereas serotonin and adenine were released by intact neutrophils in equivalent amounts, suggesting a lytic event (246). In the intact cell system, release was prevented by omission of halides, by the addition of catalase, by the use of MPO-deficient neutrophils unless MPO was added, or by the use of CGD neutrophils unless H_2O_2 was added. These data strongly suggest the involvement of the peroxidase system. Paradoxically, the heme-protein inhibitors azide and cyanide did not inhibit release, but rather increased it. This effect of heme-protein inhibitors was also observed with MPO-deficient neutrophils (but not with CGD neutrophils) or when the neutrophils were replaced by reagent H_2O_2 or an H_2O_2-generating enzyme system. It was concluded that neutrophils activated by phagocytosis induce release of platelet constituents by a lytic process through the action of the peroxidase system. However, when MPO and platelet catalase is inhibited by heme enzyme inhibitors, H_2O_2 can accumulate to levels that are lytic in the absence of peroxidase.

Spermatozoa

A number of peroxidases, including MPO when combined with H_2O_2 and a halide (or the pseudohalide thiocyanate), are toxic to spermatozoa (317,318). H_2O_2 is formed by spermatozoa in the presence of phenylalanine or certain other amino acids, and the H_2O_2 so formed is autoinhibitory in the presence of the other components of the peroxidase system (318).

Chemotactic Factors

The chemotactic factors C5a desarg and *N*-formyl-methionyl-leucyl-phenylalanine (FMLP) are inactivated by the MPO-H_2O_2-halide system (319), an effect that correlated with a decrease in binding of the peptide to the leukocyte receptor (205). The biochemical basis for the inactivation of FMLP by the peroxidase system was the oxidation of the sulfur-ether group of the methionine residue to form the corresponding sulfoxide (205). Free methionine is also oxidized by the cell-free (320,321) and cell-associated (203) MPO-H_2O_2-halide system to methionine sulfoxide.

Intact neutrophils, when exposed to a particulate or soluble stimulus, also inactivated FMLP (322–324), and the MPO-H_2O_2-halide system was implicated. As with the cell-free MPO-H_2O_2-halide system, inactivation of FMLP by intact leukocytes resulted in the oxidation of the methionine residue and was associated with decreased binding to surface receptors. The functional activity of the sulfoxide and sulfone derivatives of FMLP have been described (325). Among the stimuli that induced neutrophils to inactivate FMLP by the release of the peroxidase system was the chemotactic factor itself (326). C5a was also inactivated by the peroxidase system released from stimulated neutrophils (322).

Although oxidant damage to chemoattractants by stimulated neutrophils has been clearly demonstrated, other mechanisms of chemotactic factor degradation by phagocytes also exist. Thus, hydrolysis of chemotactic peptides by neutrophils can be induced by the stimulation of proteinase secretion at relatively high chemotactic peptide concentration (327,328), or can occur at the cell surface by a mechanism independent of degranulation (329). The latter occurred at low (0.01–1.0 mM) concentrations of the chemoattractant. Similarly, C5a can be inactivated by neutrophil granule components, presumably by proteolysis (330–332).

α_1-Proteinase Inhibitor

α_1-Proteinase inhibitor (α_1-antitrypsin) inhibits a number of serine proteinases of biologic importance and, indeed, is the major serine proteinase inhibitor of plasma. Its importance is emphasized by the increased incidence of emphysema in persons genetically deficient in this inhibitor (333). This raises the possibility that in those persons with normal production of α_1-proteinase inhibitor, its increased inactivation may contribute to uncontrolled destruction of lung elastin and other proteins by tissue proteinases. The reactive site of α_1-proteinase inhibitor contains a methionine residue (334,335) whose oxidation to the corresponding sulfoxide inhibits antiproteinase activity (335).

The MPO-H_2O_2-halide system converts the methionine residue of α_1-proteinase inhibitor to the sulfoxide with a loss of biologic activity (204,206,336–338). Intact neutrophils, when appropriately stimulated, also inactivate α_1-proteinase inhibitor through the release of the MPO system (336,337,339–341). Both HOCl and long-lived *N*-chloramines can be utilized by stimulated neutrophils to inactivate α_1-proteinase inhibitor, with HOCl being the predominant oxidant over short distances and *N*-chloramines being effective even when the neutrophils were separated from the α_1-proteinase inhibitor by a dialyzing membrane (342). Among the proteinases inhibited by α_1-proteinase inhibitor is human neutrophil elastase (342,343), and the inhibition of α_1-proteinase inhibitor by the MPO system is associated with a delay in its ability to form stable complexes with elastase (335,337, 343,344). Although recombinant α_1-proteinase inhibitor containing methionine at the active site (position 358) was more sensitive to inactivation by the MPO-H_2O_2-

halide system and activated neutrophils than was a mutant in which the methionine was replaced by valine, prolonged exposure produced partial inactivation of the mutant inhibitor (345). Thus, oxidation of sites other than methionine-358 in the inhibitor may contribute to the inactivation.

Oxidant inactivation of α_1-proteinase inhibitor can be inhibited by antioxidants such as ascorbate, cysteine, and dapsone (346); by certain antiarthritic drugs (347); by relatively high concentrations of nicotine (348); by erythrocytes (349); and by methionine or methionine-containing proteins, which compete with the methionine residues of α_1-proteinase inhibitor for the oxidant formed by phagocytes (340,350). An enzyme, methionine sulfoxide-peptide reductase, which can reduce methionine sulfoxide residues in proteins, restores the biologic activity of oxidatively inactivated α_1-proteinase inhibitor (351). This enzyme has been detected in human lung homogenates, human neutrophils, and rabbit alveolar type II cells (352).

Although the MPO system appears to be the predominant source of oxidants for the inactivation of α_1-proteinase inhibitor by neutrophils, other oxidants, specifically $\cdot$OH, have also been implicated (336,339,353). Inactivation of α_1-proteinase inhibitor by nonoxidative mechanisms, i.e., by proteolysis, may also occur (354), and this appears to be the major mechanism for its inactivation by rabbit alveolar macrophages (350), which lack a granule peroxidase. However, oxidative inactivation of α_1-proteinase inhibitor by H_2O_2 formed by stimulated human alveolar macrophages was evident when MPO released from neutrophils also was present (355). Proteolytic inactivation of α_1-proteinase inhibitor by stimulated neutrophils (342,354,356), possibly through activation of the latent metalloproteinase by the HOCl-generating MPO system (356), has also been reported.

A number of studies have suggested that oxidative inactivation of α_1-proteinase inhibitor also occurs *in vivo*. Thus, α_1-proteinase inhibitor isolated from the synovial fluid of patients with rheumatoid arthritis contained oxidized methionine residues and was unable to form complexes with elastase (357). Functionally inactive α_1-proteinase inhibitor has also been detected in the bronchoalveolar lavage fluid of patients with respiratory distress syndrome (358–362) and of smokers (363), as well as in certain animal models (364,365). In one study, no evidence was found for the enhancement of the human neutrophil elastase-induced emphysema in the hamster by the co-instillation of MPO-system–derived oxidants (366).

Leukotrienes

Leukotriene C_4 (LTC$_4$), the slow reacting substance of anaphylaxis (SRS-A), is a lipoxygenase product of arachidonic acid metabolism that contains glutathione bound covalently to C6 of the arachidonic acid backbone by a sulfur-ether bond. Crude SRS-A was inactivated by horseradish or mast cell peroxidase when combined with H_2O_2 (367), and SRS-A activity of LTC$_4$ and the chemotactic activity of LTB$_4$ was decreased by EPO or MPO when combined with H_2O_2 and a halide (368). Horse eosinophils that generated large amounts of LTC$_4$ when stimulated by the Ca^{2+} ionophore A23187 (369) also released both H_2O_2 and EPO when stimulated in this way (368). Azide, which inhibits EPO and catalase, which degrade H_2O_2, increased the amount of SRS activity detected following A23187 stimulation of intact eosinophils (368), suggesting that eosinophils may modulate the amount of LTC$_4$ at an inflammatory site by both its production and degradation. The two 6-*trans* sterioisomers of LTB$_4$, 5-(S), 12-(S)-6-*trans* LTB$_4$ and 5-(S), 12-(R)-6-*trans* LTB$_4$, were detected as products of the degradation of LTC$_4$ by PMA-stimulated human eosinophils and by the cell-free EPO-H_2O_2-iodide system (370), and a detailed study of the products formed by the degradation of LTC$_4$, LTD$_4$, or LTE$_4$ by PMA-stimulated neutrophils, by the cell-free MPO-H_2O_2-chloride system, and by HOCl indicated the formation of the corresponding S-diasterioisomeric sulfoxides in addition to the 5-(S), 12-(S), and 5-(S), 12-(R)-6-*trans* isomers of LTB$_4$ (208,209). The inhibition of degradation by peroxidase inhibitors and by catalase suggested the involvement of the peroxidase system in the degradation of LTC$_4$ by PMA- (208,209) or A23187- (371) stimulated neutrophils, and by PMA-stimulated eosinophils (370).

Other Compounds

Other compounds or systems that can be modified by the cell-free and/or cell-associated MPO system include liposomes, particularly those containing double bonds (372,373); the lysine side chains of elastin (374); prostaglandins (375); fluorescent probes of membrane polarization (376) or intravacuolar pH (377); immunoglobulins (294,295); fibronectin (378); transferrin (379,380); lactoferrin (379); hyaluronic acid (381); articular cartilage proteoglycan (382); sulfonamides (383); glutathione (197); as well as a number of other substances (196,384,385).

Stimulatory Activity of the MPO System

The peroxidase system, although predominantly inhibitory in its action, can be stimulatory under some conditions. This occurs with intact cells as targets when the concentration of the components of the peroxidase system are relatively low, so that reaction with the cell surface is sufficient to trigger a secretory response without inducing irreversible membrane damage. In addition, certain enzymes and complement can be activated by exposure to the products of the MPO system.

Platelet Secretion

The MPO-H_2O_2-halide system caused the release of the dense-granule marker serotonin from platelets to a significantly greater degree than the release of the cytoplasmic marker adenine, suggesting, in part, a nonlytic process analogous to the platelet release reaction (316). Serotonin release was rapid, reaching maximum levels at 2 to 5 minutes and was blocked by agents that inhibit the peroxidase system (azide, cyanide, catalase) and by agents that affect platelet metabolism (dinitrophenol, deoxyglucose) or chelate Mg^{2+} [ethylenediaminetetraacetic acid (EDTA) but not Mg-ethyleneglycoltetraacetic acid (EGTA)], supporting an active nonlytic secretory process. The MPO system released from stimulated neutrophils also caused release of the platelet markers (246); however, in this instance equivalent amounts of serotonin and adenine were released, suggesting a lytic process.

Mast Cell Secretion

EPO or MPO at relatively low concentrations, when combined with H_2O_2 and a halide, induced mast cell secretion as indicated by the release of the granule component histamine without the concomitant release of the cytoplasmic marker lactate dehydrogenase (LDH) (386), and by ultrastructural changes typical of those seen when mast cells are stimulated to secrete by classic secretagogues (386,387). An increase in EPO to relatively high levels when combined with H_2O_2 and a halide was cytotoxic to mast cells, as indicated by the release of both histamine and LDH and by morphologic evidence of cell damage (386,387). Intact neutrophils stimulated by the phagocytosis of zymosan also initiated mast cell degranulation through the release of the components of the peroxidase system (388,389), an effect that was inhibited by dapsone and sulfapyridine. In contrast, mast cell degranulation induced by PMA-stimulated neutrophils did not require the peroxidase system; histamine release was unaffected by azide and catalase and by the substitution of MPO-deficient for normal neutrophils.

Enzyme Activation

Neutrophils contain a collagenase that is stored in a latent, inactive form in the specific granules (390–392). It is a metalloenzyme that attacks interstitial collagens type I, II, and III. When neutrophils are stimulated, this enzyme is released and simultaneously activated, particularly under aerobic conditions (393). The activation of latent collagenase was unaffected by SOD, but was inhibited by catalase, thus implicating H_2O_2 (394). The absence of collagenase activation by CGD neutrophils unless H_2O_2 was added further supported H_2O_2 involvement. The activation of latent collagenase by neutrophils also was inhibited by the peroxidase inhibitor azide and by methionine, which can scavenge HOCl. The addition of reagent HOCl or chloramines activated the latent collagenase (393–395). These findings suggest that collagenase activation is a consequence of the formation of oxidants by the peroxidase system. Activation of collagenase by HOCl has been reported to require cathepsin G (396).

Gelatinase is a metalloenzyme different from collagenase, which is stored in a latent form in a distinct secretory granule (397). This enzyme attacks denatured collagen (gelatin) and solubilizes type IV and V collagens. Like collagenase, this latent gelatinase is activated by stimulated neutrophils in part through the formation of chlorinated oxidants (398). However, activation also occurs in part by an oxygen-independent mechanism, since some activation was observed when CGD neutrophils were employed. It has been reported that activation of gelatinase by stimulated neutrophils is induced largely by endogenous serine proteinases, particularly elastase, rather than by oxidative mechanisms (399).

The degradation of human glomerular basement membrane by stimulated neutrophils has also been reported to involve the activation of metalloproteinases by oxidants formed by the MPO system (400).

Complement Activation

MPO binds to C1q to form a complex that increases the stability of C1q; however, the further addition of H_2O_2 and chloride resulted in the complete inactivation of C1q (401). Hypochlorous acid and taurine chloramine convert C5 to an activated state (C5b), which combines with C6, C7, C8, and C9 to form the terminal complement complex C6–C9 (402).

In Vivo Effects of the MPO System

Pulmonary Injury

Instillation into rat lung of either a low dose of glucose oxidase as a source of H_2O_2, or peroxidase [lactoperoxidase (LPO), MPO] produced little lung injury; however, when both glucose oxidase and peroxidase were instilled, severe acute lung injury was observed, which progressed to interstitial fibrosis (403). The pulmonary injury could be prevented by catalase but not by SOD. Similarly, the neutrophil-mediated pulmonary injury induced by immune complexes was inhibited by catalase but not by SOD, thus implicating H_2O_2 (404). Intratracheal injection of MPO and H_2O_2 into hamsters produced a partial inactivation of α_1-proteinase inhibitor as measured by decreased binding to elastase (365), suggesting that, in addition to a direct toxic effect of the products of the MPO system, indirect toxicity may occur through the increase in proteinase activity resulting from inhibitor inactivation. Lung inflammatory cells from patients with idiopathic pulmonary fibrosis spontaneously released increased amounts of O_2^- and H_2O_2 and were toxic to alveolar epithelial cells, particularly when incubated with alveolar epithelial lining fluid (405). The lining fluid from idiopathic fibrosis patients had elevated MPO levels, and evidence was presented that implicated MPO in the toxicity. A positive correlation was found between the level of MPO in the lining fluid and the rate of deterioration of the vital capacity of the patient.

Renal Injury

MPO is a highly cationic protein that, when administered intravenously to mice, binds on the basis of charge and size to anionic sites in the glomerular capillary wall, and to mesangial cells (406). Similarly, MPO was detected in the glomerular basement membrane following infusion into the renal artery of rats, with concentration in the subepithelial space at the base of the epithelial cell foot processes (407). MPO, when administered alone, did not produce glomerular injury. However, when the MPO infusion was followed by H_2O_2 at a concentration that was not toxic alone, injury was indicated in the first few hours by proteinuria and by marked endothelial cell swelling, focal epithelial cell foot process fusion, and a marked influx of platelets (407,408). By 4 days there was marked proliferation of endothelial cells and possibly mesangial cells, and by 21 days the glomerular lesion had largely resolved (408). When radioiodide was added to the last infusion, iodination of glomerular structures was observed, with concentration in the glomerular basement membrane and mesangial cells (407). Iodination is a consequence of the oxidation of iodide by peroxidase and H_2O_2, and thus indicates the interaction of these components in the glomerular capillary wall.

The lectin concanavalin A (conA) infused into the renal artery binds to sugars in the glomerular capillary wall, thus serving as a planted antigen. When this infusion is followed by one of anti-conA antibody, an antigen-antibody complex is formed on the glomerular basement membrane that activates complement and attracts neutrophils to the region (409). Proteinuria occurs, which is decreased when the animals are neutrophil-depleted by the infusion of antineutrophil antibody. Iodination of glomeruli occurs in the neutrophil-mediated conA–anti-conA model of glomerulonephritis (409), raising the possibility of the involvement of the MPO system in the glomerular damage.

The mechanism by which the MPO system induces glomerular injury is unknown. Isolated glomerular basement membrane is degraded by proteinases released by neutrophils (300,400,410), and preincubation of the glomerular basement membrane with the MPO-H_2O_2-chloride system increases its susceptibility to proteolysis (299). The MPO system also activates endogenous glomerular basement membrane-degrading proteinases (400). Elastase alone and the MPO system alone cause degradation of the heparan sulfate proteoglycans of subendothelial matrix; however, when exposure to elastase was followed by exposure to the MPO system, degradation was greater than additive (411). The infusion of the neutral serine proteinases elastase and cathepsin G into the renal artery of rats produces marked proteinuria without evidence of morphologic damage (412). These findings raise the possibility that the MPO system combines with neutral proteinases (and perhaps other neutrophil products) to produce the damage observed in neutrophil-dependent glomerulonephritis. Neutrophils adherent to glomerular basement membrane release oxidants only at the site of attachment, in an area that is inaccessible to proteins in the medium and presumably to circulating oxidant scavengers and proteinase inhibitors (413).

Antitumor Activity

Intraperitoneal or subcutaneous injection into mice of glucose oxidase covalently coupled to polystyrene microspheres suppressed the growth of some locally transplanted tumor cells and prolonged survival (414). This protective effect of glucose oxidase was prevented by the co-injection of catalase coupled to latex beads, thus implicating H_2O_2 as the protective agent. The H_2O_2 could theoretically limit tumor cell growth directly or via the formation of a more reactive oxidant such as a product of the MPO system or $\cdot OH$. MPO injected daily into mammary tumor–bearing mice in conjunction with an antitumor agent thiotepa was shown to significantly decrease the rate of tumor growth (415,416).

Atherosclerosis

A role for reactive oxygen species in the initiation of the atherosclerotic lesion has been proposed based largely on evidence that oxidation of low-density lipoprotein (LDL) promotes uptake by macrophages, which are in this way converted to lipid-laden foam cells. Early studies suggested that free transition metal ions (copper, iron) were required for oxidation of LDL; however, horseradish peroxidase–dependent free metal–independent oxidation of LDL (417) suggested that mammalian peroxidases may be biologic catalysts of this reaction. Modification of LDL (lipid peroxidation, oxidation of amino acid residues, tyrosylation, chlorhydrin formation) by the MPO-H_2O_2-chloride system or its products (190,191,418–426) with associated increased uptake by macrophages (421) has been reported. The involvement of peroxidase-catalyzed reactions in the initiation of atherosclerosis *in vivo* has been proposed, based on the detection of MPO (427) and specific markers of MPO-catalyzed oxidation (428,429) in human atherosclerotic lesions.

Evidence for the Involvement of the MPO System in Intact Leukocytes

There are a number of lines of evidence that support the involvement of the MPO system in the toxic activity of neutrophils:

1. The components of the MPO system (MPO, H_2O_2, chloride) are present in neutrophils in adequate concentrations and the formation of H_2O_2, and the release of MPO occurs at a time appropriate to the microbicidal act.

2. Cytochemical studies have demonstrated the presence of both MPO (430) and H_2O_2 (431,432) in the phagosome following particle ingestion, and their interaction there with a halide is indicated by the iodination reaction that occurs when neutrophils ingest microorganisms (144). Iodination of the microorganisms by the cell-free MPO-H_2O_2-iodide system is evident autoradiographically (144). In intact leukocytes, the fixed iodide can be localized in part in the phagosome by autoradiographic techniques (430) and by the analysis of isolated phagosomes (433). Extracellular proteins are also iodinated when intact neutrophils ingest bacteria (434,435), and although autoradiographic studies indicate the presence of silver grains on the organism surface in the phagosome (430), other neutrophil constituents are also iodinated (430,436).

3. A high proportion of the oxygen consumed by stimulated neutrophils can be accounted for by the formation of chloride oxidation products. Estimates have varied from 28% to 72%, depending on the stimulus (162,163), and it has been emphasized that these are minimum values that do not take into account the competing effect of proteins and other HOCl scavengers in the assay system (162). Similarly, a high proportion of the H_2O_2 generated by neutrophils is utilized to generate HOCl (164). In one study (384), 88.3 nmol of HOCl/OCl- was generated by 5×10^6 human neutrophils during a 2-hour incubation at 22°C with opsonized zymosan.

4. The H_2O_2 generated by stimulated neutrophils is required for optimal microbicidal activity. Patients with CGD have severe and repeated infections due to the inability of their neutrophils to kill certain ingested organisms (6). This microbicidal defect is associated with, and is presumably a result of, the absence of a respiratory burst (7), thus emphasizing the role of the products of the respiratory burst in the killing of some organisms. The importance of H_2O_2 deficiency in the microbicidal defect has been emphasized by its partial reversal by the introduction of H_2O_2 into the cell (437,438). Glucose oxidase, an enzyme that forms H_2O_2 without an apparent O_2^- intermediate, can be employed for this purpose, emphasizing that H_2O_2 is effective even when O_2^-

remains deficient in these cells. Some microorganisms, namely lactic acid bacteria such as lactobacilli, streptococci, and pneumococci, generate H_2O_2 and are killed well by CGD leukocytes (439–441) unless mutant strains are employed that are relatively deficient in H_2O_2 production (213,442). Thus, the susceptibility of H_2O_2-generating organisms to the intracellular microbicidal systems appears to be due to the replacement of a defective leukocytic H_2O_2-generating system with H_2O_2 of microbial origin.

Finally, certain microorganisms can be protected from the microbicidal activity of neutrophils by their content of the H_2O_2-scavenging enzymes catalase and glutathione peroxidase. Thus, for example, the resistance of coagulase-positive staphylococci to killing by reagent H_2O_2 (443,444) and by intact neutrophils *in vitro* (445) is directly related to their catalase content, and strains rich in catalase are more virulent *in vivo* (445).

5. The MPO released by stimulated neutrophils is required for optimal microbicidal activity. This association is supported by a number of lines of evidence:

a. Inhibitors of peroxidase-catalyzed reactions such as azide (255,434,446–448), cyanide (434,446, 448), propylthiouracil (434), methimazole (434), and sulfonamides (449) inhibit the microbicidal activity of normal neutrophils. Although the specificity of these inhibitors for peroxidase-catalyzed reactions is not absolute, azide (446,448), cyanide (446,448), and sulfonamides (449) have little or no effect on the microbicidal activity of MPO-deficient neutrophils, suggesting that they exert their effect on normal neutrophils largely by the inhibition of MPO.

b. Neutrophil cytoplasts have decreased cytotoxic activity unless MPO is added. Neutrophil-derived cytoplasts (neutroplasts) lack nuclei and are greatly depleted of their cytoplasmic granules (and thus MPO), but have an intact respiratory burst (450,451). Whereas intact neutrophils readily kill *Staphylococcus aureus* and, when stimulated, lyse erythrocytes and inactivate α_1-proteinase inhibitor, neutroplasts phagocytose but do not kill *S. aureus* unless the bacteria are coated with MPO (452), and stimulated neutroplasts do not lyse erythrocytes (453) or inactivate α_1-proteinase inhibitor (340) unless MPO is added.

c. The neutrophils of patients with hereditary MPO deficiency have a microbicidal defect. Hereditary MPO deficiency is a genetic disorder in which MPO is absent from neutrophils and monocytes (1,454,455). It was first described in 1963 in healthy siblings (456); however, interest in this condition intensified with the finding of the microbicidal activity of MPO when combined with H_2O_2 and a halide (144,145) and the description of a patient with MPO deficiency and systemic candidiasis in whom a neutrophil microbicidal defect was demonstrated (457). Although initially the few sporadic cases of MPO deficiency described suggested a very rare condition, the introduction of an automated flow cytochemical system for routine leukocyte differential counts that used cellular peroxidase activity indicated a more frequent occurrence of this condition (458,459), with an incidence of complete deficiency of 1 in 4,000 in one study (459) and 0.15% in another (460). Individuals with this condition generally do not have an increased incidence of infection, although some have had major systemic infections (461), particularly with *C. albicans* (457,459,462–469). The genetic defect in hereditary MPO deficiency varies among patients, with some patients reported to have a defect in posttranslational processing and others having a pretranslational defect. A number of patients with hereditary MPO deficiency have an arginine 569 to tryptophane mutation, producing a novel Bgl II fragment (470–473). A 90-kd protein reacting with anti-MPO antibody but lacking heme and enzyme activity suggestive of maturation arrest at apopro-MPO has been detected (73). Partial deficiency of MPO has also been described. Partially MPO-deficient neutrophils contain MPO that is electrophoretically, functionally, and immunologically normal but in decreased amounts, whereas completely MPO-deficient neutrophils lack any evidence of mature MPO protein (474,475).

The isolated leukocytes of patients with MPO deficiency have decreased microbicidal activity (446,448, 457–459,476–478), suggesting a requirement for MPO for optimum killing. This defect is particularly severe when fungicidal activity is measured (457,479). The bactericidal defect is characterized by a lag period, which the organisms are killed (478); it is not as severe as in the leukocytes of patients with CGD, and is reported to be mild in some patients (459). These findings, although implicating MPO in the microbicidal activity of phagocytes, also indicate the presence of MPO-independent antimicrobial systems in these cells that are adequate to maintain most patients in good health.

Does the microbicidal activity of MPO-deficient neutrophils accurately reflect the relative role of MPO-dependent and MPO-independent antimicrobial systems in normal cells? A number of lines of evidence suggests that it may not:

1. Agents, such as azide or cyanide, that inhibit peroxidase-catalyzed reactions decrease the bactericidal activity of normal leukocytes to a level below that of similarly treated MPO-deficient leukocytes (446,448), suggesting that the MPO-independent antimicrobial

systems are more highly developed in MPO-deficient than in normal cells.

2. The respiratory burst is considerably greater in MPO-deficient than in normal neutrophils (292,434, 448,474,476,477,480–485). Those measures of the respiratory burst dependent in part or totally on MPO (e.g., iodination, chemiluminescence), as would be anticipated, are decreased in MPO-deficient neutrophils (292,448,477,481,483,486) unless peroxidase is added (486,487). The increased respiratory burst of MPO-deficient neutrophils is due to at least two mechanisms. First, MPO appears to be required for the termination of the respiratory burst through inactivation of the NADPH oxidase (488,489). As a result, the respiratory burst would be expected to be prolonged in the absence of MPO. Second, since H_2O_2 is degraded in part by the MPO system, the absence of MPO would be expected to result in a buildup of H_2O_2 with associated increased production of oxidants dependent on H_2O_2 for their formation. This would be particularly evident in the phagosome or extracellular fluid, since cytosolic H_2O_2-degrading systems, e.g., catalase, glutathione cycle, appear to be normal in MPO deficiency (490).

3. Degranulation following phagocytosis is greater in MPO-deficient than in normal cells (491). This effect could not be accounted for by increased ingestion, increased respiratory burst activity, or decreased inactivation of the released granule components.

4. Phagocytosis of IgG- or C3b-coated yeast particles (292), serum opsonized zymosan (484), or erythrocytes coated with either IgG or C3b plus limited IgG (492) by MPO-deficient neutrophils is enhanced. The MPO-H_2O_2-halide system appears to inhibit the phagocytosis of normal neutrophils and the increased phagocytosis of MPO-deficient neutrophils is due to the absence of this inhibition. Thus, ingestion by normal neutrophils is suppressed by the addition of MPO and H_2O_2 individually or in combination (292,492,493), and anaerobiasis and agents that scavenge H_2O_2 and/or inhibit the MPO system enhance phagocytosis (37,292,492,494). Phagocytosis by MPO-deficient neutrophils, however, is not enhanced by the peroxidase inhibitor azide, is only minimally inhibited by H_2O_2 (492), but is depressed by the addition of MPO (292). The MPO system inhibits both the attachment of the opsonized particle to the cell surface and ingestion (292,492) and can attack either the opsonin (293) or its receptor (493).

Despite functional alterations in MPO-deficient neutrophils that would be expected to increase the killing capacity of the cells, i.e., increased respiratory burst, degranulation, and phagocytosis, a microbicidal defect is present. This raises the possibility that normal neutrophils kill certain microorganisms predominantly by the

MPO system, but that, when MPO is absent, modifications occur that increase the MPO-independent antimicrobial activity to an effective level.

Studies of the degradation of LTC_4 by normal and MPO-deficient neutrophils suggests that an adaptation of this sort occurs (495). LTC_4 was degraded by the MPO-H_2O_2-chloride system and, as anticipated, this degradation was inhibited by catalase and by the heme-protein inhibitor azide at low concentration (10^{-5} M) but was unaffected by SOD or by the ·OH scavengers mannitol or ethanol. LTC_4 was also degraded by the xanthine oxidase system; however, the inhibitor profile was very different. Both catalase and SOD were strongly inhibitory, as were mannitol and ethanol. Azide was inhibitory at relatively high concentration (10^{-3} M), but not at the low concentration inhibitory to the peroxidase system. This inhibitor profile is that expected for a reaction dependent on ·OH generated by the Haber-Weiss reaction. Thus, LTC_4 is degraded both by the MPO system and by ·OH.

Intact normal neutrophils stimulated by the Ca^{2+} ionophore A23187 degrade LTC_4 and the inhibitor profile suggested the involvement of the MPO system; degradation was inhibited by catalase and by azide at concentrations down to 10^{-5} M but was unaffected by SOD, mannitol, or ethanol. MPO-deficient neutrophils stimulated with A23187 were also found to completely degrade LTC_4; however, in this instance degradation was inhibited by catalase, SOD, the ·OH scavengers mannitol and ethanol, and by azide only at high concentration (10^{-3} M). Thus, MPO-deficient neutrophils, like the xanthine oxidase system, appear to degrade LTC_4 by ·OH generated by the Haber-Weiss reaction. These findings suggest that the predominant LTC_4 degrading system in normal neutrophils is the MPO-H_2O_2-halide system, but that when MPO is absent there is an increased respiratory burst resulting in the formation of ·OH in amounts able to degrade LTC_4.

Synergism Between Reactive Oxygen Species and Other Mammalian Cell or Microbial Components

The interaction of reactive oxygen species and proteinases to produce tissue damage has been reviewed (496). As indicated above, the effect of the MPO system on the activity of proteinases is complex, with MPO-derived oxidants under some conditions increasing proteinase activity by inactivation of proteinase inhibitors, by direct activation of certain proteinases, or by modification of the substrate to make it more susceptible to proteinase digestion, and under other conditions decreasing proteinase activity by inactivation of the enzyme. A synergism also exists between H_2O_2 and proteinases. A neutral serine proteinase, present in the plasma membrane fraction of human neutrophils, was lytic to erythrocytes only following pretreatment of the target cells with nonlytic concentrations of H_2O_2 (497). H_2O_2 also acts synergistically with a neutral proteinase (cytolytic factor) released from activated macrophages to lyse tumor cells (498), with the proteinases trypsin, chymotrypsin, elastase, and cathepsin G to kill endothelial cells (499), and with the peptide defensins of neutrophil granules in the cytolysis of certain tumor cells (500). Reactive oxygen species released by neutrophil or eosinophil cytoplasts also act synergistically with eosinophil cationic protein (but not eosinophil major basic protein) to kill the schistosomula of *S. mansoni* (501). The synergism between biologic oxidants and a variety of cellular and microbial products (proteinases, cationic proteins, hemolysins, lysophosphatides, fatty acids, phospholipases, etc.) has recently been reviewed (502).

Nitric oxide (NO·) synthesis by phagocytes and its role in host defense is considered in the chapter by Moilanen et al. and will be considered here only in relation to its interaction with products of the respiratory burst and MPO. NO· reacts with O_2^- (503,504) to form peroxynitrite (ONOO–), which is a potent oxidant of sulfhydryl groups (505) and which at acid pH converts to its protonated form, peroxynitrous acid (ONOOH), which assumes some of the properties of hydroxyl radicals perhaps by decomposition (503) as follows:

$$NO· + O_2^- \rightarrow ONOO^- + H^+ \rightleftharpoons ONOOH \rightarrow ·OH + NO_2^-$$

The toxicity of NO· is believed to be due in part to this sequence of reactions. MPO can react with ONOOH to yield the inactive form of MPO, compound II (506). Nitrite, an end product of NO· metabolism, also reacts with MPO (506–508) to form an inactive product (508). Paradoxically, nitrite also can increase the microbicidal activity of MPO and H_2O_2 under some experimental conditions (508).

Apoptosis

Apoptosis is a process in which characteristic changes in cells including cytoplasmic shrinkage, membrane blebbing, chromatin condensation, and DNA fragmentation lead to programmed cell death. Neutrophils are short-lived cells particularly prone to apoptosis (509). The Fas/Fas ligand system has been implicated as an important pathway for the induction of apoptosis in a variety of cell types. Fas (APO-1, CD95) is a widely distributed 45-kd cell surface receptor that is activated to induce apoptosis by reaction with its natural ligand or anti-Fas IgM antibody. Fas ligand is a 37-kd cell component, with more restricted distribution than Fas, which can be present on the cell surface or be released in a lower molecular weight (~30 kd) soluble form. The interaction of anti-Fas IgM antibody or Fas ligand with Fas initiates a cascade of intracellular changes leading to apoptosis. Reagent H_2O_2 (510–516) and H_2O_2 released by stimulated phagocytes (515,516) can initiate apoptosis. Both spontaneous and Fas-mediated apoptosis of neutrophils is decreased when CGD neutrophils are employed, an effect that is reversed by the addition of H_2O_2 (516). This suggests that autodestruction of neutrophils by either spontaneous or Fas-induced apoptosis is potentiated by the release of H_2O_2 and perhaps other oxidants from the stimulated cells.

Hydroxyl Radical (·OH)

The further reduction of H_2O_2 can result in the formation of ·OH as follows:

$$H_2O_2 \xrightarrow{e} OH^- + \cdot OH$$

·OH is one of the most powerful oxidants known, raising the possibility that it may contribute to the toxic activity of phagocytes. Four mechanisms for the formation of ·OH are considered in this section: Fenton reagent, Haber-Weiss reaction, the autoxidation of iron, and MPO-catalyzed reactions. The interaction of O_2^- and nitric oxide to form ·OH is considered above.

Fenton Reagent

Fenton (517) described the strong oxidizing activity of a mixture of ferrous sulfate and H_2O_2 and it was subsequently proposed (518) that the powerful oxidant formed by Fenton's reagent was ·OH as follows:

$$H_2O_2 + Fe^{2+} \rightarrow Fe^{3+} + OH^- + \cdot OH$$

The formation of ·OH by Fenton's reagent requires stoichiometric amounts of Fe^{2+} and H_2O_2. The free iron concentration in biologic fluids is extremely low and would be expected to limit the formation of ·OH by this mechanism. It has been proposed that hemoglobin-Fe^{2+} can react with H_2O_2 to form ·OH as follows (519):

$$Hb\text{-}Fe^{2+} + H_2O_2 \rightarrow Hb\text{-}Fe^{3+} + OH^- + \cdot OH$$

This reaction is facilitated by the reduction of the methemoglobin formed by ascorbic acid (520). The H_2O_2 needed for this reaction can be generated by the interaction of ascorbic acid and oxyhemoglobin (520). Although this mechanism may serve to generate ·OH in erythrocytes, it cannot do so in leukocytes.

An additional potential source of iron is the microorganism. Iron is released from organisms exposed to the MPO-H_2O_2-halide system (200,521) or ingested by neutrophils (521), and the iron released by neutrophils is bound, in part, to lactoferrin (521). Bacteria grown in a high iron medium increased their iron content and were more susceptible to destruction by H_2O_2 (522,523). The inhibition of this H_2O_2-dependent toxicity by ·OH scavengers suggested the involvement of ·OH formed by the interaction of Fe^{2+} and H_2O_2. Growth of organisms in a high iron medium did not increase their susceptibility to killing by intact neutrophils (523–525), although a small but significant increase in killing by monocytes and neu-

troplasts was observed (523). Neither neutrophils nor monocytes generated levels of ·OH detected by electron paramagnetic resonance (EPR) following ingestion of iron-rich bacteria (525).

Fe^{2+}-H_2O_2-Iodide System

Iodide considerably increases the antimicrobial effect of Fenton's reagent against bacteria (526) and fungi (527,528). The properties of the Fe^{2+}-H_2O_2-iodide system differs from those of the MPO-H_2O_2-halide system in several respects (526). Both systems are inhibited by catalase and are unaffected by SOD. However, the Fe^{2+}-H_2O_2-iodide system is strongly inhibited by the ·OH scavengers mannitol and ethanol at concentrations that do not affect the MPO-dependent system. Although both systems are inhibited by azide, a considerably higher concentration is required for inhibition of the Fe^{2+} than the MPO-dependent system. The pH optimum of the Fe^{2+}-dependent system was 5.5; 0.2 M acetate buffer could be employed at this pH, whereas phosphate and lactate buffers at the same pH and molarity were ineffective, and indeed inhibited the bactericidal activity of the system in acetate buffer (or when unbuffered). In contrast, the pH optimum of the MPO-H_2O_2-iodide system was 5.0, and all three buffers could be employed at this pH with comparable results. EDTA inhibited the Fe^{2+} but not the MPO-dependent system. Whereas the MPO system was effective with iodide, bromide, or chloride as the halide, only iodide was effective when MPO was replaced by iron. Thyroxine could serve as the source of iodide for the MPO-H_2O_2-iodide system, but not for the Fe^{2+}-H_2O_2-iodide system. It was proposed that ·OH formed by Fe^{2+} and H_2O_2 reacts with iodide to form a toxic species:

$$\cdot OH + I^- \rightarrow OH^- + I^*$$

The overall reaction is

$$Fe^{2+} + H_2O_2 + I^- \rightarrow Fe^{3+} + 2OH^- + I^*$$

Haber-Weiss Reaction

When the iron concentration is limiting, the reduction of the ferric iron formed by Fenton's reagent is needed for the complete conversion of H_2O_2 to ·OH. This can be accomplished by O_2^- as follows:

$$O_2^- + Fe^{3+} \rightarrow Fe^{2+} + O_2$$

The overall reaction is

$$H_2O_2 + O_2^- \xrightarrow{Fe} O_2 + OH^- + \cdot OH$$

This iron-catalyzed interaction of H_2O_2 and O_2^- has been termed the Haber-Weiss reaction, or the superoxide-driven Fenton reaction. A direct interaction between H_2O_2

and O_2^- (actually its protonated form HO_2^-) to form ·OH was originally proposed by Haber and Weiss (518). However, there is abundant evidence that O_2^- does not react directly with H_2O_2 at an appreciable rate as compared to competing reactions such as the spontaneous dismutation of O_2^-. Thus, a rate constant of 0.50 $M^{-1}sec^{-1}$ for $HO_2^- + H_2O_2$ and 0.13 $M^{-1}sec^{-1}$ for $O_2^- + H_2O_2$ has been reported (529), which can be compared to a rate constant of 8.5×10^7 $M^{-1}sec^{-1}$ for spontaneous dismutation at pH 4.8 ($HO_2^- + O_2^-$) (11). Trace metal catalysis is now an accepted requirement for the generation of ·OH by the Haber-Weiss reaction (530–532).

Although ·OH is generally believed to be the product of the Fenton and Haber-Weiss reactions, other species functionally similar to ·OH have been suggested (533). These include the "crypto-OH radical" of unknown structure that mimics free ·OH but is more discriminating in its reactions (534,535), the ferryl radical ($FeOH^{3+}$ or FeO^{2+}) (536–538), or the perferryl radical (FeO^+ or Fe^{3+}-O_2^-). The ferryl radical has an appreciably longer lifetime than ·OH in aqueous solution when complexed with simple ligands such as hydroxide ions (537) and is more discriminating than ·OH in its actions. Its reactivity is greater than that of the perferryl radical. When xanthine oxidase was used as the source of O_2^- and H_2O_2 and Fe^{2+}-EDTA was used as the catalyst, the oxidant formed had the properties of ·OH. However, in the absence of EDTA, Fe^{2+} catalyzed the formation of an oxidant that differed from free ·OH (539). The iron bound with high affinity to the enzyme and the possibility of a bound iron-oxygen species was considered.

O_2^- Requirement

In the iron-catalyzed Haber-Weiss reaction, the Fe^{3+} formed by Fenton's reagent is reduced by O_2^-. However, under certain conditions thiols such as GSH or cysteine (540–542), the reduced pyridine nucleotides NADH and NADPH (543), paraquat (544–546), and ascorbic acid (547–552) can replace O_2^- as the reductant required for the formation of ·OH. Enzymatic reduction of Fe^{3+}-chelates also may occur (553). This prooxidant activity of the reducing agents may be offset by antioxidant activity due to the scavenging of O_2^- (554,555), ·OH (548), or H_2O_2, particularly when the concentration of the reducing agent is high. Although reductants such as GSH or ascorbic acid are present in neutrophils, their release into the phagosome has not been demonstrated (556), suggesting that they function not as prooxidants in the phagosome, but in a protective role as scavengers of reactive oxygen species in the cytoplasm (557,558). In this regard, stimulation of neutrophils with opsonized zymosan or PMA oxidized a portion (30–40%) of the cellular ascorbate to dehydroascorbate without affecting total (reduced + oxidized) ascorbate levels (556).

Metal Requirement

Iron has been most often implicated as the trace metal catalyst of the Haber-Weiss reaction (531,532,559). However, other metals may also be involved. CO^{2+} reacts with H_2O_2 to form an oxidant that can hydroxylate aromatic compounds and degrade deoxyribose (560). These reactions are stimulated by EDTA and are inhibited by scavengers of ·OH, raising the possibility that the reactive species is ·OH formed by a Fenton-type reaction:

$$H_2O_2 + CO^{2+} \rightarrow CO^{3+} + OH^- + \cdot OH$$

The addition of an O_2^--generating system did not potentiate the reactivity of H_2O_2 and CO^{2+}, suggesting that cobalt does not catalyze the Haber-Weiss reaction. Cupric ions (Cu^{2+}) appear to catalyze the formation of ·OH by a mechanism analogous to the Haber-Weiss reaction (561–564). Cu^{2+} is reduced by O_2^-:

$$Cu^{2+} + O_2^- \rightarrow Cu^+ + O_2$$

The Cu^+ formed reacts with H_2O_2 to generate ·OH:

$$Cu^+ + H_2O_2 \rightarrow Cu^{2+} + OH^- + \cdot OH$$

The overall reaction is a copper-catalyzed Haber-Weiss reaction:

$$O_2^- + H_2O_2 \xrightarrow{Cu} O_2 + OH^- + \cdot OH$$

O_2^- can be replaced by ascorbate (562,564,565) or thiols (566). When the copper is bound to certain amino acids or proteins, the release of free ·OH into solution is inhibited; however, site-specific damage to the protein, presumably by localized formation of ·OH, occurs (561,563,564). The degradation of DNA and deoxyribose by a copper-phenanthroline complex required a reductant such as NADH, 2-mercaptoethanol, or O_2^- and was inhibited by catalase but not by ·OH scavengers (567). SOD was inhibitory when O_2^- was used but not with the other reductants. It was proposed that Cu^{2+}-phenanthroline is reduced to Cu^+-phenanthroline by the reductant, and that Cu^+-phenanthroline reacts with H_2O_2 to form an oxidant that can attack DNA and deoxyribose. This oxidant did not appear to be free ·OH, since ·OH scavengers were not inhibitory; however, the formation of ·OH in close association with the DNA was not excluded.

Chelator Requirement

The catalytic effect of iron on the Haber-Weiss reaction is increased considerably under some experimental conditions by the chelator EDTA (531,532,559,568–570). Optimum catalysis occurred in the vicinity of iron and EDTA equivalence, with activity falling when either iron or EDTA is in great excess (559,569). The nature of the iron chelator complex appears to be critical for catalysis, as other chelators, e.g., diethylenetriaminepentaacetic acid (DTPA), bathophenanthrolinesulfonate, or deferoximine, decrease rather than increase the iron-catalyzed Haber-Weiss reaction (531,559,568–572). The inhibition by the latter chelators is generally believed to be due to the chelation of iron in a nonreactive form; however, inhibition by deferoxamine may be due in part to the scavenging of O_2^- (573) and ·OH (574).

Ferric iron is poorly soluble in aqueous solution at physiologic pH levels, since hydrated polynuclear iron complexes are formed which precipitate (559,575). Chelation of iron by EDTA maintains iron in solution in a form that is catalytically active, i.e., can be oxidized and reduced (532,576,577) and thus can catalyze the Haber-Weiss reaction:

$$H_2O_2 + Fe^{2+}\text{-EDTA} \rightarrow Fe^{3+}\text{-EDTA} + OH^- + \cdot OH$$
$$\underline{O_2^- + Fe^{3+}\text{-EDTA} \rightarrow Fe^{2+}\text{-EDTA} + O_2}$$
$$H_2O_2 + O_2^- \rightarrow O_2 + OH^- + \cdot OH$$

In contrast, iron chelates of DTPA, bathophenanthroline, and deferoxamine react much more slowly with O_2^- (577).

It has been proposed that the chemical basis for the reactivity of the Fe-EDTA chelate is the presence of an aquo coordination site that is catalytically active in contrast to other chelates in which all coordination sites are bound (559). Iron has six coordination sites and in aqueous solution water is bound to each to form the hexaaquo coordinate written for Fe^{3+} as $[Fe(H_2O)_6]^{3+}$. When iron is chelated, the chelator displaces water and is coordinately bound to the iron. A multidentate chelator such as DTPA or deferoxamine may bind to all six coordination sites, completely displacing water, and since a free aquo site appears to be required for catalysis, the chelated iron is in a catalytically inactive form. Although EDTA is also multidentate, it is too small to completely encompass the iron atom. As a result, there is the retention of a catalytically active aquo coordination site, possibly resulting from the distortion of the usual symmetry of coordination with the formation of a seventh coordination site to which water can bind. This hypothesis has been tested (578) using 12 different iron chelates, and a direct correlation found between the presence of at least one open coordination site (or one occupied by a readily dissociable ligand such as water) and the ability of the chelated iron to catalyze the formation of ·OH by the Haber-Weiss reaction.

Is a chelator required for iron catalysis of the Haber-Weiss reaction *in vivo* and, if so, what is its nature? The concentration of free iron in biologic fluids is very low with the bulk of the iron bound to protein either for storage and transport in a releasable form, or as a catalytic center in a more firmly bound form. The ability of a bound form of iron to catalyze the Haber-Weiss reaction in biologic fluids would increase considerably the amount of iron available for this reaction.

Most interest has centered around the iron-lactoferrin chelate as the physiologic catalyst of the Haber-Weiss reaction. Lactoferrin is present in the specific granules of neutrophils and is released into the phagosome following particle ingestion. It is an iron-binding protein that, when fully saturated, contains two Fe^{3+} atoms per molecule. Iron-saturated lactoferrin was reported to catalyze the Haber-Weiss reaction (579,580); however, lactoferrin saturated with an exact equivalence of iron was found to have little or no stimulatory effect on ·OH formation (581,582), and partially iron-saturated lactoferrin was inhibitory (581–583). Under physiologic conditions, lactoferrin is largely unsaturated, containing 20% or less of its total iron at saturation. It would therefore be expected to inhibit the Haber-Weiss reaction under these conditions, with catalysis by fully iron-saturated lactoferrin being due to excess iron bound to the protein at nonspecific sites (or released into the medium). This was supported by the finding that apolactoferrin protects rats from acute lung injury induced by systemic activation of complement with cobra venom factor, whereas infusion of iron-saturated lactoferrin had no effect, and ionic iron potentiated the tissue injury (584).

Transferrin also catalyzed ·OH formation when fully iron loaded (532,585,586), but not when partially saturated with iron (581,587). Alteration of transferrin by enzymes (e.g., *Pseudomonas* elastase), and/or oxidants (e.g., HOCl) present at an inflammatory site may increase its ·OH-generating capacity (588). When the iron concentration is low, phosphate ions can form a reactive chelate (575) and ·OH formation catalyzed by Fe^{2+} bound to α picolinic acid [an intermediate in the metabolic degradation of tryptophan (589)]; to the *Pseudomonas* siderophore pyochelin (590); to the di- and triphosphate nucleotides of adenosine, cytidine, thymidine, and guanosine (591–593); and to DNA (594) has been reported. However, iron bound to pyrophosphate, DTPA, citrate, ATP, or ADP in phosphate or Tris buffer pH 7.3 was considerably less effective than Fe^{2+}-EDTA as the catalyst of the Haber-Weiss reaction (595). Iron compounds capable of catalyzing the formation of ·OH have been detected in biologic fluids in some studies (596–598) but not in others (551).

When the pH is lowered to 5.0 to 5.5, iron-catalysis of ·OH formation can occur in the absence of a chelator (599). EDTA was inhibitory under these conditions. When the pH was increased, free iron-dependent ·OH formation by the Haber-Weiss reaction fell sharply, whereas ·OH formation in the presence of iron-EDTA rose so that at pH 7.0 the iron-EDTA chelate was considerably more effective than free iron. Thus, a low pH within the phagosome may make a chelator unnecessary or even inhibitory.

Autoxidation of Fe²⁺

Hydroxyl radicals can be generated by the aerobic oxidation of Fe^{2+} in the absence of an exogenous source of

O_2^- and H_2O_2 (552,600–607). The following sequence of reactions was proposed:

$$Fe^{2+} + O_2 \rightarrow [Fe^{3+}-O_2^-] \rightarrow Fe^{3+} + O_2^-$$
$$2O_2^- + 2H^+ \rightarrow O_2 + H_2O_2$$
$$Fe^{2+} + H_2O_2 \rightarrow O_2 + OH^- + \cdot OH$$

Certain chelating agents can stimulate the autoxidation of Fe^{2+} (608), and this occurs best when the affinity of the chelator for Fe^{3+} greatly exceeds its affinity for Fe^{2+} (609). Thus, the autoxidation of Fe^{2+} at acid pH is greatly accelerated by deferoxamine (606), apotransferrin (607), and apolactoferrin (607), with the formation of products (H_2O_2, $\cdot OH$) that are toxic to bacteria. This is in sharp contrast to the inhibitory effect of deferoxamine, apotransferrin, and apolactoferrin on $\cdot OH$ formation by the iron-catalyzed Haber-Weiss reaction. The autoxidation of Fe^{2+} can also be accelerated by phosphate (601,602, 605,608), EDTA (603,608), and certain other chelators.

MPO-Catalyzed Reactions

HOCl reacts with O_2^- at an appreciable rate with the formation of $\cdot OH$ (610,611), and it has been proposed that $\cdot OH$ can be generated by the MPO-H_2O_2-Cl^- system (612,613) by this reaction as follows:

$$H_2O_2 + Cl^- \xrightarrow{MPO} HOCl + OH^-$$
$$HOCl + O_2^- \rightarrow \cdot OH + O_2 + Cl^-$$

The degradation of hyaluronic acid by the MPO system has been reported to require the formation of $\cdot OH$ (381).

Formation by Leukocytes

The formation of O_2^- and H_2O_2 by stimulated phagocytes raises the possibility that these cells can also generate $\cdot OH$. Hydroxyl radical formation by phagocytes has been sought using a variety of techniques and, although the totality of the evidence supports the formation of this (or a functionally similar) radical under certain conditions, its formation has not been unequivocably demonstrated.

Ethylene Formation from Thiolethers

Ethylene is formed from methional by abstraction of an electron from the sulfur atom to form the radical cation, which is converted under nucleophilic attack by OH^- to form ethylene, methyldisulfide, and formic acid, with the ethylene readily detected by gas chromatography (614). 2-Keto-4-thiomethylbutyric acid (KMB) is similarly degraded, except that the final products are ethylene, methyldisulfide, and carbon dioxide (614). Hydroxyl radicals are powerful one-electron oxidants capable of the formation of ethylene from methional (615) or KMB (616), and this prompted the use of ethylene formation from these thiolethers by stimulated phagocytes as a mea-

sure of $\cdot OH$ formation. Ethylene formation by stimulated neutrophils (617–621), eosinophils (618), and mononuclear phagocytes (617,622) was demonstrated, and the partial inhibition of this reaction by SOD, catalase, and $\cdot OH$ scavengers implicated $\cdot OH$ generated by the Haber-Weiss reaction.

A number of other oxidants can initiate the formation of ethylene from methional or KMB (618,623–625). Thus, organic free radicals are effective with the relative reactivity being $\cdot OH > RO\cdot > ROO\cdot > RCO-O\cdot > R\cdot$ (624), and O_2^- reacts sluggishly with methional to form ethylene (623). Ethylene formation by neutrophils is dependent largely on MPO; it is inhibited by the peroxidase inhibitors azide and cyanide and is less than 10% of normal when neutrophils that lack MPO are employed (618), suggesting that ethylene formation by neutrophils is due predominantly to an MPO-dependent mechanism. The nature of the oxidant (or oxidants) that initiates ethylene formation by an MPO-dependent reaction in intact neutrophils is unknown.

Methane or Formaldehyde Formation from Dimethylsulfoxide (DMSO)

Hydroxyl radicals react readily with DMSO with the formation of methane, and this reaction was employed as a measure of $\cdot OH$ formation by stimulated neutrophils, monocytes, or alveolar macrophages (619). The inhibition of methane formation by SOD, catalase, and $\cdot OH$ scavengers suggested that it was due in part to $\cdot OH$ formation by the Haber-Weiss reaction. Formaldehyde is also formed by the interaction of DMSO and $\cdot OH$, and its formation is more sensitive than that of methane as a measure of $\cdot OH$ (626). It is not known whether MPO is required for methane or formaldehyde formation from DMSO by neutrophils as it is for ethylene formation from thiolethers.

CO_2 Release from Benzoic Acid

The release of $^{14}CO_2$ by the decarboxylation of carboxyl-labeled ^{14}C-benzoic acid has been employed as a measure of $\cdot OH$ formation by stimulated neutrophils (627). Decarboxylation of benzoic acid by phagocytes was inhibited by SOD, catalase, azide and mannitol, and was absent when CGD neutrophils were employed. Studies with neutrophils that lack MPO were not performed.

Deoxyribose Degradation

The formation of a thiobarbituric acid–reactive substance from deoxyribose has been proposed as a method for the detection of $\cdot OH$ (604). This method has been applied to the detection of $\cdot OH$ by stimulated phagocytes (628). Under the conditions employed, the degradation of deoxyribose required the addition of an iron-chelate, with the most effective chelator being EDTA.

Electron Paramagnetic Resonance (EPR) Spectrometry

EPR spectrometry detects free radicals, and when the radical is unstable it is often possible to trap it as a more stable radical adduct using a nitrone or nitroso compound as a spin trap. Hydroxyl radicals form an adduct with the nitrone compound 5,5-dimethylpyrroline-N-oxide (DMPO), which is sufficiently long-lived for detection by its characteristic EPR spectrum (629,630).

Neutrophils stimulated in the presence of DMPO form the $\cdot$OH adduct (631–633). The adduct is not formed by CGD neutrophils, and its formation is greater than normal when MPO-deficient leukocytes are employed (632). DMPO-OH$\cdot$ adduct formation also is increased when the peroxidase inhibitors azide and cyanide are added to normal neutrophils stimulated by phagocytosis (631). The increased DMPO-OH$\cdot$ adduct formation may reflect the greater respiratory burst of MPO-deficient leukocytes and/or the degradation of the DMPO-OH$\cdot$ adduct by the MPO system (634).

The detection of the DMPO-OH$\cdot$ adduct does not unequivocably establish the formation of $\cdot$OH by stimulated leukocytes, since the DMPO-OH$\cdot$ adduct can be formed in ways other than by the direct interaction of DMPO and $\cdot$OH. Thus, DMPO forms a radical adduct with O_2^- or HO_2^- (DMPO-OOH$\cdot$), which has an EPR spectrum distinct from that of the OH$\cdot$ adduct (629,635). The DMPO-OOH$\cdot$ adduct is formed, along with the DMPO-OH$\cdot$ adduct, by stimulated polymorphonuclear cells (PMNs) under some experimental conditions (631,636, 637). The rate constant for the reaction of DMPO with $\cdot$OH (3.4×10^9 M^{-1}sec^{-1}) is considerably greater than that for reaction with HO_2^- (6.6×10^3 M^{-1}sec^{-1}) or O_2^- (10 M^{-1}sec^{-1}) (638). The reduction or homeolytic cleavage of the DMPO-OOH$\cdot$ adduct to form DMPO-OH$\cdot$ can occur (635,638–640) and DMPO-OH$\cdot$ adduct formation thus may reflect O_2^- rather than $\cdot$OH formation. Further, the product of the MPO system of leukocytes, HOCl, reacts with DMPO to form a number of products including the DMPO-OH$\cdot$ adduct (634,641,642), and DMPO has been reported to form an adduct with $^1O_2$, which, on hydration, forms the $\cdot$OH adduct (643).

The formation of $^1O_2$ by neutrophils has not been clearly established (see below) and its role in the formation of DMPO-OH$\cdot$ thus is unclear. It is unlikely that the MPO system is involved in the formation of the DMPO-OH$\cdot$ adduct by phagocytes, since the concentration of HOCl required appears to be greater than that formed by PMNs (634) and adduct formation is not decreased, indeed, it appears to be increased when MPO-deficient PMNs are employed (632) or when the peroxidase inhibitors azide and cyanide are added to normal PMNs (631). Strong evidence has been presented, however, that suggests that the DMPO-OH$\cdot$ adduct formed by phagocytes is normally derived from the DMPO-OOH$\cdot$ adduct

and thus reflects O_2^- rather than $\cdot$OH formation (636, 644–646).

$\cdot$OH reacts with DMSO to form the methyl radical that reacts with DMPO to form the DMPO-CH$_3^-$ adduct with a characteristic EPR spectrum. This reaction has been proposed as a more specific measure of $\cdot$OH formation and when applied to stimulated PMNs suggested that $\cdot$OH is not formed unless exogenous iron is added (636,647). The iron chelator DTPA (DETAPAC) also was required for optimum DMPO-CH$_3^-$ detection. Similarly, no evidence was found, using this technique, for the formation of intraphagosomal $\cdot$OH (648).

It was concluded that the low concentration of iron normally limits the formation of $\cdot$OH by the Haber-Weiss reaction in PMNs. Hydroxyl radical formation by PMNs was found to be inhibited by lactoferrin (647,649), presumably by the chelation of iron in a nonreactive form, and by MPO (649,650) due to competition for the available H_2O_2. It has been proposed that DMPO-OOH$\cdot$ is the only spin adduct initially formed and that the formation of the $\cdot$OH adduct is associated with cell lysis, which results in the release of factors that convert the $\cdot$OOH to the $\cdot$OH adduct (637). The inhibition of PMN function by DMPO at the concentrations employed in spin trap experiments has been reported (637,651). However, toxicity to PMNs as measured by trypan blue exclusion was found in one study (637) but not in another (651).

It has been proposed that DMPO is not a suitable spin trap for the detection of radical formation by PMNs, since the DMPO spin adducts of $\cdot$OH and CH$_3^-$ are efficiently degraded by O_2^- (652–655), particularly in the presence of thiols (656,657). However, O_2^- was reported not to interfere with the use of the DMPO spin trapping method to detect $\cdot$OH formation by PMNs (657). Further, when the spin trap N-t-butyl-α-phenylnitrone (PBN) was employed, rather than DMPO, a spin adduct was formed by stimulated PMNs in the presence of DMSO, DTPA, and exogenous iron, which is stable to O_2^- (658). This adduct was not seen in the absence of added iron, supporting the thesis that neutrophils lack the endogenous capacity to form $\cdot$OH by the Haber-Weiss reaction.

Recently a new spin trap procedure for the detection of $\cdot$OH has been applied to neutrophils in which $\cdot$OH reacts with ethanol to form the α-hydroxyethyl radical that forms a measurable adduct with the spin trap 4-pyridyl 1-oxide N $tert$-butylnitrone (4-POBN) (613). This procedure was an order of magnitude more sensitive than previously employed methods and, with it, $\cdot$OH formation by PMA-stimulated PMNs could be detected in the absence of added iron. Further, evidence was presented that the formation of $\cdot$OH by stimulated PMN was by an MPO-dependent mechanism in which MPO catalyzes the H_2O_2-dependent oxidation of Cl^- to HOCl/OCl$^-$, which reacts with O_2^- to form $\cdot$OH. The evidence was as follows: $\cdot$OH formation was inhibited by SOD implicating O_2^-, catalase implicating H_2O_2, and azide implicating MPO. Further, the reaction of purified MPO with the xanthine oxidase system (which generates both O_2^- and H_2O_2) resulted in the formation of ·OH by a reaction that was dependent on Cl^- and was inhibited by SOD, catalase, and azide. Augmentation of the bactericidal activity of MPO-derived ·OH may occur when MPO binds to the surface of the organisms (659). In addition to its catalysis of ·OH formation, MPO was reported to be an effective inhibitor of the formation of ·OH by iron-supplemented phagocytes by competitive reaction with H_2O_2 (649,650). Less than 1% of PMN O_2^- production could be accounted for by the formation of ·OH, raising a question about its physiologic significance.

Role in Leukocytes

A variety of studies have implicated ·OH as a toxic species in cell-free O_2^- and H_2O_2-generating systems. In general, the evidence implicating ·OH formed by the Haber-Weiss reaction consists of the inhibition by catalase, SOD, and ·OH scavengers.

The xanthine oxidase system, with either xanthine, hypoxanthine, or acetaldehyde as substrate forms O_2^-, H_2O_2, and, in the presence of iron, ·OH (615,660–663), and thus has been employed as a model of the oxygen-dependent microbicidal mechanisms of phagocytes. In early studies of the bactericidal activity of xanthine oxidase, inhibition by catalase implicated H_2O_2 (664,665). However, the discovery of SOD and its use with catalase and ·OH scavengers to detect ·OH formation by the Haber-Weiss reaction have led to the identification of ·OH as a microbicidal product of the xanthine oxidase system (559,666,667). In some instances, the bactericidal activity of the xanthine oxidase system was inhibited by catalase but not by SOD (668,669), or by catalase and SOD but not by ·OH scavengers (668), suggesting that with some targets and under some experimental conditions, products of the xanthine oxidase system other than ·OH may be the toxic agent.

The participation of ·OH in the microbicidal activity of neutrophils has been proposed based on the inhibition of the bactericidal activity of intact leukocytes by SOD and catalase bound to latex beads (670) and by some ·OH scavengers (670,671). When DMSO was employed as the scavenger, the ·OH product, methane, was detected (671). Similarly, ·OH has been implicated in PMN-mediated tissue injury (584,672,673). The O_2^- and H_2O_2 required for ·OH formation are provided by the respiratory burst, and the iron needed for catalysis may come from leukocytic or microbial sources. However, as described above, the formation of ·OH by PMNs in significant amounts has been questioned, with the availability of iron being the limiting factor. Different mechanisms of toxicity may be operative in neutrophils depending on the target, the state of stimulation, and pathologic variations. Thus, for example, normal neutrophils degrade LTC_4 by the MPO sys-

tem, whereas when MPO is absent, as in hereditary MPO deficiency, the properties of degradation are suggestive of an ·OH-dependent mechanism (495).

·OH is an extremely powerful oxidant (674) and as such is not discriminating in its action, reacting with essentially the first molecule it meets. Therefore, it can be readily scavenged by compounds in the medium or by nonessential components of the target. It is, thus, unlikely that ·OH formed by PMNs is toxic at a distance of even a few microns from its origin, with its toxicity limited to ingested microorganisms or adherent extracellular targets. However, H_2O_2 formed by phagocytes may move to more distant sites due to its limited reactivity and may penetrate the targets to react with iron at a crucial site to form ·OH, which is toxic. MPO and EPO are strongly basic proteins that when released by phagocytes can bind to the target on a charge basis, and there react with H_2O_2 to form halide oxidation products and, in the presence of O_2^-, ·OH.

Singlet Oxygen ($^1O_2$)

Of the two forms of $^1O_2$, $^1\Sigma_g^+O_2$ has a higher energy above ground state (37.5 kcal) than does $^1\Delta_gO_2$ (22.4 kcal) but a considerably shorter lifetime. In aqueous solution the lifetime of $^1\Sigma_g^+O_2$ does not exceed 10^{-11} sec, whereas that of $^1\Delta_gO_2$ is approximately 2 msec (675). The lifetime of $^1\Delta_gO_2$ is increased considerably in a number of solvents (up to 1,000 msec with Freon) and is increased at least tenfold by the substitution of deuterium oxide (D_2O) for water (675). The increase in a chemical reaction by the substitution of D_2O for H_2O has been employed as evidence for $^1O_2$ involvement.

$^1\Delta_gO_2$, the reactive form of $^1O_2$ in solution, is a strong electrophile that reacts with compounds in areas of high electron density to form characteristic, generally oxygenated products. That such reactions can be toxic is indicated by the photodynamic action of dyes. Certain dyes in the presence of light and oxygen are toxic to cells and other targets, and one of the mechanisms proposed is the reaction of the light-sensitized dye with oxygen to form $^1O_2$, which can attack the cell or other target (676). This, together with the chemiluminescence observed when neutrophils are stimulated (677), raised the possibility of the formation of $^1O_2$ by phagocytes and its involvement in microbicidal activity. $^1O_2$ can be formed by a variety of reactions; only three of possible pertinence to the neutrophil are considered here.

Spontaneous Dismutation

It has been proposed that the oxygen formed during the spontaneous dismutation of O_2^- is in part in the excited state, that is $^1O_2$ (678). Although the evidence was initially indirect and dependent on techniques (chemiluminescence, chemical scavengers) that have been criticized due to their lack of specificity, the development of a sensitive spectrometer capable of the detection of the characteristic emission of $^1\Delta_gO_2$ decay at 1,268 nm (679) has allowed the detection of $^1O_2$ in the reaction of water with potassium superoxide suspended in chloroform (680). Although this evidence supports the generation of $^1O_2$ by the spontaneous dismutation of O_2^- under the experimental conditions employed, unequivocal evidence for its formation by spontaneous dismutation under biologic conditions has not been provided. It would seem unlikely that $^1O_2$ formed by dismutation could be responsible for the biologic toxicity of O_2^-, since in one study $^1O_2$ accounted for less than 0.2% of the oxygen produced in the dismutation reaction (681,682).

Haber-Weiss Reaction

The formation of $^1O_2$ by the Haber-Weiss reaction has been proposed (683,684). However, in subsequent studies, $^1O_2$ was found to account for no more than 0.1% of the O_2^- formed by the aerobic xanthine oxidase system and was thus at best a minor product of the Haber-Weiss reaction (685).

Peroxidase-H₂O₂-Halide System

A well-established mechanism for the formation of $^1O_2$ is by the interaction of hypochlorite and H_2O_2:

$$OCl^- + H_2O_2 \rightarrow Cl^- + H_2O_2 + {}^1O_2$$

This reaction emits a weak red chemiluminescence, and spectroscopic studies have established that the metastable product formed is $^1\Delta_gO_2$ (686,687). The formation of $^1O_2$ by the interaction of HOCl and O_2^- also has been proposed (610). The finding that HOCl is the primary product formed by the oxidation of chloride by MPO and H_2O_2 (159,161) has raised the possibility that its reaction with excess H_2O_2 or O_2^- may result in the formation of $^1O_2$.

$^1O_2$ reacts with a number of compounds to yield characteristic products whose formation has been employed for the detection of $^1O_2$. One such reaction is the conversion of 2,5-diphenylfuran to cis-dibenzoylethylene (688). The MPO-H₂O₂-halide system was found to initiate this reaction and $^1O_2$ was implicated by the stimulation of conversion by D_2O and by the inhibition of conversion by the $^1O_2$ quenchers, β-carotene, bilirubin, histidine, and 1,4-diazabicyclo[2,2,2]octane (DABCO) (689). HOCl also converted diphenylfuran to cis-dibenzoylethylene, and this reaction exhibited properties comparable to those of the enzyme system (689). Diphenylfuran conversion by HOCl at acid pH was increased by the addition of chloride but not by H_2O_2, suggesting that the classic reaction for the formation of $^1O_2$, the interaction of hypochlorite and H_2O_2, was not operative. The conversion of diphenylisobenzofuran to o-dibenzoylbenzene by the LPO-H₂O₂-bromide system has also been observed and

an $^1O_2$-dependent mechanism proposed (690,691). HOCl (692–694) or Cl_2 formed by the interaction of HOCl and chloride at acid pH (689) may initiate furan conversion directly, i.e., without $^1O_2$ involvement, thus bringing into question the validity of this reaction for the detection of $^1O_2$ formation by the MPO system.

Early studies had indicated that the MPO-H₂O₂-halide system emits light with the effectiveness of the halides decreasing in the order Br>Cl>I (483,695,696). The pH optimum of the chemiluminescence was 4.4 to 5.0 (696) and the light emission was increased by the addition of zymosan or bacteria (483). Presumably, excitation of surface components on the particle was the primary source of the chemiluminescence. The development of instrumentation for the detection of the infrared emission band at 1,268 nm characteristic of $^1\Delta_gO_2$ decay to the ground state (679,697,698) has renewed interest in the formation of $^1O_2$ by the peroxidase system (reviewed in refs. 699,700). Using this technique, $^1\Delta_gO_2$ has been detected as a product of the interaction of LPO, H_2O_2, and bromide (697,701,702); EPO, H_2O_2, and bromide (699); chloroperoxidase, H_2O_2, and chloride or bromide (701–704); bromoperoxidase, H_2O_2, and bromide (705); and horseradish peroxidase, H_2O_2, and bromide (699). The formation of $^1O_2$ with high efficiency by the MPO-H₂O₂-bromide system also has been observed by this technique (706,707). In contrast, $^1O_2$ formation by the MPO-H₂O₂-chloride system was much less efficient. It was concluded (706) that the conditions required for the formation of $^1O_2$ by PMNs were not physiologic. The poor yield of $^1O_2$ by the MPO-H₂O₂-chloride system was associated with MPO inactivation (706). The finding that ascorbic acid in micromolar quantities protected MPO from inactivation (125) prompted a study of the effect of ascorbic acid on the yield of $^1O_2$ from the MPO-H₂O₂-halide system (708). No increased production was found.

Role in Leukocytes

The formation of $^1O_2$ by intact leukocytes was first proposed by Allen et al. (677) based on the chemiluminescence of stimulated neutrophils. Chemiluminescence indicates the formation of electronically excited states but, without spectral analysis, does not indicate the nature of the excited species. Analysis of the light emitted by stimulated neutrophils revealed broad peak activity with a maximum at about 570 nm, rather than the characteristic spectrum of $^1O_2$ decay (709,710). This suggests that the light emitted by phagocytes is not due primarily to $^1O_2$ decay, but to secondary excitations that could be induced by reaction of a number of the oxidants formed by stimulated leukocytes with cellular constituents. No evidence of $^1O_2$ production by stimulated neutrophils was found using instrumentation that can detect $^1O_2$ emission at 1,268 nm (711).

Another mechanism for the detection of $^1O_2$ formation by phagocytes is by product analysis. A compound that reacts with $^1O_2$ is added to the leukocytes and the product formed by the reaction of that compound with $^1O_2$ is sought. However, the chemical traps for $^1O_2$ are generally nonspecific, leaving open the possibility that the chemical conversion is by another mechanism. Cholesterol is believed to be a specific chemical trap for $^1O_2$ with the product formed, 3β-hydroxy-5α-cholest-6-ene-5-hydroperoxide, being different from that produced by radical oxidation (712). Cholesterol, however, is an inefficient $^1O_2$ scavenger as compared to other less specific traps. Incubation of polystyrene latex microbeads or mineral oil droplets containing ^{14}C-cholesterol with neutrophils or macrophages did not result in the formation of the $^1O_2$ product, leading to the conclusion that $^1O_2$ is at best a very minor product of the respiratory burst of phagocytes (682,713). Recently it has been proposed that $^1O_2$ reacts specifically with 9,10-diphenylanthracene (DPA) to form DPA-endoperoxide and that PMN ingesting beads coated with DPA form $^1O_2$ (714). Under these conditions, up to 19% of the oxygen consumed could be accounted for by the formation of $^1O_2$. This is a very high percentage in view of the lack of success of others in the detection of $^1O_2$ formation. This may be due to the greater sensitivity of the DPA detection method. $^1O_2$ formation by the cell-free MPO-H_2O_2-Cl^- system also was detected, and it was proposed that this was the major pathway by which $^1O_2$ is generated by PMNs stimulated by phagocytosis. The observation that carotenoid-containing wild-type *Sarcina lutea* are less readily killed by neutrophils than are mutant pigmentless mutants (715) was proposed as evidence of $^1O_2$ involvement, since carotenoid pigments are very efficient $^1O_2$ scavengers. However, other interpretations are possible.

EOSINOPHIL

Eosinophils can ingest and kill microorganisms; however, in general they do this less effectively than do neutrophils (716–721), which may be related, in part, to their decreased phagocytic activity (716,717,720–722). The primary cytotoxic role of this cell thus may be against extracellular targets such as helminths and tumor cells.

Eosinophils have potent cytotoxic constituents in cytoplasmic granules (723) and, like neutrophils, respond to stimulation with degranulation and with a respiratory burst forming O_2^- (724–726), H_2O_2 (270,716,720,724, 725), and possibly $\cdot OH$ (618,727) and $^1O_2$ (728). Among the granule components are a group of basic proteins whose properties and function have been extensively studied (723) (see chapter by Rosenberg). Their cytotoxic activity is independent of oxygen and thus will not be considered here.

Respiratory Burst

With most stimuli, the respiratory burst of eosinophils is greater than that of equivalent numbers of neutrophils comparably stimulated (716,720,724,725,729–732). An NADPH oxidase similar to that present in neutrophils appears to be involved (716,724,726). NADPH oxidase activity was reported to be three to six times greater in eosinophils than in comparable neutrophil preparations (724), and eosinophils have a cytochrome b_{558} concentration that is twice that of neutrophils or monocytes (733). As with neutrophils, oxygen does not appear to be required for phagocytosis by eosinophils (718), but rather is utilized for the generation of toxic oxygen metabolites.

Eosinophil Peroxidase (EPO)-H_2O_2-Halide System

The eosinophil is exceptionally rich in peroxidase (reviewed in ref. 734). Cytochemical studies have localized the peroxidase in the matrix of the specific granules of the mature eosinophil surrounding the central crystalline core (735). These granules form during the myelocyte stage of eosinophil development, where peroxidase activity can be detected in the cisternae of the rough endoplasmic reticulum and Golgi complex, as well as in the developing granules (735). Following phagocytosis, peroxidase is detected in the phagosome surrounding the ingested organism (736). Eosinophils adherent to a target too large to be ingested release their granule components including peroxidase extracellularly, and the peroxidase can be detected on the target cell surface (234,737). The peroxidase can also be released extracellularly by soluble stimuli (371), and peroxidase-containing granules, released by lysis of eosinophils in tissues, are taken up by macrophages (738,739).

EPO has been purified from rat (740–742), guinea pig (743), horse (744), and human (745–749) eosinophils. The human enzyme is a glycoprotein of approximately 77 kd that can be separated into a large (approximately 50 kd) and small (10–15 kd) subunit under reducing conditions (745,746,750,751), with the carbohydrate associated with the large subunit and consisting of mannose and *N*-acetylglucosamine residues (751). The heme prosthetic group of EPO is a protoporphyrin (750,752), which is similar to that of LPO in optical and EPR spectra (750,752), but which differs to some degree from LPO in its resonance Raman spectrum (753). The EPO gene has been cloned and the predicted amino acid sequence revealed a precursor protein of 79,551 dalton, consisting of a prosequence at the NH_2-terminus joined to the light subunit (12,712 daltons) and then the heavy subunit (53,011 daltons) (754). Considerable homology with other peroxidases was observed, suggesting a peroxidase multigene family.

EPO, like MPO, has toxic properties when combined with H_2O_2 and a halide. In early studies, human eosinophil granules were found to be candidacidal (258) and sonicates bactericidal (755) when combined with H_2O_2 and iodide but not chloride, and this was supported by the finding that EPO did not catalyze the oxidative deamination and decarboxylation of amino acids when combined with H_2O_2 and chloride under conditions in which MPO was active (755). However, when purified EPO was employed, toxic activity was observed with chloride as well as iodide or bromide as the halide (234,269,744,756), although chloride was less effective than iodide or bromide with EPO than with MPO. The effect of chloride was more evident when the pH was lowered (234,744,757,758).

The relative ineffectiveness of chloride with EPO as compared to MPO raises the question of the physiologic halide for an EPO-mediated antimicrobial system. Chloride at physiologic concentration (0.1 M) has little effect at neutral pH but is effective at this concentration when the pH is lowered to 5.0. Since the pH within the phagosome (or in the space between an adherent eosinophil and a target too large to be ingested) may fall to this level, there may be a contribution by chloride to the effective halide pool in these locations. Iodide is the most effective halide on a molar basis; however, its concentration in biologic fluids is very low (<1 mg/100 ml), suggesting that its contribution is small. Bromide is nearly as effective as iodide in the EPO-H_2O_2-halide system and is present in biologic fluids in considerably higher concentrations. Thus, the level of bromide in blood ranges from 130 to 810 mg/100 ml and that of urine from 213 to 520 mg/100 ml (148). In one study (759) bromide was effective as a component of the EPO-mediated antimicrobial system at pH 5.0 at a concentration of 8 mg/100 ml and at pH 7.0 at 80 mg/100 ml, raising the possibility that bromide is the physiologic halide. Strong support for bromide involvement in intact cells comes from the finding that intact human eosinophils stimulated by PMA or opsonized zymosan preferentially used bromide to generate a halogenating oxidant (presumably hypobromous acid) when both bromide and chloride were present in physiologic concentrations (760,761). It has also been proposed that thiocyanate is the major (pseudo) halide for the EPO system (762). At least 25% to 35% of the oxygen consumed by stimulated eosinophils can be accounted for by the formation of halogenating species (761).

The cell-free EPO-H_2O_2-halide system is toxic to bacteria, including E. coli (744,755,758), S. aureus (755,759), L. pneumophila (253), or M. leprae (251); fungi (258); viruses including HIV-1 (763); the schistosomula of S. mansoni (234,269); the newborn larvae of T. spiralis (271,756); Trypanosoma cruzi (764,765); Toxoplasma gondii (766); tumor cells (757); human nasal epithelium (767); and mast cells (386). EPO is a highly basic protein that binds avidly to negatively charged surfaces with retention of peroxidatic activity. Among the surfaces to which it binds is that of the target cell. If H_2O_2 and a halide are added to target cells with surface-bound EPO, the target cells are rapidly killed under conditions in which control cells without bound peroxidase are unaf-

fected. This has been observed with S. aureus (759), L. pneumophila (253), T. gondii (766), T. cruzi (764), schistosomula of S. mansoni (234), and tumor cells (235) as the target. The toxicity of the EPO-H_2O_2-halide system is strongly inhibited by protein when the EPO is free in solution due to competition with the target cell for the toxic products of the peroxidase system. Protein is much less inhibitory when EPO is bound to the target cell surface (234,235), presumably due to proximity of toxic oxidant production to critical sites on the membrane. The toxic effect of intact neutrophils (234) or macrophages (see below) is considerably increased when EPO is bound to the target cell surface due to a more efficient utilization of the H_2O_2 generated by the phagocyte.

EPO binds to and is internalized by neutrophils (768), lymphocytes, monocytes, and endothelial cells (769), and thus may contribute to the toxic activity of these cells. The binding of EPO to neutrophils results in the reversible inhibition of EPO activity and in increased neutrophil aggregation and adherence to endothelial cells (770). EPO also binds to the negatively charged mast cell granule to form a complex that retains toxic activity when combined with H_2O_2 and a halide (771); indeed, the bactericidal (771) and tumoricidal (772) activity of the complex is greater than that of free EPO when standardized to the same guaiacol units of peroxidase activity. The finding that H_2O_2 alone at high concentration and the EPO-H_2O_2-halide system at lower H_2O_2 concentrations can initiate mast cell secretion with the release of mast cell granules (386) raises the possibility that, in an inflammatory lesion, mast cell granules released by the EPO system bind EPO with potentiation of their toxic activity. Mast cells contain a small amount of peroxidase in their cytoplasmic granules (367), which may be synthesized by the cell (773) or acquired by endocytosis of exogenous EPO (774,775). EPO binds to the surface of guinea pig basophils and cloned mouse mast cells and is internalized by a vesicular transport system and incorporated into cytoplasmic granules (774). Mast cells, when incubated with H_2O_2 and a halide, were toxic to tumor cells (772) or schistosomula (776), and the mechanism proposed was the initiation of mast cell secretion by H_2O_2 and the reaction of the endogenous peroxidase of the mast cell granule with H_2O_2 and a halide to form a toxic system.

When eosinophils adhere to a target, they discharge their granule contents, which include EPO (234,737,777) as well as a number of basic proteins (723). Eosinophils, when stimulated, generate H_2O_2 in large amounts and thus the interaction of EPO and H_2O_2 with a halide at the target cell surface might be anticipated. Support for the involvement of the peroxidase system in the toxicity of eosinophils against HIV-1 (763), tumor cells (757), the schistosomula of S. mansoni (270), endothelial cells (778), and myoblasts (779) has been provided, although other studies have emphasized the involvement of other basic granule proteins (723). Infusion of EPO, followed by H_2O_2 and bromide into the left ventricle of the isolated rat heart, rapidly resulted in damage suggestive of congestive heart failure (778). Although the basic proteins of eosinophils have well-recognized direct toxic properties, the major basic protein (MBP) of eosinophils can also scavenge the toxic product of the EPO-H_2O_2-halide system and in this way inhibit EPO-mediated killing (271). A comparison of the toxicity of EPO (when combined with H_2O_2 and a halide) and granule basic proteins suggested that EPO contributed to a considerably greater degree than did other granule basic proteins to the total toxic activity of the granule components (780).

Hydroxyl Radicals

Eosinophils also can form ·OH in small amounts via an EPO-dependent mechanism in which chloride or bromide is oxidized to the corresponding hypohalous acid that reacts with O_2^- to form ·OH (727).

Singlet Oxygen

The formation of small amounts of $^1O_2$ by PMA-stimulated human eosinophils has been detected by 1,268-nm chemiluminescence, and the involvement of the EPO-H_2O_2-bromide system in its production has been proposed (728).

MONONUCLEAR PHAGOCYTES

Mononuclear phagocytes are a continuum of changing cells, beginning with bone marrow precursors and continuing through the blood monocyte to the fully developed tissue macrophage. The latter vary in their morphologic and functional characteristics, depending on their location and state of activation.

All mononuclear phagocytes respond to a greater or lesser degree to stimulation with a burst of oxygen consumption. The mechanism of the respiratory burst in mononuclear phagocytes appears to be comparable to that of neutrophils. As with neutrophils and eosinophils, the respiratory burst appears to contribute oxidants required for optimum microbicidal activity. The role of toxic oxygen metabolites in the effector function of macrophages has been reviewed (781–783).

Monocyte

Of the mononuclear phagocytes, the blood monocyte most closely resembles the neutrophil in its antimicrobial systems. Monocytes respond to stimulation with a brisk respiratory burst, although its magnitude is less than that of equivalent numbers of neutrophils comparably stimulated (784). In one study in which paired measurements were made using monocytes and neutrophils from the same blood sample, oxygen consumption and H_2O_2 pro-

duction by opsonized zymosan-stimulated monocytes were 39% and 19%, respectively, of that of similarly treated neutrophils (785). The blood monocyte contains a peroxidase in cytoplasmic granules that is identical to that of the MPO of neutrophils, as indicated by comparable structural and functional properties (786) and by the absence of a granule peroxidase from both neutrophils and monocytes in hereditary MPO deficiency in which there is a genetic absence of this enzyme (456). However, monocytes contain less MPO than do neutrophils. Thus, the average number of peroxidase-positive granules in human monocytes is 34 per thin section (787) as compared to 75 per thin section in human neutrophils (45), and quantitative analysis revealed approximately three times as much MPO in neutrophils as in monocytes (786,788).

The MPO of monocytes is released into the phagosome following particle ingestion (789), where it can react with H_2O_2 and a halide to form a microbicidal system. Thus, iodination, which is a measure of the interaction of MPO, H_2O_2, and iodide, occurs in monocytes, although its level is less than that of comparably stimulated neutrophils (487,786,788,790). Further, monocytes, when stimulated, form a chlorinating species, presumably HOCl (791). The involvement of the MPO-H_2O_2-halide system in the killing of *C. albicans* (790,792) and *Aspergillus fumigatus* (793) by human monocytes was suggested by the decreased fungicidal activity induced by peroxidase inhibitors or the substitution of MPO-deficient for normal monocytes. However, MPO-independent and nonoxidative fungicidal mechanisms were also detected in monocytes. *T. gondii* were killed at a slower rate by MPO-deficient monocytes than by normal cells, and this defect was abolished by the introduction of EPO into the phagosome bound to the surface of the organisms (766). In contrast, the toxoplasmacidal defect of CGD monocytes was unaffected by surface-bound EPO. As with neutrophils, the respiratory burst of monocytes as measured by O_2^- production or by iodination in the presence of added MPO was greater in MPO-deficient than in normal monocytes (487).

Monocytes are also toxic to extracellular targets such as erythrocytes or tumor cells. In some instances, toxic oxygen species do not appear to be major contributors to the toxicity (794–796), whereas a contribution by oxygen metabolites has been proposed in other studies. The toxic oxygen metabolites primarily involved have varied with the experimental conditions; they include products of the MPO-H_2O_2-halide system (286,797), H_2O_2 operating in the absence of MPO (798), a combination of O_2^- and H_2O_2 (798,799), ·OH (308), or an unidentified oxygen product (795,800).

Macrophage

Monocytes that transform into macrophages develop multiple synthetic and secretory functions (801); however, this is associated with a decrease in microbicidal potency. Blood monocytes maintained in culture for several days to weeks acquire many of the properties of tissue macrophages and these functional changes therefore can be studied under controlled conditions *in vitro*. Thus, transformation of human monocytes to macrophages in culture results in a marked decline in antimicrobial activity against a variety of pathogens, including *Listeria monocytogenes* (802), *Cryptococcus neoformans* (254), *T. gondii* (803), *L. donovani* (804), type 1 herpes simplex virus (805), and HIV-1 (797). This presents a problem to the host, since these and other organisms may survive and replicate in macrophages, producing disease.

The basis for the decreased potency of macrophages is, in part, a decline in oxygen-dependent mechanisms of toxicity. Blood monocytes retain their granule peroxidase for a time following passage into the extravascular space (806), and this peroxidase is released into the phagosome following particle ingestion (789). Since many of the macrophages in a granulomatous lesion are relatively recent immigrants (807,808), their granule peroxidase may contribute to their antimicrobial effect. However, as tissue monocytes mature into macrophages *in vivo* (806) or *in vitro* (809–812), their granule peroxidase is lost.

The magnitude of the respiratory burst also decreases markedly when monocytes mature into macrophages. This is indicated by the weak respiratory burst of resident macrophages (813,814), and by the sharp decline in the respiratory burst when monocytes differentiate into macrophages *in vitro* (804,810,815,816). Some studies have indicated an increase in the respiratory burst at day 3 of culture (810,815,817) prior to the sharp decline with continued culture (810,815). The decreased potency is presumably due in part to the decreased respiratory burst and MPO content of the mature resident macrophage.

Activation is a process by which macrophages develop morphologic and metabolic changes associated with heightened microbicidal activity following exposure to activating agents for periods generally measured in days (see chapter by Gordon). In contrast, stimulation is an acute process, generally measured in minutes, in which phagocytes respond to phagocytosis or a soluble stimulus such as PMA with a respiratory burst and degranulation. The respiratory burst of resident macrophages in response to stimulation is increased severalfold when the macrophages are activated *in vivo* (813,814). Activation of cultured monocyte-derived macrophages also can be induced *in vitro* by the addition of granulocyte-macrophage colony-stimulating factor (GM-CSF) (818–822), tumor necrosis factor-α (TNF-α) (823,824), and particularly interferon-γ (IFN-γ) (825–827), whereas a number of other cytokines are ineffective (828). In one study, stimulated human monocytes were viricidal to HIV-1 through the release of the components of the MPO-H_2O_2-chloride system (797). When the monocytes were maintained in culture, the viricidal activity was lost

unless MPO was added to 3- to 9-day monocyte-derived macrophages, whereas loss of viricidal activity by 12-day monocyte-derived macrophages was not reversed by added MPO unless the cells were pretreated with IFN-γ. The respiratory burst of activated macrophages can be suppressed (deactivation) by exposure of the cells to a factor in the culture medium of a wide variety of malignant and some nonmalignant cells (829,830). The oxygen-dependent microbicidal activity of mature activated macrophages may be due to the formation of H_2O_2, ·OH, and/or $^1O_2$. The role of nitrogen oxides is considered in the chapter by Moilanen et al.

H_2O_2

H_2O_2 has been implicated in the toxic activity of macrophages. Thus, *Leishmania* promastigotes are readily killed by resident mouse peritoneal macrophages, and this leishmanicidal activity is inhibited by catalase or glucose deprivation (which decreases H_2O_2 production by macrophages) but not by SOD or by the ·OH scavengers mannitol or benzoate, thus implicating H_2O_2 (831). Similar findings were obtained when the lymphokine-treated macrophage cell line J744G8 was employed (832). Sensitivity to H_2O_2 is related to the level of H_2O_2 scavenging enzymes. Thus, *Leishmania* promastigotes, which are considerably more sensitive to H_2O_2 than *T. gondii,* contain lower levels of catalase and glutathione peroxidase (831). Further, *L. donovani* amastigotes are more resistant to H_2O_2 and to the toxic activity of macrophages than are promastigotes and have correspondingly higher levels of catalase (833). The killing of *L. donovani* promastigotes and amastigotes by human monocyte-derived macrophages stimulated with lymphokine (IFN-γ) also correlated with H_2O_2 production by the cells (804,826,834). However, similarly treated cells from patients with CGD retained partial leishmanicidal activity, indicating a contribution by oxygen-independent mechanisms.

T. cruzi trypomastigotes survive in normal mouse peritoneal macrophages but are killed by macrophages activated *in vitro* or *in vivo* by lymphokines, and this trypanocidal activity correlated well with the amount of H_2O_2 formed on stimulation of the macrophages with PMA (835). A variant macrophage cell line defective in the respiratory burst was unable to kill epimastigotes of *T. cruzi* unless glucose oxidase, an enzyme that generates H_2O_2 without an O_2^- intermediate, was introduced into the cell covalently bound to zymosan particles (836).

H_2O_2 has also been identified as the toxic species responsible for the killing of tumor cells by activated macrophages stimulated by PMA (237,837,838). Although an oxidative mechanism appeared to be involved in the lysis of tumor cells by activated macrophages in the presence of antitumor cell antibody, H_2O_2 was not definitively established as the product responsible, since catalase was not inhibitory (839). However, the scavenging of H_2O_2 by the glutathione oxidation-reduction cycle in murine tumor cells is important to their susceptibility to lysis by macrophages plus anti-tumor cell antibody, as well as by PMA-triggered macrophages and by H_2O_2 generated by glucose oxidase (840–842). Some human tumor cells use the glutathione redox system as the primary defense against H_2O_2, whereas others appeared to utilize catalase (843). The capacity to secrete H_2O_2 can be dissociated from the tumor cell cytolytic activity of activated macrophages under some conditions (844).

Since mature tissue macrophages in general lack a granule peroxidase, they cannot amplify the toxicity of H_2O_2 through the release of this enzyme into the phagosome (or extracellularly) by degranulation. Many resident macrophages contain cytochemically identifiable peroxidase in the perinuclear cisternae, rough endoplasmic reticulum and, in some instances, the Golgi lamellae (reviewed in refs. 845,846). Further, mononuclear phagocytes that do not contain a peroxidase in the endoplasmic reticulum can develop a peroxidase there transiently when the cells adhere to a surface in vitro (845,847,848). The nature of this peroxidase is unknown. It is not MPO, since it appears in the endoplasmic reticulum of adherent monocytes from patients with hereditary MPO deficiency (845,849). The release of prostanoids corresponded to the appearance of the peroxidase, raising the possibility that it is associated with arachidonic acid metabolism (850). The peroxidase of the endoplasmic reticulum is not packaged into granules, nor is it released into the phagosome (789), suggesting that it is not involved in microbicidal activity. Although catalase generally inhibits H_2O_2-dependent microbicidal systems, it can be microbicidal when the pH is low (i.e. 4.5), the H_2O_2 is maintained at low steady-state concentrations and iodide (or thyroxine) is added as the halide (851,852). Catalase, present in high concentration in rabbit alveolar macrophages (853), is released in part into the phagosome (854), and granule preparations from these cells are bactericidal at acid pH when combined with iodide and low levels of H_2O_2 (855). This raises the possibility that catalase may serve a microbicidal function in these cells. However, procedures that decreased the catalase content of rabbit alveolar macrophages did not decrease their bactericidal activity (852,856), suggesting that catalase is either present in considerable excess or is not involved in microbicidal activity.

Mature macrophages can acquire peroxidase by endocytosis, and this exogenous peroxidase could, theoretically, greatly amplify the toxicity of the small amount of H_2O_2 formed by these cells. Pinocytic uptake of fluid phase peroxidase (52,436,857,858) can occur via reaction with the mannose receptor (52), and peroxidase released from adjacent neutrophils, eosinophils, or monocytes in particulate form can be taken up by phagocytosis (738,739,858–862). Phagocytic cell peroxidases, especially EPO, are strongly basic proteins that bind avidly to the surface of microorganisms and mammalian cells. Peroxidase-coated targets are killed much more readily by macrophages than are uncoated targets through an H_2O_2-dependent mechanism. This has been observed with S. aureus (759), T. gondii (766), T. cruzi (764), and tumor cells (235). Alternatively the uptake of peroxidase by macrophages may serve to clear a potentially toxic enzyme from the extracellular fluid (52,858).

Hydroxyl Radicals

Hydroxyl radicals have been implicated in the toxic activity of macrophages against some targets. Thus, T. gondii are rich in catalase and glutathione peroxidase and are relatively resistant to destruction by H_2O_2 (863). T. gondii, however, are killed by the xanthine-xanthine oxidase system (666), by macrophages from immune mice chronically infected with T. gondii or from these mice immune-boosted with Toxoplasma (864), and by normal macrophages cocultivated in vitro with lymphokine and heart infusion broth (865). This toxicity is inhibited by catalase, SOD, and the ·OH scavengers mannitol and benzoate, thus implicating ·OH. Similarly, human normal or lymphokine-activated monocyte-derived macrophages kill T. gondii predominantly by an oxygen-dependent mechanism that is inhibited by glucose deprivation or by the addition of catalase, SOD, or mannitol (866). However, studies with CGD monocytes and macrophages indicated the presence in these cells of an oxygen-independent toxoplasmacidal system as well (826,866). Like neutrophils, monocytes or monocyte-derived macrophages, when stimulated, did not appear to generate ·OH, by the Haber-Weiss reaction, unless exogenous iron was added (867). When iron was added, ·OH production was more sustained than that observed with similarly treated neutrophils (867). Monocytes however, like neutrophils, can form small amounts of ·OH by an MPO-dependent reaction (613).

Singlet Oxygen

Rat peritoneal macrophages adherent to DPA-coated coverslips were reported to generate $^1O_2$ as measured by the formation of DPA-endoperoxide (868). This reaction was inhibited by SOD and an $^1O_2$ quencher histidine, suggesting that the intracellular production of $^1O_2$ by stimulated macrophages is by an O_2^--dependent mechanism. Similar findings were observed when the O_2^--generating xanthine oxidase system was used instead of macrophages.

ACKNOWLEDGMENTS

The studies from our laboratory reviewed here were supported by U.S. Public Health Service grant AI07763.

The excellent secretarial assistance of Ms. Peggy Sue O'Brien in the preparation of the manuscript is gratefully acknowledged.

REFERENCES

1. Klebanoff SJ, Clark RA. *The neutrophil: function and clinical disorders.* Amsterdam: North-Holland, 1978.
2. Hurst JK, Barrette WC Jr. Leukocytic oxygen activation and microbicidal oxidative toxins. *Crit Rev Biochem Mol Biol* 1989;24:271–328.
3. Winterbourn CC. Neutrophil oxidants: production and reactions. In: Das DK, Essman WB eds. *Oxygen radicals: systemic events and disease processes.* Basel: Karger, 1990:31–70.
4. Mandell GL. Bactericidal activity of aerobic and anaerobic polymorphonuclear neutrophils. *Infect Immun* 1974;9:337–341.
5. Vel WAC, Namavar F, Verweij A, Marian JJ, Pubben ANB, MacLaren DM. Killing capacity of human polymorphonuclear leukocytes in aerobic and anaerobic conditions. *J Med Microbiol* 1984;18:173–180.
6. Quie PG, White JG, Holmes B, Good RA. *In vitro* bactericidal capacity of human polymorphonuclear leukocytes: diminished activity in chronic granulomatous disease of childhood. *J Clin Invest* 1967;46:668–679.
7. Holmes B, Page AR, Good RA. Studies of the metabolic activity of leukocytes from patients with a genetic abnormality of phagocytic function. *J Clin Invest* 1967;46:1422–1432.
8. Babior BM, Kipnes RS, Curnutte JT. Biological defense mechanisms. The production by leukocytes of superoxide, a potential bactericidal agent. *J Clin Invest* 1973;52:741–744.
9. Ilan YA, Czapski G, Meisel D. The one-electron transfer redox potentials of free radicals. 1. The oxygen/superoxide system. *Biochim Biophys Acta* 1976;430:209–224.
10. Wood PM. The redox potential of the system oxygen-superoxide. *FEBS Lett* 1974;44:22–24.
11. Behar D, Czapski G, Rabani J, Dorfman LM, Schwarz HA. The acid dissociation constant and decay kinetics of the perhydroxyl radical. *J Phys Chem* 1970;74:3209–3213.
12. Bielski BHJ, Allen AO. Mechanism of the disproportionation of superoxide radicals. *J Phys Chem* 1977;81:1048–1050.
13. Fridovich I. Superoxide dismutases. An adaptation to a paramagnetic gas. *J Biol Chem* 1989;264:7761–7764.
14. Rabani J, Klug D, Fridovich I. Decay of the HO_2 and O_2 radicals catalyzed by superoxide dismutase. A pulse radiolytic investigation. *Isr J Chem* 1972;10:1095–1106.
15. Rest RF, Spitznagel JK. Subcellular distribution of superoxide dismutases in human neutrophils. Influence of myeloperoxidase on the measurement of superoxide dismutase activity. *Biochem J* 1977;166:145–153.
16. Roos D, Hamers MN, van Zwieten R, Weening RS. Acidification of the phagocytic vacuole: a possible defect in chronic granulomatous disease? *Adv Host Def Mech* 1983;3:145–193.
17. Segal AW, Geisow M, Garcia R, Harper A, Miller R. The respiratory burst of phagocytic cells is associated with a rise in vacuolar pH. *Nature* 1981;290:406–409.
18. Cech P, Lehrer RI. Phagolysosomal pH of human neutrophils. *Blood* 1984;63:88–95.
19. Fee JA. Is superoxide toxic? *Dev Biochem* 1980;11B:41–48.
20. Sawyer DT, Valentine JS. How super is superoxide. *Acc Chem Res* 1981;14:393–400.
21. Bielski BHJ, Arudi RL, Sutherland MW. A study of the reactivity of HO_2/O_2 with unsaturated fatty acids. *J Biol Chem* 1983;258:4759–4761.
22. Gebicki JM, Bielski BHJ. Comparison of the capacities of the perhydroxyl and the superoxide radicals to initiate chain oxidation of linoleic acid. *J Am Chem Soc* 1981;103:7020–7022.
23. Gennaro R, Romeo D. The release of superoxide anion from granulocytes: effect of inhibitors of anion permeability. *Biochem Biophys Res Commun* 1979;88:44–49.
24. Lynch RE, Fridovich I. Effects of superoxide on the erythrocyte membrane. *J Biol Chem* 1978;253:1838–1845.
25. Lynch RE, Fridovich I. Permeation of the erythrocyte stroma by superoxide radical. *J Biol Chem* 1978;253:4697–4699.
26. Roos D, Eckmann CM, Yazdanbakhsh M, Hamers MN, deBoer M. Excretion of superoxide by phagocytes measured with cytochrome c entrapped in resealed erythrocyte ghosts. *J Biol Chem* 1984;259:1770–1775.
27. Weiss SJ. Neutrophil-mediated methemoglobin formation in the erythrocyte. The role of superoxide and hydrogen peroxide. *J Biol Chem* 1982;257:2947–2953.
28. Halliwell B, Gutteridge JMC. *Free radicals in biology and medicine.* Oxford: Oxford University Press, 1985.
29. Iyer GYN, Islam DMF, Quastel JH. Biochemical aspects of phagocytosis. *Nature* 1961;192:535–541.
30. Weening RS, Wever R, Roos D. Quantitative aspects of the production of superoxide radicals by phagocytizing human granulocytes. *J Lab Clin Med* 1975;85:245–252.
31. Curnutte JT, Tauber AI. Failure to detect superoxide in human neutrophils stimulated with latex particles. *Pediatr Res* 1983;17:281–284.
32. Green TR, Wu DE. The NADPH:O_2 oxidoreductase of human neutrophils. Stoichiometry of univalent and divalent reduction of O_2. *J Biol Chem* 1986;261:6010–6015.
33. Green TR, Pratt KL. A reassessment of the product specificity of the NADPH:O_2 oxidoreductase of human neutrophils. *Biochem Biophys Res Commun* 1987;142:213–220.
34. Follin P, Dahlgren C. Altered O_2/H_2O_2 production ratio by *in vitro* and *in vivo* primed human neutrophils. *Biochem Biophys Res Commun* 1990;167:970–976.
35. Hoffstein ST, Gennaro DE, Manzi RM. Neutrophils may directly synthesize both H_2O_2 and O_2- since surface stimuli induce their release in stimulus-specific ratios. *Inflammation* 1985;9:425–437.
36. Frimer AA, Forman A, Borg DC. H_2O_2-diffusion through lysosomes. *Isr J Chem* 1983;23:442–445.
37. Baehner RL, Boxer LA, Allen JM, Davis J. Autooxidation as a basis for altered function by polymorphonuclear leukocytes. *Blood* 1977;50:327–335.
38. Tsan M. Phorbol myristate acetate induced neutrophil autotoxicity. *J Cell Physiol* 1980;105:327–334.
39. Tsan M, Denison RC. Phorbol myristate acetate-induced neutrophil autotoxicity. A comparison with H_2O_2 toxicity. *Inflammation* 1980;4:371–380.
40. Roos D, Weening RS, Wyss SR, Aebi HE. Protection of human neutrophils by endogenous catalase. Studies with cells from catalase-deficient individuals. *J Clin Invest* 1980;65:1515–1522.
41. Voetman AA, Roos D. Endogenous catalase protects human blood phagocytes against oxidative damage by extracellularly generated hydrogen peroxide. *Blood* 1980;56:846–852.
42. Roos D, Weening RS, Voetman AA, et al. Protection of phagocytic leukocytes by endogenous glutathione. Studies in a family with glutathione reductase deficiency. *Blood* 1979;53:851–866.
43. Spielberg SP, Boxer LA, Oliver JM, Allen JM, Schulman JD. Oxidative damage to neutrophils in glutatione synthetase deficiency. *Br J Haematol* 1979;42:215–223.
44. Klebanoff SJ. Myeloperoxidase: occurrence and biological function. In: Everse J, Everse KE, Grisham MB, eds. *Peroxidases in chemistry and biology,* vol 1. Boca Raton: CRC Press, 1991:1–35.
45. Bainton DF, Ullyot JL, Farquhar MG. The development of neutrophilic polymorphonuclear leukocytes in human bone marrow. Origin and content of azurophil and specific granules. *J Exp Med* 1971;134:907–934.
46. Kinkade JMJ, Pember SO, Barnes KC, Shapira R, Spitznagel JK, Martin LE. Differential distribution of distinct forms of myeloperoxidase in different azurophilic granule subpopulations from human neutrophils. *Biochem Biophys Res Commun* 1983;114:296–303.
47. Spitznagel JK, Dalldorf FG, Leffell MS, et al. Character of azurophil and specific granules purified from human polymorphonuclear leukocytes. *Lab Invest* 1974;30:774–785.
48. West BC, Rosenthal AS, Gelb NA, Kimball HR. Separation and characterization of human neutrophil granules. *Am J Pathol* 1974;77:41–66.
49. Bradley PP, Christensen RD, Rothstein G. Cellular and extracellular myeloperoxidase in pyogenic inflammation. *Blood* 1982;60:618–622.
50. Edwards SW, Nurcombe HL, Hart CA. Oxidative inactivation of myeloperoxidase released from human neutrophils. *Biochem J* 1987;245:925–928.
51. King CC, Jefferson MM, Thomas EL. Secretion and inactivation of myeloperoxidase by isolated neutrophils. *J Leukoc Biol* 1997;61:293–302.

52. Shepherd VL, Hoidal JR. Clearance of neutrophil-derived myeloperoxidase by the macrophage mannose receptor. *Am J Respir Cell Mol Biol* 1990;2:335–340.

53. Agner K. Verdoperoxidase. A ferment isolated from leucocytes. *Acta Chem Scand* 1941;2(suppl 8):1–62.

54. Rohrer GF, von Wartburg JP, Aebi H. Myeloperoxidase aus menschlichen Leukocyten. I. Isolierung und Charakterisierung des Enzyms. *Biochem Z* 1966;344:478–491.

55. Schultz J, Kaminker K. Myeloperoxidase of the leucocyte of normal human blood. 1. Content and localization. *Arch Biochem Biophys* 1962;96:465–467.

56. Chang KS, Trujillo JM, Cook RG, Stass SA. Human myeloperoxidase gene: molecular cloning and expression in leukemic cells. *Blood* 1986;68:1411–1414.

57. Yamada M, Hur S, Hashinaka K, et al. Isolation and characterization of a cDNA coding for human myeloperoxidase. *Arch Biochem Biophys* 1987;255:147–155.

58. Morishita K, Kubota N, Asano S, Kaziro Y, Nagata S. Molecular cloning and characterization of cDNA for human myeloperoxidase. *J Biol Chem* 1987;262:3844–3851.

59. Johnson KR, Nauseef WM, Care A, et al. Characterization of cDNA clones for human myeloperoxidase: predicted amino acid sequence and evidence for multiple mRNA species. *Nucleic Acids Res* 1987;15:2013–2028.

60. Weil SC, Rosner GL, Reid MS, et al. cDNA cloning of human myeloperoxidase: decrease in myeloperoxidase mRNA upon induction of HL-60 cells. *Proc Natl Acad Sci USA* 1987;84:2057–2061.

61. Venturelli D, Bittenbender S, Rovera G. Sequence of the murine myeloperoxidase (MPO) gene. *Nucleic Acids Res* 1989;17:7987–7988.

62. Hosokawa Y, Kawaguchi R, Hikiji K, et al. Cloning and characterization of four types of cDNA encoding myeloperoxidase from human monocytic leukemia cell line, SKM-1. *Leukemia* 1993;7:441–445.

63. Johnson KR, Nauseef WM. Molecular biology of MPO. In: Everse J, Everse KE, Grisham MB, eds. *Peroxidases in chemistry and biology,* vol 1. Boca Raton: CRC Press, 1991:63–81.

64. Chang KS, Schroeder W, Siciliano MJ, et al. The localization of the human myeloperoxidase gene is in close proximity to the translocation breakpoint in acute promyelocytic leukemia. *Leukemia* 1987;1:458–462.

65. Inazawa J, Inoue K, Nishigaki H, et al. Assignment of the human myeloperoxidase gene (MPO) to bands q21.3—>q23 of chromosome 17. *Cytogenet Cell Genet* 1989;50:135–136.

66. Zaki SR, Austin GE, Chan WC, et al. Chromosomal localization of the human myeloperoxidase gene by *in situ* hybridization using oligonucleotide probes. *Genes Chromosomes Cancer* 1990;2:266–270.

67. Nauseef WM, Olsson I, Arnljots K. Biosynthesis and processing of myeloperoxidase—a marker for myeloid cell differentiation. *Eur J Haematol* 1988;40:97–110.

68. Stromberg J, Persson A, Olsson I. The processing and intracellular transport of myeloperoxidase. Modulation by lysosomotropic agents and monensin. *Eur J Cell Biol* 1985;39:424–431.

69. Nauseef WM. Myeloperoxidase biosynthesis by a human promyelocytic leukemia cell line: insight into myeloperoxidase deficiency. *Blood* 1986;67:865–872.

70. Nauseef WM, McCormick SJ, Clark RA. Calreticulin functions as a molecular chaperone in the biosynthesis of myeloperoxidase. *J Biol Chem* 1995;270:4741–4747.

71. Nauseef WM, McCormick S, Yi H. Roles of heme insertion and the mannose-6-phosphate receptor in processing of the human myeloid lysosomal enzyme, myeloperoxidase. *Blood* 1992;80:2622–2633.

72. Pinnix IB, Guzman GS, Bonkovsky HL, Zaki SR, Kinkade JMJ. The post-translational processing of myeloperoxidase is regulated by the availability of heme. *Arch Biochem Biophys* 1994;312:447–458.

73. Nauseef WM, Cogley M, McCormick S. Effect of the R569W missense mutation on the biosynthesis of myeloperoxidase. *J Biol Chem* 1996;271:9546–9549.

74. Schultz J. Myeloperoxidase. In: Sbarra AJ, Strauss RR, eds. *The reticuloendothelial system. A comprehensive treatise. 2. Biochemistry and metabolism.* New York: Plenum Press, 1980:231–254.

75. Hur S, Toda H, Yamada M. Isolation and characterization of an unprocessed extracellular myeloperoxidase in HL-60 cell cultures. *J Biol Chem* 1989;264:8542–8548.

76. Yamada M, Hur S, Toda H. Isolation and characterization of extracel-

lular myeloperoxidase precursor in HL-60 cell cultures. *Biochem Biophys Res Commun* 1990;166:852–859.

77. Cully J, Harrach B, Hauser H, et al. Synthesis and localization of myeloperoxidase protein in transfected BHK cells. *Exp Cell Res* 1989;180:440–450.

78. Moguilevsky N, Garcia-Quintana L, Jacquet A, et al. Structural and biological properties of human recombinant myeloperoxidase produced by Chinese hamster ovary cell lines. *Eur J Biochem* 1991;197:605–614.

79. Taylor KL, Uhlinger DJ, Kinkade JMJ. Expression of recombinant myeloperoxidase using a baculovirus expression system. *Biochem Biophys Res Commun* 1992;187:1572–1578.

80. Andrews PC, Krinsky NI. The reductive cleavage of myeloperoxidase in half, producing enzymatically active hemi-myeloperoxidase. *J Biol Chem* 1981;256:4211–4218.

81. Harrison JE, Pabalan S, Schultz J. The subunit structure of crystalline canine myeloperoxidase. *Biochim Biophys Acta* 1977;493:247–259.

82. Olsen RL, Little C. Studies on the subunits of human myeloperoxidase. *Biochem J* 1984;222:701–709.

83. Atkin CL, Andersen MR, Eyre HJ. Abnormal neutrophil myeloperoxidase from a patient with chronic myelocytic leukemia. *Arch Biochem Biophys* 1982;214:284–292.

84. Taylor KL, Guzman GS, Burgess CA, Kinkade JMJ. Assembly of dimeric myeloperoxidase during posttranslational maturation in human leukemic HL-60 cells. *Biochemistry* 1990;29:1533–1539.

85. Andrews PC, Parnes C, Krinsky NI. Comparison of myeloperoxidase and hemi-myeloperoxidase with respect to catalysis, regulation, and bactericidal activity. *Arch Biochem Biophys* 1984;228:439–442.

86. Nauseef WM, Malech HL. Analysis of the peptide subunits of human neutrophil myeloperoxidase. *Blood* 1986;67:1504–1507.

87. Taylor KL, Guzman GS, Pohl J, Kinkade JMJ. Distinct chromatographic forms of human hemi-myeloperoxidase obtained by reductive cleavage of the dimeric enzyme. *J Biol Chem* 1990;265:15938–15946.

88. Fenna RE. Crystallization and subunit structure of canine myeloperoxidase. *J Mol Biol* 1987;196:919–925.

89. Zeng J, Fenna RE. Tetragonal crystals of canine myeloperoxidase suitable for X-ray structural analysis. *J Mol Biol* 1989;210:681–683.

90. Zeng J, Fenna RE. X-ray crystal structure of canine myeloperoxidase at 3 Å resolution. *J Mol Biol* 1992;226:185–207.

91. Fenna R, Zeng J, Davey C. Structure of the green heme in myeloperoxidase. *Arch Biochem Biophys* 1995;316:653–656.

92. Sutton BJ, Little C, Olsen RL, Willassen NP. Preliminary crystallographic analysis of human myeloperoxidase. *J Mol Biol* 1988;199:395–396.

93. Pember SO, Kinkade JMJ. Differences in myeloperoxidase activity from neutrophilic polymorphonuclear leukocytes of differing density: relationship to selective exocytosis of distinct forms of the enzyme. *Blood* 1983;61:1116–1124.

94. Pember SO, Fuhrer-Krusi SM, Barnes KC, Kinkade JMJ. Isolation of three native forms of myeloperoxidase from human polymorphonuclear leukocytes. *FEBS Lett* 1982;140:103–108.

95. Pember SO, Shapira R, Kinkade JMJ. Multiple forms of myeloperoxidase from human neutrophilic granulocytes; evidence for differences in compartmentalization, enzymic activity, and subunit structure. *Arch Biochem Biophys* 1983;221:391–403.

96. Wright J, Bastian N, Davis TA, et al. Structural characterization of the isoenzymatic forms of human myeloperoxidase: evaluation of the iron-containing prosthetic group. *Blood* 1990;75:238–241.

97. Miyasaki KT, Song J, Murthy ARK. Secretion of myeloperoxidase isoforms by human neutrophils. *Anal Biochem* 1991;193:38–44.

98. Agner K. Crystalline myeloperoxidase. *Acta Chem Scand* 1958;12:89–94.

99. Agner K. Verdoperoxidase. *Adv Enzymol* 1943;3:137–148.

100. Newton N, Morell DB, Clarke L, Clezy PS. The haem prosthetic groups of some animal peroxidases. II. Myeloperoxidase. *Biochim Biophys Acta* 1965;96:476–486.

101. Arnljots K, Olsson I. Myeloperoxidase precursors incorporate heme. *J Biol Chem* 1987;262:10430–10433.

102. Taylor KL, Pohl J, Kinkade JMJ. Unique autolytic cleavage of human myeloperoxidase. Implications for the involvement of active site Met[409]. *J Biol Chem* 1992;267:25282–25288.

103. Taylor KL, Strobel F, Yue KT, et al. Isolation and identification of a protoheme IX derivative released during autolytic cleavage of human myeloperoxidase. *Arch Biochem Biophys* 1995;316:635–642.

104. Eglinton DG, Barber D, Thomson AJ, Greenwood C, Segal AW. Studies of cyanide binding to myeloperoxidase by electron paramagnetic resonance and magnetic circular dichroism spectroscopies. *Biochim Biophys Acta* 1982;703:187–195.

105. Babcock GT, Ingle RT, Oertling WA, et al. Raman characterization of human leukocyte myeloperoxidase and bovine spleen green haemoprotein. Insight into chromophore structure and evidence that the chromophores of myeloperoxidase are equivalent. *Biochim Biophys Acta* 1985;828:58–66.

106. Sibbett SS, Hurst JK. Structural analysis of myeloperoxidase by resonance Raman spectroscopy. *Biochemistry* 1984;23:3007–3013.

107. Hurst JK. Myeloperoxidase: active site structure and catalytic mechanisms. In: Everse J, Everse KE, Grisham MB, eds. *Peroxidases in chemistry and biology,* vol 1. Boca Raton: CRC Press, 1991:37–62.

108. Sono M, Bracete AM, Huff AM, Ikeda-Saito M, Dawson JH. Evidence that a formyl-substituted iron porphyrin is the prosthetic group of myeloperoxidase: magnetic circular dichroism similarity of the peroxidase to *Spirographis* heme-reconstituted myoglobin. *Proc Natl Acad Sci USA* 1991;88:11148–11152.

109. Harrison JE, Schultz J. Myeloperoxidase: confirmation and nature of heme-binding inequivalence. *Biochim Biophys Acta* 1978;536:341–349.

110. Odajima T. Myeloperoxidase of the leukocyte of normal blood. Nature of the prosthetic group of myeloperoxidase. *J Biochem* 1980;87:379–391.

111. Agner K. Studies on myeloperoxidase activity. 1. Spectrophotometry of the MPO-H_2O_2 compound. *Acta Chem Scand* 1963;17:332–338.

112. Booth KS, Kimura S, Lee HC, Ikeda-Saito M, Caughey WS. Bovine myeloperoxidase and lactoperoxidase each contain a high affinity site for calcium. *Biochem Biophys Res Commun* 1989;160:897–902.

113. Lefkowitz DL, Mills K, Morgan D, Lefkowitz SS. Macrophage activation and immunomodulation by myeloperoxidase. *Proc Soc Exp Biol Med* 1992;199:204–210.

114. Whittenbury R. Hydrogen peroxide formation and catalase activity in the lactic acid bacteria. *J Gen Microbiol* 1964;35:13–26.

115. Cohen G, Somerson NL. Glucose-dependent secretion and destruction of hydrogen peroxide by *Mycoplasma pneumoniae. J Bacteriol* 1969;98:547–551.

116. Cole BC, Ward JR, Martin CH. Hemolysin and peroxide activity of *Mycoplasma* species. *J Bacteriol* 1968;95:2022–2030.

117. Sobeslavsky O, Chanock RM. Peroxide formation by mycoplasmas which infect man. *Proc Soc Exp Biol Med* 1968;129:531–535.

118. Somerson NL, Walls BE, Chanock RM. Hemolysin of *Mycoplasma pneumoniae:* tentative identification as a peroxide. *Science* 1965;150:226–228.

119. Danley DL, Hilger AE, Winkel CA. Generation of hydrogen peroxide by *Candida albicans* and influence on murine polymorphonuclear leukocyte activity. *Infect Immun* 1983;40:97–102.

120. Odajima T, Yamazaki I. Myeloperoxidase of the leukocyte of normal blood. I. Reaction of myeloperoxidase with hydrogen peroxide. *Biochim Biophys Acta* 1970;206:71–77.

121. Harrison JE. The functional mechanism of myeloperoxidase. In: Schultz J, Ahmad F, eds. *Cancer enzymology.* New York: Academic Press, 1976:305–317.

122. Kettle AJ, Winterbourn CC. Superoxide modulates the activity of myeloperoxidase and optimizes the production of hypochlorous acid. *Biochem J* 1988;252:529–536.

123. Kettle AJ, Winterbourn CC. Influence of superoxide on myeloperoxidase kinetics measured with a hydrogen peroxide electrode. *Biochem J* 1989;263:823–828.

124. Kettle AJ, Winterbourn CC. Superoxide enhances hypochlorous acid production by stimulated human neutrophils. *Biochim Biophys Acta* 1990;1052:379–385.

125. Bolscher BGJM, Zoutberg GR, Cuperus RA, Wever R. Vitamin C stimulates the chlorinating activity of human myeloperoxidase. *Biochim Biophys Acta* 1984;784:189–191.

126. Marquez LA, Dunford HB, Van Wart H. Kinetic studies on the reaction of compound II of myeloperoxidase with ascorbic acid. Role of ascorbic acid in myeloperoxidase function. *J Biol Chem* 1990;265:5666–5670.

127. Hoogland H, Dekker HL, van Riel C, van Kuilenburg A, Muijsers AO, Wever R. A steady-state study on the formation of compounds II and III of myeloperoxidase. *Biochim Biophys Acta* 1988;955:337–345.

128. Wittenberg JB, Noble RW, Wittenberg BA, Antonini E, Brunori M, Wyman J. Studies on the equilibria and kinetics of the reactions of

129. Yamazaki I, Yokota KN. Oxidation states of peroxidase. *Mol Cell Biochem* 1973;2:39–52.

130. Odajima T, Yamazaki I. Myeloperoxidase of the leukocyte of normal blood. III. The reaction of ferric myeloperoxidase with superoxide anion. *Biochim Biophys Acta* 1972;284:355–359.

131. Winterbourn CC, Garcia RC, Segal AW. Production of the superoxide adduct of myeloperoxidase (compound III) by stimulated human neutrophils and its reactivity with hydrogen peroxide and chloride. *Biochem J* 1985;228:583–592.

132. Metodiewa D, Dunford HB. The reactions of horseradish peroxidase, lactoperoxidase, and myeloperoxidase with enzymatically generated superoxide. *Arch Biochem Biophys* 1989;272:245–253.

133. Kettle AJ, Sangster DF, Gebicki JM, Winterbourn CC. A pulse radiolysis investigation of the reactions of myeloperoxidase with superoxide and hydrogen peroxide. *Biochim Biophys Acta* 1988;956:58–62.

134. Phelps CF, Antonini E, Giacometti G, Brunori M. The kinetics of oxidation of ferroperoxidase by molecular oxygen. *Biochem J* 1974;141:265–272.

135. Tamura M, Yamazaki I. Reactions of the oxyform of horseradish peroxidase. *J Biochem* 1972;71:311–319.

136. Yokota K, Yamazaki I. Reaction of peroxidase with reduced nicotinamide-adenine dinucleotide and reduced nicotinamide-adenine dinucleotide phosphate. *Biochim Biophys Acta* 1965;105:301–312.

137. Yokota K, Yamazaki I. The activity of the horseradish peroxidase compound III. *Biochem Biophys Res Commun* 1965;18:48–53.

138. Marquez LA, Dunford HB. Reaction of compound III of myeloperoxidase with ascorbic acid. *J Biol Chem* 1990;265:6074–6078.

139. Akazawa T, Conn EE. The oxidation of reduced pyridine nucleotides by peroxidase. *J Biol Chem* 1958;232:403–415.

140. Klebanoff SJ. An effect of thyroxine on the oxidation of reduced pyridine nucleotides by the peroxidase system. *J Biol Chem* 1959;234:2480–2485.

141. Williams-Ashman HG, Cassman M, Klavins M. Two enzymic mechanisms for hydrogen transport by phenolic oestrogens. *Nature* 1959;184:427–429.

142. Klebanoff SJ. Reduced pyridine nucleotides as activators of certain reactions catalyzed by peroxidase. *Biochim Biophys Acta* 1960;44:501–509.

143. Yamazaki I, Yokota K, Nakajima R. A mechanism and model of peroxidase-oxidase reaction. In: King TE, Mason HC, Morrison M, eds. *Oxidases and related redox systems,* vol 1. New York: Wiley, 1965:485–513.

144. Klebanoff SJ. Iodination of bacteria: a bactericidal mechanism. *J Exp Med* 1967;126:1063–1078.

145. Klebanoff SJ. Myeloperoxidase-halide-hydrogen peroxide antibacterial system. *J Bacteriol* 1968;95:2131–2138.

146. Klebanoff SJ, Luebke RG. The antilactobacillus system of saliva. Role of salivary peroxidase. *Proc Soc Exp Biol* Med 1965;118:483–486.

147. Klebanoff SJ, Clem WH, Luebke RG. The peroxidase-thiocyanate-hydrogen peroxide antimicrobial system. *Biochim Biophys Acta* 1966;117:63–72.

148. Holzbecher J, Ryan DE. The rapid determination of total bromine and iodine in biological fluids by neutron activation. *Clin Biochem* 1980;13:277–278.

149. Thomas EL, Fishman M. Oxidation of chloride and thiocyanate by isolated leukocytes. *J Biol Chem* 1986;261:9694–9702.

150. Wever R, Kast WM, Kasinoedin JH, Boelens R. The peroxidation of thiocyanate catalyzed by myeloperoxidase and lactoperoxidase. *Biochim Biophys Acta* 1982;709:212–219.

151. Andrews PC, Krinsky NI. A kinetic analysis of the interaction of human myeloperoxidase with hydrogen peroxide, chloride ions, and protons. *J Biol Chem* 1982;247:13240–13245.

152. Bakkenist ARJ, DeBoer JEG, Plat H, Wever R. The halide complexes of myeloperoxidase and the mechanism of the halogenation reactions. *Biochim Biophys Acta* 1980;613:337–348.

153. Zgliczynski JM, Selvaraj RJ, Paul BB, Stelmaszynska T, Poskitt PKF, Sbarra AJ. Chlorination by the myeloperoxidase-H_2O_2-Cl^- antimicrobial system at acid and neutral pH. *Proc Soc Exp Biol Med* 1977;154:418–422.

154. Ikeda-Saito M, Prince RC. The effect of chloride on the redox and EPR properties of myeloperoxidase. *J Biol Chem* 1985;260:8301–8305.

155. Ikeda-Saito M, Argade PV, Rousseau DL. Resonance Raman evidence

of chloride binding to the heme iron in myeloperoxidase. *FEBS Lett* 1985;184:52–55.

156. Stelmaszynska T, Zgliczynski JM. Myeloperoxidase of human neutrophilic granulocytes as chlorinating enzyme. *Eur J Biochem* 1974; 45:305–312.

157. Wever R, Bakkenist ARJ. The interaction of myeloperoxidase with ligands as studied by EPR. *Biochim Biophys Acta* 1980;612:178–184.

158. Thomas EL, Learn DB. Myeloperoxidase: catalyzed oxidation of chloride and other halides: the role of chloramines. In: Everse J, Everse KE, Grisham MB, eds. *Peroxidases in chemistry and biology,* vol 1. Boca Raton: CRC Press, 1991:83–103.

159. Agner K. Peroxidative oxidation of chloride ions. *Proc Int Congr Biochem 4th Vienna* 1958;15:64(abst).

160. Agner K. Biological effects of hypochlorous acid formed by "MPO"-peroxidation in the presence of chloride ions. In: Akeson A, Ehrenberg A, eds. *Structure and function of oxidation reduction enzymes,* vol 18. New York: Pergamon Press, 1972:329–335.

161. Harrison JE, Schultz J. Studies on the chlorinating activity of myeloperoxidase. *J Biol Chem* 1976;251:1371–1374.

162. Foote CS, Goyne TE, Lehrer RI. Assessment of chlorination by human neutrophils. *Nature* 1983;301:715–716.

163. Thomas EL, Grisham MB, Jefferson MM. Myeloperoxidase-dependent effect of amines on functions of isolated neutrophils. *J Clin Invest* 1983;72:441–454.

164. Weiss SJ, Klein R, Slivka A, Wei M. Chlorination of taurine by human neutrophils. Evidence for hypochlorous acid generation. *J Clin Invest* 1982;70:598–607.

165. Hazen SL, Hsu FF, Mueller DM, Crowley JR, Heinecke JW. Human neutrophils employ chlorine gas as an oxidant during phagocytosis. *J Clin Invest* 1996;98:1283–1289.

166. Thomas EL, Aune TM. Peroxidase-catalyzed oxidation of protein sulfhydryls mediated by iodine. *Biochemistry* 1977;16:3581–3586.

167. Thomas EL, Aune TM. Oxidation of *Escherichia coli* sulfhydryl components by the peroxidase-hydrogen peroxide-iodide antimicrobial system. *Antimicrob Agents Chemother* 1978;13:1006–1010.

168. Grisham MB, Jefferson MM, Melton DF, Thomas EL. Chlorination of endogenous amines by isolated neutrophils. Ammonia-dependent bactericidal, cytotoxic and cytolytic activities of the chloramines. *J Biol Chem* 1984;259:10404–10413.

169. Test ST, Weiss SJ. The generation and utilization of chlorinated oxidants by human neutrophils. *Adv Free Rad Biol Med* 1986;2:91–116.

170. Test ST, Lampert MB, Ossanna PJ, Thoene JG, Weiss SJ. Generation of nitrogen-chlorine oxidants by human phagocytes. *J Clin Invest* 1984;74:1341–1349.

171. Weiss SJ, Lampert MB, Test ST. Long-lived oxidants generated by human neutrophils: characterization and bioactivity. *Science* 1983; 222:625–628.

172. Soupart P. Free amino acids in blood and urine in the human. In: Holden JT, ed. *Amino acid pools.* Amsterdam: Elsevier Publishing, 1962:220–262.

173. Learn DB, Fried VA, Thomas EL. Taurine and hypotaurine content of human leukocytes. *J Leukoc Biol* 1990;48:174–182.

174. Zgliczynski JM, Stelmaszynska T, Domanski J, Ostrowski W. Chloramines as intermediates of oxidative reaction of amino acids by myeloperoxidase. *Biochim Biophys Acta* 1971;235:419–424.

175. Strauss RR, Paul BB, Jacobs AA, Sbarra AJ. Role of the phagocyte in host-parasite interactions. XXVII. Myeloperoxidase-H$_2$O$_2$-Cl$^-$-mediated aldehyde formation and its relationship to antimicrobial activity. *Infect Immun* 1971;3:595–602.

176. Thomas EL. Myeloperoxidase-hydrogen peroxide-chloride antimicrobial system: effect of exogenous amines on antibacterial action against *Escherichia coli.* *Infect Immun* 1979;25:110–116.

177. Passo SA, Weiss SJ. Oxidative mechanisms utilized by human neutrophils to destroy *Escherichia coli.* *Blood* 1984;63:1361–1368.

178. Grisham MB, Jefferson MM, Thomas EL. Role of monochloramine in the oxidation of erythrocyte hemoglobin by stimulated neutrophils. *J Biol Chem* 1984;259:6757–6765.

179. Sykes G. The halogens. In: *Disinfection and sterilization,* 2nd ed. Philadelphia: JB Lippincott, 1965:381–410.

180. Zgliczynski JM, Stelmaszynska T, Ostrowski W, Naskalski J, Sznajd J. Myeloperoxidase of human leukemic leucocytes. Oxidation of amino acids in the presence of hydrogen peroxide. *Eur J Biochem* 1968;4: 540–547.

181. Hazen SL, Hsu FF, Heinecke JW. *p*-Hydroxyphenylacetaldehyde is the major product of L-tyrosine oxidation by activated human phagocytes. *J Biol Chem* 1996;271:1861–1867.

182. Stelmaszynska T. Formation of HCN by human phagocytosing neutrophils. 1. Chlorination of *Staphylococcus epidermidis* as a source of HCN. *Int J Biochem* 1985;17:373–379.

183. Stelmaszynska T, Zgliczynski JM. N-(2-oxoacyl) amino acids and nitriles as final products of dipeptide chlorination mediated by the myeloperoxidase/H$_2$O$_2$/Cl$^-$ system. *Eur J Biochem* 1978;92:301–308.

184. Zgliczynski JM, Stelmaszynska T. Hydrogen cyanide and cyanogen chloride formation by the myeloperoxidase-H$_2$O$_2$-Cl$^-$ system. *Biochim Biophys Acta* 1979;567:309–314.

185. Thomas EL, Grisham MB, Melton DF, Jefferson MM. Evidence for a role of taurine in the *in vitro* oxidative toxicity of neutrophils toward erythrocytes. *J Biol Chem* 1985;260:3321–3329.

186. Thomas EL, Jefferson MM, Grisham MB. Myeloperoxidase-catalyzed incorporation of amines into proteins: role of hypochlorous acid and dichloramines. *Biochemistry* 1982;21:6299–6308.

187. Bearman SI, Schwarting GA, Kolodny EH, Babior BM. Incorporation of glucosamine by activated human neutrophils. A myeloperoxidase-mediated process. *J Lab Clin Med* 1980;96:893–902.

188. Turk J, Henderson WR, Klebanoff SJ, Hubbard WC. Iodination of arachidonic acid mediated by eosinophil peroxidase, myeloperoxidase and lactoperoxidase: identification and comparison of products. *Biochim Biophys Acta* 1983;751:189–200.

189. Zgliczynski JM, Stelmaszynska T. Chlorinating ability of human phagocytosing leucocytes. *Eur J Biochem* 1975;56:157–162.

190. Winterbourn CC, van den Berg JJM, Roitman E, Kuypers FA. Chlorohydrin formation from unsaturated fatty acids reacted with hypochlorous acid. *Arch Biochem Biophys* 1992;296:547–555.

191. Heinecke JW, Li W, Mueller DM, Bohrer A, Turk J. Cholesterol chlorohydrin synthesis by the myeloperoxidase-hydrogen peroxide-chloride system: potential markers for lipoproteins oxidatively damaged by phagocytes. *Biochemistry* 1994;33:10127–10136.

192. Domigan NM, Charlton TS, Duncan MW, Winterbourn CC, Kettle AJ. Chlorination of tyrosyl residues in peptides by myeloperoxidase and human neutrophils. *J Biol Chem* 1995;270:16542–16548.

193. Selvaraj RJ, Zgliczynski JM, Paul BB, Sbarra AJ. Chlorination of reduced nicotinamide adenine dinucleotides by myeloperoxidase: a novel bactericidal mechanism. *J Reticuloendothel Soc* 1980;27:31–38.

194. Bernofsky C. Nucleotide chloramines and neutrophil-mediated cytotoxicity. *FASEB J* 1991;5:295–300.

195. Albrich JM, McCarthy CA, Hurst JK. Biological reactivity of hypochlorous acid: implications for microbicidal mechanisms of leukocyte myeloperoxidase. *Proc Natl Acad Sci USA* 1981;78: 210–214.

196. Winterbourn CC. Comparative reactivities of various biological compounds with myeloperoxidase-hydrogen peroxide-chloride, and similarity of the oxidant to hypochlorite. *Biochim Biophys Acta* 1985;840: 204–210.

197. Turkall RM, Tsan M. Oxidation of glutathione by the myeloperoxidase system. *J Reticuloendothel Soc* 1982;31:353–360.

198. Sagone ALJ, Husney RM, O'Dorisio MS, Metz EN. Mechanisms for the oxidation of reduced glutathione by stimulated granulocytes. *Blood* 1984;63:96–104.

199. Rosen H, Klebanoff SJ. Oxidation of microbial iron-sulfur centers by the myeloperoxidase-H$_2$O$_2$-halide antimicrobial system. *Infect Immun* 1985;47:613–618.

200. Rosen H, Klebanoff SJ. Oxidation of *Escherichia coli* iron centers by the myeloperoxidase-mediated microbicidal system. *J Biol Chem* 1982;257:13731–13735.

201. Hurst JK, Barrette WC Jr, Michel BR, Rosen H. Hypochlorous acid and myeloperoxidase-catalyzed oxidation of iron-sulfur clusters in bacterial respiratory dehydrogenases. *Eur J Biochem* 1991;202: 1275–1282.

202. Naskalski JW. Myeloperoxidase inactivation in the course of catalysis of chlorination of taurine. *Biochim Biophys Acta* 1977;485:291–300.

203. Tsan M, Chen JW. Oxidation of methionine by human polymorphonuclear leukocytes. *J Clin Invest* 1980;65:1041–1050.

204. Matheson NR, Wong PS, Travis J. Enzymatic inactivation of human alpha-1-proteinase inhibitor by neutrophil myeloperoxidase. *Biochem Biophys Res Commun* 1979;88:402–409.

205. Clark RA, Szot S, Venkatasubramanian K, Schiffmann E. Chemotactic factor inactivation by myeloperoxidase-mediated oxidation of methionine. *J Immunol* 1980;124:2020–2026.

206. Matheson NR, Wong PS, Schuyler M, Travis J. Interaction of human alpha-1-proteinase inhibitor with neutrophil myeloperoxidase. *Biochemistry* 1981;20:331–336.

207. Matheson NR, Travis J. Differential effects of oxidizing agents on human plasma alpha$_1$-proteinase inhibitor and human neutrophil myeloperoxidase. *Biochemistry* 1985;24:1941–1945.

208. Lee CW, Lewis RA, Corey EJ, et al. Oxidative inactivation of leukotriene C$_4$ by stimulated human polymorphonuclear leukocytes. *Proc Natl Acad Sci USA* 1982;79:4166–4170.

209. Lee CW, Lewis RA, Tauber AI, Mehrotra M, Corey EJ, Austen KF. The myeloperoxidase-dependent metabolism of leukotriene C$_4$, D$_4$ and E$_4$ to 6-*trans*-leukotriene B$_4$ diastereoisomers and the subclass specific *S*-diastereoisomeric sulfoxides. *J Biol Chem* 1983;258:15004–15010.

210. Adeniyi-Jones SK, Karnovsky ML. Oxidative decarboxylation of free and peptide-linked amino acids in phagocytizing guinea pig granulocytes. *J Clin Invest* 1981;68:365–373.

211. Selvaraj RJ, Paul BB, Strauss RR, Jacobs AA, Sbarra AJ. Oxidative peptide cleavage and decarboxylation by the MPO-H$_2$O$_2$-Cl$^-$ antimicrobial system. *Infect Immun* 1974;9:255–260.

212. Anderson MM, Hazen SL, Hsu FF, Heinecke JW. Human neutrophils employ the myeloperoxidase-hydrogen peroxide-chloride system to convert hydroxy-amino acids into glycoaldehyde, 2-hydroxypropanal, and acrolein. A mechanism for the generation of highly reactive α-hydroxy and α, β-unsaturated aldehydes by phagocytes at sites of inflammation. *J Clin Invest* 1997;99:424–432.

213. Shohet SB, Pitt J, Baehner RL, Poplack DG. Lipid peroxidation in the killing of phagocytized pneumococci. *Infect Immun* 1974;10:1321–1328.

214. Stossel TP, Mason RJ, Smith AL. Lipid peroxidation by human blood phagocytes. *J Clin Invest* 1974;54:638–645.

215. Kanner J, Kinsella JE. Initiation of lipid peroxidation by a peroxidase/hydrogen peroxide/halide system. *Lipids* 1983;18:204–210.

216. Stelmaszynska T, Kukovetz E, Egger G, Schauer RJ. Possible involvement of myeloperoxidase in lipid peroxidation. *Int J Biochem* 1992;24:121–128.

217. Albrich JM, Hurst JK. Oxidative inactivation of *Escherichia coli* by hypochlorous acid. Rates and differentiation of respiratory from other reaction sites. *FEBS Lett* 1982;144:157–161.

218. Camper AK, McFeters GA. Chlorine injury and the enumeration of waterborne coliform bacteria. *Appl Environ Microbiol* 1979;37:633–641.

219. Barrette WC Jr, Albrich JM, Hurst JK. Hypochlorous acid-promoted loss of metabolic energy in *Escherichia coli*. *Infect Immun* 1987;55:2518–2525.

220. Albrich JM, Gilbaugh JHI, Callahan KB, Hurst JK. Effects of the putative neutrophil-generating toxin, hypochlorous acid, on membrane permeability and transport systems of *Escherichia coli*. *J Clin Invest* 1986;78:177–184.

221. Sips HJ, Hamers MN. Mechanism of the bactericidal action of myeloperoxidase: increased permeability of the *Escherichia coli* cell envelope. *Infect Immun* 1981;31:11–16.

222. Barrette WC Jr, Hannum DM, Wheeler WD, Hurst JK. General mechanism for the bacterial toxicity of hypochlorous acid: abolition of ATP production. *Biochemistry* 1989;28:9172–9178.

223. Barrette WC Jr, Albrich JM, Hurst JK. Hypochlorous acid-promoted loss of metabolic energy in *Escherichia coli*. *Infect Immun* 1987;55:2518–2525.

224. Rosen H, Rakita RM, Waltersdorph AM, Klebanoff SJ. Myeloperoxidase-mediated damage to the succinate oxidase system of *Escherichia coli*. *J Biol Chem* 1987;262:15004–15010.

225. Rakita RM, Michel BR, Rosen H. Myeloperoxidase-mediated inhibition of microbial respiration: damage to *Escherichia coli* ubiquinol oxidase. *Biochemistry* 1989;28:3031–3036.

226. Rakita RM, Michel BR, Rosen H. Differential inactivation of *Escherichia coli* membrane dehydrogenases by a myeloperoxidase-mediated antimicrobial system. *Biochemistry* 1990;29:1075–1080.

226a. Rakita RM, Rosen H. Penicillin-binding protein inactivation by human neutrophil myeloperoxidase. *J Clin Invest* 1991;88:750–754.

226b. Rakita RM, Michel BR, Rosen H. Inactivation of *Escherichia coli* penicillin-binding proteins by human neutrophils. *Infect Immun* 1994;62:162–165.

227. McKenna SM, Davies KJA. The inhibition of bacterial growth by hypochlorous acid. Possible role in the bactericidal activity of phagocytes. *Biochem J* 1988;254:685–692.

228. Rosen H, Orman J, Rakita RM, Michel BR, VanDevanter DR. Loss of DNA-membrane interactions and cessation of DNA synthesis in myeloperoxidase-treated *Escherichia coli*. *Proc Natl Acad Sci USA* 1990;87:10048–10052.

229. Schraufstatter IU, Browne K, Harris A, et al. Mechanisms of hypochlorite injury of target cells. *J Clin Invest* 1990;85:554–562.

230. Savenkova MI, Mueller DM, Heinecke JW. Tyrosyl radical generated by myeloperoxidase is a physiological catalyst for the initiation of lipid peroxidation in low density lipoprotein. *J Biol Chem* 1994;269:20394–20400.

231. Heinecke JW, Li W, Daehnke HL III, Goldstein JA. Dityrosine, a specific marker of oxidation, is synthesized by the myeloperoxidase-hydrogen peroxide system of human neutrophils and macrophages. *J Biol Chem* 1993;268:4069–4077.

232. Jacob JS, Cistola DP, Hsu FF, et al. Human phagocytes employ the myeloperoxidase-hydrogen peroxide system to synthesize dityrosine, trityrosine, pulcherosine, and isodityrosine by a tyrosyl radical-dependent pathway. *J Biol Chem* 1996;271:19950–19956.

233. Heinecke JW, Li W, Francis GA, Goldstein JA. Tyrosyl radical generated by myeloperoxidase catalyzes the oxidative cross-linking of proteins. *J Clin Invest* 1993;91:2866–2872.

234. Jong EC, Chi EY, Klebanoff SJ. Human neutrophil-mediated killing of schistosomula of *Schistosoma mansoni*: augmentation by schistosomal binding of eosinophil peroxidase. *Am J Trop Med Hyg* 1984;33:104–115.

235. Nathan CF, Klebanoff SJ. Augmentation of spontaneous macrophage-mediated cytolysis by eosinophil peroxidase. *J Exp Med* 1982;155:1291–1308.

236. Bass DA, Szejda P. Mechanism of killing of newborn larvae of *Trichinella spiralis* by neutrophils and eosinophils. Killing by generators of hydrogen peroxide *in vitro*. *J Clin Invest* 1979;64:1558–1564.

237. Nathan CF, Silverstein SC, Brukner LH, Cohn ZA. Extracellular cytolysis by activated macrophages and granulocytes. II. Hydrogen peroxide as a mediator of cytotoxicity. *J Exp Med* 1979;149:100–113.

238. Knowles DMI, Sullivan TJI, Parker CW, Williams RCJ. In vitro antibody-enzyme conjugates with specific bactericidal activity. *J Clin Invest* 1973;52:1443–1452.

239. Philpott GW, Bower RJ, Parker CW. Selective iodination and cytotoxicity of tumor cells with an antibody-enzyme conjugate. *Surgery* 1973;74:51–58.

240. Philpott GW, Shearer WT, Bower RJ, Parker CW. Selective cytotoxicity of hapten-substituted cells with an antibody-enzyme conjugate. *J Immunol* 1973;111:921–929.

241. Okuda K, Ishiwara K, Noguchi Y, Takahashi T, Tadokoro I. New type of antibody-enzyme conjugate which specifically kills *Candida albicans*. *Infect Immun* 1980;27:690–692.

242. Pene J, Rousseau V, Stanislawski M. In vitro cytolysis of myeloma tumor cells with glucose oxidase and lactoperoxidase antibody conjugates. *Biochem Int* 1986;13:233–243.

243. Stanislawski M, Rousseau V, Goavec M, Ito H. Immunotoxins containing glucose oxidase and lactoperoxidase with tumoricidal properties: *in vitro* killing effectiveness in a mouse plasmacytoma cell model. *Cancer Res* 1989;49:5497–5504.

244. Ito H, Morizet J, Coulombel L, et al. An immunotoxin system intended for bone marrow purging composed of glucose oxidase and lactoperoxidase coupled to monoclonal antibody 097. *Bone Marrow Transplant* 1989;4:519–527.

245. Casentini-Borocz D, Bringman T. Enzyme immunoconjugates utilizing glucose oxidase and myeloperoxidase are cytotoxic to *Candida tropicalis*. *Antimicrob Agents Chemother* 1990;34:875–880.

246. Clark RA, Klebanoff SJ. Neutrophil-platelet interaction mediated by myeloperoxidase and hydrogen peroxide. *J Immunol* 1980;124:399–405.

247. Voetman AA, Weening RS, Hamers MW, Meerhof LJ, Bot AAAM, Roos D. Phagocytosing human neutrophils inactivate their own granular enzymes. *J Clin Invest* 1981;67:1541–1549.

248. McRipley RJ, Sbarra AJ. Role of the phagocyte in host-parasite interactions. XII. Hydrogen peroxide-myeloperoxidase bactericidal system in the phagocyte. *J Bacteriol* 1967;94:1425–1430.

249. Jacobs AA, Low IE, Paul BB, Strauss RR, Sbarra AJ. Mycoplasmacidal activity of peroxidase-H$_2$O$_2$-halide systems. *Infect Immun* 1972;5:127–131.

250. Yong EC, Klebanoff SJ, Kuo C. Toxic effect of human polymor-

phonuclear leukocytes on *Chlamydia trachomatis. Infect Immun* 1982; 37:422–426.

251. Klebanoff SJ, Shepard CC. Toxic effect of the peroxidase-hydrogen peroxide-halide antimicrobial system on *Mycobacterium leprae. Infect Immun* 1984;44:534–536.

252. Miyasaki KT, Wilson ME, Genco RJ. Killing of *Actinobacillus actinomycetemcomitans* by the human neutrophil myeloperoxidase-hydrogen peroxide-chloride system. *Infect Immun* 1986;53:161–165.

253. Locksley RM, Jacobs RF, Wilson CB, Weaver WM, Klebanoff SJ. Susceptibility of *Legionella pneumophila* to oxygen-dependent microbicidal systems. *J Immunol* 1982;129:2192–2197.

254. Diamond RD, Clark RA. Damage to *Aspergillus fumigatus* and *Rhizopus oryzae* hyphae by oxidative and nonoxidative microbicidal products of human neutrophils *in vitro. Infect Immun* 1982;38: 487–495.

255. Diamond RD, Root RK, Bennett JE. Factors influencing killing of *Cryptococcus neoformans* by human leukocytes *in vitro. J Infect Dis* 1972;125:367–376.

256. Diamond RD, Clark RA, Haudenschild CC. Damage to *Candida albicans* hyphae and pseudohyphae by the myeloperoxidase system and oxidative products of neutrophil metabolism *in vitro. J Clin Invest* 1980;66:908–917.

257. Howard DH. Fate of *Histoplasma capsulatum* in guinea pig polymorphonuclear leukocytes. *Infect Immun* 1973;8:412–419.

258. Lehrer RI. Antifungal effects of peroxidase systems. *J Bacteriol* 1969; 99:361–365.

259. Lehrer RI, Jan RG. Interaction of *Aspergillus fumigatus* spores with human leukocytes and serum. *Infect Immun* 1970;1:345–350.

260. Belding ME, Klebanoff SJ, Ray CG. Peroxidase-mediated virucidal systems. *Science* 1970;167:195–196.

261. Klebanoff SJ, Coombs RW. Viricidal effect of polymorphonuclear leukocytes on HIV-1: Role of the myeloperoxidase system. *J Clin Invest* 1992;89:2014–2017.

262. Moguilevsky N, Steens M, Thiriart C, Prieels J-P, Thiry L, Bollen A. Lethal oxidative damage to human immunodeficiency virus by human recombinant myeloperoxidase. *FEBS Lett* 1992;302:209–212.

263. Chochola J, Yamaguchi Y, Moguilevsky N, Bollen A, Strosberg AD, Stanislawski M. Virucidal effect of myeloperoxidase on human immunodeficiency virus type 1-infected T cells. *Antimicrob Agents Chemother* 1994;38:969–972.

264. Thorne KJI, Svvennsen RJ, Franks D. Role of hydrogen peroxide and peroxidase in the cytotoxicity of *Trypanosoma dionisii* by human granulocytes. *Infect Immun* 1978;21:798–805.

265. Villalta F, Kierszenbaum F. Role of polymorphonuclear cells in Chagas' disease. I. Uptake and mechanisms of destruction of intracellular (amastigote) forms of *Trypanosoma cruzi* by human neutrophils. *J Immunol* 1983;131:1504–1510.

266. Chang K. Leishmanicidal mechanisms of human polymorphonuclear phagocytes. *Am J Trop Med Hyg* 1981;30:322–333.

267. Pearson RD, Steigbigel RT. Phagocytosis and killing of the protozoan *Leishmania donovani* by human polymorphonuclear leukocytes. *J Immunol* 1981;127:1438–1443.

268. Ferrante A, Hill NL, Abell TJ, Pruul H. Role of myeloperoxidase in the killing of *Neigleria fowleri* by lymphokine-altered human neutrophils. *Infect Immun* 1987;55:1047–1050.

269. Jong EC, Mahmoud AAF, Klebanoff SJ. Peroxidase-mediated toxicity to schistosomula of *Schistosoma mansoni. J Immunol* 1981;126: 468–471.

270. Kazura JW, Fanning MM, Blumer JL, Mahmoud AAF. Role of cell-generated hydrogen peroxide in granulocyte-mediated killing of schistosomula of *Schistosoma mansoni in vitro. J Clin Invest* 1981;67:93–102.

271. Buys J, Wever R, Ruitenberg EJ. Myeloperoxidase is more efficient than eosinophil peroxidase in the *in vitro* killing of newborn larvae of *Trichinella spiralis. Immunology* 1984;51:601–607.

272. Agner K. Detoxicating effect of verdoperoxidase on toxins. *Nature* 1947;159:271–272.

273. Agner K. Studies on peroxidative detoxification of purified diphtheria toxin. *J Exp Med* 1950;92:337–347.

274. Agner K. Peroxidative detoxification of diphtheria toxin studied by using I^{131}. *Rec Trav Chim* 1955;74:373–376.

275. Ooi W, Levine HG, LaMont JT, Clark RA. Inactivation of *Clostridium difficile* cytotoxin by the neutrophil myeloperoxidase system. *J Infect Dis* 1984;149:215–219.

276. Clark RA. Oxidative inactivation of pneumolysin by the myeloperox-

idase system and stimulated human neutrophils. *J Immunol* 1986;136: 4617–4622.

277. Clark RA, Leidal KG, Taichman NS. Oxidative inactivation of *Actinobacillus actinomycetemcomitans* leukotoxin by the neutrophil myeloperoxidase system. *Infect Immun* 1986;53:252–256.

278. Odajima T. Oxidative destruction of the microbial metabolite aflatoxin by the myeloperoxidase-hydrogen peroxide-chloride system. *Arch Oral Biol* 1981;26:339–340.

279. Clark RA, Klebanoff SJ, Einstein AB, Fefer A. Peroxidase-H$_2$O$_2$-halide system: cytotoxic effect on mammalian tumor cells. *Blood* 1975;45:161–170.

280. Edelson PJ, Cohn ZA. Peroxidase-mediated mammalian cell cytotoxicity. *J Exp Med* 1973;138:318–323.

281. Clark RA, Klebanoff SJ. Neutrophil mediated tumor cell cytotoxicity: role of the peroxidase system. *J Exp Med* 1975;141:1442–1447.

282. Clark RA, Klebanoff SJ. Role of the myeloperoxidase-H$_2$O$_2$-halide system in concanavalin A-induced tumor cell killing by human neutrophils. *J Immunol* 1979;122:2605–2610.

283. Clark RA, Szot S. The myeloperoxidase-hydrogen peroxide-halide system as effector of neutrophil-mediated tumor cell cytotoxicity. *J Immunol* 1981;126:1295–1301.

284. Dallegri F, Frumento G, Patrone F. Mechanisms of tumour cell destruction by PMA-activated human neutrophils. *Immunology* 1983; 48:273–279.

285. Slivka A, LoBuglio AF, Weiss SJ. A potential role for hypochlorous acid in granulocyte-mediated tumor cell cytotoxicity. *Blood* 1980;55: 347–350.

286. Weiss SJ, Slivka A. Monocyte and granulocyte-mediated tumor cell destruction. A role for the hydrogen peroxide-myeloperoxidase-chloride system. *J Clin Invest* 1982;69:255–262.

287. Learn DB, Thomas EL. Inhibition of tumor cell glutamine uptake by isolated neutrophils. *J Clin Invest* 1988;82:789–796.

288. Clark RA, Klebanoff SJ. Studies on the mechanism of antibody-dependent polymorphonuclear leukocyte-mediated cytotoxicity. *J Immunol* 1977;119:1413–1418.

289. Hafeman DG, Lucas ZJ. Polymorphonuclear leukocyte-mediated, antibody-dependent, cellular cytotoxicity against tumor cells: dependence on oxygen and the respiratory burst. *J Immunol* 1979;123: 55–62.

290. Lanza F, Fietta A, Spisani S, Castoldi GL, Traniello S. Does a relationship exist between neutrophil myeloperoxidase deficiency and the occurrence of neoplasms? *J Clin Lab Immunol* 1987;22:175–180.

291. Clark RA, Klebanoff SJ. Myeloperoxidase-H$_2$O$_2$-halide system: cytotoxic effect on human blood leukocytes. *Blood* 1977;50:65–70.

292. Stendahl O, Coble B, Dahlgren C, Hed J, Molin L. Myeloperoxidase modulates the phagocytic activity of polymorphonuclear neutrophil leukocytes. Studies with cells from a myeloperoxidase-deficient patient. *J Clin Invest* 1984;73:366–373.

293. Coble B, Dahlgren C, Hed J, Stendahl O. Myeloperoxidase reduces the opsonizing activity of immunoglobulin G and complement component C3b. *Biochim Biophys Acta* 1984;802:501–505.

294. Jasin HE. Generation of IgG aggregates by the myeloperoxidase-hydrogen peroxide system. *J Immunol* 1983;130:1918–1923.

295. Jasin HE. Oxidative cross-linking of immune complexes by human polymorphonuclear leukocytes. *J Clin Invest* 1988;81:6–15.

296. Kobayashi M, Tanaka T, Usui T. Lysosomal enzyme release from polymorphonuclear leukocytes in patients with chronic granulomatous disease: the effect of hydrogen peroxide on released enzyme activities. *Hiroshima J Med Sci* 1981;30:339–344.

297. Kobayashi M, Tanaka T, Usui T. Inactivation of lysosomal enzymes by the respiratory burst of polymorphonuclear leukocytes. Possible involvement of myeloperoxidase-H$_2$O$_2$-halide system. *J Lab Clin Med* 1982;100:896–907.

298. Clark RA, Borregaard N. Neutrophils autoinactivate secretory products by myeloperoxidase-catalyzed oxidation. *Blood* 1985;65: 375–381.

299. Vissers MCM, Winterbourn CC. The effect of oxidants on neutrophil-mediated degradation of glomerular basement membrane collagen. *Biochim Biophys Acta* 1986;889:277–286.

300. Vissers MCM, Winterbourn CC. Myeloperoxidase-dependent oxidative inactivation of neutrophil neutral proteinases and microbicidal enzymes. *Biochem J* 1987;245:277–280.

301. Zgliczynski JM. Characteristics of myeloperoxidase from neutrophils and other peroxidases from different cell types. In: Sbarra AJ, Strauss

RR, eds. *The reticuloendothelial system. A comprehensive treatise, vol 2: biochemistry and metabolism.* New York: Plenum Press, 1980: 255–278.

302. Matheson NR, Wong PS, Travis J. Isolation and properties of human neutrophil myeloperoxidase. *Biochemistry* 1981;20:325–330.

303. El-Hag A, Clark RA. Down-regulation of human natural killer activity against tumors by the neutrophil myeloperoxidase system and hydrogen peroxide. *J Immunol* 1984;133:3291–3297.

304. El-Hag A, Lipsky PE, Bennett M, Clark RA. Immunomodulation by neutrophil myeloperoxidase and hydrogen peroxide: differential susceptibility of human lymphocyte functions. *J Immunol* 1986;136: 3420–3426.

305. Smit MJ, Anderson R. Inhibition of mitogen-activated proliferation of human lymphocytes by hypochlorous acid *in vitro*: protection and reversal by ascorbate and cysteine. *Agents Actions* 1990;30:338–343.

306. El-Hag A, Clark RA. Immunosuppression by activated human neutrophils. Dependence on the myeloperoxidase system. *J Immunol* 1987;139:2406–2413.

307. Klebanoff SJ, Clark RA. Hemolysis and iodination of erythrocyte components by a myeloperoxidase-mediated system. *Blood* 1975;45: 699–707.

308. Borregaard N, Kragbelle K. Role of oxygen in antibody-dependent cytotoxicity mediated by monocytes and neutrophils. *J Clin Invest* 1980;66:676–683.

309. Dallegri F, Patrone F, Frumento G, Banchi L, Succhetti C. Phagocytosis-dependent neutrophil-mediated extracellular cytotoxicity against different target cells. *Acta Haematol* 1984;71:371–375.

310. Greene WH, Colclough L, Anton A, Root RK. Lectin-dependent neutrophil-mediated cytotoxicity against chicken erythrocytes: a model of non-myeloperoxidase-mediated oxygen-dependent killing by human neutrophils. *J Immunol* 1980;125:2727–2734.

311. Katz P, Simone CB, Henkart PA, Fauci AS. Mechanisms of antibody-dependent cellular cytotoxicity. Use of effector cells from chronic granulomatous disease patients as investigative probes. *J Clin Invest* 1980;65:55–63.

312. Simchowitz L, Spilberg I. Evidence for the role of superoxide radicals in neutrophil-mediated cytotoxicity. *Immunology* 1979;37:301–309.

313. Weiss SJ. The role of superoxide in the destruction of erythrocyte targets by human neutrophils. *J Biol Chem* 1980;255:9912–9917.

314. Clark RA. Extracellular effects of the myeloperoxidase-hydrogen peroxide-halide system. In: Weissmann G, ed. *Advances in inflammation research,* vol 5. New York: Raven Press, 1983:107–146.

315. Baehner RL, Nathan DG, Castle WB. Oxidant injury of caucasian glucose-6-phosphate dehydrogenase-deficient red blood cells by phagocytising leukocytes during infection. *J Clin Invest* 1971;50: 2466–2473.

316. Clark RA, Klebanoff SJ. Myeloperoxidase-mediated platelet release reaction. *J Clin Invest* 1979;63:177–183.

317. Smith DC, Klebanoff SJ. A uterine fluid-mediated sperm inhibitory system. *Biol Reprod* 1970;3:229–235.

318. Klebanoff SJ, Smith DC. The source of H_2O_2 for the uterine fluid-mediated sperm-inhibitory system. *Biol Reprod* 1970;3:236–242.

319. Clark RA, Klebanoff SJ. Chemotactic factor inactivation by the myeloperoxidase-hydrogen peroxide-halide system. An inflammatory control mechanism. *J Clin Invest* 1979;64:913–920.

320. Tsan M. Myeloperoxidase-mediated oxidation of methionine. *J Cell Physiol* 1982;111:49–54.

321. Tsan M. Myeloperoxidase-mediated oxidation of methionine and amino acid decarboxylation. *Infect Immun* 1982;36:136–141.

322. Clark RA, Szot S. Chemotactic factor inactivation by stimulated human neutrophils mediated by myeloperoxidase-catalyzed methionine oxidation. *J Immunol* 1982;128:1507–1513.

323. Lane TA, Lamkin GE. Myeloperoxidase-mediated modulation of chemotactic peptide binding to human neutrophils. *Blood* 1983;61: 1203–1207.

324. Tsan M, Denison RC. Oxidation of n-formyl methionyl chemotactic peptide by human neutrophils. *J Immunol* 1981;126:1387–1389.

325. Harvath L, Aksamit RR. Oxidized N-formylmethionyl-leucyl-phenylalanine: effect on the activation of human monocyte and neutrophil chemotaxis and superoxide production. *J Immunol* 1984;133: 1471–1476.

326. Clark RA. Chemotactic factors trigger their own oxidative inactivation by human neutrophils. *J Immunol* 1982;129:2725–2728.

327. Aswanikumar S, Schiffmann E, Corcoran BA, Whal SM. Role of a peptidase in phagocyte chemotaxis. *Proc Natl Acad Sci USA* 1976;73: 2439–2442.

328. Gallin JI, Wright DG, Schiffmann E. Role of secretory events in modulating human neutrophil chemotaxis. *J Clin Invest* 1978;62: 1364–1374.

329. Yuli I, Snyderman R. Extensive hydrolysis of N-formyl-L-methionyl-l-leucyl-l-[³H] phenylalanine by human polymorphonuclear leukocytes. A potential mechanism for modulation of the chemoattractant signal. *J Biol Chem* 1986;261:4902–4908.

330. Brozna JP, Senior RM, Kreutzer DL, Ward PA. Chemotactic factor inactivators of human granulocytes. *J Clin Invest* 1977;60:1280–1288.

331. Venge P, Olsson I. Cationic proteins of human granulocytes. VI. Effects on the complement system and mediation of chemotactic activity. *J Immunol* 1975;115:1505–1508.

332. Wright DG, Gallin JI. A functional differentiation of human neutrophil granules: generation of C5a by a specific (secondary) granule product and inactivation of C5a by azurophil (primary) granule products. *J Immunol* 1977;119:1068–1076.

333. Morse JO. Alpha₁-antitrypsin deficiency. *N Engl J Med* 1978;299: 1045–1048,1099–1105.

334. Johnson D, Travis J. Structural evidence for methionine at the reactive site of human α-1-proteinase inhibitor. *J Biol Chem* 1978;253: 7142–7144.

335. Johnson D, Travis J. The oxidative inactivation of human alpha-1-proteinase inhibitor. Further evidence for methionine at the reactive center. *J Biol Chem* 1979;254:4022–4026.

336. Carp H, Janoff A. Potential mediator of inflammation. Phagocyte-derived oxidants suppress the elastase-inhibitory capacity of alpha₁-proteinase inhibitor *in vitro*. *J Clin Invest* 1980;66:987–995.

337. Clark RA, Stone PJ, El Hag A, Calore JD, Franzblau C. Myeloperoxidase-catalyzed inactivation of alpha₁-protease inhibitor by human neutrophils. *J Biol Chem* 1981;256:3348–3353.

338. Maier KL, Matejkova E, Hinze H, Leuschel L, Weber H, Beck-Speier I. Different selectivities of oxidants during oxidation of methionine residues in the α-1-proteinase inhibitor. *FEBS Lett* 1989;250: 221–226.

339. Carp H, Janoff A. *In vitro* suppression of serum elastase-inhibitory capacity by reactive oxygen species generated by phagocytosing polymorphonuclear leukocytes. *J Clin Invest* 1979;63:793–797.

340. Stroncek DF, Vercellotti GM, Huh PW, Jacob HS. Neutrophil oxidants inactivate alpha-1-protease inhibitor and promote PMN-mediated detachment of cultured endothelium. Protection by free methionine. *Arteriosclerosis* 1986;6:332–340.

341. Shock A, Baum H. Inactivation of alpha-1-proteinase inhibitor in serum by stimulated human polymorphonuclear leucocytes. Evidence for a myeloperoxidase-dependent mechanism. *Cell Biochem Function* 1988;6:13–23.

342. Ossanna PJ, Test ST, Matheson NR, Regiani S, Weiss SJ. Oxidative regulation of neutrophil elastase-alpha-1-proteinase inhibitor interactions. *J Clin Invest* 1986;77:1939–1951.

343. Zaslow MC, Clark RA, Stone PJ, Calore JD, Snider GL, Franzblau C. Human neutrophil elastase does not bind to alpha 1-protease inhibitor that has been exposed to activated human neutrophils. *Am Rev Respir Dis* 1983;128:434–439.

344. Padrines M, Schneider-Pozzer M, Bieth JG. Inhibition of neutrophil elastase by alpha-1-proteinase inhibitor oxidized by activated neutrophils. *Am Rev Respir Dis* 1989;139:783–790.

345. Janoff A, George-Nascimento C, Rosenberg S. A genetically engineered, mutant human alpha-1-proteinase inhibitor is more resistant than the normal inhibitor to oxidative inactivation by chemicals, enzymes, cells, and cigarette smoke. *Am Rev Respir Dis* 1986;133: 353–356.

346. Theron A, Anderson R. Investigation of the protective effects of the antioxidants ascorbate, cysteine, and dapsone on the phagocyte-mediated oxidative inactivation of human alpha-1-protease inhibitor *in vitro*. *Am Rev Respir Dis* 1985;132:1049–1054.

347. Matheson NR. The effect of antiarthritic drugs and related compounds on the human neutrophil myeloperoxidase system. *Biochem Biophys Res Commun* 1982;108:259–265.

348. Nowak D, Ruta U. Nicotine inhibits α-1-proteinase inhibitor inactivation by oxidants derived from human polymorphonuclear leukocytes. *Exp Pathol* 1990;38:249–255.

349. Nowak D, Piasecka G. Erythrocytes protect α-1-proteinase inhibitor from oxidative inactivation induced by chemicals, the myeloperoxi-

dase-H_2O_2-halide system and stimulated polymorphonuclear leukocytes. *Exp Pathol* 1991;42:47–58.

350. Banda MJ, Clark EJ, Werb Z. Regulation of alpha$_1$, proteinase inhibitor function by rabbit alveolar macrophages. Evidence for proteolytic rather than oxidative inactivation. *J Clin Invest* 1985;75:1758–1762.

351. Abrams WR, Weinbaum G, Weissbach L, Weissbach H, Brot N. Enzymatic reduction of oxidized α-1-proteinase inhibitor restores biological activity. *Proc Natl Acad Sci USA* 1981;78:7483–7486.

352. Carp H, Janoff A, Abrams W, et al. Human methionine sulfoxide-peptide reductase, an enzyme capable of reactivating oxidized alpha-1-proteinase inhibitor *in vitro*. *Am Rev Respir Dis* 1983;127:301–305.

353. Aruoma OI, Halliwell B. Inactivation of α$_1$-antiproteinase by hydroxyl radicals. The effect of uric acid. *FEBS Lett* 1989;244:76–80.

354. Vissers MCM, George PM, Bathurst IC, Brennan SO, Winterbourn CC. Cleavage and inactivation of α$_1$-antitrypsin by metalloproteinases released from neutrophils. *J Clin Invest* 1988;82:706–711.

355. Wallaert B, Gressier B, Aerts C, Mizon C, Voisin C, Mizon J. Oxidative inactivation of α1-proteinase inhibitor by alveolar macrophages from healthy smokers requires the presence of myeloperoxidase. *Am J Respir Cell Mol Biol* 1991;5:437–444.

356. Ottonello L, Dapino P, Dallegri F. Inactivation of alpha-1-proteinase inhibitor by neutrophil metalloproteinases. Crucial role of the myeloperoxidase system and effects of the anti-inflammatory drug nimesulide. *Respiration* 1993;60:32–37.

357. Wong PS, Travis J. Isolation and properties of oxidized alpha-1-proteinase inhibitor from human rheumatoid synovial fluid. *Biochim Biophys Res Commun* 1980;96:1449–1454.

358. Bruce M, Boat T, Martin RJ, Dearborn D, Fanaroff A. Proteinase inhibitors and inhibitor inactivation of neonatal airways secretions. *Chest* 1982;81(suppl):44S–45S.

359. Cochrane CG, Spragg RG, Revak SD. Studies on the pathogenesis of the adult respiratory distress syndrome: evidence of oxidant activity in bronchoalveolar lavage fluid. *J Clin Invest* 1983;71:754–761.

360. Cochrane CG, Spragg RG, Revak SD, Cohen AB, McGuire WW. The presence of neutrophil elastase and evidence of oxidant activity of bronchoalveolar lavage fluid of patients with adult respiratory distress syndrome. *Am Rev Respir Dis* 1983;127:S25–S27.

361. Lee CT, Fein AM, Lippmann M, Holtzman H, Kimbel P, Weinbaum G. Elastolytic activity in pulmonary lavage fluid from patients with adult respiratory distress syndrome. *N Engl J Med* 1981;304:192–196.

362. Merritt TA, Cochrane C, Holcomb K, et al. Elastase and α$_1$ proteinase inhibitor activity in tracheal aspirates during respiratory distress syndrome. Role of inflammation in the pathogenesis of bronchopulmonary dysplasia. *J Clin Invest* 1983;72:656–666.

363. Carp H, Miller F, Hoidal JR, Janoff A. Potential mechanism of emphysema:α$_1$-proteinase inhibitor recovered from lungs of cigarette smokers contains oxidized methionine and had decreased elastase inhibitory activity. *Proc Natl Acad Sci USA* 1982;79:2041–2045.

364. Janoff A, Carp H, Lee DK, Drew RT. Cigarette smoke inhalation decreases α$_1$-antitrypsin activity in rat lung. *Science* 1979;206:1313–1314.

365. Zaslow MC, Clark RA, Stone PJ, Calore J, Snider GL, Franzblau C. Myeloperoxidase-induced inactivation of alpha$_1$-antiprotease in hamsters. *J Lab Clin Med* 1985;105:178–184.

366. Stone PJ, Lucey EC, Breuer R, et al. Oxidants from neutrophil myeloperoxidase do not enhance elastase-induced emphysema in the hamster. *Respiration* 1993;60:137–143.

367. Henderson WR, Kaliner M. Mast cell granule peroxidase: location, secretion and SRS-A inactivation. *J Immunol* 1979;122:1322–1328.

368. Henderson WR, Jorg A, Klebanoff SJ. Eosinophil peroxidase-mediated inactivation of leukotrienes B$_4$, C$_4$ and D$_4$. *J Immunol* 1982;128:2609–2613.

369. Jorg A, Henderson WR, Murphy RC, Klebanoff SJ. Leukotriene generation by eosinophils. *J Exp Med* 1982;155:390–402.

370. Goetzl EJ. The conversion of leukotriene C$_4$ to isomers of leukotriene B$_4$ by human eosinophil peroxidase. *Biochem Biophys Res Commun* 1982;106:270–275.

371. Henderson WR, Chi EY, Jorg A, Klebanoff SJ. Horse eosinophil degranulation induced by the ionophore A23187. Ultrastructure and role of phospholipase A$_2$. *Am J Pathol* 1983;111:341–349.

372. Sepe SM, Clark RA. Oxidant membrane injury by the neutrophil myeloperoxidase system. I. Characterization of a liposome model and injury by myeloperoxidase, hydrogen peroxide, and halides. *J Immunol* 1985;134:1888–1895.

373. Sepe SM, Clark RA. Oxidant membrane injury by the neutrophil myeloperoxidase system. II. Injury by stimulated neutrophils and protection by lipid-soluble antioxidants. *J Immunol* 1985;134:1896–1901.

374. Clark RA, Szot S, Williams MA, Kagan HM. Oxidation of lysine sidechains of elastin by the myeloperoxidase system and by stimulated human neutrophils. *Biochem Biophys Res Commun* 1986;135:451–457.

375. Paredes J, Weiss SJ. Human neutrophils transform prostaglandins by a myeloperoxidase-dependent mechanism. *J Biol Chem* 1982;257:2738–2740.

376. Whitin JC, Clark RA, Simons ER, Cohen HJ. Effects of the myeloperoxidase system on fluorescent probes of granulocyte membrane potential. *J Biol Chem* 1981;256:8904–8906.

377. Hurst JK, Albrich JM, Green TR, Rosen H, Klebanoff SJ. Myeloperoxidase-dependent fluorescein chlorination by stimulated neutrophils. *J Biol Chem* 1984;259:4812–4821.

378. Vissers MCM, Winterbourn CC. Oxidative damage to fibronectin. 1. The effects of the neutrophil myeloperoxidase system and HOCl. *Arch Biochem Biophys* 1991;285:53–59.

379. Winterbourn CC, Molloy AL. Susceptibilities of lactoferrin and transferrin to myeloperoxidase-dependent loss of iron-binding capacity. *Biochem J* 1988;250:613–616.

380. Clark RA, Pearson DW. Inactivation of transferrin iron binding capacity by the neutrophil myeloperoxidase system. *J Biol Chem* 1989;264:9420–9427.

381. Lindvall S, Rydell G. Influence of various compounds on the degradation of hyaluronic acid by a myeloperoxidase system. *Chem Biol Interact* 1994;90:1–12.

382. Katrantzis M, Baker MS, Handley CJ, Lowther DA. The oxidant hypochlorite (OCl$^-$), a product of the myeloperoxidase system, degrades articular cartilage proteoglycan aggregate. *Free Radic Biol Med* 1991;10:101–109.

383. Cribb AE, Miller M, Tesoro A, Spielberg SP. Peroxidase-dependent oxidation of sulfonamides by monocytes and neutrophils from humans and dogs. *Mol Pharmacol* 1990;38:744–751.

384. Kalyanaraman B, Sohnle PG. Generation of free radical intermediates from foreign compounds by neutrophil-derived oxidants. *J Clin Invest* 1985;75:1618–1622.

385. Odajima T. Study on the inactivation of antibiotics and hydrolases by myeloperoxidase. *Jpn J Oral Biol* 1985;27:1216–1227.

386. Henderson WR, Chi EY, Klebanoff SJ. Eosinophil peroxidase-induced mast cell secretion. *J Exp Med* 1980;152:265–279.

387. Chi EY, Henderson WR. Ultrastructure of mast cell degranulation induced by eosinophil peroxidase: use of diaminobenzidine cytochemistry by scanning electron microscopy. *J Histochem Cytochem* 1984;32:332–341.

388. Stendahl O, Molin L, Lindroth M. Granulocyte-mediated release of histamine from mast cells. Effect of myeloperoxidase and its inhibition by antiinflammatory sulfone compounds. *Int Arch Allergy Appl Immunol* 1983;70:277–284.

389. Coble B, Lindroth M, Molin L, Stendahl O. Histamine release from mast cells during phagocytosis and interaction with activated neutrophils. *Int Arch Allergy Appl Immunol* 1984;75:32–37.

390. Macartney H, Tschesche H. Latent and active human polymorphonuclear leukocyte collagenases. Isolation, purification and characterization. *Eur J Biochem* 1983;130:71–78.

391. Murphy G, Reynolds J, Bretz U, Baggiolini M. Partial purification of collagenase and gelatinase from human polymorphonuclear leukocytes. *Biochem J* 1982;203:209–221.

392. Tschesche H, Macartney H. A new principle of regulation of enzymic activity. Activation and regulation of human polymorphonuclear leukocyte collagenase via disulfide-thiol exchange as catalyzed by the glutathione cycle in a peroxidase coupled reaction to glucose metabolism. *Eur J Biochem* 1981;120:183–190.

393. Claesson R, Karlsson M, Zhang Y, Carlsson J. Relative role of chloramines, hypochlorous acid, and proteases in the activation of human polymorphonuclear leukocyte collagenase. *J Leukoc Biol* 1996;60:598–602.

394. Weiss SJ, Peppin G, Ortiz X, Ragsdale C, Test ST. Oxidative autoactivation of latent collagenase by human neutrophils. *Science* 1985;227:747–749.

395. Saari H, Suomalainen K, Lindy O, Konttinen YT, Sorsa T. Activation of latent human neutrophil collagenase by reactive oxygen species and serine proteases. *Biochem Biophys Res Commun* 1990;171:979–987.

396. Capodici C, Berg RA. Hypochlorous acid (HOCl) activation of neutrophil collagenase requires cathepsin G. *Agents Actions* 1989;27: 481–484.

397. Dewald B, Bretz U, Baggiolini M. Release of gelatinase from a novel secretory compartment of human neutrophils. *J Clin Invest* 1982;70: 518–525.

398. Peppin GJ, Weiss SJ. Activation of the endogenous metalloproteinase, gelatinase, by triggered human neutrophils. *Proc Natl Acad Sci USA* 1986;83:4322–4326.

399. Vissers MCM, Winterbourn CC. Activation of human neutrophil gelatinase by endogenous serine proteinases. *Biochem J* 1988;249: 327–331.

400. Shah SV, Baricos WH, Basci A. Degradation of human glomerular basement membrane by stimulated neutrophils. Activation of a metalloproteinase(s) by reactive oxygen species. *J Clin Invest* 1987;79: 25–31.

401. Zabucchi G, Menegazzi R, Roncelli L, Bertoncin P, Tedesco F, Patriarca P. Protective and inactivating effects of neutrophil myeloperoxidase on C1q activity. *Inflammation* 1990;14:41–53.

402. Vogt W, Hesse D. Oxidants generated by the myeloperoxidase-halide system activate the fifth component of human complement, C5. *Immunobiology* 1994;192:1–9.

403. Johnson KJ, Fantone JCI, Kaplan J, Ward PA. *In vivo* damage of rat lungs by oxygen metabolites. *J Clin Invest* 1981;67:983–993.

404. Johnson KJ, Ward PA. Role of oxygen metabolites in immune complex injury of lung. *J Immunol* 1981;126:2365–2369.

405. Cantin AM, North SL, Fells GA, Hubbard RC, Crystal RG. Oxidant-mediated epithelial cell injury in idiopathic pulmonary fibrosis. *J Clin Invest* 1987;79:1665–1673.

406. Graham RC, Karnovsky MJ. Glomerular permeability. Ultrastructural cytochemical studies using peroxidases as protein tracers. *J Exp Med* 1966;124:1123–1134.

407. Johnson RJ, Couser WG, Chi EY, Adler S, Klebanoff SJ. New mechanism for glomerular injury. Myeloperoxidase-hydrogen peroxide-halide system. *J Clin Invest* 1987;79:1379–1387.

408. Johnson RJ, Guggenheim SJ, Klebanoff SJ, et al. Morphologic correlates of glomerular oxidant injury induced by the myeloperoxidase-hydrogen peroxide-halide system of the neutrophil. *Lab Invest* 1988;5: 294–301.

409. Johnson RJ, Klebanoff SJ, Ochi RF, et al. Participation of the myeloperoxidase-H$_2$O$_2$-halide system in immune complex nephritis. *Kidney Int* 1987;32:342–349.

410. Vissers MCM, Winterbourn CC, Hunt JS. Degradation of glomerular basement membrane by human neutrophils *in vitro*. *Biochim Biophys Acta* 1984;804:154–160.

411. Klebanoff SJ, Kinsella MG, Wight TN. Degradation of endothelial cell matrix heparan sulfate proteoglycan by elastase and the myeloperoxidase-H$_2$O$_2$-chloride system. *Am J Pathol* 1993;143:907–917.

412. Johnson RJ, Couser WG, Alpers CE, Vissers M, Schulze M, Klebanoff SJ. The human neutrophil serine proteinases, elastase and cathepsin G, can mediate glomerular injury *in vivo*. *J Exp Med* 1988;168: 1169–1174.

413. Vissers MCM, Day WA, Winterbourn CC. Neutrophils adherent to a nonphagocytosable surface (glomerular basement membrane) produce oxidants only at the site of attachment. *Blood* 1985;66:161–166.

414. Nathan CF, Cohn ZA. Antitumor effects of hydrogen peroxide *in vivo*. *J Exp Med* 1981;154:1539–1553.

415. Schultz J, Baker A, Tucker B. Myeloperoxidase-enzyme therapy on rat mammary tumors. In: Schultz J, Ahmad F, eds. *Cancer enzymology.* New York: Academic Press, 1976:319–333.

416. Everse J. Tumoricidal activity of peroxidases. In: Everse J, Everse KE, Grisham MB, eds. *Peroxidases in chemistry and biology,* vol 2. Boca Raton, FL: CRC Press, 1990:239–255.

417. Wieland E, Parthasarathy S, Steinberg D. Peroxidase-dependent metal-independent oxidation of low density lipoprotein *in vitro*: a model for *in vivo* oxidation. *Proc Natl Acad Sci USA* 1993;90:5929–5933.

418. Arnhold J, Wiegel D, Richter O, Hammerschmidt S, Arnold K, Krumbiegel M. Modification of low density lipoproteins by sodium hypochlorite. *Biomed Biochim Acta* 1991;50:967–973.

419. Evgina SA, Panasenko OM, Sergienko VI, Vladimirov YA. Peroxidation of human plasma lipoproteins induced by hypochlorite. *Biol Mem* 1992;6:1247–1254.

420. Francis GA, Mendez AJ, Bierman EL, Heinecke JW. Oxidative tyrosylation of high density lipoprotein by peroxidase enhances cholesterol removal from cultured fibroblasts and macrophage foam cells. *Proc Natl Acad Sci USA* 1993;90:6631–6635.

421. Hazell LJ, Stocker R. Oxidation of low-density lipoprotein with hypochlorite causes transformation of the lipoprotein into a high-uptake form for macrophages. *Biochem J* 1993;290:165–172.

422. Hazell LJ, van den Berg JJM, Stocker R. Oxidation of low-density lipoprotein by hypochlorite causes aggregation that is mediated by modification of lysine residues rather than lipid oxidation. *Biochem J* 1994;302:297–304.

423. O'Connell AM, Gieseg SP, Stanley KK. Hypochlorite oxidation causes cross-linking of Lp(a). *Biochim Biophys Acta* 1994;1225:180–186.

424. Panasenko OM, Evgina SA, Aidyraliev RK, Sergienko VI, Vladimirov YA. Peroxidation of human blood lipoproteins induced by exogenous hypochlorite or hypochlorite generated in the system of "myeloperoxidase + H$_2$O$_2$ + Cl$^-$." *Free Radic Biol Med* 1994;16:143–148.

425. Panasenko OM, Evgina SA, Driomina ES, Sharov VS, Sergienko VI, Vladimirov YA. Hypochlorite induces lipid peroxidation in blood lipoproteins and phospholipid liposomes. *Free Radic Biol Med* 1995; 19:133–140.

426. Hazen SL, Hsu FF, Duffin K, Heinecke JW. Molecular chlorine generated by the myeloperoxidase-hydrogen peroxide-chloride system of phagocytes converts low density lipoprotein cholesterol into a family of chlorinated sterols. *J Biol Chem* 1996;271:23080–23088.

427. Daugherty A, Dunn JL, Rateri DL, Heinecke JW. Myeloperoxidase, a catalyst for lipoprotein oxidation, is expressed in human atherosclerotic lesions. *J Clin Invest* 1994;94:437–444.

428. Malle E, Hazell L, Stocker R, Sattler W, Esterbauer H, Waeg G. Immunologic detection and measurement of hypochlorite-modified LDL with specific monoclonal antibodies. *Arterioscler Thromb Vasc Biol* 1995;15:982–989.

429. Hazell LJ, Arnold L, Flowers D, Waeg G, Malle E, Stocker R. Presence of hypochlorite-modified proteins in human atherosclerotic lesions. *J Clin Invest* 1996;97:1535–1544.

430. Klebanoff SJ. Myeloperoxidase-mediated antimicrobial systems and their role in leukocyte function. In: Schultz J, ed. *Biochemistry of the phagocytic process.* Amsterdam: North Holland, 1970;89–110.

431. Briggs RT, Karnovsky ML, Karnovsky MJ. Cytochemical demonstration of hydrogen peroxide in the polymorphonuclear leukocyte phagosomes. *J Cell Biol* 1975;64:254–260.

432. Briggs RT, Drath DB, Karnovsky ML, Karnovsky MJ. Localization of NADH oxidase on the surface of human polymorphonuclear leukocytes by a new cytochemical method. *J Cell Biol* 1975;67:566–586.

433. Root RK, Stossel TP. Myeloperoxidase-mediated iodination by granulocytes. Intracellular site of operation and some regulating factors. *J Clin Invest* 1974;53:1207–1215.

434. Klebanoff SJ, Hamon CB. Role of myeloperoxidase-mediated antimicrobial systems in intact leukocytes. *J Reticuloendothel Soc* 1972;12: 170–196.

435. Odeberg H, Olofsson T, Olsson I. Myeloperoxidase-mediated extracellular iodination during phagocytosis in granulocytes. *Scand J Haematol* 1974;12:155–160.

436. Segal AW, Garcia RC, Harper AM. Iodination by stimulated human neutrophils. Studies on its stoichiometry, subcellular localization and relevance to microbial killing. *Biochem J* 1983;210:215–225.

437. Johnston RBJ, Baehner RL. Improvement of leukocyte bactericidal activity in chronic granulomatous disease. *Blood* 1970;35:350–355.

438. Root RK. Correction of the function of chronic granulomatous disease (CGD) granulocytes (PMN) with extracellular H$_2$O$_2$. *Clin Res* 1974;22:452A(abst).

439. Kaplan EL, Laxdal T, Quie PG. Studies of polymorphonuclear leukocytes from patients with chronic granulomatous disease of childhood: bactericidal capacity for streptococci. *Pediatrics* 1968;41:591–599.

440. Klebanoff SJ, White LR. Iodination defect in the leukocytes of a patient with chronic granulomatous disease of childhood. *N Engl J Med* 1969;280:460–466.

441. Mandell GL, Hook EW. Leukocyte bactericidal activity in chronic granulomatous disease: correlation of bacterial hydrogen peroxide production and susceptibility to intracellular killing. *J Bacteriol* 1969;100:531–532.

442. Pitt J, Bernheimer HP. Role of peroxide in phagocytic killing of pneumococci. *Infect Immun* 1974;9:48–52.

443. Amin VM, Olson NF. Selective increase in hydrogen peroxide resistance of a coagulase-positive staphylococcus. *J Bacteriol* 1968;95: 1604–1607.

444. Amin VM, Olson NF. Influence of catalase activity on resistance of coagulase-positive staphylococci to hydrogen peroxide. *Appl Microbiol* 1968;16:267–270.

445. Mandell GL. Catalase, superoxide dismutase, and virulence of staphylococcus aureus. *In vitro* and *in vivo* studies with emphasis on staphylococcal-leukocyte interaction. *J Clin Invest* 1975;55:561–566.

446. Klebanoff SJ. Myeloperoxidase: contribution to the microbicidal activity of intact leukocytes. *Science* 1970;169:1095–1097.

447. Koch C. Effect of sodium azide upon normal and pathological granulocyte function. *Acta Pathol Microbiol Scand* 1974;82:136–142.

448. Stendahl O, Lindgren S. Function of granulocytes with deficient myeloperoxidase-mediated iodination in a patient with generalized pustular psoriasis. *Scand J Haematol* 1976;16:144–153.

449. Lehrer RI. Inhibition by sulfonamides of the candidacidal activity of human neutrophils. *J Clin Invest* 1971;50:2498–2505.

450. Korchak HM, Roos D, Giedd KN, et al. Granulocytes without degranulation: neutrophil function in granule-depleted cytoplasts. *Proc Natl Acad Sci USA* 1983;80:4968–4972.

451. Roos D, Voetman AA, Meerhof LJ. Functional activity of enucleated human polymorphonuclear leukocytes. *J Cell Biol* 1983;97:368–377.

452. Odell EW, Segal AW. The bactericidal effects of the respiratory burst and the myeloperoxidase system isolated in neutrophil cytoplasts. *Biochim Biophys Acta* 1988;971:266–274.

453. Schock L, Vercellotti G, Stroncek D, Jacob HS. Use of lysosome-free PMN cytoplasts ("neutroplasts") uncovers the critical role of myeloperoxidase for target cell lysis. *Clin Res* 1984;32:753A(abst).

454. Nauseef WM. Myeloperoxidase deficiency. *Hematol Oncol Clin North Am* 1988;2:135–158.

455. Nauseef WM. Myeloperoxidase deficiency. *Hematol Pathol* 1990;4:165–178.

456. Grignaschi VJ, Sperperato AM, Etcheverry MJ, Macario AJL. Un nuevo cuadro citoquimico: negatividad espontanea de las reacciones de peroxidasas, oxidasas y lipido en la progenie neutrofila y en los monocitos de dos hermanos. *Rev Asoc Med Argent* 1963;77:218–221.

457. Lehrer RI, Cline MJ. Leukocyte myeloperoxidase deficiency and disseminated candidiasis: the role of myeloperoxidase in resistance to *Candida* infection. *J Clin Invest* 1969;48:1478–1488.

458. Cramer R, Soranzo MR, Dri P, et al. Incidence of myeloperoxidase deficiency in an area of northern Italy: histochemical, biochemical and functional studies. *Br J Haematol* 1982;51:81–87.

459. Parry MF, Root RK, Metcalf JA, Delaney KK, Kaplow LS, Richar WJ. Myeloperoxidase deficiency. Prevalence and clinical significance. *Ann Intern Med* 1981;95:293–301.

460. Becker R, Pfluger K-H. Myeloperoxidase deficiency: an epidemiological study and flow-cytometric detection of other granular enzymes in myeloperoxidase-deficient subjects. *Ann Hematol* 1994;69:199–203.

461. Grossl NA, Candel AG, Shrit A, Schumacher HR. Myeloperoxidase deficiency and severe sepsis. *South Med J* 1993;86:832–836.

462. Moosmann K, Bojanovsky A. Rezidivierende Candidosis bei Myeloperoxydasemangel. *Mschr Kinderheilk* 1975;123:408–409.

463. Cech P, Stalder H, Widmann J, Rohner A, Miescher PA. Leukocyte myeloperoxidase deficiency and diabetes mellitus associated with *Candida albicans* liver abscess. *Am J Med* 1979;66:149–153.

464. Robertson CF, Thong YH, Hodge GL, Cheney K. Primary myeloperoxidase deficiency associated with impaired neutrophil margination and chemotaxis. *Acta Paediatr Scand* 1979;68:915–919.

465. Kusenbach G, Rister M. Der Myeloperoxidase—Mangel als Ursache rezidivierender Infektionen. *Klin Padiatr* 1985;197:443–445.

466. Weber ML, Abela A, Derepentigny L, Garel L, Lapointe N. Myeloperoxidase deficiency with extensive candidal osteomyelitis of the base of the skull. *Pediatrics* 1987;80:876–879.

467. Okuda T, Yasuoka T, Oka N. Myeloperoxidase deficiency as a predisposing factor for deep mucocutaneous candidiasis. A case report. *J Oral Maxillofac Surg* 1991;49:183–186.

468. Ludviksson BR, Thorarensen O, Gudnason T, Halldorsson S. *Candida albicans* meningitis in a child with myeloperoxidase deficiency. *Pediatr Infect Dis* 1993;12:162–164.

469. Nguyen C, Katner HP. Myeloperoxidase deficiency manifesting as pustular candidal dermatitis. *Clin Infect Dis* 1997;24:258–260.

470. Nauseef WM. Aberrant restriction endonuclease digests of DNA from subjects with hereditary myeloperoxidase deficiency. *Blood* 1989;73:290–295.

471. Selsted ME, Miller CW, Novotny MJ, Morris WL, Koeffler HP. Molecular analysis of myeloperoxidase deficiency shows heterogeneous patterns of the complete deficiency state manifested at the genomic, mRNA, and protein levels. *Blood* 1993;82:1317–1322.

472. Nauseef WM, Brigham S, Cogley M. Hereditary myeloperoxidase deficiency due to a missense mutation of arginine 569 to tryptophan. *J Biol Chem* 1994;269:1212–1216.

473. Kizaki M, Miller CW, Selsted ME, Koeffler HP. Myeloperoxidase (MPO) gene mutation in hereditary MPO deficiency. *Blood* 1994;83:1935–1940.

474. Nauseef WM, Root RK, Malech HL. Biochemical and immunologic analysis of hereditary myeloperoxidase deficiency. *J Clin Invest* 1983;71:1297–1307.

475. Bos AJ, Weening RS, Hamers MN, Wever R, Behrendt H, Roos D. Characterization of hereditary partial myeloperoxidase deficiency. *J Lab Clin Med* 1982;99:589–600.

476. Cech P, Papathanassiou A, Boreux G, Roth P, Miescher PA. Hereditary myeloperoxidase deficiency. *Blood* 1979;53:403–411.

477. Kitahara M, Eyre HJ, Simonian Y, Atkin CL, Hasstedt SJ. Hereditary myeloperoxidase deficiency. *Blood* 1981;57:888–893.

478. Lehrer RI, Hanifin J, Cline MJ. Defective bactericidal activity in myeloperoxidase-deficient human neutrophils. *Nature* 1969;223:78–79.

479. Lehrer RI, Cline MJ. Interaction of *Candida albicans* with human leukocytes and serum. *J Bacteriol* 1969;98:996–1004.

480. Cramer R, Soranzo MR, Patriarca P. Evidence that eosinophils catalyze the bromide-dependent decarboxylation of amino acids. *Blood* 1981;58:1112–1118.

481. DeChatelet LR, Long GD, Shirley PS, et al. Mechanism of the luminol-dependent chemiluminescence of human neutrophils. *J Immunol* 1982;129:1589–1593.

482. Klebanoff SJ, Pincus SH. Hydrogen peroxide utilization in myeloperoxidase-deficient leukocytes: a possible microbicidal control mechanism. *J Clin Invest* 1971;50:2226–2229.

483. Rosen H, Klebanoff SJ. Chemiluminescence and superoxide production by myeloperoxidase-deficient leukocytes. *J Clin Invest* 1976;58:50–60.

484. Dri P, Soranzo MR, Cramer R, Menegazzi R, Miotti V, Patriarca P. Role of myeloperoxidase in respiratory burst of human polymorphonuclear leukocytes. Studies with myeloperoxidase-deficient subjects. *Inflammation* 1985;9:21–31.

485. Dri P, Cramer R, Soranzo MR, Miotti R, Menegazzi R, Patriarca P. Influence of myeloperoxidase on neutrophil functions: studies with MPO-deficient neutrophils. *Agents Actions* 1984;15:43–44.

486. Klebanoff SJ, Clark RA. Iodination by human polymorphonuclear leukocytes: a re-evaluation. *J Lab Clin Med* 1977;89:675–686.

487. Locksley RM, Wilson CB, Klebanoff SJ. Increased respiratory burst in myeloperoxidase-deficient monocytes. *Blood* 1983;62:902–909.

488. Jandl RC, Andre-Schwartz J, Borges-Dubois L, Kipnes RS, McMurrich BJ, Babior BM. Termination of the respiratory burst in human neutrophils. *J Clin Invest* 1978;61:1176–1185.

489. Edwards SW, Swan TF. Regulation of superoxide generation by myeloperoxidase during the respiratory burst of human neutrophils. *Biochem J* 1986;237:601–604.

490. Nauseef WM, Metcalf JA, Root RK. Role of myeloperoxidase in the respiratory burst of human neutrophils. *Blood* 1983;61:483–492.

491. Dri P, Cramer R, Menegazzi R, Patriarca P. Increased degranulation of human myeloperoxidase-deficient polymorphonuclear leukocytes. *Br J Haematol* 1985;59:115–125.

492. Gaither TA, Medley SR, Gallin JI, Frank MM. Studies of phagocytosis in chronic granulomatous disease. *Inflammation* 1987;11:211–227.

493. Hakansson L, Venge P. Kinetic studies of neutrophil phagocytosis. V. Studies on the co-operation between the Fc and C3b receptors. *Immunology* 1982;47:687–694.

494. Boxer LA, Allen JM, Baehner RL. Potentiation of polymorphonuclear leukocyte motile functions by 2,3-dihydroxybenzoic acid. *J Lab Clin Med* 1978;92:730–736.

495. Henderson WR, Klebanoff SJ. Leukotriene production and inactivation by normal, chronic granulomatous disease and myeloperoxidase-deficient neutrophils. *J Biol Chem* 1983;258:13522–13527.

496. Weiss SJ. Tissue destruction by neutrophils. *N Engl J Med* 1989;320:365–375.

497. Pontremoli S, Melloni E, Michetti M, et al. Cytolytic effects of neutrophils: role for a membrane-bound neutral proteinase. *Proc Natl Acad Sci USA* 1986;83:1685–1689.

498. Adams DO, Johnson WJ, Fiorito E, Nathan CF. Hydrogen peroxide and cytolytic factor can interact synergistically in effecting cytolysis of neoplastic targets. *J Immunol* 1981;127:1973–1977.

499. Varani J, Ginsburg I, Schuger L, et al. Endothelial cell killing by neutrophils. Synergistic interaction of oxygen products and proteases. *Am J Pathol* 1989;135:435–438.

500. Lichtenstein AK, Ganz T, Selsted ME, Lehrer RI. Synergistic cytolysis mediated by hydrogen peroxide combined with peptide defensins. *Cell Immunol* 1988;114:104–116.

501. Yazdanbakhsh M, Tai P, Spry CJF, Gleich GJ, Roos D. Synergism between eosinophil cationic protein and oxygen metabolites in killing of schistosomula of *Schistosoma mansoni*. *J Immunol* 1987;138:3443–3447.

502. Ginsburg I, Kohen R. Cell damage in inflammatory and infectious sites might involve a coordinated "cross-talk" among oxidants, microbial haemolysins and ampiphiles, cationic proteins, phospholipases, fatty acids, proteinases and cytokines (an overview). *Free Radic Res* 1995;22:489–517.

503. Beckman JS, Beckman TW, Chen J, Marshall PA, Freeman BA. Apparent hydroxyl radical production by peroxynitrite: implications for endothelial injury from nitric oxide and superoxide. *Proc Natl Acad Sci USA* 1990;87:1620–1624.

504. McCall TB, Boughton-Smith NK, Palmer RMJ, Whittle BJR, Moncada S. Synthesis of nitric oxide from L-arginine by neutrophils. Release and interaction with superoxide anion. *Biochem J* 1989;261:293–296.

505. Radi R, Beckman JS, Bush KM, Freeman BA. Peroxynitrite oxidation of sulfhydryls. The cytotoxic potential of superoxide and nitric oxide. *J Biol Chem* 1991;266:4244–4250.

506. Floris R, Piersma SR, Yang G, Jones P, Wever R. Interaction of myeloperoxidase with peroxynitrite. A comparison with lactoperoxidase, horseradish peroxidase and catalase. *Eur J Biochem* 1993;215:767–775.

507. Cooper CE, Odell E. Interaction of human myeloperoxidase with nitrite. *FEBS Lett* 1992;314:58–60.

508. Klebanoff SJ. Reactive nitrogen intermediates and antimicrobial activity: role of nitrite. *Free Radic Biol Med* 1993;14:351–360.

509. Liles WC, Klebanoff SJ. Regulation of apoptosis in neutrophils—Fas track to death? *J Immunol* 1995;155:3289–3291.

510. Lennon SV, Martin SJ, Cotter TG. Dose-dependent induction of apoptosis in human tumor cell lines by widely diverging stimuli. *Cell Prolif* 1991;24:203–214.

511. Pierce GB, Parchment RE, Lewellyn AL. Hydrogen peroxide as a mediator of programmed cell death in the blastocyst. *Differentiation* 1991;46:181–186.

512. Sandstrom PA, Roberts B, Folks TM, Buttke TM. HIV gene expression enhances T cell susceptibility to hydrogen peroxide-induced apoptosis. *AIDS Res Hum Retrovir* 1993;9:1107–1113.

513. Forrest VJ, Kang Y-H, McClain DE, Robinson DH, Ramakrishnan N. Oxidative stress-induced apoptosis prevented by Trolox. *Free Radic Biol Med* 1994;16:675–684.

514. Whittemore ER, Loo DT, Cotman CW. Exposure to hydrogen peroxide induces cell death via apoptosis in cultured rat cortical neurons. *NeuroReport* 1994;5:1485–1488.

515. Hansson M, Asea A, Ersson U, Hermodsson S, Hellstrand K. Induction of apoptosis in NK cells by monocyte-derived reactive oxygen metabolites. *J Immunol* 1996;156:42–47.

516. Kasahara Y, Iwai K, Yachie A, et al. Involvement of reactive oxygen intermediates in spontaneous and CD95 (Fas/APO-1)-mediated apoptosis of neutrophils. *Blood* 1997;89:1748–1753.

517. Fenton HJH. Oxidation of tartaric acid in the presence of iron. *J Chem Soc* 1894;65:899–910.

518. Haber F, Weiss J. The catalytic decomposition of hydrogen peroxide by iron salts. *Proc R Soc Lond [A]* 1934;147:332–351.

519. Sadrzadeh SMH, Graf E, Panter SS, Hallaway PE, Eaton JW. Hemoglobin. A biologic Fenton reagent. *J Biol Chem* 1984;259:14354–14356.

520. Benatti U, Morelli A, Guida L, De Flora A. The production of activated oxygen species by an interaction of methemoglobin with ascorbate. *Biochem Biophys Res Commun* 1983;111:980–987.

521. Molloy AL, Winterbourn CC. Release of iron from phagocytosed *Escherichia coli* and uptake by neutrophil lactoferrin. *Blood* 1990;75:984–989.

522. Repine JE, Fox RB, Berger EM. Hydrogen peroxide kills *Staphylococcus aureus* by reacting with staphylococcal iron to form hydroxyl radical. *J Biol Chem* 1981;256:7094–7096.

523. Hoepelman IM, Bezemer WA, Vandenbroucke-Grauls CMJE, Marx JJM, Verhoef J. Bacterial iron enhances oxygen radical-mediated killing of *Staphylococcus aureus* by phagocytes. *Infect Immun* 1990;58:26–31.

524. Repine JE, Fox RB, Berger EM, Harada RN. Effect of staphylococcal iron content on the killing of *Staphylococcus aureus* by polymorphonuclear leukocytes. *Infect Immun* 1981;32:407–410.

525. Cohen MS, Britigan BE, Chai YS, Pou S, Roeder TL, Rosen GM. Phagocyte-derived free radicals stimulated by ingestion of iron rich *Staphylococcus Aureus*: a spin trapping study. *J Infect Dis* 1991;163:819–824.

526. Klebanoff SJ. The iron-H_2O_2-iodide cytotoxic system. *J Exp Med* 1982;156:1262–1267.

527. Levitz SM, Diamond RD. Killing of *Aspergillus fumigatus* spores and *Candida albicans* yeast phase by the iron-hydrogen peroxide-iodide cytotoxic system: comparison with the myeloperoxidase-hydrogen peroxide-halide system. *Infect Immun* 1984;43:1100–1102.

528. Sugar AM, Chahal RS, Brummer E, Stevens DA. The iron-hydrogen peroxide-iodide system is fungicidal: activity against the yeast phase of *Blastomyces dermatitidis*. *J Leukoc Biol* 1984;36:545–548.

529. Weinstein J, Bielski BHJ. Kinetics of the interaction of HO_2 and O_2 radicals with hydrogen peroxide. The Haber-Weiss reaction. *J Am Chem Soc* 1979;101:58–62.

530. Czapski G, Ilan YA. On the generation of the hydroxylation agent from the superoxide radical. Can the Haber-Weiss reaction be the source of ·OH radicals? *Photochem Photobiol* 1978;28:651–653.

531. Halliwell B. Superoxide-dependent formation of hydroxyl radicals in the presence of iron chelates: is it a mechanism for hydroxyl radical production in biochemical systems? *FEBS Lett* 1978;92:321–326.

532. McCord JM, Day ED Jr. Superoxide-dependent production of hydroxyl radical catalyzed by iron-EDTA complex. *FEBS Lett* 1978;86:139–142.

533. Sutton HC, Winterbourn CC. On the participation of higher oxidation states of iron and copper in Fenton reactions. *Free Radic Biol Med* 1989;6:53–60.

534. Youngman RJ. Oxygen activation—is the hydroxyl radical always biologically relevant. *Trends Biochem Sci* 1984;9:280–283.

535. Youngman RJ, Elstner EF. Oxygen species in paraquat toxicity: the crypto-OH radical. *FEBS Lett* 1981;129:265–268.

536. Koppenol WH, Liebman JF. The oxidizing nature of the hydroxyl radical. A comparison with the ferryl ion (FeO^{2+}). *J Phys Chem* 1984;88:99–101.

537. Rush JD, Bielski BHJ. Pulse radiolysis studies of alkaline Fe (III) and Fe (VI) solutions. Observation of transient iron complexes with intermediate oxidation states. *J Am Chem Soc* 1986;108:523–525.

538. Rush JD, Koppenol WH. Oxidizing intermediates in the reaction of ferrous EDTA with hydrogen peroxide. Reactions with organic molecules and ferrocytochrome C. *J Biol Chem* 1986;261:6730–6733.

539. Winterbourn CC, Sutton HC. Iron and xanthine oxidase catalyze formation of an oxidant species distinguishable from OH·: comparison with the Haber-Weiss reaction. *Arch Biochem Biophys* 1986;244:27–34.

540. Rowley DA, Halliwell B. Superoxide-dependent formation of hydroxyl radicals in the presence of thiol compounds. *FEBS Lett* 1982;138:33–36.

541. Saez G, Thornalley PJ, Hill HAO, Hems R, Bannister JV. The production of free radicals during the autoxidation of cysteine and their effect on isolated rat hepatocytes. *Biochim Biophys Acta* 1982;719:24–31.

542. Searle AJF, Tomasi A. Hydroxyl free radical production in iron-cysteine solutions and protection by zinc. *J Inorg Biochem* 1982;17:161–166.

543. Rowley DA, Halliwell B. Superoxide-dependent formation of hydroxyl radicals from NADH and NADPH in the presence of iron salts. *FEBS Lett* 1982;142:39–41.

544. Sutton HC, Winterbourn CC. Chelated iron-catalyzed OH· formation from paraquat radicals and H_2O_2: mechanism of formate oxidation. *Arch Biochem Biophys* 1984;235:106–115.

545. Winterbourn CC. Production of hydroxyl radicals from paraquat radicals and H_2O_2. *FEBS Lett* 1981;128:339–342.

546. Winterbourn CC, Sutton HC. Hydroxyl radical production from hydrogen peroxide and enzymatically generated paraquat radicals: catalytic requirements and oxygen dependence. *Arch Biochem Biophys* 1984;235:116–126.

762 / Chapter 47

547. Breslow R, Lukens LN. On the mechanism of action of an ascorbic acid-dependent nonenzymatic hydroxylating system. *J Biol Chem* 1960;235:292–296.

548. Grinstead RR. The oxidation of ascorbic acid by hydrogen peroxide. Catalysis by ethylenediaminetetraaceto-iron (III). *J Am Chem Soc* 1960;82:3464–3471.

549. Rowley DA, Halliwell B. Formation of hydroxyl radicals from hydrogen peroxide and iron salts by superoxide- and ascorbate-dependent mechanisms: relevance to the pathology of rheumatoid disease. *Clin Sci* 1983;64:649–653.

550. Winterbourn CC. Comparison of superoxide and other reducing agents in the biological production of hydroxyl radicals. *Biochem J* 1979;182:625–628.

551. Winterbourn CC. Hydroxyl radical production in body fluids. Roles of metal ions, ascorbate and superoxide. *Biochem J* 1981;198:125–131.

552. Wong SF, Halliwell B, Richmond R, Skowroneck WR. The role of superoxide and hydroxyl radicals in the degradation of hyaluronic acid induced by metal ions and by ascorbic acid. *J Inorg Biochem* 1981;14:127–134.

553. Winston GW, Feierman DE, Cederbaum AI. The role of iron chelates in hydroxyl radical production by rat liver microsomes, NADPH-cytochrome P-450 reductase and xanthine oxidase. *Arch Biochem Biophys* 1984;232:378–390.

554. Halliwell B, Foyer CH. Ascorbic acid, metal ions and the superoxide radical. *Biochem J* 1976;155:697–700.

555. Nishikimi M. Oxidation of ascorbic acid with superoxide generated by the xanthine-xanthine oxidase system. *Biochem Biophys Res Commun* 1975;63:463–468.

556. Winterbourn CC, Vissers MCM. Changes in ascorbate levels on stimulation of human neutrophils. *Biochim Biophys Acta* 1983;763:175–179.

557. Stankova L, Rigas DA, Keown P, Bigley R. Leukocyte ascorbate and glutathione: potential capacity for inactivating oxidants and free radicals. *J Reticuloendothel Soc* 1977;21:97–102.

558. Stankova L, Bigley R, Wyss SR, Aebi H. Catalase and dehydroascorbate reductase in human polymorphonuclear leukocytes (PMN). Possible functional relationship. *Experientia* 1979;35:852–853.

559. Rosen H, Klebanoff SJ. Role of iron and ethylenediaminetetraacetic acid in the bactericidal activity of a superoxide anion-generating system. *Arch Biochem Biophys* 1981;208:512–519.

560. Moorhouse CP, Halliwell B, Grootveld M, Gutteridge JMC. Cobalt (II) ion is a promoter of hydroxyl radical and possible "crypto-hydroxyl" radical formation under physiological conditions. Differential effects of hydroxyl radical scavengers. *Biochim Biophys Acta* 1985;843:261–268.

561. Gutteridge JMC, Wilkins S. Copper salt-dependent hydroxyl radical formation. Damage to proteins acting as antioxidants. *Biochim Biophys Acta* 1983;759:38–41.

562. Rowley DA, Halliwell B. Superoxide-dependent and ascorbate-dependent formation of hydroxyl radicals in the presence of copper salts: a physiologically significant reaction? *Arch Biochem Biophys* 1983;225:279–284.

563. Samuni A, Chevion M, Czapski G. Unusual copper-induced sensitization of the biological damage due to superoxide radicals. *J Biol Chem* 1981;256:12632–12635.

564. Shinar E, Navok T, Chevion M. The analogous mechanisms of enzymatic inactivation induced by ascorbate and superoxide in the presence of copper. *J Biol Chem* 1983;258:14778–14783.

565. Samuni A, Aronovitch J, Godinger D, Chevion M, Czapski G. On the cytotoxicity of vitamin C and metal ions. A site-specific Fenton mechanism. *Eur J Biochem* 1983;137:119–124.

566. van Stevenick J, van der Zee J, Dubbleman TMAR. Site-specific and bulk-phase generation of hydroxyl radicals in the presence of cupric ions and thiol compounds. *Biochem J* 1985;232:309–311.

567. Gutteridge JMC, Halliwell B. The role of superoxide and hydroxyl radicals in the degradation of DNA and deoxyribose induced by a copper-phenanthroline complex. *Biochem Pharmacol* 1982;31:2801–2805.

568. Buettner GR, Oberley LW, Chan Leuthauser SWH. The effect of iron on the distribution of superoxide and hydroxyl radicals as seen by spin trapping and on the superoxide dismutase assay. *Photochem Photobiol* 1978;28:693–695.

569. Gutteridge JMC, Richmond R, Halliwell B. Inhibition of the iron-catalyzed formation of hydroxyl radicals from superoxide and of lipid peroxidation by desferrioxamine. *Biochem J* 1979;184:469–472.

570. Halliwell B. Superoxide-dependent formation of hydroxyl radicals in the presence of iron salts. Its role in degradation of hyaluronic acid by a superoxide-generating system. *FEBS Lett* 1978;96:238–242.

571. Buettner GR, Doherty TP, Patterson LK. The kinetics of the reaction of superoxide radical with Fe(III) complexes of EDTA, DETAPAC and HEDTA. *FEBS Lett* 1983;158:143–146.

572. Cederbaum AI, Dicker E. Inhibition of microsomal oxidation of alcohols and of hydroxyl-radical-scavenging agents by the iron-chelating agent desferrioxamine. *Biochem J* 1983;210:107–113.

573. Sinaceur J, Ribiere C, Nordmann J, Nordmann R. Desferrioxamine: a scavenger of superoxide radicals? *Biochem Pharmacol* 1984;33:1693–1694.

574. Hoe S, Rowley DA, Halliwell B. Reactions of ferrioxamine and desferrioxamine with hydroxyl radical. *Chem Biol Interact* 1982;41:75–81.

575. Flitter W, Rowley DA, Halliwell B. Superoxide-dependent formation of hydroxyl radicals in the presence of iron salts. What is the physiological iron chelator? *FEBS Lett* 1983;158:310–312.

576. Bull C, McClune G, Fee JA. The mechanisms of Fe-EDTA catalyzed dismutation. *J Am Chem Soc* 1983;105:5290–5300.

577. Butler J, Halliwell B. Reaction of iron-EDTA chelates with the superoxide radical. *Arch Biochem Biophys* 1982;218:174–178.

578. Graf E, Mahoney JR, Bryant RG, Eaton JW. Iron-catalyzed hydroxyl radical formation. Stringent requirement for free iron coordination site. *J Biol Chem* 1984;259:3620–3624.

579. Ambruso DR, Johnston RBJ. Lactoferrin enhances hydroxyl radical production by human neutrophils, neutrophil particulate fractions and an enzymatic generating system. *J Clin Invest* 1981;67:352–360.

580. Bannister JV, Bannister WH, Hill HAO, Thornalley PJ. Enhanced production of hydroxyl radicals by the xanthine-xanthine oxidase reaction in the presence of lactoferrin. *Biochim Biophys Acta* 1982;715:116–120.

581. Baldwin DA, Jenny ER, Aisen P. The effect of human serum transferrin and milk lactoferrin on hydroxyl radical formation from superoxide and hydrogen peroxide. *J Biol Chem* 1984;259:13391–13394.

582. Winterbourn CC. Lactoferrin-catalyzed hydroxyl radical production. Additional requirement for a chelating agent. *Biochem J* 1983;210:15–19.

583. Gutteridge JMC, Paterson SK, Segal AW, Halliwell B. Inhibition of lipid peroxidation by the iron-binding protein lactoferrin. *Biochem J* 1981;199:259–261.

584. Ward PA, Till GO, Kunkel R, Beauchamp C. Evidence for role of hydroxyl radical in complement and neutrophil-dependent tissue injury. *J Clin Invest* 1983;72:789–801.

585. Bannister JV, Bellavite P, Davoli A, Thornalley PJ, Rossi F. The generation of hydroxyl radicals following superoxide production by neutrophil NADPH oxidase. *FEBS Lett* 1982;150:300–302.

586. Motohashi N, Mori I. Superoxide-dependent formation of hydroxyl radical catalyzed by transferrin. *FEBS Lett* 1983;157:197–199.

587. Maguire JJ, Kellogg EW III, Packer L. Protection against free radical formation by protein bound iron. *Toxicol Lett* 1982;14:27–34.

588. Britigan BE, Edeker BL. Pseudomonas and neutrophil products modify transferrin and lactoferrin to create conditions that favor hydroxyl radical formation. *J Clin Invest* 1991;88:1092–1102.

589. Bannister WH, Bannister JV, Searle AJF, Thornalley PJ. The reaction of superoxide radicals with metal picolinate complexes. *Inorg Chim Acta* 1983;78:139–142.

590. Coffman TJ, Cox CD, Edeker BL, Britigan BE. Possible role of bacterial siderophores in inflammation. Iron bound to the *Pseudomonas* siderophore pyochelin can function as a hydroxyl radical catalyst. *J Clin Invest* 1990;86:1030–1037.

591. Floyd RA. Direct demonstration that ferrous ion complexes of di- and triphosphate nucleotides catalyze hydroxyl free radical formation from hydrogen peroxide. *Arch Biochem Biophys* 1983;225:263–270.

592. Floyd RA, Lewis CA. Hydroxyl free radical formation from hydrogen peroxide by ferrous iron-nucleotide complexes. *Biochemistry* 1983;22:2645–2649.

593. Zs-Nagy I, Floyd RA. Hydroxyl free radical reactions with amino acids and proteins studied by electron spin resonance spectroscopy and spin-trapping. *Biochim Biophys Acta* 1984;790:238–250.

594. Floyd RA. DNA-ferrous iron catalyzed hydroxyl free radical formation from hydrogen peroxide. *Biochem Biophys Res Commun* 1981;99:1209–1215.

595. Sutton HC. Efficiency of chelated iron compounds as catalysts for the Haber-Weiss reaction. *J Free Radic Biol Med* 1985;1:195–202.

596. Gutteridge JMC. Fate of oxygen free radicals in extracellular fluids. *Biochem Soc Trans* 1982;10:72–73.

597. Gutteridge JMC, Rowley DA, Halliwell B. Superoxide-dependent formation of hydroxyl radicals in the presence of iron salts. Detection of "free" iron in biological systems by using bleomycin-dependent degradation of DNA. *Biochem J* 1981;199:263–265.

598. Gutteridge JMC, Rowley DA, Halliwell B. Superoxide-dependent formation of hydroxyl radicals and lipid peroxidation in the presence of iron salts. Detection of "catalytic" iron and anti-oxidant activity in extracellular fluids. *Biochem J* 1982;206:605–609.

599. Klebanoff SJ. Iodination catalyzed by the xanthine oxidase system: role of hydroxyl radicals. *Biochemistry* 1982;21:4110–4116.

600. Cohen G, Sinet PM. Fenton's reagent—once more revisited. *Dev Biochem* 1980;11A:27–37.

601. Gutteridge JMC. Thiobarbituric acid-reactivity following iron-dependent free-radical damage to amino acids and carbohydrates. *FEBS Lett* 1981;128:343–346.

602. Gutteridge JMC. Ferrous ion-EDTA-stimulated phospholipid peroxidation—a reaction changing from alkoxyl-radical-dependent to hydroxyl-radical-dependent initiation. *Biochem J* 1984;224:697–701.

603. Gutteridge JMC. Reactivity of hydroxyl and hydroxyl-like radicals discriminated by release of thiobarbituric acid-reactive material from deoxy sugars, nucleosides and benzoate. *Biochem J* 1984;224:761–767.

604. Halliwell B, Gutteridge JMC. Formation of a thiobarbituric-acid-reactive substance from deoxyribose in the presence of iron salts. The role of superoxide and hydroxyl radicals. *FEBS Lett* 1981;128:347–352.

605. Michelson AM. Studies in bioluminescence. X. Chemical models of enzymic oxidations. *Biochimie* 1973;55:465–479.

606. Klebanoff SJ, Waltersdorph AM, Michels BR, Rosen H. Oxygen-based free radical generation by ferrous ions and deferoxamine. *J Biol Chem* 1989;264:19765–19771.

607. Klebanoff SJ, Waltersdorph AM. Prooxidant activity of transferrin and lactoferrin. *J Exp Med* 1990;172:1293–1303.

608. Harris DC, Aisen P. Facilitation of Fe(II) autoxidation by Fe(III) complexing agents. *Biochim Biophys Acta* 1973;329:156–158.

609. Kurimura Y, Ochiai R, Matsuura N. Oxygen oxidation of ferrous ions induced by chelation. *Bull Chem Soc Jpn* 1968;41:2234–2239.

610. Long CA, Bielski BHJ. Rate of reaction of superoxide radical with chloride-containing species. *J Phys Chem* 1980;84:555–557.

611. Candeias LP, Patel KB, Stratford MRL, Wardman P. Free hydroxyl radicals are formed on reaction between the neutrophil-derived species superoxide anion and hypochlorous acid. *FEBS Lett* 1993;333:151–153.

612. Bannister JV, Bannister WH, Hill HAO, Thornalley PJ. Some current aspects of oxygen radicals in biological systems. *Life Chem Rep* 1982;1:49–53.

613. Ramos CL, Pou S, Britigan BE, Cohen MS, Rosen GM. Spin trapping evidence for myeloperoxidase-dependent hydroxyl radical formation by human neutrophils and monocytes. *J Biol Chem* 1992;267:8307–8312.

614. Yang SF. Further studies on ethylene formation from keto-methyl-thiobutryric acid or β-methylthiopropionaldehyde by peroxidase in the presence of sulfite and oxygen. *J Biol Chem* 1969;244:4360–4365.

615. Beauchamp C, Fridovich I. A mechanism for the production of ethylene from methional. The generation of hydroxyl radical by xanthine oxidase. *J Biol Chem* 1970;245:4641–4646.

616. DiGuiseppi J, Fridovich I. Ethylene from 2-keto-4-thiomethyl butyric acid: the Haber-Weiss reaction. *Arch Biochem Biophys* 1980;205:323–329.

617. Drath DB, Karnovsky ML, Huber GL. Hydroxyl radical formation in phagocytic cells of the rat. *J Appl Physiol* 1979;46:136–140.

618. Klebanoff SJ, Rosen H. Ethylene formation by polymorphonuclear leukocytes. Role of myeloperoxidase. *J Exp Med* 1978;148:490–506.

619. Repine JE, Eaton JW, Anders MW, Hoidal JR, Fox RB. Generation of hydroxyl radical by enzymes, chemicals, and human phagocytes *in vitro*. Detection with the anti-inflammatory agent, dimethyl sulfoxide. *J Clin Invest* 1979;64:1642–1651.

620. Tauber AI, Babior BM. Evidence for hydroxyl radical production by human neutrophils. *J Clin Invest* 1977;60:374–379.

621. Weiss SJ, Rustagi PK, LoBuglio AF. Human granulocyte generation of hydroxyl radical. *J Exp Med* 1978;147:316–323.

622. Weiss SJ, King GW, LoBuglio AF. Evidence for hydroxyl radical generation by human monocytes. *J Clin Invest* 1977;60:370–373.

623. Bors W, Lengfelder E, Saran M, Fuchs C, Michel C. Reactions of oxygen radical species with methional: a pulse radiolysis study. *Biochem Biophys Res Commun* 1976;70:81–87.

624. Pryor WA, Tang RH. Ethylene formation from methional. *Biochem Biophys Res Commun* 1978;81:498–503.

625. Saran M, Bors W, Michel C, Elstner EF. Formation of ethylene from methionine. Reactivity of radiolytically produced oxygen radicals and effect of substrate activation. *Int J Radiat Biol* 1980;37:521–527.

626. Klein SM, Cohen G, Cederbaum AI. The interaction of hydroxyl radicals with dimethylsulfoxide produces formaldehyde. *FEBS Lett* 1980;116:220–222.

627. Sagone ALJ, Decker MA, Wells RM, DeMocko C. A new method for the detection of hydroxyl radical production by phagocytic cells. *Biochim Biophys Acta* 1980;628:90–97.

628. Greenwald RA, Rush SW, Moak SA, Weitz Z. Conversion of superoxide generated by polymorphonuclear leukocytes to hydroxyl radical: a direct spectrophotometric detection system based on degradation of deoxyribose. *Free Radic Biol Med* 1989;6:385–392.

629. Harbour JR, Chow V, Bolton JR. An electron spin resonance study of the spin adducts of OH and HO₂ radicals with nitrones in the ultraviolet photolysis of aqueous hydrogen peroxide solutions. *Can J Chem* 1974;52:3549–3553.

630. Janzen EG, Nutter DE Jr, Davis ER, Blackburn BJ, Poyer JL, McCay PB. On spin trapping hydroxyl and hydroperoxyl radicals. *Can J Chem* 1978;56:2237–2242.

631. Green MR, Hill HAO, Okolow-Zubkowska MJ, Segal AW. The production of hydroxyl and superoxide radicals by stimulated human neutrophils. Measurements by EPR spectroscopy. *FEBS Lett* 1979;100:23–26.

632. Rosen H, Klebanoff SJ. Hydroxyl radical generation by polymorphonuclear leukocytes measured by electron spin resonance spectroscopy. *J Clin Invest* 1979;64:1725–1729.

633. Kleinhans FW, Barefoot ST. Spin trap determination of free radical burst kinetics in stimulated neutrophils. *J Biol Chem* 1987;262:12452–12457.

634. Britigan BE, Hamill DR. The interaction of 5,5-dimethyl-1-pyrroline-N-oxide with human myeloperoxidase and its potential impact on spin trapping of neutrophil-derived free radicals. *Arch Biochem Biophys* 1989;275:72–81.

635. Finkelstein E, Rosen GM, Rauckman EJ, Paxton J. Spin trapping of superoxide. *Mol Pharmacol* 1979;16:676–685.

636. Britigan BE, Rosen GM, Chai Y, Cohen MS. Do human neutrophils make hydroxyl radical? Determination of free radicals generated by human neutrophils activated with a soluble or particulate stimulus using electron paramagnetic resonance spectrometry. *J Biol Chem* 1986;261:4426–4431.

637. Ueno I, Kohno M, Mitsuta K, Mizuta Y, Kanegasaki S. Reevaluation of the spin-trapped adduct formed from 5,5-dimethyl-1-pyrroline-1-oxide during the respiratory burst in neutrophils. *J Biochem* 1989;105:905–910.

638. Finkelstein E, Rosen GM, Rauckman EJ. Spin trapping. Kinetics of the reaction of superoxide and hydroxyl radicals with nitrones. *J Am Chem Soc* 1980;102:4994–4999.

639. Finkelstein E, Rosen GM, Rauckman EJ. Spin trapping of superoxide and hydroxyl radical: practical aspects. *Arch Biochem Biophys* 1980;200:1–16.

640. Finkelstein E, Rosen GM, Rauckman EJ. Production of hydroxyl radical by decomposition of superoxide spin-trapped adducts. *Mol Pharmacol* 1982;21:262–265.

641. Janzen EG, Jandrisits LT, Barber DL. Studies on the origin of the hydroxyl spin adduct of DMPO produced from the stimulation of neutrophils by phorbol-12-myristate-13-acetate. *Free Radic Res* 1987;4:115–123.

642. Bernofsky C, Bandara BMR, Hinojosa O. Electron spin resonance studies of the reaction of hypochlorite with 5,5-dimethyl-1-pyrroline-N-oxide. *Free Radic Biol Med* 1990;8:231–239.

643. Foote CS. Detection of singlet oxygen in complex systems: a critique. In: Caughey WS, ed. *Biochemical and clinical aspects of oxygen*. New York: Academic Press, 1979:603–625.

644. Britigan BE, Cohen MS, Rosen GM. Detection of the production of oxygen-centered free radicals by human neutrophils using spin trapping techniques: a critical perspective. *J Leukoc Biol* 1987;41:349–362.

645. Cohen MS, Britigan BE, Hassett DJ, Rosen GM. Do human neutrophils form hydroxyl radical? Evaluation of an unresolved controversy. *Free Radic Biol Med* 1988;5:81–88.

646. Cohen MS, Britigan BE, Hassett DJ, Rosen GM. Phagocytes, O_2 reduction, and hydroxyl radical. *Rev Infect Dis* 1988;10:1088–1096.

647. Britigan BE, Rosen GM, Thompson BY, Chai Y, Cohen MS. Stimulated human neutrophils limit iron-catalyzed hydroxyl radical formation as detected by spin-trapping techniques. *J Biol Chem* 1986;261:17026–17032.

648. Pou S, Rosen GM, Britigan BE, Cohen MS. Intracellular spin-trapping of oxygen-centered radicals generated by human neutrophils. *Biochim Biophys Acta* 1989;991:459–464.

649. Britigan BE, Hassett DJ, Rosen GM, Hamill DR, Cohen MS. Neutrophil degranulation inhibits potential hydroxyl-radical formation. Relative impact of myeloperoxidase and lactoferrin release on hydroxyl-radical production by iron-supplemented neutrophils assessed by spin-trapping techniques. *Biochem J* 1989;264:447–455.

650. Winterbourn CC. Myeloperoxidase as an effective inhibitor of hydroxyl radical production. Implications for the oxidative reactions of neutrophils. *J Clin Invest* 1986;78:545–550.

651. Britigan BE, Hamill DR. Effect of the spin trap 5,5 dimethyl-1-pyrroline-N-oxide (DMPO) on human neutrophil function: novel inhibition of neutrophil stimulus-response coupling. *Free Radic Biol Med* 1990;8:459–470.

652. Samuni A, Carmichael AJ, Russo A, Mitchell JB, Riesz P. On the spin trapping and ESR detection of oxygen-derived radicals generated inside cells. *Proc Natl Acad Sci USA* 1986;83:7593–7597.

653. Samuni A, Black CDV, Krishna M, Malech HL, Bernstein EF, Russo A. Hydroxyl radical production by stimulated neutrophils reappraised. *J Biol Chem* 1988;263:13797–13801.

654. Samuni A, Swartz HM. The cellular-induced decay of DMPO spin adducts of ·OH and ·O_2^-. *Free Radic Biol Med* 1989;6:179–183.

655. Samuni A, Krishna CM, Riesz P, Finkelstein E, Russo A. Superoxide reaction with nitroxide spin-adducts. *Free Radic Biol Med* 1989;6:141–148.

656. Rosen GM, Britigan BE, Cohen MS, Ellington SP, Barber MJ. Detection of phagocyte-derived free radicals with spin trapping techniques: effect of temperature and cellular metabolism. *Biochim Biophys Acta* 1988;969:236–241.

657. Pou S, Cohen MS, Britigan BE, Rosen GM. Spin-trapping and human neutrophils. Limits of detection of hydroxyl radical. *J Biol Chem* 1989;264:12299–12302.

658. Britigan BE, Coffman TJ, Buettner GR. Spin trapping evidence for the lack of significant hydroxyl radical production during the respiration burst of human phagocytes using a spin adduct resistant to superoxide-mediated destruction. *J Biol Chem* 1990;265:2650–2656.

659. Britigan BE, Ratcliffe HR, Buettner GR, Rosen GM. Binding of myeloperoxidase to bacteria: effect on hydroxyl radical formation and susceptibility to oxidant-mediated killing. *Biochim Biophys Acta* 1996;1290:231–240.

660. Fridovich I. Quantitative aspects of the production of superoxide anion radical by milk xanthine oxidase. *J Biol Chem* 1970;245:4053–4057.

661. Kuppusamy P, Zweier JL. Characterization of free radical generation by xanthine oxidase. Evidence for hydroxyl radical generation. *J Biol Chem* 1989;264:9880–9884.

662. Lloyd RV, Mason RP. Evidence against transition metal-independent hydroxyl radical generation by xanthine oxidase. *J Biol Chem* 1990;265:16733–16736.

663. Britigan BE, Pou S, Rosen GM, Lilleg DM, Buettner GR. Hydroxyl radical is not a product of the reaction of xanthine oxidase and xanthine. The confounding problem of adventitious iron bound to xanthine oxidase. *J Biol Chem* 1990;265:17533–17538.

664. Green DE, Pauli R. The anti-bacterial action of the xanthine oxidase system. *Proc Soc Exp Biol Med* 1943;54:148–150.

665. Lipmann F, Owen CR. The antibacterial effect of enzymatic xanthine oxidation. *Science* 1943;98:246–248.

666. Murray HW, Cohn ZA. Macrophage oxygen-dependent antimicrobial activity. I. Susceptibility of *Toxoplasma gondii* to oxygen intermediates. *J Exp Med* 1979;150:938–949.

667. Rosen H, Klebanoff SJ. Bactericidal activity of a superoxide anion generating system: a model for the polymorphonuclear leukocyte. *J Exp Med* 1979;149:27–39.

668. Babior BM, Curnette JT, Kipnes RS. Biological defense mechanisms. Evidence for the participation of superoxide in bacterial killing by xanthine oxidase. *J Lab Clin Med* 1975;85:235–244.

669. Ismail G, Sawyer WD, Wegener WS. Effect of hydrogen peroxide and superoxide radical on viability of *Niesseria gonorrhoeae* and related bacteria. *Proc Soc Exp Biol Med* 1977;155:264–269.

670. Johnston RBJ, Keele BBJ, Misra HP, et al. The role of superoxide anion generation in phagocytic bactericidal activity. Studies with normal and chronic granulomatous disease leukocytes. *J Clin Invest* 1975;55:1357–1372.

671. Repine JE, Fox RB, Berger EM. Dimethyl sulfoxide inhibits killing of *Staphylococcus aureus* by polymorphonuclear leukocytes. *Infect Immun* 1981;31:510–513.

672. Fligiel SEG, Ward PA, Johnson KJ, Till GO. Evidence for a role of hydroxyl radical in immune-complex-induced vasculitis. *Am J Pathol* 1984;115:375–382.

673. Varani J, Fligiel SEG, Till GO, Kunkel RG, Ryan US, Ward PA. Pulmonary endothelial cell killing by human neutrophils. Possible involvement of hydroxyl radical. *Lab Invest* 1985;53:656–663.

674. Dorfman LM, Adams GE. Reactivity of the hydroxyl radical in aqueous solutions. *National Standard Reference Data System National Bureau of Standards* 1973;46:1–59.

675. Kearns DR. Solvent and solvent isotope effects on the lifetime of singlet oxygen. In: Wasserman HH, Murray RW, eds. *Singlet oxygen*. New York: Academic Press, 1979:115–137.

676. Foote CS. Photosensitized oxidation and singlet oxygen: consequences in biological systems. In: Pryor WA, ed. *Free radicals in biology*, vol 2. New York: Academic Press, 1976:85–133.

677. Allen RC, Stjernholm RL, Steele RH. Evidence for the generation of an electronic excitation state(s) in human polymorphonuclear leukocytes and its participation in bactericidal activity. *Biochem Biophys Res Commun* 1972;47:679–684.

678. Khan AU. Activated oxygen: singlet molecular oxygen and superoxide anion. *Photochem Photobiol* 1978;28:615–627.

679. Khan AU, Kasha M. Direct spectroscopic observation of singlet oxygen emission at 1268 nm excited by sensitizing dyes of biological interest in liquid solution. *Proc Natl Acad Sci USA* 1979;76:6047–6049.

680. Khan AU. Direct spectral evidence of the generation of singlet molecular oxygen ($^1\Delta g$) in the reaction of potassium superoxide with water. *J Am Chem Soc* 1981;103:6516–6517.

681. Foote CS, Shook FC, Abakerli RB. Chemistry of superoxide ion. 4. Singlet oxygen is not a major product of dismutation. *J Am Chem Soc* 1980;102:2503–2504.

682. Foote CS, Abakerli RB, Clough RL, Shook FC. On the question of singlet oxygen production in leukocytes, macrophages and the dismutation of superoxide anion. *Dev Biochem* 1980;11B:222–230.

683. Kellogg EWI, Fridovich I. Superoxide, hydrogen peroxide, and singlet oxygen in lipid peroxidation by a xanthine oxidase system. *J Biol Chem* 1975;250:8812–8817.

684. Kellogg EWI, Fridovich I. Liposome oxidation and erythrocyte lysis by enzymatically generated superoxide and hydrogen peroxide. *J Biol Chem* 1977;252:6721–6728.

685. Nagano T, Fridovich I. Does the aerobic xanthine oxidase reaction generate singlet oxygen? *Photochem Photobiol* 1985;41:33–37.

686. Kasha M, Khan AU. The physics, chemistry and biology of singlet molecular oxygen. *Ann NY Acad Sci* 1970;171:5–23.

687. Nilsson R, Kearns DR. Role of singlet oxygen in some chemiluminescence and enzyme oxidation reactions. *J Phys Chem* 1974;78:1681–1683.

688. King MM, Lai EK, McCay PB. Singlet oxygen production associated with enzyme-catalyzed lipid peroxidation in liver microsomes. *J Biol Chem* 1975;250:6496–6502.

689. Rosen H, Klebanoff SJ. Formation of singlet oxygen by the myeloperoxidase-mediated antimicrobial system. *J Biol Chem* 1977;252:4803–4810.

690. Piatt J, O'Brien PJ. Singlet oxygen formation by a peroxidase, H_2O_2 and halide system. *Eur J Biochem* 1979;93:323–332.

691. Piatt JF, Cheema AS, O'Brien PJ. Peroxidase catalyzed singlet oxygen formation from hydrogen peroxide. *FEBS Lett* 1977;74:251–254.

692. Harrison JE, Watson BD, Schultz J. Myeloperoxidase and singlet oxygen: a reappraisal. *FEBS Lett* 1978;92:327–332.

693. Held AM, Hurst JK. Ambiguity associated with use of singlet oxygen trapping agents in myeloperoxidase-catalyzed oxidations. *Biochem Biophys Res Commun* 1978;81:878–885.

694. Ushijima Y, Nakano M. No or little production of singlet molecular oxygen in HOCl or HOCl/H_2O_2. A model system for myeloperoxidase/H_2O_2/Cl. *Biochem Biophys Res Commun* 1980;93:1232–1237.

695. Allen RC. Halide dependence of the myeloperoxidase-mediated antimicrobial system of the polymorphonuclear leukocyte in the phenomenon of electronic excitation. *Biochem Biophys Res Commun* 1975;63:675–683.

696. Allen RC. The role of pH in the chemiluminescent response of the myeloperoxidase-halide-HOOH antimicrobial system. *Biochem Biophys Res Commun* 1975;63:684–691.

697. Kanofsky JR. Singlet oxygen production by lactoperoxidase. Evidence from 1270 nm chemiluminescence. *J Biol Chem* 1983;258:5991–5993.

698. Krasnovsky AAJ. Photoluminescence of singlet oxygen in pigment solutions. *Photochem Photobiol* 1976;29:29–36.

699. Kanofsky JR. The detection of singlet oxygen in biochemical systems using 1268 nm chemiluminescence. In: Simic MG, Taylor KA, Ward JF, von Sonntag C, eds. *Oxygen radicals in biology and medicine.* New York: Plenum Press, 1988:211–218.

700. Kanofsky JR. Peroxidase-catalyzed generation of singlet oxygen and of free radicals. In: Everse J, Everse KE, Grisham MB, eds. *Peroxidases in chemistry and biology,* vol 2. Boca Raton: CRC Press, 1991:219–237.

701. Khan AU. Enzyme system generation of singlet ($^1\Delta$g) molecular oxygen observed directly by 1.0–1.8 μm luminescence spectroscopy. *J Am Chem Soc* 1983;105:7195–7197.

702. Khan AU. Discovery of enzyme generation of $^1\Delta$g molecular oxygen: spectra of (0,0) $^1\Delta$g→$^3\Sigma$g IR emission. *J Photochem* 1984;25:327–333.

703. Kanofsky JR. Singlet oxygen production by chloroperoxidase-hydrogen peroxide-halide systems. *J Biol Chem* 1984;259:5596–5600.

704. Khan AU, Bebauer P, Hager LP. Chloroperoxidase generation of singlet Δ molecular oxygen observed directly by spectroscopy in the 1- to 1.6 μm region. *Proc Natl Acad Sci USA* 1983;80:5195–5197.

705. Everett RR, Kanofsky JR, Butler A. Mechanistic investigations of the novel non-heme vanadium bromoperoxidases. Evidence for singlet oxygen production. *J Biol Chem* 1990;265:4908–4914.

706. Kanofsky JR, Wright J, Miles-Richardson GE, Tauber AI. Biochemical requirement for singlet oxygen production by purified human myeloperoxidase. *J Clin Invest* 1984;74:1489–1495.

707. Khan AU. Myeloperoxidase singlet molecular oxygen generation detected by direct infrared electronic emission. *Biochem Biophys Res Commun* 1984;122:668–675.

708. Kanofsky JR, Wright J, Tauber AI. Effect of ascorbic acid on the production of singlet oxygen by purified human myeloperoxidase. *FEBS Lett* 1985;187:299–301.

709. Andersen BR, Brendzel AM, Lint TF. Chemiluminescence spectra of human myeloperoxidase and polymorphonuclear leukocytes. *Infect Immun* 1977;17:62–66.

710. Cheson BD, Christensen RL, Sperling R, Kohler BE, Babior BM. The origin of the chemiluminescence of phagocytosing granulocytes. *J Clin Invest* 1976;58:789–796.

711. Kanofsky JR, Tauber AI. Non-physiologic production of singlet oxygen by human neutrophils and by the myeloperoxidase-H$_2$O$_2$-halide system. *Blood* 1983;62:82a.

712. Kulig MJ, Smith LL. Sterol metabolism. XXV. Cholesterol oxidation by singlet molecular oxygen. *J Org Chem* 1973;38:3639–3642.

713. Foote CS, Abakerli RB, Clough RL, Lehrer RI. On the question of singlet oxygen production in polymorphonuclear leucocytes. In: DeLuca MA, McElroy WD, eds. *Bioluminescence and chemiluminescence.* New York: Academic Press, 1980:81–88.

714. Steinbeck MJ, Khan AU, Karnovsky MJ. Intracellular singlet oxygen generation by phagocytosing neutrophils in response to particles coated with a chemical trap. *J Biol Chem* 1992;267:13425–13433.

715. Krinsky NI. Singlet excited oxygen as a mediator of the antibacterial action of leukocytes. *Science* 1974;186:363–365.

716. Baehner RL, Johnston RBJ. Metabolic and bactericidal activities of human eosinophils. *Br J Haematol* 1971;20:277–285.

717. Bujak JS, Root RK. The role of peroxidase in the bactericidal activity of human blood eosinophils. *Blood* 1974;43:727–736.

718. Cline MJ. Microbicidal activity of human eosinophils. *J Reticuloendothel Soc* 1972;12:332–339.

719. DeChatelet LR, Migler RA, Shirley PS, Muss HB, Szejda P, Bass DA. Comparison of intracellular bactericidal activities of human neutrophils and eosinophils. *Blood* 1978;52:609–617.

720. Mickenberg ID, Root RK, Wolff SM. Bactericidal and metabolic properties of human eosinophils. *Blood* 1972;39:67–80.

721. Yazdanbakhsh M, Eckmann CM, Bot AAM, Roos D. Bactericidal action of eosinophils from normal human blood. *Infect Immun* 1986;53:192–198.

722. Cline MJ, Hanifin J, Lehrer RI. Phagocytosis by human eosinophils. *Blood* 1968;32:922–934.

723. Gleich GJ, Adolphson CR. The eosinophilic leukocyte: structure and function. *Adv Immunol* 1986;39:177–253.

724. DeChatelet LR, Shirley PS, McPhail LC, Huntley CC, Muss HB, Bass DA. Oxidative metabolism of the human eosinophil. *Blood* 1977;50:525–535.

725. Klebanoff SJ, Durack DT, Rosen H, Clark RA. Functional studies on human peritoneal eosinophils. *Infect Immun* 1977;17:167–173.

726. Tauber AI, Goetzl EJ, Babior BM. Unique characteristics of superoxide production by human eosinophils in eosinophilic states. *Inflammation* 1979;3:261–272.

727. McCormick ML, Roeder TL, Railsback MA, Britigan BE. Eosinophil peroxidase-dependent hydroxyl radical generation by human eosinophils. *J Biol Chem* 1994;269:27914–27919.

728. Kanofsky JR, Hoogland H, Wever R, Weiss SJ. Singlet oxygen production by human eosinophils. *J Biol Chem* 1988;263:9692–9696.

729. Learn DB, Brestel EP. A comparison of superoxide production by human eosinophils and neutrophils. *Agents Actions* 1982;12:485–488.

730. Pincus SH. Peroxidase-mediated iodination by guinea pig peritoneal exudate eosinophils. *Inflammation* 1980;4:89–106.

731. Pincus SH. Comparative metabolism of guinea pig peritoneal exudate neutrophils and eosinophils. *Proc Soc Exp Biol Med* 1980;163:482–489.

732. Yamashita T, Someya A, Hara E. Response of superoxide anion production by guinea pig eosinophils to various soluble stimuli: comparison to neutrophils. *Arch Biochem Biophys* 1985;241:447–452.

733. Segal AW, Garcia R, Goldstone AH, Cross AR, Jones OTG. Cytochrome b.$_{245}$ of neutrophils is also present in human monocytes, macrophages and eosinophils. *Biochem J* 1981;196:363–367.

734. Henderson WR Jr. Eosinophil peroxidase: occurrence and biological function. In: Everse J, Everse KE, Grisham MB, eds. *Peroxidases in chemistry and biology,* vol 1. Boca Raton: CRC Press, 1991:105–121.

735. Bainton DF, Farquhar MG. Segregation and packaging of granule enzymes in eosinophilic leukocytes. *J Cell Biol* 1970;45:54–73.

736. Cotran RS, Litt M. The entry of granule-associated peroxidase into the phagocytic vacuole of eosinophils. *J Exp Med* 1969;129:1291–1306.

737. McLaren DJ, Mackenzie CD, Ramalho-Pinto FJ. Ultrastructural observations on the *in vitro* interaction between rat eosinophils and some parasitic helminths (*Schistosoma mansoni, Trichinella spiralis* and *Nippostrongylus brasiliensis. Clin Exp Immunol* 1977;30:105–118.

738. Ross R, Klebanoff SJ. The eosinophilic leukocyte. Fine structure studies of changes in the uterus during the estrous cycle. *J Exp Med* 1966;124:653–660.

739. Dvorak AM, Weller PF, Monahan-Earley RA, Letourneau L, Ackerman SJ. Ultrastructural localization of Charcot-Leyden crystal protein (lysophospholipase) and peroxidase in macrophages, eosinophils, and extracellular matrix of the skin in the hypereosinophilic syndrome. *Lab Invest* 1990;62:590–607.

740. Archer GT, Jackas M. Disruption of mast cells by a component of eosinophil granules. *Nature* 1965;205:599–600.

741. Archer GT, Air G, Jackas M, Morell DB. Studies on rat eosinophil peroxidase. *Biochim Biophys Acta* 1965;99:96–101.

742. Kariya K, Lee E, Hirouchi M, Hosokawa M, Sayo H. Purification and some properties of peroxidases of rat bone marrow. *Biochim Biophys Acta* 1987;911:95–101.

743. Desser RK, Himmelhoch SR, Evans WH, Januska M, Mage M, Shelton E. Guinea pig heterophil and eosinophil peroxidase. *Arch Biochem Biophys* 1972;148:452–465.

744. Jorg A, Pasquier J, Klebanoff SJ. Purification of horse eosinophil peroxidase. *Biochim Biophys Acta* 1982;701:185–191.

745. Carlson MG, Peterson CGB, Venge P. Human eosinophil peroxidase: purification and characterization. *J Immunol* 1985;134:1875–1879.

746. Olsen RL, Little C. Purification and some properties of myeloperoxidase and eosinophil peroxidase from human blood. *Biochem J* 1983;209:781–787.

747. Wever R, Plat H, Hamers MN. Human eosinophil peroxidase: a novel isolation procedure, spectral properties and chlorinating activity. *FEBS Lett* 1981;123:327–331.

748. Olsson I, Persson A, Stromberg K, Winqvist I, Tai P, Spry CJF. Purification of eosinophil peroxidase and studies of biosynthesis and processing in human marrow cells. *Blood* 1985;66:1143–1148.

749. Menegazzi R, Zabucchi G, Patriarca P. A simple procedure for the purification of eosinophil peroxidase from normal human blood. *J Immunol Methods* 1986;91:283–288.

750. Bolscher BGJM, Plat H, Wever R. Some properties of human eosinophil peroxidase, a comparison with other peroxidases. *Biochim Biophys Acta* 1984;784:177–186.

751. Olsen RL, Syse K, Little C, Christensen TB. Further characterization of human eosinophil peroxidase. *Biochem J* 1985;229:779–784.

752. Wever R, Hamers MN, Weening RS, Roos D. Characterization of the peroxidase in human eosinophils. *Eur J Biochem* 1980;108:491–495.

753. Sibbett SS, Klebanoff SJ, Hurst JK. Resonance Raman characterization of the heme prosthetic group in eosinophil peroxidase. *FEBS Lett* 1985;189:271–275.

754. Ten RM, Pease LR, McKean DJ, Bell MP, Gleich GJ. Molecular cloning of the human eosinophil peroxidase. Evidence for the existence of a peroxidase multigene family. *J Exp Med* 1989;169:1757–1769.

755. Migler R, DeChatelet LR, Bass DA. Human eosinophilic peroxidase: role in bactericidal activity. *Blood* 1978;51:445–456.

756. Buys J, Wever R, van Stigt R, Ruitenberg EJ. The killing of newborn larvae of *Trichinella spiralis* by eosinophil peroxidase in vitro. *Eur J Immunol* 1981;11:843–845.

757. Jong EC, Klebanoff SJ. Eosinophil-mediated mammalian tumor cell cytotoxicity: role of the peroxidase system. *J Immunol* 1980;124:1949–1953.

758. Jong EC, Henderson WR, Klebanoff SJ. Bactericidal activity of eosinophil peroxidase. *J Immunol* 1980;124:1378–1382.

759. Ramsey PG, Martin T, Chi E, Klebanoff SJ. Arming of mononuclear phagocytes by eosinophil peroxidase bound to *Staphylococcus aureus*. *J Immunol* 1982;128:415–420.

760. Weiss SJ, Test ST, Eckmann CM, Roos D, Regiani S. Brominating oxidants generated by human eosinophils. *Science* 1986;234:200–203.

761. Mayeno AN, Curran AJ, Roberts RL, Foote CS. Eosinophils preferentially use bromide to generate halogenating agents. *J Biol Chem* 1989;264:5660–5668.

762. Slungaard A, Mahoney JR Jr. Thiocyanate is the major substrate for eosinophil peroxidase in physiologic fluids: implications for cytotoxicity. *J Biol Chem* 1991;266:4903–4910.

763. Klebanoff SJ, Coombs RW. Virucidal effect of stimulated eosinophils on human immunodeficiency virus type 1. *AIDS Res Hum Retrovir* 1996;12:25–29.

764. Noqueira NM, Klebanoff SJ, Cohn ZA. *T. cruzi:* sensitization to macrophage killing by eosinophil peroxidase. *J Immunol* 1982;128:1705–1708.

765. Molina HA, Kierszenbaum F, Hamann KJ, Gleich GJ. Toxic effects produced or mediated by human eosinophil granule components on *Trypanosoma cruzi*. *Am J Trop Med Hyg* 1988;38:327–334.

766. Locksley RM, Wilson CB, Klebanoff SJ. Role for endogenous and acquired peroxidase in the toxoplasmacidal activity of murine and human mononuclear phagocytes. *J Clin Invest* 1982;69:1099–1111.

767. Ayars GH, Altman LC, McManus MM, et al. Injurious effect of the eosinophil peroxide-hydrogen peroxide-halide system and major basic protein on human nasal epithelium in vitro. *Am Rev Respir Dis* 1989;140:125–131.

768. Zabucchi G, Menegazzi R, Soranzo MR, Patriarca P. Uptake of human eosinophil peroxidase by human neutrophils. *Am J Pathol* 1986;124:510–518.

769. Zabucchi G, Soranzo MR, Menegazzi R, Bertoncin P, Nardon E, Patriarca P. Uptake of human eosinophil peroxidase and myeloperoxidase by cells involved in the inflammatory process. *J Histochem Cytochem* 1989;37:499–508.

770. Zabucchi G, Menegazzi R, Cramer R, Nardon E, Patriarca P. Mutual influence between eosinophil peroxidase (EPO) and neutrophils: neutrophils reversibly inhibit EPO enzymatic activity and EPO increases neutrophil adhesiveness. *Immunology* 1990;69:580–587.

771. Henderson WR, Jong EC, Klebanoff SJ. Binding of eosinophil peroxidase to mast cell granules with retention of peroxidatic activity. *J Immunol* 1980;124:1383–1388.

772. Henderson WR, Chi EY, Jong EC, Klebanoff SJ. Mast cell-mediated tumor-cell cytotoxicity. Role of the peroxidase system. *J Exp Med* 1981;153:520–533.

773. Escribano LM, Gabriel LC, Sainz T, Rocamora A, Arrazola JM, Navarro JL. Peroxidase activity in human cutaneous mast cells: an ultrastructural demonstration. *J Histochem Cytochem* 1984;32:573–578.

774. Dvorak AM, Klebanoff SJ, Henderson WR, Monahan RA, Pyne K, Galli SJ. Vesicular uptake of eosinophil peroxidase by guinea pig basophils and by cloned mouse mast cells and granule-containing lymphoid cells. *Am J Pathol* 1985;118:425–438.

775. Dvorak AM, Ishizaka T, Galli SJ. Ultrastructure of human basophils developing in vitro. Evidence for the acquisition of peroxidase by basophils and for different effects of human and murine growth factors on human basophil and eosinophil maturation. *Lab Invest* 1985;53:57–71.

776. Henderson WR, Chi EY, Jong EC, Klebanoff SJ. Mast cell-mediated toxicity to schistosomula of *Schistosoma mansoni*: potentiation by exogenous peroxidase. *J Immunol* 1986;137:2695–2699.

777. Khalife J, Capron M, Grzych J, Bazin H, Capron A. Extracellular release of rat eosinophil peroxidase (EPO). I. Role of anaphylactic immunoglobulin. *J Immunol* 1985;134:1968–1974.

778. Slungaard A, Mahoney JRJ. Bromide-dependent toxicity of eosinophil peroxidase for endothelium and isolated working rat hearts: a model for eosinophilic endocarditis. *J Exp Med* 1991;173:117–126.

779. Molina HA, Kierszenbaum F. Interaction of human eosinophils or neutrophils with *Trypanosoma cruzi in vitro* causes bystander cardiac cell damage. *Immunology* 1989;66:289–295.

780. Klebanoff SJ, Agosti JM, Jorg A, Waltersdorph AM. Comparative toxicity of the horse eosinophil peroxidase-H_2O_2-halide system and granule basic proteins. *J Immunol* 1989;143:239–244.

781. Klebanoff SJ. Oxygen-dependent antimicrobial systems in mononuclear phagocytes. In: Reichard S, Kojima M, eds. *Progress in leukocyte biology, vol 4. Macrophage biology.* New York: Alan R. Liss, 1985:487–503.

782. Nathan CF. Secretion of oxygen intermediates: role in effector functions of activated macrophages. *Fed Proc* 1982;41:2206–2211.

783. Nathan CF. Mechanisms of macrophage antimicrobial activity. *Trans R Soc Trop Med Hyg* 1983;77:620–630.

784. Roos D, Balm AJM. The oxidative metabolism of monocytes. In: Sbarra AJ, Strauss RR, eds. *The reticuloendothelial system. A comprehensive treatise. 2. Biochemistry and metabolism.* New York: Plenum Press, 1980:189–229.

785. Reiss M, Roos D. Differences in oxygen metabolism of phagocytosing monocytes and neutrophils. *J Clin Invest* 1978;61:480–488.

786. Bos A, Wever R, Roos D. Characterization and quantification of the peroxidase in human monocytes. *Biochim Biophys Acta* 1978;525:37–44.

787. Nichols BA, Bainton DF. Differentiation of human monocytes in bone marrow and blood. Sequential formation of two granule populations. *Lab Invest* 1973;29:27–40.

788. Baehner RL, Johnston RBJ. Monocyte function in children with neutropenia and chronic infections. *Blood* 1972;40:31–41.

789. Daems WT, Poelmann RE, Brederoo P. Peroxidatic activity in resident peritoneal macrophages and exudate monocytes of the guinea pig after ingestion of latex particles. *J Histochem Cytochem* 1973;21:93–95.

790. Lehrer RI. The fungicidal mechanisms of human monocytes. I. Evidence for myeloperoxidase-linked and myeloperoxidase-independent candidacidal mechanisms. *J Clin Invest* 1975;55:338–346.

791. Lampert MB, Weiss SJ. The chlorinating potential of the human monocyte. *Blood* 1983;62:645–651.

792. Diamond RD, Haudenschild CC. Monocyte-mediated serum-independent damage to hyphal and pseudohyphal forms of *Candida albicans in vitro*. *J Clin Invest* 1981;67:173–182.

793. Washburn RG, Gallin JI, Bennett JE. Oxidative killing of *Aspergillus fumigatus* proceeds by parallel myeloperoxidase-dependent and-independent pathways. *Infect Immun* 1987;55:2088–2092.

794. Fleer A, Roos D, von dem Borne EGK, Engelfriet CP. Cytotoxic activity of human monocytes toward sensitized red cells is not dependent on the generation of reactive oxygen species. *Blood* 1979;54:407–411.

795. Klassen DK, Sagone ALJ. Evidence for both oxygen and non-oxygen dependent mechanisms of antibody sensitized target cell lysis by human monocytes. *Blood* 1980;56:985–992.

796. Seim S, Espevik T. Toxic oxygen species in monocyte-mediated antibody-dependent cytotoxicity. *J Reticuloendothel Soc* 1983;33:417–428.

797. Chase MJ, Klebanoff SJ. Viricidal effect of stimulated human mononuclear phagocytes on human immunodeficiency virus type 1. *Proc Natl Acad Sci USA* 1992;89:5582–5585.

798. Mavier P, Edgington TS. Human monocyte-mediated tumor cytotoxicity. *J Immunol* 1984;132:1980–1986.

799. Weiss SJ, LoBuglio AF, Kessler HB. Oxidative mechanisms of monocyte-mediated cytotoxicity. *Proc Natl Acad Sci USA* 1980;77:584–587.

800. Koller CA, LoBuglio AF. Monocyte-mediated, antibody-dependent cell-mediated cytotoxicity: the role of the metabolic burst. *Blood* 1981;58:293–299.

801. Cohn ZA. The macrophage-versatile element of inflammation. *Harvey Lect* 1983;77:63–80.

802. Czuprynski CJ, Campbell PA, Henson PM. Killing of Listeria monocytogenes by human neutrophils and monocytes, but not by monocyte-derived macrophages. *J Reticuloendothel Soc* 1983;34:29–44.

803. Wilson CB, Tsai V, Remington JS. Failure to trigger the oxidative metabolic burst by normal macrophages. Possible mechanism for survival of intracellular pathogens. *J Exp Med* 1980;151:328–346.

804. Murray HW, Cartelli DM. Killing of intracellular *Leishmania donovani* by human mononuclear phagocytes. Evidence for oxygen-dependent and -independent leishmanicidal activity. *J Clin Invest* 1983;72:32–44.

805. Daniels CA, Kleinerman ES, Snyderman R. Abortive and productive infections of human mononuclear phagocytes by Type I herpes simplex virus. *Am J Pathol* 1978;91:119–136.

806. van Furth R, Hirsch JG, Fedorko ME. Morphology and peroxidase cytochemistry of mouse promonocytes, monocytes and macrophages. *J Exp Med* 1970;132:794–812.

807. Ando M, Dannenberg AMJ, Shima K. Macrophage accumulation, division, maturation and digestion and microbicidal capacities in tuberculous lesions. II. Rate at which mononuclear cells enter and divide in primary BCG lesions and those of reinfection. *J Immunol* 1972;109:8–19.

808. North RJ. The relative importance of blood monocytes and fixed macrophages to the expression of cell-mediated immunity to infection. *J Exp Med* 1970;132:521–534.

809. Johnson WDJ, Mei B, Cohn ZA. The separation, long-term cultivation and maturation of the human monocyte. *J Exp Med* 1977;146:1613–1626.

810. Nakagawara A, Nathan CF, Cohn ZA. Hydrogen peroxide metabolism in human monocytes during differentiation *in vitro*. *J Clin Invest* 1981;68:1243–1252.

811. Seim S. Role of myeloperoxidase in the luminol-dependent chemiluminescence response of phagocytosing human monocytes. *Acta Pathol Microbiol Immunol Scand (C)* 1983;91:123–128.

812. Stevenson HC, Katz P, Wright DG, et al. Human blood monocytes: characterization of negatively selected human monocytes and their suspension cell culture derivatives. *Scand J Immunol* 1981;14:243–256.

813. Johnston RBJ, Godzik CA, Cohn ZA. Increased superoxide anion production by immunologically activated and chemically elicited macrophages. *J Exp Med* 1978;148:115–127.

814. Nathan CF, Root RK. Hydrogen peroxide release from mouse peritoneal macrophages. Dependence on sequential activation and triggering. *J Exp Med* 1977;146:1648–1662.

815. Musson RA, McPhail LC, Shafran H, Johnston RBJ. Differences in the ability of human peripheral blood monocytes and *in vitro* monocyte-derived macrophages to produce superoxide anion: studies with cells from normals and patients with chronic granulomatous disease. *J Reticuloendothel Soc* 1982;31:261–266.

816. Pabst MJ, Hedegaard HB, Johnston RBJ. Cultured human monocytes require exposure to bacterial products to maintain an optimal oxygen radical response. *J Immunol* 1982;128:123–128.

817. Seim S. Production of reactive oxygen species and chemiluminescence by human monocytes during differentiation and lymphokine activation *in vitro*. *Acta Pathol Microbiol Immunol Scand (C)* 1982;90:179–185.

818. Grabstein KH, Urdal DL, Tushinski RJ, et al. Induction of macrophage tumoricidal activity by granulocyte-macrophage colony-stimulating factor. *Science* 1986;232:506–508.

819. Weiser WY, Van Niel A, Clark SC, David JR, Remold HG. Recombinant human granulocyte/macrophage colony-stimulating factor activates intracellular killing of *Leishmania donovani* by human monocyte-derived macrophages. *J Exp Med* 1987;166:1436–1446.

820. Reed SG, Nathan CF, Pihl DL, et al. Recombinant granulocyte/macrophage colony-stimulating factor activates macrophages to inhibit *Trypanosoma cruzi* and release hydrogen peroxide. *J Exp Med* 1987;166:1734–1746.

821. Denis M, Ghadirian E. Granulocyte-macrophage colony-stimulating factor restricts growth of tubercle bacilli in human macrophages. *Immunol Lett* 1990;24:203–206.

822. Bermudez LEM, Young LS. Recombinant granulocyte-macrophage colony-stimulating factor activates human macrophages to inhibit growth or kill *Mycobacterium avium* complex. *J Leukoc Biol* 1990;48:67–73.

823. De Titto EH, Catterall JR, Remington JS. Activity of recombinant tumor necrosis factor on *Toxoplasma gondii* and *Trypanosoma cruzi*. *J Immunol* 1986;137:1342–1345.

824. Shparber M, Nathan C. Autocrine activation of macrophages (Mφ) by recombinant tumor necrosis factor (rTNFα) but not recombinant interleukin-I (rIL-I). *Blood* 1986;68:86a.

825. Nathan CF, Murray HW, Wiebe ME, Rubin BY. Identification of interferon-γ as the lymphokine that activates human macrophage oxidative metabolism and antimicrobial activity. *J Exp Med* 1983;158:670–689.

826. Murray HW, Rubin BY, Rothermel CD. Killing of intracellular *Leishmania donovani* by lymphokine-stimulated human mononuclear phagocytes. Evidence that interferon-γ is the activating lymphokine. *J Clin Invest* 1983;72:1506–1510.

827. Cassatella MA, Della Bianca V, Berton G, Rossi F. Activation by gamma interferon of human macrophage capability to produce toxic oxygen molecules is accompanied by decreased Km of the superoxide-generating NADPH oxidase. *Biochem Biophys Res Commun* 1985;132:908–914.

828. Nathan CF, Prendergast TJ, Wiebe ME, Stanley ER, Platzer E, Remold HG, Welte K, et al. Activation of human macrophages: comparison of other cytokines with interferon-γ. *J Exp Med* 1984;160:600–605.

829. Szuro-Sudol A, Nathan CF. Suppression of macrophage oxidative metabolism by products of malignant and nonmalignant cells. *J Exp Med* 1982;156:945–961.

830. Szuro-Sudol A, Murray HW, Nathan CF. Suppression of macrophage antimicrobial activity by a tumor cell product. *J Immunol* 1983;131:384–387.

831. Murray HW. Susceptibility of *Leishmania* to oxygen intermediates and killing by normal macrophages. *J Exp Med* 1981;153:1302–1315.

832. Murray HW. Interaction of *Leishmania* with a macrophage cell line. Correlation between intracellular killing and the generation of oxygen intermediates. *J Exp Med* 1981;153:1690–1695.

833. Murray HW. Cell-mediated immune response in experimental visceral leishmaniasis. II. Oxygen-dependent killing of intracellular *Leishmania donovani* amastigotes. *J Immunol* 1982;129:351–357.

834. Murray HW, Byrne GI, Rothermel CD, Cartelli DM. Lymphokine enhances oxygen-dependent activity against intracellular pathogens. *J Exp Med* 1983;158:234–239.

835. Nathan C, Nogueira N, Juangbhanich C, Ellis J, Cohn Z. Activation of macrophages *in vivo* and *in vitro*. Correlation between hydrogen peroxide release and killing of *Trypanosoma cruzi*. *J Exp Med* 1979;149:1056–1068.

836. Tanaka Y, Kiyotaki C, Tanowitz H, Bloom BR. Reconstitution of a variant macrophage cell line defective in oxygen metabolism with a H₂O₂-generating system. *Proc Natl Acad Sci USA* 1982;79:2584–2588.

837. Nathan CF. The release of hydrogen peroxide from mononuclear phagocytes and its role in extracellular cytolysis. In: van Furth R, ed. *Mononuclear phagocytes—Functional aspects*. The Hague: Martinus Nijhoff, 1980:1105–1137.

838. Nathan CF, Brukner LH, Silverstein SC, Cohn ZA. Extracellular cytolosis by activated macrophages and granulocytes. 1. Pharmacologic triggering of effector cells and the release of hydrogen peroxide. *J Exp Med* 1979;149:84–99.

839. Nathan C, Cohn Z. Role of oxygen-dependent mechanisms in antibody-induced lysis of tumor cells by activated macrophages. *J Exp Med* 1980;152:198–208.

840. Arrick BA, Nathan CF, Griffith OW, Cohn ZA. Glutathione depletion sensitizes tumor cells to oxidative cytolysis. *J Biol Chem* 1982;257:1231–1237.

841. Arrick BA, Nathan CF, Cohn ZA. Inhibition of glutathione synthesis augments lysis of murine tumor cells by sulfhydryl-reactive antineoplastics. *J Clin Invest* 1983;71:258–267.

842. Nathan CF, Arrick BA, Murray HW, DeSantis NM, Cohn ZA. Tumor cell anti-oxidant defenses. Inhibition of the glutathione redox cycle enhances macrophage-mediated cytolysis. *J Exp Med* 1981;153:766–782.

843. O'Donnell-Tormey J, DeBoer CJ, Nathan CF. Resistance of human tumor cells *in vitro* to oxidative cytolysis. *J Clin Invest* 1985;76:80–86.

844. Cohen MS, Taffet SM, Adams DO. The relationship between competence for secretion of H_2O_2 and completion of tumor cytotoxicity by BCG-elicited murine macrophages. *J Immunol* 1982;128:1781–1785.

845. Bainton DF. Changes in peroxidase distribution within organelles of blood monocytes and peritoneal macrophages after surface adherence *in vitro* and *in vivo*. In: van Furth R, ed. *Mononuclear phagocytes. Functional aspects*. The Hague: Martinus Nijhoff, 1980:61–86.

846. Daems WT, van der Rhee HJ. Peroxidase and catalase in monocytes, macrophages, epithelioid cells and giant cells of the rat. In: van Furth R, ed. *Mononuclear phagocytes. Functional aspects*. The Hague: Martinus Nijhoff, 1980:43–60.

847. Bodel PT, Nichols BA, Bainton DF. Appearance of peroxidase activity within the rough endoplasmic reticulum of blood monocytes after surface adherence. *J Exp Med* 1977;145:264–274.

848. Bodel PT, Nichols BA, Bainton DF. Difference in peroxidase localization of rabbit peritoneal macrophages after surface adherence. *Am J Pathol* 1978;91:107–118.

849. Breton-Gorius J, Guichard J, Vainchenker W, Vilde JL. Ultrastructural and cytochemical changes induced by short and prolonged culture of human monocytes. *J Reticuloendothel Soc* 1980;27:289–301.

850. Deimann W, Seitz M, Gemsa D, Fahimi HD. Endogenous peroxidase in the nuclear envelope and endoplasmic reticulum of human monocytes *in vitro*: association with arachidonic acid metabolism. *Blood* 1984;64:491–498.

851. Klebanoff SJ. Antimicrobial activity of catalase at acid pH. *Proc Soc Exp Biol Med* 1969;132:571–574.

852. Klebanoff SJ, Hamon CB. Antimicrobial systems of mononuclear phagocytes. In: van Furth, R ed. *Mononuclear phagocytes in immunity infection and pathology*. Oxford: Blackwell Scientific, 1975:507–531.

853. Gee JBL, Vassallo CL, Bell P, Kaskin J, Basford RE, Field JB. Catalase-dependent peroxidative metabolism in the alveolar macrophage during phagocytosis. *J Clin Invest* 1970;49:1280–1287.

854. Stossel TP, Mason RJ, Pollard TD, Vaughan M. Isolation and properties of phagocytic vesicles. II. Alveolar macrophages. *J Clin Invest* 1972;51:604–614.

855. Paul BB, Strauss RR, Selvaraj RJ, Sbarra AJ. Peroxidase mediated antimicrobial activities of alveolar macrophage granules. *Science* 1973;181:849–850.

856. Gee JBL, Kaskin J, Duncombe MP, Vassallo CL. The effect of ethanol on some metabolic features of phagocytosis in the alveolar macrophage. *J Reticuloendothel Soc* 1974;15:61–68.

857. Mathy-Hartert M, Deby-Dupont G, Melin P, Lamy M, Deby C. Bactericidal activity against Pseudomonas aeruginosa is acquired by cultured human monocyte-derived macrophages after uptake of myeloperoxidase. *Experientia* 1996;52:167–174.

858. Shellito J, Sniezek M, Warnock M. Acquisition of peroxidase activity by rat alveolar macrophages during pulmonary inflammation. *Am J Pathol* 1987;129:567–577.

859. Atwal OS. Cytoenzymological behavior in peritoneal exudate cells of rat *in vivo* 1. Histochemical study of enzymatic function of peroxidase. *J Reticuloendothel Soc* 1971;10:163–172.

860. Heifets L, Imai K, Goren MB. Expression of peroxidase-dependent iodination by macrophages ingesting neutrophil debris. *J Reticuloendothel Soc* 1980;28:391–404.

861. Leung K-P, Goren MB. Uptake and utilization of human polymorphonuclear leukocyte granule myeloperoxidase by mouse peritoneal macrophages. *Cell Tissue Res* 1989;257:653–656.

862. Schmekel B, Hornblad Y, Linden M, Sundstrom C, Venge P. Myeloperoxidase in human lung lavage. II. Internalization of myeloperoxidase by alveolar macrophages. *Inflammation* 1990;14:455–461.

863. Murray HW, Nathan CF, Cohn ZA. Macrophage oxygen-dependent antimicrobial activity. IV. Role of endogenous scavengers of oxygen intermediates. *J Exp Med* 1980;152:1610–1624.

864. Murray HW, Juangbhanich CW, Nathan CF, Cohn ZA. Macrophage oxygen-dependent antimicrobial activity. II. The role of oxygen intermediates. *J Exp Med* 1979;150:950–964.

865. Murray HW, Cohn ZA. Macrophages oxygen-dependent antimicrobial activity. III. Enhanced oxidative metabolism as an expression of macrophage activation. *J Exp Med* 1980;152:1596–1609.

866. Murray HW, Rubin BY, Carriero SM, Harris AM, Jaffee EA. Human mononuclear phagocyte antiprotozoal mechanisms: oxygen-dependent vs. oxygen-independent activity against intracellular *Toxoplasma gondii*. *J Immunol* 1985;134:1982–1988.

867. Britigan BE, Coffman TJ, Adelberg DR, Cohen MS. Mononuclear phagocytes have the potential for sustained hydroxyl radical production. *J Exp Med* 1988;168:2367–2372.

868. Steinbeck MJ, Khan AU, Karnovsky MJ. Extracellular production of singlet oxygen by stimulated macrophages quantified using 9,10–diphenylanthracene and perylene in a polystyrene film. *J Biol Chem* 1993;268:15649–15654.

Inflammation: Basic Principles and Clinical Correlates,
3rd ed., edited by John I. Gallin and Ralph Snyderman.
Published by Lippincott Williams & Wilkins, Philadelphia 1999.

CHAPTER 48

The Respiratory Burst Oxidase

Thomas L. Leto

Neutrophils and other phagocytes are uniquely capable of generating large amounts of reactive oxidants in response to a variety of particulate or soluble inflammatory stimuli. The rapid consumption of oxygen observed during phagocytosis of microbes is attributed to the activity of a multicomponent phagocyte-specific reduced nicotinamide-adenine dinucleotide phosphate (NADPH) oxidase that uses molecular oxygen and cytosolic NADPH as a source of electrons to produce superoxide anion (1,2). This activity has been referred to as the respiratory burst (3), although the oxygen consumed is not associated with mitochondrial oxidative phosphorylation (4). Superoxide is readily converted to hydrogen peroxide, hypochlorous acid, and other potent microbicidal oxidants that are effective against bacterial and fungal pathogens. This pathway also gives rise to other reactive oxygen species (e.g., free radicals) that damage host tissues in processes that have a role in the pathogenesis of disease states associated with chronic or acute inflammation, such as rheumatoid arthritis (5), ischemia-reperfusion injury (6), septic shock (7), and adult respiratory distress syndrome (8). While the role of oxygen in the microbicidal activity of phagocytes has been appreciated for some time (9), the importance of NADPH oxidase in host defense became most dramatically evident from studies on a group of patients with chronic granulomatous disease (CGD), whose phagocytes have genetic defects in superoxide production (3,10). These defects render CGD patients susceptible to recurrent and sometimes life-threatening infections by a number of low-grade pathogenic microorganisms. In addition to their enhanced susceptibility to bacterial and fungal infections, these patients suffer from an apparent dysregulation of normal inflammatory responses, which is evident from the excessive granuloma formation that also characterizes the disease (11). Thus, in addition to their primary role as microbicidal agents, the oxidants generated in response to microbial infections appear to have a role in modulating the normal course of inflammation, conceivably serving as chemical messengers at sites of infection.

The importance of the respiratory burst oxidase in both host defense and inflammation has been recognized for decades; several excellent reviews describe many landmarks in the development of this field (1,12–16). This chapter focuses on recent advances in understanding the structural basis of NADPH oxidase function that have occurred in recent years, with only selected references to earlier work. Many of these advances have been fostered by work in three areas: (a) the development of methods for *in vitro* reconstitution of NADPH oxidase activity, (b) the delineation of NADPH oxidase genes affected in CGD, and (c) the use of recombinant DNA expression systems to examine the function of oxidase components. These advances have provided significant insights into the function and activation of the respiratory burst oxidase in molecular terms and the evolution of this important oxygen-dependent host defense system, which is used in both the plant and animal kingdoms. The regulation of the respiratory burst oxidase has also been an area of intense interest from the perspective of intracellular signal transduction mechanisms, since the oxidase is a useful paradigm for protein-protein interactions and assembly of signaling complexes through conserved protein motifs used throughout biology. The NADPH oxidase is also discussed in three other chapters of this text, in the contexts of phagocyte oxidative metabolism in general (see chapter by Klebanoff), phagocyte stimulation and upstream signaling events leading to activation of the respiratory burst (see chapter by Uhing and Snyderman), and clinical consequences of NADPH oxidase defects causing CGD (see chapter by Holland and Gallin).

T.L. Leto: Laboratory of Host Defenses, National Institute of Allergy and Infectious Diseases, National Institutes of Health, Bethesda, Maryland 20892.

DELINEATION OF NADPH OXIDASE COMPONENTS AFFECTED IN CHRONIC GRANULOMATOUS DISEASE

The activated NADPH oxidase is assembled from proteins found in both cytosolic and membranous compartments of resting neutrophils. Oxidase activation is accompanied by movement of components that assemble as a complex within specific membrane domains, such as newly forming phagosomes where superoxide is released. Much of what is known about the core components of this enzyme has been learned from analysis of biochemical or genetic defects occurring in CGD. While genetic deficiencies of NADPH oxidase causing CGD are rare, these patients represent a remarkably heterogeneous group. Any one of four distinct genes is affected in CGD and numerous genetic lesions are now recognized at each of these loci. The recent review by Roos et al. (16) provides an extensive overview of genetic defects causing CGD; only those that provide insights into the structure or function of the oxidase are mentioned in this chapter. Even before these CGD genes were described, researchers appreciated the heterogeneity of biochemical defects among CGD patients. Segal and coworkers (17) noted that most X-linked CGD patients' neutrophils lack a membrane-bound b-type cytochrome, referred to as flavocytochrome b-245 (due to its unusually low redox midpoint potential of -245 mV) or flavocytochrome b558 (based on its characteristic α-band absorbance at 558 nm). The cytochrome comprises two subunits that coisolate during purification (18,19): the β-subunit (gp91phox) is a 91-kd *ph*agocyte *ox*idase glycoprotein affected in X-linked CGD, while the α-subunit (p22phox) is affected in rare autosomal-recessive forms of CGD. Neither subunit is detected in patients with CGD lesions affecting expression of either subunit, suggesting that synthesis of both chains is required to stabilize the cytochrome heterodimer (20,21).

Neutrophils from most patients with autosomal recessive forms of CGD, however, have a normal membrane cytochrome b content and suffer from deficiencies in the neutrophil cytosolic fraction (22–25). This became apparent when methods for cell-free reconstitution of NADPH oxidase activity were described, involving use of neutrophil membranes, cytosol, and soluble anionic amphiphiles as activators (26–29). Further studies proved that at least three factors fractionated from neutrophil cytosol are needed to support oxidase activity *in vitro;* two are distinct factors (p47phox and p67phox) affected in most autosomal-recessive CGD patients (30–34). It was noted that most autosomal-recessive CGD patients lack a prominent 44- to 48-kd protein that is hyperphosphorylated during oxidase activation (25,35–37), which was later confirmed as p47phox. NADPH oxidase activity could be reconstituted *in vitro* when neutrophil membranes and CGD neutrophil cytosol deficient in p47phox

were mixed with cytosol from p67phox-deficient patients (23). Final proof of the essential roles of both factors was provided when recombinant proteins from these two distinct CGD-associated genes were shown to restore oxidase activity to defective cytosols from these patients (30–32,34). Gene defects affecting the production or function of these four of the five essential core oxidase components (gp91phox, p22phox, p47phox, and p67phox) together account for all cases of CGD described to date. The frequencies of various gene defects among CGD patients and clinical consequences of NADPH oxidase deficiency are discussed in further detail in the chapter by Holland and Gallin.

The requirement for trace amounts of cytosol for cell-free oxidase reconstitution, in addition to p47phox and p67phox, indicated involvement of yet another cytosolic factor in oxidase activation (23,34). This third cytosolic component was identified as the small molecular mass guanosine triphosphatase (GTPase) Rac, which endows the enzyme with sensitivity to guanine nucleotides *in vitro* (38–41). Rac 1 or Rac 2 were shown to enhance oxidase activity in a guanosine triphosphate (GTP)-dependent manner, and, when used in combination with purified recombinant p47phox and p67phox, were sufficient to generate high levels of superoxide in the absence of any other cytosolic factors (41–43). Involvement of Rac in whole cell oxidase activity was later demonstrated by gene transfection and antisense oligonucleotide inhibition experiments (44,45).

DEDUCED STRUCTURES OF THE CORE COMPONENTS OF NADPH OXIDASE

Cytochrome b558

The gene encoding gp91phox was cloned by reverse genetics, using subtractive hybridization methods with DNA from a patient with a major X-chromosome deletion (X-p21) resulting in CGD, Duchenne muscular dystrophy, retinitis pigmentosa, and Macleod's syndrome (46). This gene hybridized to mRNA species that exhibited limited, myeloid-specific expression and that were shown to be deficient in other X-CGD patients. The complete polypeptide sequence deduced from this gene was confirmed by direct peptide sequencing (47,48) and was shown at that time to encode a unique protein. Hydropathy analysis of the deduced gp91phox peptide sequence predicts a membrane-embedded protein with as many as six potential membrane-spanning helical segments. This notion is supported by studies that mapped sites for glycosylation (49), antibody binding (50), and interactions with cytosolic components (51–55). A large body of evidence indicates that the C-terminus of gp91phox is exposed to the cytosol, including antibody labeling (50), CGD mutation studies (51), and peptide binding and inhibition studies that suggest this domain interacts with cytosolic oxidase components through direct contacts with p47phox (52–55).

The gene encoding the small (α) subunit of the cytochrome, p22phox, was identified based on direct peptide sequence data and antibodies that selected corresponding cDNA clones from expression libraries (56). This gene was mapped to chromosome 16 and appears to be more widely expressed than the other oxidase components (57). The best available data on the membrane topology of p22phox suggest that this subunit spans the membrane twice with both the amino and carboxyl termini exposed to the cytosolic surface. Antibodies against either terminal domain react only with permeabilized cell preparations (50), while other work indicates that the carboxyl terminus of p22phox interacts with p47phox (53,58–60).

At present, cytochrome b558 is considered by most workers to represent the sole electron transporting apparatus of NADPH oxidase. A schematic illustrating features of the flavocytochrome b558 relating to its function as a transmembrane carrier of electrons is shown in Fig. 48-1. NADPH binding motifs shared by the ferrodoxin NADP+ reductase (FNR) family of flavoproteins were recognized within the C-terminal half of gp91phox (42,61–63), including the GXGXGXXP sequence thought to bind NADPH ribose phosphate in various reductases. A model based on the crystal structure of FNR has been proposed (62). These features are consistent with observations showing that the purified, relipidated cytochrome binds flavin, and that no other flavoproteins are needed to reconstitute the enzyme *in vitro* (42,43,64).

Recently, this subunit was affinity-labeled with reactive analogues of NADPH and flavin adenine dinucleotide (FAD) (61,65–67), although earlier work using various affinity probes had led previous authors astray (68–70). Evidence based on comparisons between normal and X-CGD cytochromes suggests that gp91phox is composed of two functionally separate domains, one that binds NADPH and flavin and the other a transmembrane heme-containing domain (71–73). An Arg54 to Ser mutation in gp91phox affects superoxide production and heme absorbance, while still permitting transfer of electrons from NADPH through FAD.

The comparison of gp91 phox to related cDNA sequences from yeast (74) and plant species (75) has further reinforced the notions that NADPH, flavin, and heme binding sites all reside within the gp91phox subunit, since all of the proposed cofactor binding motifs are conserved within the yeast and rice homologues (Fig. 48-2). Earlier models for heme binding suggested that at least one of the heme moieties is bound to the small subunits of the cytochrome (76,77). The sequence flanking His 94 of p22phox contains a Val-Leu-His-Leu sequence motif (VLHL) motif seen in the heme-binding subunit of cytochrome c oxidase (56). However, expression studies on the yeast gp91phox homologue, ferric reductase, revealed a b cytochrome with remarkably similar spectral properties with a low redox midpoint potential of about -250 mV, suggesting that the hemes are contained in this subunit alone (78). Furthermore, mutation studies on ferric reductase have provided strong evidence to suggest the existence of two heme binding sites in both the yeast and

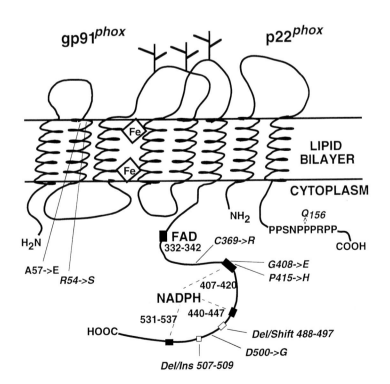

FIG. 48-1. Topology of flavocytochrome b558 with respect to the cell membrane, highlighting structural mutations in chronic granulomatous disease (CGD) *(italics)* resulting in a defective respiratory burst oxidase [reviewed by Roos et al. (16)]. The gp91phox component may span the membrane as many as six times, based on hydropathy analysis. The carboxyl terminal domains of both subunits are exposed to the cytoplasm (50), while the location of the amino terminus of gp91phox is unconfirmed. Mutations at residues Arg369, Glu408, and Asp500 of gp91phox or Pro156 of p22phox disrupt assembly of cytosolic factors. The Agr54 mutation shifts the redox midpoint potential of one of two hemes, but permits electron flow through the C-terminal, flavin-binding domain (72,73). Other mutations may affect flavin adenine dinucleotide (FAD) or NADPH binding. It is proposed that the two heme iron molecules are coordinated by four histidines located in two membrane-embedded helices (79). (See text and Fig. 48-2 for other details.)

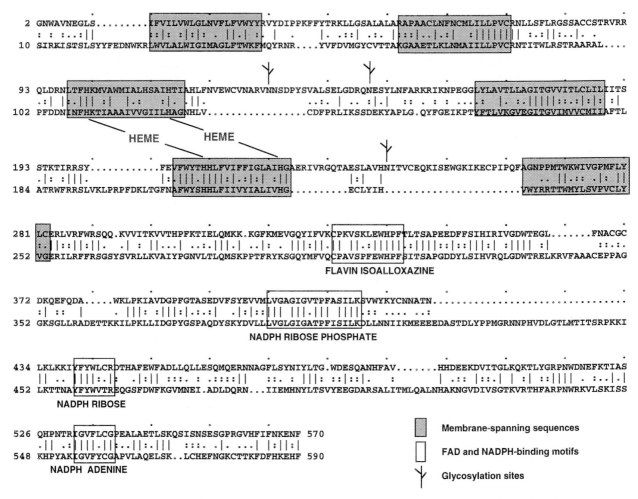

FIG. 48-2. Alignment of the amino acid sequence of human gp91phox *(upper lines)* with its closest homologue deduced from a rice cDNA *(lower lines)* (75). Numbers on the *left* indicate positions of the first amino acid in each line. The comparison across kingdoms emphasizes similarities within putative membrane-spanning sequences and motifs proposed for binding flavin and NADPH, based on similarities to the ferredoxin NADP⁺ family of flavoproteins (42,61–63). Spectroscopic studies suggest that the hemes are ligated through bisimidazole coordination (80–83); the proposed binding sites were inferred from mutagenesis studies on ferric reductase (79). N-linked glycosylation sites were mapped by site-directed mutagenesis (49).

human proteins (79). Four critical histidines were needed to observe the normal heme spectrum of ferric reductase; the locations of these regularly spaced histidines near both ends of two hydrophobic segments suggest that both hemes are sandwiched between two membrane-spanning α-helices. This intramembranous bis-heme motif would facilitate rapid transmembranous electron transport required by both ferric reductase and NADPH oxidase. All four histidines are conserved in both the plant and human gp91phox homologues (human residues 101, 115, 209, and 222) and point mutations in all but one of these codons (res. 115) have been attributed to cytochrome-deficient X-CGD (16), which would suggest that heme incorporation is required for stabilization of gp91phox. Spectroscopic studies lend further support to the model, since electron paramagnetic resonance (EPR), circular dichroism, and Raman spectroscopy were consistent with

low-spin bis-imidazole, hexacoordinate hemes (80–83). Finally, several reports claim the purified cytochrome contains two heme moieties, and two nonidentical hemes were detected in the potentiometric titration of a CGD mutant (Arg54→Ser) of gp91phox (61,73,84).

p47phox and p67phox

The identification of p47phox and p67phox and their corresponding cDNAs relied on the development of a specific antiserum against a GTP agarose-bound protein fraction from neutrophil cytosol (22). This fraction was enriched in cytosolic activity required to complement neutrophil membranes in cell-free reconstitution of NADPH oxidase. Despite the complexity of this preparation, the antiserum generated against it exhibited remarkable specificity; two of the three proteins detected were 47- and 67-

kd proteins absent from neutrophil cytosol in two distinct autosomal recessive forms of CGD (p47phox and p67phox) (22,23). These antibodies were used to select lambda phage cDNA clones encoding both p47phox and p67phox from expression libraries (30–32). Recombinant forms of both proteins were used to demonstrate cell-free NADPH oxidase activity using cytosol preparations from either p47phox or p67phox deficient CGD patients, thus establishing the identities of both proteins as essential cytosolic oxidase components affected in CGD. The recombinant proteins produced in *Escherichia coli* are proteolytically unstable; considerably more active and intact proteins are produced from recombinant baculovirus-infected *Sf9* insect cell cultures (34). Neither of the purified recombinant cytosol factors bind flavin, consistent with their primary structures that do not exhibit significant homology to flavoproteins in other electron carrier systems (34). Recombinant p47phox binds to GTP-agarose, probably by electrostatic interactions, either alone or as a noncovalent complex with recombinant p67phox (34). The p47phox cDNA encodes a basic protein of 390 amino acids with a predicted mass of 44.7 kd. The molecule exhibits a remarkable polarity in the distribution of charged amino acids, showing a concentration of acidic residues in the central region, followed by a highly basic, C-terminal domain that contains several candidate sites for phosphorylation by protein kinase C (PKC) and mitogen-activated protein (MAP) kinase (30,31). Thus, phosphorylation at multiple sites during oxidase activation would dramatically affect electrostatic interactions in this molecule.

The p67phox cDNA predicts a 526-residue protein with a mass of 60.9 kd. The recombinant protein from baculovirus systems is both chemically and thermally unstable (34,85); thus, p67phox may be subject to negative feedback regulation by the oxidase products themselves. The most remarkable feature of both cytosolic proteins is the presence of duplicated sequence motifs (~60 amino acids), known as Src homology 3 (SH3) domains that are found in a variety of intracellular signaling proteins that shuttle between the cytosol and membrane or cytoskeletal complexes (30–32). These include the Src family of nonreceptor tyrosine kinases, as well as various phosphatases, phospholipases (PLC-γ), GTPase activating proteins (GAPs), cytoskeletal proteins (α-spectrins and myosins), and adapter proteins (e.g., GRB-2) that link other intracellular signaling components (for reviews, see refs. 86–88). The SH3 domains of these diverse proteins function as recognition motifs for proline-rich peptide ligands within target proteins. In the oxidase system these domains have a central role in the interaction of several oxidase components leading to assembly of the active membrane-bound enzyme complex, since p47phox, p67phox, and p22phox also contain several proline-rich SH3-binding sequences. The roles of these specific SH3 interactions, both in maintenance of the latent states of the oxidase and in assembly of the acti-

vated complex, are discussed in detail below in the context of oxidase activation mechanisms.

Protein sequence database searches also identified another unusual relationship between the amino-terminal domain of p67phox and another group of functionally diverse proteins (89,90). These proteins contain an internally repetitive motif known as the tetratricopeptide (34 amino acid) repeat (TPR) (91,92). Proteins with these repeats exhibit a variety of subcellular localization patterns and functions, ranging from regulation of the cell cycle, gene transcription, and mitochondrial and peroxisomal protein import. Four TPR motifs were recognized within p67phox; three occur in tandem at the amino terminus, while the third and fourth repeats are interrupted by 16 intervening residues. Together, these repeats make up a major portion of the amino-terminal region of p67phox representing a minimum functional domain of p67phox that supports cell-free oxidase activation (res. 1–246) (93) and binds to Rac (res. 1–199) (94). Physical studies on other proteins containing the TPR motif in corroboration with molecular modeling suggest that the tandem repeats are amphipathic helical segments (or snap helices) that engage in homotypic interactions (95,96). The most conserved features of these repeats essential to these interactions are complementary knob and hole structures that lie on opposite hydrophobic surfaces of the helices. The repeats within p67phox may either self-associate, mediate p67phox dimerization, or bind to other TPR-containing proteins. The importance of this conserved TPR feature in p67phox structure is evident from a CGD-associated lesion, where a single Gly-78 point mutation is apparently sufficient to cause complete p67phox deficiency (97). The location of this Gly → Gln point mutation is predicted to disrupt normal TPR structure by occupying the critical hole position of the third repeat with a bulkier side chain, rendering the mutant p67phox unstable. In another p67phox-defective CGD patient, a single point deletion (lysine 58) in the second TPR repeat was recently described (98). In this case, the mutant protein was detected in the patient's neutrophils; the lesion appears to interfere with binding of p67phox to Rac. This deletion is predicted to have dramatic effects on the overall folding of this domain, since it would place the entire downstream helical segment out of phase with normal contacts with other repeats. Thus, the misfolded repeats may interfere with Rac to a distal site, rather than a disruption of binding of Rac to TPRs themselves. Other TPR-containing proteins are not known to bind Rac; p67phox lacks the CDC42-Rac interaction binding (CRIB) domain seen in other Rac targets, such as p21rac-activated kinase (PAK) (99).

Rac

While several distinct cellular functions of Rac have been described, including modulation of actin-based cytoskeleton (100), activation of various serine/threonine kinases (e.g., PAKs) (101), and signaling events linked to cell proliferation (102,103), oxidase activation was the first well-defined terminal effector system of Rac identified *in vitro*. Rac 1, which is widely expressed in many cell types, was identified as an oxidase cofactor from guinea pig peritoneal macrophages (38), while Rac 2, which is produced at high levels during myeloid differentiation, was independently identified from mature neutrophils by others (39–41). These proteins are members of the Rho subfamily of Ras-related proteins, have 92% identical sequences, and exhibit only ≈30% identity with Ras. Surprisingly, recombinant forms of both Rac proteins produced in *E. coli*, which are not posttranslationally modified by C-terminal geranylgeranylation, still support arachidonate-activated cell-free oxidase activity; this provided investigators with a relatively easy *in vitro* assay of an effector function of this Ras relative. Several groups used this system to explore structural determinants within Rac specific for oxidase activation by comparing various mutant and chimeric recombinant proteins produced in *E. coli* (94,104–109).

Comparison of chimeric proteins constructed with portions of Rac 1 exchanged with homologous regions of CDC42Hs, the closest nonfunctional relative of Rac (70% identical), revealed the importance of sequence analogous to the effector loop or switch I region of Ras (res. 30–40) (104,110). Point mutagenesis studies showed that the difference in activity between Rac 1 and CDC42Hs is due entirely to differences at positions 27 and 30. Substitution of several Rac residues within the effector loop with analogous residues of Ras confirmed the essential role of this site in Rac regulation of oxidase activity (94,104,106–109). A sequence analogous to the Ras switch II region, which also changes conformation upon binding of GTP, also appears to be involved in Rac regulation of the oxidase, since a mutation of position 61 (gln to leu) somehow compensates for disabling mutations in the switch I region (109). Comparative analysis of various Rac/Rho chimeras also revealed involvement of the less conserved C-terminal region of Rac, as well (107). Another critical site that provides specificity for effectors of members of the Rho family is an insert region (res. ~130–140) that is represented by only a short loop in the structure of Ras. Mutations in this segment of Rac distinguish between interactions of Rac with two of its effectors, PAK and NADPH oxidase (106). The recently published crystallographic structure of Rac confirmed that the most remarkable structural differences between Rac and Ras occur within two of the sites shown to be specific for oxidase activation: (a) the effector loop, which binds to p67phox and, in Rac, bears fewer charges and is likely less stable than Ras when exposed; and (b) the insert region, which is an additional helical segment presented on a distinct surface of Rac (108,111). These and other potential sites for downstream regulation of the oxidase were also identified by "peptide walking," in which a series of pentadecapeptides spanning to entire sequence of Rac were compared as inhibitors of oxidase activity *in vitro* (112). Together these studies reveal distinct structural differences between the Ras and Rho families that can account for their diverse regulatory functions.

ASSEMBLY AND ACTIVATION OF THE MEMBRANE-BOUND NADPH OXIDASE COMPLEX

The mechanisms of cellular activation leading to respiratory burst activity have been a subject of great interest in recent years, particularly since the identification of all core components of this effector system (reviewed in refs. 113 and 114). Many of the themes emerging from this work have been useful paradigms for signal transduction mechanisms encountered in other cells. In general terms, respiratory burst activation begins with cell stimulation through G-protein–coupled receptors, activation of various kinases (115) and phospholipases (A₂, C, and D) (116–118), and enhanced phosphorylation of target proteins. These events are somehow correlated with phosphorylation of several oxidase components (35–37,119–127), transmigration of these proteins to specific membrane domains where assembly of the oxidase complex occurs (128–135), and subsequent activation of the electron transport process (136). While the precise signaling pathways leading directly to oxidase activation are largely unexplained, it is clear that several distinct pathways lead to activation of the respiratory burst. Experimentally, this has been evident from the disparate effects with various oxidase inhibitors, depending on the stimulus used to elicit a burst (113–115,121,122). Phorbol myristate acetate (PMA) elicits a robust burst, although the activity is calcium independent and may involve less relevant pathways physiologically. Respiratory burst activities in response to phagocytic or chemotactic stimuli are associated with intracellular calcium transients, are less inhibited by stuarosporin (a PKC inhibitor) but more effectively inhibited by tyrosine kinase and phosphatidylinositol 3-kinase inhibitors. These agents have the opposite effects on PMA-elicited burst activity. The classical pathway of G-protein–coupled receptor activation, where extracellular ligands trigger activation of phospholipase C-B1, release of inositol triphosphate and diacyl glycerol, elevations in intracellular calcium, and activation of PKC, does not entirely explain oxidase activation by several physiologic stimuli because changes in intracellular calcium induced by these agents do not alone account for activation (137). Phospholipases A₂ and D (PLA₂ and PLD) are also activated by a variety of natural stimuli; the products of these lipases may directly or indirectly affect several oxidase components (64,84,138–141). While several protein kinases have been proposed to act directly in the phosphorylation of oxidase components during oxidase activation, the terminal mediators of oxidase activation have not been clearly identified.

Considerable attention has been focused on p47phox because this protein undergoes dramatic stepwise changes in phosphorylation state during membrane translocation and oxidase activation, suggesting that phosphorylation of this protein is closely linked to assembly of the activated oxidase complex (119–124). However, activation-dependent phosphorylation of p67phox and the cytochrome have also been noted (125–127). As many as nine phosphorylated forms of p47phox have been detected in PMA-activated neutrophils; the most heavy phosphorylated species are detected only on the membrane and depend on the presence of cytochrome b558 (119). Seven phosphorylated serines have been mapped within the highly basic C-terminal domain of p47phox in PMA-activated neutrophils (120). Mutations at some of these sites inhibit oxidase activation in whole transfected Epstein-Barr virus transformed (EBV)-B cells, suggesting that p47phox phosphorylation is a requisite of oxidase activation (124). When phosphorylated in vitro, alterations in its reactivity with N-ethylmaleimide were noted, suggestive of phosphorylation-dependent conformational changes (142). PKC was shown to activate oxidase activity in vitro, albeit at low levels (143,144). A unique phosphatidic acid (PA)-activated p47phox kinase has also been identified (145). The enzyme phosphorylates p47phox and can stimulate oxidase activity in a phosphorylation dependent manner in vitro. Thus, it is a plausible signaling intermediately downstream from phospholipase D activation, although its role in oxidase activation in whole cells has not been established. A p21rac-activated kinase (PAK) is also activated in formyl-methionyl-leucyl-phenylalanine (fMLP)-stimulated neutrophils and is thought to phosphorylate p47phox (146), although transfection studies with constitutively active PAK suggest that PAK actually downregulates oxidase activity (147).

Cell-free activation of NADPH oxidase by soluble anionic amphiphiles such as arachidonic acid (AA) and sodium or lithium dodecylsulphate (SDS or LiDS) does not require protein phosphorylation (148,149). The physiologic relevance of this process has been controversial, because these amphophiles have multiple effects on oxidase components in vitro (138–141). These amphophiles may bind p47phox and merely mimic the effects of phosphorylation in whole cells (142). Other evidence indicates that LiDS and PA can interact directly with the flavocytochrome and enable low-level production of superoxide, even in the absence of the cytosol factors (64,84). Other recent and exciting work suggests that AA acts in a final activation phase after assembly of the complex of flavocytochrome with the cytosol factors, because cell lines deficient in cytosolic PLA2 (p85) show normal translocation of oxidase components but are deficient in

oxidase activity (136). The activity is restored by addition of exogenous AA. Finally, AA is thought to activate H^+ channel activity attributed to the cytochrome. This channel was genetically reconstituted in cells producing of the amino-terminal portion (res. 1–230) of gp91phox (138). Thus, activation of PLD and PLA2 following stimulation of neutrophils with opsonized particles, PMA, or fMLF may affect flavocytochrome function through direct interactions with the lipid second messengers generated by these enzymes.

Activation-Dependent Interactions of Oxidase Components

In resting neutrophils the bulk of cytochrome b558 is found within secondary granules; upon activation the cytochrome is delivered to the plasma membrane and newly forming phagolysosomes (133–135). In resting cells, the cytosolic factors p47phox and p67phox are found in a noncovalent, high molecular weight complex of ≈250,000 daltons (150–152). Studies on CGD neutrophils have provided key insights into distinct roles of each oxidase component in the assembly of the active oxidase complex. The cytosolic proteins translocate to the membrane as a complex; this association appears to involve a primary interaction between p47phox and both subunits of cytochrome b558. The absence of cytochrome b558 associated with CGD (119,128), or specific mutations in either gp91phox (res. 500) (51) or p22phox (res. 156) (58,60), result in dramatically reduced membrane translocation of both p47phox and p67phox when compared with normal activated neutrophils. Furthermore, neutrophils from autosomal-recessive CGD patients lacking p47phox show significantly reduced translocation of p67phox, while those lacking p67phox exhibit normal translocation of p47phox (128). Thus, p47phox appears to serve as a bridge between other essential components. Studies on cell-free oxidase reconstitution involving neutrophil membranes, purified or crude cytosolic components, soluble amphophilic activators, and peptide inhibitors showed that the interaction of p47phox with cytochrome b558 is a primary event in the oxidase activation process and that assembly of p67phox and Rac into the activated complex is secondary (153). Transfection studies comparing translocation of various truncated forms of the cytosolic factors confirmed that p47phox functions as a multivalent adapter between p67phox and the flavocytochrome (154,155).

The translocation of Rac to the membrane apparently occurs independently of the other cytosolic factors, based on analysis of CGD patient neutrophils and differential effects of various oxidase inhibitors on oxidase assembly (129–131). Cell-free interactions of Rac with the membrane also appear to be independent of the other cytosolic factors (141). Like other members of the Rho family of small molecular weight GTPases, Rac is found entirely associated in a stoichiometric complex with RhoGDI [guanosine diphosphate (GDP) dissociation inhibitor] in resting cells through interactions with its geranylgeranylated carboxyterminal domain (38,40,41,156). Translocation of Rac is triggered by guanine nucleotide exchange, whereupon RhoGDI dissociates and the active Rac-GTP complex binds favorably to the plasma membrane through the same terminal domain. Consistent with such a mechanism, cell-free oxidase activity is inhibited by the GTPase activating protein RhoGAP and promoted by the guanine nucleotide exchange factor RhoGEF. This model of Rac regulation is further supported by studies on the *bcr* gene knock-out in transgenic mice, where the absence of this Rac GTPase-activating protein results in enhanced oxidative burst activity and acute sensitivity to bacterial endotoxin (7). The enhanced oxidase activity in *bcr-/bcr-* mice correlates with higher levels of membrane-bound Rac in resting neutrophils. Once membrane bound, Rac is thought to regulate the oxidase through interactions with p67phox and possibly the cytochrome (94,108). Thus, as far as assembly of the cytosolic factors is concerned, at least two independent converging pathways control oxidase activation: one regulating movement of Rac to the membrane and the other(s) independently affecting translocation and assembly of the p47phox-p67phox complex.

SH3 Domains

The SH3 domains in both p47phox and p67phox have a central role in assembly of these components into the activated, membrane-bound NADPH oxidase complex. Shortly after the roles of several SH3 domains were described as recognition motifs for proline-rich peptide ligands in other signaling systems (reviewed in refs. 86–88), several groups focused their attention on proline-rich domains found within several oxidase components, as potential targets of the SH3 domains in p47phox or p67phox (58–60,157). Based on a series of *in vitro* binding studies with engineering protein domains and synthetic peptides, in conjunction with mutagenesis and transfection experiments, several specific SH3 interactions were identified among oxidase components (Fig. 48-3) (58–60,154,155,157–162). Many of these interactions were later confirmed in yeast two-hybrid interactions (163–166). The C-terminal proline-rich domain of p22phox was of particular interest, because a single proline 156 → glutamine mutation was noted in this domain in a CGD patient with a normal membrane cytochrome content (167). This mutation proved to be the first case where a defect in an SH3 ligand has been linked to human disease (58–60). This mutation in the cytoplasmic domain of p22phox was sufficient to disrupt PMA-activated translocation of p47phox to membranes in transfected K562 cells (58) or neutrophils from the CGD patient with this defect (60).

The effects on p47phox membrane binding was correlated with a loss of binding between the core region of p47, spanning both of its SH3 domains, and the proline-rich cytoplasmic domain of p22phox (res. 149–162) (58,59). In addition to this interaction, the core of p47phox also bound to its own proline-rich C-terminal domain, suggesting that an intramolecular interaction could compete with or mask the domain in p47phox involved in binding to p22phox. Addition of SDS or arachidonate to p47phox, used to activate the oxidase *in vitro*, had the apparent effect of unmasking p47phox and allowing binding to p22phox and p67phox, as detected by exposure of occult epitopes that bind a specific monoclonal antibody directed against p47phox (59). Subsequent binding and membrane translocation studies, involving truncations or point mutations of the individual SH3 domains in p47phox, confirmed that the first SH3 domain of p47phox domain bound both to the proline-rich tail of p22phox and its own C-terminal proline-rich domain (155,159,164). The second SH3 domain of p47phox is involved in cotranslocation of p67phox to the membrane, through interactions with the N-terminal domain of p67phox (res. 1–246) (155). Thus, the central segment of p47phox (res. 151–284) containing two SH3 domains represents a bivalent functional core of this molecule capable of mediating translocation of both cytosol factors through SH3 interactions with the membrane-bound cytochrome through the first SH3 domain, and with p67phox through the second (154,155).

The C-terminal domain of p47phox, which is highly basic and contains multiple sites of phosphorylation and the proline-rich binding site for the first SH3 domain of p47phox, appears to serve in regulating access to the p22phox binding site in a phosphorylation-dependent manner. In a sense, p47phox can be viewed as a classic adapter, such as GRB-2, which functions solely in bringing other interacting partners together in response to activation through multiple interactions with separate modular domains (86,87). Consistent with such a model for p47phox function, significant levels of NADPH oxidase activity have been reconstituted *in vitro*, even in the absence of p47phox when high concentrations of p67phox and Rac are mixed with the flavocytochrome (168,169).

Other independent work in EBV-immortalized lymphoblastoid B cells from a p67phox-deficient CGD patient indicates that both the SH3 domains in p67phox are also critical to oxidase activation in whole cells (93). When comparing various truncated forms of p67phox for reconstitution of oxidase activity, deletions of sequences encoding either SH3 domain of p67phox resulted in significant reductions in whole cell oxidase activity (>90%). However, the N-terminal domain of p67phox (res. 1–246), lacking both SH3 domains, does support oxidase activity in the arachidonate-activated cell-free oxidase reconstitution assay. Studies involving truncated proteins

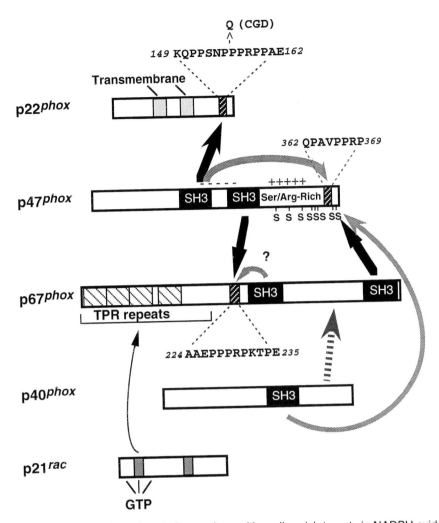

FIG. 48-3. Model of multiple SH3 domain interactions with proline-rich targets in NADPH oxidase components. Interactions that contribute to formation of the active oxidase complex are shown *(black arrows)*, as are those that inhibit or prevent oxidase assembly *(gray arrows)*. Phosphorylation of all three cytosolic phox proteins, which occurs during oxidase activation, is thought to influence several SH3 interactions. Intramolecular contacts in p47phox and p67phox are thought to maintain these proteins in latent states. The p22phox interaction has a predominant role in oxidase assembly, while there is a redundancy in contacts between p47phox and p67phox (58–60,154,155,157–166). The SH3 domain of p40phox competitively inhibits oxidase activity (163,166). The interaction of rac with p67phox is guanosine triphosphate (GTP) dependent and likely occurs after membrane translocation. For simplicity, interactions involving other domains are not shown. (See text for details.)

or proline-rich peptides corresponding to the C-terminal domain of p47phox, showed that the C-terminal SH3 domain of p67phox bound specifically to the proline-rich tail domain of p47phox (58,158,160,163–166). This interaction was readily demonstrated with native full-length proteins or crude cytosolic preparations, in contrast to the other interaction between p47phox and p67phox described above, which were only evident in activated transfected cells, suggesting that the tail-tail interaction between p47phox and p67phox also occurs in resting cells. Several observations suggest that this interaction is important in assembly of the activated, membrane-bound oxidase complex in activated cells: (a) deletion of the C-terminal domain of p67phox dramatically

affects both whole-cell oxidase activity and membrane translocation of p67phox in transfected cells (93); (b) scanning mutagenesis of this proline-rich target sequence in p47phox inhibits whole-cell oxidase activity in a manner that parallels the effects of these mutations on binding of the C-terminal p67phox SH3 domain (162); and (c) p40phox or its isolated SH3 domain, which binds competitively to the tail domain of p47phox (166), inhibits whole-cell oxidase activity in transfected cells (163).

The function of the first p67phox SH3 domain has not been clearly defined. One notion worthy of speculation is that this domain participates in intramolecular contacts that mask the proline-rich target sequence within the N-terminal domain of p67phox and prevent p47phox interaction in the latent state. The movement of p67phox to membranes of transfected K562 cells is remarkably dependent on PMA activation, particularly when coexpressed along with the core fragment of p47phox, which lacks its phosphorylated domain (and proline-rich tail) and is membrane-bound even without PMA activation (154). Thus, a PMA-dependent conformational change within p67phox would promote its interaction with p47phox and allow membrane translocation following activation. This process could involve direct phosphorylation of p67phox, which has been demonstrated in activated cells (125,126). A model in which intramolecular SH3 interactions within both p47phox and p67phox maintain these proteins in inactive or locked conformations, until cellular activation and phosphorylation promote a switching to other SH3 domain contacts, is not without precedence. Many SH3 domain-containing proteins contain proline-rich sequences that engage in intramolecular interactions. Crystallographic studies have shown that the inactive forms of Src and its close relative, Hck, involve intramolecular contacts of both the SH3 and SH2 domains of these proteins (170,171). Activation of these kinases can be induced by alterations in phosphorylation state or competitive interactions with other proline-rich target proteins.

Another inhibitory mechanism involving competing SH3 interactions was observed in studies on p40phox, which is another cytosol factor found within a high molecular weight complex with p67phox and p47phox in resting neutrophils and appears to translocate to the membrane upon activation (130,152,172,173). The importance of the p40phox-p67phox interaction is evident in p67phox-deficient CGD neutrophils, where reduced levels of p40phox are detected, although this protein is not essential for oxidase reconstitution *in vitro* (38,42). Sites for interactions of p40phox with both cytosolic proteins have been identified; p40phox binds p67phox through its C-terminal domain, while interactions with p47phox involve the SH3 domain of p40phox and the same proline-rich tail of p47phox that binds p67phox (163–166). The SH3 domain of p40phox has greatest homology with the C-terminal SH3 domain of p67phox, with 44% sequence identity (172), and the two proteins appear to bind p47phox competitively and are presumably influenced by phosphorylation (123, 163,166). Furthermore, p40phox significantly inhibits NADPH oxidase activity, either when assayed in combination with other recombinant proteins in the cell-free system or in whole transfected K562 cells that normally lack p40phox (163). Deletion studies in these cells indicated that the inhibition relates to the p40phox-p47phox interaction. Removal of the p67phox-binding domain of p40phox does not relieve the inhibition by p40phox, while the isolated SH3 domain of p40phox that binds p47phox was even more effective in inhibiting whole-cell oxidase activity.

The analysis of multiple SH3 domain interactions in NADPH oxidase illustrates a range of versatile functions that these domains can serve in signal transduction. This work has provided insights on the structural basis by which these many functions are performed. One reason for the functional versatility of SH3 interactions relates to the remarkable pseudosymmetrical structure of their proline-rich target sequences (174–176). The cores of these peptide ligands adopt a polyproline type-II helical conformation, such that the regular, three residues-per-turn helix occupies the same space profile in both the forward and backward directions. When detailed structures of several SH3 domain–proline-rich ligand complexes became available, the complexes were described in either of two separate classes, based on two entirely opposite orientations of the bound peptides with respect to the binding surfaces of the SH3 domains (174–176). It was suggested that the p22phox proline-rich target bound to the first SH3 domain of p47phox was a class I ligand, based on remarkable similarities with the proline-rich peptide, 3BP-1, bound to the SH3 domain of Abl (155), while the tail-tail interaction of p47phox and the SH3 domain of p67phox was predicted to represent a reverse orientation or class II complex, based on the effects of mutations in this SH3 domain, or its ligand, on binding (161,162). Interestingly, the opposite (in this case, forward) binding orientation is also possible for other SH3 domain complexes with the p47phox tail sequence (i.e., intramolecular contacts), which would predict distinctly different effects from phosphorylation at sites flanking this target.

Other Interactions

In addition to the SH3 interactions described above, several other sites of interaction between oxidase components have been proposed as important in assembly of the oxidase, based primarily on the effects of synthetic peptide on oxidase activation in cell-free or electropermeabilized cell systems (51–55,148,153,177–180). Most peptides were designed based on considerations of surface-exposed epitopes (52,53,55), identified as possible binding sequences by screening peptide phage display libraries (54,177,178), or corresponded to sites mutated in CGD (51). Many have cited the effects of peptides derived from gp91phox as evidence that these sequences are exposed within cytoplasmic domains of gp91phox that interact with p47phox (see Fig. 2); however, the corresponding sites of interaction with p47phox have not been defined. Inhibition of cell-free oxidase activity by all of these peptides requires the addition of peptides to p47phox prior to activation by arachidonate or SDS. These amphiphiles apparently induce formation of irreversible complexes between p47phox and gp91phox or p67phox *in vitro* that are not dissociated if the peptides are added after activation. One noteworthy feature of many of the most potent inhibitory peptides is their high content of basic or basic and hydrophobic residues, particularly since the p47phox sequence exhibits such an unusual segregation in charged amino acids. Indeed, several polybasic peptides, such as polylysine, polyhistine, and polyarginine (181), or the basic amphopathic peptides mastoparan (182) and PR-39 (183), demonstrated impressive oxidase inhibitory activities *in vitro* [concentrations that inhibit 50% (IC_{50}) were found to be ~1–2 μM]. The issue of whether the inhibitory effects of many of these basic peptides reflect disruption of specific protein-protein interactions relevant to whole-cell oxidase assembly warrants additional attention. In only a few studies were the specific contexts of peptide sequences examined with regard to oxidase inhibition and specific binding activities (51,179,180,183). Studies on the C-terminal domain of gp91phox correlated oxidase inhibition with immobilization of specific residues in gp91phox (558–RGVHFIF–564) by p47phox (180). In another study, disruption of p47phox membrane translocation in CGD neutrophils caused by a gp91phox mutation (res. 500) was correlated with inhibition of cell-free oxidase activity and p47phox translocation by a peptide corresponding to residues 491 to 504 (51).

Another cytochrome interaction representing an additional GTP-dependent control point concerns the Ras-related protein, Rap1a. Rap1a copurifies with cytochrome b558 and colocalizes with the enzyme in newly formed phagolysosomes (184). While Rap1a is not needed for cell-free reconstitution of oxidase activity, transfection studies in HL-60 and EBV-transformed B cells have implicated Rap1a in whole-cell oxidase function (45,185). Transfection of either constitutively active (G12V) and negative dominant (N17T) mutants of Rap1a inhibits whole-cell oxidase activity, suggesting that its role requires GTP hydrolysis cycling. Rap1a is phosphorylated by cyclic adenosine monophosphate (cAMP)-dependent protein kinases, and its phosphorylation appears to inhibit its association with the cytochrome (186). These observations provide one explanation for the inhibitory effects of β-adrenergic agonists on oxidase activity, since these agonists cause elevations in neutrophil cAMP levels (187).

Role of the Cytoskeleton in Oxidase Assembly

It has been suggested that the cytoskeleton has a role in oxidase assembly and activation, although most data cited in support of cytoskeleton involvements have been indirect. The active oxidase somehow becomes associated with nondenaturing detergent-insoluble residues of extracted cells, but no specific associations with cytoskeletal proteins have been identified as yet (188,189). Furthermore, the cytosolic oxidase components are rendered insoluble by soluble amphiphiles, even in the absence of membrane fractions (139). Circumstan-

tial arguments, based on the association of many SH3 domain-containing proteins with the cytoskeleton, have led many to suggest that these domains could link the cytosol factors to the cytoskeleton; however, no specific SH3 targets have been identified within cytoskeletal proteins to date. Furthermore, Rac's role in oxidase activation, where p67phox is the downstream effector of this system, has been dissociated from its role in PAK regulation or actin reorganization events (94,99–101,106–109). Recent immunoelectron-microscopy studies show that active oxidase complexes are assembled principally within membrane domains devoid of cytoskeletal structures (135). Thus, the cytochrome may have a leading role in determining the site of active oxidase assembly. According to the assembly models discussed above, translocation of the cytosol factors to the membrane may be limited solely by exposure or modification of domains that interact with the flavocytochrome; once these domains become exposed, the movement would be accomplished by diffusion to their docking sites on the cytochrome. Thus, it could be argued that the cytoskeletal matrix is an impediment to oxidase assembly, which would account for the enhancing effects of cytochalasin B on fMLP-activated respiratory burst activity (190).

CONCLUSION

Assembly and activation of phagocyte NADPH oxidase complexes involve the input of several signal transduction cascades acting in a coordinate, multistage process. This begins with the independent translocation of Rac and other cytosol factors and movement of membrane components to newly forming phagosomal membranes, assembly of the membrane bound complex, and subsequent activation of electron transfer through the flavocytochrome. While p47phox appears to play a critical role in the initiation of these events, it is thought that p67phox has a more direct role in the regulation of electron flow through direct interactions with the flavocytochrome. It is thought that p67phox or Rac induce changes in the cytochrome to permit binding of NADPH, while other evidence indicates that AA may also act directly on the cytochrome in some later stage of activation. Recent studies on the effects of arachidonic acid on cytochrome heme spectra suggest that arachidonate ultimately controls transmembrane flow of electrons through the heme-containing domain of gp91phox (83). The consumption of cytosolic NADPH and translocation of electrons to an extracytoplasmic compartment require concomitant translocation of protons to maintain a neutral cytosolic pH. Recent work involving heterologous expression of gp91phox suggests that the membrane-embedded portion of the cytochrome subunit (res. 1–230) itself constitutes an arachidonate-activated H^+ channel (138), although other mechanisms for proton translocation have been described (191).

Little is known about the mechanisms involved in termination of the respiratory burst. It has been suggested that maintenance of an active respiratory burst in whole cells reflects a continuous cycling or turnover of components in their active states (192), whereby some components are subject to control by GTP hydrolysis cycles while others are in flux between phosphorylated and dephosphorylated states (45,185). In contrast to whole-cell respiratory burst activity, such control mechanisms are not evident *in vitro,* because neither protein phosphorylation nor GTP hydrolysis are needed in most cell-free systems (148). However, oxidase activity assayed *in vitro* is also short-lived, but can be prolonged by chemical crosslinking (193), suggesting that disassembly processes also downregulate the enzyme *in vitro.* Direct negative feedback inhibition of the oxidase through oxidant-sensitive components, such as p67phox, is also a plausible mechanism of downregulation.

It is hoped that eventually knowledge about fine-structure details involved in the regulation of NADPH oxidase may serve as a basis for rational design of drugs that inhibit the oxidase in circumstances where acute or chronic inflammatory processes are undesirable. Suitable targets for such agents might include specific upstream activators of the oxidase (e.g., kinases, lipases, or GTPase) or the oxidase components themselves. In the latter case, peptidomimetics that interfere with assembly of the oxidase are good candidates, although these agents would have to reach intracellular targets to be effective. It has been suggested that the amphopathic proline-rich peptide PR-39 inhibits whole-cell oxidase activity by binding to an SH3 domain of p47phox; however, cellular uptake of this peptide inhibitor has not been directly demonstrated (183).

Exciting new research directed toward genetic correction of NADPH oxidase defects indicates that CGD is a useful model for gene therapy of hematopoietic disorders, in general. The progress here also suggests that this approach may soon provide a feasible therapeutic alternative in the management of this disease (reviewed in ref. 194). Several factors make CGD an attractive model for piloting gene therapy strategies targeted to hematopoietic cells. From a technical standpoint, sensitive methods for detecting oxidase reconstitution such as enhanced chemiluminescence and fluorescence activated cell sorting (FACS) analysis have enabled investigators to readily assess low levels of enzymatic correction, even at the level of single cells. This has allowed scientists to explore a range of parameters enhancing gene transfer and expression efficiencies. It is thought that even low levels of oxidase correction will provide clinical benefits, since X-linked CGD carriers remain healthy even in cases where only 3% to 5% of circulating neutrophils are oxidase positive. To date, the correction of all four oxidase gene defects in CGD has been achieved with a variety of gene transfer vectors. Test systems for demonstrating oxi-

dase reconstitution have been limited to cells capable of developing a myeloid phenotype, such as EBV-immortalized lymphoblastoid B cell lines from CGD patients, hematopoietic progenitor cells from bone marrow or peripheral blood from CGD patients or CGD gene knockout models in mice (p47phox and gp91phox deficient) (195,196), and human myelomonoblastic leukemia cell lines (gp91phox-deficient knock-out lines) (197). High levels of oxidase activity were also reconstituted in erythroleukemic cell lines (K562) transfected or transduced with all three of the myeloid-specific oxidase genes, p47phox, p67phox, and gp91phox (198); this system offers flexibility for testing expression vectors encoding all three oxidase genes. In many studies normal levels of oxidase restoration have been observed using either selectable expression vectors or recombinant retroviruses.

The greatest hurdles faced in developing clinically effective CGD gene therapy protocols relate primarily to two major challenges: the need for obtaining suitable, self-renewing populations of human hematopoietic stem cells as targets for gene transfer, and the need for designing efficient and stable gene expression vectors that remain transcriptionally active *in vivo.* Despite these challenges, promising results have already been obtained in correcting oxidase deficiencies in both CGD mice and humans, using murine recombinant retroviral vectors to transduce hematopoietic progenitor cells. In both p47phox- and gp91phox-deficient CGD mice, retroviral vectors were used to transduce bone marrow stem cells *ex vivo.* Transplantation of transduced cells into irradiated recipient mice resulted in significant counts of oxidase-positive neutrophils, which remained in circulation for weeks and provided significant protection against microbial challenges when compared to controls (199,200). In phase I clinical trials of gene therapy for CGD in humans, correction of the p47phox deficiency was attempted in five patients by transduction of peripheral blood–derived stem cell progenitors, which resulted in low numbers of oxidase-positive neutrophils (0.004% to 0.05%) that were detected in the circulation up to 3 to 6 months after transduction (201). Future success in this endeavor will depend on development of methods that promote stable, long-term engraftment of transduced progenitor cells. The preliminary findings confirm the safety and feasibility of gene therapy for CGD and have provided an impetus for other trials examining the efficacy of multiple cycles of gene therapy, particularly in patients with serious infections.

While the oxidase is generally considered a specialized system of myeloid cells critical in host defense, evidence is accumulating to indicate that related oxidases exist in other cells, which produce low levels of oxidants that serve as intracellular second messengers in a manner functionally analogous to nitric oxide. It is thought that in many tissues superoxide and hydrogen peroxide can transduce signals that promote processes ranging from cellular proliferation to apoptosis (103,202,203). Downstream targets of these oxidants include various kinases (204) and gene transcription factors, such as nuclear factor κB (NF-κB) (205), which can alter the gene expression pattern in response to intracellular oxidants. Thus, considerable interest is being directed at characterizing the nonmyeloid oxidase(s) that generate these redox signals. While scattered reports indicate detection of p47phox and p67phox in fibroblasts, endothelial cells, or mesangial cells by polymerase chain reaction (PCR) or immunochemical methods (206–208), these proteins have not yet been functionally implicated in these cells. In no case has a counterpart of gp91phox been identified in nonmyeloid cells. In fact, it has been argued that this cytochrome subunit in fibroblasts is genetically and immunochemically distinct from gp91phox, since fibroblasts of X-CGD patients exhibit a normal oxidative burst (209). In contrast, the two essential components of the phagocyte oxidase that are widely expressed have, in fact, been linked to redox signaling in other cell types. For example, antisense approaches suggest that p22phox participates in the oxidant-linked proliferation response to angiotensin II in vascular smooth muscle cells (202), and Rac and superoxide have been implicated in proliferation responses downstream of transforming Ras in fibroblasts (103). It will be interesting to know whether a p22phox deficiency in CGD offers any particular advantage against cardiovascular disease to those patients. The animal models of CGD should permit a direct examination of the roles of these phagocyte proteins in nonmyeloid cells.

In contrast to the animal kingdom, where high levels of NADPH oxidase activity are restricted to circulating phagocytes, most plants tissues possess an ability to mount an oxidative burst in response to pathogens or injury (210,211). Indeed, the familiar bruising of an apple can be viewed as a oxidative host defense reaction in response to traumatic injury, and it has been suggested that the hardening or lignification of tender shoots involves oxidative crosslinking of cell wall proteins and phenolics. What is most surprising about these processes in plants is that they involve an oxidase that is closely related to the neutrophil system. The closest structural homologue of gp91phox described to date was deduced from a cDNA cloned from rice (75). Furthermore, antibodies against neutrophil p47phox, p67phox, and p22phox detected proteins of the same molecular weights in various plant species (212–214). The analogy between plant and animal systems also extends to a variety of signaling systems that activate the oxidases in both kingdoms. Both systems respond to pathogen-derived elicitor molecules that bind membrane receptors linked to heterotrimeric G proteins, phospholipase C, inositol triphosphate, intracellular calcium transients, phosphorylation of intracellular proteins, and translocation of the cytosolic factors. Thus NADPH oxidase, once thought to be a unique component of the antimicrobial arsenal of circulating phagocytes, has been deeply rooted in oxygen-dependent host defense systems that have evolved before the divergence of plant and animal kingdoms.

REFERENCES

1. Rossi F. The O_2^-- forming NADPH oxidase of the phagocytes: nature, mechanisms of activation and function. *Biochim Biophys Acta* 1986; 853:65–89.
2. Babior BM, Kipnes RS, Curnutte JT. Biological defense mechanisms: the production by leukocytes of superoxide, a potential bactericidal agent. *J Clin Invest* 1973;52:741–744.
3. Holmes B, Page AR, Good RA. Studies of the metabolic activity of leukocytes from patients with a genetic abnormality in phagocyte function. *J Clin Invest* 1967;46:1422–1432.
4. Sbarra AJ, Karnovsky ML. The biochemical basis of phagocytosis. 1. Metabolic changes during phagocytosis of particles by polymorphonuclear leukocytes. *J Biol Chem* 1959;234:1355–1362.
5. Kitsis E, Weissmann G. The role of the neutrophil in rheumatoid arthritis. *Clin Orthop Rel Res* 1991;265:63–72.
6. Walder CE, Green SP, Darbonne WC, et al. Ischemic stroke injury is reduced in mice lacking a functional NADPH oxidase. *Stroke* 1997; 28:2252–2258.
7. Voncken JW, Van Schaick H, Kaatinen V, et al. Increased respiratory burst in bcr-null mutants. *Cell* 1995;70:401–410.
8. Boxer LA, Axtell R, Suchard S. The role of the neutrophil in inflammatory diseases of the lung. *Blood Cells* 1994;16:25–42.
9. Selvaraj RJ, Sbarra AJ. Relationship of glycolytic and oxidative metabolism to particle entry and destruction in phagocytosing cells. *Nature* 1966;211:1272–1276.
10. Quie PG, White JG, Holmes B, Good RA. *In vitro* bactericidal capacity of human polymorphonuclear leukocytes: diminished in chronic granulomatous disease of childhood. *J Clin Invest* 1967;46:668–679.
11. Malech HL, Gallin JI. Neutrophils in human diseases. *N Engl J Med* 1987;317:687–694.
12. Babior BM. Oxygen-dependent killing by phagocytes. *N Engl J Med* 1978;298:659–668.
13. Morel F, Doussiere J, Vignais PV. The superoxide-generating oxidase of phagocytic cells. Physiological, molecular and pathological aspects. *Eur J Biochem* 1991;201:523–546.
14. Thrasher AJ, Keep NH, Wientjes F, Segal AW. Chronic granulomatous disease. *Biochim Biophys Acta* 1994;1227:1–24.
15. Malech HL. Phagocyte oxidative mechanisms. *Curr Opin Hematol* 1993;1:123–132.
16. Roos D, de Boer M, Kuribayashi F, et al. Mutations in the X-linked and autosomal recessive forms of chronic granulomatous disease. *Blood* 1996;87:1663–1681.
17. Segal AW, Cross AR, Garcia RC. Absence of cytochrome b-245 in chronic granulomatous disease: a multicenter European evaluation of its incidence and relevance. *N Engl J Med* 1983;308:245–251.
18. Tehan C, Rowe P, Parker P, Totty N, Segal AW. The X-linked chronic granulomatous disease gene codes for the beta-chain of cytochrome b-245. *Nature* 1987;327:720–721.
19. Parkos CA, Allen RA, Cochrane CG, Jesaitis AJ. Purified cytochrome b from human granulocyte plasma membrane is comprised of two polypeptides with relative molecular weights of 91,000 and 22,000. *J Clin Invest* 1987;80:732–742.
20. Parkos CA, Dinauer MC, Jesaitis AJ, Orkin SH, Curnutte JT. Absence of both the 91kD and 22kD subunits of human neutrophil cytochrome b in two genetic forms of chronic granulomatous disease. *Blood* 1989; 73:1416–1420.
21. Segal, AW. Absence of both cytochrome b_{-245} subunits from neutrophils in X-linked granulomatous disease. *Nature* 1987;326:88–91.
22. Volpp BD, Nauseef WM, Clark RA. Two cytosolic neutrophil oxidase components absent in autosomal recessive chronic granulomatous disease. *Science* 1988;242:1295–1297.
23. Nunoi H, Rotrosen D, Gallin JI, Malech HL. Two forms of autosomal chronic granulomatous disease lack distinct neutrophil cytosol factors. *Science* 1988;242:1298–1301.
24. Curnutte JT, Scott PJ, Mayo LA. Cytosolic components of the respiratory burst oxidase: resolution of four components, two of which are missing in complementing types of chronic granulomatous disease. *Proc Natl Acad Sci USA* 1989;86:825–829.

25. Bolscher BG, van Zwieten R, Kramer IM, Weening RS, Verhoeven AJ, Roos D. A phosphoprotein of Mr 47,000, defective in autosomal chronic granulomatous disease, copurifies with one of two soluble components required for NADPH:O₂ oxidoreductase activity in human neutrophils. *J Clin Invest* 1989;83:757–763.

26. Heyneman RA, Vercauteren RE. Activation of a NADPH oxidase from horse polymorphonuclear leukocytes in a cell-free system. *J Leukoc Biol* 1984;36:751–759.

27. McPhail LC, Shirley PS, Clayton CC, Snyderman R. Activation of the respiratory burst enzyme from human neutrophils in a cell-free system. *J Clin Invest* 1985;75:1735–1739.

28. Curnutte JT. Activation of human neutrophil nicotinamide adenine dinucleotide phosphate, reduced (triphosphopyridine nucleotide, reduced) oxidase by arachidonic acid in a cell-free system. *J Clin Invest* 1985;75:1740–1743.

29. Bromberg Y, Pick E. Activation of NADPH-dependent superoxide production in a cell-free system by sodium dodecyl sulfate. *J Biol Chem* 1985;260:13539–13545.

30. Lomax KJ, Leto TL, Nunoi H, Gallin JI, Malech HL. Recombinant 47-kilodalton cytosol factor restores NADPH oxidase in chronic granulomatous disease. *Science* 1989;245:409–412.

31. Volpp BD, Nauseef WM, Donelson JE, Moser DR, Clark RA. Cloning of the cDNA and functional expression of the 47-kilodalton cytosolic component of human neutrophil respiratory burst oxidase. *Proc Natl Acad Sci USA* 1989;86:7195–7199.

32. Leto TL, Lomax KJ, Volpp BD, et al. Cloning of a 67K neutrophil oxidase factor with similarity to a noncatalytic region in p60c-Src. *Science* 1990;248:727–730.

33. Clark RA, Malech HL, Gallin JI, et al. Genetic variants of chronic granulomatous disease: prevalence of deficiencies of two cytosolic components of the NADPH oxidase system. *N Engl J Med* 1989;321:647–652.

34. Leto TL, Garrett MC, Fujii H, Nunoi H. Characterization of neutrophil NADPH oxidase factors p47-phox and p67-phox from recombinant baculoviruses. *J Biol Chem* 1991;266:19812–19818.

35. Segal AW, Heyworth PG, Cockcroft S, Barrowman MM. Stimulated neutrophils from patients with autosomal recessive chronic granulomatous disease fail to phosphorylate an Mr-44,000 protein. *Nature* 1985;316:547–549.

36. Caldwell SE, McCall CE, Hendricks CL, Leone PD, Bass DA, McPhail LC. Coregulation of NADPH oxidase activation and phosphorylation of a 48-kD protein by a cytosolic factor defective in autosomal recessive chronic granulomatous disease. *J Clin Invest* 1988; 81;1485–1496.

37. Okamura N, Curnutte JT, Roberts RL, Babior BM. Relationship of protein phosphorylation to the activation of the respiratory burst in human neutrophils. Defects in the phosphorylation of a group of closely related 48-kDa proteins in two forms of chronic granulomatous disease. *J Biol Chem* 1988;263:6777–6782.

38. Abo A, Pick E, Hall A, Totty N, Teahan CG, Segal AW. Activation of the NADPH oxidase involves the small GTP-binding protein p21rac1. *Nature* 1991;353:668–670.

39. Knaus UG, Heyworth PG, Evans T, Curnutte JT, Bokoch GM. Regulation of phagocyte oxygen radical production by the GTP-binding protein Rac 2. *Science* 1991;254(5037):1512–1515.

40. Mizuno T, Kaibuchi K, Ando S, et al. Regulation of the superoxide-generating NADPH oxidase by a small GTP-binding protein and its stimulatory and inhibitory GDP/GTP exchange proteins. *J Biol Chem* 1992;267:10215–10218.

41. Kwong CH, Rotrosen D, Malech HL, Leto TL. Regulation of the human neutrophil NADPH oxidase by rho-related G-proteins. *Biochemistry* 1993;32:5711–5717.

42. Rotrosen D, Yeung CL, Leto TL, Malech HL, Kwong CH. Cytochrome b558: the flavin-binding component of phagocyte NADPH oxidase. *Science* 1992;256:1459–1462.

43. Abo A, Boyhan A, West I, Thrasher AJ, Segal AW. Reconstitution of neutrophil NADPH oxidase activity in the cell-free system by four components: p67phox, p47phox, p21rac1, and cytochrome b₋₂₄₅. *J Biol Chem* 1992;269:22405–22411.

44. Dorseuil O, Quinn MT, Bokoch GM. Inhibition of superoxide production in B lymphocytes by rac antisense oligonucleotides. *J Biol Chem* 1992;267:20540–20542.

45. Gabig TG. Function of wild-type or mutant Rac2 and Rap1a GTPases in differentiated HL60 cell NADPH oxidase activation. *Blood* 1995; 85:804–811.

46. Royer-Pokora B, Kunkel LM, Monaco AP, et al. Cloning the gene for an inherited human disorder—chronic granulomatous disease—on the basis of its chromosomal location. *Nature* 1986;322:32–38.

47. Teahan C, Rowe P, Parker P, Totty N, Segal AW. The X-linked chronic granulomatous disease gene codes for the beta-chain of cytochrome b-245. *Nature* 1987;327:720–721.

48. Dinauer MC, Orkin SH, Brown R, Jesaitis AJ, Parkos CA. The glycoprotein encoded by the X-linked chronic granulomatous disease locus is a component of the neutrophil cytochrome b complex. *Nature* 1987; 327:717–720.

49. Wallach TM, Segal AW. Analysis of glycosylation sites on gp91phox, the flavocytochrome of the NADPH oxidase, by site-directed mutagenesis and translation *in vitro*. *Biochem J* 1997;321:583–585.

50. Imajoh-Ohmi S, Tokita K, Ochiai H, Nakamura M, Kanegasaki S. Topology of cytochrome b558 in neutrophil membrane analyzed by anti-peptide antibodies and proteolysis. *J Biol Chem* 1990;267: 180–184.

51. Leusen JHW, de Boer M, Bolscher BGJM, et al. A point mutation in gp91-phox of cytochrome b₅₅₈ of the human NADPH oxidase leading to defective translocation of the cytosolic proteins p47-phox and p67-phox. *J Clin Invest* 1994;93:2120–2126.

52. Rotrosen D, Kleinberg ME, Nunoi H, Leto TL, Gallin JI, Malech HL. Evidence for a functional cytoplasmic domain of phagocyte oxidase cytochrome b558. *J Biol Chem* 1990;265:8745–8750.

53. Nakanishi A, Imajoh-Ohmi S, Fujinawa T, Kikuchi H, Kanagegasaki S. Direct evidence for interaction between COOH-terminal regions of cytochrome b558 subunits and cytosolic 47-kDa protein during activation of an O₂⁻-generating system in neutrophils. *J Biol Chem* 1990; 267:19072–19074.

54. DeLeo FR, Yu L, Burritt JB, et al. Mapping sites of interaction of p47-phox and flavocytochrome b with random-sequence peptide phage display libraries. *Proc Natl Acad Sci USA* 1995;92:7110–7114.

55. Park MY, Imajoh-Ohmi S, Nunoi H, Kanegasaki S. Synthetic peptides corresponding to various hydrophilic regions of the large subunit of cytochrome b558 inhibit superoxide generation in a cell-free system from neutrophils. *Biochem Biophys Res Commun* 1997;234: 531–536.

56. Parkos CA, Dinauer MC, Walker LE, Allen RA, Jesaitis AJ, Orkin SH. Primary structure and unique expression of the 22-kilodalton light chain of human neutrophil cytochrome b. *Proc Natl Acad Sci USA* 1988;85:3319–3323.

57. Dinauer MC, Pierce EA, Bruns GA, Curnutte JT, Orkin SH. Human neutrophil cytochrome b light chain (p22phox). Gene structure, chromosome location and mutations in cytochrome-negative autosomal recessive chronic granulomatous disease. *J Clin Invest* 1990;86: 1729–1737.

58. Leto TL, Adams AG, de Mendez I. Assembly of the phagocyte NADPH oxidase: binding of Src homology 3 domains to proline-rich targets. *Proc Natl Acad Sci USA* 1994;91:10650–10654.

59. Sumimoto H, Kage Y, Nunoi H, et al. Role of Src homology 3 domains in assembly and activation of the phagocyte NADPH oxidase. *Proc Natl Acad Sci USA* 1994;91:5345–5349.

60. Leusen JHW, Bolscher BGJM, Hilarius PM, et al. 156Pro→Gln substitution in the light chain of cytochrome b₅₅₈ of the human NADPH oxidase (p22-phox) leads to defective translocation of the cytosolic proteins p47-phox and p67-phox. *J Exp Med* 1994;180:2329–2334.

61. Segal AW, West I, Wientjes F, et al. Cytochrome b-245 is a flavocytochrome containing FAD and the NADPH-binding site of the microbicidal oxidase of phagocytes. *Biochem J* 1992;284:781–788.

62. Taylor WR, Jones DT, Segal AW. A structural model for the nucleotide binding domains of the flavocytochrome b-245 beta-chain. *Protein Sci* 1993;2:1675–1685.

63. Sumimoto H, Sakamoto N, Nozaki M, Sakaki Y, Takeshige K, Minakami S. Cytochrome b558, a component of the phagocyte NADPH oxidase, is a flavoprotein. *Biochem Biophys Res Commun* 1992;186:1368–1375.

64. Koshkin V, Pick E. Generation of superoxide by purified and relipidated cytochrome b559 in the absence of cytosolic activators. *FEBS Lett* 1993;327:57–62.

65. Doussiere J, Buzenet G, Vignais PV. Photoaffinity labeling and photoinactivation of the O₂-generating oxidase of neutrophils by an azido derivative of FAD. *Biochemistry* 1995;34:1760–1770.

66. Ravel P, Lederer F. Affinity-labeling of an NADPH-binding site on the heavy subunit of flavocytochrome b558 in particulate NADPH oxi-

dase from activated human neutrophils. *Biochem Biophys Res Commun* 1993;196:543–552.

67. Nisimoto Y, Otsuka-Murakami H, Lambeth DJ. Reconstitution of flavin-depleted neutrophil flavocytochrome b558 with 8-mercapto-FAD and characterization of the flavin-reconstituted enzyme. *J Biol Chem* 1995;270:16428–16434.

68. Umei T, Babior BM, Curnutte JT, Smith RM. Identification of the NADPH-binding subunit of the respiratory burst oxidase. *J Biol Chem* 1991;266:6019–6022.

69. Yea CM, Cross AR, Jones OT. Purification and some properties of the 45 kDA diphenylene iodonium-binding flavoprotein of neutrophil NADPH oxidase. *Biochem J* 1990;265:95–100.

70. Smith RM, Curnutte JT, Mayo LA, Babior BM. Use of an affinity label to probe the function of the NADPH binding component of the respiratory burst oxidase of human neutrophils. *J Biol Chem* 1989; 264:12243–12248.

71. Cross AR, Curnutte JT. The cytosolic activating factors p47phox and p67phox have distinct roles in the regulation of electron flow in NADPH oxidase. *J Biol Chem* 1994;270:26543–26548.

72. Cross AR, Heyworth PG, Rae J, Curnutte JT. A variant X-linked chronic granulomatous disease patient (X91+) with partially functional cytochrome b. *J Biol Chem* 1995;270:8194–8200.

73. Cross AR, Rae J, Curnutte JT. Cytochrome b-245 of the neutrophil superoxide-generating system contains two nonidentical hemes. Potentiometric studies of a mutant form of gp91phox. *J Biol Chem* 1995;270:17075– 17077.

74. Dancis A, Roman DG, Anderson GJ, Hinnebusch AG, Klausner RD. Ferric reductase of *Saccharomyces cerevisiae:* molecular characterization, role in iron uptake, and transcriptional control by iron. *Proc Natl Acad Sci USA* 1992;89:3869–3873.

75. Groom QJ, Torres MA, Fordham-Skelton AP, Hammond-Kosack KE, Robinson NJ, Jones JD. rbohA, a rice homologue of the mammalian gp91phox respiratory burst oxidase gene. *Plant J* 1996;10: 515–522.

76. Nugent JHA, Gratzer W, Segal AW. Identification of the heme-binding subunit of cytochrome b-245. *Biochem J* 1989;264:921–924.

77. Quinn MT, Mullen ML, Jesaitis AJ. Human neutrophil cytochrome b contains multiple hemes. Evidence for heme associated with both subunits. *J Biol Chem* 1992;267:7303–7309.

78. Shatwell KP, Dancis A, Cross AR, Klausner RD, Segal AW. The FRE1 ferric reductase of *Saccharomyces cerevisiae* is a cytochrome b similar to that of NADPH oxidase. *J Biol Chem* 1996;271: 14240–14244.

79. Finegold AA, Shatwell KP, Segal AW, Klausner RD, Dancis A. Intramembrane bis-heme motif for transmembrane electron transport conserved in a yeast iron reductase and the human NADPH oxidase. *J Biol Chem* 1996;271:31021–31024.

80. Hurst JK, Loehr TM, Curnutte JT, Rosen H. Resonance Raman and electron paramagnetic resonance structural investigations of neutrophil cytochrome b558. *J Biol Chem* 1991;266:1627–1634.

81. Isogai Y, Iizuka T, Makino R, Iyanagi T, Orii Y. Superoxide-producing cytochrome b. Enzymatic and electron paramagnetic resonance properties of cytochrome b558 purified from neutrophils. *J Biol Chem* 1993;268:4025–4031.

82. Fujii H, Johnson MK, Finnegan MG, Miki T, Yoshida LS, Kakinuma K. Electron spin resonance studies on neutrophil cytochrome b558. Evidence that low-spin heme iron is essential for O2-generating activity. *J Biol Chem* 1995;270:12685–12689.

83. Doussiere J, Gaillard J, Vignais PV. Electron transfer across the O2-generating flavocytochrome b of neutrophils. Evidence for a transition from a low-spin state to a high-spin state of the heme iron component. *Biochemistry* 1996;35:13400–13410.

84. Koshkin V, Pick E. Superoxide production by cytochrome b559. Mechanism of cytosol-independent activation. *FEBS Lett* 1994;338: 285–289.

85. Erickson RW, Malawista SE, Garrett MC, Van Blaricom G, Leto TL, Curnutte JT. Identification of a thermolabile component of the human neutrophil NADPH oxidase. A model for chronic granulomatous disease caused by deficiency of the p67-phox cytosolic component. *J Clin Invest* 1992;89:1587–1595.

86. Pawson T. Protein modules and signalling networks. *Nature* 1995;373: 573–580.

87. Cohen GB, Ren R, Baltimore D. Modular binding domains in signal transduction proteins. *Cell* 1995;80:237–248.

88. Musacchio A, Wilmanns M, Saraste M. Structure and function of the SH3 domain. *Prog Biophys Mol Biol* 1994;61:283–297.

89. Leto TL. The p67phox NADPH oxidase component is composed of several tetratricopeptide repeats that are affected in a rare form of chronic granulomatous disease. *FASEB J* 1996;10:1262A.

90. Ponting CP. Novel domains in NADPH oxidase subunits, sorting nexins, and PtdIns 3-kinases: binding partners of SH3 domains? *Protein Sci* 1996;5:2353–2357.

91. Goebl M, Yanagida M. The TPR snap helix: a novel protein repeat motif from mitosis to transcription. *Trends Biochem Sci* 1991;16: 173–177.

92. Lamb JR, Tugendreich S, Hieter P. Tetratrico peptide repeat interactions: to TPR or not to TPR? *Trends Biochem Sci* 1995;20:257–259.

93. de Mendez I, Garret MC, Adams AG, Leto TL. Role of p67-phox SH3 domains in assembly of the NADPH oxidase system. *J Biol Chem* 1994;269:16326–16332.

94. Diekmann D, Abo A, Johnston C, Segal AW, Hall A. Interaction of Rac with p67phox and regulation of the phagocytic NADPH oxidase activity. *Science* 1994;265:531–533.

95. Hirano T, Kinoshita N, Morikawa K, Yanagida M. Snap helix with knob and hole: essential repeats in S. pombe nuclear protein nuc2+. *Cell* 1990;60:319–328.

96. Sikorski RS, Boguski MS, Goebl M, Hieter P. A repeating amino acid motif in CDC23 defines a family of proteins and a new relationship among genes required for mitosis and RNA synthesis. *Cell* 1990;60: 307–317.

97. de Boer M, Hilarius-Stokman PM, Hossle JP, et al. Autosomal recessive chronic granulomatous disease with absence of the 67-kD cytosolic NADPH oxidase component: identification of mutation and detection of carriers. *Blood* 1994;83:531–536.

98. Leusen JH, de Klein A, Hilarius PM, et al. Disturbed interaction of p21-rac with mutated p67-phox causes chronic granulomatous disease. *J Exp Med* 1996;184:1243–1249.

99. Burbelo PD, Drechsel D, Hall A. A conserved binding motif defines numerous candidate target proteins for both Cdc42 and Rac GTPases. *J Biol Chem* 1995;270:29071–29074.

100. Nobes CD, Hall A. Rho, rac, and cdc42 GTPases regulate the assembly of multimolecular focal complexes associated with actin stress fibers, lamellipodia, and filopodia. *Cell* 1995;81:53–62.

101. Manser E, Leung T, Salihuddin H, Zhao ZS, Lim L. A brain serine/threonine protein kinase activated by Cdc42 and Rac1. *Nature* 1994; 367:40–46.

102. Peppelenbosch MP, Qiu RG, de Vries-Smits AM, et al. Rac mediates growth factor-induced arachidonic acid release. *Cell* 1995;81: 849–856.

103. Irani K, Xia Y, Zweier JL, et al. Mitogenic signaling mediated by oxidants in Ras-transformed fibroblasts. *Science* 1997;275:1649–1652.

104. Kwong CH, Adams AG, Leto TL. Characterization of the effector-specifying domain of Rac involved in NADPH oxidase activation. *J Biol Chem* 1995;270:19868–19872.

105. Kreck ML, Uhlinger DJ, Tyagi SR, Inge KL, Lambeth JD. Participation of the small molecular weight GTP-binding protein Rac1 in cell-free activation and assembly of the respiratory burst oxidase. *J Biol Chem* 1994;269:4161–4168.

106. Freeman JL, Abo A, Lambeth JD. Rac "insert region" is a novel effector region that is implicated in the activation of NADPH oxidase, but not PAK65. *J Biol Chem* 1996;271:19794–19801.

107. Diekmann D, Nobes CD, Burbelo PD, Abo A, Hall A. Rac GTPase interacts with GAPs and target proteins through multiple effector sites. *EMBO J* 1995;14:5297–5305.

108. Nisimoto Y, Freeman JLR, Motalebi SA, Hirshberg M, Lambeth JD. Rac binding to p67(phox). Structural basis for interactions of the rac1 effector region and insert region with components of the respiratory burst oxidase. *J Biol Chem* 1997;272:18834–18841.

109. Xu X, Barry DC, Settleman J, Schwartz MA, Bokoch GM. Differing structural requirements for GTPase-activating protein responsiveness and NADPH oxidase activation by Rac. *J Biol Chem* 1994;269: 23569– 23574.

110. Milburn MV, Tong L, deVos AM, et al. Molecular switch for signal transduction: structural differences between active and inactive forms of protooncogenic ras proteins. *Science* 1990;247:939–945.

111. Hirshberg M, Stockley RW, Dodson G, Webb MR. The crystal structure of human rac1, a member of the rho- family complexed with a GTP analogue. *Nat Struct Biol* 1997;4:147–152.

112. Joseph G, Pick E. "Peptide walking" is a novel method for mapping functional domains in proteins. Its application to the Rac1-dependent activation of NADPH oxidase. *J Biol Chem* 1995;270:29079–29082.

113. McPhail LC, Strum SL, Leone PA, Sozzani S. The neutrophil respiratory burst mechanism. *Immunol Ser* 1992;57:47–76.

114. Thelen M, Dewald B, Baggiolini M. Neutrophil signal transduction and activation of the respiratory burst. *Physiol Rev* 1993;73:797–821.

115. Heyworth PG, Badwey JA. Protein phosphorylation associated with the stimulation of neutrophils. Modulation of superoxide production by protein kinase C and calcium. *J Bioenerg Biomembr* 1990;22:1–26.

116. Olson SC, Lambeth JD. Biochemistry and cell biology of phospholipase D in human neutrophils. *Chem Phys Lipids* 1996;80:3–19.

117. Henderson LM, Chappell JB, Jones OT. Superoxide generation is inhibited by phospholipase A2 inhibitors. Role for phospholipase A2 in the activation of the NADPH oxidase. *Biochem J* 1989;26:249–255.

118. Dana R, Malech HL, Levy R. The requirement for phospholipase A2 for activation of the assembled NADPH oxidase in human neutrophils. *Biochem J* 1994;297:217–223.

119. Rotrosen D, Leto TL. Phosphorylation of neutrophil 47-kDa cytosolic oxidase factor. Translocation to membrane is associated with distinct phosphorylation events. *J Biol Chem* 1990;265:19910–19915.

120. El Benna J, Faust LRP, Babior BM. The phosphorylation of the respiratory burst oxidase component p47[phox] during neutrophil activation. *J Biol Chem* 1994;269:23431–23436.

121. Lu DJ, Takai A, Leto TL, Grinstein S. Modulation of neutrophil activation by okadaic acid, a protein phosphatase inhibitor. *Am J Physiol* 1992;262:C39–C49.

122. Levy R, Dana R, Leto T, Malech HL. The requirement of p47phox phosphorylation for NADPH oxidase activation by opsonized zymosan in human neutrophils. *Biochim Biophys Acta* 1994;1220:253–260.

123. Fuchs A, Bouin AP, Rabilloud T, Vignais PV. The 40-kDa component of the phagocyte NADPH oxidase (p40phox) is phosphorylated during activation in differentiated HL60 cells. *Eur J Biochem* 1997;249:531–539.

124. Faust LR, el Benna J, Babior BM, Chanock SJ. The phosphorylation targets of p47phox, a subunit of the respiratory burst oxidase. Functions of the individual target serines as evaluated by site-directed mutagenesis. *J Clin Invest* 1995;96:1499–1505.

125. Dusi S, Rossi F. Activation of NADPH oxidase of human neutrophils involves the phosphorylation and the translocation of cytosolic p67phox. *Biochem J* 1993;296:367–371.

126. El Benna J, Dang PM, Gaudry M, et al. Phosphorylation of the respiratory burst oxidase subunit p67(phox) during human neutrophil activation. Regulation by protein kinase C-dependent and independent pathways. *J Biol Chem* 1997;272:17204–17208.

127. Garcia RC, Segal AW. Phosphorylation of the subunits of cytochrome b-245 upon triggering of the respiratory burst of human neutrophils and macrophages. *Biochem J* 1988;252:901–904.

128. Heyworth PG, Curnutte JT, Nauseef WM, et al. Neutrophil nicotinamide adenine dinucleotide phosphate oxidase assembly. Translocation of p47-phox and p67-phox requires interaction between p47-phox and cytochrome b558. *J Clin Invest* 1991;87:352–356.

129. Heyworth PG, Bohl BP, Bokoch GM, Curnutte JT. Rac translocates independently of the neutrophil NADPH oxidase components p47phox and p67phox. Evidence for its interaction with flavocytochrome b558. *J Biol Chem* 1994;269:30749–30752.

130. Dusi S, Donini M, Rossi F. Mechanisms of NADPH oxidase activation: translocation of p40phox, Rac1 and Rac2 from the cytosol to the membranes in human neutrophils lacking p47phox or p67phox. *Biochem J* 1996;314:409–412.

131. Dorseuil O, Quinn MT, Bokoch GM. Dissociation of Rac translocation from p47phox/p67phox movements in human neutrophils by tyrosine kinase inhibitors. *J Leukoc Biol* 1995;58:108–113.

132. Quinn MT, Evans T, Loetterle LR, Jesaitis AJ, Bokoch GM. Translocation of Rac correlates with NADPH oxidase activation. Evidence for equimolar translocation of oxidase components. *J Biol Chem* 1993;268:20983–20987.

133. Borregaard N, Heiple JM, Simons ER, Clark RA. Subcellular localization of the b-cytochrome component of the human neutrophil microbicidal oxidase: translocation during activation. *J Cell Biol* 1983;97:52–61.

134. Jesaitis AJ, Buescher ES, Harrison D, et al. Ultrastructural localization of cytochrome b in the membranes of resting and phagocytosing human granulocytes. *J Clin Invest* 1990;85:821–835.

135. Wientjes FB, Segal AW, Hartwig JH. Immunoelectron microscopy shows a clustered distribution of NADPH oxidase components in the human neutrophil plasma membrane. *J Leukoc Biol* 1997;61:303–312.

136. Dana R, Leto TL, Malech HL, Levy R. Essential role of cytosolic phospholipase A2 for activation of the phagocyte NADPH oxidase. *J Biol Chem* 1998;273:441–445.

137. Pozzan T, Lew DP, Wollheim CB, Tsein RY. Is cytosolic calcium regulating neutrophil activation? *Science* 1983;221:1413–1415.

138. Henderson LM, Thomas S, Banting G, Chappell JB. The arachidonate-activatable, NADPH oxidase-associated H+ channel is contained within the multi-membrane-spanning N-terminal region of gp91-phox. *Biochem J* 1997;325:701–705.

139. Chiba T, Kaneda M, Fujii H, Carrk RA, Nauseef WM, Kakinuma K. Two cytosolic components of the neutrophil NADPH oxidase, P47-phox and P67-phox, are not flavoproteins. *Biochem Biophys Res Commun* 1993;173:376–381.

140. Tyagi SR, Neckelmann N, Uhlinger DJ, Burnham DN, Lambeth JD. Cell-free translocation of recombinant p47-phox, a component of the neutrophil NADPH oxidase: effects of guanosine 5′-O-(3-thiotriphosphate), diacylglycerol, and an anionic amphiphile. *Biochemistry* 1992;31:2765–2774.

141. Chuang TH, Bohl BP, Bokoch GM. Biologically active lipids are regulators of Rac.GDI complexation. *J Biol Chem* 1993;268:26206–26211.

142. Park JW, Babior BM. Activation of the leukocyte NADPH oxidase subunit p47phox by protein kinase C. A phosphorylation-dependent change in the conformation of the C-terminal end of p47phox. *Biochemistry* 1997;36:7474–7480.

143. Park JW, Hoyal CR, Benna JE, Babior BM. Kinase-dependent activation of the leukocyte NADPH oxidase in a cell-free system. Phosphorylation of membranes and p47(PHOX) during oxidase activation. *J Biol Chem* 1997;272:11035–11043.

144. Cox JA, Jeng AY, Sharkey NA, Blumberg PM, Tauber AI. Activation of the human neutrophil nicotinamide adenine dinucleotide phosphate (NADPH)-oxidase by protein kinase C. *J Clin Invest* 1985;76:1932–1938.

145. Waite KA, Wallin R, Qualliotine-Mann D, McPhail LC. Phosphatidic acid-mediated phosphorylation of the NADPH oxidase component p47-phox. Evidence that phosphatidic acid may activate a novel protein kinase. *J Biol Chem* 1997;272:15569–15578.

146. Knaus UG, Morris S, Dong HJ, Chernoff J, Bokoch GM. Regulation of human leukocyte p21-activated kinases through G protein–coupled receptors. *Science* 1995;269:221–223.

147. de Mendez, Abo A, Leto TL. Down-regulation of a phagocyte host defense system, the NADPH oxidase, by PAK2. *Mol Biol Cell* 1997;8:133a.

148. Nauseef WM, McCormick S, Renee J, Leidal KG, Clark RA. Functional domain in an arginine-rich carboxyl-terminal region of p47phox. *J Biol Chem* 1993;268:23646–23651.

149. Peveri P, Heyworth PG, Curnutte JT. Absolute requirement for GTP in activation of human neutrophil NADPH oxidase in a cell-free system: role of ATP in regenerating GTP. *Proc Natl Acad Sci USA* 1992;89:2494–2498.

150. Park JW, Ma M, Ruedi JM, Smith RM, Babior BM. The cytosolic components of the respiratory burst oxidase exist as a M(r) approximately 240,000 complex that acquires a membrane-binding site during activation of the oxidase in a cell-free system. *J Biol Chem* 1992;267:17327–17332.

151. Iyer SS, Pearson DW, Nauseef WM, Clark RA. Evidence for a readily dissociable complex of p47phox and p67phox in cytosol of unstimulated human neutrophils. *J Biol Chem* 1994;269:22405–22411.

152. Someya A, Nagaoka I, Yamashita T. Purification of the 260 kDa cytosolic complex involved in the superoxide production of guinea pig neutrophils. *FEBS Lett* 1993;330:215–218.

153. Kleinberg ME, Malech HL, Mital DA, Leto TL. p21rac does not participate in the early interaction between p47-phox and cytochrome b558 that leads to phagocyte NADPH oxidase activation *in vitro*. *Biochemistry* 1994;33:2490–2495.

154. de Mendez I, Adams AG, Sokolic RA, Malech HL, Leto TL. Multiple SH3 domain interactions regulate NADPH oxidase assembly in whole cells. *EMBO J* 1996;15:1211–1220.

155. de Mendez I, Homayounpour N, Leto TL. Specificity of p47phox SH3

domain interactions in NADPH oxidase assembly and activation. *Mol Cell Biol* 1997;17:2177–2185.

156. Abo A, Webb MR, Grogan A, Segal AW. Activation of NADPH oxidase involves the dissociation of p21rac from its inhibitory GDP/GTP exchange protein (rhoGDI) followed by its translocation to the plasma membrane. *Biochem J* 1994;298:585–591.

157. McPhail LC. SH3-dependent assembly of the phagocyte NADPH oxidase. *J Exp Med* 1994;180:2011–2015.

158. Finan P, Shimizu Y, Gout I, et al. An SH3 domain and proline-rich sequence mediate an interaction between two components of the phagocyte NADPH oxidase complex. *J Biol Chem* 1994;269:13752–13755.

159. Sumimoto H, Hata K, Mizuki K, et al. Assembly and activation of the phagocyte NADPH oxidase. Specific interaction of the N-terminal Src homology 3 domain of p47phox with p22phox is required for activation of the NADPH oxidase. *J Biol Chem* 1996;271:22152–22158.

160. Leusen JHW, Fluiter K, Hilarius PM, Verhoeven AJ, Bolscher BJM. Interactions between the cytosolic components p47-phox and p67-phox of human NADPH oxidase not required for activation in the cell. *J Biol Chem* 1994;270:11216–11221.

161. Finan P, Ka H, Zvelebil MJ, Waterfield MD, Kellie S. The C-terminal SH3 domain of p67phox binds its natural ligand in a reverse orientation. *J Mol Biol* 1996;261:173–180.

162. Leto TL, Adams AG, de Mendez I. Activation and assembly of NADPH oxidase: role of the tail-tail interaction between cytosolic components p47-phox and p67-phox. *Mol Biol Cell* 1995;6:241a.

163. Sathyamoorthy M, de Mendez I, Adams AG, Leto TL. p40(phox) down-regulates NADPH oxidase activity through interactions with its SH3 domain. *J Biol Chem* 1997;272:9141–9146.

164. Fuchs A, Dagher MC, Faure J, Vignais PV. Topological organization of the cytosolic activating complex of the superoxide-generating NADPH-oxidase. Pinpointing the sites of interaction between p47phox, p67phox and p40phox using the two-hybrid system. *Biochim Biophys Acta* 1996;1312:39–47.

165. Fuchs A, Dagher MC, Vignais PV. Mapping the domains of interaction of p40phox with both p47phox and p67phox of the neutrophil oxidase complex using the two-hybrid system. *J Biol Chem* 1995;270:5695–5697.

166. Ito T, Nakamura R, Sumimoto H, Takeshige K, Sakaki Y. An SH3 domain-mediated interaction between the phagocyte NADPH oxidase factors p40phox and p47phox. *FEBS Lett* 1996;385:229–232.

167. Dinauer MC, Pierce EA, Erickson RW, et al. Point mutation in the cytoplasmic domain of the neutrophil p22-phox cytochrome b subunit is associated with a nonfunctional NADPH oxidase and chronic granulomatous disease. *Proc Natl Acad Sci USA* 1991;88:11231–11235.

168. Koshkin V, Pick E. The cytosolic component p47(phox) is not a sine qua non participant in the activation of NADPH oxidase but is required for optimal superoxide production. *J Biol Chem* 1996;271:30326–30329.

169. Freeman JL, Lambeth JD. NADPH oxidase activity is independent of p47phox *in vitro*. *J Biol Chem* 1996;271:22578–22582.

170. Sicheri F, Moarefi I, Kuriyan J. Crystal structure of the Src family tyrosine kinase Hck. *Nature* 1997;385:602–609.

171. Xu W, Harrison SC, Eck MJ. Three-dimensional structure of the tyrosine kinase c-Src. *Nature* 1997;385:595–602.

172. Wientjes FB, Hsuan JJ, Totty NF, Segal AW. p40phox, a third cytosolic component of the activation complex of the NADPH oxidase to contain src homology 3 domains. *Biochem J* 1993;296:557–561.

173. Tsunawaki S, Mizunari H, Nagata M, Tatsuzawa O, Kuratsuji T. A novel cytosolic component, p40phox, of respiratory burst oxidase associates with p67phox and is absent in patients with chronic granulomatous disease who lack p67phox. *Biochem Biophys Res Commun* 1994;199:1378–1387.

174. Lim WA, Richards FM, Fox RO. Structural determinants of peptide-binding orientation and of sequence specificity in SH3 domains. *Nature* 1994;372:375–379.

175. Feng S, Chen JK, Yu H, Simon JA, Schreiber SL. Two binding orientations for peptides to the Src SH3 domain: development of a general model for SH3-ligand interactions. *Science* 1994;266:1241–1247.

176. Saraste M, Musacchio A. Backwards and forwards binding. *Nat Struct Biol* 1994;1:835–837.

177. DeLeo FR, Nauseef WM, Jesaitis AJ, Burritt JB, Clark RA, Quinn MT. A domain of p47phox that interacts with human neutrophil flavocytochrome b558. *J Biol Chem* 1995;270:26246–26251.

178. De Leo FR. Assembly of the human neutrophil NADPH oxidase involves binding of p67phox and flavocytochrome b to common functional domain in p47phox. *J Biol Chem* 1996;271:17013–17020.

179. Kleinberg ME, Mital D, Rotrosen D, Malech HL. Characterization of a phagocyte cytochrome b558 91-kilodalton subunit functional domain: identification of peptide sequence and amino acids essential for activity. *Biochemistry* 1992;31:2686–2690.

180. Adams ER, Dratz EA, Gizachew D, et al. Interaction of human neutrophil flavocytochrome b with cytosolic proteins: transferred-NOESY NMR studies of a gp91phox C-terminal peptide bound to p47phox. *Biochem J* 1997;325:249–257.

181. Joseph G, Gorzalczany Y, Koskin V, Pick E. Inhibition of NADPH oxidase activation by synthetic peptides mapping within the carboxyl-terminal domain of small GTP-binding proteins. Lack of amino acid sequence specificity and importance of polybasic motif. *J Biol Chem* 1994;269:29024–29031.

182. Tisch D, Sharoni Y, Danilenko M, Aviram I. The assembly of neutrophil NADPH oxidase: effects of mastoparan and its synthetic analogues. *Biochem J* 1995;310:715–719.

183. Shi J, Ross CR, Leto TL, Blecha F. PR-39, a proline-rich antibacterial peptide that inhibits phagocyte NADPH oxidase activity by binding to Src homology 3 domains of p47 phox. *Proc Natl Acad Sci USA* 1996;93:6014–6018.

184. Quinn MT, Parkos CA, Walker L, Orkin SH, Dinauer MC, Jesaitis AJ. Association of a Ras-related protein with cytochrome b of human neutrophils. *Nature* 1989;342:198–200.

185. Maly FE, Quilliam LA, Dorseuil O, Der CJ, Bokoch GM. Activated or dominant inhibitory mutants of Rap1A decrease the oxidative burst of Epstein-Barr virus-transformed human B lymphocytes. *J Biol Chem* 1994;269:18743–18746.

186. Bokoch GM, Quilliam LA, Bohl BP, Jesaitis AJ, Quinn MT. Inhibition of Rap1A binding to cytochrome b558 of NADPH oxidase by phosphorylation of Rap1A. *Science* 1991;254:1794–1796.

187. Mueller H, Weingarten R, Ransnas LA, Bokoch GM, Sklar LA. Differential amplification of antagonistic receptor pathways in neutrophils. *J Biol Chem* 1991;266:12939–12943.

188. Nauseef WM, Volpp BD, McCormick S, Leidal KS, Clark RA. Assembly of the neutrophil respiratory burst oxidase. Protein kinase C promotes cytoskeletal and membrane association of cytosolic oxidase components. *J Biol Chem* 1991;266:5911–5917.

189. Woodman RC, Ruedi JM, Jesaitis AJ, et al. Respiratory burst oxidase and three of four oxidase-related polypeptides are associated with the cytoskeleton of human neutrophils. *J Clin Invest* 1991;87:1345–1351.

190. Lehmeyer JE, Snyderman R, Johnston RB Jr. Stimulation of neutrophil oxidative metabolism by chemotactic peptides: influence of calcium ion concentration and cytochalasin B and comparison with stimulation by phorbol myristate acetate. *Blood* 1979;54:35–45.

191. Lukacs GL, Kapus A, Nanda A, Romanek R, Grinstein S. Proton conductance of the plasma membrane: properties, regulation, and functional role. *Am J Physiol* 1993;265:C3–C14.

192. Akard LP, English D, Gabig TG. Rapid deactivation of NADPH oxidase in neutrophils: continuous replacement by newly activated enzyme sustains the respiratory burst. *Blood* 1988;72:322–327.

193. Tamura M, Takeshita M, Curnutte JT, Uhlinger DJ, Lambeth JD. Stabilization of human neutrophil NADPH oxidase activated in a cell-free system by cytosolic proteins and by 1-ethyl-3-(3-dimethylaminopropyl) carbodiimide. *J Biol Chem* 1992;267:7529–7538.

194. Malech HL, Bauer TR Jr, Hickstein DD. Prospects for gene therapy of neutrophil defects. *Semin Hematol* 1997;34:355–361.

195. Jackson SH, Gallin JI, Holland SM. The p47phox mouse knock-out model of chronic granulomatous disease. *J Exp Med* 1995;182:751–758.

196. Pollock JD, Williams DA, Gifford MA, et al. Mouse model of X-linked chronic granulomatous disease, an inherited defect in phagocyte superoxide production. *Nat Genet* 1995;9:202–209.

197. Ding C, Kume A, Bjorgvinsdottir H, Hawley RG, Pech N, Dinauer MC. High-level reconstitution of respiratory burst activity in a human X-linked chronic granulomatous disease (X-CGD) cell line and correction of murine X-CGD bone marrow cells by retroviral-mediated gene transfer of human gp91phox. *Blood* 1996;88:1834–1840.

198. de Mendez I, Leto TL. Functional reconstitution of the phagocyte NADPH oxidase by transfection of its multiple components in a heterologous system. *Blood* 1995;85:1104–1110.

199. Mardiney M, Jackson SJ, Spratt SK, Li F, Holland SM, Malech HL.

Enhanced host defense after gene transfer in the murine p47phox-deficient model of chronic granulomatous disease. *Blood* 1997;89: 2268–2275.

200. Bjorgvinsdottir H, Ding C, Pech N, Gifford MA, Li LL, Dinauer MC. Retroviral-mediated gene transfer of gp91phox into bone marrow cells rescues defect in host defense against Aspergillus fumigatus in murine X-linked chronic granulomatous disease. *Blood* 1997;89: 41–48.

201. Malech HL, Maples PB, Whiting-Theobald N, et al. Prolonged production of NADPH oxidase-corrected granulocytes after gene therapy of chronic granulomatous disease. *Proc Natl Acad Sci USA* 1997;94: 12133– 12138.

202. Ushio-Fukai M, Zafari AM, Fukui T, Ishizaka N, Griendling KK. p22phox is a critical component of the superoxide-generating NADH/NADPH oxidase system and regulates angiotensin II-induced hypertrophy in vascular smooth muscle cells. *J Biol Chem* 1996;271: 23317–23321.

203. Kane DJ, Sarafian TA, Anton R, et al. Bcl-2 inhibition of neural death: decreased generation of reactive oxygen species. *Science* 1993;262: 1274–1277.

204. Fialkow L, Chan CK, Grinstein S, Downey GP. Regulation of tyrosine phosphorylation in neutrophils by the NADPH oxidase. Role of reactive oxygen intermediates. *J Biol Chem* 1993;268:17131–17137.

205. Baeuerle PA, Henkel T. Function and activation of NF-kappa B in the immune system. *Annu Rev Immunol* 1994;12:141–179.

206. Jones SA, Wood JD, Coffey MJ, Jones OT. The functional expression of p47-phox and p67-phox may contribute to the generation of super-oxide by an NADPH oxidase-like system in human fibroblasts. *FEBS Lett* 1994;355:178–182.

207. Jones SA, Hancock JT, Jones OT, Neubauer A, Topley N. The expression of NADPH oxidase components in human glomerular mesangial cells: detection of protein and mRNA for p47phox, p67phox, and p22phox. *J Am Soc Nephrol* 1995;5:1483–1491.

208. Jones SA, O'Donnell VB, Wood JD, Broughton JP, Hughes EJ, Jones OT. Expression of phagocyte NADPH oxidase components in human endothelial cells. *Am J Physiol* 1996;271:H1626–H1634.

209. Meier B, Jesaitis AJ, Emmendorffer A, Roesler J, Quinn MT. The cytochrome b-558 molecules involved in the fibroblast and polymorphonuclear leukocyte superoxide-generating NADPH oxidase systems are structurally and genetically distinct. *Biochem J* 1993;289: 481–486.

210. Wojtaszek P. Oxidative burst: an early plant response to pathogen infection. *Biochemical J* 1997;322:681–692.

211. Shirasu K, Dixon RA, Lamb C. Signal transduction in plant immunity. *Curr Opin Immunol* 1996;8:3–7.

212. Dwyer S, Legrendre L, Heinstein PF, Low PS, Leto TL. Plant and human neutrophil oxidative burst complexes contain immunologically related proteins. *Biochim Biophys Acta* 1996;1289:231–237.

213. Tenhaken R, Levine A, Brisson LF, Dixon RA, Lamb C. Function of the oxidative burst in hypersensitive disease resistance. *Proc Natl Acad Sci USA* 1995;92:4158–4163.

214. Xing T. Race-specific elicitors of *Cladosporium fulvum* promote translocation of cytosolic components of NADPH oxidase to the plasma membrane of tomato cells. *Plant Cell* 1997;9:249–259.

Inflammation: Basic Principles and Clinical Correlates,
3rd ed., edited by John I. Gallin and Ralph Snyderman.
Lippincott Williams & Wilkins, Philadelphia © 1999.

CHAPTER 49

Nitric Oxide as a Factor in Inflammation

Eeva Moilanen, Brendan Whittle, and Salvador Moncada

The biologic actions of nitric oxide (NO) can be divided into two main categories, those involving physiologic regulation and those contributing to pathologic processes. NO acts as a labile intercellular messenger molecule regulating a range of physiologic functions including vascular tone, platelet aggregation, the immune response, and neurotransmission in the brain as well as in the periphery in the so-called NANC (nonadrenergic, noncholinergic) nerves (1). In addition, NO synthesized in high amounts by activated inflammatory cells possesses cytotoxic properties implicated in the ability of these cells to kill bacteria, viruses and protozoa as well as tumor cells. Although the latter function is an important mechanism in host defense (2), it can also have a damaging action on host tissues and thus be involved in the pathogenesis of acute and chronic inflammatory conditions.

The fundamental role of NO in the regulation of vascular tone became clear when the chemical nature of the earlier-known endothelium-derived relaxing factor (EDRF) was identified as NO (3–5). Shortly afterward, the importance of NO as an effector molecule in macrophage cytotoxicity was described (6). However, the complex role of NO in the immune response and inflammatory diseases is only recently becoming clear. This chapter gathers together the diverse and sometimes apparently contradictory data on the role of NO in the inflammatory process.

BIOSYNTHESIS AND BIOCHEMICAL ACTIONS OF NITRIC OXIDE

NO is synthesized from the amino acid L-arginine by the NO synthase enzymes (7,8). NO synthases (NOS) are a family of enzymes that oxidatively remove the terminal guanidine nitrogen from L-arginine to form citrulline and NO. Three major types of NOS have been characterized—two constitutive enzymes originally detected in endothelial cells (eNOS) or in neurons (nNOS) and an inducible isoform (iNOS) detected originally in murine macrophages.

Each NOS isoform exists as a homodimer of approximately 260 kd. Distinct genes encode each isoform of NOS and consist of either 26 exons (iNOS and eNOS) or 29 exons (nNOS) (2,7), and share 50% to 60% homology. Sequence analysis of the predicted primary structure of the NOS isoforms has indicated that all NOS proteins possess a bi-domain structure and that dimerization to homodimers is required for enzymatic activity. The C-terminal portion of the NOS protein, referred to as the reductase domain, resembles cytochrome P-450 reductase, and appears to possess the same cofactor binding sites. At the C-terminus is a reduced nicotinamide-adenine dinucleotide phosphate (NADPH)-binding region, which is conserved in all the isoforms, and is followed by flavin adenine dinucleotide (FAD) and flavin mononucleotide (FMN) consensus sequences, which comprise approximately 200 and 60 amino acids, respectively (9–11). NOS is a self-sufficient enzyme and substrate oxygenation occurs at a heme site in the N-terminal portion, or oxygenase domain of the protein. Stoichiometric amounts of heme are present in NOS and are required for its catalytic activity (10,12,13). Both L-arginine and pterin binding sites are located in the oxygenase domain, and a calmodulin binding site bridges the reductase and oxygenase domains. The eNOS isoform possesses consensus sequences for myristoylation/palmitoylation at its N-terminus.

E. Moilanen: Department of Pharmacology, University of Tampere, 33101 Tampere, Finland.

B. Whittle: William Harvey Research Institute and St. Bartholomew's and the Royal London School of Medicine and Dentistry, Charterhouse Square, London, United Kingdom.

S. Moncada: Wolfson Institute for Biomedical Research, University College London, London W1P 9LN, United Kingdom.

NO is generated via a five-electron oxidation of a terminal guanidinium nitrogen on the L-arginine molecule. This stereospecific reaction is both oxygen- and NADPH-dependent and yields the coproduct L-citrulline in addition to NO. The initial reaction involves N-hydroxylation of the guanidinium nitrogen to form N-hydroxy-L-arginine. The reaction utilizes one equivalent of NADPH and O_2 to conduct a simple two-electron oxidation of nitrogen.

It is now known that eNOS and nNOS, although first described in endothelial and neuronal cells, respectively, are present in many cell types in the body. Cells containing these constitutive isoforms of NOS produce physiologic amounts of NO, rapidly and transiently, in response to agonists such as acetylcholine in vascular endothelium, glutamate in the brain, or collagen acting on platelets. Such receptor-mediated responses result in an increase in the intracellular concentrations of calcium, known to be critical for activation of constitutive NOS.

Production of NO by the inducible isoform is not immediate, since several hours are required for the synthesis of iNOS protein. Once iNOS is expressed, this isoform of NOS can produce copious quantities of NO for prolonged periods. Widespread induction of iNOS has been detected in most organs following *in vivo* challenge with endotoxin (14). Many distinct cell types including macrophages, chondrocytes, neutrophils, hepatocytes, epithelium of lung and gut, and smooth muscle cells have been reported to express iNOS in response to inflammatory stimuli. Depending on the cell type, some bacteria, endotoxins, and certain proinflammatory cytokines such as interleukin-1 (IL-1), interleukin-6 (IL-6), tumor necrosis factor-α (TNF-α) and interferon-α and -γ induce the expression of iNOS, either alone or in combination. Other cytokines, such as IL-4, -8, -10, and -13, transforming growth factor-β, and platelet-derived growth factor can act as inhibitors of the induction of iNOS in certain cell types (15).

Control of Isoform Nitric Oxide Synthase Expression

Since iNOS possesses tightly bound calmodulin, it is virtually independent of free intracellular calcium concentrations and, therefore, once expressed, could theoretically continue to synthesize NO indefinitely until substrate and cofactors become limiting. Thus, iNOS activity is regulated by protein expression rather than functional modulation. The 5'-flanking region of iNOS contains conserved consensus sequences for nuclear factor-κB (NF-κB), interferon-γ–responsive elements (I-γ-RE), and a tumor necrosis factor responsive element (TNF-RE). An A-activator–binding site (AABS) also exists in the promoter region. The iNOS promoter possesses an NF-κB binding site at position -76 to -85 that has been shown to bind proteins of the Rel/NF-κB family in response to lipopolysaccharide (LPS) (16).

NF-κB is a transcription factor that plays a pivotal role in the expressional regulation of many genes that encode proinflammatory proteins (17) and, as such, may impose transcriptional control on iNOS expression. NF-κB is a heterodimeric protein composed of the DNA-binding proteins p50 and p65. This nuclear factor resides in the cytoplasm as a latent form stabilized by an inhibitory protein, IκB (18), but undergoes phosphorylation following cellular activation by pathophysiologic mediators, including cytokines and bacterial metabolites. Subsequent phosphorylation-regulated ubiquitination gives rise to a rapid degradation of IκB with liberation of the NF-κB heterodimer, which translocates into the nucleus and binds to appropriate regulatory elements in promoter regions on target genes. This results in gene expression and subsequent protein synthesis (19). Many of the stimuli that activate NF-κB are associated with oxidative stress and increased production of reactive oxygen species.

Modulation of NF-κB activity affects the induction of iNOS. Thus, pyrrolidinedithiocarbamate (PDTC) and diethyldithiocarbamate (DETC), which inhibit NF-κB, can attenuate iNOS expression in cultured cells (20,21). Antiinflammatory corticosteroids such as dexamethasone interfere with iNOS expression (22–24) and may do so by reducing the DNA binding capacity of NF-κB. Glucocorticoids have also been shown to induce the expression of the IκB protein, thereby preventing the liberation of free NF-κB heterodimer (25,26). Nonsteroidal antiinflammatory drugs, including aspirin and sodium salicylate, at high concentrations, also appear to downregulate iNOS expression by interfering with NF-κB activity (27,28).

Nitric Oxide Synthase Inhibitors

Arginine analogues such as N^G-monomethyl-L-arginine (L-NMMA), N^G-nitro-L-arginine methyl ester (L-NAME), and N-iminoethyl-L-ornithine (L-NIO) are widely used nonselective inhibitors of NOS enzymes (1). The identification of highly selective inhibitors of the various NOS isoforms will greatly assist in providing further analysis of the role of NO produced by these isoforms. Claims for selectivity with NOS inhibitors must be critically appraised, especially if based solely on *in vitro* data. Thus, differences in potency and activity of analogues between broken or whole-cell preparations may be anticipated because such agents can also differentially inhibit the unidirectional L-arginine transporter into endothelial cells, with L-NMMA but not L-NAME, for example, affecting L-arginine uptake (29). Indeed, selective inhibition of substrate uptake into inflammatory cells may offer another pharmacologic approach to the regulation of inappropriate NO biosynthesis. Because of pharmacokinetic and metabolic considerations, any differential potency of arginine analogues *in vitro* may not be observed *in vivo*.

L-Canavanine and aminoguanidine, compounds that are not simple arginine analogues, have been shown to inhibit iNOS in elicited or cultured neutrophils, vascular tissue, and pancreatic insulinoma cells *in vitro* (30,31). However, selectivity *in vivo* of aminoguanidine has not been confirmed (32) and these agents are likely to exert a broad range of biochemical and pharmacologic actions other than NOS inhibition. As with any pharmacologic agent, claims for selectivity of action of all novel inhibitors of the different NOS isoforms will therefore require careful consideration, especially for *in vivo* evaluation, and experimental studies will probably need judicious selection of appropriate concentrations or dosing schedules unless substantial selectivity can be achieved. More selective inhibitors of iNOS have been described such as L-*N*-iminoethyl lysine (33), 1-amino-hydroxy-guanidine, and aminoethyl isothiourea (34), and more recently *in vitro* and *in vivo* data on the highly potent and selective iNOS inhibitor 1400W have been reported (35).

Nitric Oxide Transduction

NO differs from earlier-known signaling molecules in that its action is not mediated by classical cell surface receptors. NO, being a small gaseous molecule, easily diffuses through biologic membranes. NO is highly reactive and, based on chemiluminescence techniques, it has been estimated that NO migrates only a few micrometers in cultures of activated macrophages (36). At the cellular level, NO has several potential targets for initiation of its biologic actions.

Even at low concentrations, NO activates the enzyme guanylate cyclase and thus increases the synthesis of cyclic guanosine monophosphate (cGMP). This process forms the biochemical basis for the majority of the physiologic actions of NO. Thus, increased intracellular cGMP can bring about relaxation of vascular smooth muscle, inhibition of platelet aggregation, and signal transduction in the central and peripheral nervous system (1,37).

NO also has direct actions on various other enzymes, particularly those containing an iron-sulfur moiety in their catalytic center, leading to either increased or decreased activity of those enzymes. Examples of key enzymes that are inactivated by NO are ribonucleotide reductase, which is involved in DNA synthesis (38); aconitase, an enzyme of the Krebs cycle; and complexes I and II of the respiratory chain (39). NO has direct effects on the synthesis of some inflammatory mediators, since it inhibits the activity of the 5-lipoxygenase enzymes (40) that produce leukotrienes, and also inhibits NADPH oxidase (41), which forms the superoxide anion. In contrast, there are reports of both stimulatory and suppressive action on the cyclooxygenase (COX) enzyme by NO. Thus, low concentrations of NO can increase prostanoid synthesis by affecting COX-1 and COX-2,

whereas higher concentrations may diminish COX activity (42–46).

In addition, NO may have a more widespread action on the synthesis of cytokines and other inflammatory mediators since it may regulate the function of the inflammatory transcription factors NF-activating protein-1 (AP-1) discussed previously (47,48). Thus NO can downregulate the synthesis of IL-6 yet upregulate the production of TNF-α in a macrophage cell line, exerting cytotoxic actions on the cells (49). NO may also act as a reactive radical either directly or after interacting with superoxide anions, produced at the sites of inflammation, to form peroxynitrite. In some instances this reaction could be regarded as an inactivation mechanism of both of these reactive molecules (50). However, peroxynitrite is a strong oxidant and nitrating agent itself; it can promote lipid peroxidation and cytolytic actions, and may degrade to form the highly cytotoxic hydroxyl radical (51). Thus, local intraluminal application of peroxynitrite *in vivo* produces extensive colonic injury in the rat (52). Tyrosine is readily nitrated by peroxynitrite, and the product, nitrotyrosine, has been used as a measure of its formation (53). Peroxynitrite formation has been detected at sites of inflammation in animal models and in humans (54–57).

NITRIC OXIDE IN THE VASCULAR EVENTS OF INFLAMMATION

Nitric Oxide, Vascular Permeability and Microcirculation

Studies with NOS inhibitors indicate that constitutive NOS has an important role in regulating the integrity of microvascular endothelium. Protective actions against acute microcirculatory damage can be demonstrated in the heart, lung, kidney, liver, and small and large intestine by the production of NO from eNOS. Thus, inhibition of constitutive NOS at the time of administration of LPS provokes a rapid and substantial increase in vascular permeability in these organs, an effect attenuated by the depletion of circulating neutrophils. Moreover, administration of platelet-activating factor (PAF)-receptor antagonists, thromboxane, and leukotriene synthase inhibitors protects against intestinal microvascular injury resulting from inhibition of eNOS (58,59). Such results demonstrate that NO synthesized by eNOS effectively counteracts the actions of injurious proinflammatory mediators that are released in the early phase of LPS-induced tissue inflammation.

However, several hours after LPS challenge, following expression of iNOS and the accompanying plasma leakage, NOS inhibitors such as L-NAME and L-NMMA have the converse action, preventing the microvascular injury in key organs. Pretreatment with the antiinflammatory corticosteroid dexamethasone inhibits both the induction of NOS and the vascular permeability changes (60).

The process by which excessive NO production may contribute to vascular leakage may also involve an increase in blood flow. While an increase in blood flow alone would not itself result in an increase in vascular permeability, it would augment the actions of other proinflammatory mediators that have a direct injurious action on the microvascular endothelium. Mast cells, which release a number of such mediators including histamine and 5-hydroxytryptamine, also produce NO (61). Exogenous NO can, however, modulate mast cell degranulation (62), which could therefore act as a feedback inhibitor. NO is involved in the cutaneous vascular permeability response provoked by 5-hydroxytrytamine (63).

Studies in rat skin have demonstrated that intradermal injection of endotoxin induced a time-dependent increase in blood flow that was inhibited by local administration of NOS inhibitors and by pretreatment with a corticosteroid (64). NO participates in the neurogenic inflammatory hyperemia elicited in rat skin by activation of sensory neurons (65,66). Inhibitors of NOS can also attenuate the changes in vascular permeability and edema formation induced by proinflammatory agents in rat skin, a process that may involve reduction in local blood flow (67,68). Such local microcirculatory actions of NOS inhibitors may also contribute to the reduction in leukocyte accumulation in passive cutaneous inflammatory reactions (69).

Findings from a rat model of edema evoked by carrageenan suggest that eNOS is involved in the development of this acute inflammatory response, whereas iNOS is involved in the maintenance of the inflammatory response (70). Studies with superoxide dismutase suggested a role for peroxynitrite in this model, since nitrotyrosine immunostaining was also detected (71).

That selective inhibition of iNOS with concomitant antiinflammatory actions can be achieved *in vivo* has recently been demonstrated with the novel highly potent and selective iNOS inhibitor, 1400W (35). This agent has no action in provoking an early phase of vascular injury following endotoxin challenge, yet prevents the plasma leakage associated with the expression of iNOS, even when administered concurrently with the endotoxin challenge (72).

Nitric Oxide and Leukocyte Adhesion

Activation of inflammatory cells and vascular endothelium by inflammatory mediators leads to adhesion of leukocytes to the endothelium and to their subsequent migration from the circulation at the inflammatory site. NO, formed by eNOS, acts as an endogenous inhibitor of neutrophil adhesion to vascular endothelium (73). Thus, inhibition of NOS greatly augments leukocyte adhesion, whereas NO donors have been shown to inhibit leukocyte adhesion to endothelial cells in various experimental models (73–75).

The inhibition of leukocyte adhesion to endothelium is of major importance, not only as a potential antiinflammatory mechanism, but also in modulation of ischemia-reperfusion injury and of tumor metastatic mechanisms. A reduction in myocardial necrosis and neutrophil accumulation by administration of an NO donor in acute myocardial ischemia and reperfusion has been observed in a canine model (76), which suggests a potential indication for the therapeutic use of NO-releasing compounds. The suppressive action of NO on the adhesion process is not limited to neutrophils, since NO also inhibits the adhesion of lymphocytes and monocytes (77).

The mechanisms underlying the inhibitory action of NO on leukocyte adhesion are not known, although the accelerated inactivation of superoxide anion by NO has been suggested (78,79). More recently, attenuation of adhesion molecule expression in endothelial cells has been described, with inhibitory actions of the NO superoxide donor 3-morpholinosydnonimine (SIN-1) on intracellular adhesion molecule-1 (ICAM-1) and vascular cell adhesion molecule-1 (VCAM-1) synthesis in human endothelial cells being reported (80). In addition, endogenously produced NO may downregulate the expression of VCAM-1 and monocyte binding to human aortic endothelial cells (81). Increased levels of P-selectin protein and mRNA have been found in human endothelial cells in culture, grown in the presence of L-NAME, suggesting a regulatory role of NO in the early leukocyte-endothelial interactions (82).

Nitric Oxide and Angiogenesis

Angiogenesis is a process in which growth of new microvascular blood vessels is induced; this is necessary for proliferative responses such as those in inflammation, wound repair, and the growth of solid tumors. NO has been reported to be involved in the angiogenic mechanisms of activated macrophages, since inhibitors of NOS cause an inhibition of macrophage-dependent angiogenesis (83).

Inhibitors of NOS delay healing of experimentally induced chronic gastric ulcers and reduce the number of capillaries in the granulation tissue at the ulcer bed, although this may also reflect removal of NO as a protective factor from the hostile gastric environment (84). Other studies have shown that tumors engineered to generate NO continuously grow faster and are more vascularized than their wild-type parental cells, suggesting that NO is involved in the signaling cascade for neovascularization (85).

NITRIC OXIDE IN THE CELLULAR EVENTS OF INFLAMMATION

Nitric Oxide and Macrophages

NO is considered to be an important effector molecule in macrophage-mediated host defense. In response to endotoxin LPS and interferon-γ, these cells produce high concentrations of NO, which contributes to their cytostatic-cytotoxic action against tumor cells (86–88), bacterial, helminth, fungal, or protozoan infections (15), and the replication of viruses (89,90).

The presence of iNOS and the role of NO in the function of human mononuclear phagocytes has, however, been more difficult to demonstrate. There are multiple iNOS-like sequences present in the human genome (91,92), but the mechanisms leading to induction of iNOS in human inflammatory cells seem to differ from those known for murine or rat cells. Thus, human monocyte-macrophages do not express iNOS in response to the cytokines or cytokine combinations known to induce NO synthesis in mouse macrophages (93–95). However, other pathways leading to induction of iNOS in human monocyte-macrophages have more recently been identified. Thus, immunoglobulin E (IgE) immune complexes can induce iNOS and NO synthesis in human monocytes stimulated to express the low-affinity IgE receptors FcεRII/CD23 (96,97). NO synthesis appears to be activated through CD23-ligation, since monoclonal antibodies against CD23 had a similar effect to that of IgE immune complexes. CD23 surface antigen–mediated activation of the L-arginine:NO pathway also occurs in human eosinophils (98), acute myeloid leukemia cells (99), and epidermal keratinocytes (100).

Induction of iNOS in human monocyte-macrophages has also been detected after infection with human immunodeficiency virus type 1 (101), *Mycobacterium avium* (102), and activation through surface receptor CD69 (103). Treatment of human monocytes *in vitro* with interferon-α also increased NO production and expression of iNOS protein and mRNA (104). In addition, immunohistochemical and biochemical evidence shows that induction of iNOS can occur in activated macrophages *in vivo* in human breast cancer (105) and in the aseptic foreign body inflammation in granulomatous tissue around failed prosthetic joints (106).

Activation of human monocytes through CD23-ligation results in production of a number of inflammatory mediators, including TNF-α and oxygen radicals. L-NMMA strongly inhibits the production of these mediators, suggesting that NO is involved in the IgE immune complex–triggered activation in human monocytes (96). Moreover, data are now accumulating to show that NO has a role in the antimicrobial mechanisms of human macrophages. Intracellular killing of *Leishmania major* parasite by human macrophages is mediated by NO induced after ligation of CD23 surface antigen or after treatment with interferon-γ in infected cells (97). In addition, leukocytes taken from clinically normal children living in an area of Tanzania where malaria is endemic were found to be iNOS positive. The iNOS activity was higher in those with overt clinical disease, but fell in those with advanced cerebral malaria. It was proposed that NO pro-duced by iNOS functioned to hold malaria in check, and that suppression of iNOS was a contributing factor in malaria lethality (107). The protection against severe malaria may be related to polymorphism in the promoter region of the iNOS gene (108). An earlier report indicated that TNF-α–induced killing of *Mycobacterium avium* in human macrophages was mediated by NO, since it was associated with increased production of nitrite in the culture and was inhibited by addition of NOS inhibitors to the culture medium (102). Thus NO production in human mononuclear phagocytes appears to be more rigorously regulated than in murine macrophages.

Nitric Oxide and Lymphocytes

NO production in murine lymphocytes has been demonstrated and seems to be subtype-specific. In a murine model of malaria infection, T helper type 1 (Th1) cells, but not Th2 cells, could be induced to produce NO (109).

Nitric oxide has been shown to inhibit lymphocyte proliferation. Thus, in murine models, production of large amounts of NO by activated macrophages accounts for their ability to suppress lymphocyte proliferation (110,111). There are also data supporting a mediator role for NO in the tumor-induced suppression of tumor-infiltrating lymphocytes (112) and an autoregulatory role for NO produced by Th1 cells (109). Proliferative responses of activated T lymphocytes are susceptible to NO, whereas other mediators such as prostaglandins or hydrogen peroxide, rather than NO, are responsible for the macrophage-induced inhibition of B lymphocyte proliferation (110). In experimentally induced murine trypanosomiasis, enhanced NO production has been shown to downregulate T lymphocyte proliferation, while inhibition of NOS can reverse the immunosuppression (113,114).

NO gas and NO-releasing compounds are also able to inhibit human T lymphocyte proliferation (115,116). Although lymphocytes exhibit an intact guanylate cyclase capable of producing cGMP in response to NO (116,117), the antiproliferative action of NO appears to be mediated by a cGMP-independent mechanism (118). NO does not influence IL-2 production or IL-2 receptor expression in human T cells (115,119), but has been reported to have a direct inhibitory action on ribonucleotide reductase, an enzyme involved in DNA synthesis (38,120). NO could also influence T-lymphocyte responses through antigen presentation, since NO has been reported to downregulate major histocompatibility complex (MHC) class II expression by macrophages (121).

In addition to the inhibitory action of higher concentrations of NO on T-lymphocyte proliferation described above, NO gas at nanomolar concentrations has been shown to stimulate resting human peripheral blood mononuclear cells (122,123). NO can also enhance NF-κB binding activity and TNF-α secretion in human peripheral blood mononuclear cells (123). It has been demonstrated that a monomeric G protein p21ras is a target of NO in T lymphocytes, and the activation of p21ras could explain these immunostimulatory properties of low concentrations of NO (47).

Less in known about the effects of NO on B lymphocytes. Epstein-Barr virus–transformed human B lymphocytes and Burkitt's lymphoma cell lines produce low levels of NO and express constitutive macrophage-type NO synthase (124). Under these conditions, NO appears to be involved in the inhibition of apoptosis and Epstein-Barr virus reactivation in these cell lines.

Nitric Oxide and Neutrophils

There are interspecies differences in the synthesis of NO by neutrophils. Rat neutrophils are known to produce NO in response to inflammatory stimuli (24,125–127). These neutrophils express an inducible calcium-independent form of NOS in response to LPS and cytokines, including interferon-γ and TNF-α, and antiinflammatory steroids prevent the induction of iNOS through inhibition of its mRNA transcription (24,127).

Human neutrophils have been reported to inhibit platelet aggregation by releasing a NO-like factor (128–130). NO synthesis in human neutrophils is triggered by receptor-mediated agonists such as F-met-leu-phe (FMLP) or by the activation of protein kinase C with phorbol myristate acetate (130–133). Priming of neutrophils by LPS, interferon-γ, IL-6, or adherence can increase NO production (132,134). Inflammatory stimuli known to induce iNOS in rat neutrophils do not have the same action in human neutrophils, at least under *in vitro* conditions. However, recent data show that neutrophils isolated from the oral cavity (135) do express iNOS, which could suggest that induction of iNOS is also involved in antimicrobial mechanisms of human neutrophils.

When human neutrophils are activated with FMLP, PAF, or leukotriene B4 to produce NO, the superoxide-generating system is also activated (125,131,132). NO reacts rapidly with superoxide anion to form peroxynitrite, the generation of which can be demonstrated during the respiratory burst of human neutrophils (136). In addition, NO can react with hydrogen peroxide to form peroxynitrous acid (137), which can decompose to the hydroxyl radical. Therefore, it is probable that only a minor portion of the synthesized NO is released unchanged outside the cell and can be detected by conventional methods. Addition of superoxide dismutase and catalase into suspensions of activated neutrophils increases the NO concentrations detected and is often needed to reveal the synthesis of NO (125,128,130–133, 138).

NO-releasing compounds are potent inhibitors of neutrophil function including degranulation, chemotaxis, leukotriene B4 release, and superoxide anion production *in vitro* (74,139–143). In addition, endogenously synthesized NO stimulates chemotaxis and degranulation and increases intracellular free calcium in neutrophils (144–146). NO-releasing compounds have been reported to stimulate LPS-induced TNF-α production in human neutrophils (147) and zymosan-stimulated superoxide anion release from canine neutrophils (143). Taken together, these findings indicate that NO can exert both inhibitory and stimulatory effects on neutrophil function, which may reflect a concentration-dependent biphasic action.

NO has several molecular targets relevant to the processes of neutrophil activation. The stimulatory actions of endogenously produced NO on chemotaxis and degranulation appear to be mediated by cGMP (134,144). The inhibitory actions of higher concentrations of NO-releasing compounds could be partly explained by cGMP-dependent effects, but actions of peroxynitrite cannot yet be excluded (148). NO has been reported to stimulate adenosine diphosphate (ADP)-ribosylation of actin in human neutrophils, which could also explain the modulation of actin-associated neutrophil actions of chemotaxis and phagocytosis (149).

NITRIC OXIDE IN INFLAMMATORY DISEASES

Evidence from studies using a number of animal models have suggested a pathophysiologic role of NO in a range of inflammatory diseases including rheumatoid arthritis, asthma, inflammatory bowel diseases, diabetes mellitus, and graft-versus-host disease. There is an increasing body of evidence to support the involvement of NO in the pathogenesis of human inflammatory diseases, giving rise to novel ideas for NO-targeted treatment of these diseases. The role of NO in inflammatory diseases is discussed in more detail below.

Nitric Oxide in Arthritis

The presence of elevated concentrations of nitrite (150), nitrotyrosine (53), and S-nitrosoproteins (151) in synovial fluid from patients with rheumatoid arthritis suggests an increased synthesis of NO in inflamed joints. N-hydroxy-L-arginine, an intermediate in the NO synthesis pathway from L-arginine, is increased in serum samples from patients with active rheumatoid arthritis (152). This is consistent with the finding that the urinary excretion of the stable metabolite of NO, nitrate, is increased in patients with rheumatoid arthritis, which reduces toward normal urinary excretory levels after commencement of treatment with the antiinflammatory agent prednisolone (153,154). An increased excretion of NO metabolites was also reported in animals with experimentally induced arthritis (155–157) and preceded the symptoms of the disease (156).

Synovial membranes (43,158–162) from experimental animals have been reported to express iNOS in response to inflammatory stimuli. Human chondrocytes express iNOS and produce NO following incubation with IL-1, TNF-α and LPS *in vitro* (163–166). Indeed, chondrocytes were one of the first cell types in which human iNOS was characterized and cloned (164,166). The signaling mechanisms of iNOS expression in human chondrocytes are not fully known and there are differences in those processes compared to the induction of murine macrophage iNOS. Induction of iNOS in chondrocytes in response to LPS and IL-1 is dependent on the activation of protein tyrosine kinases but not on activation of protein kinase C, protein kinase A, or calcium-calmodulin kinase (167). Increased intracellular calcium downregulates NO production in human chondrocytes by reducing the stability of mRNA for iNOS (168).

Increased production of NO has been reported in chondrocytes from patients with rheumatoid and osteoarthritis (169,170). It is possible that more than one subtype of NOS is induced in affected cartilage since, in addition to the iNOS cloned from IL-1–treated human chondrocytes (164,166), another NOS isoform subtype, provisionally called osteoarthritis-NOS (OA-NOS) has been detected (170).

Inflammatory synovium from patients with rheumatoid arthritis produces NO in *ex vivo* organ cultures (169). Immunohistochemical analysis and *in situ* hybridization showed the presence of iNOS primarily in synovial lining cells and endothelial cells and, to a lesser extent, in infiltrating mononuclear cells and synovial fibroblasts. The increased production of NO by primary synovial cultures from patients with rheumatoid and osteoarthritis has also been observed (171). In addition, NO may be involved in the pathogenesis of extraarticular manifestations of rheumatic diseases. Thus, an increased production of NO has been reported in salivary glands in patients with Sjögren's syndrome (172).

In addition to the modulatory actions on inflammatory cells, NO may be directly involved in the cartilage destruction in arthritic joints, acting to increase the activity of metalloprotease enzymes (173) and suppress the formation of novel matrix components (160,161) induced by proinflammatory cytokines. NO can induce apoptosis in chondrocytes (174) and it may be involved in the mechanism of chondrocyte loss that is typical for cartilage destruction observed in osteoarthritis. NO has also been implicated in the regulation of osteolysis caused by osteoclasts. NO can exert a biphasic effect on osteoclast function, being stimulatory at low concentrations and inhibitory at higher concentrations (175,176). NO acts as a local regulator of the complex network of cytokines and other inflammatory mediators produced in inflamed joints; thus, an increased production of the proinflamma-

tory cytokine TNF-α was reported in human synovial cells following exposure to NO (171). In human chondrocytes (45) and endothelial cells (46), exposure to NO leads to reduced production of proinflammatory prostaglandins by the inducible cyclooxygenase isoform COX-2.

Studies with experimental models of these human diseases suggest that inhibitors of NOS, most possibly selective inhibitors of inducible NOS, may have therapeutic potential in the treatment in these inflammatory arthritides. In experimentally induced arthritis, inhibitors of NO synthesis have been reported to relieve or even prevent the clinical and histologic signs of arthritis induced by injection of streptococcal cell wall fragments (158), adjuvant arthritis (156,177–179), antigen-induced arthritis (180), and spontaneous autoimmune arthritis in MRL-*lpr/lpr* mice (155). NOS inhibitors may therefore have therapeutic potential in preventing the progression of joint destruction in osteoarthritis.

Nitric Oxide in Asthma

Patients with bronchial asthma show increased concentrations of NO in exhaled air, which decrease toward normal concentrations after commencement of treatment with inhaled or oral antiinflammatory steroids (181–186). This elevated concentration of NO is also seen in pediatric patients with asthma (187,188). After allergen challenge, increased amounts of NO in exhaled air can be detected, especially with the late response (189). Increased concentrations of NO in exhaled air are not, however, specific for asthma (190–193), and samples may be contaminated by NO produced in the upper respiratory tract (194). Therefore, recommendations for the measurements of exhaled and nasal NO have recently been given by a task force of the European Respiratory Society (195).

Increased concentrations of products of NO are also found in induced sputum in patients with asthma (196). Importantly, the concentrations of NO metabolites in sputum correlate with other markers of the severity of asthma, such as the percentages of eosinophil counts, the concentrations of eosinophil cationic protein in sputum, and the degree of airflow obstruction. Whether analysis of the noninvasive samples will provide a prognostic indicator for disease progression or amelioration awaits further evaluation.

Early immunohistochemical evidence suggested that iNOS expression could be detected in bronchial biopsies from asthmatic patients but not in healthy controls (197). The ability of pulmonary epithelial cells to generate NO is supported by *in vitro* data showing that primary or immortalized bronchial epithelial cells can express iNOS in response to stimulation with microbial products or cytokines (198,199). A continuous synthesis of NO by iNOS as a function of normal human airway epithelium *in vivo* has been reported (200), suggesting a constitutive expression of iNOS in those cells. However, removal of epithelial cells from the *in vivo* airway environment led to a rapid loss of iNOS expression, which suggests that the induction is dependent on conditions or factors present in airways. It is therefore difficult to know whether iNOS in human airway epithelium is expressed constitutively or whether it is continually induced by inhaled irritants, including airborne LPS or ozone. In sites of chronic inflammation in human lungs, alveolar macrophages and vascular endothelial cells stain positively with iNOS antibodies (201).

Eosinophils have been implicated as a major inflammatory cell type involved in asthma. Human eosinophils as well as macrophages and keratinocytes have been reported to express iNOS and produce NO by an IgE-mediated mechanism (96–98,100). Thus, when the cells are treated with IL-4 or certain other cytokines to express CD23 (a low-affinity receptor for IgE) and then activated by IgE immunocomplexes, expression of iNOS and production of NO is provoked. The presence of iNOS in human eosinophils was recently confirmed by molecular techniques (202). The presence of an IgE-mediated mechanism in induction of iNOS in human inflammatory cells thus supports a role for NO in the pathogenesis of asthmatic inflammation.

NO may also have harmful effects in the lungs through augmentation of the inflammatory response by increasing pulmonary blood flow and vascular permeability and thus plasma extravasation and edema (181,203,204). Based on studies with nonhuman cells, a more profound pathophysiologic role of increased NO production in airway epithelial cells and pulmonary macrophages in asthma has also been suggested (109,205). By inactivating the functions of T helper type 1 lymphocytes, NO could lead to overactivation of T helper type 2 lymphocyte responses, which in turn results in accumulation of eosinophils in the airways and increases IgE-mediated responses.

In addition to its pathologic actions as an inflammatory mediator, NO has several physiologic roles in the lung where it serves as a neurotransmitter in the NANC nerves, and functions as a bronchodilator and vasodilator. NO has been shown to be involved in neurally mediated bronchodilatation (206). Endogenous NO may therefore provide a defense mechanism against bronchoconstrictor events in human lungs. Thus, bronchoconstriction after bradykinin challenge, and to a lesser extent after methacoline provocation, is augmented by administration of a NOS inhibitor in asthmatic patients (207). Inhaled NO had no effect on airway tone in healthy volunteers but did attenuate methacholine-induced bronchoconstriction in asthmatic patients, although the response was weak compared with that of β-agonists (208,209).

Nitric Oxide in Inflammatory Bowel Disease

Induction of iNOS has been observed in epithelial cells isolated from the rat small intestine and colon following endotoxin challenge *in vivo,* and such expression of iNOS is associated with a reduction in cell viability. Both the induction of iNOS and the cell injury is prevented by pretreatment *in vivo* with dexamethasone, while delayed administration of L-NAME *in vivo* can also prevent the epithelial damage (210,211). Induction of iNOS in intestinal epithelial cells thus provokes injury, which contrasts with the role of NO formed by the constitutive NOS isoform in maintaining epithelial integrity (212). The induction of iNOS in intestinal epithelial cells may also contribute to the accumulation of fluid within the intestinal lumen in response to exposure to bacterial toxins by disrupting electrolyte transport in the villus cells, as well as by the stimulation of crypt cell secretion.

Induction of iNOS has been observed in a model of inflammatory bowel disease induced by trinitrobenzene sulfonic acid (TNB) in the rat over the initial 3 days after challenge (213). In other studies, levels of nitrite in the luminal lavage of the inflamed guinea pig ileum are elevated when measured 7 days following TNB instillation, and iNOS gene expression has also been demonstrated. In this model, intense staining for iNOS protein was found in the ileum on immunohistochemical evaluation; this was colocalized with tyrosine nitration as an index of peroxynitrite activity (54,214). Experimental colonic inflammation provoked by a sulfhydryl blocker also appears to involve iNOS (215).

Elevated plasma concentrations of nitrate and nitrite are also observed in the chronic, but not the acute, phases of colonic inflammation induced by bacterial wall polymers in the rat (216). Increased production of nitrite and nitrate, as well as iNOS activity, has also been demonstrated in the HLA-B27 transgenic rat, which exhibits spontaneous colitis (217). In rhesus macaques displaying idiopathic colitis, increased nitrogen intermediates, gene expression, and iNOS activity have been determined (218).

Evidence for the involvement of NO in inflammatory bowel disease in humans has also accumulated. Early studies had shown that nitrite concentrations in rectal dialysates are elevated in patients with active ulcerative colitis (219) and augmented concentrations of citrulline, the coproduct of NOS activity, have been detected in biopsies of inflamed human colon (220). In more direct studies on colonic NOS in inflammatory bowel diseases, a sixfold increase in calcium-independent iNOS activity has been determined in colonic mucosal biopsies from patients with ulcerative colitis (221). Subsequent studies have also demonstrated increases in iNOS activity in colonic tissue from Crohn's patients (222), which can be localized in the epithelium, along with nitrotyrosine staining (57). In other studies, toxic megacolon in patients with inflammatory bowel disease was associated with the appearance of iNOS in the colonic muscularis propria (223). Not all the experimental findings from animal models support a pathogenic role of iNOS in inflammatory bowel disease, but the body of evidence does implicate excessive NO production in this disease (224).

The expression of iNOS may also be involved in other inflammatory diseases of the gut. Thus, experimental studies have also shown the involvement of iNOS in the chronic microvascular leakage and tissue inflammatory injury in the small intestine that follows the administration of nonsteroidal antiinflammatory agents such as indomethacin (225). This slowly developing enteropathy involves indigenous bacteria and is attenuated by inhibition of iNOS, suggesting that following ingress of bacteria, LPS is liberated in the intestinal mucosa, which brings about the induction of iNOS. It has also been demonstrated that the organism implicated in the pathogenesis of peptic ulceration, *Helicobacter pylori,* can elaborate a factor that can induce iNOS in human THP-1 and rodent macrophage cell lines (226). More recently, the purified LPS derived from *H. pylori* has been shown to be highly active *in vivo* in stimulating the expression of iNOS in epithelial cells (227). Moreover, the induction of iNOS brought about epithelial injury, as determined in the duodenum, an event that was inhibited both by inhibitors of NOS, and by superoxide dismutase. These findings point to the involvement of NO, in combination with superoxide to produce peroxynitrite, in epithelial injury associated with *H. pylori* challenge. Such mechanisms may be involved in the pathogenesis of peptic ulceration associated with infection with this organism.

CONCLUSIONS

The role of NO in inflammatory diseases is not yet completely understood and several questions remain to be answered. Depending on the type and phase of the inflammatory reaction and the individual vascular or cellular responses studied, NO can exert both proinflammatory and antiinflammatory properties. Constitutively produced NO appears to offer protection against acute inflammatory insults, whereas expression of iNOS is associated with widespread tissue injury and inflammation. In support of the proinflammatory role of iNOS, the inflammatory response to carrageenan is reduced and the susceptibility to infection with leishmania or listeria is enhanced in iNOS-gene disrupted mice (228,229). Thus NO, like many other inflammatory mediators, has a dual regulatory function in inflammation. Evidence is now accumulating to suggest that NO is indeed produced in human inflammatory cells, but in many instances its synthesis is regulated differently from that originally described in murine cells. Our knowledge of the synthesis and role of NO in human inflammatory diseases is still somewhat limited but, on the basis of experimental models of these diseases, both specific inhibitors of iNOS and NO-releasing compounds have therapeutic potential as antiinflammatory and immunomodulatory drugs.

REFERENCES

1. Moncada S, Higgs EA. Molecular mechanisms and therapeutic strategies related to nitric oxide. *FASEB J* 1995;9:1319–1330.
2. Nathan C. Nitric oxide as a secretory product of mammalian cells. *FASEB J* 1992;6:3051–3064.
3. Palmer RMJ, Ferrige AG, Moncada S. Nitric oxide release accounts for the biological activity of endothelium-derived relaxing factor. *Nature* 1987;327:524–526.
4. Khan MT, Furchgott RF. Additional evidence that endothelium-derived relaxing factor is nitric oxide. In: Rand MJ, Raper C, eds. *Pharmacology.* Amsterdam: Elsevier, 1987:341–344.
5. Ignarro LJ, Buga GM, Wood KS, Byrns RE, Chaudhuri G. Endothelium-derived relaxing factor produced and released from artery and vein is nitric oxide. *Proc Natl Acad Sci USA* 1987;84:9265–9269.
6. Hibbs JB Jr. Overview of cytotoxic mechanisms and defence of the intracellular environment against microbes. In: Moncada S, Marletta MA, Hibbs JB Jr, Higgs EA, eds. *The biology of nitric oxide: enzymology, biochemistry and immunology,* vol 2. London: Portland Press, 1992:201–206.
7. Knowles RG, Moncada S. Nitric oxide synthases in mammals. *Biochem J* 1994;298:249–258.
8. Nathan C, Xie QW. Nitric oxide synthases: roles, tolls and controls. *Cell* 1994;78:915–918.
9. Bredt DS, Hwang PM, Glatt CE, Lowenstein C, Reed RR, Snyder SH. Cloned and expressed nitric oxide synthase structurally resembles cytochrome P450 reductase. *Nature* 1991;351:714–718.
10. Stuehr DJ, Cho HJ, Kwon NS, Weise MF, Nathan CF. Purification and characterization of the cytokine-induced macrophage nitric oxide synthase; an FAD- and FMN-containing flavoprotein. *Proc Natl Acad Sci USA* 1991;86:7773–7777.
11. Chartrain NA, Geller DA, Koty PP, et al. Molecular cloning, structure and chromosomal localization of the human inducible nitric oxide synthase gene. *J Biol Chem* 1994;269:6765–6772.
12. Stuehr DJ, Ikeda-Saito M. Spectral characterization of brain and macrophage nitric oxide synthases. Cytochrome P450-like hemoproteins that contain a flavin semiquinone radical. *J Biol Chem* 1992; 267:20547–20550.
13. White KA, Marletta MA. Nitric oxide synthase is a cytochrome P450-type hemoprotein. *Biochemistry* 1992;31:6627–6631.
14. Salter M, Knowles RG, Moncada S. Widespread tissue distribution, species distribution and changes in activity of Ca^{2+}-dependent and Ca^{2+}-independent nitric oxide synthases. *FEBS Lett* 1991;291:145–149.
15. MacMicking J, Xie Q, Nathan C. Nitric oxide and macrophage function. *Annu Rev Immunol* 1997;15:323–350.
16. Xie QW, Kashiwabara Y, Nathan C. Role of transcription factor NF-κB/Rel in induction of nitric oxide synthase. *J Biol Chem* 1994;269:4705–4708.
17. Baeuerle PA. The inducible transcription factor NF-κB: regulation by distinct protein subunits. *Biochim Biophys Acta* 1991;1072:63–80.
18. Urban MB, Schreck R, Baeuerle PA. NF-κB contacts DNA by a heterodimer of the p50 and p65 subunit. *EMBO J* 1991;10:1817–1825.
19. Traenckner EB, Pahl HL, Henkel T, Schmidt KN, Wilk S, Baeuerle PA. Phosphorylation of human IκB-α on serines 32 and 36 controls IκB-α proteolysis and NF-κB activation in response to diverse stimuli. *EMBO J* 1995;14:2876–2883.
20. Sherman MP, Aeberhard EE, Wong VZ, Griscavage JM, Ignarro LJ. Pyrrolidine dithiocarbamate inhibits induction of nitric oxide synthase activity in rat alveolar macrophages. *Biochem Biophys Res Commun* 1993;191:1301–1308.
21. Mulsch A, Schray-Utz B, Mordvintcev PI, Hauschildt S, Busse R. Diethyldithiocarbamate inhibits induction of macrophage NO synthase. *FEBS Lett* 1993;321:215–218.
22. Radomski MW, Palmer RM, Moncada S. Glucocorticoids inhibit the expression of an inducible, but not the constitutive, nitric oxide synthase in vascular endothelial cells. *Proc Natl Acad Sci USA* 1990; 87:10043–10047.
23. Di Rosa M, Radomski MW, Carnuccio R, Moncada S. Glucocorticoids inhibit the induction of nitric oxide synthase in macrophages. *Biochem Biophys Res Commun* 1990;171:1246–1252.
24. Kolls J, Xie J, LeBlanc R, et al. Rapid induction of messenger RNA for nitric oxide synthase II in rat neutrophils *in vivo* by endotoxin and its suppression by prednisolone. *Proc Soc Exp Biol Med* 1994;205:220–225.

25. Auphan N, DiDonato JA, Rosette C, Helmberg A, Karin M. Immunosuppression by glucocorticoids: inhibition of NF-κB activity through induction of IκB synthesis. *Science* 1995;270:286–290.

26. Kleinert H, Euchenhofer C, Ihrig-Biedert I, Forstermann U. Glucocorticoids inhibit the induction of nitric oxide synthase II by downregulating cytokine-induced activity of transcription factor nuclear factor-κB. *Mol Pharmacol* 1996;49:15–21.

27. Aeberhard EE, Henderson SA, Arabolos NS, et al. Nonsteroidal antiinflammatory drugs inhibit expression of the inducible nitric oxide synthase gene. *Biochem Biophys Res Commun* 1995;208:1053–1059.

28. Kopp E, Ghosh S. Inhibition of NF-κB by sodium salicylate and aspirin. *Science* 1994;265:956–959.

29. Bogle RG, Baydoun AR, Pearson JD, Moncada S, Mann GE. L-arginine transport is increased in macrophages generating nitric oxide. *Biochem J* 1992;284:15–18.

30. Umans JG, Samsel RW. L-Canavanine selectively augments contraction in aortas from endotoxemic rats. *Eur J Pharmacol* 1992;210: 343–346.

31. Misko TP, Moore WM, Kasten TP, et al. Selective inhibition of the inducible nitric oxide synthase by aminoguanidine. *Eur J Pharmacol* 1993;233:119–125.

32. Laszlo F, Evans SM, Whittle BJR. Aminoguanidine inhibits both constitutive and inducible nitric oxide synthase isoforms in rat intestinal microvasculature in vivo. *Eur J Pharmacol* 1995;272:169–175.

33. Moore WM, Webber RK, Jerome GM, Tjoeng FS, Misko TP, Currie MG. L-N6-(1-iminoethyl)lysine: a selective inhibitor of inducible nitric oxide synthase. *J Med Chem* 1994;37:3886–3888.

34. Ruetten H, Southan GJ, Abate A, Thiemermann C. Attenuation of endotoxin-induced multiple organ dysfunction by 1-amino-2-hydroxyguanidine, a potent inhibitor of inducible nitric oxide synthase. *Br J Pharmacol* 1995;118:261–270.

35. Garvey EP, Oplinger JA, Furfine ES, et al. 1400W is a slow, tight binding, and highly selective inhibitor of inducible nitric oxide synthase in vitro and in vivo. *J Biol Chem* 1997;272:4959–4963.

36. Leone AM, Furst VW, Foxwell NA, Cellek S, Moncada S. Visualisation of nitric oxide generated by activated murine macrophages. *Biochem Biophys Res Commun* 1996;221:37–41.

37. Ignarro LJ. Heme-dependent activation of guanylate cyclase by nitric oxide: a novel signal transduction mechanism. *Blood Vessels* 1991;28: 67–73.

38. Lepoivre M, Chanais B, Yapo A, Lemaire G, Thelander L, Tenu JP. Alteration of ribonucleotide reductase activity following induction of the nitrite-generating pathway in adenocarcinoma cells. *J Biol Chem* 1990;265:14143–14149.

39. Drapier JC, Hibbs JB Jr. Differentiation of murine macrophages to express nonspecific cytotoxicity for tumor cells results in L-arginine-dependent inhibition of mitochondrial iron-sulfur enzymes in the macrophage effector cells. *J Immunol* 1988;140:2829–2838.

40. Kanner J, Harel S, Granit R. Nitric oxide, an inhibitor of lipid oxidation by lipoxygenase, cyclooxygenase and hemoglobin. *Lipids* 1992;27:46–49.

41. Clancy RM, Leszczynska-Piziak J, Abramson SB. Nitric oxide, an endothelial cell relaxation factor, inhibits neutrophil superoxide anion production via a direct action on the NADPH oxidase. *J Clin Invest* 1992;90:1116–1121.

42. Salvemini D, Misko TP, Masferrer JL, Seibert K, Currie MG, Needleman P. Nitric oxide activates cyclooxygenase enzymes. *Proc Natl Acad Sci USA* 1993;90:7240–7244.

43. Stadler J, Stefanovic-Racic M, Billiar TR, et al. Articular chondrocytes synthesize nitric oxide in response to cytokines and lipopolysaccharide. *J Immunol* 1991;147:3915–3920.

44. Vane JR, Mitchell JA, Appleton I, et al. Inducible isoforms of cyclooxygenase and nitric oxide synthase in inflammation. *Proc Natl Acad Sci USA* 1994;91:2046–2050.

45. Amin AR, Attur M, Patel RN, et al. Superinduction of cyclooxygenase-2 activity in human osteoarthritis-affected cartilage. *J Clin Invest* 1997;99:1231–1237.

46. Kosonen O, Kankaanranta H, Malo-Ranta U, Ristimäki A, Moilanen E. Inhibition by nitric oxide-releasing compounds of prostacyclin production in human endothelial cells. *Br J Pharmacol* 1998;125:247–254.

47. Lander HM, Ogiste JS, Pearce SFA, Levi R, Novogrodsky A. Nitric oxide-stimulated guanine nucleotide exchange on p21ras. *J Biol Chem* 1995;270:7017–7020.

48. Pilz RB, Suhasini M, Idriss S, Meinkoth JL, Boss GR. Nitric oxide

49. Deakin AM, Payne AN, Whittle BJR. The modulation of IL-6 TNF-alpha release by nitric oxide following stimulation of J774 cells with LPS and IFN-gamma. *Cytokine* 1995;7:408–416.

50. Gryglewski RJ, Palmer RMJ, Moncada S. Superoxide anion is involved in the breakdown of endothelium-derived vascular relaxing factor. *Nature Lond* 1986;320:454–456.

51. Beckman JS, Beckman TW, Chen J, Marshall PA, Freeman BA. Apparent hydroxyl radical production by peroxynitrite: implications for endothelial injury from nitric oxide and superoxide. *Proc Natl Acad Sci USA* 1990;87:1620–1624.

52. Rachmilewitz D, Stamler JS, Karmeli F, et al. Peroxynitrite-induced rat colitis—a new model of colonic inflammation. *Gastroenterology* 1993;105:1681–1688.

53. Kaur H, Halliwell B. Evidence for nitric oxide-mediated oxidative damage in chronic inflammation. Nitrotyrosine in serum and synovial fluid from rheumatoid patients. *FEBS Lett* 1994;350:9–12.

54. Miller MJ, Thompson JH, Zhang XJ, et al. Role of inducible nitric oxide synthase expression and peroxynitrite formation in guinea pig ileitis. *Gastroenterology* 1995;109:1475–1483.

55. Kooy NW, Royall JA, Ye YZ, Kelly DR, Beckman JS. Evidence for in vivo peroxynitrite production in human acute lung injury. *Am J Respir Crit Care Med* 1995;151:1250–1254.

56. Szabo C, Salzman AL, Ichiropoulos H. Endotoxin triggers the expression of an inducible isoform of nitric oxide synthase and the formation of peroxynitrite in the rat aorta in vivo. *FEBS Lett* 1995;363: 235–238.

57. Kimura H, Hokari R, Miura S, et al. Increased expression of an inducible isoform of nitric oxide synthase and the formation of peroxynitrite in colonic mucosa of patients with active ulcerative colitis. *Gut* 1998;42:180–187.

58. Laszlo F, Whittle BJR, Moncada S. Interactions of constitutive nitric oxide with PAF and thromboxane on rat intestinal vascular integrity in acute endotoxaemia. *Br J Pharmacol* 1994;113:1131–1165.

59. Laszlo F, Whittle BJ, Evans SM, Moncada S. Association of microvascular leakage with induction of nitric oxide synthase: effects of nitric oxide synthase inhibitors in various organs. *Eur J Pharmacol* 1995;283:47–53.

60. Boughton-Smith NK, Evans SM, Laszlo F, Whittle BJR, Moncada S. The induction of nitric oxide synthase and intestinal vascular permeability by endotoxin in the rat. *Br J Pharmacol* 1993;10:1189–1195.

61. Salvemini D, Masini E, Anggard E, Mannaioni PF, Vane JR. Synthesis of a nitric oxide-like factor from L-arginine by rat serosal mast cells: stimulation of guanylate cyclase and inhibition of platelet aggregation. *Biochem Biophys Res Commun* 1990;169:596–601.

62. Gaboury JP, Niu XF, Kubes P. Nitric oxide inhibits numerous features of mast cell-induced inflammation. *Circulation* 1996;93:318–326.

63. Fujii E, Irie K, Uchida Y, Tsukahara F, Muraki T. Possible role of nitric oxide in 5-hydroxytryptamine-induced increase in vascular permeability in mouse skin. *Naunyn Schmiedebergs Arch Pharmacol* 1994;350:361–364.

64. Warren JB, Coughlan ML, Williams TJ. Endotoxin-induced vasodilatation in anaesthetized rat skin involves nitric oxide and prostaglandin synthesis. *Br J Pharmacol* 1992;106:953–957.

65. Lippe I Th., Stabentheiner A, Holzer P. Participation of nitric oxide in the mustard oil-induced neurogenic inflammation of the rat paw skin. *Eur J Pharmacol* 1993;232:113–120.

66. Kajekar R, Moore PK, Brain SD. Essential role for nitric oxide in neurogenic inflammation in rat cutaneous microcirculation. Evidence for an endothelium-independent mechanism. *Circ Res* 1995;76:441–447.

67. Hughes SR, Williams TJ, Brain SD. Evidence that endogenous nitric oxide modulates oedema formation induced by substance P. *Eur J Pharmacol* 1990;191:481–484.

68. Ialenti A, Ianaro A, Moncada S, Di Rosa M. Modulation of acute inflammation by endogenous nitric oxide. *Eur J Pharmacol* 1992;211: 177–182.

69. Teixeira MM, Williams TJ, Hellewell PG. Role of prostaglandins and nitric oxide in acute inflammatory reactions in guinea-pig skin. *Br J Pharmacol* 1993;110:1515–1521.

70. Salvemini D, Wang ZQ, Wyatt PS, et al. Nitric oxide: a key mediator in the early and late phase of carrageenan-induced rat paw inflammation. *Br J Pharmacol* 1996;118:829–888.

71. Salvemini D, Wang ZQ, Bourdon DM, Stern MK, Currie MG, Man-

ning PT. Evidence of peroxynitrite involvement in the carrageenan-induced rat paw edema. *Eur J Pharmacol* 1996;303:217–220.

72. Laszlo F, Whittle BJR. Actions of isoform-selective and non-selective nitric oxide synthase inhibitors on endotoxin-induced vascular leakage in rat colon. *Eur J Pharmacol* 1997;334:99–102.

73. Kubes P, Suzuki M, Granger DN. Nitric oxide: an endogenous modulator of leukocyte adhesion. *Proc Natl Acad Sci USA* 1991;88:4651–4655.

74. Moilanen E, Vuorinen P, Kankaanranta H, Metsä-Ketelä T, Vapaatalo H. Inhibition by nitric oxide donors of human polymorphonuclear leukocyte functions. *Br J Pharmacol* 1993;109:852–858.

75. Moilanen E, Vapaatalo H. Nitric oxide in inflammation and immune response. *Ann Med* 1995;27:359–367.

76. Lefer DJ, Nakanishi K, Johnston WE, Vinten-Johansen J. Antineutrophil and myocardial protecting actions of a novel nitric oxide donor after acute myocardial ischemia and reperfusion of dogs. *Circulation* 1993;88:2337–2350.

77. Cartwright JE, Whitley GS, Johnstone AP. Endothelial cell adhesion molecule expression and lymphocyte adhesion to endothelial cells: effect of nitric oxide. *Exp Cell Res* 1997;235:431–434.

78. Kubes P, Kanwar S, Niu X-F, Gaboury JP. Nitric oxide synthesis inhibition induces leukocyte adhesion via superoxide and mast cells. *FASEB J* 1993;7:1293–1299.

79. Gaboury JP, Woodman RC, Granger DN, Reinhardt P, Kubes P. Nitric oxide prevents leukocyte adherence: role of superoxide. *Am J Physiol* 1993;265:H862–867.

80. Takahashi M, Ikeda U, Masuyama J, Funayama H, Kano S, Shimada K. Nitric oxide attenuates adhesion molecule expression in human endothelial cells. *Cytokine* 1996;8:817–821.

81. Tsao PS, Buitrago R, Chan JR, Cooke JP. Fluid flow inhibits endothelial adhesiveness. Nitric oxide and transcriptional regulation of VCAM-1. *Circulation* 1996;94:1682–1689.

82. Armstead VE, Minchenko AG, Schuhl RA, Hayward R, Nossuli TO, Lefer AM. Regulation of P-selectin expression in human endothelial cells by nitric oxide. *Am J Physiol* 1997;273:H740–H746.

83. Leibovich, Polverini PJ, Fong TW, Harlow LA, Koch AE. Production of angiogenic activity by human monocytes requires an L-arginine/nitric oxide-synthase-dependent effector mechanism. *Proc Natl Acad Sci USA* 1994;91:4190–4194.

84. Konturek SJ, Brzozowski T, Majka J, Pytko-Polonczyk J, Stachura J. Inhibition of nitric oxide synthase delays healing of chronic gastric ulcers. *Eur J Pharmacol* 1993;239:215–217.

85. Jenkins DC, Charles IG, Thomsen LL, et al. Roles of nitric oxide in tumor growth. *Proc Natl Acad Sci USA* 1995;92:4392–4396.

86. Hibbs JB Jr, Taintor RR, Vavrin Z, Rachlin EM. Nitric oxide: a cytotoxic activated macrophage effector molecule. *Biochem Biophys Res Commun* 1988;157:87–94.

87. Lorsbach RB, Murphy WJ, Lowenstein CJ, Snyder SH, Russell SW. Expression of the nitric oxide gene in mouse macrophages activated for tumour cell killing. *J Biol Chem* 1993;268:908–913.

88. Cox GW, Melillo G, Chattopadhyay U, Mullet D, Fertel RH, Varesio L. Tumor necrosis factor-alpha-dependent production of reactive nitrogen intermediates mediates IFN- plus IL-2-induced murine macrophage tumoricidal activity. *J Immunol* 1992;149:3290–3296.

89. Croen KD. Evidence for antiviral effect of nitric oxide. Inhibition of herpes. *J Clin Invest* 1993;91:2446–2452.

90. Karupiah G, Xie QW, Buller RM, Nathan C, Duarte C, MacMicking JD. Inhibition of viral replication by interferon-gamma-induced nitric oxide synthase. *Science* 1993;261:1445–1448.

91. Xu W, Charles IG, Liu L, Koni PA, Moncada S, Emson P. Molecular genetic analysis of the duplication of human inducible nitric oxide synthase (NOS2) sequences. *Biochem Biophys Res Commun* 1995;212:466–472.

92. Bloch KD, Wolfram JR, Brown DM, et al. Three members of the nitric oxide synthase II gene family (NOS2A, NOS2B, NOS2C) colocalize to human chromosome 17. *Genomics* 1995;27:526–530.

93. Bermudez LE. Differential mechanisms of intracellular killing of mycobacterium avium and listeria monocytogenes by activated human and murine macrophages. The role of nitric oxide. *Clin Exp Immunol* 1993;91:277–281.

94. Schneemann M, Schoedon G, Hofer S, Blau N, Guerrero L, Schaffner A. Nitric oxide synthase is not a constituent of the antimicrobial armature of human mononuclear phagocytes. *J Infect Dis* 1993;167:1358–1363.

95. Reiling N, Ulmer AJ, Duchrow M, Ernst M, Flad HD, Hauschildt S. Nitric oxide synthase: mRNA expression of different isoforms in human monocytes/macrophages. *Eur J Immunol* 1994;24:1941–1944.

96. Mossalayi MD, Paul-Eugene N, Ouaaz F, et al. Involvement of FceRII/CD23 and L-arginine-dependent pathway in IgE-mediated stimulation of human monocyte functions. *Int Immunol* 1994;6:931–934.

97. Vouldoukis I, Riveros-Moreno V, Dugas B, et al. The killing of Leishmania major by human macrophages is mediated by nitric oxide induced after ligation of the FceRII/CD23 surface antigen. *Proc Natl Acad Sci USA* 1995;265:C201–C211.

98. Arock M, Le Goff L, Becherel PA, Dugas B, Debre P, Mossalayi MD. Involvement of FceRII/CD23 and L-arginine dependent pathway in IgE-mediated activation of human eosinophils. *Biochem Biophys Res Commun* 1994;203:265–271.

99. Ouaaz F, Sola B, Issaly F, et al. Growth arrest and terminal differentiation of leukemic myelomonocytic cells induced through ligation of surface CD23 antigen. *Blood* 1994;84:3095–3104.

100. Becherel PA, Mossalayi MD, Ouaaz F, et al. Involvement of cyclic AMP and nitric oxide in immunoglobulin E-dependent activation of FceRII/CD23+ normal human keratinocytes. *J Clin Invest* 1994;93:2275–2279.

101. Bukrinsky MI, Nottet HSLM, Schmidtmayerova H, et al. Regulation of nitric oxide synthase activity in human immunodeficiency virus type 1 (HIV-1)-infected monocytes: implications for HIV-associated neurological disease. *J Exp Med* 1995;181:735–745.

102. Denis M. Tumor necrosis factor and granulocyte macrophage colony stimulating factor stimulate human macrophages to restrict growth of virulent Mycobacterium avium and to kill avirulent *M. avium*: killing effector mechanism depends on the generation of reactive nitrogen intermediates. *J Leukoc Biol* 1991;49:380–387.

103. De Maria R, Cifone MG, Trotta R, et al. Triggering of human monocyte activation through CD69, a member of the natural killer cell gene complex family of signal transducing receptors. *J Exp Med* 1994;180:1999–2004.

104. Sharara AI, Perkins DJ, Misukonis MA, Chan SU, Dominitz JA, Weinberg JB. Interferon (IFN)-α activation of human blood mononuclear cells *in vitro* and *in vivo* for nitric oxide synthase (NOS) type 2 mRNA and protein expression: possible relationship of induced NOS2 to the anti-hepatitis C effects of IFN-α *in vivo*. *J Exp Med* 1997;186:1495–1502.

105. Thomsen LL, Miles DW, Happerfield L, Bobrow LG, Knowles RG, Moncada S. Nitric oxide synthase activity in human breast cancer. *Br J Cancer* 1995;72:41–44.

106. Moilanen E, Moilanen T, Knowles R, et al. Nitric oxide synthase is expressed in human macrophages during foreign body inflammation. *Am J Pathol* 1997;150:881–887.

107. Anstey NM, Weinberg JB, Hassanali MY, et al. Nitric oxide in Tanzanian children with malaria: inverse relationship between malaria severity and nitric oxide production/nitric oxide synthase type 2 expression. *J Exp Med* 1996;184:557–567.

108. Kun JFJ, Mordmüller B, Lell B, Lehman LG, Luckner D, Kremsner PG. Polymorphism in promoter region of inducible nitric oxide synthase gene and protection against malaria. *Lancet* 1998;357:265–266.

109. Taylor-Robinson AW, Liew FY, Severn A, et al. Regulation of the immune response by nitric oxide differentially produced by T-helper type-1 and T-helper type-2 cells. *Eur J Immunol* 1994;24:980–984.

110. Albina JE, Henry WL. Suppression of lymphocyte proliferation through the nitric oxide synthesizing pathway. *J Surg Res* 1991;50:403–409.

111. Mills CD. Molecular basis of "suppressor" macrophages: arginine metabolism via the nitric oxide synthase pathway. *J Immunol* 1991;146:2719–2723.

112. Lejuine P, Lagadec P, Onier N, Pinard D, Ohshima H, Jeannin JF. Nitric oxide involvement in tumour-induced immunosuppression. *J Immunol* 1994;152:5077–5083.

113. Sternberg J, McGuigan F. Nitric oxide mediates suppression of T cell responses in murine *Trypanosoma brucei* infection. *Eur J Immunol* 1992;22:2741–2744.

114. Schleifer KW, Mansfield JM. Suppressor macrophages in African trypanosomiasis inhibit T cell proliferative responses by nitric oxide and prostaglandins. *J Immunol* 1993;151:5492–5503.

115. Merryman PF, Clancy RM, He XY, Abramson SB. Modulation of human T cell responses by nitric oxide and its derivative, S-nitrosoglutathione. *Arthritis Rheum* 1993;36:1414–1422.

116. Kosonen O, Kankaanranta H, Vuorinen P, Moilanen E. Inhibition of human lymphocyte proliferation by nitric oxide-releasing oxatriazole derivatives. *Eur J Pharmacol* 1997;337:55–61.

117. Vuorinen P. Exogenous modification of nitrovasodilator-induced cyclic GMP formation in human lymphocytes. *Pharmacol Toxicol* 1992;70: 463–467.

118. Kosonen O, Kankaanranta H, Lähde M, Vuorinen P, Ylitalo P, Moilanen E. Nitric oxide-releasing oxatriazole derivatives inhibit human lymphocyte proliferation by a cyclic GMP-dependent mechanism. *J Pharmacol Exp Ther* 1998;286:215–220.

119. Huot AE, Moore AL, Roberts JD, Hacker MP. Nitric oxide modulates lymphocyte proliferation but not secretion of IL-2. *Immunol Invest* 1993;22:319–327.

120. Kwon NS, Stuehr DJ, Nathan CF. Inhibition of tumor cell ribonucleotide reductase by macrophage-derived nitric oxide. *J Exp Med* 1991; 174:761–767.

121. Sicher SC, Vazquez MA, Lu CY. Inhibition of macrophage Ia expression by nitric oxide. *J Immunol* 1994;153:1293–1300.

122. Lander HM, Sehajpal P, Levine DM, Novogrodsky A. Activation of human mononuclear cells by nitric oxide-generating compounds. *J Immunol* 1993;150:1509–1516.

123. Lander HM, Sehajpal PK, Novogrodsky A. Nitric oxide signalling: a possible role for G proteins. *J Immunol* 1993;151:7182–7187.

124. Mannick JB, Asano K, Izumi K, Kieff E, Stamler JS. Nitric oxide produced by human B lymphocytes inhibits apoptosis and Epstein-Barr virus reactivation. *Cell* 1994;79:1137–1146.

125. McCall TB, Boughton-Smith NK, Palmer RMJ, Whittle BJR, Moncada S. Synthesis of nitric oxide from L-arginine by neutrophils. *Biochem J* 1989;261:293–296.

126. McCall TB, Feelisch M, Palmer RMJ, Moncada S. Identification of N-iminoethyl-L-ornithine as an irreversible inhibitor of nitric oxide synthase in phagocytic cells. *Br J Pharmacol* 1991;102:234–238.

127. McCall TB, Palmer RMJ, Moncada S. Induction of nitric oxide synthase in rat peritoneal neutrophils and its inhibition by dexamethasone. *Eur J Immunol* 1991;21:2523–2527.

128. Salvemini D, de Nucci G, Gryglewski RJ, Vane JR. Human neutrophils and mononuclear cells inhibit platelet aggregation by releasing a nitric oxide-like factor. *Proc Natl Acad Sci USA* 1989;86:6328–6332.

129. Nicolini FA, Wilson AC, Mehta P, Mehta JL. Comparative platelet inhibitory effects of human neutrophils and lymphocytes. *J Lab Clin Med* 1990;116:147–152.

130. Faint RW, Mackie IJ, Machin SJ. Platelet aggregation is inhibited by a nitric oxide-like factor released from human neutrophils in vitro. *Br J Haematol* 1991;77:539–545.

131. Schmidt HHW, Seifert R, Böhme E. Formation and release of nitric oxide from human neutrophils and HL-60 cells induced by a chemotactic peptide, platelet activating factor and leukotriene B4. *FEBS Lett* 1989;244:357–360.

132. Goode HF, Webster NR, Howdle PD, Walker BE. Nitric oxide production by human peripheral blood polymorphonuclear leucocytes. *Clin Sci* 1994;86:411–415.

133. Lärfars G, Gyllenhammar H. Measurement of methemoglobin formation from oxyhemoglobin. A real-time, continuous assay of nitric oxide release by human polymorphonuclear leukocytes. *J Immunol Methods* 1995;184:53–62.

134. Wyatt TA, Lincoln TM, Pryzwansky KB. Vimentin is transiently co-localized with and phosphorylated by cyclic GMP-dependent protein kinase in formyl-peptide-stimulated neutrophils. *J Biol Chem* 1991; 266:21274–21280.

135. Sato EF, Utsumi K, Inoue M. Human oral neutrophils: isolation and characterization. *Methods Enzymol* 1996;268:503–509.

136. Carreras MC, Pargament GA, Catz SD, Poderoso JJ, Boveris A. Kinetics of nitric oxide and hydrogen peroxide production and formation of peroxynitrite during the respiratory burst of human neutrophils. *FEBS Lett* 1994;341:65–68.

137. Carmichael AJ, Steel-Goodwin L, Gray B, Arroyo CM. Nitric oxide interaction with lactoferrin and its production by macrophage cells studied by EPR and spin trapping. *Free Radicals Res Commun* 1993; 19:s201.

138. Wright CD, Mulsch A, Busse R, Osswald H. Generation of nitric oxide by human neutrophils. *Biochem Biophys Res Commun* 1989; 160:813–819.

139. Ney P, Schröder H, Schrör K. Nitrovasodilator-induced inhibition of LTB4 release from human PMN may be mediated by cyclic GMP. *Eicosanoids* 1990;3:243–245.

140. Schröder H, Ney P, Woditsch I, Schrör K. Cyclic GMP mediates SIN-1-induced inhibition of human polymorphonuclear leukocytes. *Eur J Pharmacol* 1990;182:211–218.

141. Darius H, Grodzinska L, Meyer J. The effects of nitric oxide donors molsidomine and SIN-1 on human polymorphonuclear leukocyte function *in vitro* and *ex vivo. Eur J Clin Pharmacol* 1992;43:629–633.

142. Siminiak T, Zozulinska D, Wysocki H. Inhibition of polymorphonuclear neutrophil function by nitric oxide donor SIN-1 *in vitro*: relationship to the presence of platelets. *Pharmacol Commun* 1992;2:217–224.

143. Pieper GM, Clarke GA, Gross GJ. Stimulatory and inhibitory action of nitric oxide donor agents vs. nitrovasodilators on reactive oxygen production by isolated polymorphonuclear leukocytes. *J Pharmacol Exp Ther* 1994;269:451–456.

144. Belenky SN, Robbins RA, Rennard SI, Glossman GL, Nelson KJ, Rubinstein I. Inhibitors of nitric oxide synthase attenuate human neutrophil chemotaxis *in vitro. J Lab Clin Med* 1993;122:388–394.

145. Wyatt TA, Lincoln TM, Pryzwansky KB. Regulation of human neutrophil degranulation by LY-83583 and L-arginine: role of cGMP-dependent protein kinase. *Am J Physiol* 1993;265:C201–211.

146. Riesco A, Caramelo C, Blum G, et al. Nitric oxide-generating system as an autocrine mechanism in human polymorphonuclear leucocytes. *Biochem J* 1993;292:791–796.

147. Van Dervort AL, Yan L, Madara PJ, et al. Nitric oxide regulates endotoxin-induced TNFα production by human neutrophils. *J Immunol* 1994;152:4102–4109.

148. Pryor WA, Squadrito GL. The chemistry of peroxynitrite: a product from the reaction of nitric oxide with superoxide. *Am J Phys* 1995; 268:L699–L722.

149. Clancy RM, Leszczynska-Piziak J, Abramson SB. Nitric oxide stimulates the ADP-ribosylation of actin in human neutrophils. *Biochem Biophys Res Commun* 1993;191:847–852.

150. Farrell AJ, Blake D, Palmer RMJ, Moncada S. Increased concentrations of nitrite in synovial fluid and serum samples suggest increased nitric oxide synthesis in rheumatic diseases. *Ann Rheum Dis* 1992;51: 1219–1222.

151. Hilliquin P, Borderie D, Hernvann A, Menkes CJ, Ekindjian OG. Nitric oxide as S-nitroproteins in rheumatoid arthritis. *Arthritis Rheum* 1997;40:1512–1517.

152. Wigand R, Meyer J, Busse R, Hecker M. Increased serum N-hydroxy-L-arginine in patients with rheumatoid arthritis and systemic lupus erythematosus as an index of an increased nitric oxide synthase activity. *Ann Rheum Dis* 1997;56:330–332.

153. Stichtenoth DO, Fauler J, Zeidler H, Frölich JC. Urinary nitrate excretion is increased in patients with rheumatoid arthritis and reduced by prednisolone. *Ann Rheum Dis* 1995;54:820–824.

154. Grabowski PS, England AJ, Dykhuizen R, et al. Elevated nitric oxide production in rheumatoid arthritis. *Arthritis Rheum* 1996;39: 643–647.

155. Weinberg JB, Granger DL, Pisetsky DS, et al. The role of nitric oxide in the pathogenesis of spontaneous murine autoimmune disease: increased nitric oxide production and nitric oxide synthase expression in MRL-*lpr/lpr* mice, and reduction of spontaneous glomerulonephritis and arthritis by orally administered N-monomethyl-L-arginine. *J Exp Med* 1994;179:651–660.

156. Stefanovic-Racic M, Meyers K, Meschter C, Coffey JW, Hoffman RA, Evans CH. N-monomethyl arginine, an inhibitor of nitric oxide synthase, suppresses the development of adjuvant arthritis in rats. *Arthritis Rheum* 1994;37:1062–1069.

157. Stichtenoth DO, Gutzki FM, Tsikas D, et al. Increased urinary nitrate excretion in rats with adjuvant arthritis. *Ann Rheum Dis* 1994;53: 547–549.

158. McCartney-Francis N, Allen JB, Mizel DE, et al. Suppression of arthritis by an inhibitor of nitric oxide synthase. *J Exp Med* 1993;178: 749–754.

159. Palmer RMJ, Andrews T, Foxwell NA, Moncada S. Glucocorticoids do not affect the induction of a novel calcium-dependent nitric oxide synthase in rabbit chondrocytes. *Biochem Biophys Res Commun* 1992; 188:209–215.

160. Järvinen TAH, Moilanen T, Jarvinen TLN, Moilanen E. Nitric oxide mediates interleukin-1 induced inhibition of glycosaminoglycan synthesis in rat articular cartilage. *Mediators Inflammation* 1995;4: 107–111.

161. Taskiran D, Stefanovic-Racic M, Georgescu H, Evans C. Nitric oxide mediates suppression of cartilage proteoglycan synthesis by interleukin-1. *Biochem Biophys Res Commun* 1994;200:142–148.

162. Kondo S, Ishiguro N, Iwata H, Nakashima I, Isobe K. The effects of nitric oxide on chondrocytes and lymphocytes. *Biochem Biophys Res Commun* 1993;197:1431–1437.

163. Palmer RA, Hickery MS, Charles IG, Moncada S, Bayliss MT. Induction of nitric oxide synthase in human chondrocytes. *Biochem Biophys Res Commun* 1993;193:398–405.

164. Charles IG, Palmer RMJ, Hickery MS, et al. Cloning, characterization, and expression of a cDNA encoding an inducible nitric oxide synthase from the human chondrocyte. *Proc Natl Acad Sci USA* 1993; 90:11419–11423.

165. Rediske JJ, Koehne CF, Zhang B, Lotz M. The inducible production of nitric oxide by articular cell types. *Osteoarthritis Cartilage* 1994;2: 199–206.

166. Maier R, Bilbe G, Rediske J, Lotz M. Inducible nitric oxide synthase from human articular chondrocytes—cDNA cloning and analysis of mRNA expression. *Biochim Biophys Acta (Protein Structure and Molecular Enzymology)* 1994;1208:145–150.

167. Geng Y, Maier R, Lotz M. Tyrosine kinases are involved with the expression of inducible nitric oxide synthase in human articular chondrocytes. *J Cell Physiol* 1995;163:545–554.

168. Geng Y, Lotz M. Increased intracellular Ca^{2+} selectively suppresses IL-1-induced NO production by reducing iNOS mRNA stability. *J Cell Biol* 1995;129:1651–1657.

169. Sakurai H, Kohsaka H, Liu M-F, et al. Nitric oxide production and inducible nitric oxide synthase expression in inflammatory arthritides. *J Clin Invest* 1995;96:2357–2363.

170. Amin AR, Di Cesare PE, Vyas P, et al. The expression and regulation of nitric oxide synthase in human osteoarthritis-affected chondrocytes: evidence for up-regulated neuronal nitric oxide synthase. *J Exp Med* 1995;182:2097–2102.

171. McInnes IB, Leung BP, Field M, et al. Production of nitric oxide in the synovial membrane of rheumatoid and osteoarthritis patients. *J Exp Med* 1996;184:1519–1524.

172. Konttinen YT, Platts LAM, Tuominen S, et al. Role of nitric oxide in Sjögren's syndrome. *Arthritis Rheum* 1997;40:875–883.

173. Murrell GA, Jang D, Williams RJ. Nitric oxide activates metalloprotease enzymes in articular cartilage. *Biochem Biophys Res Commun* 1995;206:15–21.

174. Blanco FJ, Ochs RL, Schwarz H, Lotz M. Chondrocyte apoptosis induced by nitric oxide. *Am J Pathol* 1995;146:75–85.

175. Brandi ML, Hukkanen M, Umeda T, et al. Bidirectional regulation of osteoclast function by nitric oxide synthase isoforms. *Proc Natl Acad Sci USA* 1995;92:2954–2958.

176. Ralston SH, Ho LP, Helfrich MH, Grabowski PS, Johnston PW, Benjamin N. Nitric oxide: a cytokine-induced regulator of bone resorption. *J Bone Miner Res* 1995;10:1040–1049.

177. Ialenti A, Moncada S, Di Rosa M. Modulation of adjuvant arthritis by endogenous nitric oxide. *Br J Pharmacol* 1993;110:701–706.

178. Oyanagui Y. Nitric oxide and superoxide radical are involved in both initiation and development of adjuvant arthritis in rats. *Life Sci* 1994; 54:PL 285–289.

179. Connor JR, Manning PT, Settle SL, et al. Suppression of adjuvant-induced arthritis by selective inhibition of inducible nitric oxide synthase. *Eur J Pharmacol* 1995;273:15–24.

180. de Mello SB, Novaes GS, Laurindo JM, Muscara MN, Maciel FM, Cossermelli W. Nitric oxide synthase inhibitor influences prostaglandin and interleukin-1 production in experimental arthritic joints. *Inflamm Res* 1997;46:72–77.

181. Alving K, Weitzberg E, Lundberg JM. Increased amounts of nitric oxide in exhaled air of asthmatics. *Eur Respir J* 1993;6:1268–1302.

182. Persson MG, Zetterström O, Agrenius V, Ihre E, Gustafsson LE. Single-breath nitric oxide measurements in asthmatic patients and smokers. *Lancet* 1994;343:146–147.

183. Kharitonov S, Yates D, Robbins RA, Logan-Sinclair R, Shinebourne EA, Barnes PJ. Increased nitric oxide in exhaled air of asthmatic patients. *Lancet* 1994;343:133–135.

184. Kharitonov S, Yates DH, Barnes PJ. Inhaled glucocorticoids decrease nitric oxide in exhaled air of asthmatic patients. *Am J Respir Crit Care Med* 1996;153:454–457.

185. Kharitonov SA, Yates DH, Chung KF, Barnes PJ. Changes in the dose of inhaled steroid affect exhaled nitric oxide levels in asthmatic patients. *Eur Respir J* 1996;9:196–201.

186. Massaro AF, Gaston B, Kita D, Fanta C, Stamler JS, Drazen JM. Expired nitric oxide levels during treatment of acute asthma. *Am J Respir Crit Care Med* 1995;152:800–803.

187. Artlich A, Hagenah J-U, Jonas S, Ahrens P, Gortner L. Exhaled nitric oxide in childhood asthma. *Eur J Pediatr* 1996;155:698–701.

188. Nelson BV, Sears S, Woods J, et al. Expired nitric oxide as a marker for childhood asthma. *J Pediatr* 1997;130:423–427.

189. Kharitonov SA, O'Connor BJ, Evans DJ, Barnes PJ. Allergen-induced late asthmatic reactions are associated with elevation of exhaled nitric oxide. *Am J Respir Crit Care Med* 1995;151:1894–1899.

190. Kharitonov S, Yates D, Barnes PJ. Increased nitric oxide in exhaled air of normal human subjects with upper respiratory tract infections. *Eur Respir J* 1995;8:295–297.

191. Kharitonov SA, Wells AU, O'Connor BJ, Hansell DM, Cole PJ, Barnes PJ. Elevated levels of exhaled nitric oxide in bronchiectasis. *Am J Respir Crit Care Med* 1995;151:1889–1893.

192. Martin U, Bryden K, Devoy M, Howarth P. Increased levels of exhaled nitric oxide during nasal and oral breathing in subjects with seasonal rhinitis. *J Allergy Clin Immunol* 1996;97:768–772.

193. Söderman C, Leone A, Furst V, Persson MG. Endogenous nitric oxide in exhaled air from patients with liver cirrhosis. *Scand J Gastroenterol* 1997;32:591–597.

194. Kharitonov S, Barnes PJ. Nasal contribution to exhaled nitric oxide during exhalation against resistance or during breath holding. *Thorax* 1997;52:540–544.

195. Kharitonov S, Alving K, Barnes PJ. Exhaled and nasal nitric oxide measurements: recommendations. *Eur Respir J* 1997;10:1683–1693.

196. Kanazawa H, Shoji S, Yamada M, et al. Increased levels of nitric oxide derivatives in induced sputum in patients with asthma. *J Allergy Clin Immunol* 1997;99:624–629.

197. Hamid Q, Springall DR, Riveros-Moreno V, et al. Induction of nitric oxide synthase in asthma. *Lancet* 1993;342:1510–1513.

198. Robbins RA, Barnes PJ, Springall DR, et al. Expression of inducible nitric oxide in human lung epithelial cells. *Biochem Biophys Res Commun* 1994;203:209–218.

199. Asano K, Chee CB, Gaston B, et al. Constitutive and inducible nitric oxide synthase gene expression, regulation, and activity in human lung epithelial cells. *Proc Natl Acad Sci USA* 1994;91:10089–10093.

200. Guo FH, De Raeve HR, Rice TW, Stuehr DJ, Thunnissen FBJM, Erzurum SC. Continuous nitric oxide synthesis by inducible nitric oxide synthase in normal human airway epithelium *in vivo*. *Proc Natl Acad Sci USA* 1995;92:7809–7813.

201. Kobzik L, Bredt DS, Lowenstein CJ, et al. Nitric oxide synthase in human and rat lung: immunocytochemical and histochemical localization. *Am J Respir Cell Mol Biol* 1993;9:371–377.

202. del Pozo V, de Arruza-Chaves E, de Andres B, et al. Eosinophils transcribe and translate messenger RNA for inducible nitric oxide synthase. *J Immunol* 1997;158:859–864.

203. Kuo HP, Liu S, Barnes PJ. The effect of endogenous nitric oxide on neurogenic plasma exudation in guinea pig airways. *Eur J Pharmacol* 1992;221:385–388.

204. Bernareggi M, Mitchell JA, Barnes PJ, Belvisi MG. Dual action of nitric oxide on airway plasma leakage. *Am J Respir Crit Care Med* 1997;155:869–874.

205. Barnes PJ, Liew FY. Nitric oxide and asthmatic inflammation. *Immunology Today* 1995;16:128–130.

206. Belvisi MG, Stretton CD, Barnes PJ. Nitric oxide is the endogenous neurotransmitter of bronchodilator nerves in human airways. *Eur J Pharmacol* 1992;210:221–222.

207. Ricciardolo FLM, Geppetti P, Mistretta A, et al. Randomised double-blind placebo-controlled study of the effect of inhibition of nitric oxide synthesis in bradykinin-induced asthma. *Lancet* 1996;348:374–377.

208. Högman M, Frostell CG, Hedenström H, Hedenstierna G. Inhalation of nitric oxide modulates adult human bronchial tone. *Am Rev Respir Dis* 1993;148:1474–1478.

209. Kacmarek RM, Ripple R, Cockrill BA, Bloch KJ, Zapol WM, Johnson DC. Inhaled nitric oxide. A bronchodilator in mild asthmatics with methacholine-induced bronchospasm. *Am J Respir Crit Care Med* 1996;153:128–135.

210. Tepperman BL, Brown JF, Whittle BJR. Nitric oxide synthase induction and intestinal epithelial cell viability in rats. *Am J Physiol* 1993;265:G214–G218.

211. Tepperman BL, Brown JF, Korolkiewicz R, Whittle BJ. Nitric oxide synthase activity, viability and cyclic GMP levels in rat colonic epithelial cells: effect of endotoxin challenge. *J Pharmacol Exp Ther* 1994; 271:1477–1482.

212. Alican I, Kubes P. A critical role for nitric oxide in intestinal barrier function and dysfunction. *Am J Physiol* 1996;270:G225–G237.

213. Whittle BJR. Nitric oxide in gastrointestinal physiology and pathology. In: Johnson LR, ed. *Physiology of the gastrointestinal tract,* 3rd ed. New York: Raven Press, 1994:267–294.

214. Miller MJS, Sadowska-Krowicka H, Chotinaruemol S, Kakkis JL, Clark DA. Amelioration of chronic ileitis by nitric oxide synthase inhibition. *J Pharmacol Exp Ther* 1993;264:11–16.

215. Rachmilewitz D, Karmeli F, Okon E. Sulfhydryl blocker-induced rat colonic inflammation is ameliorated by inhibition of nitric oxide synthase. *Gastroenterology* 1995;109:98–106.

216. Grisham MB, Specian RD, Zimmerman TE. Effects of nitric oxide synthase inhibition on the pathophysiology observed in a model of chronic granulomatous colitis. *Pharmacol Exp Ther* 1994;271:1114–1121.

217. Aiko S, Grisham MB. Spontaneous intestinal inflammation and nitric oxide metabolism in HLA-B27 transgenic rats. *Gastroenterology* 1995;109:142–150.

218. Ribbons KA, Zhang XJ, Thompson JH, et al. Potential role of nitric oxide in a model of chronic colitis in rhesus macaques. *Gastroenterology* 1995;108:705–711.

219. Roediger WE, Lawson MJ, Nance SH, Radcliffe BC. Detectable colonic nitrite levels in inflammatory bowel disease—mucosal or bacterial malfunction. *Digestion* 1986;35:199–204.

220. Middleton SJ, Shorthouse M, Hunter JO. Increased nitric oxide synthesis in ulcerative colitis. *Lancet* 1993;341:465–466.

221. Boughton-Smith NK, Evans SM, Hawkey CJ, et al. Nitric oxide synthase activity in ulcerative colitis and Crohn's disease. *Lancet* 1993; 342:338–340.

222. Rachmilewitz D, Stamler JS, Bachwich D, Karmeli F, Ackerman Z, Podolsky DK. Enhanced colonic nitric oxide generation and nitric oxide synthase activity in ulcerative colitis and Crohn's disease. *Gut* 1995;36:718–723.

223. Mourelle M, Casellas F, Guarner F, Salas A, Riveros-Moreno V, Moncada S. Induction of nitric oxide synthase in colonic smooth muscle from patients with toxic megacolon. *Gastroenterology* 1995;109: 1497–1502.

224. Whittle BJR. Nitric oxide—a mediator of inflammation or mucosal defence. *Eur J Gastro Hepatol* 1997;9:1026–1032.

225. Whittle BJR, Laszlo F, Evans SM, Moncada S. Induction of nitric oxide synthase and microvascular injury in the rat jejunum provoked by indomethacin. *Br J Pharmacol* 1995;116:2286–2290.

226. Perez-Perez GI, Shepherd VL, Morrow JD, Blaser MJ. Activation of human THP-1 cells and rat bone marrow-derived macrophages by *Helicobacter pylori* lipopolysaccharide. *Infect Immun* 1995;63: 1183–1187.

227. Lamarque D, Kiss J, Tankovic J, Flejou JF, Delchier J-C, Whittle BJR. Induction of nitric oxide synthase *in vivo* and cell injury in rat duodenal epithelium by a water soluble extract of *Helicobacter pylori. Br J Pharmacol* 1998;123:1073–1078.

228. MacMicking JD, Nathan C, Hom G, et al. Altered responses to bacterial infection and endotoxic shock in mice lacking inducible nitric oxide synthase. *Cell* 1995;81:641–650.

229. Wei X, Charles IG, Smith A, et al. Altered immune responses in mice lacking inducible nitric oxide synthase. *Nature* 1995;375:408–411.

Inflammation: Basic Principles and Clinical Correlates,
3rd ed., edited by John I. Gallin and Ralph Snyderman.
Lippincott Williams & Wilkins, Philadelphia © 1999.

CHAPTER 50

Oxygen-Independent Antimicrobial Systems of Phagocytes

Peter Elsbach, Jerrold Weiss, and Ofer Levy

When the first edition of this book was published less than one decade ago, mammalian antimicrobial peptides and proteins were still viewed as merely a backup for oxygen-dependent antimicrobial host defenses. They have now come to be recognized as an integral part of an effective endogenous antibiotic system. Since the appearance of the second edition in 1992, further progress in the isolation, identification, and structural and functional characterization of antimicrobial peptides and proteins has been very rapid. Among the important new advances and insights are the following:

- The recognition that antimicrobial peptides and proteins have had a role in protecting all living creatures, both prokaryotic and eukaryotic, from the beginning of evolution, often based on common structural and functional features (1–6).
- The application of genetic analysis and manipulation of plants (6,7) and of insects such as *Drosophila* (4) for further dissection of individual roles of members of the antimicrobial arsenal.
- The recognition that the presence of antimicrobial polypeptides is not limited to cells traditionally associated with antimicrobial defense (professional phagocytes) but includes epithelial barriers lining internal and external surfaces (5,8–11).
- The application of the tools of molecular biology for the isolation of new and steadily expanding families of antibiotic peptides and proteins (5,10–12).
- Preliminary evidence that the host's own antimicrobial peptides and proteins may have a place as therapeutic

agents in clinical settings plagued by growing inadequacy of the existing pharmaceutical arsenal of antibiotics.

Each of these advances has reflected or has benefitted progress in the study of the antimicrobial peptides and proteins of mammalian phagocytes, the focus of this review.

Although it is now evident that skin (13), respiratory (10), intestinal (14), and probably all epithelial layers exposed to the external and internal microbial environment are endowed with antimicrobial defenses, these do not provide adequate protection against most common pathogens. Too few or defective circulating phagocytes represent a breach in innate immunity that cannot be filled by current therapeutic means and consequently is associated with unavoidable infections. It is in this context that one should see both the advances and the limits of the knowledge gained during the past 5 years concerning the antimicrobial arsenal of the mammalian phagocyte.

It is now relatively easy to identify by state-of-the-art methods molecules that have their origin in polymorphonuclear cells (PMNs) and other leukocytes and that inhibit bacterial growth as isolated agents under arbitrary *in vitro* conditions. However, a clear contribution of many of these agents to antimicrobial host defense has not yet been established. The extraordinary complexity of the interactive cellular and extracellular networks that make up host responses to microbial invaders implies that the actual role of any single component must be examined in a broad biologic context. Effective antibacterial action depends on the integration of the cellular and extracellular innate immune systems, as illustrated by a study showing that *Escherichia coli* ingested by PMNs are promptly killed only if they are first exposed to nonlethal concentrations of serum containing the membrane attack complex of complement. Without such pretreatment the bacteria, although effectively ingested and growth-arrested, could be rescued, indicating that the PMNs by themselves have a limited

P. Elsbach: Departments of Medicine and Microbiology, New York University School of Medicine, New York, New York 10016.

J. Weiss: Departments of Medicine and Microbiology, University of Iowa College of Medicine, Iowa City, Iowa 52246.

O. Levy: Department of Medicine, The Children's Hospital, Boston, Massachusetts 02115.

destructive capability (15). Such synergy among disparate host systems is also demonstrable among individual antibacterial polypeptides secreted by PMNs *in vivo* in an inflammatory setting (16,17). In contrast, other antimicrobial polypeptides are inhibited by physiologic salt concentration (11,12,18), or by interaction with other proteins in body fluids (19–21). It follows that it has not yet been established which of the many members of the polypeptide arsenal of the phagocyte fulfills a major function in host defense. To determine relative roles is not an easy task. Moreover, if it is reasonable to attribute the growing diversity during evolution of the antimicrobial equipment of the host to the need to match the enormous diversity of potential pathogens in the environment, this may imply that each antimicrobial agent, or combination of agents, is meant for a limited set of targets. Therefore, our choices of laboratory assays and test organisms (22) may not provide appropriate conditions for finding the true biologic role of a given isolated compound. Nevertheless, considerable progress has been made in assigning well-defined antimicrobial functions to several antimicrobial polypeptides that occur as natural constituents in a complex biologic setting.

ANTIMICROBIAL POLYPEPTIDES OF PHAGOCYTES

Because of space limitations and to avoid duplication, this chapter does not provide an exhaustive bibliography. The reader needing a more comprehensive list of literature references (especially of earlier publications) is referred to previous editions of this book and subsequent reviews (11,12,23,24). For purposes of organization, the antibiotic proteins of PMNs are grouped by subcellular localization and discussed in order of increasing size (Table 50-1).

PRIMARY (AZUROPHILIC) GRANULES

Defensins

The primary granules of PMNs of many mammals, including humans, contain a family of abundant 3.5- to 4.5-kd cationic peptides with broad-spectrum cytotoxic activity (11). Named *defensins* by Lehrer et al. (11), these peptides are characterized by a three-disulfide motif (Fig. 50-1) that stabilizes a three-stranded antiparallel β-sheet capable of dimerizατιον (25). Despite distinct spacing and arrangement of disulfide bonds, β defensins are similar in tertiary structure to "classic" or α defensins, possessing a triple-stranded β-sheet with cationic/hydrophobic amphiphilic character (26).

A feature common to most of the granule-associated low-molecular-weight cationic cytotoxic polypeptides of the PMNs, including the defensins and cathelicidins (discussed later), is that they are synthesized as larger, noncytotoxic preforms having little or no net charge. The primary translation products of α defensins are 93- to 95-residue preforms that include an anionic propiece that, until further processing, efficiently suppresses defensin cytotoxicity within the producing cell (27). The net charge properties of the anionic propiece and the cationic mature peptide have coevolved to maintain the charge neutrality of the proform despite wide variation in the degree of cationicity of the mature α defensins. Sites within the anionic propiece also help direct efficient granulocyte-specific subcellular sorting and cleavage to generate the mature cytotoxic peptides that are stored in the granules of differentiated cells (28). Potential toxicity of secreted defensins toward host cells may also be reduced by trapping the defensins within inactive complexes formed with various proteins in serum and other

TABLE 50-1. *Antibiotic proteins of polymorphonuclear leukocytes (PMN)*

Localization	Protein	Molecular weight (kd)	Concentration (μg/10⁶ PMN)	Animals	Activity	References
Primary granule	Defensins	4	~4 H/12 R	H, R, G, Hm, Rt, C	B±, F, EV, m, Mam	11
	Serprocidins	30	1–2.5 (each)	H, C	B±, F, m, Mam	205
	BPI	50–60	1.5	H, R, C	B–	81
Secondary granule	Cathelicidins	11–20 (2–7)[a]	2–3	H, R, M, C[b], S, P	B±, F	9
	Phospholipase	14	0.05–0.5	H, R	B+	151, 159, 206
	Lactoferrin	78	3	H, R	B±, F	207
Primary and secondary granule	Lysozyme	14.5	2	H, E	B+, F	208
Granule (unspecified)	Granulothelins	6.5	~0.005	H, E	B±	49
	Four-disulfide core	7	0.16–0.32	E	B±	209
	C3 (C6 and C7)	185 (110)	? (0.15, 0.06)	H, M	(B–)[c]	195, 210
Cytosol	Calprotectin	14 and 8	5	H, M, P	B±, F	211

BPI, bactericidal/permeability-increasing protein; H, human; R, rabbit; M, mouse; G, guinea pig; Hm, hamster; Rt, rat; E, horse; C, cow; S, sheep; P, pig; B, bacteria (Gram's stain, + and/or –); F, fungi; m, metazoan parasites; Mam, mammalian cells; EV, enveloped viruses.

[a]Most cathelicidins require proteolytic cleavage to generate active microbicidal peptides of 2–7 kd.
[b]Bactenecins are located in the large granules of bovine PMN.
[c]Bactericidal activity of complement requires assembly of the membrane attack complex.

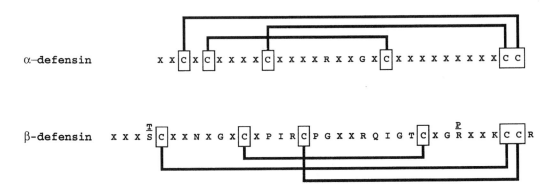

FIG. 50-1. Characteristic covalent structures of α and β defensins. Defensin consensus sequences are shown, using the single-letter amino acid code. Disulfide bonds are shown schematically as solid lines. (Adapted from ref. 204.)

body fluids (11,19–21). Both α and β defensins have been identified within the primary granules of PMNs and in mucosal secretions, but within a single animal species various defensins exhibit an almost nonoverlapping tissue-specific pattern of expression, possibly indicative of tissue-specific functions (11,29). For example, in humans, four α defensins (human neutrophil peptide [HNP] 1 through 4) are found in neutrophils, two different α defensins (HNP-5 and -6) are in small intestinal Paneth cells, and human β defensin-1 is highly expressed in kidney, pancreas, and, to a lesser extent, other epithelial cells. Mucosal β defensins are induced by inflammatory stimuli such as gram-negative bacterial lipopolysaccharides (LPS) (10) and appear to play a role in bactericidal activity of human lung fluid (18). All known human defensin genes are encoded within a cluster of genes on chromosome 8p23, suggesting that these genes evolved from a common precursor. Defensins and defensin-like cysteine-rich peptides are increasingly being recognized as widely-expressed, ancient components of antimicrobial host defenses. This includes α or β defensins in phagocytes and epithelia of many birds and mammals and less related peptides in insects, molluscs, and plants (11).

Defensins are broadly cytotoxic toward bacteria (especially gram-positive bacteria), fungi, metazoan parasites, and mammalian cells (11). Independent microbicidal effects are expressed *in vitro* at micromolar concentrations under hypotonic conditions, but much higher defensin concentrations are needed when physiologic concentrations of salts are present (11,18). However, the ability of particular defensins to act synergistically with another antibacterial PMN protein that exhibits a high degree of cytotoxic specificity for gram-negative bacteria (30)—bactericidal/permeability-increasing protein (BPI; see later discussion)—may permit these defensins to contribute to antibacterial host defense at concentrations that have no independent cytotoxic activity.

Studies with model membranes suggest that after initial electrostatic interactions of these cationic peptides with anionic surface lipids, followed by insertion driven by transmembrane potential, defensins permeabilize membranes in an all-or-none fashion through the formation of multimeric pores (31,32). Differences in effects on model membranes appear to correlate with the ability or inability of particular defensin species to form stable dimers in solution but do not obviously correlate with cytotoxic activity. Resistance of some bacteria to the actions of defensins and other microbicidal proteins has been linked to several genetic loci (33). Some of these loci may modulate defensin action by altering LPS structure, including polysaccharide chain length and the fatty acid composition of the lipid A moiety (34), and thereby altering accessibility to the bacterial target membrane. Involvement of other loci results in such pleiotropic effects that no specific mechanism of resistance can be deduced.

It has been argued that the cytotoxic action of PMN-derived defensins may be limited to the phagolysosome because (a) defensins reside in the primary granules, which release their contents into the phagosome rather than extracellularly (35); (b) microbicidal activity of defensins is limited by ambient divalent cation concentrations present in biologic fluids, which presumably are lower in the phagolysosome; and (c) defensins can be bound and inactivated by various extracellular plasma- or serum-derived proteins, including the cleaved (coagulation cascade) form of α_2-macroglobulin, complement component C1q, and certain serine protease inhibitors (19–21). However, defensins, added in micromolar concentrations, are capable of acting in anticoagulated (citrated) whole blood and plasma *ex vivo* (30) and are released extracellularly during inflammatory responses *in vivo* (36–39), leaving unsettled the extent of their contribution to extracellular microbicidal activity. The ability of defensins to bind to and neutralize the proinflammatory actions of LPS (or "endotoxin") is substantially reduced in the presence of serum, probably reflecting not only formation of defensin-protein complexes but also the relatively low affinity of defensin for LPS, compared with the affinities of LPS-binding protein (LBP) and other LPS-interactive proteins present in body fluids (23).

Defensins have been found to exert additional effects independent of their cytotoxic action. At nanomolar concentrations, defensins are chemoattractive toward T cells (40) and activate the calcium channels of villus enterocytes (41). At micromolar concentrations, these peptides reduce the barrier integrity of epithelial monolayers (42) and stimulate cell growth (43). Defensins can inhibit tissue-type plasminogen activator–mediated fibrinolysis *in vitro,* suggesting a mechanism by which PMNs may maintain a fibrin barrier at sites of infection (44). The ability of defensins to inhibit the action of corticotropin (ACTH) at its receptor (45), which is functionally expressed on leukocytes (46), has prompted some to call these peptides "corticostatins" (47). Detection of defensin NP-3A ("corticostatin I") in rabbit adrenal and pituitary glands (48) lends further credence to the notion that defensins may serve important roles as modulators of the hypophyseal-pituitary-adrenal axis.

PMNs contain other granule-associated cysteine-rich peptides that are distinct from the defensins. Although these peptides are capable of inhibiting the growth of bacteria under hypotonic conditions, they are only weakly antimicrobial and have been shown to serve additional functions with substantially greater potency. For example, the 7-kd equine neutrophil antimicrobial peptide-1 (eNAP-1; 49) is a member of the granulin/epithelin ("granulothelin") family of peptides, which potently modulate epithelial cell growth through binding to high-affinity (nanomolar) surface receptors (50). Another cysteine-rich peptide identified in equine PMNs is eNAP-2, a member of the four-disulfide core protein family, which manifests protease-inhibitory activity toward microbial proteases, including subtilisin (*Bacillus subtilis*) and proteinase K (*Tritirechium album*) (51).

As it has become evident that the defensins and related peptides can express multiple activities, caution must be exercised in focusing mainly on their role in anitimicrobial host defense. Their abundance may well imply important additional biologic functions that also may be different for the intracellular and the extracellular environment.

Lysozyme

Lysozyme, a cationic 14-kd protein found in the primary and secondary granules of PMNs (52) and also in macrophages and multiple mucosal secretions, is an enzyme that acts on substrates including the peptidoglycan polymer (GlcNAc-MurNAc) of bacterial cell walls and the chitin of phytopathogenic fungi (53). Potent independent antimicrobial action of lysozyme is generally limited to nonpathogenic gram-positive bacteria (e.g., *B. subtilis*) and some fungi with susceptible cell walls (54). High-level resistance to lysozyme, exhibited by most other gram-positive bacterial species, reflects more extensive crosslinking and greater complexity of the peptidoglycan matrix, which impedes access of lysozyme to its substrate (55). Gram-negative bacteria are further protected from lysozyme action by the barrier properties of the outer membranes of these microorganisms. Antibacterial synergy between lysozyme and other host-defense systems that disrupt the gram-negative bacterial outer membrane has been well documented in the bacteriolytic action of serum against complement-sensitive gram-negative bacteria (56) but has not been demonstrated to date under physiologic conditions for other PMN granule proteins (57). A variant form of lysozyme bearing an N-terminal hydrophobic peptide has increased bactericidal activity against gram-negative bacteria (58). Because lysozyme toxicity toward some bacteria is independent of muramidase activity, implying noncatalytic membrane-perturbing effects of this cationic protein (59), it remains to be determined whether the increased activity of the lysozyme variant is or is not linked to peptidoglycan degradation.

Multiple gene duplications have expanded the lysozyme gene family, allowing some animals such as cows to express a range of lysozyme isoforms, including tracheal and intestinal forms. In such tissue locations in ruminant animals the enzymes apparently are involved in lysis of rumen bacteria that contribute to fermentation in the foregut (60). The chicken leukocyte lysozyme gene contains a myeloid-specific enhancer that possesses an Erythroblastosis virus Twenty-six Specific (Ets) transcription factor binding site (61) as well as a distant enhancer that confers LPS-inducible expression (62). Although lysozyme can bind to and neutralize LPS in laboratory media (63,64), this activity is substantially reduced in serum, presumably because lysozyme has a lower affinity for LPS than do other LPS-binding lipoproteins in serum.

Although lysozyme was the first antimicrobial protein isolated and its structure and function have been the subject of intense scrutiny, much remains to be learned about its actual contribution to host defense.

Serprocidins

The azurophilic granules of PMNs contain a number of *ser*ine *pro*tease homologues with microbi*cidal* activity, called *serprocidins* (65), including neutrophil elastase, cathepsin G, proteinase-3/myeloblastin (PR-3), and the proteolytically inactive azurocidin/CAP-37/heparin-binding protein (AZU). The serprocidins are proteins of about 30 kd that are homologous to the granzymes of T cells and to mast cell protease (66). Genes encoding serprocidins are clustered on chromosome 19 and are expressed in a coordinated fashion during myelopoiesis (67). Many transcription factors, including CCAAT/enhancer binding protein (C/EBP), myeloblastosis (MYB), and PU.1, act in concert to regulate the neutrophil elastase promoter in ways that direct expression of neutrophil elastase specifically to immature myeloid cells (68). The same transcriptional regulation may control expression of the genes of human AZU and PR-3, which contain closely similar 5′-consensus binding sites (69,70).

The microbicidal activity of the serprocidins toward many pathogens is independent of proteolytic action. This has prompted a search for more limited (noncatalytic) regions of these proteins with antibacterial activity. A number of cathepsin G–derived synthetic peptides have been shown to be cytotoxic for a range of microbial pathogens (71). However, the activity of these peptides provides little insight into the determinants of the activity of full-length cathepsin G because (a) these peptides are orders of magnitude less potent, on a molar basis, than full-length cathepsin G; (b) the antimicrobial spectrum of the peptides differs from that of full-length cathepsin G; and (c) the crystal structure of cathepsin G suggests that several of the peptides are only partially exposed on the surface of the protein, so that their contribution to interaction with microorganisms is difficult to envision without major structural rearrangement on contact (66).

Activated PMNs and monocytes both upregulate serprocidins on their cell surfaces and release the proteins extracellularly (72). The demonstration of surface-active neutrophil elastase and cathepsin G has suggested a function in regulation of catalytic activity and in egress from the circulation into sites of inflammation (73). Examples of the diverse proinflammatory actions of serprocidins include activation and chemoattraction of monocytes by AZU (74), stimulation of acute phase response by α_1-chymotrypsin-cathepsin G complexes (75), and activation of platelet aggregation and degranulation by PR-3 (76). Whereas many other cationic proteins and peptides of PMNs bind to and neutralize LPS, AZU stimulates LPS-induced release of interleukin-6 (IL-6) and tumor necrosis factor-α (TNF-α) from human monocytes under serum-free conditions (77). It remains to be determined whether such enhancement occurs in a serum (LBP-rich) environment and whether it reflects recognition of an AZU-LPS complex or independent interactions of LPS and AZU with respective cellular (monocyte) receptors.

PR-3 is a major antigenic target of anti-neutrophil cytoplasmic antibodies (ANCA) in Wegener's granulomatosis (78). Induction of endothelial cell apoptosis by PR-3 and elastase *in vitro* suggests a mechanism by which release of these serine proteases by neutrophils activated during inflammation, including ANCA-associated vasculitis, may contribute to vascular damage during inflammation (79). PR-3 can also maintain growth of immature myeloid precursors, earning it the name "myeloblastin" (80).

The serprocidins represent yet another family of proteins with antimicrobial activity *in vitro* that clearly perform many other biologic functions that have been incompletely dissected in the complex host environment.

Bactericidal/Permeability-increasing Protein

BPI is a highly cationic, 50- to 55-kd protein remarkable for its potent (nanomolar) and selective cytotoxic activity toward gram-negative bacteria and its high affinity for LPS, unique and prominent components of the outer membrane of these bacteria (81,82). BPI is expressed solely by myeloid precursors of PMNs coincident with primary granule biogenesis (83) but has also been detected on the surfaces of PMNs (84) and monocytes (85). Initial interactions between BPI and target bacteria probably involve electrostatic interactions of basic regions of BPI with acidic moieties clustered near the highly conserved lipid A region of LPS, followed by hydrophobic interactions. Insertion of BPI into model membranes composed of asymmetric LPS/phospholipid bilayers that simulate the lipid organization of the outer membrane has been demonstrated (86). In intact bacteria, these interactions trigger rearrangement of outer membrane lipids (LPS and phospholipids) and displacement of LPS-bound Mg^{2+} and Ca^{2+}, resulting in increased permeability to small, hydrophobic molecules (including β-lactam derivatives) normally excluded by the outer membrane, increased susceptibility of phospholipids to attack by phospholipase A, and bacterial growth inhibition (81). The BPI concentration required to produce these outer envelope–associated alterations is reduced when certain other PMN granule proteins (e.g., defensins NP-1 and -2 and the 15-kd proteins [p15s] of rabbit PMNs) are present (30). This synergy may be operative in intact PMNs during phagocytosis, where initial damage to BPI-sensitive bacteria is very similar to that produced by purified BPI (15,81,87). However, greater synergy (up to 100-fold reduction in BPI concentration requirements) is possible when the molar ratio of p15s and/or defensins to BPI exceeds that present within PMNs. This is observed for the p15s in the extracellular fluid of PMN-rich rabbit peritoneal exudates and accounts in part for the potent BPI-dependent bactericidal activity of this inflammatory fluid (17).

The initial BPI-mediated alterations are potentially reversible; bacterial killing requires impairment of biochemical processes linked to the inner membrane, where much of the cell's energy-generating and biosynthetic machinery resides (81,88). Sublethal BPI effects are accompanied by increased bacterial phospholipid and LPS synthesis, which can be used for membrane repair (24), and discrete changes in protein synthesis (24,89). In the absence of other serum proteins, physiologic concentrations of albumin block progression of BPI-mediated injury from the outer to inner envelope and prevent bacterial killing (88). Nevertheless, nanomolar concentrations of extracellular BPI, resulting from secretion by PMNs in inflammatory exudates or from exogenous administration, confer potent bactericidal activity in biologic fluids against many gram-negative bacteria, including complement- and phagocytosis-resistant encapsulated organisms (17,90). BPI's potency in these settings reflects its ability to act synergistically with other protein constituents of the inflammatory environment; these include, in addition to the p15s, sublethal assemblies of the membrane attack complex of complement and group II phospholipase A_2 (PLA$_2$). Whereas the p15s (and defensins) potentiate the initial, sublethal effects of BPI, complement and PLA$_2$ promote progression of BPI-dependent injury to the bacterial inner envelope and override the inhibitory effects of albumin (90). Similar effects are observed during phagocytosis when precoating of BPI-sensitive bacteria with complement and PLA$_2$ before ingestion leads to greatly enhanced intracellular bacterial destruction (16,90,91).

Binding of BPI to either purified LPS aggregates, released outer membrane fragments (blebs), or intact bacteria potently inhibits the proinflammatory action of endotoxin (81,92,93). Several other granule-derived PMN proteins can bind LPS and modulate endotoxin activity, but these effects are greatly reduced in biologic fluids containing other LPS-interactive molecules (23,63,64,94). In contrast, the endotoxin-neutralizing activity of BPI is fully expressed in plasma, serum, or whole blood *ex vivo* (90), and protective effects of administered BPI (or a bioactive N-terminal fragment of BPI; see later discussion) against a variety of sublethal and lethal LPS and bacterial challenges have been demonstrated *in vivo* (92,95,96). BPI activity is manifested at concentrations present in inflammatory fluids of PMN-rich exudates (17,97); this suggests that released BPI at inflammatory sites could downregulate endotoxin-mediated signaling, both by promoting elimination of bacteria that produce LPS and by inhibiting endotoxin that is already present. These dual protective activities of BPI in biologic fluids have stimulated intense efforts to develop recombinant BPI derivatives for therapeutic application when endogenous defenses and conventional antibiotics are inadequate (17,92,95–97). The closely similar high-affinity binding of BPI to isolated LPS (apparent K_d, approximately 1 to 5 nmol/L) (82,98) from a variety of bacterial species, independent of polysaccharide chain length and structure, is consistent with the view that the highly conserved lipid A region is the principal site of BPI attachment. Increasing polysaccharide chain length of LPS and increasing ambient divalent cation concentrations reduce BPI binding to bacteria but not to isolated LPS, presumably reflecting the greater packing density of LPS in the bacterial envelope (93,99). The presence of capsule has no effect on BPI binding and antibacterial activity (92). BPI can bind to other acidic lipids and polysaccharides (86,100,101), but with lower affinity and uncertain physiologic significance.

BPI is most closely related (about 45% sequence identity) to another LPS-binding protein (LBP), an acute phase secretory product of hepatocytes (86,100–102).

BPI and LBP also exhibit almost 25% sequence identity with two other plasma/lipoprotein-associated lipid-transfer proteins, phospholipid transfer protein (PLTP) and cholesterol ester transfer protein (CETP) (103). BPI, LBP, and PLTP each contain 455 (or 456) amino acids (CETP contains 476 residues), and the human genes encoding BPI, LBP, and PLTP are in close proximity on chromosome 20 (q11.23–q12) (103,104), suggesting a common ancestral origin. Several pieces of biochemical evidence suggest a two-domain organization of BPI and LBP, with the N-terminal domain mediating LPS binding (and antibacterial cytotoxicity in the case of BPI) and the C-terminal domain mediating delivery of LPS or LPS-containing particles to cellular and/or extracellular acceptors (105–109). The bactericidal and endotoxin-neutralizing activities of BPI are fully expressed by an N-terminal fragment of BPI (residues 1–193) (92,106) whereas only holo BPI and not the BPI fragment can opsonize encapsulated bacteria for phagocytosis by PMNs (100). X-ray analysis of the crystal structure of human BPI at a resolution of 2.4 Å has revealed a highly elongated molecule (approximately $135 \times 35 \times 35$ Å) formed by two domains of similar size connected by a proline-rich linker (residues 230–250) (110). The structure is consistent with a requirement for almost the entire N-terminal domain (residues 12–193) to form a stable molecule with full LPS-binding and antibacterial activity (106). The one disulfide that is present (Cys 135–175) is essential for optimal stability and antibacterial function (106,111) and is conserved in LBP, PLTP, and CETP (103). The overall configuration of the N- and C-terminal domains is remarkably similar despite sequence dissimilarity, large charge differences (+17 and −2, respectively), and distinct functions. Conformationally divergent regions in the N-terminal domain map to one end of the protein, where much of the net basicity of BPI is concentrated (110; Fig. 50-2). It is likely that this end of BPI participates in LPS binding and antibacterial activity (100,112), leaving the other end free to interact with potential acceptor molecules (108). Each domain contains a molecule of phosphatidylcholine bound in apolar pockets and at surface sites near the interface of the two domains. Modeling suggests that PLTP, CETP, and especially LBP are likely to display the same overall topologic features as BPI, including the apolar binding pockets. The potential roles of these sites in lipid A binding, lipid transfer, and possibly amphiphilic transitions of BPI occurring during membrane insertion are important questions raised by these findings.

Despite their close similarity in overall structural and functional design, the biologic activities of BPI and LBP are strikingly different: whereas BPI is cytotoxic toward gram-negative bacteria and inhibits endotoxin signaling, LBP is noncytotoxic and greatly enhances the proinflammatory action of low doses of LPS (91,109,113). Membrane and soluble forms of CD14, important components

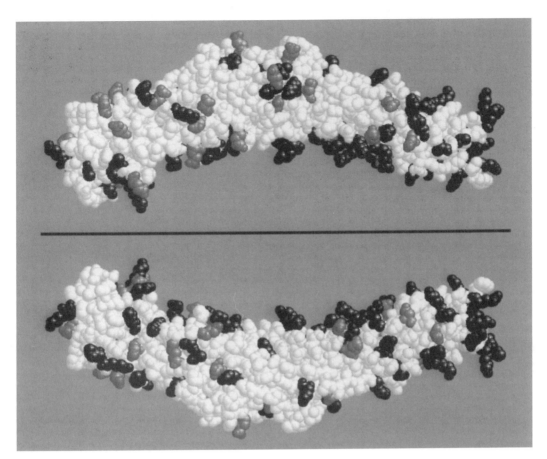

FIG. 50-2. Space-filling model of the structure of bactericidal/permeability-increasing protein (BPI), with basic (*black*) and acidic (*grey*) side chains highlighted to show spatial distribution of charged residues. The N-terminal domain is to the right, the C-terminal domain to the left; the two images represent the protein rotated by 180 degrees to show the front and back faces.

in the LPS-signaling cascade (109), are major targets of LBP-LPS (bacteria) complexes but not of BPI-LPS (bacteria) complexes, apparently explaining the opposing effects of BPI and LBP on endotoxin signaling. The physical properties of BPI-LPS and LBP-LPS complexes are also strikingly different: under the same conditions in which LBP induces LPS disaggregation, thought to be important for LPS signaling (109), BPI apparently inserts into the LPS aggregate and makes it refractory to LBP-induced disaggregation (114). The potent endotoxin-neutralizing activity of BPI in body fluids where LBP is also present is consistent with the much higher affinity of BPI (compared with LBP) for LPS and with the ability of BPI, even at very low (1 : 40) BPI-LPS molar ratios, to block LPS interactions with LBP (114,115).

SECONDARY (SPECIFIC) GRANULES

Cathelicidins

The cloning of an increasing number of mammalian cDNAs encoding the proforms of a family of structurally diverse cationic antimicrobial peptides from various mammalian species has revealed a homologous N-terminal proform domain with sequence similarity (including the positioning of the four cysteines) to the cystatin superfamily of protease inhibitors. Based on the bipartite structure (Fig. 50-3) of an N-terminal cystatin-like proform domain linked to a C-terminal peptide with antimicrobial activity, this novel family of proteins has been termed *cathelicidins* (9,116). Early reports that some of these proforms possessed cysteine protease inhibitory activity were later retracted (117,118), leaving the biologic significance of the homology to cystatins unclear.

Cathelicidins are components of PMNs that reside in membrane-bound compartments prone to extracellular secretion, including the large granules of bovine PMNs (119) and the secondary (specific) granules of human (120), rabbit (83), and mouse (121) PMNs. The detection of cathelicidin mRNA in mouse embryo and in multiple adult tissues may imply a broader range of cell types in which these proteins exist and function (122). Cathelicidins in the PMN granules are stored as 12- to 20-kd inactive proforms that require stimulus-dependent proteolytic cleavage to generate the microbicidal cationic peptide (123,124). Secretion of cathelicidins has been

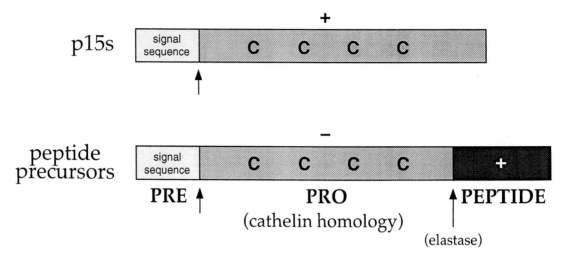

FIG. 50-3. The cathelicidin protein family.

demonstrated *in vivo* (17,125,126), suggesting that these proteins also perform extracellular functions during inflammation. This prediction is supported by the finding that the antimicrobial activity of the cathelicidins, in contrast to that of many other antimicrobial peptides, is fully expressed at physiologic sodium chloride concentrations (30,127), in serum (128), and in inflammatory fluids generated *in vivo* (17). Cathelicidin genes are located on chromosome 3 in humans (129), in a region syntenic to murine chromosome 9 (122), and contain 5'-flanking regions with consensus sequences for the transcription factors NF-κB, NF-IL6, and APRF (129–131). The NF-κB pathway has been demonstrated in mature PMNs (132), providing a possible mechanism by which PMNs at inflammatory sites might continue to transcribe cathelicidin genes (83).

The C-terminal antimicrobial peptides cleaved from the proforms of the cathelicidins are structurally highly diverse. They include linear proline- and arginine-rich peptides such as the bactenecins of bovine PMNs (133), the lysine-rich α-helical peptides derived from rabbit CAP-18 (134), the bovine peptides BMAP-27 and -28 (135), and the tryptophan-rich indolicidin also from cow neutrophils (136). Disulphide-containing cathelicidin peptides include the cyclic dodecapeptide (137) and the two-disulphide protegrins of porcine PMNs (138).

The antimicrobial activity of bactenecins is particularly pronounced toward gram-negative bacteria (133). The protegrins have been reported to be broadly cytotoxic toward both gram-negative and gram-positive bacteria; toward *Chlamydia trachomatis, Mycobacterium tuberculosis, Candida albicans,* and human immunodeficiency virus type-1 (HIV-1); and also toward mammalian cells (128,139). The antibacterial activity of protegrins depends on intact intramolecular disulphide bonds (127).

The p15s of rabbit comprise several closely similar isoforms and are divergent members of the cathelicidin family. These proteins were initially identified and isolated on the basis of their strong binding affinity for the gram-negative bacterial envelope (140). In contrast to the other known members of the cathelicidin family, the p15s apparently do not require proteolytic cleavage to manifest antimicrobial activity (141). The p15s at 0.1 to 1 mol/L are cytotoxic toward *E. coli* in isotonic laboratory media and in biologic fluids, including anticoagulated plasma, whole blood, and inflammatory fluid (17,30). Although much less potent than BPI, p15s can act in synergy with BPI to inhibit gram-negative bacterial viability (17,30) and bacterial induction of TNF-α release in whole blood *ex vivo* (23). This contribution of the p15s to antimicrobial activity is also evident *in vivo* in a model of sterile inflammation elicited in the peritoneal cavity of the rabbit. In this inflammatory site, the p15s are released by the PMNs into the cell-free ascitic fluid and contribute there to anti–gram negative bacterial activity by acting synergistically with BPI, which is also secreted (17). As has been reported for several other cathelicidins, p15s are stored in the secondary granules of PMNs (83), which readily release their contents extracellularly in response to stimuli that trigger degranulation (17).

The biologic activities of at least one cathelicidin-derived peptide, the proline- and arginine-rich PR-39 of porcine PMNs (142), are not limited to its antimicrobial function. Among the additional activities that PR-39 exhibits are the following: (a) acting as a neutrophil-specific chemoattractant (143); (b) inducing expression of cell-surface syndecans that may play important roles in wound healing (125); and (c) inhibiting the respiratory burst oxidase by binding to the cytosolic 47-kd phagocyte oxidase protein (p47-phox) via an SRC-homology domain (144). Apparently, PR-39, in unknown fashion, is capable of gaining access to p47-phox in the cytosolic compartment, because incubation of extracellular PR-39 with PMNs *in vitro* inhibits oxidase function (144). These observations on the diverse bioactivities of this one member of the cathelicidin family should stimulate exploration of a broader range of functions than has so far been recognized for the other members of this family. The function of the cathelicidin cystatin-like proregion is currently unknown. Despite the retraction of reports of anti–cysteine protease activity of cathelicidin members (117,118), the structural homology of the proregions of these molecules with the cystatins justifies further examination of the possibility that the cathelicidins do target such activity in a highly specific manner toward individual cysteine proteases.

Other features of cathelicidins that may be worthy of exploration are suggested by observations on bradykinin. This peptide is expressed N-terminal to the cystatin-like domain of high-molecular-weight kininogen. Bradykinin, once liberated by inflammatory proteinases, mediates its effects via specific cell surface receptors (145,146). Although the peptide is not known to possess antimicrobial activity, the question may be raised whether analogous cell surface receptors exist for the cathelicidin-derived peptides. Further, various cystatins have been reported to upregulate nitric oxide release from macrophages (147), leading to the question of whether cathelicidins share this ability as part of their participation in the inflammatory process.

Group II Phospholipase A$_2$

The granules of PMNs and those of at least some macrophages contain a PLA$_2$ of about 14 kd that is a member of a large family of "secretory" PLA$_2$ (sPLA$_2$) enzymes produced by both invertebrates and vertebrates (148). This family of enzymes has several highly conserved features, including size (about 14 to 16 kd), high disulfide content (more than six disulfides, six of which are invariant), a Ca^{2+}-binding loop, and closely similar catalytic machinery and secondary and tertiary structure (148). These enzymes generally show a broad substrate specificity when assayed against purified lipid dispersions. However, toward biologic targets they display significant target cell selectivity, with very wide variation among the members of this PLA$_2$ family in activity toward specific targets (87,149–151). In several instances these functional differences have been traced to compositional differences within variable surface domains of the PLA$_2$ that mediate interactions between the molecule and target sites (often not involving phospholipids) needed for subsequent (catalytic) action (87,150,152,153).

In mammals, including humans, two major subcategories of sPLA$_2$ (groups I and II) have been extensively characterized. Other related enzymes that do not fit in either group have also been discovered (154). Group II PLA$_2$ are present not only in the granules of phagocytes, but also in granules of platelets, mast cells, and Paneth cells and in the secretions of many cell types, including liver, vascular smooth muscle cells, keratinocytes, and lacrimal glands (148,155). During inflammation, production or secretion of these enzymes, originating in several cell types, is upregulated, giving rise at inflammatory sites to extracellular levels of group II PLA$_2$ of up to 1 mg/mL, 100- to 1,000-fold higher than at rest (149,151,156). Certain specialized microenvironments (e.g., tears, seminal fluid) may contain even higher levels of the enzyme.

Antibacterial actions of group II PLA$_2$ that are constituents of both inflammatory cells and the extracellular environment have been demonstrated as effects on viability or degradation of bacterial membrane phospholipids by purified enzyme with or without cofactors, in serum and inflammatory fluids, and within PMNs during phagocytosis (87,91,151,157–159). Against many strains and species of gram-positive bacteria, including multidrug-resistant *Staphylococcus aureus,* these PLA$_2$ express remarkably potent bactericidal activity, the lethal dose against 90% of bacteria (LD$_{90}$) being approximately 1 to 10 nmol/L (Fig. 50-4). Their bactericidal action depends on Ca^{2+}-independent binding (presumably to sites in the cell wall), penetration of the cell wall, and Ca^{2+}-dependent degradation of membrane phospholipids. The purified or recombinant enzyme is fully active when added to biologic fluids such as plasma. Moreover, during inflammation the levels of the enzyme mobilized both locally and systemically in extracellular fluids can account for almost all of the antibacterial activity against many gram-positive bacteria (e.g., *S. aureus,* group A streptococci) (151,156). The enzyme can produce multilog killing at PLA$_2$ concentrations present in inflammatory fluids, and its potency is further enhanced about tenfold by factors present constitutively in plasma (156).

Against gram-negative bacteria, in contrast, independent antibacterial activity of mammalian group II PLA$_2$ requires enzyme concentrations (micromolar or greater) (87,159) that greatly exceed PLA$_2$ levels at most or perhaps all body sites even during inflammation. However, other host defense agents that disrupt the bacterial outer membrane and that are present at the same intracellular (e.g., BPI, p15s) or extracellular (e.g., complement, BPI in inflammatory fluid) sites as the PLA$_2$ trigger the action of nanogram-per-milliliter amounts of the PLA$_2$ (87,91). Moreover, extracellular coating of *E. coli* with sublethal assemblies of the membrane attack complex of complement, as occurs during opsonization, greatly enhances intracellular bacterial destruction during phagocytosis by PMNs that includes phospholipolysis, in which the granule-associated PLA$_2$ participates (16,91). Intracellular destruction of ingested bacteria is further enhanced by the ability of extracellular (e.g., inflammatory fluid) group II PLA$_2$ to bind to bacteria to PMNs, or both, thus permitting internalization and intracellular action of this enzyme during phagocytosis (87,158).

The potent antibacterial activities expressed by the mammalian group II PLA$_2$s studied thus far represent unique biologic actions of these enzymes that are not

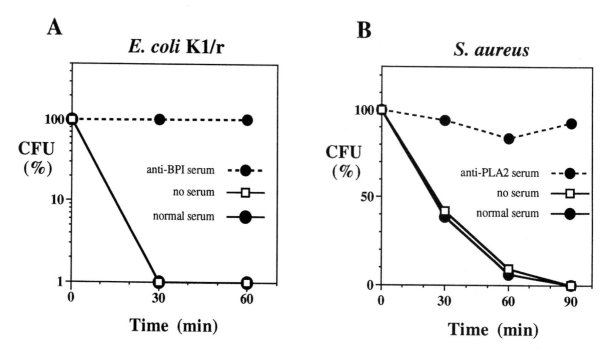

FIG. 50-4. Bactericidal/permeability-increasing (BPI)–dependent anti–*Escherichia coli* activity and phospholipase A₂ (PLA₂)–dependent anti–*Staphylococcus aureus* activity of an inflammatory fluid generated *in vivo*. A sterile inflammatory exudate was induced in New Zealand White rabbits by sterile intraperitoneal injection of glycogen in saline. Ascitic fluid (AF) was collected at 16 hours; the cells, which were more than 95% polymorphonuclear leukocytes (PMNs), were sedimented by centrifugation. The cell-free ascitic fluid is potently bactericidal toward serum-resistant encapsulated *E. coli* and *S. aureus*. The effects of a neutralizing anti-BPI serum on AF activity toward *E. coli* are shown in panel **A** and of a neutralizing anti-PLA₂ serum on AF activity toward *S. aureus* in panel **B**. (From refs. 17 and 151.)

shared by mammalian group I enzymes (even at 100,000-fold higher protein concentrations), nor by most other related sPLA₂ (87,151,160). All of the sPLA₂ display similar catalytic activity toward dispersed forms of bacterial phospholipids after extraction of the lipids from the bacterial envelope. The selective ability of the mammalian group II PLA₂ to act on phospholipids of intact bacteria correlates closely with their ability to bind to target bacteria (87,161); in the case of PLA₂ action against *E. coli* treated with purified BPI or with complement or ingested by PMNs, this ability depends on the presence of a cluster of basic amino acids along a discrete, variable surface region near the N-terminus of the protein (87,91,160). This region is functionally and topologically distinct from the highly conserved catalytic machinery of sPLA₂ and from other variable surface regions implicated in anticlotting, neurotoxic, and myotoxic actions of selected sPLA₂ (149,150) and only partially accounts for the targetting of gram-positive bacteria by mammalian group II PLA₂ (151).

Lactoferrin

Lactoferrin, a member of the transferrin family of iron-binding proteins, is an 80-kd cationic protein (isoelectric point, 8.7) that is present in the specific granules of PMNs as well as in breast milk and in all other mucosal secretions examined. The crystal structure of lactoferrin reveals a bilobed iron-binding molecule (162) in which the C-terminal domain imparts unique iron-binding stability (163).

Lactoferrin exerts antimicrobial activity both by limiting available iron needed for bacterial growth and by direct interactions with microorganisms (164,165), including alterations of the gram-negative bacterial outer membrane that may enhance the antibacterial actions of immunoglobulins, complement, and other PMN cationic granule proteins (165). In contrast, Neisseriaceae (166) and probably *Helicobacter pylori* (167,168) express receptors for lactoferrin, allowing the bacteria to use this host defense factor as an iron source, apparently without undergoing its cytotoxic effects (166). Lactoferrin manifests antiviral activity by inhibiting adsorption or penetration (or both) of HIV and cytomegalovirus in cell culture (169).

Digestion of lactoferrin by pepsin releases the antibacterial peptide lactoferricin (170). Lactoferricin consists mainly of a loop of 18 amino acids, including several basic residues, derived from the N-terminal region of the parent protein. Peptides containing the loop region of human lactoferricin (residues 20–35 and 24–35) exert antibacterial activity not shown by apolactoferrin (170).

Lactoferrin present in human milk presumably is exposed to pepsin in the neonate's digestive tract. It is unknown whether this provides the neonate with a source of protective antimicrobial lactoferrin-derived peptides, nor whether, in other *in vivo* settings, endogenous proteases cleave lactoferrin of PMNs, yielding bioactive peptides.

Like many other cationic antimicrobial proteins and peptides of PMNs (23,171), lactoferrin has the ability to neutralize LPS in artificial media by binding to the lipid A region (172). The lactoferricin loop region (residues 28–34) is required for the high-affinity (K_d approximately 4 nmol/L) binding of lactoferrin to *E. coli* LPS (173). Because the LPS-neutralizing activity of lactoferrin apparently is eliminated in the presence of serum or plasma, it is not clear whether lactoferrin contributes to inactivation of endotoxin in biologic settings (94).

In addition to its antimicrobial properties, lactoferrin has the ability to interact with and modulate the function of a variety of host cells. This includes inhibition of proinflammatory cytokine release from LPS- or TNF-stimulated monocytes (174); stimulation of lymphocyte proliferation, apparently via 100- and 110-kd lactoferrin receptors that are upregulated in phytohemagglutinin antigen–activated peripheral blood lymphocytes (175); downregulation of myelopoiesis (176); and priming of PMNs (177). Interactions of lactoferrin with nucleic acids include ribonuclease activity of some lactoferrin isoforms (178) as well as sequence-specific interactions with DNA leading to transcriptional activation (179). Lactoferrin may function in the digestive tract to deliver iron to the small intestine and enhance hepatic protein synthesis (180). In inflammatory bowel disease, release of lactoferrin into the lumen of the gastrointestinal tract has been proposed to serve as a fecal marker of disease activity, reflecting not only lactoferrin in mucosal cell secretions but also lactoferrin from infiltrating neutrophils (181).

CYTOSOLIC ANTIBIOTIC PROTEINS

Calprotectin

Calprotectin is an abundant complex of anionic 8- and 14-kd calcium-binding proteins estimated to account for 30% to 60% of the total cytosolic protein of PMNs. The protein is also a constituent of monocytes, mucosal squamous epithelia, and plasma under inflammatory conditions (182). Antimicrobial activity of calprotectin against bacteria and fungi is inhibitable by zinc and has been observed against *C. albicans* in the absence of direct contact, suggesting that calprotectin acts by depriving microorganisms of zinc (183). PMN lysates, as well as abscess and empyema fluids, possess zinc-reversible antifungal activity, prompting the view that release of calprotectin by "holocrine secretion" from disintegrating PMNs may represent an important defense against some pathogens *in vivo* (184,185). Calprotectin is also cyto-

toxic toward mammalian cells through a zinc-reversible mechanism that induces apoptosis in certain tumor cell lines (186). The calprotectin proteins may also have regulatory functions: They contain sequences of peptides that are potent neutrophil immobilizing factors, raising the possibility that accumulation of calprotectin at inflammatory sites may serve to focus the inflammatory response (182). Further, the calprotectin component proteins p8 and p14 are members of the S-100 family of calcium-binding proteins that are implicated in cell cycle progression, cell differentiation, and cytoskeletal-membrane interactions (182).

Integration of Host Defenses

The microbicidal activity of antibiotic proteins and peptides can be modulated by both intracellular and extracellular factors. Synergistic microbicidal effects have been demonstrated among serprocidins (187), among defensins (188), between lysozyme and lactoferrin (57), between apolactoferrin and bactenecin (Bac7) (189), and between BPI and p15s or defensins (30,90). PMN-derived cytoplasts that are devoid of granules but capable of generating respiratory burst oxidase activity require addition of granule components for potent fungicidal activity toward hyphae of *C. albicans,* suggesting that PMNs can deploy their oxidative and nonoxidative arsenals in synergy (190). Integration of innate and acquired immunity is suggested by the discovery in breast milk of naturally occurring covalent complexes of lactoferrin with secretory immunoglobulin A (IgA) that exhibit bactericidal activity not duplicated when uncomplexed lactoferrin and secretory IgA are combined *in vitro* (191).

Epithelial cells have been shown to release IL-8, thereby signaling for PMN influx, and PMN-derived microbicidal proteins have been detected in intestinal epithelial crypts in some inflammatory conditions (192), suggesting conditions in which antimicrobial products of mobilized PMNs and mucosal cells act in concert.

PERSPECTIVES

In the second (1992) edition of this book we pointed out that, in contrast to what had been learned about the antimicrobial polypeptides of the PMN in the preceding 5 years, not much had been added to knowledge of the antimicrobial equipment of the mononuclear phagocyte. This gap in understanding of what molecular elements this cell employs, in addition to its ability to generate nitric oxide and other toxic O_2 derivatives (see Chapter 47) in the performance of its essential role in host defense, has still not been filled. Particularly because the host relies on mononuclear phagocytes for protection against a very different spectrum of microbial pathogens, compared with PMNs, it is likely that their antimicrobial equipment is correspondingly different. In the future investigators may address what should be an exciting and as yet unmet challenge.

The foregoing review, therefore, concerns mainly the polypeptides of the PMN. Although these agents are considered to belong to the antimicrobial arsenal of this arm of the innate immune system, this classification is often based on an unproved assumption—namely, that the use of an assay that assesses bacterial growth-inhibition by a given isolated polypeptide justifiably defines what its place is in the biology of the phagocyte. There is much reason to view the bioactive peptides and proteins of the phagocytes in a much broader context. The PMN is not merely a cell that sequesters and destroys microorganisms. These highly mobile cells, whether in the circulation or migrating into the tissues at inflammatory sites, are secretory cells that contribute to and modulate the inflammatory process in many ways. Among the bioactive proteins and peptides that PMNs and mononuclear phagocytes produce, store, and secrete are known cytokines (193,194), complement components (116,195), coagulation stimulatory tissue factor and modifiers that affect adhesive properties of the PMN itself and of endothelial cells (196). The evidence suggesting that PR-39 has a role in postinflammatory tissue repair offers yet another argument for viewing the granules of the phagocyte as more than just a repository for microbicidal and enzymatically destructive polypeptides. Taken together, such observations suggest strongly that some of these polypeptides should not be regarded solely as antimicrobial agents and that other or additional functions should also be explored. A case in point is the very abundant α defensins, which lose most of their antibacterial potency and capabilities in physiologic fluids and have already been shown, at concentrations much lower than those needed for antimicrobial activity, to possess chemotactic and hormone-like properties (12).

In the years ahead the understanding of host defenses against infection should gain greatly from two rapidly developing areas of science. First, evidence is mounting that the regulatory and biochemical pathways of inflammatory responses underlying the mobilization of antimicrobial host defenses are preserved to a remarkable degree throughout evolution. It is now possible to make use of relatively primitive organisms, notably *Drosophila* (197–199), insects that can be readily manipulated genetically, as a model for the further dissection of host-microbe interactions in higher animals, including humans. Second, it is now recognized that invading microbes can become more pathogenic by adjusting their metabolism and structure to resist the antimicrobial systems of the host (34,89,200,201). It is still uncertain how promptly bacteria can adapt to a hostile environment within the host. However, if invading bacteria are indeed capable of rapid adaptation, for example by changing the structure of LPS and hence becoming less susceptible to some antimicrobial polypeptides (34), it will be important to introduce these phenotypic variables into *in vitro* assays to provide a more accurate model of host-microbe interactions *in vivo*.

Despite these remaining uncertainties, some of the proteins and peptides of PMNs have been shown to be essential participants in the destruction of a broad range of bacterial species under biologically relevant conditions. With such studies as a basis, large-scale production by recombinant DNA technology has made possible the generation of quantities of several of these polypeptides sufficient to allow exploration of their ability as administered agents to protect animals against lethal inocula of bacteria and their products. The encouraging results of some of these preclinical studies are now being followed by testing in humans (96,202,203). For example, phase I and II clinical trials with recombinant N-terminal BPI fragment (rBPI-21) have shown neither toxicity nor immunogenicity in healthy human volunteers and in patients with severe childhood meningococcemia, hemorrhagic trauma, partial hepatectomy, or serious peritoneal infections (96,202,203) (unpublished observation). Preliminary evidence of therapeutic benefit of rBPI-21 has led to accelerated further clinical testing (phase III) in patients with meningococcemia and after hemorrhagic trauma.

As expanding microbial resistance progressively limits the efficacy of conventional antibiotics, exploration of "endogenous antibiotics" as potential alternative therapeutic agents will be aided by the advancing technology of recombinant polypeptide production and delivery.

REFERENCES

1. Middlebrook JL, Dorland RB. Bacterial toxins: cellular mechanisms of action. *Microbiol Rev* 1984;48:199–221.
2. Nakamura T, Furunaka H, Miyata T, et al. Tachyplesin, a class of antimicrobial peptide from the hemocytes of the hoseshoe crab (*Tachypleus tridentatus*). *J Biol Chem* 1988;263:16709–16713.
3. Kawano K, Yoneya T, Miyata T, et al. Antimicrobial peptide, tachyplesin I, isolated from hemocytes of the horseshoe crab (*Tachypleus tridentatus*). *J Biol Chem* 1990;265:15365–15367.
4. Hoffmann JA. Innate immunity of insects. *Curr Opin Immunol* 1995; 7:4–10.
5. Boman HG. Peptide antibiotics and their role in innate immunity. *Annu Rev Immunol* 1995;13:61–92.
6. Broekaert WF, Terras FR, Cammue BP, Osborn RW. Plant defensins: novel antimicrobial peptides as components of the host defense system. *Plant Physiology* 1995;108:1353–1358.
7. Epple P, Apel K, Bohlmann H. Overexpression of an endogenous thionin enhances resistance of Arabidopsis against *Fusarium oxysporum*. *Plant Cell* 1997;9:509–520.
8. Weiss J. Leukocyte-derived antimicrobial proteins. *Curr Opin Hematol* 1994;1:78–84.
9. Zanetti M, Gennaro R, Romeo D. Cathelicidins: a novel protein family with a common proregion and a variable C-terminal antimicrobial domain. *FEBS Lett* 1995;374:1–5.
10. Diamond G, Russell JP, Bevins CL. Inducible expression of an antibiotic peptide gene in lipopolysaccharide-challenged tracheal epithelial cells. *Proc Natl Acad Sci U S A* 1996;93:5156–5160.
11. Lehrer RI, Ganz T. Endogenous vertebrate antibiotics: defensins, protegrins, and other cysteine-rich antimicrobial peptides. *Ann N Y Acad Sci* 1996;797:228–239.

12. Ganz T, Lehrer RI. Antimicrobial peptides of leukocytes. *Curr Opin Hematol* 1997;4:53–58.

13. Zasloff M. Antibiotic peptides as mediators of innate immunity. *Curr Opin Immunol* 1992;4:3–7.

14. Huttner KM, Selsted ME, Ouellette AJ. Structure and diversity of the murine cryptdin gene family. *Genomics* 1994;19:448–453.

15. Mannion BA, Weiss J, Elsbach P. Separation of sublethal and lethal effects of polymorphonuclear leukocytes on *Escherichia coli*. *J Clin Invest* 1990;86:631–641.

16. Elsbach P, Weiss J, Levy O. Integration of antimicrobial host defenses: role of the bactericidal/permeability-increasing protein. *Trends Microbiol* 1994;2:324–328.

17. Weinrauch Y, Foreman A, Shu C, et al. Extracellular accumulation of potently microbicidal bactericidal/permeability-increasing protein and p15s in an evolving sterile rabbit peritoneal inflammatory exudate. *J Clin Invest* 1995;95:1916–1924.

18. Goldman MJ, Anderson GM, Stolzenberg ED, Kari UP, Zasloff M, Wilson JM. Human beta-defensin-1 is a salt-sensitive antibiotic in lung that is inactivated in cystic fibrosis. *Cell* 1997;88:553–560.

19. Panyutich A, Ganz T. Activated α2-macroglobulin is a principal defensin-binding protein. *Am J Respir Cell Mol Biol* 1991;5:101–106.

20. Panyutich AV, Hiemstra PS, van Wetering S, Ganz T. Human neutrophil defensin and serpins form complexes and inactivate each other. *Am J Respir Cell Mol Biol* 1995;12:351–357.

21. Panyutich AV, Szold O, Poon PH, Tseng Y, Ganz T. Identification of defensin binding to C1 complement. *FEBS Lett* 1994;356:169–173.

22. Cross AS, Opal SM, Sadoff JC, Gemski P. Choice of bacteria in animal models of sepsis. *Infect Immun* 1993;61:2741–2747.

23. Levy O, Ooi CE, Elsbach P, Doerfler ME, Lehrer RI, Weiss J. Antibacterial proteins of granulocytes differ in interaction with endotoxin: comparison of bactericidal/permeability-increasing protein, p15s, and defensins. *J Immunol* 1995;154:5403–5410.

24. Elsbach P, Weiss J. Oxygen-independent antimicrobial systems of phagocytes. In: Gallin JI, Goldstein IM, Snyderman R (eds). *Inflammation: Basic Principles and Clinical Correlates*. New York: Raven Press, 1992:603–636.

25. Hill CP, Yee J, Selsted ME, Eisenberg D. Crystal structure of defensin HNP-3, an amphiphilic dimer: mechanisms of membrane permeabilization. *Science* 1991;251:1481–1485.

26. Zimmermann GR, Legault P, Selsted ME, Pardi A. Solution structure of bovine neutrophil beta-defensin-12: the peptide fold of the beta-defensins is identical to that of the classical defensins. *Biochemistry* 1995;34:13663–13671.

27. Valore EV, Martin E, Harwig SS, Ganz T. Intramolecular inhibition of human defensin HNP-1 by its propiece. *J Clin Invest* 1996;97:1624–1629.

28. Ganz T. Biosynthesis of defensins and other antimicrobial peptides. *Ciba Found Symp* 1994;186:62–71.

29. Zhao C, Wang I, Lehrer RI. Widespread expression of beta-defensin hBD-1 in human secretory glands and epithelial cells. *FEBS Lett* 1996;396:319–322.

30. Levy O, Ooi CE, Weiss J, Lehrer RI, Elsbach P. Individual and synergistic effects of rabbit granulocyte proteins on *Escherichia coli*. *J Clin Invest* 1994;94:672–682.

31. White SH, Wimley WC, Selsted ME. Structure, function, and membrane integration of defensins. *Curr Opin Struct Biol* 1995;5:521–527.

32. Hristova K, Selsted ME, White SH. Interactions of monomeric rabbit neutrophil defensins with bilayers: comparison with dimeric human defensin HNP-2. *Biochemistry* 1996;35:11888–11894.

33. Groisman EA. How bacteria resist killing by host-defense peptides. *Trends Microbiol* 1995;2:444–449.

34. Guo L, Lim KB, Gunn JS, et al. Regulation of lipid A modifications by *Salmonella typhimurium* virulence genes phoP-phoQ. *Science* 1997;276:250–253.

35. Borregaard N, Lollike K, Kjeldsen L, et al. Human neutrophil granules and secretory vesicles. *Eur J Haematol* 1993;51:187–198.

36. Panyutich AV, Panyutich EA, Krapivin VA, Baturevich EA, Ganz T. Plasma defensin concentrations are elevated in patients with septicemia or bacterial meningitis. *J Lab Clin Med* 1993;122:202–207.

37. Ashitani J, Mukae H, Ihiboshi H, et al. Defensin in plasma and in bronchoalveolar lavage fluid from patients with acute respiratory distress syndrome. *Nippon Kyobu Shikkan Gakkai Zasshi* 1996;34:1349–1353.

38. Prieto JA, Panyutich AV, Heine RP. Neutrophil activation in preeclampsia: are defensins and lactoferrin elevated in preeclamptic patients? *J Reprod Med* 1997;42:29–32.

39. Barnathan ES, Raghunath PN, Tomaszewski JE, Ganz T, Cines DB, Higazi A-R. Immunohistochemical localization of defensin in human coronary vessels. *Am J Pathol* 1997;150:1009–1020.

40. Chertov O, Michiel DF, Xu L, et al. Identification of defensin-1, defensin-2, and CAP37/azurocidin as T-cell chemoattractant proteins released from interleukin-8-stimulated neutrophils. *J Biol Chem* 1996;271:2935–2940.

41. MacLeod RJ, Hamilton JR, Bateman A, et al. Corticostatic peptides cause nifedipine-sensitive volume reduction in jejunal villus enterocytes. *Proc Natl Acad Sci U S A* 1991;88:552–556.

42. Nygaard SD, Ganz T, Peterson MW. Defensins reduce the barrier integrity of a cultured epithelial monolayer without cytotoxicity. *Am J Respir Cell Mol Biol* 1993;8:193–200.

43. Murphy CJ, Foster BA, Mannis MJ, Selsted ME, Reid TW. Defensins are mitogenic for epithelial cells and fibroblasts. *J Cell Physiol* 1993;155:408–413.

44. Higazi A, Ganz T, Kariko K, Cines DB. Defensin modulates tissue-type plasminogen activator and plasminogen binding to fibrin and endothelial cells. *J Biol Chem* 1996;271:17650–17655.

45. Zhu Q, Solomon S. Isolation and mode of action of rabbit corticostatic (antiadrenocorticotropin) peptides. *Endocrinology* 1992;130:1413–1423.

46. Smith EM, Brosnan P, Meyer WJ, Blalock JE. An ACTH receptor on human mononuclear leukocytes. *N Engl J Med* 1987;317:1266–1269.

47. Solomon S, Hu J, Zhu Q, et al. Corticostatic peptides. *J Steroid Biochem Mol Biol* 1991;40:391–398.

48. Hu J, Jothy S, Solomon S. Localization and measurement of corticostatin-I in nonpregnant and pregnant rabbit tissues during late gestation. *Endocrinology* 1993;132:2351–2359.

49. Couto MA, Harwig SS, Cullor JS, Hughes JP, Lehrer RI. Identification of eNAP-1, an antimicrobial peptide from equine neutrophils. *Infect Immun* 1992;60:3065–3071.

50. Culouscou JM, Carlton GW, Shoyab M. Biochemical analysis of the epithelin receptor. *J Biol Chem* 1993;268:10458–10462.

51. Couto MA, Harwig SS, Lehrer RI. Selective inhibition of microbial serine proteases by eNAP-2, an antimicrobial peptide from equine neutrophils. *Infect Immun* 1993;61:2991–2994.

52. Cramer EM, Breton-Gorius J. Ultrastructural localization of lysozyme in human neutrophils by immunogold. *J Leukoc Biol* 1987;41:242–247.

53. Holtje JV. Lysozyme substrates. *EXS* 1996;75:105–110.

54. Selsted ME, Martinez RJ. Lysozyme: primary bactericidin in human plasma serum active against *Bacillus subtilis*. *Infect Immun* 1978;20:782–791.

55. Johnson KG. Effect of growth conditions on peptidoglycan structure and susceptibility to lytic enzymes in cell walls of *Micrococcus sodonensis*. *Biochemistry* 1972;11:277–286.

56. Taylor PW. Bactericidal and bacteriolytic activity of serum against gram-negative bacteria. *Microbiol Rev* 1983;47:46–83.

57. Ellison RT, Giehl TJ. Killing of gram-negative bacteria by lactoferrin and lysozyme. *J Clin Invest* 1991;88:1080–1091.

58. Ibrahim HR, Yamada M, Matsushita K, Kobayashi K, Kato A. Enhanced bactericidal action of lysozyme to *Escherichia coli* by inserting a hydrophobic pentapeptide into its C terminus. *J Biol Chem* 1994;269:5059–5063.

59. Laible NJ, Germaine GR. Bactericidal activity of human lysozyme, muramidase-inactive lysozyme, and cationic polypeptides against *Streptococcus sanguis* and *Streptococcus faecalis*: inhibition by chitin oligosaccharides. *Infect Immun* 1985;48:720–728.

60. Irwin DM, Yu M, Wen Y. Isolation and characterization of vertebrate lysozyme genes. *EXS* 1996;75:225–241.

61. Ahne B, Strätling WH. Characterization of a myeloid-specific enhancer of the chicken lysozyme gene. *J Biol Chem* 1994;269:17794–17801.

62. Goethe R, van LP. The far upstream chicken lysozyme enhancer at -6.1 kilobase, by interacting with NF-M, mediates lipopolysaccharide-induced expression of the chicken lysozyme gene in chicken myelomonocytic cells. *J Biol Chem* 1994;269:31302–31309.

63. Ohno N, Morrison DC. Lipopolysaccharide interaction with lysozyme: binding of lipopolysaccharide to lysozyme and inhibition of lysozyme enzymatic activity. *J Biol Chem* 1989;264:4434–4441.

64. Takada K, Ohno N, Yadomae T. Lysozyme regulates LPS-induced interleukin-6 release in mice. *Circ Shock* 1994;44:169–174.

65. Gabay JE, Almeida RP. Antibiotic peptides and serine protease homologs in human polymorphonuclear leukocytes: defensins and azurocidin. *Curr Opin Immunol* 1993;5:97–102.

66. Hof P, Mayr I, Huber R, et al. The 1.8 angstrom structure of human cathepsin G in complex with suc-val-pro-pheP-(OPh)2: a Janus-faced proteinase with two opposite specificities. *EMBO J* 1996;15:5481–5491.

67. Zimmer M, Medcalf RL, Fink TM, Mattmann C, Lichter P, Jenne DE. Three human elastase-like genes coordinately expressed in the myelomonocyte lineage are organized as a single genetic locus on 19pter. *Proc Natl Acad Sci U S A* 1992;89:8215–8219.

68. Oelgeschlager M, Nuchprayoon I, Luscher B, Friedman AD. C/EBP, c-Myb, and PU.1 cooperate to regulate the neutrophil elastase promoter. *Mol Cell Biol* 1996;16:4717–4725.

69. Friedman AD. Regulation of immature myeloid cell differentiation by PEBP2/CBF, MYB, C/EBP, and ETS family members. In: Wolff L, Perkins AS, eds. *Molecular aspects of myeloid stem cell development*. New York: Springer, 1996:149–171.

70. Sturrock A, Franklin KF, Hoidal JR. Human proteinase-3 expression is regulated by PU.1 in conjunction with a cytidine-rich element. *J Biol Chem* 1996;271:32392–32402.

71. Shafer WM, Hubalek F, Huang M, Pohl J. Bactericidal activity of a synthetic peptide (CG 117-136) of human lysosomal cathepsin G is dependent on arginine content. *Infect Immun* 1996;64:4842–4845.

72. Campbell EJ, Silverman EK, Campbell MA. Elastase and cathepsin G of human monocytes: quantitation of cellular content, release in response to stimuli and heterogeneity in elastase-mediated proteolytic activity. *J Immunol* 1989;143:2961–2968.

73. Owen CA, Campbell MA, Sannes PL, Boukedes SS, Campbell EJ. Cell surface-bound elastase and cathepsin G on human neutrophils: a novel, non-oxidative mechanism by which neutrophils focus and preserve catalytic activity of serine proteases. *J Cell Biol* 1995;131:775–789.

74. Pereira HA, Schafer WM, Pohl J, Martin LE, Spitznagel JK. CAP37, a human neutrophil-derived chemotactic factor with monocyte specific activity. *J Clin Invest* 1990;85:1468–1476.

75. Kurdowska A, Travis J. Acute phase protein stimulation by α1-antichymotrypsin-cathepsin G complexes. *J Biol Chem* 1990;265:21023–21026.

76. Renesto P, Halbwachs-Mecarelli L, Nusbaum P, Lesavre P, Chignard M. Proteinase 3: a neutrophil proteinase with activity on platelets. *J Immunol* 1994;152:4612–4617.

77. Rasmussen PB, Bjorn S, Hastrup S, et al. Characterization of recombinant human HBP/CAP37/azurocidin, a pleiotropic mediator of inflammation-enhancing LPS-induced cytokine release from monocytes. *FEBS Lett* 1996;390:109–112.

78. Witko-Sarsat V, Halbwachs-Mecarelli L, Almeida RP, et al. Characterization of a recombinant proteinase 3, the autoantigen in Wegener's granulomatosis and its reactivity with anti-neutrophil cytoplasmic antibodies. *FEBS Lett* 1996;382:130–136.

79. Yang JJ, Kettritz R, Falk RJ, Jennette JC, Gaido ML. Apoptosis of endothelial cells induced by the neutrophil serine proteases proteinase 3 and elastase. 1996;.

80. Bories D, Raynal M, Solomon DH, Darzynkiewicz Z, Cayre YE. Down-regulation of a serine protease, myeloblastin, causes growth arrest and differentiation of promyelocytic leukemia cells. *Cell* 1989;59:959–968.

81. Elsbach P, Weiss J. The bactericidal/permeability-increasing protein (BPI), a potent element in host-defense against gram-negative bacteria and lipopolysaccharide. *Immunobiology* 1993;187:417–429.

82. Gazzano-Santoro H, Parent JB, Grinna L, et al. High-affinity binding of the bactericidal/permeability-increasing protein and a recombinant amino-terminal fragment to the lipid A region of lipopolysaccharide. *Infect Immun* 1992;60:4754–4761.

83. Zarember K, Elsbach P, Shin-Kim K, Weiss J. p15s (15-kD antimicrobial proteins) are stored in the secondary granules of rabbit granulocytes: implications for antibacterial synergy with the bactericidal/permeability-increasing protein in inflammatory fluids. *Blood* 1997;89:672–679.

84. Weersink AJ, van Kessel KP, van den Tol ME, et al. Human granulocytes express a 55-kDa lipopolysaccharide-binding protein on the cell surface that is identical to the bactericidal/permeability-increasing protein. *J Immunol* 1993;150:253–263.

85. Dentener MA, Francot GJ, Buurman WA. Bactericidal/permeability-increasing protein, a lipopolysaccharide-specific protein on the surface of human peripheral blood monocytes. *J Infect Dis* 1996;173:252–255.

86. Wiese A, Brandenburg K, Lindner B, Schromm AB, Rietschel ET, Seydel U. *Biochemistry* 1997;36:10301–10310.

87. Weiss J, Inada M, Elsbach P, Crowl RM. Structural determinants of the action against *Escherichia coli* of a human inflammatory fluid phospholipase A2 in concert with polymorphonuclear leukocytes. *J Biol Chem* 1994;269:26331–26337.

88. Mannion BA, Weiss J, Elsbach P. Separation of sublethal and lethal effects of the bactericidal/permeability increasing protein on *Escherichia coli*. *J Clin Invest* 1990;85:853–860.

89. Qi SY, Li Y, Szyroki A, Giles IG, Moir A, O'Connor CD. *Salmonella typhimurium* responses to a bactericidal protein from human neutrophils. *Mol Microbiol* 1995;17:523–531.

90. Weiss J, Elsbach P, Shu C, et al. Human bactericidal/permeability-increasing protein and a recombinant NH2-terminal fragment cause killing of serum-resistant gram-negative bacteria in whole blood and inhibit tumor necrosis factor release induced by the bacteria. *J Clin Invest* 1992;90:1122–1130.

91. Madsen LM, Inada M, Weiss J. Determinants of activation by complement of group II phospholipase A2 acting against *Escherichia coli*. *Infect Immun* 1996;64:2425–2430.

92. Elsbach P, Weiss J. Prospects for the use of recombinant BPI in the treatment of gram-negative bacterial infections. *Infect Agents Dis* 1995;4:102–109.

93. Katz SS, Chen K, Chen S, Doerfler ME, Elsbach P, Weiss J. Potent CD14-mediated signalling of human leukocytes by *Escherichia coli* can be mediated by interaction of whole bacteria and host cells without extensive prior release of endotoxin. *Infect Immun* 1996;64:3592–3600.

94. Wang D, Pabst KM, Aida Y, Pabst MJ. Lipopolysaccharide-inactivating activity of neutrophils is due to lactoferrin. *J Leukoc Biol* 1995;57:865–874.

95. Lin Y, Leach WJ, Ammons WS. Synergistic effect of a recombinant N-terminal fragment of bactericidal/permeability-increasing protein and cefamandole in treatment of rabbit gram-negative sepsis. *Antimicrob Agents Chemother* 1996;40:65–69.

96. von der Mohlen MA, Kimmings AN, Wedel NI, et al. Inhibition of endotoxin-induced cytokine release and neutrophil activation in humans by use of recombinant bactericidal/permeability-increasing protein. *J Infect Dis* 1995;172:144–151.

97. Opal SM, Palardy JE, Marra MN, Fisher CJ, McKelligon BM, Scott RW. Relative concentrations of endotoxin-binding proteins in body fluids during infection. *Lancet* 1994;344:429–431.

98. Gazzano-Santoro H, Parent JB, Conlon PJ, et al. Characterization of the structural elements in lipid A required for binding of a recombinant fragment of bactericidal/permeability-increasing protein rBPI23. *Infect Immun* 1995;63:2201–2205.

99. Capodici C, Chen S, Sidorczyk Z, Elsbach P, Weiss J. Effect of lipopolysaccharide (LPS) chain length on interactions of bactericidal/permeability-increasing protein and its bioactive 23-kilodalton NH2-terminal fragment with isolated LPS and intact *Proteus mirabilis* and *Escherichia coli*. *Infect Immun* 1994;62:259–265.

100. Little RG, Kelner DN, Lim E, Burke DJ, Conlon PJ. Functional domains of recombinant bactericidal/permeability-increasing protein (rBPI23). *J Biol Chem* 1994;268:1865–1872.

101. Jahr TG, Ryan L, Sundan A, Lichenstein HS, Skjak-Break G, Espevik T. Induction of tumor necrosis factor production from monocytes stimulated with mannuronic acid polymers and involvement of lipopolysaccharide-binding protein, CD14, and bactericidal/permeability-increasing factor. *Infect Immun* 1997;65:89–94.

102. Schumann RR, Leong SR, Flaggs GW, et al. Structure and function of lipopolysaccharide binding protein. *Science* 1990;249:1429–1431.

103. Day JR, Albers JJ, Lofton-Day CE, et al. Complete cDNA encoding human phospholipid transfer protein from human endothelial cells. *J Biol Chem* 1994;269:9388–9391.

104. Gray PW, Corcorran AE, Eddy RL, Byers MG, Shows TB. The genes for the lipopolysaccharide binding protein (LBP) and the bactericidal/permeability-increasing protein (BPI) are encoded in the same region of chromosome 20. *Genomics* 1993;15:188–190.

105. Ooi CE, Weiss J, Doerfler ME, Elsbach P. Endotoxin-neutralizing properties of the 25 kD N-terminal fragment and a newly isolated 30

kD C-terminal fragment of the 55–60 kD bactericidal/permeability-increasing protein of human neutrophils. *J Exp Med* 1991;174:649–655.

106. Capodici C, Weiss J. Both N- and C-terminal regions of the bioactive N-terminal fragment of the neutrophil granule bactericidal/permeability-increasing protein are required for stability and function. *J Immunol* 1996;156:4789–4796.

107. Abrahamson SL, Wu HM, Williams RE, et al. Biochemical characterization of recombinant fusions of lipopolysaccharide binding protein and bactericidal/permeability-increasing protein: implications in biological activity. *J Biol Chem* 1997;272:2149–2155.

108. Iovine N, Elsbach P, Weiss J. An opsonic function of the neutrophil bactericidal/permeability-increasing protein depends on both its N- and C-terminal domains. *Pro Natl Acad Sci* 1997;94:10793–10948.

109. Ulevitch RJ, Tobias PS. Receptor-dependent mechanisms of cell stimulation by bacterial endotoxin. *Annu Rev Immunol* 1995;13:437–457.

110. Beamer LJ, Carroll SF, Eisenberg D. Crystal structure of human BPI and two bound phospholipids at 2.4 angstrom resolution. *Science* 1997;276:1881–1884.

111. Horwitz AH, Leigh SD, Abrahamson S, et al. Expression and characterization of cysteine-modified variants of an amino-terminal fragment of bactericidal/permeability-increasing protein. *Protein Expr Purif* 1996;8:28–40.

112. Lamping N, Hoess A, Yu B, et al. Effects of site-directed mutagenesis of basic residues (Arg94, Lys95, Lys99) of lipopolysaccharide (LPS)-binding protein on binding and transfer of LPS and subsequent immune cell activation. *J Immunol* 1996;157:4648–4656.

113. Elsbach P, Weiss J, Doerfler M, et al. The bactericidal/permeability increasing protein of neutrophils is a potent antibacterial and anti-endotoxin agent *in vitro* and *in vivo*. *Prog Clin Biol Res* 1994;388:41–51.

114. Tobias PS, Soldau K, Iovine N, Elsbach P, Weiss J. Lipopolysaccharide (LPS) binding proteins BPI and LBP form different complexes with LPS. *J Biol Chem* 1997;272:18682–18685.

115. Gazzano-Santoro H, Meszaros K, Birr C, et al. Competition between rBPI23, a recombinant fragment of bactericidal/permeability-increasing protein, and lipopolysaccharide (LPS)-binding protein for binding to LPS and gram-negative bacteria. *Infect Immun* 1994;62:1185–1191.

116. Levy O. Antibiotic proteins of polymorphonuclear leukocytes. *Eur J Haematol* 1996;56:263–277.

117. Lenarcic B, Ritonja A, Dolenc I, et al. Pig leukocyte cysteine proteinase inhibitor (PLCPI), a new member of the stefin family. *FEBS Lett* 1993;336:289–292.

118. Storici P, Tossi A, Lenarcic B, Romeo D. Purification and structural characterization of bovine cathelicidins, precursors of antimicrobial peptides. *Eur J Biochem* 1996;238:769–776.

119. Zanetti M, Litteri L, Gennaro R, Horstmann H, Romeo D. Bactenecins, defense polypeptides of bovine neutrophils, are generated from precursor molecules stored in the large granules. *J Cell Biol* 1990;111:1363–1371.

120. Cowland JB, Johnsen AH, Borregaard N. hCAP-18, a cathelin/probactenecin-like protein of human neutrophil specific granules. *FEBS Lett* 1995;368:173–176.

121. Moscinski LC, Hill B. Molecular cloning of a novel myeloid granule protein. *J Cell Biochem* 1995;59:431–442.

122. Gallo RL, Kim KJ, Bernfield M, et al. Identification of CRAMP, a cathelin-related antimicrobial peptide expressed in embryonic and adult mouse. *J Biol Chem* 1997;272:13088–13093.

123. Zanetti M, Litteri L, Griffiths G, Gennaro R, Romeo D. Stimulus-induced maturation of probactenecins, precursors of neutrophil antimicrobial polypeptides. *J Immunol* 1991;146:4295–4300.

124. Panyutich A, Shi J, Boutz PL, Zhao C, Ganz T. Porcine polymorphonuclear leukocytes generate extracellular microbicidal activity by elastase-mediated activation of secreted proprotegrins. *Infect Immun* 1997;65:978–985.

125. Gallo RL, Ono M, Povsic T, et al. Syndecans, cell surface heparan sulfate proteoglycans, are induced by a proline-rich antimicrobial peptide from wounds. *Proc Natl Acad Sci U S A* 1994;91:11035–11039.

126. Frohm M, Gunne H, Bergman AC, et al. Biochemical and antibacterial analysis of human wound and blister fluid. *Eur J Biochem* 1996;237:86–92.

127. Harwig SSL, Waring A, Yang HJ, Cho Y, Tan L, Lehrer RI. Intramolecular disulfide bonds enhance the antimicrobial and lytic activities of protegrins at physiological sodium chloride concentrations. *Eur J Biochem* 1996;240:352–357.

128. Yasin B, Harwig SS, Lehrer RI, Wagar EA. Susceptibility of *Chlamydia trachomatis* to protegrins and defensins. *Infect Immun* 1996;64:709–713.

129. Gudmundsson GH, Magnusson KP, Chowdhary BP, Johansson M, Andersson L, Boman HG. Structure of the gene for porcine peptide antibiotic PR-39, a cathelin gene family member: comparative mapping of the locus for the human peptide antibiotic FALL-39. *Proc Natl Acad Sci U S A* 1995;92:7085–7089.

130. Zhao C, Ganz T, Lehrer RI. The structure of porcine protegrin genes. *FEBS Lett* 1995;368:197–202.

131. Gudmundsson GH, Agerberth B, Odeberg J, Bergman T, Olsson B, Salcedo R. The human gene FALL39 and processing of the cathelin precursor to the antibacterial peptide LL-37 in granulocytes. *Eur J Biochem* 1996;238:325–332.

132. McDonald PP, Bald A, Cassatella MA. Activation of the NF-κB pathway by inflammatory stimuli in human neutrophils. *Blood* 1997;89:3421–3433.

133. Gennaro R, Skerlavaj B, Romeo D. Purification, composition, and activity of two bactenecins, antibacterial peptides of bovine neutrophils. *Infect Immun* 1989;57:3142–3146.

134. Larrick JW, Morgan JG, Palings I, Hirata M, Yen MH. Complementary DNA sequence of rabbit CAP18—a unique lipopolysaccharide binding protein. *Biochem Biophys Res Commun* 1991;179:170–175.

135. Skerlavaj B, Gennaro R, Bagella L, Merluzzi L, Risso A, Zanetti M. Biological characterization of two novel cathelicidin-derived peptides and identification of structural requirements for their antimicrobial and cell lytic activities. *J Biol Chem* 1996;271:28375–28381.

136. Selsted ME, Novotny MJ, Morris WL, Tang YQ, Smith W, Cullor JS. Indolicidin, a novel bactericidal tridecapeptide amide from neutrophils. *J Biol Chem* 1992;267:4292–4295.

137. Storici P, Del SG, Schneider C, Zanetti M. cDNA sequence analysis of an antibiotic dodecapeptide from neutrophils. *FEBS Lett* 1992;314:187–190.

138. Kokryakov VN, Harwig SS, Panyutich EA, et al. Protegrins: leukocyte antimicrobial peptides that combine features of corticostatic defensins and tachyplesins. *FEBS Lett* 1993;327:231–236.

139. Tamamura H, Murakami T, Horiuchi S, et al. Synthesis of protegrin-related peptides and their antibacterial and anti-human immunodeficiency virus activity. *Chem Pharm Bull (Tokyo)* 1995;43:853–858.

140. Ooi CE, Weiss J, Levy O, Elsbach P. Isolation of two isoforms of a novel 15-kDa protein from rabbit polymorphonuclear leukocytes that modulate the antibacterial actions of other leukocyte proteins. *J Biol Chem* 1990;265:15956–15962.

141. Levy O, Weiss J, Zarember K, Ooi CE, Elsbach P. Antibacterial 15-kDa protein isoforms (p15s) are members of a novel family of leukocyte proteins. *J Biol Chem* 1993;268:6058–6063.

142. Agerberth B, Lee JY, Bergman T, et al. Amino acid sequence of PR-39: isolation from pig intestine of a new member of the family of proline-arginine-rich antibacterial peptides. *Eur J Biochem* 1991;202:849–854.

143. Huang H, Ross CR, Blecha F. Chemoattractant properties of PR-39, a neutrophil antibacterial peptide. *J Leukoc Biol* 1997;61:624–629.

144. Shi J, Ross CR, Leto TL, Blecha F. PR-39, a proline-rich antibacterial peptide that inhibits phagocyte NADPH oxidase activity by binding to Src homology 3 domains of p47phox. *Proc Natl Acad Sci U S A* 1996;93:6014–6018.

145. Hasan AA, Cines DB, Zhang J, Schmaier AH. The carboxyl terminus of bradykinin and amino terminus of kininogens comprise an endothelial cell binding domain. *J Biol Chem* 1994;269:31822–31830.

146. Bockman AA, Paegelow I. Bradykinin receptors in signal transduction pathways in peritoneal guineapig macrophages. *Eur J Pharmacol* 1995;291:159–165.

147. Verdot L, Lalmanach G, Vercruysse V, et al. Cystatins up-regulate nitric oxide release from interferon-γ-activated mouse peritoneal macrophages. *J Biol Chem* 1996;271:28077–28081.

148. Dennis EA. Diversity of group types, regulation, and function of phospholipase A2. *J Biol Chem* 1994;269:13057–13060.

149. Kudo I, Murakami M, Hara S, Inoue K. Mammalian non-pancreatic phospholipases A2. *Biochim Biophys Acta* 1993;1171:217–231.

150. Inada M, Crowl RM, Bekkers AC, Verheij H, Weiss J. Determinants of the inhibitory action of purified 14-kDa phospholipases A2 on cell-free prothrombinase complex. *J Biol Chem* 1994;269:26338–26343.

151. Weinrauch Y, Elsbach P, Madsen LM, Foreman A, Weiss J. The potent anti-*Staphylococcus aureus* activity of a sterile rabbit inflammatory fluid is due to a 14-kD phospholipase A2. *J Clin Invest* 1996;97:250–257.

152. Hanasaki K, Arita H. Characterization of a high affinity binding site for pancreatic-type phospholipase A2 in the rat: its cellular and tissue distribution. *J Biol Chem* 1992;267:6414–6420.

153. Murakami M, Nakatani Y, Kudo I. Type II secretory phospholipase A2 associated with cell surfaces via C-terminal heparin binding lysine residues augments stimulus-initiated delayed prostaglandin generation. *J Biol Chem* 1996;271:30041–30051.

154. Cupillard L, Koumanov K, Mattei M-G, Lazdunski M, Lambeau G. Cloning, chromosome mapping and expression of a novel human secretory phospholipase A2. *J Biol Chem* 1997;272:15745–15752.

155. Chilton F. Would the real role(s) for secretory PLA2s please stand up. *J Clin Invest* 1996;97:2161–2162.

156. Weinrauch Y, Abad C, Liang N-S, Lowry S, Weiss J. Mobilization of potent plasma (serum) bactericidal activity during systemic bacterial challenge: role of group II phospholipase A2. *J Invest Med* 1996;44:268A. *J Clin Invest* 1998;102:633–638.

157. Elsbach P, Weiss J. Phagocytosis of bacteria and phospholipid degradation. *Biochim Biophys Acta* 1988;947:29–52.

158. Wright GC, Weiss J, Kim KS, Verheij H, Elsbach P. Bacterial phospholipid hydrolysis enhances the destruction of *Escherichia coli* ingested by rabbit neutrophils: role of cellular and extracellular phospholipases. *J Clin Invest* 1990;85:1925–1935.

159. Harwig SS, Tan L, Qu XD, Cho Y, Eisenhauer PB, Lehrer RI. Bactericidal properties of murine intestinal phospholipase A2. *J Clin Invest* 1995;95:603–610.

160. Weiss J, Bekkers GW, van den Bergh CJ, Verheij HM. Conversion of pig pancreas phospholipase A2 by protein engineering into enzyme active against *Escherichia coli* treated with the bactericidal/permeability-increasing protein. *J Biol Chem* 1991;266:4162–4167.

161. Liang NS, Madsen LM, Weiss J. Functional bases of differences in the antibacterial activity of various purified 14 kD phospholipases A2 toward gram-positive bacteria (*in preparation*).

162. Anderson BF, Baker HM, Norris GE, Rice DW, Baker EN. Structure of human lactoferrin: crystallographic structure analysis and refinement at 2.8 Å resolution. *J Mol Biol* 1989;209:711–734.

163. Ward PP, Zhou X, Conneely OM. Cooperative interactions between the amino- and carboxyl-terminal lobes contribute to the unique iron-binding stability of lactoferrin. *J Biol Chem* 1996;271:12790–12794.

164. Arnold RR, Russell JE, Champion WJ, Brewer M. Bactericidal activity of human lactoferrin: differentiation from stasis of iron deprivation. *Infect Immun* 1982;35:792–799.

165. Ellison RT. The effects of lactoferrin on gram-negative bacteria. In: Hutchens TW, Rumball SV, Lonnerdal B, eds. *Lactoferrin: structure and function,* vol 357. New York: Plenum Press, 1994:71–90.

166. Gray-Owen SD, Schryvers AB. Bacterial transferrin and lactoferrin receptors. *Trends Microbiol* 1996;4:185–191.

167. Miehlke S, Reddy R, Osato MS, Ward PP, Conneely OM, Graham DY. Direct activity of recombinant human lactoferrin against *Helicobacter pylori*. *J Clin Microbiol* 1996;34:2593–2594.

168. Dhaenens L, Szczebara F, Husson MO. Identification, characterization, and immunogenicity of the lactoferrin-binding protein from *Helicobacter pylori*. *Infect Immun* 1997;65:514–518.

169. Harmsen MC, Swart PJ, Bethune MD, et al. Antiviral effects of plasma and milk proteins: lactoferrin shows potent activity against both human immunodeficiency virus and human cytomegalovirus replication *in vitro*. *J Infect Dis* 1995;172:380–388.

170. Yamauchi K, Tomita M, Giehl TJ, Ellison RT. Antibacterial activity of lactoferrin and a pepsin-derived lactoferrin peptide fragment. *Infect Immun* 1993;61:719–728.

171. Marra MN, Wilde CG, Griffith JE, Snable JL, Scott RW. Bactericidal/permeability-increasing protein has endotoxin-neutralizing activity. *J Immunol* 1990;144:662–666.

172. Appelmelk BJ, An YQ, Geerts M, et al. Lactoferrin is a lipid A-binding protein. *Infect Immun* 1994;62:2628–2632.

173. Elass-Rochard E, Roseanu A, LeGrand D, et al. Lactoferrin-lipopolysaccharide interaction: involvement of the 28-34 loop region of human lactoferrin in the high-affinity binding to *Escherichia coli* O55B5 lipopolysaccharide. *Biochem J* 1995;312:839–845.

174. Mattsby-Baltzer I, Roseanu A, Motas C, Elverfors J, Engberg I, Hanson LA. Lactoferrin or a fragment thereof inhibits the endotoxin-induced interleukin-6 response in human monocytic cells. *Pediatr Res* 1996;40:257–262.

175. Mazurier J, LeGrand D, Hu WL, Montreuil J, Spik G. Expression of human lactotransferrin receptors in phytohemagglutinin-stimulated human peripheral blood lymphocytes. *Eur J Biochem* 1989;179:481–487.

176. Gentile P, Broxmyer HE. Suppression of mouse myelopoiesis by administration of human lactoferrin *in vivo* and the comparative action of human transferrin. *Blood* 1983;61:982–993.

177. Kurose I, Yamada T, Wolf R, Granger DN. P-selectin-dependent leukocyte recruitment and intestinal mucosal injury induced by lactoferrin. *J Leukoc Biol* 1994;55:771–777.

178. Furmanski P, Li ZP, Fortuna MB, Swamy CV, Das MR. Multiple molecular forms of human lactoferrin: identification of a class of lactoferrins that possess ribonuclease activity and lack iron-binding capacity. *J Exp Med* 1989;170:415–429.

179. He J, Furmanski P. Sequence specificity and transcriptional activation in the binding of lactoferrin to DNA. *Nature* 1995;373:721–724.

180. Burrin DG, Wang H, Heath J, Dudley MA. Orally administered lactoferrin increases hepatic protein synthesis in formula-fed newborn pigs. *Pediatr Res* 1996;40:72–76.

181. Sugi K, Saitoh O, Hirata I, Katsu K. Fecal lactoferrin as a marker for disease activity in inflammatory bowel disease: comparison with other neutrophil-derived proteins. *Am J Gastroenterol* 1996;91:927–934.

182. Hessian PA, Edgeworth J, Hogg N. MRP-8 and MRP-14, two abundant Ca2—binding proteins of neutrophils and monocytes. *J Leukoc Biol* 1993;53:197–204.

183. Sohnle PG, Hahn BL, Santhanagopalan V. Inhibition of *Candida albicans* growth by calprotectin in the absence of direct contact with the organisms. *J Infect Dis* 1996;174:1369–1372.

184. Sohnle PG, Collins LC, Wiessner JH. The zinc-reversible antimicrobial activity of neutrophil lysates and abscess fluid supernatants. *J Infect Dis* 1991;164:137–142.

185. Santhanagopalan V, Hahn BL, Dunn BE, Weissner JH, Sohnle PG. Antimicrobial activity of calprotectin isolated from human empyema fluid supernatants. *Clin Immunol Immunopathol* 1995;76:285–290.

186. Yui S, Mikami M, Yamazaki M. Induction of apoptotic cell death in mouse lymphoma and human leukemia cell lines by a calcium-binding protein complex, calprotectin, derived from inflammatory peritoneal exudate cells. *J Leukoc Biol* 1995;58:650–658.

187. Miyasaki KT, Bodeau AL. Human neutrophil azurocidin synergizes with leukocyte elastase and cathepsin G in the killing of *Capnocytophaga sputigena*. *Infect Immun* 1992;60:4973–4975.

188. Lehrer RI, Szklarek D, Ganz T, Selsted ME. Synergistic activity of rabbit granulocyte peptides against *Candida albicans*. *Infect Immun* 1986;52:902–904.

189. Skerlavaj B, Romeo D, Gennaro R. Rapid membrane permeabilization and inhibition of vital functions of gram-negative bacteria by bactenecins. *Infect Immun* 1990;58:3724–3730.

190. Stein DK, Malawista SE, Van Blaricom G, Wysong D, Diamond RD. Cytoplasts generate oxidants but require added neutrophil granule constituents for fungicidal activity against *Candida albicans* hyphae. *J Infect Dis* 1995;172:511–520.

191. Akin DT, Lu MQ, Lu SJ, Kendall S, Rundegren J, Arnold RR. Bactericidal activity of different forms of lactoferrin. In: Hutchens TW, Rumball SV, Lonnerdal B, eds. *Lactoferrin: structure and function,* vol 357. New York: Plenum Press, 1994:61–70.

192. Monajemi H, Meenan J, Lamping R, et al. Inflammatory bowel disease is associated with increased mucosal levels of bactericidal/permeability-increasing protein. *Gastroenterology* 1996;110:733–739.

193. Altstaedt J, Kirchner H, Rink L. Cytokine production of neutrophils is limited to interleukin-8. *Immunology* 1996;89:563–568.

194. Brooks CJ, King WJ, Radford DJ, Adu D, McGrath M, Savage CO. IL-1 beta production by human polymorphonuclear leucocytes stimulated by anti-neutrophil cytoplasmic autoantibodies: relevance to systemic vasculitis. *Clin Exp Immunol* 1996;106:273–279.

195. Hogasen AKM, Wurzner R, Abrahamsen TG, Dierich MP. Human polymorphonuclear leukocytes store large amounts of terminal complement components C7 and C6, which may be released on stimulation. *J Immunol* 1994;154:4734–4740.

196. Varki A. Selectin ligands: will the real ones please stand out. *J Clin Invest* 1997;99:158–162.

197. Ip YT, Reach M, Engstrom Y, et al. Dif, a dorsal-related gene that mediates an immune response in *Drosophila*. *Cell* 1993;75:753–763.

198. Ip YT, Levine M. Molecular genetics of *Drosophila* immunity. *Curr Opin Genet Devel* 1994;4:672–677.
199. Hoffmann JA, Reichhart JM, Hetru C. Innate immunity in higher insects. *Curr Opin Immunol* 1996;8:8–13.
200. Groisman EA. Bacterial responses to host-defense peptides. *Trends Microb* 1996;4:127–128.
201. Yamamoto T, Hanawa T, Ogata S, Kamiya S. The *Yersinia enterocolitica* GsrA stress protein, involved in intracellular survival, is induced by macrophage phagocytosis. *Infect Immun* 1997;65:2190–2196.
202. von der Mohlen MA, van Deventer SJ, Levi M, et al. Inhibition of endotoxin-induced activation of the coagulation and fibrinolytic pathways using a recombinant endotoxin-binding protein (rBPI23). *Blood* 1995;85:3437–3443.
203. de Winter RJ, von der Mohlen MA, van Lieshout H, Wedel N, et al. Recombinant endotoxin-binding protein (rBPI23) attenuates endotoxin-induced circulatory changes in humans. *J Inflamm* 1995;45:193–206.
204. Tang YQ, Selsted ME. Characterization of the disulfide motif in BNBD-12, an antimicrobial beta-defensin peptide from bovine neutrophils. *J Biol Chem* 1993;268:6649–6653.
205. Gabay JE. Antimicrobial proteins with homology to serine proteases. *Ciba Found Symp* 1994;186:237–247.
206. Wright GW, Ooi CE, Weiss J, Elsbach P. Purification of a cellular (granulocyte) and an extracellular (serum) phospholipase A2 that participate in the destruction of *Escherichia coli* in a rabbit inflammatory exudate. *J Biol Chem* 1990;265:6675–6681.
207. Iyer S, Lonnerdal B. Lactoferrin, lactoferrin receptors and iron metabolism. *Eur J Clin Nutr* 1993;47:232–241.
208. Jolles P. From the discovery of lysozyme to the characterization of several lysozyme families. *EXS* 1996;75:3–5.
209. Couto MA, Harwig SS, Cullor JS, Hughes JP, Lehrer RI. eNAP-2, a novel cysteine-rich bactericidal peptide from equine leukocytes. *Infect Immun* 1992;60:5042–5047.
210. Botto M, Lissandrini D, Sorio C, Walport MJ. Biosynthesis and secretion of complement component (C3) by activated human polymorphonuclear leukocytes. *J Immunol* 1992;149:1348–1355.
211. Brandtzaeg P, Gabrielsen TO, Dale I, Muller F, Steinbakk M, Fagerhol MK. The leucocyte protein L1 (calprotectin): a putative nonspecific defence factor at epithelial surfaces. *Adv Exp Med Biol* 1995;371A:201–206.

Inflammation: Basic Principles and Clinical Correlates,
3rd ed., edited by John I. Gallin and Ralph Snyderman.
Lippincott Williams & Wilkins, Philadelphia © 1999.

CHAPTER 51

Apoptosis and Senescence of Hematopoietic and Immune Cells:

Mechanisms and Significance

Lina M. Obeid and Yusuf A. Hannun

The optimum functioning of most tissues requires the operation of sophisticated mechanisms that allow the tissue to respond and adapt to various changes in the demands made upon it. The components of hematopoietic and vascular tissues (red blood cells, neutrophils, lymphocytes, platelets, and endothelial cells) are constantly called on to deal with either acute problems, such as bleeding or vascular injury, or more long-term changes, such as infection or tissue injury. Whereas many of these responses require the operation of specific and preexisting regulatory pathways, a major component in the normal function of hematopoietic cells relies on the maintenance of a delicate balance among proliferation, differentiation, cell death, and senescence of specific cell types (Fig. 51-1). For example, short- and intermediate-term responses to infectious and inflammatory conditions may require an expansion of blood neutrophils, whereas long-term responses may require expansion of specific pools of lymphocytes and macrophages.

The influence of proliferation rates on the ultimate size of a tissue has received significant attention. Many of the growth factors, intracellular mechanisms that transduce their effects, and components of the cell cycle machinery that regulate cell division and proliferation have been defined and are becoming more clearly understood. However, control of terminal differentiation, cell senescence, and cell death are equally important in determining the net rate of tissue growth (see Fig. 51-1). The processes and mechanisms that regulate cell senescence and cell

death have received belated attention and are currently under intensive investigation. This chapter provides an overview of the mechanisms that operate in the regulation of cell death and cell senescence along with a discussion of the biologic relevance of these processes to hematopoietic systems, the effects of derangements of these processes in various pathologic situations, and the possible development of novel therapeutic approaches based on the understanding of these mechanisms.

DEFINITIONS AND SIGNIFICANCE

Programmed Cell Death or Apoptosis

The demise of most cell types under physiologic conditions and probably under a majority of pathologic conditions occurs through the operation of highly regulated biochemical processes that precisely orchestrate the orderly breakdown of the cell and its ultimate death. Although exact definitions vary, these mechanisms are referred to collectively as *programmed cell death* or *apoptosis*. The death of a cell can be initiated in response to either internal programs (the classic definition of programmed cell death), environmental factors (e.g., death-inducing cytokines), or cell injury (e.g., hypoxia, cytotoxic agents) (1–12).

During the process of apoptosis, there is an orderly breakdown of internal structures and macromolecules (3,13) (Fig. 51-2). For example, the nuclear matrix undergoes breakdown due to proteolysis of lamins, whereas chromatin is initially processed into large DNA fragments (on the order of 50 kb) and eventually these are broken down into internucleosomal fragments. The

L. M. Obeid and Y. A. Hannun: Departments of Medicine and Biochemistry, Medical University of South Carolina, Charleston, South Carolina 29425.

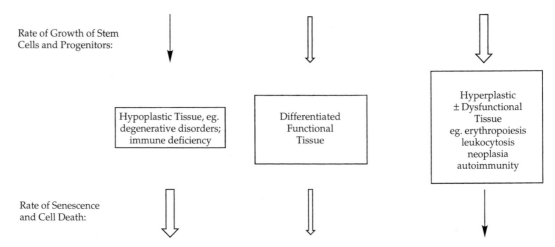

Rate of Growth of Stem
Cells and Progenitors:

Hypoplastic Tissue, eg.
degenerative disorders;
immune deficiency

Differentiated
Functional
Tissue

Hyperplastic
± Dysfunctional
Tissue
eg. erythropoiesis
leukocytosis
neoplasia
autoimmunity

Rate of Senescence
and Cell Death:

FIG. 51-1. Scheme of tissue regulation through changes in rates of growth, senescence, and cell death. Under normal homeostasis, the rate of growth is balanced by the rates of senescence and cell death. This allows for normal differentiation and function of a tissue. A decrease in the rate of growth of progenitor cells or an increase in the rate of senescence or cell death can lead to a hypoplastic tissue with decreased function. This may occur in degenerative disorders and immune deficiency disorders. On the other hand, an increase in the rate of growth or a decrease in the rate of senescence or cell death may result in tissue hyperplasia. Often, a hyperplastic response is required for normal function, as in the reactive erythropoiesis seen in response to decreased oxygen tension or the reactive leukocytosis seen in infections. Pathologically, this may result in increased immune function, as in autoimmune disorders, and in preneoplastic conditions that would provide the background for cancer development.

plasma membrane undergoes blebbing and exteriorization of phosphatidylserine from the inner leaflet to the outer leaflet. This is followed by the formation of apoptotic bodies, which contain cytoplasmic and membrane fragments. These apoptotic bodies appear to be sealed through the action of transglutaminases, which may act to prevent leakage or nonspecific release of cytoplasmic granules and contents. This may be especially important in the prevention of lysosomal release, because lysosomal hydrolases are capable of inducing a strong inflammatory response. The apoptotic bodies are then picked up by adjacent normal tissue cells, predominantly through the action of reticuloendothelial cells. Therefore, the breakdown of the cell into apoptotic bodies results in an orderly clearing of the cell.

Apoptosis is appreciated to play significant roles in a number of areas, including developmental biology, immunobiology, tissue homeostasis, reaction to injury, and cancer biology (Table 51-1).

Normal development requires the elimination of predetermined cell types, such as cells that produce interdigital webbing (14–16). Apoptosis in development is best illustrated and studied in the nematode *Caenorhabditis elegans,* in which a fixed number of cells undergo developmental elimination (17,18). Study of this organism has yielded a number of cell death genes, including homologues of the B-cell CLL/lymphoma-2 gene *BCL2* (19) and mammalian cysteine proteases (18) (see later discussion).

Self-tolerance and activation-induced cell death involve the operation of programmed cell death (14,20). Malfunctioning of this system, as occurs in mice with genetic defects in Fas or Fas ligands (regulators of apoptosis), results in hyperproliferation of immune cells and autoimmune disease (21).

The determination of the normal size and function of a tissue relies substantially on a delicate balance among cell growth, cell differentiation, and cell death. For example, in skin, the most differentiated epidermal cells undergo cell death as they provide the permeability barrier. This also allows for continuous replenishing of the epithelium and maintenance of the appropriate thickness of skin. This paradigm can be generalized to all proliferating or regenerating tissues, such as intestinal epithelium, liver, and hematopoietic cells (4,13,14).

Many noxious agents or injurious insults such as heat, ischemia, reperfusion, or hypoxia cause cell death, which can be necrotic if the insult is acute and severe or apoptotic if the insult is more gradual and less dramatic. One fundamental difference between necrosis and apoptosis relates to the orderly breakdown of apoptotic cells without the release of intracellular contents (e.g., lysosomal enzymes) that might elicit inflammatory responses. Apoptotic cell death can result in more controlled death of cells without inflammation, whereas necrosis may be accompanied by severe inflammatory reactions. It is possible that tissues strive to contain the consequences of damage by activating apoptotic programs.

Apoptosis appears to play two fundamental roles in cancer medicine. First, disturbances in apoptotic mechanisms may underlie the progression to a malignant phenotype in most cancer types (1,22,23). This is illustrated by mutations in the gene encoding p53, which plays an anti-apoptotic role in response to DNA damage (11,24).

Such mutations allow many cancer cells to grow and proliferate despite the accumulation of serious mutations. Second, it is increasingly apparent that most forms of cytotoxic chemotherapy as well as hyperthermia and ionizing radiation therapy act by eventually turning on apoptotic mechanisms of cell death (7,25).

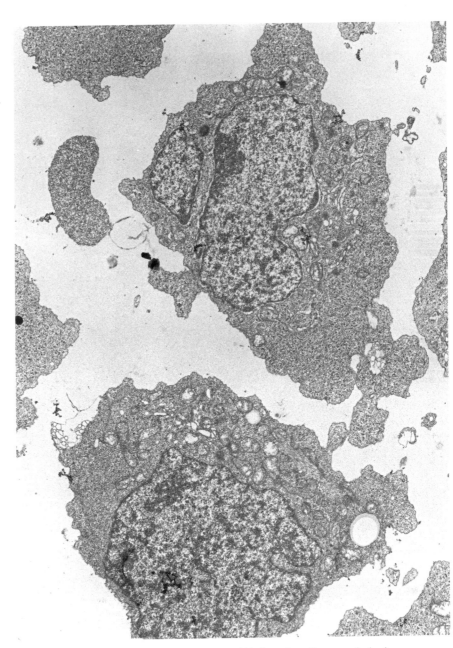

Characteristics of Apoptotic Cells:

- chromatin condensation
- nuclear collapse
- formation of apoptotic bodies
- mitochondrial fragmentation?
- formation of cytoplasmic vesicles
- cyoplasmic shrinkage

A   B

FIG. 51-2. Characteristics and morphology of apoptotic cells. The table (**A**) describes the morphologic characteristics of apoptotic cells. The electron micrographs show normal (**B**) and apoptotic (**C**) ALL-697 lymphoblasts treated with 20 μmol/L etoposide. The cells show the characteristic features of nuclear collapse, chromatin condensation, cytoplasmic blebbing, and formation of apoptotic bodies. The long arrow shows condensed chromatin, and the short arrows show apoptotic bodies at various stages of formation. *(Continued on next page)*

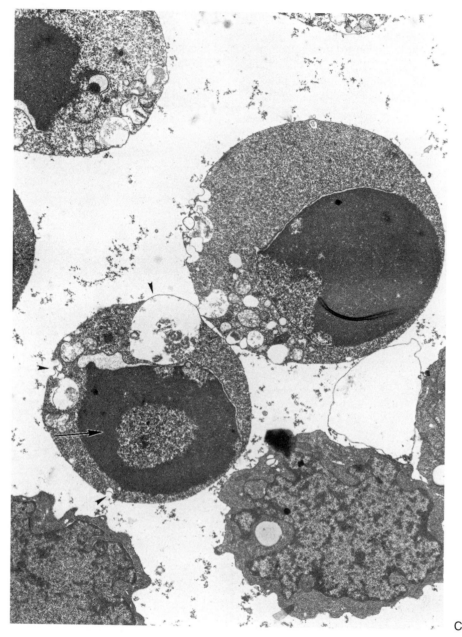

FIG. 51-2. *(Continued)*

Cell Senescence

Cell senescence is defined as the finite life span phenotype of cells in culture, beyond which cells appear to be unable to respond to growth factors and mitogens (i.e.,

unable to proliferate). Cellular senescence was initially described by Hayflick and Moorhead in reference to fibroblasts (26) in culture (Fig. 51-3*A*, *B*) but has more recently been reported for several other cell types, including melanocytes, keratinocytes, and cells of the hematopoietic and immune systems such as red blood cells, neutrophils, lymphocytes, and endothelial cells (27–30). In addition, senescence has been described across species, including mice, *Drosophila*, *C. elegans*, and yeast. Several important insights into the mechanisms of aging have been obtained from studies of conserved molecular and biochemical pathways among species. Cellular senescence is considered to be a convenient and appropriate model to study *in vivo* aging

TABLE 51-1. *Biologic functions of apoptosis and senescence*

Apoptosis	Senescense
Developmental biology	Antioncogenic function
Immune function	Response to injury
Tissue injury	
Tissue homeostasis	

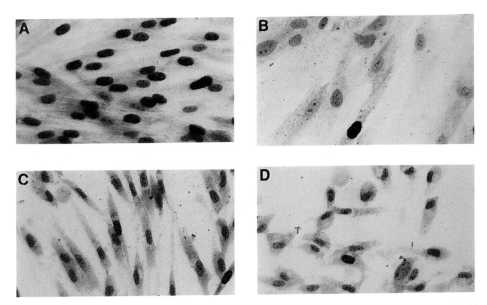

FIG. 51-3. Characteristics and morphology of senescent cells. **(A)** Normal human diploid fibroblasts in tissue culture, showing the predominance of nuclei (75%) labeled with thymidine (as an index of proliferation). **(B)** Senescent fibroblasts with near absence of labeling (<2%) and with characteristic morphologic changes. **(C and D)** Young fibroblasts treated with ceramide (10 and 15 μmol/L, respectively), mimicking senescent morphology. This figure is reproduced with permission from Venable ME, Lee JY, Smyth MJ, Bielawska A, Obeid LM. Role of ceramide in cellular senescence. *J Biol Chem* 1995;270:30701–30708.

because of an inverse correlation between the life span of the donor and the life span of the donated cells in culture. In addition, cells from organisms with a longer life span live longer in cultured conditions (31).

There are several theories pertaining to the initiation and significance of the cellular senescence programs. One theory proposes that senescence is a preprogrammed event—that is, there are specific genes that get turned on to induce the senescent phenotype. Supporting evidence includes several observations indicating that senescence is a dominant phenotype. For example, when young and senescent cells are fused, the resultant heterokaryon displays a senescent phenotype (32,33). Also, when mRNA from senescent cells is injected into young cells, it is able to induce senescence (34). According to this scenario, senescence may function as an anti-oncogenic mechanism (35). Another theory indicates that senescence occurs in response to the accumulation of environmental and toxic damage sustained during the life span (36,37). Evidence comes from the discovery of numerous insults that appear to induce a senescent phenotype. These include oxygen free radicals and ultraviolet radiation, which cause damage to DNA that may eventually be irreparable, leading to the growth arrest seen in cellular senescence (38,39). According to this hypothesis, senescence may function as a resistance to cell injury.

Some of the features that distinguish senescence are more specific to this condition than others, but taken together they lead to what has become accepted as the senescent phenotype. Senescent cells are not dead or dying cells; rather they are metabolically active cells that are larger and have larger nuclei and increased content of RNA, protein, lipid, and extracellular matrix, compared with nonsenescent cells (31). Senescent cells, however, cannot undergo DNA synthesis, and it has been proposed that this is in part caused by the existence of dominant inhibitors of DNA synthesis. Another distinguishing feature of cellular senescence is that it is irreversible except when cells have been transformed by DNA tumor viruses such as SV40 (40). This irreversible feature is shared with cells that undergo terminal differentiation; hence, the similarity between the senescent phenotype and cellular differentiation (35).

RELATION BETWEEN APOPTOSIS AND CELL SENESCENCE

Cell senescence (which in many ways resembles terminal cell differentiation) and apoptosis are intimately related as the two major forms by which cells exit permanently the proliferative life cycle. Apoptosis results in the regulated elimination of the cell, whereas cell senescence and terminal differentiation result in the formation of a metabolically active and functional cell (often with specialized function) that has lost the capacity for regeneration. These processes may be considered as programs of growth suppression that play important roles in normal tissue homeostasis. In addition, both processes appear to operate in response to various forms of stress or injury. For example, apoptosis is induced by many physical and toxic agents in the environment and by stress cytokines, whereas cell senescence has been linked to oxidative damage and possibly other forms of intracellular stress. Both processes also appear to play important roles in anti-oncogenesis, in that apoptosis provides for elimination of damaged or mutated cells and serves as a check against unrestrained growth, whereas senescent cells are incapable of the unlimited cell divisions characteristic of cancer cells.

MECHANISMS OF APOPTOSIS AND SENESCENCE

Any given cell possesses a number of biochemical and molecular mechanisms for interacting with its environment and transducing the effects of extracellular agents and stimuli. These processes, collectively called *signal transduction mechanisms,* involve the operation of receptors, transducers (e.g., G proteins), enzymes (e.g., cyclases, protein kinases), and various second messengers (e.g., cyclic adenosine monophosphate [cAMP], diacylglycerol, inositol trisphosphate) (41–45). The action of growth hormones is the best studied example. Growth factors and growth hormones interact with transmembrane receptors, resulting in the activation of a number of biochemical mechanisms of signal transduction involving various tyrosine and serine-threonine protein kinases, G proteins, lipases, lipid kinases, and other adapter and coupling proteins (41,45,46). Eventually this results in induction of gene transcription, promotion of cell cycle progression through effects on cyclin-dependent kinases, and reprogramming of the metabolic functions of the cell.

The cell contains complex machineries that monitor the activities and health of the organism, the tissue, and various components of intracellular function. These mechanisms are not as clearly defined as the transmembrane signal transduction mechanisms operating in response to mitogenic growth factors. However, it is becoming obvious that the response of cells to growth suppressor stimuli, adverse and stress stimuli in the environment, and cytotoxic agents involves biochemical pathways that monitor the level of stress or injury and activate appropriate response programs (5,6,43,47,48).

These pathways are perhaps best studied in the case of stress cytokines such as tumor necrosis factor-α (TNF-α) and the FAS ligand (Fig. 51-4A). These cytokines act on transmembrane receptors that do not appear to contain any intrinsic enzymatic activity. However, receptor occupancy leads to recruitment of a number of proteins that serve to couple the receptor to various intracellular effectors. In the case of TNF-α, occupancy of its primary pro-apoptotic receptor (p55/p60 receptor) results in association with a number of adapter proteins such as TRAF (49–52). These proteins somehow result in linking of the TNF receptor to activation of nuclear factor-κB (53,54), activation of JUN kinase (55,56) (also known as stress-activated protein

kinase, or SAPK), and the apoptotic pathway. In the case of FAS, a major component appears to be the cysteine protease Mach I/Flice (57,58). Several downstream components have been delineated, including effects on mitochondrial function, possibly mediated through the formation of oxygen radicals. TNF-α has been shown to activate sphingomyelinases, which act on membrane sphingomyelin, causing the accumulation of ceramide (59,60). In turn, ceramide has been implicated as a potential transducer/modulator of the apoptotic effects of TNF-α as well as those of FAS, dexamethasone, heat, ionizing radiation, various cytotoxic chemotherapeutic agents, and many other inducers of stress or injury (61–65). These mediators (i.e., ceramide, reactive oxygen species) somehow result in the release of cytochrome *c* from mitochondria into the cytosol (66–68). The release of cytochrome *c* is indirectly inhibited by the BCL2 anti-apoptotic protein.

BCL2 has emerged as a key regulator of the apoptotic pathway. It was originally identified as a translocated oncogene in human lymphoma and then was discovered to exert its "oncogenic" effects by inhibiting apoptosis. BCL2 belongs to an extended family of proteins, some of which are anti-apoptotic (e.g., BCL$_X$) and others pro-apoptotic (e.g., BCL2-associated X protein [BAX], BCL2-antagonist of cell death [BAD]). The precise mechanism of action of these proteins is unknown, but they have been suggested to form membrane channels or to function as regulatory proteins for several components of the apoptotic pathways, or both (66,68).

Studies suggest that the release of cytochrome *c* indirectly activates cysteine proteases of the caspase family, probably through recruitment of the protein APAF1 (69,70). Activation of proteases such as caspase-3 (CPP32) results in degradation and processing of key substrates such as lamin B or endonucleases that cause the ultimate breakdown of the cell (71–73). Studies indicate that caspases activate a specific endonuclease by cleaving an inhibitor of this endonuclease (74).

These emerging biochemical insights into the mechanisms regulating apoptosis complement genetic studies initially conducted in the nematode *C. elegans*. In this organism, programmed cell death results in a fixed number of dead cells; it is regulated primarily by two pro-apoptotic genes, *ced-3* and *ced-4*, and inhibited by *ced-9*. *Ced-3* is homologous to mammalian caspases that are activated during apoptosis, whereas *ced-9* is homologous to BCL2, and the two proteins are functionally interchangeable. Mammalian proteins that share some homology to *ced-4* have been identified (e.g., APAF1) and may function in the regulation of cytochrome *c* release (see Fig. 51-4A).

Other key proteins that have been identified in the apoptotic process include phospholipase A$_2$ (especially in the case of TNF-α) (75–77), fast kinase in the case of FAS (78), and tyrosine kinases and some of their regulators (79,80). During activation of the apoptotic program, changes occur in many of the pathways involved in

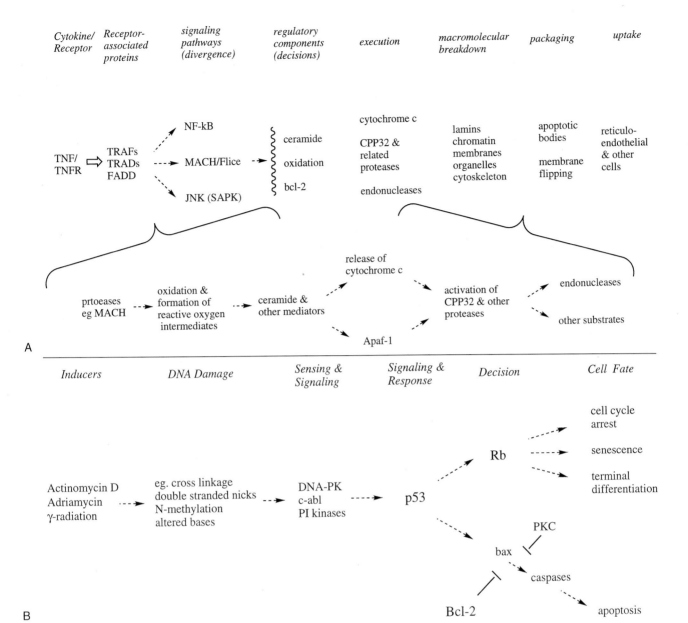

Cytokine/ Receptor	Receptor-associated proteins	signaling pathways (divergence)	regulatory components (decisions)	execution	macromolecular breakdown	packaging	uptake

TNF/ TNFR ⇒ TRAFs TRADs FADD

NF-kB

MACH/Flice

JNK (SAPK)

ceramide

oxidation

bcl-2

cytochrome c

CPP32 & related proteases

endonucleases

lamins chromatin membranes organelles cytoskeleton

apoptotic bodies

membrane flipping

reticulo-endothelial & other cells

prtoeases eg MACH → oxidation & formation of reactive oxygen intermediates → ceramide & other mediators → release of cytochrome c → activation of CPP32 & other proteases → endonucleases / other substrates

Apaf-1

A

Inducers	DNA Damage	Sensing & Signaling	Signaling & Response	Decision	Cell Fate

Actinomycin D Adriamycin γ-radiation

eg. cross linkage double stranded nicks N-methylation altered bases

DNA-PK c-abl PI kinases

p53

Rb

cell cycle arrest

senescence

terminal differentiation

bax

PKC

caspases

Bcl-2

apoptosis

B

FIG. 51-4. Schemes of apoptotic regulatory pathways. (**A**) Pathways induced by cytokines. A summary of major regulators and mediators of the effects of tumor necrosis factor-α (TNF-α) on apoptosis is shown. The action of TNF-α on its transmembrane receptor (TNFR) leads to interaction of this receptor with a family of regulatory and adapter proteins (including TRAF, TRAD, and FADD) that also interact with each other. By as yet poorly understood mechanisms, these receptor-mediated interactions cause activation of distinct pathways that can result in activation of NF-κB, which may exert an anti-apoptotic effect; activation of the stress-activated protein kinase JNK; and activation of members of the caspase family of cysteine proteases. The caspases appear to be important in launching specific apoptotic mechanisms. Somehow, activation of these proteases results in formation of the sphingolipid ceramide, in modulation of the redox status of the cell, and in the formation of reactive oxygen species. This could possibly result in mitochondrial dysfunction with involvement of some mitochondrial regulatory factors in processing the apoptotic signal. This activity appears to involve the release of cytochrome *c* from the mitochondria to the cytosol, which appears to be the major step for the action of the anti-apoptotic protein BCL2. The release of cytochrome *c*, coupled with the action of protein cofactors such as APAF-1 (possibly the mammalian homologue of the nematode gene *ced-4*), results in activation of downstream (or execution-phase) proteases such as CPP32, which in turn cause activation of endonucleases and cleavage of other protein substrates. The overall outcome of this process is the breakdown of supramolecular structures and macromolecules in the cell. These are packaged into apoptotic bodies, which are then taken up by normal cells and by cells of the reticuloendothelial system. (**B**) Scheme of induction of apoptosis in response to DNA-damaging agents. DNA-damaging agents may cause multiple forms of DNA damage. Damaged DNA is sensed by poorly defined signaling mechanisms that may involve the DNA-dependent protein kinase (DNA-PK), the ABL tyrosine kinase, and members of the phosphatidylinositol 3-kinase (PI3K) family. Many inducers of DNA damage induce or activate p53. p53 appears to function primarily as a transcription factor. Some of the genes induced by p53 cause activation of the retinoblastoma gene product (RB), which may drive the cells into cell cycle arrest, or activation of the BAX pro-apoptotic member of the BCL2 family, with subsequent activation of caspases and induction of apoptosis.

growth regulation. For example, changes in the cAMP–protein kinase A pathway have been shown to modulate apoptosis. Activation of protein kinase C has been shown to oppose apoptosis in many cell types, whereas inhibition of protein kinase C may result in loss of viability and promotion of apoptosis. Also, persistent calcium influx (as opposed to transient intracellular calcium release in response to growth factors) can result in cytotoxicity and apoptosis (81–83).

Another rapidly developing model for understanding mechanisms of apoptosis has emerged from the study of DNA-damaging agents (see Fig. 51-4B) Much of this insight came from studies of the tumor suppressor gene, *p53*. This gene is mutated in a large number of cancers, and early studies resulted in identification of an important role for the normal p53 protein in driving cells toward either apoptosis or cell cycle arrest (11,24). Many DNA-damaging agents, such as ionizing radiation or chemotherapeutic agents, cause induction and activation of p53 (11,24,84). This may involve activation of the ABL tyrosine kinase, DNA-dependent protein kinase (DNA-PK), and phosphatidylinositol 3-kinase (PI3K) (85–87). Little is known about the specific signals generated from damaged DNA and how these can regulate sensing or signaling components such as ABL (87) that somehow result in induction and activation of p53. Once induced, p53 activates growth suppressor pathways, probably by acting as a transcription factor, leading to either cell cycle arrest or apoptosis, depending on the cell type and other regulatory factors (24,88). The mechanisms involved in this action also remain poorly understood but may involve effects on the retinoblastoma gene product (RB) and on members of the BCL2 family of apoptosis regulators (89–93) (see Fig. 51-4).

In tissue culture, apoptosis also occurs when cells appear to receive two or more "conflicting" signals. For example, cells that are deprived of growth factors (which is usually a signal to undergo growth arrest) and at the same time are driven by overexpression of growth-promoting genes (such as RAS or MYC) may undergo apoptosis (94,95). This phenomenon may have *in vivo* counterparts.

The picture that is emerging reveals complicated and interacting mechanisms that allow the cell to monitor both its intracellular health and the suitability of the extracellular environment. Growth-promoting influences result in the generation of viability signals and drive the cell cycle, whereas stressful and toxic stimuli result in the generation of growth suppressor or apoptotic signals. The cell appears to possess the machinery to assess and integrate these responses and reach critical decisions. If the level of damage is tolerable and repairable (e.g., modest DNA injury), then the cell may "decide" to undergo cell cycle arrest in order to allow repair of the damage before normal cell growth and cell function resume. On the other hand, if the degree of injury is beyond repair, then the cell may decide to undergo apoptosis (possibly for the benefit of the rest of the tissue). Little is known concern-

ing these decision points and the precise mechanisms that regulate cell fate. One important factor may be RB, whose status of phosphorylation may decide whether the cell continues to undergo proliferation or undergoes cell cycle arrest (see Fig. 51-4B). Many of the same stimuli that could cause apoptosis would also result in dephosphorylation of RB. The dephosphorylated form of RB binds the E2F transcription factor and prevents it from stimulating transcription (96,97). Therefore, if this pathway of cell regulation is intact and operative, the cell may have the option of undergoing cell cycle arrest. When this system fails (for example, many apoptotic agents result in the proteolysis of RB, which is a mechanism for its inactivation), the cell may preferentially undergo apoptosis.

Once the decision for apoptosis has been established, the cell enters a series of simultaneous and sequential biochemical events that constitute the execution phase of apoptosis. One early set of cellular proteins in this phase is a group of cysteine proteases including CPP32 (apopain). Several protein substrates for these proteases have been identified, including poly-adenosine diphosphate-ribose-polymerase (PARP), nuclear lamins, RB, and protein kinase C$_\delta$. Activation of these proteolytic pathways results in nuclear collapse, internucleosomal DNA fragmentation, cytoplasmic blebbing, and formation of apoptotic bodies (see Fig. 51-4). In concert, these events define the apoptotic outcome for an individual cell. For final completion of the apoptotic process, the formation and release of apoptotic bodies, which contain debris, organelles, and degraded chromatin, are followed by uptake by neighboring cells and by cells of the reticuloendothelial system.

Much has been elucidated about the molecular characteristics of cellular senescence, but not as much is known about the mechanisms that lead to the inhibition of mitogenesis and growth arrest of senescence.

Senescent cells are characterized by their inability to respond to mitogenic stimuli. This has been demonstrated to be caused, in some cases, by decreases in cell surface receptors for certain growth factors such as epidermal growth factor (EGF), platelet-derived growth factor (PDGF), and insulin-like growth factor (IGF) (98–101) and, in other cases, by decreased responsiveness of those receptors to their extracellular ligands (despite adequate numbers of receptors and normal binding affinities). Other receptor classes (e.g., adrenergic receptors) have been demonstrated to have altered regulation in aging. Decreases are reported in agonist levels, receptor numbers, receptor affinities, G-protein activation, and levels of G protein (102). Several alterations in other signal transduction pathways have been described in senescent cells; some are cell specific, and others appear to be universally altered in senescent cells (103). For example, RAS expression is significantly decreased in senescent fibroblasts, and the activation of mitogen-activated protein (MAP) kinase is decreased in senescent melanocytes. There are age-related decreases in protein-tyrosine kinase activation in human T lymphocytes that are thought to be a consequence of dysfunction of components of the signaling cascade (104). The sphingolipid-mediated signaling pathway also has been implicated in senescence. Activity of the enzyme sphingomyelinase and levels of ceramide have been demonstrated to be significantly elevated in senescent human diploid fibroblasts and were implicated in inducing the senescent phenotype (see Fig. 51-3B) (105). Ceramide causes inhibition of DNA synthesis and transcription factor (AP1) activation, as well as dephosphorylation of RB, all accepted parameters of cellular senescence. Other lipid-mediated signaling pathways have also been investigated in senescent cells. These include the diacylglycerol–protein kinase C–phospholipid D pathway. Senescent cells are unable to respond to growth factor stimulation because they are unable to generate diacylglycerol and consequently are unable to translocate and activate protein kinase C (106). This is thought to be a result of inhibition of phospholipase D activity in senescent cells. In addition, there is crosstalk between the sphingolipid and glycerolipid signaling pathways, as seen in apoptosis. Ceramide appears to cause inhibition of phospholipase D in cells and *in vitro* (107). This inhibition is thought to be mediated by ceramide-activated protein phosphatase and to involve the protein kinase C–activatable component of phospholipase D.

Other mechanisms that occur in and may lead to cellular senescence have been investigated extensively. These are the mechanisms that regulate the cell cycle and gene expression. Alterations in cell cycle regulatory proteins in cellular senescence include marked decreases in the activity of cyclin dependent kinase 2 (CDK2) kinase and in cyclin A (CYCA) and cyclin B (CYCB) protein levels, along with overexpression of p21 and possibly p53 (108,109). RB is found predominantly in the hypophosphorylated form in senescent cells, possibly because of inhibition of CDK2 activity (110). Recent data implicate ceramide in the inhibition of CDK2, probably through activation of ceramide-activated protein phosphatase. Lee and Obeid (submitted). This leads to dephosphorylation of RB and a senescent phenotype, thus corroborating a key role for ceramide in the induction of a senescent phenotype.

The activation of transcription factor AP1 is decreased in senescent fibroblasts and in lymphocytes. This is believed to be caused by loss of c-Fos transcription in senescence (111). It could also be explained by the lack of activation of protein kinase C (because AP1 is a downstream target of protein kinase C), which in turn may be due in part to ceramide inhibition of cellular protein kinase C.

An important area in the understanding of cellular senescence involves telomeres and telomerase. Telomerase is the enzyme that is known to add telomeric DNA to the ends of chromosomes (telomeres). This enzyme activity is elevated in cancer cells. It is significantly decreased in senescent lymphocytes and absent in senescent fibroblasts, resulting in progressively shorter telom-

eres with age of these cells (112). This phenomenon has been implicated as a critical factor in leading to the growth arrest seen in senescence. Whether growth arrest occurs because shorter telomeres are interpreted as DNA damage by cells or because subtelomeric DNA encodes for genes involved in cellular senescence is not yet clearly understood.

BIOLOGIC SIGNIFICANCE OF APOPTOSIS AND SENESCENCE IN THE HEMATOPOIETIC SYSTEM

The following sections describe several examples of the operation of apoptosis and senescence in hematopoietic function.

Removal of Polymorphonuclear Leukocytes from Circulation and from Sites of Inflammation

Polymorphonuclear leukocytes (PMNs) have a finite life span on the order of a few hours in circulation, and they appear to be eliminated by the process of apoptosis. At sites of inflammation, PMNs are engulfed by macrophages, and this process appears to require that the PMNs undergo apoptosis before engulfment and clearance (113–115). The normal elimination and apoptosis of PMNs appears also to involve induction of FAS and the FAS ligand, which may then trigger apoptosis of mature PMNs (116).

Apoptosis and Granulomatous Inflammation

There is ample evidence to support the notion that giant cells, which lead to granuloma formation, undergo apoptosis and not necrosis. Evidence comes from models such as experimentally induced myocarditis in rats, in which the giant cell reaction that occurs contains chromatin fragments and is terminal deoxynucleotide transferase (TdT)-mediated duTP-digoxigenin nick-end labeling assay (TUNEL) positive and the cells appear to undergo apoptosis when viewed by electron microscopy (117). Other evidence for apoptosis in granulomatous inflammation comes from the demonstration that the giant cells formed in brains of patients with acquired immunodeficiency syndrome (AIDS) dementia show evidence of apoptotic neuronal cell death (118). Similarly, in the study of granulomas formed in cryptococcal meningitis, the dead cells have features of apoptosis (119). Finally, caseating granulomas observed in lung tissue samples from clinical cases of tuberculosis show extensive apoptosis (120).

Termination of Cellular Immune Responses

After activation of cellular immune responses with consequent fending off of the insult, and when the cells are no longer needed, they are known to disappear. The mechanism of regulation of this termination in cellular immune response is mediated by cytokine release and appears to occur by apoptosis. In addition, activation of the FAS system has been implicated in the termination of cellular immune responses (121). Stimulation by the cytokines TNF-α and interferon-γ (IFN-γ) caused marked increase in expression of FAS antigen on progenitor and stem cells, rendering them susceptible to apoptosis induced by FAS antibody (122). Other evidence implicates interleukin-2 (IL-2) in generating the signal necessary to activate FAS-mediated apoptosis in the termination response. Mice deficient in IL-2 accumulate cells that normally would have undergone termination (123). Apoptosis has also been demonstrated in pulmonary alveolar and interstitial lymphocytes of mice challenged with T cell–dependent Ag sheep erythrocytes (SRBC). When mice harboring the *lpr* or *gld* mutations were used, the pulmonary inflammation continued, indicating again that FAS-mediated apoptosis is required for termination of the immune response (124).

Erythropoiesis

During normal erythroid development and maturation, the induction of anti-apoptotic genes such as *BCLX* appears to be important in mediating the action of erythropoietin, a critical regulator of erythropoiesis (125). Thrombopoietin also stimulates erythropoiesis by inhibiting apoptosis (126). According to this scenario, one major function of erythropoietin is not only to induce differentiation of erythroid precursors but to endow them with viability and survival through the induction of these anti-apoptotic genes.

Also during erythropoiesis, the induction of the transcription factor GATA-1 appears to promote survival by preventing apoptosis (127). Taken together, these results suggest that a major mechanism for allowing the development of mature cells is the prevention of apoptosis.

The action of many stem cell factors, such as granulocyte-macrophage colony-stimulating factor (GM-CSF) and granulocyte colony-stimulating factor (G-CSF), also appears to manifest as both enhanced proliferation and enhanced survival through anti-apoptotic mechanisms (128). Similarly, the action of IL-2 on T cells appears to confer an anti-apoptotic and survival function (129). Therefore, it may be concluded that most of these cytokines and differentiation factors act not only by enhancing proliferation but also by preventing apoptosis of the mature cells.

Senescence as a Protective Mechanism against Cancer Formation

One possible biologic significance of senescence is to prevent proliferation and cancer formation. It is presumed that the accumulation of toxic environmental stimuli and oxidative stress, as well as ultraviolet radiation and other causes of DNA damage, may lead to cancer formation. Cellular senescence could be a protective mechanism whereby cells preferentially undergo growth arrest

and no longer respond to mitogenic stimuli or proliferate; that is, they turn on a gene or genes that result in induction of cell cycle arrest and are thereby protected from cancer formation.

PATHOLOGIC STATES ASSOCIATED WITH DEFECTS IN APOPTOSIS OR CELL SENESCENCE

Cancer

Defects in mechanisms regulating apoptosis or senescence appear to be of fundamental significance in the development of the malignant phenotype. Whereas enhanced growth of tumor cells (usually caused by the action of oncogenes) drives the formation of benign tumors, the deterioration into a full-fledged malignant and metastatic phenotype appears to require the ability of the cell to survive in hostile environments despite the accumulation of mutations and other derangements in the structure or function of the cell. This survival requires overcoming the intrinsic mechanisms of apoptosis that would have resulted in the elimination of cells with serious mutations or genomic instability. This ability allows malignant cells to survive and to continue to accumulate mutations at an accelerated rate. This is where mutations in tumor suppressor genes (or anti-oncogenes) appear to predominate. The most frequently mutated tumor suppressor gene is *p53*; it is either poorly expressed or mutated in 50% to 90% of tumors (11,85). Derangements in the p53 pathway result in uncoupling of DNA damage from appropriate responses that lead to repair or cell death. *RB* is another tumor suppressor gene that plays an important role in a small number of cancers (e.g., osteosarcoma, breast carcinoma, retinoblastoma, urologic malignancies) (96,130). Normal functioning of RB would ensure cell cycle arrest in response to intracellular damage or other agents of stress or toxicity. Elimination of RB would permit unchecked growth of malignant cells. Other components involved in the RB pathway of growth suppression, such as cyclins, cyclin-dependent kinases, and their inhibitors (e.g., p16), appear to be deranged in a significant proportion of malignancies (131–133).

Defects in Cell Senescence Also Appear to be Instrumental in Propagation of the Malignant Phenotype

Transformed cells in tissue culture appear to possess an infinite life span with an unlimited (or very high) number of replications, in contradistinction to the much more limited life span of normal cells (i.e., senescence). Therefore, it appears that transformed cells (at least in tissue culture) escape from the mechanisms that regulate and ensure cell senescence. This may allow tumor cells to keep multiplying even in environments that would have been considered hostile for the normal counterpart of those malignant cells (134). Indeed, senescence has been proposed to function primarily as an anti-oncogenic process. At a mechanistic level, the function of telomerase appears to connect cell senescence and oncogenesis. Telomerase is an enzyme that ensures fidelity in maintaining the length of the ends of chromosomes during successive mitotic events. In cell senescence, it has been proposed that telomerase ceases to function and that the progressive shortening of telomeres eventually results in the inability of cells to undergo cell division (135). It has been observed that transformed cells have high levels of telomerase and that they do not display progressive loss and shortening of telomeres during successive cell divisions (136). This phenomenon has also been observed in primary tumors, although perhaps not to the same extent as in transformed cells in tissue culture. This has led to the proposal that maintenance of telomeres through persistent action of telomerase is essential for allowing the growth of cancer cells.

Specific Examples of Oncogenes and Anti-oncogenes in Hematologic Malignancies

Several of the best-studied oncogenes were discovered during the investigation of hematologic malignancies (23). The most notable of these is BCR-ABL in chronic myelogenous leukemia, a stem cell malignancy characterized by hyperproliferation of leukocytes, erythroid cells, and platelet precursors. This is the initial disorder in which a unique chromosomal abnormality was identified (translocation of chromosomes 9 and 22). The result of this translocation is a fusion protein, BCR-ABL, which is formed by the joining of segments of the *BCR* and *ABL* genes (137). Studies suggest that the function of the ABL protooncogene may be to enhance apoptosis in response to DNA-damaging agents (87). On the other hand, the BCR-ABL fusion protein appears to function as a potent anti-apoptotic product (138).

The *BCL2* oncogene was described from a translocation of chromosomes 14 and 18 in follicular lymphomas (8,139). As discussed previously, the BCL2 gene product functions as a potent anti-apoptotic molecule, and this probably enhances the growth and malignant transformation of follicular lymphomas.

P53, which plays a fundamental role in the oncogenic transformation of many cancers, is also found to be mutated in a smaller number of hematologic malignancies, and such mutation is associated with poor prognosis and poor response to chemotherapy (11,140).

Homozygous deletions of the *p16* gene, which functions to suppress cyclin-dependent kinases, occur very frequently in T-cell acute leukemias (133). Homozygous deletions of the p15 gene product, which also functions to inhibit cyclic-dependent kinases, also occur with high frequency in T-cell but not in B-cell leukemias (132, 133,141).

Several other oncogenes and anti-oncogenes have been shown to be defective in several forms of hematologic malignancies, including the "deleted in colon cancer" gene (*DCC*); *BRCA2*, which is associated primarily with breast cancer; the Wilms' tumor suppressor gene (*WT1*), the neurofibromatosis-1 tumor suppressor gene (*NF1*), and RAS (131,142,143). Many of the oncogenes and tumor suppressor genes that have been described in nonhematologic malignancies also appear to malfunction or to contribute to the pathogenesis of several hematologic malignancies, although usually in only a small percentage of cases. These results suggest that dysfunction of the normal regulation of growth of cells is required for either initiation or maintenance of the malignant phenotype and that dysfunction can be achieved by interference with any of several key regulators of normal growth, apoptosis, or senescence.

A recent finding may explain why the acquired mutation in the class A phosphotidylinositol glycan gene (PIGA) that results in paroxysmal nocturnal hemoglobinuria predisposes to leukemia. Although cells with this mutation do not proliferate faster than normal cells, they acquire resistance to apoptosis, thus providing a potential survival advantage and a predisposition to leukemia (144).

Immune Deficiency Disorders

Infection with the human immunodeficiency virus (HIV), which can result in AIDS, appears to cause significant apoptosis (145–147). It has been proposed that elimination of CD4-positive T cells during HIV infection is a direct result of the activation of apoptotic pathways, and apoptosis has been shown to occur in tissue culture studies of HIV infection. More importantly, it has been demonstrated that T cells undergo apoptosis *in vivo* during ongoing HIV infection. Mechanistically, HIV infection results in elevations in cellular levels of ceramide, both in tissue culture and *in vivo*, and ceramide may mediate the effects of HIV on apoptosis (148–150). However, the mechanisms involved in formation of ceramide in response to HIV infection remain poorly determined.

Autoimmune Disorders

Studies with mice models of autoimmunity have demonstrated a close link between autoimmunity, apoptosis, and regulators of apoptosis. The *gld* mice harbor a mutation in the ligand for the Fas antigen, whereas the *lpr* mice harbor mutations in the Fas receptor (21). Both mouse models show that mutations in these regulators cause a deficiency in apoptosis and an expansion of subpopulations of lymphocytes, resulting in autoimmune disorders (21). It has been more difficult to demonstrate these connections in human disorders of autoimmunity, but the results from the mouse models suggest that one mechanism for inappropriate expansion of lymphocytes may occur as a result of interference with normal mechanisms of apoptosis.

Immunosenescence

The decline of immune function with increasing age is well known and documented (27). One of the key functions of the immune system that is affected by aging is cell-mediated immunity (i.e., T-lymphocyte senescence). T-lymphocyte senescence leads to a decreased ability to react with foreign antigens and also to increased production of autoantibodies and reactivity with autoantigens (27). This dysregulation of the immune system with aging leads to increased susceptibility to infections, autoimmune disorders, cancer, and monoclonal gammopathies. There also is an increased incidence of reactivation of some chronic infections such as herpes zoster.

Myelodysplasia

Myelodysplastic syndromes are disorders of hematopoiesis whereby various stem cells become defective, resulting in anemia, leukopenia, or thrombocytopenia. This is accompanied by disordered growth in the bone marrow of the precursors to these cell types, usually with increased proliferation. The discrepancy between the increased growth of precursor cells and decreased levels of mature progeny has been attributed to enhanced apoptosis during the development and differentiation of the various hematopoietic cell lines (23). Moreover, some forms of therapy that ameliorate myelodysplasia (e.g., cytokines, erythropoietin) have been shown to act by decreasing the level of apoptosis (151). Because the primary defects in these disorders have not been elucidated at a molecular level, it is not known whether the increased apoptosis is a primary defect or a consequence of abnormal growth regulation in hematopoietic stem cells. In any case, apoptosis in this disorder appears to play a major role in the pathogenesis of the myelodysplastic phenotype.

Ineffective Erythropoiesis

Whereas many causes of anemia (e.g., aplastic anemia) are attributed directly to decreased proliferation rates of erythroid precursors, several conditions of anemia are characterized by hyperproliferation of erythroid precursors in the bone marrow coupled with an inability to generate mature red cells. These conditions include vitamin B_{12} deficiency, iron deficiency, congenital dyserythropoietic anemias, and thalassemic disorders. This type of condition has been described as ineffective erythropoiesis, and it is characterized by the morphologic appearance of defective and dying red cell precursors. It is becoming increasingly obvious that the defective erythroid precursors undergo apoptosis instead of further development into mature red cells, resulting in the appearance of ineffective erythropoiesis (152).

There are other pathologic conditions in which dysregulation of apoptosis may play a role. The loss of proliferative capacity of many tissues during the aging process may reflect an increased or an unbalanced rate of apoptosis. This may account for the decreased hematopoiesis seen in aplastic anemia (153), poor tissue healing due to defects in fibroblast growth, and poor vascular healing due to apoptosis or senescence of endothelial cells.

Endothelial Cell Senescence and Atherosclerosis

Endothelial cell senescence has been implicated in the increased incidence of atherosclerotic and thrombotic events that occurs with aging. Senescent endothelial cells have increased levels of type I plasminogen activator inhibitor (PAI-1), which also is increased in a number of prothrombotic conditions (154). In addition, enhanced adhesion of monocytes to senescent endothelium has been demonstrated. This enhanced adhesiveness could be implicated in the formation of atherosclerotic lesions (155). Fibronectin, which is necessary for cell spreading and attachment, has been demonstrated to have increased expression in senescent endothelial cells (156).

Senescent endothelial cells have significantly decreased responsiveness to EGF and fibroblast growth factors (157,158), with consequent decreases in angiogenic and vascular responsiveness. This can, in part, explain the delayed wound healing and increased vascular stiffness seen in aging (159).

MODULATION OF APOPTOSIS OR CELL SENESCENCE AS A POSSIBLE THERAPEUTIC GOAL

Given the fundamental role of apoptosis in cell senescence in biology and the role of derangements of this mechanism in several pathologic conditions, it is plausible that modulation of these processes could have a significant impact on normal biologic responses and in rectifying pathologic conditions. This is perhaps best understood currently in the area of cancer treatment: most forms of cancer therapy, including chemotherapy, radiation therapy, and hyperthermia, appear to induce apoptosis in cancer cells (somewhat selectively). As mentioned previously, the administration of cytokines to patients with myelodysplastic syndrome may also alleviate the severity of the disorder through suppression of apoptosis. It should be noted, however, that the effects of these therapeutic manipulations on apoptosis were realized after extensive empiric use of these treatments. In a more rational approach, therapies aimed directly at modulation of apoptosis or cell senescence may result in more specific treatments and obviate some of their untoward effects. For example, if apoptosis-inducing therapy is designed with selectivity for cancer cells, it may bypass many of the mechanisms of resistance in cancer cells while sparing normal tissues. Significant investigation is required to decipher the mechanisms of apoptosis, the mechanisms that determine selectivity of response of cancer cells compared with normal cells, and key targets for manipulation.

There are other potential hematologic targets for therapies aimed at modulation of apoptosis or senescence. For example, if senescence or apoptosis underlies certain anemias or cytopenias, then agents that prevent apoptosis or senescence may result in restoration of proliferative capacity and maturation of the affected stem cells or precursor cells. Similarly, in immune deficiency disorders characterized by senescence or apoptosis, therapies aimed at preventing these processes could enhance lymphoid survival. This could be of significant application in HIV infection if, indeed, most T lymphocytes die through apoptotic mechanisms. Conversely, selective induction of apoptosis or senescence may ameliorate disorders characterized by hyperproliferation or hyperplasia, such as autoimmune disorders.

This is an area of research in its infancy, and further elucidation of mechanisms and significance should result in enhanced understanding of normal physiology and relevant pathologic processes.

ACKNOWLEDGMENTS

The work in the authors' laboratories was supported in part by NIH grants GM-43825 and AG-12467. L. M. O. is also a recipient of a Paul Beeson Physician Faculty Scholars in Aging Research Award. We also thank Jiandi Zhang for providing Figures 51-3*A* and *B*.

REFERENCES

1. Williams GT. Programmed cell death: apoptosis and oncogenesis. *Cell* 1991;65:1097–1098.
2. Carson DA, Ribeiro JM. Apoptosis and disease. *Lancet* 1993;341:1251–1254.
3. Gerschenson LE, Rotello RJ. Apoptosis: a different type of cell death. *FASEB J* 1992;6:2450–2455.
4. Wyllie AH, Kerr JFR, Currie AR. Cell death: the significance of apoptosis. *Int Rev Cytol* 1992;68:251–306.
5. McConkey DJ, Orrenius S. Signal transduction pathways to apoptosis. *Trends Cell Biol* 1994;4:370–374.
6. Hannun YA, Obeid LM. Ceramide: an intracellular signal for apoptosis. *Trends Biochem Sci* 1995;20:73–77.
7. Reed JC. BCL-2: prevention of apoptosis as a mechanism of drug resistance. *Hematol Oncol Clin North Am* 1995;9:451–473.
8. Korsmeyer SJ, Yin X-M, Oltvai ZN, Veis-Novack DJ, Linette GP. Reactive oxygen species and the regulation of cell death by the Bcl-2 gene family. *Biochem Biophys Acta* 1995;1271:63–66.
9. Martin SJ, Green DR. Protease activation during apoptosis: death by a thousand cuts? *Cell* 1995;82:349–352.
10. Jacobson MD. Reactive oxygen species and programmed cell death. *Trends Biochem Sci* 1996;21:83–86.
11. Oren M. P53: the ultimate tumor suppressor gene? *FASEB J* 1992;6:3169–3176.
12. Clarke PGH, Clarke S. Nineteenth century research on naturally occurring cell death and related phenomena. *Anat Embryol* 1996;193:81–99.
13. Kerr JFR, Harmon BV. Definition and incidence of apoptosis: an historical perspective. In: Tomei LD, Cope FO, eds. *Apoptosis: the molecular basis of cell death.* Cold Spring Harbor: Cold Spring Harbor Laboratory Press, 1991:5–29.
14. Michaelson J. The significance of cell death. In: Tomei LD, Cope FO, eds. *Apoptosis: the molecular basis of cell death.* Cold Spring Harbor: Cold Spring Harbor Laboratory Press, 1991:31–46.
15. Kruppa G, Thoma B, Machleidt T, Wiegmann K, Krönke M. Inhibition of tumor necrosis factor (TNF)-mediated NF-kappaB activation by selective blockade of the human 55-kDa TNF receptor. *J Immunol* 1992;148:3152–3157.
16. Kamada Y, Qadota H, Python CP, Anraku Y, Ohya Y, Levin DE. Activation of yeast protein kinase C by Rho1 GTPase. *J Biol Chem* 1996;271:9193–9196.
17. Hedgecock EM, Salston JE, Thomson JN. Mutations affecting programmed cell death in the nematode *Caenorhabditis elegans. Science* 1983;220:1277–1279.
18. Yuan J, Shaham S, Ledoux S, Ellis HM, Horvitz HR. The *C. elegans* cell death gene *ced-3* encodes a protein similar to mammalian interleukin-1b-converting enzyme. *Cell* 1993;75:641–652.
19. Hengartner MO, Horvitz HR. Activation of *C. elegans* cell death protein CED-9 by an amino-acid substitution in a domain conserved in Bcl-2. *Nature* 1994;369:318–320.
20. Berridge MJ. Lymphocyte activation in health and disease. *Crit Rev Immunol* 1997;17:155–178.
21. Nagata S. Apoptosis regulated by a death factor and its receptor: Fas ligand and Fas. *Philos Trans R Soc Lond [Biol]* 1994;345:281–287.
22. Kerr JFR, Winterford CM, Harmon BV. Apoptosis: its significance in cancer and cancer therapy. *Cancer* 1994;73:2013–2026.
23. DiGiuseppe JA, Kastan MB. Apoptosis in haematological malignancies. *J Clin Pathol* 1997;50:361–364.
24. Vogelstein B, Kinzler KW. p53 function and dysfunction. *Cell* 1992;70:523–526.
25. Hannun YA. Apoptosis and the dilemma of cancer chemotherapy. *Blood* 1997;89:1845–1853.
26. Hayflick L, Moorhead PS. The serial cultivation of human diploid strains. *Exp Cell Res* 1961;25:585–621.
27. Currie MS. Immunosenescence. *Compr Ther* 1992;18:26–34.
28. Saltzman RL, Peterson PK. Immunodeficiency in the elderly. *Rev Infect Dis* 1987;9:1127–1139.
29. Shinozuke T. Changes in human red blood cells during aging *in vivo. Keio J Med* 1994;43:155–163.
30. Dohi Y. Age-related changes in vascular smooth muscle and endothelium. *Drugs Aging* 1995;7:278–291.
31. Goldstein S. Replicative senescence: the human fibroblast comes of age. *Science* 1990;249:1129–1133.
32. Norwood TH, Pendergrass WR, Sprague CA, Martin GM. Dominance of the senescent phenotype in heterkaryons between replicative and post-replicative human fibroblast-like cells. *Proc Natl Acad Sci U S A* 1974;71:2231–2235.
33. Pereira-Smith OM, Smith JR. Phenotype of low proliferative potential is dominant in hybrids of normal human fibroblasts. *Somat Cell Genet* 1982;8:731–742.
34. Lumpkin CK, McClung JK, Pereira-Smith OM, Smith JR. Existence of high abundance antiproliferative mRNA's in senescent human diploid fibroblasts. *Science* 1986;232:393–398.
35. Campisi J, Dimri GP, Nehlin JO, Testori A, Yoshimoto K. Coming of age in culture. *Exp Gerontol* 1996;31:7–12.
36. Liu SC, Meagher K, Hanwalt PC. Role of solar conditioning in DNA repair response and survival of human epidermal keratinocytes following UV irradiation. *J Invest Dermatol* 1985;85:93–97.
37. Ames BN, Gold LS. Endogenous mutagens and the causes of aging and cancer. *Mutat Res* 1991;250:3–16.
38. Yaar M, Gilchrest BA. Cellular and molecular mechanisms of cutaneous aging. *J Dermatol Surg Oncol* 1990;16:915–922.
39. Bond J, Haughton M, Blaydes J, Gire V, Wynford-Thomas D, Wyllie F. Evidence that transcriptional activation by p53 plays a direct role in the induction of cellular senescence. *Oncogene* 1996;13:2097–2104.
40. Gorman SD, Cristofalo VJ. Reinitiation of cellular DNA synthesis in BrdU-selected nondividing senescent WI-38 cells by simian virus 40 infection. *J Cell Physiol* 1985;125:122–126.
41. Birnbaumer L. Receptor-to-effector signaling through G proteins: roles for bg dimers as well as a subunits. *Cell* 1992;71:1069–1072.
42. Hannun YA. Signal transduction in cancer. In: *Cancer Medicine,* 4th Ed, J.F. Holland, E. Frei, III, R.C.Bast, Jr., D.W. Kufe, D.L. Morton,

and R.R. Weichselbaum, eds. Baltimore, MD: Williams & Wilkins, 1997;65–83.

43. Obeid LM, Hannun YA. Ceramide: a stress signal and mediator of growth suppression and apoptosis. *J Cell Biochem* 1995;58:191–198.

44. Liscovitch M, Cantley LC. Lipid second messengers. *Cell* 1994;77: 329–334.

45. Davis RJ. The mitogen-activated protein kinase signal transduction pathway. *J Biol Chem* 1993;268:14553–14556.

46. Divecha N, Irvine RF. Phospholipid signaling. *Cell* 1995;80:269–278.

47. Vilcek J, Lee TH. Tumor necrosis factor: new insights into the molecular mechanisms of its multiple actions. *J Biol Chem* 1991;266: 7313–7316.

48. Bursch W, Kleine L, Tenniswood M. The biochemistry of cell death by apoptosis. *Biochem Cell Biol* 1990;68:1071–1074.

49. Beutler B, Van Huffel C. Unraveling function in the TNF ligand and receptor families. *Science* 1994;264:667–668.

50. Wallach D. Cell death induction by TNF: a matter of self control. *Trends Biochem Sci* 1997;22:107–109.

51. Hsu HL, Shu HB, Pan MG, Goeddel DV. TRADD-TRAF2 and TRADD-FADD interactions define two distinct TNF receptor 1 signal transduction pathways. *Cell* 1996;84:299–308.

52. Chinnaiyan AM, Tepper CG, Seldin MF, et al. FADD/MORT1 is a common mediator of CD95 (Fas/APO-1) and tumor necrosis factor receptor-induced apoptosis. *J Biol Chem* 1996;271:4961–4965.

53. Rothe M, Sarma V, Dixit VW, Goeddel DV. TRAF2-mediated activation of NF-kappaB by TNF receptor 2 and CD40. *Science* 1995;269: 1424–1427.

54. Cheng GH, Baltimore D. TANK, a co-inducer with TRAF2 of TNF- and CD40L-mediated NF-kappaB activation. *Genes Dev* 1996;10: 963–973.

55. Liu ZG, Hsu HL, Goeddel DV, Karin M. Dissection of TNF receptor 1 effector functions: JNK activation is not linked to apoptosis while NF-kappaB activation prevents cell death. *Cell* 1996;87:565–576.

56. Westwick JK, Weitzel C, Minden A, Karin M, Brenner DA. Tumor necrosis factor α stimulates AP-1 activity through prolonged activation of the c-jun kinase. *J Biol Chem* 1994;269:26396-26401.

57. Boldin MP, Goncharov TM, Goltsev YV, Wallach D. Involvement of MACH, a novel MORT1/FADD-interacting protease, in Fas/APO-1- and TNF receptor-induced cell death. *Cell* 1996;85:803–815.

58. Muzio M, Chinnaiyan AM, Kischkel FC, et al. FLICE, a novel FADD-homologous ICE/CED-3-like protease, is recruited to the CD 95 (Fas/APO-1) death-inducing signaling complex. *Cell* 1996;85: 817–827.

59. Kim M-Y, Linardic C, Obeid L, Hannun Y. Identification of sphingomyelin turnover as an effector mechanism for the action of tumor necrosis factor α and gamma-interferon: specific role in cell differentiation. *J Biol Chem* 1991;266:484–489.

60. Dressler KA, Mathias S, Kolesnick RN. Tumor necrosis factor-α activates the sphingomyelin signal transduction pathway in a cell-free system. *Science* 1992;255:1715–1718.

61. Hannun YA. The sphingomyelin cycle and the second messenger function of ceramide. *J Biol Chem* 1994;269:3125–3128.

62. Kolesnick R, Golde DW. The sphingomyelin pathway in tumor necrosis factor and interleukin-1 signaling. *Cell* 1994;77:325–328.

63. Lumelsky NL, Forget BG. Negative regulation of globin gene expression during megakaryocytic differentiation of a human erythroleukemic cell line. *Mol Cell Biol* 1991;11:3528–3536.

64. Liscovitch M. Crosstalk among multiple signal-activated phopholipases. *Trends Biochem Sci* 1992;17:393–399.

65. Hannun YA. Functions of ceramide in coordinating cellular responses to stress. *Science* 1996;274:1855–1859.

66. Yang J, Liu XS, Bhalla K, et al. Prevention of apoptosis by Bcl-2: release of cytochrome *c* from mitochondria blocked. *Science* 1997; 275:1129–1132.

67. Kluck RM, Bossy-Wetzel E, Green DR, Newmeyer DD. The release of cytochrome *c* from mitochondria: a primary site for Bcl-2 regulation of apoptosis. *Science* 1997;275:1132–1136.

68. Kim CN, Wang XD, Huang Y, et al. Overexpression of Bcl-x$_L$, inhibits Ara-C-induced mitochondrial loss of cytochrome *c* and other perturbations that activate the molecular cascade of apoptosis. *Cancer Res* 1997;57:3115–3120.

69. Zou H, Henzel WJ, Liu X, Lutschg A, Wang X. Apaf-1, a human protein homologous to *C. elegans* CED-4, participates in cytochrome *c*-dependent activation of caspase-3. *Cell* 1997;90:405–413.

70. Kluck RM, Martin SJ, Hoffman BM, Zhou JS, Green DR, Newmeyer DD. Cytochrome *c* activation of CPP32-like proteolysis plays a critical role in a *Xenopus* cell-free apoptosis system. *EMBO J* 1997;16: 4639–4649.

71. Rao L, Perez D, White E. Lamin proteolysis facilitates nuclear events during apoptosis. *J Cell Biol* 1996;135:1441–1455.

72. Liu XS, Zou H, Slaughter C, Wang XD. DFF, a heterodimeric protein that functions downstream of caspase-3 to trigger DNA fragmentation during apoptosis. *Cell* 1997;89:175–184.

73. Perry DK, Smyth MJ, Stennicke HR, et al. Zinc is a potent inhibitor of the apoptotic protease, caspase-3: a novel target for zinc in the inhibition of apoptosis. *J Biol Chem* 1997;272:18530–18533.

74. Enari M, Sakahira H, Yokoyama H, Okawa K, Iwamatsu A, Nagata S. A caspase-activated DNase that degrades DNA during apoptosis, and its inhibitor ICAD. *Nature* 1998;391:43–50.

75. Larrick JW, Wright SC. Cytotoxic mechanism of tumor necrosis factor-α. *FASEB J* 1990;4:3215–3223.

76. Bünemann M, Liliom K, Brandts BK, et al. A novel membrane receptor with high affinity for lysosphingomyelin and sphingosine 1-phosphate in atrial myocytes. *EMBO J* 1996;15:5527–5534.

77. Jayadev S, Hayter HL, Andrieu N, et al. Phospholipase A$_2$ is necessary for tumor necrosis factor α-induced ceramide generation in L929 cells. *J Biol Chem* 1997;272:17196–17203.

78. Tian QS, Taupin JL, Elledge S, Robertson M, Anderson P. Fas-activated serine threonine kinase (FAST) phosphorylates TIA-1 during Fas-mediated apoptosis. *J Exp Med* 1995;182:865–874.

79. Engel K, Ahlers A, Brach MA, Herrmann F, Gaestel M. MAPKAP kinase 2 is activated by heat shock and TNF-α: *in vivo* phosphorylation of small heat shock protein results from stimulation of the MAP kinase cascade. *J Cell Biochem* 1995;57:321–330.

80. Ji L, Zhang G, Hirabayashi Y. Tumor necrosis factor α increases tyrosine phosphorylation of a 23-kDa nuclear protein in U937 cells through ceramide signaling pathway. *Biochem Biophys Res Commun* 1995;215:489–496.

81. McConkey DJ, Hartzell P, Nicotera P, Orrenius S. Calcium-activated DNA fragmentation kills immature thymocytes. *FASEB J* 1989;3: 1843–1849.

82. McCabe MJ Jr, Nicotera P, Orrenius S. Calcium-dependent cell death: role of the endonuclease, protein kinase C, and chromatin conformation. *Ann N Y Acad Sci* 1992;663:269–278.

83. Rovere P, Clementi E, Ferrarini M, et al. CD95 engagement releases calcium from intracellular stores of long term activated, apoptosis-prone gamma T cells. *J Immunol* 1996;156:4631–4637.

84. Lane DP. P53, guardian of the genome. *Nature* 1992;358:15–16.

85. Morgan SE, Kastan MB. P53 and ATM: cell cycle, cell death, and cancer. *Adv Cancer Res* 1997;71:1–25.

86. Strasser A, Harris AW, Jacks T, Cory S. DNA damage can induce apoptosis in proliferating lymphoid cells via p53-independent mechanisms inhibitable by Bcl-2. *Cell* 1994;79:329–339.

87. Yuan ZM, Huang YY, Ishiko T, Kharbanda S, Weichselbaum R, Kufe D. Regulation of DNA damage-induced apoptosis by the c-Abl tyrosine kinase. *Proc Natl Acad Sci U S A* 1997;94:1437–1440.

88. Perry ME, Piette J, Zawadzki JA, Harvey D, Levine AJ. The mdm-2 gene is induced in response to UV light in a p53-dependent manner. *Proc Natl Acad Sci U S A* 1993;90:11623–11627.

89. McCurrach ME, Connor TMF, Knudson CM, Korsmeyer SJ, Lowe SW. *bax*-Deficiency promotes drug resistance and oncogenic transformation by attenuating p53-dependent apoptosis. *Proc Natl Acad Sci U S A* 1997;94:2345–2349.

90. Wang Y, Szekely L, Okan I, Klein G, Wiman KG. Wild-type p53-triggered apoptosis is inhibited by *bcl*-2 in a v-*myc*-induced T-cell lymphoma line. *Oncogene* 1993;8:3427–3431.

91. Slebos RJC, Lee MH, Plunkett BS, et al. P53-dependent G$_1$ arrest involves pRB-related proteins and is disrupted by the human papillomavirus 16 E7 oncoprotein. *Proc Natl Acad Sci U S A* 1994;91:5320–5324.

92. Caelles C, Helmberg A, Karin M. P53-dependent apoptosis in the absence of transcriptional activation of p53-target genes. *Nature* 1994; 370:220–223.

93. El-Deiry WS, Harper JW, O'Connor PM, et al. WAF1/CIP1 is induced in p53-mediated G$_1$ arrest and apoptosis. *Cancer Res* 1994;54: 1169–1174.

94. Harrington EA, Bennett MR, Fanidi A, Evan GI. c-Myc-induced apoptosis in fibroblasts is inhibited by specific cytokines. *EMBO J* 1994;13:3286–3295.

95. Wagner AJ, Kokontis JM, Hay N. Myc-mediated apoptosis requires wild-type p53 in a manner independent of cell cycle arrest and the ability of p53 to induce p21[wafl/cip1]. *Genes Dev* 1994;8:2817–2830.

96. Weinberg RA. Tumor suppressor genes. *Science* 1991;254:1138–1146.

97. Chellappan SP, Hiebert S, Mudryj M, Horowitz JM, Nevins JR. The E2F transcription factor is a cellular target for the RB protein. *Cell* 1991;65:1053–1061.

98. Tang Z, Zhang Z, Zheng Y, Corbley MJ, Tong T. Cell aging of human diploid fibroblasts is associated with changes in responsiveness to epidermal growth factor and changes in HER-2 expression. *Mech Ageing Dev* 1994;83:57–67.

99. Aoyagi M, Fukai N, Ogami K, Yamamoto M, Yamamoto K. Kinetics of ^{125}I-PDGF binding and downregulation of PDGF receptor in human arterial smooth muscle cell strains during cellular senescence *in vitro*. *J Cell Physiol* 1995;164:376–384.

100. Mori S, Kawano M, Kenzaki T, Morisaki N, Saito Y, Yoshida S. Decreased expression of the platelet-derived growth factor receptor in fibroblasts from a patient with Werner's syndrome. *Eur J Clin Invest* 1996;23:161–165.

101. Ferber A, Chang C, Sell C, et al. Failure of senescent human fibroblasts to express the insulin-like growth factor-1 gene. *J Biol Chem* 1993;268:17883–17888.

102. Insel PA. Adrenergic receptors, G proteins, and cell regulation: implications for aging research. *Exp Gerontol* 1993;28:341–348.

103. Obeid LM, Venable ME. Signal transduction in cellular senescence. *J Am Geriatr Soc* 1997;45:361–366.

104. Quadri RA, Plastre O, Phelouzat MA, Arbogast A, Proust JJ. Age-related tyrosine-specific protein phosphorylation defect in human T lymphocytes activated through CD3, CD4, CD8 or the IL-2 receptor. *Mech Ageing Dev* 1996;88:125–138.

105. Venable ME, Lee JY, Smyth MJ, Bielawska A, Obeid LM. Role of ceramide in cellular senescence. *J Biol Chem* 1995;270:30701–30708.

106. Venable ME, Blobe GC, Obeid LM. Identification of a defect in the phospholipase D/diacylglycerol pathway in cellular senescence. *J Biol Chem* 1994;269:26040–26044.

107. Venable ME, Bielawska A, Obeid LM. Ceramide inhibits phospholipase D in a cell-free system. *J Biol Chem* 1996;271:24800–24805.

108. Cristofalo VJ, Pignolo RJ. Molecular markers of senescence in fibroblast-like cultures. *Exp Gerontol* 1996;31:111–123.

109. Vaziri H, Benchimol S. From telomere loss to p53 induction and activation of a DNA-damage pathway at senescence: the telomere loss/DNA damage model of cell aging. *Exp Gerontol* 1996;31:295–301.

110. Stein GH, Beeson M, Gordon L. Failure to phosphorylate the retinoblastoma gene product in senescent human fibroblasts. *Science* 1990;249:666–669.

111. Seshadri T, Campisi J. Repression of c-*fos* transcription and an altered genetic program in senescent human fibroblasts. *Science* 1990;247: 205–209.

112. Chiu CP, Harley CB. Replicative senescence and cell immortality: the role of telomeres and telomerase. *Proc Soc Exp Biol Med* 1997;214: 99–106.

113. Newman SL, Henson JE, Henson PM. Phagocytosis of senescent neutrophils by human monocyte-derived macrophages and rabbit inflammatory cells. *J Exp Med* 1982;156:430–432.

114. Whyte MK, Meagher LC, MacDermot J, Haslett C. Impairment of function in aging neutrophils is associated with apoptosis. *J Immunol* 1993;150:5124–5134.

115. Matsuba KT, Van Eeden SF, Bicknell SG, Walker BAM, Hayashi S, Hogg JC. Apoptosis in circulating PMN: increased susceptibility in L-selectin-deficient PMN. *Am J Physiol Heart Circ Physiol* 1997;272: H2852–H2858.

116. Hsieh SC, Huang MH, Tsai CY, et al. The expression of genes modulating programmed cell death in normal human polymorphonuclear neutrophils. *Biochem Biophys Res Commun* 1997;233:700–706.

117. Suzuki K, Izumi T, Iwanaga T, Fujita T, Shibata A. Multinucleated giant cells undergoing apoptosis in experimental autoimmune myocarditis. *Arch Histol Cytol* 1995;58:231–241.

118. Lipton SA. Similarity of neuronal cell injury and death in AIDS. *Brain Pathol* 1996;6:507–517.

119. Goldman DL, Casadevall A, Cho Y, Lee SC. *Cryptococcus neoformans* meningitis in the rat. *Lab Invest* 1996;75:759–770.

120. Keene J, Balcewicz-Sablinska MK, Remold HG, et al. Infection by *Mycobacterium tuberculosis* promotes human alveolar macrophage apoptosis. *Infect Immun* 1997;65:298–304.

121. Alderson MR, Armitage RJ, Maraskovsky E, et al. Fas transduces activation signals in normal human T lymphocytes. *J Exp Med* 1993;178: 2231–2235.

122. Maciejewski J, Selleri C, Anderson S, Young NS. Fas antigen expression on CD34+ human marrow cells is induced by interferon gamma and tumor necrosis factor alpha and potentiates cytokine-mediated hematopoietic suppression *in vitro*. *Blood* 1995;85:3183–3190.

123. Kneitz B, Herrmann T, Yonehara S, Schimpl A. Normal clonal expansion but impaired Fas-mediated cell death and anergy induction in interleukin-2-deficient mice. *Eur J Immunol* 1995;25:2572–2577.

124. Milik AM, Buechner-Maxwell VA, Sonstein J, et al. Lung lymphocyte elimination by apoptosis in the murine response to intratracheal particulate antigen. *J Clin Invest* 1997;99:1082–1091.

125. Gregoli PA, Bondurant MC. The roles of Bcl-XL and apopain in the control of erythropoiesis by erythropoietin. *Blood* 1997;90:630–640.

126. Ratajczak MZ, Ratajczak J, Marlicz W, et al. Recombinant human thrombopoietin (TPO) stimulates erythropoiesis by inhibiting erythroid progenitor cell apoptosis. *Br J Haematol* 1997;98:8–17.

127. Weiss MJ, Orkin SH. Transcription factor GATA-1 permits survival and maturation of erythroid precursors by preventing apoptosis. *Proc Natl Acad Sci U S A* 1995;92:9623–9627.

128. Lotem J, Sachs L. Hematopoietic cytokines inhibit apoptosis induced by transforming growth factor β1 and cancer chemotherapy compounds in myeloid leukemic cells. *Blood* 1992;80:1750–1757.

129. Deng G, Podack ER. Suppression of apoptosis in a cytotoxic T-cell line by interleukin 2-mediated gene transcription and deregulated expression of the protooncogene *bcl-2*. *Proc Natl Acad Sci U S A* 1993;90:2189–2193.

130. Knudson AG. Antioncogenes and human cancer. *Proc Natl Acad Sci U S A* 1993;90:10914–10921.

131. Allen PD, Bustin SA, Newland AC. The role of apoptosis (programmed cell death) in haemopoiesis and the immune system. *Blood Rev* 1993;7:63–73.

132. Takeuchi S, Bartram CR, Seriu T, et al. Analysis of a family of cyclin-dependent kinase inhibitors: p15/MTS2/INK4B, p16/MTS1/INK4A, and p18 genes in acute lymphoblastic leukemia of childhood. *Blood* 1995;86:755–760.

133. Hatta Y, Hirama T, Miller CW, Yamada Y, Tomonaga M, Koeffler HP. Homozygous deletions of the p15 (MTS2) and p16 (CDKN2/MTS1) genes in adult T-cell leukemia. *Blood* 1995;85:2699–2704.

134. Campisi J. Aging and cancer: the double-edged sword of replicative senescence. *J Am Geriatr Soc* 1997;45:482–488.

135. Pan C, Xue BH, Ellis TM, Peace DJ, Diaz MO. Changes in telomerase activity and telomere length during human T lymphocyte senescence. *Exp Cell Res* 1997;231:346–353.

136. Shay JW, Wright WE. Telomerase activity in human cancer. *Curr Opin Oncol* 1996;8:66–71.

137. Witte ON. Role of the BCR-ABL oncogene in human leukemia: fifteenth Richard and Linda Rosenthal Foundation Award Lecture. *Cancer Res* 1993;53:485–489.

138. McGahon A, Bissonnette R, Schmitt M, Cotter KM, Green DR, Cotter TG. BCR-ABL maintains resistance of chronic myelogenous leukemia cells to apoptotic cell death. *Blood* 1994;83:1179–1187.

139. Reed JC. Bcl-2 and the regulation of programmed cell death. *J Cell Biol* 1994;124:1–6.

140. Faleiro L, Kobayashi R, Fearnhead H, Lazebnik Y. Multiple species of CPP32 and Mch2 are the major active caspases present in apoptotic cells. *EMBO J* 1997;16:2271–2281.

141. Hebert J, Cayuela JM, Berkeley J, Sigaux F. Candidate tumor-suppressor genes MTS1 (p16INK4A) and MTS2 (p15INK4B) display frequent homozygous deletions in primary cells from T- but not from B-cell lineage acute lymphoblastic leukemias. *Blood* 1994;84:4038–4044.

142. Profiri E. DCC (deleted in colorectal cancer) inactivation in hematological malignancies. *Leuk Lymphoma* 1995;18:69–72.

143. Gaidano G, Guerrasio A, Serra A, et al. Mutations in the p53 and RAS family genes are associated with tumor progression of BCR/ABL negative chronic myeloproliferative disorders. *Leukemia* 1993;7:946–953.

144. Brodsky RA, Vala MS, Barber JP, Medof ME, Jones RJ. Resistance to apoptosis caused by PIG-A gene mutations in paroxysmal nocturnal hemoglobinuria. *Proc Natl Acad Sci U S A* 1997;94:8756–8760.

145. Dobkin JF. Apoptosis and AIDS pathogenesis. *Complications Surg* 1993;12:16.

146. Gougeon M-L, Montagnier L. Apoptosis in AIDS. *Science* 1993;260: 1269–1270.

147. Lu W, Andrieu J-M. Apoptosis and HIV disease. *Nat Med* 1995;1: 386–387.
148. Van Veldhoven PP, Matthews TJ, Bolognesi DP, Bell RM. Changes in bioactive lipids, alkylacylglycerol and ceramide, occur in HIV-infected cells. *Biochem Biophys Res Commun* 1992;187:209–216.
149. Rivas CI, Golde DW, Vera JC, Kolesnick RN. Involvement of the sphingomyelin pathway in autocrine tumor necrosis factor signaling for human immunodeficiency virus production in chronically infected HL-60 cells. *Blood* 1994;83:2191–2197.
150. De Simone C, Cifone MG, Roncaioli P, et al. Ceramide, AIDS and long-term survivors. *Immunol Today* 1996;17:48.
151. Yoshida Y. Apoptosis as a parameter of cytokine treatment in myelodysplasia. *Leukoc Res* 1997;21:427–428.
152. Koury MJ, Horne DW, Brown ZA, et al. Apoptosis of late-stage erythroblasts in megaloblastic anemia: association with DNA damage and macrocyte production. *Blood* 1997;89:4617–4623.
153. Callera F, Falcão RP. Increased apoptotic cells in bone marrow biopsies from patients with aplastic anaemia. *Br J Haematol* 1997;98: 18–20.
154. Comi P, Chiaramonte R, Maier JA. Senescence-dependent regulation of type 1 plasminogen activator inhibitor in human vascular endothelial cells. *Exp Cell Res* 1995;219:304–308.
155. Maier JA, Statuto M, Ragnotti G. Senescence stimulates U937-endothelial cell interactions. *Exp Cell Res* 1993;208:270–274.
156. Pagani F, Zagato L, Maier JA, Ragnotti G, Coviello DA, Vergani C. Expression and alternative splicing of fibronectin mRNA in human diploid endothelial cells during aging *in vitro. Biochim Biophys Acta* 1993;1173:172–178.
157. Matsuda T, Okamura K, Sato Y, et al. Decreased response to epidermal growth factor during cellular senescence in cultured human microvascular endothelial cells. *J Cell Physiol* 1992;150:510–516.
158. Gospodarowicz D, Brown KD, Birdwell CR, Zetter BR. Control of proliferation of human vascular endothelial cells: characterization of the response of human umbilical vein endothelial cells to fibroblast growth factor, epidermal growth factor, and thrombin. *J Cell Biol* 1978;77:774–788.
159. Marin J. Age-related changes in vascular responses: a review. *Mech Ageing Dev* 1995;79:71–114.

PART IV

Responses to Inflammation

Inflammation: Basic Principles and Clinical Correlates,
3rd ed., edited by John I. Gallin and Ralph Snyderman.
Lippincott Williams & Wilkins, Philadelphia © 1999.

CHAPTER 52

Role of Interleukin-10, Interleukin-4, and Interleukin-13 in Resolving Inflammatory Responses

René de Waal Malefyt

T cells of both rodents and humans can be categorized into two mutually exclusive subsets based on the profile of cytokines they are able to produce after activation. T_H1 helper T cells secrete interleukin-2 (IL-2), interferon-γ (IFN-γ), and lymphotoxin, whereas T_H2 cells make IL-4, IL-5, IL-6, IL-10, and IL-13 (1). This subdivision has proved to be significant, because these differences in cytokine production profiles correlate with differences in function. T_H1 cells are predominantly involved in cellular immune reactions and mediate delayed-type hypersensitivity (DTH) responses, whereas T_H2 cells are involved in humoral immune reactions and provide help to B cells for immunoglobulin production (2,3). Repetitive antigenic stimulation of naive T cells, which produce initially only IL-2 (4), drives their development toward polarized T-cell subsets. This differentiation of naive T cells into T_H1 and T_H2 cells depends on the presence of specific cytokines (4–6). Priming of naive T cells in the presence of IL-12 leads to the development of T_H1 cells, whereas IL-4 is both necessary and sufficient for T_H2 development (7–9). An additional role in T_H1 cell differentiation is fulfilled by IFN-γ, which acts in two ways to aid priming. It activates monocytes/macrophages to produce IL-12 (10), and it maintains the expression of the IL-12 receptor β_2 chain (IL-12Rβ_2) on T_H1 cells, which allows these cells to respond to IL-12 (11). Expression of the IL-12Rβ_2 subunit is induced after T-cell receptor triggering. Maintenance of IL-12Rβ_2 expression on T_H1 cells is mediated by IFN-α in humans (12).

T_H1 and T_H2 subsets regulate each other's differentiation and function by several mechanisms. IL-4 and, more

importantly, IL-10 inhibit the production of IFN-γ and IL-12, thereby limiting both subsequent T_H1 differentiation and effector function (13,14). Furthermore, IL-4, IL-13, and IL-10 antagonize the function of IFN-γ on effector cells and vice-versa. For example, the production of proinflammatory cytokines by monocytes is enhanced by IFN-γ and inhibited by IL-4, IL-13, and IL-10, whereas IL-4– or IL-13–induced synthesis of immunoglobulin E (IgE) by B cells is inhibited by IFN-γ (15–18). On the other hand, IFN-γ inhibits the proliferation of T_H2 cells without affecting T_H1 cells, because these cells no longer express the IFN-γ receptor β_2 chain (19). Several T_H2-derived cytokines thus can strongly affect the development and magnitude of inflammatory T_H1 responses. The most effective cytokine in this respect is IL-10, which has potent antiinflammatory and immunosuppressive effects (20,21). Because it is produced relatively late in the immune response, it has an important role in diminishing and dampening immune and inflammatory reactions, leading the way to resolution of these reactions when antigenic stimuli are neutralized. In this chapter, the roles of IL-10, IL-4, and IL-13 in inflammatory responses are discussed. The other major antiinflammatory cytokine, transforming growth factor-β (TGF-β), discussed elsewhere, can synergize with and complement the antiinflammatory activities of IL-4, IL-13, and IL-10 in a number of experimental systems.

INTERLEUKIN-10

IL-10 was initially characterized as "cytokine synthesis inhibitory factor" by T. Mosmann and colleagues. It was produced by mouse T_H2 clones and inhibited cytokine production, in particular IFN-γ production, by activated

R. de Waal Malefyt: DNAX Research Institute, Immunobiology Department, Palo Alto, California 94304-1104.

T_H1 clones (22). The cloning of mouse and human IL-10 (mIL-10, hIL-10) revealed a high homology to an Epstein-Barr virus gene (vIL-10) (14,23); vIL-10 shared some but not all of the biologic activities of hIL-10.

The hIL-10 is a nonglycosylated 18-kd polypeptide of 178 amino acids that belongs to the "long chain" four α-helical bundle cytokine family (14,23–26). It is an acid-sensitive, noncovalent homodimer of two interpenetrating polypeptide chains (22,25–28) and contains two intrachain disulfide bonds. Although hIL-10 is active on both mouse and human cells, mIL-10 is not active on human cells.

The mIL-10 and hIL-10 genes are composed of five exons and are located on chromosome 1 in both cases (21,29). Transcription generates predominantly single mRNAs of approximately 1.4 kb (mIL-10) or 2 kb (hIL-10) (23).

The IL-10 receptor complex consists of at least two polypeptide chains, IL-10Rα and IL-10Rβ (CRF2–4), which are members of the type II cytokine receptor family. Other members of this family include the IFNα/β and IFN-γ receptors. IL-10Rα binds ligand with high affinity (K_d, approximately 35 to 200 pmol/L) (27,30–32), and its expression was detected in all IL-10–responsive cells examined, although at low levels of a few hundred IL-10R per cell (27,30–33). hIL-10Rα has a molecular size of 90 to 120 kd and consists of 578 amino acids with two intracellular tyrosine residues that are important for the initiation of signal transduction. Its gene is located on chromosome 11. IL-10Rβ has a molecular mass of 60 kd and is ubiquitously expressed; its gene is located on chromosome 21. Binding of IL-10 to the IL-10R complex results in phosporylation and activation of (Janus kinase) JAK-1 and (tyrosine kinase) TYK-2 tyrosine kinases (34,35), leading to phosphorylation, activation, and the formation of homodimeric or heterodimeric signal transducer and activator of transcription-1 (STAT-1), STAT-3, or STAT-5 complexes that translocate to the nucleus and activate transcription of IL-10–responsive genes (36–38).

INTERLEUKIN-13 AND INTERLEUKIN-4

Human IL-4 and IL-13 are proteins of 129 and 132 amino acids with molecular masses of 18 and 12 kd, respectively. IL-13 and IL-4 contain four cysteine residues, which form two intramolecular disulfide bonds (39,40). Both IL-4 and IL-13 belong to the "short chain" cytokine family characterized by a four α helical structure. The IL-13 protein is about 25% homologous to IL-4, and all residues that contribute to the hydrophobic structural core of IL-4 are conserved or have conservative replacements in IL-13, suggesting that the overall three-dimensional structures of IL-4 and IL-13 are similar (41,42). Both human and mouse IL-13 are biologically active on human and murine cells. The gene encoding

hIL-13 is located on chromosome 5q31, in the same 3,000-kb cluster of genes that encodes IL-3, IL-4, IL-5, IL-9, and granulocyte-macrophage colony-stimulating factor (GM-CSF) (43,44). The IL-13 gene is only 12 kb upstream from the gene encoding IL-4. The hIL-13 gene is composed of four exons separated by three relatively short introns, which makes the total gene size approximately 3 kb (45); the hIL-4 gene spans approximately 10 kb.

IL-13 and IL-4 share many, but not all, biologic properties, partially because of the sharing and differential expression of IL-4 and IL-13 receptor components on various cell types (42). IL-4 binds to an IL-4 receptor complex composed of a 140-kd IL-4Rα chain and the common γ-chain (γc), a shared component of receptors for IL-2, IL-4, IL-7, IL-9, and IL-15. The IL-4Rα chain alone binds IL-4 with a relatively high affinity (K_d, approximately 1 pmol/L) but does not bind IL-13. The IL-4Rα chain is expressed by B cells, T cells, natural killer cells, and monocytes.

IL-13 receptors are usually present at 200 to 3,000 sites per cell and bind IL-13 with high affinity (K_d, approximately 30 pmol/L). The high-affinity IL-13 receptor complex comprises the 140-kd IL-4Rα chain and an IL-13 binding protein. Two different cDNAs encoding IL-13 binding proteins have been cloned; they are called IL-13Rα1 and IL-13Rα2 (46–48). IL-13Rα1 consists of a 427-amino-acid protein; it binds IL-13 with low affinity (K_d, approximately 40 pmol/L) but does not bind IL-4. It is encoded by a 4-kb mRNA, and the gene is located on the X chromosome. IL-13Rα2 is a 380-amino-acid protein that binds IL-13 with high affinity (K_d, approximately 50 pmol/L) in the absence of the IL-4Rα chain (49). Human IL-13Rα1 and IL-13Rα2 are 27% homologous. Both IL-13Rα1 and IL-13Rα2 show homology to the IL-5Rα and the prolactin receptor. They contain two consensus patterns characteristic for the hematopoietic cytokine receptor family. One is the WSXWS motif in the extracellular domain, and the other is a consensus binding motif for a (STAT) protein present in their short cytoplasmic tails. The IL-13Rα chains are expressed as glycosylated molecules of about 65 to 70 kd present on monocytes and B cells.

IL-13Rα/IL-4Rα complexes can also function as a second receptor for IL-4. Binding of IL-13 and IL-4 to their receptor complexes activates the JAK-1 and TYK-2 kinases and induces tyrosine phosphorylation of the IL-4Rα chain and the 170-kd insulin receptor substrate-2/IL-4–induced phosphotyrosine substrate (50), which, in its phosphorylated state, forms a docking site for the SRC homology domain–containing 85-kd subunit of phosphatidylinositol 3-kinase in lymphohematopoietic cells (51–55). However, IL-13 did not induce activation of the JAK-3 kinase, which associates with γc of the IL-4R complex after IL-4 binding (51,55). Phosphorylation of the IL-4Rα chain after binding of IL-13 or IL-4 leads to the recruitment, phosphorylation, dimerization, and nuclear translocation of STAT-6 and activation of IL-4/IL-13–responsive genes such as the Igε promoter, in a manner independent of γc and JAK-3 (56).

EFFECTS OF IL-4, IL-13, AND IL-10 ON MONOCYTES/MACROPHAGES AND DENDRITIC CELLS

IL-10, IL-4, and IL-13 modulate the expression of cytokines, soluble mediators, and cell surface molecules on cells of myeloid origin. Such changes have important consequences for the function of these cells in activation, maintenance, or downregulation of immune and inflammatory responses. IL-10, IL-4, and IL-13 strongly inhibited production of the proinflammatory cytokines and chemokines IL-1α, IL-1β, IL-6, IL-8, IL-10, IL-12, GM-CSF, G-CSF, M-CSF, TNF-α, macrophage inflammatory protein-1α (MIP-1α), MIP-1β, MIP-2, the "regulated on activation, normally T-cell expressed and secreted" cytokine (RANTES), and leukemia inhibitory factor (LIF) by activated monocytes/macrophages (18,40, 57–69). In addition, IL-4, IL-13, and IL-10 enhanced the production of IL-1RA (57,70–75) and upregulated expression of the soluble p55 and p75 TNF receptor (76–78), indicating that these cytokines induce a shift in the production of cytokines from proinflammatory to antiinflammatory mediators. Although IL-13 and IL-4 inhibit the production of IL-12 by lipopolysaccharide (LPS)–activated monocytes, overnight priming of monocytes with these cytokines before activation with LPS or staphylococcus aureus strain cowan I (SAC) increased the production of IL-12 (79).

IL-10 also inhibits C reactive protein–induced and LPS-induced, but not CD40-induced, tissue factor expression by human monocytes, leading to a reduction in procoagulant activity (80–84). IL-13, like IL-4, also downregulates tissue factor expression on LPS-activated monocytes (85–87).

IL-10 and IL-13 inhibit the production of vascular permeability factor activity from activated monocytes and act synergistically (88).

IL-10, IL-4, and IL-13 reduce the ability of cells to kill ingested organisms by decreasing the generation of superoxide anion (O_2^-) and nitric oxide (NO) (69, 89–101). The inhibitory effects of IL-10 on the production of NO by mouse macrophages can occur by an indirect mechanism involving inhibition of cytokine synthesis, and IL-10 and IL-4 have been shown to act synergistically (102–104). Inhibition of NO production resulted in enhanced iron uptake by murine macrophages, which contributed to the downregulation of their effector functions (105). IL-13 and IL-4, but not IL-10, induce expression of 15-lipoxygenase, which catalyzes the formation of 15S-hydroxyeicosatetraenoic acid and lipoxin A₄, mediators that antagonize proinflammatory leukotrienes (106). In addition, IL-10, IL-4, and IL-13 all inhibit the formation from arachidonic acid of prostaglandin E₂ (PGE₂), another proinflammatory mediator, through the inhibition of cyclooxygenase-2 induction by LPS-stimulated monocytes (107) and osteoclasts, resulting in the latter case in inhibition of IL-1–induced bone resorption by these cells (108,109).

IL-10 and IL-4 inhibit the ability of monocytes/macrophages to modulate the turnover of extracellular matrix through their inhibitory effects on the production of gelatinase and collagenase, but only IL-10 has the ability to enhance the production of tissue inhibitor of metalloproteinases-1 (TIMP-1) (110,111). The inhibition of gelatinase and collagenase by IL-4 and IL-10 is regulated through a PGE₂– and cyclic adenosine monophosphate (cAMP)–dependent pathway and is therefore secondary to the effects of these cytokines on PGE₂ formation (112).

IL-4 and IL-13 increase the expression of mannose receptors on mouse and human monocytes and macrophages, resulting in the elimination of proteins bearing terminal mannosyl ligands, such as lysosomal hydrolases and plasminogen activators (99,113,114). In addition, enhanced expression of mannose receptors is involved in human macrophage fusion and formation of foreign body giant cells (114). IL-10 has been shown to enhance mannose receptor–mediated antigen uptake by monocytes and dendritic cells (115).

Although the activities of IL-10, IL-4, and IL-13 on cytokine and chemokine production, procoagulant activity, inflammatory mediators, and mannose receptor expression are quite similar, the expression of cell surface markers, morphology, and differentiation are affected in distinctly different ways by these cytokines. The expression of Fc receptors and co-stimulatory molecules is regulated in an antagonistic manner. IL-4 and IL-13 downregulated the expression of Fcγ receptors (CD16, CD32, and CD64) on human monocytes and induced expression of the low-affinity IgE receptor, FcεRII (CD23) (18,39). Downregulation of CD64 expression correlated with decreased antibody-dependent cell-mediated cytotoxicity (ADCC) (18). In contrast, IL-10 upregulated the expression of Fc receptors on monocytes, including CD16 and CD64 (18,116,117), but downregulated the expression of IL-4–induced CD23 (118). These activities are shared by IL-10 and IFN-γ. Functionally, the upregulation of CD64 correlated with enhanced ADCC (15). The upregulation of Fc receptors by IL-10 enhances the capacity of monocytes/macrophages to phagocytose opsonized particles, bacteria, or fungi (119,120).

IL-10, IL-4, AND IL-13 DIFFERENTIALLY AFFECT T-CELL STIMULATORY ACTIVITIES OF MONOCYTES AND MONOCYTE-DERIVED DENDRITIC CELLS

IL-4 and IL-13 upregulate the expression of various adhesion molecules on monocytes, including CD11b,

CD11c, CD18, CD29, and CD49e (very late activation antigen-5) (18). This may contribute to the changes in morphology induced in monocytes/macrophages, such as homotypic aggregation, strong adherence, and the development of long cytoplasmic processes. IL-13 and IL-4 also upregulate the expression of major histocompatibility complex (MHC) class II molecules on human monocytes and expression of CD80 and CD86, the ligands of CD28 on T cells, which leads to an enhanced capacity to stimulate alloantigen-specific T-cell responses. In contrast, IL-10 inhibited the expression of MHC class II antigens, CD54 (intercellular adhesion molecule-1 [ICAM-1]), CD80 (B7), and CD86 (B7-2) on monocytes, even after the induction of these molecules by IL-4, IL-13, or IFN-γ (121–124), resulting in a strong inhibition of T-cell proliferative responses toward alloantigens as well as soluble antigens (121,125, 126). Downregulation of MHC class II molecules by IL-10 is mediated by a novel posttranscriptional mechanism that involves the blockade of intracellular transport of mature peptide-loaded molecules from the MHC class II loading compartment to the plasma membrane (127). Long-term culture of monocytes and macrophage precursors in the presence of IL-4 or IL-13 and GM-CSF leads to differentiation of monocytes into dendritic cells and inhibition of monocyte proliferation (128–130). The addition of IL-10 inhibits such differentiation. In addition, IL-10 inhibits the production of IL-12 and the expression of co-stimulatory molecules on various types of dendritic cells (131–135), which contributes to its ability to inhibit primary alloantigen-specific T-cell responses (136,137).

The effects of IL-10 on cytokine production and function in human macrophages are generally similar to those in monocytes, although less pronounced (58,138–143).

EFFECTS OF IL-10, IL-4, AND IL-13 ON T CELLS

The effects of IL-4, IL-13, and IL-10 on T-cell functions are diverse. IL-10 has both immunostimulatory and immunosuppressive activities; IL-4 is a T-cell growth and differentiation factor; and IL-13 has not been shown to bind to or have biologic activities on T cells (42,144). IL-4 supports the proliferation of activated T cells, induces the expression of CD8a on CD4+ T cells, and drives their differentiation toward a T_H2 phenotype, indicating that this cytokine can induce and enhance inflammatory responses, especially against allergens. The lack of biologic activities of IL-13 on T cells, including the induction of differentiation of naive CD4+ cord blood T cells toward a T_H2 phenotype (9), can be explained by the absence of IL-13–binding proteins (42,144). IL-10 strongly inhibits cytokine production and proliferation of antigen-specific T cells and T-cell clones under conditions of activation by antigen-presenting cells (APCs). This effect of IL-10 occurs predominantly through its downregulation of APC functions (121,126). However, T cells do express IL-10 receptors (31), and direct inter-

action of IL-10 with the IL-10 receptor modulates T-cell function. IL-10 inhibits the production of IL-2 and TNF-α, but not that of IL-4 and IFN-γ, when T cells are stimulated in an APC-independent manner (145,146). In addition, inhibition of IL-2 production may indirectly inhibit the CD28- and phorbol myristate acetate–induced production of IL-5, which is dependent on IL-2 (147).

Activation of T cells in the presence of IL-10 can induce a long-lasting state of nonresponsiveness or anergy, which cannot be reversed by addition of IL-2 or stimulation by anti-CD3 and anti-CD28 (148). In addition, repeated antigenic activation or differentiation of T cells in the presence of IL-10 results in the generation of a subset of T cells (Tr1, T regulatory cells) that produce large amounts of IL-10 and TGF-β and act as suppressor cells *in vivo* (149,150). A role for IL-10 in the induction and maintenance of nonresponsiveness or anergy has previously been described in anti–tumor cell responses, ultraviolet (UV) radiation–induced tolerance, hapten-specific tolerance, infections by parasites or by the human immunodeficiency virus, and superantigen-induced hyporesponsiveness (151–159).

EFFECTS OF IL-10, IL-4, AND IL-13 ON GRANULOCYTES AND MAST CELLS

Cytokine and chemokine production, as well as generation of superoxide anions and survival by polymorphonuclear leukocytes or purified neutrophils (160–164), was inhibited by IL-10, IL-4, and IL-13 after activation by LPS, whereas the production of IL-1RA was enhanced (70,165). IL-10 also inhibited cytokine production by activated eosinophils (166) and the production of TNF-α and GM-CSF by mast cells after triggering of the high-affinity IgE receptor (167). IL-10 and IL-4 inhibited the LPS-induced production of PGE_2 by neutrophils through the inhibition of cyclooxygenase-2 expression (168).

In general, the inhibitory effects of IL-10, IL-4, and IL-13 on the production of chemokines, proinflammatory cytokines, mediators, and survival of granulocytes, which limit the duration of the inflammatory response, all contribute to the antiinflammatory activities of these cytokines. However, in infectious diseases the inhibitory effects of IL-10, IL-4, and IL-13 on NO and superoxide production can be counterproductive to the organism. Neutralization of IL-10 led to enhanced survival in murine models of *Klebsiella pneumoniae, Streptococcus pneumoniae,* and *Mycobacterium avium* infections, because killing of phagocytosed bacteria was partly suppressed by endogenous IL-10 (169–171).

IN VIVO EFFECTS OF IL-10

Systemic Inflammation

Based on the effects of IL-4, IL-13, and IL-10 on individual cell types, it is clear that these cytokines may have potent antiinflammatory and immunosuppressive activities *in vivo*. This theory has been tested in a variety of experimental models. IL-10 and IL-13 rescued BALB/c (*B*gg, *alb*ino) and BDF1 mice from LPS-induced lethal endotoxemia, in correlation with reduced serum levels of TNF-α, IFN-γ, and IL-12 (172–174). Both administration of IL-10 protein and IL-10 gene transfer protected mice from a lethal intraperitoneal endotoxin challenge (175). In addition, the protective effects of monocyte chemoattractant protein-1 (MCP-1) in this model correlated with an increase in serum levels of IL-10 and a decrease in TNF-α and IL-12 (176). In humans, IL-10 reduced serum levels of TNF-α, IL-6, and IL-8 as well as neutrophil accumulation, elastase production, and cortisone levels when volunteers were challenged with a low dose of endotoxin (177).

Administration of endotoxin results in the production of IL-10 in mice, chimpanzees, baboons, and humans (177–180). LPS-induced production of IL-10 by monocytes *in vitro* occurs late after activation (57), but IL-10 serum levels *in vivo* are already elevated at 3 to 6 hours after endotoxin challenge (177–180), indicating that other factors or cells may contribute to the production of IL-10 under these circumstances. Endogenously produced IL-10 confers a significant protection against endotoxin challenge and reduces TNF-α, IFN-γ, and MIP-2 production (181,182). This is also clearly observed in mice treated from birth with anti–IL-10 monoclonal antibodies (MAbs) and in IL-10−/− mice, which are susceptible to 20-fold lower doses of LPS to induce lethality (183,184). Furthermore, IL-10−/− mice were extremely vulnerable to a generalized Swartzman reaction, in which prior exposure to a small amount of LPS footpad (fp) primes the host for a lethal response to a subsequent sublethal intravenous dose of LPS (184). Priming mice with larger amounts of LPS induces LPS tolerance, in which exposure to LPS induces a downregulation of the cytokine response to a second, high dose of LPS. The induction of LPS tolerance can be prevented by anti–IL-10 and anti–TGF-β antibodies or induced by IL-10 and TGF-β in the absence of LPS, indicating that IL-10 is involved in this induction (185). Induction of LPS tolerance can be restored and prevented by IFN-γ or GM-CSF in both mice and humans (186,187). The requirement for TGF-β, and probably other factors as well, is supported by the observation that LPS tolerance can be induced in IL-10-/- mice (184). Immunosuppression of T-cell and macrophage functions is also observed in critically ill patients after sepsis or trauma, which induces a high susceptibility to infection, and is similar to LPS tolerance induced *in vitro* (188,189). IL-10 is probably involved in the induction of this state, as evidenced by the decreased expression of the human leukocyte antigen HLA-DR on monocytes (189).

IL-10 is also active in an *in vivo* model that more closely resembles human sepsis. Endogenously produced IL-10 had a protective effect on survival of mice undergoing cecal ligation and puncture, which results in septic peritonitis (190,191). Prophylactic or therapeutic administration of IL-10 strongly reduced serum levels of TNF-α, IL-1, and IL-6 (192). The protective effect of an NO inhibitor in this peritonitis model could be blocked by anti–IL-10 and anti–MCP-1 antibodies, indicating that endogenous IL-10, which may have been induced by MCP-1, was involved in the therapeutic effect (193).

IL-10 could also protect adult mice from staphylococcal enterotoxin B (SEB)–induced toxic shock (194) and neonatal mice from lethal streptococcal B infections (195). Furthermore, in a less severe model of SEB-induced shock, which depends on IL-2 and IFN-γ production by T cells, endogenous IL-10 prevented lethality (196).

In humans, IL-10 is produced during septicemia and septic shock, and serum levels correlate with the intensity of the inflammatory response (197–201). This was especially evident in patients with meningococcal infections (202–205). In contrast, IL-13 production was not detected during clinical sepsis and experimental endotoxemia in humans, indicating that endogenous IL-13 is unlikely to play an important antiinflammatory role in this form of systemic inflammation (199). However, IL-4, IL-10, and IL-13 are detected in the sera of patients with systemic sclerosis who have systemic inflammation.

An important role for IL-10 in controlling systemic inflammation is further suggested by the inhibitory effects of IL-10 on the endotoxin-induced production of proinflammatory cytokines, including indirect effects on endothelial cell activation and adhesion (206,207) and expression of monocyte tissue factor, which contributes to procoagulant activity and ultimately to disseminated intravascular coagulation (80–84). Consistent with this, many strategies to intervene in sepsis have proven to affect IL-10 production (208–211).

Localized Inflammatory Disease

In addition to the antiinflammatory effects of IL-10 in systemic inflammatory processes, IL-10 has protective effects in a variety of experimental models of local inflammation, such as pancreatitis (212), uveitis (213,214), hepatitis (215), peritonitis (190,191,195), and lung injury (216,217). Additive or synergistic effects of IL-10 and IL-4 have been reported in some models of localized inflammation. For example IL-4 and IL-10 attenuate established crescentic glomerulonephritis, a T$_H$1-dependent DTH reaction against the glomerular basement membrane (218).

The inhibitory effects of IL-4, IL-13, and IL-10 on the production of TNF-α and IL-1β by alveolar macrophages play an important role in the attenuation of IgG complex–induced lung injury by reducing the TNF-induced expression of ICAM-1 and subsequent migration of neutrophils to the lungs (216,217,219). IL-10 and IL-13 reduce TNF production by suppressing nuclear factor-κB activation through preservation of its inhibitor, IκBα (220). Reduced granulocyte migration into lungs also was observed after treatment of human volunteers with low doses of LPS combined with IL-10 (177). Another mechanism by which IL-10 reduced lung injury after LPS- or antigen-induced pulmonary inflammation was by induction of neutrophil apoptosis (164,221).

In IL-10–/– mice, a role for IL-10 as a natural suppressor of cytokine production and inflammation in allergic bronchopulmonary aspergillosis was revealed, indicating that IL-10 is able to suppress not only inflammatory T_H1 but also T_H2 responses (222).

IL-10 is more potent in its antiinflammatory activities than IL-4 or IL-13. Some of the antiinflammatory activities of IL-4 and IL-13 on cytokine production are offset by their role in promoting T_H2 inflammatory responses. IL-4 and IL-13 induce expression of vascular cell adhesion molecule-1 on human umbilical vein endothelial cells, which results in adhesion of $\alpha_4\beta_1$-positive cells, including eosinophils (223,224). This emphasizes the importance of these cytokines in the pathogenesis of allergic and asthmatic responses, since eosinophils accumulated at sites of allergic inflammation are thought to play a crucial role in the pathogenesis of lung inflammation and lung epithelial cell destruction in asthmatic patients (225). Furthermore, IL-13 acts directly on eosinophils to induce their expression of CD69 and prolonged survival (226). In addition, it upregulates GM-CSF expression by bronchial epithelial cells, which may enhance survival of eosinophils (227). The production of IL-4 and IL-13 by mast cells and basophils after crosslinking of FcεRI could also contribute to initiation and maintenance of allergic responses (228–230). Finally, IL-4 and IL-13 are able to activate B cells to proliferate, enhance immunoglobulin production, and induce switching to IgE production, which is crucial for allergic inflammation (16,231).

Cutaneous Inflammation

The role of IL-10 and IL-4 in crossregulation between T_H1 and T_H2 subsets is clearly demonstrated in models of cutaneous inflammation. IL-10 affected the initiation and effector phases of cellular (T_H1) and DTH responses (232,233) as well as the elicitation of contact hypersensitivity reactions in sensitized mice (234,235). IL-10 acted in synergy with IL-4 to inhibit tuberculin-type DTH reactions of BALB/c mice that had recovered from a *Leishmania major* infection (236). The production of endogenous IL-10 in these responses is critical because reactions to irritants, DTH, and contact hypersensitivity responses in IL-10–/– mice are exaggerated and prolonged (237). Keratinocytes or keratinocyte cell lines secrete IL-10 on exposure to UV light in mice (238,239), but not in

humans (240–242). This keratinocyte-derived IL-10 plays a major role in the UV-induced suppression of DTH, contact hypersensitivity, and antitumor responses (153,238,239,243–245), and IL-10–/– mice are completely resistant to UV-induced immunosuppression (246). IL-10 administration to patients with psoriasis, a T_H1-mediated inflammatory dermatosis, showed clinical efficacy and reduced production of TNF, IL-12, and HLA-DR expression (247). These results indicate that IL-10 plays an important role as a regulator of cutaneous immune responses.

INFLAMMATORY BOWEL DISEASE

IL-10 may be involved in the development of inflammatory bowel disease (IBD), as suggested by two *in vivo* models. First, the transfer of naive CD45RbB^{hi} T cells, which develop in T cells that produce high levels of IFN-γ and TNF-α in response to enteric antigens, from BALB/c mice into CB-17 severe combined immunodeficiency (SCID) mice resulted in the spontaneous development of IBD. This disease could be prevented by coadministration of CD45Rb^{lo} cells, which include regulatory cells able to make IL-10 and IL-4; by treatment with anti–IFN-γ or anti-TNF MAbs; or by administration of IL-10 (248–250). Disease could also be prevented by administration of a novel subset of T cells that produce high levels of IL-10 after activation and act as suppressor cells *in vivo* (150). Both CD45Rb^{hi} and CD45Rb^{lo} cells isolated from IL-10–/– mice were able to induce IBD in (rearrangement activating gene) RAG2–/– mice, suggesting that IL-10 is involved in the protective effects of the CD45Rb^{lo} cells in wild-type mice (251). In addition, IL-10–/– mice themselves spontaneously developed enterocolitis, which is more similar in histologic appearance and pathology to Crohn's disease in humans than it is to ulcerative colitis (252). More prolonged stages of the disease involved the appearance of adenocarcinomas (253). The enterocolitis in IL-10–/–mice could be prevented by administration of IL-10 from birth and treatment with anti–IFN-γ or anti–IL-12 MAbs. Once disease was established, IL-10 ameliorated but could not completely cure it. CD4$^+$ T cells isolated from diseased colon produced high levels of IFN-γ and TNF and could transfer disease, indicating that the interaction between enteric flora and inflammatory cells is dysregulated in the absence of IL-10 and leads to uncontrolled T_H1 responses (254). IL-10 was present in the sera of patients with IBD (255). IL-10 and IL-13 inhibited the pokeweed mitogen–induced production of IL-1, IL-6, and TNF by monocytes isolated from patients with inactive IBD, but not from patients with active IBD. However, in combination with IL-10, IL-13 and IL-4 acted synergistically to inhibit the production of proinflammatory cytokines even from these patients (256,257).

RHEUMATOID ARTHRITIS

A beneficial role for antiinflammatory cytokines in the pathogenesis of rheumatoid arthritis has been described. IL-10, IL-4, and IL-13 inhibited TNF, IL-1β, and IL-8 production by synovial macrophages and synoviocytes (258–261), and synergistic effects were observed in combination with IL-4 (260,262). IL-10 was demonstrated in sera, synovial fluid, and synovial explant cultures from patients with rheumatoid arthritis (263–267). Endogenously produced IL-10 had a suppressive effect on cytokine production from synovial cells, indicating that IL-10 *in vivo* may have a protective role (267). In the joint, both synovial macrophages and T cells produce IL-10 (267,268). On the other hand, IL-10 production in rheumatoid arthritis has been linked to increased autoantibody production, serum factor, and B-cell activation (265,266,269). IL-10 is protective in animal models of rheumatoid arthritis; it reduced joint swelling, infiltration, cytokine production, and cartilage degradation in collagen (CIA)–induced and streptococcal cell wall–induced arthritis (270–274), and IL-4 and IL-10 synergistically reduced joint inflammation in acute and chronic models of arthritis (275). IL-13 also reduced severity and incidence of CIA in DBA/1 mice, which correlated with a reduced production of TNF in the spleen (276).

CONCLUSIONS

The most dramatic biologic effects of IL-10 are its potent deactivating effects on monocytes/macrophages, granulocytes, and dendritic cells. These include downregulatory activities on MHC class II and accessory molecules, production of monokines and chemokines, and release of inflammatory mediators. These activities lead to inhibition of antigen presentation and accessory functions and result in abrogation of antigen-specific T-cell proliferation and cytokine production, as well as alterations in cell trafficking, survival, and migration. In addition, IL-10 has direct inhibitory effects on proliferation and IL-2 production by T cells and can induce an anergic state under physiologic conditions. Together with the observations that IL-10 is produced by multiple cell types after activation and the findings that it is indispensable, these results indicate that IL-10 plays an important role as a natural dampener of immune and inflammatory reactions (20,251,277). Although the focus here is on inflammatory responses, immunomodulating effects of IL-10, IL-4, and IL-13 have also been observed in autoimmune and infectious diseases or disease models. IL-4 and IL-13 share a number of the antiinflammatory activities of IL-10 but also possess immunostimulatory activities that do not lead to abrogation of immune or inflammatory responses but instead lead to deviation toward T_H2 responses.

ACKNOWLEDGMENT

DNAX Research Institute is supported by Schering-Plough Corporation.

REFERENCES

1. Mosmann TR, Cherwinski H, Bond M, Giedlin M, Coffman RL. Two types of mouse helper T cell clones. I. Definition according to profile of lymphokine activities and secreted proteins. *J Immunol* 1986;136:2348.
2. Mosmann TR, Schumacher JH, Street NF, et al. Diversity of cytokine synthesis and function of mouse CD4+ T cells. *Immunol Rev* 1991;123:209–229.
3. Coffman RL, Varkila K, Scott P, Chatelain R. The role of cytokines in the differentiation of CD4+ subsets *in vivo*. *Immunol Rev* 1991;123:189–207.
4. Swain SL, Bradley LM, Croft M, et al. Helper T cell subsets: phenotype, function and the role of cytokines in regulating their development. *Immunol Rev* 1991;123:115–145.
5. Seder RA, Paul WE. Acquisition of lymphokine producing phenotype by CD4+ T cells. *Annu Rev Immunol* 1994;12:635–675.
6. O'Garra A, Murphy K. Role of cytokines in development of Th1 and Th2 cells. *Chem Immunol* 1996;63:1–13.
7. Hsieh CS, Macatonia SE, Tripp CS, Wolf SF, O'Garra A, Murphy KM. Development of TH1 CD4+ T cells through IL-12 produced by *Listeria*-induced macrophages. *Science* 1993;260:547–549.
8. Kopf M, Le Gros G, Bachmann M, Lamers MC, Bluethmann H, Kohler G. Disruption of the murine IL-4 gene blocks Th2 cytokine responses. *Nature* 1993;362:245–248.
9. Sornasse T, Larenas PV, Davis KA, de VJ, Yssel H. Differentiation and stability of T helper 1 and 2 cells derived from naive human neonatal CD4+ T cells, analyzed at the single-cell level. *J Exp Med* 1996;184:473–483.
10. Kubin M, Chow J, Trinchieri G. Differential regulation of interleukin-12 (IL-12), tumor necrosis factor alpha and IL-1 beta production in human myeloid leukemia cell lines and peripheral blood mononuclear cells. *Blood* 1994;83:646–652.
11. Szabo S, Dghe A, Gubler U, Murphy K. Regulation of the Interleukin (IL)-12 Rβ2 subunit expression in developing T helper 1 (Th1) and Th2 cells. *J Exp Med* 1997;185:817–824.
12. Rogge L, Barberis-Maino L, Biffi M, et al. Selective expression of an interleukin-12 receptor component by human T helper 1 cells. *J Exp Med* 1997;185:825–831.
13. Fitch FW, McKisic MD, Lancki DW, Gajewski TF. Differential regulation of murine T lymphocyte subsets. *Annu Rev Immunol* 1993;11:1–29.
14. Vieira P, de Waal-Malefyt R, Dang M-N, et al. Isolation and expression of human cytokine synthesis inhibitory factor (CSIF/IL10) cDNA clones: homology to Epstein-Barr virus open reading frame BCRFI. *Proc Natl Acad Sci U S A* 1991;88:1172–1176.
15. te Velde AA, de Waal Malefyt R, Huijbens RJF, de Vries JE, Figdor CG. IL-10 stimulates monocyte FcγR surface expression and cytotoxic activity: distinct regulation of ADCC by IFNγ, IL-4, and IL-10. *J Immunol* 1992;149:4048–4052.
16. Pene J, Rousset F, Briere F, et al. IgE production by normal human lymphocytes is induced by interleukin-4 and suppressed by interferons alpha and gamma and prostaglandin E2. *Proc Natl Acad Sci U S A* 1988;85:6880–6884.
17. Ezernieks J, Schnarr B, Metz K, Duschl A. The human IgE germline promoter is regulated by interleukin-4, interleukin-13, interferon-alpha and interferon-gamma via an interferon-gamma-activated site and its flanking regions. *Eur J Biochem* 1996;240:667–673.
18. de Waal Malefyt R, Figdor CG, Huijbens R, et al. Effects of IL-13 on phenotype, cytokine production, and cytotoxic function of human monocytes: comparison with IL-4 and modulation by IFN-gamma or IL-10. *J Immunol* 1993;151:6370–6381.
19. Pernis A, Gupta S, Gollob KJ, et al. Lack of interferon gamma receptor beta chain and the prevention of interferon gamma signaling in TH1 cells [see comments]. *Science* 1995;269:245–247.
20. Moore KW, O'Garra A, de Waal Malefyt R, Vieira P, Mosmann TR. Interleukin-10. *Annu Rev Immunol* 1993;11:165–190.
21. de Waal Malefyt R, de Vries J. Interleukin-10. In: Aggarwal B, Gut-

terman J, eds. *Human cytokines: a handbook for basic and clinical research,* vol II. Cambridge, MA: Blackwell Science, 1996:19–42.

22. Fiorentino DF, Bond MW, Mosmann TR. Two types of mouse helper T cells. IV. Th2 clones secrete a factor that inhibits cytokine production by Th1 clones. *J Exp Med* 1989;170:2081–2095.

23. Moore KW, Vieira P, Fiorentino DF, Trounstine ML, Khan TA, Mosmann TR. Homology of cytokine synthesis inhibitory factor (IL-10) to the Epstein-Barr virus gene BCRFI. *Science* 1990;248:1230–1234.

24. Sprang SR, Bazan JF. Cytokine structural taxonomy and mechanisms of receptor engagement. *Curr Opin Struct Biol* 1993;3:815–827.

25. Walter MR, Nagabhushan TL. Crystal structure of interleukin 10 reveals an interferon γ-like fold. *Biochemistry* 1995;34:12118–12125.

26. Zdanov A, Schalk-Hihi C, Gustchina A, Tsang M, Weatherbee J, Wlodawer A. Crystal structure of interleukin-10 reveals the functional dimer with an unexpected topological similarity to interferon γ. *Structure* 1995;3:591–601.

27. Tan JC, Indelicato S, Narula SK, Zavodny PJ, Chou C-C. Characterization of interleukin-10 receptors on human and mouse cells. *J Biol Chem* 1993;268:21053–21059.

28. Windsor WT, Syto R, Tsarbopoulos A, et al. Disulfide bond assignments and secondary structure analysis of human and murine interleukin 10. *Biochemistry* 1993;32:8807–8815.

29. Kim JM, Brannan CI, Copeland NG, Jenkins NA, Khan TA, Moore KW. Structure of the mouse interleukin-10 gene and chromosomal localization of the mouse and human genes. *J Immunol* 1992;148:3618–3623.

30. Liu Y, de Waal Malefyt R, Briere F, et al. The Epstein-Barr virus interleukin-10 (IL-10) homolog is a selective agonist with impaired binding to the IL-10 receptor. *J Immunol* 1997;158:604–613.

31. Liu Y, Wei SH-Y, Ho AS-Y, de Waal Malefyt R, Moore KW. Expression cloning and characterization of a human interleukin-10 receptor. *J Immunol* 1994;152:1821–1829.

32. Ho AS-Y, Liu Y, Khan TA, Hsu D-H, Bazan JF, Moore KW. A receptor for interleukin-10 is related to interferon receptors. *Proc Natl Acad Sci U S A* 1993;90:11267–11271.

33. Carson WE, Lindemann MJ, Baiocchi R, et al. The functional characterization of interleukin-10 receptor expression on human natural killer cells. *Blood* 1995;85:3577–3585.

34. Ho AS-Y, Wei SH, Mui AL, Miyajima A, Moore KW. Functional regions of the mouse interleukin-10 receptor cytoplasmic domain. *Mol Cell Biol* 1995;15:5043–5053.

35. Finbloom DS, Winestock KD. IL-10 induces the tyrosine phosphorylation of tyk2 and Jak1 and the differential assembly of STAT1 alpha and STAT3 complexes in human T cells and monocytes. *J Immunol* 1995;155:1079–1090.

36. Lai CF, Ripperger J, Morella KK, et al. Receptors for interleukin (IL)-10 and IL-6-type cytokines use similar signaling mechanisms for inducing transcription through IL-6 response elements. *J Biol Chem* 1996;271:13968–13975.

37. Wehinger J, Gouilleux F, Groner B, Finke J, Mertelsmann R, Weber-Nordt RM. IL-10 induces DNA binding activity of three STAT proteins (Stat1, Stat3, and Stat5) and their distinct combinatorial assembly in the promoters of selected genes. *FEBS Lett* 1996;394:365–370.

38. Weber-Nordt RM, Riley JK, Greenlund AC, Moore KW, Darnell JE, Schreiber RD. Stat3 recruitment by two distinct ligand-induced, tyrosine-phosphorylated docking sites in the interleukin-10 receptor intracellular domain. *J Biol Chem* 1996;271:27954–27961.

39. McKenzie ANJ, Culpepper JA, de Waal Malefyt R, de Vries JE, Zurawski G. Interleukin-13, a T cell derived cytokine that regulates human monocyte and B cell function. *Proc Natl Acad Sci U S A* 1993; 150:5436–5444.

40. Minty A, Chalon P, Derocq JM, et al. Interleukin-13 is a new human lymphokine regulating inflammatory and immune responses. *Nature* 1993;362:248–250.

41. Bamborough P, Duncan D, Richards WG. Predictive modelling of the 3-D structure of interleukin-13. *Protein Eng* 1994;7:1077–1082.

42. Zurawski SM, Vega F Jr, Huyghe B, Zurawski G. Receptors for interleukin-13 and interleukin-4 are complex and share a novel component that functions in signal transduction. *EMBO J* 1993;12:2663–2670.

43. Morgan JG, Dolganov GM, Robbins SE, Paul W. The selective isolation of novel cDNAs encoded by the regions surrounding the human interleukin 4 and 5 genes. *Nucleic Acids Res* 1992;20:5173–5179.

44. Smirnov DV, Smirnova MG, Korobko VG, Frolova EI. Tandem arrangement of human genes for interleukin-4 and interleukin-13: resemblance in their organization. *Gene* 1995;155:277–281.

45. McKenzie AN, Li X, Largaespada DA, et al. Structural comparison and chromosomal localization of the human and mouse IL-13 genes. *J Immunol* 1993;150:5436–5444.

46. Aman MJ, Tayebi N, Obiri NI, Puri RK, Modi WS, Leonard WJ. cDNA cloning and characterization of the human interleukin 13 receptor alpha chain. *J Biol Chem* 1996;271:29265–29270.

47. Gauchat JF, Schlagenhauf E, Feng NP, et al. A novel 4-kb interleukin-13 receptor alpha mRNA expressed in human B, T, and endothelial cells encoding an alternate type-II interleukin-4/interleukin-13 receptor. *Eur J Immunol* 1997;27:971–978.

48. Miloux B, Laurent P, Bonnin O, et al. Cloning of the human IL-13R alpha1 chain and reconstitution with the IL4R alpha of a functional IL-4/IL-13 receptor complex. *FEBS Lett* 1997;401:163–166.

49. Caput D, Laurent P, Kaghad M, et al. Cloning and characterization of a specific interleukin (IL)-13 binding protein structurally related to the IL-5 receptor alpha chain. *J Biol Chem* 1996;271:16921–16926.

50. Sun XJ, Wang LM, Zhang Y, et al. Role of IRS-2 in insulin and cytokine signalling. *Nature* 1995;377:173–177.

51. Keegan AD, Johnston JA, Tortolani PJ, et al. Similarities and differences in signal transduction by interleukin 4 and interleukin 13: analysis of Janus kinase activation. *Proc Natl Acad Sci U S A* 1995;92: 7681–7685.

52. Lefort S, Vita N, Reeb R, Caput D, Ferrara P. IL-13 and IL-4 share signal transduction elements as well as receptor components in TF-1 cells. *FEBS Lett* 1995;366:122–126.

53. Smerz-Bertling C, Duschl A. Both interleukin 4 and interleukin 13 induce tyrosine phosphorylation of the 140-kDa subunit of the interleukin 4 receptor. *J Biol Chem* 1995;270:966–970.

54. Wang LM, Michieli P, Lie WR, et al. The insulin receptor substrate-1-related 4PS substrate but not the interleukin-2R gamma chain is involved in interleukin-13-mediated signal transduction. *Blood* 1995; 86:4218–4227.

55. Welham MJ, Learmonth L, Bone H, Schrader JW. Interleukin-13 signal transduction in lymphohemopoietic cells: similarities and differences in signal transduction with interleukin-4 and insulin. *J Biol Chem* 1995;270:12286–12296.

56. Izuhara K, Heike T, Otsuka T, et al. Signal transduction pathway of interleukin-4 and interleukin-13 in human B cells derived from X-linked severe combined immunodeficiency patients. *J Biol Chem* 1996;271:619–622.

57. de Waal Malefyt R, Abrams J, Bennett B, Figdor C, de Vries J. IL-10 inhibits cytokine synthesis by human monocytes: an autoregulatory role of IL-10 produced by monocytes. *J Exp Med* 1991;174: 1209–1220.

58. Berkman N, John M, Roesems G, Jose PJ, Barnes PJ, Chung KF. Inhibition of macrophage inflammatory protein-1 alpha expression by IL-10: differential sensitivities in human blood monocytes and alveolar macrophages. *J Immunol* 1995;155:4412–4418.

59. Gruber MF, Williams CC, Gerrard TL. Macrophage-colony-stimulating factor expression by anti-CD45 stimulated human monocytes is transcriptionally up-regulated by IL-1 beta and inhibited by IL-4 and IL-10. *J Immunol* 1994;152:1354–1361.

60. Marfaing-Koka A, Maravic M, Humbert M, Galanaud P, Emilie D. Contrasting effects of IL-4, IL-10 and corticosteroids on RANTES production by human monocytes. *Int Immunol* 1996;8:1587–1594.

61. Fiorentino DF, Zlotnik A, Mosmann TR, Howard M, O'Garra A. IL-10 inhibits cytokine production by activated macrophages. *J Immunol* 1991;147:3815–3822.

62. D'Andrea A, Aste AM, Valiante NM, Ma X, Kubin M, Trinchieri G. Interleukin 10 (IL-10) inhibits human lymphocyte interferon gamma-production by suppressing natural killer cell stimulatory factor/IL-12 synthesis in accessory cells. *J Exp Med* 1993;178:1041–1048.

63. Cosentino G, Soprana E, Thienes CP, Siccardi AG, Viale G, Vercelli D. IL-13 down-regulates CD14 expression and TNF-alpha secretion in normal human monocytes. *J Immunol* 1995;155:3145–3151.

64. Hart PH, Ahern MJ, Smith MD, Finlay-Jones JJ. Regulatory effects of IL-13 on synovial fluid macrophages and blood monocytes from patients with inflammatory arthritis. *Clin Exp Immunol* 1995;99: 331–337.

65. Yanagawa H, Sone S, Haku T, et al. Contrasting effect of interleukin-13 on interleukin-1 receptor antagonist and proinflammatory cytokine production by human alveolar macrophages. *Am J Respir Cell Mol Biol* 1995;12:71–76.

66. Yano S, Yanagawa H, Nishioka Y, Mukaida N, Matsushima K, Sone S.

T helper 2 cytokines differently regulate monocyte chemoattractant protein-1 production by human peripheral blood monocytes and alveolar macrophages. *J Immunol* 1996;157:2660–2665.

67. Minty A, Chalon P, Guillemot JC, et al. Molecular cloning of the MCP-3 chemokine gene and regulation of its expression. *Eur Cytokine Netw* 1993;4:99–110.

68. Berkman N, John M, Roesems G, Jose P, Barnes PJ, Chung KF. Interleukin 13 inhibits macrophage inflammatory protein-1 alpha production from human alveolar macrophages and monocytes. *Am J Respir Cell Mol Biol* 1996;15:382–389.

69. Doherty TM, Kastelein R, Menon S, Andrade S, Coffman RL. Modulation of murine macrophage function by IL-13. *J Immunol* 1993;151:7151–7160.

70. Cassatella MA, Meda L, Gasperini S, Calzetti F, Bonora S. Interleukin 10 (IL-10) upregulates IL-1 receptor antagonist production from lipopolysaccharide-stimulated human polymorphonuclear leukocytes by delaying mRNA degradation. *J Exp Med* 1994;179:1695–1699.

71. Jenkins JK, Malyak M, Arend WP. The effects of interleukin-10 on interleukin-1 receptor antagonist and interleukin-1 beta production in human monocytes and neutrophils. *Lymphokine Cytokine Res* 1994;13:47–54.

72. Muzio M, Re F, Sironi M, et al. Interleukin-13 induces the production of interleukin-1 receptor antagonist (IL-1ra) and the expression of the mRNA for the intracellular (keratinocyte) form of IL-1ra in human myelomonocytic cells. *Blood* 1994;83:1738–1743.

73. Colotta F, Re F, Muzio M, et al. Interleukin-13 induces expression and release of interleukin-1 decoy receptor in human polymorphonuclear cells. *J Biol Chem* 1994;269:12403–12406.

74. Colotta F, Saccani S, Giri JG, et al. Regulated expression and release of the IL-1 decoy receptor in human mononuclear phagocytes. *J Immunol* 1996;156:2534–2541.

75. Vannier E, de Waal Malefyt R, Salazar-Montes A, de Vries JE, Dinarello CA. Interleukin-13 (IL-13) induces IL-1 receptor antagonist gene expression and protein synthesis in peripheral blood mononuclear cells: inhibition by an IL-4 mutant protein. *Blood* 1996;87:3307–3315.

76. Hart PH, Hunt EK, Bonder CS, Watson CJ, Finlay-Jones JJ. Regulation of surface and soluble TNF receptor expression on human monocytes and synovial fluid macrophages by IL-4 and IL-10. *J Immunol* 1996;157:3672–3680.

77. Linderholm M, Ahlm C, Settergren B, Waage A, Tarnvik A. Elevated plasma levels of tumor necrosis factor (TNF)-alpha, soluble TNF receptors, interleukin (IL)-6, and IL-10 in patients with hemorrhagic fever with renal syndrome. *J Infect Dis* 1996;173:38–43.

78. Joyce DA, Steer JH. IL-4, IL-10 and IFN-gamma have distinct, but interacting, effects on differentiation-induced changes in TNF-alpha and TNF receptor release by cultured human monocytes. *Cytokine* 1996;8:49–57.

79. D'Andrea A, Ma X, Aste-Amezaga M, Paganin C, Trinchieri G. Stimulatory and inhibitory effects of interleukin (IL)-4 and IL-13 on the production of cytokines by human peripheral blood mononuclear cells: priming for IL-12 and tumor necrosis factor alpha production. *J Exp Med* 1995;181:537–546.

80. Jungi TW, Brcic M, Eperon S, Albrecht S. Transforming growth factor-beta and interleukin-10, but not interleukin-4, down-regulate procoagulant activity and tissue factor expression in human monocyte-derived macrophages. *Thromb Res* 1994;76:463–474.

81. Pradier O, Willems F, Abramowicz D, et al. CD40 engagement induces monocyte procoagulant activity through an interleukin-10 resistant pathway. *Eur J Immunol* 1996;26:3048–3054.

82. Ramani M, Khechai F, Ollivier V, et al. Interleukin-10 and pentoxifylline inhibit C-reactive protein-induced tissue factor gene expression in peripheral human blood monocytes. *FEBS Lett* 1994;356:86–88.

83. Pradier O, Gerard C, Delvaux A, et al. Interleukin-10 inhibits the induction of monocyte procoagulant activity by bacterial lipopolysaccharide. *Eur J Immunol* 1993;23:2700–2703.

84. Ramani M, Ollivier V, Khechai F, et al. Interleukin-10 inhibits endotoxin-induced tissue factor mRNA production by human monocytes. *FEBS Lett* 1993;334:114–116.

85. Herbert JM, Savi P, Laplace MC, et al. IL-4 and IL-13 exhibit comparable abilities to reduce pyrogen-induced expression of procoagulant activity in endothelial cells and monocytes. *FEBS Lett* 1993;328:268–270.

86. Del Prete G, De Carli M, Lammel RM, et al. Th1 and Th2 T-helper cells exert opposite regulatory effects on procoagulant activity and tissue factor production by human monocytes. *Blood* 1995;86:250–257.

87. Ernofsson M, Tenno T, Siegbahn A. Inhibition of tissue factor surface expression in human peripheral blood monocytes exposed to cytokines. *Br J Haematol* 1996;95:249–257.

88. Matsumoto K, Ohi H, Kanmatsuse K. Interleukin-10 and interleukin-13 synergize to inhibit vascular permeability factor release by peripheral blood mononuclear cells from patients with lipoid nephrosis. *Nephron* 1997;77:212–218.

89. Bogdan C, Vodovotz Y, Nathan C. Macrophage deactivation by interleukin 10. *J Exp Med* 1991;174:1549–1555.

90. Niiro H, Otsuka T, Abe M, et al. Epstein-Barr virus BCRF1 gene product (viral interleukin 10) inhibits superoxide anion production by human monocytes. *Lymphokine Cytokine Res* 1992;11:209–214.

91. Cunha FQ, Moncada S, Liew FY. Interleukin-10 (IL-10) inhibits the induction of nitric oxide synthase by interferon-gamma in murine macrophages. *Biochem Biophys Res Commun* 1992;182:1155–1159.

92. Gazzinelli RT, Oswald IP, Hieny S, James SL, Sher A. The microbicidal activity of interferon-gamma-treated macrophages against *Trypanosoma cruzi* involves an L-arginine-dependent, nitrogen oxide-mediated mechanism inhibitable by interleukin-10 and transforming growth factor-beta. *Eur J Immunol* 1992;22:2501–2506.

93. Wu J, Cunha FQ, Liew FY, Weiser WY. IL-10 inhibits the synthesis of migration inhibitory factor and migration inhibitory factor-mediated macrophage activation. *J Immunol* 1993;151:4325–4332.

94. Cenci E, Romani L, Mencacci A, et al. Interleukin-4 and interleukin-10 inhibit nitric oxide-dependent macrophage killing of *Candida albicans*. *Eur J Immunol* 1993;23:1034–1038.

95. Niiro H, Otsuka T, Tanabe T, et al. Inhibition by interleukin-10 of inducible cyclooxygenase expression in lipopolysaccharide-stimulated monocytes: its underlying mechanism in comparison with interleukin-4. *Blood* 1995;85:3736–3745.

96. Kuga S, Otsuka T, Niiro H, et al. Suppression of superoxide anion production by interleukin-10 is accompanied by a downregulation of the genes for subunit proteins of NADPH oxidase. *Exp Hematol* 1996;24:151–157.

97. Roilides E, Dimitriadou A, Kadiltsoglou I, et al. IL-10 exerts suppressive and enhancing effects on antifungal activity of mononuclear phagocytes against *Aspergillus fumigatus*. *J Immunol* 1997;158:322–329.

98. Vouldoukis I, Becherel PA, Riveros-Moreno V, et al. Interleukin-10 and interleukin-4 inhibit intracellular killing of *Leishmania infantum* and *Leishmania major* by human macrophages by decreasing nitric oxide generation. *Eur J Immunol* 1997;27:860–865.

99. Doyle AG, Herbein G, Montaner LJ, et al. Interleukin-13 alters the activation state of murine macrophages *in vitro*: comparison with interleukin-4 and interferon-gamma. *Eur J Immunol* 1994;24:1441–1445.

100. Saura M, Martinez-Dalmau R, Minty A, Perez-Sala D, Lamas S. Interleukin-13 inhibits inducible nitric oxide synthase expression in human mesangial cells. *Biochem J* 1996;313:641–646.

101. Sozzani P, Cambon C, Vita N, et al. Interleukin-13 inhibits protein kinase C-triggered respiratory burst in human monocytes: role of calcium and cyclic AMP. *J Biol Chem* 1995;270:5084–5088.

102. Flesch IE, Hess JH, Oswald IP, Kaufmann SH. Growth inhibition of *Mycobacterium bovis* by IFN-gamma stimulated macrophages: regulation by endogenous tumor necrosis factor-alpha and by IL-10. *Int Immunol* 1994;6:693–700.

103. Oswald IP, Wynn TA, Sher A, James SL. Interleukin 10 inhibits macrophage microbicidal activity by blocking the endogenous production of tumor necrosis factor alpha required as a costimulatory factor for interferon gamma-induced activation. *Proc Natl Acad Sci U S A* 1992;89:8676–8680.

104. Oswald IP, Gazzinelli RT, Sher A, James SL. IL-10 synergizes with IL-4 and transforming growth factor-beta to inhibit macrophage cytotoxic activity. *J Immunol* 1992;148:3578–3582.

105. Weiss G, Bogdan C, Hentze MW. Pathways for the regulation of macrophage iron metabolism by the anti-inflammatory cytokines IL-4 and IL-13. *J Immunol* 1997;158:420–425.

106. Nassar GM, Morrow JD, Roberts LJD, Lakkis FG, Badr KF. Induction of 15-lipoxygenase by interleukin-13 in human blood monocytes. *J Biol Chem* 1994;269:27631–27634.

107. Endo T, Ogushi F, Sone S. LPS-dependent cyclooxygenase-2 induc-

tion in human monocytes is down-regulated by IL-13, but not by IFN-gamma. *J Immunol* 1996;156:2240–2246.

108. Onoe Y, Miyaura C, Kaminakayashiki T, et al. IL-13 and IL-4 inhibit bone resorption by suppressing cyclooxygenase-2-dependent prostaglandin synthesis in osteoblasts. *J Immunol* 1996;156:758–764.

109. Niiro H, Otsuka T, Kuga S, et al. IL-10 inhibits prostaglandin E2 production by lipopolysaccharide-stimulated monocytes. *Int Immunol* 1994;6:661–664.

110. Mertz PM, DeWitt DL, Stetler-Stevenson WG, Wahl LM. Interleukin 10 suppression of monocyte prostaglandin H synthase-2: mechanism of inhibition of prostaglandin-dependent matrix metalloproteinase production. *J Biol Chem* 1994;269:21322–21329.

111. Lacraz S, Nicod LP, Chicheportiche R, Welgus HG, Dayer JM. IL-10 inhibits metalloproteinase and stimulates TIMP-1 production in human mononuclear phagocytes. *J Clin Invest* 1995;96:2304–2310.

112. Corcoran ML, Stetler-Stevenson WG, Brown PD, Wahl LM. Interleukin-4 inhibition of prostaglandin E2 synthesis blocks interstitial collagenase and 92-kDa type IV collagenase/gelatinase production by human monocytes. *J Biol Chem* 1992;267:515–519.

113. Stein M, Keshav S, Harris N, Gordon S. Interleukin-4 potently enhances murine macrophage mannose receptor activity: a marker of alternative immunologic macrophage activation. *J Exp Med* 1992;176:287–292.

114. DeFife KM, Jenney CR, McNally AK, Colton E, Anderson JM. Interleukin-13 induces human monocyte/macrophage fusion and macrophage mannose receptor expression. *J Immunol* 1997;158:3385–3390.

115. Morel AS, Quaratino S, Douek DC, Londei M. Split activity of interleukin-10 on antigen capture and antigen presentation by human dendritic cells: definition of a maturative step. *Eur J Immunol* 1997;27:26–34.

116. te Velde AA, de Waal Malefijt R, Huijbens RJ, de Vries JE, Figdor CG. IL-10 stimulates monocyte Fc gamma R surface expression and cytotoxic activity: distinct regulation of antibody-dependent cellular cytotoxicity by IFN-gamma, IL-4, and IL-10. *J Immunol* 1992;149:4048–4052.

117. Calzada-Wack JC, Frankenberger M, Ziegler-Heitbrock HW. Interleukin-10 drives human monocytes to CD16 positive macrophages. *J Inflamm* 1996;46:78–85.

118. Morinobu A, Kumagai S, Yanagida H, et al. IL-10 suppresses cell surface CD23/Fc epsilon RII expression, not by enhancing soluble CD23 release, but by reducing CD23 mRNA expression in human monocytes. *J Clin Immunol* 1996;16:326–333.

119. Capsoni F, Minonzio F, Ongari AM, Carbonelli V, Galli A, Zanussi C. IL-10 up-regulates human monocyte phagocytosis in the presence of IL-4 and IFN-gamma. *J Leukoc Biol* 1995;58:351–358.

120. Spittler A, Schiller C, Willheim M, Tempfer C, Winkler S, Boltz-Nitulescu G. IL-10 augments CD23 expression on U937 cells and down-regulates IL-4-driven CD23 expression on cultured human blood monocytes: effects of IL-10 and other cytokines on cell phenotype and phagocytosis. *Immunology* 1995;85:311–317.

121. de Waal Malefyt R, Haanen J, Spits H, et al. IL-10 and viral IL-10 strongly reduce antigen-specific human T cell proliferation by diminishing the antigen-presenting capacity of monocytes via downregulation of class II MHC expression. *J Exp Med* 1991;174:915–924.

122. Ding L, Linsley PS, Huang LY, Germain RN, Shevach EM. IL-10 inhibits macrophage costimulatory activity by selectively inhibiting the up-regulation of B7 expression. *J Immunol* 1993;151:1224–1234.

123. Willems F, Marchant A, Delville JP, et al. Interleukin-10 inhibits B7 and intercellular adhesion molecule-1 expression on human monocytes. *Eur J Immunol* 1994;24:1007–1009.

124. Kubin M, Kamoun M, Trinchieri G. Interleukin-12 synergizes with B7/CD28 interaction in inducing efficient proliferation and cytokine production by human T cells. *J Exp Med* 1994;180:263–274.

125. Ding L, Shevach EM. IL-10 inhibits mitogen-induced T cell proliferation by selectively inhibiting macrophage costimulatory function. *J Immunol* 1992;148:3133–3139.

126. Fiorentino DF, Zlotnik A, Vieira P, et al. IL-10 acts on the antigen-presenting cell to inhibit cytokine production by Th1 cells. *J Immunol* 1991;146:3444–3451.

127. Koppelman B, Neefjes JJ, de Vries JE, de Waal Malefyt R. Interleukin-10 downregulates MHC class II αβ peptide complexes at the plasma membrane of monocytes by affecting arrival and recycling. *Immunity* 1997;7:861–871.

128. Romani N, Reider D, Heuer M, et al. Generation of mature dendritic cells from human blood: an improved method with special regard to clinical applicability. *J Immunol Methods* 1996;196:137–151.

129. Sakamoto O, Hashiyama M, Minty A, Ando M, Suda T. Interleukin-13 selectively suppresses the growth of human macrophage progenitors at the late stage. *Blood* 1995;85:3487–3493.

130. Piemonti L, Bernasconi S, Luini W, et al. IL-13 supports differentiation of dendritic cells from circulating precursors in concert with GM-CSF. *Eur Cytokine Netw* 1995;6:245–252.

131. Buelens C, Willems F, Delvaux A, et al. Interleukin-10 differentially regulates B7-1 (CD80) and B7-2 (CD86) expression on human peripheral blood dendritic cells. *Eur J Immunol* 1995;25:2668–2672.

132. Peguet-Navarro J, Moulon C, Caux C, Dalbiez-Gauthier C, Banchereau J, Schmitt D. Interleukin-10 inhibits the primary allogeneic T cell response to human epidermal Langerhans cells. *Eur J Immunol* 1994;24:884–891.

133. Ludewig B, Graf D, Gelderblom HR, Becker Y, Kroczek RA, Pauli G. Spontaneous apoptosis of dendritic cells is efficiently inhibited by TRAP (CD40-ligand) and TNF-alpha, but strongly enhanced by interleukin-10. *Eur J Immunol* 1995;25:1943–1950.

134. Macatonia SE, Doherty TM, Knight SC, O'Garra A. Differential effect of IL-10 on dendritic cell-induced T cell proliferation and IFN-gamma production. *J Immunol* 1993;150:3755–3765.

135. Mitra RS, Judge TA, Nestle FO, Turka LA, Nickoloff BJ. Psoriatic skin-derived dendritic cell function is inhibited by exogenous IL-10: differential modulation of B7-1 (CD80) and B7-2 (CD86) expression. *J Immunol* 1995;154:2668–2677.

136. Bejarano MT, de Waal Malefyt R, Abrams JS, et al. Interleukin 10 inhibits allogeneic proliferative and cytotoxic T cell responses generated in primary mixed lymphocyte cultures. *Int Immunol* 1992;4:1389–1397.

137. Caux C, Massacrier C, Vanbervliet B, Barthelemy C, Liu YJ, Banchereau J. Interleukin 10 inhibits T cell alloreaction induced by human dendritic cells. *Int Immunol* 1994;6:1177–1185.

138. Armstrong L, Jordan N, Millar A. Interleukin 10 (IL-10) regulation of tumour necrosis factor alpha (TNF-alpha) from human alveolar macrophages and peripheral blood monocytes. *Thorax* 1996;51:143–149.

139. Park DR, Skerrett SJ. IL-10 enhances the growth of *Legionella pneumophila* in human mononuclear phagocytes and reverses the protective effect of IFN-gamma: differential responses of blood monocytes and alveolar macrophages. *J Immunol* 1996;157:2528–2538.

140. Thomassen MJ, Divis LT, Fisher CJ. Regulation of human alveolar macrophage inflammatory cytokine production by interleukin-10. *Clin Immunol Immunopathol* 1996;80:321–324.

141. Wilkes DS, Neimeier M, Mathur PN, et al. Effect of human lung allograft alveolar macrophages on IgG production: immunoregulatory role of interleukin-10, transforming growth factor-beta, and interleukin-6. *Am J Respir Cell Mol Biol* 1995;13:621–628.

142. Zissel G, Schlaak J, Schlaak M, Muller-Quernheim J. Regulation of cytokine release by alveolar macrophages treated with interleukin-4, interleukin-10, or transforming growth factor beta. *Eur Cytokine Netw* 1996;7:59–66.

143. Nicod LP, el Habre F, Dayer JM, Boehringer N. Interleukin-10 decreases tumor necrosis factor alpha and beta in alloreactions induced by human lung dendritic cells and macrophages. *Am J Respir Cell Mol Biol* 1995;13:83–90.

144. de Waal Malefyt R, Abrams JS, Zurawski SM, et al. Differential regulation of IL-13 and IL-4 production by human CD8+ and CD4+ Th0, Th1 and Th2 T cell clones and EBV transformed B cell lines. *Int Immunol* 1995;7:1405–1416.

145. de Waal Malefyt R, Yssel H, de Vries JE. Direct effects of IL-10 on subsets of human CD4+ T cell clones and resting T cells. *J Immunol* 1993;150:4754–4765.

146. Taga K, Tosato G. IL-10 inhibits human T cell proliferation and IL-2 production. *J Immunol* 1992;148:1143–1148.

147. Schandene L, Alonso-Vega C, Willems F, et al. B7/CD28-dependent IL-5 production by human resting T cells is inhibited by IL-10. *J Immunol* 1994;152:4368–4374.

148. Groux H, Bigler M, de Vries JE, Roncarolo MG. Interleukin-10 induces a long-term antigen-specific anergic state in human CD4+ T cells. *J Exp Med* 1996;184:19–29.

149. Buer J, Lanoue A, Franzke A, Garcia C, von Boehmer H, Sarukhan A. Interleukin-10 secretion and impaired effector function of major his-

tocompatibility complex class-II restricted T cells anergized *in vivo*. *J Exp Med* 1998;187:177–183.

150. Groux H, O'Garra A, Bigler M, et al. A CD4+ T cell subset inhibits antigen-specific T cell responses and prevents colitis. *Nature* 1997; 389:737–742.

151. Suzuki T, Tahara H, Narula S, Moore KW, Robbins PD, Lotze MT. Viral interleukin 10 (IL-10), the human herpes virus 4 cellular IL-10 homologue, induces local anergy to allogeneic and syngeneic tumors. *J Exp Med* 1995;182:477–486.

152. Becker JC, Czerny C, Brocker EB. Maintenance of clonal anergy by endogenously produced IL-10. *Int Immunol* 1994;6:1605–1612.

153. Enk AH, Saloga J, Becker D, B PmM, Knop J. Induction of hapten-specific tolerance by interleukin 10 *in vivo*. *J Exp Med* 1994;179: 1397–1402.

154. Flores Villanueva PO, Reiser H, Stadecker MJ. Regulation of T helper cell responses in experimental murine schistosomiasis by IL-10: effect on expression of B7 and B7-2 costimulatory molecules by macrophages. *J Immunol* 1994;153:5190–5199.

155. King CL, Medhat A, Malhotra I, et al. Cytokine control of parasite-specific anergy in human urinary schistosomiasis: IL-10 modulates lymphocyte reactivity. *J Immunol* 1996;156:4715–4721.

156. Schols D, De Clercq E. Human immunodeficiency virus type 1 gp120 induces anergy in human peripheral blood lymphocytes by inducing interleukin-10 production. *J Virol* 1996;70:4953–4960.

157. Sundstedt A, Hoiden I, Rosendahl A, Kalland T, van Rooijen N, Dohlsten M. Immunoregulatory role of IL-10 during superantigen-induced hyporesponsiveness *in vivo*. *J Immunol* 1997;158:180–186.

158. Enk AH, Angeloni VL, Udey MC, Katz SI. Inhibition of Langerhans cell antigen-presenting function by IL-10: a role for IL-10 in induction of tolerance. *J Immunol* 1993;151:2390–2398.

159. Flores VP, Chikunguwo SM, Harris TS, Stadecker MJ. Role of IL-10 on antigen-presenting cell function for schistosomal egg-specific monoclonal T helper cell responses *in vitro* and *in vivo*. *J Immunol* 1993;151:3192–3198.

160. Cassatella MA, Meda L, Bonora S, Ceska M, Constantin G. Interleukin 10 (IL-10) inhibits the release of proinflammatory cytokines from human polymorphonuclear leukocytes: evidence for an autocrine role of tumor necrosis factor and IL-1 beta in mediating the production of IL-8 triggered by lipopolysaccharide. *J Exp Med* 1993;178: 2207–2211.

161. Wang P, Wu P, Anthes JC, Siegel MI, Egan RW, Billah MM. Interleukin-10 inhibits interleukin-8 production in human neutrophils. *Blood* 1994;83:2678–2683.

162. Kasama T, Strieter RM, Lukacs NW, Burdick MD, Kunkel SL. Regulation of neutrophil-derived chemokine expression by IL-10. *J Immunol* 1994;152:3559–3569.

163. Chaves MM, Silvestrini AA, Silva-Teixeira DN, Nogueira-Machado JA. Effect *in vitro* of gamma interferon and interleukin-10 on generation of oxidizing species by human granulocytes. *Inflamm Res* 1996; 45:313–315.

164. Cox G. IL-10 enhances resolution of pulmonary inflammation *in vivo* by promoting apoptosis of neutrophils. *Am J Physiol* 1996;271: L566–L571.

165. Marie C, Pitton C, Fitting C, Cavaillon JM. IL-10 and IL-4 synergize with TNF-alpha to induce IL-1Rα production by human neutrophils. *Cytokine* 1996;8:147–151.

166. Takanaski S, Nonaka R, Xing Z, O'Byrne P, Dolovich J, Jordana M. Interleukin 10 inhibits lipopolysaccharide-induced survival and cytokine production by human peripheral blood eosinophils. *J Exp Med* 1994;180:711–715.

167. Arock M, Zuany-Amorim C, Singer M, Benhamou M, Pretolani M. Interleukin-10 inhibits cytokine generation from mast cells. *Eur J Immunol* 1996;26:166–170.

168. Niiro H, Otsuka T, Izuhara K, et al. Regulation by interleukin-10 and interleukin-4 of cyclooxygenase-2 expression in human neutrophils. *Blood* 1997;89:1621–1628.

169. Greenberger MJ, Strieter RM, Kunkel SL, Danforth JM, Goodman RE, Standiford TJ. Neutralization of IL-10 increases survival in a murine model of *Klebsiella* pneumonia. *J Immunol* 1995;155: 722–729.

170. Denis M, Ghadirian E. IL-10 neutralization augments mouse resistance to systemic *Mycobacterium avium* infections. *J Immunol* 1993; 151:5425–5430.

171. van der Poll T, Marchant A, Keogh CV, Goldman M, Lowry SF. Inter-

leukin-10 impairs host defense in murine pneumococcal pneumonia. *J Infect Dis* 1996;174:994–1000.

172. Gerard C, Bruyns C, Marchant A, et al. Interleukin 10 reduces the release of tumor necrosis factor and prevents lethality in experimental endotoxemia. *J Exp Med* 1993;177:547–550.

173. Howard M, Muchamuel T, Andrade S, Menon S. Interleukin 10 protects mice from lethal endotoxemia. *J Exp Med* 1993;177:1205–1208.

174. Muchamuel T, Menon S, Pisacane P, Howard MC, Cockayne DA. IL-13 protects mice from lipopolysaccharide-induced lethal endotoxemia: correlation with down-modulation of TNF-alpha, IFN-gamma, and IL-12 production. *J Immunol* 1997;158:2898–2903.

175. Rogy MA, Auffenberg T, Espat NJ, et al. Human tumor necrosis factor receptor (p55) and interleukin 10 gene transfer in the mouse reduces mortality to lethal endotoxemia and also attenuates local inflammatory responses. *J Exp Med* 1995;181:2289–2293.

176. Zisman DA, Kunkel SL, Strieter RM, et al. MCP-1 protects mice in lethal endotoxemia. *J Clin Invest* 1997;99:2832–2836.

177. Pajkrt D, Camoglio L, Tiel- van Buul MCM, et al. Attenuation of proinflammatory response by recombinant human IL-10 in human endotoxemia: effect of timing of recombinant human IL-10 administration. *J Immunol* 1997;158:3971–3977.

178. Durez P, Abramowicz D, Gerard C, et al. *In vivo* induction of interleukin-10 by anti-CD3 monoclonal antibody or bacterial lipopolysaccharide: differential modulation by cyclosporin A. *J Exp Med* 1993; 177:551–555.

179. Jansen PM, van der Pouw Kraan TC, de Jong IW, et al. Release of interleukin-12 in experimental *Escherichia coli* septic shock in baboons: relation to plasma levels of interleukin-10 and interferon-gamma. *Blood* 1996;87:5144–5151.

180. van der Poll T, Jansen J, Levi M, ten Cate H, ten Cate JW, van Deventer SJ. Regulation of interleukin 10 release by tumor necrosis factor in humans and chimpanzees. *J Immunol* 1994;180:1985–1988.

181. Marchant A, Bruyns C, Vandenabeele P, et al. Interleukin-10 controls interferon-gamma and tumor necrosis factor production during experimental endotoxemia. *Eur J Immunol* 1994;24:1167–1171.

182. Standiford TJ, Strieter RM, Lukacs NW, Kunkel SL. Neutralization of IL-10 increases lethality in endotoxemia: cooperative effects of macrophage inflammatory protein-2 and tumor necrosis factor. *J Immunol* 1995;155:2222–2229.

183. Ishida H, Hastings R, Thompson SL, Howard M. Modified immunological status of anti–IL-10 treated mice. *Cell Immunol* 1993;148: 371–384.

184. Berg DJ, Kuhn R, Rajewsky K, et al. Interleukin-10 is a central regulator of the response to LPS in murine models of endotoxic shock and the Shwartzman reaction but not endotoxin tolerance. *J Clin Invest* 1995;96:2339–2347.

185. Randow F, Syrbe U, Meisel C, et al. Mechanism of endotoxin desensitization: involvement of interleukin 10 and transforming growth factor beta. *J Exp Med* 1995;181:1887–1892.

186. Randow F, Docke WD, Bundschuh DS, Hartung T, Wendel A, Volk HD. *In vitro* prevention and reversal of lipopolysaccharide desensization by IFN-gamma, IL-12, and granulocyte macrophage colony-stimulating-factor. *J Immunol* 1997;158:2911–2918.

187. Bundschuh DS, Barsig J, Hartung T, et al. Granulocyte-macrophage colony-stimulating factor and IFN-gamma restore the systemic TNF-alpha response to endotoxin in lipopolysaccharide-desensitized mice. *J Immunol* 1997;158:2862–2871.

188. Ertel W, Keel M, Neidhardt R, et al. Inhibition of the defense system stimulating interleukin-12 interferon-gamma pathway during critical illness. *Blood* 1997;89:1612–1620.

189. Docke WD, Randow F, Syrbe U, et al. Monocyte deactivation in septic patients: restoration by IFN-gamma treatment. *Nat Med* 1997;3: 678–681.

190. van der Poll T, Marchant A, Buurman WA, et al. Endogenous IL-10 protects mice from death during septic peritonitis. *J Immunol* 1995; 155:5397–5401.

191. Kato T, Murata A, Ishida H, et al. Interleukin 10 reduces mortality from severe peritonitis in mice. *Antimicrob Agents Chemother* 1995; 39:1336–1340.

192. Rongione AJ, Kusske AM, Ashley SW, Reber HA, McFadden DW. Interleukin-10 prevents early cytokine release in severe intraabdominal infection and sepsis. *J Surg Res* 1997;70:107–112.

193. Hogaboam CM, Steinhauser ML, Schock H, et al. Therapeutic effects of nitric oxide inhibition during experimental fecal peritonitis: role of

interleukin-10 and monocyte chemoattractant protein 1. *Infect Immun* 1998;66:650–655.

194. Bean AG, Freiberg RA, Andrade S, Menon S, Zlotnik A. Interleukin 10 protects mice against staphylococcal enterotoxin B-induced lethal shock. *Infect Immun* 1993;61:4937–4939.

195. Cusumano V, Genovese F, Mancuso G, Carbone M, Fera MT, Teti G. Interleukin-10 protects neonatal mice from lethal group B streptococcal infection. *Infect Immun* 1996;64:2850–2852.

196. Florquin S, Amraoui Z, Abramowicz D, Goldman M. Systemic release and protective role of IL-10 in staphylococcal enterotoxin B-induced shock in mice. *J Immunol* 1994;153:2618–2623.

197. Marchant A, Deviere J, Byl B, De Groote D, Vincent JL, Goldman M. Interleukin-10 production during septicaemia. *Lancet* 1994;343: 707–708.

198. Marchant A, Alegre ML, Hakim A, et al. Clinical and biological significance of interleukin-10 plasma levels in patients with septic shock. *J Clin Immunol* 1995;15:266–273.

199. van der Poll T, de Waal Malefyt R, Coyle SM, Lowry SF. Antiinflammatory cytokine responses during clinical sepsis and experimental endotoxemia: sequential measurements of plasma soluble interleukin (IL)-1 receptor type II, IL-10, and IL-13. *J Infect Dis* 1997;175: 118–122.

200. Sherry RM, Cue JI, Goddard JK, Parramore JB, DiPiro JT. Interleukin-10 is associated with the development of sepsis in trauma patients. *J Trauma* 1996;40:613–616; discussion, 616–617.

201. Gomez-Jimenez J, Martin MC, Sauri R, et al. Interleukin-10 and the monocyte/macrophage-induced inflammatory response in septic shock. *J Infect Dis* 1995;171:472–475.

202. Frei K, Nadal D, Pfister HW, Fontana A. *Listeria* meningitis: identification of a cerebrospinal fluid inhibitor of macrophage listericidal function as interleukin 10. *J Exp Med* 1993;178:1255–1261.

203. Lehmann AK, Halstensen A, Sornes S, Rokke O, Waage A. High levels of interleukin 10 in serum are associated with fatality in meningococcal disease. *Infect Immun* 1995;63:2109–2112.

204. van Furth AM, Seijmonsbergen EM, Langermans JA, Groeneveld PH, de Bel CE, van Furth R. High levels of interleukin 10 and tumor necrosis factor alpha in cerebrospinal fluid during the onset of bacterial meningitis [see comments]. *Clin Infect Dis* 1995;21:220–222.

205. Derkx B, Marchant A, Goldman M, Bijlmer R, van Deventer S. High levels of interleukin-10 during the initial phase of fulminant meningococcal septic shock. *J Infect Dis* 1995;171:229–232.

206. Pugin J, Ulevitch RJ, Tobias PS. A critical role for monocytes and CD14 in endotoxin-induced endothelial cell activation. *J Exp Med* 1993;178:2193–2200.

207. Eissner G, Lindner H, Behrends U, et al. Influence of bacterial endotoxin on radiation-induced activation of human endothelial cells *in vitro* and *in vivo*: protective role of IL-10. *Transplantation* 1996;62: 819–827.

208. van der Poll T, Coyle SM, Barbosa K, Braxton CC, Lowry SF. Epinephrine inhibits tumor necrosis factor-alpha and potentiates interleukin 10 production during human endotoxemia. *J Clin Invest* 1996; 97:713–719.

209. Suberville S, Bellocq A, Fouqueray B, et al. Regulation of interleukin-10 production by beta-adrenergic agonists. *Eur J Immunol* 1996;26: 2601–2605.

210. Mengozzi M, Fantuzzi G, Faggioni R, et al. Chlorpromazine specifically inhibits peripheral and brain TNF production, and up-regulates IL-10 production, in mice. *Immunology* 1994;82:207–210.

211. Bourrie B, Bouaboula M, Benoit JM, et al. Enhancement of endotoxin-induced interleukin-10 production by SR 31747A, a sigma ligand. *Eur J Immunol* 1995;25:2882–2887.

212. Van Laethem JL, Marchant A, Delvaux A, et al. Interleukin 10 prevents necrosis in murine experimental acute pancreatitis. *Gastroenterology* 1995;108:1917–1922.

213. Rosenbaum JT, Angell E. Paradoxical effects of IL-10 in endotoxin-induced uveitis. *J Immunol* 1995;155:4090–4094.

214. Li Q, Sun B, Dastgheib K, Chan CC. Suppressive effect of transforming growth factor beta1 on the recurrence of experimental melanin protein-induced uveitis: upregulation of ocular interleukin-10. *Clin Immunol Immunopathol* 1996;81:55–61.

215. Arai T, Hiromatsu K, Kobayashi N, et al. IL-10 is involved in the protective effect of dibutyryl cyclic adenosine monophosphate on endotoxin-induced inflammatory liver injury. *J Immunol* 1995;155: 5743–5749.

216. Mulligan MS, Jones ML, Vaporciyan AA, Howard MC, Ward PA. Protective effects of IL-4 and IL-10 against immune complex-induced lung injury. *J Immunol* 1993;151:5666–5674.

217. Shanley TP, Schmal H, Friedl HP, Jones ML, Ward PA. Regulatory effects of intrinsic IL-10 in IgG immune complex-induced lung injury. *J Immunol* 1995;154:3454–3460.

218. Kitching AR, Tipping PG, Huang XR, Mutch DA, Holdsworth SR. Interleukin-4 and interleukin-10 attenuate established crescentic glomerulonephritis in mice. *Kidney Int* 1997;52:52–59.

219. Mulligan MS, Warner RL, Foreback JL, Shanley TP, Ward PA. Protective effects of IL-4, IL-10 , IL-12 and IL-13 in IgG immune complex induced lung injury: role of endogenous IL-12. *J Immunol* 1997; 159:3483–3489.

220. Lentsch AB, Shanley TP, Sarma V, Ward P. *In vivo* suppression of NF-κB and preservation of IκBα by interleukin-10 and interleukin-13. *J Clin Invest* 1997;100:2443–2448.

221. Zuany-Amorim C, Haile S, Leduc D, et al. Interleukin-10 inhibits antigen-induced cellular recruitment into the airways of sensitized mice. *J Clin Invest* 1995;95:2644–2651.

222. Grünig G, Corry DB, Leach MW, Seymour BWP, Kurup VP, Rennick DM. Interleukin-10 is a natural suppressor of cytokine production and inflammation in a murine model of allergic bronchopulmonary aspergillosis. *J Exp Med* 1997;185:1089–1099.

223. Sironi M, Sciacca FL, Matteucci C, et al. Regulation of endothelial and mesothelial cell function by interleukin-13: selective induction of vascular cell adhesion molecule-1 and amplification of interleukin-6 production. *Blood* 1994;84:1913–1921.

224. Bochner BS, Klunk DA, Sterbinsky SA, Coffman RL, Schleimer RP. IL-13 selectively induces vascular cell adhesion molecule-1 expression in human endothelial cells. *J Immunol* 1995;154:799–803.

225. Ying S, Meng Q, Barata LT, Robinson DS, Durham SR, Kay AB. Associations between IL-13 and IL-4 (mRNA and protein), vascular cell adhesion molecule-1 expression, and the infiltration of eosinophils, macrophages, and T cells in allergen-induced late-phase cutaneous reactions in atopic subjects. *J Immunol* 1997;158: 5050–5057.

226. Luttmann W, Knoechel B, Foerster M, Matthys H, Virchow JC Jr, Kroegel C. Activation of human eosinophils by IL-13. Induction of CD69 surface antigen, its relationship to messenger RNA expression, and promotion of cellular viability. *J Immunol* 1996;157:1678–1683.

227. Nakamura Y, Azuma M, Okano Y, et al. Upregulatory effects of interleukin-4 and interleukin-13 but not interleukin-10 on granulocyte/ macrophage colony-stimulating factor production by human bronchial epithelial cells. *Am J Respir Cell Mol Biol* 1996;15:680–687.

228. Gauchat JF, Henchoz S, Mazzei G, et al. Induction of human IgE synthesis in B cells by mast cells and basophils. *Nature* 1993;365:340–343.

229. Marietta EV, Chen Y, Weis JH. Modulation of expression of the anti-inflammatory cytokines interleukin-13 and interleukin-10 by interleukin-3. *Eur J Immunol* 1996;26:49–56.

230. Pawankar RU, Okuda M, Hasegawa S, et al. Interleukin-13 expression in the nasal mucosa of perennial allergic rhinitis. *Am J Respir Crit Care Med* 1995;152:2059–2067.

231. Punnonen J, Aversa G, Cocks BG, et al. Interleukin 13 induces interleukin 4-independent IgG4 and IgE synthesis and CD23 expression by human B cells. *Proc Natl Acad Sci U S A* 1993;90:3730–3744.

232. Li L, Elliott JF, Mosmann TR. IL-10 inhibits cytokine production, vascular leakage, and swelling during T helper 1 cell-induced delayed-type hypersensitivity. *J Immunol* 1994;153:3967–3978.

233. Schwarz A, Grabbe S, Riemann H, et al. *In vivo* effects of interleukin-10 on contact hypersensitivity and delayed-type hypersensitivity reactions. *J Invest Dermatol* 1994;103:211–216.

234. Kondo S, McKenzie RC, Sauder DN. Interleukin-10 inhibits the elicitation phase of allergic contact hypersensitivity. *J Invest Dermatol* 1994;103:811–814.

235. Ferguson TA, Dube P, Griffith TS. Regulation of contact hypersensitivity by interleukin 10. *J Exp Med* 1994;179:1597–1604.

236. Powrie F, Menon S, Coffman RL. Interleukin-4 and interleukin-10 synergize to inhibit cell-mediated immunity *in vivo*. *Eur J Immunol* 1993;23:3043–3049.

237. Berg DJ, Leach MW, Kuhn R, et al. Interleukin 10 but not interleukin 4 is a natural suppressant of cutaneous inflammatory responses. *J Exp Med* 1995;182:99–108.

238. Enk AH, Katz SI. Identification and induction of keratinocyte-derived IL-10. *J Immunol* 1992;149:92–95.

239. Rivas JM, Ullrich SE. Systemic suppression of delayed-type hypersensitivity by supernatants from UV-irradiated keratinocytes: an essential role for keratinocyte-derived IL-10. *J Immunol* 1992;149: 3865–3871.

240. Kang K, Hammerberg C, Meunier L, Cooper KD. CD11b-macrophages that infiltrate human epidermis after *in vivo* ultraviolet exposure potently produce IL-10 and represent the major secretory source of epidermal IL-10 protein. *J Immunol* 1994;153:5256–5264.

241. Enk CD, Sredni D, Blauvelt A, Katz SI. Induction of IL-10 gene expression in human keratinocytes by UVB exposure *in vivo* and *in vitro*. *J Immunol* 1995;154:4851–4856.

242. Teunissen MB, Koomen CW, Jansen J, et al. In contrast to their murine counterparts, normal human keratinocytes and human epidermoid cell lines A431 and HaCaT fail to express IL-10 mRNA and protein. *Clin Exp Immunol* 1997;107:213–223.

243. Rivas JM, Ullrich SE. The role of IL-4, IL-10, and TNF-alpha in the immune suppression induced by ultraviolet radiation. *J Leukoc Biol* 1994;56:769–775.

244. Beissert S, Ullrich SE, Hosoi J, Granstein RD. Supernatants from UVB radiation-exposed keratinocytes inhibit Langerhans cell presentation of tumor-associated antigens via IL-10 content. *J Leukoc Biol* 1995;58:234–240.

245. Yagi H, Tokura Y, Wakita H, Furukawa F, Takigawa M. TCRV beta 7+ Th2 cells mediate UVB-induced suppression of murine contact photosensitivity by releasing IL-10. *J Immunol* 1996;156:1824–1831.

246. Beissert S, Hosoi J, Kuhn R, Rajewsky K, Muller W, Granstein RD. Impaired immunosuppressive response to ultraviolet radiation in interleukin-10-deficient mice. *J Invest Dermatol* 1996;107:553–557.

247. Asadullah K, Sterry W, Stephanek K, et al. IL-10 is a key cytokine in psoriasis: proof of principle by IL-10 therapy. A new therapeutic approach. *J Clin Invest* 1998;101:783–794.

248. Powrie F, Leach MW, Mauze S, Coffman RL. Phenotypically distinct subsets of CD4+ T cells induce or protect from chronic intestinal inflammation in C. B-17 scid mice. *Int Immunol* 1993;5:1461–1471.

249. Powrie F, Leach MW, Mauze S, Menon S, Barcomb Caddle L, Coffman RL. Inhibiton of Th1 responses prevents inflammatory bowel disease in scid mice reconstituted with CD45RBhi CD4+ T cells. *Immunity* 1994;1:553–562.

250. Powrie F. T cells in inflammatory bowel disease: protective and pathogenic roles. *Immunity* 1995;3:171–174.

251. Rennick DM, Fort MM, Davidson NJ. Studies with IL-10–/– mice: an overview. *J Leukoc Biol* 1997;61:389–396.

252. Kuhn R, Lohler J, Rennick D, Rajewsky K, Muller W. Interleukin-10 deficient mice develop chronic enterocholitis. *Cell* 1993;75:263–274.

253. Berg DJ, Davidson N, Kuhn R, et al. Enterocolitis and colon cancer in interleukin-10-deficient mice are associated with aberrant cytokine production and CD4(+) TH1-like responses. *J Clin Invest* 1996;98: 1010–1020.

254. Davidson NJ, Leach MW, Fort MM, et al. T helper cell 1-type CD4+ T cells, but not B cells, mediate colitis in interleukin 10-deficient mice. *J Exp Med* 1996;184:241–251.

255. Kucharzik T, Stoll R, Lugering N, Domschke W. Circulating antiinflammatory cytokine IL-10 in patients with inflammatory bowel disease (IBD). *Clin Exp Immunol* 1995;100:452–456.

256. Kucharzik T, Lugering N, Weigelt H, Adolf M, Domschke W, Stoll R. Immunoregulatory properties of IL-13 in patients with inflammatory bowel disease: comparison with IL-4 and IL-10. *Clin Exp Immunol* 1996;104:483–490.

257. Kucharzik T, Lugering N, Adolf M, Domschke W, Stoll R. Synergistic effect of immunoregulatory cytokines on peripheral blood monocytes from patients with inflammatory bowel disease. *Dig Dis Sci* 1997;42: 805–812.

258. Hart PH, Ahern MJ, Smith MD, Finlay-Jones JJ. Comparison of the suppressive effects of interleukin-10 and interleukin-4 on synovial fluid macrophages and blood monocytes from patients with inflammatory arthritis. *Immunology* 1995;84:536–542.

259. Chomarat P, Vannier E, Dechanet J, et al. Balance of IL-1 receptor antagonist/IL-1 beta in rheumatoid synovium and its regulation by IL-4 and IL-10. *J Immunol* 1995;154:1432–1439.

260. Deleuran B, Iversen L, Kristensen M, et al. Interleukin-8 secretion and 15-lipoxygenase activity in rheumatoid arthritis: *in vitro* anti-inflammatory effects by interleukin-4 and interleukin-10, but not by interleukin-1 receptor antagonist protein. *Br J Rheumatol* 1994;33:520–525.

261. Isomaki P, Luukkainen R, Toivanen P, Punnonen J. The presence of interleukin-13 in rheumatoid synovium and its antiinflammatory effects on synovial fluid macrophages from patients with rheumatoid arthritis. *Arthritis Rheum* 1996;39:1693–1702.

262. Sugiyama E, Kuroda A, Taki H, et al. Interleukin 10 cooperates with interleukin 4 to suppress inflammatory cytokine production by freshly prepared adherent rheumatoid synovial cells. *J Rheumatol* 1995;22: 2020–2026.

263. Llorente L, Richaud-Patin Y, Fior R, et al. *In vivo* production of interleukin-10 by non-T cells in rheumatoid arthritis, Sjögren's syndrome, and systemic lupus erythematosus: a potential mechanism of B lymphocyte hyperactivity and autoimmunity. *Arthritis Rheum* 1994;37: 1647–1655.

264. Bucht A, Larsson P, Weisbrot L, et al. Expression of interferon-gamma (IFN-gamma), IL-10, IL-12 and transforming growth factor-beta (TGF-beta) mRNA in synovial fluid cells from patients in the early and late phases of rheumatoid arthritis (RA). *Clin Exp Immunol* 1996; 103:357–367.

265. Cush JJ, Splawski JB, Thomas R, et al. Elevated interleukin-10 levels in patients with rheumatoid arthritis. *Arthritis Rheum* 1995;38:96–104.

266. al-Janadi M, al-Dalaan A, al-Balla S, al-Humaidi M, Raziuddin S. Interleukin-10 (IL-10) secretion in systemic lupus erythematosus and rheumatoid arthritis: IL-10-dependent CD4+CD45RO+ T cell-B cell antibody synthesis. *J Clin Immunol* 1996;16:198–207.

267. Katsikis PD, Chu CQ, Brennan FM, Maini RN, Feldmann M. Immunoregulatory role of interleukin 10 in rheumatoid arthritis. *J Exp Med* 1994;179:1517–1527.

268. Cohen SB, Katsikis PD, Chu CQ, et al. High level of interleukin-10 production by the activated T cell population within the rheumatoid synovial membrane. *Arthritis Rheum* 1995;38:946–952.

269. Perez L, Orte J, Brieva JA. Terminal differentiation of spontaneous rheumatoid factor-secreting B cells from rheumatoid arthritis patients depends on endogenous interleukin-10. *Arthritis Rheum* 1995;38: 1771–1776.

270. Kasama T, Strieter RM, Lukacs NW, Lincoln PM, Burdick MD, Kunkel SL. Interleukin-10 expression and chemokine regulation during the evolution of murine type II collagen-induced arthritis. *J Clin Invest* 1995;95:2868–2876.

271. Persson S, Mikulowska A, Narula S, O'Garra A, Holmdahl R. Interleukin-10 suppresses the development of collagen type II-induced arthritis and ameliorates sustained arthritis in rats. *Scand J Immunol* 1996;44:607–614.

272. Tanaka Y, Otsuka T, Hotokebuchi T, et al. Effect of IL-10 on collagen-induced arthritis in mice. *Inflamm Res* 1996;45:283–288.

273. van Roon JA, van Roy JL, Gmelig-Meyling FH, Lafeber FP, Bijlsma JW. Prevention and reversal of cartilage degradation in rheumatoid arthritis by interleukin-10 and interleukin-4. *Arthritis Rheum* 1996;39: 829–835.

274. Walmsley M, Katsikis PD, Abney E, et al. Interleukin-10 inhibition of the progression of established collagen-induced arthritis. *Arthritis Rheum* 1996;39:495–503.

275. Joosten LA, Lubberts E, Durez P, et al. Role of interleukin-4 and interleukin-10 in murine collagen-induced arthritis: protective effect of interleukin-4 and interleukin-10 treatment on cartilage destruction. *Arthritis Rheum* 1997;40:249–260.

276. Bessis N, Boissier MC, Ferrara P, Blankenstein T, Fradelizi D, Fournier C. Attenuation of collagen-induced arthritis in mice by treatment with vector cells engineered to secrete interleukin-13. *Eur J Immunol* 1996;26:2399–2403.

277. de Waal Malefyt R, Yssel H, Roncarolo MG, Spits H, de Vries JE. Interleukin-10. *Curr Opin Immunol* 1992;4:314–320.

Inflammation: Basic Principles and Clinical Correlates,
3rd ed., edited by John I. Gallin and Ralph Snyderman.
Lippincott Williams & Wilkins, Philadelphia © 1999.

CHAPTER 53

Angiogenesis

Douglas A. Arenberg and Robert M. Strieter

Angiogenesis, defined as the growth of new capillaries from preexisting vessels, is a pervasive biologic phenomenon that is at the core of many physiologic and pathologic processes. Examples of physiologic processes that depend on angiogenesis include embryogenesis, wound repair, and the ovarian/menstrual cycle. In contrast, chronic inflammation as well as growth and metastasis of solid tumors are associated with improper angiogenesis. Angiogenesis is similar to but distinct from vasculogenesis, which describes the *de novo* formation of the vascular system from precursor blood islands during embryogenesis. Development of the heart and great vessels occurs by vasculogenesis, whereas organs that require invasion of blood vessels for development (brain, lung, kidney) are supplied by angiogenesis (1). Neovascularization is a term that can be used interchangeably with angiogenesis, but may be more appropriately reserved for describing aberrant angiogenesis that accompanies pathologic processes such as tumorigenesis or chronic inflammation.

Inflammation and angiogenesis, while distinct and separable, are closely related processes (2). The histologic appearance of chronic inflammation includes the presence of granulation-like tissue, a prominent feature of which is neovascularization. The marked increase in the metabolic demands of tissue that proliferates, repairs, or hypertrophies must be accompanied by a proportional increase in capillary blood supply. This absolute dependence suggests several characteristics of angiogenesis. First, the vascular system must be able to rapidly respond to increased tissue needs with increased microvasculature. Second, because of the high metabolic cost of angiogenesis, under basal conditions the process must be

tightly controlled, occurring only when necessary. Indeed, angiogenesis occurs rarely in the adult organism. Finally, in the absence of such strict control, abnormal physiology or disease is likely to result. To understand pathologic angiogenesis, it is best to start with a description of a physiologic condition, the angiogenic response to a wound (Fig. 53-1).

THE SEQUENCE OF EVENTS IN PHYSIOLOGIC ANGIOGENESIS

While endothelial cells are normally quiescent, during the angiogenic response they become activated. The rate of normal capillary endothelial cell turnover is typically measured in months or years (3,4). However, when endothelial cells of the microvasculature are stimulated, they will degrade their basement membrane and proximal extracellular matrix, migrate directionally, divide, and organize into functioning capillaries invested by a new basal lamina all within a matter of days. These steps are not sequential. Rather, they represent an orchestration of overlapping events necessary to return injured tissue to homeostasis. In each of the steps of angiogenesis, there are gaps in our knowledge of the exact mechanisms. Nevertheless, significant advances in cell and molecular biology have led to a greater understanding of angiogenesis.

The Angiogenic Signal

The signal(s) that initiate angiogenesis vary with the condition that requires angiogenesis, and may be organ specific (5). During the wound response, angiogenic factors may be released through platelet degranulation (6) or proteolytic digestion of extracellular matrix (7). The importance of these latter mechanisms may lie in the fact that they occur rapidly in response to tissue injury since they do not require new protein synthesis (8). However, many cells may be the source of angiogenic signals,

D. A. Arenberg and R. M. Strieter: Department of Internal Medicine, Division of Pulmonary and Critical Care Medicine, University of Michigan Medical School, Ann Arbor, Michigan 48109-0360.

ANGIOGENIC RESPONSE TO A WOUND

From lower left, the sequence of events must be carried out with fidelity to assure adequate wound repair.
Abnormal angiogenesis results in poor wound healing.
However, exaggerated angiogenesis is seen in chronic inflammatory conditions, as well as cancer.

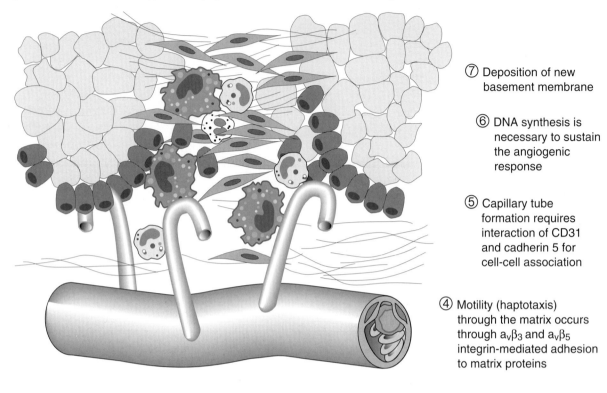

⑦ Deposition of new
basement membrane

⑥ DNA synthesis is
necessary to sustain
the angiogenic
response

⑤ Capillary tube
formation requires
interaction of CD31
and cadherin 5 for
cell-cell association

④ Motility (haptotaxis)
through the matrix occurs
through $a_v\beta_3$ and $a_v\beta_5$
integrin-mediated adhesion
to matrix proteins

① Initial angiogenic signal
  • Platelet degranulation
  • Macrophage products
  • Release of matrix bound proteins
  • Products of many cell types

② Detachment from
neighboring cells by
dissociation of adherens
junctions

③ Digestion of basement
membrane and proximal
extracellular matrix

FIG. 53-1. A schematic example of the sequence of events in tissue undergoing wound repair.

including tumor cells (9), fibroblasts (10), endothelial cells (11,12), epithelial cells (13), or activated macrophages (14). Embryonic angiogenesis is activated by genes that are transcribed in response to hypoxia and hypoglycemia in the developing embryonic tissue (15). Importantly, the signal for angiogenesis may also be initiated by a decrease in the presence of an inhibitory signal, rather than simply requiring a positive stimulus (16).

Endothelial Dedifferentiation

Once the endothelial cell receives an angiogenic stimulus, a process of dedifferentiation is initiated. For endothelium to invade into the surrounding matrix, cells must first detach from their tight association with neighboring endothelial cells. These cell-cell appositions, called adherens junctions, are composed of proteins of the cadherin family. Vascular endothelial cadherin (VE

cadherin, or cadherin 5) is highly specific for endothelial cells (17), and is associated with the cytoskeleton through other intermediate proteins, β-catenin, and plakoglobin (18,19). One of the earliest events in the angiogenic response is alteration of the adherens junction complexes, leading to increased pericellular permeability, and detachment of the endothelial cell from its neighboring cells (20).

Proteolysis and Cell Migration

To form new vessels, the existing basement membrane must be degraded. Protease activity is necessary to digest the basement membrane, and early in the angiogenic response metalloproteases are expressed (21). Inhibitors of matrix metalloproteases are capable of inhibiting angiogenesis (22). This proteolytic activity also results in the further release of growth factors and angiogenic factors that are sequestered in the basement membrane (7,12).

After proteolysis of the basement membrane, angiogenic endothelial cells must migrate through the extracellular matrix. The structural constituents of extracellular matrix consist of a variety of components, including fibrin, fibronectin, vitronectin, and hyaluronan as well as other glycosaminoglycans (23). Endothelial cells express both urokinase and tissue-type plasminogen activators during angiogenesis, which allow invasion into the surrounding matrix (24). Motility through this environment requires cell-matrix adhesion, which occurs through cell surface associated integrins.

In vitro endothelial cell chemotaxis, is typically assessed in an aqueous environment. However, endothelial cell migration *in vivo* occurs in a solid-phase environment, referred to as haptotaxis. Reversible integrin-mediated binding to matrix components allows haptotaxis of endothelial cells along a chemotactic gradient through the extracellular matrix. Since endothelial cells must respond to injury in all organs and tissues of the body, they must be capable of adherence to a variety of matrix components. The $\alpha_v\beta_3$ and $\alpha_v\beta_5$ integrins are important endothelial cell adhesion molecules that display appropriately promiscuous binding profiles, and are both involved in angiogenesis (25,26). The importance of this cell-matrix interaction in angiogenesis is demonstrated by work showing that specific inhibition of integrin binding in angiogenic endothelium leads to apoptosis of the endothelial cells (25,26). Thus, integrin binding not only facilitates adhesive and locomotive functions, but also inhibits apoptotic cell death.

Cell Proliferation

While DNA synthesis occurs early in the angiogenic response, it has been shown both *in vitro* (27) and *in vivo* (28) that vascular sprouting can occur in the absence of endothelial cell proliferation. However, when proliferation is inhibited, the angiogenic response does not progress beyond vascular sprouting, the earliest stage of neovascularization (28). Maintenance of the angiogenic response requires an increase in the number of endothelial cells to provide adequate capillary perfusion to the proliferative and repair processes of wound repair. While some angiogenic factors are only chemotactic for endothelial cells (29), most are also endothelial cell mitogens (27,29).

The signaling pathways that control cell growth are separable from those that lead to other aspects of the angiogenic response, and may be dependent on the degree of cell-matrix adhesion (30). For example, *in vitro* studies demonstrate that endothelial cell proliferation occurs in conditions of increased cell-matrix adhesiveness, whereas growth arrest and loss of viability occur in cells plated on poorly adhesive substrates (30). Interme-

diate levels of adhesiveness promote differentiation into tube-like structures (30). One might hypothesize that these *in vitro* findings have an *in vivo* correlate during wound repair. The early primordial matrix of a wound is rich in plasma proteins, which provide an abundant source of extracellular matrix to which endothelial cells may adhere, thus promoting cell migration and proliferation. As a wound matures, however, the primordial matrix is altered. Fibroblasts deposit type III collagen, and phagocytic cells remove debris, perhaps leading to reduced adhesiveness of the matrix and promoting capillary tube formation (8,14,31–33).

Additional evidence relating cell adhesion to control of proliferation is seen in studies of cadherin 5, the main component of the endothelial cell adherens junction. Homophilic cell-cell interaction through cadherin 5 inhibits endothelial cell proliferation and motility (34). Similarly, cadherin 5 expressing cells have impaired proliferation when cultured on a cadherin 5–coated substrate (34). Thus, cell-cell contact through the adherens junction and cadherin 5 may impair cell cycle progression. Early alteration of endothelial cell adherens junctions during the angiogenic response not only allows for vascular permeability and motility, but also permits endothelial cell proliferation.

Tube Formation

Once endothelial cells have invaded injured or inflamed hypoxic tissue, the integrity of the circulatory system must then be maintained. This critical process requires the formation of functioning capillaries with tight cell-cell adhesion. Investigators are beginning to define the nature of the cellular interactions underlying tube formation. In addition to the importance of cadherin 5 and the adherens junction, tube formation requires the function of CD31 (Platelet endothelial cell adhesion molecule) (PECAM-1) (35). PECAM-1 is a 130-kd membrane glycoprotein and a member of the immunoglobulin supergene family that can mediate both heterotypic and homotypic adhesion (36). The importance of this interaction was demonstrated by a study in which neutralizing antibodies to PECAM-1 inhibited tube formation *in vitro,* and angiogenesis *in vivo* (37). In a distinct *in vitro* model system, other authors have found that a combination of blocking antibodies to both CD31 and cadherin 5 were necessary to inhibit tube formation (35).

Subsequent to the formation of a continuous capillary tube, the final step in forming a new blood vessel is the deposition of a basement membrane. Similar to other steps in the sequence of events that occurs during angiogenesis, inhibition of collagen biosynthesis both prevents the *in vitro* formation of capillary-like tubes and inhibits an *in vivo* model of angiogenesis (38). The inhibition of any of the steps involved in angiogenesis appears to have a profound effect on inhibiting the process as a whole. Thus, while on a tissue level the events of angiogenesis occur in a parallel fashion, individually interrupting any of these events on a cellular level demonstrates the need for a complex orchestration of events in a serial fashion (Fig. 53-2).

Maintenance of the Angiogenic Response

Persistence of neovascularization requires a proangiogenic environment. This implies that the local expression of angiogenic factors outweighs the expression of angiostatic factors. The events that dictate this imbalance have not been fully defined. Since the number of factors capable of regulating angiogenesis is extensive (see below), it is not possible to discuss all the interactions that might affect this balance. However, there are several potential factors that may be important. First, early in the wound response, tissue injury itself leads to release of angiogenic factors from the extracellular matrix. Platelet degranulation releases both angiostatic (39) and angiogenic (40) factors. Activated macrophages release their own angiogenic factors (14,29,41–43), while macrophage-derived proteases are probably important in the generation of angiostatic factors such as angiostatin (44) and endostatin (45). Other cells that can affect this balance include fibroblasts (10), epithelial cells (13), and endothelial cells (12). These counterbalancing events that occur simultaneously during a wound response suggest the strict control that is inherent in physiologic angiogenesis.

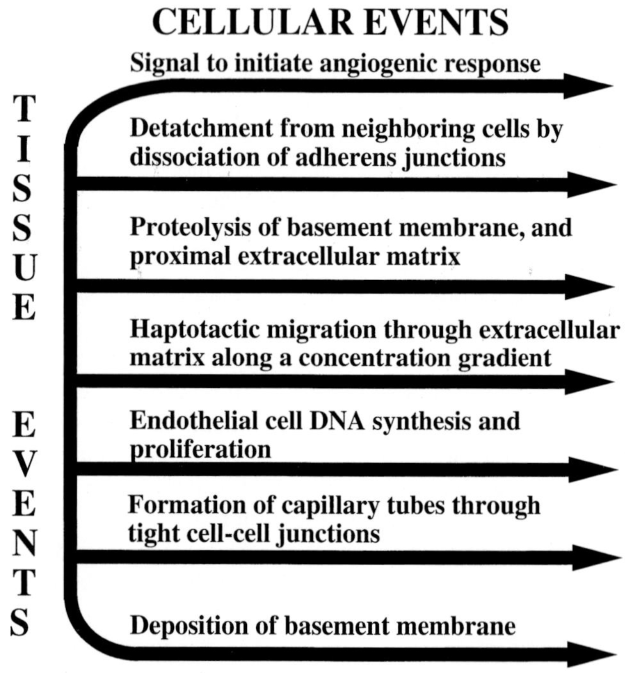

CELLULAR EVENTS

Signal to initiate angiogenic response

T
I
S   Detachment from neighboring cells by
S   dissociation of adherens junctions
U
E   Proteolysis of basement membrane, and
         proximal extracellular matrix

         Haptotactic migration through extracellular
         matrix along a concentration gradient

E   Endothelial cell DNA synthesis and
V   proliferation
E
N   Formation of capillary tubes through
T   tight cell-cell junctions
S
         Deposition of basement membrane

FIG. 53-2. From a tissue perspective, the events of the angiogenic response occur in an overlapping or parallel fashion. However, on a cellular level, the success of the angiogenic response depends on a complex orchestration of events in a serial fashion.

Termination of the Angiogenic Response

Once the balance of angiogenic and angiostatic factors favors angiostasis, the newly formed blood vessels will regress. This process has been studied in the cornea of the rabbit, and the sequence of events was similar whether the vessels formed in response to a wound or to a tumor factor (46). Regression of capillaries begins with morphologic changes of endothelial cells including mitochondrial swelling and development of cytoplasmic projections. This is followed by platelet adherence to vessel walls and platelet degranulation (46). This process is eventually accompanied by degeneration of endothelial cells and removal of debris by mononuclear cells migrating into the area. Regression first occurs in the newest vessels, and proceeds proximally to involve the earliest vessels (46). These morphologic changes described in regressing vessels probably resemble programmed endothelial cell death (apoptosis) (47).

FACTORS THAT REGULATE ANGIOGENESIS

The paradigm of a balance between angiogenic and angiostatic factors is absolutely essential to understanding net angiogenesis. There is an abundance of factors that can impact on this balance and the list continues to grow (Table 53-1). A detailed discussion of each of these is impractical in the context of this chapter, and therefore the focus will be on those factors that have been most intensely studied. These include the cytokines, acidic and basic fibroblast growth factor (aFGF, and bFGF), vascular endothelial cell growth factor (VEGF), members of the family of chemotactic cytokines known as CXC chemokines, and the angiopoietin/Tie ligand-receptor system. More recently, internal peptide fragments of larger peptides, angiostatin and endostatin, have been identified as potent angiogenesis inhibitors.

Fibroblast Growth Factors

The FGF gene family consists of nine members, the prototypes of which are aFGF and bFGF. These two members of the FGF family are distinct in that they lack a classic signal peptide to direct their processing in the golgi apparatus and eventual secretion (48). Consequently, little is known of how aFGF and bFGF become secreted into the extracellular space. Other members of the FGF family that do possess the signal peptide sequence were initially discovered as oncogenic growth factors (49). Transfection of cells with mutants of aFGF that contain a signal peptide leads to cell transformation (50,51). Thus, the lack of signal sequence in aFGF and bFGF is thought to reflect the evolution of a tighter degree of control over their secretion (50,51).

FGFs induce endothelial cell migration, proliferation, and tube formation *in vitro* (52,53). The involvement of

TABLE 53-1. *Factors that directly or indirectly regulate angiogenesis*

Angiostatic factors	Angiogenic factors
Proteins and peptides	**Proteins and peptides**
Angiopoietin-2	Angiogenin
Angiostatin	Angiopoitetin-1
Endostatin	Angiotensin II
Eosinophil major basic protein	ELR-CXC chemokines
High-molecular-weight hyaluronan	Epidermal growth factor
Interferon-α	Fibrin peptide fragments
Interferon-β	Fibroblast growth factors
Interferon-γ	Haptoglobin
Non-ELR-CXC chemokines	Plasminogen activator
Interleukin-12	Polyamines
Laminin and fibronectin peptides	Substance P
Placental RNAase inhibitor	Hepatocyte growth factor
Somatostatin	Soluble E-selectin
Thrombospondin-1	Transforming growth factor-α
Tissue inhibitors of metalloproteinases	Transforming growth factor-β
Lipids	Tumor necrosis factor-α
Angiostatic steroids	Vascular endothelial growth factor
Retinoids	**Carbohydrates and lipids**
Vitamin A	12(R)-hydroxyeicosatrienoic acid
Others	Hyaluronan fragments
Nitric oxide	Platelet activating factor
Vitreous fluids	Monobutyrin
Prostaglandin synthase inhibitor	Prostaglandins E_1 and E_2
Protamine	Urokinase
	Others
	Adenosine
	Angiotropin
	Ceruloplasmin
	Heparin
	Nicotinamide

CXC, chemokines with adjacent first two cysteines; ELR, glutamate-leucine-arginine motif.

FGFs in pathologic angiogenesis is inferred by studies of tumor associated angiogenesis. Basic FGF may influence angiogenesis associated with Kaposi's sarcoma (54), breast cancer (55), and lung cancer (56). Furthermore, FGFs have been studied in models of myocardial ischemia and may play a therapeutic role in the development of collateral circulation (57,58).

FGF Receptors

FGFs bind to glycosaminoglycans (59). Low-affinity heparin binding is necessary for FGFs to bind to their high-affinity cell surface receptors (60). Specific high-affinity FGF receptors have been cloned and exist in three different isoforms (FGFR-1, -2, and -3) that result from alternative splicing of the FGFR gene transcripts. Each receptor has three immunoglobulin (Ig)-like extracellular domains (except for FGFR-2, which has only two Ig domains), a transmembrane domain, and an intracellular tyrosine-kinase domain (61). The alternative extracellular domains confer differing ligand-binding specificity for members of the FGF family (61), and these splice variants are distributed in a tissue specific manner (62). There are several inherited disorders of

skeletal development associated with mutations of the FGF receptors (63). The multifunctional potential of the FGF family is inferred by the existence of these human disorders.

Vascular Endothelial Cell Growth Factor

Also identified as vascular permeability factor (VPF), VEGF is the initial member of a family of proteins with mitogenic and angiogenic activity (64). As its name implies VEGF also has potent effects on vessel permeability in addition to endothelial cell proliferation and migration. VEGF exists in multiple isoforms—VEGF-189, -165, and -121—distinguished by the amino acid length of the primary structure (65). These different VEGF molecules result from alternative splicing of a single gene transcript (65). VEGF-189 consists of eight exons, with VEGF-165 lacking the amino acids encoded by exon 6, whereas VEGF-121 lacks amino acids encoded by exons 6 and 7. Additionally, the VEGF family consists of two other members, VEGF B (66) and C (67) that, while closely related, map to different chromosomes (68). The more recently cloned VEGF B and C are less well characterized, but evidence suggests a critical role for VEGF C in the development of the lymphatic system (69,70). VEGF is biologically active as a dimer (71), and may require downstream activity of nitric oxide synthase and guanylate cyclase to induce angiogenesis (72). While VEGF was initially thought to be an endothelial cell specific agonist, recent evidence demonstrates expression of specific VEGF receptors on monocytes, and that VEGF induces migration of these cells (73).

VEGF-induced angiogenesis is involved in a number of physiologic and pathologic processes. VEGF is expressed in the walls of both normal and atherosclerotic coronary arteries (74), as well as in multiple experimental (75) and naturally occurring human tumors (76). A recent study has correlated the presence of increased immunostaining for VEGF with a poor prognosis in breast cancer (77). In animal models, neutralizing antibodies to VEGF are effective in inhibiting tumor growth in tumor cell lines expressing VEGF (78–80). In synovia of patients with rheumatoid arthritis, expression of VEGF mRNA is seen in macrophages, fibroblasts, and smooth muscle cells (81). Finally, in a rabbit model of hind-limb ischemia, VEGF and bFGF are synergistic in their ability to induce collateral circulation (82).

Perhaps the strongest data demonstrating a role for VEGF-induced angiogenesis is derived from mice with targeted deletion of either the VEGF gene or its receptors. Mouse embryos with a mutation in a single allele of the VEGF gene develop abnormal vessels and die at embryonic day 11 to 12 (83,84). Similarly, targeted inactivation of either of the two known receptors for VEGF results in embryonic lethality at 8 to 9 days (85,86). These findings suggest a central role of VEGF in embryonic development.

Among the factors known to regulate expression of VEGF as well as its receptors is hypoxia (87), which induces VEGF from a number of cell types (87–89). Murine embryonic stem cells genetically engineered to lack the gene for the arylhydrocarbon-receptor nuclear translocator (arnt) are unable to augment VEGF expression in response to hypoxia. Interestingly, embryos derived from these cells display a developmental phenotype similar to VEGF knock-out mice (15). This suggests that arnt is a required factor for the hypoxic induction of VEGF gene transcription. Additionally, the expression of VEGF appears to be augmented in the presence of mutant *ras* oncogenes (90). VEGF can also form heterodimers with placenta growth factor that bind and activate VEGF receptors, but have reduced angiogenic activity (91). Through this interaction, angiogenic activity of VEGF may be regulated after secretion.

VEGF Receptors

The two known receptors for VEGF, flk-1/KDR and flt-1, are both members of the tyrosine kinase family of transmembrane receptors. The receptors probably mediate different actions of VEGF. For example, studies employing VEGF mutants that retain binding to only one of the two receptors reveal that flk-1/KDR mediates VEGF-induced endothelial cell proliferation (92). In contrast, migration of monocytes in response to VEGF occurs via the flt-1 VEGF receptor (73).

Angiostatin and Endostatin

These two recently described molecules are potent inhibitors of angiogenesis (45,93). O'Reilly and colleagues (93) discovered angiostatin while studying an interesting phenomenon; the growth inhibition of tumor metastases by primary tumors. Angiostatin was isolated from the urine of tumor-bearing mice (93). Mice bearing experimental Lewis Lung carcinoma tumors typically developed extensive metastases only after removal of the primary tumor. However, in mice that received injections of purified angiostatin, growth of metastases was inhibited, even after removal of the primary tumor (93). Using a similar experimental strategy, the same group of investigators subsequently isolated a molecule with similar activity—endostatin (45).

These two molecules also share another property, in that both are internal fragments of larger peptides with neither angiogenic or angiostatic properties (45,93). Angiostatin is a 38-kd internal fragment derived from plasminogen (93), and endostatin is a 20-kd internal fragment of collagen XVIII (45). Subsequent studies revealed that macrophage metalloelastase is responsible for the proteolytic cleavage of plasminogen to yield angiostatin (94). To date, there are no studies to define an analogous mechanism for the generation of endostatin. However, the discovery of these two important inhibitors of angiogenesis will surely lead to a search for similar peptide fragments that are capable of inhibiting angiogenesis. Indeed, one of the more exciting findings about these molecules is their ability to induce and sustain dormancy of micrometastases via suppression of angiogenesis in animal models of cancer (45,95).

The Angiopoietin/Tie Receptor-Ligand System

A recently characterized receptor-ligand system appears to be very important in development of the vascular system, but is not yet widely implicated in pathologic angiogenesis. The Tie receptors (Tie-1 and Tie-2) are protein-tyrosine kinases that are expressed in the embryonic yolk sac and in areas of vascular development. Tie-1–deficient animals develop to birth, but die perinatally due to a defect in vascular integrity, with resulting hemorrhage and generalized edema (96). In contrast, Tie-2 (also known as tek)–deficient embryos die at embryonic day 10 to 11, with the most prominent abnormalities being failure of development of the endothelial lining of the heart, and failure of the early vascular system to progress beyond its earliest stages of vessel formation (96).

A search for ligands for this receptor system has led to the cloning of angiopoietin-1, which is a specific activating ligand for Tie-2 (97). Expression of angiopoietin-1 in developing embryos is localized predominantly to the myocardial tissue surrounding the endocardium, and later in mesenchymal tissue surrounding the developing vasculature (97). Angiopoietin-1 is not an endothelial cell mitogen, nor does it induce tube formation *in vitro,* but it plays a vital role in the remodeling of the vascular system during development (97,98), perhaps by facilitating communication between endothelium and the surrounding mesenchymal cells. A naturally occurring antagonist for the Tie-2 receptor exists, termed angiopoietin-2, and is expressed in areas of vascular remodeling in embryonic, as well as adult tissues (99).

While the Tie/angiopoietin system seems to have a definite role in embryonic development, the only pathologic condition in which this receptor-ligand family has thus far been implicated is a familial form of vascular malformations. In this condition a mutation of the Tie-2 receptor tyrosine kinase domain leads to its constitutive activation (100). However, high levels of mRNA for Tie-2 are found in the endothelium of malignant melanomas (101). Therefore, further study of these novel factors may uncover additional pathologic conditions in which they play a role.

CXC Chemokines

The CXC chemokine family are cytokines that in their monomeric forms are less than 10 kd and, like many regulators of angiogenesis, are characteristically basic heparin-binding proteins. This family displays four highly conserved cysteine amino acid residues, with the first two cysteines separated by one nonconserved amino acid (102–108). The CXC amino acid sequence and the generally shared property of being chemotactic factors led to the designation of these cytokines as the CXC chemokine family. In general, CXC chemokines are chemotactic for neutrophils. However, platelet factor-4 (PF-4) has potent angiostatic and antitumor activity, and was the first member of this family to be identified as a

regulator of angiogenesis (109). Subsequently, interleukin-8 (IL-8), a classic neutrophil chemotactic factor, was identified as a potent inducer of angiogenesis in the absence of inflammation (110–112). A unique aspect of the CXC chemokine family is that it displays disparate activity as regulators of angiogenesis (109–111, 113–116). This is the only family of closely related cytokines that is composed of both angiogenic and angiostatic factors (Table 53-2). This is especially important when one considers the paradigm of net angiogenic activity reflecting a balance between positive and negative regulators of angiogenesis.

The structural feature that appears to distinguish angiogenic and angiostatic CXC chemokines is the presence or absence of three conserved amino acid residues that immediately precede the first cysteine in the primary structure of these cytokines. These are the glutamic acid-leucine-arginine (ELR) motif (116). CXC chemokines containing the ELR motif are potent angiogenic factors, whereas those CXC chemokines that lack the ELR motif are angiostatic factors (110–114,116). There are several lines of evidence that support this notion. First, the ELR motif appears to be the critical structural motif that confers binding activity to neutrophils (117). Recently, more direct evidence in support of this came from the finding that angiogenic members of the CXC chemokine family not only lose their angiogenic activity, but become potent angiostatic factors when the ELR motif is mutated to contain either the TVR (from interferon gamma inducible protein 10 (IP-10)) or DLQ (from PF-4) amino acid sequences (Table 53-3) (116). In contrast, mutation of the ELR motif into the primary amino acid structure of monokine induced by interferon gamma (MIG) converted it into a potent angiogenic factor (116). These findings support the notion that the CXC chemokine family is made up of potent regulators of angiogenesis whose activity is dependent on a critical three amino acid sequence, the ELR motif.

This disparity in angiogenic activity may be important in understanding the role of interferons in regulating angiogenesis. IP-10 and MIG are non-ELR CXC chemokines that are angiostatic (113,114,116,118). The primary signal leading to expression of IP-10 and MIG is interferon-γ

TABLE 53-2. *CXC chemokines as angiogenic or angiostatic factors*

Angiogenic factors	Angiostatic factors
Interleukin-8 (IL-8)	Platelet factor-4 (PF-4)
Epithelial neutrophil-activating protein-78 (ENA-78)	Interferon-γ–inducible 10-kd protein (IP-10)
Growth-related oncogene products (GRO-α, GRO-β, and GRO-γ)	Monokine induced by interferon-γ (MIG)
Granulocyte chemotactic protein-2 (GCP-2)	Stromal cell-derived factor-1 (SDF-1)
Platelet basic protein (PBP)	
Connective tissue activating protein-III	
β-Thromboglobulin (β-TG)	
Neutrophil-activating protein-2 (NAP-2)	

CXC, chemokines with adjacent first two cysteines.

TABLE 53-3. *NH$_2$-terminal amino acid sequence alignment of wild type CXC chemokines and mutants of IL-8 with PF-4 or IP-10 motif inserted or mutants of MIG with the ELR motif*

Angiogenic factors		Angiostatic factors	
IL-8	S-A-K-**E-L-R**-C-Q-C	PF-4	E-D-G-**D-L-Q**-C-L-C
ENA-78	V-L-R-**E-L-R**-C-V-C	*IL-8/PF-4*	*S-A-K-**D-L-Q**-C-Q-C*
GRO-α	V-A-T-**E-L-R**-C-Q-C	IP-10	L-S-R-**T-V-R**-C-T-C
GRO-β	L-A-T-**E-L-R**-C-Q-C	*IL-8/IP-10*	*S-A-K-**T-V-R**-C-Q-C*
GRO-γ	V-V-T-**E-L-R**-C-Q-C	MIG	V-V-R-**K-G-R**-C-S-C
MIG/IL-8[a]	*V-V-R-**E-L-R**-C-S-C*		

CXC, chemokines with adjacent first two cysteines; ELR, glutamate-leucine-arginine (ELR) motif; ENA-78, epithelial neutrophil-activating protein-78; GRO, growth-related oncogene products; IP-10, interferon-γ–inducible 10-kd protein; MIG, monokine induced by interferon-γ; PF-4, platelet factor-4.
[a]Mutant proteins are listed in italics.

(119–121), while interferons are potent inhibitors of the production of monocyte-derived IL-8, (growth related gene) GRO-α, and (epithelial neutrophil activating peptide) ENA-78 (all ELR+ angiogenic factors) (122,123). The induction of non-ELR CXC chemokines by interferon-γ may be important in understanding the antiangiogenic properties of interferons, which are potent inhibitors of wound repair and tumor growth (8,124,125). In contrast to MIG and IP-10, the primary signal(s) for induction of the ELR CXC chemokines are tumor necrosis factor (TNF) and IL-1 (119,126–129). Thus, there appears to be signal specificity for the expression of the angiogenic (ELR) and angiostatic (non-ELR) members of the CXC chemokine family.

This family of molecules may be particularly relevant to the study of angiogenesis in chronic inflammation, given that they are produced by virtually all nucleated cells (106,108). IL-8 is an angiogenic factor in several angiogenesis-dependent chronic inflammatory conditions, including rheumatoid arthritis (111,130), psoriasis (13,131), and idiopathic pulmonary fibrosis (10). Additionally, IL-8 is an important source of angiogenic activity in human lung cancer (56,132). The non-ELR CXC chemokines IP-10, PF-4, and MIG are potent angiostatic factors that inhibit angiogenesis induced not only by the ELR CXC chemokines, but also by other classic angiogenic factors such as bFGF and VEGF. For example, IP-10 inhibits *in vitro* endothelial cell chemotaxis and proliferation, as well as *in vivo* matrigel invasion in response to bFGF (113). In the rat corneal model of neovascularization, both IP-10 and MIG inhibit angiogenesis in response to either bFGF or VEGF (118).

A growing body of evidence is supporting the notion that members of the CXC chemokine family regulate net neovascularization in angiogenesis-dependent disorders. For example, in an animal model of human lung cancer, expression of IL-8 correlated directly with tumor size, and inhibition of IL-8 led to inhibition of tumor-derived angiogenic activity and tumor growth (132). Also, IL-8 expression correlates with experimental metastatic activity of some melanoma cell lines (133). Another ELR CXC chemokine, melanoma growth stimulatory activity

(GRO-α), is expressed not only in melanomas, but also in healing human burn wounds in areas of neovascularization (134,135). These findings suggest a role for ELR CXC chemokines in a variety of angiogenesis-dependent conditions.

In contrast, the non-ELR CXC chemokines may play a role as endogenous inhibitors of angiogenic activity. For example, IP-10 is an endogenous angiostatic factor in human lung cancer (136). Expression of IP-10 had an inverse correlation with tumor size in a murine model of human lung cancer tumorigenesis (136), and intratumor administration of IP-10 in this model reduced both tumor growth and spontaneous metastases (136). IP-10 is probably one of the major mediators of the antitumor activity of IL-12 (137,138). More recently, MIG, another non-ELR CXC chemokine, was found to induce tumor necrosis *in vivo* (139). These findings suggest that IP-10 and MIG may eventually prove to be useful as therapeutic adjuncts for the treatment of solid tumors. In total, the above findings support the hypothesis that net angiogenic activity in many conditions may be dependent, in part, on the balance of expression of ELR and non-ELR CXC chemokines.

Receptors Mediating Angiogenic Activity of CXC Chemokines

The receptor(s) responsible for regulation of angiogenesis by CXC chemokines are currently unknown. However, strong indirect evidence suggests that the CXC chemokine receptor, CXCR2, is the putative receptor that mediates this activity. First, the ELR CXC chemokines are all angiogenic, and all bind to CXCR2 (140,141). Second, expression of CXCR2 has been demonstrated on angiogenic endothelium of human burn wounds, specifically at the advancing edge of the healing wound (134). Interestingly, a recent study has identified a gene encoded by human herpesvirus 8, the virus associated with Kaposi's sarcoma (142), a highly vascular neoplasm characterized by proliferating capillary-like structures. This new gene encodes a G-protein–coupled seven transmembrane-domain protein with significant homology to CXCR2 (142). Importantly, this viral CXCR2 homologue is constitutively activated, perhaps leading to ligand-independent growth signaling in the endothelial-like cells of the Kaposi's sarcoma lesion. This indirect evidence supports the contention that CXCR2 mediates the angiogenic activity of ELR CXC chemokines.

The receptor for the angiostatic activity of non-ELR CXC chemokines is also unknown. IP-10 and PF-4 can compete for binding on endothelial cells, and this binding is inhibited by pretreatment of the cells with heparinase (114). There is a specific transmembrane protein receptor for IP-10 and MIG—CXCR3 (143). This receptor has been found in endothelial cells by RT-PCR (Strieter et al., unpublished observations). The role of these receptors in regulating angiostatic activity of non-ELR CXC chemokines remains to be determined. Determining which receptor mediates this activity will be important in developing antiangiogenic therapy for angiogenesis-dependent disorders.

CLINICAL CORRELATES OF DYSREGULATED ANGIOGENESIS

Physiologic angiogenesis is rare once the adult stage of development has been achieved. Situations in which the angiogenic response is appropriate include the ovarian/menstrual cycle in the female reproductive organs and normal healing of a wound. Other than these examples, angiogenesis in an adult is usually associated with a pathologic condition. Below are examples of such conditions, and a brief review of the known regulators of angiogenesis in these conditions.

Psoriasis

Psoriasis is a skin disorder characterized by inflammatory cellular infiltration, abnormal proliferation of keratinocytes, and dermal neovascularization. While it is not clear that the angiogenesis associated with psoriasis is a primary cause of the pathogenesis of the disease, the angiogenic activity is partly due to a combination of overproduction of IL-8, and underproduction of the angiogenesis inhibitor, thrombospondin-1 (13). Other angiogenic factors have been associated with psoriasis including VEGF (144), and transforming growth factor-α (145). Additionally, the angiostatic factor IP-10 is expressed in psoriatic plaques, with expression being reduced after successful treatment of active lesions (146). The significance of this finding is not clear. However, this highlights the potential importance of endogenous angiostatic factors in angiogenesis-dependent disorders. Interestingly, many commonly used treatments for psoriasis are potentially angiostatic, including topical steroids (147,148), cyclosporine (149,150), and retinoids (151).

Rheumatoid Arthritis

The importance of angiogenesis in the pathogenesis of rheumatoid arthritis has been appreciated for many years (152). The synovial inflammation of rheumatoid arthritis leads to formation of a highly vascularized pannus, and to the eventual destruction of articular cartilage and bone. This tissue destruction may be partly dependent on proteases and collagenases that are released during the angiogenic response (153). Studies of angiogenic factors have either directly or indirectly implicated IL-8 (130), hepatocyte growth factor (154), and VEGF (81,155) in the angiogenic activity of rheumatoid arthritis. From a therapeutic standpoint, minocycline, an antibiotic with potent angiostatic activity, was beneficial in the treatment of patients with rheumatoid arthritis in a double-blind placebo-controlled study (156–158).

Pulmonary Fibrosis

As a prototypical fibroproliferative disease, the deposition of extracellular matrix seen in the lungs of patients with pulmonary fibrosis is an example of exaggerated granulation tissue. Indeed, one of the classic early reports of the pathology of pulmonary fibrosis included the description of neovascularization (159). While most studies of this disease have focused on the role of inflammatory cell infiltration and fibroblast function, recent data have suggested a role for CXC chemokines as regulators of angiogenic activity in patients with pulmonary fibrosis (10). Specifically, there appears to be overexpression of angiogenic (ELR) and underexpression of angiostatic (non-ELR) CXC chemokines during the pathogenesis of a murine model of pulmonary fibrosis (10). This imbalance is associated with increased angiogenic activity that likely supports the fibroproliferation seen in the lungs of these animals. Interestingly, angiogenic activity is found in the alveolar space early in the course of acute lung injury (160), suggesting that the process of chronic pulmonary fibrosis may be initiated soon after acute lung injury. Further investigations are needed to determine the role of angiogenesis in the pathogenesis of pulmonary fibrosis and to improve the dismal prognosis associated with fibrotic lung diseases.

Tumorigenesis and Metastasis

The dependence of tumor growth on angiogenesis was first noted by Gimbrone and Folkman (9) in 1972. This is perhaps the most fertile area of research on angiogenesis, and the one in which therapeutic advances are most needed. Early in the pathogenesis of a tumor, and before a tumor can become clinically significant, there must be a switch to an angiogenic phenotype (161). This angiogenic switch can be mediated by either an increase in expression of angiogenic factors (161,162), a decrease in the expression of angiostatic factors (16,136,163), or both. Many factors have been implicated in the control of tumor-associated angiogenic activity including VEGF (77,78,90,164,165), bFGF (164,166,167), and the CXC chemokines (132,133,135,168).

In addition to the growth of a primary tumor, the spread and growth of distant metastases can only be accomplished by individual cells capable of expressing an angiogenic phenotype (169). The population of cells in a primary tumor is heterogeneous, and only those cells that can induce angiogenesis at a distant site will form a clinically evident metastasis (169). One theory that has gained favor recently is that dormant metastases are those that have a balance of proliferation and apoptosis (9,170). Only when the metastatic deposit has made the angiogenic switch will the rate of proliferation surpass the rate of apoptosis, and the metastatic focus become clinically manifest (95,171). An effective inhibitor of tumor-derived angiogenic activity would prevent further growth of a primary tumor, and halt the development of metastases. Since tumor endothelium is not genetically abnormal, and therefore not subject to a high rate of mutation, it is unlikely to develop drug resistance to angiostatic therapy. Such an advance could render all other aspects of tumor biology irrelevant. Therefore, some investigators have proposed a two-compartment approach to tumor therapy, one targeted at the malignant cells, and one at the endothelial cells (171). This is clearly an area where research into the mechanisms of angiogenesis is potentially very beneficial.

SUMMARY

Angiogenesis is a complex process that involves the activation of normally quiescent endothelium. In the course of the angiogenic response, endothelial cells must dissociate themselves from their neighbors, digest the basement membrane and proximal matrix, migrate along a concentration gradient, divide, and reform a capillary tube. All of these functions are vital to the formation of a functioning capillary. Since angiogenesis is intricately associated with physiologic wound repair, and pathologic processes such as chronic inflammation and tumor growth, it is likely that with future study many diseases will be found to be associated with a defect in one or more of these steps.

The complex control of angiogenesis is illustrated by the ever-increasing number of molecules that can affect the response. While research has primarily focused on the discovery of angiogenic factors, recent studies have highlighted the importance of endogenous angiostatic factors in many disease states. There has been remarkable progress in the knowledge of angiogenesis in the last three decades. However, a more thorough understanding of the control of angiogenesis will allow future therapeutic advances that exploit the dependence of chronic inflammation, tumor growth, and wound repair on angiogenesis.

ACKNOWLEDGMENTS

The work was supported, in part, by National Institutes of Health grants CA66180, HL50057, 1P50HL56402 (R.M.S.), and CA72543 (D.A.A.); an American Lung Association Research grant, and the University of Michigan's Phoenix Memorial Project (D.A.A.).

REFERENCES

1. Risau W. Vasculogenesis, angiogenesis and endothelial cell differentiation during embryonic development. In: Feinberg RN, Sherer GK, Auerbach R, eds. *The development of the vascular system.* Basel: K. Karger, 1991:58–68.
2. Jackson JR, Seed MP, Kircher CH, Willoughby DA, Winkler JD. The codependence of angiogenesis and chronic inflammation. *FASEB J* 1997;11(6):457–465.
3. Engerman RL, Pfaffenenbach D, Davis MD. Cell turnover of capillaries. *Lab Invest* 1967;17:738–743.
4. Tannock IF, Hayashi HS. The proliferation of capillary and endothelial cells. *Cancer Res* 1972;32:77–82.
5. Auerbach R. Vascular endothelial cell differentiation: organ specificity and selective affinities as the basis for developing anticancer strategies. *Int J Radiat Biol* 1991;60(1–2):1–10.
6. Sato N, Beitz JG, Kato J, et al. Platelet-derived growth factor indirectly stimulates angiogenesis in vitro. *Am J Pathol* 1993;142(4):1119–1130.
7. Vlodavsky I, Korner G, Ishai-Michaeli R, Bashkin P, Bar-Shavit R, Fuks Z. Extracellular matrix-resident growth factors and enzymes: possible involvement in tumor metastases and angiogenesis. *Cancer Metastases Rev* 1990;9:203–226.
8. Clark RA. Basics of cutaneous wound repair. *J Dermatol Surg Oncol* 1993;19(8):693–706.
9. Gimbrone MA, Leapman SB, Cotran RS, Folkman J. Tumor dormancy in vivo by prevention of neovascularization. *J Exp Med* 1972;136:261–276.
10. Keane M, Arenberg D, Lynch JP III, et al. The CXC chemokines, IL-8 and IP-10, regulate angiogenic activity in idiopathic pulmonary fibrosis. *J Immunol* 1997;159:1437–1443.
11. Strieter RM, Kunkel SL, Showell HJ, Marks RM. Monokine-induced gene expression of human endothelial cell-derived neutrophil chemotactic factor. *Biochem Biophys Res Commun* 1988;156:1340–1345.
12. Vlodavski I, Folkman J, Sullivan R, et al. Endothelial cell-derived basic fibroblast growth factor: synthesis and deposition into subendothelial extracellular matrix. *Proc Natl Acad Sci USA* 1987;84:2292–2296.
13. Nickoloff BJ, Mitra RS, Varani J, Dixit VM, Polverini PJ. Aberrant production of interleukin-8 and thrombospondin-1 by psoriatic keratinocytes mediates angiogenesis. *Am J Pathol* 1994;144(4):820–828.
14. Leibovich SJ, Weisman DM. Macrophages, wound repair and angiogenesis. *Prog Clin Biol Res* 1988;266:131–145.
15. Maltepe E, Schmidt JV, Baunoch D, Bradfield CA, Simon MC. Abnormal angiogenesis and responses to glucose and oxygen deprivation in mice lacking the protein ARNT. *Nature* 1997;386:403–407.
16. Rastinejad F, Polverini PJ, Bouck NP. Regulation of the activity of a new inhibitor of angiogenesis by a cancer suppressor gene. *Cell* 1989;56(3):345–355.
17. Lampugnani MG, Resnati M, Raiteri M, et al. A novel endothelial-specific membrane protein is a marker of cell-cell contacts. *J Cell Biol* 1992;118(6):1511–1522.
18. Lampugnani MG, Corada M, Caveda L, et al. The molecular organization of endothelial cell to cell junctions: differential association of plakoglobin, beta-catenin, and alpha-catenin with vascular endothelial cadherin (VE-cadherin). *J Cell Biol* 1995;129(1):203–217.
19. Tanihara H, Kido M, Obata S, et al. Characterization of cadherin-4 and cadherin-5 reveals new aspects of cadherins. *J Cell Sci* 1994;107(6):1697–1704.
20. Dejana E. Endothelial adherens junctions: implications in the control of vascular permeability and angiogenesis. *J Clin Invest* 1996;98(9):1949–1953.
21. Pepper MS, Vassaui JD, Orci L, Montesano R. Proteolytic balance and capillary morphogenesis in vitro. In: Steiner R, Weisz PB, Langer R, eds. *Angiogenesis: key principles.* Basel: Birkhauser Verlag, 1992:137–145.
22. Takigawa M, Nishida Y, Suzuki F, Kishi J, Yamashita K, Hayakawa T. Induction of angiogenesis in chick yolk-sac membrane by polyamines

and its inhibition by tissue inhibitors of metalloproteinases (TIMP and TIMP-2). *Biochem Biophys Res Commun* 1990;171(3):1264–1271.

23. Arnold F, West DC. Angiogenesis in wound healing. *Pharmacol Ther* 1991;52(3):407–422.

24. Gross JL, Moscatelli D, Rifkin DB. Increased capillary endothelial cell protease activity in response to angiogenic stimuli *in vitro. Proc Natl Acad Sci USA* 1983;80(9):2623–2627.

25. Brooks PC, Clark RA, Cheresh DA. Requirement of vascular integrin alpha v beta 3 for angiogenesis. *Science* 1994;264(5158):569–571.

26. Brooks PC, Montgomery AM, Rosenfeld M, et al. Integrin alpha v beta 3 antagonists promote tumor regression by inducing apoptosis of angiogenic blood vessels. *Cell* 1994;79(7):1157–1164.

27. Koolwijk P, van Erck MG, de Vree WJ, et al. Cooperative effect of TNFalpha, bFGF, and VEGF on the formation of tubular structures of human microvascular endothelial cells in a fibrin matrix. Role of urokinase activity. *J Cell Biol* 1996;132(6):1177–1188.

28. Sholly MM, Fergusen GP, Seibel HR, Montour JL, Wilson JD. Mechanisms of neovascularization: vascular sprouting can occur without proliferation of endothelial cells. *Lab Invest* 1984;51:624–634.

29. Sunderkotter C, Goebeler M, Schulze-Osthoff K, Bhardwaj R, Sorg C. Macrophage-derived angiogenesis factors. *Pharmacol Ther* 1991;51(2):195–216.

30. Ingber DE, Folkman J. Mechanochemical switching between growth and differentiation during fibroblast growth factor-stimulated angiogenesis *in vitro*: role of extracellular matrix. *J Cell Biol* 1989;109(1):317–330.

31. Davidson JM. Wound repair. In: Gallin JI, Goldstein IM, Snyderman R, eds. *Inflammation: basic principles and clinical correlates.* New York: Raven Press, 1992:809–819.

32. French-Constant C, Van DWL, Dvorak HF, Hynes RO. Reappearance of an embryonic pattern of fibronectin splicing during wound healing in the adult rat. *J Cell Biol* 1989;109:903–914.

33. Kurkinen M, Vaheri A, Roberts PJ, Stenan S. Sequential appearance of fibronectin and collagen in experimental granulation tissue. *Lab Invest* 1980;43:47–51.

34. Caveda L, Martin-Padura I, Navarro P, et al. Inhibition of cultured cell growth by vascular endothelial cadherin (cadherin-5/VE-cadherin). *J Clin Invest* 1996;98(4):886–893.

35. Matsumura T, Wolff K, Petzelbauer P. Endothelial cell tube formation depends on cadherin 5 and CD31 interactions with filamentous actin. *J Immunol* 1997;158(7):3408–3416.

36. DeLisser HM CJ, Yan HC, Daise ML, Buck CA, Albelda SM. Deletions in the cytoplasmic domain of platelet-endothelial cell adhesion molecule-1 (PECAM-1, CD31) result in changes in ligand binding properties. *J Cell Biol* 1994;124(1–2):195–203.

37. Delisser HM, Christofidou-Solomidou M, Strieter RM, et al. Involvement of endothelial PECAM-1/CD31 in angiogenesis. *Am J Pathol* 1997;151(3):671–677.

38. Haralabopoulos GC, Grant DS, Kleinman HK, Lelkes PI, Papaioannou SP, Maragoudakis ME. Inhibitors of basement membrane collagen synthesis prevent endothelial cell alignment in matrigel *in vitro* and angiogenesis *in vivo. Lab Invest* 1994;71(4):575–582.

39. Hansell P, Maione TE, Borgstrom P. Selective binding of platelet factor 4 to regions of active angiogenesis *in vivo. Am J Physiol* 1995;269(3 Pt 2):H829–836.

40. Walz A, Baggiolini M. Generation of the neutrophil-activating peptide NAP-2 from platelet basic protein or connective tissue-activating peptide III through monocyte proteases. *Exp Med* 1990;171:449–454.

41. Koch AE, Leibovich SJ, Polverini PJ. Stimulation of neovascularization by human rheumatoid synovial tissue macrophages. *Arthritis Rheum* 1989;29(4):471–479.

42. Polverini PJ. How the extracellular matrix and macrophages contribute to angiogenesis-dependent diseases. *Eur J Cancer* 1996;32A(14):2430–2437.

43. Polverini PJ, Cotran PS, Gimbrone MA, Unanue ER. Activated macrophages induce vascular proliferation. *Nature* 1977;269(5631):804–806.

44. Dong Z, Kumar R, Yang X, Fidler IJ. Macrophage-derived metalloelastase is responsible for the generation of angiostatin in Lewis lung carcinoma. *Cell* 1997;88:801–810.

45. O'Reilly M, Boehm T, Shing Y, et al. Endostatin: an endogenous inhibitor of angiogenesis and tumor growth. *Cell* 1997;88(2):277–285.

46. Ausprunk DH, Folkman J. The sequence of events in the regression of corneal capillaries. *Lab Invest* 1978;38:284–296.

47. Robaye B, Mosselmans R, Fiers W, Dumont JE, Galand P. Tumor necrosis factor induces apoptosis (programmed cell death) in normal endothelial cells *in vitro. Am J Pathol* 1991;138(2):447–453.

48. Burgess WH, Maciag T. The heparin-binding (fibroblast) growth factor family of proteins. *Annu Rev Biochem* 1989;58:575–606.

49. Talarico D, Basilico C. The K-fgf/hst oncogene induces transformation through an autocrine mechanism that requires extracellular stimulation of the mitogenic pathway. *Mol Cell Biol* 1991;11(2):1138–1145.

50. Forough R, Xi Z, MacPhee M, et al. Differential transforming abilities of non-secreted and secreted forms of human fibroblast growth factor-1. *J Biol Chem* 1993;268(4):2960–2968.

51. Rogelj S, Weinberg RA, Fanning P, Klagsbrun M. Basic fibroblast growth factor fused to a signal peptide transforms cells. *Nature* 1988;331(6152):173–175.

52. Connolly DT, Stoddard BL, Harakas NK, Feder J. Human fibroblast-derived growth factor is a mitogen and chemoattractant for endothelial cells. *Biochem Biophys Res Commun* 1987;144(2):705–712.

53. Montesano R, Vassalli JD, Baird A, Guillemin R, Orci L. Basic fibroblast growth factor induces angiogenesis *in vitro. Proc Natl Acad Sci USA* 1986;83(19):7297–7301.

54. Ensoli B, Markham P, Kao V, et al. Block of AIDS-Kaposi's sarcoma (KS) cell growth, angiogenesis, and lesion formation in nude mice by antisense oligonucleotide targeting basic fibroblast growth factor. A novel strategy for the therapy of KS. *J Clin Invest* 1994;94(5):1736–1746.

55. Lewis CE, Leek R, Harris A, McGee JO. Cytokine regulation of angiogenesis in breast cancer: the role of tumor-associated macrophages. *J Leukoc Biol* 1995;57(5):747–751.

56. Smith DR, Polverini PJ, Kunkel SL, et al. Inhibition of IL-8 attenuates angiogenesis in bronchogenic carcinoma. *J Exp Med* 1994;179:1409–1415.

57. Isner JM. The role of angiogenic cytokines in cardiovascular disease. *Clin Immunol Immunopathol* 1996;80(3 pt 2):S82–S91.

58. Sellke FW, Li J, Stamler A, Lopez JJ, Thomas KA, Simons M. Angiogenesis induced by acidic fibroblast growth factor as an alternative method of revascularization for chronic myocardial ischemia. *Surgery* 1996;120(2):182–188.

59. Friesel RE, Maciag T. Molecular mechanisms of angiogenesis: fibroblast growth factor signal transduction. *FASEB J* 1995;9(10):919–925.

60. Yayon A, Klagsbrun M, Esko JD, Leder P, Ornitz DM. Cell surface, heparin-like molecules are required for binding of basic fibroblast growth factor to its high affinity receptor. *Cell* 1991;64(4):841–848.

61. Johnson DE, Williams LT. Structural and functional diversity in the FGF receptor multigene family. *Adv Cancer Res* 1993;60:1–40.

62. Orr-Urtreger A, Bedford MT, Burakova T, et al. Developmental localization of the splicing alternatives of fibroblast growth factor receptor 2 (FGFR2). *Dev Biol* 1993;158:475–486.

63. Muenke M, Schell U. Fibroblast-growth-factor receptor mutations in human skeletal disorders. *Trends Genet* 1995;11(8):308–313.

64. Tischer E, Gospodarowicz D, Mitchell R, et al. Vascular endothelial growth factor: a new member of the platelet-derived growth factor gene family. *Biochem Biophys Res Commun* 1989;165(3):1198–1206.

65. Tischer E, Mitchell R, Hartman T, et al. The human gene for vascular endothelial growth factor. Multiple protein forms are encoded through alternative exon splicing. *J Biol Chem* 1991;266(18):11947–11954.

66. Olofsson B, Pajusola K, Kaipainen A, et al. Vascular endothelial growth factor B, a novel growth factor for endothelial cells. *Proc Natl Acad Sci USA* 1996;93(6):2576–2581.

67. Joukov V, Pajusola K, Kaipainen A, et al. A novel vascular endothelial growth factor, VEGF-C, is a ligand for the Flt4 (VEGFR-3) and KDR (VEGFR-2) receptor tyrosine kinases [published erratum appears in EMBO J 1996 Apr 1;15(7):1751]. *EMBO J* 1996;15(2):290–298.

68. Wei MH, Popescu NC, Lerman MI, Merrill MJ, Zimonjic DB. Localization of the human vascular endothelial growth factor gene, VEGF, at chromosome 6p12. *Hum Genet* 1996;97(6):794–797.

69. Jeltsch M, Kaipainen A, Joukov V, et al. Hyperplasia of lymphatic vessels in VEGF-C transgenic mice. *Science* 1997;276(5317):1423–1425.

70. Kukk E, Lymboussaki A, Taira S, et al. VEGF-C receptor binding and pattern of expression with VEGFR-3 suggests a role in lymphatic vascular development. *Development* 1996;122(12):3829–3837.

71. Claffey KP, Senger DR, Spiegelman BM. Structural requirements for dimerization, glycosylation, secretion, and biological function of VPF/VEGF. *Biochim Biophys Acta* 1995;1246(1):1–9.

72. Ziche M, Morbidelli L, Choudhuri R, Zhang H-T, Donnini S, Granger HJ. Nitric Oxide synthase lies downstream from vascular endothelial growth factor-induced, but not basic fibroblast growth factor-induced angiogenesis. *J Clin Invest* 1997;99:2626–2634.

73. Barleon B, Sozzani S, Zhou D, Weich HA, Mantovani A, Marme D. Migration of human monocytes in response to vascular endothelial growth factor (VEGF) is mediated via the VEGF receptor flt-1. *Blood* 1996;87(8):3336–3343.

74. Couffinhal T, Kearney M, Witzenbichler B, et al. Vascular endothelial growth factor/vascular permeability factor (VEGF/VPF) in normal and atherosclerotic human arteries. *Am J Pathol* 1997;150(5):1673–1685.

75. Warren RS, Yuan H, Matli MR, Gillett NA, Ferrara N. Regulation by vascular endothelial growth factor of human colon cancer tumorigenesis in a mouse model of experimental liver metastasis. *J Clin Invest* 1995;95(4):1789–1797.

76. Takahashi Y, Kitadai Y, Bucana CD, Cleary KR, Ellis LM. Expression of vascular endothelial growth factor and its receptor, KDR, correlates with vascularity, metastasis, and proliferation of human colon cancer. *Cancer Res* 1995;55(18):3964–3968.

77. Toi M, Hoshina S, Takayanagi T, Tominaga T. Association of vascular endothelial growth factor expression with tumor angiogenesis and with early relapse in primary breast cancer. *Jpn J Cancer Res* 1994; 85(10):1045–1049.

78. Borgstrom P, Hillan KJ, Sriramarao P, Ferrara N. Complete inhibition of angiogenesis and growth of microtumors by anti-vascular endothelial growth factor neutralizing antibody: novel concepts of angiostatic therapy from intravital videomicroscopy. *Cancer Res* 1996;56(17): 4032–4039.

79. Claffey KP, Brown LF, del Aguila LF, et al. Expression of vascular permeability factor/vascular endothelial growth factor by melanoma cells increases tumor growth, angiogenesis, and experimental metastasis. *Cancer Res* 1996;56(1):172–181.

80. Kim JK, Li B, Winer J, et al. Inhibition of vascular endothelial growth factor-induced angiogenesis suppresses tumor growth *in vivo*. *Nature* 1993;362:841–844.

81. Nagashima M, Yoshino S, Ishiwata T, Asano G. Role of vascular endothelial growth factor in angiogenesis of rheumatoid arthritis. *J Rheumatol* 1995;22(9):1624–1630.

82. Asahara T, Bauters C, Zheng LP, et al. Synergistic effect of vascular endothelial growth factor and basic fibroblast growth factor on angiogenesis *in vivo*. *Circulation* 1995;92(suppl 9):II365–371.

83. Carmeliet P, Ferreira V, Breier G, et al. Abnormal blood vessel development and lethality in embryos lacking a single VEGF allele. *Nature* 1996;380(6573):435–439.

84. Ferrara N, Carver-Moore K, Chen H, et al. Heterozygous embryonic lethality induced by targeted inactivation of the VEGF gene. *Nature* 1996;380(6573):439–442.

85. Fong GH, Rossant J, Gertsenstein M, Breitman ML. Role of the Flt-1 receptor tyrosine kinase in regulating the assembly of vascular endothelium. *Nature* 1995;376(6535):66–70.

86. Shalaby F, Rossant J, Yamaguchi TP, et al. Failure of blood-island formation and vasculogenesis in Flk-1-deficient mice. *Nature* 1995; 376(6535):62–66.

87. Detmar M, Brown LF, Berse B, et al. Hypoxia regulates the expression of vascular permeability factor/vascular endothelial growth factor (VPF/VEGF) and its receptors in human skin. *J Invest Dermatol* 1997;108(3):263–268.

88. Brogi E, Wu T, Namiki A, Isner JM. Indirect angiogenic cytokines upregulate VEGF and bFGF gene expression in vascular smooth muscle cells, whereas hypoxia upregulates VEGF expression only. *Circulation* 1994;90(2):649–652.

89. Freeman MR, Schneck FX, Gagnon ML, et al. Peripheral blood T lymphocytes and lymphocytes infiltrating human cancers express vascular endothelial growth factor: a potential role for T cells in angiogenesis. *Cancer Res* 1995;55(18):4140–4145.

90. Rak J, Mitsuhashi Y, Bayko L, et al. Mutant ras oncogenes upregulate VEGF/VPF expression: implications for induction and inhibition of tumor angiogenesis. *Cancer Res* 1995;55(20):4575–4580.

91. Cao Y, Chen H, Zhou L, et al. Heterodimers of placenta growth factor/vascular endothelial growth factor. Endothelial activity, tumor cell expression, and high affinity binding to Flk-1/KDR. *J Biol Chem* 1996;271(6):3154–3162.

92. Keyt BA, Nguyen HV, Berleau LT, et al. Identification of vascular endothelial growth factor determinants for binding KDR and FLT-1

93. O'Reilly MS, Holmgren L, Shing Y, et al. Angiostatin: a novel angiogenesis inhibitor that mediates suppression of metastases by a Lewis lung carcinoma. *Cell* 1994;79(2):315–328.

94. Dong Z, Kumar R, Yang X, Fidler IJ. Macrophage-derived metalloelastase is responsible for the generation of angiostatin in Lewis lung carcinoma. *Cell* 1997;88(6):801–810.

95. O'Reilly MS, Holmgren L, Chen C, Folkman J. Angiostatin induces and sustains dormancy of human primary tumors in mice. *Nat Med* 1996;2(6):689–692.

96. Sato TN, Tozawa Y, Deutsch U, et al. Distinct roles of the receptor tyrosine kinases Tie-1 and Tie-2 in blood vessel formation. *Nature* 1995;376(6535):70–74.

97. Davis S, Aldrich TH, Jones PF, et al. Isolation of angiopoietin-1, a ligand for the TIE2 receptor, by secretion-trap expression cloning [see comments]. *Cell* 1996;87(7):1161–1169.

98. Suri C, Jones PF, Patan S, et al. Requisite role of angiopoietin-1, a ligand for the TIE2 receptor, during embryonic angiogenesis [see comments]. *Cell* 1996;87(7):1171–1180.

99. Maisonpierre PC, Suri C, Jones PF, et al. Angiopoietin-2, a natural antagonist for Tie2 that disrupts *in vivo* angiogenesis [see comments]. *Science* 1997;277(5322):55–60.

100. Vikkula M, Boon LM, Carraway KL III, et al. Vascular dysmorphogenesis caused by an activating mutation in the receptor tryosine kinase TIE2. *Cell* 1996;87:1181–1190.

101. Kaipainen A, Vlaykova T, Hatva E, et al. Enhanced expression of the tie receptor tyrosine kinase messenger RNA in the vascular endothelium of metastatic melanomas. *Cancer Res* 1994;54(24):6571–6577.

102. Baggiolini M, Dewald B, Walz A. Interleukin-8 and related chemotactic cytokines. In: Gallin JI, Goldstein IM, Snyderman R, eds. *Inflammation: basic principles and clinical correlates.* New York: Raven Press, 1992:247–263.

103. Baggiolini M, Walz A, Kunkel SL. Neutrophil-activating peptide-1/interleukin 8, a novel cytokine that activates neutrophils. *J Clin Invest* 1989;84:1045–1049.

104. Matsushima K, Oppenheim JJ. Interleukin 8 and MCAF: novel inflammatory cytokines inducible by IL-1 and TNF. *Cytokine* 1989;1:2–13.

105. Miller MD, Krangel MS. Biology and biochemistry of the chemokines: a family of chemotactic and inflammatory cytokines. *Crit Rev Immunol* 1992;12:17–46.

106. Strieter RM, Kunkel SL. Chemokines and the lung. In: Crystal R, West J, Weibel E, and Barnes P, eds. *Lung scientific foundations,* 2nd ed. New York: Raven Press, 1997:155–186.

107. Strieter RM, Lukacs NW, Standiford TJ, Kunkel SL. Cytokines and lung inflammation. *Thorax* 1993;48:765–769.

108. Walz A, Kunkel SL, Strieter RM. CXC chemokines—an overview. In: Koch AE, Strieter RM, eds. *Chemokines in disease.* Austin, TX: R.G. Landes, 1996:1–26.

109. Maione TE, Gray GS, Petro J, et al. Inhibition of angiogenesis by recombinant human platelet factor-4 and related peptides. *Science* 1990;247(4938):77–79.

110. Hu DE, Hori Y, Fan TPD. Interleukin-8 stimulates angiogenesis in rats. *Inflammation* 1993;17:135–143.

111. Koch AE, Polverini PJ, Kunkel SL, et al. Interleukin-8 (IL-8) as a macrophage-derived mediator of angiogenesis. *Science* 1992;258:1798–1801.

112. Strieter RM, Kunkel SL, Elner VM, et al. Interleukin-8: a corneal factor that induces neovascularization. *Am J Pathol* 1992;141:1279–1284.

113. Angiolillo AL, Sgadari C, Taub DT, et al. Human interferon-inducible protein 10 is a potent inhibitor of angiogenesis *in vivo. J Exp Med* 1995;158:155–162.

114. Luster AD, Greenberg SM, Leder P. The IP-10 chemokine binds to a specific cell surface heparan sulfate shared with platelet factor 4 and inhibits endothelial cell proliferation. *J Exp Med* 1995;182:219–232.

115. Strieter RM, Kunkel SL, Shanafelt AB, Arenberg DA, Koch AE, Polverini PJ. CXC chemokines in regulation of angiogenesis. In: Koch AE, Strieter RM, eds. *Chemokines in disease.* Austin, TX: R.G. Landes, 1996:195–210.

116. Strieter RM, Polverini PJ, Kunkel SL, et al. The functional role of the ELR motif in CXC chemokine-mediated angiogenesis. *J Biol Chem* 1995;270(45):27348–27357.

117. Hebert CA, Vitangcol RV, Baker JB. Scanning mutagenesis of interleukin-8 identifies a cluster of residues required for receptor binding. *J Biol Chem* 1991;266:18989–18994.

receptors. Generation of receptor-selective VEGF variants by site-directed mutagenesis. *J Biol Chem* 1996;271(10):5638–5646.

118. Strieter RM, Kunkel SL, Arenberg DA, Burdick MD, Polverini PJ. Interferon gamma-inducible protein 10 (IP-10), a member of the C-X-C chemokine family, is an inhibitor of angiogenesis. *Biochem Biophys Res Commun* 1995;210(1):51–57.

119. Boorsma DM, de Haan P, Willemze R, Stoof TJ. Human growth factor (huGRO), interleukin-8 (IL-8) and interferon-gamma-inducible protein (gamma-IP-10) gene expression in cultured normal human keratinocytes. *Arch Dermatol Res* 1994;286(8):471–475.

120. Farber JM. A macrophage mRNA selectively induced by gamma-interferon encodes a member of the platelet factor 4 family of cytokines. *Proc Natl Acad Sci USA* 1990;87(14):5238–5242.

121. Farber JM. HuMIG: a new member of the chemokine family of cytokines. *Biochem Biophys Res Commun* 1993;192:223–230.

122. Gusella GL, Musso T, Bosco MC, Espinoza-Delgado I, Matsushima K, Varesio L. IL-2 up-regulates but IFN-γ suppresses IL-8 expression in human monocytes. *J Immunol* 1993;151:2725–2732.

123. Schnyder-Candrian S, Strieter RM, Kunkel SL, Walz A. Interferon-α and interferon-γ downregulate the production of interleukin-8 and ENA-78 in human monocytes. *J Leukoc Biol* 1995;in press.

124. Majewski S, Szmurlo A, Marczak M, Jablonska S, Bollag W. Synergistic effect of retinoids and interferon alpha on tumor-induced angiogenesis: anti-angiogenic effect on HPV-harboring tumor-cell lines. *Int J Cancer* 1994;57(1):81–85.

125. Saiki I, Sato K, Yoo YC, et al. Inhibition of tumor-induced angiogenesis by the administration of recombinant interferon-gamma followed by a synthetic lipid-A subunit analogue (GLA-60). *Int J Cancer* 1992;51(4):641–645.

126. Kasahara T, Mukaido N, Yamashita K, Yagisawa H, Akahoshi T, Matsushima K. IL-1 and TNF-alpha induction of IL-8 and monocyte chemotactic and activating factor (MCAF) mRNA expression in a human astrocytoma cell line. *Immunology* 1991;74:60–67.

127. Standiford TJ, Kunkel SL, Basha MA, et al. Interleukin-8 gene expression by a pulmonary epithelial cell line: a model for cytokine networks in the lung. *J Clin Invest* 1990;86:1945–1953.

128. Strieter RM, Kunkel SL, Showell H, Phan DGRH, Ward PA, Marks RM. Endothelial cell gene expression of a neutrophil chemotactic factor by TNF-α, LPS, and IL-1β. *Science* 1989;243:1467–1469.

129. Strieter RM, Phan SH, Showell HJ, et al. Monokine-induced neutrophil chemotactic factor gene expression in human fibroblasts. *J Biol Chem* 1989;264:10621–10626.

130. Koch AE, Kunkel SL, Burrows JL, et al. The synovial tissue macrophage as a source of the chemotactic cytokine interleukin-8. *J Immunol* 1991;147:2187–2195.

131. Nickoloff BJ, Karabin GD, Barker JWCN, et al. Cellular localization of interleukin-8 and its inducer, tumor necrosis factor-alpha in psoriasis. *Am J Pathol* 1991;138:129–140.

132. Arenberg DA, Kunkel SL, Polverini PJ, Glass M, Burdick MD, Strieter RM. Inhibition of interleukin-8 reduces tumorigenesis of human non-small cell lung cancer in SCID mice. *J Clin Invest* 1996;97(12):2792–2802.

133. Singh RK, Gutman M, Radinsky R, Bucana CD, Fidler IJ. Expression of interleukin 8 correlates with the metastatic potential of human melanoma cells in nude mice. *Cancer Res* 1994;54(12):3242–3247.

134. Nanney LB, Mueller SG, Bueno R, Peiper SC, Richmond A. Distributions of melanoma growth stimulatory activity or growth-related gene and the interleukin-8 receptor type B in human wound repair. *Am J Pathol* 1995;147(5):1248–1260.

135. Richmond A, Thomas HG. Melanoma growth stimulatory activity: isolation from human melanoma tumors and characterization of tissue distribution. *J Cell Biochem* 1988;36:185–198.

136. Arenberg DA, Kunkel SL, Polverini PJ, et al. Interferon-γ-inducible protein 10 (IP-10) is an angiostatic factor that inhibits human non-small cell lung cancer (NSCLC) tumorigenesis and spontaneous metastases. *J Exp Med* 1996;184(3):981–992.

137. Angiolillo AL, Sgadari C, Tosato G. A role for the interferon-inducible protein 10 in inhibition of angiogenesis by interleukin-12. *Ann N Y Acad Sci* 1996;795:158–167.

138. Sgadari C, Angiolillo AL, Tosato G. Inhibition of angiogenesis by interleukin-12 is mediated by the interferon-inducible protein 10. *Blood* 1996;87(9):3877–3882.

139. Sgadari C, Farber JM, Angiolillo AL, et al. Mig, the monokine induced by interferon-gamma, promotes tumor necrosis *in vivo*. *Blood* 1997;89(8):2635–2643.

140. Lee J, Horuk R, Rice GC, Bennett GL, Camerato T, Wood WI. Char-

141. acterization of two high affinity human interleukin-8 receptors. *J Biol Chem* 1992;267:16283–16287.

141. Moser B, Schumacher C, Von Tschamer V, Clark-Lewis I, Baggiolini M. Neutrophil-activating peptide 2 and gro/melanoma growth-stimulatory activity interact with neutrophil-activating peptide 1/interleukin 8 receptors on human neutrophils. *J Biol Chem* 1991;266:10666–10671.

142. Arvanitakis L, Geras-Raaka E, Varma A, Gershengorn MC, Cesarman E. Human herpesvirus KSHV encodes a constitutively active G-protein-coupled receptor linked to cell proliferation [see comments]. *Nature* 1997;385(6614):347–350.

143. Loetscher M, Gerber B, Loetscher P, et al. Chemokine receptor specific for IP-10 and Mig: structure, function, and expression in activated T-lymphocytes. *J Exp Med* 1996;184:963–969.

144. Detmar M, Brown LF, Claffey KP, et al. Overexpression of vascular permeability factor/vascular endothelial growth factor and its receptors in psoriasis. *J Exp Med* 1994;180(3):1141–1146.

145. Elder JT, Fisher GJ, Lindquist PB, et al. Overexpression of transforming growth factor alpha in psoriatic epidermis. *Science* 1989;243 (4892):811–814.

146. Gottlieb AB, Luster AD, Posnett DN, Carter DM. Detection of a gamma interferon-induced protein IP-10 in psoriatic plaques. *J Exp Med* 1988;168(3):941–948.

147. Crum R, Szabo S, Folkman J. A new class of steroids inhibits angiogenesis in the presence of heparin or a heparin fragment. *Science* 1985;230:1375–1378.

148. Ingber DE, Madri JA, Folkman J. A possible mechanism for inhibition of angiogenesis by angiostatic steroids: induction of capillary basement membrane dissolution. *Endocrinology* 1986;119:1768–1775.

149. Norrby K. Cyclosporine is angiostatic. *Experientia* 1992;48(11–12):1135–1138.

150. Sharpe RJ, Arndt KA, Bauer SI, Maione TE. Cyclosporine inhibits basic fibroblast growth factor-driven proliferation of human endothelial cells and keratinocytes. *Arch Dermatol* 1989;125(10):1359–1362.

151. Oikawa T, Okayasu I, Ashino H, Morita I, Murota S, Shudo K. Three novel synthetic retinoids, Re 80, Am 580 and Am 80, all exhibit anti-angiogenic activity *in vivo*. *Eur J Pharmacol* 1993;249(1):113–116.

152. Harris ED. Recent insights into the pathogenesis of the proliferative lesion in rheumatoid arthritis. *Arthritis Rheum* 1976;19:68.

153. Kimball ES, Gross JL. Angiogenesis in pannus formation. *Agents Actions* 1991;34(3–4):329–331.

154. Koch AE, Halloran MM, Hosaka S, et al. Hepatocyte growth factor. A cytokine mediating endothelial migration in inflammatory arthritis. *Arthritis Rheum* 1996;39(9):1566–1575.

155. Koch AE, Harlow LA, Haines GK, et al. Vascular endothelial growth factor. A cytokine modulating endothelial function in rheumatoid arthritis. *J Immunol* 1994;152(8):4149–4156.

156. Gilbertson-Beadling S, Powers EA, Stamp-Cole M, et al. The tetracycline analogs minocycline and doxycycline inhibit angiogenesis *in vitro* by a non-metalloproteinase-dependent mechanism [published erratum appears in Cancer Chemother Pharmacol 1995;37(1–2):194]. *Cancer Chemother Pharmacol* 1995;36(5):418–424.

157. Tamargo RJ, Bok RA, Brem H. Angiogenesis inhibition by minocycline. *Cancer Res* 1991;51(2):672–675.

158. Tilley BC, Alarcon GS, Heyse SP, et al. Minocycline in rheumatoid arthritis. A 48-week, double-blind, placebo-controlled trial. MIRA Trial Group [see comments]. *Ann Intern Med* 1995;122(2):81–89.

159. Turner-Warwick M. Precapillary systemic-pulmonary anastomoses. *Thorax* 1963;18:225–237.

160. Henke C, Knighton D, Wick M, Fiegel V, Bitterman P. Mechanisms of alveolar fibrosis following acute lung injury. Presence of angiogenesis bioactivity in the lower respiratory tract. *Chest* 1991;99(suppl 3):40S.

161. Folkman J, Watson K, Ingber D, Hanahan D. Induction of angiogenesis during the transition from hyperplasia to neoplasia. *Nature* 1989;339:58–61.

162. Hanahan D, Christofori G, Naik P, Arbeit J. Transgenic mouse models of tumour angiogenesis: the angiogenic switch, its molecular controls, and prospects for preclinical therapeutic models. *Eur J Cancer* 1996;32A(14):2386–2393.

163. Good DJ, Polverini PJ, Rastinejad F, et al. A tumor suppressor-dependent inhibitor of angiogenesis is immunologically and functionally indistinguishable from a fragment of thrombospondin. *Proc Natl Acad Sci USA* 1990;87(17):6624–6628.

164. Alvarez JA, Baird A, Tatum A, et al. Localization of basic fibroblast

growth factor and vascular endothelial growth factor in human glial neoplasms. *Mod Pathol* 1992;5(3):303–307.

165. Cornali E, Zietz C, Benelli R, et al. Vascular endothelial growth factor regulates angiogenesis and vascular permeability in Kaposi's sarcoma. *Am J Pathol* 1996;149(6):1851–1869.

166. Potgens AJ, Westphal HR, de Waal Malefyt R, Ruiter DJ. The role of vascular permeability factor and basic fibroblast growth factor in tumor angiogenesis. *Biol Chem Hoppe Seyler* 1995;376(2):57–70.

167. Rogelj S, Weinberg RA, Fanning P, Klagsbrun M. Characterization of tumors produced by signal peptide-basic fibroblast growth factor-transformed cells. *J Cell Biochem* 1989;39(1):13–23.

168. Strieter RM, Polverini PJ, Arenberg DA, et al. Role of C-X-C chemokines as regulators of angiogenesis in lung cancer. *J Leukoc Biol* 1995;57(5):752–762.

169. Fidler IJ. Critical factors in the biology of human cancer metastasis: Twenty-Eighth G.H.A. Clowes Memorial Award Lecture. *Cancer Research* 1990;50:6130–6138.

170. Holmgren L, O'Reilly MS, Folkman J. Dormancy of micrometastases: balanced proliferation and apoptosis in the presence of angiogenesis suppression [see comments]. *Nat Med* 1995;1(2):149–153.

171. Folkman J. Clinical applications of research on angiogenesis. *N Engl J Med* 1995;333(26):17597.

Inflammation: Basic Principles and Clinical Correlates, 3rd ed., edited by John I. Gallin and Ralph Snyderman. Lippincott Williams & Wilkins, Philadelphia © 1999.

CHAPTER 54

Wound Repair: An Overview

Salah Chettibi and Mark W. J. Ferguson

Wound repair is a vital process for the reestablishment of normal tissue integrity following damage in both the animal and plant kingdoms. In the animal kingdom, and particularly the higher vertebrates, the body is protected from the harsh environment of the outside world by the skin. The skin in vertebrates is composed of two layers, the epidermis and dermis, with a complex nerve and blood supply. These two tissue layers play an important role in protecting the body from any mechanical damages such as wounding. Wound repair in adult skin involves a series of overlapping and highly orchestrated events involving inflammation, reepithelialization, granulation tissue formation, and finally scar formation (1).

Tissue repair begins immediately following injury with the deposition of a fibrin clot at the site of injury to prevent hemorrhage from injured blood vessels. When tissue injury occurs, blood vessels are ruptured, resulting in severe bleeding, which causes platelets to change their appearance through a rapid crawling movement and stop bleeding. Circulating platelets are tiny discoid objects; however, at the sites of injury they quickly spread into flatter shapes to plug leaks in injured blood vessels. Platelet aggregation and activation at the site of injury results in the release of inflammatory mediators, including platelet-derived growth factors (PDGFs), transforming growth factor-α (TGF-α) and -β (TGF-β), fibroblast growth factors (FGFs), epidermal growth factor (EGF), and insulin-like growth factors (IGF) (2–5). These molecules are implicated in the initiation of the inflammatory response and in orchestrating wound repair.

Inflammation and repair of epithelial and mesenchymal structures follows immediately after blood clot formation by a coordinated process of cell migration and proliferation directed by specific biochemical mediators.

The inflammatory response of adult tissues to wounding is characterized by an early influx of neutrophils whose numbers increase steadily, peaking at 24 to 48 hours postwounding. As the number of neutrophils begin to decline, the macrophage population starts to increase.

Macrophages (Mφ) continue to accumulate at the wound site by recruitment from the circulating pool of bloodborne monocytes and, unlike neutrophils, appear to be essential for effective and efficient wound healing (6). In the meantime, reepithelialization is taking place to restore the functional barrier property of the skin. Repair of the epidermis is initiated by the loss of contact with the basement membrane (7). The process of reepithelialization occurs quickly, in days over incisions, but may extend for weeks in large areas. In chronic wounds, such as venous ulcers, it may never occur. Keratinocytes from epithelial appendages deep within the dermis and from the basal cells at the wound edge elongate and migrate across the granulation tissue. Migration of marginal keratinocytes and basal cell mitosis continue until contact with opposing epithelial cells has taken place, leading to the inhibition of cell migration and proliferation. At this time, keratinocytes resume a basal cell phenotype and differentiate into a stratified squamous keratinizing epidermis (8).

The later phases of the inflammatory response and epithelialization overlap with a period of cell proliferation and differentiation that is characterized by migration of fibroblasts and endothelial cells and the formation of granulation tissue. Mφ continues to supply matrix metalloproteinases (MMPs) that participate in the early debridement of eschar or fibrinous exudate present in the wound bed, and to provide a continuous source of growth factors and cytokines, which stimulate fibroplasia and angiogenesis. Fibroblasts become the dominant cells and collagen production and deposition predominate to form the new extracellular matrix (ECM). The development of granulation tissue is characterized by an ingrowth of

S. Chettibi and M. W. J. Ferguson: School of Biological Sciences, University of Manchester, Manchester M13 9PT, United Kingdom.

endothelial cells involved in capillary formation. This angiogenic response is vigorous in the immature granulation tissue but lessens as the granulation tissue matures and remodeling of the scar begins. During this phase, fibroblasts and Mφ continue to produce MMPs, which degrade collagen, allowing a remodeling process that can continue for several months. Scarred dermis is characterized by an abnormal morphology of the extracellular matrix (collagen) fibers, which afterward results in functional defects, e.g., contraction and contractures. This chapter summarizes the sequential events that occur during wound repair such as inflammation, reepithelialization, granulation tissue formation, and remodeling, and highlights some of the clinical problems associated with wound repair, such as chronic ulcers and hypertrophic scars.

THE ROLE OF INFLAMMATION IN WOUND REPAIR

The inflammatory response, initiated in response to injury, is characterized by a network of chemical signals that initiate and maintain the host response by stimulating endothelial cells, inducing leukocyte recruitment, and activating phagocytic functions. The series of events that occurs subsequent to trauma and antigen deposition is similar, being relatively independent of the causative agent. Initially platelets, fibrinogen, fibrin, and fibronectin form a provisional wound matrix for recruited leukocytes. Platelet aggregation and activation lead to the release of granule contents (thrombin, tissue factors, and growth factors) that initiate the inflammatory response. This inflammatory response is regulated by specific interactions between activated leukocytes and vascular endothelium. These interactions are mediated by cell adhesion molecules, which are constitutively expressed or induced on both the endothelial cells and the leukocytes. The recruitment of inflammatory cells to the site of injury occurs in four steps:

1. Rolling along the vascular endothelium is mediated by members of the selectin family. The selectins comprise a group of three related molecules. L-selectin (Lam-1, LECAM-1) is constitutively expressed on leukocytes and is shed from the cell surface upon cell activation, assumed to occur immediately after rolling begins (9). Several ligands have been identified, including at least three different heavily glycosylated mucin-like proteins [CD34, glycosylation-dependent cell adhesion molecule-1, and mucosal addresin cell adhesion molecule-1 (MAdCAM-1)] (10,11). P-selectin (GMP140 or PADGEM) is found in the membrane of secretory granules in platelets and in the Weibel-Plade bodies of endothelial cells. When stimulated with growth factors, cytokines, histamine, thrombin, bradykinin, leukotriene C_4 (LTC_4), and free radicals, the Weibel-Plade bodies fuse with the plasma membrane of the endothelial cells and P-selectin and rapidly translocate to the cell surface, where they recognize glycoproteins bearing the sialyl Lewis-X carbohydrate moieties, found on the cell surfaces of all leukocytes. The *in vivo* function of P-selectin, i.e., the induction of leukocyte rolling and subsequent extravasation, has been elegantly confirmed by experimental studies in P-selectin–deficient mice that have demonstrated an almost total absence of leukocyte rolling in mesenteric venules (12). E-selectin [endothelial leukocyte adhesion molecule-1 (ELAM-1)] is expressed solely on endothelial cells, where it is synthesized rapidly after cell stimulation by cytokines.

2. Triggering of signals activates the upregulation of leukocyte integrins. This activation is mediated by cytokine and other leukocyte-activating molecules, and permits the arrest of the rolling leukocytes. Ligand interaction of L-selectin, or antibody crosslinking in neutrophils, leads to partial activation of β_2 integrins by a signal pathway involving mitogen-activated protein kinases (13,14).

3. Tight adhesion to the vascular endothelium is mediated by two main classes of integrins that immobilize rolling leukocytes on the surface of the vascular endothelium. The $\alpha_4\beta_1$ and $\alpha_4\beta_7$ integrins bind to endothelial vascular cell adhesion molecule-1 (VCAM-1) and MAdCAM-1, respectively, and the $\alpha_L\beta_2$ (leukocyte function associated molecule-1 [LAF-1]) and $\alpha_M\beta_2$ (MAC-1) (15–17) binds to endothelial intercellular adhesion molecule (ICAM) 1, 2, and 3.

4. Transmigration occurs through the endothelium and to the site of injury. This process starts with the locomotion of adherent leukocytes toward and through the endothelial cell-cell junctions and then through the ECM, a process facilitated by proteases.

The role of adhesion molecules in leukocyte accumulation and tissue necrosis following injury were recently demonstrated using antibodies to L-selectin (CD62-L) and leukocyte β_2 integrin (CD18) (18). New Zealand white rabbits were subjected to burn injury and treated randomly with either saline (control) or monoclonal antibodies to L-selectin or CD18. Animals treated with anti–L-selectin demonstrated reduced accumulation of leukocytes after 24 hours postinjury but did not show improved wound perfusion or reduced tissue necrosis. Animals treated with anti-CD18 showed significant improvement in tissue survival and tissue perfusion but had grades of leukocyte accumulation similar to those in the control.

Platelets

When a blood vessel is injured, control of bleeding starts with the rapid adhesion of circulating platelets to the site of damage and activation of the clotting cascade leading to hemostasis. Blood platelets contribute to every aspect of hemostasis, from the initial adhesion of platelets to the vessel walls and the exposed matrix via β_1 and β_3 integrins to spreading over the surface and forming a platelet aggregate. Platelet aggregation promoted by thrombin-induced activation and degranulation of platelet $\alpha_{ii}\beta_3$ provides an activated cell surface that vastly accelerates coagulation and leads to stabilization of the platelet aggregate by fibrin (19,20). Fibrin is cross-linked and protected from the fibrinolytic enzyme plasmin by blood coagulation factor XIII, which is reported to be involved in wound healing and tissue repair. The fibrin protection is achieved mainly by covalently linking α_2-antiplasmin, the most potent physiologic inhibitor of plasmin, to fibrin (for review see ref. 21).

Platelets contain a vast number of biologically active molecules within their cytoplasmic granules including α-granules, lysozomes, and dense granules. The α-granule is a unique secretory organelle that acquires its protein content via two distinct mechanisms: (a) biosynthesis predominantly at the megakaryocyte level, which results in the production of platelet factor-4 (PF4); and (b) endocytosis and pinocytosis at both the megakaryocyte and circulating platelet levels, which results in the production of fibrinogen (Fg) and immunoglobulin G (IgG).

The currently known list of α-granular proteins that play a role in wound repair continues to enlarge and includes coagulation factors (e.g., factor V), adhesive proteins (e.g., fibrinogen, von Willebrand factor, and thrombospondin), plasma proteins (e.g., IgG and albumin), cellular mitogens [e.g., PDGFs, platelet-derived angiogenesis factor (PDAF), TGF-α, TGF-β, and basic fibroblast growth factor (bFGF)], and protease inhibitors (e.g., α_2-macroglobulin and α_2-antiplasmin) (22). The content of platelets and the fibrin plug holds the wounded tissues together and provides a provisional matrix for the recruitment of inflammatory cells and later the migration of fibroblasts endothelial and other resident cells.

Polymorphonuclear Leukocytes

Polymorphonuclear leukocytes, mainly neutrophils, are the first inflammatory cells to arrive at the wound site, and are detected within the first hour of wounding, reaching a peak between 24 and 48 hours postwounding. Recruitment of these cells from the circulating blood pool is mediated by the processes of rolling (via selectins), adhesion (via integrin β_1 and β_2 subfamilies), and migration through the endothelium (23). Migration to the site of injury is stimulated and directed by chemotactic factors such as circulating complement factor 5 (C5a), bacteria products (24), and factors released by platelets such as platelet factor-4 (PF4), PDGF, and TGF-β (25,26).

The prime function of polymorphs was long thought to be the killing and ingestion of any invading foreign anti-

gens (e.g., bacteria), and clearing the wound of fibrin matrix. These processes are achieved by the release of various proteases and oxygen radicals and by phagocytosis (27). Recently studies have emerged showing that besides the above functions, these cells also play a major role in the initiation of the wound-healing process by serving as an important source of proinflammatory cytokines. *In situ* hybridization and immunocytochemistry studies showed that the expression pattern of tumor necrosis factor-α (TNF-α) mRNA and protein in mouse skin wounds was detected in a distinct layer mainly composed of neutrophils subjacent to the wound clot (28). This layer of TNF-α–positive cells extended from the margin of one advancing epithelial outgrowth to the opposing one. The mRNA of TNF-α was apparent at 12 hours postwounding, peaked after 72 hours, and remained visible up to 120 hours postwounding (28). In a separate study Hubner et al. (29) also showed that during the early stages of wound repair the proinflammatory cytokines, interleukin-1α and β (IL-1α, β) and TNF-α were predominantly expressed by polymorphonuclear leukocytes, and that their expression was significantly reduced during wound repair in healing-impaired glucocorticoid-treated mice. The specific expression of TNF-α in the margin of the epithelial outgrowth (28), the involvement of both TNF-α and IL-1α in the modulation of MMPs, and the strong induction of the expression of keratinocyte growth factor (KGF) by IL-1 (30) emphasize the important role of neutrophils in the initiation of normal wound repair.

Mononuclear Monocytes and Mϕ

Cells belonging to the mononuclear phagocyte system are derived from bloodborne myeloid precursors that originate from the bone marrow stem cell population. Macrophage progenitors, under the influence of colony stimulating factors and differentiating inducing signals, divide, differentiate, and move into the bloodstream as circulating monocytes. Monocytes form 1% to 6% of the total circulating white blood cells. In response to tissue injury, these cells migrate from the blood pool by a mechanism similar to that of neutrophils to reach the damaged site. The recruitment of monocytes to the site of injury is mediated by various chemotactic factors released by platelets and neutrophils. Such factors include PF4, growth factors (TGF-β, PDGF) (31), chemokines (monocyte-chemoattractant protein-1, -2, and -3) (32), macrophage inflammatory protein-1α and β (33), and cytokines (IL-1β and TNF-α) (34). Recruitment of monocytes/Mϕ begins at the site of injury as the number of neutrophils begins to decline and in acute dermal incisions it reaches a peak between 5 and 7 days postwounding. This organized sequence in the deployment of these inflammatory cells to the site of injury is possibly due to the slow locomotive characteristics of monocytes compared to neutrophils. An alternative view suggests that as monocytes are important cells for the repair process, the delay in their arrival at the site of injury protects them against the harsh environment created by the neutrophils through the release of destructive molecules such as oxygen species and proteases.

Once monocytes arrive at the site of injury they rapidly differentiate into Mϕ and dendritic cells (35). The mechanisms underlying this differentiation remain poorly understood; however, it has been shown recently that the *in vitro* culture of retinal pigment epithelial cells with peripheral blood mononuclear cells promotes the maturation of monocytes to M. This effect is reversed by the addition of anti–TGF-β antibodies to the culture, suggesting a role for TGF-β in monocyte differentiation into Mϕs (36,37).

Mϕs populate virtually every tissue compartment in the body, where they perform specialized functions depending on the tissue or organ in which they reside: alveolar Mϕs in the lungs, Kupffer cells in the liver, osteoclasts in the bone, intraglomerular mesangial Mϕs in the kidney, microglia in the brain, peritoneal Mϕs, synovial type A cells, Langerhans cells, and dermal dendritic cells in the skin.

The role of Mϕ in wound healing was highlighted by experiments conducted by Leibovitch and Ross (6). The authors showed that the combined depletion of blood monocytes and local tissue Mϕ in guinea pigs resulted not only in a severe retardation of tissue debridement, but also in a marked delay in fibroblast proliferation and subsequent wound fibrosis.

Wound Mϕs have been reported to be a major source of growth factors and cytokines that recruit and activate additional Mϕs and fibroblasts at the site of injury, and promote cellular proliferation and tissue remodeling (38,39). The process of tissue remodeling by Mϕs includes (a) production of proteases such as collagenase and gelatinase and their tissue inhibitors of metalloproteinases (TIMPs), (b) synthesis and secretion of ECM molecules, and (c) factors that may restrain tissue growth once repair is completed (40). The *in vivo* production of ECM by Mϕs was demonstrated using *in situ* hybridization with probes for various fibronectin mRNAs in conjunction with collagen and lysozyme probes to distinguish the cells from fibroblasts. Two-day cutaneous excisional wounds in mice contained a large number of Mϕs that were the principal cells expressing embryonic FN mRNA. This molecule provides an ECM that facilitates wound repair (41). Mϕs were reported to be involved in the regulation of urokinase-type plasminogen activator (uPA)-mediated plasminogen activation in healing human skin wounds. Immunohistologic and zymographic studies on human skin wounds revealed that uPA was found associated with cells of granulation tissue, in particular with Mϕs and fibroblasts, whereas the uPA receptor was localized in Mϕs only (42). In addition

monocytes/Mϕs are responsible for phagocytosing and clearing areas of apoptotic cells and debris. Immunocytochemical studies using monocyte/macrophage-specific monoclonal antibody F4/80 revealed a close association between areas of programmed cell death in the remodeling interdigital region of the embryonic mouse footplate and F4/80-positive cells (43). Mϕs were shown to play a pivotal role in the modulation of angiogenesis in wound repair through the production of the angiogenic modulator thrombospondin-1 (TSP-1). *In situ* hybridization studies revealed that the primary source of TSP-1 mRNA within wounds was Mϕ-like cells. Antisense-treated wounds contained 55% to 66% less TSP-1–positive Mϕs than controls and exhibited a marked delay in the repair process. This delay included a decreased rate of reepithelialization as well as a delay in dermal reorganization (44,45).

Mϕs are the major inflammatory cells responsible for cellular debridement, recruitment of other inflammatory and fibroblastic cells, and induction of reepithelialization, cell proliferation, and regrowth of peripheral nerves (46). Implantation of granulation tissue containing mainly Mϕs into a peripheral nerve induces a conditioning effect, in that it enhances the regeneration capability of peripheral nerve endings after a test crush lesion. Granulation tissue was implanted close to the sciatic nerves and test crush lesions applied after various periods of time (0–21 days) in rats. Regeneration distance was evaluated after an additional 2, 3, 4, and 6 days. Regeneration distances were longer in granulation tissue–treated nerves than in nerves treated with subcutaneous tissue. Inactivation of the granulation tissue by freezing suppressed the conditioning effect (46). This effect on nerve regeneration by granulation tissue was attributed to the presence of Mϕs.

The importance of Mϕ in relation to wound healing has become apparent in recent years, and the development of therapeutic strategies to modulate wound repair continues to use key macrophage secretary products. Recently it has been shown that immunomodulators such as glucan phosphate that enhance macrophage function increase wound tensile strength and collagen biosynthesis (47). In addition, inhibition of macrophage accumulation in adult wounds with either neutralizing antibodies for TGF-β1 and -β2 or exogenous application of TGF-β3 significantly reduced scar formation (48).

Lymphocytes

Although macrophages have been strongly implicated in mammalian tissue repair (6), less is known concerning the role of lymphocytes in the process of adult and especially fetal wound repair. Depletion of T lymphocytes *in vivo* significantly impairs wound breaking strength and wound collagen deposition. Furthermore, continued antigenic stimulation leads to excessive fibrosis via activation of T lymphocytes that secrete a fibroblast-activating factor (49). In human skin wound biopsies, T lymphocytes have been shown to be present at the wound site from the first hour postwounding and to peak between 7 and 14 days postwounding (50). T lymphocytes have been found scattered throughout the dermis of keloid and hypertrophic scars (51). These data suggest a role for lymphocytes in both normal adult wound healing and in the genesis of abnormal scars. Hypertrophic and keloid scars showed differences in the distribution of T-lymphocyte subsets (52). CD8-positive T lymphocytes (cytotoxic T cells and natural killer cells) were the predominant inflammatory cells in both normal and hypertrophic scars; however, CD4 (helper T cells)–positive cells were the predominant inflammatory cells in keloids.

REEPITHELIALIZATION AND WOUND REPAIR

Keratinocytes

During cutaneous wound repair, keratinocytes move laterally across the healing surface. For this lateral movement epidermal cells must disassemble their tenacious connections through desmosomes to their neighboring cells and hemidesmosomes to the basement membrane, and express surface receptors that permit translocation over the ECM of the granulation tissue. Keratinocyte migration over the provisional matrix that contains fibrinogen, fibronectin, vitronectin, and tenascin involves additional cellular interactions via distinct adhesion molecules. In normal skin tissue keratinocytes reside on the basement membrane, composed primarily of laminin and type IV collagen, and express a variety of integrins along their lateral borders (53). During wound healing they become activated and migratory. The process of cell migration requires enzymes that dissolve the fibrin clot. The major fibrinolytic enzyme plasmin is derived from plasminogen. The activation of plasmin is associated with an increase in the expression of uPA and tissue-type plasminogen activator (tPA) (54). Expression of uPA receptor mRNA was found in keratinocytes at the front of the regenerative epithelial outgrowths of 12-, 48-, and 96-hour-old wounds. The signal was strongest in the keratinocytes just beginning to move 12 hours after wounding (55). In transgenic mice where the gene encoding plasminogen has been knocked out, wound reepithelialization is almost completely blocked (56). Collagenases have also been associated with the initiation of wound-edge keratinocyte migration after an acute injury in human skin. *In vivo* collagenase expression peaked in migrating keratinocytes at the wound edge at day one, then gradually decreased and was undetectable at day nine when reepithelialization was complete (57). *In vitro* studies revealed that keratinocytes proliferate twofold better on collagenase-digested matrix compared to controls and that addition of collagenase to the growth medium potentiates collagenase-induced proliferation by an additional 30%. Further cell migration is markedly stimulated when keratinocytes are plated on a biomatrix previously digested with purified collagenase and is markedly potentiated when collagenase is added to the media during the migratory response to injury (58).

Another major factor in keratinocyte migration is the increase in ECM proteins such as vitronectin, fibronectin, and collagens. Stimulation of keratinocyte migration by ECM is mediated by an increase in integrin expression (59,60), in particular $\alpha_3\beta_1$ (laminin 5 receptor), which plays an important role in the migration of keratinocytes by strongly promoting their interaction with the substratum (61,62), $\alpha_v\beta_5$ (vitronectin receptor), $\alpha_v\beta_6$ (tenascin receptor) (63), and $\alpha_5\beta_1$ (fibronectin receptor) (64). Expression of these molecules disappears when a new basement membrane is formed and epithelial integrity is achieved. *In vivo* analysis of the expression and distribution of $\alpha_5\beta_1$, $\alpha_v\beta_5$, and $\alpha_v\beta_6$ was demonstrated using full-thickness 4-mm punch biopsies taken from the inner surface of the upper arm of human adult volunteers at 3, 7 and 14 days after injury. At 3 days, $\alpha_5\beta_1$ and $\alpha_v\beta_5$, but not $\alpha_v\beta_6$, appeared around the basal and suprabasalar cells of the migrating epidermis. At 7 days, $\alpha_5\beta_1$, $\alpha_v\beta_5$, and $\alpha_v\beta_6$ appeared around the perimeter of the basal cells of the migrating epidermis. By 14 days, when reepithelialization was complete, all basal and suprabasalar cells overlaying the wound expressed $\alpha_5\beta_1$ and $\alpha_v\beta_6$, but not $\alpha_v\beta_5$, suggesting a switch of α_v heterodimeric association from β_5 to β_6 subunit during reepithelialization (65).

The importance of adhesion molecules in the migration of keratinocytes was demonstrated *in vitro* using antibodies to various integrins. Migration of human keratinocytes on vitronectin was totally inhibited by the presence of argenine-glycine-aspartic acid (RGD) tripeptide or antibodies to $\alpha_v\beta_5$ receptor on keratinocytes (66). In addition, epithelial cell migration on collagen type I or fibronectin coated substrates was completely blocked by the presence of antibody to α_5 integrin (62).

Other factors that participate in the reepithelialization process are cytokines and growth factors. These molecules are considered to be key regulators of keratinocyte proliferation, migration, and differentiation. Mertz et al. (67) showed that addition of exogenous IL-1α to partial- and full-thickness wounds stimulated epidermal migration resulting in a rapid reepithelialization. TGF-α and EGF induced epidermal regeneration of partial-thickness burns on pigs and growth and proliferation of human keratinocytes (68). However, *in vitro* studies demonstrated that addition of TGF-β1 to rabbit tracheal epithelial cells plated on different ECMs resulted in an increase in cell migration but a marked inhibition of cell proliferation. Cell shape changes, including cell spreading and lack of stratification, were associated with reduced cell-cell contacts and increased cell-substratum anchorage. This observation was supported by electron microscope studies that demonstrated that TGF-β1 induced actin cytoskeleton reorganization corresponding to development of a basal stress fiber network and a decrease of the annular cell border, without affecting the tight junctions (69).

Components of the basal lamina are deposited with epithelial cell migration but it is completely mature only after epithelialization has stopped and the cells form hemidesmosomes (70).

GRANULATION TISSUE AND REMODELING

Tissue injury is followed by formation of a provisional fibrin-containing matrix that is later replaced by granulation tissue. Replacement involves extracellular proteolysis by fibrinolytic enzymes such as plasmin, a fibrinolytic proteinase generated from ubiquitous plasminogen by cell-derived uPA. The term *granulation tissue* was originally used to describe the granular appearance of the blood vessels in the wound tissue at the time. Granulation tissue develops from the connective tissue surrounding the damaged or missing area and contains many inflammatory cells, fibroblasts, and myofibroblasts and an extensive neovasculature embedded within the loosely assembled matrix component of collagens, fibronectin, and proteoglycans. The granulation tissue is gradually replaced with more organized and elastic ECM components particularly collagen I. During the transition of granulation tissue into a mature scar, collagen remodeling depends on a balance between catabolism and continued synthesis and deposition. Fibroblasts, Mφs, and keratinocytes produce MMPs that participate in the transition from provisional matrix to collagenous scar. MMPs can be divided into three subgroups: (a) Interstitial collagenases MMP-1 and MMP-8 are involved in the initial cleavage of type I collagen, the most predominant form in skin. (b) The gelatinases MMP-2 and MMP-9 further degrade the MMP-1 cleavage products of type I collagen and degrade type IV collagen, the major form of collagen in the basement membranes. (c) Stromelysins MMP-3 and MMP-10 have a broad substrate preference for the collagens and degrade proteoglycans as well (71–74). MMP activity in the wounds are regulated by growth factors and cytokines as well as by TIMPs produced by cells in the wound.

Fibroblasts

In normal wound healing, fibroblasts appear in significant numbers at the wound site between 5 and 7 days postwounding and become the predominant cells in the wounded areas by day 10 to 14 postwounding. Fibroblasts that enter and proliferate within wound sites generally have been regarded to arise from the division, recruitment, and migration of cells from the deep dermis of sub-

cutaneous tissues beneath the panniculus carnosus muscle. Once fibroblasts are at the wound site they begin to proliferate, synthesize, and remodel a new matrix to form a connective tissue scar. Some fibroblasts progress through a series of phenotypic changes and transform into myofibroblasts that participate in wound contraction (8). The processes of fibroblast migration, proliferation, differentiation, and synthesis of ECM are mediated locally by the release of growth factors, cytokines, and ECM components. Cytokines and growth factors may directly or indirectly influence fibroblast recruitment and proliferation. PDGF may act in an autocrine or paracrine fashion to regulate cell growth. TGF-β indirectly regulates fibroblast proliferation but directly stimulates matrix production. Not only is collagen synthesis upregulated by TGF-β, but fibronectin and other matrix molecules are also increased and their degradation inhibited by the induction of TIMPs (75). ECM components serve as major substrates for fibroblast adhesion. Interaction between fibroblast adhesion molecules and their ligands (ECM) results in the initiation and activation of various cellular signaling pathways that play a vital role in fibroblast behavior (76).

Fibroblasts not only function to secrete ECM but also regulate adjacent cell behavior including migration, proliferation, and differentiation. Human skin fibroblasts when cultured with bovine aortic endothelial cells in collagen gels caused the endothelial cells to become spindle shaped and to organize into capillary-like structures within the collagen gel. In addition, fibroblast-conditioned medium also induced endothelial cells initially to elongate and subsequently to organize into a capillary-like structure within collagen gels. These *in vitro* results suggested that fibroblasts secrete soluble factors that can influence endothelial cell behavior relevant to angiogenesis with possible implications for vascularization in fibroproliferative conditions (77).

Fibroblast heterogeneity in different healing wounds can be illustrated by differences between fetal, adult, and granulation tissue cell phenotypes. Fetal fibroblasts display enhanced migratory activity compared to their adult counterparts in various tissue culture assays of cell motility (78,79). The secretion of matrix-degrading proteases, namely uPA and gelatinase A and B by fetal and adult fibroblasts, appeared to differ significantly between the two cell types. The levels of uPA and its inhibitor were notably higher in media conditioned by neonatal fibroblasts in comparison with fetal samples. By contrast, the basal level of gelatinase A was the same in both types, while the level of gelatinase B was elevated in fetal fibroblasts. TGF-β reduced the level of uPA and stimulated the secretion of plasminogen activator inhibitor-1 and progelatinase B in both neonatal and fetal fibroblasts. However, only progelatinase A and an activated form of gelatinase B were significantly elevated in fetal fibroblasts. In contrast PDGF stimulated urokinase plasminogen activator, its inhibitor, and both gelatinase A and B, an effect that was more apparent in fetal fibroblasts (80). The persistence of this behavioral difference *in vitro* suggests that it is not simply a response to differences in the fetal and adult tissue environment, but rather reflects a developmentally regulated alteration in intrinsic fibroblast phenotype.

The expression of α-smooth muscle actin in fibroblastic cells in granulation results in a different fibroblast phenotype called myofibroblast. Myofibroblasts are phenotypically unique cells that play an important role in wound contraction and the development of chronic inflammatory lesions in connective tissue, and can be induced by several agents such as growth factors, cytokines, and ECM (81). Ultrastructurally myofibroblasts appear intermediary between smooth muscle cells and fibroblasts, the main characteristics being a highly indented nucleus, parallel aligned microfilaments, and abundant rough endoblastic reticulum. They are also identified on the basis of their immunolabeling pattern for intracellular contractile proteins. Thus, myofibroblasts will label positive for a smooth actin (whereas fibroblasts will label negative) and negative for desmin (smooth muscle cells are positive) (81). A significant number of myofibroblasts undergo apoptosis in the later stages of granulation tissue maturation.

Extracellular Matrix

ECM consists of a dynamic assemblage of a variety of interacting molecules capable of reorganization in response to endogenous and exogenous stimuli. The ECM regulates wound repair by modulating cellular behaviors and phenotypes. By binding specific cytokines and growth factors, the ECM serves as an important reservoir of these potent biologic response modifiers in the microenvironment of wound repair. The growth factors and cytokines organize the geometric framework that facilitates cell migration, proliferation, and differentiation, and modulates cell-cell interaction. Interactions of the individual components of the ECM with specific cell-surface molecules, integrin receptors, or proteoglycans initiate a cascade of signal transduction pathways leading to varied short-term or persistent cellular responses (82,83). Adhesive interactions between cells and ECM proteins are important in cell attachment, migration, and proliferation. Many of the adhesive glycoproteins known to be present in the ECM during wound repair (such as collagens and fibronectins, vitronectins, osteopontins, thrombospondin, fibrinogen, and von Willebrand factor) contain the amino acid sequence RGD as their cell recognition site (84). The interactions between cells and such ECM molecules are mediated by cell-surface receptor β_1 integrins. These interactions are continuously modified by growth factors and cytokines, and are subject to feedback regulation mediated by transcriptional, posttran-

scriptional, translational, and posttranslational mechanisms elaborated during wound repair. We will briefly summarize some of the ECM components that play a major role in wound repair. For further information, consult the reviews cited.

Fibronectins (FN) are a family of adhesive glycoproteins that are predominantly found in serum development and wound healing. These 540-kd glycoproteins are a dimer of two similar polypeptide chains. Each polypeptide subunit of fibronectin is made up of repeating modular domains in addition to unique modules interacting with collagen, heparin, and fibrin. FNs arise by alternative splicing of a single gene transcript at three sites, termed EIIIA, EIIIB, and V.

During wound repair the soluble blood plasma FN that lacks the EIIIA and EIIIB domains, along with fibrin, compromises the provisional matrix that forms within minutes of tissue injury. By 2 days after cutaneous excisional wounding, total FN mRNA expression is increased locally and dramatically within the surrounding dermis, in the subjacent muscle (panniculus carnosus), and notably at the wound margins. The 2-day wound-insoluble FNs, which contain EIIIA and EIIIB domains along with fibrin, have been demonstrated to be an excellent substrate for cross-linking by transglutaminase (41). Both soluble and insoluble FNs were reported to modulate alveolar epithelial wound healing *in vitro*. Serum-free medium containing soluble fibronectin decreased the half-time of alveolar epithelial wound closure and increased the internuclear distance between two adjacent cells at the migrating edge of the wound. On the other hand, insoluble FN was a potent stimulator of alveolar type II cell motility and wound healing (85). FN fragments were also reported to modulate tissue remodeling activity by inducing MMPs in synovial fibroblasts and in cells of the periodontal ligament (86).

Collagens are a family of connective tissue proteins with a rigid and durable structure and are ubiquitous components of wound ECM. Collagens may be fibrillar (types I, II, III), nonfibrillar (type IV), or the so-called FACIT (fibril-associated collagens with interrupted triple helices) (87). In response to wounding, fibroblasts migrate into the wound bed and deposit initially collagen type III, which is gradually replaced later by collagen type I. The synthesis and deposition of collagen by fibroblasts are stimulated by various growth factors and cytokines such as TGF-β1, -β2, and -β3, PDGF, IL-1α and -1β, and IL-4. Collagen type I, which is deposited by fibroblasts at later stages of wound repair, forms the major component of the ECM. Once sufficient collagen has been produced, the expression of this critical matrix protein is shut off. Thus, in wound repair collagen production is under precise spatial and temporal expression, aberrant regulation of this process may lead to abnormal healing associated with an ulcer or hypertrophic scar (88).

Laminins are a family of ECM glycoproteins localized in the basement membrane that separates epithelial cells from the underlying dermis. They are also found in basement membranes surrounding fat, muscle, and peripheral nerve cells. This major component of the basement membrane interacts with a variety of epithelial and mesenchymal cells that includes muscle cells, adipocytes, and neurons (89). Purified laminin exhibits different biologic activities, including promotion of cell proliferation, attachment and chemotaxis, inhibition or enhancement of angiogenesis, differentiation of neuronal precursor cells, and induction of collagen type IV and tyrosine hydroxylase enzymes.

Thrombospondins (TSPs) are a family of multifunctional glycoproteins that are present in connective tissues, the α-granule of platelets, wound fluid, and embryonic tissues. TSP is secreted by platelets and most epithelial and mesenchymal cells, and incorporated into the ECM *in vitro*. TSP forms specific complexes with active TGF-β and in platelet releasate, and activates endogenous latent TGF-β, secreted by endothelial cells via a cell-and-protease–independent mechanism. It also exhibits adhesive and antiadhesive properties depending on the cell type, promotes keratinocyte attachment, and inhibits the growth and adhesion of endothelial cells and therefore inhibits angiogenesis. However matrix-bound TSP can indirectly promote microvessel formation through growth-promoting effects on fibroblast-like cells (myofibroblasts) (90).

Tenascin (Tn) is a large oligomeric glycoprotein of the ECM that is expressed in a temporally and spatially restricted pattern associated with stromal-epithelial interactions. In adult human skin, the expression level of tenascin is low but tenascin is abundantly present in the dermal compartment during embryonic development, wound repair, and in skin tumors. *In situ* hybridization studies have identified that the basal layer of keratinocytes migrating over the healing wound expresses the mRNA for tenascin. Intense expression was seen during the first 3 days after wounding, but after 7 days, when the epithelium had covered the wound, no tenascin transcripts were seen in epithelial cells (74,91).

Proteoglycans are a nonfibrillar component of the ECM made up of a core polypeptide to which linear heteropolysaccharide and glycosaminoglycans (GAG) are covalently attached either through O-glycosidic linkage to serine or through N-linked asparagine residues. GAG chains, which may be heparan sulfate (HSPG, heparan sulfate proteoglycan), chondroitin sulfate (GSPG, chondroitin sulfate proteoglycan), dermatan sulfate (DSPG), or keratan sulfate (KSPG), are all covalently attached to the core proteins except for hyaluronic acid (HA), which is unattached to a polypeptide. Decorin, biglycan, and fibromodulin are additional members of the family of ECM proteoglycans. They contain small structurally related leucine-rich repeats, bind TGF-βs, and control collagen fibril formation.

During wound repair proteoglycans bind and influence the function of multiple effector molecules such as growth factors and cytokines, matrix adhesion molecules, insoluble components of the ECM, proteases, and protease inhibitors (92). Thus, alterations in the synthesis of proteoglycans and their constituent glycosaminoglycans may result in effects on the inflammatory response, cell proliferation, migration, collagen synthesis, granulation tissue, angiogenesis, and scar formation (93). Proteoglycans are particularly prominent in scarless fetal wound healing (93,94). HA, the principal GAG in fetal tissue, has been implicated in promoting regenerative-like repair in fetal wounds. In adult wounds the deposition of HA occurs in the early stages of repair, reaches a peak, and then falls in the first 2 days due to the production and secretion of hyaluronidase. HA remains elevated at a sustained high level in the fetal normal matrix, during and after healing, and hyaluronidase is reduced (94). Enzymatic degradation of HA in healing fetal wounds resulted in scar formation; therefore, intact HA may be required to maintain scarless tissue repair. The effect of HA on wound repair may be attributed to its antiadhesive property for leukocytes and to its stimulatory effect on fibroblast migration, inhibition of fibroblast-induced collagen gel contraction, and modulation of collagen synthesis (79,95).

Syndecans, another family of cell-surface proteoglycans, also play a role in adult and in fetal skin wound repair. The expression of syndecan-1 and -4 were induced in the dermis within 12 hours after incisional injury of murine or neonatal human skin. By contrast, wounded fetal skin showed no increase in expression of syndecans. This lack of expression in fetal wounds may correlate with the low inflammatory response and lack of fibrosis in fetal wound repair (96).

Endothelial Cells

Besides their role in the initiation of the inflammatory response through their interaction with leukocytes in the early stages of wound repair, microvascular endothelial cell invasion into fibrin provisional matrix is an integral component of angiogenesis during wound repair. Formation of new capillaries by endothelial cells involves complex activities, including degradation of capillary basement membrane, migration, division, and then transformation to capillary structures (97,98). Endothelial cells upregulate $\alpha_v\beta_3$ integrins, which are expressed transiently at the tips of sprouting capillaries in the granulation tissue, and the presence of blocking peptides or antibodies against these integrins causes angiogenesis to fail and result in severely impaired wound healing (99). The process of angiogenesis involves multiple interactions between endothelial cells and the proteins of the ECM. ECM proteins can regulate endothelial cell functions, such as proliferation and chemotaxis, and may play a role in stabilizing newly formed capillaries. Growth factors and cytokines such as FGF-1, FGF-2, EGF, TGF-α, TGF-β1, hepatocyte growth factor (HGF), TNF-α, and IL-8 have also been identified as potential positive regulators of angiogenesis.

Growth Factors and Cytokines

The process of wound repair is in part orchestrated by the release of and response to growth factors and cytokines. These molecules are released by most nucleated cells in the body as potent bioactive molecules responsible for the coordination of many cell functions and interactions through autocrine and paracrine mechanisms. Since these proteins are all distinct gene products, elaborate regulation can occur at the cellular level. They are often pleiotropic with multiple overlapping functions, mainly for functional redundancy. In addition, many growth factors are produced in latent forms or linked to carrier molecules. Growth factors and cytokines can be released from the ECM during turnover, and they can be sequestered by newly deposited matrix. Growth factors and cytokines exert their effects by binding to specific receptors, which can be divided into three superfamilies: the immunoglobulin superfamily, the hematopoietin family, and the tumor necrosis factor family (5,100,101). In this section we summarize some of the important growth factors that are actively involved in the processes of wound repair.

Platelet-Derived Growth Factor

The PDGF family consists of homo- or heterodimers of products of two different genes, A-chain and B-chain, which form the dimers PDGF-AA, -AB, and -BB (102–104). PDGF isoforms are produced by platelets, Mφs, fibroblasts, and vascular endothelial cells. They exert their effects on cells by interacting with two structurally similar protein tyrosine kinase receptors. The α receptor binds both A and B chains, whereas the β receptor binds only the B chain. PDGF is a potent activator for cells of mesenchymal origin, and a stimulator of chemotaxis, proliferation, and new gene expression in monocytes/Mφs and fibroblasts, and it accelerates provisional ECM deposition (105,106). A single application of PDGF-BB to incisional wounds increased the wound breaking strength to 150% to 170% of control wounds, and thus decreased the time for healing (107,108). In an excisional wound model, in which 6-mm-wide pieces of dermis were removed from the rabbit ear down to the level of the cartilage, a single application of PDGF led to an increase of granulation tissue rich in fibroblasts and glycosaminoglycans to 200% of the control wounds after 7 days (109,110). Addition of 10 ng/mL PDGF in the presence of 0.2% fetal calf serum to wounded human periodontal ligament fibroblasts stimulated their prolifer-

ation and migration and increased ECM synthesis (111). PDGF has also been used successfully to treat human diabetic ulcers, and a commercial product has been licensed for this use.

Transforming Growth Factor-βs

TGF-βs are a family of small polypeptides secreted by virtually all cell types as biologically inactive molecules. Three mammalian isoforms of TGF-β (TGF-β1, -β2, and -β3) are expressed as latent complexes, each encoded by a unique gene on different chromosomes. Three distinct latent complexes have also been described. The small latent complex contains a noncovalent complex between the proregion latency-associated protein (LAP) and the mature C-terminal of TGF-β. The large latent complex contains an additional protein-latent TGF-β–binding protein (LTBP) covalently linked to LAP. Finally a complex between α2-macroglobulin and mature TGF-β has been described (112). These latent complexes need to be converted into active forms before the TGF-β can interact with its distinct membrane-bound receptors. The activation of latent TGF-β1 involves the manose-6-phosphate receptor, plasmin, thrombospondin, and possibly an acidic microenvironment (113,114). The ability of cells to produce TGF-β or to respond to it via cell-surface receptors is conserved throughout the animal kingdom. TGF-β was first identified as an activity able to induce anchorage-independent growth of fibroblasts. Since its identification, TGF-β has been shown to possess many important biologic activities. TGF-β1 is chemotactic for various cell types, is immunosuppressive, inhibits proliferation of most cells (but can stimulate the growth of some mesenchymal cells), induces the synthesis and inhibits the degradation of ECM, and stimulates the formation of granulation tissue (115–118). TGF-β3 binds to a cell-surface receptor complex of type I, II, and III receptors, and their intracellular responses are stimulated by serine/threonine kinases and SMAD molecules.

In experimental incisions in animals, and in models of impaired wound repair, topical application of TGF-β1 increased the wound inflammatory response and breaking strength (119,120). The increase in the wound-breaking strength was attributed to the effect of TGF-β1 on the ECM in particular collagen synthesis and deposition. Addition of TGF-β1 and -β2 neutralizing antibodies to incisional wounds in rats dramatically reduced the number of inflammatory cells, ECM deposition, and scar formation (48,121,122). In chronic gastric ulcer induced in rats by 100% acetic acid, addition of TGF-β1 neutralizing antibody significantly reduced the number of Mφs at the wound site and strongly accelerated the healing process (123). Contrariwise TGF-β3 is also antiinflammatory and produces better quality scars—an effect mediated in part by its antagonism of the effects of TGF-β1 and -β2. TGF-β1 and -β2 are present at low levels in adult wound healing; however, TGF-β3 appears late, around the onset of granulation tissue resolution, and may be one of the effects of excessive repair.

Fibroblast Growth Factors

FGFs consist of a family of nine structurally related polypeptide cytokines that include acidic fibroblast growth factor (FGF-1) (124), basic fibroblast growth factor (FGF-2) (125), Int-2 protein (FGF-3) (126), Kaposi's FGF (FGF-4) (127), FGF-5 (128), Hst-2 (FGF-6) (129), keratinocyte growth factor (FGF-7) (130), androgen inducible growth factor (FGF-8) (131), and FGF-9 (132). This family of growth factors exhibits its effects on various cell types by interacting with transmembrane high-affinity FGF receptors, which consist of four homologous protein tyrosine kinases, and with the low-affinity cell-surface heparan sulfate proteoglycan receptors known as syndecans (syndecans 1, 2, 3, and 4) (94). The expression of FGF family members during wound repair was found to increase between tenfold for FGF-1, FGF-2, and FGF-5, and 160-fold for FGF-7. However, the transcripts for other FGFs were not detected in either the wounded or unwounded tissue (133,134). Both FGF-1 and FGF-5 expression was found to peak at 24 hours postwounding, but FGF-2 expression peaked at 5 days postwounding. FGF-7 expression reached its maximum at 24 hours postwounding and remained elevated after 7 days postwounding. Exogenous application of FGFs to normal and chronic wounds resulted in acceleration of wound repair by increasing the rate of reepithelialization, enhancing granulation tissue formation and ECM deposition, and increasing angiogenesis (135). Recently, Okumura et al. (136) showed that the addition of FGF-2 to wounds enhanced granulation tissue formation in subcutaneous implants of a paper disk in normal rats, and restored its formation in healing-impaired rat models treated with steroids, chemotherapy, and x-ray irradiation. Repeated applications of FGF-2 accelerated closure of full-thickness excisional wounds in diabetic mice. Different FGFs are expressed during embryogenesis, where they act as morphogens (137-140). In embryos the function of the permissive epidermis in promoting limb outgrowth can be replaced by FGF-2 and FGF-4 (141,142), and application of FGF-2–coated beads induced amphibian limb regeneration (143).

Epidermal Growth Factor

EGF is a single polypeptide containing three disulfide bridges that are required for its biologic activity. EGF exerts its effects in target cells by binding to transmembrane protein tyrosine kinase receptors that are present in high- and low-affinity classes (144). These receptors also bind to molecules with EGF-like regions such as TGF-α, heparin-binding epidermal growth factor (HB-EGF),

amphiregulin, vaccinia virus growth factor, α- and β-neuregulin, and β-cellulin (145). Ligand occupation of EGF receptors results in the induction of signal transduction pathways that lead to the regulation of multiple functions of cells and tissues (146). EGF is present in high levels in saliva and may accelerate healing of skin lesions in animals when they lick their wounds. Topical application of EGF to human donor sites appeared to accelerate wound healing (147). TGF-α is localized in developing organs during embryogenesis and in a number of normal adult tissues. It is an autocrine/paracrine regulator of normal growth and development and often considered to be a fetal EGF (148,149). It has been implicated in wound healing and homeostasis in a number of tissues including colon, skin, mammary gland, liver, and kidney (150). TGF-α is produced by activated Mφs and keratinocytes (151,152). In wound repair TGF-α was reported to induce keratinocyte migration and proliferation (68) and promote angiogenesis through its ability to induce expression of vascular endothelial growth factor (VEGF) (153,154).

SCARRING

Wound repair in adult and fetal tissues differs on a number of clinically relevant parameters. For example, adult wound healing is essentially a reparative process, normally accompanied by scar formation. By contrast, dermal wound healing in the early gestation fetus is regenerative in nature, and usually results in a unique ability to heal without scar formation, fibrosis, or contraction (155). These fundamental differences between adult and fetal wound repair have sparked investigations into the mechanisms that govern fetal scar free wound healing and adult scarring. Fetal wound repair has been investigated in a number of animal models including human (156), monkey (157), sheep (158), rabbit (159), rat (160), chicken (43), opossum (161), and mouse (162). Such studies have contributed to the development of fetal human surgery, e.g., for well-defined anatomical birth defects such as congenital diaphragmatic hernia, and to the experimental therapeutic manipulation of adult wound healing to reduce or eliminate scarring.

Numerous studies have compared embryonic and adult healing in a search for histologic, cellular, biochemical, and molecular differences between fetal scar free healing and adult scar-forming wound repair. Documented differences are numerous and include, in the fetus, minimal inflammation, different growth factor and cytokine profiles, faster reepithelialization, minimal fibroblast proliferation, accelerated angiogenesis, more rapid turnover of ECM, and minimal contraction (163–165). However, the important question is which of these numerous differences are causative of the scar-free fetal healing phenotype. One of the factors that was once believed to be associated with scarless fetal wound repair is the environment in which fetal wounds heal. Fetal skin wounds are continuously bathed in warm, sterile amniotic fluid that is rich in growth factors and ECM, such as hyaluronic acid, tenascin, and fibronectin (94,162,166). Fetal tissue oxygenation is much less than that of adult tissue, and fetal serum contains much higher levels of insulin-like growth factor II. The role of these factors in scarless fetal wounds has been ruled out by the following findings:

1. Fetuses present in the same environment but at different stages of gestation heal differently. For example, fetal wounds heal without a scar early in gestation and begin to scar late in gestation (167–169).
2. Grafting adult skin into a fetal environment and then wounding it results in healing with a scar, whereas grafting fetal skin into an adult environment and then wounding it results in healing without scars (170, 171).
3. Scarless healing occurs in postnatal marsupials like the South American opossum, *Monodelphis domestica*, which are born at developmental stages equivalent to young amniote fetuses (161).
4. Scarless healing was also demonstrated *in vitro* in isolated fetal rat, mouse, and chicken tissues grown in organ culture media (172). However, one difference that emerged as a major causative factor between fetal scar-free and adult scarred wounds is the extent and type of inflammation and some growth factors at the wound site. Adult wound healing proceeds with a maximum inflammatory response associated with scarring; by contrast, fetal wounds heal with minimal inflammation associated with an absence of scaring. When an acute inflammatory response was evoked at the site of fetal wounds by the application of diverse agents such as bacteria and bacteria products (173), cytokines such as TGF-β (174) and PDGF (175), and burns (43), fetal wounds healed in an adult-like process with the development of scar formation. Interestingly, the addition early in adult wound healing of neutralizing antibodies to growth factors such as TGF-β1 and -β2 or PDGF resulted in a diminished scarring (48,176).

Although fetal skin in early gestation heals without scarring, other fetal organs such as muscle of the diaphragm, stomach, and peritoneum are reported to heal with a scar following injury (177,178). The difference between scarless fetal skin and the scarred fetal organs could be due to differences in the inflammatory response or to the presence of phenotypically different fibroblasts. Therefore, understanding differences between fetal dermal fibroblasts and adult fibroblasts may also lead to a better understanding of adult scar formation. The role of fibroblasts in fetal and adult wound healing and scar formation was demonstrated by placing full-thickness skin grafts from human fetuses at 18 weeks' or 24 weeks' gestational age onto athymic mice in two locations: cuta-neously onto a fascial bed, and subcutaneously in a pocket under the murine panniculus carnosus muscle. Linear incisions were made in each graft 7 days after transplantation. Grafts were harvested at 7, 14, and 21 days after. Immunocytochemistry for either human collagen type I or type III or for mouse collagen type I was performed. The cutaneous grafts healed with mouse collagen in a scar pattern, whereas the subcutaneous grafts healed with human collagen types I and III in a scarless pattern (171). Fetal fibroblasts differ from adult fibroblasts in a number of parameters, including gene expression and regulation, migration, and contraction. Human fetal fibroblasts were reported to contain much greater prolyl hydroxylase activity up to 20 weeks' gestation, which gradually decreases toward adult levels in late gestation (179). In addition, they expressed high levels of transcription factors called homeobox genes (180). These genes have been associated with the regeneration of newt limbs, and their presence in fetal skin could have a major role in scarless wound healing.

ECM synthesis and deposition is different between scarless fetal wound healing and adult wound scarring. Whitby and Ferguson (162) analyzed the spatial and temporal distribution of collagen types I, III, IV, V, and VI, fibronectin, tenascin, laminin, chondroitin, and heparin sulfates in upper lip wounds of adult, neonatal, and fetal mice. The timing of appearance and the persistence of some of these ECM molecules in fetal and adult wound healing were different. The matrix also had a different organization; the lack of scarring in fetal wounds is due to a near-perfect organization of the new matrix within the wound and scarring, not simply to a lack of excess collagen formation. Other studies have also revealed that fetal wounds are characterized by persistent and higher levels of HA and tenascin when compared with adult wounds (94,162). Ashcroft et al. (181) reported that aging alters the inflammatory response and endothelial cell adhesion molecule profiles during human cutaneous wound healing, resulting in slow epithelialization but improved quality of scarring (181). Estrogen markedly affects the degree of healing especially in postmenopausal women and is associated with an alteration in the levels of TGF-β1 (182).

WOUND-HEALING PROBLEMS

Normal Scars

Scarring in adult animal tissue occurs in virtually every injury where the integrity of that tissue has been compromised either by disease or trauma. The resulting scar is characterized by a disorganized fibrous tissue replacing the original injured tissue. This may lead to an aesthetically unpleasant scar, as in the case with the majority of injuries to skin. Following severe dermal injuries, further adverse consequences may ensue, such as contractures leading to greatly reduced function or impaired growth in children. The consequences of such scarring are often highly debilitating. With neurologic tissues even a small degree of scarring can lead to a dramatic impairment of function. Numerous pathologic lesions manifest themselves as a result of impaired function caused by scar tissue. Pulmonary fibrosis, cirrhosis of the liver, glumerulonephritis, cardiac arrhythmias, posttraumatic epilepsy, intestinal obstruction due to strictures or peritoneal adhesion, and impaired vision and hearing from scarring of the cornea or tympanic membrane are only a few examples of problems caused by scarring.

Hypertrophic Scars and Keloids

Hypertrophic scars and keloids are a major clinical problem in Asians and Africans. Both scars are characterized by the presence of an increased cellular infiltrate, excessive collagen accumulation, and fibrosis, resulting in a markedly raised scar (183). Keloids are an abnormal response to wound healing distinguished by overgrowth beyond the margin of the original injury. Keloids occur predominantly in dark-skinned individuals, and have been correlated to many factors causing an aberration in the metabolism of melanocyte-stimulating hormone. Thickened bundles of collagen in the reticular dermis oriented haphazardly often in whorls in relation to the overlying epithelium are found in keloids, in contrast to thinner collagen fibers in a more orderly arrangement that are found in normal scar. Histologic analysis of dermal excisions from both normal patients and keloid patients showed a greater HA content in keloid tissue compared with normal dermal tissue. In agreement with this observation, keloid fibroblasts were found to synthesize twice as much HA as normal dermal fibroblasts (184). Keloid fibroblasts have also been shown to be defective in their regulation of TGF-β1.

The papillary dermis in hypertrophic scars and keloids contains a perivascular infiltrate of functionally activated CD4-positive T lymphocytes, LFA-1–positive cells associated with dendritic cells, and ICAM-1-positive cells. However, CD36-positive dendritic cells and CD68-positive macrophages are found in low numbers (185). Unlike hypertrophic scars, which usually regress, keloids have a tendency to outgrow their initial boundary (186). The mainstay of treatment is compression garmenting, with surgical excision as a last resort (187). However, in the case of keloids, excision usually results in recurrence and exacerbates the condition (188).

Chronic Wound Healing

Chronic wounds in skin persist because the normal process of wound healing is disrupted. Failures may occur in the inflammation and proliferation phases of wound healing that reduce formation of granulation tissue and prevent epithelial migration to close the wound. Microbial contamination of chronic wounds also contributes to their persistence and is characteristic of venous stasis, and diabetic, arterial, and decubitus ulcers (189). In slow healing wounds, i.e., those with little granulation tissue with deep necrotic tissue and exudation, complicated by inflammation, there are depolymerization and degradation of local glycosaminoglycans, especially hyaluronic acid. A local deficit of hyaluronic acid may lead to insufficient regeneration of connective tissue, poor angiogenesis, and deficient differentiation of histiocyte and fibroblast populations leading to ulceration. Chronic wound fluids are characterized by the presence of high levels of serine proteinases, metalloproteinases including 72-kd and 94-kd gelatinases (MMP-2 and MMP-9), stromolysin-1 and -2, collagenases, elastases, and low levels of glycosaminoglycan (GAG) and TIMP-1 when compared with acute wound fluids (190–193). Each chronic wound state has an underlying pathology, e.g., chronic ischemia/reperfusion in venous ulcers, altered blood sugar and microvascular lesion in diabetes, and pressure in pressure sores. Wound therapy treatment of the underlying pathology ensures that the ulcer stays healed; in practice, many chronic ulcers recur.

The distribution of inflammatory cells in chronic wounds was analyzed using immunocytochemical studies of human skin biopsies. Samples taken from the center, the edge, and 2 cm distant from the edge of venous leg ulcers showed that in the epidermis the mean number of Langerhans cells (CD1a+) were four times lower at the edge of the ulcer compared to clinically intact epidermis 2 cm distant from the edge. The area toward the center of the ulcer and the area 2 cm distant from the edge were heavily infiltrated by macrophages (CD68+) and neutrophils (NP57+). No significant differences were observed in the distribution of T cells nor in the ratio of CD4-/CD8-positive cell subsets between the different regions of the ulcer. B cells were relatively rare in all areas (194).

Antibodies capable of recognizing the three isoforms of PDGF, AA, AB, and BB dimers, and capable of discriminating between two alternatively spliced A chain transcripts, detected very little PDGF isoform expression in normal skin and in nonhealing dermal ulcer. However, human chronic dermal wounds treated with recombinant PDGF-BB show increased healing coupled with fibroblast activation and granulation tissue formation (195).

SUMMARY

In this overview we have described the various elements that are involved in mechanisms of wound repair. The overall picture emerging from available data of fetal and adult wound repair indicates that inflammation is an important first step in initiating the repair processes. As we learn more about the cellular and molecular mechanisms of inflammation in wound healing, new therapies may emerge. Alteration or manipulation of the inflammatory response by, for example, growth factors and cytokines has already provided some clues as to how we can stimulate adult wound repair and minimize the problems associated with scarring. Therefore, interfering with the recruitment and activation of leukocytes, and manipulating their growth factor and cytokine secretion and the subsequent cell-mediated events may lead to a new wound therapy.

ACKNOWLEDGMENTS

This work was supported by a grant from Smith & Nephew for which we are grateful.

REFERENCES

1. Clark RAF. Wound repair overview and general consideration. In: Clark RAF, ed. *The molecular and cellular biology of wound repair.* New York: Plenum Press, 1996:3–35.
2. Seppa H, Grotendorst G, Seppa S, Schiffmann E, Martin GR. Platelet-derived growth-factor chemotactic for fibroblasts. *J Cell Biol* 1982; 92:584–588.
3. Grotendorst GR, Chang T, Seppa HEJ, Kleinman HK, Martin GR. Platelet-derived growth-factor is a chemoattractant for vascular smooth-muscle cells. *J Cell Physiol* 1982;113:261–266.
4. Derynck R, Lindquist PB, Bringman TS, Winkler ME. Transforming growth factor-α- structure, expression and biological-activities. *Biophys J* 1988;53:207.
5. Moulin V. Growth-factors in skin wound-healing. *Eur J Cell Biol* 1995;68:1–7.
6. Leibovitch SJ, Ross R. The role of the macrophage in wound repair. A study with hydrocortisone and anti-macrophage serum. *Am J Pathol* 1975;78:71–91.
7. Saarialhokere UK, Kovacs SO, Pentland AP, Olerud JE, Welgus HG, Parks WC. Cell-matrix interactions modulate interstitial collagenase expression by human keratinocytes actively involved in wound-healing. *J Clin Invest* 1993;92:2858–2866.
8. Schaffer CJ, Nanney LB. Cell biology of wound-healing. *Int Rev Cytol Surv Cell Biol* 1996;169:151–181.
9. Kishimoto TK, Jutila MA, Berg EL, Butcher EC. Neutrophil Mac-1 and MEL-14 adhesion proteins inversely regulated by chemotactic factors. *Science* 1989;245:1238–1241.
10. Rosen SD, Bertozzi CR. The selectins and their ligands. *Curr Opin Cell Biol* 1994;6:663–673.
11. Baumheter S, Singer MS, Henzel W, et al. Binding of L-selectin to the vascular sialomucin CD34. *Science* 1993;262:436–438.
12. Mayadas TN, Johnson RC, Rayburn H, Hynes RO, Wagner DD. Leukocyte rolling and extravasation are severely compromised in P-selectin–deficient mice. *Cell* 1993;74:541–554.
13. Waddell TK, Fialkow L, Chan CK, Kishimoto TK, Downey GP. Signaling functions of L-selectin—enhancement of tyrosine phosphorylation and activation of MAP kinase. *J Biol Chem* 1995;270: 15403–15411.
14. Simon DI, Xu H, Rao NK, Meckel CR. Monoclonal-antibody directed against the platelet IIB/IIIA receptor cross-reacts with the leukocyte integrin MAC-1 and blocks adhesion to fibrinogen and ICAM-1. *Circulation* 1995;92:SS, 519.
15. Springer TA. Traffic signals for lymphocyte recirculation and leukocyte emigration—the multistep paradigm. *Cell* 1994:76:301–314.
16. Albelda SM, Smith CW, Ward PA. Adhesion molecules and inflammatory injury. *FASEB J* 1994;8:504–512.
17. Imhof BA, Dunon D. Leukocyte migration and adhesion. *Adv Immunol* 1995;58:345–416.
18. Nwariaku FE, Sikes PJ, Lightfoot E, Mileski WJ. Inhibition of selectin-mediated and integrin-mediated inflammatory response after burn injury. *J Surg Res* 1996;63:355–358.
19. Albelda SM, Buck CA. Integrins and other cell-adhesion molecules. *FASEB J* 1990;4:2868–2880.
20. Andrews RK, Lopez JA, Berndt MC. Molecular mechanisms of platelet adhesion and activation. *Int J Biochem Cell Biol* 1997;29: 91–105.
21. Muszbek L, Adany R, Mikkola H. Novel aspects of blood-coagulation factor XIII. 1. Structure, distribution, activation, and function. *Crit Rev Clin Lab Sci* 1996;33:357–42120.
22. Harrison P, Cramer EM. Platelet α-granules. *Blood Rev* 1993;7: 52–62.
23. Menger MD, Vollmar B. Adhesion molecules as determinants of disease from molecular biology to surgical research. *Br J Surg* 1996; 83:588–601.
24. Marder SR, Chenoweth DE, Goldstein IM, Perez HD. Chemotactic responses of human peripheral-blood monocytes to the complement-derived peptides c5a and c5a. *J Immunol* 1985;134;3325–3331.
25. Deuel TF, Senior RM, Chang D, Griffin GL, Heinrikson RI, Kaiser ET. Platelet factor-4 is chemotactic for neutrophils and monocytes. *Proc Natl Acad Sci USA* 1981;78:4584–4587.
26. Matsui T, Pierce JH, Fleming TP, et al. Independent expression of human alpha-derived or beta-derived platelet-derived growth-factor receptor cDNAs in a naïve hematopoietic cell leads to functional coupling with mitogenic and chemotactic signaling pathways. *Proc Natl Acad Sci USA* 1989;86:8314–8318.
27. Grinnell F, Zhu MF. Identification of neutrophil elastase as the proteinase in burn wound fluid responsible for degradation of fibronectin. *J Invest Dermatol* 1994;103:155–161.
28. Feiken E, Romer J, Eriksen J, Lund LR. Neutrophils express tumor necrosis factor-alpha during mouse skin wound-healing. *J Invest Dermatol* 1995;105:120–123.
29. Hubner G, Brauchle M, Smola H, Madlener M, Fassler R, Werner S. Differential regulation of pro-inflammatory cytokines during wound-healing in normal and glucocorticoid-treated mice. *Cytokine* 1996;8:548–556.
30. Chedid M, Rubin JS, Csaky KG, Aaronson SA. Regulation of keratinocyte growth-factor gene-expression by interleukin-1. *J Biol Chem* 1994;269:10753–10757.
31. Cromack DT, Porrasreyes B, Mustoe TA. Current concepts in wound-healing growth-factor and macrophage interaction. *J Trauma* 1990;30: S129–S133.
32. Ham JM, Kunkel SL, Dibb CR, Standiford TJ, Rolfe MW, Strieter RM. Chemotactic cytokine (IL-8 and MCP-1) gene-expression by human whole-blood. *Immunol Invest* 1991;20:387–394.
33. Sherry B, Tekampolson P, Gallegos C, et al. Resolution of the 2 components of macrophage inflammatory protein-1, and cloning and characterization of one of those components, macrophage inflammatory protein-1-beta. *J Exp Med* 1988;168:2251–2259.
34. Lake FR, Noble PW, Henson PM, Riches DWH. Functional switching of macrophage responses to tumor-necrosis-factor-alpha (TNF-alpha) by interferons: implications for the pleiotropic activities of TNF-alpha. *J Clin Invest* 1994;93:1661–1669.
35. Riches DWH. Macrophage involvement in wound repair, remodeling and fibrosis. In: Clark RAF, ed. *The molecular and cellular biology of wound repair.* New York: Plenum Press, 1996:95–135.
36. Bombara C, Ignotz RA. TGF-beta inhibits proliferation of and promotes differentiation of human promonocytic leukemia cells. *J Cell Physiol* 1992;153:30–37.
37. Osusky R, Malik P, Ryan SJ. Retinal pigment epithelium cells promote the maturation of monocytes to macrophages *in vitro. Ophthalmic Res* 1997;29:31–36.
38. Plemons JM, Dill RE, Rees TD, Dyer BJ, Ng MG, Iacopino AM. PDGF-B producing cells and PDGF-B gene-expression in normal gingiva and cyclosporine-A-induced gingival overgrowth. *J Periodontol* 1996;67:264–270.
39. Fritsch J, Simon Assmann P, Kedinger M, Evans GS. Cytokines modulate fibroblast phenotype and epithelial-stroma interactions in rat intestine. *Gastroenterology* 1997;112:826–838.
40. Pentland AP, Shapiro SD, Welgus HG. Agonist-induced expression of tissue inhibitor of metalloproteinases and metalloproteinases by human macrophages is regulated by endogenous prostaglandin E2 synthesis. *J Invest Dermatol* 1995;104:52–57.
41. Brown LF, Dubin D, Lavigne L, Logan B, Dvorak HF, Vandewater L.

Macrophages and fibroblasts express embryonic fibronectins during cutaneous wound healing. *Am J Pathol* 1993;142:793–801.

42. Schafer BM, Maier K, Eickhoff U, Todd RF, Kramer MD. Plasminogen activation in healing human wounds. *Am J Pathol* 1994;144: 1269–1280.

43. Hopkinson-Woolley J, Hughes D, Gordon S, Martin P. Macrophage recruitment during limb development and wound healing in the embryonic and foetal mouse. *J Cell Sci* 1994;107:1159–1167.

44. Dipietro LA, Nissen NN, Gamelli RL, Koch AE, Pyle JM, Polverini PJ. Thrombospondin-1 synthesis and function in wound repair. *Am J Pathol* 1996;148:1851–1860.

45. Dipietro LA. Wound healing—the role of macrophages and other immune cells. *Shock* 1995;4:233–240.

46. Miyauchi A, Kanje M, Danielsen N, Dahlin LB. Role of macrophages in the stimulation and regeneration of sensory nerves by transposed granulation tissue and temporal aspects of the response. *Scand J Plast Reconst Surg Hand Surg* 1997;31:17–23.

47. Portera CA, Love EJ, Memore L, et al. Effect of macrophage stimulation on collagen biosynthesis in the healing wound. *Am Surg* 1997;63: 125–130.

48. Shah M, Foreman DM, Ferguson MWJ. Neutralization of TGF-beta(1) and TGF-beta(2) or exogenous addition of TGF-beta(3) to cutaneous rat wounds reduces scarring. *J Cell Sci* 1995;108:985–1002.

49. Peterson JM, Barbul A, Breslin RJ, Wasserkrug HL, Efron G. Significance of T-lymphocytes in wound healing. *Surgery* 1987;102: 300–305.

50. Martin CW, Muir IFK. The role of lymphocytes in wound healing. *Br J Plast Surg* 1990;43:655–662.

51. Borgognoni L, Pimpinelli N, Martini L, Brandani P, Reali UM. Immuno-histologic features of normal and pathological scars—possible clues to the pathogenesis. *Eur J Dermatol* 1995;5:407–412.

52. Appleton I, Floyd H, Ferguson MWJ. Differential lymphocyte profiles in hypertrophic and keloid scars: implications for scar formation. Submitted.

53. Luscinskas FW, Lawler J. Integrins as dynamic regulators of vascular function. *FASEB J* 1994;8:929–938.

54. Quax PHA, Boxman LA, Vankesteren CAM, Verheijen JH, Ponec M. Plasminogen activators are involved in keratinocyte and fibroblast migration in wounded cultures *in-vitro*. *Fibrinolysis* 1994;8:221–228.

55. Romer J, Lund LR, Eriksen J, Pyke C, Kristensen P, Dano K. The receptor for urokinase-type plasminogen-activator is expressed by keratinocytes at the leading skin during reepithelization. *J Invest Dermatol* 1994;102:519–522.

56. Romer J, Bugge TH, Pyke C, et al. Impaired wound-healing in mice with a disrupted plasminogen gene. *Nature Med* 1996;2:287–292.

57. Inoue M, Kratz G, Haegerstrand A, Stahle-Bbackdahle M. Collagen expression is rapidly induced in wound edge keratinocytes after acute injury in human skin, persists during healing, and stops at reepithelialization. *J Invest Dermatol* 1995;104:1458–1469.

58. Herman IM. Stimulation of human keratinocyte migration and proliferation *in vitro* insights into the cellular responses to injury and wound-healing. *Wounds Compendium Clin Res Pract* 1996;8:33–41.

59. Watt FM, Jones PH. Expression and function of keratinocyte integrins. *Development* 1993;SS:185–192.

60. Jones PH, Watt FM. Separation of human epidermal stem-cells from transit amplifying cells on the basis of differences in integrin function and expression. *Cell* 1993;73:713–724.

61. Woodley DT. Reepithelialization. In: Clark RAF, ed. *The molecular and cellular biology of wound repair*. New York: Plenum Press, 1996; 239–308.

62. Zhang K, Maida N, Richards DW, Kramer RH. Role of alpha-6-beta-4 integrin in keratinocyte deposition of endogenous laminin-5. *J Dental Res* 1996;75:1637.

63. Haapasalmi K, Zhang K, Tonnesen M, et al. Keratinocytes in human wounds express alpha-v-beta-6 integrin. *J Invest Dermatol* 1996;106: 42–48.

64. Juhasz I, Murphy GF, Yan HC, Herlyn M, Albelda SM. Regulation of extracellular-matrix proteins and integrin cell-substratum adhesion receptors on epithelium during cutaneous human wound-healing *in-vivo*. *Am J Pathol* 1993;143:1458–1469.

65. Clark RAF, Ashcroft GS, Spencer MJ, Larjava H, Ferguson MWJ. Reepithialization of normal human excisional wounds is associated with a switch from alpha-v-beta-5 to alpha-v-beta-6 integrins. *Br J Dermatol* 1996;135:46–51.

66. Kim JP, Zhang K, Chen JD, Kramer RH, Woodley DT. Vitronectin-driven human keratinocyte locomotion is mediated by the alpha-v-beta-5 integrin receptor. *J Biol Chem* 1994;269:26926–26932.

67. Mertz PM, Sauder DL, Davis SC, Kilian PL, Herron AJ, Eaglstein WH. IL-1 as a potent inducer of wound reepithelization. In: *Clinical and experimental approaches to dermal and epidermal repair: normal and chronic wounds*. New York: Wiley-Liss, 1991:473–480.

68. Schultz G, Rotatori DS, Clark W. EGF and TGF-alpha in wound-healing and repair. *J Cell Biochem* 1991;45:346–352.

69. Boland S, Boisvieuxulrich E, Houcine O, et al. TGF-beta-1 promotes actin cytoskeleton reorganization and migratory phenotype in epithelial tracheal cells in primary culture. *J Cell Sci* 1996;109:2207–2219.

70. Grinnell F. Wound repair, keratinocyte activation and integrin modulation. *J Cell Sci* 1992;101:1–5.

71. Salo T, Makela M, Kylmaniemi M, Autioharmainen H, Larjava H. Expression of matrix metalloproteinase-2 and metalloproteinase-9 during early human wound-healing. *Lab Invest* 1994;70:176–182.

72. Polarek JW, Clark RAF, Pickett MP, Pierschbacher MD. Development of a provisional extracellular-matrix to promote wound-healing. *Wounds Compendium Clin Res Pract* 1994;6:46–53.

73. Tomasbarberan S, Schultz GS, Tarnuzzer RW, Fagerholm P. Detection and measurement of messenger RNAs for TGF-alpha, TGF-beta(1), EGF-R MMP2, MMP9, TIMP1 and collagen (alpha-1) III in normal human corneal epithelium and after myopic regression following excimer-laser photorefractive keratectomy. *Invest Ophthalmol Visual Sci* 1996;37:2097.

74. Aukhil I, Sahlberg C, Thesleff I. Basal layer of epithelium expresses tenascin messenger-RNA during healing of incisional skin wounds. *J Periodont Res* 1996;31:105–112.

75. Wahl SM. Inflammation and growth factor. *J Urol* 1997;157:303–305.

76. Ridelly AJ, Hall A. The small GTP-binding protein rho regulates the assembly of focal adhesions and actin stress fibers in response to growth factors. *Cell* 1992;70:389–399.

77. Kuzuya M, Kinsella JL. Induction of endothelial-cell differentiation *in-vitro* by fibroblast-derived soluble factors. *Exp Cell Res* 1994;215: 310–318.

78. Schor SL, Schor AM, Grey AM, et al. Mechanism of action of the migration stimulating factor produced by fetal and cancer patient fibroblasts effect on hyaluronic-acid synthesis *in vitro*. *Cell Dev Biol* 1989;25:737–746.

79. Ellis I, Banyard J, Schor SL. Differential response of fetal and adult fibroblasts to cytokines: cell migration and hyaluronan synthesis. *Development* (in press).

80. Cullen B, Silcock D, Brown LJ, Gosiewska A, Geesin JC. The differential regulation and secretion of proteinases from fetal and neonatal fibroblasts by growth factors. *Int J Biochem Cell Biol* 1997;29: 241–250.

81. Gabbiani G. Modulation of fibroblastic cytoskeletal features during wound healing and fibrosis. *Pathol Res Pract* 1994;190:851–853.

82. Raghow R. The role of extracellular-matrix in postinflammatory wound healing and fibrosis. *FASEB J* 1994;8:823–831.

83. Macneil S. What role does the extracellular-matrix serve in skin-grafting and wound healing. *Burns* 1994;20:S67–S70.

84. Polarek JW, Clark RAF, Pickett MP, Pierschbacher MD. Development of a provisional extracellular-matrix to promote wound-healing. *Wounds Compendium Clin Res Pract* 1994;6:46–53.

85. Garat C, Kheradmand F, Albertine KH, Folkesson HG, Matthay MA. Soluble and insoluble fibronectin increases alveolar epithelial wound-healing *in-vitro*. *Am J Physiol Lung Cell Mol Physiol* 1996;15: L844–L853.

86. Kapila YL, Kapila S, Johnson PW. Fibronectin and fibronectin fragments modulate the expression of proteinases and proteinase-inhibitors in human periodontal-ligament cells. *Matrix Biol* 1996;15: 251–261.

87. Eckes B, Aumailley M, Kreig T. Collagens and the reestablishment of dermal integrity. In: Clark RAF, ed. *The molecular and cellular biology of wound repair*. New York: Plenum Press, 1996:493–512.

88. Kreig T. Collagen in the healing wounds. *Wounds Compendium Clin Res Pract* 1995;7:A5–A12.

89. Malinda KM, Kleinman HK. The laminins. *Int J Biochem Cell Biol* 1996;28:957–959.

90. Nicosia RF, Tuszynski GP. Matrix-bound thrombospondin promotes angiogenesis *in-vitro*. *J Cell Biol* 1994;124:183–193.

91. Latijnhouwers M, Bergers M, Ponec M, Dijkman H, Andriessen M,

Schalkwijk J. Human epidermal keratinocytes are a source of tenascin-C during wound healing. *J Invest Dermatol* 1997;108: 776–783.

92. Reiland J, Rapraeger AC. Heparan-sulfate proteoglycan and FGF receptor target basic FGF to different intracellular destinations. *J Cell Sci* 1993;105:1085–1093.

93. Gallo RL, Bernfield M. Proteoglycans and their role in wound repair. In: Clark RAF, ed. *The molecular and cellular biology of wound repair.* New York: Plenum Press, 1996:475–492.

94. Longaker MT, Chiu ES, Adzick NS, Stern M, Harrison MR, Stern R. Studies in fetal wound-healing. 5. A prolonged presence of hyaluronic-acid characterizes fetal wound fluid. *Ann Surg* 1991;213: 292–296.

95. Dillon PW, Keefer K, Blackburn JH, Houghton PE, Krummel TM. The extracellular-matrix of the fetal wound-hyaluronic-acid controls lymphocyte adhesion. *J Surg Res* 1994;57:170–173.

96. Gallo R, Kim C, Kokenyesi R, Adzick NS, Bernfield M. Syndecan-1 and syndecan-4 are induced during wound repair of neonatal but not fetal skin. *J Invest Dermatol* 1996;107:676–683.

97. Folkman J, Klagsbrun M. Angiogenic factors. *Science* 1987;235: 442–447.

98. Folkman J, Klagsbrun M. A family of angiogenic peptides. *Nature* 1987;329:671–672.

99. Martin P. Wound healing—aiming for perfect skin regeneration. *Science* 1997;276:75–81.

100. Davidson JM. Growth-factors in wound-healing. *Wounds Compendium Clin Res Pract* 1995;7:A53–A64.

101. Feliciani C, Amerio P, Pour SM, et al. IL-1-alpha, IL-6 and TNF-alpha in cutaneous lesions of lupus-erythematosus are inhibited by topical application of calcipotriol. *Int J Immunopathol Pharmacol* 1995;8: 199–207.

102. Ross R, Bowenpope DF, Raines EW. Platelet-derived growth-factor and its role in health and disease. *Philosophic Trans R Soc Lond [B] Biol Sci* 1990;327:155–169.

103. Hart CE, Bailey M, Curtis DA, et al. Purification of PDGF-AB and PDGF-BB from human-platelet extracts and identification of all 3 PDGF dimers in human-platelets. *Biochemistry* 1990;29:166–172.

104. Meyer-Iingold W, Eichner W. Platelet-derived growth-factor. *Cell Biol Int* 1995;19:389–398.

105. Shure D, Griffin GL, Pierce GF, Deuel TF, Senior RM. Recombinant platelet-derived growth-factor (PDGF)—a chain is chemotactic for granulocytes, monocytes, and fibroblasts. *Clin Res* 1991;39:P.A 279.

106. Pierce GF, Vandeberg J, Rudolph R, Tarpley J, Mustoe TA. Platelet-derived growth-factor-BB and transforming growth factor-beta1 selectively modulate glycosaminoglycans, collagen, and myofibroblasts in excisional wounds. *Am J Pathol* 1991;138:629–646.

107. Pierce GF, Mustoe TA, Senior RM, et al. *In vivo* incisional wound-healing augmented by platelet-derived growth-factor and recombinant c-sis gene homodimeric proteins. *J Exp Med* 1988;167:974–987.

108. Pierce GF, Mustoe TA, Lingelbach J, et al. Platelet-derived growth-factor and transforming growth factor-beta enhance tissue-repair activities by unique mechanisms. *J Cell Biol* 1989;109:429–440.

109. Mustoe TA, Pierce GF, Morishima C, Deuel TF. Growth factor-induced acceleration of tissue repair through direct and inductive activities in a rabbit dermal ulcer model. *J Clin Invest* 1991;87:694–703.

110. Pierce GF, Mustoe TA, Altrock BW, Deuel TF, Thomason A. Role of platelet-derived growth-factor in wound-healing. *J Cell Biochem* 1991;45:319–326.

111. Bartold PM, Raben A. Growth-factor modulation of fibroblasts in simulated wound-healing. *J Periodont Res* 1996;31:205–216.

112. Hinck AP, Archer SJ, Qian SW, et al. Transforming growth-factor-beta-1-3-dimensional structure in solution and comparison with the x-ray structure of transforming growth-factor-beta2. *Biochemistry* 1996; 35:8517–8534.

113. Lawrence DA. Transforming growth-factor-beta—a general review. *Eur Cytokine Network* 1996;7:363–374.

114. Feige JJ, Quirin N, Souchelnitskiy S. TGF-beta, a biological peptide under control—latent forms and mechanisms of activation. *Med Sci* 1996;12:929–939.

115. Roberts AB, Sporn MB. Transforming growth factor-b. In: Clark, RAF ed. *The molecular and cellular biology of wound repair.* New York: Plenum Press, 1996:275–311.

116. Grande JP. Role of transforming growth factor-beta in tissue injury and repair. *Proc Soc Exp Biol Med* 1997;214:27–40.

117. Ferguson MWJ. Role of transforming growth-factor-beta isoforms in wound healing. *Immunology* 1996;89:So 50.

118. O'Kane S, Ferguson MWJ. Transforming growth factor betas and wound healing. *Int J Biochem Cell Biol* 1997;29:63–78.

119. Pierce GF, Mustoe TA, Lingelbach J, Masakowski VR, Gramates P, Deuel TF. Transforming growth factor-beta reverses the glucocorticoid-induced wound-healing deficit in rats—possible regulation in macrophages by platelet-derived growth-factor. *Proc Natl Acad Sci USA* 1989;86:2229–2233.

120. Pierce GF, Brown D, Mustoe TA. Quantitative analysis of inflammatory cell influx, procollagen type-i synthesis, and collagen cross-linking in incisional wounds—influence of PDGF-BB and TGF-beta-1 therapy. *J Lab Clin Med* 1991;117:373–382.

121. Shah M, Foreman DM, Ferguson MWJ. Control of scarring in adult wounds by neutralizing antibody to transforming growth-factor-beta. *Lancet* 1992;339:213–214.

122. Shah M, Foreman DM, Ferguson MWJ. Neutralizing antibody to TGF-beta(1,2) reduces cutaneous scarring in adult rodents. *J Cell Sci* 1994;107:1137–1157.

123. Ernst H, Konturek P, Hahn EG, Brzozowski T, Konturek SJ. Acceleration of wound healing in gastric ulcers by local injection of neutralizing antibody to transforming growth factor beta-1. *Gut* 1996;39: 172–175.

124. Thomas KA, Riley MC, Lemmon SK, Baglan NC, Bradshaw RAS. Brain derived fibroblast growth factor: nonidentity with myelin basic protein. *J Biol Chem* 1980;255:5517–5520.

125. Abraham JA, Whang JL, Tumolo A, et al. Human basic fibroblast growth factor: nucleotide sequence and genomic organization. *EMBO J* 1986;5:2523–2528.

126. Dickson C, Peters G. Potential oncogene product related to growth factors. *Nature* 1987;326:830–833.

127. DeliBovi P, Curatola AM, Kern FG, Greco A, Ittman M, Basilico C. An oncogene isolated by transfection of Kaposi's sarcoma DNA encodes a growth factor that is a member of the FGF family. *Cell* 1987;50:729–737.

128. Zhan XI, Bates B, Hu XG, Goldfarb M. The human FGF-5 oncogene encodes a novel protein related to fibroblast growth-factors. *Mol Cell Biol* 1988;8:3487–3495.

129. Marics I, Adelaide J, Raybaud F, et al. Characterization of the hst-related FGF-6 gene, a new member of the fibroblast growth-factor gene family. *Oncogene* 1989;4:335–340.

130. Finch PW, Rubin JS, Miki T, Ron D, Aaronson SA. Human KGF is FGF-related with properties of a paracrine effector of epithelial-cell growth. *Science* 1989;245:752–755.

131. Tanaka A, Miyamoto K, Minamino N, et al. Cloning and characterization of an androgen-induced growth of mouse mammary carcinoma cells. *Proc Natl Acad Sci USA* 1992;89:8928–8932.

132. Miyamoto M, Naruo KI, Seko C, Matsumoto S, Kondo T, Kurokawa T. Molecular cloning of a novel cytokine cDNA encoding the ninth member of the fibroblast growth factor family, which has a unique secretion property. *Mol Cell Biol* 1993;13:4251–4259.

133. Werner S, Peters KG, Longaker MT, Fullerpace F, Banda MJ, Williams LT. Large induction of keratinocyte growth factor expression in the dermis during wound healing. *Proc Natl Acad Sci USA* 1992;89:6896–6900.

134. Werner S, Smola H, Liao X, Longaker MT, Kreig T. The function of KGF in morphogenesis of epithelium and reepithelialization of wounds. *Science* 1994;266:819–822.

135. Slavin J. Fibroblast growth-factors—at the heart of angiogenesis. *Cell Biol Int* 1995;19:431–444.

136. Okumura M, Okuda T, Okamoto T, Nakamura T, Yajima M. Enhanced angiogenesis and granulation-tissue formation by basic fibroblast growth factor in healing impaired animals. *Arzneimittelforschung Drug Res* 1996;46:1021–1026.

137. Rappolee DA, Basilico C, Patel Y, Werb Z. Expression and function of FGF-4 in periimplantation development in mouse embryos. *Development* 1994;120:2259–2269.

138. Ohuchi H, Yoshioka H, Tanaka A, Kawakami Y, Nohno T, Noji S. Involvement of androgen-induced growth-factor (FGF-8) gene in mouse embryogenesis and morphogenesis. *Biochem Biophys Res Commun* 1994;204:882–888.

139. Heikinheimo M, Lawshe A, Shackleford GM, Wilson DB, Macarthur CA. FGF-8 expression in the post-gastrulation mouse suggests roles in the development of the face, limbs and central nervous system. *Mech Dev* 1994;48:129–138.

140. Niswander L, Martin GR. FGF-4 expression during gastrulation, myogenesis, limb and tooth development in the mouse. *Development* 1992;114:755–768.

141. Niswander L, Martin GR. FGF-4 and BMP-2 have opposite effects on limb growth. *Nature* 1993;361:68–71.

142. Niswander L, Tickle C, Vogel A, Booth I, Martin GR. FGF-4 replaces the apical ectodermal ridge and directs outgrowth and patterning of the limb. *Cell* 1993;75:579–587.

143. Mullen LM, Bryant SV, Torok MA, Blumberg B, Gardiner DM. Nerve dependency of regeneration—the role of distal-less and FGF signaling in amphibian limb regeneration. *Development* 1996;122:3487–3497.

144. Boonstra J, Rijken P, Humbel B, Cremers F, Verkleij A, Henegouwen PVE. The epidermal growth-factor. *Cell Biol Int* 1995;19:413–430.

145. Mutsaers SE, Bishop JE, Mcgrouther G, Laurent GJ. Mechanisms of tissue repair: from wound healing to fibrosis. *Int J Biochem Cell Biol* 1997;29:5–17.

146. Nanney LB, Sundberg JP, King LE. Increased epidermal growth-factor receptor fsn/fsn mice. *J Invest Dermatol* 1996;106:1169–1174.

147. Falanga V, Eaglstein WH, Bucalo B, Katz MH, Harris B, Carson P. Topical use of human recombinant epidermal growth-factor (H-EGF) in venous ulcers. *J Dermatol Surg Oncol* 1992;18:604–606.

148. Wilcox JN, Derynck R. Developmental expression of transforming growth factors alpha and beta in mouse fetus. *Mol Cell Biol* 1988;8:3415–3422.

149. Dixon MJ, Foreman D, Schor S, Ferguson MWJ. Epidermal growth-factor and transforming growth-factor-alpha regulate extracellular-matrix production by embryonic mouse palatal mesenchymal cells cultured on a variety of substrata. *Rouxs Arch Dev Biol* 1993;203:140–150.

150. Wilcox JN, Derynck R. Developmental expression of transforming growth factors alpha and beta in mouse fetus. *Mol Cell Biol* 1988;8:3415–3422.

151. Wong DT, Weller PF, Galli SJ, et al. Human eosinophils express transforming growth factor α. *J Exp Med* 1990;172:673–681.

152. Coffey RJ, Derynck R, Wilcox JN, et al. Production and auto-induction of transforming growth factor alpha in human keratinocytes. *Nature* 1987;328:817–820.

153. Barrandon Y, Green H. Cell-migration is essential for sustained growth of keratinocyte colonies—the roles of transforming growth factor-alpha and epidermal growth-factor. *Cell* 1987;50:1131–1137.

154. Senger DR, Vandewater L, Brown LF, et al. Vascular-permeability factor (VPF, VEGF) in tumor biology. *Cancer Metastasis Rev* 1993;12:303–324.

155. Ferguson MWJ, Whitby DJ, Shah MJ, Siebert JW, Longaker MT. Scar formation: the spectral nature of fetal and adult wound repair. *Plast Reconst Surg* 1996;97:854–860.

156. Lin RY, Sullivan KM, Argenta PA, Meuli M, Lorenz HP, Adzick NS. Exogenous transforming growth-factor-beta amplifies its own expression and induces scar formation in a model of human fetal skin repair. *Ann Surg* 1995;222:146–154.

157. Sopher DA. Study of wound healing in the fetal tissues of the cynomologus monkey. *Lab Animal Handbooks* 1975;6:327–335.

158. Burrington JD. Wound healing in fetal lamb. *J Pediatr Surg* 1971;6:523–528.

159. Krummel TM, Nelson JM, Diegelmann RF, et al. Fetal response to injury in the rabbit. *J Pediatr Surg* 1987;22:640–644.

160. Roswell AR. The intrauterine healing of fetal muscle wounds: experimental study in the rat. *Br J Plast Surg* 1984;37:635–642.

161. Ferguson MWJ, Howarth G. Marsupial models of scarless fetal wound healing. In: Adzick NS, Longaker MT, eds. *Fetal wound healing.* New York: Elsevier, 1992:95–125.

162. Whitby DJ, Ferguson MWJ. The extracellular-matrix of lip wounds in fetal, neonatal and adult mice. *Development* 1991;112:651–668.

163. Whitby DJ, Ferguson MWJ. Immunohistochemical localization of growth factors in fetal wound healing. *Dev Biol* 1991;147:207–215.

164. McCallion RL, Ferguson MWJ. Fetal wound healing and the development of antiscarring therapies for adult wounds. In: Clark RAF, ed. *The molecular and cellular biology of wound repair.* New York: Plenum Press, 1996:561–600.

165. Adzick NS, Longaker MT. Characteristics of fetal tissue repair. In: Adzick NS, Longaker MT, eds. *Fetal wound healing.* New York: Elsevier, 1992:53–70.

166. Mast BA, Flood LC, Haynes JH, et al. Hyaluronic acid is a major component of the matrix of fetal rabbit skin and wounds. Implications for healing by regeneration. *Matrix* 1991;11:63–68.

167. Longaker MT, Adzick NS. The biology of fetal wound-healing—a review. *Plast Reconstr Surg* 1991;87:788–798.

168. Longaker MT, Whitby DJ, Ferguson MWJ, et al. Studies in fetal wound healing. Early deposition of fibronectin distinguishes fetal from adult wound-healing. *J Pediatr Surg* 1989;24:799–805.

169. Ihara S, Motobayashi Y. Wound closure in fetal-rat skin. *Development* 1992;114:573–582.

170. Longaker MT, Whitby DJ, Ferguson MWJ, Lorenz HP, Harrison MR, Adzick NS. Adult skin wounds in the fetal environment heal with scar formation. *Ann Surg* 1994;219:65–72.

171. Lorenz HP, Lin RY, Longaker MT, Whitby DJ, Adzick NS. The fetal fibroblast—the effector cell of scarless fetal skin repair. *Plast Reconstr Surg* 1995;96:1251–1259.

172. Martin P, Lewis J. Actin cables and epidermal movement in embryonic wound healing. *Nature* 1992;360:179–183.

173. Frantz FW, Bettinger DA, Haynes JH, et al. Biology of fetal repair—the presence of bacteria in fetal wounds induces an adult-like healing response. *J Pediatr Surg* 1993;28:428–434.

174. Durham LA, Krummel TM, Cawthorn JW, Thomas BL, Diegelmann RF. Analysis of transforming growth-factor beta-receptor binding in embryonic, fetal, and adult-rabbit fibroblasts. *J Pediatr Surg* 1989;24:784–788.

175. Haynes JH, Johnson DE, Mast BA, et al. Platelet-derived growth-factor induces fetal wound fibrosis. *J Pediatr Surg* 1994;29:1405–1408.

176. Ferguson MWJ. Skin wound-healing-transforming growth-factor-beta antagonists decrease scarring and improve quality. *J Interferon Res* 1994;14:303–304.

177. Longaker MT, Whitby DJ, Jennings RW, et al. Fetal diaphragmatic wounds heal with scar formation. *J Surg Res* 1991;50:375–385.

178. Meuli M, Lorenz HP, Hedrick MH, Sullivan KM, Harrison MR, Adzick NS. Scar formation in the fetal alimentary-tract. *J Pediatr Surg* 1995;30:392–395.

179. Mackenzie A, Ferguson MWJ, Sharpe PT. Hox-7 expression during murine craniofacial development. *Development* 1991;113:601–611.

180. Coelho CND, Sumoy L, Rodgers BJ, et al. Expression of the chicken homeobox-containing gene GHOX-8 during embryonic chick limb development. *Mech Dev* 1991;34:143–154.

181. Ashcroft GS, Horan MA, Ferguson MWJ. Ageing alters the inflammatory and endothelial cell adhesion molecule profiles during human cutaneous wound healing. *Lab Invest* 1998;78:47–58.

182. Ashcroft GS, Dodsworth J, vanBoxtel E, et al. Estrogen accelerates cutaneous wound healing associated with an increase in TGF-beta 1 levels. *Nature Med* 1997;3:1209–1215.

183. Dicesare PE, Cheung DT, Perelman N, Libaw E, Peng L, Nimni ME. Alteration of collagen composition and cross-linking in keloid tissues. *Matrix* 1990;10:172–178.

184. Alaish SM, Yager DR, Diegelmann RF, Cohen IK. Hyaluronic-acid metabolism in keloid fibroblasts. *J Pediatr Surg* 1995;30:949–952.

185. Borgognoni L, Pimpinelli N, Martini L, Brandani P, Reali UM. Immunohistologic features of normal and pathological scars—possible clues to the pathogenesis. *Eur J Dermatol* 1995;5:407–412.

186. Rudolph R. Wide spread scars, hypertrophic scars and keloids. *Clin Plast Surg* 1991;14:253–260.

187. Linares HA, Larson DL, Willisgalstaun BA. Historical notes on the use of pressure in the treatment of hypertrophic scars or keloids. *Burns* 1993;19:17–21.

188. Murray JC, Pollack SV, Pinnelli SR. Keloids: a review. *J Am Acad Dermatol* 1981;4:461–470.

189. Boyce ST, Glatter R, Kitzmiller WJ. Treatment of chronic wounds with cultured skin substitutes. A pilot-study. *Wounds Compendium Clin Res Pract* 1995;7:24–29.

190. Rao CN, Ladin DA, Liu YY, Chilukuri K, Hou ZZ, Woodley DT. Alpha-1 antitrypsin is degraded and nonfunctional in chronic wounds but intact and functional in acute wounds. The inhibitor protects fibronectin from degradation by chronic wound fluid enzymes. *J Invest Dermatol* 1995;105:572–578.

191. Vaalamo M, Weckroth M, Puolakkainen P, et al. Patterns of matrix metalloproteinase and TIMP-1 expression in chronic and normally healing human cutaneous wounds. *Br J Dermatol* 1996;135:52–59.

192. Vaalamo M, Johansson N, Westermarck J, Kahari VM, Saarialhokere U. Collagenase-3 is expressed by stromal cells in chronic ulcers but not in normally healing wounds. *J Invest Dermatol* 1996;107:417.

193. Weckroth M, Vaheri A, Lauharanta J, Sorsa T, Konttinen YT. Matrix metalloproteinases, gelatinase and collagenase in chronic leg ulcers. *J Invest Dermatol* 1996;106:1119–1124.

194. Rosner K, Ross C, Karlsmark T, Petersen AA, Gottrup F, Vejlsgaard GL. Immunohistochemical characterization of the cutaneous cellular infiltrate in different areas of chronic leg ulcers. *APMIS* 1995;103: 293–299.

195. Pierce GF, Tarpley JE, Tseng J, et al. Detection of platelet-derived growth-factor (PDGF)-AA in actively healing human wounds treated with recombinant PDGF-BB and absence of PDGF in chronic non-healing wounds. *J Clin Invest* 1995;96:1336–1350.

Inflammation: Basic Principles and Clinical Correlates,
3rd ed., edited by John I. Gallin and Ralph Snyderman.
Published by Lippincott Williams & Wilkins, Philadelphia 1999.

CHAPTER 55

Transforming Growth Factor-β (TGF-β) in the Resolution and Repair of Inflammation

Sharon M. Wahl

Transforming growth factor-β (TGF-β) is a member of a growing superfamily of related disulfide-linked homodimeric polypeptides. Among the more than 30 family members are the bone morphogenetic proteins, mullerian inhibiting substance, activins, and inhibins, which are functionally important in differentiation and tissue morphogenesis. The family prototype TGF-β is represented by three mammalian isoforms, TGF-β1, TGF-β2 and TGF-β3, which share 70% to 80% amino acid homology and many activities, but are encoded by separate genes, and independently synthesized and secreted (1). Mechanisms for TGF-β1 synthesis allow for a rapid response, and this isoform has been likened to the "911" of cytokines, whereas TGF-β2 and TGF-β3 are synthesized and secreted in a more leisurely fashion. These differences in transcription are likely related to the differences in promoter regions and in the 5′ and 3′ untranslated regions of the isoforms (2,3). The TGF-β1 promoter contains activating protein-1 (AP-1) and early growth response-1 (Erg-1) response elements lacking in TGF-β2 and TGF-β3, whereas TGF-β2 and TGF-β3, but not TGF-β1 promoters, include TATA and CAAT boxes (3), providing for selective activation by developmental and environmental signals. Although the three isoforms have many overlapping activities, the isoform-specific knockout mice phenotypes provide compelling evidence that they also have unique and specific functions (4–8).

As a multifunctional growth factor that regulates cellular proliferation and differentiation, migration, and extracellular matrix production, TGF-β1, the most abundant isoform, is a key player in inflammatory and immune responses (9–12). The versatility of TGF-β in both positively and negatively influencing the processes of inflammation and repair underscores the essential role it plays in orchestrating these complex events. TGF-β's potent proinflammatory properties, including leukocyte recruitment, adhesion, matrix metalloproteinase secretion, and activation (10,13,14), set the stage for this molecule to then reverse its role, suppress these events, and mediate repair (15). As immune cells become activated, they alter their TGF-β receptor profile and become susceptible to TGF-β–mediated suppression. This cell activation/maturation-dependent response to TGF-β is critical in inflammation resolution. By inhibiting the proliferation of T and B lymphocytes and downregulating macrophage activation, TGF-β prepares the site for fibroblast recruitment, proliferation, and matrix synthesis. The differential activities of TGF-β are dependent on its concentration, cell type, receptor profile, differentiation status of the cell, presence of binding proteins, and a myriad of other co-regulatory molecules and events (15,16). Nonetheless, over the evolution of a physiologic inflammatory response, the conditions emerge that enable TGF-β to foster resolution and repair, which are the focus of this chapter. Dysregulation of these converging forces can lead to any number of potential aberrancies and ultimately, pathogenesis.

TGF-β PRODUCTION, RECEPTORS, AND SIGNALING PATHWAYS

Based on the potent and pleiotropic activities of TGF-β, as well as its nearly ubiquitious distribution, there are many built-in regulatory mechanisms to control its activity. As indicated, differences in regulation of transcription and translation of the three TGF-β isoforms account, in part, for their discordant spatial and temporal distribution. At an inflammatory site such as bleomycin-induced lung injury, alveolar macrophages are stimulated to

S. M. Wahl: Oral Infection and Immunity Branch, National Institute of Dental Research, National Institutes of Health, Bethesda, Maryland 20892-4352.

secrete increased quantities of TGF-β1 without concomitant enhancement of TGF-β2 and TGF-β3 (17). Under these circumstances, the control of TGF-β expression appears to occur not at the mRNA level, but rather in the selective regulation of secretion and activation of the latent isoforms of TGF-β. Differential control of macrophage isoform-specific mRNA also occurs in response to activating signals as determined *in vitro* (18).

Besides the distinct regulatory profiles of transcription and translation and the complexity and selectivity of the receptor signaling system, one of the very effective mechanisms for keeping TGF-β in check is its secretion as a latent molecule that must be activated prior to binding to the cell surface receptors (Fig. 55-1). The TGF-βs are produced as approximately 400 amino acid precursors that dimerize and are cleaved during or after secretion to release the bioactive peptides as disulfide-linked homodimers (1). For the most part, the isoforms are secreted noncovalently bound to a latency associated peptide (LAP) that blocks receptor binding and renders the

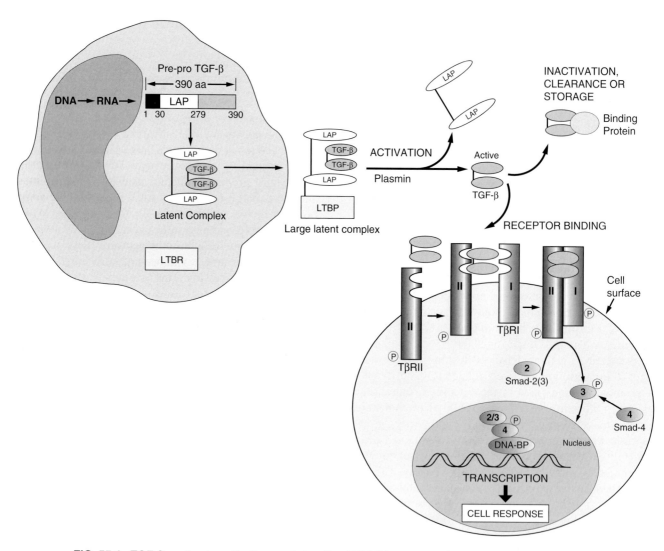

FIG. 55-1. TGF-β synthesis, activation, and signaling. TGF-β is generated as a 390 amino acid precursor molecule (pre-pro TGF-β) composed of a signal peptide, the TGF-β monomer, and the latency associated peptide (LAP). Once the signal peptide (aa 1–29) has been removed, proteolytic cleavage yields the mature TGF-β (residues 279–390) and LAP (residues 30–278), which noncovalently associate to form the small latent TGF-β complex. The latent TGF-β binding protein (LTBP) binds the small latent complex by disulfide bonds to form a large latent complex that may facilitate secretion (reviewed in refs. 1 and 3). Extracellular release of mature TGF-β from the latent complex is dependent on proteolytic cleavage (plasmin) and the active molecule can then bind to TGF-β receptors on the target cell to initiate signal transduction or become complexed with binding proteins (Table 55-1) for clearance or for storage. For signaling, TGF-β binds first to TβRII, present in the membrane as an oligomer with constitutively activated kinase. TβRII recruits and phosphorylates TβRI to initiate the signaling cascade, which involves phosphorylation of cytosolic Smad mediators to effect transcriptional regulation.

mature TGF-β biologically inactive. Posttranslational processing of the TGF-β to release it from LAP and, when present, the large latent TGF-β–binding protein (LTBP) offers an important mechanism of control, since TGF-β and its receptors are ubiquitously expressed. Once activated, the mature TGF-β avidly binds to its receptors to initiate signal transduction (Fig. 55-1) or is stored extracellularly in complexes with binding proteins (Table 55-1), where it can be accessed as needed.

Activation of TGF-β likely involves plasmin-dependent cleavage of the latent molecule, but other proteases (e.g., cathepsins), thrombospondin, and an acidic milieu may also participate in this multifactorial process (19,20). At sites of inflammation, typified by rheumatoid synovium and bleomycin-induced lung injury, activated macrophages, a source of the serine protease plasmin, secrete biologically active rather than latent TGF-β (21,22). In such macrophages, plasmin and urokinase-type plasminogen activator (uPA), together with transglutaminase and the uPA and mannose-6-phosphate receptors, may cooperate in a complex pattern to release the active form of TGF-β (23). TGF-β may itself promote this cooperative interaction by increasing uPA and its receptors (24). However, since plasmin generation in activated macrophages occurs transiently, the secretion of active TGF-β subsides, even though latent TGF-β continues to be produced (22). The cessation of plasmin-dependent cleavage of latent TGF-β may be an important contributing factor to resolution of inflammatory sequelae.

Like the three isoforms of the peptide, there are three major cell surface receptors that recognize TGF-β, but there is no correspondence between the receptor and isoform nomenclature. Of the three primary TGF-β receptors, TGF-β receptor-1 (TβR1) (55 kd) and TGF-β receptor-2 (TβRII) (70–85 kd) are involved in signaling. The function of TβRIII (β-glycan; 200–400 kd), which has a short cytoplasmic domain lacking an apparent signaling motif, appears to be concentration/presentation of ligand to TβR1 and TβRII (25,26). TβRIII, which binds all isoforms, is widely distributed, but is expressed only at low levels on hematopoietic and endothelial cells (27,28). TβRIII may also be secreted in a soluble form to function

as a reservoir for ligand retention (29). An additional receptor, endoglin, is structurally related to TβRIII, shares a high degree of identity in the transmembrane and cytoplasmic domains (~70%), and lacks a kinase domain, but has a distinct overall sequence. This molecule is predominantly expressed on endothelium and preferentially binds TGF-β1 and TGF-β3 (30,31). Moreover, endoglin expression appears to be differentiation-dependent, and is found on pre-B cells, hematopoietic stromal cells, and on activated (not resting) monocytes and tissue macrophages (30,32–34). Transfection of endoglin into the U937 monocytic cell line modulates TGF-β–dependent inhibition of proliferation, decreases c-*myc*, and increases fibronectin production and adhesion (34).

For signaling, hematopoietic cells, including monocytes and lymphocytes, rely on the high-affinity receptors, identified primarily as TβR1 by crosslinking studies (28,35–37), and also TβRII. In contrast to most growth factor receptors, TGF-β receptors possess unique transmembrane serine/threonine kinases (38) whose signal transduction pathway continues to be deciphered. Considerable enlightenment of the signaling cascade emerged from the study of the Drosophila family counterpart to TGF-β, decapentaplegic (DPP) (reviewed in ref. 29). In mammalian cells, as well as in Drosophila, TGF-β and DPP initiate signaling when they come into contact with both TβRI and TβRII, respectively. The dual receptor requirement, confirmed by signal disruption in mutations of either receptor type (39–41), involves initial recognition of ligand by TβRII, and then this complex recruits and phosphorylates TβRI to form an oligomeric complex, potentially a heterotetramer, capable of phosphorylating downstream effectors to promulgate signal transduction (Fig. 55-1). The obviousness of the critical role for TβRII in cell responsiveness is evidenced in the TGF-βRII knock-out, which is embryonically lethal (42). Moreover, inactivation or reduced expression of TβRII as well as TβRI results in diminished susceptibility to TGF-β signaling and is associated, in some cases, with tumorigenicity (43,44).

Sequential phosphorylation of TβRI catalyzed by constitutively active TβRII kinase leads to the generation of a

TABLE 55-1. *Transforming growth factor-β–binding proteins*

Protein	Isoform specificity	Activity of complexed TGF-β
Soluble betaglycan (extracellular domain)	TGF-β1 = β2 = β3	Active
α2-Macroglobulin (in serum)	TGF-β2 > TGF-β1	Inactive
Decorin (proteoglycan)	TGF-β1, β2, β3	Inactive/active
Biglycan	TGF-β1, β2, β3	Inactive
α-Fetoprotein (amniotic fluid, plasma)	TGF-β2	Active
Type IV collagen	TGF-β1, β2, β3	Inactive
Fibronectin	TGF-β1, β2, β3	Active
β-Amyloid precursor	TGF-β1, β2, β3	Active
Thrombospondin	TGF-β1, β2, β3	Active
Immunoglobulin G	TGF-β1	Active

wide range of signals that are ligand- and receptor-combination dependent (29). Translation of these receptor signals into specific responses involves products of the MAD (mothers against DPP in Drosophila or Sma in *Caenorhabditis elegans (C. elegans)* (now referred to as SMAD, for vertebrate homologues of Sma and Mad) gene family (45). The downstream substrates of TβRI kinase, the Smad proteins, of which several have been identified, are composed of ~450 amino acids with highly conserved N- and C-terminal domains and a variable protein-rich intervening region. While the full cytosolic cascade of

events for signal propagation has not yet been elucidated, pieces of the puzzle continue to be put in place (46). Evidence suggests that different TGF-β family members may signal through any of several Smad proteins, the selection of which is specified primarily by the type I receptor isoform engaged in the complex (39), which thereby provides a basis for the multifunctional nature of these growth factors. TGF-β induces phosphorylation of Smad proteins, but it is not yet known whether this is catalyzed directly by the receptor kinase, involves an intermediate kinase, or perhaps occurs following entry into the nucleus (29).

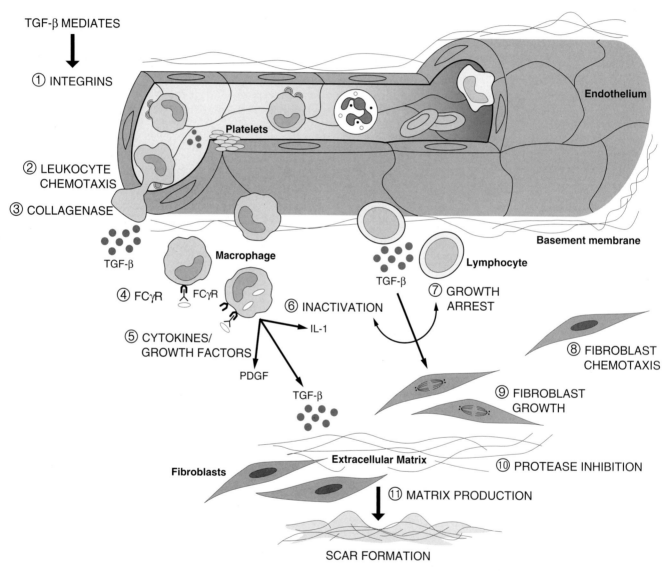

FIG. 55-2. Role of TGF-β in inflammation and repair. At sites of injury, infection or antigen deposition, platelet aggregation, and cell activation stimulate TGF-β release and synthesis. At low concentrations, TGF-β promotes leukocyte recruitment by influencing integrin expression, mediating chemotaxis, and enhancing enzymes that are important in extravasation *(1–3)*. Within the lesion site, increasing levels of TGF-β activate monocytes/macrophages and lymphocytes to clear the inciting agent *(4,5)* followed by their deactivation and growth arrest *(6,7)*. In sequence, TGF-β recruits fibroblasts and enhances their numbers by promoting growth *(8,9)*. Primed for tissue repair, these mesenchymal cells decrease protease production, increase protease inhibitors [tissue inhibitor of metalloproteinase (TIMP), plasminogen activator inhibitor-1 (PAI-1)], and synthesize matrix molecules *(10,11)*.

In mammalian cells, recent evidence suggests that TGF-β signaling protein-1 (BSP-1) or Smad 1 is rapidly phosphorylated on serine and threonine in response to TGF-β and may function as a docking protein (47). The related DPC4 (deleted in pancreatic cancer), identified as a tumor suppressor gene, or its homologue, Smad 4, reportedly associates with Smad 2/3 upon phosphorylation in response to TGF-β (46,48), whereupon the complex translocates to the nucleus (48,49) (Fig. 55-1). Once translocated to the nucleus, these evolutionarily conserved Smad family members may have transcriptional activity, but confirmation of such activity hinges on the demonstration that Smad proteins interact with specific response elements in target genes to induce their transcription in response to receptor signals (46). Dissection of the responsive signaling components subsequent to ligand-receptor interaction is essential to define the regulatory pathways whereby TGF-β mediates inflammation and repair. While considerable progress has been made in defining this novel signaling sequence, there remains a void in our understanding of these pivotal events. Nonetheless, via these signaling pathways, TGF-β orchestrates inflammatory cell recruitment and activation and then paradoxically, signals resolution and repair (Fig. 55-2).

RESOLUTION OF INFLAMMATORY EVENTS

A fundamental component of TGF-β's ability to orchestrate resolution and repair of immune and inflammatory events is its antiproliferative capacity. Suppression of cell growth generally requires that the cells be in an activated status. Progress in defining the mechanisms whereby TGF-β arrests cell cycle has revealed the intersection of TGF-β with cyclin-dependent kinases (cdks) (50,51), which are critical in G_1 progression to S phase. Guanine nucleotide (G) binding proteins, by inhibiting adenyl cyclase to reduce cyclic adenosine monophosphate (cAMP), have also been implicated in this late G_1 blockage (52). By inhibiting cdk2 and cdk4 complexes, TGF-β suppresses phosphorylation of the tumor suppressor retinoblastoma (Rb) protein, and maintenance of Rb in an underphosphorylated state prevents the cell cycle from continuing beyond G_1 (53). Inhibition of the cdks by TGF-β involves production of cdk inhibitors, including but not limited to p21-WAF and p15^{INK4B} (54). TGF-β reportedly induces phosphorylation and increases activity of a cytoplasmic 78-kd protein serine/threonine kinase (possibly TGF-β–activated kinase, TAK1), distinct and downstream from the TβRI and TβRII receptors, and postulated to be an intermediate signal involved in blocking mitogenic, but not matrix-inducing, signals (55). Differential regulation of distinct cytoplasmic kinases may underlie mediation of specific TGF-β signals and cellular responses.

Susceptibility to growth regulation is both cell-type and cell-differentiation status dependent. In B lymphocytes, exposure to TGF-β1 typically causes growth arrest and apoptosis through downregulation of cdk, pRb, the c-myc protooncogene, and nuclear factor κB (NF-κB)/Rel (56). The change in NF-κB/Rel, attributed in part to increased transcription of IκBα, leads to a drop in c-myc expression that triggers apoptosis in immature B cell lines. Moreover, TβRI has been proposed to interact with the immunophilin protein FKB12 to inhibit NF-κB/Rel expression through a calcineurin-dependent pathway (57). TGF-β also controls B-cell differentiation, and, while generally suppressing immunoglobulin synthesis, also influences isotype switching (reviewed in ref. 12).

Like most other cells, the effects of TGF-β on T cells can be either stimulatory or inhibitory. Naive T lymphocytes are susceptible to variable regulation, including enhanced growth, which is dependent on cofactors (58,59), but once activated, this population becomes subject to inhibition and cell cycle arrest (60,61). In a similar fashion, immature bloodborne monocytes, readily motivated to migrate, adhere and generate cytokines in response to TGF-β signals (13,14,18), modulate their complement of TGF-β receptors upon activation, thereby altering their response to this ligand and becoming susceptible to deactivation (9,37,62). Such bifunctional responses, although appearing contradictory, are conducive to promotion of leukocyte participation in the initiation and amplification of an inflammatory response, and reversal of this no-longer needed leukocyte accumulation and activation as the inciting agent is successfully eliminated (Fig. 55-2). In this regard, recruitment of monocytes by femtomolar levels of TGF-β at a site of injury or infection precedes their activation and production of inflammatory mediators including TGF-β (13). TGF-β, in turn, continues to recruit and activate immature leukocytes. Upon accumulation within the inflammatory lesion, the mononuclear phagocytes are influenced by picomolar levels of TGF-β to increase their FcγRIII receptors, which recognize complexed immunoglobulin G (IgG) (63), and then phagocytose pathogens, foreign molecules, and tissue debris. Clearance of the pathogen is associated with decreased recruitment and activation with a corresponding loss of plasmin production and, therefore, declining levels of active TGF-β. Besides TGF-β, inflammatory macrophages secrete both angiogenic and fibrogenic mediators including interleukin-1 (IL-1), tumor necrosis factor (TNF), platelet-derived growth factor (PDGF), and basic fibroblast growth factor (bFGF) (18,64). These growth factors not only direct fibroblast recruitment and proliferation by paracrine mechanisms, but also influence the now-expanded fibroblast population to commence activities leading to the generation of connective tissue matrix molecules essential to tissue repair.

Endogenously derived TGF-β is considered essential to the natural suppression and resolution of an inflammatory response. Although most circulating TGF-β is usually bound to latency-associated peptide, latent binding protein, or α_2-macroglobulin and thereby inactive (65,66), TGF-β can also circulate in an active form (67,68). Moreover, TGF-β complexed to IgG may be even more active than uncomplexed TGF-β (69). In tissues, TGF-β isoforms interact with matrix molecules where they can be stored in either an inactive or active state (Table 55-1), resulting in accumulated protein levels available to mediate immune function and repair.

Importantly, TGF-β is capable of positively regulating its own expression (18). As the levels of the cytokine accumulate through secretion from inflammatory and mesenchymal cells, and activated populations become susceptible to its antiproliferative and inhibitory properties, TGF-β dampens the inflammatory response (9–11) (Fig. 55-2). The essentiality of TGF-β in resolution is nowhere more graphically illustrated than in the TGF-β1 null mutant (knock-out) mouse, which, lacking the ability to generate TGF-β, is unable to reverse the autoimmune-like rampant inflammation that develops in these animals (70,71). In corroboration, systemic delivery of exogenous TGF-β can contribute to amelioration and resolution of disease in animal models of exaggerated inflammation and pathology (72,73). In recent studies, gene transfer by muscle injection of plasmid DNA encoding TGF-β resulted in elevated circulating levels of TGF-β and a striking suppression of experimental arthritis (67). With this foundation of successful experimental therapy, clinical trials in which exogenous TGF-β will be delivered systemically to patients with multiple sclerosis have been initiated (74).

Beyond the systemic delivery of exogenous TGF-β and gene therapy to promote immune suppression, it may be possible to boost the host's own production of this immunosuppressive factor to function in a similar manner. Retinoids, steroids (tamoxifen), vitamin D derivatives, and a bioflavinoid, quercetin, all reportedly enhance TGF-β secretion (75,76) with immunosuppressive consequences. Moreover, enhanced endogenous expression of TGF-β can also be triggered through the induction of oral tolerance. In an impressive series of studies, it has been shown that oral administration of antigens can evince the development of peripheral tolerance associated with inducible synthesis and secretion of TGF-β (77,78). During tolerance, TGF-β levels rise systemically, implicating endocrine-like effects and/or autoregulation of its own production. In low-dose oral tolerance, the production of TGF-β by antigen-specific T cells, recently referred to as T helper type 3 (Th3) lymphocytes (79,80), likely suppresses activated T-cell proliferation, antagonizes the Th1-derived cytokines IL-12 and interferon-γ (IFN-γ) (81), and cooperates with IL-4 to inhibit immune responses (82). Circulating TGF-β also negates the requisite chemotactic concentration gradient emanating from an inflammatory site to interrupt cell recruitment. Uptake by endothelial cells antagonizes their role

in inflammatory cell recruitment as well. The consequences of this multifactorial suppression include unresponsiveness to specific and bystander antigens with therapeutic benefit demonstrated in experimental animal models of autoimmunity and chronic inflammation and, more recently, in human diseases (77,83). Thus, TGF-β, generated endogenously or delivered exogenously, has the potential to effectively dampen immune and inflammatory pathways (9,12,15).

TISSUE REPAIR

The potential impact of TGF-β on wound healing and tissue repair was presaged by the demonstration of its abundance in blood platelets (84) and by its ability to recruit inflammatory cells and matrix-generating fibroblasts (13,36,85). Interestingly, TGF-β1, not TGF-β2, is found in human platelets (86), whereas TGF-β3 is apparent in human epidermis (87). Matrix synthesis in wound repair is highly TGF-β dependent. TGF-β1 is the predominant endogenous isoform released at sites of injury, but local administration of either isoform promotes the healing response (70,88). However, by dampening TGF-β1 and TGF-β2, wound repair without scar formation can be achieved (89). In the fetus, in contrast to adults, wound repair lacks a scarring component. In dissecting this age-dependent differential deposition of scar tissue, the fetuses were found to lack an inflammatory infiltrate and an angiogenic response, and to express TGF-β1 only transiently. Whereas TGF-β1 and TGF-β2 were identified as matrix promoters, TGF-β3 minimized scar formation (89). Based on these observations, deficient healing was reinvigorated by topical application of TGF-β1 or -β2 (reviewed in refs. 3 and 70). Collectively, the evidence is suggesting that the ratio of the three TGF-β isoforms may be decisive in determining scarring levels.

In the course of the healing response, TGF-β influences profibrotic events by regulating fibroblast growth and by inducing new matrix synthesis, while coordinately suppressing matrix degradation. Consistent with the pattern in other cell populations, the synthesis, secretion, and response to TGF-β by fibroblasts reflect their state of differentiation and the coordinate context of other factors in their microenvironment (16). In fibroblasts and other cells of mesenchymal origin (osteoblasts, chondrocytes), TGF-β may facilitate, rather than inhibit, growth (1). Growth enhancement occurs through direct signaling of mitotic pathways or indirectly, as the consequence of the induction of cofactors, notably matrix molecules and growth factors, such as PDGF (18,90). In a human embryonic fibroblast population, TGF-β decreased p21-WAF, the cdk inhibitor associated with reduced cdk2 kinase activity, and thereby enhanced growth (91). Other avenues whereby TGF-β might favor cell cycle progression include induction of c-myc (54) and increased expression of growth factor receptors, as is the case for epidermal growth factor (EGF) (92). Multiple mechanisms evidently contribute to the accumulation of fibroblasts as displayed at sites of inflammation or following local injection of TGF-β (1,3,13,93) (Fig. 55-2). Nonetheless, this is a tightly regulated process and vulnerable to miscues.

In addition to controlling fibroblast recruitment and proliferation, TGF-β regulates the expression of matrix molecules through an intricate pattern of stimulatory and inhibitory actions. Continued exploration of the signaling pathways in proliferating fibroblasts has revealed that TGF-β activates extracellular signal-regulated kinase (ERK) and the small G protein Rac in the cascade driving plasminogen activator inhibitor-1 (PAI-1) and type I collagen gene promoters (94). Among the transcription factors responsive to TGF-β is AP-1, which is apparently an important site not only on the PAI-1 promoter, but also for fibronectin and tissue inhibitor of metalloproteinases (TIMP-1), as well as TGF-β1 itself. Some studies implicate the transcription factor SP1 in mediating α_2 (I) and αI (I) collagen promoters, but it is unclear whether ERK plays a role in this pathway (94). Additionally, type I collagen regulation involves nuclear factor I promoters (95), but may also occur via posttranscriptional mechanisms (96). TGF-β–dependent transcription of fibronectin, collagens, elastin, tenascin, thrombospondin, and proteoglycans contributes to deposition of matrix needed for tissue repair. This transcriptional activation occurs in target populations beside fibroblasts, including keratinocytes, smooth muscle cells, and osteoblasts (3).

Concomitant with matrix synthesis, TGF-β prevents matrix degradation by its ability to both inhibit matrix-degrading proteases and increase production of protease inhibitors. This complex scenario involves reductions in key enzymes such as the serine proteases and matrix metalloproteinase (MMP) family. By promoting PAI production (97), the conversion of plasminogen to the active serine protease plasmin is blocked, thereby deleting a key pathway in extracellular matrix breakdown. Obstruction of plasmin not only eliminates the plasmin-dependent conversion of one of the MMP family members, procollagenase, to collagenase, but also inhibits autocrine/paracrine activation of latent TGF-β and prevents plasmin-mediated release of other matrix-bound growth factors (24) (Table 55-1). Reduced proteolysis also minimizes the liberation of matrix-derived peptides, many of which regulate cellular signaling and ecology (98). Besides PAI-1, TGF-β enhances the production of TIMPs, which neutralize the degradative activity of the MMPs (99). In this way, TGF-β shifts the balance of matrix-remodeling cofactors to one favoring matrix deposition rather than destruction. Cumulatively, TGF-β functions to increase production of matrix, the objective of which is the generation of scar tissue and restoration of tissue integrity. In the event of compromised healing, TGF-β is considered a likely candidate for restoring the deficit.

Transgenic mice in which specific cell populations are engineered to overexpress TGF-β document the direct role of TGF-β in matrix deposition. In this regard, one transgenic mouse model, characterized by astrocyte overexpression of bioactive TGF-β1, exhibits production of fibronectin, laminin, and heparan sulfate proteoglycan in the central nervous system (CNS). Matrix accumulation is particularly evident in the vicinity of the perivascular astrocytes expressing TGF-β, with the development of a hydrocephalitic phenotype (100). In an analogous fashion, hepatocytes expressing active TGF-β1 (albumin/TGF-β1 transgene) promote local fibrosis and liver pathology (101), but due to elevated systemic levels of the cytokine, distant sites (kidney) are also impacted (102). Beyond inducing fibronectin-related molecules and extracellular matrix generation by renal cells, TGF-β1 reportedly stimulated mesangial cell proliferation in the alb/TGF-β1 transgenic mice, likely through induction of PDGF receptor expression (103). In the liver of these alb/TGF-β1 transgenic mice, type I collagen was deposited around individual hepatocytes and within the space of Disse in a radiating pattern not unlike that seen in alcohol-induced liver fibrosis. Increased mitotic activity and apoptosis were also evident. In an extension of these studies, the transgenic mice were infected with *Schistosoma mansoni* and developed increased fibrotic granuloma in liver and lungs (104). In another model, TGF-β, when coupled to an insulin promoter, drove the development of chronic pancreatitis with fibrotic lesions (105). Targeting calcified tissues, osteoblast overexpression of TGF-β2 (osteocalcin promoter) resulted in bone loss and osteoporosis as the osteoblasts generated matrix, but the osteoclasts resorbed it faster (106). These transgenic studies clearly support the critical etiologic role for TGF-β1 in inflammatory and fibrotic disorders. Consequently, the relatively mild deviation from normal wound repair in TGF-β1 null mice was somewhat unanticipated (107). It appears, however, that increased expression of other isoforms (TGF-β3) may compensate, at least in part, for the absence of TGF-β1.

Converging concepts imply that the effects of TGF-β on proliferation can be uncoupled from its effects on extracellular matrix production. For example, the type II receptor reportedly orchestrates changes in cell proliferation, while TβRI promotes the induction of protein synthesis (108). Alterations in TGF-β receptor expression could yield aberrant responses to TGF-β and foster pathogenic sequelae. Consistent with this hypothesis, in atherosclerosis and postangioplasty restenosis, which may represent abnormal wound healing, smooth muscle cells decrease their TβRII without concomitant changes in TβRI or TβRIII. Functionally, this reverses the impact of TGF-β on these cells with loss of TGF-β–mediated growth inhibition and an increase in collagen synthesis (109). Together with overexpression of TGF-β in such lesions, the consequences of the emergence of a subset of receptor variant cells would be to encourage fibroproliferative vascular lesions. Whether a similar TGF-β receptor dysfunction and altered spectra of responses to TGF-β contribute to other fibroproliferative diseases remains to be established, but if such a dichotomy exists, it may allow selective manipulation of a preferred pathway.

Controlled expression of TGF-β is essential for resolution and repair. TGF-β, perhaps more than any other growth factor/cytokine, orchestrates the maturation, integrity, and strength of wounds. Although no cytokine acts alone, considerable evidence has accumulated demonstrating that dysregulation of TGF-β, either by over- or underproduction, uncontrolled activation of latent forms, dysfunctional receptor repertoire, or absence of adequate antagonists, is associated with pathologic complications. Overexuberant production of TGF-β has been linked, by association, with the emergence of fibropathology in human and in rodent models of chronic diseases (110–113). In experimental glomerulonephritis, liver fibrosis, experimental allergic encephalomyelitis (EAE), and arthritis, neutralization of TGF-β with anti–TGF-β antibodies, binding proteins (decorin), or antisense oligonucleotides has a beneficial effect, thereby establishing a cause-and-effect relationship (110–116). Thus, fibrosis, in response to uncontrolled TGF-β, represents a repair process gone awry. Moreover, direct local delivery of exogenous TGF-β or TGF-β delivered by adenoviral vectors to a tissue site confirms that TGF-β is central to the development of fibropathogenic events (3,93,117). Since excessive TGF-β may be a key factor in irreversible scar formation and disruption of tissue or organ function, it provides an important target for therapeutic consideration. Conversely, in situations characterized by insufficient amounts of this limiting cytokine, resolution and repair may be impaired and at least under certain conditions, subject to acceleration by its exogenous application.

TGF-β, acting individually, in synchrony, or in synergy with or by antagonizing other cytokines and growth factors, is clearly instrumental in initiating inflammation and subsequently in mediating resolution leading to repair. Under physiologic conditions, when these multiple factors are in harmony, the multiplicity of cellular and molecular mechanisms merge to effect successful healing of injured tissue. Inhibition, interruption or excess expression of these signals upsets the delicate balance required for successful resolution of the host response (15), and may elicit detrimental consequences. As is often the case, a little is good, but too much or even not enough can be harmful, and continued revelation of these processes will provide targets for regulation and intervention.

REFERENCES

1. Roberts AB, Sporn MB. The transforming growth factors-β: handbook of experimental pharmacology. In: Sporn MB, Roberts AB, eds. *Peptide Growth Factors and Their Receptors.* New York: Springer-Verlag, 1990:419–472.
2. Attisano L, Wrana JL. Signal transduction by members of the transforming growth factor-beta superfamily. *Cytokine Growth Factor Rev* 1996;7:327–339.
3. Roberts AB, Sporn MB. Transforming growth factor-β. In: Clark RAF, ed. *The molecular and cellular biology of wound repair.* New York: Plenum Press, 1996:275–308.
4. Kulkarni AB, Huh C-H, Becker D, et al. Transforming growth factor-β1 null mutation in mice causes excessive inflammatory response and early death. *Proc Natl Acad Sci USA* 1993;90:770–774.
5. Shull MM, Ormsby I, Kier AB, et al. Targeted disruption of the mouse transforming growth factor-beta 1 gene results in multifocal inflammatory disease. *Nature* 1992;359:693–699.
6. Sanford LP, Ormsby I, Gittenberger-de Groot AC, et al. TGF-β2 knockout mice have multiple development defects that are non-overlapping with other TGF-β knockout phenotypes. *Development* 1997; 124:2659–2670.
7. Kaartinen V, Voncken JW, Shuler C, et al. Abnormal lung development and cleft palate in mice lacking TGF-β3 indicates defects of epithelial-mesenchymal interaction. *Nat Genet* 1995;11:415–421.
8. Proetzel G, Pawlowski SA, Wiles MV, et al. Transforming growth factor-β3 is required for secondary palate fusion. *Nat Genet* 1995;11: 409–414.
9. Wahl SM. TGF-β in inflammation. A cause and a cure. *J Clin Immunol* 1992;12:61–74.
10. McCartney-Francis NL, Wahl SM. Transforming growth factor β: a matter of life and death. *J Leuk Biol* 1994;55:401–409.
11. Wahl SM. Transforming growth factor β: the good, the bad, and the ugly. *J Exp Med* 1994;180:1587–1590.
12. Letterio JJ, Roberts AB. Regulation of immune responses by TGF-β. *Annu Rev Immunol* 1998;16:137–161.
13. Wahl SM, Hunt DA, Wakefield L. Transforming growth factor β (TGF-β) induces monocyte chemotaxis and growth factor production. *Proc Natl Acad Sci USA* 1987;84:5788–5792.
14. Wahl SM, Allen JB, Weeks SB, Wong HL, Klotman PE. TGF-β enhances integrin expression and type IV collagenase secretion in human monocytes. *Proc Natl Acad Sci USA* 1993;90:4577–4581.
15. McCartney-Francis NL, Frazier-Jessen M, Wahl SM. TGF-β: a balancing act. *Int Rev Immunol* 1998;16:553–580.
16. Nathan C, Sporn MB. Cytokines in context. *J Cell Biol* 1991;113: 981–986.
17. Khalil N, Whitman C, Zuo L, Danielpour D, Greenberg AH. Regulation of alveolar macrophage transforming growth factor-β secretion by corticosteroids in bleomycin-induced pulmonary inflammation in the rat. *J Clin Invest* 1993;92:1812–1818.
18. McCartney-Francis N, Mizel D, Wong H, Wahl L, Wahl SM. TGF-β regulates production of growth factors and TGF-β by human peripheral blood monocytes. *Growth Factor* 1990;4:27–35.
19. Harpel JG, Metz NC, Kojima S, Rifkin DB. Control of transforming growth factor-β1 activity: latency vs. activation. *Prog Growth Factor Res* 1992;4:321–335.
20. Schultz-Cherry S, Chen H, Mosher DF, et al. Regulation of transforming growth factor-beta activation by discrete sequences of thrombospondin 1. *J Biol Chem* 1995;270:7304–7310.
21. Wahl SM, Wong H, Allen JB, Ellingsworth LR. Antagonistic and agonistic effects of transforming growth factor β and IL-1 in rheumatoid arthritis. *J Immunol* 1990;145:2514–2519.
22. Khalil N, Corne S, Whitman C, Yacyshyn H. Plasmin regulates the activation of cell-associated latent TGF-β1 secreted by rat alveolar macrophages after in vivo bleomycin injury. *Am J Respir Cell Mol Biol* 1996;15:252–259.
23. Nunes I, Shapiro RL, Rifkin DB. Characterization of latent TGF-beta activation by murine peritoneal macrophages. *J Immunol* 1995;155: 1450–1459.
24. Falcone DJ, McCaffrey TA, Mathew J, McAdam K, Borth W. THP-1 macrophage membrane-bound plasmin activity is up-regulated by transforming growth factor-beta 1 via increased expression of urokinase and the urokinase receptor. *J Cell Physiol* 1995;164:334–343.
25. Lopez-Casillas F, Wrana JL, Massague J. Betaglycan presents ligand to the TGF-β signaling receptor. *Cell* 1993;73:1435–1444.
26. Wang XF, Lin HY, Ng-Eaton E, Downward J, Lodish HF, Weinberg RA. Expression cloning and characterization of the TGF-beta type III receptor. *Cell* 1991;67:797–805.

27. Cheifetz S, Hernandez H, Laiho M, ten Dijke P, Iwata KK, Massague J. Distinct transforming growth factor-β (TGF-β) receptor subsets as determinants of cellular responsiveness to three TGF-β isoforms. *J Biol Chem* 1990;265:20533–20538.

28. Ohta M, Greenberger JS, Ankelsaria P, Bassols A, Massague J. Two forms of transforming growth factor-β distinguished by multipotential haemopoietic progenitor cells. *Nature* 1987;329:539–541.

29. Massague J, Weis-Garcia F. Serine/threonine kinase receptors: mediators of transforming growth factor β family signals. *Cancer Surv* 1996;27:41–64.

30. Zhang H, Shaw AR, Mak A, Letarte M. Endoglin is a component of the transforming growth factor (TGF)-beta receptor complex of human pre-B leukemic cells. *J Immunol* 1996;156:564–573.

31. Cheifetz S, Bellon T, Cales C, et al. Endoglin is a component of the transforming growth factor-beta receptor system in human endothelial cells. *J Biol Chem* 1992;267:19027–19030.

32. Rokhlin OW, Cohen MB, Kubagawa H, Letarte M, Cooper MD. Differential expression of endoglin in fetal and adult hematopoietic cells in human bone marrow. *J Immunol* 1995;154:4456–4465.

33. O'Connell PJ, McKenzie A, Fisicaro N, Rockman SP, Pearse MJ, d'Apice AJF. Endoglin: a 180-kD endothelial and macrophage-restricted differentiation molecule. *Clin Exp Immunol* 1992;90:154–159.

34. Lastres P, Letamendia A, Zhang H, et al. Endoglin modulates cellular responses to TGF-β. *J Cell Biol* 1996;133:1109–1121.

35. Kehrl JH, Taylor AS, Delsing GA, Roberts AB, Sporn MB, Fauci AS. Further studies of the role of transforming growth factor-β in human B cell function. *J Immunol* 1989;143:1868–1874.

36. Brandes ME, Mai UEH, Ohura K, Wahl SM. Human neutrophils express type I TGF-β receptors and chemotax to TGF-β. *J Immunol* 1991;147:1600–1606.

37. Brandes ME, Wakefield LM, Wahl SM. Modulation of monocyte type 1 TGF-β receptors by inflammatory stimuli. *J Biol Chem* 1991;266:19697–19703.

38. Derynck R. TGF-beta-receptor-mediated signaling. *Trends Biochem Sci* 1994;19:548–553.

39. Wrana JL, Attisano L, Wieser R, Ventura F, Massague J. Mechanism of activation of the TGF-β receptor. *Nature* 1994;370:341–347.

40. Letsou A, Arora K, Wrana JL, et al. Drosophila Dpp signaling is mediated by the punt gene product: a dual ligand-binding type II receptor of the TGF-beta receptor family. *Cell* 1995;80:899–908.

41. Ruberte E, Marty T, Nellen D, Affolter M, Basler K. An absolute requirement for both the type II and type I receptors, punt and thick veins, for dpp signaling *in vivo*. *Cell* 1995;80:889–897.

42. Oshima M, Oshima H, Taketo MM. TGF-beta receptor type II deficiency results in defects of yolk sac hematopoiesis and vasculogenesis. *Dev Biol* 1996;179:297–302.

43. Wang J, Han W, Zborowska E, et al. Reduced expression of transforming growth factor β type I receptor contributes to the malignancy of human colon carcinoma cells. *J Biol Chem* 1996;271:17366–17371.

44. Kadin ME, Cavaille-Coll MW, Gertz R, Massague J, Cheifetz S, George D. Loss of receptors for transforming growth factor beta in human T-cell malignancies. *Proc Natl Acad Sci USA* 1994;91:6002–6006.

45. Derynck R, Gelbart WM, Harlaand RM, et al. Nomenclature: vertebrate mediators of TGF-β family signals. *Cell* 1996;87:173.

46. Heldin C-H, Miyazono K, Dijke P. TGF-β signalling from cell membrane to nucleus through SMAD proteins. *Nature* 1997;390:465–471.

47. Lechleider RJ, de Caestecker MP, Dehejia A, Polymeropoulos MH, Roberts AB. Serine phosphorylation, chromosomal localization, and transforming growth factor-β signal transduction by human bsp-1. *J Biol Chem* 1996;271:17617–17620.

48. Lagna G, Hata A, Hemmati-Brivanlou A, Massague J. Partnership between DPC4 and SMAD proteins in TGF-β signaling pathways. *Nature* 1996;383:832–836.

49. Yingling JM, Datto MB, Wong C, Frederick JP, Liberati NT, Wang XF. Tumor suppressor Smad4 is a transforming growth factor beta-inducible DNA binding protein. *Mol Cell Biol* 1997;17:7019–7028.

50. McCarthy SA, Bicknell R. Responses of pertussis toxin-treated microvascular endothelial cells to transforming growth factor β 1. No evidence for pertussis-sensitive G-protein involvement in TGF-beta signal transduction. *J Biol Chem* 1992;267:21617–21622.

51. Ewen ME, Sluss HK, Whitehouse LL, Livingston DM. TGF β inhibition of Cdk4 synthesis is linked to cell cycle arrest. *Cell* 1993;74:1009–1020.

52. Howe PH, Bascom CC, Cunningham MR, Leof EB. Regulation of transforming growth factor-β1 action by multiple transducing pathways: evidence for both G protein-dependent and -independent signaling. *Cancer Res* 1989;49:6024.

53. Laiho M, DeCaprio JA, Lundlow JW, Livingston DM, Massague J. Growth inhibition of TGF-β1 linked to suppression of retinoblastoma protein phosphorylation. *Cell* 1990;62:175–185.

54. Lawrence DA. Transforming growth factor-β: a general review. *Eur Cytokine Netw* 1996;7:363–374.

55. Afti A, Lepage K, Allard P, Chapdelaine A, Chevalier S. Activation of a serine/threonine kinase signaling pathway by transforming growth factor type beta. *Proc Natl Acad Sci USA* 1995;92:12110–12114.

56. Arsura M, Wu M, Sonenshein GE. TGF-β1 inhibits NF-κB/Rel activity inducing apoptosis of B cells: transcriptional activation of IκBα. *Immunity* 1996;5:31–40.

57. Wang T, Li B-Y, Danielson PD, et al. The immunophilin FKBP12 functions as a common inhibitor of the TGF-β family type I receptors. *Cell* 1996;86:435–444.

58. Zhang X, Giangreco L, Broome HE, Dargan CM, Swain SL. Control of CD4 effector fate: transforming growth factor β1 and interleukin 2 synergize to prevent apoptosis and promote effector expansion. *J Exp Med* 1995;82:699–709.

59. Rich S, Van Nood N, Lee HM. Role of alpha 5 β 1 integrin in TGF-beta 1-costimulated CD8+ T cell growth and apoptosis. *J Immunol* 1996;157:2916–2923.

60. Ahuja SS, Paliogianni F, Yamada H, Balow JE, Boumpas DT. Effect of transforming growth factor-beta on early and late activation events in human T cells. *J Immunol* 1993;150:3109–3118.

61. Wahl SM, Hunt DA, Wong HL, et al. Transforming growth factor β is a potent immunosuppressive agent which inhibits interleukin-1-dependent lymphocyte proliferation. *J Immunol* 1988;140:3026–3032.

62. Bogdan C, Nathan C. Modulation of macrophage function by transforming growth factor beta, interleukin-4, and interleukin-10. *Ann NY Acad Sci* 1993;685:713–723.

63. Welch G, Wong H, Wahl SM. Selective induction of FcγRIII on human monocytes by transforming growth factor-β. *J Immunol* 1990;144:3444–3448.

64. Rappolee DA, Werb Z. Macrophage-derived growth factors. *Curr Top Microbiol Immunol* 1992;181:87–140.

65. Miyazono K, Ichijo H, Heldin CH. Transforming growth factor-β: latent forms, binding proteins and receptors [review]. *Growth Factors* 1993;8:11–22.

66. Allen JB, Wong HL, Guyre P, Simon G, Wahl SM. Circulating FcγRIII positive monocytes in AIDS patients. Induction by transforming growth factor β. *J Clin Invest* 1991;87:1773–1779.

67. Song X, Gu ML, Jin W, Klinman DK, Wahl SM. Plasmid DNA encoding transforming growth factor-β1 suppresses chronic disease in a streptococcal cell wall-induced arthritis model. *J Clin Invest* 1998;101:2615–2621.

68. Grainger DJ, Kemp PR, Liu AC, Lawn RM, Metcalfe JC. Activation of transforming growth factor-β is inhibited in transgenic apolipoprotein(a) mice. *Nature* 1994;370:460–462.

69. Caver TE, O'Sullivan FX, Gold LI, Gresham HD. Intracellular demonstration of active TGF-beta1 in B cells and plasma cells of autoimmune mice. IgG-bound TGF-beta1 suppresses neutrophil function and host defense against *Staphylococcus aureus* infection. *J Clin Invest* 1996;98:2496–2506.

70. Christ M, McCartney-Francis NL, Kulkarni AB, et al. Immune dysregulation in TGF-β-deficient mice. *J Immunol* 1994;153:1936–1946.

71. McCartney-Francis NL, Mizel DE, Redman RS, et al. Autoimmune Sjogren's-like lesions in salivary glands of TGF-β1-deficient mice are inhibited by adhesion-blocking peptides. *J Immunol* 1996;157:1306–1312.

72. Brandes ME, Allen JB, Ogawa Y, Wahl SM. TGF-β1 suppresses leukocyte recruitment and synovial inflammation in experimental arthritis. *J Clin Invest* 1991;87:1108–1113.

73. Kuruvilla AP, Shah R, Hochwald GM, Liggitt HD, Palladino MA, Thorbecke GJ. Protective effect of transforming growth factor β 1 on experimental autoimmune diseases in mice. *Proc Natl Acad Sci USA* 1991;88:2918–2921.

74. Rowe PM. Clinical potential for TGF-β. *Lancet* 1994;344:72–73.

75. Sporn MB. Chemoprevention of cancer. *Lancet* 1993;342:1211–1213.

76. Larocca LM, Teofili L, Sica S, et al. Quercetin inhibits the growth of leukemic progenitors and induces the expression of transforming growth factor-beta 1 in these cells. *Blood* 1995;85:3654–3661.

77. Weiner HL. Oral tolerance for the treatment of autoimmune diseases. *Annu Rev Med* 1997;48:341–351.

78. Chen W, Jin W, Cook M, Weiner HL, Wahl SM. Oral delivery of group A streptococcol cell walls augments circulating TGF-β and suppresses streptococcal cell wall arthritis. *J Immunol.* 1998;161:6297–6304.

79. Fukaura H, Kent SC, Pietrusewicz MJ, Khoury SJ, Weiner HL, Hafler DA. Induction of circulating myelin basic protein and proteolipid protein-specific transforming growth factor-β1-secreting Th3 T cells by oral administration of myelin in multiple sclerosis patients. *J Clin Invest* 1996;98:70–77.

80. Bridoux F, Badou A, Saoudi A, et al. Transforming growth factor β (TGF-β)-dependent inhibition of T helper cell 2 (Th2)-induced autoimmunity by self-major histocompatibility complex (MHC) class II-specific, regulatory CD4+ T cell lines. *J Exp Med* 1997;185: 1769–1775.

81. Strober W, Kelsall B, Fuss I, et al. Reciprocal IFN-gamma and TGF-beta responses regulate the occurrence of mucosal inflammation. *Immunol Today* 1997;18:61–64.

82. Wong HL, Welch GR, Brandes ME, Wahl SM. Interleukin-4 (IL-4) antagonizes induction of FcγRIII (CD16) expression by transforming growth factor-beta on human monocytes. *J Immunol* 1991;147: 1843–1848.

83. Trentham DE, Dynesius-Trentham RA, Orav EJ, et al. Effects of oral administration of type II collagen on rheumatoid arthritis. *Science* 1993;261:1727–1730.

84. Assoian RK, Komoriya A, Meyers CA, Miller DM, Sporn MB. Transforming growth factor-beta in human platelets. Identification of a major storage site, purification, and characterization. *J Biol Chem* 1983;258:7155–7160.

85. Postlethwaite AE, Seyer JM. Identification of a chemotactic epitope in human transforming growth factor-beta 1 spanning amino acid residues 368–374. *J Cell Physiol* 1995;164:587–592.

86. Cheifetz S, Westherbee JA, Tsang ML, et al. The transforming growth factor-beta system, a complex pattern of cross-reactive ligands and receptors. *Cell* 1987;48:409–415.

87. Cox DA. Transforming growth factor β-3. *Cell Biol Int* 1995;19: 357–371.

88. Beck LS, Deguzman L, Lee WP, Xu Y, McFatridge LA, Amento EP. TGF-β1 accelerates wound healing: reversal of steroid-impaired healing in rats and rabbits. *Growth Factors* 1991;5:295–304.

89. Shah M, Foreman DM, Ferguson MWJ. Neutralization of TGF-β1 and TGF-β2 or exogenous addition of TGF-β3 to cutaneous rat wounds reduces scarring. *J Cell Sci* 1995;108:15–17.

90. Leof EB, Proper JA, Goustin AS, Shipley GD, DiCorleto PE, Moses HL. Induction of c-sis mRNA and activity similar to platelet-derived growth factor by transforming growth factor-β: a proposed model for indirect mitogenesis involving autocrine activity. *Proc Natl Acad Sci USA* 1986;83:2453–2457.

91. Raynal S, Lawrence DA. Differential effects of transforming growth factor-β1 on protein levels of p21 WAF and cdk-2 and on cdk-4 kinase activity in human RD and CCL64 mink lung cells. *Int J Oncol* 1995;7:337–341.

92. Hou X, Johnson AC, Rosner MR. Induction of epidermal growth factor receptor gene transcription by transforming growth factor β 1: association with loss of protein binding to a negative regulatory element. *Cell Growth Differ* 1994;5:801–809.

93. Allen JB, Manthey CL, Hand AR, Ohura K, Ellingsworth L, Wahl SM. Rapid onset synovial inflammation and hyperplasia induced by TGF-β. *J Exp Med* 1990;171:231–247.

94. Mucsi I, Skorecki KL, Goldberg HJ. Extracellular signal-regulated kinase and the small GTP-binding protein, Rac, contribute to the effects of transforming growth factor-β1 on gene expression. *J Biol Chem* 1996;271:16567–16572.

95. Rossi P, Karsenty G, Roberts AB, Roche NS, Sporn MB, deCrombrugghe B. A nuclear factor I binding site mediates the transcriptional activation of a type I collagen promotor by transforming growth factor-beta. *Cell* 1988;52:405–414.

96. Penttinen RP, Kobayashi S, Bornstein P. Transforming growth factor β increases mRNA for matrix proteins both in the presence and in the absence of changes in mRNA stability. *Proc Natl Acad Sci USA* 1988;85:1105–1108.

97. Keeton MR, Curriden SA, van Zonneveld AJ, Loskutoff DJ. Identification of regulatory sequences in the type 1 plasminogen activator inhibitor gene responsive to transforming growth factor β. *J Biol Chem* 1991;266:23048–23052.

98. Werb Z. ECM and cell surface proteolysis: regulating cellular ecology. *Cell* 1997;91:439–442.

99. Edwards DR, Murphy G, Reynolds JJ, et al. Transforming growth factor β modulates the expression of collagenase and metalloproteinase inhibitor. *EMBO J* 1987;6:1899–1904.

100. Wyss-Coray T, Feng L, Masliah E. Increased central nervous system production of extracellular matrix components and development of hydrocephalus in transgenic mice overexpressing transforming growth factor-beta 1. *Am J Pathol* 1995;147:53–67.

101. Sanderson N, Factor V, Nagy P, et al. Hepatic expression of mature transforming growth factor β1 in transgenic mice results in multiple tissue lesions. *Proc Natl Acad Sci USA* 1995;92:2572–2576.

102. Kopp JB, Factor VM, Mozes M. Transgenic mice with increased plasma levels of TGF-β1 develop progressive renal disease. *Lab Invest* 1996;74:991–1003.

103. Haberstroh U, Zahner G, Disser M, Thaiss F, Wolf G, Stahl RAK. TGF-β stimulates rat mesangial cell proliferation in culture: Role of PDGF β-receptor expression. *Am J Physiol* 1993;33:F199–F205.

104. Wahl SM, Frazier-Jessen M, Jin WW, Kopp JB, Sher A, Cheever AW. Cytokine regulation of schistosome-induced granuloma and fibrosis. *Kidney Intern* 1997;51:1370–1375.

105. Lee M-S, Gu D, Feng L, et al. Accumulation of extracellular matrix and developmental dysregulation in the pancreas by transgenic production of transforming growth factor-β1. *Am J Pathol* 1995;147:42–52.

106. Erlebacher A, Derynck R. Increased expression of TGF-beta 2 in osteoblasts results in an osteoporosis-like phenotype. *J Cell Biol* 1996;132:195–210.

107. Brown RL, Ormsby I, Doetschman TC, Greenhalgh DG. Wound healing in the transforming growth factor-β1-deficient mouse. *Wound Rep Reg* 1995;3:25–36.

108. Chen RH, Ebner R, Derynck R. Inactivation of the type II receptor reveals two receptor pathways for the diverse TGF-beta activities. *Science* 1993;260:1335–1338.

109. McCaffrey TA, Consigli S, Du B, et al. Decreased type II/type I TGF-beta receptor ratio in cells derived from human atherosclerotic lesions. Conversion from an antiproliferative to profibrotic response to TGF-beta1. *J Clin Invest* 1995;96:2667–2675.

110. Border WA, Noble NA, Yamamoto T, et al. Natural inhibitor of transforming growth factor-β protects against scarring in experimental kidney disease. *Nature* 1992;360:361–364.

111. Border WA, Noble NA. TGF-β in kidney fibrosis: a target for gene therapy. *Kidney Int* 1997;51:1388–1396.

112. Bernasconi P, Torchiana E, Confalonieri P, et al. Expression of transforming growth factor-β1 in dystrophic patient muscles correlates with fibrosis. *J Clin Invest* 1995;96:1137–1144.

113. Manthey CL, Allen JB, Ellingsworth LR, Wahl SM. *In situ* expression of transforming growth factor β in streptococcal cell wall-induced granulomatous inflammation and hepatic fibrosis. *Growth Factors* 1990;4:17–26.

114. Wahl SM, Allen JB, Costa GL, Wong HL, Dasch JR. Reversal of acute and chronic synovial inflammation by anti-transforming growth factor β. *J Exp Med* 1993;177:225–230.

115. Chegini N. The role of growth factors in peritoneal healing: transforming growth factor β (TGF-beta). *Eur J Surg Suppl* 1997;577: 17–23.

116. Racke MK, Cannella B, Albert P, Sporn MB, Raine CS, McFarlin DE. Evidence of endogenous regulatory function of transforming growth factor-beta 1 in experimental allergic encephalomyelitis. *Int Immunol* 1992;4:615–620.

117. Sime PJ, Xing Z, Graham FL, Csaky KG, Gauldie J. Adenovector-mediated gene transfer of active transforming growth factor-β1 induces prolonged severe fibrosis in rat lung. *J Clin Invest* 1997;100: 768–776.

PART V

Clinical Correlates

Inflammation: Basic Principles and Clinical Correlates,
3rd ed., edited by John I. Gallin and Ralph Snyderman.
Published by Lippincott Williams & Wilkins, Philadelphia 1999.

CHAPTER 56

Disorders of Phagocytic Cells

Steven M. Holland and John I. Gallin

Ehrlich (1) and Metchnikoff (2) predicted that abnormal function of any element of the host defense system would lead to disease. Perhaps no deficiency of the host defenses dramatizes this point better than patients with absent or severely impaired inflammation due to dysfunction of the phagocytic cells. Absent inflammation causes a compromised host (3), and inadequate turnoff of inflammation contributes to diseases such as rheumatoid arthritis, vasculitis, lupus, and the adult respiratory distress syndrome (see chapters by Kavanaugh and Lipsky [Chapter 64], Sundy and Haynes [Chapter 63], and Dar and Crystal [Chapter 67]. This chapter illustrates how disease models demonstrate salient features of the role of phagocytes in inflammation. Neutropenia and monocytopenia are obvious extreme examples of absent function and demonstrate the critical importance of phagocytes in inflammation. The molecular bases for the pathologic defects listed in Table 56-1 have been defined in only a few congenital disorders of phagocyte function. Detailed understanding of several of these diseases (Table 56-2) has provided an understanding of phagocytic cell function in inflammation, including cell adherence, function of neutrophil granules (see chapter by Bainton), and the respiratory burst (hydrogen peroxide formation; see chapters by Leto and Moilanen et al.). This chapter focuses on the congenital phagocyte defects that serve as models of the physiologic processes not covered elsewhere in this book.

ABNORMAL NEUTROPHIL PRODUCTION

Neutrophil production is complexly regulated (4). It takes 4 to 6 days for maturation to pass through the mitotic phase to the myelocyte stage, and 5 to 7 days more for the myelocyte to develop into a mature neutrophil during the postmitotic phase. Following the myelocyte stage, the maturing neutrophil passes through the metamyelocyte and band stages before acquiring the fully developed neutrophil phenotype. Approximately 10^{11} neutrophils are generated daily, and this number is readily expanded in the setting of infection by another order of magnitude. Development of neutrophils through the myelocyte stage occurs exclusively in the bone marrow, where about 60% of the developing cells are in the neutrophil lineage. The calculated circulating granulocyte pool is 0.3×10^9 cells/kg blood and the marginated pool 0.4×10^9 cells/kg blood, comprising 3% and 4% of the total granulocyte pool, respectively (5). The bone marrow releases 1.5×10^9 cells/kg blood/day to this pool but keeps 8.8×10^9 cells/kg blood in the marrow in reserve. An additional reserve of immature and less competent neutrophils, 2.8×10^9 cells/kg blood, is also available.

Neutropenia is most commonly due to drugs such as chemotherapies, idiosyncratic and toxic drug reactions, and drug-associated autoimmune reactions. An absolute neutrophil count that falls below 500 cells/μL may carry a serious risk of bacterial and fungal infection (6). The rapidity of the fall in neutrophils, the extent of marrow neutrophil reserve, and the duration of neutropenia are relevant to determining the clinical importance of an episode of neutropenia.

Cyclic neutropenia or cyclic hematopoiesis is a rare disease occurring in autosomal dominant and sporadic forms and is characterized by regular 21-day oscillations in the levels of blood neutrophils, monocytes, eosinophils, lymphocytes, platelets, and reticulocytes (7). The defect in cyclic neutropenia is at the level of the hematopoietic stem cell and is associated with abnormal colony-stimulating factor responses in bone marrow precursor cells. Patients with hereditary forms of cyclic neutropenia usually present in childhood and have recurrent episodes of fever, malaise, mucosal ulcers, and occasionally, life-

S. M. Holland: Laboratory of Host Defenses, National Institute of Allergy and Infectious Diseases, National Institutes of Health, Bethesda, Maryland 20892.

J. I. Gallin: Warren G. Magnuson Clinical Center, National Institutes of Health, Bethesda, Maryland 20892.

TABLE 56-1. *Types of phagocyte dysfunction*

Function	Acquired disease	Congenital disorder
Adherence-aggregation deformability	Hemodialysis, leukemia, neonatal defects, diabetes mellitus, immature neutrophils	Leukocyte adhesion deficiency (see Chapter 37)
Chemokinesis or chemotaxis	Thermal injury, malignancy, malnutrition, periodontal disease, neonatal defects, systemic lupus erythematosus, rheumatoid arthritis, diabetes mellitus, sepsis, influenza virus infection, herpes simplex virus infection, acrodermatitis enteropathica	Down syndrome, α-mannosidase deficiency, severe combined immunodeficiency, Wiskott-Aldrich syndrome, hyper-IgE–recurrent-infection (Job's) syndrome, Chediak-Higashi syndrome, neutrophil specific-granule deficiency
Microbicidal activity	Leukemia, aplastic anemia, certain neutropenias, thermal injury, sepsis, neonatal defects, diabetes mellitus, malnutrition, corticosteroid therapy	Chediak-Higashi syndrome, neutrophil specific-granule deficiency, chronic granulomatous diseases of childhood, Interferon-γ receptor deficiency, interleukin-12 dysregulation
Neutropenia	Aplastic anemia, sepsis, drug-induced, autoimmune, large granular lymphocyte proliferation, chemotherapy-induced	Chediak-Higashi syndrome, granulocyte colony–stimulating factor receptor mutations, Kostmann syndrome, benign neutropenia of infancy

896

TABLE 56-2. *Distinguishing features of congenital phagocyte dysfunction syndromes*

Disease	Gene/inheritance/chromosomal location	Defect	Clinical manifestations
Leukocyte adhesion deficiency type 1 (iC3b-receptor [CR3] deficiency) (see Chapter 37)	CD18, β-chain integrin/AR/21q22.3	Tight adhesion, aggregation, spreading, chemotaxis	Delayed separation of umbilical stump, depressed inflammation, bacterial infections, gingivitis, periodontal disease
Leukocyte adhesion deficiency type 2 (sialyl Lewisˣ [CD15s] deficiency) (see Chapter 38)	Unknown/AR/unknown	Defective selectin ligand, rolling adhesion	Mental retardation, short stature, depressed inflammation, bacterial infections, gingivitis, periodontal disease, Bombay (Hh) blood type
Chediak-Higashi syndrome	LYST/AR/1q43	Giant lysosomal granules; neutropenia; decreased chemotaxis, degranulation, and microbicidal activity; excess O_2 consumption and H_2O_2 production; deficient neutrophil cathepsin G and elastase	Recurrent pyogenic infections, especially with *Staphylococcus aureus*; periodontal disease; partial oculocutaneous albinism; nystagmus; progressive peripheral neuropathy; many patients develop lymphoma-like illness during adolescence
Neutrophil specific-granule deficiency	C/EBPE AR/	Absent neutrophil-specific granules, decreased chemotaxis, decreased O_2 production, decreased bactericidal activity, absent neutrophil gelatinase and defensins	Recurrent cutaneous, ear, and sinopulmonary bacterial infections; diminished inflammation
Chronic granulomatous diseases			
Membrane defects			
gp91phox deficiency	gp91phox/ X-linked/Xp21.1	H_2O_2 production absent in neutrophils and monocytes, defective "turn-off" of inflammation	Severe infections of skin, ears, lungs, liver, and bone with catalase (+) microorganisms such as *S. aureus*, *Burkholderia cepacia*, *Aspergillus* species, and *Chromobacterium violaceum*; often hard to culture organism; excessive inflammation; suppuration; granulomas
p22 phox deficiency	p22phox/AR/16q24		
Cytosol defects			
p47phox	p47phox/AR/7q11-23		
p67phox	p67phox/AR/1q25		
Myeloperoxidase deficiency	MPO/AR/17q12-21	Low or absent myeloperoxidase	Minimal unless another defect, then *Candida albicans* or other fungal infections
Hyper-IgE–recurrent-infection (Job's) syndrome	Unknown/AD/ 4p12–q12	Variable chemotactic defects, very high IgE; anti-*S. aureus* IgE; low anti-*S. aureus* IgA in serum and saliva	"Coarse" facies in most patients; "cold" skin abscesses; recurrent pulmonary, bone, upper airway infections with *S. aureus* or *Haemophilus influenzae*; mild eosinophilia; mucocutaneous candidiasis; failure of primary dentition deciduation
Interferon-gamma receptor 1 deficiency	IFNGR1/AR/6q23-q24	Absent IFNGR1; no IFN-γ signaling; failure to activate monocytes and macrophages to antimycobacterial state	Disseminated nontuberculous mycobacterial infections; *Salmonella* infections; CMV infections
Interferon-gamma receptor 2 deficiency	IFNGR2/AR/21	Absent IFNGR2; no IFN-γ signaling; failure to activate monocytes and macrophages to antimycobacterial state	Disseminated nontuberculous mycobacterial infections

AR, autosomal recessive inheritance; AD, autosomal dominant inheritance; X, X-linked inheritance.

897

threatening infections associated with periods of profound neutropenia (<200/μL) (7). Neutrophil number is recurrently low in cyclic neutropenia but function is normal. The diagnosis is suspected in children or adults with recurrent stomatitis, gingivitis, cutaneous infections, lymphadenopathy, and fever. The diagnosis can only be established after repeated blood counts with differentials at least three times per week for at least 6 weeks. In congenital agranulocytosis (Kostmann's syndrome; 8), neutrophil counts are consistently low from birth and show no periodicity. Both cyclic neutropenia and congenital agranulocytosis can be successfully treated with recombinant granulocyte colony-stimulating factor (G-CSF) (9–11). Recently Dong et al. (12) described cases of profound neutropenia associated with dominant negative mutations in the G-CSF receptor. These cases had neutropenia responsive to G-CSF, but eventually developed acute myelocytic leukemia. The original cases described by Kostmann (8) were shown not to have these mutations, but subsequent cases of severe neutropenia called Kostmann's syndrome have included G-CSF receptor mutations (12).

Adult onset cases of cyclic neutropenia are associated with clonal or polyclonal proliferation of large granular lymphocytes (13). The adult form of cyclic neutropenia is less regular in its periodicity but has similar clinical features to the hereditary forms. In these cases, peripheral blood shows abnormally high levels of lymphocytes coexpressing CD8 and CD57 surface markers (13). Successful treatment of the lymphocyte proliferation with cyclosporine, chemotherapy, or steroids has been reported.

Great strides have been made recently in the dissection of the factors underlying myeloid proliferation and differentiation. The upstream promotor site CCAAT is central to myeloid growth and there are myeloid-specific proteins that bind to it. There are several members of the family of the CCAAT enhancer binding proteins (C/EBPs) that have been shown to be critical regulators of myeloid development through gene targeting experiments in mice (14). Mice deficient in C/EBPα have a maturation arrest at the myeloblast stage and express no G-CSF receptor in those cells (15). Mice deficient in C/EBPβ [nuclear factor-IL-6 (NF-IL-6)] show enhanced susceptibility to intracellular infections (16). Disruption

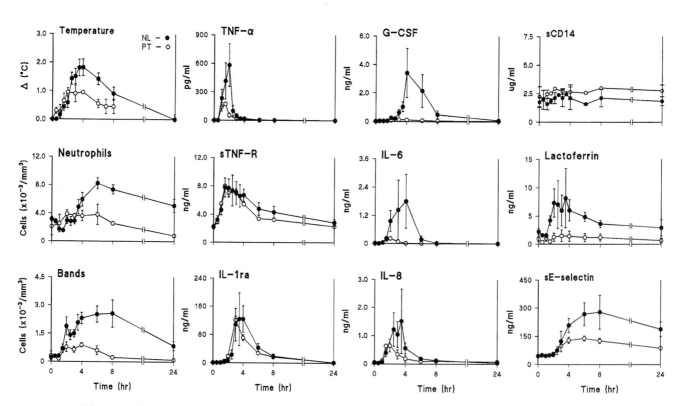

FIG. 56-1. Endotoxin-induced physiologic changes in 10 normal volunteers *(solid circles)* and a patient with endotoxin and IL-1 hyporesponsiveness *(open circles)*. There are stereotyped responses in normals that peak by 8 hours and then decline. Note the characteristic dip in peripheral blood neutrophil count immediately following endotoxin administration in normals, which is due to acute margination *(square root sign)*. Leukocytosis follows shortly after as neutrophils are mobilized from bone marrow and the marginated pool. TNF-α, tumor necrosis factor-α; sTNF-R, soluble 60-kd TNF-α receptor; IL-1ra, interleukin-1 receptor antagonist; G-CSF, granulocyte-colony stimulating factor; Il-6, interleukin-6; IL-8, interleukin-8; sCD14, soluble CD14; sE-selectin, soluble E-selectin. (From ref. 19, with permission.)

of the C/EBPε gene leads to mice unable to produce mature granulocytes. The cells that are produced are incapable of producing an oxidative burst and have incomplete nuclear segmentation (17). Further definition of this set of transcription factors will be highly informative regarding control of myeloid growth and differentiation.

Abnormal Endotoxin Responsiveness

The normal mechanisms by which neutrophils exit the bone marrow are still unclear. However, administered cytokines such as granulocyte-macrophage colony-stimulating factor (GM-CSF) and G-CSF lead to substantial increases in neutrophil production and release. Neutropenia is not always associated with an increased susceptibility to infection. In some chronic neutropenias there may be adequate marrow reserve of granulocytes to respond to infections when necessary and no need for specific therapy to increase the neutrophil count (18). Bone marrow granulocyte reserve and the marginated pool of granulocytes can be assessed by injection of low dose intravenous endotoxin. Endotoxin challenge produces stereotyped increases in body temperature, white blood cell count, and cytokine profile (Fig. 56-1) (19). Illustrative of the importance of endotoxin responsiveness, one patient hyporesponsive to endotoxin and interleukin-1 (IL-1) has been described who had recurrent life-threatening bacterial infections with minimal systemic response (Fig. 56-1). Her defect appears to be in the postbinding signal transduction pathways for endotoxin and IL-1 and may prove informative for cellular events in endotoxin activation (19).

ABNORMAL NEUTROPHIL GRANULE FORMATION AND FUNCTION

Striking morphologic derangements of neutrophils are seen in patients with abnormal neutrophil granules. The morphologic abnormalities of toxic neutrophil granulations seen with acute infection of normal subjects, Auer bodies seen in acute myelogenous leukemia, giant granules of Chediak-Higashi syndrome and leukemia, specific granule deficiency, and deficiency of all granules in a patient with leukemia have been described in depth in Chapter 2 by Bainton.

Neutrophil granule contents have potentially important roles in modulating inflammation (20–22). Discharge of specific (secondary) granule contents amplifies the function of the neutrophil and recruit inflammatory mediators. For example, the specific granules contain receptors for the chemoattractant N-formyl-methionyl-leucyl-phenylalanine (FMLP), C3bi, and laminin as well as a complement activator, a monocyte chemoattractant, gelatinase, and cytochrome b_{558} (reviewed in refs. 20 and 22–24). The presence of several receptors within the specific granule compartment has resulted in the hypothesis that the specific granules function as an important reservoir of certain plasma membrane receptors that are used during chemotaxis and phagocytosis (20). Another specific granule product, lactoferrin, may have a role in regulating neutrophil adhesiveness (25–27), myelopoiesis (28), and immunomodulation (29). Histaminase, which is important in modulating the effects of histamine on inflammation (see Chapter 7 by Nilsson, Costa and Metcalfe), has also been localized to neutrophil specific granules. Azurophil (primary) granules contain elastase and myeloperoxidase (24,30), which are potentially important modulators of inflammation. In addition, azurophil granules contain bactericidal/permeability increase (BPI) proteins and defensins, which are important antimicrobial glycoproteins (see Chapter 50 by Elsbach, Weiss, and Levy). Several diseases, in which neutrophil granules are abnormal, emphasize the importance of neutrophil granules in the regulation of inflammation.

Neutrophil Specific-Granule Deficiency

Neutrophil specific granules are the most prevalent granules within the mature cell (see Chapter 2 by Bainton), and their contents are released into the circulation in response to inflammatory stimuli (31). Absence of neutrophil specific granules has been noted in certain leukemic patients, and absence or deficiency of neutrophil specific granules has been described as a congenital deficiency in neutrophils from neonates and in neutrophils from thermally injured patients (reviewed in refs. 22 and 32; also see refs. 25, 30, and 33–36).

The depressed inflammatory response in a small group of patients congenitally deficient in neutrophil specific granules is a dramatic demonstration of the importance of these granules (32). General comments can be made about the patients (Table 56-2). Most patients are products of nonconsanguineous marriages, although the parents of one patient are first cousins once removed. Both sexes are affected about equally. There are no documented examples of siblings with the disease, but the sister of the patient whose parents were related died of infection at 1 year of age. Therefore, if the disease is inherited, it probably follows an autosomal recessive (AR) pattern of inheritance.

All patients have recurrent infections with bacteria without increased susceptibility to a particular pathogen. The peripheral white blood count is usually normal, but on smears exposed to Wright's stain, which stains specific granules, the neutrophils appear to lack granules. Azurophil granules, however, are evident on peroxidase stain (Fig. 56-2). Nuclei are frequently bilobed, and the nuclear membrane may be distorted by blebs, clefts, and pockets (see Fig. 56-3C). Normal specific granule contents such as lactoferrin, vitamin B_{12}–binding protein, and cytochrome b are either absent or markedly reduced,

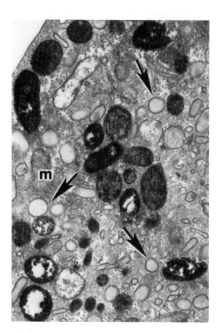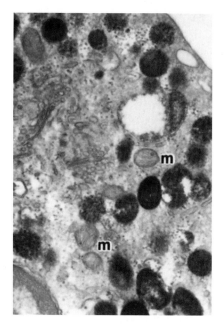

FIG. 56-2. Peroxidase stain of norm *(left)* and specific-granule-deficient *(right)* polymorphonuclear neutrophils; note darkly stained azurophil granules (×27,000). *Arrows* indicate specific granules; m, mitochondrion. (Electron micrographs courtesy of M. M. Friedman, Georgetown University. From ref. 40, with permission.)

and cells are deficient in alkaline phosphatase. Parmley et al. (37) studied neutrophils and bone marrow of a specific-granule–deficient patient using a periodic-acid–thiocarbohydrazide staining method to identify vicinal glycol-containing complex carbohydrates. It was inferred that the patient's cells contained empty specific granules, because small, abnormal, elongated organelles appeared late in neutrophil maturation and were "secreted" in response to phorbol myristate acetate. However, the underlying defect in granule genesis probably differs among patients, because ultrastructural studies have not demonstrated empty granules in neutrophils from all patients studied (Fig. 56-2).

The accumulation of neutrophils and monocytes *in vivo* into Rebuck skin windows and skin blister devices, as well as *in vitro* chemotaxis of neutrophils, is impaired in neutrophil specific-granule deficiency (32). In one patient, monocyte chemotaxis *in vitro* was normal (33), suggesting that the impaired monocyte recruitment seen *in vivo* reflects deficient release of monocyte chemoattractants or of factors capable of generating chemoattractants. In support of this, secretory products from the patient's neutrophils exposed to specific-granule secretagogues failed to generate C5a from patient serum (33). Neutrophils from patients with deficiency of specific granules also exhibit impaired upregulation of formyl peptide receptors and CR3, impaired respiratory burst to certain stimuli, and deficient bacterial killing (32). Whether the latter finding is a consequence of absent specific granules or absence of other important neutrophil components is not known. Thus, patients with neutrophil specific-granule deficiency

constitute an important model illustrating the critical role that granules normally play in modulating inflammation. Specific-granule–deficient neutrophils lack the contents of the specific granules but are also deficient in defensins (38), which are localized to the azurophil granules. The azurophil granules from patients with specific-granule–deficiency have a decreased density on sucrose gradients when compared with normal azurophil granules (33). In addition, patients with neutrophil specific-granule deficiency have abnormal platelet granules (39) and lack eosinophil specific granules (40). Thus, the abnormality in neutrophil specific-granule deficiency is not limited to neutrophils, and the secretory proteins absent from neutrophils of individuals with this disorder are not limited to specific granules.

Additional studies have provided possible mechanisms for understanding specific-granule deficiency as an abnormality with specificity for myeloid cells. A signal peptide splice variant (delta lactoferrin) has been identified that has differential tissue expression and is not expressed in tumor cell lines (41). A myeloid zinc finger protein, MZF-1, has been shown to regulate several myeloid specific genes including lactoferrin (42). Patients with neutrophil specific-granule deficiency have no immunologically detectable synthesis of lactoferrin or lactoferrin precursors in metabolically radiolabeled bone marrow. However, analysis using lactoferrin cDNA demonstrated that RNA isolated from the bone marrow of two specific-granule–deficient patients contained trace amounts of lactoferrin transcripts (43). In contrast, lactoferrin biosynthesis in nasal secretory glands and other nonmyeloid tissues was normal in these patients. Because there is only one lactoferrin gene coding for lactoferrin found in various tissues (44), the data indicate that the abnormality of lactoferrin gene expression is tissue specific and limited to cells of the myeloid lineage. The tissue specificity of the lactoferrin production defect supports the hypothesis that hereditary neutrophil specific-granule deficiency represents abnormal control of gene expression during granulopoiesis with failure to activate a specific cassette of genes normally expressed at the myelocyte/metamyelocyte stage of maturation. It is also possible that there is a general defect of a mechanism affecting the production or stability of mRNA transcripts for these secretory proteins. Elucidation of the abnormal mechanisms of regulation of granulopoiesis in these patients will have broad implications for understanding the control of coordinated gene expression during normal myeloid differentiation and in certain myeloid leukemic states.

Models of Neutrophil Specific-Granule Deficiency

Acquired forms of neutrophil specific-granule deficiency further emphasize the points observed in the congenital lesion. For example, neutrophils from patients with thermal injury are deficient in specific granules but appear "activated" with increased surface area and leukocyte adhesion receptor expression (45–47). This may represent premature granule discharge in thermal injury. The neutrophil granule defect in thermal injury is temporally associated with the appearance of a chemotactic defect, defective oxidative metabolism, and elevation of serum lysozyme and lactoferrin. The increased neutrophil surface marker expression and decreased specific-granule content correlate with the degree of neutrophil functional impairment, suggesting that the acquired deficiency of specific granules in thermal injury plays a role in the increased susceptibility of burn patients to infection.

Other models of neutrophil specific-granule deficiency include neonatal cells, normal cells experimentally depleted of organelles (cytoplasts), and HL-60 promyelocytic leukemia cells induced in vitro toward a neutrophil-like phenotype (24,48–50). Although HL-60 cells can be induced to differentiate into cells resembling granulocytes, they are not a faithful model of myeloid differentiation because they fail to produce specific granules and, in particular, do not produce lactoferrin. No lactoferrin mRNA transcripts in these cells can be detected before or after induction along granulocytic lines (44,51). Thus, HL-60 cells have an abnormality of differentiation similar to the defect in lactoferrin expression described in hereditary neutrophil specific-granule deficiency. Not enough is known to conclude that they represent the same defect. At the present time, no myeloid cell line is available that actively expresses the lactoferrin or other specific-granule genes, making it difficult to further dissect the abnormality in specific-granule deficiency.

Chediak-Higashi Syndrome

The Chediak-Higashi syndrome is a rare inherited disease (autosomal recessive) characterized clinically by partial oculocutaneous albinism, photophobia, nystagmus, progressive peripheral neuropathy, mild neutropenia, gingivitis, periodontal disease, and recurrent pyogenic infections (52,53). In many cells, giant lysosomal granules are seen (Fig. 56-3B) (see Chapter 2 by Bainton). These giant granules result from fusion of predominantly azurophilic granules, but also secondary granules, with each other (54,55). A similar disease has been described in Aleutian mink, partial albino Hereford cattle, albino whales, and beige mice. The increased susceptibility to infection is related to a depressed inflammatory response beyond that due to the mild neutropenia. During infection the patients can mount a leukocytosis, although it is somewhat less than normal. Impaired neutrophil and monocyte migration and defective degranulation are thought to be the basis for the delayed inflammatory response and increased susceptibility to infection (56-58). In addition, neutrophils from beige mice and humans with Chediak-Higashi syndrome are deficient in cathepsin G and elastase (38).

Factors underlying the abnormal phagocyte function in Chediak-Higashi syndrome include abnormal cyclic nucleotide metabolism, disorders of microtubule assembly, markedly increased tyrosinolyation of the alpha chain of tubulin, and abnormal membrane fluidity (for review see ref. 59). The abnormalities of microtubules may relate to a profound abnormality of orientation of intracellular elements of neutrophils in a gradient of chemoattractant (Fig. 56-4). Oxygen consumption and hydrogen peroxide production are greatly exaggerated for unknown reasons and may compensate, at least in part, for the compromised defenses in this disease (58).

Boxer et al. (60) noted markedly elevated levels of cyclic adenosine monophosphate (cAMP) in an 11-month-old girl who was in the accelerated (lymphoma-like) stage of Chediak-Higashi syndrome. The patient responded clinically to ascorbate. It was suggested that the improvement in neutrophil function in response to ascorbate resulted from enhanced microtubule assembly and correction of the abnormal cyclic nucleotide metabolism. However, in a study of two adult brothers with Chediak-Higashi syndrome who were not in the accelerated phase of the disease, benefit from ascorbate was not confirmed, although neutrophil function in beige mice was improved by ascorbate (61). The different results with ascorbate are not understood, but it is possible that in Chediak-Higashi syndrome the stage of the underlying disease determines responsiveness.

Lymphocytes from patients with Chediak-Higashi syndrome have impaired natural killer (NK) activity and lack antibody-dependent cell-mediated cytotoxicity (62). Cytotoxic CD8$^+$ T lymphocytes from Chediak-Higashi

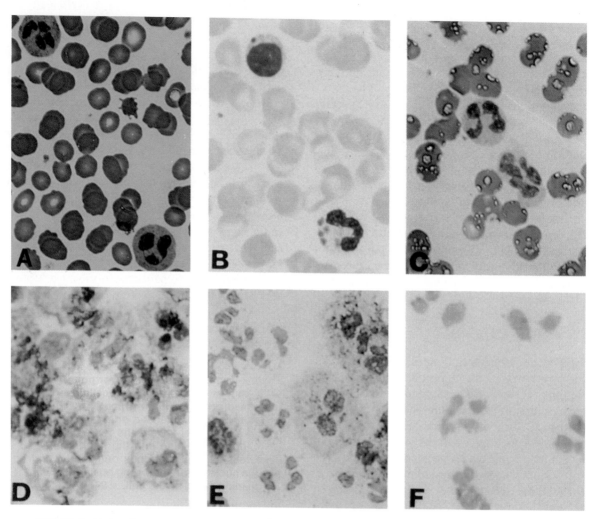

FIG. 56-3. Light microscopy (oil immersion) of peripheral blood cells. **A:** Wright's stain of normal peripheral blood. **B:** Wright's stain of peripheral blood from a patient with Chediak-Higashi syndrome. Note giant granule in the cytoplasm of a lymphocyte, and also note multiple granules in the cytoplasm of a neutrophil. **C:** Wright's stain of cells from a patient with neutrophil specific-granule deficiency. Note the bilobed nucleus with nuclear membrane distorted by blebs, clefts, and pockets. **D–F:** Nitroblue tetrazolium (NBT) dye reduction test of purified neutrophils (Hypaque-Ficoll) stimulated with phorbol myristate (20 ng/ml for 30 min at 37°C). **D:** Normal cells showing NBT reduction *(purple)*. **E:** Cells from a woman heterozygous for X-linked chronic granulomatous disease showing NBT-reducing and NBT non-reducing cells. **F:** Cells from a patient with X-linked chronic granulomatous disease showing no NBT reduction.

patients are unable to secrete lytic enzymes due to an inability to degranulate (63). However, *in vitro* exposure of the NK cells from Chediak-Higashi patients to normal cells reconstitutes the NK defect (64). Whether the absence of NK-cell activity or the increase in gamma-delta T cells in Chediak-Higashi syndrome is related to the presence of inhibitory factors or the absence of trophic factors is not known.

Genetic Studies in Chediak-Higashi Syndrome

The defective gene in Chediak-Higashi syndrome was previously mapped to human chromosome 1q42-q44 and the homologous beige locus in the mouse to chromosome

13 (65). It has been shown recently that the genes at these loci (CHS1) in human and mouse are homologous and encode the gene for lysosomal trafficking, *Lyst* (66,67). This gene encodes an mRNA of 13.5 kb and a protein of 3,801 amino acids (68). *Lyst* has motifs including carboxy-terminal prenylation, multiple phosphorylation sites, and extended helical domains consistent with a coiled-coil structure (66). Molecular genetic studies of Chediak-Higashi syndrome patients have found frameshift mutations and deletions widely spaced through the gene, suggesting that the full-length product is required for function (68). In the mouse, deletions and point mutations have been identified, indicating that multiple versions of the beige phenotype have arisen over time (68). Despite the

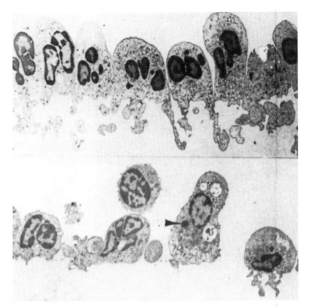

FIG. 56-4. Abnormal orientation of neutrophils from a patient with Chediak-Higashi syndrome in a gradient of *Escherichia coli* endotoxin-activated serum (5% vol/vol). Normal neutrophils **(upper panel)** or neutrophils from a patient with Chediak-Higashi syndrome **(lower panel)** were oriented for 45 min at 37°C on 0.45-μm cellulose nitrate filters. *Arrowhead* points to giant granule in Chediak-Higashi cell. Note the characteristic orientation of normal neutrophils with nuclei toward the rear; also note the long pseudopods projecting into the filter. The Chediak-Higashi cells send pseudopods out poorly, and in some cells the nucleus is in the wrong position, toward the bottom (leading edge) of the cell (×2,400).

extensive and rapidly evolving molecular understanding of this syndrome, the relationship of the defect to the described phenomena remains to be determined.

DISORDERS OF OXYGEN-DEPENDENT ANTIMICROBIAL SYSTEMS

Chronic Granulomatous Diseases (CGD) of Childhood

Since the initial descriptions of CGD in the mid-1950s, hundreds of cases have been reported (reviewed in detail in refs. 69–71). The disease represents a group of disorders of phagocyte oxidative metabolism (see chapters by Leto (48) and Klebanoff (47). for a detailed discussion of normal oxidative metabolism and the NADPH oxidase) with a common phenotype. Neutrophils, mononuclear phagocytes, and eosinophils are abnormal. In addition, oxidative metabolism is abnormal in Epstein-Barr virus–transformed B cells (72). The disease is inherited in X-linked and autosomal recessive patterns (73). Patients have recurrent infections with catalase-positive microorganisms and, in response to inflammation, develop severe chronic inflammation leading to granuloma formation. Thus, there are two clinical features to the disease: recurrent life-threatening infection and excessive inflammation with granuloma formation.

CGD is uncommon, affecting about one in 250,000 to 500,000 persons (74); nonetheless, the disease has engendered tremendous interest as a prototype for abnormalities of phagocyte oxidative metabolism. Elucidation of the underlying defects has been critical to developing an understanding of the structure, activation, and function of the reduced nicotinamide adenine oxidase, a complex enzyme system comprising membrane and cytosolic components (see Chapter 48 by Leto).

Defects of the various *phagocyte oxidase (phox)* components account for CGD (Table 56-2) (75). The most common form of CGD (occurring in about 60% of patients) is caused by an abnormality of gp91^{phox}, the membrane-associated heavy chain of cytochrome b_{558}, located at Xp21.1 (76). Deficiency of the 47-kd cytosolic protein, p47^{phox}, encoded at 7q11.23 (77), is the next most common form of CGD, accounting for about 30% of patients. Deficiency of p22^{phox}, the light chain of cytochrome b_{558}, is at 16q24 (78) and explains about 5% of cases. Deficiency of the 67-kd cytosolic protein, p67^{phox}, at 1q25 (77), accounts for the remaining 5% of patients with CGD.

Abnormalities of Membrane Components in CGD

Cytochrome b_{558} is a membrane bound heterodimer composed of gp91^{phox} and p22^{phox}. About half of the patients with X-linked CGD (X-CGD) are cytochrome b-negative (i.e., absence of cytochrome b_{558} as detected by its characteristic absorption pattern or by immunoblotting) but have relatively normal amounts of gp91^{phox} mRNA transcript of apparently normal size. An increasing number of patients with cytochrome b_{558}–positive X-CGD have been identified (i.e., gp91^{phox} mRNA present, normal results on a spectral assay for cytochrome b_{558}, and both gp91^{phox} and p22^{phox} detectable on immunoblotting) (73). The cytochrome b_{558}–positive forms of X-CGD have been highly informative as to specific binding locations for p47^{phox} to gp91^{phox}, proposed sites of heme binding, and other regions implicated in electron transfer (see Chapter 48 by Leto). Prenatal diagnosis, which previously required fetal blood sampling and the nitroblue tetrazolium dye (NBT) test in mid-gestation, can now be done early in pregnancy by chorionic villus biopsy and haplotype analysis, using either restriction fragment length polymorphism (RFLP) analysis at the X-CGD locus (79) or polymerase chain reaction (PCR) (80).

A small number of patients with autosomal recessive CGD resemble patients with X-CGD, in that their phagocytes also lack cytochrome b_{558} according to a spectral assay. Based on the structure of cytochrome b_{558} and the genetic abnormality responsible for XCGD, it was suggested that cytochrome b_{558}–negative autosomal recessive CGD represents an abnormality of the gene coding for the 22-kd small subunit: p22^{phox}. Dinauer et al. (78) studied three unrelated patients with autosomal recessive CGD for evidence of mutations in the p22^{phox} gene. One patient was shown to be a compound heterozygote for two alleles containing point mutations in the open reading frame that predicted a frame shift and a nonconservative amino acid replacement. Another patient, whose parents were first cousins, was homozygous for a different single-base substitution resulting in another nonconservative amino acid change. Leto et al. (81) showed that mutation of Pro156Gln of p22^{phox} caused ablation of the p47^{phox} binding site on p22^{phox} required for NADPH oxidase assembly, confirming the role of p22^{phox} as a docking site for the cytosolic components.

In neutrophils from both cytochrome b_{558}–negative X-CGD and cytochrome b_{558}–negative AR-CGD patients, neither large-subunit nor small-subunit peptides can be detected, despite the presence of presumably normal amounts of p22^{phox} mRNA in X-CGD and normal gp91^{phox} mRNA in cytochrome b_{558}–negative AR-CGD (82). This suggests that there is independent regulation of transcription of mRNA for the two subunits, but that translation of the two subunits is not independent. Translation of both subunits may require the presence of both normal mRNA transcripts. Alternatively, post-translational processing or stability of either subunit may be adversely affected by the absence of one of the subunit peptides.

Abnormalities of Cytosolic Factors

Most patients with AR-CGD have normal levels of cytochrome b_{558} in phagocytic cells. Studies of phosphorylation of proteins in neutrophils during activation of the respiratory burst indicated that many proteins are phosphorylated, but that one phosphoprotein at about 47 kd fails to appear in neutrophils from most patients with cytochrome b_{558}–positive AR-CGD (83). The defect in these patients was due to absence of the 47-kd cytosolic protein required for NADPH oxidase activation (84,85). The defective patient cytosol was corrected in a cell-free assay with recombinant p47^{phox} produced by baculovirus-infected cells (86). The majority of cases of p47^{phox}-deficient CGD from all races and many ethnic groups are due to a dinucleotide deletion at the beginning of exon 2 (87). The existence of a p47^{phox} pseudogene has been demonstrated, raising the possibility of a gene conversion event leading to this recurrent mutation (88).

Cytochrome b_{558}–positive CGD patients have been identified with a cytosolic defect that could complement cytochrome b_{558}–positive AR-CGD patients lacking p47^{phox} *in vitro*. The defect in these latter patients' neutrophil cytosol was shown to be due to absence of the 67-kd protein, p67^{phox} (89). p67^{phox} is not only necessary for function of the NADPH oxidase, it also is the major

binding site for one of the presumed downregulators of NADPH oxidase activity, p40^{phox} (90).

Clinical Manifestations of CGD (Table 56-2)

Patients with CGD develop serious infections early in life, usually in the first year (69–71). Common infectious syndromes include pneumonia and lung abscesses, skin and soft tissue infections, lymphadenopathy, suppurative lymphadenitis, osteomyelitis (usually involving the small bones of the hands and feet), and hepatic abscesses. Septicemia, meningitis, brain abscesses, and infection of the gastrointestinal and genitourinary tracts are not common, possibly because of high circulating immunoglobulin G (IgG) levels in CGD. Though severe, infection in CGD may follow a rather indolent course characterized initially only by malaise, low-grade fever, and a mild leukocytosis or elevation of the erythrocyte sedimentation rate (69). The diagnosis of CGD is readily established by an inability of neutrophils to reduce the dye nitroblue tetrazolium (Fig. 56-3D–F), by absence of chemiluminescence, or by failure of neutrophils to oxidize dihydrorhodamine 123 to rhodamine 123 (91). Diagnosis is often delayed because of failure to entertain CGD in the differential diagnosis or failure to obtain the appropriate confirmatory testing, sometimes with catastrophic consequences.

Staphylococcus aureus and the gram-negative bacilli *Serratia Burkholderia* account for the majority of serious infections, but infections with *Aspergillus* species and other fungi and *Nocardia* are also observed (69–71, 92–94). Organisms that produce hydrogen peroxide but that are catalase-negative (e.g., streptococci, lactobacilli) are not major pathogens. Bacterial production of hydrogen peroxide within the phagosome by catalase-negative microorganisms (no microbial catalase to break down the hydrogen peroxide) in concert with host cell myeloperoxidase may result in efficient bactericidal activity against these organisms (95) (see Chapter 48 by Leto). Alternatively, oxygen-independent microbicidal mechanisms (see Chapter 50 by Elsbach et al.) may be sufficient to kill certain pathogens by CGD phagocytes. Recent studies using genetically engineered catalase-deficient *Aspergillus nidulans* have shown that virulence is preserved in CGD mice, indicating that in the case of this fungus, which is highly pathogenic in CGD patients, catalase is not a necessary virulence factor (95a).

The granulomas characteristic of CGD can obstruct vital structures such as the gastrointestinal and genitourinary tracts. The mechanism for the granulomatous process in CGD is unknown but may relate to the inability of CGD neutrophils to inactivate leukotrienes and other mediators via the myeloperoxidase-halide–hydrogen peroxide (MPO-Cl-H$_2$O$_2$) system (96), resulting in prolonged leukocyte recruitment. In addition, inefficient degradation of antigen by the MPO-Cl-H$_2$O$_2$ system could result in chronic release of mediators, such as interferon-γ, which may play an important role in monocyte recruitment and polykaryon (giant cell) formation (see Chapter 29 by Sundy et al.). Thus, abnormal turnoff of inflammation may be a major problem in CGD. Obstruction by granulomas in CGD can be dramatically reversed by hydrocortisone (97), presumably by "turning off" the granulomatous process by affecting the production or action of cytokines such as interferon-γ, tumor necrosis factor, or interleukin-1.

Interferon-γ in the Management of CGD

Until recently, the approaches used for the management of CGD were limited to aggressive treatment of infections using antibiotics, surgical drainage, and, in some life-threatening settings, white blood cell transfusions. Prophylactic antibiotics, especially trimethoprim-sulfamethoxazole, reduced the incidence of life-threatening infections significantly (69). Recently, prophylactic interferon-γ has been shown to reduce the incidence of life-threatening infections in CGD (98). Interferon-γ not only reduced the number of serious primary infections by over 70% but also reduced their severity, as monitored by the length of hospitalization for serious infections. The mechanisms of action of interferon-γ were probably multifactorial (99). In some patients, interferon-γ stimulated macrophage oxidative metabolism through stimulation of components of the NADPH oxidase, especially the heavy chain of the b cytochrome. Interferon-γ also stimulates macrophage tryptophan metabolism, granule protein synthesis, and Fc and other receptor expression (see Chapter 29 by Sundy et al. and Chapter 33 by Bach et al.). Subcutaneous interferon-γ three times a week increased staphylococcidal activity of CGD phagocytes, which in some patients was associated with induction of the respiratory burst and superoxide production (100,101) and enhanced damage to *Aspergillus* conidia *in vitro* (102). Currently, interferon-γ is recommended in conjunction with trimethoprim-sulfamethoxazole as prophylaxis in CGD patients.

Gene Therapy for Correction of CGD

The isolation of the genetic bases of CGD raised hopes early on of definitive correction without bone marrow transplantation. Both retroviral (103) and episomal (104) correction of p47^{phox} deficient B cells *in vitro* have been performed. Retrovirus-mediated gene therapy has been successfully applied to p47^{phox}-deficient (105) and gp91^{phox}-deficient (106) mouse models of CGD, proving the feasibility of this approach *in vivo*. Recently, transient retrovirus-mediated gene therapy for p47^{phox}-deficient CGD in humans has been safely accomplished (107). Efforts to achieve long-term genetic correction *in vivo* are underway.

Myeloperoxidase Deficiency

The development in the early 1980s of an automated flow cytochemical system for performing leukocyte differential counts enabled screening of large populations for neutrophil myeloperoxidase deficiency. It is now apparent that myeloperoxidase deficiency is a relatively common disorder, occurring in approximately one in 2,000 individuals (108,109; see also Chapter 48 by Leto). Most patients with phagocyte myeloperoxidase deficiency are not at increased risk of serious infection. Disseminated infection with *Candida albicans* has been noted infrequently; in these patients, underlying immunosuppressive conditions, such as poorly controlled diabetes mellitus, probably contributed greatly to the risk of infection.

Phagocytosis in myeloperoxidase deficiency is normal or increased, probably as a result of a failure to downregulate receptor-mediated recognition mechanisms (110). Deactivation of the respiratory burst is likewise delayed, and hydrogen peroxide generation is markedly exaggerated and may compensate for the absence of myeloperoxidase-halide–hydrogen peroxide microbicidal activity. Bactericidal activity is usually normal, whereas candidacidal activity may be moderately to severely impaired (109). Unlike patients with CGD, patients with myeloperoxidase deficiency do not get granulomas as a complication of their disease. Presumably this is because, as a result of excessive hydrogen peroxide generation, patients with myeloperoxidase deficiency do not have difficulty metabolizing chemoattractants and other mediators of inflammation (96).

Approximately 50% of patients with myeloperoxidase deficiency are totally deficient in myeloperoxidase; the other patients have a partial deficiency associated with decreased amounts of structurally and functionally normal myeloperoxidase (108,109). Native myeloperoxidase consists of two heavy chain–light chain dimers, each with a heavy chain of approximately 59 kd and a light chain of about 14 kd. The interrelationships between the subunits and the location of heme groups have not been fully established (111,112).

Cloning of the cDNA for myeloperoxidase has made it possible to investigate the molecular genetics underlying hereditary myeloperoxidase deficiency (Table 56-2). Immunochemical studies of neutrophils from individuals with complete myeloperoxidase deficiency indicate that no mature myeloperoxidase protein was detectable, but that trace amounts of an 80-kd precursor peptide may be present (108). Northern blot analysis of mRNA isolated from the bone marrow of a myeloperoxidase-deficient subject demonstrated the presence of a normal-sized (3.6 kb) myeloperoxidase mRNA transcript (113). Molecular analysis of patients with both complete and incomplete forms of myeloperoxidase deficiency has shown that the most common mutation contributing to this disease is caused by a C to T substitution in exon 10 at codon 569 leading to conversion of arginine to tryptophan (114, 115), thereby disabling heme incorporation into myeloperoxidase. Although R569W is the most common mutation described in myeloperoxidase deficiency, it is not the only one, as evidenced by the fact that many patients are compound heterozygotes for R569W and other, as yet undefined, mutations (115).

HYPERIMMUNOGLOBULIN-E–RECURRENT-INFECTION SYNDROME (JOB'S SYNDROME)

In 1966, Davis et al. (116) described two girls with persistent weeping eczematoid lesions and large subcutaneous staphylococcal abscesses that were termed "cold" because they lacked typical signs of inflammation. Otitis, sinusitis, staphylococcal pneumonia, furunculosis, and cellulitis were prominent features. The severe problem with furunculosis resulted in the eponym "Job's syndrome." Patients described in subsequent reports have had similar clinical features in addition to characteristic coarse facies with hypertelorism, prominent triangular mandible, craniosynostosis, and osteoporosis (for reviews see refs. 117–120). Recurrent cutaneous and sinopulmonary infection with *S. aureus* is the major problem clinically, but pulmonary infection with *Haemophilus influenzae* is also common. Following pneumonia, these patients have difficulty healing and frequently develop pneumatoceles that may become superinfected with *Pseudomonas aeruginosa* or *Aspergillus* species. In addition, approximately 50% of the patients have mucocutaneous candidiasis. Characteristically, the patients have extreme elevation of serum IgE, particularly against *S. aureus* and *C. albicans* (121), prompting the name hyperimmunoglobulin-E–recurrent-infection syndrome (HIE). The IgE is usually higher than in patients with eczema and recurrent cutaneous *S. aureus* infection and has been shown to be related to increased IgE synthesis and decreased catabolism (122,123). In addition, in patients with HIE there is low or absent serum and salivary anti–*S. aureus* IgA, slight elevation of IgM, and normal IgD (122). The low anti–*S. aureus* IgA correlates with sinopulmonary infections (122). There is a low-grade eosinophilia and prominent eosinophil enrichment at infected foci (124).

Patients with this syndrome have a striking depression of acute inflammation, as evidenced by their "cold" abscesses despite pronounced local infection. Abnormal neutrophil and monocyte chemotaxis have been documented, and it has been argued that too few phagocytes arrive too late (125,126). A chemotactic inhibitory factor produced *in vitro* by mononuclear cells from Job's patients was partially purified and shown to be heterogeneous, with molecular weights of approximately 61,000 and 30,000 to 45,000; it was sensitive to proteolytic digestion and stable at 56°C (126,127). Although the abnormality of phagocyte chemotaxis may contribute to the recurrent infections, the chemotactic defect is variable and unlikely to fully explain the depressed inflammation (126).

Other factors may contribute to the compromised host defenses in this syndrome. Hill (118) suggested that elevated histamine, which is known to inhibit neutrophil function (128), would be released locally as organisms interacted with organism-specific IgE. Elevation of urinary histamine has been seen in only some patients, and the increased urinary histamine appears to be related to eczematoid dermatitis and not to infection (129). It is our impression that antihistamines have not helped our patients (J. I. Gallin, unpublished observations), raising some question as to the clinical importance of histamine in these patients' compromised defenses.

Lymphocyte function in HIE is abnormal (130). Delayed hypersensitivity responses to a variety of skin-test antigens are impaired in some, but not all, patients (131). Mitogen-induced and antigen-induced lymphocyte transformation is impaired, especially with regard to *Candida* antigen and tetanus toxoid, and may be related to the mucocutaneous candidiasis in many patients. Deficient suppressor T-cell numbers may account for increased IgE (130). Low or absent salivary and plasma antistaphylococcal IgA likely contributes to the propensity to mucosal infections.

Bone development and homeostasis are abnormal in HIE. Craniosynostosis has been reported at a higher than expected rate in HIE (132). In addition to bony abnormalities in early development, recurrent fractures and abnormalities of the long bones have been reported (133). Osteopenia and kyphoscoliosis are common in adult patients. Spinal deformity can be severe, especially following pulmonary surgery (119). Monocytes have been investigated for their role in bone resorption in HIE. Leung et al. (134) found an increase in bone resorbing activity in HIE monocytes compared to normal, which correlated with elevated prostaglandin E_2 (PGE_2) production and was downregulated by aspirin *in vivo*. Cohen-Solal et al. (135) confirmed the elevated PGE_2 levels in HIE cultured monocyte supernatants and found similarities in terms of *in vitro* cytokine profile to postmenopausal women. These data suggest that there is a major abnormality in bone growth and development in HIE that is cytokine mediated and may therefore be cytokine controlled.

Recently we have undertaken an extensive evaluation of 30 HIE patients and their families followed at the National Institutes of Health to better determine the disease phenotype in affected individuals and to search for extended phenotypes, since this disease appears to be autosomal dominant and there have been several reports of familial occurrences. In addition to the previously recognized facial, bony, and infection susceptibility features, we have found that patients report failure of their primary teeth to deciduate, leading to extensive extractions. We have found a significant rate of scoliosis in family members, in some cases associated with IgE elevation but not infection susceptibility. Further, we have found several obviously affected patients in whom the IgE level has fallen from very elevated to near or into the normal range. These findings show that the abnormality in HIE is genetic, that it has profound and novel dental manifestations, and that IgE is not a lifelong concomitant of disease (135a).

Interferon-γ in Hyperimmunoglobulin-E– Recurrent-Infection Syndrome Patients

Interleukin-4 (IL-4), interferon-γ, and interleukin-12 (IL-12) play central roles in regulating the IgE response (136,137; also see Chapter 29 by Sundy et al.). In both the murine and human systems, IgE production is dependent on the T-cell cytokine IL-4. In contrast, interferon-γ acts as an antagonist to IL-4 and suppresses IgE production. Based on a large body of experimental evidence, it appears that the magnitude of the IgE response to a given stimulus is, at least in part, regulated by a balance between IL-4 and interferon-γ production. When T lymphocytes from patients with HIE are exposed *in vitro* to a variety of mitogenic stimuli, they produce normal amounts of IL-4 but exhibit deficient interferon-γ production (138,139). Thus, in patients with HIE it is possible that a relative deficiency in interferon-γ production results in the unopposed action of IL-4 on B lymphocytes, which, in turn, leads to excessive IgE production (and perhaps the deficient production of other immunoglobulin isotypes). *In vitro*, B lymphocytes from HIE patients exhibit abnormally high spontaneous IgE production, which can be suppressed by the addition of exogenous interferon-γ (140). Furthermore, in a short-term (2–4 weeks) clinical trial in which five HIE patients were treated with interferon-γ three times a week, a significant decrease in *in vitro* spontaneous IgE production was seen in all patients, and two patients exhibited a fall in their serum IgE levels (140). Taken together, these findings suggested that the abnormally high IgE production in these patients may be secondary to an imbalance in IL-4 and interferon-γ production, and administration of interferon-γ may partially reverse this abnormality. In other studies, Vercelli et al. (141) found no causal relation between increased production of IgE and IL-4 secretion in HIE patients. A deficiency in local production of interferon-γ may also play a role in the abnormality of neutrophil chemotaxis described in HIE patients. In a study of seven patients with HIE who exhibited abnormal neutrophil chemotaxis, *in vitro* exposure of these patients' neutrophils to interferon-γ resulted in a significant improvement in neutrophil chemotaxis (142).

Genetic Studies in Hyperimmunoglobulin-E– Recurrent-Infection Syndrome

HIE has occurred in several kindreds in an autosomal dominant pattern with transmission from mother to daughter (143,144) and father to son (135a). Sporadic cases have been identified as well. Interest has been focused on the long arm of chromosome 5 as the locus for numerous cytokine genes (145), the locus for the control of IgE levels (146), and some forms of craniofacial malformations and craniosynostosis (147). Karyotyping has shown an anomaly involving 4q in one patient. Formal genome wide screening in multiple kindreds is under way and suggests linkage to the 4q region.

LOCALIZED JUVENILE PERIODONTITIS

In patients with neutropenia or functional phagocyte impairment, mucosal ulcerations, gingivitis, and periodontitis occur frequently and are often severe. In most cases, intraoral infection is associated with recurrent infection at other sites. In contrast, localized juvenile periodontitis is an adolescent disease of the supporting structures of the permanent dentition, characterized by severe alveolar bone loss limited primarily to the first molars and incisors. Patients are not predisposed to extraoral infection (148,149).

Genco's team (149,150) has demonstrated in patients with localized juvenile periodontitis a moderate, but reproducible, impairment of chemotaxis to formyl peptides (FMLP) and C5a; neutrophil adherence is normal. Defective chemotaxis persists following aggressive local therapy and has been demonstrated in siblings prior to the development of the clinical syndrome. Using antibodies directed against the FMLP chemoattractant receptor, De Nardin et al. (151) demonstrated differences in binding of the antibodies to neutrophils from chemotactically depressed juvenile periodontitis patients when compared with that of normal subjects. Perez et al. (152) have shown that although the FMLP receptor was of normal molecular weight and had normal N-linked glycosylation, the receptors from juvenile periodontitis patients were more resistant to papain cleavage than normal. Two-dimensional electrophoresis of normal and juvenile periodontitis neutrophil extracts demonstrated decreased amounts of FMLP receptor isoforms in patient cells. Hurttia et al. (153) showed defects in diacyl glycerol kinase activation by FMLP in the cytosol of neutrophils from some patients with localized juvenile periodontitis, suggesting that abnormal receptors or postreceptor signaling is involved in the neutrophil chemotactic defect.

NEUTROPHIL HETEROGENEITY AS A POSSIBLE EXPLANATION FOR CERTAIN ACQUIRED CHEMOTACTIC DEFECTS

Neutrophil heterogeneity was first suggested by Florence Sabin (154) in 1923. She observed that myelocytes had poor locomotory capacity and speculated that the poor movement of immature myeloid cells kept them in the marrow. The wide range of individual rates of neutrophil locomotion was described in the same year (155). Based on clot preparation studies, Howard (156) subsequently divided neutrophils into fast-moving (>7 μm/min) and slow-moving (<7 μm/min) populations. Harvath and Leonard (157) described two neutrophil populations separable on the basis of their chemotactic responsiveness. Using a fluorescence-activated cell sorter, Seligmann et al. (158) demonstrated a heterogeneous response of neutrophil binding of the chemotactic peptide FMLP. Monoclonal antibodies that bind to neutrophils in a heterogeneous fashion have been described. Ball et al. (159) reported a monoclonal antibody (AML-2-23), made against acute myelogenous leukemia myeloblasts, that labeled 85% to 90% of normal neutrophils. The fluorescence staining pattern of each individual studied showed a single peak, and nonstaining cells were defined as those cells on the peak that overlapped in the negative control range. Clement et al. (160) described two antineutrophil monoclonal antibodies (IBS and 4D1) that recognized a mean of 57% and 51% of neutrophils, respectively. The fluorescence staining pattern was that of two distinct peaks, with the more negative peak overlapping the negative control peak. A mouse IgG1 monoclonal antibody (31D8) that binds heterogeneously to neutrophils exhibiting a bright and dull staining pattern has been described (161). When neutrophils are stained with fluorochrome-labeled 31D8, the vast majority stain in a bright pattern. The dull-staining cells tend to be less capable of chemotaxis, NBT reduction, and membrane depolarization. Band forms are 31D8-dull, but many 31D8-dull–staining neutrophils appear morphologically mature. It is not clear at this point how 31D8 epitope expression relates to neutrophil maturity. Of interest, however, is the demonstration that 31D8 epitope expression becomes undetectable in a select group of chronic myelogenous leukemia patients who, within a year, develop blast crisis (162). 31D8 has recently been identified as FcRγIII, or CD16 (163).

An antineutrophil IgG monoclonal antibody C10 binds neutrophils heterogeneously, with distinct positive and negative peaks (164). Whereas variation between individuals in percent positive C10 staining of neutrophils is considerable, the variation in the same individual over time is small. Furthermore, while the negative population number and staining pattern remain constant, the positive population increases its expression of C10 with activation *in vitro* or *in vivo* in the circulation after endotoxin injec-

tion or following exudation. Studies of C10 binding to neutrophils from patients with different defects of phagocyte function indicated normal function in CGD, Chediak-Higashi syndrome, and Job's syndrome. However, there was no C10 epitope expression in two patients with neutrophil specific-granule deficiency. Although this suggests that the C10 epitope may reside in specific granules, cellular fractionation studies were not done to determine the compartmental localization in neutrophils. In one patient with idiopathic leukemoid reaction, 100% of the neutrophils expressed the C10 epitope, which was clearly abnormal. This patient had heterogeneous G6PD expression, indicating the presence of a polyclonal neutrophil population. The meaning of the uniform C10 expression in the patient with idiopathic leukemoid reaction is unknown but suggests a relation between expression of the C10 epitope and neutrophil maturation. Despite these studies, neutrophil heterogeneity has not yet been proven to be important in normal or pathologic phagocyte function. However, the possibility that shifts in the distribution of populations of neutrophils may lead to phagocyte defects emphasizes the potential importance of neutrophil heterogeneity in the pathogenesis of certain acquired phagocyte disorders (165).

DISORDERS OF THE MONONUCLEAR PHAGOCYTE SYSTEM

Many disorders of the neutrophil extend to the mononuclear phagocyte system. Thus, patients with leukocyte adhesion deficiency, Job's syndrome, Chediak-Higashi syndrome, and CGD of childhood all have abnormalities of their mononuclear phagocytes.

Investigation of nontuberculous mycobacterial infections in patients who are not human immunodeficiency virus (HIV) infected has identified disorders that have profound effects on monocyte/macrophage activation and mycobacterial killing. Frucht and Holland (166) identified IL-12 deficiency in a family with disseminated MAC infection affecting three males in two generations. Their defect appeared to be at a regulatory level since *in vitro* administration of interferon-γ was restorative. *In vivo* administration of interferon-γ was highly effective (167). Mutations in the interferon-γ receptor-1 gene, the gene for the interferon-γ binding chain of the interferon-γ receptor, have been identified in several children with severe disseminated nontuberculous mycobacterial infections (168–170). A patient with a disabling mutation of the interferon-γ signal transducing chain (IFNγR2) of the interferon-γ receptor has also been identified (171). These findings confirm interferon-γ's central role in control of mycobacterial infections (Fig. 56-5). Of note, in the patients with interferon-γ receptor-1 and interferon-γ receptor-2 deficiency identified to date, nontuberculous mycobacteria have been the predominant opportunistic infections identified, suggesting that there may be redun-

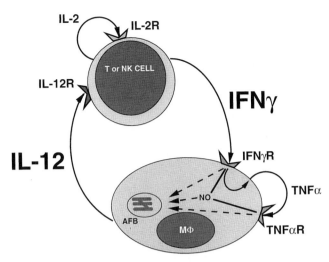

FIG. 56-5. Schematic representation of critical pathways in the control of mycobacteria. Mycobacterial infection leads to production of IL-12 leading to stimulation of T cells and natural killer (NK) cells to produce interferon-γ and IL-2. Interferon-γ binds to its cognate receptor, further activating the infected macrophage to produce tumor necrosis factor-α, to kill intracellular mycobacteria via nitric oxide (NO) and other pathways, and to drive IL-12 production forward. The *dashed lines* represent multiple direct and indirect effects of interferon-γ, tumor necrosis factor-α, and NO on killing of intracellular mycobacteria (acid fast bacilli, AFB). Not shown are numerous counterregulatory pathways (e.g., IL-4, IL-10) that work to attenuate and downregulate the inflammatory response.

dant pathways for prevention and clearance of other infections, but not for mycobacteria (172). Nitric oxide synthase is intimately involved in the control of mycobacteria. In the mouse, nitric oxide production by the macrophage-inducible nitric oxide synthase is a critical factor in protection against experimental tuberculosis (173). No lesions in human inducible nitric oxide synthase pathways have yet been identified, but if they exist, they would likely be manifest as increased susceptibility to intracellular infections. For patients with intact interferon-γ receptors and severe nontuberculous mycobacterial infections, interferon-γ has been an effective therapeutic when added to antimycobacterials (167). IL-12 is under study and may prove a useful therapeutic agent as well.

Certain viral infections impair mononuclear phagocyte function. For example, influenza and herpes simplex virus infection are associated with abnormal monocyte chemotaxis (174–176). Abnormal monocyte chemotaxis and clearance of IgG-coated erythrocytes (discussed below) are also seen in the acquired immunodeficiency syndrome (AIDS) (177). It is likely that the defects of the monocyte-macrophage system in AIDS contribute to the increased susceptibility to opportunistic infection with intracellular microorganisms such as *Pneumocystis carinii* and *Mycobacterium avium* complex (159).

Specific defects of the mononuclear phagocytes have been described in neoplasms and in certain autoimmune diseases (176). Removal of IgG-coated, radiolabeled autologous erythrocytes, presumably via the Fc receptor of splenic macrophages, is profoundly abnormal in patients with active systemic lupus erythematosus (178). Patients with other autoimmune diseases characterized by tissue deposition of immune complexes, as seen in Sjögren's syndrome, mixed cryoglobulinemia, dermatitis herpetiformis, and chronic progressive multiple sclerosis, also have defects in Fc-receptor function, as judged by clearance of IgG-coated erythrocytes. The basis for the abnormality in Fc-receptor clearance is not known. Clinically normal subjects with genetic haplotypes commonly associated with autoimmune disease (e.g., HLA-B8/DRw3) also have an increased incidence of defective Fc-receptor–specific functional activity, suggesting that this genetic profile may predispose to immune complex disease.

DIAGNOSIS AND MANAGEMENT OF PHAGOCYTE DYSFUNCTION

Most patients with disorders of phagocyte function present with clinical evidence for impaired inflammation (3). Patients often have aphthous ulcers of the mucous membranes (gray ulcers without pus). Gingivitis is common and periodontal disease is frequent in some patient groups (179). Characteristically, patients with phagocyte defects have recurrent and often severe bacterial or fungal infections that often present as difficult management problems. Patients with congenital defects can have infections within the first few days of life. In some disorders, the frequency of infection is variable, and patients may go months or even years without major infection. In recent years, with aggressive management, better diagnostic tools, and increased indices of suspicion, adults with these diseases are being seen with increasing frequency. Skin, ear, upper and lower respiratory tract, and bone infections are common. For unexplained reasons, meningitis and sepsis are rare in this group of patients.

Initial studies of white blood cell count and differential (and often bone marrow) examinations are followed by assessment of bone marrow reserves (steroid challenge test), marginated circulating pool (epinephrine challenge test), and marginating ability (endotoxin challenge test) (180). Gross abnormalities of neutrophil morphology are seen by direct examination of blood smears (e.g., Fig. 56-3B,C). *In vivo* assessment of inflammation is possible with a Rebuck skin window test, in which the ability of leukocytes to accumulate at a superficial abrasion and adhere to a glass coverslip is tested. Quantitation of neutrophil and monocyte responses, as well as of mediator production, *in vivo* is readily accomplished with a blister apparatus in which phagocyte accumulation into blisters created by suction over the forearm skin is monitored over time (181). *In vivo* clearance of IgG-coated erythrocytes provides a useful way to monitor the mono-nuclear-phagocyte system (178). *In vitro* tests of phago-cyte aggregation, adherence, chemotaxis, phagocytosis, degranulation, and microbicidal activity (for *S. aureus*) help pinpoint cellular or humoral defects that can then be characterized further at the molecular level. Deficiencies of oxidative metabolism are screened with the nitroblue tetrazolium dye (NBT) test, which is based on the ability of products of oxidative metabolism to reduce yellow, soluble NBT to blue-black formazan, an insoluble material that precipitates intracellularly and can be seen microscopically (Fig. 56-3D–F). Further aspects of neutrophil oxidative metabolism are defined by studies of super-oxide and hydrogen peroxide production. (Details of phagocyte function assays can be obtained in ref. 180). The recent development of flow cytometric detection of hydrogen peroxide detection by oxidation of dihydro-rhodamine 123 to rhodamine 123 with release of fluorescence has been effective in the diagnosis of CGD and detection of highly ionized X-linked carriers (182).

The most important aspect of patient management is to appreciate that patients with depressed phagocyte function have delayed inflammatory responses. Therefore, clinical manifestations may be minimal despite overwhelming infection, and unusual infections must always be suspected in some patients. White blood cell transfusions appear to be an important adjunct to therapy in patients with CGD (183,184). In CGD patients it has been shown that transfused phagocytes arrive at inflammatory foci functionally intact (183). Hydrogen peroxide from the normal cells diffuses into the CGD cells (185), and it is suspected that a few normal cells have the capacity to reconstitute the function of multiple CGD cells; this may explain why some CGD heterozygotes, who have only 10% normal phagocytes, live normal lives. In CGD, when excessive granulomas lead to obstruction of vital structures such as the esophagus or ureter, steroids can bring prompt relief (97). Cure of some congenital phagocyte defects has been reported by bone marrow transplantation (186–188). However, complications of bone marrow transplantation are still great, and, with rigorous medical care, many patients with disorders of phagocyte function can go for years without a life-threatening infection.

The emerging use of cytokines, especially interferon-γ, as adjunct therapy in certain patients with disorders of phagocyte function has been encouraging (189). Gene therapy for the phagocyte defects is at hand and should transform the course of these diseases in the near future (107).

REFERENCES

1. Ehrlich P. Leukocytose. In: *13th Congress of internal medicine.* Paris: 1900.
2. Metchnikoff E. *Immunity in infective diseases.* Cambridge, England: Cambridge University Press, 1905.
3. Holland SM, Gallin JI. Disorders of phagocytic cells. In: Fauci AS, Wilson JD, Braunwald E, et al., eds. *Harrison's principles of internal medicine,* 14th ed. New York: McGraw-Hill, 1998.
4. Metcalf D. Control of granulocytes and macrophages: molecular, cellular, and clinical aspects. *Science* 1991;254:529–534.
5. Athens et al. Leukokinetic studies. IV. The total blood, circulating and the granulocyte turnover rate in normal subjects. *J Clin Invest* 1961; 40:989.
6. Bodey GP, Buckley M, Sathe YS, Freireich EJ. Quantitative relationships between circulating leukocytes and infection in patients with acute leukemia. *Ann Intern Med* 1966;64:328–340.
7. Wright DG, Dale DC, Fauci AS, Wolff SM. Human cyclic neutropenia: clinical review and long term follow up of patients. *Medicine* 1981;60:1–13.
8. Kostmann R. Infantile genetic agranulocytosis: a review with presentation of ten new cases. *Acta Paediatr Scand* 1975;64:362–368.
9. Bonilla MA, Gillio AP, Ruggiero M, et al. Effects of recombinant human granulocyte colony-stimulating factor on neutropenia in patients with congenital agranulocytosis. *N Engl J Med* 1989;320: 1574–1580.
10. Welte K, Dale D. Pathophysiology and treatment of severe chronic neutropenia. *Ann Hematol* 1996;72:158–165.
11. Dale DC, Bonilla MA, Davis MW, et al. A randomized controlled phase III trial of recombinant human granulocyte colony-stimulating factor (filgrastim) for treatment of severe chronic neutropenia. *Blood* 1993;81:2496–2502.
12. Dong F, Brynes RK, Tidow N, Welte K, Lowenberg B, Tuow IP. Mutations in the gene for the granulocyte colony-stimulating-factor receptor in patients with acute myeloid leukemia preceded by severe congenital neutropenia. *N Engl J Med* 1995;333:487–493.
13. Loughran TP Jr. Clonal diseases of large granular lymphocytes. *Blood* 1993;82:1–14.
14. Lekstrom-Himes J, Xanthopoulos KG. Biological role of the CCAAT/enhancer-binding protein family of transcription factors. *J Biol Chem* 1997;273:28545–28548.
15. Zhang D-E, Nai-dy Wang PZ, Hetherington CJ, Darlington GJ, Tenen DG. Absence of granulocyte colony-stimulating factor signalling and neutrophil development in CCAAT enhancer binding protein α-deficient mice. *Proc Natl Acad Sci USA* 1997;94:569–574.
16. Screpanti I, Piero Musiani LR, Modesti A, et al. Lymphoproliferative disorder and imbalanced T-helper response in C/EBPβ deficient mice. *EMBO J* 1995;14:1932–1941.
17. Yamanaka R, Kim GD, Radomska HS, et al. CCAAT/enhancer binding protein epsilon is preferentially up-regulated during granulocytic differentiation and its functional versatility is determined by alternative use of promoters and differential splicing. *Proc Natl Acad Sci USA* 1997;94:6462–6467.
18. Pincus SH, Boxer LA, Stossel TP. Chronic neutropenia in childhood. Analysis of 16 cases and a review of the literature. *Am J Med* 1976;61: 849–861.
19. Kuhns DB, Long Priel DA, Gallin JI. Endotoxin and IL-1 hypo-responsiveness in a patient with recurrent bacterial infections. *J Immunol* 1997;158:3959–3964.
20. Gallin JI. Neutrophil specific granules: a fuse that ignites the inflammatory response. *Clin Res* 1984;32:320–328.
21. Weiss SJ. Tissue destruction by neutrophils. *N Engl J Med* 1989;320: 365–376.
22. Falloon J, Gallin JI. Neutrophil granules in health and disease. *J Allergy Clin Immunol* 1986;77:653–662.
23. Malech HL, Gallin JI. Neutrophils in human diseases. *N Engl J Med* 1987;317:687–694.
24. Borregaard N, Cowland JB. Granules of the human neutrophilic polymorphonuclear leukocyte. *Blood* 1997;89:3503–3521.
25. Boxer LA, Coates TD, Haak RA, Wolach JB, Hoffstein S, Baehner RL. Lactoferrin deficiency associated with altered granulocyte function. *N Engl J Med* 1982;307:404–409.
26. Boxer LA, Haak RA, Yang H-H, et al. Membrane-bound lactoferrin alters the surface properties of polymorphonuclear leukocytes. *J Clin Invest* 1982;70:1049–1057.
27. Oseas R, Yang H-H, Baehner RL, Boxer LA. Lactoferrin: a promoter of polymorphonuclear leukocyte adhesiveness. *Blood* 1981;57:939–948.
28. Broxmeyer HE, DeSousa M, Smithyman A, et al. Specificity and modulation of the action of lactoferrin, a negative feedback regulator of myelopoiesis. *Blood* 1980;55:324–333.

29. Brock J. Lactoferrin: a multifunctional immunoregulatory protein? *Immunol Today* 1995;16:417–419.

30. Brenton-Gorius J, Mason DY, Bruiot D, Vilde JL, Griscelli C. Lactoferrin deficiency as a consequence of a lack of specific granule in neutrophils from a patient with recurrent infection. *Am J Pathol* 1980; 99:413–419.

31. Zimmerli W, Seligmann B, Gallin JI. Exudation primes human and guinea pig neutrophils for subsequent responsiveness to the chemotactic peptide N-formylmethionylleucyl-phenylalanine and increases complement component C3bi receptor expression. *J Clin Invest* 1986; 77:925–933.

32. Gallin JI. Neutrophil specific granule deficiency. *Annu Rev Med* 1985; 36:263–274.

33. Gallin JI, Fletcher MP, Seligmann BE, Hoffstein S, Cehrs K, Mounessa N. Human neutrophil-specific granule deficiency: a model to assess the role of neutrophil-specific granules in the evolution of the inflammatory response. *Blood* 1982;59:1317–1329.

34. Komiyama A, Morosawa H, Nakahata T, Miyagawa Y, Akabane T. Abnormal neutrophil maturation in a neutrophil defect with morphologic abnormality and impaired function. *J Pediatr* 1979;94:19–25.

35. Spitznagle JK, Cooper MR, McCall AE, DeChatelet LR, Welsh IRH. Selective deficiency of granules associated with lysozyme and lactoferrin in human polymorphs with reduced microbicidal capacity. *J Clin Invest* 1972;51:93a.

36. Strauss RG, Bove KE, Jones JR, Mauer AM, Fulginiti VA. An anomaly of neutrophil morphology with impaired function. *N Engl J Med* 1974;290:478–484.

37. Parmley RT, Tzeng DY, Baehner RL, Boxer LA. Abnormal distribution of complex carbohydrates in neutrophils of a patient with lactoferrin deficiency. *Blood* 1983;62:538–548.

38. Ganz T, Metcalf JA, Gallin JI, Boxer LA, Lehrer RI. Microbicidal/cytotoxic proteins of neutrophils are deficient in two disorders: Chediak-Higashi syndrome and "specific" granule deficiency. *J Clin Invest* 1988;82:552–556.

39. Parker RI, McKeown LP, Gallin JI, Gralnick HR. Absence of the largest platelet-von Willebrand multimers in a patient with lactoferrin deficiency and a bleeding tendency. *Thromb Haemost* 1992;67:320–324.

40. Rosenberg H, Gallin JI. Neutrophil-specific granule deficiency includes eosinophils. *Blood* 1993;73:268–273.

41. Siebert PD, Huang BC. Identification of an alternative form of human lactoferrin mRNA that is expressed differentially in normal tissues and tumor derived cell lines. *Proc Natl Acad Sci USA* 1997;94: 2198–2203.

42. Hormas R, Davis B, Rauscher FJ 3rd, et al. Hematopoietic transcriptional regulation by the myeloid zinc finger gene, MZF-1. *Curr Top Microbiol Immunol* 1996;211:159–164.

43. Lomax KJ, Gallin JI, Rotrosen D, et al. Selective defect in myeloid cell lactoferrin gene expression in neutrophil specific granule deficiency. *J Clin Invest* 1989;83:514–519.

44. Lomax KJ, Malech HL, Gallin JI. The molecular biology of selected phagocyte defects. *Blood Rev* 1989;3:94–104.

45. Warden GD, Mason AD, Pruitt BA. Evaluation of leukocyte chemotaxis *in vitro* in thermally injured patients. *J Clin Invest* 1974;54: 1001–1003.

46. Davis JM, Dineen P, Gallin JI. Neutrophil degranulation and abnormal chemotaxis after thermal injury. *J Immunol* 1980;124:1467–1471.

47. Wolach B, Coates TD, Hugli TE, Baehner RL, Boxer LA. Plasma lactoferrin reflects granulocyte activation via complement in burn patients. *J Lab Clin Med* 1984;103:284–293.

48. Ambruso DR, Sasada M, Nishiyama H, Kubo A, Koiyama A, Allen RH. Defective bacterial activity and absence of specific granules in neutrophils from a patient with recurrent bacterial infections. *J Clin Immunol* 1984;4:23–30.

49. Freeman KB, Huges BJ, Buffone G, Anderson DC. Abnormal motility of neonatal PMNs: relationships to impaired "upregulation" of chemotactic factor receptors and lactoferrin secretion. *Proc Infect Immunocomp Host* 1984;3:27(abst).

50. Gallin JI, Metcalf JA, Roos D, Seligmann BE, Friedman MM. Organelle-depleted human neutrophil cytoplasts used to study fmet-leu-phe receptor modulation and cell functions. *J Immunol* 1984;133: 415–421.

51. Johnston JJ, Rintels P, Chung J, Sather J, Benz EJ Jr, Berliner N. Lactoferrin gene promoter: structural integrity and nonexpression in HL60 cells. *Blood* 1992;79:2998–3006.

52. Blume RS, Wolff SM. The Chediak-Higashi syndrome: studies in four patients and a review of the literature. *Medicine* 1972;51:247–280.

53. Wolff SM, Dale DC, Clark RA, Root RK, Kimball HR. The Chediak-Higashi syndrome: studies of host defenses. *Ann Intern Med* 1972;76: 293–306.

54. Rausch PG, Pryzwansky KB, Spitznagel JK. Immunocytochemical identification of azurophilic and specific granule markers in the giant granules of Chediak-Higashi neutrophils. *N Engl J Med* 1978;298: 693–698.

55. White JG, Clawson CC. The Chediak-Higashi syndrome: the nature of the giant neutrophil granules and their interactions with cytoplasm and foreign particulates. *Am J Pathol* 1980;98:151–167.

56. Clark RA, Kimball HR. Defective granulocyte chemotaxis in the Chediak-Higashi syndrome. *J Clin Invest* 1971;50:2645–2652.

57. Gallin JI, Klimerman JA, Padgett GA, Wolff SM. Defective mononuclear leukocyte chemotaxis in the Chediak-Higashi syndrome of humans, mink, and cattle. *Blood* 1975;45:863–870.

58. Root RK, Rosenthal AS, Balestra DJ. Abnormal bactericidal, metabolic, and lysosomal functions of Chediak-Higashi syndrome leukocytes. *J Clin Invest* 1972;51:649–665.

59. Rotrosen D, Gallin JI. Disorders of phagocyte function. *Annu Rev Immunol* 1987;5:127–150.

60. Boxer LA, Watanabe AM, Rister M, Besch HR Jr, Allen J, Baehner RL. Correction of leukocyte function in Chediak-Higashi syndrome by ascorbate. *N Engl J* Med 1976;295:1041–1045.

61. Gallin JI, Elin RJ, Hubert RT, Fauci AS, Kaliner MA, Wolff SM. Efficacy of ascorbic acid in Chediak-Higashi syndrome (CHS): studies in humans and mice. *Blood* 1979;226–234.

62. Klein M, Roder J, Haliotis T, et al. Chediak-Higashi gene in humans II. The selectivity of the defect in natural killer and antibody-dependent cell-mediated cytotoxicity function. *J Exp Med* 1980;151: 1049–1058.

63. Baetz K, Isaaz S, Griffiths GM. Loss of cytotoxic lymphocyte function in Chediak-Higashi syndrome arises from a secretory defect that prevents lytic granule exocytosis. *J Immunol* 1995;154:6122–6131.

64. Targan SR, Oseas R. The lazy NK cells of Chediak-Higashi syndrome. *J Immunol* 1983;130:2671–2674.

65. Jenkins NA, Justice MJ, Gilbert DJ, Chu M-L, Copeland NG. Nidogen/entactin (Nid) maps to the proximal end of mouse chromosome 13 linked to beige (bg) and identifies a new region of homology between mouse and human chromosomes. *Genomics* 1991;9: 401–403.

66. Barbosa MD, Nguyen QA, Tchernev VT, et al. Identification of the homologous beige and Chediak-Higashi syndrome genes. *Nature* 1996;382:262–265 (erratum *Nature* 1997;385:97).

67. Nagle DL, Karim MA, Woolf EA, et al. Identification and mutation analysis of the complete gene for Chediak-Higashi syndrome. *Nat Genet* 1996;14:307–311.

68. Karim MA, Nagle DL, Kandil HH, Burger J, Moore KJ, Spritz RA. Mutations in the Chediak-Higashi syndrome gene (CHS1) indicate a requirement for the complete 3801 amino acid CHS protein. *Hum Mol Genet* 1997;6:1087–1089.

69. Gallin JI, Buesher ES, Seligmann BE, Nath J, Gaither TE, Katz P. Recent advances in chronic granulomatous disease. *Ann Intern Med* 1983;99:657–674.

70. Tauber AI, Borregaard N, Simons E, Wright J. Chronic granulomatous disease: a syndrome of phagocyte oxidase deficiencies. *Medicine* 1983;62:286–309.

71. Gallin JI, Fauci AS, eds. *Advances in host defense mechanisms, vol 3: chronic granulomatous disease.* New York: Raven Press, 1982.

72. Volkman DJ, Buescher ES, Gallin JI, Fauci AS. B cell lines as models for inherited phagocytic diseases: abnormal superoxide generation in chronic granulomatous disease and giant granules in Chediak-Higashi syndrome. *J Immunol* 1984;133:3006–3009.

73. Roos D, de Boer M, Kuribayashi F, et al. Mutations in the X-linked and autosomal recessive forms of chronic granulomatous disease. *Blood* 1996;87:1663–1681.

74. Ahlin A, De Boer M, Roos D, et al. Prevalence, genetics and clinical presentation of chronic granulomatous disease in Sweden. *Acta Paediatr* 1995;84:1386–1394.

75. Clark RA, Malech HL, Gallin JI, et al. Genetic variants of chronic granulomatous disease: prevalence of deficiencies of two cytosolic compartments of the NADPH oxidase system. *N Engl J Med* 1989; 321:647–652.

76. Royer-Pokora B, Kunkel LM, Monaco P, et al. Cloning the gene for an inherited human disorder—chronic granulomatous disease—on the basis of its chromosomal location. *Nature* 1986;322:32–38.

77. Francke U, Hsieh C-L, Foellmer BE, Lomax KJ, Malech HL, Leto TL. Genes for two autosomal recessive forms of chronic granulomatous disease assigned to 1q25 (NCF2) and 7q11.23 (NCF1). *Am J Hum Genet* 1990;47:483–492.

78. Dinauer MC, Pierce EA, Bruns GAP, Curnutte JT, Orkin SH. Human neutrophil cytochrome b light chain (p22-phox). Gene structure, chromosome location, and mutations in cytochrome-negative autosomal recessive chronic granulomatous disease. *J Clin Invest* 1990;86: 1729–1737.

79. Francke U, Ochs HD, Darras BT, Swaroop A. Origins of mutations in two families with X-linked chronic granulomatous disease. *Blood* 1990;76:602–606.

80. De Boer M, Bolscher BG, Sijmons RH, Scheffer H, Weening RS, Roos D. Prenatal diagnosis in a family with X-linked chronic granulomatous disease with the use of the polymerase chain reaction. *Prenat Diagn* 1992;12:773–777.

81. Leto TL, Adams AG, de Mendez I. Assembly of the phagocyte NADPH oxidase: binding of Src homology 3 domains to proline-rich targets. *Proc Natl Acad Sci USA* 1994;91:10650–10654.

82. Segal AW. Absence of both cytochrome b-245 subunits from neutrophils in X-linked chronic granulomatous disease. *Nature* 1987;326:88–91.

83. Segal AW, Heyworth PG, Cockroft S, Barrowman M. Stimulated neutrophils from patients with autosomal recessive chronic granulomatous disease fail to phosphorylate a Mr-44000 protein. *Nature* 1985; 316:547–549.

84. Lomax KJ, Leto TL, Nunoi H, Gallin JI, Malech HL. Recombinant 47-kD cytosol factor restores NADPH oxidase in chronic granulomatous disease. *Science* 1989;245:409–412.

85. Volpp BD, Nauseef WM, Donelson JE, Moser DR, Clark RA. Cloning of the cDNA and functional expression of the 47-kilodalton cytosolic component of human respiratory burst oxidase. *Proc Natl Acad Sci USA* 1989;86:7195–7199.

86. Leto TL, Garrett MC, Fujii H, Nunoi H. Characterization of neutrophil NADPH oxidase factors p47phox and p67phox from recombinant baculoviruses. *J Biol Chem* 1991;266:19812–12818.

87. Casimir CM, Bu-Ganim HN, Rodaway ARF, Bentley DL, Rowe P, Segal AW. Autosomal recessive chronic granulomatous disease caused by deletion at a dinucleotide repeat. *Proc Natl Acad Sci USA* 1991;88: 2753–2757.

88. Gorlach A, Lee PL, Roesler J, et al. A p47-phox pseudogene carries the most common mutation causing p47-phox-deficient chronic granulomatous disease. *J Clin Invest* 1997;100:1907–1918.

89. Leto TL, Lomax KJ, Volpp BD, et al. Cloning of a 67 K neutrophil cytosolic oxidase factor and its similarity to a noncatalytic region of p60c-src. *Science* 1990;248:727–730.

90. Sathyamoorthy M, de Mendez I, Adams AG, Leto TL. p40(phox) down-regulates NADPH oxidase activity through interactions with its SH3 domain. *J Biol Chem* 1997;272:9141–9146.

91. Holland SM. Neutropenia and neutrophil defects. In: Rose NR, Conway de Macrio E, Folds JD, Lane HC, Nakamura RM, eds. *Manual of clinical laboratory immunology,* 5th ed. Washington, DC: American Society for Microbiology Press, 1997:855–863.

92. Forrest CB, Forehand JR, Axtell RA, Roberts RL, Johnston RB. Clinical features and current management of chronic granulomatous disease. *Hematol Oncol Clin North Am* 1988;2:253–266.

93. Muoy R, Fisher A, Vilmer E, Seger R, Griscelli C. Incidence, severity and prevention of infections in chronic granulomatous disease. *J Pediatr* 1989;114:555–560.

94. Margolis DM, Melnick DA, Alling DW, Gallin JI. Trimethoprim-sulfamethoxazole prophylaxis in the management of chronic granulomatous disease. *J Infect Dis* 1990;162:723–726.

95. Klebanoff SJ, White LR. Iodination defect in the leukocytes of a patient with chronic granulomatous disease of childhood. *N Engl J Med* 1969;280:460–466.

95a. Chang Y, Segal BH, Holland SM, Kwon-Chung J. Virulence of catalase-deficient *Aspergillus nidulans* in p47phox-/-mice. Implications for fungal pathogenicity and host defense in chronic granulomatous disease. 1998;101:1843–1850.

96. Henderson WR, Klebanoff SJ. Leukotriene production and inactivation by normal, chronic granulomatous disease and myeloperoxidase-deficient neutrophils. *J Biol Chem* 1983;258:13522–13527.

97. Chin TW, Stiehm ER, Falloon J, Gallin JI. Corticosteroids in the treatment of obstructive lesions of chronic granulomatous disease. *J Pediatr* 1987;111:349–352.

98. The International Chronic Granulomatous Disease Study Group. A controlled trial of interferon gamma to prevent infection in chronic granulomatous disease. *N Engl J Med* 1991;324:509–516.

99. Gallin JI. Interferon-gamma in the management of chronic granulomatous disease. *Rev Infect Dis* 1991;13:973–978.

100. Sechler JMG, Malech HL, White CJ, Gallin JI. Recombinant human interferon-gamma reconstitutes defective phagocyte function in patients with chronic granulomatous disease of childhood. *Proc Natl Acad Sci USA* 1988;85:4874–4878.

101. Ezekowitz RA, Dinauer MC, Jaffe HS, Orkin SH, Newburger PE. Partial correction of the phagocyte defect in patients with X-linked chronic granulomatous disease by subcutaneous interferon gamma. *N Engl J Med* 1988;319:146–151.

102. Rex JH, Bennett JE, Gallin JI, Malech HL, DeCarlo ES, Melnick DA. *In vivo* interferon gamma therapy augments the *in vivo* ability of chronic granulomatous disease neutrophils to damage Aspergillus hyphae. *J Infect Dis* 1991;163:849–852.

103. Cobbs CS, Malech HL, Leto TL, et al. Retroviral expression of recombinant p47phox protein by Epstein-Barr virus-transformed B lymphocytes from a patient with autosomal chronic granulomatous disease. *Blood* 1992;79:1829–1835.

104. Chanock SJ, Faust LRP, Barrett D, et al. O$_2$-production by B lymphocytes lacking the respiratory burst oxidase subunit p47phox after transfection with an expression vector containing a p47phox cDNA. *Proc Natl Acad Sci USA* 1992;89:10174–10177.

105. Mardiney M III, Jackson SH, Spratt SK, Li F, Holland SM, Malech HL. Enhanced host defense after gene transfer in the murine p47phox-deficient model of chronic granulomatous disease. *Blood* 1997;89: 2268–2275.

106. Bjorgvinsdottir H, Ding C, Pech N, Gifford MA, Li LL, Dinauer MC. Retroviral-mediated gene transfer of gp91phox into bone marrow cells rescues defect in host defense against Aspergillus fumigatus in murine X-linked chronic granulomatous disease. *Blood* 1997;89: 41–48.

107. Malech HL, Maples PB, Whiting-Theobald N, et al. Prolonged production of NADPH oxidase-corrected granulocytes after gene therapy of chronic granulomatous disease. *Proc Natl Acad Sci USA* 1997;94: 12133–12138.

108. Nauseef WM, Root RK, Malech HL. Biochemical and immunologic analysis of hereditary myeloperioxidase deficiency. *J Clin Invest* 1983; 71:1297–1307.

109. Nauseef WM. Myeloperoxidase deficiency. *Hematol Pathol* 1990;4: 165–178.

110. Stendahl O, Coble BI, Dahlgre C, Hed J, Molin L. Myeloperoxidase modulates the phagocytic activity of polymorphonuclear neutrophil leukocytes. Studies with cells from a myeloperoxidase-deficient patient. *J Clin Invest* 1984;73:366–373.

111. Koeffler HP, Ranyard J, Pertcheck M. Myeloperoxidase. Its structure and expression during myeloid differentiation. *Blood* 1985;65:484–491.

112. Nauseef WM. Myeloperoxidase biosynthesis by a human promyelocytic leukemia cell line: insight into myeloperoxidase deficiency. *Blood* 1986;67:965–972.

113. Nauseef WM. Aberrant restriction endonuclease digests of DNA from subjects with hereditary myeloperoxidase deficiency. *Blood* 1989;73: 290–295.

114. Kizaki M, Miller CW, Selsted ME, Koeffler HP. Myeloperoxidase (MPO) gene mutation in hereditary MPO deficiency. *Blood* 1994;83: 1935–1940.

115. Nauseef WM, Brigham S, Cogley M. Hereditary myeloperoxidase deficiency due to a missense mutation of arginine 569 to tryptophan. *J Biol Chem* 1994;269:1212–1216.

116. Davis SD, Schaller JK, Wedgewood RJ. Job's syndrome: recurrent "cold" staphylococcal abscesses. *Lancet* 1966;1:1013–1015.

117. Buckley RH, Becker WG. Abnormalities in the regulation of human IgE synthesis. *Immunol Rev* 1978;41:288–314.

118. Hill HR. The syndrome of hyperimmunoglobulin E and recurrent infections. *Am J Dis Child* 1982;136:767–771.

119. Donabedian H, Gallin JI. The hyperimmunoglobulin E recurrent infection (Job's) syndrome. *Medicine* 1983;62:195–208.

120. Geha RS, Leung DYM. Hyper immunoglobulin E syndrome. *Immunodeficiency Rev* 1989;1:155–172.

121. Berger M, Kirkpatrick CH, Goldsmith PK, Gallin JI. IgE antibodies to *Staphylococcus aureau* and *Candida albicans* in patients with the syndrome of hyperimmunoglobulin E and recurrent infections. *J Immunol* 1980;125:2437–2443.

122. Dreskin SC, Goldsmith PK, Gallin JI. Immunoglobulins in the hyperimmunoglobulin E and recurrent infection (Job's) syndrome. *J Clin Invest* 1985;75:26–34.

123. Dreskin SC, Goldsmith PK, Strober W, Zech LA, Gallin JI. The metabolism of IgE in patients with markedly elevated serum IgE levels. *J Clin Invest* 1987;79:1764–1772.

124. Buckley RH, Sampson HA. The hyperimmunoglobulinema E syndrome. In: Franklin EC, ed. *Clinical immunology update*. Amsterdam: Elsevier/North-Holland, 1981:148–167.

125. Clark RA, Root RK, Kimball HR, Kirkpatrick CH. Defective neutrophil chemotaxis and cellular immunity in a child with recurrent infections. *Ann Intern Med* 1973;78:515–519.

126. Donabedian H, Gallin JI. Mononuclear cells from patients with the hyperimmunoglobulin E-recurrent infection syndrome produce an inhibitor of leukocyte chemotaxis. *J Clin Invest* 1982;69:1155–1163.

127. Donabedian H, Gallin JI. Two inhibitors of neutrophil chemotaxis are produced by hyperimmunoglobulin E recurrent infection syndrome mononuclear cells exposed to heat-killed staphylococci. *Infect Immun* 1983;40:1030–1037.

128. Seligmann BE, Fletcher MP, Gallin JI. Histamine modulation of human neutrophil oxidative metabolism, locomotion, degranulation and membrane potential changes. *J Immunol* 1983;130:1902–1909.

129. Dreskin SC, Kaliner MA, Gallin JI. Elevated urinary histamine in the hyperimmunogobulin-E and recurrent infection (Job's) syndrome: association with eczematoid dermatitis and not with infection. *J Allergy Clin Immunol* 1987;79:515–522.

130. Geha RS, Reinherz E, Lung D, McKee KT, Schlossman S, Rosen FS. Deficiency of suppressor T cells in the hyperimmunoglobulin E syndrome. *J Clin Invest* 1981;68:783–791.

131. Gallin JI, Wright DG, Malech HL, Davis JM, Klempner MS, Kirkpatrick CH. Disorders of phagocyte chemotaxis. *Ann Intern Med* 1980;92:520–538.

132. Hoger PH, Bolthauser E, Hitzig WH. Craniosynostosis in hyper-IgE-syndrome. *Eur J Pediatr* 1985;144:414–417.

133. Brestel EP, Klingberg WG, Veltri RW, Dorn JS. Osteogenesis imperfecta tarda in a child with hyper-IgE syndrome. *Am J Dis Child* 1982; 136:774–776.

134. Leung DY, Key L, Steinberg JJ, et al. Increased *in vitro* bone resorption by monocytes in the hyper-immunoglobulin E syndrome. *J Immunol* 1988;140:84–88.

135. Cohen-Sala M, Prieur AM, Prin L, et al. Cytokine-mediated bone resorption in patients with the hyperimmunoglobulin E syndrome. *Clin Immunol Immunopathol* 1995;76:75–81.

135a. Grimbacher B, Holland SM, Gallin JI, et al. Hyper IgE recurrent infection syndrome: an autosomal dominant multisystem disorder. *N Engl J Med,* in press.

136. Delespesse G, Sarafati M, Heusser C. IgE synthesis. *Curr Opin Immunol* 1990;2:506.

137. Vercelli D, Geha RS. Regulation of IgE synthesis in man. *J Clin Immunol* 1989;9:75–83.

138. Del Prete G, Tiri A, Maggi E, et al. Defective *in vitro* production of gamma-interferon and tumor necrosis factor by circulating T cells from patients with the hyperimmunoglobulin E syndrome. *J Clin Invest* 1989;84:1830–1835.

139. Paganelli R, Scala E, Capobianchi MR, et al. Selective deficiency of interferon-gamma production in the hyper-IgE syndrome. *Clin Exp Immunol* 1991;84:28.

140. King CL, Gallin JI, Malech HL, Abramson SL, Nutman TB. Regulation of immunoglobulin production in hyperimmunoglobulin E recurrent-infection syndrome by interferon gamma. *Proc Natl Acad Sci USA* 1989;86:10085–10089.

141. Vercelli D, Jabara HH, Cuningham-Rundles C, et al. Regulation of immunoglobulin E synthesis in the hyper-IgE syndrome. *J Clin Invest* 1990;85:1666–1671.

142. Jeppson JD, Jaffe HS, Hill HR. Use of recombinant human interferon gamma to enhance neutrophil chemotactic responses in Job syndrome of hyperimmunoglobulin E and recurrent infections. *J Pediatr* 1991; 118:383.

143. Van Scoy RE, Hill HR, Ritts RE, Quie PG. Familial neutrophil chemotaxis defect, recurrent bacterial infections, mucocutaneous candidiasis, and hyperimmunoglobulinemia E. *Ann Intern Med* 1975;82:766–771.

144. Dreskin SC, Gallin JI. Evolution of the hyper immuno-globulin E and infection (HIE, Job's) syndrome in a young girl. *J Allergy Clin Immunol* 1987;80:746–751.

145. Mareni C, Sessarego M, Montera M, et al. Expression and genomic configuration of GM-CSF, IL-3, M-CSF receptor (C-FMS), early growth response gene-1 (EGR-1) and M-CSF genes in primary myelodysplastic syndromes. *Leuk Lymphoma* 1994;15:135–141.

146. Marsh DG, Neely JD, Breazeale DR, et al. Linkage analysis of IL4 and other chromosome 5q31.1 markers and total serum immunoglobulin E concentrations. *Science* 1994;264:1152–1156.

147. Lewanda AF, Jabs E. Genetics of craniofacial disorders. *Curr Opin Pediatr* 1994;6:690–697.

148. van Dyke TE. Role of the neutrophil in oral disease: receptor deficiency in leukocytes from patients with juvenile periodontitis. *Rev Infect Dis* 1985;7:419–425.

149. van Dyke TE, Levine MJ, Tabak LA, Genco RJ. Reduced chemotactic peptide binding in juvenile periodontitis: a model for neutrophil function. *Biochem Biophys Res Commun* 1981;100:1278–1284.

150. van Dyke TE, Levine MJ, Genco RJ. Neutrophil function and oral disease. *J Oral Pathol* 1985;14:95–120.

151. De Nardin E, De Luca C, Levine MJ, Genco RJ. Antibodies directed to the chemotactic factor receptor detect differences between chemotactically normal and defective neutrophils from LJP patients. *J Periodontol* 1990;61:609–617.

152. Perez HD, Kelly E, Elfman F, Armitage G, Winkler J. Defective polymorphonuclear leukocyte formyl peptide receptors in juvenile periodontitis. *J Clin Invest* 1991;87:971–976.

153. Hurttia HM, Pelto LM, Leino L. Evidence of an association between functional abnormalities and defective diacylglycerol kinase activity in peripheral blood neutrophils from patients with localized juvenile periodontitis. *J Periodontal Res* 1997;32:401–407.

154. Sabin FB. Studies of living human blood cells. *Bull Johns Hopkins Hosp* 1923;34:277–288.

155. McCutcheon M. Studies on the locomotion of leukocytes. I. The normal rate of locomotion of human neutrophilic leukocytes *in vivo. Am J Physiol* 1923;66:180–195.

156. Howard TH. Quantitation of the locomotive behavior of polymorphonuclear leukocytes in clot preparations. *Blood* 1982;59:946–951.

157. Harvath L, Leonard EJ. Two neutrophil populations in human blood with different chemotactic activities: separation and chemoattractant binding. *Infect Immun* 1982;36:443–451.

158. Seligmann B, Chused TM, Gallin JI. Differential binding of chemoattractant peptide to subpopulations of human neutrophils. *J Immunol* 1984;133:2641–2646.

159. Ball ED, Graziano RF, Shen L, Fanger MW. Monoclonal antibodies to novel myeloid antigens reveal human neutrophil hetergeneity. *Proc Natl Acad Sci USA* 1982;79:5374–5378.

160. Clement LT, Lehmeryer JE, Gartland GL. Identification of neutrophil subpopulations with monoclonal antibodies. *Blood* 1983;61:326–332.

161. Seligmann B, Malech HL, Melnick DA, Gallin JI. An antibody binding to human neutrophils demonstrates antigenic heterogeneity detected early in myeloid maturation which correlates with functional heterogeneity of mature neutrophils. *J Immunol* 1985;135:2647–2653.

162. Gallin JI, Jacobson RJ, Seligmann BE, et al. A neutrophil membrane marker reveals two groups of chronic myelogenous leukemia and its absence may be a marker of disease progression. *Blood* 1986;68: 343–346.

163. Spiekermann K, Roesler J, Elsner J, et al. Identification of the antigen recognized by the monoclonal antibody 31D8. *Exp Hematol* 1996;24: 453–458.

164. Brown CC, Malech HL, Jacobson RJ, et al. Unique human neutrophil populations are defined by monoclonal antibody ED12F8C10. *Cell Immunol* 1991;132:102–114.

165. Gallin JI. Human heterogeneity exists but is it meaningful. *Blood* 1984;63:977–983.

166. Frucht DM, Holland SM. Defective monocyte costimulation for interferon gamma production in familial disseminated *Mycobacterium avium* complex infection. *J Immunol* 1996;157:411–416.

167. Holland SM, Eisenstein E, Kuhns DB, et al. Treatment of refractory disseminated non-tuberculous mycobacterial infection with interferon gamma: a preliminary report. *N Engl J Med* 1994;330:1348–1355.

168. Newport MJ, Huxley CM, Huston S, et al. A mutation in the inter-

feron-gamma-receptor gene and susceptibility to mycobacterial infection. *N Engl J Med* 1996;335:1941–1949.

169. Jouanguy E, Altare F, Lamhamedi S, et al. Interferon-gamma-receptor deficiency in an infant with fatal bacille Calmette-Guerin infection. *N Engl J Med* 1996;335:1956–1961.

170. Holland SM, Dorman SE, Kwon A, et al. Abnormal regulation of interferon-gamma, interleukin-12, tumor necrosis factor-alpha in human interferon-gamma receptor 1 deficiency. *J Infect Dis* 1998;178:1095.

171. Dorman SE, Holland SM. Mutation in the signal transducing chain of the interferon gamma receptor and susceptibility to disseminated nontuberculous mycobacterial infection. Submitted.

172. Jouanguy E, Altare F, Lamhamedi-Chrradi S, Casanova J-L. Infections in IFNgammaR1-deficient children. *J Interferon Cytokine Res* in press.

173. MacMicking JD, North RJ, LaCourse R, Mudgett JS, Shah SK, Nathan CF. Identification of nitric oxide synthase as a protective locus against tuberculosis. *Proc Natl Acad Sci USA* 1997;94:5243–5248.

174. Kleinerman ES, Snyderman R, Daniels CA. Depression of human monocyte chemotaxis by herpes simplex and influenza viruses. *J Immunol* 1974;113:1562–1567.

175. Larson HE, Blades R. Impairment of human polymorphonuclear leukocyte function by influenza virus. *Lancet* 1976;1:283–284.

176. Snyderman R, Pike MC. Pathophysiologic aspects of leukocyte chemotaxis: identification of a specific chemotactic factor binding site on human granulocytes and defects of macrophage function associated with neoplasia. In: Gallin JI, Quie PG, eds. *Leukocyte chemotaxis: methods, physiology and clinical implications.* New York: Raven Press, 1978:357–378.

177. Smith PD, Ohura K, Masur H, Lane HC, Fauci AS, Wahl SM. Monocyte function in the acquired immune deficiency syndrome. Defective chemotaxis. *J Clin Invest* 1984;74:2121–2128.

178. Frank MM, Lawley TJ, Hamberger MI, Brown EJ. Immunoglobulin G Fc receptor-mediated clearance in autoimmune diseases. *Ann Intern Med* 1983;98:206–218.

179. Charon JA, Mergenhagen SE, Gallin JI. Gingivitis and oral ulceration in patients with neutrophil dysfunction. *J Oral Pathol* 1985;14:150–155.

180. Metcalf JA, Gallin JI, Nauseef WM, Root RK. *Laboratory manual of neutrophil function.* New York: Raven Press, 1986.

181. Zimmerli W, Gallin JI. Monocytes accumulate on Rebuck skin window coverslips but not in skin chamber fluid: a comparative evaluation of two *in vivo* migration methods. *J Immunol Methods* 1987;96:11–17.

182. Vowells SJ, Sekhsaria S, Malech HL, Shalit M, Fleisher TA. Flow cytometric analysis of the granulocyte respiratory burst: a comparison of fluorescent probes. *J Immunol Methods* 1995;178:89–97.

183. Buescher ES, Gallin JI. Leukocyte transfusions in chronic granulomatous disease. *N Engl J Med* 1982;307:800–803.

184. Quie PG. The white cells: use of granulocyte transfusions. *Rev Infect Dis* 1987;9:189–193.

185. Ohno Y, Gallin JI. Diffusion of extracellular hydrogen peroxide into intracellular compartments of human neutrophils. *J Biol Chem* 1985;260:8438–8446.

186. Anderson DC, Schmalstieg FC, Arnaout MA, et al. Abnormalities of polymorphonuclear leukocyte function associated with a heritable deficiency of high molecular weight surface glycoproteins (gp138): common relationship to diminished cell adherence. *J Clin Invest* 1984;74:536–551.

187. Fisher A, Trung PH, Descamps-Latsdra B, et al. Bone marrow-transplantation for inborn error of phagocytic cells associated with defective adherence, chemotaxis, and oxidative response during opsonized particle phagocytosis. *Lancet* 1983;2:473–476.

188. Kamani N, August CS, Douglas SD, Burkey E, Etzioni A, Lischner HW. Bone marrow transplantation in chronic granulomatous disease. *J Pediatr* 1984;105:42–46.

189. Gallin JI, Farber JM, Holland SM, Nutman TB. Interferon-g in the management of infectious diseases. *Ann Intern Med* 1995;123:216–224.

Inflammation: Basic Principles and Clinical Correlates,
3rd ed., edited by John I. Gallin and Ralph Snyderman.
Lippincott Williams & Wilkins, Philadelphia © 1999.

CHAPTER 57

Urticaria and Angioedema

Allen P. Kaplan

Urticaria and angioedema are common disorders affecting approximately 20% of the population at some time during their lifetime. Urticaria (hives) is an intensely pruritic rash that consists of a centrally raised, blanched wheal surrounded by an erythematous flare that is generally circular but can vary greatly in size and shape, depending on the particular type. It is caused by inflammation that is localized to the venular plexuses of the superficial dermis. Angioedema (except hereditary and vibratory angioedema) has the same causes and pathogenic mechanisms as does urticaria, but the reaction occurs in the deep dermis and subcutaneous tissue; swelling is the prominent manifestation, and the external appearance of the skin is normal.

Inflammatory mechanisms operative in urticaria can be divided into two types, depending on the rate at which hive formation occurs and the length of time it is evident. One form of urticaria has lesions that last 1 to 2 hours and results from degranulation of mast cells. The inciting stimulus is present only briefly, and there is no late component to the urticaria. Biopsy of such lesions reveals little or no cellular infiltrate. The second form has a prominent cellular infiltrate, and individual lesions can last from many hours to as long as 2 days. This review describes the various types of urticaria, ranging from those that are among the most fleeting (and simplest) to those of progressively longer duration. The focus is on pathogenic mechanisms and the nature of the inflammatory reaction.

THE PHYSICAL URTICARIAS

Physically induced hives or swelling share the common property of being reproducibly induced by environmental factors such as a change in temperature or by direct stimulation of the skin by pressure, stroking, vibration, or light (1). These disorders have been the subject of considerable investigation and serve as models (2) from which a great deal has been learned about pathogenic mechanisms leading to hive formation and swelling. A classification of these disorders is given in Table 57-1, which includes virtually all described types.

Cold-Dependent Disorders

Idiopathic cold urticaria is characterized by the rapid onset of pruritus, erythema, and swelling after exposure to a cold stimulus. The swelling is confined to those parts of the body that have been exposed; in this sense, it is a local rather than a systemic disorder. However, total body exposure, such as occurs with swimming, can cause massive release of vasoactive mediators, resulting in hypotension; if the subject loses consciousness, death by drowning can result. The disease can begin at any age, and there is no obvious sex predilection. When cold urticaria is suspected, an ice-cube test can be performed. An ice cube is placed on the subject's forearm for 4 to 5 minutes. Formation of a hive in the shape of the area contacted by the ice cube within 10 minutes after the stimulus is removed constitutes a positive reaction. The time course of this reaction (i.e., cold challenge followed by hive formation as the area returns to body temperature) demonstrates that a two-step reaction has occurred; exposure to cold is a prerequisite, but hive formation actually occurs as the temperature increases.

The term *idiopathic* was used originally to indicate that the cause of cold urticaria was unknown and was unassociated with abnormal circulating plasma proteins such as cryoglobulins. However, there is evidence that many of these responses are caused by an immunologic reaction. Within this group, most have been shown to depend on immunoglobulin E (IgE), based on passive transfer stud-

A. P. Kaplan: Department of Medicine, Medical University of South Carolina, Charleston, South Carolina 29425.

TABLE 57-1. *Classification of physically induced urticaria and/or angioedema*

Cold-dependent disorders
  Idiopathic cold urticaria
  Cold urticaria associated with abnormal serum proteins:
    cold agglutinins, cryoglobulin, cryofibrinogen, Donath-
    Landsteiner antibody
  Systemic cold urticaria
  Cold-induced cholinergic urticaria
  Cold-dependent dermatographism
  Delayed cold urticaria
Exercise-induced disorders
  Exercise-induced anaphylaxis: idiopathic or
    food-dependent
  Cholinergic urticaria
    (see above for cold-dependent variant)
  Exercise-induced angioedema
Local heat urticaria
  Familial variant
Dermatographism
  Urticaria pigmentosa/systemic mastocytosis
  Cold-dependent variant (see above)
  Delayed dermatographism
Pressure-induced urticaria/angioedema (delayed)
  Immediate-pressure urticaria
Solar urticaria
  Types I through VI
Aquagenic urticaria
Vibratory angioedema
  Familial
  Sporadic

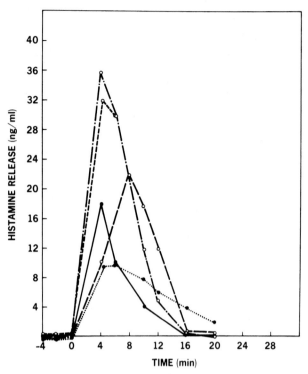

FIG. 57-1. Time course of histamine release into the venous circulation of five patients with cold urticaria. The patient's hand was placed in ice water for 5 minutes, and serial blood samples were obtained from the brachial vein draining that arm. Histamine was determined by radioenzyme assay.

ies (3). Serum of the subject is injected intradermally into a normal recipient. After 48 hours, the site is challenged with an ice cube. Although the reported incidence of positive transfer varies, experience suggests that about 10% of responses are positive. This is undoubtedly an underestimate, because passive transfer is far less sensitive than an ice-cube test in the propositus, and the reactions of only those subjects with sufficient pathogenic IgE in the circulation (rather than IgE bound to mast cells) are detected. In two cases, an IgM antibody was shown to mediate cold urticaria (4). In these cases, passive transfer was positive after a short interval of 3 to 6 hours but was negative at 48 hours, in contrast to the IgE-mediated reaction, which remains positive at 48 hours. A similar passive transfer (i.e., positive only after short-term sensitization) that seemed to be caused by an IgG antibody has also been reported (5).

Studies of the pathogenesis of cold urticaria have demonstrated release of mediators into the circulation when one of a patient's hands was placed in ice water for 5 minutes (Fig. 57-1) and serial blood samples were obtained for 20 minutes thereafter. As with the ice-cube test, swelling usually is not evident while the hand is being chilled; instead, swelling appears 4 to 8 minutes after the stimulus is removed and is associated with marked pruritus. In this case, chilling occurs in the deep dermis and subcutaneous tissue in addition to the more superficial skin layers; therefore, the entire hand swells and angioedema results. Studies have documented the release of histamine (6), eosinophilotactic peptides (7), high-molecular-weight neutrophil chemotactic factor (8), platelet-activating factor (9), and prostaglandin D_2 (10,11), into the circulation, with a time course that parallels the manifest swelling. It is envisioned that chilling initiates a reaction mediated by IgE bound to mast cells and that, on warming, mediators are released into the circulation. When skin biopsy specimens were tested by chilling and warming, histamine release also was demonstrated (12) (Fig. 57-2); however, chilling and warming of basophils of patients did not result in histamine release, even in those in whom IgE-mediated disease was documented. Therefore, it appears unlikely that the disorder is caused by a circulating IgE cryoglobulin (unless the patients' basophils are desensitized). Rather, the presence of skin or cutaneous mast cells seems essential.

One proposal to explain such a result is that patients have an IgE autoantibody to a cold-induced skin antigen; sensitization would occur in the cold condition, and release of mediators would proceed as the cells warmed. Studies to test this hypothesis have thus far been negative. High levels of IgM and IgG antibodies directed against the Fc portion of IgE were found in patients with cold urticaria (5); although the clinical significance of such autoantibodies is questionable (13), one such serum

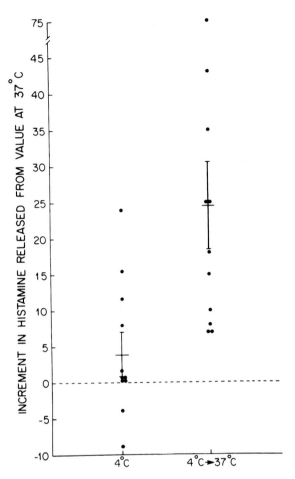

FIG. 57-2. Histamine release from skin biopsy specimens of patients with cold urticaria. Replicate skin fragments were suspended in phosphate-buffered saline and either (a) chilled for 30 minutes at 4°C and then maintained for 30 minutes at 37°C or (b) chilled for 15 minutes at 4°C and then warmed to 37°C for 15 minutes. Histamine was determined in the surrounding fluid. Samples that were chilled or chilled and then warmed were compared with those kept at 37°C, and the differences in histamine values were plotted. The mean ± 1 standard error is indicated. Samples that were chilled were not significantly different from those maintained at 37°C, whereas those that were chilled and warmed released histamine into the surrounding medium.

caused release of histamine when incubated with normal basophils. However, this reaction was demonstrable at 37°C and did not require chilling followed by warming, so its relation to the disease is not clear.

Cyproheptadine (Periactin) in divided doses is the drug of choice for cold urticaria. Histamine release is unaffected by doses that completely control symptoms (14), so the drug appears to act as a classic antihistamine (i.e., by blockade of histamine type 1 [H$_1$] receptors). However, other antihistamines of comparable potency are less effective; the reason for this is uncertain. Although cyproheptadine has antiserotonin activity, serotonin does not appear to be released in cold urticaria. Some patients do

not respond well to cyproheptadine either, and it has been reported that symptoms do not always correlate well with histamine release (15). Therefore, other vasoactive factors may make a significant contribution for some patients. Experimental cromolyn-like drugs, which inhibit mast cell degranulation, are effective in controlling symptoms and suppressing the ice-cube test reaction in patients who are poorly responsive to cyproheptadine (16). Ketotifen, in particular, has been shown to inhibit histamine release and is effective in a variety of physically induced urticarias (17).

Localized cold urticaria, in which only certain areas of the body urticate with cold contact, has been reported after predisposing conditions such as cold injury; it has also been reported at sites of intracutaneous allergen injections, ragweed immunotherapy, or insect bites. One patient has been described who had cold urticaria confined to the head and face but no identifiable antecedent or associated event (18). Such cases argue against the presence of a circulating factor and in favor of a local abnormality of mast cells.

Cold urticaria has also been described as being associated with the presence of cryoproteins such as cold agglutinins, cryoglobulins, cryofibrinogen, and the Donath-Landsteiner antibody seen in secondary syphilis (paroxysmal cold hemoglobinuria). The only reported studies that address mechanisms of hive formation are those performed in patients with associated cryoglobulins. The isolated proteins appear to transfer cold sensitivity and activate the complement cascade on *in vitro* incubation with normal plasma (19,20). Therefore, it is possible that hive formation in these subjects results from cold-dependent release of anaphylatoxin. Therapy in this case is directed toward the underlying disease plus antihistamines. It is clear that a disorder such as cryoglobulinemia can be associated with cutaneous vasculitis as well as with cold urticaria, and other associations between these two entities have been reported. Eady and Greaves (21) reported that frequent and repeated cooling of the skin in patients with idiopathic cold urticaria can cause vasculitic lesions. In one case, immune reactants (IgM and C3) were deposited in the vessels of such lesions (22). In two other patients, leukocytoclastic vasculitis was seen in association with cold urticaria, and circulating immune complexes were clearly evident (23,24). It appeared that the mediator release caused by cold challenge could localize immune complexes to cutaneous sites, where they then caused vasculitis (23). Sites of typical urticarial vasculitis independent of temperature change also were evident (24).

Other cold-dependent syndromes have been reported, but the incidence of such cases is unknown. A delayed form of cold urticaria was described (25) in which swelling appeared 9 to 18 hours after cold exposure. Studies of mediator release were unrevealing, the cold sensitivity could not be passively transferred, and biopsy of a lesion revealed edema and a mononuclear cell infiltrate. Family studies suggested a dominant mode of inheritance.

Four patients have been described in whom exercise in a cold environment induced hives similar to those seen with cholinergic urticaria; however, hive formation did not occur if exercise was performed in a heated environment. This disorder, in which the cold exposure is systemic rather than local, should be suspected in any patient whose symptoms are suggestive of either cold urticaria or cholinergic urticaria but who have negative results on standard tests for those disorders (26). Exercise in a cold room or running on a winter's day leads to generalized urticaria and confirms the diagnosis. Because of the visual resemblance of the lesions to those of typical cholinergic urticaria, the disorder has been called *cold-induced cholinergic urticaria*. A study of 13 patients with symptoms suggestive of cold urticaria and cholinergic urticaria revealed 2 who did not have both disorders but who had the cold-induced cholinergic-type hives (27).

Another related disorder, called *systemic cold urticaria*, yields severe generalized hive formation on systemic cold challenge occurring over covered or uncovered parts of the body. Symptoms are unrelated to exercise or other activities (28), and the ice-cube test is negative. Histamine release on cold challenge (with or without exercise as appropriate) has been seen in cold-induced cholinergic urticaria as well as in systemic cold urticaria. Treatment regimens of hydroxyzine plus cyproheptadine in high dosage (29) or of doxepin (30) have been used successfully.

Another disorder, called *cold-dependent dermatographism*, has been reported in which prominent hive formation is seen if the skin is scratched and then chilled (28). In this disorder, the ice-cube test and the systemic cold challenge yield no hives. Simply scratching the skin yields a weakly positive dermatographic response, but dramatic accentuation is seen when the scratched area is chilled. Treatment once again consists of high-dose antihistamines—for example, 200 mg of diphenhydramine per day or a combination of hydroxyzine (100 to 200 mg/day) and cyproheptadine (8 to 16 mg/day).

Finally, a disorder called *localized cold reflex urticaria* has been reported in which the ice-cube test is positive but hives form in the vicinity of the contact site, not where the cube is applied (31,32). The appearance of the hives resembles the punctate lesions of cholinergic urticaria, and there is no confluent hive where the ice cube is applied. A methacholine or acetylcholine skin test for cholinergic urticaria is negative, although the symptoms of one such patient resembled those of cold-induced cholinergic urticaria in that exercise-induced hives were seen in a cold environment (31).

Exercise-Induced Disorders

Cholinergic or generalized heat urticaria is characterized by the onset of small punctate wheals surrounded by a prominent erythematous flare associated with exercise, hot showers, sweating, and anxiety (33). Typically, lesions first appear about the neck and upper thorax; when viewed from a distance, hives may not be perceived and the patient appears flushed (Fig. 57-3). However, pruritus is a prominent feature of the reaction; on close inspection, small punctate wheals can be discerned that are sometimes as small as 1 mm in diameter and are surrounded by a prominent flare. Gradually, the lesions spread distally to involve the face, back, and extremities, and the wheals increase in size. In some patients, the hives become confluent and resemble angioedema (34). Also occasionally seen are symptoms of more generalized cholinergic stimulation such as lacrimation, salivation, and diarrhea. These various stimuli have the common feature of being mediated by cholinergic nerve fibers that innervate the musculature via parasympathetic neurons and innervate the sweat glands via cholinergic fibers that travel with the sympathetic nerves (35). The characteristic lesion of cholinergic urticaria can be reproduced by intradermal injection of 0.1 mg of methacholine (Mecholyl) in 0.1 mL saline. When positive, the resultant localized hive surrounded by satellite lesions is indistinguishable from the patient's spontaneously induced lesions and confirms the diagnosis. However, my colleagues and I have found that only about one third of patients give a clearly positive skin test, these generally being the most severe cases. Challenge by exercise (e.g., running in an 85°F warmed room or using a bicycle ergometer for 10 to 15 minutes) is a far more sensitive test. Therefore, the skin test can be used to confirm the diagnosis but cannot be used as a diagnostic test (6,36). Those patients who have a positive methacholine skin test demonstrate a

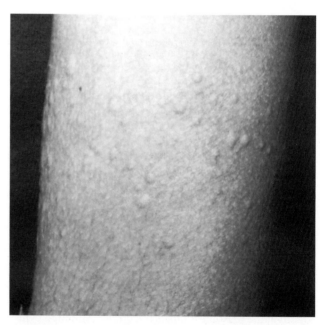

FIG. 57-3. Urticaria developing about the forearm of a patient with cholinergic urticaria.

"hypersensitivity" to cholinergic mediators, but they have no evidence of an immunoglobulin-mediated allergy to acetylcholine. It is possible that the disorder is caused by an intrinsic cellular abnormality that results in abnormal mediator release in the presence of cholinergic agents. One study addressing this issue demonstrated an increased number of muscarinic receptors in urticarial sites. These receptors were further augmented when exercise followed patch testing with copper-containing materials (37). The increased number of acetylcholine binding sites may be an important key to understanding the pathogenesis of cholinergic urticaria. The importance of copper is unclear, but it may affect ligand-receptor affinity.

There is evidence that a reflex consisting of afferent humoral and efferent neurogenic components is involved in this urticarial disorder. When a patient's hand is placed in warm water with a tourniquet tied proximal to that hand, there is no urticaria until the tourniquet is released. A generalized eruption then ensues. A central perception of temperature change transmitted via the circulation appears to be followed by an efferent reflex leading to urticaria. Such a reflex could also account for the association of hives with anxiety (38), although it should be emphasized that in these instances the emotional reaction may be completely appropriate. Cholinergic urticaria is the only form of hives in which emotional stimuli can, in some patients, initiate an urticarial reaction.

Studies of mediator release during attacks of cholinergic urticaria have demonstrated that, in most cases, the elevation in plasma histamine levels parallels the onset of pruritus and urticaria (Fig. 57-4) (6). Further studies have confirmed the presence of histaminemia in association with cholinergic urticaria (6,39), and release of eosinophilotactic peptides and neutrophil chemotactic

factor have also been observed (40). When patients were challenged while wearing a plastic occlusive suit to produce maximal changes in cutaneous and core body temperature, significant falls in 1-second forced-expiratory volumes, maximal midexpiratory flow rate, and specific conductance were seen associated with a rise in residual volume. Four of seven patients also had wheezing detected by auscultation. Therefore, under such conditions, an abnormality in pulmonary function can be detected, reflecting either primary pulmonary involvement or altered pulmonary mechanics secondary to circulating mediators. A clinically significant alteration in pulmonary function is unusual in cholinergic urticaria and has no known association with exercise-induced asthma.

Kaplan et al. (41) also described two patients with typical cholinergic urticaria in whom lesions became confluent and were associated with prominent elevation of plasma histamine as well as recurrent episodes of hypotension. Therefore, some extreme cases of cholinergic urticaria can resemble the exercise-induced anaphylactic syndrome. An important distinguishing feature is that an increase in core body temperature of more than 0.7°C, obtained with the use of hyperthermic blankets or submersion in warmed water, causes hives, histamine release, and anaphylactic symptoms in patients with cholinergic urticaria with anaphylactic-like symptoms, but not in those with the exercise-induced anaphylactic syndrome (42).

Combinations of physical urticarias can occur in the same patient—for example, cold urticaria (39) or dermatographism (40) in association with cholinergic urticaria. Furthermore, the combined response of cold and cholinergic urticaria, fulfilling separate criteria for

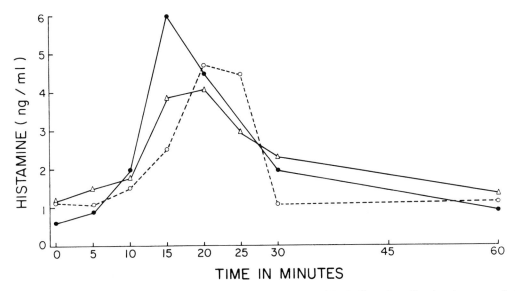

FIG. 57-4. Time course of histamine release in three patients with cholinergic urticaria who were challenged by running in a heated room (85°F) for 10 minutes.

each disorder (27,39), is to be distinguished from cold-induced cholinergic urticaria (26).

Treatment of cholinergic urticaria generally consists of hydroxyzine (100 to 200 mg/day) in divided doses (38). Many, but not all, patients respond to this regimen. Anticholinergic agents such as atropine or propantheline bromide (Pro-Banthine) have little effect, perhaps because of an inability to attain a sufficient systemic level; however, injected atropine can reverse the methacholine skin test (39).

The syndrome of exercise-induced anaphylaxis was first described in a series of patients in whom combinations of pruritus, urticaria, angioedema, wheezing, and hypotension occurred as a result of exercise. Symptoms did not occur with each exercise experience, and most of the described patients were accomplished athletes (43). The disorder is distinguished from cholinergic urticaria by the following criteria. First, although exercise is the precipitating stimulus of each disorder, hot showers, sweating in the absence of exercise, and anxiety do not trigger attacks of exercise-induced anaphylaxis as they do in cholinergic urticaria. Second, the hives seen with exercise-induced anaphylaxis are large (10 to 15 mm), in contrast to the punctate lesions that characterize cholinergic urticaria. Finally, when patients with exercise-induced anaphylaxis were challenged in an occlusive suit, no change in pulmonary function was seen, although histamine release was documented (45). Optimal therapy for the exercise-induced anaphylactic syndrome is uncertain, and attempts at prophylaxis using H_1 and H_2 antagonists have not generally been effective (46). In contrast, classic cholinergic urticaria usually is responsive to prophylactic use of hydroxyzine.

Subtypes of exercise-induced anaphylaxis that are food-related have also been described. In one case, exercise-induced anaphylaxis occurred if the exercise took place 5 to 24 hours after eating shellfish, whereas exercise alone or eating shellfish alone did not cause any symptoms (47). In five other reported cases, two patients had symptoms only if exercise followed the ingestion of any food within 2 hours (34,48). In the remaining three cases, symptoms were precipitated by the specific ingestion of celery within 2 hours of exercise (49); these patients also had positive skin tests to celery. Therefore, various forms of food-dependent exercise-induced anaphylaxis are possible, and treatment requires avoidance of specific foodstuffs before exercising or avoidance of exercise within certain time intervals after eating. Kivity et al. (50) demonstrated augmented wheal responses to skin tests of compound 48/80 (a cutaneous mast cell degranulating agent), but not of histamine, in subjects with food-induced (skin-test-positive), exercise-induced anaphylaxis. Food or exercise alone did not affect the 48/80 response, suggesting increased mast cell releasability caused by the combination of food plus exercise. In another report, one patient with cholinergic urticaria and

associated anaphylaxis was successfully treated by vigorous daily exercise: desensitization occurred within a week (41). The number of patients with cholinergic urticaria or the exercise-induced anaphylactic syndrome that might respond to such treatment is unknown, although this treatment is more likely to be effective in cholinergic urticaria (with or without hypotension) because symptoms occur reproducibly each time an exercise challenge is done.

Other Physically Induced Forms of Urticaria or Angioedema

The remaining forms of physically induced hives or swelling are, with the exception of dermatographism, relatively rare disorders. These include local heat urticaria, pressure-induced urticaria and angioedema, solar urticaria, aquagenic urticaria, and vibratory angioedema.

Localized Heat Urticaria

Localized heat urticaria is a rare disorder in which urticaria develops within minutes after exposure to applied heat (51). Sixteen patients with this disorder have been described, mostly women. When the disorder is suspected, it can be tested by application of a test tube of warm water at 44°C to the arm for 4 to 5 minutes. If the test is positive, a hive is seen a few minutes after the test tube is removed. Studies of mediator release in local heat urticaria resemble those reported in cold urticaria—plasma histamine levels peak 5 to 10 minutes after heat exposure (52,53)—but passive transfer studies have been negative. Neutrophil chemotactic factor was also found to be released in one study (52); therefore, mast cell degranulation in response to heat challenge seems likely. In one report, complement abnormalities were reported in the absence of histamine release (54). Association with other forms of physical allergy is sometimes seen—for example, combined cold urticaria and local heat urticaria (55). Therapy has been problematic, because antihistamines such as hydroxyzine or cyproheptadine, as well as oral disodium cromoglycate, have been ineffective. One patient was successfully desensitized by repeated daily immersion in hot baths, but caution is advised, because systemic reactions are possible (54).

A variant of this disorder has been described which was familial and in which urticaria occurred 1.5 to 2 hours after application of a warm stimulus (56) and persisted for 6 to 10 hours. Sunbathing with pronounced heating of skin could produce wheals as a result of the temperature effect, even though sunlight itself was tolerated. Desensitization of an area of skin could be achieved with repeated challenge every few days. Skin biopsy demonstrated a pronounced inflammatory cell infiltrate in the upper dermis and around hair follicles. The pathogenesis of this form of local heat urticaria is unknown. Partial control was achieved with oral antihistamines.

Dermatographism

The ability to write on skin, termed *dermatographism,* can occur as an isolated disorder that often manifests as traumatically induced urticaria. It can be diagnosed by observing the skin after stroking it with a tongue depressor or fingernail. In such patients, a white line secondary to reflex vasoconstriction is followed by pruritus, erythema, and a linear wheal, as in the classic wheal-and-flare reaction. It is said to be present in 2% to 5% of the population (2,57); however, only a small fraction of these cases are of sufficient severity to warrant treatment. Biopsy of the skin reveals few changes, but most occur in the epidermis and consist of vacuolation of keratinocytes and basal epidermal cell pseudopodia, along with the appearance of typical mast cell granules (58). In approximately 50% of cases, passive transfer studies have demonstrated an IgE-dependent mechanism (60). Many patients, it appears, have an abnormal circulating IgE that confers a particular form of pressure sensitivity to dermal mast cells. Such observations further suggest that histamine is one of the mediators of dermatographism, although demonstration of such release has been difficult because of the localized nature of the reaction. Early studies did suggest that histamine is released into whole blood (61); that induced blisters over lesions contain elevated histamine levels (62); that 24-hour urine histamine levels are elevated (63); and that histamine is increased in the perfusate, as shown by *in vivo* subcutaneous perfusion studies (64). In a single, unusually severe case of IgE-mediated dermatographism, elevation of plasma histamine levels was documented within 1 minute of stroking of the skin, and the baseline histamine level was abnormal in multiple determinations, suggesting that "leakage" of histamine was ongoing at all times (65).

Although the evidence is anecdotal because a formal study has not been performed, dermatographism has been observed as a consequence of drug reactions (57); in one case, dermatographism could be observed only on challenge with the offending agent—in this instance, penicillin (66). Therapy for dermatographism consists of antihistamines (67,68); for severe symptoms, high doses may be needed. The initial objective of therapy is to decrease pruritus so that the stimulation for scratching is diminished. Many patients complain of a sensation of itching or "skin crawling" that is readily relieved by antihistamines. At higher doses, the wheal-and-flare reaction to stroking also is markedly diminished.

Dermatographism also occurs in association with other disorders; for example, a mild form may be seen in some patients with chronic urticaria. Severe dermatographism is also associated with disorders in which a marked increase in dermal mast cells is seen (e.g., urticaria pigmentosa or systemic mastocytosis). Release of histamine in these disorders has been demonstrated (63). It is also

possible that other vasoactive agents released from cutaneous mast cells can be implicated in dermatographism and, in fact, in all forms of physically induced urticaria. An example is the elevation of prostaglandin D_2 metabolites in the urine of patients with systemic mastocytosis, which may contribute to the hypotension associated with this disorder (69).

Pressure-induced Urticaria and Angioedema

Pressure-induced urticaria differs from most of the aforementioned types of hives or angioedema in that symptoms typically occur 4 to 6 hours after pressure has been applied (70). The disorder is clinically heterogeneous in that some patients may complain of swelling secondary to pressure with normal-appearing skin (i.e., no erythema or superficial infiltrating hive), so that the term angioedema is more appropriate. Others reactions are predominantly urticarial and may or may not be associated with significant swelling. When urticaria is present, an infiltrative lesion is seen, characterized by a perivascular mononuclear cell infiltrate and dermal edema similar to that seen with chronic idiopathic urticaria (71). Immediate dermatographism is not present, but delayed dermatographism is seen and may represent the same disorder (29). Symptoms occur about tight clothing; the hands may swell with activity such as hammering; foot swelling is common after walking; and buttock swelling may be prominent after sitting for a few hours. Testing for pressure-induced urticaria can be done by placing a sling (with a 5- to 15-lb weight attached) over the forearm or shoulder for 10 to 20 minutes. Gradual pressure applied by devices in grams per square millimeter can also be used (71). There are few available studies regarding pathogenesis; however, mediators that cause pain rather than pruritus (e.g., kinins) have been considered, because the lesions typically are described as burning or painful. Nevertheless, induced blisters over lesions revealed histamine release following the time course of hive formation (62). Antihistamines have little effect on the disorder, and patients with severe disease often have to be treated with corticosteroids.

Although pressure urticaria or angioedema can occur as an isolated disorder, it is most often seen in association with chronic urticaria. Therapy is then usually directed toward the chronic urticaria. There are data to suggest an increased incidence of food allergy in those patients with chronic urticaria in whom pressure-induced symptoms are also prominent (72).

Immediate-pressure urticaria has been described in patients with the hypereosinophilia syndrome, characterized by an acute wheal-and-flare reaction within 1 to 2 minutes after the application of pressure (e.g., pressing on the back with one's thumb). These patients also were dermatographic, although dermatographics typically do not have immediate-pressure urticaria and require a stroking motion to produce a hive (73).

Solar Urticaria

Solar urticaria is a rare disorder in which brief exposure to light causes the development of urticaria within 1 to 3 minutes. Typically, pruritus occurs first, in about 30 seconds, followed by edema confined to the light-exposed area and surrounded by a prominent erythematous zone caused by an axon reflex. The lesions usually disappear within 1 to 3 hours. When large areas of the body are exposed, systemic symptoms may occur, including hypotension and asthma. Although most reported patients have been in their third and fourth decades, the disorder can occur in any age group and has no association with other allergic disorders.

Solar urticaria has been classified into six types, depending on the wavelength of light that induces lesions and the ability or inability to passively transfer the disorder with serum (74–76). Types I and IV can be passively transferred and therefore may be immunologically (possibly IgE) mediated; they are associated with wavelengths of 280 to 320 nm and 400 to 500 nm, respectively. An antigen has not been identified. Histamine release, mast cell degranulation (77), and formation of chemotactic factors for eosinophils and neutrophils (78) have been observed coincident with induction of lesions when ultraviolet light (type I) was shone on skin.

Type VI solar urticaria, activated at 400 nm, is clearly an inherited metabolic disorder, in which protoporphyrin IX acts as a photosensitizer, and is synonymous with erythropoietic protoporphyria. It is caused by ferrochetalase deficiency (79,80). In contrast to other forms of porphyria, the urinary porphyrin excretion is normal; however, red blood cell protoporphyrin and fecal protoporphyrin and coproporphyrin levels are elevated. Irradiation of serum samples of such patients resulted in activation of the classic complement pathway and generation of C5a chemotactic activity (81); this activity was proportional to the serum level of protoporphyrin (44). Irradiation of the forearms of two such patients also resulted in *in vivo* complement activation, as assessed by a diminution of titers of C3 and C5 and generation of C5a (82). Consistent with these observations are the facts that deposition of C3 and accumulation of neutrophils are seen in the dermis (83,84) and that complement fragments can be detected in the serum and suction blister fluid of irradiated skin (83). The condition responds to oral β-carotene, which absorbs light at the same wavelengths as protoporphyrin IX (85).

The mechanism by which urticaria is produced in types II, III, and V is unknown, but these reactions are induced by inciting wavelengths of 320 to 400, 400 to 500, and 280 to 500 nm, respectively. As a simple screen, fluorescent tubes that emit a broad, continuous spectrum can be used to test the patient, and filters can then be used to define the spectrum that causes urticaria. Therapy for this disease requires avoidance of sunlight, protective garments to cover the skin, and use of topical preparations to absorb or reflect light. A 5% solution of paraaminobenzoic acid in ethanol, as found in sunscreen lotions, can be helpful in the 280- to 320-nm range, but it is more difficult to screen out the visible spectrum. The most effective agents for this purpose contain titanium oxide or zinc oxide, or both. The efficacy of antihistamines, antimalarials, and corticosteroids in these disorders is not clear and needs to be evaluated in each case.

Aquagenic Urticaria

Thirteen cases have been reported of patients who developed small wheals after contact with water, regardless of its temperature, and who were distinguishable from patients with cold urticaria or cholinergic urticaria. This disorder has been termed *aquagenic urticaria* (86). Direct application of a compress of tap water or distilled water to the skin is used to test for its presence. The diagnosis should be reserved for those rare patients who test positively for water but negatively for all other forms of physical urticaria. Combined cholinergic and aquagenic urticaria has been reported, and histamine release into the circulation has been documented on challenge with water (87).

Hereditary Vibratory Angioedema

Hereditary vibratory angioedema has been described in a single family, in whom it was inherited in an autosomal dominant pattern. It is properly viewed as a physically induced angioedema, because patients complain of intense pruritus and swelling within minutes after vibratory stimulation (88). The patients are not dermatographic and do not have pressure-induced urticaria. Lesions can be reproduced by gentle stimulation of the patient's forearm with a laboratory vortex for 4 minutes. Rapid swelling of the entire forearm and a portion of the upper arm ensues, and histamine has been shown to be released after such a vibratory stimulus (89). With care, patients can avoid vibratory stimuli, and their symptoms can otherwise be partially relieved with diphenhydramine (Benadryl). Nonfamilial, sporadic cases have also been described.

ACUTE, NONPHYSICALLY INDUCED URTICARIA

Acute urticaria is a commonly encountered disorder that can be caused by a wide variety of agents. Most prominent are drug reactions, allergy to foods, and urticaria in association with infection or other systemic diseases. Episodes of acute urticaria usually last from a few days to 2 or 3 weeks. When the urticarial episode exceeds 6 weeks, it is arbitrarily designated "chronic."

The hive caused by a food or drug reaction differs from that seen with the various physical urticarias because individual lesions can remain prominent for many hours to 1 or 2 days. In this respect, the lesions more closely resemble those of chronic urticaria than those of the physical urticarias (90). An allergic mechanism, in the strictest sense, requires an interaction of IgE antibody with the allergen (e.g., food or drug), followed by degranulation of cutaneous mast cells. However, when an allergic person is skin-tested (e.g., intracutaneous administration of ragweed antigen to a person with ragweed-induced rhinitis), the immediate wheal-and-flare reaction lasts a few minutes and disappears; it may then be followed by a swelling, 4 to 6 hours later, which is called a late phase reaction (91). It has been shown that late phase reactions depend on the prior IgE reaction (92). They consist of a mixed cellular infiltrate containing mononuclear cells, neutrophils, eosinophils, and basophils (93,94) and are associated with a second wave of secretion of histamine (95) and other vasoactive substances.

Human mast cells have been shown to release an array of cytokines, including chemokines, that may be necessary for the late phase reaction (see Chapter 7). These include tumor necrosis factor-α; granulocyte-macrophage colony-stimulating factor; interleukins -1, -4, -5, -6, -9, and -13 (96); and chemokines such as interleukin-8 and "regulated on activation, normally T-cell expressed and secreted" (RANTES) (97). The stimulation of endothelial cells by vasoactive mediators followed by these cytokines plus priming of migrating cells, and release of chemotactic substances, may lead to the transendothelial cell migration into skin that is required for a late phase reaction to occur. Virtually all β chemokines are chemotactic for monocytes and subpopulations of T lymphocytes. Monocyte chemotactic proteins (MCP)-1, -2, -3, and -4, RANTES, and macrophage inflammatory protein-1α are chemotactic for basophils and activate them (98–102), whereas RANTES, eotaxin, MCP-3, and MCP-4 are active on eosinophils (59,102–104). The protracted histamine release associated with the late phase may be caused by basophil (rather than mast cell) infiltration and activation. Cutaneous injection of 48/80, a polypeptide that causes mast cell degranulation, can also lead to late phase reactions (105). It appears that the late phase reaction in the skin requires something besides a single burst of mast cell degranulation, but no data are available regarding this issue. It can be theorized that mast cell degranulation that persists over time or persistence of antigenic stimulation over time (or both) is the critical difference. This would be absent in virtually all the physical urticarias except delayed-pressure urticaria. Perhaps the persistence of the hive in food or drug reactions is related to this phenomenon.

Urticaria has also been well documented during viral infections such as hepatitis (106) or infectious mononucleosis (107), and a large number of helminthic parasites are associated with hives. Serum sickness reactions (including the prodrome of hepatitis B infection) can be seen as a manifestation of drug reactions, and on biopsy evidence of a small-vessel cutaneous vasculitis is observed (108). Urticaria in association with systemic lupus erythematosus (109,110) or other vasculitides appears similar. Necrosis of the vessel wall (most prominent in small venules), infiltration with neutrophils, and deposition of immunoglobulins and complement occur. It is thought that these disorders are caused by immune complex deposition in the dermal vasculature and release of histamine (and other mediators) from perivenular mast cells as a result of local formation of the anaphylatoxins C3a, C5a, and C4a (111). IgE antibody to the initiating antigen may also be contributory. Patients with systemic lupus erythematosus in particular may, alternatively, have classic chronic urticaria rather than a necrotizing angiitis, because there is now evidence that the latter disorder is autoimmune in origin and associated with Hashimoto's thyroiditis.

CHRONIC IDIOPATHIC URTICARIA AND IDIOPATHIC ANGIOEDEMA

This is a common disorder of unknown origin. Patients need not be atopic persons; that is, they do not have an increased incidence of atopic dermatitis, allergic rhinitis, or asthma compared with the incidence of these disorders in the absence of chronic urticaria. Their IgE level, as a group, is within normal limits. Some patients are dermatographic, although this condition is usually of milder degree than is seen with the IgE-dependent dermatographism described earlier. The dermatographism may wax and wane, just as the urticaria may vary from severe to mild or may intermittently subside. These patients have a normal leukocyte count and erythrocyte sedimentation rate and have no evidence of systemic disease. They do not demonstrate evidence of any of the causes of urticaria or angioedema discussed previously (i.e., foods, drugs, additives, infection, systemic disease, association with other allergic phenomena, or triggering by physical agents). Chronic urticaria therefore does not appear to be an allergic reaction in the classic sense, because IgE antibody is not involved and no external allergen is needed to initiate or perpetuate the process. It differs from allergen-induced skin reactions and from physically induced urticaria (e.g., dermatographia, cold urticaria) in that histologic studies reveal a cellular infiltrate predominantly about small venules (90). External examination reveals infiltrative hives with palpably elevated borders, sometimes varying greatly in size or shape but generally being rounded.

The typical lesion consists of a nonnecrotizing perivascular mononuclear cell infiltrate (Fig. 57-5). However, many types of histopathologic processes can occur in the skin and manifest as hives. For example, patients with hypocomplementemia and cutaneous vasculitis can have urticaria (or angioedema), and biopsy of patients with

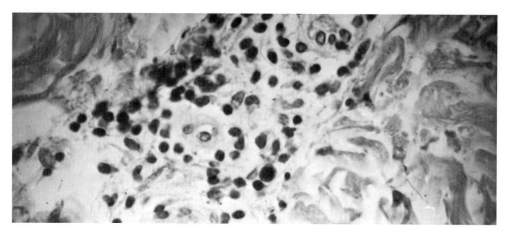

FIG. 57-5. Skin biopsy of chronic urticaria demonstrating a nonnecrotizing perivenular infiltrate consisting primarily of mononuclear cells.

urticaria, arthralgias, myalgias, and an elevated erythrocyte sedimentation rate as manifestations of necrotizing venulitis revealed fibrinoid necrosis with a predominant neutrophilic infiltrate (112,113). Yet, the urticarial lesions were indistinguishable from those seen in the more typical, nonvasculitis cases.

Other studies (114–117) have examined the incidence of vasculitis in patients with urticaria with a wide variety of results. Mathison et al. (114) found that 10 of 78 patients had hypocomplementemia, and many patients showed evidence of activation of the classic complement pathway. Six of the 10 had increased levels of circulating immune complexes. If hypocomplementemia and vasculitis are equated, the incidence of presumed vasculitis was 14%. Monroe et al. (115) found neutrophilic leukocytoclastic angiitis in 20% of patients; the other 80% had a perivascular infiltrate of mononuclear cells that was classified as dense or sparse. The vasculitis, dense infiltrate, and sparse infiltrate groups had circulating immune complex levels of 33%, 29%, and 13%, respectively, as measured by multiple assays. Phanuphak et al. (117) used the criterion of significant cellular infiltrate within vessel walls (rather than endothelial damage, nuclear dust, fibrin deposition, or red blood cell extravasation) to define vasculitis and found a 52% incidence of vasculitis (various types of predominant cells) and a 48% incidence of a perivascular mononuclear-cell infiltrate. Deposition of immune complexes in skin was seen in 18% of the vasculitis group, almost exclusively in those with an abundance of neutrophils.

My colleagues and I have reported results of a study of the histopathology of chronic idiopathic urticaria in 43 consecutive patients (116). All but one in the group had a nonnecrotizing perivascular infiltrate consisting primarily of lymphocytes. We therefore found vasculitis to be a rare cause of urticaria and believe that our group is comparable to the group without vasculitis in the study of Mathison et al. (114), to the sparse and dense infiltrate

groups of Monroe et al. (115), and to the perivasculitis group of Phanuphak et al. (117).

We also noted a tenfold increase in the number of mast cells and a fourfold increase in the number of mononuclear cells in skin biopsy specimens from the patients with chronic urticaria, compared with normal controls (Table 57-2). No increase in basophil number was seen; however, circulating basophils of chronic urticaria patients are reported to be less responsive to anti-IgE than are cells of normal subjects, suggesting *in vivo* desensitization (118) and the presence of a circulating basophil activator.

The increase in mast cells observed may be reflected in the increased amount of histamine found in blister fluid suctioned from patients with chronic urticaria compared with normal controls (62) and in the increased level of total skin histamine content reported to be present in such patients (119). A more recent study (120) did not confirm an increased number of mast cells based on tryptase staining, and the authors speculated that basophil infiltration or an increased histamine content per cell might account for the earlier observations. Differences in sampling and level of mast cell degranulation are other variables that might explain the discrepancy. Although eosinophils were not prominent in the skin biopsies of our series of patients when considered as a group, some patients had a prominent eosinophil accumulation. In one study, deposition of eosinophil major basic protein in skin specimens of 50% of patients with chronic urticaria was demonstrated, although only a fraction of them had obvious eosinophil infiltration (121). Therefore, degranulated eosinophils may be present, perhaps more commonly than previously appreciated.

A later study of the histology of chronic urticaria identified the infiltrating cells by immunoperoxidase staining of cell-surface antigens, employing monoclonal antibodies specific for monocytes, T cells, B cells, and natural killer (NK) cells, and by histochemical staining of mast

TABLE 57-2. *Infiltrating cells in skin biopsy specimens from patients with chronic urticaria and normal controls*

Cell type	Mean no. of cells (range)[a]	
	Patients (n = 43)	Controls (n = 7)
Eosinophils	1.2 (0–12)	0
Basophils	0.35 (0–2)	0
Neutrophils	3.0 (0–50)	0.14 (0–1)
Mononuclear cells	52.4 (16–247)	13.4 (3–25)
Mast cells	7.6 (0–19)	0.71 (0–3)

[a]Number counted per five reticules.

cells. The infiltrate was shown to consist of 50% T lymphocytes, 20% monocytes, 11% mast cells, and 19% unidentified infiltrating lymphocytes (122). There were no B lymphocytes or NK cells. The unidentified cells may have represented immature cells that were nonreactive within a tissue section or perhaps γδ T lymphocytes; these possibilities require reassessment with additional antisera. Chronic urticaria is most frequently characterized by a nonnecrotizing perivascular lymphocyte infiltrate with an accumulation of histamine-containing cells and augmented releasability. Patients with vasculitis and urticaria probably represent a separate subpopulation in whom the pathogenesis of hive formation probably involves immune complexes, complement activation, anaphylatoxin formation, histamine release, and neutrophil accumulation, activation, and degranulation.

There has been considerable interest in the possibility that chronic urticaria may be an autoimmune disorder. Perhaps the first suggestion for this hypothesis arose from data that demonstrated an association of chronic urticaria with autoimmune hypothyroidism (Hashimoto's thyroiditis) and, more specifically, with the presence of antibodies to peroxidase or thyroglobulin. The incidence was 12% to 14% in two studies of patients with chronic urticaria (123,124). However, it was noted that thyroid status did not relate to the occurrence of urticaria and that, typically, hives did not remit when a euthyroid status was achieved. However, thyroid autoantibodies in these patients typically persist as well.

Gruber et al. (125) reported the presence of circulating IgG or IgM anti-IgE antibodies in subjects with chronic urticaria. The incidence was approximately 10%, and the condition was not seen in normal controls or in patients with other types of urticaria, except cold urticaria. The underlying hypothesis was that such an antibody could degranulate cutaneous mast cells *in vivo* and lead to acute hives or even to a late phase reaction and its concomitant cellular infiltrate. More recently, Hide et al. (126) reported the presence of anti-IgE receptor antibodies in 30% to 40% of patients with chronic urticaria and anti-IgE antibodies in an additional 10%. These studies demonstrated autoreactivity to autologous serum in such subjects; that is, injections of serum induced a wheal-and-flare reaction (126). These sera could degranulate

basophils to release histamine, and those reactive with cells stripped of their IgE were presumed to be reactive with the IgE receptor. The sera were inhibitable either with the α subunit of the IgE receptor or with IgE itself, confirming the functional reactivity.

Fiebiger et al. (127) reported similar functional data in patients with chronic urticaria and demonstrated that the observations cannot be ascribed to IgE-containing immune complexes. They also demonstrated positive immunoblots to cloned α subunit, indicating the presence of IgG anti-FcεRIa. Functional analysis of sera capable of degranulating basophils also concluded that anti-receptor antibodies were present. IgE was removed from the cells by mild acid treatment, and most sera could still cause degranulation (128). The incidence of such antibodies is, however, uncertain, and proof of their pathogenicity requires confirmation that they are responsible for the cellular infiltrate seen as well as for the resulting symptoms.

We assessed patients with chronic urticaria for such antibodies by a variety of methods, including histamine release from human basophils, β-hexosaminodase release from Rat basophil leukemia (RBL) cells that were transfected with the α subunit of the IgE receptor (Fig. 57-6), and immunoblotting for the presence of IgG anti-FcεRIa. The results of these initial experiments suggested the presence of such antibodies in at least one third of patients with chronic urticaria (129). We subsequently enlarged this population from 50 to 83 subjects and included studies of histamine release from partially purified cutaneous mast cells, since this is clearly the relevant cell in the reaction. When all the data from these patients were combined, 46% were found to test positive for basophil histamine release and 60% were positive with cutaneous mast cells; moreover, 59% had positive immunoblots. Although all of these studies are highly correlated with each other, it is clear that a greater number of positive results are obtained when cutaneous mast cells are used, and we have identified a subgroup of

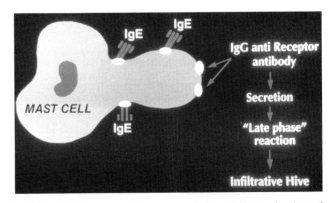

FIG. 57-6. Diagrammatic representation of the activation of cutaneous mast cells by immunoglobulin G (IgG) antibody directed to the IgE receptor.

patients with positive histamine release but negative immunoblots, suggesting an alternative pathogenic mechanism. All tests are negative in about 40% of subjects, even though these patients are clinically indistinguishable from those with positive results.

A detailed protocol for the treatment of chronic urticaria has been published (130). It consists of antihistamine therapy to maximally tolerated doses and alternate-day administration of corticosteroids. The latter regimen is recommended for some patients in whom the disease cannot otherwise be controlled; these most typically are patients with daily or almost daily generalized eruptions. They may also have associated angioedema, particularly of the face. A typical dose is 20 to 25 mg prednisone every other day, with a slow taper of 2.5 to 5.0 mg every 2 to 3 weeks, as tolerated. These most recent data provide a rationale for such an approach, although we have used it for the past 25 years. If chronic urticaria is an autoimmune disease with protracted mast cell degranulation, the cellular infiltrate may represent a late phase reaction or a cutaneous variant thereof. Like the late phase reaction observed in severe allergic rhinitis or asthma, chronic urticaria may require antiinflammatory therapy with steroids. However, typical therapy is ineffective, and use of systemic steroids is required. Since an autoantibody has now been demonstrated, experimental protocols being considered include use of cyclosporin, plasmapheresis, intravenous γ-globulin, and methotrexate. One or more of these treatments may prove to be efficacious and helpful for particularly severe cases that are poorly responsive even to corticosteroids, but their use currently should be restricted to research protocols.

REFERENCES

1. Gorevic P, Kaplan AP. The physical urticarias. *Int J Dermatol* 1980; 19:417.
2. Soter NA, Wasserman SI. Physical urticaria/angioedema: an experimental model of mast cell activation in humans. *J Allergy Clin Immunol* 1980;66:358.
3. Houser DD, Arbesman CE, Ito K, Wicher K. Cold urticaria: immunologic studies. *Am J Med* 1970;49:23.
4. Wanderer AA, Maselli R, Ellis EF, Ishizaka K. Immunologic characterization of serum factors responsible for cold urticaria. *J Allergy Clin Immunol* 1971;48:13.
5. Gruber BL, Marchese M, Ballan D, Kaplan AP. Anti IgG autoantibodies: detection in urticarial syndromes and ability to release histamine from basophils [abstract]. *J Allergy Clin Immunol* 1986;77:187.
6. Kaplan AP, Gray L, Shaff RE, et al. *In vivo* studies of mediator release in cold urticaria and cholinergic urticaria. *J Allergy Clin Immunol* 1975; 55:394–402.
7. Soter NA, Wasserman SI, Austen KF. Cold urticaria: release into the circulation of histamine and eosinophil chemotactic factor of anaphylaxis during cold challenge. *N Engl J Med* 1976;294:687.
8. Wasserman SE, Soter NA, Center DM, Austen KF. Cold urticaria: recognition and characterization of a neutrophil chemotactic factor which appears in serum during experimental cold challenge. *J Clin Invest* 1977;60:189.
9. Grandel KE, Farr RS, Wanderer AA, Eisenstadt TC, Wasserman SI. Association of platelet-activating factor with primary acquired cold urticaria. *N Engl J Med* 1985;313:405–409.
10. Ormerod AD, Black AK, Dawes J, et al. Prostaglandin D2 and histamine release in cold urticaria unaccompanied by evidence of platelet activation. *J Allergy Clin Immunol* 1988;82:586.
11. Weinstock G, Arbeit L, Kaplan AP. Release of prostaglandin D₂ and kinins in cold urticaria and cholinergic urticaria [abstract]. *J Allergy Clin Immunol* 1986;77:188.
12. Kaplan AP, Garofalo J, Sigler R, Hauber T. Idiopathic cold urticaria: *in vitro* demonstration of histamine release upon challenge of skin biopsies. *N Engl J Med* 1981;305:1074.
13. Quinti I, Brozek C, Wood N, Geha R, Leung OYM. Circulating IgG autoantibodies to IgE in atopic syndromes. *J Allergy Clin Immunol* 1986;77:586.
14. Sigler RW, Evans R III, Horakova Z. The role of cyproheptadine in the treatment of cold urticaria. *J Allergy Clin Immunol* 1980;65:309.
15. Keahey TM, Greaves MW. Cold urticaria: dissociation of cold-evoked histamine release and urticaria following cold challenge. *Arch Dermatol* 1980;116:174.
16. Petillo JJ, Natbony SK, Zisblatt M, Vukovich RA, Neiss ES, Kaplan AP. Preliminary report of the effects of tiaramide on the ice cube test in patients with idiopathic cold urticaria. *Ann Allergy* 1983;51:511.
17. Houston DP, Bressler RB, Kaliner M, Sowell LK, Baylor MW. Prevention of mast-cell degranulation by ketotifen in patients with physical urticaria. *Ann Intern Med* 1986;204:507.
18. Kurtz AS, Kaplan AP. Regional expression of cold urticaria. *J Allergy Clin Immunol* 1990;86:272.
19. Costanzi JJ, Coltman CA Jr. Kappa chain cold precipitable immunoglobulin (IgG) associated with cold urticaria: 1. Clinical observations. *Clin Exp Immunol* 1967;2:167.
20. Costanzi JJ, Coltman CA Jr, Donaldson VH. Activation of complement by a monoclonal cryoglobulin associated with cold urticaria. *J Lab Clin Med* 1969;74:902.
21. Eady RA, Greaves MW. Induction of cutaneous vasculitis by repeated cold challenge in cold urticaria. *Lancet* 1978;1:336.
22. Eady RAJ, Keahey TM, Sibbald RG, Black AK. Cold urticaria with vasculitis: report of a case with light and electron microscopic, immunofluorescence, and pharmacological studies. *Clin Exp Dermatol* 1981;6:335.
23. Soter NA, Mihm MC Jr, Dvorak HF, Austen KF. Cutaneous necrotizing venulitis: a sequential analysis of the morphological alterations occurring after mast cell degranulation in a patient with a unique syndrome. *Clin Exp Immunol* 1978;32:46.
24. Wanderer AA, Nuss DP, Tormey AD, Giclas PC. Urticarial leukocytoclastic vasculitis with cold urticaria: report of a case and review of the literature. *Arch Dermatol* 1983;119:145.
25. Soter WA, Joski NP, Twarog FJ. Delayed cold-induced urticaria: a dominantly inherited disorder. *J Allergy Clin Immunol* 1977;54:294.
26. Kaplan AP, Garofalo J. Identification of a new physically induced urticaria: cold induced cholinergic urticaria. *J Allergy Clin Immunol* 1981;68:438.
27. Ormerod AD, Kobza-Black A, Milford-Ward A, Greaves MW. Combined cold urticaria and cholinergic urticaria—clinical characterization and laboratory findings. *Br J Dermatol* 1988;118:621.
28. Kaplan AP. Unusual cold-induced disorders: cold dependent dermatographism and systemic cold urticaria. *J Allergy Clin Immunol* 1984; 73:453–456.
29. Kalz F, Bower CM, Prichard H. Delayed and persistent dermographia. *Arch Dermatol* 1950;61:772.
30. Kivity S, Schwartz Y, Wolf R, Topilsky M. Systemic cold-induced urticaria: clinical and laboratory characterization. *J Allergy Clin Immunol* 1989;85:52.
31. Czarnetzki BM, Frosch PJ, Sprekeler R. Localized cold reflex urticaria. *Br J Dermatol* 1981;104:83.
32. Ting S, Mansfield LE. Localized cold reflex urticaria. *J Allergy Clin Immunol* 1985;75:421.
33. Grant RT, Pearson RSB, Comeaw WJ. Observations on urticaria provoked by emotion, by exercise, and by warming the body. *Clin Sci (Colch)* 1935;2:253.
34. Lawrence CM, Jorizzo JL, Kobza-Black A. Cholinergic urticaria with associated angioedema. *Br J Dermatol* 1981;105:543.
35. Herxheimer A. The nervous pathway mediating cholinergic urticaria. *Clin Sci (Colch)* 1956;15:195.
36. Commens CA, Greaves CA. Tests to establish the diagnosis in cholinergic urticaria. *Br J Dermatol* 1978;98:47.
37. Shelley WB, Shelley CD, Ho AKS. Cholinergic urticaria: acetyl-

choline-receptor dependent immediate-type hypersensitivity reaction to copper. *Lancet* 1983;1:843.

38. Moore-Robinson M, Warin RP. Some clinical aspects of cholinergic urticaria. *Br J Dermatol* 1968;80:794.

39. Sigler RW, Levinson AI, Evans R III, Horokova Z, Kaplan AP. Evaluation of a patient with cold and cholinergic urticaria. *J Allergy Clin Immunol* 1979;63:35.

40. Soter NA, Wasserman SI, Austen KF, McFadden ER Jr. Release of mast-cell mediators and alterations in lung function in patients with cholinergic urticaria. *N Engl J Med* 1980;302:604.

41. Kaplan AP, Natbony SF, Tawil AP. Exercise-induced anaphylaxis as a manifestation of cholinergic urticaria. *J Allergy Clin Immunol* 1981; 68:319–324.

42. Casale TB, Keahey TM, Kaliner M. Exercise-induced anaphylactic syndromes: insights into diagnostic and pathophysiologic features. *JAMA* 1986;255:2049.

43. Sheffer AL, Austen KF. Exercise-induced anaphylaxis. *J Allergy Clin Immunol* 1980;66:106.

44. Reference moved in text.

45. Sheffer AL, Soter NA, McFadden ER Jr, Austen KF. Exercise-induced anaphylaxis: a distinct form of physical allergy. *J Allergy Clin Immunol* 1983;71:311.

46. Lewis J, Lieberman P, Treadwell G, Erffmeyer J. Exercise-induced urticaria, angioedema, and anaphylactoid episodes. *J Allergy Clin Immunol* 1981;68:432.

47. Maulitz RM, Pratt DS, Schocket AL. Exercise-induced anaphylactic reaction to shellfish. *J Allergy Clin Immunol* 1979;63:433.

48. Novey HS, Fairshter RD, Salness K. Postprandial exercise-induced anaphylaxis. *J Allergy Clin Immunol* 1983;71:498–502.

49. Kidd JM III, Cohen SH, Sosman AJ, Fink JN. Food dependent exercise-induced anaphylaxis. *J Allergy Clin Immunol* 1983;71:407.

50. Kivity S, Sneh E, Greif J, Topilsky M, Mekori YA. The effect of food and exercise on the skin response to compound 48/80 in patients with food-associated exercise-induced urticaria-angioedema. *J Allergy Clin Immunol* 1987;81:1155.

51. Greaves MW, Sneddon IB, Smith AK, Stanworth DR. Heat urticaria. *Br J Dermatol* 1974;90:L289.

52. Atkins PC, Zweiman B. Mediator release in local heat urticaria. *J Allergy Clin Immunol* 1981;68:286.

53. Grant JA, Findlay JR, Thueson DO. Local heat urticaria/angioedema: evidence for histamine release without complement activation. *J Allergy Clin Immunol* 1981;67:75.

54. Daman L, Lieberman P, Garner M, Hashimoto K. Localized heat urticaria. *J Allergy Clin Immunol* 1978;61:273.

55. Tennenbaum JI, Lowney E. Localized heat and cold urticaria. *J Allergy Clin Immunol* 1973;51:57.

56. Michaelsson G, Ros A. Familial localized heat urticaria of delayed type. *Acta Derm Venereol* 1971;51:279.

57. Mathews KP. Urticaria and angioedema. *J Allergy Clin Immunol* 1983;72:11.

58. Cauna N, Levine MI. The fine morphology of the human skin in dermographism. *J Allergy Clin Immunol* 1970;45:266.

59. Reference moved in text.

60. Newcomb RW, Nelson H. Dermographism mediated by IgE. *Am J Med* 1973;54:174.

61. Rose B. Studies on blood histamine in cases of allergy: I. Blood histamine during wheal formation. *J Allergy* 1941;12:327.

62. Kaplan AP, Horakova Z, Katz SI. Assessment of tissue fluid histamine levels in patients with urticaria. *J Allergy Clin Immunol* 1978; 61:350–354.

63. Greaves MW. Histamine excretion and dermographism in urticaria pigmentosa before and after administration of a specific histidine-decarboxylase inhibitor. *Br J Dermatol* 1971;85:467.

64. Greaves MW, Sundergoard J. Urticaria pigmentosa and factitious urticaria: direct evidence for release of histamine and other smooth muscle-contracting agents in dermographic skin. *Arch Dermatol* 1970;101:418.

65. Garofalo J, Kaplan AP. Histamine release and therapy of severe dermatographism. *J Allergy Clin Immunol* 1981;68:103.

66. Smith JA, Mansfield LE, Fokakis A, Nelson HS. Dermographism caused by IgE mediated penicillin allergy. *Ann Allergy* 1983;57:30.

67. Matthews CNA, Boss JM, Warin RP, Storari F. The effect of H1 and H2 histamine antagonists on symptomatic dermographism. *Br J Dermatol* 1979;101:57.

68. Matthews CNA, Kirby JD, James J, Warin RP. Dermographism: reduction in wheal size by chlorpheniramine and hydroxyzine. *Br J Dermatol* 1973;88:279.

69. Roberts LJI, Sweetman BJ, Lewis RA. Increased production of prostaglandin D_2 in patients with systemic mastocytosis. *N Engl J Med* 1980;303:1400.

70. Ryan TJ, Shim-Young N, Turk JL. Delayed pressure urticaria. *Br J Dermatol* 1968;80:485.

71. Estes SA, Yang CW. Delayed pressure urticaria: an investigation of some parameters of lesion induction. *J Am Acad Dermatol* 1981;5:25.

72. Davis KC, Mekori YA, Kohler PF, Schocket AL. Possible role of diet in delayed pressure urticaria [abstract]. *J Allergy Clin Immunol* 1984;73:183.

73. Parrillo JE, Lawley TJ, Frank MM. Immunologic reactivity in the hypereosinophil syndrome. *J Allergy Clin Immunol* 1979;64:113.

74. Harber LC, Holloway RM, Sheatley VR, Baer RL. Immunologic and biophysical studies in solar urticaria. *J Invest Dermatol* 1963;41:439.

75. Horio T. Photoallergic urticaria induced by visible light: additional cases and further studies. *Arch Dermatol* 1978;114:1761.

76. Sams WM Jr, Epstein JH, Winkelmann RK. Solar urticaria: investigation of pathogenic mechanisms. *Arch Dermatol* 1969;99:390.

77. Hawk JLM, Eady RAJ, Challiner AVJ. Elevated blood histamine levels and mast cell degranulation in solar urticaria. *Br J Clin Pharmacol* 1980;9:183.

78. Soter NA, Wasserman SI, Pathak MA. Solar urticaria: release of mast cell mediators into the circulation after experimental challenge. *J Invest Dermatol* 1979;72:282.

79. Bonkowsky HL, Bloomer JR, Ebert PS, Mahoney MJ. Heme synthetase deficiency in human protoporphyria: demonstration of the defect in liver and cultured skin fibroblasts. *J Clin Invest* 1975;56:1139.

80. Bottomley SS, Tanaka M, Everett MA. Diminished erythroid ferrochetalase activity in protoporphyria. *J Lab Clin Med* 1975;86:126.

81. Lim HW, Perez HD, Poh-Fitzpatrick M. Generation of chemotactic activity in serum from patients with erythropoietic protoporphyria and porphyria cutanea tarda. *N Engl J Med* 1981;304:212.

82. Lim HW, Poh-Fitzpatrick MB, Gigli I. Activation of the complement system in patients with porphyria after irradiation *in vivo. J Clin Invest* 1984;74:1961.

82a. Gigli I, Schothorst AA, Soter NA, Pathak MA. Erythropoietic protoporphyria: photoactivation of the complement system. *J Clin Invest* 1980;66:517.

83. Baart DLFH, Beerens EGJ, van Weelden H, Berens L. Complement components in blood serum and suction blister fluid in erythropoietic protoporphyria. *Br J Dermatol* 1978;99:401.

84. Epstein JH, Tuffanelli DL, Epstein WL. Cutaneous changes in the porphyrias: a microscopic study. *Arch Dermatol* 1973;107:689.

85. Moshell AN, Bjornson L. Protection in erythropoietic protoporphyria: mechanism of photoprotection by β carotene. *J Invest Dermatol* 1977; 68:157.

86. Chalamidas SL, Charles CR. Aquagenic urticaria. *Arch Dermatol* 1971;104:541.

87. Davis RS, Remigio LK, Schocket AL, Bock SA. Evaluation of a patient with both aquagenic and cholinergic urticaria. *J Allergy Clin Immunol* 1981;68:479.

88. Patterson R, Mellies CJ, Blankenship ML, Pruzansky JJ. Vibratory angioedema: a hereditary type of physical hypersensitivity. *J Allergy Clin Immunol* 1972;50:174.

89. Metzger WJ, Kaplan AP, Beaven MA. Hereditary vibratory angioedema: confirmation of histamine release in a type of physical hypersensitivity. *J Allergy Clin Immunol* 1976;57:605.

90. Kaplan AP. Urticaria and angioedema. In: Kaplan AP, ed. *Allergy.* New York: Churchill Livingstone, 1985:439–471.

91. Dolovich J, Little DC. Correlates of skin test reactions to *Bacillus subtilis* enzyme preparations. *J Allergy Clin Immunol* 1972;49:43.

92. Dolovich J, Hargreave FE, Chalmers R, Shier KJ, Gauldie J, Bienenstock J. Late cutaneous allergic responses in isolated IgE-dependent reactions. *J Allergy Clin Immunol* 1973;52:38–46.

93. Durham SR, Lee TH, Cromwell O, et al. Immunologic studies in allergen-induced late-phase asthmatic reactions. *J Allergy Clin Immunol* 1984;74:49–60.

94. Solley GO, Gleich GJ, Jordan RE, Schroeter AL. The late phase of the immediate wheal and flare skin reaction: its dependence upon IgE antibodies. *J Clin Invest* 1976;58:408–420.

95. Reshef A, Kagey-Sobotka A, Adkinson NF, Lichtenstein LM, Norman PS. The pattern and kinetics in human skin of erythema and mediators during the acute and late-phase response (LPR). *J Allergy Clin Immunol* 1989;84:678–687.

96. Schwartz LB. Basophils and mast cells. In: Kaplan AP, ed. *Allergy.* Philadelphia: WB Saunders, 1997, pp. 133–148.

97. Church MD, Levi-Schaffer F. The human mast cell. *J Allergy Clin Immunol* 1997;99:155.

98. Alam R, Forsythe P, Stafford S, et al. Monocyte chemotactic protein-2, monocyte chemotactic protein-3, and fibroblast-induced cytokine: three new chemokines induce chemotaxis and activation of basophils. *J Immunol* 1994;153:3155–3159.

99. Alam R, Forsythe PA, Stafford S, et al. Macrophage inflammatory protein Iα activates basophils and mast cells. *J Exp Med* 1992;176: 781–786.

100. Kuna P, Reddigari SR, Rucinski D, et al. Monocyte chemotactic and activating factor is a potent histamine-releasing factor for human basophils. *J Exp Med* 1992;175:489–493.

101. Kuna P, Reddigari SR, Schall TJ, et al. RANTES, a monocyte and T lymphocyte chemotactic cytokine releases histamine from human basophils. *J Immunol* 1992;149:636–642.

102. Stellato C, Collins P, Ponath PD, et al. Production of the novel C-C chemokine MCP-4 by airway cells and comparison of its biological to other C-C chemokines. *J Clin Invest* 1997;99:926.

103. Dahinden CA, Geiser T, Brunner T, et al. Monocyte chemotactic protein 3 is a most effective basophil and eosinophil-activating chemokine. *J Exp Med* 1994;179:751–756.

104. Ponath FD, Qin S, Ringler DJ, et al. Cloning of the human eosinophil chemoattractant, eotaxin: expression, receptor binding, and functional properties suggest a mechanism for the selective recruitment of eosinophils. *J Clin Invest* 1996;97:604.

104a. Alam RS, Stafford P, Forsythe R, et al. RANTES is a chemotactic and activating factor for human eosinophils. *J Immunol* 1993;150: 3442–3447.

105. Dor PJ, Vervloet D, Supene M, Andrac L, Bonerandi JJ, Charpin J. Induction of late cutaneous reaction by kallikrein injection: comparison with allergic-like late response to compound 48/80. *J Allergy Clin Immunol* 1983;71:363.

106. Koehn GG, Thorne EG. Urticaria and viral hepatitis. *Arch Dermatol* 1972;106:442.

107. Cowdry SL, Reynolds JS. Acute urticaria in infectious mononucleosis. *Ann Allergy* 1969;27:182.

108. Arbesman CE, Reisman RE. Serum sickness and human anaphylaxis. In: Samter M, ed. *Immunologic diseases,* vol 1. Boston: Little, Brown, 1971;495.

109. Paver WK. Discoid and subacute systemic lupus erythematosus associated with urticaria. *Aust J Dermatol* 1971;12:113.

110. Provost TT, Zone JJ, Synkowski D. Unusual clinical manifestations of systemic lupus erythematosus: I. Urticaria-like lesions: correlations with clinical and serological abnormalities. *J Invest Dermatol* 1980; 75:495.

111. Ghebrehiwet B. The complement system: mechanism of activation, regulation, and biological functions. In: Kaplan AP, ed. *Allergy.* New York: Churchill Livingstone, 1985:131–152.

112. Soter NA, Austen KF, Gigli I. Urticaria and arthralgias as a manifestation of necrotizing angiitis. *J Invest Dermatol* 1974;63:485.

113. Soter NA, Mihm MC Jr, Gigli I, et al. Two distinct cellular patterns in cutaneous necrotizing angiitis. *J Invest Dermatol* 1976;66:334.

114. Mathison DA, Arroyave CM, Bhat KN. Hypocomplementemia in chronic idiopathic urticaria. *Ann Intern Med* 1977;86:534.

115. Monroe EW, Schulz CI, Maize JC, Jordon RE. Vasculitis in chronic urticaria: an immunopathologic study. *J Invest Dermatol* 1981;76:103.

116. Natbony SF, Phillips ME, Elias JM, Godfrey HP, Kaplan AP. Histologic studies of chronic idiopathic urticaria. *J Allergy Clin Immunol* 1983;77:177–183.

117. Phanuphak P, Kohler PF, Stanford RE. Vasculitis in chronic urticaria. *J Allergy Clin Immunol* 1980;65:436.

118. Kern F, Lichtenstein LM. Defective histamine release in chronic urticaria. *J Clin Invest* 1977;57:1360.

119. Phanuphak P, Schocket AL, Arroyave CM. Skin histamine in chronic urticaria. *J Allergy Clin Immunol* 1980;65:371.

120. Smith CH, Kepley C, Schwartz L, et al. Mast cell number and phenotype in chronic idiopathic urticaria. *J Allergy Clin Immunol* 1995;96: 360–364.

121. Peters MS, Schroeter AL, Kephart GM, Gleich GJ. Localization of eosinophil granule major basic protein in chronic urticaria. *J Invest Dermatol* 1983;81:39.

122. Elias J, Boss E, Kaplan AP. Studies of the cellular infiltrate of chronic idiopathic urticaria: prominence of T lymphocytes, monocytes, and mast cells. *J Allergy Clin Immunol* 1986;78:914–918.

123. Leznoff A, Josse RG, Denberg J, et al. Association of chronic urticaria and angioedema with thyroid autoimmunity. *Arch Dermatol* 1983; 119:636–640.

124. Leznoff A, Sussman GL. Syndrome of idiopathic chronic urticaria and angioedema with thyroid autoimmunity: a study of 90 patients. *J Allergy Clin Immunol* 1989;84:66–71.

125. Gruber BL, Baeza M, Marchese M, et al. Prevalence and functional role of anti-IgE autoantibodies in urticarial syndromes. *J Invest Dermatol* 1988;90:213–217.

126. Hide M, Francis DM, Grattan CEH, et al. Autoantibodies against the high-affinity IgE receptor as a cause of histamine release in chronic urticaria. *N Engl J Med* 1993;328:1599—1604.

127. Fiebiger E, Maurer D, Holub H, et al. Serum IgG autoantibodies directed against the α chain of FcεRI: a selective marker and pathogenic factor for a distinct subset of chronic urticaria patients. *J Clin Invest* 1995;96:2606–2612.

128. Zweiman B, Valenzano M, Atkins PC, et al. Characteristics of histamine-releasing activity in the sera of patients with chronic idiopathic urticaria. *J Allergy Clin Immunol* 1996;98:89–98.

129. Tong LJ, Balakrishan G, Kochan JP, et al. Assessment of autoimmunity in patients with chronic urticaria. *J Allergy Clin Immunol* 1997; 99:461–465.

130. Kaplan AP. Urticaria and angioedema. In: Kapplan AP, ed. *Allergy* Philadelphia: WB Saunders, 1997, pp. 573–592.

Inflammation: Basic Principles and Clinical Correlates,
3rd ed., edited by John I. Gallin and Ralph Snyderman.
Lippincott Williams & Wilkins, Philadelphia © 1999.

CHAPTER 58

Role of Immunoglobulin E and Eosinophils in Mediating Protection and Pathology in Parasitic Helminth Infections

Amy D. Klion, Myriam A. Armant, and Thomas B. Nutman

Parasitic infections are caused by unicellular protozoa or multicellular helminths (worms), and their global prevalence imposes a major medical and economic burden (Table 58-1). These parasites have an exceedingly diverse biology. Protozoa usually are a few micrometers in size, whereas helminths are typically centimeters to meters in length. Tissue-dwelling protozoa are often intracellular parasites at some stage of infection, whereas helminths, being larger than most tissue cells, are almost always extracellular pathogens—the significant exception being *Trichinella spiralis,* which encysts within mammalian muscle cells. Protozoa usually replicate during infection of a single host; helminths do not reproduce without the assistance of intermediate hosts or passage through soil or water.

Helminths characteristically have complex life cycles with many developmental stages present during infection (1). In the course of a single infection, the host may be exposed repeatedly to larval-, adult-, or egg-stage antigens. Free-swimming cercariae of the trematode, *Schistosoma mansoni,* penetrate the skin of humans immersed in infested water and evolve into tissue-stage schistosomula, which migrate to the liver and mesenteric veins for further differentiation into sexually dimorphic adult worms. Eggs are laid and migrate through tissues into the bowel or bladder lumen for environmental release. Similarly, filarial infection involves repeated exposure to arthro-

pod-borne infective larvae and parasitization by long-lived adult worms that continuously release microfilariae that circulate in the bloodstream or migrate through subcutaneous tissues.

Because each stage of parasite development may be antigenically distinct, the host response to helminth infection is often characterized by a series of discrete immune responses that evolve at different times during the course of infection. Protective immunity directed against a single stage may be circumvented by parasite differentiation, which assists the survival of the pathogen and poses a significant challenge to immune-mediated resistance. Each stage of parasite development may also entail a change in tissue trophism, introducing a compartmental feature to immune or inflammatory responses. For example, a variety of distinct cutaneous, pulmonary, and intestinal inflammatory or hypereosinophilic syndromes are associated with different stages of *Ascaris* and *Strongyloides* as they migrate through the skin and lung before reaching adulthood in the gastrointestinal tract (2). This temporal evolution of antigenic diversity and tissue tropism is another unique aspect of parasite immunology.

Because complex parasitic life cycles can be maintained only by sequential passage through intermediate and definitive hosts, parasites have adapted methods of optimizing transmission by prolonging infection. This is critical if passage through a series of intermediate hosts depends on infrequent events, such as ingestion of excreted eggs and larvae or uptake by a biting insect. Perhaps because of this evolutionary pressure, chronicity and latency are hallmarks of helminth infections. For example, adult schistosoma and filariae may survive in host tissues for as long as 20 to 30 years, continuously

A. D. Klion: Laboratory of Parasitic Diseases, National Institutes of Health, Bethesda, Maryland 20892.

M. A. Armant and T. B. Nutman: Helminth Immunology Section, National Institute of Allergy and Infectious Diseases, National Institutes of Health, Bethesda, Maryland 20892.

TABLE 58-1. *Prevalence and distribution of common helminth infections*

Types of helminths	No. infected	Distribution
Intestinal helminths		
Ascaris lumbricoides	1,000 million	Worldwide
Hookworm spp[a]	900 million	Worldwide
Strongyloides stercoralis	75 million	Worldwide
Trichuris trichiura	500 million	Worldwide
Schistosomes		
Schistosoma mansoni	150 million	South America, Africa
Schistosoma japonicum	2 million	East Asia
Schistosoma haematobium	50 million	Africa
Filarial parasites		
Onchocerca volvulus	13 million	Africa, Central and South America
Wuchereria bancrofti	80 million	Worldwide
Brugia malayi	10 million	Asia
Loa loa	13 million	Africa
Animal parasites[b]		
Taenia solium	1 million	Worldwide
Echinococcus granulosus	1.5 million	Worldwide
Toxocara spp	7 million	Worldwide

[a]Includes both *Necator americanus* and *Ancylostoma duodenale*.
[b]Characteristically animal parasites that incidentally infect humans but cause diseases such as cysticercosis, hydatid disease, and visceral larval migrans.

producing eggs and larvae. *Strongyloides,* because of its ability to autoinfect, maintains its life cycle for decades. Chronicity may also reflect pressure toward "true parasitism," in that induction of mortality in the host before egg-laying or larval release occurs would disrupt parasite transmission. In response to the evolutionary pressure for chronic infection, a broad range of evasive and suppressive strategies have evolved among the helminth parasites to maintain long-term viability in their hosts.

Adaptations for chronicity can be so successful among parasites that naturally acquired protective immunity may be observed only rarely in areas endemic for a given disease. Specifically, schistosomiasis results in an incomplete form of protection in which reinfection is limited but adult worms are tolerated for years (concomitant immunity) (3). A similar hypothesis has been proposed for filarial infection (4).

Heterogeneity in host immune responsiveness may also serve to help maintain the parasite in animal or human reservoirs. Filarial infections, for example, have a range of clinical manifestations determined in part by the immune responses of the host. Prolonged microfilaremia reflects apparent immunologic hyporesponsiveness to the parasite, whereas other clinical states are associated with vigorous inflammatory responses that limit transmission but may cause pathology (5).

Whereas pathology and protective immunity against most protozoa are thought to reflect T-cell–, B-cell–, and macrophage-dependent (and in part cytokine-mediated) mechanisms, infection with helminth parasites induces immune effector mechanisms that are associated with immediate hypersensitivity. As in the atopic state, these are characterized by immunoglobulin E (IgE) antibody production, tissue and peripheral blood eosinophilia, and the participation of inflammatory mediator–rich basophils and mast cells. For the atopic state, these immediate hypersensitivity responses have clearly been implicated in the pathogenesis of allergic diseases. In parasitic infection, although these types of responses can certainly induce pathologic reactions, they have also been implicated in protective immunity against helminth parasites (6–8).

The responses to parasitic infection are myriad, as are the effector mechanisms operating to control these infections. The biology of the major components of the immediate hypersensitivity response are delineated elsewhere in this book (see Chapters 5, 7, 18). This chapter seeks to explore the nature of the inflammatory responses induced by parasitic helminth infection and to identify not only the effector mechanisms used by the host to control the infection but also those that result, directly or indirectly, in pathology.

IMMUNOGLOBULIN E AND HELMINTH INFECTIONS

Although IgE antibody responses in most persons are strictly regulated both quantitatively and qualitatively, the presence of the atopic state or helminth infection appears to overcome these regulatory mechanisms, so that high levels of IgE are consistently produced *in vivo* (9,10). Furthermore, in the case of helminth infection, most of the IgE produced is not antigen specific and is therefore thought to represent nonspecific potentiation of a normally well-controlled immune response (11–14). This potentiating effect seems to be selective for the IgE isotype (14), as was demonstrated most definitively in studies in which animals previously sensitized to a nonparasite antigen (e.g., ovalbumin) were subsequently infected with a helminth parasite. IgE antibodies directed not only against the parasite but also against the nonparasite antigen were detected (12,15,16).

Increased levels of total serum IgE in atopic and parasitized patients have been documented in many studies (17,18). Characteristically, patients with allergic disorders have serum IgE levels approximately ten times those of normal persons; those with invasive helminth infections have serum IgE levels approaching 100 times normal (10). The factors responsible for this degree of elevation reflect the massive clonal expansion of IgE-producing B cells, which in turn reflects a marked increase in interleukin-4 (IL-4)–producing T cells (19). There seem to be, however, not only quantitative but also qualitative differences. Although atopic patients have moderate elevations of IgE, their IgE responses are restricted to a small number of antigens. In contrast, patients with invasive helminth infection produce IgE antibodies with specificity against a very broad range of parasite antigens (20). It has been proposed that this potentiated, antigen-nonspecific response leads to the production of irrelevant IgE that saturates the mast cells' high affinity Fc Epsilon Receptor 1 (FcER1) and renders it unable to be triggered by parasite antigen. This situation is quite different from that seen in allergic disorders, in which mast cell–IgE interactions are a major initiator of the disease process.

Parasite-induced perturbations of the specific antibody isotype generated during infection may additionally diminish the effects of a given immune response. Helminth infections—particularly lymphatic filariasis and schistosomiasis—result in the production of high levels of IgE and IgG4. The expression of antibodies of distinct isotypes directed against the same antigens may be beneficial to the host when IgG4 blocks IgE-mediated allergic responses (21). However, the increased magnitude of IgG4 and IgE responses commonly seen in schistosomiasis (22) and in filariasis may also diminish the protective response mediated by other antibody isotypes directed against the parasite. Similarly, antibodies of the IgM and IgG2 isotypes have been shown to block antibody-dependent killing of schistosomula (23). Finally, the presence of these blocking antibodies is associated with susceptibility to reinfection with schistosomiasis after chemotherapy (24,25).

It has been postulated that the immediate hypersensitivity response (and particularly that of IgE) evolved as a specific effector mechanism to kill parasitic worms and prevent reinfection or hyperinfection (26). Specialized characteristics of IgE and eosinophils (see Chapters 5 and 18) can facilitate killing of large multicellular organisms. These observations were initially established by studies in vitro, and the crucial role of the IgE and eosinophil response for parasite killing in vivo has been convincingly demonstrated in only a few parasite-host models. It has become increasingly recognized that other effector arms of the immune response (e.g., monocytes, platelets, immunoglobulin isotypes other than IgE) can accomplish parasite killing with efficiencies equivalent to those classically associated with immediate hypersensitivity.

The role of IgE in protecting the host against helminth infection therefore remains unclear. The most compelling evidence comes from studies in schistosomiasis. Studies of Schistosoma haematobium in the Gambia showed that persons with high serum levels of parasite-specific IgE after antischistosomal chemotherapy were less likely to become reinfected or had lighter reinfections compared to those with lower IgE levels (27,28). Additionally, there was an associated increase in serum levels of parasitic-specific IgE with increasing age, which was closely correlated with the development of acquired resistance. This suggests that an augmented helper T cell type 2 (TH2) response, indicated by increased serum IgE, may be associated with the development of acquired immunity with age (22,29). Similar studies of S. mansoni in Brazil, Senegal, and Kenya also point to an association between increased levels of antischistosomal IgE and acquired immunity (23,25,30–36). Similar findings have been seen in Schistosoma japonicum infections as well (37). Although the mechanism by which IgE antibody mediates this protection is unknown, it has been postulated that IgE mediates the antibody-dependent cellular cytotoxicity (ADCC) reactions in concert with eosinophils, macrophages, or even platelets (38–42). Of note is the finding from field studies in a schistosomiasis-endemic region of Brazil suggesting that a gene, localized to a region of human chromosome 5 (5q31–33) which encodes many of the cytokines mediating eosinophilia and IgE, plays a major role in resistance to infection with schistosomiasis (43).

In support of these findings in humans are animal studies suggesting a protective role for IgE in rats infected with filarial parasites (44), T. spiralis (45), or S. mansoni (39). In contrast, however, are the findings that mice incapable of making IgE (from studies using anti–IL-4 monoclonal antibodies, IL-4/IL-13 knock-outs, and IL-4R knock-outs) can respond to vaccination against S. mansoni, suggesting that IgE alone is not mediating protection against schistosome infection (46). Similarly, in mice with a targeted deletion of the IgE gene, although primary infection with S. mansoni was associated with higher worm burdens, resistance to challenge infection was no different than in mice with the normal IgE gene (47). Consistent with these findings are the results in IgE-suppressed mice, in which resistance to S. japonicum was no different than in control mice with normal IgE levels (48).

Intestinal helminths have been used as the prototypical parasite infection to demonstrate the importance of IgE in mediating protection. It has been demonstrated that passive transfer of IgE antibodies can mediate the rapid-expulsion phenomenon in rats infected with *T. spiralis* (49) and that diminished levels of IgE are associated with dissemination of *Strongyloides stercoralis* (50,51) in the context of coinfection with the human T-cell lymphotrophic virus type I. Elucidation of the cytokine control of the IgE response (e.g., IL-4 and IL-13) and the fact the these cytokine activities occur in the context of a broader (T$_H$2 or type 2) response suggest that the IgE reaction itself may be merely an indicator of a more general protective response comprising many different components (52–56).

Although the IgE induced in response to parasitic helminth infections clearly helps mediate (albeit in part) resistance or protective immunity, humans with these infections can manifest symptoms suggestive of IgE-mediated pathology (10,57,58). An example is allergic reactivity (e.g., wheezing, urticaria) that occurs during the early or acute phase of infection with invasive helminth parasites such as ascaris, hookworm, schistosomes, or filariae (10). In the clinical syndromes associated with *Loa loa* infection (angioedematous Calabar swellings) (59), tropical pulmonary eosinophilia (2), and strongyloidiasis (larva currens) (60), IgE-mediated reactions are thought to reflect the underlying mechanism of the signs and symptoms. For the tropical pulmonary eosinophilia syndrome, for example, the induced IgE antibodies are cross-reactive with the human γ-glutamyl transpeptidase (61) that is localized to the lung epithelium and may mediate the bronchoreactivity seen in this disorder. Moreover, the IgE elevations seen in helminth infection occur in the context of series of cytokine-mediated (T$_H$2-type) events that often include eosinophilia, mastocytosis, and concurrent modulation of T$_H$1 responses. Therefore, a single unifying mechanism (i.e., IgE-mediated activity) for either pathologic or protective mechanisms in helminth infections is unlikely.

EOSINOPHILS AND HELMINTH INFECTION

Blood and tissue eosinophilia are also characteristic responses in both allergy and helminth infection. IL-5 has been implicated in mediating this response in bone marrow cultures *in vitro* (62), in animal models of helminth infection (63,64), and in cross-sectional studies of eosinophilic patients with filarial infection (65). Although other cytokines, including IL-3 and granulocyte-macrophage colony-stimulating factor, have been shown to stimulate eosinophilopoeisis *in vitro* and to induce eosinophilia *in vivo* (66), only IL-5 appears to be eosinophil (and probably basophil) specific in its colony-stimulating activity (67,68).

As early as 1939, eosinophils were postulated to play a role in the immune response to helminth infection (69). Such hypotheses were based primarily on histopathologic evidence of eosinophils surrounding dying parasites in tissue biopsies. More recently, *in vitro* killing of parasites by eosinophils (in the presence of antibodies or complement, or both) (70–72) and eosinophil granule products (73,74) has been demonstrated. Despite these *in vitro* findings and epidemiologic evidence correlating high eosinophil counts with resistance to posttreatment reinfection with *S. haematobium* and *S. mansoni* in humans (75,76), the *in vivo* role of eosinophils in immunity to helminth infection has been much more difficult to define.

Treatment with anti-IL-5 antibody prevents the tissue and blood eosinophilia that occurs in animal models of gastrointestinal helminth infection (63,77). However, such treatment has not been shown to increase susceptibility to infection in murine models of *T. spiralis* (78), *Trichuris muris* (79), *Nippostrongylus brasiliensis* (63), *Heligosomoides polygyrus* (52), or schistosomiasis (80). Similarly, IL-5 transgenic mice, which have persistent high levels of eosinophilia, do not demonstrate enhanced immunity to *T. spiralis* or *S. mansoni* infection (81,82).

Eosinophils do appear to play a role in the killing of some helminths, particularly those with tissue-migratory stages. Larval stages of many of the intestinal helminths, including *Strongyloides* spp., *Nippostrongylus,* and *Ascaris,* migrate through the lungs or skin on their way to the gastrointestinal tract. Although treatment with anti–IL-5 antibody had no effect on primary infection with *Strongyloides venezuelensis* in mice, recovery of worms from the lungs after challenge infection was increased in treated mice compared with controls (83). Similarly, in studies examining the survival of infective larvae of *S. stercoralis* in diffusion chambers implanted under the skin of immune mice, larval killing depended on contact with eosinophils and was reduced to control levels when eosinophil migration into the diffusion chamber was prevented or when mice were treated with antibody to IL-5 (84,85). Parasite-specific IgM antibody and complement were also necessary for larval killing in this model (86).

In *Angiostrongylus cantonensis* infection in mice, immature worms develop in the brain before migrating to the lungs. Prolonged survival of intracranial worms, resulting in a larger parasite burden in the lungs, has been demonstrated in normal mice treated with anti–IL-5 antibody (87) and in IL-5 receptor-α (IL-5Rα)–deficient mice (88), again consistent with a role for eosinophils in tissue-based larval killing.

Animal models of protective immunity to the exclusively tissue-dwelling nematode, *Onchocerca,* further support this hypothesis. In diffusion chamber studies of infective larval survival in immune mice, eosinophils were the only cell that accumulated in the chambers concomitant with larval killing (89). Furthermore, as with *Strongyloides* larvae, eosinophil-larva contact was necessary for larval destruction to occur (89). In a different murine model, mice infected with *Onchocerca lienalis* depleted of eosinophils (but not of macrophages or neutrophils) with monoclonal antibody showed delayed clearance of primary infection and abrogation of resistance to secondary infection (90).

In humans with onchocerciasis, the picture is somewhat more complex. Some studies of *in vitro* cytokine production in response to parasite antigens have demonstrated increased IL-5 production by peripheral blood mononuclear cells from putatively immune persons living in areas endemic for onchocerciasis, compared with infected persons (91); other studies have detected no difference in parasite antigen–induced IL-5 production between these groups (92).

The mechanism by which eosinophil-mediated protection against helminth infection occurs is incompletely understood, but in most cases it appears to involve antibody- or complement-induced release of toxic granule proteins and reactive oxygen intermediates by activated eosinophils. Evidence suggests that there may be significant differences in the susceptibility to and mechanisms of eosinophil-mediated killing for different life-cycle stages of the same parasite (93). These differences, as well as differences in the relative importance of eosinophils in larval killing depending on the animal model studied (38), could account for some of the controversy regarding the role of eosinophils in immunity to helminth infection.

Eosinophils have also been implicated in the pathogenesis of helminth infection (Table 58-2). Clinical similarities between the sequelae of hypereosinophilic syndrome, a syndrome characterized by extremely high levels of eosinophilia and eosinophil-mediated end-organ damage (94), and the pathologic consequences of infection with filaria (95) and Toxocara (96) suggest a role for eosinophils in the pathologic sequelae of these infections. Additional indirect support for this hypothesis is provided by the fact that increased eosinophil activation—as measured by increased responsiveness to the inflammatory mediator, platelet-activating factor (PAF)—has been described in patients with sowdah (a chronic hyperreactive form of onchocerciasis associated with severe skin pathology), compared with normal individuals or with onchocerciasis-infected patients with milder symptomatology (97).

Eosinophil cationic proteins, including major basic protein, eosinophil cationic protein, and eosinophil-derived neurotoxin, are toxic to various normal tissues and cells both *in vitro* and *in vivo* (8,98,99) (see Chapter 5). High levels of these proteins have been demonstrated in the sera of patients with filarial infections or schistosomiasis (100). Other potentially toxic inflammatory mediators that are released by activated eosinophils include leukotrienes (101), PAF (102), reactive oxygen species (103), and lysosomal hydrolases (99). These mediators not only serve to damage the parasite and surrounding tissues (reactive oxygen intermediates [104,105], hydrolases) but also play a role in the perpetuation of the local immune response (PAF, leukotrienes). In a murine model of schistosomiasis, eosinophil production of IL-4 appeared to be essential to the early induction of a T_H2-type immune response (106).

Posttreatment reactions in onchocerciasis (the Mazzotti reaction) can be severe and are thought to reflect an acute exacerbation of the host immune response to microfilariae in the skin and other organs. One of the characteristics of this response is an increase in blood and tissue levels of eosinophils and eosinophil granule proteins that is temporally related to the onset of symptomatology (107) and is preceded by an increase in serum levels of IL-5 (108). Although localization of eosinophils and their products in the skin is most pronounced at sites of microfilarial degeneration (107), consistent with the hypothesis that eosinophil-mediated parasite killing plays a major role in pathogenesis, the possibility that recruitment of eosinophils occurs secondarily in response to parasite death cannot be excluded.

More direct evidence that eosinophils mediate the pathology seen in onchocerciasis comes from animal models of corneal pathology (109,110). Eosinophil infiltration is a characteristic component of the keratitis seen in the corneas of sensitized mice injected intrastromally with onchocercal antigens (111). Sensitized IL-4 knockout mice injected intrastromally with parasite antigen

TABLE 58-2. *Role of the eosinophil in mediating protection or pathology in selected helminth infections*

Species	Protection		Pathology		References
	Animal Model	Human	Animal Model	Human	
Angiostrongylus	++				87, 88
Nippostrongylus	+/−		—		63, 112
Onchocerca	++	+/−	++	++	89–92, 97, 107–110
Schistosoma	—	++	—	++	64, 75, 76, 80, 82, 100
Strongyloides	++				83–85
Toxocara	—		++		113, 114
Trichinealla	+/−				78, 81, 115
Trichuris	—				116

+/−, conflicting information; ++, documented role; —, shown to play no role.

developed mild to no keratitis, and inflammatory cells (including eosinophils) were rarely seen in histologic sections of the corneal stroma (111). In contrast, mice treated with IL-12 at the time of corneal sensitization to onchocercal antigens developed more severe onchocercal keratitis associated with increased mononuclear and eosinophil infiltration into the corneal stroma despite decreased local expression of T$_H$2 cytokines including IL-5 (110). The presence of eosinophil infiltration in a T$_H$1 environment could be accounted for by a marked increase in corneal chemokines, including "regulated on activation, normally T-cell expressed and secreted," (RANTES) and eotaxin (110). Taken together, these data suggest that the presence of eosinophils, rather than the cytokine milieu, is crucial to the development of keratitis.

Although it seems clear that eosinophils play a role in some types of helminth-induced pathology, they do not appear to be essential to the development of pathologic sequelae in all cases. Liver granulomas in schistosomiasis typically contain a high percentage of eosinophils. However, mice infected with schistosomiasis that were treated with anti–IL-5 produced normal-sized granulomas despite the absence of eosinophils (64). Similarly, lung infiltrates in mice infected with *N. brasiliensis* that were treated with anti–IL-5 differed from infected control mice in the absence of eosinophils but not in size or number (63).

CONCLUSION

Despite many advances in the understanding of the fundamental regulation of IgE and eosinophils—two important effector arms of adaptive immune response to parasitic infection—the importance of these responses in mediating toxicity to or protection from tissue-invasive or intestinal helminths remains unclear. Given both the redundancy of the immune system—such that no single molecule or cell appears to be responsible for an observed response—and the often parallel protective and bystander pathologic outcomes of the IgE and eosinophil responses seen with helminth infections, research efforts targeted toward the elimination of these important pathogens must integrate the induction of protective responses with prevention of local pathology.

REFERENCES

1. Markell EK, Voge M. *Medical Parasitology,* 4th ed. Philadelphia: WB Saunders, 1976.
2. Neva FA, Ottesen EA. Tropical (filarial) eosinophilia. *N Engl J Med* 1978;298:1129–1131.
3. Smithers SR, Terry RJ. Concomitant immunity. *Adv Parasitol* 1976; 14:399–428.
4. Day KP, Gregory WF, Maizels RM. Age-specific acquisition of immunity to infective larvae in a bancroftian filariasis endemic area of Papua New Guinea. *Parasite Immunol* 1991;13:277–290.
5. King CL, Nutman TB. Regulation of the immune response in lymphatic filariasis and onchocerciasis. *Immunol Today* 1991;12: A54–A58.
6. Damonneville M, Auriault C, Verwaerde C, Delanoye A, Pierce R, Capron A. Protection against experimental *Schistosoma mansoni* schistosomiasis achieved by immunization with schistosomula released products antigens (SRP-A): role of IgE antibodies. *Clin Exp Immunol* 1986;65:244–252.
7. Ridel PR, Auriault C, Darcy F, et al. Protective role of IgE in immunocompromised rat toxoplasmosis. *J Immunol* 1988;141:978–983.
8. Gleich GJ, Frigas E, Loegering DA, Wassom DL, Steinmuller D. Cytotoxic properties of the eosinophil major basic protein. *J Immunol* 1979;123:2925–2927.
9. Marsh DG, Bias WB, Ishizaka K. Genetic control of basal serum immunoglobulin E level and its effect on specific reaginic sensitivity. *Proc Natl Acad Sci U S A* 1974;71:3588–3592.
10. Ottesen E. Parasite infections and allergic reaction: how each affects the other. In: S EB, Weiss MS, Stein M, eds. *Bronchial asthma: mechanisms and therapeutics,* 2nd ed. New York: Little, Brown, 1985.
11. Turner K, Fedde AL, Quinn EH. Non-specific potentiation of IgE by parasite infections in man. *Int Arch Allergy Immunol* 1979;58: 232–236.
12. Jarrett EEE, Bazin H. Elevation of total serum IgE in rats following helminth parasite infection. *Nature* 1974;251:613–614.
13. Jarrett EEE, Stewart DC. Potentiation of rat reaginic (IgE) antibody by helminth infection: simultaneous potentiation of separate reagins. *Immunology* 1972;23:749–755.
14. Jarrett E. Stimuli for the production and control of IgE in rats. *Immunol Rev* 1978;41:52–76.
15. Orr T, Riley P, Doe J. Potentiated reagin response to egg albumin in *Nippostrongylus brasiliensis* infected rats: II. Time course of the reagin response. *Immunology* 1971;20:185–189.
16. Orr T, Blair A. Potentiated reagin response to egg albumin and conalbumin in *Nippostrongylus brasiliensis* infected rats. *Life Sci* 1969;15: 1073–1077.
17. Hussain R, Hamilton RG, Kumaraswami V, Adkinson NJ, Ottesen EA. IgE responses in human filariasis: I. Quantitation of filaria-specific IgE. *J Immunol* 1981;127:1623–1629.
18. Kojima S, Yokagawa M, Tada T. Raised levels of serum IgE levels in human helminthiasis. *Am J Trop Med Hyg* 1972;21:913–914.
19. King CL, Nutman TB. Biological role of helper T-cell subsets in helminth infections. *Chem Immunol* 1992;54:136–165.
20. Hussain R, Ottesen EA. IgE responses in human filariasis: III. Specificities of IgE and IgG antibodies compared by immunoblot analysis. *J Immunol* 1985;135:1415–1420.
21. Hussain R, Ottesen E. The IgG4 isotype acts as the blocking antibody in human lymphatic filariasis. *J Immunol* 1991;148:2731–2737.
22. Hagan P, Blumenthal UJ, Dunn D, Simpson AJ, Wilkins HA. Human IgE, IgG4 and resistance to reinfection with *Schistosoma haematobium. Nature* 1991;349:243–245.
23. Butterworth AE, Taylor DW, Veith MC, et al. Studies on the mechanisms of immunity in human schistosomiasis. *Immunol Rev* 1982;61: 5–39.
24. Butterworth AE, Bensted SR, Capron A, et al. Immunity in human schistosomiasis mansoni: prevention by blocking antibodies of the expression of immunity in young children. *Parasitology* 1987; 281–300.
25. Butterworth AE, Curry AJ, Dunne DW, et al. Immunity and morbidity in human schistosomiasis mansoni. *Trop Geogr Med* 1994;46:197–208.
26. Moqbel R, Pritchard D. Parasites and allergy: evidence for a "cause and effect" relationship. *Clin Exp Allergy* 1990;20:611–618.
27. Hagan P. Immunity and morbidity in infection due to *Schistosoma haematobium. Am J Trop Med Hyg* 1996;55:116–120.
28. Hagan P, Abath FG. Recent advances in immunity to human schistosomiasis. *Mem Inst Oswaldo Cruz* 1992;87[Suppl 4]:95–98.
29. Satti MZ, Lind P, Vennervald BJ, Sulaiman SM, Daffalla AA, Ghalib HW. Specific immunoglobulin measurements related to exposure and resistance to *Schistosoma mansoni* infection in Sudanese canal cleaners. *Clin Exp Immunol* 1996;106:45–54.
30. Butterworth AE, Dalton PR, Dunne DW, et al. Immunity after treatment of human schistosomiasis mansoni: I. Study design, pretreatment observations and the results of treatment. *Trans R Soc Trop Med Hyg* 1984;78:108–123.
31. Butterworth AE, Capron M, Cordingley JS, et al. Immunity after treatment of human schistosomiasis mansoni: II. Identification of resistant individuals, and analysis of their immune responses. *Trans R Soc Trop Med Hyg* 1985;79:393–408.

32. Butterworth AE, Dunne DW, Fulford AJ, Ouma JH, Sturrock RF. Immunity and morbidity in *Schistosoma mansoni* infection: quantitative aspects. *Am J Trop Med Hyg* 1996;55:109–115.

33. Rihet P, Demeure CE, Bourgois A, Prata A, Dessein AJ. Evidence for an association between human resistance to *Schistosoma mansoni* and high anti-larval IgE levels. *Eur J Immunol* 1991;21:2679–2686.

34. Ndhlovu P, Cadman H, Vennervald BJ, Christensen NO, Chidimu M, Chandiwana SK. Age-related antibody profiles in *Schistosoma haematobium* infections in a rural community in Zimbabwe. *Parasite Immunol* 1996;18:181–191.

35. van Dam GJ, Stelma FF, Gryseels B, et al. Antibody response patterns against *Schistosoma mansoni* in a recently exposed community in Senegal. *J Infect Dis* 1996;173:1232–1241.

36. Dunne DW, Butterworth AE, Fulford AJ, Ouma JH, Sturrock RF. Human IgE responses to *Schistosoma mansoni* and resistance to reinfection. *Mem Inst Oswaldo Cruz* 1992;87[Suppl 4]:99–103.

37. Zhang Z, Wu H, Chen S, et al. Association between IgE antibody against soluble egg antigen and resistance to reinfection with *Schistosoma japonicum*. *Trans R Soc Trop Med Hyg* 1997;606–608.

38. Capron M, Capron A. Immunoglobulin E and effector cells in schistosomiasis. *Science* 1994;254:1876–1877.

39. Capron A, Dessaint JP. Effector and regulatory mechanisms in immunity to schistosomes: a heuristic view. *Annu Rev Immunol* 1985;3: 455–476.

40. Capron A, Dessaint JP, Joseph M, Rousseaux R, Capron M, Bazin H. Interaction between IgE complexes and macrophages in the rat: a new mechanism of macrophage activation. *Eur J Immunol* 1977;7: 315–322.

41. Capron M, Rousseaux J, Mazingue C, Bazin H, Capron A. Rat mast cell-eosinophil interactions in antibody-dependent eosinophil cytotoxicity of *Schistosoma mansoni* schistosomula. *J Immunol* 1978;121: 2518–2525.

42. Capron A, Ameisen JC, Joseph M, Auriault C, Tonnel AB, Caen J. New functions for platelets and their pathological implications. *Int Arch Allergy Appl Immunol* 1985;77:107–114.

43. Marquet S, Abel L, Hillaire D, et al. Genetic localization of a locus controlling the intensity of infection by *Schistosoma mansoni* on chromosome 5q31-q33. *Nat Genet* 1996;14:181–184.

44. Gusmao RD, Stanley AM, Ottesen EA. Brugia pahangi: immunologic evaluation of the differential susceptibility of filarial infection in inbred Lewis rats. *Exp Parasitol* 1981;52:147–159.

45. Grove DI, Warren KS. Effects on murine trichinosis of niridazole, a suppressant of cellular but not humoral immunological responses. *Ann Trop Med Parasitol* 1976;70:449–453.

46. Sher A, Coffman RL, Hieny S, Cheever AW. Ablation of eosinophil and IgE responses with anti–IL-5 or anti–IL-4 antibody fails to affect immunity against *Schistosoma mansoni* in the mouse. *J Immunol* 1990;145:3911–3916.

47. King CL, Xianli J, Malhotra I, Liu S, Mahmoud AA, Oettgen HC. Mice with a targeted deletion of the IgE gene have increased worm burdens and reduced granulomatous inflammation following primary infection with *Schistosoma mansoni*. *J Immunol* 1997;158:294–300.

48. Watanabe N, Janecharut T, Kojima S, Ovary Z. Acquired resistance to *Schistosoma japonicum* in IgE-deficient SJA/9 mice immunized with irradiated cercariae. *Int Arch Allergy Immunol* 1993;102:191–194.

49. Ahmad A, Wang CH, Bell RG. A role for IgE in intestinal immunity: expression of rapid expulsion of *Trichinella spiralis* in rats transfused with IgE and thoracic duct lymphocytes. *J Immunol* 1991;146: 3563–3570.

50. Robinson RD, Lindo JF, Neva FA, et al. Immunoepidemiologic studies of *Strongyloides stercoralis* and human T lymphotropic virus type I infections in Jamaica. *J Infect Dis* 1994;169:692–696.

51. Newton RC, Limpuangthip P, Greenberg S, Gam A, Neva FA. *Strongyloides stercoralis* hyperinfection in a carrier of HTLV-I virus with evidence of selective immunosuppression [see comments]. *Am J Med* 1992;92:202–208.

52. Finkelman FD, Shea-Donohue T, Goldhill J, et al. Cytokine regulation of host defense against parasitic gastrointestinal nematodes: lessons from studies with rodent models. *Annu Rev Immunol* 1997;15: 505–533.

53. Else KJ, Finkelman FD, Maliszewski CR, Grencis RK. Cytokine-mediated regulation of chronic intestinal helminth infection. *J Exp Med* 1994;179:347–351.

54. Urban JF Jr, Madden KB, Svetic A, et al. The importance of Th2

55. Grencis RK. Enteric helminth infection: immunopathology and resistance during intestinal nematode infection. *Chem Immunol* 1997;66: 41–61.

56. Grencis RK. Th2-mediated host protective immunity to intestinal nematode infections. *Philos Trans R Soc Lond B Biol Sci* 1997;352: 1377–1384.

57. Bell RG. IgE, allergies and helminth parasites: a new perspective on an old conundrum. *Immunol Cell Biol* 1996;74:337–345.

58. Lobos E. The basis of IgE responses to specific antigenic determinants in helminthiasis. *Chem Immunol* 1997;66:1–25.

59. Nutman TB, Miller KD, Mulligan M, Ottesen EA. *Loa loa* infection in temporary residents of endemic regions: recognition of a hyperresponsive syndrome with characteristic clinical manifestations. *J Infect Dis* 1986;154:10–18.

60. Neva FA. Biology and immunology of human strongyloidiasis. *J Infect Dis* 1986;153:397–406.

61. Lobos E, Zahn R, Weiss N, Nutman TB. A major allergen of lymphatic filarial nematodes is a parasite homolog of the gamma-glutamyl transpeptidase. *Mol Med* 1996;2:712–724.

62. Clutterbuck EJ, Hirst EM, Sanderson CJ. Human interleukin-5 (IL-5) regulates the production of eosinophils in human bone marrow cultures: comparison and interaction with IL-1, IL-3, IL-6 and GM-CSF. *Blood* 1989;73:1504–1512.

63. Coffman RL, Seymour BW, Hudak S, Jackson J, Rennick D. Antibody to interleukin-5 inhibits helminth-induced eosinophilia in mice. *Science* 1989;245:308–310.

64. Sher A, Coffman RL, Hieny S, Scott P, Cheever AW. Interleukin 5 is required for the blood and tissue eosinophilia but not granuloma formation induced by infection with *Schistosoma mansoni*. *Proc Natl Acad Sci U S A* 1990;87:61–65.

65. Limaye AP, Abrams JS, Silver JE, Ottesen EA, Nutman TB. Regulation of parasite-induced eosinophilia: selectively increased interleukin 5 production in helminth-infected patients. *J Exp Med* 1990;172: 399–402.

66. Rennick DM, Lee FD, Yokota T, Arai K, Cantor H, Nabel GJ. A cloned MCGF cDNA encodes a multilineage hemopoetic growth factor: multiple activities of interleukin 3. *J Immunol* 1985;134:910–914.

67. Denburg JA, Silver JE, Abrams JS. Interleukin is a human basophilopoeitin: induction of histamine content and basophilic differentiation of HL-60 cells and peripheral blood basophil-eosinophil progenitors. *Blood* 1991;77:1462–1468.

68. Saito H, Hatake K, Dvorak AM, et al. Selective differentiation and proliferation of hematopoietic cells induced by recombinant human interleukins. *Proc Natl Acad Sci U S A* 1988;85:2288–2292.

69. Taliaferro WH, Sarles MP. The cellular reactions in the skin, lungs, and intestine of normal and immune rats after infection with *Nippostrongylus brasiliensis*. *J Infect Dis* 1939;64:157–192.

70. David JR, Butterworth AE, Vadas MA. Mechanism of interaction mediating killing of *Schistosoma mansoni* by human eosinophils. *Am J Trop Med Hyg* 1980;29:842–848.

71. Haque A, Ouaissi A, Joseph M, Capron M, Capron A. IgE antibody in eosinophil- and macrophage-mediated *in vitro* killing of *Dipetalonema viteae* microfilariae. *J Immunol* 1981;127:716–725.

72. Kazura JW, Grove DI. Stage-specific antibody-dependent eosinophil-mediated destruction of *Trichinella spiralis*. *Nature* 1978;274: 588–589.

73. Hamann KJ, Gleich GJ, Checkel JL, Loegering DA, McCall JW, Barker RL. *In vitro* killing of microfilariae of *Brugia pahangi* and *Brugia malayi* by eosinophil granule proteins. *J Immunol* 1990;144: 3166–3173.

74. Butterworth AE, Wassom DL, Gleich GJ, Loegering DA, David JR. Damage to schistosomula of *Schistosoma mansoni* induced directly by eosinophil major basic protein. *J Immunol* 1979;122:221–229.

75. Sturrock RF, Kimani R, Cottrell BJ, et al. Observations on possible immunity to reinfection among Kenyan schoolchildren after treatment for *Schistosoma mansoni*. *Trans R Soc Trop Med Hyg* 1983;77: 363–371.

76. Hagan P, Wilkins HA, Blumenthal UJ, Hayes RJ, Greenwood BM. Eosinophilia and resistance to *Schistosoma haematobium* in man. *Parasite Immunol* 1985;7:625–632.

77. Rennick DM, Thompson-Snipes L, Coffman RL, Seymour BW, Jackson JD. *In vivo* administration of antibody to interleukin-5 inhibits

increased generation of eosinophils and their progenitors in bone marrow of parasitized mice. *Blood* 1990;76:312–316.

78. Herndon FJ, Kayes SG. Depletion of eosinophils by anti–IL-5 monoclonal antibody treatment of mice infected with *Trichinella spiralis* does not alter parasite burden or immunologic resistance to infection. *J Immunol* 1992;149:3642–3647.

79. Urban JFJ, Katona IM, Paul WM, Findelman RD. Interleukin 4 is important in protective immunity to a gastrointestinal nematode infection in mice. *Proc Natl Acad Sci U S A* 1991;88:5513–5517.

80. Sher A, Coffman RF, Hieny S, Cheever AW. Ablation of eosinophil and IgE responses with anti–IL-5 or anti–IL-4 antibodies fails to affect immunity against *Schistosoma mansoni* in the mouse. *J Immunol* 1990;145:3911–3916.

81. Hokibara S, Takamoto M, Tominaga A, Takatsu K, Sugane K. Marked eosinophilia in interleukin-5 transgenic mice fails to prevent *Trichinella spiralis* infection. *J Parasitol* 1997;83:1186–1189.

82. Dent LA, Munro GH, Piper KP, et al. Eosinophilic interleukin 5 (IL-5) transgenic mice: eosinophil activity and impaired clearance of *Schistosoma mansoni. Parasite Immunol* 1997;19:291–300.

83. Korenaga M, Hitoshi Y, Yamaguchi N, Sato Y, Takatsu K, Tada I. The role of interleukin-5 in protective immunity to *Strongyloides venezuelensis* infection in mice. *Immunology* 1991;72:502–507.

84. Rotman HL, Yutanawiboonchai W, Brigandi RA, et al. *Strongyloides stercoralis:* eosinophil-dependent immune-mediated killing of third stage larvae in BALB/cByJ mice. *Exp Parasitol* 1996;82:267–278.

85. Abraham D, Rotman HL, Haberstroh HF, et al. *Strongyloides stercoralis:* protective immunity to third-stage larvae in BALB/cByJ mice. *Exp Parasitol* 1995;80:297–307.

86. Brigandi RA, Rotman HL, Yutanawiboonchai W, et al. *Strongyloides stercoralis:* role of antibody and complement in immunity to the third stage larvae in BALB/cByJ mice. *Exp Parasitol* 1996;82:279–289.

87. Sasaki O, Sugaya H, Ishida K, Yoshimura K. Ablation of eosinophils with anti–IL-5 antibody enhances the survival of intracranial worms of *Angiostrongylus cantonensis* in the mouse. *Parasite Immunol* 1993; 15:349–354.

88. Yoshida T, Ikuta K, Sugaya H, et al. Defective B1-cell development and impaired immunity against *Angiostrongylus cantonensis* in IL-5R alpha-deficient mice. *Immunity* 1996;4:483–494.

89. Lange AM, Yutanawiboonchai W, Scott P, Abraham D. IL-4- and IL-5–dependent protective immunity to *Onchocerca volvulus* infective larvae in BALB/cByJ mice. *J Immunol* 1994;153:205–211.

90. Folkard SG, Hogarth PJ, Taylor MJ, Bianco AE. Eosinophils are the major effector cells of immunity to microfilariae in a mouse model of onchocerciasis. *Parasitology* 1996;112:323–329.

91. Steel C, Nutman TB. Regulation of IL-5 in onchocerciasis: a critical role for IL-2. *J Immunol* 1993;150:5511–5518.

92. Elson LH, Calvopina M, Paredes W, et al. Immunity to onchocerciasis: putative immune persons produce a Th1-like response to *Onchocerca volvulus. J Infect Dis* 1995;171:652–658.

93. Brattig NW, Tischendorf FW, Strote G, Medina-de la Garza CE. Eosinophil-larval-interaction in onchocerciasis: heterogeneity of *in vitro* adherence of eosinophils to infective third and fourth stage larvae and microfilariae of *Onchocerca volvulus. Parasite Immunol* 1991;13:13–22.

94. Weller PF, Bubley GJ. The idiopathic hypereosinophilic syndrome. *Blood* 1994;83:2759–2779.

95. Nutman TB, Miller KD, Mulligan M, Ottesen EA. *Loa loa* infection in temporary residents of endemic regions: recognition of a hyperresponsive syndrome with characteristic clinical manifestations. *J Infect Dis* 1986;154:10–18.

96. Kayes SG. Human toxocariasis and the visceral larva migrans syndrome: correlative immunopathology. *Chem Immunol* 1997;66:99–124.

97. de Krömer MT, Medina-De-la-Garza CE, Brattig NW. Differences in

eosinophil and neutrophil chemotactic responses in sowda and generalized form of onchocerciasis. *Acta Trop* 1995;60:21–33.

98. Gleich GJ, Schroeter AL, Marcoux JP, Sachs MI, O'Connell EJ, Kohler PF. Episodic angioedema associated with eosinophilia. *N Engl J Med* 1984;310:1621–1626.

99. Costa JJ, Weller PF, Galli SJ. The cells of the allergic response: mast cells, basophils , and eosinophils. *JAMA* 1997;278:1815–1822.

100. Tischendorf FW, Brattig NW, Buttner DW, Pieper A, Lintzel M. Serum levels of eosinophil cationic protein, eosinophil-derived neurotoxin and myeloperoxidase in infections with filariae and schistosomes. *Acta Trop* 1996;62:171–182.

101. Shaw RJ, Walsh GM, Cromwell O, Moqbel R, Spry CJ, Kay AB. Activated human eosinophils generate SRS-A leukotrienes following IgG-dependent stimulation. *Nature* 1985;316:150–152.

102. Cromwell O, Wardlaw AJ, Champion A, Moqbel R, Osei D, Kay AB. IgG-dependent generation of platelet-activating factor by normal and low density human eosinophils. *J Immunol* 1990;145:3862–3868.

103. McCormick ML, Metwali A, Railsback MA, Weinstock JV, Britigan BE. Eosinophils from schistosome-induced hepatic granulomas produce superoxide and hydroxyl radical. *J Immunol* 1996;157:5009–5015.

104. Thomas GR, McCrossan M, Selkirk ME. Cytostatic and cytotoxic effects of activated macrophages and nitric acid donors on *Brugia malayi. Infect Immun* 1997;65:2732–2739.

105. Yazdanbakhsh M, Tai PC, Spry CJ, Gleich GJ, Roos D. Synergism between eosinophil cationic protein and oxygen intermediates in killing of schistosomula of *Schistosoma mansoni. J Immunol* 1987; 138:3443–3447.

106. Sabin EA, Kopf MA, Pearce EJ. *Schistosoma mansoni* egg-induced early IL-4 production is dependent upon IL-5 and eosinophils. *J Exp Med* 1996;184:1871–1878.

107. Ackerman SJ, Kephart GM, Francis H, Awadzi K, Gleich GJ, Ottesen EA. Eosinophil degranulation: an immunologic determinant in the pathogenesis of the Mazzotti reaction in human onchocerciasis. *J Immunol* 1990;144:3961–3969.

108. Limaye AP, Abrams JS, Silver JE, et al. Interleukin-5 and the post-treatment eosinophilia in patients with onchocerciasis. *J Clin Invest* 1991;88:1418–1421.

109. Pearlman E. Immunopathology of onchocerciasis: a role for eosinophils in onchocercal dermatitis and keratitis. *Chem Immunol* 1997;66:26–40.

110. Pearlman E, Lass JH, Bardenstein DS, et al. IL-12 exacerbates helminth-mediated corneal pathology by augmenting inflammatory cell recruitment and chemokine expression. *J Immunol* 1997;158:827–833.

111. Pearlman E, Lass JH, Bardenstein DS, et al. Interleukin 4 and T helper type 2 cells are required for the development of onchocercal keratitis (river blindness). *J Exp Med* 1995;182:931–940.

112. Zhou Y, Bao S, Rothwell TLW, Husband AJ. Differential expression of interleukin-5 mRNA+ cells and eosinophils in *Nippostrongylus brasiliensis* infection in resistant and susceptible strains of mice. *Eur J Immunol* 1996;26:2133–2139.

113. Takamoto M, Ovington KS, Behm CA, Sugane K, Young IG, Matthaei KI. Eosinophilia, parasite burden and lung damage in Toxocara canis infection in C57Bl/6 mice genetically deficient in IL-5. *Immunology* 1997;90:511–517.

114. Cookston M, Stober M, Kayes S. Eosinophilic myocarditis in CBA/J mice infected with *Toxocara canis. Am J Pathol* 1990;136:1137–1145.

115. Grove DI, Hamburger J, Warren KS. Kinetics of immunological responses, resistance to reinfection, and pathological reactions to infection with *Trichinella spiralis. J Infect Dis* 1977;136:562–570.

116. Urban JF Jr, Katona IM, Paul WE, Finkelman FD. Interleukin 4 is important in protective immunity to a gastrointestinal nematode infection in mice. *Proc Natl Acad Sci U S A* 1991;88:5513–5517.

Inflammation: Basic Principles and Clinical Correlates,
3rd ed., edited by John I. Gallin and Ralph Snyderman.
Lippincott Williams & Wilkins, Philadelphia © 1999.

CHAPTER 59

Autoantibodies:

Their Induction and Pathogenicity

Gisele Zandman-Goddard and Betty Diamond

STRUCTURE OF AUTOANTIBODIES

Antibodies are glycoproteins that are produced in both membrane-bound and secreted forms by B lymphocytes (1) (see Chapter 18). They are composed of two heavy chains and two light chains. The association of the heavy and light chains forms two functional units, the Fab and the Fc. The Fab is responsible for antigen binding, and the Fc portion of the antibody, the constant region of the heavy chain, determines the isotype (class) of the antibody molecule (IgM, IgD, IgG, IgA, or IgE) and therefore all effector functions (1,2) (see Chapter 18).

The variable region of a heavy or light chain is divided into complementarity-determining regions (CDRs), which previously were called hypervariable regions, and framework regions (FRs). The CDRs contain most of the contact amino acids for antigen binding and therefore are the dominant regions contributing to antigenic specificity. The FRs constitute the backbone of the antigen-binding pocket. Both CDRs and FRs undergo amino acid changes during B-cell activation that may confer structural changes on the antigen-binding pockets (3,4) (Fig. 59-1).

Immunoglobulins are the only self proteins that are routinely immunogenic. The variable region of an antibody serves as an antigen during the progression of an immune response. Antigenic determinants in the variable region comprise the idiotype (Id). Anti-idiotypes are antibodies that bind to the variable region of an antibody molecule. Activation of B cells responding to foreign antigen is followed by activation of anti-idiotypic B cells. This cascade, called an *idiotypic network*, mediates some

important functions: members of the network regulate each other, which serves to control immune responses, and they link internal (self) immune responses to external (environmental) immune responses (5–8).

ANTIBODY ASSEMBLY

In most vertebrates, the genes encoding the antibody variable region are assembled during B-cell development from gene segments designated V (variable), D (diversity), and J (joining) for the heavy chain and V and J for the light chain (9). This is accomplished through site-specific recombination involving the introduction of double-stranded breaks at specific recognition signal sequences adjacent to the V, D, and J elements and the activity of the recombination-activating genes *RAG1* and *RAG2* as well as additional genes (9–16).

In humans, the heavy-chain V_H, D_H, and J_H gene segments are tandemly arrayed on chromosome 14 (17,18). The 50 to 100 functional heavy-chain V-segment genes have been divided into 7 families. Members of a V gene family share 80% homology in nucleotide sequence (19–22). There are approximately 30 functional D segments and 6 J segments. The light-chain gene segment can rearrange in either of two loci, κ or λ. The $V_κ$ locus is found on chromosome 2 (23–27). It consists of approximately 35 functional genes divided into 7 families; there are 5 J segments. The λ locus on chromosome 22 contains at least 7 V gene families with approximately 70 members (28–34).

Immunoglobulin gene rearrangement occurs in an orderly fashion, with assembly of the heavy chain first, and then the light chain. The D and J gene segments of the heavy chain rearrange first, followed by the V-to-DJ rearrangement. The μ protein produced by the productive rearrangement of V, D, and J segments inhibits further rearrangement of heavy-chain gene segments, thus

G. Zandman-Goddard: Department of Microbiology and Immunology and Medicine, Division of Rheumatology, Albert Einstein College of Medicine, Bronx, New York 10461.

B. Diamond: Department of Medicine, Albert Einstein College of Medicine, Bronx, New York 10461.

THE ANTIGEN BINDING REGION

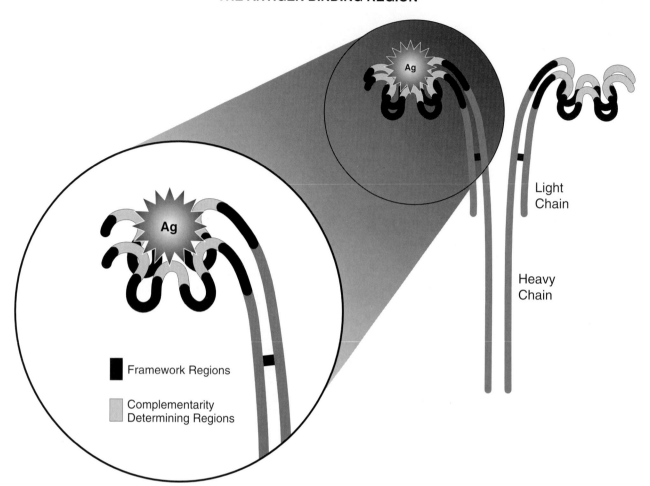

FIG. 59-1. The antigen-binding site. The binding site is a pocket into which the antigen fits. The complementarity-determining regions are the contact sites for the antigen, whereas the framework regions act as the backbone of the structure.

accounting for allelic exclusion of immunoglobulin heavy chains. This mechanism ensures that heavy-chain genes rearrange first on one chromosome, rearranging on the second chromosome only if the first rearrangement is nonproductive. As a result, in any B cell, one heavy-chain allele is productively rearranged and expressed, and the second is in germ-line configuration or is nonproductively rearranged. If both alleles undergo nonproductive rearrangements, the cell dies. This is a common occurrence and helps explain why only a small fraction of B-cell progenitors develop into mature B cells (9,35).

Another consequence of μ-chain production is the stimulation of light-chain gene rearrangement. The μ heavy chain associates first with a surrogate light chain and forms a pre-B-cell receptor. It is not clear what signaling must occur through this receptor for B-cell maturation to continue, but B cells that do not express this receptor do not undergo light-chain rearrangements. The κ light chains rearrange first, followed by λ light chains if no productive κ rearrangement has occurred (9,35).

In this way, a relatively limited set of genes can lead to the generation of a vast array of antibodies. Since this process of gene rearrangement occurs without reference to existing self or foreign antigens, autospecificities are generated.

Much work has been performed to determine whether persons who make autoantibodies do so because they generate a B-cell repertoire from a unique array of V gene segments or by abnormal mechanisms of rearrangement. Little evidence has emerged that an abnormal V-gene repertoire is associated with autoimmune disease. In an elegant study in the mouse, Gavalchin et al. (36) characterized V gene use in the production of autoantibodies. The SWR strain of mouse displays no autoimmunity. The NZB strain displays autoantibody production and hemolytic anemia. The SNR mouse is the offspring of an SWR nonautoimmune parent and an NZB autoimmune parent. The F1 offspring develop anti-DNA antibodies and a lupus-like glomerulonephritis. When the anti-DNA antibodies produced in these mice were analyzed, more than half were found to be encoded by V_H genes derived from the nonautoimmune SWR parent (36). This study demonstrated that pathogenic autoantibodies can be encoded by V genes from an animal that does not routinely display autoreactivity. There has been one report in humans of a particular V-gene repertoire potentially predisposing to autoimmunity. A member of the V_H3 gene family has been reported to be absent more commonly in persons with systemic lupus erythematosus (SLE) than in the nonautoimmune population (37). It appears that, in general, there are no polymorphisms in the available V-gene repertoire that predispose to the production of autoantibodies. Most autoantibodies are encoded by V_H genes that are present in the nonautoimmune population (38). Alternatively stated, nonautoimmune persons have the V-gene repertoire needed to encode pathogenic autoantibodies. Furthermore, V genes used in the production of autoantibodies are also used in the production of presumably protective antibodies directed against foreign antigen (39–42).

Extensive studies have also been performed to determine whether V-gene rearrangement is abnormal in the production of autoantibodies. There is little evidence to support this suggestion. Early studies on the question raised the possibility that CDR3 of the heavy chain encoded by the VDJ junction might display inverted D segments or D-D fusions more commonly in autoantibodies than in protective antibodies (43,44). As the number of analyses of protective antibodies has increased, it has become apparent that in human antibodies inverted D segments and D-D fusions are quite common (45,46).

There are some data to suggest that the CDR3s of the light chains of patients with rheumatoid arthritis may contain a larger number of amino acids than usually is seen in light chain CDR3s (47). The CDR3 of the light chain is, in general, a fairly uniform length of nine amino acids; because terminal deoxytransferase (tdt), an enzyme that adds non template encoded bases (N sequence) at the junctions of V-D and D-J heavy chain rearrangements, is no longer expressed in the B cell during light-chain rearrangement, there is rarely N-sequence addition in light-chain CDR3. The finding of longer CDR3s in light chains of patients with rheumatoid arthritis raised the possibility that light chains were rearranging while tdt was expressed, perhaps even before rearrangement of the heavy chain (46,47). Although this has been a provocative hypothesis, in general autoantibodies do not display abnormal light-chain V-J junctions (48).

Antibodies that arise in response to viral infection or to noncarbohydrate antigens in bacteria display evidence of being produced by B cells that have differentiated in germinal centers. There is extensive somatic mutation and heavy-chain class switching (38). In addition, there is evidence of antigen selection, as demonstrated by a higher-than-random ratio of replacement to silent mutations in CDRs (38). Analysis of the heavy- and light-chain genes

of autoantibodies from mice and from patients with autoimmune disease also reveals somatic mutation, isotype switching, and clustering of replacement mutations in CDRs, again indicative of antibodies arising from antigen-specific B-cell activation and selection (38,48–52). There appears to be no difference in the frequency of somatic mutations in autoantibodies, although there may be subtle alterations in the targeting of mutations to mutational hot spots in patients with SLE (53).

In summary, the majority of analyses show that the generation of autoantibodies or abnormalities in VDJ or VJ recombination does not appear to involve altered heavy- or light-chain family use (46). Furthermore, studies in mice suggest that autoantibody formation is a normal part of a developing B-cell repertoire, and that organisms have developed multiple strategies to ensure the elimination of autoantibodies (49).

REGULATION OF AUTOREACTIVE B CELLS

The immature B cell expresses IgM only. These cells do not proliferate or differentiate on encounter with antigen. In fact, antigen encounter in the bone marrow leads to tolerance induction or nonresponsiveness rather than activation. Studies of mice expressing autoantibody-encoding transgenes have provided important insights into the regulation of autoreactive B cells arising in the naive B-cell repertoire. When these transgenes are expressed in a nonautoimmune mouse strain, autoreactive B cells undergo one of three fates.

Autoreactive B cells may be anergized so that they are not deleted but cannot be induced to differentiate and secrete immunoglobulin by the usual activation signals. Alternatively, autoreactive B cells may be eliminated by a process of programmed cell death (apoptosis). It has been hypothesized that the extent of membrane-immunoglobulin cross-linking determines whether an autoreactive B cell undergoes anergy induction or apoptosis. A third option for avoiding B-cell autoreactivity is receptor editing. Receptor editing is the displacement of a productive rearrangement by an additional productive rearrangement on the same allele. It may occur at the heavy-chain locus, resulting in heavy-chain editing, or, more commonly, at a light-chain locus, resulting in light-chain editing. Mounting evidence suggests that this process is a result of receptor engagement (54), and its function may be to provide an alternative to programmed cell death or anergy of immature autoreactive B cells (55). When autoantibody-encoding transgenes are expressed in autoimmune mouse strains, the B cells do not undergo receptor editing and are not deleted or anergized. These studies have shown that defects in central tolerance or in the regulation of naive B cells can lead to autoimmunity (56–61).

Studies of human disease to date have not revealed whether defects in central tolerance account for autoantibody expression. Studies of receptor editing are few and rely on indirect evidence, because bone marrow B cells, which are the cells that undergo receptor editing, are not routinely available for study. Nevertheless, the studies that exist do not suggest a defect in receptor editing (54). It is equally difficult to determine whether a defect in deletion of naive B cells in the bone marrow contributes to autoimmune disease. Most B cells producing disease-associated autoantibodies display signs of antigen activation, and most autoantibodies that are presumed to be pathogenic are somatically mutated (see later discussion). Yet, it is possible that the mutations are not responsible for the acquisition of autoreactivity—that is, that the naive, unmutated B cell also was autoreactive, and defective tolerance induction early in its maturation led to its survival and subsequent activation.

B cells that are not deleted or tolerized migrate out of the bone marrow into the peripheral circulation and secondary lymphoid tissues, where they continue to mature in the absence of antigenic stimulation. Mature B cells coexpress μ and δ heavy chains in association with a κ or λ light chain, and therefore produce membrane-bound IgM and IgD. These cells can be activated by antigen. Unless B cells encounter antigen, they die within days to weeks (35).

On encounter with antigen, naive mature B cells become activated B cells and begin to proliferate and differentiate. Some participate in a primary immune response and are found in the periarteriolar lymphoid sheath of secondary lymphoid organs. Others migrate to germinal centers, where they may undergo somatic mutation and heavy-chain isotype switching. In the germinal center, competition for antigen leads to the selective survival of those B cells with V-region mutations that produce an antibody with increased affinity for antigen. This accounts for the phenomenon of affinity maturation. Some germinal center cells become plasma cells; others become memory cells. Memory B cells survive for weeks or months and actively recirculate in the periphery. Reencounter with antigen results in a secondary immune response, with the activation of high-affinity memory cells (62–65).

The generation of autoreactivity in the periphery has also been studied, especially in murine models. It is possible to demonstrate in mice that, during the course of a response to foreign antigen, somatic mutation of B cells responding to that antigen produces progeny with autospecificities (40,41,66,67). It is thought that these B cells are deleted within the germinal center, probably because they encounter antigen but receive no T-cell help. If the antibodies produced cross-react with both foreign antigen and self antigen, the B cells may survive selection in the germinal center, but they may be deleted or anergized after they enter the recirculating B-cell pool because of a lack of T-cell help. This generation of autospecificities occurs in nonautoimmune mouse strains and leads to large numbers of autoreactive B cells that require peripheral regulation. These autoantibodies can

be demonstrated to be pathogenic, again indicating that nonautoimmune hosts can produce disease-inducing autoantibodies (61).

In human studies, evidence is again indirect for autoreactivity arising in the periphery. Many studies of human autoantibodies, especially anti-DNA antibodies, show that somatic mutation has occurred (38,42,43,45), but in general it has not been possible to state that the autoreactivity is a consequence of mutation. Therefore, it is not possible to know with certainty whether the progenitor B cell was responding to self or foreign antigen.

B1 cells, many of which express CD5, constitute a subpopulation of B cells. It is not clear whether the B1 cells represent a separate lineage or an alternative differentiation pathway. In the mouse, B1 cells comprise 10% to 40% of peritoneal B cells and are infrequently found in the spleen and lymph nodes. In human SLE, both B1 and B2 cells have been shown to secrete IgG anti-DNA antibodies (68,69). The B1 lineage is implicated in the production of natural antibodies (69,70).

NATURAL ANTIBODIES

Historically, autoantibodies have been classified as either natural autoantibodies or pathogenic autoantibodies. Natural antibodies are defined as IgM immunoglobulins encoded by germ-line genes. They often display polyreactivity, with low-affinity interactions toward a large array of antigens. The natural antibody response may be driven by environmental antigens or by nonspecific activation of immune responses (71). Natural autoantibodies are thought to be part of a highly conserved antibody repertoire (71–73) that appears to be preferentially directed to polysaccharide or T-independent antigens. The repertoire of natural autoantibodies may be biased toward a selective set of autoantigens that includes nucleic acids (72,73).

Possible biologic roles of natural antibodies include participation in the natural defenses against infectious agents and removal of senescent or altered self molecules, cells, or tumors (74–76). The physiologic response to self antigen has also been suggested to protect against pathogenic autoreactivity (77–80). The postulated mechanism involves blockade by natural autoantibodies of immunogenic epitopes on self antigens to prevent induction of a high-affinity, potentially pathogenic response to these epitopes.

The classification of natural autoantibodies as distinct from pathogenic autoantibodies was amended after it become apparent that some pathogenic antibodies are of IgM isotype and are germ-line encoded (81–83). Nevertheless, there is a population of apparently nonpathogenic autoantibodies present in all persons. It remains controversial whether pathogenic autoantibodies often derive from these natural autoantibodies via mutation and aberrant selection or whether pathogenic and natural autoantibodies most commonly represent different B-cell responses.

PATHOGENIC AUTOANTIBODIES

In the study of disease-associated autoantibodies, particular attention has been paid to two aspects of the response: the molecular genetic origins of the autoantibodies (already described) and the determinants and mechanisms of pathogenicity.

The pathogenicity of autoantibodies can be mediated through several mechanisms, including opsonization of soluble factors or cells, activation of an inflammatory cascade via the complement system, and interference with the physiologic function of soluble molecules or cells (Table 59-1).

In idiopathic thrombocytopenic purpura, opsonization of platelets targets them for elimination by the reticular endothelial system. Likewise, in autoimmune hemolytic anemia, binding of immunoglobulin to red cell membranes leads to phagocytosis and lysis of the opsonized cell (84). Goodpasture's syndrome, a disease characterized by lung hemorrhage and severe glomerulonephritis, represents an example of antibody binding leading to local activation of complement and neutrophils. The autoantibody in this disease binds to the noncollagenous domain of type IV collagen in the basement membrane, leading to local activation of the complement cascade (84,85). In SLE also, activation of the complement cascade at sites of immunoglobulin deposition in renal glomeruli is considered to be a major mode of renal destruction.

Although it has long been known that autoantibodies can interfere with normal physiologic functions, the extent to which autoantibodies exert their pathogenic effects in this way is only now being appreciated. Autoantibodies against hormone receptors can lead to stimulation of target cells or to inhibition of target cell function through interference with receptor signaling. For example, autoantibodies to the receptor for thyroid-stimulating hormone (TSH) are present in Grave's disease and function as agonists, causing the thyroid to respond as if there were an excess of TSH (86–88). Alternatively, antibodies to the insulin receptor can cause insulin-resistant diabetes mellitus through receptor blockade. They prevent cell signaling through the insulin receptor (86,89). In myasthenia gravis, autoantibody is directed at the acetylcholine receptor (90,91). Anti–acetylcholine receptor antibodies can be detected in 85% to 90% of patients and are clearly responsible for symptomatology (90). Presumably, the exact location of the antigenic epitope, the valence and affinity of the antibody, and perhaps other characteristics determine whether activation or blockade results from antibody binding (86). The pathogenicity of many other autoantibodies has been demonstrated.

Anti-cardiolipin antibodies are associated with thromboembolic events in primary and secondary antiphospholipid syndrome (92–94) and have also been associated with fetal wastage. The major antibody specificity is the cardiolipin-β_2–glycoprotein I complex (β_2GPI) (95). The pathogenic role of these antibodies in thrombotic disease has been studied with the use of a passive transfer model in mice (96). Anti-phospholipid antibody appears to act in part by exerting a procoagulant effect that inhibits the phospholipid-dependent activation of the protein C–protein S pathway that plays a role in regulating thrombus development. The antibodies bind β_2GPI, which inhibits the thrombin-thrombomodulin activation of protein C. Furthermore, it has been shown that anti-phospholipid antibodies inhibit degradation of activated factor V by protein S (97,98).

In pemphigus, autoantibodies, primarily of the IgG4 isotype, bind to the surface of epidermal cells (99–101). These antibodies have been shown to play a role in the induction of the disease. They exert their pathologic effect by disrupting cell-cell junctions through stimula-

TABLE 59-1. *Mechanisms of autoantibody pathogenicity*

Mechanism	Autoantibody	Disease
Opsonization	Anti-gpIIa/IIIb	Idiopathic thrombocytopenic purpura
	Anti-RBC	Autoimmune hemolytic anemia
Inflammatory	Anti-glomerular basement membrane	Goodpasture's syndrome
	Anti-desmosome	Pemphigus
	Anti-DNA	Systemic lupus erythematosus
Alteration of physiologic function	Anti-Ca^{2+} channel	Myocarditis
	Anti-β-adrenergic receptor	
	Anti-MAT	
	Anti-insulin receptor	Insulin-resistant diabetes mellitus
	Anti-TSH receptor	Grave's disease, Hashimoto's thyroiditis
	Anti-acetylcholine receptor	Myasthenia gravis
	c-ANCA	Wegener's granulomatosis
	Anti-cardiolipin	Anti-phospholipid syndrome

RBC, red blood cell; MAT, mitochondrial adenosine translocator; TSH, thyroid-stimulating hormone; c-ANCA, anti-neutrophil cytoplasmic antibodies.

tion of epithelial proteases, thus leading to blister formation (102).

Anti-neutrophil cytoplasmic antibody (c-ANCA), found in Wegener's granulomatosis, is also an antibody to an intracellular antigen, the 29-kd serine protease (proteinase-3), a component of the primary lysosome of neutrophils (86,103). *In vitro* experiments have shown, however, that addition of IgG c-ANCA to neutrophils primed by tumor necrosis factor (TNF) causes cellular activation and degranulation, suggesting that the antibodies may bind a cell membrane antigen also (86,103).

Approximately 60% of patients with myocarditis have circulating heart-specific antibodies (104,105). Increasing evidence, mainly from murine models, suggests that autoreactivity against cardiac antigens has pathologic consequences (104). Patients with myocarditis display serum autoantibodies to a number of cardiac antigens, including cardiac-myosin heavy chain (104,106), Ca^{2+} channel (107), β-adrenergic receptor (108), and the mitochondrial adenosine nucleotide translocator (109). *In vitro* studies have shown that heart-specific antibodies from the sera of patients with myocarditis can induce complement-dependent and cell-mediated cytolysis of cardiac myocytes (110).

New data are suggesting that autoantibodies of a given specificity may cause disease only in genetically susceptible hosts. Studies of anti-myosin–mediated myocarditis demonstrated that a monoclonal anti-myosin antibody caused myocarditis in a mouse strain exhibiting extracellular myosin but not in a strain lacking extracellular antigen expression (111,112). Clinical studies of myasthenia gravis also suggest that antibodies cause disease only in susceptible hosts (113). Finally, some autoantibodies seem to be markers for disease but have no known pathogenic potential. It may be that, as we improve our understanding of disease pathogenesis, a function for some of these will become apparent.

INDUCTION OF AUTOANTIBODIES

The trigger for production of autoantibodies remains a controversial and unresolved question. There are several mechanisms that have been invoked. The first is molecular mimicry, in which a foreign antigen has sufficient structural homology to a self antigen to cause antibodies to the foreign antigen to cross-react with self. The second mechanism is epitope spreading or presentation of cryptic epitopes. This occurs when the immune system is confronted with antigenic epitopes of a self antigen to which it has not been tolerized, either because of enhanced presentation of an epitope that is usually presented in too small an amount to signal lymphoid cells or by presentation of an epitope that is not ordinarily processed and presented. The third mechanism is alteration of the autoantigen itself, so that it displays neoepitopes and is therefore immunogenic. A fourth possibility is that B-cell superantigens activate autoreactive B cells. Finally, it is possible that the idiotypic network gives rise to autoantibodies (Fig. 59-2).

There has been increasing evidence for molecular mimicry leading to autoantibody production. Insulin-dependent diabetes mellitus may be an example of molecular mimicry that exists between the P2-C protein of coxsackievirus B4 and glutamic acid decarboxylase (GAD), which is found in pancreatic islet cells and neurons (114,115). Even before clinical manifestations occur, autoantibodies to GAD can be found in the sera of patients (116). Perhaps the best example of autoreactivity deriving from molecular mimicry exists in rheumatic fever. Antibodies made against the M protein of streptococci cross-react with the rod portion of myosin (117–119) and sometimes with laminin and other matrix proteins as well. This cross reactivity leads to immunoglobulin deposition in the heart, with the ensuing inflammatory cascade. Examples of cross-reactivity or abnormal immune responses between viruses and self proteins have been described in rheumatoid arthritis (120), celiac disease (121), primary biliary cirrhosis (122), and multiple sclerosis (123).

Structure homology between foreign and self antigens can also lead to autoreactivity arising through somatic mutation. Mutation of an antimicrobial antibody may cause changes in the antigen-binding site. The hypothesis that somatic mutation of protective antibodies may lead to the production of antibodies displaying autoreactivity has been confirmed in an *in vivo* mouse model. Phosphorylcholine is a dominant antigen on the pneumococcal cell wall. Many years ago, it was demonstrated *in vitro* that a single amino acid substitution in an anti-phosphorylcholine antibody led to a loss of binding to phosphorylcholine and the acquisition of DNA binding (43,124). More recently, it was demonstrated that an anti-phosphorylcholine antibody can be converted into antibody with specificity to double-stranded DNA (dsDNA) by somatic mutation during the course of an *in vivo* antibody

FIG. 59-2. Triggers of autoantibody production. **(A)** Molecular mimicry. Microbial agents may induce responses that cross-react with self antigens. **(B)** Epitope spreading. The antigen is processed into fragments so that different epitopes are presented on the surface of the B cell and then recognized by the T cell. **(C)** B-cell superantigens. B cells are activated by a microbial superantigen binding outside the conventional binding site. **(D)** Idiotype network. The anti-idiotypic antibodies induce complementary antibodies with different antigenic specificities.

TRIGGERS OF AUTOANTIBODY PRODUCTION

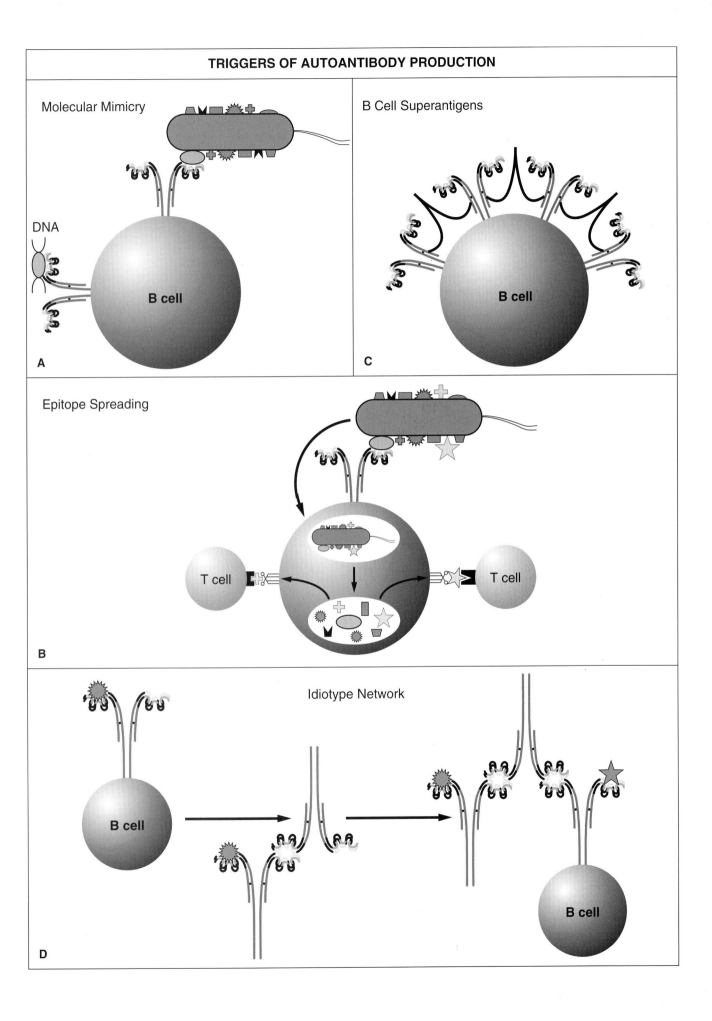

Molecular Mimicry

A

DNA

B cell

B Cell Superantigens

C

B cell

Epitope Spreading

B

T cell

T cell

Idiotype Network

D

B cell

B cell

response (39). These autoreactive B cells arise at high frequency but are usually regulated by apoptosis. By interfering with the apoptotic program, it is possible to rescue anti-DNA anti-phosphorylcholine cross-reactive antibodies. These antibodies are both protective and potentially pathogenic (39,66,125).

Persons with bacterial infections transiently make anti-DNA antibodies that are idiotypically related to the anti-DNA antibodies of SLE patients. Furthermore, nonautoimmune persons vaccinated with pneumococcal polysaccharide produce anti-pneumococcal antibodies bearing anti-DNA–associated idiotypes (43,126). These results indicate that anti-dsDNA antibodies may be produced in an anti-pneumococcal response in humans as well as in murine models.

A consequence of autoantibody formation during microbial infection is epitope (determinant) spreading as described above. This is the development of an immune response to multiple regions of an antigen once a response to one region is present, or even the development of antibody to multiple members of a macromolecular complex once antibody to one member is present. Experimental support for this phenomenon comes from animal studies in which multiple autoantibody specificities are induced after immunization with a defined epitope of a single autoantigen (127). In a rodent model of SLE, mice were immunized with an SmB peptide and were found to produce autoantibodies to multiple other spliceosomal proteins (128). Similarly, immunization of mice with a fragment of the La protein led to autoantibody responses to other non-cross-reactive components of the La/Ro ribonucleoprotein complex (129). It is thought that B cells mediate antigen-specific uptake of large complexes, leading to the presentation of multiple self epitopes from the multiple proteins that make up the complexes (127,128). These epitopes are not normally presented to T cells or are not presented in sufficient amounts to tolerize T cells.

A number of studies have shown how this phenomenon of epitope spreading could lead to autoantibody production after infection and a response to foreign antigen. For example, the large T antigen of polyoma virus binds DNA; once an immune response is mounted to this foreign antigen, the response can spread to self molecules such as DNA that associate with the large T antigen (130–132). As viruses have adapted to use cellular machinery for their own proliferation, there are many viral proteins that associate with cellular proteins during infection, and these are potential targets for autoimmune responses.

Microbial infection or environmental factors may lead to the exposure to the immune system of antigens that are normally sequestered, by inducing the translocation of intracellular antigens to the cell membrane. For example, ultraviolet irradiation has been shown to cause translocation of the La protein, which is normally intracellular, to the plasma membrane, where it can be recognized as a foreign antigen by the immune system (133,134).

B-cell superantigens are believed to bind to a segment of the immunoglobulin V region that is distinct from the conventional antigen binding site. The prototype is Ig superantigen *Staphylococcus aureus* bacterial toxin protein A (135–139), which is now known to bind specifically to members of the V_H3 family (138–140) in the CDR2 and/or FR3 domains (140,141). Another superantigen, gp120, is the outer envelope glycoprotein of the human immunodeficiency virus, HIV-1. The gp120 binds to a subpopulation of B cells expressing the V_H3 gene products and can stimulate B cells to secrete immunoglobulin (142–144). Its binding to the heavy-chain locus is independent of the light-chain isotype (142). Although the V_H3 genes in this population are diverse in their CDR regions, they share conserved peptide segments in FR1 and FR3, providing evidence for an alternative antigen binding site (142).

Binding to superantigen leads to an initial activation of the B cell, followed by cell death. For example, in patients with the acquired immunodeficiency syndrome (AIDS), there is a clonal deficit of V_H3-expressing B cells. This clonal deficit is preceded by an expansion of the V_H3 B-cell pool in earlier clinical stages of HIV infection (142). Because the V_H3 family is the largest in the expressed human repertoire, this superantigen property of gp120 is thought to have deleterious effects for the host, including a steady decline in B cells capable of mounting protective antibody responses with progression of the HIV-induced disease (144).

The idiotype network may also function to induce autoantibody production. When antibody is made to foreign antigen, an anti-idiotypic response is also induced. The anti-idiotypic antibodies bind those antibodies induced by the eliciting antigen, but they also bind a set of structurally related antibodies with different antigenic specificities. This set of antibodies may, in theory, include autospecificities (145,146). The autoantibodies that arise are idiotypically related to autoantibodies in nonautoimmune hosts. This has been demonstrated in murine models of a number of diseases, including SLE (145,146), anti-phospholipid syndrome (147,148), and Wegener's granulomatosis (149,150). It has also been speculated that anti-idiotypes can play a role in suppressing autoantibody production, and that their presence may be responsible for disease remission (151–154). Although it has not been proved that anti-idiotypic antibodies are physiologic regulators of autoimmune disease, their use as pharmacologic regulators continues to be explored.

GENETIC SUSCEPTIBILITY

Genetic susceptibility plays an important role in many autoimmune diseases, as has been shown by studies of populations and families. Elements complicating the study of susceptibility genes in genetically complex autoimmune diseases such as SLE include ethnic diversity, clinical heterogenicity, incomplete penetrance, and environmental factors. As noted previously, there may be genetic factors that determine whether autoantibodies cause target organ injury, but most genetic studies have focused on the induction of autoreactivity. Genetic studies of autoimmune disease in mice have identified susceptibility loci in several inbred strains that spontaneously develop SLE glomerulonephritis or diabetes (155,156). These studies have included genome-wide searches for evidence of linkage using backcrosses or F2 intercrosses of susceptible and nonsusceptible mice. The distal end of mouse chromosome 1 (Sle 1) was shown to predispose to a specific manifestation of SLE, including glomerulonephritis and IgG autoantibodies to chromatin, DNA, and histone (157–161). Genomic intervals on chromosome 4 (Sle2) and chromosome 7 (Sle 3) are being investigated for SLE association (162). Accelerated autoantibody production has been clearly documented in mice with defects in Fas and Fas ligand, the Y accelerator of autoimmunity, and protein-tyrosine phosphatase 1C. Polymorphisms in other immunologically relevant genes, including those encoding the T cell receptor and cytokines, have been postulated to predispose to lupus (163).

In human studies, the genetic basis for SLE is complex and polygenic. Certain major histocompatibility complex class II alleles or complement gene deficiencies (homozygous deficiency for C1q, C2, and C4) are associated with SLE in most ethnic groups studied (163,164). The FcγRIIa and FcγRIIIa genes are located at chromosome arm 1q23-24. Tsao et al. (155) tested a candidate region homologous to a murine SLE susceptibility region in 52 SLE-affected sibpairs from three ethnic groups and found evidence for linkage at 1q41-42. Serum levels of IgG antichromatin also showed evidence for linkage in that area, suggesting that this phenotype is conserved in mice and humans (155). Other candidate genes include the gene for mannose-binding protein, the Sjogren's associated autoantigen, Ro/SSA, complement receptor type 1 (CR1), interleukin-6 (IL-6), Ig heavy and light chain allotypes, TCR, TNF-α, FcγRIIa, and a heat shock protein Hsp-70 (155).

Autoantibody formation is polygenic and appears to depend on threshold effects. It is now clear from animal and human studies that both susceptibility and resistance genes exist. Multiple combinations of these genes exist in the population, and each combination determines an individual's predisposition to a breakdown in immunologic self-tolerance. Furthermore, sex hormones and neuropeptides may alter thresholds for lymphoid cell activation or tolerance induction. For example, estrogen appears to increase expression of *BCL2*, an antiapoptosis gene important in both B- and T-cell survival (165–167). Unraveling such mechanisms will reveal how environmental factors, hormones, and stress may all contribute to autoantibody formation.

ACKNOWLEDGMENTS

The authors wish to thank Dan Michaels for his help with the figures. We also thank Chaim Putterman, Linda Spatz, Philip Kuo, and Jeff Newman for their critical reading of the manuscript. We are grateful to Sylvia Jones for her help in the preparation of the manuscript.

REFERENCES

1. Putterman C, Kuo P, Diamond B. The structure and derivation of antibodies and autoantibodies. In: Wallace DJ, Hahn BH, eds. *Dubois lupus erythematosus,* 5th ed. Baltimore: Williams & Wilkins, 1997: 383–396.
2. Spiegelberg HL. Biological activities of immunoglobulins of different classes and subclasses. *Adv Immunol* 1974;19:259–294.
3. Kabat EA, Wu TT. Attempts to locate complementarity determining residues in the variable positions of light and heavy chains. *Ann NY Acad Sci* 1971;190:382–393.
4. Padlan EA. Anatomy of the antibody molecule. *Mol Immunol* 1994; 31:169–217.
5. Jerne NK. Towards a network theory of the immune system. *Annu Immunol (Paris)* 1974;125:373–389.
6. Rajewsky K, Takemori T. Genetics, expression and function of idiotypes. *Annu Rev Immunol* 1983;1:569–603.
7. Capra JD, Kehoe JM, Winchester RS, Kunkel HG. Structure function relationship among anti-gamma globulin antibodies. *Ann N Y Acad Sci* 1971;190:371–381.
8. Hahn BH, Ebling FM. Idiotypes and idiotype networks. In: Wallace DJ, Hahn BH, eds. *Dubois lupus erythematosus,* 5th ed. Baltimore: Williams & Wilkins, 1997:291–310.
9. Rajewsky K. Clonal selection and learning in the antibody system. *Nature* 1996;381:751–758.
10. Tonegawa S. Somatic generation of antibody diversity. *Nature* 1983; 302:575–581.
11. Alt F, Blackwell TK, Yancopoulos GD. Development of the primary antibody repertoire. *Science* 1987;238:1079–1087.
12. Oettinger MA, Schatz DG, Gorka C, Baltimore D. RAG-1 and RAG-2, adjacent genes that synergistically activate V(D)J recombination. *Science* 1990;248:1517–1523.
13. McBlane JF, van Gent DC, Ramsden DA, et al. Cleavage at a V(D)J recombination signal requires only RAG1 and RAG2 proteins and occurs in two steps. *Cell* 1995;83:387–395.
14. Roth DB, Lindahl T, Gellert M. Repair and recombination: how to make ends meet. *Curr Biol* 1995;5:496–499.
15. Schatz DG, Oettinger MA, Baltimore D. The V(D)J recombination activating gene, RAG-1. *Cell* 1989;59:1035–1048.
16. van Gent DC, McBlane JF, Ramsden DA, Sadofsky MJ, Hesse JE, Gellert M. Initiation of V(D)J recombination in a cell free system by RAG-1 and RAG-2 proteins. *Curr Top Microbiol* 1996;217:1–9.
17. Kodaira M, Kinashi T, Umemura I, et al. Organization and evolution of variable region genes of the human immunoglobulin heavy chain. *J Mol Biol* 1986;190:529–541.
18. Walter MA, Sorti V, Hofker MH, Cox DW. The physical organization of the human immunoglobulin heavy chain gene complex. *EMBO J* 1990;9:3303–3313.
19. Berman J, Mellis S, Pollack R, et al. Content and organization of the human immunoglobulin V$_H$ locus: definition of new V$_H$ families and linkage to the immunoglobulin C$_H$ locus. *EMBO J* 1988;7:727–738.
20. Pascual V, Capra JD. Human immunoglobulin heavy chain variable region genes: organization, polymorphism, and expression. *Adv Immunol* 1991;49:1–74.
21. Honjo T, Habu S. Origin of immune diversity: generation and selection. *Annu Rev Biochem* 1985;54:803–830.
22. Cook GP, Tomlinson IM. The human immunoglobulin repertoire. *Immunol Today* 1995;16:37–42.
23. Jaenichen HR, Pech M, Lindenmaier W, Weldgruber N, Zachau HG. Composite human Vk genes and a model of their evolution. *Nucleic Acids Res* 1984;12:5249–5263.
24. Klobeck HG, Meindl A, Combriato F, Solomon A, Zachau HG. Human immunoglobulin kappa light chain genes of subgroups II and III. *Nucleic Acids Res* 1985;13:6499–6514.

25. Klobeck HC, Bornkamm GW, Combriato G, Mocikat R, Pohlenz HD, Zachau HG. Subgroup IV of human immunoglobulin κ light chains is encoded by a single germline gene. *Nucleic Acids Res* 1985;13: 6515–6530.

26. Meindl A, Klobeck HC, Ohnheiser R, Zachau HG. The V kappa gene repertoire in the human germ line. *Eur J Immunol* 1990;20:1855–1863.

27. Schable KF, Zachau HG. The variable genes of the human immunoglobulin kappa locus. *Biol Chem* 1993;374:1001–1022.

28. Chuchana P, Blaucher A, Brockly F, Alexandre D, LeFranc G, LeFranc M. Definition of the human immunoglobulin variable lambda (IGLV) gene subgroup. *Eur J Immunol* 1990;20:1317–1325.

29. Solomon A, Weiss DT. Serologically defined V region subgroups of human lambda light chains. *J Immunol* 1987;139:824–830.

30. Lai E, Wilson RK, Hood LE. Physical maps of the mouse and the human immunoglobulin-like loci. *Adv Immunol* 1989;46:1–59.

31. Chang L-Y, Yen C-P, Besl L, Schell M, Solomon A. Identification and characterization of a functional human Ig V lambda germline gene. *Mol Immunol* 1994;31:531–536.

32. Frippiat JP, LeFranc MP. Genomic organization of 34 kb of the human immunoglobulin lambda locus (IGLV): restriction map and sequences of new V lambda III genes. *Mol Immunol* 1994;31:657–670.

33. Vasicek J, Leder P. Structure and expression of the human immuno-globulin λ genes. *J Exp Med* 1990;172:609–620.

34. Tsujimoto Y, Croce CM. Molecular cloning of human immunoglobu-lin λ chain variable sequence. *Nucleic Acids Res* 1984;12:8407–8414.

35. Abbas AK, Lichtman AH, Pober JS. *Cellular and molecular immunol-ogy*. Philadelphia: WB Saunders, 1994:66–94.

36. Gavalchin J, Nicklas JA, Eastcott JW, et al. Lupus prone (SWR × NZB) F1 mice produce potentially nephritogenic autoantibodies inherited from the normal SWR parent. *J Immunol* 1985;134: 885–894.

37. Yang PM, Olsen NJ, Siminovitch KA, et al. Possible deletion of a developmentally regulated heavy-chain variable region gene in autoimmune diseases. *Proc Natl Acad Sci U S A* 1990;87:7907–7911.

38. Diamond B, Katz JB, Paul E, Aranow C, Lustgarten D, Scharff MD. The role of somatic mutation in the pathogenic anti-DNA response. *Annu Rev Immunol* 1992;10:731–757.

39. Ray S, Putterman C, Diamond B. Pathogenic autoantibodies are rou-tinely generated during the response to foreign antigen: a paradigm for autoimmune disease. *Proc Natl Acad Sci U S A* 1996;93:2019–2024.

40. Limanasithikul W, Ray S, Diamond B. Cross reactive antibodies have both protective and pathogenic potential. *J Immunol* 1995;155: 967–973.

41. Behar SM, Scharff MD. Somatic diversification of the S107 (T15) VH11 germ-line gene that encodes the heavy chain variable region of antibodies to double-stranded DNA in (NZB × NZW) F1 mice. *Proc Natl Acad Sci U S A* 1988;85:3970–3974.

42. Davidson A, Manheimer-Lory A, Aranow C, Peterson R, Hannigan N, Diamond B. Molecular characterization of a somatically mutated anti-DNA antibody bearing the systemic lupus erythematosus-related idio-types. *J Clin Invest* 1990;85:1401–1409.

43. Manheimer-Lory A, Katz JB, Pillinger M, Ghossein C, Smith A, Dia-mond B. Molecular characteristics of antibodies bearing an anti-DNA-associated idiotype. *J Exp Med* 1991;174:1639–1652.

44. Meek KD, Hasemann CA, Capra JD. Novel rearrangements at the immunoglobulin D locus: inversions and fusions add to IgH somatic diversity. *J Exp Med* 1989;170:39–57.

45. DeMaison C, Chastagner P, Theze J, Zouali M. Somatic diversifica-tion in the heavy chain variable region genes expressed by human autoantibodies bearing a lupus-associated nephritogenic anti-DNA idiotype. *Proc Natl Acad Sci U S A* 1994;91:514–518.

46. Zouali M. The structure of human lupus anti-DNA antibodies. *Meth-ods* 1997;11:27–35.

47. Pascual C, Victor K, Randen I, et al. Nucleotide sequence analysis of rheumatoid factors and polyreactive antibodies derived from patients with rheumatoid arthritis reveals diverse use of VH and VL gene seg-ments and extensive variability in CDR-3. *Scand J Immunol* 1992;36: 349–362.

48. Radic MZ, Weigart M. Genetic and structural evidence for antigen selec-tion of anti-DNA antibodies. *Annu Rev Immunol* 1994;12:487–520.

49. Shlomchik M, Mascelli M, Shan H, Radic MZ, Pisetsky D, Marshak-Rithstein A, Weigart M. Anti-DNA antibodies from autoimmune mice arise by clonal expansion and somatic mutation. *J Exp Med* 1990; 171:265–297.

50. Behar SM, Corbet S, Diamond B, Scharff MD. The molecular origin of anti-DNA antibodies. *Int Rev Immunol* 1989;5:23–42.

51. Marion TN, Tillman DM, Jou N-T, Hill RJ. Selection of immunoglob-ulin variable regions in autoimmunity to DNA. *Immunol Rev* 1992;128:123–149.

52. Spatz L, Iliev A, Saenko V, et al. Studies on the structure, regulation and pathogenic potential of anti-DNA antibodies. *Methods* 1997;11: 70–78.

53. Manheimer-Lory A, Zandman-Goddard G, Davidson A, Aranow C, Diamond B. Lupus-specific antibodies reveal an altered pattern of somatic mutation. *J Clin Invest* 1997;100:2538–2546.

54. Radic MZ, Zouali M. Receptor editing, immune diversification, and self tolerance. *Immunity* 1996;5:505–511.

55. Rothstein T. Signals and susceptibility to programmed death in B cells. *Curr Opin Immunol* 1996;8:362–371.

56. Goodnow CC. Transgenic mice and analysis of B cell tolerance. *Annu Rev Immunol* 1992;10:489.

57. MacLennan IC. Autoimmunity: deletion of autoreactive B cells. *Curr Biol* 1995;5:103–106.

58. Radic M, Ericson J, Litwin S, Weigart M. B lymphocytes may escape tolerance by revising their antigen receptor. *J Exp Med* 1993;177: 1165.

59. Goodnow CC, Crosbie T, Adelstein S, et al. Altered immunoglobulin expression and functional silencing of self reactive B lymphocytes in transgenic mice. *Nature* 1988;334:676.

60. Tiegs S, Russell D, Nemazee D. Receptor editing in self reactive bone marrow B cells. *J Exp Med* 1993;177:1009.

61. Kuo P, Michael T, Tadmor B, Diamond B. Generation and regulation of B cell autoreactivity arising in the periphery. In: Gupta S, Cohen J, eds. *Mechanisms of lymphocyte activation and immune regulation,* VI ed. New York: Plenum Press, 1996;167–176.

62. Burrows PD, Cooper MD. B cell development and differentiation. *Curr Opin Immunol* 1997;9:239–244.

63. Abbas AK, Lichtman AH, Pober JS. *Cellular and molecular immunol-ogy*. Philadelphia: WB Saunders, 1994;199–200.

64. Kelsoe G. *In situ* studies of the germinal center reaction. *Adv Immunol* 1995;60:267–288.

65. Goodnow CC, Cyster JG, Hartley SB, et al. Self tolerance checkpoints in B lymphocyte development. *Adv Immunol* 1995;59:279–367.

66. Ray S, Diamond B. Generation of a novel fusion partner to sample the repertoire of splenic B cells destined for apoptosis. *Proc Natl Acad Sci U S A* 1994;91:5548–5551.

67. Casson LP, Manser T. Random mutagenesis of two complementarity determining region amino acids yields an unexpectedly high fre-quency of antibodies with increased affinity for both cognate antigen and autoantigen. *J Exp Med* 1995;182:743–751.

68. Suzuki N, Sakane T, Engleman EG. Anti-DNA antibody production by CD5+ and CD5− B cells of patients with SLE. *J Clin Invest* 1990;85: 238–247.

69. Kasaian MT, Casali P. Autoimmunity-prone B-1 (CD B cells, natural antibodies and self recognition. *Autoimmunity* 1993;15:315–329.

70. Hayakawa K, Hardy RR, Honda M, Herzenberg LA, Steinberg AD. Ly-1 B cells: functionally distinct lymphocytes that secrete IgM anti-bodies. *Proc Natl Acad Sci U S A* 1984;81:2494–2498.

71. Coutinho A, Kazatchkine MD, Avrameas S. Natural autoantibodies. *Curr Opin Immunol* 1995;7:812–818.

72. Mouthon L, Nobrega A, Nicolas N, et al. Invariance and restriction toward a limited set of self-antigens characterize neonatal IgM anti-body repertoires and prevail in autoreactive repertoires of healthy adults. *Proc Natl Acad Sci U S A* 1995;92:3839–3843.

73. Mouthon L, Haury M, Lacroix-Desmazes S, Barreau C, Coutinho A, Kazatchkine MD. Analysis of the normal human IgG antibody reper-toire: evidence that IgG autoantibodies of healthy adults recognize a limited and conserved set of protein antigens in homologous tissues. *J Immunol* 1995;154:5769–5778.

74. Ando K, Kikugawa K, Beppu M. Involvement of sialylated poly-*N*-acetyllactosaminyl sugar chains of band 3 glycoprotein on senescent erythrocytes in anti-band 3 autoantibody binding. *J Biol Chem* 1994; 269:19394–19398.

75. Schlesinger JS, Horwitz MA. A role for natural antibody in the patho-genesis of leprosy: antibody in nonimmune serum mediates C3 fixa-tion to the *Mycobacterium leprae* surface and hence phagocytosis by human mononuclear phagocytes. *Infect Immun* 1994;62:280–289.

76. Gruppi A, Pistoresi-Palencia MC, Ordonez P, Cerban F, Vottero-Cima

E. Enhancement of natural antibodies in mice immunized with exoantigens of pI 4.5 from *Trypanosoma cruzi*. *Immunol Lett* 1994; 42:151–159.

77. Lacroix-Desmazes S, Mouthon L, Coutinho A, Kazatchkine MD. Analysis of the natural human IgG repertoire: life long stability of reactivities towards self antigens contrasts with age dependent diversification of reactivities against bacterial antigens. *Eur J Immunol* 1995;25:2598–2604.

78. Holmberg D, Coutinho A. Natural antibodies and autoimmunity. *Immunol Today* 1985;6:356–357.

79. Huetz F, Jacquemart F, Pena-Rossi C, Varela F, Coutinho A. Autoimmunity: the moving boundaries between physiology and pathology. *J Autoimmun* 1988;1:507–518.

80. Avrameas S. Natural autoantibodies: from "horror autotoxicus" to "gnothi seauton." *Immunol Today* 1991;12:154–159.

81. Potter KN, Li Y, Pascual V, et al. Molecular characterization of a cross-reactive idiotope on human immunoglobulins utilizing the VH4-21 gene segment. *J Exp Med* 1993;178:1419–1428.

82. Pascual V, Victor K, Spellerberg M, Hamblin TJ, Stevenson FK, Capra JD. VH restriction among human cold agglutinins: the VH4-21 gene segment is required to encode anti-I and anti-i specificities. *J Immunol* 1992;149:2337–2344.

83. Kraj P, Friedman DF, Stevenson F, Silberstein LE. Evidence for the overexpression of the VH4-34 (VH4.21) Ig gene segment in the normal adult human peripheral blood B cell repertoire. *J Immunol* 1995;154:6406–6420.

84. Abbas AK, Lichtman AH, Pober JS. *Cellular and molecular immunology*. Philadelphia: WB Saunders, 1994:401–404.

85. Kelly PT, Haponik EF. Goodpasture syndrome: molecular and clinical advances. *Medicine (Baltimore)* 1994;73:171–185.

86. Naparstek Y, Plotz H. The role of autoantibodies in autoimmune disease. *Annu Rev Immunol* 1993;11:79–104.

87. Salvi M, Fukazawa H, Bernard N, Hiromatsu Y, How J, Wall JR. Role of autoantibodies in the pathogenesis and association of endocrine autoimmune disorders. *Endocrinol Rev* 1988;9:450–466.

88. Burman KD, Baker JR Jr. Immune mechanisms in Graves disease. *Endocrinol Rev* 1985;6:183–232.

89. Taylor SI, Barbetti F, Accili D, Roth J, Gorden P. Syndromes of autoimmunity and hypoglycemia: autoantibodies directed against insulin and its receptor. *Endocrinol Metab Clin North Am* 1989;18: 123–143.

90. Tzartos SJ, Barkas T, Cung MT, et al. The main immunogenic region of the acetylcholine receptor: structure and role in myasthenia gravis. *Autoimmunity* 1991;8:259–270.

91. Schonbeck S, Chrestel S, Hohlfeld R. Myasthenia gravis: prototype of the antireceptor autoimmune diseases. *Int Rev Neurobiol* 1990;32: 175–200.

92. Asherson RA. A primary antiphospholipid syndrome. *J Rheumatol* 1988;15:1742–1746.

93. Harris EN, Chan JK, Asherson RA, Aber VR, Gharavi AE, Hughes GRV. Thrombosis, recurrent fetal loss, and thrombocytopenia: predictive value of the anti-cardiolipin antibody test. *Arch Intern Med* 1986; 146:2153–2156.

94. Alarcon-Segovia D, Deleze M, Oria CV, et al. Antiphosphlipid antibodies and the antiphospholipid syndrome in systemic lupus erythematosus: a prospective analysis of 500 consecutive patients. *Medicine (Baltimore)* 1989;68:353–365.

95. McNeil HP, Simpson RJ, Chesterman CN, Krilis SA. Anti-phospholipid antibodies are directed against a complex antigen that includes a lipid-binding inhibitor of coagulation: beta 2-glycoprotein I (apolipoprotein H). *Proc Natl Acad Sci U S A* 1990;87:4120–4124.

96. Blank M, Cohen J, Toder V, Shoenfeld Y. Induction of anti-phospholipid syndrome in naive mice with mouse lupus monoclonal and polyclonal anti-cardiolipin antibodies. *Proc Natl Acad Sci U S A* 1991;88: 3069–3073.

97. Gharavi AE, Wilson WA. Antiphospholipid antibodies. In: Wallace DJ, Hahn BH, eds. *Dubois lupus erythematosus*, 5th ed. Baltimore: Williams & Wilkins, 1997:471–491.

98. Lockshin MD. Pathogenesis of the antiphospholipid antibody syndrome. *Lupus* 1996;5:404–408.

99. Berbard P, Prost C, Aucouturier P, Durepaire N, Denis F, Bonnetblanc JM. The subclass distribution of IgG autoantibodies: in cicatricial pemphigoid and epidermolysis bullosa acquisita. *J Invest Dermatol* 1991;97:259–263.

100. Kim YH, Geoghegan WD, Jordan RE. Pemphigus immunoglobulin G subclass autoantibodies: studies of reactivity with cultured human keratinocytes. *J Lab Clin Med* 1990;115:324–331.

101. Rock B, Martins CR, Theofilopoulos AN, et al. The pathogenic effect of IgG4 autoantibodies in endemic pemphigus foliaceus (fogo selvagem). *N Engl J Med* 1989;320:1463–1469.

102. Jones JC, Arnn J, Staehelin LA, Goldman RD. Human autoantibodies against desmosomes: possible causative factors in pemphigus. *Proc Natl Acad Sci U S A* 1984;81:2781–2785.

103. Ewert BH, Jennette JC, Falk RJ. The pathogenic role of anti-neutrophil cytoplasmic autoantibodies. *Am J Kidney Dis* 1991;18: 188–195.

104. Malkiel S, Kuan A, Diamond B. Autoimmunity in heart disease: mechanisms and genetic susceptibility. *Mol Med Today* 1996;8: 336–342.

105. Neumann DA, Burek CL, Baughman KL, Rose NR, Herskowitz A. Circulating heart-reactive antibodies in patients with myocarditis or cardiomyopathy. *J Am Coll Cardiol* 1990;16:839–846.

106. Lauer B, Padberg K, Schultheiss HP, Strauere BE. Autoantibodies against human ventricular myosin in sera of patients with acute and chronic myocarditis. *J Am Coll Cardiol* 1994;23:146–153.

107. Kuhl U, Melzner B, Schafer B, Schultheiss HP, Strauer BE. The Ca^{2+}-channel as cardiac autoantigen. *Eur Heart J* 1991;12[Suppl D]: 99–104.

108. Wallukat G, Morwinski M, Kowal K, Forster A, Boewer V, Wollerberger A. Autoantibodies against the β adrenergic receptor in human myocarditis and dilated cardiomyopathy: β adrenergic agonism without desensitization. *Eur Heart J* 1991;112[Suppl D]:178–181.

109. Schultheiss HP. The significance of autoantibodies against the ADP/ATP carrier for the pathogenesis of myocarditis and dilated cardiomyopathy-clinical and experimental data. *Springer Semin Immunopathol* 1989;11:15–30.

110. Beisel KW, Traystman MD. Autoimmune myocarditis: a murine model. *Immunol Ser* 1990;52:267–293.

111. Neu N, Beisel KW, Traystman MD, Rose NR, Craig SW. Autoantibodies specific for the cardiac myosin isoform are found in mice susceptible to coxsackievirus B₃-induced myocarditis. *J Immunol* 1987; 138:2488–2492.

112. Alvarez FL, Neu N, Rose NR, Craig SW, Beisel KW. Heart-specific autoantibodies induced by coxsackievirus B₃: identification of heart autoantigens. *Clin Immunol Immunopathol* 1987;43:129–139.

113. Lefvert AK, Pirskanen R, Svanborg E. Anti-idiotypic antibodies acetylcholine receptor antibodies and disturbed neuromuscular function in healthy relatives to patients with myasthenia gravis. *J Neuroimmunol* 1985;9:41–53.

114. von Herrath MG, Oldstone MBA. Virus-induced autoimmune disease. *Curr Opin Immunol* 1996;8:878–885.

115. Kaufman DL, Erlander MG, Clare-Salzler M, Atkinson MA, Maclaren NK, Tobin AJ. Autoimmunity in two forms of glutamate decarboxylase in insulin-dependent diabetes mellitus. *J Clin Invest* 1992;89:283–292.

116. Baekkeskov S, Nielson JH, Marner B, Bilde T, Ludvigsson J, Lernmark A. Autoantibodies in newly diagnosed diabetic children immunoprecipitate human pancreatic islet cell proteins. *Nature* 1982; 298:167–169.

117. Cunningham MW, McCormack JM, Fenderson PG, Ho MK, Beachey EH, Dale JB. Human and murine antibodies cross-reactive with streptococcal M protein and myosin recognize the sequence GLN-LYS-SER-LYS-GLN in M protein. *J Immunol* 1989;143:2677–2683.

118. Dell A, Antone SM, Gauntt CJ, Crossley CA, Clark WA, Cunningham MW. Autoimmune determinants of rheumatic carditis: localization of epitopes in human cardiac myosin. *Eur Heart J* 1991;12[Suppl D]: 158–162.

119. Quinn A, Adderson EE, Shackelford PG, Carroll WL, Cunningham MW. Autoantibody germ-line gene segment encodes VH and VL regions of a human anti-streptococcal monoclonal antibody recognizing streptococcal M protein and human cardiac myosin epitopes. *J Immunol* 1995;154:4203–4212.

120. Albani S, Keystone E, Nelson J, et al. Positive selection in autoimmunity: abnormal immune responses to a bacterial DNA J antigenic determinant in patients with early RA. *Nat Med* 1995;1:448–452.

121. Tuckova L, Tlaskalova M, Farre K, et al. Molecular mimicry as a possible cause of autoimmune reactions in celiac disease? *Clin Immunol Immunopathol* 1995;74:170–176.

122. Baum H, Davies H, Peakman M. Molecular mimicry in the MHC: hidden clues to autoimmunity? *Immunol Today* 1996;17:64–71.

123. Sorbel RA. The pathology of multiple sclerosis. *J Virol* 1995;13:1–21.

124. Kuo P, Kowal C, Tadmor B, Diamond B. Microbial antigens can elicit autoantibody production: a potential pathway to autoimmune disease. *Ann N Y Acad Sci* 1997;815:230–236.

125. Putterman C, Limpanisithikul W, Diamond B. The double-edged sword of the immune response: mutational analysis of a murine anti-pneumococcal, anti-DNA antibody. *J Clin Invest* 1996;97:2251–2259.

126. Paul E, Diamond B. Characterization of two human anti-DNA antibodies bearing the pathogenic idiotype 8.12. *Autoimmunity* 1993;16:13–21.

127. Vanderlugt C, Miller SD. Epitope spreading. *Curr Opin Immunol* 1996;8:831–836.

128. James JA, Gross T, Scofield RH, Harley JB. Immunoglobulin epitope spreading and autoimmune disease after peptide immunization: Sm B/B′-derived PPPGMRPP and PPPGIRGP induce spliceosome autoimmunity. *J Exp Med* 1995;181:453–461.

129. Topfer F, Gordon T, McCluskey J. Intra- and intermolecular spreading of autoimmunity involving the nuclear self-antigens La (SS-B) and Ro (SS-A). *Proc Natl Acad Sci U S A* 1995;92:875–879.

130. Rekvig OP, Fredriksen K, Hokland K, et al. Molecular analyses of anti-DNA antibodies induced by polyomavirus BK in BALB/C mice. *Scand J Immunol* 1995;41:593–603.

131. Moens U, Eternes OM, Hey AW, et al. *In vivo* expression of a single viral DNA-binding protein generates systemic lupus erythematosus-related autoimmunity to double-stranded DNA and histones. *Proc Natl Acad Sci U S A* 1995;92:12393–12397.

132. Kalden J, Marion TN. Environmental and other stimuli for DNA antibody production. *Lupus* 1997;6:324–329.

133. Casciola-Rosen LA, Anhalt G, Rosen A. Autoantigens targeted in systemic lupus erythematosus are clustered in two populations of surface structures on apoptotic keratinocytes. *J Exp Med* 1994;179:1317–1330.

134. Golan TD, Elkon KB, Gharavi AE, Krueger JG. Enhanced membrane binding of autoantibodies to cultured keratinocytes of systemic lupus erythematosus patients after ultraviolet B/ultraviolet A irradiation. *J Clin Invest* 1992;90:1067–1076.

135. Goodglick L, Zevit N, Neshat M, Braun J. Mapping the Ig superantigen-binding site of HIV-1 gp120. *J Immunol* 1995;155:5151–5159.

136. Goodglick L, Braun J. Revenge of the microbes: superantigens of the T and B cell lineage. *Am J Pathol* 1994;144:623–636.

137. Silverman GJ. Superantigens and the spectrum of unconventional B-cell antigens. *The Immunologist* 1994;2:57–64.

138. Sasso EH, Silverman GJ, Mannik M. Human IgA and IgG F(ab′)₂ that bind to staphylococcal protein A belong to the VHIII subgroup. *J Immunol* 1991;47:1877–1883.

139. Potter KN, Li Y, Capra JD. Staphylococcal protein A simultaneously interacts with framework region 1, complementarity-determined region 2, and framework region 3 on human VH3-encoded Igs. *J Immunol* 1996;157:2982–2988.

140. Hillson JL, Karr NS, Oppliger IR, Mannik M, Sasso EH. The structural basis of germline-encoded VH3 immunoglobulin binding to staphylococcal protein A. *J Exp Med* 1993;178:331–336.

141. Randen I, Potter KN, Li Y, et al. Complementarity-determining region 2 is implicated in the binding of staphylococcal protein A to human immunoglobulin VHIII variable regions. *Eur J Immunol* 1993;23:2682–2686.

142. Berberian L, Goodglick L, Kipps TJ, Braun J. Immunoglobulin VH3 gene products: natural ligands for HIV gp120. *Science* 1993;261:1588–1591.

143. Townsley-Fuchs J, Kam L, Fairhurst R, et al. Human immunodeficiency virus-1 (HIV-1) gp120 superantigen-binding serum antibodies. *J Clin Invest* 1996;98;1794–1801.

144. Karray S, Zouali M. Identification of the B cell superantigen-binding site of HIV-1 gp120. *Proc Natl Acad Sci U S A* 1997;94:1356–1360.

145. Shoenfeld Y. Idiotypic induction of autoimmunity: a new aspect of the idiotypic network. *FASEB J* 1994;8:1296–1301.

146. Shoenfeld Y, George J. Induction of autoimmunity: a role for the idiotypic network. *Ann N Y Acad Sci* 1997;815:342–349.

147. Bakimer R, Fishman P, Blank M, Sredni B, Djaldetti M, Shoenfeld Y. Induction of primary antiphospholipid syndrome in mice by immunization with a human monoclonal anti-cardiolipin antibody (H-3). *J Clin Invest* 1992;89:1558–1663.

148. Blank M, Tincani A, Shoenfeld Y. Induction of experimental anti-phospholipid syndrome in naive mice with purified IgG anti-phosphatidylserine antibodies. *J Rheumatol* 1994;21:100–104.

149. Blank M, Tomer Y, Stein M, Kapolovic J, Wiik A, Meroni PL. Immunization with anti-neutrophil cytoplasmic antibody (ANCA) induces the production of mouse ANCA and perivascular lymphocyte infiltration. *Clin Exp Immunol* 1995;102:120–130.

150. Tomer Y, Gilburd B, Blank M, et al. Characterization of biologically active antineutrophil cytoplasmic antibodies induced in mice: pathogenic role in experimental vasculitis. *Arthritis Rheum* 1995;38:1375–1381.

151. Lange H, Solterbeck M, Berek C, Lemke H. Correlation between immune maturation and idiotypic network recognition. *Eur J Immunol* 1996;26:2234–2242.

152. Pawlak L, Hart D, Nisonoff A. Requirements for prolonged suppression of an idiotypic specificity in adult mice. *J Exp Med* 1973;137:1442–1448.

153. Hahn BH, Ebling FM. Suppression of murine lupus nephritis by administration of an anti-idiotypic antibody to anti-DNA. *J Immunol* 1984;132:187–190.

154. Hahn BH, Ebling FM, Panosian-Sahakian N, et al. Idiotype selection is an immunoregulatory mechanism which contributes to the pathogenesis of systemic lupus erythematosus. *J Autoimmunity* 1989;1:673–681.

155. Tsao BP, Cantor RM, Kalunian KC, et al. Evidence for linkage of a candidate chromosome 1 region to human systemic lupus erythematosus. *J Clin Invest* 1997;99:725–731.

156. Theofilopoulos AN. The basis of autoimmunity: part II. Genetic predisposition. *Immunol Today* 1995;15:150–158.

157. Kono DH, Burlingame DH, Owens D, et al. Lupus susceptibility loci in New Zealand mice. *Proc Natl Acad Sci U S A* 1994;91:10168–10172.

158. Drake CG, Rozzo SJ, Hirschfeld HF, Smarnworawong NP, Palmer E, Kotzin BL. Analysis of the New Zealand Black contribution to lupus-like renal disease: multiple genes that operate in a threshold manner. *J Immunol* 1995;154:2441–2447.

159. Morel L, Rudofsky UH, Longmate JA, Schiffenbauer J, Wakeland EK. Polygenic control of susceptibility to murine SLE. *Immunity* 1994:1:219–229.

160. Mohan C, Alas E, Morel L, Yang P, Wakeland EK. Genetic dissection of SLE pathogenesis: Sle1 on murine chromosome 1 leads to loss of tolerance to H2A/H2B/DNA subnucleosomes (abstract). *Arthritis Rheum* 1996;39:S216.

161. Morel L, Yu Y, Blenman KR, Caldwell RA, Wakeland EK. Production of congenic mouse strains carrying genomic intervals containing SLE-susceptibility genes derived from the SLE prone NZM2410 strain. *Mamm Genome* 1996;7:335–339.

162. Morel L, Mohan C, Yu Y, et al. Functional dissection of systemic lupus erythematosus using congenic mouse strains. *J Immunol* 1997;158:6019–6028.

163. Kono DH, Theofliopoulos AN. The genetics of murine systemic lupus erythematosus. In: Wallace DJ, Hahn BH, eds. *Dubois lupus erythematosus,* 5th ed. Baltimore: Williams & Wilkins, 1997:119–132.

164. Bowness P, Davies KA, Norsworthy PJ, et al. Hereditary C1q deficiency and systemic lupus erythematosus. *Q J Med* 1994;87:455–464.

165. Verthelyi D, Ahmed SA. 17β-Estradiol, but not 5α-dihydrotestosterone, augments antibodies to double-stranded deoxyribonucleic acid in nonautoimmune C57BL/6J mice. *Endocrinology* 1994;135:2615–2622.

166. Adam L, Crepin M, Israel L. Tumor growth inhibition, apoptosis, and bcl-2 down regulation of MCF-7 ras tumors by sodium phenylacetate and tamoxifen combination. *Cancer Res* 1997;57:1023–1029.

167. Spyridopoulos I, Sullivan AB, Kearney M, Isner JM, Losordo DW. Estrogen-receptor-mediated inhibition of human endothelial cell apoptosis: estradiol as a survival factor. *Circulation* 1997;95:1505–1514.

Inflammation: Basic Principles and Clinical Correlates,
3rd ed., edited by John I. Gallin and Ralph Snyderman.
Lippincott Williams & Wilkins, Philadelphia © 1999.

CHAPTER 60

Pemphigus and Pemphigoid:

Autoantibody-Mediated Dermatoses

Hossein C. Nousari, Gerald S. Lazarus, and Grant J. Anhalt

The subject of autoimmune blistering skin diseases has been an area of intense investigation in the field of dermatology. There has been rapid advancement in the understanding of these diseases, and significant insights have been gained into the precise molecular mechanisms of tissue injury induced by binding of autoantibodies in the skin. Although there are many immunologic subgroups of intraepidermal and subepidermal autoimmune blistering diseases, the most compelling data has arisen from the study of pemphigus and bullous pemphigoid (BP). Although autoantibody binding in both diseases activates many inflammatory events, it is now realized that in pemphigus, the binding of the autoantibody to a cell adhesion molecule can be sufficient to cause the end point of tissue injury, loss of cellular adhesion, and epidermal blistering. Other inflammatory events occur but are of secondary importance. By contrast, in BP, it appears that binding of antibody alone is insufficient to cause blistering, and a sequence of additional inflammatory events must occur to cause subepidermal blistering and loss of epidermal adhesion. These two well characterized and contrasting disorders are discussed herein.

H. C. Nousari and G. J. Anhalt: Division of Dermatoimmunology, Department of Dermatology, Johns Hopkins University School of Medicine, Baltimore, Maryland 21205.

G. S. Lazarus: Department of Dermatology, University of California Davis, School of Medicine, Davis, California 95616.

PEMPHIGUS

Clinical, Histologic, and Ultrastructural Characteristics of Pemphigus Lesions

The term *pemphigus* refers to several distinct autoimmune dermatoses that share the characteristic of loss of epidermal cell-cell adhesion. The disruption in cell-cell adhesion is manifested clinically by blistering of stratified squamous epithelia (1). Frequently, even clinically normal-appearing skin adjacent to a lesion can be induced to blister by the application of gentle pressure (Nikolsky's sign) (2), indicating that epidermal cohesion can be abnormal in clinically unblistered skin (2). Autoantibodies directed against molecules of the epithelial cell surface (3) are pathogenic in all forms of pemphigus; they induce the precise clinical features of the disease *in vivo* and reproduce the histologic, immunofluorescent, and ultrastructural features both *in vitro* and *in vivo* (Table 60-1) (4).

There are three major forms of pemphigus that have distinctive clinical, histologic, and immunologic features. They are pemphigus vulgaris (PV), pemphigus foliaceus (PF), and paraneoplastic pemphigus (PNP). PF is divided into four subtypes, which have identical features but arise in unique circumstances. They are idiopathic (nonendemic) PF, drug-induced PF, pemphigus erythematosus, and a form that is endemic to regions of Brazil and Colombia, called *fogo selvagem* or endemic PF. Immunoglobulin A (IgA) pemphigus is a blistering disease that has been arbitrarily included within the pemphigus foliaceus spectrum.

PV is the most common form of pemphigus in North America, Europe, and the Middle East. Men and women are equally affected, and the disease occurs most often

TABLE 60-1. *Autoantigens in cutaneous bullous diseases[a]*

Disease	Antigen	Location/function of antigen
Pemphigus vulgaris	130-kd desmoglein-3	Stratified squamous epithelia/cell-cell adhesion
Pemphigus foliaceus	160-kd desmoglein-1	Stratified squamous epithelia/cell-cell adhesion
Paraneoplastic pemphigus	250- and 210-kd desmoplakins/ envoplakin, 230-kd bullous pemphigoid antigen, 190-kd antigen, 170-kd antigen	All epithelia/cell-cell and cell-matrix adhesion
Immunoglobulin A pemphigus	Desmocollin-1	Stratified epithelia/cell-cell adhesion
Bullous pemphigoid	230-kd antigen/BP-230/BPAG-1 (50–70%), 180-kd antigen/ BP-180/ BPAG-2(30–50%)	Stratified squamous epithelial hemidesmosome/cell-substrate adhesion, interacts with integrins and laminins
Herpes gestationis (gestational pemphigoid)	180-kd bullous pemphigoid antigen (90%), 230-kd bullous pemphigoid antigen (10%)	Same as bullous pemphigoid
Cicatricial pemphigoid	BP-180, laminin-5, laminin-6, others	Stratified squamous epithelia

[a]This table summarizes what is currently known of the antigens recognized by autoantibodies in cutaneous bullous diseases. In some cases, the function of the antigen is presumed or only partially proven. In all the listed diseases, demonstration of the presence of the specific autoantibody in the affected tissue is necessary to confirm the diagnosis.

during the fourth or fifth decade of life. All races are affected by the disease, but there are differences in incidence among populations, depending on the relative frequency of human leukocyte antigen (HLA) genes that confer susceptibility to the disease. There is a high frequency of disease among Ashkenazi Jews (Jews of eastern European origin) that is strongly linked to a rare subtype of the HLA class II gene DR4, known as DRB1*0402. In non-Ashkenazi Jews, Caucasians, and Japanese, the disease is linked to a rare subtype of DQ1, known as DQB1*0503. PV lesions usually develop first in the oral mucosa and subsequently affect upper trunk, head and neck, and intertriginous areas, especially the axillae and groin. Lesions are restricted to stratified squamous epithelia, and internal organs are not affected. Small, flaccid bullae that break easily give rise to large, denuded areas that may expand around their periphery without further formation of distinct bullae. In the absence of oral lesions, the diagnosis of PV becomes suspect. Erosions can become secondarily infected, and they require specific therapy for healing.

Before the development of oral corticosteroids in the 1950s, the disease had a 50% mortality after 2 years and almost 100% mortality at 5 years. The therapeutic goal in PV is the reduction of the synthesis of antibodies, and this most often is accomplished with the use of systemic corticosteroids alone or in conjunction with other immunosuppressive drugs.

In PV, cellular dysadhesion affects all layers of the epidermis, and the blister forms just above the least differentiated, lowest layer of basal epidermal cells. Microscopic examination of an early lesion reveals loss of adhesion of the apposed plasma membranes of adjacent epidermal cells between the focal adhesion organelles— the desmosomes (5,6). Subsequently, the desmosomes also detach, and the keratin intermediate filaments retract from their insertion into the desmosomal plaque at the

cell periphery and aggregate around the nucleus. At this point, the cells assume a rounded morphology, without cell-cell contact, recognizable at the light microscopic level as *acantholysis* (7). Despite the loss of cell-cell adhesion, the basal epithelial cells remain tightly attached to the basement membrane of the dermis, even when all cell-cell contact at the apical and lateral faces of the cells is lost. This distinctive histologic pattern has been compared to a "row of tombstones" (8). Infiltration of blisters with inflammatory cells is variable; often lesions are devoid of inflammatory cells, but early lesions may be rich in eosinophils (9).

By contrast, in PF, the intraepidermal split is high in the plane of the epidermis, involving only the more differentiated cells that comprise the granular cell layer. Acantholytic cells are present only on the floor and roof of the blister. Unlike PV, mucosal lesions in PF are rare, even though direct immunofluorescence shows that autoantibodies are bound to the oral mucosa *in vivo*. Cutaneous bullae are small, flaccid, and fragile and produce shallow erosions. Erythema, scaling, and crusting lesions are frequently present. PF is less lethal than PV, probably because of the superficial nature of the lesions and the lack of mucosal involvement.

In the pemphigus erythematosus variant (10), the features of PF coexist with clinical and immunologic features of lupus erythematosus. Brazilian pemphigus (endemic PF) is histopathologically and immunologically identical to PF (11) but is differentiated by its unique epidemiology. Its endemic occurrence in certain rural areas of South America (12) suggests that an arthropod vector may play a role in transmission of the disease, but direct proof is lacking. Drugs can also induce pemphigus; the majority of cases are identical to PF, but there are some patients in whom the disease resembles PV. The drugs that induce pemphigus are most often drugs with highly reactive sulfhydryl groups, such as D-penicillamine and captopril (13). These drugs can directly induce acantholysis *in vitro* in the absence of autoantibody (14), or, more commonly, they may initiate autoantibody-mediated disease *in vivo* that persists even after withdrawal of the implicated drug (15).

IgA pemphigus, also known as "intercellular IgA bullous dermatosis," is a cutaneous blistering condition that clinically and histologically resembles PF or subcorneal pustular dermatosis (Sneddon-Wilkinson syndrome). An association with paraproteinemia has been reported. The classification of IgA pemphigus in the PF spectrum remains controversial (16).

PNP is a variant about which less is known (17). To date, all patients have had an accompanying known or occult neoplasm. Most associated neoplasms are non-Hodgkin's lymphoma, chronic lymphocytic leukemia, thymomas, Waldeström's macroglobulinemia, Castleman's disease, and spindle cell sarcoma. Patients present with painful oral erosions that prove refractory to standard therapies and a polymorphous cutaneous eruption characterized by episodes of blistering and healing. The mucosal and cutaneous blisters show a characteristic combination of suprabasilar acantholysis, similar to that observed in PV, and keratinocyte necrosis, which may resemble erythema multiforme or a lichenoid inflammatory eruption. All patients have tissue-bound and circulating autoantibodies that bind to all epithelia *in vitro* and share a common and unique immunologic specificity. The mortality rate in cases of PNP associated with a malignant neoplasm approaches 100%. Survival of PNP occurs only in those cases associated with a benign neoplasm (e.g., thymoma, localized Castleman's disease). In such cases, complete surgical excision of the tumor carries a good prognosis in terms of reduction or elimination of the autoimmune disease. Cyclosporine in combination with systemic corticosteroids can provide some palliation of symptoms in cases associated with lymphoma or chronic lymphocytic leukemia. Other immunosuppressive or antiinflammatory drugs have little effect on the disease. Respiratory involvement, with acantholytic lesions of respiratory epithelium, has been reported as a fatal complication in PNP (18,19).

Pemphigus Autoantibodies Are Specific for Desmosomal Proteins

In all cases and all forms of idiopathic and endemic pemphigus, autoantibodies of the IgG isotype are bound *in vivo* in a characteristic pattern around the plasma membranes of affected epithelia (20,21). These antibodies are also detected in the serum (22). Each major form of pemphigus is characterized by distinct and specific autoantibodies that are directed against normal epithelial structural proteins. In PV and PF, the desmosomal antigens are expressed only in stratified squamous epithelia

(23). In PNP, the relevant antigens are found in all epithelia (24,25).

The glycoprotein recognized by PV autoantibodies is most reliably detected by immunoprecipitation of nonionic detergent extracts of metabolically labeled keratinocytes (26). The epitopes recognized by PV autoantibodies are largely conformational and are best detected by immunoprecipitation in nondenaturing conditions, as opposed to Western immunoblotting. Immunoprecipitation and cDNA cloning have shown that all PV sera immunoprecipitate a 130-kd glycoprotein, called *desmoglein-3*, also known as *PV antigen* (27). Desmoglein-3 is a desmosomal transmembrane protein that belongs to the larger family of proteins known as epithelial cadherins (*ca*lcium-*d*ependent ad*herins* proteins) (28). Desmosomal cadherins are represented by desmogleins and desmocollins (29). Desmogleins are distinguished from other epithelial cadherins by the presence of extended carboxy-terminal repeats, which are not present in other, simpler cadherins. Desmoglein-3 is located in desmosomes of the cells of the lower, less differentiated layers of the epidermis (30,31). All desmosomal cadherins are encoded on chromosome 18q12 (32). The intracellular domain of desmoglein-3 interacts directly and indirectly with desmosomal plaque proteins such as plakoglobin, desmoplakins, and envoplakin (33–36). The extracellular domains (ectodomains) of desmoglein-3 mediate adhesion by homophilic interactions with apposing desmosomal cadherins and also possess the conformational immunogenic and pathogenic epitopes of PV (37–39).

PF sera specifically recognize a 160-kd transmembrane glycoprotein, called *desmoglein-1*, which is a member of the desmosomal cadherins (40,41). Desmoglein-1, like desmoglein-3, is complexed in normal epidermis with plakoglobin and other desmosomal plaque proteins (42). Desmoglein-1 is located predominantly in upper epidermal desmosomes (43).

Desmocollins are closely related desmosomal cadherins that play a crucial role in initiating desmosome assembly. A subset of IgA pemphigus patients have circulating autoantibodies directed against desmocollin-1 (44). The pathogenic role of these antibodies has not yet been confirmed. In typical cases of PV and PF, IgG autoantibodies do not react with desmocolins.

In PNP, the humoral immune response is more complex and less well defined. Sera from patients with PNP immunoprecipitate a complex of epithelial antigens consisting of desmoplakin-1, a plaque protein common to desmosomes of all epithelia (28,29,45); desmoplakin-2, a product of alternative splicing of the desmoplakin-1 transcript; envoplakin, a desmosomal plaque protein (46); the 230-kd BP antigen, a plaque protein of hemidesmosomes (47); and at least two other antigens (a 190-kd and a 170-kd antigen) that are not yet characterized. The autoantibodies of PNP are most distinctive because they bind to the cell surfaces of all epithelia, not just stratified squamous epithelia. The implications of autoantibodies with such a broad specificity are not yet clear (48), but passive transfer of these human autoantibodies into mice reproduces characteristic acantholytic lesions in the skin and esophagus.

Pathogenicity of Pemphigus Autoantibodies

There is compelling evidence that the autoantibodies found in pemphigus patients' sera are pathogenic. Once laboratory and sampling errors are excluded, all patients have circulating and tissue-bound IgG, the levels of the circulating antibody correlate well with disease activity, and the antibodies are pathogenic by passive transfer. Pemphigus is one of the few human autoimmune diseases in which all the features of the disease can be reproduced *in vivo* in an experimental animal solely by passive transfer of human autoantibody.

The first observations that established the pathogenicity of the autoantibodies arose from *in vitro* studies in which fragments of normal human skin (which can be maintained in explant culture for approximately 2 days) were exposed to human antibody. Early experiments showed that the addition of pemphigus serum (49) or purified pemphigus IgG fractions (50) to such organ cultures led to the development of acantholytic changes that mimicked the histologic changes characteristic of pemphigus lesions (51). In explant culture, the location of the intraepidermal split was suprabasilar when PV IgG was added (52,53) and more superficial when PF IgG was employed, thus histologically and ultrastructurally mimicking the pattern observed in patients' lesions (54). The immunoglobulin fraction of human pemphigus serum was responsible for the development of the epidermal dysadhesion; it was not necessary to add a complement source to the culture medium for acantholysis to occur, and complement components were not detected in the skin explants.

Finally, development of an animal model provided unambiguous evidence for the pathogenicity of pemphigus autoantibodies. Neonatal mice, when injected parenterally with PV IgG (10 ng per gram of body weight per day), developed pemphigus-like lesions within 18 to 72 hours of the injection (55). Discrete vesicles, extensive sloughing of the epidermis, and a positive Nikolsky sign were noted. Immunofluorescence revealed binding of IgG to lesional and perilesional epidermis. Histologically, suprabasilar intraepidermal lesions were observed that precisely resembled human cutaneous lesions. Dramatic widening of the intercellular spaces was not noted at the ultrastructural level. Both noninflammatory and inflammatory lesions (containing many polymorphonuclear leukocytes [PMNs]) were observed, frequently at the same time and in the same animal.

Acantholytic lesions have also been induced in neonatal mice by injection of IgG from patients with Brazilian PF (at a dose of 40 mg per gram of body weight) (56). In contrast to the results observed with PV IgG, intraepidermal clefts developed only in the more differentiated granular cell layer of the epidermis, precisely replicating the distinctive changes of human PF. Widening of the intercellular spaces between desmosomes was the first ultrastructural change detected; this was followed by separation and then disappearance of desmosomes. The lower layers of epidermis did not show any alterations (57). Therefore, injection of neonatal mice with large doses of pemphigus IgG led to cutaneous alterations that clinically, histologically, and ultrastructurally resembled the human disease.

Early attempts at biochemical purification of the PV antigen to better define the molecular pathogenesis were intriguing but sometimes equivocal (58). Once the gene encoding desmoglein-3 was cloned, more persuasive data were obtained. Bacterial fusion proteins encoding the ectodomain of desmoglein-3 were produced, and it was found that epitopes in the distal amino-terminus of the molecule (extracellular domains EC 1–2) were more antigenic and pathogenic than those located in the more proximal portion of the molecule (EC 3–5) (59). However, it became apparent that many pathogenic epitopes were not represented in the recombinant bacterial fusion protein, because these recombinant proteins failed to completely remove the pathogenic activity of PV antibodies absorbed against these fusion proteins. An explanation for this phenomenon may be the inability of bacterial expression systems to reproduce the proper conformation of the desmoglein-3 ectodomains or even the possible absence of pathogenic epitopes in these encoded fusion proteins.

To circumvent the limitations of the bacterial expression system, Amagai et al. (60) designed a baculovirus system that produced a secreted form of the PV antigen as a chimeric molecule containing the entire ectodomain of desmoglein-3 linked to the constant region of the heavy chain of IgG1. This hybrid baculovirus fusion protein, called PVIg, was shown to contain pathogenically relevant epitopes. For example, the reactivity of PV antibodies against keratinocyte cell surfaces, as well as the titers of circulating PV antibodies, decreased significantly after preincubation of PV serum with PVIg baculovirus protein. Finally, similar preincubation of PV IgG with the baculovirus protein eliminated the ability of the human autoantibody fraction to induce blisters in the neonatal mouse model. Further, it was shown that these pathogenic epitopes of PVIg are calcium-dependent and glycosylation-independent conformational motifs.

There is evidence that these PV antigen fusion proteins may be useful in examining the initiation and propagation of the immune response against the autoantigen. One study showed that epitopes in the ectodomain of the PV antigen bacterial fusion protein selectively stimulate

HLA DR–bearing CD4-positive T cells in PV patients. This stimulation was HLA class II specific, and it was not observed on presentation to T cells bearing HLA DQ or DP. On stimulation by PVIg, the CD4$^+$ T cells secreted cytokines with a T_H2 profile—that is, they preferentially secreted IL-4, IL-6, and IL-10 (61). These findings could have relevance in the understanding of cellular immune abnormalities involved in the production of pathogenic IgG antibodies in PV patients.

Genetically engineered mice with a targeted disruption of the desmoglein-3 gene have been produced (62). These mice have apparently normal skin at birth but develop significant runting and hair thinning compared with littermates. This runting is caused by the presence of extensive intraoral acantholytic lesions, present from birth, that interfere with normal nutritional intake. Histologic examination of oral lesions show changes typical of PV, and by indirect immunofluorescence examination there is no detectable expression of desmoglein-3 in skin or oral mucosa. Cutaneous lesions do not develop in these desmoglein-3 knock-out mice, except on the muzzle, paws, and other limited areas that are subjected to repeated mechanical trauma.

Studies of the immunodominant epitopes of the PF antigen using bacterial fusion proteins have provided significant data. Immunogenic epitopes have been identified both in the amino-terminus of the desmoglein-1 molecule (EC 1–2) and in the more proximal EC 4–5 domains of the extracellular portion of the molecule. Studies using the baculovirus fusion protein system in PF have also shown that the immunogenic and pathogenic epitopes of desmoglein-1 are also calcium-dependent conformational motifs (63,64). Preincubation of PF sera with PF fusion proteins eliminated the pathogenic activity of the sera, prevented gross blister formation, and eliminated the ability of the IgG to induce typical immunohistologic findings in the neonatal mouse model. Elution of the PF antibodies from a PF antigen fusion protein column demonstrated that the purified autoantibodies are pathogenic, because they were able to induce gross blister formation and typical immunohistologic findings of PF *in vivo* in mice. These experiments clearly confirmed the pathogenicity of PF antibodies.

Passive transfer studies in PNP have demonstrated that IgG autoantibodies in PNP sera are pathogenic. Passive transfer of whole IgG fractions from patients into neonatal mice resulted in acantholytic blistering of skin and esophageal mucosa, but studies using antibodies against individual PNP antigens have not yet been performed.

Proposed Mechanisms of Acantholysis: Complement Activation and Its Relation to Cellular Dysadhesion

As noted, pemphigus autoantibodies are pathogenic and directly causative in the disease. There has, however, been considerable debate about the importance of other inflammatory events that occur after autoantibody binding to the epithelial cell surface. It was proposed that antibody binding to the pemphigus antigen or antigens alone could cause cellular detachment, but this hypothesis was greeted with some skepticism, because there is usually significant redundancy of cell adhesion molecules in any epithelial tissue, and antibodies against a single adhesion molecule are unlikely to cause detachment without other contributing factors or events. For this reason, the role of complement activation in the development of pemphigus lesions was examined, and the results of these studies have been somewhat controversial.

It seems clear that there is involvement of the complement cascade after autoantibody binding in the epidermis *in vivo*. In human biopsies, complement deposition is observed in acantholytic lesions (65,66). There is little detectable complement deposition in lesions from patients undergoing corticosteroid therapy (67,68). In biopsies taken from normal-appearing skin adjacent to pemphigus lesions, IgG deposits were present, but complement components (C1q, C3, and C3 proactivator) could not be detected. Total hemolytic complement was reduced in pemphigus blister fluids, compared with sera from the same patients or with other types of blister fluids (69). Cryoproteins are observed in sera of pemphigus patients with clinically active disease; these abnormal complexes contain pemphigus IgG and complement components C3 and C4 (70). It has been postulated that complement activation may be responsible for the influx of inflammatory cells that occurs in developing lesions. In the presence of complement, pemphigus antibodies were shown to mediate attachment of PMNs to epidermis *in vitro* (71). Furthermore, a proteinase obtained from human epidermis was shown to induce PMN chemotaxis via a complement-mediated mechanism (72). The presence of activated infiltrating cells in the epidermis and dermis of acantholytic lesions may lead to further cutaneous damage.

In Vitro Studies

Although some early studies questioned the role of complement fixation in acantholysis (73), several groups have now clearly shown that pemphigus IgG can indeed fix complement (74–76). Pemphigus sera fix complement components C1q, C4, and C3 to epidermis *in vitro*, suggesting activation of the classic pathway of complement after immune complex formation between pemphigus antibodies and epidermal antigens. In addition, purified pemphigus IgG fixed complement components C1q, C3, and C4 in murine epidermal cell monolayer cultures and human skin organ cultures.

Murine epidermal cells in culture bound pemphigus antibody at their cell surfaces, and the antibody induced detachment of the epidermal cells from their culture plates (77,78). The pemphigus antibody–induced detachment was blocked by addition of a serine protease inhibitor, soybean trypsin inhibitor, or a general proteinase inhibitor (α_2-macroglobulin). Control experiments demonstrated that complement was not required for detachment of living cells and that the binding of pemphigus IgG to the cell surface was not decreased by soybean trypsin inhibitor. These experiments demonstrated that pemphigus IgG can induce dysadhesion in tissue culture, and they suggest that a proteolytic enzyme, specifically of the serine protease family, may mediate the effect.

This view is supported by data obtained from explant culture experiments (79,80). Enhanced proteolytic enzyme activity was observed in the conditioned medium of normal human explant cultures that were incubated with pemphigus IgG. Furthermore, the conditioned medium was able to induce acantholysis in fresh explants, even when totally depleted of remaining IgG (79). Pepstatin A, an inhibitor of carboxyl-type proteases, and high concentrations of soybean trypsin inhibitor, an inhibitor of serine-type proteases, were able to prevent pemphigus IgG–induced acantholysis in organ culture. These reagents did not block binding of pemphigus IgG to the epidermal cells (79).

In Vivo Studies

Whereas *in vitro* studies show that there is activation of complement by tissue-bound autoantibodies, there is also compelling evidence that IgG binding to the cell adhesion molecules alone can cause impairment of adhesion sufficient to cause acantholysis without activation of the complement cascade. By manipulation of the *in vivo* model for PV, the following data were obtained. In the first group of experiments, neonatal mice were depleted of functional complement by pretreatment with cobra venom factor and then given intraperitoneal injections of human PV IgG in varying doses (81). In the absence of a functional complement system, human PV antibodies could induce the characteristic epidermal lesions. However, a slightly higher threshold of antibody dose was required to precipitate clinical lesions compared with that in animals that had not been depleted of complement. In a second group of experiments, bivalent Fab1 fragments of pemphigus IgG were purified and similarly were readily able to induce lesions *in vivo* without detectable complement activation within the epidermis (82).

In PF, the evidence that antibody alone can induce acantholysis is even more striking. For example, in endemic PF, the major autoantibody activity is found in the IgG4 subclass (83), which is a class of immunoglobulin that is thought to be functionally monovalent and incapable of activating complement (84,85). The IgG4 fraction of patients with PF was separated from other immunoglobulin subclasses and passively transferred into neonatal mice, inducing characteristic acantholytic

lesions (83). Monovalent Fab' fragments of the IgG4 autoantibodies were produced, and these also were capable of inducing lesions *in vivo*. There was no detectable complement activation in the lesions of animals treated with either the intact IgG4 or the monovalent Fab1 fragments. This suggests that antibodies binding to the cadherin protein (desmoglein-1) induce blister formation *in vivo*.

In summary, complement activation does occur *in vivo* after binding of pemphigus IgG to the epithelial cell surface, and this may augment acantholysis; however, if enough autoantibody attaches to the cell surface, the cells lose their adhesion in the absence of any activation of the complement system.

Plasminogen Activator Involvement in Acantholysis

Early experiments suggested that pemphigus autoantibody might function by activation of proteinase activity (77–79,86). The general hypothesis suggested that localized increases in activity or concentration of a proteinase leads to cleavage of cell-cell adhesion molecules and hence to a fragile and disrupted epidermis.

The concept that pemphigus IgG may exert its pathogenicity through one or more proteolytic enzymes, without the involvement of complement, represents a rather unconventional mode of action for an antibody. However, studies have suggested a hypothesis that accommodates both the clear pathogenic role of pemphigus antibody and the involvement of a proteinase in pemphigus. The addition of pemphigus IgG to human epidermal cells in culture induced increased activity of the proteinase plasminogen activator (PA), both in the conditioned medium and in the cell lysate (87). Addition of cycloheximide, at concentrations that blocked protein synthesis by 80%, prevented the pemphigus IgG–induced PA activation, suggesting that the antibody induced synthesis of the PA. The induction of PA by pemphigus IgG was rather specific: neither the lysosomal enzyme cathepsin D nor general protein synthesis was enhanced by addition of pemphigus antibody to epidermal cells.

The mechanisms by which pemphigus IgG increases PA in epidermal cells is unclear, but the enzyme induction is not limited to pemphigus antibody or to epidermis. Cell-surface antibodies directed against kidney cells (88) and against melanoma cells were also shown to induce enhanced PA activity on binding to their target tissues.

PA is a serine-type proteinase that converts the inactive proenzyme plasminogen into the broad-specificity protease plasmin through cleavage of a single peptide bond (89,90). Because of the high circulating levels of plasminogen and the nonselectivity of plasmin action, the PA-plasmin system represents a supply of proteolytic activity that is available and adaptable to a wide range of physiologic and pathologic functions. Historically, the PA-plasmin system has been most extensively studied for its role in fibrinolysis. However, more recent work has demonstrated the rather ubiquitous nature of the enzyme system and suggested many diverse areas of its involvement (91).

There are two types of PAs that are products of different genes (92–96); immunologically, they are not cross-reactive (97–99). The tissue-type PA (t-PA) plays a critical role in fibrinolysis (100,101) and hence in maintenance of plasma fluidity. This function is reflected by the biochemical finding that t-PA binds to fibrin (95) and is fully active in the presence of fibrin (102–104). It is likely that t-PA has physiologic roles other than fibrinolysis; other studies have shown that t-PA is made by a number of cell types (72,80), including melanoma cells in culture (95), granulosa cells (105), oocytes (106), and endothelial cells (107).

Urokinase-type PAs (u-PAs) have a very wide distribution and appear to initiate localized extracellular proteolysis for diverse physiologic and pathologic functions, including mammary gland involution (108), blastocyst implantation (109), ovulation (110,111), macrophage migration (112), and metastasis (113). In each of these cases, localized extracellular proteolysis is required during tissue degradation and remodeling or migration. A complex regulation system for urokinase yields active enzyme in the appropriate tissue at the required time for each physiologic function. Regulation of urokinase occurs at many levels: synthesis is hormonally controlled, inactive proenzyme must be converted to active enzyme by proteolytic cleavage, inhibitors of several types are present in serum and tissues, and the cell-surface urokinase receptor must be synthesized. The proteinase u-PA is made by a great many cell types, and some cells appear to make both u-PA and t-PA (114–117).

The components of the PA-plasmin system are present in human skin. Human epidermal cells in culture, under both control and pemphigus IgG–stimulated conditions, synthesized u-PA (118,119). Keratinocytes also synthesized the u-PA receptor (120). In extracts of normal epidermis, most of the PA activity was the urokinase type (121). Plasminogen is immunocytochemically detectable in the epidermis, with the highest concentration in the basal layers (122). Inhibitors of PA are found in conditioned media of keratinocyte cultures (123,124) and in low-salt extracts of normal human epidermis (125). The highest level of PA is associated with the more differentiated epidermal cells (126). It appears that t-PA is present preferentially in the differentiated cells. Compatible with this localization is evidence to implicate a role for plasmin in the nuclear dissolution that occurs during terminal differentiation of epidermal cells (127). In addition, urokinase was immunocytochemically detected in migrating epidermal cells, suggesting a role for the enzyme in the migration of keratinocytes that occurs in the early stages of cutaneous wound healing (128). Chen et al. (129), using biochemical and molecular probes in cocultures of human and human dermis at air-fluid inter-faces, demonstrated that explants mimic human skin. Both t-PA and plasminogen activator inhibitor-2 (PAI-2) are synthesized in more differentiated epidermis, whereas urokinase and PAI-1 are produced in more basal epithelium.

The hypothesis that links PA with acantholysis in pemphigus is that binding of pemphigus IgG to the surfaces of epidermal cells leads to increased PA; enhanced PA produces localized increases in epidermal plasmin levels; and plasmin cleaves one or more cell-cell adhesion molecules, producing a fragile epidermis that is easily induced to blister (130). In testing this hypothesis, experiments in skin explant culture have been informative. As described earlier, an inhibitor of serine proteases, soybean trypsin inhibitor, was able to prevent pemphigus IgG–induced acantholysis in organ culture. Because soybean trypsin inhibitor blocks many serine proteinases, this finding did not conclusively demonstrate that the PA-plasmin system was involved in acantholysis. An inhibitor that is specific for urokinase (i.e., that does not affect other proteinases) is provided by antiserum made against purified urokinase. Addition of purified antiurokinase IgG along with pemphigus IgG to explant cultures prevented the development of acantholysis. Because of the specificity of the antiurokinase IgG, this experiment provided strong evidence for the involvement of PA in pemphigus acantholysis *in vitro*.

Addition of exogenous plasminogen to explant culture was not generally required for pemphigus IgG–induced acantholysis; however, addition of plasminogen dramatically decreased the time of onset and increased the extent of acantholytic damage (130). The endogenous stores of plasminogen present in skin may be sufficient to support acantholysis in the absence of additional exogenous plasminogen. High concentrations (200 to 300 mg/mL) of plasminogen alone, in the absence of any pemphigus IgG, were able to induce foliaceus-like acantholysis in explant culture (130). Nonetheless, clinical administration of pharmacologic levels of t-PAs to humans has not resulted in blistering disease.

In a study of PV lesions (131), urokinase and urokinase receptor were found to be displayed on the surface of acantholytic cells in four of ten cases. Plasminogen was found in all ten patients, but no t-PA was detected. These data may imply that urokinase activation on the cell surface occurs as an early biologic event in acantholysis. The lack of detection of t-PA may be related to insufficient quantities of extravasted serum, which is capable of inducing synthesis of t-PA.

Studies using the neonatal mouse model of pemphigus do not demonstrate increased synthesis of PA *in vivo* by enzymologic or molecular biologic methods (Teikemeier 1988 *unpublished data*). It may be that localized activation of the PA-plasmin system is important in the early development of the pathologic changes that are characteristic of PV and PF.

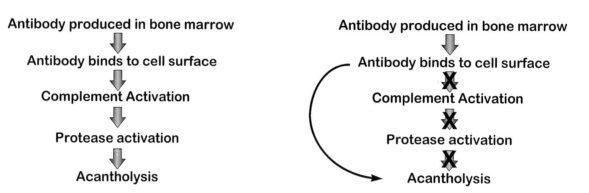

FIG. 60-1. In pemphigus, a series of events occurs after autoantibody binding to the extracellular domain of the desmoglein molecule (**A**). In experimental pemphigus *in vivo* in neonatal mice receiving passively transferred human pemphigus IgG, inhibition or ablation of any of these events does not prevent the autoantibody from producing cellular detachment (**B**). In this setting, binding of the autoantibody alone can downregulate the function of this key epidermal adhesion molecule, resulting in intraepidermal blistering (acantholysis). This may help explain why true remissions of the human disease are seen only when there is concomitant reduction in serum autoantibody levels.

Conclusion

Pemphigus is an autoimmune dermatosis in which pathogenic autoantibodies directed against desmosomal adhesion molecules can induce cutaneous lesions independent of mediators of inflammation such as complement or infiltrating cells. *In vitro* and *in vivo* experiments, as well as clinical and histologic observations, support the primary role of autoantibody in this disease, and inhibition of inflammatory events does not abolish the ability of pemphigus IgG to produce cellular dysadhesion *in vivo* (Fig. 60-1). The events that occur in the human disease are certainly more complex, and there is considerable evidence for the participation of numerous inflammatory events in the net tissue injury that occurs *in vivo*.

In epidermal cell culture, pemphigus antibody is able to induce release and activation of PA, which converts plasminogen into the broad-specificity proteinase, plasmin. Experiments in skin explant cultures provide strong evidence that PA, through plasmin, mediates the interepidermal cell dysadhesion that is characteristic of pemphigus lesions. The role of PA in pemphigus *in vivo* is under active investigation. Complement components and inflammatory cells are generally present in pemphigus lesions, especially at their earliest stages, and therefore are likely to play a role in exacerbation of the cutaneous damage.

PEMPHIGOID

BP is an acquired, blistering disease of the elderly. It is characterized histologically by subepidermal bullae and immunopathologically by *in vivo* deposition of autoantibodies and complement components along the epidermal basement membrane zone (BMZ). The majority (50% to 70%) of these patients also have detectable circulating autoantibodies directed against the BMZ of stratified squamous epithelium. Because of these observations, it was originally hypothesized that BP is an autoimmune disease in which the cutaneous lesions are a consequence of the anti-BMZ antibodies. This hypothesis has now been proved convincingly, and the molecular mechanisms of the blistering injury have been evaluated in detail.

Lever (132), in 1953, was the first to recognize that BP was a distinct bullous disease by its clinical and histologic features. He chose to call the disease *pemphigoid* because it was clinically similar to PV but histologically lacked acantholysis. In 1967, Jordon et al. (133) described the typical immunohistologic characteristics of BP, which are considered essential criteria for establishing the diagnosis. BP is considered part of the pemphigoid spectrum of diseases, which also includes herpes gestationis (HG) and cicatricial pemphigoid (CP). These diseases share clinical, histologic, and immunopathologic similarities, but their exact relations to one another remain to be determined.

The most characteristic clinical feature of BP is the presence of large, tense bullae, which can arise either on an erythematous base or on normal skin. Although the distribution is usually widespread, sites of predilection include the lower abdomen, inner thighs, groin, axillae, and flexural aspects of the arms and legs (134). Unlike PV and PNP, mucosal lesions in BP are uncommon, and when they do occur they are often transient. They usually are restricted to the mouth and are only rarely the presenting feature (135–137).

HG, or gestational pemphigoid, has some similarities with and some differences from BP. The major similarity is the presence of a mixture of urticarial and bullous lesions, and although there is more pronounced basal cell necrosis in HG, the immunochemical, immunopathologic, and clinical characteristics closely resemble those of BP (138). The unique feature of gestational pemphigoid is that it arises during pregnancy and usually remits after delivery but typically reemerges with subsequent pregnancies or on challenge with oral estrogens. The most characteristic immunologic feature of the disease is the presence of an avidly complement-fixing IgG autoantibody in the serum, originally called the "herpes gestationis factor" (139–141); this HG factor has been shown to be an autoantibody that reacts against the 180-kd BP antigen (142). It can now be reasonably assumed that HG is merely BP that occurs during pregnancy, so the term *gestational pemphigoid* is appropriate. The challenge in understanding this disorder is to determine how the pregnant state predisposes to this autoimmune phenomenon.

Finally, CP also shares similarities with BP while having some distinct differences. Whereas BP is a disorder in which lesions form predominantly or exclusively on cornified skin, in CP the lesions occur almost exclusively on mucosal stratified squamous epithelia (143), and skin involvement is often transient and trivial. In contrast to BP, mucosal lesions heal with pronounced scarring and fibrosis, and this also distinguishes CP from BP. Severe morbidity can result from ocular scarring (144). CP is characterized by subepidermal blisters and deposition of IgG and complement components along the BMZ of affected epithelia. Circulating autoantibodies are rarely detected, and they are usually present in very low titers in this disorder (145,146). This fact has delayed considerably efforts to define the disorder on an immunochemical basis (147). Until such studies can be concluded, the relation between CP and BP will remain unresolved.

BP is an autoimmune disease mediated by autoantibodies directed against an antigen or antigens in the BMZ of stratified squamous epithelia. Supportive evidence includes the presence of circulating anti-BMZ antibodies, deposition of these antibodies at the site of clinical lesion formation, association with other autoimmune diseases (148), and *in vitro* (149) and *in vivo* (148) models using BP antibody to reproduce features of the spontaneously occurring disease.

Immunopathogenesis of Bullous Pemphigoid

The BP antigens are a normal constituent of the BMZ of stratified squamous epithelia and are found in the epidermis of all vertebrates (151). Studies have shown that most of the BP antigen is found within the basilar pole of the keratinocyte, with a smaller amount in the lamina lucida immediately beneath the hemidesmosome (152). It is established that BP autoantibodies recognize more than one hemidesmosomal protein. The most frequently detected antigens are a 230-kd antigen (approximately 50% to 70% of cases), called BP-230 or BPAG1, and a 180-kd antigen (30% to 50% of cases), called BP-180 or BPAG2.

BPAG1 is a hemidesmosomal protein that is encoded in the human chromosomal locus 6p11-12 (153). BPAG1 is a plaque protein of the hemidesmosome; it is located entirely within the cytoplasm of the keratinocyte and has approximately 60% structural homology with desmoplakin-1, the major plaque protein of the epidermal desmosome. BPAG2 is a transmembrane glycoprotein of the hemidesmosome and has a very interesting structure. It has an unusual type II orientation; that is, the amino-terminal domain localizes to the intracellular hemidesmosomal plaque, while the carboxyl-terminal domain is extracellular. The extracellular portion of the molecule contains multiple triple-helical collagenous domains. A noncollagenous stretch (NC16A) is present in the ectodomain adjacent to the plasma membrane. This NC16A domain is capable of forming a stable interaction with the α subunit of the $\alpha_6\beta_4$ integrin, another protein involved in cell-matrix hemidesmosomal adhesion (154). An epitope mapping study revealed that, in both BP and HG, autoantibodies preferentially recognize a common antigenic site within the NC16A domain of the BPAG2, called the *MCW1 epitope* (155,156).

Autoantibodies from patients with the clinical phenotype of CP are more heterogenous and react against antigens in different sites within the epidermal basement membrane. These autoantigens include BPAG2, laminin-5, and laminin-6. One study showed that CP autoantibodies that react with BPAG2 recognize collagenous C-terminus ectodomains that localize to the lower lamina lucida and lamina densa, a site distant from the keratinocyte plasma membrane where the MCW1 epitope is found (157). There is convincing evidence that a group of CP patients has circulating antibodies against laminin-5 (previously named epiligrin, kalinin, nicein, or BM600) and laminin-6 (previously named k-laminin) (158–160). Laminin-5 is a protein that anchors epidermal cells to the lower basement membrane by linking $\alpha_3\beta_1$ and $\alpha_6\beta_4$ integrins and forming a complex with laminin-6. Laminin-5 is the major component of the lamina lucida and is composed of disulfide-linked α, β, and γ subunits. Some patients with anti–laminin-5 CP have circulating pathogenic antibodies against the α unit of laminin-5 and also against laminin-6 as a cotarget antigen (161).

Pathogenicity

It is now convincingly established that BP autoantibodies are pathogenic. These data are derived from extensive *in vitro* and *in vivo* studies.

Gammon et al. (162) described an *in vitro* model for BP, referred to as a leukocyte attachment assay, which has been useful for evaluating the functional properties of BP antibodies and their interactions with complement and inflammatory cells. With this assay, normal human skin is first treated with BP sera, then incubated with fresh normal human serum as a source of complement and viable leukocytes. When complement-binding BP antibodies are used, leukocytes migrate toward and attach to the BMZ. The attached leukocytes are apparently activated and, with prolonged incubation, dermal-epidermal separation, similar to that observed in early lesions of BP, occurs. Leukocyte migration and attachment depend on the presence of complement-fixing BP antibodies, complement, and viable leukocytes (163). Using direct methods, in which biopsies from BP patients are similarly incubated with complement and leukocytes, it has been shown that there is leukocyte attachment, and the degree of chemoattraction is greater in biopsies from lesional as opposed to perilesional skin (164). This functional assay suggests that immune complexes in lesional skin from BP patients have greater complement-activating capacity than do those from adjacent normal skin. This model provides functional evidence that BP antigen-antibody complexes can activate complement, produce chemotactic activity, and recruit activated leukocytes to the BMZ, and it suggests that all three events play a role in mediating the inflammatory events in BP.

Definitive evidence that BP antibodies are pathogenic has been obtained by *in vivo* passive transfer studies, although the initial studies were not entirely convincing. For example, Anhalt et al. (165) first demonstrated that purified IgG from BP patients injected into the corneal stroma of rabbits produced corneal inflammatory lesions, with visible epithelial blisters. Histologically, the lesions showed subepithelial blister formation with PMNs along the BMZ, and direct immunofluorescence demonstrated linear deposition of human IgG and rabbit C3 along the BMZ. The intensity of the inflammation correlated with the complement fixation titers of the IgG, supporting a role for complement in mediating BP lesion production. It was not possible to produce similar changes by intradermal injection into rabbit skin, and this was attributed to rapid washout of locally injected antibodies in skin, as opposed to the avascular cornea, where antibodies are retained for prolonged periods and can optimally bind to the hemidesmosomal antigens. Naito et al. (166) reported the development of dermal-epidermal separation and dermal inflammation in guinea pigs at the site of intradermally injected, concentrated sera and IgG fractions from BP patients. However, Gammon and Briggaman (167) were not able to reproduce these findings.

Definite evidence of the pathogenicity of BP antibodies was not demonstrated until the genes for BPAG1 and then BPAG2 were identified. Antibodies against BPAG1 were not pathogenic in any *in vivo* system tested, but anti-

bodies against BPAG2 were capable of inducing blistering *in vivo*. Simple passive transfer of human BP autoantibodies into neonatal mice, using the same techniques that were so successful in the study of pemphigus, failed to cause disease. Although BP antibodies were detectable in the blood of these mice, there was no binding of the human antibody into the hemidesmosomes of skin. Extensive studies by Diaz, Guidice, and Liu, showed that the cause of this failure was the fact that human anti–BPAG2 (anti–BP-180) autoantibodies preferentially recognized the MCW1 epitope of the ectodomain of the antigen and that in this key region the murine BP-180 was not homologous to the human antigen. To overcome this problem, Liu et al. (168) modified the traditional neonatal mouse model by first producing antibodies against the murine BP-180 NC16A domain by immunization of rabbits with a fusion protein. Then, instead of transferring human anti–BP-180 antibodies into neonatal mice, they infused polyclonal rabbit anti–murine BPAG2 antibodies. The injected mice developed subepidermal blistering disease that closely mimicked BP and HG. Histologic examination of the skin revealed findings typical of BP, with subepidermal blistering and a PMN infiltration along the BMZ and blister cavity. Direct immunofluorescence examination of these mice revealed linear deposition of rabbit IgG and murine C3 along the epidermal BMZ. This study clearly demonstrated that anti–BP-180 antibodies bind the extracellular domain of the BP-180 antigen and initiate a cascade of events, including the activation of complement, that leads to subepidermal blistering.

Activation of Complement in Pemphigoid

The models described suggest that complement is an important mediator of the inflammatory response, so it may be expected that BP antibodies are capable of fixing complement, but this is not universally true. Although essentially all tissue-bound antibodies fix complement *in vivo*, as evidenced by direct immunofluorescence, not all circulating antibodies are capable of fixing complement (169,170). Sams and Schur (171) suggested that complement-activating antibodies are primarily of the IgG3 subclass and may play the major role in lesion formation. However, Bird et al. (172), using monoclonal antibodies to the four subclasses of IgG, showed that IgG4, which is not capable of fixing complement, is the predominant subclass found both in sera and deposited in tissue of BP patients. The reason for this discrepancy is unclear, but IgG4 may have homocytotropic properties for mast cells (173) and therefore may play a role in mast cell degranulation, providing an additional mechanism for mediation of inflammation.

Several lines of evidence support a critical role for complement activation in the pathogenesis of BP. These include the frequent detection of C3 with direct immunofluorescence studies, the ability of most circulating anti-

BMZ antibodies to fix complement *in vitro*, and immu-noelectronmicroscopic studies showing C3 deposition at the site of blister formation (lamina lucida) (174). Levels of total hemolytic complement and of individual comple-ment components are reduced in blister fluid compared with sera of BP patients, suggesting local activation of the complement cascade (175). Additionally, *in vivo* and *in vitro* models for BP have in general required the pres-ence of complement-fixing antibodies or complement (or both) to produce positive results. Components of both the classic and alternative pathways—including C1q, C4, C3, C5, C5b–9, factor B, factor H, and properdin—have been detected in skin lesions and are fixed *in vitro* by serum anti-BMZ antibodies (176). These findings probably reflect activation of the classic pathway with amplifica-tion through the alternative pathway. Using a monoclonal antibody to a neoantigen on C9, Dahl et al. (177) demon-strated the presence of the membrane attack complex of complement at the BMZ in biopsies from BP patients. Detection of this complex in some lesions with a paucity of inflammatory cells suggested a direct cytopathic role for complement in the production of lesions.

The clearest confirmation of the critical role of com-plement activation for lesion development was obtained by the investigators who developed the experimental murine BP model (178). They showed that rabbit anti–murine BP-180 antibodies were effective in inducing blisters in a C5-sufficient mouse strain but failed to induce disease in a C5-deficient mouse strain. The anti-bodies also failed to induce disease in mice pretreated with cobra venom factor to deplete complement. They also demonstrated that F(ab')2 fragments generated from the anti–BP-180 IgG were not pathogenic. Minimal or absent neutrophilic infiltrates were present in the skin of mice pretreated with cobra venom and in mice transfused with F(ab')2 fragments of anti–BP-180 antibodies, despite strong antibody binding.

Evidence of the pathogenicity of the anti–basement membrane antibodies in the form of CP associated with antibodies against laminin-5 was demonstrated by Lazarova et al. (179). Human anti–laminin-5 autoanti-bodies do not bind murine epidermal basement mem-brane *in vitro* or after passive transfer to mice *in vivo*. A plausible explanation for this phenomenon could be that the antigenic epitopes in the α subunit of the human laminin-5 are dissimilar to those found in murine laminin-5. Although precise epitope comparisons were not done, the investigators used the murine BP model and passively transferred rabbit polyclonal antibodies against epitopes present on all subunits of human and murine laminin-5 into normal, C5-deficient or mast cell–deficient neonatal mice (179). The transfused nor-mal BALB/c mice developed gross mucocutaneous blis-ters and a noninflammatory subepidermal blistering; linear rabbit IgG and murine C3 deposition was observed on direct immunofluorescence examination.

C5-deficient and mast cell–deficient mice developed the same clinical and immunopathologic features as those observed in normal complementemic mice. The same group of investigators passively transferred human anti–laminin-5 IgG antibodies into mice with severe combined immunodeficiency disease grafted with human skin onto their backs (180). They were able to reproduce gross blisters only on the grafted human skin. Histologic examination showed noninflammatory subepidermal blisters only on the grafted human skin, and direct immunofluorescence examination revealed linear human IgG and murine C3 along the BMZ only on the grafted human skin.

This last experiment clearly demonstrated the patho-genic role of the anti–laminin-5 antibodies in a subset of patients with CP. In contrast to BP, complement activation does not seem to be required for lesion development in this subset of CP.

Inflammatory Cellular Events in Pemphigoid

The role of inflammatory cells in the induction of BP lesions has also been studied extensively. Wintroub et al. (181) reported the histologic abnormalities seen at various stages in the development of human BP lesions and pos-tulated a functional and morphologic role for mast cells in the production of these lesions. Histologic examination of clinically normal perilesional skin, which showed deposi-tion of C3 by direct immunofluorescence, revealed an increased number of mast cells in the papillary dermis. Biopsies from early erythematous macules showed mast cell degranulation and an inflammatory infiltrate consist-ing of mononuclear cells only. More advanced lesions demonstrated progressive hypogranularity of mast cells and an influx of eosinophils. The suggestion that mast cell degranulation induces an influx of eosinophils is sup-ported by the finding of an eosinophilic chemotactic fac-tor called *eotaxin* in BP lesions (182). Eotaxin is produced by leukocytes and keratinocytes. Epidermal expression of eotaxin is significantly increased in BP lesions, and it is upregulated by proinflammatory cytokines such as IL-1α (182). Increased levels of histamine in blister fluid further support a role for mast cell activation in the pathogenesis of BP (183). Connective tissue mast cells contain the pro-teolytic enzyme chymase within their granules (184). This enzyme cleaves the dermal-epidermal basement mem-brane at the level of the lamina lucida (185). It is reason-able to hypothesize that this enzyme could play a signifi-cant role in blister formation, especially in lesions that are poor in inflammatory cells. The blister fluid of BP lesions is rich in many other mediators of inflammation, includ-ing platelet-activating factor (186) and leukotrienes B₄ and C₄ (187).

Eosinophils are the predominant cell in the blister cav-ity of lesions in BP. Ultrastructural studies have shown that once eosinophils accumulate near the BMZ, they release their granules, which contain proteolytic enzymes and a cytotoxic agent, eosinophilic major basic protein (188). Blister fluid from lesions, when incubated with isolated guinea-pig eosinophils, produces increased density of Fc and complement receptors on the eosinophil cell membrane as well as increased helminthotoxic activity and amplified chemiluminescence in response to opsonized zymosan (189). Deposition of eosinophil-derived enzymes has been demonstrated on the epidermal basement membrane in perilesional skin and on the floor of blisters from BP patients (190), supporting the proposal that proteolytic enzymes of eosinophils play a role in the early stages of blister formation. Neutrophil elastase is one of the most important enzymes involved in the blistering mechanism of BP. Neonatal mice pretreated with α_1-antitrypsin, an elastase inhibitor, were resistant to induced cutaneous BP lesions after passive transfer of anti–BP-180 IgG (191). Therefore, elastase may play a crucial role in the pathogenesis of experimental BP. Elastase can degrade the extracellular portion of the BP-180 molecule in areas of collagenous repeats, and this is presumed to be important in the loss of basal cell adhesion.

Studies have shown a concentration of T cells with a phenotype of activated helper T cells (CD4$^+$CD25$^+$) at the periphery of bullous lesions in patients with BP (192). Local production of autoantibody may be most relevant to the pathogenesis of CP, in which lesions show dense lymphocytic infiltrates, local autoantibody production is uniformly present, and, in contrast to BP and HG, circulating autoantibodies are difficult to detect.

Proposed Hypothesis for the Immunopathologic Events in Bullous Pemphigoid

Current evidence has prompted the following hypothesis for molecular mechanisms that eventuate in subepidermal blister formation in BP (193). The initial event is presumed to be an alteration of the BP antigen that causes it to stimulate a clone of B cells/plasma cells that produce various classes of anti-BMZ antibodies, with the IgG class predominating. These autoantibodies attach to an extracellular domain of the BP-180 antigen in the lamina lucida and activate the complement cascade, which generates the anaphylatoxins C3a and C5a. Mast cells degranulate in response to the anaphylatoxins and possibly in response to IgG4; they also release eosinophilic chemotactic factor of anaphylaxis (ECF-A), neutrophilic chemotactic factor, eotaxin, histamine, and proteolytic enzymes. Eosinophils and neutrophils are recruited, both by mast cell factors and by C5a, adhere to the BMZ by virtue of their Fc and C3b receptors, and release tissue-destructive enzymes. Injury to the BMZ may be mediated by these enzymes, producing dermal-epidermal separation.

Conclusion

There is compelling evidence that all forms of pemphigoid require the presence of IgG autoantibodies against structural proteins of the BMZ of stratified squamous epithelia. In BP and gestational pemphigoid (HG), the key antigen is a transmembrane protein of the hemidesmosomes, BPAG2 (BP-180). The complex cascade of inflammatory events that occurs after autoanti-

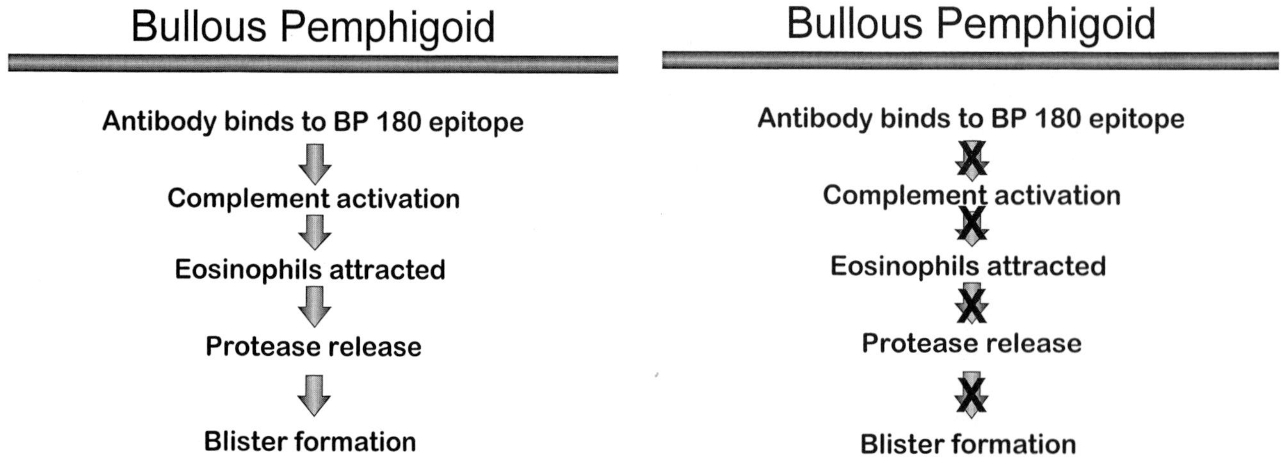

FIG. 60-2. In bullous pemphigoid, autoantibodies binding specific epitopes in the extracellular portion of the BPAG2 molecule initiate a series of inflammatory events which eventuate in subepidermal blister formation (**A**). In experimental pemphigus *in vivo*, in which neonatal mice are transfused with rabbit polyclonal antibodies against the antigen BPAG2, inhibition or ablation of any of these events inhibits blister formation completely (**B**). In contrast to pemphigus, autoantibody binding to this cellular adhesion molecule is insufficient to cause cellular detachment. In the human disease, this may help explain why pemphigoid generally responds promptly to antiinflammatory drugs such as corticosteroids and why serum antibody levels do not correlate with disease activity during treatment with these drugs.

body binding has been reasonably dissected, and the participation of mast cells, eosinophils, complement activation, and possibly other proinflammatory events is apparently required for the formation of blisters *in vivo*. In contrast to pemphigus, in which antibody binding to the relevant antigens can by itself cause the characteristic tissue injury (acantholysis), lesions in pemphigoid do not occur in the absence of a sequential series of inflammatory events (Fig. 60-2). The final key event in the pathogenesis of lesions in pemphigoid may be the degradation of the targeted antigen by proteolytic enzymes released from infiltrating PMNs.

REFERENCES

1. Lever WF. Pemphigus and pemphigoid: a review of the advances made since 1964. *J Am Acad Dermatol* 1979;1:2–31.
2. Goodman H. Nikolsky sign. *Arch Dermatol Syphilol* 1953;68: 334–335.
3. Beutner EH, Jordan RE. Demonstration of skin antibodies in sera of pemphigus vulgaris patients by indirect immunofluorescent staining. *Proc Soc Exp Biol Med* 1964;117:505–510.
4. Singer KH, Hashimoto K, Jensen PJ, Morioka S, Lazarus GS. Pathogenesis of autoimmunity in pemphigus. *Annu Rev Immunol* 1985;3: 87–108.
5. Hashimoto K, Lever WF. An electronmicroscopic study of pemphigus vulgaris of the mouth and the skin with special reference to the intercellular cement. *J Invest Dermatol* 1967;48:540–552.
6. Takahashi Y, Patel HP, Labib RS, Diaz LA, Anhalt GJ. Experimentally induced pemphigus vulgaris in neonatal BALB/c mice: a time course study of clinical, immunologic, ultrastructural and cytochemical changes. *J Invest Dermatol* 1985;84:41–46.
7. Lever WF. *Pemphigus and pemphigoid.* Springfield, IL: Charles C Thomas, 1965.
8. Director W. Pemphigus vulgaris: a clinicopathological study. *Arch Dermatol Syphilol* 1952;65:155–169.
9. Emmerson RW, Wilson-Jones E. Eosinophilic spongiosis in pemphigus. *Arch Dermatol* 1968;97:252–257.
10. Senear FE, Usher B. An unusual type of pemphigus combining features of lupus erythematosus. *Arch Dermatol Syphilol* 1926;13: 761–767.
11. Diaz LA, Sampaio SAP, Rivitti EA, et al. Endemic pemphigus foliaceous (fogo selvagem): I. Clinical features and immunopathology. *J Am Acad Dermatol* 1989;20:657–669.
12. Diaz LA, Sampaio SAP, Rivitti EA, et al. Endemic pemphigus foliaceous (fogo selvagem): II. Current and historic epidemiologic studies. *J Invest Dermatol* 1989;92:4–12.
13. Ruocco V, de Luca M, Pisana M. Pemphigus provoked by D-penicillamine: an experimental approach using *in vitro* tissue cultures. *Dermatologica* 1982;164:236–248.
14. Yokel BK, Hood AF, Anhalt GJ. Induction of acantholysis in organ explant culture by D-penicillamine and captopril. *Arch Dermatol* 1989;125:1367–1370.
15. Korman NJ, Eyre RW, Zone J, Stanley JR. Drug-induced pemphigus: autoantibodies directed against the pemphigus antigen complexes are present in penicillamine and captopril-induced pemphigus. *J Invest Dermatol* 1990;96:273–275.
16. Nousari HC, Anhalt GJ. Bullous diseases. *Curr Opin Immunol* 1995; 7:844–852.
17. Anhalt GJ, Kim SC, Stanley JR, et al. Paraneoplastic pemphigus: an autoimmune mucocutaneous disease associated with neoplasia. *N Engl J Med* 1990;323:1729–1735.
18. Fullerton SH, Woodley DT, Smoller B, Anhalt GJ. Paraneoplastic pemphigus with immune deposits in bronchial epithelium. *JAMA* 1992;267.
19. Nousari HC, Wojczak HA, Anhalt GJ. Autoantibody-mediated acantholysis of respiratory epithelium in paraneoplastic pemphigus [abstract 621]. *J Invest Dermatol* 1997;108:641.
20. Beutner EH, Jordon RE, Chorzelski TP. The immunopathology of pemphigus and bullous pemphigoid. *J Invest Dermatol* 1968;51: 64–75.
21. Jordon RE. Direct immunofluorescent studies of pemphigus and bullous pemphigoid. *Arch Dermatol* 1971;103:486–491.
22. Beutner EH, Leverm WF, Witebsky E, Jordon R, Chertock B. Autoantibodies in pemphigus vulgaris. *JAMA* 1965;192:682–688.
23. Diaz LA, Weiss HJ, Calvanico N. Phylogenetic studies with pemphigus and pemphigoid antibodies. *Acta Derm Venereol* 1979;58:537–540.
24. Franke WW, Moll R, Schiller DL, Schmid E, Kartenbeck J, Mueller H. Desmoplakins of epithelial and myocardial desmosomes are immunologically and biochemically related. *Differentiation* 1982;23:115–127.
25. Oursler JR, Ariss-Abdo L, Labib RS, O'Keefe E, Anhalt GJ. Human autoantibodies against desmoplakins in paraneoplastic pemphigus. *J Clin Invest* 1992;89:1775–1782.
26. Stanley JR, Yaar M, Hawley-Nelson P, Katz SI. Pemphigus antibodies identify a cell surface glycoprotein synthesized by human and mouse keratinocytes. *J Clin Invest* 1982;70:281–288.
27. Amagai M, Klaus KV, Stanley JR. Autoantibodies against a novel epithelial cadherin in pemphigus vulgaris, a disease of cell adhesion. *Cell* 1991;67:869–877.
28. Buxton RS, Magee AI. Structure and interactions of desmosomal and other cadherins. *Semin Cell Biol* 1992;3:157–167.
29. Amagai M. Adhesion molecules: I. Keratinocyte-keratinocyte interactions; cadherins and pemphigus. *J Invest Dermatol* 1995;104: 146–152.
30. Karpati S, Amagai M, Prussick R, Cehrs K, Stanley JR. Pemphigus vulgaris antigen, a desmoglein type of cadherin, is located within keratinocyte desmosomes. *J Cell Biol* 1993;122:409–415.
31. Amagai M, Koch PJ, Nishikawa T, Stanley JR. Pemphigus vulgaris antigen (desmoglein 3) is localized in the lower epidermis, the site of blister formation in patients. *J Invest Dermatol* 1996;106: 351–355.
32. Arnemann J, Spurr NK, Buxton RS. The human gene (DSG 3) coding for the pemphigus vulgaris antigen is, like the genes coding for the other two known desmogleins, assigned to chromosome 18. *Hum Genet* 1992;89:347–350.
33. Korman NJ, Eyre RW, Klaus-Kovtun V, Stanley JR. Demonstration of an adhering-junction molecule (plakoglobin) in the autoantigens of pemphigus foliaceous and vulgaris. *N Engl J Med* 1989;321:631–635.
34. Cowin P, Kapprell HP, Franke WW, Tamkun J, Hynes RO. Plakoglobin: a protein common to different kinds of intercellular adhering junctions. *Cell* 1986;46:1063–1073.
35. Joo-Young, Stanley JR. Plakoglobin binding by human Dsg 3 (pemphigus vulgaris antigen) in keratinocytes requires the cadherin-like intracytoplasmic segment. *J Invest Dermatol* 1995;104:720–724.
36. Troyanovsky SM, Troyanovsky RB, Eshkind LG, Krutovkikh VA, Leube RE, Franke WW. Identification of the plakoglobin-binding domain in desmoglein and its role in plaque assembly and intermediate filament anchorage. *J Cell Biol* 1994;127:151–160.
37. Lewis JE, Jensen PJ, Wheelock MJ. Cadherin function is required for human keratinocytes to assemble desmosomes and stratify in response to calcium. *J Invest Dermatol* 1994;102:870–877.
38. Amagai M, Fujimori T, Masunaga T, et al. Delayed assembly of desmosomes in keratinocytes with disrupted classic-cadherin-mediated cell adhesion by dominant negative mutant. *J Invest Dermatol* 1995;104:27–32.
39. Amagai M, Klaus KV, Udey MC, Stanley JR. The extracellular domain of pemphigus vulgaris antigen (desmoglein 3) mediates weak homophilic adhesion. *J Invest Dermatol* 1994;102:402–408.
40. Joulu L, Kusumi A, Steinberg MS, Klaus-Kovtun V, Stanley JR. Human antibodies against a desmosomal core protein in pemphigus foliaceous. *J Exp Med* 1984;160:1509–1518.
41. Stanley JR, Koulu L, Thivolet C. Distinction between epidermal antigens binding pemphigus vulgaris and pemphigus foliaceous autoantibodies. *J Clin Invest* 1984;74:313–320.
42. Mathur M, Goodwin L, Cowin P. Interaction of the cytoplasmic domain of the desmosomal cadherin dsg 1 with plakoglobin. *J Biol Chem* 1994;269:14075–14080.
43. Koch PJ, Walsh MJ, Schmelz M, Goldschmidt MD, Zimbelmann R, Franke WW. Identification of desmoglein, a constitutive desmosomal glycoprotein, as a member of the cadherin family of cell adhesion molecules. *Eur J Cell Biol* 1990;53:1–12.
44. Akiyama M, Ahshimoto T, Sugiura M, Nishikawa T. Ultrastructural localization of autoantigens of intercellular IgA vesicopustular dermatosis in cultured human squamous cell carcinoma cells. *Arch Dermatol Res* 1992;284:371–373.
45. Green KJ, Parry DAD, Steinert PM, et al. Structure of the human desmoplakin: implications for function in the desmosomal plaque. *J Biol Chem* 1990;265:2603–2612.

46. Kim SC, Young DD, Lee IJ, Chang SN, Lee TG. Envoplakin is a component of the antigen complex in paraneoplastic pemphigus [abstract 259]. *J Invest Dermatol* 1997;108:581.

47. Mutasim DF, Takahashi Y, Labib RS, Anhalt GJ, Patel HP, Diaz LA. A pool of bullous pemphigoid antigen(s) is intracellular and associated with the basal cell cytoskeleton-hemidesmosome complex. *J Invest Dermatol* 1985;84:47–53.

48. Oursler J, Ariss-Abdo L, Labib RS, O'Keefe E, Burke T, Anhalt GJ. Human autoantibodies against desmoplakins in paraneoplastic pemphigus. *J Clin Invest* 1992;89:1775–1782.

49. Bellone AG, Leone V. Richerche sull influenza esercitata da sieri di soggetti san o affetti da pemfigo su pelle umana normale e pemfigosa coltivata *in vitro*. *G Ital Dermatol Sifilol* 1956;2:97–109.

50. Schiltz JR, Michel B. Production of epidermal acantholysis in normal human skin *in vitro* by the IgG fraction from pemphigus serum. *J Invest Dermatol* 1976;67:254–260.

51. Michel B, Ko CS. An organ culture model for the study of pemphigus acantholysis. *Br J Dermatol* 1977;96:295–302.

52. Hashimoto K, Shafran KM, Webber PS, Lazarus GS, Singer KH. Anti-cell surface pemphigus autoantibody stimulates plasminogen activator inhibitor in the epidermis. *Br J Dermatol* 1983;113:523–527.

53. Morioka S, Lazarus GS, Jensen PJ. Involvement of urokinase-type plasminogen activator in acantholysis induced by pemphigus IgG. *J Invest Dermatol* 1987;89:474–477.

54. Barnett MD, Buetner EH, Chorzelski TP. Organ culture studies of pemphigus antibodies: II. Ultrastructural comparison between acantholysis changes *in vitro* and human pemphigus lesions. *J Invest Dermatol* 1977;68:265–271.

55. Anhalt GJ, Labib RS, Voorhees JJ, Beald TF, Diaz LA. Induction of pemphigus in neonatal mice by passive transfer of IgG from patients with the disease. *N Engl J Med* 1982;306:1189–1196.

56. Roscoe JT, Diaz L, Sampaio SAP, et al. Brazilian pemphigus foliaceous antibodies are pathogenic to BALB/c mice by passive transfer. *J Invest Dermatol* 1985;85:538–541.

57. Futamura S, Martins CR, Rivitti EA, Labib RS, Diaz LA, Anhalt GJ. Ultrastructural studies of acantholysis induced *in vivo* by passive transfer of IgG from endemic pemphigus foliaceus (fogo selvagem). *J Invest Dermatol* 1989;93:480–485.

58. Peterson LL, Wuepper KD. Isolation and purification of a pemphigus vulgaris antigen from human epidermis. *J Clin Invest* 1984;73:1113–1120.

59. Amagai M, Karpati S, Prussick R, Klaus KV, Stanley JR. Autoantibodies against the amino-terminal cadherin-like binding domain of pemphigus vulgaris antigen are pathogenic. *J Clin Invest* 1992;90:919–926.

60. Amagai M, Hashimoto T, Shimizu N, Nishikawa T. Absorption of pathogenic autoantibodies by extracellular domain of pemphigus vulgaris antigen (Dsg 3) produced by baculovirus. *J Clin Invest* 1994;94:59–67.

61. Lin MS, Swartz SJ, Lopez A, et al. Development and characterization of desmoglein-3 specific T cells from patients with pemphigus vulgaris. *J Clin Invest* 1997;99:31–40.

62. Koch PJ, Mahoney M, Pulkkinen L, et al. Mice with a targeted gene disruption of pemphigus vulgaris (PV) antigen (desmoglein 3, DSG3) have a phenotype similar to PV patients [abstract 41]. *J Invest Dermatol* 1997;108:544.

63. Amagai M, Hashimoto T, Green KJ, Shimizu N, Nishikawa T. Antigen-specific immunoadsorption of pathogenic autoantibodies in pemphigus foliaceus. *J Invest Dermatol* 1995;104:895–901.

64. Kowalcyk AP, Anderson JE, Borgwardt JE, Hashimoto T, Stanley JR, Green KJ. Pemphigus sera recognize conformationally sensitive epitopes in the amino-terminal region of desmoglein-1. *J Invest Dermatol* 1995;105:147–152.

65. Cormane RH, Chorzelski TP. "Bound" complement in the epidermis of patients with pemphigus vulgaris. *Dermatologica* 1967;134:463–466.

66. Van Joost TH, Cormane RH, Pondman KW. Direct immunofluorescent study of the skin on occurrence of complement in pemphigus. *Br J Dermatol* 1972;87:466–474.

67. Cram DL, Fukuyama K. Immunohistochemistry of ultraviolet-induced pemphigus and pemphigoid lesions. *Arch Dermatol* 1972;106:819–824.

68. Jordon RE, Sams WM Jr, Diaz G, Beutner EH. Negative complement immunofluorescence in pemphigus. *J Invest Dermatol* 1971;57:407–410.

69. Jordon RE, Schroeter AL, Rogers RS III, Perry HO. Classical and alternate pathway activation of complement in pemphigus vulgaris lesions. *J Invest Dermatol* 1974;63:256–259.

70. Miyagawa S, Sakamoto L. Characterization of cryoprecipitates in pemphigus: demonstration of pemphigus antibody activity in cryoprecipitates using the immunofluorescent technique. *J Invest Dermatol* 1977;69:373–375.

71. Iwatsuki K, Tagami H, Yamada M. Pemphigus antibodies mediate the development of an inflammatory change in the epidermis. *Acta Derm Venereol* 1983;63:495–500.

72. Thomas CA, Yost FJ Jr, Snyderman R, Hather VB, Lazarus GS. A cellular serine proteinase induces chemotaxis by complement activation. *Nature* 1977;269:521–522.

73. Sams WM, Schur PH. Studies of the antibodies in pemphigoid and pemphigus. *J Lab Clin Med* 1973;82:249–254.

74. Hashimoto T, Sigiura M, Kurihara S, Nishikawa T. *In vitro* complement activation by intercellular antibodies. *J Invest Dermatol* 1982;78:316–318.

75. Kawana S, Jason M, Jordon RE. Complement fixation by pemphigus antibody: I. *In vitro* fixation to organ and tissue culture skin. *J Invest Dermatol* 1984;82:506–510.

76. Nishikawa T, Kurihara S, Harrada T, Sugawara M, Hatano H. Capability of fixation of pemphigus antibodies *in vitro*. *Arch Dermatol Res* 1977;260:1–6.

77. Farb RM, Dykes R, Lazarus GS. Anti-epidermal-cell-surface pemphigus antibody detaches viable epidermal cells from culture plates by activation of proteinase. *Proc Natl Acad Sci U S A* 1978;75:459–463.

78. Schiltz JR, Michel B, Papay R. Pemphigus antibody interactions with human epidermal cells in culture: a proposed mechanism for pemphigus acantholysis. *J Clin Invest* 1978;62:778–784.

79. Morioka S, Naito K, Ogawa H. The pathogenic role of pemphigus antibodies and proteinase in epidermal acantholysis. *J Invest Dermatol* 1981;76:337–341.

80. Schiltz J, Michel B, Papay R. Appearance of "pemphigus acantholysis factor" in human skin cultured with pemphigus antibody. *J Invest Dermatol* 1979;73:575–581.

81. Anhalt GJ, Till GO, Diaz LA, Labib RS, Patel HP, Eaglstein NF. Defining the role of complement in experimental pemphigus in mice. *J Immunol* 1986;137:2835–2840.

82. Anhalt GJ, Patel HP, Labib RS, Diaz LA, Proud DA. Dexamethasone inhibits plasminogen activator activity in experimental pemphigus *in vivo* but does not block acantholysis. *J Immunol* 1986;136:113–117.

83. Rock B, Martins CR, Theofilopoulos AN, et al. The pathogenic effect of IgG4 autoantibodies in endemic pemphigus foliaceus. *N Engl J Med* 1989;320:1463–1469.

84. van der Zee JS, Alberse RC. IgG4 and hyposensitization. *N Engl Reg Allergy Proc* 1987;8:389–391.

85. Schur PH. IgG subclasses: a review. *Ann Allergy* 1987;58:89–99.

86. Singer KH, Sawka NJ, Samowitz HR, Lazarus GS. Proteinase activation: a mechanism for cellular dyshesion in pemphigus. *J Invest Dermatol* 1980;74:363–367.

87. Hashimoto K, Shafran KM, Webber PS, Lazarus GS, Singer KH. Anti-cell surface pemphigus autoantibody stimulates plasminogen activator activity of human epidermal cells: a mechanism for the loss of epidermal cohesion and blister formation. *J Exp Med* 1983;157:259–272.

88. Becker D, Ossowski L, Reich E. Induction of plasminogen activator synthesis by antibodies. *J Exp Med* 1981;154:385–396.

89. Dano J, Andreasen PA, Grondahl-Hansen J, Kristen P, Nielsen LS, Skiver L. Plasminogen activators, tissue degradation, and cancer. *Adv Cancer Res* 1985;44:139–266.

90. Reich E. Activation of plasminogen: a widespread mechanism for generating localized extracellular proteolysis. In: Ruddon RW, ed. *Biological markers of neoplasia: basic and applied aspects.* Amsterdam: Elsevier/North-Holland, 1978:491–498.

91. Salksela O. Plasminogen activation and regulation of peri-cellular proteolysis. *Biochim Biophys Acta* 1985;823:35–65.

92. Edlund T, Ny T, Ranby M, et al. Isolation of cDNA sequences coding for a part of human tissue plasminogen activator. *Proc Natl Acad Sci U S A* 1983;80:349–352.

93. Fisher R, Waller EK, Grossi G, Thompson D, Tizard R, Schleuning WD. Isolation and characterization of the human tissue-type plasminogen activator structural gene including its 5′ flanking region. *J Biol Chem* 1985;260:11223–11230.

94. Nagamine Y, Person D, Altos MS, Reich E. cDNA and gene nucleotide

sequence of porcine plasminogen activator. *Nucleic Acids Res* 1984; 12:9525–9541.

95. Pennica D, Holmes WE, Kohr WJ, et al. Cloning and expression of human tissue-type plasminogen activator cDNA in *E. coli. Nature* 1983;301:214–221.

96. Riccio A, Gormaldi G, Verde P, Sebastiao G, Boast S, Blasi F. The human urokinase-plasminogen activator gene and its promoter. *Nucleic Acids Res* 1985;13:2759–2771.

97. Bernik MD, Wijngaards G, Rijken DC. Production by human tissues in culture of immunologically distinct, multiple molecular weight forms of plasminogen activators. *Ann N Y Acad Sci* 1981;370:529–608.

98. Rijken DC, Collen D. Purification and characterization of the plasminogen activator secreted by human melanoma cells in culture. *J Biol Chem* 1981;256:7035–7041.

99. Vetterlein D, Bell TE, Young PL, Roblin R. Immunological quantitation and immunoadsorption of urokinase-like plasminogen activators secreted by human cells. *J Biol Chem* 1980;255:3665–3672.

100. Collen D. On the regulation and control of fibrinolysis. *Thromb Haemost* 1980;43:77–89.

101. Wilman B, Collen D. Molecular mechanism of physiological fibrinolysis. *Nature* 1978;272:549–550.

102. Camiolo SM, Thorsen S, Astrup T. Fibrinogenolysis and fibrinolysis with tissue plasminogen activator, streptokinase-activated human globulin, and plasmin. *Proc Soc Exp Biol Med* 1971;138:277–280.

103. Hoylaerts M, Rijken DS, Lijnen HR, Collen D. Kinetics of the activation of plasminogen by human tissue plasminogen activator. *J Biol Chem* 1982;257:2912–2919.

104. Vetterlein D, Young PL, Bell TE, Robin R. Immunological characterization of multiple molecular weight forms of human cell plasminogen activators. *J Biol Chem* 1979;254:575–578.

105. Canipari R, Strickland S. Plasminogen activator in the rat ovary. *J Biol Chem* 1985;260:5121–5125.

106. Huarte J, Belin D, Vasasalli JD. Plasminogen activator in mouse and rat oocytes: induction during meiotic maturation. *Cell* 1985;43:551–558.

107. Levin EG, Loskutoff DJ. Cultured bovine endothelial cells produce both urokinase and tissue-type plasminogen activators. *J Cell Biol* 1982;94:631–636.

108. Ossowski L, Biegel D, Reich E. Mammary plasminogen activator: correlation with involution, hormonal modulation and comparison between normal and neoplastic tissue. *Cell* 1979;16:929–940.

109. Strickland S, Reich E, Sherman MI. Plasminogen activator in early embryogenesis: enzyme production by trophoblast and parietal endoderm. *Cell* 1976;9:231–240.

110. Strickland S, Mahdavi V. The induction of differentiation in teratocarinoma stem cells by retinoic acid. *Cell* 1978;15:393–403.

111. Strickland S, Beers WH. Studies on the role of plasminogen activator in ovulation. *J Biol Chem* 1976;251:5694–5702.

112. Vassalli JD, Baccino D, Belin D. A cellular binding site for the Mr 55,000 form of the human plasminogen activator, urokinase. *J Cell Biol* 1985;100:86–92.

113. Ossowski L, Reich E. Antibodies to plasminogen activator inhibit human tumor metastasis. *Cell* 1983;35:611–619.

114. Levin EG, Loskutoff DJ. Cultured bovine endothelial cells produce both urokinase and tissue-type plasminogen activators. *J Cell Biol* 1982;94:631–636.

115. Ryan TJ, Seeger JI, Kumar A, Dickerman HW. Estradiol preferentially enhances extracellular tissue plasminogen activators of MCF-7 breast cancer cells. *J Biol Chem* 1984;259:14234–14327.

116. Vetterlein D, Young PL, Bell TE, Roblin R. Immunological characterization of multiple molecular weight forms of human cell plasminogen activators. *J Biol Chem* 1979;254:575–578.

117. Grondahl-Hansen J, Lund LR, Ralfkiaer E, Ottevanger V, Dano K. Urokinase- and tissue-type plasminogen activators in keratinocytes during wound reepithelialization *in vivo. J Invest Dermatol* 1988;90: 790–795.

118. Hashimoto K, Shafran KM, Webber PS, Lazarus GS, Singer KH. Anti-cell surface pemphigus autoantibody stimulates plasminogen activator inhibitor in the epidermis. *Br J Dermatol* 1983;113:523–527.

119. Morioka S, Jensen PJ, Lazarus GS. Human epidermal plasminogen activator: characterization, localization, and modulation. *Exp Cell Res* 1985;161:364–372.

120. McNeil H, Jensen PJ. A high-affinity receptor for urokinase plasminogen activator on human keratinocytes: characterization and potential modulation during migration. *Cell Regul* 1990;1:843–852.

121. Jensen PJ, Baird J, Morioka S, Lessin S, Lazarus GS. Epidermal plasminogen activator is abnormal in cutaneous lesions. *J Invest Dermatol* 1988;90:777–782.

122. Isseroff RR, Fusening NE, Rifkin DB. Plasminogen is present in the basal layer of the epidermis. *J Invest Dermatol* 1983;80:297–299.

123. Biekedah-Hansen H, Taylor RE. Production of three plasminogen activators and inhibitor in keratinocyte cultures. *Biochim Biophys Acta* 1983;756:308–318.

124. Hashimoto K, Wun T-C, Baird J, Morioka S, Lazarus GS, Jensen PL. Characterization of keratinocyte plasminogen activator inhibitors and demonstration of the prevention of pemphigus IgG-induced acantholysis by a purified plasminogen activator inhibitor. *J Invest Dermatol* 1989;92:310–314.

125. Isseroff RR, Fusening NE, Rifklin DB. Plasminogen activator in differentiating mouse keratinocyte. *J Invest Dermatol* 1983;80:217–222.

126. Jensen PJ, John M, Baird J. Urokinase and tissue type plasminogen activators in human keratinocyte culture. *Exp Cell Res* 1990;187: 162–169.

127. Green H. Terminal differentiation of cultured human epidermal cells. *Cell* 1977;11:405–416.

128. Morioka S, Jensen PJ, Lazarus GS. Human epidermal plasminogen activator: characterization, localization and modulation. *Exp Cell Res* 1985;161:364–372.

129. Chen C-S, Lyons-Giordano B, Lazarus GS, Jensen P. Differential expression of plasminogen activators and inhibitors in an organotypic skin co-culture system. *J Cell Sci* 1993;106:45–53.

130. Morioka S, Lazarus GS, Jensen PJ. Involvement of urokinase-type plasminogen activator in acantholysis induced by pemphigus IgG. *J Invest Dermatol* 1987;89:474–477.

131. Schaefer BM, Jaeger C, Kramer MD. Plasminogen activator system in pemphigus vulgaris. *Br J Dermatol* 1996;135:726–732.

132. Lever WF. Pemphigus. *Medicine (Baltimore)* 1953;32:1–123.

133. Jordon RE, Beutner EH, Witebsky E, et al. Basement zone antibodies in bullous pemphigoid. *JAMA* 1967;200:751–758.

134. Jordon RE. Bullous, cicatricial pemphigoid and chronic bullous dermatosis of childhood. In: Fitzpatrick TB, Eisen AZ, Wolff K, Freedberg IM, Austen KF, eds. *Dermatology in general medicine.* New York: McGraw-Hill. 1987:580–586.

135. Lever WF. *Pemphigus and pemphigoid.* Springfield, IL: Charles C Thomas, 1965:222.

136. Ahmed AR, Maize JC, Provost TT. Bullous pemphigoid. Clinical and immunologic follow-up after successful therapy. *Arch Dermatol* 1977; 113:1043–1046.

137. Person JR, Rogers RS. Bullous and cicatricial pemphigoid: clinical, histopathologic, and immunopathologic correlations. *Mayo Clin Proc* 1977;52:54–66.

138. Shornick JK, Banger JL, Freeman RG. Herpes gestationis: clinical and histologic features of 28 cases. *J Am Acad Dermatol* 1983;8: 214–224.

139. Provost TT, Tomasi TB. Evidence for complement activation via the alternative pathway in skin diseases: I. Herpes gestationis, systemic lupus erythematosus, and bullous pemphigoid. *J Clin Invest* 1973;52: 1779–1787.

140. Jordon RE, Heine KG, Tappeiner G, Bushkell LL, Provost TT. The immunopathology of herpes gestationis: immunofluorescence studies and characterization of the "HG factor." *J Clin Invest* 1976;57: 1426–1433.

141. Katz SI, Hertz KC, Yaoita H. Herpes gestationis: immunopathology and characterization of the HG factor. *J Clin Invest* 1976;57: 1434–1441.

142. Morrison LH, Labib RS, Zone JJ, Labib RS, Diaz LA, Anhalt GJ. Herpes gestationis autoantibodies recognize a 180 KD human epidermal antigen. *J Clin Invest* 1988;81:2023–2026.

143. Shklar G, McCarthy PL. Oral lesions of mucous membrane pemphigoid: a study of 85 cases. *Arch Otolaryngol* 1971;93:354–364.

144. Foster CS. Cicatricial pemphigoid. *Trans Am Ophthalmol Soc* 1986; 84:527–663.

145. Kelly SE, Wojnarowska F. The use of chemically split tissue in the detection of circuating anti-basement membrane zone antibodies in bullous and cicatricial pemphigoid. *Br J Dermatol* 1988;118:31–40.

146. Fine JD, Neises GR, Katz SI. Immunofluorescence and immunoelectron microscopic studies in cicatricial pemphigoid. *J Invest Dermatol* 1984;82:39–43.

147. Chan LS, Hammerberg C, Cooper KD. Cicatricial pemphigoid: identification of two distinct sets of epidermal antigens by IgA and IgG class circulating autoantibodies. *Arch Dermatol* 1990;126:1466–1471.

148. Dahl MV. Bullous pemphigoid. In: Ahmed AR, ed. *Clinics in dermatology*. Philadelphia: JB Lippincott, 1987:64–70.
149. Gammon WR, Merritt CC, Lewis DM. An *in vitro* model of immune complex-mediated basement membrane zone separation caused by pemphigoid antibodies, leukocytes, and complement. *J Invest Dermatol* 1982;78:285–290.
150. Anhalt GJ, Bahn CF, Labib RS, et al. Pathogenic effects of bullous pemphigoid autoantibodies on rabbit corneal epithelium. *J Clin Invest* 1978;68:1097–1101.
151. Diaz LA, Weiss HJ, Calvanico NJ, et al. Phylogenetic studies with pemphigus and pemphigoid antibodies. *Acta Derm Venereol* 1978;58:537–540.
152. Mutasim DF, Morrison LH, Takahashi Y, et al. Definition of bullous pemphigoid antibody binding to intracellular and extracellular antigen associated with hemidesmosomes. *J Invest Dermatol* 1989;92:225–230.
153. Tamai K, Sawamura D, Choi Do HY, Li K, Uitto J. Molecular biology of the 230 kd bullous pemphigoid antigen. *Dermatology* 1994;189:27–33.
154. Hopkinson SB, Baker SE, Jones JC. Molecular genetics studies of a human epidermal antigen (the 180-kd bullous pemphigoid antigen/BP 180): identification of functionally important sequences within the BP 180 molecule and evidence for an interaction between BP 180 and alpha 6 integrin. *J Cell Biol* 1995;130:117–125.
155. Liu Z, Diaz LA, Swartz SJ, Troy JL, Fairley JA, Giudice GJ. Molecular cloning of pathogenically relevant BP 180 epitope associated with experimentally induced murine bullous pemphigoid. *J Immunol* 1995;155:5449–5454.
156. Giudice GJ, Emery DJ, Zelickson BD, Anhalt GJ, Liu Z, Diaz LA. Bullous pemphigoid and herpes gestationis autoantibodies recognize a common non-collagenous site on the BP 180 ectodomain. *J Immunol* 1993;151:5742–5750.
157. Bedane C, McMillan JR, Balding SD, et al. Bullous pemphigoid and cicatricial pemphigoid autoantibodies react with ultrastructurally separable epitopes on the BP180 ectodomain: evidence that BP180 spans the lamina lucida. *J Invest Dermatol* 1997;108:901–906.
158. Domloge-Hultsch N, Anhalt GJ, Gammon WR, et al. Antiepiligrin cicatricial pemphigoid: a subepithelial bullous disorder. *Arch Dermatol* 1994;130:1521–1529.
159. Chan LS, Majmudar AA, Tran HH, et al. Laminin-6 and laminin-5 are recognized by autoantibodies in a subset of cicatricial pemphigoid. *J Invest Dermatol* 1997;108:848–853.
160. Shimizu H, Masunaga T, Ishiko A, et al. Autoantibodies from patients with cicatricial pemphigoid target different sites in epidermal basement membrane. *J Invest Dermatol* 1995;104:370–373.
161. Kirtschig G, Marinkovich P, Burgeson RE, Yancey KB. Anti-basement membrane autoantibodies in patients with anti-epiligrin cicatricial pemphigoid bind the alpha subunit of laminin 5. *J Invest Dermatol* 1995;105:543–548.
162. Gammon WR, Lewis DM, Carlo JR. Pemphigoid antibody mediated attachment of peripheral blood leukocytes at the dermal-epidermal junction of normal human skin. *J Invest Dermatol* 1980;75:334–339.
163. Gammon WR, Merritt CC, Lewis DM. Leukocyte chemotaxis to the dermal-epidermal junction of human skin mediated by pemphigoid antibody and complement: mechanisms of cell attachment in the *in vitro* leukocyte attachment method. *J Invest Dermatol* 1981;76:514–519.
164. Gammon WR, Merritt CC, Lewis DM, et al. Functional evidence for complement-activating immune complexes in the skin of patients with bullous pemphigoid. *J Invest Dermatol* 1982;78:52–58.
165. Anhalt GJ, Bahn CF, Labib RS, Voorhees JJ, Sugar A, Diaz LA. Pathogenic effects of bullous pemphigoid autoantibodies on rabbit corneal epithelium. *J Clin Invest* 1981;68:1097–1101.
166. Naito K, Morioka S, Ikeda S, et al. Experimental bullous pemphigoid in guinea pigs: the role of pemphigoid antibodies, complement, and migrating cells. *J Invest Dermatol* 1984;82:227–230.
167. Gammon RW, Briggaman RA. Absence of specific changes in guinea pig skin treated with bullous pemphigoid antibodies. *Clin Res* 1987;35:388A.
168. Liu Z, Diaz LA, Troy JL, et al. A passive transfer model of the organ specific autoimmune disease, bullous pemphigoid using antibodies generated against the hemidesmosomal antigen, BP180. *J Clin Invest* 1993;92:2480–2488.
169. Jordon RE, Nordby JM, Milstein H. The complement system in bullous pemphigoid: III. Fixation of C1q and C4 by pemphigoid antibody. *J Lab Clin Med* 1975;86:733–740.
170. Jordon RE, Sams WM, Beutner EH. Complement immunofluorescent staining in bullous pemphigoid. *J Lab Clin Med* 1969;74:548–556.
171. Sams WM, Schur PH. Studies of the antibodies in pemphigoid and pemphigus. *J Lab Clin Med* 1973;78:249–254.
172. Bird P, Friedmann PS, Ling N, et al. Subclass distribution of IgG autoantibodies in bullous pemphigoid. *J Invest Dermatol* 1986;86:21–25.
173. Nakagawa T, DeWeck AL. Membrane receptors for the IgG4 subclass on human basophils and mast cells. *Clin Rev Allergy* 1983;1:197–206.
174. Schmidt-Ullrich B, Rule A, Schaumburg-Lever G, et al. Ultrastructural localization of *in vivo*-bound complement in bullous pemphigoid. *J Invest Dermatol* 1975;65:217–219.
175. Jordon RE, Day NK, Sams WM, et al. The complement system in bullous pemphigoid: I. Complement and component levels in sera and blister fluids. *J Clin Invest* 1973;52:1207–1214.
176. Jordon RE, Kawana S, Fritz KA. Immunopathologic mechanisms in pemphigus and bullous pemphigoid. *J Invest Dermatol* 1985;85:72S–78S.
177. Dahl MV, Falk RJ, Carpenter R, et al. Deposition of the membrane attack complex of complement in bullous pemphigoid. *J Invest Dermatol* 1984;82:132–135.
178. Liu Z, Giudice GJ, Swartz SJ. The role of complement in experimental bullous pemphigoid. *J Invest Dermatol* 1995;95:1539–1544.
179. Lazarova Z, Yee C, Darling T, Briggaman RA, Yancey KB. Passive transfer of anti-laminin 5 antibodies induces subepidermal blisters in neonatal mice. *J Clin Invest* 1996;98:1509–1518.
180. Lazarova Z, Hsu R, Yee C, Yancey K. IgG from patients with anti-epiligrin cicatricial pemphigoid induces subepidermal blisters in human skin grafted onto SCID mice [abstract 131]. *J Invest Dermatol* 1997;108:559.
181. Wintroub BU, Mihm MC, Goetzl EJ, et al. Morphologic and functional evidence for release of mast-cell products in bullous pemphigoid. *N Engl J Med* 1978;298:417–424.
182. O'Toole EA, Arami S, Guitart J, Mackay CR, Woodley DT, Chan LS. Eoraxin, an eosinophil-specific chemoattractant, is upregulated in bullous pemphigoid lesional epidermis and in normal human keratinocytes stimulated by a pro-inflammatory cytokine IL-1 alfa [abstract 50]. *J Invest Dermatol* 1997;108:546.
183. Katayama I, Doi T, Nishioka K. High histamine level in the blister fluid of bullous pemphigoid. *Arch Dermatol Res* 1984;276:126–127.
184. Sayama S, Iozzo RV, Lazarus GS, Schechter NM. Human skin chymotrypsin-like proteinase chymase: subcellular localization to mast cell granules and interaction with heparin and other glucosaminoglycans. *J Biol Chem* 1987;262:6808.
185. Briggaman RA, Schechter NM, Fraki J, Lazarus GS. Degradation of the epidermal-dermal junction by proteolytic enzymes from human skin and human polymorphonuclear leukocytes. *J Exp Med* 1985;160:1027–1042.
186. Okubo K, Karashima T, Hachisuka H, Sasai Y. The existence of a platelet-activating factor (Paf-acether)-like substance in blister fluid derived from patients with bullous pemphigoid as demonstrated by *human platelet aggregation techni*ques. *Kurume Med J* 1989;36:173–179.
187. Kawana S, Ueno A, Nishiyama S. Increased levels of immunoreactive leukotriene B4 in blister fluids of bullous pemphigoid patients and effects of a selective 5-lipoxygenase inhibitor on experimental skin lesions. *Acta Derm Venereol* 1990;70:281–285.
188. Dvorak AM, Mihm MC, Osage JE, et al. Bullous pemphigoid, an ultrastructural study of the inflammatory response: eosinophil, basophil and mast cell granule changes in multiple biopsies from one patient. *J Invest Dermatol* 1982;78:91–101.
189. Miyasato M, Tsuda S, Kasada M, Iryo K, Sasai Y. Alteration in the density, morphology, and biological properties of eosinophils produced by bullous pemphigoid blister fluid. *Arch Dermatol Res* 1989;281:304–309.
190. Dubertret L, Bertaux B, Fosse M, et al. Cellular events leading to blister formation in bullous pemphigoid. *Br J Dermatol* 1980;104:615–624.
191. Liu Z, Twining S, Giudice GJ, et al. Neutrophil elastase is essential for subepidermal bullous pemphigoid [abstract 114]. *J Invest Dermatol* 1997;108:556.
192. Michalaki H, Nicolas J-F, Kanitakis J, Machado P, Roche P, Thivolet J. T cells in bullous pemphigoid: presence of activated CD4+ T cells at the basement membrane zone in pre- and peri-bullous skin. *Reg Immunol* 1991;3:151–155.
193. Sams WM, Gammon WR. Mechanism of lesion production in pemphigus and pemphigoid. *J Am Acad Dermatol* 1980;6:431–449.

Inflammation: Basic Principles and Clinical Correlates,
3rd ed., edited by John I. Gallin and Ralph Snyderman.
Published by Lippincott Williams & Wilkins, Philadelphia 1999.

CHAPTER 61

The Role of Inflammation in Sepsis and Septic Shock:

A Meta-analysis of Both Clinical and Preclinical Trials of Anti-inflammatory Therapies

Bradley D. Freeman, Peter Q. Eichacker, and Charles Natanson

While an intact host defense system is essential to survival, excessive levels of inflammation during infection have been proposed as mediating the organ dysfunction and lethality of sepsis. Based on this hypothesis, a number of agents have been developed to limit the inflammatory response in this syndrome. These agents fall into three broad categories: (a) proinflammatory mediator-specific antagonists [e.g., interleukin-1 receptor antagonists (IL-1ra), soluble tumor necrosis factor-α (TNF-α) receptors, etc.]; (b) high-dose glucocorticoids; and (c) antiendotoxin agents (e.g., antiserum and antibodies directed against epitopes on the endotoxin molecule). Early studies, evaluating these agents in animal models, suggested that they improved outcome in sepsis. These promising results prompted large numbers of clinical trials of these agents in humans with sepsis. To date, the effect on outcome of these agents in these trials has been disappointing (1–3). This has subsequently raised doubts regarding both the initial hypothesis of the role of inflammation in the sepsis syndrome, and the relevance of animal models to human sepsis. This chapter focuses on the clinical and preclinical studies evaluating the use of antiinflammatory agents in sepsis. It is our hope that this systematic review will foster better understanding of the importance of specific inflammatory mediators in pro-

ducing the sepsis syndrome, and help determine why these antiinflammatory therapies, which were founded on extensive preclinical research, failed to produce benefit when administered to septic patients.

ORIGINS OF THE HYPOTHESIS

Despite more than 40 clinical trials using multiple types of purported antiinflammatory agents in an excess of 14,000 septic patients, convincing evidence of a beneficial effect for any one agent has not been demonstrated (1–4). Thus, the strongest supporting evidence that these antiinflammatory agents improve outcome in sepsis has been derived not from human studies, but rather from animal models. More than three decades ago, Hinshaw et al. (5) first reported that inhibiting inflammation with high-dose glucocorticoids could lower mortality rates associated with endotoxin-challenge in dogs. Next, in the early 1970s, Ziegler and Braude's team (6,7) tested antibodies against epitopes on endotoxin molecules. They showed that these antibodies improved outcome in sepsis models, presumably by preventing a host inflammatory response to endotoxin. Then, in the mid-1980s, Beutler et al. (8) demonstrated that an antiserum directed against TNF-α could improve outcome in endotoxin-challenged mice. This led to a series of studies showing that inhibition of any one of a vast number of host proinflammatory mediators [e.g., IL-1, platelet activating factor (PAF), etc.] could improve outcome in sepsis models (9–33).

Animal studies have not only shown that inhibiting proinflammatory mediators is beneficial, but also that

B.D. Freeman: Department of Surgery, Section of Burns/Trauma/Critical Care, Washington University Medical Center, St. Louis, Missouri 63110.

P.Q. Eichacker and C. Natanson: Critical Care Medicine Department, National Institutes of Health, Bethesda, Maryland 20892.

administering these substances can produce shock-like states. More than 30 years ago, Weil et al. (34) demonstrated that bacterial endotoxin challenges produced cardiovascular collapse in dogs. More recently, it has been shown that giving proinflammatory mediators such as TNF-α and IL-1 produces a clinical picture mimicking bacterial septic shock (35–37).

Based in large part on these animal studies, the following hypothesis has been developed to explain the pathogenesis of sepsis and septic shock (Fig. 61-1) (1). In brief, during severe infection, the host defense system becomes overwhelmed either due to loss of protective barriers and/or increased virulence of pathogens. This results in invasive infection with release of bacteria and/or bacterial toxins into the circulation. In response, there is rapid activation of host defenses including circulating protein systems, such as the complement and coagulation cascades, and kallikrein-kinin systems. Over the ensuing hours, endothelial cells elaborate large quantities of pro- and antiinflammatory mediators. This uncontrolled activation of protein cascades and release of inflammatory mediators results in shock, organ injury, and death.

HUMAN CLINICAL TRIALS OF ANTI-INFLAMMATORY AGENTS: META-ANALYSES

Since no single anti-inflammatory agent has shown consistent benefit in human clinical trials (1–3), we combined the individual sepsis trials into broad categories to compare various classes of anti-inflammatory agents in hopes that this larger database could help us better understand why clinical trials of anti-inflammatory agents failed. We recently published a metanalysis (4) of 18 clinical trials comprising six different mediator-specific nonglucocorticoid anti-inflammatory agents: three studies examining IL-1ra (38–40), two studies of soluble TNF-α receptors (41,42), six studies of anti–TNF-α antibodies (43–48), two studies of bradykinin antagonists (49,50), two studies of PAF antagonists (51,52), and three studies of anti-prostaglandins (53–55). For this chapter, we updated this meta-analysis to include data from two recently completed clinical trials of anti–TNF-α antibodies (4) and additional data made available from a recently

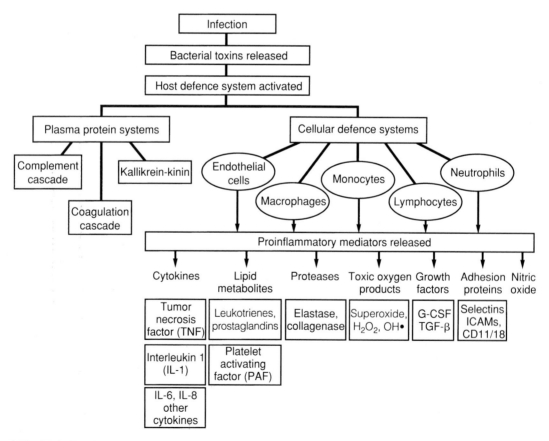

FIG. 61-1. Pathogenesis of sepsis and septic shock and potential therapeutic targets in the inflammatory cascade. This diagram illustrates a model in which the presence of infection elicits the activation of plasma protein systems and the release of complex cascades of mediators resulting in the sepsis syndrome. Many of these mediators have been targeted in clinical sepsis trials. (Reproduced with permission from BioWorld Financial Watch, American Health Consultants Inc., Atlanta, GA.)

TABLE 61-1. *Clinical trials of non-glucocorticoid mediator-specific anti-inflammatory agents in sepsis and septic shock*

Therapy Compound (company) (reference)	Study designs	Inclusion criteria	Control arm deaths/ total (percent)	Treatment arm deaths/ total (percent)
IL-1ra				
Antril (Synergen) (38)	Open-label, phase II	Severe sepsis or septic shock (68%)[a]	11/25 (44)	18/74 (24)
Antril (Synergen) (39)	Double-blinded, phase III	Severe sepsis or septic shock (79%)[a]	102/302 (34)	177/591 (30)
Antril (Synergen) (40)	Double-blinded, phase III	Sepsis with organ dysfunction and/or shock	163/456 (36)	151/450 (34)
Combined			276/783 (35)	346/1115 (31)
Anti-bradykinin				
CPO-127 (Cortech) (49)	Double-blinded, phase II	SIRS secondary to presumed infection	24/84 (29)	62/167 (37)
CPO-127 (Cortech) (50)	Double-blinded, phase II	SIRS secondary to presumed infection	52/126 (41)	150/378 (40)
Combined			76/210 (36)	212/545 (39)
Anti-PAF				
BN-52021 (Ipsen) (51)	Double-blinded, phase III	Severe sepsis or septic shock (75%)[a]	66/130 (51)	55/132 (42)
BN-52021 (Ipsen) (52)	Double-blinded, phase III	Severe sepsis or septic shock (75%)[a]	152/308 (49)	140/300 (47)
Combined			218/438 (50)	195/432 (45)
Anti-TNF				
MAK-195F (Knoll) (44)	Open-label, phase II	Severe sepsis or septic shock (69%)[a]	12/29 (41)	44/93 (47)
MAK-195F (Knoll) (43)	Open-label, phase II	Severe sepsis or septic shock	6/12 (50)	7/27 (26)
MAK-195F (Knoll) (4)	Double-blinded, phase III	Severe sepsis and elevated IL-6 levels	125/221 (57)	121/225 (54)
CDP-571 (Celltech) (46)	Open-label, phase II	Septic Shock (100%)[a]	6/10 (60)	20/32 (63)
CB-0006 (Celltech) (45)[b]	Open-label, phase II	Severe sepsis or septic shock	6/19 (32)	27/61 (44)
BAY-x1351 (Bayer/Miles) (47)	Double-blinded, phase III	Severe sepsis or septic shock (49%)[a]	108/326 (33)	196/645 (30)
BAY-x1351 (Bayer/Miles) (48)	Double-blinded, phase III	Severe sepsis or septic shock (80%)[a]	66/167 (40)	144/386 (37)
BAY-x1351 (Bayer/Miles) (58)	Double-blinded, phase III	Septic shock	398/930 (43)	382/949 (40)
Combined			727/1714 (42)	941/2418 (39)
Soluble TNF receptor				
P80 (Immunex) (41)	Double-blinded, phase II	Septic shock (100%)[a]	10/33 (30)	49/108[c] (45)
P55 (Hoffman) (42)	Double-blinded, phase II	Severe sepsis or Septic shock (44%)[a]	54/140 (39)	136/358 (38)
Combined			64/173 (37)	185/466[c] (40)
Anti-prostaglandin				
Ibuprofen (Upjohn) (54)	Double-blinded, phase II	Severe sepsis or septic shock (31%)[a]	4/13 (31)	9/16 (56)
Ibuprofen (Upjohn) (55)[c]	Double-blinded, phase II	Sepsis syndrome (50%)[a]	6/14 (43)	3/16 (19)
Ibuprofen (Upjohn) (53)[c]	Double-blinded, phase III	Sepsis syndrome (63%)[a]	92/231 (40)	83/224 (37)
Combined			102/258 (40)	95/256 (38)
All Studies	—		1463/3576 (41)	1974/5232 (38)

IL-1ra, interleukin-1 receptor antagonist; PAF, platelet-activating factor; TNF, tumor necrosis factor; SIRS, systemic inflammatory response syndrome.

[a]Percentage of participants in the control arm with septic shock.

[b]In this study, the lowest dosage treatment group was considered the control group.

[c]This study was funded by the National Institutes of Health.

From reference 4, with permission.

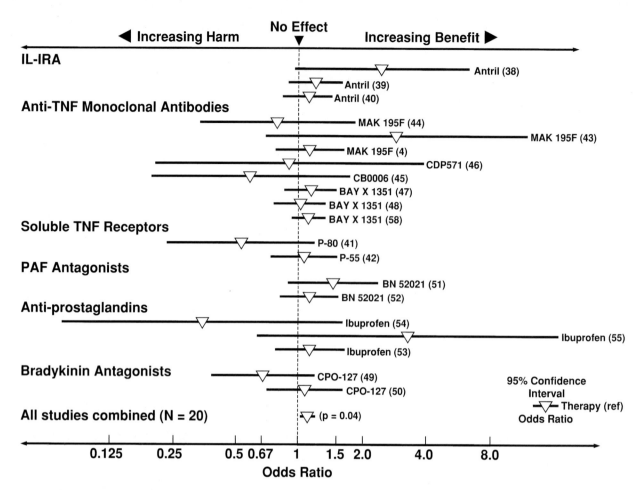

FIG. 61-2. Odds ratios and 95% confidence intervals for survival in 20 clinical trials of non-glucocorticoid mediator specific anti-inflammatory agents in patients with sepsis. The odds of surviving is the probability of surviving divided by the probability of dying. In this meta-analysis the odds ratios were determined by calculating the odds of surviving in the treatment group and dividing this by the odds of surviving in the control group. These odds ratios include all doses of soluble tumor necrosis factor-α receptors studied. IL-1ra, interleukin-1 receptor antagonist; TNF-α, tumor necrosis factor-α; PAF, platelet activating factor.) (From ref. 4, with permission.)

TABLE 61-2. *Clinical trials of high-dose glucocorticoids in sepsis and septic shock*

Therapy (reference)	Dose	Study design	Inclusion criteria	Endpoint	Control arm deaths/total (percent)	Treatment arm deaths/total (percent)
Methylprednisolone (59)	30 mg/kg (×4)	Double-blinded	Septic shock	Hospital mortality or discharge	20/37 (54)	22/38 (58)
Methylprednisolone (60)	30 mg/kg followed by 45 mg/kg	Double-blinded	Sepsis	14-day mortality	24/111 (22)	23/112 (21)
Methylprednisolone (61)	30 mg/kg (×4)	Double-blinded	Sepsis	14-day mortality	48/190 (25)	65/191 (34)
Methylprednisolone or dexamethasone (62)	30 mg/kg[a] or 6 mg/kg[a]	Double-blinded	Septic shock	Hospital mortality	11/16 (69)	33/43 (76)
Methylprednisolone (63)	30 mg/kg, repeated ×3 if in shock	Double-blinded	N/A	Hospital mortality	25/32 (78)	22/28 (79)
Dexamethasone (64)	6 mg/kg	Open-label	Septic shock	14-day mortality	5/25 (20)	5/23 (22)
Methylprednisolone or dexamethasone (65)	30 mg/kg[a] or 3 mg/kg[a]	Double-blinded	Septic shock	28-day mortality	33/86 (38)	9/86 (10)
Betamethasone (66)	1 mg/kg daily ×3	Double-blinded	Septic shock	20-day mortality	22/39 (56)	24/46 (52)
Hydrocortisone (67)	1050 mg over 6 d	Double-blinded	Severe infection	Hospital mortality	32/98 (33)	54/96 (56)
All Studies	—	—	—	—	220/634 (35)	257/663 (39)

[a]Repeated as necessary.
From reference 4, with permission.

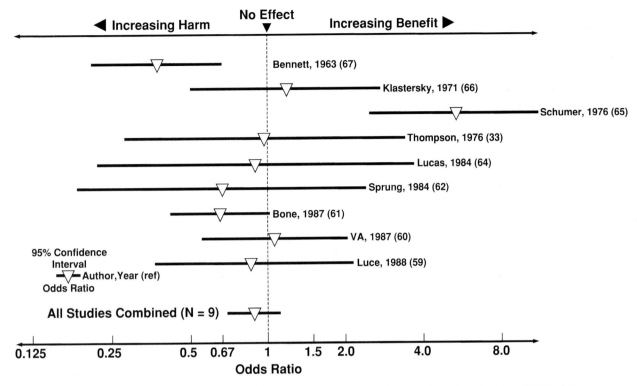

FIG. 61-3. Odds ratios and 95% confidence intervals for survival in nine clinical trials of high-dose glucocorticoids in patients with sepsis syndrome. (From ref. 4, with permission.)

published clinical trial of soluble TNF-α receptors (4,42) (Table 61-1, Fig. 61-2). In this chapter we compare these mediator-specific therapies to meta-analyses done of sepsis trials of high-dose glucocorticoids (56,57) (Table 61-2, Fig. 61-3) and anti-endotoxin agents (1) (Table 61-3, Fig. 61-4). We hope that contrasting and comparing these three different approaches of inhibiting inflammation will help clarify why each failed to show a significant beneficial effect on outcome.

TABLE 61-3. *Clinical trials of endotoxin-directed antibodies in sepsis and septic shock*

Therapy (reference)	Inclusion criteria	Control arm deaths/total (percent)	Treatment arm deaths/total (percent)
J5 antiserum (68)	Gram-negative bacteremia	42/109 (39)	23/103 (22)
J5 antiserum (69)	Prophylaxis in neutropenic patients	2/53 (4)	4/47 (9)
J5 immune plasma (70)	Prophylaxis in high-risk surgical patients	18/136 (13)	14/126 (11)
J5 immune plasma (71)	Infectious purpura in children	12/33 (36)	10/40 (25)
J5 intravenous immunoglobulin (72)	Gram-negative septic shock	20/41 (49)	15/30 (50)
J5 intravenous immunoglobulin (73)	Prophylaxis in high-risk surgical patients	22/112 (19.6)	20/108 (18.5)
E5 (74)	Gram-negative sepsis	62/152 (41)	63/164 (38)
E5 (75)	Gram-negative sepsis and non-refractory shock	69/266 (26)	79/264 (30)
HA-1A (76)	Gram-negative bacteremia	45/92 (49)	32/105 (30)
HA-1A (77)	Gram-negative bacteremia	95/293 (32)	109/328 (33)
All studies	—	387/1287 (30)	369/1315 (28)

Survival rates as reported; from reference 1, with permission.

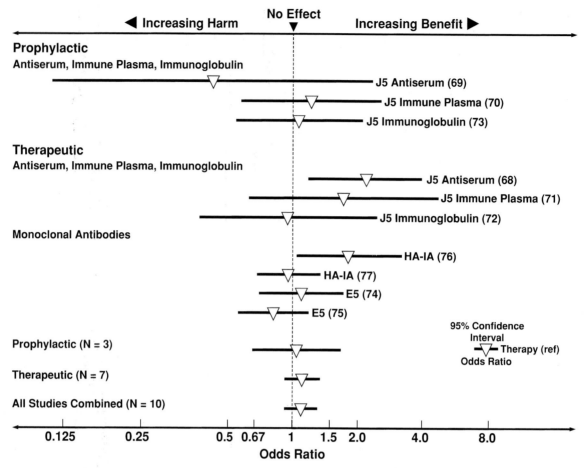

FIG. 61-4. Odds ratios and 95% confidence intervals for survival in ten clinical trials of anti-endotoxin directed antiserum and antibodies in patients with sepsis and septic shock.

MEDIATOR-SPECIFIC ANTI-INFLAMMATORY AGENTS

Analyzing all patients ($n = 6,429$) included in the 18 studies found in our original meta-analysis (4), combined with patients from the three studies that subsequently have become available ($n = 2,379$) (4,42,58), we found a small and statistically significant reduction in mortality rates for patients treated with non-glucocorticoid mediator-specific anti-inflammatory therapies (odds ratio: 1.10; 95% confidence interval: 1.01 to 1.20; $P = .044$; Fig. 61-2). We tested each dose of each agent studied for consistency to the combined data set. Of note, we found that the treatment effect of high and medium doses of the high molecular weight (P-80) soluble TNF-α receptors (41) and low doses of the low molecular weight (P-55) soluble TNF-α receptors (42), although administered to only 78 and 54 patients, respectively, were significantly different compared to the treatment effect of the agents administered to the 8,676 other patients in the metanalysis (both $P < .05$) (Fig. 61-5). The mortality rate associated with P-80 (40 deaths for a 51% mortality rate) and

P-55 (30 deaths for a 56% mortality rate) was higher than that of all other treated patients in the metanalysis (5,183 noncontrol patients receiving an antiinflammatory agent with a 37% mortality rate). If we exclude patients treated with high and medium doses of the P-80 and low doses of the P-55 soluble TNF-α receptor (the groups that constitute significant outliers), we found an even more significant reduction in mortality with non-glucocorticoid mediator-specific therapies (odds ratio: 1.12; 95% confidence interval: 1.02 to 1.22; $P = .02$) (Fig. 61-5).

For consistency, we also examined the percent mortality for control groups classified according to type of anti-inflammatory agent [bradykinin antagonist: 36% (49,50); anti–TNF-α monoclonal antibodies: 40% (43–48,58); soluble TNF-α receptors: 37% (41,42); prostaglandin antagonists: 40% (53–55); IL-1ra: 36% (38–40); and PAF antagonist: 50% (51,52)]. There was marked similarity for control group mortality, except for the PAF antagonist trials (51,52) (Table 61-1). The reason for this increased control group mortality in the PAF antagonist trials is unclear, since these patients did not differ significantly in severity of sepsis compared to septic patients enrolled in other tri-

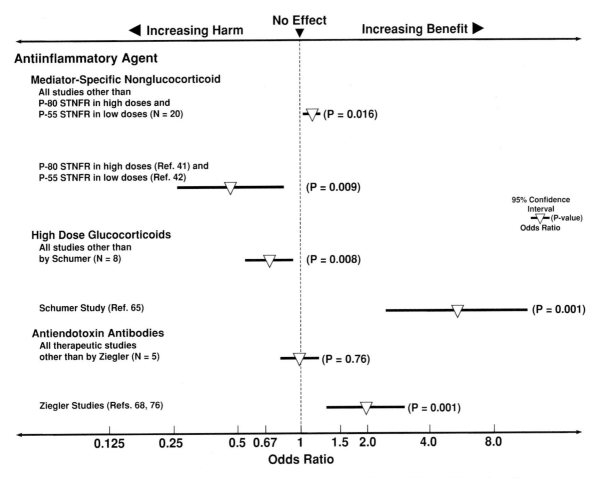

FIG. 61-5. Odds ratios and 95% confidence intervals for metanalyses of clinical trials of mediator-specific nonglucocorticoid antiinflammatory agents, high-dose glucocorticoids, and antiendotoxin therapies in patients with sepsis, comparing statistical outliers to remaining studies within each category. Odds ratios: *High-dose P-80 and low dose P-55 soluble tumor necrosis factor-α receptor vs. other nonglucocorticoids (P = .02); **Schumer et al. (65) vs. other high-dose glucocorticoid studies (P = .0001); Ziegler et al. (68,76) vs. other therapeutic antiendotoxin antiserum and antibody studies (P = .002 uncorrected; p = .04 corrected for multiple comparisons).

als (4). One of the eight anti–TNF-α antibody (MAK195F) trials (4) had an elevated control group mortality rate (57%), and was not included in the above analysis of controls. In that study, an IL-6 dipstick test was used to identify patients with a high mortality risk. IL-6–positive control patients (serum level >1,000 pg/ml) had a higher mortality rate compared to those with a negative test. The patients with low IL-6 levels (serum level <1,000 pg/ml) were not entered into the study. Interestingly, despite identifying a group of patients with high cytokine levels and increased mortality rates, the treatment effect for anti–TNF-α antibody was remarkably similar (approximately 2–3% decrease in mortality rate compared to controls) to the other anti–TNF-α antibody studies that did not use this IL-6 dipstick test (4,43–48,58).

We also compared studies that were double-blinded (n = 15) (4,39–42,47–55) to those that were open label (n = 5) (38,43–46). While single-blinded studies enrolled fewer patients and had greater variability than open label

studies, the odds ratios for treatment effect were similar between these two study designs (odds ratio for double-blind studies: 1.10; 95% confidence interval: 1.01 to 1.27; P = .052 versus odds ratio for single-blind studies: 1.09; 95% confidence interval: 0.95 to 1.30; P = .57, respectively). Of interest, analysis of the blinded studies, with or without inclusion of the open label studies, showed a statistically significant beneficial effect on survival.

In summary, our meta-analysis demonstrates the following:

• Mediator-specific non-glucocorticoid anti-inflammatory agents improve outcome, but their beneficial effect is small. Overall, these studies support a role for excessive inflammation in the pathogenesis of sepsis. However, the role for any single circulating mediator appears minimal since circulating mediator-specific inhibition has only modest effects on patients with sepsis.

- Individual sepsis trials to date appear to have overestimated the treatment effect of mediator-specific antiinflammatory therapies, and consequently did not enroll a sufficient number of patients to demonstrate a statistically significant effect on outcome. We estimate that these agents reduce mortality by approximately 7% to 10%, and would require a clinical trial enrolling 6,000 to 7,000 patients to demonstrate a statistically significant beneficial effect on survival rates.
- At specific doses, soluble TNF-α receptors appear harmful to patients with sepsis. Whether this is a reflection of an idiosyncratic drug toxicity, or a result of inhibition of host defenses and worsening of infection and thus outcome, is unclear from our analysis.
- Anti-inflammatory therapies, such as anti–TNF-α antibodies, are not necessarily more effective in subsets of patients with elevated cytokine (e.g., IL-6) levels.
- The consistent mortality rate for most of these trials (30–40%) suggests that they are well standardized. Further, the well-established practices of antibiotic administration and hemodynamic support in patients with sepsis appear to be utilized consistently and effectively.

HIGH-DOSE GLUCOCORTICOIDS

Clinical trials of high-dose glucocorticoids have spanned the last three decades and represent the first widely utilized approach to inhibit inflammation in septic patients. Two recent meta-analyses published in *Critical Care Medicine* (56,57) identified nine well designed trials (59–67) (Table 61-2). For consistency, we re-analyzed these nine trials using similar methodology to our 21 clinical trials of mediator-specific non-glucocorticoid therapies (4) (Table 61-2, Fig. 61-3). In analyzing all patients ($n = 1,297$) included in the nine studies, there was no significant beneficial effect of high-dose glucocorticoids on survival (odds ratio: 0.89; 95% confidence interval: 0.70 to 1.12; $P = .31$) (Fig. 61-3). Of note, one study by Schumer (65) had a beneficial effect that differed significantly ($P = .007$) from the other studies (Fig. 61-5). Excluding this outlier, high-dose glucocorticoids were actually significantly harmful in patients with septic shock (odds ratio: 0.70; 95% confidence: 0.543 to 0.914; $P = .008$). The increased mortality with high-dose glucocorticoids was significantly different than the reduced mortality seen with mediator-specific non-glucocorticoid anti-inflammatory therapies ($P = .001$).

For consistency, we also examined the control group mortality rate in these nine clinical trials (59–67). The average mortality rate was 35% for controls in high-dose glucocorticoid trials, similar to the average mortality rate for controls (37%) in our meta-analysis of mediator-specific non-glucocorticoid therapies (Table 61-1, Fig. 61-2). However, the mortality rate in the nine individual trials was more variable (20% to 78%) than for the six

individual classes of non-glucocorticoid mediator specific therapies (35% to 50%). This increased variability could be explained by the fact that many of these high-dose glucocorticoid trials enrolled few patients, and/or were performed more than a decade ago when the conduct of trials and treatment of sepsis may have been less well standardized (4).

These nine clinical trials of high-dose glucocorticoids (59–67), along with the previously discussed soluble TNF-α receptor data (41,42), emphasize that inhibition of inflammation can be dangerous. Either these anti-inflammatory agents were immunosuppressive and worsened infection and outcome, or they altered normal regulation of inflammation in such a way as to produce harm independent of infection, or both.

CLINICAL TRIALS OF ANTISERUM AND ANTIBODIES AGAINST ENDOTOXIN

Clinical trials of antiserum and antibodies directed against shared epitopes of endotoxin molecules found in the cell wall of gram-negative bacteria have spanned the last two decades. Initial studies used antiserum and polyclonal antibodies, but, with advances in biotechnology, monoclonal antibodies were subsequently developed and administered. In a recent review published in the *Annals of Internal Medicine* (1), we summarized the results of ten clinical trials that assessed the effects of antiendotoxin therapies in sepsis (68–77). For consistency, we performed an analysis of these ten trials similar to that done for trials of mediator-specific non-glucocorticoid and high-dose glucocorticoid therapies (Table 61-3, Fig. 61-4). In analyzing all patients ($n = 2,605$) included in these ten studies, there was no significant beneficial effect on survival with these agents (odds ratio: 1.11; 95% confidence interval: 0.934 to 1.32; $P = .24$). These ten studies included three in which the antiendotoxin therapy was given prophylactically (odds ratio: 1.05; 95% confidence interval: 0.652 to 1.701; $P = .84$) (69,70,73). Excluding these three studies and examining only the seven therapeutic studies (68,71,72,74–77), there was a beneficial effect with antiendotoxin agents that was not statistically significant (odds ratio: 1.12; 95% confidence interval: 0.927 to 1.347; $P = .23$). Examining the seven studies for consistency, we found that the two studies by Ziegler et al. (68,76) were significant outliers ($P = .04$; $P = .002$ uncorrected, and $P = .04$ corrected for multiple comparisons). The two Ziegler studies showed a marked beneficial effect (odds ratio: 1.98; 95% confidence interval: 1.31 to 3.004; $P = .001$) that was significantly different from the five other studies (71,72,74, 75,77) that showed no significant effect (odds ratio: 0.97; 95% confidence interval: 0.285 to 1.19; $P = .84$) (Fig. 61-5).

The two studies by Ziegler et al. (68,76) and the previously discussed study by Schumer (65) investigating high-dose glucocorticoids had 95% confidence intervals that overlapped, indicating that the beneficial effects of these therapies were in a similar range (Fig. 61-5). In contrast, the 95% confidence intervals for the 20 studies in our metanalysis of mediator specific antiinflammatory trials (4,38–55,58), the other eight studies in our met-analysis of high-dose glucocorticoid trials (59–64,66,67), as well as the other five studies in our meta-analysis of anti-endotoxin trials (71,72,74,75,77), did not overlap with these three clinical trials. These three studies differ so greatly from most of the work in this field that they must be considered unexplained outliers. The majority of anti-endotoxin trials suggest that the antibodies and anti-serum tested to date had no significant beneficial effect in patients with sepsis. Of note, another large phase III clinical trial of E5, a monoclonal antibody against endo-toxin, has been recently completed, and, like the two pre-vious phase III clinical trials of this antibody (74,75), showed no beneficial effect (Joseph E. Parrillo, M.D., personal communication).

WERE ANIMAL MODELS PREDICTIVE OF THE EFFECTS OF ANTI-INFLAMMATORY AGENTS IN HUMANS?

We analyzed the animal studies cited in the human clinical trials included in our meta-analysis of non-glucocorticoid mediator-specific agents [i.e., 13 studies cited examining TNF-α–directed monoclonal antibodies in animals (8,22–33), five studies cited examining solu-ble TNF-α receptors (17–21), three studies cited exam-ining IL-1ra (9–11), and five studies cited examining PAF antagonists (12–16)]. The beneficial effect of these mediator-specific agents on survival was much greater in the cited animal studies (odds ratio: 9.0; 95% confi-dence interval: 5.8 to 14.3) compared to the subsequent clinical trials (odds ratio: 1.1; 95% confidence interval: 1.01 to 1.25). One explanation for this discrepancy is that variables that potentially alter the effects of anti-inflammatory agents (e.g., type and site of bacterial infection, timing of administration of anti-inflammatory therapy, and the use of supportive measures) were not thoroughly evaluated in animal models. For example, anti-inflammatory agents in animal models were most commonly administered prior to, or immediately follow-ing, intravenous challenge with *Escherichia coli,* in the absence of supportive therapy. In contrast, in clinical studies, patients typically had extravascular sites of infection with non–*E. coli* bacteria, received the experi-mental anti-inflammatory therapy several hours after the diagnosis of sepsis had been made, and received sup-portive therapy (vasopressors, fluid resuscitation, antibi-otics, dialysis, mechanical ventilation, etc.). Of note, ani-mal studies in which these therapies were administered more than 2 hours following the onset of infection, or in the setting of non–*E. coli* extravascular challenge, found

these anti-inflammatory agents much less effective (odds ratio: 1.18; 95% confidence interval: 1.003 to 2.45) (8,13, 18,23,27,28,32,33).

We also analyzed the 18 animal studies (78–95) cited in the nine clinical trials (59–67) used in our metanalysis of high-dose glucocorticoids. The beneficial effects on survival were again greater in the animal (odds ratio: 2.2; 95% confidence interval: 2.0 to 2.5) compared to the clinical (odds ratio: 0.70; 95% confidence interval: 0.543 to 0.914) studies. This discrepancy in clinical and pre-clinical outcomes appeared to relate to the same aspects of experimental design that we identified in preclinical studies examining non-glucocorticoid mediator-specific therapies.

Lastly, we analyzed preclinical studies assessing the effects of endotoxin-directed monoclonal antibodies. While three preclinical studies demonstrated benefit for endotoxin-directed antibodies in animal models (96–98), an equivalent number of animal studies suggested that these agents lacked benefit (99–101) and one study actu-ally suggested harm (102). Further, early *in vitro* data demonstrating that these monoclonal antibodies, which were subsequently tested in patients, had specific endo-toxin-binding and -neutralizing activity, could not be reproduced by independent investigators (96,103–106). Therefore, it appears that the lack of efficacy of these endotoxin-directed therapies in humans was, in part, pre-dicted by the preclinical laboratory and animal data.

In summary, a review of preclinical studies that exam-ined the use of anti-inflammatory therapies in sepsis sug-gests the following:

- Preclinical studies examining the use of non-glucocor-ticoid mediator-specific agents and high-dose gluco-corticoids in sepsis failed to examine important vari-ables that potentially alter the effectiveness of these agents. As a consequence, these studies over-estimated the potential benefits of these agents in humans.
- The limited number of preclinical studies demonstrat-ing the beneficial effects of anti-endotoxin monoclonal antibodies were not confirmed by independent labora-tories prior to the initiation of clinical studies. This may have led to ineffective agents being tested clinically.

CONCLUSION

Excessive inflammation has been proposed as mediat-ing the organ injury and mortality of sepsis. Based on this hypothesis, one therapeutic strategy has been the admin-istration of agents to inhibit the inflammatory response. These agents, i.e., mediator-specific antagonists, high-dose glucocorticoids, and endotoxin-directed therapies, were administered initially in animal models with promising results. Their administration to humans, how-ever, proved disappointing, prompting questions regard-ing both the initial hypothesis and the value of animal studies in modeling human sepsis. We undertook a meta-analysis of both preclinical and clinical trials of these antiinflammatory agents in hopes that this larger database would allow us to better understand why these trials failed. Our analysis of human trials of endotoxin-directed antibodies as well as preclinical studies suggests that agents lacking the appropriate bioactivity were tested. Consequently, whether endotoxin is a useful therapeutic target to inhibit inflammation in sepsis remains, at present, unstudied. In contrast, our analysis of mediator-specific antagonists suggests that the use of these agents in humans with sepsis actually does produce a small beneficial effect on survival. These findings support a role for inflammation in sepsis, but suggest that inhibition of specific mediators has much less of an effect on mortality rate than first hoped (i.e., approximately a 7–8% decrease in mortality). Finally, the use of some anti-inflammatory agents (i.e., soluble TNF-α receptors or high-dose glucocorticoids) at particular doses may ultimately have adverse effects, either by excessive immunosuppression, idiosyncratic drug toxicity, or both.

Many issues pertaining to the pathophysiology and treatment of sepsis remain unresolved. Further insight is needed into the regulatory and counter-regulatory mechanisms of inflammation, and how the inflammatory response is influenced by underlying illness, patient age, and various pathogens in mediating the sepsis syndrome. In addition, the discrepancy in outcomes between animal and humans studies must be reconciled. Clearly, the use of animal models has been critical to understanding sepsis. However, to accurately assess the potential efficacy of new therapies, it is imperative that future preclinical animal studies include models that more realistically reflect conditions encountered clinically. New approaches to inhibiting inflammation are needed. Novel agents, such as those that disrupt intracellular signaling pathways utilized by bacterial toxins and host pro-inflammatory mediators (107), or agents that directly antagonize endotoxin receptors (108), appear promising. The failure in clinical trials of previously tested anti-inflammatory agents does not necessarily preclude the possibility of greater treatment effects of these new approaches to inhibit inflammation. Sustained efforts in animal and human research are essential as sepsis remains a highly lethal syndrome and one of the most clinically challenging unsolved problems in medicine today.

REFERENCES

1. Natanson C, Hoffman WD, Suffredini AF, Eichacker PQ, Danner RL. Selected treatment strategies for septic shock based on proposed mechanisms of pathogenesis. *Ann Intern Med* 1994;120:771–783.
2. Quezado ZMN, Banks SM, Natanson C. New strategies for combating sepsis: the magic bullets missed the mark...but the search continues. *Trends Biotechnol* 1995;13:56–63.
3. Freeman BD, Natanson C. Clinical trials in sepsis and septic shock. *Curr Opin Crit Care* 1995;1:349–357.
4. Zeni F, Freeman BD, Natanson C. Anti-inflammatory therapies to treat sepsis and septic shock: a reassessment. *Crit Care Med* 1997;25:1095–1100.
5. Hinshaw LB, Solomon LA, Freeny PC, Reins DA. Hemodynamic and survival effects of methylprednisolone in endotoxin shock. *Arch Surg* 1967;94:61–66.
6. Ziegler E, McCutchan J, Douglas H, Braude A. Prevention of lethal *Pseudomonas* bacteremia with epimerase-deficient *E. coli* antiserum. *Trans Assoc Am Physicians* 1975;88:101–108.
7. Ziegler E, Douglas H, Braude A. Human antiserum for prevention of the local Schwartzman reaction and death from bacterial lipopolysaccharides. *J Clin Invest* 1973;52:3236–3238.
8. Beutler B, Milsark IW, Cerami AC. Passive immunization against cachetin/tumor necrosis factor protects mice from lethal effect of endotoxin. *Science* 1995;229:869–871.
9. Ohlsson K, Björk, Bergenfeldt M, Hageman R, Thompson RC. Interleukin-1 receptor antagonist reduces mortality from endotoxin shock. *Nature* 1990;348:550–552.
10. Wakabayashi G, Gelfand JA, Burke JF, Thompson RC, Dinarello CA. A specific receptor antagonist for interleukin-1 prevents *Escherichia coli*–induced shock in rabbits. *FASEB* 1991;5:338–343.
11. Fisher E, Marano MA, Van Zee KJ, et al. Interleukin-1 receptor blockade improves survival and hemodynamic performance in *Escherichia coli* septic shock, but fails to alter host responses to sublethal endotoxemia. *J Clin Invest* 1992;89:1551–1557.
12. Rabinovici R, Yue T, Farhat M, et al. Platelet activating factor (PAF) and tumor necrosis factor (TNF) interactions in endotoxemic shock: studies with BN 50739, a novel PAF antagonist. *J Pharmacol Exp Ther* 1990;255:256–263.
13. Feuerstein G, Leader P, Siren AL, Braquet P. Protective effect of a PAF-acether antagonist, BN 52021, in trichothecene toxicosis. *Toxicol Lett* 1987;38:271–274.
14. Etienne A, Hecquet F, Guilmard C, Soulard C, Braquet P. Inhibition of rat endotoxin-induced lethality by BN 52021 and BN 52063, compounds with PAF-acether antagonist effect and protease-inhibitory activity. *Int J Tissue React* 1987;9:19–26.
15. Chang S, Fedderson CO, Henson PM, Voekel NF. Platelet activating factor mediates hemodynamic changes and lung injury in endotoxin-treated rats. *J Clin Invest* 1987;79:1498–1509.
16. Myers AK, Robey JW, Price RM. Relationships between tumor necrosis factor, eicosinoids, and platelet-activating factor as mediators of endotoxin-induced shock in mice. *Br J Pharmacol* 1990;99:499–502.
17. Van Zee KJ, Kohno T, Fischer E, Rock C, Moldawer LL, Lowrey SF. Tumor necrosis factor soluble receptors circulate during experimental and clinical inflammation and can protect against excessive tumor necrosis factor-α *in vitro* and *in vivo*. *Proc Natl Acad Sci USA* 1992;89:4845–4849.
18. Mohler KM, Torrance DS, Smith CA, et al. Soluble tumor necrosis factor (TNF) receptors are effective therapeutic agents in lethal endotoxemia and function simultaneously as both TNF carriers and antagonists. *J Immunol* 1993;151:1548–1561.
19. Jin H, Yang R, Marsters SA, et al. Protection against rat endotoxic shock by p55 tumor necrosis factor (TNF) receptor immunoadhesion: comparison with anti-TNF monoclonal antibody. *J Infect Dis* 1994;170:1323–1326.
20. Ashkenzi A, Marsters SA, Capon DJ, et al. Protection against endotoxic shock by a tumor necrosis factor receptor immunoadhesion. *Proc Natl Acad Sci USA* 1991;88:10535–10539.
21. Evans TJ, Moyes D, Carpenter A, et al. Protective effect of 55- but not 75-kd soluble tumor necrosis factor receptor-immunoadhesion G fusion proteins in an animal model of gram-negative sepsis. *J Exp Med* 1994;180:2173–2179.
22. Suitters AJ, Foulkes R, Opal SM, et al. Differential effect of isotype on efficacy of anti-tumor necrosis factor-α chimeric antibodies in experimental septic shock. *J Exp Med* 1994;179:849–856.
23. Bagby GJ, Plessala KJ, Wilson LA, Thompson JJ, Nelson S. Divergent efficacy of antibody to tumor necrosis factor-α in intravascular and peritonitis models. *J Infect Dis* 1991;163:83–88.
24. Mathison JC, Wolfson E, Ulevitch RJ. Participation of tumor necrosis factor in the mediation of gram negative bacterial lipopolysaccharide-induced injury in rabbits. *J Clin Invest* 1988;81:1925–1937.
25. Fiedler VB, Loof I, Sander E, Voehringer V, Galanos C, Fournal MA. Monoclonal antibody to tumor necrosis factor-α prevents lethal endotoxin sepsis in adult rhesus monkeys. *J Lab Clin Med* 1992;120:574–588.

26. Emerson TE, Lindsey DC, Jesmonk GJ, Duerr ML, Fournel MA. Efficacy of monoclonal antibody against tumor necrosis factor-α in an endotoxemic baboon model. *Circ Shock* 1992;38:75–84.

27. Eskandari MK, Bolgos G, Miller C, Nguyen DT, DeForge LE, Remick DG. Anti-tumor necrosis factor antibody therapy fails to prevent lethality after cecal ligation and puncture or endotoxemia. *J Immunol* 1992;9:2724–2730.

28. Silva AT, Bayston KF, Cohen J. Prophylactic and therapeutic effects of a monoclonal antibody to tumor necrosis factor-α in experimental gram-negative shock. *J Infect Dis* 1990;162:421–427.

29. Jesmok G, Lindsey C, Duerr M, Fournel M, Emerson T. Efficacy of monoclonal antibody against human recombinant tumor necrosis factor in *E. coli*–challenged swine. *Am J Pathol* 192;141:1197–1207.

30. Hinswaw LB, Tekamp-Olson P, Chang ACK, et al. Survival of primates in LD100 septic shock following therapy with antibody to tumor necrosis factor (TNF-α). *Circ Shock* 1990;30:279–292.

31. Tracey KJ, Fong Y, Hesse DG, et al. Anti-cachectin/TNF monoclonal antibodies prevent septic shock curing lethal bacteremia. *Nature* 1987; 330:662–664.

32. Hinshaw LB, Emerson TE, Taylor FB, et al. Lethal *Staphylococcus aureus*–induced shock in primates: prevention of death with anti-TNF antibody. *J Trauma* 1992;33:568–573.

33. Opal SM, Cross AS, Kelly NM, et al. Efficacy of a monoclonal antibody directed against tumor necrosis factor in protecting neutropenic rats from lethal infection with *Pseudomonas aeruginosa*. *J Infect Dis* 1990;161:1148–1152.

34. Weil MH, Maclean CD, Fisseher MB, Spink WW. Studies of the circulatory changes in the dog produced by endotoxin from gram-negative micoorganisms. *J Clin Invest* 1956;35:1191–1198.

35. Natanson C, Eichenholz PW, Danner RL, et al. Endotoxin and tumor necrosis factor challenges in dogs simulate the cardiovascular profile of human septic shock. *J Exp Med* 1989;169:823–832.

36. Waage A, Espevik T. Interleukin-1 potentiates the lethal effects of tumor necrosis factor/cachectin in mice. *J Exp Med* 1988;167: 1987–1992.

37. Okusawa S, Gelfand JA, Ikejima T, Connolly RJ, Dinarello CA. Interleukin-1 induces a shock like state in rabbits: synergism with tumor necrosis factor and the effect of cyclooxygenase inhibition. *J Clin Invest* 1988;81:1162–1172.

38. Fisher CJ, Slotman GJ, Opal SM, et al., and the IL-1ra sepsis syndrome study group. Initial evaluation of human recombinant interleukin-1 receptor antagonist in the treatment of sepsis syndrome: a randomized, open-label, placebo-controlled multicenter trial. *Crit Care Med* 1994;22:12–21.

39. Fisher CJ, Dhainaut JF, Opal SM, et al., and the Phase III rhIL-1ra Sepsis Syndrome Study Group. Recombinant human interleukin-1 receptor antagonist in the treatment of patients with sepsis syndrome. *JAMA* 1994;271:1836–1843.

40. Opal SM, Fisher CJ, Dhainaut JF. Confirmatory interleukin-1 receptor antagonist trial in severe sepsis: a phase III, randomized, double-blind, placebo-controlled, multicenter trial. *Crit Care Med* 1997;25: 1115–1124.

41. Fisher CJ, Agosti JM, Opal SM, et al. Treatment of septic shock with the tumor necrosis factor receptor: Fc fusion protein. *N Engl J Med* 1996;334:1697–1702.

42. Abraham E, Glauser MP, Butler T, et al. p55 tumor necrosis factor receptor fusion protein in the treatment of patients with severe sepsis and septic shock. *JAMA* 1997;277:1531–1538.

43. Kay CA. Can better measures of cytokine responses be obtained to guide cytokine inhibition? Knoll AG, Ludwigshafen, Germany. Presentation and handout. Cambridge Health Institutes' Designing Better Drugs & Clinical Trials for Sepsis/SIRS: Reducing Mortality to Patients and Suppliers. Washington, DC, February 20–21.

44. Reinhart K, Wiegand-Löhnert GF, Kaul M, et al., and the MAK 195F Sepsis Study Group. Assessment of the safety and efficacy of the monoclonal anti-tumor necrosis factor antibody fragment, MAK 195F, in patients with sepsis and septic shock: a multicenter, randomized, placebo-controlled, dose-ranging study. *Crit Care Med* 1996;24: 733–742.

45. Fisher CJ, Opal SM, Dhainaut JF, et al., and the CB0006 Sepsis Syndrome Study Group. Influence of an anti-tumor necrosis factor monoclonal antibody on cytokine levels in patients with sepsis. *Crit Care Med* 1993;21:318–327.

46. Dhainaut JFA, Vincent JL, Richard C, et al., and the CDP571 Sepsis

47. Abraham E, Wunderink R, Silverman H, et al. Efficacy and safety of monoclonal antibody to human tumor necrosis factor-α in patients with sepsis syndrome. *JAMA* 1995;273:934–941.

48. Cohen J, Carlet J. INTERSEPT: an international, multicenter, placebo-controlled trial of monoclonal antibody to human tumor necrosis factor-α in patients with sepsis. *Crit Care Med* 1996;26:1431–1440.

49. Rodell TC, Foster C. Sepsis data show negative trend in second phase II sepsis trial. Press Release, July 18, 1995. Cortech Inc., 7000 North Broadway, Denver, CO 80821.

50. Fein AM, Bernard GR, Criner GJ, et al. Treatment of severe systemic inflammatory response syndrome and sepsis with a novel bradykinin antagonist, Deltbant (CP-0127). *JAMA* 1997;277:482–487.

51. Dhainaut JFA, Tenaillon A, Tulzo YL, et al. Platelet-activating factor receptor antagonist BN 52021 in the treatment of severe sepsis: a randomized, double-blind, placebo-controlled, multicenter clinical trial. *Crit Care Med* 1994;22:1720–1728.

52. Dhainaut JF, Tenaillon A, Hemmer M, et al. and the BN 52021 Sepsis Study Group. Confirming phase III clinical trial to study the efficacy of a PAF antagonist, BN 52021, in reducing mortality of patients with severe gram-negative infection. *Am J Resp Crit Care Med* 1995;151: A447(abst).

53. Bernard GR, Wheeler AP, Russell JA, et al. The effects of ibuprofen on the physiology and survival of patients with sepsis. *N Engl J Med* 1997;336:912–918.

54. Haupt MT, Jastremski MS, Clemmer TP, Metz CA, Goris GB, and the Ibuprofen Study Group. Effect of ibuprofen in patients with severe sepsis: a randomized, double-blind, multicenter study. *Crit Care Med* 1991;19:1339–1347.

55. Bernard GR, Reines HD, Halushka PV. Prostacyclin and thromboxane A2 formation is increased in human sepsis syndrome. *Am Rev Respir Dis* 1991;144:1095–1101.

56. Cronin L, Cook DJ, Carlet J, et al. Corticosteroid treatment for sepsis: a critical appraisal and meta-analysis of the literature. *Crit Care Med* 1997;23:1430–1439.

57. Lefering RNEAM. Steroid controversy in sepsis and septic shock: a meta-analysis. *Crit Care Med* 1995;23:1294–1303.

58. Abraham E, and North American Sepsis Trial II (NORSEPT II) Study Group. Effect of a murine monoclonal antibody (TNF-mAb) in patients with septic shock. International Conference of Chemotherapy, Sidney, Australia, July 3, 1997 (abst).

59. Luce JM, Montgomery AB, Marks JD, Turner J, Metz CA, Murray JF. Ineffectiveness of high-dose methylprednisolone in preventing parenchymal lung injury and improving mortality in patients with septic shock. *Am Rev Respir Dis* 1988;138:62–68.

60. The Veterans Administration Systemic Sepsis Cooperative Study Group. Effect of high-dose glucocorticoid therapy on mortality in patients with clinical signs of systemic sepsis. *N Engl J Med* 1987; 317:659–665.

61. Bone RC, Fisher CJ, Clemmer TP, Slotman GJ, Metz CA, Balk RA, and the Methylprednisolone Severe Sepsis Study Group. A controlled trial of high-dose methylprednisolone in the treatment of severe sepsis and septic shock. *N Engl J Med* 1987;317:653–658.

62. Sprung CL, Caralis PV, Marcial EH, et al. The effects of high-dose corticosteroids in patients with septic shock. *N Engl J Med* 1984;311: 1137–1143.

63. Thompson WL, Gurley HT, Lutz BA, Jackson DL, Kvols LK, Morris IA. Inefficacy of glucocorticoids in shock (double-blind study). *Clin Res* 1976;24:258A(abst).

64. Lucas CE, Ledgerwood AM. The cardiopulmonary response to massive doses of steroids in patients with septic shock. *Arch Surg* 1984; 119:537–541.

65. Schumer W. Steroids in the treatment of clinical septic shock. *Ann Surg* 1976;184:333–339.

66. Klastersky J, Cappell R, Debusscher L. Effectiveness of betamethasone in management of severe infections. *N Engl J Med* 1971;284: 1248–1250.

67. Bennett IL, Finland M, Hamborger M, Kass EH, Lepper M, Waisbren BA. The effectiveness of hydrocortisone in the management of severe infection. *JAMA* 1963;183:462–465.

68. Ziegler EJ, McCutchan JA, Fierer J, et al. Treatment of gram-negative

bacteremia and shock with human antiserum to a mutant *Escherichia coli. N Engl J Med* 1982;307:1225–1230.

69. McCutchan JA, Wolf JL, Ziegler EL, Braude AI. Ineffectiveness of single-dose human antiserum to core glycolipid (*Escherichia coli* J5) for prophylaxis of bacteremic, gram-negative infection in patients with prolonged neutropenia. *Schweiz Med Wochenschr* 1983;113 (suppl):40–55.

70. Baumgartner JD, Glauser MP, McCutchan JA, et al. Prevention of gram-negative shock and death in surgical patients by antibody to endotoxin core glycolipid. *Lancet* 1985;11:59–63.

71. The J5 Study Group. Treatment of severe infectious purpura in children with human plasma from donors immunized with *Escherichia coli* J5: a prospective double-blind study. *J Infect Dis* 1992;165: 695–701.

72. Calandra T, Glauser MP, Schellekens J, Verhoef J, and the Swiss-Dutch J5 Immunoglobulin Study Group. Treatment of gram-negative septic shock with human IgG antibody to *Escherichia coli* J5: a prospective, double-blind, randomized trial. *J Infect Dis* 1988;158: 312–319.

73. The Intravenous Immunoglobulin Collaborative Study Group. Prophylactic intravenous administration of standard immune globulin as compared with core-lipopolysaccharide immune globulin in patients at high risk of postsurgical infections. *N Engl J Med* 1992;327: 234–240.

74. Greenman RL, Scein RMH, Martin MA, et al., and the XOMA Sepsis Study Group. A controlled clinical trial of E5 murine monoclonal IgM antibody to endotoxin in the treatment of gram-negative sepsis. *JAMA* 1991;266:1097–1102.

75. Bone RC, Balk RA, Fein AM, et al., and the E5 Sepsis Study Group. A second large controlled clinical study of E5, a monoclonal antibody to endotoxin: results of a prospective, multicenter, randomized, controlled trial. *Crit Care Med* 1995;23:994–1006.

76. Ziegler EJ, Fisher CJ, Sprung CL, et al., and the HA-1A Sepsis Study Group. Treatment of gram-negative bacteremia and septic shock with HA-1A human monoclonal antibody against endotoxin. *N Engl J Med* 1991;324:429–436.

77. McClosky RV, Straube RC, Sanders C, Smith SM, Smith CR, and the CHESS trial Study Group. Treatment of septic shock with human monoclonal antibody HA-1A. *Ann Intern Med* 1994;121:1–5.

78. Elinger JH, Seyde WC, Longnecker DE. Methylprednisolone plus ibuprofen increases mortality in septic rats. *Circ Shock* 1984;14:208.

79. Pitcairn M, Schuler J, Erve PR, Holtzman S, Schumer W. Glucocorticoid and antibiotic effect on experimental gram negative bacteremic shock. *Arch Surg* 1975;110:1012–1015.

80. Fabian TC, Patterson R. Steroid therapy in septic shock. Survival study in a laboratory model. *Am Surg* 1982;48:614–617.

81. Hinshaw LB, Beller-Todd BK, Archer LT, Benjamen B, Flournoy DJ, Passey R. Effectiveness of steroid antibiotic treatment in primates administered LD$_{100}$ *Escherichia coli. Ann Surg* 1981;194:51–56.

82. Hinshaw LB, Archer LT, Beller-Todd BK, Benjamen B, Flournoy DJ, Passey R. Survival of primates in lethal septic shock following delayed treatment with steroid. *Circ Shock* 1981;8:291–300.

83. Hinshaw LB, Flournoy DJ, Archer LT, White GL, Phillips RW. Recovery from lethal *Escherichia coli* shock. *Surg Gynecol Obstet* 1979; 545–553.

84. Hinshaw LB, Archer LT, Beller-Todd BK, et al. Survival of primates in LD$_{100}$ septic shock following steroid/antibiotic therapy. *J Surg Res* 1980;151–170.

85. White GL, Archer LT, Beller-Todd BK, Hinshaw LB. Increased survival with methylprednisolone treatment in canine endotoxin shock. *J Surg Res* 1978;25:357–364.

86. Beller-Todd BK, Archer LT, Passey R, Flournoy DJ, Hinshaw LB. Effectiveness of modified steroid-antibiotic therapies for lethal sepsis in the dog. *Arch Surg* 1983;118:1293–1299.

87. Schefer CF, Brackett DJ, Wilson MF. The benefits of corticosteroid given after the onset of hypotension during endotoxin shock in the conscious rat. *Adv Shock Res* 1983;10:183–194.

88. Robson HG, Cluff LE. Experimental pneumococcal and staphylococ-

cal sepsis: the effects of hydrocortisone and phenoxybenzamine upon mortality rate. *J Clin Invest* 1966;45:1432.

89. Ottoson J, Brandberg A, Erikson B, Hedman L, Davidson I, Soderberg R. Experimental septic shock: effects of corticosteroids. *Circ Shock* 1982;9:571–577.

90. Hinshaw LB, Coalson JJ, Benjamen BA, et al. *Escherichia coli* shock in the baboon and the response to adrenocorticosteroid treatment. *Surg Gynecol Obstet* 1978;147:545–557.

91. Balis J, Patterson JF, Shelly SA, Larson CH, Fareed J, Gerber LI. Glucocorticoid and antibiotic effects on hepatic microcirculation and associated host responses. *Lab Invest* 1979;55–65.

92. Lillehei RC, Lonerbeam JK, Bloch JH. Physiology and therapy of bacteremic shock: experimental and clinical observations. *Am J Cardiol* 1963;599–613.

93. Schuler JJ, Erve PR, Schumer W. Glucocorticoid effects on hepatic carbohydrate metabolism in the endotoxin shocked monkey. *Ann Surg* 1975;183:345–352.

94. Greisman SE, DuBuy JB, Woodward CL. Experimental gram-negative bacterial sepsis: prevention of mortality not preventable by antibiotics alone. *Infect Immun* 1979;538–576.

95. Greisman SE. Experimental gram negative bacterial sepsis: optimal methylprenisolone requirements for prevention of mortality not preventable by antibiotics alone. *Proc Soc Exp Biol Med* 1982;170: 436–442.

96. Teng NNH, Kaplan HS, Hebert JM. Protection against gram-negative bacteremia and endotoxemia with human monoclonal IgM antibodies. *Proc Natl Acad Sci USA* 1985;82:1790–1794.

97. Ziegler EJ, Teng NNH, Douglas H, Wunderlich A, Berger HJ, Bolmer SD. Treatment of *Pseudomonas* bacteremia in neutropenic rabbits with human monoclonal IgM antibody against *E. coli* lipid A. *Clin Res* 1987;35:J-S(abst).

98. Romula RL, Palardy JE, Opal SM. Efficacy of anti-endotoxin monoclonal antibody E5 alone or in combination with ciprofloxacin in neutropenic rats with *Pseudomonas* sepsis. *J Infect Dis* 1993;167: 126–130.

99. Baumgartner JD, Heumann D, Gerain J, Weinbreck P, Grau GE, Glauser MP. Association between protective efficacy of anti-lipopolysaccharide (LPS) antibodies and suppression of LPS-induced tumor necrosis factor-α and interleukin-6. *J Exp Med* 1990;171:896.

100. Chen TY, Zapol WM, Greene E, Robinson DR, Rubin RH. Protective effects of E5, an anti-endotoxin monoclonal antibody, in the ovine pulmonary circulation. *J Appl Physiol* 1993;75:126–130.

101. Wheeler AP, Hardie WD, Bernard G. Studies of an anti-endotoxin antibody in preventing the physiologic changes of endotoxemia in awake sheep. *Am Rev Respir Dis* 1990;142:775–781.

102. Quezado ZMN, Natanson C, Alling DW, et al. A controlled trial of HA-1A in a canine model of gram-negative septic shock. *JAMA* 1993; 269:2221–2227.

103. Gazzono-Santoro H, Parant JB, Wood OM, et al. Reactivity of E5 monoclonal antibody to smooth lipopolysaccharides. In: *Program and Abstracts of the 31st Interscience Conference on Antimicrobial Agents and Chemotherapy, Chicago, Sept. 29–Oct. 2, 1991.* Washington, DC: American Society of Microbiology, 1991:230(abst).

104. Baumgartner JD. Immunotherapy with antibodies to core lipopolysaccharide: a critical appraisal. *Infect Dis Clin North Am* 1991;5:915–917.

105. Warren HS, Amato SF, Fitting C, et al. Assessment of ability of murine and human antilipid A monoclonal antibodies to bind and neutralize lipopolysaccharide. *J Exp Med* 1993;177:89–97.

106. Chin JKS, Pollack M, Guelde G, Koles NL, Miller M, Evans ME. Lipopolysaccharide (LPS)-reactive monoclonal antibodies fail to inhibit LPS-induced tumor necrosis factor secretion by mouse-derived macrophages. *J Infect Dis* 1989;159:872–880.

107. Sevransky JE, Shaked GNA, Levitzki A, et al. Tyrphostin AG 556 improves survival and reduces multiorgan failure in canine *Escherichia coli* peritonitis. *J Clin Invest* 1997;99:1966–1973.

108. Leturcq DJ, Moriarty AM, Talbott G, et al. Winn RK, Martin TR, Ulevitch RJ. Antibodies against CD14 protect primates from endotoxinshock. *J Clin Invest* 1996;98:1533–1538.

Inflammation: Basic Principles and Clinical Correlates,
3rd ed., edited by John I. Gallin and Ralph Snyderman.
Lippincott Williams & Wilkins, Philadelphia © 1999.

CHAPTER 62

Granulomatous Inflammation:

Host Antimicrobial Defense in the Tissues in Visceral Leishmaniasis

Henry W. Murray

Recognized under the microscope more than a century ago as histopathologically distinct, granulomatous inflammation represents a specialized tissue reaction now known to be remarkably complex. While often considered associated with a select group of infections, it is quite clear that various forms of the granulomatous response can be triggered by a remarkably diverse group of signals (Table 62-1) (1–10). In addition, given the proper stimulus (exogenous, endogenous, microbial, or unrelated to infection), sufficient time, and an immunologically intact host, granulomatous inflammation can develop in virtually any organ or tissue, including the vasculature. The morphologic culmination of this reaction, the granuloma, is a metabolically and enzymatically active secretory structure (2,3,6,7) in which multiple effector cells, an array of cell-derived soluble factors, and any inflammatory mechanism can be brought together and focused.

The capacity to assemble this type of inflammatory microenvironment endows the host with the important homeostatic ability to initially contain and then ideally destroy the target stimulus within the tissues. In some instances, however, the stimulus is not entirely degraded, and although not usually considered optimal from the perspective of host antimicrobial defense, the attainment of quiescence (walling-off) may be the maximum tissue effect achieved. Moreover, this latter result may succeed in productively immunizing the host, thus providing the capacity to resist reinfection. The final expression of the granuloma's antimicrobial effects (early containment, destruction and removal, or eventual walling-off) likely

depends on several factors including both the host and the stimulus. Nonetheless, the ability to assemble granulomas is probably critical for defense against a wide spectrum of pathogenic microorganisms. For example, granulomas appear especially important in host control over certain pathogens that have evolved to produce asymptomatic but lifelong, chronic intracellular infection. It is also possible that some of the same effects of granulomatous inflammation (early containment or perhaps destruction) may be locally active against certain tumor cells as well (11,12).

Table 62-1 lists disorders associated with granuloma formation (1–22). Much of the relevant clinical (human) data has been derived from studying liver biopsies (1,9,10,14–22). As made clear by Table 62-1, stimuli other than infection or cancer, including chemicals, toxins, drugs, and identified or unidentified antigens, also provoke a granulomatous reaction. Irrespective of the trigger, this response presumably evolved to contain and limit injury, and ultimately led to tissue repair. Thus, most granulomas are not necrotic and do not show caseation. However, any homeostatic inflammatory response, including granulomatosis, can turn aberrant, escape the control normally exerted by dampening mechanisms (likely induced simultaneously), and propagate tissue injury either in a targeted organ or in a generalized fashion (13). Caseous necrosis, tissue liquefaction, and cavity formation in progressive tuberculosis reflect at least in part unregulated granulomatous inflammation (23,24). While inciting triggers have not been identified in disorders such as sarcoidosis, Crohn's disease, and most forms of vasculitis, widespread granulomas in these diseases likely reflect unrelenting antigenic stimulation rather than a failure of compensatory, dampening mechanisms (13).

H. W. Murray: Department of Medicine, Cornell University Medical College, New York, New York 10021.

TABLE 62-1. *Disorders and agents reported to provoke epithelioid granulomatous inflammation in various organs, primarily the liver*

Disease category	Specific disorder or agent[a]
Infection	
Parasitic	Schistosomiasis, visceral and cutaneous leishmaniasis, amebiasis, pneumocystosis, visceral larval migrans, ascariasis
Bacterial	Typhoid fever, brucellosis, tularemia, listeriosis, yersiniosis, actinomycosis, cat scratch disease, endocarditis, Whipple's disease, nocardiosis, osteomyelitis, abdominal abscess
Mycobacterial	Tuberculosis, atypical mycobacterial infections, tuberculoid leprosy
Viral	Cytomegalovirus, Epstein-Barr, influenza B, Sendai
Fungal	Histoplasmosis, coccidioidomycosis, blastomycosis, cryptococcosis, aspergillosis, candidiasis
Other	Q fever, lymphogranuloma venereum, syphilis
Neoplasia	Hodgkin's disease, lymphoma, adenocarcinoma, hypernephroma, chronic myelogenous leukemia
Inflammation	Sarcoidosis, inflammatory bowel disease, vasculitis and connective tissue diseases (e.g., Wegener's granulomatosis, polyarteritis nodosa, temporal arteritis, rheumatoid arthritis, allergic vasculitis), extrinsic allergic alveolitis, psoriasis with gout, erythema nodosum, hypersensitivity pneumonitis (e.g., fungi, bacteria, animal proteins, isocyanates)
Drugs	Sulfonamides, allopurinol, phenylbutazone, phenytoin, isoniazid, penicillin, methyldopa, hydralazine, procainamide, halothane, cephalexin, procarbazine, diazepam, methotrexate, oral contraceptives
Chemicals or toxins	Starch, talc, Freund's complete adjuvant, beryllium, zirconium, aluminum, titanium, barium sulfate, oil (mineral, paraffin, contrast media), carbon, lipids, mycobacterial and bacterial cell wall extracts and residues, muramyl dipeptide, immune complexes, sutures, glass coverslips
Hepatic and biliary tract disease	Primary biliary cirrhosis, idiopathic cirrhosis, hepatitis (e.g., acute viral [hepatitis C], chronic active, alcoholic), pericholangitis, fatty liver, lipogranulomas (e.g., associated with alcohol abuse, diabetes, obesity, malnutrition)

[a]Inclusion on this list does not imply that the specified disorder or agent commonly induces granuloma formation; many of the listed disorders and agents are infrequently associated with tissue granulomas (1–21). For example, in the United States (1,14–17) and United Kingdom (9,18–20), the most commonly identified inducers of granuloma formation in the liver are tuberculosis, sarcoidosis, primary biliary cirrhosis, and histoplasmosis; schistosomiasis and tuberculosis are the most common inducers in Saudi Arabia (21).

GRANULOMATOUS INFLAMMATION

Histologic definitions of granulomatous inflammation and the granuloma differ widely, and elaborate classification schemes have been devised (2–4,7,10). However, most investigators would agree that these focal collections of aggregated cells represent a chronic rather than an acute form of inflammation in which, for example, polymorphonuclear leukocytes are not as prominent as in an abscess or are altogether absent. Instead, the mononuclear phagoctye predominates in the granuloma, with the resident tissue macrophage promptly joined by the influxing blood monocyte. With time, and depending on the inflammatory stimulus, these cells move together and fuse into central cores, take on additional epithelioid cell characteristics and secretory activities (2,3,7), and develop into discrete foci. With most foreign body–type granulomas, cellular assembly typically goes no further. In contrast, in immunologically active (epithelioid-type) granulomas, additional cells, primarily T lymphocytes, are recruited over time. In some instances, plasma cells, B cells, and eosinophils may be attracted as well. The interdigitating presence of T cells among aggregated mononuclear phagocytes, however, is the main feature distinguishing the specialized epithelioid granuloma from its foreign body counterpart. The central regions of either type of tissue reaction may then become populated with multinucleated giant cells via fusion of mononuclear phagocytes. Multinucleated giant cells are classified as foreign body type or Langhans type, depending on the arrangement of cell nuclei. Both forms of giant cells may coexist in the same focus (3).

THE FUNCTIONALLY ACTIVE GRANULOMA

Of much more significance to the host, however, is how thoroughly the fused macrophage cores containing the inciting stimulus come to be infiltrated and/or encircled by tissue-homing blood monocytes and cytokine-secreting T cells, and how well such cells are retained (2,24–26). Thus, from the perspective of host defense, the well-developed, mature granuloma is not simply an inert collection of fused mononuclear phagocytes. Rather, granulomatous inflammation in general and specifically the functionally active host defense granuloma require complex chemoattractant mechanisms (27–51) resulting in carefully directed and focused assembly of at least two groups of cells: (a) antimicrobial effector cells [e.g., influxing blood monocytes, natural killer (NK) cells, cytotoxic T cells]; and (b) secretory cells (T cells, NK cells, endothelial cells, fibroblasts) fully competent in expressing and delivering activating signals. Although monocytes and macrophages are the principal targets for such activating signals (e.g., cytokines) (52,53), they also generate similar activating signals themselves (3,13,23, 24,54). The latter likely include critical homeostatic antimicrobial and antineoplastic factors such as interleukin-12 (IL-12), tumor necrosis factor-α (TNF-α), IL-1, and a diverse group of chemokines (31,55,56).

INACTIVATION OF GRANULOMATOUS INFLAMMATION

Mechanisms are also in place to inhibit granulomatous inflammation. These mechanisms suppress granuloma formation should it become excessive, help to control secondary tissue injury in a compensatory fashion, and eventually cause granulomas to involute once the inciting stimulus has been rendered inactive. Identification of the signals that naturally terminate granulomatous inflammation (and associated delayed-type hypersensitivity) would be particularly important and perhaps of therapeutic benefit in disorders such as tuberculosis, sarcoidosis, and schistosomiasis, in which the intense host response may lead to tissue destruction and/or pathologic degrees of fibrosis during repair (3,13,23,58–60). Conversely, it is also possible that compensatory dampening mechanisms may develop prematurely, accelerate inappropriately, overshoot, or become chronically dysregulated. Aberrant responses such as these might be important immunopathogenetically since they could impair host defense at the tissue level and serve to perpetuate infection.

ASPECTS TO CONSIDER IN GRANULOMATOUS INFLAMMATION

In addition to *Mycobacterium tuberculosis*, perhaps the best-studied of the granuloma-inducing microorganisms (23,24), there are many other clinically relevant microbial stimuli for granuloma induction (Table 62-1). Accordingly, there are an array of experimental models devoted to granuloma formation in which basic research has addressed cell recruitment and trafficking, the development and activity of the epithelioid cell, secretory behavior and growth factor effects within the granuloma, and molecular mechanisms involving transcription factors, receptor expression, and cell-to-cell and intracellular signaling; such topics have been addressed elsewhere (3,7,13,27,31,61,61a).

This chapter focuses on one experimental model with clear-cut clinical correlations, the granulomatous tissue response in the liver caused by the intracellular protozoan *Leishmania donovani* (52,62–76). These studies in experimental visceral leishmaniasis along with those reported from other laboratories (54,77–83) reemphasize two particular features relevant to other infectious diseases as well: first, the complex interaction of multiple cells, cytokines, and related mechanisms required in the tissues for successful host intracellular antimicrobial defense;

and second, that granulomatous inflammation can be pharmacologically manipulated in the tissues in therapeutic favor of the infected host.

HUMAN VISCERAL LEISHMANIASIS

Leishmaniasis is transmitted by the bite of an infected sandfly, and can be expressed clinically as cutaneous, mucocutaneous, or visceral disease. In the case of visceralizing strains, primarily *L. donovani*, *L. chagasi*, and *L. infantum*, the intracellular amastigote form of the parasite is largely found within macrophages of the liver, spleen, and bone marrow; lymph nodes and occasionally other tissues may also be involved. If symptomatic visceral leishmaniasis (kala-azar) develops, common clinical features include fever, weight loss, hepatomegaly, and marked splenomegaly; hypergammaglobulinemia and pancytopenia are frequent laboratory abnormalities (84). The diagnosis of visceral infection is usually made by microscopic examination of splenic, bone marrow, or lymph node aspirates that demonstrate parasitized macrophages containing replicating intracellular amastigotes (Fig. 62-1).

Immunologic Responses in Clinically Expressed Infection

During acute symptomatic visceral infection, delayed-type hypersensitivity skin testing typically reveals cutaneous anergy, circulating CD4 cells may be reduced in number and function, and *in vitro* testing can demonstrate a variety of CD4-cell–associated defects and aberrant responses (84–98). The latter include downregulated secretion of activating, Th1-cell–type host defense

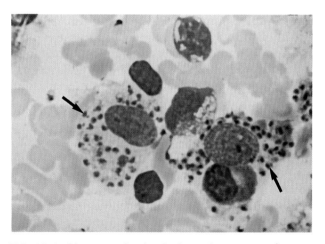

FIG. 62-1. Giemsa-stained splenic aspirate smear from an *L. donovani*–infected Indian patient with splenomegaly and symptomatic kala-azar. Two splenic macrophages in the center of the field contain numerous intracellular amastigotes *(arrows)* (×630).

cytokines [interferon-γ (IFN-γ), IL-2], and enhanced generation of deactivating, Th2-cell–associated cytokines including IL-4 and IL-10 (84–96). Similar abnormalities have also been detected in the tissues and in the peripheral circulation of infected patients in some but not all studies (97–99). CD8 cells may contribute to the Th2-cell–associated response (100). Thus, progressive visceral infection may represent the clinical expression of a net Th2 cell state associated with an overshadowed and therefore ineffective Th1 cell response (99).

The relevance of impaired IFN-γ secretion and/or reduced target cell responsiveness to IFN-γ (101) relates directly to unrestrained intracellular parasite replication in the tissues since IFN-γ, likely induced by IL-12 together with IL-2 (55,68,76), is principally responsible for activating macrophages to kill ingested *Leishmania* (102,103). This conclusion led to testing IFN-γ as therapy in kala-azar (104). TNF is capable of interacting with IFN-γ to activate macrophages and is therefore also thought to be an antileishmanial cytokine (69,105). TNF is often detected at high levels in the serum of untreated patients ill with overt kala-azar (106,107); however, infection is not controlled. Thus, in the presence of impaired secretion of or responsiveness to IFN-γ or other effects of a Th2 cell mechanism, TNF may serve more as a marker of the intense but ineffective soluble inflammatory response that develops in patients symptomatic with visceral infection.

Histologic Reactions

In contrast to the wealth of data that has been generated about the immunology of human visceral leishmaniasis, modern analytical techniques have not been brought to bear on the mechanisms of the tissue reaction in human kala-azar. Tissue imprints and smears of organ aspirates, the typical clinical samples available, yield little specific histologic information. However, previous studies have illustrated that human visceral leishmaniasis is indeed a granulomatous disease, and have provided evidence suggesting that the presence of granulomas correlates with control over infection in tissues such as the liver (108–113). Conversely, in patients with progressive, uncontrolled (symptomatic) kala-azar and in fatal infection, mature granulomas do not appear to develop (108–113).

Asymptomatic and Subclinical Infection

In the past, it was assumed that once a person was infected with *L. donovani* or other visceralizing strains, overtly progressive disease almost always followed and, left untreated, was typically fatal. These assumptions, however, overlooked isolated clinical observations that clearly documented the occurrence of asymptomatic infection. In one such study, liver biopsies demonstrated epithelioid-type granulomas in each infected but asymptomatic patient examined (109,110). More recent work

has advanced these studies by making it clear that in most areas of the world the majority of exposed individuals either remain entirely asymptomatic or develop self-limited, oligosymptomatic disease that resolves without treatment (93,94,114–117). The best correlate of spontaneous control of visceral infection appears to be the capacity to develop and express a CD4-cell–dependent Th1 type response (93,94). Estimates suggest that in some regions as many as 60% to 80% of patients infected with visceralizing strains of *Leishmania* remain asymptomatic (93,94,114–117).

Recrudescence

Nevertheless, in patients with subclinical infection as well as in those who are treated for symptomatic kala-azar, lifelong infection likely persists and remains capable of reactivating. Recrudescence may develop spontaneously for unclear reasons or if a future T-cell deficiency state intervenes (84). For example, patients with previously controlled visceral infection who are subsequently rendered T-cell deficient by advanced human immunodeficiency virus (HIV) disease or corticosteroid therapy are at predictably high risk for reactivated kala-azar (118–120). In acquired immune deficiency syndrome (AIDS) patients, visceral leishmaniasis is often diffuse with multiorgan involvement, and there is little or no evidence of macrophage activation (Fig. 62-2), granuloma-

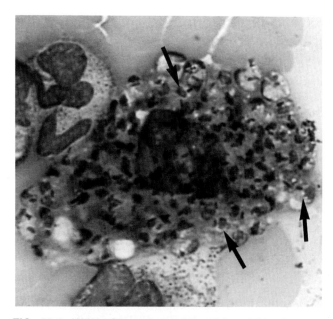

FIG. 62-2. Wright-Giemsa stained peripheral blood smear from a patient with advanced AIDS and diffuse reactivated visceral leishmaniasis (164) showing a large, remarkably heavily parasitized macrophage-like cell. Amastigotes *(arrows)* show characteristic nuclear morphology and rod-like kinetoplast (×1000). (Photograph prepared by Janice Godwin, Division of Hematology-Oncology, New York Hospital-Cornell Medical Center, New York, NY.)

tous inflammation, or functional granulomas in heavily parasitized tissues. Histologic evidence of limited granuloma formation, however, has been reported in some HIV-infected patients with other types of opportunistic infections despite the presence of the fully established AIDS T-cell defect (120–123). In addition, experimental observations also support the notion of T-cell–independent granuloma development (124–128) presumably reflecting auxiliary pathways. However, since neither AIDS patients nor T-cell–deficient animals readily control granuloma-inducing types of infections, the simple histologic presence of granulomatous inflammation should not necessarily be equated with intact antimicrobial function.

EXPERIMENTAL VISCERAL LEISHMANIASIS

A Basic Model of Acquired Resistance

L. donovani infection in BALB/c mice is a model of granulomatous inflammation and acquired resistance that probably resembles human visceral infection in the 60% to 80% of patients who show spontaneous control. In BALB/c mice, initial innate susceptibility following intravenous challenge gives way after 4 weeks to control over visceral parasite replication and by week 8 to resolution with subsequent establishment of a low-level state of chronic intracellular infection (Fig. 62-3) (129). Thereafter, these animals express solid immunity and resist rechallenge (62,67). Quiescent infection in the tissues of immune mice, however, can be induced to reactivate with immunosuppressive manipulation (130).

Participating Cells

The capacity to control *L. donovani* in the liver does not involve NK cells but is strictly T-cell dependent, requiring both antigen-sensitized CD4 and CD8 cells acting in concert (Table 62-2) (62,64,66). Athymic (nude) BALB/c mice, for example, permit uncontrolled and extraordinary visceral replication that is not appreciably reduced by reconstitution with either CD4 or CD8 cells alone (62,64). In normal mice, secretion of activating lymphokines by CD4 and perhaps CD8 cells is involved in control of infection (62,64,65,68); cytolytic destruction of parasitized resident macrophages [e.g., Kupffer cells in the case of the liver (62)] by sensitized T cells may also take place (63). The latter effect might serve to liberate amastigotes for a second round of ingestion and killing by more competent, activated mononuclear phagocytes. Influxing blood monocytes likely represent these latter cells, are critically involved in acquired resistance, and probably function not only as cytokine-generators (69,76) but as the final effector cells in the overall antileishmanial host defense response (52). CD4 and CD8 cells and immigrant monocytes are all readily assembled to support granuloma formation in the *L. donovani*–infected liver (63) (see below).

Activating Endogenous Cytokines

Initial control over visceral parasite replication, resolution of infection, and maintenance of relapse-free immunity also involves an array of well-recognized host defense cytokines (Table 62-2) (62,65,68–70,75,76,101,130). These critical factors probably act together to help attract necessary effector cells to the tissues, amplify their own secretory and inflammatory activities, induce macrophage/monocyte activation, and then perpetuate microbicidal effects. The latter appear to be mainly induced by phagocyte-derived reactive oxygen and toxic nitrogen intermediates (75,80,102,103,131,132). In the BALB/c mouse model, initial acquisition of resistance is associated

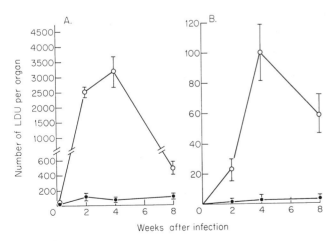

FIG. 62-3. Course of visceral *L. donovani* infection in the liver *(left)* and spleen *(right)* after intravenous challenge in innately susceptible BALB/c mice *(open circle)*. Resistance is acquired after week 4. Contrasting results in innately resistant DBA/2 mice *(filled circle)* highlight the susceptibility of BALB/c mice. LDU, Leishman-Donovan unit (129). (From ref. 129, with permission.)

TABLE 62-2. *Mononuclear cells and endogenous cytokines active in acquired resistance and granuloma assembly in experimental visceral leishmaniasis in BALB/c mice*

Cell or cytokine	Acquired resistance	Granuloma formation
CD4 cells	R	R
CD8 cells	R	R
NK cells	NR	NR
Blood monocytes	R	R
IL-12	R	R
IL-2	R	R
IFN-γ	R	R
TNF-α	R	NR
GM-CSF	R	NR
IL-1	NR	NR

GM-CSF, granulocyte-macrophage colony-stimulating factor; IFN, interferon; IL, interleukin; NK, natural killer; NR, not required; R, required; TNF, tumor necrosis factor.
Data from refs. 52, 64–66, 68–70, 75, and 76.

with induction of multicytokine mRNA expression in infected tissue (75,101), and requires an endogenous Th1-cell–associated cytokine response mediated by IL-12, IL-2, and IFN-γ (65,68,76). Studies carried out in IFN-γ gene knock-out mice have confirmed the requirement for IFN-γ (75). Additional antileishmanial inflammatory effects are also stimulated by locally induced granulocyte-macrophage colony-stimulating factor (GM-CSF) and TNF (69,70,75); endogenous IL-1 does not appear to be involved (69). Once visceral infection comes under control by week 4, the Th1 response involutes, endogenous IL-2 and IFN-γ assume minor and probably nonessential roles (65,68,75,101), and mechanisms largely dependent on TNF emerge and lead to resolution (69,75).

THE TISSUE GRANULOMATOUS REACTION TO INTRACELLULAR L. DONOVANI

Histologic Responses and Effector Cell Assembly in the Development and Expression of Acquired Resistance

Table 62-3 summarizes the overall kinetics of granuloma formation in the liver in this model. Fig. 62-4 illustrates the histologic appearance of the developing tissue reaction as it progresses from parasitized Kupffer cells to mature, functional leishmanicidal granulomas. Injecting BALB/c mice with readily degradable heat-killed L. donovani amastigotes results in no detectable histologic response.

Initial Events

Hours after intravenous inoculation, amastigotes are found in the liver, spleen, and bone marrow within their principal target cell, the resident tissue macrophage. In the liver, the sinusoidal-lining Kupffer cell [positive for F4/80 and Ia (major histocompatibility complex [MHC] class II determinant), negative for M1/70 (Mac-1), capable of ingesting injected colloidal carbon], is the target for L. donovani (62,63). In BALB/c mice, amastigotes begin replicating rapidly such that liver burdens increase by 20- to 25-fold within the first week after challenge (Fig. 62-3) (129). At this time of unrestrained intracellular growth, Kupffer cells become distended with organisms, and except for Kupffer cell fusion at one-third of infected foci (Table 62-3) and occasional granulocytes that later disappear, there is little other cellular reaction at week 1 (Fig. 62-4A,B).

Early Granuloma Development

The earliest sign of the impending granulomatous response is more widespread Kupffer cell fusion accompanied by the arrival of newly recruited inflammatory cells at >30% of infected liver foci by the end of week 2 (Table 62-3) (Fig. 62-4C) (62). At this point, influxing monocytes and T cells appear and all cellular elements at infected foci begin to rapidly increase in number (63). This quantitative effect is also joined at this stage by clear-cut evidence of focusing directed at fused cores of parasitized Kupffer cells. At week 2, the initial CD4:CD8 cell ratio in developing granulomas is 1.5. This ratio is maintained until after week 4, by which time the numbers of CD4 and CD8 cells in the infected liver have increased by 15- and 10-fold, respectively. By week 4, there has also been an overall 12-fold increase in numbers of influxing blood monocytes (63). During this same period, the logarithmic growth of L. donovani in the liver [up to a 50- to 85-fold increase in parasite burden (129)] begins to slow, plateaus, and then declines steeply as effective resistance in the tissues is expressed as leishmanicidal activity (Fig. 62-3).

TABLE 62-3. *Kinetics of the histologic response to experimental L. donovani infection in the liver in normal BALB/c mice.*

Extent of infection and cellular response[a]	Weeks after Infection			
	1	2	4	8
Liver parasite burden (LDU)	908	1867	1664	270
Infected foci (number)	61	86	81	29
No cellular reaction (%)	56	27	7	3
KC fusion alone (%)	38	39	23	17
KC fusion + infiltrate (%)	6	30	48	28
Mature granulomas (%)	0	4	23	52
Uninfected granulomas (number)	0	0	8	36

[a]Liver imprints were used to determine amastigote burdens (expressed as Leishman-Donovan units [LDU] [62]), and the number of discrete infected foci per 50 ×63 microscopic fields was counted in histologic sections. Results are mean values. The cellular reaction at each infected focus was scored as no reaction—unfused Kupffer cells (KC) with no mononuclear cell infiltrate; KC fusion alone; KC fusion with some cellular infiltrate (e.g., early granuloma formation); or mature granulomas—well-organized reaction with a mononuclear cell mantle surrounding a core of parasitized multinucleated (fused) KC (see Fig. 62-4).
From ref. 62, with permission.

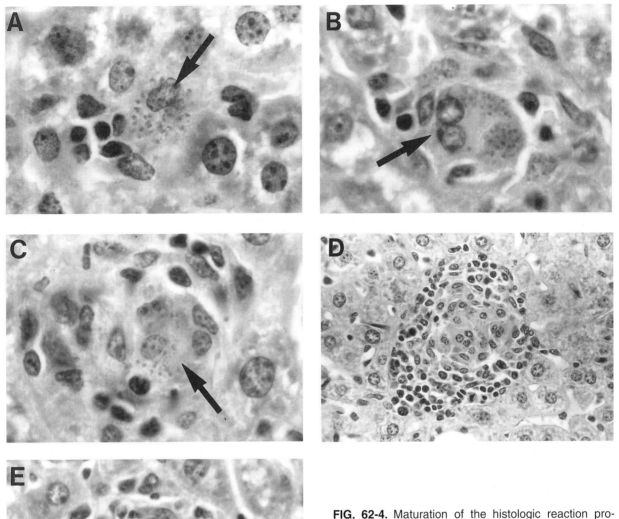

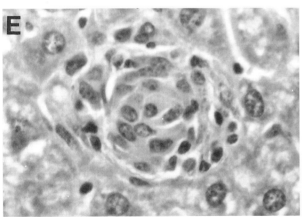

FIG. 62-4. Maturation of the histologic reaction provoked by *L. donovani* infection in the liver in BALB/c mice 1 to 8 weeks after infection. **A** and **B:** Initial parasitization of Kupffer cells (KC) with some KC fusion **(B)** and little cellular reaction (week 1). **C:** Early granuloma assembly as fused parasitized KC begin to attract mononuclear cells (week 2). **D:** Mature granuloma formation with mononuclear cell mantle encircling fused, parasitized Kupffer cell core (week 4) (also, see Fig. 62–5A). **E:** Involuting granulomas devoid of amastigotes (week 8). (**A,B,C** ×500; **D** ×315; **E** ×400). (**B** and **D** from refs. 62 and 65, respectively, with permission.)

Mature Granulomas

At the time resistance is established, the granulomas at the majority of infected foci in the liver consist of a core of fused parasitized Kupffer cells surrounded by a mononuclear cell mantle (Fig. 62-4D). Multinucleated giant cells, likely generated in part from the effects of IFN-γ (133,134), are also present. The mononuclear cell mantle is composed of nearly equal numbers of immigrant monocytes and T cells (63). This tissue response continues to mature after week 4, the critical period during which >80% of parasites are killed and removed.

Resolution of Visceral Infection and Involution of the Granulomatous Response

While initially somewhat slow, the acquired cell-mediated immune response is ultimately efficient as judged by the overall decline in organ parasite burdens largely completed by week 8 (62,129). At week 8, the principal histologic feature in the liver is still the presence of mature granulomas, but many are now devoid of amastigotes by light microscopy (Table 62-3). Scattered, partially developing foci still persist in this transition stage to chronic infection, and they contain easily visualized parasites.

After week 8, however, the majority of foci become smaller and less cellular, and the mononuclear cell mantle is the first structural component of the granuloma to recede (Fig. 62-4E). Compared to week 4, for example, the number of M1/70+ monocytes declines by >50% and the number of CD4 cells decreases by >65% by week 8 (63). Not all cell populations behave the same, however, since CD8 cell numbers remain high. At week 8, the CD4:CD8 cell ratio has declined to 0.4 (63). Thus, during the time of maximal parasite elimination (between weeks 4 and 8), the CD8 cell appears to be the principal effector T cell supporting granuloma maintenance, and it may play a major role in resolution of visceral infection.

Twelve to 18 weeks after the original challenge, only rare Kupffer cells are visibly infected, and the previously intensely inflamed liver shows only scattered aggregates of mononuclear cells. While the actual mechanism(s) of granuloma involution have not been studied, a principal factor is likely to be eradication of the bulk of the parasites. Residual amastigotes that persist in the tissues do not seem quantitatively sufficient nor perhaps in the necessary antigenic form to continue to act as inflammatory stimuli.

Recall of the Granulomatous Response in Resistance to Rechallenge

In studies carried out up to a year after resolution of primary infection, rechallenge of immune BALB/c mice with viable amastigotes results in rapid killing of the new parasite inoculum and a strikingly accelerated granulomatous reaction. The latter is fully expressed in the liver within 1 to 2, rather than 4 to 8, weeks (67). While indistinguishable by light microscopy, recall granulomas differ from those assembled in naive mice since the influx of monocytes and CD4 cells is considerably more modest while the recruitment of CD8 cells is remarkably enhanced (63). The latter observation again points to the likely key antimicrobial and granuloma-forming role for the cytotoxic CD8 cell in these parasitized tissues (135).

FUNCTIONAL ROLE OF EFFECTOR CELLS AND CYTOKINES IN GRANULOMA ASSEMBLY AND ACTIVITIES

Effector Cells

The functional relevance of the histology of acquired resistance to *L. donovani* has been clarified using tissue from mice lacking or depleted of specific effector cells and/or endogenous activating cytokines. Inspection of infected livers from T-cell–deficient nude BALB/c mice confirmed that granuloma formation in this model is T-cell dependent (Fig. 62-5B). Although the initial step, Kupffer cell fusion, did develop in a delayed fashion at about 50% of parasitized foci in nude mice, the tissue reaction failed to proceed further (Table 62-3). Reconstitution experiments demonstrated that CD4 and CD8 cells act together and both are required for mature granuloma development (64); injecting normal animals with cell-depleting anti-CD4 or anti-CD8 confirmed this finding (64). In contrast, depleting NK cells had no effect in normal mice (62,66).

Taking advantage of the differential *in situ* expression of the type 3 complement receptor (CR3) by blood monocytes (present) versus Kupffer cells (absent), monocyte recruitment into infected liver foci was blocked by injection of anti-CR3 monoclonal antibody (52). This treatment abolished granuloma formation, demonstrating that influxing blood monocytes, already identified immunohistochemically as abundant in developing granulomas (63), were critical cellular participants (52). In anti-CR3–treated mice, Kupffer cell fusion was intact; however, there was a remarkable paucity of surrounding lymphocytes (Fig. 62-5C), indicating an additional role for monocytes— directing the tissue recruitment and assembly of influxing CD4 and CD8 T cells. At the same time, as judged by the minimal tissue reaction (other than Kupffer cell fusion) in infected nude mice and in normal animals depleted of either CD4 or CD8 cells, optimal monocyte recruitment appeared to be T-cell dependent as well (62,64). Thus, while macrophage fusion can proceed independently, mature granuloma assembly in response to *L. donovani* is likely governed by the interaction of at least two cell populations, each of which may attract the other, thereby amplifying the tissue reaction.

Endogenous Cytokines

Ten to 14 days after challenge with *L. donovani*, mRNA expression for the following activating, host defense cytokines is induced or enhanced in the livers and/or spleens of BALB/c mice: IL-12, IL-2, IFN-γ, GM-CSF, and TNF (68,70,75,101). IL-4 and IL-10 mRNA expression is also induced, representing the simultaneous stimulation of what may, in this host infected with this particular strain of *Leishmania*, represent a normal dampening Th2-cell–type response (101). In contrast to the extraordinarily aberrant Th2 reaction that *L. major* triggers in BALB/c mice (136,137) and as discussed more fully below, the Th2 cell response in this model is either not functional or more likely is rapidly overshadowed by the simultaneously induced Th1 cell mechanism that goes on to mediate acquired resistance (74,101). Injecting BALB/c mice with neutralizing antibodies directed at any one of the five endogenous activating cytokines, IL-12, IL-2, and IFN-γ (Th1-cell–associated), GM-CSF, and TNF, comparably impairs the development of resistance and inhibits the capacity to kill visceral parasites (Table 62-2) (65,68–70,76). Thus, the successful response to *L. donovani* is complex and multicytokine dependent.

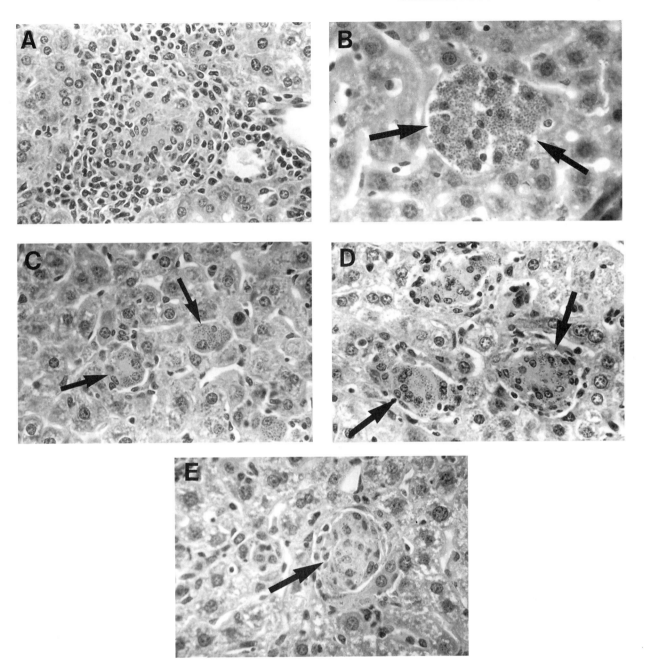

FIG. 62-5. State of granuloma development 4 weeks after *L. donovani* infection in BALB/c mice lacking or depleted of selected effector cells or endogenous activating cytokines. **A:** Normal control mice demonstrate well-developed mature granulomas and few intracellular amastigotes. **B:** Tissue in T-cell–deficient nude mice shows strikingly parasitized, fused Kupffer cell core but no surrounding mononuclear cell mantle. **C:** In anti-CR3–treated normal mice, blockade of blood monocyte recruitment to infected foci abolishes granuloma development other than initial KC fusion. Note paucity of all types of mononuclear cells including lymphocytes at infected foci. **D** and **E:** Neutralization of endogenous interferon-γ (IFN-γ) **(D)** or endogenous interleukin-12 (IL-12) **(E)** by anticytokine antibody injection also inhibits granuloma assembly in the liver. Anti–IL-2 injection produced a similar histologic effect (68). Note numerous amastigotes in **B–E** versus few in normal controls in **A.** (**A,C,D,E** ×315; **B** ×400). (With permission: **A** and **C** from ref. 52; **B** from ref. 62; **D** from ref. 65; and **E** from ref. 76.)

However, depleting these same cytokines does not necessarily inhibit granuloma formation (69,70). Anti–IL-12, anti–IL-2, and anti–IFN-γ each abolishes granuloma development, including recruitment of both monocytes and T cells (Fig. 62-5D,E), indicating the chemoattractant activities of Th1 cell cytokines. IL-12 and IL-2 are principal inducers of IFN-γ in this model (68,76). Thus, in view of the failure of IFN-γ gene knock-out mice to form granulomas in response to *L. donovani* (75), it seems likely that the capacity of anti–IL-12 and anti–IL-2 to inhibit granuloma formation relates primarily to blocking IFN-γ secretion.

Injections of anti–GM-CSF and anti-TNF also inhibit control of visceral infection, but have no discernible effect on the granulomatous response (Table 62-2) (69,70). Treatment with anti–IL-1 receptor antibody similarly produces no effect (69). However, both TNF and IL-1 have been implicated in the tissue response and granuloma formation in other experimental models (47–50,138). While the results with anti–GM-CSF and anti-TNF treatment in BALB/c mice dissociate granuloma formation and resistance in this instance (Table 62-2), they also serve to highlight the apparent requirement for a fully functional (secretory) granuloma in defense against *L. donovani* in the tissues. Thus, the histologic appearance of a mature granuloma by itself may not be sufficient to guarantee control over infection in the absence of the capacity to secrete a full complement of antileishmanial cytokines.

MODELS OF IMPAIRED GRANULOMA ASSEMBLY IN *L. DONOVANI* INFECTION

Depletion of a Cell or Cytokine

The behavior of and response to *L. donovani* infection in nude mice and in normal mice first depleted of CD4 cells alone can be viewed as models of visceral leishmaniasis in the T-cell–deficient and the CD4-cell–deficient host, respectively (62,64). The heavily parasitized tissues in both types of animals are clinically relevant since newly acquired or reactivated kala-azar is a well-recognized opportunistic infection in endemic regions in patients immunosuppressed iatrogenically or by advanced HIV infection (118,119). Both of these latter states also result in deficient generation of antigen-induced IFN-γ (104, 139), and thus, a failure of macrophage activation. Therefore, anti–IFN-γ treatment, interference with IFN-γ induction by injection of anti–IL-12 or anti–IL-2, and use of IFN-γ knock-out mice (65,68,75,76) are worth examining (Fig. 62-5) for insight into mechanisms of human disease. This latter conclusion has been strengthened considerably by the recent demonstration that patients with selective IFN-γ receptor deficiency are susceptible to mycobacterial infection and fail to assemble mature granulomas in involved tissue (140,141).

Effect of a Suppressive Th2-Cell–Associated Response

Visceralizing strains of *Leishmania* act as classic opportunistic pathogens in T-cell–deficient hosts. However, in otherwise immunologically intact patients, the failure to properly mount a Th1-cell response and/or the presence of a T-cell–suppressive, macrophage-deactivating Th2-cell–associated response can also lead to the development of kala-azar. This latter mechanism is thought to be mediated primarily by IL-4 and/or IL-10 (95–99) (and perhaps by other factors such as IL-13 (142).

To determine how the tissue granulomatous reaction may be affected by a Th2-cell response, a separate model was needed, since unlike experimental cutaneous *L. major* infection (136,137), *L. donovani* does not provoke a functionally active, disease-exacerbating Th2 mechanism in mice (74). Four once-weekly subcutaneous injections of heat-killed *L. major* promastigotes given prior to challenge with viable *L. donovani*, however, induced BALB/c mice to cross-react with an IL-4– and IL-10–dependent response. This response suppressed acquired resistance and converted mice to a noncure phenotype (74). Other than Kupffer cell fusion, mature granuloma assembly was entirely inhibited, and amastigotes were not cleared from the liver (74). Treatments designed to inhibit the Th2 cell response (injections of anti–IL-4 or anti–IL-10; prophylactic infusions of IL-12) (74) restored acquired resistance, which was simultaneously expressed in the liver by the generation of intact granulomas.

The preceding results highlight the likely immunopathogenic effects of a Th2 cell response and support the notion of active inhibition of both host defense and the tissue reaction in progressive visceral leishmaniasis. This same Th2-cell–type mechanism is also probably active in a variety of other experimental and human infections (142–145), some of which are granulomatous diseases as well. An example of this putative Th2 cell state appears to be the lepromatous form of leprosy in which the dermis typically shows sheets of *M. leprae* within macrophages, little effective inflammatory reaction, no hint of macrophage activation, and few, if any, granulomas (146). Such responses contrast with the more benign and better controlled tuberculoid form of leprosy associated with evidence of a Th1 cell response (146).

In the setting of the Th2 response in lepromatous leprosy, however, responsiveness to Th1-cell cytokines is not necessarily lost, since injections of IFN-γ induce antimycobacterial effects and modify the tissue response in favor of the host (147,148). The latter effects include widespread and marked mononuclear cell recruitment with intradermal accumulation of both CD4 and CD8 T cells and mononuclear phagocytes (147). Treatment of lepromatous leprosy patients with IL-2 can also restore granulomatous inflammation at the site of cytokine injection (149); whether this effect reflects local induction of IFN-γ and/or a separate IL-2–induced mechanism is not clear. Local injections of IL-2 can also induce similar enhancement in granulomatous inflammation in another Th2 response-associated infection, diffuse cutaneous leishmaniasis (150).

Despite the sense that a Th2 cell response is likely detrimental to the host and to the tissue reaction, in certain selected helminthic infections the opposite appears to be the case, at least as judged by experimental studies in mice and limited clinical information (60,151,152). For example, in experimental infection caused by *Schistosoma mansoni*, a trematode capable of inducing exuberant granulomatous inflammation both in animals and man, it is the Th2-cell–associated mechanism (IL-4) that seems to be largely responsible for granuloma induction, multinucleated cell formation (153), and the intense egg-provoked inflammatory reaction; the latter eventually results in widespread pathologic fibrosis during tissue repair (57–60). At the same time, however, endogenous secretion of or exogenous treatment with Th1-cell–derived cytokines may also be active in this model. For instance, IFN-γ and IL-12 can suppress the schistosome egg-induced pathology associated with an unopposed Th2-cell–dependent granulomatous reaction and

therefore presumably reduce fibrosis in a fashion beneficial to the host (57,60). This latter effect may not be produced in all instances by IL-12, however, if its capacity to simultaneously induce chemokine expression and inflammatory cell recruitment overrides inhibition of Th2-cell–derived (IL-4–related) pathology (51).

Failure of Granuloma Assembly in C57BL/6 ep/ep (Pale Ear) Mice

While normal C57BL/6 mice infected with *L. donovani* behave similarly to BALB/c animals and acquire resistance and promptly generate an appropriate granulomatous response (Fig. 62-6A), euthymic C57BL/6 pale ear mice (coat pigment mutation) do neither (66,73). Although pale ear mice are immunocompetent as judged by normal numbers of CD4 and CD8 cells, macrophage antimicrobial activity, and secretion of IL-2, IFN-γ, and TNF, they nonetheless express several suboptimal cellular immune responses. Most prominent among these lesions are the failure to respond to exogenous treatment with Th1-cell–associated cytokines and poor-to-absent granuloma formation (66,73). The latter defect in the tissue cellular immune response in these mice is not related to the failure of the proper inflammatory cells to reach

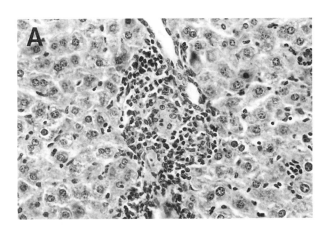

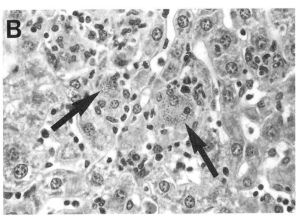

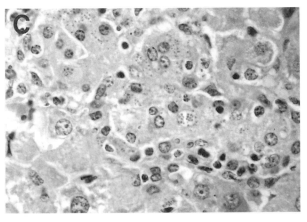

FIG. 62-6. Defective granuloma assembly in the liver of C57BL/6 ep/ep (pale ear) mice. **A:** Four weeks after *L. donovani* infection, mature granuloma formation is focal and complete in normal parent C57BL/6 mice, which acquire resistance. **B:** In contrast, in 4-week infected pale ear mice, overall mononuclear cell influx is numerically satisfactory but diffuse, and inflammatory cells have not been properly directed to, nor focused at, KC. **C:** At week 8, mature granulomas have still not developed, and the scanty mononuclear cell infiltrate has begun to recede. At week 8, liver parasite burdens are 12- to 30-fold higher in pale ear mice than in controls (66,73). (**A** ×200; **B** and **C** ×315). (**B** from ref. 73, with permission.)

the target organ (liver); instead, it lies in the subsequent failure to direct or attract sufficient numbers of influxing monocytes and T cells specifically to the parasitized Kupffer cell (Fig. 62-6B). Although an analysis of chemotactic mechanisms [adhesion molecules, chemokines (27, 31)] has not yet been carried out in this model, emerging results from other systems have implicated chemokine-mediated events, for example, the effects of macrophage inflammatory protein 1-α in both host defense and granuloma formation (37). Since the histologic abnormalities in pale ear mice point to a lesion in chemotactic mechanisms, they serve to reemphasize proper cell homing and trafficking as critical components of the granulomatous host defense response.

In addition, in *L. donovani*–infected C57BL/6 pale ear mice, rather than progressing, the scanty inflammatory infiltrate that does develop by week 4 inappropriately and prematurely recedes (Fig. 62-6C) (66). This finding suggests a related defect in the molecular signaling mechanisms (soluble, surface receptor) that act to retain attracted cells at an infected focus and maintain granulomas. While a partially active, IL-4–dependent Th2 cell reaction develops in pale ear mice, injections of anti–IL-4 do not correct the pale ear defect in granuloma assembly or enhance retention of inflammatory cells (73).

Another relevant expression of the tissue granuloma defect in pale ear mice is the inability to respond normally to conventional antileishmanial chemotherapy (pentavalent antimony) (73). Monocytes accumulate antimony, which may in part explain antimony's efficacy in the tissues in this intracellular infection (154,155). Thus, the conspicuous paucity of these effector cells in close proximity to parasitized foci in pale ear mice (Fig. 62-6B) suggests one explanation for their failure to respond to antimony treatment. The potential clinical relevance of this observation relates to the now available capacity to use cytokines such as GM-CSF (70) to pharmacologically mobilize and augment the delivery of blood monocytes to infected tissue foci (see below), thereby providing not only a key effector cell but one capable of modifying antibiotic delivery (155). Results from a recent pilot trial have demonstrated that combination treatment with antimony plus GM-CSF was well tolerated in patients with kala-azar and ameliorated the characteristic leukopenia (156). Thus, the stage is now set for additional clinical testing of this or perhaps other similar, cytokine-based interventions (considered next) designed to adjust the tissue reaction in favor of the host.

CYTOKINE-INDUCED MODIFICATION OF THE GRANULOMATOUS RESPONSE

Enhancement

In established visceral infection in normal BALB/c mice, cytokine treatment begun 2 weeks after challenge and given continuously for 7 days produced variable effects on parasite killing and the tissue reaction. While injections of TNF produced no antileishmanial effect (69), treatment with IFN-γ, IFN-γ inducers (IL-2, IL-12), or GM-CSF induced leishmanicidal activity in the liver (68,70,72,103). Neither exogenous IFN-γ nor IL-12, however, discernibly altered the developing granulomatous response already in motion in normal mice during weeks 2 to 3 (72,103).

In contrast, there were striking histologic effects induced by continuous administration of IL-2 or GM-CSF by subcutaneous osmotic pump (Fig. 62-7). After 7 days of pump-delivered IL-2, there was a remarkable influx of mononuclear cells into the liver, and these cells were particularly well focused at discrete loci of intracellular infection (Fig. 62-7C) (68). Encasement of parasitized Kupffer cells by influxing myelomonocytic cells was induced by pump-delivered GM-CSF (Fig. 62-7D) (70). The capacity of IL-2 and GM-CSF to direct cells first into the liver and then to the infected focus was strictly T-cell dependent, being absent in nude BALB/c mice. While neutrophils exert little or no antileishmanial effect in this model, substituting granulocyte colony-stimulating factor (G-CSF) for GM-CSF treatment led to population of foci of *L. donovani* infection with granulocytes (Fig. 62-7E) (70). Treatment with exogenous IL-1 has also been reported to enhance *L. donovani*–induced granuloma formation (157).

T-cell–intact 2-week infected normal BALB/c mice are already actively engaged in cytokine secretion and granuloma generation; thus, it was not surprising that treatment with IFN-γ or IL-12 failed to affect the tissue response. However, activities could be documented in deficient hosts. Thus, although IFN-γ had no effect in the tissues of nude mice [IFN-γ's actions require the presence of host T cells (71)], in partially reconstituted nude animals treatment with IFN-γ clearly promoted mononuclear cell recruitment into the infected liver and induced granuloma formation (71). Similarly, granuloma-inducing activity of exogenous IL-12 could be uncovered in IFN-γ gene knock-out BALB/c mice (75), an action presumably more easily detected in the absence of IFN-γ's own inflammatory and cell-recruiting effects (39–43,71).

Inhibition

In contrast to injections of IFN-γ, IFN-γ inducers (IL-12, IL-2), or GM-CSF into BALB/c mice with established *L. donovani* infection, treatment with exogenous TNF did not induce antileishmanial activity (69). Since endogenous TNF plays a central role in defense against this intracellular pathogen (69), a likely explanation for the lack of effect of exogenous TNF is that levels of TNF induced by infection are already optimal. However, high doses of exogenous TNF brought the progress of granuloma to a virtual standstill (Fig. 62-7F); in parallel, vis-

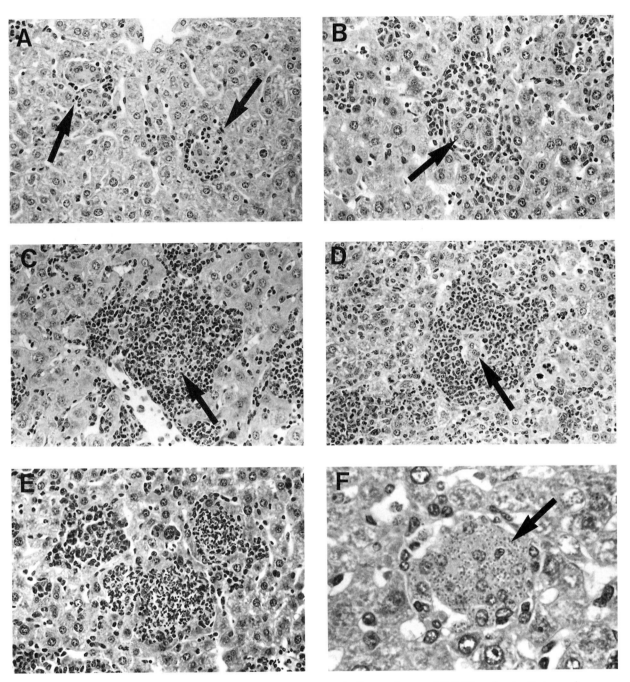

FIG. 62-7. Modification of the granulomatous response in livers of normal BALB/c mice by 7 days of exogenous treatment with recombinant cytokines. Two weeks after *L. donovani* challenge (day 14) at the time of logarithmic parasite visceral replication, osmotic pumps were implanted subcutaneously to continuously deliver saline or cytokine for 7 days. **A:** Control mouse on day 14 just prior to pump implantation. **B–F:** Histologic appearance of the granulomatous reaction on day 21 in response to 7 days of treatment with saline **(B)**, human IL-2 **(C)**, human granulocyte-macrophage colony-stimulating factor (GM-CSF) **(D)**, human granulocyte colony-stimulating factor (G-CSF) **(E)**, or murine tumor necrosis factor (TNF) **(F)** (68–70). While saline had no effect **(B)**, striking modifications in cell influx and focal recruitment to parasitized areas *(arrows)* were induced by IL-2 (mononuclear cells, **C**), GM-CSF (myelomonocytic cells, **D**), and G-CSF (granulocytes, **E**). In contrast, high-dose TNF (10 µg/day) inhibited granuloma formation **(F)**. (**A–E** ×200; **F** ×315). (With permission: **A, D**, and **E** from ref. 70; **C** from ref. 68; and **B** and **F** from ref. 69.)

ceral infection was exacerbated (69). This observation reemphasizes lessons learned from other models about the potential double-edge of a heightened inflammatory response. In addition, this finding may also have some relevance to human visceral leishmaniasis, since patients with untreated kala-azar routinely show high serum levels of TNF but nonetheless permit progressive infection (106,107). At the same time, however, TNF has also been implicated experimentally as a key initiator of granuloma formation in entirely separate models (47,48,138).

While neither IL-4 nor IL-10 has been injected in this model of visceral leishmaniasis to determine if Th2-cell–associated cytokines can directly interrupt active granuloma formation, the presence of a Th2-type of response from the outset of *L. donovani* infection clearly prevented granuloma assembly (74). Additional suppressive cytokines such as transforming growth factor-β (158) or IL-13 (142) might also downregulate the tissue reaction.

THERAPEUTIC ENTRY INTO THE GRANULOMA

Along with modifying the cellular components of the granuloma (68,70,157), the notion of delivering antimicrobial agents or perhaps microbicidal mechanisms themselves directly into a persistently infected focus, walled-off but not eradicated, has long been considered as one approach to the treatment of chronic intracellular infections. Experimental visceral leishmaniasis has been one such test system for three reasons: (a) the capacity of the targeted tissues (liver, spleen, bone marrow) to readily take up agents injected into the circulation, (b) accessibility to amastigotes replicating within highly phagocytic/endocytic cells (macrophages), and (c) the occurrence of lysosomal fusion with parasite-containing vacuoles (159). The efficacy of drugs and cytokines encapsulated in liposomes in experimental visceral infection (160,161) and that of lipid formulations of amphotericin B in human kala-azar (162) likely depend on drug delivery into parasitized tissue macrophages in the inflammatory focus.

To characterize the accessibility of the *L. donovani*-induced granulomatous reaction in the liver to an injectible microbicidal mechanism, infected mice were given intravenous injections of latex beads to which glucose oxidase had been covalently linked (163). In the presence of glucose, these beads readily generate hydrogen peroxide, to which *Leishmania* are susceptible (131). In the liver, >50% of intracellular (intragranuloma) amastigotes were killed one day after two consecutive once-daily injections of hydrogen peroxide-producing beads. The appearance of tissue imprints (Fig. 62-8) showed that beads had reached their proper target cell. These results demonstrated the accessibility of the tissue granuloma to an exogenous particulate system capable of delivering a well-defined antimicrobial activity (163).

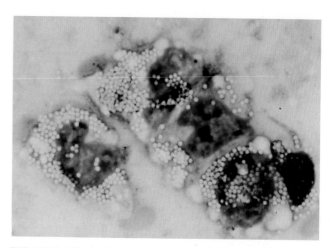

FIG. 62-8. Giemsa-stained liver imprint from 2-week infected BALB/c mouse 24 hours after intravenous injection of glucose oxidase beads (163). Imprint shows four infected granuloma mononuclear phagocytes that have ingested numerous latex beads. (×500).

SUMMARY

The studies reviewed here focus on the tissue response to one intracellular protozoan. Nevertheless, the lessons learned from this ongoing analysis of the *L. donovani*-parasitized liver are likely applicable at least in part to the diverse group of pathogens (as well as perhaps to the nonmicrobial stimuli) that similarly elicit granulomatous inflammation.

Presumably, this specialized form of chronic inflammation evolved as a host defense mechanism because certain microbial agents acquired the capacity to evade the effects of the acute inflammatory response. How and why inflammatory diseases of unknown cause provoke this same type of tissue response are not clear. Irrespective of the nature of the initiating stimulus, however, the host response that culminates in the formation of mature, functional, and secretory granulomas is dynamic and complex. At a minimum, epithelioid granuloma assembly requires orchestration of multiple soluble cytokine signals, recruitment of numerous populations of leukocytes, surface expression of diverse proteins and receptor mechanisms, and activation of effector cells. The homeostatic consequences of too exuberant a granulomatous response on the one hand and the failure to properly assemble granulomas on the other have also been well identified clinically and closely correlated with recognized human disorders. The potential to modify granulomatous inflammation via pharmacologic intervention, especially the capacity to immunologically enhance its expression, represents one future approach to strengthen host antimicrobial defense in the tissues.

ACKNOWLEDGMENT

This work was supported by National Institutes of Health research grant AI 16963.

REFERENCES

1. Guckian JC, Perry JE. Granulomatous hepatitis. An analysis of 63 cases and review of the literature. *Ann Intern Med* 1966;65: 1081–1100.
2. Adams DO. The granulomatous inflammatory response. *Am J Pathol* 1976; 84:164–191.
3. Williams GT, Williams WJ. Granulomatous inflammation—a review. *J Clin Pathol* 1983;36:723–733.
4. Warren KS. A functional classification of granulomatous inflammation. *Ann NY Acad Sci* 1976;278:7–12.
5. Deepe GS, Bullock WE. Histoplasmosis: a granulomatous inflammatory response. In: Gallin JI, Goldstein IM, Snyderman R, eds. *Inflammation: basic principles and clinical correlates.* New York: Raven Press, 1988:733–749.
6. Wahl SM. Fibrosis: bacterial cell-wall-induced hepatic granulomas. In: Gallin JI, Goldstein IM, Snyderman R, eds. *Inflammation: basic principles and clinical correlates.* New York: Raven Press, 1988: 841–860.
7. Sheffield EA. The granulomatous inflammatory response. *J Pathol* 1990;160:1–2.
8. Editorial. Granulomas and cytokines. *Lancet* 1991;337:1067–1068.
9. McCluggage WG, Sloan JM. Hepatic granulomas in Northern Ireland: a thirteen year review. *Histopathology* 1994;25:219–228.
10. Denk H, Scheuer PJ, Bapista A, et al. Guidelines for the diagnosis and interpretation of hepatic granulomas. *Histopathology* 1994;25: 209–218.
11. Lamm DL, van der Meijden PM, Morales A, et al. Incidence and treatment of complications of bacillus Calmette-Guerin intravesical therapy in superficial bladder cancer. *J Urol* 1992;147:596–600.
12. Sparks FC. Hazards and complications of BCG immunotherapy. *Med Clin North Am* 1976;60:499–510.
13. Newman LS, Rose CS, Maier LA. Sarcoidosis. *N Engl J Med* 1997; 336:12241–12234.
14. Wagoner GP, Anton AT, Gall EA, Schiff L. Needle biopsy of the liver. Experience with hepatic granulomas. *Gastroenterology* 1953; 25:487–494.
15. Mir-Madjlessi SH, Farmer RG, Hawk WA. Granulomatous hepatitis: a review of 50 cases. *Am J Gastroenterol* 1973;60:122–134.
16. Klatskin G. Hepatic granuloma: problems in interpretation. *Ann NY Acad Sci* 1976;278:427–431.
17. Sartin JS, Walker RC. Granulomatous hepatitis: a retrospective review of 88 cases at the Mayo Clinic. *Mayo Clin Proc* 1991;66:914–918.
18. Hughes M, Fox H. A histological analysis of granulomatous hepatitis. *J Clin Pathol* 1972;25:817–820.
19. Neville E, Piyasena KHG, James DG. Granulomas of the liver. *Postgrad Med J* 1975;51:361–365.
20. Cunningham D, Mills PR, Quigley EMM, et al. Hepatic granulomas: experience over a 10 year period in the west of Scotland. *Q J Med* 1982;51:162–170.
21. Satti MB, Hussein A, Ibrahim EM, et al. Hepatic granuloma in Saudi Arabia: a clinicopathological study of 59 cases. *Am J Gastroenterol* 1990;85:669–674.
22. McMaster KR, Hennigar GR. Drug-induced granulomatous hepatitis. *Lab Invest* 1981;44:61–73.
23. Dannenberg AM. Delayed-type hypersensitivity and cell-mediated immunity in the pathogenesis of tuberculosis. *Immunol Today* 1991;12:228–233.
24. Barnes PF, Rom WN. Cytokine production in tuberculosis. In: Rom WN, Garay SM, eds. *Tuberculosis.* Boston: Little, Brown, 1996:291–303.
25. Ward PA. Leukotaxis and leukocytic disorders: a review. *Am J Pathol* 1974;77:520–538.
26. Orme IM, Furney SK, Skinner PS, et al. Inhibition of growth of *Mycobacterium avium* in murine and human mononuclear phagocytes by migration inhibitory factor. *Infect Immun* 1993;61:338–342.
27. Cronstein BN, Weissmann G. The adhesion molecules of inflammation. *Arthritis Rheum* 1993;36:147–157.
28. Subramaniam M, Saffaripour S, Watson SR, Mayadas TN, Hynes RO, Wagner DD. Reduced recruitment of inflammatory cells in a contact hypersensitivity response in P-selectin-deficient mice. *J Exp Med* 1995;181:2277–2282.
29. Tedder TF, Steeber DA, Pizcueta P. L-selectin-deficient mice have impaired leukocyte recruitment into inflammatory sites. *J Exp Med* 1995;181:2259–2264.
30. Tapia FJ, Caceres-Dittmar G, Sanchez MA, Fernandez CT, Rondon AJ, Convit J. Adhesion molecules in lesions of American cutaneous leishmaniasis. *Exp Dermatol* 1994;3:17–22.
31. Adams DH, Lloyd AR. Chemokines: leucocyte recruitment and activation cytokines. *Lancet* 1997;349:490–495.
32. Gruss HJ, Brach MA, Schumann RR, Herrmann F. Regulation of MCP/JE gene expression during monocytic differentiation. *J Immunol* 1994;153:4907–4914.
33. Luo Y, Laning J, Hayashi M, Hancock PR, Rollins B, Dorf ME. Serologic analysis of the mouse B chemokine JE/monocyte chemoattractant protein-1. *J Immunol* 1994;153:3708–3716.
34. Vaddi K, Newton RC. Regulation of monocyte integrin expression by B-family chemokines. *J Immunol* 1994;153:4721–4732.
35. Clark-Lewis I, Kim KS, Rajarathnam K, et al. Structure-activity relationships of chemokines. *J Leukoc Biol* 1995;57:703–711.
36. Kasama T, Strieter RM, Standiford TJ, Burdick MD, Sunkel SL. Expression and regulation of human neutrophil-derived macrophage inflammatory protein-1α. *J Exp Med* 1993;178:63–72.
37. Lukacs NW, Kunkel SL, Strieter RM, Warmington K, Chensue SW. The role of macrophage inflammatory protein 1α in *Schistosoma mansoni* egg-induced granulomatous inflammation. *J Exp Med* 1993; 177:1551–1559.
38. Taub DD, Lloyd AR, Conlon K, et al. Recombinant human interferon-inducible protein 10 is a chemoattractant for human monocytes and T lymphocytes and promotes T cell adhesion to endothelial cells. *J Exp Med* 1993;177:1809–1814.
39. Issekutz TB, Stoltz JM, van der Meide P. Lymphocyte recruitment in delayed-type hypersensitivity. *J Immunol* 1986;140:2989–2993.
40. Issekutz TB, Stoltz JM, van der Meide P. The recruitment of lymphocytes into the skin by T cell lymphokines: the role of γ-interferon. *Clin Exp Immunol* 1988;73:70–75.
41. Nickoloff BJ. Role of interferon-γ in cutaneous trafficking of lymphocytes with emphasis on molecular and cellular adhesion events. *Arch Dermatol* 1988;124:1835–1843.
42. Kaplan G, Nusrat A, Sarno EN, et al. Cellular responses to the intradermal injection of recombinant human γ-interferon in lepromatous leprosy patients. *Am J Pathol* 1987;128:345–353.
43. Nathan CF, Squires K, Griffo W, et al. Widespread intradermal accumulation of mononuclear leukocytes in lepromatous leprosy patients treated systemically with recombinant interferon-γ. *J Exp Med* 1990;172:1509–1512.
44. Asano M, Nakane A, Minagawa T. Endogenous gamma interferon is essential in granuloma formation induced by glycolipid-containing mycolic acid in mice. *Infect Immun* 1993;61:2872–2878.
45. Issekutz TB. Effects of six different cytokines on lymphocyte adherence to microvascular endothelium and *in vivo* lymphocyte migration in the rat. *J Immunol* 1990;144:2140–2146.
46. Cooper AM, Dalton DK, Stewart TA, Griffin JP, Russell DG, Orme IA. Disseminated tuberculosis in interferon γ gene-disrupted mice. *J Exp Med* 1993;178:2243–2247.
47. Kindler V, Sappinno A, Grau GE, Piguet P, Vassalli P. The inducing role of tumor necrosis factor in the development of granulomas during BCG infection. *Cell* 1989;56:731–742.
48. Amiri P, Locksley RM, Parslow TG, et al. Tumor necrosis factor α restores granulomas and induces parasite-laying in schistosome-infected SCID mice. *Nature* 1992;356:604–606.
49. Chen W, Havell EA, Moldawer LL, McIntyre KW, Chizzonite RA, Harmsen AG. Interleukin 1: an important mediator of host resistance against *Pneumocystis carinii. J Exp Med* 1992;176:713–718.
50. Kobayashi K, Allred C, Cohen S, Yoshida T. Role of interleukin 1 in experimental pulmonary granuloma in mice. *J Immunol* 1985;134: 358–364.
51. Pearlman E, Lass JH, Bardenstein DS, et al. IL-12 exacerbates helminth-mediated corneal pathology by augmenting inflammatory cell recruitment and chemokine expression. *J Immunol* 1997;158:827–833.
52. Cervia J, Rosen H, Murray HW. Effector role of blood monocytes in experimental visceral leishmaniasis. *Infect Immun* 1993;61: 1330–1333.
53. Murray HW. Blood monocytes: differing effector roles in experimental visceral vs. cutaneous leishmaniasis. *Parasitol Today* 1994;10: 220–223.
54. Kaye PM, Cooke A, Lund T, Wattie M, Blackwell JM. Altered course of visceral leishmaniasis in mice expressing transgenic I-E molecules. *Eur J Immunol* 1992;22:357–364.

55. Trinchieri G. Interleukin 12: a proinflammatory cytokine with immunoregulatory functions that bridges innate resistance and antigen-specific adaptive immunity. *Annu Rev Immunol* 1995;13:251–262.

56. Le J, Vilcek J. Biology of disease. Tumor necrosis factor and interleukin-1: cytokines with multiple overlapping activities. *Lab Invest* 1986;55:234–252.

57. Wynn TA, Cheever AW, Jankovic D, et al. An IL-12 based vaccination method for preventing fibrosis induced by schistosome infection. *Nature* 1995;376:594–597.

58. Chensue SW, Warmington KS, Rith J, Lincoln PM, Kunkel SL. Cross-regulatory role of interferon-gamma, IL-4 and IL-10 in schistosome egg granuloma formation: *in vivo* regulation of Th activity and inflammation. *Clin Exp Immunol* 1994;98:395–400.

59. Cheever AW, Williams ME, Wynn TA, et al. Anti-IL-4 treatment of *Schistosoma mansoni*-infected mice inhibits development of T cells and non-B, non-T cells expressing Th2 cytokines while decreasing egg-induced hepatic fibrosis. *J Immunol* 1994;153:753–759.

60. Wynn TA, Cheever AW. Cytokine regulation of granuloma formation in schistosomiasis. *Curr Opin Immunol* 1995;7:505–511.

61. Barnes PJ, Karin M. Nuclear factor-KB—a pivotal transcription factor in chronic inflammatory diseases. *N Engl J Med* 1997;336:1066–1071.

61a. Locksley RM, Wilson CB. Cell-mediated immunity and its role in host defense. In: Mandell GL, Bennett JE, Dolin R, eds. *Principles and practice of infectious diseases*. New York: Churchill Livingstone, 1995:102–149.

62. Murray HW, Stern J, Welte K, Rubin BY, Carriero SM, Nathan CF. Experimental visceral leishmaniasis: production of interleukin 2 and gamma interferon, tissue immune reaction, and response to treatment with interleukin 2 and gamma interferon. *J Immunol* 1987;138:2290–2297.

63. McElrath J, Murray HW, Cohn ZA. Dynamics of granuloma formation in experimental visceral leishmaniasis. *J Exp Med* 1988;167:1927–1937.

64. Stern J, Oca M, Rubin BY, Anderson S, Murray HW. Role of L3T4+ and Lyt 2+ cells in experimental visceral leishmaniasis. *J Immunol* 1988;140:3971–3977.

65. Squires KE, Schreiber RD, McElrath MJ, Murray HW. Experimental visceral leishmaniasis: role of endogenous interferon gamma in host defense and tissue granulomatous response. *J Immunol* 1989;143:4244–4249.

66. Squires KE, Kirsch M, Silverstein SC, Acosta A, McElrath MJ, Murray HW. Defect in the tissue cellular immune response: experimental visceral leishmaniasis in euthymic C57BL/6 ep/ep mice. *Infect Immun* 1990;58:3893–3898.

67. Murray HW, Squires KE, Miralles CD, et al. Acquired resistance and granuloma formation in experimental visceral leishmaniasis. Differential T cell and lymphokine roles in initial versus established immunity. *J Immunol* 1992;148:1858–1863.

68. Murray HW, Miralles GD, Stoeckle MY, McDermott DF. Role and effect of interleukin 2 in experimental visceral leishmaniasis. *J Immunol* 1993;151:929–938.

69. Tumang M, Keogh C, Moldawer LL, Teitelbaum RF, Hariprashad J, Murray HW. The role and effect of tumor necrosis factor alpha in experimental visceral leishmaniasis. *J Immunol* 1994;153:768–775.

70. Murray HW, Cervia JS, Hariprashad J, Taylor AP, Stoeckle MY, Hochman H. Effect of granulocyte macrophage colony stimulating factor in experimental visceral leishmaniasis. *J Clin Invest* 1995;95:1183–1192.

71. Murray HW, Hariprashad J, Aguero B, Arakawa T, Yeganegi H. Intracellular antimicrobial response of the T cell deficient host to cytokine therapy: effect of interferon gamma in experimental visceral leishmaniasis in nude mice. *J Infect Dis* 1995;171:1309–3016.

72. Murray HW, Hariprashad J. Interleukin 12 is effective treatment for an established systemic intracellular infection: experimental visceral leishmaniasis. *J Exp Med* 1995;181:387–391.

73. Murray HW, Hariprashad J, McDermott DF, Stoeckle MY. Multiple host defense defects in the failure of C57BL/6 ep/ep (pale ear) mice to resolve visceral *Leishmania donovani* infection. *Infect Immun* 1996;64:161–166.

74. Murray HW, Hariprashad J, Coffman RL. Behavior of visceral *Leishmania donovani* in an experimentally-induced Th2 cell-associated response model. *J Exp Med* 1997;185:867–874.

75. Taylor A, Murray HW. Intracellular antimicrobial activity in the absence of interferon-γ: effect of interleukin 12 in experimental visceral leishmaniasis in interferon-γ gene-disrupted mice. *J Exp Med* 1997;185:1231–1239.

76. Murray HW. Endogenous interleukin 12 regulates acquired resistance in experimental visceral leishmaniasis. *J Infect Dis* 1997;175:1477–1479.

77. Bradley DJ, Kirkley J. Regulation of *Leishmania* populations within the host. I. The variable course of *L. donovani* infections in mice. *Clin Exp Immunol* 1977;30:119–129.

77a. Gutierrez Y, Maksem JA, Reiner NE. Pathologic changes in murine leishmaniasis (*Leishmania donovani*) with special reference to the dynamics of granuloma formation in the liver. *Am J Pathol* 1984;114:222–230.

78. Wilson ME, Innes DJ, de Queiroz Sousa A, Pearson RD. Early histopathology of experimental infection with *Leishmania donovani* in hamsters. *J Parasitol* 1987;73:55–63.

79. Kaye PM. Inflammatory cells in murine visceral leishmaniasis express a dendritic cell marker. *Clin Exp Immunol* 1987;70:515–519.

80. Davies EV, Singleton AMT, Blackwell JM. Differences in *Lsh* gene control over systemic *Leishmania major* and *Leishmania donovani* or *Leishmania mexicana mexicana* infections are caused by differential targeting to infiltrating and resident liver macrophage populations. *Infect Immun* 1988;56:1128–1134.

81. Laurenti DM, Scotto MN, Corbett CEP, et al. Experimental visceral leishmaniasis: sequential events of granuloma formation at subcutaneous inoculation site. *Int J Exp Pathol* 1990;71:791–797.

82. Correa EB, Cunha JMT, Bunn-Moreno MM, Madeira ED. Cyclophosphamide affects the dynamics of granuloma formation in experimental visceral leishmaniasis. *Parasitol Res* 1992;78:154–160.

83. Wilson ME, Sandor M, Blum AM, et al. Local suppression of IFN-γ in hepatic granulomas correlates with tissue-specific replication of *Leishmania chagasi*. *J Immunol* 1996;1546:2231–2239.

84. Pearson RD, de Queiroz Sousa A. Clinical spectrum of leishmaniasis. *Clin Infect Dis* 1996;22:1–13.

85. Rees PH, Kager PA, Muriithi MR, Wambua PP, Shah SD, Butterworth AE. Tuberculin sensitivity in kala-azar. *Trans R Soc Trop Med Hyg* 1981;75:630–631.

86. Saran R, Gupta AK, Sharma MC. Leishmanin skin test in clinical and subclinical kala-azar cases. *J Commun Dis* 1991;23:135–137.

87. Sciotto A, Russo-Mancuso G, Zinna CM, Comisi FF, Sciannaca RM, Schiliro G. Lymphocyte subsets in kala-azar. *Ann Allergy* 1989;63:343–346.

88. Koech DK. Subpopulations of T lymphocytes in Kenyan patients with visceral leishmaniasis. *Am J Trop Med Hyg* 1987;36:497–500.

89. Cillari E, Liew FY, Lo Campo P, Milano S, Mansueto S, Salerno A. Suppression of IL-2 production by cryopreserved peripheral blood mononuclear cells from patients with active visceral leishmaniasis in Sicily. *J Immunol* 1988;140:2721–2726.

90. Cillari E, Milano S, Dieli M, et al. Reduction in the number of UCHL-1+ cells and IL-2 production in the peripheral blood of patients with visceral leishmaniasis. *J Immunol* 1991;146:1026–1030.

91. Carvalho EM, Badaro R, Reed SG, Jones TC. Absence of gamma interferon and interleukin 2 production during active visceral leishmaniasis. *J Clin Invest* 1985;76:2066–2069.

92. Sacks DL, Lata Lal S, Shrivastava SN, Blackwell J, Neva FA. An analysis of T cell responsiveness in Indian kala-azar. *J Immunol* 1987;138:908–913.

93. Meller-Melloul C, Farnier C, Dunan S, et al. Evidence of subjects sensitized to *Leishmania infantum* on the French Mediterranean coast: differences in gamma interferon production between this population and visceral leishmaniasis patients. *Parasite Immunol* 1991;13:531–536.

94. Carvalho EM, Barral A, Pedral-Sampaio D, et al. Immunologic markers of clinical evolution in children recently infected with *Leishmania donovani chagasi*. *J Infect Dis* 1992;165:535–540.

95. Holaday BJ, de Lima Pompeu MM, Evans T, et al. Correlates of *Leishmania*-specific immunity in the clinical spectrum of infection with *Leishmania chagasi*. *J Infect Dis* 1993;167:411–417.

96. Carvalho EM, Bacellar O, Regis T, Coffman R, Reed SG. Restoration of IFN-γ production and lymphocyte proliferation in visceral leishmaniasis. *J Immunol* 1994;152:5949–5956.

97. Karp C, Wynn T, Satti M, et al. *In vivo* cytokine profiles in patients with kala-azar. Marked elevation of both interleukin-10 and interferon-gamma. *J Clin Invest* 1993;91:1644–1648.

98. Ghalib H, Piuvezam M, Siddig M, et al. Interleukin-10 production correlates with pathology in human *Leishmania donovani* infections. *J Clin Invest* 1993;92:324–329.

99. Sundar S, Reed SG, Sharma S, Mehrota A, Murray HW. Circulating Th1 cell- and Th2 cell-associated cytokines in Indian patients with visceral leishmaniasis. *Am J Trop Med Hyg* 1997;56:522–525.

100. Holaday B, de Lima Pompeu M, Jeronimo S, et al. Potential role for interleukin-10 in the immunosuppression associated with kala-azar. *J Clin Invest* 1993;92:2626–2632.

101. Miralles GD, Stoeckle MY, McDermott DF, Finkelman FD, Murray HW. Induction of Th1 and Th2 cell associated cytokines in experimental visceral leishmaniasis. *Infect Immun* 1994;62:1058–1063.

102. Murray HW, Rubin BY, Rothermel CD. Killing of intracellular *Leishmania donovani* by lymphokine-stimulated human mononuclear phagocytes: evidence that interferon-gamma is the activating lymphokine. *J Clin Invest* 1983;72:1506–1522.

103. Murray HW. Effect of continuous administration of interferon gamma in experimental visceral leishmaniasis. *J Infect Dis* 1990;161:992–994.

104. Murray HW. Interferon gamma in host antimicrobial defense: current and future clinical applications. *Am J Med* 1994;97:459–469.

105. Roach TI, Kiderlen AF, Blackwell JM. Role of inorganic nitrogen oxides and tumor necrosis factor-alpha in killing *Leishmania donovani* amastigotes in gamma-interferon lipopolysaccharide-activated macrophages from *Lsh*s and *Lsh*r congenic mouse strains. *Infect Immun* 1991;59:3935–3944.

106. Scuderi P, Lam KS, Ryan J, et al. Raised serum levels of tumour necrosis factor in parasitic infections. *Lancet* 1986;2:1364–1366.

107. Zwingenberger K, Harms G, Pedrosa C, et al. Generation of cytokines in human visceral leishmaniasis: disassociation of endogenous TNF-α and IL-1B production. *Immunobiology* 1991;183:125–131.

108. Daneshbod K. Visceral leishmaniasis (kala-azar) in Iran: a pathologic and electron microscopic study. *Am J Clin Pathol* 1972;57:156–166.

109. Pampiglione S, La Placa M, Schlick G. Studies on Mediterranean leishmaniasis. I. An outbreak of visceral leishmaniasis in northern Italy. *Trans R Soc Trop Med Hyg* 1974;68:349–359.

110. Pampiglione S, Manson-Bahr PEC, Giunti F, Giunti G, Parenti A, Trotti CG. Studies on Mediterranean leishmaniasis. II. Asymptomatic cases of visceral leishmaniasis. *Trans R Soc Trop Med Hyg* 1974;68:447–453.

111. Moreno A, Marazuela M, Yebra M, et al. Hepatic fibrin-ring granulomas in visceral leishmaniasis. *Gastroenterology* 1988;95:1123–1126.

112. El Hag IA, Hashim FA, El Toum A, Homeida M, l Kalifa M, El Hassan AM. Liver morphology and function in visceral leishmaniasis. *J Clin Pathol* 1994;47:547–551.

113. Veress B, Omer A, Satir AA, El Hassan AM. Morphology of spleen and lymph nodes in fatal visceral leishmaniasis. *Immunology* 1977;33:605–610.

114. Evans TG, Teixeira MJ, McAuliffe IT, et al. Epidemiology of visceral leishmaniasis in northeast Brazil. *J Infect Dis* 1992;166:1124–1132.

115. Saran R, Gupta AK, Sharma MC. Evidence of *Leishmania donovani* infection in household members residing with visceral leishmaniasis patients. *J Commun Dis* 1992;24:242–244.

116. Ephros M, Paz A, Jaffe CL. Asymptomatic visceral leishmaniasis in Israel. *Trans R Soc Trop Med Hyg* 1994;88:651–652.

117. Marty P, Lelievre A, Quaranta JF, Rahal A, Gari-Toussaint M, Le Fichoux Y. Use of the leishmanin skin test and Western blot analysis for epidemiological studies in visceral leishmaniasis areas: experience in a highly endemic focus in Alpes-Maritimes (France). *Trans R Soc Trop Med Hyg* 1994;88:658–659.

118. Fernandez-Guerrero M, Aguado JM, Buzon L, et al. Visceral leishmaniasis in immunocompromised hosts. *Am J Med* 1987;83:1098–1102.

119. Peters BS, Fish D, Golden R, Evans DA, Bryceson ADM, Pinching AJ. Visceral leishmaniasis in HIV infection and AIDS: clinical features and response to therapy. *Q J Med* 1990;77:1101–1111.

120. Jagadha V, Andavolu RH, Huang CT. Granulomatous inflammation in the acquired immune deficiency syndrome. *Am J Clin Pathol* 1985;34:598–602.

121. Klatt EC, Jensen DF, Meyer PR. Pathology of *Mycobacterium avium-intracellulare* infection in acquired immunodeficiency syndrome. *Hum Pathol* 1987;18:709–714.

122. Glickman RJ, Rosner F, Guaneri JJ. The diagnostic utility of bone marrow aspiration and biopsy in patients with acquired immunodeficiency syndrome. *J Natl Med Assoc* 1989;81:119–125.

123. Wilkins MJ, Lindley R, Dourakis SP, Goldin RD. Surgical pathology of the liver in HIV infection. *Histopathology* 1991;18:459–464.

124. Rothwell TLW, Spector WG. The effect of neonatal and adult thymectomy on the inflammatory response. *J Pathol* 1972;108:15–21.

125. Papadimitriou JM. The influence of the thymus on multinucleate giant cell formation. *J Pathol* 1976;118:153–156.

126. Epstein WL, Fukuyama K, Danno K, Kwan-Wong E. Granulomatous inflammation in normal and athymic mice infected with *Schistosoma mansoni*: an ultrastructural study. *J Pathol* 1979;127:207–215.

127. Tanaka A, Emori K, Hagao S, et al. Epithelioid granuloma formation requiring no T-cell function. *Am J Pathol* 1982;106:165–170.

128. Hamilton HL, Follett DM, Siegfried LM, Czuprynski CJ. Intestinal multiplication of *Mycobacterium paratuberculosis* in athymic nude gnotobiotic mice. *Infect Immun* 1989;57:225–230.

129. Murray HW, Masur H, Keithly JS. Cell-mediated immune response in experimental visceral leishmaniasis. I. Correlation between resistance to *Leishmania donovani* and lymphokine-generating capacity. *J Immunol* 1982;129:344–351.

130. Murray HW, Hariprashad J, Fichtl RE. Models of relapse of experimental visceral leishmaniasis. *J Infect Dis* 1996;173:1041–1044.

131. Murray HW. Cell-mediated immune response in experimental visceral leishmaniasis. II. Oxygen-dependent killing of intracellular *Leishmania donovani* amastigotes. *J Immunol* 1982;129:351–357.

132. Murray HW, Cartelli DM. Killing of intracellular *Leishmania donovani* by human mononuclear phagocytes: evidence for oxygen-dependent and -independent leishmanicidal activity. *J Clin Invest* 1983;72:32–39.

133. Most J, Neumayer HP, Dierich MP. Cytokine-induced generation of multinucleated giant cells *in vitro* requires interferon-γ and expression of LFA-1. *Eur J Immunol* 1990;20:1661–1667.

134. Fais S, Burgio VL, Silvestri M, Capobianchi MR, Pacchiarotti A, Pallone F. Multinucleated giant cells generation induced by interferon-γ. Changes in the expression and distribution of the intracellular adhesion molecule-1 during macrophage fusion and multinucleated giant cell formation. *Lab Invest* 1994;71:737–744.

135. Kaufmann SHE. Immunity to intracellular bacteria. *Annu Rev Immunol* 1993;11:129–164.

136. Liew FY, O'Donnell C. Immunology of leishmaniasis. *Adv Parasitol* 1993;32:162–258.

137. Reiner SL, Locksley RM. The regulation of immunity to *Leishmania major*. *Annu Rev Immunol* 1995;13:151–171.

138. van Furth R, van Zwet TL, Buisman AM, van Dissel JT. Anti-tumor necrosis factor antibodies inhibit the influx of granulocytes and monocytes into an inflammatory exudate and enhance the growth of *Listeria monocytogenes* in various organs. *J Infect Dis* 1994;170:234–237.

139. Murray HW. Gamma interferon, macrophage activation, and host defense against microbial challenge. *Ann Intern Med* 1988;108:595–604.

140. Jouanguy E, Altare F, Lamhamedi S, et al. Interferon-γ-receptor deficiency in an infant with fatal bacille Calmette-Guerin infection. *N Engl J Med* 1996;335:1956–1961.

141. Newport MJ, Huxley CM, Huston S, et al. A mutation in the interferon-γ-receptor gene and susceptibility to mycobacterial infection. *N Engl J Med* 1996;335:1941–1949.

142. Doherty T, Kastelein R, Menon S, Coffman RL. Modulation of macrophage function by IL-13. *J Immunol* 1993;151:7151–7160.

143. Yamamura M, Uyemurak F, Deans RJ, et al. Defining protective responses to pathogens: cytokine profiles in leprosy patients. *Science* 1991;254:277–279.

144. Sher A, Gazzinelli RT, Oswald IP, et al. Role of T-cell derived cytokines in the downregulation of immune responses in parasitic and retroviral infection. *Immunol Rev* 1992;127:183–205.

145. Romagnani S. Human TH1 and TH2 subsets: doubt no more. *Immunol Today* 1991;12:256–257.

146. Kaplan G. Recent advances in cytokine therapy in leprosy. *J Infect Dis* 1993;167(suppl 1):S18–S22.

147. Nathan CF, Kaplan G, Levis WR, et al. Local and systemic effects of intradermal recombinant interferon-γ in patients with lepromatous leprosy. *N Engl J Med* 1986;315:6–15.

148. Samuel NM, Grange JM, Samuel S, et al. A study of the effects of intradermal administration of recombinant gamma interferon in lepromatous leprosy patients. *Lepr Rev* 1987;58:389–400.

149. Kaplan G, Kiessling R, Teklemariam S, et al. The reconstitution of cell-mediated immunity in the cutaneous lesions of lepromatous leprosy by recombinant interleukin 2. *J Exp Med* 1989;169:893–907.

150. Akuffo H, Kaplan G, Kiessling R, Dietz M, McElrath J, Cohn ZA. Administration of interleukin-2 reduces the local parasite load of patients with diffuse cutaneous leishmaniasis. *J Infect Dis* 1990;161:775–776.

151. McCarthy JS, Nutman TB. Perspective: prospects for development of vaccines against human helminth infections. *J Infect Dis* 1996;174: 1384–1390.

152. Locksley RM. Th2 cells: help for helminths. *J Exp Med* 1994;179: 1405–1407.

153. McInnes A, Rennick DM. Interleukin 4 induces cultured monocytes/ macrophages to form giant multinucleated cells. *J Exp Med* 1988;167: 598–611.

154. Sundar S, Rosenkaimer F, Lesser ML, Murray HW. Immunochemotherapy for a systemic intracellular infection: accelerated response using interferon gamma in visceral leishmaniasis. *J Infect Dis* 1995; 171:992–996.

155. Murray HW, Berman JD, Wright SD. Immunochemotherapy for intracellular *Leishmania donovani* infection: interferon gamma plus pentavalent antimony. *J Infect Dis* 1988;157:973.

156. Badaro R, Nascimento C, Carvalho JS, et al. Recombinant human granulocyte-macrophage colony-stimulating factor reverses neutropenia and reduces secondary infections in visceral leishmaniasis. *J Infect Dis* 1994;170:413–418.

157. Curry A, Kaye PM. Recombinant interleukin-1α augments granuloma formation but not parasite clearance in mice infected with *Leishmania donovani. Infect Immun* 1992;60:4422–4424.

158. Barral-Netto M, Barral A, Brownell C, Skeiky Y, Twardizk D, Reed S. Transforming growth factor-B in leishmanial infection. *Science* 1992; 257:545–548.

159. Chang K-P., Dwyer DM. *Leishmania donovani.* Hamster macrophage interactions *in vitro:* cell entry, intracellular survival, and multiplication of amastigotes. *J Exp Med* 1978;147:515–530.

160. Reed SG, Barral-Netto M, Inverso JA. Treatment of experimental visceral leishmaniasis with lymphokine encapsulated in liposome. *J Immunol* 1984;132:3116–3120.

161. Alving CR, Steck EA, Chapman WL, et al. Therapy of leishmaniasis: superior efficacies of liposome-encapsulated drugs. *Proc Natl Acad Sci USA* 1978;75:2959–2963.

162. Sundar S, Agrawal NK, Sinha PR, Horwith GS, Murray HW. Short-course, low-dose amphotericin B lipid complex therapy for antimony-unresponsive visceral leishmaniasis in India. *Ann Intern Med* 1997; 127:133–137.

163. Murray HW, Nathan CF. *In vivo* killing of intracellular visceral *Leishmania donovani*: effect of a macrophage targeted hydrogen peroxide generating system. *J Infect Dis* 1988;158:1372–1374.

164. Parkas V, Godwin J, Murray HW. Kala-azar comes to New York. *Arch Intern Med* 1997;157:921–923.

Inflammation: Basic Principles and Clinical Correlates,
3rd ed., edited by John I. Gallin and Ralph Snyderman.
Lippincott Williams & Wilkins, Philadelphia © 1999.

CHAPTER 63

Vasculitis: Pathogenic Mechanisms of Vessel Damage

John S. Sundy and Barton F. Haynes

The necrotizing vasculitides are diseases characterized by inflammation and necrosis of blood vessels, resulting in vessel occlusion and ischemia of tissues supplied by involved vessels (1–7). The clinical spectrum of vasculitis ranges from diseases in which vessel inflammation and necrosis result in the preponderance of clinical signs and symptoms (primary vasculitis syndromes), to well-characterized diseases in which vasculitis is only one of several manifestations of a secondary disease (e.g., vasculitis associated with systemic rheumatic diseases or with malignancies). The vasculitis syndromes are commonly grouped as a single disease entity, although it is important to note that multiple pathogenic mechanisms can result in blood vessel damage (8). Although no single classification schema has been able to categorize every vasculitis syndrome, it is useful to attempt to properly classify types of vasculitis in order to design rational clinical trials and to institute appropriate treatment (Table 63-1) (4,9,10). In general, vasculitis syndromes are mediated by immunologic mechanisms (4,11,12). That immune mechanisms are operative in vasculitis has been suggested from observations in animal models of immune-complex–mediated disease, from immunologic studies of patients with vasculitis, and from the responses of vasculitis patients to various modes of antiinflammatory and immunosuppressive therapy (1,4).

This chapter reviews the mechanisms operative in the pathogenesis of vasculitis (Table 63-2). Advances in the study of the molecules involved in immune intercellular interactions and in leukocyte–endothelial cell interactions have clarified pathogenic mechanisms involved in many types of inflammation. The concept has emerged that the cytokines and adhesion molecules that mediate normal inflammation and regulate salutory protective immune responses are also the mediators of pathogenic inflammatory responses in autoimmune diseases and vasculitis syndromes. The new frontier for research on vasculitis syndromes, as well as for all inflammatory diseases, is the search for identity of host genes that predispose to the development of these diseases. Examples of host genes that might predispose to the development of inflammatory diseases are genes that regulate the timing and magnitude of cytokine production in response to immune activation.

Mediators of inflammation necessary for the full expression of immune-mediated vasculitis syndromes include activated complement components, prostaglandins, cytokines, and chemokines. Each type of mediator will be discussed in relation to the pathogenesis of specific vasculitis syndromes. Similarly, adhesion molecules and T-cell co-stimulatory molecules are discussed in the context of their involvement in vessel damage. Both immune and nonimmune pathogenic mechanisms of vessel damage in vasculitis syndromes are also reviewed (Table 63-2).

IMMUNOLOGIC AND INFLAMMATORY PROCESSES INVOLVED IN VESSEL DAMAGE

Cytokines and Other Mediators of Inflammation

Cytokines play an integral role in the initiation and maintenance of inflammation; certain cytokines also downregulate inflammatory responses (13). Expression of cytokines in inflammatory lesions is tightly regulated,

J. S. Sundy: Department of Medicine, Duke University Medical Center, Durham, North Carolina 27710.

B. F. Haynes: Departments of Medicine and Immunology, Duke University School of Medicine, Durham, North Carolina 27710.

TABLE 63-1. *Human vasculitis syndromes*

Vasculitis syndrome	Usual patient characteristics	Mechanisms of vascular damage	Common pathologic findings[#]	General treatment approach
Polyarteritis nodosa group				
Polyarteritis nodosa	Adults 5th–7th decade, male-female ratio of 2:1	Immune complex formation, cellular immune response, antilysosomal antibodies	Small to medium vessels; microaneurysms; focal, panmural, assymmetric vessel involvement; macrophages and CD4[+] T cells predominate	Glucocorticoids, cytotoxic therapy
Churg-Strauss syndrome	Adults; male-female ratio of 2:1, eosinophilia, asthma symptoms common, any age	Immune complex formation, cellular immune response, infectious agents, antilysosomal antibodies	Granulomatous or necrotizing small vessel involvement; marked eosinophilic infiltrate; extravascular eosinophilic granulomas; perinuclear anti-neutrophil cytoplasmic antibodies (p-ANCA)	Antihistamines, glucocorticoids, cytotoxic therapy
Microscopic polyarteritis	Similar to polyarteritis nodosa	Immune complex formation, cellular immune response, antilysosomal antibodies	Similar to polyarteritis nodosa; necrotizing glomerulonephritis and pulmonary capillaritis common; p-ANCA	Glucocorticoids, cytotoxic therapy
Hypersensitivity vasculitis				
Serum sickness	Heterologous serum administration, certain medications	Immune complex formation	Arterioles and venules; neutrophilic or lymphocytic infiltrates; leukocytoclasis; hypocomplementemia common	Nonsteroidal antiinflammatory drugs (NSAIDs), glucocorticoids, cytotoxic therapy, plasmapheresis
Henoch-Schönlein purpura	Usually affects children	Immune complex formation	Small vessels; purpura; gastrointestinal vasculitis; necrotizing crescentic glomerulonephritis; similar to polyarteritis nodosa; marked IgA deposition	Glucocorticoids
Essential mixed cryoglobulinemia with vasculitis	Usually associated with chronic infection by hepatitis B or C virus	Immune complex formation, infectious agents	Small vessels; leukocytoclasis, cryoglobulins	NSAIDs, glucocorticoids, interferon-α, cytotoxic therapy, plasmapheresis
Malignancy-associated vasculitis	Usually associated with chronic infection by hepatitis B or C virus	Immune complex formation, tumor cell mediated, anti-endothelial cell antibodies	Variable	Treat underlying malignancy, glucocorticoids
Vasculitis associated with systemic rheumatic disease	Correlated with patient characteristics of systemic rheumatic disease	Immune complex formation, cellular immune response, anti-endothelial cell antibodies, anti-lysosomal antibodies	Variable	Treat underlying systemic rheumatic disease, glucocorticoids, cytotoxic therapy

TABLE 63-1. *Continued*

Vasculitis syndrome	Usual patient characteristics	Mechanisms of vascular damage	Common pathologic findings#	General treatment approach
Wegener's granulomatosis	Mean age 40s; male-female ratio of 1:1, 97% Caucasian	Cellular immune response, antilysosomal antibodies, immune complex formation	Small vessels; necrotizing granulomas and vasculitis of upper and lower respiratory tract; focal segmental necrotizing glomerulonephritis; granulomatous inflammation and multinucleated giant cells common	Glucocorticoids, cytotoxic therapy
Giant cell arteritis Temporal arteritis	European descent; age >50 y	Cellular immune response	Medium to large arteries; usually external carotid distribution; panarteritis; macrophage and CD4+ cells predominate; multinucleated giant cells common	Glucocorticoids, rarely cytotoxic therapy
Takayasu's arteritis	Women of reproductive age; most common in Asia, Eastern Europe, and Latin America	Cellular immune response	Large arteries; aorta, pulmonary artery, major limb arteries; proximal carotid and coronary arteries; panarteritis similar to temporal arteritis	Glucocorticoids, rarely cytotoxic therapy, angioplasty
Kawasaki's disease	Children <5 y; slight male predominance; fever, lymphadenopathy, rash, and mucosal inflammation	Immune complex formation, cellular immune response, possible infectious agent	Small, medium, and large vessels; coronary artery aneurysms	Intravenous γ-globulin, salicylates
Thromboangiitis obliterans (Buerger's disease)	Young male smokers	? Immune complex formation, ? cellular immune response	Thrombosis, vessel obliteration	Tobacco avoidance, revascularization
Miscellaneous vasculitides Lymphomatoid granulomatosis	5th–7th decade, male-female ratio of 2:1, respiratory and constitutional symptoms	Tumor cell mediated	Angiocentric, destructive lesions, usually in pulmonary vessels; T-cell infiltrate	Glucocorticoids, cytotoxic therapy
Cogan's syndrome	Mean age 25; male-female ratio of 1:1, keratitis and audiovestibular symptoms	Cellular immune response	Interstitial keratitis; small, medium, and large artery vasculitis	Glucocorticoids, cytotoxic therapy, cyclosporin A
Behçet's disease	Adults, mean age 25–35; male-female ratio of 1:1; Mediterranean and Far East predominance; oral and gential aphthous ulcers	Cellular immune response, ? immune complex formation	Arteries and veins of all sizes, lymphohistiocytic perivascular infiltrates with thrombosis	Colchicine, glucocorticoids, cytotoxic therapy, cyclosporin A
Infection-associated vasculitis	Variable	Multiple mechanisms	Variable	Treat underlying infection

#Classification adapted from ref. 4, with permission. # Ref. 209

TABLE 63-2. *Possible mechanisms of vascular damage in vasculitic syndromes*

Pathogenic immune complex formation
Anti-endothelial cell antibody—mediated vessel damage
Vessel damage associated with antibodies against lysosomal enzymes
Vessel damage caused by pathogenic cellular immune responses and granuloma formation
Vessel damage or altered vessel function mediated directly by infectious agents
Tumor cell—mediated vessel damage

and disordered expression of cytokines may contribute to the pathophysiology of vasculitis syndromes. Studies of the role of cytokines in vasculitis syndromes initially focused on detection of cytokines in serum, whereas recent studies have used *in situ* techniques to determine the cytokines produced *in vivo* in the microenvironment of vasculitis lesions (Table 63-3).

The cytokines most frequently identified in serum or tissues of vasculitis patients are interleukin-1 (IL-1), tumor necrosis factor-α (TNF-α), and interleukin-6 (IL-6). These cytokines upregulate expression of histocompatibility antigens on leukocytes and endothelial cells, induce T- and B-lymphocyte activation, upregulate chemokine expression in numerous cell types, induce monocyte activation, and stimulate production of acute-phase reactants (reviewed in refs. 14–16). Serum levels of proinflammatory cytokines such as IL-1, TNF-α, and IL-6, have been shown to be upregulated in Wegener's granulomatosis, giant cell arteritis, Kawasaki disease, Behçet's disease, and Henoch-Schönlein purpura (17–22). In some studies, expression of proinflammatory cytokines has been correlated with vasculitis disease activity

(23). Immune complex deposition in vessels, as well as antilysosomal and antiendothelial cell antibodies, stimulate production of IL-1, TNF-α, and IL-6 by endothelial cells and leukocytes (24–26).

Among CD4$^+$ T cells, interferon-γ (IFN-γ) is produced by Th1 helper T cells (27). IFN-γ induces a wide variety of cellular immune responses, including the migration of monocytes/macrophages (28). IFN-γ has been associated predominantly with vasculitis syndromes in which T cells are thought to play a significant role. Elevated serum levels of IFN-γ have been reported in patients with Kawasaki disease, polyarteritis nodosa, and Churg-Strauss syndrome (18,29). Weyand et al. (30) have reported upregulated expression of IFN-γ mRNA *in situ* in temporal arteritis vessel lesions, but not in blood vessels in the related but less severe syndrome of polymyalgia rheumatica. IFN-γ stimulates macrophage multinucleated giant cell formation, one of the histologic hallmarks of temporal arteritis (31). Upregulated expression of IFN-γ in the setting of macrophage multinucleated giant cell formation has emerged as a common finding in a variety of granulomatous inflammatory disease states (32,33). Another vasculitis syndrome commonly associated with giant cell formation is Wegener's granulomatosis; however, to date, no studies have assessed IFN-γ production in this disease.

Interleukin-2 (IL-2) is a T-cell stimulatory cytokine produced by T cells. Inductive actions of IL-2 include T-cell activation and proliferation as well as upregulation of production by endothelial cells of the potent vasoconstrictor endothelin (34). Upregulated T-cell IL-2 mRNA or protein expression has been described in temporal arteritis and in Kawasaki disease, two conditions characterized by marked T-cell infiltration of pathologic lesions

TABLE 63-3. *Cytokines involved in the pathogenesis of vasculitis*

Cytokine	Associated vasculitis syndrome	References
TNF-α	Wegener's granulomatosis, giant cell arteritis, Kawasaki disease, Behçet's disease, Henoch-Schönlein purpura	17–22
TNF-β	Kawasaki disease	247
IFN-α	Polyarteritis nodosa	18
IFN-γ	Churg-Strauss syndrome, polyarteritis nodosa, Kawasaki disease, temporal arteritis	18, 29, 30
IL-1	Wegener's granulomatosis, giant cell arteritis, Kawasaki disease, Behçet's disease, Henoch-Schönlein purpura	17–22
IL-2	Kawasaki disease, giant cell arteritis, polyarteritis nodosa	18, 35, 36
IL-4	Kawasaki disease, Churg-Strauss syndrome	39, 40
IL-5	Churg-Strauss syndrome	40
IL-6	Wegener's granulomatosis, giant cell arteritis, Kawasaki disease, Behçet's disease, Henoch-Schönlein purpura	17–22
IL-8	Behçet's disease, Wegener's granulomatosis	42, 44, 45
IL-10	Behçet's disease, Kawasaki disease	23, 39
IL-12	Behçet's disease	23
MCP-1	Wegener's granulomatosis, mixed essential cryoglobulinemia	41
G-CSF	Cutaneous vasculitis	248
TGF-β1	Wegener's granulomatosis	249

G-CSF, granulocyte colony-stimulating factor; IFN, interferon; IL, interleukin; MCP, monocyte chemotactic protein; TGF, transforming growth factor; TNF, tumor necrosis factor.

(35,36). The presence of IL-2 mRNA expression in vessel lesion tissue correlated with symptoms of polymyalgia rheumatica in patients with temporal arteritis (37). Another T-cell–derived cytokine, interleukin-4 (IL-4), was upregulated in tissue in mercuric chloride–induced vasculitis syndrome in rats (38). IL-4 levels were elevated in the serum of children in the acute phase of Kawasaki disease (39), and elevated serum IL-4 and interleukin-5 (IL-5) levels have been reported in a patient with Churg-Strauss syndrome (40).

Chemokines are a subgroup of cytokines important in recruiting leukocytes to sites of inflammation. Expression of the chemokine interleukin-8 (IL-8) and macrophage chemotactic protein-1 (MCP-1) has been demonstrated in lesional tissue of vasculitis syndromes (41,42). Endothelial cells cultured in the presence of antiendothelial cell antibodies (AECA) from the sera of Wegener's granulomatosis patients expressed increased levels of both IL-8 and MCP-1. IL-8 expression was also increased in endothelial cells incubated with proteinase-3, a neutrophil lysosomal protein that is the target of antineutrophil cytoplasmic antibodies (c-ANCA), with a cytoplasmic staining pattern (43). Increased serum levels of IL-8 have been reported in patients with Behçet's disease, a finding that correlated with increased *in vitro* adhesion of Behçet patient polymorphonuclear cells (PMNs) to endothelial cells (44,45).

Another important mediator of inflammation is nitric oxide (NO). Inhibitors of NO production have prevented vessel damage in mouse models of vasculitis (46,47). Human temporal arteritis–severe combined immune deficiency (SCID) mouse chimeras exhibited decreased inducible nitric oxide synthase (iNOS) expression after treatment of mice with dexamethasone (48). MRL/lpr mice rendered iNOS deficient by homologous recombination were protected from the spontaneous onset of vasculitis that occurs in this autoimmune mouse strain (49). Increased NO production was detected in Kawasaki disease patients during acute disease, and levels fell after treatment (50). Finally, macrophages expressing iNOS have been detected in the intimal vessel layer of temporal arteritis tissues (51).

The prostaglandins, leukotrienes, and thromboxanes are also important mediators of vessel damage in vasculitis syndromes. Increased leukotriene levels have been detected in Kawasaki disease and Henoch-Schönlein purpura (52,53). Matrix metalloproteinases contribute to tissue injury by degrading collagen and other matrix molecules. These enzymes may also directly stimulate some of the inflammatory responses seen in vessel lesions in temporal arteritis (8).

Immune Cell Adhesion and Co-Stimulatory Molecules

Cell-cell interactions among leukocytes, and between leukocytes and endothelial cells, are critical in the development of inflammatory responses. As with cytokines, inappropriate expression or upregulation of normal cell adhesion and cell co-stimulatory molecules is thought to contribute to the clinical expression of vasculitis syndromes. Often, the binding of a leukocyte cell surface molecule to its ligand results in both cell-cell adhesion and the stimulation of specialized immune cell functions (reviewed in ref. 54). Therefore, the role of adhesion molecules as co-stimulatory molecules in the pathogenesis of vasculitis are discussed together in this section (Table 63-4).

Immune and endothelial cell adhesion molecules mediate a three-step process that enables leukocytes to migrate from the intravascular space into tissue (55). These steps are leukocyte rolling, leukocyte firm adherence, and leukocyte extravasation. Three classes of adhesion molecules mediate these leukocyte-endothelial cell interactions. The selectins mediate rolling, whereas the integrins and the immunoglobulin superfamily members mediate firm adherence and leukocyte extravasation (reviewed in ref. 54). Studies of serum and lesional tissue from patients have yielded important information on the role of adhesion molecules in the pathogenesis of vasculitis syndromes (Table 63-4) (reviewed in ref. 56).

Soluble adhesion molecules have been detected in the serum of patients with vasculitis, and in some instances serum levels of soluble adhesion molecules have been correlated with disease activity (57). However, changes in soluble adhesion molecule levels are not specific for vasculitis syndromes, thus limiting the utility of their measurement as a marker of disease activity or an indicator of disease recrudescence (58,59). Leukocytes circulating in the peripheral blood of vasculitis patients also have upregulated expression of certain adhesion molecules.

The selectins, CD62L (L-selectin), CD62E (E-selectin), and CD62P (P-selectin), mediate the initial stages of leukocyte adherence to endothelium (60). CD62L is expressed on all leukocytes, and after cell activation is shed from the cell surface (60). Soluble serum CD62L levels were found to be decreased during the acute stage of Kawasaki disease (61) followed by increased expression during the convalescent phase of the disease (62). CD62E is expressed only on activated endothelial cells and binds to CD15 on rolling leukocytes (60). IL-1, TNF-α, and IFN-γ, cytokines involved in the pathogenesis of vasculitis syndromes, upregulate CD62E expression on endothelial cells (60,63–65). Elevated soluble serum CD62E levels have been described in generalized Wegener's granulomatosis (59,66,67) and in temporal arteritis (67). During the acute phase of Kawasaki disease (58,68,69), soluble CD62E serum levels were elevated. CD62E serum levels correlated with serum TNF-α levels and were shown to decrease after treatment (68). *In situ* studies revealed upregulated CD62E expression on cutaneous vessels in leukocytoclastic vasculitis and cutaneous lymphocytic vasculitis (70,71). Neutrophil infiltra-

TABLE 63-4. *Adhesion molecules in vasculitis syndromes*

Adhesion molecule	Ligand	Disease	Cell type	References
VLA-4 (CD49d/CD29)	VCAM-1 (CD106), fibronectin	SLE with vasculitis	Blood lymphocytes	76
		WG	CD4+ cells	57
ICAM-1 (CD54)	LFA-1 (CD11a/CD18)	WG	Serum	59, 66, 86
		WG, MPA	Peripheral blood lymphocyte	57, 74
		KD	Serum	58, 69
		KD	Skin lesions	20
		GCA	Lesional granulomas	78
		Cutaneous vasculitis	Lesional endothelial cells, inflammatory cells	70, 71
VCAM-1 (CD106)	VLA-4 (CD49d/CD29), α4β7 integrin	WG	Serum	59, 66, 86
		Cutaneous vasculitis	Lesional endothelial cells, inflammatory cells	70, 71
		ANCA + vasculitis	Lesional kidney tissue	91
		KD	Serum	58
LFA-3 (CD58)	LFA-2 (CD2)	WG	Peripheral blood lymphocytes	57
		GCA	Lesional granulomas	78
ELAM-1 (CD62E)	Sialyl Lewis a,x	GCA	Serum	67
		KD	Skin lesions	20
		Cutaneous vasculitis	Lesional endothelial cells, inflammatory cells	70, 71
		WG	Serum	59, 66, 86
		KD	Serum	68
CD11a (LFA-1 subunit)	ICAM-1, ICAM-2	WG	Blood granulocytes, monocytes	75
CD11b	ICAM-1, fibrinogen	WG	Blood granulocytes, monocytes	75
CD18 (LFA-1 subunit)	ICAM-1, fibrinogen	WG	Blood granulocytes, monocytes, lymphocytes	75
LFA-1 (CD11a/CD18)	ICAM-1(CD54), ICAM-2, ICAM-3	GCA	Lesional CD3+ cells	77
CD29	VCAM-1, VLA 1-6	WG	Blood granulocytes, monocytes, lymphocytes	75
VLA-1 (CD49a/CD29)	collagen, laminin	GCA	Lesional CD3+ cells	77

GCA, giant cell arteritis; SLE, systemic lupus erythematosus; WG, Wegener's granulomatosis; MPA, microscopic polyangiitis; KD, Kawasaki disease; VLA, very late antigen of activation; VCAM, vascular cell adhesion molecule; ICAM, intercellular adhesion molecule; ANCA, anti-neutrophil cytoplasmic antibody; LFA, lymphocyte function-associated antigen; ELAM, endothelial-leukocyte adhesion molecule.

tion of cutaneous vasculitis lesions occurred only in regions of CD62E expression, and the degree of neutrophil infiltration correlated with the intensity of CD62E staining (71). CD62E was also upregulated on cutaneous vessels obtained from Kawasaki disease skin lesions (20). Biopsies of skin lesions obtained after treatment of Kawasaki disease with intravenous immunoglobulin showed reduced CD62E expression, suggesting that endothelial cell activation and upregulated CD62E expression is important in the pathogenesis of cutaneous manifestations of Kawasaki disease (20).

The integrins mediate leukocyte firm adherence and also transduce signals from the extracellular matrix and the cell membrane to the inside of the cell (reviewed in ref. 60). The β_1 and β_3 integrins are expressed by a wide variety of immune cell types and bind to ligands of the extracellular matrix such as laminin, collagen, and fibronectin. Integrins also bind to clotting factor components such as fibrinogen and von Willebrand factor (reviewed in refs. 60,72,73). The β_2 integrins [lymphocyte function antigen-1 (LFA-1), membrane attack complex-1 (MAC-1)/Mo-1, and p150,95] are expressed on leukocytes, and bind either immunoglobulin superfamily

molecules such as intracellular adhesion molecule-1 or (ICAM-1) or -2 (ICAM-2), as in the case of LFA-1, or bind complement and clotting cascade factors as do p150,95 and MAC-1/Mo-1. The β_2 integrins are key components required for normal leukocyte homing and migration, and they are essential for many leukocyte effector functions. In many types of inflammatory lesional tissue, the receptors that bind integrins are upregulated, and integrins themselves are induced to be upregulated or to be in a high-affinity state as well (60).

Increased expression of integrin adhesion molecules has been demonstrated in several vasculitis syndromes. In patients with Wegener's granulomatosis, high levels of LFA-3 were expressed on peripheral blood lymphocytes, and CD11b was upregulated on peripheral blood monocytes and granulocytes in patients with active disease (57,74,75). The β-integrin subunits, CD11a, CD18 and CD29, were upregulated on peripheral blood leukocytes of patients with active Wegener's granulomatosis (75). In some patients, CD18 levels decreased after treatment of Wegener's granulomatosis (75). Serum levels of very late activation antigen-4 (VLA-4) were increased in patients with vasculitis associated with systemic lupus erythematosus (76). Finally, CD3$^+$ cells infiltrating temporal arteritis lesions exhibited high levels of LFA-1 and VLA-1 expression (77), while granuloma cells in temporal arteritis lesions expressed high levels of LFA-3 (78).

Adhesion molecules of the immunoglobulin superfamily also play central roles in the initiation of inflammatory responses. ICAM-1 is widely distributed, and its expression is induced on endothelial cells and fibroblasts by IL-1, TNF-α, and IFN-γ (60,79). VCAM-1 is the ligand for the integrin VLA-4, and similarly is induced on endothelium by IL-1, TNF-α, and IFN-γ (80–83; reviewed in ref. 84). The induction of ICAM-1 and vascular cell adhesion molecule-1 (VCAM-1) on endothelial cells by proinflammatory cytokines (IL-1, TNF-α, and IFN-γ) is a central event in the inflammatory response and plays a major role in leukocyte binding to, and transmigration through, the endothelial-cell layer of the vessel wall—a central event in the development of necrotizing vasculitis (60,79,84). The CD2/LFA-3 ligand pair is involved in T-cell activation and cytotoxic T-cell effector function (reviewed in refs. 69 and 84). In addition, CD2 on T cells interacts with LFA-3 on fibroblasts and monocytes and mediates T-cell interactions with nonleukocyte components of inflammatory microenvironments (85).

Serum ICAM-1 and/or VCAM-1 levels were increased in the serum of patients with Wegener's granulomatosis, temporal arteritis, systemic lupus erythematosus–associated vasculitis, and Kawasaki disease (58,59,66,68,69, 76,86). ICAM-1 levels in Kawasaki disease correlated with serum TNF-α levels and decreased after therapy (58,68,69). Patients developing coronary artery aneurysms in Kawasaki disease had the highest levels of soluble ICAM-1 compared to patients without coronary artery inflammation (68,69). ICAM-1 is highly expressed on macrophages in granulomas, on intimal myofibroblasts, and on medial smooth muscle cells in temporal arteritis lesions (78). ICAM-1 levels were also increased on cutaneous vessels in skin lesions of patients with Kawasaki disease, and levels decreased after treatment with intravenous immunoglobulin (20).

Burrows et al. (70) studied vasculitic skin tissue and compared adhesion molecule expression in leukocytoclastic vasculitis versus lymphocytic vasculitis. ICAM-1 and CD62E were expressed at higher levels in lesional tissue compared to normal control tissue. However, VCAM-1 was expressed only in lesional tissues. VCAM-1 was expressed in a greater percentage of lesional tissues from patients with lymphocytic vasculitis (50%) in comparison to leukocytoclastic vasculitis (21%). In a separate study of cutaneous vasculitis tissue, neutrophil infiltration was dependent on the expression of CD62E, and the degree of infiltration correlated with the intensity of expression of CD62E (71). Conversely, endothelial expression of ICAM-1 and VCAM-1 was correlated with infiltration of mononuclear cells. These data suggest that unique inflammatory stimuli influence the types of adhesion molecules expressed on endothelial cells, which, in turn, may influence the type of immune cells that infiltrate vessel walls.

Other studies of in situ immunoglobulin superfamily adhesion molecule expression have revealed increased VCAM-1 and ICAM-1 expression in kidney tissue from patients with idiopathic glomerulonephritis, microscopic polyarteritis, and Wegener's granulomatosis (87–90). Renal glomerular VCAM-1 expression in ANCA-positive vasculitis kidney lesions was correlated with migration of macrophages into glomeruli (91). ICAM-1 was also upregulated in tissues from temporal arteritis, and in involved muscle and nerve tissue from patients with small and medium vessel vasculitis syndromes (78,92).

Co-stimulatory signals mediated by adhesion molecules are key regulatory events of T-cell activation (see chapter by Lee et al.). A critical co-stimulatory signal for T-cell activation involves the ligation of the T cell CD28 molecule by the B7 (CD80) molecule on antigen-presenting cells (93). Antigen binding to the T-cell antigen receptor does not lead to T-cell activation unless a co-stimulatory signal delivered through CD28 ligation is simultaneously received. In contrast, antigen stimulation of T cells in the absence of CD28 co-stimulation leads to T-cell anergy. Thus, CD28/CD80 binding is likely to be important in T-cell activation in vasculitis syndromes, although no studies have directly addressed this issue.

Another receptor-ligand interaction that is likely important in the pathogenesis of certain vasculitis syndromes occurs between CD154 (gp39; CD40L) on activated CD4$^+$ T cells, endothelial cells, smooth muscle cells, and macrophages, and CD40 on B cells, granulocytes, and mesenchymal cells (94,95, reviewed in ref. 96). Deficiency of CD154 on T cells leads to the X-linked hyperimmunoglobulin M (IgM) syndrome in humans, a congenital immunodeficiency disease resulting from the inability of B cells to switch immunoglobulin isotypes (96). CD40 is expressed on kidney tubules, and cross-linking of CD40 on these cells results in IL-8, MCP-1, and RANTES (regulated on activation, normally T-cell expressed and secreted) production (97). Therefore, activated T cells may trigger nephritis through CD40 ligation on tubule cells with production of inflammatory chemokines, resulting in leukocyte infiltration into the renal interstitium. CD40 ligation of CD154 by pulmonary fibroblasts can also lead to T cell activation in a CD28-independent manner (95). Interestingly, CD40 and its ligand are expressed on vascular endothelial cells and levels of surface expression are upregulated by stimulation with IL1β, TNF-α, and IFN-γ (94). The role of CD40 and CD154 in the pathogenesis of vasculitis has not been studied, but the broad distribution of these molecules suggests that they play an important role in stimulating inflammatory responses by lymphocytes and myeloid cells in vasculitis syndromes.

Finally, the Fas antigen (CD95) and its ligand are important in downregulating immune responses by inducing apoptosis. The murine strains MRL/lpr and MRL/gld encode a Fas deletion and Fas functional mutant respectively (98). Vasculitis develops spontaneously in both strains, supporting an important role for Fas-mediated apoptosis in preventing vascular inflammation.

PATHOGENIC MECHANISMS OF VESSEL DAMAGE

Pathogenic Immune-Complex Formation

Pathogenic immune complexes can activate complement components that participate in the amplification phases of the inflammatory response via generation of chemotactic factors for polymorphonuclear cells and monocytes (e.g., C5a). Further activation of complement can lead to assembly of the membrane attack complex (C5b–C9), thereby causing cellular damage. Polymorphonuclear cells and monocytes are activated to produce numerous proinflammatory cytokines (Table 63-3), adhere to activated ICAM-1+ and ELAM-1+ endothelium, extravasate, and migrate toward the site of immune-complex deposition (Fig. 63-1). Further phagocyte activation causes release of proteolytic enzymes (elastase, cathepsin G, proteinase-3), reactive oxygen metabolites, and proinflammatory substances such as platelet activating factor, leukotrienes, and prostaglandins. Platelets may (a) adhere to locally damaged endothelium via platelet gpIIb-IIIa binding to vessel von Willebrand factor, fibronectin, fibrinogen, and aggregate; (b) obstruct blood vessels; and (c) induce vessel necrosis and clot formation (Fig. 63-2). Once the vessel is damaged, production of NO is inhibited and release of endothelin is augmented, leading to vasoconstriction, larger clot formation, and eventually vascular occlusion (reviewed in ref. 99). Thus, these reactions spiral into an amplification cascade, causing damage to vessel walls and surrounding tissues (4,100,101).

The deposition of immune complexes in and around vessel walls is an important event in the genesis of vasculitis lesions in many of the syndromes listed in Table 63-1. Studies in animal models of acute serum sickness have demonstrated a series of events that lead to immune-complex–mediated vascular damage (reviewed in ref.

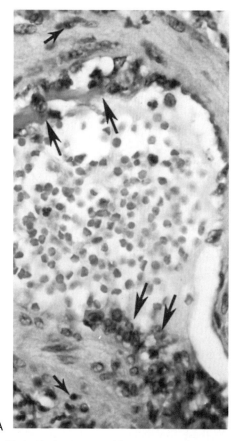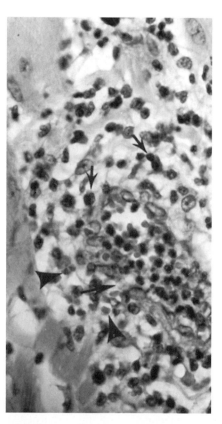

A   B

FIG. 63-1. Early stages of immune-mediated vascular damage in systemic necrotizing vasculitis. **A:** Adhesion of clumps of numerous mononuclear cells *(large arrows)* to damaged endothelium, with other mononuclear cells *(small arrows)* in and around the wall of the vessel. ×400. **B:** Small vessel with perivascular infiltration *(small arrows)* and vessel disruption *(large arrow)*, with extravasated erythrocytes *(arrowheads)* outside of the vessel lumen. ×400.

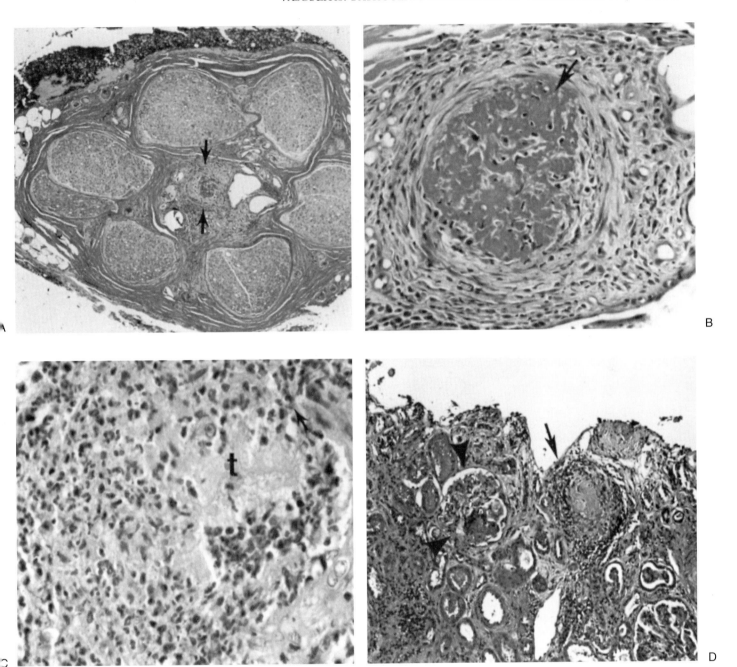

FIG. 63-2. Late stages of vessel damage in systemic necrotizing vasculitis. **A:** Low-power view of a nerve bundle with vasculitis of the central small muscular artery *(arrows)* ×100. **B:** Central clot *(arrow)* in the central small muscular artery seen in A. ×400. **C:** Thrombosis (t) and extensive vessel inflammation *(arrow)* in a gastric artery. ×400. **D:** Kidney biopsy from a patient with Wegener's granulomatosis with both renal vasculitis *(arrow)* and necrotizing proliferative glomerulonephritis *(arrowheads)* present. ×400.

102). Rabbits given a single intravenous injection of bovine serum albumin (BSA) developed necrotizing arteritis and glomerulonephritis similar to the lesions seen in humans with polyarteritis nodosa (103,104). Immunofluorescent studies of affected vessel walls and glomeruli showed immunoglobulins, BSA, and complement (105). Complement fixation, histamine release, and the presence of neutrophils were all important for induction of vessel damage in this model (106).

In 1982, Lawley et al. (107) documented the clinical and immunologic features of human serum sickness in patients with aplastic anemia who had received horse antithymocyte globulin. These patients developed fever, skin lesions, arthralgias, gastrointestinal symptoms, and proteinuria 8 to 13 days after initiation of therapy. Similar to observations in animal models, the clinical manifestations of serum sickness in humans were related to the formation of immune complexes. A rise in the level of serum immune complexes was accompanied by decreases in serum levels of C3 and C4 and increases in serum levels of C3a/C3a des Arg. In indirect immunofluorescence assays, three of five skin biopsies showed immunoglobulin and/or complement deposition in small dermal blood vessels (107). It has since been shown that immune complex deposition is dependent on increased vascular permeability and that immune complexes are directly capable of activating PMNs to induce increased vascular permeability (108).

In the early 1970s, an association between persistent hepatitis B virus infection and a systemic necrotizing vasculitic syndrome indistinguishable from classic polyarteritis nodosa was noted (109,110). Subsequently, the association of essential mixed cryoglobulinemia and vasculitis with hepatitis B and hepatitis C virus infection was described (111,112). In hepatitis B and C virus–associated vasculitic syndromes, viral antigens are present in circulating or tissue-bound immune complexes (109, 113), strongly suggesting that such immune complexes are causally related to the development of vasculitis. Antiviral therapy diminished the manifestations of hepatitis syndrome–induced vasculitis concomitant with a reduction in levels of circulating immune complexes (113). A spectrum of vasculitic syndromes ranging from urticarial vasculitis to systemic necrotizing vasculitis has been associated with hepatitis B infection (114). In polyarteritis nodosa not associated with hepatitis B or other defined antigens, immunoglobulin deposits in vascular lesions have been seen in some, but not all, patients (115–121). In a retrospective study of polyarteritis nodosa, immunoglobulin deposition was found in glomeruli and arteries in only a small percentage of cases (122). However, elevated serum immune complexes (measured by C1q binding) were present in 90% of patients, with serum cryoglobulins being present in 20%, and elevated serum rheumatoid factor in 30% (122).

Cryoglobulins are immunoglobulins that precipitate from blood at low temperatures. Elevated serum levels of cryoglobulins are found in a large variety of diseases in addition to occurring as a primary disorder (123). Type I cryoglobulins are monoclonal immunoglobulins that aggregate to form cryoprecipitates. Type II cryoglobulins consist of monoclonal immunoglobulins that bind to polyclonal IgG, whereas type III cryoglobulins generally are polyclonal rheumatoid factors (RFs) that activate complement via the classical pathway (124). In general, type I cryoproteins aggregate on a nonimmune basis and mediate vessel damage by complement activation via the alternative pathway (124). The clinical syndromes produced by type I cryoprecipitates are usually hyperviscosity syndromes or, less commonly, a hypersensitivity vasculitis (124). The most common type of cryoglobulinemia associated with systemic vasculitis is the mixed (type III) variety and is usually associated with hepatitis C virus infection (112). Type III cryoglobulinemia produces the distinctive

mixed cryoglobulinemia-purpura-nephritis-vasculitis syndrome (125,126). Recently, the neuropathy associated with mixed cryoglobulinemia was shown to be associated with immunoglobulin and complement deposition in endoneurial capillaries, while a mononuclear cell infiltrate was present in the endoneurial arterioles (127). Cryoglobulins can also directly stimulate the release of PMN lysosomal enzymes. Cold-induced cutaneous polyarteritis nodosa has been described with a mixed cryoglobulin complex containing hepatitis B surface antigen and IgG, IgA, IgM, and C3. *In vitro* studies demonstrated that these immune complexes could be phagocytosed by polymorphonuclear cells, resulting in release of lysosomal enzymes (128).

Churg-Strauss syndrome, or allergic angiitis and granulomatosis, was first described in 1950 and is considered to be a clinical subset of systemic necrotizing vasculitis syndromes (4,129). Churg-Strauss syndrome occurs in patients with a prior history of asthma or other atopic diseases and is characterized by eosinophilia, eosinophilic tissue infiltration of various organs (particularly lung), presence of extravascular granulomas, and necrotizing vasculitis of small arteries and veins (129). Elevated serum IgE levels during the vasculitic phase of the illness are typical (130), and elevated serum levels of IgE-containing immune complexes have been reported (131). In one review, two of 14 sera contained elevated immune-complex levels. In addition, renal biopsies showed IgM deposits in four patients, with C3 deposition in three and IgA in one (132).

Circulating and deposited immune complexes have been reported in some cases of Wegener's granulomatosis, a form of systemic necrotizing vasculitis characterized by granulomatous vasculitis of the upper and lower airways and crescentic glomerulonephritis (4,133–135). C3, IgM, or IgG is present in a granular pattern in Wegener's granulomatosis in less than half of renal biopsies (130,136). Rheumatoid factor is present in ~40% of patients with Wegener's granulomatosis (4). Immunofluorescence studies on lung tissues from patients with Wegener's granulomatosis have demonstrated C3 and IgG deposition in a granular pattern in alveolae as well as within medium-sized pulmonary vessels (137).

Two connective tissue diseases frequently associated with formation of immune complexes and vasculitis are rheumatoid arthritis (RA) and systemic lupus erythematosus (SLE). The spectrum of vasculitis in RA and SLE ranges from a hypersensitivity vasculitis affecting small vessels, resulting in skin and nerve involvement, to a severe systemic necrotizing vasculitis syndrome similar to that seen in classic polyarteritis nodosa (4,138). Patients with RA and vasculitis are more likely to have severe erosive joint disease, hypocomplementemia, circulating cryoglobulins, and low-molecular-weight IgM and IgG rheumatoid factors (139). In RA, elevated levels of serum immune complexes are common, and immunoglobulin and complement deposition have been found in vessels of perineural tissue, rheumatoid nodules, synovium, and skin. Immune deposits have also been found in normal skin of patients with RA (140). Immune complexes from RA patient sera have been shown to activate neutrophils, which in turn induce injury to endothelial cells (141). Histamine injected into the skin of RA patients induced leukocytoclastic vasculitis in rheumatoid factor positive patients, suggesting that vasoactive amines such as histamine contribute to the pathogenesis of immune complex vasculitis (142).

IgM rheumatoid factors have been demonstrated in cryoglobulins in rheumatoid vasculitis, and their levels have been correlated with disease activity (143). Stage and Mannik (144) found that the presence of monomeric serum IgM in RA was associated with severe articular disease, rheumatoid nodules, high erythrocyte sedimentation rate, antinuclear antibodies, and rheumatoid vasculitis. IgG rheumatoid factors have been shown to occur more frequently and in higher titer in patients with rheumatoid vasculitis and in patients with RA and active extraarticular disease (145). Studies of serum IgG RF and C4 levels showed that IgG RF levels and anticomplement activity rose while C4 fell with clinical relapse and returned to normal during remission (146). In addition, immune complexes containing complement-activating RFs have been found in sera of rheumatoid vasculitis patients (147). Some IgG RFs can form unique immune complexes (cyclic homodimers) with themselves as well with as with normal IgG; in doing so, they activate complement via the classical pathway (148).

In SLE, elevated levels of circulating immune complexes are common, and immune-complex deposition can be demonstrated in vessels in multiple organs (149). SLE vasculitis is more likely to be seen with large immune complexes, whereas smaller immune complexes are found in patients with SLE glomerulonephritis (149). The relevance of elevated serum immune complexes in SLE is strongly suggested by the common occurrence of hypocomplementemia associated with disease activity (149). Patients with SLE have abnormally long clearance times for IgG-coated erythrocytes; patients with higher immune-complex levels have a greater defect in CR1-mediated and Fc-receptor–mediated clearance (150,151).

Hypersensitivity vasculitis syndromes constitute a broad category of diseases whose clinical hallmark is necrotizing arteritis of the skin manifested clinically as palpable purpura or recurrent urticaria (4) (Table 63-1). Forms of hypersensitivity vasculitis have been associated with connective tissue diseases, certain medications, malignancies, and infections (4,152). In hypersensitivity vasculitis, the vascular lesions may remain localized to skin or involve various organ systems (152). In most forms of hypersensitivity vasculitis, immune complexes have been demonstrated in cutaneous vessels (153–156).

Henoch-Schönlein purpura (HSP) is a form of hypersensitivity vasculitis in which cutaneous palpable purpura is accompanied by arthralgias, nephritis, gastrointestinal bleeding, and abdominal pain (157). In HSP, biopsy of affected skin shows small-vessel vasculitis (158) (Fig. 63-3). Immunofluorescence of these lesions reveals granu-

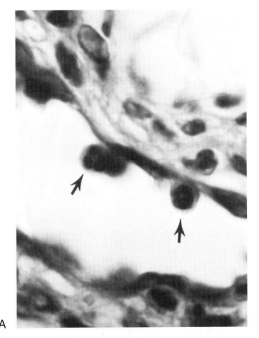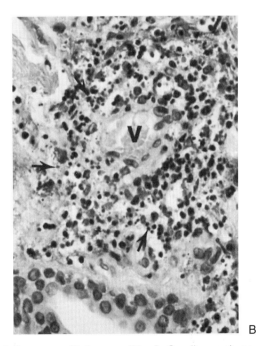

A B

FIG. 63-3. Immune-mediated small-vessel damage in hypersensitivity vasculitis. **A:** Small-vessel vasculitis in a dermal vessel in Henoch-Schönlein purpura. Note neutrophils adherent to endothelium *(arrows)*. ×1000. **B:** Extensive polymorphonuclear-cell infiltration in a skin vessel (V) with extensive necrosis (pyknotic nuclei, *arrows*) from a biopsy from a patient with Wegener's granulomatosis. ×400.

lar IgA deposition in vessel walls with C3, fibrin, and fibrinogen present (159). Immune deposits may be present in uninvolved skin as well (160). Gastrointestinal symptoms result from bowel wall small vessel vasculitis (161). Characteristic findings in kidneys range from minimal change to diffuse mesangial proliferation, with mesangial deposits of IgA1 predominating (160–162). C3, IgG, properdin, and factor B glomerular deposits have also been reported in HSP (100). Approximately 60% of patients with HSP have elevated serum IgA levels. Elevated serum immune complexes containing IgA have been documented in HSP, as have increased numbers of IgA-producing lymphocytes (163–165). Finally, many patients with HSP have low total hemolytic complement levels with decreased alternative pathway components (166). Inability of IgA to activate the classic complement pathway, as well as inefficient C3 binding by IgA immune complexes, can result in pathogenic immune-complex formation and defective C3b-mediated immune-complex clearance (167).

Antibodies Against Neutrophil Lysosomal Enzymes

Antineutrophil cytoplasmic antibodies (ANCA) were first described in 1982 (168) and were associated with vasculitis syndromes in 1984 (169). Analysis of sera from patients with primary vasculitis syndromes has led to a grouping of ANCA-associated vasculitides that includes Wegener's granulomatosis and microscopic polyangiitis (reviewed in ref. 170). While detecting ANCAs is important in the diagnosis and management of patients with vasculitis, it has also become clear that the presence of ANCA is not specific for vasculitis, and that ANCAs can be detected in a variety of infectious, neoplastic, and inflammatory disorders (170–172). Recent research has focused on identifying the potential role of ANCAs in the pathogenesis of the primary vasculitides (Fig. 63-4).

Two types of ANCAs have been described. Cytoplasmic ANCAs (c-ANCAs) react with neutrophils in a cytoplasmic pattern and usually recognize a 29-kd serine pro-

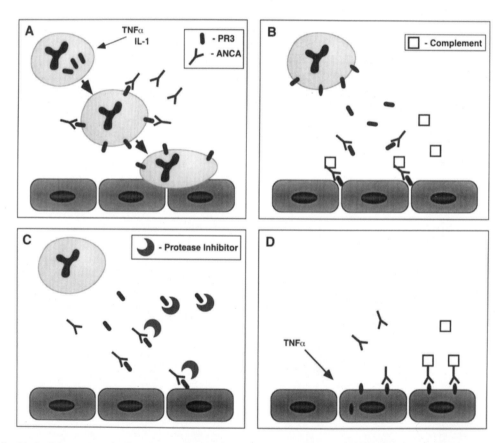

FIG. 63-4. Potential mechanisms of pathogenesis of antineutrophil cytoplasmic antibodies. **A:** Proinflammatory cytokines stimulate neutrophils [polymorphonuclear cells (PMNs)] to express surface proteinase-3. Cytoplasmic antineutrophil cytoplasmic antibody (c-ANCA) activates PMNs through cell surgace proteinase-3, leading to bystander injury of vessels. **B:** Proteinase-3 is released from PMNs, resulting in immune complex formation with ANCA. Immune complexes deposit on endothelium, leading to complement fixation and vessel damage. **C:** ANCA binds to secreted proteinase-3, preventing inactivation of proteinase-3 by protease inhibitors. Active proteinase-3 directly mediates vessel damage. **D:** ANCA antigen is directly expressed on endothelium, leading to ANCA binding and subsequent vessel damage by complement activation and inflammatory cell infiltration.

tease, proteinase-3 (Fig. 63-5) (173). c-ANCA antibodies with specificities other than proteinase-3 have been described, but they represent less than 5% of c-ANCAs and are not associated with Wegener's granulomatosis (170). Proteinase-3–specific ANCAs have 95% specificity for Wegener's granulomatosis, while the sensitivity varies from 50% to 100% depending on disease activity (172,174–176). The second type of ANCA, perinuclear ANCAs (p-ANCAs), react with neutrophils in a perinuclear pattern and bind predominantly to myeloperoxidase (Fig. 63-5) (177,178). Myeloperoxidase-specific ANCA is highly associated with microscopic polyangiitis, a pauci-immune small vessel vasculitis characterized by crescentic glomerulonephritis and/or alveolar capillaritis (10). However, the specificity of p-ANCAs for a particular vasculitis syndrome is far less than that of c-ANCA (171). The p-ANCAs are present in up to 70% of patients with ulcerative colitis, and can be detected in patients with polyarteritis nodosa, Churg-Strauss syndrome, and a variety of systemic rheumatic diseases (173,177, 179,180). The specificity of p-ANCAs in diseases other than microscopic polyangiitis varies and includes elastase, lactoferrin, β-glucuronidase, and cathepsin G (175, 181–189).

In addition to serving as markers for forms of systemic necrotizing vasculitis and idiopathic glomerulonephritis, ANCAs have been postulated to play a pathogenic role in vessel injury in these vasculitic syndromes (Fig. 63-4). It has been postulated that exogenous stimuli, such as bacterial antigens, are involved in the pathogenesis of Wegener's granulomatosis (180). In Wegener's granulomatosis, disease exacerbations are often associated with infection of the upper respiratory tract (190). Recent reports of the efficacy of antibiotics in preventing relapses in Wegener's granulomatosis lend support to this hypothesis (191,192). In response to infectious agents, neutrophils become activated and release lysosomal enzymes. Proteinase-3 and myeloperoxidase are present on the surface of activated neutrophils but not on nonactivated ones (180,193). Surface expression of proteinase-3 is induced by a combination of TNF-α and IL-8 (194). Neutrophils from Wegener's granulomatosis patients have increased surface expression of proteinase-3 (195). Falk et al. (196) demonstrated that purified anti–proteinase-3 and antimyeloperoxidase antibodies stimulated the release of toxic superoxide radicals from TNF-α–primed neutrophils. Thus, the presence of anti–proteinase-3 and antimyeloperoxidase antibodies in systemic necrotizing

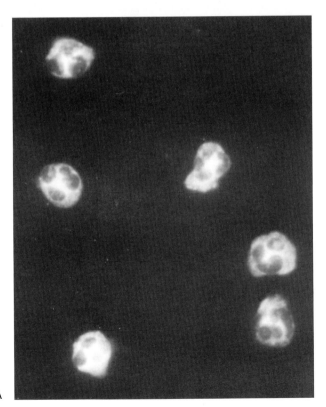 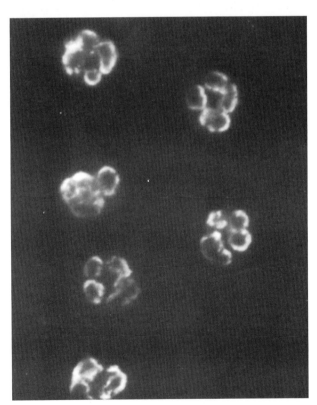

A
B

FIG. 63-5. Indirect immunofluorescence microscopy staining pattern of c-ANCA and perinuclear ANCA (p-ANCA) primary antibody, using normal human neutrophils as substrate and fluorescein-conjugated anti–human IgG as secondary antibody. **A:** Alcohol-fixed neutrophils were used as substrate and demonstrated a typical c-ANCA staining pattern with central accentuation. **B:** Alcohol-fixed neutrophils were used, thereby allowing the artifactual redistribution of nucleophilic cytoplasmic antigens (e.g., MPO) that results in p-ANCA perinuclear staining. (From ref. 250, with permission.)

vasculitides may stimulate cytokine (e.g., TNF-α) primed neutrophils to induce endothelial-cell injury (Fig. 63-4A) (180,196,197). Another mechanism by which ANCAs may further activate neutrophils is by engagement of neutrophil FcRIIa by surface-bound ANCAs (198,199).

A second role for ANCAs in the pathogenesis of systemic necrotizing vasculitides (SNV) may be formation of immune complexes with lysosomal enzymes released from neutrophils (Fig. 63-4B) (180). By activating the complement cascade, proteinase-3– and myeloperoxidase-containing immune complexes may contribute to local tissue damage in both the respiratory tract and the kidneys. That immunofluorescence studies on SNV tissue do not always reveal immune complexes in the kidney glomerular basement membrane or in vessels in other sites may be due to rapid immune-complex clearance from these sites (180). Third, anti–proteinase-3 (c-ANCA) and antimyeloperoxidase (p-ANCA) antibodies may interfere with inactivation of the enzymes (Fig. 63-4C) (180). Tissue destruction by neutrophil lysosomal enzymes is normally limited by inactivation of proteases by antiproteases. In Wegener's granulomatosis and other systemic necrotizing vasculitis syndromes, it has been postulated that lysosomal enzymes may escape their physiologic inactivation by binding to ANCAs (180). Finally, Mayet and colleagues (200,201) demonstrated that cytokine stimulated endothelial cells express proteinase-3 on their surface, thus providing a mechanism for direct binding of ANCA to endothelial cells and initiation of endothelial cell injury (Fig. 63-4D).

Antiendothelial-Cell Antibodies

Antiendothelial-cell antibodies have been described in the sera of patients with active SLE (202) and Kawasaki disease (203). Brasile et al. (204) have described a high incidence (86%) of autoantibodies against monocyte–vascular-endothelial-cell antigens in Wegener's granulomatosis, polyarteritis nodosa, and other forms of SNV. The level of these anti–monocyte/endothelial-cell autoantibodies correlated with disease activity (204). Interestingly, these antiendothelial-cell antibodies preferentially bound to splenic artery and inferior mesenteric artery endothelium and not to aortic endothelium (204), the former arteries being most commonly involved in systemic necrotizing vasculitis syndromes (4).

Heurkens et al. (205) have demonstrated antiendothelial-cell antibodies in vasculitis associated with RA; 68% of RA vasculitis patients were positive for antiendothelial-cell antibodies, whereas only 16% of RA patients without vasculitis have the antibodies. In the spontaneous polyarteritis nodosa–like disease that occurs in SL/Ni mice, vascular injury is thought to be initiated by antiendothelial-cell antibodies directed at the gp70 envelope protein of murine leukemia virus budding from the endothelium of affected vessels (206). Finally, Dami-

anovich et al. (207) have shown that antiendothelial cell antibodies induced in mice cause vascular injury in an idiotypic experimental model. Thus, evidence is emerging that antibodies to endothelial surface antigens may play pathogenetic roles leading to vessel damage in forms of systemic necrotizing vasculitis.

Cellular Immune Responses and Granuloma Formation

Temporal Arteritis

The most important advances in the understanding of cellular immune responses in vasculitis have come from the study of lesional vessel tissue from patients with temporal arteritis (8). Temporal arteritis is uniquely localized to the temporal arteries, to extracranial branches of the carotid artery, and, less commonly, to the proximal aorta, innominate arteries, and the coronary arteries (reviewed in ref. 208). Histologic analysis of temporal arteries reveals skin lesions with focal segmental involvement of affected areas (reviewed in ref. 209). The inflammatory infiltrate is composed predominantly of mononuclear cells localized to the internal elastic lamina. Multinucleated giant cells are identified in 50% of specimens (209).

Weyand and Goronzy (8) have used in situ techniques to systematically tease apart the milieu of cells, cytokines, and inflammatory mediators involved in temporal arteritis. These investigators have shown that the clinical presentation of temporal arteritis correlates with the cytokines expressed in vessel lesional tissue. This work has also demonstrated that the inflammatory infiltrate in temporal arteritis lesions follows an ordered vessel topography, and that the function of cells infiltrating affected arteries is influenced by their location within the vessel (Fig. 63-6) (8). Further, analysis of the antigen receptors of T cells infiltrating temporal arteritis lesions supports the notion that temporal arteritis is an antigen-driven disease (210).

While IFN-γ production appears to be necessary for the complete expression of temporal arteritis, only 2% to 4% of the T cells infiltrating the vessel wall expressed IFN-γ mRNA (35). Interestingly, these CD4+, IFN-γ mRNA+ T cells were localized in the arterial adventitia, remote from the primary focus of inflammatory infiltration near the internal elastic lamina (Fig. 63-6) (35). Despite residing distant from the site of vessel inflammation, IFN-γ–producing T cells appeared to be central to the pathologic process in temporal arteritis, since they had a high frequency of IL-2 receptor expression, were proliferating, and had rearranged the cytoskeletal protein talin, a finding in cells undergoing antigen presentation (35).

The location of macrophages infiltrating temporal arteritis lesions is organized according to macrophage functional capabilities (Fig. 63-6). CD68+ macrophages in the adventitia expressed IL-1β, IL-6, and transforming growth factor-β₁ (TGF-β₁) mRNA (51). IL-1 and IL-6 may augment inflammatory responses and facilitate T cell stimulation. The role of TGF-β is less clear, as this cytokine exhibits both proinflammatory and antiinflammatory properties (8). CD68⁺ macrophages in the media do not express IL-1, IL-6, or TGF-β₁. Instead, they express the matrix metalloproteinase, collagenase. The release of metalloproteinases in the media may explain the fragmentation of the internal elastic lamina seen in temporal arteritis lesions. A third type of CD68⁺ macrophage is found in the intima of temporal arteritis lesions. This macrophage population expresses inducible nitric oxide synthase (iNOS), which synthesizes nitric oxide (NO). NO has a homeostatic role in blood vessel relaxation, but also has strong proinflammatory properties (211). Some patients were found to have TGF-β₁+ macrophages in the intima in the setting of neointima formation, thus providing a potential mechanism for vessel occlusion in temporal arteritis (8).

Finally, Weyand and Goronzy (210) have presented evidence supporting the notion that temporal arteritis is an antigen-driven disease with antigen recognition, T-cell activation, and subsequent arteritis initiated within the affected artery. Most T cells infiltrating temporal arteritis lesions are CD4⁺ cells, but only a fraction of the CD4⁺ cells show signs of recent activation as determined by IL-2 receptor expression (212). CD4⁺ T cells expressing the IL-2 receptor were isolated from temporal arteritis lesions and their T-cell receptors sequenced (213). Sequence analysis revealed identical clonotypes in distinct vasculitis lesions from the same artery or from the contralateral temporal artery. Only a small percentage of the CD4⁺ T cells infiltrating the temporal artery had undergone clonal expansion, but these expanded T-cell populations were enriched in temporal artery tissue and

not peripheral blood (213). Whether the inciting antigen in temporal arteritis is an exogenous or endogenous antigen is not known.

Other Vasculitis Models and Syndromes

Animal models have been developed for investigating cell-mediated mechanisms of vascular damage. Of interest are studies in mice in which systemic vasculitis was produced by injecting animals with syngeneic T cells sensitized *in vitro* to cultured vascular smooth muscle cells (214); 20% of animals developed granulomatous inflammation of the pulmonary arterioles. Moyer and Reinisch (215) studied immune-complex–mediated vasculitis in MRL/1pr mice and found evidence for T-cell–mediated vascular damage in this model as well.

Winkleman et al. (121) examined skin biopsy specimens from four patients with forms of cutaneous granulomatous vasculitis and reported that CD4⁺ T lymphocytes were consistently found around inflamed vessel walls. Phenotypic analysis of pulmonary infiltrates in patients with Wegener's granulomatosis has demonstrated both monocytes and T lymphocytes in the vascular infiltrates with both CD4⁺ and CD8⁺ cells present (216).

Study of renal biopsy specimens from Wegener's granulomatosis patients obtained prior to initiation of therapy revealed cellular infiltrates consisting of predominantly T cells, with a CD4-to-CD8 ratio of 5:1. Ten to forty percent of infiltrating mononuclear cells were monocytes (217). A similar distribution of T-lymphocyte subtypes has been seen in cutaneous mononuclear-cell infiltrates in classic delayed-type hypersensitivity lesions (218), in RA synovial lesions (219), and in drug-induced systemic lupus erythematosus nephritis (220).

Macrophages may be directly involved in inducing vascular damage, either via direct cell cytotoxicity or via

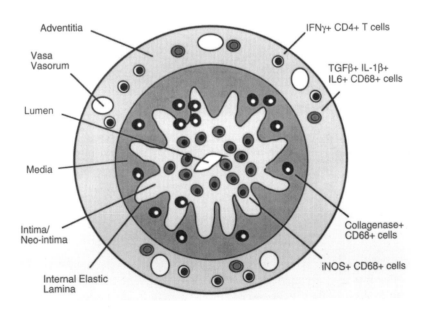

FIG. 63-6. Organization of the inflammatory lesions in giant cell arteritis. The panarteritic infiltrate in the walls of medium-sized arteries acquires a strict topographic arrangement. CD4⁺ T cells with the ability to secrete interferon-γ home to the tunica adventitia in proximity to the vasa vasorum. They are intermingled with CD68⁺ macrophages producing IL-1β, IL-6, and transforming growth factor-β. Macrophages in the tunica media are specialized to produce inducible nitric oxide synthase (iNOS). (From ref. 8, with permission.)

the production of IL-1 and TNF-α (reviewed in refs. 79 and 221). IL-1 and TNF-α have been shown to induce endothelial cells to become "procoagulant" via induction of endothelial-cell tissue factor, factor Xa, and thrombin levels (222,223). Induction of expression of procoagulant molecules and endothelial leukocyte adhesion molecule-1 (ELAM-1), ICAM-1, and ICAM-2 endothelial antigens by TNF-α and IL-1 are associated with increased platelet, mononuclear-cell, and polymorphonuclear-leukocyte adherence to endothelial cells, important events that lead to vessel inflammation and occlusion (reviewed in ref. 222). Work using the *Lactobacillus casei* cell wall–induced model of coronary arteritis in mice has demonstrated that macrophages are critical for the generation of coronary artery lesions (206). This latter model is thought to be a model of Kawasaki disease.

The occurrence of granulomas in forms of systemic necrotizing vasculitis such as Wegener's granulomatosis and Churg-Strauss syndrome clearly indicates that intense T-cell and monocyte/macrophage immune responses have occurred. Indeed, T-cell infiltrates are present throughout involved tissues in diseases associated with ANCAs (reviewed in ref. 180). Although the antigen specificities of T cells in forms of systemic necrotizing vasculitis are not known, in animal models of crescentic glomerulonephritis antigen-specific T-cell–mediated glomerular disease has been induced using trinitrophenol-albumin (224) or azobenzenearsenate (225) immunization. Thus, T-cell responses to antigens that lodge in glomeruli can induce crescentic glomerulonephritis, an important component of human systemic vasculitis (4).

Van der Woude's team (180,197) has postulated that proteinase-3 and myeloperoxidase may localize to the glomerular basement membrane, where they incite T-cell–mediated glomerular injury in Wegener's granulomatosis and other forms of systemic necrotizing vasculitis. Importantly, Wegener's granulomatosis peripheral blood T cells proliferate *in vitro* in response to the c-ANCA antigen (proteinase-3), suggesting the presence of antigen-primed memory T cells in Wegener's granulomatosis (160,107). Thus, it is most likely that in the case of ANCA-associated vasculitic syndromes, both T- and B-cell responses may act in concert to cause vessel damage. Autoantibodies to proteinase-3 and myeloperoxidase may activate neutrophils, cause persistence of the ANCA autoantigens, and form immune complexes. Response to ANCA immune complexes by macrophages induces TNF-α and IL-1, which, in turn, induce endothelial-cell ELAM-1, ICAM-1, ICAM-2, and procoagulant activity.

Vessel Damage or Altered Vessel Function Mediated Directly by Infectious Agents

In theory, any infectious agent (or antigen) that induces an immune response could cause vasculitis. Possible mechanisms of vascular damage caused by infections are (a) the presence of the organism in the vessel by direct invasion or embolization with resultant inflammatory response, (b) immune complex formation and deposition, (c) induction of cytotoxic antiendothelial-cell antibodies, (d) induction of aberrant cell-mediated immune reactions, and (e) toxin-induced vascular damage.

For instance, herpes virus infections, including varicella zoster, herpes simplex, and cytomegalovirus, have been associated with arteritis in the presence or absence of lymphoproliferative disease (4,226–228). Viral inclusion bodies in or near vessels have been described in many of these cases (229). Cines et al. (230) showed that herpes simplex virus-1 (HSV-1) infection of human endothelial cells resulted in endothelial-cell expression of C3b and Fc receptors. Glycoproteins of HSV-1 can function as Fc receptors for immunoglobulin and receptors for C3b on the surface of HSV-I–infected cells (231,232), possibly promoting the binding of immune complexes to endothelial cells.

Mycoplasma pneumoniae infections in humans can cause disease in sites distant to the lungs, and cases of meningoencephalitis with vasculitis have been reported (233–235). Two animal models of mycoplasma infection, *Mycoplasma neurolyticum* in mice and *Mycoplasma gallisepticum* in turkeys, are associated with forms of vasculitis (236,237). In both of these animal models, vascular inflammation was caused by mycoplasmal production of substances toxic for vascular endothelium (236,237).

Vasculitis involving small arterioles is characteristic of rickettsial infections in humans such as Rocky Mountain spotted fever. Endothelial cells are the primary targets of rickettsial infection leading to mural thrombus formation, vessel occlusion, and mononuclear-cell perivascular infiltrations (238).

The human retrovirus HTLV-I has been shown to infect human endothelial cells *in vitro* (239) and likely explains the clinical syndrome of cutaneous lymphomatous vasculitis seen associated with HTLV-I–induced T-cell leukemia (240). In this regard, murine leukemia virus budding from endothelial cells is responsible for induction of antiviral antibodies that induce a polyarteritis nodosa–like syndrome in SL/Ni mice (206). In human immunodeficiency virus (HIV), vasculitis and other autoimmune manifestations have been described, although the immune basis of these syndromes is not known (241). In HIV infection, lung vasculitis has been reported to occur in association with *Pneumocystis carinii* infection (242). In this setting, pulmonary vasculitis was caused by direct invasion of pulmonary vessels with pneumocystic organisms (242).

Tumor-Cell–Mediated Vascular Damage

Many vasculitis syndromes have been described in association with various malignant diseases (reviewed in refs. 4 and 243). These include the association of polyarteritis nodosa with hairy-cell leukemia, granulomatous vasculitis associated with Hodgkin's disease, and various forms of hypersensitivity vasculitis associated with a wide spectrum of malignant disease types. The pathophysiology of most vasculitic syndromes associated with malignancies has been related to the formation of immune complexes containing tumor-associated antigens. However, in some malignant diseases associated with vasculitis, tumor cells have a predilection for direct invasion of vessel walls, thereby causing vessel damage. This type of vascular damage occurs in mycosis fungoides (244), in HTLV-I–associated T-cell leukemia (240), and in the T-cell premalignant syndrome of lymphomatoid granulomatosis (245). The latter is a disease characterized by infiltration of various organs by a polymorphic cellular infiltrate of lymphoid and plasmacytoid cells together with an angiocentric, angiodestructive pattern of inflammation (245). The disease has characteristics of both a primary vasculitis and a lymphoproliferative disease and evolves into a T-cell lymphoma in approximately 50% of cases (245).

Finally, a systemic vasculitis syndrome can occur associated with (a) a cardiac left atrial myxoma with embolization of tumor from the primary source to distal arteries and (b) subsequent invasion of vessels by the malignant myxoma cells (246).

REFERENCES

1. Cupps T, Fauci AS. The vasculitides. In: *Major problems in internal medicine*, vol 21. Philadelphia: WB Saunders, 1981, pp 1–5.
2. Cupps T, Fauci AS. The vasculitis syndromes. *Adv Intern Med* 1982; 27:315–344.
3. Fauci AS. Vasculitis. *J Allergy Clin Immunol* 1983;72:211–223.
4. Fauci AS, Haynes BF, Katz P. The spectrum of vasculitis: clinical, pathological, immunologic, and therapeutic considerations. *Ann Intern Med* 1978;89:660–676.
5. Andrassy K, Darai G, Koderisch J, et al. Anti-Ro antibodies in Wegener's granulomatosis. *Klin Wochenschr* 1983;61:873–875.
6. McCluskey R, Bhan A. Cell mediated mechanisms in renal diseases. *Hum Pathol* 1983;14:305–315.
7. Haynes BF, Allen NB, Fauci AS. Diagnostic and therapeutic approach to the patient with vasculitis. *Med Clin North Am* 1986;70:355–368.
8. Weyand CM, Goronzy JJ. Multisystem interactions in the pathogenesis of vasculitis. *Curr Opin Rheumatol* 1997;9:3–11.
9. Hunder GG, and members and consultants of the American College of Rheumatology Subcommittee on Vasculitis. The American College of Rheumatology 1990 criteria for the classification of vasculitis: introduction. *Arthritis Rheum* 1990;33:1065–1067.
10. Jennette JC, Falk RJ, Andrassy K, et al. Nomenclature of systemic vasculitides. *Arthritis Rheum* 1994;37:187–192.
11. Smoller BR, McNutt NS, Contreras F. The natural history of vasculitis. What the histology tells us. *Arch Dermatol* 1990;126:84–89.
12. Smiley JD, Moore SE. Immune complex vasculitis: role of complement and IgG-Fc receptor functions. *Am J Med Sci* 1989;298:267–277.
13. Mossman TR. Properties and functions of interleukin-10. *Adv Immunol* 1994;56:1–26.
14. Dinarello CA. Biologic basis for interleukin-1 in disease. *Blood* 1996; 87:2095–2147.
15. Bazzoni F, Beutler B. The tumor necrosis factor ligand and receptor families. *N Engl J Med* 1996;334:1717–1725.
16. Kishimoto T. The biology of interleukin 6. *Blood* 1989;74:1–10.
17. Sayinalp N, Ozcebe OI, Ozdemir O, Haznedaroglu IC, Dundar S, Kirazli S. Cytokines in Behçet's disease. *J Rheumatol* 1996;23: 321–322.
18. Grau GE, Roux-Lombard P, Gysler C, et al. Serum cytokine changes in systemic vasculitis. *Immunology* 1989;68:196–198.
19. Yosipovitch G, Shohat B, Bshara J, et al. Elevated serum interleukin 1 receptors and interleukin 1B in patients with Behçet's disease: correlations with disease activity and severity. *Isr J Med Sci* 1995;31: 345–348.
20. Leung DYM, Cotran RS, Kurt-Jones E, et al. Endothelial cell activation and high interleukin 1 expression in the pathogenesis of acute Kawasaki disease. *Lancet* 1989;2:1298–1302.
21. Roche NE, Fulbright JW, Wagner AD, et al. Correlation of interleukin-6 production and disease activity in polymyalgia rheumatica and giant cell arteritis. *Arthritis Rheum* 1993;36:1286–1294.
22. Nakahama H, Yokokawa T, Okada M, et al. Distinct responses of interleukin-6 and other laboratory parameters to treatment in a patient with Wegener's granulomatosis. *Int Med* 1993;32:189–192.
23. Turan B, Gallati H, Erdi H, Gurler A, Michel BA, Villiger PM. Systemic levels of the T cell regulatory cytokines IL-10 and IL-12 in Behçet's disease; soluble TNFR-75 as a biological marker of disease activity. *J Rheumatol* 1997;24:128–132.
24. Brooks CJ, King WJ, Radford DJ, Adu D, McGrath M, Savage CO. IL-1 beta production by human polymorphonuclear leucocytes stimulated by anti-neutrophil cytoplasmic autoantibodies: relevance to systemic vasculitis. *Clin Exp Immunol* 1996;106:273–279.
25. Del Papa N, Guidali L, Sironi M, et al. Anti-endothelial cell IgG antibodies from patients with Wegener's granulomatosis bind to human endothelial cells *in vitro* and induce adhesion molecule expression and cytokine secretion. *Arthritis Rheum* 1996;39:758–766.
26. Mulligan MS, Ward PA. Immune complex-induced lung and dermal vascular injury. Differing requirements for tumor necrosis factor-alpha and IL-1. *J Immunol* 1992;149:331–339.
27. Mossman TR, Cherwinski H, Bond MW, et al. Two types of murine helper T cell clones. I. Definition according to profiles of lymphokine activities and secreted proteins. *J Immunol* 1987;136:2348–2357.
28. Boehm U, Klamp T, Groot M, et al. Cellular responses to interferon-γ. *Annu Rev Immunol* 1997;15:749–795.
29. Lin CY, Lin CC, Hwang B, Chiang BN. The changes of interleukin-2, tumour necrotic factor and gamma-interferon production among patients with Kawasaki disease. *Eur J Pediatr* 1991;150:179–182.
30. Weyand CM, Schonberger J, Oppitz U, et al. Distinct vascular lesions in giant cell arteritis share identical T cell clonotypes. *J Exp Med* 1994;179:951–960.
31. Weyand CM, Hicok KC, Hunder GM, et al. Tissue cytokine patterns in patients with polymyalgia rheumatica and giant cell arteritis. *Ann Intern Med* 1994;121:484–491.
32. Most J, Neumayer HP, Dierich MP. Cytokine-induced generation of multinucleated giant cells *in vitro* requires interferon-gamma and expression of LFA-1. *Eur J Immunol* 1990;20:1661–1667.
33. Yamamura M, Uyemura K, Deans RJ. Defining protective responses to pathogens: cytokine profiles in leprosy lesions. *Science* 1991;254: 277–279.
34. Warner TD, Klemm P. What turns on the endothelins? *Inflammation Res* 1996;45:51–53.
35. Wagner AD, Bjornsson J, Bartley GB, Goronzy JJ, Weyand CM. Interferon-gamma-producing T cells in giant cell vasculitis represent a minority of tissue-infiltrating cells and are located distant from the site of pathology. *Am J Pathol* 1996;148:1925–1933.
36. Sato N, Sagawa K, Sasaguri Y, Inoue O, Kato H. Immunopathology and cytokine detection in the skin lesions of patients with Kawasaki disease. *J Pediatr* 1993;122:198–203.
37. Weyand CM, Tetzlaff N, Bjornsson J, Brack A, Younge B, Goronzy JJ. Disease patterns and tissue cytokine profiles in giant cell arteritis. *Arthritis Rheum* 1997;40:19–26.
38. Qasim FJ, Thiru S, Gillespie K. Gold and D-penicillamine induce vasculitis and up-regulate mRNA for IL-4 in the brown Norway rat: support for a role for Th2 cell activity. *Clin Exp Immunol* 1991;108:438–445.
39. Hirao J, Hibi S, Andoh T, Ichimura T. High levels of circulating interleukin-4 and interleukin-10 in Kawasaki disease. *Int Arch Allergy Immunol* 1997;112:152–156.
40. Kojima K, Omoto E, Katayama Y, et al. Autoimmune hemolytic anemia in allergic granulomatous angitis (Churg-Strauss syndrome). *Int J Hematol* 1996;63:149–154.
41. Gesualdo L, Grandaliano G, Ranieri E, et al. Monocyte recruitment in cryoglobulinemic membranoproliferative glomerulonephritis: a pathogenetic role for monocyte chemotactic peptide-1. *Kidney Int* 1997;51: 155–163.

42. Casselman BL, Kilgore KS, Miller BF, Warren JS. Antibodies to neutrophil cytoplasmic antigens induce monocyte chemoattractant protein-1 secretion from human monocytes. *J Lab Clin Med* 1995;126:495–502.
43. Berger SP, Seelen MA, Hiemstra PS, et al. Proteinase 3, the major autoantigen of Wegener's granulomatosis, enhances IL-8 production by endothelial cells *in vitro*. *J Am Soc Nephrol* 1996;7:694–701.
44. Sahin S, Akoglu T, Direskeneli H, Sen LS, Lawrence R. Neutrophil adhesion to endothelial cells and factors affecting adhesion in patients with Behçet's disease. *Ann Rheum Dis* 1996;55:128–133.
45. al-Dalaan A, al-Sedairy S, al-Balaa S, et al. Enhanced interleukin 8 secretion in circulation of patients with Behçet's disease. *J Rheumatol* 1995;22:904–907.
46. Mulligan MS, Moncada S, Ward PA. Protective effects of inhibitors of nitric oxide synthase in immune complex-induced vasculitis. *Br J Pharmacol* 1992;107:1159–1162.
47. Woolfson RG, Qasim FJ, Thiru S, Oliveira DB, Neild GH, Mathieson PW. Nitric oxide contributes to tissue injury in mercuric chloride-induced autoimmunity. *Biochem Biophys Res Commun* 1995;217:515–521.
48. Brack A, Rittner HL, Younge BR, Kaltschmidt C, Weyand CM, Goronzy JJ. Glucocorticoid-mediated repression of cytokine gene transcription in human arteritis-SCID chimeras. *J Clin Invest* 1997;99:2842–2850.
49. Gilkeson GS, Mudgett JS, Seldin MF, et al. Clinical and serologic manifestations of autoimmune disease in MRL-lpr/lpr mice lacking nitric oxide synthase type 2. *J Exp Med* 1997;186:365–373.
50. Tsukahara H, Kikuchi K, Matsuda M, et al. Endogenous nitric oxide production in Kawasaki disease. *Scand J Clin Lab Invest* 1997;57:43–47.
51. Weyand CM, Wagner AD, Bjornsson J, Goronzy JJ. Correlation of the topographical arrangement and the functional pattern of tissue-infiltrating macrophages in giant cell arteritis. *J Clin Invest* 1996;98:1642–1649.
52. Mayatepek E, Lehmann WD. Increased generation of cysteinyl leukotrienes in Kawasaki disease. *Arch Dis Child* 1995;72:526–527.
53. Buyan N, Hasanoglu E, Oguz A, Ercan S. The role of plasma arachidonic acid metabolites in the pathogenesis and the prognosis of Henoch-Schönlein purpura. *Prostaglandins Leukot Essent Fatty Acids* 1994;50:353–356.
54. Springer TA. Traffic signals on endothelium for lymphocyte recirculation and leukocyte emigration. *Annu Rev Physiol* 1995;57:827–872.
55. Jain KK. Cutaneous vasculitis associated with granulocyte colony stimulating factor. *J Am Acad Dermatol* 1994;31:213–215.
56. Cohen-Tervaert JWC, Kallenberg CGM. Cell adhesion molecules in vasculitis. *Curr Opin Rheumatol* 1997;9:16–25.
57. Gutfleisch J, Baumert E, Wolff-Vorbeck G, et al. Increased expression of CD25 and adhesion molecules on peripheral blood lymphocytes of patients with Wegener's granulomatosis and ANCA positive vasculitides. *Adv Exp Med Biol* 1993;336:397–404.
58. Nash MC, Shah V, Dillon MJ. Soluble cell adhesion molecules and von Willebrand factor in children with Kawasaki disease. *Clin Exp Immunol* 1995;101:13–17.
59. Stegeman CA, Tervaert JW, Huitema MG, et al. Serum levels of soluble adhesion molecule intercellular adhesion molecule 1, vascular cell adhesion molecule 1, and E-selectin in patients with Wegener's granulomatosis: relationship to disease activity and relevance during followup. *Arthritis Rheum* 1994;37:1228–1235.
60. Springer TA. Adhesion receptors of the immune system. *Nature* 1990;346:425–434.
61. Spertini O, Schleiffenbaum B, White-Owen C, Ruiz P, Tedder TF. ELISA for quantitation of L-selectin shed from leukocytes *in vivo*. *J Immunol Methods* 1992;156:115–123 .
62. Takeshita S, Dobashi H, Nakatani K, et al. Circulating soluble selectins in Kawasaki disease. *Clin Exp Immunol* 1997;108:446–450.
63. Brandley BK, Swiedler SJ, Robbins PW. Carbohydrate ligands of the LFC cell adhesion molecules. *Cell* 1990;63:861–863.
64. Luscinskas FW, Cybulsky MI, Kiely JM, Peckins CS, Davis VM, Gimbrone MA. Cytokine-activated human endothelial cell monolayers support enhanced neutrophil transmigration via a mechanism involving both endothelial-leukocyte adhesion molecule-1 and intercellular adhesion molecule-1. *J Immunol* 1991;146:1617–1625.
65. Picker LJ, Kishimoto TK, Smith CW, Warnock RA, Butcher EC. ELAM-1 is an adhesion molecule for skin homing T cells. *Nature* 1991;349:796–799.
66. Mrowka C, Sieberth HG. Detection of circulating adhesion molecules

ICAM-1, VCAM-1 and E-selectin in Wegener's granulomatosis, systemic lupus erythematosus and chronic renal failure. *Clin Nephrol* 1995;43:288–296.
67. Carson CW, Beall LD, Hunder GG, et al. Serum ELAM-1 is increased in vasculitis, scleroderma, and systemic lupus erythematosus. *J Rheumatol* 1993;20:809–814.
68. Kim DS, Lee KY. Serum soluble E-selectin levels in Kawasaki disease. *Scand J Rheumatol* 1994;23:283–286.
69. Furukawa S, Imai K, Matsubara T, et al. Increased levels of circulating intercellular adhesion molecule 1 in Kawasaki disease. *Arthritis Rheum* 1992;35:672.
70. Burrows NP, Molina FA, Terenghi G, et al. Comparison of cell adhesion molecule expression in cutaneous leucocytoclastic and lymphocytic vasculitis. *J Clin Pathol* 1994;47:939–944.
71. Bradley JR, Lockwood CM, Thiru S. Endothelial cell activation in patients with systemic vasculitis. *Q J Med* 1994;87:741–745.
72. Hemler ME, Huang C, Schwarz L. The VLA protein family. Characterization of five distinct cell surface heterodimers each with a common 130,000 molecular weight β subunit. *J Biol Chem* 1987;262:3300–3309.
73. Ruoslahti E. Integrins. *J Clin Invest* 1991;87:1–5.
74. Wang CR, Liu MF, Tsai RT, et al. Circulating intercellular adhesion molecules-1 and autoantibodies including anti-endothelial cell, anti-cardiolipin, and anti-neutrophil cytoplasmic antibodies in patients with vasculitis. *Clin Rheumatol* 1993;12:375–380.
75. Haller H, Eichhorn J, Pieper K, Gobel U, Luft FC. Circulating leukocyte integrin expression in Wegener's granulomatosis. *J Am Soc Nephrol* 1996;7:40–48.
76. Takeuchi T, Amano K, Sekine H, et al. Upregulated expression and function of integrin adhesive receptors in systemic lupus erythematosus patients with vasculitis. *J Clin Invest* 1993;92:3008–3016.
77. Schaufelberger C, Stemme S, Andersson R, et al. T lymphocytes in giant cell arteritic lesions are polyclonal cells expressing alpha-beta type antigen receptors and VLA-1 integrin receptors. *Clin Exp Immunol* 1993;91:421–428.
78. Wawryk SO, Ayberk H, Boyd AW, et al. Analysis of adhesion molecules in the immunopathogenesis of giant cell arteritis. *J Clin Pathol* 1991;44:497–501.
79. Lipsky PE, Davis LS, Cush JJ, Oppenheimer Markes N. The role of cytokines in the pathogenesis of rheumatoid arthritis. *Springer Semin Immunopathol* 1989;11:123–162.
80. Holzmann B, McIntyre BW, Weissman IL. Identification of a murine Peyer's patch-specific lymphocyte homing receptor as an integrin molecule with an a chain homologous to human VLA-4a. *Cell* 1989;56:37–46.
81. Freedman AS, Munro JM, Rice GE, et al. Adhesion of human B cells to germinal centers *in vitro* involves VLA-4 and IN CAM-110. *Science* 1990;249:1030–1033.
82. Rice GE, Munro JM, Bevilacqua MP. Inducible cell adhesion molecule 110 (IN CAM-110) is an endothelial receptor for lymphocytes. *J Exp Med* 1990;171:1369–1374.
83. Elices MJ, Osborn L, Takada Y, et al. VCAM-1 on activated endothelium interacts with the leukocyte integrin VLA-4 at a site distinct from the VLA-4/fibronectin binding site. *Cell* 1990;60:577–584.
84. Singer KH. The lymphocyte surface: molecules that mediate adhesion and signaling. In: Joklik W, Willett H, Amos B, Wilfert C, eds. *Zinsser's textbook of microbiology,* 20th ed. New York: Appleton-Century-Crofts, 1992:296–310.
85. Haynes BF, Grover BJ, Whichard LP, et al. Synovial microenvironment—T cell interactions. Human T cells bind to fibroblast-like synovial cells *in vitro*. *Arthritis Rheum* 1988;31:947–955.
86. John S, Neumayer HH, Weber M. Serum circulating ICAM-1 levels are not useful to indicate active vasculitis or early renal allograft rejection. *Clin Nephrol* 1994;42:369–375.
87. Fuiano G, Sepe V, Stanziale P, et al. Expression of intercellular adhesion molecule in idiopathic crescentic glomerulonephritis. *Contrib Nephrol* 1991;94:81–88.
88. Lhotta K, Neumayer HP, Joannidis M, Geissler D, Konig P. Renal expression of intercellular adhesion molecule-1 in different forms of glomerulonephritis. *Clin Sci* 1991;81:447–481.
89. Chow J, Hartley RB, Jagger C, Dilly SA. ICAM-1 expression in renal disease. *J Clin Pathol* 1992;45:880–884.
90. Baraldi A, Zambruno G, Furci L, et al. β1 and β2 integrin upregulation in rapidly progressive glomerulonephritis. *Nephrol Dial Transplant* 1995;10:1155–1161.

91. Ristaldi MP, Ferrario F, Tunesi S, Yang L, D'Amico G. Intraglomerular and interstitial leukocyte infiltration, adhesion molecules, and interleukin 1α expression in 15 cases of antineutrophil cytoplasmic autoantibody-associated renal vasculitis. *Am J Kidney Dis* 1996;27: 48–57.

92. Panegyres PK, Faull RJ, Russ G, Appleton SL, Wangel AG, Bluberg PC. Endothelial cell activation in vasculitis of peripheral nerve and muscle. *J Neurol Neurosurg Psychiatry* 1991;55:4–7.

93. Lenschow DJ, Walunas TL, Bluestone JA. CD28/B7 system of T cell costimulation. *Annu Rev Immunol* 1996;14:233–258.

94. Mach F, Schonbeck U, Sukhova GK, et al. Functional CD40 ligand is expressed on human vascular endothelial cells, smooth muscle cells, and macrophages: implications for CD40–CD40L signaling in atherosclerosis. *Proc Natl Acad Sci USA* 1997;94:19310–19316.

95. Sempowski GD, Chess PR, Phipps RP. CD40 is a functional activation antigen and B7-independent T cell costimulatory molecule on normal human lung fibroblasts. *J Immunol* 1997;158:4670–4677.

96. Grewal IS, Flavell RA. The role of CD40 ligand in costimulation and T cell activation. *Immunol Rev* 1996;153:85–106.

97. van Kooten C, Gerritsma JS, Paape ME, van Es LA, Banchereau J, Daha MR. Possible role for CD40-CD40L in the regulation of interstitial infiltration in the kidney. *Kidney Int* 1997;51:711–721.

98. Ito MR, Terasaki S, Itoh J, Katoh H, Yonehara S, Nose M. Rheumatic diseases in an MRL strain of mice with a deficit in the functional Fas ligand. *Arthritis Rheum* 1997;40:1054–1063.

99. Conn DL. Update on systemic necrotizing vasculitis. *Mayo Clin Proc* 1989;64:535–543.

100. van Es L, Daha M, Valentijn R, Kauffman R. The pathogenetic significance of circulating immune complexes. *Neth J Med* 1984;27: 350–358.

101. Tosca N, Stratigos JD. Possible pathogenetic mechanisms in allergic cutaneous vasculitis. *Int J Dermatol* 1988;27:291–296.

102. Leber P, McCluskey R. Immune complex disease. In: Zweifach B, Grant L, McCluskey R, eds. *The inflammatory process,* vol 3, 2nd ed. New York: Academic Press, 1974:401–438.

103. Germuth FG. A comparative histologic and immunologic study in rabbits of induced hypersensitivity of the serum sickness type. *J Exp Med* 1953;97:257–281.

104. Hawn C, Janeway C. Histological and serological sequences in experimental hypersensitivity. *J Exp Med* 1947;85:571–589.

105. Cochrane CG. Mechanisms involved in the deposition of immune complexes in tissue. *J Exp Med* 1971;134:75s–89s.

106. Dixon F, Feldman J, Vazquez J. Experimental glomerulonephritis. *J Exp Med* 1961;113:899–917.

107. Lawley T, Bielory L, Gascon P, Yancey K, Young N, Frank M. A prospective clinical and immunological analysis of patients with serum sickness. *N Engl J Med* 1982;311:1407–1413.

108. Beynon HL, Davies KA, Haskard DO, Walport M. Erythrocyte complement receptor type 1 and interactions between immune complexes, neutrophils, and endothelium. *J Immunol* 1994;153:3160–3167.

109. Gocke D, Hsu K, Morgan C, et al. Association between polyarteritis and australia antigen. *Lancet* 1970;2:1149–1153.

110. Trepo C, Thivolet J. Hepatitis associated antigen and periarteritis nodosa. *Vox Sang* 1970;19:410–411.

111. Levo Y, Gorevic P, Kassab H, Zucker T, Franklin D, Franklin E. Association between hepatitis B virus and essential mixed cryoglobulinemia. *N Engl J Med* 1977;296:1501–1503.

112. Misiani R, Bellavita P, Fenili D, et al. Hepatitis C virus infection in patients with essential mixed cryoglobulinemia. *Ann Intern Med* 1992;117:573–577.

113. Nityanand S, Holm G, Lefvert AK. Immune complex mediated vasculitis in hepatitis B and C infections and the effect of antiviral therapy. *Clin Immunol Immunopathol* 1997;82:250–257.

114. Dienstag JL. Hepatitis B as an immune complex disease. *Semin Liver Dis* 1981;1:45–57.

115. Burkholder P. Immunology and immunohistopathology of renal diseases. In: Becker EL, ed. *Structural basis of renal disease.* New York: Harper & Row, 1968:211.

116. Freedman P, Peters J, Kark R. Localization of gammaglobulin in the diseased kidney. *Arch Intern Med* 1960;105:524–535.

117. Leib ES, Hibrawi H, Chia D, Blaker RG, Barnett EV. Correlation of disease activity in systemic necrotizing vasculitis with immune complexes. *J Rheum* 1981;8:258–265.

118. Mellors R, Ortega L. Analytical pathology III. New observations on pathogenesis of glomerulonephritis, lipid nephrosis, polyarteritis nodosa and secondary amyloid. *Am J Pathol* 1956;32:455–499.

119. McIntosh R, Tinglof B, Kaufman D. Immunohistology of renal disease. *Q J Med* 1971;40:385–390.

120. Paronetto F, Strauss L. Immunocytochemical observations on polyarteritis nodosa. *Ann Intern Med* 1962;56:289–296.

121. Winkleman R, Buechner S, Powell F, Banks P. The T lymphocyte and cutaneous Churg-Strauss granuloma. *Acta Derm Venereol (Stockh)* 1983;63:199–204.

122. Ronco P, Verrous T, Mignon F, et al. Immunopathological studies of polyarteritis nodosa and Wegener's granulomatosis: a report of 43 patients with renal biopsies. *Q J Med* 1983;52:121–123.

123. Brouet J, Clauvel J, Damon F, Klein M, Seligmann M. Biological and clinical significance of cryoglobulins: a report of 86 cases. *Am J Med* 1974;57:775–787.

124. Lightfoot RW Jr. Cryoglobulinemias and other dysproteinemias. In: Kelley W, Harris E, Ruddy S, Sledge C, eds. *Textbook of rheumatology,* vol 2, 2nd ed. Philadelphia: WB Saunders, 1985:1337–1350.

125. Gorevic P, Kassab J, Levo Y, et al. Mixed cryoglobulins: clinical aspects and long-term follow up of 40 patients. *Am J Med* 1980;9: 128–133.

126. Meltzer M, Franklin E. Cryoglobulinemia—a study of twenty-nine patients. *Am J Med* 1966;40:828–836.

127. Bonetti B, Invernizzi F, Rizzuto N, et al. T-cell-mediated epineural vasculitis and humoral-mediated microangiopathy in cryoglobulinemic neuropathy. *J Neuroimmunol* 1997;73:145–154.

128. Pette J, van de Jarvis J, Wilton J, MacDonald D. Cutaneous periarteritis nodosa. *Arch Dermatol* 1984;120:109–111.

129. Churg J, Strauss L. Allergic granulomatosis, allergic angiitis and periarteritis nodosa. *Am J Pathol* 1951;27:277–301.

130. Conn D, McDuffie F, Holley K, Schroeter A. Immunologic mechanisms in systemic vasculitis. *Mayo Clin Proc* 51:511–518.

131. Manger B, Krapf F, Granatzki M, et al. IgE containing circulating immune complexes in Churg-Strauss vasculitis. *Scand J Immunol* 1985;21:369–376.

132. Lanham J, Elkon K, Pusey C, Hughes G. Systemic vasculitis with asthma and eosinophilia: a clinical approach to the Churg-Strauss syndrome. *Medicine* 1984;63:65–81.

133. Horn R, Fauci A, Rosenthal A, Wolff S. Renal biopsy pathology in Wegener's granulomatosis. *Am J Med* 1974;74:423–433.

134. Howell S, Epstein W. Circulating immune complexes in Wegener's granulomatosis. *Am J Med* 1976;60:259–268.

135. Roback S, Herdman R, Hoyer J, Good R. Wegener's granulomatosis in a child: observations on pathogenesis and treatment. *Am J Dis Child* 1969;118:608–614.

136. Pinching A, Lockwood C, Pussell B, et al. Wegener's granulomatosis: observations on 18 patients with severe renal disease. *Q J Med* 1983; 208:435–460.

137. Shasby D, Schwarz M, Forstot J. Pulmonary immune complex deposition in Wegener's granulomatosis. *Chest* 1982;81:338–340.

138. Abel T, Andrews B, Cunningham P, Brunner C, Davis J, Horwitz D. Rheumatoid vasculitis: effect of cyclophosphamide on the clinical course and levels of circulating immune complexes. *Ann Rheum Dis* 1980;93:407–413.

139. Quismorio F, Beardmore T, Kaufman R, Mongan P. IgG rheumatoid factors and antinuclear antibodies in rheumatoid vasculitis. *Clin Exp Immunol* 1983;52:333–340.

140. Rapoport R, Kozin F, Mackel S, Jordon R. Cutaneous vascular immunofluorescence in rheumatoid arthritis. *Am J Med* 1980;68:325–331.

141. Breedveld FC, Heurkens AHM, Lafeber GJM, van Hinsbergh VWM, Cats A. Immune complexes in sera from patients with rheumatoid vasculitis induce polymorphonuclear cell-mediated injury to endothelial cells. *Clin Immunol Immunopathol* 1988;48:202–213.

142. Jorizzo J, Daniels J, Apisarnthanaraz P, Gonzalez B, Cavallo D. Histamine triggered localized cutaneous vasculitis in patients with seropositive rheumatoid arthritis. *J Am Acad Dermatol* 1983;9:845–851.

143. Weisman M, Zvaifler N. Cryoimmunoglobulinemia in rheumatoid arthritis. *J Clin Immunol* 1975;56:725–739.

144. Stage D, Mannik M. IgM-globulin in rheumatoid arthritis: evaluation of its clinical significance. *Arthritis Rheum* 1971;14:440–450.

145. Allen C, Elson C, Scott DGI, Bacon PA, Bucknall RC. IgG antiglobulins in rheumatoid arthritis and other arthrites: relationship with clinical features and other parameters. *Ann Rheum Dis* 1981;93: 127–131.

146. Scott D, Bacon P, Allen C, Elson C, Wallington T. IgG rheumatoid arthritis factor, complement and immune complexes in rheumatoid synovitis and vasculitis: comparative and serial studies during cytotoxic therapy. *Clin Exp Immunol* 1981;104:254–259.

147. Elson C, Scott D, Blake D, Bacon P, Holt P. Complement activating rheumatoid-factor-containing complexes in patients with rheumatoid vasculitis. *Ann Rheum Dis* 1983;42:147–150.

148. Mannik M, Nardella F. IgG rheumatoid factors and self-association of these antibodies. *Clin Rheum Dis* 1985;11:551–572.

149. Theofilopoulos A. Evaluation and clinical significance of circulating immune complexes. *Prog Clin Immunol* 1979;4:63–92.

150. Frank M, Hamburger M, Lawley T, Kimberly R, Plotz P. Defective reticuloendothelial system Fc receptor function in systemic lupus erythematosus. *N Engl J Med* 1979;300:518–523.

151. Frank M, Lawley T, Hamburger M, Brown E. Immunoglobulin G Fc receptor mediated clearance in autoimmune diseases. *Ann Intern Med* 1983;98:206–218.

152. Soter NA. Clinical presentations and mechanisms of necrotizing angiitis of the skin. *J Invest Dermatol* 1976;67:354–359.

153. Braverman I, Yen A. Demonstration of complexes in spontaneous and histamine induced lesions and in normal skin of patients with leukocytoclastic angiitis. *J Invest Dermatol* 1975;64:105–112.

154. Schoenfeld Y, Copeman P, Jordon R, Sams W, Winkelman R. Immunofluorescence of cutaneous vasculitis associated with systemic disease. *Arch Dermatol* 1971;104:254–259.

155. Abramson S, Belmont HM, Hopkins P, Buyon J, Winchester R, Weissman G. Complement activation and vascular injury in systemic lupus erythematosus. *J Rheumatol* 1987;14:43–46.

156. Sams WM. Hypersensitivity vasculitis. *J Invest Dermatol* 1989;93:785–815.

157. Saulsbury FT. Henoch-Schönlein purpura. *Pediatr Dermatol* 1984;1:195–201.

158. Gairdner D. The Schönlein-Henoch syndrome. *Q J Med* 1947;17:95–122.

159. Giangiocomo J, Tisai C. Dermal and glomerular deposition of IgA in anaphylactoid purpura. *Am J Dis Child* 1977;131:981–983.

160. Baart de la Faille-Kuyser E, Kater L, Kuitjten R. Occurrence of IgA deposits in clinically normal skin of patients with renal disease. *Kidney Int* 1976;9:424–429.

161. Stevenson J, Leong L, Cohen A, Border W. Henoch-Schönlein purpura: simultaneous demonstration of IgA deposition in involved skin, intestine and kidney. *Arch Pathol Lab Med* 1982;106:192–195.

162. Koskimies O, Rapola J, Savilahti E, Vilska J. Renal involvement in Schönlein-Henoch purpura. *Acta Paediatr Scand* 1974;63:357–363.

163. Kauffman R, Herrman N, Meyer C, Daha M, van Es L. Circulating IgA immune complexes in Henoch-Schönlein purpura. *Am J Med* 69:859–866.

164. Kuno-Sakai H, Sakai H, Nomoto V, Takakura I, Kimura M. Increase of IgA-bearing peripheral blood lymphocytes in children with Henoch-Schönlein purpura. *Pediatrics* 1979;64:918–922.

165. Trygstad CW. Elevated serum IgA globulin in anaphylactoid purpura. *Pediatrics* 1971;47:1023–1028.

166. Garcia-Fuentes M, Martin A, Chantler C, William D. Serum complement components in Henoch-Schönlein purpura. *Arch Dis Child* 1978;53:417–419.

167. Schifferli J, Yin C, Peters D. The role of complement and its receptor in the elimination of immune complexes. *N Engl J Med* 315:488–495.

168. Davies DJ, Moran JE, Nial JF, et al. Segmental necrotizing glomerulonephritis with antineutrophil antibody: a possible arbovirus aetiology. *Br Med J* 1982;2:606.

169. Hall JB, Wadham BMN, Wood CJ, et al. Vasculitis and glomerulonephritis: a subgroup with an antineutrophil cytoplasmic antibody. *Aust NZ J Med* 1984;14:277–278.

170. Gross WL. Antineutrophil cytoplasmic antibody testing in vasculitides. *Rheum Dis Clin NA* 1995;21:987–1011.

171. Peter HH, Metzger D, Rump A, et al. ANCA in diseases other than systemic vasculitis. *Clin Exp Immunol* 1993;93(suppl 1):12–14.

172. Rao JK, Weinberger M, Oddone EZ, Allen NB, Landsman P, Fuessner JR. The role of antineutrophil cytoplasmic antibody (c-ANCA) testing in the diagnosis of Wegener granulomatosis: A literature review and meta-analysis. *Ann Intern Med* 1995:123:925–932.

173. Niles JL, McCluskey RT, Ahmad MF, Arnaout MA. Wegener's granulomatosis autoantigen is a novel neutrophil serine protease. *Blood* 1989;74:1888–1893.

174. Gross WL, Csernok E, Flesch B. Classic anti-neutrophil cytoplasmic

175. Cohen-Tervaert JWC, Woude van der FJ, Fauci AS, et al. Association between active Wegener's granulomatosis and anticytoplasmic antibodies. *Arch Intern Med* 1989;149:2461–2465.

176. Nolle B, Specks U, Ludemann J, et al. Anticytoplasmic autoantibodies: their immunodiagnostic value in Wegener's granulomatosis. *Ann Intern Med* 1989;111:28–40.

177. Falk RJ, Jennette JC. Anti-neutrophil cytoplasmic autoantibodies with specificity for myeloperoxidase in patients with systemic vasculitis and idiopathic necrotizing and crescentic glomerulonephritis. *N Engl J Med* 1988;318:1651–1657.

178. Cohen Tervaert JW, Goldschmeding R, Elema JD, et al. Association of autoantibodies to myeloperoxidase with different forms of vasculitis. *Arthritis Rheum* 1990;33:1264–1272.

179. Gross WL, Schmitt WH, Csernok E. Antineutrophil cytoplasmic antibody-associated diseases: a rheumatologists view. *Am J Kidney Dis* 1991;18:157–179.

180. Kallenberg CG, Cohen Tervaert JW, van der Woude FJ, Goldschmeding R, von dem Borne AEG, Weeming JJ. Autoimmunity to lysosomal enzymes: new clues to vasculitis and glomerulonephritis? *Immunol Today* 1991;12:61–64.

181. Halbwachs-Mecarelli L, Nusbaum P, Noel LH, et al. Antineutrophil cytoplasmic antibodies (ANCA) directed against cathepsin G in ulcerative colitis, Crohn's disease and primary sclerosing cholangitis. *Clin Exp Immunol* 1992;90:79–84.

182. Klein R, Eisenburg J, Weber P, Seibold F, Berg PA. Significance and specificity of antibodies to neutrophils detected by western blotting for the serological diagnosis of primary sclerosing cholangitis. *Hepatol* 1991;14:1147–1152.

183. Mulder AH, Broekroelofs J, Horst G, Limburg PC, Nelis GF, Kallenberg CG. Anti-neutrophil cytoplasmic antibodies (ANCA) in inflammatory bowel disease: characterization and clinical correlates. *Clin Exp Immunol* 1994;95:490–497.

184. Reumaux D, Delecourt L, Colombel JF, Noel LH, Duthilleul P, Cortot A. Anti-neutrophil cytoplasmic autoantibodies in relatives of patients with ulcerative colitis. *Gastroenterology* 1992;103:1706.

185. Rump JA, Worner I, Roth M, Scholmerich J, Hansch M, Peter HH. p-ANCA of undefined specificity in ulcerative colitis: correlation to disease activity and therapy. *Adv Exp Med Biol* 1993;336:507–513.

186. Saxon A, Ke Z, Bahati L, Stevens RH. Soluble CD23 containing B cell supernatants induce IgE from peripheral blood B-lymphocytes and costimulate with interleukin-4 in induction of IgE. *J Allergy Clin Immunol* 1990;86:333–344.

187. Warny M, Brenard R, Cornu C, Tomasi JP, Geubel AP. Anti-neutrophil antibodies in chronic hepatitis and the effect of alpha-interferon therapy. *J Hepatol* 1993;17:294–300.

188. Lee SS, Lawton JW, Chan CE, Li CS, Kwan TH, Chau KF. Antilactoferrin antibody in systemic lupus erythematosus. *Br J Rheumatol* 1992;31:669–673.

189. Nassberger L, Hultquist R, Sturfelt G. Occurrence of anti-lactoferrin antibodies in patients with systemic lupus erythematosus, hydralazine-induced lupus, and rheumatoid arthritis. *Scand J Rheumatol* 1994;23:206–210.

190. Fauci AS, Haynes BF, Katz P, Wolff SM. Wegener's granulomatosis: prospective clinical and therapeutic experience with 85 patients over 21 years. *Ann Intern Med* 1983;98:76–85.

191. Specks U, DeRemee RA. Granulomatous vasculitis, Wegener's granulomatosis and Churg-Strauss syndrome. *Rheum Clin North Am* 1990;16:377–397.

192. Stegeman CA, Cohen Tervaert JW, de Jong PE, Kallenberg CG. Trimethoprim-sulfamethoxazole (co-trimoxazole) for the prevention of relapses of Wegener's granulomatosis. Dutch Co-Trimoxazole Wegener Study Group. *N Engl J Med* 1996;335:16–20.

193. Csernok E, Ludemann J, Gross WL. Ultrastructural localization of proteinase 3, the target antigen of anti-cytoplasmic antibodies circulating in Wegener's granulomatosis. *Am J Pathol* 1990;137:1113–1120.

194. Csernok E, Ernst M, Schmitt W, et al. Activated neutrophils express proteinase 3 on their plasma membrane *in vitro* and *in vivo*. *Clin Exp Immunol* 1994;95:244–240.

195. Cupps TR. Infections and vasculitis: mechanisms considered. In: LeRoy ED, ed. *Systemic vasculitis: the biologic basis*. New York: Marcel Dekker, 1992, pp. 65–92.

196. Falk RJ, Terrell RS, Charles LA, Jennette JC. Anti-neutrophil cyto-

plasmic autoantibodies induce neutrophils to degranulate and produce oxygen radicals *in vitro. Proc Natl Acad Sci USA* 1990;87:4115–4119.

197. van der Woude FJ, van Es LA, Daha MR. The role of c-ANCA antigen in the pathogenesis of Wegener's granulomatosis. A hypothesis based on both humoral and cellular mechanisms. *Neth J Med* 1990; 36:169–171.

198. Porges AJ, Redecha PB, Kimberly WT, et al. Anti-neutrophil cytoplasmic autoantibodies engage and activate human neutrophils via FcgRIIa. *J Immunol* 1994;97:48–51.

199. Mulder AHL, Heeringa P, Brouwer E, et al. Activation of granulocytes by antineutrophil cytoplasmic antibodies (ANCA): a FcgRII-dependent process. *Clin Exp Immunol* 1994;98:270–278.

200. Mayet WJ, Csernok E, Szymkowiak C, et al. Human endothelial cells express proteinase 3, the target antigen of anticytoplasmic antibodies in Wegener's granulomatosis. *Blood* 1993;82:1221–1229.

201. Mayet WJ, Meyer zum Buschendelde KH. Antibodies to proteinase 3 increase adhesion of neutrophils to human endothelial cells. *Clin Exp Immunol* 1993;94:440.

202. Cines D, Lyss A, Reeber M, Bina M, DeHoratius R. Presence complement fixing anti-endothelial cell antibodies in systemic lupus erythematosus. *J Clin Immunol* 1984;73:611–625.

203. Leung D, Collins T, LaPierre L, Geha R, Pober J. Immunoglobulin antibodies present in the acute phase of Kawasaki syndrome lyse cultured vascular endothelial cells stimulated by gamma interferon. *J Clin Immunol* 1986;77:1428–1435.

204. Brasile L, Kremer JL, Clarke JL, Cerelli J. Identification of an autoantibody to vascular endothelial cell-specific antigen in patients with systemic vasculitis. *Am J Med* 1989;87:74–80.

205. Heurkens AH, Hiemstra PS, Lafeber GJM, Daha MR, Breedveld FC. Anti-endothelial cell antibodies in patients with rheumatoid arthritis complicated by vasculitis. *Clin Exp Immunol* 1989;78:7–12.

206. Miyazawa M, Nose M, Kawashima M, Kyogoku M. Pathogenesis of arteritis of SL/Ni mice. *J Exp Med* 1987;166:890–908.

207. Damianovich M, Gilburd B, George J, et al. Pathogenic role of anti-endothelial cell antibodies in vasculitis: an idiotypic experimental model. *J Immunol* 1996;156:4946–4951.

208. Nordborg E, Nordborg C, Malmvall B-E, Andersson R, Bengtsson B-A. Giant cell arteritis. *Rheum Clin North Am* 1995;21:1014–1026.

209. Lie JT. Histopathologic specificity of systemic vasculitis. *Rheum Clin North Am* 1995;21:883–909.

210. Weyand C, Goronzy JJ. Giant cell arteritis as an antigen-driven disease. *Rheum Clin North Am* 1995;21:1027–1039.

211. Yun HY, Dawson VL, Dawson TM. Neurobiology of nitric oxide. *Crit Rev Neurobiol* 1996;10:291–316.

212. Cid MC, Campo E, Ercilla G, et al. Immunohistochemical analysis of lymphoid and macrophage cell subsets and their immunological activation markers in temporal arteritis. *Arthritis Rheum* 1989;32:884–893.

213. Weyand CM, Hicok KC, Hunder GG, Goronzy JJ. Tissue cytokine patterns in polymyalgia rheumatica and giant cell arteritis. *Ann Intern Med* 1994;121:484–491.

214. Hart M, Tassell S, Sadenwasser K, Schelper R, Moore S. Autoimmune vasculitis resulting from *in vitro* immunity of lymphocytes to smooth muscle. *Am J Pathol* 1985;119:448–455.

215. Moyer C, Reinisch C. The role of vascular smooth muscle cells in experimental autoimmune vasculitis. *Am J Pathol* 1984;117:380–390.

216. Gephardt G, Ahmad M, Tubbs R. Pulmonary vasculitis (Wegener's granulomatosis). Immunohistochemical studies of T and B cell markers. *Am J Med* 1983;74:700–703.

217. Ten Berge I, Wilmink J, Meyer C, et al. Clinical and immunologic follow up of patients with severe renal disease in Wegener's granulomatosis. *Am J Nephrol* 1985;5:21–29.

218. Willemze R, Graafereitsma C, de Cnossen J, van Vloten W, Meyer C. Characterization of T cell subpopulations in skin and peripheral blood of patients with cutaneous T cell lymphomas and benign inflammatory dermatoses. *J Invest Dermatol* 1983;80:60–66.

219. Kurosaka M, Ziff M. Immunoelectron microscopic study of the distribution of T cell subsets in rheumatoid synovium. *J Exp Med* 1983; 158:1191–1210.

220. Couser W, Salant K. *In situ* immune complex formation and glomerular injury. *Kidney Int* 1980;17:1–13.

221. Dinarello CA. An update on human IL-1: from molecular biology to clinical significance. *J Clin Immunol* 1985;5:287–297.

222. Bevilacqua MP, Gimbrone MA. Inducible endothelial functions in inflammation and coagulation. *Semin Thromb Hemost* 1987;13: 425–433.

223. Bevilacqua M, Pober J, Majeau G, Cotran R, Gimbrone M. Interleukin-1 induces biosynthesis and cell surface expression of procoagulant activity in human vascular endothelial cells. *J Exp Med* 1984; 160:618–623.

224. Oite T, Shimizu F, Kagami S, Morioka T. Hapten specific cellular immune response producing glomerular injury. *Clin Exp Immunol* 1989;76:463–468.

225. Rennke HG, Klein PS, Sandstrom DJ, Mendrick DL. Cell-mediated immune injury in the kidney: acute nephritis induced in the rat by azobenzenearsonate. *Kidney Int* 1994;45:1044–1056.

226. Doherty A, Bradfield J. Polyarteritis nodosa associated with acute cytomegalovirus infection. *Ann Rheum Dis* 1981;8:161–169.

227. Hawley D, Schaefer J, Schulz D, Mulle R. Cytomegalovirus encephalitis in acquired immunodeficiency syndrome. *Am J Clin Pathol* 1983; 80:874–877.

228. Koeppen A, Lansing L, Peng S, Smith R. Central nervous system vasculitis in cytomegalovirus infection. *J Neurol Sci* 1981;51: 395–410.

229. Reyes M, Fresco R, Chokroverty S, Salud E. Virus-like particles in granulomatous angiitis of the central nervous system. *Neurology* 1976;26:797–799.

230. Cines DB, Lyss A, Mahin B, Corkey R, Kefalides N, Friedman H. Fc and C3 receptors induced by herpes simplex virus on cultured human endothelial cells. *J Clin Immunol* 1983;63:123–128.

231. Friedman H, Cohen G, Eisenberg R, Seidel C, Cines D. Glycoprotein C of herpes simplex virus I acts as a receptor for C3b complement component in infected cells. *Nature* 1984;309:633–635.

232. Para M, Baucke R, Spear P. Glycoprotein IgE of herpes simplex virus type I: effects of anti-IgE on virion infectivity and on virus induced Fc binding receptors. *J Virol* 1982;41:129–136.

233. Dorff B, Lind K. Two fatal cases of meningoencephalitis associated with *Mycoplasma pneumoniae* infection. *Scand J Infect Dis* 1976;8: 49–51.

234. Feder H, Watkin T, Cole S, Quinfiliare R. Severe meningoencephalitis complicating *Mycoplasma pneumoniae* infection in a child. *Arch Pathol Lab Med* 1981;105:619–621.

235. Fernald GW. Immunologic interactions between host cells and mycoplasmas. *Rev Infect Dis* 1982;4:S201–S204.

236. Thomas L, Davidson M, McCluskey R. Studies of PPLO infection I. The production of cerebral polyarteritis by *Mycoplasma gallisepticum* in turkeys. The neurotoxic property of the mycoplasma. *J Exp Med* 1966;123:897–911.

237. Thomas L, Aleu F, Bitensky M, Davidson M, Gesner B. Studies of PPLO Infection. II. The neurotoxin of *Mycoplasma neurolyticum. J Exp Med* 1966;124:1067–1081.

238. Walker D, Mattern W. Rickettsial vasculitis. *Am Heart J* 1980;6: 896–906.

239. Hoxie J, Matthews D, Cines D. Infection of human endothelial cells by human T cell leukemia virus type I. *Proc Natl Acad Sci USA* 1984;81: 7591–7595.

240. Haynes BF, Miller S, Moore J, Dunn P, Bolognesi D, Metzgar R. Identification of human T cell leukemia virus in a Japanese patient with adult T cell leukemia and cutaneous lymphomatous vasculitis. *Proc Natl Acad Sci USA* 1983;80:2054–2058.

241. Schwartz ND, So YT, Hollander H, Allen S, Fye KH. Eosinophilic vasculitis leading to amaurosis fugax in a patient with acquired immunodeficiency syndrome. *Arch Intern Med* 1986;146:2059–2060.

242. Liu YC, Tomashefski JF, Tomford JW, Green H. Necrotizing *Pneumocystis carinii* vasculitis associated with lung necrosis and cavitation in a patient with acquired immunodeficiency syndrome. *Arch Pathol Lab Med* 1989;113:494–497.

243. Greer JM, Longley S, Edwards NL, El Jenbein GJ, Panush RS. Vasculitis associated with malignancy. Experience with 13 patients and literature. *Rev Med* 1988;67:220–230.

244. Granstein R, Soter N, Haynes H. Necrotizing vasculitis within cutaneous lesions of mycosis fungoides. *J Am Acad Dermatol* 1981;9: 128–133.

245. Fauci AS, Haynes BF, Costa J, Katz P, Wolff S. Lymphomatoid granulomatosis, prospective clinical and therapeutic experience over ten years. *N Engl J Med* 1982;306:68–74.

246. Huston K, Combs J, Lie J, Giuliani E. Left atrial myxoma simulating peripheral vasculitis. *Mayo Clin Proc* 1978;53:752–756.

247. Eberhard BA, Andersson U, Laxer RM, Rose V, Silverman ED. Evaluation of the cytokine response in Kawasaki disease. *Pediatr Infect Dis J* 1995;14:199–203.

248. Vidarsson B, Geirsson AJ, Onundarson PT. Reactivation of rheumatoid arthritis and development of leukocytoclastic vasculitis in a patient receiving granulocyte colony-stimulating factor for Felty's syndrome. *Am J Med* 1995;98:589–591.

249. Csernok E, Szymkowiak CH, Mistry N, Daha MR, Gross WL, Kekow J. Transforming growth factor-beta (TGF-beta) expression and interaction with proteinase 3 (PR3) in anti-neutrophil cytoplasmic antibody (ANCA)-associated vasculitis. *Clin Exp Immunol* 1996;105:104–111.

250. Jennette JC, Wilkman AS, Falk RJ. Anti-neutrophil cytoplasmic autoantibody-associated glomerulonephritis and vasculitis. *Am J Pathol* 1989;135:921–930.

Inflammation: Basic Principles and Clinical Correlates,
3rd ed., edited by John I. Gallin and Ralph Snyderman.
Lippincott Williams & Wilkins, Philadelphia © 1999.

CHAPTER 64

Rheumatoid Arthritis

Arthur F. Kavanaugh and Peter E. Lipsky

Rheumatoid arthritis (RA) is a chronic, systemic, inflammatory disorder that affects approximately 0.8% of the population. Despite intensive investigation, the precise cause of RA remains undefined. However, paralleling the important strides that have been made toward an understanding of the human immune system, the pathogenesis of RA has been increasingly well defined (1,2). It is thought that RA results from the exposure of a genetically susceptible host to the relevant but unidentified etiopathogenic antigens. Dysregulation of various components of the immune response has been demonstrated in affected patients and is thought to underlie the systemic inflammation.

The characteristic clinical presentation of RA is a symmetric polyarthritis, often associated with constitutional symptoms such as fever and malaise. The small joints of the hands and feet are preferentially affected, although any diarthrodial joint may become involved. Synovial inflammation may ultimately result in bony and cartilaginous destruction and deformity. The articular and extraarticular manifestations of RA result directly from the chronic synovial and systemic inflammation. Most of these manifestations can be ascribed in large part to the actions of various cytokines and other inflammatory mediators. The extent to which these manifestations may be expressed in a given individual depends on a variety of genetic, hormonal, and immunologic host variables.

RA was previously considered a relatively benign disease that was self-limited for most patients. However, it has become appreciated that the disease is often chronic and progressive (3). RA is associated with substantial morbidity and accelerated mortality. In concert with this modified realization of its severity, the therapeutic approach to patients with RA has undergone considerable evolution. More aggressive and earlier therapeutic intervention has become standard.

HISTORICAL ASPECTS

Unlike several other arthritides, such as osteoarthritis (OA), RA may be a relatively modern disease. There is a relative paucity of persuasive evidence of RA in archaic skeletal remains or in the art and literature of antiquity (4). Modern consideration of RA began in the early part of this century, when the distinction between purely degenerative arthropathy and inflammatory arthritis was realized (5). The inflammatory arthritides included RA and arthritis related to various microorganisms, fostering the hypothesis that some infectious agent might be the relevant etiologic factor in RA. However, despite years of investigation, no single etiologic agent has been conclusively implicated. The hypothesis that RA resulted from an infection did provide a rationale for the use of various therapeutic agents. Several of these putative antiinfectious agents, such as injectable gold salts, sulfasalazine, and tetracyclines, are still part of the modern therapeutic armamentarium. Although their mechanisms of action remain incompletely defined, it is doubtful that their antimicrobial properties contribute to their activity.

The concept that the inflammation characteristic of RA was immunologically mediated began in 1948 with the landmark observation that the sera of RA patients could cause the agglutination of immunoglobulin-coated red blood cells (6). It was soon realized that this resulted from the binding of the Fc piece of IgG by other antibodies. Such autoantibodies, which are predominantly of the IgM isotype, are known as rheumatoid factors (RFs). The large body of work since that time has further characterized numerous aspects of the immunologic abnormalities associated with RA and the inflammatory and pathologic changes characteristic of the disease (1,2,7).

A. F. Kavanaugh and P. E. Lipsky: Rheumatic Diseases Division, Department of Internal Medicine, University of Texas Southwestern Medical Center at Dallas, Dallas, Texas 75235.

EPIDEMIOLOGY

The prevalence of RA is remarkably consistent throughout the world, affecting approximately 0.8% of the population. Exceptions to this generalization include the scarcity of RA in rural sub-Saharan black African populations and a somewhat higher incidence (≥5%) of RA in certain Native-American populations. It has been suggested that the incidence and prevalence of RA may be decreasing (8). In all populations, women are affected about three times more commonly than men. The prevalence of RA increases with age, and differences in prevalence related to gender lessen with advancing age. RA develops most commonly during the fourth and fifth decades of life, with 80% of the total cases arising between the ages of 35 and 50 years.

Family studies of patients with RA suggest a genetic predisposition. Monozygotic twins have a 15% to 30% concordance for RA, contrasted with 5% for dizygotic twins and nontwin siblings. First-degree relatives of patients develop RA at approximately fourfold to sixfold the expected rate (9). Such studies highlight a genetic propensity to the development of RA, but the relatively low penetrance implies a polygenic pattern of inheritance and a potential contribution of environmental agents and other factors.

HORMONAL FACTORS

The differences in prevalence related to gender suggest that the expression of RA is influenced by various sex hormones. Additional support for this association comes from several observations. The activity of RA tends to abate during pregnancy and increase in the postpartum period, the risk of RA is higher in nulliparous women, and oral contraceptive use early in adult life appears to delay the onset of RA and to attenuate its severity. Some of the gender and reproductive associations with RA may be related to differences in prolactin synthesis (10).

In addition to the sex hormones, other endocrine factors have substantial modulatory effects on RA. The discovery of the glucocorticosteroids was prompted in part by the observation that arthritis improved in patients who had diseases that caused endogenous corticosteroid excess. The profound ability of these compounds to suppress rheumatoid inflammation prompted the hypothesis that expression of RA may be related in part to defective endogenous production of glucocorticosteroids. An intriguing animal model that may bear some relevance to this theory is the Lewis rat. These rats, which have hyporesponsive hypothalamic-pituitary-adrenal (HPA) axis function, are more susceptible to the development of inflammatory arthritis after streptococcal cell wall injection than Fisher rats, who have normal HPA axis function (11). It has been difficult to demonstrate any substantial abnormalities in HPA axis function by testing RA patients. However, it has been suggested that the beneficial therapeutic effects of low-dose corticosteroid therapy in RA provide indirect evidence of an endocrine effect on rheumatoid inflammation.

GENETICS

The genetic contribution to RA is evidenced most convincingly by the association between the expression of certain class II major histocompatibility complex (MHC) gene products (e.g., HLA-DR) and the development or severity of RA (12–17). RA patients who are homozygous for certain MHC types tend to have more extraarticular manifestations and more destructive joint involvement than those with only one allele. Those with one "at risk" allele tend to have more severe disease than those with RA who exhibit other MHC haplotypes (14).

RA is strongly associated with the presence of DR4 alleles in distinct ethnic groups, including Caucasians, Japanese, southern Chinese, and native populations in the Americas. In other ethnic groups, an association has been observed between RA and other MHC class II gene products. For example, RA has been associated with *DRB1 (DRB1*0101)* in Asian Indians and Ashkenazi Jews. Resolution of these human leukocyte antigen (HLA) associations came from molecular analysis of the MHC class II molecules (13). The HLA-DR molecule is composed of an invariant α chain and a highly polymorphic β chain. Allelic variations in the HLA-DR molecule reflect differences in the primary amino acid sequences of the chains. The preponderance of these sequence differences occurs in three hypervariable regions of the molecule. RA appears to be associated with a specific epitope of the third hypervariable region of the DR chain, which is conserved in the susceptibility-associated alleles. Each of the HLA-DR molecules that is associated with RA has the same or a very similar sequence of amino acids in positions 67 through 74 of the third hypervariable region of the chain of the molecule, the so-called shared epitope. Of particular importance are positions 71 and 74, which appear to be involved in the capacity of the molecules to bind specific peptides. Amino acid differences at position 71 may define clinical subsets of RA patients (18). Other HLA-DR chains, which are not associated with RA, have differences in the amino acid sequence in this region such that there are alterations in important physiochemical characteristics such as charge and hydrophobicity.

The association between RA and certain MHC alleles may be important in dissecting the pathogenesis of this disease. However, the mechanisms underlying this association remain unknown. MHC molecules play a pivotal role in the generation of immune responses by virtue of their ability to bind antigenic fragments and present them to T cells. The third hypervariable region of the

DR chain may serve a crucial role in antigen binding, raising the intriguing hypothesis that the genetic proclivity to RA engendered by these molecules is related to an ability to bind the etiologic antigens. Differences in peptide-binding capability have been observed between RA-associated and -nonassociated DRB1 molecules. However, several observations argue against this binding hypothesis: the infrequent development of RA among persons possessing the relevant MHC haplotypes; the relative lack of this determinant in certain RA populations, such as African Americans; and the dosage effect (i.e., patients homozygous for susceptibility epitopes have a greater severity of disease than heterozygotes) (15,16).

There are alternative explanations for the MHC associations in RA. MHC molecules play a critical role in the shaping of the T-cell repertoire during T-cell maturation in the thymus. The predisposition of certain MHC class II gene products to RA may be related to the repertoire of T-cell receptors selected (i.e., T-cell selection hypothesis). This situation may predispose to disease by several means. For example, fragments of MHC peptides may themselves be presented as antigens, particularly by dendritic cells. Thymic presentation of fragments of the "shared epitope" may select for T cells that subsequently recognize autologous antigen or cross-reactive antigen from infectious agents in the joint. Alternatively, expression of RA associated DRB alleles may represent a marker for a "hole" in the T-cell repertoire. In this model, DRB1 alleles that are not associated with RA may somehow confer protection against the etiologic agent.

Although their association with RA is important, HLA genes contribute only a portion of the genetic susceptibility to RA. Genes outside the HLA group that may also contribute include those for immunoglobulin heavy and light chains (19). Despite the correlations with HLA and non-HLA alleles, it is clear that genetic risk factors do not fully account for the incidence of RA. Environmental factors are relevant, as evidenced by the impact urbanization and climate have had on the incidence and severity of RA in Africa. Hormonal influences on disease activity have also been well established.

In addition to associations with incidence and severity of disease, there appears to be an association between genes of the MHC and the development of certain adverse reactions induced by therapeutic agents used in the management of RA (20). For example, the presence of the HLA-DR3 allele is associated with the development of thrombocytopenia, proteinuria, and dermatitis in patients treated with injectable gold compounds. Similarly, the presence of this allele appears to predispose to the development of proteinuria after therapy with D-penicillamine. In general, no association has been found between HLA type and the response to therapy with any agents.

PATHOGENESIS

Etiology

The cause of RA remains unknown. It is assumed that the pathophysiology of RA is related to a persistent immunologic response of a genetically susceptible host to one or more antigens, possibly an infectious agent (21). Given the worldwide distribution of RA, any such agents would, by necessity, be ubiquitous. Over the years, a number of potential etiologic agents have been suggested (Table 64-1). Although many of the suggested pathogens can cause arthritis, no etiologic agent has ever been conclusively implicated as the cause of RA.

The process by which an infectious agent may cause RA remains a subject of debate. Perhaps the simplest mechanism would be persistent infection of articular structures or the retention of microbial products within the synovium as causes of the chronic inflammatory response. A brisk proliferative response of rheumatoid synovial T cells to mycobacterial heat shock proteins has been observed (22). Another possibility is that the infection or the host response to the infection alters articular structures such that they become immunogenic. Reactivity to type II collagen cartilage glycoprotein gp39 and heat shock proteins has been demonstrated in RA patients (22,23). Alternatively, the infecting microorganisms may prime the host to cross-reactive determinants expressed on joint structures as a result of "molecular mimicry" (24). For example, a 5–amino acid peptide (QKRAA) common to the third hypervariable region of the DR chain of HLA-DRB1*0401, is also present in the Epstein-Barr virus glycoprotein gp110 and in a heat shock protein (DnaJ) from *Escherichia coli* (25). Products of infecting organisms such as superantigens may play a role in the induction of disease.

For alternative means of identifying the causative agents in RA, investigators have approached the question

TABLE 64-1. *Proposed etiologic agents for rheumatoid arthritis*

Bacteria
  Mycobacteria
  Escherichia coli
  Proteus mirabilis
Bacteria capable of producing superantigens
  Group A streptococci
  Staphylococci
  Mycoplasma arthritidis
  Clostridia perfringens
  Yersinia enterocolitica
Viruses
  Rubella
  Human parvovirus, strain B19
  Epstein-Barr
  Cytomegalovirus
  Hepatitis B
  Human T-cell lymphotropic virus type 1
  Various retroviruses

of cause from the standpoint of the antigen-specific cells that should respond to the inciting agents. In theory, if RA results from exposure to a certain etiologic antigen, this antigen should elicit a preferential response by a limited repertoire of T cells (26–29). T cells with antigen receptors with specificity for that antigen should be able to be identified within the synovium. Investigations along these lines have progressed over the years using the developing techniques of immunology. Such investigations have been hampered by several problems, including the need to amplify the number of cells recovered from inflammatory sites, which may introduce bias. In RA, as in other inflammatory conditions, there is extensive antigen-nonspecific recruitment of T cells into inflammatory sites. There is no consensus about the nature of restricted heterogeneity of T cells recovered from the rheumatoid synovium (27). However, there have been several provocative study findings. There may be restricted use of T-cell receptors in inflammatory sites when analysis is limited to the region that interacts with antigen, the CD3 region (27,28). Some degree of restricted heterogeneity in T-cell receptor gene usage was observed among patients with early RA (30). Oligoclonal T-cell populations have also been recovered from severe combined immune deficiency mice into which human RA synovial tissue had been placed (31). Restricted T-cell receptor gene use has also been observed among mycobacterial heat shock protein T-cell clones derived from the synovium of RA patients (32). The oligoclonality found in these studies may reflect immunoregulatory defects and not antigen-driven processes.

Evidence supporting the hypothesis that the immunologic response in RA is antigen driven is derived from analysis of intrasynovial RF. This immunoglobulin has restricted clonality in RA patients compared with controls (33,34). Evidence of somatic mutation of RF-encoding immunoglobulin genes also supports the possibility of antigen selection.

Histopathology

RA may affect any diarthrodial joints. Such articulations are movable joints in which the opposing bony surfaces are covered with cartilage, there is a joint cavity containing synovial fluid, and the joint cavity is lined by a synovial membrane that is reinforced by a fibrous capsule. In the affected joints of patients with RA, the characteristic histopathologic changes vary with the stage of the disease. The earliest discernible alterations include vascular congestion and obliteration of small vessels by inflammatory cells and thrombi (35). In addition to microvascular injury, hyperplasia and hypertrophy of the synovial lining cells and a modest perivascular accumulation of leukocytes are typical findings in the initial weeks of arthritis. At this point in the disease process, polymorphonuclear leukocytes may be seen within the

synovial tissue. As the arthritis persists, the nature of the leukocytic infiltration in the synovium evolves, and there is a preponderance of lymphocytes and other mononuclear cells. The pathologic characteristics seen in early RA are not unique to this disease process. Synovial hypertrophy, microvascular abnormalities, and leukocytic infiltration may be seen in other types of inflammatory arthritis, such as gouty arthritis, septic arthritis, systemic lupus erythematosus, and the seronegative spondyloarthropathies (36). Pathologic changes more characteristic of RA occur in the later stages of disease.

The chronic phase of RA is characterized grossly by edema and swelling of the synovium, which protrudes into the joint space predominantly as villous projections. Although a similar picture may be seen in other arthritides, exuberant synovial hypertrophy is a classic characteristic of RA (2,7). Histopathologically, there is a progression of the synovial hypertrophy and hyperplasia observed early in the disease; synoviocytes may be stratified in layers of 5 to 10 cells, compared with a normal filamentous layer of 1 to 3 cells. The synovial lining cells may be divided into two types: type A synoviocytes, with phagocytic capacity and derived from the myeloid lineage, and type B synoviocytes, with secretory features and apparently derived from fibroblasts. Subsynovial focal and segmental vascular changes observed in early RA persist in the later stages. There is also evidence of endothelial injury, thrombosis, and neovascularization (35). Neovascularization may serve a critical role in the perpetuation of the inflammatory response (37). The formation of new subsynovial vessels, which typically have large fenestrations analogous to those of the glomerulus, may facilitate the introduction of inflammatory mediators into the joint.

In the chronic phase of RA, the extravascular lymphocytic infiltration becomes more abundant. The cellular aggregates also demonstrate more organization, such that lymphoid follicles with germinal centers, similar to those in lymphoid tissue, are observed (7). This orderly aggregation of lymphoid cells, along with the presence of abundant plasma cells, is more characteristic of RA than of other arthritides. Changes in the endothelium differ in the chronic phase of RA. Earlier in the disease, the morphology of the endothelial cells is diffusely altered throughout the synovial tissue, but in the chronic phase, these changes become more localized. The synovial inflammatory cell infiltrate is particularly prominent in perivascular sites, where it consists largely of CD4$^+$ helper T lymphocytes (T$_H$1 and T$_H$2), which are in close apposition to antigen-presenting cells such as dendritic cells and macrophages (38,39) (Fig. 64-1). Pathologically, this is similar to the characteristics of cutaneous delayed-type hypersensitivity (type IV) reactions to known antigens. By extension, this pattern offers some support for the hypothesis that RA results from the exposure of a genetically susceptible host to some relevant eti-

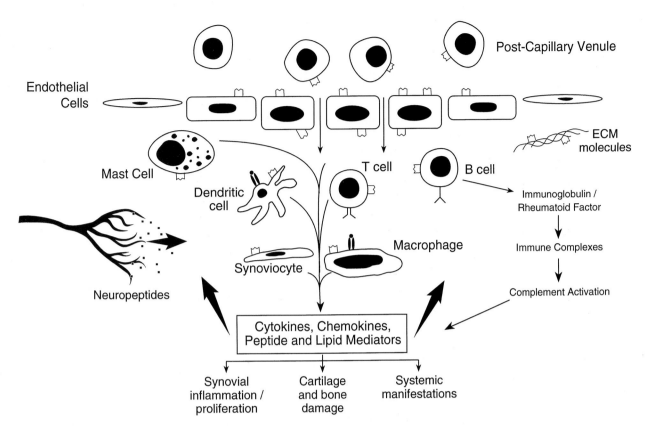

Post-Capillary Venule

Endothelial
Cells

ECM
molecules

Mast Cell

T cell

B cell

Dendritic
cell

Immunoglobulin /
Rheumatoid Factor

Macrophage

Immune Complexes

Synoviocyte

Neuropeptides

Complement Activation

Cytokines, Chemokines,
Peptide and Lipid Mediators

Synovial
inflammation /
proliferation

Cartilage
and bone
damage

Systemic
manifestations

FIG. 64-1. In the inmmunopathogenesis of rheumatoid arthritis, many cells participate in generating immunologically driven inflammation, but T cells are thought to orchestrate this response. T cells that have migrated into the synovium recognize antigen presented by specialized antigen-presenting cells (e.g., dendritic cells, monocytes, macrophages). These cells express class II major histocompatibility complex molecules, such as HLA-DR. T-cell interactions generate cytokines, and these pluripotent peptides have profound effects on many cell types in the joint. Secretion of immunoglobulin and rheumatoid factor by B cells may result in immune complex formation and activation of the complement cascade.

ologic antigens. However, the inciting agent remains undefined. The similarity to delayed-type hypersensitivity reactions also provides support for the characterization of RA predominantly as a T_H1-type lesion.

Nearly all of the synovial tissue $CD4^+$ T cells are of the memory phenotype (CD45RO-/CD29 "bright"), whereas few are of the naive phenotype (CD45RA "bright") (39). Presumably, this reflects cells that express an altered phenotype as a consequence of previous antigenic exposure. Further analysis has revealed that many of these T cells exhibit a phenotype characteristic of chronically activated or differentiated cells (40). In areas of the synovium distant from the vessels, fewer $CD4^+$ T cells are seen, and there are few aggregates of cells. These areas have a diffuse infiltrate consisting predominantly of $CD8^+$ suppressor T cells (41), although it has been suggested that these cells are largely of the cytotoxic rather than the suppressor phenotype. The rheumatoid synovium also contains populations of $\gamma\delta$ T cells, which may be present in increased numbers compared with the level in circulation. The function of this subset of T cells in RA remains unknown (42).

B cells also are present in large numbers in the rheumatoid synovium. In the follicles and germinal centers, there are large numbers of lymphoblasts and plasma cells. Presumably, small lymphoblasts migrate into the synovium, where they may differentiate into antibody secreting plasma cells. Synovial tissue is capable of secreting large amounts of immunoglobulin. Approximately 20% of the immunoglobulin recovered from synovial fluid may be locally synthesized by synovial tissue (43). An increased fraction of the synovial antibody has RF activity (44). The precise role of these autoantibodies in disease propagation is uncertain, but immune complexes containing RF may precipitate in synovial tissues, such as the superficial layers of cartilage, and activate the complement cascade (45). These antibodies may amplify the synovial inflammatory response.

The synovium in the chronic phase of RA contains many cell types other than lymphocytes. Fibroblasts are present in increased numbers and have characteristics that suggest transformed cells (46). Their numbers are increased, and they proliferate rapidly with a lack of characteristic contact inhibition. Fibroblasts may also demonstrate locally invasive behavior and may be important in the genesis of bony erosions. Macrophages are present in the perivascular infiltrates and throughout the synovial tissue. The extent to which predominantly macrophage-associated cytokines (e.g., interleukin-1 [IL-1], IL-6, tumor necrosis factor-α [TNF-α], and IL-8) are recovered from the synovium argues for an important role for these cells in the maintenance of synovial inflammation (47). Mast cells are abundant in the rheumatoid synovium, particularly in perivascular locations.

Chronic synovial inflammation in RA results in the formation of pannus. This highly vascularized granulation tissue is composed of a variety of cell types, including lymphocytes, macrophages, fibroblasts, synoviocytes, and mast cells (46–48). Pannus is found in particular at the marginal areas of diarthrodial joints, where it often impinges on articular cartilage and subchondral bone. Direct tissue invasion by pannus is one of the principal mechanisms responsible for the damage to articular cartilage, erosions in subchondral bone, and impairment of periarticular structures that are characteristic of severe RA (49). Synovial cells from patients with RA may exhibit certain phenotypic characteristics of transformed cells, such as anchorage-independent growth in vitro.

It is not clear to what extent immunologically driven inflammatory processes are necessary for the generation of pannus. Although there is evidence that T cells orchestrate rheumatoid inflammation, it has been suggested that monocyte-driven inflammation may be the central event in pannus formation (50,51). Invasion of cartilage and subchondral bone by hyperplastic synovial cells, independent of any mononuclear cell infiltrates, has also been described (49). In animal models of RA-like polyarthritis, joint destruction can develop in the absence of an inflammatory infiltrate (52). In these animals (MRL/l mice), destruction is often observed in juxtaposition to invading synoviocytes. However, in other animal models and in RA, inflammatory cells are thought to play a role in the induction of the synovial cell hyperplasia.

In addition to inflammation of rheumatoid synovial tissue, there is an acute inflammatory process in the synovial fluid of patients with RA. The typical exudative synovial fluid contains more polymorphonuclear leukocytes than mononuclear cells, unlike the histopathologic pattern of the synovial tissue. This picture may be influenced by the concurrent use of medications. Several mechanisms may play a role in stimulating the exudation of synovial fluid. For example, locally generated immune complexes may activate the complement cascade, thereby generating chemotactic products and the anaphylatoxins C3a and C5a (53). Vasoactive mediators such as histamine may subsequently be released from synovial mast cells. These mediators then facilitate synovial accumulation of fluid and accrual of inflammatory cells. Local production of factors such as IL-1,

TNF-α, and leukotriene B$_4$ by mononuclear phagocytes and other resident synovial cells may stimulate the endothelial cells of postcapillary venules to enhance their expression of adhesion receptors, enhancing the ability of the endothelium to facilitate the adherence and transendothelial migration of other leukocytes (54). Chemoattractants such as complement split products, platelet-activating factor, leukotriene B$_4$, and IL-8 and the other chemokines can enhance the accrual of inflammatory cells in the synovium through their chemotactic activity. The vasodilatory effects of locally produced prostaglandin E$_2$ may also facilitate the entry of inflammatory cells into the joint. Once in the synovial fluid, the polymorphonuclear leukocytes can ingest immune complexes, causing the neutrophils to produce reactive oxygen metabolites and other inflammatory mediators. This result can further enhance the inflammatory cascade (55). Synovial polymorphonuclear leukocytes can also be stimulated by locally generated cytokines, including TNF-α, IL-8, and granulocyte-macrophage colony-stimulating factor (GM-CSF). Generation of large amounts of products of the cyclooxygenase and lipoxygenase pathways of arachidonic acid metabolism by cells in the synovial fluid and tissue further accentuates the signs and symptoms of inflammation.

Cartilage Degeneration and Erosive Bone Disease

Maintenance of the integrity of extracellular matrix (ECM) tissue, cartilage, and bone is a dynamic process. Interference with the integrity of these structures produces several of the characteristic findings of RA.

Normally, the synthesis of ECM components such as collagen and fibronectin by fibroblasts is counterbalanced by the specific degradation of these molecules. Likewise, the continuous synthesis of proteoglycan and collagen by chondrocytes is balanced by their degradation. An analogous situation exists in bone. Synthesis of bony matrix by osteoblasts is opposed by the resorption of bone by osteoclasts.

Degradation of structural components is mediated to a large extent by a family of proteolytic enzymes commonly known as matrix metalloproteinases (MMPs) (56). Prominent enzymes in this category include collagenase, stromelysin, the cathepsins, elastase, and gelatinase (57). Several membrane-type MMPs have been described (58). Important sources of these proteases include many of the cells within the rheumatoid synovium, including synoviocytes, fibroblasts, monocytes, and chondrocytes. In the case of bone, osteoclasts are the predominant source of degradative proteases, although a substantial contribution can be made by cells of the myeloid lineage in inflammatory conditions such as RA (57,58). Because they are secreted as proenzymes, these enzymes must be activated by the proteolytic activity of other enzymes, such as trypsin and plasmin. Once activated, they can be regulated by the inhibitory influence of yet other enzymes, including the tissue inhibitors of metalloproteinases (TIMP-1 and TIMP-2), and α_2-macroglobulin.

In RA, there is an alteration in the balance of synthetic and degradative processes, producing a net loss of structural constituents. Several factors contribute to this imbalance in the normal homeostasis. Inflammatory cells, particularly cells of the monocyte-macrophage lineage, are important sources of MMPs such as elastase and cathepsin and sources of other proteases. When activated, as they are in the rheumatoid synovium, production of MMPs increases substantially. Various cytokines, many of which are also derived from monocytes and play a central role in the immunopathophysiology of RA, also contribute to this process (see Appendix B).

Cytokines have diverse effects on tissue integrity (59). IL-1, IL-6, and TNF-α may directly activate osteoclasts, whereas IL-1 and TNF-α may cause ECM degradation through their ability to stimulate collagenase and stromelysin production by synoviocytes and chondrocytes. IL-1 and TNF-α also may enhance proteoglycan production, and IL-6 may stimulate TIMP-1 production. The ultimate effect of inflammation in terms of tissue damage depends on the concentrations of these factors produced locally and on the influence of these cytokines on degradative and counterregulatory enzymes.

Although complex, it appears that the net result of chronic inflammation in RA is the degradation of articular and periarticular ECM. A decrease in the integrity of articular cartilage occurs in juxtaposition to the pannus. Activation of osteoclasts occurs with an increase in bone matrix degradation. Another role of degradative enzymes in the pathogenesis of RA may be related to the perpetuation of the immune response. Proteases may unmask epitopes on articular cartilage that could stimulate further immune responses (60).

The expression of inhibition of bone integrity has two predominant clinical expressions in RA: juxtaarticular osteopenia and marginal erosions. Juxtaarticular osteopenia is not unique to RA, but it is more characteristic of this disease than of other inflammatory arthritides and may provide a roentgenographic clue to the diagnosis. Although bone loss may be asymptomatic, the impairment in the overall structural integrity of the bone may predispose the patient to the development of fractures. Bony erosions in RA occur most commonly at the margins of joints, where the pannus is most pronounced. Osteoclasts, which may be found at the bone-pannus junction, contribute substantially to marginal erosions. When severe, excessive joint destruction may be seen as part of the erosive process (Fig. 64-2). Common locations of erosions in RA include the proximal aspect of the metacarpophalangeal (MCP) and metatarsophalangeal (MTP) joints and the wrists.

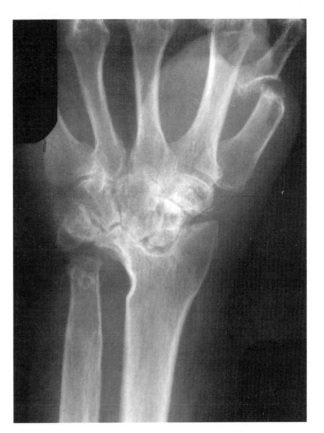

FIG. 64-2. A roentgenogram of the wrist reveals complete erosion of the distal end of the ulna in a patient with rheumatoid arthritis. The distal end of the first metacarpal bone has eroded; the radiocarpal articulation has collapsed, with erosion into the radius; and the carpal bones demonstrate ankylosis.

Immunologic Basis

Vascular Endothelium

Alterations in the vascular endothelium may be found in all stages of RA (35,61) (see Fig. 64-2). Because they are among the earliest pathologic changes, they may play an important role in the cause of RA. The endothelium appears to undergo three types of revision in RA: morphologic and phenotypic changes, evidence of endothelial injury, and neovascularization.

Under the influence of locally generated cytokines, synovial postcapillary venules undergo a morphologic alteration such that they resemble the so-called high endothelial venules (HEVs) characteristic of lymphoid tissues (35) (Fig. 64-3). These HEV-like vessels presumably serve an important role in the propagation of rheumatoid inflammation by facilitating the transvascular migration of leukocytes. In support of this, these endothelial cells have an enhanced expression of various cell surface adhesion receptors, including intercellular adhesion molecule-1 (ICAM-1, CD54), vascular cell adhesion molecule-1 (VCAM-1), E-selectin (ELAM-1, CD62E), and vascular

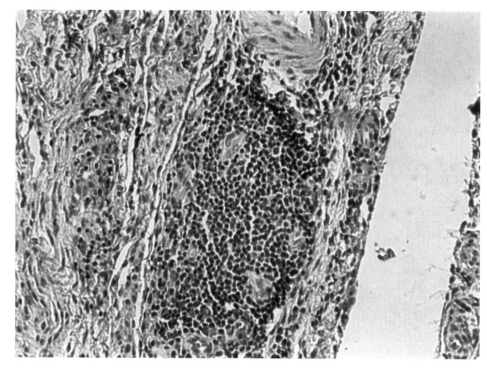

FIG. 64-3. In a patient with rheumatoid arthritis, the characteristic features include proliferation of the synovial lining layer, organized subsynovial accumulation of mononuclear cells, and endothelial cells that have assumed a high endothelial venule (HEV) phenotype.

adhesion protein-1 (VAP-1) (54). The expression of these adhesion receptors is known to be upregulated by cytokines found in the rheumatoid synovium, including IL-1, IL-4, and TNF-α. Various chemokines in the rheumatoid synovium, such as IL-8 and the monocyte chemotactic proteins, play a stimulatory role in adhesion receptor–mediated interactions. In concert, the various factors that are capable of qualitatively and quantitatively upregulating adhesion receptor function potentiate the extravasation of leukocytes into the synovium. The extravascular accrual of leukocytes in the synovium provides a basis for the sustenance of the inflammatory reaction and for the manifestations of the disease process.

In addition to these gross morphologic changes, the endothelium in RA demonstrates signs of activation and injury. Intraluminal occlusion with inflammatory cells or thrombi is common (62). The normal impermeability and barrier function of the endothelium may be compromised. As a result, there is an increased exudation of plasma and its constituents, including high-molecular-weight proteins. Vascular compromise delays the clearance of materials from the synovium. Such changes presumably result from the local generation of proinflammatory cytokines, which have profound effects on the normal anticoagulant, rheologic, and barrier functions of the endothelium (62).

Neovascularization is a common finding in the rheumatoid synovium. Various soluble mediators secreted during the local inflammatory response have the capability of stimulating new vessel growth (37). These include the cytokines TNF-α, transforming growth factor-β (TGF-β), platelet-derived growth factors A and B, fibroblast growth factor, vascular endothelial growth factor, and soluble forms of certain adhesion receptors such as VCAM-1. It can be hypothesized that the new vessel growth contributes to the propagation of the synovial inflammation, but it is also possible that the new vessel growth results from other factors such as tissue hypoxia.

T Cells

Of the melange of leukocytes recruited into the joint, T cells, particularly CD4$^+$ helper T cells, may serve a pivotal etiologic role (7). Several lines of evidence support this contention (Table 64-2). Increased numbers of activated T cells may be detected in the peripheral circulation of RA patients. Such activated T cells are also present in abundance in the rheumatoid synovium (39). These T cells are thought to represent an activated population by virtue of their cell surface phenotype. The T cells express various cell surface molecules to an extent that they approximate the phenotype of T cells that have been activated *in vitro* with various stimuli such as mitogens (41). For example, the differentiation markers CD3 and CD4 are expressed at a lower density, whereas MHC class II products (e.g., HLA-DR) and adhesion receptors such as the very late activation antigen (CD49a/CD29) and lymphocyte function antigen-1 (CD11a/CD18) are expressed

TABLE 64-2. *Role of CD4+ T cells in rheumatoid arthritis*

Evidence for
  Synovial tissue is consistently infiltrated with T
    lymphocytes, especially CD4+ T cells.
  Synovial T cells express activation markers.
  T cells are critical in certain animal models of arthritis.
  HLA-DR is associated with rheumatoid arthritis.
  Improvement in arthritis with elimination of T cells or
    suppression of T cell function by means of thoracic
    duct drainage, total lymphoid irradiation,
    lymphocytapheresis, or cyclosporine therapy.
Evidence against
  Small quantities of T-cell–derived cytokines are recovered
    from rheumatoid synovium.
  Responsiveness of synovial T cells is diminished.
  Animal models of arthritis and bony destruction can be
    T cell independent.
  Lack of effect of some T-cell–directed therapies (e.g.,
    anti-CD4, anti-CD5, anti-CD7 monoclonal antibodies).

at higher densities. The T cells express the early activation antigen CD69. The phenotype of rheumatoid synovial cells approximates that of highly differentiated memory cells (e.g., CD45RO+, CD45RB$_{dim}$, CD27-) (40). Several other cell surface markers typically expressed on T cells activated *in vitro*, such as the high-affinity receptor for IL-2 (CD25), are not typically expressed by T cells in synovial tissue. This may be a result of continuous, long-term *in vivo* stimulation (63).

Additional evidence implicating T cells in the pathogenesis of RA comes from animal studies. In experimental models of rheumatoid-like inflammatory arthritis, such as collagen-induced arthritis or adjuvant arthritis, synovitis can be generated in susceptible hosts through the transfer of T cells from affected animals (64). Transfer of T cells from RA patients into the joints of immunodeficient severe combined immune deficiency mice can result in synovitis (65). Additional evidence supporting a role for T cells in RA comes from clinical studies with various therapeutic modalities that share an ability to eliminate T cells or interfere with T-cell function. Such therapies include thoracic duct drainage (66), lymphocytapheresis (67), total lymphoid irradiation (68), and medications (e.g., cyclosporine) (69).

Among the subsets of T cells, helper T cells, characterized by the presence of the CD4 molecule on their surface, have been suggested to play an essential role in RA. CD4+ T cells are present in abundance in the rheumatoid synovium and represent the predominant T-cell subset in the organized perivascular cellular aggregates (38,39). Further evidence implicating CD4+ T cells comes from genetic studies (12,13). T cells recognize antigen only when bound to appropriate MHC antigens. The CD8+ T cells only recognize antigen that is associated with MHC class I antigens, whereas CD4+ T cells recognize antigen bound to MHC class II antigens. The association of RA with the expression of specific class II MHC molecules strongly implies a role for CD4+ T cells in RA.

The precise origin of activated synovial T cells is not entirely clear. T cells are migratory, and they perform their immunosurveillance function by constantly recirculating throughout the body. It has been demonstrated that the recirculation pattern of memory cells, as are found in the rheumatoid synovium, is distinct from naive T cells. Memory cells, in part because of their increased expression of adhesion receptors, migrate from the blood, through the tissues (including inflammatory sites), through the draining lymph nodes and vessels, and then back to the blood (40). *In vitro*, memory T cells possess an enhanced ability to migrate across endothelial monolayers. It appears that most synovial T cells are selectively recruited from a recirculating population. However, it is possible that local interactions may shape the population of synovial T cells. For example, interactions between T cells and endothelial cells can activate the T cells, resulting in increased expression of various surface markers such as CD69. It is possible that other activating interactions occur within the rheumatoid synovium. It has been shown that the expected apoptosis of synovial T cells that is mediated by specific cytokines and by fibroblast–T-cell interactions (70) is inhibited, providing a possible explanation for the persistent T-cell infiltration within the rheumatoid synovium.

On the basis of cytokines secreted, helper T cells may be subdivided into two distinct functional subsets: T$_H$1 and T$_H$2 cells. T$_H$1 cells, which predominantly secrete the cytokines interferon-γ (IFN-γ) and TNF-β, interact primarily with monocytes and serve prominent roles in delayed-type hypersensitivity reactions. T$_H$2 cells, which secrete IL-4 and IL-5 in humans, interact with B cells and play an important role in antibody-mediated immune reactions. In animal models and human disease, there is evidence for bias of the T-cell response into T$_H$1- and T$_H$2-dominant responses. In RA, a bias toward a T$_H$1 response has been shown (71). Cytokines secreted by T$_H$1 and T$_H$2 cells differentially regulate the development of cells into these subsets. For example, IL-4 and IL-10 favor the development of pluripotent T$_H$0 cells into T$_H$2 cells and away from T$_H$1 type. Manipulation of the T helper cell type may be an avenue for therapeutic intervention with cytokines in RA.

Whereas data suggest that T cells play an important role in the etiopathogenesis of RA, there is also evidence against this hypothesis (see Table 64-2). Only small quantities of predominantly T-cell–derived cytokines (e.g., IL-2, IL-3, IL-4, IFN-γ) are recovered from the rheumatoid synovium. T cells isolated from the rheumatoid synovium typically display decreased responsiveness to stimuli. Possible explanations for the observed hyporesponsiveness include the possibility that continuous *in vivo* activation has rendered the cells less active. The redox state of the inflammatory synovium may have detrimental effects on the T cells (72). Another factor arguing against the central role of T cells in RA includes animal models in which RA-like bony erosions develop without T cells. The lack of efficacy of T-cell–directed therapies, such as anti-CD4 monoclonal antibody, in human RA questions the importance of these cells in established disease (29).

In addition to lymphocytes, cells of other lineages and their secreted cytokines are involved in the pathologic changes characteristic of this disease. It has been suggested that cells other than T cells may play an etiopathogenic role in the progression of chronic rheumatoid inflammation (47), particularly at certain times during the disease course (73). Macrophages and mast cells, for example, are readily demonstrable in the rheumatoid synovium. The cytokines most reproducibly recovered from synovial fluid (e.g., IL-1, IL-6, IL-8, and TNF-α) are those typically secreted by activated macrophages or other resident synovial tissue cells rather than those typically secreted by T cells (47,59).

Macrophages in particular may play a key role in sustaining rheumatoid inflammation. After an immunologically driven inflammatory response is initiated, macrophages may have the ability to sustain the inflammation without further stimulation, in part because of the variety and amount of inflammatory mediators macrophages are capable of producing and by interactions mediated by cell surface molecules. Mediators secreted by macrophages include cytokines, chemokines, peptide mediators, and lipid mediators.

Cytokines and Chemokines

Cytokines exert a number of effector functions in normal homeostasis and in the development of immune and inflammatory responses. In autoimmune systemic inflammatory disorders such as RA, there may be an imbalance in the relative quantities of specific cytokines synthesized at sites of inflammation. Such cytokine dysregulation may be an important contributory pathophysiologic mechanism in RA (59). Many of the diverse local and systemic inflammatory manifestations of RA can be ascribed to the action of several cytokines and other soluble mediators synthesized within the rheumatoid synovium. In patients with RA, mRNAs encoding numerous cytokines have been detected in cells recovered from the inflamed synovium. Included herein are IL-1α, IL-1β, IL-2, IL-6, IL-10, GM-CSF, granulocyte colony-stimulating factor (G-CSF), TNF-α, TNF-β, IFN-γ, platelet-derived growth factor, and TGF-β. Cytokines considered to play a particularly prominent role in rheumatoid inflammation are IL-1, IL-6, and TNF-α (47).

In addition to the production of cytokines that propagate the immunologically driven inflammation, some local factors tend to dampen the inflammatory process. For example, the cytokine transforming growth factor-β (TGF-β) inhibits several of the features of synovial inflammation stimulated by other cytokines, including T-cell activation and proliferation, B-cell differentiation, and migration of leukocytes into inflammatory sites. TGF-β stimulates collagen production by fibroblasts. IL-6 may function to limit tissue damage by its ability to induce production of TIMPs (59). Other inhibitory mediators include cytokine antagonists, such as the IL-1 receptor antagonist (IL-1Ra). This cytokine, which is a member of the IL-1 family, binds the IL-1 receptor but transmits no signal, thereby acting as a competitive inhibitor (74). IL-1Ra is synthesized naturally in the rheumatoid synovium, perhaps as a means of downmodulating the activity of IL-1. Soluble forms of certain cytokine receptors, such as the receptor for TNF-α, have also been recovered from the rheumatoid synovium (75). Although their function is uncertain, it is hypothesized that they may be inhibitory or regulatory factors in the cytokine network.

Chemokines serve predominant roles by activating circulating cells and enhancing their accrual into the rheumatoid synovium. Important chemokines serving these functions include IL-8, monocyte chemotactic protein-1, and RANTES (i.e., regulated on activation, normally T-cell expressed and secreted).

Neuropeptides

Several lines of evidence support a role for the nervous system in the pathophysiology of RA (76,77). RA is usually a symmetric disease, with a predilection for specific joints. Moreover, when patients with hemiplegia develop RA, synovitis does not develop in the paretic limbs, implicating a role of innervation of the joint in the generation of inflammation. An explanation for the involvement of the nervous system in RA may be provided by neuropeptides. These small neurotransmitters may be released antidromically from the distal ends of primary sensory nerves. Substance P, a neuropeptide hypothesized to play a role in RA, is involved in the transmission of pain signals. It has multiple proinflammatory properties. Substance P causes the release of vasoactive mediators from mast cells, inflammatory cytokines from macrophages, and prostaglandins and enzymes from synoviocytes (77). Locally synthesized neuropeptides may contribute to the propagation of rheumatoid inflammation.

CLINICAL FEATURES

Onset

The onset of RA varies among patients. For approximately 55% to 70% patients, the onset is insidious (78). A symmetric arthritis developing over weeks or months typically involves the small joints of the hands and feet initially (79,80). It may be accompanied by stiffness of the involved joints in the morning, which usually lasts longer than 1 hour. The articular symptoms are often accompanied by or may be preceded by constitutional symptoms, such as fatigue, anorexia, low-grade fever, and generalized musculoskeletal pain. The slow progression of symptoms may delay the establishment of the diagnosis for some time.

Approximately 8% to 15% of patients present with a rapid onset of severe, widespread arthritis (80,81). The extent and severity of the concurrent constitutional symptoms, including fever, weight loss, and diffuse lymphadenopathy, often result in the inclusion of malignancy and infectious processes in the differential diagnosis at presentation. Although their initial presentations are flagrant, the patients with fulminant onset of disease may have a better prognosis than those whose presentation is more insidious (81).

Some patients may have a less typical presentation of RA, including palindromic rheumatism (82), in which limited disease activity waxes and wanes without specific therapy. Some patients present initially with monoarticular or oligoarticular arthritis. In both instances, patients may eventually exhibit the more typical sustained, symmetric polyarthritis.

Articular Signs and Symptoms

Pain and stiffness of the affected joints are nearly universal in patients with RA (78). Early in the course of their disease, patients may have difficulty localizing these symptoms to the joints. Joint pain, which is often aggravated by motion of the affected joints, is the most common manifestation of established RA (81). It corresponds with joint involvement but does not always correlate with the degree of apparent inflammation. Generalized stiffness is common and is usually greatest after periods of inactivity. Stiffness about the affected joints, which classically occurs in the morning and lasts for more than 1 hour, is almost a universal feature of RA. Although not specific, it may help in differentiating inflammatory arthritides such as RA from various noninflammatory joint disorders such as OA. The duration and severity of morning stiffness can provide a rough measure of disease activity and can be a useful parameter for the longitudinal assessment of patients.

In addition to articular symptoms, most patients experience a variety of constitutional symptoms such as generalized weakness, easy fatigability, malaise, anorexia, sleep disturbance, weight loss, and low-grade fever. Although these symptoms may seem relatively mild or moderate in severity, they are often of significant concern to the patients.

Clinically, synovial inflammation may be associated with all of the cardinal signs of inflammation. *Warmth* is often evident on examination, particularly during acute flares of activity. Warmth may also be a subtle finding. For example, arthritis of the knee may result in the skin over the patella being the same temperature as the rest of the leg skin, rather than feeling cooler to the touch, as it does normally. *Erythema* over affected joints is relatively infrequent in established disease, but it may be detected when patients initially present. Pain originates predominantly from the joint capsule, which is abundantly supplied with pain fibers and is exquisitely sensitive to stretching or distention. *Swelling* of the joints may result from accumulation of synovial fluid, hypertrophy of the synovium, and thickening of the joint capsule. With the advent of magnetic resonance imaging (MRI), it is possible to define the contribution of these different factors to the swelling of a particular joint, a distinction not always possible on physical examination.

Loss of function of the joints is primarily related to loss of motion. This is serious because it can quickly result in irreversible changes and significant morbidity. Initially, motion is restricted voluntarily as a response to the pain. The affected joint is usually held in slight flexion to maximize joint volume and thereby minimize joint capsule distention and pain. This decrease in motion can quickly result in muscle atrophy and tendon shortening. As these changes become chronic, the loss of motion becomes more difficult to reverse. Soft tissue contractures and even bony ankylosis may develop, resulting in fixed joint deformities.

RA can affect any diarthrodial joint, but it has a distinct predilection for certain joints, such as the small joints of the hands and feet (79,81) (Table 64-3). The reasons for the disparate involvement of various diarthrodial joints is uncertain, but the pattern of involvement is useful in establishing the diagnosis of RA and in alerting the clinician to the risk of potential functional impairments associated with synovitis of various joints.

Hands

Aside from being among the most frequently involved joints in patients with RA, inflammation of the MCP and proximal interphalangeal (PIP) joints frequently prompts patients to seek medical attention. Involvement of the dis-

TABLE 64-3. *Joint involvement in rheumatoid arthritis*

Involved joint	Approximate frequency (%)
Metacarpophalangeal	85
Wrist	80
Proximal interphalangeal	75
Knee	75
Metatarsophalangeal	75
Ankle (tibiotalar and subtalar joints)	75
Shoulder	60
Hip	50
Elbow	50
Acromioclavicular	50
Cervical spine	40
Temporomandibular	30
Sternoclavicular	30

tal interphalangeal (DIP) joints is far less common. Loss of motion because of MCP and PIP arthritis may result in atrophy of the intrinsic musculature of the hands, which tends to escalate hand weakness and further diminish functional status. With persistent inflammation, several characteristic deformities may be seen in the hands of RA patients. Pathophysiologically, these deformities represent the sum of a variety of contributory factors: muscle atrophy and therefore imbalance in forces transmitted across the joint, tendon laxity or shortening, rupture of tendons or ligaments, weakening of the joint capsule, and destruction of cartilage.

These factors may cause abnormal positioning or subluxation of the joint. Characteristic deformities of the hand include hyperextension of the PIP joints with compensatory flexion of the DIPs (i.e., swan-neck deformity); flexion of the DIP joints with extension of the PIPs (i.e., boutonniere deformity); ulnar deviation of the phalanges; and hyperextension of the first interphalangeal joint with flexion of the first MCP. All of these deformities may impair the "pincer" function of the hand, which adversely affects the performance of the activities of daily living.

Wrists

As for MCP and PIP involvement, synovitis of the wrists may be an early marker of disease and is almost uniformly present in established RA. With progressive swelling about the wrist, the median nerve may become entrapped, resulting in the symptoms of carpal tunnel syndrome. Wrist synovitis may cause decreased grip strength, which may serve as a longitudinal measure of disease activity. Active synovitis about the wrist may result in rupture of the extensor tendons, particularly those of the fourth and fifth digits.

Elbows

Involvement of the elbows is most commonly demonstrated clinically by the development of loss of extension and ultimately by flexion contractures. Because the elbow is uncommonly involved in OA, synovitis of this joint helps to differentiate RA from OA. The skin over the olecranon process is a common site for development of rheumatoid nodules.

Shoulders

Complaints generally related to the area of the shoulder are common in RA. Their cause can be discerned by history and physical examination. Shoulder pain can result from several sources, including arthritis of the glenohumeral joint, subacromial bursitis, rotator cuff dysfunction, acromioclavicular joint arthritis, sternoclavicular joint arthritis, and involvement of the cervical spine (83). A common manifestation of these diverse pathologic processes is limited range of motion of the shoulder, particularly abduction. With continued voluntary decrease in the range of motion caused by pain, the condition may become chronic.

Spine

Unlike OA and the seronegative spondyloarthropathies, spinal involvement by RA is usually restricted to the diarthrodial joints of the cervical spine (84). The prevalence of symptoms related to the neck may be greater than can be explained by demonstrable involvement, which is often greatest in the upper vertebrae. The three predominant patterns of significant cervical spine involvement are atlantoaxial subluxation, wherein involvement at the C2 level allows exaggerated motion of the odontoid process and potentially spinal cord compression; basilar invagination, with vertical subluxation of the spinal column through the foramen magnum; and subaxial subluxation, or spondylolisthesis, of vertebrae distal to C2. Complaints consistent with significant cervical spine involvement often begin insidiously and are commonly aggravated by positional change. Surgical intervention is indicated for significant neurologic deficit. Cervical spine involvement is an important prognostic factor, because severely affected patients have significantly reduced life expectancies.

Hips

The hips are involved less frequently than the small joints of the upper or lower extremities, although asymptomatic roentgenographic abnormalities are routine (85). Symptoms related to involvement of the hip become more frequent with longer duration of disease. As is true for the shoulder, complaints by the patient about the general area of the hip may be related to causes other than hip synovitis, including bursitis (e.g., trochanteric or ischial bursitis), lumbar spine pathology, neurologic dysfunction, and pelvic insufficiency fractures. True arthritis of the hip joint, unlike pain related to various periarticular structures, is classically referred to the groin area. The pain may radiate, especially to the thigh, and may also be referred to the knee. Hip arthritis may manifest with gait abnormalities and restricted range of motion on physical examination. For advanced degenerative changes of the hip, surgical replacement may provide excellent long-term results.

Knees

The knee joint commonly has synovitis and chronic effusions. Atrophy of the quadriceps muscle and periarticular ligamentous laxity related to the chronic arthritis may result in significant morbidity. The presence of hypertrophied synovium may establish a ball-valve type mechanism, such that synovial fluid is trapped in the posterior compartment of the knee. This accumulation of fluid in the popliteal space, the so-called Baker's cyst, may dissect or rupture into the calf and mimic deep vein thrombosis.

Feet and Ankles

Arthritis of the tibiotalar and subtalar ankle joints may be associated with ligamentous laxity. Chronic instability of the ankle and its resultant deformity, usually a valgus deformity, have a significant impact on patient mobility. They are often a source of substantial pain. Significant deformity of the ankle may also be associated with entrapment of the posterior tibial nerve, resulting in tarsal tunnel syndrome with dysesthesia in the foot. Arthritis of the joints of the feet is relatively common and in many ways mirrors involvement of the hands (86). Subluxation of the MTP joints results in upward movement of the phalanges, producing the "cock-up toe." Downward displacement of the metatarsal heads may cause profound pain and restricted mobility. Callous formation over the metatarsal heads should alert the clinician to these changes, which may be amenable to orthotic devices. Erosive changes of RA may be seen initially about the MTP joints (87).

Other Joints

Additional diarthrodial joints may be involved with RA. Arthritis of the temporomandibular joints (TMJ) may cause symptoms in more than half of the patients with RA. Because TMJ involvement is rare with other arthritides, TMJ arthritis may support the diagnosis of RA in difficult or unusual cases. Arthritis of the cricoarytenoid joints is not clinically apparent in most patients with RA. However, because synovitis of these joints may lead to swelling in the larynx and symptoms such as hoarseness or dyspnea, the potential for their involvement should be kept in mind for RA patients who have symptoms referable to the upper airway.

Extraarticular Manifestations

Although inflammation of the joints is the most prominent feature, RA is most properly considered a systemic inflammatory disease. RA patients experiencing flares of activity may present with symptoms such as fever, sweats, anorexia, weight loss, lymphadenopathy, weakness, and fatigue in addition to articular difficulties. Aside from these constitutional symptoms, the systemic inflammation of RA commonly causes diverse extraarticular manifestations that may be relevant to establishing the diagnosis of RA (88,89) (Table 64-4). Certain extraarticular manifestations, such as rheumatoid nodules, usu-

ally have minimal clinical significance. Others, such as rheumatoid vasculitis, may be important causes of morbidity and may require specific therapeutic intervention. In general, extraarticular manifestations occur in patients with high titers of RF.

Cutaneous Manifestations

Subcutaneous nodules develop in approximately 20% to 30% of persons with RA. Rheumatoid nodules are usually found in periarticular locations that are subject to mechanical pressure, such as the olecranon bursa. Other common locations include the Achilles tendon, the occiput, and the dorsum of the hands. Nodules may also

TABLE 64-4. *Extraarticular manifestations of rheumatoid arthritis*

Constitutional
  Fever, sweats
  Weight loss, anorexia
  Weakness, fatigue
  Lymphadenopathy
Cutaneous
  Subcutaneous nodules (i.e., rheumatoid nodules)
  Vasculitis (e.g., infarcts, ulceration)
Ocular
  Episcleritis
  Scleritis
  Scleromalacia perforans
  Keratoconjunctivitis sicca (i.e., Sjögren's syndrome)
Cardiovascular
  Pericarditis
  Myocarditis
  Vasculitis
Pulmonary
  Pleuritis
  Interstitial fibrosis
  Rheumatoid nodules
  Pulmonary arteritis and hypertension
  Caplan's syndrome (i.e., nodular pulmonary infiltrates in arthritic patients with pneumoconiosis)
Neurologic
  Myelopathy
  Entrapment neuropathy
  Neuropathy related to vasculitis
Hematologic
  Anemia (i.e., iron disuse as in anemia of chronic disease)
  Eosinophilia
  Thrombocytosis
  Felty's syndrome (e.g., neutropenia, splenomegaly)
Renal
  Interstitial nephritis
  Renal tubular acidosis (with Sjögren's syndrome)
  Membranous nephropathy
  Amyloidosis
Gastrointestinal
  Xerostomia
  Amyloidosis
  Elevated liver function test results
Miscellaneous
  Osteoporosis
  Myositis

develop in extracutaneous locations, such as the pleura, pericardium, and meninges. The presence of rheumatoid nodules is almost uniformly associated with high titers of RF, and they tend to occur more commonly in patients with erosive, deforming disease. Because they develop insidiously, they may be confused initially with other subcutaneous lesions, including gouty tophi, epidermal cysts, and xanthomas.

Biopsy of rheumatoid nodules reveals a central zone of necrotic material, including collagen fibrils, noncollagenous filaments, and cellular debris; a midzone of palisading macrophages that express HLA-DR antigens; and an outer zone of granulation tissue. Examination of early nodules suggested that the initial event may be a focal vasculitis. Unless the skin overlying the nodule breaks down, resulting in infection, rheumatoid nodules are usually asymptomatic and require no treatment. They may regress, sometimes with diminished disease activity, although in many cases, they persist. In some patients, the use of methotrexate has been associated with development or worsening of rheumatoid nodules and cutaneous vasculitis (90). The mechanisms underlying this association are unclear.

Rheumatoid vasculitis may involve vessels of various sizes, from postcapillary venules through medium-sized arteries. Almost every organ system can be affected. Case reports have described rheumatoid vasculitis affecting the heart, lungs, gastrointestinal tract, spleen, liver, lymph nodes, testes, and kidneys. However, most patients with rheumatoid vasculitis suffer predominantly cutaneous manifestations. Splinter hemorrhages, most frequently in the digital pulp or paronychial area, and palpable purpura are most common. As larger vessels are involved and the vasculitic process becomes more diffuse, ulcerations and even gangrene may occur. In addition to cutaneous involvement, rheumatoid vasculitis may affect the vasa nervosum, resulting in neuropathy. Polyneuropathy, predominantly sensory, and mononeuritis multiplex may be the sole manifestation of vasculitis. Frequently, rheumatoid vasculitis is associated with conspicuous constitutional symptoms. It has rarely been described in blacks and tends to occur in patients with high titers of RF. Rheumatoid vasculitis may require aggressive immunomodulatory therapeutic intervention and close monitoring for signs of internal organ involvement (91).

Pulmonary Manifestations

Several distinct patterns of pulmonary involvement occur in patients with RA (92) (see Table 64-4). Pleural disease may be detected in almost one half of RA patients at necropsy, but it infrequently causes significant clinical disease. Pleural effusions may be observed in as many as 5% of patients, but they rarely compromise pulmonary function. Typically, the pleural fluid is exudative, with low glucose and low complement levels.

Leukocyte counts tend to be lower than would be expected for bacterial effusions, and the percentage of lymphocytes may be somewhat higher. Although very low concentrations of glucose are suggestive, none of the results from analysis of the pleural fluid are diagnostic of rheumatoid effusions. The differential diagnosis should include neoplasm and infection causes, particularly tuberculosis. Histologic examination of pleural biopsy specimens may reveal rheumatoid nodules, but often a nonspecific inflammatory process is observed. Although usually asymptomatic, pleural nodules may rarely cavitate, resulting in pneumothorax or bronchopleural fistula.

Rheumatoid nodules may occur singly or in clusters in the pulmonary parenchyma. They often are an incidental finding on the chest roentgenogram and are not associated with specific symptoms. Although such lesions may be suspected to be rheumatoid nodules in the appropriate clinical setting, they can be differentiated form neoplastic lesions only by histologic analysis. Diffuse nodular infiltrates may also occur in RA patients in association with pneumoconiosis. Known as Caplan's syndrome, it has been described in RA patients who have been exposed to coal dust, asbestos, silica, and other pulmonary toxins. The nodules are differentiated from typical rheumatoid nodules only by the presence of the offending dust particle in the central zone.

Pulmonary manifestations of RA that are more likely to become symptomatic include interstitial disease and pulmonary arteritis (92). Evidence of interstitial disease, such as a restrictive pattern detected on pulmonary function testing, may be found in more than a third of RA patients. In some cases, this is associated with a reticular nodular pattern on chest radiographs. Patients may remain asymptomatic, but interstitial involvement of RA may become apparent when patients are subjected to additional pulmonary insults. Pulmonary arteritis, which is rare, may cause pulmonary hypertension and cor pulmonale. Chest radiographs in patients with pulmonary arteritis may be normal.

Pulmonary involvement in patients with RA may also result from the drugs used in therapy. Methotrexate can cause an acute pulmonary toxic reaction that most closely resembles hypersensitivity pneumonitis (93). After intercurrent infections have been excluded, patients are treated with high-dose corticosteroids and supplemental measures such as the administration of oxygen. Treatment with penicillamine rarely results in the development of syndromes resembling other autoimmune diseases, such as Goodpasture's disease.

Cardiac Manifestations

The most common cardiac manifestation of RA is pericarditis (94). Pericarditis may be demonstrated in approximately one half of RA patients at autopsy. It is often observed in conjunction with pleuritis, and pericardial fluid usually has low glucose concentrations and complement levels. Most patients are asymptomatic, but some present with acute pericarditis that requires specific intervention. Although pericardial tamponade is rarely seen in rheumatoid pericarditis, it may portend shortened patient survival. Less common cardiac manifestations of RA include myocarditis, coronary vasculitis, and nodular lesions of the endocardium or heart valves.

Ocular and Oral Manifestations

Ocular involvement is a frequent complaint of patients with RA (95). The most common symptom is that of a dry or gritty sensation of the eyes. Although this may result from diverse causes, such as allergies, the most common cause of these symptoms in RA is Sjögren's syndrome, which may affect 10% to 20% of patients. In this condition, lymphocytic infiltration of the lacrimal glands leads to decreased tear production. The inability to produce tears results in a loss of the protective coating of the superficial parts of the globe. When this occurs in conjunction with irritative changes in the conjunctiva, it is known as keratoconjunctivitis sicca. The diagnosis, which is usually suspected on clinical grounds, is typically made in one of two ways: the Schirmer's test, which documents decreased tear production using filter paper placed under the lower eyelid, and rose Bengal staining, which highlights desiccated corneal epithelium. Treatment is mostly supportive, with replacement of tears at regular intervals and appropriate therapy of complications, such as corneal abrasions.

The most superficial layer of the sclera, the episclera, may be involved by RA. Patients complain of discomfort, and physical examination reveals inflammatory changes of the episcleral vessels that cause a salmon pink discoloration of the globe. Episcleritis is usually self-limited, and complications are rare. In contrast, inflammation of the sclera can cause severe destruction and subsequent problems such as loss of visual acuity, cataract formation, uveitis, and glaucoma. Scleritis occurs most commonly in patients with severe systemic disease and is therefore associated with decreased survival. With repeated episodes of scleritis, thinning of the sclera reveals a bluish tint of the underlying pigmented choroid. In scleromalacia perforans, extreme destruction of the sclera allows peroration of the globe and herniation of the uveal tract.

Lymphocytic infiltration of the salivary glands is seen in Sjögren's syndrome and leads to xerostomia, or dryness of the mouth (95). In addition to causing discomfort, patients with oral dryness are also at increased risk for dental caries and periodontal disease. Management is supportive, with heightened attention to dental hygiene and the use of saliva substitutes. Oral problems in RA patients also are caused by medications. Gold compounds, penicillamine, and methotrexate have been associated with the development of stomatitis, often necessitating discontinuation of treatment.

Felty's Syndrome

Patients with long-standing, severe RA may develop splenomegaly, lymphadenopathy, and neutropenia, a constellation known as Felty's syndrome (96). This syndrome is rare in blacks with RA. Additional common findings may include anemia, thrombocytopenia, and severe constitutional symptoms. Although the hypersplenism may contribute to the neutropenia, splenectomy does not correct the abnormality in about one third of affected patients. Patients with Felty's syndrome have an increased susceptibility to infections associated with neutropenia or neutrophil dysfunction. RA patients may also have neutropenia, with or without splenomegaly, in association with the expansion of large granular lymphocytes in the peripheral blood.

Other Manifestations

Clinical weakness and atrophy of skeletal muscle are common among RA patients (88). Muscle atrophy may become evident within weeks of the onset of a flare of RA. It is most apparent in the musculature approximating affected joints. Although myositis occasionally is demonstrated on muscle biopsy, the most common histologic finding is atrophy of type II muscle fibers. This finding and the clinical weakness may be exacerbated by the chronic use of corticosteroids.

Like pulmonary and pericardial involvement, histologic examination of the kidneys from RA patients frequently demonstrates abnormalities (97). The most common findings are amyloid deposits and membranous glomerular changes. Although proteinuria can be demonstrated in many patients using sensitive detection methods, renal disease of a magnitude to be clinically significant is uncommon. More commonly, abnormalities of renal function may be ascribed to the effects of various medications used for the treatment of RA. For example, injectable gold salts and penicillamine cause reversible proteinuria in a subset of treated patients. Perhaps the most prominent cause of renal dysfunction in RA patients is the use of nonsteroidal antiinflammatory drugs (NSAIDs), which can depress the glomerular filtration rate. Patients with underlying renal disease, such as hypertensive or diabetic nephropathy, are at greatest risk. The elderly tend to be quite susceptible to such deleterious effects of the NSAIDs.

CLINICAL COURSE AND PROGNOSIS

Appreciation of the severity of RA has increased (98). Once considered largely a benign, self-limited condition, it has become clear that RA is associated with substantial morbidity and accelerated mortality. The evolution in our perception of disease severity is related to several factors.

About 25 years ago, two longitudinal, community-based surveys of the prevalence and course of RA were conducted (99,100). Both studies found that, after 3 to 5 years, most patients who were originally diagnosed with RA no longer met the diagnostic criteria. These results helped affirm the prevailing concept that spontaneous remission could be expected for most RA patients. Later clinic-based studies, in contrast, painted a different picture. In these studies, the cohort evaluated is derived from patients presenting to physicians because of articular complaints rather than from the general population. Analysis of the clinic patients showed that more than 90% of patients had disease after 3 to 5 years of follow-up (98,101,102). Spontaneous remissions are uncommon, with only approximately 10% to 15% of patients with RA having a short-lived inflammatory process that remits without sequelae.

Another factor influencing the perception of RA severity is a more sharply focused definition of the disease. Compared with previous diagnostic criteria for RA (103), the latest classification criteria (104) are more stringent. Some of the patients diagnosed with RA in earlier studies would no longer be classified as having RA using the current criteria.

Nevertheless, the course of RA can be quite variable and, for an individual patient, difficult to predict. Most patients experience persistent but fluctuating disease activity. For most affected patients, the disease is also progressive, with some degree of joint deformities developing in many patients (101). After 10 or 12 years, fewer than 20% of RA patients have no evidence of disability or deformity. Damage and disability begin early in the course of the disease. The rate of progression of joint damage is greater during the first year of observation than in the second and third years. Within 2 years of disease, approximately one half of patients have some radiographic evidence of damage to joints (105). The rate of joint destruction decreases over time. However, functional disability, which also begins early in the course of disease, continues to progress at a significant rate over time.

Disability is manifested in several ways for patients with RA. Inability to sustain employment is common. Because disease is progressive, 40% of patients are unable to work after 5 years of disease, one half at 10 years, and more than two thirds at 15 years (101,106). Employed patients have more sick days and lower income than age-matched controls. The divorce rate for patients with RA is 70% higher than that for the general population. In addition to the personal and family costs, the damage and disability of RA are associated with higher costs to society. RA patients accrue medical expenses at a rate far in excess of the general population (106). These costs come in various forms, including hospitalization,

TABLE 64-5. *Factors associated with a poor prognosis in rheumatoid arthritis*

Extraarticular manifestations
  Rheumatoid nodules
Early evidence of joint damage
  Radiologic evidence of erosions
  Development of functional disability
High titers of rheumatoid factor
Persistent evidence of active inflammation
  Elevated erythrocyte sedimentation rate
  Elevated C-reactive protein levels
  Anemia
Active disease
  More then 20 joints involved
Advanced age at onset
Comorbid conditions
Socioeconomic factors
  Lower socioeconomic status
  Lower level of formal education
Female gender

outpatient care, medication costs, surgical procedures, long-term care, and transportation.

In addition to increased disability, it has been demonstrated that mortality is accelerated for patients with RA (98). The excess mortality is more than twofold that of matched controls. The survival for patients with very severe RA has been estimated at approximately 40% to 50% at 5 years, which can be likened to the survival of patients with three-vessel coronary artery disease. In many cases, the excess mortality is related to the disease itself or to complications from therapy. Infections and gastrointestinal hemorrhage are important contributory factors.

Several features of patients with RA appear to carry prognostic significance (3,98,107) (Table 64-5). Many of these factors signify patients whose disease is active, aggressive early in its course, and persistent. Prognostic factors associated with decreased survival in other nonrheumatologic conditions, such as advanced age, are also important for RA patients.

DIAGNOSIS

Laboratory Findings

No laboratory tests can be used alone to diagnose RA. The various findings on laboratory examination can provide support for the diagnosis that is suspected on clinical grounds.

The laboratory test most closely associated with the diagnosis of RA is detection of RFs (108). These autoantibodies, which are reactive with the Fc portion of IgG, are present in 75% to 90% of RA patients. The most widely used tests largely detect IgM RF, which is the most common isotype. Approximately 5% of persons in the general population test positive for RF. The presence of RF may vary with certain factors, most importantly advancing age. As many as 10% to 20% of healthy persons older than 65 have RF. The increased prevalence of RFs with age therefore reduces its specificity in such populations. Several conditions other than RA can be associated with the presence of RF, including other systemic inflammatory diseases, infections, and neoplastic diseases (Table 64-6). Determination of RF is therefore a poor screening test for RA among unselected populations (109).

Just as the presence of RF does not establish the diagnosis of RA, its absence does not exclude it. This is especially true early in the course of disease, when clinical findings may antedate the development of RF by several months. Approximately 10% or more of patients with RA may never have detectable RF in their sera. Nevertheless, RF is a useful adjunct in the diagnosis of RA. It is also useful as a prognostic factor for patients with established disease. RA patients with high serum concentrations of RF tend to develop more severe and progressive articular disease than other patients (107,108,110). There is a correlation between RF concentration and the development of extraarticular manifestations such as rheumatoid nodules and vasculitis.

Examination of synovial fluid aspirated from affected joints is a frequently performed laboratory test in RA (111). Early in the course of RA, it can be useful in supporting the diagnosis, largely by excluding other causes. For example, a noninflammatory fluid with fewer than 2,000 leukocytes/mm^3 with normal viscosity would be unexpected in synovial effusions of RA and would rather support the diagnosis of OA. A synovial fluid leukocyte count greater than 50,000/mm^3 would be more consistent with arthritis related to infection or crystal deposition than RA. In RA, the leukocyte count usually ranges between these values. As with many inflammatory arthritides, there is usually a preponderance of neutrophilic leukocytes. The synovial fluid is usually turbid, has

TABLE 64-6. *Conditions in which rheumatoid factor may be detected*

Inflammatory diseases
   Rheumatoid arthritis
   Sjögren's syndrome
   Cryoglobulinemia
   Systemic lupus erythematosus
   Progressive systemic sclerosis (i.e., scleroderma)
   Idiopathic inflammatory myositis
Infectious diseases
   Bacterial endocarditis
   Mycobacterial infection (e.g., tuberculosis, leprosy)
   Syphilis
   Hepatitis
   Epstein-Barr virus infection
   Many other viral and parasitic infections
Neoplastic diseases
   Lymphoproliferative diseases

reduced viscosity, and has an increased protein content. In patients with established RA, analysis of synovial fluid is of greatest utility in excluding the presence of superimposed infection in a joint severely affected by RA.

Several changes in hematologic parameters are common in RA patients. A normocytic, normochromic anemia, frequently in conjunction with thrombocytosis, often accompanies active disease (111). The anemia most probably reflects ineffective erythropoiesis, which is related to the chronic systemic inflammation and cytokine generation. Bone marrow iron stores and serum ferritin concentrations are normal or increased in the absence of comorbid conditions. The peripheral white blood cell count may be normal or mildly increased. Alternatively, leukopenia may be observed in the absence of other signs of Felty's syndrome. Eosinophilia, apart from that related to medications, has been observed, most commonly in patients with severe systemic disease.

Measures of the acute phase response are often elevated in patients with RA and serve as indirect estimates of systemic inflammation (112). The erythrocyte sedimentation rate, which largely reflects serum fibrinogen concentrations, is nearly uniformly increased in affected patients. Levels of other acute phase proteins, such as C-reactive protein, are also elevated, and such elevations tend to correlate with disease activity. In conjunction with clinical assessment, these laboratory measures of the acute phase response may be useful in the longitudinal evaluation of disease activity in RA patients.

Imaging Studies

Very early in the course of the disease, plain roentgenograms of the affected joints are usually not helpful in establishing a diagnosis. They reveal only what is apparent from physical examination—evidence of joint effusion and periarticular soft tissue swelling. As the disease progresses, abnormalities become more pronounced. However, none of the radiographic findings is diagnostic of RA. The diagnosis may be supported by a characteristic pattern of abnormalities, including the tendency toward symmetric involvement (113). Juxtaarticular osteopenia may become apparent within weeks of onset. Loss of articular cartilage and bone erosions may develop after several months of sustained disease activity (see Fig. 64-2). The utility of radiography lies in the ability to assess the extent of joint damage longitudinally and the capacity to assess joint anatomy before consideration of surgical intervention.

Other commonly employed modalities of evaluating bones and joints include ^{99m}Tc-bisphosphonate bone scanning and MRI. MRI evaluation of affected joints in RA patients has demonstrated erosions at much earlier times than conventional roentgenography (114). MRI allows detailed depiction of the periarticular structures, which may be of value in planning surgical intervention,

TABLE 64-7. *1987 revised criteria for the classification of rheumatoid arthritis*

1. Stiffness in and around the joints lasting one hour before maximal improvement
2. Soft tissue swelling (arthritis) of three or more joint areas, simultaneously, observed by a physician
3. Swelling (arthritis) of the proximal interphalangeal, metacarpophalangeal, or wrist joints
4. Symmetric swelling (arthritis)
5. Rheumatoid nodules
6. Presence of rheumatoid factor
7. Radiographic erosions and/or periarticular osteopenia in hand and/or wrist joints

• Four of seven criteria are required to classify a patient as having rheumatoid arthritis.
• Criteria 1 through 4 must exist for at least 6 weeks.
• Criteria 2 through 5 must be observed by a physician.

but the expense associated with this technique is substantial. Although the images obtained are quite striking, information gleaned from them may not alter medical management of an individual patient. These considerations may preclude the widespread use of MRI in the routine assessment of joints in RA patients.

Classification Criteria

In persons with established, typical disease, the diagnosis of RA can be readily made, most often within the first year of disease onset. In other patients, the progression of symptoms may be atypical, and a more prolonged period of evaluation may be necessary before the diagnosis is confirmed. The American College of Rheumatology has developed revised criteria for the classification of RA (104) (Table 64-7). The newer criteria are simpler to apply than the previous criteria (103). For example, the results of invasive procedures such as synovial biopsy are no longer used. The previous classifications of probable, definite, and classic RA have been eliminated, and patients with more than a single diagnosis are not excluded. The new criteria demonstrate a sensitivity of 91% to 94% with a specificity of 89% when used to classify patients with RA compared with patients with rheumatic diseases other than RA. Although these criteria were developed as a means to classify patients for epidemiologic purposes, they serve as useful guidelines for the establishment of the diagnosis of RA for patients seen in the clinic. However, failure to meet these criteria, particularly during the early stages of the disease, does not exclude the diagnosis.

TREATMENT

The goals of therapy in RA are relief of pain, reduction of inflammation, preservation of functional status, prevention of complications of the disease, resolution of the etiopathogenic process, facilitation of healing, and avoidance of complications related to therapy.

Pharmacologic Therapy

Appreciation of the substantial morbidity and mortality associated with RA has spawned a reappraisal of the traditional approach to therapy. Historically, patients were treated according to the "therapeutic pyramid" (115). According to this strategy, the treating physician responded to the manifestations of the disease. Therapy was initiated with salubrious nonpharmacologic measures, such as joint rest, complemented by medications thought to have the smallest potential for injury. Historically, this meant aspirin or other NSAIDs. More "aggressive" therapies—those requiring greater care of administration and with potentially more deleterious adverse reactions—were withheld until patients clearly demonstrated significant disease related morbidity. If these treatments proved insufficient, yet more aggressive or experimental therapies were instituted. It is now understood that RA has a substantial adverse impact on the quality of life of most affected patients and that such effects begin early in the disease course. The approach to treating RA patients has changed. Although the general tenets of the pyramid are considered, treatment has become more aggressive in the hope of preventing joint damage (116). Therapies once reserved for those suffering years of destructive disease may be used for newly diagnosed patients.

Although much has been learned about the pathophysiology of RA, its cause remains undefined. Therapy of RA is aimed largely at suppressing signs and symptoms of the disease (117,118). Over the years, three categories of therapeutic modalities have emerged for this purpose:

1. Agents such as NSAIDs and low-dose corticosteroids that decrease inflammation and pain but do not appear to affect the outcome of the disease in most patients, although steroids may exert a beneficial effect on bone loss
2. Drugs that appear to be able to abate progression of disease transiently in certain patients but possess neither nonspecific antiinflammatory nor systemic immunosuppressive properties
3. Systemic immunosuppressive drugs

Nonpharmacologic Therapy

In addition to the various types of pharmacologic interventions, care of the patient with RA relies on a variety of nonpharmacologic measures. These activities may be grouped into categories such as joint protection, range of motion maintenance, and muscle strengthening. The ultimate goals are avoidance of damage to articular and periarticular structures, preservation of function, and alleviation of pain. In many cases, programs of these activities may be carried out initially with the assistance of allied health personnel. Occupational, physical, and rehabilitation therapists can be important members of the team in the care of patients with RA. Patients with RA may have psychosocial problems to an extent that specific intervention may be required.

One of the most significant developments in the care of arthritis patients over the past 3 decades has been the refinement of joint replacement surgery (119). Technical advances have resulted in substantial improvements in long-term results, and joint replacement is a reasonable option for a number of RA patients. The primary indications for surgical intervention include irreversible joint damage with functional limitation and intractable pain. Other useful surgical interventions include synovectomy (open or arthroscopic), arthrodesis, and correction of soft tissue abnormalities (120).

REFERENCES

1. Harris ED. Rheumatoid arthritis: pathophysiology and implications for therapy. *N Engl J Med* 1990;322:1277–1289.
2. Sewell KL, Trentham DE. Pathogenesis of rheumatoid arthritis. *Lancet* 1993;341:283–286.
3. Wolfe F. 50 Years of antirheumatic therapy: the prognosis of rheumatoid arthritis. *J Rheumatol Suppl* 1990;17:24–32.
4. Short CL. The antiquity of rheumatoid arthritis. *Arthritis Rheum* 1974;17:193–205.
5. Benedek TG. A century of American rheumatology. *Ann Intern Med* 1987;106:304–309.
6. Rose HM, Ragan C, Pearce E, Lipman MO. Differential agglutination of normal and sensitized sheep erythrocytes by sera of patients with rheumatoid arthritis. *Proc Soc Exp Biol Med* 1948;68:1–12.
7. Cush JJ, Lipsky PE. Cellular basis for rheumatoid inflammation. *Clin Orthop Rel Res* 1991;265:9–22.
8. Jacobsson LH, Hanson RL, Knowler WC, et al. Decreasing incidence and prevalence of rheumatoid arthritis in Pima Indians over a twenty-five-year period. *Arthritis Rheum* 1994;37:1158–1165.
9. Silman A, MacGregor A, Thomson W, et al. Twin concordance rates for rheumatoid arthritis: results of a nationwide study. *Br J Rheumatol* 1993;32:903–907.
10. Brennan P, Ollier B, Worthington J, Hajeer A, Silman A. Are both genetic and reproductive associations with rheumatoid arthritis linked to prolactin? *Lancet* 1996;348:106–109.
11. Sternberg EM, Chrousos GP, Wilder RL, Gold PW. The stress response and the regulation of inflammatory disease. *Ann Intern Med* 1992;117:854–859.
12. Stastny P. Mixed lymphocyte culture typing cells from patients with rheumatoid arthritis. *Tissue Antigens* 1974;4:572–579.
13. Wordsworth BP, Lanchbury JSS, Sakkas LI, Welsh KI, Panayi GS, Bell JI. HLA-DR4 subtype frequencies in rheumatoid arthritis indicate that DRB1 is the major susceptibility locus within the HLA class II region. *Proc Natl Acad Sci USA* 1989;86:10049–10060.
14. Weyand CM, Hicok KC, Conn DL, Goronzy JJ. The influence of HLA-DRB1 genes on disease severity in rheumatoid arthritis. Ann Intern Med 1992;117:801–809.
15. McDaniel DO, Alarcon G, Pratt P, Reveille J. Most African-American patients with rheumatoid arthritis do not have the rheumatoid antigenic determinant (epitope). *Ann Intern Med* 1995;123:181–187.
16. Weyand C, Goronzy J. Inherited and noninherited risk factors in rheumatoid arthritis. *Curr Opin Rheumatol* 1995;7:206–213.
17. Weyand CM, McCarthy TG, Goronzy JJ. Correlation between disease phenotype and genetic heterogeneity in rheumatoid arthritis. *J Clin Invest* 1995;95:2120–2126.
18. Hammer J, Gallazzi F, Bono E, et al. Peptide binding specificity of HLA-DR4 molecules: correlation with rheumatoid arthritis association. *J Exp Med* 1995;181:1847–1855.
19. Moxley G. Immunoglobulin kappa genotype confers risk of rheumatoid arthritis among HLA-DR4 negative individuals. *Arthritis Rheum* 1989;32:1365–1373.
20. Panayi GS, Wooley P, Batchelor JR. Genetic basis of rheumatoid disease: HLA antigens, disease manifestations and toxic reactions to drugs. *Br Med J* 1978;2:1326–1329.
21. Venables PJ. Infection and rheumatoid arthritis. *Curr Opin Rheumatol* 1989;1:15–30.
22. Kaufman SH. Heat shock proteins and the immune response. *Immunol Today* 1990;11:129–131.
23. Tarkowski A, Klareskog L, Carlsten H, Heberts P, Koopman W. Secretion of antibodies to type I and type II collagen by synovial tissue in patients with rheumatoid arthritis. *Arthritis Rheum* 1989;32:1087–1096.
24. Winchester RJ, Gregersen PK. The molecular basis of susceptibility to rheumatoid arthritis: the conformational equivalence hypothesis. *Springer Semin Immunopathol* 1988;10:119–127.
25. Roudier J, Petersen J, Rhodes GH, et al. Susceptibility to rheumatoid arthritis maps to a T-cell epitope shared by the HLA-Dw4 DR beta-1 chain and the Epstein-Barr virus glycoprotein gp110. *Proc Natl Acad Sci USA* 1989;86:5104–5109.
26. Paliard X, West SG, Lafferty JA, et al. Evidence for the effects of a superantigen in rheumatoid arthritis. *Science* 1991;253:325–329.
27. Struyk L, Hawes G, Chatila T, Breedveld F, Kurnick J, van den Elsen P. T cell receptors in rheumatoid arthritis. *Arthritis Rheum* 1995;38:577–589.
28. Alam A, Lambert N, Lule J, et al. Persistence of dominant T cell clones in synovial tissues during rheumatoid arthritis. *J Immunol* 1996;156:3480–3485.
29. Kavanaugh AF, Lipsky PE. The application of biotechnological advances to the treatment of rheumatoid arthritis. In: Pincus T, Wolfe F, eds. *Rheumatoid arthritis: assessment, prognosis, and therapy.* New York: Marcel Dekker, 1994:373–401.
30. Fischer D, Opalka B, Hoffman A, Mayr W, Haubeck H. Limited heterogeneity of rearranged T cell receptor Vα and Vβ transcripts in synovial fluid T cells in early stages of rheumatoid arthritis. *Arthritis Rheum* 1996;39:454–462.
31. Mima T, Sakei Y, Oshima S, et al. Transfer of rheumatoid arthritis into severe combined immunodeficient mice: the pathogenetic implications of T cell populations oligoclonally expanding in the rheumatoid joints. *J Clin Invest* 1995;96:1746–1758.
32. Celis L, Vandevyer C, Geusens P, Dequeker J, Raus J, Zhang J. Clonal expansion of mycobacterial heat-shock protein-reactive T lymphocytes in the synovial fluid and blood of rheumatoid arthritis patients. *Arthritis Rheum* 1997;40:510–519.
33. Hoffman W, Jump A, Smiley JD. Synthesis of specific IgG idiotypes by rheumatoid synovium. *Arthritis Rheum* 1990;33:1196–1204.
34. Bridges S, Lee S, Johnson M, et al. Somatic mutation and CDR3 lengths of immunoglobulin κlight chains expressed in patients with rheumatoid arthritis and normal controls. *J Clin Invest* 1995;96:831–841.
35. Yanni G, Whelan A, Feighery C, Fitzgerald O, Bresnihan B. Morphometric analysis of synovial membrane blood vessels in rheumatoid arthritis: associations with the immunohistochemical features, synovial fluid cytokine levels and the clinical course. *J Rheumatol* 1993;20:634–639.
36. Goldenberg DL, Cohen SA. Synovial membrane histopathology in the differential diagnosis of rheumatoid arthritis, gout, pseudogout, systemic lupus erythematosus, infectious arthritis, and degenerative joint disease. *Medicine (Baltimore)* 1978;57:239–248.
37. Colville-Nash PR, Scott DL. Angiogenesis and rheumatoid arthritis: pathogenic and therapeutic implications. *Ann Rheum Dis* 1992;51:919–923.
38. Kurosaka M, Ziff M. Immunoelectron microscopic study of the distribution of T cell subsets in rheumatoid synovium. *J Exp Med* 1983;158:1191–1199.
39. Cush JJ, Lipsky PE. Phenotypic analysis of synovial tissue and peripheral blood lymphocytes isolated from patients with rheumatoid arthritis. *Arthritis Rheum* 1988;31:1230–1238.
40. Kohem CL, Brezinschek RI, Wisbey H, Tortorella C, Lipsky PE, Oppenheimer-Marks N. Enrichment of differentiated CD45RBdim, CD27- memory T cells in the peripheral blood, synovial fluid, and

synovial tissue of patients with rheumatoid arthritis. *Arthritis Rheum* 1996;39:844–854.

41. Pitzalis C, Kingsley G, Murphy J, Panayi G. Abnormal distribution of the helper-inducer and suppressor-inducer T-lymphocyte subsets in the rheumatoid joint. *Clin Immunol Immunopathol* 1987;45:252–265.

42. Lunardi C, Marguerie C, Walport MJ, So AK. T γδ cells and their subsets in blood and synovial fluid from patients with rheumatoid arthritis. *Br J Rheumatol* 1992;31:527–530.

43. Sliwinski AJ, Zvaifler NJ. *In vivo* synthesis of IgG by the rheumatoid synovium. *J Lab Clin Med* 1970;76:304–309.

44. Cecere F. Evidence for the local production and utilization of immunoreactants in rheumatoid arthritis. *Arthritis Rheum* 1982;25:1307–1315.

45. Winchester RJ. Characterization of IgG complexes in patients with rheumatoid arthritis. *Ann N Y Acad Sci* 1975;256:73–90.

46. Remmers EF, Sano H, Wilder RL. Platelet-derived growth factors and heparin-binding (fibroblast) growth factors in the synovial tissue pathology of rheumatoid arthritis. *Semin Arthritis Rheum* 1991;21:191–199.

47. Firestein GS, Zvaifler NJ. How important are T cells in chronic rheumatoid synovitis? *Arthritis Rheum* 1990;33:768–769.

48. Bromley M, Fischer WD, Wooley DE. Mast cells at sites of cartilage erosions in the rheumatoid joint. *Ann Rheum Dis* 1984;43:76–80.

49. Fassbender HG. Histomorphic basis of articular cartilage destruction in rheumatoid arthritis. *Collagen Rel Res* 1983;3:141–149.

50. Fassbender HG. Is pannus a residue of inflammation? *Arthritis Rheum* 1984;27:956–962.

51. Burmester GR, Stuhlmüller B, Keyszer G, Kinne RW. Mononuclear phagocytes and rheumatoid synovitis: mastermind or workhorse in arthritis. *Arthritis Rheum* 1997;40:5–18.

52. O'Sullivan FX, Fassbender HG, Gay S, et al. Etiopathogenesis of the rheumatoid arthritis-like disease in MRL/1 mice. I. The histomorphic basis of joint destruction. *Arthritis Rheum* 1987;28:529–537.

53. Korchak HM, Vienne K, Rutherford LE, Weissman G, Neutrophil stimulation: receptor, membrane, and metabolic events. *Fed Proc* 1984;43:2749–2753.

54. Springer TA. Adhesion receptors of the immune system. *Nature* 1990;346:425–434.

55. Henson PM, Johnston RB. Tissue injury in inflammation: oxidants, proteinases, and cationic proteins. *J Clin Invest* 1987;79:669–687.

56. Firestein GS. Mechanisms of tissue destruction and cellular activation in rheumatoid arthritis. *Curr Opin Rheumatol* 1992;4:348–354.

57. Iwata Y, Mort JS, Tateishi H, Lee ER. Macrophage cathepsin L, a factor in the erosion of subchondral bone in rheumatoid arthritis. *Arthritis Rheum* 1997;40:499–509.

58. Buttner FH, Chubinskaya S, Margerie D, et al. Expression of membrane type I matrix metalloproteinase in human articular cartilage. *Arthritis Rheum* 1997;40:704–709.

59. Lipsky PE, Davis LS, Cush JJ, Oppenheimer-Marks N. The role of cytokines in the pathogenesis of rheumatoid arthritis. *Springer Semin Immunopathol* 1989;11:123–134.

60. Moreland LW, Stewart T, Gay RE, et al. Immunohistologic demonstration of type II collagen in synovial fluid phagocytes of osteoarthritis and rheumatoid arthritis. *Arthritis Rheum* 1989;32:1458–1468.

61. Rothschild BM, Masi AT. Pathogenesis of rheumatoid arthritis: a vascular hypothesis. *Semin Arthritis Rheum* 1982;12:11–22.

62. Kavanaugh A, Oppenheimer-Marks N. The role of the vascular endothelium in the pathogenesis of vasculitis. In: Leroy EC, ed. *Systemic vasculitis: the biologic basis.* New York: Marcel Dekker, 1992:27–48.

63. Pitzalis C, Kingsley G, Lanchbury JS, Murphy J, Panayi GS. Expression of HLA-DR, DQ, and DP antigens and interleukin-2 receptor on synovial fluid T lymphocyte subsets in rheumatoid arthritis: evidence for "frustrated" activation. *J Rheumatol* 1987;14:662–667.

64. Holoshitz J, Matitiau A, Cohen IR. Arthritis induced in rats by cloned T lymphocytes responsive to mycobacteria but not to collagen type II. *J Clin Invest* 1984;73:211–219.

65. Mima T, Saeki Y, Ohshima S, et al. Transfer of rheumatoid arthritis into severe combined immunodeficient mice. *J Clin Invest* 1995;96:1746–1758.

66. Ueo T, Tanaka S, Tominaga Y, Ogawa H, Sakurami T. The effect of thoracic duct drainage on lymphocyte dynamics and clinical symptoms in patients with rheumatoid arthritis. *Arthritis Rheum* 1979;22:1405–1414.

67. Karsh J, Klippel JH, Plotz PH, Decker JL, Wright DG, Flye MW. Lymphapheresis in rheumatoid arthritis. *Arthritis Rheum* 1981;24:867–871.

68. Gaston JSH, Strober S, Solvera JJ, et al. Dissection of the mechanisms of immune injury in rheumatoid arthritis using total lymphoid irradiation. *Arthritis Rheum* 1988;31:21–29.

69. Dougadas M, Awada H, Amor B. Cyclosporin in rheumatoid arthritis: a double-blind placebo controlled study in 52 patients. *Ann Rheum Dis* 1988;47:127–133.

70. Salmon M, Scheel-Toeliner D, Huisson A, et al. Inhibition of T cell apoptosis in the rheumatoid synovium. *J Clin Invest* 1997;99:439–446.

71. Dolhain R, van der Heiden A, ter Haar NT, Breedveld F, Miltenburg AMM. Shift toward T lymphocytes with a T helper 1 cytokine-secretion profile in the joints of patients with rheumatoid arthritis. *Arthritis Rheum* 1996;39:1961–1969.

72. Maurice MM, Nakamura H, van der Voort, et al. Evidence for the role of an altered redox state in hyporesponsiveness of synovial T cells in rheumatoid arthritis. *J Immunol* 1997;158:1458–1465.

73. Koopman WJ, Gay S. Do nonimmunologically mediated pathways play a role in the pathogenesis of rheumatoid arthritis? *Rheum Dis Clin North Am* 1993;19:107–120.

74. Larrick JW. Native interleukin 1 inhibitors. *Immunol Today* 1989;10:61–63.

75. Cope AP, Aderka D, Doherty M, et al. Increased levels of soluble tumor necrosis factor receptors in the sera and synovial fluid of patients with rheumatic diseases. *Arthritis Rheum* 1992;35:1160–1171.

76. Levine JD, Collier DH, Basbaum AI, Moskowitz MA, Helms CA. Hypothesis: the nervous system may contribute to the pathophysiology of rheumatoid arthritis. *J Rheumatol* 1985;12:406–408.

77. Lotz M, Carson DA, Vaughan JH. Substance P activation of rheumatoid synoviocytes: neural pathway in pathogenesis of arthritis. *Science* 1987;235:893–896.

78. Jacoby RK, Jayson MI, Cosh JA. Onset, early stages, and prognosis of rheumatoid arthritis: a clinical study of 100 patients with 11-year follow-up. *Br Med J* 1973;858:96–99.

79. Fleming A, Crown JM, Corbett M. Early rheumatoid disease. I. Onset. *Ann Rheum Dis* 1976;35:357–361.

80. Fleming A, Crown JM, Corbett M. Early rheumatoid disease. II. Patterns of joint involvement. *Ann Rheum Dis* 1976;35:361–365.

81. D'Cruz D, Hughes G. Rheumatoid arthritis: the clinical features. *J Musculoskel Med* 1993;10:85–93.

82. Schumacher HR. Palindromic onset of rheumatoid arthritis: clinical, synovial fluid and biopsy studies. *Arthritis Rheum* 1982;25:361–368.

83. Uhthoff HK, Sarkar K. Periarticular soft tissue conditions causing pain in the shoulder. *Curr Opin Rheumatol* 1992;4:241–252.

84. Morizono Y, Sakou T, Kawaida H. Upper cervical involvement in rheumatoid arthritis. *Spine* 1987;12:721–727.

85. Duthie R, Harris C. A radiographic and clinical survey of the hip joints in seropositive rheumatoid arthritis. *Acta Orthop Scand* 1969;40:346–359.

86. Vidigal E. The foot in chronic rheumatoid arthritis. *Ann Rheum Dis* 1975;34:292–296.

87. Mottonen TT. Prediction of erosiveness and rate of development of new erosions in early rheumatoid arthritis. *Ann Rheum Dis* 1988;47:648–652.

88. Hurd ER. Extra-articular manifestations of rheumatoid arthritis. *Semin Arthritis Rheum* 1979;8:151–169.

89. Hollingsworth JW, Saykaly RJ. Systemic complications of rheumatoid arthritis. *Med Clin North Am* 1977;61:217–231.

90. Segal R, Caspi D, Tishler M, Fishel B, Yaron M. Accelerated nodulosis and vasculitis during methotrexate therapy for rheumatoid arthritis. *Arthritis Rheum* 1988;31:1182–1188.

91. Vollersten RS. Rheumatoid vasculitis: survival and associated risk factors. *Medicine (Baltimore)* 1986;65:365–378.

92. Jurik AG, Davidsen D, Graudal H. Prevalence of pulmonary involvement in rheumatoid arthritis and its relationship to some characteristics of the patients. *Scand J Rheumatol* 1982;11:217–222.

93. Carson CW, Cannon GW, Egger M, Ward J, Clegg DO. Pulmonary disease during the treatment of rheumatoid arthritis with low dose pulse methotrexate. *Semin Arthritis Rheum* 1987;16:186–198.

94. John JT, Hough A, Sergent JS. Pericardial disease in rheumatoid arthritis. *Am J Med* 1979;66:385–394.

95. Fox RI, Michelson PE, Howell FV. Ocular and problems in arthritis. *Postgrad Med* 1985;78:87–97.
96. Rosenstein ED, Kramer N. Felty's and pseudo-Felty's syndromes. *Semin Arthritis Rheum* 1991;21:129–141.
97. Boers M. Renal disorders in rheumatoid arthritis. *Semin Arthritis Rheum* 1990;20:57–70.
98. Pincus T, Callahan LF. What is the natural history of rheumatoid arthritis? *Rheum Dis Clin North Am* 1993;19:123–138.
99. Mikkelsen WM, Dodge H. A four year follow-up of suspected rheumatoid arthritis: the Tecumseh, Michigan, Community Health Study. *Arthritis Rheum* 1969;12:87–96.
100. O'Sullivan JB, Cathcart ES. The prevalence of rheumatoid arthritis: follow-up evaluation of the effect of criteria on rates in Sudbury, Massachusetts. *Ann Intern Med* 1972;76:573–584.
101. Pincus T, Callahan LF, Sale WG, et al. Severe functional declines, work disability, and increased mortality in seventy-five rheumatoid arthritis patients studied over nine years. *Arthritis Rheum* 1984;27:864–874.
102. Rasker JJ, Cosh JA. The natural history of rheumatoid arthritis: a fifteen year follow-up study: the prognostic significance of features noted in the first year. *Clin Rheumatol* 1984;3:11–18.
103. Ropes MW, Bennet GA, Cobb S, Jacox R, Jessar RA. 1958 revision of diagnostic criteria for rheumatoid arthritis. *Bull Rheum Dis* 1958;9:175–176.
104. Arnett FC, Edworthy SM, Bloch DA, et al. The American Rheumatism Association 1987 revised criteria for the classification of rheumatoid arthritis. *Arthritis Rheum* 1988;31:315–324.
105. Fuchs HA, Kaye JJ, Callahan LF, et al. Evidence of significant radiographic damage in rheumatoid arthritis within the first 2 years of disease. *J Rheumatol* 1989;16:585–594.
106. Meenan RF, Yelin EH, Nevitt M, et al. The impact of chronic disease: a sociomedical profile of rheumatoid arthritis. *Arthritis Rheum* 1981;24:544–555.
107. Scott DL, Coulton BL, Symmons DP, Popert AJ. Long-term outcome of treating rheumatoid arthritis: results after 20 years. *Lancet* 1987;329:1108–1112.
108. Van Zeben D, Hazes JM, Zwinderman AH, et al. Clinical significance of rheumatoid factors in early rheumatoid arthritis: results of a follow up study. *Ann Rheum Dis* 1992;51:1029–1032.
109. Schmerling RH, DelBanco TL. The rheumatoid factor: an analysis of clinical utility. *Am J Med* 1991;91:528–534.
110. Van Schaardenburg D, Hazes JM, de Boer A, et al. Outcome of rheumatoid arthritis in relation to age and rheumatoid factor at diagnosis. *J Rheumatol* 1993;20:45–52.
111. Baum J. Laboratory tests in rheumatoid arthritis. *J Musculoskel Med* 1993;10:55–68.
112. Bull BS, Westengard JC, Farr M, Bacon PA, Meyer PJ, Stuart J. Efficacy of tests used to monitor rheumatoid arthritis. *Lancet* 1991;334:965–969.
113. Brower AC. Use of the radiograph to measure the course of rheumatoid arthritis. *Arthritis Rheum* 1990;33:316–324.
114. Corvetta A, Giovagnoni A, Baldelli S, et al. MR imaging of rheumatoid hand lesions: comparison with conventional radiology in 31 patients. *Clin Exp Rheumatol* 1992;10:217–228.
115. Hess EV, Luggen ME. Remodeling the pyramid—a concept whose time has not yet come. *J Rheumatol* 1989;16:1175–1184.
116. Wilske KR, Healey LA. Remodeling the pyramid—a concept whose time has come. *J Rheumatol* 1989;16:565–573.
117. Kavanaugh AF, Lipsky PE. Gold, penicillamine, antimalarials, and sulfasalazine. In: Gallin JI, Goldstein IM, Snyderman R, eds. *Inflammation: basic principles and clinical correlates*, 2nd ed. New York: Raven Press, 1992:1083.
118. Brooks PM. Clinical management of rheumatoid arthritis. *Lancet* 1992;341:286–290.
119. Ayers DC, Short WH. Arthritis surgery. *Clin Exp Rheumatol* 1993;11:75–83.
120. Bogoch ER. Surgery of rheumatoid arthritis in peripheral joints. *Curr Opin Rheumatol* 1992;4:191–210.

Inflammation: Basic Principles and Clinical Correlates,
3rd ed., edited by John I. Gallin and Ralph Snyderman.
Lippincott Williams & Wilkins, Philadelphia © 1999.

CHAPTER 65

Crystal-Induced Arthropathies

Shaun R. McColl and Paul H. Naccache

Crystal-induced inflammation is relevant to several acute and chronic human pathologies, namely gout and pseudogout in various joints and silicosis occurring in the lung. These diseases have as their root the deposition of crystals in tissues. Crystals implicated to date include monosodium urate (MSU), calcium pyrosphosphate dihydrate, hydroxyapatite (CPPD), and calcium oxalate in joint inflammation and silicon dioxide in the lung. This chapter focuses in particular on MSU and CPPD and describes the pathogenesis of crystal-induced arthropathies and the mechanisms involved in cellular activation leading to inflammation.

HISTORICAL OVERVIEW

Gouty arthritis is one of the best-described human diseases. Its distinctive clinical features were recognized more than 2,000 years ago by Hippocrates and were described in the oldest known medical text (1). There have been many landmarks in the understanding of this disease, as outlined in a review by Cohen and Emmerson (2). The first observation of crystals in gout was made by Van Leeuwenhoek in the 17th century (3), and over the next 100 years identification of the nature of these crystals as uric acid was achieved (4). Another landmark was the reproduction of symptoms of acute gout by injection of synthetic crystals (5), suggesting a central role for urate crystals in the triggering of acute gouty attacks. Clinical research did not progress significantly until relatively recently, when, in 1961, interest in sodium urate crystals in gouty effusions was effectively revived (6).

Pseudogout, a related disease, was effectively documented in 1962 when deposition of CPPD ($Ca_2P_2O_7 \cdot 2H_2O$) was first detected in inflammatory synovial effusions (7,8). It was subsequently appreciated that a disease known as chondrocalcinosis articularis syndrome or articular chondrocalcinosis (9) was the consequence of the deposition of CPPD crystals. As with MSU crystals, injection of synthetic CPPD crystals was shown to produce a powerful inflammatory response *in vivo*.

The mechanisms underlying gout and, to a significantly lesser extent, pseudogout have been extensively studied, and significant inroads have been made. However, despite intense research over the last decade, it is clear that the pathogenesis of these diseases is complex and many of the basic aspects remain to be elucidated.

CLINICAL ASPECTS

Formation of Crystals

The development of gouty arthritis depends on the deposition of MSU crystals. MSU crystals accumulate in the superficial layer of the synovium and articular cartilage and in the synovial fluid (10,11). Usually, crystallization of urate as a monosodium salt occurs in hyperuricemic fluids that contain increased levels of urate. Although hyperuricemia is necessary for the development of gout, not all hyperuricemic patients exhibit tissue deposits of urate or develop gout (12); in fact, acute attacks of gout can be correlated with the rate of change of serum uric acid rather than with a sustained high or low level (13).

There appear to be many factors that influence MSU crystal formation. Clearly, the effective level of supersaturation of sodium and urate ions in the surrounding milieu is important, but a variety of other factors that affect nucleation and the growth rate of the crystals are also involved. Such factors include pH, glycosaminoglycans, temperature, the rate of turnover of connective tis-

S. R. McColl: Department of Microbiology and Immunology, The University of Adelaide, Adelaide, South Australia, 5005 Australia.

P. H. Naccache: Le Centre de Recherche en Rhumatologie et Immunologie, Centre de Recherche du CHUL, Université Laval, Ste-Foy, Québec, G1V 4G2, Canada.

sue, and other solutes such as sodium or calcium (14,15). In addition, it has been suggested that urate crystals may be recognized by the immune system as conventional antigens, leading to the production of specific antibodies (16). Such antibodies could bear an imprint of the crystal surface and consequently behave as a nucleating matrix to enhance crystallization. Evidence to support this idea comes from studies in which immunoglobulin G (IgG) antibodies isolated from joint fluids of gouty patients accelerated the development of new MSU crystals *in vitro* (16). This effect was specific to gout; synovial fluids from patients with other joint diseases (e.g., pseudogout, rheumatoid arthritis, osteoarthritis) failed to facilitate crystallization. Antibodies of the IgG class isolated from rabbits injected with MSU also facilitate MSU crystallization.

CPPD crystals are frequently found in synovium or synovial fluids, extraarticular tendons, articular cartilage, ligaments, and bursae with or without clinical symptoms (11). It is currently believed that the initial formation of CPPD crystals in articular cartilage probably results from either biochemical abnormalities that lead to increased levels of calcium or inorganic pyrophosphate in serum or synovial fluid, changes in the cartilage matrix, or a combination of both. In support of a role for primary changes in cartilage matrix in CPPD deposition, there is a strong association between CPPD deposition and aging (17). Although the basis for this association is not yet clear, it has been suggested that increases in the ratio of keratin sulfate to chondroitin sulfate in human hyaline articular cartilage, as occurs with increasing age, may facilitate the deposition of CPPD crystals (18).

Description and Course of Disease

The term *gout* refers to a heterologous group of diseases observed exclusively in humans. Many excellent clinical reviews on the varying forms of this group of diseases have been published (17,19–21). Interested readers are advised to refer to these reviews.

The full development of gout may include four major phases: asymptomatic hyperuricemia, acute gout, intercritical gout, and chronic tophaceous gout. The first stage, asymptomatic hyperuricemia, occurs when the serum level of urate is increased in the absence of symptoms of arthritis, tophi, or detectable urate deposition. Acute gout is generally characterized by a rapid onset and buildup of severe pain in joints. It is usually monoarticular initially but can often become polyarticular at the latter stages. Almost any joint can be affected, although gout does not always involve articulations. Affected areas are also characterized by considerable redness and swelling, symptoms underlying the acute inflammatory nature of the disease. Most mild attacks resolve within 1 or 2 days, more severe cases within 7 to 10 days, with the characteristic severe pain being present for a significant period.

Very severe cases may take several weeks to resolve. Intercritical gout reflects the periods between gouty attacks, although clearly some patients may experience only one attack. Such periods may range from months to several years. Attacks can recur at increasingly shorter intervals, eventually resolving incompletely and potentially leading to a chronic tophaceous gout that may progress to a crippling disease state.

Treatment of the Disease

An important predisposing factor for gout is hyperuricemia. Treatment of this condition is considered to be of benefit to patients with recurrent gouty attacks. Under these circumstances, a xanthine oxidase inhibitor is usually prescribed. However, there appears to be little value in the treatment of patients with asymptomatic hyperuricemia.

Colchicine, an alkaloid extracted from the seeds and tubers of *Colchicum autumnale,* has been used in the treatment of acute gouty inflammation for centuries. It binds to the dimers of tubulin and thereby prevents the assembly of tubulin subunits into microtubules (22–24). It has been suggested that, by disrupting the microtubule network of cells such as polymorphonuclear leukocytes, colchicine can prevent extravasation, thereby reducing the accumulation of such cells in the synovial environment (25). Nonetheless, the mechanism of action of colchicine may rather relate to its effects on tyrosine phosphorylation (see later discussion). Colchicine is by no means the only form of therapy. Nonsteroidal antiinflammatory drugs such as indomethacin, naproxen, fenoprofen, piroxicam, and many others are also used to effectively treat gouty attacks, as are corticosteroids (26). Probably the two most important factors involved in effective treatment of gout are correct early diagnosis and corresponding early treatment. One of the features of the available therapy is its dramatic efficacy, provided that treatment occurs as early as possible.

Details of therapeutic intervention are available in a number of reviews (17,19–21,26).

HUMORAL ASPECTS OF PATHOGENESIS

Both MSU and CPPD crystals interact with various humoral components of the immune system. MSU crystals directly activate both the classic and alternative complement pathways *in vitro* (27–30), and activated complement components have been detected in synovial fluids from gouty patients (31). It has also been shown that a stable C5 convertase formed at the surface of the crystals cleaves the fifth component of human complement (C5) to C5a and C5b (32). MSU and CPPD crystals also can activate blood coagulation systems. Both types of crystals activate the Hageman factor (coagulation factor XII) (33,34), which then triggers the clotting cascade, the plasmin and kinin systems. This implies that crystals can initiate the generation of a variety of factors involved in vascular permeability, pain, and leukocyte chemotaxis (33,35,36).

Although both MSU and CPPD are capable of activating complement and the contact system, it appears that these events are not absolutely required for crystal-induced inflammation *in vivo*. Evidence in support of this hypothesis includes the observation that acute synovitis can be induced in chicken joints by injection of MSU crystals, even though this animal lacks Hageman factor and does not have detectable kinin activity in its synovial fluids (37). Moreover, experimental depletion of complement in dogs and in rabbits has little or no effect on synovitis induced by synthetic MSU crystals (38–41). Finally, humans with Hageman factor deficiency may still develop gout (42,43).

CELLULAR ASPECTS OF PATHOGENESIS

The basic and clinical data accumulated on crystal-induced arthropathies have made it abundantly clear that these diseases result from the interactions among crystals, the cells of the environment in which they form, and inflammatory cells (neutrophils and monocytes). These interactions result in a self-amplifying loop of cellular activation and synthesis and secretion of inflammatory cytokines and chemokines.

Interaction with Synovial Cells

It stands to reason that the initial interactions of inflammatory microcrystals would be with the cells of the synovial lining or synovial membrane where they are first detected arthroscopically. The synovial lining comprises two types of cells, type A and type B synoviocytes.

Type A Synoviocytes

Type A synoviocytes are believed to be of monocytic origin. Little, if any, direct data on their interactions with crystals exist because of the difficulty of isolating and maintaining these cells in culture. Blood monocytes have been used as an alternative model and have been shown to respond to MSU and CPPD crystals. Synthesis and secretion of interleukin-1 (IL-1), IL-6, IL-8, and tumor necrosis factor (TNF) by crystal-stimulated blood monocytes has been reported (44–46). Evidence for enhanced phospholipase A_2 activity and increased levels of phospholipase A_2 activating protein in response to MSU crystals has also been obtained (47). More recently, we have observed an induction of cyclooxygenase-2 (mRNA as well as protein) in MSU-stimulated monocytes that correlated with the production of prostanoids by these cells (Pouliot et al., 47a). These events are likely to play critical and synergistic roles in the initiation of the inflammatory reactions associated with crystal deposition diseases.

Type B Synoviocytes

One of the major cell types comprising the synovial tissue and lining layer is the type B synoviocyte, also referred to as the *synovial fibroblast*. This resident cell is likely to be one of the first cell types exposed to crystals in the joint tissue or synovial fluid. However, there have been few studies documenting the ability of inflammatory microcrystals to stimulate the release of inflammatory mediators in these cells.

Guerne et al. (44) demonstrated in 1989 the ability of both MSU and CPPD to stimulate the release of IL-6 by synovial fibroblasts. IL-6 is a mediator of acute phase protein release and can therefore contribute substantially to some of the systemic inflammatory changes observed during crystal-induced arthritis, such as leukocytosis, the hepatic acute phase response, and fever. Studies in our laboratories have focussed on the regulation of chemokine gene expression by inflammatory microcrystals and have been extended to include effects of MSU and CPPD on IL-8 production by human synovial fibroblasts (48). Both types of crystal induced the release of immunoreactive IL-8 by synovial fibroblasts in a dose- and time-dependent manner, with MSU being the more potent of the two crystals. Because IL-8 is one of the most potent chemotactic factors for neutrophils yet described, it is possible that its production by synovial fibroblasts early during the deposition of crystals may contribute substantially to the accumulation of neutrophils in the synovial fluid during gouty attacks.

Human synovial fibroblasts, or synovial fibroblasts cultured from dogs or rabbits, are a source of matrix metalloproteinases and eicosanoids in response to various inflammatory microcrystals, including CPPD and MSU. For instance, cultured canine synovial fibroblasts produce prostaglandin E_2 (PGE_2) on exposure to CPPD crystals (49), as do rabbit and human synovial fibroblasts exposed to MSU crystals (50,51). Moreover, 6-keto-$PGF_1\alpha$ and the lipoxygenase products hydroxyeicosatetraenoic acids are released (51). The eicosanoids are known to play an important role in acute inflammation by virtue of their effects on the vasculature. In addition, various prostaglandins are known to be potent nociceptive agents and therefore may contribute to the pain associated with crystal-induced inflammation.

The regulation of matrix metalloproteinase production is critical in the effective maintenance of the joint structure. Synovial fibroblasts are a major source of such enzymes. Several studies have demonstrated the ability of both MSU and CPPD crystals to induce expression of collagenase, an effect that is caused by increased transcription, RNA accumulation, and protein synthesis (52–56).

In addition to these effects on inflammatory mediator production by fibroblasts, both MSU and CPPD have been shown to stimulate proliferation of canine synovial fibroblasts and human foreskin fibroblasts (55) and to stimulate adhesion of neutrophils in an integrin-independent manner (57).

Interaction with Neutrophils

The diagnostic hallmark of gout, the demonstration of intracellular MSU crystals in synovial fluid neutrophils, underlines the central effector role of neutrophils in crystal-induced arthropathies. Systemic depletion of neutrophils abrogates MSU- and CPPD-induced synovitis, which is restored when neutrophils are replaced or allowed to reappear (58,59). Very high leukocyte counts (mostly neutrophils) are also characteristic of crystal-induced inflammatory responses. Finally, as detailed later, neutrophils actively respond to these microcrystals in an acutely proinflammatory manner.

The *in vitro* interaction of MSU or CPPD crystals with neutrophils leads to significant proinflammatory responses, including extracellular release of the constituents of their azurophil and specific granules (60) and activation of the nicotinamide-adenine dinucleotide phosphate oxidase system, resulting in the generation and extracellular diffusion of various oxygen-derived reactive metabolites (61,62). In addition, such interactions lead to lipid mediator release (63) and to inflammatory gene expression (48,64).

Signal Transduction in Neutrophils

A considerable body of work has accumulated in support of the hypothesis that MSU and CPPD crystals activate neutrophils not by nonspecific membranolytic mechanisms but by interactions with (presently undefined) surface receptors (see later discussion).

The available evidence favors the hypothesis that the major signal transduction pathway involved in the activation of human neutrophils by inflammatory microcrystals depends on the stimulation of tyrosine phosphorylation. Colchicine-inhibitable increases in the levels of tyrosine phosphorylation have been observed on stimulation of neutrophils by MSU and CPPD crystals. The patterns of tyrosine phosphorylation induced by the crystals are qualitatively different from those observed in response to G protein–dependent agonists such as chemotactic factors (including chemokines) or growth factors such as granulocyte-macrophage colony-stimulating factor (GM-CSF). Tyrosine kinase inhibitors such as erbstatin and the closely related methyl 2,5-dihydroxycinnamate (65) inhibit several of the functional responses of neutrophils induced by MSU and CPPD crystals, including mobilization of calcium, degranulation, and stimulation of the oxidative burst (62; P. H. Naccache et

al., 1993 unpublished observations). Stimulation of tyrosine phosphorylation is also critical to activation by the crystals of phosphatidylinositol 3-kinase, presumably p85/p110 (65), and of phospholipase D (65a). Inflammatory microcrystals stimulate tyrosine phosphorylation of the tyrosine kinases LYN (66) and, more prominently, SYK (66a), as well as the adaptor protein CBL (66b). These observations all support the notion that stimulation of tyrosine phosphorylation plays a critical role in the activation of the various signaling pathways such as calcium mobilization (62,63,67) and activation of phospholipase D (68).

The receptors, or surface structures, with which inflammatory microcrystals interact on the human neutrophil membranes remain to be positively identified. The relative insensitivity of most crystal-induced responses to pertussis toxin (62,67) suggests that pertussis toxin–sensitive G protein–linked receptors are not directly involved. On the other hand, data from our laboratory have provided evidence for a crucial role of Fc receptors. Antibodies to the glycosyl phosphatidylinositol–linked neutrophil FcγRIIIb receptor (CD16) specifically abrogate all the responses to the crystals tested, including the stimulation of tyrosine phosphorylation (including that of CBL and of SYK), the mobilization of calcium, and the activation of phospholipase D (66a). Evidence was also obtained indicating that signaling through CD16 requires interactions with CD11b. These data are consistent with the previous observations of Abramson et al. (69), demonstrating enhanced superoxide production of human neutrophils in response to IgG-coated (compared with uncoated) MSU crystals, and those of Jaques and Ginsberg (70), who observed an association between MSU crystals and glycoproteins Ib, IIb, and III in human platelets. In addition, these data are consistent with a central role of tyrosine phosphorylation in the mediation of neutrophil responses to MSU and CPPD crystals, because both FcγR and CD11b signaling appear to depend on tyrosine phosphorylation pathways.

Cytokine Production

It has become increasingly apparent that neutrophils may be a significant source of a wide range of cytokines during acute inflammatory responses. These cells have been shown to produce IL-1α and IL-1β, IL-1 receptor antagonist (IL-1Ra), TNF-α, IL-6, several colony-stimulating factors, and the chemokines IL-8, macrophage inflammatory protein-1α (MIP-1α), MIP-1β, and IP-10 (48,71–80). In the context of gout, the ability to produce such molecules is probably significant, because many of these extracellular messengers are known to play important amplification roles in inflammation.

When considering the ability of agonists to stimulate the production of proinflammatory agents such as IL-1α and β, consideration must also be given to regulation of the endogenous IL-1 antagonist, IL-1Ra. Both MSU and CPPD stimulate expression of IL-1α and IL-1β by neutrophils without significantly affecting the regulation of IL-1Ra (64). Neutrophils incubated with GM-CSF or TNF-α respectively produce approximately 300 and 200 times more IL-1Ra than IL-1. However, when neutrophils are co-incubated with cytokines such as GM-CSF and TNF-α in addition to MSU and CPPD, the production of IL-1 is upregulated while that of IL-1Ra is downregulated. These results demonstrate that the combined presence of inflammatory cytokines such as GM-CSF and TNF-α, which are likely to be present in inflammatory synovial fluids, and microcrystals, favors the production of biologically active IL-1 over that of IL-1Ra, with a resultant enhancement of the proinflammatory action of IL-1α and IL-1β.

In another study, the effect of MSU and CPPD on the production of the chemokines IL-8 and MIP-1α by human neutrophils was examined (48). These two chemokines are chemotactic factors for neutrophils and mononuclear cells, respectively. Both MSU and CPPD increase the secretion of IL-8 by neutrophils in a dose- and time-dependent manner but have no effect on secretion of MIP-1α. The proinflammatory cytokines TNF-α and GM-CSF, both of which are likely to be present in the joint during a gouty attack, stimulate IL-8 production, but only TNF-α exerts a significant effect on MIP-1α secretion. On co-incubation, IL-8 production induced by TNF-α and GM-CSF is synergistically enhanced in the presence of MSU or CPPD, whereas MIP-1α secretion induced by TNF-α is completely inhibited in the presence of either MSU or CPPD. These results suggest that the combination of TNF-α and GM-CSF with MSU or CPPD leads to the production of IL-8 by neutrophils and abolishes the release of MIP-1α, an event that theoretically leads to recruitment of neutrophils but not mononuclear cells. These results are in accordance with the pathologic state of gout and pseudogout, in which the predominant inflammatory cell is the neutrophil.

Other Inflammatory Mediators

Although limited, there is evidence that neutrophils exposed to MSU and CPPD produce other inflammatory mediators, including leukotriene B$_4$ (LTB$_4$) and related 5-lipoxygenase products (63,81). Other studies have shown that this is related to the ability of the crystals to induce phospholipase A$_2$ activity and phospholipase A$_2$–activating protein expression (47). Production of these lipid mediators probably plays a role in the amplification of inflammation, owing to their effects on the vasculature and their chemotactic and activating potential for phagocytes. Human neutrophils also release superoxide anion when exposed to MSU and CPPD (61,62). The production of these highly reactive oxygen-derived free radicals

may contribute to the cell and tissue destruction that occurs in gout.

Modulation of Crystal-Induced Responses by Adsorbed Proteins

The composition of the proteins coating MSU and CPPD crystals changes during the course of the inflammatory response, switching from being predominantly immunoglobulins during the early phases to including a majority of lipoproteins later on, during the resorption phases (82,83). These observations provide a basic framework to examine the relevance of the influence of opsonization by serum proteins on crystal-neutrophil interactions. As mentioned previously, IgG coating of MSU crystals enhances the production of superoxide anions by neutrophils (69,84). On the other hand, coating of MSU crystals with low-density lipoprotein, purified apo B100, or apo E inhibits their capacity to interact with neutrophils and platelets, resulting in decreased phagocytosis and decreased activating potential (85–87). Coating of MSU crystals with IgG has no qualitative effect on the ability of the crystals to stimulate tyrosine phosphorylation in neutrophils. On the other hand, opsonization with serum, which contains lipoproteins, significantly weakens this response (P. H. Naccache et al., 1997). Therefore, a close correlation exists between the known composition of the protein coating the crystals and the characteristics of the phases of the inflammatory response.

IN VIVO EXPERIMENTATION

Data accumulated from various models of crystal-induced arthritis provide support for the in vitro findings outlined previously. Several types of models have been used in the past, of which two—injection of crystals into the joints of dogs and rabbits and injection of crystals into subcutaneous air pouches raised on the backs of mice and rats—are particularly prominent. The results of these studies have implicated a number of effector molecules in the generation and modulation of acute inflammation in vivo after injection of MSU or CPPD crystals, although the data accumulated to date are limited.

Injection of inflammatory microcrystals into air pouches leads to a marked inflammatory response characterized by the accumulation of large numbers of neutrophils. The cellular exudate is generally composed of more than 97% neutrophils. The inflammation produced by MSU crystals in the rat subcutaneous air pouch is markedly reduced by simultaneous or delayed injection of transforming growth factor-β. In this model, TNF-α and various eicosanoids, including PGE$_2$ and LTB$_4$, are rapidly produced (89–91), as are the chemokines MIP-2 and MIP-1α (S.R. McColl et al., 1997, unpublished observations). When MSU or CPPD is injected into the joints of larger animals such as rabbits or dogs, a significant acute inflammatory response involving predominantly neutrophils occurs, as described previously (92,93).

CONCLUDING REMARKS

The data reported thus far are sufficient to propose a working model for the chain of events occurring during a gouty attack. Deposition of either MSU (gout) or CPPD (pseudogout) crystals in synovial tissue probably leads to the activation of the two major cell types present in this environment, namely the type A and type B synoviocytes. In addition, deposition of crystals at the junction of the tissue and joint space could lead to activation of complement and generation of humoral factors that enhance leukocyte recruitment into the joint space. *In vitro* evidence suggests that direct activation of type A and B synoviocytes leads to the production of a wide range of cytokines, including IL-1α and β and TNF-α, and chemokines, particularly IL-8. Theoretically, this in turn activates other cells in the environment, both amplifying the production of the same cytokines and initiating recruitment of large numbers of phagocytes, predominantly neutrophils, from the peripheral blood. These cells, accumulating in the synovial environment, are exposed to crystals and various cytokines. Their activation via the excitation-response coupling sequence as outlined previously, particularly in the presence of "priming" cytokines such as GM-CSF and TNF-α (94–97), amplifies the inflammatory response through the production of IL-1α, IL-1β, and IL-8, as we have previously described (48,64).

The proposed model places the neutrophil at the center of the inflammatory cycle. This is by far the major cell type present in crystal-induced arthropathies, and it has been shown to be capable of producing a wide range of inflammatory mediators that contribute to the inflammation observed in these pathologies. Colchicine, one of the more effective therapeutic interventions in crystal-induced arthropathies, profoundly inhibits neutrophil activation by either MSU or CPPD crystals. The data at hand suggest that interference with one or more tyrosine phosphorylation pathways represents a critical site of action of this alkaloid.

ACKNOWLEDGMENTS

Supported by the National Health and Medical Research Council and the Arthritis Foundation of Australia, The Medical Research Council and the Arthritis Society of Canada.

REFERENCES

1. Adams F. *The genuine works of Hippocrates.* New York: Wood, 1886.
2. Cohen MG, Emmerson BT. Crystal-induced arthropathies. In: Klippel JH, Dieppe PA, eds. *Rheumatology.* St. Louis: Mosby, 1994: 1258–1275.
3. McCarthy DJ. A historical note: Leuuwenhoek's description of crystals from gouty patients. *Arthritis Rheum* 1970;13:414.
4. Scheele KW. Examen chemicum cacculi urinarti. *Opuscula* 1776;2:73.
5. Freudweiler M. Experimentelle untersuchungen iiber das wesen der gichknoten. *Dustch Arch Klin Med* 1899;63:452.
6. McCarthy DJ, Hollander JL. Identification of urate crystals in gouty synovial fluid. *Ann Intern Med* 1961;54:266.
7. McCarthy DJ, Kohn NN, Faires JS. The significance of calcium phosphate crystals in the synovial fluid of arthritic patients: the pseudogout syndrome. I: Clinical aspects. *Ann Intern Med* 1962;56:217.
8. Kohn NN, Hughes RE, McCarthy DJ, Faires JS. The significance of calcium phosphate crystals in the synovial fluid of arthritic patients: the pseudogout syndrome. II: Identification of crystals. *Ann Intern Med* 1962;56:738.
9. Zitnan D, Sitaj S. Monohopocetna familiarna kalcifikacia ortikularynck churupick. *Bratisl Lek Listy* 1958;38:217.
10. Terkeltaub RA. Gout and mechanisms of crystal-induced inflammation. *Curr Opin Rheumatol* 1993;5:510–516.
11. Terkeltaub RA, Ginsberg MH, McCarthy DJ. *Pathogenesis and treatment of crystal-induced inflammation.* Philadelphia: Lea & Febiger, 1989.
12. Hall AP, Barry PE, Dawber TR, McNamara PM. Epidemiology of gout and hyperuricaemia: a long term population study. *Am J Med* 1967;42:38.
13. Maclachlan MJ, Rodnan GP. Effect of foods, fast, and alcohol on serum uric acid and acute attacks of gout. *Am J Med* 1967;42:38.
14. Katz WA. Deposition of urate crystals in gout. *Arthritis Rheum* 1975;18:753.
15. Wilcox WR, Khalaf AA. Nucleation of monosodium urate crystals. *Ann Rheum Dis* 1975;34:332–339.
16. Kam M, Perl Treves D, Caspi D, Addadi L. Antibodies against crystals. *FASEB J* 1992;6:2608–2613.
17. Terkeltaub RA. *Pathogenesis and treatment of crystal-induced inflammation.* Philadelphia: Lea & Febiger, 1993.
18. Hunter GK, Grynpas MD, Cheng PT, Pritzker KP. Effect of glycosaminoglycans on calcium pyrophosphate crystal formation in collagen gels. *Calcif Tissue Int* 1987;41:164–170.
19. Levinson DJ, Becker MA. Clinical gout and the pathogenesis of hyperuricemia. In: McCarty DJ, Koopman WJ, eds. *Arthritis and allied conditions: a textbook of rheumatology.* London: Lea & Febiger, 1993:1773–1805.
20. Doherty M, Dieppe P. Clinical aspects of calcium pyrophosphate dihydrate crystal deposition. *Rheum Dis Clin North Am* 1988;14:395–414.
21. Ryan LM, McCarty DJ. Calcium pyrophosphate crystal deposition disease; pseudogout; articular chondrocalcinosis. In: McCarthy DJ, Koopman WJ, eds. *Arthritis and allied conditions.* Philadelphia: Lea & Febiger, 1993:1835–1855.
22. Hastie SB. Interactions of colchicine with tubulin. *Pharmacol Ther* 1991;51:377.
23. Borisy GG, Taylor EW. The mechanism of action of colchicine: binding of ³H-colchicine to cellular proteins. *J Cell Biol* 1967;34:525.
24. Shelanski ML, Taylor EW. Isolation of a protein sub-unit from microtubules. *J Cell Biol* 1967;34:549.
25. Ehrenfeld M, Levy M, Bar Eli M, Gallily R, Eliakim M. Effect of colchicine on polymorphonuclear leucocyte chemotaxis in human volunteers. *Br J Clin Pharmacol* 1980;10:297–300.
26. Kelley WN, Fox IH, Palella TD. *Gout and related disorders of purine metabolism.* Philadelphia, WB Saunders, 1989.
27. Giclas PC, Ginsberg MH, Cooper NR. Immunoglobulin G independent activation of the classical complement pathway by monosodium urate crystals. *J Clin Invest* 1979;63:759–764.
28. Naff GB, Byers PH. Complement as a mediator of inflammation in gouty arthritis: I. Studies on the reaction between human serum complement and sodium urate crystals. *J Lab Clin Med* 1973;81:747.
29. Doherty M, Whicher JT, Dieppe PA. Activation of the alternative pathway of complement by monosodium urate monohydrate crystals and other inflammatory particles. *Ann Rheum Dis* 1983;42:285–291.
30. Fields TR, Abramson SB, Weissmann G, Kaplan AP, Ghebrehiwet B. Activation of the alternative pathway of complement by monosodium urate crystals. *Clin Immunol Immunopathol* 1983;26:249–257.
31. Hasselbacher P. Binding of immunoglobulin and activation of complement by asbestos fibers. *J Allergy Clin Immunol* 1979;64: 294–298.
32. Russell IJ, Mansen C, Kolb LM, Kolb WP. Activation of the fifth component of human complement (C5) induced by monosodium urate

crystals: C5 convertase assembly on the crystal surface. *Clin Immunol Immunopathol* 1982;24:239–250.

33. Kellermeyer RW. Activation of Hageman factor by sodium urate crystals. *Arthritis Rheum* 1965;8:741–743.

34. Ginsberg MH, Jaques B, Cochrane CG, Griffin JH. Urate crystal-dependent cleavage of Hageman factor in human plasma and synovial fluid. *J Lab Clin Med* 1980;95:497–506.

35. Kellermeyer RW, Breckenridge RT. The inflammatory process in acute gouty arthritis: II. The presence of Hageman factor and plasma thromboplastin antecedent in synovial fluid. *J Lab Clin Med* 1966;67:455–460.

36. Kellermeyer RW. Inflammatory process in acute gouty arthritis: III. Vascular permeability-enhancing activity in normal human synovial fluid; induction by Hageman factor activators; and inhibition by Hageman factor antiserum. *J Lab Clin Med* 1967;70:372–383.

37. Spilberg I. Urate crystal arthritis in animals lacking Hageman factor. *Arthritis Rheum* 1974;17:143–148.

38. Hasselbacher P. C3 activation by monosodium urate monohydrate and other crystalline material. *Arthritis Rheum* 1979;22:571–578.

39. Spilberg I, Osterland CK. Anti-inflammatory effect of the trypsin-kallikrein inhibitor in acute arthritis induced by urate crystals in rabbits. *J Lab Clin Med* 1970;76:472–479.

40. Webster ME, Maling HM, Zweig MH, Williams MA, Anderson W Jr. Urate crystal induced inflammation in the rat: evidence for the combined actions of kinins, histamine and components of complement. *Immunol Commun* 1972;1:185–198.

41. Phelps P, McCarty DJ Jr. Crystal-induced arthritis. *Postgrad Med* 1969;45:87–93.

42. Londino AV Jr, Luparello FJ. Factor XII deficiency in a man with gout and angioimmunoblastic lymphadenopathy. *Arch Intern Med* 1984;144:1497–1498.

43. Green D, Arsever CL, Grumet KA, Ratnoff OD. Classic gout in Hageman factor (factor XII) deficiency. *Arch Intern Med* 1982;142:1556–1557.

44. Guerne PA, Terkeltaub R, Zuraw B, Lotz M. Inflammatory microcrystals stimulate interleukin-6 production and secretion by human monocytes and synoviocytes. *Arthritis Rheum* 1989;32:1443–1452.

45. Terkeltaub R, Zachariae C, Santoro D, Martin J, Peveri P, Matsushima K. Monocyte-derived neutrophil chemotactic factor/interleukin-8 is a potential mediator of crystal-induced inflammation. *Arthritis Rheum* 1991;34:894–903.

46. Di Giovine FS, Malawista SE, Thornton E, Duff GW. Urate crystals stimulate production of tumor necrosis factor alpha from human blood monocytes and synovial cells: cytokine mRNA and protein kinetics, and cellular distribution. *J Clin Invest* 1991;87:1375–1381.

47. Bomalaski JS, Baker DG, Brophy LM, Clark MA. Monosodium urate crystals stimulate phospholipase A2 enzyme activities and the synthesis of a phospholipase A2-activating protein. *J Immunol* 1990;145:3391–3397.

47a. Pouliot M, James MJ, McColl SR, Naccache PH, Cleland LG. Monosodium urate micro crystals induce cyclooxygenase 2 in human monocytes. *Blood* 1998;91:1769–1776.

48. Hachicha M, Naccache PH, McColl SR. Inflammatory microcrystals differentially regulate the secretion of macrophage inflammatory protein 1 and interleukin 8 by human neutrophils: a possible mechanism of neutrophil recruitment to sites of inflammation in synovitis. *J Exp Med* 1995;182:2019–2025.

49. McCarty DJ, Cheung HS. Prostaglandin (PG) E2 generation by cultured canine synovial fibroblasts exposed to microcrystals containing calcium. *Ann Rheum Dis* 1985;44:316–320.

50. Hasselbacher P. Stimulation of synovial fibroblasts by calcium oxalate and monosodium urate monohydrate: a mechanism of connective tissue degradation in oxalosis and gout. *J Lab Clin Med* 1982;100:977–985.

51. Wigley FM, Fine IT, Newcombe DS. The role of the human synovial fibroblast in monosodium urate crystal-induced synovitis. *J Rheumatol* 1983;10:602–611.

52. Brinckerhoff CE, Mitchell TI. Autocrine control of collagenase synthesis by synovial fibroblasts. *J Cell Physiol* 1988;136:72–80.

53. Cheung HS, Halverson PB, McCarty DJ. Phagocytosis of hydroxyapatite or calcium pyrophosphate dihydrate crystals by rabbit articular chondrocytes stimulates release of collagenase, neutral protease, and prostaglandins E2 and F2 alpha. *Proc Soc Exp Biol Med* 1983;173:181–189.

54. Cheung HS, Halverson PB, McCarty DJ. Release of collagenase, neutral protease, and prostaglandins from cultured mammalian synovial cells by hydroxyapatite and calcium pyrophosphate dihydrate crystals. *Arthritis Rheum* 1981;24:1338–1344.

55. Cheung HS, Story MT, McCarty DJ. Mitogenic effects of hydroxyapatite and calcium pyrophosphate dihydrate crystals on cultured mammalian cells. *Arthritis Rheum* 1984;27:668–674.

56. Hasselbacher P, McMillan RM, Vater CA, Hahn J, Harris ED Jr. Stimulation of secretion of collagenase and prostaglandin E2 by synovial fibroblasts in response to crystals of monosodium urate monohydrate: a model for joint destruction in gout. *Trans Assoc Am Physicians* 1981;94:243–252.

57. Reinhardt PH, Naccache PH, E PP, Demedicis R, Kehrli ME, Kubes P. Monosodium urate crystals promote neutrophil adhesion via a CD18-independent and selectin independent mechanism. *Am J Physiol* 1996;39:C31–C39.

58. Chang YH, Gralla EJ. Suppression of urate crystal-induced canine joint inflammation by heterologous anti polymorphonuclear leukocyte serum. *Arthritis Rheum* 1968;11:145–150.

59. Phelps P, McCarthy DJ. Crystal-induced inflammation in canine joints: II. Importance of polymorphonuclear leukocytes. *J Exp Med* 1966;124:115–126.

60. Hoffstein S, Weissman G. Mechanism of lysosomal enzyme release from human leukocytes: IV. Interaction of monosodium urate crystals with dogfish and human leukocytes. *Arthritis Rheum* 1975;18:153–163.

61. Simchowitz L, Atkinson JP, Spilberg I. Stimulation of the respiratory burst in human neutrophils by crystal phagocytosis. *Arthritis Rheum* 1982;25:181–188.

62. Naccache PH, Grimard M, Roberge CJ, et al. Crystal-induced neutrophil activation: I. Initiation and modulation of calcium mobilization and superoxide production by microcrystals. *Arthritis Rheum* 1991;34:333–342.

63. Poubelle PE, De Medicis R, Naccache PH. Monosodium urate and calcium pyrophosphate crystals differentially activate the excitation-response coupling sequence of human neutrophils. *Biochem Biophys Res Commun* 1987;149:649–657.

64. Roberge CJ, de Medicis R, Dayer JM, Rola Pleszczynski M, Naccache PH, Poubelle PE. Crystal-induced neutrophil activation: V. Differential production of biologically active IL-1 and IL-1 receptor antagonist. *J Immunol* 1994;152:5485–5494.

65. Burt HM, Jackson JK, Dryden P, Salari H. Crystal-induced protein tyrosine phosphorylation in neutrophils and the effect of a tyrosine kinase inhibitor on neutrophil responses. *Mol Pharmacol* 1993;43:30–36.

65a. Marcil J, Harbour D, Houle MG, Naccache PH, Bourgoin SG. Monosodium urate crystal-stimulated phospholipase D in human neutrophils. *Biochem J* 1998 (in press).

66. Gaudry M, Gilbert C, Barabe F, Poubelle PE, Naccache PH. Activation of Lyn is a common element of the stimulation of human neutrophils by soluble and particulate agonists. *Blood* 1995;86:3567–3574.

66a. Barubé F, Gilbert C, Liao N, Bourgoin SG, Naccache PH. Crystal-induced neutrophil activation VI. Involvement of FcγRIIIB (CD16) and CD11b in responses to inflammatory microcrystals. *FASEB J* 1998;12:209–220.

66b. Naccache PH, Gilbert C, Barubé F, Al-Shami A, Mahana W, Bourgoin SG. Agonist-specific tyrosine phosphorylation of Cbl in human neutrophils. *J Leuk Biol* 1997;12:901–910.

67. Terkeltaub RA, Sklar LA, Mueller H. Neutrophil activation by inflammatory microcrystals of monosodium urate monohydrate utilizes pertussis toxin-insensitive and -sensitive pathways. *J Immunol* 1990;144:2719–2724.

68. Naccache PH, Bourgoin S, Plante E, et al. Crystal-induced neutrophil activation: II. Evidence for the activation of a phosphatidylcholine-specific phospholipase D. *Arthritis Rheum* 1993;36:117–125.

69. Abramson S, Hoffstein ST, Weissmann G. Superoxide anion generation by human neutrophils exposed to monosodium urate. *Arthritis Rheum* 1982;25:174–180.

70. Jaques BC, Ginsberg MH. The role of cell surface proteins in platelet stimulation by monosodium urate crystals. *Arthritis Rheum* 1982;25:508–521.

71. Cassatella MA, Gasperini S, Calzetti F, Bertagnin A, Luster AD, McDonald PP. Regulated production of the interferon-gamma-

inducible protein-10 (IP-10) chemokine by human neutrophils. *Eur J Immunol* 1997;27:111–115.

72. Bazzoni F, Cassatella MA, Rossi F, Ceska M, Dewald B, Baggiolini M. Phagocytosing neutrophils produce and release high amounts of the neutrophil-activating peptide 1/interleukin 8. *J Exp Med* 1991;173:771–774.

73. Gasperini S, Calzetti F, Russo MP, De Gironcoli M, Cassatella MA. Regulation of GRO alpha production in human granulocytes. *J Inflamm* 1995;45:143–151.

74. Cassatella MA, Meda L, Gasperini S, D'Andrea A, Ma X, Trinchieri G. Interleukin-12 production by human polymorphonuclear leukocytes. *Eur J Immunol* 1995;25:1–5.

75. Beaulieu AD, Paquin R, Rathanaswami P, McColl SR. Nuclear signaling in human neutrophils: stimulation of RNA synthesis is a response to a limited number of proinflammatory agonists. *J Biol Chem* 1992;2 67:426–432.

76. McColl SR, Paquin R, Menard C, Beaulieu AD. Human neutrophils produce high levels of the interleukin 1 receptor antagonist in response to granulocyte/macrophage colony-stimulating factor and tumor necrosis factor alpha. *J Exp Med* 1992;176:593–598.

77. Kasama T, Strieter RM, Lukacs NW, Burdick MD, Kunkel SL. Regulation of neutrophil-derived chemokine expression by IL-10. *J Immunol* 1994;152:3559–3569.

78. Kasama T, Strieter RM, Standiford TJ, Burdick MD, Kunkel SL. Expression and regulation of human neutrophil-derived macrophage inflammatory protein 1 alpha. *J Exp Med* 1993;178:63–72.

79. Tiku K, Tiku ML, Skosey JL. Interleukin 1 production by human polymorphonuclear neutrophils. *J Immunol* 1986;136:3677–3685.

80. Dubravec DB, Spriggs DR, Mannick JA, Rodrick ML. Circulating human peripheral blood granulocytes synthesize and secrete tumor necrosis factor alpha. *Proc Natl Acad Sci U S A* 1990;87:6758–6761.

81. Serhan CN, Lundberg U, Weissmann G, Samuelsson B. Formation of leukotrienes and hydroxy acids by human neutrophils and platelets exposed to monosodium urate. *Prostaglandins* 1984;27:563–581.

82. Ortiz Bravo E, Schumacher HR Jr. Components generated locally as well as serum alter the phlogistic effect of monosodium urate crystals *in vivo. J Rheumatol* 1993;20:1162–1166.

83. Ortiz Bravo E, Sieck MS, Schumacher HR Jr. Changes in the proteins coating monosodium urate crystals during active and subsiding inflammation: immunogold studies of synovial fluid from patients with gout and of fluid obtained using the rat subcutaneous air pouch model. *Arthritis Rheum* 1993;36:1274–1285.

84. Rosen MS, Baker DG, Schumacher HR Jr, Cherian PV. Products of polymorphonuclear cell injury inhibit IgG enhancement of monosodium urate-induced superoxide production. *Arthritis Rheum* 1986; 29:1473–1479.

85. Terkeltaub RA, Dyer CA, Martin J, Curtiss LK. Apolipoprotein (apo) E inhibits the capacity of monosodium urate crystals to stimulate neu-

trophils: characterization of intraarticular apo E and demonstration of apo E binding to urate crystals *in vivo. J Clin Invest* 1991;87:20–26.

86. Terkeltaub R, Smeltzer D, Curtiss LK, Ginsberg MH. Low density lipoprotein inhibits the physical interaction of phlogistic crystals and inflammatory cells. *Arthritis Rheum* 1986;29:363–370.

87. Terkeltaub R, Martin J, Curtiss LK, Ginsberg MH. Apolipoprotein B mediates the capacity of low density lipoprotein to suppress neutrophil stimulation by particulates. *J Biol Chem* 1986;261:15662–15667.

88. Liote F, Prudhommeaux F, Schiltz C, et al. Inhibition and prevention of monosodium urate monohydrate crystal–induced acute inflammation *in vivo* by transforming growth factor beta 1. *Arthritis Rheum* 1996;39:1192–1198.

89. Forrest MJ, Zammit V, Brooks PM. Inhibition of leucotriene B4 synthesis by BW 755c does not reduce polymorphonuclear leucocyte (PMNL) accumulation induced by monosodium urate crystals. *Ann Rheum Dis* 1988;47:241–246.

90. Gordon TP, Kowanko IC, James M, Roberts Thomson PJ. Monosodium urate crystal–induced prostaglandin synthesis in the rat subcutaneous air pouch. *Clin Exp Rheumatol* 1985;3:291–296.

91. Watanabe W, Baker DG, Schumacher HR Jr. Comparison of the acute inflammation induced by calcium pyrophosphate dihydrate, apatite and mixed crystals in the rat air pouch model of a synovial space. *J Rheumatol* 1992;19:1453–1457.

92. Fam AG, Morava-Protzner I, Purcell C, Young BD, Bunting PS, Lewis AJ. Acceleration of experimental lapine osteoarthritis by calcium pyrophosphate microcrystalline synovitis. *Arthritis Rheum* 1995;38: 201–210.

93. Myers SL, Brandt KD, Eilam O. Even low-grade synovitis significantly accelerates the clearance of protein from the canine knee: implications for measurement of synovial fluid "markers" of osteoarthritis. *Arthritis Rheum* 1995;38:1085–1091.

94. McColl SR, Krump E, Naccache PH, et al. Granulocyte-macrophage colony-stimulating factor increases the synthesis of leukotriene B4 by human neutrophils in response to platelet-activating factor: enhancement of both arachidonic acid availability and 5-lipoxygenase activation. *J Immunol* 1991;146:1204–1211.

95. McColl SR, Kreis C, DiPersio JF, Borgeat P, Naccache PH. Involvement of guanine nucleotide binding proteins in neutrophil activation and priming by GM-CSF. *Blood* 1989;73:588–591.

96. McColl SR, Beauseigle D, Gilbert C, Naccache PH. Priming of the human neutrophil respiratory burst by granulocyte-macrophage colony-stimulating factor and tumor necrosis factor-alpha involves regulation at a post-cell surface receptor level: enhancement of the effect of agents which directly activate G proteins. *J Immunol* 1990;145:3047–3053.

97. McColl SR, DiPersio JF, Caon AC, Ho P, Naccache PH. Involvement of tyrosine kinases in the activation of human peripheral blood neutrophils by granulocyte-macrophage colony-stimulating factor. *Blood* 1991;78:1842–1852.

Inflammation: Basic Principles and Clinical Correlates,
3rd ed., edited by John I. Gallin and Ralph Snyderman.
Lippincott Williams & Wilkins, Philadelphia © 1999.

CHAPTER 66

Reperfusion Injury

Kenneth S. Kilgore, Robert F. Todd III, and Benedict R. Lucchesi

Although tissue ischemia of sufficient duration produces irreversible injury and subsequent cell death, the rate of conversion from a viable to a nonviable state is significantly increased when the previously ischemic tissue is reperfused. A paradoxical situation develops in which reoxygenation, which is essential for survival of the tissue, may in fact be harmful. Damage caused by the restoration of blood flow is termed *reperfusion injury*. Simply defined, reperfusion injury is the conversion of reversibly injured cells to a state of irreversible injury as a result of the reintroduction of flow to an ischemic area. Associated with the restoration of flow is activation of the inflammatory response, which acts directly to extend the degree of injury in the reperfused zone. Induction of the inflammatory response is characterized by activation of the complement cascade and the adhesion and subsequent infiltration of inflammatory cell types, including neutrophils, into the previously ischemic area. Components of the complement cascade can promote tissue damage indirectly by generation of the anaphylatoxins and directly by formation of the membrane attack complex. Invading neutrophils injure the tissue through the generation of oxygen-derived free radicals and the release of proteolytic enzymes.

The ability of reperfusion to elicit additional cellular damage makes it imperative that the mechanisms of reperfusion injury be understood. A number of causative factors have been discovered, and a great deal of effort is now being devoted to the development of therapeutic approaches to limit tissue damage incurred during reperfusion. Although research in this area initially focused on the myocardium, the process is not solely limited to this organ. Any tissue or organ deprived of blood flow is subject to the events related to reperfusion injury (1). Therefore, this concept is of interest to physicians in a number of clinical settings, including organ transplantation and any surgical intervention in which blood flow to an organ is interrupted for a defined period followed by reperfusion.

NEUTROPHILS AND REPERFUSION INJURY

Role of Adhesion Molecules in Promoting Neutrophil-Mediated Tissue Damage

A substantial and convincing body of evidence indicates that neutrophils mediate tissue damage in organs subjected to ischemia followed by reperfusion. Multiple studies have demonstrated that if intact animals or perfused organs are depleted of circulating neutrophils (e.g., with the use of anti-neutrophil antiserum or myelosuppressive agents) before being subjected to regional ischemia and subsequent reperfusion, the extent of organ necrosis and other manifestations of tissue injury is reduced, compared with that observed in experimental subjects with normal neutrophil numbers (2–6). In further support of the role of the neutrophil as a mediator of ischemia-reperfusion injury are the results of other studies in which inhibitors of neutrophil activation and accumulation in ischemic organs also attenuated tissue damage after reperfusion (7). These observations have led to the concept that previously ischemic tissues elaborate chemoattractant factors such as C5a, interleukin-8 (IL-8), platelet activating factor (PAF), and leukotriene B_4 (8–12), which recruit neutrophils and activate them to release injurious products of the respiratory burst (O_2^-) and exocytosis (various proteases), thus causing tissue damage.

As detailed in Chapters 37–39, neutrophil recruitment to sites of inflammation is governed not only by chemoattractant factors but also by the regulated expression of adhesion molecules found on the surface membranes of

K. S. Kilgore and B. R. Lucchesi: Department of Pharmacology, University of Michigan Medical School, Ann Arbor, Michigan 48109-0632.

R. F. Todd III: Division of Hematology/Oncology, Department of Internal Medicine, University of Michigan Medical School, Ann Arbor, Michigan 48109-0374.

neutrophils and vascular endothelial cells (see Appendix A). Neutrophils in circulation make primary contact with injured endothelium via low-affinity interactions involving the selectins expressed by neutrophils (L-selectin [CD62L]) and by endothelium (E-selectin [CD62E], P-selectin [CD62P]) and their sialyl Lewis^X (sLe^X)–containing counterreceptors. These interactions are manifested by neutrophil "rolling" along microvessels. Exposure of rolling neutrophils to various cytokines elaborated by inflammatory tissues enhances the affinity of β_2 integrins, including lymphocyte function antigen-1 (LFA-1 [CD11a/CD18]), Mo1/Mac-1 (CD11b/CD18), and p150,95 (CD11c/CD18), for their counterreceptor intercellular adhesion molecule-1 (ICAM-1 [CD54]), which is inducibly expressed by inflamed endothelium. This high-affinity integrin–ICAM-1 interaction causes neutrophils to stop rolling, spread out on the endothelium, and migrate into subjacent tissues through endothelial cell junctions. Exposure of neutrophils to chemoattractant factors may also promote integrin-dependent homotypic adherence leading to neutrophil clumping.

The application of anti-integrin and anti-selectin monoclonal antibodies (MAbs) to various models of ischemia-reperfusion injury has contributed much to our current understanding of how adhesive interactions involving neutrophils and vascular endothelial cells result in tissue injury in the acute inflammatory response. Immunocytochemical analysis of microvessels in ischemic brain, heart, kidney, and intestine have demonstrated the endothelial cell expression of ICAM-1 and E-selectin within hours after reperfusion (13–21). Weyrich et al. (22) reported sequential expression of P-selectin, ICAM-1, and E-selectin in the coronary venules of cats subjected to myocardial ischemia followed by reperfusion.

The availability of MAbs that block integrin- or selectin-mediated binding has made it possible to assess the role of specific types of adhesive interactions in promoting various manifestations of ischemia-reperfusion injury. Representative data from experiments in which MAbs were applied to various models of ischemia-reperfusion injury that focused on the heart, nervous tissue, lung, kidney, intestine, liver, skeletal muscle, and the whole animal (resuscitation after hemorrhagic shock) are shown in Table 66-1. MAbs specific for CD11a or CD11b were used to block the adhesive function of individual members of the β_2 integrin family (LFA-1 and Mo1/Mac-1, respectively), whereas CD18 MAbs were employed to inhibit adhesive interactions mediated by all three β_2 integrin molecules (LFA-1, Mo1/Mac-1, and p150,95). MAb specific for CD54 targeted ICAM-1–dependent β_2 integrin adhesion. In the absence of blocking MAb against selectin counterreceptors, soluble forms of sLe^X carbohydrate (fucoidin) capable of inhibiting selectin-dependent adhesion were employed in certain studies.

In each of the model systems shown in Table 66–1, the administration of blocking MAbs (or soluble counterreceptor) just before or after reperfusion of ischemic tissues attenuated one or more of the manifestations of ischemia-reperfusion injury, including neutrophil infiltration, loss of vascular integrity (e.g, capillary leak of fluid, frank hemorrhage), impairment of blood flow ("no-reflow" phenomenon), tissue necrosis with impaired organ function, and mortality. The beneficial effect of inhibiting neutrophil adhesion, as demonstrated by decreased organ injury, was observed in diverse animal species including mice, rats, rabbits, dogs, cats, sheep, and nonhuman primates. In most reports, blockade of integrin or selectin-dependent adhesion resulted in reduced tissue damage of the ischemic-reperfused organ. In other studies, the lung was the target of secondary inflammatory injury, which was often attenuated by the systemic administration of blocking MAbs. Although relatively few studies directly compared the effects of multiple MAbs with specificity for distinct adhesion receptors, inspection of the data compiled in Table 66–1 suggests that interference with selectin-dependent adhesion attenuated ischemia-reperfusion injury to an extent comparable to that achieved with blocking of β_2 integrin–dependent adhesion. Moreover, despite an apparent redundancy in their adhesive function, inhibition of individual members of the β_2 integrin and selectin families was generally sufficient to produce significant reductions in tissue damage. Consistent with the inhibitory effect of MAbs that block the integrin–ICAM-1 interaction are the results of other studies in which ischemia-reperfusion injury of kidney and brain was significantly reduced in ICAM-1 knock-out mice, compared with wild-type littermates (23–25). Similarly, the administration of an anti-sense oligonucleotide to ablate ICAM-1 expression in rats resulted in diminished renal cortical damage in ischemic/reperfused kidneys (26).

Whereas most published reports describe the inhibitory (beneficial) effect of anti-adhesion reagents (as exemplified in Table 66-1), limited "negative" data also have been cited: the administration of sLe^X to dogs had no effect on myocardial infarct size or neutrophil infiltration (27); anti-CD18 MAb failed to prevent paraplegia in a rabbit model of spinal cord ischemia-reperfusion injury (28); anti-CD18 MAb had no impact on neutrophil emigration into the alveoli of rabbits subjected to pulmonary ischemia-reperfusion injury (29); and anti-CD62P failed to avert neutrophil sequestration and increases in vascular permeability in the lungs of rats subjected to intestinal ischemia-reperfusion injury (30).

Despite the appearance of isolated negative reports, the preponderance of published data supports the concept that neutrophil adhesion mediated by the selectins and by the β_2 integrins has a critical role in the recruitment of neutrophils to ischemic tissues (or to secondary target organs such as the lung) leading to neutrophil-mediated

TABLE 66-1. *Attenuation of ischemia-reperfusion injury by blockade of β_2-integrin or selectin-dependent neutrophil adhesion*

Organ (References)	β_2 Integrin–dependent adhesion				Selectin-dependent adhesion			
	CD11a	CD11b	CD18	CD54	CD62E	CD62L	CD62P	SLe^X/fucoidin
Heart (86, 109–113)	Infarct size PMN infiltration	Infarct size PMN infiltration	Infarct size PMN infiltration No reflow Contractile dysfunction	Infarct size PMN infiltration	Infarct size PMN infiltration Mortality	Infarct size PMN infiltration	Infarct size PMN infiltration No reflow Contractile dysfunction	Infarct size PMN infiltration No reflow Contractile dysfunction
Brain/spinal cord (114–119)	Infarct size Edema PMN infiltration	Infarct size Neurologic deficit	Infarct size Edema PMN infiltration No reflow	Infarct size Neurologic deficit No reflow PMN infiltration	—	—	—	Infarct size PMN infiltration
Lung (120–124)	—	—	Capillary permeability PMN infiltration	Hypoxemia Capillary permeability	Mortality	Mortality	Capillary permeability PMN infiltration	—
Kidney (31, 125–129)	Renal failure Tissue injury	Renal failure Tissue injury	No reflow PMN infiltration	Renal failure Tissue injury PMN infiltration Mortality Allograft rejection	—	—	—	—
Intestine (30, 124, 130–135)	—	Vascular permeability Lung capillary permeability Lung hemorrhage PMN vascular adherence	Vascular permeability Lung capillary permeability Lung PMN infiltration PMN vascular adherence	Vascular permeability PMN vascular adherence	—	PMN rolling + adherence Vascular permeability	PMN rolling + adherence PMN infiltration Tissue injury Lung capillary permeability	PMN rolling + adherence Lung capillary permeability
Liver (136–140)	—	—	Tissue necrosis	Tissue injury Excretory dysfunction	—	—	Tissue injury PMN infiltration Mortality	Tissue injury PMN infiltration
Skeletal muscle (141–149)	Lung capillary permeability Lung hemorrhage Lung PMN infiltration	Lung capillary permeability Lung hemorrhage Lung PMN infiltration Muscle necrosis PMN infiltration No reflow Vascular permeability	Lung capillary permeability Lung hemorrhage Lung PMN infiltration Tissue necrosis Edema	Lung capillary permeability Lung hemorrhage Lung PMN infiltration Vascular permeability No reflow	Lung capillary permeability Lung hemorrhage Lung PMN infiltration	Lung capillary permeability Lung hemorrhage Lung PMN infiltration Edema Tissue necrosis	Lung capillary permeability Lung hemorrhage Lung PMN infiltration Edema Tissue necrosis	Lung capillary permeability Lung hemorrhage Lung PMN infiltration Edema Tissue necrosis
Whole animal (150–153)	—	—	Multiorgan tissue injury Mortality	—	—	Vascular permeability Mortality	—	Mortality Intestinal PMN infiltration

PMN, polymorphonuclear leukocytes; SLe^X, sialyl, Lewis^X.

tissue damage. In addition to contributing to our understanding of the pathophysiology of ischemia-reperfusion injury, the inhibitory effect of adhesion-blocking agents (MAb and sLe^X) in animal models suggests their potential utility as therapeutic agents. Indeed, the survival of human kidney allografts appears to be improved in donors receiving anti–ICAM-1 MAb, based on the results of a phase I clinical trial (31). Another clinical trial currently in progress is designed to test the efficacy of anti–ICAM-1 MAb in reducing infarct size in patients with nonhemorrhagic strokes.

Mediators of Neutrophil-induced Cellular Injury

Activated neutrophils are able to elicit tissue injury through several different mechanisms, including generation of oxygen-derived free radicals and release of cytotoxic lysosomal enzymes. Chemotactic factors including C5a, PAF, and cytokines are capable of activating neutrophils. Stimulation of the neutrophils by one or more of these factors elicits the "respiratory burst," characterized by a sudden increase in oxygen consumption and a release of reactive oxygen intermediates into the surrounding environment. Superoxide anion (O_2^-), hypochlorous acid (HOCl), hydroxyl anion ($\cdot$OH), and chloramine (RNHCl$^-$) are oxidants produced by the stimulated neutrophil. In addition, circulating PAF stimulates neutrophils to synthesize H_2O_2 (32), which has been shown to induce a PAF-dependent adherence of neutrophils to the endothelium (33). Generation of H_2O_2 by the neutrophil thus may act as a positive feedback mechanism, allowing the neutrophil to recruit other circulating neutrophils to the injured tissue. Evidence for the role of reactive radicals in reperfusion injury, coupled with the ability of neutrophils to produce free radicals, implicates this mechanism as one way by which neutrophils elicit tissue damage.

Coinciding with the generation of oxygen-derived free radicals by the neutrophil is the release of cytotoxic proteases stored in intracellular granules. A number of these granule products have the capacity to alter vascular permeability, thereby aiding the movement of the neutrophil into the surrounding tissue. Cationic proteins and neutral proteases serve to alter vascular permeability and disrupt the basement membrane of the vascular wall. Two metalloproteases, collagenase and gelatinase, when activated by HOCl, are capable of degrading collagen and lysing endothelial cells (34). Other important lysosomal enzymes released during activation include elastase and heparinase, the latter participating in degradation of heparan and heparin sulfate associated with the extracellular matrix or glycocalyx.

It is not entirely clear whether the cells must emigrate from the endothelium into the surrounding tissue to elicit injury or whether damage to the endothelial cell is sufficient. It is likely that the neutrophil causes deleterious effects in both the vasculature and surrounding tissue. Because neutrophils can form aggregates, small capillaries may become physically plugged and represent the underlying mechanism for the no-reflow phenomenon, in which areas of the ischemic region are not reperfused adequately (35). Neutrophils also may affect larger vessels, such as arterioles and precapillary vessels. Release of vasoconstricting agents from the activated neutrophils is thought to decrease vessel diameter, resulting in decreased perfusion of the surrounding tissue (36). The decrease in perfusion may be exacerbated by release from the neutrophil of factors such as PAF, which serves to activate circulating platelets. The accumulation of platelets in the reperfused area would allow for an increase in vascular plugging in addition to release of platelet-derived factors that act on the vasculature (36).

THE COMPLEMENT SYSTEM IN REPERFUSION INJURY

The complement system is composed of two separate pathways, the classic and the alternative pathways. The classic pathway provides the "specific" adaptive response involving immune complex formation, whereas the alternative path is responsible for "nonspecific," innate immunity. Although triggered by different mechanisms, both pathways converge at the level of C3, ultimately forming the anaphylatoxins (C3a, C4a, and C5a) and the membrane attack complex (MAC). The latter consists of the distal complement components C5b–9. As described later, both the anaphylatoxins and the MAC have an important role in mediating the pathogenesis of ischemia-reperfusion injury.

Although activation of the complement system in the setting of ischemia-reperfusion injury was proposed more than 25 years ago, the exact role of complement in this type of injury has yet to be understood in detail. Studies continue to support the concept that complement activation is one of the primary mediators in the pathogenesis of ischemia-reperfusion injury. Early evidence for the role of complement was demonstrated by the observation that C1q, an early component of the classic pathway, was present after myocardial ischemia and reperfusion injury in the canine (37). The localization of complement components also was noted when sections of rat (38) or baboon (39) myocardium were obtained after regional myocardial ischemia. Localization of complement proteins in most infarcted myocardial fibers and vessels coincided with sequestration of polymorphonuclear leukocytes (37). However, neither deposition of complement proteins nor leukocytes were observed in myocardial tissue that was not subjected to an ischemic insult.

Evidence also exists for complement activation during myocardial infarction in humans (37,40,41). Analysis of serum samples from postmyocardial infarct patients has shown increased concentrations of the soluble form of the

MAC (sMAC), composed of proteins C5b–9 (40). Antibodies directed against the neoantigen of the human C5b–9 complex were used to identify MAC deposits in infarcted human myocardial tissue obtained at autopsy (42). Very little detection was observed with a monoclonal antibody to complement S-protein, indicating that the terminal complement components were deposited mainly in the form of membrane-damaging C5b–9 complexes. Localization of the MAC was limited to areas within the infarcted zone, and the surrounding tissue was free of MAC deposition. Schafer et al. (42) showed that localization of the MAC is not limited to the membranes of target cells but may also include the cytoplasmic regions. Therefore, complement components are capable of diffusing into the interstitial space, where the MAC may be assembled. The resulting deposition of C5b–9 on the cell membranes could contribute to functional disturbances (signal transduction) and irreversible damage (altered intracellular electrolyte and water balance) of cells during ischemia and reperfusion. Other studies have shown a significant increase in the deposition of C3bBb (the C3 convertase of the alternative pathway) and the degradation products of the anaphylatoxins in the plasma of patients after acute myocardial infarction, indicating that these products of complement activation, in addition to the MAC, serve an important role in ischemia-reperfusion injury (40,43,44).

Activation of Complement in the Setting of Reperfusion Injury

The mechanisms by which complement is activated on reperfusion are not clear. Because complement appears to be activated within a short time after reperfusion, it is reasonable to focus on the initial events known to occur on reperfusion of the ischemic myocardium. Vogt et al. (45,46) showed that the fifth component of complement can be converted to an active form by oxygen-derived free radicals, which rapidly appear in the extracellular milieu on reperfusion. This nonenzymatic conversion of C5 to a functionally active C5b-like form by hydroxyl radicals results in the formation of the complete, lytic MAC. Products of neutrophil activation, including superoxide anion, hydrogen peroxide, hydroxyl radical, peroxide-like radicals, and myeloperoxidase, also have been implicated in promoting complement activation (47,48). Exposure of basement membranes and subcellular organelles that may appear after an ischemic event has been shown to activate complement (49). Early investigations demonstrated that isolated myocardial membranes bind C1, leading to activation of the entire cascade. Furthermore, cytoplasmic constituents, including the mitochondria, are able to elicit activation of the complement system (50).

Damage to the cellular membrane may provide an indirect mechanism by which free radicals initiate activation of complement. Damage to the membrane may take the form of denaturation of integral proteins or altered membrane integrity, or both. Denaturation of protective membrane proteins impairs the ability of the cell to ward off injury via activation of the complement system. The expression of various membrane regulators of complement activation in normal and infarcted human tissue has been analyzed in an effort to address the question of why the strictly controlled complement system reacts against autologous tissue subjected to ischemia and reperfusion (38,51). For example, in the heart, protectin (CD59) was strongly expressed by normal myocardium but infarcted cells had a substantial decrease in the expression of this regulator of MAC formation. The expression of CD59, but not of C8 binding protein, was clearly diminished in the lesions. The results show that C8 binding protein, vitronectin, and C4 binding protein (C4bp) do not prevent complement attack against the infarcted myocardium but become codeposited with the MAC. Ischemia-induced transformation of complement-resistant viable cells into activators of complement may result from the acquired loss of resistance to the MAC by shedding of CD59 and other complement-protective proteins.

Plasmin-dependent fibrinolytic agents used for thrombolysis are known to activate complement in vitro and may contribute to its activation in vivo. The extent of complement activation in patients with an evolving acute myocardial infarction, some treated and some not treated with streptokinase, has been reported (52). Streptokinase treatment caused abrupt activation of the complement system, whereas no significant complement activation was detected in plasma of the patients not treated with fibrinolytic agents. Complement activation was accompanied by a transient leukopenia, as reported for other clinical procedures such as hemodialysis and cardiopulmonary bypass, and possibly contributed to the hypotension observed during streptokinase treatment. Similar results were reported by Agostoni et al. (53,54).

In like fashion, plasmin generation after administration of recombinant tissue plasminogen activator (rt-PA) has been associated with activation of complement (55,56). Bennett et al. (56) tested the hypothesis that rt-PA could induce in vivo activation of complement during thrombolytic therapy for management of acute myocardial infarction. The findings are suggestive of complement activation arising from the administration of rt-PA but definitely independent of reperfusion. Other investigators obtained similar results when streptokinase was used as the thrombolytic agent (52,54), thereby providing evidence that plasmin can initiate activation of the complement cascade. A direct comparison between the effects of streptokinase and rt-PA on complement activation during thrombolytic therapy demonstrated that complement activation occurs during the administration of either compound (53). However, the influence of streptokinase on the generation of complement activation products, including the anaphylatoxins, was more pronounced, compared with rt-PA.

Actions of the Anaphylatoxins

Production of the anaphylatoxins C3a and C5a occurs in both the classic and the alternative pathways, whereas C4a is produced only via the classic pathway. Both C3a and C5a are derived through the actions of convertases on the N-terminal ends of the α chain of their respective precursors. The proteolytic generation of the anaphylatoxins C3a, C4a, and C5a during the early phases of complement activation is associated with the inflammatory reaction during the evolution of a myocardial infarction. The anaphylatoxins induce localized vasoactive effects in a variety of tissues, including those damaged during the process of ischemia and reperfusion. The anaphylatoxins mediate alterations in vascular permeability, induce smooth muscle cell contraction, and release histamine from mast cells and basophils. The spasmogenic properties of C3a and C4a are regulated by plasma carboxypeptidase N, which removes from the anaphylatoxins the C-terminal arginine that is essential for activity. However, the lack of a C-terminal arginine on C5a does not reduce its chemotactic action or its facilitation of an inflammatory response. On a molar basis, C5a is tenfold more active than C3a, but there are fewer C5a molecules produced during complement activation, so the net effectiveness of C5a may be less than that of C3a (57).

Both C5a and C3a have a wide range of biologic activities that may be of importance in the setting of ischemia-reperfusion injury, including eliciting mast cell degranulation, contracting vascular smooth muscle, and increasing vascular permeability (58). The anaphylatoxins C3a and C5a not only have potent vasoactive actions on the coronary vasculature but also serve as potent chemoattractants for cellular constituents of inflammation, including neutrophils (Fig. 66-1).

Foreman et al. (59) reported that human umbilical vein endothelial cells stimulated with purified C5a exhibit an increase in P-selectin expression, demonstrating that C5a has a role in both recruitment and adhesion of neutrophils. C5a alone does not cause significant injury in the reperfused myocardium, but in the presence of neutrophils C5a promotes marked injury, suggesting that complement-derived products are required for neutrophil activation and subsequent contractile dysfunction (60). This conclusion is in agreement with other observations showing a reduction in infarct size in a pig model of myocardial infarction with the administration of a monoclonal antibody against C5a (61). These observations support the concept of an important role for the alternative com-

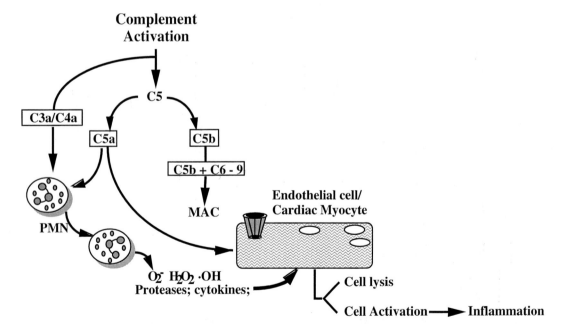

FIG. 66-1. Effects of complement activation in mediating ischemia-reperfusion injury. The anaphylatoxins generated by complement activation during reperfusion not only have potent vasoactive actions on the coronary vasculature but also serve as potent chemoattractants for inflammatory cell types, including neutrophils. The membrane attack complex (MAC), when assembled in high concentrations on the target cell membrane, may promote irreversible cell injury by altering intracellular ion and water fluxes. Nucleated cells, by virtue of possessing cell-associated complement inhibitors, have the ability to limit the degree of complement activation and subsequent deposition of the MAC. Therefore, the MAC, while not directly lysing target cells, may act to stimulate the cell, thereby enhancing the proinflammatory response.

plement pathway and C5a in the propagation of myocardial damage during reperfusion. C5a also is likely to mediate the early events of neutrophil recruitment. In a rabbit model of ischemia and reperfusion injury, greater concentrations of C5a were associated with earlier stages of reperfusion, whereas C5a was not detectable during the ischemic period (11). The increase in C5a generation correlated with increases in neutrophil accumulation within the ischemic zone during reperfusion. As C5a concentrations declined, concentrations of IL-8 in myocardial tissue increased, demonstrating a biphasic generation of neutrophil chemotactic factors (11). Uncertainty remains regarding the ability of C5a to influence the formation of IL-8.

Although little data have been reported concerning the effects of C3a and C4a in disease states, it would not be unreasonable to hypothesize that both of these complement products could elicit similar responses from endothelial cells, especially during evolution of a myocardial infarction. However, the influence of C3a on the vasculature may not result from direct actions but rather from the release of histamine by other target cells. Nevertheless, the roles that C3a and C4a play in mediating vascular changes and recruiting inflammatory cell types to the ischemic area warrant further attention.

Role of the Membrane Attack Complex

Previous studies have demonstrated that the MAC has a functional role in mediating the pathogenesis of ischemia-reperfusion injury. The presence of complement-derived factors in human tissues after an ischemic episode, coupled with the ability of cobra venom factor and the complement inhibitor soluble complement receptor-1 (sCR1) to decrease tissue injury in experimental models, provides compelling evidence for the detrimental role of complement and the MAC (62,63). The impor-

tance of reperfusion in mediating complement activation and subsequent deposition of the MAC was exemplified in a study by Mathey et al. (64) that delineated the temporal characteristics of MAC deposition in nonreperfused and reperfused myocardium. In the reperfused myocardium, MAC deposition occurred rapidly (30 minutes), compared with the 5 to 6 hours required for MAC deposition in hearts that did not undergo reperfusion. The data suggest that reperfusion is a prerequisite for rapid activation of the complement cascade and subsequent deposition of the MAC. The detrimental role of the MAC in augmenting myocardial injury after ischemia-reperfusion is substantiated further by experiments using animals deficient in the complement protein C6. Ito et al. (65) reported a decrease in myocardial infarct size and the no-reflow phenomenon in C6-deficient rabbits, compared with C6-sufficient rabbits. Subsequently it was determined that neutrophil accumulation within the area at risk in C6-deficient rabbits was decreased, compared with that in C6-sufficient animals. This observation suggests a link between deposition of the MAC and the subsequent recruitment and accumulation of leukocytes within the ischemic region. The ability of the MAC to modulate the expression of proinflammatory chemokines *in vitro* (see later discussion), suggests that, in addition to its direct lytic effects, the MAC may participate in mediation of the recruitment of neutrophils in the setting of ischemia-reperfusion injury.

Proinflammatory Effects of the MAC

The deleterious effects of MAC assembly on cellular membranes have been attributed primarily to the direct, lytic effects of the complex on nucleated cells (Fig. 66-2). Nucleated cells, by virtue of possessing cell-associated complement inhibitors, have the ability to limit the degree of local complement activation and subsequent

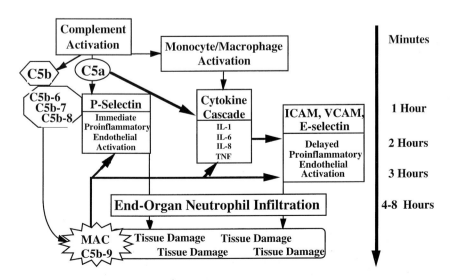

FIG. 66-2. C5a and the membrane attack complex (MAC) probably mediate various aspects of the inflammatory response by inducing the expression of proinflammatory cytokines and cellular adhesion molecules. Complement activation probably occurs rapidly (within minutes) after restoration of flow to the ischemic area and is followed by complement-mediated upregulation of numerous proinflammatory mediators. P-selectin is rapidly (30 minutes) upregulated by the endothelium on exposure to either C5a or the MAC. Other cell adhesion molecules such as intercellular adhesion molecule-1 (ICAM-1 and E-selectin) and cytokines such as interleukin-8 (IL-8) and tumor necrosis factor-α (TNF-α) require longer periods of time (hours) for full expression.

formation of the MAC. Partial formation of the terminal complex or complete assembly of the MAC, while not directly lysing target cells, may act to stimulate the cell, thereby modulating the proinflammatory response noted during the reperfusion period. There is a compelling body of data indicating that the MAC mediates various aspects of the inflammatory response by inducing the expression of proinflammatory mediators. Stimulation of granulocytes or mesangial cells with nonlytic concentrations of the MAC promotes the formation of reactive oxygen metabolites and a number of arachidonic acid metabolites (e.g., prostaglandins, leukotrienes) (66). In addition, the MAC has been shown to modulate the expression of cellular adhesion molecules including P-selectin, which is mobilized rapidly from intracellular storage granules after deposition of the MAC (67).

The MAC also may interact with other components of the inflammatory response to promote upregulation of cell adhesion molecules (see Fig. 66-2). For example, addition of tumor necrosis factor-α (TNF-α) to endothelial cells preexposed to the MAC resulted in a synergistic increase in the expression of E-selectin and ICAM-1, suggesting that the MAC may act to "prime" the cells to respond to other inflammatory mediators (68). In addition, although the MAC is important for leukocyte adhesion, it has been suggested that it has the capacity to enhance the recruitment of leukocytes by increasing the expression of cytokines from both effector cells of the immune system and nonimmune cells. Numerous proinflammatory cytokines, including TNF-α and IL-1β, are secreted by mesangial cells and monocytes after MAC deposition (69,70). The recruitment of inflammatory cells, including neutrophils and monocytes, may be increased by the assembly of sublytic concentrations of the MAC on endothelial cells as a result of the local induction of chemotactic cytokines. Both the neutrophil chemotactic cytokine IL-8 and the monocyte chemokine monocyte chemoattractant protein-1 are secreted in response to sublytic MAC formation *in vitro* (71).

The mechanisms by which assembly of the MAC promotes increased expression of proinflammatory mediators have yet to be ascertained, although initial *in vitro* studies provide some insight. The complex has been linked with a number of second messenger signaling pathways (72). Indirectly, the membrane-associated, pore-forming protein complex provides a mechanism for transmembrane ion fluxes; calcium, once brought into the cytoplasm by this mechanism, may promote activation of calcium-dependent phospholipases, increased adenosine triphosphatase activity, and the uncoupling of oxidative phosphorylation in mitochondria (73,74). The development of contracture bands and the formation of large amorphous densities within the mitochondria are examples of the marked changes in cellular ultrastructure that are mediated, in part, by calcium. The appearance of the ultrastructural markers is indicative of irreversible injury and cell death (75).

The MAC also may elicit activation of signal transduction mechanisms in a receptor-independent manner. For example, MAC formation is associated with increased intracellular levels of 2-diacylglycerol and activation of a variety of protein kinases, including protein kinase C and protein kinase A (76). An increase in protein kinase C and cyclic adenosine monophosphate activity in Ehrlich cells is noted after exposure to the "sublytic" MAC (72). Other investigators have noted that the biologic activities induced by MAC in nucleated cells may be mediated in part by activation of pertussis-sensitive G proteins (77). The interaction of the MAC with multiple signal transduction pathways suggests a possible link between MAC formation and the subsequent upregulation of proinflammatory mediators (78).

Formation of the entire MAC (C5b–9) is not required to impart second messenger activation. In addition to C5b–9, the nonlytic membrane-associated complexes C5b–7 and C5b–8 can impart a signal to the target cell in the absence of pore formation. In addition to mediating signaling events in the cytoplasm, it is known that MAC deposition modulates the activity of transcription factors, including nuclear factor-κB, which controls the expression of proinflammatory cytokines and adhesion molecules (79). These observations strengthen the hypothesis that the terminal complement complexes C5b–7, C5b–8, and C5b–9 are able to generate nonlethal and perhaps reversible cell signals independent of those arising from lethal pore formation. It is apparent therefore that MAC deposition, through its ability to alter the activation state of nucleated cells, may serve an important role in amplifying the inflammatory response.

THERAPEUTIC APPROACHES FOR REDUCING THE EXTENT OF ISCHEMIA-REPERFUSION INJURY

Although the concept of reperfusion injury has become widely accepted, the question remains to what extent reperfusion is involved in the genesis of tissue injury and whether therapeutic intervention would be beneficial. Prevention of events associated with reperfusion, including activation of complement, formation of oxygen-derived free radicals, and neutrophil accumulation, has been shown to be beneficial in preserving reperfused tissues in a number of experimental models. The possibility remains that adjunctive therapy administered at the time of restoration of flow to the ischemic area may serve to decrease the detrimental effects of reperfusion and thereby provide additional therapeutic benefits to the patient. Recognition that the inflammatory response is associated with the pathogenesis of reperfusion injury has provided a number of therapeutic targets intended to optimize salvage of otherwise jeopardized tissues. However, it is apparent that a number of contributing factors are involved in reperfusion injury, and it is likely that an effective therapeutic intervention would require interdiction of several events, including free radical formation and the inflammatory response. Although no "magic bullet" is yet available for reducing the injurious effects associated with ischemia-reperfusion, there are recognized pharmacologic approaches designed to inhibit the individual facets involved in mediating such tissue injury.

Inhibition of Neutrophil Adhesion

As discussed previously, neutrophils, the primary inflammatory cell type involved in the early inflammatory response, mediate tissue injury through the release of reactive oxygen metabolites and degradative enzymes. Therefore, inhibition of neutrophil infiltration or activation may have therapeutic benefit in the setting of reperfusion injury. The primary line of evidence implicating neutrophils in the pathogenesis of reperfusion injury is derived from studies showing that depletion of circulating neutrophils before reperfusion significantly reduces myocardial injury (2). Further support for this hypothesis is provided by the observation that infarct size is directly proportional to the degree of neutrophil infiltration (3). It has been suggested that firm attachment to the endothelium is required for the subsequent migration of the neutrophil out of the vasculature. Lawrence and Springer (80) showed that, at physiologic flow rates, selectin-mediated rolling is a prerequisite for a firm adhesion mediated by integrins. Pharmacologic agents designed to inhibit the adhesion process may reduce the degree of injury mediated by neutrophils and other inflammatory cell types. The role of the neutrophil in reperfusion injury suggests that regulation of the events orchestrating neutrophil influx within the previously ischemic region may be of benefit by preventing extension of tissue injury after reperfusion.

The multistep process by which the neutrophil adheres to the endothelium provides numerous avenues by which to intervene pharmacologically. Past data demonstrating the ability to inhibit β_2 integrin– and selectin-dependent adhesion are summarized in Table 66-1. The first efforts to suppress neutrophil adhesion focused on agents designed to inhibit the adhesive events mediated by the integrins. MAbs directed against the CD11b/CD18 adhesion complex and against ICAM-1 were shown to decrease myocardial infarct size after ischemia-reperfusion (81,82). Other studies focused on the early events of neutrophil adhesion, mediated primarily by the selectin family of adhesion molecules.

The early events of neutrophil adhesion (occurring within minutes) are characterized by "rolling" of the neutrophil along the endothelium, an interaction mediated in part by the endothelial adhesion molecule P-selectin (also known as granule membrane protein (GMP)-140 or platelet activation dependent granule external membrane (PADGEM) (83,84). A variety of approaches have been used to demonstrate that inhibition of selectin-mediated neutrophil adhesion within the previously ischemic tissue leads to a reduction in myocardial infarct size. Ma et al. (85) and Weyrich et al. (86) reported that antibodies directed against L-selectin and P-selectin, respectively, provided protection against myocardial reperfusion injury in the cat. However, the use of antibodies as therapeutic agents has a number of important limitations, including their large size and potential immunogenicity. Low-molecular-weight, synthetic oligosaccharide derivatives of one of the primary ligands for P-selectin, sLe^X, reduce the degree of neutrophil accumulation after reperfusion. However, the carbohydrate-containing synthetic sLe^X mimetics, while retaining the ability to provide protection against reperfusion injury, are costly and difficult to synthesize.

The large number of studies demonstrating a protective effect with the use of inhibitors of neutrophil adhesion suggest that this approach may be reasonable for the development of pharmacologic agents designed to modulate the inflammatory response to injury, thereby leading to maintenance of tissue viability.

The Complement System as a Therapeutic Target

The complement system has multiple roles in the pathogenesis of reperfusion injury, and inactivation or control of the cascade may afford protection against damage attributable to the anaphylatoxins and to assembly of the terminal complement components. The multiplicity of events provides a number of sites at which specific pharmacologic interventions may be targeted.

Complement activation is regulated by a number of plasma- and cell-associated proteins that function to inactivate specific steps of the complement pathway. The so-called regulators of complement activation offer a mechanism for preventing the excessive generation of activated complement products, thus confining the event near the site of injury in an effort to protect normal tissues from complement-mediated "bystander" cell lysis. The membrane-associated regulators of complement activation include complement receptor-1 (CR1), decay accelerating factor (DAF [CD55]) and membrane cofactor protein (MCP [CD56]) and are expressed by almost all cell types, including endothelium, epithelial cells, fibroblasts, and leukocytes. Plasma-associated regulators of complement activation include factor H (alternative pathway inhibitor) and C4bp. The latter, in concert with factor I, splits C4b molecules. In addition, C4bp interferes with the C2a association with C4b and promotes dissociation of C4b2a into C4b and C2a. CD59, an 18- to 20-kd glycoprotein present on many hematopoietic and nonhematopoietic cells, is involved in binding to C8 and preventing insertion of C9 to complete formation of the MAC. The expression and isolation of soluble forms of the membrane- and plasma-associated regulators of complement activation has resulted in their use in experimental models of complement-mediated tissue injury.

Pharmacologic inhibition of the complement cascade is typified by the ability of the soluble form of complement receptor 1 (sCR1) to decrease infarct size in the rat (63). sCR1 is formed by removal of the membrane-spanning and cytoplasmic regions of the protein. CR1 inhibits both the alternative and classic pathways of complement. In addition to its involvement in the processing and clearance of immune complexes with C3b or C4b on their surface, CR1 acts as a cofactor for the proteolysis of C3b and C4b by factor I. In rats subjected to coronary occlusion-reperfusion, the human sCR1 reduced infarct size, neutrophil infiltration, and assembly of cell-associated MAC (63).

In vitro and *in vivo* studies (87) have demonstrated the inhibition of complement activation using human recombinant soluble DAF. DAF accelerates inactivation of the C3 and C5 convertases, a mechanism of action resembling that of endogenous CR1. Zalman et al. (88) isolated a soluble form of homologous restriction factor (HRF, C8 binding protein), which binds C8 and C9 and regulates assembly of the MAC.

A potential disadvantage of complement inhibition during the latter portions of the cascade is that it does not prevent activation of C3 or production of the anaphylatoxins. The recently described complement activation blocker-2 (CAB-2), a molecule that makes up portions of the human complement regulatory proteins MCP and DAF, is another example of how complement-mediated tissue responses may be modulated (89). The complement regulatory proteins are most effective at controlling the activation of homologous complement and the complement of closely related species; they are much less effective regulators of complement from more divergent species (90,91). The availability of other recombinant inhibitors of the complement system is anticipated with enthusiasm.

The lack of sufficient human organs available for transplantation has increased interest in xenotransplantation, with the anticipation that the pig can serve as a source of organs. The pig is considered an attractive species because of its availability in large numbers and its many anatomic and physiologic similarities to humans. Discordant xenotransplantation is accompanied by complement activation, hyperacute rejection, and graft loss in minutes to hours. Because the major barriers in hyperacute rejection include natural antibody, complement activation, and blood coagulation, many means to inhibit these pathways have been developed. Hyperacute rejection, but not subsequent irreversible accelerated acute rejection, can be overcome in discordant cardiac xenografts by various means of complement inhibition, including use of donor organs expressing species-specific transgenic regulators of complement activation, treatment with inhibitors of C5b–9 such as antibodies to C5 and C8 or C6, and treatment with inhibitors of C3 and C5 convertases.

The use of sCR1 is one approach under consideration and has been reported to prolong xenograft survival (92). Complement inhibition with a recombinant sCR1 alone prevented hyperacute rejection of discordant pig-to-cynomolgus monkey cardiac xenografts, but not subsequent irreversible accelerated acute rejection, which occurs within 1 week. To inhibit accelerated acute rejection, which is associated with a rise in serum xenoreactive antibody and a cellular infiltrate, triple therapy with standard immunosuppressive agents (cyclosporine, cyclophosphamide, and steroids) was combined with continuous complement inhibition using sCR1. Monkeys that received sCR1 plus immunosuppressive triple therapy showed minimal evidence of rejection when euthanized on days 21 and 32, compared with controls.

In vitro expression of human regulators of complement activation, such as human DAF (hDAF) or MCP, on the surface of pig cells has been shown to protect them from lysis by human complement (93–95). Hearts from hDAF transgenic pigs are not hyperacutely rejected when they are transplanted heterotopically into the abdomen of cynomolgus monkeys, and prolonged survival can be obtained when such transplantation is combined with immunosuppression (96).

Effective inhibitors of complement are not limited to recently developed compounds. Commonly used therapeutic agents such as the anticoagulant heparin and its inactive derivative *N*-acetylheparin have been implicated in the inhibition of complement activation both *in vivo* and *in vitro* (97). The ability of glycosaminoglycans (including heparin sulfate) to modulate activation of the complement cascade was demonstrated initially by the failure of guinea pig plasma to hemolyze sheep erythrocytes in the presence of heparin sulfate (98). Other studies showed that glycosaminoglycans possessing highly sulfated structural domains are capable of regulating the complement cascade at a variety of steps (99–103). Both heparin and *N*-acetylheparin have been found to protect against tissue injury in experimental models of myocardial ischemia-reperfusion (104–106).

The observations regarding the cardioprotective effects of heparin and *N*-acetylheparin provide support for the concept involving activation of the complement system in ischemia-reperfusion injury. There is sufficient evidence to suggest that the therapeutic uses of heparin may extend beyond its traditional role as an anticoagulant, providing an opportunity to offer therapeutic benefits for a wide range of inflammatory diseases. Saliba et al. (107) demonstrated the effects of heparin in large doses on the extent of myocardial necrosis after left anterior descending coronary artery occlusion in the dog. In addition, it is reported that low-molecular-weight heparin (enoxaparin) reduced infarct size when given systemically immediately before reperfusion (108).

The cytoprotective action of glycosaminoglycans and the lack of dependence on plasma drug concentrations and anticoagulant/antithrombotic activity provide further support for the role of glycosaminoglycans as modulators of the complement cascade (106). Studies suggesting that the glycosaminoglycans inhibit complement activation *in vivo* provide a strong motivation for further examination of related compounds using experimental models of tissue injury in which complement is reported to have a deleterious role (97). Along with the aforementioned reports examining the effects of glycosaminoglycan administration beyond the clinical anticoagulant action, data suggest their potential application as modulators of the immune system in the management of inflammatory states that may involve tissue injury secondary to ischemia and reperfusion. The fact that heparin administration, for purposes of anticoagulation, is routine in the management of patients undergoing coronary artery balloon angioplasty, thrombolytic therapy, and cardiopulmonary bypass would suggest that some degree of protection against complement-mediated injury has unknowingly been put into practice. The opportunity exists to develop heparin derivatives that lack anticoagulant activity but retain other biologic properties, especially those with the potential to control the inflammatory response.

The direct and indirect involvement of complement in the development of a number of pathologies including ischemia-reperfusion injury and transplant rejection lends credence to the belief that the components of the complement system are potential therapeutic targets. Complement has gained the attention of many investigators in the field of molecular biology. New therapeutic agents based on expression of endogenous regulators of complement activation are under development. The future looks encouraging for gaining deeper insight into the importance of the complement system in molecular and cellular biology. The ability to pharmacologically modulate the complement system should provide a better appreciation of its function in health and disease with the anticipation of better management of clinical events secondary to inappropriate activation of the complement cascade.

Although the long-term effects of inhibition of the inflammatory response remain to be determined, the results derived from previous studies provide convincing arguments for limited-duration inhibition of inflammation as a therapeutic tool for the reduction of cellular injury. It should be noted that therapeutic strategies designed to inhibit one facet of inflammation may have profound effects on other aspects of the inflammatory response. For example, inhibition of complement would not only eliminate the direct effects of complement activation mediated primarily by the anaphylatoxins and MAC but also decrease the intensity of the inflammatory response. The protection afforded by inhibiting the inflammation would benefit not only the myocardium but also any tissue or organ that has been subjected to a period of ischemia followed by reperfusion. Among the areas of consideration is that which involves the inflammatory response to tissue or organ ischemia that is exacerbated further by reperfusion. The development of pharmacologic interventions to modulate inflammation represents an area of importance that is in need of continued research.

REFERENCES

1. McCord JM. Oxygen-derived free radicals in postischemic tissue injury. *N Engl J Med* 1985;312:159–163.
2. Romson JL, Hook BG, Kunkel SS, Abrams GD, Schork MA, Lucchesi BR. Reduction of the extent of ischemic myocardial injury by neutrophil depletion in the dog. *Circulation* 1983;67:1016–1020.
3. Mullane KM, Read N, Salmon JA, Moncada S. Role of leukocytes in acute myocardial infarction in anesthetized dogs: relationship to myocardial salvage by anti-inflammatory drugs. *J Pharmacol Exp Ther* 1984;228:510–522.
4. Eppinger MJ, Jones ML, Deeb GM, Bolling SF, Ward PA. Pattern of injury and the role of neutrophils in reperfusion injury of rat lung. *J Surg Res* 1995;58:713–718.
5. Forbes TL, Harris KA, Jamieson WG, DeRose G, Carson M, Potter RF. Leukocyte activity and tissue injury following ischemia-reperfusion in skeletal muscle. *Microvasc Res* 1996;51:275–287.
6. Matsuo Y, Onodera H, Shiga Y, et al. Correlation between myeloperoxidase-quantified neutrophil accumulation and ischemic brain injury in the rat: effects of neutrophil depletion. *Stroke* 1994b;25:1469–1475.
7. Zimmerman BJ, Granger DN. Mechanisms of reperfusion injury. *Am J Med Sci* 1994;307:284–292.
8. Bienvenu K, Granger DN. Leukocyte adhesion in ischemia/reperfusion. *Blood Cells* 1993;19:279–288; discussion 288–289.
9. Massey KD, Strieter RM, Kunkel SL, Danforth JM, Standiford TJ. Cardiac myocytes release leukocyte-stimulating factors. *Am J Physiol* 1995;269:H980–H987.
10. Colletti LM, Kunkel SL, Walz A, et al. The role of cytokine networks in the local liver injury following hepatic ischemia/reperfusion in the rat. *Hepatology* 1996;23:506–514.
11. Ivey CL, Williams FM, Collins PD, Jose PJ, Williams TJ. Neutrophil chemoattractants generated in two phases during reperfusion of ischemic myocardium in the rabbit: evidence for a role for C5a and interleukin-8. *J Clin Invest* 1995;95:2720–2728.
12. Yamasaki Y, Matsuo Y, Matsuura N, Onodera H, Itoyama Y, Kogure K. Transient increase of cytokine-induced neutrophil chemoattractant, a member of the interleukin-8 family, in ischemic brain areas after focal ischemia in rats. *Stroke* 1995;26:318–322; discussion 322–323.
13. Clark WM, Lauten JD, Lessov N, Woodward W, Coull BM. Time course of ICAM-1 expression and leukocyte subset infiltration in rat forebrain ischemia. *Mol Chem Neuropathol* 1995;26:213–230.
14. Haring HP, Berg EL, Tsurushita N, Tagaya M, del Zoppo GJ. E-selectin appears in nonischemic tissue during experimental focal cerebral ischemia. *Stroke* 1996;27:1386–1391; discussion 1391–1392.
15. Hawkins HK, Entman ML, Zhu JY, et al. Acute inflammatory reaction after myocardial ischemic injury and reperfusion: development and use of a neutrophil-specific antibody. *Am J Pathol* 1996;148:1957–1969.
16. Youker KA, Hawkins HK, Kukielka GL, et al. Molecular evidence for a border zone vulnerable to inflammatory reperfusion injury. *Trans Assoc Am Physicians* 1993;106:145–154.
17. Youker KA, Hawkins HK, Kukielka GL, et al. Molecular evidence for induction of intracellular adhesion molecule-1 in the viable border zone associated with ischemia-reperfusion injury of the dog heart. *Circulation* 1994;89:2736–2746.
18. Shen I, Verrier ED. Expression of E-selectin on coronary endothelium after myocardial ischemia and reperfusion. *J Card Surg* 1994;9:437–441.
19. Stokes KY, Abdih HK, Kelly CJ, Redmond HP, Bouchier-Hayes DJ. Thermotolerance attenuates ischemia-reperfusion induced renal injury and increased expression of ICAM-1. *Transplantation* 1996;62:1143–1149.

20. Billups KL, Palladina MA, Hinton BT, Sherley JL. Expression of E-selectin mRNA during ischemia/reperfusion injury. *J Lab Clin Med* 1995;125:626–633.

21. Wyble CW, Desai TR, Clark ET, Hynes KL, Gewertz BL. Physiologic concentrations of TNFalpha and IL-1beta released from reperfused human intestine upregulate E-selectin and ICAM-1. *J Surg Res* 1996; 63:333–338.

22. Weyrich AS, Buerke M, Albertine KH, Lefer AM. Time course of coronary vascular endothelial adhesion molecule expression during reperfusion of the ischemic feline myocardium. *J Leukoc Biol* 1995; 57:45–55.

23. Kelly KH, Williams WW Jr, Colvin RB, et al. Intercellular adhesion molecule-1-deficient mice are protected against ischemic renal injury. *J Clin Invest* 1996;97:1056–1063.

24. Soriano SG, Lipton SA, Wang YF, et al. Intercellular adhesion molecule-1-deficient mice are less susceptible to cerebral ischemia-reperfusion injury. *Ann Neurol* 1996;39:618–624.

25. Connolly ES Jr, Winfree CJ, Springer TA, et al. Cerebral protection in homozygous null ICAM-1 mice after middle cerebral artery occlusion: role of neutrophil adhesion in the pathogenesis of stroke. *J Clin Invest* 1996;97:209–216.

26. Haller H, Dragun D, Miethke A, et al. Antisense oligonucleotides for ICAM-1 attenuate reperfusion injury and renal failure in the rat. *Kidney Int* 1996;50:473–480.

27. Gill EA, King Y, Horwitz LD. An oligosaccharide sialyl-Lewis(x) analogue does not reduce myocardial infarct size after ischemia and reperfusion in dogs. *Circulation* 1996;94:542–546.

28. Forbes AD, Slimp JC, Winn RK, Verrier ED. Inhibition of neutrophil adhesion does not prevent ischemic spinal cord injury. *Ann Thorac Surg* 1994;58:1064–1068.

29. Thomas DD, Sharar SR, Winn RK, et al. CD18-independent mechanism of neutrophil emigration in the rabbit lung after ischemia-reperfusion. *Ann Thorac Surg* 1995;60:1360–1366.

30. Gibbs SA, Weiser MR, Kobzik L, Valeri CR, Shepro D, Hechtman HB. P-selectin mediates intestinal ischemic injury by enhancing complement deposition. *Surgery* 1996;199:652–656.

31. Haug CE, Colvin RB, Delmonico FL, et al. A phase 1 trial of immunosuppression with anti-ICAM-1 (CD54) mAb in renal allograft recipients. *Transplantation* 1993;55:766–772; discussion 772–773.

32. Ko W, Hawes AS, Lazenby WD, et al. Myocardial reperfusion injury: platelet-activating factor stimulates polymorphonuclear leukocyte hydrogen peroxide production during myocardial reperfusion. *J Thorac Cardiovasc Surg* 1991;102:297–308.

33. Gasic AC, McGuire G, Krater S, et al. Hydrogen peroxide pretreatment of perfused canine vessels induces ICAM-1 and CD-18-dependent neutrophil adherence. *Circulation* 1991;84:2154–2166.

34. Werns SW, Lucchesi BR. Myocardial ischemia and reperfusion: the role of oxygen radicals in tissue injury. *Cardiovasc Drugs Ther* 1989; 2:761–769.

35. Schmid-Schonbein GW, Engler RL. Granulocytes as active participants in acute myocardial ischemia and infarction. *Am J Cardiovasc Pathol* 1986;1:15–30.

36. Mullane K. Neutrophil and endothelial changes in reperfusion injury. *Trends Cardiovasc Med* 1991;1:282–289.

37. Rossen RD, Swain JL, Michael LH, Weakley S, Giannini E, Entman ML. Selective accumulation of the first component of complement and leukocytes in ischemic canine heart muscle: a possible initiator of an extra myocardial mechanism of ischemic injury. *Circ Res* 1985;57: 119–130.

38. Vakeva A, Morgan BP, Tikkanen I, Helin K, Laurila P, Meri S. Time course of complement activation and inhibitor expression after ischemic injury of rat myocardium. *Am J Pathol* 1994;144:1357–1368.

39. McManus LM, Kolb WP, Crawford MH, O'Rourke RA, Grover FL, Pinckard RN. Complement localization in ischemic baboon myocardium. *Lab Invest* 1983;48:436–447.

40. Langlois PF, Gawryl MS. Detection of the terminal complement complex in patient plasma following acute myocardial infarction. *Atherosclerosis* 1985;70:95–105.

41. Rus HG, Niculescu F, Vlaicu R. Presence of C5b-9 complement complex and S-protein in infarcted areas with necrosis and sclerosis. *Immunol Lett* 1987;16:15–20.

42. Schafer H, Mathey D, Hugo F, Bhakdi S. Deposition of the terminal C5b-9 complement complex in infarcted areas of human myocardium. *J Immunol* 1986;137:1945–1949.

43. Yasuda M, Kawarabayashi T, Akioka K, et al. The complement system in the acute phase of myocardial infarction. *Jpn Circ J* 1989;53: 1017–1022.

44. Semb AG, Vaage J, Sorlie D, Lie M, Mjos OD. Coronary trapping of a complement activation product (C3a des-Arg) during myocardial reperfusion in open-heart surgery. *Scand J Thorac Cardiovasc Surg* 1990;24:223–227.

45. Vogt W, von Zabern I, Hesse D, Nolte R, Haller Y. Generation of an activated form of human C5 (C5b-like C5) by oxygen radicals. *Immunol Lett* 1986;14:209–215.

46. Vogt W, Damerau B, von Zabern I, Nolte R, Brunahl D. Nonenzymatic activation of the fifth component of human complement, by oxygen radicals: some properties of the activation product, C5b-like C5. *Mol Immunol* 1989;26:1133–1142.

47. Shingu M, Nonaka S, Nishimukai H, Nobunaga M, Kitamura H, Tomo-Oka K. Activation of the complement in normal serum by hydrogen peroxide and hydrogen peroxide-related oxygen radicals produced by activated neutrophils. *Clin Exp Immunol* 1992;90:72–78.

48. Vogt W. Complement activation by myeloperoxidase products released from stimulated human polymorphonuclear leukocytes. *Immunobiology* 1996;195:334–346.

49. Williams JD, Czop JK, Abrahamson DR, Davies M, Austen KF. Activation of the alternative pathway by isolated human glomerular basement membranes. *J Immunol* 1984;133:394–399.

50. Rossen RD, Michael LH, Kagiyama A, et al. Mechanism of complement activation following coronary artery occlusion: evidence that myocardial ischemia causes release of constituents of myocardial subcellular origin which complex with the first component of complement. *Circ Res* 1988;62:572–584.

51. Vakeva A, Laurila P, Meri S. Regulation of complement membrane attack complex formation in myocardial infarction. *Am J Pathol* 1993; 143:65–75.

52. Frangi D, Gardinali M, Conciato L, Cafaro C, Pozzoni L, Agostoni A. Abrupt complement activation and transient neutropenia in patients with acute myocardial infarction treated with streptokinase. *Circulation* 1994;89:76–80.

53. Agostoni A, Gardinali M, Frangi D, et al. Activation of complement and kinin systems after thrombolytic therapy in patients with acute myocardial infarction: a comparison between streptokinase and recombinant tissue-type plasminogen activator. *Circulation* 1994b;90: 2666–2670.

54. Agostoni A, Gardinali M, Frangi D, et al. Thrombolytic treatment and complement activation. *Ann Ital Med Int* 1994a;9:178–179.

55. Bennet WR, Young DH, Migliore PJ, et al. Activation of the complement system by recombinant tissue plasminogen activator. *J Am Coll Cardiol* 1987;10:627–632.

56. Roberts R, Bolli R. Activation of the complement system by recombinant tissue plasminogen activator. *J Am Coll Cardiol* 1987;10: 627–632.

57. Walport M. Complement. In: Roitt IM, Brostoff J, Male DK, eds. *Immunology*, 2nd ed. St Louis: CV Mosby, 1985:13.1–13.16.

58. Hugli TE. The chemistry and biology of C3a, C4a and C5a and their effects on cell. In: August JT, ed. *Biological response mediators and modulators*. New York: Academic Press, 1983:99–116.

59. Foreman KE, Vaporciyan AA, Bonish BK, et al. C5a-induced expression of P-selectin in endothelial cells. *J Clin Invest* 1994;94:1147–1155.

60. Shandelya SM, Kuppusamy P, Weisfeldt ML, Zweier JL. Evaluation of the role of polymorphonuclear leukocytes on contractile function in myocardial reperfusion injury: evidence for plasma-mediated leukocyte activation. *Circulation* 1993b;87:536–546.

61. Amsterdam EA, Stahl GL, Pan HL, Rendig SV, Fletcher MP, Longhurst JC. Limitation of reperfusion injury by a monoclonal antibody to C5a during myocardial infarction in pigs. *Am J Physiol* 1995;268:H448–H457.

62. Maclean D, Fishbein MC, Braunwald E, Marko PR. Long term preservation of ischaemic myocardium after experimental coronary artery occlusion. *J Clin Invest* 1978;61:541—551.

63. Weisman HF, Bartow T, Leppo MK, et al. Soluble human complement receptor type 1: *in vivo* inhibitor of complement suppressing postischemic myocardial inflammation and necrosis. *Science* 1990;249: 146–151.

64. Mathey D, Schofer J, Schafer HJ, et al. Early accumulation of the terminal complement-complex in the ischemic myocardium after reperfusion. *Eur Heart J* 1994;15:418–423.

65. Ito W, Schafer HJ, Bhakdi S, Klask R, Hansen S. Influence of the terminal complement-complex on reperfusion injury, no-reflow and arrythmias: a comparison between C6-competent and C6-deficient rabbits. *Cardiovasc Res* 1996;32:294–305.

66. Morgan BP. Complement membrane attack on nucleated cells: resistance, recovery and non-lethal effects. *Biochem J* 1989;264:1–14.

67. Hattori R, Hamilton KK, McEver RP, Sims PJ. Complement proteins C5b-9 induce secretion of high molecular weight multimers of endothelial von Willebrand factor and translocation of granule membrane protein GMP-140 to the cell surface. *J Biol Chem* 1989;264:9053–9060.

68. Kilgore KS, Shen J, Miller BF, Ward PA, Warren JS. Enhancement by the complement membrane attack complex of tumor necrosis factor-α-induced endothelial cell expression of ICAM-1 and E-selectin. *J Immunol* 1995;155:1434–1441.

69. Lovett DG, Haensch GM, Goppelt M, Resch K, Gemsa D. Activation of glomerular mesangial cells by the terminal membrane attack complex of complement. *J Immunol* 1987;138:2473–2481.

70. Schonermark M, Deppisch R, Riedasch G, Rother K, Hansch GM. Induction of mediator release from human glomerular mesangial cells by the terminal complement components C5b-9. *Int Arch Allergy Appl Immunol* 1991;96:331–341.

71. Kilgore KS, Flory CM, Miller BF, Evans VM, Warren JS. The membrane attack complex of complement induces interleukin-8 and monocyte chemoattractant protein-1 secretion from human umbilical vein endothelial cells. *Am J Pathol* 1996;149:953–961.

72. Carney DF, Lang TJ, Shin ML. Multiple signal messengers generated by terminal complement complexes and their role in terminal complement complex elimination. *J Immunol* 1990;145:623–629.

73. Nicholson-Weller A, Happerin JA. Membrane signaling by complement C5b-9, the membrane attack complex. *Immunol Res* 1993;12:244–257.

74. Becker LC, Ambrosio G. Myocardial consequences of reperfusion. *Prog Cardiovasc Dis* 1987;30:23–44.

75. Jennings RB, Schaper J, Hill ML, Steenbergen C Jr, Reimer KA. Effect of reperfusion late in the phase of reversible ischemic injury: changes in cell volume, electrolytes, metabolites and ultrastructure. *Circ Res* 1985;56:262–278.

76. Wiedmer T, Ando B, Sims PJ. Complement C5b-9-stimulated platelet secretion is associated with a Ca2+-initiated activation of cellular protein kinases. *J Biol Chem* 1987;262:13674–13681.

77. Niculescu F, Rus H, Shin ML. Receptor-independent activation of guanine nucleotide-binding regulatory proteins by terminal complement complexes. *J Biol Chem* 1994;269:4417–4423.

78. Lenard MJ, Baltimore D. NF-κB: a pleiotropic mediator of inducible and tissue-specific gene control. *Cell* 1988;7:318–332.

79. Kilgore KS, Schmid E, Shanley TP, et al. Sublytic concentrations of the membrane attack complex of complement induce endothelial interleukin-8 and monocyte chemoattractant protein-1 through nuclear factor-kappa B activation. *Am J Pathol* 1997;150:2019–2031.

80. Lawrence MB, Springer TA. Leukocytes roll on a selectin at physiologic flow rates: distinction from and prerequisite for adhesion through integrins. *Cell* 1991;65:859–863.

81. Simpson PJ, Todd RF III, Fantone JC, Mickelson JK, Griffin JD, Lucchesi BR. Reduction of experimental myocardial reperfusion injury by a monoclonal antibody (anti-Mol, anti-CD11b) that inhibits leukocyte adhesion. *J Clin Invest* 1988;81:624–629.

82. Ma XL, Tsao PS, Lefer AM. Antibody to CD-18 exerts endothelial and cardioprotective effects in myocardial ischemia and reperfusion. *J Clin Invest* 1991;88:127–143.

83. Jutila MA, Rott L, Berg EL, Butcher EC. Function and regulation of the neutrophil MEL-14 antigen *in vivo*: comparison with LFA-1 and MAC-1. *J Immunol* 1989;143:3318–3323.

84. Kishimoto TM, Jutila MA, Berg EL, Butcher EC. Neutrophil Mac-1 and MEL-14 adhesion proteins inversely regulated by chemotactic factors. *Science* 1989;245:1238–1241.

85. Ma X-L, Weyrich AS, Lefer DJ, et al. Monoclonal antibody to L-selectin attenuates neutrophil accumulation and protects ischemic reperfused cat myocardium. *Circulation* 1993;88:649–653.

86. Weyrich AS, Ma X-L, Lefer DJ, Albertine KH, Lefer AM. *In vivo* neutralization of P-selectin protects feline heart and endothelium in myocardial ischemia and reperfusion injury. *J Clin Invest* 1993;91:2620–2629.

87. Moran P, Beasley H, Gorrell A, et al. Human recombinant soluble decay accelerating factor inhibits complement activation *in vitro* and *in vivo*. *J Immunol* 1992;149:1736–1743.

88. Zalman LS, Brothers MA, Muller-Eberhard HJ. Isolation of homologous restriction factor from human urine: immunochemical properties and biologic activity. *J Immunol* 1989;143:1943–1947.

89. Ko J-L, Lobell R, Sardonini C, Alessi MK, Yeh CG. A soluble chimeric complement inhibitory protein that possesses both decay-accelerating and factor I cofactor activities. *J Immunol* 1997;158:2872–2881.

90. Rollins SA, Zhao J, Ninomiya H, Sims PJ. Inhibition of homologous complement by CD59 is mediated by a species-selective recognition conferred through binding to C8 within C5b-8 or C9 within C5b-9. *J Immunol* 1991;146:2345–2351.

91. Ninomiya H, Sims PJ. The human complement regulatory protein CD59 binds to the α-chain of C8 and to the "b" domain of C9. *J Biol Chem* 1992;267:13675–13680.

92. Davis EA, Pruitt SK, Greene PS, et al. Inhibition of complement, evoked antibody, and cellular response prevents rejection of pig-to-primate cardiac xenografts. *Transplantation* 1996;62:1018–1023.

93. Fodor WL, Williams BL, Matis LA, et al. Expression of a functional human complement inhibitor in a transgenic pig as a model for the prevention of xenogeneic hyperacute organ rejection. *Proc Natl Acad Sci U S A* 1994;91:11153–11157.

94. Rosengard AM, Cary N, Horsley J, et al. Endothelial expression of human decay accelerating factor in transgenic pig tissue: a potential approach for human complement inactivation in discordant xenografts. *Transplant Proc* 1995;27:326–327.

95. McCurry KR, Kooyman DL, Diamond LE, et al. Human complement regulatory proteins in transgenic animals regulate complement activation in xenoperfused organs. *Transplant Proc* 1995;27:317–318.

96. Waterworth PD, Cozzi E, Tolan MJ, et al. Pig-to-primate cardiac xenotransplantation and cyclophosphamide therapy. *Transplant Proc* 1997;29:899–900.

97. Weiler JM, Edens RE, Linhardt RJ, Kapelanski DP. Heparin and modified heparin inhibit complement activation *in vivo*. *J Immunol* 1992;148:3210–3215.

98. Ecker EE, Gross P. Anticomplementary power of heparin. *J Infect Dis* 1929;44:250–253.

99. Baker PJ, Lint TF, McLeod BC, Behrends CL, Gewurz H. Studies on the inhibition of C56-induced lysis (reactive lysis): VI. Modulation of C56-induced lysis polyanions and polycations. *J Immunol* 1975;114:554–558.

100. Loos M, Volanakis JE, Stroud RM. Mode of interaction of different polyanions with the first (C1, C1), the second (C2) and the fourth (C4) component of complement—II. Effect of polyanions on the binding of C2 to EAC4b. *Immunochemistry* 1976;13:257–261.

101. Sharath MD, Merchant ZM, Kim YS, Rice KG, Linhardt RJ, Weiler JM. Small heparin fragments regulate the amplification pathway of complement. *Immunopharmacology* 1985;9:73–80.

102. Meri S, Pangburn MK. Discrimination between activators and non-activators of the alternative pathway of complement: regulation via a sialic acid/polyanion binding site on factor H. *Proc Natl Acad Sci U S A* 1990;87:3982–3986.

103. Meri S, Pangburn MK. Regulation of alternative pathway complement activation by glycosaminoglycans: specificity of the polyanion binding site on factor H. *Biochem Biophys Res Commun* 1994;198:52–59.

104. Friedrichs GS, Kilgore KS, Manley PJ, Gralinski MR, Lucchesi BR. Effects of heparin and *N*-acetyl heparin on ischemia/reperfusion-induced alterations in myocardial function in the rabbit isolated heart. *Circ Res* 1974;75:701–710.

105. Black SC, Gralinski MR, Friedrichs GS, Kilgore KS, Driscoll EM, Lucchesi BR. Cardioprotective effects of heparin or *N*-acetylheparin in an *in vivo* model of myocardial ischaemic and reperfusion injury. *Cardiovasc Res* 1995;29:629–636.

106. Gralinski MR, Driscoll EM, Friedrichs GS, DeNardis MR, Lucchesi BR. Reduction of myocardial necrosis after glycosaminoglycan administration: effects of a single intravenous administration of heparin or *N*-acetylheparin 2 hours before regional ischemia and reperfusion. *J Cardiovasc Pharmacol Ther* 1996a;1:219–228.

107. Saliba M Jr, Covell JW, Bloor CM. Effects of heparin in large doses on the extent of myocardial ischemia after acute coronary occlusion in the dog. *Am J Cardiol* 1976;37:599–604.

108. Libersan D, Khalil A, Quan E, Kallaayoune R, Tran D, Latour JG. The

low molecular weight heparin: enoxaparin reduces infarct size when given at reperfusion in untreated and streptokinase-treated dogs [abstract]. *J Mol Cell Cardiol* 1993;25(Suppl III):S90.

109. Lefer DJ, Flynn DM, Phillips ML, Ratcliffe M, Buda AJ. A novel sialyl Lewis X analog attenuates neutrophil accumulation and myocardial necrosis after ischemia and reperfusion. *Circulation* 1994;90:2390–2401.

110. Flynn DM, Buda AJ, Jeffords PR, Lefer DJ. A sialyl Lewis(x)-containing carbohydrate reduces infarct size: role of selectins in myocardial reperfusion injury. *Am J Physiol* 1996;271:H2086–H2096.

111. Buerke M, Weyrich AS, Zheng Z, Gaeta FC, Forrest MJ, Lefer AM. Sialyl Lewis x-containing oligosaccharide attenuates myocardial reperfusion injury in cats. *J Clin Invest* 1994;93:1140–1148.

112. Murohara T, Margiotta J, Phillips LM, et al. Cardioprotection by liposome-conjugated sialyl Lewisx-oligosaccharide in myocardial ischaemia and reperfusion injury. *Cardiovasc Res* 1995;30:965–974.

113. Miura T, Nelson DP, Schermerhorn ML, et al. Blockade of selectin-mediated leukocyte adhesion improves postischemic function in lamb hearts. *Ann Thorac Surg* 1996;62:1295–1300.

114. Matsuo Y, Onodera H, Shiga Y, et al. Role of cell adhesion molecules in brain injury after transient middle cerebral artery occlusion in the rat. *Brain Res* 1994a;656:344–352.

115. Chen H, Chopp M, Zhang RL, et al. Anti-CD11b monoclonal antibody reduces ischemic cell damage after transient focal cerebral ischemia in rat. *Ann Neurol* 1994;35:458–463.

116. Mori E, del Zoppo GJ, Chambers JD, Copeland BR, Arfors KE. Inhibition of polymorphonuclear leukocyte adherence suppresses no-reflow after focal cerebral ischemia in baboons. *Stroke* 1992;23:712–718.

117. Lindsberg PJ, Siren AL, Feuerstein GZ, Hallenbeck JM. Antagonism of neutrophil adherence in the deteriorating stroke model in rabbits. *J Neurosurg* 1995;82:269–277.

118. Bowes MP, Zivin JA, Rothlein R. Monoclonal antibody to the ICAM-1 adhesion site reduces neurological damage in a rabbit cerebral embolism stroke model. *Exp Neurol* 1993;119:215–219.

119. Zhang RL, Chopp M, Zhang ZG, et al. E-selectin in focal cerebral ischemia and reperfusion in the rat. *J Cereb Blood Flow Metab* 1996;16:1126–1136.

120. Adkins WK, Taylor AE. Role of xanthine oxidase and neutrophils in ischemia-reperfusion injury in rabbit lung. *J Appl Physiol* 1990;69:2012–2018.

121. Moore TM, Khimenko P, Adkins WK, Miyasaka M, Taylor AE. Adhesion molecules contribute to ischemia and reperfusion-induced injury in the isolated rat lung. *J Appl Physiol* 1995;78:2245–2252.

122. Buchanan SA, Mauney MC, deLima NF, et al. Enhanced isolated lung function after ischemia with anti-intercellular adhesion molecule antibody. *J Thorac Cardiovasc Surg* 1996;111:941–947.

123. Steinberg JB, Mao HZ, Niles SD, Jutila MA, Kapelanski DP. Survival in lung reperfusion injury is improved by an antibody that binds and inhibits L- and E-selectin. *J Heart Lung Transplant* 1994;13:306–318.

124. Carden DL, Young JA, Granger DN. Pulmonary microvascular injury after intestinal ischemia-reperfusion: role of P-selectin. *J Appl Physiol* 1993;75:2529–2534.

125. Rabb H, Mendiola CC, Dietz J, et al. Role of CD11a and CD11b in ischemic acute renal failure in rats. *Am J Physiol* 1994;267:F1052–F1058.

126. Booster M, Yin M, Kurvers HA, et al. Inhibition of CD18-dependent leukocyte adherence by mAb 6.5E does not prevent ischemia-reperfusion injury as seen in grafted kidneys. *Transplant Int* 1995;8:126–132.

127. Rabb H, Mendiola CC, Saba SR, et al. Antibodies to ICAM-1 protect kidneys in severe ischemic reperfusion injury. *Biochem Biophys Res Commun* 1995;211:67–73.

128. Linas SL, Whittenburg D, Parsons PE, Repine JE. Ischemia increases neutrophil retention and worsens acute renal failure: role of oxygen metabolites and ICAM 1. *Kidney Int* 1995;48:1584–1591.

129. Kelly KJ, Williams WW Jr, Colvin RB, Bonventre JV. Antibody to intercellular adhesion molecule 1 protects the kidney against ischemic injury. *Proc Natl Acad Sci U S A* 1994;91:812–816.

130. Kurose I, Anderson DC, Miyasaka M, et al. Molecular determinants of reperfusion-induced leukocyte adhesion and vascular protein leakage. *Circ Res* 1994;74:336–343.

131. Koike K, Moore EE, Moore FA, Francoise RJ, Fontes B, Kim FJ.

CD11b blockade prevents lung injury despite neutrophil priming after gut ischemia/reperfusion. *J Trauma* 1995;39:23–27.

132. Hernandez LA, Grisham MB, Twohig B, Arfors KE, Harlan JM, Granger DN. Role of neutrophils in ischemia-reperfusion-induced microvascular injury. *Am J Physiol* 1987;253:H699–H703.

133. Slocum MM, Granger DN. Early mucosal and microvascular changes in feline intestinal transplants. *Gastroenterology* 1993;105:1761–1768.

134. Hill J, Lindsay T, Valeri CR, Shepro D, Hechtman HB. A CD18 antibody prevents lung injury but not hypotension after intestinal ischemia-reperfusion. *J Appl Physiol* 1993;74:659–664.

135. Kubes PM, Jutila M, Payne D. Therapeutic potential of inhibiting leukocyte rolling in ischemia/reperfusion. *J Clin Invest* 1995;95:2510–2519.

136. Liu P, McGuire GM, Fisher MA, Farhood A, Smith CW, Jaeschke H. Activation of Kupffer cells and neutrophils for reactive oxygen formation is responsible for endotoxin-enhanced liver injury after hepatic ischemia. *Shock* 1995;3:56–62.

137. Vollmar B, Glasz J, Menger MD, Messmer K. Leukocytes contribute to hepatic ischemia/reperfusion injury via intercellular adhesion molecule 1-mediated venular adherence. *Surgery* 1995;117:195–200.

138. Farhood A, McGuire GM, Manning AM, Miyasaka M, Smith CW, Jaeschke H. Intercellular adhesion molecule 1 (ICAM-1) expression and its role in neutrophil-induced ischemia-reperfusion injury in rat liver. *J Leukoc Biol* 1995;57:368–374.

139. Garcia-Criado FJ, Toledo-Pereyra LH, Lopez-Neblina F, Phillips ML, Paez-Rollys A, Misawa K. Role of P-selectin in total hepatic ischemia and reperfusion. *J Am Coll Surg* 1995;181:327–334.

140. Misawa K, Toledo-Pereyra LH, Phillips ML, Garcia-Cirado FJ, Lopez-Neblina F, Paez-Rollys A. Role of sialyl Lewis(x) in total hepatic ischemia and reperfusion. *J Am Coll Surg* 1996;182:251–256.

141. Seekamp A, Mulligan MS, Till GO, et al. Role of beta 2 integrins and ICAM-1 in lung injury following ischemia-reperfusion of rat hind limbs. *Am J Pathol* 1993;143:464–472.

142. Crinnion JN, Homer-Vanniasinkam S, Parkin SM, Gough MJ. Role of neutrophil-endothelial adhesion in skeletal muscle reperfusion injury. *Br J Surg* 1996;83:251–254.

143. Nolte D, Hecht R, Schmid P, et al. Role of Mac-1 and ICAM-1 in ischemia-reperfusion injury in a microcirculation model of BALB/C mice. *Am J Physiol* 1994;267:H1320–H1328.

144. Petrasek PF, Liauw S, Romaschin AD, Walker PM. Salvage of postischemic skeletal muscle by monoclonal antibody blockade of neutrophil adhesion molecule CD18. *J Surg Res* 1994;56:5–12.

145. Seekamp A, Till GO, Mulligan MS, et al. Role of selectins in local and remote tissue injury following ischemia and reperfusion. *Am J Pathol* 1994;144:592–598.

146. Mihelcic D, Schleiffenbaum B, Tedder TF, Sharar SR, Harlan JM, Winn RK. Inhibition of leukocyte L-selectin function with a monoclonal antibody attenuates reperfusion injury to the rabbit ear. *Blood* 1994;84:2322–2328.

147. Winn RK, Liggitt D, Vedder NB, Paulson JC, Harlan JM. Anti-P-selectin monoclonal antibody attenuates reperfusion injury to the rabbit ear. *J Clin Invest* 1993;92:2042–2047.

148. Lee WP, Gribling P, De Guzman L, Ehsani N, Watson SR. A P-selectin-immunoglobulin G chimera is protective in a rabbit ear model of ischemia-reperfusion. *Surgery* 1995;117:458–465.

149. Han KT, Sharar SR, Phillips ML, Harlan JM, Winn RK. Sialyl Lewis(x) oligosaccharide reduces ischemia-reperfusion injury in the rabbit ear. *J Immunol* 1995;155:4011–4015.

150. Vedder NB, Fouty BW, Winn RK, Harlan JM, Rice CL. Role of neutrophils in generalized reperfusion injury associated with resuscitation from shock. *Surgery* 1989;106:509–516.

151. Vedder NB, Winn RK, Rice CL, Chi EY, Arfors KE, Harlan JM. A monoclonal antibody to the adherence-promoting leukocyte glycoprotein, CD18, reduces organ injury and improves survival from hemorrhagic shock and resuscitation in rabbits. *J Clin Invest* 1988;81:939–944.

152. Ramamoorthy C, Sharar SR, Harlan JM, Tedder TF, Winn RK. Blocking L-selectin function attenuates reperfusion injury following hemorrhagic shock in rabbits. *Am J Physiol* 1996;271:H1871–H1877.

153. Skurk C, Buerke M, Guo JP, Paulson J, Lefer AM. Sialyl Lewis x-containing oligosaccharide exerts beneficial effects in murine traumatic shock. *J Appl Physiol* 1994;267:H2124–H2131.

Inflammation: Basic Principles and Clinical Correlates,
3rd ed., edited by John I. Gallin and Ralph Snyderman.
Lippincott Williams & Wilkins, Philadelphia © 1999.

CHAPTER 67

Inflammatory Lung Disease:

Molecular Determinants of Emphysema, Bronchitis, and Fibrosis

Khavar J. Dar and Ronald G. Crystal

The term *inflammatory lung disease* encompasses both acute and chronic disorders that are characterized by the accumulation of inflammatory cells within the parenchyma of the respiratory tract. The inflammation is usually referred to by its major anatomic location with terms such as "alveolitis," "bronchitis," and "vasculitis." Although the lung inflammation may represent only a component of an underlying systemic inflammatory disorder such as a collagen-vascular disease, many of the inflammatory disorders of the lung are localized exclusively to lung tissues. The purpose of this chapter is to examine current principles underlying the pathogenesis of the inflammatory lung disorders and the role of these principles in the development of rational strategies for therapy. The focus is on three common chronic inflammatory lung diseases: emphysema, bronchitis, and fibrosis (Fig. 67-1).

The anatomy of the lung is similar to that of an upside-down tree: the trachea and bronchi serve as the trunk and branches, respectively, and the alveoli serve as the leaves. The tracheobronchial tree is a branching structure with an internal surface area of 1 to 2 m^2. At the 22nd to 23rd branches, the airways open into the alveoli, a 130- to 150-m^2 surface where gas exchange takes place (1,2). The pulmonary artery branches successively to form the alveolar capillaries, which then regroup to form the pulmonary veins.

It is in the context of this anatomy that the potential consequences of inflammation become apparent. The lung is chronically exposed to the outside environment with the attendant xenobiotics present in ambient air (3). Furthermore, the lung receives the entire cardiac output, constituting the venous return of all organs. Large numbers of neutrophils marginate in the pulmonary capillary bed in normal persons (4). In addition, the epithelial surface of the normal lung contains inflammatory cells in numbers comparable to those of blood (5). Normally, this population is dominated by mononuclear phagocytes (17×10^3 "alveolar" macrophages per microliter of epithelial lining fluid [ELF]), with lesser numbers of T lymphocytes (4×10^3/μL ELF) and neutrophils (150/μL ELF). Taken together, these features make it easy to conceptualize the lung as an "inflammation time bomb" awaiting the appropriate signal to initiate an inflammatory lung disorder (4,6,7).

The concept of the lung as a focus for localized inflammation was recognized by histologic studies in the 19th century. However, it was not until the late 1970s that modern biologic methods were applied to defining the character of the inflammation. With the adaptation of the fiberoptic bronchoscope and bronchoalveolar lavage to access the ELF of the human lung, it became possible to quantify the types and numbers of inflammatory cells present, the inflammatory mediators that these cells were releasing, and the defenses operating within the lung to protect the airways and alveoli from inflammatory injury (4–7).

EMPHYSEMA

Emphysema is defined as abnormal permanent enlargement of the airspaces distal to the terminal bron-

K. J. Dar and R. G. Crystal: Division of Pulmonary and Critical Care Medicine, The New York Hospital—Cornell Medical Center, New York, New York 10021.

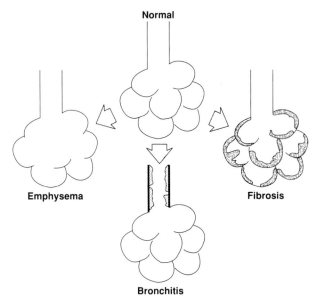

FIG. 67-1. Common forms of inflammatory lung disease. *Top:* Schematic of a portion of the normal lung with an airway and alveoli. *Left:* In emphysema, the inflammation is in the alveolar walls and in the alveolar airspaces, with resultant destruction of alveolar walls. *Bottom:* In bronchitis, the inflammation is on the epithelial surface of the airways, with consequent damage to the epithelium, production of excess mucus, and interference with host defense. *Right:* In fibrosis, the inflammation is in the alveolar walls and in the alveolar airspaces. The inflammation deranges the alveolar walls and directs the accumulation of mesenchymal cells, with resultant scarring within the alveolar walls and within the alveolar airspaces.

chioles, accompanied by destruction of their walls and without obvious fibrosis (8). Four patterns of emphysema are recognized: (a) proximal acinar (centrilobular) emphysema, in which respiratory bronchioles are abnormally enlarged and destroyed; (b) panacinar (panlobular) emphysema, in which the process of enlargement and destruction in the acinus involves the acinus more or less uniformly; (c) distal acinar (paraseptal) emphysema, in which alveolar ducts are dominantly affected; and (d) irregular emphysema, in which there is irregular enlargement and destruction of the acinus (9). Of these patterns, the two major forms are centrilobular and panacinar.

Persons with emphysema typically have difficulty exhaling, owing to the loss of elastic recoil and airway support normally provided by the alveoli. The air trapping and hyperinflation that ensue place the respiratory muscles at a disadvantage, increasing the work of both the inspiratory and the expiratory phases of respiration (10). The loss of alveolar tissue diminishes the surface area available for gas exchange, reducing the amount of oxygen that can be transferred to red blood cells. The loss of pulmonary capillaries limits the capacity of the right side of the heart to transfer the cardiac output across the lungs. Together, these pathophysiologic processes impair

the ability of the cardiopulmonary system to deliver oxygen to other organs, thus markedly reducing the ability of affected persons to exercise and placing vital organs at risk of the consequences of oxygen starvation (11).

The central concept in the pathogenesis of emphysema is that the lung destruction results from inadequate protection of the alveoli against proteolytic enzymes released by inflammatory cells in the local milieu (12,13). The alveolar walls are necessarily thin and fragile, because their major function is to bring air and blood into as close proximity as possible. In 1965, Gross et al. (14) instilled the proteolytic enzyme papain into the trachea of experimental animals. From this study the concept evolved that if proteases capable of destroying the alveolar tissues gain access to the lung parenchyma without being inhibited by the local defenses, the consequence will be emphysema.

Proteases Relevant to the Lung

In the lung, some proteases function within cells and others function after they are secreted into the extracellular environment. The secreted proteases play an important role in modifying the extracellular matrix components of the lung. The proteases that exert the most obvious effects on the lung are the extracellular endopeptidases whose catalytic site contains either serine (*serine proteases*) or zinc (*metalloproteases*). The proteases for which there is evidence of relevance to the development of emphysema are neutrophil elastase (NE), macrophage elastase, gelatinase B, and interstitial collagenase.

NE, a 29-kd glycoprotein, is the major serine protease contained within azurophilic granules of neutrophils (15,16). It is produced in the bone marrow in promyelocytes during the process of neutrophil differentiation (17,18). When neutrophils are activated or lysed, NE is released into the local milieu. It has a broad substrate specificity and is capable of degrading a wide range of extracellular matrix proteins that comprise the alveolar wall, including elastin, collagen (types I through IV), fibronectin, laminin, and proteoglycans (12,19–21). It is because of this broad activity against the connective tissue of the alveolar wall that the presence of uninhibited NE in the lower respiratory tract is so devastating, causing progressive destruction of alveoli. The concentration of NE within a single neutrophil is 36 to 58 μmol/L (22). Because of the high turnover of neutrophils, and because a large proportion of neutrophils originate in the pulmonary capillaries, the lung must maintain a significant anti-NE protective screen to protect the alveoli.

Macrophage elastase is secreted by human alveolar macrophages (23). The proenzyme form of macrophage elastase has a mass of 54 kd, but the mature form is 22 kd. It degrades insoluble elastin, and its elastolytic activity is inhibited by tissue inhibitor of metalloproteases (TIMP).

Interstitial collagenase (also called matrix metalloproteinase-1 [MMP-1]), a 56-kd enzyme, is synthesized and secreted by fibroblasts and alveolar macrophages (24). Interstitial collagenase is relatively specific, cleaving the interstitial collagens type I, II, and III at a single locus and having low activity on other matrix proteins (25).

Gelatinase B (MMP-9), a 95-kd enzyme, is released by both neutrophils and macrophages (26,27). The exact storage location of gelatinase B within the neutrophil is disputed (28–30). Like other collagenases, it is released in its latent form and subsequently activated (31). It is capable of degrading denatured collagen, type IV and V collagens, and elastin (27,32).

Antiproteases Relevant to the Lung

Antiproteases are molecules that function to prevent proteases from interacting with their natural substrates. The major antiprotease known to be relevant to lung disease is α_1-antitrypsin (α_1-AT), although other antiproteases (e.g., TIMP-1 through TIMP-4) may also play a role (33–36). None of the pulmonary protein antiproteases are protein specific; they all inhibit more than one protease. However, most are protease class specific; for example, α_1-AT and secretory leukoprotease inhibitor (SLPI) inhibit serine proteases, whereas TIMP inhibits metalloproteases.

α_1-AT is a 52-kd glycoprotein produced mainly by hepatocytes (37). It inhibits a broad range of serine proteases, but its major role is as an inhibitor of NE in the lower respiratory tract, where it provides more than 90% of the anti-NE protective screen (37–39). The α_1-AT gene, comprised of seven exons, spans 12.2 kb of chromosome 14 at q31-32.3 (Fig. 67-2A) (40). It is expressed in a manner that is typical of a secretory glycoprotein, with translation of the α_1-AT mRNA on the rough endoplasmic reticulum (RER) and secretion of the precursor protein into the cisterna of the RER, where it undergoes core glycosylation (41) (Fig. 67-2B). The N-terminal peptide is cleaved, and then the glycosylated protein folds into its three-dimensional configuration and is translocated to the Golgi apparatus, where the three carbohydrate side chains are trimmed to their final form. The mature α_1-AT protein is then secreted.

The major site of α_1-AT gene expression is the hepatocyte (37,42,43). Mononuclear phagocytes also express the α_1-AT gene, but hepatocytes contain approximately 200 times more α_1-AT mRNA transcripts per cell than do mononuclear phagocytes. The gene is also expressed in neutrophils, megakaryocytes, islet cells, intestinal cells, and, in studies in transgenic mice with the α_1-AT promoter, in kidney and brain (44,45). More than 95% of the α_1-AT in the lung is produced in the liver; from there it is secreted into plasma and then diffuses throughout the body, including into the lung (41).

Although α_1-AT inhibits many proteases, including trypsin, chymotrypsin, cathepsin G, plasmin, thrombin, tissue kallikrein, factor X, and plasminogen, its major func-

tion is to inhibit NE (46). The active site of α_1-AT is at residues Met^{358}-Ser^{359}, part of a stressed, external loop protruding from the molecule (47). The active-site bond is held under tension, and, if cleaved, the two residues separate widely. The conformation of the active-site loop gives rise to the specificity of α_1-AT for NE. The Met^{358}-Ser^{359} docks with the catalytic triad of NE, leading to formation of a tight noncovalent interaction between NE and α_1-AT that prevents NE from functioning. The interaction between α_1-AT and NE is a suicide reaction for both molecules (48). NE can cleave the Met^{358}-Ser^{359} bond of α_1-AT, but if this occurs the NE remains bound to the N-terminal portion of the α_1-AT ending with the Met^{358}, and the 36-amino acid C-terminal Ser^{359} through Lys^{394} is released. This complex is itself chemotactic for neutrophils, thereby potentially increasing the neutrophil burden and hence NE in vivo. The α_1-AT–NE complex eventually undergoes catabolism, at least in part via a specific pathway mediated by the serpin-enzyme complex receptor (41).

α_1-Antitrypsin Deficiency

The "protease-antiprotease" concept of the pathogenesis of emphysema evolved from the identification of one of the most common lethal hereditary disorders of Caucasians, α_1-AT deficiency (43). This disorder is characterized by reduced serum levels of α_1-AT, development of emphysema by the third to fourth decades, and, less commonly, liver disease in neonates, children, and adults (43,49). The emphysema associated with α_1-AT deficiency is panacinar and begins in the lower lung zones. Typically, the life expectancy of persons with α_1-AT deficiency is 10 to 15 years shorter than normal, and it is further reduced by smoking (42,50).

The basic concept of the pathogenesis of emphysema of α_1-AT deficiency is that mutations in the two parental α_1-AT deficiency genes result in a reduced secretion of α_1-AT by the liver and therefore a marked reduction of α_1-AT levels in blood and throughout the body, including the lung (13,42,43,49). This leaves the fragile alveolar walls vulnerable to proteolytic destruction by NE. Over many years, the unfettered NE slowly destroys alveoli, a process that is accelerated in cigarette smokers. By age 30 to 40 years, the lung destruction becomes clinically apparent, with the progressive loss of lung function causing a 10- to 15-year reduction in the life span compared with the general population (50–53).

The Z Mutation

The two parental α_1-AT genes are codominantly expressed, and one normal gene is sufficient to provide adequate amounts of functional α_1-AT to protect the lung. In other words, the inheritance of two abnormal α_1-AT genes is necessary to put the lung at risk for emphysema (13,43,49,54). Although more than 20 mutations of the

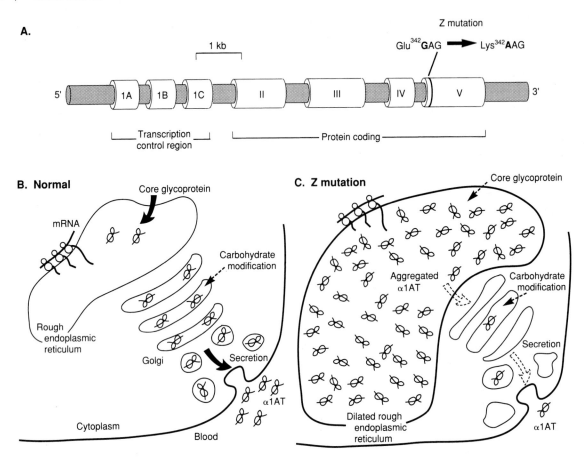

FIG. 67-2. The α₁-antitrypsin (α₁-AT) gene and consequences of the common Z mutation. (**A**) Structure of the α₁-AT gene. It includes seven exons (IA–IC, II–V) spread out over 12.2 kb of chromosome 14. Exons IA through IC include transcriptional control units, and exons II through V contain the protein-coding sequence. The common Z mutation is a single base substitution in exon V coding for residue 342. (**B**) Synthesis and secretion of α₁-AT as directed by the normal α₁-AT gene. Shown is the cytoplasm of a hepatocyte. The α₁-AT mRNA transcript is translated, and the newly synthesized α₁-AT molecule is secreted into the cisternae of the rough endoplasmic reticulum. After core glycosylation and folding of the molecule, the α₁-AT is translocated to the Golgi region, where the carbohydrates are modified to their final form. The mature α₁-AT molecule is then secreted into the circulation. (**C**) Synthesis and secretion of α₁-AT as directed by the Z-type gene. α₁-AT mRNA translation is normal, as is core glycosylation. Because of the Glu³⁴² → Lys substitution, the Z-type molecule aggregates in the rough endoplasmic reticulum, limiting translocation to the Golgi. The consequences are dilation of the rough endoplasmic reticulum and a marked reduction in the amount of α₁-AT secreted into the circulation, causing the α₁-AT deficiency state.

gene have been associated with α₁-AT deficiency (13,43,49), one mutation, referred to as the *Z mutation*, is responsible for more than 95% of all cases of α₁-AT deficiency (55).

The Z mutation (Glu³⁴² *GAG* → Lys*A*AG) produces the deficiency state because the single amino acid substitution causes the molecule to aggregate in the RER rather than being secreted (see Fig. 67-*A*, *C*). Therefore, although α₁-AT deficiency is a serum "deficiency" disorder, it actually is a hepatocyte "RER storage" disorder (56,57). The mechanisms responsible for the aggregation of the Z-type molecule are not clear. There is evidence that it results in part from the loss of an internal salt bridge (Glu³⁴² → Lys²⁹⁰) that plays a critical role in the folding of the molecule; this allows hydrophobic residues

of α₁-AT molecules in close proximity to interact, causing aggregation (41,52,58).

The Z mutation not only causes a systemic deficiency of α₁-AT; it also renders the molecule less capable of performing its function as an inhibitor of NE (59). Together, the deficiency state and dysfunction of the molecule conspire to render the lung susceptible to proteolytic destruction by NE. The normal α₁-AT molecule is a pseudoirreversible inhibitor of NE; the attraction of the two molecules is very high, and dissociation is negligible, resulting in an association rate constant of 10⁷/second per mole (38). The Z mutation of the α₁-AT molecule reduces the association rate constant to 4.5×10⁶/second per mole, making it a less effective inhibitor of NE than normal α₁-AT (59). Although the dysfunction of the Z form of α₁-

AT does not seem to be very large, when taken together with the deficiency state it is devastating to the normal anti-NE defenses of the alveolar walls.

Because its molecular mass is 52 kd, the α_1-AT molecule is able to diffuse through the endothelial and epithelial layers of the alveolar wall. The normal estimated alveolar interstitial level is 10 to 40 mol/L, and the measured alveolar ELF level is 2 to 5 mol/L (13,60). If NE levels are assumed to be in the same range, the estimated *in vivo* NE inhibition time—the time required for the amounts of α_1-AT present *in vivo* at the target organ to combine with and inhibit an equal amount of NE—is 0.12 seconds for normal persons (41). In contrast, the combined effect of a reduction in α_1-AT levels (<1 mol/L in alveolar ELF) and a reduction in the association rate constant for NE results in an *in vivo* NE inhibition time of 2.4 seconds, a 20-fold increase from normal (41). As a result, the alveoli are inadequately defended from NE, and chronic alveolar destruction occurs.

Neutrophils in the α_1-Antitrypsin–Deficient Lung

Although there is overwhelming evidence of the inadequacy of anti-NE defenses in the lungs of persons with α_1-AT deficiency, there is less information regarding the NE burden in the α_1-AT deficient lung. Neutrophils normally marginate in the pulmonary capillaries, so that even the normal lung has a potential burden of NE that is quite large (4). In α_1-AT deficiency, the number of neutrophils migrating into the lung parenchyma is increased, and there is evidence that this increase is directly linked to the α_1-AT deficiency state (61). Because of the inadequate anti-NE defenses, uninhibited NE is free to interact with receptors on the surface of alveolar macrophages (62). This results in activation of alveolar macrophages with release of neutrophil chemoattractants, such as leukotriene B$_4$ (LTB$_4$) (61). Therefore the migration of neutrophils to the lung is increased, as is the accompanying burden of NE.

Therapeutic Strategies for α_1-Antitrypsin Deficiency

In the context of the understanding of α_1-AT deficiency as an inflammatory disorder leading to an excess of NE that overwhelms the inadequate anti-NE defenses of the lower respiratory tract, rational therapy for α_1-AT deficiency would consist of either reducing the NE burden or increasing the anti-NE protection of the alveoli. Little attention has been given to the former strategy, because it is not known how to limit neutrophil access to one organ and also because neutrophils play a critical role in host defense for the lung. Three major approaches to improve anti-NE defenses have been developed: intravenous α_1-AT augmentation therapy with α_1-AT purified from human plasma, aerosol augmentation with plasma α_1-AT or recombinant α_1-AT, and gene therapy.

Intravenous Augmentation Therapy

Because α_1-AT deficiency is a systemic deficiency state, the most direct approach to therapy is to augment the blood, and hence the levels in the lung, with α_1-AT purified from pooled human plasma. This strategy was developed by Gadek et al. (39), who demonstrated that intravenous infusion of purified plasma α_1-AT into deficient persons augmented both serum and lung ELF levels of α_1-AT. In 1987, Wewers et al. (63) further evaluated this strategy in a group of α_1-AT–deficient persons over a period of 6 months, showing that the improved lung levels of α_1-AT were maintained by once-weekly intravenous infusions of 60 mg/kg of α_1-AT. This dosage provided adequate levels to protect the lung against NE. In an effort to minimize the requirement for weekly infusions of α_1-AT, Hubbard et al. (64) demonstrated that equally effective lung anti-NE protection could be achieved in α_1-AT–deficient persons with a monthly dose of 250 mg/kg. The intravenous form of therapy is now generally available and is being administered to more than 2,000 persons worldwide (53,65). The efficacy of α_1-AT augmentation therapy was evaluated in 1,129 patients as part of a multicenter, nationwide α1-Antitrypsin Deficiency Registry run by the National Heart, Lung and Blood Institute (53). With the caveat that the Registry was not designed as a controlled efficacy trial, the data demonstrated that α_1-AT augmentation therapy significantly reduces the mortality rate.

Aerosol Augmentation Therapy

Although intravenous augmentation therapy appears to be effective, it is also wasteful. The lung constitutes only 2% of body weight and is the only organ that appears sufficiently burdened by neutrophils and sufficiently fragile to put it at risk in α_1-AT deficiency. One strategy to circumvent this inefficiency is to direct therapy to the lung by aerosolization. The feasibility of this approach has been demonstrated for α_1-AT purified from human plasma (66) and for α_1-AT produced by recombinant DNA methods in yeast (67,68). Using available nebulizer systems, it is possible to aerosolize plasma α_1-AT or recombinant α_1-AT in droplets of sufficiently small diameter (0.2 to 5 μm) to reach the lower respiratory tract. Short-term studies in persons with α_1-AT deficiency have shown that with both molecules, this approach augments lower respiratory tract α_1-AT levels and anti-NE capacity (66,68).

Gene Therapy

The most direct form of therapy for any genetic disease is to augment the missing or defective gene so that the gene product can be synthesized by the body rather than being administered exogenously. Because systemic augmentation therapy with α_1-AT is sufficient to treat α_1-AT deficiency, gene therapy using placement of a recombinant α_1-AT gene with the normal coding sequence into almost any cell type should also be sufficient to treat the disorder, so long as the amount of α_1-AT that is produced is sufficient to reestablish the lung anti-NE protective screen. Several strategies have been evaluated to accomplish this aim. Together they demonstrate that gene therapy for α_1-AT deficiency is feasible, although the necessity of providing high levels of gene expression on a persistent basis continues to be a major challenge.

First, a recombinant retrovirus was used to transfer the human α_1-AT cDNA into the genome of mouse fibroblasts, with consequent production of human α_1-AT (69). When such fibroblasts were transplanted into the peritoneum of mice, human α_1-AT could be detected in serum and in the ELF of the lung (70). As an alternative approach, using a retrovirus vector, murine T lymphocytes were modified with human α_1-AT cDNA so that they produced human α_1-AT. To circumvent the problem of the relatively small amounts of protein that T lymphocytes are capable of secreting, the modified T lymphocytes were transplanted directly to the epithelial surface of the lung (71). Retrovirus vectors also have been used to transfer the α_1-AT cDNA to hepatocytes (72,73).

Second, cationic liposomes were used to deliver plasmids containing the α_1-AT cDNA to the lung endothelium and to the respiratory epithelium, with evidence of low levels of α_1-AT produced within the lung (74).

Third, replication-deficient, recombinant adenovirus vectors containing the human α_1-AT cDNA driven by a constitutive viral promoter were used to transfer the α_1-AT coding sequence to the epithelium of the respiratory tract, with local secretion of the α_1-AT into the lung (75). Alternatively, adenovirus vectors were used to transfer the α_1-AT cDNA to the peritoneal mesothelium (76) and to the liver, with consequent secretion of human α_1-AT into the circulation (77,78).

Cigarette Smoking and Emphysema

Unlike the emphysema of α_1-AT deficiency, which is based in the lower lung zones, the emphysema associated with cigarette smoking typically begins in the upper zones (42,54). Despite this anatomic difference, there is evidence that the pathogenesis of the common form of emphysema associated with cigarette smoking, like that of α_1-AT deficiency, is linked to an inflammatory process in the lung parenchyma that overwhelms the local antiprotease defenses, resulting in progressive protease-mediated destruction of alveoli. Unlike α_1-AT deficiency, which is linked to an imbalance of NE and α_1-AT, the protease-antiprotease imbalance in cigarette smoking is more complex and probably involves more than one protease-antiprotease system, with the proteases derived from both neutrophils and alveolar macrophages.

Cigarette smoking is associated with an increased recruitment of neutrophils to the lung, which exposes the alveoli to neutrophil proteases and oxidants. Smoking induces alveolar macrophages to release chemoattractants for neutrophils (79) and initiates release of inflammatory mediators by bronchial epithelial cells (80). Consistent with this concept, the levels of interleukin-8 (IL-8), a potent neutrophil chemoattractant, are higher in respiratory ELF of smokers and correlate with the amount of neutrophils in the ELF (80). It has been suggested that nicotine in cigarette smoke may upregulate the NE gene in neutrophil precursor cells, leading to an increase in neutrophil elastase protein concentration per cell, although for this to be relevant the nicotine concentration in blood would have to be sufficient to affect bone marrow precursors (81). Nicotine also prolongs neutrophil survival by suppression of apoptosis, an effect that appears to be dose-dependent (82).

Whereas NE is the major protease involved in the pathogenesis of emphysema in α_1-AT deficiency, the metalloproteases relevant to emphysema are derived from alveolar macrophages and neutrophils. The alveolar macrophage is the predominant cell recovered from the respiratory ELF of smokers, and there are several lines of evidence suggesting the importance of the alveolar macrophage in the pathogenesis of emphysema in smokers. First, like humans, mice chronically exposed to cigarette smoke develop a macrophage-predominant inflammatory infiltrate in the lungs followed by airspace enlargement (83). In contrast to wild-type littermates, mice deficient in macrophage elastase fail to recruit macrophages and do not develop pulmonary emphysema in response to cigarette smoke exposure (83). Second, alveolar macrophages from patients with emphysema secrete greater quantities of an elastolytic gelatinase B (a metalloprotease with elastolytic activity), than alveolar macrophages from control subjects (84). There is also increased release of interstitial collagenase (a collagen-degrading metalloprotease) by alveolar macrophages in persons with emphysema compared with control subjects, as well as increased amounts of collagenase activity in the ELF (84). Emphysematous macrophages also release significant quantities of NE-like activity (84). Finally, transgenic mice overexpressing interstitial collagenase in their lungs have pulmonary morphologic changes similar to those seen in human emphysema (85).

In addition to contributing to the protease burden in the lung, the alveolar macrophages of cigarette smokers are activated to release free radicals, such as superoxide anion and hydrogen peroxide (86). One consequence of this oxidant burden in the lower respiratory tract is the inactivation of α_1-AT by oxidation of the methionine residue at its active inhibitory site (Met[358]) (87). α_1-AT can be inactivated *in vitro* by oxidants in cigarette smoke and by oxidants released by inflammatory cells recovered from the lungs of cigarette smokers (86). Oxidation of the methionine residue at the active site of the molecule markedly decreases the association rate constant of α_1-AT for NE, rendering the α_1-AT impotent as an NE inhibitor (88). Confirmation that this process is ongoing in the lungs of cigarette smokers comes from observations of α_1-AT recovered by bronchoalveolar lavage of smokers: the Met[358] residue in the α_1-AT is oxidized (12), and the association rate constant of the α_1-AT for NE is markedly decreased (88).

Therefore, cigarette smoking results in the equivalent of a mild form of α_1-AT deficiency in the lungs, by virtue of an increased NE burden and a decreased anti-NE protective screen. From a therapeutic standpoint, these insights have led to the development of "oxidation-resistant" forms of α_1-AT. Using site-directed mutagenesis, the α_1-AT molecule can be modified so that residue 358 is changed from methionine to valine, leucine, or alanine. In all cases the molecule retains its ability to inhibit NE but is resistant to oxidants, including those spontaneously released by inflammatory cells recovered from the lungs of cigarette smokers (86,89). However, in regard to therapy, the complexity of the mixed protease-antiprotease imbalance in the lungs of cigarette smokers beyond that of only NE and α_1-AT suggests that anti-NE therapy by itself will probably not be sufficient to prevent the emphysema associated with cigarette smoking. For example, the TIMP class of metalloprotease inhibitors should provide protection against proteases such as interstitial collagenase and gelatinase B.

BRONCHITIS

As the term suggests, *bronchitis* is an inflammatory disorder of the airways (90). It is primarily an epithelial disorder, with the inflammation concentrated at the airway surface throughout the lung, usually involving both large and small airways to some extent. Mucus hypersecretion occurs in response to the inflammation, and persons with bronchitis produce sputum on a chronic basis. Associated dysfunction of the host defense of the tracheobronchial tree results in bacterial colonization of the retained secretions, leading to intermittent frank infection manifested by purulent sputum. In many cases chronic bronchitis is relatively mild, with little effect on lung function, but in some there is extension of inflammation into the peribronchiolar and alveolar interstitial tissue, accompanied by progressive derangement of the airway architecture, loss of lung function, and respiratory limitation (91). The worsening airflow ultimately limits the ability of the lung to transfer oxygen, owing to mismatch of ventilation and pulmonary capillary perfusion (92). The term *bronchiectasis* is applied to those cases in which progressive destruction of the components of the bronchial wall leads to bronchial dilatation.

The pathogenesis of bronchitis begins with the development of chronic inflammation on the airway epithelial surface. The airways are hardier structures than alveoli, and they can withstand the onslaught of chronic inflammation without destruction. However, significant airway distortion with attendant morbidity and mortality may follow the progressive assault on the epithelium as a result of proteases and oxidants released by inflammatory cells and interference with normal host defense processes (93).

Cystic Fibrosis

Cystic fibrosis (CF), a common hereditary disorder of Caucasians, represents the most aggressive form of bronchitis known (94). Although it is less common than the bronchitis associated with chronic cigarette smoking (95), much more is known about the pathogenesis of CF-associated bronchitis, and it used here as the major example for understanding chronic inflammation in the airways.

The respiratory manifestations of CF develop at an early age, often in the first year of life (94,96,97). Initially, frequent respiratory infections occur; they are localized to the epithelial surface of the airways. Eventually the chronic production of thick, sticky sputum develops; the sputum is colonized with bacteria, often of the *Pseudomonas* species. The clinical course is punctuated by acute exacerbations of inflammation and infection of the airways, with progressive deterioration of airway function and eventual derangement of lung parenchyma. Persons with CF usually die from respiratory failure, at an average age of 31 years (98).

Molecular Basis

CF is caused by mutations of the CF transmembrane conductance regulator (CFTR) gene, a 27-exon, 250-kb segment of chromosome 7 at q31 (99–101) (Fig. 67-3). There are more than 500 mutations of CFTR associated with CF, but the most common is Phe[508], a deletion of residue 508 of the predicted 1,480-residue CFTR protein (99,102–104). CFTR functions as a Cl$^-$ channel on the apical surface of epithelial cells capable of responding to increased intracellular levels of cyclic adenosine monophosphate (cAMP) (105,106) (Fig. 67-4). It is not clear why a mutation in this gene leads to the production of abnormal respiratory mucus and its colonization with bacteria, but these processes are thought to be related to the existence of an abnormal ionic milieu on the airway epithelial surface or within the airway epithelial cells, or both (94,107). For example, defensins, natural antibiotics of the respiratory epithelium, do not function in the abnormal ionic milieu of the CF airway ELF (108). Independent of the exact underlying mechanism, it is clear that these abnormalities are associated with a very intense, chronic, neutrophil-dominated inflammatory process on the airway epithelial surface, beginning very

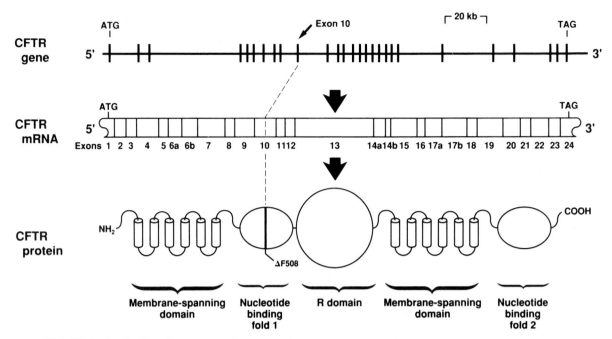

FIG. 67-3. Cystic fibrosis transmembrane conductance regulator (CFTR) gene and predicted CFTR protein. *Top:* Structure of the CFTR gene. The gene occupies 250 kb of chromosome 7 and includes 27 exons. The start (ATG) and stop (TAG) codons are indicated. Exon 10 is the site of the common ΔF508 mutation, a deletion of three nucleotides resulting in an in-phase deletion of Phe[508]. *Middle:* CFTR mRNA transcript. The 27 exons are indicated: the 6a, 6b, 14a, 14b, 17a, 17b nomenclature resulted from the identification of these as separate exons after the original description of the gene. *Bottom:* The proposed structure of the CFTR protein includes (N- to C-terminal) a membrane-spanning domain, nucleotide-binding fold 1, the R domain, a second membrane-spanning domain, and nucleotide-binding fold 2.

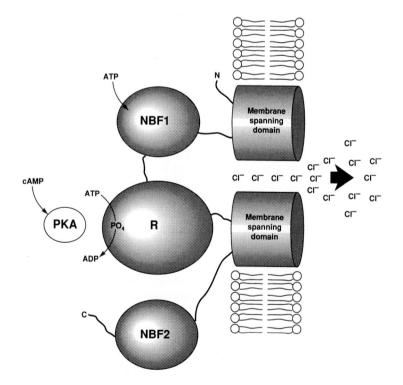

FIG. 67-4. Proposed function of the CFTR protein. CFTR functions as a Cl⁻ channel on the apical membrane of epithelial cells and possibly in organelles within the cells. The channel responds to elevations in intracellular cyclic adenosine monophosphate (cAMP) and consequent activation of protein kinase A (PKA). Adenosine triphosphate (ATP) binds to nucleotide-binding fold 1 (NBF1), and ATP is a substrate for phosphorylation of the R domain. Both ATP binding and R-domain phosphorylation are required for channel activation. The membrane-spanning domains modulate cation selectivity and, presumably, membrane insertion. The function of nucleotide-binding fold 2 (NBF2) is not known. With the ΔF508 mutation, the CFTR protein does not reach the apical membrane.

early in childhood (96,97,109,110). This inflammation leads to the derangements in airway structure and ineffective host defenses of the airway surface that are characteristic of the disease (111).

Respiratory Inflammation

The lung inflammation that typifies CF is similar to that observed in α_1-AT deficiency, in that the epithelial surface of the lung is burdened in both disorders by NE and oxidants. However, there are major differences in the intensity and anatomic location of the inflammation, factors that weigh heavily in the consequences to the lung. First, the intensity of the inflammation differs. In α_1-AT deficiency, the number of neutrophils present is increased, but at most to only a few times greater than the level observed in normal subjects (61). In CF the inflammation is much more intense; the number of neutrophils in the airway epithelial lining fluid may be 500 times greater than normal (5,111–113). Second, in α_1-AT deficiency the inflammation predominates at the alveolar level of the lower respiratory tract, whereas in CF it manifests primarily on the epithelial surface of the airways (13,111).

The pathogenesis of airway inflammation in patients with CF remains the subject of much debate. Although studies have demonstrated the presence of inflammation without infection in infants as young as 4 weeks of age (96,110), it is likely that airway inflammation follows infection and colonization with bacterial pathogens, particularly *Pseudomonas aeruginosa* (97). Colonization and frank infection with *P. aeruginosa* is closely associated with the development and progression of pulmonary disease in CF (114). Several mechanisms have been proposed to explain how the genetic defect in CF and the resultant deficiency in CFTR function lead to chronic infection.

First, the airway surface fluid of the normal airway epithelium has antimicrobial activity that is sensitive to high concentrations of salt (108). This antimicrobial activity is defective in CF, probably because antimicrobial peptides (e.g., human β defensin-1) secreted by airway epithelial cells, are inactivated in the high-salt environment of the CF airway surface fluid. If so, and if these peptides play a significant role in protecting the airways from organisms like *Pseudomonas*, this inactivation may explain the colonization in the airway with microbial pathogens early in CF (108,115). However, this view has been challenged by studies that have demonstrated no difference in the ionic constituents of airway surface fluid between normal subjects and those with CF (116).

Second, the pili of *P. aeruginosa* can mediate adhesion to the respiratory epithelium (117). CFTR dysfunction, by limiting acidification within the trans-Golgi region, can result in diminished sialylation of cell glycoconjugates (118). As a result, the CF airway epithelial cell surface has a higher than normal concentration of asialoGM1, especially in persons who are homozygous

for the CFTR ΔF508 mutation (119). This increase in surface asialoGM1 is likely to result in increased binding of *P. aeruginosa* to respiratory epithelial cells (120). Consistent with this concept, *in vitro* transfer of normal CFTR cDNA to airway epithelial cells reduced binding of *P. aeruginosa* to the CF respiratory epithelium (121).

Third, it has been suggested that, in the normal human airway, epithelial cells bind and internalize respiratory pathogens and that this mechanism for clearing these organisms from the airways may be defective in CF (122). Consistent with this concept, cultured human airway epithelial cells expressing the ΔF508 allele of the CFTR are defective in uptake of *P. aeruginosa*, compared with cells expressing the wild-type allele.

Inflammatory Mediators

A variety of inflammatory mediators have been identified in the airway secretions of persons with CF, including inflammatory cell and epithelial cell products. One group of stimuli are the bacteria colonizing the epithelial surface. In the mouse model of CF, the inflammatory response to infection is exaggerated compared with normal controls (123). During the earliest stages of infection of the CF lung, when *P. aeruginosa* organisms are transiently inspired but not cleared by the usual mucociliary mechanisms, they may attach via pili to the asialoGM1 receptors found on the airway epithelium in significantly increased numbers (120). The *Pseudomonas* binding triggers IL-8 production by respiratory epithelial cells (114). Because IL-8 is a potent neutrophil chemoattractant, the result is a self-perpetuating inflammatory process on the CF bronchial surface, whereby NE released by neutrophils induces the bronchial epithelium to secrete more IL-8, which in turn recruits additional neutrophils to the bronchial surface, whose elaboration of superoxide and NE further stimulates the epithelium to produce IL-8 (124). This cycle of inflammation persists during the later stages of infection, when the *Pseudomonas* organisms may no longer express pili or flagella, and may not even be directly apposed to the epithelium, but are enmeshed in relatively inert microcolonies surrounded by glycoconjugates of both bacterial and human origin. Under these conditions, exoproducts such as the *Pseudomonas* autoinducer, secreted during chronic infection, continue to evoke IL-8 expression (114).

Alveolar macrophages in the airways of persons with CF are another source of inflammatory mediators. They release tumor necrosis factor-α (TNF-α), IL-1β, and IL-8 in response to infection with *P. aeruginosa* (125). TNF-α enhances neutrophil adhesion and superoxide production *in vitro* and *in vivo*, and IL-1β is a potent neutrophil activator (126–128). TNF-α and IL-1β, produced by the alveolar macrophages, may also stimulate epithelial cells to produce IL-8, thereby forming a local network that amplifies their effects (129,130).

LTB$_4$, a mediator capable of recruiting neutrophils into the human airway *in vivo* (131), is also present in increased amounts in lung secretions of patients with CF, compared with healthy control subjects (132). LTB$_4$ also induces neutrophil adherence, degranulation, and superoxide generation (133–135). CF respiratory ELF also contains high levels of soluble TNF-α receptor and the interleukin-1 receptor antagonist (IL-1Ra), perhaps representing an attempt by homeostatic mechanisms to prevent the systemic effects of these potent inflammatory mediators (125). CF ELF contains depressed levels of IL-10, a mediator that normally dampens a variety of inflammatory processes, further contributing to enhanced local inflammation and tissue damage (125,136).

Airway Secretions

P. aeruginosa lipopolysaccharide (LPS) is a potent stimulus of mucin production in epithelial cells, in part because of its ability to upregulate transcription of the *MUC2* mucin gene in airway epithelial cells (137). Once airway infection has occurred, *P. aeruginosa* LPS provides a local stimulus for exaggerated airway mucin synthesis, which probably contributes to airway mucus obstruction. CF airway secretions have a high concentration of undigested DNA, derived mostly from inflammatory cells that have disintegrated, which contributes to the increased viscosity of the airway secretions (138,139). In the presence of impaired mucociliary clearance resulting from damage to the cilia by NE, this provides a favorable milieu for colonization with *P. aeruginosa*.

Protease- and Oxidant-Induced Airway Injury

As a result of the character, intensity, and location of the inflammation in CF, there are major consequences regarding the anti-NE defenses of the airway epithelium. In normal persons, the airway ELF is protected by α$_1$-AT, as is the lower respiratory tract ELF (39). However, the upper airways also possess a second, major anti-NE defense, provided by SLPI. SLPI, a 12-kd protein produced by airway secretory cells, works in concert with α$_1$-AT in normal persons to protect the airways from NE (140). In persons with CF, however, the inflammation on the airway epithelial surface is so intense that both of these anti-NE defenses are overwhelmed and rendered ineffective.

In addition to a deficiency in anti-NE protection in the CF lung, there is also a deficiency in protection against oxidants. In the normal lung, the fluid covering the respiratory epithelial surface contains a variety of enzymes and small molecules that are capable of inhibiting oxidants released by activated inflammatory cells (141). Among these molecules is glutathione, a tripeptide antioxidant that normally is present in respiratory ELF at a concentration of 300 to 450 μmol/L, levels 100- to 150-

fold higher than those observed in plasma (142). In CF, the level of glutathione in respiratory ELF is markedly decreased, for reasons that are not understood (113). Whatever the underlying mechanism, the consequences to the epithelium are significant. First, the epithelium is less able to defend itself against the intense oxidant burden of CF, with consequent development of chronic, oxidant-induced damage. Second, both α$_1$-AT and SLPI are vulnerable to damage from oxidants, and their inactivation results in a deficiency in the anti-NE protective screen of the epithelium (111,140).

Therapeutic Strategies

The conventional therapy for the respiratory manifestations of CF centered on clearing the lungs of mucus and infection using chest physiotherapy and antibiotics (141). Newer strategies based on an understanding of the molecular basis of the disease have been developed to protect the airway epithelium against the inflammation, clear the purulent mucus from the airways, reestablish the normal ionic milieu of the epithelium, and correct the fundamental abnormality causing the disease through gene therapy.

Protection against Inflammation

The two most damaging classes of mediators released by the inflammatory cells on the epithelial surface in CF are proteases and oxidants. Strategies have been developed to protect the epithelium from both.

Although other proteases may be involved, NE is probably the most harmful in the pathogenesis of CF (111). Enormous quantities of NE are present in the airways of persons with CF— so much so that their sputum is used as a commercial source of NE for laboratory studies (22). The free NE on the airway epithelial surface directly damages the epithelial cells and probably cleaves cell-cell contacts and basement membrane components. In addition, it alters the host defense system of the airways by increasing mucus production, interfering with normal ciliary function, and cleaving immunoglobulins and complement components; it also interferes with the ability of neutrophils to phagocytize and kill microorganisms such as *Pseudomonas* by cleaving complement receptors on the neutrophil surface (143). As discussed previously, free NE also amplifies the extent of the inflammation by inducing bronchial epithelial cells to release IL-8 (112).

Two strategies have been used to suppress the airway epithelial burden of NE in CF: aerosolization of α$_1$-AT purified from human plasma and aerosolization of SLPI produced by recombinant DNA technology (112,144). Both methods have been evaluated in short-term studies. Aerosolization of 1.5 to 3 mg/kg of plasma α$_1$-AT twice daily suppresses the NE in respiratory ELF of patients with CF and prevents the NE from interfering with the ability of neutrophils to phagocytize and kill *Pseudo-*

monas (111). Likewise, aerosolization of 100 mg of recombinant SLPI twice daily suppresses both the NE burden and the airway ELF concentration of IL-8, thereby probably interfering with signals that amplify the airway inflammation (112,145).

Antioxidants

Less attention has been given to augmenting the antioxidant screen of the airway epithelium, probably because there are not many options available currently in this therapeutic class. Preliminary studies with aerosolization of reduced glutathione have demonstrated that it is feasible to augment the respiratory epithelial antioxidant defense in CF and to simultaneously diminish the release of oxidants by inflammatory cells in response to activation stimuli (146). Aerosolization of recombinant SLPI to experimental animals results in augmentation of the glutathione levels in airway ELF (147). Because the pathogenesis of CF can be characterized by an increased burden of NE and a deficiency of glutathione on the respiratory epithelial surface, aerosolization of SLPI may be directed at the two major causes of airway damage in this disease.

Clearance of Purulent Mucus

A significant proportion of the purulent mucus characterizing CF consists of high-molecular-weight DNA derived from the nuclei of disintegrated neutrophils participating in the airway inflammation (148). Concentrated solutions of high-molecular-weight DNA are highly viscous and sticky, resembling the sputum of persons with CF. Addition of recombinant deoxyribonuclease (rDNase) to CF sputum *in vitro* results in the cleavage of high-molecular-weight DNA within the mucus, reducing its viscosity (148,149). A similar effect after aerosolization of rDNase to persons with CF occurs *in vivo*, with cleavage of high-molecular-weight DNA in purulent mucus associated with a significant improvement in lung function and reduction of rates of infection requiring hospitalization, and this is now standard therapy for this disorder (148,150–152).

Reestablishment of the Ionic Milieu

The discovery that epithelial cells in the airways of persons with CF reabsorb Na^+ in an enhanced fashion and also are unable to secrete Cl^- normally in response to signals that increase intracellular cAMP suggests that the abnormalities on the airway epithelial surface in CF are secondary to abnormalities in the ionic milieu on the epithelial surface or within the epithelial cells, or both. In an attempt to correct this ionic derangement, amiloride (a diuretic that blocks Na^+ reabsorption) has been administered to persons with CF by aerosol, with beneficial

effects on lung function (107,153). Alternative strategies to achieve the same goal include activation of other pathways by which airway epithelial cells secrete Cl^-, such as Ca^{2+}-dependent calmodulin pathways (154) and purinergic receptor pathways (155,156).

Gene Therapy

The most direct approach to correction of the underlying abnormality in the airway epithelium in CF would be to use gene therapy to "complement" the mutations in the two parental CFTR genes with the normal CFTR gene inserted into the airway epithelial cells *in vivo*. The feasibility of this strategy has been demonstrated by *in vitro* studies showing that transfer of the normal gene into epithelial cells derived from persons with CF results in "correction" of the inability of the cells to secrete Cl^- in response to elevation of cAMP (157–160) and by *in vivo* studies in which viral and nonviral vectors have been used to transfer genes into the airway epithelium of experimental animals (159,161–169). Human studies with CF have shown it is feasible to transfer the normal CFTR cDNA to the airway epithelium of persons with CF using adenovirus, adeno-associated virus, and liposome vectors (170–180)

Bronchitis Associated with Cigarette Smoking

Whereas the bronchitis associated with CF is the most aggressive form known, that associated with cigarette smoking is by far the most common. Few studies have been conducted to characterize the airway inflammation in humans with bronchitis, but a combination of morphologic and bronchoalveolar lavage studies has suggested that it has features similar to those of the bronchitis observed in CF, albeit in a milder form (181–183). The inflammatory population includes neutrophils and alveolar macrophages (181–183), which release an increased burden of oxidants and proteases, including NE, on the airway epithelial surface (181). It is assumed, but not proved, that the airway epithelial anti-NE and antioxidant protection mechanisms are overwhelmed by the inflammation, as in CF, but to a lesser extent. Furthermore, as occurs at the alveolar level, it is likely that smoking renders the airway epithelial anti-NE protection ineffective owing to the increased burden of oxidants associated with cigarette smoke itself and activation of the inflammatory cells with release of oxidants.

FIBROSIS

Pulmonary fibrosis is a general term used to define a class of inflammatory disorders of the lower respiratory tract associated with fibrosis of the alveoli (184,185). These disorders are also referred to as the *interstitial* lung disorders, to reflect the fact that the alveolar walls are typically thickened by scarring of the interstitium (186). More than 150 diseases of known and unknown origin are included in this classification (187).

Individuals with pulmonary fibrosis typically are dyspneic—first with exercise, but eventually at rest (186,187). Unlike patients with emphysema, who have difficulty exhaling air, persons with fibrosis experience increased work with inspiration, due to the decreased compliance of the fibrotic lung (188,189). In addition, pulmonary fibrosis is associated with reduced transfer of oxygen to the pulmonary capillaries. Therefore, oxygen delivery to other organs is limited, with consequences for exercise tolerance similar to those seen in persons with emphysema (11).

Pathogenesis

The central concept in the pathogenesis of pulmonary fibrosis, independent of the specific disease involved, is that it is primarily an inflammatory disorder, in which inflammation in the lower respiratory tract is responsible for derangement of the alveoli and resultant scarring of the lung parenchyma (184,185). Which specific inflammatory cells are involved depends on the disease, with alveolar macrophages, neutrophils, lymphocytes, and eosinophils dominating to a variable degree in the different disorders (184,185,187). It is the character and intensity of the inflammation that dictates the character and extent of the alveolar derangement and fibrosis.

Idiopathic Pulmonary Fibrosis

Idiopathic pulmonary fibrosis (IPF) is the classic clinical model of pulmonary fibrosis (190). It generally appears in middle age, although children and older adults can be affected (184). The dyspnea gradually increases, as does the limitation in exercise. The disease is usually fatal 4 to 5 years after the onset of symptoms (52,184,185).

The morphology of IPF is that of inflammation concentrated in the alveoli and, to a lesser extent, in the terminal bronchioles (189,190). The alveolar epithelium is deranged, with replacement of the normal type I epithelial cells with type II epithelial cells and migration of epithelial cells from the terminal bronchioles down to the alveoli (Fig. 67-5) (191). In addition, there is loss of endothelium and pulmonary capillaries. The interstitium is thickened with bundles of connective tissue dominated by type I collagen (185,192). Rents in the alveolar epithelial basement membrane are associated with migration of mesenchymal cells from the interstitium into the alveolar airspaces, where they may deposit components of connective tissue. This "intraalveolar" fibrosis becomes covered with epithelium and is incorporated into the mass of the thickened alveolar walls (193).

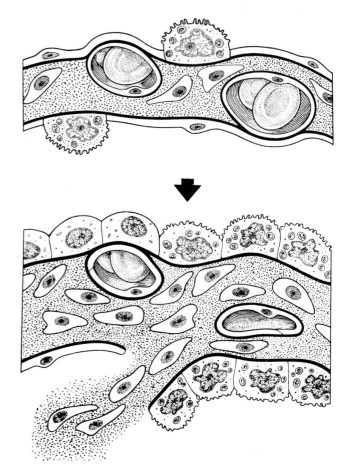

FIG. 67-5. Morphology of alveolar derangements in idiopathic pulmonary fibrosis (IPF). *Top:* Normal alveolar wall showing the flat, squamous type I epithelial cells; the cuboidal type II epithelial cells; endothelial cells lining the capillaries; and mesenchymal cells in the interstitium. The epithelial and endothelial basement membranes and the interstitial connective tissue provide architectural support and modulate the mechanical properties of the alveolar walls. *Below:* In IPF, derangements of the alveolar walls include changes in the epithelium, loss of pulmonary capillaries, and rents in the epithelial basement membrane. Mesenchymal cells expand in number and migrate into the airspaces. The result is interstitial and intraalveolar fibrosis.

Etiology

The cause of IPF is unknown. There is circumstantial evidence to suggest that it is an immune complex disorder with immunoglobulin G (IgG) immune complexes (with unknown antigens) initiating the inflammation in the alveoli (184,194–197). Families with IPF have been identified in which the disease typically manifests itself in middle age (198). Evaluation of the asymptomatic offspring of persons who have clinical evidence of such "familial IPF" has shown that some have prior evidence of inflammation in the lower respiratory tract, suggesting that the inflammation precedes the development of the fibrosis (198).

Alveolitis

The inflammation in the alveoli of persons with IPF is dominated by alveolar macrophages, but the striking component is the increase in neutrophils, which constitute 5% to 20% of the inflammatory cells in the ELF. There is also an increase in the total numbers of lymphocytes, eosinophils, basophils, and mast cells (184,186, 190,199,200). The inflammation is present on the alveolar epithelial surface and in the interstitium.

The alveolar macrophage plays a key role in the pathogenesis of alveolitis in IPF (Fig. 67-6). Increased numbers of macrophages in the lower respiratory tract result both from increased recruitment of monocytes and local proliferation (201,202). Monocyte chemotactic protein-1 is released by the injured airway epithelium and probably accounts for the enhanced recruitment of blood monocytes (203–205). The inflammatory process in IPF is driven, at least in part, by immune complexes produced within the lower respiratory tract (206–208). These immune complexes interact with alveolar macrophages, maintaining these cells in a chronic state of activation. Respiratory ELF of persons with IPF contains high levels of immune complexes (196) and activates alveolar macrophages from normal persons to release chemoattractants for neutrophils, such as LTB$_4$ and IL-8 (130,195,209). There is increased expression of E-selectin on the endothelium of small vessels of the IPF lung, resulting in the enhanced recruitment of neutrophils to the lung (210). Intercellular adhesion molecule-1, another adhesion molecule, is expressed on the type II epithelial cells and on alveolar macrophages in IPF lung (210). The mechanisms of accumulation of eosinophils, lymphocytes, basophils, and mast cells in IPF are unknown.

Mechanisms of Injury

Together, the activated inflammatory cells damage the alveolar structures by releasing oxidants and proteases (211–214), although other mediators probably also play a role.

The exaggerated release of oxidants by alveolar macrophages, neutrophils, and possibly eosinophils probably plays a major role in the injury to the epithelium and

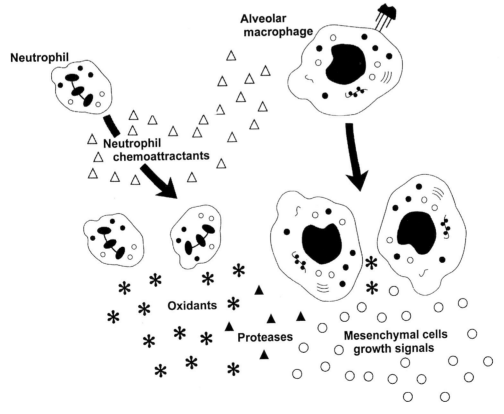

FIG. 67-6. Inflammatory mediators central to the pathogenesis of idiopathic pulmonary fibrosis (IPF). The alveolar macrophage directs the inflammatory process. Immune complexes stimulate the macrophages to release neutrophil chemoattractants, with consequent recruitment and activation of neutrophils. Together, the activated neutrophils and macrophages release oxidants and proteases that derange the alveolar walls. The activated macrophages also release mesenchymal cell growth signals, and thereby direct the fibrotic process.

endothelium in IPF. All of these cells are known to be capable of releasing oxidants, including superoxide anion, hydrogen peroxide, and the hydroxyl radical. Inflammatory cells recovered from the lung of persons with IPF are releasing exaggerated amounts of superoxide anions and hydrogen peroxide (211,213). Neutrophils contain myeloperoxidase, an enzyme capable of converting hydrogen peroxide to the highly toxic hypohalide radical (213). Consistent with the chronic burden of neutrophils in the IPF lung, the ELF of persons with IPF contains high concentrations of myeloperoxidase (211). When lung epithelial cells are exposed to inflammatory cells and to ELF recovered from the IPF lung, there is a synergistic cytotoxic effect (211). Finally, the respiratory ELF in IPF is deficient in glutathione (215). Therefore, the alveolar epithelium in IPF is confronted with an increased oxidant burden and a decreased antioxidant screen, analogous to that confronted by the airway epithelium in CF.

The fragmentation of interstitial collagen fibers and basement membrane components observed in IPF strongly suggests that proteases play a role in the injury process. The most direct evidence for this is the finding of large concentrations of collagenase, probably derived from neutrophils, in the ELF of persons with IPF (216). No active NE is detected in the IPF lung, despite the fact that neutrophils are present and probably are releasing this potent protease. Consistent with this concept, elastic fibers in the alveolar interstitium do not appear to be deranged in IPF. The most likely explanation for these observations is that NE is released but is subsequently inhibited by α_1-AT, the natural inhibitor of this enzyme. In contrast, the lung has very little defense against collagenase and therefore is susceptible to collagenolytic enzymes, even though they are generally less potent than NE.

Several other inflammatory mediators are present in the ELF of persons with IPF. Eosinophil cationic protein, a mediator capable of damaging cell membranes, has been identified on the respiratory epithelial surface in IPF (217), but its role in the pathogenesis of the disease is not clear. Histamine levels are also increased (218,219), probably reflecting the increase in mast cells in the alveolar walls (200). This might be the mechanism of the mild permeability observed in the lung parenchyma in IPF. Other mediators observed to be increased in lungs of IPF patients are plasminogen activator inhibitor-1, the plasminogen activator inhibitor-2, and procoagulant tissue factor (220). Increased amounts of TNF-α and IL-1Ra and decreased levels of interleukin-1β have been reported in the IPF lung, but it is unclear how these mediators play a role in the pathogenesis of the disease (221,222).

Mechanisms of Fibrosis

The dominant "repair" mechanism after alveolar injury is mesenchymal cell proliferation (184,223–225). This concept results from several lines of evidence. First, the parenchyma of the lung in IPF contains relatively more mesenchymal cells than other parenchymal cells (191). Second, whereas mitoses of mesenchymal cells within the alveolar wall are rarely observed, such events can be found in the IPF lung, suggesting that mesenchymal cells are proliferating at a rate higher than normal (185). Finally, alveolar macrophages removed from the lungs of persons with IPF are releasing potent polypeptide growth factors for mesenchymal cells, the same growth factors that stimulate mesenchymal cells to proliferate *in vitro* (224–231).

Among the mesenchymal cell growth signals released by the alveolar macrophages in IPF are platelet-derived growth factor (PDGF), fibronectin, and alveolar macrophage insulin-like growth factor-1 (IGF-1) (224,230,232). Among these, PDGF is probably the most important (224,229,233).

There are two PDGF genes, *PDGF-A* and *PDGF-B* (234). PDGF exists as 31-kd homodimers or heterodimers (229,235). PDGF molecules comprising two B chains are believed to be the most potent (234). Evaluation of alveolar macrophages recovered from persons with IPF has demonstrated an increased rate of transcription of the genes for the PDGF-A and -B chains, and it is the B-chain gene that is activated to a greater extent in the alveolar macrophages in IPF (229). PDGF has the ability to attract mesenchymal cells and stimulate them to enter the growth cycle. In IPF, the alveolar macrophages are releasing four times more PDGF than normal (224). Immune complexes are capable of activating normal alveolar macrophages *in vitro* to release PDGF (224).

Fibronectin, a 440-kd dimer, is generally considered to be a matrix component, with a variety of functions relevant to cell-cell and cell-matrix interactions (236). However, fibronectin can also act as a growth factor, initiating mesenchymal cells to enter the G$_1$ stage of the cell cycle (225,226,231,232,234,237). In IPF, alveolar macrophages express increased amounts of fibronectin mRNA transcripts and release increased amounts of fibronectin, and there are increased levels of fibronectin in the ELF of these persons (225,226,231,232).

Corresponding to the increase in fibronectin production by alveolar macrophages, prominent extracellular deposits of fibronectin are found in areas of intraalveolar fibrosis (238). Fibronectin mRNA is also upregulated in fibroblasts in the IPF lung, and there is a codistribution of fibronectin expression by fibroblasts with high levels of transforming growth factor-β1 (TGF-β1) and procollagen type 1 in fibrotic loci (239). The alveolar macrophage form of IGF-1 is 20 to 25 kd, much larger than the serum form of IGF-1. IGF-1 acts late in G$_1$ to take PDGF- or fibronectin-stimulated mesenchymal cells through to the S phase of the cell cycle and subsequent proliferation (210,227,230). It is unknown whether IGF-1 or other late G$_1$-acting growth signals are mandatory to drive mesenchymal cells to proliferate in the lung in IPF, because PDGF can stimulate mesenchymal cells to proliferate in the absence of such signals (185). In addition to IGF-1, there is an increase in IGF-1 binding protein-3 in ELF of IPF patients (240).

Modulation of Connective-Tissue Production and Degradation

There is no clear evidence that changes in connective tissue synthesis or degradation are important biologic processes in the pathogenesis of pulmonary fibrosis in IPF, but there are observations consistent with the concept that such processes may be ongoing. Three classes of molecules—TGF-β, prostaglandin E (PGE), and collagenases—have been implicated.

TGF-β, a 25-kd molecule, has dual effects in relation to fibrosis (241–243). In some *in vitro* systems, TGF-β decreases the rate of proliferation of mesenchymal cells, whereas in others it has the opposite effect. TGF-β is capable of upregulating genes for type I collagen and fibronectin, and therefore it may play a role in stimulating mesenchymal cells in the lung parenchyma to produce more connective tissue (244,245). TGF-β is present in the ELF of the normal lung and is expressed and released by alveolar macrophages (231,243). In homogenates of IPF lungs, the level of TGF-β is increased (222), and increased amounts of TGF-β are observed in type II pneumocytes, in honeycomb cysts, and around fibroblasts in fibrotic foci in IPF (239). Placed in the context that the respiratory ELF of the normal human lung contains large amounts of TGF-β and that alveolar macrophages are capable of expressing the TGF-β gene and releasing TGF-β (231,243), a scenario can be hypothesized whereby TGF-β in ELF gains access to mesenchymal cells after lung injury and breaks in the alveolar basement membrane, causing increased connective tissue deposition in the lung parenchyma. With the use of a replication-deficient adenovirus vector to transfer the cDNA of porcine TGF-β1 to rat lung, transient overexpression of active TGF-β1 was shown to result in prolonged and severe pulmonary fibrosis characterized by extensive deposition of collagen, fibronectin, and elastin and by emergence of cells with the myofibroblast phenotype (246).

PGE, a metabolite of arachidonic acid, has possible dual effects relevant to pulmonary fibrosis. PGE causes increased intracellular degradation of collagen as it is being synthesized by mesenchymal cells (185). PGE also suppresses the rate of mesenchymal cell proliferation in response to polypeptide growth factors (247). In the normal lung, there are large amounts of PGE in respiratory ELF (185). Therefore, it is likely that PGE normally serves as a counterbalance to signals for mesenchymal cell production of collagen and/or proliferation. In IPF, the levels of PGE in respiratory ELF are decreased sig-

nificantly, and alveolar macrophages derived from the IPF lung release decreased levels of PGE (247). Although the mechanisms causing this are unknown, the consequence may be to allow mesenchymal cells to respond to exogenous signals capable of inducing the accumulation of mesenchymal cells and their connective tissue products.

Not much is known about the normal turnover of collagen in the human lung, although the fact that the normal human lung parenchyma continually synthesizes and secretes collagen but does not accumulate collagen implies that there must be ongoing mechanisms to balance synthesis with degradation of extracellular collagen (248). Collagenase has been observed in the normal human lung, and it is produced by cells such as mesenchymal cells and inflammatory cells. Studies with fragments of lung from persons with IPF imply a decrease in collagenase activity, but it is unclear what role this may have in in the enhanced collagen accumulation observed as part of the fibrotic process (216,249).

Therapeutic Strategies

Because the pathogenesis of fibrosis in IPF involves a variety of normal but exaggerated biologic processes, therapeutic strategies in IPF are directed toward suppressing these processes.

The classic therapy for IPF is the chronic administration of corticosteroids (184,186,187). Although there has never been a blinded therapeutic trial to assess this form of therapy, it is generally accepted that corticosteroids suppress the alveolar inflammation to some degree, improving lung function in some, and slow down the progression of the disease in most cases (184,186,187). Although human alveolar macrophages have receptors for glucocorticoids, IPF patients treated with glucocorticoids generally release the same exaggerated amounts of polypeptide growth factors as do untreated IPF patients (250).

Suppression of neutrophil accumulation in the lung in IPF has been achieved by administration of cyclophosphamide (251). Small clinical trials comparing corticosteroids and cyclophosphamide in the treatment of IPF suggest that the latter may be more efficacious, a result consistent with the demonstration of a greater decrease in the number of neutrophils in the lung with cyclophosphamide therapy than with corticosteroid therapy alone (251,252).

Based on the knowledge of the pathogenesis of IPF, a rational therapeutic approach would be to enhance the antioxidant and antiprotease defense in the lung. Antioxidant therapy using a short-term trial of aerosolization of reduced glutathione was evaluated in IPF with the goal of augmenting the deficient glutathione levels on the respiratory epithelial surface (215,253). There was evidence of oxidation of some of the aerosolized glutathione *in vivo* and suppression of oxidant release by inflammatory cells in the IPF lung, suggesting that the aerosolized glutathione was utilized *in vivo* (253).

With regard to suppressing proteases in the IPF lung, the most rational approach would be to augment anticollagenase levels to protect against the fragmentation of collagen by neutrophil collagenase. One such approach would be administration of TIMP, a known collagenase inhibitor. Such studies have not been attempted, and there is a risk that enhancing anticollagenase activity may permit collagen to accumulate at a more rapid rate.

Colchicine, an inhibitor of protein secretion, has been used in an attempt to suppress the release of growth factors by alveolar macrophages. However, although suppression is possible *in vitro*, the levels required for *in vivo* suppression are not tolerated without adverse effects. PGE₁ plays an important suppressive role in respiratory ELF, decreasing the response of mesenchymal cells to exogenous growth factors and also suppressing collagen production by mesenchymal cells. The levels of PGE are reduced in the IPF lung, giving further rationale for the augmentation of PGE levels in ELF as a therapy for IPF. Studies with experimental animals have shown that it is possible to deliver PGE₁ to the respiratory epithelial surface by the aerosol route and that the respiratory ELF PGE levels can be enhanced by this approach, although interstitial levels are not significantly increased (254). Therefore, this approach may be useful for suppressing the intraalveolar component of the fibrosis of IPF but not for suppressing the interstitial component.

ACKNOWLEDGMENTS

We thank C. Jennings, who contributed to this chapter in the last edition, on which the current edition is based, and Y. Bodden, J.E. Coleman, and N. Mohamed for help in preparation of the manuscript. K.D. and R.G.C. are supported, in part, by NHLBI P01 HL51746; P01 HL59312; GenVec, Inc., Rockville, MD; and the Will Rogers Memorial Fund, Los Angeles, CA.

REFERENCES

1. Horsefield K. Pulmonary airways and blood vessels considered as confluent trees. In: Crystal RG, West JB, Weibel ER, Barnes PJ, eds. *The lung: scientific foundations.* Philadelphia: Lippincott-Raven, 1997:1073–1079.
2. Weibel ER. Design of airways and blood vessels considered as branching trees. In: Crystal RG, West JB, Weibel ER, Barnes PJ, eds. *The lung: scientific foundations.* Philadelphia: Lippincott-Raven, 1997:1061–1071.
3. Cross CE, Halliwell B. General biological consequences of inhaled environmental toxicants. In: Crystal RG, West JB, Weibel ER, Barnes PJ, eds. *The lung: scientific foundations.* Philadelphia: Lippincott-Raven, 1997:2421–2437.
4. Hogg JC. Neutrophil traffic. In: Crystal RG, West JB, Weibel ER, Barnes PJ, eds. *The lung: scientific foundations.* Philadelphia: Lippincott-Raven, 1997:891–904.
5. Rennard SI, Basset G, Lecossier D, et al. Estimation of volume of epithelial lining fluid recovered by lavage using urea as marker of dilution. *J Appl Physiol* 1986;60:532–538.
6. Reynolds HY, Fulmer JD, Kazmierowski JA, Roberts WC, Frank MM, Crystal RG. Analysis of cellular and protein content of broncho-alveolar lavage fluid from patients with idiopathic pulmonary fibrosis and chronic hypersensitivity pneumonitis. *J Clin Invest* 1977;59:165–175.
7. Reynolds HY, Newball HH. Analysis of proteins and respiratory cells obtained from human lungs by bronchial lavage. *J Lab Clin Med* 1974;84:559–573.
8. American Thoracic Society. Standards for the diagnosis and care of patients with chronic obstructive pulmonary disease. *Am J Respir Crit Care Med* 1995;152:S77–S121.
9. Thurlbeck WM. Chronic airflow obstruction. In: Thurlbeck WM, Churg AM, eds. *Pathology of the lung.* New York: Thieme Medical, 1995:739.
10. Younes M. Load responses, dyspnea, and respiratory failure. *Chest* 1990;97:59S–68S.
11. Keogh BA, Lakatos E, Price D, Crystal RG. Importance of the lower respiratory tract in oxygen transfer: exercise testing in patients with interstitial and destructive lung disease. *Am Rev Respir Dis* 1984; 129:S76–S80.
12. Janoff A. Elastases and emphysema: current assessment of the protease-antiprotease hypothesis. *Am Rev Respir Dis* 1985;132:417–433.
13. McElvaney NG, Crystal RG. Vulnerability to proteolytic injury. In: Crystal RG, West JB, Weibel ER, Barnes PJ, eds. *The lung: scientific foundations.* Philadelphia: Lippincott-Raven, 1997:2537–2553.
14. Gross P, Pfitzer E, Tolker E, Bobyak M, Kaschak M. Experimental emphysema: its production with papain in normal and silicotic rats. *Arch Environ Health* 1965;11:50–58.
15. Falloon J, Gallin JI. Neutrophil granules in health and disease. *J Allergy Clin Immunol* 1986;77:653–662.
16. Travis J. Structure, function, and control of neutrophil proteinases. *Am J Med* 1988;84:37–42.
17. Takahashi H, Nukiwa T, Basset P, Crystal RG. Myelomonocytic cell lineage expression of the neutrophil elastase gene. *J Biol Chem* 1988; 263:2543–2547.
18. Fouret P, du Bois RM, Bernaudin JF, Takahashi H, Ferrans VJ, Crystal RG. Expression of the neutrophil elastase gene during human bone marrow cell differentiation. *J Exp Med* 1989;169:833–845.
19. Gadek JE, Fells GA, Wright DG, Crystal RG. Human neutrophil elastase functions as a type III collagen "collagenase." *Biochem Biophys Res Commun* 1980;95:1815–1822.
20. Janoff A, Scherer J. Mediators of inflammation in leukocyte lysosomes: IX. Elastinolytic activity in granules of human polymorphonuclear leukocytes. *J Exp Med* 1968;128:1137–1155.
21. McElvaney NG, Crystal RG. Proteases and lung injury. In: Crystal RG, West JB, eds. *The lung: scientific foundations.* Philadelphia: Lippincott-Raven, 1997:2205–2218.
22. Travis J, Dubin A, Potempa J, Watorek W, Kurdowska A. Neutrophil proteinases: caution signs in designing inhibitors against enzymes with possible multiple functions. *Ann N Y Acad Sci* 1991;624:81–86.
23. Shapiro SD, Kobayashi DK, Ley TJ. Cloning and characterization of a unique elastolytic metalloproteinase produced by human alveolar macrophages. *J Biol Chem* 1993;268:23824–23829.
24. Welgus HG, Campbell EJ, Bar-Shavit Z, Senior RM, Teitelbaum SL. Human alveolar macrophages produce a fibroblast-like collagenase and collagenase inhibitor. *J Clin Invest* 1985;76:219–224.
25. Murphy G, Reynolds JJ. Extracellular matrix degradation. In eds., Royce PM, Steinmann B, *Connective tissue and its heritable disorders.* New York: Wiley-Liss, 1993:287–316.
26. Woessner JF. Matrix metalloproteinases and their inhibitors in connective tissue remodeling. *FASEB J* 1991;5:2145–2154.
27. Baramova E, Foidart JM. Matrix metalloproteinase family. *Cell Biol Int* 1995;19:239–242.
28. Hibbs MS, Bainton DF. Human neutrophil gelatinase is a component of specific granules. *J Clin Invest* 1989;84:1395–1402.
29. Kjeldsen L, Bjerrum OW, Askaa J, Borregaard N. Subcellular localization and release of human neutrophil gelatinase, confirming the existence of separate gelatinase-containing granules. *Biochem J* 1992; 287:603–610.
30. Murphy G, Hembry RM, McGarrity AM, Reynolds JJ, Henderson B. Gelatinase (type IV collagenase) immunolocalization in cells and tissues: use of an antiserum to rabbit bone gelatinase that identifies high and low Mr forms. *J Cell Sci* 1989;92:487–495.

31. Murphy G, Bretz U, Baggiolini M, Reynolds JJ. The latent collagenase and gelatinase of human polymorphonuclear neutrophil leucocytes. *Biochem J* 1980;192:517–525.

32. Murphy G, Reynolds JJ, Bretz U, Baggiolini M. Partial purification of collagenase and gelatinase from human polymorphonuclear leucocytes: analysis of their actions on soluble and insoluble collagens. *Biochem J* 1982;203:209–221.

33. Carmichael DF, Sommer A, Thompson RC, et al. Primary structure and cDNA cloning of human fibroblast collagenase inhibitor. *Proc Natl Acad Sci U S A* 1986;83:2407–2411.

34. Greene J, Wang M, Liu YE, Raymond LA, Rosen C, Shi YE. Molecular cloning and characterization of human tissue inhibitor of metalloproteinase 4. *J Biol Chem* 1996;271:30375–30380.

35. Miyazaki K, Funahashi K, Numata Y, et al. Purification and characterization of a two-chain form of tissue inhibitor of metalloproteinases (TIMP) type 2 and a low molecular weight TIMP-like protein. *J Biol Chem* 1993;268:14387–14393.

36. Stetler-Stevenson WG, Brown PD, Onisto M, Levy AT, Liotta LA. Tissue inhibitor of metalloproteinases-2 (TIMP-2) mRNA expression in tumor cell lines and human tumor tissues. *J Biol Chem* 1990;265: 13933–13938.

37. Travis J, Salvesen GS. Human plasma proteinase inhibitors. *Annu Rev Biochem* 1983;52:655–709.

38. Beatty K, Bieth J, Travis J. Kinetics of association of serine proteinases with native and oxidized alpha-1-proteinase inhibitor and alpha-1-antichymotrypsin. *J Biol Chem* 1980;255:3931–3934.

39. Gadek JE, Klein HG, Holland PV, Crystal RG. Replacement therapy of alpha 1-antitrypsin deficiency: reversal of protease-antiprotease imbalance within the alveolar structures of PiZ subjects. *J Clin Invest* 1981;68:1158–1165.

40. Brantly M, Nukiwa T, Crystal RG. Molecular basis of alpha-1-antitrypsin deficiency. *Am J Med* 1988;84:13–31.

41. McElvaney NG, Crystal RG. Antiproteases and lung defense. In: Crystal RG, West JB, Weibel ER, Barnes PJ, eds. *The lung: scientific foundations.* Philadelphia: Lippincott-Raven, 1997:2219–2235.

42. Brantly ML, Paul LD, Miller BH, Falk RT, Wu M, Crystal RG. Clinical features and history of the destructive lung disease associated with alpha-1-antitrypsin deficiency of adults with pulmonary symptoms. *Am Rev Respir Dis* 1988;138:327–336.

43. Crystal RG. The alpha 1-antitrypsin gene and its deficiency states. *Trends Genet* 1989;5:411–417.

44. Kelsey GD, Povey S, Bygrave AE, Lovell-Badge RH. Species- and tissue-specific expression of human alpha 1-antitrypsin in transgenic mice. *Genes Dev* 1987;1:161–171.

45. Carlson JA, Rogers BB, Sifers RN, Hawkins HK, Finegold MJ, Woo SL. Multiple tissues express alpha 1-antitrypsin in transgenic mice and man. *J Clin Invest* 1988;82:26–36.

46. Heidtmann H, Travis J. Human α1-proteinase inhibitor. In: Barrett AJ, Salvesen G, eds. *Proteinase inhibitors.* Amsterdam: Elsevier, 1986: 441–445.

47. Loebermann H, Tokuoka R, Deisenhofer J, Huber R. Human alpha 1-proteinase inhibitor: crystal structure analysis of two crystal modifications, molecular model and preliminary analysis of the implications for function. *J Mol Biol* 1984;177:531–557.

48. Banda MJ, Rice AG, Griffin GL, Senior RM. The inhibitory complex of human alpha 1-proteinase inhibitor and human leukocyte elastase is a neutrophil chemoattractant. *J Exp Med* 1988;167:1608–1615.

49. Crystal RG. Alpha 1-antitrypsin deficiency, emphysema, and liver disease: genetic basis and strategies for therapy. *J Clin Invest* 1990;85: 1343–1352.

50. Larsson C. Natural history and life expectancy in severe alpha1-antitrypsin deficiency, pi z. *Acta Med Scand* 1978;204:345–351.

51. Seersholm N, Dirksen A, Kok-Jensen A. Airways obstruction and two year survival in patients with severe alpha 1-antitrypsin deficiency. *Eur Respir J* 1994;7:1985–1987.

52. Brantly M, Courtney M, Crystal RG. Repair of the secretion defect in the Z form of alpha 1-antitrypsin by addition of a second mutation. *Science* 1988;242:1700–1702.

53. The Alpha 1-Antitrypsin Study Group. Survival and FEV₁ decline in individuals with severe deficiency of α1-antitrypsin. *Am J Respir Crit Care Med* 1998;158(1):49–59.

54. Crystal RG. α1-Antitrypsin deficiency. In: Fishman AP, ed. *Pulmonary diseases and disorders update.* New York: McGraw-Hill, 1991:19–35.

55. Nukiwa T, Satoh K, Brantly ML, et al. Identification of a second mutation in the protein-coding sequence of the Z type alpha 1-antitrypsin gene. *J Biol Chem* 1986;261:15989–15994.

56. Sharp HL, Bridges RA, Krivit W, Freier EF. Cirrhosis associated with alpha-1-antitrypsin deficiency: a previously unrecognized inherited disorder. *J Lab Clin Med* 1969;73:934–939.

57. Birrer P, McElvaney NG, Chang-Stroman LM, Crystal RG. Alpha 1-antitrypsin deficiency and liver disease. *J Inherit Metab Dis* 1991;14: 512–525.

58. Sifers RN, Hardick CP, Woo SL. Disruption of the 290-342 salt bridge is not responsible for the secretory defect of the PiZ alpha 1-antitrypsin variant. *J Biol Chem* 1989;264:2997–3001.

59. Ogushi F, Fells GA, Hubbard RC, Straus SD, Crystal RG. Z-type alpha 1-antitrypsin is less competent than M1-type alpha 1-antitrypsin as an inhibitor of neutrophil elastase. *J Clin Invest* 1987;80: 1366–1374.

60. Hubbard RC, Crystal RG. Augmentation therapy of alpha 1-antitrypsin deficiency. *Eur Respir J Suppl* 1990;9:44s–52s.

61. Hubbard RC, Fells G, Gadek J, Pacholok S, Humes J, Crystal RG. Neutrophil accumulation in the lung in alpha 1-antitrypsin deficiency: spontaneous release of leukotriene B4 by alveolar macrophages. *J Clin Invest* 1991;88:891–897.

62. Campbell EJ, White RR, Senior RM, Rodriguez RJ, Kuhn C. Receptor-mediated binding and internalization of leukocyte elastase by alveolar macrophages *in vitro. J Clin Invest* 1979;64:824–833.

63. Wewers MD, Casolaro MA, Sellers SE, et al. Replacement therapy for alpha 1-antitrypsin deficiency associated with emphysema. *N Engl J Med* 1987;316:1055–1062.

64. Hubbard RC, Sellers S, Czerski D, Stephens L, Crystal RG. Biochemical efficacy and safety of monthly augmentation therapy for alpha 1-antitrypsin deficiency. *JAMA* 1988;260:1259–1264.

65. Crystal RG. Alpha 1-antitrypsin deficiency: pathogenesis and treatment. *Hosp Pract* 1991;26:81–84,88–89,93–94.

66. Hubbard RC, Brantly ML, Sellers SE, Mitchell ME, Crystal RG. Antineutrophil-elastase defenses of the lower respiratory tract in alpha 1-antitrypsin deficiency directly augmented with an aerosol of alpha 1-antitrypsin. *Ann Intern Med* 1989;111:206–212.

67. Hubbard RC, Casolaro MA, Mitchell M, et al. Fate of aerosolized recombinant DNA-produced alpha 1-antitrypsin: use of the epithelial surface of the lower respiratory tract to administer proteins of therapeutic importance. *Proc Natl Acad Sci U S A* 1989;86:680–684.

68. Hubbard RC, McElvaney NG, Sellers SE, Healy JT, Czerski DB, Crystal RG. Recombinant DNA-produced alpha 1-antitrypsin administered by aerosol augments lower respiratory tract antineutrophil elastase defenses in individuals with alpha 1-antitrypsin deficiency. *J Clin Invest* 1989;84:1349–1354.

69. Garver RI Jr, Chytil A, Karlsson S, et al. Production of glycosylated physiologically "normal" human alpha 1-antitrypsin by mouse fibroblasts modified by insertion of a human alpha 1-antitrypsin cDNA using a retroviral vector. *Proc Natl Acad Sci U S A* 1987;84:1050–1054.

70. Garver RI Jr, Chytil A, Courtney M, Crystal RG. Clonal gene therapy: transplanted mouse fibroblast clones express human alpha 1-antitrypsin gene *in vivo. Science* 1987;237:762–764.

71. Kanno T, Fukayama M, Brody SL, Crystal RG. Retroviral transfer of the human α1-antitrypsin gene to T-lymphocytes for *in vivo* gene transfer. *Am Rev Respir Dis* 1991;143(Suppl):A325.

72. Kay MA, Li Q, Liu TJ, et al. Hepatic gene therapy: persistent expression of human alpha 1-antitrypsin in mice after direct gene delivery *in vivo. Hum Gene Ther* 1992;3:641–647.

73. Kay MA, Baley P, Rothenberg S, et al. Expression of human alpha 1-antitrypsin in dogs after autologous transplantation of retroviral transduced hepatocytes. *Proc Natl Acad Sci U S A* 1992;89:89–93.

74. Canonico AE, Conary JT, Meyrick BO, Brigham KL. Aerosol and intravenous transfection of human alpha 1-antitrypsin gene to lungs of rabbits. *Am J Respir Cell Mol Biol* 1994;10:24–29.

75. Rosenfeld MA, Siegfried W, Yoshimura K, et al. Adenovirus-mediated transfer of a recombinant alpha 1-antitrypsin gene to the lung epithelium *in vivo. Science* 1991;252:431–434.

76. Setoguchi Y, Jaffe HA, Chu CS, Crystal RG. Intraperitoneal *in vivo* gene therapy to deliver alpha 1-antitrypsin to the systemic circulation. *Am J Respir Cell Mol Biol* 1994;10:369–377.

77. Jaffe HA, Danel C, Longenecker G, et al. Adenovirus-mediated *in vivo* gene transfer and expression in normal rat liver. *Nat Genet* 1992; 1:372–378.

78. Kay MA, Graham F, Leland F, Woo SL. Therapeutic serum concentrations of human alpha-1-antitrypsin after adenoviral-mediated gene transfer into mouse hepatocytes. *Hepatology* 1995;21:815–819.

79. Hunninghake GW, Crystal RG. Cigarette smoking and lung destruction: accumulation of neutrophils in the lungs of cigarette smokers. *Am Rev Respir Dis* 1983;128:833–838.

80. Mio T, Romberger DJ, Thompson AB, Robbins RA, Heires A, Rennard SI. Cigarette smoke induces interleukin-8 release from human bronchial epithelial cells. *Am J Respir Crit Care Med* 1997;155:1770–1776.

81. Armstrong LW, Rom WN, Martiniuk FT, Hart D, Jagirdar J, Galdston M. Nicotine enhances expression of the neutrophil elastase gene and protein in a human myeloblast/promyelocyte cell line. *Am J Respir Crit Care Med* 1996;154:1520–1524.

82. Aoshiba K, Nagai A, Yasui S, Konno K. Nicotine prolongs neutrophil survival by suppressing apoptosis. *J Lab Clin Med* 1996;127:186–194.

83. Hautamaki RD, Kobayashi DK, Senior RM, Shapiro SD. Requirement for macrophage elastase for cigarette smoke-induced emphysema in mice. *Science* 1997;277:2002–2004.

84. Finlay GA, O'Driscoll LR, Russell KJ, et al. Matrix metalloproteinase expression and production by alveolar macrophages in emphysema. *Am J Respir Crit Care Med* 1997;156:240–247.

85. D'Armiento J, Dalal SS, Okada Y, Berg RA, Chada K. Collagenase expression in the lungs of transgenic mice causes pulmonary emphysema. *Cell* 1992;71:955–961.

86. Hubbard RC, Ogushi F, Fells GA, et al. Oxidants spontaneously released by alveolar macrophages of cigarette smokers can inactivate the active site of alpha 1-antitrypsin, rendering it ineffective as an inhibitor of neutrophil elastase. *J Clin Invest* 1987;80:1289–1295.

87. Johnson D, Travis J. The oxidative inactivation of human alpha-1-proteinase inhibitor: further evidence for methionine at the reactive center. *J Biol Chem* 1979;254:4022–4026.

88. Ogushi F, Hubbard RC, Vogelmeier C, Fells GA, Crystal RG. Risk factors for emphysema: cigarette smoking is associated with a reduction in the association rate constant of lung alpha 1-antitrypsin for neutrophil elastase. *J Clin Invest* 1991;87:1060–1065.

89. Courtney M, Jallat S, Tessier LH, Benavente A, Crystal RG, Lecocq JP. Synthesis in *E. coli* of alpha 1-antitrypsin variants of therapeutic potential for emphysema and thrombosis. *Nature* 1985;313:149–151.

90. Spencer H. *Pathology of the lung.* New York: Pergamon Press, 1985:131–166.

91. Burrows B, Bloom JW, Traver GA, Cline MG. The course and prognosis of different forms of chronic airways obstruction in a sample from the general population. *N Engl J Med* 1987;317:1309–1314.

92. Bates DV. Respiratory function in disease. Philadelphia: WB Saunders, 1989:192–195.

93. Higgins MW, Thom T. Incidence, prevalence, and mortality: intra- and intercountry differences. In: Helmsley MJ, Saunders NA, eds. *Clinical epidemiology of chronic obstructive lung disease.* New York: Marcel Dekker, 1989:23–29.

94. Welsh MJ, Tsui L, Boat TF, Beaudet AL. Cystic fibrosis. In: Scriver CR, Beaudet AL, Sly WS, Valle D, eds. *The metabolic and molecular basis of inherited disease.* New York: McGraw-Hill, 1995:3799–3876.

95. Troisi RJ, Speizer FE, Rosner B, Trichopoulos D, Willett WC. Cigarette smoking and incidence of chronic bronchitis and asthma in women. *Chest* 1995;108:1557–1561.

96. Khan TZ, Wagener JS, Bost T, Martinez J, Accurso FJ, Riches DW. Early pulmonary inflammation in infants with cystic fibrosis. *Am J Respir Crit Care Med* 1995;151:1075–1082.

97. Armstrong DS, Grimwood K, Carlin JB, et al. Lower airway inflammation in infants and young children with cystic fibrosis. *Am J Respir Crit Care Med* 1997;156:1197–1204.

98. The Cystic Fibrosis Foundation. *Annual Report, 1997.* Bethesda, MD: Cystic Fibrosis Foundation, 1998.

99. Kerem B, Rommens JM, Buchanan JA, et al. Identification of the cystic fibrosis gene: genetic analysis. *Science* 1989;245:1073–1080.

100. Riordan JR, Rommens JM, Kerem B, et al. Identification of the cystic fibrosis gene: cloning and characterization of complementary DNA. *Science* 1989;245:1066–1073.

101. Rommens JM, Iannuzzi MC, Kerem B, et al. Identification of the cystic fibrosis gene: chromosome walking and jumping. *Science* 1989;245:1059–1065.

102. Tsui L. The spectrum of cystic fibrosis mutations. *Trends Genet* 1992;8:392–398.

103. Dean M, Santis G. Heterogeneity in the severity of cystic fibrosis and the role of CFTR gene mutations. *Hum Genet* 1994;93:364–368.

104. Zielenski J, Tsui LC. Cystic fibrosis: genotypic and phenotypic variations. *Annu Rev Genet* 1995;29:777–807.

105. Anderson MP, Rich DP, Gregory RJ, Smith AE, Welsh MJ. Generation of cAMP-activated chloride currents by expression of CFTR. *Science* 1991;251:679–682.

106. Kartner N, Hanrahan JW, Jensen TJ, et al. Expression of the cystic fibrosis gene in non-epithelial invertebrate cells produces a regulated anion conductance. *Cell* 1991;64:681–691.

107. Knowles MR, Church NL, Waltner WE, et al. A pilot study of aerosolized amiloride for the treatment of lung disease in cystic fibrosis. *N Engl J Med* 1990;322:1189–1194.

108. Smith JJ, Travis SM, Greenberg EP, Welsh MJ. Cystic fibrosis airway epithelia fail to kill bacteria because of abnormal airway surface fluid. *Cell* 1996;85:229–236.

109. Birrer P, McElvaney NG, Rudeberg A, et al. Protease-antiprotease imbalance in the lungs of children with cystic fibrosis. *Am J Respir Crit Care Med* 1994;150:207–213.

110. Balough K, McCubbin M, Weinberger M, Smits W, Ahrens R, Fick R. The relationship between infection and inflammation in the early stages of lung disease from cystic fibrosis. *Pediatr Pulmonol* 1995;20:63–70.

111. McElvaney NG, Hubbard RC, Birrer P, et al. Aerosol alpha 1-antitrypsin treatment for cystic fibrosis. *Lancet* 1991;337:392–394.

112. McElvaney NG, Nakamura H, Birrer P, et al. Modulation of airway inflammation in cystic fibrosis: *in vivo* suppression of interleukin-8 levels on the respiratory epithelial surface by aerosolization of recombinant secretory leukoprotease inhibitor. *J Clin Invest* 1992;90:1296–1301.

113. Roum JH, Buhl R, McElvaney NG, Borok Z, Crystal RG. Systemic deficiency of glutathione in cystic fibrosis. *J Appl Physiol* 1993;75:2419–2424.

114. Di Mango E, Zar HJ, Bryan R, Prince A. Diverse *Pseudomonas aeruginosa* gene products stimulate respiratory epithelial cells to produce interleukin-8. *J Clin Invest* 1995;96:2204–2210.

115. Goldman MJ, Anderson GM, Stolzenberg ED, Kari UP, Zasloff M, Wilson JM. Human beta-defensin-1 is a salt-sensitive antibiotic in lung that is inactivated in cystic fibrosis. *Cell* 1997;88:553–560.

116. Knowles MR, Robinson JM, Wood RE, et al. Ion composition of airway surface liquid of patients with cystic fibrosis as compared with normal and disease-control subjects. *J Clin Invest* 1997;100:2588–2595.

117. Irvin RT, Doig P, Lee KK, et al. Characterization of the *Pseudomonas aeruginosa* pilus adhesin: confirmation that the pilin structural protein subunit contains a human epithelial cell-binding domain. *Infect Immun* 1989;57:3720–3726.

118. Barasch J, Kiss B, Prince A, Saiman L, Gruenert D, Al-Awqati Q. Defective acidification of intracellular organelles in cystic fibrosis. *Nature* 1991;352:70–73.

119. Zar H, Saiman L, Quittell L, Prince A. Binding of *Pseudomonas aeruginosa* to respiratory epithelial cells from patients with various mutations in the cystic fibrosis transmembrane regulator. *J Pediatr* 1995;126:230–233.

120. Saiman L, Prince A. *Pseudomonas aeruginosa* pili bind to asialoGM1 which is increased on the surface of cystic fibrosis epithelial cells. *J Clin Invest* 1993;92:1875–1880.

121. Davies JC, Stern M, Dewar A, et al. CFTR gene transfer reduces the binding of *Pseudomonas aeruginosa* to cystic fibrosis respiratory epithelium. *Am J Respir Cell Mol Biol* 1997;16:657–663.

122. Pier GB, Grout M, Zaidi TS, et al. Role of mutant CFTR in hypersusceptibility of cystic fibrosis patients to lung infections. *Science* 1996;271:64–67.

123. van Heeckeren A, Walenga RW, Konstan MW, Bonfield T, Davis PB, Ferkol T. Excessive inflammatory response of cystic fibrosis mice to bronchopulmonary infection with *Pseudomonas aeruginosa. J Clin Invest* 1997;100:2810–2815.

124. Nakamura H, Yoshimura K, McElvaney NG, Crystal RG. Neutrophil elastase in respiratory epithelial lining fluid of individuals with cystic fibrosis induces interleukin-8 gene expression in a human bronchial epithelial cell line. *J Clin Invest* 1992;89:1478–1484.

125. Bonfield TL, Panuska JR, Konstan MW, et al. Inflammatory cytokines in cystic fibrosis lungs. *Am J Respir Crit Care Med* 1995;152:2111–2118.

126. Okusawa S, Yancey KB, van der Meer JW, et al. C5a stimulates secretion of tumor necrosis factor from human mononuclear cells *in vitro*: comparison with secretion of interleukin 1 beta and interleukin 1 alpha. *J Exp Med* 1988;168:443–448.

127. Warren JS, Kunkel SL, Cunningham TW, Johnson KJ, Ward PA. Macrophage-derived cytokines amplify immune complex-triggered O2⁻ responses by rat alveolar macrophages. *Am J Pathol* 1988;130: 489–495.

128. Tosi MF, Stark JM, Smith CW, Hamedani A, Gruenert DC, Infeld MD. Induction of ICAM-1 expression on human airway epithelial cells by inflammatory cytokines: effects on neutrophil-epithelial cell adhesion. *Am J Respir Cell Mol Biol* 1992;7:214–221.

129. Standiford TJ, Kunkel SL, Basha MA, et al. Interleukin-8 gene expression by a pulmonary epithelial cell line: a model for cytokine networks in the lung. *J Clin Invest* 1990;86:1945–1953.

130. Strieter RM, Chensue SW, Basha MA, et al. Human alveolar macrophage gene expression of interleukin-8 by tumor necrosis factor-alpha, lipopolysaccharide, and interleukin-1 beta. *Am J Respir Cell Mol Biol* 1990;2:321–326.

131. Martin TR, Pistorese BP, Chi EY, Goodman RB, Matthay MA. Effects of leukotriene B4 in the human lung: recruitment of neutrophils into the alveolar spaces without a change in protein permeability. *J Clin Invest* 1989;84:1609–1619.

132. Konstan MW, Walenga RW, Hilliard KA, Hilliard JB. Leukotriene B4 markedly elevated in the epithelial lining fluid of patients with cystic fibrosis. *Am Rev Respir Dis* 1993;148:896–901.

133. Bokoch GM, Reed PW. Effect of various lipoxygenase metabolites of arachidonic acid on degranulation of polymorphonuclear leukocytes. *J Biol Chem* 1981;256:5317–5320.

134. Gay JC, Beckman JK, Brash AR, Oates JA, Lukens JN. Enhancement of chemotactic factor-stimulated neutrophil oxidative metabolism by leukotriene B4. *Blood* 1984;64:780–785.

135. Gimbrone MA Jr, Brock AF, Schafer AI. Leukotriene B4 stimulates polymorphonuclear leukocyte adhesion to cultured vascular endothelial cells. *J Clin Invest* 1984;74:1552–1555.

136. Bonfield TL, Konstan MW, Burfeind P, Panuska JR, Hilliard JB, Berger M. Normal bronchial epithelial cells constitutively produce the anti-inflammatory cytokine interleukin-10, which is downregulated in cystic fibrosis. *Am J Respir Cell Mol Biol* 1995;13:257–261.

137. Li JD, Dohrman AF, Gallup M, et al. Transcriptional activation of mucin by *Pseudomonas aeruginosa* lipopolysaccharide in the pathogenesis of cystic fibrosis lung disease. *Proc Natl Acad Sci U S A* 1997; 94:967–972.

138. Kirchner KK, Wagener JS, Khan TZ, Copenhaver SC, Accurso FJ. Increased DNA levels in bronchoalveolar lavage fluid obtained from infants with cystic fibrosis. *Am J Respir Crit Care Med* 1996;154: 1426–1429.

139. Lethem MI, James SL, Marriott C, Burke JF. The origin of DNA associated with mucus glycoproteins in cystic fibrosis sputum. *Eur Respir J* 1990;3:19–23.

140. Vogelmeier C, Hubbard RC, Fells GA, et al. Anti-neutrophil elastase defense of the normal human respiratory epithelial surface provided by the secretory leukoprotease inhibitor. *J Clin Invest* 1991;87: 482–488.

141. Davis WB, Pacht ER. Extracellular antioxidant defenses. In: Crystal RG, West JB, Weibel ER, Parnes PJ, eds. *The lung: scientific foundations*. Philadelphia: Lippincott-Raven, 1997:2271–2278.

142. Cantin AM, North SL, Hubbard RC, Crystal RG. Normal alveolar epithelial lining fluid contains high levels of glutathione. *J Appl Physiol* 1987;63:152–157.

143. Berger M, Sorensen RU, Tosi MF, Dearborn DG, Doring G. Complement receptor expression on neutrophils at an inflammatory site, the *Pseudomonas*-infected lung in cystic fibrosis. *J Clin Invest* 1989;84: 1302–1313.

144. Vogelmeier C, Buhl R, Hoyt RF, et al. Aerosolization of recombinant SLPI to augment antineutrophil elastase protection of pulmonary epithelium. *J Appl Physiol* 1990;69:1843–1848.

145. Vogelmeier C, Gillissen A, Buhl R. Use of secretory leukoprotease inhibitor to augment lung antineutrophil elastase activity. *Chest* 1996; 110:261S–266S.

146. Roum JH, Kirby M, Borok Z, Hubbard R, Crystal RG. Ability of extracellular glutathione to suppress oxidant generation in alveolar macrophages in individuals with chronic interstitial lung disease. *Am Rev Respir Dis* 1991;143(Suppl):A740.

147. Gillissen A, Birrer P, McElvaney NG, et al. Recombinant secretory leukoprotease inhibitor augments glutathione levels in lung epithelial lining fluid. *J Appl Physiol* 1993;75:825–832.

148. Hubbard RC, McElvaney NG, Birrer P, et al. A preliminary study of aerosolized recombinant human deoxyribonuclease I in the treatment of cystic fibrosis. *N Engl J Med* 1992;326:812–815.

149. Shak S, Capon DJ, Hellmiss R, Marsters SA, Baker CL. Recombinant human DNase I reduces the viscosity of cystic fibrosis sputum. *Proc Natl Acad Sci U S A* 1990;87:9188–9192.

150. McCoy K, Hamilton S, Johnson C. Effects of 12-week administration of dornase alfa in patients with advanced cystic fibrosis lung disease. Pulmozyme Study Group. *Chest* 1996;110:889–895.

151. Shah PI, Bush A, Canny GJ, et al. Recombinant human DNase I in cystic fibrosis patients with severe pulmonary disease: a short-term, double-blind study followed by six months open-label treatment. *Eur Respir J* 1995;8:954–958.

152. Shah PL, Scott SF, Knight RA, Hodson ME. The effects of recombinant human DNase on neutrophil elastase activity and interleukin-8 levels in the sputum of patients with cystic fibrosis. *Eur Respir J* 1996;9:531–534.

153. Knowles MR, Olivier K, Noone P, Boucher RC. Pharmacologic modulation of salt and water in the airway epithelium in cystic fibrosis. *Am J Respir Crit Care Med* 1995;151:S65–S69.

154. Wagner JA, Cozens AL, Schulman H, Gruenert DC, Stryer L, Gardner P. Activation of chloride channels in normal and cystic fibrosis airway epithelial cells by multifunctional calcium/calmodulin-dependent protein kinase. *Nature* 1991;349:793–796.

155. Knowles MR, Clarke LL, Boucher RC. Activation by extracellular nucleotides of chloride secretion in the airway epithelia of patients with cystic fibrosis. *N Engl J Med* 1991;325:533–538.

156. Bennett WD, Olivier KN, Zeman KL, Hohneker KW, Boucher RC, Knowles MR. Effect of uridine 5′-triphosphate plus amiloride on mucociliary clearance in adult cystic fibrosis. *Am J Respir Crit Care Med* 1996;153:1796–1801.

157. Drumm ML, Pope HA, Cliff WH, et al. Correction of the cystic fibrosis defect *in vitro* by retrovirus-mediated gene transfer. *Cell* 1990;62: 1227–1233.

158. Rich DP, Anderson MP, Gregory RJ, et al. Expression of cystic fibrosis transmembrane conductance regulator corrects defective chloride channel regulation in cystic fibrosis airway epithelial cells. *Nature* 1990;347:358–363.

159. Rosenfeld MA, Yoshimura K, Trapnell BC, et al. *In vivo* transfer of the human cystic fibrosis transmembrane conductance regulator gene to the airway epithelium. *Cell* 1992;68:143–155.

160. Rosenfeld MA, Chu CS, Seth P, et al. Gene transfer to freshly isolated human respiratory epithelial cells *in vitro* using a replication-deficient adenovirus containing the human cystic fibrosis transmembrane conductance regulator cDNA. *Hum Gene Ther* 1994;5:331–342.

161. Hyde SC, Gill DR, Higgins CF, et al. Correction of the ion transport defect in cystic fibrosis transgenic mice by gene therapy. *Nature* 1993; 362:250–255.

162. Conrad CK, Allen SS, Afione SA, et al. Safety of single-dose administration of an adeno-associated virus (AAV)-CFTR vector in the primate lung. *Gene Ther* 1996;3:658–668.

163. Goldman MJ, Litzky LA, Engelhardt JF, Wilson JM. Transfer of the CFTR gene to the lung of nonhuman primates with E1-deleted, E2a-defective recombinant adenoviruses: a preclinical toxicology study. *Hum Gene Ther* 1995;6:839–851.

164. Sene C, Bout A, Imler JL, et al. Aerosol-mediated delivery of recombinant adenovirus to the airways of nonhuman primates. *Hum Gene Ther* 1995;6:1587–1593.

165. Alton EW, Middleton PG, Caplen NJ, et al. Non-invasive liposome-mediated gene delivery can correct the ion transport defect in cystic fibrosis mutant mice. *Nat Genet* 1993;5:135–142.

166. Logan JJ, Bebok Z, Walker LC, et al. Cationic lipids for reporter gene and CFTR transfer to rat pulmonary epithelium. *Gene Ther* 1995;2:38–49.

167. McDonald RJ, Lukason MJ, Raabe OG, et al. Safety of airway gene transfer with Ad2/CFTR2: aerosol administration in the nonhuman primate. *Hum Gene Ther* 1997;8:411–422.

168. Yoshimura K, Rosenfeld MA, Nakamura H, et al. Expression of the human cystic fibrosis transmembrane conductance regulator gene in the mouse lung after *in vivo* intratracheal plasmid-mediated gene transfer. *Nucleic Acids Res* 1992;20:3233–3240.

169. Zabner J, Petersen DM, Puga AP, et al. Safety and efficacy of repetitive adenovirus-mediated transfer of CFTR cDNA to airway epithelia of primates and cotton rats. *Nat Genet* 1994;6:75–83.

170. Zabner J, Couture LA, Gregory RJ, Graham SM, Smith AE, Welsh MJ. Adenovirus-mediated gene transfer transiently corrects the chloride transport defect in nasal epithelia of patients with cystic fibrosis. *Cell* 1993;75:207–216.

171. Crystal RG, McElvaney NG, Rosenfeld MA, et al. Administration of an adenovirus containing the human CFTR cDNA to the respiratory tract of individuals with cystic fibrosis. *Nat Genet* 1994;8:42–51.

172. Welsh MJ, Smith AE, Zabner J, et al. Cystic fibrosis gene therapy using an adenovirus vector: *in vivo* safety and efficacy in nasal epithelium. *Hum Gene Ther* 1994;5:209–219.

173. Caplen NJ, Alton EW, Middleton PG, et al. Liposome-mediated CFTR gene transfer to the nasal epithelium of patients with cystic fibrosis. *Nat Med* 1995;1:39–46.

174. Crystal RG, Mastrangeli A, Sanders A, et al. Evaluation of repeat administration of a replication deficient, recombinant adenovirus containing the normal cystic fibrosis transmembrane conductance regulator cDNA to the airways of individuals with cystic fibrosis. *Hum Gene Ther* 1995;6:667–703.

175. Crystal RG, Jaffe A, Brody S, et al. A phase I study, in cystic fibrosis patients, of the safety, toxicity, and biological efficacy of a single administration of a replication deficient, recombinant adenovirus carrying the cDNA of the normal cystic fibrosis transmembrane conductance regulator gene in the lung. *Hum Gene Ther* 1995;6:643–666.

176. Hay JG, McElvaney NG, Herena J, Crystal RG. Modification of nasal epithelial potential differences of individuals with cystic fibrosis consequent to local administration of a normal CFTR cDNA adenovirus gene transfer vector. *Hum Gene Ther* 1995;6:1487–1496.

177. Flotte T, Carter B, Conrad C, et al. A phase I study of an adeno-associated virus-CFTR gene vector in adult CF patients with mild lung disease. *Hum Gene Ther* 1996;7:1145–1159.

178. Zabner J, Ramsey BW, Meeker DP, et al. Repeat administration of an adenovirus vector encoding cystic fibrosis transmembrane conductance regulator to the nasal epithelium of patients with cystic fibrosis. *J Clin Invest* 1996;97:1504–1511.

179. Porteous DJ, Dorin JR, McLachlan G, et al. Evidence for safety and efficacy of DOTAP cationic liposome mediated CFTR gene transfer to the nasal epithelium of patients with cystic fibrosis. *Gene Ther* 1997;4:210–218.

180. Zabner J, Cheng SH, Meeker D, et al. Comparison of DNA-lipid complexes and DNA alone for gene transfer to cystic fibrosis airway epithelia *in vivo*. *J Clin Invest* 1997;100:1529–1537.

181. Thompson AB, Daughton D, Robbins RA, Ghafouri MA, Oehlerking M, Rennard SI. Intraluminal airway inflammation in chronic bronchitis: characterization and correlation with clinical parameters. *Am Rev Respir Dis* 1989;140:1527–1537.

182. Balbi B, Bason C, Balleari E, et al. Increased bronchoalveolar granulocytes and granulocyte/macrophage colony-stimulating factor during exacerbations of chronic bronchitis. *Eur Respir J* 1997;10:846–850.

183. Linden M, Rasmussen JB, Piitulainen E, et al. Airway inflammation in smokers with nonobstructive and obstructive chronic bronchitis. *Am Rev Respir Dis* 1993;148:1226–1232.

184. Crystal RG, Bitterman PB, Rennard SI, Hance AJ, Keogh BA. Interstitial lung diseases of unknown cause: disorders characterized by chronic inflammation of the lower respiratory tract. *N Engl J Med* 1984;310:235–244.

185. Wolff G, Crystal RG. Biology of pulmonary fibrosis. In: Crystal RG, West JB, Weibel ER, Barnes PJ, eds. *The lung: scientific foundations.* Philadelphia: Lippincott-Raven, 1997:2509–2524.

186. Crystal RG, Gadek JE, Ferrans VJ, Fulmer JD, Line BR, Hunninghake GW. Interstitial lung disease: current concepts of pathogenesis, staging and therapy. *Am J Med* 1981;70:542–568.

187. Crystal RG. Interstitial lung disease. In: Wyngaarden JR, Smith LH Jr, eds. *The Cecil textbook of medicine.* Philadelphia: WB Saunders, 1991:421–435.

188. Fulmer JD, Roberts WC, von Gal ER, Crystal RG. Morphologic-physiologic correlates of the severity of fibrosis and degree of cellularity in idiopathic pulmonary fibrosis. *J Clin Invest* 1979;63:665–676.

189. Fulmer JD, Roberts WC, von Gal ER, Crystal RG. Small airways in idiopathic pulmonary fibrosis: comparison of morphologic and physiologic observations. *J Clin Invest* 1977;60:595–610.

190. Crystal RG, Fulmer JD, Roberts WC, Moss ML, Line BR, Reynolds HY. Idiopathic pulmonary fibrosis: clinical, histologic, radiographic, physiologic, scintigraphic, cytologic, and biochemical aspects. *Ann Intern Med* 1976;85:769–788.

191. Kawanami O, Ferrans VJ, Crystal RG. Structure of alveolar epithelial cells in patients with fibrotic lung disorders. *Lab Invest* 1982;46:39–53.

192. Crystal RG, Fulmer JD, Baum BJ, et al. Cells, collagen and idiopathic pulmonary fibrosis. *Lung* 1978;155:199–224.

193. Basset F, Ferrans VJ, Soler P, Takemura T, Fukuda Y, Crystal RG. Intraluminal fibrosis in interstitial lung disorders. *Am J Pathol* 1986; 122:443–461.

194. Hance A, Crysal RG. Idiopathic pulmonary fibrosis. In: Flenlley DC, Petty TL, eds. *Recent advances in respiratory medicine.* New York: Churchill Livingstone, 1983:249–287.

195. Hunninghake GW, Gadek JE, Lawley TJ, Crystal RG. Mechanisms of neutrophil accumulation in the lungs of patients with idiopathic pulmonary fibrosis. *J Clin Invest* 1981;68:259–269.

196. Borok Z, Trapnell BC, Crysal RG. Neutrophils and the pathogenesis of idiopathic pulmonary fibrosis. In: Baggiolini M, Pozzi E, Semenzato G, eds. *Pathophysiology of pulmonary cells: neutrophils and lymphocytes.* Milano: Masson Italia, 1990:111–122.

197. Meliconi R, Senaldi G, Sturani C, et al. Complement activation products in idiopathic pulmonary fibrosis: relevance of fragment ba to disease severity. *Clin Immunol Immunopathol* 1990;57:64–73.

198. Bitterman PB, Rennard SI, Keogh BA, Wewers MD, Adelberg S, Crystal RG. Familial idiopathic pulmonary fibrosis: evidence of lung inflammation in unaffected family members. *N Engl J Med* 1986;314: 1343–1347.

199. Fortoul TI, Barrios R. Mast cells and idiopathic lung fibrosis. *Arch Invest Med (Mex)* 1990;21:5–10.

200. Kawanami O, Ferrans VJ, Fulmer JD, Crystal RG. Ultrastructure of pulmonary mast cells in patients with fibrotic lung disorders. *Lab Invest* 1979;40:717–734.

201. Bitterman PB, Saltzman LE, Adelberg S, Ferrans VJ, Crystal RG. Alveolar macrophage replication: one mechanism for the expansion of the mononuclear phagocyte population in the chronically inflamed lung. *J Clin Invest* 1984;74:460–469.

202. Hoogsteden HC, van Dongen JJ, van Hal PT, Delahaye M, Hop W, Hilvering C. Phenotype of blood monocytes and alveolar macrophages in interstitial lung disease. *Chest* 1989;95:574–577.

203. Antoniades HN, Neville-Golden J, Galanopoulos T, Kradin RL, Valente AJ, Graves DT. Expression of monocyte chemoattractant protein 1 mRNA in human idiopathic pulmonary fibrosis. *Proc Natl Acad Sci U S A* 1992;89:5371–5375.

204. Car BD, Meloni F, Luisetti M, Semenzato G, Gialdroni-Grassi G, Walz A. Elevated IL-8 and MCP-1 in the bronchoalveolar lavage fluid of patients with idiopathic pulmonary fibrosis and pulmonary sarcoidosis. *Am J Respir Crit Care Med* 1994;149:655–659.

205. Iyonaga K, Takeya M, Saita N, et al. Monocyte chemoattractant protein-1 in idiopathic pulmonary fibrosis and other interstitial lung diseases. *Hum Pathol* 1994;25:455–463.

206. Dreisin RB, Schwarz MI, Theofilopoulos AN, Stanford RE. Circulating immune complexes in the idiopathic interstitial pneumonias. *N Engl J Med* 1978;298:353–357.

207. Hunninghake GW, Gadek JE, Fales HM, Crystal RG. Human alveolar macrophage-derived chemotactic factor for neutrophils: stimuli and partial characterization. *J Clin Invest* 1980;66:473–483.

208. Martinet Y, Haslam PL, Turner-Warwick M. Clinical significance of circulating immune complexes in "lone" cryptogenic fibrosing alveolitis and those with associated connective tissue disorders. *Clin Allergy* 1984;14:491–497.

209. Martin TR, Raugi G, Merritt TL, Henderson WR Jr. Relative contribution of leukotriene B4 to the neutrophil chemotactic activity produced by the resident human alveolar macrophage. *J Clin Invest* 1987; 80:1114–1124.

210. Nakao A, Hasegawa Y, Tsuchiya Y, Shimokata K. Expression of cell adhesion molecules in the lungs of patients with idiopathic pulmonary fibrosis. *Chest* 1995;108:233–239.

211. Cantin AM, North SL, Fells GA, Hubbard RC, Crystal RG. Oxidant-mediated epithelial cell injury in idiopathic pulmonary fibrosis. *J Clin Invest* 1987;79:1665–1673.

212. Maier K, Leuschel L, Costabel U. Increased levels of oxidized methionine residues in bronchoalveolar lavage fluid proteins from patients with idiopathic pulmonary fibrosis. *Am Rev Respir Dis* 1991;143: 271–274.

213. Strausz J, Muller-Quernheim J, Steppling H, Ferlinz R. Oxygen radical production by alveolar inflammatory cells in idiopathic pulmonary fibrosis. *Am Rev Respir Dis* 1990;141:124–128.

214. Kawakami M, Kameyama S, Takizawa T. Lipid peroxidation in bronchoalveolar lavage fluid in interstitial lung diseases in relation to other components and smoking. *Nippon Kyobu Shikkan Gakkai Zasshi* 1989;27:422–427.

215. Cantin AM, Hubbard RC, Crystal RG. Glutathione deficiency in the epithelial lining fluid of the lower respiratory tract in idiopathic pulmonary fibrosis. *Am Rev Respir Dis* 1989;139:370–372.

216. Gadek JE, Kelman JA, Fells G, et al. Collagenase in the lower respiratory tract of patients with idiopathic pulmonary fibrosis. *N Engl J Med* 1979;301:737–742.

217. Hallgren R, Bjermer L, Lundgren R, Venge P. The eosinophil component of the alveolitis in idiopathic pulmonary fibrosis: signs of eosinophil activation in the lung are related to impaired lung function. *Am Rev Respir Dis* 1989;139:373–377.

218. Casale TB, Trapp S, Zehr B, Hunninghake GW. Bronchoalveolar lavage fluid histamine levels in interstitial lung diseases. *Am Rev Respir Dis* 1988;138:1604–1608.

219. Rankin JA, Kaliner M, Reynolds HY. Histamine levels in bronchoalveolar lavage from patients with asthma, sarcoidosis, and idiopathic pulmonary fibrosis. *J Allergy Clin Immunol* 1987;79:371–377.

220. Kotani I, Sato A, Hayakawa H, Urano T, Takada Y, Takada A. Increased procoagulant and antifibrinolytic activities in the lungs with idiopathic pulmonary fibrosis. *Thromb Res* 1995;77:493–504.

221. Zhang Y, Lee TC, Guillemin B, Yu MC, Rom WN. Enhanced IL-1 beta and tumor necrosis factor-alpha release and messenger RNA expression in macrophages from idiopathic pulmonary fibrosis or after asbestos exposure. *J Immunol* 1993;150:4188–4196.

222. Smith DR, Kunkel SL, Standiford TJ, et al. Increased interleukin-1 receptor antagonist in idiopathic pulmonary fibrosis: a compartmental analysis. *Am J Respir Crit Care Med* 1995;151:1965–1973.

223. Bitterman PB, Rennard SI, Hunninghake GW, Crystal RG. Human alveolar macrophage growth factor for fibroblasts: regulation and partial characterization. *J Clin Invest* 1982;70:806–822.

224. Martinet Y, Rom WN, Grotendorst GR, Martin GR, Crystal RG. Exaggerated spontaneous release of platelet-derived growth factor by alveolar macrophages from patients with idiopathic pulmonary fibrosis. *N Engl J Med* 1987;317:202–209.

225. Rennard SI, Hunninghake GW, Bitterman PB, Crystal RG. Production of fibronectin by the human alveolar macrophage: mechanism for the recruitment of fibroblasts to sites of tissue injury in interstitial lung diseases. *Proc Natl Acad Sci U S A* 1981;78:7147–7151.

226. Adachi K, Yamauchi K, Bernaudin JF, Fouret P, Ferrans VJ, Crystal RG. Evaluation of fibronectin gene expression by *in situ* hybridization: differential expression of the fibronectin gene among populations of human alveolar macrophages. *Am J Pathol* 1988;133:193–203.

227. Bitterman PB, Wewers MD, Rennard SI, Adelberg S, Crystal RG. Modulation of alveolar macrophage-driven fibroblast proliferation by alternative macrophage mediators. *J Clin Invest* 1986;77:700–708.

228. Mornex JF, Martinet Y, Yamauchi K, et al. Spontaneous expression of the c-sis gene and release of a platelet-derived growth factor-like molecule by human alveolar macrophages. *J Clin Invest* 1986;78:61–66.

229. Nagaoka I, Trapnell BC, Crystal RG. Upregulation of platelet-derived growth factor-A and-B gene expression in alveolar macrophages of individuals with idiopathic pulmonary fibrosis. *J Clin Invest* 1990;85:2023–2027.

230. Rom WN, Basset P, Fells GA, Nukiwa T, Trapnell BC, Crysal RG. Alveolar macrophages release an insulin-like growth factor I-type molecule. *J Clin Invest* 1988;82:1685–1693.

231. Yamauchi K, Martinet Y, Crystal RG. Modulation of fibronectin gene expression in human mononuclear phagocytes. *J Clin Invest* 1987;80:1720–1727.

232. Rennard SI, Crystal RG. Fibronectin in human bronchopulmonary lavage fluid: elevation in patients with interstitial lung disease. *J Clin Invest* 1982;69:113–122.

233. Antoniades HN, Bravo MA, Avila RE, et al. Platelet-derived growth factor in idiopathic pulmonary fibrosis. *J Clin Invest* 1990;86:1055–1064.

234. Polonovsky V, Bitterman PB. Regulation of cell population size. In:

235. Ross R, Raines EW, Bowen-Pope DF. The biology of platelet-derived growth factor. *Cell* 1986;46:155–169.

236. Roman J, McDonald JA. Fibronectins and fibronectin receptors in lung development, injury and repair. In: Crystal RG, West JB, Weibel ER, Barnes PJ, eds. *The lung: scientific foundations.* Philadelphia: Lippincott-Raven, 1997:737–755.

237. Bitterman PB, Rennard SI, Adelberg S, Crystal RG. Role of fibronectin as a growth factor for fibroblasts. *J Cell Biol* 1983;97:1925–1932.

238. Fukuda Y, Basset F, Ferrans VJ, Yamanaka N. Significance of early intra-alveolar fibrotic lesions and integrin expression in lung biopsy specimens from patients with idiopathic pulmonary fibrosis. *Hum Pathol* 1995;26:53–61.

239. Broekelmann TJ, Limper AH, Colby TV, McDonald JA. Transforming growth factor beta 1 is present at sites of extracellular matrix gene expression in human pulmonary fibrosis. *Proc Natl Acad Sci U S A* 1991;88:6642–6646.

240. Aston C, Jagirdar J, Lee TC, Hur T, Hintz RL, Rom WN. Enhanced insulin-like growth factor molecules in idiopathic pulmonary fibrosis. *Am J Respir Crit Care Med* 1995;151:1597–1603.

241. Hill DJ, Crace CJ, Fowler L, Holder AT, Milner RD. Cultured fetal rat myoblasts release peptide growth factors which are immunologically and biologically similar to somatomedin. *J Cell Physiol* 1984;119:349–358.

242. Roberts AB, Anzano MA, Wakefield LM, Roche NS, Stern DF, Sporn MB. Type beta transforming growth factor: a bifunctional regulator of cellular growth. *Proc Natl Acad Sci U S A* 1985;82:119–123.

243. Yamauchi K, Martinet Y, Basset P, Fells GA, Crystal RG. High levels of transforming growth factor-beta are present in the epithelial lining fluid of the normal human lower respiratory tract. *Am Rev Respir Dis* 1988;137:1360–1363.

244. Fine A, Goldstein RH. The effect of transforming growth factor-beta on cell proliferation and collagen formation by lung fibroblasts. *J Biol Chem* 1987;262:3897–3902.

245. Roberts CJ, Birkenmeier TM, McQuillan JJ, et al. Transforming growth factor beta stimulates the expression of fibronectin and of both subunits of the human fibronectin receptor by cultured human lung fibroblasts. *J Biol Chem* 1988;263:4586–4592.

246. Sime PJ, Xing Z, Graham FL, Csaky KG, Gauldie J. Adenovector-mediated gene transfer of active transforming growth factor-beta1 induces prolonged severe fibrosis in rat lung. *J Clin Invest* 1997;100:768–776.

247. Ozaki T, Rennard SI, Crystal RG. Cyclooxygenase metabolites are compartmentalized in the human lower respiratory tract. *J Appl Physiol* 1987;62:219–222.

248. Bradley K, McConnell-Breul S, Crystal RG. Collagen in the human lung: quantitation of rates of synthesis and partial characterization of composition. *J Clin Invest* 1975;55:543–550.

249. Selman M, Montano M, Ramos C, Chapela R. Concentration, biosynthesis and degradation of collagen in idiopathic pulmonary fibrosis. *Thorax* 1986;41:355–359.

250. Lacronique JG, Rennard SI, Bitterman PB, Ozaki T, Crystal RG. Alveolar macrophages in idiopathic pulmonary fibrosis have glucocorticoid receptors, but glucocorticoid therapy does not suppress alveolar macrophage release of fibronectin and alveolar macrophage derived growth factor. *Am Rev Respir Dis* 1984;130:450–456.

251. O'Donnell K, Keogh B, Cantin A, Crystal RG. Pharmacologic suppression of the neutrophil component of the alveolitis in idiopathic pulmonary fibrosis. *Am Rev Respir Dis* 1987;136:288–292.

252. Johnson MA, Kwan S, Snell NJ, Nunn AJ, Darbyshire JH, Turner-Warwick M. Randomised controlled trial comparing prednisolone alone with cyclophosphamide and low dose prednisolone in combination in cryptogenic fibrosing alveolitis. *Thorax* 1989;44:280–288.

253. Borok Z, Buhl R, Grimes GJ, et al. Effect of glutathione aerosol on oxidant-antioxidant imbalance in idiopathic pulmonary fibrosis. *Lancet* 1991;338:215–216.

254. Borok Z, Gillissen A, Buhl R, et al. Augmentation of functional prostaglandin E levels on the respiratory epithelial surface by aerosol administration of prostaglandin E. *Am Rev Respir Dis* 1991;144:1080–1084.

Crystal RG, West JB, Weibel ER, Barnes PJ, eds. *The lung: scientific foundations.* Philadelphia: Lippincott-Raven, 1997:133–153.

Inflammation: Basic Principles and Clinical Correlates,
3rd ed., edited by John I. Gallin and Ralph Snyderman.
Lippincott Williams & Wilkins, Philadelphia © 1999.

CHAPTER 68

Atherogenesis

Russell Ross

Atherosclerosis is one of the most common diseases in Western civilization and is the principal cause of death in the United States and Western Europe (1). Contrary to earlier notions, this disease process is not just a problem of adulthood but rather begins in early childhood, since the earliest lesions of atherosclerosis can be found in young infants. When the disease progresses to the point that advanced lesions develop, these lesions protrude into the lumen of the artery and can lead to various clinical sequelae, including myocardial infarction, cerebral infarction, gangrene of the extremities, and loss of function of a given organ (1–6). The advanced, occlusive lesion of atherosclerosis represents a fibroproliferative response involving large numbers of intimal smooth muscle cells, together with numerous macrophages, varying numbers of T lymphocytes, and, if the lesion is very advanced, capillaries known as vasa vasorum (3,7–9).

The process of atherogenesis is fundamentally an inflammatory-fibroproliferative process; thus, as is the case with so many other disease entities that result from tissue injury, atherosclerosis is an inflammatory disease. When the inflammation is prolonged and excessive, it is accompanied or followed by a fibroproliferative, or healing, response. Although the inflammation may begin as a protective response, when it becomes excessive, it can cause great tissue damage. Each of the risk factors of atherogenesis is associated with substances responsible for injury to the artery wall. The inflammatory response begins and leads to characteristic changes in the artery that are manifest as the different lesions of atherosclerosis. The lesions embody phases of inflammation and repair (discussed below).

The intimal fibroproliferative response usually occurs at sites in the arteries such as branches and bifurcations,

suggesting that the rheologic properties of blood flow may have an impact at these sites and thus play an important role in lesion formation (10).

Data from experimental animals suggest that interactions among the cellular components of the lesions of atherosclerosis lead to proliferation of smooth muscle cells and monocyte-derived macrophages. This mixed proliferation of smooth muscle and macrophages culminates in the advanced, sometimes occlusive, lesions that can lead to myocardial or cerebral infarction. Thrombosis and occlusion of the affected artery usually happen to occur because of changes in the surface of the lesions, such as ulceration, erosion, fissuring, or cracking. Such changes provide sites where platelet adherence, mural thrombi, and occlusive thrombi can form. This latter series of changes sometimes happens rapidly and can lead to sudden death (11).

The most common cause of sudden death may be due to the fibrous cap covering the advanced lesion. If the fibrous cap is unusually thin, it may rupture from the activity of metalloproteases released by macrophages. These enzymes may degrade the fibrous cap covering the necrotic, lipid-rich core of the advanced lesion, exposing it to the lumen, thus leading to thrombosis or hemorrhage. If the forming thrombus occludes the artery, sudden death could occur rapidly (12,13).

When the artery wall becomes injured by various substances associated with the risk factors of atherosclerosis, for example, cigarette smoking, hyperlipidemia, the presence of free radicals associated with the formation of oxidized or modified lipoproteins, elevation of abnormal amino acids such as homocysteine, or other toxic factors, the artery wall can respond in a characteristic fashion to the injury, first by inflammation, and second by using its principal connective tissue-forming cells, the smooth muscle cells of the wall. The smooth muscle cells multiply and form a fibroproliferative response, the combination of which leads to the development of advanced

---

R. Ross: Department of Pathology, University of Washington School of Medicine, Seattle, Washington 98195.

lesions of atherosclerosis (14). The ontogeny of these lesions is presented below.

THE LESIONS OF ATHEROSCLEROSIS

The lesions of atherosclerosis have been divided somewhat arbitrarily into three categories: the early lesion, or fatty streak; the so-called intermediate or fibrofatty lesion; and the advanced, complicated lesion or fibrous plaque.

Early Lesions—The Fatty Streak

In a study of children and young adults, Stary (15) observed the presence of fatty streaks in children under 10 years of age. The fatty streaks consisted principally of intimal lipid-filled macrophages together with variable numbers of lipid-filled smooth muscle cells, which usually were found below the macrophages. Both of these cell types have been called foam cells because of their lipid content (16,17). The lesions are called fatty streaks because of their gross appearance on examination of the surface of the artery with a hand lens. This yellow discoloration is due to the lipid that accumulates in the foam cells, most of which are lipid-filled macrophages, which make up the bulk of the lesions. Most of the lipid, in the form of free cholesterol and cholesterol esters, enters the intima of the artery via the endothelial cells by active transport and usually occurs in individuals who are hypercholesterolemic.

The data of Stary (15) and others (16–18) suggest that many of the fatty streaks, particularly those located at branches and bifurcations in the artery, are converted through a series of changes into the more advanced fibroproliferative lesions of atherosclerosis. At other anatomic sites the fatty streaks may remain the same, or they may regress and disappear (11,19). Using cell-specific monoclonal antibodies, it is possible to demonstrate that the earliest fatty streaks consist entirely of lipid-laden, monocyte-derived macrophages together with variable numbers of T lymphocytes (9,20,21). With time, smooth muscle cells accumulate within the fatty streaks. In some instances, fatty streaks appear at sites of preexisting accumulations of intimal smooth muscle cells, often called diffuse intimal thickenings (22). In these thickenings, the accumulations of macrophages and T lymphocytes overlie, or are intermixed with, accumulations of smooth muscle and connective tissue.

Intermediate Lesions—The Fibrofatty Lesion

The intermediate lesions of atherosclerosis extend the process initiated with development of the fatty streak. Monocytes and lymphocytes continue their ingress; smooth muscle cells accumulate, many derived from the media of the artery. This continued expansion of cells, along with matrix formed by the smooth muscle cells, leads to a lesion resulting in a somewhat thickened intima that may begin to intrude into the lumen of the artery.

Advanced Lesions—The Fibrous Plaque

In contrast to the earlier lesions of atherosclerosis, fibrous plaques are grossly white in appearance and usually elevated, and they eventually intrude into the lumen of the artery. If the fibrous plaque becomes sufficiently large, it can compromise the flow of blood. These lesions represent the result of continued smooth muscle migration and proliferation, coupled with accumulation and proliferation of monocyte-derived macrophages and continued accumulation of T lymphocytes (8,9,18,19,23,24). The proliferating smooth muscle cells lay down large amounts of connective tissue matrix, including collagen, proteoglycan, and new elastic fibers (25,26). The advanced lesion tends to develop a luminal layer of dense connective tissue containing smooth muscle and intermixed with some macrophages (27), known as a fibrous cap. The fibrous cap overlies a deeper collection of macrophages (many of which contain lipid if the individual is hypercholesterolemic), necrotic debris, T lymphocytes, and varying numbers of smooth muscle cells. Large numbers of proliferated smooth muscle cells and macrophages can often be found deep in the lesion as well.

The amount of lipid in a fibrous plaque depends on the extent of the patient's exposure to the various risk factors associated with atherosclerosis. Some fibrous plaques are rich in connective tissue and contain relatively little lipid, whereas others are highly fatty and contain large lipid deposits (27). As noted earlier, the fibrous plaque is the lesion that usually leads to the terminal sequelae of infarction. When infarction occurs, alterations in the surface of the lesion, such as ulcerations, fissures, or erosions, usually lead to platelet adhesions that line the vessel lumen. Such adhesions can form mural thrombi and lead to arterial occlusion (Fig. 68-1).

Etiologic Factors in Atherogenesis

Numerous risk factors have been associated with the genesis of the lesions of atherosclerosis, including elevated cholesterol [increased low-density lipoprotein (LDL) and decreased high-density lipoprotein (HDL)], cigarette smoking, hypertension, diabetes mellitus, hyperhomocysteinemia, and, possibly, viral or other infectious agents such as *Chlamydia*. However, these risk factor associations are statistical, based on epidemiologic studies (14). In many cases, specific etiologic agents still need to be determined. Oxidized LDL appears to be one of the principal mediators that affects endothelial injury in hyperlipidemic individuals (discussed below). Accumulating data suggest that infectious agents may be

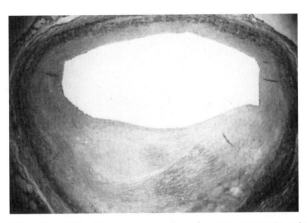

FIG. 68-1. This fibrous plaque in a human coronary artery demonstrates the asymmetric nature of the lesion, the occlusive potential of the lesion, and the marked intimal thickening that is visible in this low-power light micrograph. Characteristically, fibrous plaques are covered by a fibrous cap of dense connective tissue that surrounds flattened smooth muscle cells together with varying numbers of intermixed macrophages. This layer covers a collection of smooth muscle cells, lymphocytes, and lipid-containing macrophages, the amount of which depends on the state of hyperlipidemia of the patient. In this particular case, the fibrous plaque is densely fibrous and contains relatively little lipid. (From ref. 105, with permission.)

involved, in particular, viruses such as cytomegalovirus or other forms of herpesvirus (28), as well as a specific form of *Chlamydia*. A herpes-like virus has been shown in chickens with Marek's disease (29). Herpesvirus is ubiquitous in humans, and, although it has been found in lesions, it is also present in many tissues. A causal role has not been demonstrated. Similarly, recent studies have shown the presence of *Chlamydia twar* in lesions of atherosclerosis. Most of these data suggest "guilt by association." Nevertheless, the possibility exists that these microorganisms and possibly others, in conjunction with elevated lipid levels or factors associated with hypertension or cigarette smoking, etc., may play roles in inducing the early injurious changes to the endothelium that lead to the inflammatory-fibroproliferative responses we call atherosclerosis.

Atherosclerosis and Immunity

The ubiquitous presence of T lymphocytes in the majority of the lesions of atherosclerosis suggests that the lesions have an immune, or possibly autoimmune, component to their genesis. It has been observed that smooth muscle cells in the lesions of atherosclerosis express the human leukocyte antigen (HLA) class II gene, HLA-DR, a gene not normally expressed by smooth muscle (30). Because HLA-DR can be induced by IFN-γ derived from activated T lymphocytes, it has been suggested that expression of HLA-DR may be induced by release of this cytokine from T cells in the lesions. Approximately 20%

of the T cells in the lesions of atherosclerosis express T cell-specific antigens, such as CD4 and CD8. Experimental data support the idea that oxidized LDL and lysophosphatidylcholine derived from oxidized LDL may act as antigens, which activate endothelial cell adhesion molecules and chemoattractant expression and bring in monocytes and T lymphocytes. In the lesions monocytes and T lymphocytes interact, generating cytokines from the activated macrophages that can further activate smooth muscle cells. The smooth muscle may continue to express antigens and an autoimmune component possibly generated by modified lipoproteins or other agents (such as those discussed above), and may participate in generating this immune response in the lesions of atherosclerosis. Thus another aspect of the inflammatory response may be represented by the immune component in the lesions (31).

THE SEQUENCE OF EVENTS IN ATHEROSCLEROSIS

Chronic Inflammation—Fatty Streak Formation

Atherogenesis has been studied in a number of experimental animals, including hypercholesterolemic nonhuman primates (32–35), rabbits (36,37), swine (38–40), rats (41), and, most recently, genetically modified mice (42). The advent of a small murine model, which can be manipulated genetically, offers exciting opportunities to study the process of atherogenesis. Genetically modified mice develop lesions of atherosclerosis similar to those in humans at anatomic sites and in cell constitution, as well as histomorphology. The roles of specific components, such as growth factors and cytokines, certain apoproteins, signaling, or other molecules, can be manipulated in these models to affect the processes of inflammation and repair in very specific ways. Perhaps the best example is the apoprotein E–deficient (Apo E–/–) mouse. This animal is homozygously deficient in apoprotein E, the principal apoprotein that transports cholesterol from the plasma to the liver, and thus becomes endogenously hypercholesterolemic. This mouse model develops all of the stages of the lesions of atherosclerosis at specific branch points and arterial bifurcations, the anatomic sites essentially identical to those in humans (42). Thus, it has been possible to study the roles of etiologic factors associated with the early inflammatory response as well as those required for the fibroproliferative response. Studies using these animals should permit the development of agents that have known effects on these responses in the mouse model and that can be subsequently studied in humans.

In studies of the different experimental animals, the first change noted in the artery wall during the evolution of the hypercholesterolemic state is the entrance of large numbers of lipid moieties, or droplets, into the intima of the artery. This accumulation of lipid occurs either at sites of diffuse intimal thickening or at sites where the intima consists of merely a space between the endothelium and the internal elastic lamina, which may contain varying amounts of connective tissue matrix, principally proteoglycan. Simionescu et al. (43) observed the formation of particles, which they described as "liposomes," in this intimal space within hours to days after inducing hypercholesterolemia in experimental animals. In a series of studies of hypercholesterolemic nonhuman primates, Faggiotto et al. (32) and Masuda and Ross (34) noted that within hours to days after the entrance of lipid into the intima there was increased adherence of monocytes and lymphocytes to the endothelium at these same sites where lesions were destined to form. Similarly, increased adherence of monocytes and lymphocytes were observed in the Apo E–/– mice at lesion-prone sites. At these sites, specific adhesion molecules, such as intercellular adhesion molecule-1 (ICAM-1) and vascular cell adhesion molecule-1 (VCAM-1), are upregulated prior to the adhesion of monocytes and T cells and their subsequent entry into the artery wall. ICAM-1 is upregulated at lesion-prone sites in normal wild-type animals and in the hypercholesterolemic Apo E–/– animals. In contrast, VCAM-1 does not appear in the wild-type animals but is rapidly upregulated during the advent of endogenous hypercholesterolemia (Nakashima et al., unpublished observations).

These two adhesion molecules, with others that may include the group of carbohydrate-rich adhesion molecules, the selectins, appear to play critical roles in the early inflammatory process, which permits adhesion to endothelium and entry of monocytes and T lymphocytes into the intima to form the first lesions of atherosclerosis (Fig. 68-2). The endothelial cells display specific signals on their surfaces in the form of these adhesion molecules, which can be upregulated not only by flow and elevated levels of lipoproteins but also by inflammatory cytokines, including interleukin-1 (IL-1), tumor necrosis factor-α (TNF-α), IL-4, and interferon-γ (IFN-γ). These molecules can induce upregulation of VCAM-1 and the selectins on the endothelial cells as well as their receptors on the monocytes and T cells, permitting receptor-ligand-type interactions to occur. The ICAM and VCAM molecules will bind to integrins on the leukocytes, and the selectins can bind to carbohydrate-rich molecules, such as sialyl-Lewis-x and others, on the leukocytes or the endothelium (44). These molecules are discussed in the chapter by Muller. They function together with chemotactic molecules that are generated at the sites of lesion formation, including monocyte chemotactic protein-1 (MCP-1) and oxidized LDL.

During the process of entry of lipoproteins from the plasma into the subendothelial space, the endothelial cells are capable of modifying, or oxidizing, these lipoproteins (45–48). If oxidation of lipoproteins occurs, the macrophages that have entered the intima could be

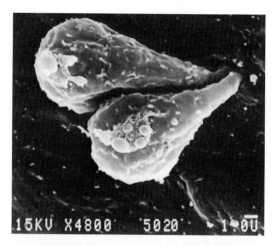

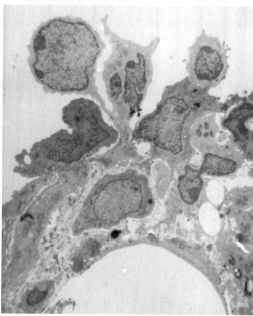

FIG. 68-2. Scanning and transmission electron micrographs demonstrating leukocytes entering into the artery wall between endothelial junctions after 6 months and 1 year on an atherogenic diet, respectively, in nonhuman primates. **A:** Thoracic aorta, 6 months. ×4000. **B:** Thoracic aorta, 1 year. ×4700. (From ref. 34, with permission.)

exposed to these modified lipoproteins, which bind to scavenger receptors on the surface of the macrophages and are ingested by them, leading to the development of foam cells (49,50). The smooth muscle cells also have the capacity to bind and take up native LDL and store them in the form of lipid droplets, and thereby also become foam cells. The LDL that is oxidized by the endothelium and the macrophages could in turn injure the endothelium, altering its permeability and activating it to form cytokines, growth factors, and vasoactive agents. As a result of these interactions, the endothelial cells can become further exposed to inciting agents, some of which can be derived from the activated monocyte-derived macrophages and T lymphocytes that have entered the intima or from platelets that form small mural thrombi on the surface (Fig. 68-3). Together with the mononuclear cells, the endothelial cells can elaborate substances that include growth-regulatory molecules such as platelet-derived growth factor (PDGF) and transforming growth factor-β (TGF-β), cytokines such as IL-1 and TNF-α, IFN-γ, and other factors such as MCP-1 (discussed below).

The Early Fibroproliferative Response— Fibrofatty Lesion Formation

The intermediate lesions also appear to develop at sites of preexisting collections of intimal smooth muscle cells and diffuse intimal thickenings, as well as in regions where no such collections exist. In the latter case, smooth muscle cells appear to migrate from the underlying media of the artery into the intima. This chemotactic response is probably due to the elaboration of substances such as PDGF by the cells that make up the fatty streak. PDGF has the ability to attract the smooth muscle cells into the intima (51–53) and can be formed by the endothelium (54), the macrophages (55,56), and the smooth muscle cells (57–60) that make up the fatty streak. The smooth muscle cells subsequently multiply and lay down connective tissues. Other growth-regulatory molecules that have been implicated in the chemotaxis of the smooth muscle cells include TGF-β (60–64), TNF-α (65), substances such as angiotensin II (AII) (66), and heparin-binding epidermal growth factor (HB-EGF) (67).

Thus the intermediate lesions represent a stage in the inflammatory-fibroproliferative process, which can resolve if the injurious factors that initiated the inflammatory response are neutralized or removed. If not, the continued inflammation and connective tissue formation lead to the development of the advanced lesions.

Continued Smooth Muscle Proliferation— Fibrous Plaque Formation

Ultimately the advanced lesions of atherosclerosis develop by the continuing migration and replication of smooth muscle cells, macrophages, and T lymphocytes. The luminal smooth muscle cells ultimately form a dense, connective-tissue–rich fibrous cap that overlies the remainder of the lesion of atherosclerosis (33,35) (Fig. 68-4). Initially it was thought that the smooth muscle cells were the principal cells that multiply in the lesions; however, it is clear that macrophages in the lesions of atherosclerosis actively replicate as well. This has been demonstrated in hypercholesterolemic rabbits given [^{3}H]thymidine, in which combined cell-specific immunohistochemistry and autoradiography showed that at least 50% of the labeled cells in advanced lesions in hypercholesterolemic rabbits were macrophages (68). Proliferating cell nuclear antigen (PCNA) was also used to identify cycling cells, and both macrophages and smooth muscle cells were identified with cell-specific monoclonal antibodies, demonstrating that both cell types replicate within human lesions as well (69).

The Role of Growth-Regulatory Molecules

Growth-regulatory molecules, including both stimulators and inhibitors, can potentially be elaborated by each of the five cell types involved in the process of atherogenesis: endothelium, monocytes/macrophages, platelets,

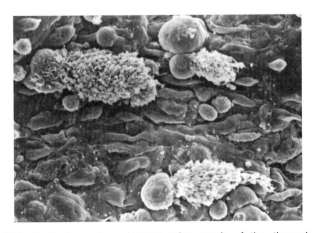

FIG. 68-3. Scanning electron micrograph of the thoracic aorta of a nonhuman primate, showing the irregular surface of a fatty streak after 2 years on an atherogenic diet. Platelet microthrombi adherent to exposed macrophages are visible at a site of endothelial retraction. Many adherent leukocytes are also seen on the intact endothelial cells. ×720. (From ref. 35, with permission.)

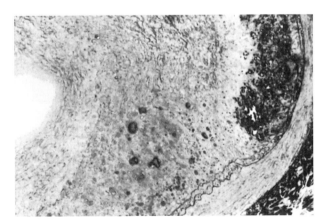

FIG. 68-4. Light micrograph demonstrating an advanced fibrous plaque that formed in the internal iliac artery of a monkey that was hypercholesterolemic for 7 months. The lesion has occluded approximately 70% of the arterial lumen and consists of numerous layers of smooth muscle cells surrounded by fibrous connective tissue. An area of lipid and necrotic tissue occupies the right side and upper portion of this lesion. (From ref. 33, with permission.)

T lymphocytes, and smooth muscle cells. Although several growth-stimulatory molecules are undoubtedly involved in this process, one of them, PDGF, probably plays a critical role in the genesis of the lesion as well as in the process of restenosis (discussed below).

The Roles of the Cells in Atherogenesis

The Endothelium

The endothelial cells play numerous roles in maintaining homeostasis in the normal artery. In addition to providing a permeability barrier, they provide a nonadhesive surface for leukocytes and platelets by generating molecules, such as prostanoids [i.e., prostacyclin (PGI_2)], heparan sulfate, and an ecto–adenosine diphosphatase (ADPase). Molecules such as nitric oxide (NO) also participate in this function, but, in addition, play a major role in the maintenance of vascular tone, which can be offset by other vasoconstrictive molecules the endothelium can also generate, including endothelin (ET) and AII. When stimulated, the endothelium can form and secrete growth factors, as well as cytokines, and they form and rest on a connective tissue matrix, consisting of specific forms of collagen that make up the basement membrane together with fibronectin. A particularly important role played by the endothelial cells in the process of atherogenesis is their ability to modify low-density lipoproteins by oxidizing or, in diabetes, glycating them (70).

These modified lipoproteins can be toxic to the endothelial cells, as well as the underlying cells of the artery wall, and eventually are taken up by scavenger receptors on the macrophages (see below). When activated, the endothelial cells can produce growth-regulatory molecules, including PDGF, which can have a profound effect on the underlying smooth muscle cells. Normally, the endothelium (as noted above) prevents leukocytes from adhering and participating in the inflammatory response. However, when they are injured, as is the case with modified lipoproteins or other injurious agents such as free radicals and homocysteine, they will upregulate genes for adhesion molecules that include VCAM-1 and P- and E-selectin, which participate in inducing monocytes and T cells to roll, attach, adhere, spread, and migrate.

Finally, the endothelial cells can also participate in the process of angiogenesis by forming new blood vessels that may play critical roles as the advanced lesions of atherosclerosis develop. These microvessels can provide oxygenation to the deeper portions of the advanced lesions. They may provide substrates that may lead to endothelial rupture, hemorrhage, and ultimately thrombosis.

Monocytes/Macrophages

Monocyte-derived macrophages, together with T cells, represent the principal leukocytes involved in the inflammatory process that leads to the advanced lesions of atherosclerosis. They can be attracted in by the adhesion molecules on the endothelium that, together with chemotactic factors, bring them into the intimal region of the artery. At least two chemotactic factors have been isolated, oxidized LDL and MCP-1, which attract the monocytes into the subendothelial region where they become activated as macrophages. They can express genes for a host of cytokines that are characteristically formed by the macrophages, including IL-1, TNF-α, TGF-β, Il-6, PDGF A- and B-chains, vascular endothelial growth factor (VEGF), HB-EGF, and numerous others (71). As noted below, the first ubiquitous lesion of atherosclerosis, the fatty streak, consists of a pure collection of monocyte-derived macrophages and T lymphocytes.

The macrophages take up modified lipoproteins via their scavenger receptors. They can present antigens to T lymphocytes during the process of lesion formation by expressing HLA-DR. They can express complement receptors and the LDL receptor-related protein (LRP), all of which may increase during their activation and in the process of foam cell formation during atherogenesis.

In addition, activated macrophages express a host of enzymes associated with lipoprotein metabolism, including lipoprotein lipase and lipoxygenases, enzymes that can degrade the extracellular matrix (e.g., collagenase, stromolysin, the metalloproteases, and inhibitors of metalloproteases, Timp-1 and-2). They are able to form enzymes that will break down fibrin, such as urokinase-type tissue plasminogen activator (uPA), tissue plasminogen activator (tPA), and inhibitors such as plasminogen activator inhibitor-1 (PAI-1). They also can express heat shock protein, which may represent a cytoprotective response to stress and lethal stimuli. All are potentially important substances formed by these cells during the process of atherogenesis (71).

Presumably, the monocyte comes in to act as a phagocytic effector cell to remove the modified lipoproteins and other foreign substances that are deposited in the evolving lesion. But in the process of continuing presentation of antigenic and deleterious substances to the artery wall, the macrophages undergo numerous changes and, in particular, begin to replicate in the lesion. One of the most common observations in the early phases of atherogenesis is the replication of macrophages that, together with smooth muscle cell replication, represents the principal means by which the lesions expand. However, the continued ingress of these cells, together with their turnover in the lesions, replication, apoptosis, necrosis, and emigration, will determine, in part, whether the lesions will continue to expand.

T Lymphocytes

The presence of CD4+ and CD8+ lymphocytes is important in the process of atherogenesis, at least in some individuals. Because endothelium and smooth muscle, as well as macrophages, can each present antigens to T lymphocytes within the lesions, their presence suggests that an immune or autoimmune component may be part of the process of atherogenesis. Hansson's team (72) has demonstrated that oxidized LDL can serve as one source of antigenic stimulation to the T lymphocytes, which can then form IFN-γ. This molecule can then further activate monocyte-derived macrophages. Many lymphocytes adjacent to smooth muscle cells in lesions express class II histocompatibility antigens in the form of HLA-DR, thus posing opportunities for smooth muscle cell interaction with lymphocytes, lymphocyte activation, and the generation of an autoimmune inflammatory response (31).

Smooth Muscle

Smooth muscle accumulation and connective tissue matrix formation by these cells are key events in the development of the advanced lesions of atherosclerosis, the fibrous plaque, and the complicated lesion. The ability of smooth muscle cells to migrate, proliferate, and lay down new collagen, elastic fibers, proteoglycans, and fibronectin represents the key to the fibroproliferative healing response that accompanies the chronic inflammatory process, an integral part of the process of atherogenesis. The smooth muscle cells lay down a uniform, thick, well-distributed fibrous cap that covers the accumulations of inflammatory cells, necrotic debris, and lipid, which aggregate in the lesions, particularly in hyperlipidemic individuals. The success of the smooth muscle cells in providing this protective cover that separates the remainder of the lesion from the flow of blood is important in lesion stability. In many instances, the fibrous cap that forms in the advanced lesion may be irregular or thinned, particularly at the margins or shoulders of the lesions. This thinning may be due to continued activation of monocyte-derived macrophages, which enter at these sites where they may make collagenolytic and stromolytic enzymes that can degrade the matrix and induce thinning and irregularity in the fibrous cap. At these sites it is common for irregular flow and areas of turbulence in the flow of blood to occur, leading to rupture of the fibrous cap and sudden death (13). Thus the ability of the smooth muscle cells to respond in an effective fashion in relation to matrix formation represents a key event in the formation of the advanced, proliferative lesions of atherosclerosis.

Platelets

Platelets may be involved in the genesis of some lesions of atherosclerosis, particularly at sites where endothelial dysfunction occurs, so that the endothelium no longer provides a nonthrombogenic surface. Platelets contain many growth factors and cytokines that are released when platelets adhere to a surface, undergo shape change, aggregate, and release their granule constituents. Thus they can be a potent source of factors that stimulate smooth muscle migration and proliferation, monocyte-derived macrophage migration and proliferation, and connective tissue formation. At sites of injury where collagen may be exposed, thrombin may be released, leading to fibrin formation. Adenosine diphosphate release also can occur, inducing platelet aggregation and thrombosis, leading to release of vasoactive, stimulatory, and proliferative agents carried in the platelets. These factors can induce vasoconstriction, smooth muscle proliferation, and thus lesion progression as well. Of course, if the thrombosis is related solely to the wall of the artery and remains a mural thrombus, there may be no other clinical sequelae, although it can play a part in lesion progression. However, if the thrombus forms on the surface of a ruptured or ulcerated lesion, it may occlude and lead to sudden death (73).

Platelet-Derived Growth Factor

PDGF is a dimeric molecule of approximately 30,000 molecular weight, highly cationic and disulfide bonded (74–77). It is a potent mitogen and chemoattractant for smooth muscle cells (51,52,78). It induces its effects by binding to a series of specific high-affinity receptors on the surface of responsive cells, such as smooth muscle. Regular binding on smooth muscle cells by the appropriate dimeric form of PDGF ultimately culminates in DNA synthesis and mitosis (79,80).

PDGF occurs in the form of three dimers of two separate chains, termed PDGF-A and PDGF-B. All three possible dimeric forms, namely PDGF-AA, PDGF-AB, and PDGF-BB, have been isolated, purified, sequenced, and cloned (81). There is a high degree of specificity of binding between each of the three different dimeric forms of PDGF and their receptors. There are two different receptor molecules, termed PDGF receptor α and PDGF receptor β. When the three different dimeric forms of the receptor (PDGF receptors αα, αβ, and ββ) bind to the appropriate form of PDGF, they generate a signal that culminates in DNA replication. The specificity of binding resides both in the receptor and the ligand. The A-chain of PDGF can only bind to the PDGF receptor α-subunit; therefore, PDGF-AA will only bind to two PDGF receptor αα-subunits. In contrast, the B-chain can bind to either PDGF receptor α or PDGF receptor β; therefore, PDGF-BB can bind to any one of the three possible dimeric forms of the PDGF receptor (82–84). Because of this specificity, there are restrictions on the types of PDGF that may be locally available, and differences in amounts of each of the two receptor molecules that may be formed by the different cells. It is important to have this information to predict the response of the smooth muscle in different regions of the arterial tree, or to determine how effective a given form of PDGF made by the local cells may be in eliciting a proliferative response.

Besides being a potent mitogen, PDGF can also specifically induce directed migration, or chemotaxis, of connective tissue cells and macrophages via the same receptor molecules (52,85). Exposure to PDGF will induce increased binding of LDL to smooth muscle cells by stimulating them to increase their number of LDL receptors (86). PDGF also induces increased synthesis of cholesterol (86), as well as increases in endocytosis (87) and in the flux of ions into the cells (88). Exposure to PDGF can also result in a reorganization of the cellular cytoskeleton and thus can induce changes in cell shape (53).

PDGF has a short half-life when injected intravenously (89), but can bind to both matrix proteoglycans and cell-surface proteoglycans such as heparan sulfate and thus probably has a reasonably long half-life in the connective tissue matrix, where it could serve as a locus for continued induction of smooth muscle replication.

With the demonstration that PDGF is such a potent chemoattractant and mitogen in vitro, it was important to determine whether this molecule was present and active in vivo as well. A monoclonal antibody has been developed that can be used immunohistochemically to demonstrate the presence of PDGF-B chain (90). cDNA probes have also been developed that can be used for in situ hybridization to determine whether or not PDGF mRNA is expressed in the cells in the lesions of atherosclerosis.

Studies using these tools have demonstrated that approximately 20% of the monocyte-derived macrophages in all phases of lesion formation of atherosclerosis have PDGF-B chain–containing protein within their cytosol (91). Sasahara et al. (unpublished observations) have observed colocalization of macrophages containing PDGF-B chain in regions of PCNA-labeled smooth muscle cells, suggesting that PDGF-containing macrophages are located in the vicinity where smooth muscle replication is taking place in both human and nonhuman lesions of atherosclerosis. Wilcox et al. (59) observed the localization of PDGF-B chain mRNA at sites in lesions of atherosclerosis that could be interpreted as endothelium, some of which may be macrophages. They also observed localization of PDGF-A chain mRNA at sites in lesions of atherosclerosis they described as "mesenchymal-appearing cells," which may in fact be smooth muscle cells.

No evidence for PDGF activity in atherogenesis has thus far been available. In contrast, evidence has been provided for a functional role for PDGF in the process of smooth muscle replication during restenosis (discussed below). Although it has not been possible to determine whether the demonstrated presence of this molecule means that it is responsible for the smooth muscle replication that occurs during atherogenesis, circumstantial evidence points to a potential role for PDGF in this process.

Transforming Growth Factor-β and Other Cytokines

TGF-β is perhaps the most potent inhibitor of cell proliferation, as well as the most potent stimulator of connective tissue formation by cells, thus far discovered. It can be formed by all of the cells involved in the process of atherogenesis (61). TGF-β has also been shown to be present within the lesions of atherosclerosis by use of monoclonal antibodies that demonstrate its presence immunohistochemically (Battegay et al., unpublished observations). Similarly, cytokines such as IL-1 and TNF-α, both of which can be produced by activated macrophages in vitro, can be shown to stimulate PDGF-A chain gene expression in smooth muscle, followed by PDGF-AA synthesis and secretion and autocrine stimulation (62). TGF-β also induces PDGF-AA synthesis and secretion by smooth muscle cells (92,93), whereas TNF-α induces PDGF-B chain synthesis and secretion by endothelial cells (94). Thus if these different cytokines and growth-regulatory molecules are also formed within the lesions of atherosclerosis in vivo, and should they elicit the same cellular responses (i.e., autocrine stimulation of smooth muscle replication via PDGF formation as in the cases of IL-1 and TGF-β), this could represent an important component of the process of lesion progression.

TGF-β is an interesting molecule in that it is probably the most potent stimulator of connective tissue formation that has thus far been discovered. At the same time, it is a potent inhibitor of smooth muscle replication. TGF-β can induce PDGF gene expression in endothelial and smooth muscle cells and is present in large quantities in lesions of atherosclerosis. Generally, it is present in the form of a latent precursor that must be activated before it becomes biologically active. As a consequence, simply measuring TGF-β mRNA may be misleading because the bulk of TGF-β present may be latent. This has provided an opportunity to look at factors responsible for TGF-β activation, which requires proteolytic cleavage of the inactive precursor and can be induced by a number of proteases. One protease in particular, plasminogen, which is subject to regulation by both activators and inhibitors of the zymogen plasmin, may be important in this process. Plasminogen is controlled by endothelium and smooth muscle. Plasminogen activation is expressed by tPA and uPA, which can be inhibited by PAI-1. Thus an elaborate mechanism has been developed to control the activation of substances such as TGF-β (92,93).

Thus growth-regulatory molecules and cytokines can be formed endogenously by the cells of the developing lesions, or they can be provided exogenously by adherent platelets that form microthrombi on the luminal surface of lesions or on injured endothelium (95). When platelet adherence occurs, release of growth-regulatory molecules could play important roles in the genesis of a lesion, which begins as a specialized type of chronic inflammatory process and culminates in a massive fibroprolifera-tive response.

The Response-to-Injury Hypothesis of Atherogenesis

The elements of the process of atherogenesis (described above) led to the development of an hypothe-sis of atherosclerosis that has been tested and, as new observations are made, revised over the past 25 years (2,3,6,7). The response-to-injury hypothesis of athero-genesis states that the lesions of atherosclerosis (depend-ing on the risk factors to which the individual has been exposed) represent specific injurious responses of the endothelial cells to different agents presented to them. For example, during hypercholesterolemia, modified LDL may be formed. Toxic factors or free radicals ema-nating from cigarette smoke or substances elaborated in individuals with diabetes, hypertension, or combinations of these injurious agents could in some fashion generate factors that are toxic to endothelium. As a result of expo-sure to these injurious agents, subtle changes may occur in the lining endothelial cells of the artery as well as in the circulating leukocytes. Such subtle forms of injury to the endothelium could lead to dysfunctional changes in these cells (making their surfaces more adhesive) and lead to increased leukocyte adherence. This is followed by entry of the adherent leukocytes into the artery, result-ing in an early, highly specialized form of chronic inflam-mation within the intima of the artery.

The inflammatory cells that interact with the overlying endothelium may also be joined by platelets if endothelial injury is sufficient to alter the nonthrombogenic charac-ter of the endothelium. When each of these different cells is activated, they can release growth-regulatory mole-cules and cytokines. When the growth-stimulatory effects exceed those of the inhibitory effects, the resulting migration and replication of macrophages and smooth muscle cells could lead to an expanding inflammatory-fibroproliferative response. Although this entire process appears to begin as a protective response, the excessive nature of the inflammatory-fibroproliferative response in itself can become the disease entity.

In the case of atherosclerosis, the resultant prolifera-tion can cause the lesion to intrude into the artery. Further changes can occur on the surface of the lesion, including erosion, ulceration, and thrombosis. The consequences can be disastrous for the patient. This hypothesis suggests that there are a number of potential sites for intervention that could result in lesion prevention and/or regression. For example, it has been shown in experimentally induced atherosclerosis that antioxidants, such as the drug probucol, vitamin E, and vitamin C, or combina-tions of these, may have a marked, inhibitory effect on the inflammatory response and, in fact, can inhibit fatty streak formation (96).

There are also epidemiologic studies that suggest that such antioxidants may inhibit the clinical sequelae of atherosclerosis in humans. Most recently, it has been shown that individuals who have a higher incidence of the sequelae of myocardial infarction or stroke also have sta-tistically significant, elevated levels of C-reactive protein within their plasma, a potent marker for the evidence of an ongoing, inflammatory process (97). Thus agents, which can modify substances such as oxidized lipoproteins that can induce this inflammatory process, or factors, which may be able to modify the inflammatory process them-selves, may be important in altering the process of athero-genesis and lesion formation. It has been demonstrated that the lesions of atherosclerosis can regress clinically (98). For example, when hypercholesterolemic individuals are placed on hypocholesterolemic-inducing regimens, their lesions of atherosclerosis have become smaller, as determined by angiography. Thus the possibility of inter-fering with the inflammatory process or with growth-regulatory molecules, particularly growth-stimulatory molecules, to prevent lesions or to induce regression rep-resents important potential approaches to the treatment of this disease entity (Fig. 68-5).

Restenosis after Angioplasty or Bypass Surgery

Two of the principal approaches that have been taken to treat the advanced occlusive lesions of atherosclerosis are angioplasty and bypass surgery. In each of these instances, there is a 30% to 40% failure rate due to either restenosis of the artery treated by angioplasty or resteno-sis at the perianastomotic site where the bypass has been anastomosed to the normal coronary artery (99,100). The restenosis probably occurs due to both migration and pro-liferation of smooth muscle cells, probably into mural thrombi, to re-form the lesion and lead to reocclusion. Using an intraarterial balloon catheter in the rat carotid artery as a model of angioplasty, it has recently been demonstrated that a specific sequence of cellular events occurs (101,102). Within the first 24 to 48 hours after ballooning, there is extensive injury to the innermost lay-ers of medial smooth muscle, leading to lysis, release of intracellular fibroblast growth factor (FGF), and a round of medial smooth muscle DNA synthesis, which can be markedly depressed with an antibody against FGF (103). Over the next 12 days there is migration of smooth mus-cle from the media into the intima, where approximately 50% of the migrated cells continue to replicate, resulting in an intima as thick as the media after 14 days (102).

Ferns et al. (104) studied this problem in the athymic nude rat. They showed that it is possible to inhibit up to 40% of the intimal thickening (restenosis) by administer-ing a neutralizing goat polyclonal antibody to PDGF beginning 24 hours prior to angioplasty and continuing for the next 8 days following angioplasty. Studies of

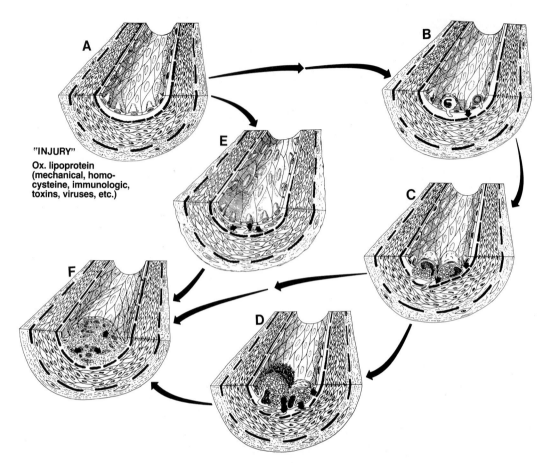

FIG. 68-5. The response-to-injury hypothesis. Advanced intimal proliferative lesions of atherosclerosis may occur by at least two pathways. The pathway demonstrated by the clockwise *long arrows* to the right has been observed in experimentally induced hypercholesterolemia. Injury to the endothelium *(A)* may induce growth factor secretion. Monocytes attach to endothelium *(B)*, which may continue to secrete growth factors *(short arrow)*. Subendothelial migration of monocytes *(C)* may lead to fatty-streak formation and release of growth factors such as platelet-derived growth factor (PDGF) *(short arrow)*. Fatty streaks may become directly converted to fibrous plaques *(long arrow* from *C* to *F)* through release of growth factors from macrophages or endothelial cells or both. Macrophages may also stimulate or injure the overlying endothelium. In some cases, macrophages may lose their endothelial cover and platelet attachment may occur *(D)*, providing three possible sources of growth factors—platelets, macrophages, and endothelium *(short arrows)*. Some of the smooth muscle cells in the proliferative lesion itself *(F)* may form and secrete growth factors such as PDGF *(short arrows)*. An alternative pathway for development of advanced lesions of atherosclerosis is shown by the arrows from *A* to *E* to *F*. In this case, the endothelium may be injured but remain intact. Increased endothelial turnover may result in growth-factor formation by endothelial cells *(A)*. This may stimulate migration of smooth muscle cells from the media into the intima, accompanied by endogenous production of PDGF by smooth muscle as well as growth factor secretion from the "injured" endothelial cells *(E)*. These interactions could then lead to fibrous-plaque formation and further lesion progression *(F)*. (From ref. 7, with permission.)

autoradiographs, made after giving [³H]thymidine 17 hours, 9 hours, and 1 hour prior to sacrificing the rats on the eighth day postangioplasty, demonstrated that the principal effect, at the doses of antibody used in these investigations, was to inhibit the chemotaxis of the smooth muscle cells from the media into the neointima. These data demonstrate a clear role for PDGF in the neointimal accumulation of smooth muscle cells postangioplasty, and they suggest possibilities for the use of specific inhibitors of PDGF in preventing this response, and thus in augmenting

the success rate of angioplasty and possibly bypass surgery as well. They also suggest that this and other growth-regulatory molecules may govern key events not only in angioplasty, but in atherosclerosis as well.

REFERENCES

1. *Report of the Working Group on Arteriosclerosis of the National Heart, Lung, and Blood Institute,* vol 2. DHEW publication no. NIH 82-2035. Washington, DC: Government Printing Office, 1981.
2. Ross R, Glomset JA. Arteriosclerosis and the arterial smooth muscle cell. *Science* 1973;180:1332–1339.

3. Ross R, Glomset JA. The pathogenesis of atherosclerosis. *N Engl J Med* 1976;295:369–377,420–425.

4. Ross R, Harker L. Hyperlipidemia and atherosclerosis. *Science* 1976;193:1094–1100.

5. Wissler RW, Vesselinovitch D, Getz GS. Abnormalities of the arterial wall and its metabolism in atherogenesis. *Prog Cardiovasc Dis* 1976;18:341–369.

6. Ross R. The pathogenesis of atherosclerosis: a perspective for the 1990s. *Nature* 1993;362:801–809.

7. Ross R. The pathogenesis of atherosclerosis—an update. *N Engl J Med* 1986;314:488–500.

8. Jonasson L, Holm J, Skalli O, Bondjers G, Hansson GK. Regional accumulations of T cells, macrophages, and smooth muscle cells in the human atherosclerotic plaque. *Arteriosclerosis* 1986;6:131–138.

9. Gown AM, Tsukada T, Ross R. Human atherosclerosis. II. Immunocytochemical analysis of the cellular composition of human atherosclerotic lesions. *Am J Pathol* 1986;125:191–207.

10. Glagov S. Hemodynamic risk factors: mechanical stress, mural architecture, medial nutrition and the vulnerability of arteries to atherosclerosis. In: Wissler RW, Geer JC, eds. *The pathogenesis of atherosclerosis.* Baltimore: Williams & Wilkins, 1972:164–199.

11. McGill HC Jr. Persistent problems in the pathogenesis of atherosclerosis. *Arteriosclerosis* 1984;4:443–451.

12. Falk E. Why do plaques rupture? *Circulation* 1992;86(suppl III):30–42.

13. Falk E, Shah PK, Fuster V. Pathogenesis of plaque disruption. In: Fuster V, Ross R, Topol EJ, eds. *Atherosclerosis and coronary artery disease.* Philadelphia: Lippincott-Raven, 1996:491–507.

14. McGill HC Jr. Overview. In: Fuster V, Ross R, Topol EJ, eds. *Atherosclerosis and coronary artery disease.* Philadelphia: Lippincott-Raven, 1996:25–41.

15. Stary HC. Macrophages, macrophage foam cells, and eccentric intimal thickening in the coronary arteries of young children. *Atherosclerosis* 1987;64:91–108.

16. Geer JC. Fine structure of human aortic intimal thickening and fatty streaks. *Lab Invest* 1965;14:1764–1783.

17. Geer JC, McGill HC Jr, Strong JP. The fine structure of human atherosclerotic lesions. *Am J Pathol* 1961;38:263–287.

18. Ghidoni JJ, O'Neal RM. Recent advances in molecular pathology—a review: ultrastructure of human atheroma. *Exp Mol Pathol* 1967;7:378–400.

19. McGill HC Jr, ed. *The geographic pathology of atherosclerosis.* Baltimore: Williams & Wilkins, 1968.

20. Munro JM, van der Walt JD, Munro CS, Chalmers JAC, Cox E. An immunohistochemical analysis of human aortic fatty streaks. *Hum Pathol* 1987;18:375–380.

21. Emeson EE, Robertson AL Jr. T lymphocytes in aortic and coronary intimas. Their potential role in atherogenesis. *Am J Pathol* 1988;130:369–376.

22. Thomas WA, Reiner JM, Florentin RA, Scott RF. Population dynamics of arterial cells during atherogenesis. VIII. Separation of the roles of injury and growth stimulation in early aortic atherogenesis in swine originating in pre-existing intimal smooth muscle cell masses. *Exp Mol Pathol* 1979;31:124–144.

23. Wissler RW, Vesselinovitch D. Atherosclerosis—relationship to coronary blood flow. *Am J Cardiol* 1983;52(2):2A–7A.

24. Strong JP, Eggen DA, Oalmann MC. The natural history, geographic pathology, and epidemiology of atherosclerosis. In: Wissler RW, Geer JC, eds. *The pathogenesis of atherosclerosis.* Baltimore: Williams & Wilkins, 1972:20–40.

25. Ross R. The smooth muscle cells. II. Growth of smooth muscle in culture and formation of elastic fibers. *J Cell Biol* 1971;50:172–186.

26. Burke JM, Ross R. Synthesis of connective tissue macromolecules by smooth muscle. *Int Rev Connect Tissue Res* 1979;8:119–157.

27. Ross R, Wight TN, Strandness E, Thiele B. Human atherosclerosis. I. Cell constitution and characteristics of advanced lesions of the superficial femoral artery. *Am J Pathol* 1984;114:79–93.

28. Kaner RJ, Hajjar DP. Viral activation of thrombo-atherosclerosis. In: Fuster V, Ross R, Topol EJ, eds. *Atherosclerosis and coronary artery disease.* Philadelphia: Lippincott-Raven, 1996:569–584.

29. Fabricant CG, Fabricant J, Minick CR, Litrenta MM. Herpes virus induced atherosclerosis in chickens. *Fed Proc* 1983;42:2476–2479.

30. Jonasson L, Holm J, Skalli O, Gabbiani G, Hansson GK. Expression of class II transplantation antigen on vascular smooth muscle in human atherosclerosis. *J Clin Invest* 1985;76:125–131.

31. Hansson GK, Libby P. The role of the lymphocyte. In: Fuster V, Ross R, Topol EJ, eds. *Atherosclerosis and coronary artery disease.* Philadelphia: Lippincott-Raven, 1996:557–568.

32. Faggiotto A, Ross R, Harker L. Studies of hypercholesterolemia in the nonhuman primate. I. Changes that lead to fatty streak formation. *Arteriosclerosis* 1984;4:323–340.

33. Faggiotto A, Ross R. Studies of hypercholesterolemia in the nonhuman primate. II. Fatty streak conversion to fibrous plaque. *Arteriosclerosis* 1984;4:341–356.

34. Masuda J, Ross R. Atherogenesis during low-level hypercholesterolemia in the nonhuman primate. I. Fatty streak formation. *Arteriosclerosis* 1990;10:164–177.

35. Masuda J, Ross R. Atherogenesis during low-level hypercholesterolemia in the nonhuman primate. II. Fatty streak conversion to fibrous plaque. *Arteriosclerosis* 1990;10:178–187.

36. Rosenfeld ME, Tsukada T, Gown AM, Ross R. Fatty streak initiation in Watanabe heritable hyperlipemic and comparably hypercholesterolemic fat-fed rabbits. *Arteriosclerosis* 1987;7:9–23.

37. Rosenfeld ME, Tsukada T, Chait A, Bierman EL, Gown AM, Ross R. Fatty streak expansion and maturation in Watanabe heritable hyperlipemic and comparably hypercholesterolemic fat-fed rabbits. *Arteriosclerosis* 1987;7:24–34.

38. Gerrity RG, Naito HK, Richardson M, Schwartz CJ. Dietary induced atherogenesis in swine: morphology of the intima in prelesion stages. *Am J Pathol* 1979;95:775–792.

39. Gerrity RG. The role of the monocyte in atherogenesis. I. Transition of blood-borne monocytes into foam cells in fatty lesions. *Am J Pathol* 1981;103:181–190.

40. Gerrity RG, Goss JA, Soby L. Control of monocyte recruitment by chemotactic factor(s) in lesion-prone areas of swine aorta. *Arteriosclerosis* 1985;5:55–66.

41. Joris I, Zand T, Nunnari JJ, Krolikowski FJ, Majno G. Studies on the pathogenesis of atherosclerosis. I. Adhesion and emigration of mononuclear cells in the aorta of hypercholesterolemic rats. *Am J Pathol* 1983;113:341–358.

42. Nakashima Y, Plump AS, Raines EW, Breslow JL, Ross R. ApoE-deficient mice develop lesions of all phases of atherosclerosis throughout the arterial tree. *Arterioscler Thromb* 1994;14:133–140.

43. Simionescu N, Simionescu M, Palade GE. Permeability of muscle capillaries to small heme-peptides: evidence for the existence of patent transendothelial channels. *J Cell Biol* 1975;64:586–607.

44. Springer TA, Cybulsky MI. Traffic signals on endothelium for leukocytes in health, inflammation, and atherosclerosis. In: Fuster V, Ross R, Topol EJ, eds. *Atherosclerosis and coronary artery disease.* Philadelphia: Lippincott-Raven, 1996:511–537.

45. Steinberg D. Lipoproteins and atherosclerosis. A look back and a look ahead. *Arteriosclerosis* 1983;3:283–301.

46. Steinberg D, Pittman RC, Carew TE. Mechanisms involved in the uptake and degradation of low density lipoprotein by the artery wall *in vivo.* *Ann NY Acad Sci* 1985;454:195–206.

47. Steinberg D, Parthasarathy S, Carew TE, Khoo JC, Witztum JL. Beyond cholesterol: modifications of low-density lipoprotein that increase its atherogenicity. *N Engl J Med* 1989;320:915–924.

48. Steinbrecher UP, Parthasarathy S, Leake DS, Witztum JL, Steinberg D. Modification of low density lipoprotein by endothelial cells involves lipid peroxidation and degradation of low density lipoprotein phospholipids. *Proc Natl Acad Sci USA* 1984;81:3883–3887.

49. Parthasarathy S, Quinn MT, Schwenke DC, Carew TE, Steinberg D. Oxidative modification of beta-very low density lipoprotein. Potential role in monocyte recruitment and foam cell formation. *Arteriosclerosis* 1989;9:398–404.

50. Carew TE, Schwenke DC, Steinberg D. Antiatherogenic effect of probucol unrelated to its hypocholesterolemic effect: evidence that antioxidants *in vivo* can selectively inhibit low density lipoprotein degradation in macrophage-rich fatty streaks and slow the progression of atherosclerosis in the Watanabe heritable hyperlipidemic rabbit. *Proc Natl Acad Sci USA* 1987;84:7725–7729.

51. Ross R, Raines EW, Bowen-Pope DF. The biology of platelet-derived growth factor. *Cell* 1986;46:155–169.

52. Grotendorst GR, Chang T, Seppa HEJ, Kleinman HK, Martin GR. Platelet-derived growth factor is a chemoattractant for vascular smooth muscle cells. *J Cell Physiol* 1982;113:261–266.

53. Ferns GAA, Sprugel KH, Seifert RA, et al. Relative platelet-derived growth factor receptor subunit expression determines cell migration

to different dimeric forms of PDGF. *Growth Factors* 1990;3: 315–324.

54. DiCorleto PE, Bowen-Pope DF. Cultured endothelial cells produce a platelet-derived growth factor-like protein. *Proc Natl Acad Sci USA* 1983;80:1919–1923.

55. Shimokado K, Raines EW, Madtes DK, Barrett TB, Benditt EP, Ross R. A significant part of macrophage-derived growth factor consists of at least two forms of PDGF. *Cell* 1985;43:277–286.

56. Martinet Y, Bitterman PB, Mornex J-F, Grotendorst GR, Martin GR, Crystal RG. Activated human monocytes express the c-sis proto-onco-gene and release a mediator showing PDGF-like activity. *Nature* 1986;319:158–160.

57. Nilsson J, Sjolund M, Palmberg L, Thyberg J, Heldin C-H. Arterial smooth muscle cells in primary culture produce a platelet-derived growth factor-like protein. *Proc Natl Acad Sci USA* 1985;82: 4418–4422.

58. Walker LN, Bowen-Pope DF, Ross R, Reidy MA. Production of platelet-derived growth factor-like molecules by cultured arterial smooth muscle cells accompanies proliferation after arterial injury. *Proc Natl Acad Sci USA* 1986;83:7311–7315.

59. Wilcox JN, Smith KM, Williams LT, Schwartz SM, Gordon D. Platelet-derived growth factor mRNA detection in human atheroscle-rotic plaques by *in situ* hybridization. *J Clin Invest* 1988;82: 1134–1143.

60. Libby P, Warner SJC, Salomon RN, Birinyi LK. Production of platelet-derived growth factor-like mitogen by smooth-muscle cells from human atheroma. *N Engl J Med* 1988;318:1493–1498.

61. Sporn MB, Roberts AB, Wakefield LM, de Crombrugghe B. Some recent advances in the chemistry and biology of transforming growth factor-beta. *J Cell Biol* 1987;105:1039–1045.

62. Raines EW, Dower SK, Ross R. IL-1 mitogenic activity for fibroblasts and smooth muscle cells is due to PDGF-AA. *Science* 1989;243: 393–396.

63. Libby P, Warner SJC, Friedman GB. Interleukin 1: a mitogen for human vascular smooth muscle cells that induces the release of growth-inhibitory prostanoids. *J Clin Invest* 1988;81:487–498.

64. Moyer CF, Sajuthi D, Tulli H, Williams JK. Synthesis of IL-1 alpha and IL-1 beta by arterial cells in atherosclerosis. *Am J Pathol* 1991; 138:951–960.

65. Sherry B, Cerami A. Cachectin/tumor necrosis factor exerts endocrine, paracrine, and autocrine control of inflammatory responses. *J Cell Biol* 1988;107:1269–1277.

66. Naftilan AJ, Pratt RE, Dzau VJ. Induction of platelet-derived growth factor A-chain and c-myc gene expression by angiotensin II in cul-tured rat vascular smooth muscle cells. *J Clin Invest* 1989;83: 1419–1424.

67. Higashiyama S, Abraham JA, Miller J, Fiddes JC, Klagsbrun M. A heparin-binding growth factor secreted by macrophage-like cells that is related to EGF. *Science* 1991;251:936–939.

68. Rosenfeld ME, Ross R. Macrophage and smooth muscle cell prolifer-ation in atherosclerotic lesions of WHHL and comparably hypercho-lesterolemic fat-fed rabbits. *Arteriosclerosis* 1990;10:680–687.

69. Gordon D, Reidy MA, Benditt EP, Schwartz SM. Cell proliferation of human coronary arteries. *Proc Natl Acad Sci USA* 1990;87: 4600–4604.

70. DiCorleto PE, Gimbrone MA Jr. Vascular endothelium. In: Fuster V, Ross R, Topol EJ, eds. *Atherosclerosis and coronary artery disease.* Philadelphia: Lippincott-Raven, 1996:387–399.

71. Raines EW, Rosenfeld ME, Ross R. The role of macrophages. In: Fuster V, Ross R, Topol EJ, eds. *Atherosclerosis and coronary artery disease.* Philadelphia: Lippincott-Raven, 1996:539–555.

72. Stemme S, Faber B, Holm J, Wiklund O, Witztum JL, Hansson GK. T lymphocytes from human atherosclerotic plaques recognize oxidized low density lipoprotein. *Proc Natl Acad Sci USA* 1995;92:3893–3897.

73. Marcus AJ. Platelet activation. In: Fuster V, Ross R, Topol EJ, eds. *Atherosclerosis and coronary artery disease.* Philadelphia: Lippincott-Raven, 1996:607–637.

74. Heldin C-H, Westermark B, Wasteson A. Platelet-derived growth fac-tor: purification and partial characterization. *Proc Natl Acad Sci USA* 1979;76:3722–3726.

75. Antoniades HN. Human platelet-derived growth factor (PDGF): purification of PDGF-I and PDGF-II and separation of their reduced subunits. *Proc Natl Acad Sci USA* 1981;78:7314–7317.

76. Huang JS, Huang SS, Kennedy B, Deuel TF. Platelet-derived growth

factor: specific binding to target cells. *J Biol Chem* 1982;257: 8130–8136.

77. Raines EW, Ross R. Platelet-derived growth factor. I. High yield purification and evidence for multiple forms. *J Biol Chem* 1982; 257:5154–5160.

78. Grotendorst G, Seppa HEJ, Kleinman HK, Martin G. Attachment of smooth muscle cells to collagen and their migration toward platelet-derived growth factor. *Proc Natl Acad Sci USA* 1981;78:3669–3672.

79. Heldin C-H, Westermark B, Wasteson A. Specific receptors for platelet-derived growth factor on cells derived from connective tissue and glia. *Proc Natl Acad Sci USA* 1981;78:3664–3668.

80. Bowen-Pope DF, Ross R. Platelet-derived growth factor. II. Specific binding to cultured cells. *J Biol Chem* 1982;257:5161–5171.

81. Raines EW, Bowen-Pope DF, Ross R. Platelet-derived growth factor. In: Sporn MB, Roberts AB, eds. *Handbook of experimental pharma-cology:* peptide growth factors and their receptors I, vol 95. New York: Springer-Verlag, 1990:173–262.

82. Hart CE, Forstrom JW, Kelly JD, et al. Two classes of PDGF receptor recognize different isoforms of PDGF. *Science* 1988;240:1529–1531.

83. Heldin C-H, Backstrom G, Ostman A, et al. Binding of different dimeric forms of PDGF to human fibroblasts: evidence for two sepa-rate receptor types. *EMBO J* 1988;7:1387–1393.

84. Seifert RA, Hart CE, Phillips PE, et al. Two different subunits associ-ate to create isoform-specific platelet-derived growth factor receptors. *J Biol Chem* 1989;264:8771–8778.

85. Deuel TF, Senior RM, Huang JS, Griffin GL. Chemotaxis of mono-cytes and neutrophils to platelet-derived growth factor. *J Clin Invest* 1982;69:1046–1049.

86. Chait A, Ross R, Bierman EL. Stimulation of receptor-dependent and receptor-independent pathways of low density lipoprotein degradation in arterial smooth muscle cells by platelet-derived growth factor. *Biochim Biophys Acta* 1988;960:183–189.

87. Davies PF, Ross R. Growth-mediated, density-dependent inhibition of endocytosis in cultured arterial smooth muscle cells. *Exp Cell Res* 1980;129:329–336.

88. Paris S, Pouyssegur J. Growth factors activate the Na+/H+ antiporter in quiescent fibroblasts by increasing its affinity for intracellular H+. *J Biol Chem* 1984;259:10989–10994.

89. Bowen-Pope DF, Malpass TW, Foster DM, Ross R. Platelet-derived growth factor *in vivo:* levels, activity, and rate of clearance. *Blood* 1984;64:458–469.

90. Shiraishi T, Morimoto S, Itoh K, et al. Radioimmunoassay of human platelet-derived growth factor using monoclonal antibody toward a synthetic 73–97 fragment of its B-chain. *Clin Chim Acta* 1989;184: 65–74.

91. Ross R, Masuda J, Raines EW, et al. Localization of PDGF-G protein in macrophages in all phases of atherogenesis. *Science* 1990;248: 1009–1112.

92. Leof EB, Proper JA, Goustin AS, Shipley GD, DiCorleto PE, Moses HL. Induction of c-sis mRNA and activity similar to platelet-derived growth factor by transforming growth factor β: a proposed model for indirect mitogenesis involving autocrine activity. *Proc Natl Acad Sci USA* 1986;83:2453–2457.

93. Battegay EJ, Raines EW, Seifert RA, Bowen-Pope DF, Ross R. TGF-β induces bimodal proliferation of connective tissue cells via complex control of an autocrine PDGF loop. *Cell* 1990;63:515–524.

94. Hajjar KA, Hajjar DP, Silverstein RL, Nachman RL. Tumor necrosis factor-mediated release of platelet-derived growth factor from cul-tured endothelial cells. *J Exp Med* 1987;166:235–245.

95. Libby P, Ross R. Cytokines and growth regulatory molecules in atherosclerosis. In: Fuster V, Ross R, Topol EJ, eds. *Atherosclerosis and coronary artery disease.* Philadelphia: Lippincott-Raven, 1996: 585–594.

96. Chang MY, Sasahara M, Chait A, Raines EW, Ross R. Inhibition of hypercholesterolemia-induced atherosclerosis in the nonhuman pri-mate by probucol: II. Cellular composition and proliferation. *Arte-rioscler Thromb Vasc Biol* 1995;15:1631–1640.

97. Ridker PM, Cushman M, Stampfer MJ, Tracy RP, Hennekens CH. Inflammation, aspirin, and the risk of cardiovascular disease in appar-ently healthy men. *N Engl J Med* 1997;336:973–979.

98. Brown BG, Albers JJ, Fisher LD, et al. Treatment study: a randomized trial demonstrating coronary disease regression and clinical benefit from lipid altering therapy among men with high apolipoprotein B. *N Engl J Med* 1990;323:1289–1298.

99. Wijns W, Serruys PW, Reiber JHC, et al. Early detection of restenosis after successful percutaneous transluminal coronary angioplasty by exercise-redistribution thallium scintigraphy. *Am J Cardiol* 1985;55: 357–361.

100. Leimgruber PP, Roubin MB, Hollman J, et al. Restenosis after successful coronary angioplasty in patients with single-vessel disease. *Circulation* 1986;73:710–717.

101. Stemerman MB, Ross R. Experimental arteriosclerosis. I. Fibrous plaque formation in primates, an electron microscope study. *J Exp Med* 1972;136:769–789.

102. Clowes AW, Reidy MA, Clowes MM. Kinetics of cellular proliferation after arterial injury. I. Smooth muscle growth in the absence of endothelium. *Lab Invest* 1983;49:327–333.

103. Lindner V, Reidy MA. Proliferation of smooth muscle cells after vascular injury is inhibited by an antibody against basic fibroblast growth factor. *Proc Natl Acad Sci USA* 1991;88:3739–3743.

104. Ferns GAA, Reidy MA, Ross R. Balloon catheter de-endothelialization of the nude rat carotid: response to injury in the absence of functional T lymphocytes. *Am J Pathol* 1991;138:1045–1057.

105. Ross R. Atherosclerosis. In: McGee JO'D, Wright NA, Isaacson PG, eds. *Oxford textbook of pathology.* Oxford: Oxford University Press, 1992:795–812.

Inflammation: Basic Principles and Clinical Correlates,
3rd ed., edited by John I. Gallin and Ralph Snyderman.
Lippincott Williams & Wilkins, Philadelphia © 1999.

CHAPTER 69

Type I Diabetes Mellitus

Charles A. Janeway, Jr. and Robert S. Sherwin

Diabetes mellitus is a common clinical syndrome characterized by alterations of the metabolism of glucose and other metabolic fuels that over time lead to the development of micro- and macrovascular and neurologic complications. It consists of a group of disorders caused by a variety of pathogenetic mechanisms in which the common denominator is hyperglycemia. Regardless of the underlying cause, the disease results from a common hormonal defect, namely, insulin deficiency, which may be total, partial, or relative when viewed in the context of coexisting insulin resistance.

Diabetes mellitus has been divided into three subclasses: (a) type I—insulin-dependent diabetes mellitus (IDDM), (b) type II—non–insulin-dependent diabetes mellitus (NIDDM), and (c) secondary diabetes (associated with another identifiable clinical condition or syndrome) (1). Type II diabetes is, by far, the most common form of diabetes in the world, comprising 85% to 90% of the diabetic population. These patients are not dependent on insulin for immediate survival as they retain some degree of endogenous secretory capacity. However, insulin levels are reduced relative to the level of glucose and insulin resistance, and they may need insulin therapy for metabolic control at some time in the course of the disease. Type II diabetes is most likely a heterogeneous disorder that (a) is commonly associated with obesity, (b) generally appears after the age of 40 years, and (c) has a high rate of genetic penetrance unrelated to human leukocyte antigen (HLA) genes or autoimmunity. It is noteworthy, however, that in some Western countries (e.g., Fin-

land), as many as 10% to 15% of patients who are classified as having type II diabetes on clinical grounds exhibit antiislet antibodies and develop the need for insulin therapy, and therefore may actually have type I diabetes (2).

This chapter focuses on type I diabetes mellitus, which affects ~10% of the diabetic population. These patients exhibit little or no insulin secretory capacity and require insulin therapy for survival. Commonly, but not always, the clinical features of the disorder appear abruptly in previously healthy children or young adults. However, a more gradual onset may occur, particularly in older adults. Studies of first-degree relatives of patients with type I diabetes have demonstrated that the disease has a long asymptomatic preclinical stage that may last months or many years, and that may be unmasked by an acute illness that superimposes an insulin resistant state (3). Once the disease first appears clinically, a so-called honeymoon period may follow, leading to a reduced-insulin or no-insulin requirement as a consequence of partial restoration of B cell function or reversal of insulin resistance with the resolution of the acute precipitating illness. Thereafter, endogenous insulin secretion is gradually lost over several years.

Estimates of prevalence rates for type I diabetes are about 0.3% (4). The disease is more prevalent in Northern European countries and Sardinia, less prevalent in Southern Europe and the Middle East, and rare in Asian countries. The annual incidence appears to have risen in the last half century, implying the influence of an undetermined environmental factor. On the other hand, the appreciation that type I diabetes has a prolonged preclinical phase has raised questions about the association of disease expression with seasonal changes, viral epidemics, or puberty, which may simply unmask B-cell deficiency by superimposing insulin resistance. The availability of methods for tracking islet autoimmunity has led to a reappraisal of the age at which the disease becomes manifest. Although type I diabetes is most com-

C. A. Janeway, Jr.: Section of Immunobiology, Yale University School of Medicine, New Haven, Connecticut 06510; Howard Hughes Medical Institute.

R. S. Sherwin: Section of Endocrinology, Department of Internal Medicine, Yale University School of Internal Medicine, New Haven, Connecticut 06510.

mon in childhood and tends to show a peak incidence in the pubertal period, it is now appreciated that incidence rates continue at a low level past middle age (5). Indeed, approximately one-third of patients who develop the disease are past the age of 20 years. Such patients tend to have a milder initial presentation and lower antibody titers, they may show different HLA haplotypes than their younger counterparts, and they may be difficult to distinguish clinically from their counterparts with type II diabetes (6,7). An important clinical issue that is unresolved is the question of whether the initiation of islet autoimmunity invariably culminates in the appearance of disease. Recent data suggest that the expression of antibodies to multiple B-cell antigens is highly predictive of type I diabetes, whereas those patients with single autoantibodies (especially with low titers) may never progress to clinical disease (8). This situation may be mimicked by rodent disease models in which islet-directed monocytic infiltration (insulitis) may be present in spite of persistent normoglycemia (9).

PATHOGENESIS OF HUMAN TYPE I DIABETES

Human type I diabetes most likely results from the interplay of genetic, environmental, and autoimmune factors, which ultimately lead to the selective destruction of B cells by T lymphocytes targeted to the islet.

Genetic Factors

The importance of genetic factors is evident from studies of identical twins in whom the concordance rates for disease are 35% to 50%, rates much higher than in HLA-identical siblings (10). While the lack of 100% concordance rates has been interpreted as indicating that environmental factors are involved, it should be noted that even identical twins do not express identical T-cell receptor and immunoglobulin genes due to random gene rearrangements, and thus one should not anticipate that autoimmune diseases such as type I diabetes should ever display 100% concordance rates.

Although current data indicate that multiple genes are linked to type I diabetes, the most dominant locus defining genetic susceptibility is found encoded within the major histocompatibility complex (MHC) or HLA region on the short arm of chromosome 6 (11). There is controversy over the exact location of the susceptibility locus and there is evidence suggesting that a single locus may not account for disease susceptibility, as the best correlation with disease occurs when a large region of the MHC is examined, which includes class I, II, and III loci (12,13). Nevertheless, the genes encoding MHC class II molecules of the D region appear to be critical. In Caucasian populations, type I diabetes has been genetically linked to the serologically defined antigens DR3 and DR4, whereas DR2 confers disease protection (14). Sub-

sequent data indicated that this is most likely due to linkage disequilibrium of these DR alleles to specific DQ alleles. This argument is strengthened by evidence that susceptibility can occur when DQA_1 and DQB_1 genes are present in the *trans* position (15). Susceptibility to diabetes in Caucasians has been associated with polymorphisms of the allele encoding the beta chain of the DQ class II molecule. Aspartic acid at position 57 appears to be protective, whereas substitution of a neutral amino acid at this position confers increased risk (16). Interestingly, an identical pattern is seen in the β-chain of the MHC class II molecule I-Ag[7] in nonobese diabetic (NOD) mice, a model of spontaneous diabetes (17; see below). However, the picture is undoubtedly more complex. Many studies suggest that a single residue does not determine susceptibility, and that the combination of DQA_1 and DQB_1 determinants is important. For example, a substitution of arginine in position 52 of the DQA_1 chain confers additional risk (18). Moreover, in studies involving diverse populations there are numerous susceptible DQ alleles and a number of distinct protective DQ alleles. Data derived from screening the entire human genome has reported that as many as 20 genes may be involved in disease susceptibility, but that linkage to MHC genes is the strongest as compared to all other genetic linkages (11).

The association of type I diabetes to particular MHC class II genes lends support for the thesis that the disease has an autoimmune component. The mature HLA-D or I-A protein is expressed on antigen-presenting cells (e.g., macrophages, dendritic cells, and B cells) where it traps antigenic peptide fragments generated in the endocytic compartment and brings them to the cell surface. Their primary role is to present these peptides in a configuration that can be recognized by CD4 T cells as well as to participate in the selection of the T-cell receptor repertoire. It has been suggested that disease-related polymorphisms of the MHC class II molecules act by altering the presentation of antigenic peptides to T cells; this view is supported by the fact that these polymorphisms occur along the binding groove of the extracellular domain of the MHC class II molecule (19). It has been hypothesized that disease-provoking peptides might bind better to disease-resistant than disease-susceptible MHC class II molecules, thereby resulting in the thymic elimination of diabetogenic T cells in the former but not in the latter.

Environmental Factors

Environmental factors have been proposed as initiating factors, including diet (e.g., milk protein in newborns), toxins, and viruses. Most attention has focused on viruses. Several systemic viral infections can destroy islets and/or induce insulitis (e.g., congenital rubella, coxsackie B4, and cytomegalovirus). Of particular interest, 12% to 20% of children afflicted with congenital rubella develop type I diabetes or abnormal glucose tolerance (20). In one instance, a coxsackie B4 virus was isolated from the pancreas of a 10-year-old child who died of diabetic ketoacidosis. Inoculation of the virus into mice resulted in the transfer of type I diabetes, thereby fulfilling Koch's postulates (21). However, viruses that produce acute, cytolytic infections are probably responsible for only an occasional case. Instead, if viruses are involved, it is more likely that they trigger autoimmune responses via molecular mimicry. For example, if a viral protein contains an epitope that resembles a B-cell protein, infection with the virus could abrogate self-tolerance, triggering autoimmunity (22). Interestingly, sequence homology has been identified between a coxsackie B virus protein and a middle region peptide from the autoantigen glutamic acid decarboxylase (GAD) (23).

Autoimmunity

The importance of autoimmunity in human type I diabetes was first suggested by the demonstration of islet cell antibodies (ICA) in sera of new-onset patients and first-degree relatives who later developed IDDM (24). Subsequently, a variety of antibodies were identified in these patients with specificity against B-cell constituents, including insulin, ICA 512 (an insulin granule-associated protein), and a 64-kd protein later shown to be GAD (24–27). The link between IDDM and GAD, an enzyme restricted mainly to brain and B cells, was uncovered by the discovery that patients with stiff-man syndrome (a rare neurologic disease) had anti-GAD autoantibodies and that many of them also had ICA and IDDM (28). Interestingly, ICA+ first-degree relatives are less likely to go on to develop IDDM if they have high-titer GAD antibodies, whereas those with lower titer and strong T-cell responses to GAD are more prone to disease (29). A similar picture has been seen with insulin as well, correlating high-titer antibodies with disease protection and strong T-cell responses to insulin with disease progression (30). This could be explained by a shift in CD4 T-cell phenotype, with high-titer antibodies reflecting a CD4 T cell expressing the CD40 ligand, and low-titer antibodies reflecting CD4 T cells expressing the Fas ligand.

Although the presence of islet-cell–directed antibodies were initially thought to be pathogenic, it is likely that they represent a reaction to epitopes exposed during the course of what appears to be a cell-mediated attack on the B cell. On the other hand, the presence of antibodies serves as a critical marker and predictor of disease. Studies examining asymptomatic first-degree relatives of patients with type I diabetes have demonstrated that about 3% are positive for islet autoantibodies (27). Current data indicate that these autoantibodies can be used to detect individuals who are at risk for the subsequent development of disease. Indeed, the predictive value for diabetes is probably >90% for patients with multiple autoantibodies (GAD, ICA 512, and insulin).

The bulk of the data indicates that islet-directed T cells rather than antibodies are the primary immune mediators of B-cell destruction, acting either via local release of cytokines or by direct cytolysis or both. Patients dying soon after the onset of IDDM who come to autopsy exhibit a cellular infiltration restricted to the islets, termed insulitis, that is mainly composed of T cells; macrophages and B cells are also present (31). A role for T cells is also supported by studies involving monozygotic twins with IDDM who received pancreas grafts from their nondiabetic but genetically identical sibling. They received little or no immunosuppression for their grafts as acceptance was anticipated, yet the pancreatic B cells were soon destroyed by infiltrating T cells, the majority of which were CD8+ (32). Further support for the role of T cells comes from another experiment of nature, namely, the adoptive transfer of diabetes following bone marrow transplantation between HLA-identical siblings who were discordant for diabetes (33).

THE CLINICAL EXPERIENCE WITH IMMUNOSUPPRESSION IN HUMAN TYPE I DIABETES

Preliminary studies have been conducted using immunosuppressive drugs (i.e., cyclosporine, azathioprine plus prednisone) to induce remissions in new-onset diabetic patients (34–36). While these studies have documented an increase in remissions (defined as lack of a requirement for exogenous insulin), the clinical improvement did not persist. The nephrotoxicity of cyclosporine, as well as concern regarding increased susceptibility to infection or neoplasia during long-term immunosuppression, have also limited the utility of these agents. Nevertheless, the clinical experience with immunosuppressive drugs has strengthened the thesis that autoimmunity causes human type I diabetes, and highlighted the need for a greater understanding of the pathogenesis of the disease so that rational, specific immunotherapies can be developed. To this end, a great deal of work has focused on the development of animal models of type I diabetes as a means of studying the immunology of this complex disease and testing potential therapies.

Animal Models of Insulin-Dependent Diabetes Mellitus, or Type I Diabetes

Early studies on spontaneous diabetes in animal models were mainly conducted in the BB/W rat model (37). This rat develops diabetes relatively readily, and has some of the hallmarks of the human disease. Early studies in the BB/W rat established that diabetes in this model was an autoimmune process, dependent on T cells of both CD4 and CD8 phenotypes. The studies showed that thymectomy at birth abrogated the disease, as did adult thymectomy, irradiation, and bone marrow reconstitution.

A striking feature was the dependence on MHC genotype and also on background genes. The main non-MHC gene contributing to disease susceptibility gives rise to lymphopenia, which raises problems with the interpretation of studies carried out in BB rats, as comparable human studies do not depend on lymphopenia. Indeed, as mentioned in the previous section, immunosuppression with cyclosporin A is a way to prevent development of chronic diabetes if administered during the so-called honeymoon period after diabetes first appears in human patients (34–36). Also missing in these rats is a subset of T cells that appear to be regulatory/suppressor T cells. These T cells are marked by expression of the RT-6 molecule. This subset has not been detected in mouse or in man. If one depletes RT-6–positive cells from animals of the same MHC genotype as the BB/W rat, then these rats become susceptible to the development of diabetes. Thus, the lymphopenia gene appears to deprive the BB/W rat of the necessary regulatory cell subset leading to spontaneous diabetes (38). This is not seen in human or mouse spontaneous diabetes, and so the BB/W rat model has been less widely exploited than the mouse model of type I diabetes, the NOD mouse (39). The rest of this section discusses studies carried out in this mouse system.

The mouse is one of the best characterized laboratory animals in terms of studies of genes and molecules, and its power is increasing as time goes by. One of the reasons for this is the ability to manipulate the mouse genome, both by transgenesis and by gene targeting. There already exist over 1,000 strains of mice with various deletions in the germ line (40), and the number is growing at an amazing rate. Some of these mutations are lethal, but their impact on immune system function can be studied by using the recombination activating gene-2 (RAG-2) blastocyst injection system. In this system, RAG-2 has been deleted, leading to the inhibition of development of both the T- and B-cell lineage, which are dependent on this gene for their formation. Thus, any mutant can in principle be tested for its impact on the adaptive immune response by reconstituting RAG-2 blastocysts with embryonal stem (ES) cells with a homozygous mutation in any gene of interest (41). These three techniques—transgenesis, gene targeting, and the RAG-2 blastocyst injection—have allowed many mutations to be tested for their effect on the adaptive immune response. In describing this model, we will frequently make use of data from transgenic and gene targeted NOD mice.

The Nonobese Diabetic Mouse Model of Human Insulin-Dependent Diabetes Mellitus

Following the discovery of a mouse that spontaneously developed IDDM, many laboratories began an intensive investigation of its genome. In the earliest studies, it became apparent that the genotype at the MHC was of paramount importance (42). Modifying this by intercrossing with mice of a different MHC genotype, it became apparent that one needed homozygosity at the MHC to get spontaneous IDDM in this mouse model (43). Nevertheless, it was possible through intensive breeding to demonstrate that genes other than the MHC also played important roles in the pathogenesis of IDDM in the NOD mouse. Particularly through the work of Todd and Wicker's team (44), it was appreciated that a minimum of 16 separable genes could be defined that contributed to susceptibility to IDDM. The genes were numbered in the order of their discovery, with the MHC-linked gene being given pride of place as *Idd-1*. The other *Idd* genes have a less dramatic effect on incidence of diabetes, but some are quite powerful in preventing IDDM. For instance, a gene tightly linked to the $C\alpha$ gene of the mouse T-cell receptor prevents diabetes sufficiently strongly that it was only after more than eight (>99.5% of the genome) backcrosses of the $C\alpha$ knock-out to NOD that it became apparent that heterozygosity at $C\alpha$ could not protect against spontaneous diabetes in NOD mice (45,46; Wong and Janeway, unpublished data; Mathis, unpublished data). Other genes must be as rigorously tested as this example before they can be seen as a true cause of protection from diabetes. As all gene knock-out mice to date have been prepared in strain 129 embryonal stem cells, there is no substitute for this rigorous back-crossing to inbreed genes on the NOD mouse genetic background. The process can be accelerated to some extent by monitoring resistance genes with microsatellite DNA for homozygosity for the NOD allele at all loci tested, but even so the process takes several crosses, with each cross requiring a minimum of 2 months. For this reason, one of the main goals of work on this mouse model is to produce ES cells from the NOD strain so that NOD alleles of susceptibility genes can be targeted.

Because of this, much of what we know about prevention of diabetes in the NOD mouse comes from inserting protective genes in the form of transgenes directly into NOD embryos. Using this approach, it has been shown that a transgenic I-$E\alpha$ gene can almost totally abolish diabetes. More importantly, changing the I-$A\beta$ chain at either position 57 or 56 can almost totally abolish IDDM susceptibility in transgenic mice. Moreover, transferring cells from such mice into NOD mice can prevent IDDM almost entirely. Thus, the MHC not only makes the mice susceptible, but it acts in a recessive manner, as shown by the dominant effect of I-E or $A\beta$ transgenes, and the protective influence of I-E$^+$ cells. The mechanism is still debated, but it appears to be related to the instability of the I-A^{g7} allele in the NOD mouse. This apparently interferes with the establishment of tolerance in the thymus, an effect that can be overcome by expressing an insulin transgene in the thymus of NOD mice (47). It should be noted that production of intrathymic insulin is also associated with diabetes resistance in humans who otherwise would be susceptible (48,49).

Many transgenes have been directed by the rat insulin promoter-1 to release cytokines and other molecules from B cells. Some of these accelerate diabetes, while others retard it. There are even cases where expression of such transgenic constructs can have both effects depending on the founder. Among the genes that have accelerated diabetes, none is quite as successful as the human CD80 (hB7.1) gene. On the first backcross to NOD, diabetes begins to appear at 3 to 4 weeks, and affects >50% of the mice before the first nontransgenic NOD mouse becomes diabetic. This transgene, however, cannot override the MHC effect, as only mice that are homozygous for H-2^{g7} are susceptible (50). This transgene has been used to map out certain features of IDDM in NOD mice. For instance, when CD4 knock-out mice are bred to mice with the RIP-CD80 transgene, no acceleration in diabetes is observed. This proves that CD4 T cells have a critical role in the accelerated diabetes seen with this transgene. Also, when the β2μ knock-out is bred to RIP-CD80 transgenic mice, there is only rarely diabetes, and on histologic inspection, only CD4 T cells are observed. Thus, CD8 T cells account for the majority of the accelerated diabetes observed in such mice, with only rare CD4 T cells able to contribute. Finally, when the immunoglobulin M (IgM) transmembrane domain is knocked out, which produces the phenotype of complete B-cell deficiency in NOD and other mice, diabetes does not occur. This could be due to a tightly linked diabetes protection gene, but this seems unlikely, as breeding NOD mice to the RIP-CD80 transgenic mice produces mice that lack B cells but develop accelerated diabetes, identical in course to the disease in RIP-CD80 transgenic normal NOD mice. This shows that the role of B cells is not to produce antibody, but presumably to play some other role in the pathogenesis of diabetes in NOD mice such as antigen presentation (Wong, unpublished data).

One of the key pathologic features of IDDM in humans is the infiltration of the islets of Langerhans with small lymphocytes. This is called insulitis, and is observed infrequently in humans, because once all the B cells are destroyed, the antigen disappears and the stimulus for recruiting and retaining these cells is lost. In the NOD mouse, insulitis appears around 3 to 5 weeks of age, and remains with subsequent invasion of the islets over the next 8 weeks, whereupon diabetes begins to emerge. This has been confirmed in mice transgenic for the receptor from a CD4 T cell clone, and appears to be due to the formation on B cells of older NOD mice of receptors for members of the tumor necrosis factor (TNF) family of cytokines, particularly p55 TNFR and Fas. These molecules appear on the B-cell surface around this age and can lead to apoptosis of B cells upon contact with their respective ligands, TNF-α or TNF-β in the case of the p55 TNFR, or Fas ligand (FasL) in the case of Fas (51). Thus, insulitis is another feature of the NOD mouse that replicates the human disease.

This insulitis is initially made up of CD8 T cells, or is dependent on their presence. The role of CD8 T cells was initially suspected from the absence of insulitis and diabetes in mice lacking the light chain of the MHC class I molecule β2μ (52–54). These mice developed neither diabetes nor insulitis, and were profoundly deficient in MHC class I expression. Subsequently, the time at which it was critical to have CD8 T cells was shown between 3 and 5 weeks by anti-CD8 monoclonal antibody treatment, during this time (55). This makes some sense, as the only MHC molecules that are expressed on the surface of the pancreatic B cell are MHC class I molecules (56). Furthermore, when RIP-CD80 mice are used, they develop diabetes at an early age, consistent with direct priming on the transgenic B cell. Thus, CD8 T cells are critical at this early phase of IDDM in NOD mice. Furthermore, it is clear that, with few exceptions, CD8 T cells are required for the final destruction of B cells in the islets of Langerhans that occurs at the end of the diabetes. This can be reiterated in recipients of human identical twin hemipancreatic islet grafts: these grafts are characterized by infiltration of mainly (but not exclusively) CD8 T cells (32), and similar behavior is seen in the requirement for CD8 T cells in adoptively transferred diabetes using spleen cells from recently diabetic NOD mice into young NOD mice (57,58).

Another feature of NOD mice that makes the study of diabetes more perplexing is the effect of the environment on the incidence of diabetes. Mice raised germ free or specific pathogen free are highly susceptible to diabetes, while mice that are deliberately exposed to various pathogens become resistant. What is not clear is the mechanism of this protection against IDDM by bacteria, but indirect evidence suggests that it is the induction of interleukin-4 (IL-4) or transforming growth factor-β (TGF-β) secretion by the mice that protects them from insulitis and diabetes. Certainly, injection with complete Freund's adjuvant, a common method for inducing many experimental autoimmune diseases, protects mice from diabetes, and this is associated with cells secreting IL-4 (59). There is also an effect of nutrition: mice fed on a regular diet get diabetes normally, while mice fed a protein-poor diet do not develop diabetes (60). Many drugs have been tested for their ability to prevent diabetes in NOD mice, and most of them work. Thus, preventing diabetes in the NOD mouse is almost too easy. This has caused many to regard them as useful tools for unraveling the pathogenesis of diabetes, but rather poor models for understanding how to prevent the disease (61).

The Cellular Pathogenesis of Diabetes in the Nonobese Diabetic Mouse

The immunology of diabetes is fairly well advanced in the study of NOD mice. However, many gaps in our knowledge still exist. The importance of MHC class II genotype to the incidence of diabetes in NOD mice has been a clear pointer that CD4 T cells must be involved. Recently, several other pieces of evidence have been added to this genetic evidence. First, CD4 T-cell clones by themselves can, on occasion, lead to IDDM (62). Transgenic mice created from one of these cloned T-cell lines develop IDDM with essentially the same kinetics as normal mice, and, when they are bred to NOD–severe combined immune deficiency (NOD-SCID) mice, which cannot rearrange their endogenous V gene segments, the incidence and the kinetics of the disease are markedly increased. Finally, it has been known for some time that anti-CD4 injection to deplete CD4 T cells is an effective therapy for NOD mice.

However, other evidence supports the importance of CD8 T cells, at least in the initiation of the cellular attack on the islets. First, in mice lacking MHC class I and CD8 T cells, diabetes and insulitis are basically entirely prevented (52–54). Second, if one treats with anti-CD8 antibody in a critical window between 3 and 5 weeks, again the occurrence of diabetes is totally abrogated (55). Third, cloned CD8 T cells can trigger acute diabetes within a week of transfer, much more rapidly than comparable transfer of CD4 T-cell clones that induce diabetes only 3 to 4 weeks after transfer (63). The importance of CD8 T cells is thought to be in initiating damage to the B cells of the islets, which only express MHC class I surface molecules. MHC class II is only found on dendritic cells and macrophages within the islets themselves. However, transferring limiting numbers of cloned CD8 T cells has not yielded a dose that causes sufficient damage to trigger diabetes, as would be predicted if their role is in the process of diabetes initiation but not in its sustaining.

Another perplexing issue is the role of B cells in the pathogenesis of IDDM in NOD mice. Several laboratories have shown that B cells play some role in diabetes, but that role is unclear. NOD mice that are bred to mice that lack B cells do not get diabetes in most cases, although this is disputed by at least one lab (64), and B cells are a prominent component of islet infiltrates. What role could B cells play in the induction of diabetes in NOD mice? One can think of several different roles, and each must be ruled in or out by experiment. It is possible that B cells play an important role as producers of serum antibodies that are specifically cytotoxic to B cells in the islets. This seems unlikely, as serum cannot transfer diabetes in NOD mice, even when given regularly. Nevertheless, this possibility is not yet ruled out. Also, the role of Fc receptors (FcR) has not yet been ruled out by breeding FcR gene deletions available to NOD mice. This will have to be done, but it seems unlikely to be a causative factor due to the ready transfer of IDDM by several different T-cell clones. However, it would be best to confirm that the infusion of B cells into young, B-less NOD mice can restore diabetes susceptibility to NOD mice. A second role is as antigen-presenting cells. This would be via direct presentation by B cells themselves, where antigen would be presented to CD4 T cells. This hypothesis would explain both the role of CD4 T cells and the role of B cells, both of which are required for spontaneous IDDM in NOD mice (65). Alternatively, an indirect role such as antibody-mediated uptake by Fc receptor–bearing cells such as macrophages could account for the importance of B cells in IDDM. This can be tested by making mice transgenic with heavy chains that are modified so that they serve as transmembrane receptors that cannot be secreted, or heavy chains that are unmodified, so that they can serve both as transmembrane and secreted Ig molecules.

The insulitis seen in NOD mice is also characterized by macrophages that appear early along with CD8 T cells, CD4 T cells, and B cells, and they are present throughout the insulitic process up to and including the destruction of all the B cells in the islets of Langerhans. Their function appears to be the ingestion of apoptotic cells, including both T cells and pancreatic B cells, but they may have other functions as well. Macrophages are difficult to deplete, so the critical role of the macrophage has not yet been convincingly tested. They are known to engulf apoptotic cells using a receptor for surface features of dead or dying cells, although the exact nature of this receptor in mammals has yet to be deciphered.

Finally, the role of various cytokines has been examined, using systemic treatment with recombinant cytokines, treatment with cytokine-specific antibodies, or transgenic mice to examine the effect of over- or underexpression of a given cytokine in the pathogenesis of diabetes. Most attention has focused on the cytokines TNF-α and TNF-β. If given to young NOD mice, TNF-α accelerates diabetes, while if given to older NOD mice, TNF-α retards development of diabetes (66). This has pointed out the diverse effects of cytokine administration, and it has led to further experimentation in these models. TNF-α expressed locally in the islets prevents diabetes, despite the presence of intense infiltration of the islets by inflammatory T cells. This is true of TNF-α driven by the rat insulin promoter, which prevents the induction of autoreactive T cells in NOD mice. However, these mice remain susceptible to transfer of cloned CD8 T cells as well as to transfer of uncloned T cells from recently diabetic NOD mice (67). Other cytokines expressed off the RIP have various effects. Interferon-γ can induce insulitis and diabetes in transgenic mice, but the diabetes in this case is due to competition for the insulin promoter at the level of transcription factors. Nevertheless, cells are generated that are autoreactive in vivo to genetically identical islets on transfer to normal hosts transplanted with normal islets (68).

In recent experiments, it was shown that the molecules Fas and FasL can be involved in a model of IDDM studied by one of the authors. Evidence for this role came from an attempt to make islets resistant to autoimmune attack by preparing NOD mice with a transgenic FasL driven by the RIP. These RIP-FasL transgenic mice were variably sensitive to IDDM; some were almost completely resistant to spontaneous IDDM, while others became diabetic in an accelerated fashion, some so early that the founders could not be bred. Upon transfer of CD8 T cell clones, which express both perforin and FasL, all of these mice got IDDM in an accelerated fashion, within 2 to 4 days of receiving the cells. It became obvious that cytokines released by the transferred cells were inducing Fas expression on the B cells of the islets of Langerhans, and this was confirmed by immunohistochemistry on the islets, demonstrating the expression of Fas in adult islet B cells within 48 hours of injecting the CD8 cytotoxic cells. After this time, the islets that were already expressing FasL endogenously due to the RIP-FasL transgene committed suicide. The importance of Fas in IDDM was confirmed by breeding the mutant Fas gene found in the lpr mouse onto the NOD background. These mice did not develop diabetes spontaneously, and they were completely resistant to the transferred cytotoxic T cells. This further demonstrated that the mode of cytotoxicity used by these CD8 T cells depended almost completely on Fas:FasL interactions (51). Furthermore, NOD mice that have a defect in their perforin genes nevertheless develop diabetes normally or nearly normally (Hengartner, personal communication). Thus, it appears that the major pathway of cell death in the islets of mice is via Fas:FasL interactions.

DIABETES PREVENTION

The ultimate goal of diabetes research is prevention of diabetes, not only in those individuals who have a family history (~10% of cases), but in the population at large. The question is how to do it, and the answer would seem to be by vaccination against diabetes. Vaccination is the only means by which the outcome of specific immune responses has been controlled, and it is unlikely that any other approach will work. So we must ask, what clues are there about antigens that can protect against diabetes in NOD mice or even people? A possible answer is insulin; but how does insulin perform as an antigen, what do we know about responses to insulin, and how can it be used to induce the necessary cells to protect mice and eventually people from diabetes?

Insulin injection was introduced by Banting and Best in the 1920s as a treatment for diabetes, and rapidly converted a disease that was uniformly fatal into a disease that was survivable. However, people with diabetes controlled by insulin still develop such complications of diabetes as renal failure, blindness, and peripheral vascular disease. These complications can be mitigated by further tightening the control of blood sugar as shown by the success of the recently completed Diabetes Control and Complications Trial (DCCT) (69). However, all this trial served to demonstrate was that costly and rigorous control of diabetes could reduce the incidence of complications, but at the cost of more frequent episodes of hypoglycemia, to say nothing of the cost in physician hours involved in keeping the trial subjects on a rigorous regimen of insulin injections and blood glucose measurements. Clearly, a vaccine directed at preventing diabetes would be far preferable.

Currently, insulin therapy is being tried to prevent diabetes in individuals who are at high risk of developing the disease. These people are identified through a variety of means, including MHC genotyping, measurement of serum antibodies to various islet autoantigens, and measurements of blood glucose. Those who meet the criteria for being at high risk are treated with daily insulin injections in the absence of overt diabetes (70). It is too early to conclude much of anything from these trials.

Another approach is to feed individual mice or people who are at risk with bovine, mouse, or human insulin. This is purported to induce a state of so-called oral tolerance, in which T cells are stimulated in the intestinal mucosa with the insulin molecules consumed by the host, and then home to the islets, where they are believed to be actively engaged in secreting TGF-β (71). TGF-β is an anti-inflammatory cytokine, well known for its ability to suppress T-cell activation. This has been shown in principle, but it has never been used as a motivation for vaccination.

Recently, one of the authors has isolated a T-cell line that responds to the β chain of insulin, residues 12-25, by producing TGF-β. The exact derivation of this line of T cells is unclear, but it clearly was produced by NOD mice undergoing autoimmune attack on the B cells. This is consistent with the origin of such cells within the context of autoimmunity, implying that such cells are always present and just need to be appropriately activated. It is interesting in this context that previous data had suggested the presence of such cells in both mice and humans, as the onset of diabetes in both species is a chronic process. However, diabetes is an acute process when either identical twin hemipancreatic grafts are placed (32), or when spleen cells from diabetic mice are transferred into nondiabetic mice (57,58). Thus, while the existence of such cells was postulated based on these kinetic differences, they had not been previously observed. It is likely that other autoimmune diseases are also accompanied by formation of such cells. The real question is, how can one generate cells with these characteristics deliberately and without provoking diabetes or other autoimmune diseases? This is especially so as insulin-reactive T-cell clones that will transfer diabetes have also been isolated (72). The answers to this and many other questions about IDDM are likely to be obtained from a thorough and meticulous analysis of the pathogenesis of IDDM first in NOD mice and then in humans, proceeding where possible in parallel, followed by attempts to induce active tolerance *in vivo,* first in NOD mice and then in people.

SUMMARY AND PERSPECTIVES

The idea that insulin-dependent diabetes mellitus may eventually be eradicated by vaccination is a long-term goal. In the short run, we will have to deal with the toll this disease exacts from all who develop it, not only in terms of reduced life expectancy but also in terms of the expense of treating it. Thus, in the short run, alternative therapies are being sought, such as transplantation with rejection-resistant islets. If this can be engineered in islets from farm animals that are free of dangerous viruses, then this will be a first step in a long road leading toward vaccination against diabetes. The ultimate goal, however, should be diabetes prevention, rather than a diabetes cure, and it is encouraging that studies in experimental animals give hope that this can be achieved. Now it is time to finish the job by making vaccination of all children a reality.

ACKNOWLEDGMENTS

The authors wish to thank their many colleagues who helped in the preparation of this chapter and whose research efforts have guided our thinking. We would also like to thank Kara McCarthy for tireless work on the manuscript for this chapter. Our work on diabetes has been supported by a Diabetes and Endocrinology Research Center Grant to Robert S. Sherwin, a diabetes program project grant to Charles A. Janeway, Jr., and the Howard Hughes Medical Institute.

REFERENCES

1. Fajans SS. Classification and diagnosis of diabetes mellitus. In: Porte D, Sherwin RS, eds. *Ellenberg and Rifkin's diabetes mellitus.* Stamford, CT: Appleton and Lange, 1997:357–372.
2. Groop L, Miettinen A, Groop PH, Seppo M, Saija K, Bottazzo GF. Organ-specific autoimmunity and HLA-DR antigens as markers for b-cell destruction in patients with type I diabetes. *Diabetes* 1988;37: 99–103.
3. Srikanta S, Ganda OP, Eisenbarth GS, Soeldner JS. Islet cell antibodies and beta cell function in monozygotic triplets and twins initially discordant for type I diabetes mellitus. *N Engl J Med* 1983;308:321–325.
4. Bennett PH, Rewers MJ, Knowler WC. Epidemiology of diabetes mellitus. In: Porte D, Sherwin RS, eds. *Ellenberg and Rifkin's diabetes mellitus.* Stamford, CT: Appleton and Lange, 1997:373–400.
5. Lorenzen T, Pociot E, Hougaard P, Nerup J. Long-term risk of IDDM in first-degree relatives of patients with IDDM. *Diabetologia* 1994;37: 321–327.
6. Caillat-Zucman A, Garchon HJ, Timsit J, et al. Age-dependent HLA genetic heterogeneity of type I insulin dependent diabetes mellitus. *J Clin Invest* 1992;90:2242–2250.
7. Schiffrin A, Suissa S, Weitzner G, Poussier P, Lalla D. Factors predicting course of β cell function in IDDM. *Diabetes Care* 1992;15: 997–1001.
8. Eizirik DL, Sandler S, Palmer JP. Repair of pancreatic beta cells. A relevant phenomenon in early IDDM? *Diabetes* 1993;43:1383–1391.
9. Garchon HJ, Bedossa P, Eloy I, Bach JF. Identification and mapping to chromosome 1 of a susceptibility locus for perinsulitis in non-obese diabetic mice. *Nature* 1991;353:260–262.
10. Pyke DA. The genetic connections. *Diabetologia* 1979;17:333–343.
11. Davies JL, Kawaguchi Y, Bennett ST, et al. A genome-wide search for human type I diabetes susceptibility genes. *Nature* 1994;371:130–136.
12. Degli-Esposti MA, Abraham LJ, McCann V, Spies T, Christiansen FT, Dawkins RL. Ancestral haplotypes reveal the role of the central MHC in the immunogenetics of IDDM. *Immunogenetics* 1992;36:345–356.
13. Fennessey M, Metcalfe K, Hitman GA, et al., and the Childhood Diabetes in Finland (DiMe) Study Group. A gene in the HLA class I region contributes to susceptibility to IDDM in the Finnish population. *Diabetologia* 1994;37:937–944.
14. Platz P, Jakobsen BK, Morling M. HLAD and DR-antigens in genetic analysis of insulin-dependent diabetes mellitus. *Diabetologia* 1981;21: 108–115.
15. Khallil I, Deschamps I, Lepage V, Al-Daccak R, Degos L, Hors J. Does effect of cis and transencoded HLA-DQab heterodimers in type I diabetes susceptibility. *Diabetes* 1992;412:378–384.
16. Todd JA, Bell JI, McDevitt HO. HLA-DQ beta gene contributes to susceptibility and resistance to insulin-dependent diabetes mellitus. *Nature* 1987;329:599.
17. Acha-Orbea H, McDevitt HO. The first external domain of the nonobese diabetic mouse class II beta chain is unique. *Proc Natl Acad Sci USA* 1987;84:2435–2441.
18. Khalil I, d'Auriol I, Gobet M, et al. A combination of HLA-DQb ASP57 negative and HLA Da Arg 52 confers susceptibility to insulin-dependent diabetes. *J Clin Invest* 1990;85:1315–1319.
19. Routsias J, Papadopoulos GK. Polymorphic structural features of modeled HLA-DQ molecules segregate according to susceptibility or resistance to IDDM. *Diabetologia* 1995;38:1251–1261.
20. Mensen MA, Forrest JM, Bransby RD. Rubella infection and diabetes mellitus. *Lancet* 1978;1:57–62.
21. Yoon JW, Austin M, Onodera T, Notkins AL. Virus-induced diabetes mellitus: isolation of a virus from the pancreas of a child with diabetic ketoacidosis. *N Engl J Med* 1979;300:173–177.
22. Oldstone MBA. Molecular mimicry and autoimmune disease. *Cell* 1987;50:819–825.
23. Kaufman DL, Erlander MG, Clare-Salzer M, Atkinson MA, Maclaren NK, Tobin AJ. Autoimmunity to two forms of glutamate decarboxylase in insulin-dependent diabetes mellitus. *J Clin Invest* 1992;89:283–287.
24. Castano L, Eisenbarth GS. Type I diabetes: a chronic autoimmune disease of human, mouse and rat. *Annu Rev Immunol* 1990;8:647–679.
25. Baekkeskov S, Nielsen JH, Marner B, Bilde T, Ludvigsson J, Lernmark A. Autoantibodies in newly diagnosed diabetic children immunoprecipitate specific human islet cell proteins. *Nature* 1982;298:169–173.
26. Baekkeskov S, Aanstoot H-J, Christgau S, et al. Identification of the 64-kd autoantigen in insulin-dependent diabetes as the GABA-synthesizing enzyme glutamic acid decarboxylase. *Nature* 1990;347:151–156.
27. Atkinson MA, MacLaren NK. Islet cell autoantigens in insulin-dependent diabetes. *J Clin Invest* 1993;92:1608–1616.
28. Solimena M, Folli F, Aparisi R, Pozza G, DeCamilli P. Autoantibodies to GABA-ergic neurons and pancreatic beta cells in stiff-man syndrome. *N Engl J Med* 1990;322:1555–1562.
29. Harrison LC, Honeyman MC, DeAizpurura HJ, et al. Inverse relationship between humoral and cellular immunity to glutamic acid decarboxylase in subjects at risk of insulin-dependent diabetes. *Lancet* 1993;341:1365–1370.
30. Ellis TM, Darrow B, Campbell L, Atkinson MA. Inverse relationship between humoral and cellular immune responses to GAD-65 and insulin in IDD. *Diabetes* 1995;41(suppl):52A.
31. Bottazzo GF, Dean BM, McNally JM, MacKay EH, Swift PGF, Gamble DR. *In situ* characterization of autoimmune phenomena and expression of HLA molecules in the pancreas in diabetic insulitis. *N Engl J Med* 1985;313:353–360.
32. Sutherland DE, Sibley R, Xu XZ, et al. Twin to twin pancreas transplantation: reversal and reenactment of the pathogenesis of type I diabetes. *Trans Assoc Am Physicians* 1984;97:80–87.
33. Lampeter EF, Homberg M, Quabeck K, et al. Transfer of insulin-dependent diabetes between HLA-identical siblings by bone marrow transplantation. *Lancet* 1993;341(8855):1243–1244.
34. Silverstein J, MacLaren N, Riley W, Spillar R, Radjenovic D, Johnson S. Immunosuppression with azathioprine and prednisone in recent-onset insulin-dependent diabetes mellitus. *N Engl J Med* 1988; 319:599–604.
35. Bougneres PF, Landais P, Boisson C, et al. Limited duration of remission of insulin dependency in children with recent overt type I diabetes treated with low-dose cyclosporin. *Diabetes* 1990;39:1264–1272.

36. Feutren G, Boitard C, Bougneres P, Assan R, Bach JF. Cyclosporin for type I diabetes: lessons from first clinical trials and new perspectives. *Immunother Diabetes Selected Autoimmune Dis* 1989;61.

37. Rossini AA, Mordes JP, Like AA. Immunology of insulin-dependent diabetes mellitus. *Annu Rev Immunol* 1985;3:289–320.

38. Mordes JP, Greiner DL, Appel MC, Rozing J, Handler ES, Rossini AA. Adoptive transfer of autoimmune diabetes and thyroiditis to athymic rats. *Proc Natl Acad Sci USA* 1990;87:7618–7622.

39. Makino S, Kunimuto K, Munaoko Y, Mizushima Y, Katagiri K, Tochino Y. Breeding of a non-obese diabetic strain of mice. *Exp Anim* 1980; 29:1–12.

40. Brandon EP. Idzerda RL, McKnight GS. Targeting the mouse genome: a compendium of knock-outs. *Curr Biol* 1995;5:625–645,728–765, 873–881.

41. Chen J, Lansford R, Steward V, Young F, Alt FW. RAG-2–deficient blastocyst complementation: an assay of gene function in lymphocyte development. *Proc Natl Acad Sci USA* 1993;90:4528–4532.

42. Todd JA, Bell JI, McDevitt HO. HLA-DQ beta gene contributes to susceptibility and resistance to insulin-dependent diabetes mellitus. *Nature* 1987;329:599–604.

43. Hattori M, Buse JB, Jackson RA, et al. The NOD mouse: recessive diabetogenic gene in the major histocompatibility complex. *Science* 1986; 231:733–735.

44. Ghosh S, Palmer SM, Rodrigues NM, et al. Polygenic control of autoimmune diabetes in nonobese diabetic mice. *Nature Genet* 1993; 404–409.

45. Elliot JI, Altmann DM. Dual T cell receptor alpha chain T cells in autoimmunity. *J Exp Med* 1995;182:953–959.

46. Elliot JI, Altmann DM. Non-obese diabetic mice hemizygous at the T cell receptor alpha locus are susceptible to diabetes and sialitis. *Eur J Immunol* 1996;26:953–957.

47. French MB, Allison J, Cram DS, et al. Transgenic expression of mouse proinsulin II prevents diabetes in nonobese diabetic mice. *Diabetes* 1997;46:34–39.

48. Pugliese A, Zeller M, Fernandez A Jr, et al. The insulin gene is transcribed in the human thymus and transcription levels correlate with allelic variation at the INS VNTR-IDDM2 susceptibility locus for type I diabetes. *Nature Genet* 1997;15:293–297.

49. Vafiadis P, Bennet ST, Todd JA, et al. Insulin expression in human thymus is modulated by INS VNTR alleles at the IDDM2 locus. *Nature Genet* 1997;15:289–292.

50. Wong S, Guerder S, Visintin I, et al. Expression of the co-stimulator molecule B7-1 in pancreatic beta cells accelerates diabetes in the NOD mouse. *Diabetes* 1995;44:326–329.

51. Chervonsky AV, Wang Y, Wong FS, et al. The role of Fas in autoimmune disease. *Cell* 1997;89:17–24.

52. Katz J, Benoist C, Mathis D. Major histocompatibility complex class I molecules are required for the development of insulitis in non-obese diabetic mice. *Nature* 1993;23:3358–3360.

53. Wicker LS, Leiter EH, Todd JA, et al. Beta 2-microglobulin-deficient NOD mice do not develop insulitis or diabetes. *Diabetes* 1994;43: 500–504.

54. Serreze DV, Leiter EH, Christianson GJ, Greiner D, Roopenian DC. Major histocompatibility complex class I-deficient NOD-beta2m^{null} mice are diabetes and insulitis resistant. *Diabetes* 1994;43:505–508.

55. Wang B, Gonzalez A, Benoist C, Mathis D. The role of CD8+ T cells in the initiation of insulin-dependent diabetes mellitus. *Eur J Immunol* 1996;26:1762–1769.

56. McInerney MF, Rath S, Janeway CA Jr. Exclusive expression of MHC class II proteins on CD45+ cells in pancreatic islets of NOD mice. *Diabetes* 1991;40:648–651.

57. Miller BJ, Apple MC, O'Neill JJ, Wicker LS. Both the Ly2+ and L3T4+ T cells subset are required for the transfer of diabetes in non-obese diabetic mice. *J Immunol* 1988;140:52–59.

58. Bendelac A, Carnaud C, Boitard C, Bach J-F. Syngeneic transfer of autoimmune diabetes from diabetic NOD mice to healthy neonates. *J Exp Med* 1987;166:823–830.

59. Quin YY, Soderlain MW, Hitchon C, Lanzon J, Singh B. Complete Freund's adjuvant-induced T cells prevent the development and adoptive transfer of diabetes in non-obese diabetic mice. *J Immunol* 1994;150: 2072–2077.

60. Pociot F, Mandrup-Poulsen T. Aetiology and pathogenesis of insulin-dependent diabetes mellitus. In: Leslie RDG, ed. *Molecular pathogenesis of diabetes mellitus.* Basel: Human Frontiers Press, 1997:1–22.

61. Bowman MA, Leither EH, Atkinson MA. Prevention of diabetes in the NOD mouse: implications for therapeutic intervention in human disease. *Immunol Today* 1994;15:115–120.

62. Katz JD, Wang B, Haskins K, Benoist C, Mathis D. Following a diabetogenic T cell from genesis through pathogenesis. *Cell* 1993;74:1089–1100.

63. Wong FS, Visintin I, Wen L, Flavell RA, Janeway CA Jr. CD8 T cell clones from young nonobese diabetic (NOD) islets can transfer rapid onset of diabetes in NOD mice in the absence of CD4 cells. *J Exp Med* 1996;183:67–76.

64. Serreze DV, Chapman HD, Varnum DS, et al. B lymphocytes are essential for the initiation of T cell-mediated autoimmune diabetes: analysis of a new speed congenic stock of NOD.Tg mu null mice. *J Exp Med* 1996;184:2049–2053.

65. Mamula MJ, Janeway CA Jr. Do B cells drive the diversification of immunological responses? *Immunol Today* 1993;14:54–56.

66. Jabob CO, Aiso S, Michie SA, McDevitt HO, Acha-Orbea H. Prevention of diabetes in nonobese diabetic mice by tumor necrosis factor (TNF): similarities between TNF alpha and interleukin 1. *Proc Natl Acad Sci USA* 1990;87:968–972.

67. Grewal IS, Greal KD, Wong FS, Picarella DE, Janeway CA Jr, Flavell RA. Local expression of transgene encoded TNF alpha in islets prevents autoimmune diabetes in nonobese diabetic (NOD) mice by preventing the development of auto-reactive islet-specific T cells. *J Exp Med* 1996;184:1963–1974.

68. Sarvetnick N, Liggit D, Pitts SL, Hansen SE, Stewart TA. Insulin-dependent diabetes mellitus induced in transgenic mice by ectopic expression of class II MHC and interferon-gamma. *Cell* 1988;52:773–782.

69. The Diabetes Control and Complications Trial Research Group. The effect of intensive treatment of diabetes on the development and progression of long-term complication in insulin-dependent diabetes mellitus. *N Engl J Med* 1993;329:979–983.

70. DPT-1 Study Group. The diabetes prevention trial-type I diabetes (DPT-1): implementation of screening and staging of relatives. *Transplant Proc* 1995;27:3377.

71. Zhang JA, Dabidson L, Eisenbarth G, Weiner HL. Suppression of diabetes in NOD mice by oral administration of insulin. *J Immunol* 1991; 145:2489–2496.

72. Daniel D, Gill RG, Schloot N, Wegmenn D. Epitope specificity, cytokine production profile, and diabetogenic activity of insulin-specific T cell clones isolated from NOD mice. *Eur J Immunol* 1995;25: 1056–1062.

Inflammation: Basic Principles and Clinical Correlates,
3rd ed., edited by John I. Gallin and Ralph Snyderman.
Lippincott Williams & Wilkins, Philadelphia © 1999.

CHAPTER 70

Persistent Mucosal Colonization by *Helicobacter pylori* and the Induction of Inflammation

Martin J. Blaser and Phillip D. Smith

In 1983, Warren and Marshall reported the first isolation of gram-negative bacteria, which we now call *Helicobacter pylori*, from the human stomach (1). This work and studies conducted by other investigators (1–4) confirmed observations made nearly a century earlier that bacteria colonize the human stomach. These observations should not have been surprising, because an indigenous biota is present in most other portions of the gastrointestinal tract of humans and because all other mammals studied have gastric microbiota. Nevertheless, finding gastric organisms launched a revolution in medical research and clinical practice, one that is continuing to evolve.

HELICOBACTER PYLORI GASTRIC COLONIZATION AND GASTROINTESTINAL DISEASES

Gastric carriage of *H. pylori* is common among persons throughout the world (5). At birth, the stomach is essentially sterile, but inoculation with *H. pylori* may lead to transient or persistent gastric colonization (6,7). After colonization is established, *H. pylori* persists for life, except when suppressed by the development of atrophic gastritis or terminated by antimicrobial chemotherapy. In this regard, *H. pylori* has many of the characteristics of a commensal. By adulthood, about 80% of persons in developing countries carry *H. pylori*, which usually is acquired by the age of 10 years. In developed countries,

carriage in childhood is much less common, and only 40% of adults on average carry the organism. Because all developed countries formerly were developing countries, there has been a gradual transition in the proportion of persons colonized by *H. pylori*. Much evidence indicates that this phenomenon reflects a birth-cohort effect in developed countries, in which the organism is acquired predominantly in childhood, but that with socioeconomic development, later birth-cohorts have grown up in periods when transmission of *H. pylori* was decreasing (5,8). This birth-cohort effect has important implications for the epidemiology of *H. pylori* colonization and for its immunologic and clinical consequences.

The presence of *H. pylori* organisms, which live in the mucous layer overlying the gastric epithelium, induces infiltration into the lamina propria by circulating inflammatory and immune cells, including polymorphonuclear leukocytes, monocytes, plasma cells, and lymphocytes (9). This lesion is called by pathologists chronic gastritis when neutrophils are not present and designated chronic active gastritis when substantial numbers of neutrophils are observed. Convincing evidence indicates that acquisition of *H. pylori* causes this histologic response and that eradication of the organism clears the cellular infiltration (10). This process is essentially asymptomatic, because most of the world's population harbors *H. pylori* for their entire lives without any clinical consequences. However, *H. pylori* is of interest to physicians and scientists because its presence is associated with increased risk for development of three important diseases: peptic ulcer disease, adenocarcinomas of the distal stomach (body and antrum), and gastric lymphomas.

Beginning with the observations of Marshall and Warren, it has become apparent that the presence of idiopathic peptic ulcer disease (i.e., gastropathy not caused by aspirin, alcohol, or nonsteroidal antiinflammatory

M. J. Blaser and *P. D. Smith: Division of Infectious Diseases, Department of Medicine, and Department of Microbiology and Immunology, Vanderbilt University School of Medicine, Nashville, Tennessee 37232, and *Division of Gastroenterology and Hepatology, Department of Medicine, and Department of Microbiology, University of Alabama School of Medicine, Birmingham, Alabama 35294.

agents) is strongly associated with the presence of *H. pylori* (2,10,11) and that the eradication of *H. pylori* cures a high proportion of peptic ulcer disease (12). As a consequence of these observations, a consensus of experts recommend that clinicians caring for patients with peptic ulcer disease attempt to diagnose the presence of *H. pylori* and, if present, to treat with appropriate antimicrobial agents to eliminate the organisms (13).

A second important clinical consequence of harboring *H. pylori* for a prolonged period is the increased risk for developing distal gastric adenocarcinomas (14–16). More than 20 years ago, Correa postulated a gradual progression from chronic gastritis to atrophic gastritis and intestinal metaplasia, leading to dysplasia and carcinoma (17). We now know that *H. pylori* is the most common cause of chronic gastritis in the world and that the presence of *H. pylori* has been associated with each step in the histologic progression to carcinoma. *H. pylori* is associated with a twofold to 12-fold increase in risk for gastric adenocarcinoma in various populations, and *H. pylori* has been designated a carcinogen by the World Health Organization (18). The presumed mechanism of carcinogenesis is the induction of chronic inflammation and the progression, in some hosts, to atrophic gastritis.

H. pylori also has been associated with the development of gastric lymphomas (19). The histopathology of these uncommon tumors ranges from high-grade malignancies to relatively low-grade processes, called gastric mucosa–associated lymphoid tumors (MALTomas). Virtually all patients with MALTomas carry *H. pylori*, and antimicrobial elimination of *H. pylori* has been associated with regression of the tumor (20,21). One hypothesis regarding the pathogenesis of *H. pylori*–associated gastric adenocarcinoma and lymphoma is that these tumors are antigen driven; recognition of and response to *H. pylori* antigens by malignant lymphoid cells is necessary for their proliferation.

The gastric diseases that affect up to 10% of persons carrying *H. pylori* are thought to be based in part on the induction of inflammation by the organism (22). An important question is why some persons become ill and others do not. A related question is how colonization by one organism results in different manifestations of disease. Understanding the relationship between mucosal inflammation and gastric physiology may provide answers to these questions.

An additional unanswered question is whether chronic carriage of *H. pylori* confers on the host any biologic advantage. In this regard, much evidence indicates that *H. pylori* organisms have colonized humans (23) and our prehuman ancestors since time immemorial (24), perhaps tens of millions of years. Examination of nonhuman primates has shown that nearly all carry *H. pylori* and other *Helicobacter* species. Based on the ancientness and ubiquity of *H. pylori* among primate species, the organism could be considered a constituent of the normal biota of the human stomach and the 20th century an aberration, because this may be the first time in human history when colonization is not essentially universal.

One implication of this interpretation is that carriage of *H. pylori* has benefits as well as the costs addressed earlier and that the loss of these organisms could lead to the rise of new diseases. There is evidence that the marked increases in the incidence of reflux esophagitis, Barrett's esophagus, and adenocarcinoma of the proximal stomach and distal esophagus may be related to lack of a protective effect by certain *H. pylori* strains, especially cytotoxin-associated gene *(cagA)* subset (25–27). The propensity of these organisms to cause or protect against disease suggests that they may best be regarded as commensals, similar to *Bacteroides* species or α-hemolytic streptococci, although with a more interactive lifestyle with the host.

PROPERTIES OF *HELICOBACTER PYLORI* THAT INDUCE GASTRIC INFLAMMATION

H. pylori are noninvasive bacteria; most organisms live in the mucous layer in the lumen of the stomach, and a small number attach to the gastric epithelium. As depicted in Figure 70-1, two major mechanisms appear to be involved in *H. pylori*–induced inflammation (28). First, the fraction of the *H. pylori* population that is adherent to the epithelium may directly signal epithelial cells. Second, the free-living *H. pylori* appear to release proinflammatory products that are absorbed into the mucosa, where resident mononuclear cells and mononuclear cells that traffic through the lamina propria can be stimulated.

Evidence indicates that both phenomena are important in *H. pylori*–induced inflammation. When *H. pylori* organisms adhere to epithelial cells, adherence pedestals may form (29,30). These are specialized responses of epithelial cells to the presence of *H. pylori* and resemble those formed in response to adherence by particular *Escherichia coli* subtypes. A large number of putative adhesins on the *H. pylori* surface have been identified (31–36). Adherence induces signal transduction, resulting in tyrosine phosphorylation, similar to that of other bacteria that signal the epithelium (37). Adherence induces epithelial cells to secrete interleukin-8 (IL-8), a proinflammatory cytokine (38–40). Transduction of the *H. pylori* signal for IL-8 induction requires activation of NF-κB, a DNA transcription factor (41–43). The production of IL-8, a mediator that recruits and activates neutrophils, is a potent mechanism for stimulating acute inflammation.

Nonadherent *H. pylori* cells that are free living in the mucous layer also appear capable of inducing an inflammatory response. The organisms release proteins, notably urease (44), which have potent chemotactic activity for inflammatory cells, including neutrophils and monocytes

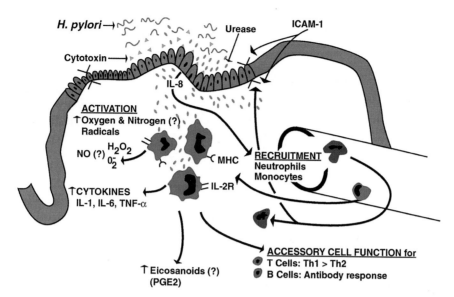

FIG. 70-1. Cellular events involved in *H. pylori* inflammation. *In vitro* and *in situ* studies suggest that *H. pylori* induce inflammation through a cascade of cellular events in the gastric mucosa. *H. pylori* bacteria colonize the mucous layer of the gastric mucosa, where they produce ammonia and release vacuolating cytotoxin, both of which are capable of damaging the gastric epithelium. As a consequence of altered epithelial barrier function, urease and possibly other proteins released or shed by the bacteria are absorbed into the lamina propria, where they act as chemotactic factors for inflammatory cells, such as monocytes and neutrophils trafficking through the mucosa. Among the absorbed proteins, urease also is capable of activating the recruited blood cells and resident tissue macrophages. The small proportion of *H. pylori* organisms that adhere to the epithelium augment or possibly initiate the recruitment and activation of neutrophils through the induction of interleukin-8 production and release. Accumulation of inflammatory cells is facilitated by the presence of adhesion molecules, such as intercellular adhesion molecule-1 (ICAM-1) on gastric epithelium, which anchor the recruited cells. The release of reactive oxygen and nitrogen intermediates, cytokines, and possibly other mediators by activated neutrophils and macrophages promotes inflammation. Chronic *H. pylori* colonization ensures continuous absorption of recruitment and activation factors to perpetuate the inflammatory response. (Adapted from ref. 28, with permission.)

(45,46). Through its urease activity and other mechanisms (47), *H. pylori* produces large amounts of ammonia, which is directly toxic to epithelial cells (48) and activates inflammatory cells (49). Urease (50) and neutrophil-activating protein (51) activate inflammatory cells. Urease activates monocytes (49,50), and evidence indicates that the molecule also activates resident mucosal macrophages (52). Urease is an internal *H. pylori* protein that is shed from organisms in culture (45) and can be released by lysis of *H. pylori* cells (53). Although *H. pylori* organisms do not invade the lamina propria, identification of urease in lamina propria inflammatory cells (45) indicates that the molecule can be absorbed into the mucosa, where it probably recruits neutrophils and monocytes. Once recruited, these cells can then be activated by urease and possibly other proteins also absorbed into the lamina propria.

An important consequence of the activation of mononuclear and epithelial cells by *H. pylori* is the production of proinflammatory and regulatory cytokines. The mechanisms by which these cytokines promote mucosal inflammation have been reviewed elsewhere (54). The ability of *H. pylori* to stimulate the production

of proinflammatory cytokines *in vivo* is supported by evidence that the levels of IL-1, IL-6, IL-8, and tumor necrosis factor-α (TNF-α) mRNA and protein are increased in the gastric mucosa in persons with *H. pylori* gastritis (39,55–61). In those with chronic active gastritis, the tissue level of IL-8 correlates with the severity of the inflammation (55–58). These findings have been extended through *in vitro* studies showing that *H. pylori* products, particularly urease, stimulate monocytes and purified primary mucosal macrophages to release IL-1, IL-6, and TNF-α in a dose-dependent manner (50,52). Exposure of epithelial cell lines to *H. pylori* results in the production of IL-8, implicating epithelial cells in the recruitment and activation of neutrophils in *H. pylori* gastritis (38,40,41). Epithelial cells express intercellular adhesion molecule-1, the counterreceptor for CD11a/CD18 on neutrophils and lymphocytes and CD11b/CD18 on neutrophils, indicating that epithelial cells express surface molecules that anchor or stabilize the adhesion of inflammatory cells after they have been recruited to the inflammatory site (40). Other proinflammatory products produced by mononuclear phagocytes in response to *H. pylori* bacteria or products include reactive oxygen intermediates (49), which promote membrane damage to gastric epithelial cells (62), and inducible nitric oxide synthase (63), which promotes the production of nitric oxide, a nitrogen radical that is cytotoxic to certain cells and is a potential mutagen.

The release of *H. pylori* constituents, such as urease, probably plays a critical role in the recruitment of inflammatory cells and the induction and maintenance of gastric inflammation (28). Chronic colonization by *H. pylori* and the presumed long survival of tissue macrophages promote the chronicity of the *H. pylori*–associated lesion. *H. pylori* also produces heat shock proteins (HSPs) that resemble the human HSP60 (64,65), raising the possibility that host responses to this protein may trigger autoimmunity, but antigenic relatedness is limited (66).

Properties That May Reduce Inflammation

For many gram-negative bacteria, lipopolysaccharide (LPS) is a powerful proinflammatory stimulus, affecting a broad array of human cells and mononuclear phagocytes in particular. The core (lipid A) structure of the *H. pylori* LPS is unique (67). Studies of its biologic activity show that *H. pylori* LPS has markedly reduced proinflammatory properties (e.g., induction of cytokine, eicosanoid, and oxygen radical production by macrophages) compared with LPS of the *Enterobacteriaceae* (68–70). Although markedly (1,000- to 30,000-fold) less efficient an activator than *E. coli* LPS, *H. pylori* LPS is recognized by LPS-binding protein, and this complex activates monocytes through the CD14 receptor (71,72). Although this is the same receptor-mediated pathway through which *E. coli* LPS activates monocytes, there is little competition by *H. pylori* LPS, presumably because of the low affinity of *H. pylori* LPS for these critical receptors (71). Unlike blood monocytes, lamina propria macrophages lack CD14 (73), rendering these cells poorly responsive to LPS from any source. For other organisms that are persistent gut colonizers, such as *Bacteroides* species, their LPS molecules also have very low biologic activity.

In 1996, Aspinall et al. (74) first reported that *H. pylori* may express the Lewis (Le) tissue antigens as part of their

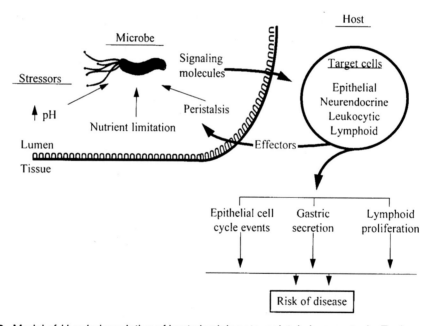

FIG. 70-2. Model of *H. pylori* regulation of host physiology to maintain homeostasis. Environmental phenomena that affect *H. pylori* populations include gastric pH, nutrient limitation, and physical removal by means of peristalsis. As with other bacteria, *H. pylori* organisms regulate gene expression in response to particular environmental signals. In the proposed model, one component of adaptation is the release of molecules that signal the host to diminish the noxious stimulus. For example, if luminal nutrients are limited, bacterial secretion of proinflammatory molecules results in greater tissue injury, permitting nutrient release. High-level (constitutive) release of proinflammatory materials results in high levels of inflammation, which quickly lead to loss of the environmental niche. Regulated inflammation best serves the needs of the microbe and the host. Similarly, secretion of *N*-α-methylhistamine stimulates the host to increase acid production when pH in a particular locale is too high for optimal microbial function. In this model, the equilibrium established by the colonizing population in each host is dynamic and unique. A consequence of these interactions is that the nature of the equilibrium determines characteristics such as epithelial cell proliferation and apoptosis, gastric secretion, and antigenic stimulation of lymphoid cell populations, and these characteristics determine the likelihood of disease under different environmental circumstances. (Adapted from ref. 85, with permission.)

terminal LPS structures. These observations of structural mimicry by colonizing bacteria have been confirmed and extended (75–79). Virtually all *H. pylori* cells have the capacity to produce Le^X, Le^Y, both, or neither (79,80). Other fucosylated blood group antigens, such as sialyl-Le^X (CD15), may be produced by the organism (79). Although one possible consequence of Le expression by *H. pylori* cells is autoimmunity (76), this hypothesis has not been confirmed. Alternatively, this structural mimicry could be a bacterial adaptation to facilitate persistent colonization. Lewis antigen expression in humans is not limited to erythrocytes but involves many epithelial cells, including those in the gastric mucosa. Because humans are polymorphic for Le expression, one hypothesis is that *H. pylori* can mimic Le expression that is specific for a particular host; observations of humans (81,82) and monkeys support the hypothesis that the host environment selects for Le expression within the colonizing *H. pylori* population. The basis for selection, whether caused by immune responses, availability of receptors for adherence, or other phenomena, is unknown.

Balance of Proinflammatory and Antiinflammatory Activities

H. pylori persist in the gastric lumen while actively replicating (i.e., not dormant like *Mycobacterium tuberculosis*) in large numbers despite an active inflammatory response by the host. Assuming a long coevolution of microbe and host, one explanation for this apparent paradox is that *H. pylori*–induced inflammation is adaptive for the organism, promoting, for example, the acquisition of nutrients (83). However, when excessive inflammation leads to atrophic gastritis, the environmental niche for *H. pylori* is lost (83,84). Over time, there has been selection for *H. pylori* strains that is able to regulate their interaction with the host to modulate the inflammatory responses (85). Nevertheless, *H. pylori* strains are highly diverse (86). Each strain may reach its own equilibrium with the host, depending on the use of nutrients and the ability to induce inflammation (Fig. 70-2). Such a model explains that, by occupying relatively exclusive ecologic niches, a host can be colonized by multiple strains of *H. pylori*. Mathematical models with feedback relationships between the host and microbe leading to equilibrium best explain the persistence of these organisms in their gastric niches (87 and M. J. Blaser and D. E. Kirschner, unpublished data, 1998). Data (88,89) further support the hypothesis that the presence of *H. pylori* and its molecular effectors lead to downregulation of inflammatory phenomena and to the more obvious proinflammatory activities.

DIVERSITY AMONG *HELICOBACTER PYLORI* STRAINS

Three different loci of diversity with pathophysiologic and clinical significance have been identified in *H.*

pylori: *vacA*, *cagA*, and *iceA* loci. *VacA* encodes a cytotoxin that induces the formation of vacuoles in eukaryotic cell lines (90–93) and primary human mucosal epithelial cells (94). In vitro, about 50% of strains express this toxin (95,96), but *in vivo* expression probably is universal, although to various degrees (97). *VacA* is polymorphic, and in Western countries, persons carrying s1 strains (referring to the signal sequence type), particularly s1a strains, are at higher risk for the development of peptic ulcer disease (98). Colonization with an s1a-type strain, which is associated with high-level toxin production *in vitro*, also is associated with a higher density of *H. pylori* colonization and with more intense gastric inflammation (99).

The *cag* locus was first identified by the cloning and characterization of *cagA*, the cytotoxin-associated gene (100,101). This locus is a 38-kb region of the *H. pylori* genome, encoding approximately 25 genes, and is present in some *H. pylori* strains (102,103). In the United States and other Western countries, about one half the strains are *cag* positive (*cag*$^+$), but in Asia, more than 80% are positive (104–106). In Western populations, carriage of a *cag*$^+$ strain is associated with a marked increase in risk for the development of peptic ulcer disease (107,108) and adenocarcinoma of the distal stomach (109,110). Compared with *cag*$^-$ strains, *cag*$^+$ strains induce increased inflammation (55,111), increase production of proinflammatory cytokines (55), more efficiently activate NF-κB (41), lead to more rapid development of atrophic gastritis (112), and re-regulate gastric acid physiology (113). Ablation of particular *cag* island genes results in diminished cytokine induction in epithelial cells (102,114), indicating the critical nature of these genes for the enhanced proinflammatory lifestyle of these strains.

The third locus, *iceA*, was identified because its transcription is induced by contact with epithelium (115). Two alleles, *iceA1* and *iceA2*, have been defined, and carriage of an *iceA1* strain is associated with enhanced risk of peptic ulceration (115). The function of *iceA* is unknown, but it has extensive homology with a restriction endonuclease and the downstream gene, *hpyIM*, which is conserved in all *H. pylori* strains, is a DNA methylase (116). One hypothesis is that the differences in the *iceA* alleles reflect differing transcription of the methylase, which is a global regulator in *H. pylori*. The *iceA1* and *iceA2* alleles may be markers for strains identified with different lifestyles.

Despite their distance on the *H. pylori* genome (117), *iceA1*, s1a *vacA*, and the *cag* island frequently coexist in the same strain. That the *cag* island is associated with proinflammatory activity (102,114), but that the linked high toxin production (s1a-type toxin) inhibits Ii-dependent antigen processing and presentation in T cells (89) is consistent with a model of balanced polymorphism that maximizes persistence of a population of organisms in a host (85). However, there are many exceptions, probably reflecting the natural competence of *H. pylori*, permitting intergenomic recombination (118,119). In any event, *H. pylori* populations are not highly clonal (120), unlike *M. tuberculosis,* for example. Differences in interactions with the host are not surprising.

IMMUNITY TO *HELICOBACTER PYLORI*

In humans (121,122) and monkeys (123), the persistence of *H. pylori* is accompanied by immune recognition but failure to eradicate the organism. Similarly, after eradication of *H. pylori*, colonization with a new or the same organism can readily occur. The presence of one *H. pylori* strain colonizing the stomach does not appear to induce sufficient immunity to prohibit the acquisition of one or more other strains. There does not appear to be any true sterilizing immunity. Nevertheless, immune cell populations are activated by the presence of *H. pylori*, and the cellular infiltrates contain T and B lymphocytes, predominantly IgA plasma cells, and macrophages (124). The specific cells involved in *H. pylori* antigen presentation have not been identified, but they probably include lamina propria macrophages, dendritic cells, and possibly epithelial cells.

The potential role of gastric epithelial cells in the presentation of *H. pylori* antigens is underscored by the ability of *H. pylori* to induce upregulation of class II major histocompatibility complex molecules (125–127) and B7-1 and B7-2 co-stimulatory molecules (128) on gastric epithelial cells. The inducible expression of stimulatory and co-stimulatory molecules in the presence of *H. pylori* equips gastric epithelium with the molecules required for activation of CD4 helper T lymphocytes.

The host immune response to microorganisms is initiated by the natural (innate) immune system when the microorganism or its products interact with a recognition molecule present in the circulation (e.g., LPS-binding protein) or on certain cells, such as macrophages (e.g., surface CD14), dendritic cells, or natural killer cells. This interaction stimulates the release of predominantly IL-12, which directs helper T cells to produce interferon-γ (IFN-γ), IL-2, and lymphotoxin (T_H1 phenotype), a cellular response; or predominantly IL-4, which directs the cells to produce IL-4, IL-5, IL-6, IL-10 and IL-13 (T_H2 phenotype), and an antibody (acquired or adaptive) response (129,130). Accumulating evidence indicates that this paradigm probably applies to the host immune response to *H. pylori* (Fig. 70-3). In the initial study addressing this topic, an increase in the number of IFN-γ–secreting cells as identified in gastric tissue from patients with *H. pylori* gastritis, suggesting a T_H1-type response (131). This finding was extended in an animal model in which *Helicobacter felis*–infected mice first developed a *Helicobacter*-independent cellular response in the stomach directed toward urease (and other proteins) and then a *Helicobacter*-dependent cellular response characterized by the local presence of IFN-γ–producing but not IL-4– or IL-5–producing cells (132). *In vivo* IFN-γ neutralization significantly reduced the *Helicobacter*-induced gastritis.

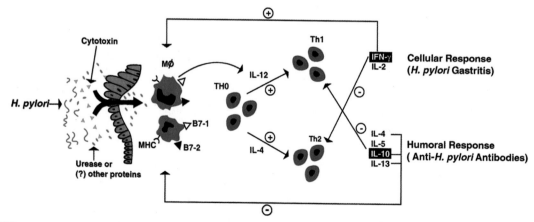

FIG. 70-3. Model for the role of T lymphocytes in the immunoregulation of the host response to *H. pylori*. Preliminary studies suggest that helper T (T_H) lymphocytes participate in the regulation of the host immune response to *H. pylori*. Bacterial products absorbed across the epithelium first interact with cells of the natural (innate) immune system, such as mucosal macrophages, dendritic cells, or possibly natural killer cells. This interaction may result in the production of interleukin-12 (IL-12), which drives T_H0 cells toward a T_H1 pathway, resulting in a predominance of cytokines (e.g., interferon-γ, IL-2) that promote a cellular response. Alternatively, the interaction may stimulate the release of predominantly IL-4, which directs the T cells toward a T_H2 pathway and the release of cytokines (e.g., IL-4, IL-5, IL-10, IL-13) that stimulate a humoral response. Although typically both cellular and humoral responses are present, one pathway may dominate, depending on the *H. pylori* constituents expressed and the relative levels of stimulatory and inhibitory cytokines in the tissue at the site of colonization.

Further evidence that *H. pylori*–associated inflammation may be mediated through a T_H1 pathway was provided by the observation that IL-12, rather than IL-10, mRNA predominated in gastric tissue from patients with *H. pylori* gastritis (133). This finding is consistent with the observation in other infectious diseases, such as tuberculoid leprosy, in which IL-12 preferentially stimulates the expansion of T_H1-type cells and is negatively regulated by IL-10 (134). T-cell clones derived from gastric mucosa from *H. pylori*–infected persons varied in their proliferative and T_H1 cytokine responses, depending on which *H. pylori* antigen was used to stimulate them (135). Moreover, T_H1-like clones were more commonly derived from gastric tissue from *H. pylori*–infected patients with peptic ulceration than from those with only gastritis (136), suggesting that the relative proportion of T_H1 cells (and therefore cytokines that promote a cellular response) *in vivo* influences the severity of the inflammatory reaction. The helper T cells probably play a fundamental role in regulating the cellular and antibody responses to *H. pylori* and the course of infection.

Although T_H1 cells predominate in *H. pylori* lesions, *H. pylori*–dependent helper (T_H2) function for B-cell proliferation and immunoglobulin production promote host B-cell responses as well. After acquisition of *H. pylori*, the host develops B-cell responses, characterized by an early rise in *H. pylori*–specific serum IgM antibodies, followed by anti-*H. pylori* IgG and IgA antibody responses (137). The latter may take several months to develop, occurring after the decline in the level of specific IgM (137). The IgG and IgA responses to *H. pylori* persist for the duration of the colonization, are remarkably stable in titer for years (138), and diminish when the organism is eradicated (122). Gastric secretions contain *H. pylori*–specific secretory IgA that generally parallels the serum responses (139). The precise role of antibody responses to *H. pylori* in protecting the host from tissue injury is unknown. However, IgA-deficient hosts (who also lack secretory IgA) have the same prevalence of *H. pylori* (140), suggesting that secretory IgA anti-*H. pylori* antibodies do not protect the host against colonization. Whether the antibody responses to *H. pylori* contribute to immunopathology leading to tissue injury has not been established (67,141,142).

CONCLUSIONS

H. pylori–induced inflammation in gastric mucosa is a major risk factor for the development of several important diseases of the stomach and duodenum. However, most persons who carry *H. pylori* for all their lives have no clinical consequences. Important emerging evidence indicates that *H. pylori* colonization may be protective against more proximal lesions involving the upper stomach and esophagus. The biology of gastric inflammation induced by *H. pylori* is complex (143–145). For highly

diverse organisms that have probably colonized outbred humans and our ancestors since time immemorial, we should not have expected otherwise. A simple model of T_H1 predominance is probably insufficient to explain the diversity of tissue responses and clinical outcomes associated with carriage of *H. pylori* (135,146). Elucidating the relationships between *H. pylori* colonization and host inflammatory cells will help us understand and approach the *H. pylori*–associated diseases of the upper gastrointestinal tract (147,148). More importantly, these relationships are models for host-microbial interactions throughout the body, especially in mucosal tissues.

ACKNOWLEDGMENTS

This work was supported in part by R01 DK53707 and R01 DK54495 from the National Institutes of Health and by the Medical Research Service of the Department of Veterans Affairs.

REFERENCES

1. Warren JR, Marshall B. Unidentified curved bacilli on gastric epithelium in active chronic gastritis. *Lancet* 1983;1:1273–1275.
2. Marshall BJ, Warren JR. Unidentified curved bacilli in the stomach of patients with gastritis and peptic ulceration. *Lancet* 1984;1: 1311–1315.
3. Langenberg ML, Tytgat GNJ, Schipper MEI, Rietra PJGM, Zanen HC. *Campylobacter*-like organisms in the stomach of patients and healthy individuals. *Lancet* 1984;1:1348.
4. Steer HW, Newell DG. Immunological identification of *Campylobacter pyloridis* in gastric biopsy tissue. *Lancet* 1985;11:38–39.
5. Pounder RE, Ng D. The prevalence of *Helicobacter pylori* infection in different countries. *Aliment Pharmacol Ther* 1995;9:S33–S39.
6. Marshall BJ, Armstrong JA, McGechie DB, Glancy RT. Attempt to fulfill Koch's postulates for pyloric *Campylobacter*. *Med J Aust* 1985; 142:436–439.
7. Morris A, Nicholson G. Ingestion of *Campylobacter pyloridis* causes gastritis and raised fasting gastric pH. *Am J Gastroenterol* 1987;82: 192–199.
8. Parsonnet J. Incidence of *H. pylori* infection. *Aliment Pharmacol Ther* 1995;9[Suppl 2]:45–51.
9. Dixon MJ. *Helicobacter pylori* and peptic ulceration: histopathological aspects. *J Gastroenterol Hepatol* 1991;6:125–130.
10. Blaser MJ. *Helicobacter pylori* and the pathogenesis of gastroduodenal inflammation. *J Infect Dis* 1990;161:626–633.
11. Rauws EA, Tytgat GN. Cure of duodenal ulcer associated with eradication of *Helicobacter pylori*. *Lancet* 1990;335:1233–1235.
12. Hentschel E, Brandstatter G, Dragoisics B, et al. Effect of ranitidine and amoxicillin plus metronidazole on the eradication of *Helicobacter pylori* and the recurrence of duodenal ulcer. *N Engl J Med* 1993;328:308–312.
13. NIH Consensus Conference. *Helicobacter pylori* in peptic ulcer disease. *JAMA* 1994;272:65–69.
14. Nomura A, Stemmermann GN, Chyou P, Kato I, Pérez-Pérez GI, Blaser MJ. *Helicobacter pylori* infection and gastric carcinoma in a population of Japanese-Americans in Hawaii. *N Engl J Med* 1991; 325:1132–1136.
15. Parsonnet J, Friedman GD, Vandersteen DP, et al. *Helicobacter pylori* infection and the risk of gastric carcinoma. *N Engl J Med* 1991;325: 1127–1131.
16. Forman D, Newell DG, Fullerton F, et al. Association between infection with *Helicobacter pylori* and risk of gastric cancer: evidence from a prospective investigation. *BMJ* 1991;302:1302–1305.
17. Correa P. Human gastric carcinogenesis: a multistep and multifactorial process—First American Cancer Society Award lecture on cancer epidemiology and prevention. *Cancer Res* 1992;52:6735–6740.

18. International Agency for Research of Cancer. Monographs on the Evaluation of Carcinogenic Risks to Humans. Infection with *Helicobacter pylori*. World Health Organization. 1994;60:177–240.

19. Parsonnet J, Hansen S, Rodriguez L, et al. *Helicobacter pylori* infection and gastric lymphoma. *N Engl J Med* 1994;330:1267–1271.

20. Wotherspoon AC, Ortiz Hidalgo C, Falzon MR, Isaacson PG. *Helicobacter pylori*–associated gastritis and primary B-cell gastric lymphoma. *Lancet* 1991;338:1175–1176.

21. Wotherspoon AC, Doglioni C, Diss TC, et al. Regression of primary low-grade B-cell lymphoma of mucosa-associated lymphoid tissue type after eradication of *Helicobacter pylori*. *Lancet* 1993;342: 575–577.

22. Blaser MJ, Parsonnet J. Parasitism by the slow bacterium *Helicobacter pylori* leads to altered gastric homeostasis and neoplasia. *J Clin Invest* 1994;94:4–8.

23. Correa P, Willis D, Allison MF, Gerszten E. *Helicobacter pylori* in pre-Columbian mummies. *Gastroenterology* 1998;114:A956.

24. Blaser MJ. Not all *Helicobacter pylori* strains are created equal: should all be eliminated? *Lancet* 1997;349:1020–1022.

25. Werdmuller BFM, Loffeld RJLF. *Helicobacter pylori* infection has no role in the pathogenesis of reflux esophagitis. *Dig Dis Sci* 1997;42: 103–105.

26. Schnell JW, Vicari JJ, Pérez-Pérez GI, et al. *Helicobacter pylori* cagA strains predominate in gastroesophageal reflux disease, Barrett's esophagus, and esophageal dysplasia/adenocarcinoma. *Gastroenterology* 1997;112:A283.

27. Chow W-H, Blaser MJ, Blot WJ, et al. *H. pylori* and *cagA* status in relation to risk of adenocarcinoma of esophagus and stomach by anatomic subsite. *Cancer Res* 1998;58:588–590.

28. Harris PR, Smith PD. The role of the mononuclear phagocyte in *H. pylori*-associated inflammation. In: Ernst PB, Michetti P, Smith PD, eds. *The immunobiology of* H. pylori—*from pathogenesis to prevention*. Philadelphia: Lippincott–Raven Publishers, 1997;127–138.

29. Smoot DT, Resau JH, Naab T, et al. Adherence of *Helicobacter pylori* to cultured human gastric epithelial cells. *Infect Immun* 1993;61:350–355.

30. Chen XG, Correa P, Offerhaus J, et al. Ultrastructure of the gastric mucosa harboring *Campylobacter*-like organisms. *Am J Clin Pathol* 1987;86:575–582.

31. Evans DG, Evans DJJ, Graham DY. Receptor-mediated adherence of *Campylobacter pylori* to mouse Y-1 adrenal cell monolayers. *Infect Immun* 1989;57:2272–2278.

32. Fauchere J, Blaser MJ. Adherence of *Helicobacter pylori* cells and superficial components to HeLa cell membranes. *Microb Pathog* 1990;9:427–439.

33. Gold BD, Huesca M, Sherman PM, Lingwood CA. *Helicobacter mustelae* and *Helicobacter pylori* bind to common lipid receptors *in vitro*. *Infect Immun* 1993;61:2632–2638.

34. Boren T, Normark S, Falk P. *Helicobacter pylori*: molecular basis for host recognition and bacterial adherence [Review]. *Trends Microbiol* 1994;2:221–228.

35. Trust TJ, Doig P, Emody L, Kienle Z, Wadstrom T, O'Toole P. High-affinity binding of the basement membrane proteins collagen type IV and laminin to the gastric pathogen *Helicobacter pylori*. *Infect Immun* 1991;59:4398–4404.

36. Lingwood CA, Wasfy G, Han H, Huesca M. Receptor affinity purification of a lipid-binding adhesin from *Helicobacter pylori*. *Infect Immun* 1993;61:2474–2478.

37. Segal ED, Falkow S, Tompkins LS. *Helicobacter pylori* attachment to gastric cells induces cytoskeletal rearrangements and tyrosine phosphorylation of host cell proteins. *Proc Natl Acad Sci USA* 1996;93: 1259–1264.

38. Sharma SA, Tummuru MKR, Miller GG, Blaser MJ. Interleukin-8 response of gastric epithelial cell lines to *Helicobacter pylori* stimulation *in vitro*. *Infect Immun* 1995;63:1681–1687.

39. Crabtree JE, Wyatt JI, Trejdosiewicz LK, et al. Interleukin-8 expression in *Helicobacter pylori* infected, normal, and neoplastic gastroduodenal mucosa. *J Clin Pathol* 1994;47:61–66.

40. Crowe SE, Alvarez L, Dytoc M, et al. Expression of interleukin-8 and CD54 by human gastric epithelium after *Helicobacter pylori* infection *in vitro*. *Gastroenterology* 1995;108:65–74.

41. Sharma SA, Tummuru MKR, Blaser MJ, Kerr LD. Activation of interleukin-8 gene expression by *Helicobacter pylori* is regulated by transcription factor NF-κB in gastric epithelial cells. *J Immunol* 1998;160: 2401–2407.

42. Keates S, Hitti YS, Upton M, Kelly CP. *Helicobacter pylori* infection activates NF-κB in gastric epithelial cells. *Gastroenterology* 1997; 113:1099–1109.

43. Munzenmaier A, Lange C, Glocker E, et al. A secreted/shed product of *Helicobacter pylori* activates transcription factor nuclear factor-κB. *J Immunol* 1997;159:6140–6147.

44. Dunn BE, Campbell GP, Pérez-Pérez GI, Blaser MJ. Purification and characterization of *Helicobacter pylori* urease. *J Biol Chem* 1990;265: 9464–9469.

45. Mai UE, Pérez-Pérez GI, Allen JB, Wahl SM, Blaser MJ, Smith PD. Surface proteins from *Helicobacter pylori* exhibit chemotactic activity for human leukocytes and are present in gastric mucosa. *J Exp Med* 1992;175:517–525.

46. Craig PM, Territo MC, Karnes WE, Walsh JH. *Helicobacter pylori* secretes a chemotactic factor for monocytes and neutrophils. *Gut* 1992;33:1020–1034.

47. Ricci V, Sommi P, Fiocca R, et al. Cytotoxicity of *Helicobacter pylori* on human gastric epithelial cells *in vitro*: role of cytotoxin(s) and ammonia. *Eur J Gastroenterol Hepatol* 1993;5:687–694.

48. Smoot DR, Mobley HL, Chippendale GR, Lewison JF, Resau JH. *Helicobacter pylori* urease activity is toxic to human gastric epithelial cells. *Infect Immun* 1990;58:1992–1994.

49. Mai UEH, Pérez-Pérez GI, Wahl LM, Wahl SM, Blaser MJ, Smith PD. Soluble surface proteins from *Helicobacter pylori* activate monocytes/macrophages by lipopolysaccharide-independent mechanism. *J Clin Invest* 1991;87:894–900.

50. Harris PR, Mobley HL, Pérez-Pérez GI, Blaser MJ, Smith PD. *Helicobacter pylori* urease is a potent stimulus of mononuclear phagocyte activation and inflammatory cytokine production. *Gastroenterology* 1996;111:419–425.

51. Evans DJ, Evans DG, Takemura T, et al. Characterization of a *Helicobacter pylori* neutrophil-activating protein. *Infect Immun* 1995;63: 2213–2220.

52. Harris PR, Ernst PB, Kawabata S, Kiyono H, Graham MF, Smith PD. Recombinant *Helicobacter pylori* urease activates primary mucosal macrophages. *J Infect Dis* 1998;178:1516–1520.

53. Phadnis SH, Parlow MH, Levy M, et al. Surface localization of *Helicobacter pylori* urease and a heat shock protein homolog requires bacterial autolysis. *Infect Immun* 1996;64:905–912.

54. Sartor RB. Cytokines in intestinal inflammation: pathophysiological and clinical considerations. *Gastroenterology* 1994;106:533–539.

55. Peek RM, Miller GG, Tham KT, et al. Heightened inflammatory response and cytokine expression to *cagA⁺ Helicobacter pylori* strains. *Lab Invest* 1995;73:760–770.

56. Fan X-G, Chua A, Fan X-J, Keeling PWN. Increased gastric production of interleukin-8 and tumour necrosis factor in patients with *Helicobacter pylori* infection. *J Clin Pathol* 1995;48:133–136.

57. Ando T, Kusugami K, Ohsuga M, et al. Interleukin-8 activity correlates with histological severity in *Helicobacter pylori*–associated antral gastritis. *Am J Gastroenterol* 1996;91:1150–1156.

58. Yamaoka Y, Kita M, Kodama T, Sawai Imanishi J. *Helicobacter pylori* cagA gene and expression of cytokine messenger RNA in gastric mucosa. *Gastroenterology* 1996;110:1744–1752.

59. Crabtree JE, Shallcross TM, Heatley RV, Wyatt JI. Mucosal tumour necrosis factor alpha and interleukin-6 in patients with *Helicobacter pylori* associated gastritis. *Gut* 1991;32:1473–1477.

60. Moss SF, Legon S, Davies J, Calam J. Cytokine gene expression in *Helicobacter pylori* associated antral gastritis. *Gut* 1994;35: 1567–1570.

61. D'Ellos MM, Manghetti M, Almerigogna F, et al. Different cytokine profile and antigen-specificity repertoire in *Helicobacter pylori*-specific T cell clones from the antrum of chronic gastritis patients with or without peptic ulcer. *Eur J Immunol* 1997;27:1751–1755.

62. Bagchi D, Bhattacharya G, Stohs SJ. Production of reactive oxygen species by gastric cells in association with *Helicobacter pylori*. *Free Radic Res* 24:439–450.

63. Wilson KT, Ramanujam KS, Mobley HLT, Musselman RF, James SP, Meltzer SJ. *Helicobacter pylori* stimulates inducible nitric oxide synthase expression and activity in a murine macrophage cell line. *Gastroenterology* 1996;1524–1533.

64. Dunn BE, Roop RM, Sung C, Sharma SA, Pérez-Pérez GI, Blaser MJ. Identification and purification of a cpn 60 heat shock protein homolog from *Helicobacter pylori*. *Infect Immun* 1992;60:1946–1951.

65. Evans DJJ, Evans DG, Engstrand L, Graham DY. Urease-associated

heat shock protein of *Helicobacter pylori*. *Infect Immun* 1992;60:
2125–2127.

66. Sharma SA, Miller GG, Peek RA, Pérez-Pérez GI, Blaser MJ. T cell,
antibody, and cytokine responses to 60-kDa heat shock protein
homologs in *Helicobacter pylori* infection. *Clin Diagn Lab Immunol*
1997;4:440–446.

67. Moran AP, Helander IM, Kosunen TU. Compositional analysis of
Helicobacter pylori rough-form lipopolysaccharides. *J Bacteriol*
1992;174:1370–1377.

68. Muotiala A, Helander IM, Pyhälä L, Kosunen TU, Moran AP. Low
biological activity of *Helicobacter pylori* lipopolysaccharide. *Infect
Immun* 1992;60:1714.

69. Pérez-Pérez GI, Shepherd VL, Morrow JD, Blaser MJ. Activation of
human THP-1 and rat bone marrow–derived macrophages by *Helicobacter pylori* lipopolysaccharide. *Infect Immun* 1995;63:
1183–1187.

70. Nielsen H, Birkholz S, Andersen LP, Moran AP. Neutrophil activation
by *Helicobacter pylori* lipopolysaccharides. *J Infect Dis* 1994;170:
135–139.

71. Kirkland T, Viriyakosol S, Pérez-Pérez GI, Blaser MJ. *Helicobacter
pylori* lipopolysaccharide can activate 70Z/3 cells via CD14. *Infect
Immun* 1997;65:604–608.

72. Cunningham MD, Seachord C, Ratcliffe K, Bainbridge B, Aruffo A,
Darveau RP. *Helicobacter pylori* and *Porphyromonas gingivalis* lipo-
polysaccharides are poorly transferred to recombinant soluble CD14.
Infect Immun 1996;64:3601–3608.

73. Smith PD, Janoff EN, Mosteller-Barnum M, et al. Isolation and purification of CD14-negative mucosal macrophages from normal human
intestine. *J Immunol Methods* 1997;202:1–11.

74. Aspinall GO, Monteiro MA, Pang H, Walsh EJ, Moran AP. Lipopolysaccharide of the *Helicobacter pylori* type strain NCTC 11637
(ATCC 43504): structure of the O antigen and core oligosaccharide
regions. *Biochemistry* 1996;35:2489–2497.

75. Aspinall G, Monteiro MA. Lipopolysaccharides of *Helicobacter
pylori* strains P466 and MO19: structures of the O antigen and core
oligosaccharide regions. *Biochemistry* 1996;35:2498–2504.

76. Appelmelk BJ, Simoons-Smit I, Negrini R, et al. Potential role of molecular mimicry between *Helicobacter pylori* lipopolysaccharide and
host Lewis blood group antigens in autoimmunity. *Infect Immun*
1996;64:2031–2040.

77. Sherbourne R, Taylor DE. *Helicobacter pylori* expresses a complex
surface carbohydrate, Lewis X. *Infect Immun* 1995;63:4564–4568.

78. Simoons Smit IM, Appelmelk BJ, Verboom T, et al. Typing of *Helicobacter pylori* with monoclonal antibodies against Lewis antigens in
lipopolysaccharide. *J Clin Microbiol* 1996;34:2196–2200.

79. Wirth H-P, Yang M, Karita M, Blaser MJ. Expression of the human
cell surface glycoconjugates Lewis X and Lewis Y by *Helicobacter
pylori* isolates is related to *cagA* status. *Infect Immun* 1996;64:
4598–4605.

80. Appelmelk BT, Shiberu B, Trinks C, et al. Phase variation in *Helicobacter pylori* lipopolysaccharide. *Infect Immun* 1998;66:70–76.

81. Wirth HP, Yang M, Peek RM, Tham KT, Blaser MJ. *Helicobacter
pylori* Lewis expression is related to the host Lewis phenotype. *Gastroenterology* 1997;113:1091–1098.

82. Wirth H-P, Yang M, Peek R, Höök-Nikanne J, Blaser MJ. Phenotypic
diversity in Lewis expression of single *H. pylori* colonies derived from
the same biopsy. *Gastroenterology* 1997;112:A331.

83. Blaser MJ. Hypotheses on the pathogenesis and natural history of
Helicobacter pylori–induced inflammation. *Gastroenterology* 1992;
102:720–727.

84. Karnes WE, Samloff IM, Siurala M, et al. Positive serum antibody and
negative tissue staining for *Helicobacter pylori* in subjects with
atrophic body gastritis. *Gastroenterology* 1991;101:167–174.

85. Blaser MJ. Ecology of *Helicobacter pylori* in the human stomach. *J
Clin Invest* 1997;100:759–762.

86. Logan RH, Berg DE. Genetic diversity of *Helicobacter pylori*. *Lancet*
1996;348:1462–1463.

87. Kirschner DE, Blaser MJ. The dynamics of *Helicobacter pylori* infection of the human stomach. *J Theor Biol* 1995;176:281–290.

88. Shirai M, Arichi T, Nakazawa T, Berzofsky JA. Persistent infection by
Helicobacter pylori down-modulates virus-specific CD8+ cytotoxic T
cell response and prolongs viral infection. *J Infect Dis* 1998;177:
72–80.

89. Molinari M, Salio M, Galli C, et al. Selective inhibition of Ii-depen-

dent antigen presentation by *Helicobacter pylori* toxin VacA. *J Exp
Med* 1998;187:135–140.

90. Cover TL, Tummuru MKR, Cao P, Thompson SA, Blaser MJ. Divergence of genetic sequences for the vacuolating cytotoxin among *Helicobacter pylori* strains. *J Biol Chem* 1994;269:10566–10573.

91. Phadnis SH, Ilver D, Janzon L, Normark S, Westblom TU. Pathological significance and molecular characterization of the vacuolating
toxin gene of *Helicobacter pylori*. *Infect Immun* 1994;62:1557–1565.

92. Schmitt W, Haas R. Genetic analysis of the *Helicobacter pylori* vacuolating cytotoxin: structural similarities with the IgA protease type
of exported protein. *Mol Microbiol* 1994;12:307–319.

93. Telford JL, Ghiara P, Dell Orco M, et al. Gene structure of the *Helicobacter pylori* cytotoxin and evidence of its key role in gastric disease. *J Exp Med* 1994;179:1653–1658.

94. Harris PR, Cover TL, Crowe DR, et al. *Helicobacter pylori* cytotoxin
induces vacuolation of primary human mucosal epithelial cells. *Infect
Immun* 1996;64:4867–4871.

95. Leunk RD, Johnson PT, David BC, Kraft WG, Morgan DR. Cytotoxic
activity in broth-culture filtrates of *Campylobacter pylori*. *J Med
Microbiol* 1988;26:93–99.

96. Figura N, Guglielmetti P, Rossolini A, et al. Cytotoxin production by
Campylobacter pylori strains isolated from patients with peptic ulcers
and from patients with chronic gastritis only. *J Clin Microbiol* 1989;
27:225–226.

97. Cover TL, Cao P, Murthy UK, Sipple MS, Blaser MJ. Serum neutralizing antibody response to the vacuolating cytotoxin of *Helicobacter
pylori*. *J Clin Invest* 1992;90:913–918.

98. Atherton JC, Cao P, Peek RM, Tummuru MKR, Blaser MJ, Cover TL.
Mosaicism in vacuolating cytotoxin alleles of *Helicobacter pylori*:
association of specific *vacA* types with cytotoxin production and peptic ulceration. *J Biol Chem* 1995;270:17771–17777.

99. Atherton JC, Peek RM, Tham KT, Cover TL, Blaser MJ. The clinical
and pathological importance of heterogeneity in *vacA*, encoding the
vacuolating cytotoxin of *Helicobacter pylori*. *Gastroenterology* 1997;
112:92–99.

100. Tummuru MKR, Cover TL, Blaser MJ. Cloning and expression of a
high molecular weight major antigen of *Helicobacter pylori*: evidence
of linkage to cytotoxin production. *Infect Immun* 1993;61:1799–1809.

101. Covacci A, Censini S, Bugnoli M, et al. Molecular characterization of
the 128-kDa immunodominant antigen of *Helicobacter pylori* associated with cytotoxicity and duodenal ulcer. *Proc Natl Acad Sci USA*
1993;90:5791–5795.

102. Censini S, Lange C, Xiang J, et al. *Cag*, a pathogenicity island of
Helicobacter pylori, encodes type I-specific and disease-associated
virulence factors. *Proc Natl Acad Sci USA* 1996;93:14648–14653.

103. Akopyanz N, Kersulyte D, Berg DE. CagII, a new multigene locus
associated with virulence in *Helicobacter pylori*. *Gut* 1995;37 (Supplement 1):A1.

104. Pérez-Pérez GI, Bhat N, Gaensbauer J, et al. Country-specific con-
stancy by age in *cagA*+ proportion of *Helicobacter pylori* infections.
Int J Cancer 1997;72:453–456.

105. Pan Z-J, vam der Hulst RWM, Feller M, et al. Equally high preva-
lences of infection with *cagA*-positive *Helicobacter pylori* in Chinese
patients with peptic ulcer disease and those with chronic gastritis-
associated dyspepsia. *J Clin Microbiol* 1997;35:1344–1347.

106. Mitchell HM, Hazell SL, Li YY, Hu PJ. Serological response to specific *Helicobacter pylori* antigens: antibody against CagA antigen is
not predictive of gastric cancer in a developing country. *Am J Gastroenterol* 1996;91:1785–1788.

107. Weel JFL, Vanderhulst RWM, Gerrits Y, et al. The interrelationship
between cytotoxin-associated gene A, vacuolating cytotoxin, and
Helicobacter pylori–related diseases. *J Infect Dis* 1996;173:
1171–1175.

108. Cover TL, Glupczynski Y, Lage AP, Burette A, Tummuru MKR, Pérez-
Pérez GI. The high molecular weight *CagA* protein as a marker for
ulcerogenic strains of *Helicobacter pylori*. *J Clin Microbiol* 1995;33:
1496–1500.

109. Blaser MJ, Pérez-Pérez GI, Kleanthous H, et al. Infection with *Helicobacter pylori* strains possessing *cagA* associated with an increased
risk of developing adenocarcinoma of the stomach. *Cancer Res* 1995;
55:2111–2115.

110. Parsonnet J, Friedman GD, Orentreich N, Vogelman H. Risk for gastric cancer in people with *CagA* positive or *CagA* negative *Helicob-
ter pylori* infection. *Gut* 1997;40:297–301.

111. Crabtree JE, Taylor JD, Wyatt JL, et al. Mucosal IgA recognition of *Helicobacter pylori* 120 kDa protein, peptic ulceration, and gastric pathology. *Lancet* 1991;338:332–335.

112. Kuipers EJ, Pérez-Pérez GI, Meuwissen SGM, Blaser MJ. *Helicobacter pylori* and atrophic gastritis: importance of the *cagA* status. *J Natl Cancer Inst* 1995;87:1777–1780.

113. Peterson W, Feldman M, Cryer B, Lee E, Perez G, Blaser M. Correlation of *H. pylori*–related *CagA* with severity of fundic gastritis and gastric secretion. *Gastroenterology* 1998;114:A258.

114. Tummuru MKR, Sharma SA, Blaser MJ. *Helicobacter pylori* picB, a homolog of the *Bordetella pertussis* toxin secretion protein, is required for induction of IL-8 in gastric epithelial cells. *Mol Microbiol* 1995;18:867–876.

115. Peek RM, Thompson SA, Atherton JC, Blaser MJ, Miller GG. Expression of *iceA*, a novel ulcer-associated *H. pylori* gene, is induced by contact with gastric epithelial cells and is associated with enhanced mucosal IL-8. Abstract presented at the European Workshop on *Helicobacter* Infections; Copenhagen, Denmark, October 1996.

116. Xu Q, Peek RM, Miller GG, Blaser MJ. The *Helicobacter pylori* genome is modified at CATG by the product of *hpyIM*. *J Bacteriol* 1997;179:6807–6815.

117. Tomb J-F, White O, Kerlavage AR, et al. The complete genome sequence of the gastric pathogen *Helicobacter pylori*. *Nature* 1997; 388:539–547.

118. Nedenskov I, Sorensen P, Bukholm G, Bovre K. Natural competence for genetic transformation in *Campylobacter pylori*. *J Infect Dis* 1990; 161:365–366.

119. Wang Y, Roos KP, Taylor DE. Transformation of *Helicobacter pylori* by chromosomal metronidazole resistance and by a plasmid with a selectable chloramphenicol resistance marker. *J Gen Microbiol* 1993; 139:2485–2493.

120. Go MF, Kapur V, Graham DY, Musser JM. Population genetic analysis of *Helicobacter pylori* by multilocus enzyme electrophoresis: extensive allelic diversity and recombinational population structure. *J Bacteriol* 1996;178:3934–3938.

121. Pérez-Pérez GI, Dworkin BM, Chodos JE, Blaser MJ. *Campylobacter pylori* antibodies in humans. *Ann Intern Med* 1988;109:11–17.

122. Kosunen TU, Seppala K, Sarna S, Sipponen P. Diagnostic value of decreasing IgG, IgA, and IgM antibody titres after eradication of *Helicobacter pylori*. *Lancet* 1992;339:893–895.

123. Dubois A, Fiala N, Heman-Ackah LM, et al. Natural gastric infection with *Helicobacter pylori* in monkeys: a model for human infection with spiral bacteria. *Gastroenterology* 1994;106:1405–1417.

124. Kirchner T, Melber A, Fischbach W, Heilmann KL, Muller-Hermelink HK. Immunohistological patterns of the local immune response in *Helicobacter pylori* gastritis. In: Malfertheiner P, Ditschuneit H, eds. *Helicobacter pylori*, gastritis and peptic ulcer. Berlin: Springer-Verlag, 1991;213–222.

125. Engstrand L, Scheynius A, Pahlson C, Grimelius L, Schwan A, Gustavsson S. Association of *Campylobacter pylori* with induced expression of class II transplantation antigens on gastric epithelial cells. *Infect Immun* 1989;57:827–832.

126. Valnes K, Huitfeldt HS, Brandtzaeg P. Relation between T cell number and epithelial HLA class II expression quantified by image analysis in normal and inflamed human gastric mucosa. *Gut* 1990;31:647–652.

127. Wee A, The M, Kang JY. Association of *Helicobacter pylori* with HLA-DR antigen expression in gastritis. *J Clin Pathol* 1992;45:30–33.

128. Ye G, Barrera C, Fan X, et al. Expression of B7-1 and B7-2 costimulatory molecules by human gastric epithelial cells. *J Clin Invest* 1997; 99:1628–1636.

129. Marrack P, Kappler J. Subversion of the immune system by pathogens. *Cell* 1994;76:323–332.

130. Fearon DT, Locksley RM. The instructive role of innate immunity in the acquired immune response. *Science* 1996;272:50–54.

131. Karttunen R, Karttunen T, Ekre H-PT, MacDonald TT. Interferon gamma and interleukin 4 secreting cells in the gastric antrum in *Helicobacter pylori* positive and negative gastritis. *Gut* 1995;36: 341–345.

132. Mohammadi M, Czinn S, Redline R, Nedrud J. *Helicobacter pylori*-specific cell-mediated immune responses display a predominant $T_H 1$ phenotype and promote a delayed-type hypersensitivity response in the stomachs of mice. *J Immunol* 1996;156:4729–4735.

133. Haeberle HA, Kubin M, Bamford KB, et al. Differential stimulation of interleukin-12 (IL-12) and IL-10 by live and killed *Helicobacter pylori in vitro* and association of IL-12 production with gamma interferon-producing T cells in the human gastric mucosa. *Infect Immun* 1997;4229–4235.

134. Sieling PA, Wang X-H, Gately MK, et al. IL-12 regulates T helper type 1 cytokine responses in human infectious disease. *J Immunol* 1994;153:3639–3647.

135. Elios MM, Manghetti M, De Carli M, et al. T helper 1 effector cells specific for *Helicobacter pylori* in the gastric antrum of patients with peptic ulcer disease. *J Immunol* 1997;158:962–967.

136. Elios MM, Manghetti M, Almerigogna F, et al. Different cytokine profile and antigen-specificity repertoire in *Helicobacter pylori*-specific T cell clones from the antrum of chronic gastritis patients with or without peptic ulcer. *Eur J Immunol* 1997;27:1751–1755.

137. Morris AJ, Ali MR, Nicholson GI, Pérez-Pérez GI, Blaser MJ. Long-term follow-up of voluntary ingestion of *Helicobacter pylori*. *Ann Intern Med* 1991;114:662–663.

138. Parsonnet J, Blaser MJ, Pérez-Pérez GI, Hargrett-Bearn N, Tauxe RV. Symptoms and risk factors of *Helicobacter pylori* infection in a cohort of epidemiologists. *Gastroenterology* 1992;102:41–46.

139. Pérez-Pérez GI, Tham KT, Peek RM, Atherton JC, Blaser MJ. Not all *Helicobacter pylori*–infected persons produce specific IgA in gastric juice. *Gastroenterology* 1997;112:A1061.

140. Bogstedt AK, Nava S, Wadstrom T, Hammarstrom L. *Helicobacter pylori* infections in IgA deficiency: lack of role of the secretory immune system. *Clin Exp Immunol* 1996;105:202–204.

141. Negrini R, Lisato L, Zanella I, et al. *Helicobacter pylori* infection induces antibodies cross-reacting with human gastric mucosa. *Gastroenterology* 1991;101:437–445.

142. Negrini R, Savio A, Poiesi C, et al. Antigenic mimicry between *Helicobacter pylori* and gastric mucosa in the pathogenesis of body atrophic gastritis. *Gastroenterology* 1996;111:655–665.

143. Kartunnen R. Blood lymphocyte proliferation, cytokine secretion and appearance of T cells with activation surface markers in cultures with *Helicobacter pylori*: comparison of the responses of subjects with and without antibodies to *H. pylori*. *Clin Exp Immunol* 1991; 83:396–400.

144. Birkholtz S, Knipp U, Nietzki C, Adamek RJ, Opferkuch W. Immunological activity of lipopolysaccharide of *Helicobacter pylori* on human peripheral mononuclear blood cells in comparison to lipopolysaccharides of other intestinal bacteria. *FEMS Immunol Med Microbiol* 1993;6:317–324.

145. Sharma SA, Miller GG, Pérez-Pérez GI, Gupta RS, Blaser MJ. Humoral and cellular immune recognition of *Helicobacter pylori* proteins are not concordant. *Clin Exp Immunol* 1994;97:126–132.

146. Di Tommaso A, Xiang Z, Bugnoli M, et al. *Helicobacter pylori*–specific CD4$^+$ T-cell clones from peripheral blood and gastric biopsies. *Infect Immun* 1995;63:1102–1106.

147. Engstrand L, Scheynius A, Pahlson C. An increased number of gamma/delta T-cells and gastric epithelial cell expression of the groEL stress-protein homologue in *Helicobacter pylori*-associated clinical gastritis of the antrum. *Am J Gastroenterol* 1991;86:976–980.

148. Tarkkanen J, Kosunen TU, Saksela E. Contact of lymphocytes with *Helicobacter pylori* augments natural killer cell activity and induces production of gamma interferon. *Infect Immun* 1993;61:3012.

Inflammation: Basic Principles and Clinical Correlates,
3rd ed., edited by John I. Gallin and Ralph Snyderman.
Lippincott Williams & Wilkins, Philadelphia © 1999.

CHAPTER 71

Inflammation and Cancer

Hans Schreiber and Donald A. Rowley

The functional relationship between inflammation and cancer has been the subject of considerable discussion and speculation for more than a century. Rudolf Virchow suggested that certain irritants and inflammation caused by the irritants could lead to cellular proliferation and be important in the pathogenesis of cancer (1,2). He also observed the frequent occurrence of cancers at sites of chronic irritation. Today, we know that cancer is caused by mutational changes and that proliferation of cells alone is usually not sufficient to cause cancers. Proliferation of cells occurs during physiologic regeneration and in response to tissue destruction and the inflammatory response associated with it. Although inflammatory and reparative cellular proliferation subsides after the injurious agent is removed or the damage is repaired, malignant cells continue to proliferate and to be surrounded by inflammatory cells, even when the agents that caused the development of the cancer are removed. Nevertheless, there is an intricate relationship between inflammatory reactions, stimulation of proliferation, and cancer development (i.e., carcinogenesis). Specific examples suggest an important causal relationship between inflammation and cancer.

INITIATION, PROMOTION AND PROGRESSION

Peyton Rous et al. (3,4) recognized in early studies that cancers developed from "subthreshold neoplastic states" (now referred to as the initiation stage) caused by viral or chemical carcinogens that induced somatic mutations. They showed experimentally that these cellular changes were irreversible and could persist in apparently normal tissues for years until nonspecific stimulation (now referred to as promotion) such as wounding caused these

cells to multiply and become tumors. In a way, Rous distinguished between initiation and promotion of cancer, although these terms were only coined later to describe "two-stage carcinogenesis" (5). Today it is assumed that as many as 10 or more mutations are required for a cell to become fully malignant. Nevertheless, a single initiating mutation may be sufficient to make a cell prone to become malignant after promotion. The reasons for a particular somatic or germ-line mutation to predispose to cancer development are not understood, but some of these mutations result in a reduced ability of the initiated cells to recognize and repair DNA mismatches, a process essential for maintaining genomic stability.

Promotion may result from exposure of initiated cells to chemical irritants such as phorbol esters or from exposure to factors released at the site of wounding, partial organ resection, or chronic irritation. Promoters such as phorbol esters cause cellular proliferation, increased production of reactive oxygen species (ROS) by many cells types, oxidative DNA damage, and reduced DNA repair. Which of these functions is critical for promotion is unclear. There is no convincing evidence that chemical promoters such as 12-O-tetradecanoylphorbol-13-acetate (TPA) can induce cancers in normal cells without previous or simultaneous exposure of the cells to carcinogens. The relative importance of the proposed mutational mechanisms remains unclear, even though the result of tumor promotion may be an accumulation of additional mutations that are required for initiated cells to become cancer cells. Alternatively, ROS also alter the structure and function of proteins and lipids that may cause epigenetic changes in gene expression and cellular metabolism that help carcinogenesis. In any case, counteracting tumor promotion is almost as important as eliminating exposure to carcinogenic mutagens, because initiated cells are innocuous until promotion occurs. Additional mutations can result from continued exposure of the initiated cells to carcinogenic mutagens, such as additional

H. Schreiber and D. A. Rowley: Department of Pathology, Division of Biological Sciences, The University of Chicago, Chicago, Illinois 60637.

exposure to a second carcinogen or continued exposure to the original carcinogen. Such a process is sometimes referred to as cocarcinogenesis rather than promotion.

The third stage of tumor development, tumor progression, originally described the progression of a noninvasive precursor lesion (e.g., a papilloma) to invasive cancer (6); the definition was widened later (7) to refer to any irreversible increase in malignant behavior after the first invasive cancer cells have appeared (e.g., by gaining independence of various host controls such as hormone dependence). These changes during progression may affect growth rate, invasiveness, metastatic behavior, hormone dependence, or susceptibility to drugs. The additional changes observed during tumor progression are mostly attributed to the accumulation of additional mutations rather than to epigenetic changes, but the molecular basis of these changes is often not understood. Inflammation can have a critical influence on initiation, promotion, and progression of cancer. Although inflammation may be advantageous to the cancer or the precursor cells by helping to add mutations or support malignant growth by various other mechanisms, inflammation also may destroy malignant cells or arrest their growth.

ROLE OF CELL PROLIFERATION IN CARCINOGENESIS

It has long been known that mutagens are far more effective as carcinogens when exposure is at levels that also causes cell proliferation (8,9). Chronic mitogenesis due to inflammation has been proposed to be a mechanism leading to carcinogenic mutations (8–11). Chemical changes of DNA are caused by a large number of exogenous and endogenous chemical and physical agents. Among the latter, endogenous oxidants whose production is increased markedly in inflamed tissues may play a critical role in carcinogenesis. For example, uncontrolled oxidative damage can lead to DNA alterations through the formation of oxidation DNA adducts such as 8-hydroxy-2-deoxyguanosine (12–14). Nitric oxide (NO) reacts with superoxide to yield peroxynitrite ($ONOO^-$), which has multiple genetic and epigenetic effects.

DNA damage also occurs under physiologic conditions, and it is estimated that more than 100 DNA adducts are formed per cell each day (10). Cell proliferation is needed to convert these "promutagenic" DNA alterations to mutations (8–10), and proliferating cells must repair the DNA adducts before replication, or mutations occur. The promutagenic damage must be repaired, or damaged cells must apoptose to prevent mutant cells from surviving and potentially propagating (15). An impediment to repair or apoptosis may occur in inflamed tissues, and if cells in this tissue are forced into DNA replication and mitosis, the risk of mutagenesis and the development of cancer may be increased. For example, tumor promoters

such as phorbol esters can interfere with apoptosis and DNA repair while stimulating proliferation (16).

TUMOR STROMA

Mutual Dependence of Cancer Cells and Stromal Cells

Unlike a parasite, which consists entirely of foreign cells, a cancer contains mutant malignant cells and large numbers of nonmalignant cells and tissue components that provide blood supply and other structural and nonstructural support, collectively forming the stroma or the bed in which cancer cells grow. The functional importance of this stroma is indicated by the fact that cancer cells removed from the tumor stroma and cultured with normal adult serum usually do not grow. For proliferation *in vitro*, most cancer cells require fetal serum, which replaces the milieu of growth factors and cytokines provided *in vivo* by the stroma. Extracellular matrix, sessile host cells, and mobile bone marrow–derived leukocytes recruited to tumor sites appear to be involved in various types of functionally important interactions that influence cell adhesion, growth factor release, and cellular proliferation (17) (see Chapter 17).

The importance of the mesenchyme (i.e., the stroma of normal tissues) in regulating differentiation and growth of normal epithelia in specific sites is well recognized. Studies by oncologists and embryologists indicate that stroma or mesenchyme from different sites of the body is morphologically indistinguishable but can differ in function. Mesenchyme from a particular location can force epithelia from a different location to assume the phenotype characteristic for the site from which this "inductive" mesenchyme was derived (18). Site-specific differences in mesenchyme are also postulated to be a reason for the finding that several human and murine tumor cell lines are transplanted much more effectively when injected at an orthotopic site (i.e., into the type of organ from which the tumor originated) (19). Difference in stromal environment may also determine whether disseminated cancer cells develop metastases at a particular organ site. Several lines of evidence show that the tumor stroma is essential for angiogenesis (see Chapter 53) and for the provision or activation of growth and angiogenic factors that are needed at the site of tumor cell growth (19–28). The reciprocal paracrine interactions between tumor cells and endothelial cells have been reviewed elsewhere (29).

During the multiple, consecutive stages of cancer development, the relationship between stromal and cancer cells is likely to change. For example, melanoma cells from primary early stage lesions may be inhibited by IL-6 secreted from dermal fibroblasts; melanoma cells from more advanced lesions can become resistant and may even be stimulated by IL-6, although the most malignant melanoma cells can produce IL-6 and use it as an autocrine growth stimulator (20–22).

The stroma of tumors also seems to counteract immunologic rejection of cancer cells. Tumor cells embedded in syngeneic stroma are rejected much less efficiently by T cells than tumor cell suspensions (30). It is unknown whether inactivation, apoptosis, or prevention of attraction of tumor-antigen–specific T cells or other mechanisms is responsible for this "stromal barrier." The importance of stroma in regulating the growth or immunologic rejection of cancer cells was suggested in studies in which tumors were manipulated so that the stroma was allogeneic and therefore a target for T-cell–mediated destruction (30,31). Destruction of the stroma was shown to help the eradication of the embedded cancer cells and lead to the rejection of the tumor (30). However, incomplete destruction of the stroma can select for more aggressively growing cancer cells, resulting in faster tumor progression (31).

Inflammatory Infiltrates in Tumor Stroma

Inflammatory infiltrates are commonly observed in the stroma of premalignant epithelial lesions and cancers, but the magnitude and cell types in the infiltrates vary greatly. The rejection of transplanted cancers cells is usually cell mediated but not antibody mediated, even though passive antibody may be useful therapeutically. The presence and magnitude of nonlymphoid inflammatory cells may not readily be recognized without the use of special histochemical stains. Dense cellular infiltrates of granulocytes, lymphocytes, macrophages, or several cell types may be present in or around aggressive tumors that show no evidence of necrosis. Malignant growth can destroy surrounding tissue that by itself causes an inflammatory response. Distinguishing by morphology inflammatory cells that cause tumor destruction from inflammatory cells that have no effect or promote tumor growth is impossible. Inflammatory infiltrates in tumors remain a histopathologic variable that is notable but not interpretable (32–35).

The problem is exemplified by melanomas. Regressive melanoma, a primary progressive melanoma with histologically "regressive" areas, may be infiltrated by oligoclonal T cells, suggesting the selective recognition of specific antigen (36); vitiligo, a depigmentation of normal skin at the site of tumor growth also may be observed. Both findings are consistent with a specific immune response against melanocytes. However, infiltrating lymphocytes are only associated with a good prognosis for lesions in the horizontal growth phase and 4 mm deep or less (37), whereas prognosis for melanomas in vertical growth phase that have invaded deeper than 4 mm is the same whether or not lymphocyte infiltration is observed (37). Because melanomas in the horizontal growth phase do not metastasize (38), it is difficult to see how inflam-

matory infiltrates or the regression of these lesions can affect melanoma survival (35). Melanoma cells at the early horizontal growth phase may be infiltrated because they still depend on a paracrine stimulatory circuit involving lymphocytes or other leukocytes and stromal cells, but melanoma cells in the vertical growth phase are no longer under paracrine control and have acquired autocrine stimulation of growth (21,22,31). These melanoma cells are more malignant, which is consistent with the adverse prognosis of finding partial regression of melanomas in the radial growth phase (32). The better prognosis of lymphocytic infiltration of earlier, less invasive melanomas may indicate that the tumor is still under paracrine control rather than being a sign of a destructive immunologic antitumor response (39).

Regression of other skin tumors and vitiligo can occur by mechanisms that do not require T lymphocytes (34,39,40). Inflammatory breast cancer is an aggressive malignant disease characterized by red, tender, swollen skin of the breast and caused by dermal lymphatic invasion by breast cancer cells, mostly in the absence of inflammatory cellular infiltrates (41).

INFLAMMATORY CELLS

Macrophages

The number of macrophages in tumors is usually underestimated because these cells are particularly difficult to recognize in tissue sections as usually stained. Macrophages and other leukocytes may be essential for tumor angiogenesis to occur (42–45), and prevention of infiltration of these cells by local release of IL-10 may prevent tumor growth (46,47). There is a direct correlation between macrophage chemoattractant activity produced by tumor cells *in vitro* and the percentage of macrophages found in the tumor *in vivo* (48). Several different macrophage chemoattractants are released by tumor cells *in vitro* (49), but most of the chemokines responsible for this attraction *in vivo* have not been identified (50).

Macrophages can produce more than 100 biologically relevant substances, including angiogenic factors such as basic fibroblast growth factor and vascular endothelial cell growth factor and growth factors such as platelet-derived growth factor and transforming growth factor-β (TGF-β) (42,49). Macrophages are also major producers of prostaglandins which may stimulate tumor cells and act as angiogenic factors (51). Macrophages can also secrete antiangiogenic substances such as thrombospondin and tumor growth inhibitory substances such as tumor necrosis factor-α (TNF-α) and IL-12 (42,50) (see Chapter 53). Although we know much about what macrophages can do, it is unclear what these cells are actually doing in the tumors. Macrophages unfortunately look morphologically identical even though they may secrete different cytokines that have opposite effects on tumor growth. Tumor growth *in vivo* selects for resistance to cytotoxicity by macrophages (52–56). However, T cells were needed for this selection (52), and T-cell–derived TNF or lymphotoxin may have provided the selective pressure rather than TNF released by macrophages.

Macrophages and neutrophils can be activated to be cytotoxic and cytostatic for tumor cells *in vitro*, but invariably elicitation with chemicals (i.e., pyran copolymers or thioglycolate) or exposure to bacteria or bacterial products is needed for this activation even though certain tumor cells, particularly those of hematopoietic origin, may contribute to the production and release of TNF-α by macrophages (57). There is no evidence that tumor cells alone, uncontaminated by mycoplasma, can activate naive residential macrophages or granulocytes *in vitro* to become tumoricidal or that macrophages are activated to be tumoricidal or tumoristatic in uninfected cancers. Because tumor cells alone seem not to be sufficient and because tumors are usually sterile, tumoricidal activation of macrophages may not occur *in vivo* without treatment with macrophage activators.

The instillation of bacille Calmette-Guérin (BCG) into the bladder cavity seems to be effective in reducing the rate of recurrence of invasive bladder cancer after surgery (58). The mechanism probably is related to the local activation of inflammatory cells, including macrophages and granulocytes to tumoricidal activity. However, systemic activation of macrophages to tumoricidal activity by systemic drug delivery is problematic. For example, the macrophage activator muramyl dipeptide is highly effective in inducing tumoricidal activity in macrophages *in vitro*, but the effects of this compound when given systemically *in vivo* are uncertain. The question remains whether or how, other than by local application of activators, macrophages in tumors can be activated to become tumoricidal.

Neutrophils and Other Granulocytes

Similar to macrophages, neutrophils activated *in vitro* with bacteria or their products can destroy human and murine cancer cells *in vitro* (59,60). Neutrophils can also kill tumor cells *in vitro* when sensitized by antibody specifically bound to the tumor cells (61). Neutrophils also have antitumor activity *in vivo* under certain experimental conditions. For example, growth of tumor cells engineered to produce artificially high levels of IL-4 (62,63) or granulocyte colony-stimulating factor (G-CSF) was arrested *in vivo* by a mechanism that appears to involve granulocytes (64,65). Neutrophils infiltrating the stroma of the cytokine secreting tumor cells may be activated *in vivo* to become tumoricidal or destroy the capillary bed of the tumor, because neutrophils can kill endothelial cells when activated by phorbol esters or bac-

terial products *in vitro* (59,60,66). Treatment with an antibody that depletes granulocytes causes the engineered tumor cells to grow, and neutrophils, not eosinophils, are responsible for IL-4–mediated growth inhibition *in vivo*, because inhibition is also observed in knock-out mice that lack eosinophils (67).

Neutrophils may also attract antigen-presenting cells (e.g. by producing granulocyte-macrophage colony-stimulating factor) to the site of inflammation (68,69), which may be important for the generation of a tumor-specific T-cell response by the host. Such a mechanism may explain the finding that the induction of CD8+ T-cell responses in a rat fibroscarcoma model was abrogated by depletion of neutrophils (70). In this model, the depletion of granulocytes led to a failure to develop tumor-specific immunity.

These findings suggest that granulocytes can be manipulated to have a role that is advantageous to the host. Many lines of evidence suggest, however, that without such manipulations granulocytes in tumors may be ineffective or even advantageous to the growth of the cancer cells. There is no evidence that neutrophils are activated by tumor cells alone, that neutrophils as they occur in tumor stroma are tumoricidal, or that granulocytes counteract the development, growth, or progression of primary cancers in humans or mice. Certain human tumors, such as squamous cell carcinomas of the head and neck, are often abundantly infiltrated by granulocytes, particularly neutrophils (71). Granulocyte infiltration is also found in murine squamous cell carcinomas from transgenic cancer-prone mutant mice carrying the viral *ras* gene (72,73). Granulocyte infiltration into these tumors occurs in the absence of any infection or necrosis and is found in proximity to highly proliferative areas of tumor growth. This contradicts any suggestion that these neutrophils are tumoricidal or tumoristatic, but the findings are consistent with the possibility that granulocytes can aid tumor growth as suggested by another tumor model.

Ultraviolet light (UV)–induced tumors in mice are often regressor tumors; the tumors regress when transplanted into normal mice but grow when transplanted into nude mice, whereas progressor tumors grow progressively in nude and normal mice. Transplantation of regressor tumors into normal hosts can lead to selection of progressor variants. These variants show a more prominent infiltration with granulocytes, primarily neutrophils. Depletion of granulocytes in mice with a granulocyte-specific antibody reduced the growth rate of the transplanted progressor tumors in nude mice (74,75) and resulted in rejection of these tumors by normal euthymic mice (76). Earlier experiments indicated that granulocytosis can correlate with enhanced growth of lung metastases after intravenous injection of tumor cells (77,78). In another model, application of phorbol esters to initiated (carcinogen-pretreated) skin is associated with dense neutrophilic infiltration and tumor promotion (79). It appears possible that neutrophils infiltrating the sites of tumor promotion or progression are not cytotoxic or cytostatic for malignant or premalignant cells but rather help promotion or progression. This could, for example, occur because the granulocytes may be needed to attract macrophages that are critical for neovascularization of the growing tumor (42), or neutrophils, by releasing platelet-activating factor, induce the release of platelet-derived growth factor, which can provide a powerful stimulating substance for cancer and normal cell growth. Many other mechanisms are possible because neutrophils can produce many other proteins and mediators (68,80,81). It appears that neutrophils in different states of activation or metabolic secretory activity may be advantageous to the tumor cells or the host.

Natural Killer Cells

Natural killer (NK) cells, particularly when activated, can kill tumor cells *in vitro*, enter solid tumors *in vivo*, and migrate to sites of metastases (82). Experimental evidence shows that this cell type eliminates intravenously injected NK-sensitive cancer cells. In animal experiments NK cells are effective in very early stages of solid tumor growth or metastatic spread (82), but little is known about the role of this cell type in the development of primary cancers. Beige mice, which have a granule exocytosis defect that decreases the lytic activity of NK cells, are not particularly susceptible to viral or chemical carcinogenesis (83). NK cells may represent a functional bridge between the early nonspecific (innate) immune response and subsequent antigen-specific (acquired) immunity (84).

Interferon-α (IFN-α) and IFN-β are potent inducers of NK activity (Chapter 8), and the proinflammatory cytokine IL-12 acts as a growth factor, increases the cytotoxic activity, and induces INF-γ production by NK cells (84) (see Chapter 34). *In vitro*, NK cells kill selectively tumor cells that have lost major histocompatibility complex (MHC) class I antigens (85), and loss of MHC class I alleles is commonly observed *in vivo* during tumor progression (86). High-dose IL-2 therapy, as it is used in patients with metastatic renal cancer, activates NK cells, and this action of IL-2 may contribute to the occasional therapeutic successes (87). However, similar therapy for malignant melanoma has not clearly improved the treatment of this cancer (88).

Lymphocytes

The significance of lymphoid infiltrates in cancers was discussed earlier, and the roles of T and B lymphocytes in cancer have been discussed in detail elsewhere (89). Tumor antigen–specific T cells can infiltrate tumors; specific priming or expansion of such T cells *in vivo* can be shown. These T cells may lyse tumor cells *in vitro* after culturing with growth factors, but none of these findings indicates that these T cells inhibit tumor growth *in vivo,* have a role in immune surveillance, or recognize antigens that are targets for tumor rejection. Epidemiologic studies indicate that T-cell–mediated immune surveillance against the development of primary cancers is restricted to certain virally associated malignancies and possibly certain UV-induced (nonmelanoma) cancers, even though T-cell–mediated, tumor-antigen–specific responses may be observed in patients with other cancers.

Fibroblasts and Fibrocytes

In areas of infections fibroblasts and fibrocytes are a significant source of proinflammatory and immunomodulatory cytokines. In response to injury, these cells provide growth factors and matrix components needed for tissue repair and remodeling (see Chapter 16). Fibrocytes may represent a key sentinel cell population that acts as an early warning system for tissue damage and infection (90–92). For example, there is a rapid response of fibroblasts to injury by production of IFN-α and IFN-β. A subpopulation of these cells may have important antigen-presenting function (93). Fibroblasts and fibrocytes also seem to play a critical role in controlling the invasiveness and growth of cancer cells *in vivo* by producing cytokines and growth factors (20,22,24,26). For example, IL-6 produced by dermal fibroblasts is a growth inhibitor for melanoma cells at an early stage, but IL-6 provides paracrine stimulation of the cancer cells at later stages of the malignancy (20–22). Conversely, tumor cells can control the responsiveness of fibroblasts to growth factors, such as by inducing receptors for growth factors on the stromal fibroblasts (27).

The REL/NF-κB family of transcription factors and their regulatory I-κB subunits play an important role in controlling inflammation, including the transcription of cytokine and cytokine receptor genes in fibroblasts and other cells of the immune system (94,95), but the same factors and proteins may also play an important role in cancer (96). Discussion of these factors is beyond the scope of this chapter.

INFLAMMATION MEDIATORS PRODUCED BY INFLAMMATORY AND CANCER CELLS

Reactive Oxygen Species

In health the small amount of ROS (e.g., superoxide, hydrogen peroxide, hydroxyl radicals, NO) produced during physiologic processes is balanced by antioxidant defenses of the cell. However, during inflammation, this balance is broken by increased production of these substances. Leukocytes and tumor cells produce reactive oxygen intermediates (ROIs) at the sites of inflammation and express the inducible nitric oxide synthase (iNOS). Antioxidant defenses may no longer suffice to cope with high levels of ROS and NO caused by increased endogenous production or secretion by leukocytes (97). The resulting uncontrolled oxidative stress may result in DNA damage or cellular destruction.

However, ROS and NO may have a dual role in carcinogenesis (98–100). High concentrations cause lipid peroxidation, DNA fragmentation, and cell death; whereas ROS and NO at orders of magnitude lower levels can cause signaling, increased intracellular second messengers, neovascularization, and promutagenic DNA damage. In one tumor model, nonmetastatic cells were found to respond to chemical inducers with high levels of iNOS and apoptosis, whereas highly metastatic cells did not (101). In several studies, low levels of NO production were positively correlated with tumor grade (98, 102–104). Malignant or premalignant cells that survive damage by NO may be more resistant to host-mediated controls and grow more aggressively. Although cancer cells transfected to produce very high levels of iNOS can kill neighboring untransfected cells *in vivo* (105), this strategy represents a considerable technical challenge for eliminating primary or metastatic cancers.

Cyclooxygenase-2 Reaction Products

Bacteria and their products such as lipopolysaccharide (LPS), growth factors, and chemical tumor promoters such as TPA induce cyclooxygenase-2 (COX-2, also called prostaglandin synthase) in macrophages and in parenchymal cells (106–111) (see Chapter 74). This inducible enzyme is overexpressed in experimental and human colonic tumors (112–114). The importance of COX-2 reaction products in tumor development is suggested by the finding (115) that knocking out this enzyme prevents cancer in mice that carry one mutant and one wild-type adenomatous polyposis coli (*APC*) gene (116); mutations in the human *APC* gene cause familial adenomatous polyposis in humans. A drug selectively inhibiting COX-2 suppressed the growth of human colon carcinoma cells in nude mice (117).

Epidemiologic and experimental studies show that nonsteroidal antiinflammatory drugs reduce the incidence and mortality from colorectal cancers (118–120). It has been proposed that some of the COX-2 reaction products contribute to carcinogenesis by producing intermediary products that break down into direct mutagens or by activating certain carcinogens. During the production of prostaglandins from arachidonic acid, oxygen is incorporated to produce prostaglandin G_2; this intermediate is reduced by the peroxidase activity of COX-2 to prostaglandin H_2. During this reaction, oxygen-derived free radicals are produced that can cause oxidative DNA adducts; procarcinogens (e.g., xenobiotics such as afla-

toxin) also may be oxidized and thereby activated to become proximate or ultimate carcinogens. Prostaglandin H_2 can be converted into different terminal prostaglandins and into malondialdehyde, a direct mutagen that forms DNA adducts. Even though oxygen-derived free radicals act at extremely short range, it has been suggested that inflammatory cells can cause oxidative DNA damage or mutations in neighboring parenchymal cells (97).

There are several alternative or additional mechanisms whereby COX-2 reaction products may contribute to tumorigenesis. Prostaglandin E_2 (PGE_2) and other products of the COX-2 pathway modulate signal transduction in various cell types (121), including lymphocytes (see Chapter 42), and PGE_2 may stimulate directly the growth of epithelial cells by an autocrine mechanism or (if PGE_2 is released preferentially from interstitial inflammatory cells) by a paracrine mechanism (115,122). Overexpression of COX-2 also leads to decreased apoptosis with increased BCL2 expression and reduced TGF-β2 receptor expression (121). Prolonged survival resulting from inhibition of apoptosis increases the time for initiated cells (e.g., for colonic cells) that have acquired one mutant allele to acquire a mutation in the remaining wild-type allele. COX-2 overexpression also leads to increased production of matrix-degrading metalloproteinases that may increase the invasive and metastatic potential of tumor cells (13). PGE_2 clearly has angiogenic activity (51), and increased release of this eicosanoid is likely to help establish neovascular support needed for growth, invasion, and metastasis of cancers.

Cytokines

Most tumor cells produce constitutively one or more cytokines or chemokines (123). This production can be regulated by the organ environment in which the tumor cells grow (124). These factors may promote the growth of tumor cells in an autocrine way or by attracting macrophages and other cells important for angiogenesis and growth. During the long clonal evolution of a cancer in an individual, subpopulations are likely to be selected that have escaped a cytokine environment that normally controls cellular growth. For example, neoplastic colon epithelial cells may have mutant TGF-β receptors to escape the negative growth-regulatory effect of this cytokine on normal colonic epithelial cells (125). Subpopulations of cancer cells may be selected producing cytokines and chemokines optimal for a vigorous angiogenesis and growth factor production (21,31).

Cytokines elicited by experimental manipulations or used as recombinant proteins can have powerful antitumor effects. For example, BCG-infected mice, when injected 2 to 3 weeks later with LPS, release a factor into the serum within minutes to a few hours; when injected into large established tumors, this factor causes central hemorrhagic necrosis, usually leaving behind a viable margin. This observation led to the discovery of TNF (126). The powerful effects of cytokines on tumors have been demonstrated using tumor cells transfected to secrete particular cytokines; this subject has been reviewed elsewhere (123).

The general observation is that genetic transduction leading to production of high levels of a cytokine often results in the rejection of the tumor cells by the syngeneic host. This rejection is usually followed by T-cell–mediated immunologic protection against rechallenge with unmodified tumor cells. Surprisingly similar antitumor effects were found with transfection of quite different cytokines such as IL-2, IL-4, IL-6, IL-12, IFN-γ, TNF, and G-CSF. The similarity of the effect may be explained by the substantial local inflammation produced at the site of injection of the cytokine-secreting tumor cells. The proinflammatory cellular and cytokine environment may activate non-T, non-B effector cells to become tumoricidal or tumoristatic. The inflammatory infiltrate may also act as an adjuvant by attracting antigen-presenting cells to the site and by releasing various cytokines there. The resulting growth arrest and ultimate rejection of the transfected but metabolically viable cancer cells may result in a prolonged antigen exposure that allows T-cell immunity to develop. Surgical removal after temporary tumor growth followed by a resting period can alone be effective in a large variety of tumor models for immunization of mice or rats against rechallenge with the same line of unmodified tumor cells.

Secretion of certain cytokines by tumor cells after transfection may lead to growth arrest *in vivo* in the absence of T-cell or B-cell immunity. For example, tumor cells transfected to produce TNF grow at the same rate as untransfected cells *in vitro* but show remarkable long-term growth arrest *in vivo* (127). For many weeks, the subcutaneous injection site of tumor cells in nude mice is a small, pale, gray-yellow, disk-like lesion slightly elevated above the skin surface. Histologically necrotic areas and areas with dense chronic inflammatory infiltrates are present, and tumor cells are difficult to detect. However, neutralization of the secreted TNF by anti-TNF antibodies or soluble TNF receptor-immunoglobulin results in rapid growth of the tumor (128). Unfortunately, the cellular or humoral mechanism responsible for the growth arrest of TNF-resistant tumor cells in the absence of B- or T-cell immunity is unknown. Tumor cells genetically engineered to release very large amounts of G-CSF, IL-2, or IL-4 also show significant inhibition of growth *in vivo* in the absence of T cells (63,64,129).

Cells transfected to produce IL-10 also fail to grow *in vivo,* even in nude or severe combined immune deficiency mice (46). Histologically, the tumors fail to be infiltrated by macrophages that are normally attracted and are part of the stroma. This absence appears to result in a failure of angiogenesis and therefore tumor growth

presumably because this cytokine may prevent the stromal inflammatory response of macrophages needed for neovascularization. Regressor tumors transfected to secrete TGF-β grew progressively, indicating that some cytokines secreted by tumor cells may interfere with the host's T-cell response against cancer (130).

Angiogenic and Antiangiogenic Factors

Tumor cells and nonmalignant cells of the tumor stroma play a central role in creating the milieu that favors or suppresses angiogenesis. This important topic is discussed in Chapter 53.

INFECTIONS AND CANCER INDUCTION

Bacteria

Epidemiologic evidence supports a linkage between certain bacterial infections and the development of specific types of cancers (131). For example, *Helicobacter pylori* infections are linked to adenocarcinoma of the stomach (see Chapter 70). The mechanisms involved are unclear. There is no evidence that *H. pylori* bacteria are directly carcinogenic, although this bacterium has been declared by the International Agency for Research on Cancer to be a group 1 carcinogen and therefore to be a definite cause of cancer. Mutagenic bacterial metabolites such as *N*-nitroso compounds are suspected as the carcinogens, and there is evidence that bacterial flora cause the formation of these carcinogenic nitrosamines in the stomach.

Infection with *H. pylori* results in a chronic inflammatory response with activated macrophages that convert nitrates to nitrites. Nitrites probably are converted to *N*-nitrosamines, and *in vitro* activated macrophages can form *N*-nitroso compounds from appropriate amines. Despite these links, chronic infection with *H. pylori* usually is insufficient to cause cancer. At least 50% of the world's population carries this organism, and the rarity of gastric cancer among *H. pylori*–infected individuals indicates that other factors must be involved. For example, prior exposure to other carcinogens may be required for *H. pylori* to "cause" cancer, and it is uncertain what the roles are of length of infection, genetic predisposition, or virulence of different strains of *H. pylori*. Parsonnet (131) suggested that *H. pylori* infection causes chronic inflammation that acts as a promoter in gastric carcinogenesis by increasing epithelial cell proliferation by direct stimulation or indirectly by damage to the gastric epithelium. Antibiotic therapy of certain high-risk patients seems reasonable (132), and prevention by the elimination of *H. pylori* would confirm an essential role of the organism in gastric cancer.

A link between bacterial flora and colon cancer has been suggested because the ileum does not have bacterial flora and is rarely a primary site for cancer. Although no specific organisms have been implicated in colon carcinogenesis in humans, the normal bacterial flora may activate exogenous carcinogen precursors such as aromatic amines or polycyclic hydrocarbons. Bacterial flora may also play a major role in tumor promotion, because bacteria can deconjugate bile acids or ferment polysaccharides and glycoproteins to produce agents that promote cell proliferation.

There is epidemiologic evidence that chronic and recurrent urinary tract infections increase the risk of bladder carcinoma; the additional presence of kidney and ureter stones increases further the risk of cancer of the renal pelvis, ureters, and bladder (133). Experimental studies have demonstrated that LPS-induced inflammation or heat-killed *E. coli* can markedly enhance urinary bladder carcinogenesis by the carcinogen *N*-methyl-*N*-nitroso-urea in rats (134,135). Instillation of the *E. coli* or the chemical carcinogen induced tumors in 10% to 16% of bladders, and 100% of bladders had tumors when treated with both agents. LPS alone did not induce tumors. The bacteria clearly synergized with the chemical carcinogen to induce bladder cancer.

Chronic bacterial respiratory infection increases the incidence of experimental lung cancer induced by a chemical carcinogen (136,137).

Parasites

Chronic parasitic infections can play a critical role in the development of malignancies. In Egypt, for example, bladder carcinomas account for about one half of all malignancies and are regularly associated with schistosomiasis that results in chronic inflammation and is associated with increased "genetic damage" of the bladder epithelium (138,139). However, the same patients usually have a history of smoking, bacterial bladder infections, or exposure to environmental carcinogens that may also contribute to development of bladder cancer (140). Chronic infections with the parasite *Opisthorchis viverrini* are important in the development of cholangiocarcinoma in Thailand (141). It is uncertain whether chronic epithelial injury and the inflammation caused by the fluke has a promoting role or the metabolites excreted by the parasites play an additional role as carcinogens or promoters (142).

Viruses

Because of substantial epidemiologic evidence for an association of hepatitis B virus (HBV) and hepatitis C virus (HCV) with hepatocellular carcinoma, these two viruses have been declared group 1 human carcinogens by the International Agency for Research on Cancer. However, the molecular mechanisms leading to cancer are uncertain. Although there is evidence for clonal integration of viral DNA in the tumors and surrounding parenchyma cells, there are no defined transforming sequences that can act as viral oncogenes. There is no evidence that viral integration activates a cellular oncogene. Chronic viral replication in hepatocytes may cause cell death continuously, with a compensatory reparative regeneration of lost parenchyma. The immune response to the viral protein may cause a chronic inflammation.

Support for such an inflammation-related pathway contributing to hepatocellular carcinogenesis comes from the study of transgenic mice that express the large HBV envelope protein on hepatocytes (169). These mice develop a chronic hepatitis similar to human HBV-induced disease and subsequently develop hepatocellular carcinomas. This chronic inflammation probably is caused by oxidative damage; however, there is no evidence that the HBV infection or the associated chronic inflammation is sufficient to induce the mutations required for hepatocytes to become malignant. Nevertheless, HBV or HCV infection appears to be critically important for the development of hepatocellular carcinoma, and it is likely that intervention by immunization can reduce the incidence of this type of cancer.

Epstein-Barr virus (EBV) immortalizes human B cells *in vitro*. *In vivo*, EBV causes polyclonal B-cell proliferation, whereas T-cell immunity against EBV antigens regularly "cures" the acute infection. After the initial phase of acute infection, the virus usually becomes latent in the host, and latently infected cells only express LMP-2a and EBNA-1 (143), which are poor targets for cytolytic T lymphocytes (144–147). Patients with suppressed T-cell immunity frequently develop EBV-associated lymphomas that express the entire array of EBV antigens (144). Such lymphomas can be rejected after immune suppression is reversed (148). EBV is also regularly associated with endemic Burkitt's lymphoma, but this tumor only expresses the EBNA-1 antigen and apparently has undergone some additional transforming events, making expression of the other EBV genes unnecessary for transformation (144). Because Burkitt's lymphoma occurs in children in tropical Africa with endemic malaria, the malarial infection has been proposed to cause constant mitogenic stimulation of the infected B lymphocytes and acquisition of additional mutations, but the relevance of such a mechanism remains unknown.

Another link between a human herpesvirus infection and cancer has been found. Kaposi's sarcoma–associated herpesvirus (KSHV) is found in dendritic cells of the bone marrow in patients with multiple myeloma, a malignancy of antibody-producing B cells (i.e., plasma cells). KSHV-infected cells produce viral IL-6, which is a growth factor for myeloma (149). The current notion is that KSHV-infected nonmalignant stromal dendritic cells produce viral IL-6, which drives the neighboring plasma cells into malignancy by paracrine stimulation (150).

Certain strains of human papillomaviruses (HPV) appear to be central etiologic agents causing cervical cancer in women. The factors that lead from initial infection to precancerous lesions and cancer are still unclear. However, the growth of HPV-immortalized cells or cervical carcinoma cells *in vitro* is stimulated by proinflammatory cytokines such as IL-1 and TNF-α (151). These cytokines appear to induce expression of amphiregulin, an epidermal growth factor ligand. The release of amphiregulin causes autocrine stimulation of growth of the HPV-transformed cells.

Intraepithelial neoplasia and invasive cancer are commonly associated with inflammatory leukocytic infiltrates (152). These leukocytes may release proinflammatory cytokines such as IL-1 and TNF-α, which act as paracrine factors to induce the release of autocrine growth factors such as amphiregulin, although local inflammation may aid cervical cancer development by other mechanisms (153).

Wounding, Scars, and Mechanical Irritation

Deelman (154) provided the first convincing evidence that papillomas and carcinomas often appear at the healing edge of scars in the tarred skin of mice. However, some investigators trying to repeat Deelman's experiments found the opposite result: prevention of tumor formation by wounding. MacKenzie and Rous (4) explained these discrepancies in an insightful discussion of the extensive early literature on skin wounding and tumor induction. These investigators correctly pointed out that intense inflammation leading to destruction of the initiated cells would decrease tumor development but that nondestructive inflammatory responses might promote tumor growth. By analogy, mutagens that are also strong cellular toxins (e.g., formaldehyde) are inefficient carcinogens because they kill the initiated or transformed cells.

A most impressive example of promotion by wounding or mechanical irritation is shown in mutant *ras* transgenic mice (72). Male transgenic mice fight and develop squamous papillomas at the site of skin injury. Even in the absence of fighting, older mice develop tumors at sites of chronic skin abrasions of the genitalia and mouth. Wounding transgenic young mice by skin incisions usually results in the formation of some papillomas along the scars. Similar to wounding, chronic application of traditional promoters such as TPA leads consistently to the development of multiple papillomas in the transgenic skin beginning 5 weeks after repeated application of this chemical; no tumors develop in control skin exposed to the same chemical.

Wounding, scarring, and chronic mechanical irritation have been postulated to play a role in the development of certain lung cancers (155,156). Other examples are cancers of the kidney and ureter associated with kidney and bladder stones and cancers of the skin associated with burn scars observed in underdeveloped areas of the world where adequate therapy is lacking (133,157). There is evidence that the environment of a healing scar can favor implantation or reimplantation of cancer cells (158). It is likely that scarring and chronic irritation can promote the development of cancer from initiated cells at any site in the body. However, the tumor-promoting effects of wound healing, scars, and chronic irritation seem to depend on the persistence of the preexisting initiating event. There is no evidence that wounding or the resulting scar by itself leads to malignancy, even though wounding and scarring in certain organs such as lung may lead to reduced clearance of inhaled carcinogens and thereby help the initiating event. Because a predisposing initiating event can rarely be excluded and may be not be easily prevented, avoiding injury or the resulting inflammation should be important in reducing the occurrence of certain cancers.

Although scars may help carcinogenesis for certain initiated tissues, scars found in cancers may or may not have a causal relation to carcinogenesis. Scars may often be the result of the cancer rather than a contributor to carcinogenesis. Scarring observed in certain cancers, such as those of the breast, may be caused by induction of intense connective tissue formation (i.e., a "desmoplastic reaction") by the tumor cells (159,160). A meaningful dissection of the cause and effect relationship of scars and cancers is often impossible in clinical settings. This is exemplified in the long-standing discussions about the concept of scar cancer of the lung (156,161) first proposed in 1939 (155).

CANCER DESTRUCTION AND PREVENTION: PROINFLAMMATORY AND ANTIINFLAMMATORY AGENTS

Destroying established cancers by injection of live bacteria into tumors was first attempted more than 100 years ago (162–164). Despite occasional successes, such treatments were usually ineffective and sometimes fatal. Safer killed bacteria (e.g., vaccines of *Corynebacterium parvum*) were found to have limited clinical use (165). Recombinant proinflammatory cytokines have been given to cancer patients systemically at doses required to induce tumoricidal effector cells, but these treatments commonly caused severe toxic reactions. Some of these cytokines, such as IL-12, are being tested at lower doses for their potential to aid T-cell–mediated tumor destruction. No therapies have achieved high cytokine levels localized at sites of malignant cells that were tumoricidal but avoided life-threatening toxicity. Despite these difficulties, one treatment has proven to be effective and safe: the topical application of live mycobacteria (BCG) for treating residual superficial bladder cancer. This cancer typically recurs after surgery. Repeated instillation of live BCG into the bladder by catheter is the treatment of choice for this cancer after surgery.

Results of experimental and epidemiologic studies support the hope that certain antiinflammatory agents can be effective in reducing the incidence of colon cancer and possibly of several other malignancies (118–120, 166–168) by using inhibitors of COX-2. Preventing or eliminating chronic infections or eliminating sources of chronic mechanical irritation should also be highly effective in preventing certain cancers. Even though inflammation may not alone be sufficient to cause cancer, preventing the cancer-promoting effects of inflammation may well be sufficient to prevent many cancers.

CONCLUSIONS

Inflammation may enhance cancer development at the initiation, promotion, and progression stages. Inflammation can result from infections, mechanical injury, or chemical injury. Inflammation may also be caused by factors released from the cancer or precancerous cells. Inflammation may help cancer cells or their precursors to acquire additional mutations needed to become fully malignant. Inflammatory cells may provide or induce important growth factors and help induce the vascular support for growth of cancers. The inflammatory response can have stimulatory effects on tumor growth, and there is no evidence for surveillance against cancer by inflammation or non-B and non-T leukocytes. Acquired immunity by T cells provides immune surveillance in cases of viral carcinogenesis, particularly by preventing EBV-associated lymphomas and possibly certain UV-induced cancers. However, non-T, non-B inflammatory cells such as macrophages and neutrophils can become powerful tumoricidal effector cells when stimulated by bacterial substances or pharmacologic doses of certain cytokines.

From this knowledge, two very different but equally important and valid concepts for counteracting cancer have evolved. One is to prevent inflammation that helps cancer development and growth (e.g., preventing colonic neoplasia by inhibiting COX-2). The other is to increase the inflammatory response to destroy rather than help tumor cells (e.g., the treatment of superficial bladder cancer by intravesicular instillation of BCG). As the specific molecules and pathways in inflammation are identified, the intricate relationship between inflammation and carcinogenesis may be untangled so that powerful new strategies will evolve for preventing and treating cancer.

ACKNOWLEDGMENTS

This work was supported by the Corinne Kreissl Foundation grant of the American Cancer Society IM773 and by U.S. Public Health Service grants RO1-CA22677, RO1-CA37156 and PO174182. The authors also gratefully acknowledge support by a gift from the Passis family.

REFERENCES

1. Virchow R, Reizung U, Reizbarkeit. *Arch Pathol Anat Klin Med* 1858; 14:1–63.
2. Virchow R. Die krankhaften Geschwülste. In: *Erster Band, Fünfte Vorlesung, Pathogenie der neoplastischen Geschwülste.* Berlin: Verlag von August Hirschwald, 1863:72–101.
3. Rous P, Kidd JG. Conditional neoplasms and subthreshold neoplastic states: a study of the tar tumors of rabbits. *J Exp Med* 1941;73: 365–389.
4. MacKenzie I, Rous P. The experimental disclosure of latent neoplastic changes in tarred skin. *J Exp Med* 1941;73:391–415.
5. Berenblum I. A re-evaluation of the concept of cocarcinogenesis. *Prog Exp Tumor Res* 1969;11:21–30.
6. Rous P, Beard JW. The progression to carcinoma of virus-induced rabbit papillomas (Shope). *J Exp Med* 1935;62:523–528.
7. Foulds L. The experimental study of tumor progression: a review. *Cancer Res* 1954;14:327–339.
8. Cohen SM, Ellwein LB. Cell proliferation in carcinogenesis. *Science* 1990;249:1007–1011.
9. Preston-Martin S, Pike MC, Ross RK, Jones PA, Henderson BE. Increased cell division as a cause of human cancer. *Cancer Res* 1990; 50:7415–7421.
10. Ames BN, Gold LS, Willett WC. The causes and prevention of cancer. *Proc Natl Acad Sci USA* 1995;92:5258–5265.
11. Butterworth BE, Goldsworthy TL. The role of cell proliferation in multistage carcinogenesis. *Proc Soc Exp Biol Med* 1991;198:683–687.
12. Feig DI, Reid TM, Loeb LA. Reactive oxygen species in tumorigenesis. *Cancer Res* 1994;54:1890s–1894s.
13. Marnett LJ, Ji C. Modulation of oxidant formation in mouse skin *in vivo* by tumor-promoting phorbol esters. *Cancer Res* 1994;54: 1886s–1889s.
14. Simic MG. DNA markers of oxidative processes *in vivo*: relevance to carcinogenesis and anticarcinogenesis. *Cancer Res* 1994;54: 1918s–1923s.
15. Lindahl T, Satoh MS, Dianov G. Enzymes acting at strand interruptions in DNA. *Philos Trans R Soc Lond B Biol Sci* 1995;347:57–62.
16. Birnboim HC. DNA strand breaks in human leukocytes induced by superoxide anion, hydrogen peroxide and tumor promoters are repaired slowly compared to breaks induced by ionizing radiation. *Carcinogenesis* 1986;7:1511–1517.
17. Nathan C, Sporn M. Cytokines in context. *J Cell Biol* 1991;113: 981–986.
18. Cunha GR, Hayashi N, Wong YC. Regulation of differentiation and growth of normal adult and neoplastic epithelia by inductive mesenchyme. *Cancer Surv* 1991;11:73–90.
19. Fidler IJ, Wilmanns C, Staroselsky A, Radinsky R, Dong Z, Fan D. Modulation of tumor cell response to chemotherapy by the organ environment. *Cancer Metastasis Rev* 1994;13:209–222.
20. Cornil I, Theodorescu D, Man S, Herlyn M, Jambrosic J, Kerbel RS. Fibroblast cell interactions with human melanoma cells affect tumor cell growth as a function of tumor progression. *Proc Natl Acad Sci USA* 1991;88:6028–6032.
21. Lu C, Vickers MF, Kerbel RS. Interleukin-6: a fibroblast-derived growth inhibitor of human melanoma cells from early but not advanced stages of tumor progression. *Proc Natl Acad Sci USA* 1992; 89:9215–9219.
22. Lu C, Kerbel RS. Interleukin-6 undergoes transition from paracrine growth inhibitor to autocrine stimulator during human melanoma progression. *J Cell Biol* 1993;120:1281–1288.
23. Chung LW. The role of stromal-epithelial interaction in normal and malignant growth. *Cancer Surv* 1995;23:33–42.
24. Singer C, Rasmussen A, Smith HS, Lippman ME, Lynch HT, Cullen KJ. Malignant breast epithelium selects for insulin-like growth factor II expression in breast stroma: evidence for paracrine function. *Cancer Res* 1995;55:2448–2454.
25. Westerlund A, Hujanen E, Puistola U, Turpeenniemi-Hujanen T. Fibroblasts stimulate human ovarian cancer cell invasion and expression of 72-kDa gelatinase A (MMP-2). *Gynecol Oncol* 1997;67: 76–82.
26. Inoue T, Chung YS, Yashiro M, et al. Transforming growth factor-beta and hepatocyte growth factor produced by gastric fibroblasts stimulate the invasiveness of scirrhous gastric cancer cells. *Jpn J Cancer Res* 1997;88:152–159.
27. Sundberg C, Branting M, Gerdin B, Rubin K. Tumor cell and connec-

tive tissue cell interactions in human colorectal adenocarcinoma: transfer of platelet-derived growth factor-AB/BB to stromal cells. *Am J Pathol* 1997;151:479–492.

28. Dvorak HF. Tumors: wounds that do not heal: similarities between tumor stroma generation and wound healing. *N Engl J Med* 1986;315: 1650–1659.

29. Rak J, Filmus J, Kerbel RS. Reciprocal paracrine interactions between tumour cells and endothelial cells: the "angiogenesis progression" hypothesis. *Eur J Cancer* 1996;32A:2438–2450.

30. Singh S, Ross SR, Acena M, Rowley DA, Schreiber H. Stroma is critical for preventing or permitting immunological destruction of antigenic cancer cells. *J Exp Med* 1992;175:139–146.

31. Mintz B, Silvers WK. Accelerated growth of melanomas after specific immune destruction of tumor stroma in a mouse model. *Cancer Res* 1996;56:463–466.

32. Balch CM, Soong S, Shaw HM, Urist MM, McCarthy WH. An analysis of prognostic factors in 8500 patients with cutaneous melanoma. In: Balch CM, Soong S, Shaw HM, Urist MM, McCarthy WH, eds. *Cutaneous melanoma,* 2nd ed. Philadelphia: JB Lippincott, 1992: 165–187.

33. Barnhill RL, Mihm MC. Histopathology of malignant melanoma and its precursor lesions. In: Barnhill RL, Mihm MC, eds. *Cutaneous melanoma,* 2nd ed. Philadelphia: JB Lippincott, 1992:234–263.

34. Berd D, Mastrangelo MJ, Lattime E, Sato T, Maguire HC Jr. Melanoma and vitiligo: immunology's Grecian urn. *Cancer Immunol Immunother* 1996;42:263–267.

35. Cook MG. The significance of inflammation and regression in melanoma. *Virchows Arch A Pathol Anat Histopathol* 1992;420: 113–115.

36. Mackensen A, Carcelain G, Viel S, et al. Direct evidence to support the immunosurveillance concept in a human regressive melanoma. *J Clin Invest* 1994;93:1397–1402.

37. Clemente CG, Mihm MC Jr, Bufalino R, Zurrida S, Collini P, Cascinelli N. Prognostic value of tumor infiltrating lymphocytes in the vertical growth phase of primary cutaneous melanoma. *Cancer* 1996;77:1303–1310.

38. Clark WH. Tumour progression and the nature of cancer. *Br J Cancer* 1991;64:631–644.

39. Prehn RT. The paradoxical association of regression with a poor prognosis in melanoma contrasted with a good prognosis in keratoacanthoma. *Cancer Res* 1996;56:937–940.

40. Andrews EJ. Evidence of the nonimmune regression of chemically induced papillomas in mouse skin. *J Natl Cancer Inst* 1971;47: 653–665.

41. Bonnier P, Charpin C, Lejeune C, et al. Inflammatory carcinomas of the breast: a clinical, pathological, or a clinical and pathological definition? *Int J Cancer* 1995;62:382–385.

42. Sunderkotter C, Steinbrink K, Goebeler M, Bhardwaj R, Sorg C. Macrophages and angiogenesis. *J Leuk Biol* 1994;55:410–422.

43. Evans R. Effect of X-irradiation on host-cell infiltration and growth of a murine fibrosarcoma. *Br J Cancer* 1977;35:557–566.

44. Gutman M, Singh RK, Yoon S, Xie K, Bucana CD, Fidler IJ. Leukocyte-induced angiogenesis and subcutaneous growth of B16 melanoma. *Cancer Biother* 1994;9:163–170.

45. Ellis LM, Fidler IJ. Angiogenesis and metastasis. *Eur J Cancer* 1996; 32A:2451–2460.

46. Richter G, Kruger-Krasagakes S, Hein G, et al. Interleukin 10 transfected into Chinese hamster ovary cells prevents tumor growth and macrophage infiltration. *Cancer Res* 1993;53:4134–4137.

47. Bogdan C, Vodovotz Y, Nathan C. Macrophage deactivation by interleukin 10. *J Exp Med* 1991;174:1549–1555.

48. Bottazzi B, Polentarutti N, Acero R, et al. Regulation of the macrophage content of neoplasms by chemoattractants. *Science* 1983; 220:210–212.

49. Mantovani A, Bottazzi B, Colotta F, Sozzani S, Ruco L. The origin and function of tumor-associated macrophages. *Immunol Today* 1992;13: 265–270.

50. Seljelid R, Busund LT. The biology of macrophages: II. Inflammation and tumors. *Eur J Haematol* 1994;52:1–12.

51. Form DM, Auerbach R. PGE₂ and angiogenesis. *Proc Soc Exp Biol Med* 1983;172:214–218.

52. Urban JL, Schreiber H. Selection of macrophage-resistant progressor tumor variants by the normal host: requirement for concomitant T cell–mediated immunity. *J Exp Med* 1983;157:642–656.

53. Urban JL, Shepard HM, Rothstein JL, Sugarman BJ, Schreiber H. Tumor necrosis factor: a potent effector molecule for tumor cell killing by activated macrophages. *Proc Natl Acad Sci USA* 1986;83: 5233–5237.

54. Nestel FP, Casson PR, Wiltrout RH, Kerbel RS. Alterations in sensitivity to nonspecific cell-mediated lysis associated with tumor progression: characterization of activated macrophage- and natural killer cell–resistant tumor variants. *J Natl Cancer Inst* 1984;73:483–491.

55. Yamamura Y, Fischer BC, Harnaha JB, Proctor JW. Heterogeneity of murine mammary adenocarcinoma cell subpopulations: *in vitro* and *in vivo* resistance to macrophage cytotoxicity and its association with metastatic capacity. *Int J Cancer* 1984;33:67–72.

56. Lattime EC, Stutman O. Tumor growth *in vivo* selects for resistance to tumor necrosis factor. *J Immunol* 1989;143:4317–4323.

57. Hasday JD, Shah EM, Lieberman AP. Macrophage tumor necrosis factor-alpha release is induced by contact with some tumors. *J Immunol* 1990;145:371–379.

58. Morales A, Eidinger D, Bruce AW. Intracavitary bacillus Calmette-Guerin in the treatment of superficial bladder tumors. *J Urol* 1976;116:180–183.

59. Lichtenstein A. Granulocytes as possible effectors of tumor immunity. In: *Immunology and Allergy Clinics of North America.* Human Cancer Immunology I. H.F. Oettgen, ed. Philadelphia: W.B Saunders, 1990: 731–746.

60. Dallegri F, Ottonello L. Neutrophil—mediated cytotoxicity against tumour cells: state of art. *Arch Immunol Ther Exp* 1992;40:39–42.

61. Dallegri F, Patrone F, Frumento G, Saccheti C. Antibody-dependent killing of tumor cells by polymorphonuclear leukocytes. Involvement of oxidative and nonoxidative mechanisms. *J Natl Cancer Inst* 1984; 73:331–339.

62. Tepper RI, Coffman RL, Leder P. An eosinophil-dependent mechanism for the antitumor effect of interleukin-4. *Science* 1992;257:548–551.

63. Tepper RI, Pattengale PK, Leder P. Murine interleukin-4 displays potent anti-tumor activity *in vivo. Cell* 1989;57:503–512.

64. Colombo MP, Ferrari G, Stoppacciaro A, et al. Granulocyte colony-stimulating factor gene transfer suppresses tumorigenicity of a murine adenocarcinoma *in vivo. J Exp Med* 1991;173:889–897.

65. Colombo MP, Lombardi L, Stoppacciaro A, et al. Granulocyte colony-stimulating factor (G-CSF) gene transduction in murine adenocarcinoma drives neutrophil-mediated tumor inhibition *in vivo.* Neutrophils discriminate between G-CSF–producing and G-CSF–nonproducing tumor cells. *J Immunol* 1992;149:113–119.

66. Ward PA, Varani J. Mechanisms of neutrophil-mediated killing of endothelial cells. *J Leukoc Biol* 1990;48:97–102.

67. Noffz G, Qin Z, Kopf M, Blankenstein T. Neutrophils but not eosinophils are involved in growth suppression of IL-4–secreting tumors. *J Immunol* 1998;160:345–350.

68. Cassatella MA. The production of cytokines by polymorphonuclear neutrophils. *Immunol Today* 1995;16:21–26.

69. Chertov O, Ueda H, Xu LL, et al. Identification of human neutrophil-derived cathepsin G and azurocidin/CAP37 as chemoattractants for mononuclear cells and neutrophils. *J Exp Med* 1997;186:739–747.

70. Tanaka E, Sendo F. Abrogation of tumor-inhibitory MRC-OX8⁺ (CD8⁺) effector T-cell generation in rats by selective depletion of neutrophils *in vivo* using a monoclonal antibody. *Int J Cancer* 1993;54:131–136.

71. Young MR, Wright MA, Lozano Y, Matthews JP, Benefield J, Prechel MM. Mechanisms of immune suppression in patients with head and neck cancer: influence on the immune infiltrate of the cancer. *Int J Cancer* 1996;67:333–338.

72. Leder A, Kuo A, Cardiff RD, Sinn E, Leder P. v-Ha-*ras* transgene abrogates the initiation step in mouse skin tumorigenesis: effects of phorbol esters and retinoic acid. *Proc Natl Acad Sci USA* 1990;87: 9178–9182.

73. Cardiff RD, Leder A, Kuo A, Pattengale PK, Leder P. Multiple tumor types appear in a transgenic mouse with the ras oncogene. *Am J Pathol* 1993;142:1199–1207.

74. Pekarek LA, Starr BA, Toledano AY, Schreiber H. Inhibition of tumor growth by elimination of granulocytes. *J Exp Med* 1995;181:435–440.

75. Seung LP, Seung SK, Schreiber H. Antigenic cancer cells that escape immune destruction are stimulated by host cells. *Cancer Res* 1995;55: 5094–5100.

76. Seung L, Rowley DA, Dubey P, Schreiber H. Synergy between T cell immunity and inhibition of paracrine stimulation causes tumor rejection. *Proc Natl Acad Sci USA* 1995;92:6254–6258.

77. Milas L, Faykus MH Jr, McBride WH, Hunter N, Peters LJ. Concomitant development of granulocytosis and enhancement of metastases formation in tumor-bearing mice. *Clin Exp Metast* 1984;2: 181–190.

78. Ishikawa M, Koga Y, Hosokawa M, Kobayashi H. Augmentation of B16 melanoma lung colony formation in C57BL/6 mice having marked granulocytosis. *Int J Cancer* 1986;37:919–924.

79. DiGiovanni J, Imamoto A, Naito M, et al. Further genetic analyses of skin tumor promoter susceptibility using inbred and recombinant inbred mice. *Carcinogenesis* 1992;13:525–531.

80. Lloyd AR, Oppenheim JJ. Poly's lament: the neglected role of the polymorphonuclear neutrophil in the afferent limb of the immune response. *Immunol Today* 1992;13:169–172.

81. Wei S, Blanchard DK, Liu JH, Leonard WJ, Djeu JY. Activation of tumor necrosis factor-alpha production from human neutrophils by IL-2 via IL-2-R beta. *J Immunol* 1993;150:1979–1987.

82. Whiteside TL, Herberman RB. The role of natural killer cells in immune surveillance of cancer. *Curr Opin Immunol* 1995;7:704–710.

83. Kärre K, Klein GO, Kiessling R, Argov S, Klein G. The beige model in studies of natural resistance to syngeneic, semisyngeneic, and primary tumors. In: Herberman RB, ed. NK cells and other natural effector cells. New York: Academic Press, 1982:1369–1378.

84. Trinchieri G. Interleukin-12: a proinflammatory cytokine with immunoregulatory functions that bridge innate resistance and antigen-specific adaptive immunity. *Annu Rev Immunol* 1995;13:251–276.

85. Leibson PJ. Signal transduction during natural killer cell activation: inside the mind of a killer. *Immunity* 1997;6:655–661.

86. Garrido F, Cabrera T, Lopez-Nevot MA, Ruiz-Cabello F. HLA class I antigens in human tumors. *Adv Cancer Res* 1995;67:155–159.

87. Canobbio L, Miglietta L, Boccardo F. Medical treatment of advanced renal cell carcinoma: present options and future directions. *Cancer Treat Rev* 1996;22:85–104.

88. Philip PA, Flaherty L. Treatment of malignant melanoma with interleukin-2. *Semin Oncol* 1997;24:S32–S38.

89. Schreiber H. Tumor immunology. In: Paul, W, ed. *Fundamental immunology,* 4th ed. Philadelphia: Lippincott-Raven Publishers, 1997.

90. Smith RS, Smith TJ, Blieden TM, Phipps RP. Fibroblasts as sentinel cells: synthesis of chemokines and regulation of inflammation. *Am J Pathol* 1997;151:317–22.

91. Xia Y, Pauza ME, Feng L, Lo D. RelB regulation of chemokine expression modulates local inflammation. *Am J Pathol* 1997;151: 375–387.

92. Chesney J, Metz C, Stavitsky AB, Bacher M, Bucala R. Regulated production of type I collagen and inflammatory cytokines by peripheral blood fibrocytes. *J Immunol* 1998;160:419–425.

93. Chesney J, Bacher M, Bender A, Bucala R. The peripheral blood fibrocyte is a potent antigen-presenting cell capable of priming naive T cells *in situ. Proc Natl Acad Sci USA* 1997;94:6307–6312.

94. Wulczyn FG, Krappmann D, Scheidereit C. The NF-kappa B/Rel and I kappa B gene families: mediators of immune response and inflammation. *J Mol Med* 1996;74:749–769.

95. Barnes PJ, Adcock IM. NF-kappa B: a pivotal role in asthma and a new target for therapy. *Trends Pharmacol Sci* 1997;18:46–50.

96. Gilmore TD, Koedood M, Piffat KA, White DW. Rel/NF-kappaB/I-kappaB proteins and cancer. *Oncogene* 1996;13:1367–1378.

97. Shacter E, Beecham EJ, Covey JM, Kohn KW, Potter M. Activated neutrophils induce prolonged DNA damage in neighboring cells. *Carcinogenesis* 1988;9:2297–2304.

98. Vamvakas S, Schmidt HH. Just say NO to cancer? *J Natl Cancer Inst* 1997;89:406–407.

99. Cerutti PA. Oxy-radicals and cancer. *Lancet* 1994;344:862–863.

100. Cerutti PA. Oxidant stress and carcinogenesis. *Eur J Clin Invest* 1991; 21:1–5.

101. Xie K, Dong Z, Fidler IJ. Activation of nitric oxide synthase gene for inhibition of cancer metastasis. *J Leukoc Biol* 1996;59:797–803.

102. Thomsen LL, Lawton FG, Knowles RG, Beesley JE, Riveros-Moreno V, Moncada S. Nitric oxide synthase activity in human gynecological cancer. *Cancer Res* 1994;54:1352–1354.

103. Jenkins DC, Charles IG, Thomsen LL, et al. Roles of nitric oxide in tumor growth. *Proc Natl Acad Sci USA* 1995;92:4392–4396.

104. Duenas-Gonzalez A, Isales CM, del Mar Abad-Hernandez M, Gonzalez-Sarmiento R, Sangueza O, Rodriguez-Commes J. Expression of inducible nitric oxide synthase in breast cancer correlates with metastatic disease. *Mod Pathol* 1997;10:645–649.

105. Xie K, Huang S, Dong Z, Juang SH, Wang Y, Fidler IJ. Destruction of bystander cells by tumor cells transfected with inducible nitric oxide (NO) synthase gene. *J Natl Cancer Inst* 1997;89:421–427.

106. Kujubu DA, Fletcher BS, Varnum BC, Lim RW, Herschman HR. TIS10, a phorbol ester tumor promoter–inducible mRNA from Swiss 3T3 cells, encodes a novel prostaglandin synthase/cyclooxygenase homologue. *J Biol Chem* 1991;266:12866–12872.

107. Lee SH, Soyoola E, Chanmugam P, et al. Selective expression of mitogen-inducible cyclooxygenase in macrophages stimulated with lipopolysaccharide. *J Biol Chem* 1992;267:25934–25938.

108. DeWitt DL, Meade EA. Serum and glucocorticoid regulation of gene transcription and expression of the prostaglandin H synthase-1 and prostaglandin H synthase-2 isozymes. *Arch Biochem Biophys* 1993; 306:94–102.

109. Ristimaki A, Garfinkel S, Wessendorf J, Maciag T, Hla T. Induction of cyclooxygenase-2 by interleukin-1 alpha: evidence for post-transcriptional regulation. *J Biol Chem* 1994;269:11769–11775.

110. Coffey RJ, Hawkey CJ, Damstrup L, et al. Epidermal growth factor receptor activation induces nuclear targeting of cyclooxygenase-2, basolateral release of prostaglandins, and mitogenesis in polarizing colon cancer cells. *Proc Natl Acad Sci USA* 1997;94:657–662.

111. Williams CS, DuBois RN. Prostaglandin endoperoxide synthase: why two isoforms? *Am J Physiol* 1996;270:G393–G400.

112. Williams CS, Luongo C, Radhika A, et al. Elevated cyclooxygenase-2 levels in Min mouse adenomas. *Gastroenterology* 1996;111: 1134–1140.

113. DuBois RN, Radhika A, Reddy BS, Entingh AJ. Increased cyclooxygenase-2 levels in carcinogen-induced rat colonic tumors. *Gastroenterology* 1996;110:1259–1262.

114. Eberhart CE, DuBois RN. Eicosanoids and the gastrointestinal tract. *Gastroenterology* 1995;109:285–301.

115. Oshima M, Dinchuk JE, Kargman SL, et al. Suppression of intestinal polyposis in Apc delta716 knockout mice by inhibition of cyclooxygenase 2 (COX-2). *Cell* 1996;87:803–809.

116. Oshima M, Oshima H, Kitagawa K, Kobayashi M, Itakura C, Taketo M. Loss of Apc heterozygosity and abnormal tissue building in nascent intestinal polyps in mice carrying a truncated Apc gene. *Proc Natl Acad Sci USA* 1995;92:4482–4486.

117. Sheng H, Shao J, Kirkland SC, et al. Inhibition of human colon cancer cell growth by selective inhibition of cyclooxygenase-2. *J Clin Invest* 1997;99:2254–2259.

118. Thun MJ, Namboodiri MM, Heath CW Jr. Aspirin use and reduced risk of fatal colon cancer. *N Engl J Med* 1991;325:1593–1596.

119. Rao CV, Rivenson A, Simi B, et al. Chemoprevention of colon carcinogenesis by sulindac, a nonsteroidal anti-inflammatory agent. *Cancer Res* 1995;55:1464–1472.

120. Smalley WE, DuBois RN. Colorectal cancer and nonsteroidal anti-inflammatory drugs. *Adv Pharmacol* 1997;39:1–20.

121. Tsujii M, DuBois RN. Alterations in cellular adhesion and apoptosis in epithelial cells overexpressing prostaglandin endoperoxide synthase 2. *Cell* 1995;83:493–501.

122. Prescott SM, White RL. Self-promotion? Intimate connections between APC and prostaglandin H synthase-2. *Cell* 1996;87:783–786.

123. Blankenstein T, Cayeux S, Qin Z. Genetic approaches to cancer immunotherapy. *Rev Physiol Biochem Pharmacol* 1996;129:1–49.

124. Gutman M, Singh RK, Xie K, Bucana CD, Fidler IJ. Regulation of interleukin-8 expression in human melanoma cells by the organ environment. *Cancer Res* 1995;55:2470–2475.

125. Tannergard P, Liu T, Weger A, Nordenskjold M, Lindblom A. Tumorigenesis in colorectal tumors from patients with hereditary non-polyposis colorectal cancer. *Hum Genet* 1997;101:51–55.

126. Carswell EA, Old LJ, Kassel RL, Green S, Fiore N, Williamson B. An endotoxin-induced serum factor that causes necrosis of tumors. *Proc Natl Acad Sci USA* 1975;72:3666–3670.

127. Teng MN, Park BH, Koeppen HKW, Tracey KJ, Fendly BM, Schreiber H. Long-term inhibition of tumor growth by tumor necrosis factor in the absence of cachexia or T-cell immunity. *Proc Natl Acad Sci USA* 1991;88:3535–3539.

128. Teng MN, Turksen K, Jacobs CA, Fuchs E, Schreiber H. Prevention of runting and cachexia by a chimeric TNF receptor-Fc protein. *Clin Immunol Immunopathol* 1993;69:215–222.

129. Bubenik J, Voitenok NN, Kieler J, et al. Local administration of cells containing an inserted IL-2 gene and producing IL-2 inhibits growth of human tumours in nu/nu mice. *Immunol Lett* 1988;19:279–282.

130. Torre-Amione G, Beauchamp RD, Koeppen H, et al. A highly immunogenic tumor transfected with a murine transforming growth factor type beta 1 cDNA escapes immune surveillance. *Proc Natl Acad Sci USA* 1990;87:1486–1490.

131. Parsonnet J. Bacterial infection as a cause of cancer. *Environ Health Perspect* 1995;8:263–268.

132. Lee J, O'Morain C. Who should be treated for helicobacter pylori infection? A review of consensus conferences and guidelines. *Gastroenterology* 1997;113:S99–S106.

133. Chow WH, Lindblad P, Gridley G, et al. Risk of urinary tract cancers following kidney or ureter stones. *J Natl Cancer Inst* 1997;89:1453–1457.

134. Yamamoto M, Wu HH, Momose H, Rademaker A, Oyasu R. Marked enhancement of rat urinary bladder carcinogenesis by heat-killed Escherichia coli. *Cancer Res* 1992;52:5329–5333.

135. Kawai K, Yamamoto M, Kameyama S, Kawamata H, Rademaker A, Oyasu R. Enhancement of rat urinary bladder tumorigenesis by lipopolysaccharide-induced inflammation. *Cancer Res* 1993;53:5172–5175.

136. Schreiber H, Nettesheim P, Lijinsky W, Richter CB, Walburg HE Jr. Induction of lung cancer in germ-free, specific-pathogen-free, and infected rats by N-nitrosoheptamethyleneimine: enhancement by respiratory infection. *J Natl Cancer Inst* 1972;49:1107–1114.

137. Nettesheim P, Schreiber H, eds. *Respiratory infections and the pathogenesis of lung cancer*, vol 44. New York: Springer-Verlag, 1974:138–157.

138. Rosin MP, Saad el Din Zaki S, Ward AJ, Anwar WA. Involvement of inflammatory reactions and elevated cell proliferation in the development of bladder cancer in schistosomiasis patients. *Mutat Res* 1994;305:283–292.

139. Rosin MP, Anwar WA, Ward AJ. Inflammation, chromosomal instability, and cancer: the schistosomiasis model. *Cancer Res* 1994;54:1929s–1933s.

140. Parsonnet J. Molecular mechanisms for inflammation-promoted pathogenesis of cancer—the Sixteenth International Symposium of the Sapporo Cancer Seminar. *Cancer Res* 1997;57:3620–3624.

141. Haswell-Elkins MR, Satarug S, Tsuda M, et al. Liver fluke infection and cholangiocarcinoma: model of endogenous nitric oxide and extragastric nitrosation in human carcinogenesis. *Mutat Res* 1994;305:241–252.

142. Satarug S, Haswell-Elkins MR, Tsuda M, et al. Thiocyanate-independent nitrosation in humans with carcinogenic parasite infection. *Carcinogenesis* 1996;17:1075–1081.

143. Chen F, Zou JZ, di Renzo L, et al. A subpopulation of normal B cells latently infected with Epstein-Barr virus resembles Burkitt lymphoma cells in expressing EBNA-1 but not EBNA-2 or LMP1. *J Virol* 1995;69:3752–3758.

144. Rickinson AB, Murray RJ, Brooks J, Griffin H, Moss DJ, Masucci MG. T cell recognition of Epstein-Barr virus associated lymphomas. *Cancer Surv* 1992;13:53–80.

145. Levitskaya J, Coram M, Levitsky V, et al. Inhibition of antigen processing by the internal repeat region of the Epstein-Barr virus nuclear antigen-1. *Nature* 1995;375:685–688.

146. Khanna R, Burrows SR, Steigerwald-Mullen PM, Thomson SA, Kurilla MG, Moss DJ. Isolation of cytotoxic T lymphocytes from healthy seropositive individuals specific for peptide epitopes from Epstein-Barr virus nuclear antigen 1: implications for viral persistence and tumor surveillance. *Virology* 1995;214:633–637.

147. Mukherjee S, Trivedi P, Dorfman DM, Klein G, Townsend A. Murine cytotoxic T lymphocytes recognize an epitope in an EBNA-1 fragment, but fail to lyse EBNA-1–expressing mouse cells. *J Exp Med* 1998;187:445–450.

148. Smith CA, Ng CY, Loftin SK, et al. Adoptive immunotherapy for Epstein-Barr virus-related lymphoma. *Leuk Lymphoma* 1996;23:213–220.

149. Rettig MB, Ma HJ, Vescio RA, et al. Kaposi's sarcoma–associated herpesvirus infection of bone marrow dendritic cells from multiple myeloma patients. *Science* 1997;276:1851.

150. Pattengale PK. Role of interleukin-6 in the pathogenesis of murine plasmacytoma and human multiple myeloma. *Am J Pathol* 1997;151:647–649.

151. Woodworth CD, McMullin E, Iglesias M, Plowman GD. Interleukin 1 alpha and tumor necrosis factor alpha stimulate autocrine amphiregulin expression and proliferation of human papillomavirus-immortalized and carcinoma-derived cervical epithelial cells. *Proc Natl Acad Sci USA* 1995;92:2840–2844.

152. Davidson B, Goldberg I, Kopolovic J. Inflammatory response in cervical intraepithelial neoplasia and squamous cell carcinoma of the uterine cervix. *Pathol Res Pract* 1997;193:491–495.

153. Bornstein J, Rahat MA, Abramovici H. Etiology of cervical cancer: current concepts. *Obstet Gynecol Surv* 1995;50:146–154.

154. Deelman HT, van Erp JP. Beobachtungen an experimentellem Tumorwachstum: uber den Zusammenhang zwischen Regeneration und Tumorbildung. *Z Krebsforsch* 1926–1927;24:86–98.

155. Friedrich G. Periphere Lungenkrebse auf dem boden pleuranaher Narben. *Virchows Arch Pathol Anat* 1938;304:230–247.

156. Flance JI. Scar cancer of the lung. *JAMA* 1991;266:2003–2004.

157. Harland DL, Robinson WA, Franklin WA, Deletion of the *p53* gene in a patient with aggressive burn scar carcinoma. *J Trauma* 1997;42:104–107.

158. Murthy MS, Reid SE Jr, Yang XF, Scanlon EP. The potential role of integrin receptor subunits in the formation of local recurrence and distant metastasis by mouse breast cancer cells. *J Surg Oncol* 1996;63:77–86.

159. Toikkanen S, Joensuu H. Long-term prognosis of scar and non-scar cancers of the breast. *APMIS* 1990;98:1033–1038.

160. Partanen S, Hyvarinen H. Scar and non-scar ductal cancer of the female breast: observations on patient age, tumour size, and hormone receptors. *Virchows Archiv A Pathol Anat Histopathol* 1987;412:145–149.

161. Madri JA, Carter D. Scar cancers of the lung: origin and significance. *Hum Pathol* 1984;15:625–631.

162. Fehleisen F. Über die Züchtung der Erysipel-Kokken auf künstlichen Nährböden und die Übertragbarkeit auf den Menschen. *Dtsch Med Wochenschr* 1882;8:553–554.

163. Bruns P. Die Heilwirkung des Erysipels auf Geschwülste. *Beitr Klin Chir* 1887–1888;3:443–466.

164. Coley WB. The treatment of malignant tumors by repeated inoculations of erysipelas: with a report of ten original cases. *Am J Med Sci* 1893;105:487–511.

165. Oettgen HF, Old LJ. The history of cancer immunotherapy. In: DeVita VT, Hellman S, Rosenberg SA, eds. *Biologic therapy of cancer* Philadelphia: JB Lippincott, 1991:87–119.

166. Subbaramaiah K, Zakim D, Weksler BB, Dannenberg AJ. Inhibition of cyclooxygenase: a novel approach to cancer prevention. *Proc Soc Exp Biol Med* 1997;216:201–210.

167. Furstenberger G, Gross M, Marks F. Eicosanoids and multistage carcinogenesis in NMRI mouse skin: role of prostaglandins E and F in conversion (first stage of tumor promotion) and promotion (second stage of tumor promotion). *Carcinogenesis* 1989;10:91–96.

168. Vainio H, Morgan G, Kleihues P. An international evaluation of the cancer-preventive potential of nonsteroidal anti-inflammatory drugs. *Cancer Epidemiol Biomarkers Prev* 1997;6:749–753.

169. Nakamoto Y, Guidotti LG, Kuhlen CV, Fowles P, Chisari FV. Immune pathogenesis of hepatocellular carcinoma. *J Exp Med* 1998;188:341–350.

Inflammation: Basic Principles and Clinical Correlates,
3rd ed., edited by John I. Gallin and Ralph Snyderman.
Lippincott Williams & Wilkins, Philadelphia © 1999.

CHAPTER 72

Cancer Immunology

Drew M. Pardoll

NATURAL IMMUNE RESPONSE TO CANCER: SURVEILLANCE VERSUS TOLERANCE

For more than a century, investigators have sought to understand the interaction between the immune system and cancer cells so that antitumor immunity could be amplified as a means of cancer therapy. The potential for tumor specificity afforded by the immune system was most clearly embodied in Paul Ehrlich's term *magic bullet,* which referred to the ability of antibodies to selectively recognize and destroy tumor cells (1). Inherent in this concept was that tumors must express chemically distinct structures, called tumor antigens, that the immune system could use to differentiate them from their normal counterparts, thereby providing a therapeutic window.

William Coley, a New York surgeon, was the first to recognize that the occasional spontaneous regression of tumors could be mediated by immunologic mechanisms. Noting that these spontaneous regressions were often associated with host responses to an infection, Coley began to treat cancer patients with bacterial extracts, called Coley's toxins, to activate general systemic immunity, a portion of which might be directed against the tumor. Coley's toxins induced some tumor regressions, even in patients with advanced cancer, and these results represent the first clear-cut demonstration that antitumor immunity could be induced or amplified with a therapeutic outcome (2). Unfortunately, the inconsistency of the preparations and clinical results, together with the prohibitive toxicity of Coley's toxins, precluded their sustained application.

A more formal description of the immune system's capacity to recognize tumors was the *immune surveillance hypothesis,* originally put forward by Lewis Thomas and updated by McFarlane Burnet (3,4). In its pure form, the immune surveillance hypothesis posits that one of the fundamental functions of the immune system is to recognize and eliminate newly developing tumors *in situ* based on recognition of neoantigens that arise as part of the transformation process. It was imagined that this spontaneous transformation process occurred with high frequency and that, because the immune system dealt with these *de novo* tumors with similar efficiency as with infections, clinically evident cancers represented exceptions that slipped through the immunologic net. A correlate of the immune surveillance hypothesis was the idea that a tumor evading surveillance and becoming clinically apparent needed to develop resistance to recognition or killing by the elements of the immune system participating in immune surveillance.

A major prediction of the immune surveillance hypothesis is that the incidence of tumors in animals and humans with defective immune responses would be greatly increased. Careful analysis of immunodeficient mice followed over their natural lifespans did not reveal an increase in the incidence of common epithelial tumors (5–8). For example, nude mice, which do not have a thymus and therefore lack functional T-cell immunity and T-cell–dependent humoral immunity, are highly susceptible to viral infections but do not have an increased incidence of cancer nor shortened latency in the development of chemically induced cancers. However, the incidence of lymphoreticular cancers secondary to activation of RNA tumor viruses does increase (9). Several studies of patients with hereditary immune deficiencies, persons with acquired immunodeficiency syndrome, and immunosuppressed transplant patients demonstrate that, although they have increased numbers of certain cancers, the common epithelial cancers of adults are not observed at increased frequencies (10–14) (Tables 72-1 and 72-2).

In humans, virtually all cancers associated with immunodeficiency are virus induced (Table 72-3). The most common tumors in immunodeficient individuals are

D. M. Pardoll: Johns Hopkins University School of Medicine, Baltimore, Maryland 21205.

TABLE 72-1. *Cases of cancer (excluding cervix cancer in situ) in transplant patients from entry to study*

| | Years from Entry to Study | | | | | | | |
| | Less than 2 | | 2 to 3 | | 4 or More | | Total | |
Type of cancer	No.	Expected	No.	Expected	No.	Expected	No.	Expected
Non-Hodgkin's lymphoma	19	0.26	6	0.16	9	0.16	34	0.58
Skin: (U.K. only) basal cell carcinoma	0	0.38	1	0.24	0	0.23	1	0.85
Skin: (U.K. only) squamous cell carcinoma	0	0.06	1	0.04	2	0.03	3	0.13
Skin: (U.K. only) melanoma	0	0.05	0	0.03	1	0.03	1	0.12
Other (excluding skin cancer in Australia)	13[a]	7.85	6[b]	5.06	11[c]	4.88	30	17.79
Total	32	8.61	14	5.53	23	5.33	69	19.46

[a]Rhabdomyosarcoma (1), hypernephroma (2), ovary (1), lung (1), vulva (1), colon (1), esophagus (1), urethra (1), thyroid (1), carcinomatosis (1), acute leukemia (1), and Kaposi sarcoma.
[b]Renal pelvis (1), stomach (1), colon (1), lung (1), mesothelioma (1), and hepatoma (1).
[c]Colon (1), rectum (1), lung (1), prostate (1), bladder (1), vulva (1), cervix (1), acute leukemia (1), myeloid leukemia (1), metastasizing carcinoid (1), and renal pelvis (1).

lymphomas (13,14). Most lymphomas are associated with Epstein-Barr virus (EBV) infection of B cells (15–17). In humans exposed to EBV infection, a few B cells of infected individuals harbor EBV in a latent state. Intact T-cell immunity appears to be critical in eliminating B cells that become transformed on activation of transforming EBV-encoded antigens. Successful reconstitution of T-cell immunity or infusion of T cells specific for the EBV nuclear antigens causes rapid regression of EBV-associated lymphomas (18).

Other tumors seen at increased frequency in immunodeficient patients, such as Kaposi's sarcoma and cervical cancer, are also linked to viral infection. Most Kaposi's sarcoma is linked to infection with a human herpesvirus 8 (also called Kaposi's sarcoma–associated herpesvirus) (19,20), and most cervical cancers are linked to infection with high-risk strains of human papillomavirus (HPV) (21–25). The increased incidence of gastric carcinoma in immunosuppressed patients may be linked to the failure of regulation of *Helicobacter pylori,* a bacterium that colonizes the stomach and is linked to ulcer disease and gastric cancer (26).

The conclusion from these analyses of immune-deficient mice and humans is that immune surveillance of cancer as it was originally envisioned is critical for virus-associated and possibly bacteria-associated cancers, but it does not appear to be an important factor in regulating the development of tumors that arise from accumulation of genetically inherited or somatically acquired mutations associated with the development of common adult cancers.

Even though the common adult cancers are not associated with viral infections, they should express multiple potential antigens recognizable by T cells. All tumors possess hundreds and possibly thousands of mutations and other chromosomal aberrations. Virtually all cancers can be expected to present peptides that are derived from somatically acquired mutations. It is therefore unreasonable to propose that the absence of a robust immune surveillance of nonviral tumors results from an absence of antigens potentially recognizable by T cells. An alternative idea, which represents the opposite end of the spectrum of immune surveillance, is that the natural response of the immune system to a tumor antigen that arises *de novo* during transformation is tolerance rather than activation.

TABLE 72-2. *Immunodeficiency cancer registry*

| | | Type of malignancy | | | | | | |
Immunodeficiency disease	Total cases	N-HL	HD	LL	ML	OL	ET	Others
Ataxia telangiectasia	101	49	10	20	0	4	17	1
Common variable	74	32	5	3	1	0	33	0
Wiskott-Aldrich syndrome	52	36	4	0	6	2	1	3
Selective IgA deficiency	16	5	1	1	0	0	8	1
X-linked (Bruton's) hypogammaglobulinemia	15	4	1	3	2	2	2	1
Severe combined	13	8	1	1	3	0	0	0
Isolated IgM deficiency	8	5	1	0	0	0	2	0
Immunodeficiency with normal/elevated serum globulins	3	3	0	0	0	0	0	0
Other disorders	10	2	2	1	0	0	4	1
Total	292	144	25	29	12	8	67	7

N-HL, non-Hodgkin's lymphoma; OL, other leukemia; HD, Hodgkin's disease; ET, epithelial tumors; LL, lymphocytic leukemia; ML, myeloid leukemia.

TABLE 72-3. *Cancers at increased incidence in immunocompromised patients*

Cancer	Infectious agent
Lymphoma	Epstein-Barr virus
Kaposi sarcoma	Human herpesvirus 8 (Kaposi sarcoma–associated herpesvirus)
Gastric carcinoma	*Helicobacter pylori*
Cervical carcinoma	Human papillomavirus

When the immune system encounters a new antigen in the periphery, the outcome is not necessarily activation. Numerous experimental examples demonstrate that encounter of antigens in the periphery by mature T cells can result in tolerance induction because of ignorance, anergy, or physical deletion (27–32). What appears to determine the outcome of antigen encounter in the periphery is the context in which that antigen is presented to the immune system. In the presence of inflammatory or tissue-destructive processes, such as those that occur during viral or bacterial infection or when antigen is mixed with the appropriate adjuvant, the outcome is typically activation. When antigen is expressed endoge-

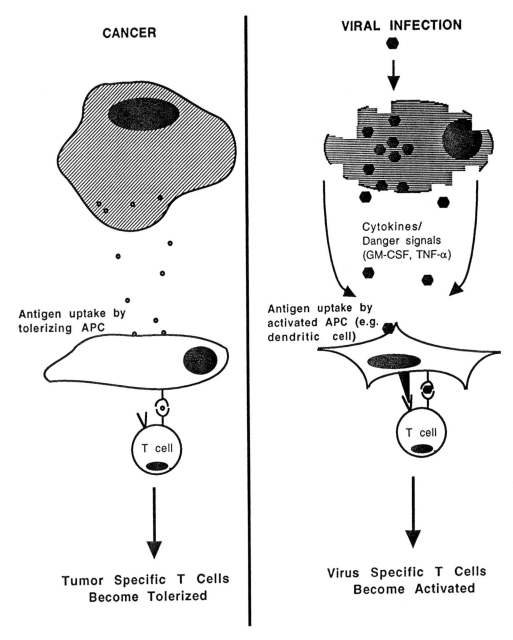

FIG. 72-1.

nously in the absence of the danger signals that accompany tissue destruction and inflammation, or when it is injected or released into the bloodstream in a soluble form, the typical outcome is immunologic tolerance.

Ultimately, it appears that the outcome at the T-cell level depends on the co-stimulatory signals present at the time of antigen recognition. In response to certain inflammatory cytokines such as granulocyte-macrophage colony-stimulating factor (GM-CSF), interferon-γ (IFN-γ) and tumor necrosis factor-α (TNF-α), antigen-presenting cells (APCs) express co-stimulatory molecules such as B7, thereby promoting T-cell activation. In the absence of the appropriate co-stimulatory signals, engagement of the T-cell receptor itself typically leads to ignorance, anergy, or apoptotic death of the antigen-specific T cell. It is reasonable to imagine that, as tumors accumulate neoantigens through mutation during the initiation of transformation, the absence of associated inflammatory or tissue-destructive processes at these early stages produces a circumstance in which neoantigens are viewed by the immune system in the same fashion as self antigens, thereby inducing tolerance (33–37) (Fig. 72-1).

The ability of tumors to induce T-cell tolerance against their antigens was demonstrated using adoptive transfer experiments with T-cell receptor (TCR) transgenic T cells. When tagged CD4+ TCR transgenic T cells specific for a model tumor antigen were cotransferred into mice together with a lymphoma expressing the cognate tumor antigen, antigen-specific anergy induction occurred in vivo (38). Anergy induction in this particular example might not have been expected, because the lymphoma efficiently presented antigen to and stimulated CD4+ cells in vitro. Tumors capable of presenting antigen to and stimulating T cells in vitro may induce tolerance in vivo for several reasons. First, the co-stimulatory signal requirements for activation of naive T cells are qualitatively and quantitatively different from those of previously stimulated T cells. Second, although it has been assumed that the initiation of T-cell responses to tumor antigens occurs through recognition of antigen directly presented by the tumor, it is possible that the response of the immune system to tumor antigens is based on transfer of antigen and processing by specialized bone marrow–derived cells. Evidence indicates that tolerance induction to parenchymal antigens also involves processing and presentation by a subset of bone marrow–derived APCs (39). Tumors arising de novo may release their antigen to bone marrow–derived APCs, which present them to T cells in a fashion that induces tolerance. In some experimental models, tumor antigens are ignored by the immune system; they neither induce active tolerance nor activation of T cells specific for their antigens.

In other murine tumor systems, antigenic tumor cells can grow progressively in immunocompetent hosts without inducing deletion or anergy of T cells specific for their antigens (40). Still other systems have demonstrated

transient stimulation of antitumor T-cell responses that fail to be maintained and do not generate memory (41). Although multiple outcomes of the interaction between the immune system and tumors have been observed, a common theme is that tumors are not good stimulators of immune responses and may be able to actively induce tolerance. Failure to observe deletional tolerance to tumor antigens provides encouragement that tumor-specific T cells exist in individuals with cancer.

TUMOR RESISTANCE TO IMMUNE RECOGNITION

The capacity of tumors to induce antigen-specific tolerance or ignorance is an area of active investigation. Circumstantial evidence supports the notion that the nature of the endogenous immune responses to antigens expressed by tumors often lies somewhere between the two extremes of immune tolerance and immune surveillance. The development of resistance mechanisms to immunologic recognition or killing by tumors can be taken as presumptive evidence for selective pressure placed on the tumor by the immune system. Several putative immunologic resistance mechanisms have been described in murine and human tumors (Table 72-4).

Defects in the expression of gene products necessary for the processing and presentation of major histocompatibility complex (MHC) class I–restricted tumor antigens are among the most commonly observed candidate mechanisms for resistance to immunologic recognition. In several experimental models, tumor variants that have lost MHC class I expression are more tumorigenic in immunocompetent animals than the parental line, whereas induction of MHC class I expression or transfection with MHC class I genes under constitutive promoter control reduces tumorigenicity in immunocompetent animals (42–44). Numerous analyses of human cancer have documented the frequent loss of MHC class I alleles on tumors (45–52). Expression of MHC class I antigens on tumors can also be lost through defects in expression of gene products involved in antigen processing and delivery of peptides to the MHC class I molecule. In particular, loss of expression of the *TAP* genes and downregulation of the MHC-encoded chromosome subunits *LMP2* and *LMP7* have been observed (53,54). Defects in other genes such as β_2-microglobulin have

TABLE 72-4. *Mechanisms of tumor resistance to immunologic recognition*

Decreased MHC class I expression
Decreased β_2-microglobulin expression
Decreased TAP expression
Antigen loss
Local production of inhibitory cytokines (e.g., TGF-β)
FASL expression
Mechanical (e.g., increased interstitial pressure)

been documented as a mechanism for loss of surface MHC class I expression (43,52).

T-cell responses against tumors appear to focus on a limited number of immunodominant antigens. Downmodulation of these immunodominant antigens, as opposed to downregulation of the antigen-presenting system, can also account for the outgrowth of resistant variants. Antigen-loss variants have been documented readily in murine tumor systems (55–60), and preliminary evidence for the selection of antigen-loss variants in human melanoma has been observed in association with peptide vaccines (61), suggesting that induced immunity can place selection pressures on tumors at the level of antigen expression.

Although it is tempting to conclude that downregulation of antigen processing and presentation molecules in the MHC class I pathway is a common mechanism used by tumors to cloak themselves from T-cell–dependent immune surveillance, other findings contradict this interpretation. Karre et al. documented experimental examples in which tumors lacking MHC class I expression are less tumorigenic than their MHC class I$^+$ counterparts (62,63). Immune surveillance of MHC class I$^-$ tumors is mediated by natural killer (NK) cells, which express killer inhibitory receptors (KIR) specific for MHC class I molecules (64,65). NK cells recognize a wide variety of cell types through incompletely defined receptors, and they become activated to kill them. However, activation is inhibited by the expression of MHC class I molecules that bind to constitutively expressed KIRs. Engagement of KIRs blocks NK activation. This recognition system whereby cells with low MHC class I expression are selectively recognized by NK cells probably represents a generalized counterresistance mechanism to attack viruses that interfere with antigen processing and MHC class I expression by infected cells.

Expression of FAS ligand (FASL) by tumor cells represents another potential mechanism of tumor resistance to T-cell attack (66,67). In some murine systems, FASL$^+$ tumors demonstrate decreased tumorigenicity in FAS-mutant mice, suggesting a functional role for FASL expression analogous to immunologically privileged tissues such as the testis and ovary. Secretion of cytokines by the tumor that inhibit immunologic priming can protect tumors from immune responses. One of the best examples of such a cytokine is transforming growth factor-β (TGF-β), a cytokine that checks inflammatory responses. Production of TGF-β by otherwise immunogenic tumors can drastically suppress priming of antitumor immunity (68). In the case of human tumors, the ultimate role of these mechanisms in providing resistance to endogenous immune surveillance requires confirmation.

TUMOR ANTIGENS RECOGNIZED BY THE IMMUNE SYSTEM

One of the most important endeavors in cancer immunology is the molecular definition of tumor antigens capable of being targeted by the immune system. In addition to helping understand mechanisms of interaction between immune system components and tumor cells, identification of tumor antigens provides the basis for antigen-specific immunotherapy.

Cancer genetics provide a molecular explanation for the existence of tumor antigens. Tumors arise from the accumulation of genetic alterations in genes that regulate cellular behavior such as cell cycle control and apoptosis. Alterations in critical "guardians of the genome" such as p53 provide tumors with an inherent genetic instability that causes them to accumulate large numbers of mutations and other genetic alterations, some of which contribute to the pathophysiology of tumor progression (69–71). Most of the genetic alterations in tumors probably do not affect the biology of the tumor but nonetheless provide potentially unique biochemical structures capable of being recognized by the immune system.

In addition to antigens derived from genetically altered gene products, epigenetic changes in gene expression within tumors provide an addition source of potential tumor antigens. These represent an important category of tumor antigens because their expression is common to many tumors rather than being unique to an individual tumor.

Shared tumor antigens can be categorized as shown in Table 72-5. One group of shared antigens is represented

TABLE 72-5. *Potential source of shared tumor antigens*

Category of antigen	Example
Oncogene product	HER-2/NEU (breast Ca, ovarian Ca)
	RAS codon 12 mutation (pancreas Ca, colon Ca)
	BCR/ABL rearrangement product (CML)
Reactivated embryonic gene products	SART-1 (squamous Ca)
	MAGE family (melanoma and breast Ca)
Viral gene products	EBV (Burkitt's lymphoma, nasopharyngeal Ca)
	HPV (cervical Ca)
	HBV (hepatocellular Ca)
Tissue-specific antigens	MART-1/Melan-A, gp1a, tyrosinase (melanoma)
Tumor suppressor gene product	P53

Ca, cancer; CML, chronic myelogenous leukemia; EBV, Epstein-Barr virus; HPV, human papillomavirus; HBV, hepatitis B virus.

by genes normally silent in most adult tissues (including the tissue of origin of the tumor) but transcriptionally activated in the tumor. Some genes in this category, such as *MAGEA1* through *MAGEA3* (formerly designated *MAGE1, MAGE2,* and *MAGE3*), are transcriptionally activated in subsets of tumors of diverse histologic type. Another group of shared tumor antigens is represented by tissue-specific antigens expressed by tumors arising from that tissue. Even when active antitumor immunity can be generated, only a few of the total set of antigens selectively or specifically expressed by a tumor are likely to be recognized by the immune system. Viral antigens associated with virus-induced cancer represent a growing category of candidate shared antigens as it becomes clear that a number of cancers in immunocompetent individuals are virus associated. As the study of cancer genetics defines critical mutations and alterations in expression of oncogenes or tumor suppressor genes, the products of these genes that are overexpressed in cancers or demonstrate mutations at common positions represent potential antigenic targets.

Tumor Antigens Recognized by Antibodies

Antibodies against tumor antigens are commonly observed in patients with cancer, as revealed by screening of phage display libraries with their antisera (72,73). Although the repertoire of tumor antigens recognized by antibodies from cancer patients appears to be diverse, most of these antibodies occur in low titers. Many are specific for intracellular antigens and therefore would not be of direct relevance in mediating an antitumor response. Almost all antibodies of defined specificity identified from cancer patients are against epitopes on self antigens (74), even those directed against mutant oncogene or tumor suppressor gene encoded proteins. The diversity of self-specific antibodies found in cancer patients probably indicates that self-tolerance is not stringently maintained in the humoral arm of the immune response. Self-specific antibodies are frequently observed transiently after infections and rarely have pathologic consequences. Similarly, there is little evidence that the broad spectrum of antitumor antibodies found in cancer patients participates in antitumor immunity. Nonetheless, because most antitumor antibodies are of IgG isotype, their induction reflects the participation of CD4$^+$ helper T cells (i.e., T$_H$1 and T$_H$2), and the set of antigens recognizable by antitumor antibodies may represent a useful group among which to identify a limited set of antigens recognized by T cells.

Tumor Antigens Recognized by T Cells

During the past 2 decades, there has been a shift of emphasis from humoral antitumor immunity to T-cell–dependent immunity. Much of the focus has been on MHC class I–restricted CD8$^+$ T-cell responses to tumors, because activated CD8$^+$ T cells are immunologic effectors for recognition of cell-associated antigens. The fact that CD8$^+$ T cells recognize small peptides derived from proteins presented by MHC class I molecules endows them with the potential to recognize epitopes derived from any protein expressed by the tumor cell. CD8$^+$ T cells are critical in most adoptive immunotherapy approaches that use tumor-specific T-cell lines, clones, or tumor-infiltrating lymphocytes. In animal models of antitumor immunity, many cancer vaccines display diminished efficacy in animals depleted of CD8$^+$ T cells or in CD8$^+$ knock-out mice (75–77).

Although most investigations of T-cell–dependent antitumor immunity have focused on CD8$^+$ cells and MHC class I–restricted antigens, experiments in CD4$^+$ cell–depleted or CD4$^+$ knock-out mice indicate that CD4$^+$ MHC class II–restricted responses are equally important in antitumor immunity (75–82). CD4$^+$ cells are critical in priming immune responses for virtually all antitumor vaccines. Even in tumors that are MHC class II$^-$, CD4$^+$ cells specific for MHC class II–restricted tumor antigens presented on bone marrow APCs are critical mediators of multiple effector functions besides induction of cytotoxic T lymphocytes (CTLs). For MHC class I$^-$ tumors, CD4$^+$ cells are important in ultimately generating NK-dependent responses. CD4$^+$ cells also activate antigen nonspecific effector arms, including generation of reactive oxygen intermediates by macrophages and T$_H$2-dependent eosinophil activation (76,83–86). It is important to identify MHC class I– and MHC class II–restricted antigens recognized by CD8$^+$ and CD4$^+$ cells, respectively.

Unique Tumor Antigens Recognized by T Cells

The first clear-cut evidence for tumor-specific rejection antigens came from the studies of Gross (87) and Prehn and Main (88), who worked with chemically induced murine tumors. They demonstrated that mice could be immunized against tumor challenge by vaccines employing the autologous tumor cells while normal cells from the tissue of origin failed to vaccinate against the tumor. These immunization and transplantation experiments demonstrated that the strongest immunologic protection against challenge with cancer cells was individually tumor specific. Immunization with one tumor protected most effectively against challenge with the same tumor, whereas protection against challenge with other tumors was absent or significantly diminished. These findings held even for cancers of the same histologic type induced by the same carcinogen. Old et al. first began to define these tumor rejection antigens on chemically induced tumors (89). Subsequently, Schreiber et al. generated CD8$^+$ and CD4$^+$ T-cell clones specific for a number of these tumors (90). They used the CTL clones to demonstrate formally that specificity was uniquely encoded by the immunizing tumor, because the CTLs did not recognize other tumors derived from the same strain of mouse.

Genetic and biochemical approaches have been used to identify the genes and peptides on tumor cells recognized by tumor-specific CTLs. A genetic approach pioneered by Boon and colleagues involves the screening of genomic or cDNA libraries derived from the tumor (91). Generally, the screening of cDNA libraries is now done by transient cotransfection of cDNA pools together with the gene encoding the restricting MHC class I molecule, followed by testing with tumor-specific CTLs. A biochemical strategy pioneered by Rotzschke et al. (92) and Van Bleek and Nathanson (93) employs acid elution of peptides from tumor MHC class I molecules and subsequent fractionation over a reversed-phase high-performance liquid chromatography (RP-HPLC) column using a gradient of hydrophobic solvent. Diluted peptide fractions are assayed for bioactivity by pulsing onto surrogate target cells that express the same MHC molecules as the tumor. Fractions containing peptides that sensitize the surrogate target cell for killing by the tumor-specific CTLs are then further purified by RP-HPLC and sequenced. Sequence is performed by mass spectrometry methods as applied by Cox et al. (94).

As predicted by cross-immunization and CTL recognition experiments, most of the MHC class I–restricted murine tumor antigens that have been identified are peptides containing altered amino acid sequences derived from mutations specific to the tumor. Two such unique antigens identified by Boon and colleagues in murine P815 mastocytoma cells illustrate the ability of point mutations to affect MHC and TCR binding. The P91A antigen is represented by a mutation in a housekeeping gene that changes arginine to histidine and confers *de novo* binding of the peptide to the MHC class I presenting molecule L^d (95). A second antigen, P198, creates a new epitope by an amino acid alteration directly affecting TCR interaction with the antigen bound to the MHC molecule (96). Mandelbaum et al. later identified a peptide antigen from Lewis lung carcinoma derived by a point mutation in the self protein connexin-37 (97), and Dubey et al. identified a tumor antigen derived from a mutation of a DNA helicase (98).

Using classic biochemical approaches for protein purification, a unique MHC class II–restricted antigen recognized by CD4 cells has been identified from a murine tumor. This antigen represents the product of a point mutation in the gene encoding a ribosomal subunit (99).

For human cancers, most information about tumor antigens recognized by endogenous T cells comes from melanoma, because tumor-reactive T cells are more easily cultured from melanoma patients than from patients with other tumors. This fact, together with the frequent responses of human melanoma to many immunothera-

pies, has earned it the label of *immunogenic tumor.* The relative immunogenicity of melanoma remains to be defined at the cellular and molecular levels.

The first identified MHC class I–restricted human melanoma antigen derived from the product of a mutated gene, was an HLA-B44–restricted peptide donated by the MUM1 gene. This gene product contained a point mutation within the region encoding the T-cell epitope and involving a residue responsible for TCR rather than MHC binding. The T-cell epitope was encoded by sequences spanning an intron-exon boundary derived from an incompletely spliced message (100).

Another melanoma-specific CD8$^+$ T-cell clone was found to recognize a peptide derived from a mutation in the cyclin-dependent kinase-4 (CDK4) gene and was restricted by HLA-A2. This gene product contained a point mutation that appeared to enhance the affinity of the T-cell epitope for HLA-A2 (101). Because CDK4 appears to play a major role in cell cycle regulation, the mutated CDK4 protein that donated the T-cell epitope was analyzed for its ability to bind the tumor suppressor gene *p16*^{INK4a} (102). The recognized mutation was found to be physiologically relevant in that it interfered with binding of p16^{INK4a}. This mutation in CDK4 was identified in a second melanoma and therefore appears to be an infrequent alternative mechanism for inactivation of the p16/CDK4 pathway in melanoma.

A third unique MHC class I–restricted melanoma antigen derives from a mutation in the β-catenin gene that donates an altered peptide restricted by HLA-A24 (103). β-catenin has been implicated in tumorigenesis based on its binding to E-cadherins and to the adenomatous polyposis coli *(APC)* tumor suppressor gene (104–106). The mutation in β-catenin recognized by the HLA-A24–restricted melanoma T-cell clone affected its biologic function within this pathway (107).

A unique MHC class I–restricted antigen has been identified from a squamous cell carcinoma of the head and neck. This unique antigen, restricted by HLA-A31, represents a point mutation in a critical regulator of apoptosis, the caspase-8 gene *(CASP8)* (108). The mutant caspase-8 gene was demonstrated to be functionally impaired in its ability to mediate apoptosis and therefore may represent a genetic alteration relevant to the biology of the tumor.

A high proportion of unique tumor-specific antigens identified as recognized by T cells represents mutations that may have direct functional relevance to neoplasia. Because there are presumably far more "neoantigens" in tumors created by nonphysiologically relevant genetic alterations, it is hard to imagine that the preponderance of functionally relevant mutations among the pool of tumor antigens recognized by tumor-specific T cells is coincidence. One intriguing explanation is related to the concept of immune surveillance. If the immune system is at least partially able to respond to new epitopes arising during the transformation process, clones that accumulate mutations that generate a strong neoantigen may be selected against. For these clones to survive in the face of an antagonistic immune response, the mutation would have to confer a biologic advantage that would counterbalance the negative selective pressure conferred by immunologic recognition of the neoantigen.

Nonmutated Shared Tumor Antigens

Although cross-protection experiments with murine tumors suggested that the most immunogenic tumor antigens were unique, lower levels of cross-protection are observed in a number of instances, suggesting the existence of shared tumor antigens. Most "shared" tumor antigens isolated from murine tumors arise from reactivation of genes normally not expressed in adult tissues. The first of this type to be isolated was the P1A antigen from the P815 murine mastocytoma (109). P1A appears to be transcriptionally activated in certain murine tumors and in transformed mast cell lines through demethylation at the promoter region.

A second example of a shared tumor antigen in this category is the gp70 gene identified as an immunodominant MHC class I–restricted antigen in the carcinogen-induced murine colorectal carcinoma CT26 (110). This gp70 is derived from one of two *env* genes from an endogenous retrovirus. It is transcriptionally silent in most tissues in BALB/c mice (the strain of origin of CT26) and appears to be reactivated in several BALB/c-derived tumors and in tumors derived from other mouse strains. Endogenous retroviral gene products are frequent targets of antitumor immune responses in murine models (111–115). The documented existence of endogenous human retroviral sequences (116–119), some of which become transcriptionally activated in human cancer (120–122), make these an intriguing set of candidate, nonmutated, shared, human tumor antigens. Although antibodies against human endogenous retroviral antigens have been observed in some patients with cancer (120,123), T-cell responses against them have not been documented.

In humans, this category of shared antigen has been identified by a number of melanoma-specific CD8⁺ T-cell clones. The best characterized example is the *MAGEA* gene family. This is a multigene family containing at least 12 members whose expression in normal adult tissues appears to be restricted to the testis. A number of family members are transcriptionally active in melanoma and other tumors (124–128). *MAGEA1* and *MAGEA3* encode peptides recognized by melanoma-specific CD8⁺ T cells. MAGEA-3–specific CD4⁺ cells have also been identified. The *MAGEA* gene family represents a prototype for a number of tumor antigens recognized by T cells whose expression is largely restricted to tumor and testis (sometimes referred to as cancer-testis antigens). Other examples of this category of tumor antigens, called BAGE and GAGE, have been identified (129,130).

All the shared melanoma antigens of this type have been identified with T cells of a single patient. Reactivity in most melanoma patients to this category of antigen is relatively infrequent, even though these antigens are commonly expressed in the melanoma. The basis for the uniquely frequent T-cell reactivity against this category of antigen in the one patient from which MAGEA, BAGE, and GAGE were identified is unknown, but it may be related to the fact the this patient was vaccinated with a mutagenized autologous melanoma vaccine before deriving the melanoma-specific T cells (131). The vaccination process might have revealed T-cell reactivities normally cryptic in unvaccinated melanoma patients.

Tissue-Specific Antigens Expressed by Tumors

One of the greatest surprises to come from identification of melanoma-specific antigens recognized by T cells is that most T-cell lines and clones derived from melanoma patients recognize nonmutated peptides derived from melanocyte-specific antigens. This was unexpected for two reasons. First, this category of antigen has infrequently been detected in antigen screens in murine models. Second, T cells specific for self antigens could be deleted or functionally tolerated.

The first tissue-specific antigen identified by MHC class I–restricted melanoma-reactive CD8⁺ cells was the melanosomal protein tyrosinase, which is the central enzyme in melanin biosynthesis (132–137). Subsequently, other melanosomal proteins were identified as antigens. HLA-A2–restricted peptides from two of these melanosome-associated antigens, MART-1/Melan-A and gp100, appear to be recognized by T cells from a high percentage of HLA-A2 patients and often represent dominant reactivities within CTL lines derived by *in vitro* stimulation by HLA-A2⁺ tumors (94,138–144). Two overlapping peptide epitopes have been identified from the MART-1/Melan-A molecule, one of which was isolated by elution from the surface of melanoma cells. Five HLA-A2 epitopes have been identified from gp100, one by elution of peptides from the melanoma cell surface. Other melanosome proteins, TRP-1 and TRP-2, have also been identified by melanosome-specific MHC class I–restricted T cells (145,146).

Analysis of binding affinities of MHC class I–restricted melanoma peptides reveals that the peptides derived from the melanocyte-specific antigens display significantly lower affinity for their MHC-restricting element than do classic viral antigens (94). In most cases, this can be attributed to nondominant MHC anchor residues at the second or last position. Modification of the anchor residues within peptide epitopes from gp100 were found to significantly increase binding affinity for HLA-A2. These modified anchor peptides appear to be more immunogenic *in vitro* than the wild-type gp100 peptide (147).

Tyrosinase is a shared MHC class II–restricted human melanoma antigen recognized by CD4+ T cells (148). Tyrosinase-specific CD4+ T cells recognize at least two distinct HLA-DR4–restricted tyrosinase peptides. Similar to the case of many CD8+ T-cell–recognized melanocyte antigens, high concentrations of peptides were required to stimulate the MHC class II–restricted tyrosinase CD4+ T cells described earlier, whereas modification of potential anchor residues to conform to DR4 binding motifs enhanced binding and shifted the dose response curve for T-cell recognition by 100- to 1,000-fold relative to the wild-type unmodified peptides (149). As these results suggest, even though T cells specific for tissue antigens are the most commonly observed specificity in melanoma patients, those that can be grown *in vitro* represent subsets specific for peptide antigens that are inefficiently presented on self MHC molecules. This low-reactivity T-cell population may represent a functionally cryptic population that escapes immune tolerance, whereas T-cell populations reactive with high-affinity tissue-specific self peptides may have been actively tolerated *in vivo* and unable to be established as long-term lines or clones *in vitro*.

Oncogene and Tumor Suppressor Gene Products as Tumor Antigens

Because of their central role in tumorigenesis, commonly altered oncogene and tumor suppressor gene products (150–153) represent tantalizing targets for antitumor immunity. Antibody and T-cell responses to oncogene and tumor suppressor gene products have been documented. The most intensively studied tumor suppressor gene product as a candidate tumor antigen is p53, the most commonly altered gene in cancer (154–161). It has been well documented that the immune system is capable of responding to p53. In the same year that p53 was discovered as a cellular protein that specifically binds viral oncogenes, it was also discovered as a tumor antigen in a murine sarcoma recognized by serum antibodies from mice inoculated with the sarcoma (162–164). Subsequent studies demonstrated a high prevalence of anti-p53 antibodies in cancer patients (165–169). Because p53 is an intracellular protein, anti-p53 antibodies do not have direct therapeutic relevance for intact tumors. However, their existence can be taken as a sign that immunologic tolerance to p53 as a self antigen can at least be partially disrupted in cancer patients.

Studies using animal models have focused on the T-cell response to p53 (170–172). In the original murine sarcoma from which p53 was identified serologically, there is a mutant p53 gene. The sarcoma could be recognized by MHC class I–restricted CD8+ T cells specific for a peptide that encompasses the mutation (173). Noguchi et

al. have shown that immunization of animals with this mutant peptide mixed with the QS21 adjuvant together with interleukin-12 (IL-12) protects against challenge with the sarcoma (174). However, cancer immunotherapy aimed specifically at p53 mutations would be impractical. Although there are hot-spot regions of mutation for p53, any single p53 mutation is present in a very small fraction of human cancers. The idea of wild-type p53 as a potential target for T-cell immunotherapy has gained attention (175).

At first glance, a ubiquitous protein such as p53 may seem to be a terrible target because of its expression in normal tissues. However, many of the p53 mutations found in cancer result in a protein that, although inactive, is expressed at significantly higher levels than in normal tissues. This is because p53 protein levels are highly regulated posttranslationally through proteolysis. Although wild-type p53 protein has a very short half-life and is usually undetectable or barely detectable in normal cells, many of the mutations of p53 found in tumors interfere with its degradation, leading to significantly elevated levels of protein.

Vierboom et al. demonstrated experimentally that cytotoxic T lymphocytes specific for an MHC class I–restricted wild-type peptide can create a therapeutic window when adoptively transferred into animals bearing a p53-overexpressing tumor (175). They were able to show eradication of established tumor on adoptive transfer of p53 specific CTL clones, and despite persistence of the p53 specific CTL, there was no evidence of autoimmune attack against normal tissues. Producing specific T-cell responses against nonmutated p53 epitopes in an individual with a p53-expressing tumor could have significant therapeutic benefit with tolerable collateral damage to normal tissues expressing lower levels of p53.

Although demonstrating a potential window at the effector phase, the murine study described points out an important barrier to immunotherapy involving self antigens such as p53 or tissue-specific antigens: tolerance. To produce p53-specific T-cell clones for the adoptive transfer experiments, they had to immunize p53−/− mice. The same immunization procedure in wild-type mice fails to produce p53-specific T cells. In p53−/− mice, p53 is recognized as a foreign antigen by the immune system, whereas in wild-type mice, tolerance to p53 as a self antigen precludes the generation of p53-specific responses.

The most extensively studied oncogene product as a candidate tumor antigen is RAS. Mutations in RAS are less complex than in p53, and most activate mutations falling at residues 12, 13, or 61 (151,152). The high frequency of these mutations in colon cancer (40%) and pancreatic cancer (90%) makes them promising targets if T-cell responses against peptides containing the mutations could be elicited. Previous studies showed that T-cell immunity to RAS could be elicited by immunization to RAS peptides spanning the mutant segment. CD4+ and

CD8$^+$ T-cell responses and responses to mutant peptides have been identified in murine and human model systems. In one study, 32% of patients with colon cancer and 3% of controls produced anti-RAS antibodies. As with p53, most recognized wild-type epitopes.

Antibodies and T cells specific for mutant RAS have been identified in patients with gastrointestinal cancer (176–183). In one patient with colon cancer, CD4$^+$ and CD8$^+$ T cells responding to the less frequent RAS ^{13}Gly→Asp mutation were identified (179). However, this mutation was not identified in the patient's tumor, implying that RAS ^{13}Gly→Asp$^+$ cells had been eliminated or that the immune responses were unrelated to the cancer. Another study detected CD4 T cells specific for the common position 12 mutation found in the patient's cancer, suggesting that T-cell responses can be primed against the patient's mutant RAS protein expressed in autochthonous tumor cells (181). These findings are reminiscent of the melanoma specific T-cell responses specific for CDK4 or β-catenin.

One additional oncogene that is being evaluated as a target for antitumor immunity is *HER2/NEU,* a membrane tyrosine kinase receptor in the epidermal growth factor receptor (EGFR) family. The HER2/NEU product is normally expressed at relatively low levels on mammary, ovarian, and other epithelium. Its expression is significantly increased on a number of carcinomas, particularly breast and ovarian cancer (184). In contrast to p53, HER2/NEU is not mutated in most cancers; the basis for HER2/NEU upregulation on tumors is increased transcription or gene amplification. Nonetheless, the same arguments for differential recognition of cancer cells based on increased expression are valid with HER2/NEU as with p53. CD8$^+$ T cells specific for HLA-A2–restricted HER2/NEU peptides can be grown from cancer patients, and in some cases, they can be shown to recognize HER2/NEU$^+$ tumor cells of many types *in vitro* (185–188). In addition to classic cell-mediated immunity, HER2/NEU represents an uncommon example of a tumor associated antigen for which humoral immunity may provide clinical benefit. The cell membrane location provides access to antibodies, and ligation of HER2/NEU with antibody appears to trigger signaling with resultant growth inhibition (189). This property has provided the basis for treatment of HER2/NEU$^+$ cancers with monoclonal anti-HER2/NEU antibodies (190).

Viral Antigens as Tumor Antigens in Virus-Associated Tumors

As an increasing number of human cancers have been associated with specific viruses, viral antigens have reemerged as important tumor associated antigens. Most cancers in immunodeficient individuals are virus associated; EBV-associated lymphoma and human herpesvirus 8–associated Kaposi's sarcoma are the most common.

Several important cancers that develop in immunocompetent individuals are associated with viral infections. In individuals with no obvious immunodeficiency, EBV infection has been linked to cancers such as Burkitt's lymphoma (191,192), Hodgkin's lymphoma (193–196), and nasopharyngeal carcinoma (197–200).

The two most common cancers worldwide, hepatoma and cervical cancer, are clearly associated with viral infection. In the case of hepatoma, hepatitis B virus (HBV) (201,202) has been implicated as the etiologic agent. Expression of viral gene products within hepatomas is variable and inconsistent (203,204), and it is unresolved whether HBV-induced carcinogenesis involves oncogene activation by integrated virus, direct effects of viral gene products, or chronic hepatitis with cycles of hepatocellular injury and regeneration that increase the number of hepatocytes at risk for subsequent transformation events. In contrast, 80% to 90% of cervical cancers express the E6 and E7 antigens from one of four so-called high-risk human papillomavirus types: HPV-16, HPV-18, HPV-31, and HPV-45 (23–25).

For virus-associated cancers in immunocompetent individuals, the E6 and E7 antigens in HPV-associated cervical cancer provide the most promising targets for a number of reasons. First, they are expressed by most cervical cancers. Second, because E6 and E7 are oncogenes essential to the transformed phenotype, tumors must maintain their expression. E6 binds p53 (205) resulting in inactivation and enhanced degradation (206,207) while E7 binds and inactivates a second tumor supresor pRb (208). The propensity of a particular HPV type to cause cervical cancer is in part related to the ability of its E6 and E7 to bind p53 and pRb, respectively. p53 and pRb inactivation, because of initial HPV infection, cause precancerous squamous intraepithelial lesions (23). These represent the *in vivo* correlate of *in vitro* immortalization of cells by E6 and E7 (209). In some individuals, additional transformation events produce invasive cervical cancer.

Critical questions surrounding virus-associated cancers in immunocompetent individuals are how the virus avoids immunologic elimination at the time of initial infection and the mechanism of immune tolerance to viral antigens that are persistently expressed in the tumor. Undoubtedly, the answers to these questions vary for different viruses and different target tissues. In the case of HPV, virtually all infected women develop antibody responses to capsid antigens, to E7, and to a variable extent, E6 (210–221). Most infected women ultimately clear their HPV and do not develop cervical cancer. In a fraction of infected women, HPV integration into cervical epithelial cells occurs and E6 and E7 expression increases (because of disruption of the E2 gene, whose product negatively regulates E6 and E7 gene transcription), causing precancerous proliferative foci called squamous intraepithelial lesions (SILs) (222,223). Most low-grade SILs heal without intervention, but roughly 10%

progress to more dysplastic, high-grade SILs, which are likely to progress to invasive cancer. E6- and E7-specific antibody titers are not predictive. Despite reports of the ability to generate *in vitro* CTL responses against E7 (including specific peptides presented by common HLA types such as HLA-A2), it is unclear whether clearance or progression correlates with activation or tolerance induction among HPV-specific T cells (224–231).

Loss of transporter associated with antigen processing (TAP-1) expression is fairly common in cervical cancers (232), but it remains to be determined how important this mechanism is in resistance to endogenous or vaccine-induced antitumor immunity. A small study of vaccinated patients with advanced cervical cancer with recombinant vaccinia-expressing E6 and E7 showed increased HPV-specific antibody responses attributable to vaccination in three of eight vaccinees, with one of three evaluable patients generating HPV-specific CTL responses post-vaccination (233). In contrast, a clinical trial using two HLA-A2–restricted E7 peptides plus a helper peptide in adjuvant failed to demonstrate induction of enhanced CTL responses against the vaccinating peptides (234). More extensive vaccination studies of patients with earlier-stage lesions are critical for determining whether therapeutically useful responses to HPV E6 and E7 can be elicited.

A different situation is found in EBV-associated Hodgkin's disease. EBV DNA has been observed in mixed cellularity and nodular sclerosing Hodgkin's disease. Polymerase chain reaction analysis of Reed-Sternberg cells, the true neoplastic cell in Hodgkin's disease, reveals that only one EBV gene product, LMP-1, is expressed (235). EBV-specific CTLs have been generated that recognize Reed-Sternberg cells (236). Regression of EBV lymphomas on immune reconstitution of immunodeficient patients depends largely on T-cell responses to multiple additional EBV gene products expressed in these tumors (237,238).

TUMOR ANTIGEN IMMUNODOMINANCE AND THE TUMOR REJECTION ANTIGEN

The obvious therapeutic implications of tumor antigen identification are related to the development of cancer vaccines. There is increasing interest in the development of antigen-specific vaccines for cancer that use shared tumor antigens rather than the tumor cell itself in creating the vaccine. The development of tumor vaccines can be operationally divided into identification of the most potent "tumor rejection antigens" and the route or vehicle (i.e., adjuvant) by which the antigen is delivered to the immune system. The concept of tumor rejection antigens originally arose in the context of early murine tumor transplant studies using relatively immunogenic tumors (239–243). The most highly immunogenic tumors, called regressor tumors, displayed a phenotype of immunologi-

cally mediated regression after a period of growth in unvaccinated syngeneic animals. The existence of tumor rejection antigens was surmised from studies in which variants of these tumors could be generated that displayed decreased immunogenicity and were postulated to represent antigen-loss variants (56–59).

The notion that loss of tumor rejection antigens was responsible for the generation of tumor variants with lower immunogenicity was confirmed at the cellular level. CD8+ CTL clones specific for the original tumor failed to recognize the "antigen loss" variant even when levels of surface of MHC class I were unchanged (57). Ultimately, the direct molecular identification of CTL recognized antigens in the P815 tumor system by Van den Eynde et al. (109) allowed for the direct demonstration of correlation between loss of expression of particular antigens and loss of immunogenicity.

A related concept to emerge from the analysis of murine tumors recognized by T cells is that of antigen immunodominance. The concept of immunodominance refers to the phenomenon that the immune response induced by immunization or infection with a complex set of antigens is largely restricted to a very small number of the total potentially recognizable epitopes (244). Immunodominance has been observed in many systems, ranging from homogeneous protein antigens to complex viruses to the most complex set of antigens of all—a tumor cell. An example of immunodominance can be seen in the murine CT26 tumor. When mice are immunized with genetically modified CT26 vaccines, virtually all of the antitumor CD8 response is directed toward a single peptide derived from the gp70 antigen and presented on L^d (110).

Several parameters can affect immunodominance (244) (Fig. 72-2). The most obvious is the affinity of the peptide epitope for MHC alleles expressed by the host. More important than overall affinity, the dissociation constant k_{off} of the peptide is the most important variable in determining the density of peptide–MHC complex on the surfaces of a tumor or APC available for recognition by T cells. Mere MHC binding fails to predict immunodominance. The immunodominant epitopes from many protein antigens are not the peptides with the highest affinity for MHC.

Another variable that influences immunodominance is antigen processing. Not all regions of a particular protein are processed equally by the proteolytic machinery responsible for a generation of MHC class I– and class II–restricted peptides. The sites of cleavage by the proteosome (for MHC class II–restricted antigens) and the endosomal acid proteases (for MHC class I–restricted peptides) relative to a potential epitope can affect the availability of that epitope for association with MHC molecules. The repertoire of T cells expressing TCRs with moderate to high affinity for a particular peptide–MHC complex is an important parameter in immunodominance. The available T-cell repertoire is determined

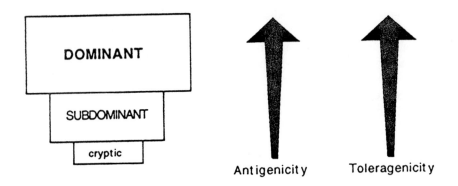

Determinants of Antigenicity

1) Processing
2) k_{on}/k_{off} for peptide and MHC
3) k_{on}/k_{off} for peptide/MHC and TCR
4) T cell repertoire (freq of moderate - high affinity TCR)

FIG. 72-2. Parameters that define the potency of a tumor rejection antigen.

by the forces of positive and negative selection in the thymus and for self antigens is further modified by peripheral mechanisms of tolerance induction.

Although the spectrum of tumor antigens recognized by antibodies appears to be much broader than that recognized by T cells, there is nonetheless evidence for a relatively small number of tumor antigens against which high-titer antibodies are generated. For example, when antiserum from rats immunized for the Dunning prostate tumor was used to probe Dunning tumor lysates by Western blotting, a single dominant protein from the Dunning tumor was recognized (245).

It is often assumed that the immunodominant tumor antigens recognized by antibodies or T cells from the tumor-bearing host or from vaccinated patients represent the best tumor rejection antigens, but this may not be the case. For example, one of the immunodominant antigens recognized by CD8+ T cells after vaccination with P815 vaccines is the P1A antigen. However, vaccination against P1A fails to generate strong systemic anti-P815 immunity despite the elicitation of CTLs specific for P1A (246). Likewise, the melanosomal antigens gp100 and MART-1/Melan-A would be considered immunodominant in human melanoma based on the high frequency of patients containing T cells specific for them. However, because the immunodominant epitopes bind relatively poorly to HLA-A2, these antigens may not elicit high-affinity T-cell responses capable of rejecting tumors. MART-1/Melan A– and gp100-specific CD8+ T cells can be readily grown from tumor-infiltrating lymphocytes and peripheral blood of patients with progressive melanoma (247), indicating that the mere presence of detectable endogenous CTL activity is insufficient to control the tumor. In considering the concept of tumor rejection antigens and tumor rejection, it must be remembered that CD4+ MHC class II–restricted T cells are a critical mediator of effector responses and that they must effectively collaborate with CD8+ T cells in providing appropriate help.

PRINCIPLES OF CANCER VACCINATION

Most efforts to enhance antitumor immunity fall into the category of "active immunotherapy," commonly referred to as cancer vaccines. Cancer vaccines involve the presentation of a cancer antigen or antigens to a patient in a way that activates immunity against these antigens *in vivo*.

There are several important differences between cancer vaccines and the standard infectious disease vaccines that are widely administered (248). First, infectious disease vaccines are prophylactic, inducing protective immunity in an immune system not previously exposed to the antigen. In contrast, current cancer vaccination uses therapeutic vaccines for which the patient's immune system has for years been exposed to the same antigens in the vaccine. High-affinity T cells specific for these tumor antigens may be functionally tolerated (249). Second, generation of neutralizing humoral immunity is the most important feature for virtually all effective prophylactic vaccines against infectious agents. In contrast, although antibodies against antigens in the tumor are often observed in cancer patients without vaccination and are sometimes boosted after vaccination, humoral immunity plays a much smaller role in overall antitumor immunity. Most of the focus in cancer vaccine development has been on the generation of antigen-specific T-cell responses. Third, by their very nature, infectious organisms represent a much smaller and simpler set of antigens. It is therefore relatively easy to identify immunodominant antigens within the set of expressed gene products for a virus or simple bacterium. In contrast, the complexity of potential antigenic epitopes provided by a tumor presents a much greater challenge in the identification of relevant immunodominant tumor rejection antigens.

One of the central principles in any vaccine is that the quantitative and qualitative nature of the elicited immune response depends on targeting of the immunizing antigen to appropriate APCs. This follows from the general principle that T-cell responses depend on the co-stimulatory signals provided by the APCs. To successfully activate antigen-specific immunity, the vaccinating antigen must be efficiently targeted to activated bone marrow–derived APCs that effectively process and present peptides and express co-stimulatory molecules such as B7 and IL-12. In addition to determining quantitative parameters of T-cell activation, characteristics of the APCs and the priming environment also probably determine qualitative aspects of T-cell activation. For cancer vaccines, there has been much focus on the activation of T_H1-type responses that lead to CTL generation. Although CTLs are important antitumor effectors, evidence is mounting that other effector arms, such as macrophage activation (through an IFN-γ–dependent T_H1 pathway) and eosinophil activation (through an IL-4/IL-5–dependent T_H2 pathway) are equally important in antitumor immunity (86). The most effective cancer vaccines probably simultaneously activate multiple effector pathways that act in concert.

Depending on the type of vaccine, targeting antigens to appropriate APCs can be accomplished through several pathways. The first pathway for targeting vaccinating antigen to bone marrow–derived APCs is the exogenous pathway of antigen uptake. This pathway, operative with most cell-based and protein-based vaccines, depends largely on the adjuvant with which the tumor cell or tumor antigen is formulated. The adjuvant is a critical component of a vaccine. It is the vaccine component that attracts and activates APCs to the site of vaccination, which they process the antigen. The original complex adjuvants, such as bacillus Calmette-Guérin (BCG) and *Corynebacterium parvum*, are beginning to be replaced by more defined chemical entities, including cytokines. Enhanced understanding of how particular cytokines and other signals mediate differentiation of APCs allows design of molecular adjuvants that can activate more potent and qualitatively distinct immune responses.

Studies have demonstrated that tumor antigens endocytosed by bone marrow–derived APCs are introduced into the MHC class II processing pathway and the MHC class I processing pathway, a system called *cross-priming* (250). The mechanism by which exogenous antigens taken up by bone marrow–derived APCs are transferred to the MHC class I processing pathway remains to be elucidated. *In vitro* and *in vivo* experiments suggest a pathway whereby antigens are transferred from the endosomal compartment to the cytosol, allowing them to be processed and presented through the standard proteosome/TAP pathway (251,252). Antigens in particulate form, such as those associated with dying tumor cells, may preferentially enter the cross-priming pathway. There is also evidence to support the idea that association with certain heat shock proteins, such as gp96, may facilitate cross-priming (253,254). The ability of endocytosed antigen to be targeted to the MHC class I and class II processing pathways enables a single APC to present antigenic epitopes to CD4$^+$ and CD8$^+$ T cells, thereby facilitating provision of CD4$^+$ help to CD8$^+$ cells. This occurs through CD4$^+$-derived lymphokines and through the APC itself by means of the CD40L-CD40 pathway (255).

A second pathway for introduction of antigen into appropriate bone marrow–derived APCs is by direct transduction. This pathway probably is operative in recombinant viral and bacterial vaccines and nucleic acid vaccines. For viruses and intracellular bacteria, infection of APCs allows the endogenous production of antigen directly within the APC. The design of recombinant viruses and bacteria must reflect the relationship between the cellular compartment to which the nascent antigen will be targeted and the consequent processing pathway. For example, a cytoplasmic antigen produced by a recombinant viral vaccine infecting an APC can be efficiently processed through the MHC class I pathway but not the MHC class II pathway.

A third pathway for targeting antigens to APCs is putatively operative in peptide vaccines. In this case, peptide can load empty MHC molecules on the surface of APCs, thereby bypassing the processing steps. For all of the pathways of APC loading, the two interrelated parameters that determine outcome in terms of immunologic priming are the density of peptide–MHC complexes able to be displayed on the APC and the particular co-stimulatory molecules (membrane and secreted) expressed by the APC.

Cell-Based Cancer Vaccines

We do not know which tumor rejection antigens are critical for most human cancers. For this reason, most cancer vaccine approaches have employed tumor cells themselves as a source of antigen, modified in various ways to enhance immunity. The validity of cell-based cancer vaccine approaches depends on the idea that, if the entire set of potential tumor antigens is presented to the immune system in an immunogenic fashion, stronger immunity can develop against tumor-specific or tumor-selective antigens than against ubiquitously expressed self antigens within the tumor. For any cell-based vaccine to provide selective antitumor immunity without concomitant induction of unacceptable autoimmunity, immune tolerance against tumor-specific or tumor-selective antigens must be inherently less stringent and therefore more easily broken by appropriate immunization than tolerance against the ubiquitous self antigens expressed by the tumor.

Early generations of cell-based cancer vaccines have consisted of killed tumor cells or tumor cell lysates mixed with adjuvants such as BCG and *C. parvum* in an attempt to amplify tumor-specific immune responses enough to produce a therapeutically relevant tumoricidal effect (256–259). Subsequently, genetically modified tumor vaccines replaced tumor-BCG mixtures. The forerunner to these studies involved the genetic modification of tumor cells by the introduction of "foreign antigens." The first studies demonstrating enhanced immunogenicity of genetically altered tumor cells were performed 25 years ago by Lindenman and Klein (260). They showed that vaccination with influenza virus–infected tumor cell lysates generated enhanced systemic immune responses against a challenge with the original tumor cells, an effect often referred to as *xenogenization.*

A later version of this approach involved the transduction of tumor cells with specific viral genes such as influenza hemagglutinin. Hemagglutinin-expressing tumor clones were capable of being rejected by their syngeneic hosts, whereas the nontransduced cells formed tumors without any evident immunologic response. In some cases, animals that had rejected the tumor transfectants became immune to challenge with nontransfected tumor cells (261). A variation on this theme involved the introduction of allogeneic MHC genes into tumor cells (262,263). Originally, investigators invoked the associative recognition theory to explain this effect, proposing that weak antigens derived from the tumor cells might become associated with or somehow linked to the more potent viral antigen and thereby elicit immunologic responses against them (261). However, the associative recognition theory has not found a molecular basis. The revised concept is that the xenogenization effect occurs because of induction of helper lymphokines in response to the strong foreign antigens expressed in the vicinity of the tumor.

The most actively studied form of genetically modified cell-based vaccine takes advantage of the large set of cytokine genes (75–77,81,264–275) and genes encoding co-stimulatory molecules such as B7 (276–278). The first cytokine genes to be introduced into tumor cells were IL-2 and IL-4. The inflammatory responses induced by the high local secretion of cytokines in these models often result in the ultimate destruction of the transduced tumor cells. Over the past few years, numerous reports have analyzed various biologic effects of injections of tumors transduced with multiple different cytokine genes. Among the most important features emphasized by all of these studies is that the locally sustained release of cytokines produces dramatic local inflammatory effects without significant evidence of systemic effects or toxic-

ity. Although the pharmacokinetics of different cytokines vary tremendously, it is rare to detect significant amounts of cytokine in the serum, even after injection of large numbers of transduced cells secreting high amounts of cytokine.

Because of the wide range of local inflammatory and vaccine effects of cytokine-secreting tumors and other parameters such as secretion rate affecting experimental outcome, a study was done using retroviral vectors to screen the immunologic effects of a large range of cytokine genes introduced into tumor cells (77). This comparative study demonstrated that GM-CSF–transduced tumor vaccines generated the most potent systemic immunity against tumor challenge. The uniquely enhanced immunologic effect of paracrine GM-CSF in multiple tumor vaccine models was related specifically to its role in inducing local dendritic cell differentiation at the vaccine site. GM-CSF has been identified as a factor critical in inducing the differentiation of primitive hematopoietic precursors into APC-type dendritic cells, distinct from macrophages and granulocytes, that are most potent at initiating T-cell responses (279–281). *In vitro* differentiation of hematopoetic progenitors into dendritic cells generally requires at least 6 days of culture in the presence of GM-CSF. Because dendritic cells are thought to be the primary cell necessary for activating virgin T cells, their role in priming immunologic responses is considered central.

Antigen-Specific Cancer Vaccines

Virus-induced tumors can display a variety of MHC-bound peptides of viral origin on their cell surface. Likewise, the shared melanoma antigens against which T-cell responses have been identified provide the bases for antigen-specific melanoma vaccines. During the past 10 years, a rapidly expanding set of peptide-based, protein-based, and recombinant antigen-specific approaches have been developed and are being tested in animal models of cancer and early-stage clinical trials in human cancer.

Vaccination with Major Histocompatibility Complex Class I Binding Peptides

The first form of antigen-specific cancer vaccine to be tested clinically used specific peptides presented by common human leukocyte antigen (HLA) alleles. Almost all peptide-based vaccines employ MHC class I–restricted antigenic peptides. Protective CTL responses induced by vaccination with MHC class I binding peptides were first reported for viruses such as lymphocytic choriomeningitis virus (LCMV) and Sendai virus (282,283). In these studies, the antiviral effect was obtained by subcutaneous vaccination with single MHC class I binding peptides in incomplete Freund's adjuvant (IFA). When applied to certain murine tumor models, vaccination with MHC class I binding immunogenic peptides resulted in induction of protective immunity. For example, prevention of outgrowth of an HPV-16–induced tumor was achieved by vaccination with an MHC class I–restricted HPV-16 E7 peptide in IFA (284). Similarly, vaccination with either of two tumor-associated mutant connexin-37 peptides from Lewis lung carcinoma emulsified in IFA or loaded on to RMA-S cells as a vaccine induced protection against metastatic tumor spread (285).

The basis for peptide vaccination is the administration of high doses of peptide that could load empty MHC molecules on APCs *in vivo*. However, simple administration of peptide without a means of targeting APCs can potentially lead to loading of MHC class I molecules on "nonprofessional" APCs, which could induce tolerance. Administration of some peptides at high doses by an intraperitoneal route induced immunologic tolerance rather than protective immunity. This was first shown with an LCMV peptide (286), and this principle has been used to prevent autoimmune diabetes in a transgenetic mouse model (287). Although some peptides can induce protective immunity when introduced in IFA, other peptides failed to produce protective immunity across a wide dose range. This phenomenon was observed in a murine tumor model for two adenoviral derived peptides that constitute major T-cell epitopes of adenovirus-induced tumors in C57BL/6 mice. CTLs against these peptides raised by immunization with irradiated tumor cells were capable of eradicating large, established tumors after intravenous infusion into tumor-bearing nude mice (288). In contrast, vaccination with a wide range of doses of the same adenoviral peptide caused enhanced outgrowth of subsequently transplanted tumors. The increased tumor growth was paralleled by specific tolerance induction for the injected peptide epitope (289).

Based on these mixed results, a number of efforts are underway to present peptides in a more immunogenic fashion. Several groups have attempted to modify peptides through conjugation to lipids as a means of preferential targeting to APCs (290,291). One of the most active approaches has been to combine the use of dendritic cells with culture in GM-CSF and IL-4 with peptide loading. Successful immunization with this approach depends on efficient homing of *ex vivo* peptide-loaded dendritic cells back to lymph nodes. At least some level of lymph node homing of *ex vivo* generated dendritic cells subsequent to reinjection has been demonstrated in murine and primate models (292,293), providing a basis for *ex vivo* peptide-loaded dendritic cell vaccines.

Recombinant Viral Vaccines

The intrinsic immunogenicity of viruses together with the development of standard techniques to engineer recombinant viruses has engendered broad interest in recombinant viral vaccines. Based on the early work of Moss' and Paoletti's groups (294,295), recombinant vaccinia and other poxviruses have been the lead agents in cancer vaccines (296–298). Adenoviral and other viruses are being applied for cancer immunotherapy (299–301). The common denominator for all recombinant viral vaccines involves introduction of the genes encoding the antigen into the viral genome using standard recombination and selection approaches adapted to the virus of interest.

Two principles underlie the capacity of recombinant viral vaccines to initiate antigen-specific immune responses. First, the cellular damage induced by viral infection produces danger signals that attract and activate bone marrow–derived APCs, which tend to present antigens in the context of co-stimulatory signals, leading to T-cell activation. A second mechanism for some recombinant viral vaccines involves direct infection of bone marrow–derived APCs. Direct infection of bone marrow–derived APCs allows for efficient processing of endogenously synthesized antigens into the MHC class I pathway.

The concept of direct infection of APCs led to various modifications of recombinant viral vaccines that enhance the processing and presentation of encoded antigens or incorporate genes encoding co-stimulatory molecules into the recombinant virus. For example, infection with recombinant vaccinia virus expressing genes encoding minimal MHC class I–restricted peptides can lead to enhanced MHC class I presentation of antigen *in vivo* (302,303). Grafting of endosomal or lysosomal sorting signals from lysosome-associated membrane protein-1 (LAMP-1) onto the gene encoding antigen has resulted in enhanced MHC class II processing and presentation and in enhanced CD4$^+$ T-cell activation by recombinant poxviruses (304,305). Incorporation of the B7 co-stimulatory gene and cytokine genes into recombinant poxviruses also has enhanced vaccine potency (306). An admixture of poxvirus expressing the GM-CSF gene together with poxvirus expressing antigen leads to enhanced vaccine potency, apparently based on enhanced dendritic cell differentiation at foci of infection (307).

Recombinant Bacterial Vaccines

One recombinant vaccine approach uses engineered bacteria. A number of bacterial strains, including *Salmonella* (308–312), BCG (313,314), and *Listeria monocytogenes* (315–320), display two characteristics that make them promising vaccine vectors. First, they possess enteric routes of infection, providing the possibility of oral vaccine delivery. Second, they have significant cellular tropism for monocytes and macrophages. They therefore have the capacity to target antigens to professional APCs.

Recombinant *L. monocytogenes* vaccines have been specifically tested in animal models of cancer. *L. monocytogenes* is a particularly interesting vector because of its two-phase intracellular life cycle (321–323). When *L. monocytogenes* first infects monocytes or macrophages, it occupies the phagolysosome for a period of hours. *L. monocytogenes* then secretes listerialysin O (LLO), which destabilizes the phagolysosomal membrane and allows transit of the bacteria into the cytoplasm. The dual phagolysosomal-cytoplasmic life cycle of *L. monocytogenes* results in efficient processing and presentation of its antigens into the MHC class II pathway during the phagolysosomal phase and into the MHC class I pathway during its cytosolic phase.

Recombinant *L. monocytogenes* can be engineered to secrete antigens by linking them to the LLO signal sequence. Vaccination with these recombinant *L. monocytogenes* engineered to secrete antigens has resulted in *in vivo* activation of antigen-specific CD4+ helper cells and CD8+ CTLs. When recombinant *L. monocytogenes* expressing a model tumor antigen was tested intraperitoneally or orally as a tumor vaccine, it proved extremely effective in generating antigen-specific antitumor immunity capable of inducing rejection of palpable established tumors (319,320). Although the mechanism by which recombinant *L. monocytogenes* induces effective immunity against large established tumors remains elusive, it is likely that potent activation of components of the innate immune response (324–326) through induction of cytokines such as IL-12 contributes to the effective access of antigen-specific T cells into established tumor beds.

Nucleic Acid Vaccines

Vaccines composed of "naked" DNA have engendered tremendous interest because, after intramuscular injection, pure recombinant DNA was shown to persist for long periods and mediate stable expression of encoded genes (327). Subsequently, DNA injection was shown to mediate antibody and cellular immune responses against encoded gene products, raising the prospects for naked DNA as a recombinant vaccine (328). Since the original report by Montgomery et al. that naked DNA vaccines encoding influenza nucleoprotein could protect animals from influenza challenge (329), naked DNA vaccines have been employed in animal models of many infectious diseases and are entering clinical testing (330). Naked DNA vaccines encoding model tumor antigens have provided some degree of protection against challenge by tumors expressing the immunizing antigen (331).

In general, the potency of naked DNA vaccines is significantly less than that of other recombinant vaccines such as recombinant vaccinia. This decreased potency probably occurs because naked DNA vaccines do not undergo a replicative amplification, as occurs with live recombinant viral and bacterial vaccines, thereby limiting the amount of antigen ultimately presented to the immune system. Naked DNA vaccines generate a much smaller inflammatory or danger response than a live viral infection, thereby limiting the amount of co-stimulation available in the priming environment. Nonetheless, injection of nucleic acid does induce local inflammation and some activation of bone marrow–derived APCs.

Chimera experiments have proven definitively that it is bone marrow–derived APCs that present the antigens encoded by naked DNA vaccines (332,333). It remains to be determined whether the pathway of antigen presentation in bone marrow–derived cells is the result of direct transduction or transfer of antigen in protein or RNA form to bone marrow–derived APCs, similar to the cross-priming observed with whole cell tumor vaccines. The appreciation that bone marrow–derived APCs are the critical presenting cells for nucleic acid vaccines allows incorporation of modifications affecting antigen processing and co-stimulation similar to those employed in recombinant viral vaccines. A mixture of plasmids encoding GM-CSF and B7 has been shown to enhance the generation of cellular immune responses induced by DNA vaccines.

An important feature of nucleic acid vaccines comes from the discovery that unmethylated CpG tracts found in bacterial DNA (the source of most recombinant nucleic acid vaccine material) is intrinsically inflammatory and activating to macrophages and other bone marrow–derived APCs (334,335). It has been demonstrated that unmethylated CpG tracts directly stimulate macrophages to produce proinflammatory cytokines such as IL-12 (336). It is likely that the proinflammatory effects of unmethylated CpG tracts in nucleic acid vaccines are critical to their vaccine capabilities.

Dendritic Cell Vaccines

Dendritic cells are a form of activated APC and are 100- and 1,000-fold more potent than macrophages in simulating antigen-specific T cells. The classic activated dendritic cell represents a state of differentiation of bone marrow–derived mononuclear cells induced by certain cytokines associated with inflammatory responses. The most important cytokine responsible for inducing differentiation to the dendritic cell lineage is GM-CSF (279–281). Other cytokines such as IL-4 and TNF-α synergize with GM-CSF in inducing dendritic cell differentiation from CD34+ precursors (337).

The potency of dendritic cells in presenting antigens to and activating T cells appears to be related to many factors. Dendritic cells express high levels of surface MHC molecules, particularly MHC class II (roughly 50-fold more than activated macrophages). The density of peptide–MHC ligand on the surface of a dendritic cell is much higher than on other cells, and this is a critical parameter for T-cell receptor engagement. Dendritic cells express extremely high levels of intercellular adhesion molecule and B7, important adhesion and co-stimulatory molecules, respectively, for T-cell activation. Other dendritic cell-specific genes, such as one encoding a T-cell–specific chemokine (338), add to the list of features that give dendritic cells their unique prowess in initiating T-cell responses.

Based on fundamental studies of dendritic cell biology, a number of groups have used dendritic cells grown by culture of bone marrow progenitors in GM-CSF, followed by loading of the dendritic cell with antigen in various forms and injection of loaded dendritic cells back into the cancer-bearing animal. The form of antigen with which dendritic cells have been loaded ranges from minimal MHC class I–restricted peptides (339) to protein (340,341) to fusion with whole tumor cells (342). Others have explored *ex vivo* transduction of dendritic cells using RNA (343) or replication-defective recombinant viral vectors (344,345) to introduce genes encoding antigen.

Heat Shock Proteins as Adjuvants

The properties of adjuvanticity are related to the recruitment and activation of appropriate forms of bone marrow APCs and to enhanced targeting of antigens into MHC processing pathways within these APCs. One form of natural biologic adjuvant displaying great promise is the heat shock protein. The pioneering studies of Srivastava et al. demonstrated that an ER-resident heat shock protein, gp96, and a cytosolic heat shock protein, HSP70, can act as immunologic adjuvants (346–349). These heat shock proteins, or chaperonins, have the capacity to bind a wide array of peptides (350,351). Immunization with native gp96 or HSP70 purified from tumor cells generates systemic antitumor immunity specific for the tumor from which the gp96 or HSP70 was extracted (352). Further analysis of this phenomenon demonstrated that tumor-specific immunity is provided by specific peptides associated with the extracted gp96 or HSP70. It is also possible to strip heat shock proteins of endogenously bound peptides and then load them with a specific peptide of interest (353). Immunization with these peptide loaded heat shock proteins generates CTL responses *in vivo*.

Adjuvanticity of certain selected heat shock proteins probably can be attributed to two features. First, peptide-loaded gp96 has been shown *in vitro* to effectively introduce antigens into the MHC class I processing pathway. Gp96 and possibly other heat shock proteins may represent important molecular conduits for antigens into the MHC class I and class II pathways of APCs. Second, there is evidence that binding of gp96 to macrophages induces them to secrete proinflammatory cytokines. The heat shock proteins may augment the function of cells to which they are targeting peptides.

CONCLUSIONS

It appears that the character of the antitumor immune response is closer to an anti-self response than to immune responses against foreign antigens. This can be seen in the ability of tumor cells to tolerize immune responses and in the high proportion of observed antitumor responses that recognize self antigens. Nonetheless, there are unique aspects to the biology of tumors that distinguish them from self tissues. For example, the loss of genomic integrity in cancer from the loss of function of critical guardians of the genome, such as p53, continuously generates and eliminates neoantigenic structures. These unique genetic and biologic features of cancer probably produce unique aspects of the antitumor immune response. This idea has already been demonstrated by identification of T-cell responses specific for peptides derived from biologically relevant mutations in cancer cells. Ultimately, as we understand more about how the antigenic variability of tumors and other aspects of tumor biology affect the interaction between the cancer cell and components of the immune system, it should be possible to develop more selective and potent approaches to cancer immunotherapy.

REFERENCES

1. Ehrlich P. Ueber den jetzigen Stand der Karzinomforschung. *Ned Tijdschr Geneeskd* 1909;5:273–290.
2. Nauts HC. Bacteria and cancer—antagonisms and benefits. *Cancer Surv* 1989;8:713–723.
3. Thomas L. *Discussion of cellular and humoral aspects of the hypersensitive states.* New York: Hoeber-Harper, 1959.
4. Burnet FM. The concept of immunological surveillance. *Prog Exp Tumor Res* 1970;13:1–27.
5. Stutman O. Tumor development after 3-methylcholanthrene in immunologically deficient athymic nude mice. *Science* 1979;183: 534–536.
6. Outzen HC, Custer RP, Eaton GJ, Prehn RT. Spontaneous and induced tumor incidence in germfree "nude" mice. *J Reticuloendothel Soc* 1975;17:1–9.
7. Rygaard J, Povlsen CO. The nude mouse vs. the hypothesis of immunological surveillance. *Transplant Rev* 1976;28:43–61.
8. Moller G. Experiments and the concept of immunological surveillance. *Transplant Rev* 1976;28:1–97.
9. Holland JM, Mitchell TJ, Gipson LC, Whitaker MS. Survival and cause of death in aging germfree athymic nude and normal inbred C3Hf/He mice. *J Natl Cancer Inst* 1978;61:1357–1361.
10. Good RA. Relations between immunity and malignancy. *Proc Natl Acad Sci USA* 1972;69:1026–1032.
11. Groopman JE. Neoplasms in the acquired immune deficiency syndrome: the multidisciplinary approach to treatment. *Semin Oncol* 1987;14:1–6.
12. Klein G. Immunological surveillance against neoplasia. *Harvey Lect* 1975;69:71–102.
13. Purtilo DT. Defective immune surveillance in viral carcinogenesis. *Lab Invest* 1984;51:373–385.
14. Penn I. Tumors of the immunocompromised patient. *Annu Rev Med* 1988;39:63–73.
15. List AF, Greco FA, Vogler LB. Lymphoproliferative diseases in immunocompromised hosts: the role of Epstein-Barr virus. *J Clin Oncol* 1987;5:1673–1689.
16. Gaidano G, Dalla FR. Biologic aspects of human immunodeficiency virus-related lymphoma. *Curr Opin Oncol* 1992;4:900–906.
17. Frizzera G. A typical lymphoproliferative disorder. In: Knowles DM, ed. *Neoplastic Hematopathology.* Baltimore: Williams & Wilkins, 1992:459–495.
18. Heslop HE, Ng CY, Li C, et al. Long-term restoration of immunity against Epstein-Barr virus infection by adoptive transfer of gene-modified virus-specific T lymphocytes. *Nat Med* 1996;2:551–555.
19. Chang Y, Cesarman E, Pessin MS, et al. Identification of herpesvirus-

like DNA sequences in AIDS-associated Kaposi's sarcoma. *Science* 1994;266:1865–1869.

20. Mesri EA, Cesarman E, Arvanitakis L, et al. Human herpesvirus-8/Kaposi's sarcoma-associated herpesvirus is a new transmissible virus that infects B cells. *J Exp Med* 1996;183:2385–2390.

21. Durst M, Gissmann L, Ikenberg H, zur Hausen H. A papillomavirus DNA from a cervical carcinoma and its prevalence in cancer biopsy samples from different geographic regions. *Proc Natl Acad Sci USA* 1983;80:3812–3815.

22. Boshart M, Gissmann L, Ikenberg H, Kleinheinz A, Scheurlen W, zur Hausen H. A new type of papillomavirus DNA, its presence in genital cancer biopsies and in cell lines derived from cervical cancer. *EMBO J* 1984;3:1151–1157.

23. Gissmann L, Schwarz E. Persistence and expression of human papillomavirus DNA in genital cancer. *Ciba Found Symp* 1986;120:190–207.

24. Beaudenon S, Kremsdorf D, Croissant O, Jablonska S, Wain HS, Orth G. A novel type of human papillomavirus associated with genital neoplasias. *Nature* 1986;321:246–249.

25. Beaudenon S, Kremsdorf D, Obalek S, et al. Plurality of genital human papillomaviruses: characterization of two new types with distinct biological properties. *Virology* 1987;161:374–384.

26. McFarlane GA, Munro A. *Helicobacter pylori* and gastric cancer. *Br J Surg* 1997;84:1190–1199.

27. Ohashi PS, Oehen S, Buerki K, et al. Ablation of "tolerance" and induction of diabetes by virus infection in viral antigen transgenic mice. *Cell* 1991;65:305–317.

28. Hanahan D, Jolicouer C, Alpert S, Skowronski J. Alternative self or nonself recognition of an antigen expressed in a rare cell type in transgenic mice: implications for self-tolerance and autoimmunity. *Cold Spring Harb Symp Quant Biol* 1989;54:821–835.

29. Lo D, Freedman J, Hesse S, Palmiter RD, Brinster RL, Sherman LA. Peripheral tolerance to an islet cell-specific hemagglutinin transgene affects both CD4$^+$ and CD8$^+$ T cells. *Eur J Immunol* 1992;22:1013–1022.

30. Miller JF, Morahan G, Allison J. Extrathymic acquisition of tolerance by T lymphocytes. *Cold Spring Harb Symp Quant Biol* 1989;2:807–813.

31. Lo D, Burkly LC, Widera G, et al. Diabetes and tolerance in transgenic mice expressing class II MHC molecules in pancreatic beta cells. *Cell* 1988;53:159–168.

32. Burkly LC, Lo D, Kanagawa O, Brinster RL, Flavell RA. T-cell tolerance by clonal anergy in transgenic mice with nonlymphoid expression of MHC class II I-E. *Nature* 1989;342:564–566.

33. Jenkins MK, Schwartz RH. Antigen presentation by chemically modified splenocytes induces antigen-specific T cell unresponsiveness *in vitro* and *in vivo*. *J Exp Med* 1987;165:302–319.

34. Linsley PS, Brady W, Grosmaire L, Arffo A, Damle NK, Ledbetter JA. Binding of the B cell activation antigen B7 to CD28 costimulates T cell proliferation and interleukin 2 mRNA accumulation. *J Exp Med* 1991;173:721–730.

35. Janeway CAJ. The immune system evolved to discriminate infectious nonself from noninfectious self. *Immunol Today* 1992;13:11–16.

36. Guerder S, Matzinger P. Activation versus tolerance: a decision made by T helper cells. *Cold Spring Harb Symp Quant Biol* 1989;2:799–805.

37. Schwartz RH. Costimulation of T lymphocytes: the role of CD28, CTLA-4, and B7/BB1 in interleukin-2 production and immunotherapy. *Cell* 1992;71:1065–1068.

38. Staveley-O'Carroll K, Sotomayor E, Montgomery J, et al. Induction of antigen-specific T cell anergy: an early event in the course of tumor progression. *Proc Natl Acad Sci USA* 1998;95:1178–1183.

39. Adler AJ, Marsh DW, Yochum GS, et al. CD4$^+$ T cell tolerance to parenchymal self-antigens requires presentation by bone marrow-derived antigen presenting cells. *J Exp Med* 1998;187:1555–1564.

40. Wick M, Dubey P, Koeppen H, et al. Antigenic cancer cells grow progressively in immune hosts without evidence for T cell exhaustion or systemic energy. *J Exp Med* 1997;186:229–238.

41. Speiser DE, Miranda R, Zakarian A, et al. Self antigens expressed by solid tumors do not efficiently stimulate naive or activated T cells: implications for immunotherapy. *J Exp Med* 1997;186:645–653.

42. Hui K, Grosveld F, Festenstein H. Rejection of transplantable AKR leukaemia cells following MHC DNA-mediated cell transformation. *Nature* 1984;311:750–752.

43. Wallich R, Bulbuc N, Hammerling GJ, Katzav S, Segal S, Feldman M. Abrogation of metastatic properties of tumour cells by *de novo* expression of H-2K antigens following H-2 gene transfection. *Nature* 1985;315:301–305.

44. Haywood GR, McKhann CF. Antigenic specificities on murine sarcoma cells. Reciprocal relationship between normal transplantation antigens (H-2) and tumor-specific immunogenicity. *J Exp Med* 1971;133:1171–1187.

45. Trowsdale J, Travers P, Bodmer WF, Patillo RA. Expression of HLA-A, -B, and -C and beta 2-microglobulin antigens in human choriocarcinoma cell lines. *J Exp Med* 1980;152:11s–17s.

46. Doyle A, Martin WJ, Funa K, et al. Markedly decreased expression of class I histocompatibility antigens, protein, and mRNA in human small-cell lung cancer. *J Exp Med* 1985;161:1135–1151.

47. Lampson LA, Fisher CA, Whelan JP. Striking paucity of HLA-A, B, C and beta 2-microglobulin on human neuroblastoma cell lines. *J Immunol* 1983;130:2471–2478.

48. Natali PG, Giacomini P, Bigotti A, et al. Heterogeneity in the expression of HLA and tumor-associated antigens by surgically removed and cultured breast carcinoma cells. *Cancer Res* 1983;43:660–668.

49. Travers PJ, Arklie JL, Trowsdale J, Patillo RA, Bodmer WF. Lack of expression of HLA-ABC antigens in choriocarcinoma and other human tumor cell lines. *Natl Cancer Inst Monogr* 1982;60:175–180.

50. Stein B, Momburg F, Schwarz V, Schlag P, Moldenhauer G, Moller P. Reduction or loss of HLA-A, B, C antigens in colorectal carcinoma appears not to influence survival. *Br J Cancer* 1988;57:364–368.

51. Smith ME, Bodmer WF, Bodmer JG. Selective loss of HLA-A, B, C locus products in colorectal adenocarcinoma [Letter]. *Lancet* 1988;1:823–824.

52. Kaklamanis L, Gatter KC, Hill AB, et al. Loss of HLA class-I alleles, heavy chains and beta 2-microglobulin in colorectal cancer. *Int J Cancer* 1992;51:379–385.

53. Restifo NP, Esquivel F, Asher AL, et al. Defective presentation of endogenous antigens by a murine sarcoma: implications for the failure of an anti-tumor immune response. *J Immunol* 1991;147:1453–1459.

54. Restifo NP, Esquivel F, Kawakami Y, et al. Identification of human cancers deficient in antigen processing. *J Exp Med* 1993;177:265–272.

55. Urban JL, Burton RC, Holland JM, Kripke ML, Schreiber H. Mechanisms of syngeneic tumor rejection: susceptibility of host-selected progressor variants to various immunological effector cells. *J Exp Med* 1982;155:557–573.

56. Ward PL, Koeppen HK, Hurteau T, Rowley DA, Schreiber H. Major histocompatibility complex class I and unique antigen expression by murine tumors that escaped from CD8$^+$ T-cell–dependent surveillance. *Cancer Res* 1990;50:3851–3858.

57. Uyttenhove C, Maryanski J, Boon T. Escape of mouse mastocytoma P815 after nearly complete rejection is due to antigen-loss variants rather than immunosuppression. *J Exp Med* 1983;157:1040–1052.

58. Ward PL, Koeppen H, Hurteau T, Schreiber H. Tumor antigens defined by cloned immunological probes are highly polymorphic and are not detected on autologous normal cells. *J Exp Med* 1989;170:217–232.

59. Wortzel RD, Philipps C, Schreiber H. Multiple tumour-specific antigens expressed on a single tumour cell. *Nature* 1983;304:165–167.

60. Urban JL, Kripke ML, Schreiber H. Stepwise immunologic selection of antigenic variants during tumor growth. *J Immunol* 1986;137:3036–3041.

61. Jager E, Ringhoffer M, Altmannsberger M, et al. Immunoselection *in vivo*: independent loss of MHC class I and melanocyte differentiation antigen expression in metastatic melanoma. *Int J Cancer* 1997;71:142–147.

62. Ljunggren HG, Karre K. Host resistance directed selectively against H-2–deficient lymphoma variants. Analysis of the mechanism. *J Exp Med* 1985;162:1745–1759.

63. Karre K, Ljunggren HG, Piontek G, Kiessling R. Selective rejection of H-2–deficient lymphoma variants suggests alternative immune defense strategy. *Nature* 1986;319:675–678.

64. Storkus WJ, Howell DN, Salter RD, Dawson JR, Cresswell P. NK susceptibility varies inversely with target cell class I HLA antigen expression. *J Immunol* 1987;138:1657–1659.

65. Yokoyama WM, Seaman WE. The Ly-49 and NKR-P1 gene families encoding lectin-like receptors on natural killer cells: the NK gene complex. *Annu Rev Immunol* 1993;11:613–635.

66. Hahne M, Rimoldi D, Schroter M, et al. Melanoma cell expression of Fas (Apo-1/CD95) ligand: implications for tumor immune escape. *Science* 1996;274:1363–1366.

67. O'Connell J, O'Sullivan GC, Collins JK, Shanahan F. The Fas counterattack: Fas-mediated T cell killing by colon cancer cells expressing Fas ligand. *J Exp Med* 1996;184:1075–1082.

68. Torre AG, Beauchamp RD, Koeppen H, et al. A highly immunogenic tumor transfected with a murine transforming growth factor type beta 1 cDNA escapes immune surveillance. *Proc Natl Acad Sci USA* 1990; 87:1486–1490.

69. Kuerbitz SJ, Plunkett BS, Walsh WV, Kastan MB. Wild-type p53 is a cell cycle checkpoint determinant following irradiation. *Proc Natl Acad Sci USA* 1992;89:7491–7495.

70. Kastan MB, Zhan QEL, Deiry WS, et al. A mammalian cell cycle checkpoint pathway utilizing p53 and GADD45 is defective in ataxia-telangiectasia. *Cell* 1992;71:587–597.

71. Lu X, Lane DP. Differential induction of transcriptionally active p53 following UV or ionizing radiation: defects in chromosome instability syndromes? *Cell* 1993;75:765–778.

72. Sahin U, Tureci O, Schmitt H, et al. Human neoplasms elicit multiple specific immune responses in the autologous host. *Proc Natl Acad Sci USA* 1995;92:11810–11813.

73. Gure AO, Tureci O, Sahin U, et al. SSX: a multigene family with several members transcribed in normal testis and human cancer. *Int J Cancer* 1997;72:965–971.

74. Old LJ. Cancer immunology: the search for specificity—G. H. A. Clowes Memorial lecture. *Cancer Res* 1981;41:361–375.

75. Fearon ER, Vogelstein B. A genetic model for colorectal tumorigenesis. *Cell* 1990;61:759–767.

76. Golumbek PT, Lazenby AJ, Levitsky HI, et al. Treatment of established renal cancer by tumor cells engineered to secrete interleukin-4. *Science* 1991;254:713–716.

77. Dranoff G, Jaffee E, Lazenby A, et al. Vaccination with irradiated tumor cells engineered to secrete murine granulocyte-macrophage colony-stimulating factor stimulates potent, specific, and long-lasting anti-tumor immunity. *Proc Natl Acad Sci USA* 1993;90:3539–3543.

78. Levitsky HI, Lazenby A, Hayashi RJ, Pardoll DM. *In vivo* priming of two distinct antitumor effector populations: the role of MHC class I expression. *J Exp Med* 1994;179:1215–1224.

79. Ostrand-Rosenberg S. Tumor immunotherapy: the tumor cell as an antigen-presenting cell. *Curr Opin Immunol* 1994;6:722–727.

80. Topalian SL. MHC class II restricted tumor antigens and the role of CD4+ T cells in cancer immunotherapy. *Curr Opin Immunol* 1994;6: 741–745.

81. Pulaski BA, McAdam AJ, Hutter EK, Biggar S, Lord EM, Frelinger JG. Interleukin 3 enhances development of tumor-reactive cytotoxic cells by a CD4-dependent mechanism. *Cancer Res* 1993;53: 2112–2117.

82. Cavallo F, Giovarelli M, Gulino A, et al. Role of neutrophils and CD4+ T lymphocytes in the primary and memory response to nonimmunogenic murine mammary adenocarcinoma made immunogenic by IL-2 gene. *J Immunol* 1992;149:3627–3635.

83. Tepper RI, Coffman RL, Leder P. An eosinophil-dependent mechanism for the antitumor effect of interleukin-4. *Science* 1992;257: 548–551.

84. Bosco M, Giovarelli M, Forni M, et al. Low doses of IL-4 injected perilymphatically in tumor-bearing mice inhibit the growth of poorly and apparently nonimmunogenic tumors and induce a tumor-specific immune memory. *J Immunol* 1990;145:3136–3143.

85. Tepper RI, Pattengale PK, Leder P. Murine interleukin-4 displays potent anti-tumor activity *in vivo*. *Cell* 1989;57:503–512.

86. Hung K, Hayashi R, Levitsky HI, Pardoll DM. The central role of CD4+ T cells in the antitumor immune response. *J Exp Med* 1998;188:2357–2368.

87. Gross L. Intradermal immunization of C3H mice against a sarcoma that originated in an animal of the same line. *Cancer Res* 1943;3:326–333.

88. Prehn RT. Immunity to methylcholanthrene-induced sarcomas. *J Natl Cancer Inst* 1957;18:769–778.

89. Old LJ, Boyle EA, Clark DA, Carswell EA. Antigenic properties of chemically induced tumors. *Ann N Y Acad Sci* 1962;101:80–106.

90. Schreiber H, Ward PL, Rowley DA, Stauss HJ. Unique tumor-specific antigens. *Annu Rev Immunol* 1988;6:465–483.

91. De Plaen E, Lurquin C, Van Pel A, et al. Immunogenic (tum-) variants of mouse tumor P815: cloning of the gene of tum-antigen P91A and identification of the tum-mutation. *Proc Natl Acad Sci USA* 1988;85: 2274–2278.

92. Rotzschke O, Falk K, Deres K, Schild H, Norda M, Metzger J, Jung G, Rammensee HG. Isolation and analysis of naturally processed viral peptides as recognized by cytotoxic T cells. *Nature* 1990;348:252–254.

93. Van Bleek G, Nathanson S. Isolation of an endogenously processed immunodominant viral peptide from the class I H-2kb molecule. *Nature* 1990;348:213–216.

94. Cox AL, Skipper J, Chen Y, et al. Identification of a peptide recognized by five melanoma-specific human cytotoxic T cell lines. *Science* 1994;264:716–719.

95. Lurquin C, Van Pel A, Mariame B, DePlaen E, Szikora JP, Janssens C, Reddehase MJ, Lejeune J, Boon T. Structure of the gene of tum- transplantation antigen P91A: the mutated exon encodes a peptide recognized with Ld by cytolytic T cells. *Cell* 1989;58:293–303.

96. Sibille C, Chomez P, Wildmann C, et al. Structure of the gene of tum-transpantation antigen P198: a point mutation generates a new antigenic peptide. *J Exp Med* 1990;172:35–45.

97. Mandelboim O, Berke G, Fridkin M, Feldman M, Eisenstein M, Eisenbach L. CTL induction by a tumor-associated antigen octapeptide derived from a murine lung carcinoma. *Nature* 1994;369:67–71.

98. Dubey P, Hendrickson RC, Meredith SC, et al. The immunodominant antigen of an ultraviolet-induced regressor tumor is generated by a somatic point mutation in the DEAD box helicase p68. *J Exp Med* 1997;185:695–705.

99. Monach PA, Meredith SC, Siegel CT, Schreiber H. A unique tumor antigen produced by a single amino acid substitution. *Immunity* 1995; 2:45–59.

100. Coulie PG, Lehmann F, Lethe B, et al. A mutated intron sequence codes for an antigenic peptide recognized by cytolytic T lymphocytes on a human melanoma. *Proc Natl Acad Sci USA* 1995;92:7976–7980.

101. Wolfel T, Hauer M, Schneider J, et al. A p16INK4a-insensitive CDK4 mutant targeted by cytolytic T lymphocytes in a human melanoma. *Science* 1995;269:1281–1284.

102. Kamb A, Gruis NA, Weaver T, et al. A cell cycle regulator potentially involved in genesis of many tumor types. *Science* 1994;264:436–440.

103. Robbins PF, El GM, Li YF, et al. A mutated beta-catenin gene encodes a melanoma-specific antigen recognized by tumor infiltrating lymphocytes. *J Exp Med* 1996;183:1185–1192.

104. Grunwald GB. The structural and functional analysis of cadherin calcium-dependent cell adhesion molecules. *Curr Opin Cell Biol* 1993; 5:797–805.

105. Vleminckx K, Vakaet LJ, Mareel M, Fiers W, Van Roy F. Genetic manipulation of E-cadherin expression by epithelial tumor cells reveals an invasion suppressor role. *Cell* 1991;66:107–119.

106. Su LK, Vogelstein B, Kinzler KW. Association of the APC tumor suppressor protein with catenins. *Science* 1993;262:1734–1737.

107. Rubinfeld B, Robbins P, El Gamil M, Albert I, Porfiri E, Polakis P. Stabilization of beta-catenin by genetic defects in melanoma cell lines. *Science* 1997;275:1790–1792.

108. Mandruzzato S, Brasseur F, Andry G, Boon T, van der Bruggen P. A CASP-8 mutation recognized by cytolytic T lymphocytes on a human head and neck carcinoma. *J Exp Med* 1997;186:785–793.

109. Van den Eynde B, Lethe B, Vel Pel A, De Plaen E, Boon T. The gene coding for a major tumor rejection antigen of tumor P815 is identical to the normal gene in syngeneic DBA/2 mice. *J Exp Med* 1991;173: 1373–1384.

110. Huang AYC, Gulden PH, Woods AS, et al. The immunodominant major histocompatibility complex class I-restricted antigen of a murine colon tumor derives from an endogenous retroviral gene product. *Proc Natl Acad Sci USA* 1996;93:9730–9735.

111. Hartley JW, Wolford NK, Old LJ, Rowe WP. A new class of murine leukemia virus associated with development of spontaneous lymphomas. *Proc Natl Acad Sci USA* 1977;74:789–792.

112. Hayashi H, Matsubara H, Yokota T, et al. Molecular cloning and characterization of the gene encoding mouse melanoma antigen by cDNA library transfection. *J Immunol* 1992;149:1223–1229.

113. O'Donnell PV, Stockert E, Obata Y, Old LJ. Leukemogenic properties of AKR dual-tropic (MCF) viruses: amplification of murine leukemia virus-related antigens on thymocytes and acceleration of leukemia development in AKR mice. *Virology* 1981;112:548–563.

114. Bookman MA, Swerdlow R, Matis LA. Adoptive chemoimmunotherapy of murine leukemia with helper T lymphocyte clones. *J Immunol* 1987;139:3166–3170.

115. Matis LA, Ruscetti SK, Longo DL, et al. Distinct proliferative T cell clonotypes are generated in response to a murine retrovirus-induced syngeneic T cell leukemia: viral gp70 antigen-specific MT4+ clones and Lyt-2+ cytolytic clones which recognize a tumor-specific cell surface antigen. *J Immunol* 1985;135:703–713.

116. Ono M, Kawakami M, Takezawa T. A novel human nonviral retroposon derived from an endogenous retrovirus. *Nucleic Acids Res* 1987; 15:8725–8737.

117. Ono M. Molecular cloning and long terminal repeat sequences of human endogenous retrovirus genes related to types A and B retrovirus genes. *J Virol* 1986;58:937–944.

118. Medstrand P, Blomberg J. Characterization of novel reverse transcriptase encoding human endogenous retroviral sequences similar to type A and type B retroviruses: differential transcription in normal human tissues. *J Virol* 1993;67:6778–6787.

119. Ono M, Yasunaga T, Miyata T, Ushikubo H. Nucleotide sequence of human endogenous retrovirus genome related to the mouse mammary tumor virus genome. *J Virol* 1986;60:589–598.

120. Sauter M, Schommer S, Kremmer E, et al. Human endogenous retrovirus K10: expression of Gag protein and detection of antibodies in patients with seminomas. *J Virol* 1995;69:414–421.

121. Wahlstrom T, Suni J, Nieminen P, Narvanen A, Lehtonen T, Vaheri A. Renal cell adenocarcinoma and retrovirus p30-related antigen excreted to urine. *Lab Invest* 1985;53:464–469.

122. Moshier JA, Luk GD, Huang RC. mRNA from human colon tumor and mucosa related to the pol gene of an endogenous A-type retrovirus. *Biochem Biophys Res Commun* 1986;139:1071–1077.

123. Vogetseder W, Dumfahrt A, Mayersbach P, Schonitzer D, Dierich MP. Antibodies in human sera recognizing a recombinant outer membrane protein encoded by the envelope gene of the human endogenous retrovirus K. *AIDS Res Hum Retroviruses* 1993;9:687–694.

124. Van der Bruggen P, Traversari C, Chomez P, et al. A gene encoding an antigen recognized by cytolytic T lymphocytes on a human melanoma. *Science* 1991;254:1643–1647.

125. Traversari C, Van der Bruggen P, Luescher IF, et al. A nonapeptide encoded by human gene MAGE-1 is recognized on HLA-A1 by cytolytic T lymphocytes directed against tumor antigen MZ2-E. *J Exp Med* 1992;176:1453–1457.

126. Van der Bruggen P, Szikora JP, Boel P, et al. Autologous cytolytic T lymphocytes recognize a MAGE-1 nonapeptide on melanomas expressing HLA-Cw*1601. *Eur J Immunol* 1994;24:2134–2140.

127. Gaugler B, Van den Eynde B, Van der Bruggen P, et al. Human gene MAGE-3 codes for an antigen recognized on a melanoma by autologous cytolytic T lymphocytes. *J Exp Med* 1994;179:921–930.

128. Van der Bruggen P, Bastin J, Gajewski T, et al. A peptide encoded by human gene MAGE-3 and presented by HLA-A2 induces cytolytic T lymphocytes that recognize tumor cells expressing MAGE-3. *Eur J Immunol* 1994;24:3038–3043.

129. Boel P, Wildmann C, Sensi ML, et al. *BAGE*: a new gene encoding an antigen recognized on human melanomas by cytolytic T lymphocytes. *Immunity* 1995;2:167–175.

130. Van den Eynde B, Peeters O, De Backer O, Gaugler B, Lucas S, Boon T. A new family of genes coding for an antigen recognized by autologous cytolytic T lymphocytes on a human melanoma. *J Exp Med* 1995;182:689–698.

131. Van den Eynde B, Hainaut P, Herin M, et al. Presence on a human melanoma of multiple antigens recognized by autologous CTL. *Int J Cancer* 1989;44:634–640.

132. Brichard V, Van PA, Wolfel T, et al. The tyrosinase gene codes for an antigen recognized by autologous cytolytic T lymphocytes on HLA-A2 melanomas. *J Exp Med* 1993;178:489–495.

133. Wolfel T, Van Pel A, Brichard V, et al. Two tyrosinase nonapeptides recognized on HLA-A2 melanomas by autologous cytolytic T lymphocytes. *Eur J Immunol* 1994;24:759–764.

134. Robbins PF, El Gamil M, Kawakami Y, Stevens E, Yannelli JR, Rosenberg SA. Recognition of tyrosinase by tumor-infiltrating lymphocytes from a patient responding to immunotherapy [published erratum appears in *Cancer Res* 1994;15:3952]. *Cancer Res* 1994;54:3124–3126.

135. Kang X, Kawakami YEL, Gamil M, et al. Identification of a tyrosinase epitope recognized by HLA-A24–restricted, tumor-infiltrating lymphocytes. *J Immunol* 1995;155:1343–1348.

136. Brichard VG, Herman J, Van Pel A, et al. A tyrosinase nonapeptide presented by HLA-B44 is recognized on a human melanoma by autologous cytolytic T lymphocytes. *Eur J Immunol* 1996;26:224–230.

137. Skipper JC, Hendrickson RC, Gulden PH, et al. An HLA-A2-restricted tyrosinase antigen on melanoma cells results from post-translational modification and suggests a novel pathway for processing of membrane proteins. *J Exp Med* 1996;183:527–534.

138. Kawakami Y, Eliyahu S, Delgado CH, et al. Identification of a human melanoma antigen recognized by tumor-infiltrating lymphocytes associated with *in vivo* tumor rejection. *Proc Natl Acad Sci USA* 1994; 91:6458–6462.

139. Coulie PG, Brichard V, Van PA, et al. A new gene coding for a differentiation antigen recognized by autologous cytolytic T lymphocytes on HLA-A2 melanomas. *J Exp Med* 1994;180:35–42.

140. Kawakami Y, Eliyahu S, Delgado CH, et al. Cloning of the gene coding for a shared human melanoma antigen recognized by autologous T cells infiltrating into tumor. *Proc Natl Acad Sci USA* 1994;91:3515–3519.

141. Bakker AB, Schreurs MW, de Boer AJ, et al. Melanocyte lineage-specific antigen gp100 is recognized by melanoma-derived tumor-infiltrating lymphocytes. *J Exp Med* 1994;179:1005–1009.

142. Kawakami Y, Eliyahu S, Sakaguchi K, et al. Identification of the immunodominant peptides of the MART-1 human melanoma antigen recognized by the majority of HLA-A2–restricted tumor infiltrating lymphocytes. *J Exp Med* 1994;180:347–352.

143. Kawakami Y, Eliyahu S, Jennings C, et al. Recognition of multiple epitopes in the human melanoma antigen gp100 by tumor-infiltrating T lymphocytes associated with *in vivo* tumor regression. *J Immunol* 1995;154:3961–3968.

144. Bakker AB, Schreurs MW, Tafazzul G, et al. Identification of a novel peptide derived from the melanocyte-specific gp100 antigen as the dominant epitope recognized by an HLA-A2.1–restricted anti-melanoma CTL line. *Int J Cancer* 1995;62:97–102.

145. Wang RF, Parkhurst MR, Kawakami Y, Robbins PF, Rosenberg SA. Utilization of an alternative open reading frame of a normal gene in generating a novel human cancer antigen. *J Exp Med* 1996;183: 1131–1140.

146. Wang RF, Appella E, Kawakami Y, Kang X, Rosenberg SA. Identification of TRP-2 as a human tumor antigen recognized by cytotoxic T lymphocytes. *J Exp Med* 1996;184:2207–2216.

147. Parkhurst MR, Salgaller ML, Southwood S, et al. Improved induction of melanoma-reactive CTL with peptides from the melanoma antigen gp100 modified at HLA-A-A*0201–binding residues. *J Immunol* 1996;157:2539–2548.

148. Topalian SL, Rivoltini L, Mancini M, et al. Human CD4+ T cells specifically recognize a shared melanoma-associated antigen encoded by the tyrosinase gene. *Proc Natl Acad Sci USA* 1994;91:9461–9465.

149. Topalian SL, Gonzales MI, Parkhurst M, et al. Melanoma-specific CD4+ T cells recognize nonmutated HLA-DR–restricted tyrosinase epitopes. *J Exp Med* 1996;183:1965–1971.

150. Bishop JM. Molecular themes in oncogenesis. *Cell* 1991;64:235–248.

151. Cantley LC, Auger KR, Carpenter C, et al. Oncogenes and signal transduction [published erratum appears in *Cell* 1991;65:following 914]. *Cell* 1991;64:281–302.

152. Hunter T. Cooperation between oncogenes. *Cell* 1991;64:249–270.

153. Fearon ER, Vogelstein B. A genetic model for colorectal tumorigenesis. *N Engl J Med* 1988;319:525–560.

154. Nigro JM, Baker SJ, Preisinger AC, et al. Mutations in the p53 gene occur in diverse human tumour types. *Nature* 1989;342:705–708.

155. Kupryjanczyk J, Thor AD, Beauchamp R, et al. *P53* gene mutations and protein accumulation in human ovarian cancer. *Proc Natl Acad Sci USA* 1993;90:4961–4965.

156. Iggo R, Gatter K, Bartek J, Lane D, Harris AL. Increased expression of mutant forms of p53 oncogene in primary lung cancer. *Lancet* 1990;335:675–679.

157. Kishimoto Y, Murakami Y, Shiraishi M, Hayashi K, Sekiya T. Aberrations of the p53 tumor suppressor gene in human non-small cell carcinomas of the lung. *Cancer Res* 1992;52:4799–4804.

158. Prosser J, Thompson AM, Cranston G, Evans HJ. Evidence that p53 behaves as a tumour suppressor gene in sporadic breast tumours [published erratum appears in *Oncogene* 1991;6:2161]. *Oncogene* 1990;5: 1573–1579.

159. Brash DE, Rudolph JA, Simon JA, et al. A role for sunlight in skin cancer: UV-induced p53 mutations in squamous cell carcinoma. *Proc Natl Acad Sci USA* 1991;88:10124–10128.

160. Marshall CJ. Tumor suppressor genes. *Cell* 1991;64:313–326.

161. Weinberg RA. Tumor suppressor genes. *Science* 1991;254: 1138–1146.

162. DeLeo AB, Jay G, Appella E, Dubois GC, Law LW, Old LJ. Detection of a transformation-related antigen in chemically induced sarcomas and other transformed cells of the mouse. *Proc Natl Acad Sci USA* 1979;76:2420–2424.

163. Lane DP, Crawford LV. T antigen is bound to a host protein in SV40-transformed cells. *Nature* 1979;278:261–273.

164. Linzer DI, Maltzman W, Levine AJ. The SV40 A gene product is required for the production of a 54,000 MW cellular tumor antigen. *Virology* 1979;98:308–318.

165. Winter SF, Minna JD, Johnson BE, Takahashi T, Gazdar AF, Carbone DP. Development of antibodies against p53 in lung cancer patients appears to be dependent on the type of p53 mutation. *Cancer Res* 1992;52:4168–4174.

166. Schlichtholz B, Legros Y, Gillet D, et al. The immune response to p53 in breast cancer patients is directed against immunodominant epitopes unrelated to the mutational hot spot. *Cancer Res* 1992;52:6380–6384.

167. Houbiers JG, Van der Burg SH, Van de Watering LM, et al. Antibodies against p53 are associated with poor prognosis of colorectal cancer. *Br J Cancer* 1995;72:637–641.

168. Lubin R, Zalcman G, Bouchet L, et al. Serum p53 antibodies as early markers of lung cancer. *Nat Med* 1995;1:701–702.

169. Green JA, Mudenda B, Jenkins J, et al. Serum p53 auto-antibodies: incidence in familial breast cancer. *Eur J Cancer* 1994:580–584.

170. Yanuck M, Carbone DP, Pendleton CD, et al. A mutant p53 tumor suppressor protein is a target for peptide-induced CD8$^+$ cytotoxic T-cells. *Cancer Res* 1993;53:3257–3261.

171. Tilkin AF, Lubin R, Soussi T, et al. Primary proliferative T cell response to wild-type p53 protein in patients with breast cancer. *Eur J Immunol* 1995;25:1765–1769.

172. Houbiers JG, Nijman HW, Van der Burg SH, et al. *In vitro* induction of human cytotoxic T lymphocyte responses against peptides of mutant and wild-type p53. *Eur J Immunol* 1993;23:2072–2077.

173. Noguchi Y, Chen YT, Old LJ. A mouse mutant p53 product recognized by CD4$^+$ and CD8$^+$ T cells. *Proc Natl Acad Sci USA* 1994;91:3171–3175.

174. Noguchi Y, Richards EC, Chen YT, Old LJ. Influence of interleukin 12 on p53 peptide vaccination against established Meth A sarcoma. *Proc Natl Acad Sci USA* 1995;92:2219–2223.

175. Vierboom MP, Nijman HW, Offringa R, et al. Tumor eradication by wild-type p53-specific cytotoxic T lymphocytes. *J Exp Med* 1997;186:695–704.

176. Abrams SI, Dobrzanski MJ, Wells DT, et al. Peptide-specific activation of cytolytic CD4$^+$ T lymphocytes against tumor cells bearing mutated epitopes of K-ras p21 [published erratum appears in *Eur J Immunol* 1995;25:3525]. *Eur J Immunol* 1995;25:2588–2597.

177. Fenton RG, Keller CJ, Hanna N, Taub DD. Induction of T-cell immunity against Ras oncoproteins by soluble protein or Ras-expressing *Escherichia coli. J Natl Cancer Inst* 1995;87:1853–1861.

178. Takahashi M, Chen W, Byrd D, et al. Antibody responses to ras proteins in patients with colon cancer. *Clin Cancer Res* 1995;1:1071–1077.

179. Fossum B, Gedde, Dahl TR, et al. P21-ras-peptide-specific T-cell responses in a patient with colorectal cancer: CD4$^+$ and CD8$^+$ T cells recognize a peptide corresponding to a common mutation (^{13}Gly→Asp). *Int J Cancer* 1994;56:40–45.

180. Fossum B, Breivik J, Meling GI, et al. A K-ras ^{13}Gly→Asp mutation is recognized by HLA-DQ7 restricted T cells in a patient with colorectal cancer: modifying effect of DQ7 on established cancers harbouring this mutation? *Int J Cancer* 1994;58:506–511.

181. Qin H, Chen W, Takahashi M, et al. CD4$^+$ T-cell immunity to mutated ras protein in pancreatic and colon cancer patients. *Cancer Res* 1995;55:2984–2987.

182. Van Elsas A, Nijman HW, Van der Minne CE, et al. Induction and characterization of cytotoxic T-lymphocytes recognizing a mutated p21ras peptide presented by HLA-A*0201. *Int J Cancer* 1995;61:389–396.

183. Fossum B, Olsen AC, Thorsby E, Gaudernack G. CD8$^+$ T cells from a patient with colon carcinoma, specific for a mutant p21-Ras-derived peptide (Gly^{13}→Asp), are cytotoxic towards a carcinoma cell line harbouring the same mutation. *Cancer Immunol Immunother* 1995;40:165–172.

184. Slamon DJ, Godolphin W, Jones LA, et al. Studies of the HER-2/neu proto-oncogene in human breast and ovarian cancer. *Science* 1989;244:707–712.

185. Fisk B, Blevins TL, Wharton JT, Ioannides CG. Identification of an immunodominant peptide of HER-2/neu protooncogene recognized by ovarian tumor-specific cytotoxic T lymphocyte lines. *J Exp Med* 1995;181:2109–2117.

186. Peoples GE, Goedegebuure PS, Smith R, Linehan DC, Yoshino I, Eberlein TJ. Breast and ovarian cancer-specific cytotoxic T lymphocytes recognize the same HER2/neu-derived peptide. *Proc Natl Acad Sci USA* 1995;92:432–436.

187. Peoples GE, Smith RC, Linehan DC, Yoshino I, Goedegebuure PS, Eberlein TJ. Shared T cell epitopes in epithelial tumors. *Cell Immunol* 1995;164:279–286.

188. Brossart P, Stuhler G, Flad T, et al. Her-2/neu-derived peptides are tumor-associated antigens expressed by human renal cell and colon carcinoma lines and are recognized by *in vitro* induced specific cytotoxic T lymphocytes. *Cancer Res* 1998;58:732–736.

189. Katsumata M, Okudaira T, Samanta A, et al. Prevention of breast tumour development *in vivo* by downregulation of the p185neu receptor. *Nat Med* 1995;1:644–648.

190. Weiner LM, Clark JI, Davey M, et al. Phase I trial of 2B1, a bispecific monoclonal antibody targeting c-erbB-2 and Fc gamma RIII. *Cancer Res* 1995;55:4586–4593.

191. Epstein MA, Barr YM. Cultivation *in vitro* of human lymphoblasts from Burkitt's malignant lymphoma. *Lancet* 1964;1.

192. Mann RB, Bernard CW. Burkitt's tumor: lessons from mice, monkeys, and man. *Lancet* 1979;2:84–88.

193. Weiss LM, Movahed LA, Warnke RA, Sklar J. Detection of Epstein-Barr viral genomes in Reed-Sternberg cells of Hodgkin's disease. *N Engl J Med* 1989;320:502–506.

194. Weiss LM, Strickler JG, Warnke RA, Purtilo DT, Sklar J. Epstein-Barr viral DNA in tissues of Hodgkin's disease. *Am J Pathol* 1987;129:86–91.

195. Wu TC, Mann RB, Charache P, et al. Detection of EBV gene expression in Reed-Sternberg cells of Hodgkin's disease. *Int J Cancer* 1990;46:801–804.

196. Staal SP, Ambinder R, Beschorner WE, Hayward GS, Mann R. A survey of Epstein-Barr virus DNA in lymphoid tissue: frequent detection in Hodgkin's disease. *Am J Clin Pathol* 1989;91:1–5.

197. zur Hausen H, Schulte-Holthausen H, Klein G. EBV DNA in biopsies of Burkitt tumors and anaplastic carcinomas of the nasopharynx. *Nature* 1970;228:1056–1059.

198. Andersson-Anvret M, Forsby N, Klein G, Henle W. Relationship between the Epstein-Barr virus and undifferentiated nasopharyngeal carcinoma: correlated nucleic acid hybridization and histopathological examination. *Int J Cancer* 1977;20:486–494.

199. Raab TN, Flynn K, Pearson G, et al. The differentiated form of nasopharyngeal carcinoma contains Epstein-Barr virus DNA. *Int J Cancer* 1987;39:25–29.

200. Pagano JS, Sixbey JW, Lin JC. Acyclovir and Epstein-Barr virus infection. *J Antimicrob Chemother* 1983:113–121.

201. Beasley RP, Hwang LY, Lin CC, Chien CS. Hepatocellular carcinoma and hepatitis B virus: a prospective study of 22,707 men in Taiwan. *Lancet* 1981;2:1129–1133.

202. Szmuness W. Hepatocellular carcinoma and the hepatitis B virus: evidence for a casual association. *Prog Med Virol* 1987;24:40–46.

203. Brechot C. What is the role of hepatitis B virus in the appearance of hepatocellular carcinomas in patients with alcoholic cirrhosis? *Gastroenterol Clin Biol* 1982;6:727–730.

204. Shafritz DA, Shouval D, Sherman HI, Hadziyannis SJ, Kew MC. Integration of hepatitis B virus DNA into the genome of liver cells in chronic liver disease and hepatocellular carcinoma: studies in percutaneous liver biopsies and post-mortem tissue specimens. *N Engl J Med* 1981;305:1067–1073.

205. Werness BA, Levine AJ, Howley PM. Association of human papillomavirus types 16 and 18 E6 proteins with p53. *Science* 1990;248:76–79.

206. Mietz JA, Unger T, Huibregtse JM, Howley PM. The transcriptional transactivation function of wild-type p53 is inhibited by SV40 large T-antigen and by HPV-16 E6 oncoprotein. *EMBO J* 1992;11:5013–5020.

207. Scheffner M, Werness BA, Huibregtse JM, Levine AJ, Howley PM. The E6 oncoprotein encoded by human papillomavirus types 16 and 18 promotes the degradation of p53. *Cell* 1990;63:1129–1136.

208. Munger K, Werness BA, Dyson N, Phelps WC, Harlow E, Howley PM. Complex formation of human papillomavirus E7 proteins with

the retinoblastoma tumor suppressor gene product. *EMBO* 1989;8: 4099–4105.

209. Hudson JB, Bedell MA, McCance DJ, Laiminis LA. Immortalization and altered differentiation of human keratinocytes *in vitro* by the E6 and E7 open reading frames of human papillomavirus type 18. *J Virol* 1990;64:519–526.

210. Galloway DA, Jenison SA. Characterization of the humoral immune response to genital papillomaviruses. *Mol Biol Med* 1990;7:59–72.

211. Tindle RW, Frazer IH. Immunology of anogenital human papillomavirus (HPV) infection. *Aust N Z J Obstet Gynaecol* 1990;30: 370–375.

212. Viscidi R. Immune response to genital tract infections with human papillomaviruses. In: Quinn TC, ed. *Sexually transmitted diseases.* New York: Raven Press, 1992:239–260.

213. Gissmann L, Jochmus I, Nindl I, Muller M. Immune response to genital papillomavirus infections in women: prospects for the development of a vaccine against cervical cancer. *Ann N Y Acad Sci* 1993;690: 80–85.

214. Jochmus I, Altmann A. Immune response to papillomaviruses: prospects of an anti-HPV vaccine. *Papillomavirus Rep* 1993;4: 147–151.

215. Dillner J. Responses to defined HPV epitopes in cervical neoplasia. *Papillomavirus Rep* 1994;5:35–41.

216. Jochmus KI, Schneider A, Braun R, et al. Antibodies against the human papillomavirus type 16 early proteins in human sera: correlation of anti-E7 reactivity with cervical cancer. *J Natl Cancer Inst* 1989;81:1698–1704.

217. Mann VM, de LSL, Brenes M, et al. Occurrence of IgA and IgG antibodies to select peptides representing human papillomavirus type 16 among cervical cancer cases and controls. *Cancer Res* 1990;50: 7815–7819.

218. Muller M, Viscidi RP, Sun Y, et al. Antibodies to HPV-16 E6 and E7 proteins as markers for HPV-16–associated invasive cervical cancer. *Virology* 1992;187:508–514.

219. Kanda T, Onda T, Zanma S, et al. Independent association of antibodies against human papillomavirus type 16 E1/E4 and E7 proteins with cervical cancer. *Virology* 1992;190:724–732.

220. Onda T, Kanda T, Zanma S, et al. Association of the antibodies against human papillomavirus 16 E4 and E7 proteins with cervical cancer positive for human papillomavirus DNA. *Int J Cancer* 1993;54: 624–628.

221. Viscidi RP, Sun Y, Tsuzaki B, Bosch FX, Munoz N, Shah KV. Serologic response in human papillomavirus-associated invasive cervical cancer. *Int J Cancer* 1993;55:780–784.

222. Howley PM. Papillomavirinae and their replication. In: Fields BN, Knipe DM, eds. *Fundamental virology.* New York: Raven Press, 1991: 743–763.

223. Cripe TP, Haugen TH, Turk JP, et al. Transcriptional regulation of the human papillomavirus-16 E6-E7 promoter by a keratinocyte-dependent enhancer, and by viral E2 trans-activator and repressor gene products: implications for cervical carcinogenesis. *EMBO J* 1987;6: 3745–3753.

224. Ressing ME, Van Driel WJ, Celis E, et al. Occasional memory cytotoxic T-cell responses of patients with human papillomavirus type 16–positive cervical lesions against a human leukocyte antigen-A*0201-restricted E7-encoded epitope. *Cancer Res* 1996;56:582–588.

225. De Gruijl TD, Bontkes HJ, Stukart MJ, et al. T cell proliferative responses against human papillomavirus type 16 E7 oncoprotein are most prominent in cervical intraepithelial neoplasia patients with a persistent viral infection. *J Gen Virol* 1996;77:2183–2191.

226. Nakagawa M, Stites DP, Farhat S, et al. T-cell proliferative response to human papillomavirus type 16 peptides: relationship to cervical intraepithelial neoplasia. *Clin Diagn Lab Immunol* 1996;3:205–210.

227. Evans C, Bauer S, Grubert T, et al. HLA-A2–restricted peripheral blood cytolytic T lymphocyte response to HPV type 16 proteins E6 and E7 from patients with neoplastic cervical lesions. *Cancer Immunol Immunother* 1996;42:151–160.

228. Luxton JC, Rowe AJ, Cridland JC, Coletart T, Wilson P, Shepherd PS. Proliferative T cell responses to the human papillomavirus type 16 E7 protein in women with cervical dysplasia and cervical carcinoma and in healthy individuals. *J Gen Virol* 1996;77:1585–1593.

229. Jochmus I, Osen W, Altmann A, et al. Specificity of human cytotoxic T lymphocytes induced by a human papillomavirus type 16 E7-derived peptide. *J Gen Virol* 1997;78:1689–1695.

230. Navabi H, Jasani B, Adams M, et al. Generation of *in vitro* autologous human cytotoxic T-cell response to E7 and HER-2/neu oncogene products using ex-vivo peptide loaded dendritic cells. *Adv Exp Med Biol* 1997;417:583–589.

231. Evans EM, Man S, Evans AS, Borysiewicz LK. Infiltration of cervical cancer tissue with human papillomavirus-specific cytotoxic T-lymphocytes. *Cancer Res* 1997;57:2943–2950.

232. Cromme FV, Airey J, Heemels MT, et al. Loss of transporter protein, encoded by the TAP-1 gene, is highly correlated with loss of HLA expression in cervical carcinomas. *J Exp Med* 1994;179:335–340.

233. Borysiewicz LK, Fiander A, Nimako M, et al. A recombinant vaccinia virus encoding human papillomavirus types 16 and 18, E6 and E7 proteins as immunotherapy for cervical cancer. *Lancet* 1996;347: 1523–1527.

234. Ressing ME, Sette A, Brandt RM, et al. Human CTL epitopes encoded by human papillomavirus type 16 E6 and E7 identified through *in vivo* and *in vitro* immunogenicity studies of HLA-A*0201–binding peptides. *J Immunol* 1995;154:5934–5943.

235. Palleson G, Hamilton-Dutoit SJ, Rowe M. Expression of Epstein-Barr virus latent gene products in tumour cells of Hodgkin's disease. *Lancet* 1991;337:320–323.

236. Sing AP, Ambinder RF, Hong DJ, et al. Isolation of Epstein-Barr virus (EBV)–specific cytotoxic T lymphocytes that lyse Reed-Sternberg cells: implications for immune-mediated therapy of EBV⁺ Hodgkin's disease. *Blood* 1997;89:1978–1986.

237. Campos LP, Levitsky V, Imreh MP, Gavioli R, Masucci MG. Epitope-dependent selection of highly restricted or diverse T cell receptor repertoires in response to persistent infection by Epstein-Barr virus. *J Exp Med* 1997;186:83–89.

238. Rickinson AB, Moss DJ. Human cytotoxic T lymphocyte responses to Epstein-Barr virus infection. *Annu Rev Immunol* 1997;15:405–431.

239. Gorer PA. Some recent work on tumor immunity. *Adv Cancer Res* 1956;4:149–186.

240. Foley EJ. Antigenic properties of methylcholanthrene-induced tumors in mice of the strain of origin. *Cancer Res* 1953;13:835–837.

241. Baldwin RW. Immunity to methylcholanthrene-induced tumors in inbred rats following atrophy and regression of implanted tumors. *Br J Cancer* 1955;9:652–665.

242. Klein G, Sjogren HO, Klein E, Hellstrom KE. Demonstration of resistance against methylcholanthrene-induced sarcomas in the primary autochthonous host. *Cancer Res* 1960;20:1561–1572.

243. Globerson A, Feldman M. Antigenic specificity of benzo(a) pyrene-induced sarcomas. *J Natl Cancer Inst* 1964;32:1229–1243.

244. Sercarz EE, Lehmann PV, Ametani A, Benichou G, Miller A, Moudgil K. Dominance and crypticity of T cell antigenic determinants. *Annu Rev Immunol* 1993;11:729–766.

245. Liu KJ, Chatta GS, Twardzik DR, et al. Identification of rat prostatic steroid-binding protein as a target antigen of experimental autoimmune prostatitis: implications for prostate cancer therapy. *J Immunol* 1997;159:472–480.

246. Ramarathinam L, Sarma S, Marie M, et al. Multiple lineages of tumors express a common tumor antigen, PIA, but they are not cross-protected. *J Immunol* 1995;155:5323–5329.

247. Kawakami Y, Robbins PF, Wang RF, Rosenberg SA. Identification of melanoma antigens recognized by T lymphocytes and their use in the immunotherapy of cancer. *Princip Pract Oncol* 1996;10:1–20.

248. Ada GL. Vaccines. In: Paul WE, ed. *Fundamental immunology.* New York: Raven Press, 1993:1309–1352.

249. Morgan DJ, Kreuwel HCT, Fleck S, Levitsky HI, Pardoll DM, Sherman LA. Activation of low avidity CTL specific for a self epitope results in tumor rejection but not autoimmunity. *J Immunol* 1998;160: 643–651.

250. Huang AY, Golumbek P, Ahmadzadeh M, Jaffee E, Pardoll D, Levitsky H. Role of bone marrow-derived cells in presenting MHC class I-restricted tumor antigens. *Science* 1994;264:961–965.

251. Kovacsovics-Bankowski M, Rock KL. A phagosome-to-cytosol pathway for exogenous antigens presented on MHC class 1 molecules. *Science* 1995;267:243–246.

252. Huang AYC, Bruce AT, Pardoll DM, Levitsky HI. *In vivo* cross-priming of MHC class I-restricted antigens requires the TAP transporter. *Immunity* 1996;4:349–355.

253. Suto R, Srivastava PK. A mechanism for the specific immunogenicity of heat shock protein-chaperoned peptides. *Science* 1995;269: 1585–1588.

254. Arnold D, Faath S, Rammensee H, Schild H. Cross-priming of minor histocompatibity antigen-specific cytotoxic T cells on immunization with the heat shock protein gp96. *J Exp Med* 1995;182:885–889.

255. Schoenberger SP, Toes REM, Van der Voort EIH, Offringa R, Melief CJM. T help for CTL is mediated by CD40-CD40L interactions. *Nature* 1998;393:480–483.

256. Berd D, Maguire HCJ, Mastrangelo MJ. Induction of cell-mediated immunity to autologous melanoma cells and regression of metastases after treatment with a melanoma cell vaccine preceded by cyclophosphamide. *Cancer Res* 1986;46:2572–2577.

257. Livingston PO, Albino AP, Chung TJ, et al. Serological response of melanoma patients to vaccines prepared from VSV lysates of autologous and allogeneic cultured melanoma cells. *Cancer* 1985;55: 713–720.

258. Berd D, Maguire HCJ, McCue P, Mastrangelo MJ. Treatment of metastatic melanoma with an autologous tumor-cell vaccine clinical and immunologic results in 64 patients. *J Clin Oncol* 1990;8:1858–1867.

259. McCune CS, O'Donnell RW, Marquis DM, Sahasrabudhe DM. Renal cell carcinoma treated by vaccines for active specific immunotherapy: correlation of survival with skin testing by autologous tumor cells. *Cancer Immunol Immunother* 1990;32:62–66.

260. Lindenmann J, Klein PA. Viral oncolysis: increased immunogenicity of host cell antigen associated with influenza virus. *J Exp Med* 1967; 126:93–108.

261. Fearon ER, Itaya T, Hunt B, Vogelstein B, Frost P. Induction in a murine tumor of immunogenic tumor variants by transfection with a foreign gene. *Cancer Res* 1988;48:2975–2980.

262. Itaya T, Yamagiwa S, Okada F, et al. Xenogenization of a mouse lung carcinoma (3LL) by transfection with an allogeneic class I major histocompatibility complex gene (H-2Ld). *Cancer Res* 1987;47: 3136–3140.

263. Plautz GE, Yang ZY, Wu BY, Gao X, Huang L, Nabel GJ. Immunotherapy of malignancy by *in vivo* gene transfer into tumors. *Proc Natl Acad Sci USA* 1993;90:4645–4649.

264. Restifo NP, Spiess PJ, Karp SE, Mule JJ, Rosenberg SA. A nonimmunogenic sarcoma transduced with the cDNA for interferon gamma elicits CD8+ T cells against the wild-type tumor: correlation with antigen presentation capability. *J Exp Med* 1992;175:1423–1431.

265. Gansbacher B, Zier K, Daniels B, Cronin K, Bannerji R, Gilboa E. Interleukin 2 gene transfer into tumor cells abrogates tumorigenicity and induces protective immunity. *J Exp Med* 1990;172:1217–1224.

266. Bubenik J, Simova J, Jandlova T. Immunotherapy of cancer using local administration of lymphoid cells transformed by IL-2 cDNA and constitutively producing IL-2. *Immunol Lett* 1990;23:287–292.

267. Asher M, Mule J, Kasid A. Murine tumor cells transduced with the gene for tumor necrosis factor-α. *J Immunol* 1991;146:3227–3229.

268. Bannerji R, Arroyo CD, Cordon CC, Gilboa E. The role of IL-2 secreted from genetically modified tumor cells in the establishment of antitumor immunity. *J Immunol* 1994;152:2324–2332.

269. Gansbacher B, Bannerji R, Daniels B. Retroviral vector-mediated gamma-interferon gene transfer into tumor cells generates potent and long lasting antitumor immunity. *Cancer Res* 1990;50:7820–7826.

270. Li WQ, Diamantstein T, Blankenstein T. Lack of tumorigenicity of interleukin 4 autocrine growing cells seems related to the anti-tumor function of interleukin 4. *Mol Immunol* 1990;27:1331–1337.

271. Hock H, Dorsch M, Diamantstein T, Blankenstein T. Interleukin 7 induces CD4+ T cell-dependent tumor rejection. *J Exp Med* 1991;174: 1291–1298.

272. Colombo MP, Ferrari G, Stoppacciaro A, et al. Granulocyte colony-stimulating factor gene transfer suppresses tumorigenicity of a murine adenocarcinoma *in vivo*. *J Exp Med* 1991;173:889–897.

273. Rollins BJ, Sunday ME. Suppression of tumor formation *in vivo* by expression of the JE gene in malignant cells. *Mol Cell Biol* 1991;11: 3125–3131.

274. Porgador A, Tzehoval E, Katz A, et al. Interleukin 6 gene transfection into Lewis lung carcinoma tumor cells suppresses the malignant phenotype and confers immunotherapeutic competence against parental metastatic cells. *Cancer Res* 1992;52:3679–3686.

275. Blankenstein T, Qin Z, Uberla K. Tumor suppression after tumor cell-targeted tumor necrosis factor via gene transfer. *J Exp Med* 1991;173: 1047–1052.

276. Townsend SE, Allison JP. Tumor rejection after direct costimulation of CD8+ T cells by B7-transfected melanoma cells. *Science* 1993;259: 368–370.

277. Chen L, Ashe S, Brady WA, et al. Costimulation of antitumor immunity by the B7 counterreceptor for the T lymphocyte molecules CD28 and CTLA-4. *Cell* 1992;71:1093–1102.

278. Baskar S, Ostrand-Rosenberg S, Nabavi N, Nadler LM, Freeman GJ, Glimcher LH. Constitutive expression of B7 restores immunogenicity of tumor cells expressing truncated major histocompatibility complex class II molecules. *Proc Natl Acad Sci USA* 1993;90:5687–5690.

279. Inaba K, Steinmann RM, Witmer-Pack M, et al. Identification of proliferating dendritic cell precursors in mouse blood. *J Exp Med* 1992; 175:1157–1167.

280. Inaba K, Inaba M, Romani N, et al. Generation of large numbers of dendritic cells from mouse bone marrow cultures supplemented with granulocyte/macrophage colony-stimulating factor. *J Exp Med* 1992; 176:1693–1702.

281. Caux C, Dezutter-Dambuyant C, Schmitt D, Bancherau J. GM-CSF and TNF-alpha cooperate in the generation of dendritic Langerhans cells. *Nature* 1992;360:258–261.

282. Schulz M, Zinkernagel RM, Hengartner H. Peptide-induced antiviral protection by cytotoxic T cells. *Proc Natl Acad Sci USA* 1991;88: 991–993.

283. Kast WM, Roux L, Curren J, et al. Protection against lethal Sendai virus infection by *in vivo* priming of virus-specific cytotoxic T lymphocytes with a free synthetic peptide. *Proc Natl Acad Sci USA* 1991;88:2283–2287.

284. Feltkamp MC, Smits HL, Vierboom MP, et al. Vaccination with cytotoxic T lymphocyte epitope-containing peptide protects against a tumor induced by human papillomavirus type 16–transformed cells. *Eur J Immunol* 1993;23:2242–2249.

285. Mandelboim O, Vadai E, Fridkin M, et al. Regression of established murine carcinoma metastases following vaccination with tumour-associated antigen peptides. *Nat Med* 1995;1:1179–1183.

286. Aichele P, Brduscha RK, Zinkernagel RM, Hengartner H, Pircher H. T cell priming versus T cell tolerance induced by synthetic peptides. *J Exp Med* 1995;182:261–266.

287. Aichele P, Kyburz D, Ohashi PS, et al. Peptide-induced T-cell tolerance to prevent autoimmune diabetes in a transgenic mouse model. *Proc Natl Acad Sci USA* 1994;91:444–448.

288. Kast WM, Offringa R, Peters PJ, et al. Eradication of adenovirus E1–induced tumors by E1A-specific cytotoxic T lymphocytes. *Cell* 1989;59:603–614.

289. Toes RE, Blom RJ, Offringa R, Kast WM, Melief CJ. Enhanced tumor outgrowth after peptide vaccination. Functional deletion of tumor-specific CTL induced by peptide vaccination can lead to the inability to reject tumors. *J Immunol* 1996;156:3911–3918.

290. Vitiello A, Ishioka G, Grey HM, et al. Development of a lipopeptide-based therapeutic vaccine to treat chronic HBV infection. I. Induction of a primary cytotoxic T lymphocyte response in humans. *J Clin Invest* 1995;95:341–349.

291. Schild H, Norda M, Deres K, et al. Fine specificity of cytotoxic T lymphocytes primed *in vivo* either with virus or synthetic lipopeptide vaccine or primed *in vitro* with peptide. *J Exp Med* 1991;174:1665–1668.

292. Ingulli E, Mondino A, Khoruts A, Jenkins MK. *In vivo* detection of dendritic cell antigen presentation to CD4(+) T cells. *J Exp Med* 1997;185:2133–2141.

293. Barratt-Boyes SM, Watkins SC, Finn OJ. Migration of cultured chimpanzee dendritic cells following intravenous and subcutaneous injection. *Adv Exp Med Biol* 1997;417:71–75.

294. Mackett M, Smith GL, Moss B. Vaccinia virus: a selectable eukaryotic cloning and expression vector. *Proc Natl Acad Sci USA* 1982;79:7415–7419.

295. Panicali D, Paoletti E. Construction of pxoviruses as cloning vectors: insertion of the thymidine kinase gene from herpes simplex virus into the DNA of infectious vaccinia virus. *Proc Natl Acad Sci USA* 1982;79:4927–4931.

296. Lathe R, Kieny MP, Gerlinger P, et al. Tumour prevention and rejection with recombinant vaccinia. *Nature* 1987;326:878–880.

297. Bernards R, Destree A, McKenzie S, Gordon E, Weinberg RA, Panicali D. Effective tumor immunotherapy directed against an oncogene-encoded product using a vaccinia virus vector. *Proc Natl Acad Sci USA* 1987;84:6854–6858.

298. Wang M, Bronte V, Chen PW, et al. Active immunotherapy of cancer with a nonreplicating recombinant fowlpox virus encoding a model tumor-associated antigen. *J Immunol* 1995;154:4685–4692.

299. Juillard V, Villefroy P, Godfrin D, Pavirani A, Venet A, Guillet JG.

Long-term humoral and cellular immunity induced by a single immunization with replication-defective adenovirus recombinant vector. *Eur J Immunol* 1995;25:3467–3473.

300. Chen PW, Wang M, Bronte V, Zhai Y, Rosenberg SA, Restifo NP. Therapeutic antitumor response after immunization with a recombinant adenovirus encoding a model tumor-associated antigen. *J Immunol* 1996;156:224–231.

301. Xiang ZQ, Yang Y, Wilson JM, Ertl HC. A replication-defective human adenovirus recombinant serves as a highly efficacious vaccine carrier. *Virology* 1996;219:

302. Minev BR, McFarland BJ, Spiess PJ, Rosenberg SA, Restifo NP. Insertion signal sequence fused to minimal peptides elicits specific CD8+ T-cell responses and prolongs survival of thymoma-bearing mice. *Cancer Res* 1994;54:4155–4161.

303. Restifo NP, Bacik I, Irvine KR, et al. Antigen processing *in vivo* and the elicitation of primary CTL responses. *J Immunol* 1995;154:4414–4422.

304. Wu TC, Guarnieri FG, Staveley-O'Carroll KF, et al. Engineering an intracellular pathway for major histocompatibility complex class II presentation of antigens. *Proc Natl Acad Sci USA* 1995;92:11671–11675.

305. Lin KY, Guarnieri FG, Staveley-O'Carroll K, et al. Treatment of established tumors with a novel vaccine that enhances major histocompatibility class II presentation of tumor antigen. *Cancer Res* 1996;56:21–26.

306. Bronte V, Tsung K, Rao JB, et al. IL-2 enhances the function of recombinant poxvirus-based vaccines in the treatment of established pulmonary metastases. *J Immunol* 1995;154:5282–5292.

307. Hung K, Fein S, Beckerleg AM, Levitsky HI, Wu T-C, Pardoll DM. Enhancement of recombinant vaccinia-induced anti-tumor immunity by coadministration of vaccinia expressing the GM-CSF gene. *Cancer Res* 1998;submitted:

308. Hoiseth SK, Stocker BA. Aromatic-dependent *Salmonella typhimurium* are non-virulent and effective as live vaccines. *Nature* 1981;291:238–239.

309. Curtiss R. Attenuated *Salmonella* strains as live vectors for the expression of foreign antigens. In: Woodrow GC, Levine MM, eds. *New generation vaccines.* New York: Mercel Dekker, 1990:161–188.

310. Strugnell RA, Maskell D, Fairweather N, et al. Stable expression of foreign antigens from the chromosome of *Salmonella typhimurium* vaccine strains. *Gene* 1990;88:57–63.

311. Poirier TP, Kehoe MA, Beachey EH. Protective immunity evoked by oral administration of attenuated aroA *Salmonella typhimurium* expressing cloned streptococcal M protein. *J Exp Med* 1988;168:25–32.

312. Sadoff JC, Ballou WR, Baron LS, et al. Oral *Salmonella typhimurium* vaccine expressing circumsporozoite protein protects against malaria. *Science* 1988;240:336–338.

313. Stover CK, De La Cruz VF, Fuerst TR, et al. New use of BCG for recombinant vaccines. *Nature* 1991;351:456–460.

314. Aldovini A, Young RA. Humoral and cell-mediated immune responses to live recombinant BCG-HIV vaccines. *Nature* 1991;351:479–482.

315. Schafer R, Portnoy DA, Brassell SA, Paterson Y. Induction of a cellular immune response to a foreign antigen by a recombinant *Listeria monocytogenes* vaccine. *J Immunol* 1992;149:53–59.

316. Ikonomidis G, Paterson Y, Kos FJ, Portnoy DA. Delivery of a viral antigen to the class I processing and presentation pathway by *Listeria monocytogenes. J Exp Med* 1994;180:2209–2218.

317. Shen H, Slifka MK, Matloubian M, Jensen ER, Ahmed R, Miller JF. Recombinant *Listeria monocytogenes* as a live vaccine vehicle for the induction of protective anti-viral cell-mediated immunity. *Proc Natl Acad Sci USA* 1995;92:3987–3991.

318. Goossens PL, Milon G, Cossart P, Saron MF. Attenuated Listeria monocytogenes as a live vector for induction of CD8+ T cells *in vivo*: a study with the nucleoprotein of the lymphocytic choriomeningitis virus. *Int Immunol* 1995;7:797–805.

319. Pan ZK, Ikonomidis G, Lazenby A, Pardoll DM, Paterson Y. A recombinant *Listeria monocytogenes* vaccine expressing a model tumour antigen protects mice against lethal tumour cell challenge and causes regression of established tumours. *Nat Med* 1995;1:471–477.

320. Pan ZK, Ikonomidis G, Pardoll D, Paterson Y. Regression of established tumors in mice mediated by the oral administration of a recombinant *Listeria monocytogenes* vaccine. *Cancer Res* 1995;55:4776–4779.

321. Falkow S, Isberg RR, Portnoy DA. The interaction of bacteria with mammalian cells. *Annu Rev Cell Biol* 1992;8:333–363.

322. Tilney LG, Portnoy DA. Actin filaments and the growth, movement, and spread of the intracellular bacterial parasite, *Listeria monocytogenes. J Cell Biol* 1989;109:1597–1608.

323. Brunt LM, Portnoy DA, Unanue ER. Presentation of *Listeria monocytogenes* to CD8+ T cells requires secretion of hemolysin and intracellular bacterial growth. *J Immunol* 1990;145:3540–3546.

324. Newborg MF, North RJ. On the mechanism of T cell-independent anti-*Listeria* resistance in nude mice. *J Immunol* 1980;124:571–576.

325. Portnoy DA. Innate immunity to a facultative intracellular bacterial pathogen. *Curr Opin Immunol* 1992;4:20–24.

326. Scott P, Kaufmann SH. The role of T-cell subsets and cytokines in the regulation of infection. *Immunol Today* 1991;12:346–348.

327. Wolff JA, Malone RW, Williams P, et al. Direct gene transfer into mouse muscle *in vivo. Science* 1990;247:1465–1468.

328. Tang DC, DeVit M, Johnston SA. Genetic immunization is a simple method for eliciting an immune response. *Nature* 1992;356:152–154.

329. Montgomery DL, Shiver JW, Leander KR, et al. Heterologous and homologous protection against influenza A by DNA vaccination: optimization of DNA vectors. *DNA Cell Biol* 1993;12:777–783.

330. Donnelly JJ, Ulmer JB, Shiver JW, Liu MA. DNA vaccines. *Annu Rev Immunol* 1997;15:617–648.

331. Irvine KR, Chamberlain RS, Shulman EP, Surman DR, Rosenberg SA, Restifo NP. Enhancing efficacy of recombinant anticancer vaccines with prime/boost regimens that use two different vectors. *J Natl Cancer Inst* 1997;89:1595–1601.

332. Pardoll DM, Beckerleg AM. Exposing the immunology of naked DNA vaccines. *Immunity* 1995;3:165–169.

333. Fu TM, Ulmer JB, Caulfield MJ, et al. Priming of cytotoxic T lymphocytes by DNA vaccines: requirement for professional antigen presenting cells and evidence for antigen transfer from myocytes. *Mol Med* 1997;3:362–371.

334. Sato Y, Roman M, Tighe H, et al. Immunostimulatory DNA sequences necessary for effective intradermal gene immunization. *Science* 1996;273:352–354.

335. Weiner GJ, Liu HM, Wooldridge JE, Dahle CE, Krieg AM. Immunostimulatory oligodeoxynucleotides containing the CpG motif are effective as immune adjuvants in tumor antigen immunization. *Proc Natl Acad Sci USA* 1997;94:10833–10837.

336. Chace JH, Hooker NA, Mildenstein KL, Krieg AM, Cowdery JS. Bacterial DNA-induced NK cell IFN-gamma production is dependent on macrophage secretion of IL-12. *Clin Immunol Immunopathol* 1997;84:185–193.

337. Steinman RM. The dendritic cell system and its role in immunogenicity. *Annu Rev Immunol* 1991;9:271–296.

338. Adema GJ, Hartgers F, Verstraten R, et al. A dendritic-cell-derived C-C chemokine that preferentially attracts naive T cells. *Nature* 1997;387:713–717.

339. Mayordomo JI, Zorina T, Storkus WJ, et al. Bone marrow-derived dendritic cells pulsed with synthetic tumour peptides elicit protective and therapeutic antitumour immunity. *Nat Med* 1995;1:1297–1302.

340. Hsu FJ, Benike C, Fagnoni F, et al. Vaccination of patients with B-cell lymphoma using autologous antigen-pulsed dendritic cells. *Nat Med* 1996;2:52–58.

341. Paglia P, Chiodoni C, Rodolfo M, Colombo MP. Murine dendritic cells loaded *in vitro* with soluble protein prime cytotoxic T lymphocytes against tumor antigen *in vivo. J Exp Med* 1996;183:317–322.

342. Gong J, Chen D, Kashiwaba M, Kufe D. Induction of antitumor activity immunization with fusion of dendritic and carcinoma cells. *Nat Med* 1997;3:558–561.

343. Boczkowski D, Nair SK, Snyder D, Gilboa E. Dendritic cells pulsed with RNA are potent antigen-presenting cells *in vitro* and *in vivo. J Exp Med* 1996;184:465–472.

344. Specht JM, Wang G, Do MT, et al. Dendritic cells retrovirally transduced with a model tumor antigen gene are therapeutically effective against established pulmonary metastases. *J Exp Med* 1997;186:1213–1221.

345. Song W, Kong H, Carpenter H, et al. Dendritic cells genetically modified with an adenovirus vector encoding the cDNA for a model tumor antigen induce protective and therapeutic antitumor immunity. *J Exp Med* 1997;186:1247–1256.

346. Srivastava PK, Heike M. Tumor-specific immunogenicity of stress-

induced proteins: convergence of two evolutionary pathways of antigen presentation? *Semin Immunol* 1991;3:57–64.

347. Udono H, Levey DL, Srivastava PK. Cellular requirements for tumor-specific immunity elicited by heat shock proteins: tumor rejection antigen gp96 primes CD8[+] T cells *in vivo*. *Proc Natl Acad Sci USA* 1994;91:3077–3081.

348. Udono H, Srivastava PK. Comparison of tumor-specific immunogenicities of stress-induced proteins gp96, hsp90, and hsp70. *J Immunol* 1994;152:5398–5403.

349. Udono H, Srivastava PK. Heat shock protein 70-associated peptides elicit specific cancer immunity. *J Exp Med* 1993;178:1391–1396.

350. Lammert E, Arnold D, Nijenhuis M, et al. The endoplasmic reticulum-resident stress protein gp96 binds peptides translocated by TAP. *Eur J Immunol* 1997;27:923–927.

351. Srivastava PK. Peptide-binding heat shock proteins in the endoplasmic reticulum: role in immune response to cancer and in antigen presentation. *Adv Cancer Res* 1993;62:153–177.

352. Tamura Y, Peng P, Liu K, Daou M, Srivastava PK. Immunotherapy of tumors with autologous tumor-derived heat shock protein preparations. *Science* 1997;278:117–120.

353. Blachere NE, Li Z, Chandawarkar RY, et al. Heat shock protein-peptide complexes, reconstituted *in vitro*, elicit peptide-specific cytotoxic T lymphocyte response and tumor immunity. *J Exp Med* 1997;186:1315–1322.

PART VI

Therapeutic Modulation of Inflammation

Inflammation: Basic Principles and Clinical Correlates,
3rd ed., edited by John I. Gallin and Ralph Snyderman.
Lippincott Williams & Wilkins, Philadelphia © 1999.

CHAPTER 73

Agents Targeting Transcription Factors

Anthony M. Manning and Anjana Rao

Over the past decade it has become clear that altered gene expression plays a key role in the pathogenesis of many inflammatory diseases, including rheumatoid arthritis, asthma, inflammatory bowel disease, and sepsis. Simultaneous with this has been an explosion in our understanding of signal transduction mechanisms that regulate inflammatory gene transcription. The efficacy of several well-established antiinflammatory agents is now known to be mediated through their ability to modulate gene transcription. This chapter discusses our current understanding of the mechanisms of inflammatory gene transcription, including descriptions of several gene regulation pathways that appear central to the inflammatory process. Novel agents that modulate the activities of these pathways provide examples of the potential of gene-regulating drugs.

INFLAMMATION: A DISEASE OF ABERRANT GENE EXPRESSION

Inflamed tissues invariably contain many activated cells, including T and B cells, monocytes/macrophages, fibroblasts, and endothelium (1). These activated cells are characterized by elevated expression of many genes encoding inflammatory molecules, including cytokines, growth factors, cell adhesion molecules, and degradative enzymes (Fig. 73-1). Indeed, altered expression of a variety of proinflammatory genes appears fundamental to the etiology of inflammatory diseases.

Overexpression of inflammatory cytokines is thought to be consequential to most inflammatory disease (Fig. 73-1). In rheumatoid arthritis (RA), for example, elevated mRNAs for interleukin-1α (IL-1α), IL-1β, IL-6,

IL-8, IL-10, granulocyte-macrophage colony-stimulating factor (GM-CSF), granulocyte colony-stimulating factor (G-CSF), macrophage colony-stimulating factor (M-CSF), tumor necrosis factor-α (TNF-α), epidermal growth factor (EGF), platelet-derived growth factor (PDGF), and transforming growth factor-β (TGF-β) are detected in synovial cells or fluid from RA patients (2). TNF-α and IL-1, in particular, appear to play a key role in RA disease progression, and in other inflammatory conditions (3). In the RA joint, both cytokines stimulate leukocyte recruitment, osteoclast activation, cartilage degradation, synovial cell and fibroblast proliferation, and the enhanced production of inflammatory mediators from a large number of different cell types. Antagonism of these cytokines using either antibodies, soluble receptors, or receptor antagonists results in clinical improvement (4,5), providing further validation for their pivotal role in joint inflammation. TNF-α also appears to play a key role as a mediator of asthma (6). TNF-α is present within mast cells in the asthmatic lung (7), and elevated levels of TNF-α are present within the bronchoalveolar lavage from atopic asthmatics following experimental challenge with allergen, and in symptomatic versus asymptomatic asthmatics (8). In animal models of allergic disease, TNF-α gene transcription is enhanced and neutralization of TNF-α dramatically suppresses the recruitment of neutrophils and eosinophils to the lung (9).

In response to tissue injury or infection, resident tissue cells such as mast cells or tissue macrophages release cytokines capable of activating the transcription of genes encoding endothelial cell adhesion molecules, including P-selectin, E-selectin, vascular cell adhesion molecule-1 (VCAM-1), and intercellular adhesion molecule-1 (ICAM-1) (10). Endothelial cell adhesion molecules play a key role in inflammation through their ability to enhance recruitment of blood leukocytes to inflamed tissues. In the RA joint, there is elevated expression of E-selectin, VCAM-1, and ICAM-1 (11),

A. M. Manning: Immunology and Preclinical Development, Signal Pharmaceuticals, San Diego, California 92121.

A. Rao: Department of Pathology, Harvard Medical School and the Center for Blood Research, Boston, Massachusetts 02115.

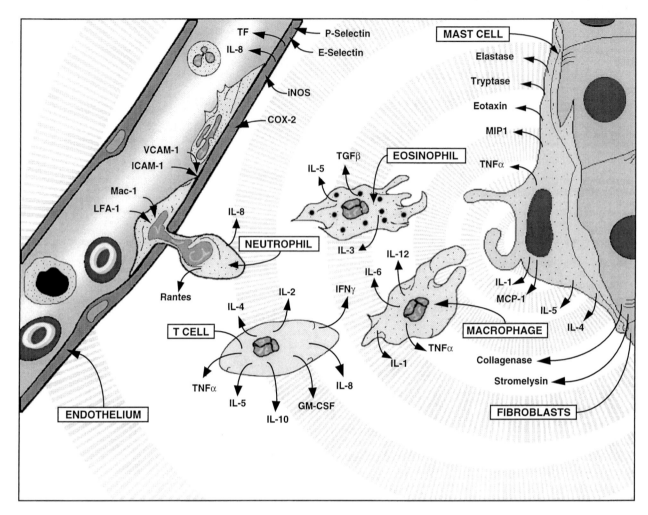

FIG. 73-1. The key role of gene expression in the inflammatory response. Circulating leukocytes are recruited to sites of inflammation by the gene products of activated vascular endothelium and tissue mast cells. Activated leukocytes express specific sets of cytokines, chemokines, growth factors, and degradative enzymes that contribute to resolution of the inflammatory insult. Perturbations in this program of gene expression are responsible for chronic inflammatory disease.

correlating with enhanced recruitment of blood leukocytes and the perpetuation of chronic joint inflammation (12). Antagonism of ICAM-1 function using monoclonal antibodies results in clinical improvement in RA (13). In Crohn's disease, a form of inflammatory bowel disease, antisense inhibition of ICAM-1 production results in clinical improvement and a reduction in the need for glucocorticoid therapy (14), again confirming the critical role of adhesion molecules in inflammation. In RA joints, treatment with monoclonal antibody to TNF-α decreased adhesion molecule expression, T cell infiltration, and joint inflammation, thus demonstrating a link between this proinflammatory cytokine, adhesion molecule expression, and RA (15). Such findings reinforce the integrated nature of inflammatory processes, and suggest the possibility for development of disease-modifying agents that act at points critical to inflammatory gene expression.

Leukotriene synthetic enzymes and other metabolic enzymes, including cyclooxygenase 2 (COX2) and inducible nitric oxide synthase (iNOS), are responsible for the enhanced production of inflammatory mediators at sites of inflammation (reviewed in ref. 16). Transcriptional activity of the genes encoding these enzymes is also elevated in inflamed tissues (17). In many inflammatory diseases, specific matrix degrading enzymes, such as stromelysin or collagenase, or protein-degrading enzymes such as tryptase, are also overexpressed and contribute to irreversible joint and tissue destruction (18).

New technologies for the large-scale analysis of gene expression in cultured cells and tissue samples have highlighted the dramatic changes in gene transcription that occur during the initiation and progression of inflammatory disease. Using cDNA microarray analysis (19) the relative expression of 96 genes, including cytokines, chemokines, growth factors, cell adhesion molecules, matrix degrading enzymes, and transcription factors, was determined in cultured macrophages, synoviocytes, and chondrocytes, and in biopsies from RA and inflammatory bowel disease patients (20). Enhanced transcription of many of these genes was revealed, and differences between RA and inflammatory bowel disease samples were noted. Such analyses support and extend earlier reports of upregulation of inflammatory gene transcription at sites of inflammation.

Because the products of multiple genes contribute to tissue destruction indicative of inflammatory disease, altered gene transcription must be considered as a fundamental process promoting the etiology of these diseases. As described in earlier chapters, several classes of agents with well-established clinical utility, including corticosteroids, cyclosporin A, and gold, are known to mediate their antiinflammatory effects through modulating gene transcription. These agents, discovered through serendipity, exhibit a number of undesirable side effects primarily due to the cellular processes they inhibit. Molecular definition of the mechanisms by which specific genes are turned on or off offers the opportunity for the discovery of novel agents with enhanced efficacy and reduced side effects.

MECHANISMS OF INFLAMMATORY GENE REGULATION

Transcription Factors as Regulators of Inducible Gene Expression

Gene transcription is defined as the copying of DNA encoding a gene into mRNA, which serves as the template for subsequent protein production. This process is regulated by the binding of *trans*-acting factors, including transcription factors, the RNA polymerase complex, and various coactivator proteins, to specific DNA elements located in gene regulatory regions (21). Typically, gene regulatory regions include a promoter region (often with a TATA box) that binds the basal transcription complex, and one or more distal enhancer elements that may be located near the proximal promoter or far distant from it. These elements provide a characteristic array of binding sites for the subset of transcription factors controlling expression of the gene. Examples of promoter-proximal regulatory elements are shown in Fig. 73-2 for the IL-2, TNF-α, and E-selectin genes. Binding of the transcription factors to proximal or distal enhancer regions facili-

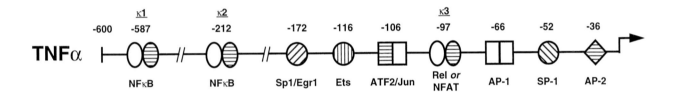

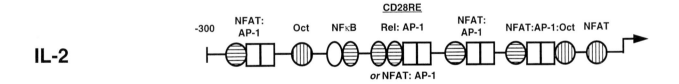

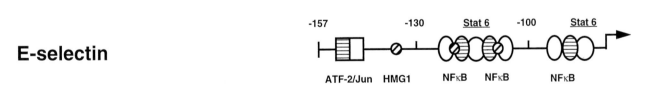

FIG. 73-2. Transcription factor binding sites within the tumor necrosis factor-α (TNF-α), interleukin-2 (IL-2), and E-selectin gene promoters. In many cases, there is highly cooperative binding of different transcription factors to adjacent sites, as seen for nuclear factor of activated T cells/activator protein-1 (NFAT:AP-1) complexes on the IL-2 promoter (29). In other cases, different transcription factors may bind to the same sites, as observed for NFAT and NF-κB on the k3 site of the TNF-α promoter (48), and NFAT and c-Rel/RelA complexes on the CD28 response element (CD28RE) of the IL-2 promoter (29). Overlapping binding sites have also been observed as illustrated for the E-selectin promoter, and may lead to synergy as demonstrated for NF-κB and HMG (I/Y) (75), or to competition as demonstrated for STAT6 and NF-κB (153). Indeed, IL-4 suppresses TNF-α–induced E-selectin gene transcription through this mechanism of STAT6–NF-κB competition.

tates their interaction with the basal transcription complex, either directly or via coactivator proteins. This interaction modulates the activity of RNA polymerase II. The summed activity of the transcription factors binding to the regulatory regions specifies the level of mRNA transcription, and hence the level of the protein product encoded by the gene.

Transcription factors can bind as monomers, dimers, or higher-order multimers to their cognate DNA motifs, which are typically 7 to 20 base pairs in length. In many cases, the transcription factors form heterodimers with other members of their own transcription factor family, and/or cooperative multimers with members of other unrelated families of transcription factors. Individual members of a given transcription factor family may be expressed in a tissue- and cell lineage–specific manner, potentially modulating the expression of specialized cell- and organ-specific genes.

The ability of transcription factors to bind DNA and modulate gene transcription is tightly regulated in normal cells. Specific intracellular signal transduction pathways regulate transcription factor activity through changes in the level of phosphorylation of key residues and domains within the transcription factor (22). These intracellular signal transduction systems transduce extracellular signals from the cell surface to the nucleus, where they are integrated at the level of transcription factor activity (Fig. 73-3). The signaling pathways are highly diverse, yet display an extraordinary degree of specificity for a given transcription factor or transcription factor family. The

identification and molecular cloning of multiple regulatory enzymes that control key steps of these signal transduction pathways have sparked a new wave of drug discoveries, based on using these regulatory enzymes and the transcription factors themselves as targets. The expectation is that these approaches will identify disease-modifying drugs, capable of regulating the expression of genes implicated in the pathogenesis of inflammatory disease.

The rational approach to the discovery of gene-regulating drugs has resulted from an enhanced understanding of specific mechanisms regulating inflammatory gene transcription (23). In particular, the four transcription factor families shown in Fig. 73-3—activator protein-1 (AP-1)/activating transcription factor-2 (ATF-2), nuclear factor-κB (NF-κB), nuclear factor of activated T cells (NFAT), and signal transducers and activators of transcription (STAT)—are likely to be critical regulators of inflammatory gene expression. Their members, upstream activators, and target genes are listed in Table 73-1. Nuclear hormone receptors are covered in another chapter and are not discussed here. The activity of at least three of these transcription factors is regulated, directly or indirectly, by mitogen-activated protein (MAP) kinase pathways, which are discussed in the next section. In subsequent sections we discuss individually the four classes of transcription factors, emphasizing the MAP kinase pathways and other signal transduction pathways that regulate their properties and functions. Where applicable, we discuss selected inhibitors that have emerged as a consequence of using these transcription factors and their

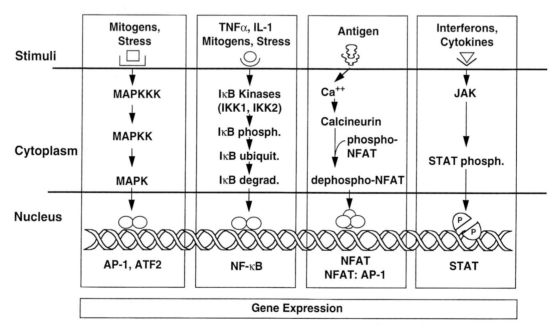

FIG. 73-3. Gene regulation pathways critical to the inflammatory response. Extracellular signals modulate gene expression by activating specific intracellular signal transduction pathways, which in turn regulate transcription factors of the AP-1, activating transcription factor-2 (ATF2), NF-κB, NFAT, and signal transducers and activators of transcription (STAT) families.

TABLE 73-1. *Characteristics of transcription factors*

Transcription factor	Members	Known activators	Products of genes regulated
AP-1/ATF	Jun and Fos JunB and FosB JunD and Fra1/2	TNF, IL-1, UV, H_2O_2, LPS, GFs, stress, T-cell receptor	TNF, IL-1, IL-2, IL-5, IFN-γ, ICAM-1, E-selectin, GM-CSF, MMPs
NF-κB/REL	Rel A p50/105 p52 Rel RelB	TNF, IL-1, UV, H_2O_2, LPS	IL-1, IL-2, IL-6, IL-8, TNF-α, E-selectin, VCAM-1, ICAM-1, MIP-1, MCP-1, eotaxin, RANTES, COX2, MYC, iNOS, cPLA$_2$
NFAT	NFAT 1/p NFAT 2/c NFAT 3 NFAT 4/x	T-cell receptor, B-cell receptor, FCϵ receptors, FCγ receptors, histamine and thrombin receptors	IL-2, IL-3, IL-4, IL-5, IL-8, IL-13, TNF-α, GM-CSF, IFN-γ, CD4OL, FASL
STAT	STATs 1–6	IFNs, CSFs, GFs, IL-1 thru IL-15	FOS, E-selectin, MYC, ICAM-1, FCγRI

AP-1, activator protein-1; CSF, colony-stimulating factor; GF, growth factor; GM-CSF, granulocyte-macrophage colony-stimulating factor; ICAM, intercellular adhesion molecule; IFN, interferon; IL, interleukin; LPS, lipopolysaccharide; MCP, monocyte chemotactic protein; MIP, macrophage inflammatory protein; MMP, matrix metalloproteinases; NF-κB, nuclear transcription factor-κB; NFAT, nuclear factor of activated T cells; RANTES, regulated on activation, normally T-cell expressed and secreted; STAT, signal transducers and activators of transcription; TNF, tumor necrosis factor; UV, ultraviolet light; VCAM, vascular cell adhesion molecule.

upstream activators as targets for the discovery of novel antiinflammatory drugs.

MAP Kinase Pathways and the Regulation of Transcription Factor Function

Diverse extracellular stimuli modulate inflammatory gene transcription via phosphorylation cascades that utilize MAP kinases (22,24). MAP kinase cascades consist of three- or four-tiered signaling modules in which the MAP kinase (MAPK) is activated by a MAP kinase kinase (MAPKK), which in turn is activated by a MAP kinase kinase kinase (MAPKKK) (Fig. 73-4). The MAP-KKK is itself activated by a small G protein such as Ras, either directly or via another upstream kinase (25). Three such MAPK signaling cascades, culminating in activation of the ERK, JNK, and p38 MAP families of MAP kinases, have been investigated in detail. ERKs are activated by mitogens and growth factors via a Ras-dependent pathway, while the JNKs and p38 kinases are activated in response to the proinflammatory cytokines TNF-α and IL-1, and by cellular stress (e.g., heat shock, osmotic shock, reactive oxygen metabolites, protein synthesis inhibitors, UV irradiation) (Fig. 73-4). The MAPKs are proline-directed serine/threonine kinases, which are activated by phosphorylation on closely spaced threonine and tyrosine residues within the activation loop; the activation sequences characteristic of the ERK, JNK, and p38 MAP kinase families are TEY, TPY, and TGY, respectively. These sequences are targets for phosphorylation by specific MAPKKs, dual specificity threonine/tyrosine kinases that are themselves activated by MAPKKK-mediated phosphorylation at a pair of serine residues in the activation loop (22,24,25).

Some features of MAP kinase pathways remain to be elucidated. For instance, while there is some crosstalk between the three major MAPK pathways (see Fig. 73-4), there is also a considerable amount of specificity, the basis for which is not yet understood. Clearly, the greater the specificity, the smaller the likelihood of unwanted side effects from pharmaceutical agents designed to target individual MAP kinase pathways. A related point is that the degree of amplification achieved in MAP kinase signaling is moderate, resembling that achieved in other pathways by the use of a single enzyme, and thus the use of a complex three-kinase cascade does not appear to be warranted on this basis alone (26). Rather, it has been postulated that MAP kinase cascades have evolved to filter out signals of insufficient magnitude or duration while making a strong response to suprathreshold stimuli, thus converting graded extracellular inputs into switch-like (all-or-nothing) intracellular responses (26). If correct, this feature would make MAP kinase pathways even more attractive as targets for pharmacologic modulation, since even partial inhibition of a step in the pathway might abrogate the intracellular response by decreasing the input stimulus to below threshold levels.

MAP kinase pathways regulate the transcriptional activities of a variety of transcription factors, as well as the activities of a number of other cellular proteins involved in gene expression. The effects on AP-1/ATF-2, NF-κB, NFAT, and STAT transcription factors are detailed in the individual sections below. Briefly, MAP kinase pathways directly regulate AP-1–dependent transcription, both at the level of de novo synthesis of AP-1 family proteins and by controlling their transactivation functions (22,24,27,28). AP-1 is a nuclear partner of

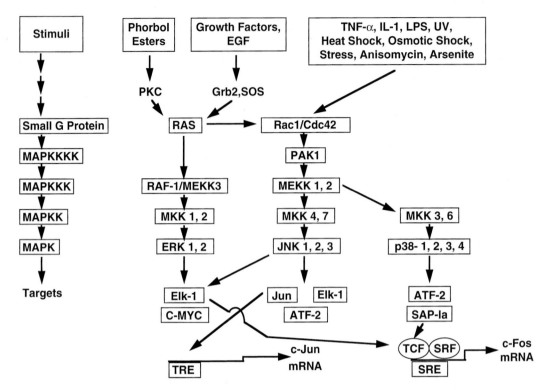

FIG. 73-4. Mitogen-activated protein (MAP) kinase regulation of AP-1, ATF-2, and other transcription factors. Extracellular stimuli activate the ERK, JNK, and p38 MAPK pathways through Ras and Rac-mediated processes. The ERK, JNK, and p38 MAPKs phosphorylate the Elk-1 and SAP-1 transcription factors, resulting in enhanced transcription of the c-Fos and c-Jun genes and protein production. In addition, JNK 1, 2, and 3 phosphorylate ATF-2 and the Jun subunit of AP-1 and directly enhance the transactivating potential of both ATF-2 and AP-1.

NFAT proteins (29), and MAP kinase pathways both indirectly and directly regulate NFAT activity (30,31). Recent work suggests that MAPK pathways are also intimately involved in NF-κB activation, although the mechanistic basis for this crosstalk has not been elucidated (32–34). Lastly, MAP kinase pathways may be implicated in modulating the transcriptional functions of some STAT-family proteins, which are activated in response to cytokine stimulation of cells (35–37). Activation of MAP kinase pathways has been repeatedly documented in inflammatory settings *in vitro* and *in vivo,* and therefore these pathways have become the focus of attention for drug discovery.

REGULATION OF AP-1 AND ATF-2 BY MAP KINASE PATHWAYS

AP-1 Regulation by MAP Kinase Cascades

AP-1 is a pivotal transcription factor that regulates T-cell activation, cytokine production, and production of matrix metalloproteinases (38). The activity of AP-1 can be stimulated by a variety of extracellular signals including cytokines, growth factors, tumor promoters, and the Ras oncoprotein (Table 73-1). AP-1 includes members of

the Jun and Fos families of transcription factors, which are characterized by basic region-leucine zipper (bZIP) DNA-binding domains (39). AP-1 proteins bind to DNA and activate transcription as Jun homodimers, Jun-Jun heterodimers, or Jun-Fos heterodimers. There are multiple Jun and Fos family members (c-Jun, JunB, JunD, and c-Fos, FosB, Fra-1, Fra-2) that are expressed in different cell types and mediate the transcription of both unique and overlapping genes (39).

AP-1 is also a component of the NFAT complex responsible for the transcription of the IL-2 gene and other cytokine genes in activated T cells (29).

All three MAP kinase pathways are involved in the transcriptional regulation of Fos- and Jun-family genes (Fig. 73-4). The ERKs, JNKs, and p38 MAP kinases each contribute to upregulation of c-*fos* gene transcription, by phosphorylating and activating the Ets-family transcription factors Elk-1 and SAP-1 (28,40). These proteins are components of the ternary complex factor (TCF), which binds cooperatively with the serum response factor (SRF) to the serum response element (SRE) of the c-Fos promoter (Fig. 73-4). Elk-1 is phosphorylated by ERK as well as JNK, while SAP-1 is a target of p38 MAPK (28,40). Transcription of the c-*jun* gene is primarily controlled by c-Jun itself via a positive autoregulatory loop

(41); thus upregulation of c-Jun expression in stimulated cells is presumed to be indirectly dependent on the JNK signaling pathway.

A major component of AP-1 regulation is a consequence of posttranslational modification (Fig. 73-4). As mentioned above, Fos activation is primarily regulated at the level of transcription and de novo protein synthesis by mechanisms involving all three MAP kinase pathways, although a yet-uncharacterized Fos-regulating kinase (FRK) that modulates c-Fos transcriptional activity has been described (42). While the c-Jun and JunB genes are also transcriptionally induced, and c-Jun and JunB are synthesized de novo in stimulated cells, a major mode of c-Jun regulation is by phosphorylation at two N-terminal serines in the transactivation domain (amino acids 63 and 73). This is accomplished by the c-Jun N-terminal kinases JNK1 and JNK2, the terminal members of a MAP kinase cascade (Fig. 73-4). Both JNK1 and JNK2 are activated via the Ras pathway by TNF-α, IL-1, T-cell receptor activation, UV irradiation, and other stimuli listed in Fig. 73-4 (43–45). However, JNK2 binds c-Jun with a tenfold higher affinity than JNK1 (45), and may be the physiologically relevant activator of AP-1. N-terminal phosphorylation of c-Jun by JNKs enhances the inducible transcriptional activity of c-Jun by at least 30-fold, with little effect on its basal transcriptional activity. Mutations at the c-Jun phosphorylation sites (serines 63 and 73) have no effect on basal transcriptional activity or DNA binding, but these mutants do not respond to cell activators such as cytokines, growth factors, and UV light (45). Therefore, two distinct forms of AP-1 appear to be responsible for constitutive and inducible gene expression, with JNK playing a critical role in activating c-Jun during the inflammatory response.

ATF-2 and Stress-Activated Kinases

Like Jun and Fos proteins, ATF-2 is a member of the bZIP family of transcription factors (39). ATF-2 is constitutively expressed and its activity is regulated primarily by modulation of its transactivation function. ATF-2 binds to DNA as a homodimer or as a heterodimer with c-Jun and other members of the bZIP family (46). ATF-2 binds sites within the TNF-α, E-selectin, and other gene promoters (47,48) (see Fig. 73-2). In ATF-2–deficient mice, endotoxin-induced E-selectin transcription in the lung is impaired, whereas VCAM-1 transcription is unaffected (49), suggesting that ATF-2 is critical for full induction of E-selectin during an inflammatory response.

ATF-2 is phosphorylated, and its transcriptional function is activated, by JNK1, JNK2, and p38 MAPKs (50). Thus ATF-2 is a direct target for the JNK and p38 signal transduction cascades (Fig. 73-4). The p38 family of MAPKs is activated in a similar fashion to JNKs in endothelial cells stimulated with TNF-α, and in neutrophils and monocytes stimulated with lipopolysaccha-

ride (LPS), platelet-activating factor, or the neutrophil chemoattractant peptide formyl-methionyl-leucyl-phenylalanine (FMLP) (51). Indeed, p38 MAPKs are activated by many of the same stimuli that activate the JNK pathway (52); since these include heat shock, osmotic shock, reactive oxygen metabolites, inhibition of protein synthesis, UV irradiation, and other stressful stimuli (see Table 73-1), the p38 and JNK kinase families have collectively been termed stress-activated protein kinases (SAPKs) (53).

Inhibitors of MAP Kinase Pathways as Antiinflammatory Agents

The ERK Pathway Inhibitor PD98059

Because all three MAP kinase pathways contribute to upregulating c-*fos* gene expression (Fig. 73-4), inhibitors of any of the three MAPK pathways might be expected to inhibit AP-1 upregulation and thus ameliorate the inflammatory response. However, the inhibitor PD98059 (Fig. 73-5), which was discovered in a screen for inhibitors of the ERK cascade (54), does not clearly function as an inhibitor of inflammatory gene transcription. PD98059 binds to the inactive form of MEK1, a primary MAPKK in the ERK cascade, with a concentration that inhibits 50% (IC$_{50}$) of ~4 μM and blocks the phosphorylation required for MEK activation. Specificity of action was indicated by the inability of PD98059 to inhibit phosphorylation mediated by c-Raf, JNK, p38, PKA, PKC, v-Src, active MEK1, and several other serine/threonine and protein tyrosine kinases (including receptor tyrosine kinases) (54). Studies in human endothelial cells confirmed that PD98059 inhibited, in a dose-dependent manner, the phosphorylation and activation of ERK1 in response to thrombin or cytokine activation (55). No inhibition of E-selectin gene expression was seen, however, suggesting that MEK1 inhibition may not affect adhesion molecule expression and leukocyte recruitment to sites of inflammation. However, the ability of PD98059 to modulate cell growth and proliferation of ras-transformed fibroblast cells (54) suggests that this compound, or derivatives thereof, could have potential in treating dysregulated cellular proliferation as seen in RA or other chronic inflammatory diseases. Additional studies using compounds of the PD98059 series will be instrumental in defining the potential role of MEK1 in inflammatory and autoimmune disease.

JNK Pathway Inhibitors

The data discussed above suggest that inhibitors of JNK-mediated AP-1 activation may prove to be novel antiinflammatory/immunosuppressive agents that will inhibit the inducible expression of inflammatory genes, without affecting AP-1–mediated housekeeping func-

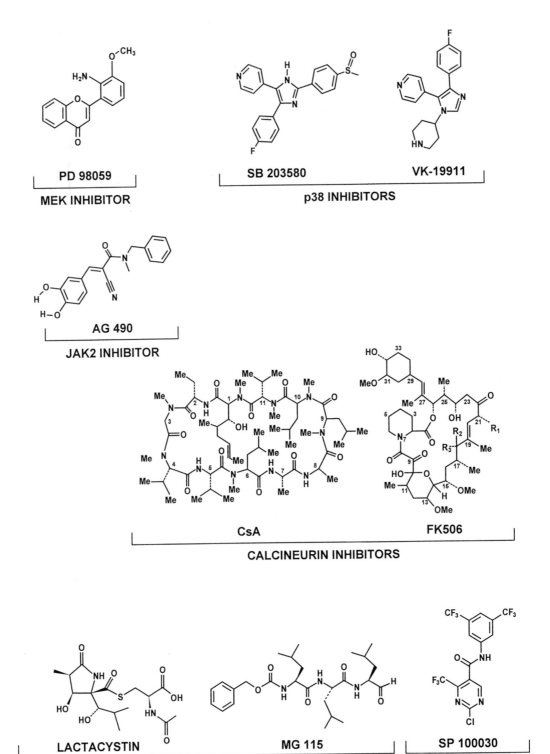

FIG. 73-5. Selected agents regulating inflammatory gene transcription. (For details see text.)

tions. As a result, JNK-1 and JNK-2 are being widely used as targets in inflammatory drug discovery programs. JNKs are activated by ischemia and reperfusion *in vivo* (56), and so could potentially be activated in the rheumatoid joint in the setting of transient ischemia. In T cells, JNK activation by stimulation through the antigen and CD28 receptors correlates with IL-2 induction (44). Similarly, JNK activation in fibroblasts in response to TNF-α and IL-1 correlates with AP-1–dependent transcriptional activation of the collagenase and stromelysin genes (57). It is hoped that JNK inhibition will result in coordinate repression of multiple matrix metalloproteinases in the rheumatic joint, potentially overcoming the overlapping pathologic roles of these enzymes. The upstream MAPKK and MAPKKK activators of JNK (58) represent additional molecular targets for the discovery of JNK inhibitors (Fig. 73-4). However, specific small molecule inhibitors of the JNK pathway have not yet been reported.

Natural inhibitors of transcription factor activation may play a critical role in regulating inflammatory gene expression. An endogenous JNK inhibitor protein, JIP, has been identified based on its ability to bind to JNK and inhibit JNK activity (59). Overexpression of JIP in cells resulted in strong inhibition of JNK-mediated cellular transformation. The identification of endogenous inhibitors, coupled with advances in technologies for gene delivery, suggests the possibility of gene therapy as an approach to modulate transcription factor activity in inflamed tissues.

Inhibitors of p38 MAP Kinases

Indirect evidence for a role of p38 MAPKs in inflammation comes from experiments utilizing a series of bicyclic imidazole derivatives, exemplified by SK&F 86002, SB 203580, and SB 210313 (Fig. 73-5). These compounds were originally termed cytokine-suppressive antiinflammatory drugs (CSAIDs) due to their inhibition of IL-1 and TNF production by human monocytes (60,61). They are potent inhibitors of p38 activity; in fact an analogue of these compounds was used in an affinity purification protocol that led to the molecular cloning of human p38 (62). SB 203580, a triarylimidazole analogue, is a selective p38 inhibitor ($IC_{50} = 0.5$ μM) that has been reported to have no effect on JNK or ERK activity. SB 203580 inhibits p38 kinase activity through direct binding to the adenosine triphosphate (ATP) pocket, thereby inhibiting the phosphorylation and activation of known substrates such as ATF-2 (63). CSAIDs inhibit TNF production following LPS administration *in vivo* and significantly reduce edema and increase bone density in animal models of arthritis (64,65). CSAIDs modulate TNF-α and IL-1 production at the translational as well as the transcriptional level, suggesting that p38 serves multiple roles in addition to activation of ATF-2 and other transcription factors. Unlike earlier compounds in this class,

the more advanced members of the CSAID series have no effect on arachidonate metabolism, demonstrating that it is possible to modulate the arthritic disease process by mechanisms distinct from those used by nonsteroidal antiinflammatory drugs (NSAIDs). However, CSAIDs do downregulate inducible COX2, hence reducing the production of inflammatory prostaglandins.

The basis for the p38 selectivity of the CSAIDs was investigated using the related, highly potent pyridinylimidazole inhibitor VK-19,911 (66). VK-19,911 binds to both unphosphorylated and phosphorylated (active) p38 with similar affinity (kd 12–15 nM). X-ray crystallographic analysis of the structure of VK-19,911–bound p38 indicated that the compound bound in the ATP pocket and contacted, as expected, many residues conserved among other MAP kinases. An exception was threonine-106, a residue in the p38 ATP-binding pocket that is substituted by methionine in the JNKs and by glutamine in the ERKs. Site-directed mutagenesis to replace Thr-106 with Met in p38 had no effect in the overall activity of p38 or its susceptibility to activation *in vitro* by MKK6; however the mutant enzyme was resistant to inhibition by VK-19,911. The results indicate that a single residue difference between p38 and other MAP kinases is sufficient to confer selectivity of inhibition by pyridinylimidazole compounds, and by extension SB 203580 and related triarylimidazole derivatives. More generally, these results, taken together with those obtained for the FGF receptor kinase (67), demonstrate that despite the structural similarity of ATP-binding pockets within different kinase classes, it is feasible to design or screen for inhibitors that selectively target individual kinases within each class.

REGULATION OF NF-κB ACTIVITY BY THE IκB KINASE COMPLEX

Role of NF-κB in Inflammation

NF-κB was first described as a B-cell–specific factor that bound to a short DNA sequence motif located in the immunoglobulin κ light chain enhancer, but it is now clear that NF-κB is expressed in all cell types and plays a broader role in gene transcription (68–70). Members of the NF-κB (also known as Rel) family (see Table 73-1) share a highly homologous N-terminal region of about 300 amino acids known as the Rel homology domain, which mediates dimerization and DNA binding. The classical NF-κB dimer (p50/p65) contains RelA (p65) and NF-κB1 (p50), but a variety of other Rel-containing dimers are also known to exist (68–70; see Table 73-1). The dimeric structure of NF-κB provides for the potential that each family member and Rel dimer serves a distinct biologic function.

NF-κB plays a key role in the expression of many genes central to the inflammatory response (70–72). Participation of this transcription factor in the expression of TNF-α in monocytes, and ICAM-1, TNF-α, and IL-6 in rheumatoid synoviocytes, has been demonstrated (73,74). Inhibition of NF-κB activity in synoviocytes inhibits their proliferation. Also, NF-κB regulates inducible expression of the cell adhesion molecules E-selectin, VCAM-1, and ICAM-1 in vascular endothelial cells, and NF-κB inhibition results in reduced leukocyte adhesion and transmigration (75,76). Activated NF-κB has been detected in a variety of inflammatory settings *in vivo,* including in atherosclerotic and restenotic lesions (77), in septicemia in humans (78), in rheumatoid synovium (79), and in UV-damaged skin (80). NF-κB is rapidly activated in the lung following administration of bacterial endotoxin, an event associated with the transcriptional activation of the P-selectin, E-selectin, VCAM-1, and ICAM-1 genes and the recruitment of leukocytes (81). Activated NF-κB is present within type A synoviocytes, CD14-positive macrophage-like subsynovial cells, and vascular endothelium in the rheumatoid joint (82). Of note, the distribution of NF-κB staining appears to be related to the clinical diagnosis, with enhanced vascular endothelial staining being observed in patients with acute RA. The distribution of activated NF-κB in the rheumatoid joint is consistent with the pattern of expression of NF-κB–dependent genes, including endothelial cell adhesion molecules and macrophage-derived TNF-α and IL-1.

The efficacy of aspirin, gold compounds such as aurothioglucose, and glucocorticosteroids in the treatment of RA correlates with their inhibitory effects on NF-κB (83–86), further validating the role of NF-κB as

an important transcription factor in the rheumatoid joint. A number of other pharmacologic inhibitors of NF-κB activation in cell culture have also been reported, including antioxidants, proteasome inhibitors, and microbial metabolites (reviewed in refs. 70 and 71). However, because these agents exert effects on multiple signaling pathways in cells, it is difficult to ascribe a causal relationship of NF-κB inhibition with any potential disease-modifying effect. Elucidation of components of the signal transduction pathway leading to NF-κB activation offers the best opportunity for the development of selective inhibitors of this transcription factor.

Activation of NF-κB

NF-κB is activated by an extraordinarily large number of different signals, ranging from ultraviolet light to T-cell activation (69,71). Notably, the same cellular stress signals that activate the JNK and p38 MAP kinase pathways also activate NF-κB (see Table 73-1). Nevertheless, the basic steps of NF-κB activation appear similar in all cases (Fig. 73-6). NF-κB exists in the cytoplasm in an inactive form associated with inhibitory proteins termed IκB, of which the most important may be IκBα, IκBβ, and IκBε (68,87). The IκB family members, which share common ankyrin-like repeat domains, regulate the DNA binding and subcellular localization of Rel/NF-κB proteins by masking a nuclear localization signal (NLS) located near the C-terminus of the Rel homology domain (88). NF-κB activation is achieved through the signal-induced proteolytic degradation of IκB in the cytoplasm

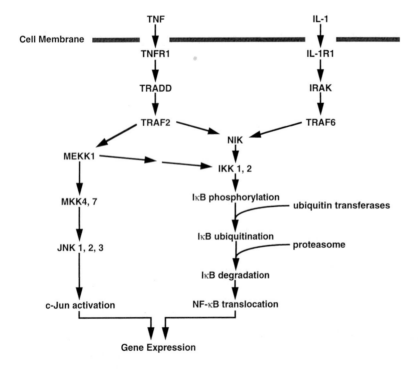

FIG. 73-6. Signal transduction pathways potentially regulating NF-κB activation by TNF-α and IL-1. Activation of the TNF receptor type 1 (TNFR1) leads to recruitment of the TNF receptor–associated proteins TRADD and TRAF2, resulting in activation of the MAPKKKs MEKK1 and NIK, which have both been implicated in activation of the IκB kinases IKK-1 and IKK-2. NIK is also activated by IL-1 through the IL-1 receptor–associated kinase IRAK and TRAF6. Phosphorylation of the cytoplasmic inhibitor of NF-κB, IκB, leads to its ubiquitination and proteolytic degradation by components of the ubiquitin-proteasome system. Free NF-κB within the cytoplasm is rapidly translocated to the nucleus where it modulates gene transcription.

(Fig. 73-6). Extracellular stimuli initiate a signaling cascade leading to activation of two IκB kinases, IKK-1 (IKKα) and IKK-2 (IKKβ), which phosphorylate IκB at specific N-terminal serine residues (S32 and S36 for IκBα, S19 and S23 for IκBβ) (89–93, reviewed in refs. 31–33). Phosphorylated IκB is then selectively ubiquitinated, presumably by an E3 ubiquitin ligase, the terminal member of a cascade of ubiquitin-conjugating enzymes (94,95). In the last step of this signaling cascade, phosphorylated and ubiquitinated IκB, which is still associated with NF-κB in the cytoplasm, is selectively degraded by the 26S proteasome (96). This process exposes the NLS, thereby freeing NF-κB to interact with the nuclear import machinery and translocate to the nucleus, where it binds its target genes to initiate transcription.

The IκB kinases IKK-1 and IKK-2 are related members of a new family of intracellular signal transduction enzymes, containing an amino-terminal kinase domain and a C-terminal region with two protein interaction motifs, a leucine zipper, and a helix-loop-helix motif. These motifs mediate the heterodimerization of IKK-1 and IKK-2, but it is not yet known whether heterodimerization is essential for function. There is strong evidence that IKK-1 and IKK-2 are themselves phosphorylated and activated by one or more upstream activating kinases, which are likely to be members of the MAPKKK family of enzymes (89–93,97,98). One such upstream kinase, NIK, was identified by its ability to bind directly to TRAF2, an adapter protein thought to couple both TNF-α and IL-1 receptors to NF-κB activation (98). A second MAPKKK, MEKK-1, was shown to be present in the IKK signalsome complex (92,97). Coexpression of either NIK or MEKK enhances the ability of the IKKs to phosphorylate IκB and activate NF-κB (89,90,92,93). The likely sites of activating phosphorylation on the IKKs have been identified as two serine residues within the kinase activation loop, which lie within a short region of homology to the MEK (MAPKK) family of proteins (92). Phosphorylation of these two serine residues in the MEKs is required for their activation. In IKK-2, mutation of the two corresponding serine residues to alanine yields an inactive, "dominant-negative" protein capable of blocking the activation of endogenous NF-κB (92); in both IKK-1 and IKK-2, mutation of these residues to glutamate yields a constitutively active kinase, presumably because the glutamate residues mimic to some degree the phosphoserines obtained after phosphorylation by the upstream activating kinase (92).

IκB phosphorylation serves as a molecular tag leading to rapid ubiquitination and degradation of IκB by components of the ubiquitin-proteasome system. The sites of ubiquitin conjugation are two adjacent lysine residues (Lys-20 and Lys-21 in IκBα) located just N-terminal to the two serines that are targets for phosphorylation by the IKKs (94,95,99). Using peptides as substrate mimics, it was established that IκBα phosphorylation generates a binding site for the specific ubiquitin ligase(s) responsible for conjugation of ubiquitin to IκBα, and that microinjection of these phosphopeptides into cells could interfere with NF-κB activation (95). These results emphasize the importance of the ubiquitin ligase system in IκB degradation. However, the IκB-specific E3 ligase remains to be molecularly identified.

The IκB kinases IKK-1 and IKK-2, their upstream activating kinases MEKK and NIK, and their downstream effector, the putative E3 ligase, all represent attractive targets for the discovery of drugs that selectively regulate NF-κB function. These proteins may all be part of a large 600- to 800-kd protein complex, the IKK signalsome (89–97). Particularly interesting is the crosstalk between the NF-κB and AP-1 activation pathways, exemplified by the homology between IKKs and MEKs, the presence of MEKK in the IKK signalsome complex, and the fact that the upstream kinases of the IKKs are members of the MAPKKK family (Fig. 73-6). Certain dual NF-κB/AP-1 inhibitors, which appear to function by inhibiting both pathways simultaneously, are discussed below.

NF-κB Inhibitors

Two recent excellent reviews have summarized the effects and (where known) the mechanism of action of many compounds reported to inhibit the activation or function of NF-κB (70,71). Here we focus on three classes of NF-κB inhibitory compounds: proteasome inhibitors, antioxidants, and dual NF-κB/AP-1 inhibitors with specificity for T cells.

Proteasome Inhibitors

As detailed in the previous section, IκB degradation is mediated by the 26S proteasome, the organelle thought to be responsible for the degradation of abnormal and denatured proteins in the cytoplasm. The 20S proteasome is a large multicatalytic protease complex that forms the core of the 26S proteasome. The 20S proteasome was identified as the specific cellular target of lactacystin, a streptomyces metabolite that inhibits cell cycle progression and promotes neurite outgrowth in a murine neuroblastoma cell line (100,101). Proteasome inhibitors such as lactacystin, MG115, and MG341 have been shown to inhibit NF-κB activation (102,103), and a subset of these (lactacystin, MG341) has been shown to inhibit the transcriptional activation of endothelial cell adhesion molecules as well as leukocyte adhesion (104). Proteasome inhibitors also induce cell cycle arrest and apoptosis (105), making them potentially useful agents in the treatment of proliferative diseases. Note, however, that tyrosine phosphorylation of IκB at Tyr-42 has been reported to induce IκB dissociation and NF-κB activation by a mechanism not involving the proteolytic degradation of IκB (106), and inhibitors of IκB degradation would not be expected to block NF-κB activation via this mechanism.

Antioxidants

Inflammatory reactions are generally accompanied by the local production of reactive oxygen metabolites, including hydroxy and nitroxy radicals, hydrogen peroxide, and superoxide. Although the exact role of these metabolites in the pathogenesis of inflammatory disease is controversial, there is extensive evidence for their role as second messengers regulating NF-κB expression (107) and Ras-mediated mitogenesis (108). Reactive oxygen activates NF-κB in cultured cells, and antioxidants such as pyrrolidone dithiocarbamate (PDTC) can inhibit NF-κB activation by a range of stimuli (109). Several antioxidants have been tested *in vivo* and found to modulate NF-κB activation and endothelial cell adhesion molecule gene transcription (110). It should be noted, however, that antioxidants exert a plethora of effects on cells, including activation of MAP kinases and other transcription factors such as AP-1 (111–113). It is unlikely that antioxidants could be developed as specific inhibitors of NF-κB activation, although their potential as antiinflammatory agents may be realized because of their pleiotropic effects on inflammatory gene expression.

Dual Inhibitors of NF-κB and AP-1

A novel class of T-cell–specific inhibitors of NF-κB and AP-1 activity was recently identified in a cell-based screening effort to identify modulators of inflammatory gene expression (114). The most potent inhibitor in this series, SP100030, inhibits NF-κB– and AP-1–dependent reporter gene expression in stably transfected Jurkat T cells with an IC$_{50}$ of 30 nM. In stimulated Jurkat T cells, SP100030 inhibited the induced transcription of the IL-2, IL-8, TNF-α, and GM-CSF genes with a similar IC$_{50}$. The effects of SP100030 were specific for human T cells, demonstrating activity in four separate T cell lines and in primary T cells isolated from whole human blood. SP100030 displayed no activity in non–T-cell lines, including monocytes, epithelial cells, fibroblasts, synoviocytes, osteoblasts, and endothelial cells. SP100030 demonstrated efficacy in preclinical models of autoimmune disease, including adjuvant-induced arthritis, delayed-type hypersensitivity, inflammatory bowel disease, and allograft rejection. SP100030 represents a new class of T-cell–specific dual inhibitors of NF-κB– and AP-1–mediated inflammatory gene expression, and suggests that cell-specific inhibitors of inflammatory gene expression can indeed be identified. An interesting implication, possibly related to the cross-regulation of NF-κB and AP-1 activity by MAP kinase pathways, is that T cells

possess a common target protein that controls the functions of both NF-κB and AP-1.

REGULATION OF NFAT ACTIVITY BY CALCINEURIN AND AP-1

Activation of Nuclear Factor of Activated T Cells (NFAT)

Proteins belonging to the NFAT family of transcription factors play a central role in inducible gene expression during the immune response (reviewed in ref. 29). NFAT is encoded by at least four genes, each expressed as several alternatively spliced isoforms (see Table 73–1). NFAT proteins are expressed and functional in several immune-related cells, including T cells, B cells, natural killer (NK) cells, mast cells, macrophages, and endothelial cells (115,116). NFAT is activated by stimulation of receptors coupled to calcium mobilization, such as the antigen receptors on T and B cells, the Fcε receptors on mast cells and basophils, the Fcγ receptors on macrophages and NK cells, and the histamine and thrombin G-protein–coupled receptors on endothelial cells. Ligand binding to these receptors leads, via activation of phospholipase C and generation of inositol trisphosphate (IP$_3$), to calcium mobilization and activation of the calcium- and calmodulin-dependent phosphatase calcineurin, a major upstream regulator of NFAT (29).

The functions of NFAT proteins are regulated by calcineurin-mediated dephosphorylation (115,117–122). In resting cells, NFAT proteins are phosphorylated and reside in the cytoplasm; in activated cells, they become dephosphorylated by calcineurin and translocate into the nucleus. Regulation of NFAT by calcineurin is a completely reversible process: in stimulated cells, inhibition of calcineurin activity [by removal of the calcium-mobilizing stimulus, chelation of extracellular calcium, treatment with inhibitors of capacitative calcium entry, or treatment with the immunosuppressive agents cyclosporin A (CsA) and FK506] permits NFAT rephosphorylation by constitutive NFAT kinases and results in nuclear export of NFAT (118,121,122). Calcineurin regulates NFAT function by binding to the NFAT regulatory domain, a conserved region of ~300 amino acids that contains the phosphoserine residues that are substrates for dephosphorylation by calcineurin (120,121). The regulatory domain controls all calcineurin-dependent functions of NFAT proteins, including the accessibility of the conserved nuclear localization signal (NLS), the accessibility of the N-terminal transactivation domain, and the stimulation-dependent increase in DNA binding (120,121,123). Fusion of the NFAT regulatory domain to unrelated proteins confers calcineurin responsiveness on the chimeric proteins (121,123,124).

The nuclear functions of NFAT proteins are regulated by cooperative interactions with AP-1 (reviewed in refs.

29 and 125). The strongly conserved DNA-binding domains of NFAT proteins are structurally similar to those of Rel/NF-κB proteins (29,125,126). Unlike Rel proteins, however, NFAT proteins bind as monomers to DNA. The majority of identified NFAT sites, described in the regulatory regions of diverse inducible genes, are composite elements containing an NFAT binding site (consensus sequence GGAAAANN) adjacent to an AP-1 binding site (consensus sequence TGAC/GTCA) (29). The affinity of the individual sites can vary widely, with a moderate- to high-affinity NFAT site juxtaposed to a low-affinity AP-1 site and vice versa (29). The affinity of the cooperative complex for the composite DNA element is at least 10 to 20 times greater than that of the individual transcription factors for their individual sites (127–129). This is explained by x-ray crystallographic analysis of the NFAT-Fos-Jun-DNA complex, which shows the existence of multiple protein-protein contacts between NFAT and the Fos-Jun dimer (130). The specificity of interaction is emphasized by the observation that when adjacent to NFAT, the Fos-Jun dimer is frozen in one of two possible orientations on the AP-1 site (129). The question of whether there are functional sites at which NFAT does not cooperate with AP-1 is not yet resolved. A fraction of NFAT sites bind NFAT with very high affinity, and there is no indication of an adjacent AP-1 site, whereas other NFAT sites, especially those in the TNF-α and IL-8 promoters, resemble NF-κB sites and bind (noncooperatively) two molecules of NFAT (29).

NFAT has been implicated in the inducible expression of a growing number of genes induced during the immune/inflammatory response (see Table 73-1). In peripheral blood mononuclear cells from RA patients, enhanced levels of nuclear NFAT DNA binding activity are observed, correlating with disease activity (131). In patients with early RA, low-dose CsA is as effective as traditional disease-modifying antirheumatic drugs (DMARDs) in controlling clinical symptoms and decreasing the rate of further joint damage in previously involved joints as well as the rate of new joint involvement (132).

Inhibitors of Calcineurin and NFAT

The potent immunosuppressive agents CsA and FK506 inhibit the expression of many cytokine genes and other inducible genes during the immune response (reviewed in refs. 29 and 133). CsA and FK506 each bind with high affinity to distinct intracellular immunophilin receptors, cyclophilins, and FK-binding proteins (FKBPs). The drug-immunophilin complexes, rather than the drugs themselves, are the active immunosuppressive agents; they bind calcineurin and inhibit its ability to dephosphorylate NFAT, thereby inhibiting NFAT activation. In T cells, CsA and FK506 also inhibit NF-κB activation (134), as well as JNK activation and thereby AP-1 activity (44).

Over the last 15 years, organ transplantation has been established as a viable medical alternative for patients facing imminent organ failure. This is entirely attributable to the clinical use of CsA, and more recently FK506, to combat transplant rejection (135). However the toxicity of these drugs, which arises from their ability to inhibit calcineurin in cells outside the immune system (136), has limited their use in clinical situations such as asthma, inflammation, and autoimmune disease, where immunosuppressive regimens might be warranted. Pharmacologic agents that targeted NFAT independently of calcineurin might lack the toxicity of CsA and FK506 while retaining their antirheumatic activity.

Potential noncalcineurin targets in the NFAT pathway include the Lck and ZAP-70 tyrosine kinases, which play a critical role in calcium mobilization and therefore NFAT activation (137). The NFAT kinases that counteract the action of calcineurin are also interesting targets, since agents that enhanced NFAT kinase activity would be expected to limit the total time spent by NFAT proteins in the nucleus. These NFAT kinases have been variously proposed to be JNK kinases (30,31) and GSK-3 (138), but the real candidate may not yet have been identified. Inhibitors of AP-1 would be expected to inhibit NFAT transcriptional activity by interfering with the activity of cooperative NFAT:AP-1 complexes. In this regard, it is interesting that PDTC and other dithiocarbamates greatly upregulate JNK activity in T cells (113) but downregulate NFAT activity (30), apparently by enhancing the activity of a kinase (potentially JNK itself) that mediates the nuclear export of NFAT (30,31). Further elucidation of the NFAT regulatory pathway will enhance the potential for new immunosuppressive drug discovery.

SIGNAL TRANSDUCERS AND ACTIVATORS OF TRANSCRIPTION (STATS)

Like NF-κB and NFAT, the STATs are a family of latent cytoplasmic transcription factors that are activated in response to stimulation of cells through various cytokine receptors (see Table 73–1). STAT proteins play a critical role in mediating the intracellular effects of many cytokines (139,140), and as such represent potential drug targets in RA (141). Seven mammalian STAT proteins, whose genes map to three chromosomal clusters, have been identified (139). In addition to their centrally located DNA-binding domains and their C-terminal transactivation domains, STAT proteins contain SH2 domains that serve a dual function, promoting the specific docking of each STAT protein to the appropriate tyrosine-phosphorylated cytokine receptor as well as the homodimerization and (in some cases) the heterodimerization of activated STAT proteins themselves. The STATs are activated by a novel family of cytoplasmic tyrosine kinases, termed Janus kinases (JAKs), that associate with cell-surface cytokine receptors and are catalytically activated by transphosphorylation following ligand binding and receptor heterodimerization (139,140). The activated JAKs phosphorylate tyrosine residues on the receptors, thus recruiting STATs; subsequently, the STATs themselves are phosphorylated, leading to their release from the receptor docking sites and the formation of dimers that then translocate to the nucleus.

There are indications that serine phosphorylation of certain STAT proteins is required for their optimal function. Phosphoserine residues have been detected in activated STATs 1, 3, 4, 5A, and 5B, but not in activated STAT2 (139). In STATs 1 and 3, phosphorylation occurs on a single serine in a conserved Pro-Met-Ser-Pro sequence in the C-terminal transactivation domain (35,36). In STAT3 and STAT5, serine phosphorylation is reported to be required for optimal DNA binding, while in STAT1, serine phosphorylation does not influence DNA binding but enhances transactivation function (35–37). The Pro-Met-Ser-Pro sequence is similar to the consensus sequence for phosphorylation by MAP kinases, and it is possible that STAT function is influenced by MAP kinase activation in cytokine-stimulated cells. However, the ERK pathway does not contribute to serine phosphorylation of STAT5 in IL-2–stimulated cells (37).

STATs have been implicated in the expression of many inflammatory effector genes, including various immunoglobulin receptors and cell surface proteins, including ICAM-1 (Table 73-1). Active STAT3 was detected in cells from inflamed joints (142), and synovial fluid from RA patients can activate STAT3 but not STAT1 (143). Although no small molecule inhibitors of the STATs themselves have yet been reported, the JAK2 antagonist AG-490 (Fig. 73-5) selectively inhibits leukemic cell growth *in vitro* and *in vivo* (144), suggesting a role for STATs in unregulated growth. The activity of this compound in an arthritis model has not been reported, but it is tempting to suggest that chronic JAK/STAT activation may play a role in synovial hyperplasia or the persistence of inflammatory cells in the inflamed joint. STAT proteins play a key role in lymphocyte differentiation and proliferation, with STAT4 and STAT6 being functionally important for Th1 and Th2 helper cell differentiation, respectively (145,146). The role of T cells in established RA is incompletely understood, and disappointing results with agents designed to diminish T-cell function in late-stage patients suggests that T-cell–directed immunotherapy may be clinically ineffective. A more complete understanding of the phenotype of T cells in the RA joint may substantiate the potential of STAT modulation to influence T-cell functions in this setting.

A family of endogenous inhibitors of STAT signaling pathways has recently been identified. Its members are the cytokine-induced SH2-binding protein CIS (147), and the suppressors of cytokine signaling SOCS-1, SOCS-2, and SOCS-3 (148–150). The SOCS proteins are also induced at the mRNA level by specific cytokines (149). SOCS-1 is also known as JAB [JAK-binding protein (149)] and SSI-1 [STAT-induced STAT inhibitor-1 (150)]. The family is characterized by the presence of an SH2 domain and a C-terminal "SOCS-box" containing a potential JAK pseudosubstrate sequence (150). SOCS-1 and CIS appear to be components of a cytokine-induced negative feedback pathway that limits the magnitude and duration of cytokine-mediated responses. CIS binds the tyrosine-phosphorylated forms of the EPO receptor and the IL-3 receptor β chain, and is thought to function by masking the docking sites on these receptors for JAKs, STATs, and other signaling proteins (147). In contrast, SOCS-1/JAB/SSI-1 is proposed to function by binding the JAK kinases JAK2 and Tyk2 and inhibiting their kinase activity, thereby inhibiting the activation of signaling intermediates such as the STATs (148–150). A similar negative feedback function, operating at the level of the IL-3 and EPO receptors, has been ascribed to the tyrosine phosphatase SHP-1 (151,152). Agents that induce or upregulate the functions of these inhibitory proteins may suppress the cytokine-induced component of the inflammatory response.

CONCLUSION

Clearly, inducible gene expression plays a fundamental role in the initiation of inflammatory responses. The protein products of newly induced genes promote the recruitment of leukocytes from the circulation to injured or infected tissues, the differential activation of leukocyte types and their effector functions, and the final resolution of the inflammatory injury. Alterations in this program of inflammatory gene expression lead to a plethora of chronic inflammatory and autoimmune diseases. We now appreciate that the efficacy of many established immunomodulatory therapeutics is due to their ability to modulate inflammatory gene transcription. Enhanced understanding of the key pro- and antiinflammatory cytokines, and of the signaling pathways and transcription factors that regulate their expression and that they in turn regulate, is laying the foundation for a new era in antiinflammatory drug discovery. Several initial successes in the identification of gene-regulating agents have been reviewed here, but these most likely represent only the first wave of promising new agents to come. Two areas do require further investigation: the mechanisms of cell-specific regulation of inflammatory gene transcription, and the mechanisms by which different gene-regulating pathways are integrated to modulate transcription at sites of inflammation. Regulation of inflammatory gene transcription holds great promise in the search for novel agents with the potential to revolutionize the treatment of inflammatory and autoimmune diseases.

ACKNOWLEDGMENTS

The authors thank Deborah Higginbottom and Nathan Eller for their assistance with figures and manuscript preparation. This work was supported in part by National Institutes of Health grants CA42471 and AI40127 to A.R. A.R. is a scholar of the Leukemia Society of America.

REFERENCES

1. Feldmann M, Brennan FM, Maini RN. Rheumatoid arthritis. *Cell* 1996;85:307–310.
2. Firestein GS. Cytokine networks in rheumatoid arthritis: implications for therapy. *Agents Actions* 1995;S47:37–51.
3. Arend WP, Dayer J. Inhibition of the production and effects of interleukin-1 and tumor necrosis factor α rheumatoid arthritis. *Arthritis Rheum* 1995;38(2):151–160.
4. Elliott MJ, Maini RN, Feldmann M, et al. Treatment of rheumatoid arthritis with chimeric monoclonal antibodies to tumor necrosis factor alpha. *Arthritis Rheum* 1993;12:1681–1690.
5. Campion GV, Lebsack ME, Lookabaugh J, Gordon G, Catalano M, The IL-1Rα Arthritis Study Group. Dose-range and dose-frequency study of recombinant human interleukin-1 receptor antagonist in patients with rheumatoid arthritis. *Arthritis Rheum* 1996;39(7):1092–1101.
6. Shah A, Church MK, Holgate ST. Tumor necrosis factor alpha—a potential mediator of asthma. *Clin Exp Allergy* 1995;25:1038–1044.
7. Bradding P, Roberts JA, Britten KM, et al. Interleukin-4, -5 and -6 and tumor necrosis factor-α in normal and asthmatic airways: evidence for the human mast cell as a source of these cytokines. *Am J Respir Cell Mol Biol* 1994;10:471–480.
8. Konno S, Gonokami Y, Kurokawa M, et al. Cytokine concentrations in sputum of asthmatic patients. *Int Arch Allergy Immunol* 1996;109:73–78.
9. Lukacs NW, Streiter RM, Chensue SW, Widmer M, Kunkel SL. TNF-α mediates recruitment of neutrophils and eosinophils during airway inflammation. *J Immunol* 1995;154:5411–5417.
10. Carlos T, Harlan JM. Leukocyte-endothelial adhesion molecules. *Blood* 1994;84:2068–2101.
11. Johnson BA, Haines GK, Harlow LA, Koch AE. Adhesion molecule expression in human synovial tissue. *Arthritis Rheum* 1993;36:137–146.
12. Tak PP, Thurkow EW, Daha MR, et al. Expression of adhesion molecules in early rheumatoid synovial tissue. *Clin Immunol Immunopathol* 1995;77(3):236–242.
13. Kavanaugh AF, Davis LS, Nichols LA, et al. Treatment of refractory rheumatoid arthritis with a monoclonal antibody to intercellular adhesion molecule 1. *Arthritis Rheum* 1994;37:992–999.
14. Isis' positive Crohn's disease trial. *SCRIP* 1997;2212:23.
15. Tak PP, Taylor PC, Breedveld FC, et al. Decrease in cellularity and expression of adhesion molecules by anti-tumor necrosis factor α monoclonal antibody treatment in patients with rheumatoid arthritis. *Arthritis Rheum* 1996;39(7):1077–1081.
16. Lewis AJ, Keft AF. A review on the strategies for the development and application of new anti-arthritic agents. *Immunopharmacol Immunotoxicol* 1995;17(4):607–663.
17. Seibert K, Zhang Y, Leahy K, et al. Pharmacological and biochemical demonstration of the role of cyclooxygenase 2 in inflammation and pain. *Proc Natl Acad Sci USA* 1994;91:12013–12017.
18. Firestein GS, Paine MM, Littman BH. Gene expression (collagenase, tissue inhibitor of metalloproteinases, complement, and HLA-DR) in rheumatoid arthritis and osteoarthritis synovium: quantitative analysis and effect of intraarticular corticosteroids. *Arthritis Rheum* 1994;34:1094–1105.
19. Schena M, Shalon D, Heller R, Chai A, Brown PO, Davis RW. Parallel human genome analysis: microarray-based expression monitoring of 1000 genes. *Proc Natl Acad Sci USA* 1996;93:10614–10619.
20. Heller RA, Schena M, Chai A, et al. Discovery and analysis of inflammatory disease-related genes using cDNA microarrays. *Proc Natl Acad Sci USA* 1997;94:2150–2155.
21. Tjian R, Maniatis T. Transcriptional activation: a complex puzzle with few easy pieces. *Cell* 1994;77:5–8.
22. Karin M, Hunter T. Transcriptional control by protein phosphorylation: signal transmission from the cell surface to the nucleus. *Curr Biol* 1995;5:747–757.
23. Manning AM, Mercurio F. Transcription inhibitors in inflammation. *Exp Opin Invest Drugs* 1997;6:555–567.
24. Su B, Karin M. Mitogen-activated protein kinase cascades and the regulation of gene expression. *Curr Opin Immunol* 1996;8:402–411.
25. Fanger GR, Gerwins P, Widmann C, Jarpe MB, Johnson GL. MEKKs, GCKs, MLKs, PAKs, TAKs, and Tpls: upstream regulators of the c-Jun amino-terminal kinases? *Curr Opin Genet Dev* 1997;7:67–74.
26. Ferrell JE. Tripping the switch fantastic: how a protein kinase cascade can convert graded inputs into switch-like outputs. *Trends Biochem Sci* 1996;252:460–466.
27. Karin M. The regulation of AP-1 activity by mitogen-activated protein kinases. *J Biol Chem* 1995;270:16483–16486.
28. Whitmarsh AJ, Davis RJ. Transcription factor AP-1 regulation by mitogen-activated protein kinase signal transduction pathways. *J Mol Med* 1996;74:589–607.
29. Rao A, Luo C, Hogan PG. Transcription factors of the NFAT family: regulation and function. *Annu Rev Immunol* 1997;15:707–747.
30. Martinez-Martinez S, Gomez P, Armesilla AL, et al. Blockade of T-cell activation by dithiocarbamates involves novel mechanisms of inhibition of nuclear factor of activated T cells. *Mol Cell Biol* 1997;17:6437–6447.
31. Chow CW, Rincon M, Cavanagh J, Dickens M, Davis RJ. Nuclear accumulation of NFAT4 opposed by the JNK signal transduction pathway. *Science* 1997;278:1638–1641.
32. Stancovski I, Baltimore D. NF-κB activation: the IκB kinase revealed? *Cell* 1997;91:299–302.
33. Maniatis T. Catalysis by a multiprotein IκB kinase complex. *Science* 1997;278:818–819.
34. Verma IM, Stevenson J. IκB kinase: beginning, not end. *Proc Natl Acad Sci USA* 1997;94:11758–11760.
35. Zhang X, Blenis J, Li HC, Schindler C, Chen-Kiang S. Requirement of serine phosphorylation for formation of STAT-promoter complexes. *Science* 1995;267:1990–1994.
36. Wen Z, Zhong Z, Darnell JE. Maximal activation of transcription by STAT1 and STAT3 requires both tyrosine and serine phosphorylation. *Cell* 1995;82:241–250.
37. Beadling C, Ng J, Babbage JW, Cantrell DA. Interleukin-2 activation of STAT5 requires the convergent action of tyrosine kinases and a serine/threonine kinase pathway distinct from the Raf1/ERK2 MAP kinase pathway. *EMBO J* 1996;15:1902–1913.
38. Angel P, Karin M. The role of Jun, Fos and the AP-1 complex in cell proliferation and transformation. *Biochim Biophys Acta* 1991;1072:129–157.
39. Kerppola TK, Curran T. Transcription factor interactions: basics on zippers. *Curr Opin Struct Biol* 1991;1:71–79.
40. Whitmarsh AJ, Shore P, Sharrocks AD, Davis RJ. Integration of MAP kinase signal transduction pathways at the serum response element. *Science* 1995;269:403–407.
41. Angel P, Hattori K, Smeal T, Karin M. The jun proto-oncogene is positively autoregulated by its product, Jun/AP-1. *Cell* 1988;55:875–885.
42. Deng T, Karin M. c-Fos transcriptional activity stimulated by H-Ras-activated protein kinase distinct from JNK and ERK. *Nature* 1994;371:171–175.
43. Hibi M, Lin A, Smeal T, Minden A, Karin M. Identification of an oncoprotein and UV-responsive protein kinase that binds and potentiates the c-Jun activation domain. *Genes Dev* 1993;7:2135–2148.
44. Su B, Jacinto E, Hibi M, Kallunki T, Karin M, Ben-Neriah Y. JNK is involved in signal integration during co-stimulation of T lymphocytes. *Cell* 1994;77:727–736.
45. Kallunki T, Su B, Tsigelny I, et al. JNK2 contains a specificity-determining region responsible for efficient c-Jun binding and phosphorylation. *Genes Dev* 1994;8:2996–3007.
46. Hai T, Curran T. Cross-family dimerization of transcription factors Fos/Jun and ATF/CREB alters DNA binding specificity. *Proc Natl Acad Sci USA* 1991;88:3720–3724.
47. Kaszubska W, Hooft van Huijsduijnen R, Ghersa P, et al. Cyclic AMP-independent ATF family members interact with NF-κB and function in the activation of the E-selectin promoter in response to cytokines. *Mol Cell Biol* 1993;13:7180–7190.
48. Tsai EY, Jain J, Pesavento PA, Rao A, Goldfeld AE. Tumor necrosis factor alpha gene regulation in activated T cell involves ATF-2/Jun and NFATp. *Mol Cell Biol* 1996;16:459–467.
49. Reimold AM, Grusby MJ, Kosaras B, et al. Chondrodysplasia and

neurological abnormalities in ATF2-deficient mice. *Nature* 1996;379:
262–265.

50. Gupta S, Campbell D, Derijard B, Davis RJ. Transcription factor ATF2
regulation by the JNK signal transduction pathway. *Science* 1995;267:
389–393.

51. Modur V, Zimmerman GA, Prescott SM, McIntyre TM. Endothelial
cell inflammatory responses to tumor necrosis factor. *J Biol Chem*
1996;271:13094–13102.

52. Han J, Lee JD, Bibbs L, Ulevitch RJ. A MAP kinase targeted by endotoxin and hyperosmolarity in mammalian cells. *Science* 1994;265:
808–811.

53. Lee JC, Young PR. Role of CSB/p38/RK stress response kinase in LPS
and cytokine signalling mechanisms. *J Leukoc Biol* 1996;59:152–157.

54. Dudley DT, Pang L, Decker SJ, Bridges AJ, Saltiel AR. A synthetic
inhibitor of the mitogen-activated protein kinase cascade. *Proc Natl
Acad Sci USA* 1995;92:7686–7689.

55. Wheeler-Jones CP, May MJ, Houliston RA, Pearson JD. Inhibition of
MAP kinase kinase (MEK) blocks endothelial PGI2 release but has no
effect on von Willebrand factor secretion or E-selectin expression.
FEBS Lett 1996;388:180–184.

56. Pombo CM, Bonventre JV, Avruch J, Woodgett JR, Kyriakis JM, Force
T. The stress-activated protein kinases are major c-Jun amino-terminal
kinases activated by ischemia and reperfusion. *J Biol Chem* 1994;269:
26546–26551.

57. Okamoto K, Fujisawa K, Hasunuma T, Kobata T, Sumida T, Nishioka
K. Selective activation of the JNK/AP-1 pathway in Fas-mediated
apoptosis of rheumatoid arthritis synoviocytes. *Arthritis Rheum* 1997;
40:919–926.

58. Tournier C, Whitmarsh A, Cavanagh S, Barrett T, Davis RJ. Mitogen
activated kinase kinase 7 is an activator of the c-jun NH2-terminal
kinase. *Proc Natl Acad Sci USA* 1997;94:337–7342.

59. Dickens M, Rogers JS, Cavanagh J, et al. A cytoplasmic inhibitor of
the JNK signal transduction pathway. *Science* 1997;277:693–696.

60. Boehm JC, Smietana JM, Sorenson ME, et al. 1-substituted 4-aryl-5-
pridinylimidazoles: a new class of cytokine suppressive drugs with
low 5-lipoxygenase and cyclooxygenase inhibitor potency. *J Med
Chem* 1996;39:3929–3937.

61. Lantos I, Bender PE, Razgaitis KA, et al. Antiinflammatory activity of
5,6-diaryl-2,3-dihydroimidazo[2,1-b]thiazoles. Isomeric 4-pyridyl
and 4-substituted phenyl derivatives. *J Med Chem* 1984;27:72–75.

62. Lee JC, Laydon JT, McDonnell PC, et al. A protein kinase involved in
the regulation of inflammatory cytokine biosynthesis. *Nature* 1994;
372:739–746.

63. Tong L, Pav S, White DM, et al. A highly specific inhibitor of human
p38 MAP kinase binds in the ATP pocket. *Nature Struct Biol* 1997;
4:311–316.

64. Badger AM, Bradbeer JN, Votta B, Lee JC, Adams JL, Griswold DE.
Pharmacological profile of SB203580, a selective inhibitor of
cytokine suppressive binding protein/p38 kinase, in animal models of
arthritis, bone resorption, endotoxin shock and immune function. *J
Pharmacol Exp Ther* 1996;279:1453–1461.

65. Griswold DE, Hillegass LM, O'Leary-Bartus J, Lee JC, Laydon JT,
Trophy TJ. Evaluation of human cytokine production and effects of
pharmacological agents in a heterologous system *in vivo*. *J Immunol
Methods* 1996;195:1–5.

66. Wilson KP, McCaffrey PG, Hsiao K, et al. Structural basis for specificity of pyridinylimidazole inhibitors of p38 MAP kinases. *Chem
Biol* 1997;4:423–431.

67. Mohammadi M, McMahon G, Sun L, et al. Structures of the tyrosine
kinase domain of the fibroblast growth factor receptor in complex
with inhibitors. *Science* 1997;276:955–960.

68. Baeuerle PA, Baltimore D. NF-κB: ten years after. *Cell* 1996;87:13–20.

69. Baeuerle PA, Henkel T. Function and activation of NF-κB in the
immune system. *Annu Rev Immunol* 1994;12:141–179.

70. Baldwin AS. The NF-κB and IκB proteins: new discoveries and
insights. *Annu Rev Immunol* 1996;14:649–681.

71. Baeuerle PA, Baichwal VR. NF-κB as a frequent target for immunosuppressive and anti-inflammatory molecules. *Adv Immunol* 1997;65:
111–137.

72. Manning AM, Anderson DC. Transcription factor NF-κB: an emerging regulator of inflammation. *Ann Rep Med Chem* 1994;29:235–244.

73. Ziegler-Heitbrock HWL, Sternsdorf T, Liese T, et al. Pyrrolidine
dithiocarbamate inhibits NF-κB mobilization and TNF production in
human monocytes. *J Immunol* 1993;151:6986–6993.

74. Fujisawa K, Aono H, Hasunuma T, Yamamoto K, Mita S, Nishioka K.
Activation of transcription factor NF-κB in human synovial cells in
response to tumor necrosis factor α. *Arthritis Rheum* 1996;39:
197–203.

75. Collins T, Read MA, Neish AS, Whitley MZ, Thanos D, Maniatis T.
Transcriptional regulation of endothelial cell adhesion molecules: NF-
κB and cytokine-inducible enhancers. *FASEB J* 1995;9:899–909.

76. Chen CC, Rosenbloom CL, Anderson DC, Manning AM. Selective
inhibition of E-selectin, vascular cell adhesion molecule-1, and intercellular adhesion molecule-1 expression by inhibitors of IκB-α phosphorylation. *J Immunol* 1995;155:3538–3545.

77. Brand K, Page S, Rogler G, et al. Activated transcription factor NF-
κB is present in the atherosclerotic lesion. *J Clin Invest* 1996;97:
1715–1722.

78. Bohrer H, Qiu F, Zimmerman T, et al. Role of NF-κB in the mortality
of sepsis. *J Clin Invest* 1997;100:972–985.

79. Handel ML, McMorrow LB, Gravallese EM. NF-κB in rheumatoid
synovium: localization of p50 and p65. *Arthritis Rheum* 1996;38:
1762–1770.

80. Fisher GJ, Datta SC, Talwar HS, et al. Molecular basis of sun-induced
premature skin aging and retinoid antagonism. *Nature* 1996;379:
335–339.

81. Manning AM, Bell FP, Rosenbloom CL, et al. NF-κB is activated during acute inflammation *in vivo* in association with elevated endothelial cell adhesion molecule gene expression and leukocyte recruitment. *J Inflammation* 1995;45:283–296.

82. Marok R, Winyard PG, Coumbe A, et al. Activation of the transcription factor nuclear factor-κB in human inflamed synovial tissue.
Arthritis Rheum 1996;39:583–591.

83. Kopp E, Ghosh S. Inhibition of NF-κB by sodium salicylate and
aspirin. *Science* 1994;265:956–959.

84. Yang JP, Merin JP, Nakano T, Kato T, Kitade Y, Okamoto T. Inhibition
of the DNA-binding activity of NF-κB by gold compounds *in vitro*.
FEBS Lett 1995;361:89–96.

85. Auphan N, DiDonato JA, Rosette C, Helmberg A, Karin M. Immunosuppression by glucocorticoids: inhibition of NF-κB activity through
induction of IκB-α synthesis. *Science* 1995;270:286–290.

86. Scheinman RI, Crosswell PC, Loftquist AK, Baldwin AS. Role of
transcriptional activation of IκB-α in mediation of the immunosuppression by glucocorticoids. *Science* 1995;270:283–286.

87. Whiteside ST, Epinat JC, Rice NR, Israel A. IκB epsilon, a novel
member of the IκB family, controls RelA and cRel NF-κB activity.
EMBO J 1997;16:1413–1426.

88. Henkel T, Zabel U, Van Zee K, Muller JM, Fanning E, Baeuerle P.
Intramolecular masking of the nuclear location signal and dimerization domain in the precursor for the p50 NF-κB subunit. *Cell*
1992;68:1121–1133.

89. Regnier CH, Song H, Gao H, Goeddel DV, Cao Z, Rothe M. Identification and characterization of an IκB kinase. *Cell* 1997;90:373–383.

90. DiDonato JA, Hayakawa M, Rothwarf DM, Zandi E, Karin M. A
cytokine-responsive IκB kinase that activates the transcription factor
NF-κB. *Nature* 1997;388:853–862.

91. Zandi E, Rothwarf DM, Delhasse M, Hayakawa M, Karin M. The IκB
kinase complex (IKK) contains two kinase subunits, IKKα and IKKβ,
necessary for IκB phosphorylation and NF-κB activation. *Cell* 1997;
91:243–252.

92. Mercurio F, Zhu H, Murray BW, et al. IKK-1 and IKK-2: cytokine-
activated IκB kinases essential for NF-κB activation. *Science* 1997;
278:860–866.

93. Woronicz JD, Gao X, Cao Z, Rothe M, Goeddel DV. IκB kinase-β:
NF-κB activation and complex formation with IκB kinase-α and NIK.
Science 1997;278:866–869.

94. Alkalay I, Yaron A, Hatzubai A, Orian A, Ciechanover A, Ben-Neriah
Y. Stimulation-dependent IκBα phosphorylation marks the NF-κB
inhibitor for degradation via the ubiquitin-proteasome pathway. *Proc
Natl Acad Sci USA* 1995;92:10599–10603.

95. Yaron A, Alkalay I, Hatzubai A, et al. Inhibition of NF-κB cellular
function via specific targeting of the IκBα ubiquitin ligase. *EMBO J*
1997;16:101–107.

96. Chen Z, Hagler J, Palombella VJ, et al. Signal-induced site-specific
phosphorylation targets IκBα to the ubiquitin-proteasome pathway.
Genes Dev 1995;9:1586–159.

97. Lee FS, Hagler J, Chen ZJ, Maniatis T. Activation of the IκBα complex by MEKK1, a kinase of the JNK pathway. *Cell* 1997;88:213–222.

98. Malinin NL, Boldin MP, Kovalenko AV, Wallach D. MAP3K-related kinase involved in NF-κB induction by TNF, CD95 and IL-1. *Nature* 1997;385:540–544.

99. Orian A, Whiteside S, Israel A, Stancovski I, Schwartz AL, Ciechanover A. Ubiquitin-mediated processing of NF-κB transcriptional activator precursor p105. Reconstitution of a cell-free system and identification of the ubiquitin-carrier protein, E2, and a novel ubiquitin-protein ligase, E3, involved in conjugation. *J Biol Chem* 1995;270: 21707–21714.

100. Fenteany GF, Standaert RF, Lane WS, Choi S, Corey EJ, Schreiber SL. Inhibition of proteasome activities and subunit-specific amino-terminal threonine modification by lactacystin. *Science* 1995;268:726–731.

101. Omura S, Fujimoto T, Otoguro K, et al. Lactacystin, a novel microbial metabolite, induces neuritogenesis of neuroblastoma cells. *J Antibiot* 1991;44:113–116.

102. Palombella VJ, Rando OL, Goldberg AL, Maniatis T. The ubiquitin-proteasome pathway is required for processing the NF-κB1 precursor protein and the activation of NF-κB. *Cell* 1994;78:773–785.

103. Traenckner B-ME, Wilk S, Baeuerle PA. A proteasome inhibitor prevents NF-κB activation and stabilizes a newly phosphorylated form of Iκ-Bα that is still bound to NF-κB. *EMBO J* 1995;13:5433–5441.

104. Read MA, Neish AS, Luscinskas FW, Palombella VJ, Maniatis T, Collins T. The proteasome pathway is required for cytokine-induced endothelial leukocyte adhesion molecule expression. *Immunity* 1995; 2:493–506.

105. Maki CG, Huibregtse JM, Howley PM. *In vivo* ubiquitination and proteasome-mediated degradation of p53. *Cancer Res* 1996;56:2649–2654.

106. Imbert V, Rupec RA, Livolsi A, et al. Tyrosine phosphorylation of IκB-α activates NF-κB without proteolytic degradation of IκB-α. *Cell* 1996;86:787–798.

107. Schreck R, Rieber P, Baeuerle PA. Reactive oxygen intermediates as apparently widely used messengers in the activation of the NF-κB transcription factor and HIV-1. *EMBO J* 1991;10:2247–2258.

108. Irani K, Xia Y, Zweier JL, et al. Mitogenic signaling mediated by oxidants in Ras-transformed fibroblasts. *Science* 1997;275:1649–1652.

109. Ziegler-Heitbrock HWL, Sternsdorf T, Liese J, et al. Pyrrolidine dithiocarbamate inhibits NF-κB mobilization and TNF production in human monocytes. *J Immunol* 1993;151:6986–6993.

110. Gerritsen ME, Carley WW, Ranges GE, et al. Flavonoids inhibit cytokine-induced endothelial cell adhesion protein gene expression. *Am J Pathol* 1995;147:278–292.

111. Coso OA, Chiariello M, Yu JC, et al. The small GTP-binding proteins Rac1 and Cdc42 regulate the activity of the JNK/DAPK signaling pathway. *Cell* 1995;81:1137–1146.

112. Meyer M, Schreck R, Baeuerle PA. H₂O₂ and antioxidants have opposite effects on activation of NF-κB and AP-1 in intact cells: AP-1 as secondary antioxidant-responsive factor. *EMBO J* 1993;12:2005–2015.

113. Gomez del Arco P, Martinez-Martinez S, Calvo V, Armesilla AL, Redondo JM. JNK is a target for antioxidants in T lymphocytes. *J Biol Chem* 1996;271:26335–26340.

114. Goldman ME, Ransone LJ, Anderson DW, et al. SP100030 is a novel T-cell-specific transcription factor inhibitor that possesses immunosuppressive activity *in vivo*. *Trans Proc* 1996;28:3106–3109.

115. Shaw KTY, Ho AM, Raghavan A, et al. Immunosuppressive drugs prevent a rapid dephosphorylation of transcription factor NFAT1 in stimulated immune cells. *Proc Natl Acad Sci USA* 1995;92:11205–11209.

116. Cockerill GW, Bert AG, Ryan GR, Gamble JR, Vadas MA, Cockerill PN. Regulation of granulocyte-macrophage colony-stimulating factor and E-selectin expression in endothelial cells by cyclosporin A and the T cell transcription factor NFAT. *Blood* 1995;86:2689–2698.

117. Loh C, Carew JA, Kim J, Hogan PG, Rao A. T-cell receptor stimulation elicits an early phase of activation and a later phase of deactivation of the transcription factor NFAT1. *Mol Cell Biol* 1996;16: 3945–3954.

118. Loh C, Shaw KT-Y, Carew J, et al. Calcineurin binds the transcription factor NFAT1 and reversibly regulates its activity. *J Biol Chem* 1996; 271:10884–10891.

119. Luo C, Burgeon E, Carew JA, et al. Recombinant NFAT1 (NFATp) is regulated by calcineurin in T cells and mediates transcription of several cytokine genes. *Mol Cell Biol* 1996;16:3955–3966.

120. Luo C, Shaw KTY, Raghavan A, et al. Interaction of calcineurin with a domain of the transcription factor NFAT2 that controls nuclear import. *Proc Natl Acad Sci USA* 1996;93:8907–8912.

121. Shibasaki F, Price ER, Milan D, Mckeon F. Role of kinases and the phosphatase calcineurin in the nuclear shuttling of transcription factor NF-AT4. *Nature* 1996;382:370–373.

122. Timmerman LA, Clipstone NA, HO SN, Northrop JP, Crabtree GR. Rapid shuttling of NF-AT in discrimination of Ca²⁺ signals and immunosuppression. *Nature* 1996;383:837–840.

123. Luo C, Burgeon E, Rao A. Mechanisms of transactivation by nuclear factor of activated T Cells-1. *J Exp Med* 1996;184:141–147.

124. Beals CR, Clipstone NA, Ho SN, Crabtree GR. Nuclear localization of NF-ATc by a calcineurin-dependent, cyclosporine-sensitive intramolecular interaction. *Genes Dev* 1997;11:824–834.

125. Chytil M, Verdine GL. The Rel family of eukaryotic transcription factors. *Curr Opin Struct Biol* 1996;6:91–100.

126. Jain J, Burgeon E, Badalian TM, Hogan PG, Rao A. A similar DNA-binding motif in NFAT family proteins and the rel homology region. *J Biol Chem* 1995;270:4138–4145.

127. Jain J, McCaffrey PG, Miner Z, et al. The T-cell transcription factor NFATp is a substrate for calcineurin and interacts with Fos and Jun. *Nature* 1993;365:352–355.

128. Jain J, Miner Z, Rao A. Analysis of the preexisting and nuclear forms of nuclear factor of activated T cells. *J Immunol* 1993;151:837–848.

129. Lin C, Oakleyt MG, Glover JNM, et al. Only one of the two DNA-bound orientations of AP-1 found in solution cooperates with NFATp. *Curr Biol* 1995;5:882–889.

130. Chen L, Glover JNM, Hogan PG, Rao A, Harrison SC. Structure of the DNA binding domains of NFAT, Fos, and Jun bound to DNA. *Nature* (submitted).

131. Becker H, Stengl G, Stein M, Federlin K. Analysis of proteins that interact with the IL-2 regulatory region in patients with rheumatic diseases. *Clin Exp Immunol* 1995;99:325–330.

132. Pasero G, Priolo F, Marubini E, et al. Slow progression of joint damage in early rheumatoid arthritis treated with cyclosporin A. *Arthritis Rheum* 1996;39:1006–1015.

133. Crabtree GR, Clipstone NA. Signal transmission between the plasma membrane and nucleus of T lymphocytes. *Annu Rev Biochem* 1994; 63:1045–1083.

134. Frantz B, Nordby EC, Bren G, et al. Calcineurin acts in synergy with PMA to inactivate IκB/MAD3, an inhibitor of NF-κB. *EMBO J* 1994; 13:861–870.

135. Wiederrecht G, Lam E, Hung S, Martin M, Sigal N. The mechanism of action of FK-506 and cyclosporin A. *Ann NY Acad Sci* 1993;696: 9–19.

136. Dumont FJ, Staruch MJ, Koprak SL, et al. The immunosuppressive and toxic effects of FK-506 are mechanically related: pharmacology of a novel antagonist of FK-506 and rapamycin. *J Exp Med* 1992; 176:751–760.

137. Cantrell D. T cell antigen receptor signal transduction pathways. *Annu Rev Immunol* 1996;14:259–274.

138. Beals CR, Sheridan CM, Turck CW, Gardner P, Crabtree GR. Nuclear export of NF-ATc enhanced by glycogen synthase kinase-3. *Science* 1997;275:1930–1933.

139. Darnell J. STATs and gene regulation. *Science* 1997;277:1630–1635.

140. Ihle JN. Cytokine receptor signalling. *Nature* 1995;377:591–594.

141. Rosen J, Day A, Jones TK, Jones ETT, Nadzan AM, Stein RB. Intracellular receptors and signal transducers and activators of transcription superfamilies: novel targets for small molecule drug discovery. *J Med Chem* 1995;38:4855–4874.

142. Wang F, Sengupta TK, Zhong Z, Ivashkiv LB. Regulation of the balance of cytokine production and the signal transducer and activator of transcription (STAT) transcription factor activity by cytokines and inflammatory synovial fluids. *J Exp Med* 1995;182:1825–1831.

143. Sengupta TK, Chen A, Zhong Z, Darnell JE, Ivashkiv LB. Activation of monocyte effector genes and STAT family transcription factors by inflammatory synovial fluid is independent of interferon. *J Exp Med* 1995;181:1015–1025.

144. Meydan N, Grunberger T, Dadi H, et al. Inhibition of acute lymphoblastic leukemia by a JAK-2 inhibitor. *Nature* 1996;379: 645–648.

145. Thiefelder WE, van Deursen JM, Yamamoto K, et al. Requirement for STAT4 in interleukin-12-mediated responses of natural killer and T cells. *Nature* 1996;382:171–174.

146. Shimoda K, van Deursen J, Sangster MY, et al. Lack of IL-4–induced Th2 response and IgE class switching in mice with disrupted STAT6 gene. *Nature* 1996;380:630–633.

147. Yoshimura A, Ohkubo T, Kiguchi T, et al. A novel cytokine-inducible

gene CIS encodes an SH2-containing protein that binds to tyrosine-phosphorylated interleukin 3 and erythropoietin receptors. *EMBO J* 1995;14:2816–2826.

148. Starr R, Willson TA, Viney EM, et al. A family of cytokine-induced inhibitors of signalling. *Nature* 1997;387:917–921.

149. Endo TA, Masuhara M, Yokouchi M, et al. A new protein containing an SH2 domain that inhibits JAK kinases. *Nature* 1997;387: 921–924.

150. Naka T, Narazaki M, Hirata M, et al. Structure and function of a new STAT-induced STAT inhibitor. *Nature* 1997;387:924–929.

151. Yi T, Mui Al, Krystal G, Ihle JN. Hematopoietic cell phosphatase associates with the interleukin-3 (IL-3) receptor beta chain and down-regulates IL-3 induced tyrosine phosphorylation and mitogenesis. *Mol Cell Biol* 1993;13:7577–7586.

152. Klingmuller U, Lorenz U, Cantley LC, Neel BG, Lodish HF. Specific recruitment of SH-PTP1 to the erythropoietin receptor causes inactivation of JAK2 and termination of proliferative signals. *Cell* 1995;80: 729–738.

153. Bennett BL, Cruz R, Lacson RG, Manning AM. Interleukin-4 suppression of tumor necrosis factor α-stimulated E-selectin gene transcription is mediated by STAT6 antagonism of NF-κB. *J Biol Chem* 1997;272:10212–10217.

Inflammation: Basic Principles and Clinical Correlates,
3rd ed., edited by John I. Gallin and Ralph Snyderman.
Lippincott Williams & Wilkins, Philadelphia © 1999.

CHAPTER 74

Inhibitors and Antagonists of Cyclooxygenase, 5-Lipoxygenase, and Platelet Activating Factor

Henry J. Showell and Kelvin Cooper

There have been several recent noteworthy discoveries and developments pertinent to the field of research covered in this chapter: (a) the discovery of the existence of a second enzyme, prostaglandin endoperoxide synthase-2 (PGHS-2) also known as cyclooxygenase-2 (COX-2), that catalyzes the conversion of arachidonate to prostaglandin H_2, the precursor of biologically active prostaglandins; (b) the discovery and demonstration of the preclinical and clinical efficacy of selective COX-2 inhibitors; (c) the development and demonstration of clinical efficacy and regulatory approval of compounds that either block the 5-lipoxygenase pathway of arachidonic acid metabolism or antagonize receptors for its metabolites, i.e., cysteinyl leukotriene (LTD_4); (d) the development and demonstration of the clinical efficacy of platelet-activating factor (PAF) receptor antagonists; (e) the discovery and demonstration of the efficacy of selective leukotriene B_4 (LTB_4) receptor antagonists in a variety of preclinical animal disease models; and (f) via specific gene deletion experiments [e.g., 5-LO, 5-lipoxygenase activating protein (FLAP), COX-1 and -2 knock-out mice] and specific antibodies [e.g., anti–prostaglandin E_2 (PGE_2)], the pathologic role of these enzymatic pathways and their products has been confirmed in a variety of preclinical animal models of disease.

Altogether, this has been an extremely exciting period in the history of inflammation research, which has allowed this field to move forward in a highly positive way. Not only have these new preclinical findings offered promise for the successful clinical development of new agents with either a greater efficacy or better safety profile, but the extant clinical data now support this notion and already indicate that some of these compounds will undoubtedly find a place in the modern armamentarium of drugs that will be available to treat a variety of inflammatory diseases.

DISCOVERY OF MOLECULAR TARGETS

Prostaglandin Endoperoxide Synthase-1 and -2 (Cyclooxygenase-1 and -2)

Inhibitors of cyclooxygenase (COX) have been the mainstay of treatment for the symptoms of rheumatoid arthritis, osteoarthritis, gout, and other inflammatory conditions for the last 100 years or so, although the basis for their activity has only been understood since the early 1970s (1). The recent discovery that there are two distinct COX enzymes, however, has excited a rebirth of interest in the inhibition of COX that is based on the differential expression of the two isozymes and an associated deeper understanding of the pharmacology of the currently available COX inhibitors (2) (see chapter by Griffiths). Thus, COX-1 is constitutively and widely expressed and involved in the release of prostaglandins involved in physiologic processes. COX-2, however, has a much more restricted expression pattern, e.g., in neutrophils, macrophages, endothelial cells, and fibroblasts after induction by an inflammatory event, and in the kidney and brain, constitutively (2). The fact that the currently available inhibitors are in general nonselective explains the occurrence of side effects, and therefore the current focus of research is to identify COX-2 selective agents that would afford all the symptomatic benefits of COX inhibition without the side effects. In addition, the role of COX-2 in cell proliferation, cell adhesion, and apoptosis,

H. J. Showell: Genomics, Targets and Cancer Research, Central Research Division, Pfizer, Groton, Connecticut 06340.

K. Cooper: Candidate Synthesis, Enhancement and Evaluation, Central Research Division, Pfizer, Groton, Connecticut 06340.

as well as the expression of COX-2 in the brain, have raised the possibilities for the use of COX-2 selective agents for the treatment of certain types of cancer (3) and Alzheimer's (4).

5-Lipoxygenase (5-LO) and 5-Lipoxygenase Activating Protein (FLAP)

The first description of the 5-LO pathway of arachidonic acid metabolism came from the work two decades ago of Borgeat et al. (5), who found rabbit neutrophils could metabolize arachidonic acid into 5-hydroxyeicosatetraenoic acid (5-HETE). This observation subsequently led to the discovery of the dihydroxyeicosatetraenoic acid, LTB_4, and the cysteinyl leukotriene, LTC_4, as products of the 5-LO pathway with potent biologic activities (see chapter by Penrose et al.). 5-LO was first purified from a variety of mammalian sources and subsequently cloned in 1988 (reviewed in ref. 6). The discovery of FLAP occurred from elucidation of the mechanisms of action of the leukotriene biosynthesis inhibitor MK-886 (reviewed in ref. 7).

Leukotriene Receptors (LTD_4 ($CysLT_1$) and LTB_4 (BLT))

The first description of the existence of receptors for LTD_4 on smooth muscle came from the original observations of Feldberg and Kellaway (8) in 1938, who were studying the pharmacologic principal product from tissues perfused with cobra venom. Subsequent studies by Kellaway and Trethewie (9) on pharmacologic activities released from antigen-challenged guinea pig lung gave rise to description of a slow-reacting smooth muscle stimulant substance (SRS). This was ultimately shown to contain a mixture of cysteinyl leukotrienes (Cys LTs) (see chapter by Penrose et al.). In 1973, prior to the structural elucidation of the Cys LTs, a selective antagonist (FPL55712) of slow-reacting substance of anaphylaxis (SRSA) was discovered by Augstein et al. (10), and this discovery formed the basis of early attempts to uncover more potent compounds.

LTB_4 receptors on leukocytes were first appreciated based on the observation by Bray et al. (11) that ionophore-stimulated neutrophils released a compound that caused chemotaxis and aggregation of isolated leukocytes. Subsequent work showed that this substance was LTB_4 (12), and through the synthesis of isotopically labeled LTB_4 the existence of specific high-affinity receptors on leukocytes (13,14) and membranes derived from animal tissue such as spleen (15) was established. The receptor for LTB_4, which is a G-protein–coupled receptor and weakly homologous (~30%) to other chemotactic factor receptors, was recently cloned (16).

Platelet Activating Factor (PAF) and Its Receptor

PAF was first identified over 25 years ago as a factor involved in hypersensitivity reactions (17,18). Its struc-

tural elucidation occurred in 1979 (19–21) and again through the use of radiolabeled PAF the existence of specific high-affinity receptors on leukocytes was established (22). The receptor for PAF was cloned in 1991 (23).

THE DISCOVERY AND CLINICAL DEVELOPMENT OF CYCLOOXYGENASE-1 AND -2 INHIBITORS

Cyclooxygenase Inhibitors

There are several potential modes for inhibition of COX, including limiting substrate concentrations, preventing the obligatory oxidative activation, reducing the catalytically active enzyme, and inhibiting arachidonic acid (AA) binding, but the vast majority of known inhibitors block AA binding. The inhibitors have been further classified into three types on the basis of their mode of action at the AA-binding site: simple competitive inhibitors; competitive, time-dependent, reversible inhibitors; and irreversible inhibitors. The various modes of inhibition have led to difficulties in establishing a universal methodology for the measurement of inhibitor potency and selectivity. Thus, depending on the assay conditions, enzyme source, and whether the assay is in vitro or in vivo, different selectivities can be obtained (24). Accordingly, comparison of IC_{50} values (concentration that inhibits 50%) should be used as a rough guide only. The availability of x-ray coordinates for the ovine COX-1 has led to a model for inhibitor docking, which has as its key features a lipid-binding domain for anchoring the enzyme to the lipid bilayer; the peroxidase-binding site; and the hydrophobic channel for AA, at the end of which is the COX active site held in close proximity to the peroxidase active site (25). More recently, x-ray structures of the COX-2 enzyme with bound inhibitors have become available and the basis for rational design of selective inhibitors established (26,27).

Nonselective Cyclooxygenase Inhibitors

Most of the currently available, nonselective COX inhibitors contain an acidic functionality that is thought to bind to Arg 120 midway down the hydrophobic channel, placing the molecule into the active site and preventing access by AA to Tyr385, the presumed radical donor site. Ibuprofen, naproxen, and piroxicam are all examples of simple competitive inhibitors (see Table 74-1 for these structures and other COX-1 and COX-2 inhibitors). Ibuprofen is a relatively weak COX inhibitor and used primarily for its analgesic properties (28). Naproxen and piroxicam are more potent and used widely for their anti-inflammatory, analgesic, and antipyretic properties (29). Indomethacin and diclofenac are examples of competitive, time-dependent, reversible inhibitors, but they have

TABLE 74-1. *Cyclooxygenase-1 and -2 inhibitors*

Compound, generic name (trade name)	Structure	Reference
Ibuprofen		28
Naproxen		29
Piroxicam		29
Diclofenac		—
Indomethacin		—
X = S, L-745,337		36, 37
X = O, flosulide		
SC-58635, celecoxib (Celebrex)		38, 39, 202, 203
L-761,066		40
RS-57067		26

essentially the same pharmacologic profiles as naproxen and piroxicam. All carry the toxicology burden of nonselective COX inhibition, gastrointestinal (GI) irritation, ulceration, and bleeding (30), and the potential for renal insufficiency (31), particularly in patients with compromised renal function (32).

Selective Agents

The drive for COX-2 selective agents has led to the profiling of previously described agents and the discovery of modest selectivities in some. For example, nabumetone, the prodrug of 6-methoxy-2-naphthyl acetic acid (6-MNA) (1.5-fold COX-2 selective), and meloxicam (3-fold COX-2 selective) have shown reduced potential for GI side effects in clinical studies (33,34), which has been attributed to their moderate selectivities. Nimesulide, an *N*-aryl sulfonamide, is more selective (approx-

imately 50-fold) and in the small number of comparative trials has shown a lower tendency for GI side effects (35). However, the most impressive gains in COX-2 selectivity have been obtained with targeted drug discovery programs, and a number of COX-2 selective agents are now poised for phase III trials, with the promise of delivering potent agents with all the beneficial effects of the COX inhibitors but without the associated side effects. These new agents are based on three major structural classes; the *N*-aryl sulfonamides, the tricyclics, and modified nonsteroidal antiinflammatory drugs (NSAIDs). The *N*-aryl sulfonamides, of which L-745,337 (36) and flosulide (37) are good examples, are based on nimesulide and show greater than a 1000-fold selectivity for COX-2 inhibition. Flosulide has been withdrawn from clinical development, and the clinical status of L-745,337 is unknown. The tricyclics are the most extensively studied class of COX-2 selective inhibitors (38) and are best represented by celecoxib, which is currently in phase III trials. Celecoxib (Celebrex) is 400-fold selective and in early studies has shown promising efficacy and no GI disturbances (39,202,203). The final class of inhibitors, modified NSAIDs, is represented by L-761,066 (40), a modified indomethacin, and RS-57067 (26), a modified zomepirac, with >170- and >1000-fold selectivity for COX-2, respectively.

THE DISCOVERY AND CLINICAL DEVELOPMENT OF 5-LIPOXYGENASE INHIBITORS AND 5-LIPOXYGENASE ACTIVATING PROTEIN INHIBITORS

5-Lipoxygenase Inhibitors

The demonstration of the existence of a nonheme iron atom in 5-LO, which was recognized to be important for 5-LO catalytic activity, suggested that compounds that bind to this Fe^{+3} atom would likely inhibit its enzymatic activity. This concept was first proven by Corey et al. (41), who found arachidonohydroxamic acid to be a 5-LO inhibitor *in vitro*. Subsequent to this demonstration, key compounds, acetyl hydroxamates, synthesized by chemists at Burroughs Wellcome (BWA4C) and Abbott (A-63162) (for structures of 5-LO inhibitors see Table 74–2) were shown to be 5-LO inhibitors both *in vitro* and *in vivo* (42,43). While the clinical development of the initial BW hydroxamate series (BWA4C) was halted due to metabolic problems in humans, conversion of this series into *N*-hydroxyureas led to the synthesis of BWB70C, which had a more desirable pharmacokinetic profile (44). Preclinical toxicologic findings of renal toxicity in rats precluded further clinical development of this compound (45). Abbott's *N*-hydroxyurea A-64077, however, progressed through preclinical evaluation successfully and was the first orally active 5-LO inhibitor to show biochemical evidence of reversible 5-LO inhibitory activity in humans (46,47). More important was the proof of the concept that inhibiting 5-LO in a patient population where 5-LO products were thought to be contributing to the disease process (e.g., bronchoconstriction in asthma) would afford clinical benefit. Several clinical studies have been performed with A-64077 (zileuton, Leutrol) and have obtained positive data, which contributed to its approval in 1996 for the treatment of asthma. These studies have included efficacious effects in clinical studies involving cold air challenge (48), exercise challenge (49), and aspirin challenge (50,51), which were all thought to have LTs as a contributing factor.

More significant were the effects of zileuton in chronic asthma. Several placebo-controlled trials in chronic asthma have demonstrated a clinical benefit, where improvements in the forced expiratory volume in 1 second (FEV_1), decreased β-agonist use, reduced steroid rescue, and improved overall symptom scores have been measurable after zileuton treatment (52,53). While the effects of zileuton on airway function parameters in asthma are clearly evident and beneficial, only modest inhibitory effects of zileuton on eosinophil infiltration and albumin leakage have been demonstrated in a segmental antigen-challenge study in asthmatics (54). It is currently unknown if this effect will have any bearing on the inflammation associated with chronic asthma. Only long-term treatment with zileuton will allow us to determine if chronic inhibition of 5-LO will afford any positive effect on the inflammatory process.

Perhaps related to this issue are the published clinical studies of the effects of zileuton in a disease, ulcerative colitis, that is believed to have neutrophilic inflammation as a significant etiologic component. In placebo-controlled clinical trials in this disease only, equivocal efficacy (disease symptoms, histologic assessment of mucosa), when compared to current therapies, e.g., sulfasalazine, has been demonstrated (55,56). As rectal dialysis fluids showed LTB_4 inhibition was in the range of 70% to 80%, it is suggested that higher levels of inhibition of LTB_4 formation may be required in order to see a more robust clinical effect (57). The current dosage form of zileuton is 600 mg q.i.d., and using this regimen, inhibition of 5-LO—reflected by inhibition of LTB_4 synthesis in blood *ex vivo*—is in the range of 70% to 80%. It has therefore been the goal of Abbott to find a compound with greater potency and duration of action. Currently, a second-generation hydroxyurea, ABT-761, has reached the phase II stage of clinical development. As revealed by the *ex vivo* whole blood assay, a single 200-mg dose of ABT-761 caused >90% inhibition of LTB_4 synthesis for 9 hours post-dosing and in addition showed protective effects in exercise- and adenosine-challenge protocols (58).

Alternative strategies to finding potent 5-LO inhibitors led to the discovery of a series of nonredox, active-site 5-LO inhibitors (59). A prototype of this series (ZM 211965) had respectable potency in *in vitro* whole blood assays; however, it lacked suitable oral bioavailability in animals. Attempts to improve bioavailability in this series ultimately led to the synthesis of the clinical candidate ZD 2138 (60). In humans, after a single oral dose of 350 mg, ZD 2138 was found to completely block LTB_4 formation in the *ex vivo* blood assay for 24 hours (61). Phase II clinical studies with ZD 2138 have shown protective effects in an aspirin-induced bronchoconstriction protocol (62) but no attenuation of bronchoconstriction induced by antigen (63).

5-Lipoxygenase–Activating Protein Inhibitors

A series of indole-2-alkanoic acids were found to be inhibitors of 5-LO activity in whole cells; however, using cell free 5-LO assays, these compounds were found to be inactive (64). It was subsequently shown that the molec-

TABLE 74-2. *5-Lipoxygenase inhibitors and 5-lipoxygenase–activating protein (FLAP) antagonists*

Compound, generic name (trade name)	Structure	Reference
BWA4C		42
A-63162		43
A-64077, zileuton (Leutrol)		46–57
ABT-761		58
ZM-211965		59
ZD-2138		60–63
MK-886		66
MK-0591		67–71
WY-50295		72, 74
BAY-X1005		73, 75–77

ular target for these compounds was a novel 18-kd protein that was given the name 5-lipoxygenase activating protein (FLAP) (65). MK-886 (for structures of FLAP antagonists, see Table 74-2) was the first prototype FLAP inhibitor to enter human clinical trials (66), but it was subsequently replaced with MK-0591 a second-generation, quinolylmethoxy-substituted compound shown to have improved potency (67). In allergen-challenge studies in asthmatics, orally dosed MK-0591 effectively blocked early-phase and late-phase bronchoconstriction, and using the *ex vivo* whole blood assay inhibited LTB_4 production by 98% over a 24-hour period (68). A series of clinical studies in both chronic asthma and ulcerative colitis with MK-0591 has provided mixed results with respect to efficacy. In a 4-week (125 mg b.i.d.) asthma study in patients already using inhaled steroids, improve-

ments in FEV_1 and, decreased β-agonist use were noted (69). Additionally, in a 6-week dose-ranging study (25 mg q.d., 25, 50, 125 mg b.i.d.) in mild to moderate asthma, improvements in pulmonary function and decreased β-agonist use were noted, although overall the degree of efficacy was not robust (70). However, in an 8-week placebo-controlled, dose ranging (12.5, 50, 100 mg b.i.d.) efficacy trial in ulcerative colitis, although MK-0591 blocked LT synthesis (rectal dialysis LTB_4, urinary LTE_4) significantly, there was no correlation between reduction of LTB_4 synthesis and disease remission (71). Other quinolylmethoxy-containing FLAP inhibitors that have entered clinical trials are WY 50295 (72) and BAY-X1005 (73). WY 50295 failed to inhibit LT synthesis in blood *ex vivo* in phase I clinical studies (74), and BAY-X1005 at doses up to 750 mg p.o. has shown efficacy in both acute allergen and cold dry air challenge studies (75,76). In a 4-week study (250 mg b.i.d. p.o.) in chronic asthma, significant improvements in FEV_1 vs. placebo were seen (77).

THE DISCOVERY AND CLINICAL DEVELOPMENT OF LTD_4 RECEPTOR (Cys LT_1) ANTAGONISTS

As discussed above, the pharmacologic effect of a novel hydroxyacetophenone (FPL-55712) (for structures of LTD_4 antagonists see Table 74-3) that antagonized the action of SRSA provided early insight into a prototypical chemical series with selective actions on Cys LT_1 receptors prior to the structural elucidation of the Cys LTs (78). The Cys LT_1 receptor itself has yet to be cloned. Early clinical trials of aerosolized FPL-55712 suggested that this compound caused some improvement in lung function in asthmatics (79); however, it is only a weak antagonist of Cys LT_1 receptor ($pA_2 = 6.0$) and a search for more potent compounds began in earnest in the early 1980s. In general, guinea pig tissue (LTD_4-induced tracheal concentration) and ^3H LTD_4 binding to lung membranes was used for *in vitro* screening purposes. LY 171883 (tomelukast) was the first LTD_4 antagonist to be clinically evaluated in a variety of acute protocols involving airway challenge in asthmatics. It too was rather weak ($pA_2 = 6.0$) and had only modest effects in these clinical tests (80–82) as well as in a 6-week study (600 mg p.o.) in mild to moderate asthmatics (83). LY 171883 was dropped from clinical development as it induced peroxisome proliferation in rodents (84). A series of compounds that had respectable affinity ($pA_2 = 7.5$–8.5) for the LTD_4 receptor was designed around the stereochemistry of LTD_4 itself, e.g., SKF104353 (pobilukast), LY 170680 (sulukast), SKF 106203, and BAY-X7195. Except for BAY-X7195, poor oral bioavailability precluded administration by this route in humans and these compounds were only evaluated by the aerosol route. Airway-challenge studies with LTD_4 suggested that these compounds caused five- to tenfold shifts in LTD_4-challenge dose-response curves and, where studied, blocked antigen- and exercise-induced bronchoconstriction (probilukast) and afforded FEV_1 improvement in asthmatics (BAY-X7195) (85–87).

A structurally novel series of LTD_4 antagonists emerged from a synthetic program that explored Structure Activity Relationships (SAR) around the hydroxy-acetophenones (FPL 55712) as well as LTD_4 itself and culminated in the discovery of a highly potent ($pA_2 = 9.5$) compound ICI-204,219 (zafirlukast, Accolate) (88). In humans, ICI-204,219 potently blocked LTD_4-induced bronchoconstriction (89) and was subsequently shown to block bronchoconstriction induced by allergen, exercise, cold air, and PAF (90–94). In trials in asthma, treatment periods of up to 13 weeks with ICI-204,219 led to signif-

icant improvements in lung function (95–97, for review, see ref. 204). Accolate was approved for the treatment of asthma in 1996.

A series of compounds that combined the quinolone moiety of the FLAP inhibitors with the thioacetal unit of the LTD_4 analogues as found to have affinity approaching that of the natural ligand. Optimization of this series led to compounds with respectable oral bioavailability (98). In clinical evaluation, when administered either parenterally or orally, MK-571 produced significant antagonism of LTD_4-induced bronchoconstriction (99) and, in antigen and cold-air challenge studies, more impressive inhibitory effects than those obtained previously with weaker compounds (100–102). In addition, in patients with asthma, MK-571 caused improvements in baseline lung function after either intravenous or oral administration (103,104). MK-571 was a racemic compound and in toxicology studies in animals it was found to cause peroxisome proliferation in mice (105), an effect potentially linked to the development of liver tumors in rodents (84). Resolution of its enantiomers indicated that the peroxisome proliferating activity was specifically associated with the S-enantiomer (106), and the R-enantiomer (MK-679) was subsequently chosen for longer term trials in asthma. As previously seen with MK-571, MK-679, when evaluated in a 6-week trial in chronic asthma, caused improvements in both FEV_1 and nocturnal asthma, as well as decreased β-agonist use (107); however, it was discontinued due to abnormalities in liver function occurring in 5% of patients (108). Further work in this chemical series led to the discovery of MK-0476, which was devoid of peroxisome proliferating activity in rodents and in addition maintained potency in *in vitro* lig- and bioassays when performed in the presence of protein (109–110). Clinical evaluation of MK-0476 has shown robust effects in a variety of either airway challenge (e.g., LTD_4, exercise, allergen) or bronchodilation studies in asthmatics with daily oral doses of MK-0476 as low as 5 mg (111–115). The New Drug Application (NDA) for MK-0476 (montelukast, Singulair) was filed early in 1997 and subsequently approved.

ONO-1078 (pranlukast) (116) is a relatively weak ($pK_B = 7.5$) antagonist of LTD_4 receptors, but its development (117,118) has proceeded in Japan, where it was approved for the treatment of asthma in 1995 (119). In a recently published randomized, double blind, placebo-controlled 6-week study in asthmatics requiring high-dose steroids, ONO-1078 was shown to prevent asthma deterioration resulting from reduction of the steroid dose (120). Phase III clinical evaluation of ONO-1078 is currently proceeding elsewhere (121–124). RO-24-5913 (cinalukast) is a highly potent ($pA_2 = 9.6$) LTD_4 antagonist that was uncovered from a unique series of styryl thiazoles (125). In clinical trials in exercise-induced bronchoconstriction, oral doses as low as 10 mg were shown to be inhibitory; however, when dosed daily for 1 week,

TABLE 74-3. *Leukotriene D_4 (CysLT) receptor antagonists*

Compound, generic name (trade name)	Structure	Reference
FPL-55712		78, 79
LY-171883, tomelukast		80–84
LY-170680, sulukast		
SKF-104353, pobilukast		85, 86
SKF-106203		
BAY-X7195		87
ICI-204,219, zafirlukast (Accolate)		88–97,204
MK-571		99–105
MK-679, verlukast (Venzair)		107, 108
MK-0476, montelukast (Singulair)		109–115
ONO-1078, pranlukast, Onon		116–124
RO24-5913, cinalukast		125, 126

protective effects were lost at the lower dose, but maintained at higher doses (50, 200 mg) (126).

THE DISCOVERY AND CLINICAL DEVELOPMENT OF LEUKOTRIENE B$_4$ (BLT) ANTAGONISTS

Early attempts to discover antagonists of LTB$_4$ receptors involved derivitization of LTB$_4$ itself, e.g., diacetyl-LTB$_4$ (127) and LTB$_4$ dimethylamide (128), as well as synthesis of a series of compounds that incorporated structural features of LTB$_4$ such as the substituted pyridines, e.g., U-75302 (129) and omega substituted compounds, e.g., SM-9064 (130). These compounds, however, had varying degrees of agonist activity, and the first bona fide examples of specific antagonists came from derivatives of the hydroxyacetophenone series of LTD$_4$ antagonists, e.g., SC-41930 (131) and LY255283 (132) (for structures of LTB$_4$ antagonists, see Table 74-4). Early *in vivo* evaluation of SC-41930 indicated that in addition to blocking intradermal challenge with LTB$_4$ (133), this compound also provided protection in a variety of acute models of colonic inflammation (134). Extended evaluation of SC-41930, however, indicated that in a similar range of concentrations that inhibited LTB$_4$, it also blocked 5-LO as well as neutrophil functional responses mediated by alternate chemotactic receptors (135), and therefore questions were raised regarding its primary mechanism of action *in vivo*.

TABLE 74-4. *Leukotriene B$_4$ (BLT) receptor antagonists*

Compound	Structure	Reference
SC-41930		131
SC-53228		136–138
LY-223982		139, 140
LY-255283		132
LY-293111		141–144
SB-201993		145
SB-209247		146
ONO-4057		147
CGS-25019C		148–152
CP-105696		153, 155–159, 161, 162

Subsequent extended synthetic efforts around SC-41930 led to the discovery of SC-53228 with much improved selectivity and potency for the LTB$_4$ receptor (136). *In vivo* evaluation of SC-53228 has shown it to be highly potent as an inhibitor of LTB$_4$-mediated cell infiltration (137), and, more importantly, when administered orally to cotton-top tamarin monkeys with spontaneous colitis—a primate model of human ulcerative colitis—led to improvement in symptomatic disease scores, and as revealed in a histologic assessment of colonic tissue, a significant reduction in the colonic, neutrophilic inflammation (138). Attempts to explore benzophenones as surrogates for acetophenones (as exemplified by LY255283) led to the synthesis of LY223982 (139). However, although this compound exhibited respectable *in vitro* potency, it lacked oral bioavailability and was therefore only evaluated topically in a phase I safety/efficacy trial in human psoriatics (140). Further efforts to find more potent, orally bioavailable compounds from the above two chemical series led to the discovery of LY-293111 (141). In phase I safety studies a b.i.d. dose of 200 mg has been reported to inhibit LTB$_4$-mediated CD11b upregulation on neutrophils in whole blood *ex vivo* by 90% at trough levels of drug (142). In a small, allergen-challenge study in a group of atopic asthmatics, LY293111 was found to suppress neutrophil infiltration (measured in bronchoalveolar lavage fluid) but to have no effect on either early- or late-phase bronchoconstrictive responses measured as decrements in FEV$_1$ (143). In skin challenge studies in humans, LY293111 was found to suppress leukocyte infiltration and epidermal hyperproliferation mediated by epicutaneous application of LTB$_4$ (144). LY293111 is currently undergoing phase II clinical trials in inflammatory bowel disease and psoriasis.

Other compounds related to the benzophenone LY223982 include SB-201993 (145), SB-209247 (146), and ONO-4507 (147), and all of these compounds are reported to be potent inhibitors of LTB$_4$ receptor binding *in vitro*. SB-209247 and ONO-4057 are currently in early stages of clinical development. In contrast to all other LTB$_4$ antagonists, which have an acidic functionality, CGS 25019C has a basic amidine. CGS 25019C potently blocked LTB$_4$ binding to neutrophils and LTB$_4$-mediated functional responses *in vitro* (148), and, *in vivo,* after oral administration, inhibited cell infiltration mediated by arachidonic acid (149). In phase I clinical evaluation the maximum tolerated dose of CGS 25019C appears to be 300 mg/day and at this dose significant inhibition of LTB$_4$-mediated CD11b upregulation on neutrophils in whole blood *ex vivo* was achieved (150–152). CP-105,696, a novel hydroxychroman, was designed from a series of prototype LTD$_4$ antagonists using LTB$_4$ as a structural template and optimized for potency using a three-point attachment model as was previously proposed for the NK1 receptor antagonist CP-96,345 (153,154). Preclinical evaluation of this compound provided evi-

dence of high intrinsic potency for the LTB$_4$ receptor on human neutrophils and on neutrophils from animal species used for efficacy evaluation (155,156). Importantly, the potency and pharmacokinetics in mice allowed the compound to be orally dosed using a once-a-day regimen. When tested in a variety of disease models in mice, e.g., collagen-induced arthritis (CIA) (157), experimental allergic encephalomyelitis (158), and cardiac allograft rejection (159), CP-105,096 was shown to be efficacious, providing compelling evidence that LTB$_4$ or alternate ligands (e.g., 12-R-HETE) that may interact with this receptor are involved in the pathogenesis of these diseases. Independent evidence of a role for 5-LO products in murine CIA has recently been obtained using mice deficient in FLAP (160). In addition to showing efficacy in several murine models of inflammation, CP-105,696 was also shown to block the development of antigen-induced airway hyperreactivity in a primate model of experimental asthma (161). In phase I clinical evaluation, CP-105,696 was found to have an exceptionally long plasma half-life (t$^1/_2$ ~400 hours) (162) and this led to suspension of further development of this compound. Other compounds related to CP-105,696 have been designed to address the unfavorable pharmacokinetics of CP-105,696, and one of these compounds, CP-195,543, is currently in early stages of clinical development (205).

THE DISCOVERY AND DEVELOPMENT OF PLATELET-ACTIVATING FACTOR ANTAGONISTS

The PAF antagonists can be classified into four distinct classes (163) according to their key structural features: PAF-analogue antagonists and other quaternary nitrogen containing compounds; sp^2-nitrogen (sp^{2}N) antagonists; diaryl antagonists; and miscellaneous antagonists.

The first antagonists to appear were structural analogues of PAF itself. These compounds were constructed with a quaternary nitrogen contained within a heterocycle, a phosphate bioisostere, a glycerol mimetic, and a replacement for the lipophilic alkyl chain. In general, these compounds were not orally active in animal models and have been targeted as intravenous therapy for shock. CV-3988 (for structures of PAF antagonists see Table 74-5), the forerunner of the class, is a weak antagonist but has been evaluated in humans, showing inhibition of platelet aggregation *ex vivo.* (164). TCV-309, a more potent PAF-analogue antagonist, also showed inhibition of PAF-induced platelet aggregation *ex vivo* (165). E-5880 is perhaps the most potent PAF-analogue antagonist and is being developed for the treatment of disseminated intravascular coagulation (DIC) (166).

The second class of PAF antagonists, the sp^{2}N antagonists, can be further divided into three subclasses; heterodiazepines, pyridines, and imidazoles. The heterodiazepines were founded on the empirical finding that the

TABLE 74-5. *Platelet-activating receptor antagonists*

Compound, generic name	Structure	Reference
CV-3988		164
TCV-309		165, 199
E-5880		166
WEB-2086, apafant		184–187
Y-24180		169, 188
Ro 24-4736		168, 198
RP-48740		170
RP-59227, tulopafant		189
ABT-299		171
SR-27417		172, 173

TABLE 74-5. *Continued*

Compound, generic name (trade name)	Structure	Reference
UK-74,505, modipafant		174, 190–191
BB-882, lexipafant (Zacutex)		175, 200
MK-287		176, 192, 193
BN-52021		179, 180, 201
Sch-37370		177

triazolobenzodiazepine triazolam is a weak PAF antagonist (167). Triazolam, however, is also a potent benzodiazepine receptor agonist, and the first compound to exhibit selective action against the PAF receptor was WEB 2086 (apafant). Further potency enhancements in different research groups led to the antagonists Ro 24-4736 (168) and Y-24180 (169). The prototype antagonist of the pyridine class, RP-48740, which blocked *ex vivo* PAF-induced platelet aggregation in phase I trials (170), was quickly followed by the much more potent compound RP-59227 (tulopafant). Additional structural variants of this class include ABT-299 (171) (a water-soluble prodrug of A-85783) and SR-27417, a very potent, orally active antagonist. SR-27417 is unusual in that it is a slowly irreversible antagonist at the PAF receptor, and after prolonged exposure to platelets the compound cannot be dissociated from the receptor. This property may explain its long-lasting inhibition of *ex vivo* PAF-induced platelet aggregation in humans, where a dose of 2.5 mg provides for 24-hour blockade and a 100-mg dose gives up to 7 days of blockade (172,173). The third subclass is the imidazole derived antagonists, which are represented by UK-74,505 (174) (modipafant) and BB-882 (175) (lexipafant). Both contain the imidazo[4,5-*c*]pyridine substructure, which is a key structural determinant for PAF antagonist activity.

The third major class of PAF antagonists is the diaryl compounds, which feature two aryl rings, substituted with at least one alkoxy group, and attached to a five- or six-membered heterocycle. The prime example of this class is MK-287, featuring a trimethoxyphenyl substituent on a tetrahydrofuran ring (176).

The fourth class, the miscellaneous antagonists, includes all the antagonists that do not fit into the former three well-defined classes. The most studied representative of this class, and arguably the most studied PAF antagonist of all, is BN-52021, a natural product isolated from the roots of the ginkgo biloba tree. It is a relatively weak antagonist, but has been advanced into several clinical trials. Sch-37370, a derivative of the antihistamine loratadine, was found to have weak PAF antagonist activity and has also been studied clinically (177).

Several pharmacophore models have been developed in an attempt to explain the activity of the immense structural diversity of the PAF antagonists. The most comprehensive model that has been published is based on the sp²N-based antagonists and provides for three main electronegative zones in the proposed pharmacophore (178).

Several antagonists have been studied for their efficacy in atopy and asthma but, with few exceptions, these clinical trials have proven to be extremely disappointing. For example, BN-52063 (a mixture of ginkgolides including BN-52021) blocked the wheal and flare to intradermal PAF (179) but not intradermal antigen (180) in atopic individuals. In a small trial in children, BN-52063 blocked PAF- (181) and antigen- (182) induced bronchoconstriction, but there was no benefit to adults challenged with either cold air or exercise (183). Apafant also blocked intradermal PAF-induced wheal and flare (184) and PAF-induced bronchoconstriction (185) but failed to protect mild atopics in an antigen challenge study (186). Asthma studies failed to show reduced inhaled corticosteroid use in atopics (187). Encouragingly, Y-24180 reduced the bronchial hyperresponsiveness to methacholine in asthmatics in a double-blind crossover study, but the compound did not affect baseline pulmonary function (188). Tulopafant also failed to show any effect on either the early or late phase in an antigen challenge study (189). Modipafant completely blocked the PAF-induced bronchoconstriction and neutropenia in normal volunteers (190), but had no effect on allergen-induced bronchoconstriction in atopic asthmatics (191). MK-287 failed to provide any protection in antigen challenge studies in atopics, although it did shift the dose response to inhaled PAF (192). In longer term studies of natural asthma, MK-287 also failed to show any improvement in lung function or other clinical parameters (193). Sch-37370, when studied in either cold air challenge in asthmatics or a 6-week natural asthma trial, did not show any improvement over the efficacy seen with antihistamine alone (194,195). Ro 24-0238, a combined PAF/TXA$_2$ antagonist applied topically in atopic eczema, showed no improvement over placebo on erythema, scaling, induration, and exudation, although a trend to reduction in pruritus was noted (196).

More encouraging results have been observed in the use of PAF antagonists for the treatment of septic shock. Thus, in a large septic shock trial with BN-52021, reduced mortality was observed in the severe gram-negative subgroup (197), although there was no improvement in overall mortality. Ro 24-4736 reduced the severity of the symptoms (rigors, myalgias, headache, and nausea) in an endotoxemia study in humans (LPS challenge in normal volunteers), although there was no improvement in mean arterial pressure, heart rate, or febrile response (198). TCV-309 failed to produce an improvement in organ failure rate in systemic inflammatory response syndrome, although there was a trend to improved survival during drug treatment (199). Lexipafant, given as an intravenous infusion over several days, significantly reduces multiple organ failure in acute pancreatitis, and the compound is proceeding into phase III trials for this indication (200).

Many animal studies show that PAF antagonists are effective in the protection and reversal of ischemia-reperfusion induced injury in a range of organ systems including the heart, kidney, brain, and liver. Excitingly, BN52021 improved posttransplant renal function in patients receiving cadaveric kidney transplants (201), but no other human studies with PAF antagonists have been published.

SUMMARY

The recent discovery of the COX-2 pathway has allowed the discovery and development of a new generation of potent inhibitors with high degrees of selectivity for COX-2 inhibition over COX-1. It is anticipated that this class of compounds will provide a new class of drugs that will be used to treat the symptoms of a variety of inflammatory diseases and afford a significant advance in tolerability when compared to currently used NSAIDs. The utility of COX-2 inhibitors in the treatment of certain forms of cancer and Alzheimer's disease remains to be established.

The contribution of leukotrienes (LTD$_4$) in asthma has been confirmed through the demonstration of efficacy of 5-LO inhibitors and Cys LT$_1$ antagonists in this disease. The ultimate utility of these classes of drugs in the long-term management of asthma will come from the clinical experience with these compounds now that they have gained regulatory approval. Based on available published clinical findings, the utility of 5-LO inhibitors/FLAP antagonists in the treatment of other inflammatory diseases, however, looks decidedly less promising. Preclinically, LTB$_4$ receptor antagonists hold promise as novel antiinflammatory agents; however, pivotal phase II clinical studies are currently ongoing and it is anticipated that results from these studies will be forthcoming in the next 2 years.

PAF antagonists overall have been disappointing when evaluated in asthma trials; however, their use in the treatment of reperfusion injury in kidney transplantation, pancreatitis, and shock states holds promise. Again, only extended clinical evaluation in these diseases will provide confidence of these early encouraging results.

ACKNOWLEDGMENTS

The authors would like to thank Ms. Doreen Gale for her excellent assistance in manuscript preparation, Ms. Robbin Breslow Alpert for her help with literature searches, and Dr. Richard Griffiths for his helpful comments on chapter content.

REFERENCES

1. Vane JR. Towards a better aspirin. *Nature* 1971;231:232–235.
2. Smith WL, Dewitt DL. Prostaglandin endoperoxide H synthases-1 and -2. *Adv Immunol* 1996;62:167–215.
3. Levy GN. Prostaglandin H synthases nonsteroidal anti-inflammatory drugs and colon cancer. *FASEB J* 1997;11:234–247.
4. Tocco G, Freive-Moar J, Schreiber SS, Sakhi SH, Aisen PS, Pasinetti GM. Maturational regulation and regional induction of cyclooxygenase-2 in rat brain. Implications for Alzheimer's disease. *Exp Neurol* 1997;144:339–349.
5. Borgeat P, Hamberg M, Samuelsson B. Transformation of arachidonic acid and homo-alpha-linolenic acid by rabbit polymorphonuclear leukocytes. *J Biol Chem* 1976;251:7816–7820.
6. Ford-Hutchinson AW, Gresser M, Young RN. 5-Lipoxygenase. *Annu Rev Biochem* 1994;63:383–417.

7. Petpiboon P, Vickers PJ. Development of MK0591: an orally active leukotriene biosynthesis inhibitor with a novel mechanism of action. In: Merlussi VJ, Adams J, eds. *The search for anti-inflammatory drugs.* Boston: Birkhauser, 1995:233–251.

8. Feldberg W, Kellaway CH. Liberation of histamine and formation of lysocithin-like substances by cobra venom. *J Physiol* 1938;94:187–226.

9. Kellaway CH, Trethewie ER. The liberation of a slow reacting, smooth muscle-stimulating substance in anaphylaxis. *Q J Exp Physiol* 1940;30:121–145.

10. Augstein J, Farmer JB, Lee TB, Sheard P, Tattersall ML. Selective inhibitors of slow reacting substance of anaphylaxis. *Nature (Lond) New Biol* 1973;245:215–217.

11. Bray MA, Ford-Hutchinson AW, Shipley ME, Smith MJH. Calcium ionophore A23187 induces release of chemotactic and aggregating factors from polymorphonuclear leukocytes. *Br J Pharmacol* 1980;71:507–512.

12. Ford-Hutchinson AW, Bray MA, Doig MV, Shipley ME, Smith MJH. Leukotriene B: a potent chemokinetic and aggregating substance released from polymorphonuclear leukocytes. *Nature (Lond)* 1980;286:264–265.

13. Goldman DW, Goetzl EJ. Specific binding of leukotriene B_4 to receptors on human polymorphonuclear leukocytes. *J Immunol* 1982;129:1600–1604.

14. Lin A, Ruppel PL, Gorman RR. Leukotriene B_4 binding to human neutrophils. *Prostaglandins* 1984;28:837–849.

15. Cheng JB, Cheng EI-P, Kohi F, Townley RG. [^{3}H] Leukotriene B_4 binding to guinea pig spleen membrane preparation: a rich source of high affinity leukotriene B_4 receptor site. *J Pharmacol Exp Ther* 1986;236:126–132.

16. Yokomizo T, Izumi T, Chang K, Takuwa Y, Shimizu T. A G-protein-coupled receptor for leukotriene B_4 that mediates chemotaxis. *Nature* 1997;387:620–624.

17. Siriganian RP, Osler AG. Destruction of rabbit platelets in the allergic response of sensitized leukocytes. 1. Demonstration of a fluid phase intermediate. *J Immunol* 1971;106:1244–1251.

18. Benveniste J, Henson PM, Cochrane CG. Leukocyte-dependent histamine release from platelets. The role of IgE, basophils and a platelet activating factor. *J Exp Med* 1972;131:1356–1377.

19. Beveniste J, Tence N, Varenne P, Bidault J, Boulet C, Polonsky J. Semi-synthese et structure purposee du facteur activant les plaquettes (PAF): PAF-aceter, un alkyl ether analogue de la phosphatidylcholine. *C R Acad Sci (Paris)* 1979;289:1037–1040.

20. Blank ML, Snyder F, Byers LW, Brooks B, Muirhead FF. Antihypertensive activity of an alkyl ether analog of phosphatidylcholine. *Biochem Biophys Res Commun* 1979;90:1194–1200.

21. Demopolus CA, Pinckard RN, Hanahan DJ. Platelet-activating factor. Evidence of 1-0-alkyl-2-acetyl-sn-glycero-3-phosphocholine as the active component. A new class of lipid chemical mediators. *J Biol Chem* 1979;254:9355–9358.

22. Valone F, Goetzl EJ. Specific binding by human polymorphonuclear leukocytes of the immunological mediator 1-0-hexadecyl/octadecyl-2-acetyl-sn-glycero-3-phosphorylcholine. *J Immunol* 1983;48:141–149.

23. Honda Z, Nakamura M, Miki I, et al. Cloning by functional expression of platelet-activating factor receptor from guinea pig lung. *Nature* 1991;349:342–346.

24. Battistini B, Botting R, Bakhlev S. COX-1 and COX-2: toward the development of more selective NSAIDs. *Drug News Perspect* 1994;7:501–512.

25. Loll PJ, Picot D, Ekabo O, Garavito RM. Synthesis and use of iodinated nonsteroidal anti-inflammatory drug analogs as crystallographic probes of the prostaglandin H2 synthase cyclooxygenase active site. *Biochemistry* 1996;35:7330–7340.

26. Luong C, Miller A, Barnett J, Chow J, Ramesha C, Browner MF. Flexibility of the NSAID binding site in the structure of human cyclooxygenase-2. *Nature Struct Biol* 1996;3:927–933.

27. Kurumbail RG, Stevens AM, Gierse JK, et al. Structural basis for selective inhibition of cyclooxygenase-2 by anti-inflammatory agents. *Nature* 1996;384:644–648.

28. Roth SH. *New directions in arthritis therapy.* Littleton, MA: PSG, 1980.

29. Brooks PM, Kean WF, Buchanan WW. *The clinical pharmacology of anti-inflammatory agents.* London: Taylor and Francis, 1986.

30. Langman MJS, Weil J, Wainwright P, et al. Risk of bleeding peptic ulcer associated with individual nonsteroidal antiinflammatory drugs. *Lancet* 1994;343:1075–1078.

31. Murray MD, Brater DC. Renal toxicity of the nonsteroidal anti-inflammatory drugs. *Annu Rev Pharmacol Toxicol* 1993;32:435–465.

32. Kleinknecht D. Interstitial nephritis, the nephrotic syndrome, and chronic renal failure secondary to non-steroidal anti-inflammatory drugs. *Semin Nephrology* 1995;15:228–235.

33. Roth SH, Bennet R, Caldron P, Mitchell C, Swenson C, Koepp R. A long term endoscopic evaluation of patients with arthritis treated with nabumetone vs. naproxen. *J Rheumatol* 1994;21:1118–1123.

34. Schattenkircher M. Meloxicam: a selective COX-2 inhibitor nonsteroidal anti-inflammatory drug. *Exp Opin Invest Drugs* 1997;6:321–334.

35. Rabasseda X. Safety profile of nimesulide: ten years of clinical experience. *Drugs Today* 1997;33:41–50.

36. Prasit P, Black WC, Chan C-C, et al. L-745,337: a selective cyclooxygenase-2 inhibitor. *Med Chem Res* 1995;5:364–374.

37. Klein T, Nusing RM, Pfeilschifter J, Ullrich V. Selective inhibition of cyclooxygenase-2. *Biochem Pharmacol* 1994;48:1605–1610.

38. Talley JJ. Selective inhibitors of cyclooxygenase-2. *Exp Opin Ther Pat* 1997;7:55–62.

39. Penning TD, Talley JJ, Bertenshaw SR, et al. Synthesis and biological evaluation of the 1,5-diarylpyrazole class of cyclooxygenase-2 inhibitors: identification of 4-[5-(4-methylphenyl)-3-(trifluoromethyl)-1*H*-pyrazol-1-yl]benzenesulfonamide (SC-58635, celecoxib). *J Med Chem* 1997;40:1347–1365.

40. LeBlanc Y, Black WC, Chann CC, et al. Synthesis and biological evaluation of both enantiomers of L-761,000 as inhibitors of cyclooxygenase-1 and -2. *Bioorg Med Chem Lett* 1996;6:731–736.

41. Corey EJ, Cashman JR, Kanter SS, Corey DR. Rationally designed, potent competitive inhibitors of leukotriene biosynthesis. *J Am Chem Soc* 1984;106:1503–1504.

42. Jackson WP, Islip PF, Kneen G, Pugh A, Water PJ. Acetohydroxyamic acids as potent selective orally active 5-lipoxygenase inhibitors. *J Med Chem* 1988;31:499–500.

43. Summers JB, Gunn BP, Martin JG, et al. Structure activity analysis of a class of orally active hydroxamic acid inhibitor of leukotriene biosynthesis. *J Med Chem* 1988;31:1960–1964.

44. Garland LG, Salmon JA. Hydroxamic acids and hydroxyureas as inhibitors of arachidonate 5-lipoxygenase. *Drugs Future* 1991;16:547–558.

45. Reed NG, Astberry P, Evans GO, Goodwin DA, Rowlands A. Nephrotic syndrome associated with N-hydroxyureas, inhibitors of 5-lipoxygenase. *Arch Toxicol* 1995;69:480–490.

46. Rubin P, Dubé L, Braeckman R, et al. Pharmacokinetics, safety and ability to diminish leukotriene synthesis by zileuton, an inhibitor of 5-lipoxygenase. In: Ackerman NR, Bonney RJ, Welton AF, eds. *Progress in inflammation research and therapy.* Basel: Birkhauser Verlag, 1991.

47. Awni WM, Braeckman RA, Granneman GR, Witt G, Dubé LM. Pharmacokinetics and pharmacodynamics of zileuton after oral administration of single and multiple dose regimens of zileuton 600 mg in healthy volunteers. *Clin Pharmacokinet* 1995;29:(suppl 2)22–33.

48. Israel E, Dermarkarian R, Rosenberg M, et al. The effects of a 5-lipoxygenase inhibitor on asthma induced by cold dry air. *N Engl J Med* 1990;323:1740–1744.

49. Meltzer SS, Hasday JD, Cohn J, Bleecker ER. Inhibition of exercise-induced asthma by zileuton, a 5-lipoxygenase inhibitor. *Am J Respir Crit Care Med* 1996;153:931–935.

50. Israel E, Fischer AR, Rosenberg MA, et al. The pivotal role of 5-lipoxygenase products in the reaction of aspirin-sensitive asthmatics to aspirin. *Am Rev Respir Dis* 1993;148:1447–1451.

51. Dahlen SE, Nizankowska E, Dahlen B, et al. The Swedish-Polish treatment study with the 5-lipoxygenase inhibitor zileuton in aspirin intolerant asthmatics. *Am J Respir Crit Care Med* 1995;151:A376.

52. Israel E, Cohn J, Dubé L, Drazen JM. Effect of treatment with zileuton, a 5-lipoxygenase inhibitor in patients with asthma. *JAMA* 1996;275:931–936.

53. Liu MC, Dubé LM, Lancaster J, and the Zileuton Study Group. Acute and chronic affects of a 5-lipoxygenase inhibitor in asthma: a 6-month randomized multicenter trial. *J Allergy Clin Immunol* 1996;98:859–871.

54. Kane GC, Pollice M, Kim C-J, et al. A controlled trial of the 5-lipoxy-

genase inhibitor zileuton on lung inflammation produced by segmental antigen challenge in human beings. *J Allergy Clin Immunol* 1996; 97:646–654.

55. Rask-Madsen J, Bukhave K, Laursen LS, Lauritsen K. 5-Lipoxygenase inhibition for the treatment of inflammatory bowel disease. *Agents Actions* 1992;C37–C45.

56. Laursen LS, Lauritsen K, Bukhavr K, et al. Selective 5-lipoxygenase inhibition by zileuton in the treatment of relapsing ulcerative colitis. A randomised double blind placebo controlled multicenter trial. *Eur J Gastroenterol Hepatol* 1994;6:209–215.

57. Hawkey CJ, Dubé LM, Rountree LV, Linnen PJ, Lancaster JF, and the European zileuton study group for ulcerative colitis. A trial of zileuton versus mesalazine or placebo in the maintenance of remission of ulcerative colitis. *Gastroenterology* 1997;112:718–724.

58. van Schoor J, Joos GF, Kips JC, Prajesk JF, Carpentier PJ, Pauwels RA. The effect of ABT-761, a novel 5-lipoxygenase inhibitor, on exercise- and adenosine-induced bronchoconstriction in asthmatic subjects. *Am J Respir Crit Care Med* 1997;155:875–880.

59. McMillan RM, Walker ERH. Designing therapeutically effective 5-lipoxygenase inhibitors. *Trends Pharmacol Sci* 1992;13:323–330.

60. Crawley GC, Foster SJ, McMillan RM, Walker ERH. Discovery of ZD 2138, a potent, selective, well-tolerated, nonredox inhibitor of the enzyme 5-lipoxygenase. In: Merluzzi VJ, Adams J, eds. *The search for antiinflammatory drugs.* Boston: Birkhauser, 1995:191–231.

61. Yates RA, McMillan RM, Ellis SH, Hutchinson M, Culmore EM, Wilkinson DM. A new non-redox 5-lipoxygenase inhibitor ICI D2138 is well tolerated and inhibits leukotriene synthesis in healthy volunteers. *Am Rev Respir Dis* 1992;145:A745.

62. Nasser SM, Bell GS, Foster SJ, et al. Effect of the 5-lipoxygenase inhibitor ZD 2138 in aspirin-induced asthma. *Thorax* 1994;49: 749–756.

63. Nasser SM, Bell GS, Hawksworth RJ, et al. Effect of the 5-lipoxygenase inhibitor ZD 2138 an allergen-induced early and late asthmatic responses. *Thorax* 1994;49:743–748.

64. Young RN, Gillard JW, Hutchinson JH, Leger S, Prasit P. Discovery of inhibitors of the 5-lipoxygenase-activating protein (FLAP). *J Lipid Mediators* 1993;6:233–238.

65. Dixon RAF, Diehl RE, Opas E, et al. Requirement of a 5-lipoxygenase-activating protein for leukotriene synthesis. *Nature (Lond)* 1990; 343:282–284.

66. Friedman BS, Bel EH, Buntinx A, et al. Oral leukotriene inhibitor (MK-886) blocks allergen-induced airway responses. *Am Rev Respir Dis* 1993;147:839–844.

67. Brideau C, Chan C, Denis D, et al. Pharmacology of MK-0591 (3-[1-(4-chlorobenzyl)-3-(t-butylthio)-5-(quinolin-2-yl-methoxyindol-2-yl]-2,2-dimethylpropanoic acid) a potent, orally active leukotriene biosynthesis inhibitor. *Can J Physiol Pharmacol* 1992;70:799–807.

68. Diamasst Z, Timmers MC, Van der Veen H, et al. The effect of MK-0591, a novel 5-lipoxygenase activating protein inhibitor, on leukotriene biosynthesis and allergen-induced airway responses in asthmatic subjects *in vivo*. *J Allergy Clin Immunol* 1995;95:42–51.

69. Chapman, KR, Friedman BS, Shingo S, Heyes J, Reiss T, Spectro R. The efficacy of an oral inhibitor of leukotriene synthesis (MK-0591) in asthmatics treated with inhaled steroids. *Am J Respir Crit Care Med* 1994;149:A215.

70. Storms W, Friedman BS, Zhang J, et al. Treating asthma by blocking the lipoxygenase pathway. *Am J Respir Crit Care Med* 1995;151: A377.

71. Roberts WG, Simon TJ, Berlin RG, et al. Leukotrienes in ulcerative colitis: results of a multicenter trial of a leukotriene biosynthesis inhibitor, MK-591. *Gastroenterology* 1997;112:725–732.

72. WY-50295 Tromethanine. *Drugs Future* 1992;17:761–762.

73. Dahlen S-E, Dahlen B, Ihre E, et al. The leukotriene biosynthesis inhibitor BAY-X1005 is a potent inhibitor of allergen-induced airway obstruction and leukotriene formation in man. *Am Rev Respir Dis* 1993;147:A837.

74. Fisher AR, Drazen JM, Roth M, et al. The effect of a leukotriene synthesis inhibitor, BAY-X1005 on bronchoconstriction induced by cold, dry air hyperventilation in asthmatics. *Am J Respir Crit Care Med* 1994;149:A1056.

75. Virchow JC, Wolter PS, Wesbmann KJ, et al. Multicenter trial of BAY X1005, a new 5-lipoxygenase activating protein (FLAP) inhibitor in the treatment of chronic asthma. *Am J Respir Crit Care Med* 1995; 151:A377.

76. Kreft AF, Marshall LA, Wong A. Structure-activity relationships in the quinolone-containing class of inhibitors of 5-lipoxygenase (5-LO) enzyme translocation and activation. *Drugs Future* 1994;19:255–264.

77. Hatzelmann A, Fruchtman R, Mohrs K-H, Raddatz S, Müller-Peddinghaus R. Mode of action of new selective leukotriene biosynthesis inhibitor BAY X1005 and structurally related compounds. *Biochem Pharmacol* 1993;45:101–111.

78. Lee TH, Walpat MJ, Wilkinson AH, Turner-Warwick M, Kay AB. Slow-reacting substance of anaphylaxis antagonist FPL55712 in chronic asthma. *Lancet* 1981;2:304–305.

79. Appleton RA, Bantick JR, Chamberlain TR, Hardern DN, Lee TB, Pratt AD. Antagonists of slow reacting substance of anaphylaxis. Synthesis of a series of chromone-2-carboxylic acids. *J Med Chem* 1977; 20:371–379.

80. Shaker G, Glovsky MM, Selso D, Glovsky S, Dowell A. Reversal of exercise induced asthma by the LTD$_4$, LTE$_4$ antagonist LY 171883. *J Allergy Clin Immunol* 1988;81:315.

81. Israel E, Juniper EF, Callaghan JT, et al. Effect of a leukotriene antagonist LY 171883 on cold air induced bronchoconstriction in asthmatics. *Am Rev Respir Dis* 1989;140:1348–1353.

82. Fuller RW, Black PN, Dollery CT. Effect of the oral leukotriene D$_4$ antagonists LY 171883 on inhaled and intradermal challenge with antigen and LTD$_4$ in atopic subjects. *J Allergy Clin Immunol* 1989;83: 939–944.

83. Cloud ML, Enas GC, Kemp J, et al. A specific LTD$_4$/E$_4$ receptor antagonist improves pulmonary function in patients with mild, chronic asthma. *Am Rev Respir Dis* 1989;140:1330–1339.

84. Bendele AM, Hoover DM, van Lier RB, Foxworthy PS, Eacho PI. Effects of chronic treatment with leukotriene D$_4$-antagonist compound LY171883 on B6C3F1 mice. *Fundam Appl Toxicol* 1990;15: 676–682.

85. Torphy TJ, Faiferman I, Gleason JG, et al. The preclinical and clinical pharmacology of SK&F 104353, a potent and selective peptidoleukotriene receptor antagonist. *Ann NY Acad Sci* 1991;629: 157–167.

86. Robuschi M, Riva E, Fuccella LM, et al. Prevention of exercise-induced bronchoconstriction by a new leukotriene antagonist (SKF-104353). A double blind study vs. disodium cromoglycate and placebo. *Am Rev Respir Dis* 1992;145:1285–1288.

87. Wisniewski PL, Busse WW, Meltzer SS, et al. Bronchodilatory effects of BAY-X7195 a selective leukotriene receptor antagonist. *J Allergy Clin Immunol* 1995;95:300.

88. Krell RD, Aharony D, Buckner CK, et al. The preclinical pharmacology of ICI 204,219. A peptide leukotriene antagonist. *Am Rev Respir Dis* 1990;141:978–987.

89. Smith LJ, Geller S, Ebright L, Glass M, Thyrum PT. Inhibition of leukotriene D4-induced bronchoconstriction in normal subjects by the oral LTD$_4$ antagonist ICI 204,219. *Am Rev Respir Dis* 1990;141: 988–992.

90. Taylor IK, O'Shaughnessy KM, Fuller RW, Dollery CT. Effect of cysteinyl-leukotriene receptor antagonist ICI 204,219 on allergen-induced bronchoconstriction and airway hyperreactivity in atopic subjects. *Lancet* 1991;337:690–694.

91. Dahlen B, Zetterstrom O, Bjorck T, Dahlen SE. The leukotriene-antagonist ICI-204,219 inhibits the early airway reaction to cumulative bronchial challenge with allergen in atopic asthmatics. *Eur Respir J* 1994;7:324–331.

92. Finnerty JP, Wood-Baker R, Thomson H, Holgate ST. Role of leukotrienes in exercise-induced asthma. Inhibitory effect of ICI 204219, a potent leukotriene D4 receptor antagonist. *Am Rev Respir Dis* 1992;145:746–749.

93. Glass M, Snader LA, Israel E. Effect of the inhaled LTD$_4$ receptor antagonist, ICI 204,219 on cold-air-induced bronchoconstriction in patients with asthma. *J Allergy Clin Immunol* 1994;93:295.

94. Kidney JC, Ridge SM, Chung KF, Barnes PJ. Inhibition of platelet-activating factor-induced bronchoconstriction by the leukotriene D4 receptor antagonist ICI 204,219. *Am Rev Respir Dis* 1993;147:215–217.

95. Spector SL, Smith LJ, Glass M. Effects of 6 weeks of therapy with oral doses of ICI 204,219, a leukotriene D$_4$ receptor antagonist in subjects with bronchial asthma. *Am J Respir Crit Care Med* 1995;150: 618–623.

96. Lockey RF, Lavins BJ, Snader L. Thirteen weeks of treatment with zafirlukast (Accolate) in patients with mild to moderate asthma. *J Allergy Clin Immunol* 1995;95:350.

97. Spector SL. Management of asthma with zafirlukast. *Drugs* 1996; 52(suppl 6):36–46.

98. Zamboni R, Belley M, Champion E, et al. Development of a novel series of styrylquinoline compounds as high-affinity leukotriene D4 receptor antagonists: synthetic and structure-activity studies leading to the discovery of (+−)-3-[[[3-[2-(7-chloro-2-quinolinyl)-(E)-ethenyl]phenyl][[3-(dimethylamino)-3-oxopropyl]thio]methyl]thio] propionic acid. *J Med Chem* 1992;35:3832–3844.

99. Kips JC, Joos GF, De Lepeleire I, et al. MK-571, a potent antagonist of leukotriene D4-induced bronchoconstriction in the human. *Am Rev Respir Dis* 1991;144:617–621.

100. Rasmussen JB, Eriksson LO, Margolskee DJ, Tagari P, Williams VC, Andersson KE. Leukotriene D4 receptor blockade inhibits the immediate and late bronchoconstrictor responses to inhaled antigen in patients with asthma. *J Allergy Clin Immunol* 1992;90:193–201.

101. Hendeles L, Davison D, Blake K, Harman E, Cooper R, Margolskee D. Leukotriene D₄ is an important mediator of antigen-induced bronchoconstriction: attenuation of dual response with MK-571, a specific LTD₄ receptor antagonist. *J Allergy Clin Immunol* 1990;85, 197A.

102. Manning PJ, Watson RM, Margolskee DJ, Williams VC, Schwartz JI, O'Byrne PM. Inhibition of exercise-induced bronchoconstriction by MK-571, a potent leukotriene D4-receptor antagonist. *N Engl J Med* 1990;323:1736–1739.

103. Gaddy JN, Margolskee DJ, Bush RK, Williams VC, Busse WW. Bronchodilation with a potent and selective leukotriene D4 (LTD₄) receptor antagonist (MK-571) in patients with asthma. *Am Rev Respir Dis* 1992;146:358–363.

104. Gaddy J, McCreedy W, Margolskee D, Williams V, Busse W. A potent leukotriene D4 antagonist (MK-571) significantly reduces airway obstruction in mild to moderate asthma. *J Allergy Clin Immunol* 1991; 87:308.

105. Grossman SJ, DeLuca JG, Samboni RJ, et al. Enantioselective induction of peroxisomal proliferation in CD-1 mice by leukotriene antagonists. *Toxicol Appl Pharmacol* 1992;116:217–224.

106. Margolskee D, Bodman S, Dockhorn R, et al. The therapeutic effects of MK-571, a potent and selective LTD₄ receptor antagonist in patients with chronic asthma. *J Clin Allergy Immunol* 1991;87:309.

107. Ford-Hutchinson AW. Leukotriene antagonists and biosynthesis inhibitors: novel therapies for the treatment of human bronchial asthma and other diseases. *Ninth International Conference on Prostaglandins and Related Compounds, Florence, Italy.* 1994:3.

108. Labelle M, Belley M, Gareau Y, et al. Discovery of MK-0476, a potent and orally active leukotriene D₄ receptor antagonist devoid of peroxisomal enzyme induction. *Bioorg Med Chem Lett* 1995;5:283–288.

109. Jones TR, Labelle M, Belley M, et al. Pharmacology of montelukast sodium (SINGULAIR), a potent and selective leukotriene D₄-receptor antagonist. *Can J Physiol Pharmacol* 1995;73:191–201.

110. Botto A, Delepeleir I, Tochette R, et al. MK-0476 causes prolonged, potent LTD₄ receptor antagonism in the airways of asthmatics. *Am J Respir Crit Care Med* 1994;149:A465.

111. Sorkness CA, Reiss TF, Zhang J, et al. Bronchodilation with a selective and potent leukotriene D4 antagonist (MK-476). *Am J Respir Crit Care Med* 1994;149:A216.

112. Reiss TF, Bronsky E, Hendeles L, et al. MK-0476, a potent leukotriene D₄ receptor antagonist, inhibits exercise induced bronchoconstriction in asthmatics at the end of a once daily dosing interval. *Am J Respir Crit Care Med* 1995;151:A377.

113. Reiss TF, Sorkness CA, Strickner W, et al. Effects of montelukast (MK-0476), a potent cysteinyl leukotriene receptor antagonist, on bronchodilation in asthmatic subjects treated with and without inhaled corticosteroids. *Thorax* 1997;52:45–48.

114. Reiss TF, Altman LC, Munk ZM, et al. MK-0476, an LTD₄ receptor antagonist, improves the signs and symptoms of asthma with a dose as low as 10 mg, once daily. *Am J Respir Crit Care Med* 1995;151:A378.

115. Delepeleire I, Reiss TF, Rochette F, et al. Montelukast causes prolonged, potent leukotriene D₄ receptor antagonism in the airways of patients with asthma. *Clin Pharmacol Ther* 1997;61:83–92.

116. ONO-1078. *Drugs Future* 1988;13:317–320.

117. Taniguchi Y, Tamura G, Honma M, et al. The effect of an oral leukotriene antagonist, ONO-1078, on allergen-induced immediate bronchoconstriction in asthmatic subjects. *J Allergy Clin Immunol* 1993;92:507–512.

118. Fujimura M, Sakamoto S, Kamio Y, Matsuda T. Effect of a leukotriene

119. Barnes NC, de Jong B, Miyamoto T. Worldwide clinical experience with the first marketed leukotriene receptor antagonist. *Chest* 1997; 111(suppl 2):525–605.

120. Tamaoki J, Kondo M, Sakai N, et al. Leukotriene antagonist prevents exacerbation of asthma during reduction of high-dose inhaled corticosteroid. *Am J Respir Care Med* 1997;155:1235–1240.

121. O'Shaughnessy TC, Georgiou P, Howland K, Barnes NC. The effect of pranlukast, an oral leukotriene antagonist, on leukotriene D₄ challenge in normal male subjects. *Am J Respir Crit Care Med* 1995;151: A378.

122. Yamamoto H, Nagata M, Kuramitsu K, et al. Inhibition of analgesic-induced asthma by leukotriene receptor antagonist ONO-1078. *Am J Respir Crit Care Med* 1994;150:254–257.

123. Barnes NC, Pujet J-C. First clinical experience with the oral leukotriene receptor antagonist, pranlukast in northern European patients with mild to moderate asthma. *Am J Respir Crit Care Med* 1995;151:A378.

124. Grossman J, Bronsky E, Busse W, et al. A multicenter, double-blind, placebo controlled study to evaluate the safety tolerability and clinical activity of oral twice daily LTA, pranlukast in patients with mild to moderate asthma. *J Allergy Clin Immunol* 1995;95:352.

125. O'Donnell M, Crowley HJ, Yaremko B, O'Neill N, Welton AF. Pharmacologic actions of RO-24-5913, a novel antagonist of leukotriene D. *J Pharmacol Exp Ther* 1991;259:751–758.

126. Adelroth E, Inman MD, Summers E, Pace D, O'Byrne PM. Prolonged protection against exercise-induced bronchoconstriction by the leukotriene D₄-receptor antagonist cinalukast. *J Allergy Clin Immunol* 1997;99:210–215.

127. Goetzl EJ, Pickett WC. Novel structural determinants of the human neutrophil chemotactic activity of leukotriene B. *J Exp Med* 1981; 153:482–487.

128. Showell HJ, Otterness IG, Marfat A, Corey EJ. Inhibition of leukotriene B4-induced neutrophil degranulation by leukotriene B4-dimethylamide. *Biochem Biophys Res Commun* 1982;106:741–747.

129. Lin AH, Morris J, Wishka DG, Gorman RR. Novel molecules that antagonize leukotriene B4 binding to neutrophils. *Ann NY Acad Sci* 1988;524:196–200.

130. Namiki M, Igarashi Y, Sakamato K, Nakamura T, Koga Y. Pharmacological profiles of potential LTB₄-antagonist, SM-9064. *Biochem Biophys Res Commun* 1986;138:540–546.

131. Tsai BS, Price D, Keith R. SC-41930: an inhibitor of LTB₄-stimulated human neutrophil functions. *Prostaglandins* 1989;38:655–674.

132. Schultz RM, Marder P, Spaette SM, Herron DK, Sofia MJ. Effects of two leukotriene B4 (LTB₄) receptor antagonists (LY255283 and SC-41930) on LTB₄-induced human neutrophil adhesion and superoxide production. *Prostaglandins Leukoc Essent Fat Acids* 1991;43: 267–271.

133. Fretland DJ, Widomski DL, Zemaitis JM, Djuric SW, Shone RL. Effect of a leukotriene B₄ receptor antagonist on LTB₄-induced neutrophil chemotaxis in cavine dermis. *Inflammation* 1989;13:601–605.

134. Fretland DJ, Widomski D, Tsai B, et al. Effect of the leukotriene B₄ receptor antagonist SC-41930 on colonic inflammation in rat, guinea pig and rabbit. *J Pharmacol Exp Ther* 1990;255:573–576.

135. Villani-Price D, Yang DC, Walsh RE, et al. Multiple actions of the leukotriene B₄ receptor antagonist SC41930. *J Pharmacol Exp Ther* 1992;260:187–191.

136. Djuric SW, Docter SH, Yu SS, et al. Synthesis and pharmacological activity of SC-53228, a leukotriene B₄ receptor antagonist with high intrinsic potency and selectivity. *Bioorg Med Chem Lett* 1994;4: 811–816.

137. Yu SS, Djuric SW, Dygos JH, et al. SC-53228. *Drugs Future* 1994;19: 1093–1097.

138. Fretland D, Sanderson T, Smith P, et al. Oral efficacy of an LTB₄ receptor antagonist in cotton-top tamarins. *Gut* 1995;37:702–707.

139. Herron DK, Goodson T, Bolinger NF, et al. Leukotriene B₄ receptor antagonists: the LY255283 series of hydroxyacetophenones. *J Med Chem* 1992;35:1818–1828.

140. DeLong AF, Oldham SW, Wiltse CG, Epinette WW, McDonald CJ, Callaghan JT. HPLC assay of LY223982 in plasma and urine during phase I safety and topical activity evaluation in psoriasis. *Pharmacologist* 1991;33:497.

141. Sawyer JS, Bach NJ, Baker SR, et al. Synthetic and structure activity

studies on acid substituted 2-aryl phenols: discovery of 2-(2-propyl-3-(3-(2-ethyl-4-(4-fluorophenyl)-5-hydroxyphenoxy)-propoxy)phenoxy)benzoic acid, a high affinity leukotriene B$_4$ receptor antagonist. *J Med Chem* 1995;38:4411–4432.

142. Marder P, Spaethe SM, Froelich LL, et al. Inhibition of *ex vivo* neutrophil activation by oral LY293111, a novel leukotriene B$_4$ receptor antagonist. *Br J Clin Pharmacol* 1996;42:457–464.

143. Evans DJ, Barnes PJ, Spaethe SM, van Alstyre EL, Mitchell MI, O'Connor BJ. Effect of a leukotriene B$_4$ receptor antagonist, LY293111, on allergen-induced responses in asthma. *Thorax* 1996;51:1178–1184.

144. van Pelt JPA, de Jong EMGJ, van Erp EJ, et al. The regulation of CD11b integrin levels on human blood leukocytes and leukotriene B$_4$-stimulated skin by a specific leukotriene B$_4$ antagonist (LY293111). *Biochem Pharmacol* 1997;53:1005–1012.

145. Daines RA, Chambers PA, Pendrak I, et al. (E)-3-[[[[6-(2-carboxyethenyl)-5-[[8-(4-methoxyphenyl)octyl]oxy]-2-pyrindinyl]methyl]thio]methyl]benzoic acid: a novel high affinity leukotriene B$_4$ receptor antagonist. *J Med Chem* 1993;36:2703–2705.

146. Sarau HM, Foley JJ, Schmidt DB, et al. SB209247, a high affinity LTB$_4$ receptor antagonist demonstrating potent antiinflammatory activity. *Adv Prostaglandin Thromboxane Leukotriene Res* 1995;23:275–277.

147. Kishikawa K, Tateishi N, Maruyama R, Seo R, Toda M, Miyamoto T. ONO-4057, a novel, orally active leukotriene B$_4$ antagonist: effects on LTB$_4$-induced neutrophil functions. *Prostaglandins* 1992;44:261–275.

148. Fujimoto RA, Main AJ, Barsky LI, et al. Aryl amidines: a new class of potent orally active leukotriene B$_4$ antagonists. *7th International Conference on Inflammation Research Association.* White Haven, PA: 1994:P29.

149. Raychandhuri A, Kotyuk B, Pellas TC, et al. Effect of CGS25019C and other LTB$_4$ antagonists in the mouse ear edema and rat neutropenia models. *Inflam Res* 1995;44:S141–S142.

150. Morgan J, Stevens R, Uziel-Fusi S, et al. Pharmacokinetics of a mono-aryl-amidine compound (CGS-25019C) and its inhibition of dihydroxy leukotrienes (LTB$_4$)-induced CD11b expression. *Clin Pharmacol Ther* 1994;55:199.

151. Uziel-Fusi S, Stevens R, Morgan J, et al. CGS25019C inhibits LTB$_4$-stimulated CD11b upregulation *in vitro* and *ex vivo*. *7th International Conference on Inflammation Research Association.* White Haven, PA: 1994:24.

152. Morgan J, Stevens R, Uziel-Fusi S, et al. Multiple dose pharmacokinetics of a mono-aryl-amidine compound (CGS25019C) and its inhibition of dihydroxy leukotrienes (LTB$_4$)-induced CD11b expression. *Clin Pharmacol Ther* 1995;57:153.

153. Koch K, Melvin LS, Reiter LA, et al. (+)-1-(3S,4R)-[3-(4-Phenylbenzyl)-4-hydroxychroman-7-yl)]cyclopentane carboxylic acid, a highly potent selective leukotriene B$_4$ antagonist with oral activity in the murine collagen-induced arthritis model. *J Med Chem* 1994;37:3197–3199.

154. Lowe III JA, Drozda SE, Snider RA, et al. The discovery of (2S, 3S)-cis-2-(diphenylmethyl)-N-[(2-methoxyphenyl)methyl]-1-azabicyclo[2.2.2]-octan-3-amine as a novel, nonpeptide substance P antagonist. *J Med Chem* 1992;35:2591–2600.

155. Showell HJ, Pettipher ER, Cheng JB, et al. The *in vitro* and *in vivo* pharmacologic activity of the potent and selective leukotriene B$_4$ receptor antagonist CP-105,696. *J Pharmacol Exp Ther* 1995;273:176–184.

156. Showell HJ, Breslow K, Conklyn MJ, Hingorami GP, Koch K. Characterization of the pharmacological profile of the potent LTB$_4$ antagonist CP-105,696 on murine LTB$_4$ receptor *in vitro*. *Br J Pharmacol* 1996;117:1127–1132.

157. Griffiths RJ, Pettipher ER, Koch K, et al. Leukotriene B4 plays a critical role in the progression of collagen-induced arthritis. *Proc Natl Acad Sci USA* 1995;92:517–521.

158. Gladue RP, Carroll LA, Milici AJ, et al. Inhibition of leukotriene B$_4$-receptor interaction suppresses eosinophi infiltration and disease pathology in a murine model of experimental allergic encephalomyelitis. *J Exp Med* 1996;183:1893–1898.

159. Weringer EJ, Perry BD, Sawyer PS, Gilman SC, Showell HJ. Acceptance of cardiac allografts after treatment with a potent LTB$_4$ receptor antagonist. *Transplantation* 1998; in press.

160. Griffiths RJ, Smith MA, Roach ML, et al. Collagen-induced arthritis

is reduced in 5-lipoxygenase-activating protein-deficient mice. *J Exp Med* 1997;185:1123–1129.

161. Turner CR, Breslow R, Conklyn MJ, et al. *In vitro* and *in vivo* effects of leukotriene B$_4$ antagonism in a primate model of asthma. *J Clin Invest* 1996;97:381–387.

162. Liston TE, Conklyn MJ, Houser J, et al. Pharmacokinetics and pharmacodynamics of the leukotriene B$_4$ receptor antagonist CP-105,696 in man following single oral administration. *Br J Clin Pharmacol* 1998;45:115–121.

163. Whittaker M. PAF receptor antagonists: recent advances. *Curr Opin Ther Pat* 1992;2:583–623.

164. Arnout J, van Hecken A, DeLepeleire I, et al. Effectiveness and tolerability of CV-3988, a selective PAF antagonist, after intravenous administration to man. *Br J Clin Pharmacol* 1988;25:445–457.

165. Stockmans F, Arnout J, Depré M, Schepper P, Anghrn JC, Vermylen J. TCV-309, a novel PAF antagonist, inhibits PAF-induced platelet aggregation *ex vivo*. *Thromb Hemostasis* 1991;65:1108.

166. Companies. *Script* 1992;1728:12.

167. Kornecki E, Ehrlich YH, Lenox RH. Platelet-activating factor-induced aggregation of human platelets specifically inhibited by triazolobenzodiazepenes. *Science* 1984;226:1454–1456.

168. Crowley HJ, Yaremko B, Selig WM, et al. Pharmacology of a potent platelet-activating factor antagonist: Ro 24-4736. *J Pharmacol Exp Ther* 1991;259:78–85.

169. Terasawa M, Aratain H, Setoguchi M, Tahara T. Pharmacological actions of Y-24180: a potent and specific antagonist of platelet activating factor. *Prostaglandins* 1990;40:553–569.

170. Pinquier JL, Sedivy P, Bruno R, et al. Inhibition of *ex vivo* PAF-induced platelet aggregation by the PAF-antagonist RP 48740: relationship to plasma concentrations in healthy volunteers. *Eur J Clin Pharmacol* 1991;41:141–145.

171. Davidsen SK, Summers JB, Albert DH, et al. N. (acyloxyalkyl) pyridinium salts as soluble products of a potent platelet activating factor antagonist. *J Med Chem* 1994;37:4423–4429.

172. Wyld P, Nimmo W, Holland T, Herbert J-M, Cluzel M. Single rising oral dose of SR 27417A, a specific PAF receptor antagonist in humans: tolerability and pharmacological assessment. *J Lipid Mediators Cell Signal* 1994;10:155–157.

173. Cluzel M, Nimmo W, Herbert J-M, Wyld P. Single rising dose of SR-27417, a specific PAF receptor antagonist in humans: tolerability and pharmacological assessment. *Fourth International Congress on PAF and Related Lipid Mediators.* Snow Bird, UT: 1992:C4.1.

174. Parry MJ, Alabaster VA, Cheesman HE, Cooper K, deSouza RN, Keiv RF. Pharmacological profile of UK-74,505, a novel and selective PAF antagonist with potent and prolonged oral activity. *J Lipid Mediators Cell Signal* 1994;10:251–268.

175. Formela LJ, Wood LM, Whittaker M, Kingsnorth AN. Amelioration of experimental acute pancreatitis with a potent platelet-activating factor antagonist. *Br J Surg* 1994;81:1783–1785.

176. Hwang SB, Lam MH, Szalkowski DM, et al. MK287: a potent, specific, and orally active receptor antagonist of platelet-activating factor. *J Lipid Mediators* 1993;7:115–134.

177. Billah MM, Chapman RW, Watnick AS, Egan RW, Siegel MI, Kreutner W. Sch 37370: a new drug combining antagonism of platelet-activating factor (PAF) with antagonism of histamine. *Agents Actions* 1991;34:313–321.

178. LeSollen H, Laguerre M, Saux M, Dubost JP. A pharmacophore for high affinity PAF antagonists. 1. Electronic model using molecular electrostatic potential. *J Lipid Mediators Cell Signal* 1996;13:249–282.

179. Roberts NM, McCusker M, Chung KF, Barnes PJ. Effect of a PAF antagonist, BN52063, on PAF-induced bronchoconstriction in normal subjects. *Br J Clin Pharmacol* 1988;26:65–72.

180. Markey AC, Barker JN, Archer CB, Guinot P, Lee TH, MacDonald DM. Platelet activating factor-induced clinical and histopathologic responses in atopic skin and their modifications by the platelet factor antagonist BN 52063. *J Am Acad Dermatol* 1990;23:263–268.

181. Hsieh KH. Effects of PAF antagonist, BN 52021, in the PAF-, methacholine- and allergen-induced bronchoconstriction in asthmatic children. *Chest* 1991;99:877–882.

182. Guinot P, Brambilla C, Duchier J, Braquet P, Bonvoisin B, Cournot A. Effects of BN 52063, a specific PAF-acether antagonist, in bronchial provocation test to allergens in asthmatic patients. A preliminary study. *Prostaglandins* 1987;34:723–731.

183. Wilkens JH, Wilkens H, Uffmann J, Bovers J, Fabel H, Frolich JC. Effects of a PAF-antagonist (BN 52063) on bronchoconstriction and platelet activation during exercise-induced asthma. *Br J Clin Pharmacol* 1990;29:85–91.

184. Hayes JP, Ridge SM, Griffith S, Barnes PJ, Chung KF. Inhibition of cutaneous and platelet responses to platelet-activating factor by oral WEB 2086 in man. *J Allergy Clin Immunol* 1991;88:83–88.

185. Adamus WS, Heuer HO, Meade CJ, Schilling JC. Inhibitory effects of the new PAF acether antagonist WEB-2086 on pharmacologic changes induced by PAF inhalation in human beings. *Clin Pharmacol Ther* 1990;47:456–462.

186. Freitag A, Watson RM, Matsos G, Eastwood C, O'Byrne PM. Effect of platelet activating factor antagonist, WEB 2086, in allergen-induced asthmatic responses. *Thorax* 1993;48:594–598.

187. Spence DP, Johnston SL, Calverley PM, et al. The effect of the orally active platelet-activating factor antagonist WEB 2086 in the treatment of asthma. *Am J Respir Crit Care Med* 1994;149:1142–1148.

188. Hozawa S, Haruta Y, Ishioka S, Yamakido M. Effects of a PAF antagonist, Y-24180, on bronchial hyperresponsiveness in patients with asthma. *Am J Respir Crit Care Med* 1995;152:1198–1202.

189. Townley RG, Eda R, Hopp RJ, Bewtra AK, Gillen MS. The effect of RP 59227, a platelet-activating factor antagonist, against antigen challenge and eosinophil chemotaxis in asthmatics. *J Lipid Mediators Cell Signal* 1994;10:345–353.

190. O'Connor BJ, Uden S, Carty TJ, Eskra JD, Barnes PJ, Chung KF. Inhibitory effect of UK-74,505, a potent and specific oral platelet-activating factor (PAF) receptor antagonist, in airway and systemic responses to inhaled PAF in humans. *Am J Respir Crit Care Med* 1994;150:35–40.

191. Kuiterk LM, Hui KP, Uthayarkumar S, et al. Effect of the platelet-activating factor antagonist UK-74,505 on the early and late response to allergen. *Am Rev Respir Dis* 1993;147:82–86.

192. Bel EH, DeSmet M, Rossing TH, Timmers MC, Dijkman JH, Sterk PJ. The effect of a specific oral PAF-antagonist, MK-287, on antigen-induced early and late asthmatic reactions in man. *Am Rev Respir Dis* 1991;143:A811.

193. Pinquier JL, Lurie A, Impens N, et al. Effect of the PAF-antagonist MK-287 in moderate asthmatic patients. *Clin Pharmacol Ther* 1993;53:202.

194. Dermarkarian RM, Israel E, Rosenberg MA, et al. The effect of Sch-37370, a dual PAF and histamine antagonist, on the bronchoconstric-tion induced in asthmatics by cold, dry air isocapnic hyperventilation. *Am Rev Respir Dis* 1991;143;A812.

195. Israel E, Chervinsky P, Rosenthal R, et al. The effect of SCH-37370(SCH), a dual platelet-activating factor (PAF) and histamine antagonist, in patients with mild chronic asthma. *J Allergy Clin Immunol* 1993;91:224.

196. Schmidt T, Abeck D, Grosshans E, et al. Topical application of a platelet-activating factor (PAF-) antagonist in atopic eczema. *J Allergy Clin Immunol* 1996;97:369.

197. Dhainaut JF, Tenaillon A, LeTulzo Y, et al. Platelet-activating factor receptor antagonist BN 52021 in the treatment of severe sepsis: a randomized, double-blind, placebo-controlled, multicenter clinical trial. BN 52021 Sepsis Study Group. *Crit Care Med* 1994;22:1720–1728.

198. Thompson WA, Coyle S, VanZeek, et al. The metabolic effects of platelet-activating factor antagonism in endotoxemic man. *Arch Surg* 1994;129:72–79.

199. Froon AMF, Grere JWM, Buurmann WA, et al. Treatment with the platelet-activating factor antagonist TCV-309 in patients with severe systemic inflammatory response syndrome: a prospective, multicenter, double-blind, randomized phase II trial. *Shock* 1996;5:313–319.

200. Kingsforth AM. Early treatment with lexipafant, a platelet activating factor antagonist reduces mortality in acute pancreatitis: a double-blind, randomized, placebo controlled study. *Gastroenterology* 1997;112(suppl):A453.

201. Grino JM. BN 52021: a platelet-activating factor antagonist for preventing post-transplant renal failure. A double-blind, randomized study. The BN 52021 study group in renal transplantation. *Ann Intern Med* 1994;121:345–347.

202. Simon LS, Lanza FL, Lipsky PE, et al. Preliminary study of the safety and efficacy of SC-58635, a novel cyclooxygenase 2 inhibitor: efficacy and safety in two placebo-controlled trials in osteoarthritis and rheumatoid arthritis, and studies on gastrointestinal platelet effects. *Arthritis and Rheumatism* 1998;41:1591–1602.

203. Graul A, Martel AM, Castaner J. Celecoxib. *Drugs of the Future* 1997;22:711–714.

204. Barnes PJ, Chung KF. Zafirlukast (Accolate™). *Drugs of Today* 1998;34:375–388.

205. Showell HJ, Conklyn MJ, Alpert R, et al. The preclinical pharmacological profile of the potent and selective Leukotriene B₄ antagonist CP-195,543. *J Pharmacol Exp Ther* 1998;285:946–954.

Inflammation: Basic Principles and Clinical Correlates,
3rd ed., edited by John I. Gallin and Ralph Snyderman.
Lippincott Williams & Wilkins, Philadelphia © 1999.

CHAPTER 75

Complement Inhibitors

Jeffrey L. Platt

The complement system provides what is arguably the most rapid and potent line of defense against invasive microorganisms. However, the activation of complement leads to formation in solution of active C3 convertase complexes and C5b67 complexes, which could in turn cause injury to autologous cells, just as they do foreign organisms. To avoid such toxic "bystander" effects of complement activation, the complement system includes a series of regulatory proteins that limit or inhibit complement activation on autologous cells. How these regulatory proteins control complement reactions in health and how various pharmaceutical agents might be used to control complement reactions in disease are the subjects of this chapter. The reader is referred to the chapter by Cooper for detailed discussion of the components of the complement system, and the biochemical pathways through which complement is activated and mediates effector functions.

PHYSIOLOGIC REGULATION OF THE COMPLEMENT SYSTEM

The complement system consists of more than 20 proteins that can assemble into biochemically active complexes, mediate opsonization, activation of phagocytic cells and endothelial cells, and cause cell lysis (Fig. 75-1). Activation of complement and manifestation of effector functions involves reactions in the solution phase of plasma and on the cell surface; the cell surface reactions involving C3 convertases and terminal complement complexes are generally targeted to foreign cells or cells that have sustained some form of injury, while the action of anaphylotoxins is targeted to healthy autologous cells bearing appropriate receptors. Thus, the separation of the cytotoxic effects of complement that are directed at

invading organisms, from the promoting of cellular activation, which is directed at autologous cells, is a significant biochemical challenge.

The need for complement regulation has been obvious for some time (1–3). For example, the cytotoxic properties of complement inspired the concept of *horror autotoxicus*, which Ehrlich thought might arise if the immune system were to turn against self. Recent studies by Matsui et al. (4) and Nishikawa et al. (5) support this dramatic view. Injection of antibodies specific for membrane inhibitors of complement in rats was found to cause the loss of vascular integrity and severe tissue reactions. Similarly, Miyagawa et al. (6) found that activation of complement of the rat on the blood vessels of a guinea pig heart transplanted into the rat [presumably caused by the failure of rat factor H to control rat C3b formation on guinea pig cell surfaces (7)] leads within 10 minutes to loss of vascular integrity and destruction of the graft (Fig. 75-2).

It is presumably because the toxic effects of complement are so considerable, that complement activation is controlled very tightly and redundantly (Fig. 75-3). This control is exerted through three general mechanisms: (a) activation of complement, especially the classical pathway, is specifically targeted to foreign organisms or foreign cell surfaces by the binding of antibodies or by spontaneous activation; (b) reactive complement complexes spontaneously dissociate or lose enzymatic activity; and (c) activation of complement is inhibited in the plasma and on autologous cell surfaces by complement regulatory proteins, the properties of which are summarized in Table 75-1 and Fig. 75-3 and described in detail in recent reviews (8–11). The need for constitutive control of complement is heightened because the complement system is continuously activated, albeit at a slow rate, by spontaneous hydrolysis of C3, and because foreign organisms invade the body under physiologic conditions. In addition to the constitutive mechanisms of

J. L. Platt: Departments of Surgery, Pediatrics, and Immunology, Mayo Clinic, Rochester, Minnesota 55905.

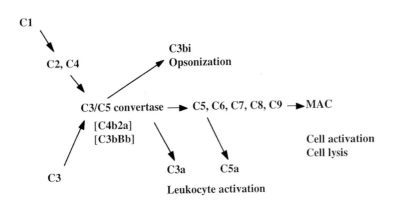

FIG. 75-1. A diagrammatic summary of the complement system and its effector functions. Activation of complement through the classical pathway (C1) or alternative pathway (C3) leads to formation of C3/C5 convertases. These convertases amplify complement reactions leading to formation of the membrane attack complex (MAC). The components and complexes of complement that bring about effector functions include the following: (a) the C3bi fragment of C3 attached to a target provides a ligand for leukocytes bearing C3 receptors (opsonization); (b) anaphylotoxins generated by cleavage of C3 and C5 bind to specific receptors on leukocytes and endothelial cells and smooth muscle cells causing activation of the cells; and (c) MAC induces activation or lysis of target cells.

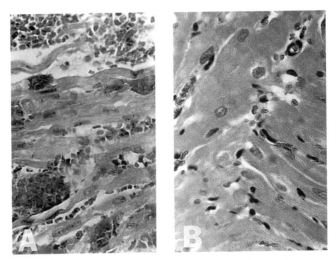

FIG. 75-2. Hyperacute rejection of guinea pig heart transplanted into a rat. **A:** A guinea pig heart transplanted heterotopically into a rat undergoes rejection within 10 to 30 minutes. Rejection is caused by the formation of terminal complement complexes on the endothelial surfaces of the transplant (78). **B:** Hyperacute rejection is prevented by the administration of cobra venom factor as shown here, by other inhibitors of C3 convertases, or potentially by anti-C5 antibodies C5 (65) (not shown).

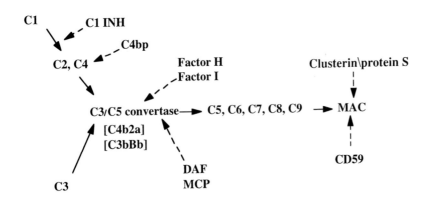

FIG. 75-3. Regulation of the complement cascade. The complement cascade is regulated by plasma proteins *(upper part dashed arrows)* and cell membrane proteins *(below, dashed arrows).* C1 inhibitor (C1 INH) interferes with the protease activity of C1. C4 binding protein serves as a cofactor for cleavage of C4. Factors H and I inhibit C3/C5 convertases, as described in the text. Clusterin and protein S inhibit the membrane attack complex (MAC) in the fluid phase. Cell membrane regulators of complement include decay accelerating factor (DAF), membrane cofactor protein (MCP; CD46), and membrane inhibitor of reactive lysis (CD59).

TABLE 75-1. *Regulators of complement*

Complement regulator	Site	Molecular mass (kd)	Target	Mechanism
C1NH	Plasma	90	C1rs	Protease inhibitor
Factor H	Plasma	160	C3b	Prevents association with factor B; cofactor for factor I
C4bp	Plasma	560	C4b	Cofactor for factor I
Factor I	Plasma	90	C3b, C4b	Cleaves to yield inactive proteins
MCP	Cell membrane	60	C4b, C3b	Cofactor for factor I
DAF	Cell membrane	70	C4b2a, C3bBb	Dissociates complex
CD59	Cell membrane	20	MAC	Prevents polymerization of C9

C1INH, C1 inhibitor; C4bp, C4 binding protein; MCP, membrane cofactor protein; DAF, decay-accelerating factor; MAC, membrane attack complex.

complement control there are adaptive mechanisms, which is to say mechanisms by which cells adapt to complement activation. For example, formation of the membrane attack complex on cell surfaces causes cells to acquire resistance to complement-mediated lysis over a period of hours (12,13). In addition to the physiologic mechanisms for the control of complement, a number of pharmaceutical and experimental agents have been developed to bring about control of complement (Table 75-1). This chapter summarizes the properties of the physiologic molecules and pharmacologic agents that inhibit the complement cascade.

MODELS FOR INVESTIGATING THE CONTROL AND INHIBITION OF COMPLEMENT

The study of complement inhibitors is facilitated by use of experimental models of complement mediated injury. The sections that follow describe some of the models more commonly in use.

Forssman Reaction

The injection of antiserum or purified antibodies specific for the Forssman antigen [GalNAc(α1–3)GalNAc] into guinea pigs leads within minutes to pulmonary failure, shock, and death (14,15). This model, known as the Forssman reaction, is thought to be mediated by the activation of complement on pulmonary endothelium. In addition to complement-mediated endothelial damage, the Forssman reaction is associated with influx of leukocytes. Pulmonary endothelial damage may be mediated (a) directly by the membrane attack complex, (b) by invading leukocytes that have been activated by anaphylotoxins, and/or (c) by leukocytes that adhere to C3bi formed on the surface of endothelial cells. It will be seen that the Forssman reaction can be prevented by treatment of the guinea pigs with any one of a variety of complement inhibitors.

Ischemia Reperfusion

The tissue injury that follows temporary disruption of blood flow is known as ischemia-reperfusion injury. It is commonly seen following coronary thrombosis, angioplasty, and organ transplantation. Ischemia-reperfusion injury may be modeled by surgical ligation of coronary or other arterial vessels or by the intentional delay in the anastomosis and reperfusion of experimental organ transplants. It is mediated at least in part by oxidants released from invading leukocytes (16). The release of oxidants is in turn driven by complement activation, particularly the generation of (C5a and C3a). Adhesion of leukocytes is thought to be caused by activation of C3, leading to formation of C3bi on affected. Which factor(s) trigger activation of the complement system in ischemia reperfusion is the subject of debate. Some evidence points to activation of the alternative pathway on the surface of damaged cells; other evidence supports activation of the classical pathway. Regardless of the mechanisms that initiate damage, there is clear evidence from many experimental systems that ischemia-reperfusion injury can be limited by therapies that interfere with complement activation or with neutrophil adhesion (17,18).

Xenograft Rejection

Organs transplanted between phylogenetically disparate species are subject to hyperacute rejection (19). Hyperacute rejection depends absolutely on activation of the complement system of the recipient on blood vessels in the newly transplanted organ (20). Complement activation may in turn be triggered by activation of the alternative pathway of complement on foreign endothelium or by the binding of xenoreactive natural antibodies that activate the classical pathway. Complement activation through either pathway leads to formation of terminal complexes on the endothelium of the graft, which in turn causes loss of endothelial integrity, hemorrhage, thrombosis, and destruction of the graft within minutes to hours, as illustrated in Fig. 75-2. Susceptibility of xenografts to hyperacute rejection reflects in part the failure of complement regulatory proteins of the foreign organ to control the complement system of the recipient (21). Inhibition of complement by any means reliably prevents hyperacute rejection.

Anaphylotoxin Lung Injury

Various models have been used to evaluate the effects of anaphylotoxins *in vivo*. In some cases such as ischemia-reperfusion injury, the effects of anaphylotoxins may be difficult to separate from other consequences of complement activation. Perhaps the most frequently used models involve analysis of the effects of anaphylotoxin generation on pulmonary structure and function. For example, infusion of anaphylotoxins (C5a) induces dramatic changes in pulmonary blood flow (22) and systemic hypotension (23). Some of these changes reflect the direct action of anaphylotoxins on blood vessels and some the systemic effects of eicosanoids, the synthesis of which is stimulated by anaphylotoxins. Administration of cobra venom factor to rats or mice generates anaphylotoxins and leads to sequestration of leukocytes in the pulmonary circulation and severe lung damage (24,25).

REGULATION AND CONTROL OF C1

The classic pathway of the complement system is activated by complement-fixing antibodies that, when bound to appropriate targets, interact with globular domains of C1. Under some circumstances C1 directly fixes to cells, leading to classical pathway activation. C1 consists of 18 chains of C1q associated via collagenous domains with C1rs, a tetramer consisting of two chains each of C1r and C1s. When activated by C1r, C1s is a serine protease that cleaves and thereby activates C4 and C2.

The protease activity of C1rs is regulated by C1 inhibitor (C1 INH), a 90-kd serum protein. C1 INH is a protease inhibitor of the serpin class. Although the inhibitory activity of C1 INH might be considered weak, it is enhanced by the presence of heparin, a component of mast cell granules, and heparan sulfate, a component of eukaryotic cell surfaces and extracellular matrices (26,27). The rich supply of heparan sulfate on endothelial cell surfaces may help protect the cells from inadvertent injury induced by fixation of C1. The importance of C1 INH is suggested by the very dramatic consequences of C1 INH deficiency, including angioneurotic edema characterized by profound swelling in the head, neck, and extremities, and obstruction of the airways at the level of the larynx. It is not clear yet whether symptoms and signs associated with C1 INH deficiency reflect unfettered activation of C1 leading to the generation of anaphylotoxins or whether it reflects a byproduct of C1 INH activity, which is control of the kinin-kininogen system (Fig. 75-2).

Therapeutic Considerations

Because the alternative pathway is more vital than the classical pathway for host defense, the development of therapeutics directed at the classical pathway is one goal (Fig. 75-4) (Table 75-2). Among the pharmacologic approaches proposed for the C1 step in complement activation have been the use of purified C1 inhibitor for administration to patients with C1 inhibitor deficiency or complement-mediated autoimmune diseases, and the administration of heparin for similar purposes. The susceptibility of the C1 system to depletion by autoantibodies is especially great because complement reactions may be limited by the relatively low concentration of C2 (~20 µg/mL). Under development are various inhibitors of C1q. Such agents may help to interfere with the interaction of C1q with receptors on cell surfaces or with β-amyloid. Advantages to focusing therapeutics on C1 include the sparing of the alternative pathway for host defense against extracellular pathogens.

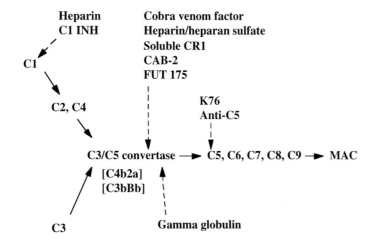

FIG. 75-4. Therapeutic agents used to control complement reactions. Some therapeutic agents used to control complement reactions are listed, and the site of action indicated *(dashed arrows)*. The function of the agents is described in the text.

TABLE 75-2. *Some inhibitors of the complement system*

Complement inhibitor	Target	Mechanism
CVF	C3/factor B	Initiatese alternative pathway, consuming complement
sCR1	C3bBb, C4b2a	Accelerates dissociation of complexes; cofactor for factor I
Heparin	C1, factor H, ATIII, C1rs, C3/5 convertases	Promotes activity of C1In, factor H, and ATIII; inhibits complement proteases
Gamma globulin	C3b, C4b	Alternative acceptor for targets
CAB-2	C3bBb, C4b2a	DAF and MCP activity (see Table 75–1)
FUT175	C1r, C1s, C3/C5 convertases	Protease inhibitor
Anti-C5	C5	Inhibits C5 cleavage

CVF, cobra venom factor; sCR1, soluble complement receptor type 1; ATIII, antithrombin III; CAB-2, complement activation blocker-2; DAF, decay-accelerating factor; MCP, membrane cofactor protein; FUT175, 6-amino-2-naphthyl-4-guanidinobenzoate.

REGULATION AND CONTROL OF C3/C5 CONVERTASE

The main enzyme mediating activation and amplification of the complement system is C3 convertase. The alternative pathway C3 convertase is activated by the spontaneous hydrolysis of C3 to yield C3(H_2O), which, like C3b, can associate with factor B to yield alternative pathway C3 convertase, an enzyme that catalyzes the cleavage of C3 to yield C3b. The classical pathway C3 convertase is formed by the association of C4b with a cleavage product of C2 (C2a). C4b2a, like the alternative pathway C3 convertase, catalyzes cleavage of C3. Association of C3b with the alternative or classic pathway convertases facilitates cleavage of C5.

Regulators of Complement Activation (RCA)

Of special importance in the regulation of C3 convertase activity are members of the RCA family. This series of proteins is encoded by a gene family located on chromosome 1 and includes factor H, C4 binding protein, decay accelerating factor, membrane cofactor protein, and complement receptors types 1 and 2. The proteins in this family have globular domains consisting of 4 to 59 cysteine-rich short consensus repeats of ~60 amino acids. The reader is referred to the chapter by Cooper and to recent reviews (10,28,29) for detailed description of the gene family and structures of the corresponding proteins.

Factor H

Alternative pathway C3 convertases [C3(H_2O)Bb and C3bBb] are regulated by factor H (Table 75-1). Factor H is a 160-kd plasma protein that recognizes C3b and mediates the dissociation of factor B and serves as a cofactor for the cleavage of C3b. Factor H confers specificity on the alternative complement pathway activation because while it regulates C3b on autologous surfaces, it may fail to interact with C3b on foreign surfaces, such as the walls of certain microorganisms and the cells of certain foreign species. The function of factor H is enhanced by the presence of negative charges on the cell surface. Thus, cells lacking polyanions such as heparan sulfate or anionic molecules such as sialic acid, on cells from which these molecules have been released, are particularly susceptible to the alternative pathway of complement. Moreover, the binding of antibodies or other proteins that counter the negative charges tend to inhibit the functional effects of factor H and allow alternative pathway activation to proceed. The importance of factor H in maintaining the control of complement and tissue homeostasis is suggested by models in which regulation of the alternative pathway fails (7). For example, guinea pig hearts transplanted into rats are destroyed within minutes because of alternative pathway activation (6), presumably reflecting failure of rat factor H to control rat C3b on guinea pig cell surfaces. In this experimental model, complement activated in the xenografts through the alternative pathway causes loss of vascular integrity and destruction of the grafts within 20 to 30 minutes (Fig. 75-2).

Membrane Cofactor Protein (MCP)

Membrane cofactor protein or CD46 is a 60-kd integral membrane protein (30). MCP regulates C3b and C4b by serving as a cofactor for factor I–mediated cleavage of these proteins (Table 75-1). MCP may function in a species-specific manner, contributing to the susceptibility of cells to lysis by heterologous complement. MCP can serve as a receptor for the measles virus.

Decay Accelerating Factor (DAF)

C3 convertase complexes are also controlled by DAF or CD55 (31), a 70-kd protein anchored to cell membranes by phosphatidyl inositol modification. DAF accelerates the dissociation of C3bBb and C4b2a complexes. It may function in a species-specific manner (32), contributing to the susceptibility of cells to lysis by heterologous complement (Table 75-1).

C4 Binding Protein (C4bp)

C4 binding protein is a large, 560-kd serum protein. Upon binding to C4, C4bp regulates classical pathway convertase activity by accelerating the dissociation of C2a and by serving as a cofactor for factor I–mediated cleavage of C4b (Table 75-1).

Complement Receptor Type 1 (CR1)

CR1 is a 200-kd protein expressed on phagocytic cells, B cells, and erythrocytes (33). CR1 is thought to be important in clearing complement complexes from the blood (34). CR1 exhibits a variety of biochemical effects, including the hastening of the decay of C3 convertase complexes, and the ability to serve as a cofactor for factor I–mediated cleavage of C3b and C4b. CR1 is particularly effective at aiding in the cleavage of C3bi to C3dg, a biologically inert form of C3.

Complement Receptor Type 2 (CR2)

CR2 is a 140-kd protein expressed on antigen presenting cells, especially dendritic cells, and on some B cells (33). CR2 can serve as a cofactor for factor I–mediated cleavage C3b; however, its main function may be related to generation of complement complexes on antigen presenting cells and the co-stimulation of B cells. Thus, perturbation of CR2 on B cells generates a signal that contributes to activation and proliferation of the cells (35,36). CR2 is a receptor for the Epstein-Barr virus, perhaps accounting in part for the lymphoproliferative effect of infection with that virus.

Factor I

The alternative pathway convertase is also regulated by factor I, a 90-kd plasma protein. Not a member of the RCA family, factor I cleaves C3b and C4b in the presence of a suitable cofactor such as factor H, C4 binding protein, membrane cofactor protein (CD46), or complement receptor type 1 (CR1) (Table 75-1).

Heparin and Heparan Sulfate

Heparin and heparan sulfate are acidic polysaccharides that may contribute to the regulation of complement at various points in the cascade. Heparin derives from the granules of mast cells and is used as an anticoagulant agent because of its ability to bind to and activate antithrombin III. Heparan sulfate is an extracellular molecule related structurally and biosynthetically to heparin, and it has less anticoagulant activity. In addition to enhancing the activity of C1 INH as discussed above, heparin and heparan sulfate can interfere with C3 convertases through various mechanisms (37,38). For example, heparan sulfate contributes to the net negative charge on cellular surfaces and thus to the functional activity of factor H. As another example, heparin and presumably heparan sulfate increase the functional activity of factor H and factor I. Heparin and heparan sulfate also bind to and activate antithrombin III, a serine protease inhibitor that in addition to inhibiting thrombin may provide potent regulation of complement at the level of C3.

Immunoglobulin

Among the molecules that regulate the function of complement at various levels of the cascade is immunoglobulin (Ig). While Ig is generally considered to initiate complement activation through the classical and/or alternative pathways as discussed in the chapter by Cooper, antibodies of IgG2 subclass may inhibit the initiation of complement by blocking the binding of complement fixing Ig (39). In addition to these properties, however, Ig also regulates complement through several mechanisms at the level of C3/C5 convertase. First, Ig can enhance alternative pathway activity by interacting with negatively charged moieties on the cell surface. Ig can interfere with the generation of C3 convertase complexes by serving as an alternative acceptor for C4b and C3b, thus diverting convertase complexes away from cell surfaces (40). For reasons yet uncertain, Ig does not inhibit formation of alternative pathway convertase complexes on bacterial surfaces (41).

THERAPEUTIC CONSIDERATIONS (FIG. 75-4)

Cobra Venom Factor (CVF)

One of the first complement inhibitory molecules discovered was a protein from the venom of cobra snakes (42). This protein, CVF, acts like C3b, forming a complex with factor B (CVFBb) to yield C3 and/or C5 convertase activity (Table 75-2) (43). The active complex induces the activation of complement in solution, leading to consumption of complement. The ability of CVF to consume complement reflects in part the stability of the CVFBb complex, which exceeds that of C3bBb and in part the resistance of CVFBb to regulation by factors H and I. CVF from the *Naja haje* cobra supports the cleavage mainly of C3 while CVF from the *Naja naja* cobra supports the cleavage of both C3 and C5. Cleavage of C5 in the latter case can give rise to formation of C5b67 complexes in solution, which in turn can mediate reactive lysis of erythrocytes into which these complexes insert.

CVF has been a standard for complement inhibition for the past 30 years. The early studies on CVF also established some of the models now commonly used for *in vivo* testing of complement inhibitors. One such model is hyperacute rejection of organ xenografts (44). The administration of CVF to xenograft recipients prevents this immediate form of tissue injury in guinea pig organs transplanted into rats (6) (Fig. 75-2) and in pig organs transplanted into nonhuman primates (45) (not shown).

If CVF is a standard complement inhibitor in the laboratory, several considerations would argue against the clinical use of CVF. First, while CVF can now be efficiently separated from phospholipases and other contaminating toxic substances, its administration is still potentially associated with toxic reactions owing to the generation of anaphylotoxins. Second, inhibition of alternative pathway C3 convertase activity deprives the individual of the most potent defense against extracellular pathogens. Third, the administration of CVF gives rise within a few days to a humoral immune response that includes the formation of neutralizing antibodies.

Soluble Complement Receptor Type 1 (sCR1)

Soluble CR1 is a recombinant form of CR1 that was engineered to eliminate the transmembrane and cytoplasmic domains (Table 75–2) (46). It is produced as a soluble, nonaggregating protein. Soluble CR1 functions as the membrane form of the protein is presumed to function in the inhibition of C3 convertases; however, in contrast to the membrane-bound form of this protein, sCR1 is free to act on complement complexes at any location. Administration of sCR1 to experimental animals leads to dose-dependent inhibition of C3b and C4b activity, promoting through cofactor activity the generation of C3d and C4d.

Soluble CR1 has been tested in a number of experimental models. The earliest studies found that administration of sCR1 to rats significantly reduced myocardial injury induced by coronary artery occlusion (46). Subsequent studies demonstrated significant efficacy in preventing hyperacute rejection of cardiac xenografts in rodents and nonhuman primates (47,48).

Soluble Complement Receptor Type 2 (sCR2)

Another pharmacologically active complement inhibitor deriving from the RCA family is sCR2. A recombinant, truncated form of the complement receptor type 2 (49), sCR2 presumably mediates cofactor activity similar to the membrane form of the molecule. In addition, sCR2 may compete with the membrane-associated receptor for recognition of C3d, and thus it may inhibit signaling by CR2, the C3d receptor. Since this signaling provides an important co-stimulus for activation of B cells, the administration of sCR2 has been found to have a potent inhibitory effect on elicited B-cell responses.

Other Regulators of Complement Activation (RCA) Constructs

The well-defined functional activity of various RCA protein domains has led to the development of several completely novel complement inhibitors. For example, Higgens et al. (50) developed a construct consisting of coding sequences for portions of MCP and DAF, which was called complement activation blocker-2 (CAB-2) (Table 75-2). The 110-kd soluble protein accelerates the dissociation of C3 and C5 convertases and mediates cofactor activity for factor I. The potential therapeutic activity of CAB-2 was approximately comparable to CVF in the Forssman model in guinea pigs. Injecting anti-Forssman serum causes guinea pigs to rapidly undergo pulmonary injury, shock, and death; pretreatment of guinea pigs with CAB-2 largely prevents the pulmonary changes. Another recombinant protein with functional domains of DAF and a terminal complement complex regulator, CD59, has been reported (51) and is described below.

Nonanticoagulant Heparin and Other Polyanions

Removal of anticoagulant heparin chains or chemical modification of heparin yields a polysaccharide that has anticomplement activity through the mechanisms discussed above, but little or no anticoagulant activity. The potential anticomplement effects of such chains have been studied extensively *in vitro* (37,52) and are summarized in Table 75-2. There is limited information regarding the anticomplement effects of polyanions in *in vivo* systems. Nonanticoagulant heparin was found to delay or prevent hyperacute rejection in a guinea pig-to-rat xenotransplant model (53); however, it is not unlikely that the polyanion acted in ways unrelated to the complement system.

FUT175 (6-Amino-2-Naphthyl-4-Guanidinobenzoate)

FUT175 is a protease inhibitor with anticoagulant and anticomplement activity. The compound inhibits C1r, C1s, and C3/C5 convertases (Table 75-2). The compound has been found to have a limited ability to inhibit hyperacute rejection of xenografts (54).

K76

Among the various products of microorganisms that can regulate the complement cascade is a protein derived from the fungus *Stachybotrys complementi*. This protein, called K76, is thought to bind and inhibit C5 and possibly C2 and C4 K76 by itself has relatively weak inhibitory activity in the severe, guinea pig-to-rat xenotransplant model and in the less severe hamster-to-rat xenograft model (55). However, there is evidence that the agent can be used to advantage in combination with FUT175 or perhaps other agents (56).

Intravenous Immunoglobulin

Although the inhibitory effects of Ig on C3 convertase activity described above are exerted at physiologic concentrations, most of the studies on the regulatory properties of Ig have been in pathologic models. For example, whereas the administration of anti-Forssman antibodies to guinea pigs leads to profound shock and death within minutes, the administration of these antibodies to animals given therapeutic concentration of Ig leads to only mild physiologic changes (40). Similarly, administration of gamma globulin to nonhuman primates prevents the hyperacute rejection of subsequently implanted pig kidneys (57). The potent effects of Ig on the complement cascade and the relative safety of administering large amounts of Ig may encourage use of gamma globulin as a therapeutic agent for humoral disease. Thus, in addition to the experimental models discussed above, gamma globulin is increasingly a standard therapy for the treatment of immune idiopathic thrombocytopenic purpura (58), although efficacy may be attributed to several mechanisms. Of importance is the ability of gamma globulin to promote host defense while preventing complement fixation on host cells. Thus, gamma globulin contains antibodies that target invasive organisms for complement-mediated injury, yet it also diverts C3 convertase activity away from autologous cells.

REGULATION AND CONTROL OF TERMINAL COMPLEMENT COMPLEXES

Clusterin and S Protein (Vitronectin)

The formation of terminal complement complexes and lytic activity of those complexes is regulated by several means. Clusterin, an 80-kd dimer also known as SP-40-40, and S protein, a 75-kd protein, bind to C5b67 complexes in solution and inhibit insertion of the complexes into cell membranes. The importance of these proteins in the regulation of the membrane attack complex in physiology has not been absolutely established, although clusterin has been observed in association with the membrane attack complex in glomerulonephritis and myocardial infarction, raising the possibility that expression of the molecule may occur in response to injury (10).

CD59

CD59, or membrane inhibitor of reactive lysis, provides constitutive protection against complement-mediated lysis (Table 75-1) (59). An 18-kd protein, CD59 is expressed on most nucleated cells, tethered by a phosphatidyl inositol (PI) anchor. CD59 binds to C8 or C9, preventing polymerization of C9 and formation of the membrane attack complex. The importance of CD59 in the homeostasis of normal tissues is suggested by the manifestation of paroxysmal nocturnal hemoglobinuria, an acquired failure to synthesized PI-linked proteins such as CD59 in cells of erythroid lineage. Patients with this disease have hemolytic anemia and consequent renal and

vascular disease (59). CD59 exhibits dramatic species specificity in some systems. For example, rabbit CD59 functions poorly against the human membrane attack complex (60). Thus, formation of the membrane attack complex in a xenograft can be inhibited by even low levels of expression of recipient CD59 as a transgene (61). Interestingly, inhibition of membrane attack complex formation by this approach does not prevent the main pathologic changes associated with hyperacute xenograft rejection. Thus, the development of hyperacute rejection (which definitively requires C5 and C6) may be brought about by C5b67 complexes (62). The species specificity of CD59 is not observed in all species combinations or on all cells (63,64), suggesting the function of CD59 may depend in part on cell membrane composition.

Because of the intrinsic ability of cells to adapt to the presence of terminal complement complexes, especially the membrane attack complex, the biologic efficacy of terminal complexes depends on both the number and the rate of complex formation. For example, the lytic effects of the membrane attack complex can be vitiated in part by slowing complex formation. To what extent regulation of terminal complexes relies on inhibition of complex formation versus slowing of complex formation is yet uncertain.

Therapeutic Considerations (Fig. 75-4)

If the major function of complement in host defense depends on the activation of C3 leading to opsonization of invasive microorganisms, and if the autoimmune properties of complement reflect in some cases the membrane attack complex, it may be possible to inhibit the complement cascade at the level of the terminal complement complexes without impairing the major contribution of complement to host defense. Consistent with this idea, individuals with deficiencies of terminal complex components do not exhibit a pronounced increase in susceptibility to most types of pyogenic infections. Accordingly, there is some impetus toward the design of therapeutics that would interfere with the terminal steps in the complement cascade.

Anti-C5 Antibodies

One promising approach toward the inhibition of terminal complex assembly is the administration of antibodies specific for C5 (Table 75-2). Anti-C5 antibodies have been shown to prevent cleavage of C5 and thus inhibit the generation of C5a and the membrane attack complex. For example, administration of monoclonal anti-C5 monoclonal antibodies to New Zealand black mice delays the onset of lupus-like renal disease. Addition of anti-C5 antibodies to human blood prevents injury to porcine organs perfused by that blood, recapitulating the circumstances that might occur in a pig-to-human xenograft

(65). To minimize the potential immune response that would be generated by administration of the murine antibody, Thomas et al. (66) engineered the constant regions and portions of the variable regions of the antibody to provide predominantly human in lieu of murine sequences.

REGULATION AND CONTROL OF ANAPHYLOTOXINS

The third step at which the complement system is regulated is at the level of anaphylotoxins. The anaphylotoxins are approximately 10-kd polypeptides generated by proteolytic cleavage of C3, C4, or C5 (C3a, C4a, C5a), as discussed in the chapter by Cooper. Binding of anaphylotoxins to specific receptors leads to activation and migration of phagocytic cells, activation of endothelial cells and smooth muscle cells, and degranulation of mast cells (22,67). The anaphylotoxins exhibit profound biologic activity at nanomolar concentrations, and therefore activity of the peptides must be strictly delimited. Human plasma contains a variety of proteases that may cleave and thus inactivate anaphylotoxins. Of greatest import may be carboxypeptidase-N, an exopeptidase synthesized in the liver and found in plasma and a few other tissues. Carboxypeptidase-N cleaves the terminal arginine residue of C3a and C5a, leading to the formation of C3a des arg, which is completely inactive, and C5a des arg, which retains some ability to activate leukocytes. As C5a des arg is not entirely devoid of biologic activity, other mechanisms must contribute to inactivation of these molecules. Owing to the action of proteases and perhaps by clearance through other means, the duration of activity of anaphylotoxins in plasma is very low, thus limiting the systemic effects of localized activation of complement.

Under some conditions, however, the local generation of anaphylotoxins can lead to profound systemic consequences. For example, during the course of hemodialysis, the contact of blood with dialysis membranes leads to generation of C5a, which in turn can cause bronchoconstriction, pulmonary failure, and hypotension (68). Similarly, the routing of blood through cardiopulmonary bypass apparatus may generate C3a and C5a, causing leukocyte sequestration in the lung following reperfusion (69). As another example, the rapid administration of CVF to rodents induces profound pulmonary failure owing to the activation of neutrophils in pulmonary blood vessels (70–72).

Therapeutic Considerations

Until recently, the therapeutic approach to anaphylotoxin-mediated pathophysiology has been relatively non-specific. For example, in the experimental model in which cobra venom factor is administered to rats, the pulmonary injury has been abrogated by administration of antibodies that block the adhesion of phagocytic cells to lung endothelium (25). Similarly, the systemic effects of anaphylotoxins have been inhibited by administration of agents that control C3/C5 convertases such as soluble CR1. Recently, however, some effort has been made to generate specific inhibitors of the anaphylotoxins. One approach has involved the administration of anti-C5a antibodies (73). Another useful approach may involve the development of soluble anaphylotoxin receptor antagonists.

TRANSGENIC ANIMALS FOR XENOTRANSPLANTATION

An archetypic manifestation of complement-mediated injury is the rejection of xenografts. The rejection of a xenograft occurs in part because of the activation of complement on foreign surfaces through the classical and/or alternative pathways and owing to incompatibility of complement regulatory proteins in the graft with the complement system of the recipient, as discussed above. One approach to the prevention of complement-mediated injury in the clinical setting would be to express human complement regulatory proteins in xenograft donors (21). This concept has been pursued by expressing human DAF, or the combination of human DAF and human CD59 in transgenic pigs (74,75). Organs from pigs expressing these human complement regulatory proteins do not undergo hyperacute rejection when transplanted into nonhuman primates (76,77). On the other hand, preliminary studies suggest that expression of human CD59 alone may not prevent hyperacute rejection (61). One important advantage to the inhibition of complement in this way is that complement control is restricted to the surface of cells in the xenotransplant, and the complement system of the recipient is spared to provide a defense against invasive organisms. The results of the studies using transgenic pigs are generally seen as a significant step toward the clinical application of xenotransplantation.

CONCLUSION

The complement system has long been appreciated to be the major system involved in defense against extracellular microorganisms in the blood and more recently as a potent system involved in the regulation of humoral and cellular immune responses. The complement system has also been seen to provide an important mechanism of tissue injury and disease. The principal challenge, then, in modulating the effects of complement is to preserve or enhance the ability of the complement system to protect the host against infection, while interfering with the ability of the complement system to attack normal cells. Until recently, most of the agents identified as complement inhibitors were naturally occurring products, and these products focused inhibition at the level of C3 with predictable consequences for the subject receiving the agents. Greater understanding of the relationship between the structure and the function of components of the complement system and the ability to deliver therapeutic agents to specific locations raises the possibility that a new series of active agents will emerge. To a certain extent this goal has already been achieved by the development of animals transgenic for human complement regulatory proteins for use as sources of xenografts, as described above. However, there is also progress in approaches that might be applied in human disease. For example, Fodor et al. (51) describe a chimeric protein with functional domains of DAF and CD59 that might be introduced through gene transfer.

ACKNOWLEDGMENT

Work in the author's laboratory is supported by the National Institutes of Health and by Nextran.

REFERENCES

1. Pillemer L, Blum L, Lepow IH, Ross OA, Todd EW, Wardlaw AC. The properdin system and immunity: demonstration and isolation of a new serum protein, properdin, and its role in immune phenomena. *Science* 1954;120:279–285.
2. Fearon DT, Austen KF. The alternative pathway of complement: a system for host resistance to microbial infection. *N Engl J Med* 1980;303:259–263.
3. Muller-Eberhard HJ. Complement: chemistry and pathways. In: Gallin JI, Goldstein IM, Snyderman R, eds. *Inflammation: basic principles and clinical correlates*, 2nd ed. New York: Raven Press, 1992:33–61.
4. Matsuo S, Ichida S, Takizawa H, et al. *In vivo* effects of monoclonal antibodies that functionally inhibit complement regulatory proteins in rats. *J Exp Med* 1994;180:1619–1627.
5. Nishikawa K, Matsuo S, Okada N, Morgan BP, Okada H. Local inflammation caused by a monoclonal antibody that blocks the function of the rat membrane inhibitor of C3 convertase. *J Immunol* 1996;156:1182–1188.
6. Miyagawa S, Hirose H, Shirakura R, et al. The mechanism of discordant xenograft rejection. *Transplantation* 1988;46:825–830.
7. Horstmann RD, Pangburn MK, Müller-Eberhard HJ. Species specificity of recognition by the alternative pathway of complement. *J Immunol* 1985;134:1101–1104.
8. Kalli KR, Hsu P, Fearon DT. Therapeutic uses of recombinant complement protein inhibitors. *Springer Semin Immunopathol* 1994;15:417–431.
9. Moore FD. Therapeutic regulation of the complement system in acute injury states. *Adv Immunol* 1994;56:267–299.
10. Liszewski MK, Farries TC, Lublin DM, Rooney IA, Atkinson JP. Control of the complement system. *Adv Immunol* 1996;61:201–283.
11. Morgan BP. Intervention in the complement system: a therapeutic strategy in inflammation. *Biochem Soc Transactions* 1995;24:224–229.
12. Shin ML, Carney DF. Cytotoxic action and other metabolic consequences of terminal complement proteins. *Progin Allergy* 1988;40:44–81.
13. Morgan BP. Complement membrane attack on nucleated cells: resistance, recovery and non-lethal effects. *Biochem J* 1989;264:1–14.
14. Forssman J. Die heterogenetischen antigene, besonders die sog: Forssman-antigene und ihre antikorper. In: Kolle W, Kraus R, Uhlenhuth B, eds. *Handbuch der pathogenen microorganismen*, 3rd ed. Berlin: Fisher und Urban & Schwarzenberg, 1930.
15. Nagai H, Kurimoto Y, Koda A. Immunopharmacological approach to Forssman shock. *Microbiol Immunol* 1980;24:649–655.
16. Klebanoff SJ. Oxygen metabolites from phagocytes. In: Gallin JI, Goldstein IM, Snyderman R, eds. *Inflammation: basic principles and clinical correlates*, 2nd ed. New York: Raven Press, 1992:541–588.
17. Maroko PR, Carpenter CB, Chiariello M, et al. Reduction by cobra venom factor of myocardial necrosis after coronary artery occlusion. *J Clin Invest* 1978;61:661–670.
18. Crawford MH, Grover FL, Kolb WP, et al. Complement and neutrophil activation in the pathogenesis of ischemic myocardial injury. *Circulation* 1988;78:1449–1458.
19. Platt JL. *Hyperacute xenograft rejection*. New York: Springer-Verlag, 1995.
20. Gewurz H, Clark DS, Cooper MD, Varco RL, Good RA. Effect of cobra venom-induced inhibition of complement activity on allograft and xenograft rejection reactions. *Transplantation* 1967;5:1296–1303.
21. Platt JL, Vercellotti GM, Dalmasso AP, et al. Transplantation of discordant xenografts: a review of progress. *Immunol Today* 1990;11:450–456.
22. Lundberg C, Marceau F, Hugli TE. C5a-induced hemodynamic and hematologic changes in the rabbit. Role of cyclooxygenase products and polymorphonuclear leukocytes. *Am J Pathol* 1987;128:471–483.
23. Hugli TE, Marçeau F, Lundberg C. Effects of complement fragments on pulmonary and vascular smooth muscle. *Am Rev Respir Dis* 1987;135:S9–S13.
24. Morganroth ML, Till GO, Kunkel RG, Ward PA. Complement and neutrophil-mediated injury of perfused rat lungs. *Lab Invest* 1986;54(5):507–513.
25. Till GO, Ward PA. Complement-induced lung injury. In: Said SI, ed. *The pulmonary circulation and acute lung injury*, 2nd ed. Mount Kisco, NY: Futura, 1991:381–401.
26. Caughman GB, Boackle RJ, Vesely J. A postulated mechanism for heparin's potentiation of C1 inhibitor function. *Mol Immunol* 1992;19:287–295.
27. Wuillemin WA, te Velthuis H, Lubbers YTP, de Ruig CP, Eldering E, Hack CE. Potentiation of C1 inhibitor by glycosaminoglycans. *J Immunol* 1997;159:1953–1960.
28. Atkinson JP, Oglesby TJ, White D, Adams EA, Liszewski MK. Separation of self from non-self in the complement system: a role for membrane cofactor protein and decay accelerating factor. *Clin Exp Immunol* 1991;86(suppl 1):27–30.
29. Hourcade D, Holers VM, Atkinson JP. The regulators of complement activation (RCA) gene cluster. *Adv Immunol* 1989;45:381–416.
30. Oglesby TJ, Allen CJ, Liszewski MK, White DJG, Atkinson JP. Membrane cofactor protein (CD46) protects cells from complement-mediated attack by an intrinsic mechanism. *J Exp Med* 1992;175:1547–1551.
31. Nicholson-Weller A, Burge J, Fearon DT, Weller PF, Austen KF. Isolation of a human erythrocyte membrane glycoprotein with decay-accelerating activity for C3 convertases of the complement system. *J Immunol* 1982;129:184–189.
32. Medof ME, Kinoshita T, Nussenzweig V. Inhibition of complement activation on the surface of cells after incorporation of decay-accelerating factor (DAF) into their membranes. *J Exp Med* 1984;160:1558–1578.
33. Ahearn JM, Fearon DT. Structure and function of the complement receptors, CR1 (CD35) and CR2 (CD21). *Adv Immunol* 1989;46:183–219.
34. Frank MM. Complement. In: Frank MM, Austen KF, Claman HN, Unanue ER, eds. *Samter's immunological diseases*, 5th ed. Boston: Little, Brown, 1995.
35. Wilson BS, Platt JL, Kay NE. Monoclonal antibodies to the 140,000 mol wt glycoprotein of B lymphocyte membranes (C3d receptor) initiates proliferation of B cells *in vitro*. *Blood* 1985;66:824–829.
36. Dempsey PW, Allison ME, Akkaraju S, Goodnow CC, Fearon DT. C3d of complement as a molecular adjuvant: bridging innate and acquired immunity. *Science* 1996;271:348–350.
37. Weiler JM, Yurt RW, Fearon DT, Austen KF. Modulation of the formation of the amplification convertase of complement, C3b, Bb, by native and commercial heparin. *J Exp Med* 1978;147:409–421.
38. Weiler JM, Linhardt RJ. Antithrombin III regulates complement activity *in vitro*. *J Immunol* 1991;146:3889–3894.
39. Yu PB, Holzknecht ZE, Bruno D, Parker W, Platt JL. Modulation of natural IgM binding and complement activation by natural IgG antibodies. *J Immunol* 1996;157:5163–5168.
40. Basta M, Kirshbom P, Frank MM, Fries LF. Mechanism of therapeutic effect on high-dose intravenous immunoglobulin: attenuation of acute, complement-dependent immune damage in a guinea pig model. *J Clin Invest* 1989;84:1974–1981.

41. Wagner E, Platt JL, Frank MM. High-dose intravenous immunoglobulin does not affect complement-bacteria interactions. *J Immunol* 1997; 160:1936–1943.

42. Flexner S, Noguchi H. Snake venom in relation to haemolysis, bacteriolysis, and toxicity. *J Exp Med* 1903;6:277–301.

43. Von Zabern I. Effects of venoms of different animal species on the complement system. In: Sim RB, ed. *Activators and inhibitors of complement.* Dordrecht: Kluwer Academic, 1993:127–135.

44. Nelson RA Jr. A new concept of immunosuppression in hypersensitivity reactions and in transplantation immunity. *Surv Ophthalmol* 1966; 11:498–505.

45. Leventhal JR, Dalmasso AP, Cromwell JW, et al. Prolongation of cardiac xenograft survival by depletion of complement. *Transplantation* 1993;55:857–866.

46. Weisman HF, Bartow T, Leppo MK, et al. Soluble human complement receptor type 1: *in vivo* inhibitor of complement suppressing postischemic myocardial inflammation and necrosis. *Science* 1990;249: 146–151.

47. Pruitt SK, Baldwin WM III, Marsh HC Jr, Lin SS, Yeh CG, Bollinger RR. The effect of soluble complement receptor type 1 on hyperacute xenograft rejection. *Transplantation* 1991;52:868–873.

48. Pruitt SK, Kirk AD, Bollinger RR, et al. The effect of soluble complement receptor type 1 on hyperacute rejection of porcine xenografts. *Transplantation* 1994;57:363–370.

49. Hebell T, Ahearn JM, Fearon DT. Suppression of the immune response by a soluble complement receptor of B lymphocytes. *Science* 1991;254: 102–105.

50. Higgins PJ, Ko J, Lobell R, Sardonini C, Alessi MK, Yeh CG. A soluble chimeric complement inhibitory protein that possesses both decay-accelerating and factor I cofactor activities. *J Immunol* 1997;158: 2872–2881.

51. Fodor WL, Rollins SA, Guilmette ER, Setter E, Squinto SP. A novel bifunctional chimeric complement inhibitor that regulated C3 convertase and formation of the membrane attack complex. *J Immunol* 1995; 155:4135–4138.

52. Weiler JM, Linhardt RJ. Comparison of the activity of polyanions and polycations on the classical and alternative pathways of complement. *Immunopharmacology* 1989;17:65–72.

53. Stevens RB, Wang YL, Kaji H, et al. Administration of nonanticoagulant heparin inhibits the loss of glycosaminoglycans from xenogeneic cardiac grafts and prolongs graft survival. *Transplant Proc* 1993;25:382.

54. Miyagawa S, Shirakura R, Matsumiya G, et al. Prolonging discordant xenograft survival with anticomplement reagents K76COOH and FUT175. *Transplantation* 1993;55:709–713.

55. Tanaka M, Murase N, Ye Q, et al. Effect of anticomplement agent K76 COOH on hamster-to-rat and guinea pig-to-rat heart xenotransplantation. *Transplantation* 1996;62:681–688.

56. Kaji H, Platt JL, Inoue K, Setoyama H, Imamura M. Effect of MX-1 and FOY on survival of discordant cardiac xenograft. *Transplant Proc* 1997;29:3024–3026.

57. Magee JC, Collins BH, Harland RC, et al. Immunoglobulin prevents complement mediated hyperacute rejection in swine-to-primate xenotransplantation. *J Clin Invest* 1995;96:2404–2412.

58. Frank MM, Milan B, Fries LF. The effects of intravenous immune globulin on complement-dependent immune damage of cells and tissues. *Clin Immunol Immunopathol* 1992;62:S82–S86.

59. Holguin MH, Wilcox LA, Belnshaw NJ, Rosse WF, Parker CJ. Relationship between the membrane inhibitor of reactive lysis and the erythrocyte phenotypes of paroxysmal nocturnal hemoglobinuria. *J Clin Invest* 1989;84:1387–1394.

60. Davies A, Simmons DL, Hale G, et al. CD59, an LY-6-like protein expressed in human lymphoid cells, regulates the action of the complement membrane attack complex on homologous cells. *J Exp Med* 1989; 170:637–654.

61. Diamond LE, McCurry KR, Oldham ER, et al. Characterization of transgenic pigs expressing functionally active human CD59 on cardiac endothelium. *Transplantation* 1996;61:1241–1249.

62. Saadi S, Platt JL. Transient perturbation of endothelial integrity induced by antibodies and complement. *J Exp Med* 1995;181:21–31.

63. Van den Berg CW, Morgan BP. Complement-inhibiting activities of human CD59 and analogues from rat, sheep, and pig are not homologously restricted. *J Immunol* 1994;152:4095–4101.

64. Miyagawa S, Shirakura R, Matsumiya G, et al. Test for ability of decay-accelerating factor (DAF, CD55) and CD59 to alleviate complement-mediated damage of xeno-erythrocytes. *Scand J Immunol* 1993;38: 37–44.

65. Kroshus TJ, Rollins SA, Dalmasso AP, et al. Complement inhibition with an anti-C5 monoclonal antibody prevents acute cardiac tissue injury in an *ex vivo* model of pig-to-human xenotransplantation. *Transplantation* 1995;60:1194–1202.

66. Thomas TC, Rollins SA, Rother RP, et al. Inhibition of complement activity by humanized anti-C5 antibody and single-chain Fv. *Mol Immunol* 1996;33:1389–1401.

67. Goldstein IM. Complement: biologically active products. In: Gallin JI, Goldstein IM, Snyderman R, eds. *Inflammation: basic principles and clinical correlates,* 2nd ed. New York: Raven Press, 1992:63–80.

68. Craddock PR, Fehr J, Dalmasso AP, Brigham KL, Jacob HS. Hemodialysis leukopenia. Pulmonary vascular leukostasis resulting from complement activation by dialyzer cellophane membranes. *J Clin Invest* 1977;59:879–888.

69. Chenoweth DE, Cooper SW, Hugli TE, Stewart RW, Blackstone EH, Kirklin JW. Complement activation during cardiopulmonary bypass: evidence for generation of C3a and C5a anaphylatoxins. *N Engl J Med* 1981;304:497–503.

70. Till GO, Johnson KJ, Kunkel R, Ward PA. Intravascular activation of complement and acute lung injury. *J Clin Invest* 1982;69:1126–1135.

71. Tvedten HW, Till GO, Ward PA. Mediators of lung injury in mice following systemic activation of complement. *Am J Pathol* 1985;119: 92–100.

72. Ward PA, Till GO, Hatherill JR, Annesley TM, Kunkel RG. Systemic complement activation, lung injury, and products of lipid peroxidation. *J Clin Invest* 1985;76:517–527.

73. Jacobsen N, Taaning E, Ladefoged J, Kristensen JK, Pedersen FK. Tolerance to an HLA-B, DR disparate kidney allograft after bone-marrow transplantation from same donor. *Lancet* 1994;343:800.

74. Cozzi E, White DJG. The generation of transgenic pigs as potential organ donors for humans. *Nature Med* 1995;1:964–966.

75. Kooyman DL, Byrne GW, McClellan S, et al. *In vivo* transfer of GPI-linked complement restriction factors from erythrocytes to the endothelium. *Science* 1995;269:89–92.

76. McCurry KR, Kooyman DL, Alvarado CG, et al. Human complement regulatory proteins protect swine-to-primate cardiac xenografts from humoral injury. *Nature Med* 1995;1:423–427.

77. Cozzi E, Yannoutsos N, Langford GA, Pino-Chavez G, Wallwork J, White DJG. Effect of transgenic expression of human decay-accelerating factor on the inhibition of hyperacute rejection of pig organs. In: Cooper DKC, Kemp E, Platt JL, White DJG, eds. *Xenotransplantation: the transplantation of organs and tissues between species,* 2nd ed. Berlin: Springer, 1997:665–682.

78. Brauer RB, Baldwin WM III, Daha MR, Pruitt SK, Sanfilippo F. Use of C6-deficient rats to evaluate the mechanism of hyperacute rejection of discordant cardiac xenografts. *J Immunol* 1993;151:7240–7248.

Inflammation: Basic Principles and Clinical Correlates,
3rd ed., edited by John I. Gallin and Ralph Snyderman.
Lippincott Williams & Wilkins, Philadelphia © 1999.

CHAPTER 76

Cytokine Inhibitors: Biologics

Marc Feldmann

Subsequent to the characterization of the cytokines, cytokine inhibitors were discovered. We are now aware that there is a wide spectrum of endogenous cytokine inhibitors that are of importance in the partial homeostasis that occurs in chronic inflammatory diseases such as rheumatoid arthritis (RA). Among the most important of these cytokine inhibitors are soluble tumor necrosis factor (TNF) receptors (sTNF-R) and the interleukin-1 receptor antagonist (IL-1ra). Cytokines can also be important cytokine inhibitors, and in diseases such as RA, IL-10 appears to be an important immunoregulatory cytokine.

Cytokine inhibitory biologics have been used in clinical trials as therapeutic agents since 1992, and have had clinical success. The blockade of TNFα by antibodies to TNFα or by TNF receptor IgG-Fc fusion proteins has been very effective in reducing disease activity in RA and Crohn's disease. These results and others have demonstrated that biologic agents can be useful therapeutic agents, even in chronic diseases, and suggest that biologics will be a part of the therapeutic armamentarium in the future.

ENDOGENOUS CYTOKINE INHIBITORS

Two classes are known: soluble cytokine receptors, and the IL-1 receptor antagonist.

Soluble Cytokine Receptors

The larger class of cytokine inhibitors is soluble cytokine receptors, comprising the extracellular cytokine binding domain of the receptor. These entities have been described for essentially all single transmembrane

M. Feldmann: Kennedy Institute of Rheumatology, London W6 8LH, England.

cytokine receptors, e.g., for IL-2, IL-4, TNFα, interferon-γ (IFN-γ), IL-6 (1). The seven spanning (serpentine) receptors for chemokines do not generate soluble receptors.

Two mechanisms have been described for the generation of soluble receptors. Alternative splicing of the cytokine receptor gene has been described in a minority of instances, e.g., for IL-4 (2). In the majority of cases the soluble receptor is formed by proteolytic cleavage of the membrane full-length receptor by enzymes. These enzymes are inhibitable by nonselective matrix metalloproteinase (MMP) inhibitors (3), and so a membrane-bound MMP enzyme is involved in the process of receptor shedding. Whether the MMP inhibitable enzymes actually cleave the cytokine receptors or are part of an enzyme cascade activating the actual cleavage enzyme is not known. The recent cloning of an enzyme capable of cleaving membrane TNF, a member of the "ADAMS" (A Disintegrin and metalloproteinase) family, and a disintegrin metalloproteinase, has suggested that the MMP activity directly cleaves membrane TNF, and that related enzymes may be responsible for cleaving the membrane cytokine receptors (4,5).

The function of soluble cytokine receptors is not entirely clear. We and others have focused on their inhibitory effects (6,7). It is possible that the major inhibitory effect of cytokine receptor cleavage is reducing receptor expression by decapitation, and possibly also by having excess cytoplasmic domains competing for intracytoplasmic signaling molecules.

A number of soluble receptors, such as that for TNFα, which has four cysteine-rich domains, retain their ligand-binding activity, and the soluble receptor for TNF has been reported to be an endogenous inhibitor. Its production reflects disease activity in RA and other diseases (6,8). While most studies *in vitro* or *in vivo* document an inhibitory effect on TNF, there is a report that soluble TNF-R may also be able to protect TNF and stabilize it

(9). This has been shown *in vitro* only, and there is no evidence that the protective effect operates *in vivo*. Another TNF inhibitory mechanism proposed for soluble TNF receptors is by augmenting clearance of the cytokine-soluble receptor complex, via the kidney (10). There is evidence *in vitro* and *in vivo* that the production of soluble TNF-R is regulated by inflammatory mediators, including TNF.

However, not all cytokine receptors have inhibitory capacity. IL-6 binds to a membrane receptor with a small cytoplasmic domain, and the signaling function involves another receptor protein gp130, now termed CD130. Soluble IL-6R has been shown to be able to replace full-length IL-6R, and thus it acts as a co-agonist (11). The co-agonist function of soluble IL-6R can be demonstrated *in vivo* also, in transgenic mice overexpressing soluble IL-6R (12). The lack of inhibitory capacity of soluble IL-6R is consistent with the capacity of IL-6 to act hormonally at a distance, for example to induce acute-phase protein production from the liver (13).

A particularly important endogenous cytokine inhibitor is the type II IL-1 receptor. This does not signal (14), since it has a very short cytoplasmic domain and, either on the cell surface or in biologic fluids, acts as a decoy, limiting access of IL-1 to the signaling type I IL-1 receptor (15).

Cytokine Receptor Antagonist

There is only one cytokine receptor antagonist described so far, the IL-1 receptor antagonist (IL-1ra). This was first described as a secretory molecule released from macrophages (16), but more recently two cytoplasmic splice forms were described (17). The function of the secreted form is clear, if present at 30- to 100-fold molar excess; it is to prevent IL-1α or IL-1 from being able to bind effectively to IL-1R type I and induce signaling (16). In inflammatory states, soluble IL-1ra levels in biologic fluids, such as serum and synovial fluid (18), are augmented. The appreciable blood levels suggest that it is an effective inhibitor *in vivo* (18). The function of the intracytoplasmic IL-1ra is not clear, but it may be released on cell lysis.

Inhibitory Cytokines

While the functions of most cytokines are very complex and none is purely pro- or antiinflammatory (19), there is a cluster of chiefly antiinflammatory cytokines, such as IL-10, IL-4, and transforming growth factor-β (TGF-β). Like the proinflammatory cytokines, these are upregulated in inflammatory diseases, and there is evidence, for example in rheumatoid joint cell cultures, that the amounts of these cytokines produced (e.g., of IL-10) are acting as endogenous regulators (20). Neutralizing antibodies to IL-10 lead to augmented levels of

TABLE 76-1. *Cytokine inhibitors*

Inhibitor type	Examples
Endogenous	
Soluble cytokine receptors	Tumor necrosis factor receptor (TNF-R), IL-1 receptor (IL-1R) type II
Cytokine receptor antagonist	IL-1 receptor antagonist (IL-1Ra)
Inhibitory cytokines	IL-4, IL-10, IL-11, IL-13, IL-6, transforming growth factor-α (TGF-α)
Exogenous	
Antibodies	Anti-TNFα
Fusion proteins	p55 TNF-R IgG1Fc p75 TNF-R IgG1Fc

IL, interleukin; IgG1Fc, crystallizable fragment of immunoglobulin G1.

TNFα and IL-1 (20), and in animal models anti–IL-10 can exacerbate disease (21). In IL-10 knockout mice, there is inflammatory bowel disease, which is dependent on the presence of the gut flora (22), and there is a greatly augmented skin response to both irritants or antigens (23).

Table 76-1 summarizes the more common cytokine inhibitory biologics. Chronic diseases such as RA involve an equilibrium, tilted toward the proinflammatory side of both pro- and antiinflammatory mediators (Fig. 76-1).

Natural Antibodies to Cytokines

Antibodies to IL-1α and IL-6 have been found in the sera of normal individuals (24). The function of these antibodies appears to be inhibitory, and some of the effects of high-dose immunoglobulin G (IgG) used in therapy has been attributed to these antibodies (25). The levels of natural antibodies detected differ greatly between individuals. While antibodies to other cytokines have been detected, these appear to react only with the denatured plastic bound form and not to soluble cytokines, and so are unlikely to be of physiologic relevance.

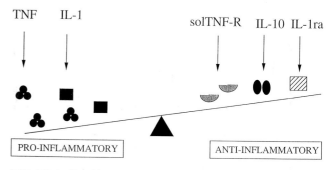

FIG. 76-1. Cytokine disequilibrium. (Reprinted, with permission, from Feldmann et al., *Cell* 1996;85:307–310.)

EXOGENOUS CYTOKINE INHIBITORS: THERAPEUTICS

Anticytokine Antibodies

Anti TNFα

Antibodies to TNFα were initially developed by a number of companies for use in sepsis, but the results for this indication have been negative (26–28). The beneficial use of anti–TNFα in RA and Crohn's disease has been much easier to demonstrate than clinical benefit in sepsis.

The rationale for the use of anti–TNFα in RA was multifactorial. In RA joint cell cultures of all the cells present, anti–TNFα antibody was found to diminish the production of other proinflammatory cytokines in these cultures, for example IL-1 (29), granulocyte-macrophage colony-stimulating factor (GM-CSF) (30), and IL-8 (31). Also, immunohistologic, *in situ,* and other studies showed that TNFα production is upregulated in synovium, as is TNF receptor expression (32). The beneficial effects of monoclonal anti–TNFα antibody in animal models of arthritis such as collagen induced arthritis verified this concept *in vivo* (33,34).

Based on the above rationale, anti–TNFα antibody (cA2, from Centocor Inc., Malvern, PA) was first infused into long-standing RA patients who were doing poorly on existing therapy. Twenty mg/kg (the effective animal model dose) was given in two or four divided doses over

2 weeks. The results showed a rapid onset of benefit in all parameters of the disease process, including tender and swollen joint counts, pain, morning stiffness, the serum markers of inflammation, C reactive protein (CRP), and the erythrocyte sedimentation rate (ESR). The duration of clinical benefit ranged from 8 to 26 weeks in 20 patients, but all eventually relapsed in this first open study (35). Most patients improved by over 50% by the Paulus criteria (36).

To determine whether this inflammatory disease remained TNFα–dependent after treatment with anti–TNFα and subsequent relapse, retreatment studies were performed in some patients. In a total of 28 relapses, among seven patients, all were treatable with anti–TNFα, demonstrating that the cytokine network in RA remains TNFα–dependent, and that other proinflammatory cytokines do not take over and replace its function (37).

The formal proof of efficacy for a therapeutic is a randomized, placebo-controlled, double-blind clinical trial, and this has been accomplished for anti–TNFα antibody, using human albumin as the placebo, and doses of 1 and 10 mg/kg of cA2. In this trial, 48% and 79% of the patients responded using the 20% Paulus criteria (36) to the low and high dose of cA2 anti–TNFα antibody, respectively, compared to an 8% response in the placebo group (38) (Fig. 76-2).

Other anti-TNF biologics have subsequently been successfully used. CDP571, a humanized antibody produced

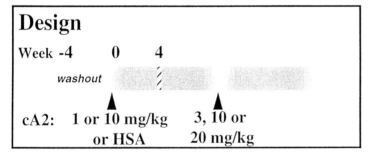

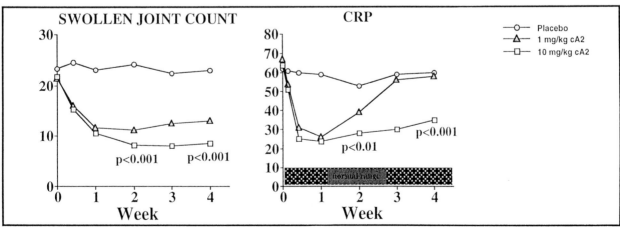

FIG. 76-2. Randomized, placebo-controlled trial of cA2 in rheumatoid arthritis. (From ref. 38.)

by Celltech, Slough, UK, was efficacious in a randomized trial, but needed higher doses than cA2 for a comparable clinical effect (39). A dimeric p75 TNF-R-IgG1Fc fusion protein developed by Immunex, Seattle, WA, has been used in RA patients (40). This material is injected subcutaneously twice weekly, and has been very effective (15). Dimeric p55 TNF-R-IgG1Fc fusion protein has been developed by Roche, Basel, Switzerland, and used in a wide variety of regimes, some of which have been efficacious (15).

Based on the success of the open trial of cA2 (35), and the likely similarities in pathogenesis, anti–TNFα antibody was also successfully used in Crohn's disease. There were excellent results using cA2 and CDP571 in placebo-controlled randomized trials in patients doing poorly on existing treatment, even with corticosteroids (41). Most notably, there has been significant healing of fistulas in Crohn's disease using cA2. The results of anti–TNFα therapy in other diseases is eagerly awaited. A comprehensive review of anti–TNFα therapy has recently been published (42).

For antibodies to be a realistic therapy, regular treatment in the long term needs to be possible, without allowing the patients to relapse and flare. A longer term (6-month) multiple-dose treatment clinical trial of anti–TNFα (cA2) has been successfully completed (43), and this was shown to be effective over this time frame. Currently a 1-year multiple treatment phase III trial has been initiated.

Interleukin-1 Receptor Antagonist (IL-1ra)

IL-1ra was also first used clinically in sepsis, and the results were initially encouraging in open studies (44). However, they were not reproducible in larger controlled studies, and these trials have been abandoned (45). Currently, IL-1ra is in clinical trials in RA, and the results indicate some but not marked effects on the inflammatory signs and symptoms (46). However, in relatively early RA patients there was evidence of joint protection on x-ray (P <.04). Further results are eagerly awaited. Probably because of the presence of two isoforms of IL-1 (α and β), there are no reports of the use of anti–IL-1 antibodies in the clinic.

Anti–Interleukin-6

Murine antibody to IL-6 has been injected into a small cohort of five RA patients. A moderate degree of benefit was noted, which lasted up to 4 weeks (47). The brief duration was probably related to the shorter half-life and greater immunogenicity of murine antibodies, compared to the chimeric or humanized antibodies that have been used for anti–TNFα therapy. The reason why anti–IL-6 is beneficial is not entirely clear, as IL-6 itself may be antiinflammatory, reducing *in vitro* the lipopolysaccharide (LPS)-induced production of TNF and IL-6 from monocytes/macrophages (48).

Interleukin-10

The endogenous immune suppressor, interleukin-10 (IL-10), inhibits both T-cell and macrophage functions, such as the production of IFN-γ, IL-1, TNFα, IL-6, and IL-12 (49). *In vitro* studies showed that despite its presence in RA synovial cultures, additional IL-10 was antiinflammatory and thus may be a useful therapeutic agent for a variety of T-cell–dependent inflammatory diseases. This concept was supported by animal model studies in which IL-10 injection ameliorates collagen-induced arthritis (50). Phase I trials of IL-10 in both diseases have been successfully completed (Maini et al., in preparation, Van Deventer et al., submitted).

Interleukin-11

While the platelet-restoring function of IL-11 has been well documented, its antiinflammatory effect is not as known (51). Based on its reduction of TNFα and IL-1 production *in vitro,* and beneficial effects in animal models such as the B27 transgenic rat, IL-11 is being investigated in Crohn's disease, and has successfully completed phase I clinical trials.

What Can We Learn from the Use of Biologics as Therapeutics?

The safety of biologic agents is one of their major features. Unlike low molecular mass organic chemical drugs, they do not enter cells, and so cannot interact with the body's entire range of approximately 100,000 expressed genes. Thus, conventional high-dose toxicity tests of biologics reveal less toxicity than conventional drugs. However, some cytokines may cause lethal shock (e.g., TNFα and IL-12). Biologic agents need to be repeatedly injected, but, depending on efficacy, this may be tolerable to patients. The problems of using biologics are likely to be mechanism related, such as the induction of IgM double-stranded DNA antibodies in 6% of patients treated with either anti–TNFα antibodies (52) or TNF-R fusion proteins. The mechanism of this effect is unclear, but a plausible hypothesis would be interference with TNF-induced apoptosis.

The concept of TNFα–dependent proinflammatory cytokine cascade, which was a major part of the rationale for anti–TNFα therapy (53), was confirmed *in vivo* (35,52). For example, the elevated IL-6 levels detected in RA patients' serum fell within 24 hours to less than 50% of their pretreatment levels. This is a more rapid effect than noted *in vitro* in RA joint cell cultures, and is probably explicable by cytokine excretion *in vivo*. The concept of cytokine cascade is summarized in Fig. 76-3.

Analysis of the duration of clinical response to anti–TNF-α revealed that the clinical response as judged by the composite criteria of Paulus (36) or the more recent American College of Rheumatology (ACR) criteria out-

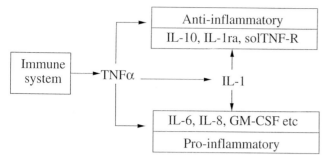

FIG. 76-3. Cytokine cascade in rheumatoid arthritis. (Reprinted, with permission, from Feldmann et al., *Cell* 1996; 85:307–310.)

lasted neutralizing levels of cA2 (approximately 1 µg/ml) in the blood. The reasons for this were investigated, and it appears likely that trafficking of leukocytes to joints is reduced by cA2 therapy. While much of the published evidence is still circumstantial, e.g., reduced expression of E selectin and intracellular adhesion molecule-1 (ICAM-1) in joints (54), as well as the soluble forms of these molecules assayed by enzyme-linked immunosorbent assay (ELISA) (55) in serum, augmented lymphocyte counts within 24 hours after infusion, and reduced serum levels of some chemokines. To prove effects on leukocyte trafficking, there is currently an open trial of infusing labeled white blood cells (WBCs) into RA patients before and after cA2 therapy, which documents the reduced trafficking into joints after cA2 (Taylor et al., unpublished data).

The rheumatoid synovium is infiltrated by a large mass of leukocytes, chiefly T lymphocytes and macrophages. Due to the volume of cells, neovascularization is necessary to sustain this mass, and this led us to investigate angiogenic factors. It was found that vascular endothelial cell growth factor (VEGF) levels in RA patients, initially elevated in active RA patients, were reduced after TNFα therapy. Thus, the inflammatory process influences VEGF production and thus probably also regulates the angiogenic process (56,57).

REFERENCES

1. Fernandez-Botran R. Soluble cytokine receptors: their role in immunoregulation. *FASEB J* 1991;5:2567–2574.
2. Mosley B, Beckmann MP, March CJ, et al. The murine interleukin-4 receptor: molecular cloning and characterization of secreted and membrane bound forms. *Cell* 1989;59:335–348.
3. Williams L, Gibbons DL, Gearing A, Feldmann M, Brennan FM. Paradoxical effects of a synthetic metalloproteinase inhibitor which blocks both p55 and p75 TNF receptor shedding and TNF-α processing. *J Clin Invest* 1996;97:2833–2841.
4. Black RA, Rauch CT, Kozlosky CJ, et al. A metalloproteinase disintegrin that releases tumour-necrosis factor α from cells. *Nature* 1997; 385:729–732.
5. Moss ML, Jin S-L, Milla ME, et al. Cloning of a disintegrin metalloproteinase that processes precursor tumour-necrosis factor α. *Nature* 1997;385:733–736.
6. Cope AP, Aderka D, Doherty M, et al. Increased levels of soluble tumor necrosis factor receptors in the sera and synovial fluid of patients with rheumatic diseases. *Arthritis Rheum* 1992;35:1160–1169.
7. Seckinger P, Isaaz S, Dayer JM. A human inhibitor of tumor necrosis factor α. *J Exp Med* 1988;167:1511–1516.
8. Aderka D, Wysenbeek A, Engelmann H, et al. Correlation between serum levels of soluble tumour necrosis factor receptor and disease activity in systemic lupus erythematosus. *Arthritis Rheum* 1993;36: 1111–1120.
9. Aderka D, Engelmann H, Maor Y, Brakebusch C, Wallach D. Stabilization of the bioactivity of tumour necrosis factor by its soluble receptors. *J Exp Med* 1992;175:323–329.
10. Bemelmans MHA, Gouma DJ, Buurman WA. Influence of nephrectomy on TNF receptor clearance in a murine model. *J Immunol* 1993; 150:2007–2017.
11. Tamura T, Udagawa U, Takahashi N, et al. Soluble interleukin-6 receptor triggers osteoclast formation by interleukin 6. *Proc Natl Acad Sci USA* 1993;90:11924–11928.
12. Peters M, Schirmacher P, Goldschmitt J, et al. Extramedullary expansion of hematopoietic progenitor cells in interleukin-6-sIL-6R double transgenic mice. *J Exp Med* 1997;185:755–766.
13. Steel DM, Whitehead AS. The major acute phase reactants: C-reactive protein, serum amyloid P component and serum amyloid A protein. *Immunol Today* 1994;15:81–88.
14. Dinarello CA. Biologic basis for interleukin-1 in disease. *Blood* 1996; 87:2095–2147.
15. Colotta F, Dower SK, Sims JE, Mantovani A. The type II "decoy" receptor: a novel regulatory pathway for interleukin-1. *Immunol Today* 1994;15:562.
16. Arend WP. Interleukin-1 receptor antagonist. *Adv Immunol* 1993;54: 167–227.
17. Haskill S, Martin G, Van Le L, et al. cDNA cloning of an intracellular form of the human interleukin 1 receptor antagonist associated with epithelium. *Proc Natl Acad Sci USA* 1991;88:3681–3685.
18. Firestein GS, Boyle DL, Yu C, et al. Synovial interleukin-1 receptor antagonist and interleukin-1 balance in rheumatoid arthritis. *Arthritis Rheum* 1994;37:644–652.
19. Wahl SM. Transforming growth factor β: the good, the bad, and the ugly. *J Exp Med* 1994;180:1587–1590.
20. Katsikis P, Chu CQ, Brennan FM, Maini RN, Feldmann M. Immunoregulatory role of interleukin 10 (IL-10) in rheumatoid arthritis. *J Exp Med* 1994;179:1517–1527.
21. Kasama T, Strieter RM, Lukacs NW, Lincoln PM, Burdick MD, Kunkel SL. Interleukin-10 expression and chemokine regulation during the evolution of murine type II collagen-induced arthritis. *J Clin Invest* 1995;95:2868–2876.
22. Kuhn R, Lohler J, Rennick D, Rajewsky K, Muller W. Interleukin-10–deficient mice develop chronic enterocolitis. *Cell* 1993;75:263–274.
23. Berg DJ, Leach MW, Kuhn R, et al. Interleukin 10 but not interleukin 4 is a natural suppressant of cutaneous inflammatory responses. *J Exp Med* 1995;182:99–108.
24. Bendtzen K, Svenson M, Jonsson V, Hippe E. Autoantibodies to cytokines—friends or foes? *Immunol Today* 1990;11:167–169.
25. Abe Y, Horiuchi A, Miyake M, Kimura S. Anti-cytokine nature of natural human immunoglobulin: one possible mechanism of the clinical effect of intravenous immunoglobulin therapy. *Immunol Rev* 1994;139: 5–19.
26. Wherry JC, Pennington JE, Wenzel RP. Tumor necrosis factor and the therapeutic potential of anti-tumor necrosis factor antibodies. *Crit Care Med* 1993;21:S436–S440.
27. Fisher CJ, Agosti JM, Opal SM, et al. Treatment of septic shock with the tumor necrosis factor receptor: Fc fusion protein. The soluble TNF receptor sepsis study group. *N Engl J Med* 1996;334:1697–1702.
28. Agosti JM, Fisher CJ, Opal SM, Lowry SF, Balk RA, Sadoff JC. Treatment of patients with sepsis syndrome with soluble TNF receptor (sTNFR). In: American Society for Microbiology, Washington DC, *Proceedings of the 34th Annual Interscience Conference on Antimicrobial Agents and Chemotherapy (ICAAC),* vol 34. 1994:65.
29. Brennan FM, Chantry D, Jackson A, Maini R, Feldmann M. Inhibitory effect of TNF-α antibodies on synovial cell interleukin-1 production in rheumatoid arthritis. *Lancet* 1989;2:244–247.
30. Haworth C, Brennan FM, Chantry D, Turner M, Maini RN, Feldmann M. Expression of granulocyte-macrophage colony-stimulating factor in rheumatoid arthritis: regulation by tumor necrosis factor-α. *Eur J Immunol* 1991;21:2575–2579.
31. Butler DM, Maini RN, Feldmann M, Brennan FM. Modulation of proinflammatory cytokine release in rheumatoid synovial membrane cell

cultures. Comparison of monoclonal anti-TNF-α antibody with the IL-1 receptor antagonist. *Eur Cytokine Network* 1995;6:225–230.

32. Chu CQ, Field M, Feldmann M, Maini RN. Localization of tumor necrosis factor α in synovial tissues and at the cartilage-pannus junction in patients with rheumatoid arthritis. *Arthritis Rheum* 1991;34:1125–1132.

33. Thorbecke GJ, Shah R, Leu CH, Kuruvilla AP, Hardison AM, Palladino MA. Involvement of endogenous tumour necrosis factor α and transforming growth factor β during induction of collagen type II arthritis in mice. *Proc Natl Acad Sci USA* 1992;89:7375–7379.

34. Williams RO, Feldmann M, Maini RN. Anti-TNF ameliorates joint disease in murine collagen-induced arthritis. *Proc Natl Acad Sci USA* 1992;89:9784–9788.

35. Elliott MJ, Maini RN, Feldmann M, et al. Treatment of rheumatoid arthritis with chimeric monoclonal antibodies to TNF-α. *Arthritis Rheum* 1993;36:1681–1690.

36. Paulus HE, Egger MJ, Ward JR, Williams HJ, and the Group CSSoRD. Analysis of improvement in individual rheumatoid arthritis patients treated with disease-modifying anti-rheumatic drugs, based on the findings in patients treated with placebo. *Arthritis Rheum* 1990;33:477–484.

37. Elliott MJ, Maini RN, Feldmann M, et al. Repeated therapy with monoclonal antibody to tumour necrosis factor α (cA2) in patients with rheumatoid arthritis. *Lancet* 1994;344:1125–1127.

38. Elliott MJ, Maini RN, Feldmann M, et al. Randomised double blind comparison of a chimaeric monoclonal antibody to tumour necrosis factor α (cA2) versus placebo in rheumatoid arthritis. *Lancet* 1994;344:1105–1110.

39. Rankin ECC, Choy EHS, Kassimos D, et al. The therapeutic effects of an engineered human anti-tumour necrosis factor alpha antibody (CD571) in rheumatoid arthritis. *Br J Rheumatol* 1995;34:334–342.

40. Baumgartner S, Moreland LW, Schiff MW, et al. Double-blind placebo-controlled trend of tumor necrosis factor receptor (p80) fusion protein (TNF-R:Fc) in active rheumatoid arthritis. *Arthritis Rheum* 1996;39:S74(abst).

41. Van Dullemen HM, Van Deventer SJH, Hommes DW, et al. Treatment of Crohn's disease with anti-tumor necrosis factor chimeric monoclonal antibody (cA2). *Gastroenterology* 1995;109:129–135.

42. Feldmann M, Elliott MJ, Woody JN, Maini RN. Anti tumour necrosis factor α therapy of rheumatoid arthritis. *Adv Immunol* 1997;64:283–350.

43. Maini RN, Breedveld FC, Kalden JR, et al. Therapeutic efficacy of multiple intravenous infusions of anti-TNFα monoclonal antibody combined with low-dose weekly methotrexate in rheumatoid arthritis. *Arthritis and Rheumatism* 1998;41:1552–1563.

44. Fisher CJJ, Slotman GJ, Opal SM, et al. Initial evaluation of human recombinant interleukin-1 receptor antagonist in the treatment of sepsis syndrome: a randomized, open-label, placebo-controlled multicenter trial. *Crit Care Med* 1994;22:12–21.

45. Pribble J, Fisher C, Opal S. Human recombinant interleukin-1 receptor antagonist (IL-1ra) increases survival time in patients with sepsis syndrome and end organ dysfunction. *Crit Care Med* 1994;22:A192(abst).

46. Bresnihan B, Lookabaugh J, Witt K, Musikic P. Treatment with recombinant human interleukin-1 receptor antagonist (rhuIL-1ra) in rheumatoid arthritis: results of a randomized double-blind, placebo-controlled multicenter. *Arthritis Rheum* 1996;39(suppl 9):S73.

47. Wijdenes J, Racadot E, Wendling D. Interleukin 6 antibodies in rheumatoid arthritis. *J Interferon Res* 1994;14:297–298.

48. Aderka D, Le J, Vilcek J. IL-6 inhibits lipopolysaccharide-induced tumor necrosis factor production in cultured human monocytes, U937 cells, and in mice. *J Immunol* 1989;143:3517–3523.

49. Moore KW, O'Garra A, de Waal Malefyt R, Vieira P, Mosmann TR. Interleukin-10. *Annu Rev Immunol* 1993;11:165–190.

50. Walmsley M, Katsikis PD, Abney E, et al. Interleukin-10 inhibition of the progression of established collagen-induced arthritis. *Arthritis Rheum* 1996;39:495–503.

51. Trepicchio WL, Bozza M, Pedneault G, Dorner AJ. Recombinant human interleukin-11 attenuates the inflammatory response through down-regulation of proinflammatory cytokine release and nitric oxide production. *J Immunol* 1996;157:3627–3634.

52. Maini RN, Elliott MJ, Charles PJ, Feldmann M. Immunological intervention reveals reciprocal roles for TNF-α and IL-10 in rheumatoid arthritis and SLE. *Springer Semin Immunopathol* 1994;16:327–336.

53. Feldmann M, Brennan FM, Maini RN. Role of cytokines in rheumatoid arthritis. *Annu Rev Immunol* 1996;14:397–440.

54. Tak PP, Taylor PC, Breedveld FC, et al. Decrease in cellularity and expression of adhesion molecules by anti-tumor necrosis factor α monoclonal antibody treatment in patients with rheumatoid arthritis. *Arthritis Rheum* 1996;39:1077–1081.

55. Paleolog EM, Hunt M, Elliott MJ, Feldmann M, Maini RN, Woody JN. Deactivation of vascular endothelium by monoclonal anti-tumor necrosis factor α antibody in rheumatoid arthritis. *Arthritis Rheum* 1996;39:1082–1091.

56. Paleolog EM, Young S, Stark AC, McCloskey RV, Feldmann M, Maini RN. Modulation of angiogenic vascular endothelial growth (VEGF) factor by TNFα and IL-1 in rheumatoid arthritis. *Arthritis and Rheumatism* 1998;41:1258–1265.

57. Williams RO, Mason LJ, Feldmann M, Maini RN. Synergy between anti-CD4 and anti-TNF in the amelioration of established collagen-induced arthritis. *Proc Natl Acad Sci USA* 1994;91:2762–2766.

Inflammation: Basic Principles and Clinical Correlates,
3rd ed., edited by John I. Gallin and Ralph Snyderman.
Lippincott Williams & Wilkins, Philadelphia © 1999.

CHAPTER **77**

Emerging Technologies for the Discovery of Small-Molecule Therapeutics

Ian A. MacNeil and Mark J. Zoller

Many of the molecular interactions that follow engagement of an extracellular receptor during an inflammatory response are now at least partially understood. Many of the proteins involved in these cellular signaling pathways have been identified, the genes encoding them have been cloned and sequenced, and the molecular details of their functions have been determined by x-ray crystallography and nuclear magnetic resonance studies (1–3). The result is a complex picture in which the type and magnitude of an inflammatory response is determined by multiple signaling pathways that converge and modulate the response. The mechanisms by which current antiinflammatory and immunosuppressive drugs function and the nature of their limitations are now beginning to be understood. Because many immunosuppressive drugs increase the susceptibility to viral and other infections, patients with diseases such as rheumatoid arthritis and those receiving organ transplants, who are treated with immunosuppressive agents for years, are at a high risk for debilitating infections. The toxic effects of these drugs and their metabolites can cause nephrotoxicity, liver damage, pneumonitis, bone marrow suppression, and an increase in the risk of malignancy (4–8). The primary reason for the associated toxicity is that many of the drugs are nonselective. Therefore, there is a need for new immunosuppressive drugs that are selectively potent on specific cell types and that are free of serious side effects. Targeting proteins that mediate intracellular signaling pathways represents a unique opportunity to achieve this selectivity (9).

This chapter focuses on the proteins that make up major signaling pathways in the hematopoietic cells responsible for initiating and maintaining an inflammatory response, particularly those signaling proteins that

I. A. MacNeil and M. J. Zoller: ARIAD Pharmaceuticals, Cambridge, Massachusetts 02139.

are part of drug discovery programs in pharmaceutical companies. Where possible, references to human patient data and to mouse models using targeted disruption of specific genes encoding signaling molecules are used to point out approaches for target validation. This type of knowledge will be used in the future to design new drugs targeted specifically to certain signaling pathways.

T-CELL ACTIVATION: AFFERENT PATHWAY

To illustrate the extent to which signaling pathways are interconnected, the intracellular events occurring during an immune response by T cells can be used as a model system. The discussion here highlights specific immune dysfunctions caused by mutations in the components of these pathways, both in human patients and in animal models.

The T cell receptor (TCR) complex is made up of several distinct transmembrane proteins termed the α, β, and ζ subunits. These components are in turn associated with the CD3 complex of transmembrane proteins, which is made up of γ, δ, and ε subunits. The α and β subunits are responsible for recognition and binding to specific antigens in association with a major histocompatibility complex (MHC) molecule. The transduction of the extracellular binding event to the intracellular compartment is carried out by the other associated polypeptides (10). Many signaling pathways in eukaryotic cells use tyrosine kinases to link extracellular receptor engagement with subsequent intracellular responses. For example, the tyrosine kinase activity of the epidermal growth factor (EGF) receptor exists as an integral part of the receptor molecule and can be activated by ligand binding to the receptor or by artificial crosslinking of the receptor by antibodies (11). Alternatively, as in the case of the TCR, tyrosine kinase activity can be recruited to the membrane receptor by a unique class of protein domains called SRC homology 2 (SH2) domains (12). SH2 domains were first identified as a conserved sequence within the SRC family of tyrosine kinases (13). Subsequently, SH2 domains have been found in a wide variety of intracellular signaling proteins and are classified based on their sequence homology as well as the specificity of their preferred phosphotyrosine tetrapeptide ligand (14). These domains, as regions of larger proteins, mediate interactions between signaling proteins by binding to phosphotyrosine-containing peptide sequences with specificity and high affinity (15–17). This ability to recognize phosphotyrosine allows these proteins to monitor the phosphorylation state of various intracellular proteins and places them in a central role for the regulation of tyrosine kinase signaling pathways.

There are two families of SH2 domain–containing proteins that initially bind to the phosphorylated tyrosine residues on the TCR receptor intracellular domain. The SRC family members LCK and FYN contain an SH2 domain, an SH3 domain, and a kinase domain. The SYK family, made up of the tyrosine kinases SYK and ζ-associated protein-70 (ZAP-70), consists of a tandem SH2 domain and a kinase domain. Engagement of immunoreceptors in hematopoietic cells leads to activation of SRC family tyrosine kinases as well as SYK or ZAP-70 (18,19). Current models propose that SRC family kinases are critical in immune response signal transduction through their role in phosphorylation of tyrosine residues within receptor immunoreceptor tyrosine-based activation motifs (ITAMs), which are found within the intracellular domains of the TCR; the ITAMs recruit the SH2 domains of SYK or ZAP-70 and phosphorylate SYK and ZAP-70 (20).

To address the question of how phosphorylation and subsequent signaling events are generated, we must first introduce additional cell surface components that act as obligatory coreceptors and accessory molecules for T-cell activation (21). The cell surface glycoproteins CD4 and CD8 play an important role in initiating the signaling cascade and act by binding to the same class II or class I MHC molecules that are engaged by the TCR. Coaggregation of these receptors with the TCR brings the cytoplasmic tails of these molecules into close proximity with each other and with any associated signaling molecules. The SRC family member LCK has been found to be associated with the cytoplasmic domain of both CD4 and CD8 in a noncovalent fashion (22,23). The importance of CD4 in T-cell activation is illustrated by mouse strains that have a targeted disruption of the CD4 gene (CD4 knock-out mice) (24). These mice have an impairment of helper T-cell function, and the defect can be isolated to the portion of the CD4 molecule that has been shown to be associated with LCK. Mice in which the LCK gene is disrupted have a substantial inhibition of T-cell function (25). There have also been reports of a novel natural product (lymphostin), derived from *Streptomyces*, that inhibits

the enzymatic activity of LCK *in vitro* and the activation of T cells in a tissue culture model *in vitro* and in tissue culture (26). In addition to LCK, the SRC family member FYN has also been shown to play an important role in T-cell activation on receptor binding. FYN knock-out mice have also been shown to have a suboptimal immune response (27,28).

Phosphorylation of the various ITAMs in the TCR complex by SRC family kinases creates docking sites for SH2 domain–containing intracellular proteins. Early work suggested this was necessary for recruitment of ZAP-70 (10,29), but more recent evidence suggests that ZAP-70, an essential component of TCR-mediated signaling, is preassociated with the receptor complex in resting T cells (30). This would imply that some low level of phosphorylation exists in the resting state and that receptor engagement leads not only to phosphorylation of ITAM regions but to activation of ZAP-70. Activated T cells do not show this preassociated event, possibly because of higher levels of phosphatase activity (see later discussion). The central role of ZAP-70 in T-cell activation is displayed in animal models and in human patients. Loss of ZAP-70 function in humans results in a severely immunocompromised state (31,32). These patients lack peripheral CD8+ T cells (cytotoxic T cells), and their small number of circulating CD4+ T cells (helper T cells) are unresponsive. The presence of CD4+ T cells is thought to be a result of the compensatory function of the related kinase SYK. This tyrosine kinase does not normally play a role in T-cell activation but, at least in humans, may function partially during T-cell development. In mature T cells, the levels of SYK are greatly diminished, and it is therefore unable to function in place of the missing ZAP-70. In mice in which ZAP-70 has been deleted, both subsets of T cells are missing from the periphery, and therefore T-cell function is absent (33).

In addition to coreceptor molecules that recruit tyrosine kinases to the TCR complex, there is also an associated phosphatase (CD45) that serves to remove phosphates from tyrosine. Contrary to the role phosphatases may play in downregulating an ongoing immune response by removing potential docking sites for SH2-containing proteins, CD45 serves to activate the SRC family kinase members (34,35). Members of this family have a negative regulatory tyrosine that, when phosphorylated, allows for intramolecular binding of the SH2 domain, effectively rendering it unable to interact with ITAMs on the receptor tails or to phosphorylate any of its substrates. Removal of this phosphate activates SRC members LCK and FYN. Mice deficient in CD45 have defective LCK function and a resulting defect in T-cell activity (36).

A final accessory pathway that is necessary to initiate a full T-cell response begins with the cell surface molecule CD28. Many cell surface proteins on T cells have

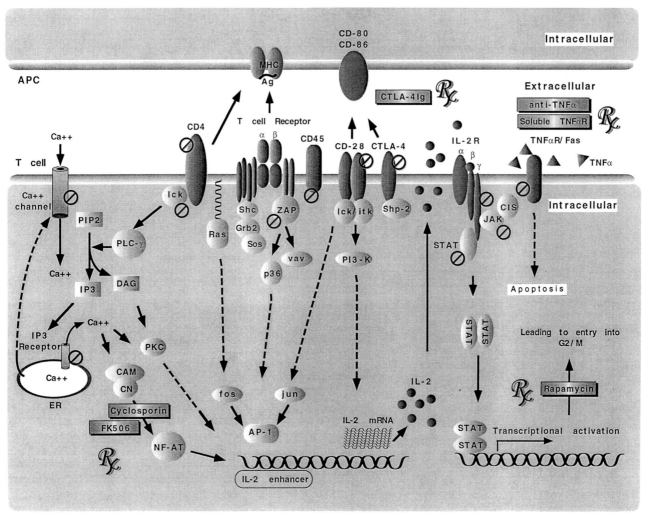

FIG. 77-1. Intracellular signaling pathways in T cells. ∅ indicates animal models or human diseases where the function of this protein has been disrupted or altered. R_x indicates examples of current pharmaceuticals used to modulate inflammatory responses both in humans and animal models. Membrane receptors and ligands: TCR, T-cell receptor complex, composed of multiple polypeptides, some of which serve to recognize external ligands and others to transduce signals into the cytoplasm; MHC, major histocompatibility complex, composed of two membrane polypeptides; CD4, accessory membrane molecule that interacts with MHC class II; CD45, membrane tyrosine phosphatase that activates SRC family kinases by removing a negative regulatory tyrosine; CD28, coreceptor that binds to CD80 and CD86 and serves to upregulate the T-cell response; CTLA-4, coreceptor related to CD28 but with opposing negative regulation function; CD80/CD86, membrane proteins that are expressed on antigen-presenting cells and bind to CD28 and CTLA-4; IL-2R, interleukin-2 receptor, expressed predominantly on T cells; IL-2, soluble cytokine that binds to IL-2R and causes T-cell proliferation and activation; TNF-αR, membrane receptor for tumor necrosis factor-α and members of the FAS family; TNF-α, soluble cytokine that is secreted by monocytes/macrophages and mediates many inflammatory processes. Cytoplasmic signaling molecules: ZAP, protein tyrosine kinase with two SH2 domains, found associated with the TCR; LCK, SRC family protein tyrosine kinase associated with CD4 and CD28; ITK, protein tyrosine kinase that is found only in T cells and associates with CD28; SHP2, protein tyrosine phosphatase containing an SH2 domain; VAV, an adaptor molecule containing an SH3 domain that is an exchange factor for RHO family guanosine triphosphate (GTP)–binding proteins; SOS, an adaptor molecule containing an SH3 domain that is an exchange factor for RAS; GRB-2, growth factor receptor–bound protein containing an SH2 domain and two SH3 domains; p36, an SH2 domain–containing protein that associates with GRB-2 in activated T cells; PLCγ, phospholipase C_γ, cleaves PIP_2 to IP_3 and DAG; PIP_2, phosphatidylinositol 4,5-bisphosphonate; IP_3, inositol 1,4,5-trisphosphate; DAG, diacylglycerol; PKC, protein kinase C, exists as several isoforms and is activated in T cells by Ca^{2+} and DAG; CAM, calmodulin, activates calcineurin; CN, calcineurin, a Ca^{2+}- and calmodulin-dependent protein phosphatase; PI3K, phosphatidylinositol 3-kinase, made up of a regulatory (p85) and a catalytic (p110) subunit; FOS, nuclear transcription factor that is required for IL-2 gene transcription, component of AP-1; JUN, nuclear transcription factor that is required for IL-2 gene transcription, component of AP-1; STAT, signal transducer and activator of transcription, involved in cytokine and growth factor receptor signaling; JAK, Janus family of protein tyrosine kinase, involved in cytokine and growth factor receptor signaling; CIS, cytokine-inducible signaling inhibitor, downregulates JAK/STAT pathway.

been shown to enhance T-cell responsiveness, and CD28 is included in this group. However, CD28 also performs an additional function in preventing the onset of anergy or unresponsiveness (37–41). CD28 is a membrane glycoprotein that exists as a homodimer on the surface of all $CD4^+$ T cells and most $CD8^+$ T cells. The extracellular ligands for CD28 are CD80 and CD86, which exist on the surface of antigen-presenting cells (APCs) and are engaged in parallel with the TCR complex. These ligands are shared by a second, related T-cell molecule that has opposing functions to CD28, called CTLA-4 (cytolytic T lymphocyte associated antigen) (see later discussion). There have been many observations that point toward the importance of CD28 in T-cell activation. CD28-deficient mice have a variety of immune defects, including decreased antigen responsiveness, limited helper functions (e.g., class switching of immunoglobulins), and, most importantly, decreases in a variety of T cell–derived cytokines that have wide effects in inflammatory responses (42). These cytokines include interleukin-2 (IL-2), IL-3, IL-4, tumor necrosis factor-α (TNF-α), and interferon-γ (IFN-γ). The inability to produce these cytokines, especially IL-2, results in a profound state of anergy. This has prompted the use of soluble portions of the related receptor CTLA-4 (known as CTLA-4Ig) as an immunosuppressive agent in a variety of experimentally induced models for human autoimmune diseases (43) (Fig. 77-1). This agent functions by binding to CD80 and CD86 and blocking the ability of CD28 to bind to the APC. Because it is postulated that the interaction of CD28 with its ligands occurs only during antigen recognition, this type of treatment would selectively inhibit only activated T cells. In the case of autoimmune diseases or anti-graft responses, only those destructive T cells would be inhibited.

The intracellular signaling proteins that interact directly with the cytoplasmic region of CD28 are not fully defined. However, several of the proteins involved in the membrane proximal steps have been identified and illustrate the crosstalk that occurs between this pathway and the TCR-mediated signaling events (see later discussion) (44,45). There are putative SH2-binding motifs on the cytoplasmic domain CD28 that are phosphorylated on receptor aggregation. There are also possible proline-rich SH3-binding motifs that may recruit kinase families containing this domain. The activation of the CD28 pathway eventually leads to activation of the transcription factor AP-1, which is also regulated by a TCR-mediated signaling cascade and therefore represents a point of signal integration.

As pointed out previously, the CD28 molecule shares its ligands with CTLA-4. However, the expression patterns of these two molecules are distinct. CD28 is expressed on most T cells, but CTLA-4 is expressed only on activated T cells, usually 24 to 48 hours after TCR activation (46). The function of this molecule is illustrated in CTLA-4–deficient mice. These mice develop an extreme lymphoproliferative disorder that eventually leads to death (47). The most likely explanation for this phenomenon is an inability to downregulate peripheral T-cell responses. This has also been demonstrated in mice receiving blocking antibodies for CTLA-4, in which anti-tumor responses are greatly enhanced. This suggests the possibility of a clinical application of CTLA-4 inhibition where an enhancement of the native T-cell response is required, as in the acquired immunodeficiency syndrome (AIDS). Several tentative associations with known autoimmune dysfunctions, including Graves' disease and diabetes mellitus, have suggested a CTLA-4 defect as a possible factor in disease severity (48).

As with CD28, the signaling pathway initiated by CTLA-4 is not fully characterized. Both SH2- and SH3-binding motifs are present on the cytoplasmic tail of CTLA-4. CTLA-4–deficient mice display hyperphosphorylated FYN, LCK, and ZAP-70, as well as other intracellular proteins. Evidence suggests that SH2-containing tyrosine phosphatase-2 (SHP-2) is associated with the cytoplasmic domain of CTLA-4, implying that this molecule could dephosphorylate TCR-associated kinases, thus downregulating the response (49).

SECONDARY MESSENGERS

T-cell activation initiates a series of signaling pathways that converge on the nucleus and affect gene transcription. Many of these pathways are not unique but serve as general second messengers in a variety of cell types. In addition, in T cells, these pathways are used by receptor systems other than the TCR complex. What is important is to understand that the nature and magnitude of the inflammatory response is a result of the synthesis of many signaling pathways. What follows is a brief outline of several of the major pathways that lie downstream of the membrane proximal TCR-signaling apparatus.

Calcium-mediated Events

Calcium plays a central role in many cellular responses, most notably in muscle and nervous tissue, where it serves as a cofactor for a variety of intracellular enzymes. The ability of calcium to regulate many responses depends not on absolute calcium levels inside a cell but on the ratio of various intracellular stores with the concentration of calcium in the extracellular environment. This is also the case for T cells, in which fluctuations in intracellular calcium mark the extremes of T-cell responses ranging from activation to anergy to apoptosis.

The release of calcium from intracellular stores within the endoplasmic reticulum and influx from the extracellular medium are linked to another signaling pathway downstream of the enzyme phospholipase C_γ (PLCγ) (50–53). PLCγ is recruited to the TCR complex after initial activation and phosphorylation of tyrosine residues (probably via its SH2 domain). Its function is in the catalysis of phosphatidylinositol 4,5-bisphosphate (PIP_2) to diacylglycerol (DAG) and inositol 1,4,5-trisphosphate (IP_3). These two products initiate several independent pathways leading to gene transcription and cellular activation. Their immediate function is to release calcium from intracellular stores (IP_3) and to activate protein kinase C (DAG), both of which are essential components of a T-cell response. In fact, combinations of a calcium ionophore (causing an influx of calcium) and phorbol ester (an activator of protein kinase C) can substitute for these secondary messengers and cause full activation of T cells. After cleavage of PIP_2, IP_3 binds to a receptor on the surface of the endoplasmic reticulum (IP_3R), causing release of its calcium stores. This release of calcium is inhibited, in some forms of common variable immunodeficiency, because of a defect in the generation of the IP_3 molecule (54). In addition, experiments in cell lines in which the IP_3R was blocked showed inhibition of T-cell activation (55).

The release of calcium from internal stores sets in motion several events. One of the first is the activation of calcineurin, a calcium-dependent phosphatase that is necessary for the activation of transcription factors central to T-cell activation. This enzyme, in the presence of calcium and calmodulin, dephosphorylates the cytoplasmic component of the transcription complex known as nuclear factor of activated T cells (NF-AT) (56,57). This allows its entry in the nucleus, where assembly with a variety of nuclear factors causes gene transcription. Understanding of the nature of this pathway has been aided by knowledge of the mechanism by which several immunosuppressive agents work to inhibit T-cell responses.

Cyclosporin A is a natural product that has been used as an immunosuppressive agent for more than a decade (58). In the late 1980s two other immunosuppressive natural products, FK506 and rapamycin, were identified; they had 10 to 100 times the activity of cyclosporine. The mechanisms by which these agents work have now been elucidated, and they show unique but related features (59–63). Both cyclosporine and FK506, although chemically distinct, were found to inhibit the phosphatase activity of calcineurin. This was accomplished only in the presence of a third class of proteins, called *immunophilins,* which themselves catalyze the isomerization of peptide bonds. FK506 and cyclosporine both bind to immunophilins, creating in essence a new molecule with a novel activity (i.e., a gain of function). This new complex binds to calcineurin and inhibits its activity, thereby inhibiting T-cell activation. The activity of rapamycin has some similarities; it binds to the same immunophilin as FK506, but this complex then interacts with FKBP-12 (FK506 Binding Protein) rapamycin-associated protein (FRAP) (59). As with FK506 and cyclosporine, the resulting complex creates a novel intracellular structure that subsequently binds to and inhibits a kinase involved in progression through G_1 of the cell cycle,

inhibiting growth factor-regulated proliferation of T cells (see later discussion). The molecular details of the FK506-immunophilin-calcineurin complex have been uncovered by x-ray crystallography, and an attempt has been made to generate synthetic FK506 analogues that possess the immunosuppressive activity of these agents but none of their associated kidney toxicity. This attempt has so far been unsuccessful, because it appears that the toxicity of FK506 is caused by its inhibition of calcineurin activity in that organ and cannot be separated from its immunosuppressive activity.

Calcium levels must be maintained for relatively long periods to ensure effective activation. Once internal stores are depleted by IP_3 binding to the endoplasmic reticulum, extracellular calcium channels must be activated. This is accomplished via signaling proteins that are released from the endoplasmic reticulum on depletion of internal stores to activate calcium channels in the plasma membrane. If these channels are blocked, then T-cell activation is inhibited. One type of severe T-cell immunodeficiency appears to be caused by a defect in this membrane channel (64).

RAS-Mediated Events

As pointed out previously, ligation of the TCR complex by antigen results in the phosphorylation of multiple tyrosines in the cytoplasmic domains of the transmembrane proteins and associated kinases (LCK, ZAP), creating essentially new docking sites for other proteins that contain SH2 domains. Some of these proteins are kinases themselves which phosphorylate substrates further downstream; others have been shown to be adapter proteins that have no intrinsic enzymatic activity but serve to direct the association of other intracellular proteins. Growth factor receptor–bound protein-2 (GRB-2) is a well described adapter protein that contains a single SH2 domain flanked by two SH3 domains (65–68). This protein is involved in the regulation of Ras, (product of the ras proto-oncogene), a membrane-bound kinase that requires guanosine triphosphate to function and involves a wide array of other intracellular proteins [son of sevenless, SH2 containing transforming protein, product of vav proto-oncogene, casitas B lymphoma, 36 kd phosphoprotein (SOS, SHC, VAV, CBL, pp36)]. Many of these proteins contain SH2 and SH3 domains and would serve as likely targets for pharmaceutical intervention. Subsequent activation of RAS initiates a phosphorylation cascade leading to activation of the mitogen-activated protein (MAP) kinase pathway and ends in the stimulation of the AP-1 DNA-binding complex and IL-2 gene transcription. The final result of this pathway, IL-2 gene transcription, is therefore the product of at least two separate signaling pathways: the TCR-mediated events and the CD28 coreceptor pathway. Other crosstalk between these two important pathways has been suggested to occur at the membrane proximal end (69). This underscores the complexity of T-cell activation and subsequent inflammatory events mediated via T cells. In addition, it illustrates the necessity for understanding the molecular events within cellular pathways to effectively design targeted pharmaceutical inhibitors with a predicted function.

T-CELL ACTIVATION: EFFERENT PATHWAY

Activation of gene transcription after the initial T-cell response causes the secretion of T cell–specific cytokines (70–73), including IL-2, IL-4, IL-9, IL-10, and IFN-γ. In addition, a variety of cytokine receptors for these molecules and other cytokines (IL-7, IL-12, and IL-15) are upregulated. Finally, there is a class of T cell–secreted cytokines that affect other cell types and modulate the immune response. These include IL-3 in mast cells, IL-4 in T cells and B cells, and granulocyte-macrophage colony-stimulating factor (GM-CSF) in granulocytes and macrophages. The following section highlights several of the soluble mediators and their receptors that drive the second phase of T-cell activation and subsequently an inflammatory response. Many of these cytokines and cytokine receptors are targets for current immunotherapy using either recombinant soluble receptors or specific antibodies. Future pharmaceuticals will use small molecules designed to interfere with these signaling pathways.

CYTOKINES AND THEIR RECEPTORS

Cytokine receptors can be divided into several families based on homologous domains in the extracellular portions of these molecules (74,75). Like the TCR, the cytoplasmic domains of these receptors are lacking in enzymatic activity but instead contain binding motifs for a variety of intracellular signaling molecules. In addition, many cytokine receptors share one common subunit (76). For example, the receptor for IL-2 is made up of three heterologous subunits: IL-2Rα, IL-2Rβ, and IL-2Rγ. The IL-2Rβ chain is found in the IL-15R, and the IL-2Rγ chain is a component of the receptors for IL-2, IL-4, IL-7, IL-9, and IL-15 (77). Other shared chains include the β subunit of the IL-3R, which is shared with the receptors for IL-5 and GM-CSF, and the γ chain of the IL-6R, which is found in the receptors for leukemia inhibitory factor (LIF) and oncostatin M (OSM). As outlined later, many of these receptor systems mediate their intracellular effects via two major signaling protein families: JAKs and STATs.

JAK/STAT

The immediate cytoplasmic protein that initiates signals from the IL-2 receptor is a member of the *Ja*nus family of intracellular *k*inases (JAK) (72,78). Triggering of cytokine receptors containing the common γ chain (γc) initiates a complex signal transduction program, including tyrosine phosphorylation of both the receptor chains

and receptor-associated proteins. The phosphorylation of receptor-associated JAK kinases is one of the first detectable events after receptor ligation. JAK kinases are then thought to phosphorylate the receptor chains, creating docking sites for SH2-containing *s*ignal *t*ransducers and *a*ctivators of *t*ranscription (STAT proteins) (78–83). STAT proteins are the natural substrates for JAK kinases, and after phosphorylation STATs dimerize and translocate to the nucleus, where they activate gene transcription. It is believed that JAKs phosphorylate STAT proteins relatively nonspecifically and that specificity is provided instead by the selective recruitment of STATs to individual phosphorylated cytokine receptor subunits. Therefore, the particular STAT proteins activated depend not on the JAK kinase involved but on the identity of the cytokine receptor subunits.

Members of this family bind to the cytoplasmic domains of many cytokine receptors and are activated on receptor crosslinking. The JAK family of kinases is composed of at least four members, JAK-1, JAK-2, JAK-3, and TYK-2 (non-receptor tyrosine kinase). All of the family members show similarity in overall organization, with a carboxyl-terminal kinase domain, a pseudokinase domain, and a conserved amino-terminal domain. This last domain is presumably the structure that binds to the intracellular portions of the various cytokine receptor molecules. Both JAK-1 and JAK-3 have been implicated in signaling via receptors for IL-2, IL-4, IL-7, IL-9, and IL-15, all of which use the cytokine receptor γc (84–87). Unlike JAK-2 and JAK-1, JAK-3 expression is restricted to lymphoid and myeloid cell lines and hematopoietic tissues such as thymus, bone marrow, fetal liver, and spleen (84–90). Mice deficient in JAK-3 expression by gene targeting have been produced and are immunocompromised (91). These animal models provide compelling evidence for a pivotal role of JAK-3 in a T-lymphocyte signaling pathway determining activation versus inactivation (anergy).

Studies of human patients with severe combined immunodeficiency (SCID) also demonstrate an essential role for JAK-3 in the immune system. Several human disease conditions demonstrate the importance of JAK-3, and JAK-3 binding to γc, in the immune system (92,93). At the most severe level, patients who completely lack expression of JAK-3 or γc have SCID. They generally have normal numbers of B cells but lack T cells. An X-linked form of combined immunodeficiency (CID) has been identified in which the affected person has normal numbers of B cells and natural killer (NK) cells, a slight reduction in the number of T cells, and defects in T-cell function (86,94). These patients were found to have a point mutation in the cytoplasmic tail of γc that reduced JAK-3 binding. Therefore, a substantially less severe disease state is manifested by a genetic defect that reduces, but does not completely abolish, the JAK-3/γc interaction.

As with any pathway leading to cellular proliferation, there exists an important inhibitory arm that controls the magnitude of the response to avoid hyperactivation. A family of proteins containing SH2 domains that are expressed after cytokine receptor engagement has been identified (95). These proteins, which go by several designations (cytokine-inducible signaling inhibitors, suppressor of cytokine signaling, JAK-binding protein), all have been shown to downregulate the JAK/STAT pathway, either by binding to the JAK proteins themselves or by interfering with the ability of the JAKs to activate STAT proteins. Some of these molecular interactions are mediated via SH2, others via protein domains not yet characterized. The discovery of this pathway has suggested another area in which pharmaceutical intervention may allow the modulation of T-cell inflammatory responses.

THE TUMOR NECROSIS FACTOR FAMILY

TNF plays a central role in driving the inflammatory process (96). In this case, the major source for this family of cytokines is cells of the monocyte/macrophage lineage. Receptors for this cytokine, on the other hand, can be found in T cells, B cells, monocytes, endothelial cells, fibroblasts, adipocytes, osteoclasts, muscle cells, and liver. This underscores the wide range of effects that can be mediated by this cytokine during inflammation. Although TNF has been shown to be important in several infectious animal models, the clinical focus has been on alleviating the effects caused by TNF in a variety of diseases, including rheumatoid arthritis, sepsis, and AIDS (97,98). In addition, the inflammatory side effects that occur during immunotherapy (such as use of anti-CD3 antibodies to suppress graft-versus-host disease) can be partially attributed to the release of TNF. Several approaches have been used to downregulate TNF levels and the subsequent inflammatory sequelae associated with its release (99). These include antibodies directed against TNF, soluble TNF receptors, small molecules that inhibit TNF synthesis (e.g., corticosteroids), and phosphodiesterase inhibitors (e.g., pentoxifylline) (100). Many of the present clinical applications of anti-TNF therapy use antibodies and recombinant soluble receptors (101). However, as more of the details of TNF production and TNF receptor signaling are revealed, it is clear that the design of small molecules that can specifically modulate this pathway will be pursued.

The receptor for TNF is part of a family of cell surface receptors that includes the FAS receptor (CD95) and the TNF-related apoptosis-inducing ligands (TRAIL) receptor, all of which can transduce a "death" signal in cells leading to apoptosis (102–104). The importance of regulated cell death in the control of an expanding inflammatory response is illustrated by examining the kinetics of FAS ligand and CD95 expression. CD95 can be found on most activated T cells in culture. However, in nonactivated cells, CD95 expression is divided into two groups: CD45RA$^+$ (naive) cells, which have little or no CD95, and CD45RO$^+$ (memory) cells, which have high levels of CD95. Neither of these groups expresses FAS ligand. FAS ligand is found on activated CD8$^+$ cells as well as all T$_H$1 cells and a small subset of T$_H$2 cells. B cells also express CD95, and their expression can be upregulated by TNF-α and IFN-γ. Early in an immune response, the low level of T cell–T cell interaction results in stimulation. As the response progresses, more FAS ligand is being expressed, and there is increased CD95 expression and differentiation of T cells into effector cells. Under these conditions, the more frequent T cell–T cell interaction leads to cell death and a decrease in the immune response. As the antigen disappears, FAS ligand expression goes down and therefore so does apoptosis. The cells that escape cell death presumably become memory cells. In addition, studies have shown the importance of these receptors and ligands for the maintenance of immune-privileged sites such as the testes and the eyes (105,106). Expression of the FAS ligand in these sites causes the death of FAS$^+$ activated T cells.

DISCOVERY OF NEW DRUGS FOR IMMUNE AND INFLAMMATORY DISEASE

In the past, most drugs were discovered without prior knowledge of their cellular target. Drugs were identified from a series of compounds tested in assays using cells or animals. For example, the immunosuppressant FK506 was identified by adding fungal extracts to a mixed-lymphocyte-response assay for T-cell function. As outlined previously, FK506 blocks T-cell activation and has been used to prevent rejection of transplanted organs, but its therapeutic usefulness is complicated by an associated renal toxicity. Until the therapeutic target and mechanism for FK506 was discovered in 1991, the molecular basis for the toxicity was not known (62,107). FK506 forms a complex with FKBP and calcineurin, thereby blocking TCR-mediated activation of calcineurin phosphatase activity. Calcineurin is not localized to T cells but is broadly expressed throughout the body, including the kidney, where interference in its activity causes renal toxicity.

The approach to drug discovery has undergone a major paradigm shift over the past 10 years, largely because of the increased understanding of disease mechanisms. As described in earlier sections, a number of proteins have been shown to play critical roles in immune and inflammatory signal transduction pathways. Armed with knowledge about these key proteins and their function, pharmaceutical researchers have begun to develop *mechanism-based* drugs for treatment of immune disorders and for use in transplantation. These new drugs promise to be highly effective with no or reduced side effects. In addition, knowledge of the target greatly aids the drug discovery process. In the remaining sections, the rationale for choosing drug targets and the approaches to drug discovery when the target is known are reviewed (108). In this discussion, the focus is on intracellular targets and drugs that inhibit the function of the target protein (9).

Choosing the Target

Much of this chapter has summarized the experiments that have led to the current understanding of the proteins involved in immune cell signal transduction. The results of these experiments and a number of other criteria are used to choose a drug target. Examples of these criteria are the following:

1. Demonstration in cellular or animal models (or both) that the protein plays a critical role in the disease process
2. Evidence that the protein target is not critically involved in other cellular processes
3. Understanding of where the target is expressed during development and in the adult
4. Expectation that inhibition of the target would not be lethal
5. Genetic evidence concerning the target from human patients in whom the function of the target protein is defective
6. Expectation that a drug against the target would treat an unmet medical need or provide a meaningful improvement in current therapies
7. Information about the target that facilitates drug discovery or helps to define an approach to drug discovery
8. Knowledge of related members of the target family and their roles in cellular processes.

Using these criteria, pharmaceutical researchers have begun to develop drugs against key proteins that function in inflammatory signal transduction pathways. A representative set of potential intracellular drug targets is listed in Table 77-1.

ZAP-70: AN EXAMPLE OF A DRUG TARGET FOR IMMUNE AND INFLAMMATORY DISEASES

ZAP-70 may be used as an example protein target to illustrate several approaches to drug discovery. As described previously, ZAP-70 is a protein that plays a key role in TCR-mediated signal transduction. Drugs that block ZAP-70 function would be potentially useful to prevent rejection of transplanted organs and to treat patients with autoimmune diseases. ZAP-70 is an example of a selective target, because its expression is restricted to T cells and NK cells. For this reason, a specific ZAP-70 inhibitor would be predicted to selectively affect only these two cell types and therefore would not be expected to exhibit the toxic effects of FK506 or cyclosporine.

Initiating the Drug Discovery Process

Before initiating drug discovery, it is important to assemble certain information about the target and the potential drug—for example, what is known about the target's mechanism of action, natural substrates, inhibitors, associated proteins, three-dimensional structure, gene expression profile, and related family members.

ZAP-70 is composed of three functional domains: two tandemly positioned SH2 domains followed by a tyrosine

TABLE 77-1. *Selected targets of drugs to treat immune and inflammatory disease*

Target	Signaling pathway	Desired mechanism	Therapeutic indication	Functional domains
ZAP-70	TCR signaling	Inhibitor	Immunosuppression	SH2 binding domain Protein kinase domain
LCK	TCR signaling	Inhibitor	Immunosuppression	SH3 binding domain SH2 binding domain Protein kinase domain
JAK-3	Cytokine signaling	Inhibitor	Immunosuppression	Receptor association domain Protein kinase domain
IκB kinase	NP-κB signaling	Inhibitor	Antiinflammatory??	Protein kinase domain
STAT-6	IL-4, IL-13 signaling	Inhibitor	Atopic allergy/asthma Other	SH2 binding domain DNA binding domain
STAT4	IL-12 signaling	Inhibitor	TH1-dependent disease	SH2 binding domain DNA binding domain
SOCS/CIS	Cytokine signaling	Inhibitor	Increased cytokine action	SH2 binding domain JAK-association domain
CD45	TCR signaling	Inhibitor	Immunosuppression	Phosphatase domain
TEC	CD28, B cell	Inhibitor	Immunosuppression	PH binding domain SH3 binding domain SH2 binding domain Protein kinase domain

ZAP-70, ζ-associated protein-70; TCR, T-cell antigen receptor; SH, SRC homology domain; LCK, lymphocyte-specific protein tyrosine kinase; JAK3, Janus kinase-3; IκB, inhibitor factor kappa B cells; NF-κB, nuclear factor kappa B cells; signal transducer and activator of transcription; IL, interleukin; T$_H$1, helper T cell; SOCS/CIS, suppressor of cytokine signaling/cytokine-inducible signaling inhibitor; TEC, tyrosine kinase expressed in hepatocellular carcinoma; PH, pleckstrin homology domain.

kinase domain (109). SH2 domains bind to tyrosine phosphorylated proteins. As discussed previously, ZAP-70 binds to the cytoplasmic tails of the activated TCR via its two SH2 domains (Fig. 77-2). ZAP-70 kinase activity becomes activated, leading to the phosphorylation of a number of proteins on tyrosine. The structure of the tandem SH2 domains of ZAP-70 when bound to a phosphorylated peptide from the TCR ζ chain has been solved by x-ray crystallography (1). This structure provides a detailed view of the SH2-peptide binding interaction. On the other hand, there is limited information on natural and synthetic peptide substrates of ZAP-70 kinase. In addition, unlike the SH2 domains, the three-dimensional structure of the kinase domain has not yet been solved. However, the identification of inhibitors that block ZAP-70 function by acting on either the SH2 or the kinase domain is a current area of investigation by pharmaceutical researchers.

Assays for Drug Discovery of ZAP-70 Inhibitors

Before the drug discovery process is initiated, a series of biochemical, cellular, and animal assays is established to be used to test the effectiveness and specificity of compounds. Biochemical assays have been developed based on SH2 binding and ZAP-70 protein kinase activities. These assays are used to measure the ability of compounds to compete with peptide binding or phosphorylation. Often it is easier to establish an assay using only part of the protein. For example, the SH2 domains can be expressed in *Escherichia coli,* whereas the complete protein is highly insoluble in *E. coli.* The kinase domain of ZAP-70, as well as the entire molecule, can be expressed in an insect cell system. The amount of specific protein that can be recovered from the insect cell systems may be 100- to 1000-fold lower than that obtained from *E. coli,* and this is one of the major reasons why only a few kinase domain structures have been solved. Counterscreens are assays for related proteins designed to test compounds for specificity against ZAP-70. For example, assays of SH2-binding and kinase activities of SYK, a structurally related kinase, are used to test compounds developed against ZAP-70.

Generally, biochemical assays are used to identify initial "hits," the first set of compounds that exhibit activity

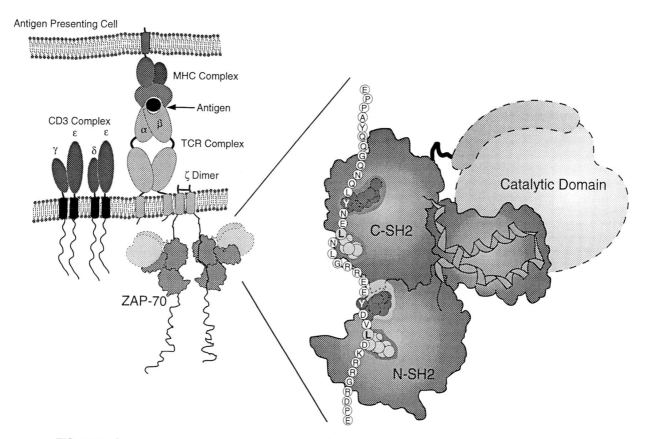

FIG. 77-2. Schematic view of ZAP-70 bound to the ζ₁ chain of the activated TCR. Activation of T cells is initiated by association of the TCR with peptide antigen bound to MHC molecules on an antigen-presenting cell. TCR-MHC association stimulates phosphorylation of the TCR subunits on tyrosines within the ITAMs. ZAP-70 binds to the phosphorylated ITAM by means of its SH2 domains (residues 1–259). The position of the other domains of ZAP-70, including the catalytic domain (residues 311–620), have not been determined, and their positions as shown are hypothetical.

against the target. Hits generally function only in bio-chemical assays, but they provide information about the chemical structures that bind to the target protein. Hits are then converted to "leads," which begin to show activity in cell culture and animal models.

Several cellular assays are being employed to identify ZAP-70 inhibitors. The first set uses the target cell, T cells, and examines the ability of compounds to block TCR-mediated IL-2 production and T-cell proliferation (10,110). Because a compound could block these processes by inhibiting a number of proteins, it is important to develop methods to demonstrate that ZAP-70 is the intracellular target. For example, a ZAP-70 inhibitor would prevent ZAP-70 from forming a complex with the active TCR, and, in fact, peptide-based SH2 inhibitors that are artificially introduced into the intracellular compartment of T cells have been shown to block the association of ZAP-70 with the activated TCR. A kinase inhibitor would prevent downstream substrates from being phosphorylated; this should also inhibit T-cell activation. Although current general kinase inhibitors do decrease the T-cell response, their nonspecificity makes it difficult to determine the magnitude of their effect on ZAP-70. A ZAP-70–specific kinase inhibitor would selectively inhibit only T cells and only their response through the TCR complex. Along with assays designed to measure specific inhibition of ZAP-70, another set of cellular assays has been developed as counterscreens. For example, compounds are tested on cellular activities that are independent of ZAP-70 to assess specificity for ZAP-70. Finally, other assays measure the general cellular toxicity of ZAP-70 inhibitory compounds.

As compounds become more potent and more specific, they are tested in animal models of the disease state. For example, a number of transplantation assays have been developed to test the ability of drugs to prevent graft rejection (111). In addition, lead compounds are tested for toxicity and pharmacologic properties such as bioavailability and pharmacokinetics.

Approaches to Drug Discovery

Screening Compound Libraries

The most widely used approach for drug discovery is screening of a diverse library of compounds against the target protein in a biochemical functional assay. The libraries are generally collections of synthetic organic compounds representing drug-like molecules. Typical chemical collections in major pharmaceutical companies contain between 100,000 and 1 million compounds. In the past, this collection was slowly built by adding compounds that were synthesized one at a time for ongoing projects. More recently, chemists developed a method, termed *combinatorial chemistry,* by which mixtures of reactants for a particular synthetic step are used to create a library of compounds with many different structures (112). The synthetic reactions can be carried out in solution or on a solid support such as glass beads. By this approach, a single chemist can synthesize millions of different compounds in about 1 week. Combinatorial chemical libraries containing more than 100,000 compounds are now being applied to the early phases of drug discovery to identify an initial hit. A third source of compounds for hit identification is natural sources. Microorganisms and plants naturally manufacture a rich variety of compounds, often as natural protection mechanisms. These compounds, termed *natural products,* are obtained from bacterial, fungal, and plant extracts. Cyclosporine, FK506, and rapamycin are examples of natural products.

The chemical and natural product libraries are used to identify the first set of compounds that show some inhibitory activity toward the target. The next step involves improving them by making new molecules derived from the structures of the original hits. Compounds that exhibit improved inhibitory activity are compared with compounds that exhibit weaker or no activity to decipher structure-activity relations. This helps the chemist to identify modifications that will lead to the most potent drug. A screening approach can be applied to identify ZAP-70 inhibitors. The availability of high-throughput assays that use multiwell plates and robotics makes this approach feasible. A high-throughput SH2 assay based on fluorescence polarization has been reported (16). Similarly, high-throughput assays for protein kinases have been established.

Peptidomimetic Approach

A second approach, termed the *peptidomimetic approach,* involves designing organic molecules based on a peptide ligand or inhibitor of the target. Generally, peptides make poor drugs because they are weakly inhibitory, are proteolytically degraded in the bloodstream, and poorly penetrate the cell membrane. However, organic compounds derived from peptides have improved stability and permeability and therefore can be effective drugs. Having a set of peptides that bind to a target protein and another set of peptides that do not bind helps to focus the design of organic inhibitors and to identify structure-activity relations. Lead molecules are generated and optimized in much the same fashion as described previously. Before solving the ZAP-70 SH2 structure, researchers had only the sequence of peptide ligands to guide drug discovery. This approach was superseded by a structure-guided approach.

Structure-Guided Design

A third approach, termed *structure-guided design,* uses knowledge of the three-dimensional structure of the target, often with a bound ligand or inhibitor, to develop drugs against the target (113). In this case, the interaction between the target and a ligand is known on a molecular level. Structural information is obtained by x-ray crystallography or nuclear magnetic resonance studies. With the use of computational and graphics programs, the interactions between target and ligand can be analyzed and organic molecules can be designed to bind to the active site of the target. Generally, a series of compounds is generated and tested in functional assays. In parallel, information on structures of the target when bound to these organic molecules are generated. The activity results are then examined in the context of the structures for each compound. This process is repeated several times in an iterative fashion, each time with changes made to the compound design to create molecules with improved inhibitory activities. Not only is structural information important for optimizing inhibition of the target, but knowledge of regions of the drug that do not contact the target can be exploited to add modifications that affect other properties of the drug, such as oral activity or cellular permeability. As with the peptidomimetic approach, the number of compounds generated is much smaller than in random screening; often, fewer than 100 compounds are tested in the progression from hit to drug candidate.

The structure of the ZAP-70 tandem SH2 domains bound to a 19-amino-acid phosphopeptide revealed a number of surprising features of the ZAP-ζ interaction. The segment of the receptor that binds ZAP-70 contains two phosphotyrosine residues. The structure clearly showed that this segment binds to ZAP-70 in an extended fashion, with the two phosphotyrosines binding to a pocket of the two SH2 domains. The extended nature of the peptide made it clear that it would be extremely difficult to design an organic drug that could fit into both SH2-binding pockets at once. A second surprising feature was that the phosphotyrosine-binding pocket of the N-terminal SH2 domain was completed by two residues from the C-terminal SH2 domain. In contrast, the phosphotyrosine-binding pocket of the C-terminal SH2 domain was intact. These details are now being used by pharmaceutical researchers to design organic small-molecule drugs to bind to one or the other of the ZAP-70 SH2 domains to block its interaction with the activated TCR.

Targeting the Protein Kinase Domain

Inhibitors of ZAP-70 kinase activity have yet to be reported in the literature. Theoretically, compounds that selectively block the protein kinase activity of ZAP-70 could be identified by similar approaches to those used to discover SH2-domain inhibitors. The first approach uses a high-throughput protein kinase assay to screen compound libraries for inhibitors; second would be a structure-guided approach. To date, the three-dimensional structure of the ZAP-70 protein kinase domain has not been solved. Model structures can be generated by

homology to protein kinases with known structures, such as insulin receptor kinase, SRC, and cyclic adenosine monophosphate–dependent protein kinase (114–116). The known protein kinase structures and the ZAP-70 model structures serve as templates for the design of ZAP-70 kinase inhibitors. Generally, model structures lack the molecular detail necessary for structure-guided design of inhibitors. Therefore, work is in progress in a number of laboratories to solve the crystal structure of the ZAP-70 kinase domain. As with the approach toward the ZAP-70 SH2 domains, protein kinase–based counterscreens are needed to test compounds for selectivity against ZAP-70. The SYK protein kinase exhibits the closest sequence homology to the ZAP-70 kinase domain and is likely to be used as a counterscreen.

Many of the known protein kinase inhibitors are adenosine triphosphate (ATP) analogues. Because virtually all protein kinases use ATP as a cosubstrate, it is important to test ZAP-70 kinase inhibitors against a broad spectrum of protein kinases. Although a number of protein kinase inhibitors are in clinical trials, there are no approved protein kinase inhibitor drugs. One reason may be that these compounds bind to the ATP-binding sites of many kinases. The challenge for the future is to develop inhibitors of ZAP-70 kinase activity that compete with the peptide substrate.

Systematization of Drug Discovery Research

The approaches taken for the discovery of ZAP-70 inhibitors can also be applied to other targets such as those listed in Table 77-1. For example, the SH2 domain of STAT-6 is necessary for binding to the IL-4R and for DNA-binding activity. A STAT-6 inhibitor may be useful for treatment of asthma. JAK-3 can potentially be blocked by interfering with its ability to associate with the IL-2R or by blocking its protein kinase activity. Other domains, such as the PH or SH3 domain, function to regulate protein localization and activity and therefore are potential targets for drug intervention.

As drugs are developed against one member of a protein family, information about the inhibitory molecules can be applied to develop drugs against other members. In this way, drugs to treat a variety of unmet medical problems can be developed. This systematization of drug discovery has been facilitated by the application of molecular biology techniques, the rapidly expanding field of genomics, and advances in chemistry and automation (108). For example, libraries of combinatorial compounds developed for one target can be useful to screen a related family member. The speed with which compound libraries can be assayed continues to increase as automation systems move toward higher-density arrays of assay plates.

Advances in structural biology also facilitate drug discovery. Nuclear magnetic resonance and x-ray structures for previously uncharacterized protein domains lay the groundwork for structure-guided drug discovery. As methods to derive homology models improve, structure-guided drug discovery may be possible with only a single structure of a related family member. In addition, structural models of related proteins can help in the design of compounds with high selectivity for a desired target, thereby eliminating or reducing toxicity due to cross-reactivity.

This wealth of information on targets, their structures, substrates, and inhibitors can no longer be easily tracked simply by memory or even by standard databases. The field of bioinformatics aims to develop relational databases so that information about one protein target will be useful for projects involving related proteins. These new databases and other bioinformatics tools will aid all stages of drug discovery, from gene sequencing of protein targets to obtaining structural information on chemical inhibitors. All of these advances promise to improve the speed with which new drugs are discovered, to increase the selectivity of drugs, and to identify drugs for unmet medical needs.

REFERENCES

1. Hatada MH, Lu X, Laird ER, et al. Molecular basis for interaction of the protein tyrosine kinase ZAP-70 with the T-cell receptor. *Nature* 1995;377:32–38.
2. Narula SS, Yuan RW, Adams SE, et al. Solution structure of the C-terminal SH2 domain of the human tyrosine kinase Syk complexed with a phosphotyrosine pentapeptide. *Structure* 1995;3:1061–1073.
3. Waksman G, Kominos D, Robertson SC, et al. Crystal structure of the phosphotyrosine recognition domain SH2 of v-src complexed with tyrosine-phosphorylated peptides. *Nature* 1992;358:646–653.
4. Baker GL, Kahl LE, Zee BC. Malignancy following treatment of rheumatoid arthritis with cyclophosphamide: a long term case-control follow-up study. *Am J Med* 1987;83:1–12.
5. Bennett WM, Pulliam JP. Cyclosporin nephrotoxicity. *Ann Intern Med* 1983;99:851–859.
6. De Neve W, Valeriote F, Edelstein M, Everett C, Bischoff M. *In vitro* DNA cross-linking by cyclophosphamide: comparison of human chronic lymphocytic leukaemia cells with mouse L1210 leukemia and normal bone marrow cells. *Cancer Res* 1989;49:3452–3465.
7. Jolivet J, Cowan KH, Curt GA, Clendeninn NJ, Chabner BA. The pharmacology and clinical use of methotrexate. *N Engl J Med* 1983;309:1094–1097.
8. Korsmeyer SS. Chromosomal translocations in lymphoid malignancies reveal novel protooncogenes. *Annu Rev Immunol* 1992;10:785–804.
9. Brugge JS. New intracellular targets for therapeutic drug design. *Science* 1993;260:918–919.
10. Weiss A, Littman DR. Signal transduction by lymphocyte antigen receptors. *Cell* 1994;76:263–274.
11. Cadena DL, Chan CL, Gill GN. The intracellular tyrosine kinase domain of the epidermal growth factor receptor undergoes a conformational change upon autophosphorylation. *J Biol Chem* 1994;269:260–265.
12. Pawson T. Protein modules and signaling networks. *Nature* 1995;373:573–580.
13. Sadowski I, Stone JC, Pawson T. A noncatalytic domain conserved among cytoplasmic protein-tyrosine kinases modifies the kinase function and transforming activity of Fujinami sarcoma virus P130gag-fps. *Mol Cell Biol* 1986;6:4396–4408.
14. Koch CA, Anderson D, Moran MF, Ellis C, Pawson T. SH2 and SH3 domains: elements that control interactions of cytoplasmic signaling proteins. *Science* 1991;252:668–674.
15. Felder S, Zhou M, Urena J, et al. SH2 domains exhibit high-affinity binding to tyrosine-phosphorylated peptides yet also exhibit rapid dissociation and exchange. *Mol Cell Biol* 1993;13:1449–1455.
16. Lynch BA, Loiacono K, Tiong C, Adams S, MacNeil IA. A fluorescence-polarization based Src-SH2 binding assay. 1996. *Anal Biochem* 1997; 247:77–82.
17. Songyang Z, Shoelson SE, Chaudhuri M, et al. SH2 domains recognize specific phosphopeptide sequences. *Cell* 1993;72:1–20.
18. Cooke MP, Abraham KM, Forbush KA, Perlmutter RM. Regulation of T cell receptor signaling by a src family protein tyrosine kinase (p59fyn). *Cell* 1991;65:281–291.
19. Eck MJ, Atwell SK, Shoelson SE, Harrison SC. Structure of the regulatory domains of the Src-family tyrosine kinase Lck. *Nature* 1994; 368:764–769.
20. Zoller KE, MacNeil IA, Brugge JS. Protein tyrosine kinases Syk and ZAP-70 display distinct requirements for Src family kinases in immune response receptor signal transduction. 1996. *J Immunol* 1997; 158:1650–1659.
21. Janeway CA Jr, Rojo J, Saizawa K, et al. The co-receptor function of murine CD4. *Immunol Rev* 1989;109:77–92.
22. Luo K, Sefton BM. Cross-linking of T cell surface molecules CD4 and CD8 stimulates phosphorylation of the lck tyrosine protein kinase at the autophosphorylation site. *Mol Cell Biol* 1990;10:5305–5313.
23. Vignali DAA, Doyle C, Kinch MS, Shin J, Strominger JL. Interactions of CD4 with MHC class II molecules, T cell receptors and p56lck. *Philos Trans R Soc Lond B Biol Sci* 1993;342:13–24.
24. Mak TW, Rahemtulla A, Schilham M, Koh DR, Fung-Leung WP. Generation of mutant mice lacking surface expression of CD4 or CD8 gene targeting. *Adv Exp Med Biol* 1992;323:73–77.
25. Molina TJ, Kishihara K, Siderovski DP, et al. Profound block in thymocyte development in mice lacking p56lck. *Nature* 1992;357:161–164.
26. Nagata H, Ochiai K, Aotani Y, et al. Lymphostin (LK6-A), a novel immunosuppressant from *Streptomyces* sp. KY11783: taxonomy of the producing organism, fermentation, isolation and biological activities. *J Antibiot (Tokyo)* 1997;50:537–542.
27. Appleby MW, Gross JA, Cooke MP, Levin SD, Qian X, Perlmutter RM. Defective T cell receptor signaling in mice lacking the thymic isoform of p59fyn. *Cell* 1992;70:571–763.
28. Stein PL, Lee HM, Rich S, Soriano P. pp59fyn mutant mice display differential signaling in thymocytes and peripheral T cells. *Cell* 1992; 70:741–750.
29. Wange RL, Malek SN, Desiderio S, Samelson LE. Tandem SH2 domains of ZAP-70 bind to T cell antigen receptor zeta and CD3e from activated Jurkat T cells. *J Biol Chem* 1993;268:19797–19801.
30. van Oers NSC, Killeen N, Weiss A. ZAP-70 is constitutively associated with tyrosine-phosphorylated TCR ζ in murine thymocytes and lymph node T cells. *Immunity* 1994;1:675–685.
31. Chan AC, Kadlecek TA, Elder ME, et al. ZAP-70 deficiency in an autosomal recessive form of severe combined immunodeficiency. *Science* 1994;264:1599–1601.
32. Elder ME, Lin D, Clever J, et al. Human severe combined immunodeficiency due to a defect in ZAP-70, a T cell tyrosine kinase. *Science* 1994;264:1596–1599.
33. Arpaia E, Shahar M, Dadi H, Cohen A, Roifman CM. Defective T cell receptor signaling and CD8+ thymic selection in humans lacking zap-70 kinase. *Cell* 1994;76:947–958.
34. Mustelin T, Coggeshall KM, Altman A. Rapid activation of the T cell tyrosine protein kinase pp56lck by the CD45 phosphotyrosine phosphatase. *Proc Natl Acad Sci U S A* 1989;86:6302–6306.
35. Ostergaard HL, Trowbridge IS. Coclustering CD45 with CD4 or CD8 alters the phosphorylation and kinase activity of p56lck. *J Exp Med* 1990;172:347–350.
36. Kishihara K, Penninger J, Wallace VA, et al. Normal B lymphocyte development but impaired T cell maturation in CD45-exon 6 protein tyrosine phosphatase-deficient mice. *Cell* 1993;74:143–156.
37. August A, Gibson S, Kawakami Y, Kawakami T, Mills GB, Dupont B. CD28 is associated with and induces the immediate tyrosine phosphorylation and activation of the Tec family kinase ITK/EMT in the human Jurkat leukemic T cell line. *Proc Natl Acad Sci U S A* 1994;91:9347–9351.
38. Harding FA, McArthur JG, Gross JA, Raulet DH, Allison JP. CD28-mediated signalling co-stimulates murine T cells and prevents induction of anergy in T cell clones. *Nature* 1992;356:607–609.
39. June CH, Ledbetter JA, Linsley PS, Thompson CB. Role of the CD28 receptor in T cell activation. *Immunol Today* 1990;11:211–216.

40. Lu Y, Granelli-Piperno A, Bjorndahl JM, Phillips CA, Trevillyan JM. CD28-induced T cell activation: evidence for a protein-tyrosine kinase signal transduction pathway. *J Immunol* 1992;149:24–29.

41. Thompson CB, Lindsten T, Ledbetter JA, et al. CD28 activation pathway. *Proc Natl Acad Sci U S A* 1989;86:1333.

42. Daikh D, Wofsy D, Imboden JB. The CD28-B7 costimulatory pathway and its role in autoimmune disease. *J Leukoc Biol* 1997;62:156–162.

43. Onodera K, Chandraker A, Schaub M, et al. CD28-B7 T cell costimulatory blockade by CTLA4Ig in sensitized rat recipients: induction of transplantation tolerance in association with depressed cell-mediated and humoral immune responses. *J Immunol* 1997;159:1711–1717.

44. Kim HH, Tharayil M, Rudd CE. Growth factor receptor-bound protein: SH2/SH3 domain binding to CD28 and its role in co-signaling. *J Biol Chem* 1998;273:296–301.

45. Raab M, Heyeck SD, Bunnell SC, Cai YC, Berg LJ, Rudd CE. p56lck and p59fyn regulation of CD28 binding to PI 3-kinase, GRB-2 and ITK: implications for T cell anergy. *Proc Natl Acad Sci U S A* (*in press*).

46. Linsley PS, Brady W, Urnes M, Grosmaire LS, Damle NK, Ledbetter JA. CTLA-4 is a second receptor for the B cell activation antigen B7. *J Exp Med* 1991;174:561–569.

47. Tivol EA, Borriello F, Schweitzer AN, Lynch WP, Bluestone JA, Sharpe AH. Loss of CTLA-4 leads to massive lymphoproliferation and fatal multiorgan tissue destruction, revealing a critical negative regulatory role of CTLA-4. *Immunity* 1995;3:541–547.

48. Awata T, Kurihara S, Iitaka M, et al. Association of CTLA-4 gene A-G polymorphism (IDDM12 locus) with acute-onset and insulin-depleted IDDM as well as autoimmune thyroid disease (Graves' disease and Hashimoto's thyroiditis) in the Japanese population. *Diabetes* 1998;47:128–129.

49. Zhang Y, Allison JP. Interaction of CTLA-4 with AP50, a clathrin-coated pit adaptor protein. *Proc Natl Acad Sci U S A* 1997;94:9273–9278.

50. Fujii S, Tani T, Hada S, et al. Role of Ca2+ in the binding of phospholipase A2 with a monomeric substrate and with its amide-type analog. *J Biochem (Tokyo)* 1994;116:870–876.

51. Graves JD, Cantrell DA. An analysis of the role of guanine nucleotide binding proteins in antigen receptor/CD3 antigen coupling to phospholipase C. *J Immunol* 1991;146:2102–2107.

52. Marshall CJ. Specificity of receptor tyrosine kinase signaling: transient versus sustained extracellular signal-regulated kinase activation. *Cell* 1995;80:179–185.

53. Nel AE, Gupta S, Lee L, Ledbette RJA, Kanner SB. Ligation of the T-cell antigen receptor (TCR) induces association of hSos1, ZAP-70, phospholipase C-gamma 1, and other phosphoproteins with Grb2 and the zeta-chain of the TCR. *J Biol Chem* 1995;270:18428–18436.

54. Fischer MB, Wolf HM, Hauber I, et al. Activation via the antigen receptor is impaired in T cells, but not in B cells from patients with common variable immunodeficiency. *Eur J Immunol* 1996;26:231–237.

55. Jayaraman T, Ondriasova E, Ondrias K, Harnick DJ, Marks AR. The inositol 1,4,5-trisphosphate receptor is essential for T-cell receptor signaling. *Proc Natl Acad Sci U S A* 1995;92:6007–6011.

56. McCaffrey PG, Jain J, Jamieson C, Sen R, Rao A. A T cell nuclear factor resembling NF-AT binds to an NF-kappa-B site and to the conserved lymphokine promoter sequence "cytokine-1." *J Biol Chem* 1992;267:1864–1871.

57. Northrop JP, Ullman KS, Crabtree GR. Characterization of the nuclear and cytoplasmic components of the lymploid-specific nuclear factor of activated T cells (NF-AT) complex. *J Biol Chem* 1993;268:2917–2923.

58. Shevach EM. The effects of cyclosporin A on the immune system. *Annu Rev Immunol* 1985;3:397–423.

59. Bierer B. Cyclosporin A, FK506, and rapamycin: binding to immunophilins and biological action. *Chem Immunol* 1994;59:128–155.

60. Jenkins MK, Schwartz RH, Pardoll DM. Effects of cyclosporine A on T cell development and clonal deletion. *Science* 1988;241:1655–1658.

61. Kosugi A, Zuniga-Pflucker JC, Sharrow SO, Kruisbeek AM, Shearer GM. Effect of cyclosporin A on lymphopoiesis: II. Developmental defects of immature and mature thymocytes in fetal thymus organ cultures treated with cyclosporin A. *J Immunol* 1989;143:3134–3140.

62. Schreiber SL, Crabtree GR. The mechanism of action of cyclosporin A and FK506. *Immunol Today* 1992;13:136–142.

63. Takahashi N, Hayano T, Suzuki M. Peptidyl-prolyl cis-trans isomerase is the cyclosporin A-binding protein cyclophilin. *Nature* 1989;337:473–475.

64. Partiseti M, Le Deist F, Hivroz C, Fischer A, Korn H, Choquet D. The calcium current activated by T cell receptor and store depletion in human lymphocytes is absent in a primary immunodeficiency. *J Biol Chem* 1994;269:32327–32335.

65. Buday L, Egan SE, Viciana Rodriguez P, Cantrell DA, Downward J. A complex of Grb2 adaptor protein, Sos exchange factor, and a 36kDa membrane-bound tyrosine phosphoprotein is implicated in ras activation in T cells. *J Biol Chem* 1994;269:9019–9023.

66. Pumiglia K, Chow YH, Fabian J, Morrison D, Becker S, Jove R. Raf-1 N-terminal sequences necessary for Ras-Raf interaction and signal transduction. *Mol Cell Biol* 1995;15:398–406.

67. Skolnik EY, Lee CH, Batzer A, et al. The SH2/SH3 domain-containing protein GRB2 interacts with tyrosine-phosphorylated IRS1 and Shc: implications for insulin control of ras signalling. *EMBO J* 1993;12:1929–1936.

68. Stowers L, Yelon D, Berg LJ, Chant J. Regulation of the polarization of T cells toward antigen-presenting cells by Ras-related GTPase CDC42. *Proc Natl Acad Sci U S A* 1995;92:5027–5031.

69. Barinaga M. Cell biology: two major signaling pathways meet at MAP-kinase [news; comment]. *Science* 1995;269:1673.

70. Briscoe J, Guschin D, Muller M. Signal transduction: just another signalling pathway. *Curr Biol* 1994;4:1033–1035.

71. Edwards DR. Cell signalling and the control of gene transcription. *Trends Pharmacol Sci* 1994;15:239–244.

72. Ihle JN. The Janus kinase family and signaling through members of the cytokine receptor superfamily. *Proc Soc Exp Biol Med* 1994;206:268–272.

73. Taga T, Kishimoto T. Signaling mechanisms through cytokine receptors that share signal transducing receptor components. *Curr Opin Immunol* 1995;7:17–23.

74. Bazan JF. Structural design and molecular evolution of a cytokine receptor superfamily. *Proc Natl Acad Sci U S A* 1990;87:6934–6938.

75. Falus A. Cytokine receptor architecture, structure and genetic assembly. *Immunol Lett* 1995;44:221–223.

76. Taniguchi T. Cytokine signaling through nonreceptor protein tyrosine kinases. *Science* 1995;268:251–255.

77. Leonard WJ, Shores EW, Love PE. Role of the common cytokine receptor γ chain in cytokine signaling and lymphoid development. *Immunol Rev* 1996;148:97–114.

78. Ihle JN, Witthuhn BA, Quelle FW, et al. Signaling by the cytokine receptor superfamily: JAKs and STATs. *Trends Biochem Sci* 1994;19:222–227.

79. Beadling C, Guschin D, A. Witthuhn BA, et al. Activation of JAK kinases and STAT proteins by interleukin-2 and interferon alpha, but not the T cell antigen receptor, in human T lymphocytes. *EMBO J* 1994;13:5605–5615.

80. Beadling C, Ng J, Babbage JW, Cantrell DA. Interleukin-2 activation of STAT5 requires the convergent action of tyrosine kinases and a serine/threonine kinase pathway distinct from the Raf1/ERK2 MAP kinase pathway. *EMBO J* 1996;15:1902–1913.

81. Darnell JE, Kerr IM, Stark GR. Jak-STAT pathways and transcriptional activation in response to IFNs and other extracellular signaling proteins. *Science* 1994;264:1415–1421.

82. Hou J, Schindler U, Henzel WJ, Wong SC, McKnight SL. Identification and purification of human Stat proteins activated in response to interleukin-2. *Immunity* 1995;2:321–329.

83. Lin JX, Migone TS, Tsang M, et al. The role of shared receptor motifs and common Stat proteins in the generation of cytokine pleiotropy and redundancy by IL-2, IL-4, IL-7, IL-13, and IL-15. *Immunity* 1995;2:331–339.

84. Johnston JA, Kawamura M, Kirken RA, et al. Phosphorylation and activation of the JAK3 kinase in response to interleukin-2. *Nature* 1994;370:151–153.

85. Musso T, Johnston JA, Linnekan D, et al. Regulation of JAK3 expression in human monocytes: phosphorylation in response to interleukins 2, 4, and 7. *J Exp Med* 1995;181:1425–1431.

86. Russell SM, Johnston JA, Noguchi M, et al. Interaction of IL-2Rβ and γc chains with Jak1 and Jak3: implications for XSCID and XCID. *Science* 1994;266:1042–1045.

87. Witthuhn BA, Silvennoinen O, Miura O, et al. Involvement of the JAK3 Janus kinase in signalling by interleukins 2 and 4 in lymphoid and myeloid cells. *Nature* 1994;370:153–157.

88. Kawamura M, McVicar DW, Johnston JA, et al. Molecular cloning of L-JAK, a Janus family protein tyrosine kinase expressed in natural

killer cells and activated leukocytes. *Proc Natl Acad Sci U S A* 1994; 91:6374–6378.

89. Kirken RA, Rui H, Malabarba MG, Farrar WL. Identification of interleukin-2 receptor associated tyrosine kinase p116 as novel leukocyte-specific Janus kinase. *J Biol Chem* 1994;269:19136–19141.

90. Rane SG, Reddy EP. JAK3: a novel JAK kinase associated with terminal differentiation of hematopoietic cells. *Oncogene* 1994;9:2415–2423.

91. Thomis DC, Gurniak CB, Tivol E, Sharpe AH, Berg LJ. Defects in B lymphocyte maturation and T lymphocyte activation in mice lacking JAK3. *Science* 1995;270:794–797.

92. Macchi P, Villa A, Giliani S, et al. Mutations of JAK3 gene in patients with autosomal severe combined immune deficiency (SCID). *Nature* 1995;377:65–68.

93. Russell SM, Tayebi N, Nakajima H, et al. Mutation of JAK3 in a patient with SCID: essential role of JAK3 in lymphoid development. *Science* 1995;270:797–800.

94. Brooks EG, Schmalstieg FC, Wirt DP, et al. A novel X-linked combined immunodeficiency disease. *J Clin Invest* 1990;86:1623–1631.

95. Aman MJ, Leonard WJ. Cytokine signaling: cytokine-inducible signaling inhibitors. *Curr Biol* 1997;7:784–788.

96. Vassalli P. The pathophysiology of tumor necrosis factors. *Annu Rev Immunol* 1992;10:411–452.

97. Dinarello CA. Proinflammatory and anti-inflammatory cytokines as mediators in the pathogenesis of septic shock. *Chest* 1997;112: 321S–329S.

98. Eigler A, Sinha B, Hartmann G, Endres S. Taming TNF: strategies to restrain this proinflammatory cytokine. *Immunol Today* 1997;18: 487–492.

99. Tracey KJ, Cerami A. Tumor necrosis factor: a pleiotropic cytokine and therapeutic target. *Annu Rev Med* 1994;45:491–503.

100. Maini RN, Brennan FM, Williams R, et al. TNF-alpha in rheumatoid arthritis and prospects of anti-TNF therapy. *Clin Exp Rheumatol* 1993;11:S173–S175.

101. Feldmann M, Brennan FM, Williams R, Elliott MJ, Maini RN. Cytokine expression and networks in rheumatoid arthritis: rationale for anti-TNF alpha antibody therapy and its mechanism of action. *J Inflamm* 1995;47:90–96.

102. Golstein P. Cell death: TRAIL and its receptors. *Curr Biol* 1997;7: 750–753.

103. Nagata S, Suda T. Fas and fas ligand: lpr and gld mutations. *Immunol Today* 1995;16:39–43.

104. van Parijs L, Abbas AK. Role of Fas-mediated cell death in the regulation of immune responses. *Curr Opin Immunol* 1996;8: 355–361.

105. Bellgrau D, Gold D, Selawry H, Moore J, Franzusoff A, Duke RC. A role for CD95 ligand in preventing graft rejection. *Nature* 1995; 377:630–632.

106. Yamagami S, Kawashima H, Tsuru T, et al. Role of Fas-Fas ligand interactions in the immunorejection of allogeneic mouse corneal transplants. *Transplantation* 1997;64:1107–1011.

107. Schreiber SL. Chemistry and biology of the immunophilins and their immunosuppressive ligands. *Science* 1991;251:283–287.

108. Anonymous. Redesigning drug discovery. *Nature* 1996;384:1–5.

109. Chan AC, Iwashima M, Turck CW, Weiss A. ZAP-70: a 70-kDa protein-tyrosine kinase that associates with the TCR ζ chain. *Cell* 1992; 71:649–662.

110. Weiss A. T cell antigen receptor signal transduction: a tale of tails and cytoplasmic protein tyrosine kinases. *Cell* 1993;73:209–212.

111. Gardner CR. The pharmacology of immunosuppressant drugs in skin transplant rejection in mice and other rodents. *Gen Pharmacol* 1995; 26:245–271.

112. Gordon EM, Barrett RW, Dower WJ, Fodor SP, Gallop MA. Applications of combinatorial technologies to drug discovery: 2. Combinatorial organic synthesis, library screening strategies, and future directions. *J Med Chem* 1994;37:1385–1401.

113. Blundell TL. Structure-based drug design. *Nature* 1996;384:23–26.

114. Hubbard SR. Crystal structure of the activated insulin receptor tyrosine kinase in complex with peptide substrate and ATP analog. *Embo J* 1997;16:5572–5581.

115. Koide K, Bunnage ME, Gomez Paloma L, et al. Molecular design and biological activity of potent and selective protein kinase inhibitors related to balanol. *Chem Biol* 1995;2:601–608.

116. Xu W, Harrison SC, Eck MJ. Three-dimensional structure of the tyrosine kinase c-Src. *Nature* 1997;385:595–602.

Inflammation: Basic Principles and Clinical Correlates,
3rd ed., edited by John I. Gallin and Ralph Snyderman.
Lippincott Williams & Wilkins, Philadelphia © 1999.

CHAPTER 78

Second-Line Antirheumatic Drugs

Bruce N. Cronstein

Treatment of inflammatory diseases such as rheumatoid arthritis (RA) has changed dramatically over the past two decades, but all of the new drugs used to treat these diseases have been introduced empirically, without much understanding of their mechanisms of action. Perhaps the most successful antiinflammatory drugs introduced (or reintroduced) during the past two decades are methotrexate, sulfasalazine (reintroduced for the treatment of inflammatory arthritis although long in use as therapy for inflammatory bowel disease), and hydroxychloroquine (introduced and approved for use in the treatment of RA). In addition, azathioprine continues to be used extensively for the treatment of inflammatory disease. Of these agents methotrexate, given weekly in low doses (1 to 2 log orders lower than the doses used to treat malignancies), has been the most successful, and more is understood about its molecular mechanism of action than for the other agents listed. This chapter discusses the clinical uses and the mechanisms of action of methotrexate, sulfasalazine, hydroxychloroquine, and azathioprine (Fig. 78-1).

METHOTREXATE

Methotrexate was first developed as a folic acid antagonist for the treatment of malignancies, and it is a component of chemotherapy regimens used to treat a variety of solid tumors and leukemias. As an inhibitor of dihydrofolate reductase and the reactions that depend on reduced folate, methotrexate is a potent inhibitor of purine and pyrimidine synthesis required for cellular proliferation. In the treatment of malignancies, methotrexate is administered in very high doses; for patients with inflammatory diseases, the doses are 10- to 100-fold lower.

B. N. Cronstein: Department of Medicine, New York University Medical Center, New York, New York 10016.

Clinical Pharmacology

Methotrexate, in doses of 7.5 to 25 mg/week, is usually administered by the intramuscular or oral route to patients with inflammatory disease. Peak serum levels are achieved within a few hours; the main catabolic product is 7-hydroxymethotrexate, which possesses activity similar to that of the parent compound. Methotrexate and 7-hydroxymethotrexate compete with folic acid for active transport into cells, where the drug undergoes polyglutamation (1). The polyglutamated forms of methotrexate also retain activity, perhaps even greater than that of the parent compound, and they remain for extended periods within the intracellular compartment (2). Excretion of methotrexate is primarily renal; toxicity of methotrexate correlates best with decreased clearance of the compound rather than with peak serum levels (1).

The efficacy of methotrexate in the treatment of inflammatory arthritis has been proved in many studies conducted throughout the world (3–10). In general, a response to methotrexate is noted within weeks after administration of the drug begins, and if the drug is discontinued for any reason a flare usually follows within a few weeks. The drug maintains its antiinflammatory efficacy over time; at 5 years, significantly more patients are still receiving methotrexate therapy than other forms of antiinflammatory therapy (3,4,8,9). For most patients with inflammatory arthritis, methotrexate is combined with nonsteroidal antiinflammatory drugs (NSAIDs) or low doses of corticosteroids (usually 5 to 10 mg of prednisone or equivalent per day), or both. Combining methotrexate with other second-line antiinflammatory agents is a therapeutic strategy that is now being investigated with some success (11).

Toxicity of low-dose, weekly methotrexate in the treatment of inflammatory arthritis is less than was expected when its use was first proposed for the treatment of inflammatory arthritis. Alarcon (12) noted that there are four categories of methotrexate-induced toxicity: (a) adverse

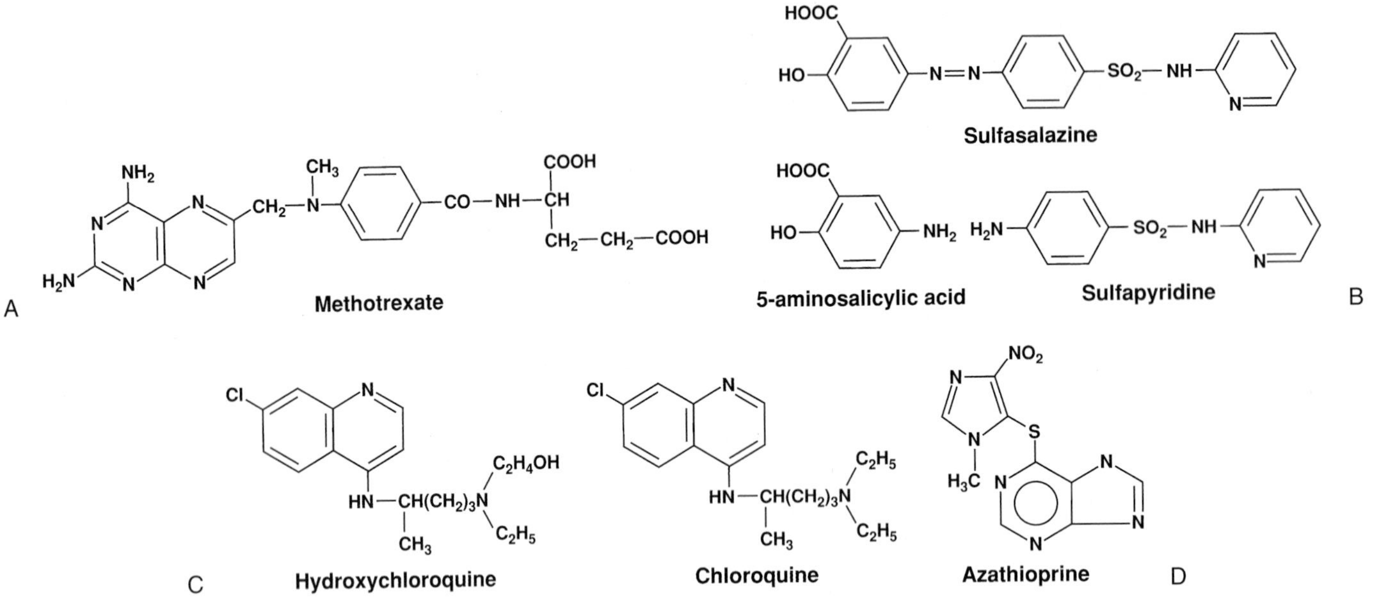

FIG. 78-1. Chemical structures of second-line antirheumatic drugs.

effects (e.g., macrocytic anemia, stomatitis), which can be alleviated by administration of the fully oxidized form of folate; (b) toxicities (e.g., moderate to severe bone marrow suppression) that are reversed by reduced folate (folinic acid); (c) idiosyncratic or allergic reactions (e.g., pneumonitis), which respond to discontinuation of the drug; and (d) irreversible toxicities, most notably hepatic fibrosis and cirrhosis.

A wide variety of methotrexate-induced toxicities have been described affecting nearly every system. The most common toxicities affect the gastrointestinal tract (nausea, stomatitis, dyspepsia and abdominal pain, diarrhea and gastrointestinal bleeding) and the hematopoietic system (macrocytic anemia and marrow suppression). The most feared toxicity of methotrexate is the development of hepatic fibrosis, cirrhosis, and liver failure. However, methotrexate-induced liver disease occurs rarely, one estimate being 1 case per 1,000 patients treated for 5 years (13). Methotrexate is an abortifacient and teratogen and should not be used in women who are contemplating pregnancy. Use of methotrexate may increase the incidence of opportunistic infections, although its effect on the incidence of serious infections is probably slight (12). Methotrexate is a cocarcinogen in animal studies, although no consistent increase in the rate of development of malignancies has been observed in patients treated for RA (12). The relation of methotrexate therapy to the development of lymphoproliferative malignancies is more problematic: patients with RA have a greater predilection to develop lymphomas, and the additional effect of methotrexate is difficult to assess. In some patients who were diagnosed with lymphoma while taking methotrexate, withdrawal of the drug led to regression of the lym-

phoma (14). One unexpected side effect of methotrexate therapy is nodulosis, the development of multiple rheumatoid nodules in the subcutaneous fascia or in the viscera (15,16). Nodulosis has also been reported to occur in patients with RA or juvenile RA (17,18). Although methotrexate, like all drugs, has its toxicity, the risk of toxicity is far lower than the benefits of this therapy.

As discussed previously, some of the toxicities observed in patients taking low-dose methotrexate can be reversed by either folic acid or folinic acid supplements. This observation led to trials of the prophylactic use of oral folic acid supplementation in patients taking methotrexate. Folic acid supplements were clearly shown to prevent methotrexate-induced toxicity, most notably stomatitis and macrocytic anemia, without diminishing the therapeutic efficacy of the drug, and folic acid supplements are now standard therapy for patients treated with methotrexate in the United States (19–21). Moderate daily doses of folinic acid, the reduced form of folic acid, formation of which is inhibited by methotrexate and its metabolites, also prevent methotrexate-induced toxicity without decreasing the beneficial effects of the drug. High doses of folinic acid administered at or near the time of administration of methotrexate diminish the effect of methotrexate on RA, but this may be a result of competitive inhibition of cellular uptake or polyglutamation of methotrexate rather than bypass of the metabolic block induced by methotrexate (22–29).

Mechanism of Action

The initial rationale for the use of low-dose methotrexate for the treatment of inflammatory arthritis was that methotrexate, by preventing synthesis of purines and pyrimidines required for cellular proliferation, would inhibit proliferation by the most rapidly dividing lymphocytes or other cells that putatively were responsible for the synovial inflammation. There is little evidence to support this hypothesis, and two different lines of evidence suggest that alternative mechanisms of action may better explain the antiinflammatory activity of methotrexate. First, inhibition of normal rapid proliferation of the cells of the gastrointestinal tract (stomatitis) or bone marrow (cytopenias) usually is an indication to stop or diminish the dose of methotrexate or to add folic acid or folinic acid to the therapeutic regimen. Second, addition of daily doses of folic acid or folinic acid to weekly methotrexate therapy prevents methotrexate-induced toxicity (cytopenias and stomatitis) but does not interfere with the antiinflammatory effect of the drug. Therefore, the beneficial effects of methotrexate in inflammatory disease may be mediated by mechanisms other than cytotoxicity caused by folate antagonism.

Phenomenology of the Antiinflammatory Effects

It is generally thought that T cells play a central role in the pathogenesis of RA and other inflammatory diseases, although specific therapy directed at modulation of cellular immunity has yielded disappointing results (30,31). There is very little evidence that methotrexate alters cellular immunity, either in patients or in experimental models of RA. Two groups have reported that there is no change in the concentration of immunoglobulin M (IgM) rheumatoid factor after successful methotrexate therapy; however, Alarcon et al., using a more sensitive assay, found a strong correlation between methotrexate therapy and diminished levels of rheumatoid factor (32–34). The effect of methotrexate on rheumatoid factor may be secondary (i.e., diminished inflammation provides less stimulus for the production of rheumatoid factor), although the correlation between rheumatoid factor levels and improvement in disease activity during methotrexate therapy is not as impressive as that between methotrexate therapy and diminished rheumatoid factor levels (33). Studies of the effect of methotrexate on *in vitro* rheumatoid factor production demonstrate a more consistent effect: methotrexate, at relatively high concentrations, inhibits rheumatoid factor production by stimulated peripheral blood mononuclear cells (35). Furthermore, Olsen et al. observed that treatment of patients with methotrexate was associated with diminished production of rheumatoid factor by their peripheral blood mononuclear cells cultured *ex vivo* (32). Although the effect of methotrexate therapy on rheumatoid factor production may be relevant to the drug's therapeutic effects in the treatment of RA, it probably is not relevant to the antiinflammatory effects of methotrexate in the treatment of such diseases as juvenile RA or inflammatory bowel disease.

Methotrexate therapy has been reported to affect the concentration or secretion of both lipid-derived and peptide inflammatory mediators. Sperling et al. reported that oral methotrexate inhibits secretion of leukotriene B$_4$ (LTB$_4$) by peripheral blood or synovial fluid neutrophils (36,37). This effect appears to be both indirect and specific, because incubation of neutrophils with methotrexate does not modulate subsequent LTB$_4$ secretion and there is no effect on synovial fluid monocyte LTB$_4$ production. Other reports have described the same or opposing effects (38,39). Nonetheless, inhibition of LTB$_4$ production probably does not account for the antiinflammatory effects of methotrexate, because similar reductions of synovial fluid LTB$_4$ concentration have been observed in patients treated with fish oil, a form of therapy that is much less effective than methotrexate in the treatment of RA (40).

Methotrexate has been reported to diminish the production of interleukin-1 (IL-1), the response to IL-1, or both, by an unknown mechanism (41–47). One group observed that methotrexate itself interferes with the binding of IL-1 to its receptor; however, it is difficult to understand how IL-1 receptor blockade of several hours' duration every week can diminish inflammation, since other agents known to block IL-1 receptors must be administered at least daily (48). *In vitro* studies of human and animal cells have demonstrated little direct effect of methotrexate on secretion of tumor necrosis factor-α (TNF-α), but methotrexate profoundly decreases synovial fluid concentrations of TNF-α in the adjuvant arthritis model of inflammatory arthritis (49). This effect has not been explored in patients with RA, although it is likely that there is a disparity between the effects of methotrexate on synovial fluid and on peripheral blood cytokine concentrations. Methotrexate has been reported to modulate levels of other inflammatory cytokines in fluids or cells from patients with RA; methotrexate therapy diminishes serum concentrations of IL-6 (50–53), increases IL-1 receptor antagonist and soluble TNF receptor levels (54), and diminishes IL-8 production by peripheral blood mononuclear cells but not synoviocytes (55,56).

Molecular Mechanisms

The antiinflammatory effects of methotrexate are best explained by two complementary hypotheses. One hypothesis, supported by *in vitro* and *in vivo* data, posits that chronic inflammation is associated with, and mediated in part by, accumulation of a variety of potentially toxic compounds (polyamines such as spermine and spermidine), the synthesis of which is inhibited by methotrexate therapy. An alternative hypothesis, also supported by *in vitro* and *in vivo* data, holds that methotrexate therapy leads to the enhanced release of an endogenous antiinflammatory compound, adenosine.

Methotrexate Inhibits Transmethylation Reactions

Methotrexate inhibits dihydrofolate reductase, an enzyme that reduces dihydrofolate to tetrahydrofolate, which, when N-methylated, donates a methyl group to homocysteine to form methionine. Methionine can be further converted to S-adenosyl-methionine (SAM), which acts as a methyl donor in a large number of cellular reactions (Fig. 78-2). In particular, SAM donates a methyl group during the synthesis of the polyamines spermine and spermidine. Increased polyamine concentrations are found in urine, synovial fluid, synovial tissue, and peripheral blood mononuclear cells from patients with RA (57–60). Monocytes metabolize polyamines to form, among other molecules, NH_3 and H_2O_2, which may be toxic to lymphocytes (59,60). When cultured *in vitro*, peripheral blood lymphocytes from RA patients secrete less IL-2 than cells from normal subjects, and this defect can be corrected by inhibitors of polyamine metabolism (59–62). The investigators inferred from these results that the lymphocytes were injured by the release of these toxic substances generated by the metabolism of the polyamines. Methotrexate prevents the synthesis of polyamines and thereby prevents the synthesis of the toxic agents. Although it is an attractive explanation for the effects of methotrexate on IL-2 production, this hypothesis essentially adds one more source of toxic agents to the inflamed synovium. But in the joints of patients with RA there are already large numbers of cells (neutrophils, monocytes) that are stimulated to produce large quantities of toxic oxygen metabolites, derivatives of nitric oxide, and other injurious substances.

In support of the hypothesis that the antiinflammatory action of methotrexate results from diminished accumulation of polyamines, Nesher et al. (63) noted that methotrexate inhibited the production of IgM rheumatoid factor by cultured peripheral blood mononuclear cells. Folinic acid, methionine, and spermidine all reversed the effect of methotrexate on IgM rheumatoid factor production, suggesting that the folinic acid–dependent accumulation of polyamines was responsible for the production of IgM rheumatoid factor and that the capacity of methotrexate to diminish IgM rheumatoid factor production was mediated by the inhibition of polyamines. In a subsequent study this same group demonstrated that methotrexate inhibited monocyte function and that the effect of methotrexate was reversed by SAM and folinic acid (but not by spermidine) (64). Although the concentrations of methotrexate required to inhibit polyamine synthesis were high in these studies, probably higher than those achieved with low-dose weekly methotrexate administration, these data do tend to support the hypothesis that inhibition of transmethylation reactions contributes to the antiinflammatory effect of methotrexate in RA. An agent that inhibits transmethylation reactions, 3-deazaadenosine, showed some promise as an antiinflammatory drug in *in vitro* and *in vivo* studies (65–72). The drug was administered to patients with RA, and evidence was published to indicate that transmethylation reactions were indeed inhibited (66). Apparently the drug was not an effective antiinflammatory agent in these patients with RA, although no further reports of its efficacy have appeared in the literature.

Increased Extracellular Adenosine Concentrations Mediate the Antiinflammatory Effects of Methotrexate

Methotrexate and its major metabolite, 7-hydroxymethotrexate, are taken up by cells and polyglutamated (2). Methotrexate polyglutamates are even more active than the parent drug as inhibitors of a variety of folate-dependent enzymes, but the enzyme inhibited most effectively by methotrexate polyglutamates is 5-aminoimidazole-4-carboxamide ribonucleotide (AICAR) transformylase (73,74) (Fig. 78-3). The inhibition of AICAR transformylase could lead to intracellular accumulation of AICAR. Because AICAR inhibits adenosine monophosphate (AMP) deaminase and its dephosphorylated metabolite (AICARiboside) directly inhibits adenosine deaminase, AICAR accumulation could lead to the

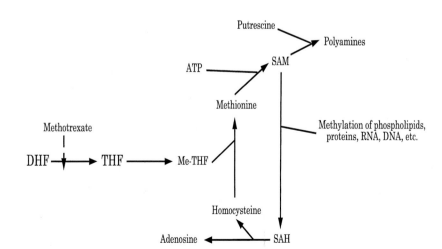

FIG. 78-2. Methotrexate inhibits transmethylation reactions required for synthesis of polyamines and methylation reactions. DHF, dihydrofolic acid; THF, tetrahydrofolic acid (folinic acid); Me, methyl; SAM, S-adenosylmethionine; SAH, S-adenosyl-homocysteine.

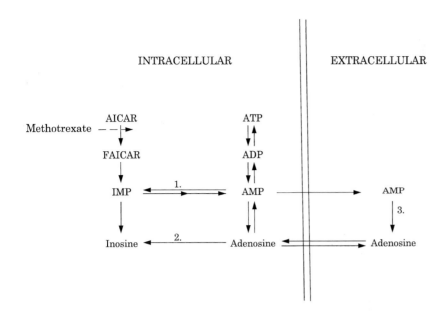

FIG. 78-3. Methotrexate promotes adenosine release: potential sites of action. AICAR, aminoimidazolecarboxamide ribonucleotide; FAICAR, formyl-AICAR; IMP, inosine monophosphate; 1., adenosine monophosphate (AMP) deaminase; 2., adenosine deaminase; 3., ecto-5′ nucleotidase.

release of AMP (which may be dephosphorylated to adenosine) or of adenosine, or both (74,75). In previous studies, patients taking large doses of methotrexate for the treatment of cancer excreted increased concentrations of aminoimidazolecarboxamide in their urine, consistent with the notion that AICAR accumulates intracellularly in patients treated with methotrexate (76).

The demonstration by Gruber et al. (77) that intracellular AICAR accumulation (induced by infusion of AICARiboside) is associated with increased adenosine release *in vivo* and the earlier observation that adenosine is a potent antiinflammatory autocoid suggested the hypothesis that adenosine might mediate the antiinflammatory effects of methotrexate treatment. In support of this hypothesis, it was found that treatment of endothelial cells and fibroblasts with methotrexate promoted release of adenosine (78), particularly after exposure to a noxious stimulus (stimulated neutrophils). The adenosine released from these cells was both necessary and sufficient to diminish the interaction of stimulated neutrophils with the methotrexate-treated cells, a surrogate antiinflammatory effect. In subsequent studies in a murine model of acute inflammation, treatment of mice with pharmacologically relevant doses of methotrexate induced intracellular AICAR accumulation, increased adenosine concentrations in inflammatory exudates, and diminished leukocyte accumulation at an inflamed site (79). Adenosine mediated the inhibition of leukocyte accumulation, since the addition of adenosine deaminase reversed the antiinflammatory effects of methotrexate. Identical observations of the effects of methotrexate-induced adenosine release on leukocyte extravasation were made by Asako et al. in a different animal model of inflammation (80). These studies clearly demonstrate that the antiinflammatory effects of methotrexate in these models of inflammation are mediated by adenosine.

A large number of antiinflammatory effects of adenosine and adenosine receptor agonists have been described, all of which appear to be mediated via occupancy of adenosine receptors on the surface of inflammatory cells. There are four different adenosine receptor subtypes (A_1, A_{2A}, A_{2B}, A_3); all are members of the family of seven transmembrane spanning receptors related to the adrenergic receptors (81). Adenosine, via interaction with A_{2A} receptors, inhibits stimulated neutrophil adhesion, generation of toxic oxygen metabolites, phagocytosis, and neutrophil-mediated cell injury (82–87). Adenosine also inhibits lymphocyte proliferation and induces suppressor function and phenotype (88–93). Occupancy of adenosine A_3 receptors on monocytes inhibits production of cytokines (TNF-α, IL-6, and IL-8) and enhances release of the antiinflammatory cytokine IL-10 (94–100). Adenosine, acting at A_{2B} receptors, inhibits synoviocyte collagenase production without affecting production of either stromelysin or tissue inhibitor of metalloprotease (101). Various adenosine receptor agonists are antiinflammatory in animal models. In the early studies, A_1 adenosine receptor agonists were found to be the most antiinflammatory; later studies suggested that the effects of A_1 receptor agonists are mediated through the central nervous system (CNS) and CNS-stimulated release of adenosine in the inflamed tissues (102).

Corroborating evidence that methotrexate therapy induces adenosine release in patients and that adenosine mediates some of the antiinflammatory effects of methotrexate has been published. As noted, patients treated with methotrexate excrete increased quantities of aminoimidazolecarboxamide in their urine (76). Bernini et al. (103) reported that children treated with methotrexate for leukemia had higher adenosine concentrations in their cerebrospinal fluid, and the highest concentrations were observed in those patients who exhibited CNS toxicity (lethargy and coma). In those patients with CNS toxicity, administration of an adenosine receptor antagonist rapidly reversed the toxicity, indicating that the adenosine released into the CNS is sufficient to occupy adenosine receptors in such a way as to lead to functional changes.

In addition to the beneficial effects of methotrexate therapy, adenosine, acting via its cell surface receptors, may also account for some of methotrexate's toxicity. Methotrexate causes mild, reversible renal dysfunction which is thought to be vascular in origin (104), and adenosine acting at A_1 receptors in the kidney is a renal vasoconstrictor (105) capable of inducing the changes observed in patients taking methotrexate. From 8% to 11% of patients with RA treated with methotrexate develop nodulosis, with an increased number of subcutaneous rheumatoid nodules, despite good control of synovial inflammation (15,16). Studies by Merrill et al. (106) indicate that methotrexate promotes release of adenosine from macrophages *in vitro*, and the released adenosine occupies macrophage A_1 adenosine receptors to promote nodule formation.

SULFASALAZINE

Of the drugs considered in this chapter, sulfasalazine is the only one designed specifically for the treatment of RA (107). It was introduced in the 1940s but was dropped as an antirheumatic drug despite early reports of good responses to therapy after publication of a single small study, the results of which did not support the previous demonstrations of therapeutic efficacy (108). Sulfasalazine was reintroduced in 1980 for the treatment of inflammatory arthritis and it is now accepted as effective therapy for both seronegative and seropositive arthritis. It is clear that the metabolite 5-aminosalicylate is the active agent in the therapy of inflammatory bowel disease, because administration of 5-aminosalicylate (Fig. 78-1*B*) yields similar therapeutic benefits. The active metabolite in the treatment of inflammatory arthritis appears to be sulfapyridine (109–112), although this is less well established. The antibiotic effects of sulfasalazine or sulfapyridine (Fig. 78-1*B*) probably are not involved in the antiinflammatory effects of the drug (113), although the actual mechanism of action is not fully understood.

Clinical Pharmacology

After oral administration of sulfasalazine, only 10% to 20% of the administered dose is taken up intact, although there is much individual variation (114). Some of the absorbed sulfasalazine reenters the colon as a result of biliary excretion; most of the rest is excreted in the urine. In the gut, most of the remainder of the sulfazine is metabolized by the intestinal bacteria to sulfapyridine and 5-aminosalicylate. Sulfapyridine is well absorbed, and measurable sulfapyridine concentrations are present

in the circulation. Only 20% to 30% of the 5-aminosalicylic acid generated in the gut is absorbed; 5-aminosalicylic acid is acetylated and excreted in the urine.

In general sulfasalazine is a safe drug, and most of its toxicity is reversed on discontinuation of the drug. Two broad categories of sulfasalazine-mediated toxicity occur, however. Dose-related toxicity includes nausea, vomiting, headache, malaise, methemoglobinemia, and hemolytic anemia. Hypersensitivity or idiosyncratic reactions include rash (including Stevens-Johnson syndrome), aplastic anemia, and autoimmune hemolysis. These latter reactions tend to occur early in the course of therapy (115).

Sulfasalazine has been used extensively as therapy for inflammatory bowel disease, but the drug has received renewed attention during the past two decades as an antirheumatic agent. Although sulfasalazine is effective in RA, it has received particular attention for treatment of the seronegative spondyloarthropathies (psoriatic arthritis, Reiter's syndrome, and the peripheral arthritis associated with ankylosing spondylitis) (116–118). Although inflammatory arthritis has always been treated with combinations of drugs (e.g., NSAIDs plus steroids or a second-line antiinflammatory agent, or both), it has recently become more acceptable to combine second-line antiinflammatory agents such as methotrexate and sulfasalazine to maximize therapeutic response and, presumably, diminish the toxic effects of the individual drugs (11).

Mechanism of Action

The search for a mechanism of action for sulfasalazine has been hindered by ignorance of the active agent involved. As noted, it is not entirely clear whether sulfasalazine or its metabolites, sulfapyridine and 5-aminosalicylic acid, mediate the antiinflammatory effects of sulfasalazine therapy. In the treatment of inflammatory bowel disease, 5-aminosalicylic acid is probably the active agent, because 5-aminosalicylic acid is as effective therapeutically as sulfasalazine. Although it has been proposed that alteration of gut flora by sulfasalazine contributes to the antiinflammatory effects of the drug, there is no evidence to support this contention. Sulfasalazine diminishes total immunoglobulin and rheumatoid factor levels in the circulation and inhibits T-cell and B-cell proliferation (119–121). Others have reported that sulfasalazine diminishes binding of TNF to its receptor (perhaps by binding to TNF itself) and decreases TNF production (121–123). Sulfasalazine (but not sulfapyridine) inhibits folate metabolism and, like methotrexate, inhibits AICAR transformylase (see previous discussion). As with methotrexate, sulfasalazine (but not sulfapyridine or 5-aminosalicylic acid) causes intracellular AICAR accumulation in experimental animals that is associated with enhanced adenosine release, and increased adenosine concentrations in the inflammatory exudates of sulfasalazine-treated animals mediates the antiinflammatory effects of oral sulfasalazine (124,125). The effects of sulfasalazine on purine release are noted at doses somewhat higher than those commonly used to treat patients.

ANTIMALARIALS (HYDROXYCHLOROQUINE AND CHLOROQUINE)

The synthesis and trial of new and effective antimalarial drugs during and after the second world war led to the anecdotal observation that patients with systemic lupus erythematosus (SLE) improved while taking quinacrine. Subsequently the safer, better-tolerated antimalarial agents chloroquine and hydroxychloroquine were introduced and shown to be effective antirheumatic agents (126). These agents were introduced empirically with no understanding of their mechanism of action, and not much greater insight was gained during the subsequent half century. Currently, hydroxychloroquine is the favored antimalarial; it is used in the treatment of discoid lupus erythematosus, SLE, and RA (127).

Clinical Pharmacology

Both chloroquine and hydroxychloroquine are rapidly but variably absorbed from the gastrointestinal tract and, after appearing in the circulation for 1 to 3 hours, are ultimately concentrated in the tissues. In particular, the antimalarial agents deposit in pigmented tissues such as melanocytes and retinal cells. Although some chloroquine and hydroxychloroquine (Fig. 78-1C) is lost in the urine, the tissue-associated drug is excreted at a much slower rate, with a half-life estimated to be 45 days. Initially relatively high doses of chloroquine and hydroxychloroquine (10 to 15 mg/kg per day) were administered to patients, but at these high doses deposition in the retina was noted with a number of reports of delayed retinopathy. Subsequently, lower doses (6 to 7 mg/kg per day) were found to be effective as antiinflammatory agents, and there was a marked reduction in the incidence of retinopathy (128).

In general, chloroquine and hydroxychloroquine exhibit relatively little toxicity as they are used to treat inflammatory disorders. However, retinopathy with blindness has been reported, primarily in patients receiving chloroquine in high daily doses (>500 mg/day), and the retinopathy may progress even after the drug has been discontinued. It is thought that chloroquine is more toxic than hydroxychloroquine. Although the actual incidence of retinopathy remains controversial, the potential for serious ocular toxicity has mandated close monitoring of patients taking hydroxychloroquine. Other toxicities include a vacuolar myopathy, rashes, neuropathy, leukopenia, and aplastic anemia (128).

Mechanism of Action

The antiinflammatory effects of antimalarials are not well understood. These agents have been reported to

inhibit production of cytokines (TNF-α, IL-1, and interferon-γ) (129–131), production of oxidants by neutrophils (132), phospholipase A_1 activity, and DNA polymerase (131). Perhaps the best explanation for the antiinflammatory action of these drugs is their capacity to buffer the acidic pH in lysosomes. The antimalarials are lipophilic agents that are taken up by cells and may be concentrated in lysosomes. By raising the pH in the lysosomes, a variety of reactions important for immunologic and inflammatory responses may be altered. Most notably, antigen processing and presentation by macrophages may be affected, resulting in modulation of immunologic responses. No critical demonstration of this hypothesis has yet been reported (131).

AZATHIOPRINE

6-Mercaptopurine (6-MP) was introduced for the treatment of malignant disease in the 1950s and was reported to be useful for autoimmune diseases in the 1960s. Azathioprine is the result of research directed at developing an orally available, more slowly metabolized form of 6-MP. Originally widely used for prevention of rejection in patients receiving transplants, its effectiveness has also been demonstrated in the treatment of RA and SLE (114).

Clinical Pharmacology

Azathioprine is taken up well from the gastrointestinal tract and is metabolized to the active compound, 6-MP, in the liver. Because 6-MP is metabolized to 6-thiouric acid by xanthine oxidase, azathioprine and its active agent accumulate in patients taking allopurinol, which inhibits xanthine oxidase. Although the drug is metabolized primarily in the liver, the effects of liver disease on azathioprine and 6-MP metabolism are not consistent; some patients accumulate toxic levels of the drug and its active metabolite, and others do not (133).

Azathioprine has been approved by the U.S. Food and Drug Administration for the treatment of RA. Usually it is given at a dose of 1.25 to 2.5 mg/kg per day. Like all of the drugs discussed in this chapter, azathioprine has a slow onset of action. Azathioprine is probably as effective as methotrexate in the treatment of RA, and the number of adverse events is probably similar. Early studies demonstrated that azathioprine is effective in the treatment of SLE, and subsequent reports appear to confirm the impression that azathioprine plus corticosteroids is better than corticosteroids alone in the prevention of end-stage renal disease in SLE patients. However, azathioprine appears to be less effective than cyclophosphamide for the treatment of SLE. Other studies demonstrate that azathioprine is useful in the treatment of inflammatory muscle disease and may also be useful for psoriasis, psoriatic arthritis, and various vasculitides (133).

Although azathioprine is generally well tolerated, it does lead to a variety of toxic reactions. Bone marrow toxicity (pancytopenia, leukopenia, thrombocytopenia, or severe anemia) is common in patients treated with azathioprine. Similarly, nausea, vomiting, and epigastric pain frequently accompany azathioprine therapy. Liver toxicity ranges from mild liver enzyme abnormalities to, rarely, fibrosis and cirrhosis. Although there are reports of pregnancies carried to term without complication despite azathioprine therapy, it is best to counsel patients to avoid pregnancy while taking this drug. Azathioprine therapy has been associated with development of lymphomas in transplantation patients, but it has been difficult to document a marked increase in the incidence of lymphomas, or malignancies in general, in RA patients treated with azathioprine.

Mechanism of Action

As with most of the other drugs discussed here, the mechanism by which azathioprine suppresses inflammation is not totally clear. The drug has immunosuppressive properties when studied *in vitro*, including suppression of natural killer cell activity, antibody production, antibody-dependent cellular cytotoxicity, and cellular immune responses. It has been much more difficult to demonstrate immunosuppressive effects *in vivo*, although azathioprine therapy suppresses autoantibody production in animal models of SLE and diminishes rheumatoid factor levels in patients with RA (this effect may be nonspecific). The active agent, 6-MP, is metabolized by hypoxanthine phosphoribosyl transferase to 6-thioIMP (inosine monophosphate), accumulation of which suppresses the interconversion of inosine monophosphate to AMP and guanosine monophosphate that is required for generation of RNA and DNA. 6-MP may also be incorporated into RNA and DNA as 6-thioguanine (134).

CONCLUSION

The treatment of RA, SLE, and other inflammatory diseases has undergone a marked change in the past two decades, in large part as a result of the introduction or reintroduction of second-line agents for the treatment of these inflammatory diseases. These effective therapeutic agents were introduced empirically, and, despite great advances in our understanding of the molecular pathogenesis of inflammation, for the most part little insight into their mechanisms of action has been added over the years. Improvement in the understanding of the molecular mechanisms of action of these drugs should allow us to maximize the antiinflammatory efficacy of the currently available second-line antirheumatic drugs and to design new agents for the treatment of inflammatory diseases.

REFERENCES

1. Furst DE. Practical clinical pharmacology and drug interactions of low-dose methotrexate therapy in rheumatoid arthritis [review]. *Br J Rheum* 1995;34(Suppl 2):20–25.
2. Chabner BA, Allegra CJ, Curt GA, et al. Polyglutamation of methotrexate: is methotrexate a prodrug? *J Clin Invest* 1985;76:907–912.
3. Weinblatt ME, Weissman BN, Holdsworth DE, et al. Long-term prospective study of methotrexate in the treatment of rheumatoid arthritis: 84-month update. *Arthritis Rheum* 1992;35:129–137.
4. Kremer JM, Phelps CT. Long-term prospective study of the use of methotrexate in the treatment of rheumatoid arthritis: update after a mean of 90 months. *Arthritis Rheum* 1992;35:138–145.
5. Weinblatt ME, Coblyn JS, Fox DA, et al. Efficacy of low-dose methotrexate in rheumatoid arthritis. *N Engl J Med* 1985;312:818–822.
6. Williams HJ, Wilkens RF, Samuelson CO Jr, et al. Comparison of low-dose oral pulse methotrexate and placebo in the treatment of rheumatoid arthritis: a controlled clinical trial. *Arthritis Rheum* 1985;28:721–730.
7. Weinblatt ME, Kaplan H, Germain BF, et al. Low-dose methotrexate compared with auranofin in adult rheumatoid arthritis: a thirty-six-week, double-blind trial. *Arthritis Rheum* 1990;33:330–338.
8. Kremer JM, Lee JK. The safety and efficacy of the use of methotrexate in long-term therapy for rheumatoid arthritis. *Arthritis Rheum* 1986;29:822–831.
9. Wein Flatt ME, Trentham DE, Fraser PA, et al. Long-term prospective trial of low-dose methotrexate in rheumatoid arthritis. *Arthritis Rheum* 1988;31:167–175.
10. Wein Flatt ME, Kaplan H, Germain BF, et al. Methotrexate in rheumatoid arthritis: effects on disease activity in a multicenter prospective study. *J Rheumatol* 1991;18:334–338.
11. O'Dell JR, Haire CE, Erikson N, et al. Treatment of rheumatoid arthritis with methotrexate alone, sulfasalazine and hydroxychloroquine, or a combination of all three medications. *N Engl J Med* 1996;334:1287–1291.
12. Alarcon GS. Methotrexate: its use for the treatment of rheumatoid arthritis and other rheumatic disorders. In: Koopman WJ, ed. *Arthritis and allied conditions: a textbook of rheumatology.* Baltimore: Williams & Wilkins, 1997:679–698.
13. Kremer JM, Lee RG, Toman C. Liver histology in rheumatoid arthritis patients receiving long-term methotrexate therapy: a prospective study with baseline and sequential biopsy samples. *Arthritis Rheum* 1989;32:121–127.
14. Moder KG, Tefferi A, Cohen MD, Menke DM, Luthra HS. Hematologic malignancies and the use of methotrexate in rheumatoid arthritis: a retrospective study [review]. *Am J Med* 1995;99:276–281.
15. Combe B, Didry D, Gutierrez M, Anaya JM, Sany J. Accelerated nodulosis and systemic manifestations during methotrexate therapy for rheumatoid arthritis. *Eur J Med* 1993;2:153–156.
16. Kerstens PJ, Boerbooms AM, Jeurissen ME, Fast JH, Assmann KJ, van de Putte LB. Accelerated nodulosis during low dose methotrexate therapy for rheumatoid arthritis: an analysis of ten cases. *J Rheum* 1992;19:867–871.
17. Falcini F, Taccetti G, Ermini M, et al. Methotrexate-associated appearance and rapid progression of rheumatoid nodules in systemic-onset juvenile rheumatoid arthritis [review]. *Arthritis Rheum* 1997;40:175–178.
18. Muzaffer MA, Schneider R, Cameron BJ, Silverman ED, Laxer RM. Accelerated nodulosis during methotrexate therapy for juvenile rheumatoid arthritis. *J Pediatr* 1996;128:698–700.
19. Morgan SL, Baggott JE, Vaughn WH, et al. Supplementation with folic acid during methotrexate therapy for rheumatoid arthritis: a double-blind, placebo-controlled trial. *Ann Intern Med* 1994;121:833–841.
20. Dijkmans BA. Folate supplementation and methotrexate [review]. *Br J Rheum* 1995;34:1172–1174.
21. Morgan SL, Alarcon GS, Krumdieck CL. Folic acid supplementation during methotrexate therapy: it makes sense [editorial]. *J Rheumatol* 1993;20:929–930.
22. Wein Flatt ME, Maier AL, Coblyn JS. Low dose leucovorin does not interfere with the efficacy of methotrexate in rheumatoid arthritis: an 8 week randomized placebo controlled trial. *J Rheumatol* 1993;20:950–952.
23. Shiroky JB, Neville C, Esdaile JM, et al. Low-dose methotrexate with

leucovorin (folinic acid) in the management of rheumatoid arthritis: results of a multicenter randomized, double-blind, placebo-controlled trial [see comments]. *Arthritis Rheum* 1993;36:795–803.

24. Joyce DA, Will RK, Hoffman DM, Laing B, Blackbourn SJ. Exacerbation of rheumatoid arthritis in patients treated with methotrexate after administration of folinic acid. *Ann Rheum Dis* 1991;50:913–914.

25. Buckley LM, Vacek PM, Cooper SM. Administration of folinic acid after low dose methotrexate in patients with rheumatoid arthritis [see comments]. *J Rheumatol* 1990;17:1158–1161.

26. Hanrahan PS, Russell AS. Concurrent use of folinic acid and methotrexate in rheumatoid arthritis. *J Rheumatol* 1988;15:1078–1080.

27. Polk JR. Beneficial effects of leucovorin after methotrexate treatment in rheumatoid arthritis: a case report [letter]. *Arthritis Rheum* 1988; 31:1587–1588.

28. Tishler M, Caspi D, Fishel B, Yaron M. The effects of leucovorin (folinic acid) on methotrexate therapy in rheumatoid arthritis patients. *Arthritis Rheum* 1988;31:906–908.

29. Shiroky J, Allegra C, Inghirami G, Chabner B, Yarboro C, Klippel JH. High dose intravenous methotrexate with leucovorin rescue in rheumatoid arthritis. *J Rheumatol* 1988;15:251–255.

30. Moreland LW, Pratt PW, Mayes MD, et al. Double-blind, placebo-controlled multicenter trial using chimeric monoclonal anti-CD4 antibody, cM-T412, in rheumatoid arthritis patients receiving concomitant methotrexate. *Arthritis Rheum* 1995;38:1581–1588.

31. van der Lubbe PA, Dijkmans BA, Markusse HM, Nassander U, Breedveld FC. A randomized, double-blind, placebo-controlled study of CD4 monoclonal antibody therapy in early rheumatoid arthritis. *Arthritis Rheum* 1995;38:1097–1106.

32. Olsen NJ, Callahan LF, Pincus T. Immunologic studies of rheumatoid arthritis patients treated with methotrexate. *Arthritis Rheum* 1987;30: 481–488.

33. Alarcon GS, Schrohenloher RE, Bartolucci AA, Ward JR, Williams HJ, Koopman WJ. Suppression of rheumatoid factor production by methotrexate in patients with rheumatoid arthritis. Arthritis Rheum 1990;33:1156–1161.

34. Spadaro A, Riccieri V, Sili Scavalli A, Taccari E, Zoppini A. One year treatment with low dose methotrexate in rheumatoid arthritis: effect on class specific rheumatoid factors. *Clin Rheum* 1993;12:357–360.

35. Nesher G, Moore TL. The *in vitro* effects of methotrexate on peripheral blood mononuclear cells: modulation by methyl donors and spermidine. *Arthritis Rheum* 1990;33:954–959.

36. Sperling RI, Coblyn JS, Larkin JK, Benincaso AI, Austen KF, Wein Flatt ME. Inhibition of leukotriene B4 synthesis in neutrophils from patients with rheumatoid arthritis by a single oral dose of methotrexate. *Arthritis Rheum* 1990;33:1149–1155.

37. Sperling RI, Benincaso AI, Anderson RJ, Coblyn JS, Austen KF, Wein Flatt ME. Acute and chronic suppression of leukotriene B4 synthesis *ex vivo* in neutrophils from patients with rheumatoid arthritis beginning treatment with methotrexate. Arthritis Rheum 1992;35:376–384.

38. Leroux JL, Damon M, Chavis C, rastes de Paulet A, Blotman F. Effects of a single dose of methotrexate on 5- and 12-lipoxygenase products in patients with rheumatoid arthritis. *J Rheum* 1992;19:863–866.

39. Hawkes JS, Cleland LG, Proudman SM, James MJ. The effect of methotrexate on *ex vivo* lipoxygenase metabolism in neutrophils from patients with rheumatoid arthritis. *J Rheum* 1994;21:55–58.

40. Kremer JM. The mechanism of action of methotrexate in rheumatoid arthritis: the search continues. *J Rheumatol* 1994;21:1–5.

41. Chang DM, Baptiste P, Schur PH. The effect of antirheumatic drugs on interleukin 1 (IL-1) activity and IL-1 and IL-1 inhibitor production by human monocytes. *J Rheumatol* 1990;17:1148–1157.

42. Hu SK, Mitcho YL, Oronsky AL, Kerwar SS. Studies on the effect of methotrexate on macrophage function. *J Rheumatol* 1988;15:206–209.

43. Segal R, Mozes E, Yaron M, Tartakovsky B. The effects of methotrexate on the production and activity of Il-1. Arthritis Rheum 1989; 32:370–377.

44. Chang DM, Wein Flatt ME, Schur PH. The effects of methotrexate on interleukin 1 in patients with rheumatoid arthritis. *J Rheumatol* 1992; 19:1678–1682.

45. Segal R, Yaron M, Tartakovsky B. Rescue of interleukin-1 activity by leucovorin following inhibition by methotrexate in a murine *in vitro* system. *Arthritis Rheum* 1990;33:1745–1748.

46. Segal R, Mozes E, Yaron M, Tartakovsky B. The effects of methotrexate on the production and activity of interleukin-1. *Arthritis Rheum* 1989;32:370–377.

47. Connolly KM, Stecher VJ, Danis E, Pruden DJ, La Frie T. Alteration of interleukin-1 production and the acute phase response following medication of adjuvant arthritic rats with cyclosporin-A or methotrexate. *Int J Pharmacol* 1988;10:717–728.

48. Brody M, Bohm I, Bauer R. Mechanism of action of methotrexate: experimental evidence that methotrexate blocks the binding of interleukin 1 beta to the interleukin 1 receptor on target cells. *Eur J Clin Chem Clin Biochem* 1993;31:667–674.

49. Smith-Oliver T, Noel LS, Stimpson SS, Yarnall DP, Connolly KM. Elevated levels of TNF in the joints of adjuvant arthritic rats. *Cytokine* 1993;5:298–304.

50. Lacki JK, Klama K, Mackiewicz SH, Mackiewicz U, Muller W. Circulating interleukin-10 and interleukin-6 serum levels in rheumatoid arthritis patients treated with methotrexate or gold salts: preliminary report. *Inflamm Res* 1995;44:24–26.

51. Crilly A, McInness IB, McDonald AG, Watson J, Capell HA, Madhok R. Interleukin 6 (IL-6) and soluble IL-2 receptor levels in patients with rheumatoid arthritis treated with low dose oral methotrexate. *J Rheumatol* 1995;22:224–226.

52. Barrera P, Boerbooms AM, Janssen EM, et al. Circulating soluble tumor necrosis factor receptors, interleukin-2 receptors, tumor necrosis factor alpha, and interleukin-6 levels in rheumatoid arthritis: longitudinal evaluation during methotrexate and azathioprine therapy [see comments]. *Arthritis Rheum* 1993;36:1070–1079.

53. Barrera P, Haagsma CJ, Boerbooms AMT, et al. Effect of methotrexate alone or in combination with sulphasalazine on the production and circulating concentrations of cytokines and their antagonists: longitudinal evaluation in patients with rheumatoid arthritis. *Br J Rheum* 1995;34:747–755.

54. Seitz M, Loetscher P, Dewald B, et al. Methotrexate action in rheumatoid arthritis: stimulation of cytokine inhibitor and inhibition of chemokine production by peripheral blood mononuclear cells. *Br J Rheum* 1995;34:602–609.

55. Seitz M, Dewald B, Ceska M, Gerber N, Baggiolini M. Interleukin-8 in inflammatory rheumatic diseases: synovial fluid levels, relation to rheumatoid factors, production by mononuclear cells, and effects of gold sodium thiomalate and methotrexate. *Rheum Int* 1992;12:159–164.

56. Loetscher P, Dewald B, Baggiolini M, Seitz M. Monocyte chemoattractant protein 1 and interleukin 8 production by rheumatoid synoviocytes: effects of anti-rheumatic drugs. *Cytokine* 1994;6:162–170.

57. Furumitsu Y, Yukioka K, Kojima A, et al. Levels of urinary polyamines in patients with rheumatoid arthritis. *J Rheumatol* 1993;20:1661–1665.

58. Yukioka K, Wakitani S, Yukioka M, et al. Polyamine levels in synovial tissues and synovial fluids of patients with rheumatoid arthritis. *J Rheumatol* 1992;19:689–692.

59. Flescher E, Bowlin TL, Talal N. Regulation of IL-2 production by mononuclear cells from rheumatoid arthritis synovial fluids. *Clin Exp Immunol* 1992;87:435–437.

60. Flescher E, Bowlin TL, Ballester A, Houk R, Talal N. Increased polyamines may downregulate interleukin 2 production in rheumatoid arthritis. *J Clin Invest* 1989;83:1356–1362.

61. Flescher E, Fossum D, Talal N. Polyamine-dependent production of lymphocytotoxic levels of ammonia by human peripheral blood monocytes. *Immunol Lett* 1991;28:85–89.

62. Flescher E, Bowlin TL, Talal N. Polyamine oxidation down-regulates IL-2 production by human peripheral blood mononuclear cells. *J Immunol* 1989;142:907–912.

63. Nesher G, Moore TM. The *in vitro* effects of methotrexate on peripheral blood mononuclear cells: modulation by methyl donors and spermidine. Arthritis Rheum 1990;33:954–959.

64. Nesher G, Moore TM, Dorner RW. *In vitro* effects of methotrexate on peripheral blood monocytes: modulation by folinic acid and S-adenosylmethionine. *Ann Rheum Dis* 1991;50:637–641.

65. Krenitsky TA, Rideout JL, Chao EY, et al. Imidazo[4,5-c]pyridines (3-deazapurines) and their nucleosides as immunosuppressive and anti-inflammatory agents. *J Med Chem* 1986;29:138–143.

66. Smith DM, Johnson JA, Turner RA. Biochemical perturbations of BW 91Y (3-deazaadenosine) on human neutrophil chemotactic potential and lipid metabolism. *Int J Tissue React* 1991;13:1–18.

67. Jurgensen CH, Huber BE, Zimmerman TP, Wolberg G. 3-Deazaadenosine inhibits leukocyte adhesion and ICAM-1 biosynthesis in tumor necrosis factor-stimulated human endothelial cells. *J Immunol* 1990;144:653–661.

68. Jurgensen CH, Wolberg G, Zimmerman TP. Inhibition of neutrophil adherence to endothelial cells by 3-deazaadenosine. *Agents Actions* 1989;27:398–400.

69. Fantone JC, Duque RE, Davis BH, Phan SH. 3-Deaza-adenosine inhibition of stimulus-response coupling in human polymorphonuclear leukocytes. *J Leukoc Biol* 1989;45:121–128.

70. Prytz S, Loennechen T, Johansson A, Larsen LB, Slordal L, Aarbakke J. Effects of 3-deazaadenosine, an inducer of HL-60 cell differentiation, on human blood cells *in vitro*. *Pediatr Hematol Oncol* 1989;6:173–179.

71. Leonard EJ, Skeel A, Chiang PK, Cantoni GL. The action of the adenosylhomocysteine hydrolase inhibitor, 3-deazaadenosine, on phagocytic function of mouse macrophages and human monocytes. *Biochem Biophys Res Commun* 1978;84:102–109.

72. Zimmerman TP, Wolberg G, Duncan GS. Inhibition of lymphocyte-mediated cytolysis by 3-deazaadenosine: evidence for a methylation reaction essential for cytolysis. *Proc Natl Acad Sci U S A* 1978;75:6220–6224.

73. Allegra CJ, Drake JC, Jolivet J, Chabner BA. Inhibition of phosphoribosylaminoimidazolecarboxamide transformylase by methotrexate and dihydrofolic acid polyglutamates. *Proc Natl Acad Sci U S A* 1985;82:4881–4885.

74. Baggott JE, Vaughn WH, Hudson BB. Inhibition of 5-aminoimidazole-4-carboxamide ribotide transformylase, adenosine deaminase and 5′-adenylate deaminase by polyglutamates of methotrexate and oxidized folates and by 5-aminoimidazole-4-carboxamide riboside and ribotide. *Biochem J* 1986;236:193–200.

75. Ha T, Morgan SL, Vaughan WH, Baggott JE. Inhibition of adenosine deaminase and S-adenosyl homocysteine hydrolase by 5-aminoimidazole-4-carboxamide riboside. *FASEB J* 1992;6:1210–1215.

76. Luhby AL, Cooperman JH. Aminoimidazole carboxamide excretion in vitamin B12 and folic acid deficiencies. *Lancet* 1962;2:1381–1382.

77. Gruber HE, Hoffer ME, McAllister DR, et al. Increased adenosine concentration in blood from ischemic myocardium by AICA riboside: effects on flow, granulocytes and injury. *Circulation* 1989;80:1400–1411.

78. Cronstein BN, Eberle MA, Gruber HE, Levin RI. Methotrexate inhibits neutrophil function by stimulating adenosine release from connective tissue cells. *Proc Natl Acad Sci U S A* 1991;88:2441–2445.

79. Cronstein BN, Naime D, Ostad E. The antiinflammatory mechanism of methotrexate: increased adenosine release at inflamed sites diminishes leukocyte accumulation in an *in vivo* model of inflammation. *J Clin Invest* 1993;92:2675–2682.

80. Asako H, Wolf RE, Granger DN. Leukocyte adherence in rat mesenteric venules: effects of adenosine and methotrexate. *Gastroenterology* 1993;104:31–37.

81. Tucker AL, Linden J. Cloned receptors and cardiovascular responses to adenosine. *Cardiovasc Res* 1993;27:62–67.

82. Cronstein BN, Levin RI, Belanoff J, Weissmann G, Hirschhorn R. Adenosine: an endogenous inhibitor of neutrophil-mediated injury to endothelial cells. *J Clin Invest* 1986;78:760–770.

83. Cronstein BN, Kramer SB, Weissmann G, Hirschhorn R. Adenosine: a physiological modulator of superoxide anion generation by human neutrophils. *J Exp Med* 1983;158:1160–1177.

84. Cronstein BN, Duguma L, Nicholls D, Hutchison A, Williams M. The adenosine/neutrophil paradox resolved: human neutrophils possess both A1 and A2 receptors which promote chemotaxis and inhibit O2⁻ generation, respectively. *J Clin Invest* 1990;85:1150–1157.

85. de la Harpe J, Nathan CF. Adenosine regulates the respiratory burst of cytokine-triggered human neutrophils adherent to biologic surfaces. *J Immunol* 1989;143:596–602.

86. Salmon JE, Cronstein BN. Fcgamma receptor-mediated functions in neutrophils are modulated by adenosine receptor occupancy: A1 receptors are stimulatory and A2 receptors are inhibitory. *J Immunol* 1990;145:2235–2240.

87. Cronstein BN, Levin RI, Philips MR, Hirschhorn R, Framson SBA, Weissmann G. Neutrophil adherence to endothelium is enhanced via adenosine A1 receptors and inhibited via adenosine A2 receptors. *J Immunol* 1992;148:2201–2206.

88. Kammer GM, Birch RE, Polmar SH. Impaired immunoregulation in systemic lupus erythematosus: defective adenosine-induced suppressor T lymphocyte generation. *J Immunol* 1983;130:1706–1712.

89. Schultz LA, Kammer GM, Rudolph SA. Characterization of the human T lymphocyte adenosine receptor: comparison of normal and systemic lupus erythosus cells. *FASEB J* 1988;2:244–250.

90. Mandler R, Birch RE, Polmar SH, Kammer GM, Rudolph SA. Abnormal adenosine-induced immunosuppression and cAMP metabolism in T lymphocytes of patients with systemic lupus erythematosus. *Proc Natl Acad Sci U S A* 1982;79:7542–7546.

91. Kammer GM, Rudolph SA. Regulation of human T lymphocyte surface antigen mobility by purinergic receptors. *J Immunol* 1984;133:3298–3302.

92. Kammer GM, Smith JA, Mitchell R. Capping of human T-cell specific determinants: kinetics of capping and receptor re-expression and regulation by the cytoskeleton. *J Immunol* 1983;130:38–44.

93. Dong RP, Kameoka J, Hegen M, et al. Characterization of adenosine deaminase binding to human CD26 on T cells and its biologic role in immune response. *J Immunol* 1996;156:1349–1355.

94. Parmely MJ, Zhou WW, Edwards CK III, Borcherding DR, Silverstein R, Morrison DC. Adenosine and a related carbocyclic nucleoside analogue selectively inhibit tumor necrosis factor-alpha production and protect mice against endotoxin challenge. *J Immunol* 1993;151:389–396.

95. Bouma MG, Stad RK, van den Wilden Ferg FAJM, Buurman WA. Differential regulatory effects of adenosine on cytokine release by activated human monocytes. *J Immunol* 1994;153:4159–4168.

96. Sajjadi FG, Takabayashi K, Foster AC, Domingo RC, Firestein GS. Inhibition of TNFα expression by adenosine: role of A3 adenosine receptors. *J Immunol* 1996;156:3435–3442.

97. Le Moine O, Stordeur P, Schandene L, et al. Adenosine enhances IL-10 secretion by human monocytes. *J Immunol* 1996;156:4408–4414.

98. Fouma MG, van den Wilden Ferg FAJM, Buurman WA. Adenosine inhibits cytokine release and expression of adhesion molecules by activated human endothelial cells. *Am J Physiol* 1996;39:C522–C529.

99. Mountz JD, Borcherding DR, Zhou BF, Edwards CK III. Increased susceptibility of fas mutant MRL-lpr/lpr mice to staphylococcal enterotoxin B-induced septic shock. *J Immunol* 1995;155:4829–4837.

100. McWhinney CD, Dudley MW, Bowlin TL, et al. Activation of adenosine A₃ receptors on macrophages inhibits tumor necrosis-α. *Eur J Pharmacol* 1996;310:209–216.

101. Boyle DL, Sajjadi FG, Firestein GS. Inhibition of synoviocyte collagenase gene expression by adenosine receptor stimulation. *Arthritis Rheum* 1996;39:923–930.

102. Bong GW, Rosengren S, Firestein GS. Spinal cord adenosine receptor stimulation in rats inhibits peripheral neutrophil accumulation: the role of *N*-methyl-D-aspartate receptors. *J Clin Invest* 1996;98:2779–2785.

103. Bernini JC, Fort DW, Griener JC, Kane BJ, Chappell WB, Kamen BA. Aminophylline for methotrexate-induced neurotoxicity. *Lancet* 1995;345:544–547.

104. Seideman P, Muller-Suur R, Ekman E. Renal effects of low dose methotrexate in rheumatoid arthritis [see comments]. *J Rheumatol* 1993;20:1126–1128.

105. Osswald H, Gleiter C, Muhlbauer B. Therapeutic use of theophylline to antagonize renal effects of adenosine [review]. *Clin Nephrol* 1995;43(Suppl 1):S33–S377.

106. Merrill JT, Shen C, Schreibman D, Coffey D, Zakharenko O, Fisher R, Lahita, RG, Salmon J, Cronstein BN. Adenosine A₁ receptor promotion of multinucleated giant cell formation by human monocytes: a mechanism for methotrexate-induced nodulosis in rheumatoid arthritis. *Arth Rheum* 1997;40:1308–1315.

107. Svartz N. Salazopyrin, a new sulfanilamide preparation. *Acta Med Scand* 1942;110:577–598.

108. Sinclair RJG, Duthie JJR. Salazopyrin in the treatment of rheumatoid arthritis. *Ann Rheum Dis* 1949;8:226–231.

109. Taggart AJ, Neumann VC, Hill J, Astbury C, Le Gallez P, Dixon JS. 5-Aminosalicylic acid or sulphapyridine: which is the active moiety of sulphasalazine in rheumatoid arthritis? *Drugs* 1996;32(Suppl 1):27–34.

110. Neumann VC, Taggart AJ, Le Gallez P, Astbury C, Hill J, Bird HA. A study to determine the active moiety of sulphasalazine in rheumatoid arthritis. *J Rheumatol* 1986;13:285–287.

111. Pullar T, Hunter JA, Capell HA. Which component of sulphasalazine is active in rheumatoid arthritis? *BMJ* 1985;290:1535–1538.

112. Farr M, Brodrick A, Bacon PA. Plasma and synovial fluid concentrations of sulphasalazine and two of its metabolites in rheumatoid arthritis. *Rheum Int* 1985;5:247–251.

113. Astbury C, Hill J, Bird HA. Co-trimoxazole in rheumatoid arthritis: a comparison with sulphapyridine. *Ann Rheum Dis* 1988;47:323–327.

114. Gardner G, Furst DE. Disease-modifying antirheumatic drugs: potential effects in older patients [review]. *Drugs Aging* 1995;7:420–437.

115. Clegg DO. Sulfasalazine. In: Koopman WJ, ed. *Arthritis and allied conditions.* Philadelphia: Lea & Febiger, 1997:699–707.

116. Clegg DO, Reda DJ, Weisman MH, et al. Comparison of sulfasalazine and placebo in the treatment of reactive arthritis (Reiter's syndrome): a Department of Veterans Affairs Cooperative Study. *Arthritis Rheum* 1996;39:2021–2027.

117. Clegg DO, Reda DJ, Mejias E, et al. Comparison of sulfasalazine and placebo in the treatment of psoriatic arthritis: a Department of Veterans Affairs Cooperative Study. *Arthritis Rheum* 1996;39:2013–2020.

118. Clegg DO, Reda DJ, Weisman MH, et al. Comparison of sulfasalazine and placebo in the treatment of ankylosing spondylitis: a Department of Veterans Affairs Cooperative Study. *Arthritis Rheum* 1996;39: 2004–2012.

119. Imai F, Suzuki T, Ishibashi T, Dohi Y. Effect of sulfasalazine on B cells. *Clin Exp Rheumatol* 1991;9:259–264.

120. Symmons DPM, Salmon M, Farr M, Bacon PA. Sulfasalazine treatment and lymphocyte function in patients with rheumatoid arthritis. *J Rheum* 1988;15:575–579.

121. Comer SS, Jasin HE. *In vitro* immunomodulatory effects of sulfasalazine and its metabolites. *J Rheum* 1988;15:580–586.

122. Shanahan F, Niederlehner A, Carramanzana N, Anton P. Sulfasalazine inhibits the binding of TNF alpha to its receptor. *Immunopharmacology* 1990;20:217–224.

123. Bissonnette EY, Enciso JA, Befus AD. Inhibitory effects of sulfasalazine and its metabolites on histamine release and TNF-alpha production by mast cells. *J Immunol* 1996;156:218–223.

124. Baggott JE, Morgan SL, Ha T, Vaughn WH, Hine RJ. Inhibition of folate-dependent enzymes by non-steroidal anti-inflammatory drugs. *Biochem J* 1992;282:197–202.

125. Gadangi P, Longaker M, Naime D, et al. The antiinflammatory mechanism of sulfasalazine is related to adenosine release at inflamed sites. *J Immunol* 1996;156:1937–1941.

126. Wallace D. Antimalarial agents and lupus. *Rheum Dis Clin North Am* 1994;20:243–263.

127. Fox R. Antimalarial drugs. In: Koopman WJ, ed. *Arthritis and allied conditions: a textbook of rheumatology.* Baltimore: Williams & Wilkins, 1997:671–678.

128. Titus ED. Recent developments in the understanding of the pharmacokinetics and mechanism of action of chloroquine. *Ther Drug Monit* 1989;11:369.

129. Rordorf-Adam C, Lazdins J, Woods Cook K, et al. An assay for the detection of interleukin-1 synthesis inhibitors: effects of antirheumatic drugs. *Drugs Exp Clin Res* 1989;15:355–362.

130. DiMartino MJ, Johnson WJ, Votta B, Hanna N. Effect of antiarthritic drugs on the enhanced interleukin-1 (IL-1) production by macrophages from adjuvant-induced arthritic (AA) rats. *Agents Actions* 1987;21: 348–350.

131. Fox R. Anti-malarial drugs: possible mechanisms of action in autoimmune disease and prospects for drug development [review]. *Lupus* 1996;5(Suppl 1):S4–S10.

132. Hurst NP, French JK, Gorjatschko L, Betts WH. Studies on the mechanism of inhibition of chemotactic tripeptide stimulated human neutrophil polymorphonuclear leucocyte superoxide production by chloroquine and hydroxychloroquine. *Ann Rheum Dis* 1987;46: 750–756.

133. Cannon GW, Ward JR. Cytotoxic drugs and combination drug therapy. In: Koopman WJ, ed. *Arthritis and allied conditions: a textbook of rheumatology.* Baltimore: Williams & Wilkins, 1997:709–729.

134. Fox DA, McCune WJ. Immunosuppressive drug therapy of systemic lupus erythematosus. *Rheum Dis Clin North Am* 1994;20:265–299.

Inflammation: Basic Principles and Clinical Correlates,
3rd ed., edited by John I. Gallin and Ralph Snyderman.
Lippincott Williams & Wilkins, Philadelphia © 1999.

CHAPTER 79

Peptide-Induced Tolerance

Halina Offner and Arthur A. Vandenbark

Although the immune system normally functions to protect the body against invading microorganisms and tumors, it may in some instances be misdirected against self tissues, causing inflammation, organ damage, and even death. During development, T and B cells are highly selected to distinguish self from nonself. Most self-reactive T cells are deleted in the thymus before they ever reach the circulation or lymphatics. Such central tolerance is guided by recognition and loss of T cells specific for immunodominant epitopes, but it may not extend to "cryptic" determinants that are not preserved during natural processing of self proteins or to even slightly altered self determinants (1). The potential for self recognition and damage persists in all of us.

In most normal individuals, potentially dangerous autoreactive T cells never exceed a critical threshold frequency because of efficient peripheral regulatory mechanisms or the lack of sufficient activation. However, in those who do develop autoimmune disease, activation and expansion of pernicious T cells may occur through exposure to cross-reactive peptide determinants on microorganisms, by release of cryptic self determinants in organs damaged by trauma or infection, or possibly by microbial superantigens that cross-link selected T-cell receptor (TCR) Vβ and major histocompatibility complex (MHC) class II molecules. The target tissues affected and extent of damage probably depend on the efficiency of inducing organ-specific inflammatory type 1 helper T cells (T_H1), a process that is influenced by genetic and environmental factors. Many human autoimmune diseases (Table 79-1) probably involve T_H1 cells directed at tissue- or organ-specific antigens.

This chapter focuses on multiple sclerosis (MS), a paralytic demyelinating disease characterized by perivascular inflammation and gliosis, leading to the formation of scarified plaques. Clinical and histologic similarities between patients with MS and animals with experimental autoimmune encephalomyelitis (EAE) raise the strong possibility that MS, like EAE, results from immune-mediated damage directed at myelin antigens capable of inducing encephalitogenic T_H1 cells.

Exploiting natural regulatory mechanisms that prevent the induction or inhibit the function of tissue-specific T_H1 cells holds promise as therapy for autoimmune diseases. Many such approaches have been proposed and have in common the use of peptides that can activate natural tolerance mechanisms (Table 79-2). We discuss several of these approaches as they have been applied to the EAE model, including our own use of TCR peptides to target potentially pathogenic T cells.

H. Offner and A. A. Vandenbark: Departments of Neurology and Molecular Microbiology and Immunology, Oregon Health Sciences University, Portland, Oregon 97201; and Neuroimmunology Research, Veterans Affairs Medical Center, Portland, Oregon 97201.

TABLE 79-1. *Human autoimmune diseases with an inflammatory T-cell component*

Disease	Target tissue	Suspected autoantigen
Multiple sclerosis	Central nervous system myelin	MBP, PLP, MOG
Myasthenia gravis	Nerve and muscle synapses	Nicotinamide acetylcholine receptor (NAChR)
Rheumatoid arthritis	Connective tissue	Collagen, heat shock protein
Insulin-dependent diabetes mellitus	Pancreatic beta cells	Glutamate decarboxylase (GADP)
Systemic lupus erythematosus	DNA, other tissues	DNA, DNA receptor

MBP, myelin basic protein; MOG, myelin oligodendroglial glycoprotein; PLP, proteolipid protein.

TABLE 79-2. *Tolerogenic approaches using peptides*

Approach	Effect on T cells	References
Direct effect on pathogenic T cells		
High-dose tolerance (oral feeding, intravenous or intrathymic injection)	Deletion or anergy	13–19
Neonatal injection	Deletion/T$_H$1 → T$_H$2 switch	20–23
ECDI/Ag conjugated APC	Anergy/T$_H$1 → T$_H$2 switch	24–27
Liposomes/Ag	Anergy	28
Soluble MHC/Ag	Anergy	29–31
Modified peptides	T$_H$1 → T$_H$2 switch/anergy	32–38
Intraocular injection	Anergy/T$_H$1 → T$_H$2 switch	39
Induction of regulatory cells		
Soluble Ag (IV, IP)	Suppression	40–42
Low-dose oral feeding	Suppression	42–45
Nasal inhalation	Suppression	46–47
TCR peptides (SC, ID)	Suppression/deletion	48–51

Ag, antigen; APC, antigen-presenting cell; ECDI, ethylene carbodiimide; MHC, major histocompatibility complex; TCR, T-cell receptor; T$_H$1 and T$_H$2, types of helper T cells.

LESSONS FROM THE EXPERIMENTAL AUTOIMMUNE ENCEPHALOMYELITIS MODEL FOR MULTIPLE SCLEROSIS

The Model

The EAE model has provided insight into autoimmune disease processes and intervention strategies. EAE can be induced by immunizing susceptible animal strains with crude central nervous system (CNS), purified myelin, myelin proteins including myelin basic protein (MBP) (2), proteolipid protein (PLP) (3), and myelin oligodendroglial glycoprotein (MOG) (4) or their peptide determinants. MBP, PLP, and MOG are widely encephalitogenic among mammalian species and strains when injected in adjuvants, inducing clinical and histologic sequelae ranging from self-limiting paralysis without demyelination (e.g., Lewis rats) to relapsing disease with extensive demyelination similar to MS (e.g., PL and SJL mice, marmosets, monkeys). In each strain, there are one or two immunodominant regions selected from a larger set of epitopes (10 to 12 on MBP) that associate with MHC class II molecules to stimulate encephalitogenic CD4$^+$ T$_H$1 cells (5).

The pathogenic contribution of the T$_H$1 cells can be further documented by induction of passive EAE after transfer of activated T-cell lines or clones (6). After activation in the periphery, these T$_H$1 cells upregulate adhesion molecules, including $\alpha_4\beta_1$ integrin (7); migrate across the blood-brain barrier (8); and on encountering specific myelin antigen fragments presented by CNS phagocytes (predominantly microglial cells), release inflammatory cytokines including interferon-γ (IFN-γ) and macrophage activating factors (9). Chemokines released in the CNS tissue (10) attract additional inflammatory cells from the circulation (11), and effector molecules such as tumor necrosis factor-α (TNF-α) or TNF-β may cause demyelination (12) or otherwise affect the function of oligodendroglial cells, resulting in neuronal dysfunction.

Tolerance Induction with Peptides

There have been many successful intervention strategies for preventing or treating EAE or other T-cell–mediated autoimmune diseases using native or modified peptides from encephalitogenic molecules to induce peripheral tolerance. These strategies can be categorized as those in which the antigenic peptide directly inhibits the function of the encephalitogenic T cells and those that induce a separate set of regulatory T cells (see Table 79-2).

The first category includes high-dose tolerance, in which MBP fragments are ingested or injected intravenously or intrathymically, and intraperitoneal injection of antigenic peptides in incomplete Freund's adjuvant into neonates. These approaches can cause a peptide-specific deletion that may be accompanied by anergy. Anergy may also be induced by activating T cells through the TCR with antigen plus MHC molecules (Ag/MHC) in the absence of co-stimulatory signals (i.e., Ag cross-linked to antigen-presenting cells [APCs], liposomes, and soluble MHC/Ag complexes). A T$_H$1 to T$_H$2 switch may be induced by using modified peptides or by injection of the peptides into the anterior chamber of the eye, where local APCs present the peptide with high concentrations of transforming growth factor-β (TGF-β).

The second category involves vaccination with peptides to expand regulatory cells that can inhibit the pathogenic T$_H$1 cells. Peptides representing the encephalitogenic determinant can be administered intravenously in soluble form, intraperitoneally with incomplete Freund's adjuvant, or given intranasally or orally (see Chapter 80) to induce peptide-specific T$_H$2 or T$_H$3 cells. These cells recirculate, and when they are stimulated with the encephalitogenic determinant in the tissues, they release soluble factors, including interleukin-10 (IL-10) and TGF-β that can locally inhibit the activation of T_H1 cells specific for the same or different antigens (i.e., bystander suppression). We have proposed a similar bystander suppression mechanism for regulatory T cells specific for TCR peptides.

Biased T-cell Receptor V Genes

One of the striking features of encephalitogenic and other pernicious T cells is their tendency to express the products of a limited set of V region genes in forming functional TCRs specific for defined epitopes on the tar-

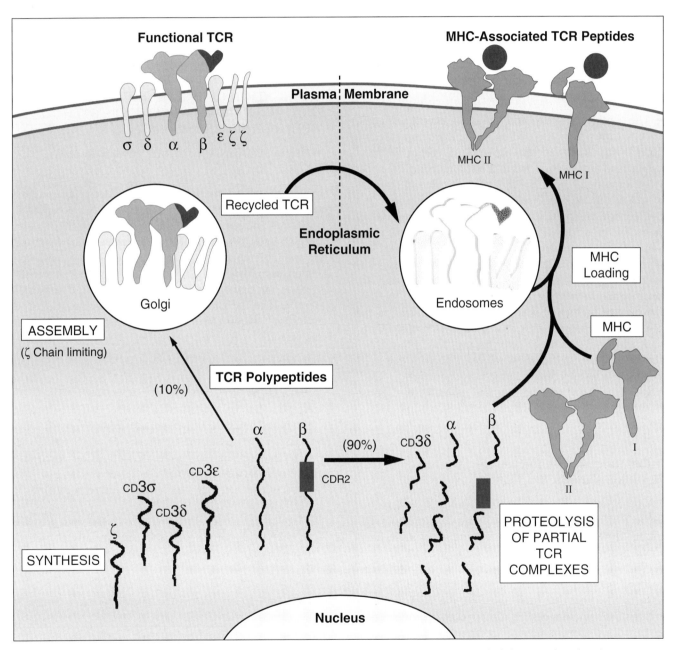

FIG. 79-1. Assembly or degradation of T-cell receptor (TCR) chains determines their fates as functional receptors or as potential major histocompatibility complex (MHC)–restricted antigenic fragments. The TCR complex, an octamer composed of five different chains, is assembled within the Golgi apparatus and transported to the external membrane. The ζ chain, which is synthesized at 10% of the rate of other chains, limits the formation of the TCR complex in the Golgi. The remaining unassembled or partially assembled chains may be digested into component peptides within the endoplasmic reticulum (ER) or lysosomes, where they may associate with MHC I or II molecules that are then expressed on the T-cell surface. Alternatively, recycled TCR chains contained within endosomes may interact predominantly with MHC II molecules.

get autoantigen (52). Perhaps the most clear-cut examples of V gene bias are in the Lewis rat (53), in which most of the encephalitogenic T cells specific for the 72–89 determinant of MBP express TCR Vβ8.2 and, to a lesser extent, TCR Vα2, and in the PL/J mouse (54–55), in which encephalitogenic T cells specific for the NAc-1–9 determinant also express Vβ8.2 and Vα2. Transgenic mice expressing an encephalitogenic Vβ8.2/Vα2 chain combination spontaneously develop EAE (56), indicating the pathogenic importance of this V gene combination.

Vaccination with T-Cell Receptor Peptides to Prevent or Treat Experimental Autoimmune Encephalomyelitis

The common expression of Vβ8.2 by encephalitogenic T cells from Lewis rats led us to identify immunogenic peptides for use as vaccines against EAE. The most interesting candidate peptide was in the second complementarity-determining region (CDR2) and consisted of residues 39–59 of the rat Vβ8.2 sequence. Preimmunization with this peptide completely prevented the subsequent induction of EAE with MBP/CFA (Complete Freund's adjuvant) (57). Moreover, the Vβ8.2-39–59 peptide had potent therapeutic effects when injected at low doses (10 to 100 μg/rat) after onset of clinical EAE, limiting the severity and shortening the duration of disease (58). Similar clinical protection was subsequently localized to the Vβ8.2-71–90 peptide (59), indicating two immunodominant and EAE-protective determinants within the Vβ8.2 sequence. The rapid clinical effect induced by the TCR peptides was apparently caused by boosting of anti-Vβ8.2 T cells and antibodies raised naturally in response to the encephalitogenic Vβ8.2$^+$ T cells (58), implicating these sequences in network regulation.

T-Cell Receptor Determinants as Targets of Autoregulation

The expression of particular V genes by autopathogenic T cells provides a potential target for immunoregulation. However, it is unlikely that the intact TCR functions as an efficient immunogen for inducing cytotoxic, regulatory, or antibody helper T cells, because T-cell recognition requires interaction with processed peptides associated with MHC molecules. For the TCR chains to function as immunogens for other T cells, they must first be processed into component peptides that are bound and expressed with MHC molecules.

Expression may occur naturally in APCs that have phagocytosed TCR molecules shed from activated or dying T cells. Alternatively, TCR peptides may be processed internally and expressed with MHC on the T-cell surface. Internal processing of TCR chains is a likely source of antigen, because up to 90% of the TCR α and β chains are not expressed on the cell surface as part of the

TCR octamer but are instead degraded in the endoplasmic reticulum, where they have access to nascent MHC class I molecules (60). TCR chains may be recycled from the surface within the endosomal compartment that also contains MHC class II molecules (61). These proposed pathways for the natural expression of TCR determinants with MHC on the T-cell surface are illustrated in Figure 79-1. Although the formal demonstration of naturally processed, MHC-associated TCR peptides is still lacking, their occurrence is strongly implied by functional studies showing that attenuated T-cell targets can stimulate TCR peptide-specific T cells.

APPLICATION OF T-CELL RECEPTOR PEPTIDE THERAPY TO PATIENTS WITH MULTIPLE SCLEROSIS

Multiple Sclerosis May Involve Myelin-Reactive T Cells

Because of its widespread encephalitogenicity in animals, MBP has been studied extensively as a potential T-cell target antigen in MS (62,63). Although other myelin antigens such as PLP and MOG deserve similar attention, the available data have focused predominantly on T-cell responses to MBP. Collectively, the data support a role for MBP in the pathogenesis of MS, at least in a subset of about half of the patients. Results implicating MBP as a prototypic myelin target antigen are listed in Table 79-3 and include

Increased frequency of MBP-specific T cells in the blood and cerebrospinal fluid (CSF) of MS versus control patients (64,65)

Increased state of activation of MBP-specific T cells in the blood and CSF of MS patients (64–66)

Sporadic increases in the frequency of MBP-specific T cells that correlate with disease activity in about one half of MS patients (67,68)

Therapeutic efficacy of intervention strategies directed at MBP-specific T cells (68–70)

Demonstrated encephalitogenicity of MBP and transfer of EAE with MBP-specific T cells in animal models representing a wide variety of MHC backgrounds (2)

TABLE 79-3. *Evidence implicating myelin basic protein as a target antigen in multiple sclerosis*

Increased frequency of MBP-specific T cells in blood and cerebrospinal fluid (64,65)
Increased expression of activation markers by MBP-specific T cells (64,65,66)
Sporadic increases in MBP-specific T cells during periods of increased clinical activity (67,68)
Apparent clinical benefit for multiple sclerosis patients from intervention strategies directed at MBP (68,69,70)
Widespread encephalitogenic activity of MBP in many mammalian species (2)

What is the nature of the response to MBP? We have observed substantial fluctuations in the frequency of MBP-specific T cells over time (67,68,71). Single time point assays have usually been unable to discern differences in MBP responses between MS patients and controls. Longitudinal assays have confirmed, that like EAE, surges in the frequency of MBP-specific T cells occur spontaneously and sporadically from a baseline of less than 1 cell per million blood mononuclear cells to more than 15 cells/million. Comparatively, frequencies of MBP-specific T cells of 8 cells/million are sufficient to induce clinical EAE in rats (72). We believe that surges in MBP activity may account for clinical changes in some (at least 50%) MS patients.

T-Cell Receptor V Gene Use by Peripheral Myelin Basic Protein–Specific T Cells

Results from the MS TCR workshop (73) indicated that there were no significant differences in Vβ gene usage among MBP-specific T-cell clones from MS patients and healthy donors or in T-cell clones from MS brains (with uncharacterized antigen specificity). Moreover, choice of a particular Vβ gene could not be associated with the MBP epitope recognized. However, MHC restriction was not considered in this analysis and conceivably could influence the selection of V genes. We decided to reevaluate the expression of putative MS-associated V genes, including Vα8 (74) and Vβ5 and 6 (75), and to determine if human leukocyte antigen DR2 (HLA-DR2) affected the selection of TCR V genes used in response to MBP. In this analysis, we reviewed data on the use of these selected V genes from a total of 654 clones specific for MBP or a variety of other autoantigens and exogenous antigens from 20 different reports (76).

As is shown in Table 79-4, MBP-specific T-cell clones from MS patients used TCR chains from the Vα8 and Vβ5 families (not necessarily together), although not the Vβ6 family, significantly more often than MBP-specific clones from non-MS patients and healthy controls. How-ever, there was no difference in the use of Vα8 or Vβ5 in DR2+ or DR2− donors. Thirty-six percent of the MS clones specific for MBP expressed Vα8, whereas only 15% of MBP-specific clones from non-MS donors used this V gene. T clones from non-MS donors (especially those who were DR2−) that were specific for certain other antigens also tended to use Vα8, including responses to DNA in lupus patients and to house dust mite allergens. There was a tendency for DR2− MS patients to use Vα8 more frequently than DR2+ MS patients, and DR2− non-MS donors did use Vα8 more often than DR2+ non-MS donors. However, more observations are needed to clarify this point. MBP-specific T-cell clones from MS patients also used Vβ5 significantly more often (23%) than MBP-specific clones (13%) or other antigen-specific clones (11%) from non-MS patients (see Table 79-4). However, the percentage of clones expressing Vβ5 was the same in DR2+ and DR2− donors within each group. In contrast to the increased usage of Vα8 and Vβ5 by MBP-specific T cells from MS patients, there was no significant difference in usage of Vβ6 (except for a slightly *lower* use in DR2+ MS patients).

In most clones, Vα8 and Vβ5 genes were not expressed on the same MBP-specific clone. At least one of these two V genes was expressed by more than one half of the total MBP-specific clones analyzed. This strongly biased use of only two V genes could provide a suitable target for TCR-based therapies, especially TCR peptides that induce regulatory T$_H$2 cells that can apparently inhibit T$_H$1 cells bearing different V genes by a bystander suppression mechanism.

More Evidence Implicating Vβ5 in Multiple Sclerosis

The potential importance of Vβ5 expression by MS T cells specific for MBP (or other antigens) is further supported by several independent studies. Rearranged Vβ5.1 or Vβ5.2 genes were found significantly more often in the plaque regions of brains from DR2+ than those from DR2− MS patients (77). Five motifs were found among

TABLE 79-4. *Increased use of Vα8 and Vβ5 in mylelin basic protein–specific T-cell clones*

Donor	Ag	DR2+			DR2−			Total		
		Vα8	Vβ5	Vβ6	Vα8	Vβ5	Vβ6	Vα8	Vβ5	Vβ6
MS	MBP	11/37 (30)[a]	47/208 (23)	16/208 (8)	6/10 (60)	20/86 (23)	8/86 (9)	17/47 (36)	67/294 (23)	24/294 (8)
Non-MS	MBP	11/71 (15)	15/106 (14)	17/106[b] (16)	7/46[c] (15)	12/103 (12)	10/103 (10)	18/117[c] (15)	27/209[c] (13)	27/209 (13)
Non-MS	Other	1/26[b] (4)	4/29 (14)	6/29 (21)	29/87[d] (33)	10/94[b] (11)	12/94 (13)	30/113 (27)	14/123[b] (11)	18/123 (13)

Ag, antigen; DR2, human leukocyte antigen DR2; MBP, myelin basic protein; MS, multiple sclerosis; Vα8, Vβ5, and Vβ6, expressed chains of the T-cell receptor.
[a]Numbers within parentheses indicate the percentage of clones expressing the V gene.
[b]$P < 0.05$ compared with MS clones responsive to MBP.
[c]$P < 0.01$ compared with MS clones responsive to MBP.
[d]Significantly higher ($P < 0.01$) in DR2− than in DR2+ non-Ms donors.

the Vβ5.2 CDR3 sequences, one of which was identical to a human MBP-specific T-cell clone (78), and was similar to encephalitogenic rat T-cell clones specific for MBP 87–99 peptide (79). CDR3 sequences putatively reactive to MBP 87–99 comprised 40% of the Vβ5.2 rearrangements in MS lesions. Another study reported a heterogeneous expression of Vα and Vβ families (including Vα8, Vβ5, and Vβ17) in acute MS brain plaques (80), but the HLA types of the donors were not presented.

In an autopsy study, direct evaluation of brain from a DR2⁺ patient with a short and aggressive course of MS revealed enhanced expression of Vβ5.2/3 in 32% of CSF cells and 11% of white matter cells (81). Moreover, IL-2–expanded Vβ5.2⁺ T cells from white matter showed limited CDR3 diversity, suggesting oligoclonality. One clone cultured successfully from white matter responded specifically to human MBP peptide 84–102, expressed Vα8 and Vβ5.2, and had a CDR3 sequence similar to a mouse T-cell clone specific for the same region of MBP (82). Other CDR3s from the Vβ5.2⁺ clones also were similar to motifs from Vβ5.2⁺ clones described earlier (77). Vβ6, Vβ5, and Vβ2 were found to be dominant in activated (IL-2 expanded) MS CSF T cells (83).

Use of Vβ5 in the TCR of MBP-specific T cells may be engendered in part by the DRB1*1501 molecule. One study (84) found a marked expansion of peripheral CD4⁺ T cells expressing Vβ5.3JB1.4 chains, with apparent specificity for MBP in five recently diagnosed and untreated DR2⁺ MS patients and in one of three progressive MS patients. A homologous sequence was not found in MS patients with other DR types, although it was detected but not expanded in healthy DR2⁺ individuals. These provocative findings suggest that T cells expressing this Vβ5.3JB1.4 combination may be involved in the onset of MS.

Rationale for Using Peptide for Vaccinating Multiple Sclerosis Patients

Based on the ability of CDR2 peptides to prevent and treat EAE, we evaluated peptides from the CDR2 loop of human Vβ3, Vβ5.2, Vβ6.1, Vβ9, and Vβ12.2 for immunogenicity (85). These peptides that encompass residues 38–58 typically have residues that interact with other regions of the folded Vα or Vβ chains or that are solvent exposed (Fig. 79-2) and may interact with the MHC/Ag complex on APCs. These characteristics of loop structures may favor binding of cytoplasmically processed CDR2 peptides to MHC in a manner that enhances immunogenicity.

Substituted Vβ5.2 CDR2 Peptide is Most Active

Based on the overexpression of Vβ5.2 by MBP-specific T cells, we identified a slightly modified CDR2 peptide, (Y49T)Vβ5.2-38–58 (ALGQGPQFIFQ*T*YEEEERQRG),

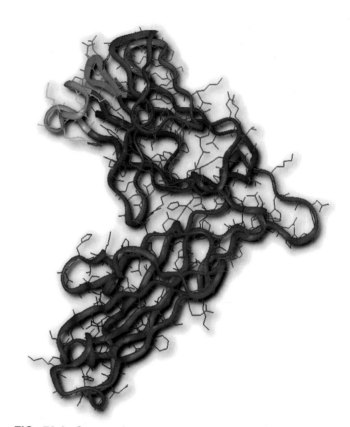

FIG. 79-2. Structural representation of the β chain of a murine T-cell antigen receptor determined at a resolution of 1.7 Å (0.17 nm). Atomic coordinates were obtained from the Brookhaven Protein Data Bank (PDB) and modeled using the Insight II program. Cβ (constant region) residues are depicted in red, and Vβ framework residues in blue. Loop structures for CDR1 (green), CDR2 (fuschia), CDR3 (yellow), and HV4 (orange) are also shown.

that significantly boosted TCR peptide–specific T cells in 7 of 11 progressive MS patients (71). However, other regions of the Vβ5.2 sequence may also be immunogenic. To identify immunogenic regions, we synthesized overlapping Vβ5.2 peptides, vaccinated MS patients using a protocol similar to that in the phase 1 trial, and monitored changes in the frequency of responding T cells (85). We found that the (Y49T)Vβ5.2-38–58 CDR2 peptide was more immunogenic than the native Vβ5.2-38–58 peptide, inducing significant changes in T-cell frequency in about 60% of the patients tested, compared with only 13% for the native sequence. Of the other peptides, only Vβ5.2-25–41 and Vβ5.2-33–52 were weakly immunogenic. These data suggest that several Vβ5.2 peptides can induce significant T-cell responses, but that the slightly altered germ-line CDR2 sequence was the most immunogenic of the peptides tested. The enhanced immunogenicity of the Y49T substitution was reflected by the increased binding affinity of the (Y49T)Vβ5.2-38–58 peptide compared with that of the native sequence for both of the DR2 alleles, suggesting that residue 49 contributed to MHC binding.

Receptor Peptide Vaccination Can Inhibit T-Cell Responses to Myelin Basic Protein and Reverse Clinical Progression

We carried out a pilot double-blind, placebo-controlled phase II trial to evaluate the ability of the native and Y49T-substituted Vβ5.2-38–58 peptides to induce TCR-specific T cells, inhibit MBP-specific T cells, and effect clinical changes (68). The results of this trial indicated that only patients who were vaccinated with peptides had significant increases in T-cell response to peptides (as assessed by frequency of peripheral blood mononuclear cells); a significant inverse correlation between response to peptide and response to MBP; a significant correlation between response to peptide and lack of disease progression; and a significant inverse correlation between response to MBP and lack of clinical progression. These changes in immunologic and clinical parameters induced by TCR peptide vaccination are illustrated for one MS patient in Figure 79-3.

Response to Vβ5.2-38–58 Correlates with Clinical Benefit

To better view the collective effects of TCR peptide vaccination directed at Vβ5.2⁺ T cells, we assembled a composite analysis of 32 DR2⁺ patients with progressive MS from the phase I and phase II trials, comparing the degree of response to the substituted or native Vβ5.2-38–58 peptide with clinical outcome (86). We found a highly signifi-

cant correlation ($P < 0.001$) between degree of response to the Vβ5.2 peptide and clinical benefit. That there was measurable clinical improvement in three of the patients with strong T-cell responses to peptide vaccination (≥8 cells/million mononuclear cells) and arrested disease progression in 7 of 9 patients with moderate T-cell responses (2 to 8 cells/million mononuclear cells) underscores the exciting clinical potential of this approach, even in this group of patients with rather advanced disease.

Mechanism of Inhibition Involves T_H2 Regulatory Cells and Bystander Suppression

To develop a rational strategy for optimizing the TCR peptide vaccine, it is important to consider the biologic characteristics of Vβ5.2-38–58-specific T cells and their mode of action for regulating neuroantigen-specific T_H1 cells, which are thought to contribute to the disease process. We have isolated and characterized more than 80 clones responsive to Vβ5.2-38–58, Vβ6.1-38–58, or Vβ9-39–59 (68,87,88). Most of these clones were CD4⁺, and about 75% produced T_H2 lymphokines, including IL-4, IL-5, and IL-10, but not T_H1 lymphokines such as IFN-γ, IL-2, or TNF. The remainder produced T_H2 and T_H1 lymphokines. Supernatants from these TCR peptide–reactive cultures had potent inhibitory properties when incubated with autologous or heterologous T_H1 clones specific for MBP or herpes simplex virus. The supernatants inhibited antigen-specific and mitogen-induced proliferation and

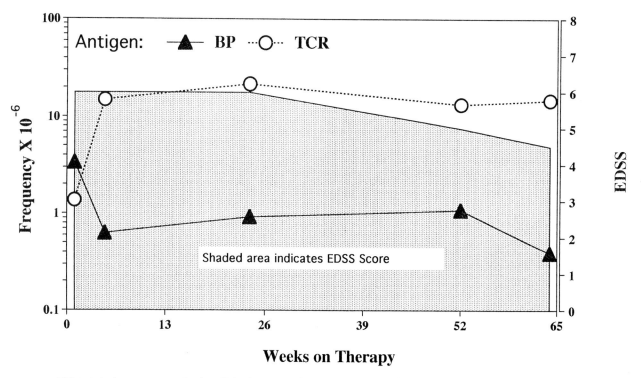

FIG. 79-3. Improvement in the clinical course of multiple sclerosis (MS) is reflected by decreased T-cell frequency in response to myelin basic protein and increased T-cell frequency in response to the TCR (Y49T) Vβ5.2-38–58 peptide during treatment of an MS patient with the Vβ5.2 peptide.

inhibited IFN-γ release in a dose-dependent, TCR V gene–independent manner (88).

Careful titration of IL-10 in the supernatants revealed that the detectable levels (1.1±0.7 ng/mL) could account for inhibition produced by similar levels of recombinant human IL-10, and the involvement of IL-10 was demonstrated by neutralizing the inhibitory properties of the supernatant with anti-IL-10 antibody (68). No inhibition of T$_H$1 cells was observed when supernatants from T$_H$1 cultures were added or when free TCR peptides were added. Conversely, no inhibition of T$_H$2 cells was observed when supernatants from T$_H$2 cells (which inhibited T$_H$1 cells) were added. Regional activation of the TCR peptide–specific T cells (i.e., by T$_H$1 cells expressing Vβ5.2 or APC presenting soluble substituted or native Vβ5.2-38–58 peptide after vaccination) would be expected to induce relatively high concentrations of soluble IL-10, which would inhibit activation of any T$_H$1 cells, including those that expressed V genes different than the target T cell (e.g., Vβ5.2$^+$) in the nearby vicinity.

This concept of *bystander suppression,* illustrated in Figure 79-4, is an attractive feature of regulation induced

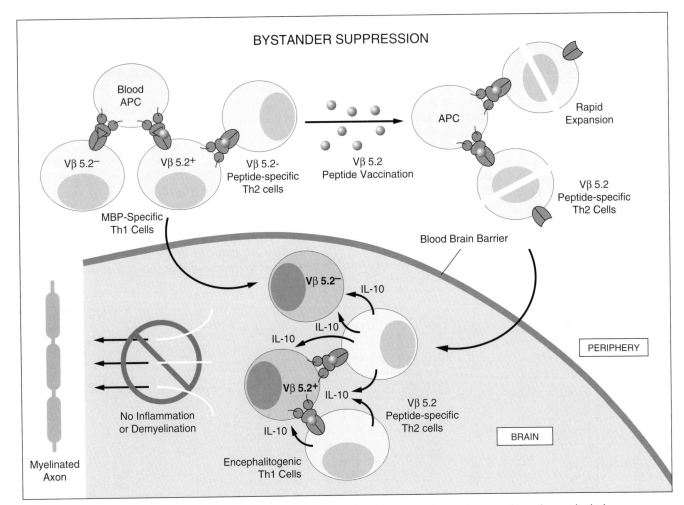

FIG. 79-4. Proposed bystander suppression mechanism. T$_H$1 cells directed at myelin antigens, including myelin basic protein (MBP), may cause or perpetuate multiple sclerosis (MS). MBP-specific T cells expressing Vβ5.2 in their receptor for HLA-DR2/MBP are thought to naturally induce T$_H$2 cells specific for naturally processed Vβ5.2 peptides, which are associated with HLA class II molecules and expressed on the T$_H$1 cell's surface. This natural network regulation seems insufficient to control encephalitogenic T$_H$1 cells in MS. However, injection of soluble Vβ5.2 peptides can boost the frequency of Vβ5.2-reactive T$_H$2 cells through blood or tissue antigen-presenting cells (APCs) to a level that can seek out and efficiently regulate the MBP-reactive T cells in the brain. Encephalitogenic MBP$^-$ or other myelin-reactive T$_H$1 cells that migrate to the central nervous system (CNS) may be inhibited by TCR peptide–specific T cells that are also able to recirculate throughout the CNS. Vβ5.2$^+$ T$_H$1 cells may activate the Vβ5.2-specific T$_H$2 cells, causing the release of inhibitory local concentrations of interleukin-10 (IL-10) that prevent activation, release of interferon-γ (IFN-γ) and other inflammatory or toxic cytokines, and proliferation of T$_H$1 cells. Local triggering of Vβ5.2-specific T$_H$2 cells may inhibit the Vβ5.2$^+$ T$_H$1 target cells and bystander Vβ5.2$^-$ T$_H$1 cells in the vicinity that are specific for MBP or other encephalitogenic determinants, preventing further inflammation or demyelination.

by TCR peptide vaccination, because it allows for localized suppression of any number of specificities of potentially encephalitogenic T_H1 cells, regardless of their V gene expression, provided that there are sufficient target (e.g., $V\beta5.2^+$) T_H1 cells present to stimulate infiltrating $V\beta5.2$-specific T_H2 cells. A critical unknown variable is how many $V\beta5.2^+$ target T_H1 cells are needed in an inflammatory lesion to trigger regulation by $V\beta5.2$-38–58 peptide-specific T_H2 cells. There is an overall increase in the use of $V\beta5$ by MBP-specific T cells in MS patients (23%) compared with that of controls (13%) (see Table 79-4). However, individual variation in use of $V\beta5$ and the use of $V\beta5.1/4$ or $V\beta5.2/3$ by some patients may explain the observed 60% rate of vaccination with $V\beta5.2$ peptides.

Effective regulation could be related to the product of frequencies of the target T_H1 cells and the regulatory T_H2 cells. When there is a low frequency of $V\beta5.2^+$ encephalitogenic T cells, a high frequency of $V\beta5.2$-reactive T cells would be required, only some of which might be activated in the tissue; when there is a substantial bias of $V\beta5.2^+$ target cells present, a lower frequency of these more efficiently activated $V\beta5.2$-reactive T cells might be sufficient for regulation. Bystander suppression may function better in localized regions of tissue (e.g., brain parenchyma), where fluid dynamics could minimize dispersion of the IL-10, than in the bloodstream. Systemic suppression due to activation of the T_H2 cells in the periphery would not be anticipated.

CONCLUSIONS AND FUTURE DIRECTIONS

Peptides that represent essential T-cell epitopes found within larger protein autoantigens have therapeutic potential for human autoimmune diseases when presented to the immune system as tolerogens. In this respect, much has been learned about using different routes of injection, complexing peptides to altered MHC molecules, or altering the peptide itself to delete inflammatory T cells or to induce regulatory T cells that limit the activation or effector function of the inflammatory T cells. Peptide-induced deletional mechanisms are highly specific for the peptide epitope and are not expected to affect the function of T cells recognizing other pathogenic determinants, even those found within the same parent protein. Although this form of tolerance is extremely selective, we need to know the range of T-cell determinants involved in the disease to effectively eliminate a pathogenic response. Mechanisms that involve release of soluble inhibitors have the potential advantage of suppressing bystander T cells in addition to the targeted T-cell specificity. The disadvantage, however, is that the pathogenic T specificities may persist and sporadically escape suppression. Optimally, peptides could be used to induce deletional and suppressive mechanisms.

The strong correlation between the T_H2 response to TCR peptide vaccination and clinical benefit in MS

patients poses an important challenge about how to enhance the overall rate of response to vaccination and the immunogenicity of the peptides *in vivo*. Our future studies will focus on defining immunogenic peptides from $V\alpha8$ (see Table 79-4), which is also overexpressed by MBP-specific T cells from MS patients, for use in conjunction with $V\beta5.2$ peptides. We also will evaluate the use of adjuvants; changes in the route, dose, and timing of injections; preparation of cocktails of TCR peptides from different V regions associated with different autoimmune diseases; and the effects of producing slight alterations in the TCR peptides (i.e., altered self sequences). Identification of TCR determinants that associate with MHC class I molecules may allow induction of cytotoxic T cells that delete pathogenic target T-cell subpopulations. We anticipate that a thorough evaluation of these parameters will improve the 60% response rate in TCR peptide–vaccinated MS patients and the degree and efficacy of response. Productive changes leading to improved immunogenicity of TCR peptides should also lead to a broadly active vaccine that can reverse immune-mediated damage in MS and other human autoimmune diseases.

ACKNOWLEDGMENTS

The authors wish to thank Ms. Eva Niehaus for preparation of the manuscript, Ms. Laura Unsicker for preparation of Figure 79-1, and Dr. Abigail Buenafe for preparation of Figure 79-2. This article was supported by NIH grants NS23444 and NS23221, the Department of Veterans Affairs, and Connetics Corporation, Palo Alto, CA.

REFERENCES

1. Moudgil KD, Sercarz EE. The T cell repertoire against cryptic self determinants and its involvement in autoimmunity and cancer. *Clin Immunol Immunopathol* 1994;73:283–289.
2. Alvord EC Jr. Species-restricted encephalitogenic determinants. In: Alvord EC Jr, Kies MW, Suckling AJ, eds. *Experimental allergic encephalomyelitis: a useful model for multiple sclerosis.* New York: Alan R Liss, 1984;523–537.
3. Tuohy VK, Lu Z, Sobel RA, Lauresen RA, Lees MB. Identification of an encephalitogenic determinant of myelin proteolipid protein for SJL mice. *J Immunol* 1989;142:1523–1527.
4. Linington C, Berger T, Perry L, et al. T cells specific for the myelin oligodendrocyte glycoprotein mediate an unusual autoimmune inflammatory response in the central nervous system. *Eur J Immunol* 1993; 23:1364–1372.
5. Bernaud E, Reshef T, Vandenbark AA, et al. Experimental autoimmune encephalomyelitis mediated by T lymphocyte lines: genotype of antigen presenting cells influences immunodominant epitope of basic protein. *J Immunol* 1986;136:511–515.
6. Ben-Nun A, Wekerle H, Cohen IR. The rapid isolation of clonable antigen-specific T lymphocyte lines capable of mediating autoimmune encephalomyelitis. *Eur J Immunol* 1981;11:195–199.
7. Yednock TA, Cannon C, Fritz LC, Sanchez-Madrid F, Steinman L, Karin N. Prevention of experimental autoimmune encephalomyelitis by antibodies against A4/B1 integrin. *Nature* 1992;356:63–66.
8. Hickey WF, Hsu BL, Kimura H. T-lymphocyte entry into the central nervous system. *J Neurosci Res* 1991;28:254–260.
9. Offner H, Buenafe AC, Vainiene M, et al. Where, when and how to detect biased expression of disease-relevant $V\beta$ genes in rats with experimental autoimmune encephalomyelitis. *J Immunol* 1993;151: 506–517.

10. Ransohoff RM, Hamilton TA, Tani M, et al. Astrocyte expression of mRNA encoding cytokines IP-10 and JE/MCP-1 in experimental autoimmune encephalomyelitis. *FASEB J* 1993;7:592–600.

11. Weinberg AD, Wyrick G, Celnik B, et al. Lymphokine mRNA expression in the spinal cords of Lewis rats with EAE is mainly associated with a host recruited CD45R hi/CD4$^+$ population during recovery. *J Neuroimmunol* 1993;48:105–118.

12. Selmaj KW, Raine CS. Tumor necrosis factor mediates myelin and oligodendrocyte damage *in vitro*. *Ann Neurol* 1988;23:339–346.

13. Critchfield JM, Racke MK, Zuniga-Pflucker JC, et al. T cell deletion in high antigen dose therapy of autoimmune encephalomyelitis. *Science* 1994;263:1139–1142.

14. Whitacre CC, Bitar DM, Gienapp IE, Orosz GC. Oral tolerance in experimental autoimmune encephalomyelitis. III. Evidence for clonal anergy. *J Immunol* 1991;147:2155–2161.

15. Gregerson DS, Orbitsch WF, Donoso LA. Oral tolerance in experimental autoimmune uveoretinitis: distinct mechanisms of resistance are induced by low dose vs high dose feeding protocols. *J Immunol* 1993;151:5751–5761.

16. Kearney ER, Pape KA, Loh DY, Jenkins MK. Visualization of peptide-specific T cell immunity and peripheral tolerance induction *in vivo*. *Immunity* 1994;1:327–339.

17. Khoury SJ, Gallon L, Chen W, et al. Mechanisms of acquired thymic tolerance in experimental autoimmune encephalomyelitis: thymic dendritic-enriched cells induce specific peripheral T cell unresponsiveness *in vivo*. *J Exp Med* 1995;182:357–366.

18. Falb D, Briner TJ, Sunshine GH, et al. Peripheral tolerance in T cell receptor-transgenic mice: evidence for T cell anergy. *Eur J Immunol* 1996;26:130–135.

19. Gaur A, Wiers B, Liu A, Rothbard J, Fathman CG. Amelioration of autoimmune encephalomyelitis by myelin basic protein synthetic peptide-induced anergy. *Science* 1992;258:1491–1494.

20. Clayton JP, Gammon GM, Ando DG, Kono DH, Hood L, Sercarz EE. Peptide-specific prevention of experimental allergic encephalomyelitis: neonatal tolerance induced to the dominant T cell determinant of myelin basic protein. *J Exp Med* 1989;169:1681–1691.

21. Qin Y, Sun D, Goto M, Meyermann R, Wekerle H. Resistance to experimental autoimmune encephalomyelitis induced by neonatal tolerization to myelin basic protein: clonal elimination vs. regulation of autoaggressive lymphocytes. *Eur J Immunol* 1989;19:373–380.

22. Vandenbark AA, Vainiene M, Celnik B, Hashim GA, Buenafe A, Offner H. Definition of encephalitogenic and immunodominant epitopes of guinea pig myelin basic protein (Gp-BP) in Lewis rats tolerized neonatally with Gp-BP or Gp-BP peptides. *J Immunol* 1994;153:852–861.

23. Singh RR, Hahn BH, Sercarz EE. Neonatal peptide exposure can prime T cells and, upon subsequent immunization, induce their immune deviation: implications for antibody vs. T cell-mediated autoimmunity. *J Exp Med* 1996;183:1613–1621.

24. Miller SD, Karpus WJ. The immunopathogenesis and regulation of T-cell–mediated demyelinating diseases. *Immunol Today* 1994;15:356–360.

25. Jenkins MK, Schwartz RH. Antigen presentation by chemically modified splenocytes induces antigen-specific T cell unresponsiveness *in vitro* and *in vivo*. *J Exp Med* 1994;165:302–308.

26. Peterson JD, Karpus WJ, Clatch RJ, Miller SD. Split tolerance to Th1 and Th2 cells in tolerance to Theiler's murine encephalomyelitis virus. *Eur J Immunol* 1993;23:46–51.

27. Vandenbark AA, Celnik B, Vainiene M, Miller SD, Offner H. Myelin antigen-coupled splenocytes suppress experimental autoimmune encephalomyelitis in Lewis rats through a partially reversible anergy mechanism. *J Immunol* 1995;155:5861–5867.

28. Strejan GH, St. Louis J. Suppression of experimental allergic encephalomyelitis by MBP-liposomes: a comparison. *Cell Immunol* 1990;127:284–290.

29. Quill H, Schwartz RH. Stimulation of normal inducer T cell clones with antigen presented by purified Ia molecules in planar lipid membranes: specific induction of a long-lived state of proliferative nonresponsiveness. *J Immunol* 1987;138:3704–3712.

30. Sharma SD, Nag B, Su X-M, et al. Antigen-specific therapy of experimental allergic encephalomyelitis by soluble class II major histocompatibility complex–peptide complexes. *Proc Natl Acad Sci USA* 1991;88:11465–11469.

31. Spack EG, McCutcheon M, Corbelletta N, Nag B, Passmore D, Sharma SD. Induction of tolerance in experimental autoimmune myasthenia gravis with solubilized MHC class II: acetylcholine receptor peptide complexes. *J Autoimmunity* 1995;8:787–807.

32. Evavold BD, Sloan LJ, Allen PM. Tickling the TCR: selective T-cell functions stimulated by altered peptide ligands. *Immunol Today* 1993;14:602–609.

33. Windhagen A, Scholz C, Hollsberg P, Fukaura H, Sette A, Hafler DA. Modulation of cytokine patterns of human autoreactive T cell clones by a single amino acid substitution of their peptide ligand. *Immunity* 1995;2:373–380.

34. Karin N, Mitchell DJ, Brocke S, Ling N, Steinman L. Reversal of experimental autoimmune encephalomyelitis by a soluble peptide variant of a myelin basic protein epitope: T cell receptor antagonism and reduction of interferon gamma and tumor necrosis factor alpha production. *J Exp Med* 1994;180:2227–2237.

35. De Magistris MT, Alexander J, Coggeshall M, et al. Antigen analog–major histocompatibility complexes act as antagonists of the T cell receptor. *Cell* 1992;68:625–634.

36. Gautam AM, Pearson CI, Smilek DE, Steinman L, McDevitt HO. A polyalanine peptide with only five native myelin basic protein residues induces autoimmune encephalomyelitis. *J Exp Med* 1992;176:605–609.

37. Nihira S-I, Falcioni F, Juretic A, Bolin D, Nagy ZA. Induction of class II major histocompatibility complex blockade as well as T cell tolerance by peptides administered in soluble form. *Eur J Immunol* 1996;26:1736–1742.

38. Kumar V, Urban JL, Horvath SJ, Hood L. Amino acid variations at a single residue in an autoimmune peptide profoundly affect its properties: T-cell activation, major histocompatibility complex binding, and ability to block experimental allergic encephalomyelitis. *Proc Natl Acad Sci USA* 1990;87:1337–1341.

39. Streilein JW, Ksander BP, Taylor AW. Immune deviation in relation to ocular immune privilege. *J Immunol* 1997;158:3557–3560.

40. Gershon RK, Kondo K. Infectious immunological tolerance. *Immunology* 1971;21:903–914.

41. Karpus WJ, Swanborg RH. CD4- suppressor cells inhibit the function of effector cells of experimental autoimmune encephalomyelitis through a mechanism involving transforming growth factor-beta. *J Immunol* 1991;146:1163–1168.

42. Miller A, Zhang ZJ, Sobel RA, Al-Sabbagh A, Weiner HL. Suppression of experimental autoimmune encephalomyelitis by oral administration of myelin basic protein. VI. Suppression of adoptively transferred disease and differential effects of oral vs. intravenous tolerization. *J Neuroimmunol* 1993;46:73–82.

43. Mattingly JA, Waksman BH. Immunologic suppression after oral administration of antigen. I. Specific suppressor cells formed in rat Peyer's patches after oral administration of sheep erythrocytes and their systemic migration. *J Immunol* 1978;121:1878–1883.

44. Lider O, Santos LMB, Lee CSY, Higgins PJ, Weiner HL. Suppression of experimental autoimmune encephalomyelitis by oral administration of myelin basic protein. II. Suppression of disease and *in vitro* immune responses is mediated by antigen-specific CD8$^+$ T lymphocytes. *J Immunol* 1989;142:748–752.

45. Weiner HL, Friedman A, Miller A, et al. Oral tolerance: immunologic mechanisms and treatment of animal and human organ-specific autoimmune diseases by oral administration of autoantigens. *Annu Rev Immunol* 1994;12:809–837.

46. Metzler B, Wraith DC. Inhibition of experimental autoimmune encephalomyelitis by inhalation but not oral administration of the encephalitogenic peptide: influence of MHC binding affinity. *Int Immunol* 1993;5:1159–1165.

47. Tian J, Atkinson MA, Clare-Salzler M, et al. Nasal administration of glutamate decarboxylase (GAD65) peptides induces Th2 responses and prevents murine insulin-dependent diabetes. *J Exp Med* 1996;183:1561–1567.

48. Offner H, Hashim GA, Vandenbark AA. Immunity to T cell receptor peptides: theory and applications. *Regul Pept* 1994;51:77–90.

49. Kumar V, Stellrecht K, Sercarz E. Inactivation of T cell receptor peptide-specific CD4 regulatory T cells induces chronic experimental autoimmune encephalomyelitis (EAE). *J Exp Med* 1996;184:1609–1617.

50. Falcioni F, Vidovic D, Ward ES, et al. Self tolerance to T cell receptor Vβ sequences. *J Exp Med* 1995;182:249–254.

51. Kuhrober A, Schirmbeck R, Reimann J. Vaccination with T cell receptor peptides primes anti-receptor cytotoxic T lymphocytes (CTL) and anergizes T cells specifically recognized by these CTL. *Eur J Immunol* 1994;24:1172–1180.

52. Heber-Katz E, Acha-Orbea H. The V-region disease hypothesis: evidence from autoimmune encephalomyelitis. *Immunol Today* 1989;10:164–169.

53. Burns FR, Li X, Shen N, et al. Both rat and mouse T cell receptors specific for the encephalitogenic determinant of myelin basic protein use similar Vα and Vβ chain genes even though the major histocompatibility complex and encephalitogenic determinants being recognized are different. *J Exp Med* 1989;169:27–39.

54. Acha-Orbea H, Mitchell DJ, Timmermann L, et al. Limited heterogeneity of T cell receptors from lymphocytes mediating autoimmune encephalomyelitis allows specific immune intervention. *Cell* 1988;54:263–273.

55. Urban JL, Kumar V, Kono DH, et al. Restricted use of T cell receptor V genes in murine autoimmune encephalomyelitis raises possibilities for antibody therapy. *Cell* 1988;54:577–592.

56. Goverman J, Woods A, Larson L, Weiner LP, Hood L, Zaller DM. Transgenic mice that express a myelin basic protein-specific T cell receptor develop spontaneous autoimmunity. *Cell* 1993;72:551–560.

57. Vandenbark AA, Hashim G, Offner H. Immunization with a synthetic T-cell receptor V-region peptide protects against experimental autoimmune encephalomyelitis. *Nature* 1989;341:541–544.

58. Offner H, Hashim GA, Vandenbark AA. T cell receptor peptide therapy triggers autoregulation of experimental encephalomyelitis. *Science* 1991;251:430–432.

59. Vainiene M, Gold DP, Celnik B, Hashim GA, Vandenbark AA, Offner H. Natural immunodominant and EAE-protective determinants within the Lewis rat Vβ8.2 sequence include CDR2 and framework 3 idiotopes. *J Neurosci Res* 1996;43:137–145.

60. Klausner RD, Lippincott-Schwartz J, Bonifacino JS. The T cell antigen receptor: insights into organelle biology. *Annu Rev Cell Biol* 1990;6:403–431.

61. Jiang H, Sercarz E, Nitecki D, Pernis B. The problem of presentation of T cell receptor peptides by activated T cells. *Ann N Y Acad Sci* 1991;636:28–32.

62. Hafler DA, Weiner HL. Immunologic mechanisms and therapy in multiple sclerosis. *Immunol Rev* 1995;144:75–107.

63. Vandenbark AA, Hashim GA, Offner H. T cell receptor peptides in treatment of autoimmune disease: rationale and potential. *J Neurosci Res* 1996;43:391–402.

64. Chou YK, Bourdette DN, Offner H, et al. Frequency of T cells specific for myelin basic protein and myelin proteolipid protein in blood and cerebrospinal fluid in multiple sclerosis. *J Neuroimmunol* 1992;38:105–114.

65. Zhang J, Markovic-Plese S, Lacet B, Raus J, Weiner HL, Hafler DA. Increased frequency of interleukin 2–responsive T cells specific for myelin basic protein and proteolipid protein in peripheral blood and cerebrospinal fluid of patients with multiple sclerosis. *J Exp Med* 1994;179:973–984.

66. Allegretta M, Nicklas JA, Sriram S, Albertini RJ. T cells responsive to myelin basic protein in patients with multiple sclerosis. *Science* 1990;247:718–721.

67. Vandenbark AA, Bourdette DN, Whitham R, Hashim GA, Chou YK, Offner H. Episodic changes in T cell frequencies to myelin basic protein in patients with multiple sclerosis. *Neurology* 1993;43:2416–2417.

68. Vandenbark AA, Chou YK, Whitham R, et al. Treatment of multiple sclerosis with T-cell receptor peptides: results of a double-blind pilot trial. *Nature Med* 1996;2:1109–1115.

69. Weiner HL, Mackin GA, Matsui M, et al. Double-blind pilot trial of oral tolerization with myelin antigens in multiple sclerosis. *Science* 1993;259:1321–1324.

70. Zhang J, Medaer R, Stinissen P, Hafler D, Rauss J. MHC-restricted depletion of human myelin basic protein-reactive T cells by T cell vaccination. *Science* 1993;261:1451–1454.

71. Bourdette DN, Whitham RH, Chou YK, et al. Immunity to TCR peptides in multiple sclerosis. I. Successful immunization of patients with synthetic Vβ5.2 and Vβ6.1 CDR2 peptides. *J Immunol* 1994;152:2510–2519.

72. Vandenbark AA, Vainiene M, Celnik B, Hashim G, Offner H. TCR peptide therapy decreases the frequency of encephalitogenic T cells in the periphery and the central nervous system. *J Neuroimmunol* 1992;39:251–260.

73. Hafler DA, Saadeh MG, Kuchroo VK, Milford E, Steinman L. TCR usage in human and experimental demyelinating disease. *Immunol Today* 1996;17:152–159.

74. Utz U, Biddison WE, McFarland HF, McFarlin DE, Flerlage M, Martin R. Skewed T-cell receptor repertoire in genetically identical twins correlates with multiple sclerosis. *Nature* 1993;364:243–247.

75. Kotzin BL, Karuturi S, Chou YK, et al. Preferential T cell receptor Vβ gene usage in myelin basic protein reactive T cell clones from patients with multiple sclerosis. *Proc Natl Acad Sci USA* 1991;88:9161–9165.

76. Offner H, Vandenbark AA. T cell receptor V genes in multiple sclerosis: increased use of Vα8 and Vβ5 in MBP-specific clones. *Int Rev Immunol* In press, 1999.

77. Oksenberg JR, Panzara MA, Begovich AB, et al. Selection of T-cell receptor Vβ-DB-JB gene rearrangements with specificity for a myelin basic protein peptide in brain lesions of multiple sclerosis. *Nature* 1993;362:68–70.

78. Martin R, Howell MD, Jaraquemada D, et al. A myelin basic protein peptide is recognized by cytotoxic T cells in the context of four HLA-DR types associated with multiple sclerosis. *J Exp Med* 1991;173:19–24.

79. Gold DP, Vainiene M, Celnik B, et al. Characterization of the immune response to a secondary encephalitogenic epitope of basic protein in Lewis rats. II. Biased T cell receptor Vβ expression predominates in spinal cord infiltrating T cells. *J Immunol* 1992;148:1712–1717.

80. Wucherpfennig KW, Newcombe J, Li H, Keddy C, Cuzner ML, Hafler DA. T cell receptor Vα-Vβ repertoire and cytokine gene expression in active multiple sclerosis lesions. *J Exp Med* 1992;175:993–1002.

81. Shimonkevitz R, Murray R, Kotzin B. Characterization of T-cell receptor Vβ usage in the brain of a subject with multiple sclerosis. *Proc N Y Acad Sci* 1995;756:305–306.

82. Shimonkevitz R. Personal communication.

83. Wilson DB, Golding AB, Smith RA, et al. Results of a phase I clinical trial of a T cell receptor peptide vaccine in patients with multiple sclerosis. I. Analysis of T cell receptor utilization in CSF cell populations. *J Immunol* 1997;in press.

84. Musette P, Dequet D, Delarbre C, Gachelin G, Kourilsky P, Dormont D. Expansion of a recurrent Vβ5.3⁺ T-cell population in newly diagnosed and untreated HLA-DR2 multiple sclerosis patients. *Proc Natl Acad Sci USA* 1996;93:12461–12466.

85. Bourdette DN, Whitham RH, Chou YK, et al. Successful immunization of multiple sclerosis patients with synthetic TCR Vβ peptides. *J Neuroimmunol* 1994;54:154(abst).

86. Vandenbark AA, Chou YK, Bourdette DN, Whitham R, Offner H. Immunogenicity is critical to the therapeutic application of T cell receptor peptide. *Drug News Perspect* 1997;10:341.

87. Chou YK, Morrison WJ, Weinberg AD, et al. Immunity to TCR peptides in multiple sclerosis. II. T cell recognition of Vβ5.2 and Vβ6.1 CDR2 peptides. *J Immunol* 1994;152:2520–2529.

88. Chou YK, Weinberg AD, Buenafe A, et al. MHC-restriction, cytokine profile, and immunoregulatory effects of human T cells specific for TCR Vβ CDR2 peptides: comparison with myelin basic protein-specific T cells. *J Neurosci Res* 1996;45:838–851.

Inflammation: Basic Principles and Clinical Correlates,
3rd ed., edited by John I. Gallin and Ralph Snyderman.
Lippincott Williams & Wilkins, Philadelphia © 1999.

CHAPTER 80

Oral Tolerance

Howard L. Weiner

Orally administered antigen encounters the gut-associated lymphoid tissue (GALT), which has the inherent properties of protecting the host from ingested pathogens and preventing the host from reacting to ingested proteins. Orally administered antigens induce systemic hyporesponsiveness to fed proteins, a phenomenon called *oral tolerance*. It was first described in 1911, when Wells fed hen egg proteins to guinea-pigs and found they were resistant to anaphylaxis when challenged. In 1946, Chase fed guinea-pigs the contact-sensitizing agent dinitrochlorobenzene (DNCB) and observed that animals had decreased skin reactivity to DNCB. It has also been observed in humans fed and immunized with keyhole limpet hemocyanin (KLH) (1).

Many studies have tried to elucidate the mechanisms of oral tolerance (2,3), and it has become clear that oral tolerance is mediated by T cells through different mechanisms, depending on the dose of antigen fed. Low-dose antigen favors the induction of regulatory helper T cells that suppress T_H1-cell–mediated responses, and high-dose antigen induces T-cell clonal anergy or deletion (Fig. 80-1). Oral tolerance has been used successfully to treat autoimmune diseases in animal models and is being applied to the treatment of human diseases (3).

MECHANISMS OF ORAL TOLERANCE

Inductive Phase of Oral Tolerance

Orally administered antigens are handled by GALT. The GALT consists of lymphoid nodules called Peyer's patches, villi containing epithelial cells, intraepithelial lymphocytes (IELs), and lymphocytes scattered throughout the lamina propria. Although dietary antigens are degraded by the time they reach the small intestine, stud-

ies in humans and rodents have indicated that degradation is partial and that some intact antigen is absorbed as well, especially when large doses of antigen are fed (4,5). High-dose oral antigen may result in systemic antigen presentation, which induces hyporesponsiveness through clonal T-cell anergy or clonal deletion.

In animals fed low-dose antigen, oral tolerance probably is induced in the gut, with a major component occurring in the Peyer's patches. Several cells capable of antigen presentation exist in the GALT, including macrophages, dendritic cells, B cells and epithelial cells. Macrophage-enriched cells obtained from mice fed ovalbumin (OVA) are able to stimulate antigen-primed lymph node T cells *in vitro* in an antigen-specific fashion without further exposure to antigen (6). Dendritic cells are the major intestinal antigen-presenting cell (APC) that can acquire and process orally administered antigen (7). Epithelial cells may preferentially trigger the activation of $CD8^+$ regulatory T cells. In rats, these epithelial cell-induced $CD8^+$ T cells are antigen specific (8), whereas in humans, they were found to be antigen nonspecific (9). Major histocompatibility complex (MHC) class II–positive intestinal epithelial cells from 2,4-DNCB–fed mice could induce anergy of DNCB-primed T cells (10). Lamina propria cells (LPCs) may be involved with APCs in oral tolerance (11). Antigen-pulsed splenic APCs stimulated antigen-specific T_H0 cytokine production, and Peyer's patch APCs induced a profile consistent with the provision of T-cell help for IgA production. Presentation of antigen by LPCs stimulated high levels of interferon-γ (IFN-γ) and transforming growth factor-β (TGF-β), and adoptive transfer of antigen-pulsed LPCs induced oral tolerance to that antigen in the recipients (11). However, the type of APC responsible for the effect of LPC was not resolved.

Type 2 helper T (T_H2) cells are preferentially generated in the GALT (12,13). T_H2 cell differentiation depends on the cytokine microenvironment or cytokine milieu the T_H

H. L. Weiner: Center for Neurologic Diseases, Brigham and Women's Hospital and Harvard Medical School, Boston, Massachusetts 02115.

precursor cells are exposed to during their activation (14). If interleukin-12 (IL-12) is present during activation, T_H1 cells are differentiated, but IL-4 induces T_H2 cell differentiation. Intestinal mucosa has high basal levels of IL-4, IL-10, and TGF-β expression, and shortly after oral administration of antigen, their expression is upregulated (15). This cytokine microenvironment may be crucial for the induction of T_H2 or T_H3 (i.e., TGF-β–secreting cells). We have shown that dendritic cells, when exposed to IL-10, can drive T_H2 cell differentiation of naive OVA T-cell receptor (TCR) CD4+-transgenic T cells (16).

The influence of cytokine milieu on the antigen presentation by dendritic cells has also been demonstrated *in vivo*. Dendritic cells exposed to IL-10 *in vitro,* when injected into the footpads of mice, can prime for T_H2 cell–type responses (17). It has also been shown in the human system that prostaglandin E_2 (PGE2)–treated dendritic cells can produce IL-10 and can prime naive human T cells for T_H2 cell differentiation (18). Dendritic cells from Peyer's patches preferentially stimulate T_H0 clones to produce large amounts of IL-4, and dendritic cells from spleen induce high IFN-γ production (19). There is also evidence that dendritic cells may be involved in oral tolerance induction in that expansion of dendritic cells *in vivo* with Flt3 ligand, a stimulator of dendritic cells, enhances oral tolerance (20). Dendritic cells, the most potent APC in activating resting T cells, under the influence of gut cytokine milieu, may present antigen for T_H2 or T_H3 cell differentiation.

APCs provide co-stimulatory signals required for the activation of T cells. B7-1 and B7-2 are the most important co-stimulatory molecules. B7-2 is critical for T_H2 cell differentiation (21). To determine the role of co-stimulatory molecules in the induction of oral tolerance, we tested the effect of anti-B7-1 and anti-B7-2 monoclonal antibodies on the induction of tolerance by high- and low-dose antigen feeding (22). *In vivo* in the experimental autoimmune encephalopathy (EAE) model, injection of anti–B7-2, but not anti–B7-1, inhibited the induction of oral tolerance to low-dose (0.5 mg) but not high-dose (20 mg) myelin basic protein (MBP). We have found that the costimulatory molecule CTLA-4 is important for high-dose oral tolerance (23). Class II molecules on the APCs also appear to be critical for the induction of oral tolerance, because oral tolerance cannot be induced in class II–deficient mice (24). Our studies also suggest that B cells may be required for low-dose oral tolerance (25) and for the induction of active TGF-β (26).

Effector Phase of Oral Tolerance

Depending on the dose of the antigen fed, there are two effector mechanisms. High dose favors T-cell clonal anergy or deletion, and low dose generates regulatory T cells that mediate active suppression (see Fig. 80-1).

Anergy and Deletion

Anergy as a mechanism for oral tolerance has been demonstrated indirectly and directly (27,28). A single feeding of 20 mg of OVA induced a state of anergy in OVA-specific T cells (29). Anergy as a mechanism also has been shown in a transfer system with OVA TCR transgenic T cells (28). In the studies demonstrating anergy as a tolerance mechanism, relatively high doses of antigen were fed. Feeding high doses of antigen can also induce T-cell clonal deletion, as shown in the OVA TCR transgenic model (30,31).

Active Suppression

Active suppression is mediated by the induction of regulatory T cells in the GALT, as in the Peyer's patches (32), and the cells then migrate to the systemic immune system. Although active cellular suppression of immune responses has been studied extensively over the years, it has remained ill defined because of difficulties in cloning suppressor cells and defining their mechanisms of action. However, evidence indicates that one of the primary mechanisms of active cellular suppression is by secretion of suppressive cytokines such as TGF-β, IL-4, and IL-10 after antigen-specific triggering (33). TGF-β is produced by CD4+ and CD8+ GALT-derived T cells (33,34) and is an important mediator of the active suppression component of oral tolerance. TGF-β–secreting CD4+ cells specific for MBP have been cloned from the mesenteric lymph nodes of SJL mice (33). These clones were found to be structurally identical to T_H1–disease-inducing clones with respect to TCR usage, MHC restriction, and epitope recognition, but they suppressed rather than

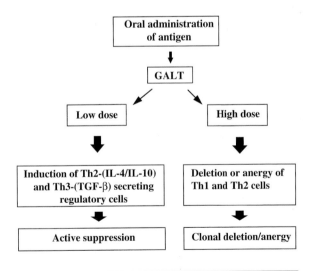

ORAL TOLERANCE

FIG. 80-1. Effector mechanisms of oral tolerance. GALT, gut-associated lymphoid tissue; IL, interleukin; TGF-β, transforming growth factor-β; T_H, helper T cell.

TABLE 80-1. *Characteristics of T-cell subsets*

	T$_H$1	T$_H$2	T$_H$3	T$_R$1
Cytokine profile				
IFN-τ	++++	–	+/–	+
IL-4	–	++++	+/–	–
TGF-β	+/–	+/–	++++	++
IL-10	–	++	+/–	++++
Growth/differentiation factors	IL-2	IL-2/IL-4	IL-4/TGF-β	IL-10
Functions				
Help	DTH/IgG2a	IgG1/IgE	IgA	?
Suppression	T$_H$2	T$_H$1	T$_H$1/T$_H$2	T$_H$1

DTH, delayed-type hypersensitivity; IFN, interferon; Ig, immunoglobulin; IL, interleukin; TGF, transforming growth factor; T$_H$, helper T cell; T$_R$, regulatory T cell.

induced disease. TGF-β–secreting CD4$^+$ cells were also cloned from MBP-TCR transgenic mice by culturing in the presence of IL-4 but not IL-2. These clones did not secrete IL-2, IFN-γ, IL-4, or IL-10 (35).

CD4$^+$ cells that primarily produce TGF-β appear to be a unique T-cell subset that includes mucosal helper T-cell function and downregulatory properties for T$_H$1 and other immune cells called T$_H$3 cells. In contrast to T$_H$1 and T$_H$2 cells, T$_H$3 cells provide help for IgA production and primarily secrete TGF-β (33) (Table 80-1). T$_H$3 cells appear distinct from T$_H$2 cells, because CD4$^+$ TGF-β–secreting cells that suppress a form of colitis have been generated from IL-4–deficient mice (36), and TGF-β–secreting cells have been observed in multiple sclerosis (MS) patients after oral administration of myelin proteins (37). Another type of regulatory T cell, which is driven by IL-10 and secretes primarily IL-10 and some TGF-β, is the T$_R$1 cell (38). In some situations, especially with high antigen doses, oral feeding has been able to suppress the T$_H$2 response (39). Feeding allergen could also suppress subsequent T$_H$2-driven allergen-specific IgE and IgG1 responses (40).

Bystander Suppression

Bystander suppression is a concept that regulatory cells induced by a fed antigen can suppress immune responses stimulated by different antigen as long as the fed antigen is present in the anatomic vicinity. It was demonstrated *in vitro* when it was shown that cells from animals fed MBP suppressed proliferation of an OVA-specific cell line across a transwell, although only when triggered by the fed antigen (41). The soluble factor was identified as TGF-β. Bystander suppression has since been demonstrated in several autoimmune and other models (Table 80-2).

Bystander suppression solves a major conceptual problem in the design of antigen- or T cell–specific therapy for inflammatory autoimmune diseases such as MS, type I diabetes, and rheumatoid arthritis (RA), in which the autoantigen is unknown or there are reactivities to multiple autoantigens in the target tissue. During the course of chronic inflammatory autoimmune processes in animals, there is intraantigenic and interantigenic spread of autoreactivity at the target organ (42). In human autoimmune diseases, there are reactivities to multiple autoantigens in the target tissue. In MS, there is immune reactivity to at least three myelin antigens: MBP, proteolipid protein (PLP), and myelin oligodendrocyte glycoprotein (43,44). In type I diabetes, there are multiple islet-cell antigens that could be the target of autoreactivity, including glutamic acid decarboxylase (GAD), insulin, and heat shock proteins (HSPs) (45). For a human organ-specific inflammatory disease, it is not necessary to know the specific antigen that is the target of an autoimmune response; it is only necessary to administer orally an antigen capable of inducing regulatory cells, which then migrate to the target tissue and suppress inflammation. Bystander suppression has been demonstrated by IL-10–secreting T$_R$1 cells, in which an OVA-specific T$_R$1 clone could suppress a murine model

TABLE 80-2. *Models of autoimmune diseases that demonstrate bystander suppression*

Autoimmune disease	Immunizing antigen	Oral antigen	Target organ
Arthritis	BSA, mycobacteria	Type II collagen	Joint
EAE	PLP	MBP	Brain
EAE	MBP peptide 71–90	MBP peptide 21–40	Brain
EAE	MBP	OVA	Lymph node, DTH response
Diabetes	LCMV	Insulin	Pancreatic islets
IBD	CD4$^+$ CD45RBhi T-cell transfer	OVA	Intestine

BSA, bovine serum albumin; DTH, delayed-type hypersensitivity; EAE, experimental allergic encephalomyelitis; LCMV, lymphocytic choriomeningitis virus; MBP, myelin basic protein; OVA, ovalbumin; PLP, proteolipid protein; IBD, inflammatory bowel disease.

of inflammatory bowel disease *in vivo* when fed OVA (38). In arthritis, bystander suppression was demonstrated by feeding type II collagen (CII) in the antigen arthritis model (46), the adjuvant arthritis model (47), and the streptococcal cell wall arthritis model (48).

Modulation

Several factors have been reported to modulate oral tolerance. Because oral tolerance has usually been defined in terms of T_H1 responses, anything that suppresses T_H1 or enhances T_H2 or T_H3 cell development would enhance oral tolerance (Table 80-3). T_H3 cells appear to use IL-4 as one of its growth and differentiation factors (35). Seder et al. found that IL-4 and TGF-β may promote growth of TGF-β–secreting cells (49). Intraperitoneal IL-4 administration enhances low-dose oral tolerance to MBP in the EAE model and is associated with increased fecal IgA anti-MBP antibodies (35). Oral IL-10 and IL-4 can also enhance oral tolerance when coadministered with antigen (50). Large doses of IFN-γ abrogate oral tolerance (51), and anti-IL-12 enhances oral tolerance and is associated with increased TGF-β production and T-cell apoptosis (31).

In the uveitis model, IL-2 potentiates oral tolerance and is associated with increased production of TGF-β, IL-10, and IL-4 (52). Lipopolysaccharide enhances oral tolerance to MBP (53) and is associated with increased expression of IL-4 in the brain. IFN-β synergizes with the induction of oral tolerance in SJL/PLJ mice fed low doses of MBP (54) Cholera toxin is one of the most potent mucosal adjuvants, and feeding cholera toxin abrogates oral tolerance when fed with an unrelated protein antigen (55). However, when a protein is coupled to recombinant cholera toxin B subunit and given orally, peripheral immune tolerance is enhanced (56). Oral administration of corneal epithelial cells markedly enhanced the corneal allograft survival (57). Antibody to chemokine monocyte chemotactic protein-1 abrogates oral tolerance (58). Oral antigen delivery using a multiple emulsion system also enhances oral tolerance (59). The γδ T cells may have an important role in oral tolerance induction, because of the apparent difficulty of inducing oral tolerance in animals depleted of such cells (60) or in δ-chain–deficient animals (61).

TREATMENT OF AUTOIMMUNE DISEASES IN ANIMALS

Several studies have demonstrated the effectiveness of orally administered myelin antigens in rodent models of autoimmune disease, including several arthritis models (Table 80-4).

Arthritis Models

Animal models of arthritis include collagen-induced arthritis (CIA), adjuvant arthritis (AA), pristane-induced arthritis (PIA), antigen-induced arthritis (AIA), silicone-induced arthritis, and streptococcal cell with arthritis. One of the first studies to demonstrate that an orally administered autoantigen can suppress an autoimmune disease was the use of oral CII in CIA (62). Oral administration of CII and other antigens has been effective in suppression of other types of arthritis.

Collagen-Induced Arthritis

Immunization with heterologous or homologous species of CII produces autoimmune responses to CII that leads to development of arthritis in susceptible mouse strains (63). CIA has been used as an animal model for RA and is characterized by chronic inflammation within the joints associated with synovitis and erosion of cartilage and bone (64). One of the first experiments of oral tolerance using rat CIA was done by Thompson et al. (62). They immunized WA/KIR rats with CII in incomplete Freund's adjuvant after oral

TABLE 80-3. *Modulation of oral tolerance*

Augments	Decreases
IL-2	IFN-γ
IL-4/IL-10	IL-12
Anti–IL-12 Ab	CT
CTB	Anti–MCP-1
LPS	Anti-γδ Ab
INF-β	GVH
Multiple emulsions	Anti-B7.2-mAb (low-dose tolerance)

Ab, antibody; CT, cholera toxin; CTB, cholera toxin B subunit; GVH, graft-versus-host; IFN, interferon; IL, interleukin; LPS, lipopolysaccharide; MCP-1; monocyte chemotactic protein-1.

TABLE 80-4. *Suppression of autoimmunity by oral tolerance*

Model or disease trial	Protein orally delivered
Animal model	
EAE	MBP, PLP, MOG
Uveitis	S-Ag, IRBP
Myasthenia gravis	AchR
Diabetes (NOD mouse)	Insulin, GAD
Transplantation	Alloantigen, MHC peptide
Thyroiditis	Thyroglobulin
Colitis	Haptenized colonic proteins
Human disease trials	
Multiple sclerosis	Bovine myelin
Rheumatoid arthritis	Chicken and bovine CII
Uveitis	Bovine S-Ag
Type I diabetes	Human insulin

AchR, acetylcholine receptor; EAE, experimental allergic encephalomyelitis; GAD, glutamic acid decarboxylase; HSP, heat shock protein; IRBP, inter-photoreceptor retinoid-binding protein; MBP, myelin basic protein; MHC, major histocompatibility complex; NOD, nonobese diabetic; PLP, proteolipid protein; S-Ag, S antigen.

administration of 2.5 or 25 µg of CII per gram of body weight. They found the disease onset was delayed and the severity was reduced at both dosages. At the same time, Nagler-Anderson et al. induced CIA in DBA/1 mice by immunizing with 300 µg of CII in complete Freund's adjuvant (65). Oral administration of CII before immunization suppressed the incidence of CIA. There was a tendency toward reduced IgG2 responses in the CII-fed mice.

Collagen peptides are also capable of inducing CIA. Immunodominant collagen peptides have been used to suppress CIA by oral or nasal administration. Kahre et al. induced CIA to DBA/1 mice by immunizing with human CII peptide (250–270) in complete Freund's adjuvant (66). Human peptide CII (250–270)–tolerized mice showed diminished T-cell proliferation. Oral tolerance with human peptide CII (250–270) abolished anti-human and anti-mouse CII antibody and markedly reduced the disease severity at early and effector phases. Staines et al. showed that CIA induced by whole bovine CII was suppressed by nasal administration of bovine CII peptide (184–198) (67). Nasal peptide administration was found to delay the onset of disease, reduce the severity, and shift the anti-CII antibody response from IgG2b to IgG1 isotype.

Other groups have shown that nasally administered CII effectively suppressed CIA in the mouse or rat. Myers et al. reported that nasal administration of intact CII or synthetic peptide reduced the incidence and severity of arthritis (68). They also showed that lymph node and spleen cells from treated mice secreted more IL-4 or IL-10 in response to CII than nontolerized mice. Al-Sabbagh et al. found that aerosolization of CII suppressed CIA in Wister/Furth rats to a degree similar to that seen with oral administration (69).

Analysis of cytokine expression in joint tissue of arthritis showed that proinflammatory cytokines such as tumor necrosis factor-α (TNF-α), IL-1, IL-6, granulocyte-macrophage colony-stimulating factor (GM-CSF), and chemokines such as IL-8 are abundant (70). We have found that mice treated with CII nasally showed diminished expression of mRNA of TNF-α and IL-6 locally (Garcia et al., 1998 unpublished observations,). We also established cell lines producing anti-inflammatory cytokines such as IL-4 and IL-10 from mice treated with CII orally or nasally.

Systemic anti–IL-4 treatment during oral administration of CII blocked the suppression of CIA by oral tolerance (71). This blockade of suppression of CIA was associated with the blockade of IL-4 secretion, decreases in anti-CII IgG2a antibody, and proliferation of lymphoid cells responsive to CII in CII-fed mice.

Adjuvant Arthritis

Another major model for RA is AA, which is a well-characterized and fulminant form of experimental arthritis. Oral administration of chicken CII consistently suppressed the development of AA in Lewis rats (47). A decrease in the delayed-type hypersensitivity (DTH) responses to CII was observed in tolerized animals. Oral type I collagen was also shown to suppress AA. Suppression of AA could be adoptively transferred by T cells from CII-fed animals. Suppression was observed at doses of 3 µg and 30 µg, but not at 300 µg or 1000 µg, suggesting that the mechanism involved the generation of suppressive regulatory T cells rather than clonal anergy, because active suppression may be lost at higher doses.

HSPs play an important role in the AA model (72). Oral administration of mycobacterial 65-kd HSPs suppressed the development of AA in rats (73). Suppression of AA was adoptive transferred by spleen cells from orally tolerized rats. Higher amounts of TGF-β were detected in the culture supernatant of spleen cells from HSP-fed rats when cultured with HSP. Prakken et al. showed that HSP peptide (176–190) that includes the arthritogenic epitope could induce nasal tolerance for AA (74). This peptide could also inhibit nonmicrobially induced experimental arthritis (avridine-induced arthritis) (74).

Other Arthritis Models

Oral tolerance is also effective in PIA (75). Immunizing mice twice with 2,6,10,14-tetramethylpentadecane (pristane) twice leads to arthritis after 100 to 200 days. Increasing doses of orally administered CII lowered the incidence and severity of PIA. Conversely, increasing dose of intraperitoneal administration worsened PIA.

Yoshino et al. induced AIA in Lewis rats by systemic immunization with methylated bovine serum albumin (mBSA) in complete Freund's adjuvant, followed by intraarticular injection of mBSA 2 weeks later (76). Orally administered CII at lower, but not higher, doses significantly reduced joint swelling, whereas oral KLH had no effect. These results demonstrate the biologic relevance of bystander suppression associated with oral tolerance. The same group reported that oral tolerance in AIA might also be mediated by clonal anergy (77). Other animal models of arthritis that have been successfully treated by mucosal tolerance include streptococcal cell wall arthritis (48), silicone-induced arthritis (78), and avridine-induced arthritis (74).

Methotrexate is a widely used drug in treating RA. We tested the effect of oral collagen on oral tolerance in animals treated with methotrexate. We previously found a synergistic effect between methotrexate and orally administered antigens such as MBP (79). A synergistic effect with oral methotrexate was also observed in the adjuvant arthritis model.

Experimental Autoimmune Encephalopathy

In the Lewis rat, high doses of MBP can suppress EAE through the mechanism of T-cell clonal anergy (80), whereas multiple lower doses prevent EAE by transferable active cellular suppression (81). In the nervous system of low-dose antigen-fed animals, inflammatory cytokines such as TNF and IFN-γ are downregulated, and TGF-β is upregulated (82). Oral MBP partially suppresses serum antibody responses, especially at higher doses (83). Administration of myelin to sensitized animals in the chronic guinea-pig model or larger doses of MBP in the murine EAE model is protective and does not exacerbate disease (84,85). Long-term (6-month) administration of myelin in the chronic EAE model was beneficial (86). EAE can also be suppressed in animals transgenic for an MBP-specific TCR after feeding with MBP (87). Nasally administered MBP peptides have been reported to suppress EAE (88).

Uveitis

Oral administration of S antigen (S-Ag), a retinal autoantigen that induces experimental autoimmune uveitis (EAU), or S-Ag peptides prevents or markedly diminishes the clinical appearance of S-Ag–induced disease, as measured by ocular inflammation (89). S-Ag–induced EAU can also be suppressed by feeding an HLA peptide (90). Feeding interphotoreceptor binding protein (IRBP) suppresses IRBP-induced disease and is potentiated by IL-2 (91). Oral feeding of retinal antigen can prevent acute disease and can effectively suppress a second attack in chronic-relapsing EAU, demonstrating that oral tolerance may have practical clinical implications in uveitis, which is predominantly a chronic-relapsing condition in humans (92,93).

Myasthenia Gravis

Although myasthenia gravis is an antibody-mediated disease, oral and nasal (94) administration of the Torpedo acetylcholine receptor (AchR) to Lewis rats prevented or delayed the onset of myasthenia gravis (95,96). The levels of anti-AchR antibodies in the serum were lower in orally tolerized animals than in control animals. The effect was dose dependent, and large doses of antigen (at least 5 mg of AchR) plus soybean trypsin inhibitor (96) were required, suggesting that anergy may be the primary mechanism.

Colitis

Oral feeding of haptenized colonic protein effectively prevents 2,4,6-trinitrobenzene sulfonic acid (TNBS)–induced granulomatous colitis through the generation of TGF-β–secreting T cells (97). Feeding OVA to mice given an OVA-specific IL-10–secreting T_R1 regulatory clone suppresses colitis (38).

Diabetes

Oral insulin can delay and, in some instances, prevent diabetes in the nonobese diabetic (NOD) mouse model.

Such suppression is transferable (98), primarily with $CD4^+$ cells (99). Immunohistochemical analysis of pancreatic islets of Langerhans isolated from insulin-fed animals demonstrated decreased insulitis associated with decreased IFN-γ and increased expression of TNF, IL-4, IL-10, TGF-β, and PGE_2 (100). It was also reported that nasal administration of the insulin B chain or GAD and aerosol insulin suppresses diabetes in the NOD mouse (101–103). Under special experimental conditions, large doses of OVA given to OVA double-transgenic mice resulted in diabetes mediated by OVA-specific cytotoxic T lymphocytes (CTLs) (104). These animals expressed OVA on the islets under the rat insulin promoter and were made chimeric to enrich for OVA-specific transgenic TCR CTLs.

Oral insulin suppressed diabetes in a virus-induced model of diabetes in which lymphocytic choriomeningitis virus (LCMV) was expressed under the insulin promoter and animals infected with LCMV to induce diabetes (105). Protection was associated with anti-inflammatory protective cytokine shifts (IL-4/IL-10, TGF-β) in the islets. Oral administration of the B chain of insulin, a 30–amino acid peptide, slowed development of diabetes and prevented diabetes in some animals (106). This effect was associated with decreased IFN-γ and increased IL-4, TGF-β, and IL-10 expression. Oral administration of recombinant GAD from plant sources suppressed the development of diabetes in NOD mice (107).

Transplantation and Other Models

Oral administration of allogeneic cells prevents sensitization by skin grafts and changes accelerated rejection of vascularized cardiac allografts to an acute form typical of unsensitized recipients (108). Orally administered allopeptides in the Lewis rat reduces DTH responses to the peptide (109). Oral, but not intravenous, alloantigen was accompanied by elevation of intragraft levels of IL-4 (110). Oral alloantigen enhanced corneal allograft survival even in preimmune hosts (57). Oral thyroglobulin has been shown to suppress autoimmune thyroiditis (111) and feeding peptides of the der pI allergen suppressed responses to the whole allergen (112). Experimental granulomatous colitis in mice is abrogated by TGF-β–mediated oral tolerance after administration of haptenized colonic proteins (97). Oral tolerization to adenoviral antigens permitted long-term gene expression using recombinant adenoviral vectors (113).

TREATMENT OF AUTOIMMUNE DISEASES IN HUMANS

Investigators have shown that exposure to a contact-sensitizing agent through the mucosa before subsequent skin challenge can lead to unresponsiveness in a portion of patients studied (114). KLH administered orally to human subjects has decreased subsequent cell-mediated immune responses, although antibody responses were not affected (1). Nasal KLH also has induced tolerance in humans (115).

On the basis of the long history of oral tolerance and the safety of the approach, human trials have been initiated with MS, RA, uveitis, and diabetes patients (see Table 80-4). The initial trials suggest that there is no systemic toxicity or exacerbation of disease, although reproducible clinical efficacy has yet to be demonstrated. Results in humans, however, have paralleled several aspects of what has been observed in animals.

MBP- and PLP-specific TGF-β–secreting T_H3-type cells have been observed in the peripheral blood of MS patients treated with an oral bovine myelin preparation and not in patients who were untreated (37). There was no increase in MBP- or PLP-specific IFN-γ–secreting cells in treated patients. These results demonstrate that it is possible to immunize through the gut for autoantigen-specific TGF-β–secreting cells in a human autoimmune disease by oral administration of the autoantigen. However, a 515-patient, placebo-controlled, double-blind phase III trial (AutoImmune Inc., Lexington, MA) of single-dose bovine myelin in relapsing-remitting MS did not show differences between placebo and treated groups in the number of relapses; a large placebo effect was observed. The 300-mg dose of myelin was given in capsule form and contained 8 mg of MBP and 15 mg of PLP. Preliminary analysis of magnetic resonance imaging data showed significant changes favoring oral myelin in certain patient subgroups. Based on the results of oral tolerance in uveitis in humans (116), it appears that protein mixtures may not be as effective oral tolerogens as purified proteins, and future trials in MS are being planned with purified myelin proteins or their analogues.

A 280-patient, double-blind phase II dosing trial of chicken CII in liquid doses ranging from 20 μg to 2500 μg per day for 6 months demonstrated statistically significant positive effects in the RA group treated with the lowest dose (117). Oral administration of larger doses of bovine CII (1 to 10 mg) did not show a significant difference between tested and placebo groups, although a higher prevalence of responders was reported for the groups treated with CII (118). These results are consistent with animal studies of orally administered CII in which protection against adjuvant- and antigen-induced arthritis and bystander suppression was observed only at the lower doses (47,76). An open-label pilot study of oral collagen in the treatment of juvenile RA produced positive results with no toxicity (119). This lack of systemic toxicity is an important feature for the clinical use of oral tolerance, especially in children for whom the long-term effects of immunosuppressive drugs are unknown.

Five phase II randomized studies of oral CII have been performed, and based on the results obtained, a multicenter, double-blind phase III trial study of oral CII (Col-

TABLE 80-5. *Oral collagen type II (Colloral) double-blind phase II studies*

Pilot
Dose ranging
Dose refinement
Abrupt methotrexate withdrawal
Hydroxychloroquine comparison

loral) is underway (AutoImmune Inc.). The five double-blind phase II studies are listed in Table 80-5, and they involved a total of 805 patients treated with oral CII and 296 treated with placebo. Two of the studies have been published (117,120). The other three studies were included in a integrated analysis that led to the decision to carry out a phase III trial. The dose refinement study tested doses of 5, 20, and 60 μg. The abrupt methotrexate withdrawal study tested the effect of 20 μg of oral CII in patients abruptly withdrawn from methotrexate, and the hydroxychloroquine comparison trial compared 20 μg of oral CII with hydroxychloroquine. Analysis of study interactions suggested that integrating clinical data was appropriate to gain information to decide on a phase III trial. Using linear logistic regression, it was found that a statistically significant effect favored patients treated on oral CII compared with those on the placebo, as measured by attaining a Paulus 20 response at any time during the study (cumulative Paulus). The effectiveness of individual Colloral doses was tested, checking cumulative Paulus 20, 50, and 70 criteria. Colloral at 60 μg was found to be the most significant dose compared with other doses. Weighted averages for the Paulus 20 and Paulus 50 responses were calculated for the 60 μg dose and placebo.

A significant effect favoring 60 μg was observed for the Paulus 20 and the Paulus 50 response (Fig. 80-2). Integrated efficacy analysis of predictors of response, including human leukocyte antigen (HLA), phenotype, rheumatoid factor, CII antibodies, duration of disease, and tender and swollen joint count, was performed, but no predictors were identified. Nonsteroidal antiinflammatory drugs (NSAIDs) did not appear to affect the clinical response of RA patients to oral CII. Safety analysis demonstrated that Colloral was extraordinarily safe, with no side effects, and appears to be the safest of the current medicines given to RA patients. The magnitude of the clinical responses of Colloral appear to be on the same level as NSAIDs for most patients. However, a subgroup of patients appear to have a more significant response to the medication. Based on these data, a phase III trial has been initiated; the phase III trial design is contained in Table 80-6. The study results are encouraging for the potential use of oral collagen in the treatment of rheumatoid arthritis in the future.

A pilot trial of S-Ag and an S-Ag mixture for the treatment of uveitis at the National Eye Institute showed positive trends with oral bovine S-Ag but not the retinal

% of Patients Achieving Paulus 20 Response

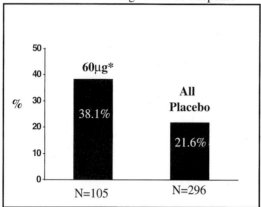

% of Patients Achieving Paulus 50 Response

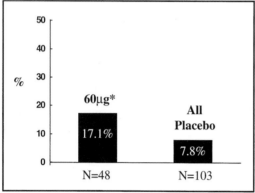

*Statistically Significant vs. placebo

FIG. 80-2. Integrated analysis of clinical response to oral type II collagen.

mixture (116). Feeding of peptide derived from patient's own HLA antigen appeared to have effect on uveitis in that patients could discontinue their steroids because of reduced intraocular inflammation mediated by oral tolerance (93).

Trials have been initiated with persons with new-onset diabetes in which recombinant human insulin is administered orally, and trials are underway using subjects at risk for diabetes as part of the diabetes prevention trial

TABLE 80-6. Colloral phase III trial design

Treatment	Colloral, 60 µg/day, vs. placebo
Study duration	8-week DMARD washout, 6-month treatment
Entry criteria	Joint count
	Class II/III
	Stable concomitant meds
Efficacy end point	Statistically significantly improvement in three of the following: tender joint count, swollen joint count, physician's global score, patient global score
Safety end points	Adverse events
	Clinical laboratory results*

(DPT-1). Preliminary analysis of a randomized, double-blind, placebo-controlled study of oral insulin in newly diagnosed immune-mediated (type I) diabetes demonstrated preserved beta cell function as measured by endogenous C-peptide insulin responses in adult new-onset diabetics fed 10 mg of recombinant human insulin compared with those fed placebo (121).

Oral desensitization to nickel allergy in humans induces a decrease in nickel-specific T cells and affects cutaneous eczema (122), and positive effects were reported in an open-label pilot study of oral type I collagen in patients with systemic sclerosis (123). A pilot immunologic study of oral MHC peptides has been initiated in transplantation patients. Based on results in humans, it appears that the clinical application of oral antigen for the treatment of human conditions will depend on the specific disease, on the nature and dosages of proteins administered, and perhaps on the use of synergists or mucosal adjuvants to enhance biologic effects. Recombinant human proteins may be more efficacious than animal proteins (124).

FUTURE DIRECTIONS

Although it is clear that oral antigen can suppress autoimmunity in animals, much remains to be learned. Under certain experimental conditions worsening of autoimmune diseases in animals by oral antigen has been reported (85,104,125,126), although this has not been observed in human trials. Cell surface molecules and cytokines associated with inductive events in the gut that generate and modulate oral tolerance are not completely understood. Important areas of investigation include cytokine milieu, antigen presentation and co-stimulation requirements, routes of antigen processing, form of the antigen, role of the liver, effect of oral antigens on antibody and IgE responses and on CTLs, and the role of $\gamma\delta$ T cells. As the molecular events associated with the generation and modulation of oral tolerance are better understood, the ability to apply mucosal tolerance successfully for the treatment of human autoimmune and other diseases will be further enhanced.

REFERENCES

1. Husby S, Mestecky J, Moldoveanu Z, Holland S, Elson CO. Oral tolerance in humans. T cell but not B cell tolerance after antigen feeding. *J Immunol* 1994;152:4663–4670.
2. Mowat AM. The regulation of immune responses to dietary protein antigens. *Immunol Today* 1987;8:93–98.
3. Weiner HL. Oral tolerance: immune mechanisms and treatment of autoimmune diseases. *Immunol Today* 1997;18:335–343.
4. Bruce MG, Ferguson A. Oral tolerance to ovalbumin in mice: studies of chemically modified and 'biologically filtered' antigen. *Immunology* 1986;57:627–630.
5. Bruce MG, Ferguson A. Oral tolerance induced by gut-processed antigen. *Adv Exp Med Biol* 1987:721–731.
6. Richman LK, Graeff AS, Strober W. Antigen presentation by

macrophage-enriched cells from the mouse Peyer's patch. *Cell Immunol* 1981;62:110–118.

7. Liu LM, MacPherson GG. Antigen acquisition by dendritic cells: intestinal dendritic cells acquire antigen administered orally and can prime naive T cells *in vivo. J Exp Med* 1993;177:1299–1307.

8. Bland PW, Warren LG. Antigen presentation by epithelial cells of the rat small intestine. II Selective induction of suppressor T cells. *Immunology* 1986;58:9–14.

9. Mayer L, Shlien R. Evidence for function of Ia molecules on gut epithelial cells in man. *J Exp Med* 1987;166:1471–1483.

10. Galliaerde V, Desvignes C, Peyron E, Kaiserlian D. Oral tolerance to haptens: intestinal epithelial cells from 2,4-dinitrochlorobenzene–fed mice inhibit hapten-specific T cell activation *in vitro. Eur J Immunol* 1995;25:1385–1390.

11. Harper HM, Cochrane L, Williams NA. The role of small intestinal antigen-presenting cells in the induction of T-cell reactivity to soluble protein antigens: association between aberrant presentation in the lamina propria and oral tolerance. *Immunology* 1996;89:449–456.

12. Daynes R, Araneo B, Dowell T, Huang K, Dudley D. Regulation of murine lymphokine production *in vivo.* III. The lymphoid tissue microenvironment exerts regulatory influences over T helper cell function. *J Exp Med* 1990;171:979–996.

13. Xu-Amano J, Aicher WK, Taguchi T, Kiyono H, McGhee JR. Selective induction of Th2 cells in murine Peyer's patches by oral immunization. *Int Immunol* 1992;4:433–445.

14. Abbas AK, Murphy KM, Sher A. Functional diversity of helper T lymphocytes. *Nature* 1996;383:787–793.

15. Gonnella PA, Chen Y, Inobe J-I, Quartulli M, Weiner HL. *In situ* immune response in gut associated lymphoid tissue (GALT) following oral antigen in TcR transgenic mice. *J Immunol* 1998;160:4708–4718.

16. Liu L, Rich BE, Inobe J-I, Chen W, Weiner HL. Induction of T helper 2 cell differentiation in the primary immune response: dendritic cells isolated from adherent cell culture treated with interleukin-10 prime naive CD4+ T cells to secrete interleukin-4. *Int Immunol* 1998;10:1017–1026.

17. DeSmedt T, Van Mechelen M, De Becker G, Urbain J, Leo O, Moser M. Effect of interleukin-10 on dendritic cell maturation and function. *Eur J Immunol* 1997;27:1229–1235.

18. Kalinski P, Hilkens CM, Snijders A, Snijdewint FG, Kapsenberg ML. IL-12 deficient dendritic cells, generated in the presence of prostaglandin E2, promote type 2 cytokine production in maturing human naive T helper cells. *J Immunol* 1997;159:28–35.

19. Everson MP, Lemak DG, McGhee JR, Beagley KW. FACS-sorted spleen and Peyer's patch dendritic cells induce different responses in Th0 clones. *Adv Exp Med Biol* 1997;417:357–362.

20. Viney JL, Mowat AM, O'Malley JM, Williamson E, Fanger NA. Expanding dendritic cells *in vivo* enhances the induction of oral tolerance. *J Immunol* 1998;160:5815–5825.

21. Freeman GJ, Boussiotis VA, Anumanthan A, et al. B7-1 and B7-2 do not deliver identical costimulatory signals, since B7-2 but not B7-1 preferentially costimulates the initial production of IL-4. *Immunity* 1995;2:523–532.

22. Liu L, Kuchroo VK, Weiner HL. B7.2 but not B7.1 costimulation is required for the induction of low dose oral tolerance. *FASEB J* 1998; I:A597.

23. Samoilova EB, Horton JL, Zhang H, Khoury SJ, Weiner HL, Chen Y. CTLA4 is required for the induction of high dose oral tolerance. *Int Immunol* 1998;10:491–498.

24. Desvignes C, Bour H, Nicolas JF, Kaiserlan D. Lack of oral tolerance but oral priming for contact sensitivity to dinitrofluorobenzene in major histocompatibility complex class II–deficient mice and in CD4+ T cell–depleted mice. *Eur J Immunol* 1996;26:1756–1761.

25. Gonnella P, Slavin A, Garcia G, Liu L, Weiner HL. Absence of low-dose oral tolerance in B cell deficient μ mice. *FASEB J* 1998:A599.

26. Komagata Y, Liu LM, Weiner HL. B cells are important for the production of active TGF-β. *FASEB J* 1998;1:A308.

27. Whitacre CC, Gienapp IE, Orosz CG, Bitar D. Oral tolerance in experimental autoimmune encephalomyelitis. III. Evidence for clonal anergy. *J Immunol* 1991;147:2155–2163.

28. Van Houten N, Blake SF. Direct measurement of anergy of antigen-specific T cells following oral tolerance induction. *J Immunol* 1996; 157:1337–1341.

29. Melamed D, Friedman A. Direct evidence for anergy in T lymphocytes tolerized by oral administration of ovalbumin. *Eur J Immunol* 1993; 23:935–942.

30. Chen Y, Inobe J-I, Marks R, Gonnella P, Kuchroo VK, Weiner HL. Peripheral deletion of antigen-reactive T cells in oral tolerance. *Nature* 1995;376:177–180.

31. Marth T, Strober W, Kelsall BL. High dose oral tolerance in ovalbumin TCR-transgenic mice: systemic neutralization of IL-12 augments TGF-beta secretion and T cell apoptosis. *J Immunol* 1996;157:2348–2357.

32. Santos LMB, Al-Sabbagh A, Londono A, Weiner HL. Oral tolerance to myelin basic protein induces regulatory TGF-β–secreting T cells in Peyer's patches of SJL mice. *Cell Immunol* 1994;157:439–447.

33. Chen Y, Kuchroo VK, Inobe J-I, Hafler DA, Weiner HL. Regulatory T cell clones induced by oral tolerance: suppression of autoimmune encephalomyelitis. *Science* 1994;265:1237–1240.

34. Chen Y, Inobe J, Weiner HL. Induction of oral tolerance to myelin basic protein in CD8-depleted mice: both CD4+ and CD8+ cells mediate active suppression. *J Immunol* 1995;155:910–916.

35. Inobe J, Slavin AJ, Komagata Y, Chen Y, Liu L, Weiner HL. IL-4 is a differentiation factor for transforming growth factor-beta secreting Th3 cells and oral administration of IL-4 enhances oral tolerance in experimental allergic encephalomyelitis. *Eur J Immunol* 1998;28:2780–2790.

36. Powrie F, Carlino J, Leach MW, Mauze S, Coffman RL. A critical role for transforming growth factor-beta but not interleukin 4 in the suppression of T helper type 1–mediated colitis by CD45RB (low) CD4+ T cells. *J Exp Med* 1996;183:2669–2674.

37. Fukaura H, Kent SC, Pietrusewicz MJ, Khoury SJ, Weiner HL, Hafler DA. Induction of circulating myelin basic protein and proteolipid protein-specific transforming growth factor-beta1–secreting Th3 T cells by oral administration of myelin in multiple sclerosis patients. *J Clin Invest* 1996;98:70–77.

38. Groux H, O'Garra A, Bigler M, Rouleau M, Antonenko S, de Vries JE, Roncarolo MG. A CD4+ T-cell subset inhibits antigen-specific T-cell responses and prevents colitis. *Nature* 1997;389:737–742.

39. Mowat AM, Steel M, Worthy EA, Kewin PJ, Garside P. Inactivation of Th1 and Th2 cells by feeding ovalbumin. *Ann N Y Acad Sci* 1996;778: 122–132.

40. van Halteren AG, van der Cammen MJ, Cooper D, Savelkoul HF, Kraal G, Holt PG. Regulation of antigen-specific IgE, IgG1, and mast cell responses to ingested allergen by mucosal tolerance induction. *J Immunol* 1997;159:3009–3015.

41. Miller A, Lider O, Weiner HL. Antigen-driven bystander suppression following oral administration of antigens. *J Exp Med* 1991;174: 791–798.

42. Cross AH, Tuohy VK, Raine CS. Development of reactivity to new myelin antigens during chronic relapsing autoimmune demyelination. *Cell Immunol* 1993;146:261–270.

43. Kerlero de Rosbo N, Milo R, Lees MB, Burger D, Bernard CCA, Ben-Nun A. Reactivity to myelin antigens in multiple sclerosis: peripheral blood lymphocytes respond predominantly to myelin oligodendrocyte glycoprotein. *J Clin Invest* 1993;92:2602–2608.

44. Zhang J, Markovic S, Raus J, Lacet B, Weiner HL, Hafler DA. Increased frequency of IL-2 responsive T cells specific for myelin basic protein and proteolipid protein in peripheral blood and cerebrospinal fluid of patients with multiple sclerosis. *J Exp Med* 1993; 179:973–984.

45. Harrison LC. Islet cell antigens in insulin-dependent diabetes: Pandora's box revisited. *Immunol Today* 1992;13:348–352.

46. Yoshino S. Antigen-induced arthritis in rats is suppressed by the inducing antigen administered orally before, but not after immunization. *Cell Immunol* 1995:163:55–58.

47. Zhang JZ, Lee CSY, Lider O, Weiner HL. Suppression of adjuvant arthritis in Lewis rats by oral administration of type II collagen. *J Immunol* 1990;145:2489–2493.

48. Chen W, Jin WW, Xiao-Yu S, Wahl SM. Oral administration of streptococcal cell walls (SCW) induces mucosal cytokines and suppresses SCW arthritis. *Arthritis Rheum* 1997;40:S55.

49. Seder RA, Marth T, Sieve MC, Strober W, Letterio JJ, Roberts AB, Kelsall B. Factors involved in the differentiation of TGF-β–producing cells from naive CD4+ T cells: IL-4 and IFN-γ have opposing effects, while TGF-β positively regulates its own production. *J Immunol* 1998; 160:5719–5728.

50. Slavin AJ, Maron R, Garcia G, Gonnella P, Weiner HL. Oral administration of IL-4 and IL-10 enhances the induction of low dose oral tolerance. *FASEB J* 1998;II:A599.

51. Zhang Z, Michael JG. Orally inducible immune unresponsiveness is abrogated by IFN-γ treatment. *J Immunol* 1990;144:4163–4165.

52. Rizzo LV, Miller-Rivero NE, Chan C-C, Wiggert B, Nussenblatt RB, Caspi RR. Interleukin-2 treatment potentiates induction of oral tolerance in a murine model of autoimmunity. *J Clin Invest* 1994;94: 1668–1672.

53. Khoury SJ, Lider O, al-Sabbagh A, Weiner HL. Suppression of experimental autoimmune encephalomyelitis by oral administration of myelin basic protein. III. Synergistic effect of lipopolysaccharide. *Cell Immunol* 1990;131:302–310.

54. Nelson PA, Akselband Y, Dearborn S, et al. Effect of oral beta interferon on subsequent immune responsiveness. *Ann N Y Acad Sci* 1996; 778:145–155.

55. Elson CO, Ealding W. Cholera toxin feeding did not induce oral tolerance in mice and abrogated oral tolerance to an unrelated protein antigen. *J Immunol* 1984;133:2892–2897.

56. Sun J-B, Holmgren C, Czerkinsky C. Cholera toxin B subunit: an efficient transmucosal carrier-delivery system for induction of peripheral immunological tolerance. *Proc Natl Acad Sci USA* 1994;91: 10795–10799.

57. Ma D, Mellon J, Niederkorn JY. Oral administration as a strategy for enhancing corneal allograft survival. *Br J Ophthalmol* 1997;81: 778–784.

58. Karpus WJ, Kennedy KJ, Kunkel SL, Lukacs NW. Monocyte chemotactic protein 1 regulates oral tolerance induction by inhibition of T helper cell-related cytokines. *J Exp Med* 1998;187:733–741.

59. Elson CO, Tomasi M, Dertzbaugh MT, Thaggard G, Hunter R, Weaver C. Oral antigen delivery by way of a multiple emulsion system enhances oral tolerance. *Ann N Y Acad Sci* 1996;778:156–162.

60. Ke Y, Pearce K, Lake JP, Ziegler HK, Kapp JA. γδ T lymphocytes regulate the induction and maintenance of oral tolerance. *J Immunol* 1997;158:3610–3618.

61. Spahn TW, Weiner HL. γδ T cells are necessary for low dose but not high dose oral tolerance. *FASEB J* 1998;12:A597, 3464.

62. Thompson HSG, Staines NA. Gastric administration of type II collagen delays the onset and severity of collagen-induced arthritis in rats. *Clin Exp Immunol* 1986;64:581–586.

63. Courtenay JS, Dallman MS, Dayan AD, Martin A, Mosedale B. Immunization against heterologous type II collagen induces arthritis in mice. *Nature* 1980;283:666–668.

64. Trentham DE, Townes AS, Kang AS. Autoimmunity to type II collagen: an experimental model of arthritis. *J Exp Med* 1977;146: 857–868.

65. Nagler-Anderson C, Bober LA, Robinson ME, Siskind GW, Thorbeke FJ. Suppression of type II collagen-induced arthritis by intragastric administration of soluble type II collagen. *Proc Natl Acad Sci USA* 1986;83:7443–7446.

66. Khare SD, Krco CJ, Griffiths MM, Luthra HS, David CS. Oral administration of an immunodominant human collagen peptide modulates collagen-induced arthritis. *J Immunol* 1995;155:3653–3659.

67. Staines NA, Harper N, Ward FJ, Malmström V, Holmdahl R, Bansal S. Mucosal tolerance and suppression of collagen-induced arthritis (CIA) induced by nasal inhalation of synthetic peptide 184–198 of bovine type II collagen (CII) expressing a dominant T cell epitope. *Clin Exp Immunol* 1996;103:368–375.

68. Myers LK, Seyer JM, Stuart JM, Kang AH. Suppression of murine collagen-induced arthritis by nasal administration of collagen. *Immunology* 1997;90:161–164.

69. Al-Sabbagh A, Nelson P, Sobel RA, Weiner HL. Antigen-driven peripheral immune tolerance: suppression of experimental autoimmune encephalomyelitis and collagen induced arthritis by aerosol administration of myelin basic protein or type II collagen. *Cell Immunol* 1996;171:111–119.

70. Feldman M, Brennan FM, Maini RN. Role of cytokines in rheumatoid arthritis. *Annu Rev Immunol* 1996;14:397–440.

71. Yoshino S. Treatment with an anti-IL-4 antibody blocks suppression of collagen-induced arthritis in mice by oral administration of type II collagen. *J Immunol* 1998;160:3067–3071.

72. van Eden W, Thole JE, van der Zee R, et al. Cloning of the mycobacterial epitope recognized by T lymphocytes in adjuvant arthritis. *Nature* 1988;331:171–173.

73. Haque MA, Yoshino S, Inada S, Nomaguchi H, Tokunaga O, Kohashi O. Suppression of adjuvant arthritis in rats by induction of oral tolerance to mycobacterial 65-kDa heat shock protein. *Eur J Immunol* 1996;26:2650–2656.

74. Prakken BJ, van der Zee R, Anderton SM, van Kooten PJS, Kuis W, van Eden W. Peptide-induced nasal tolerance for a mycobacterial heat shock protein 60 T cell epitope in rats suppresses both adjuvant arthritis and nonmicrobially induced experimental arthritis. *Proc Natl Acad Sci USA* 1997;94:3284–3289.

75. Thompson SJ, Thompson HSG, Harper N, et al. Prevention of pristane-induced arthritis by the oral administration of type II collagen. *Immunology* 1993;79:152–157.

76. Yoshino S, Quattrocchi E, Weiner HL. Oral administration of type II collagen suppresses antigen-induced arthritis in Lewis rats. *Arthritis Rheum* 1995;38:1092–1096.

77. Inada S, Yoshino S, Haque MA, Ogata Y, Kohashi O. Clonal anergy is a potent mechanism of oral tolerance in the suppression of acute antigen-induced arthritis in rats by oral administration of the inducing antigen. *Cell Immunol* 1997;175:67–75.

78. Yoshino S. Downregulation of silicone-induced chronic arthritis by gastric administration of type II collagen. *Immunopharmacology* 1995;31:103–108.

79. Al-Sabbagh AM, Garcia G, Slavin AJ, Weinerx HL, Nelson PA. Combination therapy with oral myelin basic protein and oral methotrexate enhances suppression of experimental autoimmune encephalomyelitis. *Neurology* 1997;48:A421.

80. Javed NH, Gienapp IE, Cox KL, Whitacre CC. Exquisite peptide specificity of oral tolerance in experimental autoimmune encephalomyelitis. *J Immunol* 1995;155:1599–1605.

81. Miller A, Al-Sabbagh A, Santos L, Das MP, Weiner HL. Epitopes of myelin basic protein that trigger TGF-β release following oral tolerization are distinct from encephalitogenic epitopes and mediate epitope driven bystander suppression. *J Immunol* 1993;151:7307–7315.

82. Khoury SJ, Hancock WW, Weiner HL. Oral tolerance to myelin basic protein and natural recovery from experimental autoimmune encephalomyelitis as associated with downregulation of inflammatory cytokines and differential upregulation of transforming growth factor β, interleukin 4, and prostaglandin E expression in the brain. *J Exp Med* 1992;176:1355–1364.

83. Higgins P, Weiner HL. Suppression of experimental autoimmune encephalomyelitis by oral administration of myelin basic protein and its fragments. *J Immunol* 1988;140:440–445.

84. Brod SA, Al-Sabbgh A, Sobel RA, Hafler DA, Weiner HL. Suppression of experimental autoimmune encephalomyelitis by oral administration of myelin antigens. IV. Suppression of chronic relapsing disease in the Lewis rat and strain 13 guinea pig. *Ann Neurol* 1991;29: 615–622.

85. Meyer AL, Benson JM, Gienapp IE, Cox KL, Whitacre CC. Suppression of murine chronic relapsing experimental autoimmune encephalomyelitis by the oral administration of myelin basic protein. *J Immunol* 1996;157:4230–4238.

86. Al-Sabbagh AM, Goad MEP, Weiner HL, Nelson PA. Decreased CNS inflammation and absence of clinical exacerbation of disease after six months oral administration of bovine myelin in diseased SJL/J mice with chronic relapsing experimental autoimmune encephalomyelitis. *J Neurol Res* 1996;45:424–429.

87. Chen Y, Inobe J, Kuchroo VK, Baron JL, Janeway CA Jr, Weiner HL. Oral tolerance in myelin basic protein T-cell receptor transgenic mice: suppression of autoimmune encephalomyelitis and dose-dependent induction of regulatory cells. *Proc Natl Acad Sci USA* 1996;93: 388–391.

88. Metzler B, Wraith DC. Inhibition of experimental autoimmune encephalomyelitis by inhalation but not oral administration of the encephalitogenic peptide: influence of MHC binding affinity. *Int Immunol* 1993;5:1159–1165.

89. Nussenblatt RB, Caspi RR, Mahdi R, et al. Inhibition of S-antigen induced experimental autoimmune uveoretinitis by oral induction of tolerance with S-antigen. *J Immunol* 1990;144:1689–1695.

90. Wildner G, Thurau SR. Cross-reactivity between an HLA-B27–derived peptide and a retinal autoantigen peptide: a clue to major histocompatibility complex association with autoimmune disease. *Eur J Immunol* 1994;24:2579–2585.

91. Wildner G, Thurau SR. Orally induced bystander suppression in experimental autoimmune uveoretinitis occurs only in the periphery and not in the eye. *Eur J Immunol* 1995;25:1292–1297.

92. Thurau S, Chan C-C, Nussenblatt R, Caspi R. Oral tolerance in a murine model of relapsing experimental autoimmune uveoretinitis (EAU): induction of protective tolerance in primed animals. *Clin Exp Immunol* 1997;109:370–376.

93. Thurau SR, Diedrichs-Mohring M, Fricke H, Arbogast S, Wildner G. Molecular mimicry as a therapeutic approach for an autoimmune disease: oral treatment of uveitis patients with an MHC-peptide crossreactive with autoantigen—first results. *Immunol Lett* 1997;57: 193–201.

94. Ma C-G, Zhang G-X, Xiao B-G, Link J, Olsson T, Link H. Suppression of experimental autoimmune myasthenia gravis by nasal administration of acetylcholine receptor. *J Neuroimmunol* 1995;58:51–60.

95. Wang H-M, Smith KA. The interleukin-2 receptor: functional consequences of its bimolecular structure. *J Exp Med* 1987;166:1055.

96. Wang Z-Y, Qiao J, Link H. Suppression of experimental autoimmune myasthenia gravis by oral administration of acetylcholine receptor. *J Neuroimmunol* 1993;44:209–214.

97. Neurath MF, Fuss I, Kelsall BL, Presky DH, Waegell W, Strober W. Experimental granulomatous colitis in mice is abrogated by induction of TGF-β–mediated oral tolerance. *J Exp Med* 1996;183:2605–2616.

98. Zhang JZ, Davidson L, Eisenbarth G, Weiner HL. Suppression of diabetes in NOD mice by oral administration of porcine insulin. *Proc Natl Acad Sci USA* 1991;88:10252–10256.

99. Bergerot J, Fabien N, Maguer V, Thivolet C. Oral administration of human insulin to NOD mice generates CD4+ T cells that suppress adoptive transfer of diabetes. *J Autoimmun* 1994;7:655–663.

100. Hancock WW, Polanski M, Zhang ZJ, Blogg N, Weiner HL. Suppression of insulitis in NOD mice by oral insulin administration is associated with selective expression of IL-4, IL-10, TGF-β and prostaglandin-E. *Am J Pathol* 1995;147:1193–1199.

101. Harrison LC, Collier-Dempsey M, Kramer DR, Takahashi K. Aerosol insulin induces regulatory CD8 γδ T cells that prevent murine insulin-dependent diabetes. *J Exp Med* 1996;184:2167–2174.

102. Daniel D, Wegmann DR. Protection of nonobese diabetic mice from diabetics by intranasal or subcutaneous administration of insulin peptide B-(9-23). *Proc Natl Acad Sci USA* 1996;93:956–960.

103. Tian J, Atkinson MA, Clare-Salzler M, Herschenfeld A, et al. Nasal administration of glutamate decarboxylase (GAD65) peptides induces Th2 responses and prevents murine insulin-dependent diabetes. *J Exp Med* 1996;183:1561–1567.

104. Blanas E, Carbone FR, Allison J, Miller JFAP, Heath WR. Induction of autoimmune diabetes by oral administration of autoantigen. *Science* 1996;274:1707–1709.

105. von Herrath MG, Dyrberg T, Oldstone MBA. Oral insulin treatment suppresses virus-induced antigen-specific destruction of beta cells and prevents autoimmune diabetes in transgenic mice. *J Clin Invest* 1996;98:1324–1331.

106. Polanski M, Blogg NS, Zhang J, Weiner HL. Oral administration of the immunodominant B-chain of insulin suppresses diabetes in NOD mice and is associated with a switch from Th1 to Th2 cytokines. *J Autoimmun* 1997;10:339–346.

107. Ma SW, Zhao DL, Yin ZQ, et al. Transgenic plants expressing autoantigens fed to mice to induce oral immune tolerance. *Nat Med* 1997;3:793–796.

108. Sayegh MH, Zhang ZJ, Hancock WW, Kwok CA, Carpenter CB, Weiner HL. Down-regulation of the immune response to histocompatibility antigen and prevention of sensitization by skin allografts by orally administered alloantigen. *Transplant* 1992;53:163–166.

109. Sayegh MH, Khoury SJ, Hancock WH, Weiner HL, Carpenter CB. Induction of immunity and oral tolerance with polymorphic class II

110. Hancock W, Sayegh M, Kwok C, Weiner H, Carpenter C. Oral, but not intravenous, alloantigen prevents accelerated allograft rejection by selective intragraft Th2 cell activation. *Transplantation* 1993;55:1112–1118.

111. Guimaraes VC, Quintans J, Fisfalen M-E, et al. Suppression of experimental autoimmune thyroiditis by oral administration of thyroglobulin. *Endocrinology* 1995;136:3353–3359.

112. Hoyne GF, Callow MG, Kuo MC, Thomas WR. Inhibition of T-cell responses by feeding peptides containing major and cryptic epitopes: studies with the der pI allergen. *Immunology* 1994;83:190–195.

113. Ilan Y, Prakash R, Davidson A, et al. Oral tolerization to adenoviral antigens permits long-term gene expression using recombinant adenoviral vectors. *J Clin Invest* 1997;99:1098–1106.

114. Lowney ED. Immunologic unresponsiveness to a contact sensitizer in man. *J Invest Dermatol* 1968;51:411–417.

115. Waldo FB, Van Den Wall Bake AWL, Mestecky J, Husby S. Suppression of the immune response by nasal immunization. *Clin Immunol Immunopathol* 1994;72:30–34.

116. Nussenblatt RB, Gery I, Weiner HL, et al. Treatment of uveitis by oral administration of retinal antigens: results of a phase I/II randomized masked trial. *Am J Opthalmol* 1997;123:583–592.

117. Barnett ML, Kremer JM, St Clair EW, et al. Treatment of rheumatoid arthritis with oral type II collagen: results of a multicenter, double-blind, placebo-controlled trial. *Arthritis Rheum* 1998;41:290–297.

118. Sieper J, Kary S, Sörensen H, Alten R, et al. Oral type II collagen treatment in early rheumatoid arthritis. *Arthritis Rheum* 1996;39: 41–51.

119. Barnett ML, Combitchi D, Trentham DE. A pilot trial of oral type II collagen in the treatment of juvenile rheumatoid arthritis. *Arthritis Rheum* 1996;39:623–628.

120. Trentham D, Dynesius-Trentham R, Orav E, et al. Effects of oral administration of type II collagen on rheumatoid arthritis. *Science* 1993;261:1727–1730.

121. Coutant R, Zeidler A, Rappaport R, et al. Oral insulin therapy in newly diagnosed immune mediated (type I) diabetes: preliminary analysis of a randomized double blind placebo controlled study. *Diabetes* 1998; 47[Suppl 1]:A97.

122. Bagot M, Charue D, Flechet ML, Terki N, Toma A, Revuz J. Oral desensitization in nickel allergy induces a decrease in nickel-specific T-cells. *Eur J Dermatol* 1995;5:614–617.

123. McKown KM, Carbone LD, Bustillo J, Sever JM, Kang AH, Postlethwaite AE. Open trial of oral type I collagen in patients with systemic sclerosis. *Arthritis Rheum* 1997;40:S100.

124. Miller A, Lider O, Al-Sabbagh A, Weiner H. Suppression of experimental autoimmune encephalomyelitis by oral administration of myelin basic protein. V. Hierarchy of suppression by myelin basic protein from different species. *J Neuroimmunol* 1992;39:243–250.

125. Terato K, Xiu JY, Miyahara H, Cremer MA, Griffiths MM. Induction of chronic autoimmune arthritis in DBA/1 mice by oral administration of type II collagen and *Escherichia coli* lipopolysaccharide. *Br J Rheumatol* 1996;35:1–11.

126. Miller A, Lider O, Abramsky O, Weiner HL. Orally administered myelin basic protein in neonates primes for immune responses and enhances experimental autoimmune encephalomyelitis in adult animals. *Eur J Immunol* 1994;24:1026–1032.

Inflammation: Basic Principles and Clinical Correlates,
3rd ed., edited by John I. Gallin and Ralph Snyderman.
Lippincott Williams & Wilkins, Philadelphia © 1999.

CHAPTER 81

Immunomodulation by Intravenous Immune Globulin

Richard I. Schiff

The protective effect of antibodies was first demonstrated before the turn of the 19th century, but the nature of these protective substances in serum was not understood until Tiselius isolated what he called the gamma fraction by electrophoresis. It was shown that the gamma could neutralize and protect against a variety of toxins and microorganisms such as tetanus, diphtheria, measles, polio, and hepatitis. However, the early preparations of gammaglobulin often were contaminated with endotoxin, and the routine use of gammaglobulin was not practical until Cohn and Oncley developed the ethanol precipitation process that is the basis for nearly all of the intravenous gammaglobulin preparations in use today.

The discovery of the first immunodeficiency disease in 1952, X-linked agammaglobulinemia, led to the widespread use of gammaglobulin to replace antibodies in patients with defective antibody production. These early preparations contained aggregates of immunoglobulin G (IgG), and only intramuscular injection was possible; intravenous administration led to severe, sometimes catastrophic reactions, especially in patients who were infected. Preparations of gammaglobulin that could be administered intravenously were developed in the 1970s, but it was not until 1981 that the first preparation was available in the United States. It was the availability of intravenous forms of immunoglobulin (IVIG) that allowed large doses of IgG to be administered and made it possible to use gammaglobulin as an immunomodulating agent.

The discovery of the immunomodulating properties of IVIG is attributed to Imbach et al., who observed that several children with hypogammaglobulinemia and thrombocytopenia had a rapid and dramatic rise in the platelet

count after he infused them with IVIG (1). Although Imbach began the modern era of the use of IgG for immunomodulation, the immunosuppressive effects had been known for more than 10 years. The Hellströms observed that antitumor antibodies promoted tumor growth (2,3), which was studied by others who demonstrated that the antibody interacted with the effector lymphocytes (4). Voisin, Kinsky, and others (5) discovered that antitumor antibodies suppressed specific immunity and enhanced tumor growth, leading to the term *enhancing antibodies* or *immunologic enhancement.*

The immunosuppressive effect was not confined to the tumor system. Plasma and IgG from postpartum women was capable of suppressing mixed lymphocyte responses and proliferation induced by mitogens *in vitro* (6). These antibodies were used in an attempt to prevent graft-versus-host disease (GVHD) when babies with severe combined immune deficiency were transplanted with bone marrow from their human leukocyte antigen (HLA)–incompatible mothers. Although successful in some patients, the effects were inconsistent, and the use of plasma to prevent GVHD was abandoned (7).

The early attempts to use IgG for immunosuppression differed in that the IgG was obtained from a single donor, rather than a pool of several thousand donors, and the doses of IgG used were considerably lower than that used when IVIG is used for immunomodulation. The use of IgG to promote tumor growth did not generate much enthusiasm among clinicians, and the inconsistent benefit when it was used to prevent GVHD led to disillusionment. The potential of IgG as an immunomodulator was largely forgotten until rediscovered by Imbach, who showed that the effect on the platelet count was not specific to immunodeficient patients. The possibility of using IgG instead of immunosuppressive drugs was appealing, and within a few years, IVIG was

R. I. Schiff: Clinical Immunology, Miami Children's Hospital, Miami, Florida 33155.

used routinely for immune thrombocytopenic purpura (ITP) and for many other autoimmune and inflammatory diseases.

CHARACTERISTICS OF INTRAVENOUS IMMUNE GLOBULIN PREPARATIONS

All of the intravenous gammaglobulin preparations are based on Cohn-Oncley fractionation (8,9) or the modification by Kistler and Nitschmann (10). The Cohn fraction 2 can be administered intramuscularly as immune serum globulin (ISG), but it contains aggregates that preclude intravenous infusion. A variety of techniques has been employed to modify the ISG to prevent adverse reactions. Initial modification with proteolytic enzymes reduced side effects but also cleaved the molecule, markedly reducing the half-life in the patient and destroying much of the biologic activity. Similarly, chemical modification altered the Fc portion of the molecule, reducing its ability to fix complement and to bind to Fc receptors on monocytes and neutrophils. The latest generation of IVIG preparations employ ion exchange chromatography, low pH with or without traces of proteolytic enzymes, and stabilizing agents such as sugars, amino acids, and albumin to prevent aggregation of the IgG and to allow safe intravenous administration.

The properties of the currently available IVIG preparations are summarized in Table 81-1. The pH varies from 4.25 to 7.2, and the osmolarity also varies significantly. All contain excipients such as sugars, amino acids, or albumin to stabilize the preparation, and these may be responsible for some of the side effects such as headache and muscle aches. Most of the IVIG preparations contain significant amounts of IgA but only trace amounts of IgM. All are free of vasoactive amines such as prekallikrein activator and proteases (11). Most of the IgG is monomeric, but some is dimeric, and the percentage of dimers increases with the number of donors in the pool (12) and with storage. No large aggregates are present that could nonspecifically activate complement. IVIG contains antibodies to a wide variety of microorganisms, representing the spectrum found in normal individuals. It contains antibodies to cytokines (13,14); cell surface receptors (CD5, CD4, and HLA) (15–17); and a variety of disease-specific antiidiotype antibodies (18). Less well appreciated, IVIG also contains significant amounts of non-IgG molecules, such as soluble HLA antigens (19,20) and soluble CD4 and CD8 (20). It is likely that these antibodies and soluble receptors are responsible for much of the immunomodulating effects of IVIG.

IVIG is a biologic product derived from blood, and therefore its use entails some risk. The various IVIG preparations have had a remarkably good safety profile, considering the millions of grams infused. Some serious adverse events have occurred, however, and these must be considered when contemplating the use of IVIG for autoimmune diseases. Fortunately, IVIG has never transmitted human immunodeficiency virus (HIV). The virus is readily destroyed by the ethanol in the Cohn fractionation process. A solvent-detergent process that inactivates enveloped viruses (21) has been added to several of the products. The transmission of hepatitis B virus has been

TABLE 81-1. *Intravenous gammaglobulin preparations available in the United States*

Brand name	Method of preparation	pH	Osmolality (mOsm)	IgA content (μg/mL)[a]	Additives	Form	Viral inactivation	Conc. (%)	Manufacturer
Gamimune N S/D	pH 4.25	4.25	335	270	10% maltose	Liquid	S/D, low pH	5	Bayer
Gamimune N, 10% S/D	pH 4.25	4.25	375	NA	0.2 mmol/L glycine	Liquid	S/D, low pH	10	Bayer
Gammagard S/D	DEAE-Sephadex polyethylene glycol (PEG)	6.8	630	<2	2% glucose, 0.2% PEG, 0.3 mmol/L glycine, 0.3% albumin	Lyophilized	SD	5, 10	Baxter
Gammar-P IV	Low ionic strength	7.0	333	20[b]	5% sucrose, 2.5% albumin	Lyophilized	Pasteurized	5	Centeon
Iveegam	Low pH, PEG, immobilized trypsin	6.8	375	≤2[b]	5% glucose 0.5% PEG	Lyophilized	Enzyme	5	Immuno-US
Polygam S/D	DEAE-Sephadex PEG	6.8	630	<2	Same as Gammagard	Lyophilized	S/D	5	Baxter/ American Red Cross
Sandoglobulin	Low pH, trace pepsin	6.6	375 (6%)	720	10% sucrose (6%)	Lyophilized	Low pH, enzyme	3, 6, 12	Sandoz
Venoglobulin-I	DEAE-Sephadex, PEG	6.8	225	20–24[b]	2% D-mannitol, 1% albumin, <0.6% PEG	Lyophilized		2.5, 5	Alpha Therapeutics
Venoglobulin-S	DEAE-Sephadex, PEG, detergent	5.2	302	10–27[b]	5% D-sorbitol, ≤0.2% albumin, ≤0.6% PEG	Liquid	S/D	5, 10	Alpha Therapeutics

S/D, solvent/detergent; N/A, not available.
[a]Concentrations approximate; there is much lot-to-lot variability.
[b]Data provided by the manufacturer.

prevented by a combination of screening for antigen-positive units, partitioning of the virus during fractionation, and neutralizing antibody in the gammaglobulin.

The history for hepatitis C is not so positive. Several sporadic cases of non-A, non-B hepatitis reported in the 1980s were associated with a variety of different IVIG preparations in England, Sweden, Norway, and Scotland (22–25). Each outbreak was acute and associated with high morbidity and mortality rates. There also was a report of several patients who developed hepatitis after being infused with an experimental lot of Gammagard (26), but there were no cases in the United States associated with a licensed product until 1993 (27). During late 1993 and early 1994, there was a worldwide outbreak associated with several lots of Gammagard. Approximately 116 cases have been reported in the United States, and an equal number has been reported throughout the rest of the world, with nearly all cases identified by September, 1994. It is believed that the outbreak was caused by removal of hepatitis C antibody-positive donors from the pool, allowing small amounts of virus to be unmasked (28). Since that episode, Gammagard has included a solvent-detergent step to inactivate the virus. Other preparations include solvent-detergent, incubation at low pH, enzyme treatment, or pasteurization to reduce the risk of viral transmission. Nonetheless, concern still exists for nonenveloped virus and the prion agent of Creutzfeldt-Jacob disease, although the transmission of Creutzfeldt-Jacob disease has never been documented or even suspected (29).

Infusions of IVIG have been associated with a variety of other, perhaps less serious, adverse reactions (30,31). Nearly all of the early products were associated with a high incidence of what were called phlogistic or inflammatory reactions: fever, chills, nausea, vomiting, headache, muscle aches, and less commonly, chest tightness or wheezing. More serious anaphylactic reactions are rare but potentially fatal, and they are thought to be caused by infusion of IgA-containing gammaglobulin into IgA-deficient patients (32). The currently available products are much better tolerated, but they still may be associated with headache, urticaria, chest tightness, fever, and aseptic meningitis (33). The cause of the meningitis is unknown, but it is more common in patients treated with larger doses of IVIG (2 g/kg), and the risk is said to be highest in patients treated for neurologic disorders. Other adverse reactions that rarely have been reported include hemolytic anemia (34,35), thrombosis (36), stroke (37), renal failure (38), myocardial infarction, and uveitis (39). In most of these reports, the patients had underlying disease, and it is not clear whether the IgG itself or one of the excipients was responsible for the reaction. Although these reactions are uncommon, they reinforce the need to carefully evaluate each patient before initiating therapy with IVIG and to consider whether the potential benefit outweighs the risks.

CLINICAL APPLICATIONS FOR IMMUNOMODULATION

Hematologic Disorders

The first widespread clinical use of IVIG for autoimmune disease was for ITP (40–43). After the initial observations of Imbach (44), several controlled studies confirmed its efficacy, especially in children with acute ITP (45–47). IVIG may prevent or at least defer the need for splenectomy in children, although it has this effect less often in adults (41). IVIG is effective in other forms of thrombocytopenia, such as that caused by alloimmunization (48–50), neonatal thrombocytopenia (51,52), or thrombocytopenia associated with HIV infection (53,54). Patients with ITP respond as well to an anti-Fc receptor monoclonal antibody (55) or to anti-Rh(D) antibody, now marketed as WinRho (56). Although the effectiveness of IVIG in these conditions is well documented and supported by placebo-controlled trials, many patients recover spontaneously or respond rapidly to conventional, less expensive therapy. The decision to use IVIG should be given careful consideration.

After the success of IVIG for ITP, it was tried in a variety of autoimmune and inflammatory diseases (30), as listed in Table 81-2. The effectiveness of IVIG is not as

TABLE 81-2. *Clinical uses of intravenous gammaglobulin for immunomodulation*

Clearly indicated and approved
  Kawasaki disease
  Idiopathic thrombocytopenic purpura
Supported by controlled clinical trials
  Bone marrow transplantation
  Neurologic diseases
    Multiple sclerosis
    Guillain-Barré syndrome
    Myasthenia gravis
    Chronic inflammatory demyelinating polyneuropathy
  Dermatomyositis
  Hemophilia caused by anti-factor VIII
Supported only by anecdotal reports or uncontrolled trials
  Hematologic disorders
    Neutropenia
    Hemolytic anemia
    Red cell aplasia
  Neurologic diseases
    Intractable seizures
    Collagen-vascular disease
    Systemic lupus erythematosus
    Systemic vasculitis
    Rheumatoid arthritis
    Anticardiolipin or recurrent abortions
  Miscellaneous inflammatory disorders
    Diabetes mellitus
    Bullous pemphigoid
    Birdshot retinopathy
Not supported or controversial data
  Collagen-vascular disease
    Inflammatory bowel disease
  Miscellaneous inflammatory disorders
    Asthma

great for the other autoimmune hematologic disorders as it is for ITP, although it has been shown to be effective if given in sufficiently high doses. Bussell et al. (57) treated four patients with refractory hemolytic anemia with 5 g/kg over 5 days, producing a sustained response in two and a transient response in another two. Several anecdotal reports describe partial responses in patients with hypogammaglobulinemia (58), thalassemia major (59), and allosensitization (60).

Others report the use of IVIG in neutropenia (61,62). In one study, six children with neutrophil counts less than 300/mm^3 and severe infections were treated with an average of 3 g/kg of IVIG, given as 1 g/kg until the neutrophil count exceeded 1,000/mm^3 (63,64).

Doses of 2 g/kg have been used to treat red cell aplasia with some success (65–67); the best responses were seen in patients with red cell aplasia associated with parvovirus B19 infection (68,69). Patients with thymoma or HIV infection also had an improvement in red blood cell production after therapy with IVIG (70).

Antibodies to factor VIII can arise spontaneously and cause acquired hemophilia or can develop in patients with congenital hemophilia as a result of therapy with factor VIII concentrates. At least 10% of patients treated with factor VIII develop antibodies that neutralize and reduce the effectiveness of the exogenous factor VIII. IVIG is not as effective for the alloimmune patients as it is for the patients with autoantibodies. Patients with autoantibodies that developed in association with pregnancy or with other autoimmune disorders responded rapidly to infusions of IVIG and went into a sustained remission that was associated with the development of antiidiotype antibodies to the anti-factor VIII antibody (71–73). Others have shown that the titers of anti-factor VIII decreases in nearly all patients treated with IVIG, although in a few it required weeks to months of therapy before the antibody was not detectable (74). However, only 6 of 16 patients were thought to have a clinical remission induced by the therapy.

Kawasaki Disease

The treatment of Kawasaki disease is one of the few absolute indications for the use of IVIG. Kawasaki disease is an acute inflammatory disorder that was initially called acute febrile mucocutaneous lymph node syndrome. It occurs predominantly in young children and is most prevalent in Japan. The cause is unknown, but it occurs in epidemics, often in the spring and fall, leading to speculation that it is caused by an infectious organism. It is thought to be the result of a superantigen because of massive T-cell activation involving Vβ2 and Vβ8.1 T cells (75). The most serious consequence of Kawasaki disease is the development of coronary aneurysms. Several controlled trials have conclusively demonstrated that IVIG reduces the incidence of coronary artery aneurysms compared with patients treated with aspirin alone (75–83). The inflammatory symptoms such as fever often resolve during the first infusion of the IVIG.

Neurologic Disorders

One of the major uses of IVIG in the 1990s is the treatment of autoimmune neurologic diseases. Study of animal models has indicated that seizures could be related to the presence of autoimmune disease, often precipitated by viral infections. Neurologic disease can be induced by immunization with myelin basic protein, such as in experimental autoimmune encephalopathy. In some diseases, such as myasthenia gravis, Rasmussen's syndrome, or chronic inflammatory polyneuropathy, autoantibodies can be identified that are pathologic when injected into experimental animals. Other diseases are thought to be mediated by T cells. The mechanism by which IVIG may modulate these diseases is unknown, but receptors for IgG have been identified in the central and peripheral nervous system (84), and IgG given intravenously passes through the blood-brain barrier to interact with the central nervous system (85).

Refractory Seizures

Ariizumi et al. first tried to treat patients with refractory seizures in 1984 (86). Eight patients who had seizures for less than 2 years improved significantly, but another eight who had seizures of longer duration did not improve. Patients were treated with only 100 to 200 mg/kg, a low dose by contemporary standards. In a study of 12 patients with intractable seizures, six were found to have IgG2 subclass deficiency. All were treated with IVIG, and whereas none of the patients with normal subclass levels improved, five of the six with IgG2 subclass deficiency had a marked reduction in the frequency of seizures after doses of 400 mg/kg (87). Neither infection nor autoimmune disease could be identified as a cause of seizures in these patients, and the relationship to the IgG2 subclass deficiency still is unknown. However, it is believed that the seizures are caused by immune dysregulation and that the IVIG restores normal immune function (88).

Guillain-Barré Syndrome

IVIG has been particularly effective in the treatment of the inflammatory polyneuropathies. This includes Guillain-Barré syndrome (GBS), chronic inflammatory polyneuropathy (CIDP), multiple sclerosis (MS), myasthenia gravis, and inflammatory myopathies. GBS is a subacute inflammatory polyneuropathy that leads to severe quadriparesis. Nearly 5% die of the disease, and 10% to 15% are permanently disabled. It is characterized by a lymphocytic infiltration of the myelin sheath that leads to segmental demyelination. About 60% of patients with GBS have antibodies that bind to neuroblastoma cells (89,90), and the serum of patients with GBS can induce demyelination when injected into animals. The binding of antibodies to the cell line was inhibited by IVIG, and recovery from GBS is associated with the presence of an antiidiotype antibody recognizing a cross-reactive epitope on anti-neuroblastoma cells (89,90). A large, multicenter study in the Netherlands comparing IVIG with plasmapheresis showed a more rapid improvement in the IVIG group. One hundred and forty patients were randomly assigned to five sessions of plasma exchange or 5 days of 400 mg/kg of Gammagard. The median time to improve one grade was 27 days in the IVIG group and 41 days in those treated with plasma exchange (91). Fewer complications such as pneumonia, thrombosis, or atelectasis occurred in the IVIG group.

Some smaller studies confirmed these results (92,93), but another study suggested that more patients relapsed after IVIG treatment (94). Although it appears that only a subset of patients show a sustained clinical response, IVIG is considered the treatment of choice by most neurologists, although it is clear that more research is needed to determine which patients are most likely to benefit.

Chronic Inflammatory Demyelinating Polyneuropathy

Chronic inflammatory demyelinating polyneuropathy is considered the chronic form of GBS. Many patients have anti-GM_1 autoantibodies, but there does not seem to be an association between the presence or the class of the antibody and severity or response to therapy (95). The benefit of plasma exchange and IVIG was shown as early as 1985 (96) and was supported by a small but placebo-controlled study in 1990 (97). An open study of 52 patients in the Netherlands showed that 32 patients improved after 2 g/kg of IVIG, and 30 of the patients had a sustained improvement of one to four grades on the Rankin scale (98). Unfortunately, a double-blind, placebo-controlled study of 15 patients by the same group did not show any benefit (99). Despite its widespread use, more research is needed before we can determine the optimal dose and treatment schedule and which patients are most likely to respond.

Multiple Sclerosis

Multiple sclerosis is a severe, relapsing and remitting demyelinating disease that is similar to an animal model in which autoimmune disease in induced by immunization with neural tissue. Patients have antibody and T cells directed against axon sheaths or the axons themselves. In an early, uncontrolled study of 31 patients, 11 patients improved, and 9 remained stable after therapy with intramuscular immunoglobulin or IVIG (100). In a study of 51 chronic patients who were treated with 2 g/kg of IVIG

every 2 months for 2 years, 71% had at least a 50% reduction in the frequency of acute exacerbations and stability or improvement in neurologic disability (101). The patients with the most active disease and with no sensory deficit were the most likely to respond. Although there are no controlled studies, most of the open-label studies show significant improvement. In Theiler's virus-induced demyelination, which is an animal model of multiple sclerosis, IVIG induces remyelination (102), lending support to the use of IgG in this disorder.

Myasthenia Gravis

Myasthenia gravis is one of the better-characterized autoimmune neuropathies. It is caused by an antibody to the acetylcholine receptor and may be associated with thymoma. Edan and Landgraf (103) summarized the use of IVIG for MG in 1994. They reviewed six studies plus their own experience for a total of 86 patients who had a 78% rate of improvement. In a study by Arsura et al. of 9 patients who were given repeated infusions of IVIG, 20 of 23 courses resulted in satisfactory improvement (104). Improvement lasted 106±49 days. In another study of 12 patients, 2 of whom did not have detectable anti-cholinergic receptor antibodies, 10 patients improved (105). There was no association with the titer of autoantibody, although others had demonstrated that IVIG contains antibodies that bind to anti-acetylcholine receptor antibodies (106). The best responses were in those patients who received concomitant immunosuppressive drugs such as steroids or azathioprine. In a prospective randomized trial of 87 patients treated with IVIG or plasma exchange, the improvement was similar with both therapies, but the incidence of side effects was less with the IVIG (107).

Inflammatory Myopathies

IVIG has been used for inflammatory myopathies and a variety of other neurologic disorders. The inflammatory myopathies include dermatomyositis, polymyositis, and multifocal motor neuropathy. Roifman et al. (108) reported improvement of polymyositis after treatment of a 15-year-old girl who failed therapy with steroids, methotrexate, and cyclophosphamide. After 6 months of therapy, her muscle strength improved in hip or shoulder muscles from one to three grades. Cherin et al. treated 20 patients with dermatomyositis or polymyositis who had failed immunosuppression and plasmapheresis with 2 g/kg each month for an average of 4 months (109). Fifteen of the 20 patients had statistically significant improvement in motor strength. An additional 5 patients with dermatomyositis were treated with 2 g/kg over 2 days monthly for 9 months (110). All patients had improvement in motor strength and decreased rash; many of the patients were able to discontinue their prednisone therapy.

A double-blind, placebo-controlled study enrolled 15 dermatomyositis patients who were unresponsive to immunotherapeutic agents or who had unacceptable side effects (111). Patients were treated with 2 g/kg of IVIG or placebo for 3 months, with an option to crossover to the other therapy for an additional 3 months. Patients who were randomized to receive IVIG had a significant improvement in muscle strength on the MRC scale from 76.6±5.7 to 84.6±4.6 and in neuromuscular symptom score from 44.0±8.2 to 51.4±6. In contrast, those receiving placebo had no change in either score. In addition to these parameters, the rash also improved, and the creatine kinase decreased 50%.

Multifocal motor neuropathy is often associated with high levels of antibodies to ganglioside GM_1, or asialo-GM_1 (112). Several open, uncontrolled studies and one placebo-controlled study of patients with chronic disease showed significant improvement in strength in most patients that lasted up to 2 months (112–115). There did not appear to be an association with the presence of anti-GM_1 antibodies, and response to therapy and the titer of the antibodies did not change during therapy with IVIG. However, treatment with IVIG was particularly effective in those with motor neuropathy associated with monoclonal gammopathy (114).

Miscellaneous Neurologic Disorders

Human T-cell lymphotrophic virus type I (HTLV-I)–associated myelopathy can result in spastic quadriparesis. Fourteen patients were treated with IVIG in a single dose of 10 g or 400 mg/kg/d for 5 days (116). Ten had significant improvement within 7 days. A beneficial response was found in patients having a high cerebrospinal fluid (CSF) titer of anti–HTLV-I antibodies, a high CSF IgG level, and a marked abnormality on magnetic resonance imaging of the brain.

IVIG was also found to be of benefit in inclusion-body myositis (117). Three of four patients who were treated monthly with 2 g/kg had improvement or normalization on nonatrophied muscles after 2 months that lasted another 2 to 4 months. Because no controlled studies have been done, the overall effectiveness is unknown.

Collagen-Vascular Disease

Infusions of IVIG have been of some benefit in the collagen-vascular diseases, but the results are not dramatic. The use of other therapy, such as anti-cytokine antibodies or soluble cytokine receptors, probably will be more effective and make the use of IVIG uncommon.

A few patients with systemic lupus erythematosus (SLE) have improved after infusions of IVIG (118–122), but others have experienced worsening of their renal disease (119,121). There have been no controlled studies, and the use of IVIG for SLE is still experimental.

Women with antiphospholipid antibodies and spontaneous abortions have been treated with IVIG during pregnancy with a successful outcome in 82%, but these were uncontrolled case reports and the effectiveness of the gammaglobulin is not clear (123–126). Further studies are underway to determine the effectiveness of IVIG in patients with recurrent abortions (127).

IVIG was effective in 23 patients with ANCA-positive vasculitis in open studies (128,129) and in Churg-Strauss syndrome (130). There was some improvement in joint symptoms at the highest doses of IVIG in several trials for rheumatoid arthritis, although the data are not strong enough to encourage widespread use in this disease (131–137). Ten patients with severe rheumatoid arthritis unresponsive to conventional therapy improved significantly during a 6-month trial of IVIG (137). All relapsed after the immunoglobulin was discontinued. Clinical response paralleled a decrease in the $CD4^+CDw29^+$: $CD4^+CD45RA^+$ subset. In the only placebo-controlled study of IVIG for rheumatoid arthritis, 31 children with active arthritis were treated with 1.5 g/kg every 2 weeks for 2 months and then monthly for 4 months (136). Fourteen patients, seven in each group, withdrew from the study prematurely; of the remaining patients, 50% in the IVIG group improved, compared with 27% in the placebo group. Despite the trend, the study did not have sufficient power to demonstrate that IVIG is effective for children with arthritis.

Miscellaneous Autoimmune and Inflammatory Disorders

IVIG has been used in a variety of other inflammatory and autoimmune disorders, including asthma, inflammatory bowel disease, atopy, bullous pemphigoid, and diabetes mellitus. There have been anecdotal reports of improvement of asthma after therapy with IVIG (138), perhaps as a result of reducing infections that could precipitate an asthma attack. An open-label study of IVIG in treating asthma (139) suggested that there was a reduction of steroid dose in the treated patients. Pulmonary functions were stable, and skin test reactivity decreased (140). However, a placebo-controlled trial did not show any benefit because all of the patients were able to reduce their dose of steroids while given intensive conventional therapy during the study (141).

IVIG was not particularly effective in a small trial of inflammatory bowel disease (142) although a few of the patients improved. A trial of IVIG in severe atopic dermatitis and the hyper-IgE syndrome did not show any benefit (143). Treatment with IVIG did allow a reduction in steroid dose in six patients with various forms of pemphigus and pemphigoid (144).

IVIG reduced the insulin requirements of most newly diagnosed children with diabetes (145), although the difference was not seen after 1 year (146). A review of six studies of the use of IVIG for children with diabetes (147) concluded that although some patients showed improvement with a prolongation of remissions or a reduction in insulin requirements, further studies are necessary before IVIG can be recommended for treatment of diabetes.

MECHANISMS OF ACTION

IVIG acts through many different mechanisms, some of which are listed in Table 81-3. Blockade of the reticuloendothelial system may be effective to prevent phagocytosis of platelets or neutrophils, but does not explain the prolonged remission that ensues. Inhibition of complement deposition can prevent cell damage and may be important in preventing vascular damage in dermatomyositis or Kawasaki disease. IVIG downregulates immunoglobulin production by B cells directly and by interfering with cytokine production by T cells and macrophages. IVIG contains antiidiotypic antibodies that can bind to free IgG molecules but also to immunoglobulin on B cells and most likely to the immunoglobulin-like T-cell receptor. These antibodies have been effective in treating hemophilia caused by factor VIII deficiency and are present in patients recovering from GBS. Modulation of T cells by direct

TABLE 81-3. *Possible mechanisms of action of intravenous gammaglobulin for immunomodulation*

Proposed mechanism	Clinical example
Inhibition of Fcγ receptors	ITP (immediate effect)— phagocytes ITP (remission)—B-cell FcγRIIb Neutropenia Hemolytic anemia ANCA+ vasculitis
Inhibition of complement (C3b)	ITP Vasculitis
Regulation of idiotype/ anti-idiotype antibodies	Hemophilia due to anti-factor VIII Guillain-Barré syndrome Polyneuropathy (CIDP) Multiple sclerosis ANCA + vasculitis
Modulation of cytokine production	Kawasaki disease Graft-versus-host disease Multiple sclerosis
Modulation of lymphocyte activation	Kawasaki disease Remission in ITP Cytopenias Graft-versus-host disease Uveitis

ANCA, anti-neutrophil cytoplasmic antibodies; CIDP, chronic inflammatory polyneuropathy; ITP, immune thrombocytopenic purpura.

interaction with cell surface receptors and by inhibiting cytokine production may prove to be the most important mechanism for most autoimmune diseases.

Effects on Fc Receptors

Inhibition of phagocytosis by blockade of Fc receptors was postulated as the mechanism by which IVIG increases the platelet count in ITP. It was known that ITP was associated with anti-platelet antibodies and that the antibody-coated platelets were taken up by the reticuloendothelial system. The increase in the platelet count occurs rapidly, making other mechanisms, such as immune modulation, less likely.

The process by which IVIG impairs Fc receptor activity is not fully elucidated. Human leukocytes have three types of Fcγ receptors (FcγR) (148). Two high-affinity receptors exist for monomeric IgG: FcRI (CD64), which is present on mononuclear phagocytes and cytokine-activated neutrophils, and FcRII (CD32), which is present on mononuclear phagocytes, neutrophils, eosinophils, and platelets. A low-affinity receptor that binds aggregated IgG and immune complexes (FcRIII, CD16) is present on neutrophils, natural killer (NK) cells, and macrophages but not on monocytes. Binding to these receptors elicits a variety of biologic responses, including antibody-dependent, cell-mediated cytotoxicity, phagocytosis, release of inflammatory mediators, and regulation of lymphocyte proliferation and differentiation. Treatment of monocytes with 10 mg/mL of IgG inhibited Fc receptor–mediated phagocytosis of IgG-coated red blood cells (149). Loss of function is energy dependent, involving ingestion, shedding, or internalization and degradation of receptors; recovery requires protein synthesis, suggesting that new receptors are generated (150).

Several lines of evidence support the role of Fc receptor blockade as a possible mechanism to account for some of the effects of IVIG. First, the clearance of IgG-coated red blood cells is impaired after administration of IVIG (151). Second, Fc fragments of IgG are as capable of increasing the platelet count as is intact IgG (152). Third, anti-Rh(D) is effective in ITP, presumably by overwhelming the phagocytic system with antibody-coated red blood cells (56). Fourth, monoclonal antibody to FcRII (153) inhibited phagocytosis in mice, and antibody to the low-affinity FcRIII was effective clinically in a patient with refractory ITP (154). IVIG and anti-Rh(D) contain anti-Fc antibodies (155,156). Soluble CD16 was detected in the serum of patients with ITP who were treated with IVIG (152). The soluble CD16 was not present in the IVIG, and the increase in the soluble receptor correlated with the rise in the platelet count. These receptors could bind to the antibody-coated platelets and competitively inhibit binding to the phagocytic cells. IVIG may inhibit Fc receptors by several mechanisms: binding of Fc by monomeric IgG, specific binding of antibody to the receptor, and shedding of receptors.

Inhibition of complement activity

IgG activates complement when complexed or bound to cells. IVIG may interact with activated complement components to prevent binding to their target cells. IgG interferes with the formation of complexes of human albumin with rabbit anti-albumin (157) and reduces the level of circulating C1q binding immune complexes in patients with SLE (158). Infusions of IVIG do not alter levels of complement components or activate complement, but very high levels of IgG could bind C3b in solution, preventing formation of C3b/IgG complexes on opsonized particles (159). IVIG significantly inhibits deposition of C3 on red blood cells sensitized with IgM and prolongs the survival of these cells *in vivo* (160). Guinea-pigs infused with anti-Forssman antibodies die within minutes unless they are complement deficient. The Forssman antigen is a lipopolysaccharide present on endothelial cells, and the antibody, in the presence of complement, destroys the endothelium, leading to pulmonary edema, hemorrhage, and death. Normally, 100% of the animals die within minutes, but up to 40% of the animals treated with 1.8 g/kg of IVIG before the IVIG survived (160,161). The effect was dose dependent, and it was shown *in vitro* that the complement binding on the endothelial cells was reduced to zero.

There is some indirect evidence that IVIG interferes with complement activation in human disease (160). The number of C3 molecules was greatly reduced on the surface of red blood cells in hemolytic anemia and on platelets in a patient with thrombocytopenia. Paroxysmal nocturnal hemoglobinuria is an acquired hemolytic process in which the red blood cells are abnormally sensitive to lysis by complement because they are lacking one of several membrane-bound proteins (e.g., decay accelerating factor, homologous restriction factor) that inactivate complement as it binds to the cells. *In vitro,* IgG can protect the red blood cells from acid lysis, suggesting that it may be interfering with deposition of complement on the surface.

Dermatomyositis has some similarities to the Forssman shock model in that both are complement-mediated angiopathies. Terminal complement components C5 through C9 are deposited on the intramuscular capillaries, leading to muscle ischemia and subsequent necrosis. IVIG is effective clinically, leading to improved muscle strength (111). After treatment with IVIG, the ability of sera from dermatomyositis patients to deposit C3 onto particular immune complexes was inhibited (160), and C3b and membrane attack complexes were no longer present on capillary endothelium (162). There is clinical and laboratory evidence that IVIG can interfere with the deposition of complement on the surface of target cells.

Modulation of the idiotype network

Idiotype-antiidiotype interactions are part of the normal regulatory mechanism, so it should not be surprising that IVIG contains antiidiotypic antibodies. Kazatchkine et al. isolated antibodies from IVIG that could bind to Fab fragments from a variety of autoantibodies, including anti-factor VIII, anti-thyroglobulin, anti-DNA, anti-FcγR, anti-neutrophil cytoplasmic antigen, and anti-actin and tubulin (163). These antiidiotype antibodies regulate the levels of autoantibody to prevent them from attaining levels that could cause disease. Recovery from anti-factor VIII (72) and from GBS (89) is associated with the appearance of antiidiotype antibodies directed against the pathogenic autoantibody. Preparations of F(ab')₂ fragments from the postrecovery sera were shown to interact with F(ab')₂ fragments of the anti-factor VIII antibody (72). Patients who respond to treatment with IVIG have a rapid fall in their levels of anti-factor VIII antibody, but treatment failures do not (73). IVIG binds to the F(ab')₂ fragments of anti-factor VIII in a manner that is similar to the binding of postrecovery sera. In another example, anti-ANCA antibodies exist in IVIG (18) and may neutralize the autoantibody to prevent damage to the endothelial cells. Levels of the autoantibody fall after treatment with IVIG (128,129).

Antiidiotype antibodies have been identified in a variety of diseases that have been shown to respond to IVIG. These include ITP, autoimmune erythroblastopenia, myasthenia gravis, chronic inflammatory demyelinating polyneuropathy, systemic vasculitis, bird-shot retinopathy, and anti-factor VIII disease (164). If autoimmune disease results from a defective idiotypic network, the IVIG may contain a wide spectrum of idiotypes and antiidiotypes expressed in normal people (163). The proportion of dimers increases as the pool size increases, suggesting that the number of idiotype-antiidiotype interactions increases. Rather than simply neutralizing the abnormal autoantibody, the IVIG probably restores the normal physiologic network (12).

Modulation of B-cell, T-cell, and Natural Killer Cell Functions

Normal human serum contains a variety of antibodies capable of interacting with lymphocytes. The antiidiotype antibodies discussed in the previous section are normally thought to interact with the V region of antibody molecules. B cells carry immunoglobulin molecules on their surface and could be targets for antiidiotype antibodies. The T-cell receptor is an immunoglobulin-like molecule that can interact with antiidiotype antibodies. Autoantibodies against the T-cell receptor β chain have been described (165), but the regulatory effects of these antibodies remain speculative. It has been known for many years that normal sera, particularly from parous women, contain agglutinating and cytotoxic antibodies that can interact with T lymphocytes (166). Many studies demonstrated that the sera of pregnant women are inhibitory to T lymphocytes (6).

An antibody to the CD5 molecule on T cells and a subset of B cells was discovered in IVIG (16). The effect of anti-CD5 has not yet been elucidated, but other anti-T-cell antibodies have been shown to have inhibitory effects. For example, a rabbit antibody directed against a lymphocyte function antigen-1–like molecule on the surface of T cells and NK cells inhibited proliferation and cytotoxic activity (167). Antibodies directed against class II HLA antigens are present in placenta-eluted gammaglobulin and are very inhibitory *in vivo* and *in vitro* (168).

Regulation of T- and B-cell function does not require antibodies to be directed against cellular components. IVIG preparations contain soluble CD4, CD8, and HLA molecules that could interfere with T-cell activation. Takei et al. described several antibodies in IVIG preparations that are directed against staphylococcal superantigens (169). These superantigens have a dual affinity for the class II MHC antigens and the relatively invariant sequence of the variable (V) β region of the T-cell receptor. Superantigens are capable of stimulating large numbers of T cells independently of the antigen specificity of the T cell. Superantigen stimulation has been implicated in diseases such as Kawasaki syndrome, in which massive T-cell stimulation occurs. Antibodies to the superantigens could block such stimulation and indirectly inhibit T-cell activation.

Another potential mechanism of action for IVIG was described by Honda et al. (170). They described a sialic acid–like substance in IVIG that could bind to the surface of platelets and prevent recognition by monocytes and macrophages. The importance of this unique inhibitory substance must be confirmed by additional studies.

Inhibition of B-cell Function

Durandy, Fischer, and Griscelli (171) treated immunologically normal children who had recurrent infections with intramuscular injections of IgG and observed that their B cells failed to produce plasma cells when stimulated with pokeweed mitogen *in vitro*. They found that, when the IgG preparations were added to cultures of normal cells, lymphocytes were unable to proliferate, and maturation of B cells was abolished. Inhibition resulted from development of suppressor activity that depended on the presence of monocytes and was mediated through prostaglandin E_2 (PGE_2). After T-cell suppressor activity developed, the monocytes were no longer necessary. They did not show a direct effect of the IgG on the B lymphocytes.

Several subsequent studies confirmed the inhibitory effects of IgG on B-cell maturation and immunoglobulin synthesis. Stohl (172,173) reported that Sandoglobulin in

concentrations of 300 mg/mL inhibited the development of pokeweed mitogen–induced plaque-forming cells. He found that the IgG had to be present at the initiation of the culture to exert its suppressive effect and that $F(ab')_2$ fragments were not effective. Removal of the IgG after 24 hours in culture did not permit the B cells to mature normally. In this system, the IgG appeared to affect the B cells directly, and no augmentation of T-cell suppressor activity or inhibition of T-cell help could be demonstrated.

Hashimoto et al. (174) also demonstrated inhibition of B-cell maturation, although they reached different conclusions regarding the mechanism of action. They evaluated ISG and several different IVIG preparations and found that the ISG was most inhibitory, followed by the sulfonated and polyethylene glycol preparations, but that a pepsin-treated IVIG preparation was not inhibitory. Their results confirmed those of Stohl (172) that an intact Fc portion of the IgG molecule was necessary for it to inhibit B-cell maturation. They incubated the IgG preparations with subsets of mononuclear cells and found that pretreatment of the B cells or T cells resulted in inhibition, but that T cells depleted of $CD8^+$ cells were not effective. Unlike Durandy et al. (171), Hashimoto et al. were not able to demonstrate a role for monocytes or PGE_2 in the development of suppression. Kondo et al. (175) also showed inhibition of immunoglobulin production by IVIG preparations that had intact Fc activity but did not get suppression at all if only the T cells were preincubated in the IgG. They did find that the suppression could be blocked by antibody to the Fc portion of IgG, suggesting that the IVIG was exerting its effect by binding to Fcγ receptors.

The best evidence that IVIG directly interacts with the B lymphocytes comes from the study of binding to the Fcγ receptors (174,176–178). B cells have the high-affinity FcγRIIb receptors, and simultaneous binding of this receptor and the antigen receptor induces a negative signal (179). Inhibition can be prevented by treatment with interleukin-4 (IL-4) or blocking the Fcγ receptor with antibody (180). Co-ligation of the Fcγ and antigen receptor can initiate apoptosis (181), which explains the lack of reversibility observed by Stoll (172,173).

Induction of Suppressor T-cell Activity

Several studies have reported that infusions of IVIG can alter the numbers and percentages of lymphocytes and NK cells in the peripheral blood and that the activity of the remaining cells is altered. One of the first was the observations of Durandy et al., who found that injections of gammaglobulin into normal children impaired the ability of B cells to mature into plasma cells when stimulated *in vitro* with pokeweed mitogen (171). They attributed this to an increase in a suppressor T cell that lacked Fcγ receptors and believed that activation of the suppressor T cells was induced by excessive PGE_2 production by monocytes.

Delfraissy et al. (182) measured suppressor activity in adult patients with ITP before and after treatment with IVIG. In the five of seven patients who responded to therapy, there was an increase in concanavalin A (Con A)–induced suppressor activity for autologous in vitro B-cell immunoglobulin production. The two patients who failed to respond had no alteration in suppressor activity. There was no alteration in lymphocyte subpopulations in any patient.

Similar results were obtained by Tsubakio et al. in five adult patients with ITP. The proportion of CD3 cells did not change, but the CD4:CD8 ratio decreased significantly and there was a 78%, 48%, and 66% suppression of in vitro synthesis of IgG, IgA, and IgM, respectively. They also observed a decrease in the titers of various autoantibodies in addition to the antiplatelet antibodies involved in the ITP.

White et al. (183) showed that IVIG could induce changes in suppressor T-cell activity in patients with common variable immune deficiency (CVID). When adult patients with CVID were infused for several months, the absolute number of CD3 and CD4 cells decreased, with a relative increase in CD8 cells and suppressor activity measured against normal B lymphocytes. Similar changes were found by Leung et al. (184) in patients with Kawasaki disease. Before treatment with IVIG, patients had elevated numbers of activated CD4[+] cells with a relative and absolute decrease in the number of CD8[+] suppressor cells. There also was a polyclonal activation of B cells to produce IgG and IgM. By the fourth day of therapy, there was a significant decrease in CD4[+] cell activation, an increase in CD8[+] cells, and a reduction in immunoglobulin production. IVIG exerts its effects in Kawasaki disease by inducing profound changes in cytokine production by monocytes and lymphocytes.

Most studies suggest that suppressor activity is increased after therapy with IVIG, and that autoantibodies and, in some cases, nonspecific immunoglobulin production are decreased. However, conflicting results have been reported. In some reports, suppressor cells increase after IVIG therapy, but in others, total T cells and NK cells are reduced. Interpretation is difficult, because patients may not have normal subsets or in vitro immunoglobulin production before therapy because of their disease or therapy with drugs such as corticosteroids. The response of patients with one disease may not be representative of all patients or normal individuals.

Inhibition of T-cell Proliferation

The immunosuppressive effects of IgG on T-cell proliferation have been known for more than 25 years. Buckley et al. (6) reported the inhibitory effects of pregnancy sera and IgG fractions obtained from those sera on lymphocyte proliferation induced by mitogens, antigens, and allogeneic cells. Subsequent studies indicated that IgG from normal donors had similar properties (185,186). Concentrations of IgG from 1 to 10 mg/mL inhibited lymphocyte proliferation in a dose-dependent manner. Proliferation induced by allogeneic cells and anti-CD3 monoclonal antibody was particularly sensitive. Inhibition was reversible if the IgG was washed out of the cultures within 48 hours, indicating that it did not result from a cytotoxic effect.

Kawada and Terasaki published the first detailed reports of the inhibitory effects of IgG (187). They demonstrated that IgG concentrations of 20 to 30 mg/mL inhibited phytohemagglutinin antigen (PHA) stimulation, mixed lymphocyte culture, NK cytotoxicity, antibody-dependent cell-mediated cytotoxicity, and cell-mediated lympholysis. The also showed that Fc fragments were more effective than intact IgG molecules.

A study by van Schaik et al. confirmed the inhibitory effects of IVIG on in vitro proliferation and examined the kinetics of the inhibition (188). Concentrations of IVIG from 1 to 50 mg/mL inhibited the response to allogeneic cells up to 80%. IL-2–stimulated cells were maximally inhibited by 15 mg/mL and PHA stimulation by 35 mg/mL. Preincubation of stimulator and responder cells and washing before culture did not result in inhibition. However, if IgG was added at the beginning of mixed lymphocyte cultures and washed out at various times after initiation of culture, no inhibition was observed if IgG was removed after 2 to 4 hours, but proliferation was inhibited if IgG was present for 12 to 24 hours. If addition of IgG was delayed until the cultures were established, inhibition of allogeneic cell or PHA-induced proliferation was observed even if addition of IgG was delayed until 4 hours before addition of ^{3}H-thymidine.

The IgG had an inhibitory effect on a variety of spontaneously growing cell lines, independent of the species of origin or the source of the cells. The IgG was not cytotoxic for the cells that were found to be arrested in the G_0/G_1 phase and not able to progress to the S phase. Taken together, these experiments suggest that IgG inhibits late in the proliferative phase rather than during initial stimulation. Much of the inhibition can be attributed to alteration in cytokine production.

Klaesson et al. (189) also found that the inhibitory effects of IgG were nonspecific, but unlike Kawada and Terasaki (187), their results showed that F(ab')$_2$ fragments were as effective as intact IgG. They were able to show inhibition of T cells stimulated with PHA, Con A, pokeweed mitogen, allogeneic cells, and Staphylococcus aureus protein A. They also investigated responses to specific antigen and showed inhibition of stimulation by herpesvirus. They compared 12 different commercial preparations and found inhibition of PHA response, ranging from 4% to 35%, and of mixed lymphocyte response, ranging from 0% to 66%. Three of five single donors were more inhibitory than the commercial pools, which is contrary to the theory that inhibition is mediated by dimers formed from idiotype-antiidiotype complexes.

Although these studies showed that IgG could inhibit a wide spectrum of T-cell activities, they did not address the mechanism of action. IVIG is a complex biologic material that contains a wide spectrum of antibodies and soluble cell receptors and cytokines. IgG obtained from placental blood has high levels of antibody to class II HLA antigens (168) and soluble Fcγ receptors (190). The inhibitory effects of the IgG preparation correlated with the levels of the soluble receptor. Blasczyk et al. (191) detected class I and class II HLA molecules and found soluble CD4 and CD8. IVIG also contains antibodies to CD5, a surface molecule on T cells, and a subset of autoantibody-producing B cells (16). The potential of this antibody to modulate T-cell activity has not been evaluated.

Vuist et al. (192) identified an antibody to a unique cell surface molecule, a glycolipid isolated from a B-cell line. It is found on B and T lymphocytes and a number of hematopoietic cell lines. The antibody eluted from the cell membranes was 1,000- to 10,000-fold more inhibitory than the initial IVIG preparation.

IVIG also contains antibodies to cytokines. Tiberio et al. (14) detected antibodies to IL-2 and antibodies to IL-1α, but neither IL-1β or tumor necrosis factor-α (TNF-α) were detected by Schifferli et al. (193). Bendtzen et al. (194) also detected antibodies to IL-1α and antibody to IL-6. Ross et al. found high-avidity neutralizing antibodies to interferon-α (IFN-α) and IFN-β (13). Lam et al. (195) detected class II antigens and anti-IFN-α but not TNF-α, IL-1R antagonist, soluble IL-2, or soluble IL-4.

Antiidiotypic antibodies react with the variable regions of immunoglobulins in solution and with immunoglobulin on B cells and the T-cell receptor. Kaveri et al. (15,196) demonstrated that IVIG contains antibody to CD4, which can suppress mixed lymphocyte responses, and antibodies to the constant and variable regions of the β chain of the T-cell receptor. Antibody directed against a highly conserved region of the α1 helix of the class I HLA molecule binds to class I antigens and inhibits CD8-mediated cytotoxicity (15). These antibodies have the potential for nonspecific inhibition and specific blocking of antigen responses, depending on whether they are directed against the constant or variable regions on the HLA molecule or T-cell receptors.

Effects on Cytokine Production and Binding

The effects of IVIG on cytokine expression were first observed in the treatment of Kawasaki syndrome (197). Kawasaki syndrome is an acute systemic vasculitis characterized immunologically by hypergammaglobulinemia, activation of T lymphocytes, production of IL-1 and IL-6, and cytotoxic antibodies directed against endothelial antigens. It is suggestive of superantigen stimulation (169) with a selective increase in Vβ2+ and Vβ8+ T cells.

Administration of IVIG results in a rapid reversal of all of these immunologic changes. The effect of IVIG depends on the clinical situation. Others found upregulation of IL-6 and IFN-γ after patients with intractable seizures were infused with IVIG. Infusion of IVIG into patients with hypogammaglobulinemia also results in changes in cytokine secretion and release of soluble cytokine receptors (198). Single infusions of IVIG were given to 12 patients, who demonstrated a rapid rise in plasma levels of IL-6, IL-8, and TNF-α within 1 hour. This was followed by a more profound elevation in the levels of TNF-α receptors, which remained elevated for at least 44 hours, which was the last time point tested. There was only a slight increase in the IL-1β level in the plasma, but it was accompanied by a marked increase in the IL-1 receptor concentration.

The *in vitro* effects of IVIG on cytokine production have been studied in detail. Mononuclear cells were stimulated with immobilized anti-CD3 monoclonal antibody or a combination of a protein kinase C activator and a calcium ionophore (199). IVIG induced a marked inhibition of T-cell proliferation. The T-cell cytokines IL-2, IL-10, IFN-γ, and TNF-β were all significantly inhibited. In contrast, IL-8 was not suppressed, and TNF-α was only moderately inhibited. IVIG profoundly inhibits synthesis of IL-2 (13200), and addition of IL-2 to the cultures reverses most of the inhibition of proliferation. The mechanism of the inhibition appears to be a change in posttranscriptional modification (13,200), because the levels of protein decrease in IVIG-treated cultures, but the levels of IL-2 mRNA remain unchanged. Neither group observed a change in the monokines TNF-α or IL-8, and they did not see a change in the levels of IL-2 receptor.

There is evidence of alteration in monokine production. Toungouz et al. observed strong inhibition of IL-6 and TNF-α when mononuclear cells were stimulated with staphylococcal enterotoxin B (201). Another potential mechanism is the production of IL-1 receptor antagonist by monocytes (202,203). IVIG selectively induced gene transcription and secretion of IL-1 receptor antagonist and IL-8 (203). In their studies, only intact IgG molecules were effective. These results are not universally accepted, however. Okitsu-Negishi et al. did not see a decrease in the synthesis or release of IL-1, even though the levels were decreased. They speculated that IVIG might act to neutralize the cytokines as they are produced (204). Dinarello (205) reviewed the effects of IVIG on IL-1 activity and concluded that more studies would be necessary before the effect of IVIG on monokines could be determined.

Inhibition of Natural Killer Cell Effector Function

NK cells have characteristics of T cells and neutrophils. They have CD16 (FcRIII) on their surface, and many are positive for CD8. Percentages of NK cells increased from 11% to 24% in patients treated with IVIG for myasthenia gravis (206), although this may have been caused by decreased numbers of T cells rather than increased numbers of NK cells. The absolute number of NK cells and B and T lymphocytes was decreased for nearly 3 weeks in patients treated for multiple sclerosis (207). NK cell activity was markedly reduced in patients treated with IVIG for hypogammaglobulinemia or ITP (208). They also found that addition of IVIG *in vitro* inhibited NK cell killing of K562 targets. Finberg et al. (209) found a transient decrease in NK activity immediately after an infusion of IVIG into patients with Kawasaki disease. That was followed by a marked increase in the absolute numbers of CD16+ NK cells and NK activity. Treatment of preterm infants with enough IVIG to bring their IgG levels to that of a term infant did not alter NK activity in these neonates (210). Although it is clear that IVIG can inhibit NK effector function *in vitro*, the clinical consequences are unknown.

CONCLUSIONS

Therapy with gammaglobulin has moved from simple replacement of antibody in patients with congenital immune defects to modulation of a large number of autoimmune and inflammatory disorders. Gammaglobulin is effective in many disorders that are unresponsive to more conventional therapy with immunosuppressive agents. Many mechanisms of action have been proposed, and it is likely that several are functional, even in a single disease.

Intravenous gammaglobulin contains antibodies that interact with cell surface molecules, cytokines, and toxins. It also contains other molecules, such as soluble receptors and cytokines, that have immunomodulating potential. There is strong evidence that IVIG interacts with immunoglobulins and cell receptors to restore the normal idiotypic network. Antibodies to specific cell receptors downregulate cytokine production and decrease proliferation and cytotoxic effector function.

For any disease, the amount of relevant antibody probably is very small, which may explain why doses in excess of 2 g/kg are necessary. As we gain a better understanding of how IVIG exerts its immunomodulating effect and are able to isolate and purify specific immunomodulating antibodies, it will be possible to treat with greater efficacy using much smaller amounts of this important yet scarce biologic product.

REFERENCES

1. Imbach P, Barandun S, Baumgartner C, Hirt A, Hofer F, Wagner HP. High-dose intravenous gammaglobulin therapy of refractory, in particular idiopathic thrombocytopenia in childhood. *Helv Paediatr Acta* 1981;46:81–86.
2. Hellström I, Hellström KE, Sjögren HO. Some recent information on "blocking antibodies" as studied *in vitro*. *Transplant Proc* 1971;3:1221–1227.
3. Hellström I, Hellström KE, Sjögren HO. Serum mediated inhibition of cellular immunity to methylcholanthrene-induced murine sarcomas. *Cell Immunol* 1970;1:18–30.
4. Möller G. Studies on the mechanism of immunological enhancement of tumor homografts. III. Interaction between humoral isoantibodies and immune lymphoid cells. *J Natl Cancer Inst* 1963;30:1205–1226.
5. Voisin GA. Immunological facilitation, a broadening of the concept of the enhancement phenomenon. *Progr Allergy* 1971;15:328–485.
6. Buckley RH, Schiff RI, Amos DB. Blocking of autologous and homologous leukocyte responses by human alloimmune plasmas: a possible *in vitro* correlate of enhancement. *J Immunol* 1972;108:34–44.
7. Buckley RH, Amos DB, Kremer WB, Stickel DL. Incompatible bone marrow transplantation in lymphopenic immunologic deficiency: circumvention of fatal graft-versus-host disease by immunologic enhancement. *N Engl J Med* 1971;285:1035–1042.
8. Cohn EJ, Strong LE, Hughes WL, et al. Preparation and properties of serum plasma proteins. IV. A system for the separation into fractions of the protein and lipoprotein components of biological tissues and fluids. *J Am Chem Soc* 1946;68:459–475.
9. Oncley JL, Melin M, Richert DA, Cameron JW, Gross PM. The separation of the antibodies, isoagglutinins, prothrombin, plasminogen, and β1-lipoprotein into subfractions of human plasma. *J Am Chem Soc* 1949;71:541–550.
10. Kistler P, Nitschmann HS. Large scale production of human plasma fractions: eight years' experience with the alcohol fractionation procedure of Nitschmann, Kistler, and Lergier. *Vox Sang* 1962;7:414–424.
11. Gardi A. Quality control in the production of an immunoglobulin for intravenous use. *Blut* 1984;48:337–344.
12. Tankersley DL. Dimer formation in immunoglobulin preparations and speculations on the mechanism of action of intravenous immune globulin in autoimmune diseases. *Immunol Rev* 1994;139:159–172.
13. Ross C, Svenson M, Hansen MB, Vejlsgaard GL, Bendtzen K. High avidity IFN-γ neutralizing antibodies in pharmaceutically prepared human IgG. *J Clin Invest* 1995;95:1974–1978.
14. Tiberio L, Caruso A, Pozzi A, et al. The detection and biologic activity of human antibodies to IL-2 in normal donors. *Scand J Immunol* 1993;38:472–476.
15. Kaveri S, Vassilev T, Hurez V, Lengagne R, LeFranc C, Cot S. Antibodies to a conserved region of HLA class I molecules, capable of modulating CD8 T cell–mediated function, are present in pooled normal immunoglobulin for therapeutic use. *J Clin Invest* 1996;97:865–869.
16. Vassilev T, Gelin C, Kaveri SV, Zilber MT, Boumsell L, Kazatchkine MD. Antibodies to the CD5 molecule in normal human immunoglobulins for therapeutic use (intravenous immunoglobulins, IVIg). *Clin Exp Immunol* 1993;92:369–372.
17. Hurez V, Kaveri SV, Mouhoub A, Dietrich G, Mani JC, Klatzmann D. Anti-CD4 activity of normal human immunoglobulin G for therapeutic use (intravenous immunoglobulin, IVIg). *Ther Immunol* 1994;1:269–277.
18. Rossi R, Kazatchkine MD. Antiidiotypes against autoantibodies in pooled normal human polyspecific IgG. *J Immunol* 1989;143:4104–4109.
19. Grosse-Wilde J, Blasczyk R, Westoff U. Soluble HLA class I and class II concentrations in commercial immunoglobulin preparations. *Tissue Antigens* 1992;39:74–77.
20. Blasczyk R, Westhoff U, Grosse Wilde H. Soluble CD4, CD8, and HLA molecules in commercial immunoglobulin preparations. *Lancet* 1993;341:789–790.
21. Horowitz B, Wiebe ME, Lippin A, Stryker MH. Inactivation of viruses in labile blood derivatives. I. Disruption of lipid-enveloped viruses by tri(n-butyl)phosphate detergent combinations. *Transfusion* 1985;25:516–522.
22. Lever AML, Webster ADB, Brown D, Thomas HC. Non-A, non-B hepatitis occurring in agammaglobulinaemic patients after intravenous immunoglobulin. *Lancet* 1984;2:1062–1064.
23. Björkander J, Cunningham-Rundles C, Lundin P, Olsson R, Söderström R, Hanson LÅ. Intravenous immunoglobulin prophylaxis causing liver damage in 16 of 77 patients with hypogammaglobulinemia or IgG subclass deficiency. *Am J Med* 1988;84:107–111.
24. Bjøro K, Froland SS, Yun Z, Samdal HH, Haaland T. Hepatitis C infection in patients with primary hypogammaglobulinemia after treatment with contaminated immune globulin. *N Engl J Med* 1994;331:1607–1611.
25. Williams PE, Yap PL, Gillon J, Crawford RJ, Urbaniak SJ, Galea G.

Transmission of non-A, non-B hepatitis by pH4-treated intravenous immunoglobulin. *Vox Sang* 1989;57:15–18.

26. Ochs HD, Fischer SH, Virant FS, et al. Non-A, non-B hepatitis after intravenous gammaglobulin. *Lancet* 1986;1:322–323.

27. Bresee J, Mast E, Coleman P, et al. Hepatitis C virus infection associated with administration of intravenous immune globulin. *JAMA* 1996;276:1563–1567.

28. Slade HB. Human immunoglobulins for intravenous use and hepatitis C viral transmission. *Clin Diagn Lab Immunol* 1994;1:613–619.

29. Heye N, Hensen S, Muller N. Creutzfeldt-Jakob disease and blood transfusion. *Lancet* 1994;343:296–299.

30. Schiff RI. Intravenous gammaglobulin, 2: pharmacology, clinical uses and mechanisms of action. *Pediatr Allergy Immunol* 1994;5:127–156.

31. Duhem C, Dicato MA, Ries R. Side-effects of intravenous immune globulins. *Clin Exp Immunol* 1994;97[Suppl 1]:79–83.

32. Burks AW, Sampson HA, Buckley RH. Anaphylactic reactions after gamma globulin administration in patients with hypogammaglobulinemia. *N Engl J Med* 1986;314:560–564.

33. Ozsoylu S. Aseptic meningitis and intravenous gammaglobulin treatment [Letter]. *Am J Dis Child* 1993;147:129–130.

34. Kim HC, Park CL, Cowan JH, Fattori FD, August CS. Massive intravascular hemolysis associated with intravenous immunoglobulin in bone marrow transplant recipients. *Am J Pediatr Hematol Oncol* 1988;10:69–74.

35. Barbolla L, Nieto S, Llamas P, et al. Severe immune haemolytic anaemia caused by intravenous immunoglobulin anti-D in the treatment of autoimmune thrombocytopenia [Letter]. *Vox Sang* 1993;64:184–185.

36. Woodruff RK, Grigg AP, Firkin FC, Smith IL. Fatal thrombotic events during treatment of autoimmune thrombocytopenia with intravenous immunoglobulin in elderly patients. *Lancet* 1986;2:217–218.

37. Silbert PL, Knezevic WV, Bridge DT. Cerebral infarction complicating intravenous immunoglobulin therapy for polyneuritis cranialis. *Neurology* 1992;42:257–258.

38. Tan E, Hajinazarian M, Bay W, Neff J, Mendell JR. Acute renal failure resulting from intravenous immunoglobulin therapy. *Arch Neurol* 1993;50:137–139.

39. Ayliffe W, Haeney M, Roberts SC, Lavin M. Uveitis after antineutrophil cytoplasmic antibody contamination of immunoglobulin replacement therapy. *Lancet* 1992;339:558–559.

40. Bussel J. Intravenous immune serum globulin in immune thrombocytopenia: clinical results and biochemical evaluation. *Vox Sang* 1985;49:44–50.

41. Bussel JB. Intravenous immunoglobulin therapy for the treatment of idiopathic thrombocytopenic purpura. *Prog Hemost Thromb* 1986;8:103–125.

42. Lusher JM, Warrier I. Use of gamma globulin in children and adolescents with idiopathic thrombocytopenic purpura and other immune thrombocytopenias. *Am J Med* 1987;83:10–16.

43. Buchanan GR. Overview of ITP treatment modalities in children. *Blut* 1989;59:96–104.

44. Imbach P. Intravenous immunoglobulin therapy for idiopathic thrombocytopenic purpura and other immune-related disorders: review and update of our experiences. *Pediatr Infect Dis J* 1988;7:S120–125.

45. Bussel JB, Kimberly RP, Inman RD, et al. Intravenous gammaglobulin treatment of chronic idiopathic thrombocytopenic purpura. *Blood* 1983;62:480–486.

46. Bussel JB, Goldman A, Imbach P, Schulman I, Hilgartner MW. Treatment of acute idiopathic thrombocytopenia of childhood with intravenous infusions of gammaglobulin. *J Pediatr* 1985;106:886–890.

47. Vos JJE, Van Aken WG, Engelfriet CP, von dem Borne AEGK. Intravenous gammaglobulin in idiopathic thrombocytopenic purpura: results with the Netherlands Red Cross immunoglobulin preparation. *Vox Sang* 1985;49:92–100.

48. Kurtzberg J, Friedman HS, Kinney TR, Chaffee S, Falletta JM. Treatment of platelet alloimmunization with intravenous immunoglobulin. *Am J Med* 1987;83:30–33.

49. Schiffer CA, Hogge DE, Aisner J, Dutcher JP, Lee EJ, Papenberg D. High-dose intravenous gammaglobulin in alloimmunized platelet transfusion recipients. *Blood* 1984;64:937–940.

50. Kickler T, Braine HG, Piantadosi S, Ness PM, Herman JH, Rothko K. A randomized, placebo-controlled trial of intravenous gammaglobulin in alloimmunized thrombocytopenic patients. *Blood* 1990;75:313–316.

51. Besa EC, MacNab MW, Solan AJ, Lapes MJ, Marfatia U. High-dose

52. Derycke M, Dreyfus M, Ropert JC, Tchernia G. Intravenous immunoglobulin for neonatal isoimmune thrombocytopenia. *Arch Dis Child* 1985;60:667–669.

53. Kurtzberg J, Friedman HS, Kinney TR, et al. Management of human immunodeficiency virus-associated thrombocytopenia with intravenous gamma globulin. *Am J Pediatr Hematol Oncol* 1987;9:299–301.

54. Rarick MU, Montgomery T, Groshen S, et al. Intravenous immunoglobulin in the treatment of human immunodeficiency virus-related thrombocytopenia. *Am J Hematol* 1991;38:261–266.

55. Hollenberg JP, Subak LL, Ferry JJ, Bussel JB. Cost-effectiveness of splenectomy versus intravenous gamma globulin in treatment of chronic immune thrombocytopenic purpura in childhood. *J Pediatr* 1988;112:530–539.

56. Bussel JB, Graziano JN, Kimberly RP, Pahwa S, Aledort LM. Intravenous anti-D treatment of immune thrombocytopenic purpura: analysis of efficacy, toxicity, and mechanism of effect. *Blood* 1991;77:1884–1893.

57. Bussel JB, Cunningham-Rundles C, Abraham C. Intravenous treatment of autoimmune hemolytic anemia with very high dose gammaglobulin. *Vox Sang* 1986;51:264–269.

58. Leickly FE, Buckley RH. Successful treatment of autoimmune hemolytic anemia in Common Variable Immunodeficiency with high-dose intravenous gamma globulin. *Am J Med* 1987;82:159–381.

59. Argiolu F, Diana G, Arnone M, Batzella MG, Piras P, Cao A. High-dose intravenous immunoglobulin in the management of autoimmune hemolytic anemia complicating thalassemia major. *Acta Haematol* 1990;83:65–68.

60. Woodcock BE, Walker S, Adams K. Haemolytic transfusion reaction—successful attenuation with methylprednisolone and high dose immunoglobulin. *Clin Lab Haematol* 1993;15:59–61.

61. Pollack S, Cunningham-Rundles C, Smithwick EM, Barandun S, Good RA. High dose intravenous gamma globulin for autoimmune neutropenia. *N Engl J Med* 1982;307:253.

62. Mascarin M, Ventura A. Anti-Rh(D) immunoglobulin for autoimmune neutropenia of infancy. *Acta Paediatr* 1993;82:142–144.

63. Bussel J, Lalezari P, Fikrig S. Intravenous treatment with γ-globulin of autoimmune neutropenia or infancy. *J Pediatr* 1988;112:298–301.

64. Hilgartner MW, Bussel J. Use of intravenous gamma globulin for the treatment of autoimmune neutropenia of childhood and autoimmune hemolytic anemia. *Am J Med* 1987;83:25–29.

65. Needleman SW. Durable remission of pure red cell aplasia after treatment with high-dose intravenous gammaglobulin and prednisone. *Am J Hematol* 1989;32:150–152.

66. Vukelja SJ, Krishnan J, Link CM, Salvado AJ, Knight RD. Resolution of pure red cell aplasia and lymphoma: response to intravenous gammaglobulin and combination chemotherapy. *Am J Hematol* 1989;32:129–133.

67. Clauvel JP, Vainchenker W, Herrera A, et al. Treatment of pure red cell aplasia by high dose intravenous immunoglobulins. *Immunology* 1990;69:380–381.

68. Kurtzman G, Frickhofen N, Kimball J, Jenkins DW, Neinhuis AW, Young NS. Pure red-cell aplasia of 10 years' duration due to persistent parvovirus B19 infection and its cure with immunoglobulin therapy. *N Engl J Med* 1989;321:519–523.

69. Raghavachar A. Pure red cell aplasia: review of treatment and proposal for a treatment strategy. *Blut* 1990;61:47–61.

70. Ballester OF, Saba HI, Moscinski LC, et al. Pure red cell aplasia: treatment with intravenous immunoglobulin concentrate. *Semin Hematol* 1992;29:106–108.

71. Sultan Y, Maisonneuve P, Kazatchkine MD, Nydegger UE. Anti-idiotypic suppression of autoantibodies to Factor VIII (antihaemophilic factor) by high-dose intravenous gammaglobulin. *Lancet* 1984;2:765–768.

72. Sultan Y, Rossi F, Kazatchkine MD. Recovery from anti-VIII:C (antihemophilic factor) autoimmune disease is dependent on generation of antiidiotypes against anti-VIII:C autoantibodies. *Proc Natl Acad Sci* 1987;84:828–831.

73. Sultan Y, Kazatchkine MD, Nydegger U, et al. Intravenous immunoglobulin in the treatment of spontaneously acquired factor VIII:C inhibitors. *Am J Med* 1991;91[Suppl 5A]:35–39.

74. Schwartz RS, Gabriel DA, Aledort LM, Green D, Kessler CM. A prospective study of treatment of acquired (autoimmune) factor VIII

inhibitors with high-dose intravenous gammaglobulin. *Blood* 1995; 86:797–804.

75. Leung DYM. Kawasaki disease. *Curr Opin Rheumatol* 1993;5:41–50.

76. Furusho K, Nakano H, Shinomiya K, et al. High-dose intravenous gammaglobulin for Kawasaki disease. *Lancet* 1984;2:1055–1058.

77. Nakashima L, Edwards DL. Treatment of Kawasaki disease. *Clin Pharmacol* 1990;9:755–762.

78. Newburger JW, Takahashi M, Burns JC, et al. The treatment of Kawasaki syndrome with intravenous gamma globulin. *N Engl J Med* 1986;315:341–347.

79. Melish ME. Intravenous immunoglobulin in Kawasaki syndrome: a progress report. *Pediatr Infect Dis J* 1986;5:S211–S215.

80. Plotkin SA, Daum RS, Giebink GS, et al. Intravenous γ-globulin use in children with Kawasaki disease. *Pediatric* 1988;82:122.

81. Engle MA, Fatica NS, Bussel JB, O'Laughlin JE, Snyder MS, Lesser ML. Clinical trial of single-dose intravenous gamma globulin in acute Kawasaki disease. *Am J Dis Child* 1989;143:1300–1304.

82. Newburger JW, Takahashi M, Beiser AS, et al. A single intravenous infusion of gamma globulin as compared with four infusions in the treatment of acute Kawasaki syndrome. *N Engl J Med* 1991;324: 1633–1639.

83. Barron KS, Murphy DJ, Silverman ED, et al. Treatment of Kawasaki syndrome: a comparison of two dosage regimens of intravenously administered immune globulin. *J Pediatr* 1990;117:638–644.

84. Vedeler C, Ulvestad E, Nyland H, Matre R, Aarli JA. Receptors for gammaglobulin in the central and peripheral nervous system. *J Neurol Neurosurg Psychiatry* 1994;57:9–10.

85. Wurster U, Haas J. Passage of intravenous immunoglobulin and interaction with the CNS. *J Neurol Neurosurg Psychiatry* 1994;57:21–25.

86. Ariizumi M, Shiihara H, Hibio S, et al. High dose gammaglobulin for intractable childhood epilepsy. *Lancet* 1983;2:162–163.

87. Duse M, Tiberti S, Plebani A, et al. IgG2 deficiency and intractable epilepsy of childhood. *Monogr Allergy* 1986;20:128–134.

88. van Engelen BGM, Renier WO, Weemaes CMR. Immunoglobulin treatment in human and experimental epilepsy. *J Neurol Neurosurg Psychiatry* 1994;57:72–75.

89. Lundkvist I, van Doorn PA, Vermeulen M, Brand A. Spontaneous recovery from the Guillain-Barré syndrome is associated with antiidiotypic antibodies recognizing a cross-reactive idiotype on anti-neuroblastoma cell line antibodies. *Clin Immunol Immunopathol* 1993; 67:192–198.

90. Ronda N, Hurez V, Kazatchkine MD. Intravenous immunoglobulin therapy of autoimmune and systemic inflammatory diseases. *Vox Sang* 1993;64:65–72.

91. van der Meché FGA, Schmitz PIM. A randomized trial comparing intravenous immune globulin and plasma exchange in Guillain-Barré syndrome. *N Engl J Med* 1992;326:1123–1129.

92. Notarangelo LD, Duse M, Tiberti S, et al. Intravenous immunoglobulin in two children with Guillain-Barré syndrome. *Eur J Pediatr* 1993; 152:372–374.

93. Jackson MC, Godwin Austen RB, Whiteley AM. High-dose intravenous immunoglobulin in the treatment of Guillain-Barré syndrome: a preliminary open study. *J Neurol* 1993;240:51–53.

94. Irani DN, Cornblath DR, Chaudhry V, Borel C, Hanley DF. Relapse in Guillain-Barré syndrome after treatment with human immune globulin. *Neurology* 1993;43:872–875.

95. Van Schaik IN, Vermeulen M, van Doorn PA, Brand A. Anti-GM1 antibodies in patients with chronic inflammatory demyelinating polyneuropathy (CIDP) treated with intravenous immunoglobulin (IVIg). *J Neuroimmunol* 1994;54:109–115.

96. Vermeulen M, van der Meche FGA, Speelman JD, Weber A, Busch HFM. Plasma and gamma-globulin infusion in chronic inflammatory polyneuropathy. *J Neurol Sci* 1985;70:317–326.

97. Van Doorn PA, Brand A, Strengers PFW, Meulstee J, Vermeulen M. High-dose intravenous immunoglobulin treatment in chronic inflammatory demyelinating polyneuropathy. A double-blind placebo-controlled crossover study. *Neurology* 1990;40:209–212.

98. van Doorn PA, Vermeulen M, Brand A, Mulder PGH, Busch HFM. Intravenous immunoglobulin treatment in patients with chronic inflammatory demyelinating polyneuropathy. *Arch Neurol* 1991;48: 217–220.

99. Vermeulen M, van Doorn PA, Brand A, Strengers PFW, Jennekens FGI, Busch HFM. Intravenous immunoglobulin treatment in patients with chronic inflammatory demyelinating polyneuropathy: a double

blind, placebo controlled study. *J Neurol Neurosurg Psychiatry* 1993; 56:36–39.

100. Schuller E, Govaerts A. First results of immunotherapy with immunoglobulin G in multiple sclerosis patients. *Eur Neurol* 1983;22: 205–212.

101. Achiron A, Barak Y, Sarova-Pinhas I, et al. Intravenous immunoglobulin in relapsing-remitting multiple sclerosis. In: Kazatchkine MD, Morell A, eds. *Intravenous immunoglobulin research and therapy.* New York: Parthenon Publishing Group, 1996:289–293.

102. van Engelen BGM, Miller DJ, Pavelko KD, Hommes OR, Rodriguez M. Promotion of remyelination by polyclonal immunoglobulin in Theiler's virus-induced demyelination and in multiple sclerosis. *J Neurol Neurosurg Psychiatry* 1994;57:65–68.

103. Edan G, Landgraf F. Experience with intravenous immunoglobulin in myasthenia gravis: a review. *J Neurol Neurosurg Psychiatry* 1994;57: 55–56.

104. Arsura EL, Bick A, Brunner NC, Grob D. Effects of repeated doses of intravenous immunoglobulin in myasthenia gravis. *Am J Med Sci* 1988;295:438–443.

105. Evoli A, Palmisain MT, Bartoccioni E, Padua L, Tonali P. High-dose intravenous immunoglobulin in myasthenia gravis. *Ital J Neurol Sci* 1993;14:233–237.

106. Liblau R, Gajdos P, Bustarret FA, el Habib R, Bach JF, Morel E. Intravenous γ-globulin in myasthenia gravis: interaction with anti-acetylcholine receptor antibodies. *J Clin Immunol* 1991;11:128–131.

107. Gajdos P, Clair B, Annane D, et al. Intravenous gammaglobulin in myasthenia gravis. In: Kazatchkine MD, Morell A, eds. *Intravenous immunoglobulin research and therapy.* New York: Parthenon Publishing Group, 1996:285–288.

108. Roifman CM, Schaffer FM, Wachsmuth SE, Murphy G, Gelfand EW. Reversal of chronic polymyositis following intravenous immune serum globulin therapy. *JAMA* 1987;258:513–515.

109. Cherin P, Herson S, Wechsler B, et al. Efficacy of intravenous gammaglobulin therapy in chronic refractory polymyositis and dermatomyositis: an open study with 20 adult patients. *Am J Med* 1991;91: 162–168.

110. Lang BA, Laxer RM, Murphy G, Silverman ED, Roifman CM. Treatment of dermatomyositis with intravenous gammaglobulin. *Am J Med* 1991;91:169–172.

111. Dalakas MC, Illae I, Dambrosia JM, et al. A controlled trial of high-dose intravenous immunoglobulin infusions as treatment for dermatomyositis. *N Engl J Med* 1993;329:1993–2000.

112. Nobile Orazio E, Meucci N, Barbieri S, Carpo M, Scarlato G. High-dose intravenous immunoglobulin therapy in multifocal motor neuropathy. *Neurology* 1993;43:537–544.

113. Chaudhry V, Corse AM, Cornblath DR, et al. Multifocal motor neuropathy: response to human immune globulin. *Ann Neurol* 1993;33: 237–242.

114. Leger JM, Younes-Chennoufi AB, Chassande B, et al. Human immunoglobulin treatment of multifocal motor neuropathy and polyneuropathy associated with monoclonal gammopathy. *J Neurol Neurosurg Psychiatry* 1994;57:46–49.

115. Azulay JP, Blin O, Pouget J, et al. Intravenous immunoglobulin treatment in patients with motor neuron syndromes associated with anti-GM1 antibodies: a double-blind, placebo-controlled study. *Neurology* 1994;44:429–432.

116. Kuroda Y, Takashima H, Ikeda A, et al. Treatment of HTLV-1–associated myelopathy with high-dose intravenous gammaglobulin. *J Neurol* 1991;238:309–314.

117. Soueidan SA, Dalakas MC. Treatment of inclusion-body myositis with high-dose intravenous immunoglobulin. *Neurology* 1993;43: 876–879.

118. Gaedicke G, Teller WM, Kohne E, Dopfer R, Niethammer D. IgG therapy in systemic lupus erythematosus—two case reports. *Blut* 1984;48:387–390.

119. Corvetta A, Bitta RD, Gabrielli A, Spaeth PJ, Danieli G. Use of high-dose intravenous immunoglobulin in systemic lupus erythematosus: report of three cases. *Clin Exp Rheumatol* 1989;7:295–299.

120. Jordan SC, Toyoda M. Treatment of autoimmune diseases and systemic vasculitis with pooled human intravenous immune globulin. *Clin Exp Immunol* 1994;97:31–38.

121. Jordan S. Intravenous γ-globulin therapy in systemic lupus erythematosus and immune complex disease. *Clin Immunol Immunopathol* 1989;53:S164–S169.

122. Winder A, Molad Y, Ostfeld I, Kenet G, Pinkhas J, Sidi Y. Treatment of systemic lupus erythematosus by prolonged administration of high dose intravenous immunoglobulin: report of 2 cases. *J Rheumatol* 1993;20:495–498.

123. Carreras LO, Perez GN, Vega HR, Casavilla F. Lupus anticoagulant and recurrent fetal loss: successful treatment with gammaglobulin. *Lancet* 1988;2:393–394.

124. Wapner RJ, Cowchock FS, Shapiro SS. Successful treatment in two women with antiphospholipid antibodies and refractory pregnancy losses with intravenous immunoglobulin infusions. *Am J Obstet Gynecol* 1989;161:1271–1272.

125. Mueller-Eckhardt G, Heine O, Neppert J, Kunzel W, Meuller-Eckhardt C. Prevention of recurrent spontaneous abortion by intravenous immunoglobulin. *Vox Sang* 1989;56:151–154.

126. Kaaja R, Julkunen H, Ammala P, Palosuo T, Kurki P. Intravenous immunoglobulin treatment of pregnant patients with recurrent pregnancy losses associated with antiphospholipid antibodies. *Acta Obstet Gynecol Scand* 1993;72:63–66.

127. Heine O, Mueller-Eckhardt G. Intravenous immune globulin in recurrent abortion. *Clin Exp Immunol* 1994;97:39–42.

128. Jayne DR, Esnault VL, Lockwood CM. ANCA anti-idiotype antibodies and the treatment of systemic vasculitis with intravenous immunoglobulin. *J Autoimmun* 1993;6:207–219.

129. Jayne DRW, Davies MJ, Fox CJV, Black CM, Lockwood CM. Treatment of systemic vasculitis with pooled intravenous gammaglobulin. *Lancet* 1991;337:1137–1139.

130. Hamilos DL, Christensen J. Treatment of Churg-Strauss syndrome with high-dose intravenous immunoglobulin. *J Allergy Clin Immunol* 1991;88:823–824.

131. Sany J, Clot J, Bonneau M, Andary M. Immunomodulating effect of human placenta-eluted gamma globulins in rheumatoid arthritis. *Arthritis Rheum* 1982;25:17–24.

132. Sany J, Jorgensen C, Anaya JM, et al. Arthritis associated with primary agammaglobulinemia: new clues to its immunopathology. *Clin Exp Rheumatol* 1993;11:65–69.

133. Webster AD, Loewi G, Dourmashkin RD, Golding DN, Ward DJ, Asherson GL. Polyarthritis in adults with hypogammaglobulinaemia and its rapid response to immunoglobulin treatment. *BMJ* 1976;1:1314–1316.

134. Struillou L, Fiks-Sigaud M, Barrier J, Blat E. Acquired haemophilia and rheumatoid arthritis: success of immunoglobulin therapy. *J Intern Med* 1992;232:304–305.

135. Silverman ED, Laxer RM, Greenwald M, et al. Intravenous gamma globulin therapy in systemic juvenile rheumatoid arthritis. *Arthritis Rheum* 1990;33:1015–1022.

136. Silverman ED, Cawkwell GD, Lovell DJ, et al. Intravenous immunoglobulin in the treatment of systemic juvenile rheumatoid arthritis: a randomized placebo controlled trial. *J Rheumatol* 1994;21: 2353–2358.

137. Tumiati B, Casoli P, Veneziani M, Rinaldi G. High-dose immunoglobulin therapy as an immunomodulatory treatment of rheumatoid arthritis. *Arthritis Rheum* 1992;35:1126–1133.

138. Page R, Friday G, Stillwagon P, Skoner D, Caliguiri L, Fireman P. Asthma and selective immunoglobulin subclass deficiency: improvement of asthma after immunoglobulin replacement therapy. *J Pediatr* 1988;112:127–131.

139. Mazer BD, Gelfand EW. An open-label study of high-dose intravenous immunoglobulin in severe childhood asthma. *J Allergy Clin Immunol* 1991;87:976–983.

140. Mazer BD, Giclas P, Gelfand EW. Immunomodulatory effects of intravenous immunoglobulin in severe steroid-dependent asthma. *Clin Immunol Immunopathol* 1989;53:S156–S163.

141. Kishiyama JL, Shames RS, Cunningham-Rundles C, et al. A multicenter, randomized, placebo-controlled trial of high dose intravenous gammaglobulin (IVIG) for oral corticosteroid-dependent asthma. *J Allergy Clin Immunol* 1997;99:S268(abst 1093).

142. Levine DS, Fischer SH, Christie DL, et al. Intravenous immunoglobulin therapy for active, extensive, and medically refractory idiopathic ulcerative or Crohn's colitis. *Am J Gastroenterol* 1992;87:91–100.

143. Wakim MA, Alazard M, Yajima A, Speights D, Saxon S, Stiehm ER. High dose intravenous immunoglobulin (IVIG) in atopic dermatitis and hyper-IgE syndrome. *J Allergy Clin Immunol* 1997;99:S332(abst 1357).

144. Beckers RCY, Brand A, Vermeer BJ, Boom BW. Adjuvant high-dose intravenous gammaglobulin in the treatment of pemphigus and bullous pemphigoid: experience in six patients. *Br J Dermatol* 1995;133: 289–293.

145. Heinze E, Thon A, Vetter U, Gaedicke G, Zuppinger K. Gamma-globulin therapy in 6 newly diagnosed diabetic children. *Acta Paediatr Scand* 1985;74:605–606.

146. Pocecco M, de Campo C, Cantoni L, Tedesco F, Panizon F. Effect of high doses intravenous IgG in newly diagnosed diabetic children. *Helv Paediatr Acta* 1987;42:289–295.

147. Heinze E. Immunoglobulins in children with autoimmune diabetes mellitus. *Clin Exp Rheumatol* 1996;14[Suppl 15]:S99–S102.

148. Raghavan M, Bjorkman PJ. Fc receptors and their interactions with immunoglobulins. *Annu Rev Cell Dev Biol* 1996;12:181–220.

149. Salmon JE, Kapur S, Kimberly RP. Gammaglobulin for intravenous use induces an Fc γ receptor-specific decrement in phagocytosis by blood monocytes. *Clin Immunol Immunopathol* 1987;43:23–33.

150. Kurlander RJ. Reversible and irreversible loss of Fc receptor function of human monocytes as a consequence of interaction with immunoglobulin G. *J Clin Invest* 1980;66:773–781.

151. Kimberly RP, Salmon JE, Bussel JB, Crow MK, Hilgartner MW. Modulation of mononuclear phagocyte function by intravenous γ-globulin. *J Immunol* 1984;132:745–750.

152. Debré M, Bonnet M-C, Fridman W-H, et al. Infusion of Fcγ fragments for treatment of children with acute immune thrombocytopenic purpura. *Lancet* 1993;342:945–949.

153. Kurlander RJ, Hall J. Comparison of intravenous gamma globulin and a monoclonal anti-Fc receptor antibody as inhibitors of immune clearance *in vivo* in mice. *J Clin Invest* 1986;77:2010–2018.

154. Clarkson SB, Bussel JB, Kimberly RP, Valinsky JE, Nachman RL, Unkeless JC. Treatment of refractory immune thrombocytopenic purpura with an anti-Fcγ-receptor antibody. *N Engl J Med* 1986;314: 1236–1239.

155. Templeton JG, Cocker JE, Crawford RJ, Forwell MA, Sandilands GP. Fcγ-receptor blocking antibodies in hyperimmune and normal pooled gammaglobulin. *Lancet* 1985;1:1337.

156. Petri IB, Lorinez A, Berek I. Detection of Fc-receptor blocking antibodies in anti-Rh(D) hyperimmune gammaglobulin. *Lancet* 1984;2: 1478–1479.

157. Andersson K, Hansson U-B, Alkner U. The effect on non-immune IgG on antigen-antibody complexation. *Scand J Immunol* 1992;35:703–710.

158. Lin RY, Racis SP. *In vivo* reduction of circulating C1q binding immune complexes by intravenous gammaglobulin administration. *Int Arch Allergy Appl Immunol* 1986;79:286–290.

159. Frank MM, Basta M, Fries LF. The effects of intravenous immune globulin on complement-dependent immune damage of cells and tissues. *Clin Immunol Immunopathol* 1992;62:S82–S86.

160. Basta M. Modulation of complement-mediated immune damage by intravenous immune globulin. *Clin Exp Immunol* 1996;104[Suppl 1]: 21–25.

161. Basta M, Kirshbom P, Frank MM, Fries LF. Mechanism of therapeutic effect of high-dose intravenous immunoglobulin: attenuation of acute, complement-dependent immune damage in a guinea pig model. *J Clin Invest* 1989;84:1974–1981.

162. Basta M, Dalakas MC. High-dose intravenous immunoglobulin exerts its beneficial effect in patients with dermatomyositis by blocking endomysial deposition of activated complement fragments. *J Clin Invest* 1994;94:1735(abst).

163. Dietrich G, Kaveri SV, Kazatchkine MD. Modulation of autoimmunity by intravenous immune globulin through interaction with the function of the immune/idiotypic network. *Clin Immunol Immunopathol* 1992; 62:S73–S81.

164. Kazatchkine MD, Dietrich G, Hurez V, et al. V region-mediated selection of autoreactive repertoires by intravenous immunoglobulin (i.v.Ig). *Immunol Rev* 1994;139:79–107.

165. Marchalonis JJ, Daymaz H, Dedeoglu R, et al. Human autoantibodies reactive with synthetic autoantigens from T-cell receptor β chain. *Proc Nat Acad Sci USA* 1992;89:3325–3329.

166. Williams RC, Emmons JD, Yunis EJ. Studies of human sera with cytotoxic activity. *J Clin Invest* 1971;50:1514–1524.

167. Berzins T, Axelsson B, Hammarström L, Hammarström S, Perlmann P. Inhibition of proliferative and cytotoxic activities of human T lymphocytes with rabbit antibodies directed against leucoagglutinin-reactive T cell surface components. *Eur J Immunol* 1984;14: 1145–1152.

168. Moynier M, Cosso B, Brochier J, Clot J. Identification of class II HLA

alloantibodies in placenta-eluted gamma globulins used for treating rheumatoid arthritis. *Arthritis Rheum* 1987;30:375–381.

169. Takei S, Arora YK, Walker SM. Intravenous immunoglobulin contains specific antibodies inhibitory to activation of T cells by staphylococcal toxin superantigens. *J Clin Invest* 1993;91:602–607.

170. Honda J, Natori H, Oizumi K, Yokoyama M. A new action mechanism of intravenous immunoglobulin for idiopathic thrombocytopenic purpura [Letter]. *Vox Sang* 1993;64:186–187.

171. Durandy A, Fischer A, Griscelli C. Dysfunctions of pokeweed mitogen-stimulated T and B lymphocyte responses induced by gammaglobulin therapy. *J Clin Invest* 1981;67:867–877.

172. Stohl W. Modulation of the immune response by immunoglobulin for intravenous use. I. Inhibition of pokeweed mitogen-induced B cell differentiation. *Clin Exp Immunol* 1985;62:200–207.

173. Stohl W. Cellular mechanisms in the *in vitro* inhibition of pokeweed mitogen-induced B cell differentiation by immunoglobulin for intravenous use. *J Immunol* 1986;136:4407–4413.

174. Hashimoto F, Sakiyama Y, Matsumoto S. The suppressive effect of gammaglobulin preparations on *in vitro* pokeweed mitogen-induced immunoglobulin production. *Clin Exp Immunol* 1986;65:409–415.

175. Kondo N, Ozawa T, Mushiake K, et al. Suppression of immunoglobulin production of lymphocytes by intravenous immunoglobulin. *J Clin Immunol* 1991;11:151–158.

176. Mannhalter JW, Ahmad R, Wolf HM, Eibl MM. Effect of polymeric IgG on human monocyte functions. *Int Arch Allergy Appl Immunol* 1987;82:159–164.

177. Heyman B. Fc-dependent IgG-mediated suppression of the antibody response: fact or artefact? *Scand J Immunol* 1990;31:601–607.

178. Fridman WH. Regulation of B-cell activation and antigen presentation by Fc receptors [Review]. *Curr Opin Immunol* 1993;5:355–360.

179. Phillips N, Parker D. Cross-linking of B lymphocyte Fcγ receptors and membrane immunoglobulin inhibits anti-immunoglobulin-induced blastogenesis. *J Immunol* 1984;132:627–632.

180. Phillips N, Gravel K, Tumas K, Parker D. IL-4 overcomes Fcγ receptor-mediated inhibition of mouse B lymphocyte proliferation without affecting inhibition of c-myc mRNA expression. *J Immunol* 1988;141:4243–4249.

181. Ashman R, Peckham D, Stunz L. Fc receptor off-signal in the B-cell involves apoptosis. *J Immunol* 1996;157:5–11.

182. Delfraissy JF, Tchernia G, Laurian Y, Wallon C, Galanaud P, Dormont J. Suppressor cell function after intravenous gammaglobulin treatment in adult chronic idiopathic thrombocytopenic purpura. *Br J Haematol* 1985;60:315–322.

183. White WB, Desbonnet MR, Ballow M. Immunoregulatory effects of intravenous immune serum globulin therapy in common variable hypogammaglobulinemia. *Am J Med* 1987;83:431–436.

184. Leung DYM, Burns JC, Newburger JW, Geha RS. Reversal of lymphocyte activation *in vivo* in the Kawasaki syndrome by intravenous gammaglobulin. *J Clin Invest* 1987;79:468–472.

185. Papadopoulos S, Schiff RI. Modulation of the immune responses by intravenous gammaglobulin (IVIG). *J Allergy Clin Immunol* 1989;83:274A.

186. Chander R, Papadopoulos S, Schiff RI. Suppression of cellular immune responses by intravenous gammaglobulin (IVIG). *J Allergy Clin Immunol* 1990;85:220A.

187. Kawada K, Terasaki PI. Evidence for immunosuppression by high-dose gammaglobulin. *Exp Hematol* 1987;15:133–136.

188. Van Schaik IN, Lundkvist I, Vermeulen M, Brand A. Polyvalent immunoglobulin for intravenous use interferes with cell proliferation *in vitro*. *J Clin Immunol* 1992;12:325–334.

189. Klaesson S, Ringden O, Markling L, Remberger M, Lundkvist I. Immune modulatory effects of immunoglobulins on cell-mediated immune responses *in vitro*. *Scand J Immunol* 1993;38:477–484.

190. Aarli Å, Jensen TS, Ulvestad E, Matre R. Suppression of mitogen-induced lymphoproliferation by soluble IgG Fc receptors in retropla-

cental serum in normal human pregnancy. *Scand J Immunol* 1993;37:237–243.

191. Grosse-Wilde H, Blaczyk R, Westhoff U. Soluble HLA class I and class II concentrations in commercial immunoglobulin preparations. *Tissue Antigens* 1992;39:34–37.

192. Vuist WM, Van SI, Van LM, Brand A. The growth arresting effect of human immunoglobulin for intravenous use is mediated by antibodies recognizing membrane glycolipids. *J Clin Immunol* 1997;17:301–310.

193. Schifferli JA, Didierjean L, Saurat JH. Immunomodulatory effects of intravenous immunoglobulin G. *J Rheumatol* 1991;18:937–939.

194. Svenson M, Hansen MB, Bendtzen K. Binding of cytokines to pharmaceutically prepared human immunoglobulin. *J Clin Invest* 1993;92:2533–2539.

195. Lam L, Whitsett CF, McNicholl JM, Hodge TW, Hooper J. Immunologically active proteins in intravenous immunoglobulin. *Lancet* 1993;342:67–81.

196. Kaveri SV, Mouthon L, Kazatchkine MD. Immunomodulating effects of intravenous immunoglobulin in autoimmune and inflammatory diseases. *J Neurol Neurosurg Psychiatry* 1994;57:6–8.

197. Leung DY. Kawasaki syndrome: immunomodulatory benefit and potential toxin neutralization by intravenous immune globulin. *Clin Exp Immunol* 1996;104:49–54.

198. Aukrust P, Froland SS, Liabakk N-B, et al. Release of cytokines, soluble cytokine receptors, and interleukin-1 receptor antagonist after intravenous gammaglobulin administration *in vivo*. *Blood* 1994;84:2136–2143.

199. Andersson UG, Bjork L, Skansen-Saphir U, Andersson JP. Down-regulation of cytokine production and interleukin-2 receptor expression by pooled human IgG. *Immunology* 1993;79:211–216.

200. Nachbaur D, Herold M, Eibl B, et al. A comparative study of the *in vitro* immunomodulatory activity of human intact immunoglobulin (7S IVIG), F(ab')2 fragments (5S IVIG) and Fc fragments: evidence for post-transcriptional IL-2 modulation. *Immunology* 1997;90:212

201. Toungouz M, Denys CH, De Groote D, Dupont E. *In vitro* inhibition of tumor necrosis factor-α and interleukin-6 production by intravenous immunoglobulins. *Br J Haematol* 1995;89:698–703.

202. Arend WP, Leung DYM. IgG induction of IL-1 receptor antagonist production by human monocytes. *Immunol Rev* 1994;139:71–78.

203. de Souza VR, Carreno M-P, Kaveri SV, et al. Selective induction of interleukin-1 receptor antagonist and interleukin-8 in human monocytes by normal polyspecific IgG (intravenous immunoglobulin). *Eur J Immunol* 1995;25:1267–1273.

204. Okitsu-Negishi S, Furusawa S, Kawa Y, et al. Suppressive effect of intravenous immunoglobulins on the activity of interleukin-1. *Immunol Res* 1994;13:49.

205. Dinarello CA. Is there a role for Interleukin-1 blockade in intravenous immunoglobulin therapy? *Immunol Rev* 1994;139:173–188.

206. Cook L, Howard JF, Folds JD. Immediate effects of intravenous IgG administration on peripheral blood B and T cells and polymorphonuclear cells in patients with myasthenia gravis. *J Clin Immunol* 1988;8:23–31.

207. Tenser RB, Hay KA, Aberg JA. Immunoglobulin G immunosuppression of multiple sclerosis: suppression of all three major lymphocyte subsets. *Arch Neurol* 1993;50:417–420.

208. Engelhard D, Waner JL, Kapoor N, Good RA. Effect of intravenous immune globulin on natural killer cell activity: possible association with autoimmune neutropenia and idiopathic thrombocytopenia. *J Pediatr* 1986;108:77–81.

209. Finberg RW, Newburger JW, Mikati MA, Heller AH, Burns JC. Effect of high doses of intravenously administered immune globulin on natural killer cell activity in peripheral blood. *J Pediatr* 1992;120:376–380.

210. Chirico G, Maccario R, Montagna D, Chiara A, Gasparoni A, Rondini G. Natural killer cell activity in preterm infants: effect of intravenous immune globulin administration. *J Pediatr* 1990;118:465–466.

Inflammation: Basic Principles and Clinical Correlates,
3rd ed., edited by John I. Gallin and Ralph Snyderman.
Lippincott Williams & Wilkins, Philadelphia © 1999.

CHAPTER 82

Antimicrobial Peptides:

Complementing Classical Inflammatory Mechanisms of Defense

Mark Anderson and Michael Zasloff

Over the past 15 years, a great diversity of peptide antibiotics has been discovered. Although antibiotic peptides have been identified throughout nature, in both plants and animals, our focus will be limited principally to the vertebrate families, and except for a discussion of the African clawed toad *(Xenopus laevis)* we will highlight studies in mammalian species. This review will focus on epithelial defenses.

A basic theme is that these antibiotic agents appear to provide an animal with a defensive shield against environmental microbes that suffices in large part to prevent infection as a clinically silent first line of defense. We will also suggest that these molecules are important for coordination and regulation of immune and inflammatory responses.

MAGAININS AND FROGS: SOME LESSONS ABOUT VERTEBRATE INNATE IMMUNITY OF RELEVANCE TO HUMANS

Our involvement in this area arose through a realization that an aquatic frog, *X. laevis,* healed surgical wounds in a medically remarkable fashion. Sutured full-thickness skin wounds healed within several weeks in animals swimming in nonsterile aquaria, even in the presence of decaying meat (food). Wounds healed without gross evidence of inflammation (redness and edema) at the margins as well as within the suture tracks as shown in Figure 82-1. This observation, from a physician's point of view, provoked the very general question: How does a vertebrate defend delicate mucous membranes in the

presence of an unlimited environmental microbial assault without exhibiting any of the clinical signs to be expected from a dependence on classic immune system defense? Microscopic examination confirmed that although a few scattered phagocytic cells could be identified at the wound site, the degree of response was far less impressive than what would have been anticipated from the nature of the wound healing environment.

A series of experiments led to the discovery of a family of antibiotics in the skin of *Xenopus* (1). Through extraction of the skin followed by standard techniques of purification, two 23 amino acid peptides, magainins 1 and 2, were isolated. Subsequently, at least 12 additional antibiotics have been isolated from this species (2). The primary sequences of the five most abundant are shown in Table 82-1. Each peptide is produced as a precursor, containing a signal sequence and an acidic spacer peptide (2). Specific protease cleavage signals precede and generally follow the peptide in the polyprotein. In the case of CPF and XPF, a hormone is also expressed on the polyprotein (caerulein and xenopsin, respectively), processed, and stored and released from the granular gland (see below).

While both magainins 1 and 2 are synthesized on a multiple copy polyprotein, containing one magainin 1 sequence and between three and eight copies of magainin 2, each of the other peptides is expressed from a different gene. What is curious is that although each of these peptides functions in a similar fashion mechanistically, they exhibit no significant homology in either amino acid sequence or nucleic acid sequence. Certain elements of the precursors, including the translated signal sequence and the 5′ nontranslated portion of the polyprotein mRNA, along with the basic design of the polyprotein,

M. Anderson and M. Zasloff: Magainin Research Institute and Magainin Pharmaceuticals, Plymouth Meeting, Pennsylvania 19462.

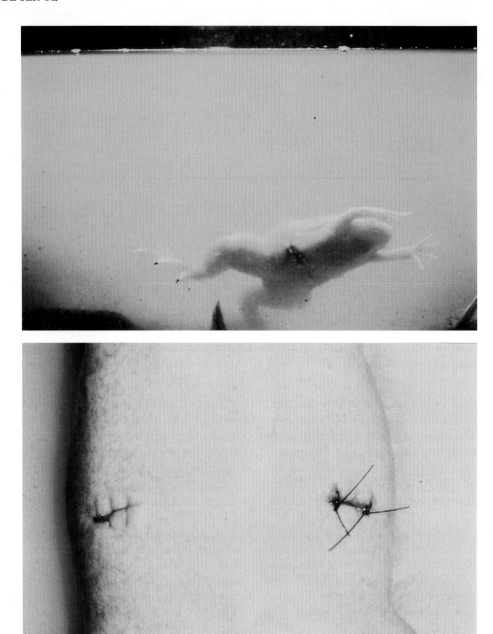

FIG. 82-1. *Xenopus laevis* in aquarium following abdominal surgery. Manner of healing of surgical wounds in the ventral surface of *X. laevis* following a sutured full-thickness epidermal incision. Animal *(top)*, 1 week after surgery; animal *(bottom)*, 1 month after surgery. Gross signs of inflammation are not observed during this healing process.

have been highly conserved. This suggests that these antibiotic sequences have been given the opportunity to undergo variation within a conserved genetic framework that preserves the function of the peptide. In a teleologic sense, variation would seem an advantage if it permitted the animal to match the precise microbiologic profile of the environment (see below).

Magainin and its relatives exhibit broad-spectrum activities against gram-negative and gram-positive bacteria, anaerobes, fungi, yeast, protozoa, and enveloped viruses (1,3–5). This extensive spectrum characterizes

many of the antibiotics found in animals, including the human defensins (6). In addition, many of these peptides exhibit activity against transformed cells, both *in vitro* and *in vivo* (7,8). Strikingly, the magainin peptides are nonhemolytic at concentrations at which they exhibit antimicrobial action (1).

In frog skin, many peptides including the magainins are stored in granules in a structure called the granular gland. Stress, injury, or direct adrenergic stimulation leads to discharge of these granules onto the skin surface. The granules then undergo osmotic rupture, creating a hydrophobic

TABLE 82-1. *Sequences of the major antibiotics found in skin of Xenopus laevis*

Magainin 1	GIGKFLHSAGKFGKAFVGEIMKS
Magainin 2	GIGKFLHSAKKFGKAFVGEIMNS
XPF	GWASKIGQTLGKIAKVGLKQLIQPK
PGLa	GMASKAGAIAGKIAKVALKAL (NH$_2$)
CPF	GFGSFLGKALKAALKIGANALGGSPQQ

XPF, Xenopsin Precursor Fragment; PGLa, Peptide-Glycine-Leucineamide; CPF, Caerulein Precursor Fragment.

gel containing high concentrations of antibiotics as shown in Figure 82-2. Epithelial repair then ultimately reseals the wound. One might reasonably expect that a system used so successfully to defend the skin would also be found to operate at other epithelial surfaces in the animal and this is indeed the case. Magainins are also produced in the gut of the frog, again in granular glands (9). These structures are interesting in that they are neuroepithelial in nature and represent an example of the interrelationship between the nervous system and immune response.

Conclusions: Exposed surfaces are invested with secretory structures that discharge active antibiotics to the surface. A single such agent can effectively kill an enormous range of microbes. It can be stored safely as a long-lived gene product and is sufficiently unreactive to permit persistence at the site of release. It exhibits specificity for microbes over host cells. The antibiotic does not flood the surrounding surface, but remains constrained within a diffusional barrier created on the epithelial surface. The system is present on both external and internal mucosal surfaces.

Antimicrobial peptides of animals are characterized by great diversity within a site of expression. Although they are usually related structurally and common motifs are recognizable, their primary amino acid sequences are very diverse. This variety is usually the result of distinct genetic loci coding for each peptide. For example, in the human phagocyte at least four major defensins have been identified (6), in the bovine neutrophil over 12 (10), and in the Paneth cells of the mouse at least 20 different but related molecules have been reported (11). Why does this diversity occur? At least several reasons can be deduced from a simple demonstration involving the five major antibiotic peptides present in the skin of *X. laevis,* as

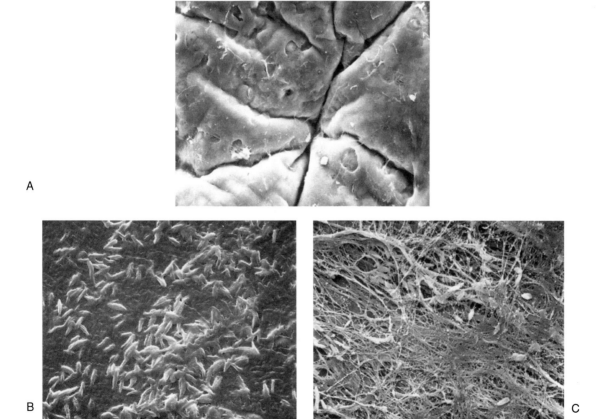

FIG. 82-2. Expression of antibiotic rich secretions from *X. laevis* skin. Granular gland secretion was induced by gentle rubbing of powdered norepinephrine over the skin surface. **A:** Untreated skin. **B:** Secretion expressed in 150 mM NaCl, where osmotic lysis of the granules does not occur, permitting visualization of the intact granules. **C:** One minute after transfer of the specimen to distilled water, demonstrating lysis of granules and formation of an adherent gel. Scanning electron micrograph (× 200).

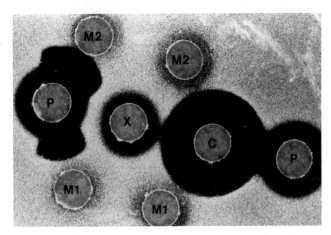

FIG. 82-3. Synergy between *X. laevis* antimicrobial peptides against *S. aureus*. Paper discs impregnated with 1 μM each of the major antimicrobial peptides of *X. laevis* were placed on a lawn of *S. aureus* grown on agarose as described in ref. 1. M1, M2, magainin 1 and 2; P, PGLa; C, CPF; X, XPF. The zone of clearing between P and M1 or P and M2 arises due to the synergistic activities of these molecules.

shown in Figure 82-3. Each disc has been impregnated with an identical molar concentration of synthetic antibiotic peptide and has been placed onto a lawn of *Staphylococcus aureus*. First, one notices that each of the peptides exhibits a somewhat different potency against this bacterial species. Thus, magainin 1 and 2 (M1 and M2) are essentially inactive against this strain of *S. aureus*, while PGLa (P) shows considerable activity. Second, if one examines the zone between the disc containing magainin and that containing PGLa, it is clear that these peptides, in combination, produce a profound synergy. Indeed, the activity of magainin and PGLa in an equimolar combination exceeds by tenfold the potency against *S. aureus* exhibited by either peptide alone. The basis of synergy is the formation of a heterodimer with unique membrane interacting characteristics (12).

In addition to the diversity of molecules found in a single species, as described above for *Xenopus*, there is even greater diversity between species. We and others have extensively surveyed the antimicrobial peptides to be found in the skin of different frog species. The surprising conclusion reached is that, so far, in no two species of frog have the same peptides been isolated. The use of either immunologic tools searching for conserved epitopes or the application of nucleic acid hybridization to identify related nucleic acid sequences would not have allowed the discovery of homologous peptides due to this significant sequence variation. In contrast, peptide hormones also contained in these skins are highly conserved and frequently identical (2).

Conclusions: Antibiotic peptides are typically expressed as families of related but distinctly different gene products. The antimicrobial spectra of these related peptides usually differ substantially. Synergies between these antimicrobial agents occur and can be impressive. In addition, as one examines the antimicrobial peptides from different animal species, extreme diversity is again observed, with no two species expressing the same array of antimicrobial peptides.

Most antimicrobial peptides are membrane active agents that lyse their targets by inserting into the lipid bilayer and forming pores or holes. This breach of the structural integrity of the membrane disrupts the ability of the pathogen to maintain homeostasis and results in cell death (13–15), as illustrated schematically in Figure 82-4. Antimicrobial peptides tend to share several important physical and structural characteristics that are critical to their specificity and activity. These features include a highly positive net charge and the ability to adopt ordered amphipathic conformations. The amphipathic nature of most antimicrobial peptides is probably necessary for integration of the charged molecule into hydrophobic target membranes. The role of the positive charges is to attract the peptide to the membrane of the target cell via electrostatic

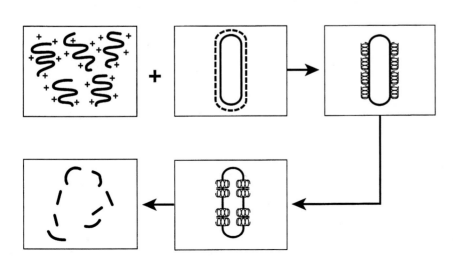

FIG. 82-4. Mechanism of antimicrobial action of magainin peptides. In solution, peptides exist as random coils. In the presence of cells displaying a sufficient surface density of acidic phospholipids on the exterior leaflet of the cytoplasmic membrane, the peptides contact the bilayer through electrostatic interactions. Once in the bilayer they undergo a change in secondary structure, adopting an alpha-helical conformation. Several peptides subsequently organize to form higher-order structures which disturb the permeability of the bilayer, resulting in cell rupture.

interactions. The basis for the surprising selectivity of these peptides is thought to be due to the relative abundance of negative charges in the outer leaflet of microbial cell membranes compared to those of the host's cells (15,16). This selectivity is innate rather than adaptive and represents an interesting example of the pattern-recognition concept elaborated by Medzhitov and Janeway (17).

It has been observed that synthetic, all D amino acid–containing magainins exhibit biologic activity equivalent to natural, L amino acid–containing peptides. This result demonstrates that chiral interactions are not necessary for full antibiotic activity (18). It also underscores the uniqueness of the mechanism of action of antimicrobial peptides as compared to traditional antibiotics, which are typically direct inhibitors of enzymes with chiral active sites.

Although animal antimicrobial peptides typically share the physicochemical features described above, they vary considerably in primary and secondary structure. Subtle variations in sequence can have substantial effects on antibiotic spectrum and potency (11,19). The mechanistic basis for these differences in activity remains poorly understood.

Conclusions: Antimicrobial peptides recognize primitive microbial markers (pattern recognition), which is characteristic of the innate arm of the immune system. The target is a membrane that is organized fundamentally differently from that of a normal host cell in its lipid composition and topology. In addition, once having recognized their targets, antimicrobial peptides lyse them directly, distinguishing them from antibodies, complement, and opsonins.

ANTIBIOTIC PEPTIDES OF MAMMALS, INCLUDING HUMANS

Antimicrobial Peptides of Phagocytic Cells

Mammalian antimicrobial peptides were first discovered in white blood cells, including neutrophils and macrophages (Table 82-2). Here they represent an important component of the nonoxidative killing pathway. They are present at high concentrations in the neutrophil granules, representing at least 30% of total granular protein and 5% to 7% of total cellular protein (42). After phagocytosis, the vesicle containing the ingested pathogen is fused with the granules, exposing the invaders to very high local concentrations of antimicrobial peptides (20). Thus far, four defensins have been described in human neutrophils and they have been designated human neu-

TABLE 82-2. *Mammalian antimicrobial peptides*

Species	Peptide	Class	Tissue	References
Human	HNP-1	α-Defensin	Granulocytes	20
	HNP-2	α-Defensin	Granulocytes	20
	HNP-3	α-Defensin	Granulocytes	20
	HNP-4	α-Defensin	Granulocytes	20
	HD-5	α-Defensin	Paneth cells	21
	HD-6	α-Defensin	Paneth cells	22
	HBD-1	β-Defensin	Epithelia	23
	HBD-2	β-Defensin	Epithelia	24
	LL-37/hCAP-18	α-helical	Granulocytes, epithelia	25, 26, 27
Cow	TAP	β-Defensin	Epithelia	28
	LAP	β-Defensin	Epithelia	29
	EBD	β-Defensin	Epithelia	30
	BNBD-1 through -13	β-Defensin	Granulocytes	10
	Indolicidin	Tryptophan-rich	Granulocytes	31
	Bac5	Proline/arginine-rich	Granulocytes	32
	Bac7	Proline/arginine-rich	Granulocytes	32
Pig	PR-39	Proline/arginine-rich	Intestine	33
	Protegrin	β-Sheet	Granulocytes	34
	Cecropin P1	α-Helical	Intestine, bone marrow	35
	PMAP 37	α-Helical	Bone marrow	36
Mouse	Cryptdins	α-Defensin	Paneth cells	11
	MBD-1	β-Defensin	Epithelia	37
	CRAMP	α-Helical	Granulocytes	38
Rabbit	CAP-18	α-Helical	Granulocytes	39
	NP-1 through -6	α-Defensin	Granulocytes	20
Horse	eNAP-1	Granulin-like	Granulocytes	40
	eNAP-2	Protease inhibitor	Granulocytes	41

HNP, human neutrophil peptide; HD, human defensin; HBD, human beta defensin; CAP, cationic antimicrobial protein; TAP, tracheal antimicrobial protein; LAP, lingual antimicrobial protein; EBD, enteric beta defensin; BNBD, bovine neutrophil beta defensin; Bac, bactenecin; PMAP, pig myeloid antibacterial peptide; MBD, mouse beta defensin; CRAMP, cathelin-related antimicrobial peptide; NP, neutrophil peptide; eNAP, equine neutrophil antimicrobial peptide.

trophil peptides (HNP) 1 to 4. Interestingly, mouse neutrophils lack defensins (43). In humans, genetic diseases in which phagocytes are deficient in defensins have been described. One of these is specific granule disease (20). In one case of this rare disease, mRNA levels coding for the defensins were also very low, consistent with a transcriptional defect as a possible cause (44). The observation that these patients are prone to frequent and severe infections suggests an important role for phagocyte antimicrobial peptides in human host defense. However, the deficiency in these cells is not limited to defensins.

Conclusions: Antimicrobial peptides are critical effector molecules in the nonoxidative cell killing pathway of mammalian phagocytes.

Enteric Defensins

In mammals, the first evidence for antimicrobial peptide production in nonphagocytic cells was uncovered in the intestinal crypts of the mouse (45). These molecules have the same basic disulfide pairing structure as the earlier discovered mammalian white cell defensins. The cellular site of production is the Paneth cell, a specialized secretory cell residing in the base of the crypts of the small intestine. Paneth cells contain secretory granules and are known to produce other defensive molecules such as lysozyme and phospholipase A_2 (11). Because of their primary site of expression, these intestinal mouse defensins have been termed cryptdins. In humans, two defensins have been described in the crypts. These also exhibit the same basic disulfide bonding pattern as the white cell defensins HNP 1 to 4 and have been named HD-5 and HD-6 (21,22). These molecules, as well as the cryptdins, are often referred to as enteric defensins. Paneth cell specific expression of HD-5 is illustrated in Figure 82-5.

In phagocytic cells, the physiologic role and mechanism of deployment of antimicrobial peptides to kill pathogens seems obvious. In nonphagocytic cells such as the Paneth cell, this is much less clear. Paneth cells discharge their contents in response to insult, much like the granular gland of the frog described above. The role and exact site of action of the secreted contents remain to be determined. One hypothesis is that secretion of these molecules is in part responsible for the relative sterility of the small bowel, where the Paneth cells reside. In the mouse, cryptdin antigen has indeed been detected in the luminal contents of the small intestine (11). Alternatively, they may be deployed locally to defend the crypt itself.

In addition to being antimicrobial, some enteric defensins may perform additional functions in intestinal homeostasis. Cryptdins 2 and 3 have been reported to form anion conductive channels in cultured human intestinal epithelial cells (46). Cryptdins 1, 4, 5, and 6 showed no activity despite having sequences that are very

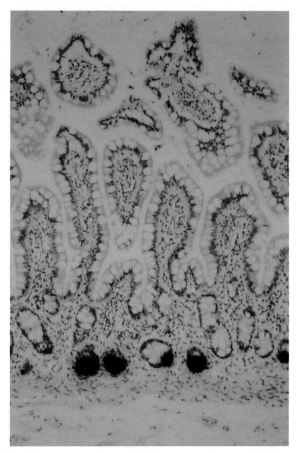

FIG. 82-5. Localization of HD-5 message to the intestinal crypt by *in situ* hybridization. (From ref. 21, with permission.)

similar to the active molecules. Formation of these channels in epithelial cells results in chloride secretion and consequently water secretion. These authors hypothesize that *in vivo* these molecules insert into epithelial cells adjacent to discharged Paneth cells, eliciting fluid secretion that effectively flushes the crypt.

Conclusions: Antimicrobial peptides are also produced in cells that are not traditionally appreciated as immune effector cells. In mammals, this includes the Paneth cells of the small intestine. Their role in health and disease remains to be determined. They may play a role in control of bacterial flora in certain portions of the gastrointestinal tract.

ANTIBIOTIC PEPTIDES IN WIDELY DISTRIBUTED EPITHELIA IN MAMMALS

The enteric defensins, though produced in the epithelium, are the products of highly specialized cells that probably defend a limited portion of the gut. However, all of the epithelial surfaces of the mammalian body that lack Paneth cells, consisting of broad sheets of barrier cells, must similarly defend themselves against microbes. The lung is a classic example in that it contains huge epithelial surfaces that are in continual contact with inhaled environmental flora. The lung does indeed use chemical defenses, and the first mammalian antimicrobial peptide found in this context was tracheal antimicrobial peptide (TAP) (12). TAP is a defensin class molecule containing three disulfide bonds, but the position of its cysteines and their connectivity differ from the conserved pattern observed in the defensins described in phagocytes and Paneth cells. TAP was therefore the defining member of a new structural class of molecules, the β-defensins (12,19). It is, like other defensins, a broad-spectrum antimicrobial peptide with activity against gram-negative and gram-positive bacteria and yeast.

Importantly, TAP is inducible in epithelial cells. Lipopolysaccharide (LPS) and tumor necrosis factor-α (TNF-α) both induce TAP RNA levels and the TAP promoter contains an NF-κB binding site (47). One imagines a scenario where bacterial debris at the site of a local injury induce both epithelial defensin expression and macrophage secretion of cytokines such as TNF. As a result of the chemoattractant activity of defensins (see below), migration of macrophages to the site of injury increases. Secretion of increasing amounts of TNF locally leads to further induction of defensin gene expression, resulting in a robust response supported by several positive feedback mechanisms. Thus, this system of defense is dynamic rather than static and passive. Further, its activity is coordinated by known inflammatory response stimulators and regulators.

Antibiotic Response to Epithelial Injury or Infection

Epithelial surfaces are exposed to environmental microbes, and despite repeated injury, rarely develop suppurative infection, and clinical inflammation is the exception. Sites that are striking in this regard include the tongue and the rectal mucosa. How does the tongue, then, deal with microbial assault in so "benign" a fashion? Although saliva has been shown to contain antimicrobial peptides, such as the histatins (48), the mouth is by no means sterile.

One simple hypothesis is that the epithelium expresses antibiotics that serve to "preserve" the covering. In this regard, a search for antibiotic substances expressed in the bovine lingual epithelium successfully yielded an abundant, novel β-defensin—lingual antibiotic peptide (LAP). This molecule is expressed on both dorsal and ventral surfaces of the tongue and it or closely related defensins are expressed widely throughout most of the exposed epithelial surfaces of the cow (29). Like other defensins, LAP is both antibacterial and antifungal.

What happens regarding the expression of this antibiotic after the tongue epithelium is injured? To answer this question, acute wounds (grazing injuries) were examined for their expression of LAP. These wounds exhibited hallmarks of acute inflammation, characterized by neutrophils, mononuclear cells, and erythrocytes. Using a nucleic acid probe specific for LAP, we demonstrated that LAP gene expression was robustly upregulated in the epithelium in the immediate anatomic vicinity of the ulcer (Fig. 82-6).

The conclusion reached from these studies is that on certain epithelial surfaces, antibiotic expression is constitutive. After injury, in a time frame that kinetically matches acute inflammation, the regenerating epithelium expresses yet higher levels of this (and most likely other) antimicrobial agents. Expression is localized; the wound is almost "painted" in the immediate area of the injury with antibiotic. We have suggested that because this antibiotic barrier deepens after injury, the tongue and other exposed surfaces rarely are forced to call into action the full support of the inflammatory cascade.

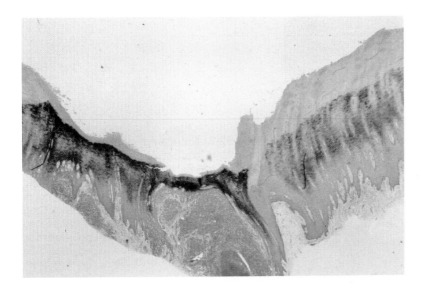

FIG. 82-6. Induction of lingual antibiotic peptide (LAP) expression in the injured tongue. *In situ* hybridization of a grazing wound of bovine tongue tissue with a LAP probe reveals induced expression (dark staining) surrounding the inflamed site. (From ref. 29, with permission.)

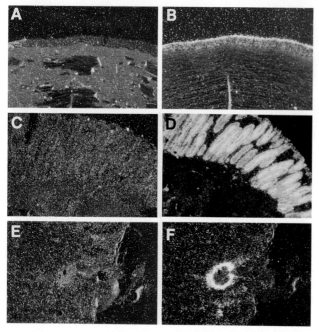

FIG. 82-7. *In situ* hybridization of LAP probe to bovine tissues. The *left* panel of each pair **(A,C,E)** represents tissue probed with the sense negative control; the second **(B,D,F)** is hybridized with the antisense LAP probe. **B:** The constitutive expression of β-defensins in the epithelial monolayer covering the eye. **D:** Induced expression of β-defensins in injured rectal tissue. **F:** A dermal abscess surrounded by epithelial cells that are producing very high levels of β-defensin RNA. (From ref. 49, with permission.)

These principles extend to other tissues in the cow (49). *In situ* hybridization experiments indicate that β-defensins are expressed at virtually every epithelial barrier in mammals. This includes the airway, the digestive tract from the mouth to the anus, the skin, and the conjunctiva (Fig. 82-7). Inducibility seems also to be a general feature. Panel D shows induction near a leukocyte-filled rectal abscess. Similarly, panel F shows a dermal abscess in which the focal infection is surrounded by epithelial cells that are producing high levels of β-defensin, presumably creating a chemical antibiotic barrier to the spread of the infection.

To understand the early responses of the epithelium a series of experimental infections were studied (Fig. 82-8). *Pasteurella haemolytica* is a gram-negative pathogen that causes acute pneumonia in the cow. In the experiment shown in Figure 82-8, sterile saline was instilled in one lung of a cow, whereas an infectious inoculum of *P. haemolytica* was placed in the other lung of the same animal. Assessment of the β-defensin RNA level in the epithelia of the two lungs highlights basic features of epithelial antimicrobial peptide response. The response is fast, in this case within 4 hours, in keeping with an innate immune response. Also, the response is local; the epithelium of the contralateral lung in the same animal is not induced. Here, the inoculum was great enough to overwhelm the system and resulted in a frank clinical infection. This type of immune mechanism is probably most accurately viewed as a first line of defense, with constitutive expression making the moist, nutrient-rich surface of the epithelium as inhospitable as possible to the small inocula of microorganisms that are constantly being deposited there. When this fails and larger numbers of organisms are present, the dose of antibiotic delivered by the epithelial cells is rapidly increased. If this is still insufficient, additional defenses, both innate and adaptive, are brought to bear.

Conclusions: Widely distributed epithelial cells such as those lining the lung are protected at their surfaces by chemical defenses, including antimicrobial peptides such as defensins. This antibiotic shield is dynamic and responsive to insult rather than passive. Its activity is controlled at least in part by well-known inflammatory response mediators.

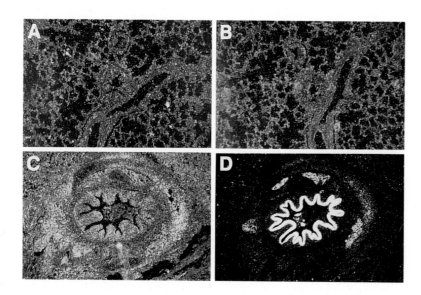

FIG. 82-8. Expression of β-defensins in the respiratory tract of *P. haemolytica* inoculated cattle. **A** and **B:** Healthy control lung tissue that was instilled with a sterile saline solution. **C** and **D:** Lung tissue from an infected lung 4 hours after inoculation. Panels **A** and **C** were probed with control sense LAP; **B** and **D** were probed with antisense LAP probe. The bright areas in **D** indicate robust expression of β-defensins in the infected airway epithelium. (From ref. 49, with permission.)

Human Antimicrobial Peptides of Epithelia

Human β-Defensin-1 (HBD-1)

Extending observations made in mammals such as the cow to human host defense has proved difficult because of the limited sequence homology among antimicrobial peptides and their genes across species. This lack of conservation makes it difficult to clone human antimicrobial peptides by standard molecular biologic techniques. Despite this, progress has been made recently in identifying new effector molecules in human epithelia. HBD-1 was discovered through a random search of peptides purified from hemofiltrate of patients undergoing dialysis treatment. Comparison of the peptide sequence to existing sequences in a database revealed the similarity to the bovine β-defensins (23). HBD-1 represents the first of the β-defensin class to be discovered in humans. HBD-1 is widely expressed in epithelia that are directly exposed to the environment or are exposed to microbial flora via ducts. Expression is observed in the lung, mammary gland, salivary gland, kidney, pancreas, and prostate, among others (50,51). In contrast to the highly inducible bovine epithelial defensins, HBD-1 thus far does not appear to be inducible at the mRNA level.

Human β-Defensin-2 (HBD-2)

The second human β-defensin was isolated, based on its antimicrobial activity, from psoriatic scale (24). HBD-2 is, like other described mammalian defensins, a broad-spectrum antibiotic with activity against Gram-negative and gram-positive bacteria as well as the yeast *Candida albicans*. Expression of HBD-2 is also widespread in epithelia, including those of the lung, gut, urogenital system, pancreas, and skin. HBD-2 also appears to be expressed in leukocytes and the bone marrow. In contrast to HBD-1, HBD-2 is highly inducible in epithelial cells.

Both heat-killed microorganisms and inflammatory cytokines such as TNF-α are potent inducers (24). Thus the system of antimicrobial peptide defense discovered in the epithelia of the cow indeed exists in a very similar configuration in humans.

LL-37/hCAP 18

LL-37/hCAP18 is a human antimicrobial peptide found both in granulocytes and epithelial cells (25–27). It differs dramatically from the defensins in that it lacks disulfide bonds and forms an alpha-helical structure in its active form. It is similar to CAP-18, a rabbit molecule that binds LPS (39). It is the only known human member of the cathelicidin family of antimicrobial peptides (52). Cathelicidins include PR-39 from the pig and the cathelin-related antimicrobial peptide (CRAMP) from the mouse (33,38). This family features a large, conserved pro-piece connected to a highly variable antibiotic portion that is liberated by proteolytic cleavage. LL-37 is expressed in epithelial cells of the skin and is induced there in inflammatory conditions such as psoriasis and nickel allergy (53).

Epithelial Defenses in Human Disease

The activities and expression patterns of antimicrobial peptides strongly suggest that they play an important role in host defense. However, due to the redundancy of these systems and their tremendous variability among species it may be difficult to draw conclusions about their *in vivo* functions by, for example, gene knock-out technology. Despite this, several recent studies support a critical role for these molecules in human health and disease.

Accumulating evidence points to the importance of antimicrobial peptides and possibly other epithelial defensive molecules in the etiology of lung disease in cystic fibrosis. Cystic fibrosis is an autosomal recessive genetic disease resulting from a defect in the cystic fibrosis transmembrane conductance regulator (CFTR). CFTR acts as an ion channel regulating the flux of chloride ions across epithelial cell sheets. The most salient clinical features of cystic fibrosis are chronic inflammation of the lungs and persistent pulmonary infections. The two most common bacterial pathogens in CF lung infections are *Pseudomonas aeruginosa* and *S. aureus*. The molecular chain of events connecting a defect in ion transport to local immunodeficiency of the lung has never been clear, and a variety of hypotheses have been put forth in an attempt to reconcile the two observations. Smith et al. (54) performed a series of experiments indicating a profound difference in the defensive capabilities of wild-type versus CF primary lung epithelial cells. In culture the wild-type cells were able to kill a small inoculum of *P. aeruginosa* placed on their apical surfaces, whereas the CF cells could not. Further, the surface fluid of both cell types contained a salt-sensitive antimicrobial substance with properties similar to those of antimicrobial peptides. This suggests that the ion channel defect leads indirectly to immune compromise by altering the normal ionic milieu of the airway surface fluid and thereby preventing the proper function of host defense molecules in that fluid. This model is represented in Figure 82-9.

The antimicrobial activity of defensins is known to be extremely salt sensitive. Further work has shown that defensins (HBD-1 and HBD-2) are in fact expressed in human lung epithelial cells (24,51,55). Localization of HBD-1 expression to the airway epithelium is shown in Figure 82-10. Human airway epithelial cells can be used to repopulate a denuded rat trachea implanted on the back of an immunocompromised mouse. The cells differentiate and form submucosal glands. Similar to what was observed in cultured cells, fluid derived from CF grafts was unable to kill bacteria, but that obtained from wild-type grafts could. Further, antisense oligonucleotides that

Normal

Cystic Fibrosis

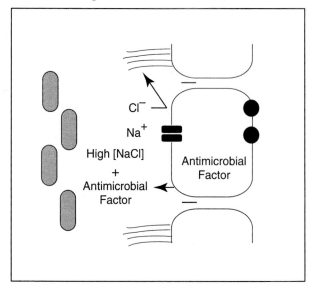

FIG. 82-9. Model of impaired pulmonary barrier defenses in cystic fibrosis. A defect in ion transport, blocking the flow of chloride ions, leads to a proposed increase in the salt concentration of the airway surface fluid. This in turn leads to inactivation of salt-sensitive epithelial antimicrobial factors such as defensins, resulting in impaired local immunity. (From ref. 71, with permission.)

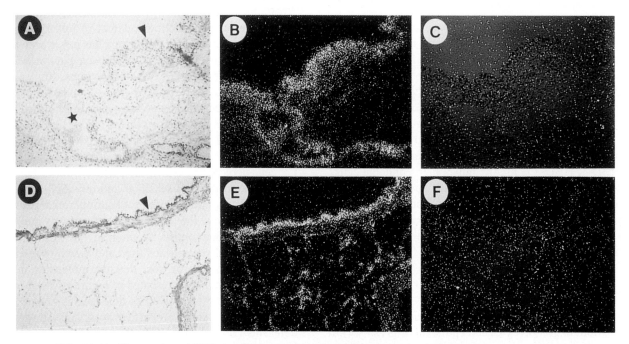

FIG. 82-10. Expression of HBD-1 mRNA in human lung epithelium. **A** and **D:** Epithelium *(arrows)* and a submucosal gland *(star)*. *In situ* hybridization with an HBD-1 probes reveals expression of HBD-1 in proximal **(B)** and distal **(E)** human airway epithelium. Negative control hybridizations with the sense probe do not stain the tissue **(C** and **F).** (From ref. 51, with permission.)

specifically ablated HBD-1 expression almost eliminated the measured antimicrobial activity (55). These observations serve to confirm the host defense function of antimicrobial peptides in epithelia in general and implicate them in the mechanism of CF lung infection specifically. Many other antimicrobial substances are present in airway surface fluid, including lactoferrin, lysozyme, and lipids. These molecules likely defend the epithelium in an additive or synergistic fashion that may also be sensitive to the ionic composition of the airway surface fluid.

Conclusions: Host defense is compromised locally in the lungs of cystic fibrosis patients, and recent evidence points to deficient innate immune function of airway epithelial cells as a critical factor. A change in the composition of the airway surface fluid in cystic fibrosis may lead indirectly to impaired lung defense by inactivating effector molecules such as antimicrobial peptides. This suggests the critical importance of innate epithelial defenses in maintaining human health.

Other Antimicrobial Peptides and Proteins

The majority of antimicrobial proteins that we have not discussed are proteins larger than the antimicrobial peptides and are found principally in circulating blood cells. Included in this group are antimicrobial proteins of the neutrophil, such as Bactericidal/Permeability Increasing Protein (BPI) (56) and the serprocidins (57); eosinophil major basic and cationic proteins (58); and NK-lysin of the lymphocyte (59). In each case, the antimicrobial activity of the protein results from its cationic net charge and its disruption of microbial membrane permeability; the proteins function either within the milieu of a phagocytic vacuole or are secreted from the cell in the vicinity of the microbial target.

Of particular interest is a family of recently described antimicrobial proteins secreted by the human platelet (59a). Just as epithelial barriers are logical sites for the deployment of chemical antimicrobial defenses, so too the site of a breach in the epithelium, such as a wound, would be expected to evolve this type of defensive mechanism. Activated platelets can be argued to be the first defensive elements deployed at a vascular injury, puncture, or wound, and their role in clotting to stop blood loss is well known. As expected, platelets also contain antimicrobial peptides and small proteins. These compounds are not yet as well characterized as other classes of antimicrobial peptides. However, they appear to kill target pathogens by disrupting membranes as do most previously described antimicrobial peptides. Curiously a comparable system was discovered several years ago in the horseshoe crab, where circulating blood cells involved in hemostasis (hemocytes) were found to discharge a potent 17 amino acid antimicrobial peptide (tachyplesin) on adherence to a site of vascular injury (59b).

Secretory leukocyte protease inhibitor (SLPI) is a 12-kd protein that inhibits the activity of proteases such as neutrophil elastase. It therefore helps to modulate inflammatory responses to prevent damage to host tissues. It is present in mucosal fluids of the lung and genital tract, and in colostrum (60,61). SLPI also acts as an antimicrobial protein with activity against *Escherichia coli, S. aureus,* some fungi, and human immunodeficiency virus (HIV) (60–62). This is another example of a host defense molecule that serves multiple roles in immune response and integration.

Lysozyme and lactoferrin are two proteins long associated with antimicrobial defense. In contrast to the antibiotic agents synthesized by the epithelium itself, high concentrations of these proteins are produced by the exocrine glands, which bathe the surrounding epithelial surfaces. Of great interest will be studies that delineate the many obvious synergies that could be imagined to occur in a setting where antimicrobial peptides are released into a fluid containing these and other antibacterial substances.

ANTIBIOTIC PEPTIDES HAVE ASSOCIATED PHARMACOLOGIC ACTIVITIES

The antibiotics from animals have been discovered largely on the basis of their activity in killing or suppressing the growth of various microbes. However, successive studies have demonstrated, principally *in vitro,* that several of these molecules exhibit other curious biologic properties. The presumption is that antibiotic peptides, although designed to attack microbes directly, also communicate with other systems in the body of the animal. By interacting with neighboring epithelial cells or the immune system they assist in the orchestration of a coordinated response to microbial invasion and injury. For example, the human defensins HNP-1 and HNP-2 have been reported to be chemotactic for monocytes (63). These same molecules are also chemotactic for T cells (64). Such activities are logical extensions of the host defense functions of defensins, serving to promote immune cell attack at sites of wounding or infection where they are released. Supporting this view is the clinical observation that patients with specific granule deficiency, who lack neutrophil defensins, fail to normally recruit monocytes to wound sites (65). Defensins, at low concentrations, also stimulate the growth of cultured fibroblasts and epithelial cells (66). Two rabbit defensins as well as HNP-1, -2, and -3 induce DNA synthesis at physiologically relevant concentrations. Again, this activity is consistent with a host defense role in promoting the healing and closure of wounds.

Another immune response–related activity of defensins is the ability to inhibit production of corticosteroid production by adrenal cells. This activity was first demonstrated for cultured cells, but rabbit defensins have also been shown to inhibit stress induced adrenocorticotropic hormone (ACTH) and corticosterone production in rodents (67,68). In cellular studies this inhibition is observed at nanomolar concentrations and is likely explained by competitive inhibition of ACTH binding to its receptor.

The porcine peptide PR-39 has several activities in addition to its direct antibiotic effects. It also stimulates cultured fibroblast cells to produce syndecans (69). Syndecans are cell surface proteoglycans that are necessary for cells to respond to certain polypeptide growth factors and extracellular matrix proteins. PR-39 was identified as the factor present in wound fluid responsible for syndecan-inducing activity. Induction of syndecans is a marker for an active state of wound healing and closure. Interestingly, another nonantibiotic activity of PR-39 may be involved in the down modulation of inflammatory responses. PR-39 is a direct inhibitor of reduced nicotinamide-adenine dinucleotide phosphate (NADPH) oxidase, which is responsible for the production of the reactive oxygen intermediates that constitute the oxidative branch of phagocytic cell killing (70). These species are also destructive to the host's tissues, and PR-39 may be an important player in regulating this system.

Conclusions: In many cases antimicrobial peptides exhibit activities beyond the direct inactivation of pathogens. In general, these activities are involved in immune regulation and integration of host defense responses.

SUMMARY

We have focused on the response of the epithelium to injury and microbial assault. We denote this arm of immunity as "barrier defense," distinguishing it from "systemic immunity," as depicted in Figure 82-11. The barrier defenses, as represented by antimicrobial peptides, are innate in the sense that they are not apparently adaptive to specific antigens. In contrast, they are designed to kill a broad range of microbes, including most known classes of pathogens ranging from bacteria, to fungi, to protozoa, including viruses. The response is rapid and is highly localized to the immediate site of

injury, no further than millimeters from the site of insult.

The systemic immune system is composed of its innate components, including complement and opsonins like the maltose binding protein. However, it is dominated by its adaptive arm. This system exerts an anatomically diffuse response around a site of injury, frequently provoking generalized systemic reactions. The system is relatively slow, highly networked, and capable of great selectivity. The pathogen binding structures are generally antibodies or cell-associated receptors, which in and of themselves are not intrinsically destructive. In addition, the equipment of the adaptive immune system is highly conserved with respect to genetic organization and sequence among mammalian species. In striking contrast to the components of the systemic immune system, the antimicrobial peptides of one mammalian species are considerably divergent in sequence, and frequently peptides present in one species in a particular location are replaced by completely different proteins in another species.

Since antimicrobial peptides exert cytokine and chemoattractant activity, we speculate that injury of an epithelial surface in each of two species, inducing different gene products, might communicate different signals to the systemic arm of the immune system. If so, then upon infection or injury of the epithelium, different systemic immune responses might ensue. Thus, as regards epithelial injury or infection, immunologically analogous animal models of human disease might not exist.

REFERENCES

1. Zasloff M. Magainins, a class of antimicrobial peptides from Xenopus skin: isolation, characterization of two active forms, and partial cDNA sequence of a precursor. *Proc Natl Acad Sci USA* 1987;84:5449–5453.
2. Bevins CL, Zasloff M. Peptides from frog skin. *Annu Review Biochem* 1990;59:395–414.
3. Soravia E, Martini G, Zasloff M. Antimicrobial properties of peptides from Xenopus granular gland secretions. *FEBS Lett* 1988;228:337–340.
4. Schuster FL, Jacob LS. Effects of magainins on ameba and cyst stages of Acanthamoeba polyphaga. *Antimicrob Agents Chemother* 1992;6:1263–1271.
5. Aboudy Y, Mendelson E, Shalit I, Bessalle R, Fridkin M. Activity of two synthetic amphilic peptides and magainin-2 against herpes simplex virus types 1 and 2. *Int J Peptide Protein Res* 1994;43:573–582.
6. Lehrer RI, Lichtenstein AK, Ganz T. DEFENSINS: antimicrobial and cytotoxic peptides of mammalian cells. *Annu Rev Immunol* 1993;11:105–129.
7. Cruciani RA, Barker JL, Zasloff M, Chen HC, Colamonici O. Antibiotic magainins exert cytolytic activity against transformed cell lines through channel formation. *Proc Natl Acad Sci USA* 1991;88:3792–3796.
8. Baker MA, Maloy WL, Zasloff M, Jacob LS. Anticancer efficacy of magainin 2 and analogue peptides. *Cancer Res* 1993;53:3052–3057.
9. Reilly DS, Tomassini N, Bevins CL, Zasloff M. A Paneth cell analogue in Xenopus small intestine expresses antimicrobial peptide genes: conservation of an intestinal host-defense system. *J Histochem Cytochem* 1994;42:697–704.
10. Selsted ME, Tang YQ, Morris WL, et al. Purification, primary structures, and antibacterial activities of β-defensins, a new family of antimicrobial peptides from bovine neutrophils. *J Biol Chem* 1993;263:9573–9575.

Barrier Defense
Innate
Localized
Rapid response time
Broad spectrum
Antimicrobial peptides differ between mammalian species

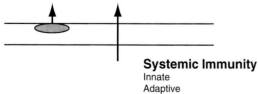

Systemic Immunity
Innate
Adaptive
  - Anatomically diffuse
  - Relatively slow response
  - High specificity for microbe
  - Conserved within mammals

FIG. 82-11. Barrier defenses vs. systemic immunity.

11. Ouellette AJ, Selsted ME. Paneth cell defensins: endogenous peptide components of intestinal host defense. *FASEB J* 1996;10:1280–1289.

12. Westerhoff HV, Zasloff M, Rosner JL, et al. Functional synergism of the magainins PGLa and magainin-2 in *Escherichia coli,* tumor cells and liposomes. *Eur J Biochem* 1995;228:257–264.

13. Cruciani RA, Barker JL, Durell SR, et al. Magainin 2, a natural antibiotic from frog skin, forms ion channels in lipid bilayer membranes. *Eur J Pharmacol* 1992;226:287–296.

14. Ludtke S, He K, Huang H. Membrane thinning caused by magainin 2. *Biochemistry* 1995;34:16764–16769.

15. White SH, Wimley WC, Selsted ME. Structure, function, and membrane integration of defensins. *Curr Opin Struct Biol* 1995;5:521–527.

16. Matsuzaki K, Sugishita K, Fujii N, Miyajima K. Molecular basis for membrane selectivity of an antimicrobial peptide, magainin 2. *Biochemistry* 1995;34:3423–3429.

17. Medzhitov R, Janeway CA. Innate immunity: the virtues of a nonclonal system of recognition. *Cell* 1997;91:295–298.

18. Wade D, Boman A, Wahlin B, et al. All-D amino acid containing channel-forming antibiotic peptides. *Proc Natl Acad Sci USA* 1990;87:4761–4765.

19. Selsted ME, Tang Y-Q, Morris WL, et al. Purification, primary structures, and antibacterial activities of β-defensins, a new family of antimicrobial peptides from bovine neutrophils. *J Biol Chem* 1993;268:6641–6648.

20. Ganz T, Lehrer RI. Defensins. *Pharmacol Ther* 1995;66:191–205.

21. Jones DE, Bevins CL. Paneth cells of the human small intestine express an antimicrobial peptide gene. *J Biol Chem* 1992;267:23216–23225.

22. Jones DE, Bevins CL. Defensin-6 mRNA in human Paneth cells: implications for antimicrobial peptides in host defense of the human bowel. *FEBS Lett* 1993;315:187–192.

23. Bensch KW, Raida M, Magert H-J, Schulz-Knappe P, Forssmann W-G. hBD-1: a novel β-defensin from human plasma. *FEBS Lett* 1995;368:331–335.

24. Harder J, Bartels J, Christophers E, Schroder J-M. A peptide antibiotic from human skin. *Nature* 1997;387:861.

25. Agerberth B, Gunne H, Odeberg J, Kogner P, Boman HG, Gudmundsson GH. FALL-39, a putative human peptide antibiotic, is cysteine-free and expressed in bone marrow and testis. *Proc Natl Acad Sci USA* 1995;92:195–199.

26. Larrick JW, Hirata M, Balint RF, Lee J, Zhong J, Wright SC. Human CAP18: a novel antimicrobial lipopolysaccharide-binding protein. *Infect Immun* 1995;63:1291–1297.

27. Cowland JB, Johsen AH, Borregaard N. hCAP18, a cathelin/probactenecin-like protein of human neutrophil specific granules. *FEBS Lett* 1995;368:173–176.

28. Diamond G, Zasloff M, Eck H, Brasseur M, Maloy WL, Bevins CL. Tracheal antimicrobial peptide, a cysteine-rich peptide from mammalian tracheal mucosa: peptide isolation and cloning of a cDNA. *Proc Natl Acad Sci USA* 1991;88:3952–3956.

29. Schonwetter BS, Stolzenberg ED, Zasloff MA. Epithelial antibiotics induced at sites of inflammation. *Science* 1995;267:1645–1648.

30. Tarver AP, Clark DP, Diamond G, et al. Enteric β-defensin: molecular cloning and characterization of a gene with inducible intestinal epithelial cell expression associated with *Cryptosporidium parvum* infection. *Infect Immun* 1998;66:1045–1056.

31. Selsted ME, Novotny MJ, Morris WL, Tang YQ, Smith W, Cullor JS. Indolicidin, a novel bactericidal tridecapeptide amide from neutrophils. *J Biol Chem* 1992;267:4292–4295.

32. Frank RW, Gennaro R, Schneider K, Przybylski M, Romeo D. Amino acid sequences of 2 proline rich bactenecins-antimicrobial peptides of bovine neutrophils. *J Biol Chem* 1990;265:18871–18874.

33. Agerberth B, Lee YJ, Bergman T, et al. Amino acid sequence of PR-39: isolation from pig intestine of a new member of the family of proline-arginine rich antibacterial peptides. *Eur J Biochem* 1991;202:849–854.

34. Kokryakov VN, Harwig SS, Panyutich EA, et al. Protegrins: leukocyte antimicrobial peptides that combine features of corticostatic defensins and tachyplesins. *FEBS Lett* 193;327:231–236.

35. Lee J-Y, Boman A, Chuanxin S, et al. Antibacterial peptides from pig intestine: isolation of a mammalian cecropin. *Proc Natl Acad Sci* 1989;86:9159–9162.

36. Tossi A, Scocchi M, Zanetti M, Storici P, Genarro R. PMAP-37, a novel antibacterial peptide from pig myeloid cells, cDNA cloning, chemical synthesis and activity. *Eur J Biochem* 1995;228:941–946.

37. Huttner KM, Kozak CA, Bevins CL. The mouse genome encodes a single homolog of the antimicrobial peptide human β-defensin 1. *FEBS Lett* 1997;413:45–49.

38. Gallo RL, Kim KJ, Bernfield M, et al. Identification of CRAMP, a cathelin-related antimicrobial peptide expressed in the embryonic and adult mouse. *J Biol Chem* 1997;272:13088–13093.

39. Larrick JW, Hirata M, Shimomoura Y, et al. Antimicrobial activity of rabbit CAP18-derived peptides. *Antimicrob Agents Chemother* 1993;37:2534–2539.

40. Couto MA, Harwig SS, Cullor JS, Hughes JP, Lehrer RI. Identification of eNAP-1, an antimicrobial peptide from equine neutrophils. *Infect Immun* 1992;60:3065–3071.

41. Couto MA, Harwig SS, Lehrer RI. Selective inhibition of microbial serine proteases by eNAP-2, an antimicrobial peptide from equine neutrophils. *Infect Immun* 1993;61:2991–2994.

42. Lehrer RI, Ganz T, Selsted ME. Defensins: endogenous antibiotic peptides of animal cells. *Cell* 1991;64:229–230.

43. Eisenhauer PB, Lehrer RI. Mouse neutrophils lack defensins. *Infect Immun* 1992;60:3446–3447.

44. Tamura A, Agematsu K, Mori T, et al. A marked decrease in defensin mRNA in the only case of congenital neutrophil-specific granule deficiency reported in Japan. *Int J Hematol* 1994;59:137–142.

45. Ouellette AJ, Greco RM, James M, Frederick D, Naftilan J, Fallon JT. Developmental regulation of cryptdin, a corticostatin/defensin precursor mRNA in mouse small intestinal crypt epithelium. *J Cell Biol* 1989;108:1687–1695.

46. Lencer WI, Cheung G, Strohmeier GR, et al. Induction of epithelial chloride secretion by channel-forming cryptdins 2 and 3. *Proc Natl Acad Sci USA* 1997;94:8585–8589.

47. Diamond G, Russell JP, Bevins CL. Inducible expression of an antibiotic peptide gene in lipopolysaccharide-challenged tracheal epithelial cells. *Proc Natl Acad Sci USA* 1996;93:5156–5160.

48. Tsai H, Raj PA, Bobek LA. Candidacidal activity of recombinant human salivary histatin-5 and variants. *Infect Immun* 1996;64:5000–5007.

49. Stolzenberg ED, Anderson GM, Ackermann MR, Whitlock RH, Zasloff M. Epithelial antibiotic induced in states of disease. *Proc Natl Acad Sci USA* 1997;94:8686–8690.

50. Zhao C, Wang I, Lehrer RI. Widespread expression of β-defensin hBD-1 in human secretory glands and epithelial cells. *FEBS Lett* 1996;396:319–322.

51. Goldman MJ, Anderson GM, Stolzenberg ED, Kari UP, Zasloff M, Wilson JM. Human β-defensin I is a salt sensitive antibiotic in lung that is inactivated in cystic fibrosis. *Cell* 1997;88:553–560.

52. Gudmundsson GH, Agerberth B, Odeberg J, Bergman T, Olsson B, Salcedo R. The human gene FALL39 and processing of the cathelin precursor to the antibacterial peptide LL-37 in granulocytes. *Eur J Biochem* 1996;238:325–332.

53. Frohm M, Agerberth B, Ahangari G, et al. The expression of the gene coding for the antibacterial peptide LL-37 is induced in human keratinocytes during inflammatory disorders. *J Biol Chem* 1997;272:15258–15263.

54. Smith JJ, Travis SM, Greenberg EP, Welsh MJ. Cystic fibrosis airway epithelia fail to kill bacteria because of abnormal airway surface fluid. *Cell* 1996;85:229–236.

55. McCray PB Jr., Bentley L. Human airway epithelia express a beta-defensin. *Am J Respir Cell Mol Biol* 1997;16:343–349.

56. Elsbach P, Weiss J, Levy O. Integration of antimicrobial host defenses: role of the bactericidal/permeability-increasing protein. *Trends Microbiol* 1994;2:324–328.

57. Gabay JE. Antimicrobial proteins with homology to serine proteases. *Ciba Found Symp* 1994;186:237–249.

58. Lehrer RI, Szklarek D, Barton A, Ganz T, Hamann KJ, Gleich GJ. Antibacterial properties of eosinophil major basic protein and eosinophil cationic protein. *J Immunol* 1989;142:4428–4434.

59. Andersson M, Gunne H, Agerberth B, Boman A, Bergman T, Sillard R, Jornvall H, Mut V, Olsson B, Wigzell H, et al. NK-lysin, a novel effector peptide of cytotoxic T and NK cells. Structure and cDNA cloning of the porcine form, induction by interleukin 2, antibacterial and antitumour activity. *EMBO J* 1995;14:1615–1625.

59a. Yeaman MR, Tang Y-Q, Shen A, Bayer AS, Selsted ME. Purification and in vitro activities of rabbit platelet microbicidal proteins. *Infect Immun* 1997;65:1023–1031.

59b. Iwanaga S, Muta T, Shigenaga T, Seki N, Kawano K, Katsu T, Kawabata S. Structure-function relationships of tachyplesins and their analogues. *Ciba Found Symp* 1994;186:160–175.

60. Wahl SM, McNeely TB, Janoff EN, et al. Secretory leukocyte protease inhibitor (SLPI) in mucosal fluids inhibits HIV-1. *Oral Dis Suppl* 1997;1:S64–S69.

61. Tomee JF, Hiemstra PS, Heinzel-Wieland R, Kauffman HF. Antileukoprotease: an endogenous protein in the innate mucosal defense against fungi. *J Infect Dis* 1997;176:740–747.

62. Hiemstra PS, Maassen RJ, Stolk J, Heinzel-Wieland R, Steffens GJ, Dijkman JH. Antibacterial activity of antileukoprotease. *Infect Immun* 1996;64:4520–4524.

63. Territo MC, Ganz T, Selsted ME, Lehrer R. Monocyte-chemotactic activity of defensins from human neutrophils. *J Clin Invest* 1989;84: 2017–2020.

64. Chertov O, Michiel DF, Xu LL, et al. Identification of defensin-1, defensin-2, and CAP37/azurocidin as T-cell chemoattractant proteins released from interleukin-8 stimulated neutrophils. *J Biol Chem* 1996; 271:2935–2940.

65. Ganz T, Metcalf JA, Gallin JI, Boxer LA, Lehrer RI. Microbicidal/ cytotoxic proteins of neutrophils are deficient in two disorders: Che-

diak-Higashi syndrome and "specific" granule deficiency. *J Clin Invest* 1988;82:552–556.

66. Murphy CJ, Foster BA, Mannis MJ, Selsted ME, Reid TW. Defensins are mitogenic for epithelial cells and fibroblasts. *J Cell Physiol* 1993; 155:408–413.

67. Zhu QZ, Hu J, Mulay S, Esch F, Shimasaki S, Solomon S. Isolation and structure of corticostatin peptides from rabbit fetal and adult lung. *Proc Natl Acad Sci USA* 1988;85:592–596.

68. Shamova OV, Lesnikova MP, Kokryakov VN, Shkhinek EK, Korneva EA. Effect of defensins on the blood level of corticosterone and the immune response during stress. *Bull Exp Biol Med* 1993; 6:728–731.

69. Gallo RL, Ono M, Povsic T, et al. Syndecans, cell surface heparin sulfate proteoglycans, are induced by a proline-rich antimicrobial peptide from wounds. *Proc Natl Acad Sci USA* 1994;91:11035–11039.

70. Shi J, Ross CR, Leto TL, Blecha F. PR-39, a proline-rich antibacterial peptide that inhibits phagocyte NADPH oxidase activity by binding to Src homology 3 domains of p47 phox. *Proc Natl Acad Sci USA* 1996; 93:6014–6018.

71. Rosenstein BJ, Zeitlin PL. Cystic fibrosis. *Lancet* 1998;351:277–282.

Inflammation: Basic Principles and Clinical Correlates,
3rd ed., edited by John I. Gallin and Ralph Snyderman.
Lippincott Williams & Wilkins, Philadelphia © 1999.

APPENDIX A

Human Leukocyte Surface Antigens

Dhavalkumar D. Patel and Barton F. Haynes

APPENDIX A. *Human leukocyte surface antigens: the CD classification of leukocyte differentiation antigens*

Surface antigen	Family	M_r	Distribution	Ligands	Function
CD1a (T6, HTA-1)	Ig	49	DC, cortical thymocytes	Not known	Possible role in T-cell development
CD1b	Ig	45	DC, cortical thymocytes	Not known	Antigen presentation of lipids
CD1c	Ig	43	DC, cortical thymocytes, subset of B cells	Not known	Unknown
CD1d	Ig	?	Cortical thymocytes, intestinal epithelium	Not known	Presentation of peptide antigens
CD2 (T12, LFA-2)	Ig	50	T, NK	CD58, CD48, CD59, CD15	Alternative T-cell activation, T-cell anergy, T-cell cytokine production, T- or NK-mediated cytolysis, T-cell apoptosis, cell adhesion
CD3 (T3, LEU-4)	Ig	γ 25–28, δ 21–28, ϵ 20–25, η 21–22, ζ 16	T	Associates with the TCR	T-cell activation and function; ζ is the signal transduction component of the CD3 complex
CD4 (T4, LEU-3)	Ig	55	T, myeloid	MHC-II, HIV gp120, IL-16, SABP	T-cell selection, T-cell activation, signal transduction with p56^{LCK}, primary receptor for HIV
CD5 (T1, LEU-1)	SRCR	67	T, subset of B cells, B-CLL	?CD72, gp35–37	Costimulatory for T cells
CD6 (T12)	SRCR	100–130	T, subset of B cells, B-CLL	ALCAM (CD166)	Cell adhesion, co-stimulatory molecule for T cells
CD7 (3A1, LEU-9)	Ig	40	T, NK	Not known	T-cell signal transduction and regulation of IFN-γ production
CD8 (T8, LEU-2)	Ig	34	T	MHC-I	T-cell selection, T-cell activation, signal transduction with p56^{LCK}
CD9 (MRP-1)	Tetraspan	24, 26	Broad	Associates with CD63, CD81, CD82	Modulate cell adhesion/ migration, platelet activation, myeloid development
CD10 (CALLA, enkephalinase)	Zinc metallo-protease	100	Early T and B precursors, G, fibroblasts, epithelia	Not known	Possible role in B-cell development, zinc metalloprotease
CD11a (LFA-1 α, α_L integrin)	Integrin α	170–180	All leukocytes	CD54, CD102, CD50	Cell adhesion, co-stimulation
CD11b (α_M integrin Mac-1, CR3)	Integrin α	165–170	G, M, NK, subset of B and T	iC3b, fibrinogen, CD23	Cell adhesion, phagocytosis, absent in patients with LAD-1
CD11c (α_X integrin, CR4)	Integrin α	145–150	G, M, NK, subset of B and T	iC3b, fibrinogen, CD23	Cell adhesion, phagocytosis, absent in patients with LAD-1
CDw12	Unknown	150–160	M, G (except basophils), NK	Not known	Unknown

D. D. Patel and B. F. Haynes: Department of Medicine, Duke University School of Medicine, Durham, North Carolina 27710.

APPENDIX A. *Continued.*

Surface antigen	Family	M$_r$	Distribution	Ligands	Function
CD13 (amino-peptidase N)	Unknown	150	CFU-GM, G, M, EC, subset of epithelia, osteoclasts, subset LGL	Not known	Trimming of peptides bound to MHC-II
CD14 (LPS receptor)	LRG	53–55	M, G (weak), not by myeloid progenitors	Endotoxin (lipopolysaccharide), lipoteichoic acid, PI	Endotoxin (LPS) receptor
CD15 (LewisX, lacto-N fucopentaose III)	Poly-N-acetyl-lactosamine	Broad	M, G, DC	Selectins	Cell adhesion
CD15s (sialyl LewisX)	Poly-N-acetyl-lactosamine	Broad	M, G, NK, subset of T, activated T and B, HEV	CD62E	Cell adhesion
CD16a (FcγRIIIa, LEU-11)	Ig	50–65	NK, G, M, subset of T	IgG	Low-affinity receptor for IgG; ADCC, activation of cytotoxicity, cytokine production
CD16b (FcγRIIIb)	Ig	50–65	G	IgG	Low-affinity IgG receptor, GPI-linked
CDw17 (lactosylceramide)	LacCer	150–160	M, G, P, CD19$^+$ B cells, DC, activated T	Not known	Unknown; may function in phagocytosis
CD18 (β$_2$ integrin)	Integrin β	95	All leukocytes	See CD11a, CD11b, CD11c	Associates with CD11a, CD11b, and CD11c; defect in CD18 causes LAD-1
CD19 (B4)	Ig	95	B (except plasma cells), FDC	Not known	Associates with CD21 and CD81 to form a complex involved in signal transduction in B-cell development, activation and differentiation
CD20 (B1)	Unassigned	33–37	B (except plasma cells)	Not known	Cell signaling; may be important for B-cell activation and proliferation
CD21 (B2, CR2, EBV receptor, C3dR)	RCA	145	Mature B, FDC, subset of thymocytes	C3d, C3dg, iC3b, CD23, EBV	Associates with CD19 and CD81 to form a complex involved in signal transduction in B-cell development, activation and differentiation, EBV receptor
CD22 (BL-CAM)	Ig	130–140	Mature B	CDw75	Cell adhesion, signaling through association with p72^{SKY}, p53/56^{LYN}, PI3 kinase, SHP1, PLCγ
CD23 (FcεRII, B6, LEU-20, BLAST-2)	C-type lectin	45	B, M, FDC	IgE, CD21, CD11b, CD11c	Regulates IgE synthesis, cytokine release by monocytes
CD24 (BA-1, HSA)	HSA	35–45	B (except plasma cells), mature G, epithelial cells	P-selectin (CD62P)	Unknown; possible role in signal transduction and cell adhesion
CD25 (IL-2Rα, TAC)		55	Stimulated B, T, M	IL-2	Low-affinity IL-2R α chain
CD26 (dipeptidyl-peptidase IV, ADA binding protein)	Prolyl-oligopep-tidase	110–120	Mature thymocytes, activated T, B, NK, M, certain epithelia	ADA, collagen, CD45	Exopeptidase, costimulatory for T-cell activation
CD27	TNFR	55	T, B, mature thymocytes, subset NK	CD70	Costimulatory for T-cell activation
CD28	Ig	44	T, plasma cells	CD80, CD86	Co-stimulatory for T-cell activation; involved in the decision between T-cell activation and anergy
CD29 (β$_1$ integrin)	Integrin β	130	Broad	See CD49a–f	Associates with CD49a–f to function in cell adhesion
CD30 (Ki-1 antigen)	TNFR	105–120	M; activated T, B, NK; Hodgkin's cells, certain non-Hodgkin's lymphomas	CD153	TCR-mediated cell death, activates NF-κB, thymocyte negative selection
CD31 (PECAM-1, GPiia′, endocam)	Ig	130	M, G, naive T, NK, P, EC	CD31, α$_v$β$_3$ integrin	Homophilic and heterophilic cell adhesion
CD32 (FcγRII)	Ig	40	M, MP, G, B, P, DC, subset EC	IgG	Low-affinity receptor for IgG mediates endocytosis, cytotoxicity, and immunomodulation

APPENDIX A. *Continued.*

Surface antigen	Family	M_r	Distribution	Ligands	Function
CD33	Sialoadhesin	67	M, MP, G, myeloid progenitors, subset DC	Not known	Unknown
CD34	Sialomucin	90	Hematopoietic progenitor cells, endothelium	L-selectin (controversial)	Cell adhesion
CD35 (CR1, C3bR, C4bR)	RCA	160–255	G, M, E, B, subset T, RBC, FDC, others	C3b, C4b, iC3b, C3dg, iC3, iC4	Binding of C4b/C3b-coated particles, removing and processing immune complexes
CD36 (GPIV, GPIIIb)	Unassigned	78–90	P, mature M, MP, subset EC, subset MP-derived DC	Oxidized LDL, collagen, thrombospondin, long-chain fatty acids	Scavenger receptor for oxidized LDL, cell adhesion
CD37	Tetraspan	40–52	Mature B; low on T, G, M	Not known	Signal transduction, marker for mature B-cell malignancies (B-CLL, HCL, B-NHL)
CD38 (T10)	Unassigned	45	Early B and T, activated B and T, thymocytes, GC B cells, plasma cells	Not known	Co-stimulatory for T-cell and B-cell activation, ADP ribosyl cyclase activity
CD39	Ecto-apyrase	80	Mantle zone B, activated T, NK, M, DC, EC	Not known	May protect cells from the toxic effects of extracellular ATP
CD40	TNFR	48–50	B, DC, EC, thymic epithelium, MP, cancers	CD154	B-cell activation, proliferation and differentiation, formation of GCs, isotype switching, rescue from apoptosis
CD41 (α_{IIb} integrin, GPIIb)	Integrin α	125, 22	P, megakaryocytes	vWF, fibrinogen, fibronectin, vitronectin, thrombospondin	Platelet aggregation, combined with CD61 forms a receptor for vWF, fibrinogen, fibronectin, vitronectin, and thrombospondin
CD42a (GPIX)	LRG	135, 25	P, megakaryocytes, subset EC	vWF, thrombin	Platelet aggregation
CD42b (GPIb-α)	LRG	22	P, megakaryocytes, subset EC	vWF, thrombin	Platelet aggregation
CD42c (GPIb-β)	LRG	23	P, megakaryocytes, subset EC	vWF, thrombin	Platelet aggregation
CD43 (sialophorin, leukosialin)	Sialomucin	95–135	All leukocytes except resting B cells	?CD54	Cell adhesion, antiadhesion, possible role in T-cell activation
CD44 (H-CAM, Pgp-1, Hermes, In(Lu)-related)	Hyaladherin	85	Broad	Hyaluronan, MIP-1β, osteopontin, ankyrin	Cell adhesion, signaling, activation
CD44R (CD44v)	Hyaladherin	85–250	Epithelia, M, activated leukocytes	Hyaluronan, MIP-1β, b-FGF, osteopontin, ankyrin	Unclear, but possibly mediates cell movement through ECM and the metastasis of certain epithelial malignancies
CD45 (LCA, T200, B220)	PTP	180, 200, 210, 220	All leukocytes	Galectin-1, CD2, CD3, CD4	T- and B-cell activation, thymocyte development, signal transduction, apoptosis
CD45RA	PTP	210, 220	Subset T, medullary thymocytes, naive T	Galectin-1, CD2, CD3, CD4	Isoforms of CD45 containing exon 4 (A), restricted to a subset of T cells
CD45RB	PTP	200, 210, 220	All leukocytes	Galectin-1, CD2, CD3, CD4	Isoforms of CD45 containing exon 5 (B)
CD45RC	PTP	210, 220	Subset T, medullary thymocytes, naive T	Galectin-1, CD2, CD3, CD4	Isoforms of CD45 containing exon 6 (C), restricted to a subset of T cells
CD45RO	PTP	180	Subset T, cortical thymocytes, memory T	Galectin-1, CD2, CD3, CD4	Isoforms of CD45 containing no differentially spliced exons, restricted to a subset of T cells
CD46 (MCP)	RCA	52–58	Epithelia, T, B, NK, EC, muscle	C3b, C4b, serum factor I protease, measles virus hemagglutinin	Cofactor for C3b, C4b, serum factor I protease; protects against inappropriate complement activation or deposition

APPENDIX A. *Continued.*

Surface antigen	Family	M_r	Distribution	Ligands	Function
CD47 (neurophilin, IAP)	Ig	50	Hematopoietic cells, EC, fibroblasts, epithelial tumors		An integrin associated protein that is involved in cell adhesion
CD48 (BLAST-1)	Ig	45	All leukocytes except P and G	CD2	Cell adhesion, associates with LCK and FYN
CD49a (VLA-1, α_1 integrin)	Integrin α	200–210	M, activated T, NK, subset EC, fibrobalsts, neuronal cells	Laminin, collagen I, collagen IV	Cell adhesion, associates with integrin β_1 (CD29)
CD49b (VLA-2, α_2 integrin, GPIa)	Integrin α	155–165	T and B, P, EC, fibroblasts, subset epithelia	Collagen I, II, III, IV; laminin	Cell adhesion, regulation of matrix metalloproteinase I and collagen I expression, associates with integrin β_1 (CD29)
CD49c (VLA-3, α_3 integrin)	Integrin α	145–150	B, subset epithelia, fibroblasts	Fibronectin, collagen, laminin	Cell adhesion, associates with integrin β_1 (CD29)
CD49d (VLA-4, α_4 integrin)	Integrin α	145–150	B, T, M, NK, DC, subset cancers	CD106, MAdCAM-1, fibronectin, invasin, thrombospondin	Cell adhesion, lymphocyte migration, associates with integrin β_1 (CD29)
CD49e (VLA-5, α_5 integrin, FNRα)	Integrin α	160	T, M, P, EC, fibroblasts, muscle cells, subset epithelia, progenitor cells	L1, fibronectin	Cell adhesion, migration, matrix assembly, associates with integrin β_1 (CD29)
CD49f (VLA-6, α_6 integrin)	Integrin α	150	T, M, eosinophils, P, epithelia	Laminin	Cell adhesion, spreading and migration, associates with integrin β_1 (CD29)
CD50 (ICAM-3)	Ig	110–135	Leukocytes, EC	CD11a/CD18 (LFA-1), $\alpha_d\beta_2$ integrin	Co-stimulation, cell adhesion
CD51 (α_v integrin, VNR-α)	Integrin α	150	M, P, subset B, activated T, EC, osteoclasts	Vitronectin, fibrinogen, vWF, thrombospondin, fibronectin, collagen	Platelet aggregation, cell adhesion, associates with CD61 (β_3 integrin)
CD52 (CAMPATH-1)	HSA	25–29	B, T, M, subset epithelia	Not known	Unknown; antibodies to CD52 have been used in clinical trials for CLL and as immunosuppressants
CD53	Tetraspan	32–42	Leukocytes	Tetraspanins, CD49d/CD29, HLA-DR	B-cell activation, signal transduction
CD54 (ICAM-1)	Ig	75–115	M, activated T and B, activated EC, activated fibroblasts, subset epithelia	CD11a/CD18, CD11b/CD18, rhinovirus	Cell adhesion, receptor for rhinovirus
CD55 (DAF)	RCA	70–80	Broad, low on NK	C3b/C3bBb convertase, C4b/C4b2a convertase, CD97, echovirus, coxsackie B, enterovirus 70	Complement regulation, receptor for echovirus, and coxsackie B virus
CD56 (NCAM, NKH-1, LEU-19)	Ig	175–220	NK, subset T, neural cells, subset cancers	CD56	Homophilic and heterophilic cell adhesion, implicated in neural development, marker of NK cells
CD57 (HNK-1, LEU-7)	Unassigned	110	NK, mature T	Unknown	MHC nonrestricted cytotoxicity
CD58 (LFA-3)	Ig	40–70	Broad	CD2	Cell adhesion
CD59 (protectin, MACIF)	Ly6	18–25	Broad	C8α, C9	Inhibits formation of the membrane attack complex, T-cell activation
CDw60 (9-o-acetyl GD3)	Glycolipid	120	Subset T, subset P, subset epithelia, fibroblasts	Unknown	Costimulatory for T-cell activation
CD61 (β_3 integrin, GPIIb/IIIa)	Integrin β	105	M, P, subset B, activated T, EC, osteoclasts	Vitronectin, fibrinogen, vWF, thrombospondin, fibronectin, collagen	Platelet aggregation, cell adhesion, associates with CD51
CD62E (E-selectin, ELAM-1, LECAM-2)	Selectin	97–115	Activated EC	CD15s, sialyl Lewis a, CLA, CD162	Leukocyte rolling on activated EC, possible role in angiogenesis

APPENDIX A. *Continued.*

Surface antigen	Family	M_r	Distribution	Ligands	Function
CD62L (L-selectin, LAM-1, LECAM-1, LEU-8)	Selectin	65–95	PBB, PBT, G, subset NK, subset hematopoietic malignancies	GlyCAM-1, MAdCAM-1, CD34	Lymphocyte homing, rolling on activated EC
CD62P (P-selectin, PADGEM GMP-140)	Selectin	140	Activated P, activated EC	CD162	Cell adhesion, leukocyte rolling on activated EC
CD63 (LIMP, LAMP-3, NGA)	Tetraspan	40–55	M, activated P, fibroblasts, degranulated neutrophils, muscle, neural cells	Unknown	Unknown
CD64 (FCγR1)	Ig	72	Myeloid cells	IgG	Bind IgG
CD65, CD65s (Ceramide dodecasaccharide)	Poly-*N*-acetyl-lactosamine	Broad	M, G, myeloid leukemias	Unknown	Unknown
CD66a (BGP, NCA-160)	Ig, CEA	140–180	G, epithelia	CD62E, CD66a, CD66c, CD66e	Cell adhesion signaling, receptor for *Neisseria*
CD66b (CD67, CGM6, NCA-95)	Ig, CEA	95–100	G	CD66c	Cell adhesion and signaling
CD66c (NCA-50/90)	Ig, CEA	90	G, epithelia	CD62E, galectins, CD66a, CD66b, CD66c, CD66e	Cell adhesion and signaling
CD66d (CGM1)	Ig, CEA	35	G	None known	Receptor for *Neisseria*
CD66e (CEA)	Ig, CEA	180–200	Epithelia	CD66a, CD66c, CD66e	Cell adhesion
CD66f (PSG)	Ig, CEA	54–72	Placenta, fetal liver, myeloid cell lines	None known	Unclear, but necessary for successful pregnancy
CD68 (macrosialin)	Sialomucin	110	M, DC, G, activated T, subset B, myeloid progenitors	Oxidized LDL	Unknown
CD69 (AIM, MLR3, EA-1)	C-type lectin	60	Subset medullary thymocytes, subset B, DC, activated leukocytes	Unknown	Signal transduction; lymphocyte, monocyte, and platelet activation
CD70 (CD27L, Ki-24 antigen)	TNF	55–170	Activated T and B, Hodgkin's cells, anaplastic large cell lymphoma	CD27	Antibodies inhibit T-cell proliferation in some systems, used for typing lymphomas
CD71 (T9, transferrin R)	Unassigned	190	Erythroid cells, all proliferating cells	Transferrin	Mediates uptake of iron
CD72 (LYB-2)	C-type lectin	43	B except plasma cells, subset MP	CD5 (controversial)	May be involved in B-cell activation and proliferation
CD73 (ecto 5′ nucleotidase)	Unassigned	69–72	Subset of T and B, FDC, EC, epithelia	AMP	Costimulatory molecule, may be involved in B-FDC interactions
CD74 (invariant chain, Ii)	Unassigned	33–41	B, activated T, M, activated EC and epithelia	Unknown	Intracellular sorting of MHC class II molecules, associated with HLA-DR
CDw75	Sialoglycan	Broad	Mature sIg+ B, subset T, RBC	CD22	Cell adhesion
CDw76	Sialoglycan	Broad	Mature sIg+ B, subset T, subset EC and epithelia	Unknown	Unknown
CD77 (globotriacyl-ceramide, Gb3, BLA)	Carbohydrate	Broad	Germinal center B cells, Burkitt's lymphoma	CD19, Shiga toxin	Cross-linking induces apoptosis in Burkitt's lymphoma cells
CDw78	Unassigned	Unknown	B, MP, EC	Not known	Possible role in B-cell proliferation
CD79a	Ig	47	B	Not known	Complexes with sIg to form the BCR
CD79b	Ig	37	B	Not known	Complexes with sIg to form the BCR
CD80 (B7-1, BB1)	Ig	60	Activated B and T, MP, DC	CD28, CD152	Coregulator of T-cell activation, signaling through CD28 stimulates and through CD152 inhibits T-cell activation
CD81 (TAPA-1)	Tetraspan	26	T, B, FDC, NK, eosinophils, subset of EC and epithelia	Unknown	Regulation of cell growth, part of complex with CD19, CD21, and LEU-13

APPENDIX A. *Continued.*

Surface antigen	Family	M_r	Distribution	Ligands	Function
CD82	Tetraspan	45–90	Activated hematopoietic cells, EC, epithelia, fibroblasts	MHC-I, MHC-II, β_1 integrins, CD4, CD8	Signal transduction
CD83	Ig	43	DC	Unknown	Unknown
CD84	Unknown	68–86	Mature B, thymocytes, subset PB T, M, P	Unknown	Unknown
CD85	Unknown	110	Plasma cells, subset B, subset T and NK, high on hairy cell leukemia	Unknown	Unknown, but is a useful marker for hairy cell leukemia
CD86 (B7-2, B70)	Ig	80	Subset B, DC, EC, activated T, thymic epithelium	CD28, CD152	Coregulator of T-cell activation, signaling through CD28 stimulates and through CD152 inhibits T-cell activation
CD87 (UPAR)	GPI-anchored	35–68	T, NK, M, G, broadly on nonhematopoietic cells	u-PA, vitronectin	Receptor-bound u-PA is active and may facilitate cell migration and invasion; possible role in cell adhesion
CD88 (C5aR)	GPCR	43	G, M, DC, astrocytes, microglia	C5a, anaphylatoxin	Granulocyte activation, signal transduction
CD89 (FcαR)	Ig	45–100	Myeloid lineage cells	IgA	Phagocytosis, degranulation, respiratory burst, killing of microorganisms
CD90 (THY-1)	Ig	25–35	Hematopoietic progenitor cells, neurons, fibroblasts, lymph node HEV	Unknown	May mediate proliferation and differentiation of hematopoietic progenitor cells
CD91 (α_2-M-R, LDL-R)	LDLR	85, 515	M, fibroblasts, neurons, smooth muscle, hepatocytes	α_2-macroglobulin, plasminogen activator complex	Endocytosis of α_2-macroglobulin, plasminogen activator complexes, chylomicrons, and lipoprotein lipase
CDw92	Unknown	70	M, G, weak on many other cell types	Unknown	Unknown
CD93	Unknown	110	M, G, myeloid blasts, EC	Unknown	Unknown
CD94	C-type lectin	30	NK, subset CD8$^+$ T	CD94/NKG2-A/p39 complex specific for MHC class I	Covalently associated with NKG2-A and p39 to form an inhibitory complex specific for MHC-I
CD95 (APO-1, FAS)	TNFR	135	Activated T and B	FAS ligand	Mediates apoptosis
CD96 (TACTILE)	Ig	160	Activated T and NK	Unknown	Cell adhesion of activated T and NK at the late stages of immune responses
CD97 (BL-KDD/F12)	Unknown	74–89	Activated B and T, M, NK, G	Unknown	Unknown
CD98 (4F2)	Unassigned	125	Broad	Unknown	Regulates cell activation; integrin-associated protein that regulates expression of the high-affinity binding forms of integrins
CD99 (E2, MIC2)	Unassigned	32	Thymocytes	Unknown	Cell adhesion and apoptosis
CD100	Ig	150–300	Hematopoietic cells	CD45	Co-stimulatory for T cells, cell adhesion
CD101	Ig	120	M, G, DC, activated T,	Unknown	Unknown
CD102 (ICAM-2)	Ig	55–65	EC, subset PBL, M, P	CD11a/CD18	Cell adhesion, co-stimulation
CD103 (α_E integrin)	Integrin α	175	IEL, subset PBT, subset T-cell leukemia/lymphoma	E-cadherin	Associates with integrin $\alpha E\beta7$ to form cell adhesion molecule
CD104 (β_4 integrin)	Integrin β		M, epithelia, CD4$^-$CD8$^-$ precursor T cells	Laminin-1, -4, -5	Cell adhesion, migration
CD105 (endoglin)	TGF-βR	90	EC, activated M, subset stromal cells	Unknown	Modulates cell responses to TGF-β1, target for HHT-I
CD106 (VCAM-1, INCAM-110)	Ig	90–110	M, DC, stromal cells, activated EC	VLA-4 (CD49d/ CD29, $\alpha_4\beta_1$), $\alpha_4\beta_7$	Cell adhesion, lymphocyte migration, recruitment and activation
CD107a (LAMP-1)	Unassigned	100–120	Degranulated P, activated T, activated EC, activated G	Unknown	Unknown, lysosome associated

APPENDIX A. *Continued.*

Surface antigen	Family	M_r	Distribution	Ligands	Function
CD107b (LAMP-2)	Unassigned	100–120	Degranulated P, activated EC, activated G	Unknown	Unknown, lysosome associated
CDw108 (JMH blood group antigen)	Unknown	76–80	RBC, low on PBL	Unknown	Unknown, but deficiency of CDw108 has been associated with a rare form of congenital dyerythropoietic anemia
CD109	Unknown	170	EC, activated P, activated T, epithelia	Unknown	Unknown
CD114 (CSFR, G-CSFR)	Class I CKR	130	Broad not on RBC or lymphocytes	G-CSF	Regulates myeloid proliferation and differentiation
CD115 (CSF-1R, FMS, MCSFR)	RTK	150	Monocyte lineage cells	M-CSF	Differentiation, survival, and growth of monocytes and macrophages
CD116 (GM-CSFR-α)	Class I CKR	80	Myeloid cells, DC	GM-CSF	Differentiation, survival, and growth of myeloid lineage cells
CD117 (SCFR, KIT)	RTK	145	Hematopoietic progenitors, mast cells, AML, subset epithelial, embryonic brain	SCF	Growth and differentiation of erythrocytes, mast cells, melanocytes, and the reproductive system
CDw119 (IFNγR-α)	Class II CKR	95	Most leukocytes	IFN-γ	Associates with IFN-γRII (β chain) to form the IFN-γ receptor
CD120a (TNFR type 1)	TNFR	55	Subset G, FDC, EC, activated M	TNF	Upregulation of adhesion molecules, induction of inflammatory mediators
CD120b (TNFR type 2)	TNFR	75	M, activated G and M	TNF	Upregulation of adhesion molecules, induction of inflammatory mediators
CD121a (IL-1R type 1)	Ig	75–85	All leukocytes	IL-1α, IL-1β, IL-1Ra	Mediates the effects of IL-1α and β
CDw121b (IL-1R type 2)	Ig	60–68	B, M, subset T, some basal epithelia	IL-1β, IL-1Ra, IL-1α	Apparently acts as a negative regulator of IL-1 in either the surface-bound or shed forms
CD122 (IL-2R-β)	CKR	70–75	T, B, NK, M	IL-2, IL-15	Forms the high-affinity IL-2R with CD25 and CD132
CDw123 (IL-3R-α)	Class I CKR	70	Myeloid-lineage cells and progenitors, EC	IL-3	Low-affinity receptor for IL-3, forms high-affinity receptor with CDw131
CD124 (IL-4R-α)	CKR	140	Low levels on many cell types, high on activated B and T	IL-4, IL-13	Forms high-affinity IL-4R with CD132, IL-13R, IL-13R with IL-13R β chain. TH2 cell induction, IgE class switching
CDw125 (IL-5R-α)	CKR	60	Activated B, eosinophils, basophils	IL-5	Forms high-affinity receptor with CDw131; eosinophilic inflammation
CD126 (IL-6R)	Class I CKR	80	T, M, activated B, hepatocytes, other cell types	IL-6	Forms IL-6R with CD130; inflammation, hematopoiesis
CD127 (IL-7R-α)	CKR	65–90	T, B cell precursors	IL-7	Forms high-affinity IL-7R with CD132; lymphocyte development
CDw128 (IL-8R types A and B, CXCR1, CXCR2)	CXCR	A, 44–59; B, 67–70	G, M, subset NK, CD8⁺ T	IL-8 (type A, CXCR1); IL-8, GRO, NAP-2, ENA 78 (type B, CXCR2)	Chemotaxis and activation
CD130	Class I CKR	130–140	Broad	Oncostatin M, IL-6, IL-11, LIF, CNF, cardiotropin-1	Signal transduction component of the IL-6, IL-11, oncostatin M, leukemia inhibitory factor, ciliary neurotrophic factor and cardiotropin-1 receptors
CDw131 (common β chain)	Class I CKR	120–140	Most myeloid cells, early B cells	IL-3, IL-5, GM-CSF	Signal transduction subunit of the IL-3, IL-5, and GM-CSF receptors
CD132 (common γ chain)	Class I CKR	64–70	T, B, MK, M, G	IL-2, IL-4, IL-7, IL-9, IL-15	Signal transduction component of the IL-2, IL-4, IL-7, IL-9, and IL-15 receptors
CD134 (OX40)	TNFR	50	Activated T	gp34	Cell adhesion and T-cell co-stimulation

APPENDIX A. *Continued.*

Surface antigen	Family	M$_r$	Distribution	Ligands	Function
CD135 (FLT3, FLK-2, STK-1)	RTK	130–160	Primitive hematopoietic progenitors	FL (FLT3 ligand)	Growth of early hematopoietic progenitors
CD136 (MSP-R, RON)	RTK	180	Epithelia, subset neuroendocrine cells	MSP, HGF-1	Cell migration, morphologic change and proliferation
CDw137 (4-1BB, ILA)	TNFR	39	Activated T, B, M, epithelial and hepatoma cells	4-1BB ligand	Co-stimulatory for T cells
CD138 (syndecan)	Syndecan	80–300	Epithelia, developing neuronal cells	Collagens, fibronectin, thrombospondin, tenascin, FGF	Coreceptor for growth factor receptors, maintenance of cell morphology through ECM interactions
CD139	Unknown	209, 228	B, M, G, weak on RBC, FDC	Unknown	Unknown
CD140a (PDGFRa)	Split-tyrosine kinase	160, 175	P, fibroblasts, smooth muscle	PDGF-α, PDGF-β	Signal transduction, cell proliferation, migration
CD140b (PDGFRb)	Split-tyrosine kinase	160, 180	M, G, subset EC, fibroblasts, smooth muscle	PDGF-β	Signal transduction, cell proliferation, migration
CD141 (thrombomodulin, fetomodulin)	C-type lectin	75–105	EC, P, megakaryocytes, M, G, epithelia, smooth muscle	Thrombin	Cofactor for thrombin-mediated activation of protein C and anticoagulation
CD142 (tissue factor)	Serine protease cofactor	45–47	Epithelia, stromal cells, activated M and EC	Factor VIIa, factor Xa/TFPI	Associated with factor VIIa forms an enzyme involved in initiation of the clotting cascade, procoagulant
CD143 (ACE, peptidyl dipeptidase A)	Peptidyl-peptidase	170	Broad	Angiotensin I, bradykinin, substance P, LR-RH	Metabolism of angiotensin I and bradykinin
CD144 (VE-cadherin)	Cadherin	130–135	EC	VE-cadherin	Homotypic cell adhesion, organizes adherin junctions
CDw145	Unknown	110, 90, 25	EC, bladder cancer	Unknown	Unknown
CD146 (MUC18, S-endo)	Ig	118–130	EC, subset activated T, subset epithelia	Unknown	Possible cell adhesion molecule
CD147 (neurothelin, basigin, EMMPRIN, M6)	Ig	50–65	All leukocytes, RBC, P, EC	Unknown	Potential cell adhesion molecule, stimulates expression of collagenase by fibroblasts
CD148 (HPTP-eta)	PTP	240–260	Broad	Unknown	Tyrosine phosphatase
CDw149	Unknown	120	PBL, M, G, P	Unknown	Unknown
CDw150 (SLAM, IPO-3)	Ig	65–95	Thymocytes, CD45RO$^+$ PBT, B, DC, EC	CDw150	Costimulatory for B and DC
CD151 (PETA-3)	Tetraspan	32	EC, P, megarkaryocytes, epithelia	Unknown	Unknown
CD152 (CTLA-4)	Ig	30–33	Activated T	CD80, CD86	Inhibits T-cell proliferation
CD153 (CD30L)	TNF	38–40	Activated T	CD30	T-cell proliferation and cytokine production
CD154 (CD40L)	TNF	33	Activated CD4$^+$ T, subset CD8$^+$ T, NK, M, basophil	CD40	Co-stimulatory for T-cell activation, B-cell proliferation, and differentiation
CD155 (poliovirus receptor)	Ig	80–90	M	Poliovirus	Poliovirus receptor
CD156 (ADAM-8)	ADAM	69	G, M	None known	Possibly involved in extravasation of leukocytes
CD157 (Mo5, BST-1)	ADP-ribosyl cyclase	42–50	Myeloid, subset of lymphocytes	NAD, cyclic ADP-ribose	ADP-ribosyl cyclase
CD158a	Ig	50–58	NK, subset T	HLA-Cw4	Regulates NK-cell–mediated cytolytic activity on interaction with HLA-Cw4 and other alleles with Asn[77] and Lys[80]
CD158b	Ig	50–58	NK, subset T	HLA-Cw3	Regulates NK-cell–mediated cytolytic activity on interaction with HLA-Cw3 and other alleles with Ser[77] and Asn[80]
CD161 (NKRP1)	C-type lectin	40	NK, subset T	Unknown	Unknown but postulated to regulate NK-cell–mediated cytotoxicity
CD162 (PSGL-1)	Sialomucin	110–120	T, M, G, subset B	CD62P, CD62E	Rolling of leukocytes on EC, P, and other leukocytes
CD163 (M130)	SRCR	110	MP, activated M	Unknown	Unknown
CD164	Unassigned	80	M, BM stroma, epithelia	Unknown	Possible role in cell adhesion

APPENDIX A. *Continued.*

Surface antigen	Family	M_r	Distribution	Ligands	Function
CD165 (AD2)	Unknown	37–42	Subset PBL, immature thymocytes, M, P, subset epithelia, neurons	Unknown	Cell adhesion
CD166 (ALCAM, CD6L)	Ig	100–105	Activated leukocytes, epithelia, fibroblasts	CD6, CD166	Cell adhesion

Abbreviations: α2M-R, α2-macroglobulin receptor; ACE, angiotensin converting enzyme; ADA, adenosine deaminase; ADAM, a disintegrin and metalloproteinase; ADCC, antibody-dependent cellular cytotoxicity; ADP, adenosine diphosphate; AIM, activation inducer molecule; ALCAM, activated leukocyte cell adhesion molecule; AML, acute myelogenous leukemia; AMP, adenosine monophosphate; ATP, adenosine triphosphate; bFGF, basic fibroblast growth factor; BGP, biliary glycoprotein; BL-CAM, B-lymphocyte cell adhesion molecule; BLA, Burkitt's lymphoma antigen; BLAST, B-cell specific activation antigen; BST, bone marrow stroma cell antigen; CALLA, common acute lymphoblastic leukemia antigen; CEA, carcinoembryonic antigen; CKR, cytokine receptor; CLA, cutaneous lymphocyte antigen; CLL, chronic lymphocytic leukemia; CNF, ciliary neurotrophic factor; CSF-1 R, colony stimulating factor-1 receptor; CSFR, colony stimulating factor receptor; CTLA, cytotoxic T lymphocyte-associated protein; CXCR1, CXC chemokine receptor 1; DAF, decay accelerating factor; DC, dendritic cells; EC, endothelial cells; ECM, extracellular matrix; ELAM, endothelial leukocyte adhesion molecule; EMMPRIN, extracellular matrix metalloproteinase inducer; ENA, epithelial derived neutrophil-activating peptide; FcγRIIIA, low-affinity IgG receptor isoform A; FDC, follicular dendritic cells; FGF, fibroblast growth factor; FLK, fetal liver kinase; FLT-3 FMS-like tyrosine kinase 3; FNR, fibronectin receptor; G, granulocytes; G-CSF, granulocyte colony stimulating factor; G-CSFR, granulocyte colony stimulating factor receptor; Gb3, globotriaosylceramide; GC, germinal center; GlyCAM, glycosylation-dependent cell adhesion molecule; GM-CSF, granulocyte-macrophage colony-stimulating factor; GM-CSFR, granulocyte-macrophage colony-stimulating factor receptor; GMP, granule membrane protein; GPCR, G-protein coupled receptor; GPI, glycosyl phosphotidylinositol; GRO, growth-related peptide; H-CAM, homing-associated cell adhesion molecule; HCL, hairy cell leukemia; HEV, high endothelial venules; HGF, hepatocyte growth factor; HIV, human immunodeficiency virus; HLA, human leukocyte antigen; HNK, human natural killer cell antigen; HPTP-eta, human protein tyrosine phosphatase eta; HSA, heat stable antigen; HTA, human thymocyte antigen; ICAM, intercellular adhesion molecule; IEL, intraepithelial lymphocytes; IFNγRII, interferon γ receptor type II; IgG, immunoglobulin G; IL-1RA, IL-1 receptor antagonist; IL-1RI, IL-1 receptor type I; ILA, induced by lymphocyte activation; INCAM, inducible cell adhesion molecule; LacSer, lactosylceramide; LAD, leukocyte adhesion deficiency; LAM, leukocyte adhesion molecule; LAMP, lysosome-associated membrane protein; LCA, leukocyte common antigen; Lck, lymphocyte-specific protein-tyrosine kinase; LDL, low density lipoprotein; LDLR, low density lipoprotein receptor; LECAM, lectin cell adhesion molecule; LFA, lymphocyte function antigen; LGL, large granular lymphocyte; LH-RH, leuteinizing hormone releasing hormone; LIF, leukemia inhibitory factor; LIMP, lysosomal integral membrane protein; LPS, lipopolysaccharide; LRG, leucine rich repeats; M, monocytes; M-CSF, macrophage colony-stimulating factor; M-CSFR, macrophage colony-stimulating factor receptor; MACIF, membrane attack complex inhibitory factor; MAdCAM, mucosal addressin cell adhesion molecule; MCP, membrane cofactor protein; MHC-1, major histocompatibility complex class I; MIP-1β, macrophage inflammatory protein-1β; MP, macrophages; Mr, relative molecular mass; MRP, motility related protein; MSP, macrophage-stimulating protein; MSPR, macrophage-stimulating protein receptor; NAD, nicotinamide-adenine dinucleotide; NAP, neutrophil-activating protein; NCA, nonspecific cross-reacting antigen; NCAM, neural cell adhesion molecule; NFκB, nuclear factor κB; NGA, neuroglandular antigen; NHL, non-Hodgkin's lymphoma; NK, natural killer cells; NKG2, natural killer cell gene 2; NKH, natural killer cell H antigen; NKRP1, natural killer cell receptor P1; P, platelets; PADGEM, platelet activation dependent granule-external membrane protein; PBB, peripheral blood B cells; PBL, peripheral blood lymphocytes; PBT, peripheral blood T cells; PDGFα, platelet-derived growth factor α; PDGFRα, platelet-derived growth factor α receptor; PECAM, platelet/endothelial cell adhesion molecule; PETA, platelet-endothelial cell tetraspan antigen; PI, phosphotidylinositol; PI3K, phosphotidylinositol 3-kinase; PLCβ, phospholipase C β; PSG, pregnancy-specific glycoprotein; PSGL, P-selectin glycoprotein ligand; PTP, protein tyrosine phosphatase; RBC, red blood cells; RCA, regulators of complement activation; RTK, receptor tyrosine kinase; SABP, secretory actin-binding protein; SCF, stem cell factor; SCFR, stem cell factor receptor; sIg, surface immunoglobulin; SLAM, signalling lymphocyte activation molecule; SRCR, scavenger receptor cysteine rich; STK, stem cell tyrosine kinase; Tac, T cell activation; TACTILE, T cell activation increased late expression; TAPA, target for anti-proliferative antigen; TCR, T cell receptor; TGF, transforming growth factor; TGFR, transforming growth factor receptor; TFPI, tissue factor pathway inhibitor; TNF, tumor necrosis factor; TNFR, tumor necrosis factor receptor; u-PA, urokinase plasminogen activator; UPAR, urokinase plasminogen activator receptor; VCAM, vascular cell adhesion molecule; VE-cadherin, vascular endothelial cadherin; VLA, very late activation antigen; VNR, vitronectin receptor; vWF, von Willebrand's factor.

Compiled with permission from Kishimoto TH, Kikutani AEG, von dem Borne SM, et al., eds. *Leukocyte typing VI*. New York: Garland Publishing, 1997; Brines R, Ager A, Callard R, Ezine S, Goyert SM, Todd RF, eds. Immune receptor supplement, 2nd ed. *Immunology Today* 1997;18S:1–34; and Shaw S, ed. *Protein reviews on the Web*. Available at http://www.ncbi.nlm.nih.gov/prow. Accessed between March 15, 1997 and October 20, 1998.

Inflammation: Basic Principles and Clinical Correlates,
3rd ed., edited by John I. Gallin and Ralph Snyderman.
Lippincott Williams & Wilkins, Philadelphia © 1999.

APPENDIX B

Cytokines and Cytokine Receptors

John S. Sundy, Dhavalkumar D. Patel, and Barton F. Haynes

APPENDIX B. *Cytokines and cytokine receptors*

Cytokine	Receptor	Cell source	Cell target	Biologic activity	Selected reference
IL-1α,β	Type I IL-1R, type II IL-1R	Monocytes/macrophages, B cells, fibroblasts, most epithelial cells including thymic epithelium, endothelial cells	All cells	Upregulated adhesion molecule expression, neutrophil and macrophage emigration, mimics shock, fever, upregulated hepatic acute phase protein production, facilitates hematopoiesis	1
IL-2	IL-2R α,β, common γ	T cells	T cells, B cells, NK cells, monocytes/ macrophages	T-cell activation and proliferation, B-cell growth, NK-cell proliferation and activation, enhanced monocyte/macrophage cytolytic activity	2
IL-3	IL-3R, common β	T cells, NK cells, mast cells	Monocytes/macrophages, mast cells, eosinophils, bone marrow progenitors	Stimulation of hematopoietic progenitors	3
IL-4	IL-4R α, common γ	T cells, mast cells, basophils	T cells, B cells, NK cells, monocytes/macrophages, neutrophils, eosinophils, endothelial cells, fibroblasts	Stimulates T_H2 differentiation and proliferation, stimulates B-cell Ig class switch to IgG_1 and IgE, antiinflammatory action on T cells, B cells, monocytes	4
IL-5	IL-5Rα, common β	T cells, mast cells, eosinophils	Eosinophils, basophils, murine B cells	Regulates eosinophil migration and activation	5
IL-6	IL-6R, gp130	Monocytes/macrophages, B cells, fibroblasts, most epithelium including thymic epithelium, endothelial cells	T cells, B cells, epithelial cells, hepatocytes, monocytes/macrophages	Induction of acute phase protein production, T- and B-cell differentiation and growth, myeloma cell growth, osteoclast growth and activation	6
IL-7	IL-7R α, common γ	Bone marrow, thymic epithelial cells	T cells, B cells, bone marrow cells	Differentiation of B, T and NK cell precursors, activation of T and NK cells	7
IL-8	CXCR1, CXCR2	Monocytes/macrophages, T cells, neutrophils, fibroblasts, endothelial cells, epithelial cells	Neutrophils, T cells, monocytes/macrophages, endothelial cells, basophils	Induces neutrophil, monocyte and T-cell migration, induces neutrophil adherance to endothelial cells, histamine release from basophils, stimulates angiogenesis, suppresses proliferation of hepatic precursors	8

J. S. Sundy: Division of Rheumatology, Allergy and Clinical Immunology, Department of Medicine, Duke University Medical Center, Durham, North Carolina 27710.

D. D. Patel: Division of Rheumatology, Allergy and Clinical Immunology, Department of Medicine, and the Department of Immunology, Duke University School of Medicine, Durham, North Carolina 27710.

B. F. Haynes: Department of Medicine, Duke University School of Medicine, Durham, North Carolina 27710.

APPENDIX B. *Continued.*

Cytokine	Receptor	Cell source	Cell target	Biologic activity	Selected reference
IL-9	IL-9R α, common γ	T cells	Bone marrow progenitors, B cells, T cells, mast cells	Induces mast cell proliferation and function, synergizes with IL-4 in IgG and IgE production, T-cell growth, activation, and oncogenesis	9
IL-10	IL-10R	Monocytes/macrophages, T cells, B cells, keratinocytes, mast cells	Monocytes/macrophages, T cells, B cells, NK cells, mast cells	Inhibits macrophage proinflammatory cytokine production, downregulates cytokine class II antigen and B7-1 and B7-2 expression, inhibits differentiation of T_H1 cells, inhibits NK-cell function, stimulates mast cell proliferation and function, B-cell activation and differentiation	10
IL-11	IL-11, gp130	Bone marrow stromal cells	Megakaryocytes, B cells, hepatocytes	Induces megakaryocyte colony formation and maturation, enhances antibody responses, stimulates acute phase protein production	11
IL-12 (35- and 40-kd sub-units)	IL-12R	Activated macrophages	T cells, NK cells	Induces T_H1 formation, stimulates proinflammatory cytokine expression in PBMCs, lymphokine-activated killer cell formation	12
IL-13	IL-13/IL-4	T cells (T_H2)	Monocytes/macrophages, B cells, endothelial cells, keratinocytes	Upregulation of VCAM-1 and CC chemokine expression on endothelial cells, B-cell activation and differentiation, inhibits macrophage proinflammatory cytokine production	13
IL-14	Unknown	T cells	Normal and malignant B cells	Induces B cell proliferation	14
IL-15	IL-15R α, common γ, IL-2R β	Monocytes/macrophages, epithelial cells, fibroblasts	T cells	T-cell activation and proliferation, promotes angiogenesis	15
IL-16	CD4	Mast cells, eosinophils, CD8+ T cells, respiratory epithelium	CD4+ T cells, monocytes/ macrophages, eosinophils	Chemoattraction of CD4+ T cells, monocytes, and eosinophils; inhibits HIV replication; inhibits T-cell activation through CD3/T-cell receptor	16
IL-17	IL-17R	CD4+ T cells	Fibroblasts, endothelium, epithelium	Enhanced cytokine secretion	17
IL-18	IL-18R (IL-1R related protein)	Keratinocytes	T cells, B cells, NK cells	Upregulated IFN-γ production, enhanced NK-cell cytotoxicity	18
IFN-α	Type I IFN receptor	All cells	All cells	Antiviral activity; stimulates T-cell, macrophage, and NK-cell activity; direct antitumor effects; upregulates MHC class I antigen expression; used therapeutically in viral and autoimmune conditions	19,20
IFN-β	Type I IFN receptor	All cells	All cells	Antiviral activity; stimulates T-cell, macrophage, and NK-cell activity; direct antitumor effects; upregulates MHC class I antigen expression; used therapeutically in viral and autoimmune conditions	19,20
IFN-γ	Type II IFN receptor	T cells, NK cells	All cells	Regulates macrophage and NK-cell activation, stimulates immunoglobulin secretion by B cells, induction of class II histocompatibility antigens, T_H1 cell differentiation	21

APPENDIX B. *Continued.*

Cytokine	Receptor	Cell source	Cell target	Biologic activity	Selected reference
TFN-α	TNF-RI, TNF-RII	Monocytes/macrophages, mast cells, basophils, eosinophils, NK cells, B cells, T cells, keratinocytes, fibroblasts, thymic epithelial cells	All cells except erythrocytes	Fever, anorexia, shock, capillary leak syndrome, enhanced leukocyte cytotoxicity, enhanced NK-cell function, acute phase protein synthesis, proinflammatory cytokine induction	22
TNF-β	TNF-RI, TNF-RII	T cells, B cells	All cells except erythrocytes	Cell cytotoxicity, lymph node and spleen development	22
LTβ	LTβR	T cells	All cells except erythrocytes	Cell cytotoxicity, normal lymph node development	22
G-CSF	G-CSFR; gp130	Monocytes/macrophages, fibroblasts, endothelial cells, thymic epithelial cells, stromal cells	Myeloid cells, endothelial cells	Regulates myelopoiesis, enhances survival and function of neutrophils, clinical use in reversing neutropenia after cytotoxic chemotherapy	23
GM-CSF	GM-CSFR; common β	T cells, monocytes/ macrophages, fibroblasts, endothelial cells, thymic epithelial cells	Monocytes/macrophages, neutrophils, eosinophils, fibroblasts, endothelial cells	Regulates myelopoiesis, enhances macrophage bactericidal and tumoricidal activity, mediator of dendritic cell maturation and function, upregulates NK-cell function, clinical use in reversing neutropenia after cytotoxic chemotherapy	24
M-CSF	M-CSFR (FMS protooncogene)	Fibroblasts, endothelial cells, monocytes/ macrophages, T cells, B cells, epithelial cells including thymic epithelium	Monocytes/macrophages	Regulates monocyte/ macrophage production and function	25
LIF	LIFR; gp130	Activated T cells, bone marrow stromal cells, thymic epithelium	Megakaryocytes, monocytes, hepatocytes, possibly lymphocyte subpopulations	Induces hepatic acute phase protein production, stimulates macrophage differentiation, promotes growth of myeloma cells and hematopoietic progenitors, stimulates thrombopoiesis	26,27
OSM	OSMR; LIFR; gp130	Activated monocytes/ macrophages and T cells, bone marrow stromal cells, some breast carcinoma cell lines, myeloma cells	Neurons, hepatocytes, monocytes/macrophages, adipocytes, alveolar epithelial cells, embryonic stem cells, melanocytes, endothelial cells, fibroblasts, myeloma cells	Induces hepatic acute phase protein production, stimulates macrophage differentiation, promotes growth of myeloma cells and hematopoietic progenitors, stimulates thrombopoiesis, stimulates growth of Kaposi's sarcoma cells	27
SCF	SCFR (KIT protooncogene)	Bone marrow stromal cells and fibroblasts	Embryonic stem cells, myeloid and lymphoid precursors, mast cells	Stimulates hematopoietic progenitor cell growth, mast cell growth, promotes embryonic stem cell migration	28
TGF-β (Three isoforms)	Type I, II, III TGF-β receptor	Most cell types	Most cell types	Downregulates T-cell, macrophage, and granulocyte responses; stimulates synthesis of matrix proteins; stimulates angiogenesis	29
Lympho- tactin/ SCM-1	Unknown	NK cells, mast cells, double negative thymocytes, activated CD8+ T cells	T cells, NK cells	Chemoattractant for lymphocytes, only known chemokine of C class	30

APPENDIX B. *Continued.*

Cytokine	Receptor	Cell source	Cell target	Biologic activity	Selected reference
MCP-1	CCR2	Fibroblasts, smooth muscle cells, activated PBMCs	Monocytes/macrophages, NK cells, memory T cells, basophils	Chemoattractant for monocytes, activated memory T cells, and NK cells; induces granule release from CD8[+] T cells and NK cells; potent histamine releasing factor for basophils; suppresses proliferation of hematopoietic precursors; regulates monocyte protease production	31
MCP-2	CCR1, CCR2	Fibroblasts, activated PBMCs	Monocytes/macrophages, T cells, eosinophils, basophils, NK cells	Chemoattractant for monocytes, memory and naïve T cells, eosinophils, ? NK cells; activates basophils and eosinophils; regulates monocyte protease production	32
MCP-3	CCR1, CCR2	Fibroblasts, activated PBMCs	Monocytes/macrophages, T cells, eosinophils, basophils, NK cells, dendritic cells	Chemoattractant for monocytes, memory and naïve T cells, dendritic cells, eosinophils, ? NK cells; activates basophils and eosinophils; regulates monocyte protease production	33
MCP-4	CCR2, CCR3	Lung, colon, small intestinal epithelial cells, activated endothelial cells	Monocytes/macrophages, T cells, eosinophils, basophils	Chemoattractant for monocytes, T cells, eosinophils, and basophils	34
Eotaxin	CCR3	Pulmonary epithelial cells, heart	Eosinophils, basophils	Potent chemoattractant for eosinophils and basophils, induces allergic airways disease, acts in concert with IL-5 to activate eosinophils, antibodies to eotaxin inhibit airway inflammation	35
TARC	CCR4	Thymus, dendritic cells, activated T cells	T cells, NK cells	Chemoattractant for T and NK cells	36
MDC	CCR4	Monocytes/macrophages, dendritic cells, thymus	Activated T cells	Chemoattractant for activated T cells, inhibits infection with T-cell tropic HIV	37
MIP-1α	CCR1, CCR5	Monocytes/macrophages, T cells	Monocytes/macrophages, T cells, dendritic cells, NK cells, eosinophils, basophils	Chemoattractant for monocytes, T cells, dendritic cells, NK cells, and weak chemoattractant for eosinophils and basophils; activates NK-cell function; suppresses proliferation of hematopoietic precursors; necessary for myocarditis associated with coxsackievirus infection; inhibits infection with monocytotropic HIV	38
MIP-1β	CCR5	Monocytes/ macrophages, T cells	Monocytes/macrophages, T cells, NK cells, dendritic cells	Chemoattractant for monocytes, T cells, and NK cells; activates NK-cell function; inhibits infection with monocytotropic HIV	39
RANTES	CCR1, CCR2, CCR5	Monocytes/macrophages, T cells, fibroblasts, eosinophils	Monocytes/macrophages, T cells, NK cells, dendritic cells, eosinophils, basophils	Chemoattractant for monocytes/ macrophages, CD4[+] CD45RO[+] T cells, CD8[+] T cells, NK cells, eosinophils, and basophils; induces histamine release from basophils; inhibits infection with monocytotropic HIV	40
LARC/ MIP-3α/ Exodus	CCR6	Dendritic cells, fetal liver cells, activated T cells	T cells, B cells	Chemoattractant for lymphocytes	41
ELC/ MIP-3β	CCR7	Thymus, lymph node, appendix	Activated T cells and B cells	Chemoattractant for B and T cells, receptor upregulated on EBV-infected B cells and HSV-infected T cells	42

APPENDIX B. *Continued.*

Cytokine	Receptor	Cell source	Cell target	Biologic activity	Selected reference
I-309/ TCA-3	CCR8	Activated T cells	Monocytes/macrophages, T cells	Chemoattractant for monocytes, prevents glucocorticoid-induced apoptosis in some T cell lines	43
SLC/ TCA-4/ Exodus-2	Unknown	Thymic epithelial cells, lymph node, appendix and spleen	T cells	Chemoattractant for T lymphocytes, inhibits hematopoiesis	44
DC-CK1/ PARC	Unknown	Dendritic cells in secondary lymphoid tissues	Naïve T cells	May have a role in the induction of immune responses	45
TECK	Unknown	Dendritic cells thymus, liver, small intestine	T cells, monocytes/ macrophages, dendritic cells	Thymic dendritic cell-derived cytokine, possibly involved in T-cell development	46
GRO-α/ MGSA	CXCR2	Activated granulocytes, monocytes/macrophages, and epithelial cells	Neutrophils, epithelial cells, ? endothelial cells	Neutrophil chemoattractant and activator, mitogenic for some melanoma cell lines, suppresses proliferation of hematopoietic precursors, angiogenic activity	47
GRO-β/ MIP-2α	CXCR2	Activated granulocytes and monocytes/macrophages	Neutrophils and ? endothelial cells	Neutrophil chemoattractant and activator, angiogenic activity	48
NAP-2	CXCR2	Platelets	Neutrophils, basophils	Derived from platelet basic protein, neutrophil chemoattractant and activator	49
IP-10	CXCR3	Monocytes/macrophages, T cells, fibroblasts, endothelial cells, epithelial cells	Activated T cells, tumor infiltrating lymphocytes, ? endothelial cells, ? NK cells	IFN-γ–inducible protein that is a chemoattractant for T cells, suppresses proliferation of hematopoietic precursors	50
MIG	CXCR3	Monocytes/macrophages, T cells, fibroblasts	Activated T cells, tumor infiltrating lymphocytes	IFN-γ–inducible protein that is a chemoattractant for T cells, suppresses proliferation of hematopoietic precursors	51
SDF-1	CXCR4	Fibroblasts	T cells, dendritic cells, ? basophils, ? endothelial cells	Low-potency, high-efficacy T-cell chemoattractant, required for B-lymphocyte development, prevents infection of CD4+, CXCR4+ cells by T-cell tropic HIV	52
Fractalkine	CX3CR1	Activated endothelial cells	NK cells, T cells, monocytes/ macrophages	Cell surface chemokine/mucin hybrid molecule that functions as a chemoattractant, leukocyte activator, and cell adhesion molecule	53
PF-4	Unknown	Platelets, megakaryocytes	Fibroblasts, endothelial cells	Chemoattractant for fibroblasts, suppresses proliferation of hematopoietic precursors, inhibits endothelial cell proliferation and angiogenesis	54

IL, interleukin; NK, natural killer; T$_H$1 and T$_H$2, helper T cell subsets; Ig, immunoglobulin; CXCR, CXC-type chemokine receptor; B7-1, CD80; B7-2, CD86; PBMC, peripheral blood mononuclear cells; VCAM, vascular cell adhesion molecule; IFN, interferon; MHC, major histocompatibility complex; TNF, tumor necrosis factor; G-CSF, granulocyte colony-stimulating factor; GM-CSF, granulocyte-macrophage CSF; M-CSF, macrophage CSF; HIV, human immunodeficiency virus; LIF, leukemia inhibitory factor; OSM, oncostatin M; SCF, stem cell factor; TGF, transforming growth factor; MCP, monocyte chemotactic protein; CCR, CC-type chemokine receptor; TARC, thymus and activation-regulated chemokine; MDC, macrophage-derived chemokine; MIP, macrophage inflammatory protein; RANTES, regulated on activation, normally T-cell expressed and secreted; LARC, liver and activation-regulated chemokine; EBV, Epstein-Barr virus; ELC, EBI1 ligand chemokine (MIP-1β); HSV, herpes simplex virus; TCA, T-cell activation protein; DC-CK, dendritic cell chemokine; PARC, pulmonary and activation regulated chemokine; SLC, secondary lymphoid tissue chemokine; TECK, thymus expressed chemokine; GRP, growth-related peptide; MGSA, melanoma growth-stimulating activity; NAP, neutrophil-activating protein; IP-10, IFN-γ–inducible protein-10; MIG, monoteine induced by IFN-γ; SDF, stromal cell–derived factor; PF, platelet factor.

REFERENCES

1. Dinarello CA. Biologic basis for interleukin-1 in disease. *Blood* 1996; 87:2095–2147.

2. Theze J, Alzari PM, Bertoglio J. Interleukin 2 and its receptors: recent advances and new immunological functions. *Immunol Today* 1997;17: 481–486.

3. Lindemann A, Mertelsmann R. Interleukin-3: structure and function. *Cancer Invest* 1993;11:609–623.

4. Paul WE. Interleukin 4: signalling mechanisms and control of T cell differentiation. *Ciba Found Symp* 1997;204:208–216.

5. Egan RW, Umland SP, Cuss FM, Chapman RW. Biology of interleukin-5 and its relevance to allergic disease. *Allergy* 1996;51:71–81.

6. Akira S, Taga T, Kishimoto T. Interleukin-6 in biology and medicine. *Adv Immunol* 1993;54:1–78.

7. Komschlies KL, Grzegorzewski KJ, Wiltrout RH. Diverse immunological and hematological effects of interleukin 7: implications for clinical application. *J Leukoc Biol* 1995;58:623–633.

8. Murphy PM. Neutrophil receptors for interleukin 8 and related CXC chemokines. *Semin Hematol* 1997;311–318.

9. Renauld J-C, Kermouni A, Vink A, Louahed J, Van Snick J. Interleukin 9 and its receptor: involvement in mast cell differentiation and T cell oncogenesis. *J Leukoc Biol* 1995;57:353–360.

10. Mossman TR. Properties and functions of interleukin-10. *Adv Immunol* 1994;56:1–26.

11. Du XX, Williams DA. Interleukin-11: a multifunctional growth factor derived from the hematopoietic microenvironment. *Blood* 1994;83: 2023–2030.

12. Trinchieri G, Scott P. Interleukin-12: a proinflammatory cytokine with immunoregulatory functions. *Res Immunol* 1995;146:423–431.

13. McKenzie AN, Zurawski G. Interleukin-13: characterization and biologic properties. *Cancer Treat Res* 1995;80:367–78.

14. Ford R, Tamayo A, Martin B, et al. Identification of B-cell growth factors (interleukin-14; high molecular weight-B-cell growth factors) in effusion fluids from patients with aggressive B-cell lymphomas. *Blood* 1995;86:283–293.

15. Kennedy MK, Park LS. Characterization of interleukin-15 (IL-15) and the IL-15 receptor complex. *J Clin Immunol* 1996;16:134–143.

16. Center DM, Kornfeld H, Cruikshank WW. Interleukin 16 and its function as a CD4 ligand. *Immunol Today* 1996;17:476–481.

17. Yao Z, Fanslow WC, Seldin MF, et al. Herpesvirus Saimiri encodes a new cytokine, IL-17, which binds to a novel cytokine receptor. *Immunity* 1995;3:811–821.

18. Torigoe K, Ushio S, Okura T, et al. Purification and characterization of the human interleukin-18 receptor. *J Biol Chem* 1997;272:25737–25742.

19. Viscomi GC. Structure-activity of type I interferons. *Biotherapy* 1997; 10:59–86.

20. Belardelli F, Gresser I. The neglected role of type I interferon in the T-cell response: implications for its clinical use. *Immunol Today* 1996;17: 369–372.

21. Boehm U, Klamp T, Groot M, Howard JC. Cellular responses to interferon-gamma. *Annu Rev Immunol* 1997;15:749–795.

22. Armitage RJ. Tumor necrosis factor receptor superfamily members and their ligands. *Curr Opin Immunol* 1994;6:407–413.

23. Tkatch LS, Tweardy DJ. Human granulocyte colony-stimulating factor (G-CSF), the premier granulopoietin: biology, clinical utility, and receptor structure and function. *Lymphokine Cytokine Res* 1993;12:477–488.

24. Tarr PE. Granulocyte-macrophage colony-stimulating factor and the immune system. *Med Oncol* 1996;13:133–140.

25. Roth P, Stanley ER. The biology of CSF-1 and its receptor. *Curr Top Microbiol Immunol* 1992;181:141–167.

26. Hilton DJ, Gough NM. Leukemia inhibitory factor: a biological perspective. *J Cell Biochem* 1991;46:21–26.

27. Taga T, Kishimoto T. Gp130 and the interleukin-6 family of cytokines. *Annu Rev Immunol* 1997;15:797–819.

28. Broudy VC. Stem cell factor and hematopoiesis. *Blood* 1997;90: 1345–1364.

29. Lawrence DA. Transforming growth factor-beta: an overview. *Kidney Int* 1995;49:S19–S23.

30. Kelner GS, Kennedy J, Bacon KB, et al. Lymphotactin: a cytokine that represents a new class of chemokine. *Science* 1994;266:1395–1399.

31. Jiang Y, Beller DI, Frendl G, Graves DT. Monocyte chemoattractant protein-1 regulates adhesion molecule expression and cytokine production. *J Immunol* 1992;148:2323.

32. Gong X, Gong W, Kuhns DB, Ben-Baruch A, Howard OM, Wang JM. Monocyte chemotactic protein-2 (MCP-2) uses CCR1 and CCR2b as its functional receptors. *J Biol Chem* 1997;272:11682–11685.

33. Dahinden CA, Geiser T, Brunner T, et al. Monocyte chemotactic protein-3 is a most effective basophil- and eosinophil-activating chemokine. *J Exp Med* 1994;179:751–756.

34. Uguccioni M, Loetscher P, Forssmann U, et al. Monocyte chemotactic protein 4 (MCP-4), a novel structural and functional analogue of MCP-3 and eotaxin. *J Exp Med* 1996;183:2379–2384.

35. Collins PD, Marleau S, Griffiths-Johnson DA, Jose PJ, Williams TJ. Cooperation between interleukin-5 and the chemokine eotaxin to induce eosinophil accumulation *in vivo*. *J Exp Med* 1995;182:1169–1174.

36. Imai T, Yoshida T, Baba M, Nishimura M, Kakizaki M, Yoshie O. Molecular cloning of a novel T cell–directed CC chemokine expressed in thymus by signal sequence trap using Epstein-Barr virus vector. *J Biol Chem* 1996;271:21514–21521.

37. Godiska R, Chantry D, Raport CJ, et al. Human macrophage-derived chemokine (MDC), a novel chemoattractant for monocytes, monocyte-derived dendritic cells, and natural killer cells. *J Exp Med* 1997;185: 1595–1604.

38. Wolpe SD, Davatelis G, Sherry B, et al. Macrophages secrete a novel heparin-binding protein with inflammatory and neutrophil chemokinetic properties. *J Exp Med* 1988;167:570–581.

39. Taub DD, Conlon K, Lloyd AR, Oppenheim JJ, Kelvin DJ. Preferential migration of activated CD4+ and CD8+ T cells in response to MIP-1 alpha and MIP-1 beta. *Science* 1993;260:355–358.

40. Schall TJ, Bacon K, Toy KJ, Goeddel DV. Selective attraction of monocytes and T lymphocytes of the memory phenotype by cytokine RANTES. *Nature* 1990;347:669–671.

41. Baba M, Imai T, Nishimura M, et al. Identification of CCR6, the specific receptor for a novel lymphocyte-directed CC chemokine LARC. *J Biol Chem* 1997;272:14893–14898.

42. Yoshida R, Imai T, Hieshima K, et al. Molecular cloning of a novel human CC chemokine EBI1-ligand chemokine that is a specific functional ligand for EBI1, CCR7. *J Biol Chem* 1997;272: 13803–13809.

43. Miller MD, Hata S, De Waal Malefyt R, Krangel MS. A novel polypeptide secreted by activated human T lymphocytes. *J Immunol* 1989;143: 2907–2916.

44. Nagira M, Imai T, Hieshima K, et al. Molecular cloning of a novel human CC chemokine secondary lymphoid-tissue chemokine that is a potent chemoattractant for lymphocytes and mapped to chromosome 9p13. *J Biol Chem* 1997;272:19518–19524.

45. Adema GJ, Hartgers F, Verstraten R, et al. A dendritic-cell-derived C-C chemokine that preferentially attracts naive T cells. *Nature* 1997;387: 713–717.

46. Vicari AP, Figueroa DJ, Hedrick JA, et al. TECK: a novel CC chemokine specifically expressed by thymic dendritic cells and potentially involved in T cell development. *Immunity* 1997;7:291–301.

47. Moser B, Clark-Lewis I, Zwahlen R, Baggiolini M. Neutrophil activating properties of the melanoma growth-stimulating activity, MGSA. *J Exp Med* 1990;171:1797–1802.

48. Haskill S, Peace A, Morris J, et al. Identification of three related human GRO genes encoding cytokine functions. *Proc Natl Acad Sci U S A* 1990;87:7732–7736.

49. Walz A, Baggiolini M. A novel cleavage product of β-thromboglobulin formed in cultures of stimulated mononuclear cells activates human neutrophils. *Biochem Biophys Res Comm* 1989;159:969–975.

50. Luster AD, Unkeless JC, Ravetch JV. Gamma-interferon transcriptionally regulates an early-response gene containing homology to platelet proteins. *Nature* 1985;315:672–676.

51. Liao F, Rabin RL, Yannelli JR, Koniaris LG, Vanguri P, Farber JM. Human Mig chemokine: biochemical and functional characterization. *J Exp Med* 1995;182:1301–1314.

52. Nagasawa T, Hirota S, Tachibana K, et al. Defects of B-cell lymphopoiesis and bone-marrow myelopoiesis in mice lacking the CXC chemokine PBSF/SDF-1. *Nature* 1996;382:635–638.

53. Fong AM, Robinson LA, Steeber DA, Tedder TF, Yoshie O, Imai T, Patel DD. Fractalkine and CX3CR1 mediate a novel mechanism of leukocyte capture, firm adhesion and activation under physiologic flow. *J Exp Med* 1998;188:1413–1419.

54. Maione TE, Gray GS, Petro J, et al. Inhibition of angiogenesis by recombinant human platelet factor 4 and related peptides. *Science* 1990;247:77–79.

Subject Index